SELECTED NURSING DIAGNOSES/CARE PLANS

NURSE–CLIENT MANAGEMENT/CARE PLANS

Fundamentals of Nursing

Collaborating for Optimal Health

Fundamentals of Nursing

Collaborating for Optimal Health

Edited by

Karen J. Berger, RN, MS, EdD (c)
Doctoral Candidate
University of San Diego
San Diego, California

Formerly Professor and Assistant Director
Department of Nursing Education
Grossmont College
El Cajon, California
and Adjunct Instructor of Nursing
Pepperdine University, Vista Campus
Vista, California

Marilyn Brinkman Williams, RN, MN
Professor, Department of Nursing Education
Grossmont College
El Cajon, California

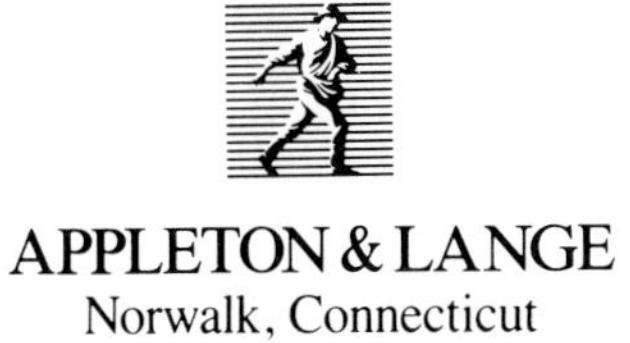

APPLETON & LANGE
Norwalk, Connecticut

Notice: The authors and the publisher of this volume have taken care to make certain that the doses of drugs and schedules of treatment are correct and compatible with the standards generally accepted at the time of publication. Nevertheless, as new information becomes available, changes in treatment and in the use of drugs become necessary. The reader is advised to carefully consult the instruction and information material included in the package insert of each drug or therapeutic agent before administration. This advice is especially important when using new or infrequently used drugs. The publisher disclaims any liability, loss, injury, or damage incurred as a consequence, directly or indirectly, of the use and application of any of the contents of this volume.

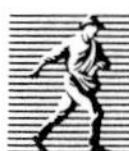

92 93 94 95 96 / 10 9 8 7 6 5 4 3 2

Prentice Hall International (UK) Limited, *London*
Prentice Hall of Australia Pty. Limited, *Sydney*
Prentice Hall Canada, Inc., Toronto
Prentice Hall Hispanoamericana, S.A., *Mexico*
Prentice Hall of India Private Limited, *New Delhi*
Prentice Hall of Japan, Inc., *Tokyo*
Simon & Schuster Asia Pte. Ltd., *Singapore*
Editora Prentice Hall do Brasil Ltda., *Rio de Janeiro*
Prentice Hall, *Englewood Cliffs, New Jersey*

Library of Congress Cataloging-in-Publication Data

Berger, Karen J.
Fundamentals of nursing : collaborating for optimal health / Karen J. Berger, Marilyn Brinkman Williams.
p. cm.
Includes index.
ISBN 0-8385-1213-5
1. Nursing. 2. Nurse and patient. 3. Nursing—Practice.
I. Williams, Marilyn Brinkman. II. Title.
[DNLM: 1. Nurse–Patient Relations. 2. Nursing Care. WY 100 B496f]
RT41.B37 1992
610.73—dc20
DNLM/DLC
for Library of Congress 91-33329

Chapter Opener Photography Credits

Pages 190 and 412: From Block GJ, Nolan JW. *Health Assessment for Professional Nursing: A Developmental Approach*, 2nd ed. Norwalk, CT: Appleton-Century-Crofts; 1986.

Page 210: Courtesy of Carol Weingarten.

Page 698: Courtesy of International Business Machines Corporation.

Page 968: From Flynn JBMcCann, Hackel R. *Technological Foundations in Nursing*. Norwalk, CT: Appleton & Lange; 1990.

Page 1676: Courtesy of IMED Corporation, San Diego, CA.

Cover art: *Gemini*, 1979, John Farnham; Courtesy of the Yale Center for British Art, New Haven, Conn. Gift of Jeffrey H. Loria.

Executive Editor, Nursing: William Brottmiller
Senior Developmental Editor: Donna Frassetto
Senior Managing Editor: John Williams
Production Editor: Elizabeth C. Ryan
Designers: Steve Byrum, Michael J. Kelly
Artists: Kathy Parks, Hal Keith, Penny Kindzierski

PRINTED IN THE UNITED STATES OF AMERICA

We dedicate this book to those who have inspired us and who have given unfailing support and encouragement:
John A. Berger, MD
Joseph Rost, PhD
Grace M. Sarosi, RN, MS
Marilyn J. Rummerfield, RN, MA
Jeffery Wohler, JD

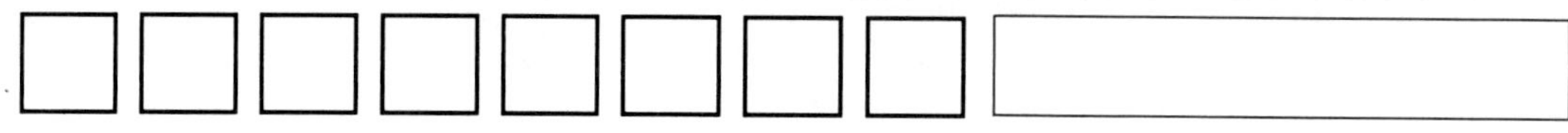

Contributors

Constance J. Adams, RN, MPH, DrPH
Associate Dean for Nursing Practice
Indiana University School of Nursing
Assistant Director for Nursing Practice
Indiana University Hospitals
Indianapolis, Indiana

Donna L. Algase, RN, PhD
Assistant Professor of Nursing and Assistant Research Scientist
University of Michigan School of Nursing
Division of Acute, Critical, and Long-term Care Programs
Ann Arbor, Michigan

Christine Alster, RN, EdD.
Associate Professor
College of Nursing
University of Massachusetts
Boston, Massachusetts

Ann N. Baker, RNCS, PhD
Clinical Director, Critical Care and Psychiatric Nursing and Adjunct Assistant Professor, Nursing
School of Nursing
Medical College of Ohio
Toledo, Ohio

Martha G. Barry, RN, MSN
Formerly, School of Nursing
University of Maryland
Baltimore, Maryland

Ruth Ann Benfield, RNCS, MSN
Associate Professor of Nursing
Montgomery County Community College
Blue Bell, Pennsylvania

Ellen W. Bernal, PhD
Hospital Ethicist
St. Vincent Medical Center
Toledo, Ohio

Bobbie Bloch, RN, MSN
Doctoral Candidate
College of Education and Allied Professions
University of Toledo
Toledo, Ohio

Keith E. Boles, PhD
Associate Professor Health Services Management
University of Missouri, Columbia
Columbia, Missouri

Nancy L. Bradley, RN, MEd
Assistant Professor of Nursing
Coordinator, Sophomore Nursing
School of Nursing
Kent State University
Kent, Ohio

Karen Brasfield, RN, MSN
Nephrology Nurse Consultant
Formerly, College of the Nazarene
Point Loma, California

Jane Edmiston Buhr, RN, MHA, MBA
St. Louis University Hospital
St. Louis, Missouri

Carolyn Spence Cagle, RN, PhD
Associate Professor
Harris College of Nursing
Texas Christian University
Fort Worth, Texas

Verna Benner Carson, RN, PhD
Assistant Professor, Psychiatric/Community Health Nursing
School of Nursing
University of Maryland
Baltimore, Maryland

Barbara A. Casey, RN, MS, CS
Clinical Nurse Specialist
Psychiatric-Mental Health Nursing
Veteran's Administration Medical Center
San Diego, California

Deanna F. Cedargren, RN, PhD
Associate Professor, Nursing
School of Nursing
Medical College of Ohio
Toledo, Ohio

JoAnn M. Clark, RN, MSN
Professor, Department of Nursing Education
Grossmont College
El Cajon, California

Mary Jo Clark, RN, MS, PhD
Assistant Professor, Philip Y. Hahn School of Nursing
University of San Diego
San Diego, California

Joseph K. Davie, RN, MSN
Dean, School of Nursing
The Long Island College Hospital
Brooklyn, New York
Member, Diagnosis Review Committee
North American Nursing Diagnosis Association

Janet-Beth McCann Flynn, RN, PhD
Writer/Editor
Nursewrite
Great Falls, Virginia

Kathleen Mary Hannon, MSN, RN
Clinical Nurse Specialist
Orthopedics/Neuroscience Unit
Fairview Southdale Hospital
Edina, Minnesota
Formerly, Associate Clinical Specialist
School of Nursing
University of Minnesota
Minneapolis, Minnesota

Dolores J. Harkins, RN, C, MS
Associate Professor of Nursing
School of Nursing
Medical College of Ohio
Toledo, Ohio

Lanis L. Hicks, PhD
Associate Professor
School of Health Services Management
University of Missouri, Columbia
Columbia, Missouri

Linda M. Hollinger, RN, MS, PhD
Assistant Chairperson for Education and Associate Professor
College of Nursing
Rush University
Chicago, Illinois

Julie E. Johnson, RN, PhD
Associate Dean and Associate Professor
College of Nursing
Montana State University
Bozeman, Montana

Judith A. Lewis, RNC, PhD
Assistant Professor
Graduate Program in Nursing
MGH Institute of Health Professions
Boston, Massachusetts

Ruth Ludwick, RN, MSN
Assistant Professor
School of Nursing
Kent State University
Kent, Ohio

Susan L. MacLean, RN, PhD
College of Nursing
Rush University
Chicago, Illinois

Janet A. McNelly, RN, MS
Nurse Manager
Orthopedics Neuroscience Unit
Fairview Southdale Hospital
Edina, Minnesota

Sharon L. Merritt, RN, EdD
Assistant Professor and Interim Director, Narcolepsy Research
Department of Medical-Surgical Nursing
College of Nursing
University of Illinois at Chicago
Chicago, Illinois

Sherry L. Merrow, RN, EdD
Associate Professor
College of Nursing
University of Massachusetts at Boston
Boston, Massachusetts

Ngozi O. Nkongho, RN, PhD
Assistant Professor, Division of Nursing
Herbert N. Lehman College
The City University of New York
Bronx, New York

Ashley E. Phillips, MA, C. Phil.
Lecturer, Department of Women's Studies
San Diego State University
Executive Director, Womancare Clinics
San Diego, California

Sheila M. Pickwell, CFNP, PhD
Associate Clinical Professor and Director, Nurse-Practitioner Program
UCSF/UCSD Intercampus Graduate Studies
Department of Community and Family Medicine
University of California, San Diego
La Jolla, California

Georgine Redmond, RN, EdD
Associate Professor and
Assistant Dean, Student Affairs
School of Nursing
George Mason University
Fairfax, Virginia

Connie Vaughn Roush, RN, MSN
Formerly, Assistant Professor
Point Loma Nazarene College
San Diego, California

Coralease Cox Ruff, RN, DNSc, FNP-C
Program Director, Family Nurse Practitioner Program
Chairperson, Graduate Program
College of Nursing
Howard University
Washington, DC

Barbara Sarter, RN, FNP, FANN, PhD
Associate Professor
Department of Nursing
University of Southern California
Los Angeles, California

Patricia F. Schmidt, RN, EdD
Associate Professor
Nursing Education Department
Palomar College
San Marcos, California

Carol A. Sedlak, RN, MSN, CCRN, ONC
Associate Professor
School of Nursing
Kent State University
Kent, Ohio

Carol A. Stephenson, RN, EdD
Associate Professor
Harris College of Nursing
Texas Christian University
Fort Worth, Texas

Jane C. Swart, RN, PhD
Dean and Professor
School of Nursing
Wright State University, Miami Valley
Dayton, Ohio

Karen Szafran, RN, MS
Lecturer, School of Nursing
San Diego State University
San Diego, California

Donna F. Ver Steeg, RN, FAAN, PhD
Maternal-Child Health/Primary Ambulatory Care Section
School of Nursing
University of California, Los Angeles
Los Angeles, California

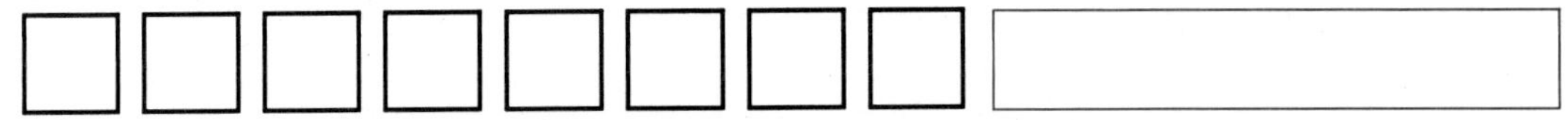

Reviewers and Consultants

Joan Arnold, RN, MA
Assistant Professor, School of Nursing, Adelphi University, Garden City, New York

Roberta M. Burris, RN, MS
College of Nursing, Texas Women's University, Denton, Texas

Catherine A. Bevil, RN, EdD
Associate Professor and Director, Baccalaureate Division, Department of Nursing, Thomas Jefferson University, Philadelphia, Pennsylvania

Peggy O'Bryan Doheny, RN, PhD, ONC
Assistant Professor, School of Nursing, Kent State University, Kent, Ohio

Marylee Evans, RN, MS
Assistant Professor, College of Nursing, University of Rhode Island, Kingston, Rhode Island

Sondra Flemming, RN, MS
Associate Dean, Health Occupations Division, El Centro College, Dallas, Texas

Shirley Ann Lewis, RN
Associate Professor, School of Nursing, Albert B. Chandler Medical Center, University of Kentucky, Lexington, Kentucky

Sandy Oestreich, RNC, MS (consultant)
Professor Emerita, School of Nursing, Adelphi University, Garden City, New York

Norma N. Pinnell, RN, MSN
Instructor, Level III Coordinator, School of Nursing, Southern Illinois University, Edwardsville, Illinois

Mary Radatovich Price, RN, EdM
Computer Education Consultant, Hunter-Bellevue School of Nursing, New York, New York

Cheryl V. Ratliff, RN, MN, MS
Vice President, Child Health Corporation of America, Shawnee Mission, Kansas

Mary Sampel, RN, MSN
Associate Professor, School of Nursing, St. Louis University, St. Louis, Missouri

Rachel Taylor, RN
College of Nursing, University of Tennessee, Memphis, Tennessee

Anna Bernadette Tritak, RN, EdD
Assistant Professor, Department of Nursing, Fairleigh Dickinson University, Teaneck, New Jersey

Ann Windsor, RN, DNS
Clinical Associate Professor, School of Nursing, Center for Health Sciences, University of Wisconsin, Madison, Wisconsin

Mary Ann (Sandy) Wyper, RN, PhD
Assistant Professor, Nursing of the Adult, Graduate Program, School of Nursing, Kent State University, Kent, Ohio

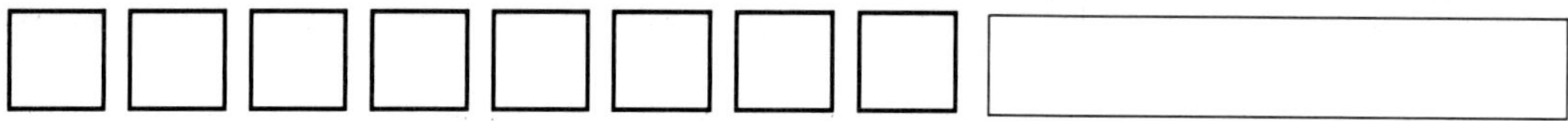

Preface

The 1990s could prove to be one of the most auspicious periods in the history of nursing. The nation seeks change in its health care system, and nursing is well positioned to make a major contribution toward society's goals of universal access and affordable health care for all Americans. At no time in recent history have the conditions been as favorable for nursing as they are today. Major reforms seem likely and nursing stands ready to act and is likely to benefit from the changes that are sure to come. Nursing's themes—prevention and community-based health care, recognition of the diverse needs of a multicultural population, personal responsibility for health based on informed decision making and consent, and cost-efficiency—are in concert with those of the nation's population and policymakers. Clearly, the time is right for nursing to realize its long-held objectives of professional autonomy and social acknowledgment of its contributions to health care.

Recognizing that today's fundamentals students are tomorrow's practitioners, we have structured this text around the values, content, and skills we believe are necessary to prepare students for the challenges ahead. Nurses' ability to initiate and influence new modes of organization in health care and to participate successfully in the reforms confronting the health care delivery system will to a large extent depend on the strength and quality of nurses' transactions within a complex and volatile environment. We believe those transactions will be enhanced by a philosophy of collaboration that emphasizes working together with others, using persuasion and influence to attain mutually beneficial and socially important goals. Collaboration both within and outside of nursing will be necessary to secure changes that reflect nursing's values and serve the public's needs for health care.

Approach

In this text, we endorse the collaborative philosophy—expressed by the phrase "partnerships in health care"—as a philosophy for health care encounters. Collaboration is compatible not only with environmental trends, but with nursing's central values and ideals. Ours is a multicultural society, characterized by diversity. Clients bring varying paradigms of health and illness to their health care encounters, and these are frequently critical to the outcomes of health care. Collaboration accommodates client diversity by bringing clients into caregiving partnerships with nurses. This promotes client self-determination and dignity, hallmarks of caring.

To equip students with a professional value system that fosters partnerships in health care, this text integrates the collaborative philosophy into the structure of helping relationships and clinical decision making. This provides a foundation for students to master the traditional cognitive skills of practice—professional decision making and the nursing process—from a person-centered perspective and a social framework that promotes caring.

The environment of nursing is growing more challenging day by day; nursing curricula in the 1990s will need to realign content to accommodate the driving forces of change. Scientific advances, ever-changing technology, and specialization are familiar health care trends. Their benefits are offset by the fragmentation of services they promote. The constant need for economy is certain to factor ever more prominently in the future of nursing practice. Managed care and case management undoubtedly will have a central place in the design of health care reforms and in all probability will become a cornerstone of provider education.

These conditions demand that during their basic education nursing students develop an economic perspective on their role that is nurtured throughout the curriculum. For that reason, *Fundamentals of Nursing: Collaborating for Optimal Health* introduces students to the essentials of economics, management, and leadership within the framework of collaboration, depicting the relevance of collaboration to the optimal use of scarce resources in practice.

Depending on the extent and rapidity of health care reform, it is likely that the environment of health care will grow ever more turbulent in the years to come. The changes that lie ahead will undoubtedly bring conflict. Interests are certain to collide. Consequently, practitioners in the future will benefit from a philosophy of interaction that serves to build important political and interdisciplinary bridges; collaboration embodies such a philosophy. In the 1990s, nurses will need to assert their interests, negotiate, lobby, exchange ideas, and compromise with colleagues to achieve consensus-building without sacrificing their own principles and ideals. This text introduces these arts and skills, which are integral to professional collaboration.

Organization

This text includes eight units that may be used in any sequence a particular curriculum dictates. Extensive content guides and cross-references help readers locate specific topics.

Unit I, The Nurse and the Nursing Profession, introduces readers to the roles, functions, and professional responsibilities of the nurse from a collaborative perspective and focuses on legal considerations, politics, and policymaking in nursing.

Unit II, Health and Health Care, introduces the topics of health and illness, stress, adaptation, and change, with emphasis on collaborating for health promotion. It orients readers to the essential concepts of family, community, sociocultural, and spiritual aspects of health.

Unit III, The Client, integrates collaboration with concepts about individuality, sexuality, growth and development, and the transition to the client role.

Unit IV, Nurse–Client Collaboration, focuses on the nurse–client relationship and identifies the essential features of communication in collaborative relationships.

Unit V, The Nursing Process as Collaboration, explores professional decision making within the framework of collaboration. Individual chapters focus on the nursing process, health history and examination, nursing diagnosis, and making, writing, and evaluating client care plans. Client teaching and learning is presented from a collaborative perspective, as is health care teamwork. Unit V also explores the role of computers as a clinical tool and an aid to collaboration, introducing computerized hospital information systems for decision support and care documentation.

Unit VI, Fundamental Nursing Assessment and Management, addresses ten functional dimensions of health that reflect the holistic nature of human functioning. Each chapter is organized around the nursing process and emphasizes the development of clinical skills. The unit includes three functional dimensions not usually found in fundamentals texts: wellness/well-being, self-expression, and neurosensory integration. Each chapter presents concepts essential to defining and understanding a functional dimension, and guidelines for collaborative health assessment with a strong emphasis on nursing diagnosis. Nurse–client management sections are divided into subsections on planning, implementation, and evaluation. Each nursing implementation section incorporates four levels of client care: preventive, supportive, restorative, and rehabilitative. This format highlights the many health care settings in which contemporary nurses practice, including school, clinic, community, and home, as well as acute and long-term care facilities.

Unit VII, Scientific and Philosophical Foundations of Nursing Practice, orients readers to the essential concepts of science and research, nursing theory, philosophy, and ethics as they relate to nursing practice.

Unit VIII, Nursing and Health Care as Business, addresses content not typically found in fundamentals texts but highly relevant to nursing in the 1990s and beyond. Chapters on the health care delivery system and economics in health care and nursing highlight strengths and weaknesses in the current health care system and the role of economics and consumerism in health care. The final chapter, Health Care as a Transaction, also provides an orientation to mutual interaction, a model of collaboration in nurse–client encounters.

Noteworthy Features

Several unique features add value to this textbook:

- Consistent emphasis on health care as a collaborative endeavor, one in which clients are empowered as full participants in decision making and in which nurses work collaboratively with each other and with other providers to promote clients' health.
- A noticeable lack of paternalistic approaches and language without losing sight of nurses' responsibilities in caregiving.
- Detailed content and guidelines on the cognitive processes of care planning and on the mechanics and pitfalls of translating care plan decisions into written documents.
- Integration of conceptually related content into single chapters. For example, Chapter 7 explores the concept of community, including the idea of hospital as community, and health as a community phenomenon; it emphasizes health promotion, but also stresses disease prevention based on an understanding of the essentials of epidemiology.
- Chapter 22, Wellness and Well-being, presents the basic concepts and dimensions of wellness, discussing problems in wellness and reiterating the themes of health promotion and disease prevention from a clinical standpoint. It builds on the Chapter 7 discussion of health as a community phenomenon and the chain of infection by translating these ideas into an understanding of medical and surgical asepsis and the role in disease prevention of related procedures.

  Chapter 24, Skin and Tissue Integrity, presents basic hygiene and wound care skills as a means of supporting optimum skin and tissue function.

  Chapter 30, Mobility, combines content on the role of exercise in promoting and improving health for all age groups with content specific to enhancing mobility in clients experiencing health alterations.
- Unique chapters that highlight a holistic perspective on nursing. Chapter 22, Wellness and Well-being, examines factors such as lifestyle, person–environment fit, spirituality, and self-responsibility and translates these into clinical implementation. It also points out the negative impact of certain practices and habits on wellness and well-being.

  Chapter 23, Self-Expression, explores the nature of self-expression, encompassing its relationship to self-concept, identity, sexuality, self-presentation, and self-disclosure. It also presents guidelines for assessing self-expression and for assisting clients with problems in self-expression.

Learning Aids

The chapters in this text all include carefully chosen pedagogical elements that promote student learning.

- *Chapter Outlines*
- *Key Vocabulary Terms*
- *Behavioral Objectives*
- Boxed *Implications for Nurse–Client or Professional Collaboration* that highlight the collaborative approach
- Boxed summaries of contemporary nursing literature, entitled *Building Nursing Knowledge* that are designed to stimulate students critical thinking about content issues related to nursing and health care.
- *Chapter Summaries* that reprise important chapter themes.
- *Illustrated Procedure Tables and Boxes.* Coverage of fundamental nursing procedures, most of which appear in the assessment and management sections of Unit VI, is detailed and heavily illustrated. Uniquely designed procedure tables provide actions with explanatory rationales. These tables contain numerous illustrations, color-toned for emphasis, that provide the student with a step-by-step visual guide to key actions. Note boxes in procedure tables remind readers of special considerations or cautions relevant to particular actions. Marginal tabbing bars on the edge of each page containing a procedure allow quick location of procedures.

  A chapter-by-chapter directory of procedures appears at the end of the table of contents to enable readers to quickly locate procedures included in the text.
- *Sample Assessment Questions, Diagnostic Tables, and Nurse–Client Management Plans.* These features in each Unit VI chapter reinforce the nursing process. Sample assessment questions guide beginning students' data gathering. Examples of nursing diagnoses associated with each functional dimension include hypothetical assessment data to illustrate how each diagnosis illustrated is derived. Correlated management tables, or care plans, provide students with an understanding of the translation of diagnoses into implementation plans.

Teaching–Learning Package

A complete ancillary package is provided for the text, including:

- An *Instructor's Manual* supplements the text chapter-by-chapter and provides a concepts directory, learning assignments, clinical experiences, discussion guide, recommendations for audiovisual aids, and suggestions for content approaches.
- A *Study Guide* for students provides a chapter overview, review questions, enrichment activities, self-examination questions, and supplemental diagnostic tables and nurse–client management plans.
- A set of two-color *Transparencies* selected from the text illustrations enhances classroom instruction.
- A *Computerized Testbank* tests students' knowledge of essential chapter content.

It is with enthusiasm that we put forth this textbook. We see it as a values-based approach, unique in the area of fundamentals nursing education, that is appropriate not only to the times, trends, and challenges nurses and nursing will face in the 1990s and beyond, but that also serves to translate the enduring ideal of caring into an operational framework for the future.

Karen J. Berger
Marty Williams

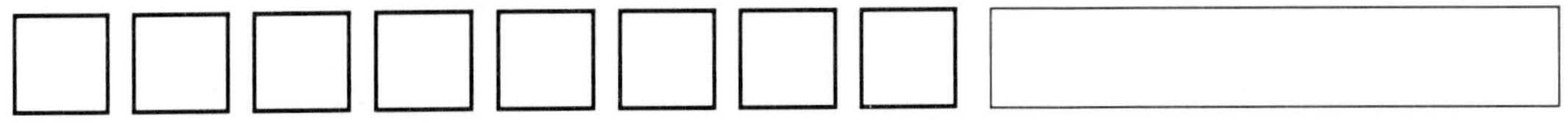

Acknowledgments

We would like to recognize and express our appreciation to many individuals whose participation in this project was pivotal to its successful completion:

- Our reviewers and contributors, for their energy, commitment, and expertise.
- The clinical facilities that served as sites for photographs: Harborview Medical Center, San Diego Rehabilitation Institute, Kaiser Permanente Mission Bay Obstetrics and Gynecology Clinic, and the Kaiser Permanente Wellness Caravan.
- Cookie Gender, MSN, CCRN, Director of Nursing/Assistant Administrator, San Diego Rehabilitation Institute, and Ann Reynolds, for their assistance with coordinating our photography session; the patients and staff at San Diego Rehabilitation Institute, the Grossmont College nursing students, and family and friends who graciously participated as models; and Diane Leong and Linda Goodwin, Grossmont College Health Science Technicians, for their assistance in obtaining and loaning equipment for photographs.
- Photographer Pat Watson, for assisting us to obtain effective and sensitive photographs to enhance the expression of our ideas.
- Illustrator Kathy Parks, for her spirit, enthusiasm, and skill. Her drawings added a critical element to the presentation of clinical procedures and enhanced the discussion of theoretical concepts.
- Stuart Horton, for his assistance through many transitions and organizational changes.
- Claude Sweet, for his generous technical assistance.
- David Knetzer, Executive Director, San Diego Medical Center, a valuable resource for up-to-date information on a variety of health care delivery topics.
- The staff at Appleton & Lange, whose expertise, ideas, and perseverance helped make *Fundamentals of Nursing: Collaborating for Optimal Health* a reality; in particular, John Williams, Senior Managing Editor; Janet Foltin, Developmental Editor; and Elizabeth Ryan, Production Editor. To Donna Frassetto, Senior Developmental Editor, we extend special appreciation and respect. Without her guidance, insight, commitment, and dedication to our ideas for a unique and quality textbook we would never have realized our goal.

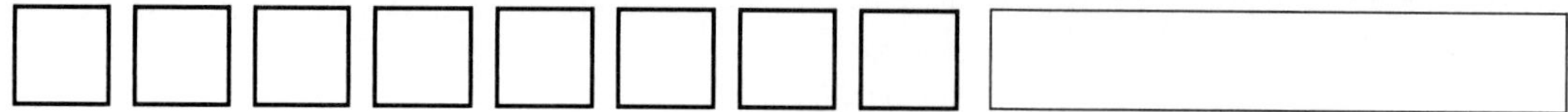

Contents in Brief

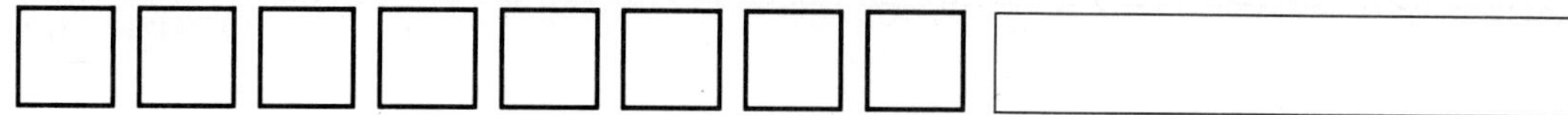

Contents in Detail

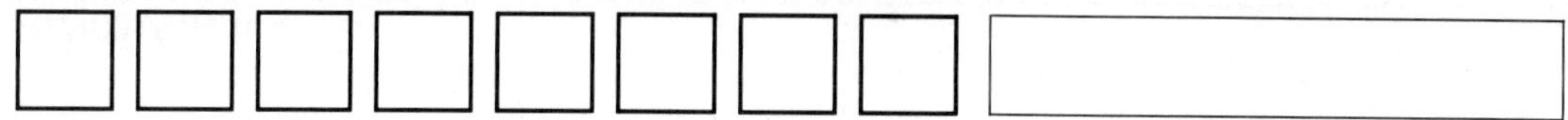

Procedures Directory

Chapter 16. Client History and Health Examination

Procedures

Procedures Presented in Narrative

Basic health assessment including measurements (height, weight, circumferences); general survey; integument; head, eye, ear, nose, throat (including face, mouth and neck); breasts and axillae (including breast self-examination; thorax and lungs; cardiovascular system; abdomen and gastrointestinal system; anus and rectum; genitourinary system; musculoskeletal system; and neurological system.

Chapter 22. Wellness and Well-being

Procedures

Procedures Presented in Narrative and Guidelines

Assessing for well-being problems, admitting a client to a health care facility, universal precautions, preparing clients for diagnostic tests, preparing clients for surgery, post-operative care, setting up a sterile field, pouring sterile solutions, opening sterile packages, using sterile forceps, use of isolation gowns and masks, promoting safety (fires, electrical hazard, radiation), managing fever, calculating drug dosages, administering topical medications, administering medications vaginally, administering medications via a nasogastric tube, troubleshooting nasogastric decompression systems.

Chapter 24. Skin and Tissue Integrity

Procedures

Procedures Presented in Narrative and Guidelines

Assessing for skin and mucosal problems; assessing wounds; treating minor skin injuries; assisting with hygiene, including early morning care, AM care, showers, tub baths, and HS care; use of special dressings for pressure ulcers; bandaging; and managing wound drainage systems.

Chapter 25. Nutrition

Procedures

Procedures Presented in Narrative and Guidelines

Assessing nutritional status, presenting meal trays, positioning for eating, assisting dysphagic clients to eat, and monitoring clients receiving tube feedings.

Chapter 26. Elimination

Procedures Presented in Narrative and Guidelines

Assessing elimination problems, assessing urine and stool characteristics, assessing ostomy stomas and peristomal skin, use of a rectal tube, removing a fecal impaction, assessing urine specific gravity, open and closed irrigation of Foley catheter, catheter care, and bowel and bladder training.

Chapter 27. Oxygenation

Procedures

Procedures Presented in Narrative and Guidelines

Assessing oxygenation problems, exercises to stimulate leg circulation (post surgical and in vascular disease), using incentive spirometers, using a variety of coughing techniques, using a pulse oximeter, and using a croupette for oxygen delivery.

Chapter 28. Sleep–Rest Patterns

Procedures

Procedures Presented in Narrative and Guidelines

Assessing sleep pattern disturbances and comparing effects of various sleeping medications.

Chapter 29. Neurosensory Integration

Procedures

Procedures Presented in Narrative and Guidelines

Assessing neurosensory integration, including cranial nerve function, orientation, memory, sensory function, coordination, reflexes, and pain; assisting clients with visual impairments; approaches to the care of clients who are blind; care of contact lenses; assisting clients with hearing loss; loss of smell or taste, and loss of peripheral sensation; techniques for relief of mild to severe pain; assisting clients with neurosensory deficits; caring for comatose clients; caring for clients during seizures; caring for clients with sensory deprivation or overload.

Chapter 30. Mobility

Procedures

Procedures Presented in Narrative and Guidelines

Assessing mobility problems, assessing activity tolerance, treating minor exercise-related injuries, protective body mechanics, assessing for appropriate transfer and ambulation techniques, using gait belts and sliding boards, using protective positioning aids, fall prevention..

Chapter 31. Fluid and Electrolyte Balance

Procedures

Procedures Presented in Narrative and Guidelines

Assessing fluid problems, calculating fluid needs, monitoring and recording intake and output, assessing and maintaining integrity of venipuncture sites, calculating and regulating IV flow rates, trouble-shooting intravenous infusions, assessing for complications of IV and transfusion therapy, and monitoring clients receiving total parenteral nutrition.

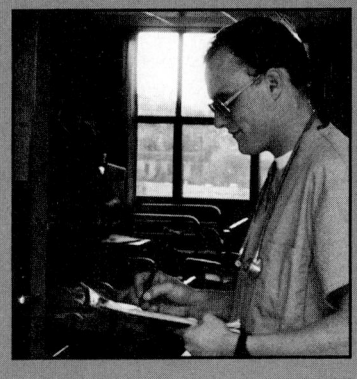

UNIT ONE
The Nurse and the Nursing Profession

CHAPTER 1

The Professional Nurse

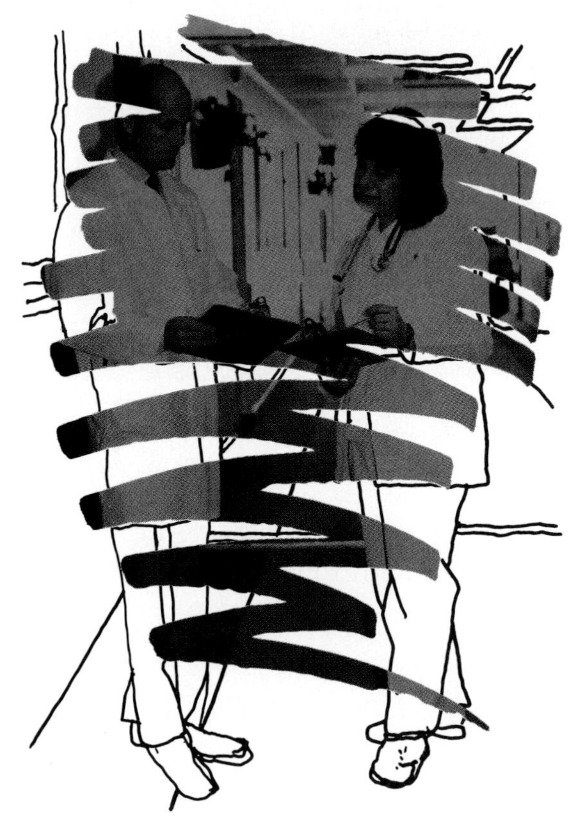

Behavioral Objectives

Upon completion of this chapter, the student will be able to:

1. Define nursing according to the ANA *Social Policy Statement* and the models of caring, collaboration, and professionalism.
2. Describe the current role of the nurse in health care delivery.
3. Describe the typical nurse profile in the United States and Canada. Discuss trends influencing changes in these profiles.
4. Describe educational programs for generalist or specialist nursing practice.
5. Identify three credentialing mechanisms that are important to the education and practice of the nurse.
6. Describe major practice settings for nurses.
7. Discuss the roles of the nurse as caregiver, advocate, health care team member, manager, and decision-maker.
8. Describe the emerging role and functions of the nurse as entrepreneur.
9. Discuss ways in which the nurse collaborates with others to achieve optimal client health.

KEY TERMS

accreditation
case management
case nursing
certification
certified nurse-midwife
clinical nurse specialist
collaboration
credentialing
functional nursing
licensed practical (vocational) nurse
licensure
nurse anesthetist
nurse practitioner
nursing
primary care
primary nursing
registered nurse
team nursing

The professional nurse of today is a versatile and unique health care provider. The practice of nursing—even the concept of what nursing is—has undergone significant evolution over time. The settings in which nurses practice, the roles in which they function, and their relationships to other health care providers are also changing and expanding. These changes have stimulated new approaches to basic nursing education, and to the development of more and varied programs for preparation for advanced and specialty practice. An understanding of the myriad roles, functions, and responsibilities of professional nurses in the current health care delivery system is an important part of nursing students' orientation to their future career.

This chapter will explore definitions of nursing and the qualities and characteristics of professional nurses. Patterns of nursing education, settings for nursing practice, and nursing roles, both current and emerging, are identified and examined. The concept of collaboration in health care is introduced, with special emphasis on nursing as collaboration. Collaboration implies partnership, equality. A collaborative approach to nursing and health care recognizes clients' rights to make decisions regarding their health care and emphasizes their role as equal and active participants on the health care team.

■ CURRENT DEFINITIONS OF NURSING

Nursing literature offers a variety of definitions for what nursing is. Those definitions that seem most relevant emphasize the social context of nursing. They clarify the relationships between client and caregivers and among the various health care providers. Notable among these definitions are the American Nurses' Association *Social Policy Statement* and the conceptualizations of nursing as caring, nursing as collaboration, and nursing as professionalism.

Social Policy Statement

The American Nurses' Association (ANA) is considered the professional association for nursing, comparable to the American Medical Association (AMA) for physicians. The ANA's *Nursing: A Social Policy Statement*[1] describes the social context of nursing and the nature and scope of nursing practice, and provides a perspective on specialization in nursing practice. The definition of nursing presented in the *Social Policy Statement* is solidly grounded in history. It also reflects the influence of nursing theory development (which is discussed in Chap. 32 of this text) and a recognition of future directions for nursing. **Nursing** is defined as "the diagnosis and treatment of human responses to actual or potential health problems."[1]

This definition encompasses a wide range of health- and illness-related human responses, such as pain and discomfort following surgery, or self-image changes and impaired sexual functioning following a mastectomy. Further, the definition indicates that it is the nurse's responsibility to identify (diagnose) the nature of a person's response to a health problem and to use appropriate nursing implementation (treatment). Nursing diagnoses influence the selection of nursing implementation: client care that is most appropriate to the situation and needs of individuals. Planning and delivering client care represents the application of nursing knowledge, art, and theory.

The emphasis in the *Social Policy Statement* definition of nursing is on the human response to health problems rather than on the health problems themselves. The health problem or disease is perceived as the focus for medicine. These foci complement each other and support the importance of collaboration between nursing and medicine in achieving optimal health for all.

Nursing as Caring

The Concept of Caring. The notion of caring always has been implicit in definitions of nursing. In its generic sense, caring refers to having regard for, or giving attention to, the needs or wants of others; it also involves a willingness to be responsible for another or to provide for others. In a fuller sense, caring combines a belief or value with ability and willingness to act. It is not enough to feel kindness toward others. Having the knowledge and skills to translate valued behavior and willingness to care into action is critical if caring is to become reality for nurses, and not merely rhetoric.

Conceptual Analysis of Caring. Although the concept of caring has been synonymous with nursing, its meaning frequently has been taken for granted. In textbooks, nursing education and health care facility philosophy statements, and research, nurses are described as providing care for others, giving nursing care, or caring for clients. Usually this care implies a one-sided relationship in which nurses provide for the basic survival needs of people who are unable to help themselves. It is only within the past decade that nurse theorists and researchers have begun to analyze and study the concept of caring as it relates to nursing. The work of three of these theorists is summarized here.

> **IMPLICATIONS FOR NURSE–CLIENT COLLABORATION**
>
> **Caring as a Transaction**
>
> Some authorities describe caring as a *transaction* between nurse and client, introducing notions of reciprocity and collaboration into the caring relationship. In the case of nurse–client relationships, clients offer information about their personal values, while nurses offer professional knowledge for solving health care problems. Transactions in a caring relationship thus benefit both parties.

Paterson and Zderad[2] describe caring as a transaction between nurse and client, introducing notions of reciprocity or collaboration to the caring relationship established between them. A transaction refers to an exchange or an agreement between two parties, in this case between nurse and client. Reciprocity infers that each party has something valued by the other to contribute or bring to the relationship, that a mutual exchange to the advantage of both characterizes the transaction.

In a transaction, a client's right to refuse care is recognized. Instead of "doing to" or "doing for" clients, nurses "do with" by facilitating and expanding clients' abilities to help themselves. Although nurses still provide assistive and supportive care when it is needed, in a reciprocal relationship, "taking care of" is not viewed as the primary focus of the nurse's role, but rather as one element among many.

Madeline Leininger,[3] a transcultural nursing expert, views caring as the central unifying concept of nursing. Her transcultural model of nursing has provided a starting place for many other researchers in the study of transcultural and caring concepts in nursing. Leininger emphasizes that caring behaviors, as well as the underlying beliefs and values about caring, vary from culture to culture. She has developed a list of "ethnocaring" constructs: traits or behaviors that she believes are elements of caring.[4] They are listed in Box 1–1. Leininger stresses that for nurses to communicate caring effectively, they must grasp the meaning of these components of caring from the point of view of the one being cared for.

Similar concepts form the basis for Jean Watson's contribution to the definition of nursing as caring. Watson, a creative nurse scholar and theorist, describes what she calls "carative" factors as essential ingredients for professional nursing. These carative factors serve as a foundation for nursing's efforts to help others maintain or attain a high level of health or die a peaceful death.[5]

The "ethnocaring" constructs and carative factors listed in Box 1–1 provide a base on which other nurse theorists and researchers are building to add a scientific dimension to the development of caring as an explicit and critical concept for defining nursing.[6–8] This evolving caring perspective contributes a unique conception of nursing as the science of caring, as encompassing but moving beyond the

BOX 1–1. CONCEPTS OF CARING IN NURSING

"Ethnocaring" Concepts

- Caring
- Compassion
- Concern
- Coping behaviors
- Empathy
- Enabling
- Facilitating
- Interest
- Involvement
- Health consultative acts
- Health instruction acts
- Health maintenance acts
- Helping behaviors
- Love
- Nurturance
- Presence
- Protective behaviors
- Restorative behaviors
- Sharing
- Stimulating behaviors
- Stress alleviation
- Succorance
- Support
- Surveillance
- Tenderness
- Touching
- Trust

Carative Factors

- Humanistic altruistic system of values
- Faith–hope
- Sensitivity to self and others
- Helping–trusting human care relationship
- Expressing positive and negative feelings
- Creative problem-solving caring process
- Transpersonal teaching–learning
- Supportive, protective, and/or corrective mental, physical, societal, and spiritual environment
- Human needs assistance
- Existential–phenomenological–spiritual forces

Data from Leininger MM. Caring: An Essential Human Need. *Thorofare, NJ: Slack; 1981:13. Watson J.* Nursing: Human Science and Human Care: A Theory of Nursing. *Norwalk, CT: Appleton-Century-Crofts; 1985:75.*

traditional meaning of caring for others that has marked nursing over time.

Nursing as Collaboration

Collaboration in nursing is a process in which clients assume primary responsibility for health-related decisions and in which nurses and clients share responsibility for planning care as equal partners. Collaboration implies mutual respect. The collaborative approach to nursing practice used as the theme for this book builds on the idea of nursing as the philosophy and science of caring. Moreover, it extends the notion of collaboration beyond nurse–client transaction and applies it to the context of interactions among health professionals as well.

The collaborative approach used in this text is conceptually consistent with Williamson's model of mutual interaction[9] (see Chap. 37). In this model, each person who participates in an interaction is assumed to have a right to self-direction. The model also focuses on reciprocity: free exchange between persons who can choose to accept or reject what the other offers; personal responsibility for health-related behaviors; and legitimization of individual conceptions of health.

The need for collaboration, or two-way exchange, in nurse–client and nurse–colleague relationships, is stressed throughout this text. This focus is essential for the successful practice of professional nursing today. Collaborative transactions are most effective when based on mutual understanding, mutual trust, mutual control, and mutual responsibility. When applied to client care the outcome of a transaction is a plan of action that reflects in a most profound way the health needs, rights, and preferences of the client, while expressing the professional responsibilities and ethics of the nurse (Fig. 1–1).

Nursing as Professionalism

Professionalism is another variable essential to the definition of nursing. The minimal qualifications for professional status include a prescribed program of advanced education, concern with matters of significance, continuing intellectual pursuits, and self-regulation of entry and practice within the profession. These issues are discussed more fully in Chapter 2. The long-standing debate about whether nursing is a profession, a technical occupation, or a vocation within the health field is no longer of concern. Nurses must take a unified position, starting with the premise that nursing is a profession, and act accordingly.

Acting as professionals is necessary and justified for nurses. When described in terms of their highest achievements in education and practice, their level of responsibility for matters of human urgency and significance, and their development of systems to safeguard the public welfare and to gain control of their practice, nurses have earned the right to call themselves professionals. Accepting this premise moves the focus from debating the issue of professional status to the individual nurse's responsibility to consistently behave as a professional. Box 1–2 summarizes the definitions of nursing discussed here.

■ QUALITIES AND CHARACTERISTICS OF THE PROFESSIONAL NURSE

Current Role in Health Care Delivery Systems

The current role of nurses in health care is based on individual professional responsibility. The functions of today's professional nurse are a unique blend of the old and the

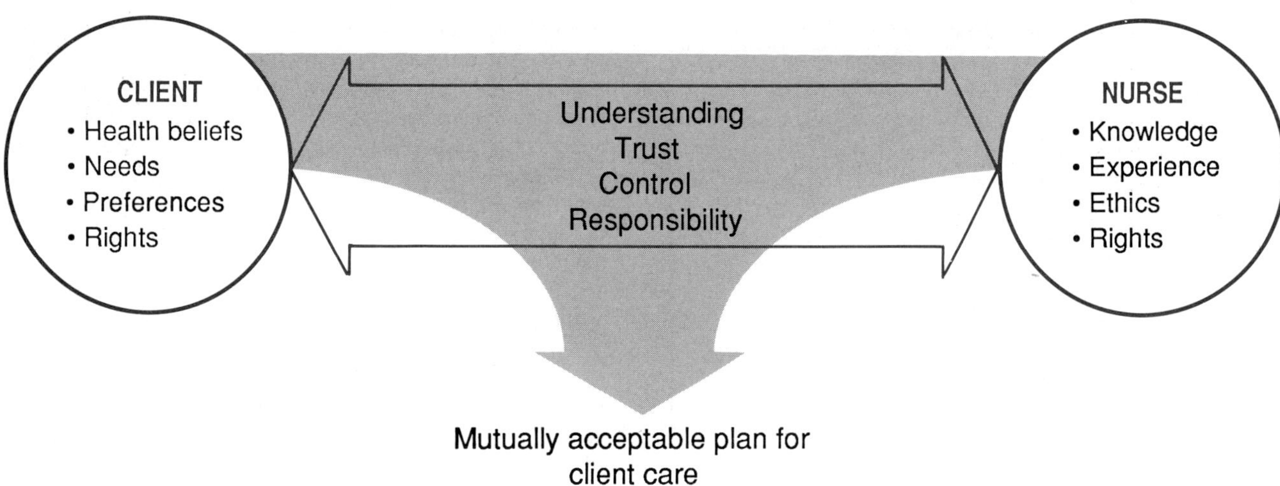

Figure 1–1. Nursing as collaboration.

new. Nursing embodies the traditional values of caring, concern for others and for the world in which we live, humility, selflessness, and altruism. At the same time, the professional nurse demonstrates strength, commitment to self, pride in knowledge and expertise, career orientation, and future vision. Nurses who demonstrate these qualities command recognition and respect from professional colleagues and clients. They embody the unique mission and role of nurses as autonomous and valued professional health care providers.

Nurses are essential in the day-to-day delivery of health care. They, more than any other team members, are the caregivers who are present around the clock in most health care institutions. Nurses frequently are the health care providers first seen by clients when they enter the health care delivery system for any type of care. Nurses influence the way in which clients and families perceive, experience, and evaluate what happens to them in hospitals, nursing homes, clinics, community health, or primary care settings. Nurses are the providers who follow clients into their homes to deliver care, help them obtain community resources, and assess their continuing health care needs. In all types of health care settings, nurses collaborate with clients and their families to identify health needs and problems. They help them to select from among alternative approaches, balance health needs with other life priorities, and work to achieve optimal health. Nurses collaborate with other health care team members to meet client needs.

This flexibility and scope of nursing are reflected in the preparation of new nurses. Nursing education is grounded in the liberal arts, as well as socio-behavioral and physical sciences. Building on this broad foundation and applying nursing science and art through clinical experiences has produced a health care provider who is versatile and unique. Professional nurses are prepared to function in all types of health care delivery systems, with all types of clients from all age groups.

In contacts with clients, nurses emphasize health promotion, wellness, health protection and disease prevention, and self-care. Nurses collaborate with other health care providers and with clients and their support persons to deliver illness care when it is needed. However, the broader vision—encompassing health and wellness as well as self-care—persists. Professional nurses organize practice around concepts of caring, collaboration, wellness, and holistic individuals in interaction with their environments. The nursing focus is on promoting optimal health for all people, regardless of health status, developmental level, sociocultural background or health needs.

BOX 1–2. DEFINITIONS OF NURSING

ANA *Social Policy Statement*	The identification and treatment of human responses to health problems.
Nursing as Caring	Selecting one's caring behaviors (caring constructs) by determining the meaning of caring for the one cared for.
Nursing as Collaboration	A transaction based on mutual trust and mutual respect that facilitates individual independence in meeting health care needs.
Nursing as Professionalism	Addressing matters of concern and significance to society using a specific body of knowledge and a self-enforced code of ethics.

In all types of health care settings, nurses are held accountable for providing high-quality client care. Using their educational preparation and experience, nurses carry out professional clinical assessments that are the basis for client care. Nurses make clinical judgments to plan and use nursing implementation that promotes optimal health. They anticipate and divert crises, and collaborate with colleagues, clients, and others to promote client well-being and access to a broad continuum of health care services. In addition, nurses assume responsibility for the administration of systems of care delivery, and for the day-to-day management of client services. They assist clients with activities of daily living and promote healthy behavior.

Nurses also facilitate the practice of other health care professionals with whom they collaborate to meet the full range of client health needs. For example, nurses make equipment available and provide appropriate support services to help physicians and other health care professionals carry out diagnostic and therapeutic procedures. Nurses also may arrange to transport clients to various appointments with other members of the health care team. In addition to delivering direct client care based on their own assessments and judgments, nurses assist in implementing the clinical plans of health care colleagues when appropriate. By collaborating in assessment, diagnosis, and client care activities, nurses function as the critical link between clients and other health care providers.

There is growing recognition among professional colleagues and consumers that nursing is essential to the success of the health care delivery system. At the same time there is confusion about the nature of nurses and nursing, and a lack of understanding about differences in levels of educational preparation and levels of nursing practice. Nursing and its role in health care delivery can be clarified by considering the characteristics, education, and responsibilities of nurses as individuals, as well as demographic data about nurses as a professional group.

Demographics and Statistics

Number, Age, and Gender. Nurses are the largest group of health care providers in the country, numbering more than 2 million, with 80 percent or over 1.6 million currently employed in nursing positions.[10] Nurses also are predominantly female (96.7 percent), despite a steady increase, from 5.7 to 9.2 percent, in admissions of men to basic registered nurse education programs between 1981 and 1989. As of 1989 close to 55,000, or 3.3 percent, of registered nurses were males.[11] The median age of US nurses is 39; less than 16 percent are under the age of 30.[10]

In contrast, in 1989, Canadian nurses numbered 251,000, with 88 percent employed in nursing. Less than 1 percent (7316) of employed nurses in Canada are males. Statistics related to age groups of practicing nurses in Canada are very similar to US statistics: 34 percent are under 34, while 53 percent are under 39.[12]

Employment Status. Of the 1,687,100 persons reported employed in nursing in 1990, 61 percent were prepared in either diploma or associate degree programs, and 31 percent received their basic nursing education in baccalaureate programs. About 7 percent of registered nurses hold master's or doctoral degrees.[10] Contrary to popular belief, those educated and licensed as registered nurses tend to remain active in the field. According to 1989 unpublished data from the Division of Nursing's National Sample Survey of Registered Nurses, only 20 percent of the total number of licensed registered nurses were not employed in nursing. A majority of those not employed in nursing were not seeking employment at the time they were surveyed.

As depicted in Figure 1–2, the majority of registered nurses, 67.9 percent, continue to work in acute care settings. Much smaller numbers are employed in community health, long-term care, primary care, and educational settings, or serve in the military. Comparatively few nurses are self-employed, although entrepreneurial nurse-owned or nurse-managed businesses are beginning to gain in number and type.

In Canada, 86 percent of persons employed in nursing hold diplomas or postbasic certificates. Baccalaureate-prepared nurses comprise 13 percent of employed nurses, while .01 percent hold master's or doctoral degrees. Only 6 percent of licensed registered nurses were not employed in nursing in 1989. A significant percentage, 72 percent, of actively employed nurses in Canada work in acute care settings; 10 percent work in community health and smaller numbers in long-term care facilities, educational settings, or physicians' offices (Fig. 1–3). No statistics are available for Canadian nurses working in entrepreneurial endeavors.[12]

Certification. A growing number of nurses are certified for specialty and advanced practice roles, such as nurse practitioners, nurse-midwives, nurse anesthetists, nurse administrators, and clinical nurse specialists in a variety of clinical areas.[13] The rationale and processes for certification are discussed at the end of this chapter.

Typical Nurse Profile. The registered nurse in the United States is most likely to be a white female, around 39 years of age, whose basic nursing preparation was in a diploma school of nursing. She works full-time in a hospital and is a staff nurse on a general medical-surgical unit. The number of registered nurses who have obtained their basic nursing preparation in diploma or associate degree programs and have returned to school to obtain a baccalaureate or higher degree has doubled in the last decade. The typical nurse, however, has not returned to school for a higher degree in nursing.[10,11] This profile will alter over the next few years, as the profession feels the impact of major changes that have occurred in nursing education and practice during the past two decades.

Trends Influencing Typical Nurse Profile for the Future. Data suggest a gradual, but distinct trend toward more males and minorities entering nursing. Also, more nurses are receiving their basic nursing education in associate de-

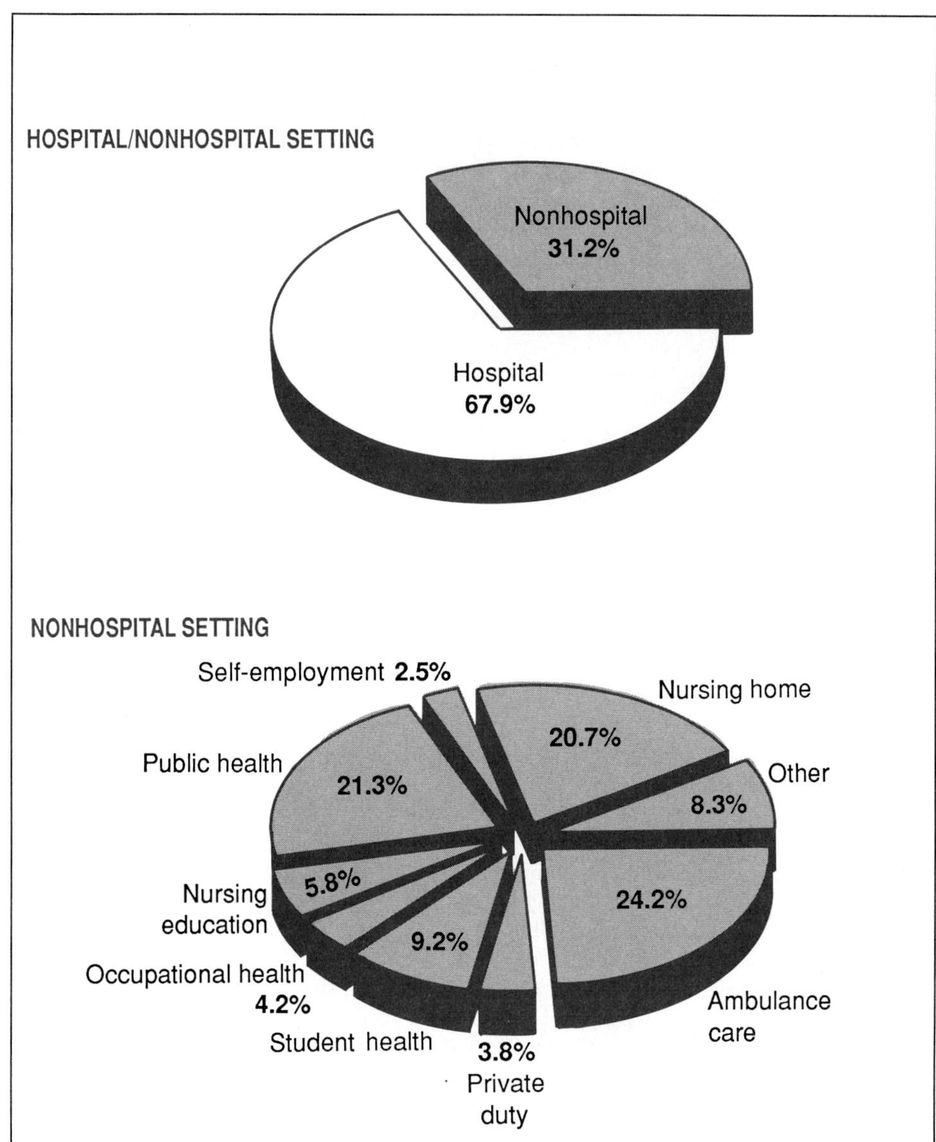

Figure 1–2. Estimated percentages of nurses employed in hospital and nonhospital settings in the United States (N = 1,627,035). (*From Division of Nursing, Bureau of Health Professions, U.S. Department of Health and Human Services, National Sample Survey of Registered Nurses, Unpublished data, 1989.*)

gree and baccalaureate programs. The number of diploma schools of nursing in the United States decreased from 721 in 1968 to 157 in 1989. During the same period, associate degree programs increased from 324 to 812 and baccalaureate programs increased from 233 to 488.[11] In 1968, US diploma schools of nursing graduated almost 68 percent of new nurse graduates, while associate degree programs graduated 15 percent and baccalaureate programs slightly over 17 percent. By 1989, more than 61 percent of new graduates were prepared in associate degree programs, 30.8 percent in baccalaureate programs, and 7.9 percent in diploma programs.[11]

An increasing number of nurses are seeking higher education, particularly master's degrees in nursing with a focus on advanced clinical practice. In 1978, 4878 full-time and 6544 part-time students were enrolled in master's programs. By 1989 the number of master's programs had increased from 117 to 212; full-time enrollment had decreased to 5860, but part-time student enrollment had increased to 16,727.[11] Doctoral programs increased from 6 in 1968 to 47 in 1989; full-time enrollment increased from 103 to 987 and part-time from 156 to 1430.[11]

These trends may be related to the growing acceptance of the baccalaureate as the basic preparation for entry into professional nursing and the associate degree as basic preparation for entry into the technical level of nursing practice (see Patterns of Education for Nursing, later in this chapter). Contributing factors also include the increasing complexity of care that clients require, hiring preferences of nurse administrators who are seeking to develop new models of professional practice, increasing nurse power accompanying stronger bases of theoretical expertise, political

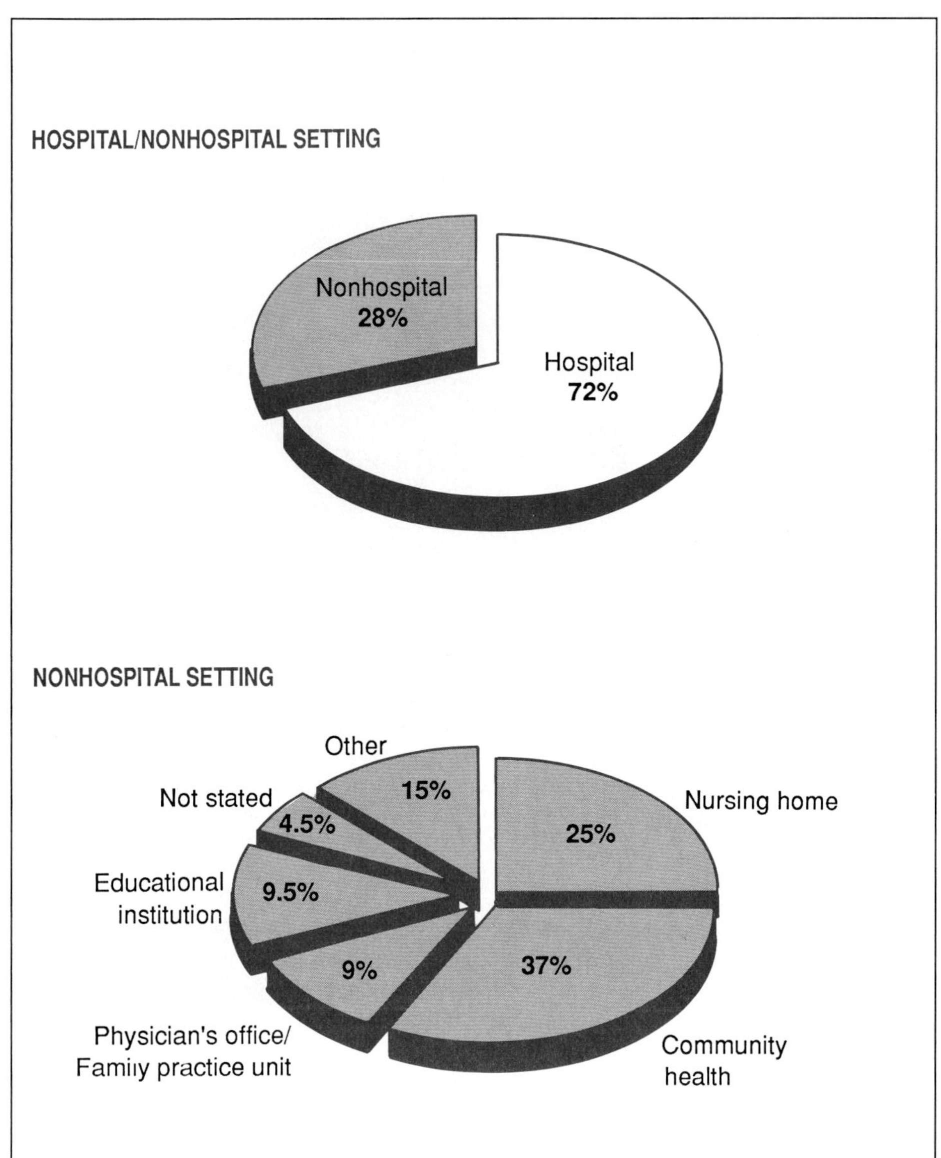

Figure 1–3. Estimated percentages of nurses employed in hospital and nonhospital settings in Canada. (*From Statistics Canada, Canadian Centre for Health Information, Registered Nurses Management Data, 1989.*)

awareness and organizational insight, and strong external pressures for change in health care delivery systems.

The Professional and Public Images of the Nurse

The image of nursing has an impact on the recruitment of new practitioners into the field and on the status and rewards accorded nurses by our society. The image of nursing has undergone considerable change over time. However, the current public perception of nursing remains colored by tradition, history, and sexism. It has been strongly influenced by the presentation of nurses in the media, which with few exceptions have portrayed nurses as one-dimensional characters.

During certain periods in history, notably the late 19th century and during the first and second world wars, nurses were viewed as "angels of mercy"—women in white whose characters and motives were pure. Even then, nursing was viewed as a "calling" rather than a profession. It often was seen as a temporary activity that women willingly gave up for marriage and family. Those who elected to remain in nursing were perceived as stern, elderly, and autocratic, sublimating their "natural womanly instincts" to serve husband and children and, instead, dedicating themselves to serving mankind (Fig. 1–4).

During times of war the profession of nursing was valued highly by society. Themes of patriotism, self-sacrifice, and the nurse as the embodiment of idealized womanhood—pure, brave, maternal, caring—provided a basis for World War I films and novels. Nursing emerged "as women's natural and most noble wartime work."[14] The World War II era saw an activist element added to the media's

BUILDING NURSING KNOWLEDGE

Do Nursing Students Change As They Go Through Nursing School?

Weller L, Harrison M, Katz Z. Changes in the self and professional images of student nurses. *J Adv Nurs.* 1988; 13:179–184.

These researchers were interested in the changes that occur in the self-images and professional images held by nursing students as they progressed through nursing school. Using two questionnaires, one to measure self-image and one to measure images of the professional nurse, they assessed the attitudes of students. Data were collected on entry into nursing school and after 3 months of studies. They also compared the attitudes of first-year, second-year, and third-year students.

The researchers predicted that differences between students' self-image and their image of the nurse would decline with time spent in nursing school. The results obtained only partially confirmed this relationship, suggesting that the self-image of students may be more clearly formed prior to entering nursing school than expected. The researchers also predicted that the students' images of the nurse would become more like the images held by their instructors. This hypothesis was confirmed. The finding was interesting in view of the fact that the researchers found a difference between the professional images held by the instructors in the two schools studied. One group held a more idealistic, and the other a more realistic, view of the nurse. The researchers concluded that the congruence between students' and instructors' professional images, whatever those images are, results from students' acceptance of their instructors' values about nursing as they advance through the program.

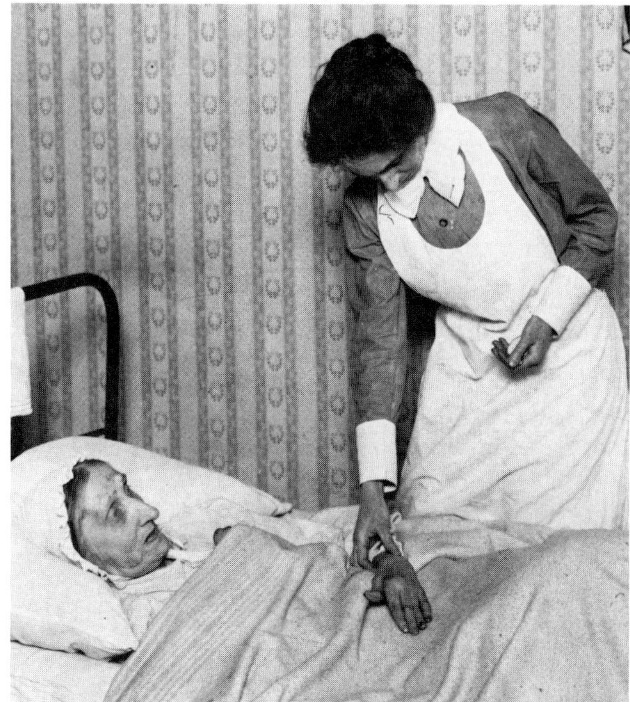

Figure 1–4. Nurse, circa 1910. The stiff, starched uniform matched the general public's view of nurses. (*From the Center for the Study of the History of Nursing, University of Pennsylvania, School of Nursing, Philadelphia, PA.*)

image of nursing, with nurses portrayed as courageous and competent. Nursing was depicted as having educational requirements for entry into practice as well as professional and moral standards for nursing practitioners.

Unfortunately this dash of realism was not strong enough to survive the next few decades. Filmmakers repeatedly cast female characters, including nurses, as passive, docile, stay-at-home creatures, willing to live vicariously through the exploits of their men.[14] This emphasis ended with the overwhelming response of nurses to the call for service in Korea and Vietnam. Responding again to the demands of war, nurses advanced their practice into areas where previously they had functioned as assistants—assessment, trauma and wound care, clinical decision making, independent judgment, and case management.

Given the directions that more recent television, films, adult novels, and even greeting cards have taken, it might have been preferable to continue living with an image that idealized nurses for their humanitarianism, selflessness, good morals, and womanly virtues, even though portraying them as nonprofessional, flighty, subservient to physicians, and operating more out of intuition than education. Instead, nurses are faced with the negative images growing out of the 1960s and 1970s media portrayals of nurses as lacking in morals, sexually promiscuous, objects of sexual diversion for physicians and male clients, authoritarian, narrow minded, sadistic, and sometimes criminally lethal.

Negative images continue to surface in the media, although a few notable efforts have been made to present nurses in a more positive light. The television series "China Beach," which focused on the role of women in Vietnam is an excellent example of a positive media image for nursing. The primary female character was a nurse portrayed as a multidimensional human being, capable of heroic action and human failures. She made mistakes and frequently lost objectivity, but was consistently presented as intelligent, competent, mature, assertive, caring, and compassionate, with a strong sense of self and ethics. On the negative side, the greeting card industry remains a serious offender where nursing's public image is concerned. In the guise of comic pornography and sadism, nurses are portrayed as sex objects or battle-axes, intent on providing sexual titillation or harassing clients.

The exaggerated images of the nurse presented by the media damage the credibility of nursing with colleagues, consumers, and impressionable young people considering career choices. The media in this country have a profound impact on the values, beliefs, and behaviors of the general public. Nurses can use this fact to the profession's advantage by focusing their efforts on influencing the media to bring to the public a professional image of nursing that emphasizes education, competence, caring, ethics, and accountability.

Characteristics of Successful Nursing Practice

How nursing is practiced and how that practice is perceived and evaluated forms nursing's current reality and future potential. Working through professional organizations and associations, nurses have exercised responsibility for self-regulation by designing standards for nursing practice. Nursing standards such as the ANA *Social Policy Statement* and the National League for Nursing's statement on competencies of graduates of nursing programs are based on the state of the art of nursing science, knowledge, and technology, and are designed to ensure that clients receive the highest quality of nursing care possible. The consistent delivery of high-quality care is a mark of success.

Nurses who are perceived as successful by clients, colleagues, and peers share certain basic characteristics. They are caring individuals who respect the rights of others. They want each client to have the best health care that technology and knowledge can offer. At the same time, they recognize clients' right to informed consent—to know the potential consequences of proposed health care interventions and to make choices. They also accept the need for cost-effective practice, for balancing outcomes for clients with cost of care.

The practice of successful nurses is guided by a code of ethics through which personal and societal values aid in critical analyses of moral dilemmas. Values, ethics, and ethical dilemmas are discussed in Chapter 34. Successful nurses have knowledge and skills, based on appropriate levels of liberal and professional education, to meet the changing health care needs of a diverse population and a health care system in transition. They recognize that nursing is an autonomous and unique health profession, and that nursing care is based on a philosophy that emphasizes caring over curing. Successful nurses value the contributions of other health care disciplines and strive to establish effective working relationships with peers and colleagues. Most importantly, successful nurses provide excellence in direct client care.

■ PATTERNS OF EDUCATION FOR NURSING

Those interested in nursing careers today can obtain basic nursing education through a variety of programs offered by different types of institutions, discussed below. Each of these entry-level programs qualifies graduates to sit for the same licensing examinations and practice under the same title—registered nurse. As a result, these graduates tend to be viewed as interchangeable by many employing institutions, other health professionals, and the general public. The result is that differences in their competencies become blurred, as does the overall image of nurses. Moreover, nursing is the only occupation claiming professional status that does not require the baccalaureate degree as the minimum education for entry into practice. Many professions require graduate degrees, at either the master's or doctoral level, for entry into professional practice.

Many professional nursing organizations, including the ANA[15] and the CNA,[16] have issued statements in recent years clarifying and supporting an official distinction between nurses with different basic educational preparation. Although no formal consensus has been reached, two levels of basic practitioners are most commonly described: technical (or associate) and professional. Generally, a diploma or associate degree is described as the minimum preparation for technical nursing, and a baccalaureate degree in nursing as the minimum for professional nursing. General role categories for associate degree (technical) and baccalaureate (professional) graduates are perceived as essentially the same, with specific functions within each role varying by level of preparation. Table 1–1 outlines a summary of the associate degree and baccalaureate graduate roles and competencies identified by four professional organizations.

Clearly distinguishing the competencies of "technical" and "professional" graduates is a first step toward officially establishing two levels of basic nursing practice. Modification of Nurse Practice Acts (the laws by which states and provinces regulate the practice of nursing) to provide separate titles, separate licensing, and separate job descriptions for the two levels of practitioners is the ultimate goal of the ANA and other professional organizations. To date, North Dakota is the only state to have modified its Nurse Practice Act to require a baccalaureate degree as minimum preparation for registered nursing practice, although several other states are considering a similar change. Grandfather clauses, permitting currently licensed associate degree graduates to continue to practice as registered nurses, and ladder programs to provide associate degree graduates easy access to higher education programs, are generally included in plans to officially designate the baccalaureate degree as minimum entry preparation for registered nursing practice.

Entry-level Education

Curently there are six different types of educational programs that prepare new practitioners for entry into nursing. Licensed vocational or practical nurse programs are typically 1 year or less in length, and prepare nurses who will have a limited scope of technical or vocational level practice that is under the direction or supervision of registered nurses. Graduates of these programs are eligible for a vocational nursing license (LVN or LPN). In Canada, graduates of such programs are eligible for licensure or certification as registered nurse assistants (RNAs). The other five patterns of basic nursing education prepare graduates who are eligible for licensure as registered nurses (RNs), all of

TABLE 1–1. COMPETENCIES EXPECTED OF GRADUATES FROM BACCALAUREATE AND ASSOCIATE DEGREE NURSING PROGRAMS

Role and Function	Baccalaureate Graduate	Associate Degree Graduate
Communicator	1. Establishes and maintains communication with individual clients, families, groups, and health care team members. 2. Incorporates interviewing techniques and communication skills in data collection, intervention, and evaluation of care. 3. Analyzes overt and covert verbal and nonverbal communication of individual clients, families, and groups. 4. Establishes and monitors the use of protocols for communicating and recording assessments, nursing care plans, implementations, and evaluation. 5. Evaluates and makes provision for the improvement of communication patterns for self, clients, and colleagues.	1. Uses communication skills in data collection, intervention, and evaluation of care. 2. Establishes and maintains communication with individual clients and health care team members. 3. Communicates and records assessments, nursing care plans, implementation, and evaluation according to established protocols. 4. Assesses overt verbal and nonverbal communication of individual clients 5. Evaluates and modifies personal communication patterns with clients and colleagues.
Client Teacher	6. Assesses learning needs, readiness, and motivation of individual clients, families, and groups in relation to health promotion, maintenance, and restoration. 7. Analyzes existing support systems and the need for support of individuals, families, and groups. 8. Develops and implements comprehensive teaching plans based on long- and short-range goals for individual clients, families, and groups. 9. Evaluates client learning, revises teaching plans, and makes referrals as needed.	6. Identifies situations in which individual clients need information and support to promote, maintain, and restore health, and follows established protocols in collecting data relevant to client need and readiness. 7. Develops and implements short-term teaching plans within the context of an established comprehensive teaching plan. 8. Participates in the evaluation of client learning and the modification of teaching plans.
Discipline of Nursing	10. Is responsible and accountable for the entire scope of nursing practice. 11. Works within established policy and procedures of employing agency, recognizing policies and protocols that may impede client care and works within the organizational framework to initiate change. 12. Functions as an advocate for clients and members of the health care team. 13. Bases practice upon the legal boundaries and ethical frameworks within the scope of own practice. 14. Assumes responsibility for continued learning as a means of growth, development, and maintenance of competence within the scope of own practice. 15. Evaluates own performance. 16. Participates in quality assurance programs. 17. Serves as a role model within context of own practice. 18. Is aware of impact of numerous systems that affect nursing, and participates in activities. 19. Participates in fashioning new nursing roles to meet the community health and societal care needs. 20. Assumes responsibility for maintaining a learning environment for nursing staff and students.	9. Is responsible and accountable for limited scope of nursing practice. 10. Functions within the legal boundaries and ethical framework consistent with the scope of own practice. 11. Assesses own performance using established criteria. 12. Participates in quality assurance programs. 13. Works within established policy and procedures of employing agency, recognizing and reporting procedures that impede client care. 14. Assumes responsibility for continued learning as a means of growth, development, and maintenance of competence within the scope of own practice. 15. Serves as a role model within context of own practice. 16. Is aware of the impact of numerous systems that affect nursing, and participates in activities to facilitate changes in these systems.
Provider of Care	21. Assesses health status and health potential of individual clients, families, and groups. 22. Establishes nursing diagnosis based upon client needs within a theoretical framework of nursing.	17. Uses knowledge, skills, and established protocols to provide an environment conducive to optimum restoration and maintenance of client's normal ability to meet basic human needs.

(continued)

TABLE 1–1. (continued)

	23. Makes decisions using scientific principles and published literature in planning nursing care with clients, families, or groups. 24. Provides nursing care for individuals, families, and communities according to priority of needs. 25. Analyzes changes in client status. 26. Synthesizes knowledge and skills in providing an environment conducive to optimum restoration and maintenance of client's normal ability to meet basic human needs. 27. Evaluates responses of clients and groups to nursing care plans and makes changes independently or in consultation with nursing colleagues. 28. Collaborates with other health care team disciplines to promote health care needs of clients and groups. 29. Identifies the need to establish protocols for groups of clients with similar health care problems. 30. Participates in identifying community and societal health care needs.	18. Collects data according to established protocols utilizing available resources. 19. Selects a nursing diagnosis from an established list. 20. Provides nursing care for individual clients based on the nursing diagnosis, and plans interventions that follow established protocols. 21. Identifies and documents changes in client status that interfere with the ability to meet basic needs. 22. Participates with other health care disciplines in meeting client needs. 23. Participates with client and members of the nursing team in evaluating the client's response to care in the modification of plan of care. 24. Consults with the baccalaureate or higher degree prepared nurse with client problems that are not within the scope of own practice.
Investigator	31. Reads, interprets, and evaluates research for applicability to own nursing practice. 32. Uses nursing practice as a means of gathering data for refining and extending practice. 33. Uses findings of nursing and other health-related research in own nursing practice. 34. Shares published research findings with colleagues. 35. Identifies nursing problems that need to be investigated. 36. Participates in the conduct of scientific study.	25. Assists in identifying problem areas in nursing practice. 26. Demonstrates awareness of the value or relevance of research in nursing. 27. Assists in collection of data within an established structured format.
Planner and Coordinator of Client Care	37. Assumes responsibility for coordinating care for a group of clients in a variety of settings. 38. Analyzes nursing care requirements of clients and determines priorities. 39. Guides and directs other nursing personnel in planning, organizing, implementing, and evaluating nursing care provided to clients. 40. Promotes a climate that fosters supportive communication and problem solving. 41. Delegates nursing responsibilities based on assessment of competencies and abilities of other nursing personnel. 42. Promotes cost-effective care through appropriate use of human, physical, and fiscal resources. 43. Participates in evaluation of other nursing personnel according to established protocols and using predetermined criteria. 44. Facilitates changes within the health care delivery system in collaboration with nursing colleagues and other health care personnel. 45. Assesses learning needs of health care personnel, and makes provision for needs to be met.	28. Assesses and establishes nursing care priorities for assigned clients. 29. With guidance, provides client care using resources and other nursing personnel commensurate with their educational preparation and experience. 30. Contributes to the promotion of a climate that fosters supportive communication and problem solving. 31. Seeks guidance to assist other nursing personnel to develop skills in giving nursing care. 32. Participates in promoting cost-effective care. 33. Participates in identification of need for change in the delivery of nursing care.

Data from Uris P, Bransletter E, Terrell M, et al. Associate and Baccalaureate Degree Nursing Graduates: Perceptions of and Recommendations for Their Preparation and Utilization. *Boulder, CO: WICHE, 1986. American Nurses' Association Commission on Nursing Education.* Educational Preparation for Nursing: A Course Book 1980. *Kansas City, MO: ANA; 1981. National League for Nursing.* Competencies of Graduates of Nursing Programs. *New York: NLN; 1983. Orange County/Long Beach Nursing Consortium.* Expected Educational Competencies of Nursing Graduates. *Long Beach, CA: Orange County/Long Beach Nursing Consortium; 1981.*

whom traditionally have perceived themselves as professional nurses.

Diploma Programs. Diploma nursing programs in the United States are usually 3 years in length. They focus on preparing nurses for technical level practice through educational programs that retain some of the elements of the traditional apprenticeship model espoused by Florence Nightingale. Building on a foundation of content from the physical and behavioral sciences, but not necessarily college courses, nursing students receive formal classes and extensive clinical experience in each of the major areas of medical-surgical, obstetrical, pediatric, and psychiatric nursing. Currently, graduates of diploma schools of nursing are eligible to take state board examinations for registered nurse licensure.

Diploma nursing programs in Canada are either hospital or college based. Most programs are 2 years in length. The college-based programs are similar to associate degree programs in the United States, discussed below. Graduates of diploma programs are eligible to take the registered nurse licensure examination. Many Canadian universities offer programs for registered nurses with diplomas to obtain baccalaureate degrees. These programs are 2 to 3 years in length.

Associate Degree Programs. Associate degree programs were developed in the United States as a solution to the nursing shortage growing out of World War II. Canada has no associate degree programs, but as indicated above, does have college-based diploma programs that are similar to US associate degree programs. Associate degree nursing programs are typically 2 years in length. Selected physical and social science courses provide a base for the study of nursing at the technical level. Focusing on the nursing process, the curriculum emphasizes both classroom and clinical learning with clients across the life span, experiencing health problems requiring general medical-surgical, obstetrical, or psychiatric nursing interventions. Although the associate degree in nursing was designed and continues to be implemented as a terminal degree, baccalaureate and higher degree nursing education programs have developed options for continued professional learning for qualified associate degree graduates. Graduates of associate degree programs are eligible to sit for the registered nurse licensure examination.

Baccalaureate Degree Programs. Baccalaureate nursing programs in the United States and Canada provide 4 years of undergraduate study, 2 of which focus on nursing education, usually at the upper division level. Some programs begin earlier, admitting students to the nursing major in the freshman or sophomore year. The first 2 years are dedicated primarily to learning in the liberal arts, humanities, and social and physical sciences. Upper division electives also may be taken in these disciplines. The focus is on achieving the level of critical inquiry, clinical judgment, and decision making, as well as clinical knowledge and skills that are critical for beginning professional practice. Theoretical concepts such as holistic health, wellness, self-help, and health promotion, as well as nursing diagnosis, interventions, evaluation, and leadership/management, usually figure prominently in baccalaureate curricula. Graduates are eligible to sit for the registered nurse licensure examination.

Master's and Doctoral Entry-level Programs. There are those who believe that entry into professional nursing requires more than baccalaureate education. The rationale offered is that the level of judgment required of professional nurses can be gained only through a complete liberal education followed by graduate-level preparation in the discipline of nursing. The direct entry master's program, exemplified by the Yale University model and offered by several other universities, and the nurse doctorate (ND) program, initiated by Case-Western Reserve University and offered by two others, prepare college graduates who have degrees in disciplines other than nursing as entry-level nurse generalists, with advanced knowledge and skill levels. Such programs may offer optional tracks for specialization as nurse-midwives, nurse practitioners, nurse administrators, and clinical specialists. Graduates are eligible to sit for the registered nurse licensure examination.

Education for Advanced Practice

Nursing has become a complex and highly varied practice discipline, with a rapidly growing, well-developed, and well-documented scientific and humanistic knowledge base. According to the Health and Human Services Report to Congress and the President in the summer of 1990, increasing numbers of nurses prepared at the master's and doctoral levels are needed to continue the expansion of this knowledge base, and to provide the leadership in health policy-making, clinical practice, and administration that is so critical to the advancement of the nursing profession and the improvement of client care.

In 1990, 124,000 (7 percent) of employed nurses were educated at the master's or doctoral level. The projected need for nurses with advanced educational preparation by the year 2020 is 392,000, but the anticipated supply is only 317,000, leaving a shortfall of 74,500.[10]

In Canada, even smaller numbers of nurses are prepared at the master's level or higher. In 1989, the total number of nurses with a master's or higher degree was 2524, of which 2238 were employed in nursing. This number represents approximately 10 percent of all employed nurses in Canada.[12]

Master's Degree Programs. Nursing education programs at the master's level usually prepare clinical specialists or advanced clinical practitioners. Some programs continue to focus on preparing graduates for functional roles in administration or education. Master's programs in nursing are offered by institutions of higher education and are built on knowledge and competencies of baccalaureate education.

Theory and research in nursing and related disciplines,

as well as other relevant information, form the basis for curriculum. Particular emphasis is given to advanced scientific concepts and guided clinical practice, which contribute to the focused body of knowledge the clinical nurse specialist uses for making clinical judgments. Graduates have the foundation for continued professional learning and doctoral study in nursing, as well as for advanced practice.

Doctoral Programs. The need for doctoral-level education is receiving greater recognition from both nursing education and service. Nurses may pursue a doctorate in nursing science (DNS, DNSc, or DSN), a doctor of philosophy in nursing (PhD), a doctorate in education (EdD), or a doctorate in public health (DrPH), public administration, communication, higher education administration, or a number of other fields. Doctoral programs produce nurse philosophers, ethicists, theorists, and researchers, who contribute to the development of new knowledge for nursing and the advancement of the nursing profession. More frequently, colleges and universities are requiring that nursing faculty members have doctorates, in keeping with their academic colleagues in other disciplines. Clinical agencies are beginning to seek doctorally prepared nurses to serve as nurse executives or directors of education and research. Nurse entrepreneurs are seeking doctorates to increase their credibility with professional colleagues and clients, and professional organizations are turning to doctorally prepared nurses to represent them to consumer groups and health policy decision makers.

Alternative Access to Nursing Education

Nursing has been making great strides in moving its educational programs into the mainstream of higher education. There has been a steady decline in the number of diploma schools of nursing over the past decade, while the number of both community college and senior college and university nursing programs has increased. In its standards for nursing education, the American Nurses' Association continues to stress that nursing programs leading to baccalaureate and higher degrees should be located in accredited institutions of higher education that offer degrees in several disciplines, including programs of study in the biological, social, and physical sciences, and in the humanities.[17]

Societal and professional demands are motivating increasing numbers of registered nurses to seek advanced education in the form of baccalaureate and higher degrees. At the same time, economic conditions, the nursing shortage and other employment problems, and personal circumstances serve as constraints to nurses' access to traditional degree programs. Many nurses live far from colleges and universities that offer undergraduate and graduate nursing programs. They are involved in their families, communities, and jobs; they are neither mobile nor wealthy enough to pull up roots and move to another area to attend a degree program. In many instances, their communities would be unable to replace them if they left to attend school.

The concept of "distance education" has evolved from the needs of learners such as these, and also from the growing emphasis on collaboration among education, business, industry, and service organizations. A variety of educational models and technologies are used to deliver needed programs to areas that are distant from the college or university campus. Among these is the external degree assessment model developed under the auspices of the New York Regents External Degree Program. This model offers learners who are distant from a traditional degree-granting campus the opportunity to earn an associate or baccalaureate degree in nursing, as well as many other disciplines. The focus of such a model is on assessment, on validating learning through testing and demonstration, rather than on instruction. It is the responsibility of the student to find learning opportunities to meet specified objectives. The learning is self-designed and self-directed. The degree program faculty provide a framework of objectives and study guides for examinations to help students meet the assessment requirements. The students are fully accountable and responsible for deciding when they are ready to complete the designated assessment processes.[18] The Statewide Nursing Program offered by the California State University system expanded this concept to develop a mediated learning model, which allows students the option of instruction, assessment, or a combination approach to achieving a baccalaureate in nursing.

Another innovation in access to nursing education called Project LINC (Ladders in Nursing Careers) was recently developed in New York City as a collaborative effort between health care facilities and nursing schools, including practical nurse, associate degree and baccalaureate degree programs.[19] The purpose of Project LINC is to provide educational advancement opportunities for individuals in entry-level or mid-level jobs in nursing. The program targets nurse aides and LPNs who are interested in upgrading within the nursing profession. Special support services are offered in addition to nursing coursework to eliminate financial, social, educational or other barriers.

A number of diploma programs have developed yet another alternative to traditional academic institutions. The actual structure of this alternative varies, but its purpose is to accommodate the trend toward moving nursing education into institutions of higher education. Some diploma programs are formally linking with colleges and universities. They continue to provide the nursing education, while the higher education institutions provide the sciences and humanities and award the baccalaureate. In other instances, diploma schools of nursing are seeking accreditation as single-purpose, degree-granting institutions, which have the right to award their own baccalaureate degrees in nursing.

Continuing Professional Education

Continuing education is a critical component of professional nursing education. Both baccalaureate and graduate nursing programs emphasize the need for lifelong learning. Schools of nursing focus on the need for continuing professional development in their educational goals and objectives. A number of states have legislated or enabled state boards of nursing to mandate continuing education as a requirement for renewing licensure. Continuing education builds on previous preservice education and on learning in the clinical practice environment. It is designed to help nurses enhance knowledge and skills in practice, education, administration, and research; modify or strengthen values and attitudes; and maintain competency and currency in a rapidly changing world. The underlying purpose is to promote optimal health and quality of life for the public and for the nurse. Assuming responsibility for one's own continuing learning is characteristic of a professional.

■ CREDENTIALING IN NURSING

Credentialing in nursing is based on the assumption that consumers have a right to expect health professionals to provide high-quality care. **Credentialing** is the process whereby qualified agents, based on a variety of measures and assessment strategies, certify that individual nurses or the institutions and programs that prepare them for entry or advanced practice meet minimum standards at specified times. Credentialing protects both the public and the profession by regulating entry into nursing and by ensuring that the programs preparing graduate nurses meet predetermined structure, process, and outcome criteria.

Licensure

Licensure is a formal mandatory process through which a government agency grants an individual the right to provide certain services. State governments protect the basic safety of the public by legislating licensing boards that set minimum requirements for entry into practice and use of the title of registered nurse (RN). In the United States, licensure as an RN requires graduation from a State Board of Nursing approved educational program and successful completion of the National Council of State Boards of Nursing Licensure Examination (NCLEX). In Canada, graduates of all registered nursing programs take the Canadian Nurses' Association Testing Service (CNATS) examination. See Chapter 3 for further discussion of the licensing process. In some states this regulatory process also extends to advanced nursing practice roles. RNs who meet specified additional educational requirements for advanced nursing practice are approved to use such titles as nurse practitioner, nurse-midwife, nurse anesthetist, or clinical nurse specialist.

Certification

Certification is a credentialing mechanism that is being used increasingly by licensed registered nurses, state regulatory bodies, and clinical agencies to validate achievement of a level of clinical specialty or functional expertise and competence that goes beyond the level required for basic licensure. **Certification** is a voluntary, nongovernmental process that attests that a nurse has met certain predetermined educational and experience standards specified by a professional certifying agency or professional association. The American Nurses' Association operates the most comprehensive certification program, offering certification examinations in 20 areas. Most major specialty nursing associations, such as the American College of Nurse-Midwives (ACNM), the American Association of Critical Care Nurses (AACN), and the American Association of Nurse Anesthetists (AANA), also offer certification programs for registered nurses.

The Canadian Nurses Association approved a three-phase plan for a certification process in 1986. The plan identified procedures for designating nursing specialties, developing certification examinations, and certifying individuals.[20]

Credentialing of Programs: Accreditation

Accreditation is a method of evaluating an institution by an officially recognized outside agency. The accreditation of nursing education programs can be either a legal requirement or a voluntary process. In the first instance, all programs must meet minimum standards within their state to obtain approval of the educational program and eligibility for graduates to sit for the registered nurse licensure examination. In addition to this legal requirement, many nursing education programs voluntarily seek accreditation, a status granted by a voluntary, nongovernmental agency or organization to educational programs that meet predetermined structure, process, and outcome criteria.

Program accreditation assures students trying to make choices among programs and employers hiring graduates that the program has successfully demonstrated high quality in a rigorous peer review process, and that the program undergoes periodic reassessment to ensure continuing acceptable quality. The National League for Nursing is the only nationally recognized accrediting agency for diploma, associate, baccalaureate, and master's degree educational programs. The American College of Nurse-Midwives and the American Association of Nurse Anesthetists offer accreditation services for programs that prepare nurses for practice in their specialty areas.

From the perspective of the profession, credentialing serves as a mechanism for unification and for improving the image of nursing with its various constituencies—collegial, public, and political. It also provides an impetus for improving the quality of nursing education and, subsequently, nursing practice, interdisciplinary collaboration, and client outcomes.

■ SETTINGS FOR NURSING PRACTICE

The settings in which nursing is practiced are varied. Ideally, they are limited only by the imagination and creativity of today's nurses. In reality, they also are constrained by other factors, including the medical community, economics, increasing malpractice insurance rates for advanced nurse practitioners, and limited access to direct reimbursement from third-party payers for nursing services. Traditional practice settings in the hospital still employ the greatest number of registered nurses. The next largest practice setting is in the community, including school nursing, public health nursing, occupational health nursing, or office nursing.

Nursing homes, private duty settings, nursing education, and other structured settings account for most of the remaining nursing positions. Nurses listed as self-employed number 2.5 percent. Based on trends, it is anticipated that the number of positions available for nurses in home health care, other community care settings, long-term care, and private practice will increase, while the staff positions in hospitals will decrease as new staffing models evolve to meet the current nursing shortage.

Hospitals

Historically, hospitals were regarded as places to die rather than places in which to regain health. Nursing changed that by improving sanitary conditions and quality of care for hospitalized clients, thereby reducing mortality rates and enhancing the image of the hospital. Today hospitals are extremely complex, labor-intensive organizations, in which nurses are the largest group of health care providers. Hospitals represent a major investment for the American public. In 1987, hospital care accounted for nearly 44 percent of health care expenditures;[21] however, during the 1980s more community hospitals closed than in any previous decade, decreasing from 5851 in 1980 to 5533 in 1989. Trends in government payment, and unsponsored care were felt to account for the decline.[22]

Hospitals differ on many variables, all of which need to be taken into account when making decisions about where to practice nursing. Size varies from those with fewer than 25 to more than 1000 beds. Services range from simple, same-day procedures to complex acute care. Organizational structures vary in acute care general hospitals, chronic care or rehabilitation hospitals, teaching hospitals and psychiatric hospitals. A hospital may emphasize a service, teaching, or research mission. The hospital's focus will influence the type of clients accepted, categories of staff employed, and professional competencies expected of staff members.

Health care services in the future will look very different. Hospitals are in transition from health care delivery systems focused on medical treatment and nursing care into a technological industry emphasizing increasing needs for capital funds and high profit margins. This will require broad diversification into a range of inpatient and outpatient services as well as real estate and other related investments.

Nurses working in the hospitals of the future may find themselves faced with resolving conflicts between ethics and finance (see Chap. 37), between client needs and corporate needs, and between competing health disciplines and consumer demands. Clients in hospitals will have more complex and critical care needs; nurses will require more specialized and advanced education to meet those needs and to deal effectively with multicorporate and economics-driven health care institutions. Nurses may need to design new structures, organizations, and models for delivering nursing care and establishing their unique role and mission within the health care delivery system of the future. Well-defined personal and professional ethics will be of paramount importance as nurses and other health care professionals struggle with the problems generated by increasing technology and diminishing health care resources.

Communities

Community Health Nursing. The community offers a wide range of employment opportunities for nurses. The minimum entry requirement for employment in public health and school settings within the community is usually the baccalaureate in nursing, although some smaller communities employ nurses prepared at the diploma or associate degree levels for these positions if baccalaureate or higher degree graduates are not readily available.

There has been a long-standing debate in nursing about whether community health is a distinct area of clinical specialization.[23] It has been suggested that the primary focus of community health nurses should be the health of population groups, or aggregates, and that the unique activities of community health nurses are assessment or definition of problems and identification of solutions or treatments at the aggregate level.[24]

This model for community health nursing practice involves a different level of decision making than is used by nurses involved in the direct delivery of care on a one-to-one basis between nurse and client. Assessment, planning, intervention, and evaluation at the aggregate rather than individual level requires a whole range of different kinds of knowledge and skills, including group process and management of systems. It also demands that nurses understand and become involved in the organization and politics of health planning and policy making, and in the general life of the community. (Concepts related to community health are discussed further in Chap. 7.)

Home Health Care. A subfield of community health, home health care provides an employment opportunity for those nurses who want to maintain a practice caring directly for individual clients, but prefer to be based in the community rather than the hospital. Since the advent of Medicare in 1965 the home health care industry has become the fastest growing component of the US health care delivery system. Home health agencies provide a range of services, including illness prevention and health maintenance, acute care follow-up, maternal-fetal care, and hospice care. Although there are some nurse owned agencies, the majority of home health agencies are owned by multi-institutional corporations or by other clinical agencies, such as acute care hospitals and nursing homes.

Nurses practice as direct care providers, supervisors, and agency administrators in home health care settings. Because today's home health clients are in general sicker and in need of more complex care than clients of the past, nurses with baccalaureate or higher degrees often are preferred for these positions. Many agencies, however, employ nurses with all levels of preparation to provide care to clients.

Other Community Settings. Clinics, physicians' offices, and business and industry are also settings for nursing practice in the community. Nurses in these settings provide direct client services, with an emphasis on assessment, health education, health promotion, and referral. In addition to providing client care services for workers, nurses also function as consultants to or public liaisons for business and industry. Professional nurses are beginning to develop entrepreneurial practices within the community, which will be discussed in the section on nursing roles later in this chapter.

Long-term Rehabilitation and Hospice Care

The needs of the elderly, the chronically ill, the disabled, and the dying provide a context within which nursing can demonstrate the strength of its humanistic philosophy and traditional emphasis on the value of caring, particularly for those least able to care for themselves without help. Nurses have practice opportunities as administrators, supervisors, instructors, head nurses, nurse practitioners, clinical nursing specialists, and staff nurses in long-term care settings.

Nurses have traditionally been the primary caregivers for the elderly, the chronically ill and disabled, and the dying. The continuum of care needed by these clients provides exciting opportunities for nursing practice. According to the Health Care Finance Administration, a long-term care system consists of those services designed to provide diagnostic, preventive, therapeutic, rehabilitative, supportive, and maintenance services for individuals with chronic physical or mental impairment, in a variety of institutional and noninstitutional health settings, with the goal of promoting the optimum level of physical, social, and psychological functioning.

Nurses can assume leadership roles in both planning and providing care within such a continuum. Although constrained by economics, employment opportunities are extensive and varied. Nurses work directly with clients to identify individual needs, and collaborate with an interdisciplinary team to meet those needs. Practice roles are available for nurses to provide a variety of services, including:

1. Rehabilitation—restoring the individual to some previous level of functioning that can be sustained.
2. Maintenance—ensuring the maximum possible independence, even if there are limitations in activity or deterioration of functions.
3. Illness prevention and health promotion—slowing of deterioration or anticipating and taking action on psychological, physiological, social, and environmental concerns that may avoid or reduce the impact of health-related problems.
4. Protection—providing humanistic care for persons who may be functionally and permanently dependent.
5. Prolonging longevity—providing services necessary to maintain life.

The ideal long-term care system provides options based on individual needs that allow persons to be treated in the least restrictive setting and to continue as long as possible to live in the communities with which they are familiar and comfortable. The ultimate aim for nursing is to become involved in caring interactions, transactions, and collaboration with clients, colleagues, and systems that contribute to the quality of life for the elderly, and the chronically ill or disabled, and that provide for comfort and dignity in the process of dying and death.

Correctional Settings

Practice roles for nurses in correctional settings are increasing, both in institutional and community-based services. Nurses provide primary care for adult and juvenile offenders in clinic and other service settings and also assume administrative and supervisory roles with correctional health services.

■ CURRENT AND EMERGING ROLES AND FUNCTIONS OF THE PROFESSIONAL NURSE

The Nurse as Caregiver

Giving care to others is the essence of nursing. The role of caregiver is fundamental for nurses. It supersedes and underlies all other nursing roles and functions. It is nursing's unique reason for being and the rationale for nursing decisions and actions. Traditionally, the concept of caring has been associated with those nurturing characteristics and behaviors generally perceived as most desirable in women and mothers: comforting, soothing, protecting, keeping clean and safe, feeding, gratifying needs, easing pain, listening, touching, being there when needed or wanted, and giving rather than taking.

In today's nursing practice, caring means purposeful, intentional human action that brings about change for the better. Dolores Gaut identifies three conditions for an interaction between nurse and client to qualify as caring: (1) the caregiver must have appropriate knowledge to identify a need and to recognize that something can be done to improve the situation; (2) the caregiver must take action after choosing among alternatives, with the intent to bring about change for the better; and (3) change is evaluated solely on the basis of the welfare of the one being cared for.[8] There are several levels of caregiving roles in nursing, related to the level of professional knowledge and expertise of the practitioner.

Nurse Generalist. Nurses are initially prepared for basic entry into practice as generalist caregivers. Nurse generalists have a broad knowledge base for practice in a variety of settings; however, the majority of nurses practicing as generalists provide bedside care for clients in hospitals. The focus for the generalist nurse is on meeting clients' basic needs and assisting with activities of daily living through nursing assessment, diagnosis, and implementation.

Nurse generalists are accountable practitioners who collaborate with clients, families, and other health care team members in health promotion and disease prevention, as well as acute and rehabilitative care. The ability to function in various clinical areas is a strength offered to cost-conscious employers by nurses prepared as generalist caregivers.

Nurse Specialist. The *Social Policy Statement* of the American Nurses' Association describes the specialist in nursing practice as

> a nurse who, through study and supervised practice at the graduate level (master's or doctorate), has become expert in a defined area of knowledge and practice in a selected clinical area of nursing. Specialists in nursing practice are also generalists, in that they hold a baccalaureate in nursing, and therefore are able to provide the full range of nursing care.[1]

A different level of professional expertise is provided by nurses prepared for the caregiver role as specialists. Specialist preparation builds on the generalist base and develops depth of knowledge in a nursing specialty, usually a defined area of clinical practice such as critical care nursing or gerontological nursing. Profound changes in health care delivery are creating a new demand for nurse specialists. Hospitals now provide care for clients who are sicker than those in the past and who are discharged earlier because of changes in the way that health care costs are reimbursed. Nurses with advanced specialty preparation are able both to provide and to guide the delivery of expert clinical care. They can offer creative solutions to problems and contribute to the development of a strong, collegial, and professional nursing staff, ensuring optimal care for all clients. Several different nurse specialist credentials are available. Four examples are discussed below.

Clinical nurse specialist (CNS) practice includes the roles of caregiver, educator, counselor, consultant, liaison, and researcher. The CNS as educator accepts responsibility for providing informal and formal education for other nurses and health care providers, as well as client groups. The aim is to help others develop new perspectives and approaches to client problems and bring a new depth to nursing care. The CNS counselor role is carried out on a personal level, involving one-on-one counseling with nurses and clients about problems that concern them. In the counselor role, the CNS provides support and demonstrates expertise in collaborating with others to address issues of concern to them.

As a consultant, the CNS serves as a catalyst and problem solver, helping others perform their caregiving roles more efficiently and effectively. The liaison role represents a more formal consultative role, whereby the CNS is responsible for support and consultation to a specified clinical area.

IMPLICATIONS FOR NURSE–CLIENT COLLABORATION

The Nurse's Client Advocate Role

It is not enough for nurses to collaborate with clients. Once a nurse and client have entered into a caregiving transaction, the nurse must be prepared to assert the rights of the client—to act on behalf of the client's legitimate interests even when these place the client in conflict with the health care institutions or other health care providers. This is the nurse's client advocate role. It is a role nurses are uniquely well prepared to play by virtue of the close contact maintained with the client during the caregiving relationship.

The researcher role is increasingly important for specialist caregivers. Clinical nurse specialists are accountable for remaining informed about the state of the art of research in their area of expertise, and for finding ways to evaluate and use research findings in their practice. They also have a responsibility to use scientific methods of inquiry to examine clinical problems and generate research questions. The specialist helps to link new knowledge with current practice.

Nurse practitioners provide primary care to clients across the life span. **Primary care** refers to the care provided at client's first contact with the health care system. Nurse practitioners diagnose and treat acute, episodic and chronic health problems, usually in an outpatient, ambulatory care, or community setting. Many nurse practitioners establish independent practices or work in partnership with a physician.

Nurse anesthetists administer surgical anesthesia under the supervision of an anesthesiologist and monitor clients' responses to anesthetic medications. Nurse anesthetists may work in ambulatory care or acute care settings.

Certified nurse-midwives provide primary health care for women. Although major emphasis is on assessment and care during pregnancy, labor, and delivery, many nurse-midwives also provide gynecological health maintenance.

The Nurse as Client Advocate

Nurses are involved in client advocacy. Advocacy derives from the ethical principle of beneficence, which underlies the nurse's duty to protect clients from harm. To be a client advocate means being assertive, sometimes being in conflict with the health care institution or other providers, and ensuring that clients and families are adequately informed to take an active role in making decisions about issues related to their own health and health care. It means recognizing that the rights and values of clients and their families must take precedence when they conflict with those of health care providers or health care delivery systems.

The Nurse as Health Care Team Member

More than ever before, contemporary health care requires teamwork. The increasing complexity of both client prob-

BUILDING NURSING KNOWLEDGE

Are There Problems With the Client Advocacy Role?

Robinson MB. Patient advocacy and the nurse: Is there a conflict of interest? *Nurs Forum.* 1985; 22:58–63.

The author's purpose in this article is to point out problems with the client advocacy role. In client advocacy, nurses take responsibility for protecting the rights of clients being cared for. Tasks include (1) helping clients to interpret agency policies, procedures, and services; (2) taking assertive action to help clients; and (3) helping other agency health care professionals understand clients' perceptions of the hospital experience.

Robinson suggests that this model of advocacy is humanitarian, but also has adversarial characteristics. For example, protecting the rights of one client can bring a nurse into conflict with the interests of the institution or coworkers, with providing for the welfare of other clients, or even with meeting the other needs of this client! Ideally, according to Robinson, the focus of the nurse advocacy role should be on taking the welfare of all into account and balancing individual client's welfare against the needs of others.

Under an adversarial model, this is not always possible. Other models, according to Robinson, emphasize compromise rather than "taking sides." One alternative model places nurses in the role of counselors whose objective is to alleviate client fear and reestablish feelings of autonomy and self-control. Under this model, the advocate is an educator. Another model involves nurse advocates as delegators. The nurse delegates client complaints to others with special expertise and authority to act on the client's behalf, usually the client ombudsman or representative. The use of these models, according to the author, protects clients' rights while also protecting nurses from the complications that can arise from conflict situations.

lems and health care systems requires collaboration among many different professionals and allied health workers to achieve the best possible outcomes in the most cost-effective manner. Establishing successful collaborative relationships is not an easy task. It requires give and take from all participants, as well as recognition of the valuable qualities and expertise of each team member.

The unique perspective that professional nurses bring to the health care team is one that humanizes and personalizes the caring process. Professional nurses, more than any other caregivers, emphasize care for the total person and collaborate with clients to determine the best choices among health care options. This broad focus contributes to nursing's potential for leadership among health care team members, many of whom have less comprehensive objectives for client care. Collaborating with the health care team is discussed in greater detail in Chapter 19.

The Nurse as Manager and Executive

Nurses act as managers of care at all levels of nursing practice. Staff nurses function as managers of client care. In a different way, nurse administrators function as managers and executives for all types of health care delivery systems. Depending on practice setting and role, nurses may emphasize one or more of the basic managerial functions of planning, leading, organizing or coordinating, and controlling. Table 1–2 provides descriptions of the basic functions and activities involved in managing.

Manager of Client Care. The role of the staff nurse includes managing the direct care of an assigned number of clients. The model or pattern of nursing practice in use—case, functional, team, primary nursing, or case management—influences the style and the level of management skills that can be used by staff nurses in a given setting.

Case Nursing. In **case nursing** one nurse is assigned to provide total care for one client for the period of a single work shift. Based on acuity and case mix, a nurse may be given responsibility for several clients at the same time. Nurses may or may not be assigned to the same clients on subsequent work days. Planning is more process oriented (focusing on how to get things done) than client oriented. Being able to organize one's work and accomplish assigned tasks in a timely manner is necessary for case nursing practice. The oldest pattern of nursing care, case nursing is the usual assignment pattern for private duty, intensive care units, and nursing students.

Functional Nursing. The functional model of client care delivery has its roots in industry and is based on duties or responsibilities. **Functional nursing** uses an assembly line approach, in which the major tasks that must be accomplished to meet client needs are delegated by the nurse in charge to individual nurses. For example, one nurse may be responsible for dispensing medications to all the clients on the unit; other nurses may be assigned to assist clients with hygiene. There is little opportunity for collaborative planning. Management activities and nursing care are task specific rather than client centered.

TABLE 1–2. BASIC MANAGERIAL FUNCTIONS AND ACTIVITIES

Planning	Making decisions about what needs to be done and what will be done Designing a course of action
Leading	Getting people to work Influencing the behavior of others to get them to do what needs to be done
Organizing	Establishing structure to get things done Coordinating integration of individual efforts and resources to bring about group efficiency and effectiveness
Controlling	Exercising power to ensure that what happens is what is planned Exercising power through evaluation and corrective measures to ensure plans are achieved.

Data from Marquis B, Huston C. Management Decision Making for Nurses. *Philadelphia; Lippincott; 1987. Marriner A.* Guide to Nursing Management. *St. Louis: Mosby; 1984. Swart J. Unpublished papers.*

Team Nursing. In **team nursing** a registered nurse serves as leader and manager for a group of nurses and allied health care personnel who assume responsibility for meeting the health care needs of a group of clients through cooperation and collaboration. The team leader typically uses a participatory management strategy to develop, implement, and evaluate client care plans. The team leader may also provide part of the direct client care. All team members participate in planning client care assignments and team goals for the day. Management aspects of the team leader's role include delegation of specific tasks to team members, as well as supervision, coordination, and evaluation of care provided by team members.

Primary Nursing. **Primary nursing** is a model that exemplifies a more professional level of nursing practice than those discussed above. It has enjoyed widespread acceptance by nurses. It was designed as a response to complaints by staff nurses about fragmentation of care and the lack of meaningful contact with clients in the previously discussed care delivery models. In primary nursing, one nurse, called the primary nurse, provides client assessment and care at the time of admission to the facility and is accountable for the full range of management functions (planning, coordinating, directing, and controlling) for comprehensive twenty-four hour care for that client throughout the stay. Other nurses, called associate nurses, collaborate in planning and provide care when the primary nurse is not on duty. Leadership and management activities are used on a small group scale. Each primary nurse is responsible for a small group of clients and for the nurse associates assisting in the care of that client group. Research indicates that nurses feel they have more autonomy and greater decision-making power in primary nursing than in the other models discussed.[25]

Case Management. Recently nurses have begun to participate in a pattern of care known as managed care or **case management.** This model involves collaborative nurse-physician joint practice. All clients are assigned to a nurse-physician team upon entry into the health care system. The nurse-physician team is then responsible for the overall health care outcomes for clients assigned to their practice and receives direct reimbursement from clients or third-party payers such as insurance companies. The case manager (nurse or physician) assumes responsibility for comprehensive care through delegation to direct caregivers, and manages the progress of their clients through the system. This involves collaboration with other health care team members and planning for discharge and follow-up. Case management involves application of the full range of management functions and activities. It also facilitates involvement of clients and their families in decision making about health care.[26] Table 1–3 summarizes models of client care delivery in nursing.

TABLE 1–3. MODELS OF CLIENT CARE DELIVERY

Case nursing	One nurse gives total care to one or more clients for an entire shift.
Functional nursing	Work assignments are organized according to tasks, rather than total care to a client.
Team nursing	Care planning and work assignments are collaboratively carried out by the team leader (RN), and team members (RNs, LVNs, nurse's aides).
Primary nursing	Primary nurse (RN) assumes responsibility for care planning and around-the-clock coordination of care for one or more clients during their entire hospital stay, as well as providing care when on duty. Associate nurses (RNs) provide care when primary nurse is not on duty.
Case management	Nurse-physician teams assume collaborative responsibility for planning, coordinating, and providing care for groups of clients from admission to discharge, and are directly reimbursed for care.

Manager of Nursing Services. Nurses also function in formal management positions in health care delivery systems. Depending on their location within the organizational hierarchy, nurses can be classified as top-level managers or executives, midlevel managers, and lower, or first-level managers.

Traditionally, the organizational design of client care units has focused on the head nurse or unit administrator as the key manager for day-to-day operations. This first-level manager decides who will provide care to which clients and how all the myriad nursing tasks associated with caring for clients on a day-to-day basis will be carried out. Ideally, first-level managers are educated at the baccalaureate level or above.

Supervisors and assistant or associate directors of nursing are midlevel managers of nursing systems with responsibility for coordinating and monitoring the operations of a prescribed group of nursing staff and services. These positions report to a director of nursing or top nurse executive. The appropriate level of education for such positions is a master's degree.

Roles of top-level nursing administrators are changing in health care institutions. Movement of nurses into more responsible positions within the corporate structure is reflected in nursing's new place on the organizational chart. Previously, many directors of nursing functioned as midlevel managers of nursing services and allocated resources. Today nurse managers are nurse executives, with a corresponding increase in power and prestige within the institution. In many ways the top nurse executive sets direction for the development of the corporate structure—the vision, values, norms, and attitudes about clients and practice. Preparation for the nurse executive role requires higher education at the master's degree or doctoral level and strong business orientation and skills.

The Nurse as Entrepreneur

The past decade could be called the age of the nurse entrepreneur. Increasingly, nurses are seeking to expand their control over professional practice and to improve their income by establishing and operating nurse-owned and managed businesses. Nurses have opened businesses such as primary care clinics and home health agencies, which provide direct client care and case management services for clients of all ages. Nurses offer independent nurse-midwifery services and care for persons with psychosocial problems. They market and operate consultant and continuing education services, temporary employment services, and agency contract services, to name a few. In addition, they are paid directly for the services they provide. In some cases payment is made by clients. Contracts with health agencies and health maintenance organizations (HMOs) represent another source of payment.

Successful nurse entrepreneurs need a whole range of skills not normally included in basic nursing education programs, so it may be necessary to seek continuing education to prepare for practice in entrepreneurial settings. Small business management skills are critical for entrepreneurs; these include strategic planning, obtaining capital, defining, pricing, packaging, and marketing services or a product, and designing efficient and cost-effective health care delivery systems.

The rewards may well be worth the effort needed to overcome obstacles. Increased autonomy, control of practice, and the opportunity for profit-sharing are strong motivators for nurse entrepreneurs. Entrepreneurial practice may become more prevalent in the future as nurses organize into corporate structures and contract to provide services for clinical agencies, physicians, and other health care providers.

Nurses entering the various current and emerging professional nursing roles often encounter challenges and role-related problems. How nurses respond to these problems will have important implications for the way in which nurses will be viewed in a future world, the world in which today's students will practice as professional nurses. Role problems in nursing are discussed in Chapter 2.

SUMMARY

Nurses are vital members of the health care team who work collaboratively with clients and colleagues to promote health, prevent illness, and implement care to treat client responses to health problems. The collaborative approach to client care used in this text is based on the recognition of nurses as responsible professionals and incorporates concepts of caring, respect for client autonomy, and rights to self-determination.

Entry into the practice of nursing may be accomplished via several types of educational preparation. Successful completion of a diploma, associate degree, baccalaureate, or generic higher degree program confers the right to sit for the registered nurse licensure examination. Alternative access to nursing education is available through external degree programs as well. There are also a variety of routes through which nurses may pursue advanced education, such as specialty certification, master's and doctoral degrees. Social and professional changes are escalating the demand for nurses with advanced educational preparation. Projections by agencies such as the National League for Nursing (NLN) and the Department of Health and Human Services indicate that this trend will continue into the 20th century.

Nurses practice in many settings. Acute care, home and community-based care, and long-term care offer a wide range of possible roles, challenges, and opportunities for professional development. Besides the roles such as caregiver and health care team member traditionally associated with nursing, emerging roles such as client advocate, manager, executive, and nurse entrepreneur reflect the growing numbers of options available to nurses with vision, creativity, and commitment to personal and professional advancement.

REFERENCES

1. American Nurses' Association. *Nursing: A Social Policy Statement.* Kansas City, MO: ANA; 1980.
2. Paterson J, Zderad L. *Humanistic Nursing.* New York: Wiley; 1976.
3. Leininger M. Caring: The essence and control focus of nursing. *Am Nurs Found Res Rep.* 1977; 12:2.
4. Leininger M. *Caring: An Essential Human Need.* Thorofare, NJ: Slack; 1981:3–15.
5. Watson J. *Nursing: The Philosophy and Science of Caring.* Boston: Little, Brown; 1979.
6. Bevis E. Caring: A life force. In: Leininger M. *Caring: An Essential Human Need.* Thorofare, NJ: Slack; 1981.
7. Ray M. A philosophical analysis of caring within nursing. In: Leininger M, ed. *Caring: An Essential Human Need.* NJ: Slack; 1981: 25–36.
8. Gaut D. Development of a theoretically adequate description of caring. *West J Nurs Res.* 1983; 5:313–324.
9. Williamson J. Mutual interaction: A model of nursing practice. *Nurs Outlook.* February 1981; 104–107.
10. News: Projected RN population decrease after the year 2000. *Am J Nurs.* 1990: 9(90):97.
11. National League for Nursing. *Nurs Data Rev.* New York: NLN; 1991.
12. Statistics Canada, Canadian Centre for Health Information, Registered Nurses Management Data, 1989.
13. Sweet J. Cost effectiveness of nurse practitioners. *Nurs Econom,* 1986; 4:190–193.
14. Kalisch P, Kalisch B. Nurses on prime time television. *AM J Nurs.* 1982; p. 606.
15. American Nurses' Association. *Educational Preparation for Nursing Competency.* Kansas City, MO: ANA; 1981.
16. Canadian Nurses' Association. *A Brief History.* Ottawa: CNA, n.d.
17. American Nurses' Association. *Standards for Professional Nursing Education.* Kansas City, MO: ANA; 1986.
18. Lenburg C. The external degree in nursing: An alternative ready for adoption. In: McClosky J, Grace H, eds. *Current Issues in Nursing.* Boston: Blackwell; 1981:177–196.

19. Dixon, AY. Project L.I.N.C.: An innovative model in educational mobility. *Nursing and Health Care.* 1989; 10(7):399–402.
20. Canadian Nurses' Association. *CNA Certification Program*, 3rd ed. Ottawa: CNA; 1989.
21. Division of National Cost Estimates. National health expenditures 1966–2000. *Health Care Financing Review.* 1987; 8(4):3.
22. Current Health News. *Sigma Theta Tau Reflections.* 1990; 16(2):5.
23. Sills G, Goeppinger J. The community as a field of inquiry in nursing. In: Herley H, Fitzpatrick J, eds. *Annual Review of Nursing Research;* 1985.
24. Wold S. *Community Health Nursing: Issues and Trends.* Norwalk, CT: Appleton & Lange; 1990.
25. Giovannetti P. Evaluation of primary nursing. In: Werley H, et al, eds. *Annual Review of Nursing Research.* New York: Springer; 1986: 127–151.
26. Zander K. Case management: A golden opportunity for whom? In: McCloskey JC, Grace HK, eds. *Current Issues in Nursing.* St. Louis: Mosby; 1990:203.

BIBLIOGRAPHY

Ayedelotte MK, et al. *Nursing Centers: Meeting the Demand for Quality Health Care.* NLN Publ #21. 1989; 2311:1–20.

Benner P, Wrubel J. *The Primacy of Caring: Stress and Coping in Health and Illness.* Menlo Park, CA: Addison-Wesley; 1988.

Briggs NA. The nurse practitioner: An expanded role within nursing. *Image.* 1990; 37:31–33.

Briggs NA. Nurse entrepreneurs/intrapreneurs changing health care (interview). *Am Nurs.* 1989; 21:9, 10.

Bunting S, et al. Feminism and nursing: Historical perspectives. *Adv Nurs Sci.* 1990; 13:41–48.

Clifford JC, et al. *Advancing Professional Nursing Practice: Innovations at Boston's Beth Israel Hospital.* New York: Springer; 1990.

delBueno DJ. Nurse-managed care: One approach. *J Nurs Admin.* 1990; 19:24–25.

Doheney M, Cook C, Stopper SM. The Discipline of Nursing. Norwalk, CT: Appleton & Lange; 1987.

Elder G, et al. Nurse practitioners and clinical nurse specialists: Are the roles merging? *Clin Nurs Spec.* 1990; 4:78–84.

Garner JF. *Strategic Nursing Management: Power and Responsibility in a New Era.* Rockville, MD: Aspen; 1990.

Gillis A. Beyond the Rhetoric: Benefits of a baccalaureate education for nursing. *Can J Nurs Admin.* 1989;2:5–8.

Hammond M. Is nursing a semi-profession? *Can Nurs.* 1990; 86:20–23.

Hawkens PL. Promoting nursing's health care agenda through collaboration. *Nurs Health Care.* 1990; 11:16–19.

Houston CJ. What makes the difference? Attributes of the exceptional nurse. *Nursing.* 1990; 20:170, 173.

Hughes L. Professionalizing domesticity: A synthesis of selected nursing historiography. *Adv Nurs Sci.* 1990; 12:25–31.

La Monica EL. *Strategic Nursing Management: An Experimental Approach that Makes Theory Work for You.* New York: Springer; 1990.

Lewis JD, et al. Men in nursing: Some troubling data. *Am J Nurs.* 1990; 90:30.

Manion J. Nurse intrapreneurs: Heroes of health care's future. *Nurs Out.* 1991; 21:50–53.

Mayer GG, et al. *Patient Care Delivery Models.* Rockville, MD: Aspen; 1990.

McKenzie CB, et al. Care and cost: Nursing case management improves both. *Nurs Manage.* 1989; 20:30–34.

McVeigh D, et al. Career liability for all RNs. *Nurs Out.* 1991; 39: 30–31.

Meloshi B. Not merely a profession: Nurses' resistance to professionalism. *Am Behav Sci.* 1989; 32:668–679.

Mittelstadt P. Reimbursement extended to NPs. *Am Nurse.* 1990; 22:2, 10.

Moore S. Thoughts on the discipline of nursing as we approach the year 2000. *J Adv Nurse.* 1990: 15:825–828.

Norris DA. Nurse entrepreneurs: The quiet revolution. *Imprint.* 1989–1990; 36:56–59.

Porter-O'Grady. *Reorganization of Nursing Practice: Creating the Corporate Venture.* Rockville, MD: Aspen; 1990.

Rawnsley M. Of human bonding: The context of nursing as caring. *Adv Nurs Sci.* 1990; 13:41–48.

Ritchie J. A framework for caring practice. *Can Nurs.* 1990; 86:28–31.

Smith LS. Nurses and the media. *Nurs Manage.* 1989; 20:13.

Stein L, Watts OT, Howell T. The doctor–nurse game revisited. *Nurs Out.* 1990; 38:264–268.

Swansburg RC. *Management and Leadership for Nurse Managers.* Boston: Jones & Bartlett; 1990.

Vestal KW. *Management Concepts for the New Nurse.* New York: Lippincott; 1987.

Wake NM. Nursing care delivery systems status and vision. *J Nurs Admin.* 1990; 20:47–51.

CHAPTER 2

Nursing as a Profession

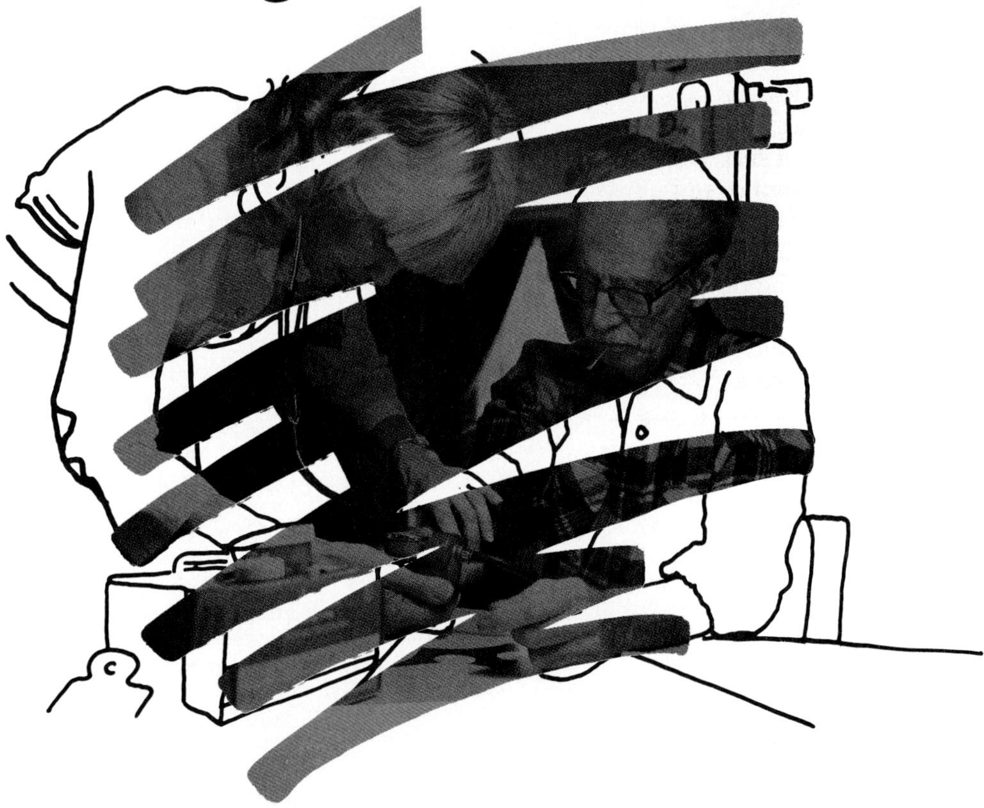

Behavioral Objectives

Upon completion of this chapter, the student will be able to:

1. Identify at least four characteristics of a profession.
2. Discuss the significance of professionalism to collaborative, collegial practice in health care.
3. Discuss the development of nursing from pre-Christian times to the present.
4. Identify at least six persons who have made significant contributions to nursing.
5. Name at least three professional nursing organizations and identify a major contribution each has made to the development of nursing as a profession.
6. Identify four role problems faced by nurses in today's health care system.
7. Describe at least three rights and three responsibilities of nurses.
8. List five current socio-political, economic, or professional trends and describe their influence on nursing and collaborative health care practice.
9. Discuss strategies by which nurses can develop their power bases to achieve a preferred future for nursing.
10. Discuss the significance of collaboration in health care practice for health care clients and the discipline of nursing.

KEY TERMS

accountability
American Academy of Nursing
American Association of Colleges of Nursing
American Nurses' Association
applied science
autonomy
body of knowledge
Canadian Nurses' Association
control
ethics
International Council of Nurses
National Black Nurses' Association
National Federation for Specialty Nursing Organizations
National League for Nursing
National Student Nurses' Association
paternalism
profession
professional values
role transition
sexism
Sigma Theta Tau

The development of nursing as a profession has been influenced by social, cultural, scientific, and technological changes. Although in its earliest history nursing was considered a calling, it is now achieving recognition not only as a practice occupation but as a scholarly discipline. Nurses are involved in research and theory building. They participate in political activity and professional organizations as well as in the delivery of health care. Issues such as professional autonomy in practice, equality, and interdependence with other health professionals and the political empowerment of nursing confront the profession and demand creative and responsible resolution. An examination of the history of nursing and the social and technological events that have had a continuing impact on the profession is an effective way to identify strategies to resolve these issues in a way that will further the development of the profession.

This chapter presents a historical overview of nursing, identifying significant individuals, organizations, issues, and trends. Role problems related to changes in the profession, and the rights and responsibilities of professional nurses, are addressed. Finally, the chapter describes the nurse of the future and strategies to achieve an ideal role for the nursing profession.

■ CHARACTERISTICS OF A PROFESSION

According to scholarly literature,[1–3] the characteristics defining a **profession** are:

- Intellectual pursuit of a body of knowledge
- Practice guided by a body of theory
- A community of shared values

- A code of ethics
- Focus on matters of human urgency and significance
- Autonomy, control, and accountability in practice

Attaining professional status is generally considered to be a worthy accomplishment. Professionals are respected by colleagues in other disciplines and by the public at large. Although nursing has not historically been accorded professional status, it has in recent times demonstrated significant achievements in each of these areas required for recognition as a profession, as discussed below.

Body of Knowledge

The term **body of knowledge** refers to the collected information that defines a discipline's overall areas of interest and reflects its philosophy. In the past few decades, nursing has made tremendous progress in articulating its specific body of knowledge and establishing that continuing to refine and organize that body of knowledge is a legitimate activity for its members.

Nursing is generally considered an **applied science**—that is, a discipline using knowledge to solve problems in a practice setting. Interdisciplinary coursework in the arts and humanities, as well as in the behavioral, social, and physical sciences, provides a general foundation of information and reasoning skills necessary for professional nursing practice. The core knowledge that is more specifically related to nursing practice is comprised of theories of nursing, information related to human functioning in health and illness, and content related to the direct care of clients. Acquisition of this knowledge base begins upon enrollment in a program of nursing education and continues throughout professional life.

Nursing research and theory development by nursing scholars and clinicians is continually refining the unique body of knowledge that is the basis for nursing practice. Reviews of published nursing research by O'Connell,[4] Brown, Tanner, and Patrick,[5] and Jacox[6] showed that nursing research has steadily increased in methodological sophistication, is increasingly focused on clinical problems and evidences a strong theory base. *The Annual Review of Nursing Research,* published annually since 1983, demonstrates a discernible increase in the volume and scope of nursing research since the journal's inception.[7] Nursing research contributes to the development of nursing theory. Nursing theory acts as an organizing framework for nursing knowledge and stimulates further research.

Body of Theory

Theories are ways of organizing knowledge in a manner that is relevant to a given discipline. A growing body of nursing theory is being generated to serve as a basis for organizing nursing knowledge. Nursing is beginning to amass an impressive body of literature through research and scholarly achievements. This is evidenced by the proliferation of nursing journals dedicated to disseminating research and theory development, and to the growing number of national and international nursing research conferences held annually. Box 2–1 provides a representative list of nursing journals whose focus is on theory and research. Nursing theory and nursing research are discussed further in Chapter 32.

Matters of Human Concern and Urgency

Nursing focuses on the human condition, quality of life, quality of care, and cost-effective health care delivery—all matters of urgency and significance. Nursing also has focused on such issues as how to support client involvement in self-care, how to improve adaptation and coping with chronic illness, and how to promote wellness.

Nursing directs attention to critical health policy issues and the development of a safe, efficient, and cost-effective health care delivery system that offers consumers viable options and optimal health outcomes. Among accomplishments relating to this effort is nursing's achievement of

IMPLICATIONS FOR PROFESSIONAL COLLABORATION

Collaboration As a Tool of Professionalization

Collaboration is the act of working jointly with others, especially in an intellectual endeavor. Collaboration at many levels is involved in achieving and sustaining professional status. For example, collaboration among nursing scientists, and between nursing scientists and scientists from other disciplines, is necessary to build a body of professional knowledge that addresses the vast array of health needs of a divergent population. Collaboration between nurses and other health professionals is important to safeguard professional standards and enforce accountability in the increasingly difficult and demanding health care environment. Collaboration with policy-makers is necessary to ensure that health policy supports nursing's unique and significant contribution to client care. And lastly, collaboration among nurses themselves is needed to disseminate nursing knowledge and reinforce nursing's shared values. Collaboration is thus an essential tool of the professionalization of nursing.

BOX 2–1. REPRESENTATIVE LIST OF NURSING JOURNALS PUBLISHING NURSING RESEARCH AND THEORY

Advances in Nursing Science
Applied Nursing Research
Canadian Journal of Nursing Research
Image: Journal of Nursing Scholarship
Inquiry in Nursing
International Journal of Nursing Studies
Nursing Scan in Research: Application for Clinical Practice
Nursing Science Quarterly
Nursing Research
Research in Nursing and Health
Research Review: Studies for Nursing Practice
Review of Research in Nursing Education
Scholarly Inquiry for Nursing Practice
Western Journal of Nursing Research

statutory support for the practice of the profession and the safety of clients through licensure and Nurse Practice Acts in each state. The vital significance of nursing's perspective, its concern with human health and well-being, and its growth through research and scholarly work, ensure that nursing will in time gain full acceptance as a profession.[8]

Self-enforced Code of Ethics

Ethics attempts to discern which actions are correct in a given situation. Ethics and ethical conduct are critical components of professionalism. Nursing practice today occurs in an atmosphere of advancing technology and diminishing financial and human resources. Nurses must confront complex questions and frequently are faced with a need to make choices between various courses of action. Often, none of the options is clearly the only right choice, and each choice has some undesirable consequences. This is called an ethical dilemma. As a member of a profession, a nurse has a responsibility to apply broad ethical principles rather than personal values and beliefs to resolve such conflicts. Many professions develop guidelines, or codes of ethics, to assist their members to deal with the types of conflicts that are typical in that profession. The American Nurses' Association (ANA) offers such a guide, the ANA Code for Nurses. The Canadian Nurses' Association Code of Ethics for Nursing is another example. They are reproduced in Chapter 34, which provides a detailed discussion of ethics in nursing.

Shared Values

All professions have **professional values,** that is, beliefs or concepts that influence practice and are generally acclaimed as being important to the discipline. Individuals who enter a profession undergo a socialization process during which they are introduced to the values of the profession and gradually integrate these values into their personal philosophy.

For members of a profession to have shared values, there must be consensus between those who educate and those who employ members of the discipline. When the primary site for nursing education moved from hospitals to universities and colleges, an ideological split occurred between the educational and practice arms of the profession that only recently has begun to heal. Nursing service personnel, for example, frequently express dissatisfaction with the competency of new nurse graduates and the cost of extended orientation periods. Nursing educators, on the other hand, contend that service expectations are too high and that new graduates need time and guidance from mentors before they can achieve the level of competency demanded by the clinical setting.

Collaborative efforts are underway to bridge the perceived gap between the "theoretical" world of nursing education and the "real" world of nursing service. For example, some faculty and nursing service personnel have joint appointments to clinical and educational settings. These individuals have role responsibilities and work relationships in both settings, making them more sensitive to the needs and perceptions of colleagues from each. Nurse educators and nursing service representatives also are collaborating to design various types of fellowship, externship, and internship programs for nursing students and graduates, enhancing the development of shared values.[9,10]

Clarity about educational preparation for the profession is generally considered an important professional value. The nursing profession has not currently identified a specific educational standard as the required preparation for practice. Individuals with an associate degree, a baccalaureate degree, or a diploma in nursing are eligible to be licensed as registered nurses. Many nursing groups have made proposals to clearly identify one specific degree as the minimal preparation for professional practice, but no consensus has been reached to date.

As described above, nursing has had less success in unifying its membership in a community of shared values and goals than it has had in fulfilling other criteria for a profession. Although the goal of service to clients—a critical human concern—remains paramount, nursing at the present time continues to be characterized by fragmentation in education and practice models, uncertainty, and frequently a sense of powerlessness. Confusion and disunity remain challenges for nursing as it concentrates efforts on strengthening the community of nurses and gaining full responsibility and accountability for its own practice.

Autonomy, Control, and Accountability in Practice

Autonomy, control, and accountability are related concepts. **Autonomy** is independence or freedom to choose one's actions. **Control** implies regulation or direction over something or someone. For a profession to be autonomous, it must have the authority to control its practice: to determine the roles, functions, and responsibilities of its members. **Accountability** means taking responsibility for one's actions. Desiring autonomy or control without accountability is irresponsible.

Professional autonomy for individual nurses means self-directed clinical practice. Professional accountability means that nurses are directly responsible to their clients for the quality of nursing care they provide. Presently, nurses do not experience self-directed clinical practice although shared governance and participative management are being introduced in some health care organizations. Nurses are the only caregivers having 24-hour responsibility for institutionalized clients, but they are rarely accorded staff and practice privileges in health care institutions—that is, the right to admit and discharge clients and to use the resources of the institution in prescribing for, treating, and referring their clients. Nurses provide essential client services, yet are unable to obtain direct reimbursement (payment for nursing services) from most insurance plans.

To have real autonomy in practice and be fully accountable, nurses also need some measure of control over the resources (personnel and material) needed to deliver quality care. Through shared governance, professional collaboration with physicians and hospital administrators in making decisions about resource allocations, in particular the resources that support nursing practice, some nurses are gaining greater autonomy and control in the clinical setting.

Nursing has the potential to become a strong and respected professional group having a significant influence in health care. It is not enough for nurses to be caring, compassionate, competent practitioners. If nurses are to have their concerns for their own profession, the health care system, the consumer, and society heard, they must speak with a unified voice from a position of power. Nurses comprise the largest group of health care providers, but have not used their numbers effectively to achieve positive change. A key issue is how to obtain the power—the ability to act, to influence others—necessary to achieve these ends. Gaining and using power effectively will increase the nursing profession's autonomy, enhance its credibility, and support collaborative and collegial practice. One way for nursing to gain this strength is for individual nurses to become involved in professional nursing organizations and participate in politics to influence public policy. These issues are discussed in greater detail in Chapter 4.

HISTORICAL PERSPECTIVES ON THE DEVELOPMENT OF NURSING

A review of nursing history will help the reader to understand the current role of the profession in the health care delivery system. Knowledge of historical influences also aids in gaining a more realistic perspective on the status and image of nursing, its achievements, and the significant current issues that are relevant to the profession.

Table 2–1 outlines significant points and people in early nursing history. It also provides a chronological context for some of the major themes that have been important in nursing's evolution.

Early History

Pre-Christian to Early Christian Era (Prehistory to 500 AD). From its earliest history, nursing has idealized the nurturing instinct attributed to the mother figure. Over time, nursing incorporated notions of waiting upon or tending the sick, the infirm, and the handicapped. Part of the value attributed to women historically lay in their skills at managing a home for their families, which included the expectation that the woman in a house would care for the sick within the family. It was an obvious progression for women who developed skills in caring for the sick to be called upon to provide the same type of care for guests in their homes who became ill, and eventually for persons in neighboring areas, usually relatives or dependents, who needed care.[11]

References to nursing prior to Christianity are sporadic. Depending on the prevailing culture and belief systems, nurses were healers, priestesses, slaves, or domestic servants. They also served as midwives, wet nurses, and children's nurses.

Christianity promoted the concept of pure altruism. Religious brothers and priests dedicated to the ideal of Christian charity assumed responsibility for care of the poor and the sick, eventually building almshouses and sick wards. The early Christian era marked the beginning of organized nursing: groups of individuals joined together in monasteries whose purpose in life was the physical care of the sick and the poor. In approximately 300 AD, women entered organized nursing.[12] The acceptance of the strict discipline inherent in monasticism as a way of life trained those involved in nursing to be subservient and to give unquestioning obedience to the decisions of those in higher positions, usually priests or physicians. Nursing was viewed as an honorable calling whose practitioners carried out the work of God. Providing care for the sick and the poor was perceived as a chosen way of life, a vocation, or a way of atoning for sins. Single-minded dedication was a prerequisite, because nursing required unceasing effort, with little or no expectations for earthly rewards.[13]

Early Middle Ages (500–1000 AD). Barbarian onslaughts and moral decay led the Western world into the Dark Ages. Women were relegated to a subordinate position as feudalism and monasticism evolved. The care of the sick occurred principally in monasteries. In the sixth and seventh centuries, nursing flourished through the efforts of wealthy women who sought protection and the opportunity to pursue studies and careers in monastic houses.[14] Nursing was still the primary type of care available for the sick in the Western world during this period because medicine was just beginning to develop as a rational discipline; however, in the East, Islam supported the study of medicine and the building of large hospitals, where both men and women practiced nursing.

Late Middle Ages (1000–1500 AD). Changes in society in the late Middle Ages produced a mobile population, less dependent on the extended family as the traditional protective and economic unit of society, and gave rise to a middle class of workers and merchants. Extensive population growth led to crowding, poor sanitation, contaminated water and food supplies, and increasing violence and disease. These conditions brought nurses out of the monasteries and hospitals and back into the community.[15]

The Crusades gave rise to nursing orders, including orders of knights, priests, and religious brothers. Some members of these orders established hospitals, while mendicant orders—those whose members took vows of poverty and depended on begging for sustenance—organized to take nursing out into the community.[16,17] Secular groups banded together to provide nursing for the poor, the sick, and foundlings. Following the Crusades, hospitals were built in European cities, and medical schools in universities thrived. University-trained physicians were successful in gaining control of hospitals.[18] Then the bubonic plague (Black Death) swept Europe in the 14th century, causing certain and terrible death for one quarter of the world's population. Sheer numbers of those afflicted with the dis-

TABLE 2–1. EARLY HISTORY OF NURSING

Prehistory	Mother care of helpless infants.
	Preservation and protection of the tribe and its members.
	Phenomenon of nature-directed life.
	Magic, religion, and naturalistic remedies, with a focus on purging the body of evil spirits, which "caused" illness.
	Legends and myths of deities who watched over health and had power over life and death; development of temples to the gods, which later became sanctuaries for the sick.
3000 BC	Advanced civilization in the Near East, with religious beliefs and myths providing foundation for practice of healing by religious leaders.
	In the Far East (China, India, and Japan), illness viewed as the result of demons invading the body. Disease prevention emphasized.
2800 BC	Medical papyri document two types of practitioners in ancient Egypt, priest-magicians and priest-physicians.
	Imhotep identified as greatest priest-physician of Egypt.
	No evidence of nursing or early hospitals.
1900 BC	Code of Hammurabi addressed medical and surgical practice, with control of the surgeon based on "eye for an eye" philosophy.
600 BC	Emperor Darius established school for training of priest-physicians.
500 BC	Ancient Jewish medicine emphasized hygiene, sanitation, and the systematic and organized prevention of disease through dietary and social regulations; viewed disease as a punishment for sin.
	Deborah was the first nurse to be recorded in history in the 24th chapter of Genesis in the Old Testament.
400 BC	Hippocrates established scientific medicine. Literature of Greece contained references to children's nurses, wet nurses, and midwives.
200 BC–200 AD	Indian Laws of Manu outlined moral and practical standards for those choosing the care of the sick as their life work.
	History of India describes nursing principles and practices and existence of hospitals.
	Greek physicians who were slaves did medical work for the Romans. Military hospitals erected. Nursing provided by orderlies and slaves. Children's nurses and midwives remained chief nursing roles for women.
	Parabolani brotherhood, an organization of men in early Rome, provided nursing care for plague victims.
300 AD	Entry of women into nursing, a humanitarian approach to the care of the sick and poor, and the beginning of organized systems for caring for the sick.
390 AD	Fabiola founded first free Christian hospital in Rome; viewed almost as patron saint of early nursing.
	Paula built hospices and hospitals for the sick along the road to Bethlehem; was the first to train nurses in a systematic way, and to teach nursing as an art distinct from generalized care of the poor.
500–1000 AD	Nursing became a penitential activity used as a means of purification and atoning for sin. During the feudal era, nursing was the responsibility of the lord's wife, the lady of the manor.
	In the era of monasticism, nursing of the sick became a chief function and duty of the monastic communities, each of which provided hospices and hospitals to care for the poor and the sick.
1000–1500 AD	Crowded living conditions and the spread of disease brought nurses out of the monastic nursing institutions and back into the homes.
	Military brotherhood nursing orders responded to the Crusades; some formed women's orders that were subordinated to the men's communities.
	Mendicant nursing orders took nursing back out into the community among the poor and sick, and secular nursing orders developed outside the religious orders to care for the sick.
	Plagues and epidemics created chaos.
1500–1860 AD	The Renaissance created a rebirth in science and art. The Reformation initiated the destruction of the system of health care and nursing based in religious orders, creating a "dark age of nursing" that lasted until 1860.

ease and inability to halt the progress of the epidemic overwhelmed medicine and nursing.[13] Confusion, terror, and panic led to a breakdown in morality and human decency, with many people seeking only to save themselves and abandoning care of others. By the last centuries of the Middle Ages the need for reforms in the care of the sick opened the doors for change.

Renaissance, Reformation, and New Directions (1500–1850 AD). The rebirth of interest in the arts and sciences during the Renaissance in the early 1500s initiated scientific inquiry, which led to the development of new knowledge and technology for care of the sick. During the same period, the Protestant Reformation changed the way in which people perceived themselves and their world. The result

IMPLICATIONS FOR PROFESSIONAL COLLABORATION

The Contrast Between Collaborative and Traditional Models of Nursing

The historical pattern of nurses as subservient and obedient functionaries operating under the authority of those in higher positions contrasts sharply with the collaborative image of nursing. In the collaborative image, nurses are independent, professional decision-makers who themselves have authority over the practice decisions that are within their professional domain, and they have substantial social and political influence in defining that domain. Further, nurses have a primary ethical and legal responsibility to their clients rather than to other health care professionals. Relationships between nursing and practitioners from other disciplines, moreover, are characterized not by obedience or subservience but by collegiality, the quality of shared authority, and a mutual respect for the varying but significant roles played by each practitioner.

was a denial of the importance of religion in everyday life, an increased emphasis on the individual and on the rewards one could accrue in this world, along with a rebirth of paganistic rituals and the belief in magic and witchcraft. Poverty and illness were seen as punishments. Religious orders were suppressed and their property confiscated, preventing their members from caring for the sick and poor.[15] In those countries where this occurred, notably England, hospitals could no longer meet even minimal care needs of the sick. There were no organized groups to take over the care that had been given by religious nursing orders.[17]

By the mid-16th century the secularization of nursing—that is, the removal of nursing from connection or protection of religious orders—made it an unacceptable occupation for respectable women. A growing number of women of the lower stata of society—prisoners, gamblers, drunkards, and prostitutes—were recruited as nurses, with many more assigned nursing duties in lieu of prison sentences.

By the 1700s, the scientific mode of inquiry, coupled with advances in technology, encouraged some physician-scientists to move into the mainstream of social change and to use new discoveries to explore bodily responses to illness and treatment. It took considerable time for advances in medicine to be translated into standards of practice, and even longer for those advances to affect nursing. Almost a century and a half elapsed before nursing began to incorporate the beginnings of a scientific base into its practice. This may have been due to the prevailing thought that nursing was not an intellectual activity, and to the continuing secularization of nursing that defined care of the sick as punishment for those employed to do it. No intelligent person would willingly work in the horrors that hospitals run by cities had become if they could earn a living in any other way.[17] The move out of the resulting "dark age of nursing" took three centuries, until the mid-1800s.

The Development of Modern Nursing

Nightingale Era (1850–1900). The last half of the 19th century marked what is commonly recognized as the beginning of modern nursing. Two seemingly incompatible social trends existed at the time: the dominance of Victorian society, which expected a passive, dependent role for women, and the growing demand for the emancipation of women. This was the context within which Florence Nightingale (1820–1910), a scientifically minded, dedicated, and stubborn English gentlewoman, introduced reforms and ideas that changed the care of the sick throughout the world (Fig. 2–1). She perceived nursing as that which put "the patient in the best condition for nature to act upon,"[19] an idea that underlies many modern views of nursing.

Nightingale's contributions to nursing are almost immeasurable. Trained by the Sisters of Charity in Paris and at Deaconess Institute in Kaiserswerth, Germany, Nightingale was later named superintendent of the English General Hospitals in Turkey. She trained women for nursing in mil-

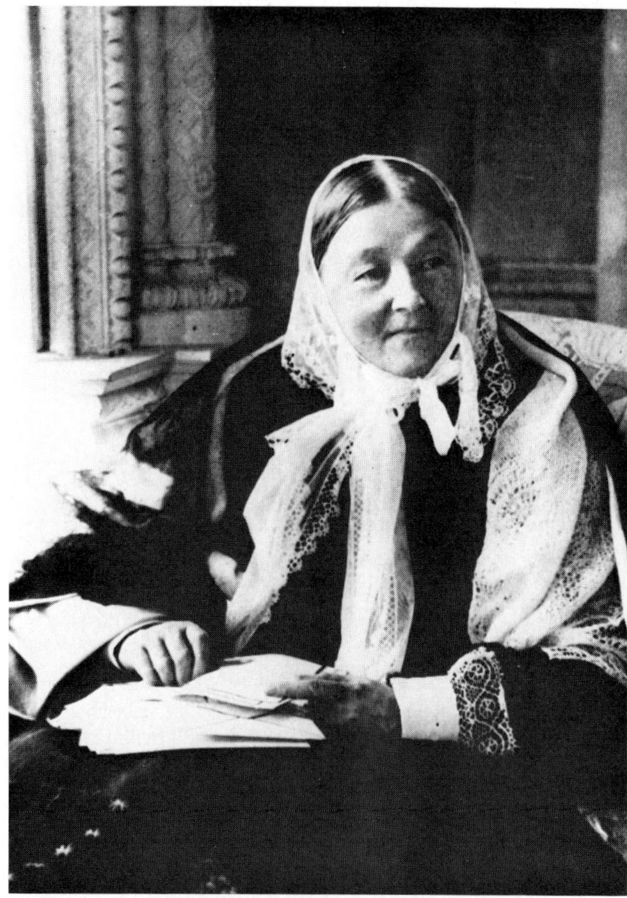

Figure 2–1. Florence Nightingale (1820–1910) introduced reforms that changed the care of the sick throughout the world. *(From the Center for the Study of the History of Nursing, University of Pennsylvania, School of Nursing, Philadelphia, PA.)*

itary hospitals and introduced sanitary science to those institutions, reducing the death rate of the British Army in the hospital at Scutari during the Crimean War from 42.7 to 2.2 percent in 6 months.[20] This gained her the gratitude and support of the English people and the power to effect much-needed change in nursing.

Nightingale wrote the first authoritative text on nursing, *Notes on Nursing,* in 1859, and founded the first training school for nurses at St. Thomas Hospital in 1860.[18] Consistent with the prevailing attitudes of the times regarding education for women, Nightingale supported apprenticeship training programs in hospitals for nurses.

Nightingale's influence extended to the United States in the early part of the 1870s. Three schools of nursing based on her training school model opened in New York, Connecticut, and Boston. These schools graduated many of the women who led nursing into the 20th century. Refer to Table 2–2 for a chronological history of modern nursing.

Nursing in the United States. Pioneers of American nursing added important dimensions to the nursing practice that helped clarify its unique contributions to the health care system. Dorothea Lynde Dix (1802–1887) fought to change care for the mentally ill in America, and in 1861 became Superintendent of the Female Nurses of the Union Army. During the same period, Clara Barton (1821–1912) nursed in federal hospitals and also cared for Confederate soldiers as a lay nurse. In 1881 she developed the American Red Cross.

When the Civil War broke out there was no organized nursing service for the country's military. Nursing was desperately needed by the wounded on both sides, and the need could only be met by voluntary religious nursing groups and laypersons, some with nursing experience but many with none.[21,22] The inadequacy of nursing during the Civil War demonstrated the need for formal training for nursing. Hospitals in New York and Philadelphia responded to the need.

Isabel Adams Hampton Robb, a forward-thinking nursing leader in the late 19th century (1859–1910), differed with the dominant social perspective of nurses as caregivers and identified teaching as a critical component of nursing. She was among the strongest supporters of the development of nursing as a scientifically based practice discipline.[23]

Lillian Wald (1867–1940) also extended the domain of nursing (Fig. 2–2). Her development of nursing settlements—neighborhood organizations dedicated to health and social welfare for all persons in the community regardless of ability to pay—supported autonomy for the practice of nursing and established the concept that community health should be a nursing concern.[24] Wald believed that nurses could make a unique and significant contribution to the health of the people. In 1912, she founded the National Organization of Public Health Nursing.

Wald and Annie Warburton Goodrich (1866–1954), the first dean of the Yale School of Nursing, added the dimension of prenatal care and health promotion to their dedicated fight against disease in the community. Both saw nursing as involved in social issues and policy-making related to social problems, such as child labor and health risks to men and women in the workplace, thus contributing to human welfare.

As Nightingale had done at Scutari during the Crimean War, nurses responded to the call of duty during World War I and demonstrated that well-trained nurses could make a difference in relieving suffering, changing sanitary conditions, improving postsurgery outcomes, and helping to reduce mortality among the wounded. They earned an "angel of mercy" image that supported the development of the fledgling profession.

The 1920s and 1930s marked significant steps forward for nursing education. In 1923, the Rockefeller Foundation funded a major survey of nursing education, the Goldmark Report, which encouraged the trend toward professionalism. The key recommendations were that standards for nursing education be raised, and that nursing education be separated from nursing service and be supported at the university level. In the early 1930s Mary Adelaide Nutting (1858–1948), Isabel Maitland Stewart (1878–1963), and Annie Goodrich assumed leadership positions in developing collegiate education programs for nurses, promoting the concept of educating nurses rather than training them. Nutting also promoted educational preparation of nurses for work in the complex field of community health.[25] The work of these pioneers in nursing set the stage for educating new nurses as generalists who could practice effectively with various client populations and in diverse clinical practice settings.

The 1930s also marked the growing emphasis by nursing leaders on a humanistic perspective for nursing practice as well as a scientific basis for nursing knowledge. A popular textbook of the time described nursing as "that service to the individual that helps him to attain or maintain a healthy state of mind or body; or where a return to health is not possible, the relief of pain and discomfort."[26]

During the 1940s, the development of nursing as a science was put on temporary hold as the first half of the decade was marked by another world war. As usual in times of crisis, nurses responded in large numbers to the call for service. In so doing they left civilian hospitals with serious nurse shortages, and the domain of nursing was radically changed. Paraprofessional workers were hired to fill the gap, marking the end of nurses' exclusive role in the care of the sick in hospitals. Lack of agreement regarding differentiation of functions continues to plague nursing, particularly when related to the controversy surrounding preparation for entry into professional nursing practice.[27]

The concept of nursing diagnosis, introduced in the 1950s, was a significant contribution to the development of nursing as a science. The process of identifying and defining nursing diagnoses continues to evolve to the present time.

The 1950s also brought another war, this time in Korea, which exacerbated the shortage of registered nurses for the homefront as nurses again responded to the call to duty. The injuries suffered by fighting men and women, and the

TABLE 2–2. HISTORY OF MODERN NURSING

1809	Mother Elizabeth Seton founded the Sisters of Charity to provide care for the poor and the sick in hospitals and homes in the United States.
	Demands for nursing religious orders increased, and Catholic and Protestant nursing orders responded rapidly and established extensive networks throughout the country. Such groups as the Sisters of Mercy, the Dominicans, the Sisters of the Poor of St. Francis, the Episcopal Sisterhood of the Communion, and the English All Saints Sisterhood were among those providing nursing care for the poor, sick, and wounded during the Civil War.
1836	Deaconess Institute established at Kaiserwerth, Germany, with a training program for nursing deaconesses that prepared them for both teaching and nursing.
	Growth of Protestant deaconesses for nursing services.
1839	The Philadelphia Dispensary established a training program to prepare competent nurses to supply maternity services in homes under the auspices of the Nurse Society of Philadelphia.
1847	Florence Nightingale enrolled in Kaiserwerth for a 3-month training program in nursing.
1853	Nightingale studied nursing in Paris under the Sisters of Charity at the Maison de la Providence.
1854	Nightingale was appointed superintendent of the Female Nursing Establishment of the English General Hospitals in Turkey. Introduced methods of sanitary care that reduced the death rate at Scutari Hospital from 42.7 to 2.2 percent within 6 months.
1859	Nightingale's *Notes on Nursing* published.
1860	Nightingale Training School for Nurses opened.
1861	Dorothea Lynde Dix appointed superintendent of the Female Nurses of the Union Army, providing for a corps of volunteer women to be organized for nursing services.
	Well-known lay nurses during the Civil War included Clara Barton (1821–1912), Mother Mary Ann Bickerdyke (1817–1901), Louisa May Alcott (1832–1888), Walt Whitman (1819–1892), Harriet Tubman (1820–1913), and Sojourner Truth (1797–1883). Sally Louisa Tompkins (1833–1916), the only woman to hold a commission in the Army of the Confederacy, organized nursing services for the South.
1864	Treaty of Geneva established principles to govern and protect those wounded in war, the supplies needed to care for them, and those providing care. National Red Cross societies established in many European countries.
1872	Women's Hospital of Philadelphia became the first endowed school for nurses in the United States.
1873	Appearance of three nursing schools in the United States: Bellevue Training School in New York City, the Connecticut Training School in New Haven, and the Boston Training School (later the Massachusetts General Hospital Training School for Nurses).
	Melinda Ann (Linda) Richards (1841–1930) became the first nurse trained in the United States when she received her certificate from the New England Hospital for Women and Children.
1879	Mary Eliza Mahoney (1845–1926) completed the 16-month program to become known as the first black nurse to graduate from a school of nursing.
1882	Clara Barton instrumental in getting the United States to ratify the Geneva Treaty and establish the American Red Cross.
1886	Beginning of the Settlement House movement in the United States.
1889	Hull Settlement House in Chicago founded by Jane Addams became typical model for others founded in the United States and provided a base for the development of public health nursing.
1893	Formation of the American Society for Superintendents of Training Schools for Nurses under the leadership of Isabel Adams Hampton, which was open to both Canadian and American membership and became an accrediting body for nursing curricula.
	Henry Street Settlement House established by Lillian D. Wald, who became known as the founder of what is now known as public health or community nursing.
1897	Creation of the Nurses' Associated Alumnae of the United States and Canada for the rank and file of nurses.
1899	International Council of Nurses (ICN) founded.
1900	Evidence of the superiority of trained nurses over volunteers or corpsmen during the Spanish-American War led to the establishment of the U.S. Army Nurse Corps.
	American Journal of Nursing, the first nursing journal to be owned and published by nurses, is established.
1902	Lillian Wald initiated public school nursing in the United States.
1903	The first nurse practice acts were passed in 4 states: North Carolina, New York, New Jersey, and Virginia.
1907	Canadian nurses formed their own independent organization, the Canadian Society of Superintendents of Training Schools.
	Mary Adelaide Nutting joined Teachers' College in New York and became the first professor of nursing in the world. Teachers' College fostered the initial movement toward undergraduate and graduate degrees for nurses.
1908	U.S. Navy Nurse Corps founded as integral unit of the Navy.
1909	American Red Cross reorganized under Jane Delano, developing a corps of graduate nurses to act as supplement to the regular army and navy nurses as needed.

TABLE 2–2. (continued)

1911	The American Nurses' Association (ANA) became the successor to the Nurses' Associated Alumnae of the United States.
	Bellevue Hospital established school of midwifery.
1912	The American Society of Superintendents became known by a new name, the National League of Nursing Education.
	Lillian Wald became the first president of the National Organization for Public Health Nursing.
1922	Sigma Theta Tau, national honor society for nursing, established at Indiana University.
1923	Goldmark Report on Nursing Education.
1925	The Frontier Nursing Service in Kentucky, founded by Mary Breckinridge, provided the first organized midwifery service in the country.
1930s	Mary Adelaide Nutting, Isabel Stewart, and Annie Goodrich assumed leadership roles in developing collegiate nursing education.
	Weir report recommended integration of Canadian Nursing Education into the provincial education system.
1940s	World War II led to the establishment of the Cadet Nurse Corps, which subsidized students and accelerated nursing programs to meet the demand for nurses. Although it was disbanded in 1945, it set a precedent that supported later development of ADRN programs.
1948	Brown Report on nursing education critical of hospital-based programs. Recommended that schools of nursing be established throughout college and university systems.
1950s	All 50 states using the State Board Test Pool Exam (SBPTE) for Registered Nursing Licensure.
	Experimental project at Columbia University Teachers College that led to the development of associate degree nursing programs for technical nursing. First program opened in 1952 at Teachers College, Columbia University, New York. Curriculum developed by Mildred Montag.
1952	National League of Nursing Education reorganized into the National League for Nursing (NLN).
1953	National Student Nurses' Association established.
1960s	Growth of master's degree programs in nursing; development of nurse practitioner role and educational programs.
	A body of theory unique to nursing established.
1965	ANA's first position paper calling for all nursing education to take place in institutions of higher learning. Called for baccalaureate degree as minimum preparation for professional nursing practice, associate degree for technical nursing practice.
1969	Establishment of the American Association of Colleges of Nursing (AACN).
1970	Canadian Nurses' Association established a national testing service (CNATS).
1971	Lucille Kinlein, first nurse to establish a practice as an independent practitioner.
1972	First nursing political action committee established by ANA.
1973	ANA began certifying nurses for specialty practice.
	First meeting of the National Conference on Classification of Nursing Diagnosis called by Kristine Gebbie and Mary Ann Lavin. Led to the development of the North American Nursing Diagnosis Association (NANDA).
1978	ANA "1985 Resolution" set a goal that minimum preparation for "entry into professional practice" be a baccalaureate degree in nursing.
1980s	Growth of doctoral programs in nursing.
	Numbers of nurse-run clinics and nurse entrepreneurs increase.
	Growing nursing shortage spurs growth of professional practice models, intensified focus on nursing recruitment and retention.
	Nurse executives becoming more common in hospitals and other health care agencies.
	Shared governance/participative management gaining support as preferred form of organizational management in health care agencies.
	Professional nursing organizations becoming more unified and politically active.
1981	National Council Licensure Exam (N-CLEX) replaces State Board Test Pool Exam.
1982	ANA adopted a federation model, increasing autonomy of state nurses' associations.
	Canadian Nurses' Association resolution calling for baccalaureate degree as minimum preparation for entry into professional nursing.
1983	Diagnostic Related Groups (DRGs) patient classification system for prospective payment established by Medicare to contain health care costs.
1986	National Center for Nursing Research established under National Institutes of Health (NIH).
1987	ANA task force on the Scope of Nursing Practice Report: defines two levels of practice under one scope of practice; levels designed for use as guidelines for changing state nurse practice acts.
1988	Secretary's Commission on Nursing. Department of Health and Human Services Secretary's Commission on Nursing report lists recommendations for improved recruitment and retention to maintain adequate supply of RNs.

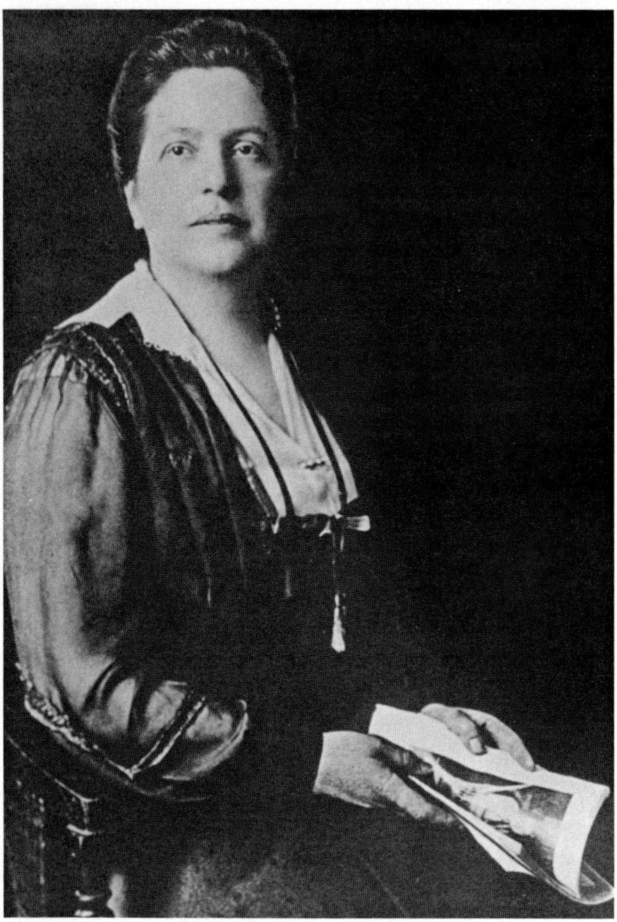

Figure 2–2. Lillian Wald. (*Courtesy of The Visiting Nurse Service of New York.*)

extensive reconstructive surgery and rehabilitation demands, stimulated rapid advances in technology to meet changing health care needs. The nurse shortage coupled with an increasing demand for nursing care motivated the development of a system of technical education for nursing. Technical nursing programs were college based, but only 2 years in length. They were intended to produce "nurse technicians" who would work under the supervision of professional nurses.

Nursing in the 1960s evolved within a society marred by violence and civil unrest, the assassination of a president, and involvement in an unpopular war in Vietnam. The nursing issues whose seeds were sown in the 1950s blossomed into full-blown conflicts. Primary among these was the need to differentiate professional and technical nursing, which was deemed critical for nursing's future as a profession. The American Nurses' Association issued a position statement in 1965 defining professional nurses as those prepared in baccalaureate nursing education programs, and technical nurses as those prepared in associate degree programs.[28] Issues relating to entry into practice, including differentiation of competencies, titling, and licensure, have yet to be resolved.

Throughout the 1960s, nursing enjoyed a time of tremendous growth, in proliferation and federal support of educational programs, and in the expansion of scope of practice for nursing. The first nurse practitioner programs, which prepared registered nurses for advanced practice roles in primary health care, were developed at the University of Colorado. Graduate programs preparing clinical specialists became common nationally. The development of nursing theory began in earnest, marking the emergence of nursing as an established academic discipline and beginning a new era for nursing education and practice. The theories of major nursing scholars are discussed in Chapter 32.

The 1970s and 1980s marked the extensive growth of doctoral education programs in nursing. Directors of nursing service moved into executive level positions in many hospitals and other health care systems. Increasingly, professional practice models guided the organization and implementation of nursing service delivery. Community nursing centers were piloted and nurse-managed clinics were developed to serve vulnerable and underserved populations, such as the elderly, the homeless, inner city and rural poor, and women and children. More nurses initiated entrepreneurial businesses to manage and broker nursing personnel or to provide consultation to health care systems and direct services for clients.[29]

Recognizing the need for survival in an increasingly economically driven health care system, nursing began to identify the costs for delivering nursing services in different settings and to establish itself as a revenue as well as cost center for hospitals and other service areas. Advanced nursing practitioners gained prescriptive privileges and the right to reimbursement for nursing services in some states. The nursing shortage focused the public on nursing recruitment and retention issues. The American Medical Association responded to the nursing shortage by developing a proposal for a new practitioner called a registered care technician, who would be certified by medicine to provide bedside nursing care in the hospital. This proposal generated organized opposition by nurses and many of their constituencies, including consumer groups and physicians, who recognized the threats to quality of care and client outcomes as well as nurse autonomy and accountability.[30] Professional nursing organizations began to recognize the power inherent in working together to accomplish nursing's goals.

■ PROFESSIONAL NURSING ORGANIZATIONS AND THE DEVELOPMENT OF NURSING

The rise of professional nursing organizations was a strong element in the development of nursing. The ability of a profession to gain control of its practice and support for its concerns, and to develop a power base for influencing the direction of change in the health care delivery system, rests on the strength of an organized membership with shared values and goals. A group is stronger than an individual; it is more than the sum of its parts and can accomplish things that an individual working alone cannot. A number of organizations continue to play important roles in nursing.

National League for Nursing

Founded in 1893, the American Society of Superintendents of Training Schools for Nurses strove to achieve high educational standards for schools of nursing based on universal standards for admission, a sound program of theory and practice, and improved working conditions. It essentially became an accrediting agency for schools of nursing in the United States and Canada.[31] In 1912, the Society became the National League of Nursing Education. It reorganized in 1952 into the **National League for Nursing** (NLN). In 1989, the "new" NLN structure included a holding company, the National League for Health (NLH), to serve as an umbrella for a variety of diversified services.

Today, the NLN holds a unique position of power within the profession by virtue of its control over the accreditation of basic entry-level and master's degree nursing education programs. The League has been responsible for much of the progress made in establishing standards and criteria for nursing education. It has taken a leadership role in the development of testing and measurement services for nursing. Current NLH activities include a nationally recognized accreditation program for home health agencies.

American Nurses' Association

Established in 1897, Nurses' Associated Alumnae of the United States and Canada provided an organization for the rank and file in nursing. It began with a primary goal to gain legislation to differentiate between nurses prepared in a program offering appropriate education for practice, and those inadequately or untrained women who claimed the title of nurse.

The organization became the **American Nurses' Association** (ANA) in 1911, following the formation of the Canadian National Association of Trained Nurses in 1908. By 1912 state nurses' associations began to form. These became the power bases for unifying nurses in eventually successful efforts to achieve state licensure for nursing. In 1982, the ANA changed its organizational structure from an organization of individual members to a federation of state associations. State nurses' associations function with greater autonomy in a federation model. Individual nurses hold membership in state associations and participate at the national level as state representatives to the ANA House of Delegates.

The ANA has been responsible for initiating and supporting much of the action that led to legal protection for the public and limited access into nursing to persons educated as nurses. Current emphases include improving economic and general welfare of nurses, establishing standards for nursing education and practice, and credentialing for specialty and advanced nursing practice. The ANA has taken a leadership role in attempting to differentiate professional and technical nursing education and practice.

American Association of Colleges of Nursing

Established in 1969, the **American Association of Colleges of Nursing** (AACN) is the third member of the triumvirate of nursing organizations consistently perceived as speaking for the profession by legislators and various policy-makers. This organization was created initially to provide deans and assistant deans of baccalaureate and higher degree programs in colleges and universities with a forum for discussing issues of common concern to nursing education and the profession. Currently its membership is limited to deans or principal heads of such nursing education programs. AACN has been instrumental in improving the practice of professional nursing by increasing the quality of baccalaureate and higher degree granting programs. Major recent projects include the development of a document outlining essential knowledge and values for baccalaureate nursing education and a series of annual forums designed to support the development of high quality in doctoral education in nursing.

American Academy of Nursing

Developed under the auspices of the ANA in 1978, **American Academy of Nursing** membership is limited to ANA members who have made significant and sustained contributions to nursing and nursing research or practice. Being elected to fellowship in the American Academy of Nursing (FAAN) by the members is an honor.

Canadian Nurses' Association

The **Canadian Nurses' Association** (CNA) was founded in 1908. It is a federation of territorial and provincial nurses' associations. CNA seeks to actively promote high standards of nursing practice, education, administration, and research. Since 1970, the CNA, through its National Testing Service, has developed and administered examinations for applicants desiring licensure as registered nurses. In 1982, CNA adopted a resolution calling for the baccalaureate degree as minimum preparation for entry into professional nursing. The organization is also developing a certification program for various nursing specialties.

International Council of Nurses

The **International Council of Nurses** (ICN) was founded in 1899 by nurses from the United States and Canada. Today, it is a federation of nearly 100 national nurses' associations worldwide, including the ANA and CNA. Among its purposes are promoting communication among nurses throughout the world, assisting national nursing organizations to develop and promote health services for all, and advancing the practice of nursing and the welfare of nurses.

Sigma Theta Tau

Sigma Theta Tau was founded in 1922 as the national honor society for nursing, focusing on the promotion of research and leadership in nursing. Membership is attained through scholastic or professional achievement. Sigma Theta Tau is now an international organization and has established a Center for Nursing Knowledge in Indiana.

National Student Nurses' Association

Established in 1953, the **National Student Nurses' Association** (NSNA) is modeled after the American Nurses' Association. It has state level associations that involve students in issues relevant to nursing education, student support, and the profession. It has state and national officers and conventions, and encourages active participation of nursing students in politics and policy development to promote a sense of professional collegiality and commitment to nursing.

Other Professional Nursing Organizations

Throughout the history of nursing, special interest groups have perceived themselves as having unique problems that could only be addressed through separate organizations.

The National Association of Colored Graduate Nurses (NACGN) was established in 1908 to achieve higher professional standards, break down discriminatory practices in education and service, and develop Negro nurse leadership.[32] The organization was phased out when members perceived that its purpose had been met in the ANA's 1948 platform supporting elimination of discrimination in the professional association and the practice arena; however, another organization, the **National Black Nurses Association,** was formed in 1971, when concerns again began to surface regarding absence of black nurses in leadership and policy positions within ANA, loss of identity, and limited recognition of contributions of black nurses.[33] Other nursing organizations have developed around race, sex, clinical specialization, research, and regional concerns. There are national organizations for Hispanic nurses, Native American nurses, and men in nursing, among others.

In addition to the groups discussed above, there are more than 30 clinical specialty nursing associations organized around every conceivable practice specialty, area of interest, special position, and branch of the military. The largest among these are the American Association of Critical Care Nurses (AACN), American College of Nurse-Midwives (ACNM), American Association of Nurse Anesthetists (AANA), and American Organization of Nurse Executives (AONE). The fragmentation of nurse membership across so many specialty organizations could lead to divisiveness and the loss of a solid power base to work toward full professionalization. This trend was offset somewhat by the convening of the National Congress of Nursing and the development of the Federation of Specialty Nursing Organizations in collaboration with the ANA in 1972. The purpose of the group was to provide a forum and an opportunity for communication and discussion so that nursing could have at least a potential for speaking out on matters of concern with a unified voice. The name of the organization was changed in 1981 to the **National Federation for Specialty Nursing Organizations** (NFSNO).

The existence of one professional association that can represent the full membership of a discipline is critical to full professionalization. Out of approximately 2.1 million registered nurses in the country, only about 10 percent belong to the American Nurses' Association. Approximately 12 percent hold membership in any nursing organization. However, even without the true mandate that comes from representing all professional nurses, the ANA, NLN, and AACN have established themselves as the three organizations recognized by the federal government and others as speaking for nursing on the significant issues facing health care today.

The challenge for today's nursing students is to strengthen the effectiveness of organized nursing by increasing involvement and active participation. This is a major concern for the development of a strong collaborative position for nursing in the health care system of the future.

■ SOCIAL AND TECHNOLOGICAL DEVELOPMENTS AND NURSING

Several major influences have had historical and contemporary impact on the evolution of nursing as a profession and a discipline. These include social influences, such as sexism and paternalism, the feminist movement, and wars; advances in science and technology; and changing health problems.

Sexism and Paternalism

Sexism is defined as the social domination and economic exploitation of members of one sex by the other. **Paternalism** refers to the system of governing or controlling a group of people in a manner suggesting a father's relationship with his children. Both concepts have their roots in the same phenomenon, the assumption that certain behaviors and attributes are defined on the basis of gender, and that those behaviors and attributes defined as male are more highly valued than those characterized as female.

The value placed on nursing by society today appears to be a historical phenomenon, closely linked to the development of woman's role in society. This included a process of socialized feminine subservience, which is grounded in the myth of male superiority. Believers of the myth perceive that more highly valued "male" characteristics of strength, aggressiveness, self-control, leadership, persistence, competence, organization, and dominance are unattainable by the warm, caring, nurturing, supportive, sensitive, less creative, more passive, noncompetitive, and illogical female of the species.[34] Nursing is a profession comprised predominantly of women, who have historically emphasized the use of traditionally "feminine" caring and nurturing behaviors.

As discussed earlier, nursing was viewed as moving traditional women's activities of caring for the sick from home to community. This perception was reinforced by the way in which institutions to care for the sick and the homeless evolved, using female servants and nuns to provide much of the direct care in monastic institutions.[15] The traditional subservience of these caregivers set the stage for male domination of the institutions providing care for the sick.

When nursing moved out of the home and community into the hospital during the late Middle Ages, and later during the 19th and 20th centuries, the dependency characterizing female roles moved as well. In many ways the hospital became a home away from home, extending the paternal protection of the traditional home environment to the work setting. It controlled the lives of nurses, provided their housing, and monitored their morals into the early 1960s. Further, the hospital rounded out the picture with authoritarian male physician and administrator figures who reinforced the dependent role enacted by nurses.

Nursing's "dark age," when the care of the sick was left to women of ill repute, only reinforced the perception that women were not suited for independence of thought or action, and needed appropriate male guidance and control. Conversely, the recurrent view of nursing as an honorable altruistic calling for women also supported the perpetuation of paternalism. It was reasoned that someone stronger—a father-figure—needed to take charge of the more pragmatic and worldly aspects of organization, direction, and control necessary for survival of the health care institutions and providers. The notion that nursing is its own reward continues to play a part in the problems nurses experience when they try to obtain compensation appropriate to their educational preparation, scope of practice, and responsibility.

Sexism and paternalism have inhibited the professionalization of nursing, and have contributed to nursing's perceived position of relative powerlessness within the health care sphere. For many years, functions carried out by nurses were primarily dependent ones, based on following orders of a physician and acting as assistant and supporter.

IMPLICATIONS FOR PROFESSIONAL COLLABORATION

The Effect of Paternalism on Professionalism

One of the most significant deterrents to professionalism in health care is paternalism. A paternalistic relationship can be autocratic and harsh or benevolent and protecting, but whatever its style, it always represents a skewing of power among the participants to favor whoever plays the "father" role. Paternalism can operate at different levels. For example, paternalism can characterize relationships between occupational groups; this has been the traditional relationship between physicians and nurses in the history of health care. Paternalism can also exist in the relationship between professionals and those they serve; for example, between nurses and their clients. Whatever the level, paternalism is ineffective over the long term because it fails to encourage and support the motivation and the development of the full potential of those placed in the "child" role.

Although not usually on site, physicians carried authority, influence, and dominance. Male physicians, hospital administrators, and trustees of boards formulated policies and made decisions about how nursing was to be practiced. The sex role and socialization of women in society became confused with the occupational role in nursing.

Despite the fact that nursing has changed, the public does not generally perceive nursing as a discipline separate and distinct from medicine. Nurses rarely receive public recognition for their unique accomplishments and expertise. Health care continues to be physician dominated and predominantly disease focused. Some physicians continue to subscribe to the 1970 American Medical Association statement that described nursing's "logical place (as being) at the physician's side," practicing "under the supervision of physicians" in order to "extend the hands of the physician."[35] There is evidence, however, that this attitude is currently less prevalent than in the past. A growing number of physicians recognize the benefits to clients, physicians, and nurses of a more mutually dependent physician–nurse relationship.[36,37]

The collaborative theme of this text, in keeping with this view, offers a means of putting to rest issues stemming from sexism and paternalism. Professional nurses who bring expert knowledge and skill to health care, and who conduct themselves with confidence and competence, demonstrate an expectation that they will be treated as professionals. The underlying assumption is that mutual respect, collegiality, and collaboration go hand in hand with recognition of the unique expertise, roles, and functions of each health care team member.

The Feminist Movement

The feminist movement has been both boon and barrier to nursing's efforts to develop a strong collaborative position. On the positive side, the women's movement has raised the consciousness of the American public about issues that principally concern women. Among these issues are society's views of women, the socialization of women, equal opportunities and right to work, the right to define one's own sexuality, and the right to be free from sexual harassment.

Despite the fact that nursing historically has been affected by all the types of social and occupational discrimination on which the feminist movement has focused its efforts, nursing frequently has been adversely affected by feminist action. Initially, the woman's movement denied or devalued that which was traditionally perceived as female in its efforts to gain equal access for women to those areas dominated by men. During the late 1960s and early 1970s, bright young women were encouraged by feminist leaders to avoid occupations such as nursing and elementary-school teaching, which primarily employed females, and seek entry into predominantly male fields such as engineering, business, law, and medicine. Traditional female roles of mother, wife, homemaker, nurse, and teacher were denigrated.

Whether that initial devaluing of the feminine image

was necessary is open to debate. It did enable women to concentrate on getting a foot in the door of traditionally male strongholds. Many women chose alternative life-styles that involved higher education; the pursuit of careers in business, the professions, and politics; and decreased dependence on home, husband, and children for self-fulfillment. Expanded opportunities and more varied options for women became available.

Feminism is now concerned with gaining social acceptance and value for those activities, characteristics, and behaviors that are traditionally defined as female qualities, and recognition by society that such qualities are not gender specific. Men as well as women can be caring and nurturing. Women as well as men can be decisive administrators. Increased awareness of these facts in society at large has had a positive impact on the development of nursing as a profession.

War

War too has influenced nursing's development. War graphically represents man's inhumanity to man. At the same time it brings forth the best in terms of courage and caring that one person can offer to others. Conditions of war create an environment and the impetus for change. The public outcries when the plight of British soldiers at Scutari became known paved the way for the Nightingale era. The Civil War, at a later point in time, also provided a proving ground on which the fledgling discipline of nursing could demonstrate its value to society. Many of the pioneers of American nursing began on the battlefields of that war to develop creative movements that changed the face of health care in this country.

Subsequent wars continued to provide a climate for nursing to grow as a profession. As more sophisticated technologies for killing and maiming were developed, health care providers were challenged to come up with new methods of treatment, care, and rehabilitation—methods that would not only sustain life but ensure some level of acceptable quality for that life. Many advances in technology and in the practice of nursing and medicine emerged from such challenges, as did radical changes in the way that care of the sick and wounded was organized and delivered. Advanced aid stations, field hospitals, evacuation hospitals, mobile army surgical hospitals, and flight nursing brought care closer to the front (Fig. 2–3). The rapidity with which treatment and care could be provided dramatically reduced mortality rates and increased the need for advances in rehabilitation.

In times of war, public concern about the quality of care available to the fighting troops heightened. Nursing gained greater visibility as a highly prized and valued service considered indispensable by both the general public and the soldier. During wartime, nurses have been accorded high status and the power to extend the boundaries of their practice to meet the demands of war as well as the accompanying shortages that develop at home.

One indirect effect of the domestic nursing shortages engendered by wars was the development of ADRN programs. Acceleration of nursing programs to meet the expanded demand during World War II demonstrated that competent practitioners could be prepared in less than the three calendar years required by diploma programs, then the most common route to practice. Some nursing historians see this change as having been detrimental to progress toward a professional image for nursing, in that it contributed to the controversy surrounding entry into practice discussed in Chapter 1.[27] Others believe that this alternative path to nursing practice contributed to professionalization because it generated progress toward the goal of establishing nursing education in institutions of higher learning rather than service-dominated hospital schools.[38]

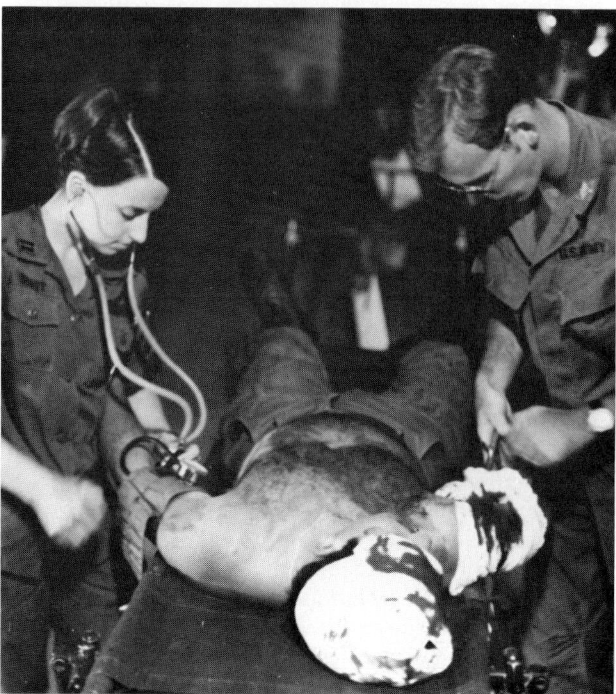

Figure 2–3. Capt. Bernice Scott, a member of the medics team, treating a wounded soldier at the 2nd Surgical Hospital, Vietnam, September, 1969. (*Courtesy of the Department of the Army, The Center of Military History, Washington, D.C.*)

Whether the changes in patterns of nursing education related to wartime nursing shortages are seen as positive or negative, the overall impact of war on nursing has been to highlight the competence and commitment of nurses, and therefore improve both the self-image and public image of nurses as professionals.

Advances in Technology

Advances in technology have changed the practice of medicine and nursing. Sophisticated equipment can prolong life. Babies born prematurely or with critical developmental problems, who in the past would have died, now can be kept alive. Transplantation of organs has become commonplace. Procedures such as computerized tomography (CT) scans, and ultrasound facilitate noninvasive diagnosis (that is, without the use of surgical techniques or probes). Computers can be used to diagnose, treat, and evaluate a client's health care needs, to organize and manage the delivery of services, and to evaluate the outcomes of care. See also Chapter 23.

The list of technological advances that are changing health care delivery is growing daily. Nurses have been both fascinated and intimidated by these changes.[39] The complex needs of clients whose hope of survival rests with advanced technology have opened a whole new field of advanced critical care to nursing. Critical care nurses—those nurses with advanced specialty preparation for providing care to critically ill adults, children, and neonates in hospital intensive care units—are essential to the successful integration of technology with client care. They are the persons who provide the 24-hour care and monitoring that can mean the difference between survival and death or chronic disability for the client.

Such expert knowledge and skills provide a power base that can further the development of nursing as a profession. At the same time, fascination with technology can tempt nurses to focus on the machines that are tools to help clients, rather than on the clients themselves. The resulting emphasis on the ability to control technology as the source of status and reward for nurses could become incompatible with their continuing professionalization. Nursing may be at risk of becoming a mechanistic, technical, supporting occupation rather than developing into an autonomous profession.

Rapid advances in technology create a further dilemma for the health care professions, including nursing. The ability to prolong life, or to improve the survival rate for people who, without the use of extraordinary measures, would not live, carries with it an awesome responsibility. The use of advanced technology is tremendously costly. Health care resources are limited. The need to make choices about when to use expensive procedures and technology in sustaining life raises ethical questions that are not easily answered.

The humanistic, caring philosophy that underlies nursing demands that each human life be valued and nurtured. Reality limits the human, technological, and economic resources available to translate that philosophy into action. There are many human lives in this world, each with competing needs that can only be met by the expenditure of the same scarce resources.

This dilemma underscores the need for a profession to have a code of ethics to serve as a guide for practice. It also increases the demand for extensive and effective collaboration among health care professionals faced with making hard decisions about who gets health care, or who has the right to scarce resources that may mean the difference between life or death for a client.

Changing Health Problems

Over the years major epidemics—diseases that broke out at specific times and affected large numbers of people—as well as wars and developing technology created not only the greatest challenges for medicine and nursing, but also provided opportunities for nursing to make its most extensive gains as a developing profession. Up through the 1800s, for example, the predominant health problems were major epidemics of acute infections, such as plague, influenza, typhoid, smallpox, and syphilis.[12] There were no cures for these diseases and no social organization responsible for providing care. Sick people were left to their own resources and to charity. Medical treatment was ineffective for the most part. The sheer number of persons affected by epidemics far outnumbered the available physicians, making it virtually impossible for physicians to treat those affected even if they had possessed the technology and scientific knowledge to make a difference.

Treating the human responses to the infectious diseases, maintaining cleanliness, and easing suffering were the only measures that offered any hope to epidemic victims. Nurses accepted the challenge of providing such care. Their ability to develop a health care delivery system without physicians' direction that was able to ease suffering and focus on the health care needs of the public marked a major step toward development of the profession of nursing.

During the first half of the 20th century, the predominant health problems were accidents or infections affecting individuals rather than large groups of people.[40] This era saw the beginning and rapid growth of basic medical sciences and technologies, which evolved to handle the health problems of the times. In the United States, it marked the beginning of governmental and societal efforts to care for persons who could not care for themselves.[41] Medicine had the technology and science to diagnose and treat individual illness and injuries, and was politically organized to solidify its control of health care policies and economics. Nursing during this period lost autonomy in the practice area and accepted a subordinate role to medicine.

In the last 40 years, trauma and chronic diseases such as coronary disease, cancer, and strokes have become the predominant health problems faced by the American people.[40] Through an explosive growth of medical and nursing sciences, technology became the focus, rather than the tool, of health care. Despite the greater emphasis on technology, however, the growing recognition that major health problems are influenced by life-style choices, supported the nursing focus on caring for the whole client.

During this same period, health care has come to be perceived by some as a universal right, with the government having responsibility to organize and regulate a system to ensure access to health care for all, regardless of age or ability to pay. Although universal access to care has not occurred, some steps in that direction have been taken with a variety of social service and welfare programs. The development of third-party reimbursement systems including both government and private insurers has helped to transform health care delivery into big business.[42] Nursing, despite its large numbers, lacked the organizational focus to obtain inclusion of nursing services in the reimbursement system established for health care or to influence the social organization of that system.

Currently chronic diseases, particularly those involving emotional and behaviorally related conditions, continue to be predominant health problems in the United States. For some age groups, accidents, substance abuse, and suicide are major health problems.[43] Rapid growth and expansion of technology continues, but now there are attempts, particularly by nursing, to return humanistic caring to technological health care.[44]

Increasing responsibility for and control of decisions that affect the organized delivery of health care is now being assumed by federal and state government in an attempt to contain escalating public health care costs.[45] Employers and unions also exercise power in setting directions for health care delivery by defining in contracts those services and providers for which they will pay. However, both nurses and health care clients are organizing to seek a greater share in controlling the development of health care delivery systems.[46]

A collaborative approach involving all concerned providers and consumers of health care offers the strongest potential for ensuring optimal health care for all in a changing world. The ability of nurses to function as true colleagues within the health care system depends in part on developing a sense of professional competence and pride in nursing as well as confidence in being able to implement nursing roles in a variety of settings. Understanding the problems that may be encountered by nurses involved in the many current and emerging roles of the nurse is a beginning step in developing the characteristics needed for effective collegiality with other health care providers.

■ ROLE PROBLEMS

Role problems are experienced when persons are faced with conflicting expectations relating to values, norms, standards, and usual behavior for a given role. How nurses respond to role problems encountered in nursing practice will have major implications for the way nursing will be viewed in a future world, the world in which today's students will practice as professional nurses.

Role Transition

Among the problems facing nurses in our rapidly changing world are those related to **role transition:** moving from one set of values, responsibilities, and functions to another. Role transition is both a fact of life and a problem faced by students and practicing nurses alike.

From Student to Nurse. Nursing is an exciting and dynamic profession. Moving from the student role to practicing nurse can be frightening, confusing, exhilarating, demanding, and highly rewarding all at the same time. Students learn and work in a protected environment. The clinical setting is used as a laboratory, in which students are assigned limited numbers of clients in order to meet specific clinical learning objectives. Clinical experiences are designed by faculty members to allow students to develop, implement, and evaluate care plans for clients with a variety of health problems.

Students are given assignments to talk with clients and families; to develop a thorough understanding of medical and nursing diagnoses, pharmacology, and other therapeutic regimens of their clients. They are given opportunities to explore the theory and research underlying nursing practice. Students test nursing interventions with support from faculty or nurse preceptors and the collaboration of staff nurses. In short, throughout the educational process students are socialized to value those elements and processes of practice that constitute professional nursing and that provide high personal satisfaction. Students usually are not required to cope with the volume and scope of client care and staffing problems that practicing nurses face every day.

New nursing graduates bring with them to the clinical scene a set of values and ideals about the way in which nursing should be practiced. They believe in the autonomy of nursing and take pride in the significance of nursing for the health and well-being of clients. They can accept accountability for their practice and, although they may be a little anxious at first, are confident that they are ready to begin practicing their chosen profession. These new nurses bring an enthusiasm and commitment to the practice setting, as well as new ideas and knowledge that are critical for the continuing vitality of nursing.

To make the transition to professional practice, however, students must be prepared to cope with the real time and workload expectations for practicing nurses. A variety of strategies can help. These include developing problem-solving skills, flexibility, and understanding of the change process. Awareness of the implications for nursing of changing demographic, economic, social, and health trends and of the influences of history and contemporary issues also are critical for understanding how nursing is practiced now. Students will need a sound foundation of ethics and professional values that can stand up to working environments that are of necessity economically driven and not always ideally staffed.

Students preparing for professional practice need to learn stress management and coping skills so that they can face the world of practice with equanimity. Successful transition from student to nurse requires that students have confidence in their basic philosophy, values, knowledge, skills, and competence. They must also develop an ability to learn new ways and new systems, and the wisdom to begin to differentiate between those things that can be tolerated and those that must be changed. New nurses need enough assertiveness to seek out those many practicing nurses who are caring, nurturing, and willing to share their experience and knowledge of the system and their support, and to serve as mentors for other nurses and students.

It is also important that both students and practicing nurses learn to accept the limitations of their education. The rapidly expanding knowledge base and changing technology in health care and nursing mean that students cannot learn everything there is to know in a basic undergraduate nursing program. Students are prepared to be creative problem solvers and continuing learners, not finished clinicians. New graduates need time to grow and mature, time to learn the roles of practicing nurses in a supportive and caring environment. With realistic performance expectations from self and others, the transition from student to professional can be made without the extreme stress level that Kramer calls reality shock.[47] Reality shock is the reaction that occurs when an individual who has been nurtured and educated in the protected environment of the nursing school suddenly discovers that nursing as practiced in the world of work is very different.

Changing Practice Roles. Throughout their careers nurses will continue to cope with role transition. In most cases, nurses move from one practice role to another by choice. As nurses gain experience and discover which areas and types of practice best fit their career goals and professional values, they move into new specialty areas or new locations, seek advanced or continuing education, and accept greater responsibility for the systems in which they work. Each change, voluntary or not, has problematic aspects.

Nursing is not practiced within a vacuum; it is dynamic. As nurses function within the environmental context—the intangible cultural values and the psychosocial, organizational, and physical characteristics of a new work setting—it is often necessary to alter the way in which they practice nursing. With each change to a different practice role, nurses have to learn new cultural values, new ways of doing things, new sets of resources, and new power and organizational structures within which they will have to function.

Changing Functional Roles. At some time in their careers, many nurses also move between different functional roles, such as teaching, administration, or research. Although some follow a path to formal academic and research careers, most nurses practice such roles within the clinical setting in which they function as caregivers. These roles are an integral part of all nursing practice, and to some extent are part of every staff nurse role. However, when a previously secondary role becomes the focus of a new position, a nurse is faced with an entirely new set of performance expectations. Thus the role change can be stressful, even as it is exciting and challenging. The dynamic and rapidly changing field of nursing presents other role-related challenges besides those related to role transition.

High Touch—High Tech: Care versus Cure Roles for Nurses

One of the most pervasive role problems facing nursing is how to balance the use of advanced technology in health care with the human needs of health care consumers. In recent years new technology has improved the potential for treatment and cure in health care. These technological advances frequently improve the level of treatment available for persons with health problems previously considered terminal or untreatable. However, the time and attention demanded to operate, monitor, and maintain the technology can dehumanize client care and decrease the level of caring by health professionals, who may find themselves focusing more on the machinery than the individual.[48]

An increase in the ability to cure may be accompanied by a decrease in quality of life for many clients. This situation has been interpreted by some as a conflict between caring and curing that marks the essential difference between nursing and medicine. More realistically, it should be viewed as an opportunity for nursing to take a leadership role among health professions in ensuring that humanizing, "high-touch" care is blended with "high-tech" intervention to meet the needs of the total client. In the neonatal intensive care unit, for example, the focus on precise physiological monitoring and support of basic life functions by technical equipment may overshadow the infants' more subtle human needs, as well as the needs of their parents. Nurses can balance the attention focused on physiological and psychological needs by such simple actions as touching, stroking, holding, and talking to the infant and by actively and supportively facilitating similar activities by the parents (Fig. 2–4).

Nursing is uniquely suited to ensure the survival of humanistic, personalized care in an increasingly technolog-

BUILDING NURSING KNOWLEDGE

How Can Nurses Smooth Problems Created by the Expansion of Technology in Health Care?

Zwolski K. Professional nursing in a technical system. *Image: Journal of Nursing Scholarship.* Winter 1989; 21(4):238–242.

Zwolski points out that health technology is expanding in all Western industrialized nations. Science is associated with technology in the minds of most individuals as the solution to health care problems. However, science and technology do not always offer solutions. Zwolski identifies several problems, among them:

1. Providers and clients have different points of view on technology. There is a danger that in the use of technology, the client's point of view may be ignored.
2. When the development of technology is in its incomplete stage, it may actually cause illness.
3. Technology creates pressure for the specialization of health professionals and this fragments care. Each specialty brings its own language and values and focuses on only a limited aspect of the client's health. Specialties even subdivide the physical plants of health facilities and create new bureaucratic structures and competition. This depersonalizes health care. Attention to the individual client's overall uniqueness is thus diminished.

Zwolski asserts that nurses have a strong role to play in assuring that clients' needs are not overlooked. Nurses are valuable in assessing clients' responses to technology and when to use alternate health promoting approaches. To do this, however, nurses need an education that includes courses in philosophy and anthropology, and other courses that stress human values and holism.

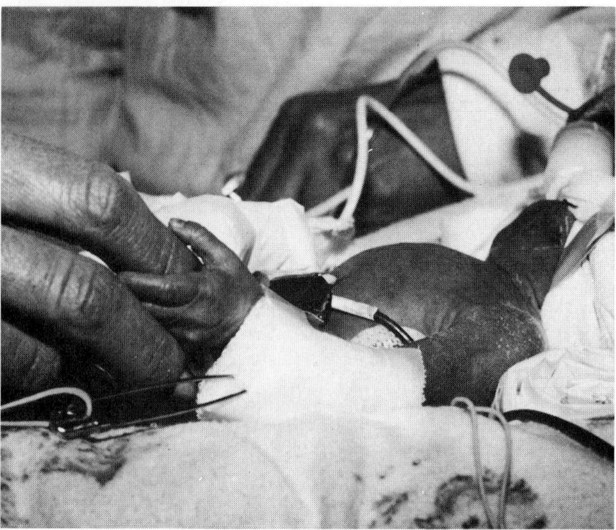

Figure 2–4. The nurse can be instrumental in providing humanizing "high touch" care for the premature infant in an NICU (*From Sherwen L. N., et al.* Nursing Care of the Childbearing Family. *Norwalk, CT: Appleton & Lange, 1991.*)

ical world. It is the only health profession that has developed around the concept of caring for the total person. Curricula for nursing education programs are grounded in philosophy and the social sciences, as well as the basic and biomedical sciences, thus laying the foundation for blending high-tech and high-touch activities.

Autonomy, Interdependence, and Competition

The increasing professional autonomy demanded and earned by nursing is changing the pattern of nurse–physician transactions.[49,50] Nurses and physicians are more likely to interact as equals than as subordinate and superior, as in the past. The emphasis on greater nursing autonomy is positive, but has the potential to produce an overreaction. Some nurses may become overly aggressive, some physicians defensive; however, interdependence need not be a barrier to autonomy. Responsible nurses recognize that a balance between autonomy and interdependence is critical for establishing stronger collaborative relationships with other providers and for helping clients to achieve optimal health.

Another effect of increasing autonomy for nurses is a growing recognition that nurses are legally accountable health practitioners. Accountability is defined as both legal and ethical responsibility, and is expected of professional practitioners from any discipline. Ability, responsibility, and authority are considered by Bergman[51] to be the preconditions leading to accountability. The willingness of nurses to exercise discretion and to answer for the consequences of discretionary judgment are necessary conditions for autonomy and accountability to exist.[52,53]

The move toward nurse autonomy and the shrinking nurse dependence on physicians have also contributed to increasing competition between medicine and nursing for power and control in health care systems. The projected surplus of physicians in the 1990s, and the growing shortage of nurses, are conditions that could escalate competition between medicine and nursing as nurses attempt to expand their scope of practice and physicians work to retain dominance over nursing education and practice. Collaboration for optimal health care appears to offer the best option for defusing the competitive time-bomb by improving quality of care for the health care consumer, and cost-effective models of service delivery for a health system that is increasingly driven by economics. Collaboration allows clients to benefit from the combined strengths of all health care disciplines, and involves clients in making decisions about health care options.

Profession versus Job

Nurses also develop role problems because of differing perceptions about what nursing is and what it means to be a nurse among different persons and groups. Some people, among them some health care colleagues, some of the public, and some nurses, perceive nursing as a job—a combination of routine and frequently tedious tasks that are done repetitively by persons with no long-range goals or real commitment to an institution or its clients—solely for the purpose of earning a salary. Those who hold this position often see no justification for developing higher education programs for nursing. They believe that persons with limited education can be trained to carry out nursing tasks. Those who view nursing as a job consider the professionalization of nursing to be unnecessary and costly, offering no major benefits to the health care system.

A profession, on the other hand, is a career. It demands long-term commitment and a pattern of behavior and choices that furthers personal and professional growth, makes a contribution to the profession, and leads to personal recognition and rewards other than just monetary compensation. Professional nurses plan a career and move through a series of nursing positions in order to accomplish established goals for the future.[54] The role of the professional nurse demands a career orientation in nursing. Without it, nurses will be unable to command the respect and achieve the power necessary to influence health policy—the accepted political positions that govern decisions about health care practices, programs, and funding—or to gain consumer support for nursing's health care agenda.

■ NURSES' RIGHTS AND RESPONSIBILITIES

Rights and responsibilities are two sides of the same coin. The privileges that accrue from education and recognized position in the community carry with them responsibilities. The American Nurses' Association Code for Nurses, discussed earlier in this chapter, summarizes the responsibilities of the professional nurse (see also Fig. 34–1). This code provides a framework within which nurses can make ethical decisions and discharge their responsibilities to the public, to other members of the health care team, and to the profession. It reflects the multiple role responsibilities that professional nurses must recognize and accept. Among these are the need for cooperation, collaboration, and joint practice among professional health care disciplines to achieve optimal health for clients.

To achieve these rights and responsibilities, professional nurses must understand and become involved in current issues that have major significance for nursing and health care.[55,56] Being able to critically analyze and clearly state a position on an issue significant to nursing and to clients is the first step to gaining support for nursing from health policy decision-makers.[57] This and other responsibilities related to the advancement of nursing as a profession are listed in Box 2–2 and discussed below.

Responsibility to Address Crucial Issues

Many crucial issues demand attention from nursing. Quality of life and quality of care are of highest priority.[58] Both are threatened by cuts in federal funding and indiscriminate use of advanced technology in the delivery of health care—that is, the use of technology simply because it is available even though the client may have no hope of recovery.

Nursing is also vulnerable to other external and internal stresses at this point in its development. These include economic constraints, image problems with colleagues and consumers, the nursing shortage and more effective use of available nurses, inadequate nurse compensation, and insufficient differential between beginning salaries and those of nurses with years of experience, and the deteriorating public health of our country's citizens.[59]

Currently, nurses are claiming greater accountability for client and professional outcomes than have nurses in the past. They are developing new nursing roles and professional practice models; to improve quality of care they are taking control of nursing practice. In some cases, these efforts have resulted in legislative and court challenges to nursing practice and the control of nursing.[60]

At the same time that nurses have made gains in professionalization, the priority given cost containment by the health care delivery system is threatening the social and economic welfare of nurses. Nurses are the largest group of health care providers in most health care institutions, and their salaries therefore represent a significant portion of institutional budgets. As institutions seek ways to contain escalating costs, nursing is often scrutinized.[61] Nursing can take a justifiably self-promotional stance, gathering data to document positive outcomes of nursing care and justify costs. Nurses also need to show that nursing is revenue generating, not only a cost center for health care institutions.[62]

Lack of consensus on entry education is another issue that needs resolution. It hampers clear definition of what competencies nurses bring to the practice arena that other health care providers do not, and encourages the development of new health care workers to substitute for nurses. It dissipates political clout and power.

BOX 2–2. NURSES' RESPONSIBILITIES FOR THE ADVANCEMENT OF NURSING AS A PROFESSION

- Address crucial current issues
- Model a professional image
- Educate consumers
- Be active in professional organizations
- Collaborate with other providers to influence health policy

BUILDING NURSING KNOWLEDGE

What Lies Ahead for the Nursing Profession?

Moccia P. Shaping a human agenda for the nineties. *Nurs Health Care.* January 1989: 15–17.

Moccia presents an optimistic view of the future of nursing. The years ahead, in this author's view, will present an opportunity in nursing to assume leadership on important questions with lasting repercussions. These include questions about who will or will not receive health care, which health care services will or will not be available, and with what degree of quality. Moccia believes that the particular skills of nurses will be in demand, because health care will increasingly focus on the well-being of those with chronic illness and on the promotion of health in the community.

Consumerism and other trends, the author notes, are creating vast changes in health care delivery systems. Traditional providers are no longer in control of decision-making in health care. Power is shifting to consumer groups that demand, among other things, information to use in making their own independent evaluation of health agencies.

The seat of power is also shifting because of changing population demographics, changes in service needs, and the diffusion of technology out of hospitals. As a consequence, nurses will be employed increasingly in out-of-hospital careers. They will have a major role to play in the new system of managed care, a system that emphasizes efficient packages of services for specific populations at the most reasonable costs. Nursing's contribution lies in preserving the quality of services for consumers while costs are being reduced. Moccia notes that there will be an increased need for collaboration. The effect of moving health care out of hospitals into homes and community-based facilities will be to make health care part of the everyday experience of a growing number of people who have ideas, questions, opinions, and criticisms about health care.

Responsibility to Model a Professional Image for Nursing

Despite its increasing strength in many areas, nursing retains an image of disunity and fragmentation that limits its power to confront crucial issues. It has been said that perception is reality. To the extent that that is true, how nurses are viewed by other health care providers, consumers, clients, the general public, and policy-makers will affect political decision-making regarding the allocation of increasingly scarce health care resources. Nurses must be aware of how their self-presentation affects the perceptions others develop of nursing, and accept the responsibility to model a professional image for nursing.[63] The extent to which nurses are able to demonstrate the knowledge, skills, critical judgment, and competence necessary for delivering care that is helpful to clients is the essence of the nursing image. Professional image also includes assertiveness and confidence that nurses communicate during the practice of nursing or when interacting with others interested in health care.

Responsibility to Educate Consumers

Nurses who believe that collaboration is essential to the achievement of optimal health must help consumers develop the skills and opportunity to participate actively in decisions affecting their health. Participation in health education for consumers of all ages is one strategy for meeting this responsibility. Children as well as adults can learn about healthy life-styles, how to "just say no" to high-risk behaviors such as smoking and substance abuse, and how to be more involved in self-care.[64] Consumer education by nurses can be accomplished by developing special programs in health care institutions and schools as well as in informal teaching as part of nurse–client interactions.

Responsibility to Get Involved

Professional nurses have a responsibility to get involved. Nurses must contribute to the discipline of nursing through their practice and research. Change to accomplish the goal of improving access to high-quality health care requires organization and collaboration. For nurses, this means accepting the responsibility to join together with other nurses in professional associations to gain the power needed to accomplish change.[55,56] Collaborating with other health professionals and public groups in seeking improvement of client care and health care delivery systems is equally important. Responsible professional nurses will be active members of a professional association and engage in collective action to influence policy and politics for optimal health care. The role of nurses in politics and policy-making is further discussed in Chapter 4.

The Rights of Nurses

As members of a profession, nurses have earned certain rights—those privileges to which a professional has claim based on law, tradition, accepted standards, or a sense of what is just (Box 2–3). Nurses have the right to regulate entry into practice. They have the right to review and sanction members of the profession, and to receive adequate compensation commensurate with professional preparation and responsibilities. They have the right to direct access to their clients and to provide direct client services for reimbursement from consumers and third-party payers. Nurses are deserving of respect and support from peers and colleagues as they work to expand the boundaries of nursing practice and to improve nursing's image, autonomy, and satisfaction with nursing. These efforts support the right to pride in their profession.

BOX 2–3. RIGHTS OF PROFESSIONAL NURSES

- Regulate entry into nursing practice
- Review and sanction peers
- Receive fair compensation for service
- Provide direct service to clients for direct reimbursement
- Pride in nursing as a profession

THE NURSE OF THE FUTURE

Margaret Mead, the noted anthropologist, once said that no one lives in the world in which he is born. The health care system in which nurses practice reflects the larger society. Thus, the rapid and continual change taking place in the world in which we live has major implications for nursing.

Nursing today is at a decisive point in its development. Nursing must become visionary. The choices made in meeting current challenges will determine nursing's position in the health care system of the future.

Today the discipline of nursing must establish its unique mission and place in a world that is undergoing change in its technology and all its major institutions at an unprecedented rate. Nursing history reveals that a time of rapid transition is also a time of great opportunity. Established systems and patterns are opened to change and it is up to nursing to take advantage of them. Nursing leaders must place themselves in a position to be involved in shaping policy for the future.[55,63]

Social Trends Shaping Future Practice

Current societal trends offer the promise of exciting new opportunities for nursing in the future.

Changing Economic Context. Health care costs are rising rapidly, and consumers are being compelled to pay more out of their own pockets for the health care they receive.[65] Demands for cost containment have led to a major change in health care reimbursement that is increasing the rate of change in health care delivery systems.[66] These economic pressures are forcing health care providers to take a closer look at what they do, how they do it, where health care is delivered and to whom, and who pays and is paid for health related services. Nursing development of more entrepreneurial, innovative, cost-effective models for health care delivery that are responsive to consumer needs will ensure that nursing becomes one of the primary solutions to problems facing future health care systems.

Changing Consumers. Consumers are becoming better informed and more assertive and participative in making choices about health and health care. Consumer demands for high-quality, efficient, accessible, and cost-effective services are setting the stage for competition among providers. Health care decisions in the future will call for increasing collaboration with consumers. The growing involvement and visibility of nurses in health education, prevention, and health promotion activities and the improving media image of nurses is contributing to consumers' seeking primary health care services from nurses.[67–69]

High Technology. Today's health care system is technologically sophisticated. Priority has been on developing the technology to treat previously incurable health problems. Biomedical and technological advances now enable us to keep alive persons at both ends of the life span, and all points in between, who only a few years ago would have died.

Treatment and technology are very expensive, and costs rarely end with the immediate hospitalization. The lives saved are often diminished in quality by chronic disease or disability. Long-term commitment of a large proportion of increasingly scarce health care resources is required to help such persons and their families overcome or accommodate the problems that accompany keeping tiny preterm infants alive, saving the life of major trauma victims, or prolonging the life of elderly cancer victims. Often, continuing care in skilled nursing facilities or at home is needed when the need for acute care is past. Nurses can play a major role in developing systems to organize and deliver care in postacute settings.

Limited Access to Health Care. Presently, a growing segment of the population, mostly poor, has no health insurance coverage. An increasing part of the working population also has limited or no health insurance, as more companies and businesses find it impossible to support the increasing cost of group health insurance for employees.[70] Under a retrospective payment system, where health care agencies were reimbursed what they billed for health care delivered, costs for indigent care could be covered by a process of cost shifting or distributing charges across other clients and cost centers. The move to prospective payment with preestablished rates of payment based on externally designated criteria (diagnosis-related groups, or DRGs) limits the ability of health care institutions to use internal accounting mechanisms to fund care for the increasing numbers of uninsured or underinsured clients in America.[71]

These groups constitute a high-risk and vulnerable population that must have access to the health care system. Ensuring access to health care for underserved populations will move health care inevitably toward some form of rationing, either through pricing in a competitive marketplace, regulation, or the nationalization of health care.[72,73] This probability will increase demands on nursing to provide a cost-effective alternative to traditional medical models for health care.

Increasing Number of Elderly. The "graying of America," the increasing proportion of the population in the group aged 65 and older, will require fuller involvement of nurses in the development of the range of health care services that will be needed by an aging population. In primary care, acute care, home health, and long-term care services, greater emphasis will be directed toward improving quality of life for the elderly and on promoting healthy aging. More social and health care resources will have to be directed toward health problems that affect older adults—namely chronic disease, coronary and respiratory problems, cognitive dysfunction, and diminished capacity for physical activities of daily living.

The changing nature of the age structure in the United States has been a dominant factor contributing to the nursing shortage and will continue to be. It has also influenced the creation of new roles for nurses, such as private geriatric case managers,[74] and stimulated moves to use new models of delivering nursing care.[75]

These societal trends have a major impact on the professional preparation needed for future practice. Increasingly, critical thinking and creative problem solving will be required of nurses. Skill in analyzing trends and issues that will influence the structure and scope of practice for health care professionals, and understanding the economics and politics of health care, will be crucial. A sound foundation in philosophy and ethics will be necessary for dealing with the critical decisions related to consumer rights, access to health care, cost, alternative treatments, use of technology, quality of care, and allocation of health care resources. These issues are discussed more fully in Chapters 33, 34, and 37.

The Nurse in the 21st Century

Picture this scenario. Nursing in the 21st century is a professional discipline with its own defined practice and nursing art and science base. It is on the cutting edge of science and knowledge development. It is implemented within the context of the marketplace, where health care consumers make choices among competitive alternative providers and types of care, and nurses as well as other health care professionals are paid directly for the services they provide. Hospitals are trauma centers and intensive care units, where high technology receives priority. Noninvasive and elective surgeries are predominantly outpatient services. Much of the primary care sought by the general population is provided through community nursing clinics and urgent-care centers. Families and clients actively participate in health care planning and choices. Although there is more competition between physicians and nurses for control of health care services and clients than there was in the past, there also is greater collaboration. Health care professionals value each other as colleagues. They recognize the distinctions between separate, autonomous professions and the importance of collaboration for optimal health outcomes for clients.

In this future scenario, funding of health care plays at least as great a role in decisions about access and quality of care as do client needs. There is more individual responsibility for health care, and greater use of alternatives to traditional medical services by the poor and the elderly. More outreach and occupational health systems are directed by professional nurses. More physicians and nurses are salaried by hospitals and corporate community health centers. There is a growing trend for hospitals to contract with nurse-owned and managed businesses to provide nursing care for units within the institution as a cost-saving measure.

Nurses in this future world are strong enough in their sense of autonomy to accept the necessity for professional and societal interdependence in identifying and meeting clients' health care needs. They maintain strong roles in health care policy development and carry out corporate roles in consulting, coordinating, monitoring, and administering client services. Nurses accept and facilitate change. They control their own practice and are paid directly for their services.

In this projected future, salaries are commensurate with preparation, scope of practice, and accountability. Practice is research based and nurses consistently contribute to the development of new nursing knowledge. Nurses share commitment to unified goals and a well-grounded socialization and educational process. They can articulate a clear vision of nursing's future and know how to carry out the strategic planning necessary to bring that vision to reality.

Strategies for Achieving a Preferred Future for Nursing

Nursing needs to set high goals for change in education; practice; research; relationships with colleagues, consumers, and other constituents; and professional organization for collective action. To ensure nursing's preferred future, professional nurses need to take risks and move out of the comfortable niches into which they have allowed themselves to be pushed by the problems that have accompanied nursing's development. They need to resolve differences among nurses, build collaborative models between education and service, and accept the need for appropriate levels of education to ensure that new nurses are prepared to meet the challenges of the future. It is crucial that nurses reach consensus about the parameters of nursing as a practice discipline.

The formation of coalitions and alliances with consumers will be a critical strategy for nurses who want to take charge of their practice. Consumer support will help nurses to eliminate barriers and constraints to full professional practice. It also will help them move into the corporate world and the boardroom, where many economic decisions that affect the delivery of health care are made. Consumer support constitutes a power base that needs to be recognized and nurtured by nursing.

Greater involvement by nurses in professional organizations and in health care policy development is essential. Better understanding of concepts of power, influence, and change will increase the willingness of nurses to consciously seek and use power and to be openly competitive to achieve goals for improving access to high-quality health care for all clients[76] (see also Chapter 4). Nurses must take charge of those aspects of health care that have long been the focus and responsibility of nursing: health promotion and health maintenance, organization and management of client care delivery, client teaching and counseling, client advocacy, and care of the elderly. Nurses are already demonstrating that they can provide alternative models for the delivery of high-quality, cost-effective health care. These models need to be moved into the mainstream of American health care.

Assuming administrative control of skilled nursing facilities and home health care services as well as nursing units in acute care institutions is a logical step toward accomplishing this. These are primary practice sites for nursing. Nurses should be making decisions about client access, quality of care, range of services, organization, structure, and the business operation of their practice settings. Collaboration with other health care providers enriches and strengthens client care. When the emphasis is on issues involving day-to-day client care, on managing care, or on human responses to health and illness, it is appropriate for nurses to assume a leadership role in the collaborative process.

Nurses must be vigilant reformers of both health care systems and nursing practice to ensure the continuing viability of high-quality health care services for vulnerable consumers. They need to synthesize the values of humanism and caring with the dictates of an increasingly economically driven delivery system.

SUMMARY

Nursing is a professional discipline, with its own practice and science base. It meets the criteria for a profession and is grounded in humanism, caring, and collaboration. The profession is on the cutting edge of development of both its scientific base and its practice.

Nursing's historical origins strongly influence the issues facing nursing today.

Professional organizations, such as the American Nurses' Association, the National League for Nursing, and others have shaped the history of nursing and continue to prevail upon its present development and future possibilities. Wars, the feminist movement, advancing technology, and changing health problems are some other phenomena that have affected what nursing is today.

Role conflicts often accompany change, even positive change. Nursing has not escaped role-related struggles in the course of its development, neither as a discipline, nor as members of that discipline. Continued progress toward a preferred future for nursing is likely to engender further role conflict as the profession pushes for amplified autonomy and effectiveness. Conflict need not be seen as negative, in fact, positive outcomes, such as unity, cohesion and growth can succeed conflict.

For nursing to attain its full potential as a profession, cohesion and unity are essential. Nurses must develop stronger bonds with one another as individuals and as practitioners. They must accept their responsibility to influence health care and public policy, recognizing and exploiting the social trends that are shaping future practice.

These challenges, although daunting, are not insurmountable. They are, rather, an invitation to all members of the profession to allow themselves to become inspired and show their commitment to self, profession and humanity.

REFERENCES

1. Kelly LY. *Dimensions of Professional Nursing*. New York: Macmillan; 1985:676.
2. McGlothin WJ. *The Professional Schools*. New York: Center for Applied Research in Education; 1964.
3. Friedson E. *Professional Dominance*. New York: Atherton Press; 1970.
4. O'Connell KA. Nursing practice: A decade of research. In Chaska, NLN (ed). The Nursing Profession: A Time to Speak Out. New York: McGraw-Hill; 1983.
5. Brown J, Tanner C, Padrick K. Nursing's search for scientific knowledge. *Nurs Res*. 1984; 33:26–32.
6. Jacox A. The coming of age of nursing research. *Nurs Outlook*. 1986; 34:276.
7. Annual Review of Nursing Research. New York: Springer Pub. Co. 1983–1991.
8. Roberts C, Burke S. *Nursing Research: A Quantitative and Qualitative Approach*. Boston: Jones and Bartlett; 1989: 6.
9. Uris Patricia, et al. *Associate and Baccalaureate Degree Nursing Graduates: Perceptions of and Recommendations for Preparation and Utilization*. Boulder: Western Interstate Commission on Higher Education; 1986.
10. Boggs D, Baker B, Price G. Determining two levels of nursing competency. *Nurs Outlook*. 1987; 35:34–37.
11. Walsh J. *The History of Nursing*. New York: P.J. Kenedy and Sons; 1929.
12. Shryock R. *The History of Nursing: An Interpretation of the Social and Medical Factors Involved*. Philadelphia: Saunders; 1959.
13. Jamieson EM, Sewall ME. *Trends in Nursing History*. Philadelphia: Saunders; 1950.
14. Dolan JA, Fitzpatrick ML, Hermann EK. *Nursing in Society: A Historical Perspective*. 15th ed. Philadelphia: Saunders; 1983.
15. Donahue MP. *Nursing: The Finest Art*. St. Louis: Mosby; 1985.
16. Frank C. *The Historical Development of Nursing*. Philadelphia: Saunders; 1953.
17. Nutting M, Dock L. *A History of Nursing*. New York: Putnam's; 1937; 1.
18. Robinson V. *White caps: The Story of Nursing*. Philadelphia: Lippincott; 1946.
19. Nightingale F. *Notes on Nursing*. New York: D. Appleton; 1859.
20. Cohen IB. Florence Nightingale. *Sci Am*. 1984; 250:137.
21. Baker N. *Cyclone in Calico: The Story of Mary Ann Bicderdyke*. Boston: Little, Brown; 1952.
22. Austin A. *History of Nursing Source Book*. New York: Putnam; 1957.
23. Dock LL, Stewart IM. *A Short History of Nursing*, 3rd ed. New York: Putnam's, 1925.
24. Woolfe SV. Miss Wald at 70 sees dreams realized. *New York Times Magazine*. March 7, 1937.
25. Nutting MA. The future. *AM J Nurs*. 1929; 29: 903–910.
26. Harmer B, Henderson V. *Textbook of the Principles and Practice of Nursing*. 4th ed. New York: Macmillan; 1939.
27. Aynes E. *From Nightingale to Eagle*. New Jersey: Prentice-Hall; 1973.
28. American Nurses' Association. First position paper on education for nurses. *Am J Nurs*. 1965; 65:106.
29. Fritsch R. Considerations on corporate consulting. *Nurs Admin*. 1986; 10:17–23.
30. Frels L, Straub L, Goldsteen R. RCTs: Not the answer to the nursing shortage. *Nurs Econ*. 1989; 7:136–141.
31. Stewart IM, Austin AL. *A History of Nursing*. 5th ed. New York: Putnam's; 1962.
32. Staupers M. *No Time for Prejudice*. New York: Macmillan; 1961.
33. Smith GR. From invisibility to blackness: The Story of the National Black Nurses' Association. *Nurs Out*. 1975; 23:225.
34. Broveman IK, Voget SR, Broveman DM., et al. Sexual stereotypes: A current appraisal. *J Soc Issues*. 1972; 282:59–78.
35. American Medical Association; 1970.
36. Stein L, Watts OT, Howell T. The doctor–nurse game revisited. *N Engl J Med*. 1990; 322:546–49.
37. Mechanic D, Aiken LH. A cooperative agenda for medicine and nursing. *N Engl J Med*. 1982; 307:747–50.
38. Kalisch P, Kalisch B. *The Advance of American Nursing*. Boston: Little, Brown; 1978.
39. Pillar B, Jacox A, Redman B. Technology, its assessment, and Nursing. *Nurs Out*. 1990; 38:16–19.
40. Starr P. *The Social Transformation of American Medicine*. New York: Basic Books; 1984.
41. Hirt EJ. *The Health Policy Agenda for the American People*. Washington, DC: US Government Printing Office; 1987.
42. Fuchs V. *The Health Economy*. Cambridge: Harvard University Press; 1986.
43. Lee P, Estes C, Ramsay N. *The Nation's Health*. San Francisco, CA: Boyd and Fraser Publishing Co; 1984.
44. Carter S. Rehumanizing the nursing role. *Top Clin Nurs*. 1983; 5:11–17.
45. Litman T, Robins L. *Health Politics and Policy*. New York: Wiley; 1984.
46. Culbert-Hinthorn PC, Fiscella KD, Shortridge LM. A nurse-managed center: The problems. *Nurs Health Care*. 1986; 7:490–494.
47. Kramer M. Philosophical foundations of baccalaureate nursing education. *Nurs Out*. 1981; 19:224–228.
48. Dracup K. Are critical care units hazardous to health? *Appl Nurs Res*. 1988; 1:14–21.
49. Porter-O'Grady T. Shared governance and new organizational models. *Nurs Econ*. 1987; 5:281–286.
50. Chavigny K. Coalition building between medicine and nursing. *Nurs Econ*. 1988; 6:179–183.
51. Bergman R. Accountability—definition and dimensions. *Int Nurs Rev*. 1981; 28:53–59.
52. McClure ML. The long road to accountability. *Nurs Out*. 1978; 5:47–51.
53. Sliefert MK. Debate quality control: Professional or institutional responsibility? In: McClosky JC, Grace HK, eds. *Current Issues in Nursing*. St. Louis: Mosby; 1990:237.
54. Fawcett J, Carino C. Hallmarks of success in nursing practice. *Adv Nurs Sci*. 1989; 11:1–8.
55. White SKO. Involvement: Influencing the delivery of health care and the future of critical care nursing. In: McClosky JC, Grace HK, eds. *Current Issues in Nursing*. Boston: Blackwell; 1983:406–412.
56. Beyers M. Public policy issues: Will they be resolved? In: *The Nurse's Legal Advisor*. Philadelphia: Lippincott; 1989:493–500.

57. Cohen WJ, Milburn LT. What every nurse should know about political action. In: McCloskey JC, Grace HK, eds. *Current Issues in Nursing*. Boston: Blackwell; 1983:401.
58. Bocchino C. An interview with President Lucille Joel: Perspectives from the ANA. *Nurs Econ*. 1989; 7:6–14.
59. Medical Economics Company. RN: Profile of the nurse. *RN*. 1989; 52:18.
60. Goldstein A, Perdew S, Pruitt S. *The Nurse's Legal Advisor*. Philadelphia: Lippincott; 1989:35.
61. Davis CK. Financing of health care and its impact on Nursing. In McCloskey JC, Grace HK, eds. *Current Issues in Nursing*. St. Louis: C.V. Mosby; 1990: 354.
62. Scherubel J. Costing out nursing services. In: *The Nurse's Legal Advisor*. Philadelphia: Lippincott; 1989:393–398.
63. Donley R, Flaherty M. Strategies for Changing Nursing's Image. *The Nurse's Legal Advisor*. Philadelphia: Lippincott; 1989: 431–439.
64. Kubok P, Earls F, Montgomery C. Life style and patterns of health and social behavior in high risk adolescents. *Adv Nurs Sci*. 1988; 11:22–35.
65. Gabel J, Jajick-Toth C, de Lissovoy. The changing world of group health insurance. *Health Affairs*. 1988; 1:48–65.
66. Bocchino C. An interview with Bruce Vladeck: Perspectives on prospective payment and medical gridlock. *Nurs Econ*. 1989; 7:71–78.
67. Eck S, Meehan R, Zigmund D, Pierro L. Consumerism, nursing and the reality of the resources. *Nurs Admin*. 1988; 12:1–11.
68. Woods N, Fugate N, Laffrey S, et al. Being healthy: women's images. *Adv Nurs Sci*. 1988; 11:36–46.
69. Walker S, Voldan K, Sechrist K, et al. Health promoting lifestyles of older adults: Comparisons with young and middle-aged adults, correlates and patterns. *Adv Nurs Sci*. 1988; 1:76–90.
70. Wilensky G. Filling the gaps in health insurance: Impact on competition. *Health Affairs*. 1988; 7:133–149.
71. Goldsmith J. Competition's impact: A report from the front. *Health Affairs*. 1988; 7:162–173.
72. Alfano GJ. Payment for health services in long term care. *The Nurse's Legal Advisor*. Philadelphia: Lippincott; 1989:405–409.
73. Russell S. High cost may lead to rationed medicine. In: *Current Issues in Nursing*. Boston: Blackwell; 1983:428–436.
74. Parker M, Second L. Case managers: Guiding the elderly through the health care maze. In: *Current Issues in Nursing*. Boston: Blackwell; 1983:271–274.
75. Floyd J, Buckle J. Nursing Care of the Elderly: The DRG Influence. In: *Current Issues in Nursing*. Boston: Blackwell; 1983:275–282.
76. Sweeney S. Traditions, transitions, and transformations of power in nursing. In: *The Nurse's Legal Advisor*. Philadelphia: Lippincott; 1989:459–465.

BIBLIOGRAPHY

Ackerman WB. Technology and nursing education: A scenario for 1990. *J Adv Nurs*. 1982; 7:59–68.

American Nurses' Association. *Codes for Nurses*. Kansas City, MO: ANA; 1980.

Ashley J. *Hospitals, Paternalism and the Role of the Nurse*. New York: Teachers College Press; 1976.

Bocker B, Frost AD, Mason D. High tech–high touch: It's high time for nursing. *Nurs Health Care*. 1985; 6:263–266.

Chaska, NL. *The Nursing Profession: Turning Points*. St. Louis: Mosby; 1990.

Chibuye PS. Nursing in action. Nurses influence in research and health policy development. *J Prof Nurs*. 1989; 5:326–329.

Donahue MP. *Nursing: The Finest Art*. St. Louis: Mosby; 1985.

Eisenhauer LA. Health care brokering—A career option for changing times. *Nurs Health Care*. 1986; 7:417–419.

Egeland JW, Brown JS. Sex role stereotyping and role strain of male registered nurses. *Res Nurs Health Care*. 1988:11:257–267.

Goldstein A, Perdew S, Pruitt S. *The Nurse's Legal Advisor*. Philadelphia: Lippincott; 1989.

Gordon S. *Prisoners of Men's Dreams: Striking Out for a New Feminine Future*. Boston: Little, Brown; 1991.

Gortner S. Nursing research: Out of the past and into the future. *Nurs Res*. 1980; 29:204–207.

Harrington C, Calbertson R. Nurses left out of reimbursement reform. *Nurs Out*. 1990; 38:156–158.

Henderson V. *The Nature of Nursing*. New York: Macmillan; 1966.

Holzemer W. *Review of Research in Nursing Education*. New York: National League for Nursing; 2; 1989.

Kalisch P, Kalisch B. The image of the nurse in motion pictures. *Am J Nurs*. 1982.

Kelly LY. *Dimensions of Professional Nursing*. New York: Macmillan; 1985.

Kidd PS, Morrison EF. The progression of knowledge in nursing: A search for meaning. *Image: J Nurs Scholar*. 1988; 20:222–224.

King IM. *Toward a Theory of Nursing*. New York: Wiley; 1971.

King IM. *Theory for Nursing*. New York: Wiley; 1981.

Kramer M, Schmalenberg C. Job satisfaction and retention in the '90s. *Nursing 1991*. 1991; 21:50–55.

Lancaster J. 1986 and beyond: Nursing's future. *J Nurse Admin*. 1986; 16:31–37.

McManus RL. Isabel M. Stewart—Foremost researcher. *Nurs Res*. 1951; 2:6.

Mitchell M. The power standards: The glory days of nursing yet to come. *Nurs Health Care*. 1989; 10:306–309.

Muff J. Myth and image of the female in nursing. *Imprint*. 1990; 37:96–98.

Neuman B. *The Neuman Sustems Model: Application to Nursing Education and Practice*. Norwalk, CT: Appleton-Century-Crofts; 1982.

Newman MA. *Theory Development in Nursing*. Philadelphia: Davis; 1979.

Norman E. The wartime experience of military nurses in Vietnam. *West J Nurs Res*. 1989; 11:219–233.

Nutting MA, Dock LL. *A History of Nursing: The Evaluation of Nursing Systems from Earliest Times to the Foundations of the First English and American Training Schools for Nurses*. (4 vols.) 1907 & 1912.

Orem DE. *Nursing: Concepts of practice*. New York: McGraw-Hill; 1985.

Orlando IJ. *The Dynamic Nurse–Patient Relationship: Function, Process, and Principles*. New York: Putnam's; 1961.

Parse RR. *Man-Living-Health: A Theory of Nursing*. New York: Wiley; 1981.

Peplau H. *Interpersonal Relations in Nursing*. New York: Putnam's; 1952.

Powell D. High touch entrepreneurs. *Nurs Econ*. 1984; 2:33–36.

Roberts C, Burke S. *Nursing Research: A Quantitative and Qualitative Approach*. Boston: Jones and Bartlett; 1989.

Rogers ME. *An Introduction to the Theoretical Basis of Nursing*. Philadelphia: Davis; 1970.

Peterson M, Allen D. Shared governance strategies for transforming organizations. *J Nsg Admin*. 1986; 16(1):9–12/16(2):11–16 (2 parts).

Porter-O'Grady T. *Shared Governance for Nursing*. Rockville, MD: Aspen; 1984.

Porter-O'Grady T. *Creative Nursing Administration: Participative Management into the 21st Century*. Rockville, MD: Aspen; 1986.

Ronceli M, Whitney J. The limits of medicine spell opportunities for nursing. *Nurs Health Care*. 1986; 7:531–534.

Roy C Sr. *Introduction to Nursing: An Adaptation Model*. Englewood Cliffs, NJ: Prentice-Hall; 1976.

Sampselle, CM. The Influence of Feminist Philosophy on Nursing Practice. *Image*, 1990. 22(4): 243–7.

Scherubel J, ed. *Patients and Purse Strings II*. New York: National League for Nursing; 1988.

Schultz PR, Meleis AI. Nursing epistemology: Traditions, insights, questions. *Image: J Nurs Scholar*. 1988; 20:217–221.

Schutzenhofer K. Measuring professional autonomy in nurses. In: Strickland O, Waltz C, eds. *Measurement of Nursing Outcomes*. New York: Springer; 1988; 2:3–18.

Sepic FT. Do you know a quitter when you see one? *Health Care Supervisor*. 1986; 4:65–74.

Shryock RH. *The History of Nursing: An Interpretation of the Social and Medical Factors Involved*. Philadelphia: Saunders; 1959.

Sliefert MK. Debate quality control: Professional or institutional responsibility? In: McCluskey JC, Grace HK, eds. *Current Issues in Nursing*. St. Louis: Mosby; 1990:234–241.

vanMaanen HMT. Nursing in transition: An analysis of the state of the art in relation to society's expectations. *J Adv Nurs*. 1990; 15:914–924.

Walsh JJ. *The History of Nursing*. New York: P. J. Kennedy and Sons; 1929.

Watson J. *Nursing: The Philosophy and Science of Caring*. Boston: Little, Brown; 1979.

Watson J. *Nursing: Human Science and Human Care: A Theory of Nursing*. New York: National League for Nursing; 1988.

Weidenback E. *Clinical Nursing: A Helping Art*. New York: Springer; 1989.

Wilson HS. *Research in Nursing*. Menlo Park, CA: Addison-Wesley; 1989.

Zwolski K. Professional nursing in a technical system. *Image: J Nurs Scholar*. 1989; 21:238–242.

CHAPTER 3

Legal Considerations

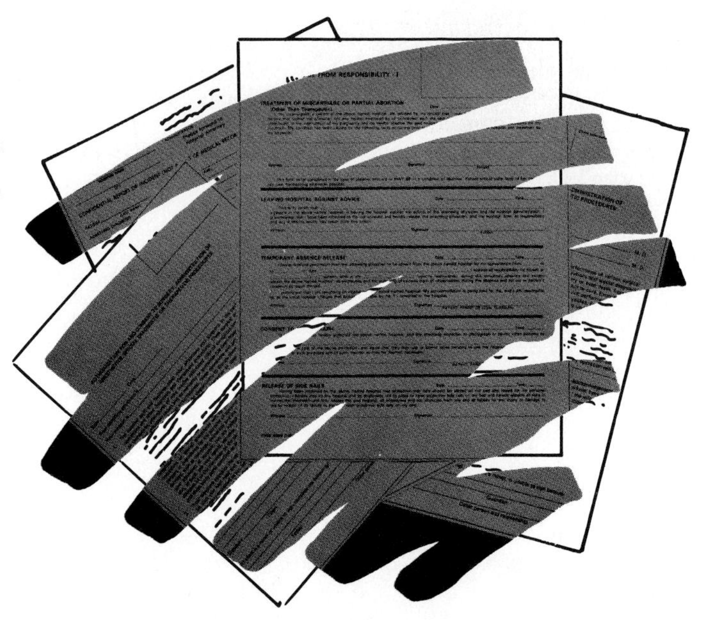

Overview of Law and Nursing Practice
- CATEGORIES OF LAW
- A BRIEF HISTORY OF LICENSURE

Nurse Practice Acts
- DEFINITION OF NURSING
- INDEPENDENT AND DEPENDENT FUNCTIONS
- RELATIONSHIP TO OTHER PRACTICE ACTS
- LIMITATIONS
- ADVANCED PRACTICE OF NURSING
- ADMINISTRATION

Requirements for Licensure and Renewal
- BASIC NURSING EDUCATION
- NATIONAL COUNCIL LICENSURE EXAMINATION
- RECIPROCITY BETWEEN STATES
- CONTINUING EDUCATION
- EXCEPTIONS
- OPTIONS

Loss of License or Limitation of Scope of Practice
- NEGLIGENCE AND INCOMPETENCE
- FALSE REPRESENTATION, FRAUD, AND DECEIT
- SUBSTANCE ABUSE
- OTHER CRIMINAL BEHAVIOR

Civil and Criminal Law
- TORTS, MISDEMEANORS, AND FELONIES
- LEGAL ACTION IN CIVIL AND CRIMINAL OFFENSES
- EVIDENCE
- MALPRACTICE SUITS

Historical and Current Trends in Liability
- RESPONDEAT SUPERIOR, CAPTAIN OF THE SHIP, BORROWED SERVANT
- CHARITABLE IMMUNITY, CORPORATE LIABILITY
- REASONABLE PRUDENT PRACTITIONER, COMMUNITY OR LOCALITY STANDARD, EXPERT WITNESS

Other Local, State, and Federal Laws Affecting Nursing Practice
- PRACTICE ACTS OF OTHER PROFESSIONS
- HOSPITAL AND OTHER HEALTH FACILITY LICENSING LAWS
- PUBLIC HEALTH AND SAFETY CODES
- INSURANCE CODES
- EDUCATION CODES
- LAWS RELATING TO WILLS AND INHERITANCE
- ANTITRUST ACT
- LAWS RELATING TO EMPLOYMENT RIGHTS

Laws Relating to the Rights of Clients
- INFORMED CONSENT, ASSAULT AND BATTERY
- UNLAWFUL IMPRISONMENT, RIGHT TO TREATMENT
- RIGHT TO DIE AND RIGHT TO LIFE
- DO NOT RESUSCITATE ORDERS
- ACCESS-TO-CARE LEGISLATION

Impact of Law on Collaboration for Optimal Health

Summary

Behavioral Objectives

Upon completion of this chapter, the student will be able to:

1. Describe in general terms the functions of licensure for a profession.
2. Compare and contrast the Nurse Practice Act for the state in which the student's school is located to the more general discussion in the chapter.
3. Describe the principles of client rights within the health care system.
4. Describe the usefulness of collaboration among health care team members and with clients in preventing misunderstandings and lawsuits.
5. Describe the principles involved in a living will and durable power of attorney for health care for clients and health care professionals.
6. Discuss the role of accurate record-keeping as a nursing responsibility as demonstrated by completing examples of actual chart and incident report forms from the student's clinical facility.
7. List the resources available to nurses for advice regarding legal and/or ethical problems in general and in the student's current practice location.
8. List seven examples of actions by nurses that will result in discipline by their state licensing board.
9. Compare and contrast the collaborative responsibilities of health care professionals and clients in the delivery of health care.

KEY TERMS

accreditation
administrative regulation
assault
battery
civil law
common law
community/locality standard
constitutional law
criminal law
dependent functions
durable power of attorney
expert witness
employment contract
felony
good samaritan laws
incompetence
independent functions
informed consent
informed dissent
intentional tort
law
licensure
living will
malpractice suit
misdemeanor
negligence
nurse practice act
protocol
reciprocity
respondeat superior
slow code
statutory law
sunset laws
sunshine laws
tort
unintentional tort

A general knowledge of the law is important to nurses because it provides a framework for describing the rights, privileges, and responsibilities that exist between nurses and clients, nurses and other health care workers, and nurses and employers. In this chapter beginning students will find a brief overview of the legal considerations important to the practice of nursing. This is the beginning of a lifelong involvement with the law as it relates to nurses and their clients, and the delivery of nursing services.

Laws constitute the written rules under which a society has agreed to function. Law as it relates to the practice of nursing and other professions has its roots in the necessity for professionals to have special access to personal and private information about clients in order to practice. Thus attorneys, clergy, physicians, nurses, and members of some other professions will know things about a client, or will function in relation to a client in ways that are forbidden to nonmembers of their professions. Professional practice is assumed to require both special knowledge and a special responsibility for the welfare of clients. When the potential for harm by an unskilled or unscrupulous professional is high, society resorts to the law (eg, licensure) to protect its interest in the public good (minimum safe practice).

A consideration of the legal aspects of practice must begin with the understanding that different professions ask different questions and use different theories and rules of proof to reach conclusions. Nurses use the nursing process to guide their questions and arrive at diagnoses and plans for treatment of human responses to health and illness. The authority to use the nursing process in the nursing care and treatment of individuals is the social mandate (license) given to professional nursing. The mandate given by society to lawyers is that of peacemaking—the prevention or resolution of conflicting demands of individuals or institutions.[1] Lawyers accomplish this through the legal process. The legal process begins with the written law, considers the established facts, and proceeds to the resolution of particular cases. Laws are established through formal means and codified in writing using the political process described in Chapter 4. Laws are not, however, cast in stone. The rules set down in laws provide only the basis or starting place from which the legal process begins.

■ OVERVIEW OF LAW AND NURSING PRACTICE

Categories of Law

There are four categories of law: constitutional law, statutory law, administrative regulation, and common law (Fig. 3–1). In general, federal law is superior to state law, and state law is superior to local law. In other words, a lower level of government may not create laws that are in conflict with the laws of higher levels of government.

Constitutional Law. The constitution of a state or nation is a system of fundamental laws that establishes the overall structure and powers of government and the rights of the citizenry under that government. The constitution is a single document, generally difficult to change, which carries the ultimate authority for the law of the government it describes. All other laws must be consistent with the **constitutional law** that authorizes them. The US Constitution creates a tripartite system based on a series of checks and balances between the legislative, executive (administrative), and judicial branches of government. Each of these three branches has lawmaking functions. Similar structures exist at the state and local level.

Statutory Law. Statutory law consists of the statutes (laws) enacted by the legislative arm of government at the federal, state, or local level. Statutes are constrained by the particular constitution that authorizes their creation. Nurse practice acts (which provide the authority for the practice of nursing) are written into state statute under the state constitution, because the US Constitution does not mention professional licensure.

Administrative Regulations. Administrative regulations are enacted by the agencies of the executive branch of government to guide the implementation of statutes. Regula-

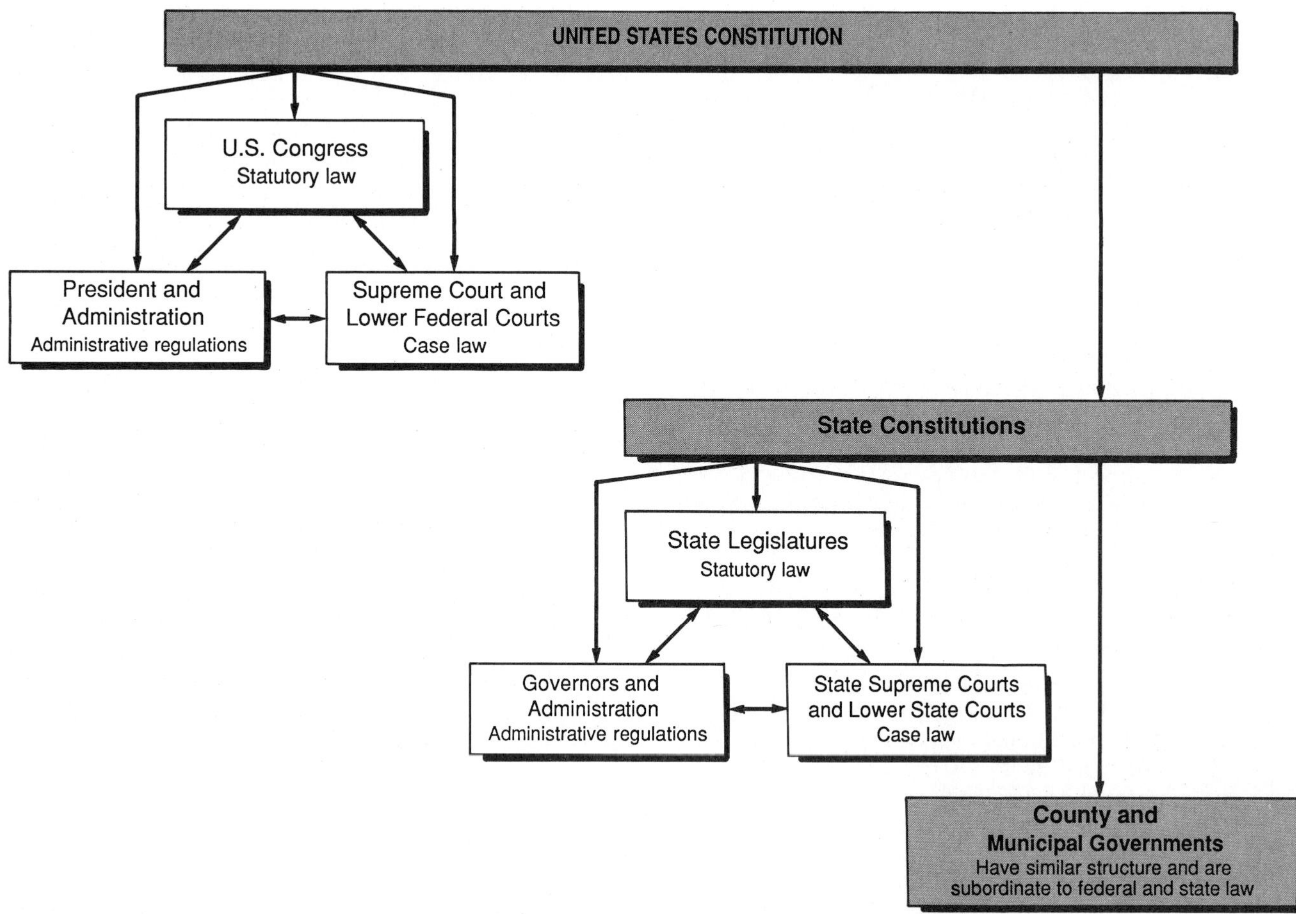

Figure 3–1. Structure of governmental system of laws in the United States.

tions define terms and establish standards. Thus the state board of registered nursing, an administrative agency, is authorized by legislative statute to write regulations to implement the Nurse Practice Act. For example, the curriculum of an approved nursing program in a state is defined in regulation. The board as an agency of the executive branch may not, however, go beyond the powers delegated to it in the statute that created it.

Common Law. **Common law,** sometimes referred to as case law, is the oldest and ultimate form of law. Common law is the body of judicial decisions rendered in specific cases. Common law interprets the constitution and statutes for its particular level of government. Decisions made in particular cases establish the precedent for future interpretation. Judicial decisions are subject to appeal to higher courts (assuming there is some element of the case that is covered under the federal law or constitution or that crosses state lines). On appeal, a higher court may support a lower court decision, may refuse to hear the case because other remedies have not yet been exhausted, may send the case back for retrial because of an error in procedure, or may overturn the decision of the lower court. In the United States, the highest court (the court of last resort) is the Supreme Court.

A Brief History of Licensure

Licensure is a mandatory process through which a government agency grants an individual the right to provide certain services. Professional licensure is a state rather than a federal function. Historically, this stemmed in part from the need to take into account regional resources, cultural norms, and local requirements for practice. The social mandate for practice in one state might differ in significant ways from the mandate in another state in another region. Ultimately licensure is one of the rights reserved to the states because it is not covered by the US Constitution. In recent years, rapid communication and national standards have reduced the importance of regional or community standards of practice. Periodically there is a drive to move licensure to the federal government. Support of federal licensure is based on the perceived value of standardization and recognition of the mobility of the population. The states have so far been successful in resisting this effort.

Licenses vary in the strength of the mandate they provide, which ranges from very weak to almost absolute. An example of a very limited (weak) form of license is a registration act such as those originally covering nursing practice. Registration protects only the right to a title. A list is created by law of qualified practitioners who may "hold out" to be, for example, registered nurses. Registration does not limit the rights of others to engage in the scope of practice—only the right to use a protected title. It is up to clients to make the choice between a registered or nonregistered practitioner. It should be noted that not all registration is based in the law. Registration can also be a function of a professional organization acting in its role of peer review.

Medical practice acts for physicians and surgeons are examples of very strong acts. Strong acts restrict not only the use of a title but the performance of various professional services, such as the delivery of babies or the writing of prescriptions for drugs. Nurse Practice Acts have become much stronger than the early nurse registration acts but are not yet as strong as medical practice acts, for reasons cited below.

Licensing as a device for the protection of the public good has proven to be a double-edged sword. In the recent past, criticisms have been levied at licensing boards, claiming that they served to protect the practitioner rather than the public.[2] Some professions have attempted to use licensing to protect their own livelihood by unnecessary restriction of public choice. When this happens, the public eventually protests, and the law is changed to reduce the rights of the licensees and increase public choice. For example, nurse-midwifery, a long established area of advanced nursing practice, only became legal in California in 1974, long after nurse-midwifery had legal standing in other parts of the country. In this case, the California medical practice act prevented the licensure of nurse midwives, thereby providing the public no other legal alternative in the choice of birthing attendant than a physician. This situation prevailed because of the nature of the definition of the scope of medical practice in the California medical practice act.

Medical practice acts have used a definition of the scope of medical practice that has been all inclusive.[3] Practicing medicine without a license was and is a legally serious offense. The practice of health professions other than medicine was originally legitimized "by exception." Their scopes of practice were all considered to be subsets of medical practice. They were not allowed to practice except in the limited area described in their own practice act. Over time, professions such as dentistry and pharmacy have succeeded in limiting the authority of physicians to practice dentistry and pharmacy, but these restrictions are built into the practice acts of dentistry and pharmacy, not medicine.

The nature of much of nursing practice requires a very close relationship to medicine. When nursing moved to licensure, it took a different approach to defining its practice than did dentistry or pharmacy. Nurse Practice Acts were apt to include language that specifically stated that the statute conferred no authority to practice medicine.[4] Nurse leaders apparently saw this strategy as a means of defining nursing as a discipline separate from medicine without antagonizing medicine. Unfortunately, nurses failed to foresee the significant overlap between the two professions that would develop with advancing technology.

Beginning in the late 1950s, the practice of nursing began to expand significantly into areas that had previously been the exclusive domain of medicine. By 1965, the development of intensive care units made visible the fact that nurses were quite capable of taking on many new responsibilities. Although some nurses had long been doing similar work, it was never seen as the legitimate practice of nursing. From the legal standpoint, the situation was serious because of the manner in which medical and Nurse Practice Acts had been written. Making diagnoses was seen as a function limited to physicians. Nurses were also not entitled by law to make decisions about the administration of emergency drugs. The effective functioning of critical care units required that nurses routinely make diagnostic and drug administration decisions.

By the early 1970s, the strain between the legal definitions and the realities of actual nursing practice reached the point of legal crisis. For the third time, it became necessary to modify Nurse Practice Acts. Major changes were required to make the everyday practice of nursing legal. Conviction of "aiding and abetting the illegal practice of medicine" carries penalties as serious as actually practicing illegally. In order to protect its own licensees the medical profession found it necessary to assist in broadening the definition of the scope of nursing practice. Medicine worked very hard, however, to maintain restrictions on the diagnosis of disease, the prescription of drugs, and the reimbursement for services to physicians. Nurses struggled to redefine nursing practice in such a way as to allow for the continuing changes in the delivery of health care. At the same time it was essential for nurses to maintain a definition of scope of practice that clearly delineated the special domain of nursing. This definition included nursing diagnoses and independent nursing practice.[5]

A fourth phase of nurse licensure began in the 1980s. The courts recognized that nursing practice could legally compete with medical practice in areas where there was overlap in the two scopes of practice. These court decisions brought into play regulations of the Federal Trade Commission, which is charged with protecting the practice rights of one group (eg, nurses) from being interfered with by another group (eg, physicians).[6] This issue is discussed in greater detail in a later section of this chapter, *Other Local, State, and Federal Laws Affecting Nursing Practice.*

NURSE PRACTICE ACTS

A **Nurse Practice Act** includes a definition of nursing, the requirements for licensure (initial and renewal), exceptions to the practice act, options that apply in special circumstances, actions or conditions that can cause the loss or limitation of a license, and the administrative structure that implements and administers the practice act.

As we have seen, a practice act for nursing or any other profession changes over time to meet the needs of society and/or the profession it regulates. Licensed practitioners are held accountable for keeping abreast of the proposed changes in their practice acts, and may participate in deciding what changes are made. This can best be done through the professional organization (eg, the state nurses' association). Changes in law or regulation involve application of the political process, which will be discussed further in Chapter 4.

The laws that regulate nursing practice are unique for each state. Each law reflects the legal and social history of its own particular government. All nursing practice may be covered in one practice act, or there may be a separate section of the law and a second board to oversee "practical" or "vocational" nursing as opposed to "professional" nursing. In some states certain areas of advanced practice such as nurse-midwifery, school nursing, or nurse anesthesiology are also regulated by other sections of the law and administered under agencies other than the board of registered nursing.

It is the responsibility of each nurse to become familiar with the practice acts of the state in which he or she is licensed (Box 3–1). This is particularly important as the profession moves to academically based post-high-school education for all licensed nurses. Professional nurses, who are ultimately responsible for all nursing practice, must concern themselves with the requirements for knowledge and skills for all categories of nursing practice. Because the general concerns of the nursing profession are common across state boundaries, it is possible to discuss the elements generally found in Nurse Practice Acts across the United States (Fig. 3–2).

Definition of Nursing

Nightingale, in *Notes on Nursing*,[7] advised women caring for their ill at home that it was the function of the nurse to "put the patient in the best condition for nature to cure him." The classic post-Nightingale definition of nursing was written by Henderson in her nursing fundamentals

BOX 3–1. GUIDELINES FOR PROFESSIONAL NURSING PRACTICE: NURSE PRACTICE ACTS

1. Obtain a current copy of your Nurse Practice Act. This may easily be done by writing or contacting the state board of nursing or by contacting the local or state office of the state nurses' association. Additionally, copies may also be available at a bookstore specializing in medical and nursing literature or at the local medical library.
2. Read the act carefully for the following elements, ensuring that you understand what each element means to you as a professional nurse.
   a. Definition of professional nursing
   b. Requirements for licensure
   c. Exemptions
   d. Grounds for disciplinary actions
   e. Criteria for out-of-state licensure
   f. Creation of the state board of nursing
   g. Penalties for practicing without a license
3. Know the state board of nursing rules and regulations regarding professional standards of care and dishonorable conduct. As you read the rules and regulations, know what each enumerated rule and regulation means, and apply each to your individual nursing practice.
4. Know who to contact and what to do if the Nurse Practice Act is violated by licensed or unlicensed practitioners. Remember, you have an obligation to uphold the state Nurse Practice Act and to see that others likewise uphold the act.

Source: *Guido G.* Legal Issues in Nursing: A Source Book for Practice. *E. Norwalk, CT: Appleton & Lange; 1988:139.*

New York Education Law, Article 139		California Business and Professions Code, Chapter 6, Article 2
	1	The Legislature recognizes that nursing is a dynamic field, the practice of which is continually evolving to include more sophisticated patient care activities. It is the intent . . . to provide clear legal authority for functions and procedures which have common acceptance and usage, . . . also to recognise the existence of overlapping functions between physicians and registered nurses and to permit additional sharing of functions within organized health care, systems which provide for collaboration between physicians and registered nurses. . . .
The practice of the profession of nursing as a registered professional nurse is defined as diagnosing and treating human responses to actual or potential health problems through such services as casefinding, health teaching, health counseling, and provision of care supportive to or restorative of life and well-being, and executing medical regimens prescribed by a licensed or otherwise legally authorized physician or dentist. A nursing regimen shall be consistent with and shall not vary any existing medical regimen. (From Section 6902.)	2	The practice of nursing within the meaning of this chapter means those functions, including basic health care, which help people cope with difficulties in daily living, which are associated with their actual or potential health or illness problems or the treatment thereof, which require a substantial amount of scientific knowledge or technical skill and includes all of the following:
As used in Section 6902: 1. "Diagnosing" in the context of nursing practice means the identification and discrimination between physical and psychological signs and symptoms essential to effective execution and management of the nursing regimen. Such diagnostic privilege is distinct from a medical diagnosis. 2. "Treating" means selection and performance of those therapeutic measures essential to the effective execution and management of the nursing regimen, and execution of any prescribed medical regimen. 3. "Human Responses" means those signs, symptoms and processes which denote the individual's interaction with and actual or potential health problem. (Section 6901.)	3	(a) Direct and indirect patient care services that insure the safety, comfort, personal hygiene, and protection of patients; and the performance of disease prevention and restorative measures. (b) Direct and indirect care services, including but not limited to, the administration of medications and therapeutic agents, necessary to implement a treatment, disease prevention, or rehabilitative regimen ordered by and within the scope of licensure of a physician, dentist, podiatrist, or clinical psychologist, as defined in Section 1316.5 of the Health and Safety Code. (c) The performance of skin tests, immunization techniques, and the withdrawal of human blood from veins and arteries. (d) Observation of signs and symptoms of illness, reactions to treatment, general behavior, or general physical condition, and (1) determination of whether such signs, symptoms, reactions, behavior, or general appearance exhibit abnormal characteristics; and (2) implementation, based on observed abnormalities, of appropriate reporting, or referral, or standardized procedures, or changes in treatment regimen according to standardized procedures, or the initiation of emergency procedures. (From Section 2725.)
Special provision 2. Nothing in this article shall be construed to confer the authority to practice medicine or dentistry. (From Section 6909.)	4	Except as otherwise provided herein, this chapter confers no authority to practice medicine or surgery. (Section 2726.)

Figure 3–2. Comparison of definitions of nursing, California and New York Nurse Practice Acts. (*California Business and Professions Code, Chapter 6, Article 2; and New York Education Law, Article 139, Sections 6902 and 6901.*)

text. This definition was accepted by the International Congress of Nursing in 1960.

> The unique function of the nurse is to assist the individual, sick or well, in the performance of those activities contributing to health or its recovery (or to a peaceful death) that he would perform unaided if he had the necessary strength, will or knowledge. And to do this in such a way as to help him gain independence as rapidly as possible.[8]

Some states have had a fairly elaborate definition of nursing in their practice acts. Other states traditionally had no definition in the law, concerning themselves not with the scope but the qualifications for practicing nursing. In 1980, following several years of dialogue, the American Nurses' Association published *Nursing: A Social Policy Statement* as a guide for the profession in developing appropriate credentialing and qualifications for entry into nursing practice.[9] According to this statement "Nursing is the

IMPLICATIONS FOR NURSE–CLIENT COLLABORATION

Nurse Practice Acts

Nurse Practice Acts contain a definition of nursing and guidelines that indicate the scope of nursing practice. They also identify exceptions to the law and options that apply under special circumstances. Nurse Practice Acts thus create the legal context and set the statutory boundaries for decision-making by nurses. These boundaries limit the type of health care decisions on which nurses and clients may collaborate. Although such limits restrict options available to both nurse and client, they also protect the public good by mandating certain qualifications for actions within the scope of practice.

diagnosis and treatment of human responses to actual or potential health problems." The nurses of many states, beginning with New York in 1972, have incorporated this language directly or paraphrased it in their revised practice acts.

Independent and Dependent Functions

A particularly troublesome component of most Nurse Practice Acts is the matter of specifying independent and dependent functions. Some nursing activities are initiated and performed by nurses independently; hence the term **independent functions.** Other activities require that someone else, typically a physician, write an order for the activity that a nurse then carries out. Following orders is considered a **dependent function.** Knowing what is independent and what is dependent and under what circumstances is critical to legal practice.

For example, in an emergency nurses may, under some practice acts, initiate activities that would be illegal at other times. (See discussion of "Good Samaritan laws" in *Requirements for Licensure* later in this chapter.) It is important to remember that such exceptions are limited. The emergency must be unexpected and unpredictable, involve a threat to life or function, and not be for compensation. An emergency room nurse on duty is not covered by such an exception. Even in an emergency, licensed persons are held responsible for not exceeding their knowledge and skills.[10]

Increasingly, the performance of "dependent" activities may be done under protocol. A **protocol** is a written guideline for what to do in a given situation. Protocols are modern descendants of standing orders. They differ in that standing orders were written by physicians. Protocols represent the joint efforts of nurses, physicians, and sometimes health care administrators, who collaborate to specify the appropriate nursing responses to problem situations. A protocol typically defines who is qualified by education or experience to carry out the activity described as well as under what conditions and in what settings the activity may take place. Also included are the nature and content of decision-making, reporting, and documentation, and conditions under which there should be immediate consultation or referral to an identified individual with superior expertise.

It must be emphasized that merely because the law entitles a nurse to do something does not mean that all nurses should do it. Nurses are responsible for knowing their limitations. If a nurse lacks knowledge or skill to perform an activity, it is ultimately that nurse's responsibility not to attempt the activity without competent supervision or assistance. This is true not only for students but for licensed nurses as well.

Relationship to Other Practice Acts

In some Nurse Practice Acts there is reference to other licensed professions, usually by name and sometimes by reference to specific sections of the legal code. These references typically define the authority relationship between nursing and the other professions. Such a section might direct nurses to carry out the orders of a physician or dentist. Or it might indicate that nurses are responsible for the actions of others such as licensed practical nurses who must practice under the supervision of a professional nurse.

Limitations

Limitations on the practice of nursing may be found in the Nurse Practice Act itself or in the practice acts of other professions. For example, the pharmacy practice act may prohibit a physician from delegating certain activities relating to the packaging and labeling of drugs to nurses or other nonphysicians.

A different kind of "limitation" is a listing of those activities that constitute negligent or unprofessional conduct on the part of a nurse. Examples are discussed later in this chapter. Such activities will certainly lead to discipline and may lead to the loss of a nurse's license to practice. A malpractice suit against the nurse is also a strong possibility. In general, the laws regarding negligence and unprofessional conduct are becoming more specific so that there can be no doubt in the mind of nurses as to what activities are prohibited.

Advanced Practice of Nursing

The rapidly increasing knowledge base for nursing practice has led to the formalization of areas of advanced practice in nursing. Nurse-midwives and nurse anesthetists were engaged in advanced practice early on, as were public health nurses. Although public health nurses have always been considered part of the nursing profession, nurse-midwives and nurse anesthetists, at least in some parts of the United States, were at one time considered outside the mainstream of nursing and outside the nursing practice act. The development of the nursing role in critical care units and ambulatory care clinics, the increase in clinical specialization, and the nurse practitioner movement have facilitated the recognition of nurse-midwives and nurse anesthetists as advanced-level nurses. Whether advanced practitioners should be recognized solely by professional certification or whether they should also carry specific licensure requirements under statute is a matter of continuing debate. Professional certification (ie, credentialing), carried out by professional nursing organizations is not in itself a legal process, although the criteria for such certification are sometimes incorporated into law (Fig. 3–3).

Professional certification for physicians is adequate to define "advanced practice" because, unlike nursing, medical licensure already encompasses the right to practice any branch of medicine regardless of the expertise of the practitioner. The limitations on advanced medical practice are primarily from peer pressure. Although some laws for institutional licensure, some accreditation standards, and some requirements of insurance companies specify certification for advanced practice in medicine, the medical practice acts have not yet made this distinction. Nurses engaged in collaborative practice arrangements with physicians need to keep this distinction in mind.

Increasingly, categories of advanced nursing practice are receiving legal recognition in Nurse Practice Acts because of problems arising out of the overlap between nursing and medical practice. Nurses have needed legal sanc-

IMPLICATIONS FOR PROFESSIONAL COLLABORATION

Advanced Nursing Practice

Growth of advanced nursing practice in the many specialty areas of health care has produced a new form of practice for nurses called collaborative practice. The term "collaborative practice" as it is used in reference to advanced nursing practice refers not only to the way nurses interact with clients and other professionals, but also to the scope of functions nurses in advanced practice perform. In a collaborative practice, nurses practice together with physicians and carry out many of the functions ordinarily restricted by medical practice acts to physicians alone, such as diagnosing and treating routine illnesses. Nurses who are educated and certified for the advanced role are supervised by physicians, who retain legal responsibility for nurses' actions. The decisions made by a nurse in collaborative practice are guided by a series of protocols and by consultations with a physician.

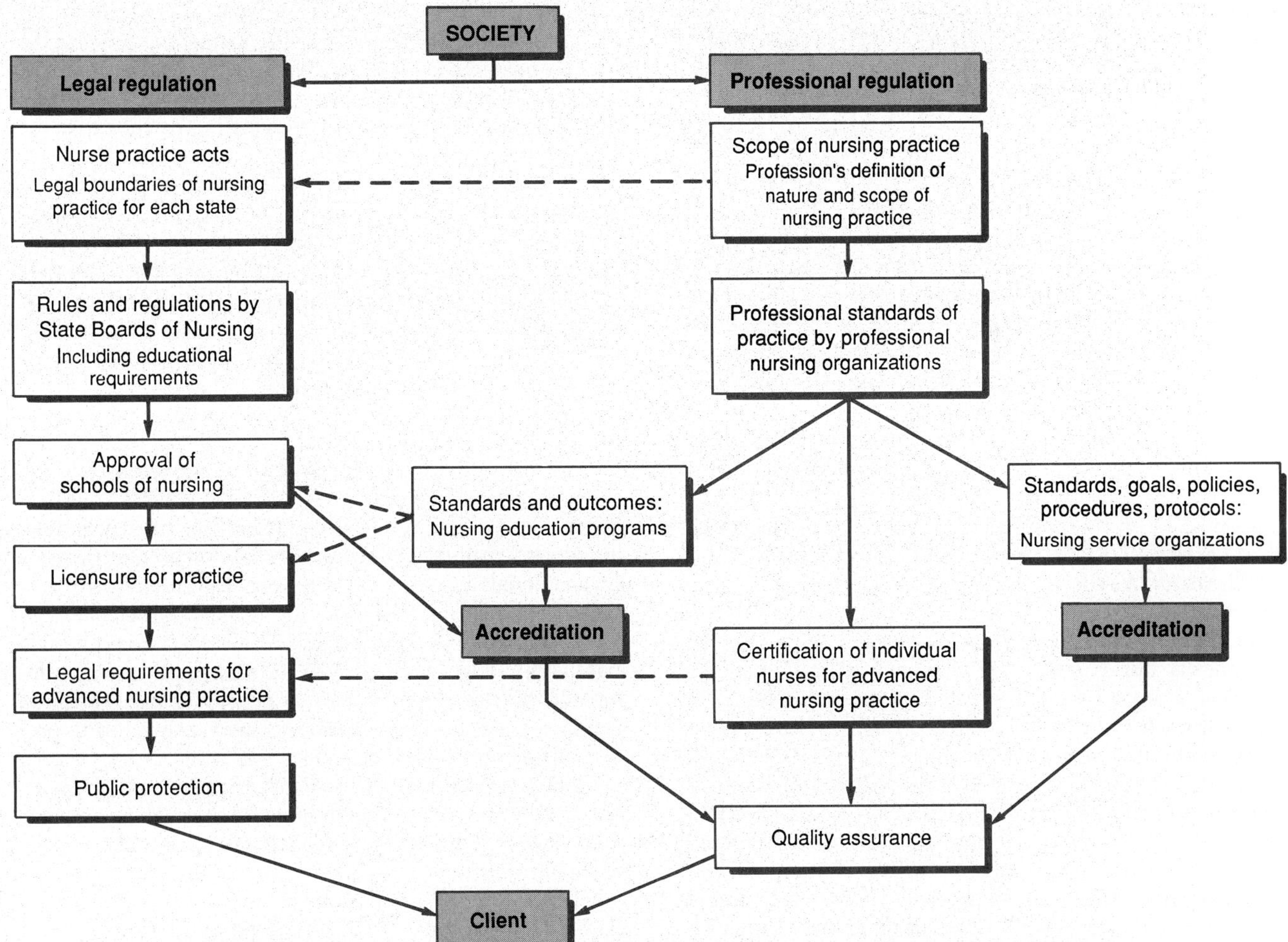

Figure 3–3. Professional and legal credentialing of nursing practice. (*Adapted from American Nurses' Association,* Scope of Nursing Practice. *Kansas City, MO: ANA, 1987.*)

tions to protect their right to engage in advanced nursing practice because of the principle of "exception" described earlier, which is inherent in many Nurse Practice Acts. Nurse Practice Acts that describe their authority as an exception to the medical practice act must add new exceptions as they broaden the scope of nursing practice. Not surprisingly, some physicians see new exceptions as an invasion of territory and vigorously oppose changes in the law. Nursing cannot, therefore, rely on professional certification in the same fashion as medicine.

Administration

Included within each Nurse Practice Act are the mechanisms for enforcing it. The number and qualifications of members of the board of nursing, who appoints them, and their term of office will be found here. The authority of the board to examine, license, and discipline practitioners is defined, as is the authority to regulate schools that prepare nurses.

The administrative section of the practice act also describes the process for creating regulations. The regulations that implement the Nurse Practice Act include such things as definitions of words found in the statute. Guidelines for determining what constitutes illegal practice, directions for applying for a license, and rules for curricula and faculty qualifications for schools of nursing may also be found here if they are not in the statute itself.

Rules requiring meeting in public (**"sunshine laws"**) may be here or elsewhere in the statutes of the state. Sunshine laws are so called because they prohibit secret ("in-the-dark") meetings for the conduct of public business.

In recent years, state legislatures concerned with the rapid proliferation of licensing boards and categories of licensure have written **"sunset laws."** These laws require licensing boards to justify their existence at regular intervals. Failure to do so results in the board's termination. Although the threat is real, there is no evidence that this strategy has actually succeeded in permanently eliminating any boards.[11]

■ REQUIREMENTS FOR LICENSURE AND RENEWAL

Basic Nursing Education

Historically, the curriculum for nursing education in the United States was defined in terms based on the needs of the hospital where the education generally took place and the availability and time commitments of physician "faculty." In 1923, the so-called Goldmark Report[12] revealed that nursing education in the United States was nearly as disorganized and lacking in standards as the medical education of the time. The report led to the development of national guidelines for nursing curriculum content written in terms of specific clinical topics to be covered over a 3-year training period. These guidelines persisted until the next major revolution in nursing education in the late 1940s.

Medicine had been able to use the earlier Flexner Report[13] as a springboard for placing medical education in the mainstream of university education. Nursing was not so fortunate, possibly because university education for women was a low priority of society at that time. Nursing had to wait until World War II, with the resulting nursing shortage and the infusion of federal funds, for the necessary resources and support. Standards for nursing educational facilities and faculty qualifications were developed as criteria for federal funding. The new standards then provided the basis for a system of national accreditation of schools of nursing. The newly organized National League for Nursing (NLN) became the accrediting body.[14] (**Accreditation** is a system for review and approval of institutions that meet professional standards. Nurses use NLN accreditation standards as a basis for lobbying for the required content of nursing education programs at the state level.)

By 1950 a number of diploma programs in the country had begun to affiliate with baccalaureate-degree-granting institutions to meet student demands for academically based education. The baccalaureate programs of the day were often 5 years in length (2 years of general education followed by 3 years of nursing). In the early 1950s, state laws that had previously required 3 years of education and training prior to licensure began to change to allow for the new Associate Degree in Nursing (ADN) programs. The 3-year requirement was replaced with one stating "not less than 2 academic years" or the equivalent. The change in the law meant that students could chose between a 2-, 3-, or 5-year program to prepare for licensure as a registered nurse. It is safe to say that no other change in nursing education has created such prolonged dissension in the nursing profession. By 1987 nearly 55 percent of all new graduates of registered nursing programs were prepared in associate-degree-granting programs. More than one third were prepared in baccalaureate degree programs which by that time were generally 4 years in length.[15]

It was not until 1985 that the two major nursing organizations, the American Nurses' Association (ANA) and the NLN, could adopt a position on what to do with the 2-year category of nursing education. In 1985, the ANA decided that the ADN nurse would be titled associate nurse, a separate title from the baccalaureate-prepared (professional) nurse. How this would be implemented in nursing licensure laws was left to the individual states. In 1987, the ANA House of Delegates decided that both associate (AN) and registered (RN) nurses would be full members of the state nurses' associations. The ANA House of Delegates also adopted a statement that technical and professional practice are differentiated not by scope but by role, by knowledge base, and by client population within a practice environment.[16,17] The NLN position in support of two categories of nursing continued under attack until, in 1987, the issue was tabled.

National Council Licensure Examination

Although licensure is a state function, all US nurses currently take the same national licensing examination after completing the required educational program. This examination, developed by the National Council of State Boards of Nursing, is the National Council Licensure Examination (NCLEX). Each state administers the test to its own applicants and establishes its own passing score and other requirements for licensure. States depend on the schools of nursing to certify psychomotor skills. The national examination is paper and pencil, multiple choice, and takes 2 days under conditions of high security.

Reciprocity Between States

Because the licensing examination is nationwide, it is not difficult for registered nurses in good standing to obtain licensure by reciprocity in states other than where they were first licensed. **Reciprocity** exists where two licensing agencies (in this instance states) have mutually agreed to recognize and accept the licenses granted by the other. In general, a nurse's educational program and score on the national examination must meet the standards of the second state, and the nursing license in his or her home state must be in good standing. The fees required and the method of application are outlined in regulations in each state.

Continuing Education

Professional licensure has traditionally been awarded for life as long as the holder paid the renewal fees and did not commit illegal actions. Recognition of the rapid changes in nursing brought with it concerns about whether or not professionals were "keeping up" with current practice. Mandatory continuing education laws are an attempt by some states to assure that members of a profession are maintaining their professional knowledge in the interests of their clients. These laws vary from state to state and may include requirements for number of hours, required subjects, approval of courses, record-keeping, and so forth.

Exceptions

Certain groups may be exempt from the practice act requirements of a particular state. Practitioners of religions which qualify their own healers may be exempt. Family members and others who are not paid for their nursing services are exempt. Traditionally, federal employees have been exempt from the license requirements of a given state so long as they were licensed in some state. A nurse who enters a state briefly while traveling with a client may be exempt so long as that nurse cares only for the traveling client.

Nursing students are exempt from licensure because they must practice under the direct supervision of their licensed instructors. Nevertheless, professional liability for what the practitioner knows or should have known begins at the student level. Many schools require students to carry their own liability insurance.

The responsibility for knowing one's own limitations is key to all professional practice.[18–21] The principle applies throughout one's professional career. Nurses' (including student nurses') accountability and personal liability increase as their knowledge and skills increase. The state holds instructors responsible for the safe assignment of students. A student who is unsure about performing a certain activity is responsible for consulting the supervising faculty before proceeding. Licensed nurses are not protected from liability by the excuse of "following orders." Faced with an order to engage in an activity outside his or her expertise or legal scope of practice, the nurse's first line of defense is to document in writing the reasons for refusing to carry out the assignment.

Options

Practice acts commonly recognize that there are situations in which normal rules may not prevail in the best interest of nurses or clients. **"Good Samaritan" laws** provide that if a health care professional stops to give aid at an accident scene, that professional is ordinarily immune from being sued. The professional must have acted in good faith and not for compensation. Such laws do not, however, excuse gross negligence or intentional misconduct by the professional. These laws also do not apply to regular emergency personnel.[18]

Another option included in some practice acts recognizes that not all people share the same belief systems. In some states, for example, nurses may file with their employer notice of refusal to participate in the performance of abortions, based on religious convictions regarding the sanctity of life.

There are areas in which the resolution of moral dilemmas have not yet been codified into law. The withholding or withdrawing of nutrition and hydration is an area still going through the courts. Where state laws have not provided direction, institutional ethics committees are an important resource to concerned health professionals in clarifying the issues to be considered.

■ LOSS OF LICENSE OR LIMITATION OF SCOPE OF PRACTICE

A license to practice carries responsibilities as well as rights and privileges. Society expects licensed professionals to monitor the quality and safety of their own practice and the practice of their peers. Suspicion of unethical, illegal, and unsafe practice, or failure to report such practice, is cause for investigation. Taking away or limiting the right to practice a profession is a serious matter, because it interferes with the ability of an individual to earn a living in that profession. The licensing board must follow due process, protecting the rights of both clients (the public) and licensees. The actual language describing grounds for discipline varies from state to state (Table 3–1).[18] The role of professional peers in this process is discussed under the section on expert witnesses later in this chapter.

Negligence and Incompetence

The exact definitions of negligence and incompetence vary from state to state. In principle, **negligence** is a crime of *omission*. A negligent nurse has failed to do something that should have been done for a client—that is, has not maintained basic standards of care. Deferring repositioning of a

TABLE 3–1. GROUNDS FOR DISCIPLINARY ACTION AGAINST NURSES CITED IN ONE OR MORE OF 53 US LEGAL JURISDICTIONS

Grounds for Disciplinary Action	Number of States
Fraud and Deceit	
Fraud or deceit in securing or attempting to secure a license	51
Fraud or deceit relating to professional services	13
Impersonation of a nurse (RN or LPN)	10
Conduct likely to deceive, defraud, or harm the public	9
Falsification of patient records	8
Criminal Activity	
Conviction or being found guilty of a felony	33
Being found guilty of moral turpitude or gross immorality	22
Conviction or being found guilty of a crime	16
Drug or Alcohol Use	
Habitual intemperateness due to use or abuse of alcohol	30
Addiction to habit-forming drugs	30
Use of alcohol or drugs resulting in unsafe practice	20
Sale or distribution of controlled substances	5
Conviction or violation of federal or state controlled-substances law	5
Illegal use of controlled substances	4
Negligence, Risk to Client, and Impaired Physical or Mental Ability	
Physical or mental illness interfering with nursing	24
Negligence	12
Gross negligence	9
Conduct resulting in risk to client or to public health	4
Immoral conduct	2
Violation of the Nurse Practice Act or Rules	
Violation of provisions of the nursing practice act	45
Revocation or suspension of license in another jurisdiction	27
Violation of rules related to nursing practice act	24
Permitting another person to use license	10
Exceeding scope of practice	8
Incompetence	
Incompetence	23
Being unfit or incompetent due to negligence, habits, or other causes	22
Mental incompetence	17
Failure to meet standards of practice	11
Unethical Practice	
Unethical practice	7
False or deceptive advertising	6
Violation of confidentiality	3
Fraud in attempting to obtain reimbursement	2
Other	2

Source: *Adapted from Clara La Bar.* Enforcement of the Nursing Practice Act. *Kansas City, MO: American Nurses' Association;* 1986.

BUILDING NURSING KNOWLEDGE

Can Laws Aid in Nurse Practice Act Enforcement?

Luckenbill-Brett L, Stuhler-Schlag K. Mandatory reporting: Legal and ethical issues. *J. Nurs Admin.* 1987; 17: 32–38.

Although professional practice acts are meant to protect the public from unsafe practitioners, voluntary professional self-policing has not proved a sufficient means of regulating conduct. This article suggests that mandatory reporting laws may help remedy the problem. Mandatory reporting of Nurse Practice Act violations requires that nurses by law must inform the regulatory board when they observe violations by other nurses. The idea behind mandatory reporting is that the withholding of information about violations is as inappropriate as the violation itself. In order to satisfy the requirements of mandatory reporting, nurses need access to information regarding the laws that govern their practice. Mandatory reporting laws have not yet been established in every state, but have proved beneficial because they clearly outline the legal responsibilities of the nurse in relation to reporting the violations of other nurses. The most commonly reported violations are associated with substance abuse. The authors also review the ethics of mandatory reporting and examine the problems and consequences of whistle-blowing.

paralyzed client, neglecting to use siderails, or overlooking frequent reassessment of a client whose clinical condition is changing, would constitute negligence. It is also considered negligent to fail to report substandard care by others.

Incompetence is a crime of *commission.* The incompetent nurse has committed an error that has harmed or could have harmed a client. Giving the wrong medication, changing surgical dressings without sterile gloves, or preparing the wrong client for surgery are examples of acts that may be considered incompetent.

The deciding factor in finding negligence or incompetence is the standard of practice of "a reasonable, prudent registered nurse" who, by definition, is expected to know the limits of his or her professional knowledge and skill.

Negligence and incompetence can be the bases for malpractice suits or even criminal charges against nurses. These topics are discussed further in the section on civil and criminal law.

False Representation, Fraud, and Deceit

A licensed professional may not pretend or assist someone else to pretend to be what he or she is not professionally. Someone who takes a licensing examination in place of another person is guilty of false representation. Someone who attempts to practice under the license of another or allows his or her own nursing license to be used by someone else is also guilty of false representation. Falsifying client records, while not specifically mentioned in all Nurse Practice Acts, is of major importance in legal actions. In all cases, the care of the client is endangered by false, inaccurate, or incomplete records.

Substance Abuse

Nurses and other health professionals are particularly vulnerable to substance abuse. Easy access to restricted drugs provides a ready opportunity for abuse. The excessive use of drugs such as alcohol, stimulants, antidepressants, and narcotics will seriously degrade the safe performance of a health care professional. Substance abuse by a nurse is a betrayal of the trust of clients and is cause for legal penalty up to and including loss of the license to practice. Beginning in the early 1980s, the American Nurses' Association publicly recognized the scope of the problem and encouraged the development of rehabilitation programs for nurses who have become substance abusers. Impaired nurse programs have been instituted by several state boards of nursing.[18,22] Similar programs have been developed in other health professions. Such programs both support professionals who need help and protect clients who would otherwise be endangered by unsafe practice. Knowing that there is help available also encourages others to carry out their own professional responsibility to report impaired colleagues to the proper authorities.

Other Criminal Behavior

In general, a crime must be substantially related to the practice of the profession before conviction will lead to loss or suspension of the license to practice. Examples of other criminal behavior for which nurses are held particularly accountable include physical (including sexual) abuse of clients, failure to maintain proper records, misrepresentation on an application for a license, failure to report abuse by others, practicing medicine without a license, and procuring or aiding in an illegal abortion.

As a rule of thumb, actions that endanger the license of nurses are also not in the best interests of clients. It is possible, although rare, for nurses to find that employment in a particular setting will require them to engage in behavior that they believe to be unsafe or criminal. An example might be a hospital where elective surgeries are scheduled even when it is known ahead of time that there will not be enough nurses available to provide safe postoperative care. Nurses may even be told that without their continued participation the clients will be abandoned. Condoning such a situation by continuing to practice in it is not in the best interests of either nurses or clients. Nurses also have an ethical or moral obligation to report such situations to the proper authorities. Depending on the situation, the proper authority might be a licensing board or an agency responsible for monitoring a particular kind of facility (eg, a department of health).

There are instances where it might appear that the interests of the state and a client are in conflict. The right to privacy of a client with an infectious disease, for example, might be in conflict with the concern of the state to protect the public and prevent the spread of disease. Such conflicts are likely to have ethical as well as legal implications. In such instances, it is important to seek the counsel of more knowledgeable persons such as faculty, nursing supervisors, and the hospital ethics committee. The ANA *Code for*

Nurses[23] (see Chap. 34) also provides guidance. In addition, the NLN, the American Hospital Association, and some state legislatures have adopted *Patients' Bills of Rights* (Fig. 3–4) that spell out the rights of clients in receiving care. Many hospitals and other institutions have adopted their own versions of these bills of rights as institutional policy. Laws relating to client rights are discussed in more detail later in this chapter.

CIVIL AND CRIMINAL LAW

Torts, Misdemeanors, and Felonies

When a wrong has been committed, action may be taken under civil law, criminal law, or both. **Civil law** protects the rights belonging to an inhabitant of a state or country by virtue of being a citizen. Rights of property, marriage, protection under the law, trial by jury, and freedom of contract are examples of civil rights. A violation of a civil right is a **tort** and the perpetrator is a tort-feasor. An **intentional tort** exists when there is provable intent to harm. An **unintentional tort** is one in which harm occurred, but there is evidence that the harm was unintentional. Table 3–2, provides examples of torts related to nursing. Civil law is concerned with providing redress to the wronged person. A civil suit is instituted by one private individual against another. Box 3–2 describes guidelines for avoiding negligent torts related to nursing practice.

Criminal law, on the other hand, is concerned with punishing the perpetrator of a crime. In a criminal suit, the party seeking relief is the government entity whose laws are alleged to have been violated. Under criminal law, a wrong may be classified as a misdemeanor or a felony. **Misdemeanors** are less serious than felonies and are usually punished by fines or imprisonment in a jail. A **felony** is a more serious crime and is punishable by imprisonment in a penitentiary or by execution. What constitutes a felony and what is a misdemeanor is determined by law.[24] Most unprofessional conduct is defined as a misdemeanor.

Legal Action in Civil and Criminal Offenses

Legal action against a licensee for committing negligence or unprofessional conduct is brought by the local or state authorities. Conviction in court is considered presumption of guilt. The state licensing board then suspends the license or

1. The patient has a right to considerate and respectful care.
2. The patient has a right to obtain from his physician complete current information concerning his diagnosis, treatment, and prognosis in terms the patient can be reasonably expected to understand. When it is not medically advisable to give such information to the patient, the information should be made available to an appropriate person in his behalf. He has the right to know, by name, the physician responsible for coordinating his care.
3. The patient has the right to receive from his physician information necessary to give informed consent prior to the start of any procedure and/or treatment. Except in emergencies, such information for informed consent should include but not necessarily be limited to the specific procedure and/or treatment, the medically significant risks involved, and the probable duration of incapacitation. Where medically significant alternatives for care or treatment exist, or when the patient requests information concerning medical alternatives, the patient has the right to such information. The patient also has the right to know the name of the person responsible for the procedures and/or treatment.
4. The patient has the right to refuse treatment to the extent permitted by law and to be informed of the medical consequences of his action.
5. The patient has the right to every consideration of his privacy concerning his own medical care program. Case discussion, consultation, examination, and treatment are confidential and should be conducted discreetly. Those not directly involved in his care must have the permission of the patient to be present.
6. The patient has the right to expect that all communications and records pertaining to his care should be treated as confidential.
7. The patient has the right to expect that within its capacity a hospital must make reasonable response to the request of a patient for services. The hospital must provide evaluation, service and/or referral as indicated by the urgency of the case. When medically permissible, a patient may be transferred to another facility after he has received complete information and explanation concerning the needs for and alternatives to such a transfer. The institution to which the patient is to be transferred must first have accepted the patient for transfer.
8. The patient has the right to obtain information as to any relationship of his hospital to other health care and educational institutions insofar as his care is concerned. The patient has the right to obtain information as to the existence of any professional relationships among individuals, by name, who are treating him.
9. The patient has the right to be advised if the hospital proposes to engage in or perform human experimentation affecting his care or treatment. The patient has the right to refuse to participate in such research projects.
10. The patient has the right to expect reasonable continuity of care. He has the right to know in advance what appointment times and physicians are available and where. The patient has the right to expect that the hospital will provide a mechanism whereby he is informed by his physician or a delegate of the physician of the patient's continuing health care requirements following discharge.
11. The patient has the right to examine and receive an explanation of his bill, regardless of source of payment.
12. The patient has a right to know what hospital rules and regulations apply to his conduct as a patient.

Figure 3–4. Patient's bill of rights. (*Reprinted with permission of the American Hospital Association, copyright 1972.*)

TABLE 3–2. VIOLATION OF CIVIL RIGHTS (TORTS) RELATED TO NURSING PRACTICE

Tort	Sample Description of Offense
Fraud	Misrepresentation of credentials, falsification of a client's records
Invasion of privacy	Sharing confidential information, refusing to allow use of personal clothing when it would not interfere with procedures, demonstrating a procedure on a client without permission
Slander (Defamation of character)	Making a false verbal statement about a client having a socially unacceptable disease (eg, AIDS) to another health professional
Libel (Defamation of character)	Making a false statement about a client in writing or making such a statement to mass media (press, television)
Assault	Threatening or appearing to threaten to provide treatment without consent
Battery	Treating a client without consent
False imprisonment	Restraining a client inappropriately, detaining a client in a treatment facility against his or her will
Negligence	Negligence is the tort—but with licensed providers it is often called malpractice
Malpractice (Negligence)	Failure to maintain expected standards of care[a].

[a] See "Loss of License or Limitation of Scope of Practice" earlier in this chapter, and "Malpractice Suits" later in this chapter.

places the convicted person on probation. Terms and conditions are attached that must be met if the license is to be restored or retained. Where there has been a flagrant violation of safe practice or a pattern of bad outcomes, the licensing board may suspend the license to practice pending legal proof of guilt or innocence. Examples of behavior leading to disciplinary action against nurses are given in Table 3–1.

In the past, action by a licensing board against a licensee relative to a criminal offense was sometimes delayed until after a client had sued the licensee for damages in civil court. The defending licensee in such a situation was left free to continue to practice while the civil trial went through the courts. The effect was to protect the civil rights of the licensee at the risk of serious harm to the public. Recently there has been a trend toward immediate suspension of practice privileges where there is potential for public harm.

It is important to remember that even good practitioners get sued by unhappy clients. Clients who have been treated respectfully and with concern are less likely to sue even a negligent professional. A client who is kept informed and whose questions and preferences are solicited is a partner rather than a receiver of care.

BOX 3–2. GUIDELINES FOR AVOIDING NEGLIGENT TORTS

1. Treat clients and their families with respect and honesty. Communicate in a truthful, open, and professional manner.
2. Respect clients' rights to education about their illness. Collaborate with other health team members to assure that clients and their families are taught what they desire to know about their health problems, planned therapy, and possible complications related to therapy.
3. Make nursing diagnoses on all clients and implement appropriate care. Nurses have an affirmative duty not only to make diagnoses, but to take action to alleviate the conditions diagnosed. Document the diagnoses and the anticipated nursing implementation by recording them on the client care plan form provided by the health care facility.
4. Clearly, completely, and concisely document all nursing care and clients' responses to care. Make chart entries as soon as possible after care while facts and observations are clearest in your mind.
5. Delegate client care with discretion. Know the scope of practice for those whom you supervise. Never allow others to accept more responsibility than their ability or the law allow.
6. Remember that you are accountable for all medical orders that you carry out, whether or not they are appropriate. Question all orders that are ambiguous or unclear. When taking telephone orders, repeat the transcribed order before hanging up to verify accuracy or clarify ambiguities. Do not carry out orders that are outdated or that may be inappropriate because of a change in a client's condition. If a physician is unresponsive to a change in a client's condition or unwilling to order therapy you consider critical, contact your supervisor. Notify the physician of any orders refused by a client.
7. Adhere to your facility's policies and procedures and insist that personnel whom you supervise do the same. Help to revise any policies that are outdated.
8. Know the scope of nursing practice in the state in which you practice and adhere to its mandates and limits of practice.
9. Remain current and up to date in your skills and education by taking advantage of continuing education programs and reading professional journals. Do not attempt to perform a procedure with which you are unfamiliar.
10. Keep your malpractice insurance current. Although this will not prevent negligent torts, it will help you should you be named in a malpractice lawsuit.

Source: *Adapted from Guido G.* Legal Issues in Nursing: A Source Book for Practice. *E. Norwalk, CT: Appleton & Lange; 1988: 47–48.*

Evidence

Both civil and criminal law depend on evidence. Evidence in health care cases is often in the form of documents that describe such things as the care given, condition of a client, sequence of events, persons present, and who was notified and when. Nurses carry a major responsibility for the quality of health care records. Accurate, succinct, complete records protect both client and health care provider. Where harm is not claimed until some future time, the usual records are the only evidence of what occurred. When an untoward event is recognized at the time of its occurrence, it is essential that an incident report be filed to give the most accurate picture of what occurred while memories are fresh. Undocumented memories of past events are a poor substitute for good charting. Records such as charts are legal documents and may not be erased without legal penalty. There are specific rules for handling errors in charting, which must be followed if the chart is to be a credible legal document. Refer to Chapter 18 for a detailed discussion of charting.

Malpractice Suits

When a client or client's family believes that harm has been caused to them by nurses or other health care providers, they may file a malpractice suit. A **malpractice suit** is an assertion by a client (the plaintiff) that a wrong has been done against him or her by a professional (the defendant). The circumstances under which such a suit may be brought against a health care professional vary from state to state, but in order to prevail in the lawsuit, the plaintiff must demonstrate four things: (1) that the defendant had a legally recognized duty to provide health care to the client; (2) that the duty was breached—that is, that the care was substandard; (3) that damages (physical harm, mental anguish) to the plaintiff resulted; and (4) that the direct cause of the damages was the breach of care by the defendant.

Examples of situations that frequently result in malpractice suits against nurses include medication errors, client falls, burns related to therapeutic application of heat, failure to take appropriate action in response to client's symptoms, and mistaken identity (providing treatment to the wrong person).

The increasing recognition of nurses as professionals brings with it the increasing risk of being sued for malpractice. Defense against such a suit requires the services of a knowledgeable attorney, expert witnesses (see later section), and often considerable expense. It is therefore essential that all nurses realize that malpractice insurance is one of the necessary costs of practice.[25]

■ HISTORICAL AND CURRENT TRENDS IN LIABILITY

In reviewing the history of liability, it is important to remember that the law reflects society. Rules of liability reflect the social order of the time, available technology, expected roles of professionals and clients, and facilities within which most of the interaction between the two take place. The slowly changing organization of society is reflected even more slowly in the law.

Respondeat Superior, Captain of the Ship, Borrowed Servant

Respondeat superior, meaning "let the master answer," also reflects the assumptions inherent in the doctrines of "captain of the ship" and "borrowed servant." Under this approach, it is assumed that the captain or master is responsible for the physical acts of the crew or servant. It is based on the presumed superior moral and technical knowledge of the one over the other. In a hospital setting, the surgeon has been held responsible for the acts of those assisting in the surgery even when they were employees of the hospital rather than of the surgeon. The surgeon was presumed to have "borrowed" them as servants and therefore to be responsible for their acts. Over the years this doctrine has led some physicians and some nurses to believe that nurses should do whatever a physician orders without exercising independent responsibility for the rightness of the order. However, the courts have disagreed, holding that nurses as licensed professionals are personally responsible for the rightness of their acts. This is true regardless of any concurrent responsibility on the part of the physician giving the order.[5] It should also be noted here that registered nurses have a responsibility for the tasks they assign to those they supervise. The supervising RN must always be certain that the person assigned is qualified to perform the work safely. For example, an untrained person changing a sterile dressing would likely contaminate the wound. The resulting infection could cause serious harm to the client.

Charitable Immunity, Corporate Liability

When hospitals were charitable institutions, they were given immunity from being sued. As hospitals depended less and less on charitable donations and more on direct and third-party (insurance) payment for their operating expenses, they lost their protection from liability. The liability of the corporation, already a principle in manufacturing, became important in health care. Hospital trustees found themselves held responsible both for the qualifications of their employees and for the care provided in their hospitals. The means for "punishing" a corporation under criminal law and providing redress for injured parties under civil law (malpractice suits) are still imperfect but, in the United States, progress is being made toward an appropriately balanced system.

Reasonable Prudent Practitioner, Community or Locality Standard, Expert Witness

In the days before modern communication systems, professionals were judged against the prevailing standards in their own community. Under this rule, the reasonable prudent practitioner in a remote rural area would be judged by different standards from a practitioner in a major teaching hospital. **Community** or **locality standards** are standards established within a fixed geographic area. These are now being replaced by regional and national standards because of faster communications, greater standardization of educational programs, and stronger involvement by the nursing community in supporting its membership.

There is still some variation between states regarding standards of care and qualifications for being an expert witness.[18] An **expert witness** possesses specialized knowledge of a profession; his or her testimony is used to establish standards of care against which the actions of an accused licensee can be judged in a court of law. These witnesses should be of the same profession as the accused. Expert witnesses commonly cite the standards of practice promulgated by their national professional organizations. The American Nurses' Association has been a leader in sponsoring the publication of such standards of care for nursing.

Because professional practice is an art as much as it is a science, proving that a practitioner has been negligent or incompetent may be difficult except in extreme cases. For example, there may be a choice between several acceptable treatments and the wisdom of choosing one over the other only becomes clear after the fact. Other members of the same profession may be reluctant to testify on the basis of hindsight. Sometimes the reluctance is a matter of fear of being later sued by the defendant. Sometimes the prospective witness identifies with or feels sorry for the defendant. Rarely, it appears to be a case of misplaced loyalty to the profession as opposed to loyalty to the client. Rising malpractice awards and professional standards review legislation have made it clear to all professionals that the public will find a way to protect itself from incompetence and negligence with or without the assistance of the concerned professions to serve as expert witnesses.

OTHER LOCAL, STATE, AND FEDERAL LAWS AFFECTING NURSING PRACTICE

Nursing is by its nature involved with broad issues of public welfare. Nursing practice therefore affects and is affected by a wide range of laws outside the Nurse Practice Act. Nursing leaders have been a major force in drafting and supporting or opposing legislation affecting the health and welfare of their clients.[14] Nurses have a long history of activism at both the state and national level. How this comes about will be discussed more fully in Chapter 4. The organization of the laws (codes) of each state is different. Code used in this sense is an organized body of law on a given subject that can be referenced by chapter, article, and section. The following sections give some examples of codes where relevant laws and regulations are likely to be found.

Practice Acts of Other Professions

As noted previously in this chapter, the language of the practice acts of other professions may influence the scope of nursing practice. Constant vigilance is required to stay informed. In general, new laws supersede laws previously written. A section of the law written later into another practice act may be interpreted to override a section of the Nurse Practice Act in that state. The most cost-effective way to monitor practice act legislation is through the service of a government relations representative or lobbyist regularly assigned that responsibility. Usually, the state nurses' association will perform this function or see that it is done. Adequate government relations activities are costly of time, money, and energy. Both the active participation and the money of nurse members in the professional organization are essential.

Hospital and Other Health Facility Licensing Laws

Laws that govern the facilities in which nurses are employed commonly address the qualifications and supervisory relationships between the various professions practicing in that facility. There is a dynamic tension between employers, employees, independent practitioners, and consumers regarding what is contained in these laws and the regulations that result. Examples of practice-related statutes and regulations in this area include the services to be provided, staffing ratios, specialty preparation, staff privileges, lines of authority, and patients' bills of rights. These codes may, in effect, expand or restrict the practice of a given professional group. Again, vigilance is required.

Public Health and Safety Codes

Facility licensing may be included in the health and safety codes, as may sanitation laws, laws regarding attendance at the birth of infants, reportable diseases, building safety, and so forth. Familiarity with the relevant codes will assist nurses in assuring client safety. A law is only effective if it is enforced.

Insurance Codes

Insurance has become a matter of paramount importance in modern society. It provides a way to share risks among policyholders and provide financial support in time of need. The insurance codes define the rules under which insurance is written, what services must be provided, and how insurance is to be paid for. In the 1980s the costs of malpractice insurance were becoming prohibitive. Efforts to control those costs led nursing and other health professions to seek changes in the law to allow professions to self-insure their members.

Health insurance, private or governmental (Medicare, Medicaid), has become the "third party" in professional–client relationships. Rising costs led both government and private insurers to take an active role in deciding what services would be covered for which clients. These "third-party payers" also became concerned with the level of payment and the designation of professionals eligible to receive payment. Not infrequently, such issues became a matter of law.

Nursing services, including advanced nursing services, have been added slowly to the insurance codes covering both private and government funded programs. Nurses will be able to demonstrate the value of nursing practice only as their services are recognized as reimbursable and discrete from those of the physician or the "room rate" of the facility. The documented use of the nursing process and the significance of nursing assessment and nursing diagnoses are important steps in this direction.

Education Codes

The education codes govern the system of public and private education in a state. They affect the structure, financing, and function of schools, including schools of nursing. The education codes affect the quality of education and may have important implications for the rights of students and faculty. In some states, such as New York, the Nurse Practice Act is located in the education code.

Laws Relating to Wills and Inheritance

The laws of each state set out the requirements for a valid will. Specific requirements, such as the responsibilities of witnesses and who may inherit, vary among states. Beginning students should therefore consult with nursing faculty if the subject of a will is brought up by a client. Students should not agree to witness a document without first seeking advice as to hospital policy, and should not give advice to a client on the wording of any legal document.

Antitrust Act

The enforcement of antitrust legislation is a federal responsibility. In general terms, antitrust laws forbid corporations or other entities from conspiring to prevent competition by engaging in restraint of trade. As nurses provide more and more reimbursable services they enter into competition with other groups for the health care dollar. Thus, antitrust legislation is assuming increased importance to the nursing profession. The ability to earn a living is an important legal right in the United States. A license to practice may not be lightly interfered with. Under the antitrust legislation, the right of one group to prevent the practice of another is severely restricted by law.[6] This law only works if the harmed person is willing to go to court. Without a court determination of harm, there is not likely to be relief. This is another instance where nurses must work together assertively to assure professional rights.[6]

Laws Relating to Employment Rights

Both state and federal laws protect the rights of employees in relation to their employers. Workman's compensation is an example of a state law that covers care for a worker injured on the job. Unemployment compensation is also regulated by state law. Both federal and state laws govern wages, overtime, and fringe benefits. Equal opportunity laws and laws against sexual harrassment in the workplace are designed to protect the right to work of all citizens.

The National Labor Relations Act is a federal law that guarantees the right of groups of employees to organize unions and engage in collective bargaining to obtain an **employment contract.** Such a contract is a legally binding document that describes rights and responsibilities of both the employer and the employee. Although some nurses are protected by contracts negotiated via the collective bargaining process, many are not. The reasons for this are complex. For further discussion of collective bargaining and nursing, refer to Chapter 4.

It is in the best interest of all employees, including nurses, to have an employment contract. This is true whether a nurse is working for an agency, such as a hospital or clinic, or for an individual, such as in a private duty situation. Contracts may be created without unions or collective bargaining, as long as both parties mutually agree to do so. However, an effective contract that covers all likely contingencies is not a simple document to develop. It is advisable to obtain assistance from a qualified professional, usually an attorney, to develop an employment contract if collective bargaining is not an option in a specific situation.

Contract law and other laws relating to employment are especially likely to depend upon precedent-setting decisions for their interpretation. Nurses seeking redress under the laws discussed in this section need the early guidance of a lawyer experienced in employment law.

The content of a contract depends on the efforts of the individuals who negotiate it. If an employment contract is to protect quality of care, it is up to the negotiating team to see that protection is included in the language of the contract. One aspect of a contract that relates to quality of care is nurse–client ratio (the number of nurses that must be scheduled for a given number of clients). This ratio not only has a direct impact on the quality of care in general, but it may also determine whether staff can effectively use a collaborative approach to care.

Contracts are designed to assure that both parties understand what has been agreed to. We live in a very complex and rapidly changing society. As the capabilities and the costs of health care have risen, the bureaucratic structure in which care is given has expanded into a tangled web of laws and regulation. In this environment, the responsibility of professionals toward clients depends on a delicate balance between client needs and bureaucratic rules. This balance is best maintained by a formal contract that spells out in writing the rights and responsibilities of all the parties involved.

■ LAWS RELATING TO THE RIGHTS OF CLIENTS

Certain laws have been used to protect the rights of clients in a professional–client relationship. Some have been written specifically with this relationship in mind, while others have been interpreted for that purpose. Civil rights laws are one example of laws interpreted to protect the health care client.

Informed Consent, Assault and Battery

Clients have the right to be given sufficient understandable information about the risks and benefits of and alternatives to proposed treatments. **Informed consent** refers to the right of the client, based on this information, to *voluntarily* consent to or to refuse treatment (Fig. 3–5). A client who lacks the capacity or competence (because of age or disabil-

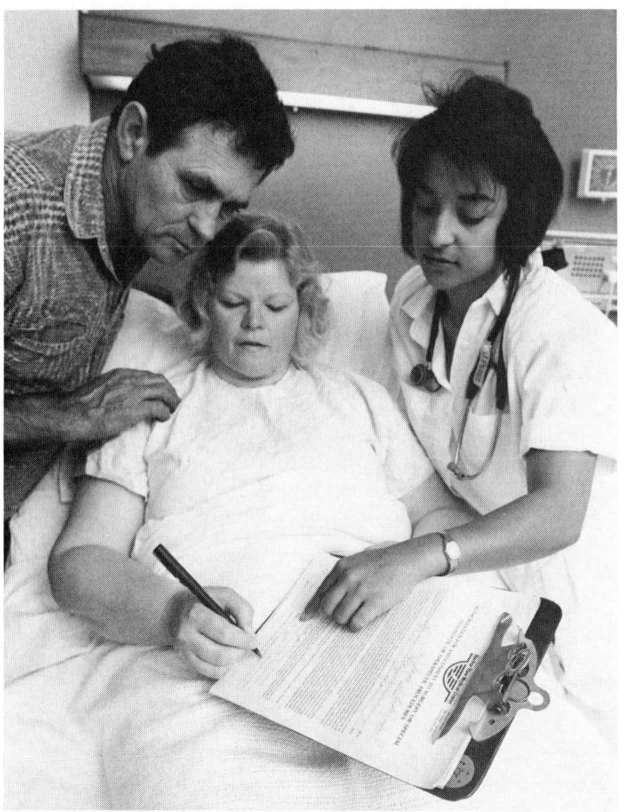

Figure 3–5. Nurses who obtain a client's signature on an informed consent document should strive to ensure that the client understands the risks and benefits of the treatment.

ity) to understand is not capable of giving an informed consent. In such instances, consent must be obtained from a guardian or the courts. State laws vary as to the fine points of informed consent. It is important to be aware of the laws in the state where a nurse is practicing. In this as in other areas of nursing practice, there are ethical as well as legal concerns that must be met.

Obtaining informed consent is the responsibility of the physician planning the treatment. Not infrequently, a nurse signs as witness to a client's signature on the informed consent form. Signing as a witness on an informed consent document involves legal and ethical responsibilities. In effect, the witness is validating that proper consent procedures were followed. In the case of later litigation regarding inappropriate consent for the treatment in question, both the witness and the physician could be considered at fault.

It is also a nurse's ethical responsibility as client advocate to be certain that clients actually understand and agree to the treatment before they sign. This can best be accomplished by a collaborative approach. In a collaborative relationship, trust is developed, making open communication more likely. In a noncollaborative, paternalistic atmosphere, a client may not feel free to voice concerns or questions about the procedure, but may still sign the consent.

IMPLICATIONS FOR NURSE–CLIENT COLLABORATION

The Right to Refuse Treatment

The mutual interaction model of client care discussed in Chapter 37 and throughout this text explicitly acknowledges the client's inalienable right to self-determination, including the right to refuse care and treatment. Health care professionals who insist on treating or providing unwanted care risk being charged with the violation of laws against assault and battery.

Even with a collaborative approach to obtaining consent clients may have second thoughts after signing as they reconsider all of the information shared about the proposed treatment. These misgivings will more likely be expressed when a collaborative tone has been established. In some cases, a nurse may decide to verify a client's understanding by initiating conversation with the client about the treatment. Doubts or misconceptions can be discovered by this approach.

Nurses have a collaborative responsibility to both client and physician when witnessing the signature on a consent form. Collaboration with a client in this instance involves answering the client's questions in a way that encourages further mutual exploration. Mutual exploration facilitates a client's becoming truly aware of the purpose, risks, and anticipated benefits of the treatment and therefore, more confident about making a decision. Collaboration with physicians involves making them aware of a client's concerns. The physician can then personally verify informed consent, if necessary.

Another possible dilemma related to informed consent can occur when a client suffering from a life-threatening disease refuses treatment. Informed, competent clients have a legal and ethical right to decline therapy regardless of the seriousness of the illness. However, it is especially important when the illness is life threatening to ascertain that the dissent was based on accurate perceptions. A client must be fully cognizant of the seriousness of the illness, all the possible options for treatment, and the probable outcome if treatment is foregone. Such an **informed dissent** must then be respected by all providers.

Except in a life-threatening emergency, a health professional who treats a client without explicit consent or against that client's wishes may be charged with assault and battery. (**Assault** is the apparent imminent threat of physical harm while **battery** is the actual touching with apparent intent to harm; see Table 3–2). Even when the situation is grave, it may be necessary to have a court authorize care if a client is unable or unwilling to make a decision to consent. The right of a client to refuse treatment even when that treatment is life saving or life sustaining must be respected. The responsibility of society must also be taken into consideration. For example, society may choose to protect the life of a minor against the wishes of the parent, or the life of a mother over the life of an unborn child.

Unlawful Imprisonment, Right to Treatment

Clients may not be detained against their will unless they are under a court order and have been properly documented to be a danger to themselves or others. Clients have a right to sign themselves out of a hospital "against medical advice" if they are not satisfied that they are receiving proper care or if they chose to end care. A terminally ill client, for example, may chose to go home to die and avoid the possibility of being kept alive by extraordinary means. On the other hand, a client who has been lawfully detained because of illness has a right to receive treatment. Otherwise there is no legal justification for keeping that client in a health care institution. For example, a client detained because of mental illness has a right to receive treatment for that illness.

Restraint is a serious and dangerous practice, both legally and physically. The use of chemical or physical restraints can only be justified to protect a client from injury to self or others and for a very limited period of time. Restraints may only be used after all other remedies have been exhausted. State regulations and institutional policies that protect the rights and safety of the client must be followed.

Right to Die and Right to Life

Right to Die. One of the dilemmas created by the technological advances in health care has to do with the increasing ability to preserve life under adverse circumstances. It is now possible to maintain heart and lung function long past the point where the quality of life has any objective meaning.

Persons who fear that they or their loved ones may be subjected to such artificial prolongation of life have lobbied successfully in many states for legislation supporting the right to create a **living will** (Fig. 3–6) to protect the wishes of clients who may later become incapable of expressing those wishes for themselves.[26] This document, prepared by clients who are of sound mind, directs that when death is inevitable, no unusual or extraordinary measures be taken to prolong life and delay a "natural death."

The definition of unusual or extraordinary is changing. As cases come before the courts, and states adopt natural death acts, the public is forced to consider the implications of traditional practice. It is generally agreed that usual and ordinary includes attempting to keep clients warm and dry and nourished. Questions arise, however, even at this presumably basic level.[27,28] How does the right to comfort or freedom from pain fit in? For example, if a client is in such pain that only life-threatening amounts of narcotics will relieve the pain, is the client entitled to be pain free? At what point on the continuum from spoon-feeding a reluctant client to nasogastric tubes to high-technology hyperalimentation (high nutrient intravenous feeding) does nourishment cease to be ordinary?

Although a living will is considered a legally binding document in many states, the response of health care professionals to living wills has been varied. In some cases this is because of conflicts with personal belief systems. In other instances health care professionals fear the possibility of later suits by a family member who did not agree with the decision. Because of the variability among state laws covering living wills and "natural death," it is essential that all nurses be aware of the relevant laws in the state where they practice. An option available in most states is **durable power of attorney** for health care (Fig. 3–7), which allows clients to communicate their wishes regarding treatment prior to becoming ill or at any time during the course of an illness. The durable power of attorney also gives a specific person the authority to make health care decisions if a client becomes unable to do so. This is a more flexible approach and can be tailored to changing situations over time. Many clients may be unaware of this option or may need assistance to explore pertinent issues. As of December, 1991, health care professionals are legally required to ensure that clients understand their options regarding advance directives such as living wills and durable powers of attorney under the Patient Self-Determination Act. This federal law mandates health care facilities such as hospitals, home health agencies, and hospices to provide this information and education to clients, staff, and community as a condition of Medicare reimbursement.[36]

The importance of encouraging individuals to create concrete evidence of their wishes regarding termination of life-sustaining treatment is illustrated by the recent US Supreme Court decision regarding Nancy Cruzan.[31] She had been left in a permanent vegetative state as a result of an automobile accident in 1983. The Court upheld the rights of the state of Missouri to prevent termination of her tube feedings without "clear and convincing evidence" of Cruzan's wishes. In this situation the testimony of her parents attesting to Cruzan's prior statements that she would not want to live under such circumstances were not considered by the state as sufficient evidence of Cruzan's expressed wishes while competent. Although similar cases in other states have upheld a decision to refuse treatment by surrogate decision-makers, much heartache can be avoided by creating a living will or durable power of attorney for health care in advance of circumstances creating a need for them.

Right to Life. At the other end of the continuum, technological advances now also make it possible to save the lives of infants who would previously have died because of prematurity or congenital malformation. In some of these cases, there is serious concern about the quality of life preserved.[32] In addition, the commitment of scarce economic resources required to save and maintain these infants can be extraordinary.

Whether the issue involved is the right to die or the right to life, there are some who feel that the increasing cost of care must be weighed against the benefits to be gained. How, asks this group, do we weigh the benefits in such a case against the alternative use of scarce resources for purposes with wider impact? Prenatal and well-child care programs for the medically indigent are examples in which many would benefit by the money that it required to pre-

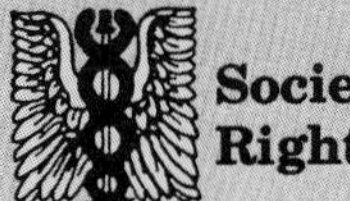

Society for the Right to Die

250 West 57th Street/New York, NY 10107

Living Will Declaration

INSTRUCTIONS ***Consult this column for help and guidance.***	To My Family, Doctors, and All Those Concerned with My Care
This declaration sets forth your directions regarding medical treatment.	I, ________________________, being of sound mind, make this statement as a directive to be followed if I become unable to participate in decisions regarding my medical care. If I should be in an incurable or irreversible mental or physical condition with no reasonable expectation of recovery, I direct my attending physician to withhold or withdraw treatment that merely prolongs my dying. I further direct that treatment be limited to measures to keep me comfortable and to relieve pain.
You have the right to refuse treatment you do not want, and you may request the care you do want.	These directions express my legal right to refuse treatment. Therefore I expect my family, doctors, and everyone concerned with my care to regard themselves as legally and morally bound to act in accord with my wishes, and in so doing to be free of any legal liability for having followed my directions.
You may list specific treatment you do not want. For example: ***Cardiac resuscitation*** ***Mechanical respiration*** ***Artificial feeding/fluids by tube*** ***Otherwise, your general statement, top right, will stand for your wishes.***	I especially do not want: ________________________
You may want to add instructions for care you do want—for example, pain medication; or that you prefer to die at home if possible.	Other instructions/comments: ________________________
If you want, you can name someone to see that your wishes are carried out, but you do not have to do this.	**Proxy Designation Clause:** Should I become unable to communicate my instructions as stated above, I designate the following person to act in my behalf: Name ________________________ Address ________________________ If the person I have named above is unable to act on my behalf, I authorize the following person to do so: Name ________________________ Address ________________________
Sign and date here in the presence of two adult witnesses, who should also sign.	Signed: ________________ Date: ________ Witness: ____________ Witness: ____________ Address: ____________ Address: ____________ *Keep the signed original with your personal papers at home. Give signed copies to doctors, family, and proxy. Review your Declaration from time to time; initial and date it to show it still expresses your intent.*

Figure 3–6. Living will declaration. (*Courtesy of the Society for the Right to Die, New York.*)

1. DESIGNATION OF HEALTH CARE AGENT. I, ________

____

(Insert your name and address) do hereby designate and appoint

____

(Insert name, address, and telephone number of one individual only as your agent to make health care decisions for you. None of the following may be designated as your agent: (1) your treating health care provider, (2) a nonrelative employee of your treating health care provider, (3) an operator of a community care facility, or (4) a nonrelative employee of an operator of a community care facility,) as my attorney in fact (agent) to make health care decisions for me as authorized in this document. For the purposes of this document, "health care decision" means consent, refusal of consent, or withdrawal of consent to any care, treatment, service, or procedure to maintain, diagnose, or treat an individual's physical or mental condition.

2. CREATION OF DURABLE POWER OF ATTORNEY FOR HEALTH CARE. By this document I intend to create a durable power of attorney for health care as allowed by the California Civil Code. This power of attorney shall not be affected by my subsequent incapacity.

3. GENERAL STATEMENT OF AUTHORITY GRANTED. Subject to any limitations in this document, I hereby grant to my agent full power and authority to make health care decisions for me to the same extent that I could make them for myself if I had the capacity to do so. In exercising this authority, my agent shall make health care decisions that are consistent with my desires as stated in this document or otherwise made known to my agent, including but not limited to my desires concerning obtaining or refusing or withdrawing life-prolonging care, treatment, services, and procedures.

4. STATEMENT OF DESIRES, SPECIAL PROVISIONS, AND LIMITATIONS. (If you do not state any limits, your agent will have broad powers to make health care decisions for you, except to the extent that there are limits provided by law.)

In exercising the authority under this durable power of attorney for health care, my agent shall act consistently with my desires as stated below and is subject to the special provisions and limitations stated:

(a) Statement of desires concerning life-prolonging care, treatment, services, and procedures: ________

(b) Additional statemenmt of desires, special provisions, and limitations: ________

____

5. INSPECTION AND DISCLOSURE OF INFORMATION RELATING TO MY PHYSICAL OR MENTAL HEALTH. Subject to any limitations in this document, my agent has the power and authority to do all of the following:

(a) Request, review, and receive any information, verbal or written, regarding my physical or mental health, including, but not limited to, medical and hospital records.

(b) Execute on my behalf any releases or other documents that may be required in order to obtain this information.

(c) Consent to the disclosure of this information.

6. SIGNING DOCUMENTS, WAIVERS, AND RELEASES.

7. AUTOPSY; ANATOMICAL GIFTS; DISPOSITIONS OF REMAINS.

8. DURATION.
(Unless you specify a shorter period in the space below, this power of attorney will exist for seven years from the date you execute this document and, if you are unable to make health care decisions for yourself at the time when this seven year period ends, the power will continue until the time when you become able to make health care decisions for yourself.)

9. DESIGNATION OF ALTERNATE AGENTS.

10. NOMINATION OF CONSERVATOR OF PERSON.
(A conservator of the person may be appointed for you if a court decides that one should be appointed. The conservator is responsible for your physical care, which under some circumstances includes making health care decisions for you. You are not required to nominate a conservator but you may do so. The court will appoint the person you nominate unless that would be contrary to your best interests. You may, but are not required to, nominate as your conservator the same person you name in paragraph 1 as your health care agent.)

Figure 3–7. Durable power of attorney. (*Excerpted from California Civil Code, Section 2500.*)

serve one life of doubtful quality. This group also points to the severe hardship and suffering sometimes caused both to clients and families.

Critics of the cost–benefit perspective state that there is no clear dividing line between what is acceptable taking of life and what is not. Their view is that the preservation of all life is mandatory and that the issue of money is, in a sense, irrelevant. This view has been criticized for not addressing those situations in which there is no access to the high technology that would make preservation of life possible.

Another argument in the issue of keeping vulnerable clients of any age alive centers on whether there is a moral difference between withholding (never starting) and withdrawing (starting and later stopping) life-sustaining treatment. Some argue that withholding is clearly the most merciful when death is inevitable. This alternative prevents the issue of the right to terminate treatment being raised, but presents the question: on what grounds does one decide that death is inevitable or how imminent it is likely to be.[29] Others believe that withdrawing allows for a more reasoned approach because it not only allows a trial for determining possible effectiveness of treatment, but also provides time for all concerned to be involved in the decision.

It is important to remember that the legal system was not designed to resolve such ethical and moral dilemmas (see also Chap. 34). The law reflects the wishes of society, and where society is in disarray on a particular issue, the legal system will reflect that disarray. Resolution will only come when consensus has been achieved in the larger society as to what constitutes the greater good.[29,32]

Do Not Resuscitate Orders

A brief history of the evolution of decisions not to resuscitate in the hospital setting will serve to illustrate the process. Once the technique of cardiopulmonary resuscitation was understood, hospitals set up systems for using the technology. Crash carts, loaded with the necessary equipment and drugs, were set up. Teams of qualified health care professionals were trained. Every television viewer has seen the dramatic response to the emergency call on a cardiac arrest. Initially, every client who suffered a cardiac arrest was treated to attempted cardiopulmonary resuscitation. As time went on it became clear that not all clients *should* be resuscitated and various strategies were used to avoid resuscitation in selected situations. Informal agreements were made that no code would be attempted or that a slow code would be performed. A **slow code** occurred when the team went through the motions of a cardiopulmonary resuscitation but responded slowly and with no expectation of success. With experience it became clear that both the informal no code, and the slow code, created serious problems both legally and ethically. Eventually it was determined that under certain specified conditions, a DNR (do not resuscitate) order could legally be written in the client's chart.

In January 1988, the Joint Commission on Accreditation of Healthcare Organizations (JCAHO, formerly JCAH) began requiring that each hospital have a DNR policy. The chief executive officer of the hospital, in consultation with the medical, nursing, and other appropriate staffs, is responsible for developing a hospital-wide DNR policy that clearly defines criteria for use of DNR orders. The policy must then be adopted by the medical staff and approved by the governing body (the board of trustees).[33] A DNR policy must, of course, be consistent with the relevant state natural death act, if one exists.

Access-to-Care Legislation

Health care is a costly commodity. Given the recognition of that cost, the question then arises of who has access to health care. Among the rich access is not a problem. In the early history of the United States, the poor were provided access through charitable clinics and hospitals. Later, the development of teaching hospitals in conjunction with schools for the health professions provided a place where care could be given by students under the supervision of their professors. The poor in effect paid for their care by allowing themselves to be used as teaching material.

For a variety of reasons, discussed more fully in Chapter 35, legislation was introduced over the years to improve access to care both geographically and economically. The Hill-Burton Act of 1946, for example, provided federal money for the construction of hospitals in areas where there was a shortage of hospital beds. The most telling advances in health care access legislation, however, were created by the Social Security Act Amendments of 1965. The systems of Medicare and Medicaid were set up to provide payment for health care for the aged and the poor, respectively. Although there had been previous experiments in such legislation (eg, the Shepherd-Towner Act of 1920 for prenatal care and child health), the Medicare and Medicaid legislation was the first to have widespread support.[34] The intent of Medicare and Medicaid was to provide one standard of care to all citizens regardless of means. As originally conceived, this legislation empowered clients to go to the physician of their choice for care. The federal government, with some assistance from the states, would subsidize the care to the extent that clients were unable to do so.

The combination of increased access to care and rapidly escalating technology had an impressive effect on the overall cost of care in the United States. In 1960 (before Medicare and Medicaid), national health care expenditures represented 5.3 percent of the Gross National Product

BUILDING NURSING KNOWLEDGE

How Can the Client Advocacy Role Smooth Implementation of Laws on the Care of the Terminally Ill?

Martin DA, Redland AR. Legal and ethical issues in resuscitation and withholding of treatment. *Crit Care Nurs Q.* 1988; 10:1–8.

This article discusses the legal issues in giving cardiopulmonary resuscitation and other life-saving treatment to terminally ill clients. Martin and Redland note that it is important for nurses to understand the laws on withholding treatment because nurses often bear the primary responsibility for implementing "do not resuscitate" orders. The authors add that the nurse frequently faces situations that require decisions on the limits of treatment. Even though it is the physician's responsibility to give the order, the nurse's role in decision-making is increasingly important because the nurse often has intimate knowledge of the client's wishes.

The authors note that since the Karen Ann Quinlan case, the courts have recognized the right of adults to forego life-sustaining treatment if there is little chance of recovery. The courts have also recognized the right of families to make treatment decisions for their adult relatives when the relative is incapacitated.* Moreover, legal safeguards have been developed for special populations such as the mentally ill, the mentally retarded, and children.

Legal opinion, developed since the Quinlan case, is now reflected in the professional standards promulgated by the Joint Commission on Accreditation of Healthcare Organizations (JCAHO). Nevertheless, decisions to withhold treatment can become very complicated, especially if there is disagreement among the client, family, and professional caregivers. The authors state that hospital rules and procedures based on professional standards simplify decision-making and that nurses should be involved in both shaping and implementing these policies.

* This right, according to the US Supreme Court decision in the case of Nancy Cruzan, may be limited by state statutes requiring particular evidence of the client's preferences. See Annas GJ. Sounding board: Nancy Cruzan and the right to die. *N Engl J Med.* 1990: 323: 670–673.

(GNP). By 1965, health care was consuming 6.1 percent. Currently, the cost has risen to 12.7 percent and is expected to rise to 15 percent by the end of the century.[35] Various efforts have been launched to bring cost under control. Some legislation resulted in restricting the amount of payment for services. This indirectly affected access to care, because some providers would not participate given the low level of reimbursement. Other legislation provided for alternative organizations of health care delivery. This directly affected access by limiting the choice of provider based on the system of reimbursement for services.

To date, an affordable solution for the problem of equal access to quality care has not been found. Efforts by the health care industry and the government to confront this complex issue continue.

■ IMPACT OF LAW ON COLLABORATION FOR OPTIMAL HEALTH

The laws of the state in which a nurse is licensed to practice dictate the limits as well as the mandates for client care. Therefore, while collaboration as a philosophy may underlie a nurse's approach to professional responsibilities and relationships with clients and colleagues, any specific actions carried out by that nurse must fall within the definition of the scope of nursing practice provided by the state Nurse Practice Act. Similarly, the practice acts of other health care professionals determine what would be acceptable collaborative actions for them. For example, a nurse and physician may wish to collaborate with a terminally ill client to facilitate the client's attaining a peaceful, dignified death. Despite the client's expressed wishes to receive a lethal dose of medication to end the suffering, neither practitioner could provide it. The practice acts of both nurses and physicians forbid such action. This particular example would also violate criminal law.

Laws also determine appropriate collaboration between health care professionals. The definitions of the scope of practice contained in each professional practice act create role boundaries and clarify respective responsibilities. These definitions must be respected. Collaborative decision-making cannot supersede the limits of practice set down by law.

Laws protecting clients' rights also affect nurse–client collaboration. As shown in this chapter, these laws often emphasize the professional's responsibility to be a client advocate—that is, to facilitate communication between a client and an institution. This role is philosophically compatible with collaboration or mutual interaction. Informed consent, the legal foundation of client self-determination, is the conceptual and moral basis for many laws relating to client rights. Informed consent is grounded in a belief that the client should participate fully in health care decision-making, and so is fundamental to a philosophy of collaboration.

The National Labor Relations Act is another law that is supportive of nurse–client collaboration. Although originally construed to protect the rights of employees, when the employees (eg, nurses) are responsible for the welfare of others (eg, clients), both groups can be served by a well-conceived contract. Nurses who believe that collaboration is central to quality care will strive to negotiate an employment contract that mandates working conditions conducive to collaboration.

It can be seen from the above discussion that law can both limit and support collaboration. It is as much a responsibility of nurses to be informed about relevant laws as it is to be skilled at carrying out nursing care techniques. Both are requisites for expert professional practice.

SUMMARY

The profession of nursing operates under a social mandate to provide nursing care. The formal outlines of this mandate are included in the state Nurse Practice Acts. The practice statutes and regulations that implement them provide the guidelines for minimum safe nursing practice in a given state. Beyond the law, however, are professional standards and ethical considerations that provide guidelines for the best possible nursing practice. The nursing profession expects that practicing nurses will not only avoid falling below the minimum standards of safe practice but will continually strive to advance professional standards and to practice in an ethical manner.

The first responsibility of nurses is to the clients who depend on them for advocacy, support, and protection in responding to actual or potential health problems. In fulfilling that responsibility, nurses collaborate with clients in determining how best to meet clients' needs. Nurses also collaborate with other members of the health care team to assure that clients will benefit from the expertise of all members of the team. Increasing technology and bureaucratization of the delivery of health care have created new problems requiring new solutions. These solutions must evolve over time until society reaches consensus. In the meantime, nurses and their colleagues in other health professions must work together with their clients in seeking the best solutions available in the existing environment.

The privileged nature of the professional–client relationship places clients in a vulnerable position. Over time a variety of laws beyond those of the practice act are interpreted to protect the rights of clients. The rights of professionals to provide care are also protected by laws. Although there is no expectation that nurses will become legal experts, it is essential for nurses to be sensitive to the legal environment in which they practice.

The professional nurses' associations at the state and national level provide the vehicle through which nurses can most effectively determine the appropriate role of the profession in delivering care. The professional organizations provide the mechanism for establishing standards, adopting a code of ethics, and supporting nurses in their efforts to establish supportive legal environments and adequate resources to provide the best possible care.

REFERENCES

1. Carter LH. *Reason in Law.* 2nd ed. Boston: Little, Brown; 1987.
2. Dvorak EM, Schowalter JM. The role of the National Council of State Boards of Nursing in consumer protection. In McCloskoy JM, Grace HK, eds. *Current Issues in Nursing.* St. Louis: C.V. Mosby; 1990.
3. Forgotson EH, Roemer R, Newman RW. Licensure of physicians. *Washington U Law Q.* 1967; 250.
4. ANA board approves a definition of nursing practice. *Am J Nurs.* 1955; 55:1474.
5. Eccard WT. A revolution in white: New approaches in treating nurses as professionals. *Vanderbilt Law Rev.* 1977; 30:839.
6. *Vinod C Bhan, CRNA, v NME Hospitals, Inc.* No. 84-2256, U.S. Court of Appeals, 9th Circuit, Oct. 2, 1985 (slip opinion).
7. Nightingale F. *Notes on Nursing: What It Is and What It Is Not.* London: Harrison and Sons; 1859. (Facsimile edition, Philadelphia: Lippincott; 1946).
8. Henderson V. *Basic Principles of Nursing Care.* London: International Council of Nurses; 1961.
9. American Nurses' Association. *Nursing: A Social Policy Statement.* Kansas City, MO: ANA; 1980.
10. *Nurses Legal Handbook.* Springhouse, PA: Springhouse; 1985.
11. Fellmeth C. A theory of regulation. *Cal Reg Law Rep.* 1985; 5:3.
12. Committee for the Study of Nursing Education, *Nursing and Nursing Education in the United States.* New York: Macmillan; 1923.
13. Flexner A. *Medical Education in the United States and Canada: A Report to the Carnegie Foundation for the Advancement of Teaching.* Boston: D.B. Updike, The Merrymount Press; 1910. Reproduced, New York: Arno Press; 1972.
14. Kalisch PA, Kalisch BJ. *The Advance of American Nursing.* Boston: Little, Brown; 1978.
15. National League for Nursing. *Nursing Data Review.* New York; NLN; 1989:55.
16. Minarik P. Ana adopts scope of practice document. *California Nurse.* 1987; 83:10.
17. Stephany T. House opens membership to associate nurses. *California Nurse.* 1987; 83:9.
18. Northrop CE, Kelly ME. *Legal Issues In Nursing.* St. Louis: Mosby; 1987.
19. Bellocq J. Protecting your license. *Journal of Professional Nursing.* 1989; 5:8.
20. LaBar C. *Enforcement of the Nursing Practice Act.* Kansas City, MO: American Nurses' Association; 1986.
21. Feutz SA. *Nursing and the Law.* Eau Claire, WI: Professional Educational Systems; 1989.
22. Swenson J, Havens B, Champagna M. State Boards and Impaired Nurses. *Nurs Out.* 1989; 37:94–96.
23. *Code for Nurses with Interpretive Statements.* Kansas City, MO: American Nurses' Association; 1986.
24. *Black's Law Dictionary.* 4th ed. St. Paul: West; 1968.
25. Feutz SA. Do you need liability insurance? *Nursing.* 1991; 21: s6–7.
26. Anderson D. Death and dying: Ethics at the end of life. In Lindeman CA, McAthie M. *Nursing Trends and Issues.* Springhouse, PA: Springhouse; 1989:480–487.
27. American Nurses' Association, Committee on Ethics. *Guidelines on Withdrawing or Withholding Food and Fluid.* Kansas City, MO: The Association. Jan. 22, 1988.
28. Fry, Sara. New ANA guidelines on withdrawing or withholding food and fluid from patients. In Lindeman CA, McAthie M. *Nursing Trends and Issues.* Springhouse, PA: Springhouse; 1989: 499–507.
29. President's Commission for the Study of Ethical Problems in Medicine and Biomedical and Behavioral Research. Deciding to Forego Life-Sustaining Treatments. Washington, DC: US Government Printing Office; 1983.
30. US Congress, Office of Technology Assessment. *Life Sustaining Technologies and the Elderly.* Washington, DC: US Government Printing Office; 1987.
31. *Cruzan v. Director, Missouri Dept. of Health,* 110 S. Ct 2841 (1990).
32. Murphy CP. Technological Advances and Ethical Dilemmas. In McCloskey JM, Grace HK, eds. *Current Issues in Nursing.* St Louis: CV Mosby; 1990: 587–589.
33. Adams R. The development and implementation of a do not resuscitate policy. *J Nurs Admin.* 1988; 3:18–21.
34. Starr P. *The Social Transformation of American Medicine.* New York: Basic Books; 1982.
35. Grace HK. Can Health Care Costs Be Contained? In McCloskey JM, Grace HK, eds. *Current Issues in Nursing.* St Louis: CV Mosby; 1990: 380–386.
36. Markus K. Durable power of attorney for health care. *Calif Nurs.* 1991; 13(4):20.

BIBLIOGRAPHY

Bailey-Allen M. Changing liability of the nurse over the past decade. *Orthop Nurs.* 1990; 9:13–15.

Brill JM. Informed consent may entail risks. *Am Nurs.* 1990; 22:42.

Creighton H. Legal implications of the impaired nurse. Part I. *Nurs Manage.* 1988; 19:21–23.

Creighton H. Legal implications of the impaired nurse. Part II. *Nurs Manage.* 1988; 19:20–21.

Goldstein A, Perdew S, Pruitt S. *The Nurse's Legal Advisor.* Philadelphia: Lippincott; 1989.

Guido GW. *Legal Issues in Nursing: A Source Book for Practice.* Norwalk, CT: Appleton & Lange; 1988.

Hogue E. *Nursing and Informed Consent: A Case Study Approach.* Owings Mills, MD: National Health Publishing, 1985.

Maher VF. Dear Florence: Legal musings for the 1990's. *Adv Clin Care.* 1990; 5:20–21.

Quinley KM. Legal side: Defending yourself against a malpractice suit. *Am J Nurs.* 1990; Jan(1): 37–38, 40.

Redman E. *Dance of Legislation.* New York: Simon & Schuster; 1974.

Steinbrook R, Lo B. Artificial feeding—Solid ground, not a slippery slope. *N Engl J Med.* 1988; 318:286.

CHAPTER 4

Politics, Policy-making, and Nursing

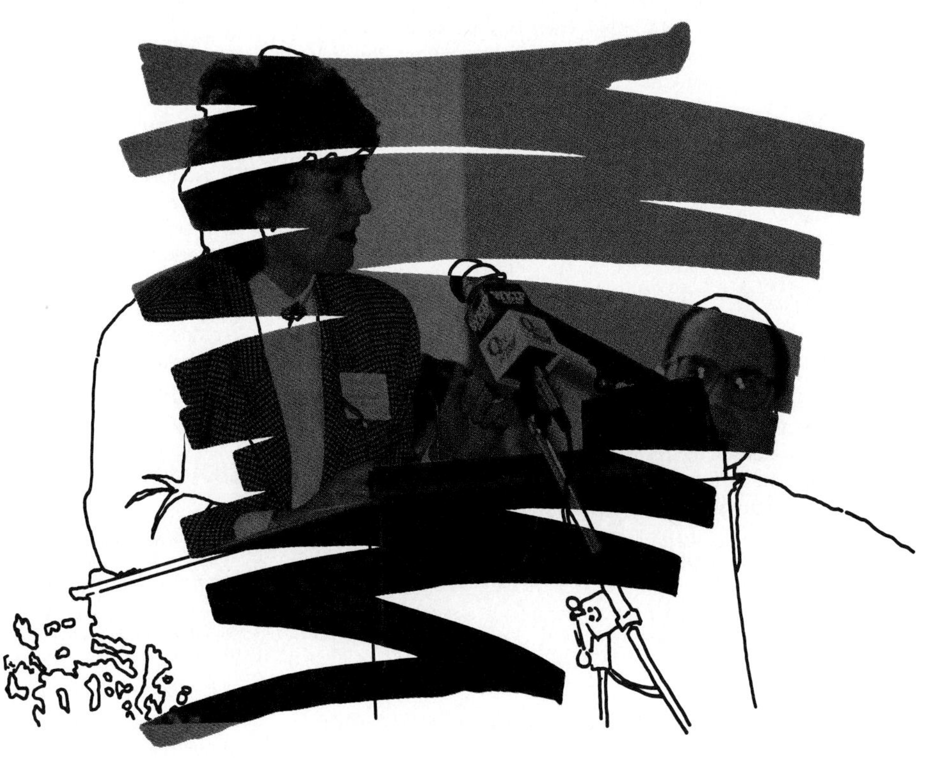

Objectives

Upon completion of this chapter, the student will be able to:

1. Describe the steps in the policy-making process.
2. Discuss the relevance of the policy-making process to the practice of professional nursing.
3. Discuss the responsibility of nurses in the policy-making process.
4. Discuss the strategies available to nurses to influence the outcome of the policy-making process.
5. Describe the modes of lobbying nurses can use to influence public policy.
6. List the "do's" and "don'ts" of successful lobbying.
7. Discuss the current and potential role of professional nursing organizations in the policy arena.
8. Identify governmental agencies that affect nursing practice.
9. Discuss ways in which nurses collaborate to effect political change.

KEY TERMS

agencies
appropriating legislation
authorizing legislation
boards
boycott
change
coalition
coercive power
collective bargaining
collective power
commissions
expert power
incremental change
legislative process
legitimate power
lobbying
personal power
policy
policy evaluation
policy implementation
policy-making
political action committee
politics
power
public policy
radical change
referent power
regulation
reward power
special interest group
testimony

In an ideal world where resources are plentiful, decisions on how to use resources are usually unnecessary. In reality, however, resources are almost always scarce and must be rationed among a large number of important uses. Many groups within society differ in their views of how resources, and particularly public resources, should be used. Conflicts exist about how much to spend and on what. Public welfare demands that these conflicts be resolved and that priorities be established. Priorities for the use of public resources are developed through the process of governmental policy-making. The political arena is where governmental policy is made.

Because of the keen competition for government funding, legislators must frequently address the question of what amount of public resources to devote to health care. The amount of resources allocated to health care fluctuates depending on the prevailing expression of public wants and needs. Changes in resource allocation are reflected in the availability and accessibility of health care services for some groups in our society, in the nation's ability to educate health care providers, and in our means for advancing health care through scientific inquiry.

Nurses are increasingly recognizing their ability to influence how policy-makers set priorities for the use of resources for health care. Nursing is a large profession and its members represent a substantial amount of political power. As a collective body, nursing has a powerful voice for influencing health care policy. Moreover, that voice is amplified whenever nurses collaborate with other groups that have similar policy interests. For these reasons, nurses are participating in politics as never before. They are involving themselves because of their awareness that through political activisim, they can influence not only health care but also their own professional goals and the interests of nursing. This chapter presents concepts and strategies to aid the nursing student's understanding of how nurses enter into and function within the political arena.

POLICY-MAKING

What Is Policy?

Definition of Policy. A **policy** is a set of plans or a course of action designed to guide and determine present and future decisions. A retail clothing store may have a return policy that states whether it allows customers to exchange items they have purchased for different items, for credit vouchers, or for cash refunds. A corporation may have personnel policies that determine employees' vacation benefits, compensation for overtime worked, and criteria for promotions. A school of nursing may have policies that describe grading practices, expectations for class attendance, and proper attire for clinical practice.

Public policy is the culmination of society's decisions on how to allocate scarce resources for reaching common goals, and usually embodies a plan for solving public problems. Public policy affects many aspects of everyone's life. Individuals have the option of selecting from whom to purchase long-distance telephone services because of a policy decision that demonopolized telephone communications. The increase in the number of homeless persons in urban areas has been attributed by some to the government's housing policy. The United States has a foreign policy that guides its relationships with other nations and that may include directives relating to tariffs on imported goods, trade agreements, and military alliances.

Health care decisions constitute a large part of the public policy agenda. In 1964 a policy was adopted that provided for federal payment for health care needs of persons receiving Social Security benefits. The ensuing program, Medicare, has dramatically changed the entire health care financing system. Public policy decisions also determine such issues as whether the government should pay for abortions, how much funding should be appropriated for AIDS research, and whether nurse practitioners should be directly reimbursed for their services.

Policy Versus Politics. Policy is related to, but not synonymous with, politics. As described later in this chapter, politics, the art or science of government, refers to the ability to guide or influence policy decisions. Politics involves the use of power for change.[1] Box 4–1 highlights the difference between policy and politics.

Policy-making is the process by which goals, purposes, and strategies are identified and priorities defined. The political process then is invoked to enact laws or regulations to formally legitimize policy initiatives. Policy issues deal with "shoulds" and "oughts"; politics translates these into "wills" and "musts."[1]

Levels of Government and Policy Issues

The various levels of government are responsible for different types of policy decisions. It is important to understand which issues are decided at what levels of government so that attempts to influence the policy-making process can be directed to the appropriate location.

BOX 4–1. THE DIFFERENCE BETWEEN POLICY AND POLITICS

Policy

The government's decisions on how to allocate scare resources for reaching common goals: federal, state, and municipal laws and regulations that specifically define the government's course of action.

Politics

The use of power for change: the process whereby individuals and groups influence policy decisions at all levels of government.

Federal Level. Policy decisions made at the federal level of government affect all citizens of our country. Issues decided here may include questions such as the future directions of the space exploration program, what types of national defense systems to fund, whether to alter current immigration quotas, and whether to subsidize farmers for surplus crops. Health care policy decisions made at the federal level include how much money to allocate for such programs as Medicare, whether to provide stipends for individuals pursuing advanced nursing education, and how much money to devote to specific types of basic and clinical health care research.

State Level. Policy decisions made at the state level of government affect citizens who reside, work, or visit in the specific state. Issues decided here may include matters such as whether to have state income or sales taxes, speed limits on state highways, and who is eligible to receive public assistance or welfare. Health care policy decisions made at the state level include determining who is eligible for Medicaid, what optional services to include in Medicaid coverage, which individuals are eligible for licensure as health care professionals, and whether state funds should be used to pay for abortions.

County Level. Policy decisions made at the county level of government affect citizens who live within the county limits. Some states have strong, highly organized county governance while other states have a less well-established structure. Policy decisions made at the county level may include issues related to law enforcement and criminal justice, water and pollution control, highway maintenance, and social services. Health care policy at the county level may include public hospital organization and management, public health nursing services, and school health regulations.

Municipal Level. Policy decisions made at the municipal level of government affect citizens living or working within a specific city or town. Issues decided here may include items such as whether to have a separate tax for individuals who are employed, but do not reside, within city limits;

whether to change local zoning regulations; how to operate the public transportation system; and whether to provide specific additional services such as trash collection. Health care policy at the municipal level may include matters such as health insurance for city or town employees, control of communicable disease, public smoking and drinking ordinances, and surveillance of restaurants and schools for compliance with Board of Health requirements.

Types of Policy and Policy-makers

Policy decisions are made by those with the formal authority to choose which, if any, course of action to follow in order to achieve a specific goal. At every level of government, a variety of individuals may have authority or leverage on a particular type of policy.

Policy and the Chief Executive. A major role of the president or the governor of any state is that of chief executive. As chief executive, the president plays a leading role in the domestic policy-making process, and is a significant actor in the legislative process. Although not involved in passing legislation until the end of the process when a bill is signed or vetoed, the president, nevertheless, takes an active role by using the influence of the executive position to persuade the legislature to enact the policies the administration favors, including health policies. The power to veto legislation is also a significant power. A presidential veto usually acts to defeat a bill. It is possible for congress to override a veto, but the two-thirds vote necessary is difficult to obtain. The role of governor in state policy-making is analogous to the role of president at the federal level. Governors also have a significant role in influencing state legislatures to pass the legislation favored by the governor's administration.

Legislation and Legislators. Legislators are elected officials who represent groups of citizens. They vote on behalf of their constituents to enact laws within the area over which they have jurisdiction. While most municipal legislation is enacted by a single group of legislators, the federal government and all states, with the exception of Nebraska, have two groups of elected legislators. The so-called bicameral structure of federal and state legislative bodies commonly divides a legislature into two chambers, a Senate and a House of Representatives or Assembly. The passage of legislation generally depends on the approval of a majority of the members of each chamber.

Regulations and Public Administrators. Public administrators and public regulatory board members exist at all levels of government. Because of their specific areas of expertise, these individuals often recommend policy initiatives to legislators who then consider them for enactment. After a law is passed, public administrators and regulatory board members are usually responsible for interpreting broadly formulated laws and writing regulations to effect policy implementation.

Judicial Decisions and Judges. Judges also exist at all levels of government. They make decisions on the constitutionality of laws and on the interpretation of regulations when those are disputed. A judge may not influence the policy-making process by proposing legislation directly. Judges are also not involved in writing the regulations that guide policy implementation. The judicial system does not become involved in the policy process until *after* the constitutionality of a law or regulation is questioned by a citizen or a group of citizens. Thus the judicial system serves as one of the "checks and balances" on the legislative branch of government.

Legal Opinions and Attorneys General. Attorneys general exist at the federal and state levels of government. They offer interpretations of laws and often are called upon to assist in writing implementation regulations when clarification is requested by the responsible authorities. Attorneys general are also responsible for prosecuting those who have disregarded existing laws and regulations.

Values As the Basis for Policy

Policy decisions are based on relative rather than absolute values. While the rules of democracy determine the procedures for making policy in our society, values provide the foundation for the content of policy.

Groups within society often hold differing values. At times, the values of one group are in direct conflict with those held by a different group. For example, the values of the liquor industry are quite different from those held by the Mothers Against Drunk Driving; values held by those promoting a smoke-free society are in opposition to values held by tobacco manufacturers. Property owners often hold values that differ from members of rent-control coalitions.

Expedience, compromise, and trade-offs are important parts of the policy-making process. Members of special interest groups often concede portions of their policy platforms in return for concessions from groups with differing values and interests. Thus, policy formation is often incremental—a process of small, slow changes—rather than comprehensive in scope.

How Policy is Made

The process by which policy is made begins when, somewhere in society, an individual or a group of individuals with a common interest decide that a problem exists. The process ends when a solution is adopted and there is general agreement that the problem has been solved. The many small, important steps along the way can be grouped into four broad categories: policy formation, the legislative process, policy implementation, and policy evaluation.

Policy Formation. Because public policy deals with large, often multifaceted issues, policy decisions usually go through a seemingly complex series of political compromises and negotiations. Individuals who understand the steps in the process are better equipped to influence the outcome.

How Issues Arise. Many policy changes begin with an individual or group of individuals, perhaps with a common

IMPLICATIONS FOR PROFESSIONAL COLLABORATION

Collaborating on Legislation

One important way policy is made is through the legislative process. It is through this process that laws are enacted in a democratic system. For bills to pass successfully into law, a legislative sponsor is often necessary. A sponsor is a legislator who acts as a proponent for a bill as it moves through the legislative process. When a bill has a highly respected sponsor, it acquires prestige, and the influence of the sponsor makes it more likely that the bill will gain support. By getting to know their legislators, nurses are able to identify those who will act as proponents for nursing bills. Nurses are then in a position to collaborate with those who act as sponsors, and through mutual effort, move toward a successful policy outcome.

purpose, who note that a problem exists and determine that something ought to be done about it. Recent health care issues that were identified in this way include the American Medical Association's policy initiative to create a new category of health care providers, registered care technicians, as a possible solution to the problem created by the shortage of registered nurses. Another example is the effort by some citizens and government leaders in the United States to revitalize the issue of national health insurance, which, although it was high on the policy agenda in the 1960s, had not been a major policy concern for several years. With the increase in the number of people who lack private health insurance and the escalating costs of health care, the idea that the government should provide some level of basic health insurance for all US citizens has again become a health care issue.

Consensus Building. Once an issue is defined, the concerned individual or group of citizens then must find others who share the same concern. Locating others who agree with the policy initiative is called consensus-building. The greater the degree of initial agreement and the fewer competing interests, the easier it is to reach consensus. It is important to build a consensus that includes as many diverse groups as possible so that the issue becomes attractive to many segments of the population. For example, the WIC program—which provides supplemental nutrition to pregnant and nursing women, infants, and children up to 5 years of age—became a reality through the united efforts of two diverse groups: health care activists who sought to improve the nutrition of women and children, and farmers who sought to find a market for surplus crops.

Setting the Agenda. The next step in the policy process is to get an issue placed high enough on the policy agenda that it receives sufficient attention. In a world where many groups compete to have their issue receive highest priority, it is not possible for all issues to receive equal attention. Issues that rise to prominence on the policy agenda are those that receive attention; those that do not attract sufficient public interest remain in the background.

Because policy is made through a democratic process of incremental change, broad-sweeping, radical reforms are usually destined to fail. Good working relationships with key players and excellent group process skills are essential to a successful outcome. Rigid, all-or-nothing positions are almost certain to be unsuccessful. If change is to be meaningful and lasting, it comes as the result of consensus-building and compromise. Changes that are supported by a broad constituency are more likely to survive the legislative and implementation processes without major modification.

The Legislative Process. One important way in which policy is made is through the legislative process. The **legislative process** is the process through which policy ideas are converted into law. The authority for making law rests with the Congress of the United States and the state legislatures. While the precise steps of the legislative process differ at the local level from those at the federal level and from state to state, the general procedure is similar. Nurses need to know how the legislative process works in order to plan and implement strategies for influencing its outcome. Figure 4–1 illustrates the legislative process.

Ideas for Legislation. Every piece of legislation starts with an idea or a policy initiative. The idea for legislation may originate with the president of the United States, a legislator, an individual citizen, or a special interest group. Ideas for legislation pertaining to nursing often originate with the members of a professional nurses' association such as the American Nurses' Association at the federal level, or any of its state counterparts at the state level. Ideas may be vague

BUILDING NURSING KNOWLEDGE

How Is Nursing Research Important to Health Care Policy-making?

Hinshaw AS. Using research to shape health policy. *Nurs Outlook.* 1988; 36:21–24.

Research, Hinshaw contends, is one of the major tools nurses have for shaping health policy. Nursing is committed as a discipline to conduct research as a means of improving practice, but research is also one of nursing's major resources for influencing public policy on health care.

Hinshaw states that nursing research on the effect of health care policy on the individual client can be applied to influence policies in health care settings. Nursing research can also be used to change state, regional, or national rules that guide the delivery of health care.

For nurses to influence health policy, they must have certain values and perspectives concerning nursing research. They must value the use of research findings for policy objectives, be able to synthesize findings from narrow and broad areas of research, and assess the major concerns and health care needs of society and state nursing's particular perspective on those concerns and needs.

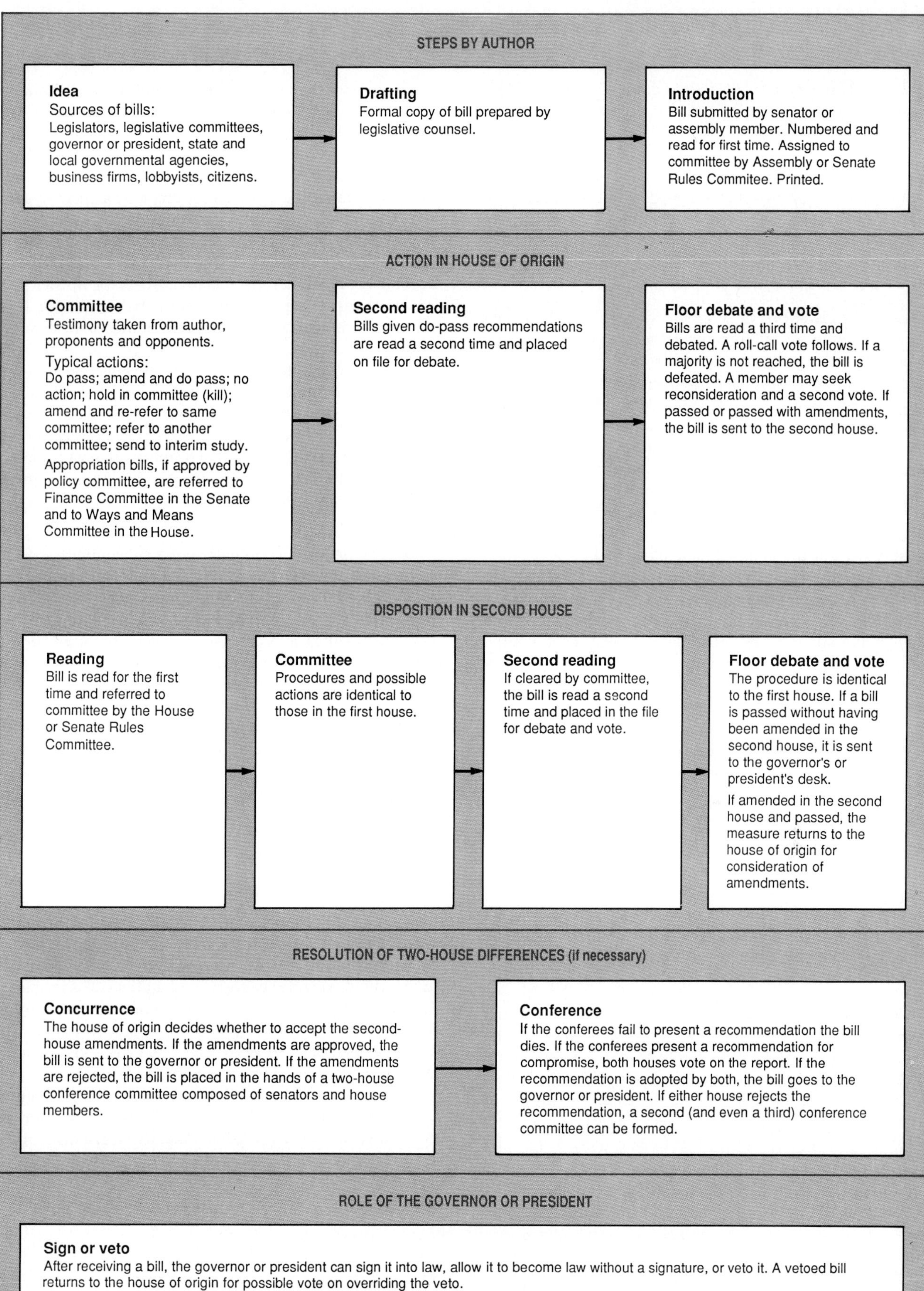

Figure 4–1. Legislative process.

initially, or they may be controversial, but an idea is always necessary to initiate the legislative process.

The development of ideas for legislation takes time, particularly when an idea is controversial. Generally, there is a period of germination during which the public becomes aware of the need for action.[2] It is during this period that professional associations can be helpful. Through the forum that associations give to legislative ideas, these ideas become developed into specific proposals, and public awareness and consensus are promoted.

Initiating Legislation. In some jurisdictions, a private citizen can introduce a bill into either house of the legislature; in others, bills must be sponsored by at least one legislator before they can be formally considered for adoption. It is wise to seek sponsors among members of the legislature, whether they are required or not, because legislators are unlikely to consider a bill seriously if it does not have support within the chamber. Seeking sponsors for a piece of legislation is an important step in the legislative process. Some members of congress have more power and evoke more respect than others. A highly respected sponsor adds prestige to a bill and makes it more likely that the legislation will gain additional sponsors.[3] On the other hand, a prestigious senator or representative may be a cosponsor of many bills and, unless he or she has a personal vested interest in a specific piece of legislation, may have limited time and energy to devote to any one bill. Sometimes a less well-known, but still respected, member of congress may have the necessary interest, time, and energy to devote to a piece of legislation to secure its passage. Many bills have multiple sponsors. When nurses know the members of their legislature well, they can identify which legislators would be the most effective sponsors of policy initiatives that are submitted as bills.

Drafting Legislation. Before a bill is formally introduced into the legislature it must be written in appropriate language. Legislative drafters, individuals with legal backgrounds, are responsible for ensuring that initiatives are worded correctly. These drafters may be employed by the federal or state governments, or may work for industry or special-interest groups.

Introducing Legislation. Bills may be introduced in either house of the legislature. Bills are numbered sequentially by the clerk of the appropriate chamber, and are usually referred to by either their number or working title. The letters preceding a bill's number indicate the chamber—house or senate—into which the piece of legislation was introduced.

Acting on Legislation

Legislative Committees. Each chamber has a defined committee structure to allow it to transact its business in an orderly fashion. The number and types of committees vary from one legislature to another.

Committees are the first bodies to formally consider a policy proposal. After a bill is introduced, it is referred to a committee. If more than one committee might appropriately consider the bill, the presiding officer of the chamber decides where it will go. This can be a crucial decision; where possible, it is important to enlist the support of the presiding officer. Committee chairs are always members of the party that holds a majority of seats in that chamber. They determine the agendas for committee meetings; thus they can, to a large degree, control how soon each piece of legislation reaches the committee floor for discussion and action. If a chairperson so chooses, he or she can refer a specific bill to numerous subcommittees for further study, effectively ensuring that it will never be voted upon by the entire committee. This is the fate of the vast majority of bills.

Nurses can follow the status of the bills that are important to them through identifying chairs of key legislative committees. By contacting the chairperson's office on a regular basis nurses gain critical information about when a bill might come up and who the proponents and opponents are. Committee chairs promote bills in a timely manner if they know that interested individuals are monitoring the status of a bill.

Public Hearings. If a committee or a subcommittee decides to consider a piece of legislation, it schedules public hearings on the bill. Proponents and opponents of the legislation present written and oral testimony to committee members at these hearings. Legislators have the opportunity to ask questions and seek clarification at this time. It is important for citizens to be present at public hearings when the issues being considered are vital to their personal interests. For example, when a public hearing is being held on a proposed housing development, those citizens who live in the immediate area should attend the hearing and present testimony on concerns they may have regarding the environmental impact of the proposed development, increased traffic on their streets, and inconveniences they anticipate during construction. Nurses' testimony is important on bills that directly or indirectly affect the practice of professional nursing.

In addition to information gained in public testimony, many legislators rely heavily on their staff to investigate policy proposals. Most representatives have legislative aides who deal with health-related matters. These aides are important persons for nurses to know because they may influence the legislator's opinion on a specific policy. Good working relationships with legislative aides can be as important as good relationships with legislators.

After legislators hear testimony and read staff reports, the entire committee votes on the bill. If a bill is defeated in committee it goes no further, and the legislative process stops. The bill can be reintroduced in a subsequent legislative session, but no action is possible until then. If the bill is passed, it is sent to the second house for consideration.

Floor Debate. Once all subcommittees and committees charged with considering a bill approve it, the bill comes to the floor of the chamber. Further debate is held at this time, and members may speak for or against the bill. Individuals and groups usually lobby key legislators to enlist their support for the bill at this time. Because all members of the legislature are not equally knowledgeable about all areas of public policy, they often depend on those with more expertise to guide them on specific issues. Specifically, legislators may seek professional opinions. Many nurses who have formed effective working relationships with their legislators report that, after a while, their legislators began consulting them about how to vote on health-related legislation.

Conference Committees. If the bill is passed by the first chamber of the legislature, it is then sent to the second chamber, where the process is repeated. Changes are often made in bills when they are considered by the second chamber. This is especially true when the same political party does not hold a majority of seats in both houses. If different versions of a bill are passed in each house, the bill is then referred to a joint conference committee, consisting of members of both chambers specifically appointed to resolve differences between the two versions of the bill. The members of the conference committee often must make compromises in the bill to ensure its passage by both chambers. At this time, proponents and opponents of the bill stay in close contact with members of the conference committee to lobby for or against proposed compromises in the legislation. It is important to remember that points often must be ceded both by proponents and opponents in order to ensure passage of the bill. After a bill is revised and agreed to by the members of the conference committee, it is returned to each chamber for a final vote. The revised bill must pass both chambers with the identical language.

Signing Legislation. After a bill is passed by both chambers it is sent to the chief executive for signature. A governor or the president may sign a bill into law or may elect to veto it. Vetoes may be overridden if the legislation is subsequently passed with a two-thirds majority in both branches of the legislature.

Authorizing and Appropriating Legislation. If a bill has a fiscal impact, money must be appropriated in the budget for any costs associated with the legislation. The legislation creating the program is called **authorizing legislation,** and the legislation providing the funds is called **appropriating legislation.** Many programs that are authorized by congress never come to fruition because opponents are successful in defeating fiscal appropriations. Funds for a program must be included in the appropriate budget every fiscal year in order to ensure that the program continues. Some legislatures have "sunset" provisions that automatically terminate programs if they are not reviewed and resubmitted to the legislature after a designated period of time.

Policy Implementation. Once a bill is enacted into law and funds for its programs are appropriated, it must be placed into action. **Policy implementation** is the process by which changes mandated by legislation become incorporated into society. After a bill becomes a law, it is assigned to an appropriate federal or state agency for implementation. The responsible agency develops implementation regulations for each program or law that it is responsible for administering.

> **IMPLICATIONS FOR PROFESSIONAL COLLABORATION**
>
> **Collaborating on Regulations**
>
> Regulations are prescribed rules of conduct or procedure. Laws are often broad and general, but regulations are specific and define how the principles of the law are to be incorporated into our lives. Most states have one or more bodies or agencies responsible for formulating regulations to implement health care policy decisions. The state board of nursing is one of those bodies. Often the state board's decisions influence some aspect of the nurse's role and thus bear on professional collaboration. By presenting testimony to the state board of nursing, nurses can share their concerns and ideas about issues before the board and help to shape the regulatory policies that affect them.

What is a Regulation? A **regulation** is a prescribed rule of conduct or procedure. While the wording of a law is often broad and general, regulations specify how the principles of the law are to be incorporated into our lives. Regulations implement and supplement legislation. The Medicare program was enacted in 1964. After its passage, the Social Security Administration was given the responsibility for developing the regulations necessary to implement the program. The regulations are very specific and define who is eligible for benefits, describe how individuals apply for entry into the program, delineate how individuals and health care providers submit claims, and determine how rates of payment are calculated.

Why are Regulations Necessary? A great deal of discussion, negotiation, and compromise occurs during the policy-making process. Many bills must be introduced during several legislative sessions before they become laws. Often the language of the final bill is the result of concessions negotiated in a conference committee hearing. While laws are general, regulations clearly delineate how the various stipulations of law are to be enacted, who must comply with its provisions, and what penalties will be levied on those who do not conform to the rules. Thus, without accompanying regulations, the practical implementation of laws would be very difficult.

Role of Regulatory Bodies in Policy Implementation. Regulatory agencies, boards, and commissions exist at all levels of government and are responsible for implementing and enforcing policy decisions. Nurses should be especially interested in those agencies and boards concerned with policy decisions on health care.

Federal and State Agencies. **Agencies** are departments within the government's organizational structure. The officials employed by agencies are appointed and often have civil service appointments. Many key workers within agencies remain in their positions beyond the terms of those of elected officials, and thus are less sensitive to political pressures than are representatives who must seek reelection to their positions on a periodic basis. There are a variety of important agencies that are responsible for implementing and enforcing health policy decisions.

The federal agency responsible for health policy is the Department of Health and Human Services. This large, complex agency develops regulations and monitors compliance with the majority of federal health policy decisions. The department official responsible for drafting regulations may consult with congressional staff, officials of other federal, state, and local agencies, and representatives from appropriate professional and consumer groups. Draft regulations are printed in the *Federal Register,* a publication that informs the public about federal activities. Interested persons may submit written comments to suggest revisions in the draft regulations. These comments are reviewed and may result in changes in the draft regulations. The final regulations are then published in the *Federal Register* 1 month before their effective date.

Most states have one or more agencies responsible for implementing health policy decisions. In many states this responsibility is delegated to the Department of Public Health. While the specific steps in the process will vary from state to state, regulations are almost always drafted, reviewed, and revised to ensure that they accurately reflect the intent of the legislation they are implementing.

Federal and State Boards and Commissions. **Boards** and **commissions** are composed of appointed individuals who are charged with the responsibility of overseeing a specific activity. Many times the creation of the board or commission is one part of the legislation enacting the policy decision. The National Labor Relations Board is one example of a federal board. This board is responsible for issuing and overseeing regulations related to unions and collective bargaining activities. The board defines who may belong to unions, the rights of labor and management, under what conditions strikes may occur, and rules governing the arbitration of employer–employee disagreements. Nurses who work in jobs regulated by collective bargaining contracts agree to abide by the rulings of the National Labor Relations Board.

Every state, district, and US territory has a board of nursing registration. The state board of nursing formulates regulations to implement statutes in the state's Nurse Practice Act. The authority of the board of nursing is prescribed by the state legislature and is defined in the state's Nurse Practice Act. By presenting testimony to the state board, nurses can share their concerns and constructive criticism about issues before the board and, in so doing, may influence formulation and interpretation of regulations. In this way, nurses ensure that their nurse practice acts accurately reflect the current status of professional nursing practice.

The Citizen's Role in Policy Implementation. As it formulates regulations, an agency may be subject to strong pressure from individuals and groups that desire the development of regulations that would substantially modify the intent of the original sponsors of the bill. Federal agency regulations are published in the *Federal Register* and may be responded to by groups that have an interest in how a law is implemented. Each state has its own mechanism for developing implementation regulations. Figure 4–2 illustrates the process for formulating regulations.

Nurses can benefit when they monitor legislation that affects them as it goes through the regulatory process. It is often possible to alter the original intent of a law substantially through the wording of regulations. For example, in recent years, the regulations for family-planning programs mandated that parental consent be obtained from all adolescents who sought contraception at federally funded clinics. Family planning program activists were dismayed at the wording and expended considerable effort in attempts to change the regulations. The autonomy of the board of nursing has been challenged in several states; to date nurses have lobbied successfully to prevent the dissolution of discrete boards of nursing.

Governmental bodies that interpret laws, issue regulations, and evaluate citizens' compliance with the law have enormous power. Having collegial relationships with state and federal bureaucrats can be valuable for nursing groups that wish to ensure that laws and regulations affecting nursing are interpreted and enforced appropriately.

The Judicial Process and Policy Implementation. Even after the implementation criteria are adopted, funding is ensured, and the program has begun, stumbling blocks may still exist. Local bureaucrats may choose to ignore the new legislation or may place it low on their list of priorities. Citizens sometimes need to seek legal recourse to ensure that they receive their legislated benefits. Opponents frequently challenge the rights of the local authorities to enforce legislation that they see as infringing upon their individual rights. For example, recent no-smoking legislation has angered smokers who feel that their individual freedom has been violated. Many communities have actively enforced smoke-free environments; others have adopted a more laissez-faire approach. If a piece of legislation is highly controversial, it may end up in judicial hearings for several years.

Opponents of a law may question its constitutionality and request a hearing before the appropriate judicial authority. A court may decide whether or not to hear arguments challenging the constitutionality of a law. Such "test cases" are often widely publicized. Individuals may appeal judicial decisions up to the level of the US Supreme Court.

Policy Evaluation. **Policy evaluation** is the process by which a policy is examined to determine whether or not the regulations in force are adequately addressing the problem they were created to solve. For example, when the speed limit on federal highways was reduced to a maximum of 55 miles per hour, it was anticipated that this policy would reduce gasoline consumption and the number of fatal motor vehicle accidents.

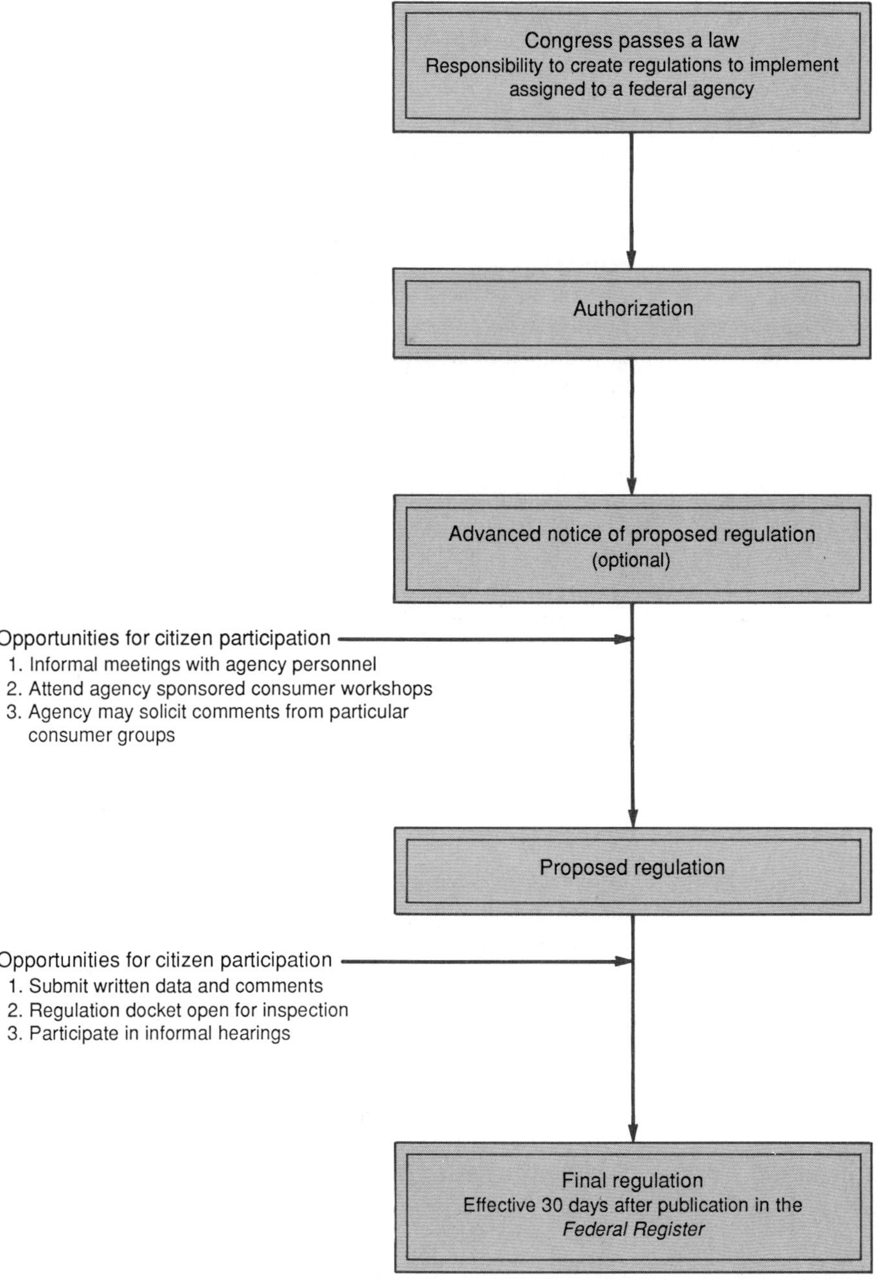

Figure 4–2. The process of making federal regulations.

Importance. It is important to know whether a policy works. Most policies have a cost associated with their implementation. Dollars spent on any particular policy initiative are unavailable for other uses. Citizens need to know that their taxes are being spent prudently. In the previous example of the 55-mile-per-hour speed limit, was the speed limit change effective in reducing gasoline consumption and did it prevent deaths associated with high-speed motor vehicle accidents? Was it an effective policy, or should it be changed? For example, if law enforcement officers were monitoring compliance with the speed limit and were therefore unavailable for other police activities, it would be necessary to hire additional police officers and purchase additional patrol cars to enforce the 55-mile-per-hour speed limit. Unless taxes were raised, less money would then be available for fire fighting, school teachers' salaries, and other municipal expenses. On the other hand, if the law was not enforced and drivers were allowed to exceed the federally mandated speed limit, the municipality might be ineligible for federal highway funds.

Health Care Policy Evaluation. Health care is second only to national defense in its cost to the public. It is important to continually determine whether current health care policies are achieving the goals they were intended to accomplish. Does the current health care financing system ensure that those who provide health care are reimbursed appropriately? Do those who pay for health care get the most benefit from the dollars they spend? Is the current system working? Where are the problems? These are all questions that might be asked as health care policies are evaluated.

On a smaller scale, individual programs must be evaluated periodically, particularly laws enacting specific programs that have "sunset" clauses in their provisions. Failing reauthorization, these programs cease to exist. Thus, sunset laws require that programs be examined periodically. Nurses can assist policy evaluation when they are aware of their role in collaborating with consumers and other health care providers. By virtue of their professional experience, nurses are in a good position to evaluate the utility of current health care policies. Such professional appraisals are valuable to the legislators and government officials who are responsible for deciding the fate of public programs.

Levels of Government, Types of Policy-makers and Policy-making in Canada

The Canadian system of government is similar to the system in the United States in that it is a democratic system with certain structural counterparts to US bodies such as a large federal government and a series of 10 regional, state-like governments, called provinces. The Canadian system differs from that of the United States, however, in that it is a parliamentary system, a feature derived from Canada's history as part of the British Commonwealth of Nations. A parliamentary system is characterized by a split in the executive aspect of government between the formal executive (the governor general) and the political executive (the prime minister). The parliamentary system is also characterized by the fact that there is a fusion between the executive and the legislative aspect of government, and the principle of the separation of powers that operates in the US system does not apply in Canada.[4]

Similar to the US, the Canadian system has federal, provincial, and municipal levels, which, as in the US, form the policies governing their respective jurisdictions. The federal government is bicameral, and is comprised of a Senate and a House of Commons. Although a recent proposal would make the Canadian Senate an elected body, its members traditionally have been appointed by the governor general on the advice of the prime minister.

The House of Commons, which is much more important than the Senate legislatively, has its members elected directly by the voters. Similar to the houses of the US Congress, the House of Commons has a series of standing committees, including one for health, that considers legislation in the bill-to-law process. All legislation undergoes six stages: first reading, second reading, committee stage, third reading, consideration by the other house, and royal assent. Any member of parliament of either house can introduce legislation; however, it is the bills introduced by the ruling party that are usually passed. Once a bill is passed by one of the houses of the legislature, the same basic steps are repeated by the other house. Rarely is there conflict, however, and, if there is, the House of Commons usually asserts its power and carries the decision. Royal assent is the approval given by the governor general to legislation once it is passed, and has never been refused to a piece of federal legislation.[4]

Canadians vote for representatives of the political party of their choice, who then become members of parliament (MPs). The leader of the party winning the majority of the parliamentary seats becomes the prime minister, the key political actor in Canadian politics. The prime minister not only leads the ruling party in establishing its policy agenda, he or she also recommends individuals to the British Monarch for appointment to the office of governor general, and is responsible for selection and organization of the ministerial cabinet (including the federal ministry of health), which under the influence of the prime minister, directs public policy. As the Canadian system has evolved, power over public policy is decidedly concentrated in the role of the prime minister.[4]

Canada's provincial parliaments each have a single house which works much like the federal parliament. Representatives to the provincial parliaments are elected. The lieutenant governors who head the provincial parliaments are appointed by the federal government. The Canadian provinces have broad constitutional authority to tax citizens and corporations, and to spend revenues on programs such as provincial health insurance plans, and play a substantial role in the administration of these programs through the provincial ministeries of health[5] (see Chapter 37 for more on the Canadian system of health finance).

The Canadian judicial system, federal and provincial, plays a role in policy-making that is similar to the role of the US judiciary. Since 1949, the Supreme Court of Canada has been the highest court of appeal. As in the United States, judicial decisions are an important ingredient in the evolution of public policy.

■ POLITICS AND POLICY-MAKING

What is Politics?

Politics refers to activities used by groups to exert control over their common affairs. Politics involves the use of power for change.[1] Because several constituencies compete for the same resources in the policy arena, the political process is necessary to determine who gets what, and in what amount. The political process is the means by which conflicting demands and desires for the allocation of resources are resolved.

Importance of the Vote in Establishing Public Policy

Voting may be viewed as the way decisions are made in our political system. Most members of congress wish to be returned to their seats in future elections, and know that in order to do so they must preserve support among their constituents. Voting is also the way our elected officials make allocation decisions. Influencing officials who do the voting, or lobbying, is one way in which citizens determine the outcome of the policy process.

Majority Rule in a Democracy

Importance of Numbers. In the democratic political system, the majority rules and no single vote counts more than any other vote. While the role of individuals cannot be underestimated there is also truth in the statement that there is strength in numbers. When nurses, as members of professional organizations, unite as special interest groups, their impact is great. The entire political system is sensitive to numbers. Hunter and Berger note that "the political impact of any special interest group rests with its ability to get out a sizable vote and to mobilize its members when critical issues are at stake."[6] There are, on average, 5000 registered nurse voters in every congressional district. Many congressional seats are won or lost by fewer than 5000 votes. If a congressional candidate were able to win the unified support of registered nurses in his or her district, the outcome of the election could shift. It is just within the past decade that nurses have become active in local and national politics. As the largest group of health care professionals in the country, nurses as a collective can have a powerful voice in deciding how public policy is made and implemented.

Importance of the Individual. Although the majority rules in a democracy, it is individuals that make up majorities. No collective voice is possible without the participation of each member. For a collective voice to be established it takes the commitment of individuals who, one by one, let their wishes be known. In a democracy, power is established by the accumulation of votes—one man or woman, one vote. Thus the role of the individual in a democracy is extremely important.

Political Tools for Influencing Policy-makers

Lobbying. Lobbying may be defined as actions that are undertaken in an effort to influence the outcome of a decision. In the political process, lobbying is the attempt to influence public policy.

Lobbying is a visible, effective way for individuals or a group of citizens to have an impact on issues affecting them. Legislators are elected to represent their constituents. Lobbying is one way constituents have of sharing their views with their elected representative. It is important that legislators be aware of constituents' perspectives so that they can make policy decisions that accurately reflect the view of those the legislator has been elected to represent.

Types of Lobbying. Lobbying may be done by individual citizens or by professional lobbyists. Citizen lobbying is accomplished by individual citizens who voluntarily contact legislators to share their views on specific policy issues that are being considered by the legislature. Because of their professional expertise, nurses are excellent citizen lobbyists, and this activity is an integral part of the role of the professional nurse.

Professional lobbying is performed by individuals who are employees of public relations or law firms, or by individuals who are self-employed as independent lobbyists. The professional lobbyist is paid to represent the concerns of a particular constituency within society. The responsibility of the professional lobbyist is to monitor political activity that may have a potential effect on that constituency's interests and to attempt to influence the outcome of the policy-making process in a way that is advantageous to the group employing the professional lobbyist.

Forms of Lobbying. Lobbyists use a variety of ways to attempt to influence policy-makers. One of the most effective ways is by giving testimony at public hearings. **Testimony,** which may be written or oral, is a public means of sharing information with all of those who will be involved in the policy-making process. Written testimony becomes a part of the permanent record of the public hearing. Oral testimony, which is often a verbal emphasis of key points in the written testimony, is transcribed into the record of the hearing as well. Legislators have the opportunity to ask questions of the lobbyist who is presenting oral testimony.

Meeting with policy-makers is another effective form of lobbying. Legislators welcome the opportunity to meet their constituents and hear their views on policy issues. Policy-makers know that, in order to maintain their positions, they must have the support of their constituency. They welcome the opportunity to learn the views of their constituents on policy issues. A personal visit to a local policy-maker, an elected state legislator, or a national representative gives the lobbyist the opportunity to share individual or organizational perspectives on policy issues.

Writing and calling policy-makers are also effective lobbying strategies. Policy-makers, in an attempt to accurately reflect the interests of their constituents, often make voting decisions based on the volume of letters and telephone calls from voters in their home district.

Special Interests and Lobbying. A group that has a vested interest in the outcome of policy decisions is called a **special interest group.** These groups maintain ongoing lobbying relationships with policy-makers. An example of one such group is the tobacco industry. There is clear evidence that cigarette smoking is unhealthy. Many citizen groups have lobbied for a smoke-free society and would favor legislation prohibiting the use of cigarettes. If this legislation were passed, the tobacco industry would be substantially weakened. Lobbyists representing the special interests of this industry maintain a constant presence in Washington, and attempt to prevent antismoking legislation by informing representatives of the economic ruin that would occur in tobacco-growing and manufacturing states if such laws were passed. Many other special interest groups maintain active lobbying presences in Washington. Special interest groups also maintain visible lobbying profiles in state capitals and, to lesser degrees, in local communities.

Coalitions. A **coalition** is a group of individuals or organizations that has temporarily come together for the purpose of collectively working toward a common policy goal. Groups often form coalitions around issues in which they have a collective interest. Because coalition members have unique, as well as common, interests, they often have spheres of influence that surpass those of any single member of the coalition. Thus coalitions often have enhanced ability to influence policy-makers.

Political Favors/Boycotts. Political favors are given by individuals and groups when they contribute to campaign funds, volunteer to work in campaigns, or vote for candidates for public office. Requesting returns on favors previously given is a common and highly effective way of influencing policy-makers. Another highly visible and effective way of influencing policy-makers is through a boycott or the threat of a boycott. A **boycott** is the organized refusal to deal with a person or organization to achieve certain goals. Recently the Massachusetts state legislature cut the budget of public colleges and universities in the state. Students boycotted classes and demonstrated at the state capitol in an effort to curb the budget cuts. Their message to the state legislature was delivered clearly and effectively.

The Electoral Process and Policy-making

Policy is made by elected public officials. Individual citizens who vote to elect officials to public office are selecting those individuals who will be making policy decisions during the time they remain in office.

Importance of a Candidate's Policy Positions. During political campaigns, candidates develop political platforms that delineate their positions on a variety of issues. Citizens read these platforms to identify each candidate's position on policy areas that are important to them. Citizens then vote for the candidate who is most likely to have a suitable position on issues that are most important to that individual citizen.

IMPLICATIONS FOR PROFESSIONAL COLLABORATION

Coalitions

Nursing is a large profession, and its 1.7 million members represent a substantial amount of political power. As a collective body, nursing has a powerful voice for influencing health care policy. When nurses speak with one voice they are often successful in achieving their policy goals. Whenever nurses collaborate with others who have a similar policy interest and join with them in coalitions around a common issue, their voice is amplified.

Incumbent candidates running for reelection know that their voting record is available for public scrutiny. Representatives cannot misrepresent the interests of their constituents on a regular basis and expect to be returned to office.

There are several ways to become informed about the differences among several candidates' positions on public policy issues. Community groups such as the League of Women Voters often sponsor gatherings at which citizens can meet candidates for public office and hear them present their platforms. Televised debates have become a routine part of political campaigns in many national and regional contests. Candidates often attend nonpolitical community functions in order to have the opportunity to meet with constituents and share their positions on policy issues.

Tools for Influencing the Electoral Process. Individuals and citizens have a variety of vehicles they may use to influence the outcome of the electoral process.

Political Action Committees. **Political action committees** are groups of individuals who agree to work together to elect candidates who agree to support the policy interests of the group in return for the support. Many state nurses' associations have independent political action committees that work to elect candidates who have policy positions supportive of nurses' interests. Many major industries and labor groups also have political action committees that work to ensure the election of candidates with compatible policy positions.

Campaign Contributions. Another way to influence the outcome of the electoral process is through campaign contributions. Political campaigns, especially for statewide or national office, are extraordinarily expensive, and candidates need broad-based financial support in order to be successful. Donors of any amount often find that their names have been placed on candidates' mailing lists, and they will continue to receive communication from the candidate for prolonged periods of time.

Grass-roots Campaign Participation. One of the most personally rewarding ways to influence the electoral process is through grass-roots campaign participation. Stuffing envelopes, answering telephones at campaign headquarters, distributing leaflets, and soliciting support for candidates make the political process personal and alive. Working together with others who share the same goal can be exciting and enjoyable.

■ EFFECTING CHANGE THROUGH USE OF POWER

What is Change?

Change is the process by which the normal course of events is altered. While change is constantly occurring in our environment, planned change is courageous, and involves risk-taking behavior. The steps in the change process are quite similar to the steps in the nursing process; indeed, application of the nursing process is an example of a planned change (see Chap. 15).

Problem-solving and the Need for Change

The Process of Change. Lippitt and associates[7] have developed a theory of change that depicts change as rational. This rational model of change characterizes change as a methodical, rational process. Natapoff and Loetterle[8] note that change theory is the basis of the nursing process, the decision-making framework upon which nursing practice is built. Thus, in order to effectively practice the profession of nursing, it is important for nurses to understand the rational process of change.

The first step of the process, assessment, is what Lippitt and associates describe as identifying the need for change, and clarifying and diagnosing a system's problem. During this phase, the scope of the problem is recognized.

The planning phase may be likened to what Lippitt and co-workers refer to as examining alternative routes and establishing goals. During this phase, alternative solutions are identified and the consequences of implenting each alternative are weighed.

Implementation occurs during the stages that transform intentions into actual change efforts. It is during this stage of the change process that the preferred solution is put into action.

BUILDING NURSING KNOWLEDGE

How Effective Are Nursing Organizations in the Political Arena?

Burda D. Nursing lobby exerting newfound power in Washington. *Mod Healthcare.* 1987; 28–30.

This article discusses nursing organizations and their ability to influence public policy, and notes that the unity developing within nursing organizations is changing the way health care politics is played at the national level. Burda states that professional groups in nursing are now more effective because they have learned to speak with one voice to the federal government. Historically, nurses have not been able to reach a consensus on the key issues affecting the profession and have focused on internal conflicts rather than national concerns. Nursing organizations are now having more influence on legislators and more success in getting legislation passed. Nursing organizations' effectiveness also has been enhanced by their ability to work with other health care groups to build coalitions.

Burda argues that ongoing success in policy-making will depend on nursing's continued solidarity; however, unity is likely to be challenged again by internal pressures. One pressure that is particularly divisive is the struggle over the appropriate education of entry-level nurses. This issue has the potential to cause a decline in the membership of nursing's major lobbying group, the American Nurses' Association.

BUILDING NURSING KNOWLEDGE

What Political Skills Do Nurses Have for Facilitating Social Change?

Rains JW. Nursing and politics: Adapting skills to spark social change. *Nurs Health Care.* 1988; 299–301.

This article notes that without special training nurses already possess many of the political skills required to produce social change. Rains argues that nurses have the skills to contribute knowledge to health care policy-making, are uniquely well prepared to discern the underlying values in complicated health care issues, generate new knowledge on such issues through their research, and communicate health care needs convincingly. Rains also asserts that nurses are more savvy in providing information to the right people through their writing and speaking skills.

Rains notes that building power is the one skill nurses need to acquire. Some nurses have personal or professional aversions to power, yet power is a necessary ingredient for social change. Power can be built through establishing relationships with legislators, maintaining memberships in professional organizations, and gaining public offices themselves. The power of office is extremely important to promoting health issues in society. Rains concludes that nurses have the opportunity to see a vision of a healthier way of life and that the political means to pursue that vision is within their reach.

Finally, evaluation occurs during the phases of generalization and stabilization of change and termination of the relationship. During this stage of the process the results are reviewed to assess whether the solution that was implemented solved the original problem in a satisfactory manner.

Models of Change. There are two basic models of change, the rational model and the political model. The rational approach to change assumes that for any situation that requires action or for any problem that requires a solution, there is a single, "best" plan that can be identified by rigorously studying the situation and examining alternatives. It is apparent in understanding the rational process that it would require time and resources to formulate an ideal approach for every problem or situation requiring action, and resources are often scarce. Moreover, seldom is there only one answer to a problem, and in a pluralistic society where people and groups differ in their values, there is often disagreement about whose plan is truly rational.[9] Therefore, another approach to change, the political approach, is also important whenever people interact to effect change—in organizations, in the workplace, and in government.

The political model of change depicts change as occurring as the result of a political or democratic process. Thus, those who wish to effect change formulate a "good enough" plan—one that may not be the product of meticulous study, but that is thought to be workable. They then endeavor to influence others to accept their plan.[10] Change occurs through a process of consensus or majority rule. Bennis and associates state that the effectiveness of political change depends on the quality of the democratic process to reflect accurately the wishes and desires of those governed.[11]

In *The Dance of Legislation*,[12] Redman describes the process of political change. Using the example of the National Health Service Bill, Redman discusses how change is enacted through politics. The maneuvering, scheming, and give-and-take of the political process are likened to the steps of a minuet.

Types of Change.

Radical Change. As described by Kuhn,[13] **radical change** occurs when current explanations for how things should work no longer adequately explain what is occurring. When this happens, according to Kuhn, people tend to reject the entire political order and search for a completely new system. During the period of transition from one system to its successor, chaos and disorganization often prevail.

Incremental Change. A second type of change is **incremental change.** With the incremental model, change occurs in a small, step-by-step fashion. Marginal changes are made to the existing model without radically altering the entire infrastructure. Many individuals feel that it is easier to deal with change when it happens in small steps because they have the opportunity to adapt to each small change before the next one occurs. Incremental change is a characteristic of the policy-making process in a democratic system.

Resistance to Change and the Role of Power

Reasons Change is Resisted. By nature, most people are resistant to change. One of the major reasons is fear of the unknown. Most people have achieved a level of comfort with that which they know. If change occurs, people are not always sure what the consequences of that change will be. Predictability is more comfortable and less stressful than the unpredictability and uneasiness of the yet-to-be tried.

A second reason why change is resisted is that people have a vested interest in the status quo. Those who benefit from the current system may fear that they will benefit less if change occurs. Resistance to change may be for political, economic, or personal reasons. It is often hard to see how one might benefit from a new system if the impression is that the current one is working to one's advantage. Even those who apparently are not receiving maximum benefits from the present system may feel that their interests will be less well served were the system to change.

Importance of Power in Achieving Change. **Power** is the ability to do or act. Bagwell and Clements[14] define power as "the ability to influence the behavior of other people" (p. 5). Powerful people have the ability to control and influence other people in ways that produce desired effects. In politics, power includes the ability to mobilize individuals, special interest groups, and legislators to support a policy initiative from the time of its conceptualization through the political process until it achieves its desired effect.

Sources of Power. Power is derived from a variety of sources. Wieland and Ullrich[15] propose five possible sources of power: legitimate power, reward power, coercive power, expert power, and referent power.

Legitimate Power. **Legitimate power** is that power inherent in a particular role or position. For example, the dean of a school of nursing may, since he or she is the dean, have the power to hire a new faculty member and determine the salary that the instructor will receive.

Reward Power. **Reward power** is defined as the ability of the person in power to grant benefits to achieve a desired result. A politician may appoint individuals who have supported his or her campaign to positions within government. These rewards would not be available for distribution if the politician were not in power.

Coercive Power. **Coercive power,** or the use of punishments, is the opposite of reward power. Parents may use either reward or coercive power in an attempt to achieve desired modifications of their children's behavior. Elected officials have the power to remove from office officials appointed by previous office-holders.

Expert Power. **Expert power** is the ability to influence knowledge and information. Politicians, while expected to vote on a wide variety of issues, often do not have sufficient information to make knowledgeable decisions. Those from whom they seek advice have expert power derived from professional knowledge. Nurses, by virtue of their education and experience, have considerable expert power.

Referent Power. **Referent power** is the power to influence based on the force of a person's or an organization's reputation. It is the power ascribed to an individual or group by external sources such as the media. Thus, although a particular group may not have legitimate or expert power, the public's perception of that group as powerful may be due to the public image the group has acquired over time.

There are other sources of power as well as those described by Wieland and Ullrich.

Personal Power. Many individuals have great personal power. **Personal power** is an ability to influence derived from the force of an individual's personality. Charismatic and convincing speakers who are able to influence others often possess this type of power. Some individuals believe that, due to the increasing prominence of television coverage of political campaigns, we are more likely to elect candidates who exude personal power.

Collective Power. **Collective power,** manifested in professionalism and social unity, can be a significant source of power. Considerable social change may be derived from organized group efforts. Civil rights, the women's movement, and efforts to ban cigarette smoking in public places are some examples of policy initiatives that have been furthered by the concerted efforts of groups of individuals who have rallied to support a common concern.

Use of Power for Changing Nursing and Health Care

Power is most productive when it is used to effect positive change. There are many spheres in which nurses can exercise power to effect change. Local, state, and federal governmental regulations affect almost all aspects of our lives. This is especially true of our professional practice. Selected examples of how government affects nursing practice are given below, along with suggested ways nursing can influence public policy. An exhaustive list would be impossible, and the reader is challenged to identify additional areas in which nursing might successfully influence policy decisions.

Third-party Payment for Nurses. The federal government, through its Medicare and Medicaid expenditures, is currently the largest third-party payer for health care. Like other third-party payers, the federal government decides what services it will cover, which providers it will reimburse, and what share of health care must be borne by consumers. Nursing has, for several years, been seeking direct third-party reimbursement for nurses practicing in certain expanded roles. Through this change the delivery of nursing services could be substantially expanded.

Government Subsidies for Nursing Education. When the demand for professional nursing services exceeds the supply of available nurses, a shortage exists. During previous nursing shortages the federal government has subsidized nurses' education in an effort to encourage more women and men to enter the profession or to pursue advanced education. Because policy initiatives such as affirmative action have succeeded in making more prestigious, higher-paying, previously male-dominated occupations more accessible to women, fewer women are opting for careers in nursing. The number of men choosing nursing as a profession has not increased in corresponding numbers. Many nursing leaders believe that the federal government should intervene to make nursing education an attractive alternative through tuition subsidies and grants to schools of nursing. Nurses can use their organizational power to further the expansion of this policy initiative.

Funding of Nursing Research. The establishment of the Center for Nursing Research within the National Institutes of Health has placed nursing research in close proximity to other health-related research. This move should increase the quantity of nursing research directed toward clinical problems, and will certainly influence the future direction of nursing practice. Nurses can exert influence to secure sufficient funding for the Center for Nursing Research to operate at a level comparable to other centers within the National Institutes of Health.

Health and Safety Law. Power can be executed to effect change at the state level as well. Nurses have an interest in social change that promotes the health and well-being of clients. Professional associations use their power to support health care initiatives. For instance, infant car-seat laws, seat belt legislation, and laws regulating smoking in enclosed public spaces are all examples of legislative initiatives for social change that nurses have vigorously supported.

Community Health. Nurses can also exert power in the local community. County health services, environmental protection and hazardous waste disposal, after-school activities for children, and community day care for children of working parents are all issues in which nurses, in collaboration with their clients, can use their power to ensure that the public's health is maintained and enhanced.

Changes in the Workplace. Nurses can exert power in other local spheres as well. Serving on an interdisciplinary committee within a hospital or a collegiate setting enables individual nurses to influence those who make decisions that affect nursing practice either directly or indirectly. A physician who admits clients to a hospital unit, a university dean who allocates faculty resources in a large university, or a social worker who helps coordinate client discharges, can all be the targets for political action by an individual nurse.

■ POWER AND POLITICS IN THE WORKPLACE

Need for Change in the Workplace

Many of the issues and strategies discussed above are just as applicable in the workplace as in the legislature. Policy initiatives may arise with individual nurses or interdisciplinary teams at the organization or unit level, or may emanate from the director's office. Change at any level in the system may give rise to new policies, and change from outside the system may require policy initiatives to implement new regulations. Political activity within the workplace is, for many nurses, the first step to involvement in the external political arena.

Employer–Employee Relations

Within the workplace, nurses often have the opportunity to become politically active. Nurses, as professionals, are granted a certain measure of autonomy in their practice by society. Autonomous professionals are expected to use independent judgment to control the scope of professional practice and to negotiate with clients on an individual basis. In reality, however, most nurses work for bureaucracies which exercise significant control over working conditions and professional practice.

Before 1974, the National Labor Relations Act specifically excluded nurses and other professional groups from bargaining collectively for working conditions. The act was changed in 1974, allowing nurses and other health care professionals to organize as labor collectives.

Collective Bargaining. The process by which an organized group of employees negotiates with an employer to define the conditions of employment is called **collective bargaining.** Nurses who are members of collective bargaining units select a bargaining agent (sometimes called unions) to represent them during negotiations where representatives of management are present. Issues negotiated in contracts include such items as salary, working conditions, employee benefits, retirement benefits, seniority rights, and other clauses important to both parties.

Who Should Represent Nurses? When an institution's nurses decide to become members of a collective bargaining unit, they often have several choices for representation. Many nurses are represented by the Professional Economic and General Welfare (PE & GW) division of their state Nurses' Association. Other nurses elect professional labor unions as their bargaining agents. The selection of a bargaining agent may be even more critical than the decision to organize a collective bargaining unit. Professional nursing organizations may not have the years of experience and fiscal resources of traditional unions, but collectives that represent nurses together with truck drivers, meat packers, and paper hangers may be concerned only with salary and benefits issues. Issues relating to the practice of professional nursing within bureaucratic settings may be best represented to management by agents that exclusively represent professional nurses.

Should Nurses Organize Collectively? This question has been debated among nurses for over a decade. Jacox[16] believes that collective bargaining through a professional association is one way for the profession to gain control over practice issues. While there is no agreement on this issue, the number of nurses who work in institutions where they are members of collective bargaining units is substantial. Nurses have successfully used the tools of collective bargaining, including striking, to significantly improve salaries and working conditions.

The regulations governing the formation, organization, and operation of collective bargaining units are contained in the National Labor Relations Act. Nurses who elect to work in agencies where collective bargaining exists need to be informed about the contractual agreement between the bargaining unit and the institutional management.

The Process of Collective Bargaining. The process of collective bargaining is similar to other political processes. Negotiation and compromise are key elements in achieving any type of mutually satisfactory agreement. The role of power in achieving change is directly related to the resources controlled by each unit involved in the negotiating process. These resources include money, numbers of members, willingness to withhold services, and solidarity among members. It is clear that nurses who bargain as a unit for a commonly held group of demands will have more leverage than an individual nurse who confronts management with a similar list of requests.

The Impact of Collective Bargaining on Client Care. Historically, nurses were reluctant to withhold services from clients in order to improve their own working conditions because of their commitment to ensuring adequate care to clients. Current regulations require that bargaining units provide management with ample notice (usually 10 days) of any job action so that alternate arrangements for client care can be made. Any strike by nurses is also accompanied by provisions for emergency care to those clients who, in the opinion of the bargaining unit leadership, would be harmed without such care.[17] Because of these safeguards, clients have not suffered a complete lack of access to nursing care because of any job actions. Clients have, on the other hand, indirectly benefitted as a result of the improved working conditions achieved for nursing through collective action by nurses.

Issues in the Workplace

The interdisciplinary nature of the health care team often creates differing perspectives about the solution of a health care problem. Those collaborating for optimal health often have to use the political process to negotiate, compromise, and lobby to have the best possible outcome for clients. Whether the issue is primary nursing, the use of the registered care technician in the inpatient setting, the allocation of scarce resources such as donated organs, or the right of a client to refuse treatment, members of the health care team have the responsibility to use their lobbying skills to shape institutional policy, to effect change, and advocate for the best possible outcome for clients.

Nurses are challenged to become politically active in the workplace as well as the political arena. As a student, the reader is challenged to become involved in student associations, local politics, and faculty–student governance (Fig. 4–3). The rewards are great, and if nursing is to achieve the professional recognition it deserves, each nurse must assume this role as a required part of his or her professional accountability.

■ THE ROLE OF THE NURSE IN POLITICS AND POLICY-MAKING

The Nurse and Politics

The Nurse as Political Participant. Political involvement is an essential part of every nurse's professional role. Lobbying is an important way for a nurse to express professional values and identity. It is an essential component of the nurse's role as a client advocate. This is especially true for client groups such as the very young, the very old, and those who have traditionally been underrepresented in the policy arena, such as the poor and members of minority groups.

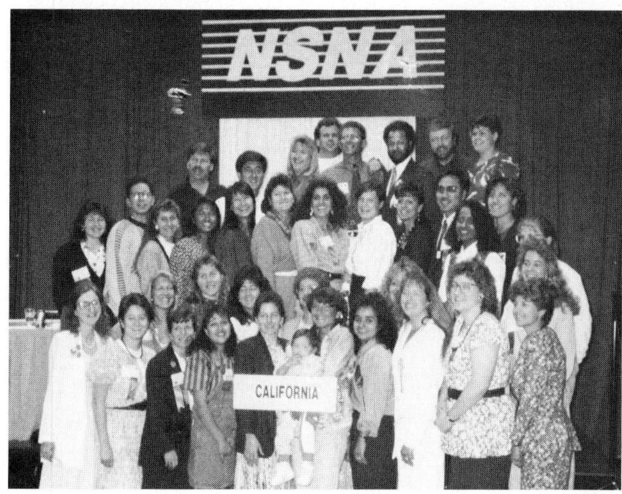

Figure 4–3. Nursing students involved in a preprofessional organization. (*Source: California Nursing Student Association.*)

Senator Edward Kennedy has noted that "the monumental contribution that nursing makes to health care in America is probably the profession's best kept secret."[18] Historically, nurses have been reticent about publicizing their accomplishments. They also have failed to educate other health care professionals and the general public about the changes that have occurred in the scope of practice during the last quarter century. Instead, all too often nurses have allowed others to debate and decide policy issues that directly affect the practice of nursing.

In the past, many nurses were hesitant to become involved in politics. As more nurses are educated about the skills involved, they are beginning to understand the nature of power and the importance of individual participation. Consequently, many nurses have experienced the excitement and professional benefits of political engagement. Nurses experiencing the rewards of political participation frequently become enthusiastic and encourage their professional colleagues to become involved. This serves to form organized alliances of involved nurses that become networks of professional collaboration and satisfying professional relationships.

It is not necessary to be an elected official to have an impact on public policy. Individual nurses can become professionally active by electing legislators and then lobbying them on issues that affect nursing and the nursing profession. Members of the legislature are elected by their constituents; they know that, if they wish to be reelected, they must accurately represent the will of their electorate. Legislators value input from their constituents and will weigh constituents' opinions when deciding whether to support or oppose a specific piece of legislation.

Professional Organizations as Special Interest Groups. Nurses may belong to one or more professional organizations, each of which represents a specific constituency within the registered nurse community. The American Nurses' Association (ANA) in the United States, and the Canadian Nurses' Association (CNA) in Canada are the organizations with the largest membership. They are the "official" organizations for nursing practice. The ANA has a political action committee, ANA-PAC, which endorses candidates who have exhibited voting records and demonstrated leadership consistent with the ANA's political agenda. Endorsement by a group that represents 1.7 million potential voters is important to any candidate; however, because numerous professional organizations represent constituencies within the nursing community, nursing's political message is seldom delivered with one voice. It is not uncommon for one nursing organization to favor a proposed piece of legislation while another organization testifies against the same bill. As a result, legislators who are sympathetic to nursing may feel unsure about what course of action will be in the best interests of the profession.

Collaborating Through Nursing Coalitions. In an effort to resolve some of the intraprofessional conflict, leaders of the major nursing associations have formed the Tri-Council. Composed of leaders from the ANA, the National League for Nursing (NLN), the Association of Nursing Executives (AONE), and the American Association of Colleges of Nursing (AACN), the Tri-Council meets regularly to discuss issues important to nursing practice. In addition, representatives of the various nursing specialty organizations such as the Association of Operating Room Nurses (AORN), the Organization for Obstetric, Gynecologic and Neonatal Nurses (NAACOG), and the American Association of Critical-Care Nurses (AACN) have likewise joined forces as the National Federation for Specialty Nursing Organizations so that they can better address issues relating to nurses who practice within a specialty area. It is clear that if nursing associations present a united front, their ideas will carry more weight.

Nursing organizations may often form coalitions with other groups that share similar perspectives on policy issues. Examples of such groups include the March of Dimes, Children's Defense Fund, and National Perinatal Association, all of which are interested in health care issues affecting pregnant women and children.

Individual nurses have the responsibility to join those professional associations that are relevant to their particular area of practice. Any organization is only as strong as its membership. If nurses want their professional associations to have an impact on public policy, they must support them and participate in their activities.

Conflict and Policy Disputes as a Barrier to Collaboration. Coalitions are born out of political expedience and necessity. Because no two organizations or associations share similar views on all issues, it is important to identify areas of potential conflict and dispute. Collaboration may be possible on some issues, but is probably impossible on all issues. It is critical that collaborators, either individuals or associations, identify which issues have potential for joint action. If there are issues upon which consensus cannot be reached, these may be acknowledged as areas in which individual efforts may be more appropriate. Often, individuals or groups agree not to issue public policy statements on matters of concern to other coalition members during the time period the coalition is working toward a common policy direction on a more pressing issue.

Nurses and the Electoral Process. Individual nurses may become involved directly in the electoral process in several ways. Many nurses begin active involvement by working for candidates who are seeking local, state, or national office. Involvement may be in the form of financial contributions to campaigns, or more active grass-roots involvement, such as volunteering at campaign headquarters, publicly supporting a candidate's position, or sponsoring a political debate among candidates. Some elected officials attribute a substantial part of their campaign successes to nurses.[19]

More and more, nurses are seeking direct involvement in politics. The ultimate level of involvement is for a nurse to successfully seek election to local, state, or federal office. Shirley Girouard, a nurse turned politician, credits much of the success of her campaign to a well-organized staff composed entirely of nurses.[20] After winning a seat in the New Hampshire House of Representatives, she found that her expert knowledge as a nurse served her well and that she quickly became an effective and valued member of the legislature. Other nurses have had equally positive experiences as legislators at all levels of government.

The Nurse as Lobbyist

During the last 25 years, nurses, as well as other groups in society, have come to appreciate the importance of political involvement to achieving their policy goals. Lobbying is a visible, effective way to have an impact on those issues about which nurses care the most: preventing illness, providing nursing care to those who are in need, defining the scope of nursing, ensuring professional competency, and improving nursing practice through research and education.

Nurses act as lobbyists when they contact policy-makers to make their positions known on legislation. For example, if the legislature is debating an act to limit the availability of abortions to those whose health care is financed by state funds, nurses can assist the development of a rational policy by individually and collectively sharing their opinions with their representatives.

Expertise and the Authority of Nurses

Initiating Legislation. Special knowledge gives the nurse expert power and validates the nurse's role in collaborating with lawmakers to facilitate change. There are several ways in which nurses, as individuals and as members of professional associations, collaborate with policy-makers to influence the public policy agenda. One of the most fundamental means of exerting influence is by suggesting legislation. Because they are comprised of individuals with expert knowledge about nursing, state nursing associations often introduce legislation to amend a Nurse Practice Act. While the act is intended to ensure the public of the safety and competence of those practicing professional nursing, it is the members of the profession who are best equipped to delineate the scope of that practice.

IMPLICATIONS FOR PROFESSIONAL COLLABORATION

The Nurse as Lobbyist

Lobbying refers to actions that are meant to influence the outcome of a decision. Political lobbying is done by citizens and by professional lobbyists. National and state nursing organizations hire professional lobbyists to promote their policy interests among legislators. As citizens and as professionals, individual nurses also lobby for important health care decisions. The nurse as lobbyist can have a significant impact on the issues and policies that are important to the nursing profession. As individual nurses make their opinions known to policy-makers, they mount a force to influence policy. The professional knowledge of nurses is a valuable source of power in policy-making, and is the basis of the collaborative exchanges the nurses have with policy makers.

Testifying Before Legislative Committees. Testifying before legislative committees or regulatory boards on important policy proposals is another way nurses act as lobbyists. In 1981, when the New Hampshire law authorizing the state board of nursing expired, nurses were able to secure renewal of the legislation. Nurses have also presented testimony across the country on proposed legislation to aid the homeless and others who lack the means to lobby effectively on their own behalf.

Belonging to Professional Organizations. Nurses are successful in using power to create positive change. Individual nurses create power when they join a professional nursing association. This form of professional activism often begins when, as students, nurses join the National Student Nurses' Association and become politically involved as a health care professional in training.

As members of a professional association, individual nurses can work in support of the organization's plan to influence policy. This is accomplished by organizing and participating in letter-writing campaigns, and by working to build coalitions with other professional groups. Members of professional associations support the organization's political action committee (PAC) by donating both time and money to support the PAC's efforts. The individual nurse may support the selection and appointment of members of the association to important boards and commissions and can work toward the election of politically active candidates to office within the association.

Shaping Public Opinion. Another important way of influencing public policy is through public opinion. Nurses need to educate the public to their unique and expert role, so that the individual who is a consumer of nursing care can collaborate with, and support, nursing's efforts in the policy arena. This education can be done through popular media such as newspapers and magazines, through public service spots on television and radio, by nurses' involvement in community activities, and by face-to-face interactions of one individual with another.

Establishing Lobbying Relationships. Individual nurses may also develop ongoing collaborative relationships with local lawmakers and others who hold influential policy-making positions. Many nurses find that working on a political campaign is an exciting and rewarding way to make initial political contacts with local politicians. Periodic telephone contact to discuss specific policy initiatives is an effective way to maintain relationships. Another valuable way to maintain collaborative relationships is to invite policy-makers to speak at local meetings of professional organizations. This may have the additional benefit of broadening the scope of political involvement of other members of the association through increasing their political activism and commitment.

Knowledge Needed to Influence Health Policy

Knowledge of the Policy Process. It is important to know the process by which health policy is made before attempting to exert influence on the outcome. To effectively lobby nurses need to know how the legislative process works. As discussed earlier in this chapter, there is a specific route that a bill must traverse as it moves through the legislature. During the process there are key times at which different lobbying efforts will be the most effective in influencing the outcome of the proposed legislation. For example, it is important to communicate factual material to legislative aides when they are performing background research on a bill. It is much easier to get a key point written into a representative's briefing while the aide is still writing the briefing than it is to get it added after the aide has completed the research. If testimony is to be effective, it must be ready for presentation when public hearings are being held. It is often necessary to register to present testimony several days beforehand. Knowing when key votes are scheduled will enable nurse lobbyists to make telephone contacts with undecided representatives. A nurse who, through an effective legislative network, knows when and how to intervene will be much more likely to affect the outcome of policy initiatives in the desired manner.

Knowledge of Government Organization. It is important to be knowledgeable about the political process in the specific jurisdiction where lobbying efforts will be directed. It is also important that nurses know whom to lobby. Although it might seem like a simple matter to identify jurisdictions, often it is not. Legislative districts, for example, often overlap. The district of a state senator may take in the districts of several state assembly or house legislators. Usually, citizens direct their opinions on policy matters to the legislators in the districts where they are registered to vote. When lobbying, nurses need to know their districts and who the elected officials are in those districts. Such information can be obtained easily from the Registrar of Voters in one's community. Sometimes, however, it is appropriate to direct policy opinions to the members of the specific legislative committee that is considering the legislation. The names, addresses, and telephone numbers of legislative committee members are available through the local public library.

Knowledge of the Legislators. Some legislators will be firm supporters of the bill in question. Although it is important to thank them for their efforts, and to remind them of the importance of their support, the lobbyist need not attempt to convince them to support the issue. Similarly, lobbyists usually know which representatives are vehemently opposed to the proposed legislation. If a legislator is firmly in opposition to a bill, it is often best not to attempt to change his or her mind. Lobbying efforts often have the most effect when directed towards those who marginally support the bill or those who have yet to decide how to vote.

Knowledge of the Issues. All effective lobbyists follow several important rules. The first is that the lobbyist must be well informed on all aspects of the issue under consideration. There are many effective techniques of compiling knowledge and information. Nurses may obtain copies of legislation that have been filed from the state or federal legislature. Single copies of bills are available free of charge. Often many issues are combined in a single bill, and it is to the nurse's advantage to understand the full scope of the proposed legislation. It is important to read bills carefully so that all aspects of the bill can be fully understood.

Local newspapers, news magazines, television, and radio can be important sources of information. The editorial pages of newspapers often contain opinion pieces that analyze controversial policy initiatives. Professional journals and nursing association newsletters often contain information on bills that have direct impact on nursing and nursing practice. Nursing research articles also provide useful information for shaping one's policy opinions.[21]

In addition, many state nurses' associations employ legislative liaisons who have responsibility for monitoring legislation and developing written fact sheets outlining the association's official position. These position papers, after being endorsed by the board of directors, are available to association members for their information and use in lobbying key representatives.

Guidelines for Lobbying. To be an effective lobbyist nurses should be well informed on the issues and able to present their professional perspective in a context that demonstrates understanding of how all components of the legislation are interrelated. It is important to discuss issues objectively and to respect the rights of others to disagree. It is also important to lobby legislators from both professional parties, because bipartisan support often portends a more positive outcome for the policy initiative. Table 4–1 presents general guidelines for lobbying public officials.

TABLE 4–1. GENERAL GUIDELINES FOR LOBBYING PUBLIC OFFICIALS

1. Prepare ahead.	Your time spent with officials is often very limited. In order to make the greatest impact, carefully prepare clear, concise statements ahead of time.
2. Never exaggerate, mislead, or lie.	Remember, you want to maintain your credibility, honesty, and integrity. Misrepresentation has a way of coming back to haunt you, and you may do irreparable damage to your cause.
3. When introducing yourself, offer the official a mutual point of reference to which he or she can relate.	Identify yourself as a constituent, member of a group the official supports or is familiar with, a friend of a friend, and any family, business, social, or political ties.
4. Do not focus your energies on officials who have already publicly stated their positions.	It is more productive to focus efforts on those officials who claim to be keeping an open mind or to be neutral and to support those who hold a position similar to yours.
5. Be courteous.	Do not lose your temper or use harsh or profane words; you may well alienate them or be labeled as a crackpot.
6. Let them know whom you are representing.	This will help the official to identify you and your cause. Also, let them know how many people you are representing.
7. Express appreciation for past services or support.	By maintaining a positive attitude, you are more likely to achieve what you want in the end. If not, you will at least leave a good impression. Reminders of past favors may trigger a sense of generosity again.
8. If further information is requested, be prepared to supply it quickly.	Legislation often moves quickly. By preparing and submitting information speedily you will make a good impression, help establish your reliability, and you may be called upon again.
9. Be discrete.	It *never* pays to gossip or make personal remarks, true or otherwise, about a public official.

From Burgess W, Ragland EC. Community Health Nursing: Philosophy, Process, Practice. *Norwalk, CT: Appleton-Century-Crofts; 1983: 213.*

A great deal of the success of lobbying efforts depends on the nurse's ability to accept incremental change. Compromise is the essence of successful policy-making. A successful lobbyist knows ahead of time which points he or she is willing to negotiate and which are essential to preserve. It is important to remember that those issues relinquished during negotiation can be readdressed at a later date.

Strategies for Lobbying. Lobbying can be accomplished through a variety of types of direct communication. Letters, telegrams, mailgrams, phone calls, oral and written testimony, and personal visits can obtain effective results. It is important to be clear, brief, specific, and accurate in all forms of direct communication.

Nurses can write, phone, or visit their legislators to make their views known. A legislator, once he or she knows the identity of interested and involved citizens, often consults them to gain a local perspective on an issue about which he or she has limited knowledge.

Letters. When writing letters, several particulars will increase the effectiveness of the communication. Individually written letters are much more valuable than petitions or form letters. Letters should clearly and concisely present two or three reasons why the legislator should support the particular issue. Letters should highlight benefits of the policy initiative for constituents in the representative's home district. Any personal connections that the letter-writer has with the legislator should be mentioned in a factual manner, and the representative should be told how to contact the letter-writer should additional information be necessary. Letters should be typed on plain paper or personal letterhead; the nurse is writing as an individual, not as an official spokesperson of an agency. Box 4–2 outlines specific dos and don'ts of letter-writing.

Telephone Calls. Telephone calls should be brief, professional, and polite. The caller should be prepared to answer any questions posed by the legislator or aide in a brief, objective, efficient manner. If the question posed is one the caller is unable to answer, the caller should acknowledge this and offer to obtain the requested information and forward it by telephone or by mail.

Personal Visits. Personal visits to legislators should be scheduled by calling ahead for an appointment. Timing of visits is important; visits should be scheduled well in advance of the date of action on the issue the lobbyist wishes to discuss. It may be better to schedule visits on issues that involve long-range plans when the legislature is not in session.[22]

It may not be possible to visit with the legislator in person, and the lobbyist should be reassured that visits with legislative aides often prove more effective than those with the representative. Aides are often extremely knowledgeable about the specifics of a piece of legislation, and may become valuable allies. Visits should be brief, courteous, and professional. Lobbyists should dress and act decorously, avoiding such activities as smoking, gum chewing, and overly familiar behavior.

BOX 4–2. DO'S AND DON'TS OF LETTER WRITING

DO	spell your legislator's name correctly and know whether he or she is a senator or representative.
DO	try to send a typewritten personal letter. Handwritten letters are fine as long as they are legible.
DO	include your name and the address at which you prefer to be contacted so your legislator can answer you. Be sure this address is within the legislator's district.
DO	use the number assigned to the bill or use its popular name so that your legislator knows exactly to which bill you are referring.
DO	be timely in your letter writing. Time your letter to arrive while the issue is still alive, preferably while the bill is in committee.
DO	be concise. Be sure to cover all your points, but be brief. With the volume of mail received daily, longer letters are read last.
DO	be sure to write a follow-up letter to thank your legislator for his or her support of your position, especially if the vote on the bill is in your favor.
DO	be sure to mention helpful and courteous staff personnel by name in the follow-up letter.
DO	draw attention to the fact that you know your legislator personally, if you do. This is one way to be sure that he or she will get to see the letter almost immediately.
DO	address the letter to a staff member you know personally or send a copy of the original. This will ensure that your letter is read by someone immediately.
DON'T	resort to name-calling. This will only detract from the validity of your letter. Be courteous in your categorization of those holding the opposing viewpoint.
DON'T	threaten your legislator.
DON'T	pretend to possess more political influence than you do.
DON'T	make promises that you know you cannot keep.
DON'T	demand that your legislator take a certain stance on an issue and neglect to give supporting evidence.
DON'T	write to a legislator who is not from your state or district.
DON'T	send form letters or petitions.
DON'T	write to your legislator on every issue being considered. You will make a nuisance of yourself.
DON'T	write more than one letter on the same issue.

Testimony. Giving testimony at a public hearing is a particularly effective way to influence legislators' opinions. Oral testimony should be brief, concise, and articulate. It is more effective to present cogent arguments on one or two key points than to present a comprehensive discourse on all possible aspects of a bill. A more extensive, although still pointed, argument can be offered in accompanying written testimony. Experienced lobbyists often prefer to offer their written testimony after they have presented oral testimony to make sure that the committee members do not ignore their verbal presentation. If, however, the oral testimony contains a great deal of technical information or statistical data, it may be more effective to distribute the written testimony ahead of time.

Attending Hearings. Nurses' physical presence is vital at hearings of bills that have the potential to affect nursing practice. Many groups of nurses who share common interests have an organized network to notify their members when debate is scheduled and plan in advance which members are best prepared to testify. Those who do not testify attend the hearing and lend support to the bill by their presence, and perhaps by submitting additional written testimony.

Maintaining the Relationship. An often-overlooked technique to maximize the effectiveness of lobbying is the thank-you note. A short written note to a legislator at the conclusion of the vote on a bill reminds the representative that you appreciate his or her efforts. This note is important regardless of the final outcome of the voting. Even if a bill was defeated, it is important to thank those who extended efforts on its behalf. The representative who knows that his or her efforts were appreciated will be more willing to offer support in the future.

Nurses, after having repeatedly contacted a legislator to share their views on health-related matters, have been offered positions as legislative aides for health affairs. These individuals, through interacting with other congressional aides, have been able to exert influence in far-reaching circles.

When planning strategies for lobbying, it is very important to be timely and to use strategies appropriately. There are various strategies that are particularly useful at each phase of the legislative process. Figure 4–4 depicts these strategies and the point in the bill-to-law process at which they are useful.

SUMMARY

Public policy is the culmination of society's decisions on how to allocate scarce resources for reaching common goals. In a democratic society, policy is formed through the policy-making process, which includes the formation, implementation, and evaluation of policy. One of the most important mechanisms for establishing policy is the legislative process, which, because of its importance, is the focal point for people's efforts to influence policy outcomes. Politics, the use of power to effect change, is the term that refers to those efforts. The legislative process provides citizens, including nurses, with many opportunities to effect policy decisions. It involves a series of steps or phases through which policy ideas are converted into law. Once laws are made, the policies they contain are refined by drafting of regulations which are the rules or guidelines for policy implementation. Drafting and evaluating regulations gives citizens additional opportunities to influence policy. When controversial policies are implemented, they are frequently brought to the attention of the courts; thus judicial review also contributes to the refinement of public policy.

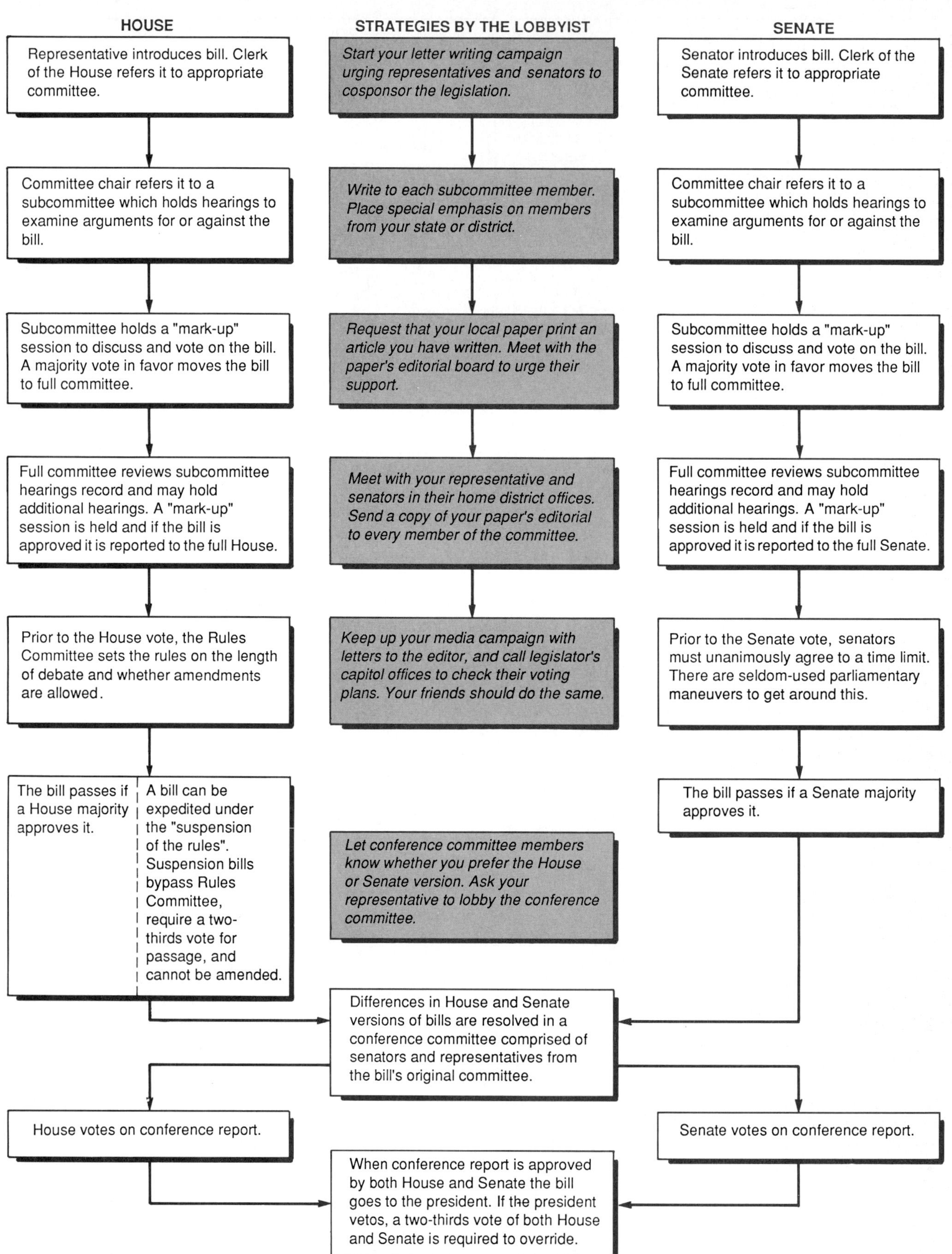

HOUSE
STRATEGIES BY THE LOBBYIST
SENATE
Representative introduces bill. Clerk of the House refers it to appropriate committee.
Start your letter writing campaign urging representatives and senators to cosponsor the legislation.
Senator introduces bill. Clerk of the Senate refers it to appropriate committee.
Committee chair refers it to a subcommittee which holds hearings to examine arguments for or against the bill.
Write to each subcommittee member. Place special emphasis on members from your state or district.
Committee chair refers it to a subcommittee which holds hearings to examine arguments for or against the bill.
Subcommittee holds a "mark-up" session to discuss and vote on the bill. A majority vote in favor moves the bill to full committee.
Request that your local paper print an article you have written. Meet with the paper's editorial board to urge their support.
Subcommittee holds a "mark-up" session to discuss and vote on the bill. A majority vote in favor moves the bill to full committee.
Full committee reviews subcommittee hearings record and may hold additional hearings. A "mark-up" session is held and if the bill is approved it is reported to the full House.
Meet with your representative and senators in their home district offices. Send a copy of your paper's editorial to every member of the committee.
Full committee reviews subcommittee hearings record and may hold additional hearings. A "mark-up" session is held and if the bill is approved it is reported to the full Senate.
Prior to the House vote, the Rules Committee sets the rules on the length of debate and whether amendments are allowed.
Keep up your media campaign with letters to the editor, and call legislator's capitol offices to check their voting plans. Your friends should do the same.
Prior to the Senate vote, senators must unanimously agree to a time limit. There are seldom-used parliamentary maneuvers to get around this.
The bill passes if a House majority approves it.
A bill can be expedited under the "suspension of the rules". Suspension bills bypass Rules Committee, require a two-thirds vote for passage, and cannot be amended.
The bill passes if a Senate majority approves it.
Let conference committee members know whether you prefer the House or Senate version. Ask your representative to lobby the conference committee.
Differences in House and Senate versions of bills are resolved in a conference committee comprised of senators and representatives from the bill's original committee.
House votes on conference report.
Senate votes on conference report.
When conference report is approved by both House and Senate the bill goes to the president. If the president vetos, a two-thirds vote of both House and Senate is required to override.

Figure 4–4. Influencing the bill-to-law process. (*Source: Ellis JR, Hartley CL.* Nursing in Today's World: Challenges, Issues, and Trends. *3rd ed. Philadelphia: Lippincott; 1988: 314–315.*)

Public policies usually embody a plan for change of some sort. Change is the alteration of the normal course of events. People frequently meet change with resistance, whether out of fear of the unknown or from a vested interest in the status quo. Thus, power, the ability to do or act, becomes an important part of the political equation. In politics, power encompasses the ability to mobilize people as individuals or as groups with a special interest to assert their will. Power from various sources, legitimate, reward, coercive, expert, referent and personal, is used to accomplish policy objectives. However, power in policy making most frequently derives from the vote and the will of the majority. In a democratic society, there are many strategies for mobilizing political power. The most important strategy is the electoral process. The lobbying of elected representatives by citizens and special interest groups is another important strategy.

Nurses have an important stake in public policy and especially in health policy. Political engagement by nurses is essential to ensure that nursing receives the resources and support necessary to meet its objectives of improving care and achieving professional self-determination. Participation in politics influences how nurses interact and collaborate with other health care professionals. As public priorities are determined through public policy, the active involvement of nurses will be an important factor in determining what opportunities nursing will gain for itself. Policy decisions will influence how, where, and to what extent nurses will gain the opportunities and the resources necessary for collaborating with clients for the achievement of optimal health. Thus, lobbying to influence public policy is an aspect of the professional responsibility of every nurse. Only through political participation can nurses expect to play a role in the vital decisions that bear on their self-interests, but more importantly, that shape the health of the nation.

REFERENCES

1. Diers D. Policy and politics. In: Mason DJ, Talbott SW. *Political Action Handbook for Nurses.* Reading, MA: Addison-Wesley; 1986; 53–59.
2. Cohen WJ, Milburn LT. What every nurse should know about political action. *Nurs Health Care.* 1988; 9:295–297.
3. Takach MB. A recipe for political action. *Nurs Econ:* 1989; 7(5): 273–275.
4. Landes RG. *The Canadian Policy.* Scarborough, Ontario: Prentice-Hall Canada.
5. Inglehart JK. Canada's health care system. *New Engl J Med;* 1986; 315:202–208.
6. Hunter PR, Berger KJ. Nurses and the political arena: Lobbying for professional impact. *Nurs Admin Quart.* 1984; 8(4):67.
7. Lippitt R, Watson J, Westley B. *The Dynamics of Planned Change.* New York: Harcourt, Brace; 1958.
8. Natapoff JN, Loetterle BC. Making a Difference: The Courage to Change. In: Mason DJ, Talbott SW. *Political Action Handbook for Nurses.* Reading, MA: Addison-Wesley; 1986:101–114.
9. Lindbloom EC. *The Policy-Making Process.* 2nd ed. Englewood Cliffs, NJ: Prentice-Hall; 1980.
10. Schuman D. *Bureaucracies, Organizations, and Administration: A Political Primer.* New York: Macmillan; 1976.
11. Bennis WG, Benne KD, Chin R, Corey KE. *The Planning of Change.* 3rd ed. New York: Holt, Rinehart & Winston; 1976.
12. Redman E. *The Dance of Legislation.* New York: Simon & Schuster; 1973.
13. Kuhn TS. *The Structure of Scientific Revolution.* Chicago: University of Chicago Press; 1970.
14. Bagwell M, Clements S. *A Political Handbook for Health Professionals.* Boston: Little, Brown; 1985.
15. Wieland GF, Ullrich RA. *Organizations: Behavior, Design, and Change.* Homewood, IL: Irwin; 1976.
16. Jacox A. Collective action: The basis for professionalism. *Super Nurs.* 1980; 11: 22–24.
17. Foley ME. The politics of collective bargaining. In: Mason DJ, Talbott, SW. *Political Action Handbook for Nurses.* Reading: MA: Addison-Wesley; 1986.
18. Mason DJ, Talbott SW. *Political Action Handbook for Nurses.* Reading, MA: Addison-Wesley; 1986.
19. Wakefield MK. Perspectives on health policy. *Nurs Econ.* 1990; 8(5): 352–353.
20. Girouard SA. The Nurse Politician. In: Mason DJ, Talbott SW. *Political Action Handbook for Nurses.* Reading, MA: Addison-Wesley; 1986.
21. Hinshaw AS. Using research to shape health policy. *Nurs Outlook.* 1988; 36(1):21–24.
22. McIntosh D. Grassroots lobbying. *Am J Nurs.* 1989; 89(11): 1515–1516.

BIBLIOGRAPHY

Aiekn LH, Mullinx CF. The nurse shortage: Myth or reality? *N Engl J Med.* 1987; 317:641–645.

American Nurses' Association. *Nursing: A Social Policy Statement.* Kansas City, MO: ANA; 1980.

Archer SE. Political involvement by nurses. *Recent Adv Nurs.* 1987; 18:25–45.

Archer SE, Goehner PA. *Nurses: A Political Force.* Monterey, CA: Wadsworth; 1982.

Aroskar MA. The interface of ethics and politics in nursing. *Nurs Outlook.* 1987;35(6):268–272.

Barry CT. Profiles of nurses professionally involved in public policy. *Nurs Econ.* 1990;8(3):174–176.

Bresler K. *Citizen's Guide to Drafting Legislation.* Boston: Office of the Massachusetts Secretary of State; 1986.

Bushy A, Smith TO. Lobbying: The hows and wherefores. *Nurs Management.* 1990;21(4):39–41.

Donaho BA. Creating wider circles of influence. Nurs Outlook. 1990;38(3):134–135.

Ellis JR, Hartley CL. *Nursing in Today's World: Challenges, Issues, and Trends.* Philadelphia: Lippincott; 1988.

Fagin C. When national health insurance comes: Where will nursing be? *Nurs Health Care.* 1989; February: 68–69.

Flynn BC. Demystifying political involvement. In: Lambert CE Jr, Lambert VA, eds. *Perspectives in Nursing: The Impacts on the Nurse, the Consumer, and Society.* Norwalk, CT: Appleton & Lange; 1989: 453–475.

Girourard SA. Health policy: Implications for the CNS. In: Hamric AB, Spross JA. *The Clinical Nurse Specialist in Theory and Practice.* 2nd ed. Philadelphia: Saunders; 1989: 363–378.

Inglehart JK. Problems facing the nursing profession. *N Engl J Med.* 1987; 317:646–651.

Johnson-Brown HW. To understand and participate in public policy formation: A challenge to nursing. In: Lambert CE Jr, Lambert VA, eds. *Perspectives in Nursing: The Impacts on the Nurse, the Consumer, and Society.* East Norwalk, CT: Appleton & Lange; 1989: 433–452.

Kalisch BJ, Kalisch PA. *Politics of Nursing.* Philadelphia: Lippincott; 1982.

Kelly LY. *The Nursing Experience: Trends, Challenges, and Transitions.* New York: Macmillan; 1987.

London HI. The phenomenon of change. *Futurist.* 1988; July–August:64.

MacPherson KI. Health care policy, values, and nursing. *Advances in Nursing Science.* 1987;9(3):1–11.

Maraldo PJ, Solomon S. *Talking Points.* New York: National League for Nursing; 1986.

Mason DJ. Nursing and politics: A profession comes of age. *Orthopedic Nurs.* 1990;9(5):11–17.

Mason DJ, Backer BA, Georges CA. Toward a feminist model for the political empowerment of nurses. *Image.* 1991;23(2):72–77.

Mason DJ, Costello-Nickitas DM, Scanlan JM, Magnuson BA. Empowering nurses for politically astute change in the workplace. *Nurs.* 1991;22(1):5–10.

Milburn LT, Hayes K, Griffith H. The information-seeker's guide to health policy news. *Nurs Outlook.* 1989; 9:307–309.

Rains JW. Nursing and politics: Adapting skills to spark social change. *Nurs Outlook.* 1989; 9:299–301.

Sharp N, Biggs S, Wakefield M. Public policy: New opportunities for nurses. *Nurs Health Care.* 1991;12(1):16–22.

Smith JP. The politics of American health care. *J Adv Nurs.* 1990; 15(4):487–497.

Solomon SB, Roe SC. *Key Concepts in Public Policy: Student Workbook.* New York: National League for Nursing; 1986.

Takach MB. A recipe for political action. *Nurs Econ.* 1989;7(5):273–275.

Wasserman G. *The Basis of American Politics.* Boston: Little, Brown; 1982.

White DL, Hamel PK. National Center for Nursing Research: How it came to be. *Nurs Econ.* 1986;4(1):19–22.

White R, ed. *Political Issues in Nursing.* New York: Wiley; 1985 and 1986 (2 vols).

Wieczorek RR, ed. *Power, Politics, and Policy in Nursing.* New York: Springer; 1984.

Wildavsky A. *The Politics of the Budgetary Process.* 4th ed. Boston: Little, Brown; 1984.

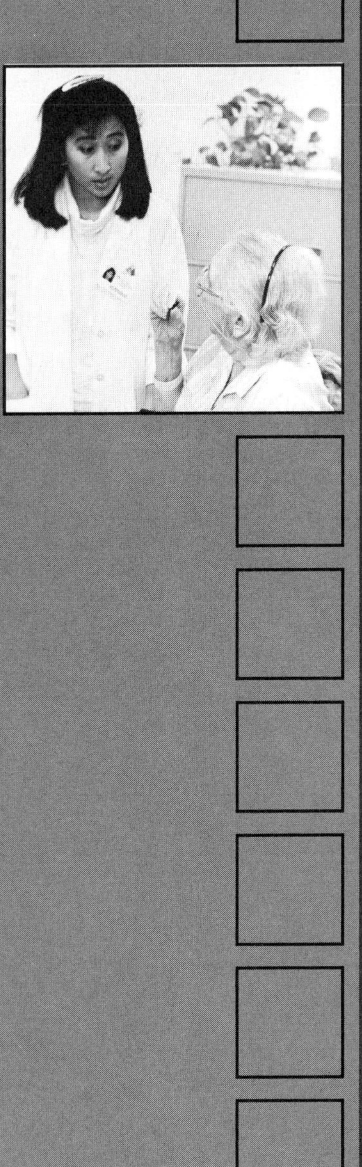

UNIT TWO
Health and Health Care

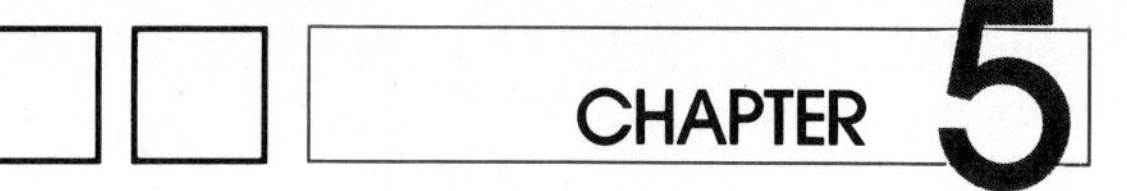

Health and Illness

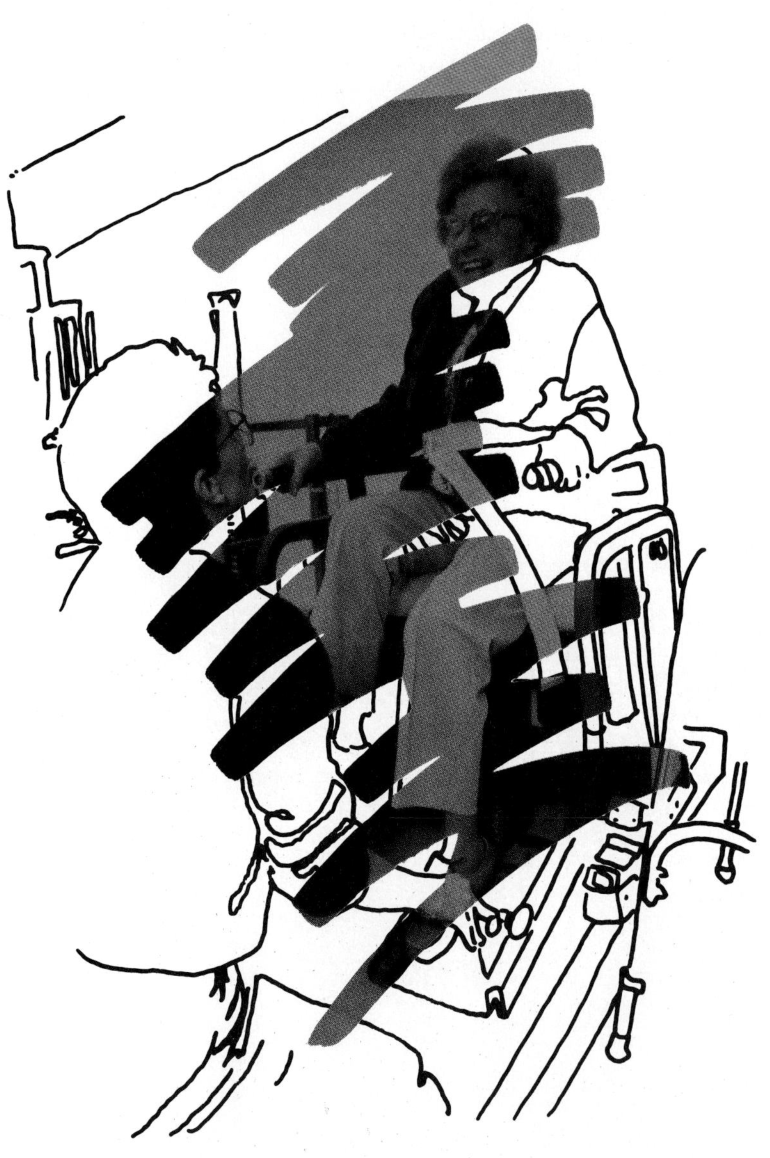

Behavioral Objectives

Upon completion of this chapter, the student will be able to:

1. Discuss why it is important to develop clear definitions of health and wellness, disease and illness.
2. Describe the role-performance, clinical, adaptive, and eudaimonistic models of health.
3. State the distinction between health and wellness.
4. Define optimal health.
5. List several health promotion measures.
6. State the distinctions among illness, disease, and deviance.
7. Discuss the concept of a health–illness continuum. Contrast 2 models of health continuua.
8. Discuss the ways in which theories of disease causation influence health behavior.
9. Give examples of primary, secondary, and tertiary measures for disease prevention.
10. Identify factors that may prevent clients from adopting positive health behaviors.
11. Outline the roles of both nurse and client when collaborating on health promotion and disease prevention.

KEY TERMS

adaptation
at-risk role
deviance
disease
disease prevention
etiology
eudaimonistic
health–illness continuum
health maintenance
health promotion
high-level wellness
holistic health
informed dissent
maladaptation
multiple-causation theory
optimal health
primary prevention
role-modeling
secondary prevention
tertiary prevention
wellness

Few people would deny that they wish to be healthy. Most desire good health and regret its loss; many actively seek to maintain or improve their health by exercising, attending to diets, obtaining adequate sleep, and by other means. Health is taught in the schools, people read about it in the press, and people purchase products that promise to enhance or restore health. Smoking cessation clinics are flourishing and health and fitness clubs advertise for new members. It may reasonably be claimed that health is nearly a universal value in today's society.

Yet there is little agreement about what actually constitutes health. A small child, for example, might describe health as "feeling good." Personal definitions may be considerably more complex, although they are likely to incorporate the child's description of a sensation of well-being.

A neighbor, on the other hand, may have a definition totally at odds with one's own personal definition. Perhaps she is a person whose religious beliefs include an understanding of health not as physical well-being, but as a correct relationship with God. She may consider herself healthy even though she experiences chronic pain from rheumatoid arthritis and suffers from frequent upper respiratory infections.

Indeed, it is unlikely that two individuals will have precisely the same definitions of health and illness. Definitions of these terms are fluid and vary among individuals and cultures (Fig. 5–1). Furthermore, they can change over time. A person's childhood notions of health as "feeling good" will probably be greatly altered by the time he or she reaches adolescence, and may continue to be modified well into adulthood. Understandings of health and illness common to particular cultures have changed over time as supernatural theories of disease causation have given way to germ theory and other explanations of modern medicine. Chapters 9 and 12 present detailed discussions of the personal and social variables influencing an individual's ideas about health and illness.

Health professionals also have various and sometimes

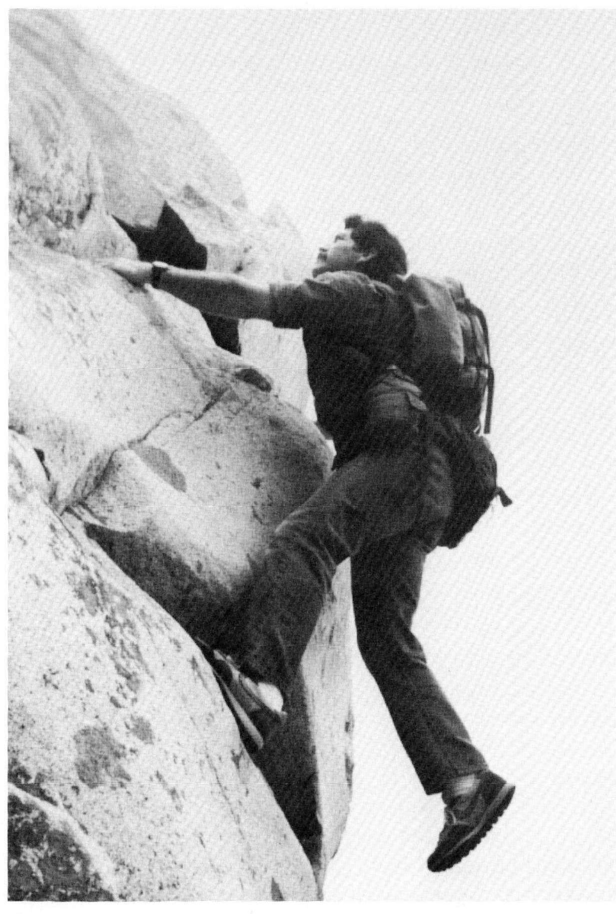

A

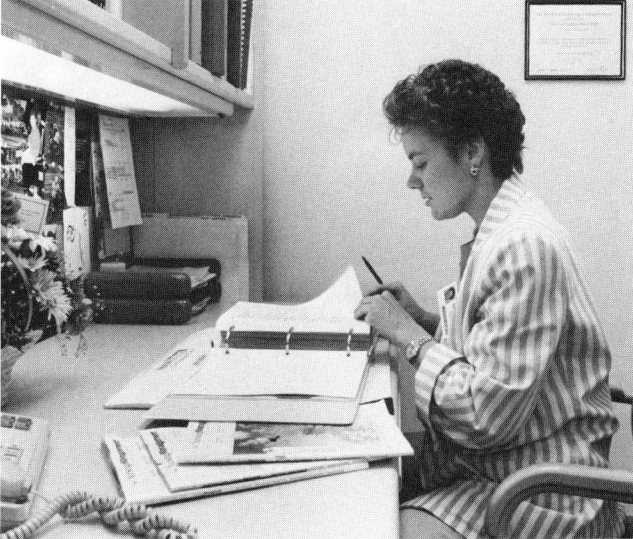

B

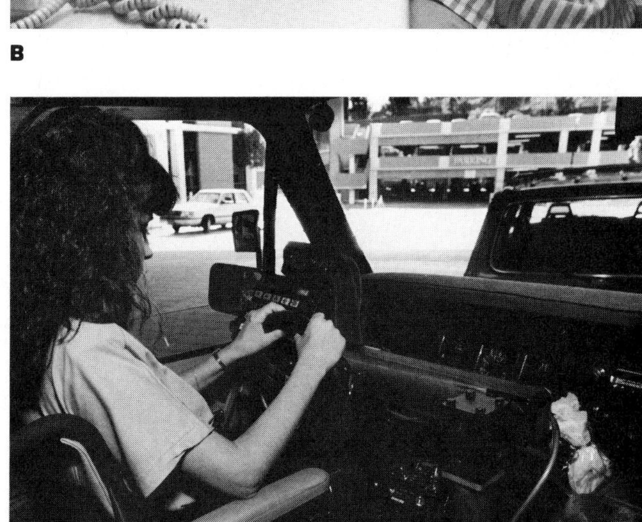

C

Figure 5–1. The concept of health varies among individuals. (**A** courtesy of Stephen Simpson, Inc. and UCSD Medical Center Nurse Recritment Office.)

conflicting interpretations of health and illness. A physician, for example, may consider a client to be in good health. A dentist, finding dental caries in the same client, may consider this evidence of inadequate dental health. There is lack of agreement over which physical conditions may be regarded as disease. Is a temporary rash resulting from exposure to poison ivy a disease? What about chronic constipation? Similarly, certain behaviors, such as use of illicit drugs, are regarded by some practitioners as illnesses and by others as social problems.

Although no consensus has yet been reached regarding how best to define health and illness, health professionals continue to examine the concepts and to propose definitions. Nurses have made significant contributions to this effort. It is important that nurses continue to clarify and refine their understanding of health and illness for two reasons. First, health beliefs influence health practices.[1] Thus, nurses' definitions of health and illness largely determine the nature and scope of nursing practice. Consider the fact that the concept of health is central to most definitions of nursing. The American Nurses' Association, for example, has defined nursing as "the diagnosis and treatment of human responses to actual or potential health problems."[2] Nurses using this definition must be able to describe both health and health problems when making decisions regarding which problems are treatable by nurses. If health is defined narrowly, as a measurable deviation in physical functioning, then nurses would confine themselves to assisting clients to regain normal physical functioning. If, on the other hand, health is defined more broadly, then the scope of nursing practice would increase correspondingly. Therefore, if a particular occurrence—say an increase in the rate of teenage pregnancies—is considered to be a problem, but not a health problem, it would be regarded as outside the scope of nursing.

A second reason for seeking clarity regarding the concepts of health and illness is that problems frequently arise when there is a discrepancy between the nurse's perspectives and values and those of the client. Baumann notes that some persons fail to respond to health care regimens simply because they do not see a relationship between the plan of care and their conception of health.[3] If nurses do not understand the reason for a person's behavior, they may become frustrated and believe that the person is being deliberately defiant or is not intelligent enough to understand the instructions. In such instances, a client may be labeled "uncooperative" or "noncompliant."

Nursing practice, then, can improve when practitioners are clear about their own ideas concerning health and illness, and when they are aware that their views may not be shared by all clients. It is not necessary for the nurse to be aware of every concept of health and illness—indeed, this would be impossible, given the great variety—but it will be helpful to have knowledge of some of the prevalent views of these concepts. This chapter discusses definitions of and factors relating to health and illness as well as health promotion and disease prevention.

BOX 5–1. SMITH'S MODELS OF HEALTH

Role Performance Model

- Health seen as the ability of a person to carry out the expected functions.
- A "common-sense" model often used by nonprofessionals.

Clinical Model

- Health seen as the absence of signs and symptoms of pathology.
- Similar to the "medical" model.

Adaptive Model

- Health seen as the ability to respond successfully to challenging stimuli, including social, environmental, and physical threats.
- Often used by health professionals because it addresses many extraphysical variables affecting health.

Eudaimonistic Model

- Health seen as the full expression of a person's physical, emotional, and social potential; a vibrant state of well-being.
- Broadest of the four models. Preferred by many nurses because of its focus on the person as a complex being.

HEALTH AND WELLNESS

Definitions of Health and Wellness

Because concepts of health are so numerous and varied, ranging from the personal meaning to complex theoretical models, it is useful to have a means of organizing them for study and discussion. Judith Smith has developed a taxonomy, that is, a scientific classification, for ideas about health.[4] She describes four models: (1) the role performance model, (2) the clinical model, (3) the adaptive model, and (4) the eudaimonistic model. Each model is described below, and a summary of the four is presented in Box 5–1.

The Role Performance Model. This model incorporates definitions and concepts that regard the ability of a person to carry out expected functions as a prime indicator of health. For example, a young man, whose roles include those of father and worker, would not be considered healthy if his physical condition prevented him from appearing for work regularly, or from interacting with and providing for his child. Smith refers to role performance as a "common-sense" measure of health, and it is a criterion used by many people.[4,5] Even the nursing student may have said "But I *can't* get sick—I have to study for my final exams." In so doing, the student was using role performance as a measure of health. In this case, being sick meant interference with the ability to carry out the responsibilities associated with the role of student.

Health care professionals also make use of this model, although seldom exclusively. A physician treating a client with chest pain will be interested in knowing if episodes of pain have prevented the client from participating in his or her usual activities. In chronic diseases—that is, diseases that are of indefinite duration—role performance may be used to differentiate between "sick with chronic condition" and "healthy with chronic condition." Thus, a clinic nurse who sees a young mother with multiple sclerosis will want to inquire about the woman's ability to care for her children and maintain her home.

Virginia Henderson, a nurse theorist, has defined health in role performance terms. She identifies 14 areas in which persons must be able to function independently if they are to be healthy.[6] The activities she lists are prerequisite to the fulfillment of familial, occupational, and civic roles.

1. Breathe normally.
2. Eat and drink adequately.
3. Eliminate body waste.
4. Move and maintain desirable postures.
5. Sleep and rest.
6. Select suitable clothes—dress and undress.
7. Maintain body temperature within normal range by adjusting clothing and modifying the environment.
8. Keep the body clean and well groomed and protect the integument.
9. Avoid changes in the environment (that is, do not disrupt the natural ecological balance) and avoid injuring others.

10. Communicate with others expressing emotions, needs, fears, or opinions.
11. Worship according to one's faith.
12. Work in such a way that there is a sense of accomplishment.
13. Play or participate in various forms of recreation.
14. Learn, discover, or satisfy the curiosity that leads to normal development and health, and use the available health facilities.[6]

Note that Henderson does not refer to the way a person feels, or to the lack of signs and symptoms, but to what a person is able to do.

The Clinical Model. Proponents of the clinical model define health as the lack of signs and symptoms of pathology. Indicators of pathology may include mental and emotional symptoms or may be restricted to physical aberrations. Thus, health is defined in negative terms. That is, if a client cannot be determined to have a disease, he or she is considered healthy. Smith points out that this is a minimal conception of health.[4] It differs from the role-performance model in that even a person who is unable to meet role expectations would be designated healthy as long as there was no evidence of pathology. People make use of this framework when they seek clinical indicators of illness. It is a common practice to require employees to "call in sick" if illness necessitates absence from work. A report of illness to the office may bring the response "Oh? What seems to be the problem?" The questioner is asking the employee to name the illness or its indicators. The statement "I'm ill" must be supported by specifics of pain, nasal congestion, rash, or other markers of deviation from health. Similarly, a parent may seek to validate a child's complaints by measuring his or her body temperature. In the absence of fever, illness may be doubted. Signs and symptoms, in the clinical model, serve to ratify claims of illness.

The clinical model has provided an extremely useful way of studying health and disease. It is compatible with the scientific mode of inquiry, and investigators operating within the framework of the model have made outstanding contributions to the understanding of ways in which health is maintained and threatened. A frequently cited example is the development of the germ theory, which states that certain diseases are caused by particular microorganisms. Using the germ theory, for instance, one is able to explain why persons exposed to the varicella virus may develop chickenpox.

The clinical model has been used in nursing practice. Bandman and Bandman[7] suggest that it was in general use until Florence Nightingale introduced a broader view, which took numerous environmental factors into account. Few nurses writing or practicing today advocate use of the clinical model, except as a subcategory of health. For many years the clinical model was dominant among physicians, the term being nearly synonymous with the "medical model." Robert Veatch stated that a health deviation is incorporated within the medical model if it has four essential characteristics. It must be: (1) nonvoluntary, (2) organic, (3) treatable by physicians, and (4) below some socially minimal standard of acceptability.[8] Many physicians, however, have broadened their understanding of health and few confine their practices to this narrow framework.

In spite of its usefulness, the clinical model has been the subject of considerable criticism in recent years, both by the public and by health care practitioners.[9] A major concern is that the model is too limited, and that health is best conceived in broader terms rather than as the mere absence of signs and symptoms. Within the medical profession itself, there is vigorous debate over the uses and limits of the model. Some feel that, for the purposes of the medical profession, health is best described simply as a state of physical well-being[10]; others believe that the model is much too limited and should be altered to incorporate social and psychological concerns. In the middle ground are practitioners who suggest that the model itself is basically sound, and not incompatible with psychosocial concerns.

The Adaptive Model. René Dubos conceived of health as a process rather than a state. To Dubos, the healthy organism was one that successfully responded to stimuli in the environment; he described this as adaptive behavior.[11, 12] Thus, **adaptation** is a process through which individuals accommodate changes in the environment in such a way that their functioning is preserved and their general goals—survival, growth, and reproduction can be pursued. Illness is viewed as a failure of adaptation, or **maladaptation.** This concept of health has been attractive to a number of practitioners because it addresses many of the extraphysical variables affecting health. The stimuli to which people must adapt include challenging environmental and social conditions as well as physical threats.[13] Therefore, the adaptive model employs a concept of health that is larger in scope than either the role performance or clinical models.

Adaptive behavior may be deliberate and purposeful, as in putting on warm clothing when the air becomes chilly. Other adaptive behavior, such as the operation of homeostatic mechanisms governing the control of body temperature, function below the level of conscious awareness.

Florence Nightingale endorsed many of the ideas within the adaptive model. She spoke of disease as a "reparative process" and noted the effect of environmental and social factors on health.[14] Sister Callista Roy is a contemporary nurse who has formulated a nursing model based on the idea of health as adaptation. It is her belief that nurses can promote health by supporting and promoting the client's own adaptation in the areas of physiologic needs, self-concept, role mastery, and interdependence relations.[15]

The Eudaimonistic Model. This is the broadest of the four models. The term **eudaimonistic** refers to happiness or well-being. In this model, health is regarded as the full expression of a person's physical, emotional, social, and spiritual potential. Some of the key concepts within this model were derived from the thinking of Abraham Maslow, who believed that human nature is innately good or neutral, and that illness is a consequence of suppressing a person's natural tendency toward growth, individuality, and wholeness.[16]

Smith regards this model as encompassing the concepts of the first three.[4] In order to be healthy in this context, then, one must be able to meet one's role obligations, be free of evidence of disease, and successfully adapt to changing conditions. Moreover, the healthy person strives to use his or her full human potential in positive ways. Health is experienced not as the lack of pathology, but as a vibrant state of well-being in which a sense of self-esteem is maintained, allowing effective interaction with family and community. In the eudaimonistic model, for example, a physically well person who carried out work responsibilities efficiently but without enthusiasm, and who dreaded going to the office each day, would not be considered healthy. This model is particularly attractive to those who regard the clinical model as excessively narrow.

In the late 1940s the World Health Organization published its now-famous definition of health: "Health is a state of complete physical, mental, and social well-being and not merely the absence of disease or infirmity."[17] This definition, clearly within the eudaimonistic framework, has provided a rallying cry for those who advocate a comprehensive understanding of health. Critics of the definition, however, have characterized it as unnecessarily broad, vague, and even dangerous because they believe it to be unrealistic and ultimately unachievable.[18–20] Nevertheless, it remains a standard, or at least an ideal, for many health care providers.

The eudaimonistic model has also been adopted by practitioners and laypersons within the holistic health movement. Braillier offers the following definition of holistic health. (Observe the parallels between her definition and the WHO definition of health.)

> **Holistic health** is an ongoing sense of finely tuned wellness, which involves not only excellent care of the physical body but also care of ourselves in such a way that we nurture our capacity to be mentally alert and creative as well as emotionally stable and satisfied. It involves the feeling of wholeness we can gain from having defined our philosophy of life and purpose in life.[21]

Braillier, like many who advocate holism as a frame of reference, views health as a way of being rather than as a state or goal. Hildegard Peplau also described health as a way of being, saying that the term health referred to "forward movement of personality and other ongoing human processes in the direction of creative, constructive, productive, personal and community living."[22]

The eudaimonistic model has also been central to what has been termed the "wellness movement." Although the terms are often used interchangeably, some writers make a distinction between health and wellness, indicating that the latter is a way of life rather than a measurable state. It encompasses the concepts of health and well-being. **Wellness** is a lifestyle that promotes optimum functioning and a sustained zest for life. The wellness movement focuses on healthy living rather than on the treatment of disease.[23] Perhaps for this reason, it has created great interest among the general population. Participants in the wellness movement suggest that individuals must not rely exclusively on health professionals to maintain health, but must take personal responsibility for this matter.

Halbert Dunn's theory of high-level wellness was the seminal work of the wellness movement. His description of high-level wellness echoes Peplau's definition of health:

> **High-level wellness** for the individual is defined as an integrated method of functioning which is oriented toward maximizing the potential of which the individual is capable. It requires that the individual maintain a continuum of balance and purposeful direction within the environment where he is functioning.[24]

Because advocates of the wellness movement, like members of the holistic health movement, believe that wellness is largely a matter of personal initiative, they emphasize nonmedical techniques for the practice of wellness. Longe and Ardell, for instance, suggest that wellness is achieved through personal responsibility and attention to nutrition, physical fitness, stress management, and the creation of a supportive environment.[25]

Of the four models described by Smith, the eudaimonistic model probably enjoys the highest favor among nurses writing today. It speaks to the concern many nurses express for the person as a complex being. And, as earlier noted, by enlarging the definition of health, nurses are effectively enlarging the scope of nursing practice. The present interest in the eudaimonistic model may lead some to believe that its key concepts are new to nursing. They are not, nor are they inventions of the holistic health or wellness movements. Interest in health as well as illness, and in the extraphysical variables affecting health, have long been part of the heritage of professional nursing.

Optimal Health

Nurses and clients, then, make use of all four models described by Smith. Individuals choose the model or models that best represent their ideas about health. The eudaimonistic model, in particular, represents an ideal that is possible only for the most fortunate individual in the most favorable circumstances. When working with a client, however, nurses must recognize that for most individuals, perfect health is not a realistic goal.

In assessing a client, nurses seek to understand that person's potential for health. Nurses need to ask not only what is desirable, but also what is possible. The term **optimal health** is used to indicate the best health possible for a particular individual. Thus, the term has not one meaning, but many. Consider, for example, the client with severe, chronic heart disease. Fatigue and shortness of breath may prevent him from seeking employment and engaging in social activities outside the home. Optimal health for this client may mean that he has adequate strength to move from his bed to a chair and to receive visitors. For a young man with no chronic diseases, however, such an existence would not indicate optimal health.

Optimal health, then, is a relative term. As with all such terms, it can become meaningless if used carelessly. It is not helpful to talk about optimal health for a particular individual without describing what would constitute that level of health. It is possible to either overestimate or underestimate a client's health potential. Therefore, it is important that nurses assess each client and each situation thoughtfully. The model of health with which a client is most closely aligned can provide one useful point of reference. Nurses may wish to introduce concepts from their own model, if it differs from that of the client. Through this kind of collaboration, a new model that has been enriched by the values of both nurse and client may emerge. The client's status can be compared to the ideal of the model, and factors that interfere with achieving that ideal can be identified. Some of these factors are subject to modification; others are not. Optimal health is achieved when all of the former are successfully eliminated. To return to the example of the man with heart disease, his underlying disease process cannot be changed by therapies presently available and prevents him from achieving excellent health. He may be able to achieve his own optimal level of health by eating nutritious foods, obtaining adequate sleep, using energy conservation measures in his daily activities, and emotionally accepting the reality of the limitations his disease imposes. Other individuals may have different factors that limit or enhance their health. The following section will review some of the factors that affect a person's health status.

Factors Contributing to Health

Health—by any definition—is a complex phenomenon. Many variables affecting health have been identified; many others remain unknown. Four factors that have a significant influence on health are genetic identity, environment, social and cultural factors, and individual behavior.

Genetic Identity. Every individual is born with a unique genetic identity. Some genetic disorders result in congenital diseases, such as Tay-Sachs disease and Down's syndrome. A person may also inherit a predisposition to develop a disease later in life, as in certain forms of cancer. In some families, there is a marked tendency *not* to develop certain diseases, such as coronary artery disease. Race and sex are also genetic variables that may influence health.

Environment. Clear air, pure water, safe housing, and uncontaminated foodstuffs are among the environmental requisites for good health. Some environmental hazards, such as air pollution, threaten entire communities. Others, such as lead paint, threaten individuals or families within a community. There is not always agreement as to what constitutes an environmental health hazard. Nuclear power plants are considered safe by some people and are regarded as serious hazards by others.

The concept of environment can be broadened to encompass one's immediate surroundings. Home, work, or school environments can contribute to overall health if they provide challenges to individual development while offering support and room to maximize one's potential. These environments can also be detrimental to health. For example, many people work in high stress jobs where expectations of performance are high but little personal recognition is offered. Others perform mundane repetitive tasks that offer no challenge or stimulation. Either situation can compromise health. A home environment in which there is conflict and dissension rather than nurturing support can be a negative influence on the health of the family. A school environment in which gang activity threatens social relationships and extracurricular events jeopardizes the emotional, social, and physical health of the students.

Social and Cultural Factors. Social and cultural factors such as income, ethnicity, and the accessibility of health care resources within the community will affect clients' views of themselves as healthy or ill, the kind of care they will seek, and their ability to pay for it. These factors will also affect the likelihood of clients having a particular health problem. A man who lives in a community in which cigarette smoking is a common and even expected adult male behavior is likely to smoke and therefore to be at increased risk for a number of respiratory and cardiac disorders. He may not regard the development of a chronic cough as a matter for concern because it is commonplace among his acquaintances.

Individual Behavior. An individual significantly affects personal health by such practices as eating nutritious foods, obtaining adequate rest, and wearing a seat belt in an automobile. A person also influences personal health by refraining from certain behaviors, such as smoking or using drugs. The following section will look at the role of the individual in health maintenance and promotion. Later in the chapter, disease prevention will be discussed.

Health Promotion

What kind of health-promoting measures are part of people's lives? Engaging in exercise on a regular basis is one kind. Selecting healthy foods to eat, or practicing some form of meditation as a method of dealing with stress are other

IMPLICATIONS FOR NURSE–CLIENT COLLABORATION

Assessment of Optimal Health

Assessment of a client's optimal health focuses not simply on what is *desirable* but what is *possible* for the client. The successful outcome of client care may be determined to a large extent by a mutual understanding held by nurse and client of what health goals are possible for the client. Their consensus on the possibilities for the client's health and the goals for client care is facilitated by the sharing of ideas that occurs in a collaborative relationship.

kinds. Many people participate in these and other health-promotion activities. There is an increasing sense among the public that health must be actively attended to, that "letting well enough alone" is not an appropriate maxim where health is concerned.

Many health professionals, too, are committed to the idea that health promotion is an important professional responsibility. If health is in fact more than the absence of disease, then health care is necessarily more than the treatment of disease. In spite of the great interest in health promotion, however, the term itself is not well understood. Reviews of the literature indicate that health professionals assign a number of vague, often contradictory meanings to the term health promotion.[23,26,27]

Brubaker describes **health promotion** as "health care directed toward high-level wellness through processes that encourage alteration of personal habits or the environment in which people live."[27] She states that health promotion takes place only after the client has resolved any active disease and is in stable health. She makes distinctions, therefore, among health promotion, health maintenance, and disease prevention. Whereas the goal of health promotion is high-level wellness, the goal of **health maintenance** is the preservation of the status quo—neutral or average health. **Disease prevention** is an activity undertaken to prevent a specific disease or disorder. Some people use exercise as a means of health promotion, hoping to go beyond neutral health to a higher level of health. By exercising vigorously, they seek to improve stamina, strength, and flexibility and to achieve a sense of well-being. Many people, however, get just enough exercise to allow for health maintenance—that is, enough to enable them to participate in routine activities of daily living. Exercise can also be a means of disease prevention, for example when a nurse provides range-of-motion exercises to a client who is partially paralyzed after a stroke, in the hope of preventing joint contractures.

It is not always clear, of course, to which of the three categories a particular activity belongs. A given activity may, in fact, qualify as an example of all three categories. If you add an additional source of vitamin C to your diet, are you improving your general nutritional status (health promotion), maintaining the integrity of vessel walls (health maintenance), or preventing scurvy (disease prevention)? Keeping in mind that distinctions among the categories are not clearly delineated, the part that nurses play in promoting good health is presented below.

The Nurse's Role. Professional nurses have long been concerned with assisting clients to improve their health. They act as resources, educators, role models, and motivators.

Although clients frequently seek assistance from nurses for purposes of disease treatment or prevention, they may not think of nurses as resources for help with health promotion. Therefore, it is often nurses who initiate this type of interaction. Consider a clinic nurse who is examining a young boy for a camp physical. The nurse discovers no evidence of disease, but finds the boy to be slightly irritable. Upon questioning, the boy's mother states that since summer vacation began, she has allowed her son to stay up later than usual, and that he has been getting fewer hours of sleep than he is accustomed to having. The nurse might use this opportunity to explain to mother and son the importance of regular sleep in adequate amounts and to collaborate with them to plan some changes in the boy's schedule.

Sometimes it is clients who identify an area for improvement. In this case, the client may come to a nurse for specific suggestions. Regardless of who suggests the possibility, one of a nurse's most useful tools for assisting clients toward improved health is client education. With some people, simply providing information will be sufficient. Others may need or desire further assistance to become motivated, to set goals, and to plan and implement specific health promotion strategies.

Nurses need to be committed to health promotion as an appropriate nursing function if they are to be effective in helping clients to improve their health. They need to be knowledgeable about factors that contribute to good health and skillful in conveying that information to clients in a useful way. Nurses also need to demonstrate by personal behavior that they value health promoting measures.

Role-modeling, or personal example, is an indirect form of client education that is frequently overlooked (see also Chap. 20). **Role-modeling** is teaching by demonstrating examples of new behaviors. Role-modeling can be focused on a specific skill or action in a circumscribed time frame, or it can be ongoing. Parents are role models for their children, often without being aware that their children are imitating behaviors they witness in their homes. In the same fashion, nurses are often role models for clients. Nurses should always be aware of the image of healthy behavior that a client might form by observing nurses' examples. Does the nurse, like other busy professionals, try to save time by sleeping less and eating fast food? Does the nurse relax by having a cigarette in the nurses' station? Does the nurse's appearance imply a sedentary lifestyle? If so, these nurses' behaviors may be diminishing their credibility as health educators.

In addition to providing specific information about health-promoting practices, nurses seek to motivate clients to seek health-promoting measures independently that are

IMPLICATIONS FOR NURSE–CLIENT COLLABORATION

Health Promotion Through Role-Modeling

The personal example of healthful living patterns the nurse projects to the client is sometimes overlooked as an important form of client education and health promotion. In a collaborative relationship, the nurse not only shares information and professional opinions with the client verbally but also models, or lives by, the principals espoused. The client is frequently aware of the nurse's habits as well as the nurse's advice, and decides whether the nurse presents an image of health that merits personal imitation.

congruent with their own values and beliefs about health. Finally, nurses need to be effective in encouraging and supporting clients' independent efforts at health promotion.

Factors other than individual nurses' efforts also influence the possibility of incorporating health promotion into nursing practice. These factors include time, agency constraints, limits to nursing practice, and cost.

Nurses have many demands on their time; it seems that there is never enough time to do all that they would like. Time given to one activity necessarily limits the amount available to spend on another. A nurse will need to make decisions on a client-by-client basis regarding how much time is to be spent on health promotion.

Because most nurses are employees, they are responsible to the agency that employs them as well as to their clients. A nurse working with acutely ill surgical clients will be expected to spend most of the work day attending to problems relating to their surgical disorders. A nurse working on a postpartum floor, on the other hand, may be expected to be quite involved with health teaching. Nurses are sometimes frustrated when they find that their beliefs regarding the value of health promotion are at odds with the expectations of the agency that employs them.

In determining how the limits of nursing practice affect health promotion activities, the definition of health must be considered. The broader the definition of health, the larger the number of activities that are designated "health promotion." It has been suggested that equating health with total well-being can create problems for health care providers if they are then expected to attend to the total well-being of clients.[28,29] Having an adequate income contributes to one's well-being, as does living in a low-crime neighborhood. To what extent, however, is a nurse responsible for assuring that clients obtain these things? Not everything that is life-enhancing is health promoting. The nurse's role in health promotion is an extremely important aspect of professional nursing practice. Health promotion activities planned, carried out or supported by nurses can have a significant impact on client health. It is important, then, that nurses establish clear boundaries for the concept of health so that determinations can be made as to which activities may legitimately be considered health promotion.

Smith's taxonomy of models can provide direction in this endeavor. Many would agree that health promotion includes those activities that increase the probability that clients carry out usual activities, remain free of signs and symptoms of pathology, and adapt successfully to stressors. A nurse planning a health promotion program for a client may wish to choose activities that fall within this framework. Nutrition counseling, for example, may help a client to avoid clinical signs associated with an inadequate diet, and childbirth preparation classes may help a pregnant woman cope with the stress of delivery.

The eudaimonistic model, however, is more problematic. This model's broad definition of health requires an equally broad definition of health promotion activities. Not everyone would agree that any activity that promotes the full expression of a client's potential is a health promotion activity. Education in the humanities, for instance, can enrich a person's life considerably, but it is more difficult to show how it improves health. When planning health promotion activities, the nurse should be aware that controversy exists in nursing regarding the use of the eudaimonistic model.

Health care is expensive. For many persons it is altogether unaffordable. Individuals, hospitals, and third-party payers are all seeking ways to control the cost of health care. Health promotion programs and services will be scrutinized to determine whether they are cost-effective. Nurses seeking to establish or maintain health promotion programs in the agencies in which they are employed may find funds budgeted for these activities shrinking or disappearing. Moreover, nurse staffing on acute care units is often limited by cost constraints, which may make it more difficult for nurses to engage in informal health promotion efforts with individual clients.

The Client's Role. Increasingly, health is regarded not as a right or as good fortune, but as an obligation of the individual.[30,31] People are expected to take active measures aimed at maintaining and promoting health. A health professional's best efforts at providing information about a sound diet are wasted if they are disregarded by the client. It is not a simple matter, however, for individuals to know which behaviors are health promoting; even health professionals are occasionally unsure. Health is so ill-defined and hard to measure that clear guidelines for promoting it have not been established.[32,33] Until such guidelines are available, it is unfair to suggest that clients could be held entirely responsible for their health. The efficacy of some health practices, however, has been established. In a well-known study by Belloc and Breslow, seven behaviors were identified that were found to have a significant positive influence on physical health.

1. Eating breakfast
2. Eating regular meals without snacking
3. Maintaining normal weight for height
4. Not smoking cigarettes
5. Drinking alcohol moderately, if at all
6. Exercising at least moderately
7. Sleeping 7 to 8 hours per night[34]

The researchers found that these behaviors were cumulative; the more of them a person maintained, the healthier he or she was likely to be. Clearly, these are practices that require the active participation of clients. A nurse may suggest them to a person, and help to plan ways of incorporating them into daily life, but clients are ultimately accountable for carrying them out. Box 5–2 gives examples of health promoting measures for clients.

Nurse–Client Collaboration for Health Promotion. The health practices listed above may provide a good starting point for a discussion of health promotion between nurse and client because they relate to a minimal definition of health; that is, physical well-being. But before beginning

BOX 5–2. EXAMPLES OF HEALTH PROMOTING MEASURES FOR CLIENTS

Sleep and Rest

- Avoid excess intake of caffeine.
- Establish regular times for sleeping and rising.
- Obtain 7 to 8 hours of sleep per night.

Nutrition

- Plan a diet according to individual needs (height and weight, developmental level, activity level.)
- Eat regular meals at regular times and limit snacking.
- Limit junk foods to occasional treats.

Exercise

- Find a form of exercise that you enjoy doing.
- Plan regular time for exercising.
- Include activities that increase endurance and flexibility.

Habits

- Drink alcohol moderately or not at all.
- Quit smoking or do not start.

actual planning for health promotion, nurses need to ascertain clients' understanding of health, because it will significantly affect their health goals. A person who defines health in terms of the clinical model, for example, would be unlikely to participate in a biofeedback program for the purpose of enhancing relaxation. This person might, on the other hand, wish to learn biofeedback techniques in order to manage hypertension.

Nurses will sometimes find that their goals for clients differ from clients' personal goals and may feel that a client's goals are unrealistic, as in the case of a woman with advanced lung disease who wishes to begin a program of strenuous exercise. Occasionally, nurses will consider a client's goals to be inappropriate. This would be the case if a nurse were working with a young woman who regarded her health status to be inversely related to her body weight and who planned to continue dieting even though her friends had expressed alarm at how much weight she had lost. Or perhaps nurses may feel that some clients' goals are too limited. In any case, nurses need to share their thoughts with clients as they work together and to invite clients' opinions and collaboration. Consider the following example. An elderly woman, seeing her nurse at a health maintenance organization, relates proudly that she stays very fit for her age by walking 3 miles per day. The nurse, after praising the woman's initiative, points out that flexibility is another parameter of fitness. Together, nurse and client conclude that the woman's joints are rather stiff, especially in her torso and upper extremities, and the client agrees to include some mild stretches into her daily exercise routine. In this situation, nurse and client had different goals initially, but were able to formulate a common goal after collaborating on the problem.

At times, individuals set realistic goals for themselves, but are unable to achieve them. There are a number of reasons why people find themselves unable to practice healthy behaviors.[26] Some do not have access to accurate information about healthful practices. Others may be aware of such practices, but do not carry them out because of pressure from peer groups or advertising to behave differently. A teenage boy, for example, may have been instructed by his athletic coach on the ill effects of alcohol consumption. Nevertheless, the boy drinks because other boys on the team do, and he wishes to fit in with the group. This behavior is reinforced by advertising, which portrays alcohol consumption as a sophisticated social activity. Finally, some people do not practice health promotion because of the cost involved, as in purchasing nutritious foods. The influence of some of these constraining factors may be diminished by nursing interventions. At times, however, clients will be unwilling or unable to adopt certain health promotion measures. Nurse and client may decide to discontinue the relationship or to work on other aspects of the client's health. They may return to the original problem at a later date if the client so chooses.

Others Who Contribute to Health Promotion. Other health care providers are also active in health promotion. Physicians, physical therapists, and nutritionists, among others, use their expertise to assist clients toward improved health. Those in the field of community health, particularly, have a history of interest in health promotion.

Some persons who offer health promotion services do not have conventional credentials. They may specialize in a particular therapy, such as massage or herbal treatments. Because the practice of these persons is unregulated and many of their claims are undocumented, some health care providers regard them as quacks or charlatans and advise clients to be wary of them.[35]

In addition to clients and providers, various groups have an interest in health promotion. Insurance companies, of course, are concerned about health, and use advertising to encourage people to engage in healthy behavior. Businesses are concerned about the health of their employees because they require a stable workforce and because they carry some of the cost of employee health insurance. Many businesses have employee health clinics and some offer fitness programs for their workers.

DISEASE AND ILLNESS

Just as there are many understandings of health and wellness, there are also many ways of describing disease and illness. Think back to a time when you were not feeling well. How did you determine that you were actually "sick"? Did you look for signs and symptoms? For some people, simply feeling unwell is enough to establish sickness, while others need to have their status confirmed by friends or family. Some persons do not consider themselves sick unless they have been so designated by a health care professional. More detail on how individuals come to define themselves as ill is provided in Chapter 12.

Health professionals, of course, must make determinations about who is healthy and who is not. But they, too, have many differing ideas as to what constitutes an illness. Although it may seem reasonable to suggest that an illness is a state identifiable by measurable deviations from the norm, this definition is often too limited to be useful. For example, a woman with an amputated leg deviates from the physical norm. If this woman adapts successfully to the use of a prosthesis, she is no longer regarded as ill, and may hardly consider herself disabled. Besson describes six situations in which a person's health status is ambiguous:

1. The person who feels well, but is in the early stages of an illness that will eventually manifest symptoms.
2. The person who feels well, but is exposed to risk factors, such as smoking.
3. The person who is temporarily overwhelmed by life's problems.
4. The physically well person who prefers the sick role.
5. The physically unwell person who refuses the sick role.
6. The person who cannot be determined to be either sick or well, because he or she never presents for examination.[36]

It is clear that coming to a conclusion about whether or not a person is sick is not a simple matter. It is, however, a most important judgment. A person's status as sick or healthy may determine eligibility for sick leave, insurance coverage, and health care. It may influence a decision to participate in a therapeutic plan and in everyday activities. The "sick" designation may affect how individuals feel about themselves and may also influence the way in which others relate to them. Therefore, it is important that health professionals give consideration to the terms illness and disease.

Distinguishing Among Illness, Disease, and Deviance

Although some persons may regard "disease" and "illness" as synonyms, health professionals often assign distinct meanings to the two terms. Illness is a subjective state; only the individual can determine that he or she is ill. When individuals perceive that their comfort is disturbed or that they are unable to engage in their usual activities, they will view the experience as **illness.**[3,4,5,37,38] **Disease,** on the other hand, is not a feeling state but a condition in which there is an observable disruption of structure or function. Eisenberg points out that "disease and illness do not stand in a one-to-one relation."[39] That is, a person may be ill, but have no identifiable disease. Conversely, it is possible to have a disease without being ill. Many persons with chronic diseases, for example, do not regard themselves as ill. It is necessary to consider whether *every* deviation of structure and function from the norm is a disease. Caplan notes that the aging person experiences many physical changes from what was normal for that person in earlier years, and asks if aging, then, is to be considered a disease.[40]

There is further distinction to be made between disease and deviance. **Deviance** is a term used to describe behaviors that depart from established social norms. Some deviant behaviors may be regarded as disease, according to the definition given above, if the observer assumes that the function that is being disrupted is not the function of an organ or a system, but the person's function as a member of a family or community. However, the line between disease and social deviance is not always clear. Use of illicit drugs may be labeled a crime or a disease, depending on the perspective of the observer. The designation of a behavior may change. Alcoholism, once regarded as a sin or moral weakness, is now categorized as a disease.

The reasons for calling a behavior a disease may be as much social as they are medical. There has been pressure from groups outside the health professions to remove the disease label from such behavior as homosexuality. The term disease can be used in a disparaging sense, to connote weakness and unwholesomeness, and some persons wish to dissociate themselves from these connotations. Some groups, on the other hand, have lobbied to have a behavior, such as compulsive gambling, labeled a disease. The person demonstrating such behavior would then be regarded as deserving of help and sympathy. Further, behavior designated as sick may not be regarded as criminal, although it deviates from societal norms. The criminal is punished; the sick person is treated. In recent years, many deviant behaviors have been reclassified as diseases.[19] Although some regard this as a humane approach, others believe that the "medicalization" of society can lead to other problems.[41] As social problems are redefined as health problems, for example, health professionals may be expected to deal with issues outside their area of expertise. The Surgeon General has called violence a health problem, but how many health care professionals are prepared to treat violence, as opposed to treating victims of violence?[42]

The distinctions among illness, disease, and deviance, then, are not insignificant. They influence decisions about who receives help and what kind of help is offered, and they determine to some extent the boundaries of the health care professions.

The Health–Illness Continuum

As the previous discussion illustrates, health and wellness, illness and disease are closely related concepts. Definitions vary, and there is some overlap. It is not always clear where health ends or illness begins. In order to illustrate the relationship among the concepts, models have been developed showing health status on a continuum. A continuum is a continuous whole or series containing many elements. A **health–illness continuum,** then, is a continuum that depicts health and illness as extreme elements of a unified concept. Although these models are referred to as health–illness continua, they also incorporate the concepts of wellness and disease. The simplest model depicts health status as a point on a line (Fig. 5–2). Health and illness are at

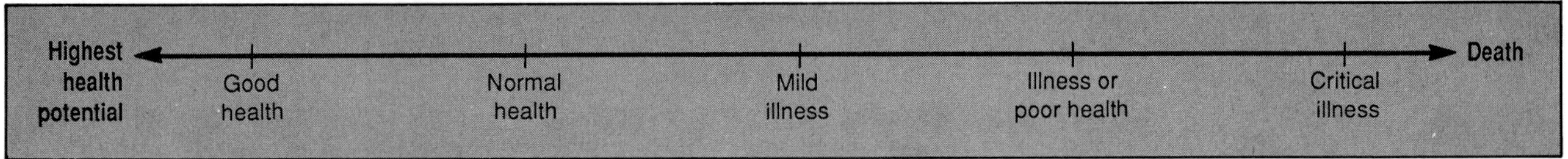

Figure 5–2. A simple health-illness continuum. (*Adapted from Flynn J, Heffron P.* Nursing: From Concept to Practice. *2nd ed. Norwalk, CT: Appleton & Lange; 1988.*)

either extreme and are considered opposites. Even in this simple model, health and illness are not represented as absolute states. Degrees of relative health and illness are recognized. For example, a person who is at a point of good health on the continuum may go on to achieve a state of even greater health.

Brubaker[27] has modified this model to illustrate the types of health care appropriate to each area of the continuum (Fig. 5–3). Health maintenance and disease prevention are required to maintain neutral health. As the person moves toward high-level wellness, he or she will need to engage in health promotion activities. The person on the illness side of the continuum is in need of cure and rehabilitation.

Conceptualizing health as occurring on a continuum reinforces that health and illness are relative terms, and that a person's health status is not fixed, but is always changing. A limitation of the model is that it does not account for the possibility that individuals may be moving toward greater health in one aspect of their lives, and lesser health in others.[43] For instance, a client may be pleased that her gums have shown improvement since she began flossing her teeth regularly. At the same time, however, she is eating an increasingly restricted diet because pain from a hiatus hernia prevents her from consuming many of her usual foods. Her dental health is improving while her nutritional health is deteriorating.

Etiologies of Disease

Etiology refers to the cause or origin of a disease. An understanding of the etiologies of diseases is important to health care providers. The etiology assigned to a disease or a symptom significantly affects both treatment and preventive measures. Heart palpitations that are believed to be the result of anxiety will be treated differently from those thought to be a side effect of medication.

Conflicts may arise between health care providers and clients when they do not share similar beliefs about disease causation. Betz describes a situation in which researchers were investigating Chagas' disease in a Native American population. The researchers believed the disease was caused by a microbe, whereas the Native Americans thought it was a consequence of disturbing the power residing in plants, animals, and other natural phenomena, and were resentful of the investigators.[44] When providers and clients are in conflict over the question of etiology, clients may feel angry or patronized if their own strongly held beliefs are not given respectful consideration. Clients may secretly substitute other treatment for the one prescribed by the provider, or may withdraw from treatment altogether. When working with a client, therefore, nurses need to understand what the client believes has caused the disease in order to enhance motivation to participate in the plan of care.

Among health professionals, the belief that a single

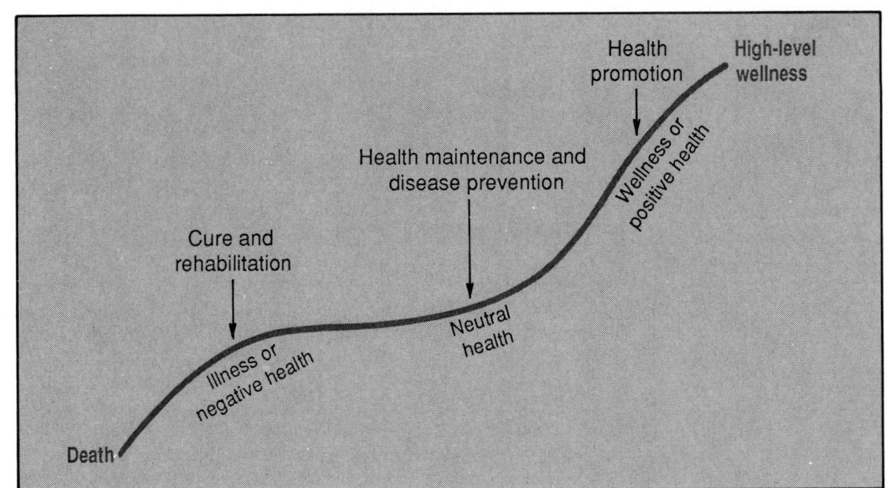

Figure 5–3. Brubaker's health–illness continuum. (*From Brubaker BH. Health promotion: A linguistic analysis.* Adv Nurs Sci. *1983; 5:13. Reprinted with permission of Aspen Systems Corporation, copyright 1983.*)

agent is responsible for a particular disease has largely given way to **multiple causation theory,** which suggests that disease is usually the result of the interaction of a number of factors. It is noted that although several people may be exposed to a disease-causing agent—such as the tubercle bacillus—not all will become infected. A distinction is sometimes made between necessary and sufficient causes of disease. In the case just mentioned, exposure to the bacillus is a necessary but perhaps not sufficient cause of tuberculosis, because not all individuals exposed to the bacillus develop the infection.

One way of analyzing the multiple factors that can contribute to disease is to study the separate and combined effects of host, agent, and environment[45] (see Chap. 7). To investigate the cause of tuberculosis, then, one would establish that the agent (bacillus) was present. The individual or host would be examined for evidence of susceptibility to the disease, perhaps by virtue of having a preexisting chronic condition such as diabetes. Additionally, the person's environment would be considered, as the incidence of tuberculosis is known to be related to environmental factors such as crowded housing.

Anthropologist George Murdock conducted a worldwide survey of theories of disease causation.[46] He identified several theories, which he divided into two categories, natural and supernatural (Box 5–3). While supernatural theories are frequently associated with primitive societies, many persons in developed societies attribute disease to a provoked deity. They may reconcile this belief with a coexisting belief in the theories of modern medicine by assuming that the causative agent—for example, a carcinogen—is but the indirect cause of illness, with the direct cause designated "God's will."

Murdock lists five theories in the natural category. Some of the societies he studied subscribed to only one of the theories. Conventional Western health professionals, however, use any or all of them in a given situation.

1. *Infection.* This classification includes any disease that results from the invasion of the body by pathogenic organisms. In Western health care, this has been developed as the germ theory.
2. *Stress.* Murdock refers to both emotional and physical stress factors. Physical stressors include such things as hunger, fatigue, and exposure to cold. In recent years, emotional stressors have received a great deal of attention. A number of investigators have sought to demonstrate a causal relationship between emotional stress and physical disease.[47–51]
3. *Organic deterioration.* Diseases associated with organic deterioration are physical, and may be related to aging or to hereditary factors. Decline of a particular organic function is unexplained in some people.
4. *Accident.* Accidents involve injury to a person without willful intent, such as motor vehicle accidents, accidental poisonings, or falls.
5. *Overt human aggression.* This involves instances of injury deliberately inflicted by others or oneself. Examples include injuries secondary to crime, warfare, domestic violence, and suicide.

Murdock's taxonomy provides large and general categories for organizing disease etiologies. In practice, health professionals may use many subcategories. Accidents, for example, may be broken down into smaller classifications such as motor vehicle accidents and industrial accidents. Diseases may be further classified as either chronic or acute, and life-threatening or non-life-threatening.

Disease Prevention

Many diseases are potentially preventable. Lead poisoning in children, for example, may be prevented by removing sources of lead from their environment. Table 5–1 lists statistics for the leading causes of death in the United States. In many instances, these diseases or the problems contributing to them are preventable. Although the treatment of existing diseases is clearly a major task, prevention of disease is an important concern of health care professionals.

Some actions are aimed at averting disease entirely, as in the administration of polio vaccine to increase immunity to polio. In other situations, disease is already present, and action is taken to prevent it from becoming worse or leaving a permanent disability. Practices directed toward preven-

BOX 5–3. MURDOCK'S SURVEY OF THEORIES OF DISEASE CAUSATION

Supernatural
- Soul loss
- Spirit aggression
- Mystical retribution
- Provoking deity
- God's (Allah's, etc) will

Natural
- Infection
- Stress
- Organic deterioration
- Accident
- Human aggression

TABLE 5–1. LEADING CAUSES OF DEATH IN THE UNITED STATES: 1987

Cause	Number of Deaths
Cardiovascular Disease	974,045
Cancer	476,927
Accidents	95,020
Chronic Obstructive Pulmonary Disease	78,380
Pneumonia and Influenza	69,225
Suicide	30,796
AIDS	13,468

From the National Center for Health Statistics, US Public Health Service, DHHS and Recommendations for Human Blood Pressure Determination by Sphygmomanometers, *Copyright American Heart Association; 1987.*

tion of disease and reduction of the negative consequences of disease have been described at three levels of prevention[45]:

1. **Primary prevention.** Efforts are aimed at improving general health and at specific protection from diseases. Fluoridation of drinking water is an example of specific protection. Nurses engage in primary prevention when they provide information to the public on how to avoid sexually transmitted diseases.
2. **Secondary prevention.** Activities include early diagnosis and prompt treatment of disease. Screening measures such as tuberculosis testing fall within this category. A nurse who monitors and controls fluid intake of a burn client is promoting secondary prevention.
3. **Tertiary prevention.** The focus is on disability limitation and rehabilitation. Teaching a client who has lung disease how continuing to smoke will increase the seriousness of the disease is an example of tertiary prevention.

Preventive measures at any of the three levels may be undertaken by clients or by health care professionals (see also Chapter 7). Institutions such as government agencies also play a role in preventive health care by providing for such things as safe waste disposal, clean water supplies, and insect control.

Influences on Individual Disease Prevention Behaviors. The availability of social support is an important variable affecting health behavior. Social support is the availability of individuals who can be relied upon for assistance and caring. Hubbard and associates identified a strong positive relationship between health practices and the presence of a spouse or confidant.[52] Schafer and colleagues found that adult diabetics who lacked support from family members were less likely to adhere to diabetes control practices.[53]

Social factors also influence health behaviors. Peer groups establish and communicate acceptable standards of behavior, and have a marked effect on an individual's decisions about weight control, alcohol consumption, and other health behaviors. In the larger social environment, government policies such as subsidies to tobacco farmers and communications from the mass media are part of the milieu in which personal health decisions are made. Finally, health behaviors are affected by the value that an individual places on health. Health is sometimes sacrificed to another goal. A father with little money may care less for his own welfare than for his children's and may see that they have enough to eat even when he does not. Some persons are willing to sacrifice health for less worthy goals, such as altered personal appearance, periodically embarking on extreme weight loss diets.

A number of theories have been proposed to explain why people fail to practice recommended health behaviors. Baric describes the **at-risk role** in which a client agrees to take steps to reduce known risk factors.[54] An example in which this role is applicable is the individual who frequently drives home from a bar where he has stopped for a few drinks. He is at risk for serious injury or death in a motor vehicle accident. If this person decides to refrain from drinking and driving after having been apprised of the risks, he is said to have assumed the at-risk role. Baric concedes that few people are willing to assume the at-risk role because it carries only responsibilities and no rights, and because it must be maintained indefinitely without immediate reward.

According to Rosenstock's health belief model, the probability that one will engage in a particular health behavior is related to one's beliefs about the seriousness of the potential illness and one's susceptibility to it, to the perceived costs and benefits of the behavior, and to the availability of cues prompting the behavior.[55] Thus, a woman who believes herself to be at high risk for lung cancer may be willing to quit smoking. Cues such as the advice of a nurse may prompt her to try quitting. She may not do so, however, if she thinks that quitting smoking will be too difficult or will be ineffective because she has already smoked for too many years. When a health benefit is to be obtained by giving up a habit, such as smoking or excessive consumption of rich foods, the likelihood that a person will discontinue the habit depends in part on its psychological

BUILDING NURSING KNOWLEDGE

What Effect Does Psychological Well-being Have on Health Behavior?

Muhlenkamp AF, Sayles A. Self-esteem, social support, and positive health practices. *Nurs Res.* 1986; 35:334–338.

Although many health professionals agree that there is a relationship between physical health and psychological well-being, there is no concensus on what the relationship is and how it works. Muhlenkamp and Sayles looked for an explanation in the connection between attitudes and health behavior. In this study, the researchers sought to determine how social support and self-esteem are related and how they influence health practices.

The researchers studied 55 men and 43 women with an average age of 29 years who were residents of a large apartment complex in a southwestern city. They gave each subject three questionnaires: one measuring self-esteem (Coopersmith Self-Esteem Inventory); one measuring perceptions of social support (Personal Resources Questionnaire); and one measuring positive health practices such as nutrition, exercise, relaxation, safety, substance use, and health promotion (Personal Lifestyle Questionnaire).

The researchers found a correlation between self-esteem and social support and found that both were related to positive health behavior; the higher the self-esteem and social support, the more positive the life-style. Findings showed that a person's perceptions of adequate social support do not affect life-style directly, but rather act to increase self-esteem, which is directly related to positive health behaviors. The researchers concluded that their findings suggest that professional efforts should incorporate creative approaches and flexible attitudes toward involving significant others in helping clients to make life-style changes.

utility. Habits such as smoking or overeating may serve such purposes as controlling anxiety or increasing pleasurable stimulation. In this case, the perceived costs of giving up the pleasurable behavior outweigh its perceived benefits.

The Nurse's Role. Nursing practice incorporates all three levels—primary, secondary, and tertiary—of disease prevention. Even when concentrating on supporting clients coping with serious, acute illnesses, nurses may act to prevent new problems from arising. Nurses participate in disease prevention both directly and indirectly. Direct participation includes such activities as administering measles vaccine to children, feeding a client who is too weak to eat, and providing skin care to a client confined to bed. In each of these situations, the nurse's action is intended to avert a potential problem.

Nurses participate indirectly in disease prevention by providing client education. Nurses are in a position to advise clients about the health consequences of particular behaviors, to help them identify risk factors, and to assist them in planning strategies to decrease their risk for disease. Initially—especially if clients are acutely ill—nurses may assume much of the responsibility for preventive measures. Later, as the illness begins to resolve, clients may be encouraged to become more active in using these measures. For example, a nurse uses tertiary preventive measures for a client with recently diagnosed diabetes by taking responsibility for ordering meals that comply with the prescribed diabetic regimen, and later, initiating teaching to promote the client's self-management of dietary restrictions.

Even in situations in which health hazards are created by complex social and economic factors, individuals may be helped to realize that they may have contributed to the development of the hazard and that they might make some contribution toward alleviating it as well. For example, no single person can eradicate air pollution; nevertheless, the collective efforts of many individuals to reduce the use of fossil fuels would go a long way toward reducing air pollution.

A final, and extremely important, responsibility of nurses with regard to disease prevention is to encourage clients to explore the limits of personal responsibility. Some clients may not accept that they are not entirely in control of their own health. They may have been exposed to family values of independence and to messages in the media emphasizing the importance of personal preventive measures and admonishments not to abdicate responsibility for health. The familiar slogan "You are responsible for your own health" is used frequently in the literature of the holistic and wellness movements and is often interpreted quite literally. Nurses have an obligation to help clients recognize that the personal responsibility for health, although significant, has limitations. It is true that some diseases are the result of individual neglect or abuse of health, but it is also true that many health hazards, such as toxic waste in the environment, are largely beyond the control of individuals.[31] In some instances, the etiology of disease is unknown; therefore, preventive measures are unavailable. Primary hypertension, or high blood pressure, is a condition for which, by definition, there is no known etiology. In other situations, disease develops in spite of preventive measures. Lung cancer, for example, may occur in individuals who have never smoked.

Preventive health care is far from being an exact science. Although health care professionals have learned a great deal about preventing disease, much remains to be discovered. The relationship between emotions and disease, in particular, remains unclear. There is controversy, for example, about the significance of emotional status in a person with cancer. Some investigators believe that psychosocial factors, particularly feelings of hope, can affect the course of the disease.[56,57] They suggest that clients may affect the disease process by learning to control their feelings and thoughts. However, results of a study by Cassileth and co-workers showed no relation between psychosocial factors such as life satisfaction and hopelessness/helplessness, and length of survival, in newly diagnosed clients with advanced metastatic disease.[58]

Such controversy illustrates that generalizations about personal responsibility for diseases are inadvisable. Overemphasis on the significance of variables such as emotions, which are not really completely under personal control, can lead to feelings of guilt, hopelessness, or depression when a person becomes ill.[59,60] Sensitive nurses can help clients reach a realistic understanding of the role they can play in disease prevention while recognizing that other factors often have significant impact as well.

The Client's Role. Even though individuals cannot influence their risk for all diseases, personal behavior is regarded as an important factor in disease prevention.[30,31,61] The beneficial effects of effective health care services and a congenial social and environmental milieu may be inadequate to counter the problems that can arise from unhealthy habits. Indeed, several of the diseases listed as leading causes of death in Table 5–1, such as lung cancer, certain cardiovascular diseases, chronic lung disease, and AIDS, are considered largely a consequence of personal behavior.[62,63]

Clients can play an important role at every level of disease prevention. An individual may take measures such as wearing a seat belt in automobiles (primary prevention), practicing monthly breast self-examination (secondary prevention), or regulating the diet to avert the complications of diabetes (tertiary prevention).

The issue, then, becomes how can clients decide what behaviors are likely to be effective in preventing disease. One factor is an effective collaborative relationship with health care providers, such as nurses. However, advice as to just what constitutes healthy or unhealthy behaviors is available to individuals from many other sources: neighbors and family, the media, self-help groups, self-styled healers, and even quacks. Some of the advice about disease prevention is dubious—there is no evidence that hanging garlic from the neck prevents colds. Some advice is potentially dangerous—for example, the recommendation of megadoses of vitamins to prevent certain diseases. The client, therefore, must carefully evaluate the credibility of such advice.

One source clients may look to is *Healthy People: The Surgeon General's Report on Health Promotion and Disease Prevention.*[64] It offers specific suggestions by age group. For infants, recommendations include such items as breastfeeding when possible, regular pediatric examinations, and immunizations. Suggestions for adolescents and young adults include attention to roadway safety, education about sexually transmitted diseases, and measures to prevent firearm accidents. The following measures are recommended for adults:

1. Stop or decrease smoking.
2. Use alcohol wisely.
3. Adopt prudent dietary measures, such as consumption of:
   a. Only sufficient calories to meet dietary needs (fewer if person is overweight).
   b. Less saturated fat and cholesterol.
   c. Less salt.
   d. Less sugar.
   e. Relatively more complex carbohydrates (whole grains, cereals, fruits, and vegetables.
   f. Relatively more fish, poultry, and legumes, and less red meat.
4. Participate in regular, vigorous exercise at least three times a week for 15 to 30 minutes each time.
5. Detect and reduce exposure to environmental hazards.
6. Detect and reduce work site hazards.
7. Have blood pressure screening every 5 years, and then every 2 to 3 years after age 40. Follow prescribed medication plan for hypertension.
8. Women: Have three Pap smears at 1-year intervals beginning at age 20 or upon becoming sexually active; and then every 3 years. Increase frequency of screening if abnormalities are found, or if taking estrogens or oral contraceptives.
9. Women: Perform breast self-examination monthly after menstrual period. Have periodic mammography after age 50, or after age 40 for women with a family history of breast cancer.
10. Watch for and report early warning signs of cancer.
11. Seek professional help for serious difficulty in coping with a life event.
12. Brush and floss teeth daily. Have a yearly dental examination.

Although these behaviors seem reasonable and even commonsensical, adopting them may require major life-style changes for some persons, and resistance to change may be high. Others may already be practicing these behaviors and may wish to go beyond them.

Nurse–Client Collaboration in Disease Prevention. As in any nurse–client interaction, mutuality is of critical importance when planning for disease prevention. Either the client or the nurse may identify a potential problem. The nurse may have a great deal of information about strategies, but will need to work closely with the client to select the ones most appropriate to the client and the situation. For example, a woman with a family history of heart disease may choose to adopt a low-fat diet. If the nurse knows that the woman travels frequently on business and eats most of her meals in restaurants, he or she will be able to offer realistic suggestions on meal planning and menu selections. For a summary of nurse and client roles in health promotion and disease prevention, see Figure 5–4.

Keep in mind that both nurse and client will have goals, and that they may or may not be similar. Generally, nurses hope that clients will adopt prudent preventive measures of known efficacy and usefulness. Two extremes present challenges to collaboration. At one extreme are persons who become excessively anxious about their well-being, and spend a great deal of energy monitoring their health status and engaging in preventive practices of dubious value. They may raise health to an ultimate value, and pursue it at the cost of neglecting other aspects of their lives. This kind of "healthism," to use Crawford's term, can lead the client to set unrealistic goals.[41]

At the other extreme are those individuals who show little concern for their health and who practice few or no preventive measures. These persons may have no particular health goals and may visit a health care provider only for treatment of acute illness.

Most persons, however, fall somewhere in the middle ground between these extremes, and are willing to adopt some preventive practices, but not others. A client with a history of heart disease may make an effort to lose weight, but may not be willing to quit smoking.

Clearly, choices regarding health behaviors are complex and influenced by many variables. Nurses will encounter many clients who will not accept their recommendations. To simply dismiss clients as "noncompliant," a disparaging reference to a client's lack of cooperation with the health professional's advice, is to ignore the possible reasons informing their decisions. In nurses' discussions with clients, they may identify variables subject to intervention. Consider the case of a man who is neglecting to take his medication for high blood pressure. In talking to him, the nurse learns that his uncle became impotent while taking antihypertensive drugs. For this client, the perceived cost of complying is too high. The nurse may help by discussing client concerns with the client and with his physician. By providing information and exploring clients' feelings, nurses can enhance clients' ability to make informed, thoughtful choices about health behaviors and can tailor client care plans to clients' desires and life-style.

At times the result of a client's thoughtful consideration is a decision not to participate in a course of action recommended by a nurse. The right of clients to refuse treatment is generally recognized by the health care professions and upheld by the courts.[65] It is also acknowledged by the mutual interaction model of nurse–client relations (see Chap. 37). This is not to suggest that the nurse's responsibility to the client ends when the client says "No."

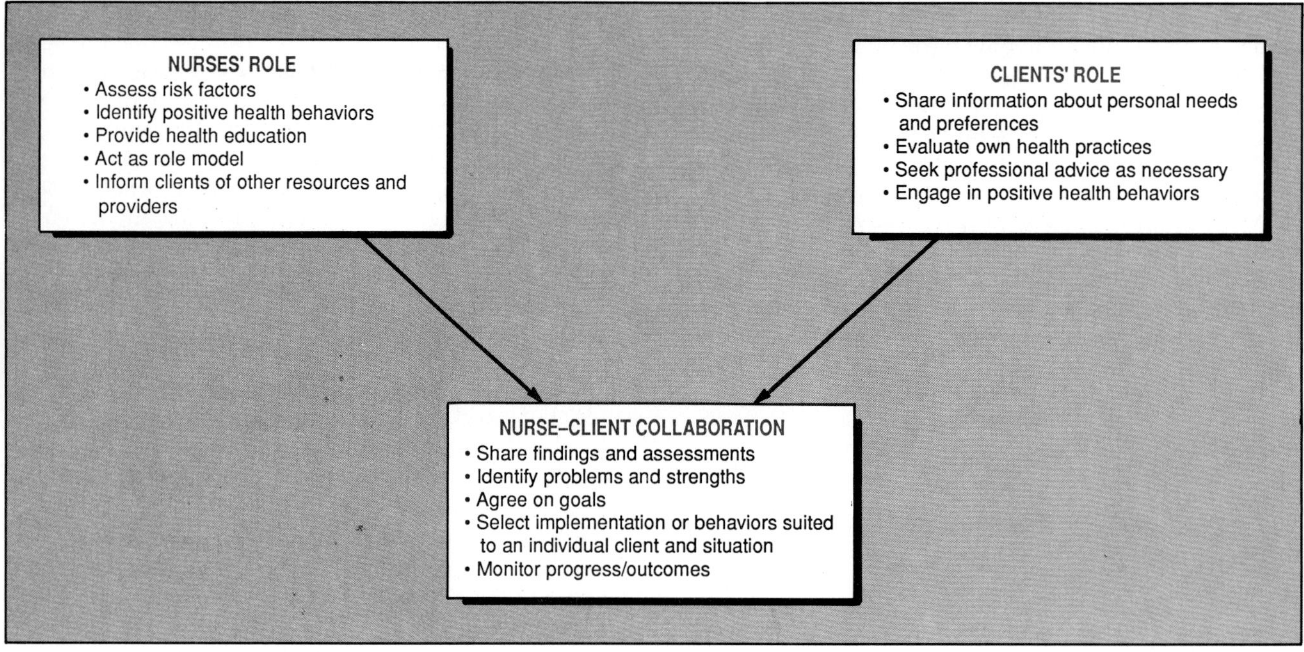

Figure 5–4. Client and nurse roles in health promotion and disease prevention.

Although obligated to respect clients' rights to autonomy and self-determination, nurses are also obligated to facilitate their making thoughtful choices regarding their own health care. Bandman and Bandman discuss several errors made by health care providers relative to clients' rights to self-determination in health care decisions, including a paternalistic approach in which providers dominate decision-making, a manipulative approach in which providers strongly imply which decision a client should make while presenting information, and an indifferent approach, in which little or no information is provided.[66] Each of these approaches ignores clients' rights to essential information related to personal health care decisions.

It has been suggested that just as clients have the right to give informed consent, so too do they have the right to **informed dissent.**[67] That is, clients have the right to expect that, regardless of the ultimate decision, providers will offer support in the decision-making process. An extreme example of the right to refuse treatment, even when it includes death, is the Nancy Cruzan case.[68] Dissent may be voiced at any point in the process. A nurse and client may not agree that a particular issue—such as a weight loss of 10 pounds—is a problem; or they may agree on the nature of the problem, but disagree on goals or strategies. The nurse's responsibility is to assure that clients are aware of the nature of potential and actual problems, the possible ways of dealing with these problems, and the probable consequences of their choices. It is necessary to avoid any semblance of coercion. Only then will the client be in a position to offer a truly informed dissent.

Because nurses and clients often work on several problems simultaneously, dissent on one issue will not necessarily signal an end to the relationship. They will likely continue to work on other issues. Further, work on a particular problem may not end when dissent is voiced. Nurses may often find that a client's choice is acceptable, even if it does not seem to be the "best" choice. Indeed, dissent may actually serve to strengthen the nurse–client relationship if clients see that nurses are respectful of them as individuals with the right to make choices regarding health care and personal health behaviors.

SUMMARY

Health and wellness, illness and disease are critical concepts in nursing. The more clearly nurses define these concepts, the better able they will be to define nursing practice and describe it to others. Little children, when asked what nurses do, sometimes reply, "They help sick people." Indeed they do. And beyond that, they seek to prevent illness and to help persons who are not ill to achieve even better health.

One of the most significant tasks of nursing, then, is the promotion of optimal health. The term "optimal" is not to be understood in ideal terms, as the absence of all disease, discomfort, and human misfortune. Rather, it refers to the greatest degree of health possible at a particular time for a particular individual. Optimal health for one person may allow him or her to participate in vigorous exercise. For another, it may mean using adaptive devices to accomplish the activities of daily living.

Physical problems, of course, can limit the possibilities for health. But other factors, such as economic and social considerations and the client's personal health beliefs, may be equally constraining. It is important to keep these considerations in mind when establishing health goals. When nurses and clients share an understanding of the meaning of optimal health, they can work together most effectively toward that goal.

Integration of the concepts presented in this chapter, including various definitions of health, illness, disease, wellness, and factors that influence their incidence, are important to an individual nurse's development of an effective collaborative role with clients in preventing disease and promoting optimal health.

REFERENCES

1. Breslow. A quantitative approach to the World Health Organization definition of health: Physical, mental and social well-being. *Int J Epidemiol.* 1972; 1:347–355.
2. American Nurses' Association. *Nursing: A Social Policy Statement.* Kansas City, MO: ANA; 1980.
3. Brauman B. Diversities in conceptions of health and physical fitness. *J Health Hum Behav.* 1961; 2:39–46.
4. Smith A. The idea of health: A philosophic inquiry. *Adv Nurs Sci.* 1981; 3:43–50.
5. Pender NJ, Pender AR. Attitudes, subjective norms and intentions to engage in health behavior. *Nurs Reas.* 1986; 35:90.
6. Henderson V. *The Nature of Nursing: A Definition and Its Implications for Practice, Research and Education.* New York: MacMillan; 1966.
7. Bandman EL, Bandman BE. Health and disease: A nursing perspective. In: Caplan AL, ed. *Concepts of Health and Disease.* Reading, MA: Addison-Wesley; 1981: 677–692.
8. Veatch RM. The medical model: Its nature and problems. *Hastings Cent Stud.* 1973; 1:59–76.
9. Kestenbaum V. The experience of illness. In: Kestenbaum V, *The Humanity of the Ill.* Knoxville: University of Tennessee Press; 1982: 3–38.
10. Callahan D. The WHO definition of health. *Hastings Cent Stud.* 1973; 1:77–87.
11. Dubos R. *Man Adapting.* New Haven: Yale University Press; 1965.
12. Dubos R. *Mirage of Health.* New York: Harper; 1959.
13. Lazarus RS, Folkman S. *Stress Appraisal and Coping.* New York: Springer; 1984.
14. Nightingale F. *Notes on Nursing: What it is and What it is Not.* New York: Dover; 1969. (Originally published, 1860).
15. Roy C. The Roy adaptation model. In: Riehl JP, Roy C, eds. *Conceptual Models for Nursing Practice,* 2nd ed. New York: Appleton-Century-Crofts; 1980.
16. Maslow AH. *Toward a Psychology of Being,* 2nd ed. New York: Van Noestrand; 1968.
17. World Health Organization. *Constitution: World Health Organization.* Geneva: WHO; 1971.
18. Callahan D. Health and society: Some ethical imperatives. In: Knowles JH, ed. *Doing Better and Feeling Worse.* New York: Norton; 1977: 23–33.
19. Mechanic D. *Medical Sociology,* 2nd ed. New York: Free Press; 1978.
20. Engelhardt HT Jr. The concepts of health and disease. In: Caplan AL, Englehardt TH Jr., McCartney JJ, eds. *Concepts of Health and Disease.* Reading, MA: Addison-Wesley; 1981: 31–75.
21. Brallier LW. The nurse as holistic health practitioner. *Nurs Clin North Am.* 1978; 13:643–655.
22. Peplau HE. *Interpersonal Relations in Nursing.* New York: Putnam's; 1952.
23. Moore V, Williamson C. Health promotion: Evolution of a concept. *Nurs Clin North Am.* 1984; 19:195–206.
24. Dunn HL. *High-Level Wellness.* Arlington, VA: R.W. Beatty; 1961.
25. Longe ME, Ardell DB. Wellness programs attract new markets for hospitals. *Hospitals* 1981; 55:115–119.
26. Grasser C, Craft BJG. The patient's approach to wellness. *Nurs Clin North Am.* 1984; 19:207–218.
27. Brubaker BH. Health promotion: A linguistic analysis. *Adv Nurs Sci.* 1983; 5:1–14.
28. Kopelman L, Moskop J. The Holistic health movement: A survey and critique. *J Med Philosophy.* 1981; 6:209–235.
29. Francis G. Gesellschaft and the hospital: Is total care a misnomer? *Adv Nurs Sci.* 1980; 2:9–13.
30. Orem DE. *Nursing: Concepts of Practice.* New York: McGraw Hill; 1985.
31. Maglacas AM. Health for all, nursing's role. *Nurs Outlook.* 1988; 36:266–271.
32. Denyes MJ. Orem's model used for health promotion: Directions from research. *Adv Nurs Sci.* 1988; 11:1, 13–21.
33. Donoghue J, Duffield C, Pellatier D, et al. Health promotion as a nursing function: Perceptions held by university students of nursing. *Int J Nurs Stud.* 1990; 27:51–60.
34. Belloc NB, Breslow L. Relationship of physical health status and health practice. *Prevent Med.* 1972; 1:409–421.
35. Todd MC. Interface: Holistic health and traditonal medicine. *West J Med.* 1979; 131:464–465.
36. Besson G. The health–illness spectrum. *Am J Pub Health.* 1967; 57:1901–1905.
37. Horgan H. Health status perceptions affect health-related behavior. *J Geron Nurs.* 1987; 13:30–35.
38. Mechanic D. Health and illness behavior. In: Last J, ed. *Public Health and Preventative Medicine.* Norwalk, CT: Appleton & Lange; 1991.
39. Eisenberg L. What makes persons "patients" and patients "well"? *Am J Med.* 1980; 69:277–286.
40. Caplan AL. The unnaturalness of aging—A sickness unto death? In Caplan AL, ed. *Concepts of Health and Disease.* Reading, MA: Addison-Wesley; 1981: 725–737.
41. Crawford R. Healthism and the medicalization of everyday life. *Int J Health Serv.* 1980; 10:365–388.
42. Will GF. Dr. Koop's Rx for violence. *Boston Sunday Globe.* November 14, 1982; p 27.
43. Wu R. *Behavior and Illness.* Engelwood Cliffs, NJ: Prentice-Hall; 1973.
44. Betz TG. Conflicts in the study of Chagas' disease between a Southwestern Indian population and the staff of a Southwestern university college of medicine. In: Bauwens EE, ed. *The Anthropology of Health.* St. Louis: Mosby; 1978:88–94.
45. Leavell HR. *Preventative Medicine for the Doctor in His Community,* 3rd ed. New York: McGraw-Hill; 1965.
46. Murdock GP. *Theories of Illness: A World Survey.* Pittsburgh: University of Pittsburgh Press; 1980.
47. Selye H. *The Stress of Life.* New York: McGraw-Hill; 1956.
48. Egger J. Psychosocial risk factors in cardiovascular diseases. *Theor Med.* 1987; 7:319.
49. Friedman M, Rosenman R. *Type A Behavior and Your Heart.* New York: Knopf; 1974.

50. Syme SL. Social determinants of health and disease. In Last J, ed. *Public Health and Preventative Medicine.* Norwalk, CT: Appleton & Lange; 1991: 953–970.
51. Hurst MW, Jenkins DC, Rose RM. The relation of psychosocial stress to onset of medical illness. In: Garfield CA, ed. *Stress and Survival.* St. Louis: Mosby; 1979:17–32.
52. Hubbard P, Muhlenkamp AF, Brown N. The relationship between social support and self-care practices. *Nurs Res.* 1984; 33:266–270.
53. Schafer L, McCaul K, Glasgow R. Supportive and nonsupportive family behaviors: Relationships to adherence and metabolic control with Type I diabetes. *Diabetes Care.* 1986; 9:179–185.
54. Baric L. Recognition of the "at-risk" role—A means to influence health behavior. *Int J Health Ed* 1969; 12:24–34.
55. Rosenstock IM. Historical origins of the health belief model. In: Becker MH, ed. *The Health Belief Model and Personal Behavior.* Thorofare, NJ: Charles B. Slack; 1974.
56. Siegel BS, Siegel BH. Holistic medicine. *Connecticut Med.* 1981; 45:441–442.
57. Simonton OC, Mathews-Simonton S, Creighton JL. *Getting Well Again.* New York: Bantam; 1980.
58. Cassileth BR, Lusk EJ, Miller DS, et al. Psychological correlates of survival in advanced metastatic disease? *N Engl J Med.* 1985; 312:1551–1555.
59. Shapiro J, Shapiro DH. The psychology of personal responsibility. *N Engl J Med.* 1979; 301:211–212.
60. Sontag S. *Illness as Metaphor.* New York: Vintage; 1979.
61. Pender N. *Health Promotion in Nursing Practice.* Norwalk, CT: Appleton & Lange; 1987.
62. Friedland GH, Klein RS. Transmission of the human immunodeficiency virus. *N Engl J Med.* 1987; 317:1125.
63. American Heart Association. *1991 Heart and Stroke Facts.* Dallas, TX: AHA; 1991.
64. US Department of Health, Education and Welfare/Public Health Service. *Healthy People: The Surgeon General's Report on Health Promotion and Disease Prevention.* DHEW (PHS) 79-55071. Washington, D.C.; 1983.
65. Potter D. The patient who refuses treatment. In: *Practices.* Springhouse, PA: Nursing 84 Books; 89–94.
66. Bandman EL, Bandman B. *Nursing Ethics Through the Life Span.* Norwalk, CT: Appleton & Lange; 1990.
67. Berger K. Williams M. Personal communication, November 1985.
68. Sounding Board: Nancy Cruzan and the Right-to-Die. *N Engl J Med.* 1990; 323:670–673.

BIBLIOGRAPHY

Alexy B. Goal setting and health risk reduction. *Nurs Res.* 1985; 34:283.

Baranowski T. Toward the definition of concepts of health and disease, wellness and illness. *Health Values.* 1981; 5:155–163.

Brown N. The relationship among health beliefs, health values, and health promotion activity. *West J Nurs Res.* 1983; 5:155–163.

Champion VL. The relationship of breast self-examination to health belief model variables. *Res Nurs Health.* 1987; 10:375–382.

Clark SR. Compliance and health behaviors. *Top Clin Nurs.* 1986; 7:39–46.

Colantino A. Lay concepts of health. *Health Val.* 1988; 12:3–7.

Donaghue J, Duffield C, Pelletier D, et al. Health promotion as a nursing function: Perceptions held by university students of nursing. *Int J Nurs Stud.* 1990; 27:51–60.

Fries JF. The future of disease and treatment, changing health conditions, changing behaviors, and new medical technology. *J Prof Nurs.* 1986; 2:10.

Hill L, Smith N. *Self Care Nursing.* Englewood Cliffs, NJ: Prentice-Hall; 1985.

Hadley, BJ. Current concepts of wellness and illness. *Image.* 1974; 6:24.

Hibbard JH. Age, social ties and health behaviors: An exploratory study. *Health Ed Res.* 1988; 3:131–139.

Kim MJ. Physiologic responses in health and illness: An overview. *Ann Rev Nurs Res.* 1987; 5:79–104.

Lowery BJ. Psychological stress, denial, and myocardial infarcation outcomes. *Image.* 1990; 23:51–55.

Molzahn AT, Northcott NC. The social bases of discrepancies in health/illness perceptions. *J Adv Nurs.* 1989; 14:132.

Philips BU. Cost containment and health promotion. *Health Values.* 1988; 12:30–31. Editorial.

Prentice-Dunn S, Rogers RW. Protection motivation theory and preventative health: Beyond the health belief model. *Health Edu Res.* 1989; 1:153.

Reynolds CL. The measurement of health in nursing research. *Adv Nurs Sci.* 1988; 10:23–31.

Shaver JF. A biopsychosocial view of human health. *Nurs Outlook.* 1985; 33:186–191.

Trice LB. Meaningful life experience to the elderly. *Image.* 1989; 22:248–255.

Tzirides E. Health outreach program: Marketing the "health way." *Nurs Man.* 1988; 19:55–57.

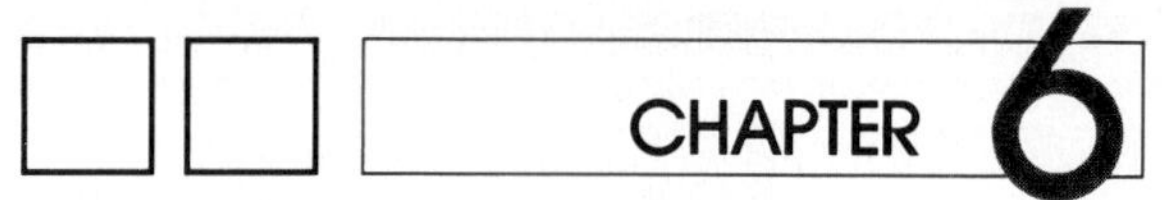

Homeostasis, Homeodynamics, and Change

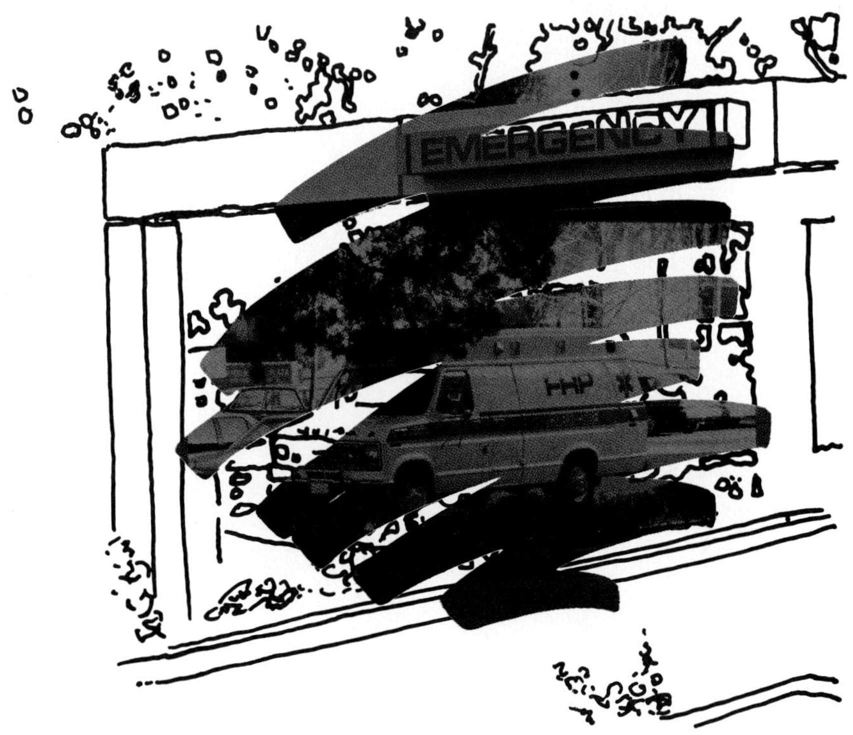

Behavioral Objectives

Upon completion of this chapter, the student will be able to:

1. Define human change.
2. Describe Lewin's three phases of change.
3. Give an example of each of the following patterns of change: maturational, situational, planned, unplanned, physiological, psychological, and social.
4. Define homeostasis and identify the two major homeostatic regulatory systems in the body.
5. Describe the effects of the two components of the autonomic nervous system on body systems and outline the "fight-or-flight" response.
6. Identify the components of a control mechanism, and give an example of a negative feedback system.
7. Compare homeostasis and adaptation and state their significance to health.
8. Define stressor and give examples of physiological, psychological, and social stressors.
9. Explain what is meant by stress as a transaction.
10. Identify the factors that regulate the cognitive appraisal of stress, and the physiological and psychological manifestations of stress.
11. Differentiate stress and crisis, and give examples of maturational and situational changes that may be experienced as crisis.
12. Identify six stress management techniques and describe how they work to neutralize stress.
13. Compare and contrast homeostatic and homeodynamic views of human change.
14. Describe the collaborative view of facilitating growth.
15. Discuss the nurse's role as participant in client change and the promotion of optimal health.

KEY TERMS

adaptation
alarm stage
anxiety
burnout
change
closed systems
cognitive appraisal
comparator
coping
crisis
defense mechanism
effector
exhaustion stage
fear
general adaptation syndrome
growth
hardiness
homeodynamics
homeostasis
maturational changes
maturational crises
mutual process
negative feedback
open systems
panic
planned change
positive feedback
receptor
resistance stage
response
situational changes
situational crises
stability
stress
stressor
system
unplanned change

Change is a constant and pervasive force in the life process. Change may occur without being noticed, or may be experienced as a life crisis. A change may be permanent or temporary, conscious or automatic. Changes may occur in an individual's physical and psychological makeup, or in the situation in which a person lives and works. Although change affects all living species, humans have a special relationship to change. As O'Connell and co-workers have noted, "Unlike any other earth species (which remain essentially the same after they reach maturity) human beings grow, learn, and change throughout their lives in their interests, in their values, in their joys, and sadnesses, and in their needs and attitudes" (p. 13).[1]

It is important for nurses to be able to understand change as they collaborate with clients in the process of promoting optimal health. Nurses often care for individuals and their families at times when they are experiencing significant life changes. Nurses are present at the birth and death of loved ones, and at the scene of a disaster or an emergency. Nurses care for clients experiencing changes in body function due to disease or injury. All of these are types of changes that affect the health status of clients.

People may welcome or resist change. Routines and rituals provide for predictable events in daily life. A person knows what to expect and derives a certain sense of security or comfort from the regularly repeated patterns of behavior represented in rituals and routines. Some people resist changes to daily routines because of the uncertainty and anxiety that may follow. Others seem to enjoy taking risks and trying new things. They seem to welcome change, and actually thrive on breaking the routines. In both cases, nurses must be ready to participate in the change process and work with clients to promote a healthy response to change.

This chapter focuses on change as it relates to individuals in health and illness situations. The broad notion of change is defined and described in the first section. Following sections discuss the nature of change, and describe human responses that resist and facilitate change. Change is then related to the classic concepts of homeostasis and adaptation to stress. The more contemporary concept of homeodynamics is also introduced and related to individual growth as a healthy process of change.

CHANGE AND HUMAN RESPONSES TO CHANGE

The term "change" has been defined by psychologists, social scientists, physicists, economists, and many others. The definition in this chapter focuses on change as it relates to individuals and the environments in which they exist.

Change as a Concept

Change can be defined as an alteration, modification, deviation, variation, or even transformation of something. Webster's Dictionary defines change simply as "making or becoming different."[2] Human beings become different as they grow and mature, and as they respond to the influence of family, friends, society, and the physical environment in which they live and work.

Defining change is difficult because of the many perspectives that can be taken. Physicists, psychologists, and economists, for example, each have different views of change. For the purposes of this chapter, **change** in individuals is defined as a continuous process in which differences in ways of being or functioning occur relative to past ways of functioning. The following discussion expands upon this definition to consider change as a relative phenomenon, process, life constant, and the opposite of stability.

Change as Relative. Change is a relative term.[3,4] It is always described in relation to past ways of being or functioning. For example, it is necessary to know an individual's past eating habits to be able to say that they have changed. Nurses recognize a change in clients' blood pressure or pulse based on past measurements. Therefore individual changes are described as differences relative to past ways of being or functioning.

Change as a Process. Change is a process.[4] It requires movement from past ways of being or functioning to different ways of being or functioning. This process is illustrated in Lewin's description of the three phases of behavioral change: unfreezing, movement, and refreezing.[4] In other words, for change to take place, the current pattern of behavior must be disrupted, the new pattern must be tried, and the new pattern adopted for consistent use (Table 6–1).

Consider the example of changing eating habits. In the unfreezing step, a client assesses his or her own diet, compares it with dietary recommendations, and decides to change to a more healthy diet. The client must be ready and willing to disrupt the current life-style or habits and make a change. In the moving step, the client actually makes the changes: all at once, or in small increments such as cutting out salt one week and limiting consumption of eggs the next week. In the refreezing phase, the client maintains the dietary changes over time, rather than slipping back into old habits. The new behavior becomes the habit. Anyone who has tried to change dietary habits realizes that this process of change is not as simple as it sounds. Dietary habits are linked to traditions, culture, and emotions. Often, the person will go through these steps a number of times before refreezing takes place.

These three phases of change illustrate the point that change is a process. Although these phases were originally used to describe behavioral change, it is important to remember that any type of change is a process that is a movement from one way of being or functioning to another.

Change as a Constant. Change occurs within and around the person in a continuous, ongoing fashion. Sarter, in her analysis of Rogers' theory of nursing, refers to this phenomenon as "the stream of becoming, . . . the continuous flow of change in the world."[5] Consider that life is a process in which the person is always changing and becoming dif-

TABLE 6–1. THE PROCESS OF CHANGE

Phase	Definition	Example
Unfreezing	Readiness or motivation to change	Assessment of diet Learning about a healthy diet Decision to change current eating habits
Moving	Disruption of past behavior patterns	Actual change in eating habits Taking salt off the table Cutting out foods high in fat Increasing high-fiber foods
Refreezing	Adopting new behavior patterns	New behavior maintained for 1 year or more Changes are now the current habits

Adapted from Lewin K: Field Theory in Social Science. *New York: Harper; 1951.*

ferent. Human beings grow and develop and accumulate many experiences along the way. If this is so, then change is the only thing that can be counted on: change is a constant in the life process. Change is always occurring in some form.

Change and Stability. Change can be characterized by its relationship to **stability.**[6,7] Even though change is constantly occurring within the life process, many routines and rhythms of life remain stable for varying periods of time. For example, people eat meals at the same time every day, work at the same occupation for several years, socialize with the same group of friends and relatives over the period of a lifetime. The pattern of life is usually disrupted only during vacations or crises such as illness or death.

The term "stable" means "firmly established" or "well-balanced."[2] Stability is reflected in the rhythms of life in which patterns of function remain relatively the same. Individuals derive a sense of security and comfort from the predictability of daily routines and habits.[8] In fact, a balance between change and stability must be maintained in the promotion of optimal health. Individuals and families tend to develop patterns of sleeping, eating, working, and playing. The rhythms of life can be seen in the cycle of sleep and activity, the regularity of the heartbeat, and the daily fluctuations of body temperature. These unchanging ways of being and functioning provide continuity to the individual in the face of constant change.

Consider a mother with a newborn child. Her body is undergoing physical changes as she recovers from pregnancy and childbirth. Her health habits and daily routines must change to provide for her own health and the health of the child. She changes her diet to accommodate the nursing child and promote healing in her own body, developing a different but stable pattern of food intake. The child awakens her during the night, interrupting her sleep–wake cycle. She accommodates by trying to maintain a regular feeding schedule for the child so that she herself can settle into a new, but predictable, sleep pattern. Her life has changed and she is seeking to establish new routines and rhythms that will balance this change with a sense of stability.

Levels of Change

Within the context of stable life rhythms and routines, change arises out of the interaction between individuals and the environment. Change in individuals has been defined as a continuous process in which differences in ways of being or functioning occur relative to past ways of functioning. New ways of being and functioning take place within and arise in response to an environment that includes home, family, workplace, school, church, and health care facilities. As individuals come in contact with people and places, an interaction takes place. Individuals influence, and are influenced by, the context in which they live at all levels of functioning: physiological, psychological, and social (Fig. 6–1).[9–11]

Physiological Change. Physiological change includes the changes that take place within the body as it adjusts and adapts to the demands of daily life. Patterns of change and stability characterize the physiological changes that maintain the life process. Within cells and organ systems, the body strives to maintain stability or balance in functioning. For example, the body maintains a balance of fluids and electrolytes and balances the intake of nutrients and output of waste products.

Physiological change patterns include growth and development throughout the life span. The changes in hormonal balance and body structure that characterize adolescence occur concurrently with the stabilizing tendencies described above.

Psychological Change. Individuals change by exhibiting different behaviors while retaining the same basic identity.[1] People change in knowledge, feelings, and ability. These changes are balanced by stability in certain personality traits. Consider the example of the changes that occur in adolescence. Changes in hormone balance cause changes in physical characteristics and behavior. Adolescents may become more moody or irritable, or they may challenge authority. But all of these changes are variations of the individual's unique identity. As individuals, we all retain a basic sense of identity and sameness that allows us to be recognized at a 20-year high school reunion. Again, stability and change coexist within an individual.

Social Change. Groups, like individuals, change while retaining the unique identity that sets them apart from other groups. All individuals belong to a number of groups, but the group with the most powerful influence is the family. The family group transmits cultural values and beliefs that will remain with family members throughout their lifetimes (see Chap. 8).

A family member's roles in the household change over time as the family changes, or as the result of a crisis. For example, a son may be expected to take on the duties of the father who is no longer in the home due to death or divorce. Changes in individuals influence group members, and changes in group members influence individuals.

The family group exists within the context of other social groups in the community and the larger society. Social groups collectively define "normal" or acceptable behavior—that is, they establish the social expectations that guide individual behavior. Behavioral norms change as individual and group values change. New expectations then filter down through the levels of society to influence individuals. For example, recent changes in societal norms in the United States have made it acceptable and even desirable for individuals to be health conscious. More and more people are concerned about what they eat and how they exercise. A family group may decide to take the salt shaker off the kitchen table and give up desserts. These changes affect the health of the individuals who are members of these groups.

Samuels and Bennett,[12] authorities on environmental health, state that the health of individuals can be seen as a measure of the health of the larger society. Therefore, in-

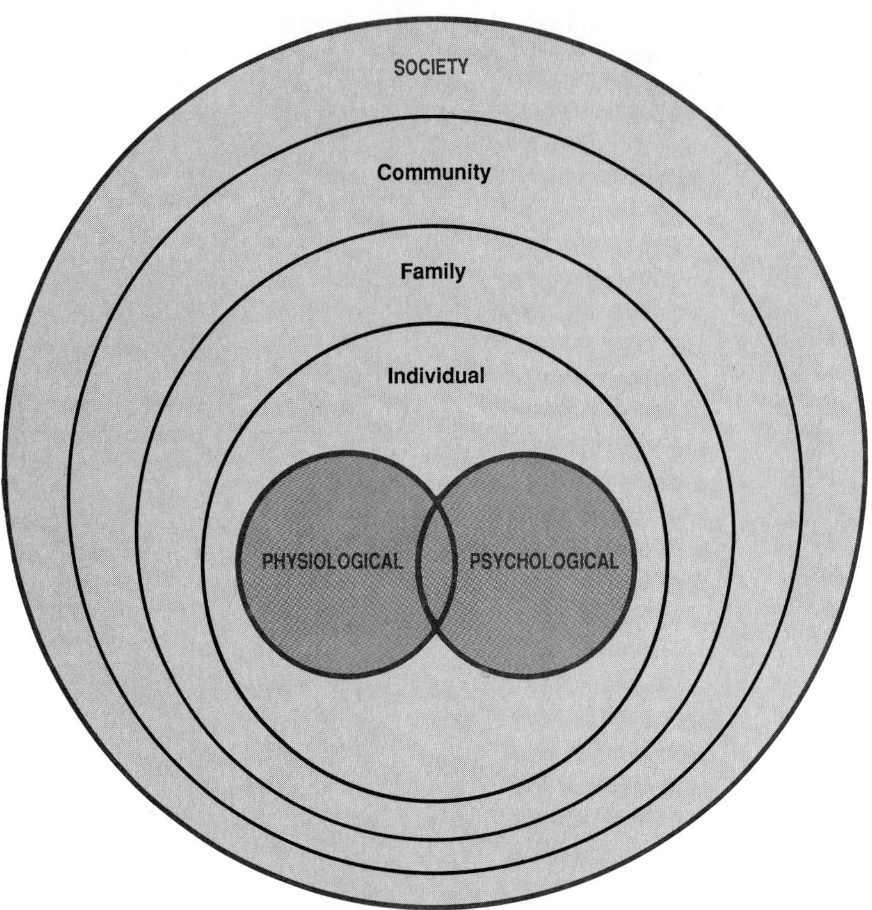

Figure 6–1. Levels of change.

dividuals must be viewed within the context of these groups when nurses plan for and effect care that promotes change toward optimal health.

Patterns of Change

Individuals and groups follow certain patterns of behavior while they are in the process of change. This section discusses two of these common patterns: maturational and situational change, and planned and unplanned change. Although these patterns of change will be discussed separately, it is important to remember that they can and often do occur simultaneously as individuals move through their life processes.

Maturational and Situational Change. Maturational and situational change coexist within the life process.[3,13] **Maturational changes** occur as a result of the process of human development. They occur as a sequence of physiological and psychological changes that progress in a fairly predictable course over the life span. The pace of developmental change slows down and speeds up as growth and aging occur. In their first year of life, infants triple their birth weight. Teenagers have growth spurts in which they may grow 1 to 2 inches in a few months. These accelerated periods of growth are complemented by slower periods of change, such as when gradual changes in skin elasticity produce wrinkles in middle-aged adults. Chapters 10 and 11 provide additional discussion of maturational change.

Maturational changes proceed at varying speeds and tend to accumulate in small increments over months and years. They can be predicted based upon the normal patterns of growth and development. In contrast, situational changes often occur unpredictably, disrupt life abruptly, and may happen in a brief period of time. **Situational changes** arise from the interaction between individuals and the environment. They include the events unrelated to an individual's age that disrupt life and threaten or challenge the person's ability to resolve them. Examples of situational changes include moving to a different home or community, losing or gaining a job, making new friends, or going away to college.

Consider the example of a change in job. An individual's interaction with the workplace stimulates the change and shapes its characteristics. The person who is abruptly fired from a position is unable to predict the event. Individuals who plan for a job change, on the other hand, take time to consider job options before resigning. Either way, a change in work situation takes place, but the special conditions of each may affect persons' capacity to adapt. Job change takes on new meaning when considered within the context of maturational change. Indeed, it is important to keep in mind that situational change occurs within the context of maturational change. For example, an individual can change jobs as a young adult without family responsibilities, or as a middle-aged adult who is trying to send children to college. The consequences of the same situational change are thus influenced by the individual's maturational stage.

Maturational change is a relatively predictable phenomenon. Nurses identify delays in maturational change—that is, the failure of individuals to accomplish developmental tasks within the expected time allotment—and collaborate with clients to help them respond in a healthy manner to both predictable and unpredictable situational changes.

Planned and Unplanned Change. Nurses in the emergency room or the intensive care unit often care for clients who are undergoing unplanned change. Accidental injury or the sudden onset of illness are examples of unplanned change. **Unplanned change** is unpredictable because it occurs spontaneously and outside the individual's control. Other options are unavailable; thus, no choices can be made.

Planned change involves choices and allows individuals to make decisions ahead of time and to maintain some control over their life situations.[14,15] A client may deliberately decide to change his eating habits and exercise schedule to lose 20 pounds. To do this, the client must take control of his behavior and make new choices that differ from past choices. The client may reduce calorie intake by choosing to broil food instead of frying it, or increase energy use by walking up the stairs instead of taking the elevator. The ability to control life situations and choose one's behavior is a common characteristic of individuals who cope with life stressors in a healthy manner.[16] Nurses are constantly collaborating with clients to assist clients to control their own behavior and make healthy choices.

Human Responses to Change

Although the focus of nursing assessment includes the change itself, clients' response to change is often the focus of nursing intervention. Clients exhibit a wide range of responses to change. This section describes the specific types of response to change that will be the focus of the rest of the chapter.

Adaptation. Adaptation, coping, and growth are terms commonly used to describe specific types of responses to change. **Adaptation** is a term often used to describe individuals' responses to environmental change.[17] Individuals adapt by accommodating to changes in the environment. For example, people don coats and scarves in the winter to ward off the cold air and maintain a stable body temperature. The general goal of adaptation is the maintenance of stability in the face of environmental change. Adaptation is often equated with health, as described in Chapter 5.

Physiological adaptation seeks to maintain a stable internal state. For example, the kidneys adapt continuously to maintain a balance of fluids and electrolytes within the body. Individuals adapt psychologically to preserve the self and maintain self-esteem. Individuals adapt to work stress by planning relaxation activities to maintain psychological balance. Social adaptation is determined by individuals' "fit" with surrounding social norms and expectations. Individuals who move to a foreign country must adapt to the social norms dictated by a different cultural group.

Stress and Coping. Because change disrupts an individual's life rhythms and routines, it can be stressful. **Stress** is experienced when change is considered to be threatening, harmful, or overly challenging.[18] The human response to stress is referred to as **coping.** Mengel,[19] a nursing authority on stress, states that coping behaviors are "part of the person's attempt to change the situation for the better, to manage the stress-resultant emotions." For a student, tests may be viewed as stressful disruptions in the usual pattern of college life. Some students cope with tests by cramming the night before. Others may cope by studying at intervals throughout the quarter and getting 8 hours of sleep on the night before the test.

Growth. Coping behaviors can be either adaptive or growth-producing. Coping behaviors that are adaptive work to resist or accommodate change and promote stability. **Growth** is a response to change that leads beyond adaptation to the achievement of personal changes that bring a new and healthier state of functioning.[1,20] Students who learn to study at intervals and get enough rest the night before a test may have learned a new and healthier way to cope with the stress of test-taking. When growth occurs, the person changes and moves to a new and better status quo.

Classic and Contemporary Views of Change

The concept of homeostasis presents a classic view of change, that change as a state requires some kind of response to correct or offset it. **Homeostasis** actually refers to a human response to change in which the desired outcome is the maintenance of a stable state of functioning.[21] The precise meaning of homeostasis is limited to the internal physiological responses—that is, to the automatic biochemical and biophysical adjustments that the body makes to maintain a stable internal environment. However, some writers have applied the term to psychological responses as well. Homeostasis as a concept is akin to adaptation. Adaptation[17] refers to behavior exhibited by a person as a whole, including the individual's emotional and social responses.

The abstract ideas of homeostasis and adaptation have been criticized by scientists and philosophers as having no real counterparts in human reality; rarely, according to the critique, is a steady state ever achieved.[22,23] This argument has led to a more contemporary view of change, that change is a constant feature of human existence in that individuals are always changing and developing. Nurse theorist Martha Rogers proposed the term **homeodynamics** as a new and more comprehensive view of human change. In Rogers' view, people do not respond to change; rather, individuals and their environments change together, each continuously affecting the other.[22,24] The focus is on the human–environment interaction as continuously creating new and different ways of being in the world. The concept of growth, as discussed earlier, fits with this view if the new and different way of functioning is better or healthier than past ways of functioning. See Table 6–2 for a comparison of homeostasis, adaptation, and homeodynamics.

The classic concepts of adaptation and homeostasis reflect a relatively static view of the life process, one in which balance and resistance or accommodation to change are the themes, while homeodynamics incorporates a more dynamic view of the life process in which the promotion of and engagement in change is the theme. Both views of human change are relevant for contemporary nursing practice. Knowledge of homeostasis is required for an understanding of the biophysical and biochemical processes that maintain a stable and healthy internal state. And yet, individuals as living systems are growing and changing within a wide and constantly changing environment. Maintaining optimal health requires both the resistance to change and the promotion of healthy change.

Human Change: Implications for the Nurse

Clients enter the health care system because of disruptions in life's routines and rhythms. When a nurse admits a client to the hospital, the health history identifies a significant change that has taken place. It could be a broken bone, pain, flu symptoms, a need for surgery or other therapy, or psychological distress. In any case, the nurse's first step is to identify the type of change taking place and the significance of that change for the client.

After identifying the change, nurses assess clients' response to the change. Does the client welcome the change or see it as threatening? Is the client trying to facilitate or resist the change? Is the client's response to change healthy for this situation? How does the change affect the individual's interaction with family and community?

Using this information, nurses works with clients to plan for a healthy response to change. The degree of client involvement in care planning and implementation is based on clients' ability to participate. Some clients take on responsibility for their care, while others are unable to do so because of physical or mental dysfunction. In review, nurses identify the change that has occurred and assess clients' responses. After judging the response to be relatively healthy or ill, nurses collaborate with clients to promote optimal health.

The rest of this chapter explores the nature of homeostasis and homeodynamics in more detail. Nurses must be aware of both views of change if they are to help clients to understand, plan for, and promote change toward optimal health.

■ HOMEOSTASIS AND ADAPTATION TO PRESERVE A STEADY STATE

In response to change, homeostatic and adaptive behaviors maintain the constancy of living conditions both inside and outside the body. Homeostatic self-regulation occurs within the body and is related to physiological functioning. The concept of adaptation refers to self-regulation of the whole person in relation to environmental change (physical and social forces).

In this section, the discussion of homeostasis and adaptation begins with a description of the physiological process of homeostasis. The discussion is then expanded to describe adaptation of the human being to the experience of stress.

The Concept of Homeostasis

The term "homeostasis" is used to describe collectively the automatic processes within the body that maintain stable functioning.[21] Other terms have been used to describe this constancy of the internal body, including "steady state," "balance," and "equilibrium." These processes occur within the systems of the body; the cells, organs, and organ systems. These systems have the task of maintaining the right conditions for optimal cellular functioning. For example, the body self-regulates blood pressure, pulse, and respirations in response to the person's activity level. To maintain an optimum supply of oxygen and nutrients to the cells, these functions increase when the person exercises. This is done automatically; the individual is not consciously aware that these processes are taking place.

TABLE 6–2. A COMPARISON OF HOMEOSTASIS, ADAPTATION, AND HOMEODYNAMICS

	Homeostasis	Adaptation	Homeodynamics
Focus	Internal physiological processes	Whole person	Whole person and environment
Control	Automatic self-regulation	Automatic self-regulation and conscious choice	Automatic self-regulation and conscious choice
Response to change	Resistance	Resistance	Resistance and facilitation
Goal	Stability	Stability	Health interaction and growth

From Barrett EAM. Visions of Rogers' Science-based Nursing. *New York: National League for Nursing; 1990. Pender NJ.* Health Promotion in Nursing Practice. *2nd Ed. Norwalk, CT: Appleton & Lange; 1987.*

Walter Cannon coined the term "homeostasis," and referred to this response as the "wisdom of the body" in his book of the same name first published in 1932.[21] Cannon was the first to detail the way that the body's internal processes automatically self-regulate to preserve the constancy of the internal environment. Current descriptions of homeostasis depart from the notion of homeostasis as a steady state. The term "steady state" refers to the maintenance of constancy of body composition at a particular moment in time. A steady state can be thought of as analogous to a snapshot of the body's internal function. This concept carries with it the connotation of no change, when in fact temporary changes or adjustments do take place. Changes related to growth and development also take place as individuals age. According to McCance, homeostasis should be described as a "dynamic steady state."[23] The description "dynamic steady state" refers to the constancy of body composition over a longer period of time, and takes into account temporary adjustments and maturational changes.

Physiology of Homeostasis

The purpose of homeostasis is to regulate the body's internal environment through a coordinated body-organ response.[23,25] All of the body's organs and tissues participate in this regulatory process. For example, in the circulatory system, homeostatic responses maintain a constant flow of the body fluids that carry nutrients to the cells and transport waste products away from the cells. Blood flows continuously, as it is pumped by the heart to the lungs, and then to the systemic circulation. Fluid and dissolved nutrients continuously diffuse back and forth between capillaries and tissue spaces to nourish cells and receive the cells' waste products. The continuous mixing of blood plasma and body fluids preserves the homogeneity or balance in the composition of these body fluids.[25] This process, known as oxygenation, illustrates the homeostatic response at the cellular, organ, and organ-system levels within the body. In order to understand the coordination of this response, it is important to understand the regulators and control mechanisms of homeostasis.

Homeostatic Regulators. Homeostatic regulators within the body automatically control organ responses to changes within the body. Homeostatic regulators are present within body organs and the organ systems they regulate. The autonomic nervous system and the endocrine system are the major regulators of organ responses.

Autonomic Nervous System. The autonomic nervous system (ANS) automatically regulates oxygenation, elimination, and glandular secretions to maintain stability and resist change outside of a healthy range of functioning. No conscious effort is required to create this regulation.

The ANS has two major branches: sympathetic and parasympathetic. Stimulation of the sympathetic division serves to mobilize energy stores in times of need, while parasympathetic stimulation functions to conserve and restore energy.[25,26] Most body organs are innervated by both sympathetic and parasympathetic fibers. The interaction of these two branches of the autonomic nervous system automatically balances organ responses and maintains healthy functioning (see Chap. 29 for further information).

Sympathetic stimulation of various organs mobilizes energy stores by bolstering the function of the heart, lungs, and large muscle groups and increasing the amount of glucose available for energy. In addition, the pupils dilate, profuse sweating occurs, and function of the stomach, intestine, and kidneys is decreased. In contrast, parasympathetic stimulation promotes digestion, intestinal peristalsis, and urinary elimination while decreasing the rate and force of heart contraction. When the body is at rest, nerve impulses from the parasympathetic division prevail. A comparison of sympathetic and parasympathetic effects on breathing, circulation, elimination, vision, and glandular secretions is presented in Table 6–3.

The organ responses related to parasympathetic and sympathetic divisions of the ANS are opposite or complementary. The functioning of both branches is necessary for the body to protect and renew itself. In response to changes in the environment, the sympathetic response mobilizes energy to protect the body. This response is self-limiting because, eventually, energy stores become exhausted. The parasympathetic response quiets the body and allows for rest and renewal, allowing the person time to store up energy reserves.

The sympathetic response, also called the "fight-or-flight" response, is considered to be a remnant of our early evolution. Flynn describes this response in terms of its original purpose:

> Let us imagine a primitive hunter in his cave. Suddenly, in the light of his fire he glimpses the shadow of a tiger. His body undergoes a torrent of changes through the complex transmissions of his sympathetic and parasympathetic nervous systems. Stored sugar and fats pour into his bloodstream to provide more oxygen, and red cells flood the bloodstream to carry more oxygen to the brain and limb muscles. The heart speeds up and blood presure soars to insure sufficient blood supply to needed areas. Blood clotting mechanisms are activated to protect against blood loss in case of injury. Muscles tense in preparation for strenuous activity, and digestion ceases so blood may be diverted to the muscles and brain. Bowel and bladder muscles release to lessen the weight the body carries, the pupils dilate to allow more light to enter, the senses are heightened, and epinephrine and norepinephrine pour into the system.[27]

Clients may demonstrate this response when faced with a diagnosis of cancer or the threat of surgery. A nursing student may experience the fight-or-flight response on the first day of a new clinical experience. The experiences are different but the response is the same. Activation of this response is described further in the discussion of the stress response later in this chapter.

Endocrine System. The endocrine system chemically regulates cellular metabolism.[25,28] Upon stimulation, the endocrine glands secrete hormones into the bloodstream for transport to the individual cells. These hormones regulate

TABLE 6–3. AUTONOMIC REGULATION AND SELECTED PHYSIOLOGICAL EFFECTS

	Sympathetic Effect	Parasympathetic Effect
Breathing	Bronchodilation Increased oxygen supply	Bronchoconstriction
Circulation	Increased rate and force of cardiac contraction Peripheral vasoconstriction or vasodilation	Decreased heart rate and contractility Vasodilatation in skeletal muscles and salivary glands
Elimination	Decreased intestinal motility	Increased intestinal motility
Stomach and intestine	Contraction of sphincters	Relaxation of sphincters
Urinary tract	Increased ureter motility Detrusor relaxation Trigone and sphincter contraction	Increased ureter motility Detrusor contraction Trigone and sphincter relaxation
Vision	Pupil dilation	Pupil constriction
Glandular secretions		
Adrenal medulla	Secretion of epinephrine and norepinephrine	No effect
Pancreas	Secretion of insulin	No effect
Sweat glands	Localized secretion	Generalized secretion

Adapted from McCance KL. Stress and disease. In: McCance KL, Huether SE. Pathophysiology: The Biologic Basis for Disease in Adults and Children. *St. Louis: Mosby; 1990:279–291. Guyton AC.* Textbook of Medical Physiology. *Philadelphia: Saunders; 1986.*

the chemical reactions within the cells. Secretion of hormones may occur in response to the level of circulating body substances, such as glucose or calcium, or in response to direct stimulation from the nervous system (electrical stimulation). In either case, hormones maintain a constancy in body composition, whether of fluids, electrolytes, or nutrients.[24,27]

Homeostatic endocrine regulation begins in the hypothalamus, a brain structure with some endocrine function. The hypothalamus receives signals that cause it to secrete hormones that excite or inhibit endocrine gland secretion. According to Guyton, the hypothalamus is a collecting center for information on the internal well-being of the body.[25]

The pituitary gland is directly connected to the hypothalamus by the pituitary stalk, a thin isthmus of tissue. The gland is divided into anterior and posterior lobes, each with different functions related to homeostatic regulation. Releasing and inhibiting factors from the hypothalamus act upon the pituitary gland to increase or decrease the release of pituitary hormones, which in turn stimulate other endocrine glands. The hormonal chain reaction eventually leads to action at the cellular level. The homeostatic functions of the endocrine hormones are presented in Table 6–4 and described below.[25,28] This discussion is limited to the endocrine hormones that function to maintain physiological homeostasis.

The anterior pituitary gland initiates the homeostatic chain reaction by secreting adrenocorticotropic hormone (ACTH) and thyroid-stimulating hormone (TSH) in response to substances released from the hypothalamus. ACTH and TSH stimulate the adrenal cortex and the thyroid, respectively, to produce hormones that maintain homeostasis by regulating metabolic rate and growth processes.

The posterior pituitary gland secretes antidiuretic hormone (ADH). ADH is formed in the hypothalamus and then transported to the posterior pituitary for secretion. This hormone acts on the kidneys to increase water reabsorption, thereby maintaining homeostasis by regulating fluid balance.

Several different hormones are secreted from the cortex (the outer layer) and the medulla (the inner core) of the two adrenal glands. The adrenal cortex secretes the hormones cortisol and aldosterone. Cortisol affects carbohydrate, protein, and fat metabolism, thereby regulating blood levels of glucose, amino acids, and free fatty acids to maintain a constant supply for energy.

Although the immediate effects of cortisol secretion help individuals adapt to stress, continued elevation of cortisol levels can have harmful effects. In addition to supplying energy needs, cortisol also suppresses the immune and inflammatory responses and promotes gastric secretion. Cortisol causes lymphocytes, monocytes, macrophages, and eosinophils to be shifted out of the circulatory system to other sites. With the decrease in macrophages, individuals' ability to make antibodies to specific antigens is reduced, thereby depressing the immune response. Also, cortisol inhibits the production of fibrin in connective tissue, reducing blood-clotting ability. All of these effects lead to poor wound healing, increased susceptibility to infection, and depression of the inflammatory response.[25,29] Cortisol affects gastrointestinal function by causing an increase in the secretion of gastric acid, which when excessive may cause gastric ulceration.[30]

Aldosterone helps regulate fluid and electrolyte balance by acting on the kidneys to reabsorb water, retain sodium, and excrete potassium. Aldosterone and ADH work to maintain homeostatic fluid balance.

The adrenal medulla secretes epinephrine and norepinephrine, and is under autonomic control. These hormones regulate the fight-or-flight response, described previously.

The thyroid gland secretes several hormones that primarily function to control the metabolic rate, or the speed of chemical reactions in the body. One thyroid hormone, calcitonin, acts to regulate the concentration of calcium in the blood by promoting the uptake of calcium by the bones,

TABLE 6–4. HOMEOSTATIC FUNCTIONS OF ENDOCRINE HORMONES

Endocrine Gland	Hormone	Homeostatic Function
Pituitary gland		
Anterior	Adrenocorticotropic hormone (ACTH)	Production of cortisol by the adrenal cortex
	Thyroid-stimulating hormone (TSH)	Production of thyroxine and triiodothyronine by the thyroid gland
Posterior	Antidiuretic hormone (ADH)	Increased water reabsorption by the kidneys to maintain fluid balance
Adrenal glands Medulla	Epinephrine and norepinephrine (catecholamines)	Fight-or-flight response
Cortex	Aldosterone	Sodium retention, potassium excretion, water reabsorption to maintain fluid and electrolyte balance
	Cortisol	Regulates blood glucose levels through gluconeogenesis; increases resistance to infection
Thyroid gland	Thyroxine and triiodothyronine	Regulates metabolic rate and growth processes
	Calcitonin	Regulates blood calcium levels by decreasing the concentration
Parathyroid glands	Parathormone	Regulates blood calcium by increasing concentration; decreasing plasma phosphate concentration
Pancreas—islets of Langerhans		
Alpha cells	Glucagon	Regulates blood glucose: stimulates glycogenolysis and increases concentration
Beta cells	Insulin	Regulates blood glucose: decreases concentration by promoting uptake of glucose, amino acids, and fatty acids into the cells

Adapted from McCance KL, Stress and disease. In: McCance KL, Huether SE. Pathophysiology: The Biologic Basis for Disease in Adults and Children. *St. Louis: Mosby; 1990:279–291. Guyton AC.* Textbook of Medical Physiology. *Philadelphia: Saunders; 1986.*

thereby maintaining optimal bone density. This action serves to decrease the level of calcium in the blood.[25,28]

The four parathyroid glands are located behind the thyroid gland. They secrete parathormone, which acts to mobilize calcium and phosphorus from the bones and decrease the excretion of calcium by the kidneys. These actions increase the level of calcium in the blood.[25,28] Thyroid and parathyroid hormones work together to homeostatically regulate levels of blood calcium and phosphorus necessary for muscle and nerve function, while maintaining optimal bone density and strength.

Within the pancreas, the cells of the islets of Langerhans secrete two hormones that regulate blood levels of glucose: insulin and glucagon. Secretion of glucagon causes an increase in blood glucose by stimulating glycogenolysis, the formation of glucose from glycogen (glucose is stored as glycogen in the liver). Insulin has the opposite effect, causing a decrease in blood glucose by promoting the uptake of glucose, amino acids, and fatty acids into the cells. Insulin and glucagon function together to regulate blood glucose levels in response to the body's changing demand for energy.

These endocrine hormones function to maintain homeostasis in interaction with each other and with many other body systems. The stability of internal environment is maintained as ADH and aldosterone regulate fluid balance; cortisol, glucose, and insulin regulate the storage and mobilization of glucose for energy; and calcitonin and parathormone maintain optimal blood calcium levels. Endocrine glands regulate homeostasis and other body processes such as growth and development.

In summary, the autonomic branch of the nervous system regulates homeostatic mechanisms through the reciprocal responses of the sympathetic and parasympathetic branches of the autonomic nervous system. The endocrine system regulates homeostasis at the cellular level through the action of hormones on cellular metabolism. The function of these regulatory mechanisms is to resist changes that lead to behaviors occurring outside a healthy range of functioning.

Control Mechanisms. The endocrine and autonomic systems use common control mechanisms to regulate homeostasis. Homeostatic control systems function to resist change and maintain constancy of body composition. Changes in body function are taken into the control system as input in the form of nerve impulses. Homeostatic control systems are varied in types and limit their input to certain specific variables such as blood pressure, pulse, or blood osmolarity. Each system processes specific information, acts on it if necessary, and responds with output.[25,28]

Homeostatic control systems rely on three components, referred to as receptor, comparator, and effector. The **receptor** receives and senses input. The input can be related to any of a number of physical or chemical variables such as heat, pressure, or concentration. The body has many types of receptors. The level or amount of input to a receptor is evaluated by a **comparator,** which determines whether there is a deviation of the input from the desired level or condition. In physiological systems, the desired level is an operating point that is genetically set and intrinsic to the specific system. The comparator functions like a thermostat, which checks the actual temperature of a room against the thermostat setting. If there is a deviation, an error signal is generated, which in turn activates or shuts off the furnace or air conditioner. In the body, error signals are transmitted to the **effectors,** the muscles and glands that perform body functions. The effectors respond by correcting their function to offset the error in the system. This kind of system correction is termed negative feedback. **Negative feedback** can be viewed as a series of changes initated by a control system that cause a return to a more normal state. Negative feedback is a characteristic of control system functioning, and in the body is an essential mechanism of homeostasis.[25]

It is important to remember that homeostasis is an automatic response to change. This means that the control operates, for the most part, outside of conscious awareness. People would have little time for other activity if they were required to consciously direct the adjustments that regulate blood pressure, fluid and electrolyte balance, or blood levels of glucose and calcium.

Figure 6–2 illustrates the automatic control of blood pressure as an example of a simple negative feedback control system. The input into the control system is the amount of stretch of arterial wall muscle fibers, which is an indicator of blood pressure. The baroreceptor, the receptor for this input, sends the information regarding arterial stretch to the cardiovascular center in the medulla of the brain. The center serves as the comparator in the control system as it interprets the information. In this case the blood pressure is determined to be high, above the normal range. An error signal results that is transmitted to the effector, in this case by the autonomic nervous system. Messages from the centers in the medulla decrease sympathetic stimulation and increase parasympathetic stimulation. The rate and strength of heart contractions decrease and the skeletal muscle vessels dilate in response. These actions have the combined effect of decreasing blood pressure. The output of the control system is to automatically decrease blood pressure value. This new information, or negative feedback, is fed back into the system as input.[25]

In reality, control mechanisms often overshoot when they correct homeostatic values, and the amount of error must then be corrected again to the acceptable range.[23] For example, adjustment in sympathetic and parasympathetic stimulation may lower blood pressure too far, requiring further adjustment to increase the blood pressure to within a normal range.

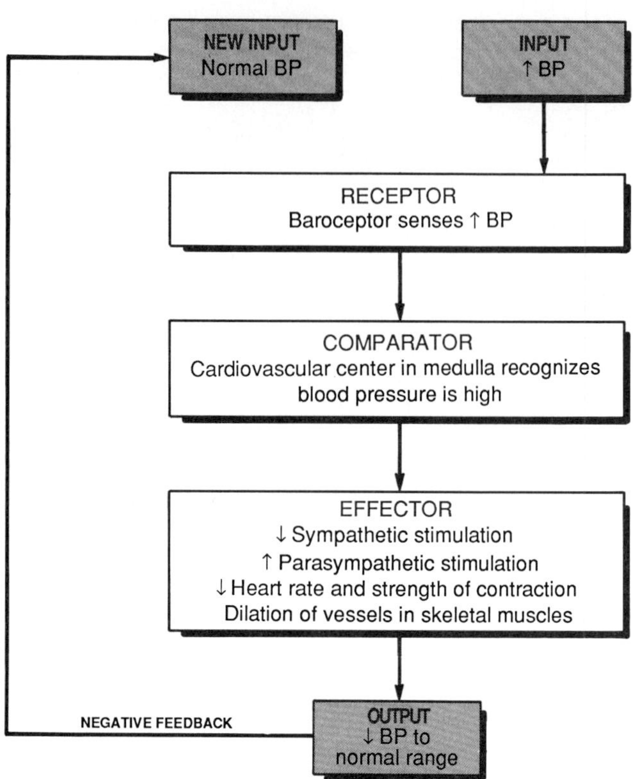

Figure 6–2. Negative feedback control system: Autonomic control of blood pressure.

Control systems operate at different levels within the body. For example, autonomic control of blood pressure is only one of the many feedback loops involved in the control of blood pressure and the blood's circulation through the body. The overall control of circulation is referred to as multiple-organ feedback.

Endocrine regulation of homeostasis is another example of multiple-organ feedback. Consider the release of the hormone thyroxine from the thyroid gland. As illustrated in Figure 6–3, hormone release occurs as a part of a chain reaction involving the hypothalamus, anterior pituitary gland, and thyroid gland.[25,28] The hypothalamus senses a drop in thyroxine level and responds with the release of thyrotropin-releasing factor (TRH). This sets up a multiple-organ chain reaction in which TRH acts on the anterior pituitary gland to stimulate secretion of thyroid-stimulating hormone (TSH), and TSH then stimulates the thyroid gland to produce thyroxine. This increase in the level of thyroxine is sensed by the thyroid, which acts on the anterior pituitary and the hypothalamus to inhibit TRH and TSH and thus decrease thyroid hormone synthesis and secretion. The amount of error is decreased; hence this is negative feedback. The continuous interaction among the three organs and their output maintains an optimum level of thyroxine.

Conversely, **positive feedback** occurs when effector mechanisms cause the error to increase and the value or

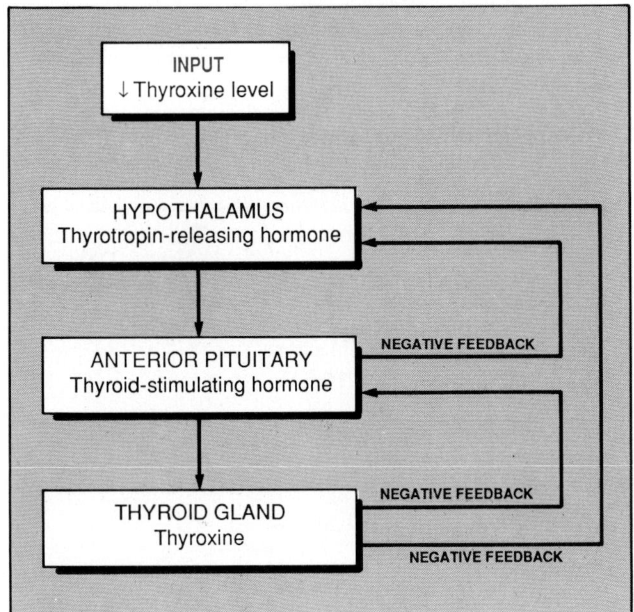

Figure 6–3. Complex multiple-organ feedback: Regulation of thyroxine level.

level to move farther from the acceptable level. Positive feedback in system function is often related to illness. For example, a condition called malignant hyperthermia occurs when the body temperature continues to increase, even though the body senses that it is already above 98.6F. This condition, which can occur postoperatively, becomes life threatening if uncontrolled.[23]

Both positive and negative feedback occur within the regulatory systems. Negative feedback is the primary means of promotion of homeostasis. Positive feedback occurs only in self-limiting situations; otherwise, it might result in death of the system.

Significance of Homeostasis

Knowledge of internal homeostatic mechanisms is necessary in order to plan interventions that support health. For example, nurses administer intravenous fluids to replace body fluids lost during surgery. This intervention supports homeostasis by maintaining an optimal balance of fluids within the body. Monitoring of vital signs, intake and output, and laboratory tests give the nurse an indication of the body's internal stability. Abnormal readings indicate that the body is having difficulty maintaining homeostasis. Nurses monitor indicators of homeostasis and intervene to promote healthy homeostatic function.

Adaptation to Stress

Pender, an expert on health promotion, describes adaptation as "the human stabilizing tendency against environmental change."[20] For example, human beings adapt to an infectious process inside the body by activating the inflammatory and immune responses. They adapt to a drop in the temperature of the air outside the body by shivering to produce heat and by putting on warmer clothing. People are continually adapting to changes in the environment.[17] Homeostasis is but one type of adaptive response to change. Remember that homeostasis refers to physiological stabilizing tendencies that take place automatically. Adaptation, on the other hand, includes all stabilizing tendencies: physiological, psychological, and social; automatic and consciously controlled.

Researchers have been particularly interested in studying human adaptation to stress, primarily because of the link found between stress and disease. This link is a connection between the mind and the body, a connection between emotions and physiological processes.

Mind–Body Connection. Prior to the 19th century, Western philosophers viewed the mind and body as separate entities. Changes in body function were not thought to affect the mind, and vice versa. Interaction between the mind and body, however, was demonstrated in the 1800s by Mesmer and Charcot, who used hypnotic suggestion to control physical symptoms. During this same period of history, Freud described the hysterical conversion of repressed anxiety into physical symptoms such as blindness or paralysis.[31]

During the 20th century, study of mind–body connections has been focused on the stress–disease link. Physicians and researchers began to identify stress-linked diseases such as ulcers and asthma, and symptoms such as headaches and hyperactivity. Selye,[32] a physician, described physiological stress as being triggered by psychological factors. Wolff,[30] a psychiatrist, conducted an extensive study on stress and disease, describing stress-linked diseases in every major body system. Scientists, also recognizing the importance of the mind–body connection, began to incorporate Eastern philosophy and meditation techniques in the control of stress. For example, Benson[33] taught people to meditate to control high blood pressure. Gradually nurses, too, recognized the importance of integrated, holistic human functioning and intervened to manage stress by facilitating control of this mind–body connection.

The Stimulus–Response Model of Stress. Early stress research defined stress as either a stimulus or a response. A stimulus, also known as as **stressor**, is something that triggers stress. A **response** is any of the physiological changes and behavioral manifestations of stress, such as fear, anxiety, or increased blood pressure. As the reader can see, it is difficult to describe one without the other. In the stimulus–response model, the stimulus is identifiable and is thought to be the direct cause of the response. This model of stress makes the assumptions that certain situations are inherently stressful, and that people respond to stress in generally the same way.[1,18] Much of the stimulus–response research provides foundational information in the study of stress. For the purposes of this chapter, the general term "stress" refers to the experience that includes both the stressor and the stress response.

Stress as a Stimulus. Theories of stress as a stimulus describe stress as a disturbance in the environment or within the body. These disturbances are also known as stressors. Selye[32] described physiological stressors as disturbances in homeostasis. Environmental stressors have been described as major life changes, or minor daily irritations.[34]

Life Change Theory. Life change theory attempts to quantify the stress of life in terms of units of life change. Holmes and Rahe[35] did extensive research that led them to the conclusion that life change is stress. Through their studies, they linked clusters of social events (life changes), such as death in the family or changing occupations, to the onset of illness. They focused on the number and types of life changes necessary to exhaust the stress response and lead to illness and crisis. Their Social Readjustment Rating Scale (SRRS) is a popular research tool that ranks life events according to their potential to cause stress (Fig. 6–4). Each life event is assigned a stress unit value that ranks that event relative to other events in the scale. A total score over 300 indicates high stress and is associated with high rates of illness.

The SRRS includes both positive and negative events. Anyone who has gone through changes in life-style that take place during the first year of marriage, or during the addition of a new baby to the household, can attest to the fact that even these positive events can be very stressful. They disrupt the person's habit patterns and often require the person to learn new coping skills.

Daily Hassles Theory. Daily hassles theory was developed by Lazarus and colleagues in response to questions about the ability of the SRRS to predict illness onset.[36] They designed a tool to measure stress in terms of daily hassles rather than major life events. Lazarus defines hassles as "the irritating, frustrating, distressing demands that to some degree characterize everyday transactions with the environment."[36] Examples of daily hassles include having too many things to do, misplacing or losing things, and worrying about a family member. The amount of life stress is measured as a proportion of hassles to uplifts. Uplifts are positive emotional experiences that may work to resist stress. Examples of uplifts include eating out and completing a task. Lazarus and his colleagues believe that negative experiences may cause illness, while positive experiences may prevent it.

The Everyday Hassles Scale can also be used in nursing practice and research. On the Everyday Hassles Scale (EHS), hassles and uplifts are listed in rank order, and the client chooses those that apply from the list, and then rates them in terms of severity. In this way, it is possible to identify patterns of hassles and uplifts that are common to people in different ages and stages of life (Fig. 6–5). For example, Lazarus and associates[36] found that the behavior patterns of middle-aged subjects included the hassles of economic concerns, too many things to do, too many re-

Select the life events that have occurred during the last year. Sum the stress unit values for the events that you have chosen. Interpret your score according to the following scale:

150–199, mild stress.
200–299, moderate stress.
300+, high stress—most likely to be related to high rates of illness.

Life Event	Stress Unit Value	Your Score
Death of a spouse	100	
Divorce	73	
Marital separation	65	
Jail term	63	
Death of a close family member	63	
Personal injury or illness	53	
Marriage	50	
Fired at work	47	
Marital reconciliation	45	
Retirement	45	
Change in health of a family member	44	
Pregnancy	40	
Sexual difficulties	39	
Gain of a new family member	39	
Business readjustment	39	
Change in financial status	38	
Death of a close friend	37	
Change to a different line of work	36	
Arguments with spouse	35	
Mortgage or loan > $10,000	31	
Foreclosure of mortgage or loan	30	
Change in responsibilities at work	29	
Children leaving home	29	
Trouble with inlaws	29	
Outstanding personal achievement	28	
Spouse begins or stops work	26	
Begin or end school	26	
Change in living conditions	25	
Revision of personal habits	24	
Trouble with boss	23	
Change in work hours or conditions	20	
Move or change in residence	20	
Change in schools	20	
Change in recreation	19	
Change in church activities	19	
Change in social activities	18	
Mortgage or loan < $10,000	17	
Change in sleeping habits	16	
Change in number of family gatherings	15	
Change in eating habits	15	
Vacation	13	
Christmas	12	
Minor law violations	11	
		TOTAL

Figure 6–4. Social Readjustment Rating Scale. (*From Holmes TH, Rahe RF. The social readjustment rating scale. J Psychosomat Res. 1967; 11:213–217.*)

The following is an abbreviation of the original hassles scale. This scale ranks hassles and uplifts in middle-aged client groups.

Hassles (in rank order)	Uplifts (in rank order)
1. Feeling concern about weight	1. Relating well to spouse or lover
2. Worrying about health of a family member	2. Relating well with friends
3. Worrying about rising cost of living	3. Completing a task
4. Dealing with home maintenance	4. Feeling healthy
5. Having too many things to do	5. Getting enough sleep
6. Misplacing or losing things	6. Eating out
7. Doing yard work or outside home maintenance	7. Meeting responsibilities
8. Worrying about property, investment, or taxes	8. Visiting, telephoning, or writing someone
9. Worrying about crime	9. Spending time with family
10. Feeling concern about physical appearance	10. Home pleasing to you

Figure 6–5. Everyday Hassles and Uplifts Scale. (*Adapted from Lazarus RS. Little hazards can be hazardous to your health. Psychology Today. 1981; 15:58–62.*)

sponsibilities, and having trouble relaxing. Uplifts reported for this group included pleasure and satisfaction from good health and spending time at home with family. In contrast, college students reported hassles such as wasting time, concerns about meeting high standards, and feeling lonely, and uplifts such as having fun, laughing, entertainment, and music. Both groups reported that completing a task and relating well with friends were uplifts.

Uses and Limitations of Stressor Scales. Both the SRRS and the EHS scales have limited usefulness because the significance of specific life events, hassles, and uplifts varies from culture to culture, and even from one stage of the life span to the next. These tools, however, help nurses identify each client's patterns of life change and adjustment. This type of information is useful in assessing individuals' risk for future development of illness and crisis.

Characteristics of Stressors. The SRRS and EHS identify specific situations that may be stressful. Stressors can also be categorized according to type. Cohen[37] describes four types of stressors, based on the duration of the event:

1. *Immediate situation stressors.* These events are stressful only for the immediate situation. For example, when a person breaks a leg, the event is stressful for a limited period of time: as it happens and during the immediate treatment.
2. *Sequences of stressors.* The second type is characterized by a sequence of stressful events. For example, being fired from a job can be a stressor in and of itself, but can also lead to a host of financial and family stressors.
3. *Intermittent stressors.* This type happens intermittently over a period of time. An example of this would be ongoing difficulties with relatives one does not see on a daily basis. The individual deals with the same stressor intermittently over many years.
4. *Chronic stressors.* This type of stressor affects that individual daily over time. An example is the stress experienced by families of Alzheimer's victims. Every day, current and new behavior patterns contribute to the cumulative stress of caring for someone who is unable to participate fully in life and may resist supportive efforts.

Stressors can be either actual or potential environmental changes.[37] The examples cited above are actual changes that can trigger a stress response if they are perceived to be threatening or harmful. Potential or anticipated changes can also trigger the stress response. Consider the burn victim who knows that the dressing will have to be changed within the next hour. Anticipation of this painful event is enough to trigger a stress response. Lack of change can also cause stress. An example of this is the person who anticipates a job promotion that does not take place. In this case, there is stress but no change.

Different events or problems cause stress in different people. For one person, speaking in front of a group may lead to cool, clammy hands, a stiff neck, and an upset stomach. For another person, speaking in front of a group may be a pleasurable experience, but taking an essay examination may be terrifying. Whatever a person perceives as stressful is a stressor. The perception of stress is what defines the stressor.[18,37]

Changes that are stressful can occur in a person's internal state or external environment. Internally, physiological and psychological processes are threatened. Massive internal bleeding and feelings of anxiety are both stressors. Bleeding is a physiological stressor, and anxiety is a psychological stressor. Community change such as gang activity in the neighborhood, or family change such as death of a loved one, are both social stressors. Box 6–1 presents some examples of possible physiological, psychological, and social stressors. The reader should remember that these situations or feelings are not stressful for everyone. They are stressors only if they are perceived to be stressors by the individual encountering them.[37,38]

The Stress Response. A great deal of research has accumulated over the years on the stress response. The **general**

BOX 6–1. POTENTIAL PHYSIOLOGICAL, PSYCHOLOGICAL, AND SOCIAL STRESSORS

Physiological Stressors

- Trauma
- Surgery
- Oxygen deprivation
- Fatigue
- Infectious processes
- Pain
- Sleep deprivation

Psychological Stressors

- Fear
- Anxiety
- Helplessness
- Powerlessness
- Loneliness
- Poor self-esteem
- Spiritual distress

Social Stressors

- Pollutants
- Urbanization
- Relocation
- Poverty
- Loss of privacy
- Family problems
- Child-rearing

From Lazarus RS, Folkman S. Stress, Appraisal, and Coping. *New York: Springer; 1984. Guzetta CE, Forsyth GL. Nursing diagnostic pilot study: Psychophysiologic stress.* Adv Nurs Sci. *1979; 2: 27–44.*

adaptation syndrome (GAS) was first described by Hans Selye as the physiological response to stress.[32] Seyle suggested in his classical work that, no matter what the stressor, all individuals have the same nonspecific physiological response to stress. He described this response as occurring in three successive stages: alarm, resistance, and exhaustion.

- The **alarm stage** is characterized by a "call to arms" in which the central nervous system is aroused and the physiological defense is mobilized. Individuals' response to a stressor is to send messages to the sympathetic nervous system and the pituitary gland to activate the fight-or-flight response.
- The **resistance** (or adaptation) **stage** follows, in which the fight-or-flight response is actually carried out. In this stage, the hormones cortisol, norepinephrine, and epinephrine set off a chain of responses that enable the body to adapt to the stressor.
- The **exhaustion stage** is reached when attempts to adapt are unsuccessful. In this stage, individuals' ability to adapt is exceeded or exhausted. Physiological signs of exhaustion include heart failure, renal failure, and impairment of the immune response.[23] Without outside intervention, death may result.

Selye initially described the GAS as a reaction to chemical or physical changes in individuals' internal or external environment. He also felt that a certain amount of stress or tension was necessary for life, that harmful effects were the result of stress that was too intense or prolonged.

Research in the past 25 years has challenged the notion that the GAS is a response to chemical or physical stressors alone, with Selye himself finding that psychological and social stressors also trigger the stress response. In addition, the idea of a nonspecific stress response has been challenged, as it has been shown that the perception of stress and the stress response differ from one person to another.[18] However, Selye's work was a starting point in stress research, and continues to provide the basic knowledge necessary to understand the stress response. Knowledge of the GAS gives nurses an idea of the possible physiological manifestations of stress and the stages of the response. With this knowledge, nurses know what to look for when assessing each client's unique experience of stress.

The Transactional Model of Stress. The stimulus–response model of stress outlined by Selye explains commonalities in the stress experience, but fails to explain individual differences in responding to events. The work of Lazarus and associates endeavors to explain these differences.[18] For example, why are some events stressful for one person and not another? Why are some people better able to resist stress and cope over longer periods of time?

According to Lazarus and Folkman,[18] the activation of the stress response depends upon the conscious appraisal of the environmental change taking place. Thus, **cognitive appraisal** or evaluation of events is an essential transaction between the person and the environment. If evaluation of this change evokes feelings of threat, harm, or challenge, then the transaction is stressful and the stress response is activated (Fig. 6–6).

Cognitive appraisal explains variations in individual responses to events. An individual's cognitive appraisal may or may not signal alarm in a situation. For example, an experienced camper is comfortable with the usual noises of the forest, while an inexperienced camper experiences fear or anxiety at these sounds. Events that stimulate anxiety or fear are stressors.

In the cognitive appraisal of a potential stressor, individuals consider two major evaluative questions:

- What does this mean to me? Is it threatening, harmful, challenging, benign, or irrelevant?
- What abilities and resources do I have to deal with this? Can I cope with this? What choices do I have?[18]

Individuals may or may not be aware of the evaluative process, they may or may not be in conscious control of this process, and it may not be rational. In addition, the evaluative questions may be considered in any order, or even at

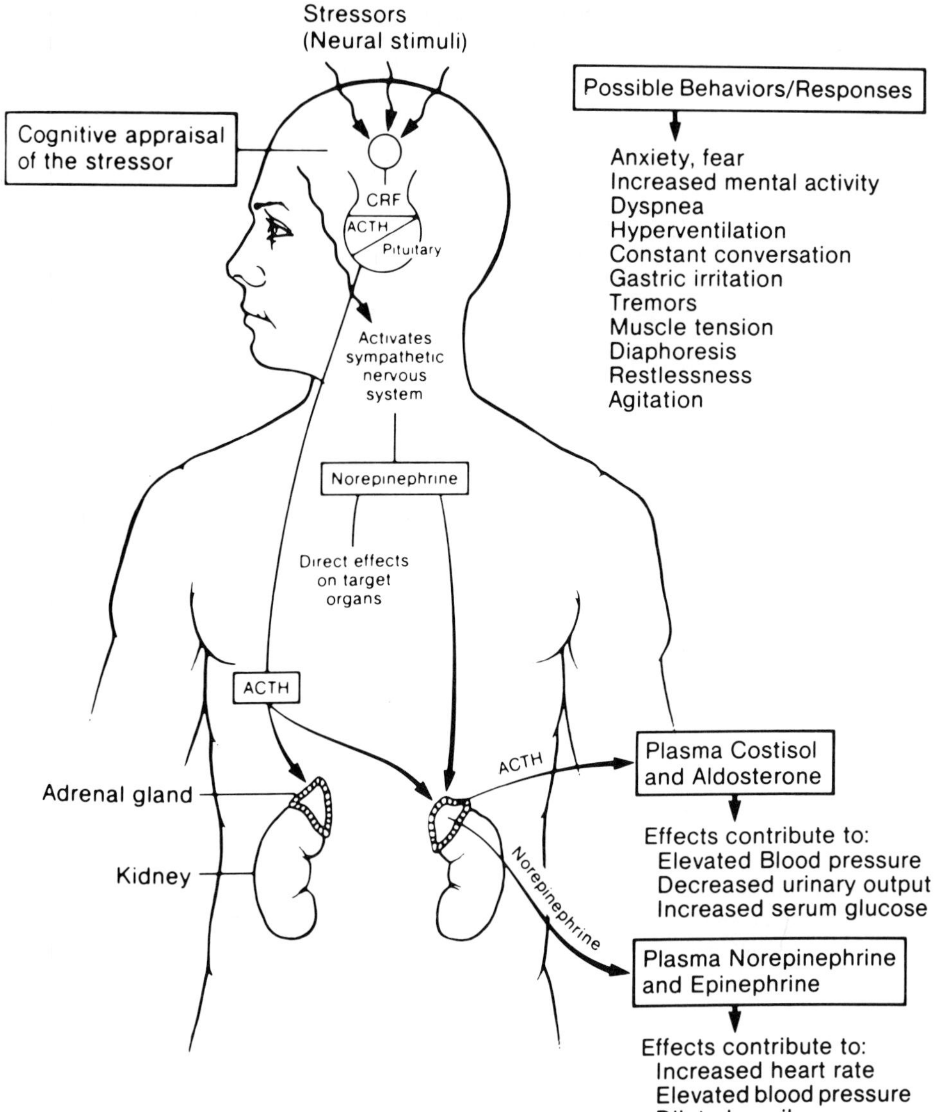

Figure 6–6. Stress as a transaction. (*Adapted from Fuller J, Schaller-Ayers JS. Assessing coping and stress tolerance. In: Fuller J, Schaller-Ayers JS, eds. Health Assessment: A Nursing Approach. Philadelphia: Lippincott; 1990; 463.*)

the same time. Individuals may not even be aware of the stress. Whether or not a person is aware, rational, or in control, an initial appraisal of stress triggers a physical and emotional response. Once initial appraisal takes place, however, individuals continually reappraise the situation and may reinterpret events to be more or less stressful, or even to be beneficial. This reappraisal may lead the individual to change and grow psychologically and reduce the threat.

Cognitive appraisal defines the stressor for individuals and through mind modulation directs the brain and body to activate a coordinated response. Dossey, an authority on holistic nursing, describes **mind modulation** as "the natural process by which thoughts, feelings, attitudes, and emotions—neural messages—are converted in the brain into neurohormonal "messenger molecules" and sent to all body systems—autonomic, endocrine, immune, and neuropeptide."[39] Research shows that stressors initiate not only sympathetic and endocrine responses, but also neurochemical responses.[26,29,40] Cognitive appraisal is neurologically mediated by brain connections between the cerebral cortex, which is the seat of logical thinking; the limbic system, which is the seat of emotions; and the hypothalamus, which responds to limbic stimuli to set off sympathetic and endocrine responses. Neuropeptides, special proteins in the brain that turn on or off physiological responses, are the chemical factors that modulate all other responses to stress—autonomic, endocrine, and immune—stimulating or inhibiting them in response to external events and the emotions that they evoke.

Beta-endorphins are one of a number of neuropeptides

that work to modulate the function of the autonomic nervous system, endocrine system, and immune system. As yet, it is not known whether the beta-endorphins are secreted in the pituitary gland or the central nervous system. Beta-endorphins act like opiates to increase individuals' ability to withstand pain. In addition, they have been associated with the generation of positive feelings such as excitement and an overall sense of well-being. They affect immune function by their close relationship with monocytes, as they work to identify foreign substances in the body and locate areas needing repair. There is much more to learn about the neuropeptides and the stress response, but it is thought that they function to modulate the body–mind transaction.[26,29,40]

Factors that Mediate Cognitive Appraisal. Cohen[37] defines **mediating factors** as those factors affecting the cognitive appraisal of an environmental change as a stressor. In other words, mediating factors are the circumstances that make this particular change threatening, harmful, or challenging. The following list includes some common mediating factors.

- *Number of potential stressors.* A particular situation may or may not be stressful, depending on when it occurs. A move to a new community may not be stressful with adequate planning and support, but if it coincides with the birth of a baby or the sudden death of a family member, the accumulation of life changes may become stressful.
- *Duration of the event or situation.* An event may be more or less stressful depending upon how long it lasts. For example, a brief illness such as a common cold may not be appraised as stressful, but chronic illness such as diabetes mellitus or arthritis challenges and threatens the person's coping skills every day over many years.
- *Intensity of the event or situation.* Some situtaions are experienced more intensely than others. For example, a minor cut on the arm requiring a Band-Aid is a less intense situation than the experience of surgery. With surgery clients feel more discomfort, and life's rhythms and routines are disrupted.
- *Availability of social and financial resources.* Individuals' social and financial resources are necessary for survival and growth. Illness often keeps people from working or caring for other family members. Comprehensive health insurance and help from reliable friends and family keep these situations from becoming stressful. On the other hand, a lack of money to pay for services or a lack of reliable help adds to the stress of the situation.

Manifestations of Stress. The transactional model of stress focuses on individual differences, not only in the appraisal of stress but in the manifestations of stress. This section reviews possible physical, emotional, and cognitive manifestations of stress, emphasizing that the patterns of response vary from person to person.

Physical Manifestations. Physical manifestations of stress are primarily a result of sympathetic and adrenal stimulation, the fight-or-flight response.[23] Common physical manifestations exhibited by the person experiencing stress include pale, cold, clammy skin; dilated pupils; heart palpitations; increased blood pressure; stomach upset; trembling; sweating; hyperventilation; decreased resistance to infection; poor wound healing; increased energy; increased pain tolerance; decreased bowel and bladder elimination; and elevated blood glucose.

One manifestation of stress that receives a lot of media attention is that of superhuman strength. The bolstering of the cardiovascular system, combined with a surge of energy from an increase in available oxygen and glucose, has been known to allow people to lift heavy objects or run faster than they normally could. Under extreme stress individuals may for a time perform better and manifest physical enhancement rather than physical deterioration.

If the stress response is prolonged to the point of exhaustion or is very severe, the immune system is depressed and individuals are susceptible to development of stress-linked disease.[30,32] Chronic suppression of the immune system may place individuals at risk for developing autoimmune diseases such as rheumatoid arthritis. Continued elevation of levels of fatty acids such as cholesterol may place individuals at risk for developing coronary artery disease. Common stress-linked diseases or conditions are presented in Table 6–5.[23,30] Thus the presence of a disease known to be stress linked may be a physical manifestation of severe stress in an individual life.

Psychological Manifestations. Psychological manifestations of stress involve emotions and cognition—that is, a person's ability to feel and know. Common emotional responses include anxiety, fear, anger, aggression, and defensive behavior. These responses affect cognition and therefore learning and problem-solving.[18,41]

Anxiety is defined by Carpenito as "a state in which the individual experiences feelings of uneasiness (apprehension)" (p. 128).[41] Anxious individuals may feel nervous, helpless, keyed up, or unable to relax; familiar surroundings may seem unreal. They may feel a loss of control over the situation or a sense of doom. Anxiety may range from moderate to severe depending on the effect on an individual's ability to function and learn.[41]

1. Mild anxiety heightens awareness and facilitates learning. A student with mild anxiety before a major examination may not sleep well, but memory and learning may be positively affected. These positive effects of anxiety begin to diminish as severity increases.
2. With moderate anxiety, individuals' perceptual field begins to narrow and concentrating becomes difficult. At this point, learning is slightly impaired. The student would now have trouble focusing attention on anything other than the situation at hand and would begin to appear nervous and shaky.
3. Severe anxiety is manifested by highly distractable behavior with severe learning impairment. Individuals find it impossible to concentrate. The student at this point

BUILDING NURSING KNOWLEDGE

What Is the Relationship Between Stress and Chronic Illness?

Leidy NK. A physiologic analysis of stress and chronic illness. *J Adv Nurs.* 1989; 14:868–876.

Selye's general adaptation syndrome (GAS) provides a useful model for understanding the relationship between stress and acute illness. In this report, however, the author explores the use of the GAS for understanding the role of stress in chronic illness—that is, illness that cannot be cured and that usually progresses in severity.

Leidy points out that both Cannon's description of the fight-or-flight response and Selye's GAS acknowledge the role of strong emotions to elicit internal responses. Under this perspective, the symptoms of disease can be looked upon as expressions of ongoing stress. For example, diabetes, a chronic metabolic disease, arises from the nutritional imbalances of obesity; while emphysema, a chronic lung disease, evolves from physical stressors such as smoking and environmental irritants. Psychosocial stressors are thought to play a role in diseases such as coronary artery disease and cancer.

Leidy proposes that clients with chronic illness are at increased risk for a progression of their disease in response to stress. He finds support for this idea in Selye's GAS stages of alarm, resistance, and exhaustion. During the alarm stage, the activation of the fight-or-flight defenses causes added stress on oxygenation mechanisms. This added stress may be harmful to clients with chronic respiratory disease. The fight-or-flight response also increases skeletal muscle tone, sometimes resulting in muscle tremor, joint pain, and backache. These problems exact a toll on clients who have chronic musculoskeletal conditions such as arthritis. Leidy also traces the relationship between psychosocial factors and cancer and autoimmune disorders—chronic diseases in which the body's immune factors attack its own tissue—to the alterations in immune response that occur in the later stages of the GAS.

Leidy notes that according to Selye, every individual is endowed with a predetermined quantity of adaptation energy. When this is drained, further resistance is limited, and the situation finally becomes irreversible. The effects of stress become pernicious and the final stage of stress—exhaustion—ensues. The author concludes that the client's stress, often manifested through body symptoms, is an important indicator of a need for supportive nursing care. Strengthening the client's resources should alter the client's concept of self and environment, thereby reducing feelings of threat and minimizing the subsequent internal stress response.

may experience somatic symptoms such as heart palpitations, dizziness, nausea, and hyperventilation.

4. The **panic** level is reached when individuals' perception of the situation is distorted, like a camera out of focus. At this level, the individuals are unable to function. Learning stops and communication is difficult. Somatic signs may progress to shortness of breath, sweating, dizziness, fainting, choking, and trembling.

Anxiety is a response to a stressor that is vague or undefined. When the threat is well defined, the response is known as fear. Carpenito defines **fear** as a "state in which an individual experiences a feeling of physiological or emotional disruption related to an identifiable source that is perceived as dangerous" (p. 324).[41] Feelings of fear are focused on the threat and, like anxiety, are manifested in a narrowing of focus and attention deficits. Fear is a feeling of being unable to control the threatening situation. Both anxiety and fear are emotional responses to a stressor that is threatening or challenging.

Individuals experiencing stress have difficulty meeting social role requirements.[37] The deficits in concentration and attention and the narrowing of perceptual focus that accompany anxiety make it difficult for individuals to be an effective family and community member. Parents may find it difficult to meet the needs of their children, work performance may suffer, and individuals may not be able to participate in school or church activities as before.

The experience of anxiety and fear can have positive or negative effects on significant others and the surrounding environment.[37] Anger and aggression are examples of negative behaviors that people under stress direct to other persons or objects in the environment.[40] Anger is an emotion felt in response to frustration and anxiety. It is short-lived and can be expressed in overt or covert ways. Overt expressions of anger include hitting, fighting, glaring, and verbal attack. Covert expression, a result of anger directed inward, may be manifested in somatic signs of stress, depression, or even suicide. Controlled expressions of anger can facilitate problem solving and help neutralize stress.

Aggression is the use of verbal or physical action to relieve tension.[41] It can range from irritation to rage, and if unchecked may progress to long-term hostility toward others. Anger and aggression may help individuals relieve anxiety, but they can have negative effects on others. Verbal and physical aggression may result in abuse of family members and friends. Families living in highly stressful situations are considered to be at high risk for abuse.

Anger and aggression are ways that people defend themselves from threat, harm, or challenge. Another way people protect themselves is through the use of defense mechanisms. **Defense mechanisms** are emotional defenses that are commonly used by people to allay painful or stressful feelings. Some commonly used defense mechanisms are listed below:[1]

1. Repression takes place when individuals prevent stressful thoughts and feelings from entering conscious awareness.
2. Denial occurs when individuals avoid the threat of a stressor by reinterpreting the event. For example, a client with chest pain may attribute it to sore muscles to deny the pain and avoid facing the threat of heart disease.
3. Rationalization takes place when individuals give a reasonable-sounding explanation that is untrue.[1] The client may rationalize that chest pain is really indigestion

TABLE 6–5. STRESS-LINKED DISEASES AND CONDITIONS

Body System	Stress-linked Disease or Condition
Pulmonary system	Asthma and hay fever (as a hypersensitivity reaction)
Circulatory system	Coronary artery disease Hypertension Stroke Arrhythmias
Musculoskeletal system	Tension headaches Backache
Gastrointestinal system	Curling's ulcer Irritable bowel syndrome Diarrhea Nausea and vomiting Ulcerative colitis
Immune system	Immunosuppression or deficiency Rheumatoid arthritis Inflammatory diseases of the connective tissue
Endocrine system	Diabetes mellitus
	Genitourinary system Diuresis Impotence Frigidity
Integumentary system	Acne Eczema Neurodermatitis

From McCance KL. Stress and disease. In: McCance, KL, Huether SE. Pathophysiology: The Biologic Basis for Disease in Adults and Children. *St. Louis: Mosby; 1990:279–291.*

even though the diagnosis of heart disease as the cause has been confirmed.

4. Regression is exhibited when individuals revert to less mature behavior. For example, an adult client may act like a child and refuse to take responsibility for his or her health when ill. A child may again wet the bed, even though bladder control had been attained.
5. Displacement occurs when individuals direct anger and aggression toward innocent people (see above discussion of anger and aggression).
6. Projection takes place when individuals attribute their own feelings to another person. A client may accuse a nurse or a family member of being threatened by a situation when, in fact, it is the client who feels threatened.

Defense mechanisms serve to protect individuals from threat for a limited period of time. Although defense mechanisms are often necessary for survival, continued use can block one's ability to change and grow. For a healthy resolution of stress, these defenses must be replaced by effective coping strategies.

Coping with Stress. Lazarus and Folkman[18] define coping as an individual's attempts to master conditions of harm, threat, or challenge when an automatic response is not immediately available. Ego defense mechanisms help people avoid threats, while coping behaviors help people adapt to the stressor and return to a stable state. People develop habitual patterns of coping behaviors. Coping patterns usually include specific strategies that help resolve the situation and reduce tension.

Modes of Coping. Modes of coping have been categorized by Folkman and Lazarus[18,42] as emotion- and problem-focused. Emotion-focused coping attacks the meaning of the stressor, thereby reducing the tension of the situation. For example, information-seeking is a coping strategy that reduces tension by clearing up any misconceptions about the stressor. Problem-focused coping resolves the stressful situation itself, thereby directly neutralizing the stressor. If the stressor is the threat of illness related to obesity, then problem-focused coping would include following a weight reduction diet and exercising regularly. This strategy attacks the stressor directly to resolve the stress of situation.

Not all coping mechanisms are positive or healthy. Box 6–2 presents a variety of coping strategies for tension reduction and problem-solving. Folkman and Lazarus[42] found problem-focused coping mechanisms to be the most effective means of resolving stress in most situations. Tension reduction through information-seeking, sharing concerns, humor, or even crying can be very healthy behaviors. The use of mind-altering drugs such as alcohol, and coping by overeating, may reduce tension temporarily, but may ultimately become sources of further stress.

Coping patterns include both tension-reduction and problem-solving strategies. The effectiveness of a particular

BOX 6–2. WAYS OF COPING WITH STRESS

Tension Reduction

- Sharing concerns with others
- Self-pity
- Crying
- Abuse of alcohol, other drugs
- Overeating
- Humor
- Self-control
- Swearing
- Boasting
- Thinking it through
- Working off energy

Problem-solving

- Seeking information about the situation
- Exploring alternatives
- Taking firm action
- Being open to assistance from others
- Redefining the situation
- Accepting the inevitable
- Accepting and finding something favorable in the situation

From Lazarus RS, Folkman S. Stress, Appraisal, and Coping. *New York: Springer; 1984. Fuller J, Schaller-Ayers JS. Assessing coping and stress tolerance. In: Fuller J, Schaller-Ayers Js.* Health Assessment: A Nursing Approach. *Philadelphia: Lippincott; 1990.*

BUILDING NURSING KNOWLEDGE

Does Social Support Diminish Stress?

Yarcheski A, Mahon NE. Perceived stress and symptom patterns in early adolescents: The role of mediating variables. *Res Nurs Health.* 1986; 9:289–297.

Yarcheski and Mahon sought to investigate stress in early adolescence to identify the stress symptoms in this age group, how children in this age group cope, and whether factors such as social support reduce stress and improve health outcomes.

The researchers studied 136 seventh and eighth graders. Each subject was asked to complete four questionnaires: an adolescent life change events questionnaire, a symptom pattern scale measuring anxiety and physical bodily complaints, a coping scale, and a social support questionnaire. The coping scale asked students to rate various coping strategies, such as daydreaming, crying, and worrying, according to how frequently they used them.

The findings showed a positive relationship between stress and symptoms: The higher the reported stress, the greater the number of symptoms. High stress also resulted in the use of emotional coping strategies such as crying and worrying. The more often the early adolescent subjects used emotional coping strategies, the more they experienced symptoms of stress, suggesting that such strategies are ineffective. Social support was also found to be related to symptoms. Subjects who perceived life events as highly stressful and who experienced low social support had more symptoms. Subjects who perceived life events as stressful, but also perceived high social support, had fewer symptoms. The investigators concluded that nurses need to identify the sources of social support that are available to adolescents and also to identify the specific types of support that children in this age group find beneficial to themselves as individuals.

coping strategy is measured by its ability to neutralize the stressor and inhibit the physiological stress response. When coping strategies are ineffective in dealing with stressors, then psychological crisis and illness may occur.

In a positive light, a stress experience may lead a person to cope by seeking out others undergoing the same experience and participating in self-help groups.[43] In these groups, people cope with a stressful experience such as chronic illness of a family member by meeting with others with a similar experience. The group members work together to problem solve and reduce tension and, while helping themselves, help others as well. In this way, individuals may be able not only to adapt to the stress of the situation, but also to grow and find new ways to cope.

Crisis: Coping With Overwhelming Stress. A stressful situation becomes a **crisis** when usual coping attempts fail; the situation is experienced as overwhelming.[44,45] Disaster and sudden death are commonly thought of as crisis situations, but any life change can be a crisis if it is a source of overwhelming stress for the individual involved.

Crisis can be described in terms of maturational (also called developmental) and situational (also called accidental) life changes (see also Chap. 8).[45] During normal growth and development, life transitions normally occur at set periods. To make the transition from one developmental stage to the next, individuals must complete certain life tasks. Successful completion of these tasks requires energy and support from family and friends. Failure to cope with the anxiety and stress that often accompany these tasks may result in **maturational crises.**

Persons with knowledge of normal growth and development can anticipate maturational crises and take measures to guide the changes involved and prevent the development of a crisis situation. In contrast, **situational crises** occur as a result of traumatic events that are beyond individual control and cannot be anticipated. Examples include natural disasters, diagnosis of chronic or fatal illness, loss of job, or death of a close relative. Many of these examples are included in the Social Readjustment Rating Scale (see Fig. 6–5). A situational crisis may be an overwhelming stressor by itself, or may occur in conjunction with a maturational crisis. The adolescent who seems to be coping with the stress of this life transition may experience crisis on receiving the news of the suicide of a close friend. Successful resolution of both situational and maturational crises requires the support of family, friends, and community.

Caplan[44] describes four phases of crisis development

(Table 6–6). These phases illustrate how the tension of a situation mounts as coping strategies fail and circumstances become overwhelming. The crisis state does not last long and is self-limiting. The overwhelming nature of the crisis requires that there be some response to it. There are three possible outcomes for the person in crisis:

- A return to the precrisis state as a result of effective problem-solving.
- Avoidance behavior such as withdrawal, depression, or substance abuse.
- Psychological growth through change to more effective coping patterns.

In the example presented in Table 6–6, developing new sources of psychological support such as joining a self-help group for parents of diabetic children would be a way to experience psychological growth. The parents could also learn more about the adjustments that their child will have to make as he or she grows and develops, and how to prevent crisis or negative outcomes from crisis in the future.

Stress Resistance. Stress resistance has been studied in an attempt to find out what factors make one individual better able to deal with stress than another.[46] In the course of this study, stress resistance has been linked with individual physical, psychological, and social factors. Some factors can be controlled or enhanced; others cannot.

Stress resistance involves the whole person: mind, body, and physical and social environment. Stress-resistant individuals have been found to be healthy in all of these dimensions.[16,47,48] Some of the factors affecting stress resistance include:

- *Genetics.* Genetic factors make individuals vulnerable to certain stressors. For example, some people are born with heart defects, or defective immune systems. The presence or absence of these genetic factors makes individuals more or less vulnerable to the negative effects of stress.
- *Healthy life-style.* Stress-resistant individuals eat a healthy diet, exercise regularly, get enough rest, and avoid destructive habits such as smoking and the abuse of alcohol or drugs. In addition, a healthy life-style includes the maintenance of regular family routines. Stress develops when family members cannot predict when daily activities such as meals, work, shopping, and bathing will take place.
- *Sense of humor.* Stress resistance involves relaxing and not taking life so seriously, being able to laugh at oneself and enjoy others.
- *Self-confidence.* Stress-resistant individuals feel good about themselves, about their abilities, accomplishments, and relationships with others. For example, it is stressful for a person to take a job for which he or she is ill-prepared because the person will lack confidence in his or her abilities. Conversely, a person with the necessary skills and knowledge to complete an assigned job is likely to feel confident and stimulated by it.
- *Safety and security.* Individuals are better able to resist stress when they feel secure with others and safe in their home and community. A lack of safety at home or in the community can lead to anxiety and fear.
- *Adequate social and material resources.* Stress resistance involves having enough help from others, enough money, adequate food, shelter, and clothing.

In addition to the factors mentioned above, the research of Kobasa[16,47] has led to the characterization of the stress-resistant personality. The term **hardiness** is used to describe the three personality characteristics that are likely to make an individual more resistant to stress and illness: control, commitment, and challenge. Hardy people view potentially stressful situations as challenging rather than threatening.[48] They control their own destiny by participat-

TABLE 6–6. PHASES OF CRISIS DEVELOPMENT

Phase	Description	Example
1	Initial rise in anxiety level Appraisal of stress Use of familiar patterns of coping	Child is diagnosed with diabetes. Family feels stress but able to cope by adjusting diet and learning to give insulin injections.
2	Usual problem-solving strategies fail Tension continues to mount	Child becomes angry about dietary restrictions and injections and acts out anger and aggression with family. Mother takes time off work to be with the child, and risks losing her job.
3	Person uses every resource available to cope with the situation Tension continues to mount	The child continues to resist the treatment for diabetes. Other family members and friends are no longer supportive. Finances become a problem as the mother loses her job.
4	Actual crisis state Usual coping mechanisms are ineffective Coping and resources are overwhelmed State does not last long, is self-limiting	Family members feel overwhelmed, that the tension is unbearable, the situation hopeless, and do not know what else to do or where to turn.

Adapted fronm Caplin G. Principles of Preventive Psychiatry. *New York: Basic Books; 1964. Hoff LA.* People in Crisis: Understanding and Helping. *3rd ed. Menlo Park, CA: Addison-Wesley; 1989.*

IMPLICATIONS FOR NURSE–CLIENT COLLABORATION

Stress Resistance and Hardiness

Stress resistance refers to those factors that make one individual better able than another to deal with stress. Research shows that several factors enhance an individual's ability to resist stress: genetics, healthy life-style, sense of humor, self-confidence, safety and security, and social and material resources. The term "hardy" describes people who possess these factors. Hardy people look at potentially stressful situations as challenges rather than threats.

ing in making choices for health. They anticipate the potential stressors of maturation and make plans for healthy transitions. Hardy individuals exhibit commitment through their active participation in activities that promote their own health and that of their family and community.

Homeostasis and Adaptation to Stress: Implications for the Nurse

Nurses use their knowledge of homeostasis and adaptation to stress to support clients in the prevention of stress and disease, the maintenance of physiological homeostasis, and the promotion of optimal health of the body and the mind. The following discussion describes how nurses help clients to manage stress.

Stress Management. Stress management involves both controlling the sources of stress in the environment and regulating the stress response.[49] It is important to note that the stress transaction is complex, involving multiple personal and environmental factors. Nurses help clients to resist stress and manage the factors that can be controlled in order to reduce stress.

Nurses assist clients to control sources of stress in the environment by a number of means.[40,49–52] Some of these include teaching clients to avoid unnecessary change, helping clients to manage their time more effectively in the pursuit of personal goals, modifying the environment in stress-reducing ways, and using techniques to mediate or control the stress response—that is, to balance the fight-or-flight defensive reaction with relaxation. Detailing the techniques of stress management is beyond the scope of this text, but guidelines to specific procedures can be found in Chapter 22. Some general tips for assisting clients include the following:

1. View each client as a unique individual. Remember that each person experiences stress differently. Elicit clients' perspective of the situation and do not assume that it will match yours. Determine what this illness or hospitalization means to a client and the effect that it has on family and work.
2. Assess clients' recent life stresses. Ask about major life changes that they have experienced in the last year. Ask about daily hassles in clients' lives both at home and in the hospital.
3. Monitor physiological parameters for signs of stress, such as increase in heart rate or blood pressure, hyperventilation, delayed healing, and increased blood glucose. Teach clients to be aware of their physical and psychological manifestations of stress.
4. Assess clients' support systems. Do they have supportive family and friends? Are there people that they count on to help out during this time of need? Are they able to ask for assistance?
5. Encourage client participation in care planning and intervention. This facilitates client control of the situation and encourages commitment to participate in the healing process.
6. Assist clients to manage their time to maintain familiar habits and routines when possible. Upon admission, ask clients about usual schedules for bathing, meals, and sleep, and try to fit these in with the hospital routine. For example, if a client is accustomed to bathing in the evening, adjust your schedule to include this rather than insisting on a morning bath like the rest of your clients.
7. As much as possible, accept and support clients' efforts to control the environment. Try to honor requests for a bed next to the window or a new roommate. Rearrange the room if necessary.
8. Teach clients and their families about their health problems, tests, and treatments. Fear of the unknown can be a source of stress. Assess whether clients' levels of anxiety affect learning and problem-solving.
9. Be alert to clients' coping patterns. Are they effective in dealing with the stress of this situation? Do they avoid stress rather than coping with it? How do they reduce tension and solve problems? Help clients to identify options for effective coping and to learn new coping skills when necessary.
10. Promote balance in daily activities. Encourage physical activity as tolerated. Teach relaxation techniques to calm clients' anxiety and increase parasympathetic activity and the release of beta-endorphins. Give backrubs, and talk clients through deep breathing, progressive relaxation, or guided imagery to promote sleep, decrease pain and discomfort, and increase their sense of well-being (see Chap. 22).
11. Encourage reappraisal of the stressful experience in a positive light. Work with clients to reinterpret the threat as challenge. Help clients to perceive the benefits they will receive as a result of this experience.
12. Maintain a calm environment to help clients rest and relax. Perform your work with a sense of self-confidence. This is communicated to clients and eases their anxiety. Avoid using a loud voice in the hallway to signal co-workers and encourage them to do the same. Play soft music.

Job Stress in Nursing. Nurses are also subject to stress and need to recognize that they are involved in a profession that can be highly stress-producing. Nursing professionals are themselves individuals. Moreover, they work in a variety of settings and care for a diverse population. Therefore, job stress will vary from setting to setting, client to client, and nurse to nurse.

The nature of job stress in nursing is partly related to social values in the Western world that rank technology above nurturing and caring. Because the nursing profession is primarily female, nurses' work is traditionally viewed as women's work, which remains socially undervalued. This means added stress and role confusion for many nurses, but particularly for nurses who are men as they struggle to prove to clients and other nurses that they can be nurturing and caring individuals.

Work conditions and work hours in nursing are often a source of stress. In addition, there is currently a shortage of nurses that creates an even greater burden on those who elect to go into or stay in nursing. The shortage is due, in part, to the opportunities now available for women in professions that were traditionally male dominated. Women are choosing professions in which they perceive they will have more control and recognition for what they do than has been afforded nurses.

Besides these social factors, there are other sources of stress in nursing. Nurses work with many needy, suffering people, and in so doing are often forced to confront their own mortality. This may disrupt nurses' feelings of safety and security and cause anxiety. In addition, nurses currently practice in a time of rapidly advancing technology and expanding knowledge. They feel pressed to keep up with volumes of new information that could help them give better client care.[53,54] Moreover, the nature of nursing creates a strong sense of responsibility for the welfare of others, but nurses are not always able to provide the kind of care they desire to all clients. Constraints of time and resources create pressures and difficult choices. Additionally, many nurses work in situations in which clients' lives are at stake, in which a medication or treatment error can be life threatening. Intensity of this nature can be highly stressful. Other stressors cited by nurses include:[53–56]

- The "reality shock" experienced by new nurses when they make the transition from the school to the workplace environment.
- Lack of control over the client care environment.
- Inadequate staffing and work overload.
- Poor communication among nurses.
- Conflict between nurses and other health care professionals.
- Poor or unresponsive leadership.
- Inadequate workspace: poorly designed, hot, cold, cramped, inconvenient.
- Disturbances in sleeping and social life related to shift work.
- Client factors such as difficult personalities, suffering, and death.
- Emotional overinvolvement with clients.
- Guilt related to emotional distancing from clients.[53–56]

When job stress becomes overwhelming, when the stress response moves to the stage of exhaustion, nurses experience the **burnout** syndrome. Nurses with burnout manifest an apathetic attitude toward their job: they are no longer able to care about clients or care about the job. Physical manifestations of burnout syndrome are those of intense or prolonged stress: stomach disorders, headaches, rashes, fatigue, depression, irritability, and insomnia, among others.[53–55]

In the context of nursing care, the term "care" means more than providing physical treatment for clients. According to Benner and Wrubel, caring "means that persons, events, projects, and things matter to people" (p. 1).[57] It means becoming involved, being connected with the client and the workplace. When nurses feel personal concern for clients and work, they also feel stress when they cannot control the work environment or provide for client needs. Burnout is a way of coping by distancing oneself from the stress of caring. Burnout in a sense is the antithesis of caring. And yet, to be an effective nurse, one must care. Benner[58] has conducted extensive research on the nature of nursing practice and has determined that the nurses identified by others as "expert," as the most effective in their practice, manifest this ability to care for others, including clients and co-workers. Therefore, nurses must learn to effectively cope with the stress of caring and to prevent burnout if they are to be effective in their practice. According to Benner and Wrubel, nurses need to find the "right level and kind of involvement" (p. 373).[57]

Nurses become overinvolved when they try to help clients by rescuing them. Benner and Wrubel indicate that "the overinvolved caregiver takes over the patient's burdens and problems" (p. 365).[57] Overinvolved nurses help too much, denying clients the right to be involved in their own care and to take a significant measure of responsibility for it. Overinvolved nurses place clients' needs above their own. This overinvolvement can be a way of avoiding relationships outside of nursing, and leads to professional relationships which lack the *mutual benefits* characteristic of collaborative interaction (see Chap. 37).

According to Smythe,[53] nurses expect some negative factors in their job, but many are stressed by the lack of positive factors, and the lack of opportunities they find to achieve job satisfaction and personal growth. They want more control over their practice. Box 6–3 lists stress management techniques that can aid nurses in learning to resist and manage this stress, and prevent burnout.[53,54]

Nurses and clients alike need to acknowledge the stress of life as well as cultivate options for coping and promoting optimal health. Change is stressful; it disrupts life's rhythms and routines and creates tension. Homeostatic mechanisms automatically regulate internal physiological functions to offset this tension and maintain a stable internal state. As a whole, individuals adapt to stressors by resisting change and seeking stable physiological, psychological, and social function. And yet, the disruption of stability sets up an opportunity for new ways of being and functioning to be created that often are better and healthier than those they replace.

BOX 6–3. STRESS MANAGEMENT TECHNIQUES FOR NURSES

1. *Take stock of yourself.* Examine your own values and personal goals related to nursing. Are they reflected in what you do? Are they unrealistic, setting you up for failure? Are you expecting to be an expert while still learning? Are you accomplishing what you set out to do? Do you feel good about your progress or are you frustrated and uncomfortable? What is helping you to accomplish your career goals? What is keeping you from it?
2. *Identify your own strengths and weaknesses.* What do you do well? Are you good at communicating with clients or performing technical procedures? What is difficult for you? Do you have trouble calculating drug dosages or remembering the functions of the 12 cranial nerves? By determining what you do well, you can feel good about these accomplishments and focus on mastery of the difficulties. Resist stress by thinking of difficulties as challenges rather than threats.
3. *Take care of yourself.* It is difficult to care for others when your own life-style keeps you off balance. Maintain a healthy life-style and make this a priority. Do not become so overinvolved with clients and work responsibilities that you deny your own health needs. Eat right, get enough rest, avoid smoking and the abuse of alcohol and drugs, and maintain healthy routines and habits. Keep yourself physically fit and allow time to relax.
4. *Take stock of your stressors.* What is stressful for you at work and at home? Is your life stress too much or too intense? How do you manifest stress? Do you have headaches or stomach upset? Do you feel anxious or angry? Does it affect your ability to think and learn? Does it affect your ability to work and attend to clients?
5. *Cultivate effective coping skills.* How do you cope with stress? Do you try to avoid stressors, or do you try to neutralize them in some way? Is your usual style of coping effective in dealing with your current life stress? Find ways to cope that reduce the tension and solve the stress-producing problems rather than avoiding them.
6. *Develop a network of friends and co-workers* who support each other during difficult times. Find the good in your co-workers and support their efforts. Learn to seek out and accept help when you need it.
7. *Take control of your work situation as much as possible.* Participate on committees that regulate client care standards or workplace rules and regulations. Approach problems at work systematically, analyzing the situation and developing ideas for change. Discuss your concerns in a nonthreatening way with the appropriate personnel. Be assertive, not aggressive, as you interact with others. Try to see the other side of the situation, the perceptions of the other people involved. Be willing to compromise. Accept what cannot be changed.
8. *Manage your time effectively,* so that you can complete as much work as possible in the time allotted. Try not to waste time at work with social activities, or with work that should be performed by someone else. Personal time management is especially important when working shift rotations. Structure your time so that you have adequate sleep and still maintain some social activities.
9. *Continue to be wary of making mistakes.* The fear of making a mistake can be stressful if it becomes an obsessive fear. On the other hand, this fear can be adaptive if it stimulates you to be diligent in seeking out the necessary information to avoid the mistake. Learn from your own mistakes and the mistakes of others so that they will not be repeated.
10. *Avoid emotional overinvolvement.* Find the "right level and kind of involvement" that allows you to simply accept clients and provide care without sacrificing yourself. Vowing to keep work from affecting your home life may be unrealistic. Caring nurses cannot help being involved and changed by their relationships with clients and co-workers. Find a balance so that work does not completely take over and supersede your own needs and the needs of your family.
11. *Acknowledge the meaning of caring.* Find the meaning in your work and concentrate on its benefits to clients and to you.

HOMEODYNAMICS: CREATING NEW WAYS OF BEING

In the discussion of change at the beginning of this chapter, homeodynamics is described as a contemporary view of change and the human condition. Martha Rogers, a nurse theorist,[22,24] found discussions of homeostasis and adaptation to be inadequate in describing the dynamic or constant nature of change and the phenomenon of psychological growth. Homeostatic and adaptive views of change are limited by their goal of stability. The homeodynamic view of change encompasses all of these ideas about change and optimal health: homeostasis, adaptation, and growth.

Homeodynamics are principles that describe the nature and direction of change. These principles were proposed by Rogers as "fundamental guides to the practice of nursing."[24] They are principles that are exclusive to nursing theory, not borrowed from theories of medicine, physics, psychology, or sociology. Homeodynamic principles describe change from a holistic viewpoint, one in which people respond as unitary beings that cannot be reduced to psychological or physiological entities.

Theoretical Basis of Homeodynamics

General systems theory serves as a basis for the principles of homeodynamics. A **system** is an organized set of components or parts that mutually interact to form an integrated whole. Systems behave as wholes, as more than the sum of their parts.[9,11] According to von Bertalanffy,[9] a systems theorist, human beings function as **open** (or living) **systems,** openly interacting with, influencing, and being influenced by their environment.

IMPLICATIONS FOR PROFESSIONAL COLLABORATION

Hardiness and Caring

Nursing is an inherently stressful job. Work conditions and the intrinsic nature of nursing, which demands continuous caring, lead easily to burnout. The hardy nurse looks upon the potentially stressful aspects of nursing as challenges. Rather than stresses, these experiences are perceived as rewards and as evidence of good work. For example, the sight of blood, which is frightening to many people, is welcomed by the nurse who endeavors to slip an IV catheter into the vein of a critically ill client. Nevertheless, to continue caring over the long term, it is necessary for even the hardiest nurses to apply the principles of stress management to their own personal involvement in nursing.

Because of their open interaction with the environment, open systems evolve and change, developing and becoming increasingly complex. This can be contrasted with **closed systems,** which limit their interaction with the environment. Closed systems function much as a homeostatic control system, monitoring input from feedback mechanisms and making adjustments in order to maintain stable functioning. A thermostat is an example of a closed system. The input into this closed system is limited to the temperature of the air. It does not process other information such as humidity or barometric pressure. Closed systems function to maintain stable states, while open systems have the ability to transform themselves, to change their character as they evolve in interaction with the environment.[9,11]

Living open systems exist in a hierarchical order, from the unit of the smallest cell to the planet as a whole (Figure 6–7). Any of these unitary entities can be viewed as a system in that they are all made up of component parts that are interrelated in some way and function together as a whole.[9,11] In this chapter, the focus is on the individual as a system. In Chapters 7 and 8, community and family systems are also discussed. The concept of a system is a unifying one in that it is a way of looking at individuals or groups as wholes, interacting with other systems. People who view the world as a hierarchy of interrelated systems view their own actions as both influencing and influenced by other systems. They see their own health as related to the health of their families, of their communities, and of the planet itself. Rogers builds on these core ideas of systems to describe homeodynamic principles of human change.

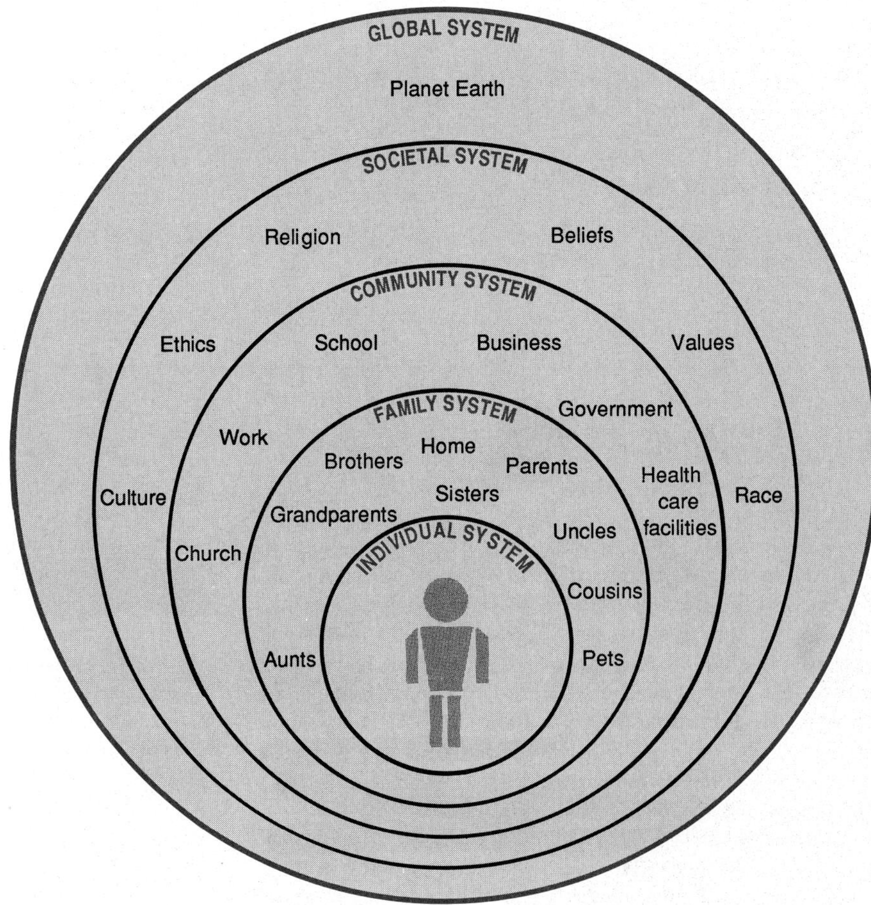

Figure 6–7. The hierarchy of living systems.

Basic Assumptions of Homeodynamics

Humans and Environments Are Unified Wholes. To understand homeodynamic change, it is necessary to understand what is meant by the description of the individual as a unified whole.[24] A unified whole is an entity that cannot be divided or reduced in any way. Human beings as unified wholes cannot be predicted to behave in certain ways from the behavior or functioning of their specific component parts. Individuals as unified wholes are different from, and more than, the sum of their physiological, psychological, and social aspects. These aspects are organized in a specific way and have an interdependent relationship with each other. A change in any one part causes change in the whole.

Lazlo,[59] a systems theorist, explains this concept by describing wholes versus heaps. Heaps are like piles of trash. If you add or take away any of the pieces of trash, the identify or function of the heap does not change, it is still a pile of trash. There is no organization or interdependence of its parts. An individual is unlike a heap, however. One cannot add, take away, or change parts of an individual without creating a new individual. This is because individuals are wholes; their parts are interrelated. If one trait of an individual, say for example a person's eating habits, is changed, there are likely to be corresponding changes in the individual's physical appearance, attitude toward self, and perhaps even patterns of social interaction as a result. Likewise, illness in any part of an individual affects the function of all other parts: organs, organ systems, emotions, cognition, and socialization. This was illustrated in the discussion of stress as a transaction. Human behavior can be broken down into categories for study, but in reality the person responds as a unitary being.[22,24]

In considering clients as unitary beings, nurses must look at all behavior as manifestations of the whole person. These manifestations should be seen as patterns of behavior that result from integrated functioning of the person as a unit.[22,24] Nurses assess clients' patterns of temperature or blood pressure change, patterns of sleep and activity, patterns of communication, or patterns of coping with stress. These patterns of behavior are actually coordinated, whole-person responses and are not caused by and cannot be predicted by the behavior of any specific body system.

The environment is also a unified whole. The environment consists of everything external to the individual; each individual's environment is therefore unique to his or her experience.[22,24] The environment includes other people (including nurses), physical structures such as home and geographic location, and abstract entities such as society and culture. Each person's environment differs in the organization and interdependence of its parts. Environments cannot be viewed as heaps. If any part is taken away or changed, the experience of the whole is affected. For example, a spouse is a person who is a significant part of an individual's environment. The loss of a spouse changes the way that the widow or widower perceives and interacts with the rest of his or her unique environment. The house seems empty at first, and patterns of social activity and work roles change. The individual's perception of the whole environment changes with the loss of this one very significant part. Nurses assess environmental patterns such as communication and transportation, community service and politics, and patterns of cultural and societal influence. These patterns are manifestations of the whole environment, with a change in any one causing change in all the others.

Humans Interact Openly With Their Environments. The relationship between human beings and their environments is characterized by openness. Individuals and their environments openly interact to simultaneously and continuously influence each other. This interaction is called **mutual process.**[24] For example, nurses, as part of clients' environment, influence clients' behaviors by teaching them new skills; guiding them through a maze of tests, treatments, and choices; and interjecting their own moods and attitudes. At the same time, clients influence nurses' behaviors by making them aware of their own vulnerabilities, making them sad or joyful or frustrated, making them hurry up or slow down. This happens simultaneously, not in sequence. Individuals and their environment are open to each other and they exist in mutual process. Individuals and their environments change as a unit, with change in one always including change in the other.

In this context, nurses realize that they are always changed by nurse–client interactions, and that clients are changed as well. For example, patterns of activity on a hospital unit change as the client population changes. Some clients require more assistance with bathing, feeding, and exercises than others. Nurses adjust their own activities to meet client needs. Sustained patterns of high need can exhaust nursing personnel, leading to frustration. This sense of frustration may be communicated to clients as brusque or uncaring behavior, thereby changing client feelings toward nurses.

Humans and Their Environments Change Continuously and Creatively Toward Increasing Complexity. As a result of this open, mutual human–environmental interaction, change proceeds as a continuous and unpredictable creative process.[24] Consider the unpredictable nature of human change. Because a person does not exist in a controlled environment, it is impossible to predict future change. For example, it is impossible to predict adult behavior from the behavior patterns of the child. While the exact nature of change cannot be predicted, it is possible to mold or guide behavior toward healthy patterns. Parents teach their children to eat healthy food and exercise regularly. They teach them about love, trust, and responsibility by giving them verbal and physical signs of affection and by setting limits in the form of discipline. They involve them in community activities such as scouting and church groups. They guide the child's behavior change by controlling factors in the child's unique environment. Healthy people participate in the change process by striving to change toward new and healthier ways of being.

The term "creativity" applies to the process of making

something new and different.[2] With the accumulation of experiences, and through interactions with a changing environment, individuals become different from what they were before. An individual can become taller, thinner, healthier, sadder, or more anxious than in the past. These changes are creative in that they are new and different behavior. Consider the example of the pain experience. Each time the individual experiences pain, it is experienced in a new way, a way that is influenced by the characteristics of the individual and the environment at that point in time. Thus, a new experience is created that is related to both past feelings and the current situation. Each experience is new and different because individuals are always evolving and creating new and different ways of experiencing their world.

Even though people and events seem to stay the same, patterns of behavior never repeat themselves exactly the same way from one time to the next. Human beings and their environments go through cycles in that they repeat similar experiences or behaviors.[22,24] For example, individuals have certain sleeping and waking cycles, fluctuating work shifts, and highs and lows in energy level. Environments exhibit rhythms in the change of seasons, the movements of the stars, and the occurrence of wars and economic recession. These patterns can be traced. Each occurrence is similar to but a little different from the previous occurrence, a variation on a theme. Rogers refers to this phenomenon as that of "nonrepeating rhythmicities" in human–environmental patterns of interaction.[22] This idea explains the person's sense of stability within a world of continuous change. The cycles or rhythms are the stabilizing forces, but they exist only as themes, with continuous change being the actuality.[12]

The direction of change, as individuals age, is toward the development of increasingly complex and diverse behavior patterns. This happens as life experiences accumulate.[22,24] For example, a client's first experience with pain may be a spontaneous withdrawal from the source of the pain. The next experience is more complex because it combines the experience of the current pain episode with memories of the past experience. During the second experience, the client anticipates the pain, based on the past experience, and may feel stress even before encountering the physical source of pain. This accumulation of experience continues to make each event more complex, and as the result of accumulated experience, the individual becomes more complex.

Humans Have the Capacity to Influence and Shape Change. According to Rogers,[22,24] people have the capacity for thinking and self-reflection and the capacity to knowingly participate in the process of change. Individuals can consciously consider their own actions and reflect upon how they feel about these actions. They can consider options and make use of the power of choice to control and shape their lives.

For example, people often reflect upon their symptoms of stress and knowingly choose whether or not to manage this stress in some way. People can shape their lives by considering their options and making choices. One person may choose to manage stress by avoiding the circumstances, while another person may choose to learn new relaxation techniques. People can continue to make the same choices, continuing their usual patterns of behavior, or they can grow and choose new and better ways to function or cope with stress. Nurses work with clients to assist them to make healthy choices, choices that help them to achieve their maximum health potential.

Limitations of Homeostasis and Adaptation Views of Human Change

Theories of homeostasis and adaptation describe change as a disruption that upsets the natural balance or equilibrium. Individuals seek stability and balance within a particular level of functioning. This perspective fails to address the fact that people do change. They change the way they look and feel about others and themselves. Sometimes they are forced to change by circumstances out of their control, and sometimes they choose to change out of a desire to be better or healthier in some way. The homeodynamic view of human change helps nurses to look at change as an option rather than a disruption.[13]

The concepts of homeostasis and adaptation describe certain aspects of human behavior and response to change, but they lead one to believe that true balance and stability can be attained and that this should be the goal of human behavior. The homeodynamic view of change acknowledges that this goal is unattainable, that change is inevitable, and that balance and stability in life are really just a series of nonrepeating rhythmicities, a repetition of similar but different behavior patterns. Change becomes the fundamental fact, with homeostasis, adaptation, coping, and growth as different aspects of and possibilities for change.[13]

Human Growth and Collaboration for Optimal Health

General Contributions of Growth Psychology. Growth is a response to change that leads beyond adaptation to the achievement of personal changes that bring a new and healthier state of functioning.[1,19] Growth psychologists—those psychologists who study the nature and dynamics of human growth—look at people as "persons in process."[60] They study the ways that people live, the choices that they make, and the meanings that they attach to their experiences. Growth psychologists believe that all people have the potential for change and the ability to make choices to make a change. They look at people as seeking new and better ways of functioning.

How does growth take place? Maslow states that people grow upward through a "hierarchy of needs," meeting lower-level needs before proceeding to higher-level needs.[1,61] Growth requires meeting lower-level needs. For example, the individual must meet needs for safety and security, love and belonging, self-esteem and recognition, before reaching the highest need for self-actualization. Self-actualization is individuals' need to achieve their highest potential, to be the best they can be.[1,61] (Further discussion of self-actualization can be found in Chapter 10.)

Maslow described "self-actualized" individuals as people who know what they want to do with their lives and are able to achieve their goals; people who have reached their highest potential.[1,61] He also noted that change proceeds both up and down this hierarchy. People change in their ability to meet these needs depending upon the circumstances of their lives. For example, in times of war, people's lives are turned upside down and they must focus on survival needs. People achieve growth when they move up the hierarchy toward self-actualization.

Carl Rogers[1,62] believed that all people have the capacity for growth, but that this capacity can become buried under layers of defense mechanisms or hidden behind an outer facade. According to Rogers, through the use of the therapeutic relationship, "the other person will discover within himself the capacity to use that relationship for growth, and change and personal development will occur" (p. 33).[62] He characterizes this relationship as honest, genuine, accepting, and understanding. Rogers stated that, as people grow, they become "fully functioning" individuals.

Allport[1] stated that people experience growth when they strive to live a life that is appropriate to their own goals, not the goals of others. He found that to grow, one must be open to change, to continually reach toward a higher level of self-awareness and achievement. He viewed people not as human beings, but as "human becomings."

These and other growth psychologists have found the following factors[1] to facilitate the process of growth:

- *Intellectual curiosity.* In order to change and grow, people need to be willing to learn more about a situation, to consider other ideas and other ways of doing things; they must be open-minded. People cannot grow if they are limited by prejudice or the opinions of others. They must have confidence in their own knowledge and make judgments and choices accordingly, even if it means going against the norm.
- *Emotional openness.* Growth is not always a pleasant experience. People often close themselves off to experiences that are uncomfortable or emotionally difficult. Individuals must be willing to experience all emotions, whether conflictual, pleasant, or unpleasant, in order for growth to take place. They must be flexible in their emotional responses and feel free to learn from their experiences and change for the better as a result.
- *Energetic motivation.* In order to grow, people must be willing to take control of their lives, take responsibility for their actions, and be motivated to continue the quest for their goals. They must learn from their mistakes and continue to strive despite setbacks or tragedy in their lives. Crisis can be an opportunity for growth when individuals are motivated to learn new and better ways of coping.
- *Spiritual compassion.* People are often motivated to grow by a sense of mission, reaching toward a higher meaning in life. Growth is facilitated when people have a highly ethical sense, a sense that all life is sacred. In this way, people are able to transcend difficulties and grow because of the meaning that they attach to their own lives and to the lives of others. People are able to transcend suffering and grow because of their beliefs.

In contrast, growth is hindered when individuals close themselves to knowledge and emotions, when they let the opinions of others dictate their life choices, when they lack a sense of higher meaning in life. DeFeo states that "to choose is to give up the old and comfortable for the questionable new."[13] To grow, individuals must make choices to participate in and control the change in their lives.

Growth and Optimal Health. Clients strive for optimal health by choosing that which is desirable and possible for them, reaching for their highest potential. Clients have different definitions of optimal health based on their own values, beliefs, and personal goals. Optimal health is an experience of being the best that one can be, living up to one's expectations, being in harmony with the self.[1,24,49]

Clients differ in what they desire in life and in their personal goals. One client may desire to achieve a healthy routine of diet and exercise while another may desire to maintain control over a chronic disease. Possibilities also differ from one person to the next. It is impossible for paraplegics, individuals paralyzed from the waist down, to be able to walk again, but it is possible for them to be independently functioning persons who use a wheelchair for mobility.

Nurses care for clients as individuals, respecting their values and beliefs and their definitions of health. Often clients view health merely as the absence of disease, without realizing their potential to be better or the options they have to choose from. Nurses can influence this definition of health in the mutual process of nurse–client interaction, helping clients to realize their own potential, their possibilities for growth, and their opportunities to be better in some way.

Illness as an Opportunity for Growth. Illness can be more than a disruption in an individual's life rhythms and routines; it can be an opportunity for growth.[1,44] During times of illness, clients are forced to step out of their daily habits and routines and reevaluate their lives. They have time to think and reflect upon their goals and achievements, and upon their weaknesses and failures.

The illness experience can be a turning point that initiates a series of fundamental changes in an individual. As individuals cope with illness, they may make changes in habits, life-style, or self-concept. These changes may occur by choice or necessity. Either way, people grow as they learn new and better ways to deal with adversity. For example, individuals who develop a chronic disease such as diabetes are forced to change their diet, learn new skills such as the injection of insulin, and employ the self-discipline required to follow a rigorous health care plan.

People who are in treatment for addiction to drugs or alcohol must change their self-concept and acknowledge their addiction in order to be able to realize their potential for change. Acknowledgement of their illness gives them the opportunity to grow and to change their self-destructive behavior.

Collaborative View of Growth. According to the principles of homeodynamics, individuals and their environments exist in mutual process, changing together through the life process. Nurses, as part of the client's environment, collaborate with clients in mutual process to promote growth toward optimal health. The collaborative relationship is one that makes the most of the nurse–client mutual process for mutual benefit.[63–65] There is mutual sharing of opinions, attitudes, and emotions. Clients are not objects of care, but are actively involved in and responsible for their own health. In the collaborative relationship, nurses are caring and compassionate companions, sharing themselves and assisting clients with the knowing participation in change.[13] Nurses do not seek to control or make choices for clients, or to rescue clients by solving their problems for them.

Collaborative Approach to Facilitating Growth. Nurses work with clients to shape the change in their lives for their benefit. Mathwig, Young, and Pepper, nurse educators who subscribe to Rogers' principles of homeodynamics, describe the goal of nursing care as participation "with the person to continuously pattern the environment to achieve the maximum health potential of that person."[66] Nurses enable clients to grow by heightening their awareness of their own potential, and the options they have to choose from in order to reach toward that goal. They assist clients to knowingly participate in the continuous process of change and growth toward optimal health.

Behavior Pattern Appraisal. How does this translate into actual nursing practice? Nurses collaborate with clients by first appraising or assessing clients' behavior patterns and the environment, and then enhancing the client's power to promote optimal health.[67]

In behavior pattern appraisal, nurses assess patterns of behavior that are a manifestation of the whole person in mutual process with the environment. The chapters that follow in this text introduce many assessment tools. The choice of appropriate tools for assessment will depend upon the client and the environment in which care is taking place.

Because change is a mutual process of client–environment reciprocity, it is also necessary to assess environmental patterns. Nurses assess the patterns of the environment, including an appraisal of the nurse's own relationship with clients and, equally important, the physical surroundings, culture, and social influences, clients' families and friends, and other health care professionals involved in care.

Deliberative Mutual Patterning. Deliberative mutual patterning occurs when nurses assist clients to grow toward optimal health. After appraisal of client behavior pattern and environmental pattern, nurses pattern the environment for healing and encourage client participation.[67] In this way, nurses facilitate change and growth toward health. However, it is important to point out that although nurses endeavor to facilitate growth, nurses do not require it. The process of growth is deliberative because it involves clients' conscious choice. Clients participate knowingly and voluntarily in the process of growth, and must be self-motivated to achieve the objective of growth.

Nurses collaborate with clients to identify and choose from options that facilitate desired change. Examples of options include health education to help clients make informed choices. For example, clients are taught about the benefits of deep breathing to prevent pneumonia. It has been found that clients are more likely to participate knowingly in this activity after surgery if they have had preoperative instruction. Often, an increase in awareness can lead to appropriate action. But ultimately the decision to participate is the client's.

Nurses also pattern the environment through the use of self.[66,67] Because nurses are a part of the environment, the nurse's mood, attentiveness, projection of self-confidence, and feelings about clients are part of the environmental pattern. Nurses deliberately change their emotional response to clients as part of patterning the environment. To better understand nursing care as deliberative mutual patterning, consider the following example.

Case Situation:

Jo is the nurse assigned to care for Mr. Bolling, a client who has extensive burn wounds that require painful dressing changes every day. Jo and Mr. Bolling collaborate to assess client and environmental patterns as they relate to the dressing change experience. Jo encourages Mr. Bolling to describe his perception of the experience and the environment in which it takes place. He states that the anticipation of the pain is almost as bad as the pain itself, and that he feels helpless because he cannot control the pain. In addition, Mr. Bolling shares his feel-

IMPLICATIONS FOR NURSE-CLIENT COLLABORATION

Homeodynamics and Mutual Process

People have the capacity for thinking and self-reflection. They can consider options and make use of the power of choice to control and shape their lives. During illness, clients are forced to step out of their daily habits and routines and reevaluate their lives. They have time to think, reflect, and make new choices. The illness experience can be a turning point.

According to the principles of homeodynamics, human beings and their environments change together in a mutual, continuous process. They change as a unit, with change in one always involving change in the other. Nurses as part of clients' environment during illness collaborates in the mutual process to promote clients' growth toward optimal health. Mutual process is synonymous with collaboration.

ings that the nurses often seem distant and unfriendly during the procedure, and that the room temperature is uncomfortably cold.

Jo has observed that Mr. Bolling becomes distracted, breathes rapidly, and talks incessantly while the nurses prepare the dressings. His heart rate and blood pressure go up. During the dressing change, he requires strong doses of pain medication just to take the edge off the pain, and often is unable to cooperate in the experience, resisting the efforts of the nurses. Jo realizes that Mr. Bolling's response to the pain changes with each experience, becoming more complex as he assimilates past experiences with the present. She shares these observations with Mr. Bolling. Mr. Bolling shares that his personal goals are to decrease pain during the dressing change and to be able to control his own behavior.

Jo and Mr. Bolling use the information obtained from their assessment to mutually plan to repattern the environment and facilitate growth toward optimal health. Jo participates with Mr. Bolling in the process, presenting him with options to decrease pain and increase self-control, and explaining how they work. They prepare the following plan:

1. Mr. Bolling will choose the time for the dressing change, in collaboration with Jo's schedule
2. Jo will assist Mr. Bolling in muscle relaxation and breathing techniques to counteract the stress response and facilitate the action of the pain medication
3. Mr. Bolling will have the power to stop the dressing change briefly at any time when the experience becomes overwhelming
4. Jo will repattern the environment by playing music of Mr. Bolling's choice to distract him from the pain, and turning up the heat in the room to promote comfort.

In addition, Jo uses herself to repattern the environment by speaking in soft, calm tones and by paying attention to Mr. Bolling's needs during the procedure, rather than distancing herself from this unpleasant experience.

After the next dressing change, Jo and Mr. Bolling are both satisfied with their plan. Mr. Bolling's tolerance of the pain has increased and his self-esteem is bolstered, as he is able to be in control of the situation and participate in rather than resist the process. He is able to grow as he learns new and better ways to cope with the pain and helplessness. Joe feels satisfied in her work and grows in her ability to connect with clients in an accepting and nonjudgmental way, guiding change and promoting growth toward optimal health.

This example illustrates the positive effect of nursing care that facilitates client change, rather than resisting it. The reader can also apply the following guidelines to his or her own practice:

1. Think of yourself as a caring companion to clients rather than as caring for clients.
2. Do not be afraid to become involved in the relationship with clients, to share your own relevant experiences.
3. Accept clients simply, without judging them. Try to put yourself in their shoes.
4. Begin by eliciting clients' perspectives of the situation. Also, discuss your own observations with clients, thereby increasing their awareness of their own situation.
5. Guide clients toward identification of their strengths and potentials, focusing on the positive and boosting self-esteem.
6. Elicit clients' perceptions of optimal health or well-being. Work toward clients' goals for optimal health, not yours.
7. Encourage clients to clarify personal values and set realistic goals accordingly. Realistic goals are more often met with success.
8. Empower clients to choose by offering information about options for care.
9. Involve family and community resources in plans for care. They are all part of a client's unique environment and are mutually changed by the experience.
10. Use your own mood and actions to repattern the environment, consciously using self to benefit clients.
11. Remember to repattern the physical environment for maximum client benefit, rearranging furniture and possessions, adjusting room temperature, providing a view out the window, or providing for privacy.
12. Let clients solve their own problems. You cannot choose for them.
13. Encourage clients to welcome change as part of the process of growth toward optimal health.
14. Remember that clients may not be able to control all factors that lead to health. Help clients to accept those things that cannot be changed and find meaning in the experience.
15. Respect clients' choices, even if you do not agree.
16. Mutually evaluate clients' progress toward optimal health, acknowledging success and growth, and learning from mistakes.
17. Be aware of how you change as a result of your relationships with clients. Take credit for your own growth toward becoming an expert, caring nurse.

Nurses and clients collaborate to appraise the client–environment behavior pattern and, from those observations, work together to select a variety of treatment modalities. Clients participate in the mutual process by making choices about their care. This results from nurses' empowerment of clients. Environmental patterning by nurses enables clients' health patterns to change and grow toward healing.[67] Human growth is a collaborative process that facilitates change and promotes health from clients' perspectives.

SUMMARY

Homeostasis and homeodynamics are classic and contemporary views of change and the human condition. Homeostasis is the automatic self-regulatory response to physiological change. This response resists major change in the functioning of physiological control systems. Negative feedback mechanisms make minor adjustments and keep functioning within a healthy range.

Adaptation is a concept similar to homeostasis, but goes beyond it, describing the physiological, psychological, and social responses to environmental change. Adaptation is the response of human beings as psychophysiological wholes, to stress. Cognitive appraisal of an experience as threatening, harmful, or challenging defines individuals' unique experiences of stress and triggers a response. Physical and psychological manifestations of the stress response vary with each person. People use coping mechanisms to neutralize the stress. When usual coping mechanisms fail, individuals may experience crisis or overwhelming stress. The crisis situation offers people the opportunity to grow, learning new and better ways to cope.

The ideals of holism and the facilitation of change characterize the concept of homeodynamics, as described by Martha Rogers. The principles of homeodynamics are based in systems theory and describe the nature of change as a mutual process between clients and their unique environment. This continuous change is manifested in patterns of behavior and is creative, unpredictable, and increasingly complex. Healthy clients participate in the change process to grow and become congruent with a self-ideal. This self-ideal is equated with optimal health for that individual. The basic tenets of growth psychology support this view of health.

Nurses can use this information to promote optimal health through nurse–client collaboration. Mutual process is synonymous with collaboration. The view of change as mutual process underscores the importance of the collaborative interaction. With this view, nurses are part of clients' environment and affect clients' health through the mutual process of client–environmental change. Nurse and client collaborate to appraise a client's behavior patterns and the behavior pattern of the environment. Nurse and client then facilitate positive change toward growth through deliberative mutual patterning. Nurses repattern the environment, including their own responses to clients. Nurses empower clients to know, and to make choices toward optimal health.

REFERENCES

1. O'Connell A, Whitmore J, O'Connell V. *Choice and Change: The Psychology of Adjustment, Growth, and Creativity*. 3rd ed. Englewood Cliffs, NJ: Prentice-Hall; 1985.
2. *Webster's Third New International Dictionary of the English Language, Unabridged*. Chicago: Encyclopedia Britannica; 1986.
3. Lippitt GL. *Visualizing Change: Model Building and the Change Process*. La Jolla, CA: University Associates; 1973.
4. Lewin K. *Field Theory in Social Science*. New York: Harper; 1951.
5. Sarter B. *The Stream of Becoming: A Study of Martha Rogers's Theory*. New York: National League for Nursing; 1988.
6. Watzlawick P, Weakland J, Fisch R. *Change: Principles of Problem Formation and Problem Resolution*. New York: Norton; 1974.
7. Hall BA. The change paradigm in nursing: Growth versus persistence. *Adv Nurs Sci*. 1981; 3:1–6.
8. Jensen EW, James SA, Boyce WT, Hartnett SA. The family routines inventory: Development and validation. *Social Sci Med*. 1983; 17:201–211.
9. Von Bertalanffy L. *General System Theory: Foundations, Development, Applications*. New York: Braziller; 1968.
10. Dossey L. Care giving and natural systems theory. *Top Clin Nurs*. 1982; 21–27.
11. Putt AM. *General Systems Theory Applied to Nursing*. Boston: Little, Brown; 1978.
12. Samuels M, Bennett HZ. *Well Body, Well Earth: The Sierra Club Environmental Health Sourcebook*. San Francisco: Sierra Club Books; 1983.
13. DeFeo DJ. Change: A central concern of nursing. *Nurs Sci Q*. 1990; 3:88–94.
14. Martel L. *Mastering Change: The Key to Business Success*. New York: Simon & Schuster; 1986.
15. Bennis WG, Benne KD, Chin R, Corey KE, eds. *The Planning of Change*. 3rd ed. San Francisco: Holt, Rinehart & Winston; 1976.
16. Kobasa SC. Stressful life events, personality, and health: An inquiry in hardiness. In: Monat A, Lazarus RS, eds. *Stress and Coping: An Anthology*. 2nd ed. New York: Columbia University Press; 1985.
17. Dubos R. *Man Adapting*. New Haven: Yale University Press; 1965.
18. Lazarus RS, Folkman S. *Stress, Appraisal, and Coping*. New York: Springer; 1984.
19. Mengel A. The concept of coping. *Top Clin Nurs*. 1982; 4:1–3.
20. Pender NJ. Stress management. In: Pender NJ, ed. *Health Promotion in Nursing Practice*. 2nd ed. Norwalk, CT: Appleton & Lange; 1987.
21. Cannon WB. *The Wisdom of the Body*. 2nd ed. New York: Norton; 1939.
22. Rogers ME. *An Introduction to the Theoretical Basis of Nursing*. Philadelphia: FA Davis; 1979.
23. McCance KL. Stress and disease. In: McCance KL, Huether SE, eds. *Pathophysiology: The Biological Basis for Disease in Adults and Children*. St. Louis: Mosby; 1990:279–291.
24. Rogers ME. Nursing: Science of unitary, irreducible, human beings: Update 1990. In: Barrett EAM, ed. *Visions of Rogers' Science-Based Nursing*. New York: National League for Nursing; 1990:5–11.
25. Guyton AC. *Textbook of Medical Physiology*. Philadelphia: Saunders; 1986.
26. Sunderland PM. Structure and function of the neurologic system. In: McCance KL, Huether SE, eds. *Pathophysiology: The Biological Basis for Disease in Adults and Children*. St. Louis: Mosby; 1990:279–291.
27. Flynn PAR. *Holistic Health: The Art and Science of Care*. Bowie, MD: Brady; 1980:97.
28. Gray PD. Mechanisms of hormonal regulation. In: McCance KL, Huether SE, eds. *Pathophysiology: The Biological Basis for Disease in Adults and Children*. St. Louis: Mosby; 1990:564–593.
29. Rossi EL. *The Psychobiology of Mind–Body Healing*. New York: Norton; 1986.
30. Wolff HG. *Stress and Disease*. 2nd ed. Springfield, IL: Thomas; 1968.
31. Freedman AM, Kaplan HI, Saddock BJ. *Comprehensive Textbook of Psychiatry*. 2nd ed. Baltimore: Williams & Wilkins; 1975; 1.
32. Selye H. History and present status of the stress concept. In: Monat A, Lazarus RS, eds. *Stress and Coping: An Anthology*. 2nd ed. New York: Columbia University Press; 1985.
33. Benson H. *The Relaxation Response*. New York: Morrow; 1975.
34. Dohrenwend BS, Dohrenwend BP, eds. *Stressful Life Events: Their Nature and Effects*. New York: Wiley; 1974.

35. Holmes TH, Rahe RH. The social readjustment rating scale. *Psychosomat Res.* 1967; 11:213–217.
36. Kanner AD, Coyne JC, Schaefer C, Lazarus RS. Comparison of two modes of stress measurement: Daily hassles and uplifts versus major life events. *J Behav Med.* 1981; 4:1–29.
37. Cohen F. Stress and bodily illness. In: Monat A, Lazarus RS, eds. *Stress and Coping: An Anthology.* 2nd ed. New York: Columbia University Press; 1985.
38. Guzetta CE, Forsyth GL. Nursing diagnostic pilot study: Psychophysiologic stress. *Adv Nurs Sci.* 1979; 2:27–44.
39. Dossey BM. The psychophysiology of bodymind healing. In: Dossey BM, Keegan L, Guzzetta CE, Kolkmeier LG, eds. *Holistic Nursing: A Handbook for Practice.* Rockville, MD: Aspen; 1988:78.
40. Dossey BM, Keegan L, Guzzetta CE, Kolkmeier LG, eds. *Holistic Nursing: A Handbook for Practice.* Rockville, MD: Aspen; 1988.
41. Carpenito LJ. *Nursing Diagnosis: Application to Clinical Practice.* 3rd ed. Philadelphia: Lippincott; 1989.
42. Folkman S, Lazarus RS. An analysis of coping in a middle-aged community sample. *J Health Soc Behav.* 1980; 21:219–239.
43. Braden CJ. A test of the self-help model: Learned response to chronic illness experience. *Nurs Res.* 1990; 39:42–47.
44. Caplan G. *Principles of Psychiatry.* New York: Basic Books; 1964.
45. Aguilera DC, Messick JM. *Crisis Intervention.* 2nd ed. St. Louis: Mosby; 1974.
46. Holahan CJ, Moos RH. Life stress and health: Personality, coping and family support in stress resistance. *J Personality Soc Psych.* 1985; 49:739–747.
47. Kobasa SCO, Pucetti MC. Personality and social resources in stress resistance. *J Personality Soc Psych.* 1983; 45:839–850.
48. Pollack SE. The hardiness characteristic: A motivating factor in adaptation. *Adv Nurs Sci.* 1989; 11:53–62.
49. Pender NJ. *Health Promotion in Nursing Practice.* 2nd ed. Norwalk, CT: Appleton & Lange; 1987.
50. Davis M, Eschelman ER, McKay M. *The Relaxation and Stress Reduction Workbook.* 3rd ed. Oakland, CA: New Harbinger; 1988.
51. Pender NJ. Stress management. In Pender NJ, ed. *Health Promotion in Nursing Practice.* 2nd ed. Norwalk, CT: Appleton & Lange; 1987:386.
52. Pender NJ. Exercise and physical fitness. In Pender NJ, ed. *Health Promotion in Nursing Practice.* 2nd ed. Norwalk, CT: Appleton & Lange; 1987:295–296.
53. Smythe EEM. *Surviving Nursing.* Reading, MA: Addison-Wesley: 1984.
54. Benner P, Wrubel J. *The Primacy of Caring: Stress and Coping in Health and Illness.* Menlo Park, CA: Addison-Wesley; 1989.
55. Harris RB. Reviewing nursing stress according to a proposed coping-adaptation framework. *Adv Nurs Sci.* 1989; 11:12–28.
56. Allanach EJ. Perceived supportive behaviors and nursing occupational stress: An evolution of consciousness. *Adv Nurs Sci.* 1988; 10:73–82.
57. Benner P, Wrubel J. The primacy of caring. In: Benner P, Wrubel J, eds. *The Primacy of Caring: Stress and Coping in Health and Illness.* Menlo Park, CA: Addison-Wesley; 1989.
58. Benner P. *From Novice to Expert: Excellence and Power in Clinical Nursing Practice.* Menlo Park, CA: Addison-Wesley; 1984.
59. Laszlo E. *The Systems View of the World.* New York: Braziller; 1972.
60. O'Connell A, Whitmore J, O'Connell V. *Choice and Change: The Psychology of Adjustment, Growth, and Creativity.* 3rd ed. Englewood Cliffs, NJ: Prentice-Hall; 1985:15
61. Maslow AH. *Motivation and Personality.* New York: Harper; 1954.
62. Rogers CR. *On Becoming a Person.* Boston: Houghton Mifflin; 1961.
63. Kasch CR. Establishing a collaborative nurse-patient relationship: A distinct focus of nursing action in primary care. *Image.* 1986; 18:44–47.
64. Pesznecker BL, Zerwekh JV, Horn BJ. The mutual participation relationship: Key to facilitating self-care practices in clients and families. *Pub Health Nurs.* 1989; 6:197–203.
65. Marck P. Therapeutic reciprocity: A caring phenomenon. *Adv Nurs Sci.* 1990; 13:49–59.
66. Mathwig GM, Young AA, Pepper JM. Using Rogerian science in undergraduate and graduate nursing education. In: Barrett EAM, ed. *Visions of Rogers' Science-based Nursing.* New York: National League for Nursing; 1990:319–333.
67. Barrett EAM. Rogers' science-based nursing practice. In: Barrett EAM, ed. *Visions of Rogers' Science-based Nursing.* New York: National League for Nursing; 1990:31–44.

BIBLIOGRAPHY

Bennis WG, Benne KD, Chin R, Corey KE, eds. *The Planning of Change.* 3rd ed. New York: Holt, Rinehart & Winston; 1976.

Bullock BL, Rosendahl PP. *Pathophysiology: Adaptations and Alterations in Function.* 2nd ed. Glenview, IL: Scott, Foresman; 1988.

Cook ND. *Stability and Flexibility: An Analysis of Natural Systems.* Elmsford, NY: Pergamon; 1980.

Dixon JP, Dixon JK, Spinner J. Perceptions of life-pattern disintegrity as a link in the relationship between stress and illness. *Adv Nurs Sci.* 1989; 1:1–11.

Donnelly GF. Consciousness: The brain and self-regulation modalities. *Top Clin Nurs.* 1982; 13–20.

Dossey L. Care giving and natural systems theory. *Top Clin Nurs.* 1982; 21–27.

Dunn HL. High-level wellness for man and society. *Am J Pub Health.* 1959; 49:786–792.

Edelman CL, Mandle CL. *Health Promotion Throughout the Lifespan.* 2nd ed. St. Louis: Mosby; 1990.

Fagin CM. Stress: Implications for nursing research. *Image.* 1987; 19:38–41.

Frain M, Valiga TM. The multiple dimensions of stress. *Top Clin Nurs.* 1979; 1:43–52.

Goosen GM, Bush HA. Adaptation: A feedback process. *Adv Nurs Sci.* 1979; 1:51–65.

Gordon M. *Nursing Diagnosis: Process and Application.* 2nd ed. New York: McGraw-Hill; 1988.

Helson H. *Adaptation-Level Theory.* New York: Harper & Row; 1964.

Johnson JE, Lauver DR. Alternative explanations of coping with stressful experiences associated with physical illness. *Adv Nurs Sci.* 1989; 11:39–52.

Kemp Vh. An overview of change and leadership. *Top Clin Nurs.* 1984; 6:1–9.

Lambert CE, Lambert VA. Hardiness: Its development and relevance to nursing. *Image.* 1987; 19:92–95.

Lowenberg JS. *Caring and Responsibility: The Crossroads Between Holistic Practice and Traditional Medicine.* Philadelphia: University of Pennsylvania Press; 1989.

Mauksch IG, Miller MH. *Implementing Change in Nursing.* St. Louis: Mosby; 1981.

Moch SD. Health within illness: Conceptual evolution and practice possibilities. *Adv Nurs Sci.* 1989; 11:23–31.

Monat A, Lazarus RS. *Stress and Coping: An Anthology.* 2nd ed. New York: Columbia University Press; 1985.

Moos RH. Context and coping: Toward a unifying conceptual framework. *Am J Community Psych.* 1984; 12:1–25.

Muir BL. *Pathophysiology: An Introduction to the Mechanisms of Disease.* 2nd ed. New York: Wiley; 1988.

Panzarine S. Coping: conceptual and methodological issues. *Adv Nurs Sci.* 1985; 7:49–57.

Pollock SE. Adaptive responses to diabetes mellitus. *West J Nurs Res.* 1989; 11:265–280.

Porth CM. *Pathophysiology: Concepts of Altered Health States.* 2nd ed. Philadelphia: Lippincott; 1986.

Roy C. *Introduction to Nursing: An Adaptation Model.* 2nd ed. Englewood Cliffs, NJ: Prentice-Hall; 1984.

Scott DW, Oberst MT, Dropkin MJ. A stress-coping model. *Adv Nurs Sci.* 1980; 3:9–22.

Smith MJ. Human-environment process: A test of Rogers' principle of integrality. *Adv Nurs Sci.* 1986; 9:21–28.

Szasz TS, Hollender MH. A contribution to the philosophy of medicine. *Arch Int Med.* 1956; 97:585–592.

Thomas SA, Friedman E. Type A behavior and cardiovascular responses during verbalization in cardiac patients. *Nurs Res.* 1990; 39:48–53.

Toffler A. *The Third Wave.* New York: Morrow; 1980.

Watson J. *Nursing: Human Science and Human Care.* New York: National League for Nursing; 1988.

Wegman JA. Measuring coping. In: Frank-Stromborg M, ed. *Instruments for Clinical Nursing Research.* Norwalk, CT: Appleton & Lange; 1988.

Zaltman G, Duncan R. *Strategies for Planned Change.* New York: Wiley; 1977.

Ziemer MM. Coping behavior: A response to stress. *Top Clin Nurs.* 1982; 4:4–12.

CHAPTER 7

Community Health

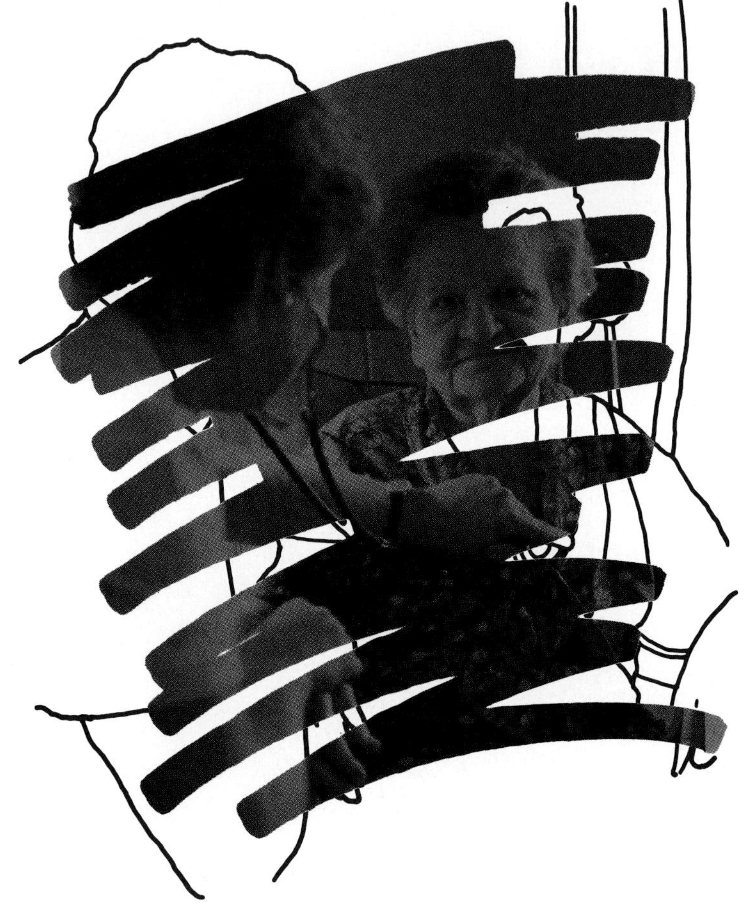

Behavioral Objectives

Upon completion of this chapter, the student will be able to:

1. Define the term "community" and identify several characteristics of a community.
2. Define the term "community health."
3. Distinguish among primary, secondary, and tertiary prevention.
4. List the members of the community health team.
5. Describe the components of the epidemiological triad.
6. List the steps of the epidemiological method.
7. Differentiate between mortality and morbidity, and between incidence and prevalence of disease.
8. Describe the chain of infection and state several ways that it can be broken.
9. Describe factors influencing the development of chronic diseases.
10. Discuss control strategies for communicable and chronic diseases and other community health problems.
11. State the importance of the concept of the community as client and describe the nurse's role in addressing the health needs of the community.
12. Discuss the role of the community health nurse as collaborator in community health nursing.

KEY TERMS

acquired immunity
active immunity
agent
carrier
chain of infection
clinical stage
communicable disease
community
community health
community health nursing
direct transmission
discharge planning
epidemiological triad
epidemiology
health education
health promotion
host
immunity
immunization
incidence
indirect transmission
infectivity
morbidity rate
mortality rate
multiple causation
natural immunity
passive immunity
pathogenicity
portal of entry
portal of exit
preclinical stage
preexposure stage
prevalence
primary prevention
rate
reservoir
resolution stage
risk
risk factor
screening
secondary prevention
target group
tertiary prevention
vaccine
vector
vehicle
virulence

Human beings are communal by nature. They live and work in communities, and provide for their common good by helping one another. General systems theory, the science of wholes, provides a way to understand this interdependence. General systems theory simply says that units or systems at all levels in nature—physical, biological, environmental—are organized and linked in a functional way.[1,2] This idea helps us understand that the needs of people who comprise a community are inevitably tied together and tied to the community itself, in health and illness as in other aspects of life. The health of one group of people affects the health of other groups: the health of individuals is linked to the health of the groups they are part of, whatever their nature. Moreover, to improve the health of people in the community, it is necessary to first address the needs and patterns of the community as a whole. This is the essence of a community perspective on health.

A community perspective on health is important because it permits a more complete understanding of health and how it is achieved and maintained. With a community perspective, broad categories rather than narrow classes of factors are considered in the search for explanations of health and illness. As the individual, social, and environmental aspects of health are understood, new and more effective approaches to health promotion and disease prevention become available. A community perspective is also important because it encourages better use of resources for health care. Health practices and procedures can be aimed at groups with common problems, thus increasing overall efficiency.

The changing environment of health care makes it urgent for nurses in all settings to grasp the application of a community perspective to nursing practice. Population growth and diversity, dwindling resources, and health care cost inflation place pressures on nurses to maximize their own efficiency and effectiveness. Sharing a community perspective on health, as they collaborate with other health care professionals and with those they serve, can help.

This chapter discusses health from a community perspective. It explores the concepts of community and community health and depicts the organization of health care in the community. It also describes the health problems prevalent in the community and the concepts necessary to understand them. Finally, the practice of nursing in the community and its roles and emphasis are discussed.

■ COMMUNITY AND COMMUNITY HEALTH

Community

A community is *not* just a geographic location with precisely stated boundaries, although this is one meaning of the term. A **community** is *any* group of people who have common problems or interests and who work together to solve those problems. By this definition, Los Angeles and New York City are "communities," but so is an ethnic group or a suburban neighborhood or the homeless population in either of these cities. By the same definition, nurses, as a professional group, form a community. In all of these instances, the groups designated as communities are bound by common interests and needs and by collective action to meet those needs.

Subgroups as Communities. Within larger population groups or communities, there may be smaller aggregates, or subgroups, that can also be considered communities. For example, within the homeless population of a city there are often subgroups made up of families that are homeless, elderly persons who are homeless, teenage runaways, or mentally ill people who are homeless. These subgroups have somewhat different health care needs, and any of them can also be the subject of health care programs.

The Hospital as a Community. A hospital might also be considered a community, because it consists of a group of people who are bound by their presence within the institution and their concern with illness and who take collective action with respect to that concern. Both hospital staff and clients are members of the community for as long as they remain within the community system. The interaction that takes place between members of the community is focused on achievement of the community's primary function, that of restoring client health as far as possible. Members of the community work together to foster achievement of this purpose. For instance, housekeeping staff abide by principles that reduce the potential for hospital-induced infection, while dietary personnel work to improve client health status through adequate nutrition.

Within the hospital community, there are subgroups that may have unique health needs. For example, housekeeping and nursing staff need protection from communicable diseases. Maintenance staff, as well as nurses, need to be protected from injuries due to heavy lifting, while clerical staff may have increased health risks related to the noise of printers or the glare of computer monitors. Hospital clients require physical care and planning to meet their needs when they are discharged from the hospital.

Community Health

How do we define "community health?" The most obvious answer is that the health of the community is the equivalent of the health of the community or group members. As is frequently the case, however, the obvious answer is not the correct one. It is possible for individual members of a community to be ill and for the community itself to be healthy. Conversely, it is possible to have healthy community members and an unhealthy community. For example, a town that is slowly dying out because young people are moving away is not a healthy community, whatever the health status of the people remaining there. Similarly, an industry plagued with safety hazards is not a healthy community.

Community health, then, is a composite of the health status of individuals, families, and groups within the population and the ability of the group to carry out certain necessary functions. These functions include the production and distribution of goods and services, member socialization, social control, provision of opportunity for member participation in community activities, and provision of support. Population groups that have inequities in the distribution of goods and services, or that cannot adequately socialize new members, or keep the behavior of members within acceptable limits, have a poorer state of health than those that more adequately fulfill these functions. Likewise, a community that denies participation to one or more segments of the population or cannot provide the support necessary to ensure members' survival is not a particularly healthy community.

■ COMMUNITY HEALTH AND THE HEALTH CARE SYSTEM

Community Health or Public Health?

Some people use the term "community health" to refer to health care services provided outside of an institutional setting such as a hospital or nursing home. This is *not* how the term is used by community health professionals. Community health refers to the overall health status of a group of people as a unit, and particularly to the health of the general public. Thus, the term can be applied to a community or to one of its subgroups. Because the term "community health" is used to mean the health of the public as a whole, the older term "public health" is considered synonymous. However, "public health" is used less frequently than "community health" because, for some people, it has connotations of an association with official government health agencies or the care of the indigent who cannot afford "private" health care. Again, this is *not* how the term "public health" is used in this chapter. Rather, public health conveys a concern for the health of the general public or populace, rich or poor, well or ill. In this chapter, the terms "public health" and "community health" are used interchangeably. Community health or public health practice, moreover, takes place in a variety of settings, including homes, clinics, physicians' offices, industry, prisons, schools—and even hospitals. The differentiating factor is not the setting, but the type of practice that takes place there, and a focus on the health of the group even while dealing with individual clients.

Components of the Health Care System

The health care delivery system is composed of two sectors: the acute care sector and the community health sector. The goal of both is the health of clients, but the two sectors differ in terms of emphasis and focus of care.

The Acute Care Sector. The acute care sector of the health care system refers to those health professionals in hospitals, clinics, and other settings who treat people who become ill. The primary emphasis of the acute care sector is on the cure of disease and the restoration of health. For example, a physician or nurse practitioner might give antibiotics to cure a child's ear infection or a teenager's gonorrhea. The focus of care in the acute care sector is on the individual. Services are provided primarily to individuals, although assistance may be given to family members as part of an overall effort to restore the individual's health. For example, the physician might have to deal with a mother's anxiety before she can be helped to understand how to give the antibiotic for her child's ear infection.

The Community Health Sector. The community health sector refers to those health professionals whose focus is on keeping people from becoming ill, and who work in various settings—such as schools, homes, clinics of various types, and hospitals. The community health sector emphasizes health promotion and illness prevention rather than cure of illness. For instance, where the health care provider in the acute care sector treats an individual's gonorrhea with antibiotics, the community health provider develops educational programs to promote condom use to prevent gonorrhea in the community.

Community health involves efforts designed to keep people healthy and to enable them to achieve their full potential. This is not to say that community health does not deal with existing health problems, but that it deals with them at a group rather than an individual level.

The primary focus of care in the community health sector, then, is the health of the total population rather than the health of the individual. The community health sector may provide services to individuals and families, but does so because such services enhance the health of the overall group.

Priorities in Health Care

Health care activities in either the acute care or community health sectors may take place at several levels. These levels are termed "levels of prevention." Each level of prevention receives a different priority in the two sectors of the health care delivery system.

Levels of Prevention in the Community Health Sector. The goal of community health is to achieve the highest level of health possible within the population. A variety of activities are employed to achieve this goal. Such activities take place at three levels of prevention: primary prevention, secondary prevention, and tertiary prevention (Box 7–1). The levels are differentiated by the time at which intervention takes place.

Primary Prevention. **Primary prevention** takes place before a health problem occurs and is aimed at preventing its occurrence. It has two major thrusts. The first thrust is **health promotion,** which refers to general strategies to maintain or enhance health. The second thrust is the prevention of specific diseases.

Health Promotion. Health promotion strategies fall into five categories: education for a healthier life, health appraisal, life-style modification, providing a healthy environment, and developing coping strategies. The process of **health education** provides people with the knowledge and skills needed to make informed health care decisions. These decisions may be related to self-care and personal health habits; the use of health resources such as insurance, entitlements, and benefits; choice of a source of health care; and decisions about which facility or professional to go to, and whether or not to follow through with health recommendations. For example, clients may need information to decide where to seek care or whether or not to follow through with the recommendations of the professional provider.

Health appraisal is the evaluation of an individual's health status and the identification of factors that interfere with optimal health. Such evaluation is necessary before the third strategy, life-style modification, can be undertaken. Health appraisal assists clients to identify personal

BOX 7–1. LEVELS OF PREVENTION

Primary Prevention

- Health promotion: health education, health appraisal, promoting life-style modification, maintaining a healthy environment, and fostering development of positive coping skills.
- Disease prevention: immunization, using protective devices, fostering modification of contributing factors in risk population, and eliminating environmental hazards.

Secondary Prevention

- Screening for health problems.
- Diagnosis of health problems.
- Treatment of health problems.

Tertiary Prevention

- Assisting with adaptation to residual consequences.
- Preventing recurrence.
- Preventing complications.

behaviors that are undermining health, hopefully resulting in adoption of a healthier life-style. Life-style modification involves changes in one's personal behaviors to replace those that undermine those that promote or enhance health.

Provision of a healthy environment, an environment that is as free as possible from hazards, is important to the promotion of health. It necessitates a concern for the quality of individuals' personal environments as well as the quality of the overall environment. For instance, use of seat belts and other safety devices contributes to a safe personal environment, while attention to environmental pollution contributes to a safe environment for all.

Attention must not be limited to the physical environment, however. Efforts may also be needed to provide a social environment conducive to health. For example, an environment that creates stress or encourages smoking, substance abuse, or unprotected sexual activity is not an environment conducive to health. Efforts to create a social environment that enhances health can also include planning and implementing programs to provide financial support or food supplements for the poor, advocacy to ensure health care for special groups, or support of social policies that have a positive effect on health. Such policies are important to promoting the health of the population.

The last strategy for health promotion is the development of positive coping skills. This should be a focus of health education at all levels, but particularly among school children. Effective coping abilities help people to live healthier lives and to avoid many stress-related health problems. Chapters 6 and 22 deal with coping strategies in greater detail.

Disease Prevention. Disease prevention is the second aspect of primary prevention. Again, there are a variety of strategies that can be used to prevent problems. A major strategy in this area is **immunization,** the process of protecting people from infectious disease by inoculating them with immunity-producing vaccines (Fig. 7–1). Polio vaccine and diphtheria vaccine are examples.

The use of protective devices is another approach to disease prevention. Protective devices are devices that reduce the likelihood of injury. For example, employees in noise-polluted plants might use ear plugs in high-noise areas to prevent noise-related stress and the hearing loss that certain kinds of noise can cause.

Elimination or modification of the factors that contribute to specific health problems is also a preventive strategy. Contributing factors are factors that enhance the chance of illness. For example, obesity and high blood pressure are known to contribute to the development of heart disease. Thus the elimination of contributing factors in heart disease might involve programs for weight reduction or control of high blood pressure, among adults, as well as programs for educating children and adults about the relationship between diet and heart disease.

The last major strategy for preventing disease is the elimination of environmental hazards, conditions in the environment that contribute to illness or injury. Cleaning up radioactive waste sites is one example of a strategy to eliminate environmental hazards. Other examples are the rebuilding of water and sewer systems in cities that have aging infrastructures, or the redesign of old highways to prevent motor vehicle accidents.

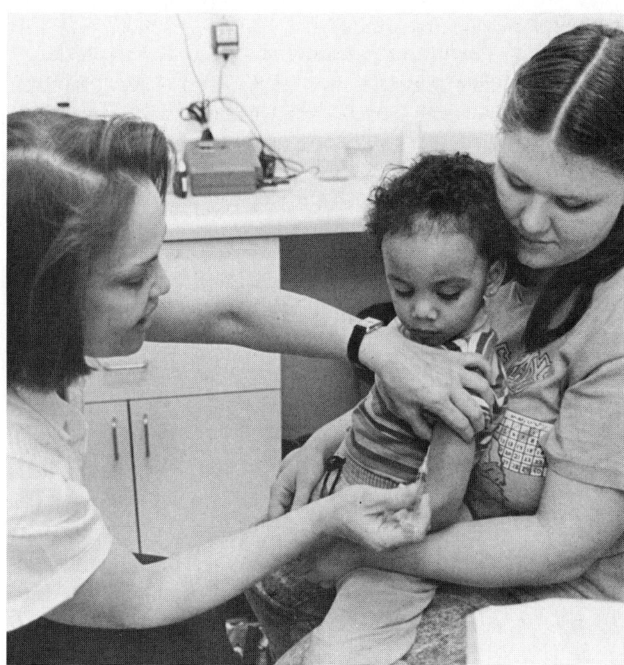

Figure 7–1. Immunization is a major strategy in disease prevention. (*Source: Clark MJ.* Nursing in the Community. *Norwalk, CT: Appleton & Lange; 1992.*)

Secondary Prevention. **Secondary prevention** takes place after a problem has occurred. It involves the recognition and resolution of existing health problems. This contrasts with primary prevention, which is aimed at preventing the occurrence of problems in the first place. Secondary prevention activities include screening, diagnosis, and treatment for specific diseases.

Screening is particularly important. It involves the examination of subgroups in the population for specific illnesses. For example, Pap smears are used to screen women for possible cancer of the cervix. Women with abnormal Pap smears can then be tested further to detect if cancer of the cervix exists, and if so, treatment for the condition can be rendered. The Pap smear and other diagnostic tests and treatment for cancer are all secondary preventive measures to control the problem of cancer of the cervix in women.

Tertiary Prevention. Tertiary prevention is carried out after the acute phase of the problem has been resolved through secondary preventive measures. In **tertiary prevention,** activities are designed to assist clients to deal with residual consequences of a health problem or to prevent its recurrence. If the problem is one that can be cured, the emphasis in tertiary prevention is on preventing recurrence. For example, once gonorrhea, a sexually transmitted disease, has been cured with antibiotics (a secondary preventive measure), attention would shift to focus on the client's habits and knowledge to prevent the person from getting the disease again.

When the health problem cannot be cured, but can be controlled or stabilized, tertiary prevention is geared to help people adjust to the disease and prevent further complications. For example, secondary preventive measures cannot cure arthritis, but can help to control the pain. Tertiary prevention measures for arthritis would focus on helping a person to live with the disease and meet the demands of daily living while preventing further immobilization of the joints affected.

Preventing the occurrence of a problem, or primary prevention, is most desirable. However, primary prevention is not possible for some problems or may not be employed soon enough to prevent a problem from occurring. In such cases, secondary and tertiary preventive activities are necessary and appropriate.

The Community Health Care Team

Community health services are planned and provided by a number of different persons who comprise the community health care team. This team consists of health care professionals and professionals outside of health care.

Health Care Professionals. Traditionally, health care professionals included physicians, dentists, community health nurses, nutritionists or dieticians, sanitarians, statisticians, administrators, social workers, and veterinarians. More recently, health educators and nurse practitioners have been added to the team.

Each of these people engages in activities related to his or her area of expertise. Physicians and nurse practitioners deal with human health problems, while community health veterinarians are concerned with animal health problems that may endanger human health. Similarly, community health dentists are concerned with preventing and treating dental problems in the population. Sanitarians or health inspectors are responsible for ensuring safe food and water supplies, and may engage in such activities as inspection of restaurants or food-processing plants, testing water supplies, and eliminating insects or animals that cause disease.

Social workers deal with clients' social problems such as housing and financial problems, and often make referrals for services to resolve such problems. Psychiatric social workers may also engage in counseling. Dieticians and nutritionists are concerned with meeting the dietary needs of groups of people and may do individual diet counseling, menu planning for school lunch or senior citizens' lunch programs, and public education regarding nutrition. Statisticians collect data and interpret health trends in the population, while administrators and clerical staff aid in the smooth operation of community health services. Health educators provide educational programs related to health and illness, and community health nurses engage in a variety of roles to be discussed later in this chapter.

Professionals Outside of Health Care. In addition to their individual functions related to expertise, the health care professionals on the team also provide consultation to each other and collaborate in efforts to resolve health problems in the population. This collaboration in planning to meet group health needs is also the function of the other members of the team who are not health care professionals. While the health care professionals on a team remain relatively constant, the other members may change depending upon the nature of problems to be solved. For example, if the problem is one of widespread drug use, law enforcement officials and substance abuse counselors are part of the team. If the problem involves school-age children, school officials and teachers may be involved. Individual clients, who are consumers of community health services and members of the population subgroup affected by the problem, are also important members of the team.

Organization for Health Care Delivery. Health care delivery in the community health sector is organized into two components, official and voluntary. The official component consists of government agencies, those agencies that have primary responsibility for health at the national, state, and local levels. At the national level, the major health-related agency is the United States Department of Health and Human Services. At the state level, all states have some form of state health department that oversees state efforts to promote and protect the health of its citizens. The local health department serves the same purpose for the local jurisdiction, which may be a county, parish, or city health department. These official agencies make and implement health policies related to the health of the general public. They may also offer direct services to clients. Official agencies are supported by tax revenues.

The other component of the community health sector includes a variety of voluntary agencies, nongovernmental agencies that assist official agencies in promoting the health of the public. Examples of such agencies are the American Red Cross, the American Heart Association, and the American Diabetes Association. These and other similar agencies engage in activities that may be beyond the capabilities of official agencies, usually because of budgetary constraints. Voluntary agencies usually focus on one aspect of health or one disease entity. For example, the American Diabetes Association focuses on the prevention and treatment of diabetes and engages in research and public education related to this disease. Voluntary agencies are supported by donations and provide a valuable adjunct to the activities of official agencies.

■ EPIDEMIOLOGY

Epidemiology is one of the tools used by community health professionals to identify and solve the health problems of population groups. **Epidemiology** is the study of factors that affect the occurrence of disease. Epidemiology is used to identify causal relationships between health problems and the multitude of etiological factors that initiate them. The ultimate purpose is to prevent and control disease. Physicians, nurses, or other professionals who are educated in the principles of epidemiology may function as epidemiologists. In large hospitals, one important nursing position is that of infection control nurse, whose primary job is to apply epidemiological principles to control the spread of infection within the hospital.

The application of epidemiology is not limited to infectious disease, however, and in fact enhances the understanding of all types of illnesses. Epidemiological concepts are equally appropriate and helpful to aid an understanding of chronic illnesses, congenital illnesses, psychosomatic illnesses, and even illnesses that result from accidents and environmental hazards. By understanding the principles of epidemiology, health care professionals, including nurses in every setting, are able to take an intelligent approach to both disease prevention and health promotion.

The Epidemiological Triad

There are several models of epidemiology from which health professionals can choose; however, the classical model is especially useful to nurses. The classical model is known as the epidemiological triad. The **epidemiological triad** examines health problems in terms of three categories of contributing factors: agent factors, host factors, and environmental factors. The model implies that each component, agent, host, and environment must be analyzed and understood to comprehend and predict patterns of disease and to devise strategies for disease control. The epidemiological triad model is depicted in Figure 7–2.

Agent Factors. The **agent** is the cause of a health problem. It is the factor that *must* be present for a disease to develop. Commonly, the agent is a living organism or a substance of some kind that has an etiologic effect without which the disease will not develop. For example, the human immunodeficiency virus (HIV) is the agent for acquired immune deficiency syndrome (AIDS). Without the virus, the disease does not develop. Likewise, lead is the causative agent in lead poisoning; without exposure to lead, lead poisoning does not occur.

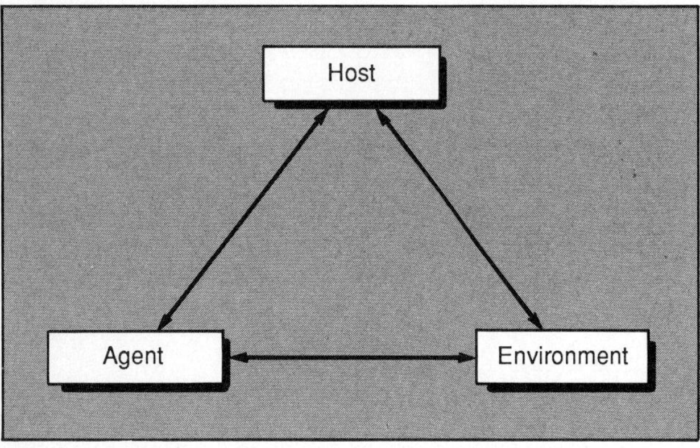

Figure 7–2. Epidemiological triad model.

Agents are of two general types, noninfectious and infectious. Noninfectious agents are often toxic but inanimate chemical substances, gases, dusts, liquids, and vapors that have a harmful effect on the body. Noninfectious agents can also be physical in nature. Temperature extremes, noise, and radiation are physical agents that cause or contribute to human disease.

Infectious agents, on the other hand, are living organisms that invade other living species to cause disease. Infectious agents live and multiply at the expense of the species they invade. Infectious agents are of various types; parasites, bacteria, and viruses are general categories of infectious organisms that produce disease in humans.

Agents do not exist separate from the environment and, in fact, are an important part of the environment. For agents to cause disease, there must be a source of the agent and a sufficient quantity of the agent present in the environment. Living agents in particular require a habitat, places where they can live and multiply for their perpetuation; such places are called **reservoirs.**

Host Factors. The **host** is the person or group of people upon whom the agent acts and who, as a result, develops a health problem or contracts a specific disease. Individuals vary in their vulnerability and resistance to particular agents. Characteristics that are important in determining whether illness develops include intrinsic factors such as age, sex, and race; socioeconomic factors; and general health.

Age, overall, is one of the most important determinants among the personal variables and is an important factor in disease and death rates within the population at large.[3] Age is related not only to the frequency but to the severity of illness; the very young and the very old are the most vulnerable to disease among the population subgroups.

Sex, race, and various social characteristics are also important determinants. Disease and death rates for various types of illness vary by gender throughout the life cycle.[4] These differences may be related to sex-linked inheritance, hormonal differences, or social and personal habit patterns. Whatever the explanation, the vulnerability of individuals to disease is considerably affected by their sex. Ethnicity also plays a role in the vulnerability of individuals to health problems.[5,6] A portion of this influence is explained by genetic variations that contribute to the development of certain diseases, but cultural differences also coexist and contribute. Socioeconomic characteristics such as occupation, income, and marital status are factors in disease, because they relate to individuals' life-style, ability to provide for self-care, and access to medical assistance. Socioeconomic characteristics also influence the individual's pattern of exposure to disease. For example, unmarried individuals—whether single, separated, divorced, or widowed—statistically are more susceptible to illness and death because of life-style factors that are common to the single population.[4]

Environmental Factors. The environment is important because it provides conditions that affect agent and host either beneficially or adversely, altering their respective capacities to cause or resist disease. The environment is also important because it can bring the agent and host together or keep them apart. The interaction of agent and host is a necessary condition to the development of any disease or health problem. This principle provides the rationale for many important strategies of disease control. Although the interaction of agent and host may be necessary, it is often an insufficient condition for disease to result. Features of the environment either suitable to the agent or harmful to the host may be required as supporting conditions.

The environment can be conceptualized as having three distinct aspects: the physical environment, the biological environment, and the social environment.

The Physical Environment. The physical environment includes meteorological and geophysical features such as climate, terrain, atmospheric conditions, and chemical and physical agents of all kinds. Characteristics of the physical environment contribute to a variety of environmental hazards. For example, the presence of a river may result in a high incidence of drowning.

The Biological Environment. The biological environment consists of living organisms that contribute to the development of disease in man and animals. This sector of the environment includes (1) the infectious agents of disease; (2) the reservoirs of infection (such as other humans, animals, or soil); (3) factors that act as the transmitters of disease (flies, mosquitos); and (4) plants and animals that serve as sources of drugs that deter the development of disease.

The Social Environment. The social environment refers to the overall economic and political organization of a society and the institutions within it. Social organization is important because it affects the quality and availability of health care in a society. For example, public funding for biomedical research and health care programs is an outgrowth of the public policy created by government entities. Moreover, government regulations and enforcement procedures control public behavior and create health standards. These are all important aspects of the social environment that relate to health.

The social environment also includes the family and the surrounding culture, which influences family life and family health practices. Social norms and customs affect health. For example, the foods people eat and the cooking practices they follow may determine whether a family is exposed to various disease-producing microorganisms.

The development of technology is also an important factor in the social environment. Technology sometimes operates to influence social attitudes and customs that in turn affect health. For example, with the development, distribution and use of contraceptives in the 20th century, reproductive freedom became a social reality, particularly for women.[7] However, along with the expansion of social options created by technological change came the risk of sexually transmitted disease. This same dilemma is now faced by people in other societies as the availability of contraceptives increases in developing countries.[8]

BUILDING NURSING KNOWLEDGE

Is Housing Important to Assess?

Sargis NM, Jennrich JA, & Murray KM. Housing Conditions and Health: A Crucial Link. *Nurse Health Care.* 1987: 335–338.

These authors stress that community health nurses have traditions of acknowledging the importance of living conditions to the quality of individuals' lives. They argue that while community health nurses have paid attention to the importance of the home when they plan care, hospital-based nurses generally have not considered the habitats from which clients come and to which they return as a factor in health.

However, the trend to earlier hospital discharge has made it imperative for nurses in the hospital to begin planning for a client's discharge on the day of admission. Home care may include the presence of highly technical equipment such as respirators, intravenous, and dialysis equipment.

Knowledge of home assessment is therefore essential. The investigators designed a study to poll nursing faculty about what home assessment should entail. They asked faculty to identify key variables. Subjects identified sanitation, safety, mobility, temperature, and space as the major housing variables that affect clients' abilities to maintain health and prevent illness.

The investigators emphasize that hospital-based nurses are in a good position to make the important housing assessments by talking with clients and families. They can gather information on clients' socioeconomic level, ethnic group, density of social network, safety, and resources available to them. The authors recommend that nurses ask questions about type of dwelling, number of floors, cooking facilities, refrigeration, plumbing, electrical, waste disposal, laundry facilities, access, heating, cooling, alarm and safety systems.

The Epidemiological Triad and Disease Prevention and Control. The essence of the epidemiological triad is that the development of disease almost never depends on a single isolated cause. Rather, disease results from chains of causation in which necessary and supporting conditions interact to form critical links. The reality that more than one factor is usually required for a disease to develop is referred to as the **multiple causation** of illness. Acceptance of this multifactorial view of the etiology of health problems is consistent with an ecological approach to understanding health and illness. The ecological approach, like general systems theory, stresses the complexities of the interdependence of living beings with each other and with the environment.[9]

Information about the relationships among agent, host, and environment is extremely useful for the development of strategies to control health problems. Once health care professionals understand how agent, host, and environment link to produce or prevent a particular disease, control measures can be aimed specifically at those relationships. For example, the malaria parasite is spread from human to human by the *Anopheles* mosquito. A mosquito bites an individual who has malaria, drawing infected blood into its stomach; organisms concentrate in the mosquito's salivary glands and are injected into the next individual the mosquito bites. With this information, control strategies have been developed that focus on the mosquito rather than the parasite.[10] Marshes are drained to eliminate mosquito breeding grounds. Insecticides are employed on a large scale to reduce or eradicate the mosquito population. When outbreaks of malaria occur, the public is warned to avoid contact with mosquitos by staying inside at night or by using insect repellents when going out. In these selective ways the balance of forces that favors health and deters the spread of malaria is supported.

The Epidemiological Method

Epidemiology is a systematic approach to identify and solve community health problems. This approach, also known as the epidemiological method, consists of the seven steps listed in Box 7–2. By applying this method, community health professionals are able to analyze the health problems that confront a community.

BOX 7–2. STEPS OF THE EPIDEMIOLOGICAL METHOD

1. Defining the problem under study.
2. Determining the natural history of the problem.
3. Determining the extent of the problem.
4. Planning a control strategy.
5. Implementing the control strategy.
6. Evaluating the effectiveness of control strategies.
7. Performing research.

Defining the Problem. The first step of the epidemiological method is to define the health problem and specify its size, scope, and parameters. Defining parameters of the problem aids health care professionals in determining the type of information needed and potential sources for that information. For example, communicable diseases are a frequent community health problem. Data may be obtained from the Centers for Disease Control (CDC), the national agency that collects such data. This national data may be used to compare with community statistics, and a determination can be made about the relative seriousness of the community's problem.

Determining the Natural History. Diseases generally develop over a period of time. While they develop, they often go through a predictable cycle or a typical sequence of stages. This sequence is created by the interaction of the agent, host, and environment and is referred to as the natural history of the disease or health problem.

Information about the natural history of a health problem provides direction for developing the strategies needed to prevent or control the illness. For example, with the problem of teenage pregnancy, understanding the factors involved may help a community to develop sex education or birth control programs specifically focused on the high-risk teenage population.

Stages of Illness. The natural history of an illness can be divided into four stages: (1) the preexposure stage, (2) the preclinical stage, (3) the clinical stage, and (4) the resolution stage (Fig. 7–3).

The Preexposure Stage. The **preexposure stage** encompasses those factors that exist prior to an individual's or group's exposure to a health problem. For example, an expanding number of unimmunized individuals in a community increases the potential for an outbreak of a communicable disease such as measles or diphtheria. On the other hand, getting immunized may prevent an individual from contracting a communicable disease.

The Preclinical Stage. The **preclinical stage** is the period of time from exposure to the agent to the manifestation of the disease itself. The preclinical period for communicable diseases is the incubation period. The amount of time that incubation takes varies with the microorganism. The incubation period is important in the natural history of a communicable disease because some infections are highly contagious during this period and can be unknowingly transmitted to others.

Factors in the preclinical stage may support, slow, or prevent the development of a health problem. If an individual is careful to get adequate rest and nourishment after exposure to an infection, natural immunity may be sufficient to prevent the illness or reduce its severity.

The Clinical Stage. In the **clinical stage,** the signs and symptoms of the health problem begin to appear. Individuals who have an infectious illness develop whatever signs and symptoms are typical of the disease.

Factors occurring in the clinical stage may influence the outcome of the illness. Proper self-care or nursing care can prevent or minimize the complications of communicable disease.

The Resolution Stage. The **resolution stage** is the stage in which the health problem has reached an outcome. The resolution of a communicable disease is signaled by the abatement of all of the signs and symptoms that appeared in the clinical stage. In some cases, complications produce permanent sequelae. These are the ongoing problems or disabilities that are sometimes part of the aftermath of disease.

Determining the Extent of the Problem. Determining the extent of a problem is important because it indicates how

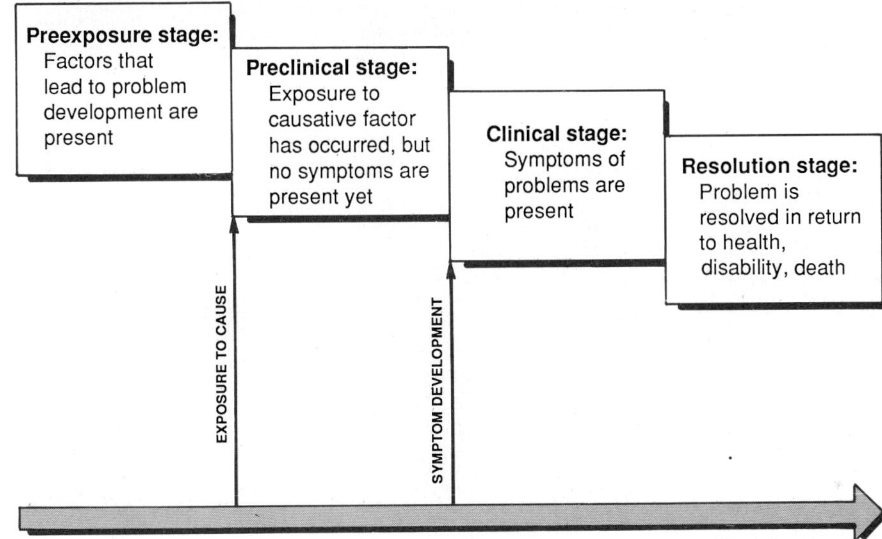
Preexposure stage:
Factors that lead to problem development are present
Preclinical stage:
Exposure to causative factor has occurred, but no symptoms are present yet
Clinical stage:
Symptoms of problems are present
Resolution stage:
Problem is resolved in return to health, disability, death
EXPOSURE TO CAUSE
SYMPTOM DEVELOPMENT

Figure 7–3. Stages of the natural history of disease.

much effort should be made to control the problem. Determining the extent of the problem involves four specific considerations: the proportion of the population affected, the severity of the problem, geographic distribution, and time relationships and trends.

Proportion of the Population Affected. The proportion of the population affected by a particular health problem is determined from records of the number of occurrences of the problem identified in the population. Such figures may be compiled by local agencies or may need to be gathered by community health professionals themselves. A problem that affects a large segment of the population is usually of greater concern than one that affects only a few.

Severity of the Problem. The second consideration in the extent of the problem is the severity of its effects for individuals and for the community. A problem with serious consequences, such as HIV infection, or AIDS, which is usually fatal to the individuals who contract it, is of greater concern than a problem with relatively minimal consequences (eg, anemia). Some problems have particularly serious consequences for the community. For example, in addition to being a fatal disease, HIV infection has serious consequences for society in terms of costs of care for victims, the cost of research for prevention and cure, and the psychological costs in the terms of fear and anxiety.

Geographic Distribution. The geographic distribution of the problem is another aspect of its extent. Geographically isolated problems can be solved by local efforts, while national or global problems require collaborative efforts on the part of many agencies and individuals.

Time Relationships and Trends. Finally, one should consider time relationships and trends in the occurrence of a problem. If the problem occurs every 10 years, or its incidence has been declining steadily over several years, there is less need for concern about it than for a problem that occurs frequently or for which the incidence is rising dramatically. HIV infection is a good example of a problem of great concern because of the tremendous increase in the number of cases over the last few years. Knowledge of the extent of the health problem within the population allows the determination of priorities among problems, and priorities assist health care professionals to make decisions on the allocation of resources that can then be directed toward those problems with the greatest impact on the health of the community.

Planning a Control Strategy. The next step in the epidemiological method is planning a control strategy. This involves determining strategic points at which the problem can be prevented. Prevention involves the modification or elimination of contributing factors in the preexposure stage. If the problem cannot be prevented completely, it may be possible to reduce its severity by interventions in the preclinical or clinical stages. Knowledge of the natural history of a problem, number of people affected, geographic distribution, and any time relationships and trends involved helps target interventions to the people at greatest risk for the problem.

Implementing a Control Strategy. Once the strategic points at which intervention is possible have been identified, a control strategy can be planned and implemented. This may involve a variety of activities such as sanitation or immunization that are designed to change the natural history. For example, this might involve developing an educational program to acquaint people with measures to prevent HIV infection, and then putting that program into operation.

Evaluating the Control Strategy. Following implementation, interventions are evaluated in terms of their effectiveness. One indicator is whether or not the incidence of the problem has decreased as a result of the control strategy. A classical example of the effectiveness of a control program is the virtual eradication of smallpox that followed worldwide immunization.

Performing Research. While research is the last step in the list in Figure 7–3, it is not the last step performed. Research contributes to all of the other steps of the method. Research determines the criteria by which a particular problem is defined and contributes to knowledge of the natural history and scope of the problem. Control strategies may also be identified through research. Moreover, intervention plans and implementation programs are tested in research studies. Finally, research methods can be used to evaluate the effectiveness of control strategies.

Statistics in Epidemiology

Statistics are an important tool of the health care professions and they are especially useful in the study of community health. Statistics reveal the existence, and depict the extent and distribution, of community health problems, and thus comprise a substantial part of the data used within the context of the epidemiological method. Nurses in hospitals and communities find an understanding of health statistics useful in their roles as practitioners and users of health information. Four general types of statistics are particularly helpful: demographic statistics, vital statistics, health and disease statistics, and utilization statistics.

Demographic Statistics. Demographic statistics provide a numerical picture of a community, a picture that shows the various groups of people within the community and their size. Community residents have various important characteristics. The characteristics that health care professionals are most interested in are the number of people in a community; the age, sex, and occupational composition of the population; and the size of the ethnic and religious groups represented. Knowing about the characteristics of a population enables health care professionals to anticipate the needs of the various groups for type and quantity of health care services. For example, a population with a large number of elderly people will often create a greater demand for home nursing services, whereas a heavily industrialized area will require more occupational health services.

Vital Statistics. Vital statistics are statistics about the number of vital events in a community. Vital events are those that are officially recorded and registered, such a births, deaths, adoptions, marriages, divorces, legal separations, and annulments. Vital statistics also aid health care professionals to understand community needs and to determine requirements for specific services. For example, a high birth rate within a community might suggest a need for family planning services; it also suggests that the important health problems within the community will be those common to pregnant women and young children. From this information, it can be inferred that the community will require both prenatal and child health care services.

IMPLICATIONS FOR PROFESSIONAL COLLABORATION

Epidemiology and Health Statistics

Community health assessment is a responsibility of all the health care professionals that comprise the community health sector, and nurses are important contributors to the overall team effort. As participants in the assessment process, nurses in the community must be familiar with the tools needed to fulfill this responsibility, including a knowledge of the importance and use of the principles of epidemiology and health statistics. This knowledge enables nurses to identify health problems that are of a general significance in the population or groups nurses serve. In turn, nurses are able to use health statistics to provide a justification for special programs to address these needs and to influence collaborative efforts among fellow health care professionals and community officials to devote the necessary resources to correcting the identified problems.

Health and Disease Statistics. Health and disease statistics are of particular interest to health care professionals because they suggest the presence or absence of specific health problems in the population. Morbidity and mortality rates are two of the statistics used to assess the health status of communities (Box 7–3).

The **mortality rate** reflects the number of deaths in the population from a specific cause and is usually broken down by age. For example, a high rate of death due to suicide is a community problem. The fact that suicide rates are higher among teenagers suggests that interventions should be directed toward this age group.

The **morbidity rate** reflects the number of people in the population who are ill with certain diseases or have other health problems. Two specific morbidity statistics are important, incidence rates and prevalence rates. **Incidence** is the number of new cases of a specific health problem that have occurred in the population in a given time period; **prevalence** reflects the total number of people affected by a particular problem at any point in time. For example, 20 new cases of tuberculosis may have been identified in the community during the previous year. This is the annual incidence of tuberculosis. However, the current total of 75 people in the community who have tuberculosis is the prevalence of tuberculosis for the community.

Statistics are also a source of information on factors influencing the occurrence of a health problem. In examining the natural history of a problem, statistics may indicate relationships between various factors and the occurrence of a problem. For example, the statistical correlation between the prevalence of smoking and the incidence of lung cancer, consistently demonstrated in research studies, indicates that smoking is a causative factor in lung cancer. (Such statistical relationships do not, of themselves, prove a causal relationship and should be interpreted with caution.)

BOX 7–3. HEALTH AND DISEASE STATISTICS

Mortality Rate: Number of deaths in a population, broken down by age and cause of death.

Morbidity Rate: Number of people in a population group with a specific disease or health problem.

Incidence: New cases in population in a given time period.

Prevalence: Total number of people affected at a given time.

Statistics that suggest relationships between specific factors and certain health problems are important because they also suggest strategic points of control. In fact, the decline in smoking rates in the population has led to a reduction in mortality from both lung cancer and coronary artery disease, which is also linked to smoking.[11]

Utilization Statistics. Utilization statistics are statistics on the extent to which health care resources and services are used. They provide additional information on the health status of the population. Examples of such statistics are the percentage of women who receive prenatal care or the average number of days each resident stays in the hospital during the year. Utilization statistics indicate whether health care resources are underused or are sufficient or insufficient to meet the demand. If resources are underused, community members may need to be educated regarding their use, or perhaps the services are not needed. If they are not needed, resources can be redirected to meet other needs. Thus, efficiency is promoted by the use of utilization statistics. Such statistics indicate the areas of gaps and overlaps in existing health care services and where changes might be needed.

Calculation of Rates. Most statistics in epidemiology are reported in terms of rates that allow comparisons between groups of different sizes. **Rates** reflect the number of occurrences of a specific event per 1000 people in the population (or 100,000 if the event occurs rather infrequently). The general formula for the calculation of any rate is the number of occurrences of the event, divided by the number of people at risk for the event, times the population base of 1000 or 100,000. The annual rate of incidence for adolescent pregnancy would be calculated by dividing the number of teenage pregnancies occurring in a year by the number of teenage girls in the population (because they are all at risk for teenage pregnancy) and multiplying the result by 1000. This formula would be as follows:

$$\frac{\text{Number of pregnancies among teenage girls}}{\text{Number of teenage girls in the population}} \times 1000$$

If the number of teenage girls in the population is 5000 and 50 of them became pregnant last year, the calculation for the adolescent pregnancy rate would look like this:

$$\frac{\text{50 teenage pregnancies}}{\text{5000 teenage girls in the population}} \times 1000 = \text{10 per 1000 population}$$

In discussing this rate, one could say that "10 out of every 1000 teenage girls in the population became pregnant," or "the incidence rate for teenage pregnancy is 10 per 1000 population." Other rates are calculated with the same general formula.

HEALTH PROBLEMS IN THE COMMUNITY

There are several categories of health problems that are frequently encountered in community health practice. Communicable and chronic diseases, and mental health problems, are the most common categories. Other categories are accidents and environmental hazards.

Communicable Disease

A **communicable disease** is an infectious disease that spreads from person to person. As an outgrowth of population density, communities have conditions that favor the transmission of communicable disease. It is not surprising, then, that the control of communicable disease often requires community measures. Despite the considerable progress in prevention and treatment made in this century, communicable diseases unfortunately persist as a problem in community health. Nurses and other health care professionals are therefore rightly concerned about the control of communicable disease in the community.

Contributing Factors—The Chain of Infection. The epidemiology of infection gives attention to the agent, host, and environmental factors that contribute to the morbidity and mortality associated with communicable disease. Of particular interest are the complex causal relationships in communicable disease, collectively referred to as the **chain of infection.** The concept of the chain of infection implies that communicability rests on the connections between the factors that cause infection. These connections are similar to the links of a chain. Factors must link together for infection to result, and breaking the chain at any point diminishes the likelihood that disease will develop.

The chain of infection consists of six factors that influence the spread of infection: the infectious agent, reservoir, portal of exit, mode of transmission, portal of entry, and new host. These are summarized in Figure 7–4.

Infectious Agent. The first link in the chain is the infectious agent, a microorganism. Microorganisms have individual properties and characteristics that influence their ability to cause disease. Three characteristics—infectivity, pathogenicity, and virulence—are particularly important. However, the relationship of the agent to the environment is also an important factor.

Infectivity. **Infectivity** is the ability of a microorganism to gain entry into the host. Some agents can easily invade the

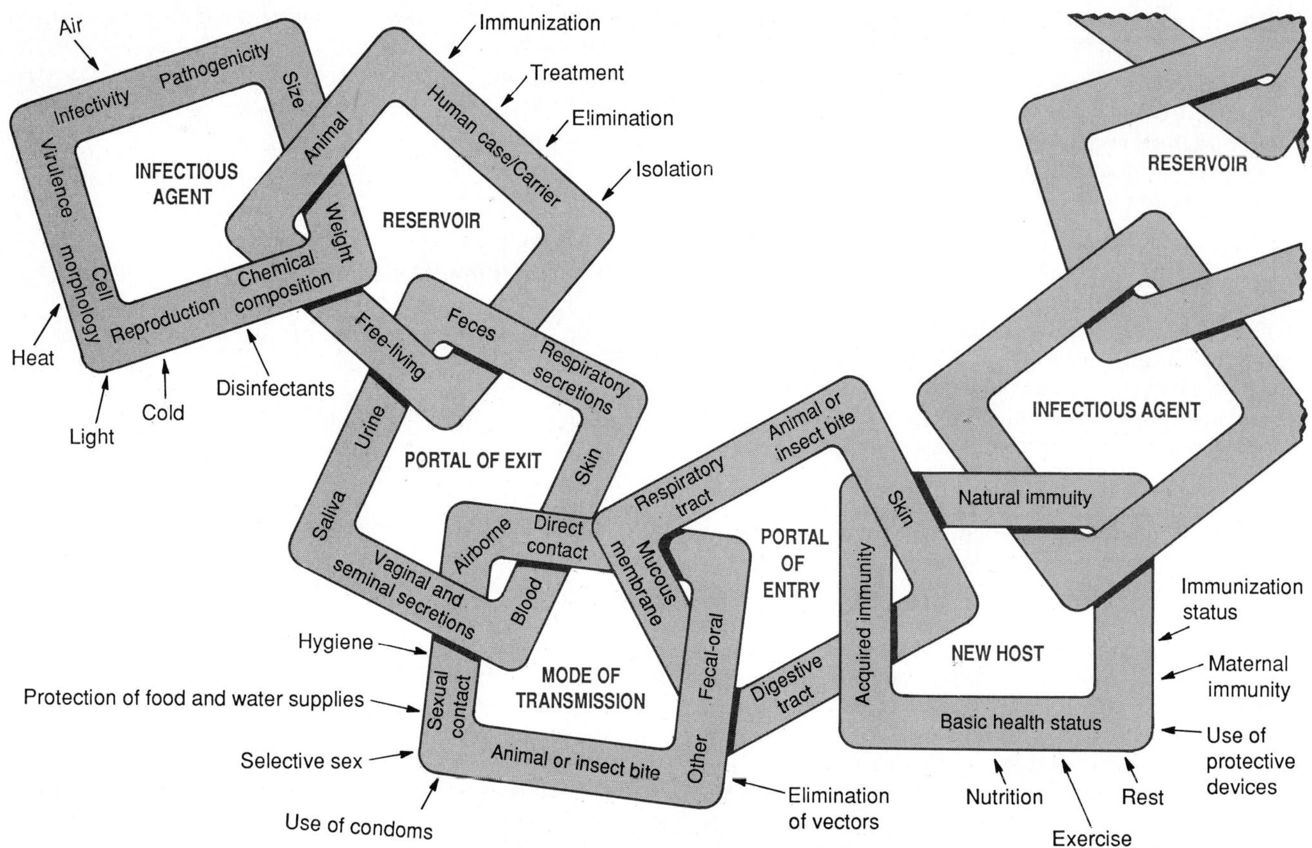

Figure 7–4. Chain of infection.

host and are highly infective, while others have a more difficult time gaining entry or are unable to do so without an artificial means of transmission. For example, polio viruses, which are airborne organisms, enter easily as the host inhales the surrounding air. The virus that causes HIV infection, however, is less infective. It requires contact with infected blood (often by transfusion or the reuse of contaminated hypodermic needles), or with infected seminal or vaginal secretions (through sexual intercourse) or other infected body fluids.

Pathogenicity. **Pathogenicity** is the ability of the agent to cause disease once it enters the host. Some agents, such as the measles virus, cause disease in virtually all susceptible individuals who are exposed. Other agents, such as the tuberculosis organism, have low pathogenicity and cause disease in only a few who are exposed.

Virulence. **Virulence** refers to the severity of disease caused by a microorganism. While the HIV virus does not have high infectivity, it is nevertheless extremely virulent and causes very severe and usually fatal disease. The virus that causes the common cold, on the other hand, has high infectivity but low virulence, and generally results in mild symptoms that abate after a week to 10 days.

Agent–Environment Relationship. Agents are affected by the conditions of the environment. Some microorganisms require highly select conditions for their growth and reproduction and are inhibited when those conditions are absent. Several, for example, require dark, moist environments and are easily killed by exposure to air and light; some, called anaerobes, grow best in an environment with little or no oxygen. In fact, agents can be killed or inactivated by a variety of physical conditions. Heat, cold, and a host of chemical substances may adversely affect agent growth and reproduction.

The Reservoir. The second link in the chain is the reservoir, animate or inanimate, where the microorganism is found. Human reservoirs are the most common sources of human pathogens. Human reservoirs fall into two categories, cases and carriers. Cases are those individuals who are obviously ill from an infectious disease. **Carriers** are those individuals who have been infected but have no symptoms, have infections that are mild enough to escape recognition, or have recovered from a disease but continue to harbor and shed the organism causing it.

Animal reservoirs also act as sources of human pathogens. For example, cows are the reservoir for bovine tuberculosis; dogs, bats, foxes, and other wild animals are the reservoirs for rabies. Diseases that are spread from animal reservoirs to human hosts are called zoonoses.

Portal of Exit. The third link in the chain of infection is the portal of exit from the reservoir. The **portal of exit** is the route by which the microorganism leaves the reservoir. Without a portal of exit, the chain of infection is broken. Human reservoirs offer a variety of portals of exit. Microorganisms leave the body with urine, feces, vomitus, drainage of intestinal fluids, respiratory secretions, vaginal and seminal secretions and discharges, blood, and wound drainage.

Respiratory Tract. Probably the most common portal of exit from the human reservoir is the respiratory tract, the passages from the nose and sinuses to the lungs. Many potentially infectious organisms live and grow in various parts of the respiratory tract. These are spewed into the environment from the nose and mouth with droplets of moisture as individuals exhale, sneeze, cough, or talk. Although the respiratory passages are normally moist, in the presence of infection the amount of moisture increases and large quantities of organism containing droplets may be expelled many feet from the body.

Gastrointestinal Tract. Another common portal of exit from the human reservoir is the intestinal tract. The principal means of escape from the intestinal tract is with the feces. The feces contain large amounts of bacteria, most varieties of which are nonpathogenic. However, the feces can also harbor the organisms for intestinal diseases which may or may not manifest themselves by the presence of diarrhea or other symptoms.

Material discharged from the intestinal tract often finds its way to new hosts. Disease from this source is diminished by hygiene practices and public health measures for sanitation and sewage disposal. These reduce the spread of infection from the intestinal tract by interfering with contact between agent and host. Public health measures are not uniform among all cultures and geographic areas, however, and in some regions intestinal organisms are a significant source of disease.

Urinary Tract. The urine can also provide a route of escape for infectious organisms. Urine, which is ordinarily sterile, is less likely than feces to carry pathogenic organisms. However, once the urinary tract becomes infected, the urine will carry the pathogens involved.

Reproductive Tract. Vaginal secretions from the female reproductive tract, and seminal secretions ejected from the male urethra, may carry a variety of microorganisms. These secretions can be important sources of pathogens for sexually transmitted diseases (STDs).

Integument and Wounds. Ordinarily, the intact skin offers an effective barrier to the spread of infection. However, interruption of skin integrity is common and the underlying tissues sometimes serve as a reservoir for pathogens. Open wounds allow the exit of these organisms. Wounds also provide a route of escape for blood, which can harbor microorganisms. Thus, it is not surprising that an important control strategy for communicable disease involves the careful discarding of bandages and dressings used to cover open wounds.

Mode of Transmission. Mode of transmission is the fourth link in the chain. The mode of transmission is the way in which the microorganism finds its way to a new host. It is a very important consideration in the control of communicable diseases.

Concepts of Transmission. There are two general methods for transmitting human infection: direct and indirect transmission. In **direct transmission,** also referred to as contact transmission, the infectious agent is transmitted immediately from the reservoir of the infected host to a new host without the intervention of intermediate objects.

In **indirect transmission,** the agent is transmitted via an intermediary, a physical or biological factor that enhances the transmission of an agent. The intermediary does not have the disease, but serves to spread it from one host to another.

There are two general types of intermediaries, vectors and vehicles. **Vectors** are living intermediaries, usually arthropods, that mechanically transmit infectious agents. In vector-borne transmission, the infectious agent is carried by a fly, for example, that soils its feet on feces or other filth, and then conveys the pathogens it contacts to a new host.

Vehicles, on the other hand, are nonliving intermediaries. Vehicles include bedding, toys, surgical instruments, contaminated food, water, hypodermic needles, and a variety of other items that serve as transmitters for microorganisms.

Transmission Modes. Along with these general concepts of transmission, there are six specific transmission modes that are particularly important for nurses to keep in mind. These are (1) airborne transmission, (2) fecal–oral transmission, (3) direct skin contact, (4) sexual transmission, (5) transmission by insect or animal bite, and (6) transmission by other means such as by injection into the bloodstream.

Airborne transmission occurs directly with the spewing of droplets, but also indirectly through dusts and droplet nuclei. Droplet nuclei are tiny particles that are the residue of evaporated droplets. They remain suspended in the air for long periods. Measles, rubella, chickenpox, tuberculosis, influenza, and polio are all serious diseases that are spread by airborne transmission. Because the control of airborne transmission is difficult, an important strategy for preventing airborne illnesses is to enhance host immunity, discussed below.

Hepatitis A, typhoid, and many intestinal diseases are spread by fecal–oral transmission. Pathogens from the feces reach the mouths of new hosts by a variety of means, either directly by person-to-person contact or indirectly by ingesting fecally contaminated food or water. Contamination occurs when cooking or eating utensils are used that harbor intestinal organisms. Pathogens are also spread directly by putting contaminated fingers into the mouth. Handwashing, therefore, is an important practice in the control of disease spread by fecal–oral transmission.

Other specific routes are implicated in other diseases. Impetigo is a very contagious disease of the skin that is spread by direct skin-to-skin contact. Syphilis, gonorrhea, and a variety of other sexually transmitted diseases are spread by direct sexual contact. Rabies, as already noted, is spread directly by animal bite. Blood transfusion can be responsible for the spread of bloodborne diseases such as hepatitis B and HIV infection. In all of these cases, understanding the mode of transmission suggests important measures of disease control, as summarized in Table 7–1.

Portal of Entry. The fifth link in the chain of infection is the portal of entry. The **portal of entry** is the route by which microorganisms gain access to the host. In humans, portals of entry are the same routes that serve as portals of exit. Blocking portals of entry is another way of protecting the host and breaking the chain of infection. For example, surgical masks protect by blocking the inhalation of pathogens.

TABLE 7–1. SPECIFIC CONTROL MEASURES FOR ROUTES OF DISEASE TRANSMISSION

Route of Transmission	Potential Control Measures	Typical Diseases
Airborne	Respiratory isolation, hygiene (eg, disposal of soiled tissues), special screening procedures (TB skin test), immunization as appropriate	Scarlet, fever, polio, tuberculosis, exanthemata, upper respiratory infection
Fecal–oral	Hygiene (eg, handwashing, disposal of feces), enteric isolation, gamma globulin for contacts to hepatitis	Hepatitis A, salmonellosis, shigellosis, typhoid
Direct contact	Wound and skin isolation, avoid sharing clothing, hats, etc	Impetigo, scabies, lice
Insect or animal bite	Eradication of vector, vaccination of domestic animals for rabies	Malaria, plague, rabies
Sexual contact	Selective sexual activity, screening of populations at risk, prophylactic treatment of contacts, use of condoms	Gonorrhea, syphilis, herpes genitalis, HIV infection, *Trichomonas*
Other	Use of protective clothing (eg, shoes for hookworm), immediate cleansing of wounds with soap and water Immunization for tetanus	Tetanus, hookworm

From Clark MJ. Nursing in the Community. *Norwalk, CT: Appleton & Lange; 1992.*

The New Host. A variety of host factors influence the development of communicable disease. A major factor is host resistance. Human hosts are more or less always in contact with sources and reservoirs of the agents of disease. Under ordinary circumstances, good general health is sufficient to protect an individual from the pathogens that gain entry. However, when general health is impaired, host resistance is weakened and individuals become vulnerable to the development of diseases.

Many preexisting conditions contribute to a deterioration of an individual's ability to resist disease. Poor nutritional status or stress, for example, interfere with resistance. The presence of other diseases also interferes with resistance. Even psychological states contribute to accidents, injury, and disease. Immunity is one of the most important host factors that affect host resistance. **Immunity** refers generally to protection against disease. Box 7–4 depicts the types of immunity. **Natural immunity** is the inherent resistance of the body to disease. It comprises all of the anatomical and physiological barriers. Natural immunity includes intact skin and mucous membranes; the acid pH of gastric juice, which inactivates many infectious agents; the presence of normal bacterial flora in the intestine, which impedes the growth of some pathogens; and a functioning immune system to produce the macrophages and nonspecific antibodies necessary to protect the body against a variety of invading organisms. Natural immunity is referred to as nonspecific because it operates against virtually any foreign substance.

Acquired immunity refers to the presence in the blood of specific antibodies for certain communicable diseases. These protective antibodies inactivate infectious agents on a highly selective basis and thus prevent the development of disease. Acquired immunity is referred to as active immunity when the body is involved in producing its own antibodies. **Active immunity** is developed by having an infectious disease that stimulates antibody production, by having a related disease that stimulates cross-immunity, or by immunization. With immunization, antigenic substances are deliberately introduced into the body to promote the development of antibodies. The antigenic substance, called a **vaccine,** may be a product secreted by a bacterium or it may be a biological preparation derived from the bacterium itself. Vaccines may be introduced into the body by an intramuscular injection or orally (for example, the polio vaccine). Because the body develops its own antibodies, active immunity is long standing, although booster doses of some vaccines are required periodically.

Acquired immunity is referred to as passive immunity when the body itself is not involved in producing the antibodies. In **passive immunity,** protective antibodies from another host are introduced into a susceptible person. The transfer of maternal antibodies from mother to fetus through the placenta is an example of passive immunity.

BOX 7–4. TYPES OF IMMUNITY

Natural: Normal body defenses.

Acquired: Production of disease-specific antibodies as a result of either having the disease or through immunization.

Active: Exposure to antigen in the environment or via vaccination results in production of antibodies by individuals.

Passive: Externally produced antibodies are given to susceptible individuals.

Antibody preparations from an external source can also be artificially instilled into the body to provide passive immunization. Immune serum globulin (ISG) is such a preparation. It may be used to provide immunity when unimmunized individuals are exposed to measles or hepatitis A. Once in the body, such antibodies are treated as other foreign substances and are destroyed fairly rapidly. Passive immunity is therefore of short duration and is used only when protection is necessary and time is insufficient to allow for the natural development of antibodies.

Control Strategies—Breaking the Chain of Infection. Control measures may be classified as primary, secondary, or tertiary prevention.

Primary Prevention. Strategies in the primary prevention of communicable disease may be directed at agent, reservoir, host, or environment.

Primary prevention directed at the agent makes use of knowledge about agent factors. One of the most important strategies is to treat cases of communicable disease whenever possible. Antibiotic therapy is commonly employed in infectious disease not only to cure the individual of illness, but also for the good of the rest of the community as a primary preventive measure to reduce the number of human reservoirs. Treating cases to eradicate the agent diminishes the likelihood that susceptible individuals will be exposed. In the hospital, moreover, a variety of agent-oriented measures are practiced that reflect an understanding of agent factors. For example, the procedure of heat-sterilizing surgical instruments acknowledges the susceptibility to infection of individuals undergoing surgery.

Host strategies are those that are aimed at individuals, families, and other groups that can benefit from various measures to promote good general health and fitness. Host strategies also include specific education in the various means people can use to avoid exposure to communicable disease or enhance their resistance to it. For example, teaching people about the importance of immunization is an important host strategy to prevent communicable disease. Nurses take an active role in applying control measures. Additionally, nurses are frequently called upon in clinical practice to educate clients about specific measures, including immunization, for keeping healthy and preventing disease.

Primary prevention also extends to the environment and underlies vital public health measures. A major aspect of primary prevention is environmental sanitation. Environmental sanitation seeks to prevent the spread of communicable disease by interrupting the transfer of infectious agents to potential new hosts or eradicating the reservoir. A variety of community measures make up an overall program of environmental sanitation. Sewage disposal, aside from its aesthetic value, is critical to prevent the transfer of contaminants into community water and food supplies. Water purification—including the sedimentation, filtration, and chlorination of water—helps to destroy the pathogens that do find their way into the water supply. Food sanitation—including cleanliness in food processing, refrigeration, and milk pasteurization—protects or rids the food supply from contamination. Pest control, which may involve the fumigation of buildings, is another measure. All of these strategies are ways in which communities break the chain of infection and prevent the spread of communicable disease.

Secondary Prevention. Screening and diagnosis are important so that treatment can be instituted early in the process of infectious disease. Ideally, treatment should commence in the preclinical stage, but this is often difficult because people usually do not seek medical attention until they reach the clinical stage. Treatment of infected people, particularly when begun early, often limits the length and severity of disease and reduces the likelihood of costly complications. Screening and diagnosis also serve the objective of primary prevention by enabling the early treatment of cases.

Tertiary Prevention. The tertiary prevention of communicable disease is directed toward preventing a recurrence of the problem. Often the strategies are host-oriented. For the person who has been treated for gonorrhea or syphilis, education on the use of condoms can help prevent reinfection. Tertiary measures may also be applied to the contact of those infected. Contacts are persons who have been exposed to a disease by their interaction with an infected person or who may have infected the person in the first place. Contact follow-up may be done in cases of sexually transmitted disease. Contact follow-up is the practice of asking infected individuals about their contacts and locating those individuals to inform them of the need for treatment. Contact follow-up reduces the potential for reexposure to a disease. It is also one of the reasons for the mandatory reporting of certain communicable diseases. Box 7–5 lists some of the reportable communicable diseases. Contact follow-up is part of the role of community health professionals and is an important way in which the chain of infection is broken. Primary, secondary, and tertiary prevention measures for communicable disease are summarized in Table 7–2. Table 7–3 presents the chain of infection, prevention, and treatment of several communicable diseases.

Trends in Communicable Disease. Patterns of disease change over time as the scientific understanding of health

BOX 7–5. REPORTABLE COMMUNICABLE DISEASES

Cholera	Rabies
Diphtheria	Rheumatic fever, acute
Food poisoning	Rocky Mountain spotted fever
Gonorrhea	Salmonella infections
Malaria	Scarlet fever
Measles	Smallpox
Meningitis, viral	Syphilis
Mumps	Tetanus
Newborn diarrhea	Tuberculosis
Pertussis	Typhoid fever (cases and carriers)
Poliomyelitis	

and illness advances and as controls are instituted to prevent the spread of disease. Among Western nations, a great deal of progress has been made in the 20th century in reducing the incidence of some communicable diseases. To a large extent, this is a result of improved public health conditions in the modern world. In general, better living conditions serve to decrease the opportunities for the spread of disease that occur when people live and work in close proximity to one another. Good housing, better nutrition, and improved sanitation are important aspects of a rising standard of living that have contributed to lowering the incidence of disease and fatalities from many kinds of communicable disease.

In addition to a rising standard of living, however, specific advances in the prevention and treatment of communicable disease also have made a substantial contribution. Changing patterns of morbidity and mortality in the population reflect the success of immunization and treatment programs for many diseases. For example, the incidence rates for measles, rubella, mumps, tetanus, pertussis, diphtheria, polio, and influenza have all dropped dramatically in correspondence to the widespread use of vaccines to prevent these illnesses.[12] Tuberculosis, once a rampant communicable disease, is now virtually unknown among many groups in the population, in part because of better living conditions but also because of the development and use of antitubercular drugs and because of a massive public health effort to find and treat individuals with the disease. Likewise, the discovery and use of penicillin decreased the morbidity of a variety of infectious illnesses including sexually transmitted diseases such as syphilis and gonorrhea.

Unfortunately, progress is not constant, and has not been uniform for all social groups. As a consequence, the incidence rates for some preventable communicable dis-

TABLE 7–2. PRIMARY, SECONDARY, AND TERTIARY CONTROL STRATEGIES FOR COMMUNICABLE DISEASES

Level of Prevention	Control Strategies	Applicable Diseases
Primary prevention	Immunization of groups at risk	Diphtheria, hepatitis B, influenza, measles, mumps, pertussis, pneumonia, poliomyelitis, rubella, tetanus, typhoid
	Immunization of contacts	Hepatitis A and B, rubella (for pregnant women), typhoid
	Prophylactic treatment of contacts	Scarlet fever, diphtheria, rabies, tuberculosis, syphilis, gonorrhea
	Use of condom and spermicide during intercourse Selective sexual activity	Sexually transmitted diseases including gonorrhea, syphilis, hepatitis B, HIV infection, herpes
	Use of disposable needles or careful sterilization after use Not sharing needles for drug use	HIV infection, hepatitis B
	Good handwashing after toileting Protection of food and water supplies Cooking food at adequate temperatures Adequate sanitation, waste removal, etc	Hepatitis A, typhoid, cholera
	Adequate nutrition and rest	Tuberculosis, influenza, childhood illnesses, penumonia
	Elimination of vectors	Malaria, hepatitis A
	Treatment or elimination of reservoirs	Typhoid, scarlet fever, rabies, tuberculosis, gonorrhea, syphilis
	Not sharing clothing, combs, etc	Lice, scabies
Secondary prevention	Screening	Tuberculosis, gonorrhea, syphilis, HIV infection
	Diagnosis and medical treatment	Scarlet fever, tuberculosis, gonorrhea, syphilis, impetigo, lice, scabies, tetanus, tuberculosis, HIV infection, diphtheria, pertussis
Tertiary prevention	Contact follow-up	Gonorrhea, syphilis, tuberculosis, hepatitis A and B, HIV infection

TABLE 7–3. CHAIN OF INFECTION, PREVENTION, AND TREATMENT OF SELECTED COMMUNICABLE DISEASES

Disease	Infectious Agent	Mode of Transmission	Portal of Entry	Portal of Exit	Prevention	Treatment
AIDS/HIV infection	Human immunodeficiency virus (HIV)	Sexual, blood products, injection	Mucosa, needle prick	Blood, vaginal and seminal secretions	Safe sex, not sharing needles	Symptomatic; AZT in asymptomatic persons (?)
Chickenpox	Varicella zoster virus	Airborne, direct contact	Respiratory tract, skin	Respiratory secretions, lesions	None	Symptomatic[a]
Diphtheria	*Corynebacterium diphtheriae*	Airborne	Respiratory	Respiratory	Immunization	Diphtheria antitoxin, penicillin
Gonorrhea	*Neisseria gonorrhoeae*	Sexual contact, passage through birth canal	Mucosa	Vaginal and seminal secretions	Selective sex, use of condoms	Penicillin or other antibiotic
Hepatitis A	Hepatitis A virus	Fecal–oral	Digestive tract	Feces	Handwashing	Symptomatic[a]
Hepatitis B	Hepatitis B virus	Sexual contact, blood products, injection, fecal–oral	Mucosa, needle prick, digestive tract	Vaginal and seminal secretions, blood, feces	Immunization, not sharing needles	Symptomatic[a]
Herpes	Herpes simplex virus, type II	Sexual contact, passage through birth canal	Mucosa, skin	Herpetic lesions	Selective sex, use of condoms, cesarean section	Symptomatic[a]
Impetigo	*Staphylococcus,* Streptococcus	Direct contact Airborne	Skin	Skin lesions, nose and throat	Hygiene	Antibiotics
Lice	Adult lice and eggs	Direct contact with person or clothing, combs, etc	Skin	Skin	Hygiene	Kwell or similar preparation
Malaria	*Plasmodium*	Insect bite	Skin	Skin, blood	Eradicate mosquito vector, remove breeding areas, protective clothing	Chloroquine

Continued

[a] Symptomatic treatment is directed at the symptoms the individual presents (eg, fever, cough).

TABLE 7–3. (continued)

Disease	Infectious Agent	Mode of Transmission	Portal of Entry	Portal of Exit	Prevention	Treatment
Measles (rubeola)	Measles virus	Airborne	Respiratory tract	Respiratory secretions	Immunization	Symptomatic[a]
Mumps	Mumps virus	Airborne	Respiratory tract	Respiratory secretions	Immunization	Symptomatic[a]
Pertussis (whooping cough)	*Bordetella pertussis*	Airborne	Respiratory tract	Respiratory secretions	Immunization	Symptomatic[a]
Polio	Poliovirus	Airborne, fecal–oral	Respiratory tract, digestive tract	Respiratory secretions, feces	Immunization	Symptomatic[a]
Rabies	A neurotrophic virus	Human or animal bite or scratch	Broken skin	Saliva	Immunization of pets and/or people, destruction of infected animals	Symptomatic[a]
Rubella (German measles)	Rubella virus	Airborne, across placenta	Respiratory tract, fetal circulation	Respiratory secretions, maternal blood	Immunization	Symptomatic[a]
Scabies	Adult scabies or eggs	Direct contact with person or clothing	Skin	Skin	Hygiene	Kwell or similar preparation
Streptococcal sore throat/scarlet fever	Beta-hemolytic *Streptococcus*	Airborne, direct contact	Respiratory tract, skin	Respiratory secretions, skin lesions	Isolation of infected person	Penicillin or other antibiotic
Syphilis	*Treponema pallidum*	Sexual contact, across placenta, circulation	Mucosa, intact skin, fetal	Skin lesions, blood	Selective sex, use of condoms	Penicillin or other antibiotic
Tetanus	*Clostridium tetani*	Open skin injury	Lacerated skin or mucosa	Soil and other inanimate objects	Immunization	Tetanus antitoxin
Tuberculosis	*Mycobacterium tuberculosis*	Airborne, milk	Respiratory tract, digestive tract	Respiratory secretions, unpasteurized milk	Antituberculin medications, pasteurization of milk	Antituberculin medications

[a] Symptomatic treatment is directed at the symptoms the individual presents (eg, fever, cough).

eases are on the rise again. For example, death rates for influenza and pneumonia—which had been decreasing—began to increase again in 1982, suggesting that susceptible persons are not being immunized.[13] Moreover, improved living standards have not been available to all segments of the population, and that is reflected in recent increases in the incidence rates for three preventable childhood diseases: measles, pertussis, and mumps. One explanation of this trend is that the immunization rates among minority children are poor.[14] Unemployment, lack of health insurance, and cuts in government subsidies put even basic health procedures out of the financial reach of many minority families. Others, particularly undocumented aliens, fear deportation and decline to expose themselves and their children by entering the mainstream of the health care system.[14] Living standards are also implicated in the resurgence of other diseases. Tuberculosis is a significant public problem among undernourished refugee and homeless populations and among Native American and migrant farm worker populations.[11] Trends in communicable disease are also subject to patterns of social behavior. While penicillin reduced the incidence of gonorrhea and syphilis for many years, there is a resurgence of both diseases.[12] Moreover, large-scale use of antibiotics to control sexually transmitted disease in the community unfortunately has resulted in the proliferation of antibiotic-resistant strains of the organisms that cause them.[15]

Finally, the forces of nature also act to change the patterns of communicable disease. As old diseases wane, new diseases appear to replace them. The historical scourge of diseases like plague, rampant in the Middle Ages; typhoid, common in the 19th century; and polio, a problem in the mid-20th century; now has been supplanted by a contemporary threat: HIV infection, or AIDS. The Centers for Disease Control (CDC) estimates that 750,000 persons in the United States were infected with HIV at the beginning of 1986 and that there are at least 1 million persons with the disease in 1991.[16,17] At least 40,000 new HIV infections occur each year among adults and adolescents, and an estimated 1500 to 2000 new infections occur each year among newborns. Some estimates suggest that these figures are low, and that a total of 1.2 to 1.5 million HIV infections with more than 80,000 new infections occurring each year since 1986 is more plausible. These adjusted figures suggest that 98,000 new cases will be diagnosed in 1993.[16]

Of all of the communicable diseases discussed in this chapter, and summarized in Table 7–3, HIV infection is the greatest public health problem because of its high fatality rate (almost 100 percent within 3 years of diagnosis), its potential to spread within the population, and its tremendous cost to society. In 1989, private insurers paid an estimated $1 billion for reimbursement in HIV-related claims for life and health insurance.[17] This figure does not take into account the tremendous personal medical costs (estimated at $8.5 billion in 1991), nor the cost to productivity (estimated to be $55.6 billion in 1991), nor the use of public hospitals.[18] Nurses have a particularly important contribution to make by educating clients and the public about the transmission and prevention of this and other communicable diseases.

Chronic Disease

Improved longevity in the population, an outcome of the decline of the childhood communicable diseases, has led to an increase in the number of elderly persons in the population and, with that increase, a marked rise in the incidence of long-term or chronic diseases. Chronic diseases are diseases caused by nonreversible pathologic alterations of the body that leave individuals with disabilities and a need for rehabilitation or self-care or, if self-care is impossible, a long period of medical supervision and a need for direct nursing care. Cardiovascular diseases, cancer, arthritis, and schizophrenia are examples of chronic diseases that are difficult to control and seriously disabling. Although communicable diseases remain a public health concern, with the exception of AIDS, it is the chronic diseases that provide the major challenges in health care today.

Contributing Factors in Chronic Disease. A significant concept in the understanding of any health problem is the concept of risk. In general, **risk** refers to the chances of exposure to a specific hazard or danger. The risk of disease is the probability (likelihood) that any person will contract a given disease, whether communicable or chronic, based on membership in a particular population subgroup. Probabilities are derived from community health statistics that show the patterns of morbidity and mortality of communicable and chronic diseases among large population subgroups.

Risk appraisal, a related concept, is the practice of estimating an individual's risk of disease based on a complete health assessment, including a nutritional and fitness evaluation. From this information personal risk factors are identified. A **risk factor** is a characteristic associated with a high probability of developing a specific health problem. Statistical correlation studies, for example, show that smoking is a common practice among individuals who develop lung cancer. Thus, smokers, even those who have no signs of disease, are considered to have a personal risk factor for lung cancer. People with risk factors have a higher probability of developing a problem than if the risk factors were not present.

Risk factors are of four types: (1) intrinsic factors such as age, sex, and race; (2) bodily changes as precursors to disease; (3) genetic factors; and (4) behavioral factors such as life-style and health habits.

The evaluation of risk factors enables health professionals to target their efforts in disease prevention. Nurses have an important role to play in the identification of risk factors. One of nurses' goals in performing client health assessments is to identify risk factors of disease. Once risk factors are identified, clients can be counseled on how to modify poor health habits, and they can be encouraged to seek medical treatment for physiological changes such as high blood pressure. Risk appraisal is particularly important in dealing with chronic diseases, the hope for which rests largely on prevention.

Control Strategies in Chronic Disease. Strategies for controlling chronic diseases are based primarily on eliminating or modifying risk factors. Public education is a particularly important part of the effort to reduce risk factors, because it enables people to make informed health decisions and to take responsibility for their own health. Both are essential aspects of chronic disease control.

Primary Prevention. Primary prevention of chronic diseases takes the form of community-based prevention programs that endeavor to check chronic disease before it develops. Stop-smoking campaigns and dietary education programs are part of that effort. Nurses and other health professionals are frequently involved in public education and life-style modification programs that teach the public about risk factors.

Secondary Prevention. Early diagnosis and treatment can limit the morbidity and mortality associated with chronic disease. Secondary prevention strategies aim to identify disease in their early stages to reduce the severity and the extent of disability as a consequence of chronic conditions. Screening is thus a particularly important aspect of secondary prevention. Chronic conditions usually have an insidious (undetected) onset and develop slowly over time. Early indicators of disease that appear at the onset can be viewed as risk factors for the development of a more severe or widespread disease. They permit diagnosis and treatment before substantial damage has occurred. By the use of the Pap smear as a screening test, for example, cervical cancers can be identified in their very early stages before they spread to other parts of the body.

Sometimes, however, the onset of disease is sudden and early indicators are unavailable. One important development in community programs for secondary prevention is the proliferation of community paramedic services; 911 emergency units bring emergency personnel and equipment to the site of life-threatening situations. For individuals who experience the sudden onset of a potentially fatal episode of disease, such as a sudden heart attack or seizure, an immediate response with life-sustaining technology can make the difference between survival and death.

Tertiary Prevention. Many chronic diseases have a natural history that includes periods of relative dormancy, during which symptoms do not progress in severity; and periods of exacerbation, during which symptoms become dramatically more severe. Tertiary prevention endeavors to prevent recurrent episodes of disease for as long as possible. Host-oriented rehabilitative measures are vital for the tertiary prevention of some illnesses. For example, emphysema is a chronic and serious respiratory disease that progresses over time. Individuals who have emphysema are taught, often by the nurses who care for them, to stop smoking, avoid air pollution (both of which aggravate respiratory disease), and improve pulmonary ventilation through the use of special breathing techniques. All of these tertiary means stave off further exacerbations of disease and a general deterioration of the individual's condition.

Community programs are also important in tertiary prevention. Community mental health clinics, for example, help individuals with chronic schizophrenia, a particularly debilitating mental illness, to remain independent by dispensing drugs for the control of mental symptoms and by providing counseling and therapy services. Such prevention limits the extent of personal suffering and also minimizes the cost of disease and disability to the community. Table 7–4 summarizes some important risk factors and control measures in chronic disease.

Trends in Chronic Disease. Progress has been made in controlling some risk factors for the chronic diseases. The quit ratio for smokers (the percentage of ever smokers [persons having smoked at least 100 cigarettes] who are former smokers) increased from 29.6 percent in 1965, to 44.8 percent in 1987. By 1987, 38 million Americans—nearly one half of all living adults who had ever smoked—had quit smoking cigarettes due primarily to public education.[19] Control of hypertension has also achieved a certain degree of success through secondary prevention measures, and there is evidence that the general public is more knowledgeable about the consequences of hypertension.[20] Behavioral risk factors such as overweight and inactivity, however, have been less successfully addressed.[21]

Overall, control efforts have resulted in a decline in mortality from several chronic diseases. From 1979 to 1987, death rates declined for several chronic diseases, including heart disease (15 percent), cerebrovascular disease (27 percent), and chronic lung disease (28 percent). Although deaths from cancer had been increasing since 1950, the death rate declined for two consecutive years, 1985 to 1987.[22] However, these declines do not indicate that efforts to control chronic diseases should be discontinued. There is still significant cost to society from chronic disease. The health care cost estimate for major cardiovascular diseases in 1991 was projected to be $83 billion. When lost productivity is considered, the cost would be $101 billion.[23] These figures also fail to consider the family and societal burdens from the loss of life associated with chronic disease. Nurses in the hospital and community have a particularly important role to play in reducing these costs by educating clients and the public about the importance of prevention.

Other Health Problems

Aside from communicable and chronic diseases, there are also other significant health problems in the community. Accidents, violent and abusive behavior, and substance abuse are among the most important of these.

Accidents. Accidents—nonintentional injuries resulting in death and disability—have led all other health problems in total years of life lost since 1979.[24] The primary cause of accidental death is from motor vehicle accidents. While this has been an important health problem for many years, as recently as 1983 there was evidence that efforts to control automobile mortality were succeeding. Mortality rates, for example, dropped from 27.4 per 100,000 to 18.5 per

TABLE 7–4. RISK FACTORS AND PRIMARY, SECONDARY, AND TERTIARY PREVENTION STRATEGIES FOR SELECTED CHRONIC DISEASES

Disease	Risk Factors	Primary Prevention	Secondary Prevention	Tertiary Prevention
Cancer	Exposure to carcinogens, smoking, low dietary fiber, radiation exposure, genetic predisposition	Prevent exposure to carcinogens, no smoking or stop smoking, increase dietary fiber, prevent radiation exposure through environmental control	Screening (breast self-examination, Pap smear, rectal examination, stool blood examination); early diagnosis; treatment with surgical removal, radiation therapy, chemotherapy	Prevent subsequent exposure to carcinogens, stop smoking, assist with peaceful death
Chronic lung disease	Smoking, air pollution	No smoking or stop smoking, reduce air pollution	Symptomatic, respiratory therapy	Prevent overexertion, stop smoking, respiratory rehabilitation
Diabetes mellitus	Overweight, genetic predisposition	Maintain appropriate body weight, exercise	Screening urine or blood sugar diagnosis, treatment with insulin or oral hypoglycemics	Prevent complications through adequate control of blood sugar
Heart disease	Smoking, sedentary life-style, high-cholesterol diet, type A personality, overweight, hypertension, genetic predisposition	No smoking or stop smoking, adequate exercise, low-cholesterol diet, stress management and positive coping skills, weight control, control of hypertension	Diagnosis, treatment with antiarrythmics, cardiotonics, etc	Prevent recurrence through modification of diet, life-style, stress management, etc
Hypertension	Smoking, overweight, high-cholesterol diet	No smoking or stop smoking, weight control, low-cholesterol diet	Screening, dietary control, antihypertensives	Prevent complications through adequate control of blood pressure
Schizophrenia	Family history, unstable family environment	Create adequate self-image, establish stable family environment	Medication, psychotherapy	Continued psychotherapy
Stroke	Smoking, high-cholesterol diet, hypertension	No smoking or stop smoking, low-cholesterol diet, control of hypertension	Anticoagulants and other medications, maintain respiration	Rehabilitation to regain function

100,000.[25] This decline was primarily due to the use of seat belts, particularly in states where they became a legal requirement. Nevertheless, in 1987, deaths from motor vehicle accidents caused more than one half of all accidental deaths,[22] and driving while intoxicated is a particularly significant host factor in the etiology of this health problem. Despite recent efforts to enforce sobriety laws, the percentage of people who drink and drive has actually increased.[26]

Another significant contribution to accident mortality rates comes from accidental poisonings and falls. Poisoning is a particularly serious problem among young children. The American Association of Poison Control Centers reported more than 500,000 exposures of children to toxic substances during 1985. Many of these cases involved prescription drugs, a substantial proportion of which were packaged in "child-resistant" containers.[27] Falls, on the other hand, are an important cause of injury among the elderly and are the second greatest cause of accident-related deaths. While the mortality rate from falls seems to be declining gradually, at 5.1 per 100,000 it remains high enough to necessitate continued work on prevention.[28]

Estimates of the direct and indirect costs of death from accidents place the amount at $75 to $100 billion per year. By continued efforts at prevention these figures could be substantially reduced.

Violence. Violence is another significant community health problem. Homicide, suicide, and abuse are all serious problems that cause a substantial loss of life in the community and are a particular problem among some subgroups. Homicide among 15 to 19 year olds, for example, is a growing problem among the general population, but among young blacks the rate is about 5 times that of whites.[29] Likewise, suicide is the leading cause of childhood fatal injuries in the general population, but age-specific rates among white children are 1.5 to 2.5 times those for blacks.[29] Most often, firearms are involved in homicides and suicides.[29] Unfortunately, many states have failed to limit access to handguns through permit and licensure requirements, and a federal gun control law was not enacted until 1991. The result has been that availability has expanded even into the school-age population. The National Adolescent Student Health Survey of 1987 reported, for example, that 41 percent of the adolescent boys and 24 percent of the girls surveyed indicated they had access to handguns.[30]

Abuse is another form of violent behavior that is perpetrated on many groups in society, such as children, the elderly, parents, spouses, and often within families. Reports of child abuse, for example, are on the rise. Child abuse is a major contributor to childhood injuries. In 1986, an estimated 1.6 million children were abused or neglected.[31] Violence between spouses, people who share a household, or those who are otherwise intimate with each other is a widespread public health problem and a substantial contributor to the public health impact of injuries, in particular injuries to women. In one study, battering was responsible for more injuries to women than were motor vehicle accidents and mugging combined.[32]

Substance Abuse. Probably one of the most costly of all public health problems is substance abuse, including alcohol and drugs of many types. Alcohol abuse is responsible for a large proportion of the loss of life in the population, even when deaths attributed to drinking and driving are factored out. In 1987, 4.9 percent of all deaths were alcohol-related.[33] In the same year, alcohol-related mortality accounted for more than 2.7 million years per life lost (YPLL) before life expectancy.[33] While there is evidence that alcohol consumption is declining slightly, high consumption remains prevalent.

Control Strategies. The stress of everyday life undoubtedly plays a very significant role in the etiology of this group of health problems. Not surprisingly, primary prevention strategies are aimed at helping people deal with stress without resorting to violence or substance abuse. Stress reduction, moreover, indirectly helps to prevent those accidents that happen while individuals are in a highly emotional state.

In all settings, nurses are involved in teaching clients about ways of coping with stress, and nurses also have a responsibility to model positive coping behavior. Chapter 6 discusses stress in depth. Nurses also participate in primary prevention by educating people on drug and alcohol use and abuse.

Nowhere is such education more important than within families. The combined approach of teaching family members about effective family communication and the importance of limiting alcohol and drugs in the family environment is important for reducing family violence. Another aspect is education in the parenting techniques that can assist parents to cope with the behavior of their children. Education on accident prevention is also important for families. Addressing the need to wear seat belts or identifying strategies for childproofing homes, for example, are important aspects of a family-oriented primary prevention plan. When nurses find that family members are in a high-stress state and have needs that go beyond an educational approach, however, referral for counseling becomes part of primary prevention. Professional counseling is always appropriate when individuals are not coping well with the stress of their lives.

Secondary prevention rests on identifying clients with drug and alcohol problems before these problems lead to accidents or violence, and recognizing cases of abuse by taking action to educate violence victims about community shelters. Counseling is also clearly an appropriate secondary prevention measure. Tertiary prevention to prevent the recurrence of violence or accidents employs the same strategies that are used at the primary and secondary prevention levels.

Finally, political involvement may be necessary to advance community programs not only for substance abuse, violence, and accident prevention, but also in the control of communicable and chronic disease. Because of their fundamental understanding of these and other community health problems, nurses make good lobbyists for community primary prevention programs.

■ HEALTH PROMOTION IN THE COMMUNITY

Much of the information in the previous sections emphasizes concepts basic to the control and prevention of disease. This information is of fundamental importance to health care professionals because it provides them with a framework for understanding their responsibilities related to health protection. Certainly, the control and prevention of disease are central to community health. However, as the section on priorities in health care established, disease prevention is only one aspect of the first-level priority of health care professionals. Health promotion, the strategies to maintain and enhance health, are also of paramount importance.

How Does Health Promotion Differ from Disease Prevention?

While disease prevention activities focus on threats to health and the need to protect people in the community from such threats, health promotion efforts focus on the well-being of individuals and the population at large. Experts have pointed out that even dictionary definitions reinforce a distinction between health promotion and disease prevention.[34,35] To "promote" means to help to exist or flourish, while to "prevent" means to keep from occurring. Pender, a leading authority on health promotion, summarizes the distinction by observing that health promotion is "approach" behavior, whereas disease prevention is "avoidance" behavior.[35]

Health promotion, according to Shamansky and

Clausen, also authorities on the subject, consists of efforts to enhance the well-being and actualize the health potential of individuals, families, communities, and society.[36] Pender points out that health promotion is not disease- or health-problem specific. Rather, health promotion seeks to expand the positive potential for health.[35] Efforts at health promotion therefore address general issues related to nutrition and fitness, stress, the environment, and habits for healthful living. To be effective, health promotion, like disease prevention, requires a focus on the individual, family, and community levels.

The Development of Interest in Health Promotion

Growing professional and social recognition that many chronic conditions result from life-style factors related to diet, exercise, stress, and substance use has led policy officials, health care professionals, and the public to acknowledge the central importance of health promotion.

Professional Interest. Professional interest in health promotion in the United States and elsewhere gained considerable momentum in the 1980s. To a substantial degree this interest was an acknowledgement of certain important trends in the characteristics of the population, trends that resulted from the success of measures to prevent and control d:sease.[37] As public health and medical care improved in the pre- and post-World-War-II eras, death rates dropped. One outcome is that the proportion of older people in society gradually expanded and continues to rise. By 2030, according to the US Census Bureau, the elderly may represent as much as 21 percent of the population.[38] Moreover, the "baby boomers," those born between 1945 and 1960 who comprise more than one third of the total US population, are becoming middle aged. These demographic facts have created the potential for a drastic impact on the health care system, as health care professionals anticipate increasing numbers of aging individuals to seek help for chronic conditions that not only reduce the quality of life but are costly to treat.

Over the last decade, considerable effort has been made by policy-makers and professionals to transform the health care delivery system from one that concentrates heavily on the problems of disease to a system that balances its emphasis on treatment, prevention, and health promotion. Interest in keeping the aging society healthy first crystallized in a 1979 landmark document called "Healthy People" published by the surgeon general of the United States.[39] This paper advanced the idea that health gains for the remainder of the 20th century would come from improvement in life-style, the environment, and from individual nutrition and fitness. This was followed in 1980 by a statement from the US Department of Health and Human Services that outlined health promotion as a national objective. The goal was to enhance the health of the population by any combination of educational, organizational, environmental, and economic interventions aimed at (1) smoking and health, (2) misuse of alcohol and drugs, (3) nutrition, (4) physical fitness and exercise, and (5) control of stress and violent behavior.[40]

Since the appearance of these official statements, a variety of public and private agencies have begun work to promote this national objective. The insurance industry and hospitals both have established organizations to advance the goal of health promotion. Worksite health promotion programs have appeared and rapidly increased in number.[41] Even churches are offering behavior change and wellness programs to their congregations.[42] Moreover, health promotion has become institutionalized in the health care delivery system. Health maintenance organizations (HMOs), organizations that assure the delivery of a range of health services to enrollees for a fixed cost, are growing in number and have become a significant force as an alternative delivery system. The HMO concept is based on the premise that the most cost-effective approach to health care is to keep the population healthy. Since 1980, federal regulations have required HMOs to provide health promotional assistance as part of their service to enrollees.[43] HMO activities generally focus on health education programs that include instruction in personal health care measures, nutrition education, and counseling.[44]

Public Interest. Fortunately, the general public seems to share the substantial professional interest in health promotion that exists. Public interest was first nurtured by a shift in American values that occurred in the 1960s and 1970s. This change redirected national emphasis on the traditional work ethic, the value of working hard to achieve the "American Dream," into a new interest in the fulfillment of personal goals through enhancement of one's "quality of life."[45] A public awakening to health as a valuable asset accompanied the new view. As many Americans reordered their personal priorities, self-actualization pursuits became as important as economic pursuits.

Public interest in personal health persists and today focuses on leisure activities, self-development, fitness, nutrition, and healthful habits. Public interest has in fact spawned industries that cater to life-style enhancement and self-help of all kinds. One need only look around to see commercial evidence of the interest in health and the "good life." The proliferation of travel agencies and sports equipment outlets, the growing number of fitness centers, weight reduction products and services, and the expansion of clinics for altering substance use habits are all expressions that the public is concerned about and willing to put its resources into improved health. As time goes on, moreover, American concern about health promotion is spreading to other countries. Japan, for example, is also enjoying a fitness boom and there is mounting pressure on business and government to increase leisure time for the Japanese worker.[46]

Cultural changes and the public interest in health have had important effects. Many Americans pursue self-development and leisure activities with the same dedication and enthusiasm they once devoted only to their careers. Habits such as smoking, drinking, and substance use are on the downslide,[19,47,48] reinforced by health promotion efforts and increasingly restrictive public policies. More and more, public attitudes are reflected in personal preferences for lighter foods and beverages, in individual concern for keeping weight down and strength and fitness up through a balance of diet and exercise, and in people's search for ways to manage stress that enhance rather than threaten health.

A Model of Health Promotion

The fundamental model around which health promotion efforts in the United States have been structured is the self-care model. This is the concept that people can help themselves in health matters by making the right choices. Self-care is not a new idea, but actually has roots in ancient cultures in which self-care was valued for religious and pragmatic reasons. Religious food laws, for example, were promulgated in biblical times not only to please God but also to ensure health. As the science of medicine developed, interest in self-care waned, only to reappear as the limits of medicine in the achievement of health have become clear. The basic idea of self-care as a model for health promotion is the belief that given the right information, people will act "rationally," often in collaboration with their health care professionals, to promote and protect their own health.

The self-care model is the predominant model of health promotion currently used by health care professionals. Under this model, the emphasis is placed on providing clients with information on nutrition, exercise, and personal habits as part of an overall life-style to achieve health. There is also emphasis on the role of stress and stress reduction and the use of substances and their relationship to health. Instruction is undertaken either through individual counseling or by providing formal health education courses to clients.

Current Issues and Trends

The most important issues in health promotion concern the effectiveness of programs designed to disseminate health promotion knowledge and skills to the public and the extent to which these programs are available to population subgroups. Unfortunately, the reality is that health promotional activities are not yet a part of the day-to-day life of all citizens. The factors that create this reality are complex. Social and cultural forces have a powerful effect on a group's approach to health. Cultures, societies, and subgroups differ in their views about health and disease and about the appropriateness of activities to achieve health. Although strategic planning has been found to be a prime factor in the success of health promotion efforts,[49] as yet not enough is understood about how to develop health educational messages that will convince people from diverse segments of the population to adopt activities that are important to health.[50]

The quality of health education programs is another factor. Experts on health promotion have identified deficiencies that are common to many health education programs and that need to be addressed if programs are to be effective. These include lack of systematic planning, including failure to consider the needs and health risks of the target population; poor curriculum content; lack of effective marketing strategies; and lack of financial resources.[51]

There are new trends to offset the organizational problems that contribute to these deficiencies. Agencies are joining with one another to improve health promotion efforts. This is reflected in numerous descriptions in the literature of the work of health coalitions, consortia, networks, and multi-institutional arrangements for health promotion. All of these represent efforts at the agency level to overcome problems of financing and coordination.[52]

Another approach, one stressing community-wide organization, seeks to avoid the problems of other programs through involving community members. This approach has been taken by the Centers for Disease Control (CDC), the federal government's health surveillance organization. The CDC's Division of Health Education developed an intervention effort for the coordination of health promotion at the local level. The program is called PATCH (planned approach to community health).[53] PATCH, which has been implemented in several states, is grounded on the concept that health promotion programs should be carried out comprehensively through the involvement of local community planners who survey the community and design programs to specifically accommodate the priority needs of the community.

Even with the trends and innovations, health promotion in the United States may fail to meet the needs of many in the population. Williams, a critic of current approaches, argues that the problem lies in the underlying philosophy of health promotion in the United States.[54] That philosophy stresses individualism and self-responsibility for health. The discussion of the self-care model above reflects the underlying assumptions that health is determined primarily by personal behavior, and life-style is brought about by the rational and free choices of the individual. Even when a "community approach" to health promotion is taken, the ultimate responsibility for change remains an individual one.

Williams disputes the individualist approach, arguing that it assumes that people understand health to be a matter of self-interest and that people have the resources needed to achieve health.[54] Williams points to research showing that the adoption of health promoting behavior is in actuality related to income, education, and occupational status, and suggests that this makes being and staying healthy more likely for some than for others. The answer, in Williams' view, lies not in the dissemination of health information but in political activism to change the way society as a whole distributes the resources that are necessary to achieve health.

■ COMMUNITY HEALTH NURSING

Nurses have long worked to promote the health of the community, and have done so in many settings, the most traditional setting being at the bedside in the hospital. Over the last two decades, however—and particularly since the implementation of Medicare's prospective payment system—the demand for home health care and community nursing service has exploded.[55] One consequence of this is that as we move into the 21st century more and more nurses will work outside of the hospital,[56] perhaps to a point to where those in other community settings will outnumber those in the hospital. New roles, responsibilities, and rewards will accompany this fundamental change in the environment for nursing care. Autonomy will increase, but so will the need for professional collaboration. An understanding of the nature, emphasis, and roles of nursing in the community will aid nurses in all settings to prepare themselves for the changes in practice that have already begun.

What is community health nursing? **Community health nursing** involves promotion of the health of groups of people. The American Public Health Association Public Health Nursing Section[57] defined community or public health nursing as follows:

> The specialty of public health nursing is professional nursing directed toward a total community or population group. Consideration is given to environmental, social, and personal health factors affecting health status. Its practice includes identification of subgroups or aggregates within the community who are at higher risk of illness or poor recovery and targeting its resources toward those groups and the families and individuals who comprise them. Emphasis is placed on planning for the community as a whole rather than on individual health care. Its purpose . . . is achieved by working with and through community leaders, health related groups, groups at risk, families, and individuals and by becoming involved in relevant social action (p. 5).

As is evident in this definition, the community health nurse is concerned with the health of population groups. Although community health nurses frequently provide care for individuals and families, the primary purpose for such care is the improvement of the health status of the total community. Thus it can be said that community health nursing is the application of the concepts and methods of community health to nursing practice.

IMPLICATIONS FOR PROFESSIONAL COLLABORATION

The Focus of Community Health Nursing

Community health nursing is a collaborative endeavor in the broadest sense. To a large extent, this is because the focus is always on the group: the family, the neighborhood, the work group, the school cohort, and the therapy group. Community health nursing places a strong emphasis on the social dynamics of health and illness, because the group is a social as well as a biophysical occurrence. Groups vary in the social values that they bring to health issues. Identification of group values is a necessary part of assessing the health needs of a group. The values of any particular group became apparent in the give and take of a collaborative exchange of information, opinions, attitudes, desires, and preferences that occurs as nurses and group members work together in a joint effort to identify and plan for the group's health needs.

Historical Perspectives

Along with her other efforts to improve nursing care, Florence Nightingale, in the mid-19th century, was instrumental in the creation of the first district public health nursing association in England. She also recognized community health nursing as a distinct area of practice requiring specialized educational preparation. Home nursing services for the sick in the United States were begun as early as 1813 with the establishment of the Ladies Benevolent Society of South Carolina.

Organized nursing efforts at the group level were pioneered by Lillian Wald in the establishment of the Henry Street Settlement in New York City in 1893. This agency also started the first school health program in 1902. Operation of the program was later taken over by the New York City Department of Health in 1903. In 1898 Los Angeles became the first municipality to employ a community health nurse, and in 1909 the Metropolitan Life Insurance Company included home nursing services in its insurance benefits. Health care in rural communities was spearheaded by the establishment of the Rural Nursing Service by the American Red Cross in 1912.

In 1923 the Goldmark Report reinforced the need for specialized education for nurses engaged in community health practice, and the first two schools of nursing housed in institutions of higher learning (Yale University School of Nursing and the Frances Payne Bolton School of Nursing at Case Western Reserve University) included community health content in their curricula.

More recently, a movement to change the national emphasis from the cure of illness to health promotion and illness prevention has made the community health nurse role even more important in today's society. In 1962 the Neighborhood Health Center Act was passed, providing federal assistance to community-based health care activities. Community health nurses have been an integral part of such service.

The Concept of the Client in Community Health Nursing

A client is someone who receives goods or services from another person. In health care, the client is the recipient of the health care services provided by health professionals. In most areas of nursing, the client is an individual, a person who faces a health problem. The focus of nursing action is on individuals and their needs for assistance. The role of nurses is to provide the care necessary to raise the individual client's level of health; depending on the situation, nurses may perform a variety of services, ranging from client education to complicated intensive care procedures, in order to achieve this objective. Even when the health problem is complex and the involvement of the family is necessary, it is the individual who is the client. Family members participate in their relatives' health care, but their own health is not an issue.

Community health nursing is similar to other areas of nursing in that the client may be, and often is, an individual (Fig. 7–5). Just as often, however, services are rendered to an entire family or to a group of people who have common or interrelated health problems. The focus of nursing action, then, is on the group as a unit, and the group is defined as the client. Under this concept, nurses are concerned both with the health of each individual within the group and with the health of the group as a whole. For example, nurses may direct nursing actions such as teaching or counseling to individual family members, but in so doing are always cognizant of how each member affects the health of the other members and, in turn, the functioning of the group as a whole. Moreover, some nursing actions in community health nursing are actually oriented to the group as a whole. Family therapy, for example, which is done by some community health nurses, is a form of group counseling aimed at helping the entire family function more effectively.

Community health nursing also embraces the concept of the *community* as client, as the introduction to this chapter highlighted. Under this concept, nurses take various actions to improve the health of the community as a whole.

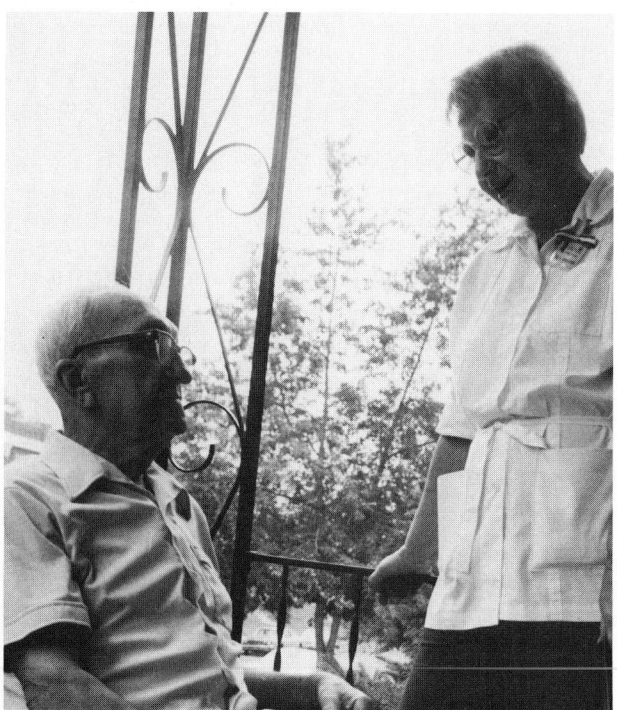

Figure 7–5. Even though community health nurses provide care to individuals, the focus of the community health nurse is on the community as client, and the nursing care benefits the community as a whole. (*Source: Clark MJ.* Nursing in the Community. *Norwalk, CT: Appleton & Lange; 1992.*)

IMPLICATIONS FOR PROFESSIONAL COLLABORATION

The Community As Client

The concept of the community as client is complex. It means that individual health can only be served by addressing the health needs and problems of the community as a whole. Approaching health at a community level is not only a complex concept, it is a complex undertaking, one that demands a strong team effort by health care providers. The need for teamwork underscores the special importance of collaboration in community health. Professionals from all the health care occupations are important to the goal of achieving health, each contributing different, but equally important, perspectives and skills. Through collaboration, providers come together to share their expertise for the good of the community and to plan the health programs needed to protect the health of community residents.

In community health nursing, the entire community or any of the various populations that comprise the community can be the client, and nurses give attention to assessing the features of the community that contribute to the health and illness of all community residents. Nursing actions may include community assessment based on statistical and other data, and, in relation, the development and implementation of health programs that benefit the community or its subgroups, such as school children, the elderly, or the homeless.

Thus, in community health nursing, all units, individuals, families, groups, and entire communities are served, and the unit is the client. The broad focus of community health nurses on the group or community as a client is particularly important and distinguishes community health nursing from other areas of nursing.

Roles in Community Health Nursing

Community health nurses engaged in primary, secondary, or tertiary prevention of health problems perform a wide variety of roles. The extent to which any single role is carried out in a particular setting depends upon the needs of the clients and the setting. Possible roles of community health nurses described by Clark[58] are listed in Box 7–6.

Client-oriented Roles. The first category of roles relates directly to the care of clients, whether individual, family, or group.

Health Educator. Because community health nursing emphasizes primary prevention of health problems, much of its practice involves education for a healthier life-style. As health educators, community health nurses help clients acquire the insights and skills needed to maintain and safeguard health (Fig. 7–6). While much of health education is related to primary prevention, it may also involve education of clients about the treatment of illness and prevention of complications.

BOX 7–6. ROLES OF COMMUNITY HEALTH NURSES

Client-oriented Roles

- Health educator
- Counselor
- Referral resource
- Liaison
- Advocate
- Role model
- Direct care provider

Delivery-oriented Roles

- Coordinator
- Collaborator
- Discharge planner
- Supervisor

Community-oriented Roles

- Case finder
- Community assessor, program planner, and evaluator

General Roles

- Researcher
- Research utilizer

Counselor. The counseling role of community health nurses is closely related to that of health educators, but is not the same thing. In counseling, community health nurses help clients to solve problems and make decisions. Community health nurses consequently counsel clients to help them identify alternative courses of action and their possible consequences.

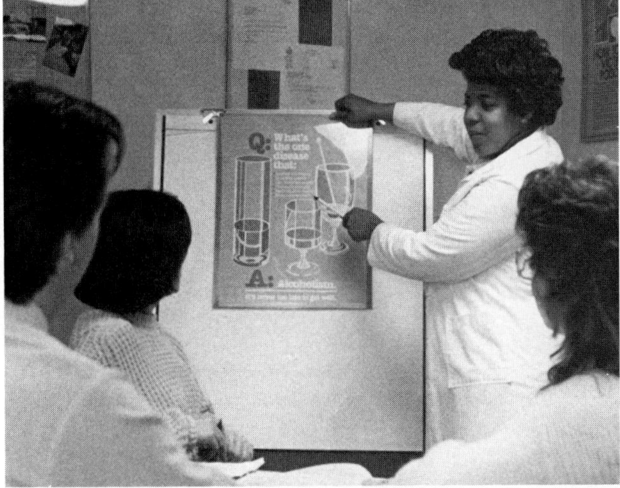

Figure 7–6. The community health nurse performs the role of health educator in providing clients with the knowledge and skills needed to maintain and enhance health.

Referral Resource. Referral is another function frequently performed by community health nurses. A referral is a formal recommendation to clients to seek health services from another agency or health care professional. Community health nurses provide clients with information about services that are available from other agencies or providers.

Liaison. Community health nurses also act as liaisons between clients and other components of the health care system. Community health nurses may make initial contact with needed services for clients when they are unable to do so themselves. Nurses may also act as go-betweens, informing others of clients' needs and circumstances. Additionally, nurses may explain the instructions of other health care providers if clients do not understand what has been said or what is required.

Advocate. Client advocacy involves speaking for clients who are unable to speak for themselves or to make their needs and desires known to others either because of fear or inability to articulate their needs. Advocacy is a critical part of every nurse's role. It is a particularly important role in the community, because community health nurses so often work with disadvantaged clients. Community health nurses are frequently aware of the unmet needs of individuals and groups within the community and can bring these needs to the attention of health care policy-makers.

Role Model. Another function of community health nurses is role-modeling. Community health nurses model healthy behaviors for clients by using effective coping strategies and problem-solving processes that assist clients to engage in such behavior themselves.

Direct Care Provider. Community health nurses give direct, hands-on care to individuals, families, and other groups of clients. Direct care refers to the assessment and management of client care problems; often this means observing clients and their environment to identify health needs. Direct care to help clients may involve assisting clients with self-care activities such as feeding, bathing, and ambulating; performing skilled nursing procedures such as dressing changes; or supervising some aspect of the medical regimen such as medication administration. Direct care is not limited to the technical tasks involved in caregiving, however, and incorporates those other functions (teaching, counseling, and role-modeling) that nurses perform while interacting with clients. Thus, demonstrating infant care techniques to a new mother, or counseling a parent on where to find help for a troubled child, are also applications of direct care.

Direct care by community health nurses is initiated by referral. Many health care providers and community health care agencies refer clients to community nursing agencies for direct care services. Referrals are also initiated by the police, concerned neighbors, church members, or others who indicate that an individual or family needs direct care services of some type. Self-referral is also common; people who are experiencing health problems may request nursing services themselves. Case finding is another source of referral. In the course of their work, community health nurses often come into contact with individuals or families who they identify as needing direct care service.

Delivery-oriented Roles. The community health nursing roles in this category promote the organization and efficiency of care given to clients.

Coordinator. Coordination is an activity performed by nurses in many areas of practice. This role is especially important in the community setting because of the number of health care providers and agencies that are often involved in a client's care. Community health nurses often with with clients who have multiple problems and require the assistance of a number of persons in addition to nurses. In such instances, nurses coordinate the services of several professionals, making needed contacts to assure that all dimensions of clients' health problems are addressed.

Coordination is also important at the community level. When the client is the community, nurses may find themselves working with politicians and government officials, police, and school officials to resolve such community problems as teenage alcoholism, drunk driving, or tobacco-related illnesses.

Collaborator. The importance of collaboration in community health nursing cannot be overestimated. Collaboration involves joint decision-making on the problems nurses and clients will address and the course of action they will take. There are two aspects to the collaboration function of community health nurses: (1) collaboration with clients and (2) collaboration with others including other health care professionals whose activities may influence the health of clients. For the most part, in the home, school, or work setting, clients have a great deal of control over the health care situation. Close collaboration with clients is important because planned interventions are frequently carried out by clients. If an individual client needs to reduce sodium intake to help control hypertension, a nurse educates the client about foods high in sodium; but food selection, preparation, and consumption are the province of the client. Nurses can suggest action, but the decision to act and the action itself are usually carried out by clients rather than nurses. The likelihood that planned interventions will be carried out is enhanced when clients (individual, family, or community) are involved in the development of the plan. Thus, in a very real sense, clients are a part of the community health team.

Collaboration with others influencing client health is also important, as the discussion of the role of coordinator suggests. Community health nurses usually collaborate with a variety of other persons in resolving health problems. These may include other health care professionals, school personnel, or protective services personnel. When the community is the client, community health nurses may collaborate with community leaders, elected officials, religious leaders, businesspeople, engineers, city planners, and media representatives.

IMPLICATIONS FOR PROFESSIONAL COLLABORATION

The Community Health Nurse As Collaborator

The importance of collaboration in community health nursing cannot be overestimated. Collaboration involves joint decision-making on health problems and the course of action for their resolution. There are two aspects to the collaboration function of the community health nurse, collaboration with clients and collaboration with others whose activities may influence the health of clients.

BUILDING NURSING KNOWLEDGE

What Role Does Collaboration Play in Nurse–Client Relationships in the Community?

Pesznecker BL, Zerwekh JV, Horn, BJ. The mutual-participation relationship: Key to facilitating self-care practices in clients and families. *Pub Health Nurs.* 1989; 6:197–203.

The authors state that collaboration is vital to nursing in the home. In their view, clients must be involved in mutual decision-making with the professional caregiver if client and family are to become able to promote, maintain, and restore their own health.

According to the authors, the home as a site for care giving contrasts to institutional sites such as hospitals. In the hospital, clients are frequently expected to conform to the institution's rules and to comply with the medical regimen prescribed. In the home, clients are consumers who are independent or interdependent agents. Even though clients may be recovering from an acute illness, they are expected to assume obligations and responsibilities.

The impact of managing illness in the home is powerful. Clients must learn the medical regimen, control symptoms, and manage crises. These responsibilities have a major effect on identity and life-style, causing a loss of time, comfort, energy, money, and human contact. When care is provided in the home, the health care professional must facilitate families' efforts to handle these issues. A major problem is integrating prescribed treatments into the family life-style, particularly in cases when there are cultural conflicts.

According to the authors, a collaborative relationship can assist nurses to facilitate client's adaptation to caring for themselves at home. Nurses encourage clients and families to share their perspective of their situation. Nurses also facilitate joint decision-making by identifying factors such as role expectations and attitudes, knowledge, personal traits, and how each party interprets the meaning of the situation. Nurses can help persuade clients to accept treatment by focusing on clients' interests and by broadening clients' choices for solutions to the problems they perceive. Ultimately, nurses must accept that clients may make decisions based on quality of life rather than survival, and may reject aspects of the medical plan.

Discharge Planner. The collaborative effort in many community health nursing situations begins with discharge planning. In **discharge planning,** clients and their families collaborate with health care providers to identify and plan for the client's needs during and after the transition from an acute care setting out into the community. Discharge planning provides an interface between the acute care setting and community. This interface is essential to assure that care is continuous during the transition and that clients' needs after discharge are adequately addressed. Ideally, planning for discharge should begin when clients are admitted to the acute care setting and should involve hospital personnel and community health nurses, and other health care and home care personnel who will be involved in the client's care after discharge.

Discharge planning entails the identification of factors that will influence health status after discharge. Because discharge plans are initiated by the institution that discharges a client, hospitals frequently employ community health nurses to coordinate discharge planning. Community health nurses' input is particularly valuable because community health nurses usually have the opportunity to view and evaluate the home situation to which the individual will be returning. Moreover, discharge plans frequently result in referral to outside agencies for services needed by individuals or families. Because of their knowledge of community resources, community health nurses can ensure that such referrals are appropriate. When a referral is made early enough, it may be possible for personnel from the referral agency to make initial contact with clients before they leave the hospital. This reassures individuals or families that someone will be available to continue to help them meet their needs.

Finally, discharge planning includes plans for client follow-up. Together, clients and other health care team members determine what follow-up is needed and when it should be undertaken. For example, a client may be told to return to see the physician in a month, or sooner if problems arise. When community health nurses are involved in discharge planning, they are able to reinforce the need for follow-up and remind individuals or families of return appointments.

Supervisor. Community health nurses frequently find themselves supervising care provided by other nursing personnel, student professionals, or even by family members. Many nursing actions are delegated to others. For instance, range-of-motion exercises might be delegated to a home health aide. Community health nurses supervise the person performing the exercises to be sure that they are being performed correctly. Community health nurses are responsible for evaluating the effects on clients of actions carried out by others.

Community-oriented Roles. The third category of community health nursing roles are those related to the care of the community as a unit. The two community-oriented roles are those of (1) case finder and (2) community assessor, program planner, and evaluator.

Case Finder. Case finding is an important function of community health nurses. As mentioned earlier, because community health nurses work with individuals and their families, they often uncover additional health problems among family members.

Interactions with clients may also suggest health problems present in the larger society. For example, a nurse might notice that many recent referrals are new mothers who show indications of drug abuse and whose newborns exhibit signs of drug toxicity. These observations suggest that there could be a community problem with drug abuse and that preventive action should be taken. Based on the results of case finding, this nurse might approach local officials to conduct a full assessment and consider establishing a substance abuse prevention program.

Community Assessor, Program Planner, and Evaluator. Community health nurses act as community assessors. Community assessment begins with the collection of information about the community. Several categories of information are needed to create a complete picture of community health status. These categories and some of the specific information included in them are presented in Box 7–7. There are a variety of sources of information for community assessment. For example, data from the most recent national census are found in libraries that function as repositories of government documents. Local planning agencies also provide a wide variety of data related to community health. The local health department and local hospitals are good sources of data on health indicators. The phone book is also a source of information about available health services. Government officials and other community leaders also provide information about the community and its health status. Once the data are obtained, community health nurses and other community health professionals analyze the data to determine community health problems. Such an analysis usually involves comparison with state or national norms to determine the scope and severity of the

BOX 7–7. CATEGORIES OF DATA FOR COMMUNITY ASSESSMENT

- General description in terms of location, size, population density, type of community, history, future prospects.
- Population characteristics: age, sex, and racial composition; religion; ethnicity; income levels; educational levels; marital status and typical family composition; employment levels; occupations.
- Community systems: governmental structure, educational system, communication network, protective services, health care system.
- Environmental characteristics: topography, housing, water supply, waste management, transportation, recreation, presence of nuisance factors.
- Health indicators: birth rates, death rates, morbidity rates, immunization rates, use of health services, attitudes toward health.

local problem. Problems are also identified from the perspective of community members. This necessitates obtaining residents' perceptions of community health problems during the assessment.

When the community's health problems are identified, nurses, together with other community health professionals and community members, plan interventions to solve those problems. Community health nurses participate in health program planning. Plans are then put into effect and their outcome evaluated.

General Roles. The last category of community health nursing roles includes two roles that cut across all of the other categories.

Researcher and Research User. Research is important in all areas of nursing, including community health nursing. The extent of individual nurses' involvement in research varies, but all community health nurses are responsible for critically reviewing research in the field and applying it to their practice. Community health nurses are also in a unique position to identify research problems related to the health of groups of people and are frequently involved in the design and implementation of research projects. Concepts related to nursing research will be addressed in greater detail in Chapter 32.

Settings for Community Health Nursing

Community health nurses practice in a variety of health care settings. The most familiar settings are the official government health agencies or health departments. There are also many other settings in which community health nurses practice. Among these are schools, industries, rehabilitation facilities, correctional institutions, ambulatory health centers, emergency centers, nurse-managed clinics, and hospitals (Box 7–8). Probably one of the most important settings for community health nursing, however, is in the home.

The Home Setting. Community health nurses have a long history of making home visits. In fact, the home is the most traditional setting for the practice of community health nursing.

BOX 7–8. SETTINGS FOR COMMUNITY HEALTH NURSING

- Government health agency
- Home
- School
- Industry
- Rehabilitation facility
- Correctional institution
- Community disaster site
- Ambulatory health center
- Emergency center
- Nurse-managed clinic
- Hospitals

Trends in Home Care. During the 1980s, the delivery of health care in the home underwent significant changes and expansion. Change was driven by health care cost inflation and the impact of a new federal hospital reimbursement policy (prospective payment) instituted by the Tax Equity and Fiscal Responsibility Act of 1982 (Public Law 97-248). As a result of these factors, hospital stays shortened and clients remained acutely ill on discharge. Thus, a strong demand developed for home health nurses who could care for acutely ill clients in their homes.

Sources of Home Nursing Services. As the demand for home nursing services has grown, so have the number and variety of agencies providing services. In the past, home nursing service was most often provided by voluntary visiting nurse associations funded by welfare or by direct payment, and by public health nursing departments, as a component of government-funded local public health services. Private duty nurses—nurses who contracted directly with clients to render nursing service in the home or hospital—were also available and could be hired from a local registry of independent nurses. But by the early 1980s, the predominance of these sources diminished as other sources rapidly expanded, particularly home care agencies.[55] The introduction of Medicare in 1965 provided payment for services to homebound clients with acute conditions requiring skilled nursing. Over the next 20 years, the number of home care agencies quadrupled.[55] The expansion of hospital-based, and for-profit home care agencies was particularly rapid in the 1980s as a direct response to the growing need for comprehensive services and the economic squeeze that caused hospitals to seek alternative sources of revenue.[55]

Nursing Services Available in the Home. Services available through most home health agencies include skilled nursing services (eg, wound dressing, intravenous infusion management, medication administration, vital signs monitoring, client assessment and client care planning) and personal care services (feeding, bathing, toileting). Physical, occupational, respiratory, and speech therapy services are also available from many agencies, as are social services. Assistance with aspects of household maintenance (housekeeping, shopping, other chores, and transportation) may also be available.

To provide these services, agencies have various types of professional and nonprofessional personnel. Professional and vocational nurses, home health aides, homemakers, therapists, and social workers may all be on staff and available to provide the level of services required by the client's health needs.

Professional nurses employed by home care agencies may or may not be educated for community health practice, which requires special training. When they have a community health background, home care nurses are more likely to share the broad perspectives of community health for health promotion, disease prevention, and health of the family as a unit, and the focus of care is usually expanded to include issues other than acute illness needs.[57] In many home care agencies, it is community health nurses who coordinate comprehensive home health services.

Funding for Home Nursing. Sources of funding for home nursing are similar to those for other types of health care. Third-party payors through a variety of insurance plans, Medicare, Medicaid, city and county programs for low-income residents, and the private payment by the care recipient are all ways in which home care is funded. Funding under insurance plans or under Medicare and Medicaid or other programs may be limited to certain types of care or for limited periods of time.

The Home Visit. A home visit is a professional encounter between nurse and client in the home setting. Home visits are important in community health because they bring nurses into contact with clients in the context of clients' own environment. A home visit occurs in three phases: (1) preparation, (2) the actual visit, and (3) documentation of the visit.

Preparation for the home visit is particularly important. Adequate preparation entails a number of activities on the part of community health nurses. Client referral data are reviewed and possible health problems identified. Nurses consider the totality of the data to identify all types of potential needs—physical, emotional, social, developmental, nutritional, educational, and motivational.

Once potential problems are identified, tentative priorities for resolving them are set. Some problems may be dealt with during the first visit, while other less pressing problems are deferred. Planning for the visit also includes identifying available resources to meet clients' needs and selecting the equipment and supplies needed for the visit.

The next stage is the visit itself. Nurses validate the accuracy of the initial assessment, collect additional data, and together with clients validate problems anticipated and identify other problems that also need to be addressed. Nurse and client exchange ideas on the goals and strategies for problem resolution. As a nurse comes to understand a client's perspective, priorities sometimes require restructuring. During the visit, nurses undertake the direct care required by clients (Fig. 7–7). As the visit concludes, nurse and client evaluate the effectiveness of the interventions to date. Nurses share observations with clients, obtain the clients' point of view, and together they draw a conclusion on what changes are necessary.

Documentation is the last phase of the home visit. In documenting the visit, nurses chart the data obtained from the visit, changes in clients' condition and situation, the actions taken, and clients' response to those actions. Plans for subsequent visits are also included.

Target Groups of Special Concern to Community Health Nurses

Community health nurses deal with a number of special target groups including parents and children, adolescents, older people, employees, the poor and the homeless, migrants, members of subcultural groups, and persons in disaster situations. A **target group** is a group of people with special needs for whom specific health programs are designed.

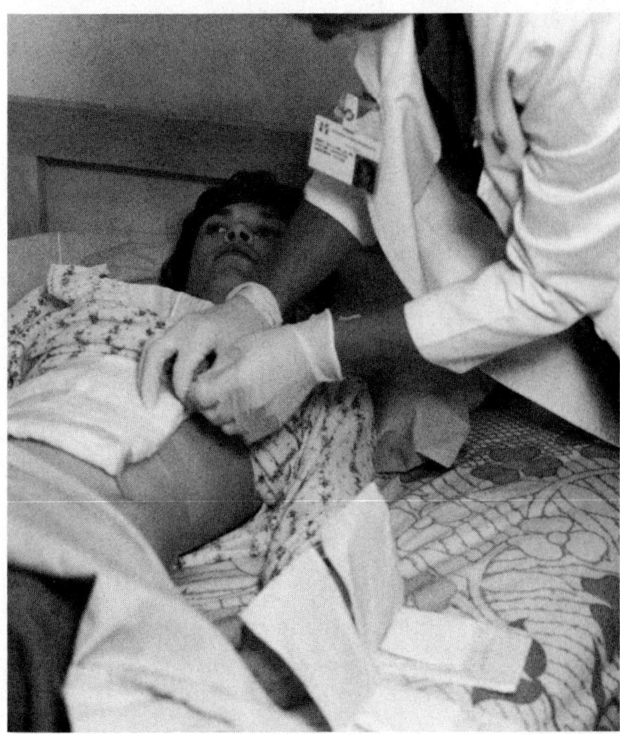

Figure 7–7. During the home visit, the community health nurse validates the accuracy of the initial assessment, collects additional data, identifies new problems, and performs direct care required by the client.

Parents and Children. Community health nurses have a number of objectives in dealing with parents and children. These include supporting the establishment of a stable family by helping new couples adjust to the demands and roles of marriage or cohabitation. Family planning is another major concern.

Parents may need help to prepare for the advent of children. They may need to learn the skills of good parenting as well as those for taking care of the physical needs of children. Parents may also need help in adjusting to the changes that pregnancy and childbirth bring to the family and may benefit from discussing anticipated changes in living arrangements, schedules, and roles.

Most parents benefit from anticipatory guidance in child development. Community health nurses provide information on child behavior expected at specific ages and counsel parents in dealing with developmental crises that occur as children mature. Tips on how to deal with toilet training or teenager rebellion can smooth some of the difficult times in raising children.

Some families need assistance to achieve effective family communication. Community health nurses can help family members develop effective ways of communicating with each other.

Families in which both parents work are increasingly common. These families may need assistance from nurses to identify appropriate child care facilities. Nurses may help by suggesting factors to be considered or by assisting parents to deal with guilt feelings about delegating childcare to others.

Parents may also need help caring for ill children or assistance to obtain a regular source of health care and basic well-child services (Fig. 7–8). Nurses initiate referrals for such services and help families find financial resources from entitlement programs such as Medicaid, that will help them provide adequate health care for family members.

Of particular concern in working with parents and children is the problem of abuse and family violence. In most states, nurses are required by law to report suspected child abuse. However, community health nurses must be alert to signs of abuse in other family members. With respect to abuse, community health nurses function as family support persons. Their primary function is to help the family change the circumstances that contribute to abuse, to develop more appropriate coping mechanisms, and to deal with the physical and psychological consequences of abuse.

Adolescents. Adolescents are a particularly vulnerable client group because of the difficult developmental tasks they face. This makes them particularly susceptible to a variety of health problems.

Major health problems among adolescents are alcoholism and drug abuse, sexually transmitted diseases, pregnancy, and suicide. Community health nurses assist teenagers by providing information on these problems and by counteracting the misinformation garnered from peers and the media. Community health nurses participate in sex education and drug education for adolescents.

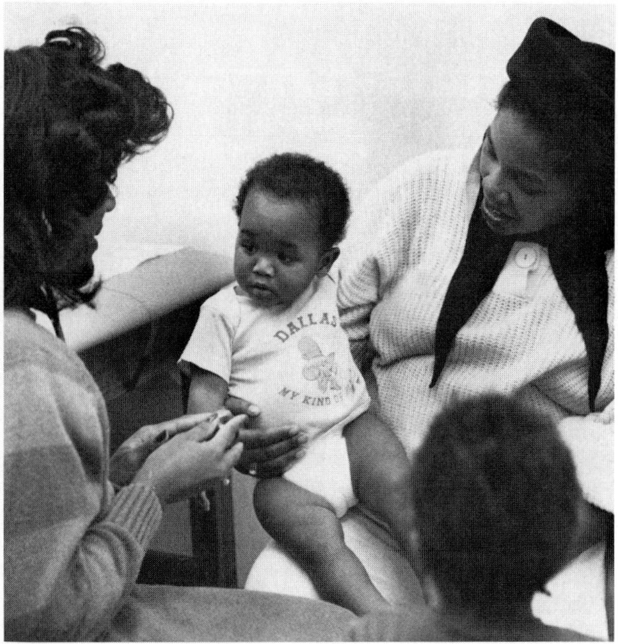

Figure 7–8. Community health nurses help parents and children identify regular sources of health care and provide them with information relating to health promotion. (*Source: Clark MJ.* Nursing in the Community. *Norwalk, CT: Appleton & Lange; 1992.*)

One of the many services that community health nurses provide for adolescents is that of acting as a sounding board for their exploration of themselves and their world. Teenagers need a safe environment in which to reflect upon their feelings and activities. Community health nurses help to provide that environment for teenagers. Adolescents need to be encouraged to discuss important matters with an understanding adult, who in turn encourages them in responsible decision-making by helping them to explore the consequences of alternative actions. Decisions thus reached are much more likely to be carried out than are those imposed from without by parents and other authority figures.

Teenagers also need opportunities to come to grips with their own sexuality and to discover that they are not alone in their fears and feelings. Community health nurses can assist in the formation of teen groups that encourage discussion of such issues and support individuals in their search for identity.

The Elderly. There are growing numbers of elderly persons in the population. The older population has a number of unique needs that often go unmet. In working with older clients, community health nurses address physical health needs created by a variety of chronic health problems as well as by the aging process itself.

Social and economic needs are also of concern. Isolation is a social problem among older adults, frequently caused by the death of a spouse or friends. It may be compounded by the fact that family members may live a great distance away. Community health nurses help older clients to find avenues for social interaction that fit their economic circumstances and personalities (Fig. 7–9).

Nurses also help elderly clients adjust to changes in income and living arrangements. Older people can be assisted with budgeting or referred for financial assistance. There may be a need to work with families to ensure that older members can maintain a desirable level of independence. Families may also need assistance in dealing with the strains of having an older family member living in the home. Areas of concern in such situations include privacy and living space, financial considerations, and incorporation of the elderly person into the life of the family.

Abuse of older persons is of growing concern across the nation, and nurses should be alert to signs of abuse in elderly clients. Abuse may involve physical mistreatment or neglect, psychological abuse, and social isolation. Nurses work with families to identify and deal with factors contributing to abuse. At a societal level, nurses work for laws protecting the elderly and services needed by the abused.

The Poor and the Homeless. Community health nurses provide services to the poor and the homeless. Common health problems encountered in these groups include chronic and communicable disease, mental health prob-

BUILDING NURSING KNOWLEDGE

How Can Nurses Determine the Health Needs of the Elderly in a Community?

Schultz PR, Magilvy JK. Assessing community health needs of elderly populations: Comparison of three strategies. *J Adv Nurs.* 1988; 13:193–202.

In this report, Schultz and Magilvy focused on the methods of assessing the needs of the elderly population, one of which is through community research. Their study incorporated a survey of elderly people from one urban neighborhood, a neighborhood census data analysis, and interviews with elderly residents to learn their ideas on what it is like to live in the community. The aim of the project was "community health diagnosis," a process of identifying health problems in communities or populations for the purpose of preventing those problems through community action.

Findings from the census data showed that at the beginning of one 10-year period, the population in the neighborhood was 25 percent elderly. Twenty-five percent were on social security payments, for a mean income of $140 a month. Over half (63 percent) had finished high school, 65 percent were single, 12 percent widowed, 3 percent separated, and 12 percent divorced. Ninety-three percent rented their housing and 69 percent had lived in the unit 2 years or less. Ten years later, the population was 20 percent elderly. Fewer were on social security (22 percent), with a mean monthly income of $303. Seventy-five percent rented their housing. From the census information, the researchers concluded that the neighborhood had a mobile population of large numbers of elderly single, widowed, and divorced people with fairly low incomes. This information raised relevant questions about the general health of the elderly population, their sources of income, and their access to health services.

The health survey provided some answers with regard to the elderly. It showed that 19 percent reported being ill enough during the past year to require care by someone else; 40 percent needed general health services; 14 percent reported needing home nursing services; and 75 percent used Medicare coverage for health insurance. Interviews were conducted with community leaders and older adults active in community organizations to determine their perceptions of their health, health needs, and services.

The researchers found that there were three distinct groups of elderly, classified by life-style. The first group was people who occupied single rooms, had low incomes, lacked social support, were marginally mentally ill, and were often lonely. The second group consisted of fairly healthy retired people with limited resources, who were able to afford subsidized senior housing, apartments, or their own homes. This group participated in a variety of religious, recreational, and social activities and meal programs. The third group included retired, well, older adults who sought high-quality housing and had a high degree of social support, were interested in community organizations, and took leadership roles. Many were retired professionals.

The researchers were able to determine from their investigation that in general the acute and chronic health problems of older residents in the neighborhood were being met by the traditional health care system and that needed services were available.

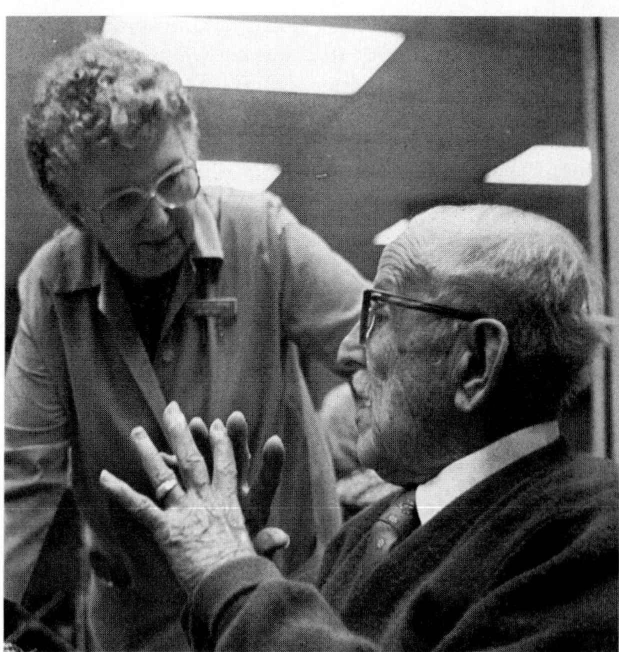

Figure 7–9. Isolation resulting from the death of spouses and friends, and changes in living arrangements, create special needs for the elderly that are recognized and met by community health nurses.

lems, malnutrition, obesity, accidents, and lack of a source of health care.

Community health nurses use three strategies to help meet the health needs of the poor and the homeless. The first is to provide access to health care so often lacking among the poor and homeless. The second major thrust lies in education to promote healthier life-styles. Community health nurses teach these clients how to use the resources available to them to improve their health status. Third, community health nurses endeavor to improve the general social and economic conditions of the poor and homeless by actively working for public policies that address these needs.

SUMMARY

A community is a group of people among whom there is some form of bond and interaction, and who act collectively with respect to common problems. The health of a community is a composite of the health status of its individual members and the ability of the community itself to carry out its designated functions.

Efforts to maintain and improve health occur at any of three levels of prevention. Primary prevention is aimed at preventing the occurrence of health problems, while secondary prevention is directed toward timely resolution of a problem once it has occurred. Tertiary prevention seeks to prevent lasting consequences of the problem and to prevent its recurrence.

Community health professionals, including nurses,

employ the concepts of epidemiology and the epidemiological method in the effort to promote health and prevent disease. The epidemiological method is used to investigate factors involved in the development of health problems and to design control strategies that will prevent or eliminate these problems. Health statistics, vital statistics, demographic statistics, and utilization statistics are helpful tools in community health decision-making. Nurses and other community health professionals use a variety of statistical information in identifying the needs of population groups and in determining factors involved in health problems.

Several general categories of health problems are of concern to community health professionals. These include communicable and chronic disease, accidents, substance abuse, and violence.

Community health nursing looks at health and illness from a community perspective, and consequently its primary focus is on health promotion and disease prevention for groups of people in the community and for the community at large. Care is provided to individuals, families, and other groups, but the ultimate aim is always the improvement of the health of the total population.

Community health nurses engage in primary, secondary, and tertiary preventive measures to promote health. In doing so, they engage in a variety of role functions. These roles include client-oriented roles, delivery-oriented roles, community-oriented roles, and general roles that influence performance of other categories of functions.

Community health nursing takes place in a variety of settings, such as schools, clinics, homes, business and industry, prisons, and hospitals or other acute health care agencies that have an objective to promote health as well as to relieve illness. Community health nurses may also be actively involved in preparing for and responding to disaster.

While the focus of community health nursing is on the health of the total population, there are several subgroups within the population that are of particular concern to community health nurses. These target groups include parents and children, adolescents, the elderly, and the poor and homeless.

Community health nurses play an important role in maintaining and improving the health of the community. They are actively involved in the health promotion and prevention of community health problems, an endeavor that requires specific knowledge of the factors that affect health in the community.

REFERENCES

1. Von Bertalanffy L. *General System Theory.* New York: Braziller; 1968.
2. Laszlo E. *The Systems View of the World.* New York: Braziller; 1972.
3. Last J. Epidemiology and health information. In: Last J, ed. *Public Health and Preventive Medicine.* 13th ed. Norwalk, CT: Appleton & Lange; 1991; 9–74.
4. Syme SL. Social determinants of health and disease. In: Last J, ed. *Public Health and Preventive Medicine.* 13th ed. Norwalk, CT: Appleton & Lange; 1991; 953–970.
5. Mechanic D. Health and illness behavior. In: Last J, ed. *Public Health and Preventive Medicine.* 13th ed. Norwalk, CT: Appleton & Lange; 1991; 971–981.
6. McKusick VA. *Mendelian Inheritance in Man.* 9th ed. Baltimore: Johns Hopkins University Press; 1990.
7. Spicker SF, Bondeson WB, Englehardt HT. *The Contraceptive Ethos.* Boston: Reidel; 1987.
8. Cates W, Holmes KK. Sexually transmitted diseases. In: Last J, ed. *Public Health and Preventive Medicine.* 13th ed. Norwalk, CT: Appleton & Lange; 1991; 257–281.
9. Commoner B. *The Closing Circle: Nature, Man, and Technology.* New York: Knopf; 1971.
10. Monath TP, Johnson KM. Diseases transmitted primarily by anthropod vectors. In: Last J, ed. *Public Health and Preventive Medicine.* 13th ed. Norwalk, CT: Appleton & Lange; 1991; 323–389.
11. Fielding JE. Smoking: Health effects and control. In: Last J, ed. *Public Health and Preventive Medicine.* 13th ed. Norwalk, CT: Appleton & Lange; 1991; 999–1033.
12. Summary of Notifiable Diseases: United States, 1987. *MMWR.* 1988; 36:54.
13. Pneumonia and influenza mortality on the increase. *Stat Bull.* 1987; April-June:10–16.
14. Measles—Los Angeles County, California, 1988. *MMWR.*1989; 38:49–57.
15. Progress toward achieving the national 1990 objectives for sexually transmitted diseases. *MMWR.* 1987; 36:173–175.
16. HIV prevalence estimates and AIDS case projections for the United States. *MMWR.* 1990; 39(RR-16):1–16.
17. Mortality attributable to HIV infection/AIDS—U.S., 1991–1990. *MMWR.* 1991; 40(3):41–44.
18. Scitovksy AA, Rice DP. Estimates of the direct costs of acquired immunodeficiency syndrome in the United States, 1985, 1986, and 1991. *Pub Health Rep.* 1987; 102:5–17.
19. The Surgeon General's 1990 report on the health benefits of smoking cessation: Executive summary. *MMWR.* 1990; 39(RR-12):2–12.
20. Advancements in meeting the 1990 hypertension objectives. *MMWR.* 1987; 36:144–151.
21. Behavioral Risk Factor Surveillance, 1988. *MMWR.* 1990; 39(SS-2):1–6.
22. Mortality patterns—United States, 1987. *MMWR.* 1990; 39(12): 193–196, 201.
23. American Heart Association. 1991 Heart and Stroke Facts. Dallas: American Heart Association; 1991.
24. Years of potential lives lost before ages 65 and 85—United States, 1987 and 1988. *MMWR.* 1990; 39(2):20–22.
25. *Statistical Abstract of the United States.* 107th ed. Washington, DC: US Department of Commerce; 1987.
26. Alcohol-related mortality and years of potential life lost—United States, 1987. *MMWR.* 1990; 39(11):173–178.
27. Unintentional ingestions of prescription drugs in children under five years old. *MMWR.* 1987; 36:124–126.
28. Centers for Disease Control. Deaths from falls, 1978–1984. In: CDC Surveillance Summaries, February. *MMWR.* 1988; 37:21.
29. Fatal injuries to children—United States, 1986. *MMWR.* 1990; 39(26):442–450.
30. Lessons in violence. *US News & World Report.* 1989; 106:84.
31. Fatal injuries to children—1986. *MMWR.* 1990; 39(26):442–450.
32. Family and other intimate assaults. *MMWR.* 1990; 39(31):525–529.
33. Alcohol-related mortality and years of potential life lost—United States, 1987. *MMWR.* 1990; 39(11):173–175.

34. Brubaker BH. Health promotion: A linguistic analysis. *Adv Nurs Sci.* 1983; 5:1–14.
35. Pender NJ. *Health Promotion in Nursing Practice.* 2nd ed. Norwalk, CT: Appleton & Lange; 1987.
36. Shamansky SL, Clausen CL. Levels of prevention: Examination of the concept. *Nurs Outlook.* 1980; 28:104–108.
37. Smith DL. Health promotion for older adults. *Health Values.* 1988; 12:46–51.
38. Fowles DG. *A Profile of Older Americans: 1989.* Washington DC: Administration on Aging, U.S. Department of Health and Human Services; 1989:2.
39. US Public Health Service. *Healthy People: The Surgeon General's Report on Health Promotion and Disease Prevention.* Washington: US Department of Health, Education, and Welfare: (PHS) 79-55071; 1979.
40. US Public Health Service. *Promoting Health/Preventing Disease: Objectives for the Nation.* Washington: US Department of Health and Human Services; 1980.
41. Eddy JM, Gold RS, Zimmerli WH. Evaluation of worksite health enhancement programs. *Health Values.* 1989; 13:3–9.
42. Miller JT. Wellness programs through the Church: Available alternative for health education. *Health Values.* 1987; 11:3–6.
43. US Public Health Service. *Health Maintenance Organizations: Requirements for a Health Maintenance Organization.* Washington: US Department of Health and Human Services, Federal Register 45:72524; 1980.
44. Wilson SL, Rudmann SV, Snyder JR. Health educators in HMOs: A study of utilization and effectiveness. *Health Values.* 1989; 13:9–14.
45. American Nurses' Association. *Environmental Assessment: Factors Affecting Long-Range Planning for Nursing and Health Care.* Kansas City, MO: ANA; 1985.
46. Wilson BRA, Wagner DI. Fitness and health promotion in Japan. *Health Values.* 1990; 14:27–31.
47. Trends in mortality from cirrhosis and alcoholism—United States, 1945–1984. *MMWR.* 1986; 35:703–704.
48. Fiore M, Novotny T, Pierce JP. Trends in cigarette smoking in the United States: The changing influence of gender and race. *JAMA.* 1989; 261:49–55.
49. Green LW, Kreuter MW, Deeds SC. *Health Education Planning: A Diagnostic Approach.* Palo Alto, CA: Mayfield; 1980.
50. Nemeck MA. Health beliefs and breast self-examination among black women. *Health Values.* 1990; 14:41–52.
51. Sevel F. Designing effective health promotion and disease prevention programs: A course model. *Health Values.* 1990; 14:32–37.
52. Fuchs JA. Planning for community health promotion: A rural example. *Health Values.* 1988; 12:3–8.
53. Nelson CF, Stoddard RP, Watkins NB. *Planned Approach to Community Health.* Atlanta: Centers for Disease Control, Division of Health Education; 1985.
54. Williams DM. Political theory and individualistic health promotion. *Adv Nurs Sci.* 1989; 12:14–25.
55. Burbach CA, Brown BE. Community health and home health nursing: Keeping the concepts clear. *Nurs Health Care.* 1988; Feb:97–100.
56. Moccia P. Shaping a human agenda for the nineties. *Nurs Health Care.* 1989; Jan:15–17.
57. Public Health Nursing Section of the American Public Health Association. The definition and role of public health nursing in the delivery of health care. Washington: APHA; 1980.
58. Clark MJ. *Nursing in the Community.* Norwalk, CT: Appleton & Lange; 1992.

BIBLIOGRAPHY

American Nurses' Association. *Standards of Community Health Nursing Practice.* Kansas City, MO: ANA; 1986.

Brandt EN, Mayer WN, Mason JO, et al. Designing a national disaster medical system. *Pub Health Rep.* 1985; 100:455–461.

Cervantes NN, Kaulukukui M, Poulson J, Kaufman H. Diverting the mentally ill from a county jail. *Am J Pub Health.* 1987; 77:367–368.

Chronic disease reports: Mortality trends—United States, 1979–1986. *MMWR.* 1989; 38:189–193.

Cleary PD, et al. Sociodemographic and behavioral characteristics of HIV antibody-positive blood donors. *Am J Pub Health.* 1988; 78:853–957.

Condoms for prevention of sexually transmitted diseases. *MMWR.* 1988; 37:133–137.

DiClemente RJ, Boyer CB, Morales ES. Minorities and AIDS: Knowledge, attitudes, and misconceptions among black and Latino adolescents. *Am J Pub Health.* 1988; 78:55–57.

Feldblum PJ, Fortney JA. Condoms, spermicides, and the transmission of human immunodeficiency virus: A review of the literature. *Am J Pub Health.* 1988; 78:52–54.

Hutt A. What exactly is the "team approach"? *Midwife, Health Vis, Comm Health Nurse.* 1986; 22:340–342.

Lesser AJ. The origin and development of maternal and child health programs in the United States. *Am J Pub Health.* 1985; 75:590–598.

MacKensie JA. Efficient home care for today's society. *Nurs Health Care.* 1985; 6:37–40.

Mason JO, Koplan JP, Layde PM. The prevention and control of chronic diseases: Reducing unnecessary deaths and disability. *Pub Health Rep.* 1987; 102:17–20.

NIOSH recommendations for occupational safety and health standards. *MMWR.* 1986; 35:1S.

Progress toward achieving the national 1990 objectives for injury prevention and control. *MMWR.* 1988; 37:138.

Purtilo RB. Ethical issues in teamwork: The context of rehabilitation. *Arch Phys Med Rehabil.* 1988; 69:318–322.

Roberts DE, Heinrich J. Public health nursing comes of age. *Am J Pub Health.* 1985; 75:1162–1172.

Schoenborn CA, Stephens T. Health promotion in the United States and Canada: Smoking, exercise, and other health related behaviors. *Am J Pub Health.* 1988; 78:983–985.

Traumatic occupational fatalities. *MMWR.* 1987; 36:461.

US Department of Health and Human Services. *Consensus Conference on the Essentials of Public Health Nursing Practice and Education.* Rockville, MD: Bureau of Health Professions, Division of Nursing; 1985.

US Department of Health and Human Services. *Setting Nationwide Objectives in Disease Prevention and Health Promotion: The United States Experience.* Washington: US Government Printing Office; 1987.

US Department of Health and Human Services. *The 1988 Report of the Joint National Committee on Detection, Evaluation, and Treatment of High Blood Pressure.* Washington: US Public Health Service; 1988.

Waller AE, Baker SP, Szocka A. Childhood injury deaths: National analysis and geographic variations. *Am J Pub Health.* 1989; 79: 310–315.

Whitman D. America's hidden poor. *U.S. News & World Report.* January 11, 1988; 106:18–24.

Wing S, Casper M, Riggan W, et al. Socioenvironmental characteristics associated with the onset of decline of ischemic heart disease mortality. *Am J Pub Health.* 1988; 78:923–926.

CHAPTER 8

Family Health

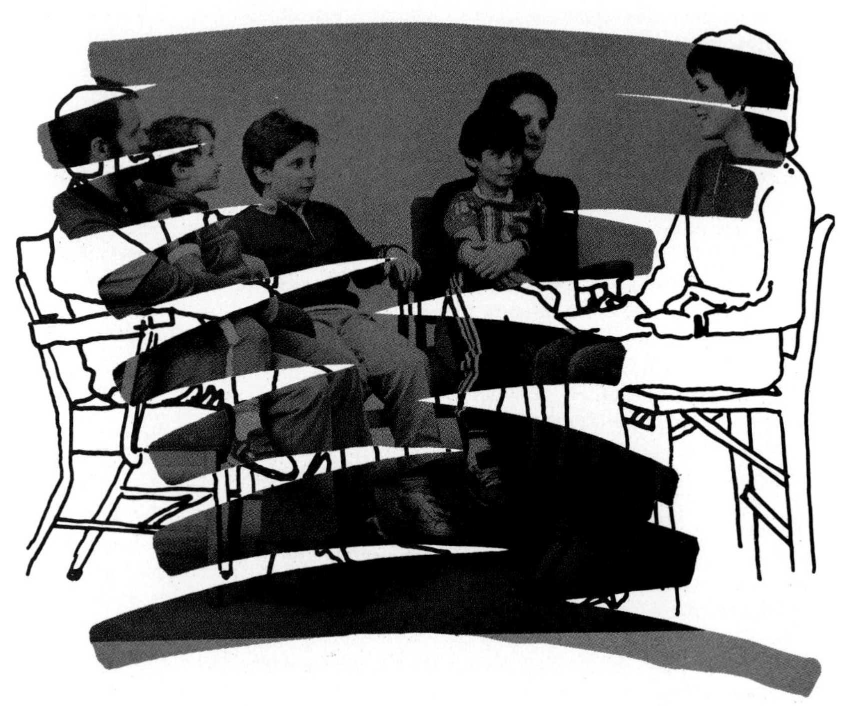

Behavioral Objectives

Upon completion of this chapter, the student will be able to:

1. Discuss the importance of the family in nursing.
2. Describe the relationship between the health of the individual and the health of the family.
3. Define the family in broad terms and as a health care unit.
4. List and describe various family forms.
5. Describe the structural and functional elements of the family.
6. List the eight stages of Duvall's family life cycle and discuss the developmental tasks involved in each stage.
7. Discuss crisis within a family and identify examples of developmental and situational crises experienced by families.
8. Describe the components of family assessment.
9. Discuss the role of family systems and self-care theories in collaborating with families.
10. Describe the nurse's role in comprehensive care of the family.

KEY TERMS

affective function
blended family
communal family
comprehensive family care
crisis
extended family
family
family assessment
family function
family life cycle
family of origin
family of procreation
family power structure
family structure
family value system
gay or lesbian family
maturational crisis
nuclear family
plural family
reproductive function
role
role complementarity
role set
single-parent family
situational crisis
socialization and social placement function

Most people grow and develop as part of a family and remain as part of some type of family throughout their lives. Despite rising divorce rates and the resultant increase in the number of single-parent and blended families, the family unit continues to survive and surmount the predictions of its demise. The family is the basic unit in our society. It is the primary socializing agent; it influences its members more than any other societal unit. All individuals learn values, health beliefs, and behaviors within a family context. The family is the system within which members must interpret changing societal values and norms. Frequently, the family serves as a buffer between its members and the stresses of modern day life. It is ideally a "port in the storm," where each member is accepted for his or her uniqueness.

Since the time of Florence Nightingale,[1] nurses instructed families in their homes about hygiene and child care. Nightingale recognized the importance of family participation in maintaining health and treating illness. Today, schools of nursing offer graduate programs in family nursing, nursing symposia are convened on both illness and health promotion in families, and recent nursing literature includes a review of both family research and family nursing research.

The entire family is often a nursing client.[2,3] Some practitioners view the family, not its members, as the sole unit of service.[4] In fact, scientific theory supports the view that illness in one family member is symptomatic of a disorder within the total family. Thus, interventions with one member are often aimed at creating change in the entire family. Family-centered nursing focuses on both the individual and the family.[5] Both must be assessed in order to assist the family and its members to achieve their ultimate health potential.

Collaboration as a client care approach is an effective way of working with clients and families to assist them with their health problems. The nurses' special knowledge of the family as a social unit can help in the effort to define family health needs and find strategies to achieve health. The family, in turn, can assist the nurse to better understand its patterns and health requirements. This chapter focuses on the relationship between the family and the health of its members and describes the implications of this relationship for the role of the nurse.

FAMILY FORMS

Definitions of Family

Today many different family forms fulfill the major family functions. Therefore, a contemporary definition of family that includes all family forms is needed. Two broad definitions of **family** are:

1. Two or more people who are emotionally involved with each other and live in close geographical proximity.[5]
2. A small social system made up of individuals related to each other by reason of strong reciprocal affection and loyalties, and comprising a permanent household (or cluster of households) that persists over years.[6]

Essential elements in these definitions include attachment and loyalty, physical proximity, two or more persons, and an enduring quality that persists over time. Situational factors sometimes alter these elements; for example, military families may be separated by distant assignments. Broad definitions are important, because people tend to define their families in unique ways and to act on these definitions. Nurses must determine their clients' definitions of family if they are to engage in collaboration with clients. Nurses may do this through observation and questioning, such as asking clients directly who they consider to be family, or observing with whom clients live, spend time, and share confidences. Validating observations with clients gives nurses valuable information about clients' perceptions of family. Nurses who are beginning their practice must be aware that they may not share clients' perceptions of family. Clients' perceptions, however, supersede nurses' perceptions in determining nursing actions. A nurse who wishes to mobilize a client's family as a resource in planning nursing care must begin with understanding the family's structure and functions.

IMPLICATIONS FOR NURSE–CLIENT COLLABORATION

Working With Families

Collaboration as a client care approach is an effective way of working with clients and families to assist them with their health problems. The nurse's special knowledge of the family as a social unit can help in the effort to define family health care needs and find strategies to achieve health. The family, in turn, can assist the nurse to better understand its patterns and health care requirements.

Contemporary family life takes many forms. During the last part of the 20th century, the "traditional" family of provider husband, homemaker wife, and two or three children makes up only a small minority of all families. Married-couple families with their own children under 18 accounted for 27 percent of households in 1988, down from 40 percent of all households in 1970.[7] There are a number of patterns of relationships that, as perceived by individuals, constitute their family form. These include married couples without children, single-parent families, and couples who have children but are not married, and couples who neither marry nor have children. They also include people who form blended families after death or divorce. There are also homosexual unions and communal families that meet the broad definitions of family just given.

Some common terms used when discussing family forms are family of origin and family of procreation. Each person has a **family of origin**, the family into which an individual is born or adopted and socialized; and most have a **family of procreation**, the family created by marriage, childbearing, and childrearing. In addition, there are several types of family forms, as discussed in the following sections (Box 8–1).

Types of Family Forms

Nuclear Family. The **nuclear family** is usually considered to be the traditional family form composed of mother, father, and children by birth or adoption. This family form is considered to be the family of origin for the children and the family of procreation for the parents. However, many couples today do not plan to include reproduction as a part of their family function. They, along with couples unable to have children, are nevertheless nuclear families.

Although the nuclear family is not necessarily the dominant family form today, it is frequently considered the ideal form by society. Nurses need to be sensitive to their clients' concepts of "ideal" family form, because families involved in nontraditional forms may experience some sense of loss of this societal ideal.

BOX 8–1. TYPES OF FAMILY FORMS

Nuclear Family: Husband, wife and children by birth or adoption.
Extended Family: Close relatives of a nuclear family, such as grandparents, uncles, aunts, and cousins.
Single-parent Family: One parent of either sex and a child or children.
Blended Family: Husband, wife, and children of either or both by previous marriages, plus children they produce.
Gay or Lesbian Family: Two parents of the same sex with or without children.
Communal Family: Group of unrelated adults and children committed to living as a family.
Plural Family: Husband, wives and their collective children by birth or adoption.

Extended Family. The **extended family** includes close relatives such as grandparents, aunts, uncles, cousins, and various other kinfolk who may, but do not necessarily, live with the family. Historically, couples shared living expenses with parents, siblings, and other close relatives. Children reared by several generations had the opportunity to pattern their behavior after several different role models. Presently, the need to move to seek employment or educational opportunities often separates extended families by hundreds or even thousands of miles. Advances in communication and transportation have served, however, to strengthen the special affection and power associated with kinship ties. Also, many families today supplement kinship ties by including friends and neighbors in their current environments as part of their "adopted" extended families. Nurses should assess the importance of extended family in clients' lives, as it may be an important resource during health and illness.

Single-parent Family. A **single-parent family** consists of one parent, either father or mother, and one or more children. Such arrangements usually result from death, divorce, or desertion of one parent. There are also increasing numbers of single-parent adoptions, particularly of older, foreign, or "special-need" children. Many single-parent families are also headed by teenage girls or women who have never been married. Finances, day-care, and problems of loneliness in our couple-oriented society are examples of common functional problems for these families. Single parents who receive help and support from their extended families and the community are more likely to be successful at the complex economic and personal challenges involved in parenting without a partner's assistance while trying simultaneously to achieve personal satisfaction in other aspects of life.

BUILDING NURSING KNOWLEDGE

How Do Different Family Types Compare in Their Ability to Cope With the Stress of Having a Handicapped Child?

McCubbin A. Family stress and family strengths: A comparison of single- and two-parent families with handicapped children. *Res Nurs Health.* 1989; 12:101–110.

Research has documented the stresses and hardships faced by families that have a handicapped child. With the rising divorce rates, the number of single-parent families with handicapped children may increase. Are single-parent families able to cope?

Using a family stress model, McCubbin studied 27 single-parent families and 27 two-parent families whose children had handicaps of similar severity. The researcher used four questionnaires to measure the variables in the study, one each for family stressors, family resources, parental coping, and family cohesion.

Contrary to expectations, McCubbin failed to find a significant difference in family stress between the single-parent and two-parent families. There were also no significant differences in family cohesion and resources. Single-parent families, however, were more adaptable than two-parent families and were more flexible in family rules, power structure, and role relationships and better able to alter their patterns to the needs of the situation.

Two areas of vulnerability in single-parent families were found: financial well-being and the mother's coping. Mothers in these families had more difficulty facilitating family togetherness, unity, and positive outlook. However, there was evidence that single mothers develop and use support networks. McCubbin concluded that the health of children in single-parent families is not compromised, although resources are needed to aid families financially and provide other sources of support.

Blended Family. The **blended family**, also referred to as a stepfamily or reconstituted family, consists of husband and wife, either or both of whom have been married before and bring one or more children from the previous marriage to the present family. Experts in family life agree that the manner in which the previous marriage ended is an important determinant of how the relations between the stepparent and stepchildren will develop. For example, if the previous marriage ended with a great deal of disagreement between the couple, children may experience ambivalence toward the missing parent. It is then difficult for the child to form affectional bonds with the new parent without experiencing guilty feelings. Some of the issues that blended families must negotiate include (1) change in the family structure, (2) unrealistic expectations on the part of parents and children regarding how family members will behave, (3) a feeling of being unwanted by all those involved, (4) the creation of many legal questions regarding adoption, and (5) sensitive and ambivalent feelings concerning surname use.[8]

Gay or Lesbian Family. A **gay or lesbian family** is formed by two adults of the same sex who share an intimate relationship with each other and who live together with or without children. Because of the minority status of gay and lesbian families, they frequently experience some of the same problems of other minority groups, such as stress, disapproval, and alienation. Some are also dealing with traumatic divorces or separations. In addition, the adult members may experience sexual role problems in relation to role enactment and adoption. For example, a woman involved in a lesbian relationship may be taking on a role that is different from the one she enacted in her previous husband–wife relationship. Nurses need to be sensitive to all of these families' concerns. Like other families, gay and lesbian families with children face many of the same developmental issues related to childrearing that are discussed next in the section on developmental stages.

Communal Family Arrangements. The **communal family** is made up of a group of unrelated adults and their children who make a commitment to each other to live together in a simulated family form. Communal family arrangements were at their peak during the 1960s and 1970s and range from formal to informal. In some ways these arrangements possess some of the attributes of the extended family; however, they differ in that they are frequently countercultural and are perceived as a rejection of more common family forms.

Initially the emphasis of childrearing is on the mother and infant, but eventually, as the child grows, the focus moves to building relationships with other adults. In loosely formed groups with members continually joining and leaving, it is difficult for a child to build a strong relationship with adults other than the mother.

Plural Family Arrangements. A **plural** (or polygamist) **family** is made up of a man, his wives, and their collective children. All family members may reside within one home or share contiguous, but separate homes. Although plural families are not legal in the United States, recent attention to the practice of polygamy in Utah has resulted in efforts by the Utah chapter of the American Civil Liberties Union to legalize polygamy in that state.[9] Moreover, a March, 1991, decision by the Utah Supreme Court struck down a trial court's ruling that a polygamist couple could not adopt a child because of their marital status.[9] It is unlikely, however, that this family form will become prevalent outside Utah, even if it is legalized there. Its proponents claim that it meets all of the needs of its members that prompt individuals to join in other family forms, while reducing the stress associated with the multiple responsibilities of managing career, family, and personal needs that face adults in many families presently. The almost uniformly negative reaction of society to polygamy is likely to create stress among those who practice it. Nurses who care for members of polygamous families need sensitivity and openness, remembering that they must defer making personal judgments and recognize families' perceptions of their own needs must be considered primary.

FAMILY STRUCTURE AND FUNCTION

Two approaches for understanding the family are the structural-functional and developmental approaches. These approaches help the beginning student to view the family from two different perspectives. The structural-functional approach looks at the arrangement of the parts that make up the family as a whole and the function the family carries out for society and for its members. The developmental approach looks at the family and its progress through normal developmental periods from its establishment in marriage through the death of one or both spouses.

Family Structure

Family structure refers to the family organization and the relationships between its members. The elements of family structure include roles, value systems, communication patterns, and power structure.[5]

Roles. Individuals within the family occupy many positions. A **role** is a set of behaviors, attitudes, beliefs, principles, and values that characterize the occupant of a given social position or status.[6] For example, "mother" is a family role that in traditional families carries expectations of child care, child socialization, housekeeper, and so forth.

A role prescribes a set of cultural expectations and gives direction to the behavior of the individual in certain situations (Fig. 8–1). Roles are understood through the lens of the family's sociocultural orientation. A given role, such as "mother" or "father," differs depending on the family's sociocultural status. For example, childrearing is becoming a shared parental role in middle-class families, but it is predominantly associated with the maternal role in working-class families. One can acquire roles in several different ways:

1. They can be ascribed based on age, sex, or birth order (eg, youngest child, mother).
2. They can be achieved by personal choice or accomplishment (eg, wife, parent, architect).
3. They can serve a special purpose (meeting a specific need; managing a problem).
4. They can be assumed through play-acting or pretense.[6]

People have many different roles in varied situations. Roles may be associated with an occupation or social position (son, lawyer, church deacon). Frequently they are reciprocal, or paired (mother–daughter, husband–wife). Alternatively, they may be part of a **role set**, a group of roles that are related to each other (eg, mother–father–daughter). One cannot look at a role in isolation, since all persons in a set are necessary for each to function. Roles change as individuals move in and out of social situations. An individ-

BUILDING NURSING KNOWLEDGE

What Is the Impact of Illness on Family Structure?

Griffith L, Griffith E. Structural family therapy in chronic illness. *Psychosomatics.* 1987; 28:202–205.

Chronic illness—illness in which there is no expectation that problems will disappear—can have a major impact on family structure. Chronic illness may change the enduring interaction patterns that are part of the family's constant relationships. Griffith and Griffith studied a series of families struggling to cope with chronic illness.

The authors found that chronic illness can change the boundaries between subunits within the family—for instance, between parents and children. Changes in boundaries affect the privacy of family members and the effectiveness of their communication. The power structure within the family can be affected by chronic illness. Family power hierarchies may become inverted, with children by virtue of their illness symptoms gaining control over parents. This situation can have a maladaptive effect on the family. Alliances may form between members. The primary caretaker may form special bonds with the ill member, and this can serve to control other facets of the family's life. The family's achievement of developmental tasks may be complicated by chronic illness.

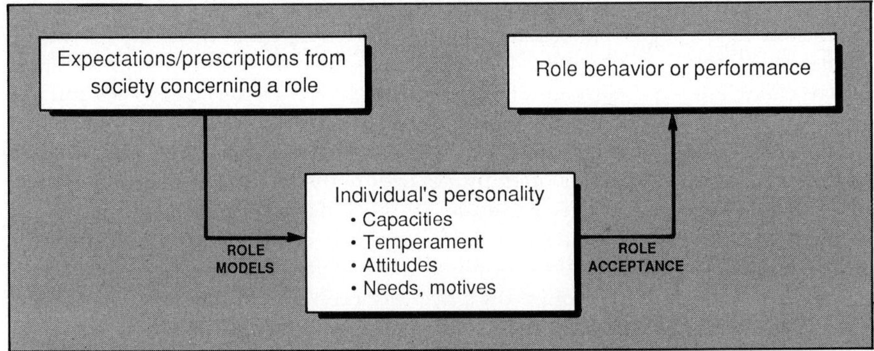

Figure 8–1. Development of role behavior. (*Source: Adapted from Friedman MM.* Family Nursing: Theory and Assessment. *2nd ed. Norwalk, CT: Appleton-Century-Crofts, 1986; 159.*)

ual may be a leader in one community group and a follower in another.

Roles are dynamic and often balance or complement one another. All participants in a role set have perceptions and role expectations of themselves and of all other people in the set. When the performance of one member of the set matches the expectations of the other members, **role complementarity** exists and family equilibrium is maintained. However, dissimilarity in expectations or performance of family roles—whether due to culture, social class or individual differences—yields noncomplementarity of roles and therefore imbalance and family conflict. For example, a wife who goes to work outside the home may expect her husband to take on new roles such as child care and household maintenance. If the husband does not perceive these roles as appropriate for him, noncomplementarity of roles would cause a disturbance in the equilibrium of the entire family. It would be important in this situation for both spouses to discuss their perceptions and expectations in order to resolve this family conflict.

Value Systems. The **family value system** refers to the conscious and unconscious ideas, attitudes, and beliefs by which family members are bound together in a common culture. Values influence the way roles are allocated and how each family member performs his or her role. For example, a father who values close relationships with his children will make time to read bedtime stories and listen to them report their daily activities.

Family values also determine how all members of the family assess their own degrees of wellness or illness. Values regarding preventive health care also determine health behavior in family members. Individuals whose parents did not have regular physical and dental examinations and who were not taught the value of frequent checkups are not likely to have them. Children whose parents go to work when they are ill are unlikely to value early treatment for signs of illness. Good nutrition is another family value that will determine the future health behavior of family members. Children who are provided with nutritious foods and healthful snacks are likely to prefer these foods in their adult lives.

Communication Patterns. Effective communication within a family is important for it to achieve its purpose as a primary socializing agent. Clear communication in families exists when what members say accurately reflects their feelings. As discussed in Chapter 14, communication involves sending and receiving messages, expressing feelings, expressing power, and resolving conflicts. Analysis of interaction within a family focuses on aspects of family communication that are functional and growth producing and those that are dysfunctional and growth inhibiting. After analyzing family interaction patterns, a nurse can point out to family members inconsistencies between observed behaviors and verbal messages, as well as examples of effective communication.

Value systems, socioeconomic situation, and ethnicity significantly influence the family's communication patterns. Families from different economic, ethnic, and racial backgrounds communicate differently within the family and within the larger society. For example, families from Caribbean countries communicate their likes and dislikes for others' behavior very directly. Within the culture and family this type of communication is understood, but in North American society it may be viewed as rude and insensitive. Families whose members come from different cultural backgrounds are becoming more common in today's society. This situation can complicate communication within the family itself, as well as influence the way individual members communicate with others. There may be a blending of cultural communication styles with a resulting pattern that is unique. Nurses must be sensitive to a family's cultural orientation to avoid potential misinterpretation of communication patterns, but must also avoid assuming that communication will be determined solely by culture.

Power Structure. Power is a dimension of the family system. The **family power structure** is the ability of one family member to influence the behavior of another.

Power influences decision-making in families. For example, if the mother is the most influential member of the family, the children's career choices may be shaped by her expectations. In assessing a family, it is important for nurses to determine with whom the power resides concerning particular issues, since this has implications for the health decisions the family will make. For example, among Hispanic families, men generally have the most power to make family decisions. Therefore, choices regarding type of health care provider and health care facility would probably be made by a male family member. As with communication, culture is not the sole determinant of family power structure. Exposure to other cultures and other values concerning relationships may alter traditional power relationships in families. Moreover, power in families may be issue related, rather than absolute. For example, one family member may have the strongest decision-making power regarding finances, another regarding health care decisions.

Family Function

Family function refers to what the family does; for example, how the family protects its members from stresses of modern day life. What the family does is based on structural elements: roles, values, communication patterns, and power.[5] Family functions are outcomes of the family structure, or how the family is organized. Family functions are not just the tasks performed by the family members, but the consequences that a family's interrelated motives and subsequent behaviors have on the family as a totality.[6] For example, the feelings of affection and care that each member has for another affect the family as a unit. These functions are both manifest (consequences intended by the family, such as the mother returning to college for a degree) and latent (consequences unintended but nonetheless beneficial, such as the children becoming more independent and assuming responsibility for household chores previously done by the mother). Families may be said to have five functions, which serve various purposes for the family members, the family unit, and the society (Table 8–1).

Affective Function. The **affective function** is focused on meeting the needs of family members for affection and understanding. It is central both to the establishment of the family through the marital union as well as the continuance of the family unit.[5] The family must meet the affectional needs of its members to maintain family integrity. These socio-emotional needs include building self-esteem and morale, as well as creating a loving environment in which members are nurtured and feel secure. The affective function is often influenced by the family's socioeconomic conditions. For example, more affluent families have the luxury of placing greater emphasis on companionship and love, while poorer families must place greater emphasis on work to acquire the physical necessities of life.

Socialization and Social Placement Function. The **socialization and social placement function** of the family is the process by which the child learns attitudes, behaviors, skills, and the interpretation of social norms from significant others. Social placement refers to the conferring of status; that is, the socialization of the child into the family's social class and the instillation of relevant aspirations and values.[5] The family provides learning experiences for its members so that they can function effectively both within the family and in the larger society. In the family, children learn language, roles, and understanding of right and wrong. The individual's sexual role patterning and development of initiative and creativity are also part of the socialization process.[5] In today's society, the socialization function is shared more and more with schools and child-care facilities because of the increasingly common need for both parents to work to meet the family economic function.

Reproductive Function. The **reproductive function** is the process by which the family perpetuates itself. Reproduction is a basic function of the family, although it is no longer limited to nuclear families in our society. There are many single-parent families and many pregnancies outside of marriage, especially among teenagers. Couples whose reproductive ability is complicated by physical and social barriers may seek solutions to accomplish this function through other means such as adoption, artificial insemina-

TABLE 8–1. FAMILY FUNCTIONS

Function	Definition	Behavioral Examples
Affective	Stabilizing adult personalities and meeting the psychological needs of the family.	Actively listening to a teenager's concerns.
Socialization and social placement	Preparing children for their expected role in society and helping them to become productive societal members. Instilling family's value system.	Involving children in community projects that assist the poor or homeless.
Reproductive	Continuing family lines and providing future citizens.	Pregnancy and childbearing.
Economic	Providing financial resources to meet the family needs and allocating them wisely.	Budgeting for effective use of finances.
Health care	Providing health care and physical necessities such as food and housing.	Providing nutritional meals for the family.

IMPLICATIONS FOR NURSE–CLIENT COLLABORATION

The Health Care Function

The health care of the family is significantly related to family structure and function. Health beliefs and values are related to the family's level of knowledge about health and illness and to what is considered normal or usual within the socioeconomic or cultural group. Family deterioration is often related to poor health of family members. The nurse may be able to help the family with an ill member to prevent further disruption of family functioning, by assisting them to clarify their values and roles and by working with them to improve their communication skills and modify their roles if necessary.

tion, and the use of surrogate parents. Teaching about safe, effective contraception to assist couples to determine the timing of family expansion is one way nurses may facilitate this family function. It is worth noting that not all couples today accept the reproductive function as a basic responsibility or reason for creating a relationship. It is becoming more common for couples to delay or permanently defer reproduction.

Economic Function. The economic function refers to the provision and allocation of sufficient material resources to meet the family's needs for food, clothing, shelter, and health care. Nurses are often involved in helping families to find resources for healthful living when they are poor or unemployed,[5] such as by assisting families to apply for food stamps or make contact with community resources for other types of assistance.

Health Care Function. The health care function refers to the ways the family protects the health of its members. The health care of the family is significantly related to family structure and function. For example, the health beliefs and values are related to the family's level of knowledge about health and illness and what is considered normal or usual within the socioeconomic or cultural group. In low-income groups many people do not consider themselves ill unless they can no longer work. In high-income groups people are more aware of symptoms as indicators of illness.

Family deterioration is often related to poor health of family members. When a family member becomes ill, nurses may be able to help other family members clarify their values and roles, or work with them on improving their communication skills and power balances to prevent deterioration of family functioning.

■ FAMILY LIFE CYCLE AND DEVELOPMENTAL STAGES

Another approach to viewing the family unit is the developmental approach. This approach studies the family and its normal developmental crises from its establishment in marriage through the death of one or both spouses. The successive stages of growth and development that families go through as a unit are referred to as the **family life cycle.**[5] Knowledge of the family life cycle prepares nurses to be aware of the developmental crises a family may face. Although each family is unique, there are universal characteristics of each developmental period.

One model commonly used for viewing family development was proposed by Duvall.[10] The model addresses the life cycle of the traditional nuclear family. The reader should be aware that the developmental approach may also be applied to viewing other family forms as they encounter family-life-cycle tasks. Table 8–2 details the family life cycle and development tasks. Like the life cycle of the individual (see Chaps. 10 and 11), each stage of the family life cycle includes a specific developmental task or milestone to be accomplished. If there is conflict between individual developmental tasks and family developmental tasks, compromises must be made. For example, in the case of teenagers who become parents, there is frequently a conflict between the adolescent developmental task of establishing personal identity and the needs of the infant for consistent nurturing care. These families need the support of their extended families and kinship networks or, in the absence of such support, nurses and other caregivers and social service agencies to learn to balance their personal needs and the needs of their infant.

Many developmental stages alter family membership, and therefore change the role individuals perform in the family. For example, the birth of a first child adds the new roles of mother and father. The family developmental stages relate to life events of members and thus sometimes may overlap. For example, a family may be in the "launching stage" by virtue of sending the first child off to college, while simultaneously in the "teenage stage" with the younger sibling. During these developmental family stages, other unpredictable events create family crises[11] (eg, stillbirth, divorce, separation, or changes in socioeconomic status). Frequently nurses meet families during a crisis, when family members are adapting to new situations. From a developmental viewpoint, the first occurrence of an event is usually the most difficult (for example, the birth of the first child, or the first child leaving home for college). If more than the usual amount of family disruption occurs when these events take place, nurses must carefully assess the family's stresses and coping patterns to determine whether other problems also exist.

■ FAMILY CRISIS

A **crisis** occurs when a family encounters problems and obstacles to the achievement of important life goals that for a time seem insurmountable and with which the family is unable to cope in its usual ways. Usually a period of disorganization follows as the family makes abortive attempts at solving the problem or overcoming the obstacle.[12]

TABLE 8–2. DUVALL'S EIGHT-STAGE FAMILY LIFE CYCLE AND DEVELOPMENTAL TASKS

Stage	Developmental Task
I Married couple (without children)	Establishing mutually satisfying relationships and establishing relationships with members of each other's families
II Childbearing family (oldest child between birth and 30 months)	Adjusting to parenthood and creating a home for the family
III Families with preschool children (oldest child 2½ to 6 years old)	Nurturing children and learning skills for effective socialization of children
IV Families with school-age children (oldest child 6 to 13 years old)	Educating and socializing the children and establishing social relationships with other families
V Families with teenagers (oldest child 13 to 20 years old)	Helping children to balance freedom and responsibility
VI Families launching young adults (first child gone to last child's leaving home)	Releasing children and developing spousal interests; continuing to provide support to children
VII Middle-aged parents (empty nest to retirement)	Solidifying the marital relationship and maintaining contacts with other generations
VIII Aging family members (retirement to death of both spouses)	Adjusting to multiple losses: spouse, job, friends

From Duvall E. Marriage and Family Development. *5th ed. Philadelphia: Copyright © 1957, 1962, 1971, 1977 by Harper & Row, Publishers, Inc. Reprinted by permission of HarperCollins Publishers.*

Types of Family Crises

There are two types of family crises: situational (or accidental) and maturational (or developmental). **Situational crisis** occurs suddenly in response to an external event or conflict involving a specific event (for example, destruction of the family home in a disaster, birth of a handicapped child, or divorce). **Maturational crisis** relates to the change involved in the developmental stages and the accomplishment of developmental tasks discussed in the previous section. This type of crisis occurs when the family is unable to complete the developmental task of one stage, creating a deficit that interferes with completing the tasks of the next stage. For example, a family in which a teenager is chronically mentally ill may be unable to assist the teenager to balance freedom and responsibility, later preventing "launching" from occurring smoothly. (Maturational and situational crises are discussed in detail in Chap. 6.)

IMPLICATIONS FOR NURSE–CLIENT COLLABORATION

Family Crisis

There are two types of family crises: (1) situational crises, which occur suddenly in response to some external event; and (2) maturational crises, which occur as an outcome of the changes in families that are related to the life cycle. Family crisis can be understood by looking at the crisis-producing situation, the family's understanding of the situation, its resources for dealing with it, and the degree of disorganization the family is experiencing as a result. The nurse facilitates family coping by being sensitive to family members' needs for reassurance about their ability to manage the crisis and providing resources for assistance for meeting the everyday requirements of living such as food, transportation, and child care.

Family crisis can be understood by looking at the crisis-producing situation, the family's perception of the situation, the family resources that can be used to deal with the situation, and the degree of disorganization the family is experiencing.[13] The family's interpretation of the meaning of the event and the presence of resources are key factors in whether a crisis evolves. For example, in a family going through divorce, disruption of family roles and relationships can create crisis conditions that may or may not be reduced by the family's resources, including financial reserves and the presence of other family members or friends who can step in to assume important roles. These factors influence the family's interpretation of the event as a crisis. Family members will balance perceived losses with their resources for coping. If the equation is positive—that is, if coping resources are adequate and the divorce actually relieves pressure on family members—then the event will likely not be perceived as a crisis and family functions will not become disorganized. On the other hand, if the family does not have the resources to make up the losses created by the change, then the divorce will likely create crisis conditions. Thus, situations that are often defined as socially negative—divorce, death in the family, separation, or job loss—may not be experienced as crises or cause family disorganization if the family's coping resources are sufficient.

However, situations that are defined as socially positive, such as marriage and birth of a new baby, may be experienced as crises if the family has either a negative perception of the experience or if there are inadequate family resources to deal with the event.

Family Crisis Intervention

The goal of crisis intervention is to restore the family to its precrisis state, or to raise it to a higher level of coping. Intervention includes helping the family to:

1. Confront the crisis in manageable increments.
2. Identify the facts to clarify the event.
3. Find and accept help, thereby acknowledging that trouble exists.

Nurses need to be sensitive to family members' needs for reassurance about their ability to manage crisis. At the same time, nurses may need to provide concrete assistance to help families meet their everyday needs for food, transportation, and child care. Crisis disorganizes families and depletes members of the energy needed to resolve the problem. Energy is lost through high anxiety levels caused by feelings of lack of control and abortive attempts to resolve the crisis. Blaming should be discouraged, as it is frequently a way of avoiding the truth and decreases the likelihood of a healthy adaptation.

BUILDING NURSING KNOWLEDGE

What Is the Effect of Having a New Baby?

Pridham KF, Egan KB, Change AS, Hansen MF. Life with a new baby: Stressors, supports, and maternal experience. *Pub Health Nurs.* 1986; 3:225–239.

The impact of having a new baby is examined in this report. The investigators focused on the day-to-day stressors, the role problems, and unpredictable crises that are part of having a new baby. They also dealt with the day-to-day supports that counter stressors; that is, the positive or satisfying experiences that act as "uplifts." The purpose of the study was to determine how the mothers' day-to-day experiences change over the first 3 months after birth, the period when mothers and infants adapt to each other.

Sixty-two women participated in the study. All were over 17 years of age, 39 percent had other children, and 96 percent were married. Subjects used a log to record demands and hassles (stressors) and the things that made things easier (supports). Log entries were sorted into categories by the researchers. Categories included mothers' mental and physical status, their responsibilities and tasks to be accomplished, activities and plans such as visits to friends, conditions such as time pressure or unusual events, and resources such as available services. Entries in each category were tallied for all subjects over a 3-month period.

The researchers found that the mothers' mental and physical status was the most frequent stressor reported in the first 15 days. Tasks and responsibilities were the most frequent stressor reported for the remainder of the study. Resources were the most frequent support reported during the first 45 days. Activities and plans were the most frequent support reported during the remainder of the time. Most significant, both stressors and supports were almost equivalent in frequency and both decreased over the 3-month period.

This finding on the effect of time, the researchers suggested, was an indication of changes both in mothers' circumstances and their perceptions of them. The researchers suggested that it is related to adaptation and mothers' changing expectations of themselves.

Crisis resolution occurs when a family perceives the stressful event realistically and, by means of appropriate support services and adequate coping mechanisms, solves its problems. However, crisis resolution is a complex phenomenon; resolution of long-standing individual and personal problems that sometimes contribute to crisis may require extended psychotherapy.

Families experience many different developmental and situational crises throughout their life cycle. The following discussion focuses on two common examples: (1) separation and divorce (a situational crisis), and (2) care of aging family members (a maturational crisis).

Separation and Divorce. The stress and emotional disruption created by separation and divorce are becoming common phenomena. Although separation and divorce are not health problems, they affect the health of the whole family. Divorce places both the separating adults and their children at risk. Divorced men frequently experience more accidents and health problems, while divorced women may experience depression and live in impoverished economic circumstances.[14] Children of divorce experience an increased probability that the following problems may occur: anger and depression, low self-esteem and depression, impaired academic performance, and difficulty with close relationships in adolescence and adulthood. There is increased evidence that 30 or 50 percent of the children in divorced families experience the pain of divorce for years.[14]

Children experience parental divorce from the perspective of their age and developmental level. For example, preschoolers experience the separation as abandonment and blame themselves for the failure of the parental union.[15]

Family members must adjust to the loss caused by the separation. They frequently go through a period of grief and mourning for the loss of past relationships and the integrity of the family unit. Early classic work done by Engle[16] on grief and grieving can be used as a framework to view divorce and the grieving process that the family must work through. Engle divided the grieving process into three stages: (1) shock and disbelief, (2) developing awareness, and (3) reorganization and restitution.

In the first stage, the family often denies the reality of the impending divorce. After separation the spouses may withdraw from contact with friends and family, and the children may deny the event and speak about the reunion of the parents. Physical symptoms such as nausea, diarrhea, fainting, restlessness, fatigue, and insomnia are not uncommon.

In the second stage, family members experience the loss more acutely. They may feel overwhelmed, angry, guilty, and depressed. Crying is common, as the individual family members begin to come to terms with the divorce.

In the third stage, family members acknowledge the inevitability of the loss and begin to reorganize their lives and move forward. Each family member moves through this grieving process according to his or her own timetable. The nurse must not only be aware of the dynamics of the grieving process but also provide support to family members that is appropriate to their stage of grief. At times nurses help individuals in the family to accept the notion that each family member's responses are individual and each needs support to proceed with grief work at an individual pace.

Recently, there has been an increasing trend in child custody proceedings to award custody of the children jointly to both parents. Frequently children live with one parent for 6 months and the other for 6 months. This allows both parents equal access to their children. This works well if parents are committed to joint custody and they work together to develop consistent rules and practices between the two households.[14]

Adult Children and Care of Elderly Family Members. Another family crisis is exemplified by middle-aged families who are involved in caring for elderly parents. According to Brody and associates,[17] this responsibility has become a common family stressor. Families are a major source of emotional, financial, and physical support for elderly family members.[18]

Even the care of healthy aged parents can be difficult for their adult children. If a parent is ill and dependent on children, the burden may become overwhelming and create the potential for abuse, neglect, and inadequate care.[19] The most stable families can be disrupted by attempts to maintain supportive relationships under this kind of stress. Unresolved family and emotional conflicts and problems in intergenerational communication contribute to the family's tension.[20]

Assessment of sources of stress is important when a nurse encounters a family caring for an elderly family member. By examining information about both generations, a nurse can predict the well-being of the elderly person. Areas of assessment include family environment (family relationships, personal growth, and maintenance of the unit); degree of impairment (the elderly person's ability to perform activities of daily living); self-worth (acceptance of positive feelings about oneself); and perceived support (knowledge that one is cared for, loved, esteemed, valued, and belongs to a network of communication and mutual obligation).[20]

This type of assessment reveals family strengths as well as sources of stress and guides identification of realistic goals and strategies for resolution of the conflict. Nurses can help the family to capitalize on family resources that will balance the negative effects of stressors. For example, grandparents and grandchildren can be wonderful resources to each other because they are not encumbered by the worries of the middle-generation parents (Fig. 8–2). These relationships should be facilitated and called upon as a source of strength for the family.[21] The focus of treatment for families in this kind of crisis is for all parties to recognize and take advantage of individual and group capacities and cooperate to achieve a positive outcome. Table 8–3 lists general treatment goals that are appropriate for families caring for elderly parents.

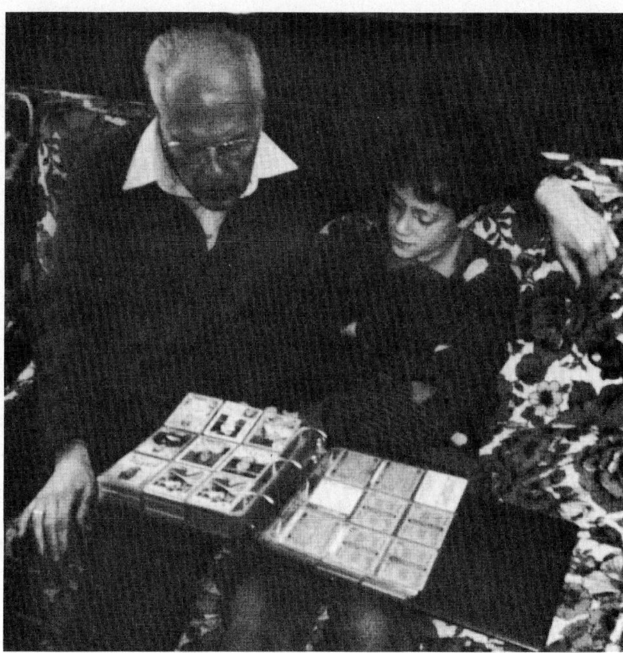

Figure 8–2. Grandparents and grandchildren can be wonderful resources to each other, as they are unencumbered by the worries of the middle-generation parents. *Source: Yurick AG, Spier BE, Robb SS, Ebert NJ.* The Aged Person and the Nursing Process. *3rd ed. Norwalk, CT: Appleton & Lange; 1989.*)

Much of the nurse's work with families involves assisting them to confront situational and maturational crises. Crises are disorganizing to families and strain their physical and emotional health. Nurses working with families in crisis need to build relationships with family members that are characterized by mutual trust and respect (Fig. 8–3). Such

TABLE 8–3. TREATMENT GOALS FOR FAMILIES CARING FOR ELDERLY PARENTS

1. Helping each person retain, regain, or develop a positive sense of self within the family.
2. Helping family members maintain or assume control of their lives and protect what they feel is theirs (physical, psychological, or social).
3. Establishing or encouraging an appropriate family role structure that allows members to meet personal needs within the family framework.
4. Resolving specific family problems arising from strained relationships or unresolved conflicts.
5. Teaching problem-solving skills.
6. Exploring institutionalization, continuing intergenerational living arrangements, or alternative life-styles.
7. Focusing on the future; developing the perspective and direction required to continue positive interaction despite physical or mental deterioration.[18]

From Miller J, Feinauer L, Lund D. Assessing families of the chronically ill aged in their homes. In: Wright L, Leahey M, eds. Families and Chronic Illness. *Springhouse, PA: Springhouse; 1987.*

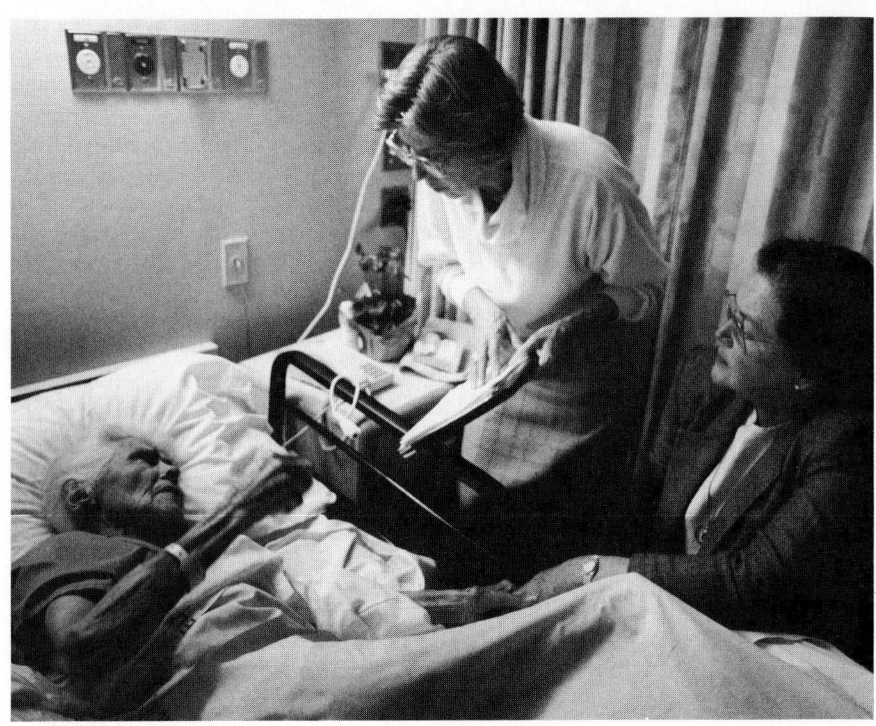

Figure 8–3. Care of an elderly client involves building a relationship of trust and respect with both generations.

collaborative relationships are effective for establishing specific goals for crisis and may make it easier for a family to accomplish necessary changes. Successful crisis intervention has long-term effects on family health—both that of individual members and on the unit as a whole. Positive crisis resolution strengthens current coping strategies, teaches new ways to deal with problems, and positively affects the family's ability to cope and withstand future crisis events.

■ THE FAMILY AS A HEALTH CARE UNIT

Because the family is the basic socializing unit in society, it has a tremendous impact on the health of individual members. Individuals learn health values and behaviors within a family unit that exists in a particular society or culture. Ethnicity, race, and social class have a profound effect on a family's attitudes regarding health and illness as well as on a family's access to health care. Education and economics also play an important role in the development of health-related behavior.

Family Health Promotion

Family health promotion is an integral component of family life-style. Family influences the health-related behavior of its members and is responsible for 75 percent of all health care provided to its members.[22] Life-style factors that contribute to family wellness include self-responsibility, nutritional awareness, stress management, physical fitness, and concern about environmental effects on health and illness (see also Chaps. 5 and 22).

Self-responsibility. Family self-responsibility is essential to carrying out any of the aspects of life-style that promote wellness. Family members must assume responsibility for avoiding unhealthy behaviors such as smoking and inadequate rest, and seeking healthy behaviors such as regular exercise and eating nutritional foods. One factor that affects the assumption of self-responsibility is the availability of education for self-care.[5] Recently the availability of these programs has increased. Schools, hospitals, adult education programs, and park and recreation associations offer a broad range of wellness programs for families. A part of self-responsibility and learning to care for oneself is knowing of community resources to meet the family's need for preventive and illness care as well as the knowledge and ability to work within the health care system to meet these needs. Nurses can provide families with this information by demonstrating how to move through the system to get appointments and referrals. Creating a life-style that keeps members well and out of the health care system is as important to family welfare as learning how to negotiate the system.[23]

Nutritional Awareness. Dietary patterns, whether healthful or unhealthful, are influenced by maturation; family, social, and cultural patterns; learned psychosocial associations between food and basic needs; and environmental availability of foods. Family influence is an especially important factor in dietary patterns. Nurses can develop insights into a family's dietary patterns by discussing what types of foods are purchased; how often the family relies on fast food; the function of mealtime in the family's life; and how and to whom tasks related to food purchase, preparation, and serving are delegated or distributed. The development of good nutritional habits is essential to the maintenance of family health and prevention of health problems.

Stress Management. Stress is a common experience for families in today's society. Some of the stressors are external to family relationships, others relate to family processes. Many families develop effective day-to-day strategies for stress management, such as open communication among family members, collaborative problem solving, and shared physical activities. These kinds of approaches build trust and resilience, so that when more challenging difficulties arise, family members can work together to meet them. Mutual effort of this nature can strengthen the family and foster the personal growth of individual members as well.[11]

Physical Fitness. The benefits of regular exercise are often learned within the context of family life. Regular exercise as part of a healthy life-style can lead to an overall feeling of healthfulness and exhilaration as well as improved physical strength and stamina. Family recreational time can be spent in physical exercise, such as biking, skating, walking or other sports (Fig. 8–4). These activities not only build physical health but bring the family together emotionally. Nurses can serve both as role models for and facilitators of physical fitness. Efforts to teach the importance of exercise will be more effective if the nurse's appearance and habits suggest that he or she is physically fit.

Environmental Effects. The environment either enhances or diminishes the family's health and well-being. In the immediate environment, the availability of sufficient space to meet the family members' needs for privacy is a significant factor. In the larger environment, both families and nurses must address more pervasive problems, such as poverty, homelessness, and substance abuse. Family health promotion at the environmental level means more than eliminating health problems such as lead poisoning and automobile accidents in communities; the underlying social structure that causes the stressors that lead to the health problems must be addressed.[22] This type of stressor includes economic and social policies that affect the distribution of basic resources such as food, shelter, sanitation, and safety. Poor children and their families frequently have more health problems because of poor nutrition, living conditions, and lack of access to preventative health care. Consequently, these families are frequently very ill when they enter the health care system.[20] Nurses and families can be active in promoting a healthful environment through their involvement in schools, churches, and the political process (see Chap. 4).

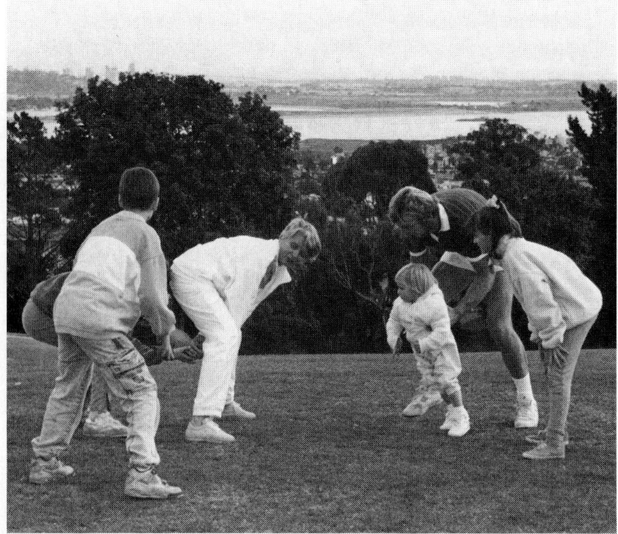

Figure 8–4. Exercising together helps to promote family health and physical fitness.

Family Health Tasks

Each family cares for its health in a way that is consistent with its values, capabilities, resources, and life-styles. All families face certain tasks regarding the health of their members (Box 8–2).

Freedman and Heinrich[24] identify these family health tasks as: (1) recognizing interruptions of health or development (for example, identification of the symptoms of illness); (2) seeking health care (for example, making the decision to see a physician or to try home remedies); (3) managing health-related and other crises (for example, managing the incapacitating illness of a family member, or moving to an unfamiliar community); (4) providing nursing care to sick, disabled, or dependent members of the family (for example, providing care to ambulatory sick family members or care after hospitalization); (5) maintaining a home environment that promotes good health and development (for example, providing physical safety for elderly persons and small children); and (6) maintaining relationships with health care facilities and community agencies (for example, maintaining the family's involvement with its children's schools).

Nurses help families achieve these family tasks by providing information appropriate to each family's need and

BOX 8–2. FAMILY TASKS RELATED TO HEALTH

- Recognizing interruptions in development or diminished wellness.
- Seeking appropriate health care
- Managing crises related to illness
- Providing care to dependent or sick family members
- Maintaining a healthful home environment
- Maintaining relationships with health care providers for wellness and illness care.

providing guidance and support for the health and illness decisions it makes. For example, a nurse may provide home safety information for the parents of a toddler and help the family "child proof" its home.

■ FAMILY ASSESSMENT

Family assessment in nursing is the collection and analysis of data relative to family health. Family assessment is concerned with family structure, function, and environment, particularly as these factors influence the health of individual members and the family as a whole. In any setting where nurses care for clients, family assessment is one of the more important functions that nurses carry out because of the interrelatedness of individual health and family health. An understanding of how family assessment is performed is therefore important knowledge for the nurse to have. General concepts related to assessment are presented in greater detail in Chapter 16.

Purposes of Family Assessment

Nurses carry out family assessment for several important reasons. These include: (1) promoting awareness of positive health practices; (2) raising the family's consciousness regarding its own organizational structure and functioning and how these relate to the health of the family; (3) providing an opportunity to collaborate with the family by listening to its concerns about health; (4) identifying the family's needs for referral to other professionals or agencies; (5) individualizing care to be given by health care professionals; and (6) promoting family responsibility for improving health.

Characteristics of Healthy Families

In assessing families, nurses need to identify the healthy aspects of each family and capitalize on these family strengths when planning care. Family theory literature concurs on the following five characteristics of healthy families.[5,11,25]

- *Mutual respect and support.* Mutual respect and support is the basis for healthy family processes. Each of the other characteristics of healthy families that follows depends on mutual respect. Respect implies valuing other family members for who they are and recognizing the unique importance of each family member to the integrity of the family as a whole. It implies an atmosphere of acceptance, not a controlling environment. When there is respect, support flows naturally. To families that respect each other, relying on one another for assistance or encouragement does not imply weakness, but rather recognition of a healthy mutual dependency.
- *Open communication.* Open communication in a family is the ability and willingness to honestly discuss all issues of concern to the family. Open communication can involve routine family decisions or matters of greater significance; for example, a child talking about school problems, a teenager sharing thoughts about experimenting with drugs, or a couple speaking with one another about sexual concerns. Open communication involves self-disclosure, sharing aspects of self that may be personal or private (see also Chap. 23). This kind of openness involves risk of rejection or punishment. Therefore, it requires self-confidence and trust in other family members. Not all families that function well operate under conditions of complete openness, but it is generally agreed that the fewer the areas of closed communication, the healthier the family.
- *Shared problem solving.* Shared problem solving implies that family decisions are made with input from all family members. Mutual trust and open communication make shared problem solving more effective. Families may address day-to-day problems, such as allocation of responsibility for household chores, or more serious problems that threaten family structure or functioning, such as serious illness of a family member.
- *Flexibility.* Flexibility implies willingness among family members to adjust family process or roles to accommodate changes in the needs of individual members. For example, children may agree to switch household chores with each other so one of them can attend team practices that conflict with chores.
- *Enhancement of personal growth.* A healthy family recognizes the needs of individual members to experience growth toward their full potential. This may require temporary or long-term adjustments in family process to accommodate the needs of a particular member. For example, the husband/father may desire a career change that requires returning to school, which in turn may create a financial burden that necessitates family life-style changes such as omitting a family vacation or limiting the number of family outings. Or, one parent may take on an extra part-time job to help with a child's college expenses. Enhancement of personal growth of individual family members also incorporates maintaining a balance between shared activities and separate activities. Each member is recognized as an individual, as well as a family member.

Families may exhibit each of these traits to a greater or lesser degree and still fall within the definition of a healthy family. The extent to which day-to-day family processes are healthy predicts the amount of disruption family stressors or family crises may cause.

Often, nurses encounter a family when one family member is ill. Nurses can help families to recognize their family strengths to cope with a family member's health problem. The same approach is effective when collaborating with families facing maturational stressors, such as dealing with a teenager learning to balance freedom and responsibility with the family automobile.

Components of Family Assessment

To assess the family, nurses collect data related to three different categories: environment, family structure, and family function. The data collected assists nurses to make appropriate nursing diagnoses with the family's input (see Chap. 17).

Environmental Data. The assessment of the environment is crucial to determining family health and health practices. This includes characteristics of the immediate home environment such as ventilation and privacy; characteristics of the neighborhood such as pollution, parks, and traffic; and the family's history of geographic mobility. Assessment of the family environment includes both the information that nurses gain from the family as well as the observations and impressions nurses make relative to the environment.

Family Structure. As discussed earlier in this chapter, the structural characteristics of the family are roles, value system, communication patterns, and power structure.[5] Family members actively participate in the assessment as they share their perceptions of these structural elements. Nurses help the family clarify problems and issues related to family structure.

Family Function. Reutter[25] divides family function into two broad categories: those meeting self-care requirements of individual members, and those needed to adapt to change.

Self-care Requirements. The self-care requirements of individual family members can be met by means of the five family functions discussed earlier in this chapter (affective, socialization and social placement, reproductive, economic, and health care).

- *Affective function.* The family's ability to meet the needs of its members for affection and understanding is assessed in this area. In addition, promotion of emotional growth and development, which results in the development of a healthy personality for family members, is a focus.
- *Socialization and social placement function.* The self-care requirement assessed here is solitude versus social interaction.[25] The family's ability to provide solitude and privacy for its members, as well as its ability to promote interaction among the family members and between the family and other social units in the community, is a key issue. Educational goals, religious values, and recreation are related factors.
- *Reproductive function.* The family function of reproduction ensures the perpetuation of society. Gender-specific role modeling is seen as part of this function.
- *Economic function.* This refers to the provisions of economic resources and the allocation of those resources to meet the basic needs of the family.
- *Health care function.* This refers to the way a family meets its members' physical needs (food, clothing, shelter, safety) and coordinates meeting its health care needs. Health beliefs, knowledge about healthful practices and hazards to health and safety, availability of health services, and presence of disease or disability in the family influence family effectiveness in this function.

Adapting to Change. Adapting to change involves the family's ability to maintain itself despite internal and external demands for change such as those that occur during situational and maturational crises. The family strengths, resources, and previous coping patterns are assessed in order to help members use those assets both to resolve the present crisis and to learn to use them in future crises. The characteristics of healthy families identified earlier in this chapter can be used to identify family strengths. This assessment may also motivate members to develop new coping mechanisms.

Throughout the family assessment, the family remains an active participant in its care. If the family members do not identify strengths, nurses can point them out and help the family build on these strengths. The family's perception of its limitations also provides nurses with relevant data. Table 8–4 suggests some appropriate assessment questions for each component of family assessment.

Nursing Diagnoses in Family Assessment

The data gathered during the family assessment is used to identify family problems that can be alleviated by nurse–client collaboration. These problems are called nursing diagnoses. The concept of nursing diagnosis and the analytic and reasoning processes that are used to generate nursing diagnoses are discussed in detail in Chapters 15 and 17. Table 8–5 presents some common nursing diagnoses that apply to families. Making these diagnoses is a relatively complex process, because of the many factors that influence family relationships and family functioning. The diagnoses are presented here not with the expectation that beginning nursing students will diagnose families, but to increase their awareness of ways in which nurses assist families.

■ COMPREHENSIVE FAMILY CARE

Comprehensive family care is generally accepted to mean providing care to the integrated physical, emotional, social, cultural, and spiritual needs of individual family members and the family as a unit. Nurses and other health care professionals provide such care directly or assist families to seek help through family support networks and other community helping agencies.

Physical, Social, Emotional, Cultural, and Spiritual Aspects of Care

Nurses have historically cared for the body, but with the increase in knowledge about the relationship between body and spirit, there is an increased emphasis on other needs. This emphasis on meeting families' spiritual, sociocultural, and emotional needs occurred partially because of the increasing stress in contemporary society. More attention is given to nontraditional methods for coping with stress. These methods involve active participation of families in such stress-reduction methods as meditation, biofeedback,

TABLE 8–4. COMPONENTS OF FAMILY ASSESSMENT

Family Assessment Component	Assessment Questions
Environmental data	1. What is the physical condition of your family's housing? 2. Does your home have a safe, reliable water supply? Waste disposal method? 3. Are you bothered by any rodent or insect pests in your home? How do you deal with these? 4. What is the surrounding neighborhood like? 5. Are the houses and property nearby well kept? 6. Is there evidence of garbage or trash not in trashcans? 7. Are there nearby community resources such as child care facilities and playgrounds?
Family structure	1. How does your family express emotion? 2. Is there a primary decision-maker in your family? 3. How does your family solve problems? 4. What kinds of things are most important to your family?
Family functions Self-care requirement Affective	1. How do family members express their affection for each other in your family? 2. Do you and your spouse experience satisfying interpersonal and sexual relationships with each other?
Socialization and social placement	1. Does each family member have adequate living space and the opportunity for privacy? 2. What kinds of planned recreational activities do family members participate in together? 3. What are your family's attitudes toward education, reading, and intellectual pursuits? 4. Do family members respect each other's needs to balance privacy and social interaction?
Reproduction	1. What are your family's feelings about family size? 2. Are you and your spouse in general agreement about the ideal number of children? 3. How do you and your spouse share parenting responsibilities?
Economic	1. Does your family have adequate income to meet basic needs? 2. Is income sufficient to meet special needs?
Health care	1. What acute and chronic health problems do members of your family experience? 2. Do any family members require each other's assistance because of these health problems? How often do family members seek health care? 3. How close do you live to health care services? Is transportation readily available?
Adapting to change	1. What do you feel are your family's strengths? 2. What resources (financial, interpersonal) are available to your family? 3. How has your family coped with changes and crises in their lives? 4. What would you say you and your family have learned in the resolution of past crises?

yoga, and fitness exercise programs. Nurses are helping clients to take charge of their own health care through client education activities and referral to community agencies.

Family Support Networks

Many support networks are available to family members. Some of these arise from extended families, kinship networks, or religious groups. In addition, there are many voluntary organizations for families of individuals who are affected by specific illnesses or other problems. Some examples of self-help groups include the National Association of Parents and Friends of Mentally Retarded Children, Mothers Against Drunk Driving, Compassionate Friends, Alcoholics Anonymous, Al-Anon, and Ala-Teen.

Community Helping Networks

Churches, social welfare organizations, and community mental health centers are more important today than during any previous period in our history. In the past few years, government aid for the chronically ill and disabled has been drastically cut, and communities have developed many private support networks. These organizations usually are dependent on multiple sources of funding, such as government contracts, foundation grants, local fund-raising, client fees, and insurance payments. The Community Chest or United Way Appeal drives have been helpful in providing additional funding for these organizations. Families may feel more welcome in small community-based organizations than in large organizations as they have less bureaucratic red tape to work through in order to receive service.

■ COLLABORATING WITH FAMILIES

Nurses need to collaborate closely with families in order to help achieve goals that are mutually determined and consistent with the family's belief system. If the family "owns" the goals, the likelihood of successful achievement is enhanced. A review of recent nursing research indicates that one future direction for family research should be toward identifying family strengths[26] and capacity for coping. In

TABLE 8–5. EXAMPLES OF FAMILY NURSING DIAGNOSES

Nursing	Explanation
Ineffective Family Coping: Compromised	A usually supportive family member provides insufficient, ineffective, or compromised support, comfort, or assistance to another family member experiencing a health challenge when support, comfort, or assistance is needed to master the challenge. For example, a client who is facing a difficult decision about treatment alternatives at the same time that his partner, who usually supports him in a shared decision-making process, is experiencing an intense emotional response to the situation and is unable to participate in shared decision-making.
Alteration in Family Processes	A family that has been functioning well experiences a stressor and has difficulty functioning. For example, a family who experiences a death of one of its members and is temporarily unable to carry on the activities of daily living.
Impaired Home Maintenance Management	A family is unable to maintain a safe home environment because of illness in a family member, poor hygienic practices, an impaired caregiver, or lack of support from family and friends. For example, alcoholic parents who are unable to maintain a physically safe environment for their children.
Alterations in Parenting	A real or potential inability of one or more adult members of the family to provide a positive environment that facilitates the growth and development of children. For example, an emotionally disturbed adult caregiver in a family who is unable to meet the children's needs for affection.
Family Coping: Potential for Growth	Family member(s) has (have) effectively adapted to a health challenge of one family member, and is (are) exhibiting desire and readiness for enhanced health and growth for self and affected family member. For example, the family of a handicapped child who exhibits readiness to use community and health resources to promote optimal social, emotional, and physical development of the child.

the past, nurses and other health care professionals often treated clients and their families paternalistically, assuming that professionals had if not all, at least most, of the right answers. Families were frequently given little choice about treatment options or even the right to refuse treatment, and thus were not involved in making health care decisions. If they tried to exercise choice, family members were labeled "noncompliant," because their point of view differed from that of the health care professional. Today, however, individuals are seen as having a right to self-determination. This point of view recognizes that families and their members have the ultimate right and responsibility for making family health choices. Nurses facilitate this process by providing the necessary information and resources as well as support and guidance that the family needs to make appropriate choices.

In order to provide optimum health care to families, nurses must understand not only the premises of the mutual interaction model but also family systems and self-care theory.

The Family As a System

Systems theory helps one to understand that individuals are inseparable from the groups of which they are a part. It proposes that all elements of the environment are interdependent, and the health implications of family relationships are important. In society, groups provide the environment in which the individuals live out their lives. The most important group is usually the family because it is most often the one with which the individual has the strongest personal ties. The family and the individual are bound by physical heritage, by strong emotional and spiritual ties, and often by economic necessity. The family is thus the nurturant environment that provides the support needed by the individual to adapt to the stresses of everyday life. To the extent that it influences the individual's ability to adapt to stress, the family is a crucial variable to achieving health.

Self-care Theory

The presuppositions underlying self-care theory are important to understanding family health. Individuals are viewed as decision-makers and problem-solvers who accomplish goals through deliberate action. Most importantly, individuals are viewed as having the right to self-determination. Major health problems in our society are frequently related to life-style or environment.[27] For example, unhealthy dietary patterns and sedentary life-styles contribute to heart disease, and environmental pollution affects clients with chronic lung diseases. Prevention or redirection of life-style problems occurs when individuals engage in healthy behaviors in order to meet their requirements for self-care. Self-care actions are activities individuals perform to contribute to their physical, psychological, and social functioning and to their development.[28] Self-care requirements common to all people are activities that everyone performs in order to meet basic needs for air, food, water, elimination, rest, activity, solitude, social interaction, protection from hazards, and maintenance of normalcy.[28]

Orem[28] contends that the family is an important resource to its members in meeting their self-care requirements. For example, the family provides a nutritionally adequate diet and role models of healthy exercise behaviors. The family provides a developmental environment for individual growth and self-actualization by promoting open communication, mutual respect, support, and flexibility in allowing for individual growth.

■ THE HEALTH CARE TEAM IN FAMILY CARE

Urban families have many choices of health care providers and settings for health care (for example, health maintenance organizations [HMOs], acute care clinics). These choices may include private physicians (generalists or family health specialists), nurse practitioners, social workers, and physician's assistants. Many of these specialists have advanced educations in family health or preventive medicine.

Nurses meet the special needs of families in various ways. For example, support groups like Make the Day Count have been organized for cancer clients and their families by nurses. Classes related to specific illnesses have been organized, such as those for postcoronary clients and their families or the families of the chronic mentally ill. Nurses have also been involved in developing family health promotion programs in local communities. Small group techniques are frequently used in these educational endeavors. Nurses now participate directly in the development of media programs geared toward community health education for families.

SUMMARY

The family is the primary socializing agent of society. The contemporary definitions of the family have been presented, as well as discussions of several family forms. Family structure is determined by its units such as roles, value systems, communication patterns, and power structure. What the family does as a basic unit of society is seen through its affective, socialization and social placement, reproductive, economic, and health care functions. In addition, family life cycle and specific developmental tasks are associated with each life stage. Family crisis, both situational and maturational, is exemplified by events such as divorce and care of elderly parents. Health promotion of families is achieved through self-responsibility, nutritional awareness, stress management, physical fitness, and environmental management. The family has certain health tasks to achieve, and family assessment and collaboration among nurses and families aids in this process. Collaborative health care must draw on all available resources, but families are the primary resource to their members.

REFERENCES

1. Nightingale F. Sick nursing and health nursing. In: Petry L, ed. *Hospitals, Dispensaries, and Nursing: Papers and Discussions from the International Congress of Charities, Corrections and Philanthropy,* Section III. Chicago: 1893; June 12–17.
2. American Nursing Association. *A Social Policy Statement.* Kansas City, MO: ANA; 1980.
3. World Health Organization. *A Guide to Curriculum Review for Basic Nursing Education: Orientation to Primary Health Care and Community Health.* Geneva: World Health Organization; 1985.
4. Frank S. The unit of care revisited. *J Fam Practice.* 1985; 21:2.
5. Friedman M. *Family Nursing: Theory and Assessment.* 2nd ed. Norwalk, CT: Appleton-Century-Crofts; 1986.
6. Heinrich K. Refocused family study program sharpens student's assessment skills. *Nurs Health Care.* 1987; 8:74–79.
7. US Dept of Commerce, Bureau of the Census: Households, Families, Marital Status and Living Arrangements, March, 1988 (Advance Report) Series p–20, No. 432. Washington D.C.: US Govt Printing Office, 1988.
8. Bryan G, Grover D. Stepfamilies: A concern health education should address. JOSH, 1984; (2)8–11.
9. Joseph E. My husband's eight other wives . . , Another view. *The San Diego Union.* 1991; 9 June, p C3.
10. Duvall E. *Marriage and Family Development.* 5th ed. Philadelphia: Lippincott; 1977.
11. Glick P. The family life cycle and social change. *Fam Relat.* 1989; 38:123.
12. Aquilera D, Messick J. *Crisis Intervention: Theory and Methodology.* 6th ed. St. Louis: Mosby; 1989.
13. Hill R. *Families Under Stress.* New York: Harper & Row; 1949.
14. Kalter N. *Growing Up With Divorce.* New York: Free Press; 1990.
15. Amato P. Family processes in one-parent, stepparent, and intact families: The child's point of view. *J Mar Fam.* 1987; 49:327.
16. Engle G. Grief and grieving. *Am J Nurs.* 1964; 64:93.
17. Brody E, et al. Parent care as a normative family stress. *Gerentol.* 1985; 25:19–29.
18. Miller J, Feinauer L, Lund D. Assessing families of the chronically ill and aged in their homes. In: Wright L, Leahey M, eds. *Families and Chronic Illness.* Springhouse, PA: Springhouse; 1987.
19. Steinmetz S, Ansden D. Dependent elders, family stress and abuse. In: Brubaker T, ed. *Family Relationships in Later Life.* Beverly Hills: Sage; 1983.
20. Murray RB, Zentner JP. *Nursing Assessment and Health Promotion Strategies Throughout the Life Span.* 4th ed. Norwalk, CT: Appleton & Lange; 1989.
21. Smoyak S. Assessing aging families and their caretakers. In: Wright L, Leahey M, eds. *Families and Chronic Illness.* Springhouse, PA: Springhouse; 1987.
22. Duffy M. Health promotion in the family: Current findings and directives for nursing research. *J Adv Nurs.* 1988; 13:109–117.
23. Bradshaw MJ. *Nursing of the Family in Health and Illness.* Norwalk, CT: Appleton & Lange; 1988.
24. Freedman R, Heinrich J. *Community Health Nursing Practice.* 2nd ed. Philadelphia: Saunders; 1981.
25. Reutter L. Family health assessment—An integrated approach. *J Adv Nurs.* 1984; 9:391–399.
26. Gilliss CL. Family nursing research, theory, and practice. *Image.* 1991; 23:19–22.
27. Ardell D. *High Level Wellness—An Alternative to Doctors, Drugs and Disease.* Emmaus, PA: Rodale Press; 1977.
28. Orem D. *Nursing: Concepts of Practice.* 4th ed. New York: McGraw-Hill; 1990.

BIBLIOGRAPHY

Austin JK. Assessment of coping mechanisms used by parents and children with chronic illness. *MCN.* 1990; 15(2):98–102.

Bell JM, Wright LM. Flaws in family nursing education. *Canadian Nurse.* 1990; 86(6):28–30.

Birenbaum LK. Measurement of family coping. *J Pediatr Oncol Nurs.* 1991; 8(1):39–42.

Campbell DW. Family paradigm theory and family rituals: Implications for child and family health. *Nurse Pract.* 1991; 16(2):22, 25–26, 31.

Clark MJ. *Nursing in the Community.* 2nd ed. Norwalk, CT: Appleton & Lange; 1992.

Doane JA, Hill WL, Kaslow N, Quinlan D. Family system functioning: Behavior in the laboratory and the family treatment setting, *Family Process.* 1988; 27:213–227.

Feeman DJ, Hagen JW. Effects of childhood chronic illness on families. *Soc Work Health Care.* 1990; 14(3):37–53.

Friedman MM. Transcultural family nursing: Application to Latino and black families. *J Pediatr Nurs.* 1990; 5(3):214–222.

Friedemann M, et al. Advanced family nursing with the control-congruence model. *Clin Nurs Specialist.* 1989; 3(4):164–170.

Friedemann M. The Concept of family nursing. *J Adv Nurs.* 1989; 14(3):211–216.

Gallo AM. Family adaptation in childhood chronic illness: A case report. *J Pediatr Health Care.* 1991; 5(2):78–85.

Haller KB. Problems in family assessment. *MCN.* 1990; 15(5):338.

Hill JP, Holmbeck GN. Disagreement about rules in families with seventh-grade girls and boys. *J Youth Adolescence.* 1987; 16:221–246.

Loos F, Bell JM. Circular questions: A family interviewing strategy. *Dimensions Crit Care Nurs.* 1990; 9(1):46–53.

Leahey M, Stout L, Myrak I. Family systems nursing: How do you practice it in an active community hospital? *Can Nurs.* 1991; 87(2): 31–33.

Mercer RT, May KA, Ferketch S, DeJoseph J. Theoretical models for studying the effect of antepartum stress on the family. *Nurs Res.* 1986; 35:339–345.

Norris MKG. Applying Orem's theory to the long-term care of adolescent transplant recipients. *ANNA J.* 1991; 18(1):45–47.

Prout V. Family influence on the child. In Mott S, Fazkas N, James S, eds. *Nursing Care of Children and Families.* 2nd ed. Menlo Park, CA: Addison-Wesley; 1990.

Stenrig TE. External structure and cohesion: Nursing perspectives. *Public Health Nurs.* 1990; 7(3):161–168.

Watson WL, Nanchoff G, Glatt M. A family systems nursing approach to premenstrual syndrome. *Rehabilitation Nurs.* 1990; 4(1): 3–9.

Wright LM, Leahey M. Trends in nursing of families. *Jnl Adv Nurs.* 1991; 15:148–154.

Wright LM, Leahey M. *Families and Chronic Illness.* Springhouse, PA: Springhouse; 1987.

Yurick AG, Spier BE, Robb SS, Ebert NJ. *The Aged Person and the Nursing Process.* 3rd ed. Norwalk, CT: Appleton & Lange; 1989.

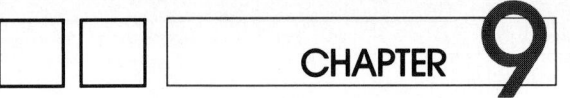

Sociocultural and Spiritual Dimensions of Health

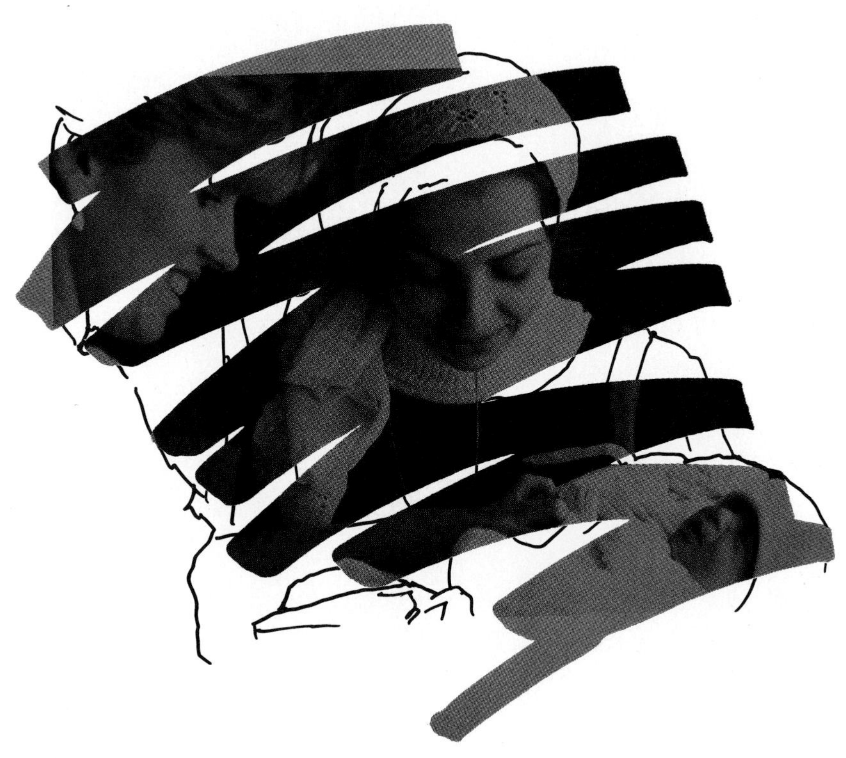

Behavioral Objectives

Upon completion of this chapter, the student will be able to:

1. Define the concept of culture.
2. Discuss the impact of culture on attitudes and habits.
3. Discuss ethnocentrism, and identify ways of becoming culturally sensitive.
4. State the relationship of cultural beliefs to health care practices.
5. Contrast the traditional and the modern health care cultures.
6. Discuss health beliefs and practices of several major cultural groups in the United States.
7. Discuss the relationship between the concepts of religion and spirituality.
8. Describe how spirituality, religion, and health interrelate with culture.
9. Discuss the relationship of religion to health practices.
10. Discuss the beliefs and practices of five prevalent religions in the United States.
11. Describe how intercultural collaboration between nurse and client promotes effective client care.
12. Define the principles of cultural relativism, cultural sensitivity, and transcultural reciprocity in nursing collaboration.
13. Identify the essential components of a cultural assessment.
14. Identify the nurse's role in planning care based on cultural differences.

KEY TERMS

acculturation
assimilation
cultural conflict
cultural relativism
cultural sensitivity
culture
culture shock
discrimination
dominant culture
enculturation
ethnicity
ethnocentrism
ideology
minority culture
prejudice
race
racism
religion
social relationships
social structure
society
spirituality
stereotyping
subculture
transcultural reciprocity

Culture plays a major role in all aspects of human life. It influences how people perceive objects, other people, and events and how they react to them. It determines individual values and often involves behaviors, values, and attitudes that are shared with other members of one's cultural group. Culture influences our health and illness behavior, communication patterns, religious practices, diet, attitudes toward family and work, gender roles, and illness. To understand a client's view of life, a nurse must have knowledge of that client's culture.

Cultural awareness is an essential part of nursing care. Such an understanding enables a nurse to interpret a client's specific ways of acting, thinking, and feeling. It also helps a nurse design an appropriate plan of care for a client. Nurses' awareness of their own cultural background helps them recognize personal beliefs, biases, and prejudices. This prevents nurses from being judgmental and nonaccepting, and thus makes nurses more supportive in a therapeutic nurse–client relationship.

In addition, nurses must know about the rich traditions present among the diverse cultures in the United States. Most nurses care for clients outside of their own cultural group. When nurses interact with individuals of another culture, the experience can lead to both personal and professional enrichment as both nurses and clients grow and expand beyond their own cultural boundaries. As language usage is culturally defined, it is necessary to understand culture to communicate effectively. Because all nurse–client interactions are based on communication, it is necessary to assess the differences and similarities between nurses' and clients' communication patterns. The goal is to establish a common approach to communication between nurse and client.

This chapter discusses sociocultural and spiritual factors in health care and their application to nursing. The chapter begins with an overall definition of culture, including components, characteristics, and modes of transmission. This is followed by a discussion of the diverse cultures in the United States and their unique perspectives on health and illness. Implications for nurse–client collaboration are included for each of these cultural groups. Implications of spiritual and religious beliefs for health care are also described. The final section focuses on collaborating with clients, with an emphasis on cultural and spiritual assessment and implications for nursing care.

■ CONCEPTS OF CULTURE AND ETHNICITY

Culture is a pattern of learned behaviors and values that are shared among members of a designated group. For example, in the United States, many people share a common language, value freedom and democracy, and share common habits, such as eating three meals a day. The attitudes that characterize a particular society or culture are a design for living, or a blueprint for how people think and act. They are therefore important in determining health and illness behavior.[1] Culture is not observable itself, but rather is a constellation of values and beliefs that people use to interpret their experience. Culture is manifested in social behavior.

Culture is related to, but different from, society in that culture is a set of rules or standards that produce socially acceptable behavior. **Society,** on the other hand, is a group of people in a specific locality that share a common culture and are dependent on each other for survival. Members of the society have a sense of group identity and depend on each other in economic and family relationships. These relationships that hold a society together are known as **social structure,** or social organization. Culture exists within society; thus there can be no culture without society and no society without individuals. All human societies exhibit culture, and every group is a culture.[2] Group in this context refers to a collection of people linked through common characteristics such as physical attributes, ideology, values, beliefs, or behaviors.

Components of Culture

Culture has three essential components: technoeconomic, social, and ideological.[2,3]

The technoeconomic component of culture refers to the way people deal with and adapt to the environment. This includes obtaining and preparing food, clothing, and shelter, as well as defending against enemies.

The social component of culture refers to **social relationships,** which include behavior between and among people, behavior toward possessions, work, learning, worshipping, and other processes. Social behavior also includes the feelings that are attached to the behaviors. This can be seen in a person's feelings toward another person or group.

The third component of culture is **ideology,** which refers to all concepts and their relationships within a cultural system. These concepts label concrete or material objects and their boundaries and attach a word or symbol to them. The material objects include art, religious artifacts, eating utensils, dress, and their use. These concepts are organized and form proverbs, folklore, myths, codes of etiquette and law, technical manuals, religious and scientific doctrines, and philosophies. For example, the Navajo Indian language reflects the concept of the universe being in motion; a withdrawal from motion, or a state of being "at rest," defines any position. Navajo mythology also depicts cultural heroes moving restlessly about trying to perfect the universe.[4]

Characteristics of Culture

Several characteristics determine what is "cultural" about a behavior or activity. Cultural behaviors and activities are shared, learned, social, and adaptive. These characteristics are summarized in Box 9–1.

Even though culture is shared, it is not completely uniform. Within cultural groups, there are value differences that are typically based on gender, age, educational background, or occupation. Subgroups that share these value differences and customs constitute a **subculture.**

Transmission of Culture

Culture is transmitted from generation to generation through enculturation. **Enculturation** is the process by which one learns appropriate ways of acting and meeting one's needs. It refers to the development of behavioral patterns in children that conform to norms of the culture. Enculturation is communicated in childrearing and through education, religion, and art. Through enculturation children are introduced to the concept of self and the behavioral environment characteristic of their culture, thus producing a unique personality. This process, which begins soon after birth, involves parents, siblings, and grandparents. As children grow up, persons outside the family, including extended family members, peers, and educational systems, become involved in enculturation.[2]

Childrearing patterns are culturally defined and variable. Differences in childrearing account, in part, for personality differences. In childrearing, children learn the cultural patterns for specific tasks and rules regarding kinship, religious beliefs, and language. They also learn about personal and social rights and duties. For example, Japanese-Americans place great emphasis on manners and etiquette in disciplining children. Japanese children are trained to address parents and elders as superiors. Apologizing for one's wrongdoings and expressing thanks for and return of favors are consistently emphasized by Japanese parents. There is also a sexual differentiation regarding appropriate social behaviors. For girls, there is emphasis on poise, grace, and control, and for boys, emphasis on determination, manliness, and the will to overcome all obstacles blocking success.[9] These cultural patterns may be implicit or explicitly stated in informal law, myths, folk tales, songs, jokes, riddles, proverbs, puns, and ideology.

Religion is a part of all cultures and is involved in en-

BOX 9–1. CHARACTERISTICS OF CULTURE

Characteristic	Explanation/Example
Culture is shared	Individuals within a culture share ideals, values, and standards of behavior. EXAMPLE: Timing and preparation of meals are shared and culturally determined.[5] In the United States, people commonly cook their food and eat three meals per day.
Culture is learned	Cultural ideals and behaviors are shared and learned, rather than inherited. People learn by growing up within a group. Children and other newcomers to the group learn the culturally determined behavior of the group through observation, discussion, and formal teaching. EXAMPLE: Hispanic-American children learn early that family rules are organized around age and gender in determining lines of authority. In family relationships, the older Hispanic male is given the greatest authority.[6]
Culture is social	Members of the cultural group share interactions and communicate ideas, emotions, and desires between generations. Culture determines how people behave toward each other, individually and in groups. EXAMPLE: Black English or dialect, which is spoken or understood by 80 to 90 percent of black Americans, is a key factor in depicting black social life.[7,8] Black dialect often conveys shared feelings of hardship, hopes, reality, and possibilities, as evident in the dialogue of young black "rappers" today.

culturation. It defines right and wrong behavior, and defines acceptable conduct as well as social bonds. Religion, an organized system of worship, consists of the beliefs, rituals, prayers, songs, dances, offerings, and sacrifices by which people seek supernatural assistance, solace, personal acceptance, or answers about the infinite. Religious beliefs and practices influence how a client responds to health care interventions. Later discussion will identify additional examples of how religion affects specific health care interventions.

Art reflects the cultural values and concerns of people. A culture's oral and written traditions—myths, legends, and tales—teach people how to order their universe and provide information about history. Music and visual arts, such as sculpture and painting, also provide insights into a culture's world view and some suggestions about their history. In addition to adding enjoyment to everyday life, art also transmits and preserves values that set standards for orderly behavior in the society.[2]

Communication is of primary concern in transmitting culture from one generation to another. Communication occurs primarily through language, but also through facial expressions, nonlinguistic noises, physical appearance, clothes, and posture (see Chapter 14). Language is the use of words and symbols to communicate and share experiences, concerns, and beliefs. All cultures have a unique common language. The use of language is influenced by social variables, including the speaker's class and status. Communication and use of language thus affect and are affected by culture.

Cultural Uniformity and Diversity

The United States is a multicultural society, consisting of dominant and minority groups. The **dominant culture** is the group that functions as guardian and sustainer of the controlling value system and allocates rewards and punishments.[10] A **minority culture** is a group that is singled out from the rest of society based on their physical appearance or cultural practices. Minority groups in the United States include African-Americans, Hispanic-Americans, Native Americans, and Asian-Americans, among others (Fig. 9–1).

Acculturation and Assimilation. All cultures change over time, making it necessary to modify behavior and values within the group. This process, **acculturation,** refers to the partial change of a group or individual's culture as a result of contact with a different culture. For example, a Vietnamese immigrant may speak English and eat hamburgers, but may still believe in "ancestor worship" as a means of protecting descendents from a harmful world.[6]

The United States was once considered the great melting pot because many of the European immigrants who came to this country in the 19th and early 20th centuries adopted dominant American habits of dress, language, and food. This process is referred to as **assimilation.**[10] Through assimilation, a group gradually gives up its traditional ways of life and conforms to the standards of the dominant group.

Rapid cultural change can be disorienting. The term **culture shock** is used to refer to the difficulties that people experience in adjusting to life in a foreign culture. For example, many people experience difficulties related to speaking the language, adjusting to the pace of life, and adjusting to the general standard of living, when they live in or work in a foreign culture.

Culture and Identity

Ethnicity and race are two ways of providing a cultural identity. **Ethnicity** refers to affiliation with a group based on hereditary and cultural traditions, such as language and religion.[11] For example, Hispanics and Irish are classified as ethnic groups. **Race** refers to a group of people (family, tribe, or nation) who are descended from a common ancestor and possess common interests, appearance, or habits. Blacks and Caucasians are examples of races of people.

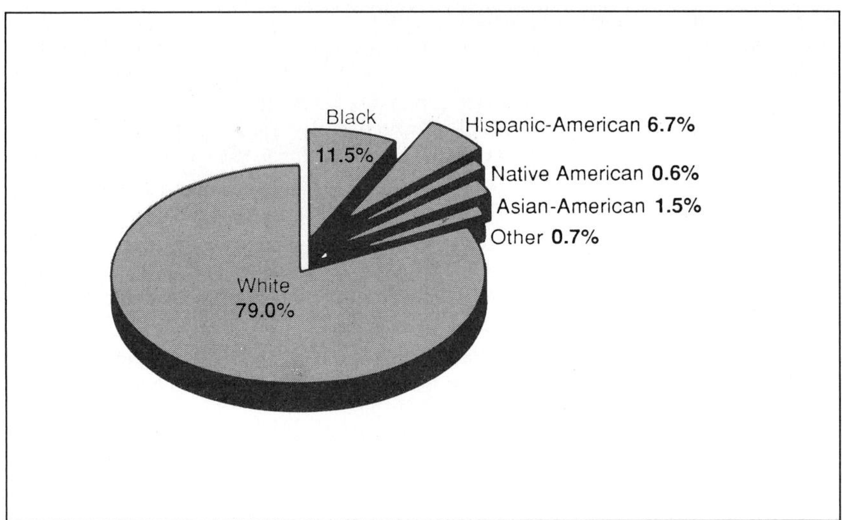

Figure 9–1. Ethnic and racial composition of the United States. (*Based on* Statistical Abstracts of the United States: 1988, *108th ed. Washington, DC; US Bureau of the Census, 1987:Table 20.*)

Cultural identity is also influenced by personality, attitudes, and habits.

Attitudes Influenced by Culture

Culture influences most attitudes. These include time orientation, personal space and territoriality, gender role behavior, and attitudes toward aging and the family.

Time Orientation. Time orientation determines an individual's actions today and in preparation for the future. For example, some cultures, such as Native Americans, are more present-oriented rather than future-oriented; members of such cultures would rather live for today than plan for tomorrow.

Territoriality. Territoriality refers to a person's perceptions of space in relationship to other people. Territoriality is related to trust and distrust, to privacy and modesty. For example, standing too close to a person can violate his or her territory; so can touching an individual or asking probing questions before trust is gained. Asian clients may feel uncomfortable if others come too close. On the other hand, Hispanic clients interpret standing away from people when talking to them as a sign of unfriendliness or haughtiness.[10] Thus, it is of paramount importance that nurses assess the specific practices of each client's cultural group.

Gender Role Behavior. Gender role behavior is ascribed or assigned to individuals based on their sex. The male or female role is culturally determined in terms of division of labor, contributions to subsistence, childrearing, and socialization. These roles often differ for men and women. For example, in Indochinese culture, men are expected to support the family and women to prepare food and care for children.

A culture also provides standards for attire, behavior, rights, and responsibilities based on sexual identity. In addition many cultures ascribe status based on gender, with men often being accorded a higher status than women.

Attitudes Toward Aging. Attitudes toward aging also are influenced by culture. For example, in African-American culture, the elderly are part of an extended family network whose members depend on one another for survival. Thus, grandmothers often care for children through informal adoption; in turn, relatives may care for elderly family members who are ill, rather than place them in a nursing home. African-American culture has also traditionally respected the elderly as possessors of a rich oral history of the black life experience. In the dominant American culture, however, modernization and rapid social change have altered extended kin networks, reduced the dependency on oral tradition, and contributed to a loss of economic and political control by the elderly. This has led to low self-esteem and depression in the elderly, as well as societal anxiety about growing old.[12]

Attitudes Toward Family. Attitudes toward family include beliefs about family structure and function. The basic family, though by no means the only unit, consists of husband, wife, and children. In many parts of the world, however, the extended family is more important than this simple or nuclear family. The extended family consists of several generations, held together either patrilineally (through the male line) or matrilineally (through the female line).

Habits Influenced by Culture

Some of the habits influenced by culture include diet, substance use (alcohol, drugs), work habits, and religious practices.

Diet. Diet and nutritional practices are culturally defined. Different groups attach different symbolic values to food. Custom specifies what foods may be eaten, when to eat, and where to eat. Custom identifies foods that are taboo. For example, Black Muslims who adhere to Islamic religious beliefs do not consume any pork. Jews who follow kosher dietary laws do not serve milk or milk products along with meat at the same meal.[13] Hispanics and Chinese both refer to foods as being "hot" (acidic and spicy) or "cold" (vegetables and dairy products) and use specific foods to treat hot or cold physical conditions. Native Americans use corn meal as a sacred food with curative powers.[10] The specific role that food plays in health and disease prevention is discussed elsewhere in this chapter.

Substance Use. Substance use is culturally influenced. Alcohol use and abuse are shaped by the culture. In many ways the culture shapes drinking behavior and the recognition of drinking as a problem. For instance, conventional therapy has been shown to be ineffective among Native American alcoholics. The difficulty in educating this group has been the denial of high-risk behavior in the Native American community. Traditional community healers have been more effective in decreasing alcoholic rates because of their shared cultural values and beliefs.[14]

Drug use and abuse are also influenced by culture. Crack, a cheap synthetic form of cocaine, is an illicit drug in the United States that has had a devastating effect on low-income urban Americans. Drug use is viewed as an undesirable and illegal behavior. By contrast, some Native Americans use peyote dust, a hallucinogenic drug, as a medium for seeking communion with God, forgiveness of sins, and cure of illness.[15,16]

Work Habits. Work habits and the division of labor, as well as differentiation of work from play, are culturally determined. In all cultures there is an acceptable division of labor that specifies who performs what duties. In most societies, men do the fighting and hunting, whereas women keep house, prepare food, and care for children.[17] With the exception of childbearing and breastfeeding, there are no universal tasks identified as women's work.

An individual perceives work activities differently depending on the cultural context in which they occur. In other words, what is considered work in one context may be considered play in another context. For example, the professional entertainer is performing work in his job, but is also providing play or recreation for the audience. Such activities as hunting, fishing, cycling, or horseback riding are considered fun and recreation. But to many people, hunting and fishing are ways to get food, and the bicycle and horse are means of transportation.

Religious Practices. Historically, a principal source of values has been religion. People have used religion to explain existence, birth, death, illness, and health. Religious practices are based on cultural beliefs about the nature of human beings in the environment.[15] For example, Mexican-Americans who believe illness is caused by evil spirits or the wrath of God may use magico-religious practices such as using holy water, visiting shrines, offering medals and candles, and offering prayers as curative measures.[10,18]

Cultural healers such as *curanderos* or medicine men may also use religious practices to cure illness. Religious practices related to cultural beliefs about health and illness are described later in the chapter.

BUILDING NURSING KNOWLEDGE

What Are Some of the Cultural Barriers That Health Professionals Encounter?

Dawes T. Multicultural nursing. *Int Rev Nurs.* 1986;33(5): 148–150.

Dawes describes a health care project in Oslo, Norway, developed by the Norwegian health authorities to deal with the health problems of foreign immigrants. One focus of the project was the experiences of the health care workers who worked with the immigrant clients. Many of the problems described by the health care workers related to communication barriers with the immigrant clients.

Dawes points out that communication goes beyond technical language problems and involves all aspects of a person's thoughts, feelings, understanding, interpretations, and responses to the environment. Culture is an important factor in communications. Culture shapes social expectations and manners, the various forms of communication, and the conditions under which they are used. Differences in habits and customs between two cultures can lead to misunderstandings among individuals who do not understand these differences. The divergent worlds of health care workers and foreign clients offer many opportunities for misunderstanding. Often immigrants do not understand the routines and expectations that go with taking on the client role in a foreign land. Staff may become irritated because they feel the foreign client has too many visitors. They may fail to understand the concern and sense of responsibility an immigrant's family feels. The client, in turn, may not be accustomed to the isolated, sterile environment encountered in the hospital.

In the Norwegian project, the experience of pain was an area of cultural conflict. Health care workers often saw immigrant clients as being less tolerant of pain than nonimmigrant clients. Immigrant women delivering babies were found to scream and cry more than Norwegian women. Staff expressed reproachful attitudes, implying the women should show more self-control. Yet Dawes notes that physical pain is expressed differently in different cultural contexts. This was difficult for Norwegian health care workers to understand. They took the "stiff upper lip" approach to pain expression.

Ethnocentrism and Cultural Conflicts

Ethnocentrism refers to the belief that one's culture or way of life is superior to that of other cultural groups. This leads one to judge another culture by one's own cultural standards and to perceive the other culture negatively or as

IMPLICATIONS FOR NURSE–CLIENT COLLABORATION

Culture and Cultural Conflict

Culture, as shared values, ideals, and standards of behavior, provides the social context within which nurse and client collaborate. Shared values facilitate understanding and understanding promotes important exchanges between the nurse and client, exchanges that ultimately bear on the client's health. Conflict in values, by contrast, can impede collaboration. When values are not held in common, it is important for the nurse to actively seek to understand the client's perspective, particularly as it pertains to the meanings the client holds for health and health care.

inferior.[1] Traditionally, nurses and other health care providers have largely provided care based on the philosophy of ethnocentrism. For example, an ethnocentric nurse might immediately view all non-Western healing methods as primitive and ineffective.

Ethnocentrism may lead to stereotyping, prejudice, discrimination, racism, and cultural conflict. **Stereotyping** is a response to a person or group based on preconceived negative labels without an objective assessment of the individual or group. Closely related to stereotyping is prejudice. **Prejudice** is a negative attitude acquired without any prior adequate evidence or experience with a group. Stereotyping and prejudice can lead to **discrimination,** or differential unequal behavioral treatment based solely on ethnic, racial or religious group affiliation.[10] These beliefs and attitudes, in turn, can lead to racism. **Racism** is any ethnocentric activity—cultural, individual, or institutional, deliberate or not—that is based on the belief that one racial group is superior to another. Racism is often the basis for oppression and control of groups of people. **Cultural conflict** occurs when there is a lack of awareness, understanding, acceptance, or responsiveness between members of different cultural groups concerning their distinct cultural experience. For example, cultural conflict may result when the beliefs of members of the Hispanic culture that leaving a candle burning at the bedside of family members who are ill will protect them from evil clash with the hospital culture's beliefs that this activity is a fire hazard.

CULTURE AND HEALTH

All cultures have specific, individualized ways of defining health and illness. They also have ways of promoting health and of caring for and curing different illnesses. Recurring traditional customs and their arrangement form cultural patterns of health and illness behavior.[3]

The patterned behaviors of a group not only affect the state of health or disease in a society, but also reveal the attitudes, beliefs, and customary actions of the group.[19] Bruhn defined health behavior as those actions (or inactions) that directly or indirectly affect health status or well-being.[3]

Patterned behaviors among many cultured groups in the United States include preventive and protective behaviors undertaken to remain well. These include, but are not limited to, proper sleep, eating habits, weight control, exercise, recreation, and choices to limit smoking, alcohol, and drug use. Other preventive behaviors include wearing seat belts and motorcycle helmets, obeying traffic regulations, and health care screening, such as regular examinations for signs of cancer, heart disease, and dental problems. Examples of protective health behaviors include praying; fixing things around the house; taking laxatives, cold showers, or hot baths; and consuming vitamins.

Subgroups within a society often demonstrate specific cultural patterns related to ethnic background, religion, and race. For instance, middle-class, Catholic Italian-Americans living in New York City share distinct cultural patterns or characteristics that distinguish them from non-middle class, non-Catholic individuals who have a differing ethnic background.

Cultural patterns were identified in a study of Mexican, black, and white Americans that demonstrated clear differences in the decisions of members of these groups to seek medical care when ill. These differences were based on fear of unfair treatment in health care institutions, reliance on cultural healing systems, and socioeconomic issues.[10]

Cultural Variability in Defining Health

All cultures characterize health as "good," "potent," and "active"; however, cultures may define health in different ways. For example, health may be represented by one's role enactment and participation in social processes. In this example, persons who do not perform their social roles are considered deviant or ill. Another example is the personal experience of general well-being. According to this definition, persons who feel well are considered healthy, whereas those who feel distressed or impaired are considered ill. (Definitions of health and illness are discussed in more detail in Chapter 5.)

Culture and Physical Health

The relationship of culture to health is demonstrated by the prevalence of disease within certain cultures. For example, Japanese-Americans have a high incidence of cancer of the stomach, which has been linked to a traditional diet of talc-treated rice. The talc treatment contains asbestos, a known carcinogen.[10]

Disease is distributed in a society based on cultural, biological, and social factors in relationship to age, sex, ethnicity, life-style, and occupation. Many acute infections occur with a higher incidence in children, suggesting that as people grow older they develop certain immunities and decrease their vulnerabilities to infectious disease. Indications are that biological factors play a role in sexual differences in mortality, with women living longer than men.

Ethnic differences also exist in the prevalence and etiology of certain diseases, among them genetic disorders, nutritional maladies, heart disease, and various forms of cancer. Sickle-cell anemia, Tay-Sachs disease, and thalassemia are examples of genetic disorders associated with specific racial and ethnic backgrounds: sickle-cell anemia, which causes destruction of red blood cells and clot formation, with black Americans;[10] Tay-Sachs disease, which is characterized by degeneration of nervous system cells, with Ashkenazic Jews; and thalassemia, a type of anemia caused by a defect in the rate of hemoglobin development, with persons of Mediterranean ancestry.[20]

Life-style also influences health and health behavior. Life-style is a broad concept that encompasses health behavior, attitudes, and outlook or philosophy of life. It also includes geographical area or residence, the way a room is decorated, the type of car driven, the type of food eaten, the kind of clothes worn, the kind of entertainment and leisure activities engaged in, and the choice of a marriage partner. Life-style is modeled and learned, but also has many components that are acquired and changed as one moves through the life cycle.

Life-style and health are closely related, so changes in one usually affect the other.[19] For example, a change in residence from rural to urban will influence how, when, and where an individual eats, sleeps, worships, and works. A change in employment will influence what, where, and with whom an individual eats. Consequently, as changes occur throughout the life cycle, modifications are made in both life-style and health behavior to accommodate the life changes. The relationship between life-style and health is discussed further in Chapter 22.

Culture and Healing

Culture plays a significant role in healing and treating disease. Every culture provides a mechanism for promoting healing that provides solutions to basic human problems related to birth, death, health, and disease. These solutions may explain the culturally defined state or condition, rules for attaining and maintaining a state of well-being, definitions of the processes and methods for care of clients, and definitions of the cultural healers.[15,21,22]

Many familial and cultural health practices in the United States derive from belief systems and practices that have historical roots and origins around the world. Cultural traditions related to health practices and healing offer a variety of approaches that have been proven effective based on empirical studies and personal reports.[23–25] Traditional practices used to maintain health include protective objects, substances, diet regimens, and religious practices and rituals. These, and other cultural beliefs and practices, are discussed in more detail in the following sections.

Religious beliefs may strongly affect people's interpretation and responses to disease, treatment, and the healing process. Many religions also dictate social, moral, and dietary practices that are designed to keep a person healthy and in balance. Religion also determines rituals and the role of faith in recovery from illness.

Rituals are an integral part of religion and healing. They are often used to defeat evil spirits or to remove them from a person's body, for example, through a process of gift giving, magical ceremonies, and rites. Baptism is a religious ritual used for cleansing and to prevent evil from harming a person.[18]

■ TRADITIONAL HEALTH CARE VERSUS THE MODERN HEALTH CARE CULTURE

A culture's beliefs about health and illness serve as the foundation for all health care. Both traditional and modern health care cultures are based on the interdependent variables of beliefs, values, attitudes, practices, and roles related to concepts of health and disease. These variables generate patterns of diagnosis and treatment.[15] To understand why persons from one culture treat an illness with medication and those from another culture call on a spiritual healer requires an understanding of the belief systems of each culture.

For instance, a belief in magic is based on an assumption that disease is due to human behavior and can be cured through sorcery (magic performed with the aid of evil spirits). A religious world view assumes that disease is due to supernatural forces and must be cured by supernatural methods (methods that are beyond the natural). A scientific view assumes that disease results from a cause-and-effect relationship among natural phenomena and that curing is effected by scientific problem solving and intervention.[15,26,27]

The traditional health care culture includes the folk health beliefs and practices that have been passed down through tradition in many societies, and that continue to be practiced as an alternative to, or in addition to, the practices of the modern health care culture. Traditional health practices include home remedies and reliance on cultural and spiritual healers who may use herbal, magical, or religious remedies.

Health and disease are typically viewed as representing either a balance or an imbalance. Diseases are often diagnosed as "hot" or "cold" and treated with herbs, drugs, or foods believed to have opposing qualities, with the aim of restoring balance.[15,26]

Illness is often viewed as a result of sorcery, failure to obey cultural norms, intrusion of harmful objects into the body, spirit intrusion (eg, devil possession), and soul loss.[27] Disease may also be viewed as "God's will" in response to sins or failure to follow religious norms.

Spiritual protection may be used to ward off or to cure illness, with prayers, saints, or spirits to provide "faith healing." Herbalism or herbal medicine is a traditional treatment method prescribed by cultural healers to cure illness. Historically, on the basis of their actual or perceived attributes, plants have been used to treat illness. The ginseng root is the most famous herb used for medicinal purposes.

Many of the cultural groups discussed later in this chapter maintain traditional, or folk, health care beliefs and practices. Examples of common beliefs and practices in traditional health care culture include:

- Holistic approach and concern with the whole client
- Search for patterns and causes
- Concern with human values
- Caring viewed as part of the healing process
- Traditional healer viewed as therapeutic partner; minimal scientific intervention; focus on noninvasive procedures

- Disease or dysfunction viewed as a process, with pain and disease denoting possible internal conflicts
- Body seen as a complex system of energy
- Emphasis on achieving maximum body, mind, and spirit health with prevention being synonymous with harmony among relationships, activities, and life goals
- Reliance on qualitative information from client, family, or traditional curer's intuition[27,28]

The modern health care culture, in contrast, is based on a scientific model in which disease is explained by a cause-and-effect relationship. This scientific model holds that (1) disease can be treated "best" by applying scientific knowledge and method; (2) the germ theory of disease explains the process of infection; and (3) illness prevention is based on proper hygiene, public sanitation, and personal and environmental restraints.[27]

Disease, in the modern health care culture, is viewed as a maladaptation or malfunctioning of biological or psychological processes in a person. Modern health care professionals thus perceive disease as having scientifically based signs, symptoms, diagnosis, and treatment. The predominant treatment method in modern health care is "allopathic medicine" based on the principle that when a substance deviates from the normal, a procedure to counteract its effects should be applied.[26,28] Such counteracting procedures include drug therapy, medical and surgical interventions, and scientific therapies such as radiation therapy for cancer.

Nurses, as participants in this modern health care culture, share to some extent its beliefs, practices, and language, as well as an institutionalized system for practice. The following beliefs and behaviors characterize the modern health care culture:

- Concern with clients in a specialized way
- Treatment of symptoms
- Emphasis on efficiency
- Role of health care professional historically seen as that of emotional neutrality and authority over dependent client
- Disease or disability viewed as a distinct entity, with pain viewed as negative
- Body viewed as a machine in good or bad repair
- Body and mind perceived as separate, with psychological illnesses seen as mental disorders requiring psychiatric or psychological services
- Prevention viewed as behavioral or environmental (eg, vitamins, rest, exercise, immunizations, avoidance of smoking, nonuse of alcohol and drugs)
- Reliance on quantitative data from physical examination and diagnostic tests[27]

■ HEALTH BELIEFS AND PRACTICES OF SPECIFIC CULTURAL GROUPS

This section discusses the health beliefs and practices of several cultural groups with whom nurses may come in contact. The cultural groups presented are African-American, Hispanic-American, Chinese-American, Japanese-American, Indo-Chinese, Native American, and low-income groups. Table 9–1 presents a comparative overview of the health beliefs and practices for these cultural groups.

The beliefs and practices discussed for each group are presented in a generalized way to facilitate discussion; however, it is important to remember that there are subcultural variations within each group. The extent to which members of a culture conform to beliefs and practices common to the culture as a whole is related to the degree of acculturation and assimilation, geographic location, and demographic variables such as age, education, socioeconomic status, and religious affiliation. Thus, not all of the descriptive statements will apply to all families or individuals of a particular culture at all times.

A holistic framework is used to describe the following factors for each cultural group: (1) family concepts, (2) definition of health and illness, (3) beliefs and practices about health and illness, (4) health problems, and (5) implications for nurse–client collaboration. The holistic approach views the client as autonomous, and the health professional as a therapeutic partner who offers "caring" as a component of healing. Using this approach, nurses collaborate with clients and families to determine and assess culturally defined health beliefs and practices. This assists nurses in planning and implementing holistic care based on culturally appropriate interventions.

African-Americans (Blacks)

The terms *black, African-American,* and *black American* are used interchangeably to refer to this cultural group, which includes persons of African descent, as well as West Indians, Haitians, and Jamaicans. The cultural roots of African-Americans are strongly entrenched in the black life experience in the United States, which has shaped their views of the external world and their internal attitudes and belief systems, and has influenced their interactions with others. The health care experiences of African-Americans reflect social injustices in American society.[29–31]

Initially, African-Americans came to the United States involuntarily as slaves. This significant fact has shaped and continues to influence all aspects of black family life. Racism and discrimination denied black Americans entry into mainstream American society. Black Americans today continue to struggle to overcome these barriers.

Family. Historically, African-American family life has been viewed from a pathological and dysfunctional perspective, emphasizing poverty, welfare dependency, illegitimacy, and matriarchal households.[32,33] This perspective assumed that universal norms exist for cultural behavior, and it viewed black families that deviated from the dominant white Anglo norm as dysfunctional.[34] This perspective has been challenged by others who emphasize the black family's ability to adapt to cultural demands and to experience growth despite persistent social, political, and economic struggles in the United States.[35–37] This latter view reflects the influence of the black family's African heritage, which-emphasizes the values of group orientation, sharing, kinship, obedience to authority, belief in spirituality, and respect for the elderly and the past.[29]

Although the African-American family is often discussed as a single entity, no single family pattern represents all families. Various factors, in particular geographical origin and location (urban north versus rural south) and socioeconomic status, influence each family's organization and adherence to cultural traditions. For instance, upper-middle-class African-American families are closer in organization and social structure to upper-middle-class white families than to black families living in poverty. Despite these variations, however, a traditional pattern can be described for black family life that is representative of families whose origins were in rural communities in the southern United States.

The African-American family is often a multigenerational, extended family, with a network of relatives connected by a strong kinship network. These strong family and kinship ties provide mutual aid for individuals within the extended family.[37] This sense of interdependence results in reliance on family resources for support rather than seeking outside assistance. The black family is also characterized by a flexibility of family roles and responsibilities. For example, if a family member cannot take care of a young child, the child may be informally adopted by another family member. Not all African-American families demonstrate an extended family pattern. Although extended kinship bonds continue to be strong, many black families now form nuclear family units because they live long distances from their extended families.

Definition of Health and Illness. Some black Americans view life as a process versus a state. When a person is in harmony with nature, he or she experiences health; disharmony with nature results in illness. Issues related to illness tend to evolve out of the everyday experiences and circumstances of a person. Health is defined as feeling good (ie, "nothing hurts me"), a happy person with no problems, or the ability to go to work. In contrast, illness is associated with feeling bad, inability to do physical activity, or bad luck.[29]

Beliefs and Practices About Health and Illness. The health beliefs of some rural blacks have been found to contain elements of African beliefs, folk and formal medicine of the 19th century, and certain contemporary health beliefs, interwoven with components of Christianity, voodoo, and magic.[38] Rural black Americans may use herbs or home remedies such as peppermint, nutmeg, and clove to cure an upset stomach or a raw potato placed on the body to treat fevers.[10,25,38] Oils, candles, or incenses may be used to repel the evil effects of unnatural illnesses.

Traditionally, the black church has helped blacks to solve problems, define values, and develop standards or patterns of behavior. Religious beliefs of black Americans help them to understand themselves in relation to life, death, health, and illness.[39] Black clergy not only serve as teachers and politicians, but also minister to those facing illness and suffering. Black clergy can often help bridge the gap between black clients and family health care professionals. Prayer is used both by and on behalf of the sick.

Urban black clients may seek health care often and practice preventive medicine in contrast to rural black clients, who may not seek health care until too late. The reasons for this unwillingness to seek health care include discrimination in the health care system, economic factors, child-care problems, fear of hospitals or death, and fear of experimentation. In addition, traditional folk healing continues to be important in both rural and urban black communities. Although upper-middle-class, well-educated blacks have predominantly abandoned most home remedies, poor clients often exhaust these measures before seeking professional medical care.[30,40]

Health Problems. There is a continuing disparity in health status of black Americans compared with that of the nation as a whole. Life expectancy for black men and women remains significantly lower than for white men and women. Higher death rates for black Americans are a result of increases in (1) cardiovascular and cerebrovascular diseases, in particular, hypertension; (2) homicide and unintentional injuries; (3) cancer, particularly esophageal, prostate, colon, rectal, urinary, laryngeal, breast, cervical, and uterine; (4) infant mortality; (5) drug or alcohol dependency; and (6) diabetes, linked to higher rates of obesity for black women versus white women.[20,41–43] Contributing factors related to premature deaths in the black community include poverty, inadequate housing, psychological stress, substance abuse, gang activity, malnutrition, inadequate access to medical care, lack of prenatal care, and lack of early detection and illness prevention techniques.[41]

Other major health problems for blacks include sickle-cell disease and acquired immunodeficiency syndrome (AIDS). Sickle-cell disease is a genetic blood disorder prevalent among blacks. Approximately 10 percent of black Americans are carriers of the sickle-cell trait, and 1 in 500 have sickle-cell anemia.[44] AIDS is currently among the nation's major health concerns. Black Americans, especially women and children, have been among those hardest hit by the deadly epidemic.

Implications for Nurse–Client Collaboration. Nurses' familiarity with black cultural traditions is an important factor influencing nurse–client collaboration. Black-American clients differ in their reliance on traditional health beliefs and remedies depending on age, socioeconomic status, and geographical location (urban north, rural south). Upper-middle-class black Americans are less likely to exhibit the traditional health beliefs and practices.

The extended family structure and role flexibility common to many black families mean that the term *significant others* often takes on a different meaning for black clients. For example, during childbearing and childrearing, an aunt or grandmother may share or assume responsibilities for child care that would otherwise fall to parents.[45] Nurses

TABLE 9–1. COMPARISON OF HEALTH BELIEFS AND PRACTICES OF SPECIFIC CULTURAL GROUPS

Subculture	Concepts of Health	Origins of Illness	Type of Healer, Prevention and Healing Practices
African-American	Health is measured by one's ability to work. React to poor health only when there is a crisis, such as high fever or bleeding.	Illness may be punishment from God for wrongdoing, or is due to voodoo, spirits, or demons.	Prevention through good diet, rest, cleanliness, and laxatives to clean the system. Wear copper and silver bracelets to prevent illness. Also use some herbs. Some believe in voodoo and religious healing.
Hispanic-American	Health is a gift from God, and is also due to good luck. Healthy person has robust appearance and feels well.	Illness may be punishment from God for wrongdoing; or caused by an imbalance between "hot" and "cold" properties of the body.	*Curandero* cures hot illness with cold medicine and vice versa. Illness is prevented by eating well, praying, being good, working, and wearing religious medals.
Chinese-American	Health involves the balance of *yin* and *yang* (negative and positive energy forces). Healthy body is gift from parents and ancestors.	Illness is caused by imbalance of *yin* and *yang.*	Healers include herbalist, spiritual healer, and physician. Food is essential for harmony with nature and is important in cause and treatment of disease. Acupuncture and moxibustion restore balance of *yin* and *yang.* Herbal remedies, such as ginseng, are also used.
Japanese-American	Health viewed as a state of harmony and balance. Healing involves reestablishing balance between the body and the universe.	Illness is due to an imbalance between positive and negative energy forces; results when the flow of energy stops along meridians of the body. Physical contact with blood, skin diseases, and corpses will cause illness, as will improper care of the body, including poor diet and lack of sleep. Also ascribe to germ theory of disease causation.	Herbalists, spiritual healers, and physicians are consulted for healing. Energy flow can be restored with acupuncture, massage, and acupressure. Kampo medicine uses natural herbs having fewer side effects than Western medicine. Purification rites are used to remove "evil" effects on the body. Cultural foods like miso soup and tofu are used to ensure health. Scientific methods include immunizations and surgery.
Indo-Chinese	Health is living in harmony with the environment.	Illness is a manifestation of supernatural powers, gods, demons, and spirits, and humoral beliefs. Also subscribe to the hot and cold theory of disease and treatment.	Use hot and cold therapy for care and treatment. Use herbs and teas. Believe in and use self-help.
Native American	Health is harmony between the individual, earth, and the supernatural, as well as the ability to survive difficult circumstances.	Illness is disharmony and can be caused by violation of taboos, witchcraft, displeasing holy people, annoying the elements, disturbing plant and animal life, neglecting the celestial bodies, or misusing sacred Native American ceremony.	Healer is the medicine man. Illness is prevented through elaborate religious rituals and charms consisting of fetishes and pollen carried in a bag. Medicine and religion are closely related. Do not believe in the germ theory.
Low-income groups	Health is often defined in terms of work. People who can work are healthy.	Believe illness is inevitable (fatalistic attitude).	Use self-care treatment to avoid high cost of health care. Regular preventive health care is seldom practiced. It is more important to work than to lose a paycheck, especially if a person is not ill.

Personal Care and Family Life	Use of Health Care Delivery System	Health Problems	Death and Dying
African-based family with large extended families, flexible family roles, and responsibilities. Strong religious orientation.	May receive inadequate health care. May experience segregation and racism when seeking care. Often use home remedies often because of effectiveness and also because they are less expensive.	Hypertension, sickle-cell anemia, some cancers (eg, lung, oral). High infant-maternal mortality, drug and alcohol abuse, obesity, and AIDS.	Believe in life after death.
Extended family is important. Value helping each other. Patriarchal family, with men making all decisions. Family honor is important. Children are a great source of pride.	Experience barriers to health care because of language (inability to speak English). May seek care from a physician, a folk practitioner, or both. May be late or miss appointments for care because of present time orientation.	Poverty-related diseases, such as tuberculosis, malnutrition, lead poisoning, and drug addiction.	View death and dying as "God's will." Believe in rewards from God in afterlife for good behavior.
Patriarchal family. Women are subservient to men. Ancestor worship and respect and obedience to parents are observed. Divorce is considered a disgrace.	Language barriers may exist; family spokesman may accompany client to Western physician. Prefer Chinese physicians if available in the community. May resist painful diagnostic tests. Having to have blood drawn is upsetting.	Respiratory diseases, immunization deficiencies, dental caries, tuberculosis, lactose intolerance.	Believe in reincarnation.
Roles are stratified in a hierarchy of old to young, man to woman, superior to subordinate. Traditional beliefs emphasize a fatalistic attitude in acceptance of roles and position in life. *Koko,* or filial piety, is demonstrated when children are faithful to parents and their teachings.	Rely on group decision making about health concerns. Will often seek both Western and Asian physicians during illness. Because of the value placed on *jaman,* or self-control, may be reluctant to seek mental health or community resources.	High incidence of stress-related conditions, such as colitis, ulcers, psoriasis, and depression. High incidence of stomach, liver, and biliary cancers. High rate of hypertension and cerebrovascular problems related to salt intake and psychological stress. Lactose intolerance common.	Older generations (*Issei* and *Nisei*) adhere strongly to the idea that life is suffering and all human lives will inevitably deteriorate and come to an end. Artificial means of prolonging life unacceptable to older generations. Younger generations (*Sansei* and *Yonsei*) are similar to their Western peers in attitudes toward death and dying.
Very close family ties. Patriarchal and extended family is important.	Rarely accept hospitalization, except in emergencies. Seek care only after much delay. Will check out of the hospital at first sign of improvement. Usually are noncompliant to medical regimen.	Malnutrition, anemia, intestinal parasites, emotional and stress-related problems, tuberculosis, resettlement problems.	Strong desire to die at home to prevent wandering soul after death.
Extended family and tribal ties are strong. Cooperation is emphasized within the family and tribe.	Speak tribal language and may not understand English. Often seek care from medicine man first. General beliefs incompatible with those of health care system. Native Americans living in the eastern United States and most urban areas are not covered by the Indian Health Service.	Cirrhosis of the liver, alcoholism, high infant mortality, shortened life span, suicide, homicide, domestic violence. Leading causes of death are heart disease, accidents, malignant neoplasms, and cirrhosis.	Fear spirits of the dead. Children and family should be with dying person. Many rules and customs surround the dying. Do not believe in life after death.
Economic and social stressors influence attitudes and behaviors toward self and children.	Underutilization of subsidized health care services despite higher disease rates. Often rely on emergency rooms in urban hospitals for health care services.	Health status depends on quality of environment. Overcrowded living conditions can lead to higher incidence of communicable diseases (eg, tuberculosis). High incidence of drug and alcohol abuse. High infant mortality rates related to lack of prenatal care. Chronic diseases such as heart disease, hypertension, diabetes, AIDS, or cancer often go unchecked because of lack of accessibility to or cost of health care.	Death and dying are believed to be the inevitable result of a life of poverty.

should therefore explore role responsibilities with each client and family to determine who fulfills what roles and to whom health teaching should be directed.

Because of the important role of religion in the black community, nurses should inquire about clients' religious support (eg, minister, cultural healer, family practices). Nurses should also respect any ornaments, charms, or objects worn or brought to the hospital by black clients.

Nurses need to be knowledgeable about physical norms for black clients. The detection of significant changes in the health status of blacks often depends on the ability to recognize skin color changes. Vasomotor dilation is not easily recognized in black skin. An ashen gray color of the skin can denote vasoconstriction and anemia. Black hair texture is distinctively different from the hair texture of nonblacks. The skin of black clients may be ashy or dry and some clients may use lotions, oils, or petroleum to remedy this jelly condition. Nurses should consult clients about methods of hair and skin care that will enable them to provide appropriate care.[29]

Nurses also need to be familiar with the dietary habits of African-Americans and the potential effects of food choices on health status. Historically, the diet of African-Americans has interwoven dietary patterns of many cultures, supplementing traditional African foods (such as yams, cassava, rice, and peanuts) with foods from French, English, Spanish, and Native American cultures.[10] Europeans contributed the "porker" used to season vegetable dishes; Native Americans contributed foods such as corn, herbs, wild game (squirrel, possum, rabbit), and fish (catfish).[10] Today, pork is still one of the main food staples, prepared in many ways (fried, barbecued, roasted, smoked, or pickled). However, dietary patterns of African-Americans are influenced by geographic location and socioeconomic status. For example, black Americans from the rural South may consume mainly traditional foods, whereas the diet of those who live in urban communities is often more strongly influenced by the dominant culture. Nurses need to consider how cultural food choices, such as highly salted foods, may affect the care of clients with hypertension. (Refer to Chapter 25 and Box 25–3 for further information about cultural dietary patterns.)

Hispanic-Americans

Hispanic-Americans originated in such Spanish-speaking countries as Puerto Rico and the countries of Central and South America. The Hispanic population today is young, growing, mainly urban, and multiracial. Hispanic-Americans are concentrated in major cities, particularly Los Angeles, Miami, and New York City, and in Texas. Although they are predominantly Roman Catholic and share a common language, Hispanic-Americans are a diverse cultural group. Traditions and beliefs, along with demographics and socioeconomic status, differ depending on country of origin[46]; however, attachment to the Spanish language and to Hispanic culture is strong. This discussion focuses on Mexican-American culture as an example of one Hispanic-American cultural tradition.

Family. Mexican-American families have strong ties characteristic of an extended family. The source of identity and security for an individual is the family. Family members demonstrate a sense of duty toward one another, and members provide support with the idea that reciprocal help will be given in the future.[10,47]

The family, as a unit, is involved in decision making, and interpersonal interactions are conducted with a sense of *respecto*: from younger to older, woman to man, and subordinate to superior. The father is the head of the family and makes the decision about therapeutic interventions when an illness occurs. *Compadres* (godparents) are also consulted for home treatment advice and to help decide whether to seek health care. Families often seek professional health care only after all other resources have been exhausted.[47] Educational background, socioeconomic status, age, gender, and primary language of Mexican-American clients influence their use of health care services.

Definition of Health and Illness. To Mexican-Americans, good health means that one is behaving in accordance with one's conscience, God's mandate, and the norms and customs of the family, church, and local community. There is no separation between the psychological and total well-being of the individual. Good health is also related to the ability to work and fulfill family and social roles, as one gains and maintains respect by meeting one's responsibilities. Criteria for health are sturdy body, maintenance of normal physical activity, and the absence of pain. Hardship and suffering are part of life and must be endured as one's destiny; rewards for being submissive to God's will and doing good will come in the afterlife.

Illness is seen as resulting from (1) psychological states, such as envy, anger, fear, fright, embarrassment, excessive worry, family turmoil, improper behavior, or misconduct related to moral and ethical codes; (2) environmental or natural conditions, such as bad air, germs, bad food, excess of cold or heat, or poverty; (3) dislocation of internal organs; and (4) supernatural causes, such as evil spirits, bad luck, witchcraft, or living enemies who cause harm as a result of vengeance or envy.[10,15,47,48]

Beliefs and Practices About Health and Illness. Mexican-Americans believe in the "hot and cold theory" of disease, which views health as a "temperate" condition or a balanced state between "hot" and "cold" elements. Illness is an imbalance among these elements, and treatment involves restoring balance.[10,47] For example, penicillin is classified as a "hot" substance because it may cause a rash or diarrhea, which are hot conditions. Hot illnesses are treated with cold or cool substances. In contrast, a cold disease, such as an earache or common cold, is treated with hot substances. All foods, beverages, animals, and people possess the characteristics of hot and cold on a continuum. Hot and cold do not refer to temperature, but are descriptive of a substance itself. Hot foods include beef, most oils, and chili peppers; cold foods include fresh vegetables, milk products, and citrus fruits.[10,15,48]

Other Mexican-American beliefs about disease causation include the following:

1. *Caida de la mollera* (fallen fontanelle): This infant condition is characterized by diarrhea, restlessness, inability to suck, and occasional fever, and is believed to be caused by bouncing or dropping an infant or touching the head. Treatment includes prayers, pushing the palate up inside the mouth, or applying eggs and warm salted olive oil to the skull.[18,48]
2. *Empacho* (intestinal blockage): The symptoms of this disease of dislocation include abdominal pain, vomiting, and lack of appetite. Treatment consists of massage and drinking herbal cathartics.[10]
3. *Mal de ojo* (evil eye): Children and pregnant women are most susceptible to *mal de ojo,* although it can affect all ages. It is caused by a person's admiration for or envy of another. Symptoms include weeping, headaches, high fever, irritability, aches, and pains. Having the admirer touch the victim is supposed to break the evil bond and alleviate symptoms. If the admirer cannot be found, placing an egg in water under the bed of the victim will draw out the evil.[18,48]
4. *Susto* (fright sickness): A frightening or upsetting experience causes the soul to leave the body and wander freely. Symptoms include listlessness, loss of appetite and sleep, depression, and indifference to personal hygiene and dress. Treatment is performed by a cultural healer who rubs the client's body with special herbs and provides prayers, herbal teas, and sugar water.[10,18,48,49]

These beliefs about disease causation are most prevalent among Mexican-Americans in the lower classes, although middle- or upper-class families may also adhere to similar health beliefs. Elderly persons tend to adhere most strongly to these health traditions.

Women in Mexican-American families usually provide primary care for illness in the home. In cases of severe or persistent illness, a folk or religious healer may be consulted.[48]

Curanderismo is a system of folk medicine used by Mexican-Americans that combines Aztec, Spanish, spiritualistic, homeopathic, and scientific elements.[18] *Curanderos* (religious healers) attempt to correct imbalances by using prayers, pledges (*mandas*) to religious or supernatural forces, and rituals. *Yerberos* (herbalists) use home remedies, such as diets and herbs. *Sobadoras* (folk chiropractors) massage or manipulate bones and joints to correct musculoskeletal imbalances. *Parteras* are lay midwives. *Espiritualistas* (spiritualists) are consulted to counteract witchcraft.[10,18] These cultural healers offer tremendous emotional support to Mexican-American clients and their families and offer inexpensive services as compared with the scientific health care community.

Health Problems. Language barriers, traditional values and beliefs, and socioeconomic status contribute to the underutilization of health care services by Mexican-Americans. Many communities lack bilingual health services, which limits access to health services.

The serious health problems experienced by Mexican-Americans include hypertension, an incidence of diabetes that is five times the national average, increasing suicide rates, high infant mortality rates, malnutrition, increased respiratory problems caused by overcrowded living conditions, and increased risk of parasitic conditions among migrant workers.[47,48] Inaccessibility to health services, especially for migrant workers who are highly mobile, weakens preventive and follow-up health care services.

Obesity is a problem among Mexican-American children. Alexander and Blank[50] found that 13.3 percent of 2- to 5-year-old Mexican-American children were overweight, in contrast to 8.9 percent in the general population. Childhood obesity is more apt to be followed by obesity as an adult, which becomes more chronic and resistant to treatment.

For Hispanic-Americans who live in the barrios of large urban centers, alcohol and drug abuse is a major health problem. Factors that contribute to high drug abuse rates are the stresses of acculturation, socioeconomic conditions, availability of illicit drugs, and peer pressure.[47] Drinking with friends is a widely accepted social practice among Hispanic men. The ability to consume substantial quantities of alcohol without intoxication or showing ill effects reinforces the concept of *machismo* (strong male image).[6]

AIDS is also a major health concern for Hispanic-Americans, who account for 15 percent of US cases.[51] *Machismo,* homophobia (fear of homosexuality), and Catholic sexual taboos, combined with poverty and poor education, have hindered the response of the Hispanic community to the threat of AIDS. It has been recommended that an intensive Spanish-language campaign be presented to combat the fatalism about AIDS characteristic of the Hispanic culture.

Implications for Nurse–Client Collaboration. Hispanic families vary in their adherence to traditional health beliefs and practices depending on their degree of acculturation. Recent immigrants follow traditional practices more strongly than those who were born in or educated in the United States. Adherence to the hot and cold theory of disease similarly varies; nurses should therefore question clients individually to determine their health beliefs. Nurses should also verify with clients what they deem appropriate foods and beverages for their illnesses. Nursing collaboration is facilitated if the nurse or other staff member speaks and understands Spanish.

Hispanic clients who wear amulets or religious objects to protect themselves from evil should not be expected to remove these articles. If it becomes necessary to remove an article, for example to facilitate care, nurses should place it close to the client. Practices that are not harmful should not be interfered with, including wearing religious jewelry (cross, medals) and prayer sessions among clients, their families, and folk healers; however, health care providers should also inquire about any herbal medicines that may have been prescribed by a folk healer, as these may interfere with a client's drug regimen.

Hispanic clients value modesty and privacy and may be embarrassed when it is necessary to undress for an examination. They often are reluctant to be examined by health care providers of the opposite sex. The nurse can respect clients' privacy by ensuring that only those areas of the body that must be exposed are uncovered during each part of the examination. Nurses should remain continuously respectful of clients' traditional beliefs and values.

Because Mexican-Americans are present-oriented, little emphasis is given to exact time of day. This creates a barrier to health care as clients may not keep important clinical appointments or may arrive late for scheduled tests. Nursing interventions should be directed toward the present without neglecting to educate toward the future.

Hispanic clients often believe that disease is related to the supernatural and to imbalances in the environment; this influences their acceptance of treatment methods. For instance, clients with cancer often do not agree to chemotherapy or radiation regimens because they view their illness as punishment for their sins. If clients believe that illness is a punishment for wrongdoing, they may believe that to alleviate their sins, they must accept pain and suffering. Clients who hold traditional beliefs often will consult a Western health care provider only if they are not cured by a traditional healer.

Chinese-Americans

Chinese-Americans are the largest group of Asian-Americans in the United States. Most Chinese-Americans reside in large urban centers of the West and East coasts, as well as in Hawaii and Chicago. They can be categorized into four groups: (1) those born in China who immigrated to the United States 40 to 50 years ago; (2) those who immigrated about 20 years ago; (3) recent immigrants; and (4) first- and second-generation Chinese-Americans. The first group identifies strongly with traditional health practices; the other three groups generally accept Western health practices, but are influenced to varying degrees by traditional practices.[52]

Family. Traditional Chinese families are patriarchal and patrilineal with strong extended family clans. There is marked role differentiation based on age, gender, and generation among members of the family. Parents, especially the father, are honored, respected, and obeyed. Grandparents also hold a special place of honor and esteem in the family. Children are involved in family activities, and strong emphasis is placed on learning about their cultural heritage (eg, Chinese-language classes after school). Many Chinese-Americans still adhere to these values.[52] Many others, however, leave their childhood environments and their extended families, often adopting a nuclear family system.[53]

In Chinese-American families, each member is expected to work hard and contribute to the success of the group. This is manifested by the high regard for education for its own sake and as a key to social and economic advancement. As a result, second-generation and younger first-generation immigrants are highly educated and many have achieved middle-class status.[53,54] On the other hand, not all Chinese-Americans have these successes, as many continue to experience racial discrimination.

Confucianism teaches that filial piety is the basis of all conduct, and children are educated along this principle. That is, children are taught to show respect and deference to parents and persons in authority. It is a son's moral obligation to serve the parents with sincerity. A hierarchy of seniority is followed: a child obeys the parents, a wife obeys her husband, and a younger brother obeys an older brother. Older adults expect to be respected and supported by their children.[54] Nurses should consider this hierarchy when establishing lines of communication with Chinese-American clients.

Children learn the value of self-discipline and self-control. Thus, negative feelings, anger, and pain may be suppressed. It is important that nurses look for emotional and physical cues to pain and discomfort in Chinese-American clients. The belief in moderation and harmony encourages politeness and restraint. As a result, open confrontation, conflict, and disagreements are discouraged.[53] A nurse working with a Chinese-American client should explore whether the client approves of the plan of care, as the client may suppress signs of disapproval, particularly because nurses and physicians are viewed as authority figures.

Definition of Health and Illness. Chinese medicine is derived from the Taoist religion (the Right Way), which is based on a theory that nature maintains a balance in all things. The concepts of health and illness are based on *yin* and *yang* energies. *Yin* represents the female, negative, force of darkness, cold, and emptiness; *yang* represents the masculine, positive, force of light, warmth, and fullness. Everything in the universe consists of these positive and negative energy forces. The balance of energy means that the body is in a healthy state. If there is an imbalance of *yin* and *yang*, then the body is susceptible to disease or illness. Thus, health is a state of spiritual and physical harmony with nature, and illness is a state of imbalance and disharmony. Healing aims to reestablish the balance.[10,18,55]

Beliefs and Practices About Health and Illness. Chinese-Americans believe when they do not feel well, the body is lacking *chi* (innate energy) and blood. A young person is considered strong and full of *chi;* an aging person has diminished *chi* and blood. When a person is fatigued or overworked, *chi* and blood are believed to be low. Therefore, Chinese-Americans do not donate blood and are hesitant to have blood drawn for fear of causing body weakness. *Chi* moves within the human body following specific pathways. This innate energy enters and exits the body through the mouth, nose, and ears. Acupressure is finger pressure applied to the focal points, or meridians, of the body to reestablish balance.[56]

An excess of *yang* causes fever, dehydration, irritability, and tension; an excess of *yin* causes nervousness, apprehension, and a predisposition to gastric disorders. The body surface, considered *yang*, protects the body from outside infiltration; inside, the body is *yin*, the vital strength of life. *Yang* is "hot"; *yin* is "cold." Similar to the Hispanic beliefs described earlier, "hot" and "cold" are specific properties and conditions and are unrelated to the concept of temperature. For example, a "hot" condition is usually caused by an imbalance between "hot" (spicy, fried, rich) and "cold" (green leafy vegetables) foods. A sore throat and fever (*yang*) may be treated with watercress or watermelon soup (*yin*). A cold condition, such as a respiratory problem, is caused by exposure to cold weather or too many "cold" foods. Ginger root, a hot food, is used to treat heart problems, because the heart is a *yang* organ.[18,56] Thus, food and nutritional practices are most important in keeping harmony with nature. Health practices emphasize moderation to prevent excesses that bring on illness.

Chinese-Americans may go to a Western physician or to a practitioner of Chinese medicine or to both. The Chinese cultural healer may be a Chinese physician, acupuncturist, herbalist, or herb pharmacist. Health-seeking behavior of Chinese-American clients is based on what works. Clients may go to a Western physician for acute illnesses and see a cultural healer for chronic conditions.

Traditional Chinese medicine is a preventive process that includes certain foods, herbs, meditation, martial arts, and acupuncture. The following are examples of treatment techniques:

1. *Diet Therapy.* Concepts of *yin* and *yang* determine which foods are prescribed and eaten. *Yin* foods, such as fish, broccoli, and bland foods, treat *yang* conditions, such as infection and upset stomach; *yang* foods, such as chicken, eggs, and spicy foods, treat *yin* conditions, such as cancer, pregnancy, and postpartum problems.
2. *Herbs.* Herbs are classified by function or actions on the body that increase, decrease, or neutralize imbalances of *yin* and *yang*: emetics, purgatives, supplementary tonics, diuretics, detoxins, neutralizers, or heat inducers. Herbs are mainly boiled down to a tea, as in ginseng.[52]
3. *Cupping.* Cupping consists of heating a bamboo cup and placing it on the skin, to which it adheres. This method is used to treat stress, headaches, abdominal pain, and arthritis.[52,55]
4. *Martial Arts. Tai chi chaun* and *kung fu* are based on an energy exchange system located in the vital points of the body.[55]
5. *Acupuncture.* This method is classified as a cold treatment and is used in diseases with excessive *yang* (stroke, deafness, facial paralysis) or to relieve pain. It involves inserting needles into the skin at body areas called meridian points, which extend in a network throughout the body and merge on the skin at the point of needle insertion.[18,52]

Health Problems. Many of the pressing health problems among Chinese-Americans are related to living conditions in the overcrowded Chinatowns of large cities. For example, San Francisco's Chinatown has the highest suicide and tuberculosis rates in the nation, and many older residents suffer from general malnutrition.[54] More immigrants than native-born Chinese-Americans suffer from tuberculosis, and stresses of survival exacerbate the disease. A high proportion of elderly men among first-generation immigrants are socially isolated and in declining health. Many elderly Chinese-Americans experience depression and stress related to lack of respect and support from their adult children, who are assuming the values of the dominant culture. Because of language barriers, lack of accessibility and familiarity with public services, and the absence of bilingual and culturally sensitive staff at extended care facilities, elderly Chinese-Americans often are reluctant to use social and health care services.[10,52,54]

As Chinese-Americans continue to assimilate, cultural conflicts can lead to stress and behavioral problems. According to Flaskerud,[57] Chinese-Americans underuse mental health services and have severe forms of mental illness when they do seek therapy. Mental illness is considered a stigma among Chinese. To save face, the family will deny that a member is mentally ill as long as they can cope. Thus, when they do seek services, the client often exhibits severe personality disorganization. Those who do not seek services may commit suicide.[10,52]

Other health problems among Chinese-Americans include lactose intolerance (94 percent of population); respiratory diseases; a high incidence of nasopharyngeal, esophageal, and liver cancers; and hypertension, especially prevalent among those immigrating from Taiwan.[20,56]

Implications for Nurse–Client Collaboration. Nurses must first assess Chinese-American clients' cultural beliefs and practices, including language spoken; birthplace; number of years in the United States; place of residence; social, family, and community resources; dietary patterns; ceremonies and rituals performed; use of herbs and traditional Chinese medicine and treatments; and previous experience with the health care system.[52,56]

Clients who retain traditional values may become upset by painful procedures and the drawing of blood. They may refuse surgery, as they wish to die with their bodies intact. Thus, health care providers should limit diagnostic tests to those that are essential. If amputation is necessary, the body part should be returned to the client or family.[18]

Nurses should strive to accommodate the food preferences of Chinese-Americans. For example, clients may prefer warm water and beverages to cold water at the bedside, may avoid dairy products, may desire high-sodium products, such as soy sauce and other condiments, and may find hospital food bland, unfamiliar, and unpalatable. A client's family can be encouraged to bring in preferred foods if they are not contraindicated in the care plan (Fig. 9–2). If a client is placed on a low-sodium diet, consult with the dietitian to see if reduced-sodium soy sauce can be provided.[52,58]

To eliminate communication barriers, the nurse should seek an interpreter who is compatible in age, sex, and social status with the client. The Chinese-American's respect and deference to those in authority may require nurses to probe for hidden feelings in a nonthreatening manner. For example, nurses should not assume that clients are not in pain because they do not complain; the nurse must ask directly about pain.[58]

Chinese-Americans may bring valuable jewelry to the hospital as evidence of status. Many bring jade for good luck. Elderly clients may hide large sums of money in their clothes and be reluctant to part with it. Traditional medicine differs from Western medicine in may ways, and health care providers' directions may be difficult for clients to follow. A client may be reluctant to tell the physician she or he is being seen by a traditional practitioner; nurses should obtain the client's permission to inform the physician of this fact.[59,60]

Japanese-Americans

Japanese Americans are the only immigrant group in the United States that defines each generation of its descendants based on their geographical location and distance from Japan; for example, the *Issei* (first generation) are the original immigrants who were born in Japan; the *Nisei* (second generation) were born in the United States between 1924 and 1945; and the *Sansei* (third generation) were born between World War II and 1965. The *Yonsei* and *Gosei* are the fourth and fifth generations. As new generations are added, further categories are developed. *Nikkei* is the collective term used for all generations of Japanese born in America.[9]

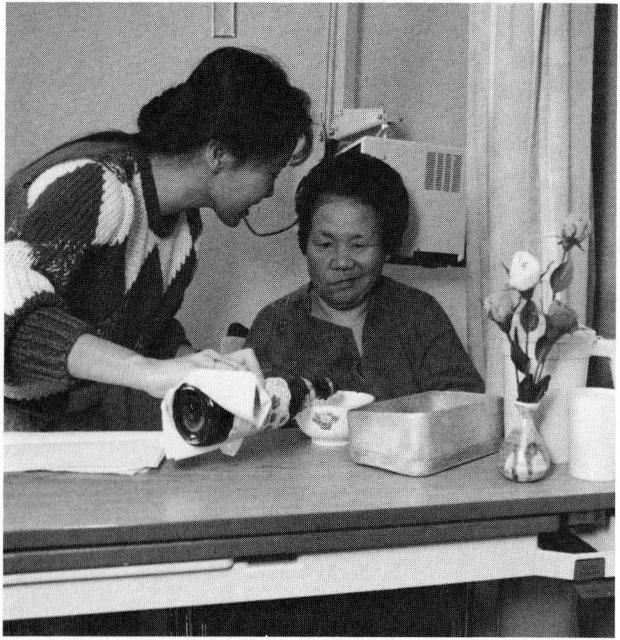

Figure 9–2. Family member bringing in traditional food for Chinese client.

Family. Like the Chinese-American family, the Japanese-American family is the major unit establishing a person's values and beliefs. Roles are stratified in a hierarchy from old to young, man to woman, and superior to subordinate. Within the family there is extreme sensitivity to words and actions with an attendant fear of disapproval. Family members rely on and expect kindness from others. This sense of interdependency in self-concept supports group decision making about health concerns rather than independence.[61] Those who hold traditional beliefs possess a fatalistic attitude in their acceptance of their role in society and position in life, and a tranquility developed through patience and self-control.

Traditionally, a Japanese wife's status is lower than that of her husband, his parents, and older siblings. In later years a mother is expected to follow the commands of her oldest son. Sons are more highly valued than daughters, but all children are viewed as owing an obligation to their parents that can never fully be repaid.

Other cultural values that influence the relationship of Japanese-Americans with health care providers include the values of *gaman, haji, enryo,* and *koko. Gaman* is self-control and is displayed by clients who are stoic in response to pain. *Haji* refers to shame. Unacceptable behavior can cause shame. Thus, attempts are made to avoid behavior that brings shame to oneself or one's family. *Enryo* is a type of behavioral politeness, respect, deference, reserve, and humility. *Koko,* or filial piety, is demonstrated when children are faithful to their parents and obedient to parental teachings.[62] Japanese-American families display these cultural values to varying degrees depending on their degree of assimilation and acculturation.

Definition of Health and Illness. The Japanese-American view of health as a state of harmony and balance and illness as a state of disharmony is similar to the Chinese definition of health and illness. Again, healing involves reestablishing balance between the body and the universe; however, illness is also viewed as being caused by germs, which coincides with the Western definition of illness.[61,62]

Beliefs and Practices About Health and Illness. Health beliefs and practices of Japanese-Americans are influenced by Shinto and Buddhist religious beliefs and by Asian medical tradition.

The Shinto religion emphasizes that all humans are

basically "good" and that "evil" is caused by outside spirits as retribution for humans who have yielded to temptation. This situation is temporary and can be removed by purification rites. Disease may also occur if a person comes into contact with polluting agents such as blood, skin diseases, and corpses. The use of natural purgatives and the emphasis on "cleanliness" by Japanese are based on this philosophy.

Asian medical traditions emphasize states of harmony and disharmony as the basis for health and illness. Improper care of the body, such as poor diet, lack of sleep, and inactivity, results in illness. Associated with this concept of imbalance is the belief that illness results when the flow of energy slows or stops along the meridians of the body. Energy flow can be restored through acupuncture, massage, and acupressure, processes also used by the Chinese. Natural herbs such as *kampo* are believed to have fewer side effects than Western medicines.[62] Japanese-Americans also use cultural foods such as miso soup (made of soya bean paste) and tofu (soya bean curd), which are believed to be responsible for good health.[9]

Japanese-Americans subscribe to a "germ theory" of disease causation and support the use of immunizations and surgery to remove diseased organs. They also view cancer as the result of external causes such as diet, smoking, and toxic substances.[61] Thus, many clients will seek both Asian and Western physicians during illness.

Buddhist thought influences ideas about sickness and dying. Older generations of immigrants adhere strongly to the idea that life is suffering and that one has a responsibility to fulfill one's role in life and to depart when that role is completed. Thus, for the elderly, the prolongation of life by artificial means is not considered a viable choice.

Health Problems. Lactose intolerance is prevalent in Japanese-Americans, as in other Asian-Americans. The incidence of stress-related conditions, such as colitis, ulcers, psoriasis, and depression, is high. Like the Chinese, Japanese-Americans are often reluctant to use mental health services and tend to keep family stresses of acculturation and intergenerational conflicts to themselves, practicing the value of *gaman*.[57] Because it is not considered acceptable to express anger, clients with serious illnesses will hold their feelings inside. Clients worry about the burden that they will be to their family and how to maintain harmony in carrying out their role responsibilities. Intergenerational conflicts and heightened anxiety levels have also contributed to an increase in suicide, drug use, and psychological problems.

Japanese-Americans have a higher incidence of stomach, liver, and biliary passage cancers. In the past the higher incidence of stomach cancers had been linked to the asbestos-containing talc used in preserving rice. They also experience a higher rate of hypertension and cerebrovascular problems than other Americans, which has been related to higher salt intake and psychological stress.[20,61,62]

Implications for Nurse–Client Collaboration. Care of Japanese-American clients requires a keen awareness and understanding of traditional health beliefs and practices. As with all cultural groups adherence to traditional cultural beliefs and practices varies depending on how many generations have lived in the United States. Most third-, fourth-, and fifth-generation Japanese-Americans are well assimilated; however, the degree of assimilation depends on socioeconomic status, geographical location, and whether an individual was educated in Japan or the United States. It is important to include the family in health care decisions whenever possible.

Communication patterns among Japanese-Americans present several challenges for nurse–client collaboration. For example, out of respect and "deference," clients may not voice their feelings about pain or disagree with the choice of therapeutic interventions. They may feel that questions present challenges to the authority of the health care professional, and are therefore to be avoided. Nurses need to carefully assess clients for knowledge deficits and internal stressors related to illness and offer information that would seem appropriate to their conditions.

As Japanese-Americans value time and use it well, they tend to follow medication schedules precisely and are compliant with medical regimens. Because of the broad health belief system in Japanese culture, clients may seek care from both Western and Asian care providers concurrently.

Indo-Chinese

Five distinct ethnic groups constitute the Indo-Chinese culture: Vietnamese, Kampuchian, Laotian, Hmong, and Chinese. Each of these groups has its own language and culture. Most Indo-Chinese came to the United States as refugees rather than immigrants. This section focuses on Vietnamese-Americans, currently the largest group of Indo-Chinese in the United States.

After the fall of the Saigon government in 1975, thousands of Vietnamese fled their homeland to seek refuge in other countries, including the United States. Although dispersed around the United States, the majority of Vietnamese settled in California, Texas, Washington, and Minnesota. The Vietnamese came to the United States in two distinct groups. The first immigrants were mainly highly urbanized educated persons with professional, technical, and managerial skills. A second group, known as the "boat people," were less educated fishermen, farmers, and traders. These immigrants, predominantly young males without their families, have had the greatest difficulties adjusting to life in the United States.[63,64]

Family. In the traditional Vietnamese family, the father is the head of the household and the decision-maker; the mother handles all household activities. As in other Asian cultures, males are valued and females are subordinate. The extended family, often consisting of three generations, is the basic unit of society. Obligation to family supersedes obligation to self, religion, and country, and a person's behavior reflects shame or honor on the entire family. The elderly are valued and respected for their wisdom and cared for by children at home until their death.

A strong family support system has helped ease the transition of Vietnamese resettlement in the United States; however, with this transition have come many social stressors. Many women have taken jobs to help support their families, causing marital conflict as traditional roles are challenged. Many Vietnamese men have had to take positions that are lower in status than those they held in Vietnam. Children attending school often learn English more quickly than parents and must serve as translators, which can lead to intergenerational conflicts. Despite these social stressors, the family unit has tended to remain strong, and many older children stay in the home until marriage to help run family businesses.[63,64]

Definition of Health and Illness. In accordance with Asian philosophy, Vietnamese view health as part of a unified, comprehensive scheme. The human body requires a balance between the opposite elements of *am* (*yin*) and *duong* (*yang*); an excess of either may lead to discomfort and illness. Illness is a direct result of disharmony with the universe.[65,66]

Beliefs and Practices About Health and Illness. The Vietnamese world view stems from the religions of Taoism, Confucianism, and Buddhism, in which the universal order of the cosmos influences a person's destiny. Spirits of dead relatives, who continue to dwell in the home, protect their descendants. Thus, ancestors are worshipped and honored for their protection and powers they bestow on the living. A person's head is not touched, as it is linked to one's ancestors.[64–66]

Vietnamese believe that illness can be caused by gods, spirits, or demons representing supernatural powers. Illness is seen as punishment for offending a god or spirit or violating a religious code. Naturalistic causes of illnesses include cold drafts, air, or the effects of bad weather (*gio*). For example, pustules or pox in children are caused by "ill winds"; thus, children must be wrapped in scarves before playing with others. Vietnamese women do not take baths after childbirth, as "air" may overcome the body's defenses. "Hot" and "cold" are used to refer to physical conditions and dietary prescriptions, and Asian herbs are used for treatment of illness. *Caogio* (rubbing out the wind) is used to treat minor ailments. In this practice a coin or fingers are dipped in tiger balm and forcefully rubbed on the chest, back, or neck (Fig. 9–3). Cultural healers provide traditional acupuncture, cupping, or moxibustion. Prayers and offerings may be made at a local temple to appease an evil spirit.[65,66]

Vietnamese tend to fear invasive procedures and mutilation, as souls are attached to body parts and can leave with a part, causing death. There is a strong aversion to hospitals and Western medicine, and hospitals are often

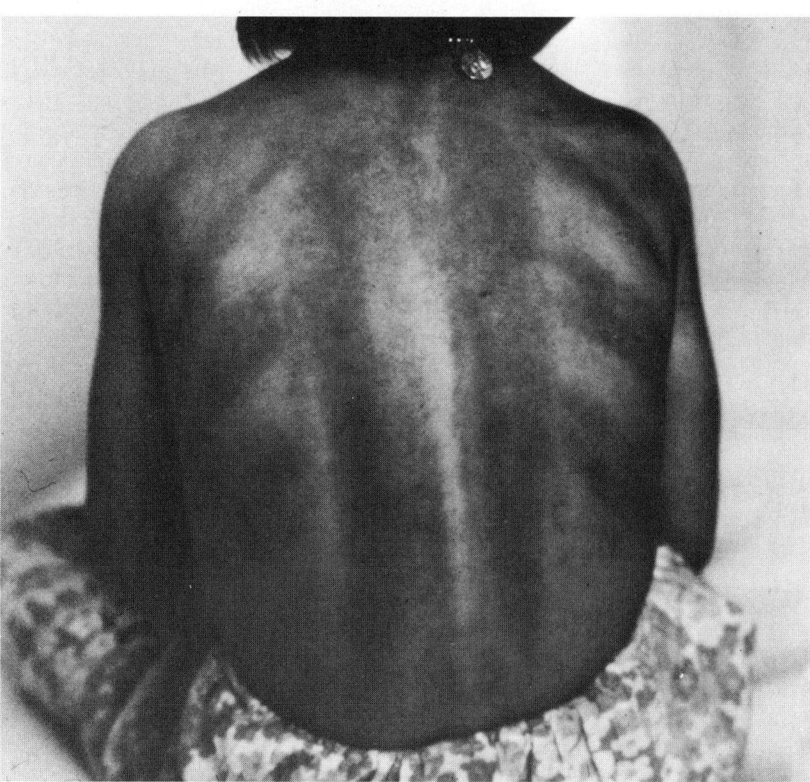

Figure 9–3. *Caogio*, "coin rubbing," is used by traditional Vietnamese to treat minor ailments. (*From Yeatman GW, et al.* Pediatrics. *1976;* **58**(*4*)*:617. Copyright American Academy of Pediatrics, 1976, with permission.*)

the last resort when a family member is too ill to be cared for at home.[65] Sometimes the use of an interpreter can reduce the stress associated with Western style health care (Fig. 9–4).

Vietnamese will not seek mental health services, which may cause embarrassment for the family, as mental illness is viewed as an offense against a deity or a moral indiscretion.[57] Instead, a sorcerer may be called in to rid the client of the illness. Value is placed on being "stoic," and endurance indicates a strong character.[65]

Health Problems. Many Indo-Chinese demonstrate a variety of physical and emotional problems resulting from the traumas of war and evacuation and the disruptions of encampment and resettlement in the United States. Tuberculosis is a major health problem that has required extensive screening and follow-up. Intestinal parasites such as hookworm, whipworm, and roundworm are frequently found among Vietnamese refugees. Malnutrition and stunted growth also frequently are noted. A high incidence of dental caries and periodontal disease is the result of malnutrition and lack of dental care.[64]

Vietnamese youth who are placed in foster homes may be at risk for posttraumatic stress syndrome as a result of loss or separation from family members, refugee flight, and acculturation problems.[67] The occurrence of depression among Vietnamese youth placed in foster families is three times higher than that for adolescents in the overall US population. Depression is also a major problem for refugees, who may experience a delayed reaction known as the "survivor syndrome" after emigrating to the United States. Elderly Vietnamese often feel alienated from the younger generation, who are becoming more Westernized.[64]

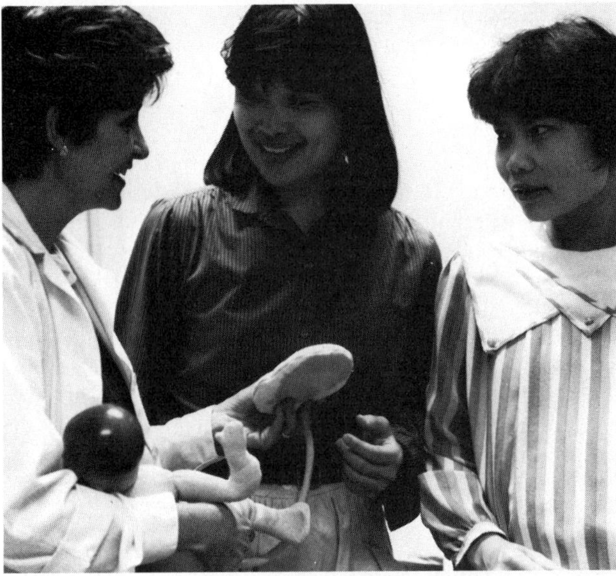

Figure 9–4. An interpreter facilitates the nurse–client relationship when primary languages differ. (*From Sherwen LN, Scoloveno MA, Weingarten CT.* Nursing Care of the Childbearing Family. *Norwalk, CT: Appleton & Lange; 1991.*)

A high dietary intake of sodium results in an increased incidence of hypertension in Vietnamese-Americans, as in other Asian populations. Lactose intolerance is a genetic problem, and low vitamin D and calcium levels may place Vietnamese at higher risk for rickets.[64]

Implications for Nurse–Client Collaboration. Indo-Chinese clients may not adhere to treatment regimens prescribed by health care providers. This leads to ineffective use of services. Self-help and use of traditional treatment methods are common.

Nurses should involve family members in client care plans, as the family, particularly the father or other male figures of authority, is viewed as the decision-making unit. Nurses should also become familiar with community resources that are used in the resettlement of Vietnamese refugees (eg, job placement, housing, funding, church organizations). These resources can aid the health care team in planning follow-up care for clients and their families.

Native Americans

Native Americans include American Indians, Aleuts, and Eskimos. There are approximately 270 tribes, each with its own dialect, philosophy, beliefs, and customs. The largest tribes are the Navajo, Cherokee, Sioux, Chippewa, and Pueblos. Native Americans live predominantly in the western United States and Alaska, although they also live in upper New York State, Maine, Florida, and North Carolina.[68] Many live on reservations or in rural areas, but increasing numbers have moved to large urban areas, especially Denver, Chicago, and the West Coast cities.[69]

Native Americans are often referred to as the "original" Americans because they inhabited North America prior to the arrival of Europeans in the 15th century. As European settlers colonized North America, much of the Native American population died. Wars, resettlement policies, and communicable diseases spread by settlers resulted in the extermination of entire tribes. To survive, many Native American tribes gave up their land in exchange for treaty rights that established reservations (land held in trust) by the US government.

Because the Native American cultural group encompasses a wide range of individual tribes, each with its own subculture, health care professionals who practice with Native Americans must learn about the particular culture of the clients with whom they practice. Every client and family must be individually assessed for unique characteristics and the degree to which they adhere to traditional beliefs and practices. For the purposes of this discussion, however, several broad cultural patterns and characteristics of Native Americans can be identified.

Family. The family is highly valued in Native American culture. Traditionally, children and elders are supported and always cared for by the group. Many tribes are matrilineal, placing women, in particular the grandmother, in a position of power and decision making. Many Native American households comprise a three-generation extended family. Individuals within the family live for the group, feel free to ask for help, and do not approach problems or successes alone. Native Americans believe possessions are to be used, not preserved, and are to be shared with the group. This contrasts with the dominant society's views, which emphasize the individual and often equate success with material wealth.

Traditionally, the spoken word is considered a sacred component of human nature. Language promotes the values of generosity, bravery, compassion, respect for elders, and concern for the tribal entity. Nonverbal communication is a highly practiced art. The importance of observing periods of silence is also a cultural trait. A person who interrupts, interjects, or hurries is considered immature.

Traditionally, Native American children were not physically punished but were taught to respect their parents. Children were encouraged to be independent and to learn to live by their own decisions. They were given much freedom to explore their environment to develop skills and confidence to function as an adult; however, in contemporary Native American families, women and children are more vulnerable to abuse and neglect.[16,18]

Definition of Health and Illness. Native Americans consider all aspects of a person—physical, mental, and spiritual—to be equal in value and interrelated. Health is defined as being in harmony with nature.[70] Native Americans believe that if people harm nature, they harm themselves, and vice versa. Health also reflects the ability to survive in exceedingly difficult circumstances.

Conversely, a person who is in disharmony with nature is considered ill.[18,71] Illness is also associated with supernatural causes. Traditionally illness, disharmony, and sadness were seen by the Navajo as the result of either displeasing the holy people, disturbing the elements, disturbing animal and plant life, neglecting celestial bodies, misusing a sacred Native American ceremony, or witchcraft.[18] Thus, illness is an imbalance between the ill person and the surrounding natural or supernatural forces.

Beliefs and Practices About Health and Illness. Healing practices differ among tribes, but their common goal is to restore the client's harmony with nature. Each tribe has its own ceremony, ritual, or religious service for the ill to support and influence the healing process. The most important factor in the healing process is for the individual to make a conscious effort to get well; without this effort, healing will not occur.

One way to maintain harmony is through purification by totally immersing the body in water for physical and spiritual cleansing.[55] Preventive measures are used to ward off the effects of witchcraft and prevent possession by evil spirits. For example, children may wear a talisman, or a buckskin herbal bag, for preventive or curative powers. The use of "sweat lodges" to "purify the body" is a form of prevention, as is the use of certain foods (such as corn meal) to ensure good health. Health maintenance may involve the use of herbs or substances that are ingested or rubbed on the body to maintain harmony. For example *yerba del la negrita,* a member of the mallow family, is given to mothers as a hot cleansing drink after childbirth and is also used for treating diarrhea.

In times of illness, family members become caretakers. They also participate in traditional healing ceremonies in the home. Friends and relatives who visit and provide comfort believe that being present is generally more important than talking.[18]

The traditional healer in Native American culture is the medicine man. Because the causes of physical illness are of a spiritual nature, the medicine man looks for the spiritual cause of the health problem.[18] All medicine men are believed to possess extrasensory powers that enable them to divine (or diagnose) and cure illnesses.

The practices of motion-in-hand, stargazing, or listening may be used to divine the cause of illness. In motion-in-hand, the diagnostician sprinkles pollen or sand around the sick person and sits with eyes closed and face turned away from the patient. He moves his hand and begins to think of various diseases and various causes. When his hands begin to move in a prescribed manner he knows he has discovered the proper disease and its cause. Then he is able to prescribe the proper treatment. In stargazing and listening, a ray of light or a specific sound signals the cause of illness.[18]

Medicine men may prescribe herbs for curative and other procedures or conduct healing ceremonies (or "sings") to restore and maintain the harmony, balance, and equilibrium of the client. The singer uses prayers, songs, corn pollen, and sand paintings in ceremonies, and may paint symbols on the client to provide protection and enable the sacredness to enter the client's body. The singer can also remove "objects" causing disease by the laying on of hands.[70–72]

Native Americans who live on reservations tend to rely on traditional medicine to a greater extent than those who live in urban areas. There is, however, a wide variation in the extent of use and many Native Americans combine traditional medicine and practices with Western medicine.[71,73]

Native Americans view death as part of the life cycle. The dead person is believed to go to another world of the long-ago ancestors. Thus, the Native American is not concerned with the future or with death and tends to live in the present and take each day as it comes. Native Americans believe that the quality of life is more important than longevity.

Health Problems. Today Native Americans who live on tribal reservations lead an isolated, rural type of existence. Those who relocate to urban areas for better opportunities often experience culture shock related to a rapid change in environment and loss of family and community support, which results in loss of identity and self-esteem. Many find difficulty in coping with the social and economic stresses, and this has led to increased morbidity and mortality.

Low socioeconomic status contributes to major health problems for most Native Americans. Poor housing, nutrition, sanitation, and health care contribute to high rates of communicable diseases (eg, tuberculosis) and high infant mortality and morbidity rates. Children 1 to 14 years of age have a high incidence of gastroenteritis and dysentery, impetigo, and pneumonia and influenza.[70] Lack of resources, such as money and transportation, may be a barrier for Native Americans living on the reservation who cannot get to health care facilities. This may result in delays in diagnosing serious conditions.

The leading causes of death for Native Americans are heart disease, accidents, malignant neoplasms, and chronic liver disease and cirrhosis.[18] Many Native American health problems are directly related to alcohol abuse, which is endemic among the Native American community. According to Long, the incidence of alcohol-related cirrhosis is eight to nine times that of the dominant population in the northwestern United States.[74] Homicide and suicide rates on the reservations are two to three times the national average, especially among males 15 to 24 years of age.[74] Suicide rates are highest among those tribes with loose social integration emphasizing a high degree of individuality, and among tribes undergoing rapid social and economic change, which often leads to acculturation stress, anxiety, and family disruption. These stressors also contribute to a high incidence of domestic violence and battering of women.[18]

In addition to alcohol-related problems, cancers of the gallbladder, lung, breast, nasopharynx, testis, cervix, kidney, and female thyroid are prevalent. Many Native American clients present with more advanced disease and have a lower 5-year survival rate than the general population. Native American women are modest about pelvic examinations and reluctant to have Pap smears, which leads to higher mortality for cervical cancer. The increased risk for nasopharyngeal cancer stems from tobacco use and, among Alaskan Native groups, consumption of salt fish. Navajo who work as uranium miners tend to have a higher incidence of lung cancer.[69]

Native Americans also demonstrate different patterns for some illnesses. For example, a Native American may have a high blood sugar level, but no symptoms of diabetes; however, it is known that diabetes causes a large number of deaths among pregnant women.[18] The highest known prevalence of non-insulin-dependent diabetes and associated obesity is found in the Pima Indians.[20]

BUILDING NURSING KNOWLEDGE

What Is the Key to Combatting Health Problems Among Native Americans?

Lamarine RJ. Self-esteem, health locus of control, and health attitudes among Native American children. *J School Health.* 1987;57(9):371–374.

Observing that traditional educational interventions have not been successful in combatting health problems afflicting Native American adolescents, Lamarine measured variables known to affect health behavior to see if these factors influenced the health attitudes of preadolescent Native American children.

Lamarine gave a series of three questionnaires to 291 fourth-, fifth-, and sixth-grade Native American children. Fifty-six percent of the children were Navajo; 35 percent were Pueblo, and 9 percent were Apache. The questionnaires focused on three classic variables that previous research on other cultural groups had shown to be related: health locus of control, self-esteem, and health attitudes.

Lamarine's findings showed a small but positive correlation between self-esteem and health attitudes. The correlation was stronger among girls and decreased as the age of subjects increased, suggesting that younger children may be more amenable to interventions.

The strongest correlations between health attitudes and self-esteem were noted for Pueblo and Navajo children. Lamarine notes that Pueblo and Navajo tribes have a higher degree of social organization than Apaches. He indicated that if this relationship is borne out by future research, it may corroborate the theory of other researchers that the degree of social organization of a culture is related to the integration of personality constructs by its members.

No significant correlation was found between health locus of control and health attitudes. Lamarine points out that powerful cultural forces influence the responses of Native Americans to questions that measure Western personality constructs. The applicability of such concepts as locus of control must be viewed with a degree of skepticism. Western values emphasize independence, assertiveness, competitiveness, time consciousness, postponement of gratification, and questioning of tradition, whereas Native American values stress cooperation, docility, lack of emphasis on time, adherence to tradition, and indifference to ownership, saving, and the work ethic.

Implications for Nurse–Client Collaboration. Collaboration with Native Americans is aided if nurses consider the following general guidelines. First, establish rapport by listening carefully, as silence is of great importance and patience is valued in the Native American culture. In taking the health history, ask one question at a time and explain why the information is needed. Avoid direct eye contact as this may be considered disrespectful. A strong and vigorous handshake may be viewed as a display of aggression. Involve the family in care and remember that one person cannot speak for another, nor can he or she reveal personal information. It is important to respect clients' privacy and understand that certain information at certain seasons of the year cannot be shared with non-Native Americans.[18,69] Attitudes toward people are not based on role and status; thus, being a physician or nurse does not in itself elicit cooperation from a Native American client. An individual must relate through his or her personal integrity to be accepted and honored.[18,69]

Nursing collaboration includes being sensitive to the important relationship between religion and medicine within the Native American culture. Nurses should provide space and privacy in the hospital for religious ceremonies and sings. Medicine persons should be welcomed as necessary collaborators in health care of Native Americans. One author has suggested that the relationship between the modern health care provider and the Native American medicine person is akin to that between the provider and the clergy.[45]

Nurses should respect rituals that are carried out by family members. Corn meal is a sacred food in Native American culture and is used in various curative ceremonies. For example, a grandmother may sprinkle corn meal around an ill child's bed. It is also important to determine what drugs or herbs a client is taking as a home remedy or from a traditional healer. Knowledge about the type, amount, and frequency of traditional remedies will help prevent overdoses from concurrently prescribed drugs.

Nurses must also recognize that Native Americans view time as a continuum, with no beginning or end. In this view, completion of a task is more important than punctuality. Some Native Americans have no clocks, as time is considered to be relative to what needs to be accomplished. This poses problems for Western health care providers, as clients may arrive late or completely miss scheduled appointments. Nurses who are unaware of this cultural belief may misinterpret clients' actions as demonstrating lack of interest or motivation in their own health care.

Finally, nurses need to be aware of the pressing psychological and physiological problems facing Native Americans today and be abreast of available resources. The lack of utilization of the Indian Health Services is a significant factor influencing the health of the Native American population. Contributing to this situation has been the insensitivity of some health care providers to Native American cultural beliefs and practices. This has led to a mistrust of staff and an environment of "their medicine" versus "our medicine." Access to health services in the rural communities has also been hindered by shortages of health care professionals in these areas. Cultural sensitivity on the part of health care professionals and increased tribal control of health care services are some of the strategies that can begin to remedy these problems.

Low-Income Groups

The concept of a "culture of poverty" was first described by anthropologist Oscar Lewis in 1966.[75] Lewis viewed the poor, or low-income groups, as a subculture of Western society. In Lewis' view, poverty or low-income status, like other cultures, provides a life-style, attitudes, behaviors, and values that allow individuals to adapt and survive within the culture.

According to this view, the poor are characterized by feelings of despair and resignation, inferiority, inability to plan for the future or to delay gratification, and a life-style of violence, unstable family structure, and abandonment. These values, beliefs, and behaviors are passed from one generation to another, cutting across ethnic and regional boundaries.[75]

This stereotypical picture has been much criticized. For one thing, poverty is a relative term that reflects changes in standards and the definition according to place and time.[18,76] For another, attitudes and beliefs of individuals vary as a result of both economic level and ethnicity; however, this portrayal of a low-income subculture does point out that the life-style, values, beliefs, and behaviors of people living in poverty may be quite different from those of their largely middle-class caregivers.[45]

Family. Proponents of the "culture of poverty" view contend that low-income families are authoritarian, are headed by women, and made up of children who have been abandoned by their fathers. Children in these families are not valued and are disciplined by physical punishment. Family life generally lacks privacy and is oriented to the present. As a result, family members manifest fatalistic attitudes and strong feelings of helplessness, dependence, and inferiority.[15,75,77]

Opponents of this view contend that this negative perception does not consider why these characteristics exist nor does it recognize the role of the larger society in perpetuating poverty. For instance, research has shown that the poor have the same values as the rest of society and that the negative traits identified by Lewis are not cultural but rather are responses to situational circumstances.[78] The poor have been found to possess a strong work ethic and to work when given the opportunity.[17] In fact, opponents of Lewis' view maintain that if society would abolish poverty, the formerly poor would demonstrate middle-class attitudes and behaviors.[79]

These researchers view the attitudes of the poor as adaptational responses enabling them to survive in a disadvantaged social situation. For example, all family members have to "pitch in" economically to make ends meet or try to avoid crisis situations. Many parents are unable to spend as much time with their children as they would like because they are preoccupied with issues of survival for the family (eg, providing food, clothing, and housing).

Definition of Health and Illness. Low-income families often define health in terms of work: when they can work they are healthy. They tend to be fatalistic and to believe that illness is inevitable. Because their current problems are great, requiring all of their efforts to ensure survival, they are often oriented more to the present than to the future. Most low-income people do not receive regular preventive medical care. To the poor, it is more important to work than to lose a day's pay to see a health care provider, especially if one is not ill. Access to health care is limited by inability to afford health care and dependence on public assistance.

Beliefs and Practices About Health and Illness. Statistically, subsidized health care services that are provided for the poor continue to be underused, despite the higher disease rates among the poor. Factors that affect the use of health care services by the poor include (1) language and communication barriers, (2) lack of familiarity with the environment of modern health care institutions, (3) work patterns based on seasonal migrations, and (4) institutional sexism, prejudice, insensitivity, and depersonalization.[18]

Low-income clients may fear being used for diagnostic experimentation for the sake of medical advancement. Clients also choose to employ "self-care" treatment to avoid the high cost of health care.

Health Problems. The health status of low-income groups is influenced to a great extent by environmental factors. Overcrowded living conditions produce lower self-esteem and alienation, and a higher incidence of illness and disease.[18] Overcrowded living conditions also result in a higher incidence of communicable diseases, such as tuberculosis. Inadequate sanitation, lead poisoning, fire hazards, and violent crime are also threats.

According to the Children's Defense Fund, poverty kills more children in the United States than accidents and suicide combined.[77] The leading causes of death are inadequately treated pneumonia, homicide resulting from child abuse and random violence, malnutrition causing failure to thrive, and high infant mortality rates related to lack of prenatal care.[77]

The poor often rely on the emergency rooms in urban hospitals for health care services. This results in fragmented, episodic treatment, lacking client follow-up and continuity, with little concern for chronic but nonthreatening health problems.[80]

Implications for Nurse–Client Collaboration. Low-income clients who seek care often face embarrassment, insensitivity, and prejudice from health care providers. Nurses who work with these clients must first identify their own attitudes and opinions about the poor and any stereotypes about their behavior.

Nursing assessment can often help to identify a family's strengths as well as its weaknesses. Nursing care can then be directed at reinforcing these strengths. Nurses should also be aware of resources available to assist low-income families in problem resolution. These include shelters for the homeless and those experiencing physical abuse, prenatal care, alcohol/substance abuse therapy, family counseling, and food services (eg, Meals on Wheels for the elderly).

SPIRITUALITY, RELIGION, AND HEALTH

Although many people use the terms *spirituality* and *religion* interchangeably, they are not identical concepts. **Spirituality** can be defined as a belief in or relationship with a higher power, divine being, or creative life force.[81] **Religion** refers to an organized system of worship with central beliefs, rituals, and practices.[82] Religion can be characterized as having four dimensions: (1) theoretical, consisting of myths, beliefs, and doctrines; (2) practical, consisting of rites, prayers, and moral codes; (3) sociological, relating to churches, leaders, and functionaries; and (4) experiential, pertaining to emotions, visions, and various sentiments.

Religion provides a framework for spiritual belief, but many people express their spiritual beliefs outside the framework of organized religion. The spiritual dimension in human beings goes beyond religious affiliation, seeking harmony with the universe and striving for inspiration, reverence, awe, meaning, and purpose and for answers about the infinite.[81]

Spirituality, religion, and health have traditionally been intertwined with culture. Spiritual and religious beliefs and practices often overlap with cultural beliefs about illness causation and methods of curing.[83,84] Religion can influence life-style, attitudes, and feelings about illness and death. Religious beliefs sometimes conflict with health care practices. For example, the practice of blood transfusion is unacceptable to Jehovah's Witnesses. In these instances, health care providers may need to adjust standard treatment regimens to accommodate clients' religious beliefs.

Spiritual and religious beliefs and practices are an important component of many people's lives. In particular, spiritual beliefs can help people find solace and strength to cope with life stresses and crises. Spiritual needs may increase during crisis situations such as birth, death, and major health problems. Clients may demonstrate a need for spiritual support by mentioning the subject of religion, asking nurses to be listeners during stressful periods, or avoiding discussion of suffering related to their health problem.[85] However, clients who do not consider themselves "religious" may also benefit greatly from spiritual support during periods of crisis. Spirituality as an aspect of well-being

IMPLICATIONS FOR NURSE–CLIENT COLLABORATION

Spiritual Beliefs

Many of the meanings that people hold about health and illness are derived from their religious or spiritual beliefs. Notions about what constitutes health are frequently linked to spiritual ideas about healthy living and "being good." Likewise, notions about illness may be linked through spiritual beliefs to one's outlook on personal responsibility. The beliefs people hold for health are closely linked to the action they take to achieve, maintain, or regain health. Thus, as nurses pursue the goal of optimal health for the client, it is imperative that they gain an understanding of the client's spiritual beliefs. This understanding can be gained through collaborative exchanges that review the connections between belief and action from the client's perspective.

is discussed in Chapter 22. Chapter 23 addresses spirituality and self-expression.

RELIGIOUS BELIEFS INFLUENCING HEALTH CARE

Nurses, as well as chaplains, clergy, and other pastoral care representatives, often assist clients in meeting their spiritual needs. Most hospitals have programs through which chaplains and other clergy visit hospitalized clients. Nurses should become familiar with these spiritual resources.[45] Nurses also need to become knowledgeable about the specific tenets of particular religions to better understand the meaning of religious beliefs and practices for care of their clients.[85]

A thorough discussion of religious faiths is beyond the scope of this text; however, this discussion provides an overview of five prevalent religions in the United States—Christianity, Judaism, Islam, Hinduism, and Buddhism. Atheism and agnosticism are also briefly considered.

Christianity

Christianity is the religion founded on the teachings of Jesus Christ. The three major branches of Christianity are Roman Catholicism, Eastern Orthodoxy, and Protestantism. Most Christians in the United States are Roman Catholic or Protestant.

Roman Catholicism. The Catholic sacraments of baptism, holy communion (holy eucharist), and anointing of the sick are of special significance to Roman Catholic clients.

Baptism is usually performed on infants from one to several months after birth, although it may be performed on any unbaptized child or adult who is in danger of death. Because Catholics believe that an infant has a soul from the beginning of conception, unless a fetus is born dead a baptism is performed. If a priest is unavailable, a nurse or another person may perform the baptism. It is preferable, but not essential, for the person performing the rite to be a Roman Catholic. It *is* essential that the person be baptized themselves. The baptism ceremony involves pouring water over the head of the infant or person being baptized while repeating the words, "I baptize you in the name of the Father, and of the Son, and of the Holy Spirit." The baptism should then be recorded on the chart and the family and priest notified.

Holy communion, or the holy eucharist, is the central act of the Catholic liturgy. The sacrament of communion may be requested by Roman Catholic clients who are acutely ill and in danger of death. When communion is planned, the nurse should tidy and arrange an area including a table for the client's use. The table may be covered with a linen hand towel if one is available. Privacy is necessary because the client may wish to make a confession at this time. Clients preparing to receive communion may abstain from solid food and alcohol for 15 minutes before receiving the consecrated bread wafer.

The sacrament of anointing the sick may be requested by ill persons who seek healing or strength to endure suffering. The priest anoints the person with oil, a sign of curing. While anointing, the priest prays that the person will receive the grace of the Holy Spirit, so that he or she may be freed from sin, comforted and strengthened in soul, and restored to health.[86] Roman Catholic clients may request the sacraments of anointing of the sick as well as holy communion and confession before death. After death, the body must not be shrouded until all of the sacraments have been performed. All body parts must be preserved for burying or cremation.

The Roman Catholic church prohibits the use of birth control, except for abstinence and natural family planning. Religious laws also prohibit sterilization and abortion, even when the mother's life is in danger.

To Roman Catholics, the rosary is a very important religious symbol. Clients may bring a rosary with them to the hospital or wear a religious medal (Fig. 9–5). Every

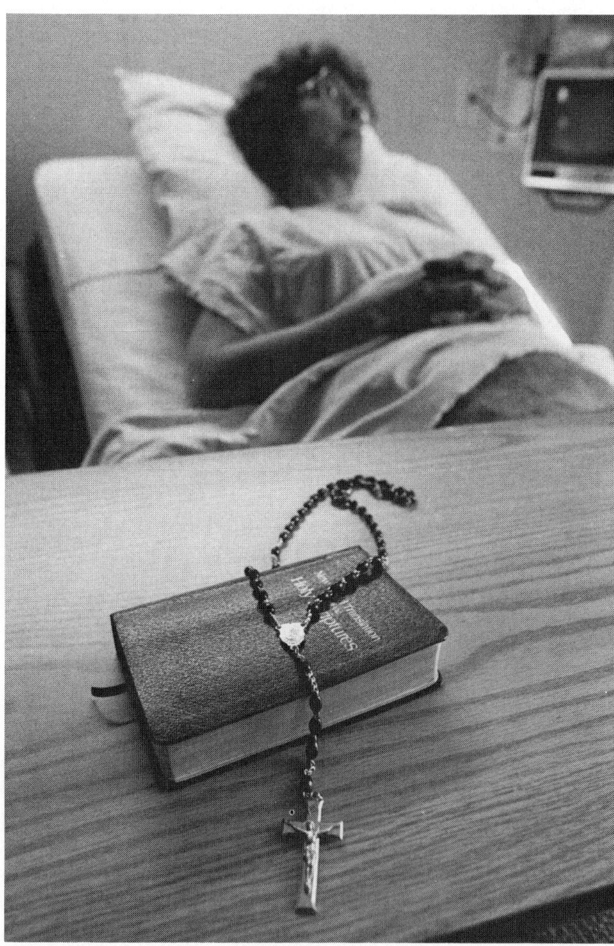

Figure 9–5. Many clients bring items with them to the hospital to use in prayer or other religious rituals. Caregivers should show respect and care for these objects for they usually have great personal significance.

effort should be made to ensure that these items are not misplaced. Occasionally, a client will request permission to take a religious object to the operating room. Although this is not a common practice, arrangements can be made with the surgeon or operating and recovery room staff. This often reduces the client's anxiety about the procedure.

Eastern Orthodoxy. Eastern Orthodoxy is divided into several denominations by nationality, among them Greek, Armenian, Ukrainian, and Syrian. Although similar in many ways to Roman Catholicism, Eastern Orthodoxy has no pope. The sacraments of Eastern Orthodoxy include baptism, communion, and unction of the sick.

Infants must be baptized within 40 days of birth. Baptism involves immersing the infant in water, pouring water on the forehead three times, and anointing with holy oil. If sprinkling or immersion in water is not possible, the infant is moved in the air in the sign of the cross by a priest or deacon.

BOX 9–2. BASIC TENETS OF SEVERAL PROTESTANT DENOMINATIONS

Baptist

Baptism is deferred until children reach the age of responsible decision making (usually at 12 or 13 years of age). Some members believe in and practice healing by the laying on of hands. Family planning choices are left to individuals. The clergy ministers to and supports individuals at times of illness. Bible reading is often desired, and nurses should provide an opportunity for clients to read or be read to if requested. Artificial prolongation of life is discouraged.

Church of Christ, Scientist (Christian Science)

Christian Scientists have an adult dedication service rather than infant baptism. Members do not usually seek medical care, turning instead to spiritual means for healing and to Christian Science "practitioners" who help them apply natural and spiritual healing. Parents do not permit their children to have physical examinations, health screenings, or immunizations.

Espiscopalian (Anglican)

Infant baptism is practiced and is considered urgent if an infant is critically ill. A nurse may baptize in an emergency. Ministers administer the rite of anointing the sick when death is imminent, but this is not considered mandatory. Nurses should notify a priest if clients wish to receive holy communion. Church members may abstain from meat on Friday and fast before receiving communion. Birth control, sterilization, and abortion are considered matters of personal choice.

Jehovah's Witness

Members refuse to accept blood transfusions, although they may accept alternatives such as intravenous fluids and nonblood plasma expanders. The law requires that blood transfusions not be withheld from minor children during a medical emergency; however, adults do have the right to refuse blood transfusions under a US Supreme Court ruling. Autopsies are accepted as required by law, but no body parts may be removed. Although abortion is prohibited, birth control and sterilization are left to individual discretion.

Lutheran

Only living infants are baptized, 6 to 8 weeks after birth. Adults may also be baptized. Clergy should be notified if a client desires communion. Most synods do not practice rites for the dying. Although prayers are offered for those who are dying, Lutherans do not pray for the dead. Decisions about medical or surgical treatments, including abortions and birth control are not dictated by the church.

Methodist

Clergy should be notified if baptism, holy communion, or anointing of the sick is requested. Donation of the body or a body part is encouraged at death.

Mormons (Church of Jesus Christ of Latter-Day Saints)

Members disapprove of alcohol, tobacco, and caffeinated beverages, limit meat consumption, and encourage intake of fruits, grains, and herbs. Personal hygiene is important and a special undergarment, which may be worn by some members, should be removed only in an emergency. Abortion is allowed to save the life of the mother. Birth control is a matter of personal conscience.

Pentecostal (Assemblies of God)

Pentecostals emphasize a postconversion experience called baptism in the Holy Spirit, which is accompanied by speaking in tongues. Members believe in divine healing through prayer and the laying on of hands.

Quakers (Friends)

Members oppose all ceremonial forms of worship including sacraments, churches, and ministers, and demonstrate diversity of personal beliefs.

Seventh-Day Adventists (Church of God, Advent Christian Church)

Members practice adult rather than infant baptism (dedication service). Sabbath day is Saturday. Some members follow a lacto-ovo-vegetarian diet, which includes milk and eggs. Alcohol, tobacco, and caffeine-containing beverages are prohibited. Birth control is not restricted by the church; abortion is allowed only in cases of rape, incest, or to save a woman's life.

Unitarian (Universalist Association)

Reason, individual responsibility, and personally established values are emphasized. Members do not oppose abortion. Cremation is preferred to burial, and donation of the body or a body part is encouraged.

Data from References 13 and 81.

The sacrament of the holy eucharist, or communion, may be conducted by a priest in the hospital room if a client wishes. Some followers of Eastern Orthodoxy practice fasting from the last meal in the evening until after communion.

The sacrament of holy unction is a blessing of the sick, rather than a last rite. The priest reads lessons about the miracle of Jesus and anoints parts of the client's body with oil. Last rites consist of obligatory administration of the holy eucharist.

The Eastern Orthodox church prohibits abortion and birth control, and discourages autopsies that cause dismemberment. Burial is preferred to cremation.[87]

Protestantism. The Protestant faith has the largest membership of any religion in the United States. Some representative Protestant denominations are listed in Box 9–2 with a summary of the major tenets of each. Because these denominations vary in specific religious beliefs and practices, it is important that nurses consult individual clients about their denomination, beliefs, and practices.

Protestant sacraments are baptism and communion. Some Protestant denominations practice infant baptism and may wish to have a seriously ill infant or child baptized. Others, for instance Baptists, believe that baptism should be deferred until the child reaches the age of responsible decision making, at about 12 or 13 years. Thus, health care providers should not undertake infant baptism without explicit instructions from the family. Protestant baptism is performed by ordained clergy.[86]

Communion, a sacrament in a majority of Protestant denominations, is usually conducted at a church in the presence of a congregation; however, it may also be performed for an individual client in the hospital, if desired. Most Protestant denominations do not routinely anoint the sick, but some may do so in special cases.

Some Protestant denominations emphasize Bible reading. Members of these churches are comforted by Bible reading, and it is common practice for family and friends to visit and pray with a sick member of the congregation who is hospitalized. At times, clients may request a nurse to read a scripture with them. Nurses who are uncomfortable with such requests might offer, instead, to find a volunteer or a member of the client's congregation to read the scripture.

Judaism

There are three main groups in Judaism: Orthodox, Conservative, and Reform. These groups differ in their interpretation of the Torah (the holy book containing early Jewish history and God's law), adherence to dietary laws, and celebration of holy days and Sabbath worship. The spiritual leader is the rabbi.

Orthodox Jews strictly interpret the Torah. They apply all of the ancient rules of worship including home rituals. Kosher dietary laws are practiced, including prohibitions against food from animals that do not chew cud and do not have cloven hoofs (eg, pig and horse), fish without fins and scales (eg, clams and shrimp), and all fowl enumerated in the Old Testament. Dietary law requires that animals and birds be ritually slaughtered by a specially trained person so that all of the blood drains from the body. Kosher food preparation also requires that meat and milk products not be mixed, and separate sets of utensils and dishes are used for these foods.

Reform Jews accept less restrictive interpretations of religious law and usually do not observe Kosher dietary regulations. Conservative Jews try to maintain a balance between the traditional ways of Judaism and the modernist spirit of Reform.

Other religious beliefs and practices include the circumcision of male infants on the eighth day of life and observance of the Sabbath from sundown on Friday to sundown on Saturday. Rosh Hashanah, the first day of the Jewish New Year, occurs in September. Yom Kippur, the "day of atonement," occurs 10 days later and is the holiest of Jewish holidays, a time to reflect on one's life.[82,88] Observant clients may wish to avoid scheduling hospital admission or medical procedures during the holy days or on the Sabbath.

Transplants and donation of body parts are prohibited. Autopsy and cremation are not acceptable because Jews believe that the body given by God must be returned to the earth intact. Conservative and Reform groups may adhere less rigidly to these restrictions.

Islam

The Islamic faith, which includes numerous sects, is a major religion in the Middle East and North Africa. Its followers, called Muslims, adhere to strict religious and dietary practices. The Koran is the Muslim holy book. It is considered sacred and must not be touched by persons who are ritually unclean.

Muslim dietary practices include restrictions against the use of alcohol and pork, and fasting from sunrise until sunset during the month of Ramadan (the ninth month of the Muhammadan year). Ill persons are usually exempted from fasting. Use of tobacco is also prohibited.

Islam emphasizes precise individual rituals and prayers, and Muslim clients wish to carry out these devotions in private. Conservative Muslims maintain traditional restrictions on the freedom of women. Women are not allowed to be seen unveiled by men other than members of the family. Health care for these women should be provided by female physicians and staff. Muslim women cannot sign consent forms; their husbands should therefore be present when consent is necessary.

Confession of sins and begging for forgiveness are characteristic behavior for a dying Muslim. After death, the family prefers to wash, prepare, and place the body in a position facing Mecca. If non-Muslim health care givers prepare the body, they must wear gloves. Burial takes place as soon as possible. Autopsy is forbidden unless required by law.[87,88] If an autopsy is performed, all body parts must be returned for burial. Cremation is forbidden.

Nation of Islam (Black Muslims). The Nation of Islam was originally an independent black religious movement that affiliated with the worldwide Islamic community. Many of its beliefs and practices are similar to those of Islam.

Dietary regulations are Kosher in origin and involve prohibitions against eating pork, shellfish, and certain vegetables (peas, beans). A diabetic Muslim will refuse porcine insulin because the pig is considered unclean. Alcohol is also prohibited. Members fast during daylight hours during the month of Ramadan, although ill Muslims are exempted.

Members of the Nation of Islam assume a Muslim name and women often wear long clothing and head coverings, following traditional Islamic practice. There are many subsects, which may follow different practices.

Hinduism

Hinduism is the third largest and the oldest major world religion. The Hindu religion does not have a strong central organization. Ceremonies are conducted by priests in temples but followers attend these ceremonies only to watch them. A Hindu's devotions are performed mainly at home.

Hindus consider certain animals and things holy, including cattle, monkeys, water in any form, the Ganges River, and the city of Benares on the Ganges. Most Hindus are vegetarian, and believe in cremation of the dead and reincarnation. Hindus perform special rituals after death. The priest may tie a thread around the neck or wrist of the dead person to represent blessing; this thread should not be removed. The priest also pours water into the mouth of the corpse immediately after death, and the family then washes the body.[87,88]

Buddhism

Buddhists believe that a person's current actions affect his or her later life and rebirth. They calmly accept whatever life has to offer and thus may not express their needs or ask for care. Consequently, nurses must be alert to nonverbal indications of clients' needs and problems. Beliefs and practices do not conflict with most modern health care practices. Some Buddhists adhere to a vegetarian diet, and many avoid the use of alcohol and tobacco. Often, last rite chanting is practiced at the bedside soon after death.[87]

Atheism and Agnosticism

Some people do not base their moral and ethical standards on a particular religion or theism (belief in a god). They may consider themselves atheists or agnostics. An atheist denies the existence of God and rejects all religious belief. An agnostic does not deny the existence of God or a supreme being, but doubts God's existence or believes that God's existence cannot be proven.

NURSING COLLABORATION IN AN INTERCULTURAL CONTEXT

The collaborative relationship between nurses and clients and between nurses and other members of the health care team is characterized by mutual trust and mutual interaction. These qualities are particularly important in an intercultural context. A client's cultural and religious beliefs and practices must be considered when planning and providing care if an effective treatment plan is to be developed. A collaborative relationship between nurse and client provides an optimal environment for identifying and incorporating cultural values, beliefs, and practices that influence client care.

To facilitate intercultural collaboration, nurses must be knowledgeable about a client's cultural background and free of ethnocentric behaviors and attitudes. The principles of cultural relativism, cultural sensitivity, and transcultural reciprocity provide a foundation for collaborative client care in an intercultural context.

Cultural relativism asserts that any culture is different from, but not superior or inferior to, any other culture. This perspective encourages nurses to view their own beliefs, values, and behaviors objectively, as one of many cultural traditions. **Cultural sensitivity** refers to an individual's awareness of which issues or concerns are important to one's own culture and the culture of others. This is a first step in transcending ethnocentric biases; however, to become culturally sensitive nurses also need to become familiar with other cultures. Nurses can begin this educational process by reading about other cultures, attending seminars and continuing education programs, attending cultural events, and meeting with members of cultural groups in their communities. Discussions with colleagues provide an opportunity to share and identify personal feelings, learn from one another, clarify information, and together plan strategies that address the health problems of a particular ethnic client or cultural group. These activities are first steps to gaining cultural sensitivity. Interacting with individuals of other cultures in their own communities is even more valuable. Firsthand experience with varied cultural, ethnic, or religious groups in a setting in which group members are comfortable not only provides a more accurate picture of who they are as people, but the experience of being a minority or an "outsider" can enlighten nurses about the feelings these individuals experience when entering the health

IMPLICATIONS FOR NURSE–CLIENT COLLABORATION

Mutual Interaction

Mutual interaction, the approach to caregiving that emphasizes the client's participation in health care decisions, embodies a set of values, ideals, and standards of behavior, and rules for nurse–client interaction. Mutual interaction can be looked on as creating a culture for caregiving. The nurse must recognize that some clients may hold values at odds with those of mutual interaction. Some clients, for example, may prefer a more traditional model of caregiving. It is important that the nurse understand the client's perspective, not only about the goals of health care, but also about the process by which those goals are to be reached.

care culture. This kind of personal experience can mitigate judgmentalness and stereotyping.

Collaborating in an intercultural context requires that nurses acknowledge the relevance of cultural beliefs and practices for client care. Dobson uses the term **transcultural reciprocity** to refer to collaborative interaction based on an exchange of cultural respect and understanding between nurse and client. Transcultural reciprocity, as Dobson describes it, is a process in which both client and nurse are equal participants, with nurses shaping care to the parameters of a client's culture. It involves an ongoing, intentional bridging of cultural disparities between nurses and clients and a recognition that providing culturally sensitive care is a central rather than a peripheral concern for nursing.[89]

IMPLICATIONS FOR CLIENT CARE

Cultural and spiritual data are relevant, even central to providing individualized client care. Cultural sensitivity is required in all contacts with clients. Nurses who lack awareness of their own personal beliefs and biases related to ethnic, cultural, and religious differences will be unable to develop sufficient rapport and trust to conduct effective and sensitive client assessments. Without accurate assessment, appropriate nursing care cannot be planned or delivered.

Cultural and spiritual assessment is usually integrated into the overall data gathering processes of obtaining a client history and examination (see Chap. 16). Figure 9–6 illustrates the types of questions that can be incorporated into a cultural assessment. Tripp-Reimer and colleagues point out that a cultural assessment need not address all elements of culture, but should include information on clients' major values, beliefs, and behaviors that influence health and health behaviors.[90] Box 9–3 lists several questions that can be used to obtain information about traditional or home remedies and health care practices.

Effective nursing assessments generate accurate nursing diagnoses. Nursing diagnoses are the basis for care plans that guide collaborative client care and its evaluation (see Chaps. 17, 18, and Unit VI). Without nurses' recognition of the importance of integrating cultural concerns and preferences into the assessment and care of all clients, the needs of many clients will go unmet. Moreover, a negative experience with insensitive health care providers contributes to avoidance of the health care system and reliance on self-care or traditional medicine, even when these are not effective. In contrast, intercultural collaboration based on cultural sensitivity and transcultural reciprocity results in care that is acceptable to clients and nurses.

Intercultural collaboration is most effective with participation of other members of the health care team. For example, social workers who make referrals for community services are often aware of the cultural networks available as resources (eg, churches, community action groups). Dietitians in clinical settings can provide assistance in developing dietary plans that incorporate a client's individual or cultural food preferences. Traditional cultural or spiritual healers are also excellent resources who can be enlisted as resources for developing a client's treatment plan.

Hospital chaplains or pastoral counselors have special training to assist clients with spiritual crises such as facing death and dying and coping with complex medical procedures. Chaplains may assist clients by talking with them about their concerns or providing spiritual support when clients seek comfort. They also support clients by performing or enabling clients to participate in religious observances and rituals in the hospital setting.[13]

BUILDING NURSING KNOWLEDGE

What Role Does Reciprocity Play in Transcultural Health Care Relationships?

Dobson SM. Conceptualizing for transcultural health visiting: The concept of transcultural reciprocity. *J Adv Nurs.* 1989; 14:97–102.

Dobson is interested in the concept of reciprocity as it applies to nursing in the community, where transcultural relationships are involved. She asserts that reciprocity is fundamental to transcultural health nursing.

The term *reciprocity* refers to a relationship in which there is mutual action, influence, giving, and taking between two parties. What does reciprocity involve? Dobson refers to the work of several authors who highlight the reciprocation of trust and information and the fulfillment of each other's needs—the nurse's need to help and the client's need for help.

In Dobson's view, transcultural nursing involves ongoing, intentional bridging of cultures to reduce the disparities that exist between nurse and client. Transcultural reciprocity is an intercultural process rooted in the reciprocation of cultural respect and understanding between nurse and client. By extending a warm, active interest in discovering the client's ethnic identity, nurses hope the client will discuss his or her needs in cultural terms so that, in turn, nurses may shape their guidance to the parameters of the client's culture. To do this requires empathy, adaptability, and awareness of one's own ethnocentricity. The nurse must be able to transcend self to some extent, to perceive the uniqueness of the other person.

IMPLICATIONS FOR NURSE–CLIENT COLLABORATION

Culture and Optimal Health

A client's potential to achieve optimal health and well-being is centered to a large extent on the values, knowledge, and resources conferred by cultural heritage. To maximize that potential, the nurse's challenge is to collaborate with the client in such a way as to blend culture into care.[89] This means that the nurse takes an active interest in the client's cultural identity and that the relationship between nurse and client is based on a reciprocation of cultural respect.

Personal
Primary Language ______________ Speaks English Yes ☐ No ☐
Time orientation: ______________
Territoriality/personal space: ______________
Touch permitted? Yes ☐ No ☐
Physical examination permitted? Yes ☐ No ☐
By whom: ______________
Specific requirements: ______________
____
Personal belongings: ______________
Other: ______________

Diet
Ethnic preferences: ______________
Religious preferences/prohibitions: ______________
____
Diet modifications due to illness: ______________
____
Likes/dislikes: ______________

Religion
Affiliation: ______________
Level of participation: ______________
Baptism required in illness: ______________ Type: ______________
By whom: ______________
Rituals necessary in illness: ______________
Religious symbols used: ______________
Religious leaders: ______________ Role in illness: ______________
Medications acceptable: ______________
Blood transfusions acceptable: ______________
Special rituals: ______________
Other requirements: ______________
Omissions required: ______________
Do family health practices conflict with current medical practices? If so, how? ______________
____

Health Beliefs/Practices
Health–illness beliefs: ______________
Beliefs about cause of illness: ______________
____
Traditional (folk) treatments used: ______________
____
Where obtained: ______________
How prepared: ______________
Traditional (cultural/spiritual) practitioner: ______________
____
Family caregiver: ______________
Treatments used: ______________
____
Beliefs about amputations, circumcision, autopsy, etc: ______________
____

Death and Dying Beliefs/Practices
Dominant practices: ______________
Who should be called: ______________
Last rites: ______________
Family members' roles: ______________
Special rituals required: ______________
Preparation for burial: ______________
Rituals regarding death: ______________
Who performs rituals/rites: ______________

Figure 9–6. Data collection form for cultural assessment.

BOX 9–3. CULTURAL ASSESSMENT OF HEALTH CARE PRACTICES

1. What has made you ill?
2. What do you ordinarily do to keep well or take care of yourself?
   - Special diet?
   - Herbs?
   - Rituals?
   - Amulets?
   - Other?
3. What drugs, tablets, or foods did you use or are you using? What did you use them for?
4. What ceremonials or rituals do you perform to get well?
5. Who took care of you when you were sick?
6. What did he or she do for you when you were sick?
7. When did you last see this person?
8. Will you take medications from me today?

Effective client care depends on an environment of mutual respect and cultural sensitivity. Nurses must recognize that each person is unique, and that individuals who share a cultural or ethnic background or religious affiliation do not necessarily share values, beliefs, or cultural traditions. Nurses must continually reassess their own behaviors and evaluate how clients respond to these behaviors. Validation of culturally sensitive care approaches is provided by feedback from clients and families and observation of positive changes in clients' condition or behavior.

SUMMARY

Culture influences peoples' values, behaviors, and attitudes, and therefore how they perceive the world. Culturally influenced values and beliefs, in turn, influence health and illness behavior, communication patterns, diet, lifestyle, and religious practices. Knowledge of a client's culture enables the nurse to interpret the client's attitudes and behaviors, and facilitates development of a plan of care appropriate to that client. Cultural awareness is therefore a necessary component of nursing care.

Understanding the underlying assumptions of both the traditional and modern health care cultures can assist the nurse in developing cultural awareness. The traditional health care culture includes folk health beliefs and practices that tend to view the client holistically and often attribute disease causation to imbalances in forces within the body or to magical, supernatural, or religious influences. In contrast, the modern health care culture views scientific knowledge as the basis for treatment; the focus of care is on resolving symptoms. The differing views of these health care cultures may lead to conflicts between clients who adhere to traditional cultural practices and health professionals who adhere to scientific treatment approaches. Nurses, as members of the modern health care culture, need to assess their cultural views of health and illness and guard against ethnocentric behavior (the belief that their own cultural beliefs and practices are superior to those of other cultures).

This chapter presented a survey of selected cultural groups in the United States: African-American, Hispanic-American, Chinese-American, Japanese-American, Indo-Chinese, Native American, and low-income groups. To provide culturally sensitive care, nurses need to be familiar with the cultural beliefs and practices of clients in their communities. Discussion of family patterns, definitions of health and illness, health beliefs and practices, and common health problems for each group has been, by necessity, selective and generalized. When caring for clients from a particular ethnic or cultural background, nurses must remember that each client is an individual and that the degree of adherence to traditional cultural beliefs and practices differs for each individual.

Spirituality and religion also play an important role in the lives of many people, especially during illness. Spiritual and religious beliefs and practices often overlap with cultural beliefs about illness causation and methods of curing.

BUILDING NURSING KNOWLEDGE

How Can Nurses Identify a Client's Ethnicity?

Sorofman B. Research in cultural diversity: Unidimensional measures of ethnicity. *West J Nurs Res.* 1986;8(4):467–468.

In this report, Sorofman addresses the problem of defining or categorizing an ethnic population for the purpose of research. He stresses that data must be collected to allow differentiation of one group from another; however, the issue he raises is also a problem in clinical practice. What indicators does the nurse use to classify a client's ethnicity?

Sorofman observes that nationality has commonly been used to describe the ethnic identity of a population. There is an inherent weakness in this method. The individual may have no affiliation with the culture of the region where he or she was born.

Kinship is another approach to ethnic identification. A client might be born in Mexico, but have parents who emigrated from Poland. Is the client ethnically Mexican, Polish, or both? Still another approach is religious heritage, but it too can be deceiving when geopolitical boundaries are considered. Being Israeli does not mean the person is Jewish.

Lastly, language is an indicator and one of the most common and reliable measures of ethnic identity. The language an individual uses usually relates to countless acts of everyday life, according to Sorofman. Other indicators include participation in ethnically specific events, consumption of ethnic diets, association with ethnic organizations, self-reported identification with a specific ethnic group, selecting friends predominantly from one ethnic group, choosing ethnic music and literature for personal enjoyment, wearing ethnic clothing, and selecting residence patterns and political affiliations that suggest ethnic identification. Sorofman suggests that multidimensional measures of ethnicity may have value for differentiating ethnic identity.

During crisis situations such as birth, death, and major health problems, religion may provide solace and strength for coping. Nurses therefore should be knowledgeable about the basic tenets of major religions in their communities to be sensitive to the spiritual needs of their clients and the implications of religious beliefs and practices for client care. This chapter presented an overview of five religions that are prevalent in the United States: Christianity, Judaism, Islam, Hinduism, and Buddhism.

The principles of cultural relativism, cultural sensitivity, and transcultural reciprocity provide a foundation for collaborative client care. Nurses who collaborate with clients from diverse ethnic and cultural populations must first become familiar with their own culture and with their culturally influenced values, beliefs, and behaviors to avoid ethnocentric biases. They must also become familiar with the values, beliefs, and practices of other cultures. Intercultural collaboration depends on the nurse's recognition that the client's cultural values, beliefs, and practices have relevance for care. Nurses who understand and respect a client's culture and are able to bridge cultural differences are able to provide culturally sensitive care. Incorporating cultural and spiritual assessment into the overall client assessment is essential for providing care to a diverse population.

REFERENCES

1. Leininger M. *Transcultural Nursing*. New York: John Wiley & Sons; 1978.
2. Haviland WA. *Cultural Anthropology*, 3rd ed. New York: Holt, Reinhart & Winston; 1981.
3. Anderson R. *The Cultural Context: An Introduction to Cultural Anthropology*. Minneapolis, MN: Burgess; 1976.
4. Sobralske MC. Perceptions of health: Navajo Indians. *Top Clin Nurs*. 1985;7:32–39.
5. Ember CR, Ember M. *Cultural Anthropology*, 3rd ed. Englewood Cliffs, NJ: Prentice-Hall; 1981.
6. *The Governor's Task Force on Black and Minority Health. Final Report*. Columbus, OH: April 1987.
7. Smitherman G. *Talkin' and Testifyin': The Language of Black America*. Detroit, MI: Wayne State University Press; 1986.
8. Gray SS, Nybell LM. Issues in African-American family preservation. *Child Welfare*. 1990;49:513–523.
9. Sodetani-Shibata AE. The Japanese American. In: Clark AL, ed. *Culture and Childrearing*. Philadelphia: FA Davis; 1981:96–138.
10. Orque MS, Bloch B, Monrroy LA. *Ethnic Nursing Care: A Multicultural Approach*. St. Louis, MO: CV Mosby; 1983.
11. US Bureau of the Census. *Statistical Abstracts of the US: 1988*, 108th ed. Washington, DC: 1987:Table 20.
12. Matteson MA, McConnell ES. *Gerontological Nursing: Concepts and Practice*. Philadelphia: WB Saunders; 1988.
13. Giger JN, Davidhziar R. Contextual care: Religious considerations for culturally appropriate nursing care. *Adv Clin Care*. 1990;5:48–51.
14. Breda VA. Health issues facing Native-American children. *Pedidatr Nurs*. 1989;15:575–577.
15. Henderson G, Primeaux M, eds. *Transcultural Health Care*. Menlo Park, CA: Addison-Wesley; 1981.
16. Farris CE, Farris LL. The American Indian. In: Clark AL, ed. *Culture and Childrearing*. Philadelphia: FA Davis; 1981: 56–67.
17. Spindler GD, ed. *The Making of Psychological Anthropology*. Los Angeles, CA: University of California Press; 1978.
18. Spector RE. *Cultural Diversity in Health and Illness*, 3rd ed. Norwalk, CT: Appleton & Lange; 1991.
19. Brown IC. *Understanding Other Cultures*. Englewood Cliffs, NJ: Prentice-Hall; 1963.
20. Overfield T. *Biologic Variation in Health and Illness: Race, Age, and Sex Differences*. Menlo Park, CA: Addison-Wesley; 1985.
21. Aamodt A. Culture. In Clark AL, ed. *Culture, Childrearing, Health Professionals*. Philadelphia: FA Davis; 1978:2–9.
22. Moore LG, Van Arsdale PW, Glittenberg JE, Aldrich RA. *The Biocultural Basis of Health*. St. Louis, MO: CV Mosby; 1980.
23. Powers BA. The use of orthodox and Black American folk medicine. *Adv Nurs Sci*. 1982;4:35–47.
24. Foreman JT. Susto and the health needs of the Cuban refugee population. *Top Clin Nurs*. 1985;7:40–47.
25. Roberson MHB. Home remedies: A cultural study. *Home Health Care Nurse*. 1987;5:35–40.
26. Whorton JC. Traditions of folk medicine in America. *JAMA*. 1987;257:1632–1635.
27. Moore LG, Van Arsdale PW, Glittenberg JE, Aldrich RA. *The Biocultural Basis of Health*. St. Louis, MO: CV Mosby; 1980.
28. La Fargue JP. Mediating between two views of illness. *Top Clin Nurs*. 1985;7:70–77.
29. Bloch B. Nursing care of black patients. In Orque, MS, Bloch B, Monrroy LA, eds. *Ethnic Nursing Care: A Multi-cultural Approach*. St. Louis, MO: CV Mosby; 1983:81–113.
30. Bullough VL, Bullough B. *Health Care for the Other Americans: Black Americans*. New York: Appleton-Century-Crofts; 1982.
31. Capers CF. Nursing and the Afro-American client. *Top Clin Nurs*. 1985;7:11–17.
32. Myrdal G. *An American Dilemma*. New York: Harper & Brothers; 1944.
33. Moynihan DP. *The Negro Family: A Case for National Action*. Washington, DC: Office of Planning and Research, U.S. Department of Labor; 1965.
34. Dodson J. Conceptualizations of black families. In McAdoo HP, ed. *Black Families*. Beverly Hills, CA: Sage; 1981:23–36.
35. Hill R. *The Strengths of Black Families*. New York: Emerson Hall; 1972.
36. Staples R, ed. *The Black Family: Essays and Studies*, 2nd ed. Belmont, CA: Wadsworth; 1978.
37. Bloch B. The black family: Rules and modes of communication. In Wang F, Nath CL, Simoni PS, eds. *Living With Change and Choice in Health*. Morgantown, WV: Sigma Theta Tau, Alpha Rho Chapter; 1986:275–280.
38. Snow L. Folk medical beliefs and their implications for care of patients: A review based on studies among black Americans. *Ann Intern Med*. 1974;81:82–96.
39. Foy S, Kunkle S, et al. Health care and illness in the black culture. *Cultural Connect*. 1985;5:1–2.
40. Guillory J. Ethnic perspectives of cancer nursing: The black American. *Oncol Nurs Forum*. 1987;14:66–69.
41. Savage DD. Highlights from the Department of Health and Human Services task force on black and minority health. *J Nat Black Nurse's Assoc*. 1987;1:16–23.
42. McCord C, Freeman HP. Excess mortality in Harlem. *N Engl J Med*. 1990;322:173–177.

43. Bloom JR, Hayes WA, Saunders F, Flatt S. Cancer awareness and secondary prevention practices in black Americans: Implications for intervention. *Fam Community Health.* 1987;10:19–29.
44. Pernoll ML. *Current Obstetric & Gynecologic Diagnosis & Treatment*, 7th ed. Norwalk, CT: Appleton & Lange; 1991.
45. Sherwen LN, Scoloveno MA, Weingarten CW. *Nursing Care of the Childbearing Family.* Norwalk, CT: Appleton & Lange; 1991.
46. Ford Foundation. *Hispanics: Challenges and Opportunities.* New York: Ford Foundation, Office of Reports; 1984:Publication 436.
47. Giachello AL. Hispanics and health care. In Cafferty PSJ, McCready WC, eds. *Hispanics in the United States.* New Brunswick, NJ: Transaction Books; 1985:159–188.
48. Reinert BR. The health care beliefs and values of Mexican-Americans. *Home Healthcare Nurse.* 1986;4:23–31.
49. Kleinman A. Folk illness. *JAMA.* 1986;255:3310–3311.
50. Alexander MA, Blank JJ. Factors related to obesity in Mexican-American preschool children. *Image.* 1988;20:79–82.
51. Flaskerud JH. Prevention of AIDS in blacks and Hispanics. *Cultural Connect.* 1987;1:3.
52. Louie KB. Providing health care to Chinese clients. *Top Clin Nurs.* 1985;7:18–25.
53. Char EL. The Chinese American. In Clark AL, ed. *Culture and Childrearing.* Philadelphia: FA Davis; 1981:140–164.
54. Chae M. Older Asians. *J Gerontol Nurs.* 1987;13:11–17.
55. Branck MR, Paxton PP, eds. *Providing Safe Nursing Care for Ethnic People of Color.* Englewood Cliffs, NJ: Prentice-Hall; 1974.
56. Chen-Louie T. Nursing care of Chinese American patients. In Orque, MS, Bloch B, Monrroy LA, eds. *Ethnic Nursing Care: A Multicultural Approach.* St. Louis, MO: CV Mosby; 1983:183–218.
57. Flaskerud JH. A proposed protocol for culturally relevant nursing psychotherapy. *Clin Nurse Specialist.* 1987;1:150–157.
58. Tien-Hyatt JL. Keying in on the unique care needs of Asian clients. *Nurs Health Care.* 1984;32:78–82.
59. Campbell T, Chang B. Health care of the Chinese in America. *Nurs Outlook.* 1973;21:245–249.
60. Hess P. Chinese and Hispanic elders and OTC drugs. *Geriatr Nurs.* 1986;7:314–318.
61. Kagawa-Singer M. Ethnic perspectives of cancer nursing: Hispanics and Japanese-Americans. *Oncol Nurs Forum.* 1987;14:59–65.
62. Takano J, Hashizume S. Nursing care of Japanese American patients. In Orque, MS, Bloch B, Monrroy LA, eds. *Ethnic Nursing Care: A Multicultural Approach.* St. Louis, MO: CV Mosby; 1983:219–243.
63. Gold SJ. Differential adjustment among new immigrant family members. *J Contemp Ethnogr.* 1989;17:408–434.
64. Orque MS. Nursing care of South Vietnamese patients. In Orque, MS, Bloch B, Monrroy LA, eds. *Ethnic Nursing Care: A Multicultural Approach.* St. Louis, MO: CV Mosby; 1983:245–269.
65. Calhoun MA. Providing health care to Vietnamese in America: What practitioners need to know. *Home Health Care Nurse.* 1986; 4:14–22.
66. Stringfellow L, Liem DN, Liem DL. The Vietnamese in America. In Clark AL, ed. *Culture and Childrearing.* Philadelphia: FA Davis; 1981:228–241.
67. Egan MG. A family assessment challenge: Refugee youth and foster family adaptation. *Top Clin Nurs.* 1985;7:64–69.
68. Attneane C. American Indians and Alaska Native families: Emigrants in their own homeland. In McGoldrick M, et al, eds. *Ethnicity and Family Therapy.* New York: Guilford; 1982.
69. Antle A. Ethnic perspectives of cancer nursing: The American Indian. *Oncol Nurs Forum.* 14:70–73.
70. Wilson UM. Nursing care of American Indian patients. In Orque, MS, Bloch B, Monrroy LA, eds. *Ethnic Nursing Care: A Multicultural Approach.* St. Louis, MO: CV Mosby; 1983:271–295.
71. Orgel J, Benson W, Knudson K, et al. The health practices of Native American Indians. *Cultural Connect.* 1985;5:3–4.
72. Coulehan JL. Navajo Indian medicine: Implications for healing. *J Fam Practice.* 1980;10:55–61.
73. Sobralske MC. Perceptions of health: Navajo Indians. *Top Clin Nurs.* 1985;7:32–39.
74. Long KA. Suicide intervention and prevention with Indian adolescent populations. *Issues Mental Health Nurs.* 1986;8:247–253.
75. Lewis O. The culture of poverty. *Sci Am.* 1966;215:19–25.
76. Kosa J, Zola I, eds. *Poverty and Health: A Sociological Analysis.* Cambridge, MA: Harvard University Press; 1975.
77. Wilson WJ. The urban underclass. In Dunbar LW, ed. *Minority Report.* New York: Pantheon Books; 1984.
78. Harrington M. *The New American Poverty.* New York: Holt, Rinehart & Winston; 1984.
79. Pesznecker BL. The poor: A population at risk. *Pub Health Nurs.* 1984;1:237–247.
80. Weaver JL. *National Health Policy and the Underserved.* St. Louis, MO: CV Mosby; 1976.
81. Murray RB, Zentner JP. *Nursing Assessment and Health Promotion Strategies Through the Life Span.* Norwalk, CT: Appleton & Lange; 1989.
82. Sutherland S, Houlden L, Clarke P, Friedhelm H, eds. *The World's Religions.* Boston, MA: GK Hall & Co; 1988.
83. Barnard D. Religion and religious studies in health care and health education. *J Allied Health.* 1983;12:192–201.
84. Harmon Y. The relationship between religiousity and health. *Health Values: Achieving High Level Wellness.* 1985;9:23–25.
85. Peterson EA. The physical . . . the spiritual . . . can you meet all of your patient's needs? *J Gerontol Nurs.* 1985;11:23–27.
86. Hutchinson JA. *Paths of Faith*, 3rd ed. New York: McGraw-Hill; 1980.
87. Pumphrey JB. Recognizing your patient's spiritual needs. *Nursing '77.* 1977;7:64–70.
88. Bach M. *Major Religions of the World.* Marina del Ray, CA: Devorss & Company; 1984.
89. Dobson SM. Conceptualizing transcultural health visiting: The concept of transcultural reciprocity. *J Adv Nurs.* 1989;14:97–102.
90. Tripp-Reimer T, Brink P, Saunders JM. Cultural assessment: Content and process. *Nurs Outlook.* 1984;32:78–82.

BIBLIOGRAPHY

Anderson JM. Health care across cultures. *Nurs Outlook.* 1990;38: 136–139.

Ashworth P. Hospital chaplains—A neglected resource? *Intensive Care Nurs.* 1990;6:165–166.

Baldwin JA, Hopkins R. African-American and European-American cultural differences as assessed by the worldviews paradigm: An empirical analysis. *West J Black Studies.* 1990;14:38–52.

Barge FC, Norr KF. Homeless shelter policies for women in an urban environment. *Image.* 1991;23:145–149.

Cerhan JU. The Hmong in the United States: An overview for mental health professionals. *J Counsel Dev.* 1990;69:88–92.

Champion VL, et al. Relationship between cross-cultural health attitudes and community health indicators. *Pub Health Nurs.* 1991; 7:243–250.

Clark CC, et al. Spirituality: Integral to quality care. *Holistic Nurs Practice.* 1991;5:67–76.

DiMeo E. RX for spiritual distress . . . a guide to religious practices. *RN.* 1991;54:22–24.

Fountain DE. Battle between the Gods: The challenge of transcultural communication. *J Christian Nurs.* 1991;8:26–30, 32–34.

Fox PG. Stress related to family change among Vietnamese refugees. *J Community Health Nurs.* 1991;8:45–56.

Friedman MM. Transcultural family nursing: Application to Latino and black families. *J Pediatr Nurs.* 1990;5:214–222.

Frye BA. Cultural themes in health-care decision making among Cambodian refugee women. *J Community Health Nurs.* 1991;8: 33–44.

Frye BA. The Cambodian refugee patient: Providing culturally sensitive rehabilitation nursing care. *Rehab Nurs.* 1990;15:156–158.

Henkle JO, et al. Cultural diversity: A resource in planning and implementing nursing care. *Pub Health Nurs.* 1990;7:145–149.

Johnson SD Jr. Toward clarifying culture, race, and ethnicity in the context of multicultural counseling. *J Multicult Counseling Dev.* 1990;18:41–50.

Kuhni CQ. When cultures clash at the bedside. *RN.* 1990;53:23–24.

LaFromboise TD. Counseling intervention and American Indian tradition: An integrative approach. *Counseling Psychol.* 1990;18: 628–654.

Lawson LV. Culturally sensitive support for grieving parents. *Am J Matern Child Nurs.* 1990;15:76–79.

Marshall PA. Cultural influences on perceived quality of life. *Semin Oncol Nurs.* 1990;6:278–284.

Nelson-Conley CL. Role development of the clinical nurse specialist within the Indian Health Service. *Clin Nurse Specialist.* 1990; 4:142–146.

Piles CL. Providing spiritual care. *Nurse Educator.* 1990;15:36–41.

Scaffa ME, et al. Culturai considerations in the treatment of persons with AIDS. *Occup Ther Health Care.* 1990;7:69–85.

Smith MA. Psychiatric function and roles in an Indian health program context. *Am Indian Alaska Native Mental Health Res.* 1990;4: 41–52.

Stiles MK. The shining stranger: Nurse–family spiritual relationship. *Cancer Nurs.* 1990;13:235–245.

Swaby-Ellis D. Why worry about cultural differences? *J Christian Nurs.* 1990;7:31,40.

Ting-Toomey S, Korzenny F. Cross-cultural interpersonal communication. *Int Intercult Annu.* 1991;15:1–296.

UNIT THREE
The Client

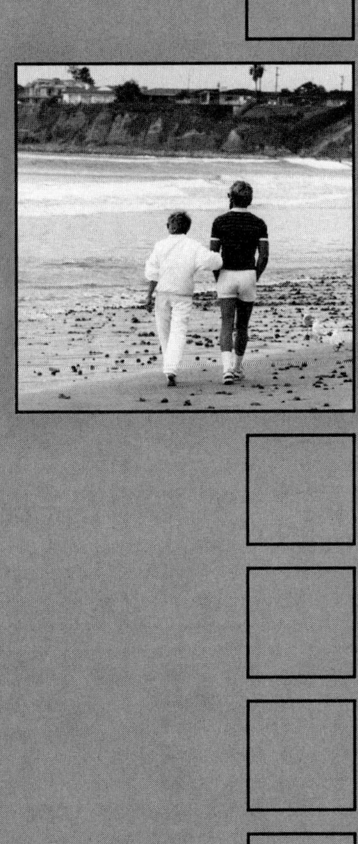

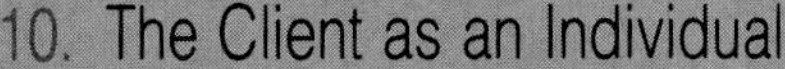

10. The Client as an Individual
11. Growth and Development Across the Life Span
12. Becoming a Client

CHAPTER 10

The Client as an Individual

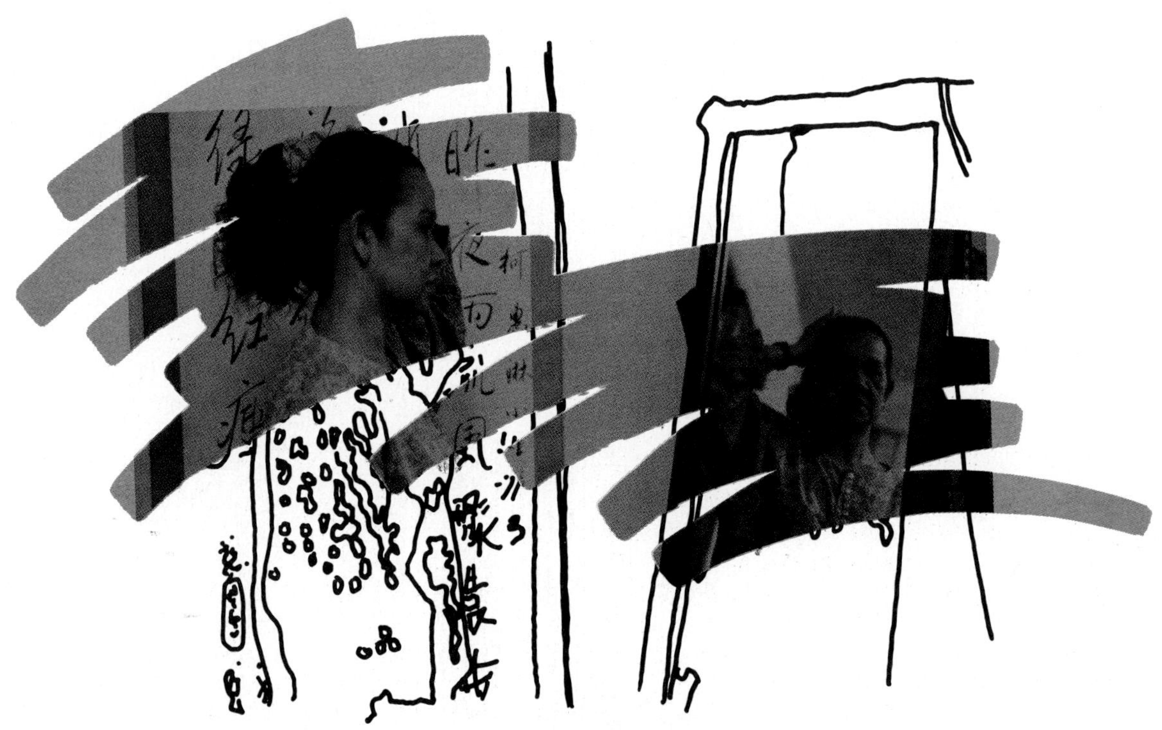

Behavioral Objectives

Upon completion of this chapter, the student will be able to:

1. Define the term "individuality."
2. Describe the phenomenologic view of perception.
3. Outline the five levels of basic human needs proposed by Maslow.
4. Describe five positive characteristics likely to be exhibited by a self-actualizing person.
5. Define the concept of identity and its component parts.
6. List six criteria useful for assessing the state of an individual's emotional health.
7. List the eight stages of psychosocial development proposed by Erikson.
8. Outline the major tasks to be accomplished during each of the four transitional periods in one's life structure.
9. Explain how a collaborative approach to health care facilitates self-actualization.

KEY TERMS

body image
coping
development
developmental task
ego
fixation
gender
gender identity
gender role
growth
human needs
id
identity
individuality
integration
life structure
life-style
maturation
perceptions
perceptual field
personality
phenomenal self
regression
role performance
self
self-acceptance
self-concept
self-esteem
stress
stressors
superego

Each client is a human being who is different from every other human being. This uniqueness is the result of a variety of complex interactions constantly taking place within the physiological and psychological dimensions of the individual, as well as the dynamic and personal interactions of the individual with the environment. Individuality results from the interaction of individual perceptions about reality with personal needs and manner of coping with stress. This individuality is reflected as one's personality. Identity is the persistent consciousness that an individual has of self, separate and distinct from others.

In order to assist clients in maintaining, attaining, or regaining an optimal level of wellness, nurses must understand clients as individuals. Clients' perceptions about themselves and their environment, as well as their stage of growth and development, have an impact on their basic needs and their reaction to stress. The most viable mechanism available to nurses to gain information about clients as individuals is collaboration with clients and other people significant in their lives. Such information is necessary for development of effective nursing implementation to help clients experience optimal wellness.

This chapter focuses on the dimensions of individuality, the components of identity, and the parameters of growth and development, including sexuality, that are part of understanding clients as individuals. Healthy individuals share certain characteristics that are reflected in the attitudes they hold about themselves and the degree of success they experience in mastering their own environments. Informed observers can note the presence or absence of these characteristics. Also, individuals must attain certain levels of growth and development at various stages in their lives in order to have the ability to master their own environment successfully. Nurses can assess levels of individuals' growth and development at any given point and compare them with norms that have been established for healthy individuals at comparable developmental stages. Several developmental theories are presented herein to provide a basis for understanding, assessing, and supporting individuality.

DIMENSIONS OF INDIVIDUALITY

Each individual is a unique being who is separate and distinct from all other human beings. Developmental theorists disagree about the degree to which the variation that exists between individuals is due to genetic makeup or heredity, and the degree to which it is influenced by environmental interactions, or life experiences. The few quantitative estimates of genetic influence indicate that at least half of the observed variation existing between individuals is due to genetic makeup.[1,2] Individual variation that is not genetically predetermined is heavily influenced by environmental interactions, which are extremely complex and variable from one individual to another. Because of the complexity and variability of individual life experiences, no two individuals are identical. Even identical twins—individuals who came from the same single fertilized ovum and who have the same genetic makeup—are not truly identical.

Individuality is the total character peculiar to an individual that distinguishes that individual from all other people.[3,4] This total character, or **personality,** encompasses the whole of an individual's behavioral and emotional tendencies, including attitudes, habits, values, motives, abilities, appearances, and psychic state. As a result, it influences how the individual will think, feel, and act in any given situation. Individuality is the result of interactions between genetic makeup and life experiences, and is intimately associated with an individual's perceptions and needs, as well as personal stress when needs are unmet.

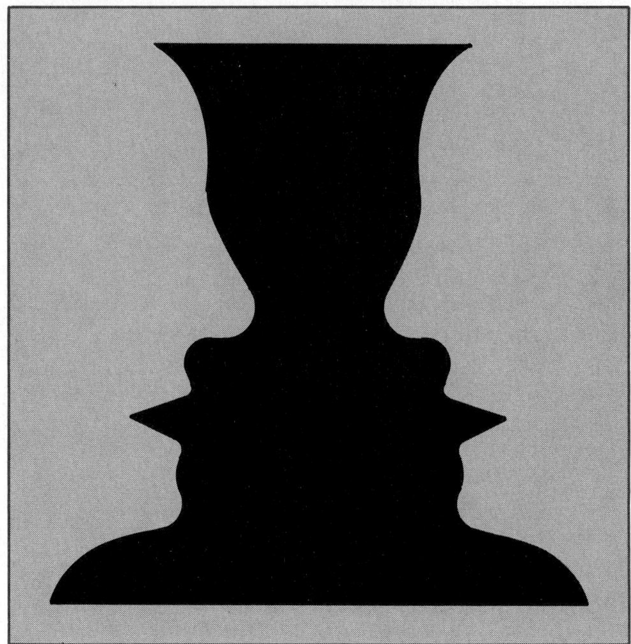

Figure 10–1. Figure–ground relationships. Is the illustration a vase, a candlestick, two faces in profile, or of an undifferentiated object? The meaning changes with the individual's interpretation.

Perceptions

Perceptions are mental images that individuals have of their environment.[3,5,6] These mental images result from personal experiences with the environment and serve as subjective interpretations of reality for the individual. When observing a cup half filled with water, for instance, one individual may consider the cup to be half full while another may consider the same cup to be half empty, depending upon prior personal experiences. Figure 10–1 demonstrates the possibilities for perceptual variation. Factors that control or limit the process of perceiving include the effects of individual need, the human organism itself, time, opportunity, goals, learning, and self-awareness (sometimes called the phenomenal self).

The concept of perception has been described in detail by phenomenologic psychologists. Phenomenologists are interested in the personal meaning of behavior from the viewpoint of the person behaving. They attempt to make observations that reflect such an understanding of the behavior they observe.[3–6] Phenomenologists believe that individuals behave according to their own interpretation of the facts rather than according to the facts as other people interpret them. Typical questions of interest to phenomenologists include "What is he thinking?" "What does this mean to her?" "How does he feel about this?" The major focus of phenomenology is to determine how an individual's environment is interpreted by that individual.

Phenomenologists use the concepts of a **perceptual field** or phenomenal field to reflect the sum total of an individual's conscious experience at any given moment. The perceptual field is composed of the individual's perceptions, beliefs, imaginings, and memories. All behavior exhibited by an individual is completely determined by the perceptual field of that individual, and no two individuals have identical perceptual fields. A good example of this concept was published by Combs and Snygg[3]:

> Several years ago a friend of mine was driving a car at dusk along a Western road. A globular mass, about two feet in diameter, suddenly appeared directly in the path of the car. A passenger screamed and grasped the wheel attempting to steer the car around the object. The driver, however, tightened his grip on the wheel and drove directly into the object. The behavior of both the driver and the passenger was determined by his own phenomenal field. The passenger, an Easterner, saw the object in the highway as a boulder and fought desperately to steer the car around it. The driver, a native Westerner, saw it as a tumbleweed and devoted his efforts to keeping his passenger from overturning the car. (p. 20)

In this example, the individuals perceived the globular mass to be a boulder or a tumbleweed based on prior life experiences with globular masses.

Factors Affecting Perceptions

Definition of Personal Adequacy. Each individual has a fundamental need for feelings of adequacy and continually searches throughout life for ways to satisfy this need. Perceptions of the environment and the self in that environment enable an individual to behave in ways that lead to satisfaction of this fundamental need. A woman, for example, who perceives that she must be slender in order to receive social approval as a female may survive on a low-calorie diet. She has determined, based on perceptions about her environment, that this action will ensure fulfillment of her need for feelings of adequacy as a female.

Sensory Function. Sensory function refers to functioning of the human sensory organs. Only those things that an organism has the equipment to perceive can be perceived. Dogs, for instance, react to high-frequency sounds that humans cannot hear because dogs have the "equipment" to hear those sounds. Although human perception extends beyond physiological limitations, the quality of functioning of the sensory organs—such as the eyes, ears, taste buds, and olfactory ends—as well as the brain and nervous system, sets broad limits on how and what an individual can perceive. A smooth-running body in good physical and mental condition is most likely to give an individual a feeling of adequacy and a sense of control over the environment. Compromises in functioning tend to limit individual ability to perceive the environment and one's role in that environment in a manner that allows for optimal adaptation.

Time and Opportunity. Time and opportunity have a direct impact on perceptions. An individual must have an opportunity to perceive an event or object to form perceptions. Without opportunity to observe a painting, for example, one cannot develop perceptions about it. That which an individual is able to perceive in any given situation also depends on the length of time he or she has been exposed to it. Often the longer one observes a painting, the more one is able to perceive in it. Although time and opportunity both affect the development of perceptions, the perceptions of two people with equivalent exposure to an event will differ because perceptions are based on prior personal experiences and unique characteristics. The perceptual fields of two different individuals will always differ.

Goals. Goals are important throughout the process of growth and development. Certain objects, feelings, or events become more or less important depending upon how they are related to an individual's goals. A teenager whose goal is to go to college is likely to perceive that studying to achieve good grades is important. Another, whose goal is to have many friends, may perceive that devoting time to social activities instead of studying is a better choice. In order for individuals to achieve the goals valued most highly, they develop techniques that provide some measure of assurance for success in attaining those goals. An individual who highly values a goal of mastery over others may perceive that aggressive physical force or athletic competition are viable techniques for helping to achieve the goal. Another individual for whom social approval is very important may work hard for a career as a physician in order to achieve that approval.

Learning. An individual must be able to adapt behavior to fit the moment if he or she is to live effectively and efficiently in modern society. This requires that the individual has access to the widest possible field of perceptions from which to draw. Learning, the process by which an individual is able to change behavior constructively, and retention of that learning over time, facilitate development of a wide perceptual field. Factors that restrict or inhibit development of the field will have negative effects on the individual's ability to deal with life successfully.

The Phenomenal Self. This is a term used by phenomenologists to describe the way in which individuals perceive themselves. In fact, all individuals have many separate perceptions about themselves—perceptions about who they are as people, their strengths and weaknesses, how they look, how effectively they manage their lives, among many other perceptions. **Phenomenal self** is each individual's unique way of organizing these myriad perceptions of self. The phenomenal self is the most stable part of the perceptual field. It gives continuity and consistency to an individual's personality and provides the central core around which all other perceptions are organized and prioritized. The manner in which individuals decide to act in any given situation depends upon how they perceive the self in that situation. If a man believes that he is Napoleon, he will behave like he thinks Napoleon would behave in the same situation. Self and self-perceptions are discussed in greater detail in a later section of this chapter.

Needs

Human needs are physiological or psychological conditions that must be met in order for an individual to achieve well-being.[7] Although some needs are basic for all human beings, others vary in their degree of urgency among different individuals. Needs are key to understanding individual behavior, because they determine how individuals perceive the world and, therefore, how they interact with that world. One woman who has ample access to food may choose to consume a low-calorie diet and remain relatively comfortable both physically and psychologically. Another woman who is forced to be on a low calorie diet because she does not have access to sufficient amounts of food may eat excessively if given access to large quantities of food. The first woman's basic need for food has always been met, so she is not concerned about a potential lack of food. The second woman, however, is insecure about future access to food based on prior experiences in meeting her basic need for food. Understanding an individual's personal needs helps to clarify individual behavior.

Maslow's Hierarchy of Needs. Maslow[7] developed a system for classifying human needs in a hierarchy, or ranking. He views a human need as a phenomenon arising from an internal tension caused by some change in the relationship between an individual and that individual's surroundings. This tension results in goal-directed behavior that persists until the tension is reduced and need is satisfied.

In an effort to provide a framework for understanding

human needs, Maslow proposed a hierarchy of needs that consists of five different levels (Fig. 10–2). As an individual progresses through life there is movement up and down within this hierarchy, as well as an overlapping of needs, and specific needs change due to alterations in the human organism and the environment.

First-level Needs. First-level needs, or the most basic level of needs in this hierarchy, are comprised of needs that stem from the physiological requirements of the human organism for survival. Needs requiring satisfaction at this level include needs for food, oxygen, water, and sleep. Participation in a sexual relationship is also considered by some authorities to be such a basic need that it should be categorized in this first level.[8,9] The physiological needs within Maslow's first level are the most prepotent of all needs. If all needs within this level are unsatisfied, the human organism will be dominated by physiological needs alone and all other needs will seem nonexistent. If an individual is starving, needs for respect or a personal philosophy will be forgotten. Once basic physiological needs have been reasonably well met, they no longer remain needs, and other, higher-level needs emerge to drive the human organism.

Second-level Needs. Second-level needs in Maslow's hierarchy are categorized as safety needs, for example, security, stability, order, and physical safety. Infants in particular demonstrate safety needs quite obviously when these needs have not been met. If suddenly dropped or startled by a loud noise, an infant will exhibit a total body reaction that includes vocal cries and muscular action.

Third-level Needs. Third-level needs are categorized as love and belonging needs. If physiological and safety needs have been fairly well gratified, this level of needs will emerge and become dominant. Individuals then strive with great intensity to develop relationships based on love and affection with mutual giving and receiving, as well as to establish recognition from their peers. Absence of friends, a sweetheart, a spouse, or children is felt deeply. Love is not synonymous with sex, yet love and affection, including their expression in sexuality, are often confronted with restrictions and inhibitions. Thwarting of the need for love and belonging has been found to be associated with maladjustment or severe psychopathology in some individuals.

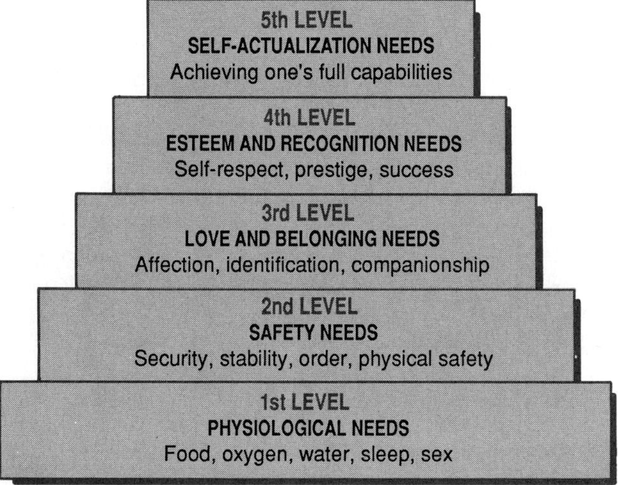
5th LEVEL
SELF-ACTUALIZATION NEEDS
Achieving one's full capabilities
4th LEVEL
ESTEEM AND RECOGNITION NEEDS
Self-respect, prestige, success
3rd LEVEL
LOVE AND BELONGING NEEDS
Affection, identification, companionship
2nd LEVEL
SAFETY NEEDS
Security, stability, order, physical safety
1st LEVEL
PHYSIOLOGICAL NEEDS
Food, oxygen, water, sleep, sex

Figure 10–2. Maslow's hierarchy of needs. (*From Maslow AH.* Motivation and Personality. *2nd ed. New York: Harper & Row; 1970. Copyright 1954 by Harper & Row, Publishers, Inc. Copyright 1970 by Abraham H. Maslow. Reprinted by permission of HarperCollins Publishers.*)

IMPLICATIONS FOR NURSE–CLIENT COLLABORATION

Human Needs

Needs are the driving force that motivates behavior because they determine how an individual perceives, and thus interacts with, the world. Through nurse–client collaboration, the nurse gains an understanding of the client's needs and thus an understanding of the reasons for the client's behavior. This understanding enables the nurse to anticipate how the client might react to his or her health care. Caregiving based on the individual needs is more likely to be effective because such care relates directly to the forces motivating the behavior.

Fourth-level Needs. Fourth-level needs are esteem needs. Individuals in modern society desire stable, firmly based, high evaluations of themselves; self-respect or self-esteem; and esteem from others. Based on the work of several theologians and psychologists, Maslow warns against the dangers of basing self-esteem on the opinions of others rather than on real capability, competence, and adequacy. He has taken the position that the most stable and healthy self-esteem is based on deserved genuine respect from others rather than on unwarranted adulation.

Fifth-level Needs. Fifth-level needs in Maslow's hierarchy are the highest level of needs, those for self-actualization. The concept of self-actualization was first published in the literature around 1940.[10] It has dominated the thinking of authors such as Carl Rogers, Erich Fromm, and Gordon Allport, as well as Abraham Maslow.

The process of self-actualization has been described in rather global terms. Rogers[11] referred to the self-actualizing individual as a "fully functioning person." Fromm[12] equated self-actualization with the act of living itself, which from his perspective is the only meaning to life. Maslow[7] describes the process as the full use of one's talents, capacities, and potentialities. He also suggests that a self-actualizing person experiences pleasurable tensions in realizing his or her own potentials.[13] The greater the amount of tension, the greater the motivation for growth and the healthier the person. Allport[14] described the self-actualizing individual as one who maintains tension in the interest of distant and often unattainable goals. The concept of self-actualization has also been linked to the concept Freud identified as "life instinct."[15] Freud used this term to reflect his concept that there are forces that tend to upset established levels of equilibrium and move the individual toward new and more complex equilibria.

Maslow's interpretation of basic human needs is that there are definite psychological and operational differences

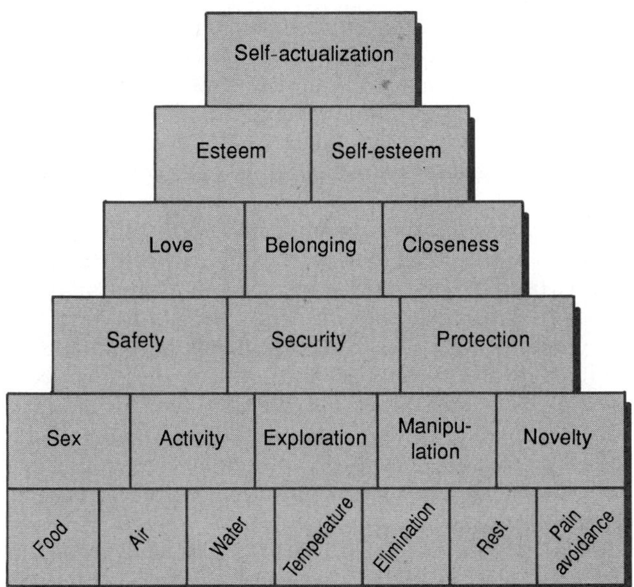

Figure 10–3. Maslow's hierarchy of needs as modified by Kalish. (*From Kalish RA.* The Psychology of Human Behavior. *5th ed. Monterey, CA: Wadsworth; 1983.*)

between needs referred to as "higher" and those referred to as "lower" needs. The human organism attaches values to needs within the hierarchy according to personal perceptions of relative potency. In spite of individual variation, physiological needs are stronger than safety needs, which in turn are stronger than love needs, which are stronger than esteem needs. The need for self-actualization has the least strength and emerges only after physiological, safety, love, and esteem needs have been relatively well satisfied. Maslow contends that when all other needs have been met, individuals become discontent and restless unless they are doing what they are most fitted for. To become self-actualized means that an individual becomes everything that he or she is capable of becoming. The specific form that gratification of this need takes varies greatly from one individual to another. One individual may desire to be an ideal parent while another may desire to be an outstanding athlete, artist, inventor, or nurse.

According to Maslow, self-actualizing individuals have a firm foundation for development of a personal value system because of their philosophical acceptance of themselves and the environment. These people are able to discriminate between means and ends in terms of goal satisfaction. As a result, conflict and struggle, or uncertainty, over choices lessen or disappear in many areas of life.

Kalish's Hierarchy of Needs. Kalish[16] adapted Maslow's hierarchy of needs into six levels rather than five (Fig. 10–3). First-level needs are physiological needs described as survival needs, or needs that must be satisfied in order for the organism to stay alive. Survival needs, the motives for satisfying those needs, and an explanation for each motive are presented in Table 10–1. Second-level needs—such as sex, activity, exploration, manipulation, and novelty—are referred to as "stimulation needs." According to Kalish, the function of stimulation needs is not well understood but appears to be more closely related to appreciation of life than to the maintenance of life.

Kalish's point of view is that the need for sex is more difficult to satisfy than other lower-level, or basic, needs. One does not need to learn to breathe, eliminate, or sleep, and satisfaction of other physiological needs for food, water, temperature control, and pain avoidance are easily learned by most individuals. The desire for sex results from biochemical changes in the body that are often triggered by visual, auditory, or other sensory stimuli that have sexual meaning for the individual. Each individual, therefore, must learn how to satisfy his or her need for sex.

Third- through sixth-level needs in Kalish's hierarchy are comparable to Maslow's second- through fifth-level needs. Needs for self-actualization are considered to be the highest level by both psychologists.

Jourard's Basic Human Needs. Jourard[17] acknowledged that biologists and psychologists vary in their opinions about the precise number of basic needs. Although there is consensus on what needs must be satisfied for sheer human survival, wide variations exist in understanding what needs will lead to achievement of unfathomed human po-

TABLE 10–1. SURVIVAL NEEDS AND MOTIVES FOR MEETING THOSE NEEDS

Survival Need	Motive for Satisfying	Reason for Motive
Food	Hunger	Initial signs of starvation are irritability, reduced level of activity, constant thoughts of food, and apathy.
Air	Air hunger	A very brief period without oxygen will produce permanent brain damage and death will result after only a few minutes of deprivation.
Water	Thirst	The motivating qualities of acute thirst are overwhelming.
Temperature	Temperature regulation demands	Human beings have ability to adjust physiologically to variations in heat and cold only up to certain limits.
Elimination	Elimination pressures	Waste products must be excreted successfully in order for human survival to be maintained.
Rest	Fatigue	Rest and sleep are required for renewal of vitality.
Pain avoidance	Pain avoidance	Pain is a signal that something has gone wrong with the human organism.

Adapted from Kalish RA. The Psychology of Human Behavior. *Belmont, CA: Wadsworth; 1966.*

tentialities if fulfilled. The basic needs proposed by Jourard are outlined in Table 10–2. The terminology used for designating the nature of these needs is different than that used by Maslow and Kalish; however, the concepts are not inconsistent with the concepts inherent in their hierarchies of needs. For example, Jourard's need to value life could be viewed as a safety need while his needs for meaning and purpose could be viewed as self actualization needs.

Coping

Coping is the manner in which an individual responds to stress. Patterns of coping developed in response to stress are another dimension of individuality and are, therefore, unique to each individual.

Stressors, or conditions that lead to stress, are external situations that disrupt internal equilibrium within the human organism and interfere with the meeting of needs.[18] **Stress** is the nonspecific systemic adaptive response of the body to a stressor or multiple stressors.[18,19] It results in a constraining force, or tension, which is felt by the individual when certain basic needs have not been met and the individual perceives potential threat to his or her own well-being as a result.[20–24] Unmet personal needs also result in an altered perception of reality.

Individuals react to stressful situations in a variety of ways. These reactions are complex and highly individualized. Innate characteristics, past life experiences, and personal goals affect an individual's adaptation to stress. Some individuals cope with stress by "superficial adaptation," or adaptation in small quantities at a time, requiring a small amount of energy that is regenerated rapidly; while others are only able to cope with stress by "deep adaptation," which results in excessive emotional strain and, eventually, irreparable degeneration of the organism.[25] It appears that the more perceived control individuals have over stressful situations, the less severe their actual reaction to the stress will be.[21,26]

Reactions to stress are physical as well as emotional. Because of the continuous interaction between mind and body, psychological stress can lead to illness and disease.[27] Development of illness or disease and degree of success in coping with these conditions are highly individualized and depend on the level of stress, personal susceptibility, and the environment.[28] Situations resulting in mild levels of stress, such as minor irritations with other individuals or with circumstances, seldom produce long-lasting physiological damage. Severe or chronic stressful situations, however, such as continued marital discord or lack of job satisfaction, frequently result in compromised health and well-being. Levels of tension that produce stress and inability to cope with stress vary greatly from one individual to another.[17] A grade of D in a chemistry course will likely cause more stress for a high school student who hopes to be admitted to medical school than it will for a student who does not wish to attend college.

Indications of difficulty in coping with stress may be behavioral, physical, or emotional.[29] Common indicators of problematic coping are outlined in Table 10–3. Stress, coping, and adaptation are discussed further in Chapter 6.

TABLE 10–2. JOURARD'S BASIC HUMAN NEEDS

Needs	Characteristics
Value life itself	Healthy individuals will do almost anything under threat—such as break laws, kill others, or sacrifice wealth—to preserve their existence.
Physical needs	Threat to availability of supplies, such as food, air, or water, for meeting basic physiological needs will result in desperate measures.
Love	Love is a need that requires willingness to give love first, or at least reciprocally.
Status, success, and self-esteem	Recognition and approval from others offset feelings of inferiority.
Freedom and space	Varying degrees of freedom are needed to conduct life according to personal wishes and goals.
Challenge	Deprivation of challenge is usually experienced as boredom or emptiness in one's existence.
Meditation and disengagement	The healthy individual needs intense involvement in life to foster full functioning, but also needs periodic freedom from the customary consciousness, such as a vacation, for renewal of vitality.
Cognitive clarity	One cannot function efficiently with ambiguity or contradiction. In the face of uncertainty, the healthy individual will construct answers perceived to be satisfactory for interacting successfully with the environment.
Meaning and purpose	One's life goals and daily actions toward meeting those goals reflect a personal understanding of meaning and purpose. Depression and neurotic suffering often result when meaning in life is not defined by an individual.
Varied experience	Multiple and varied experiences are needed to expand the scope of one's perceptual field and allow for multiple choices in interacting with the environment.
Contact with nature and own body	Contact with nature, such as the seaside, forests, or animals, allows an individual to understand that he or she does not simply have a body, but is an embodied being who is part of nature.

Adapted from Jourard SM. Healthy Personality: An Approach from the Viewpoint of Humanistic Psychology. *New York: Macmillan; 1974.*

TABLE 10–3. INDICATIONS OF DIFFICULTY IN COPING WITH STRESS

Behavioral Indications
- Decreased productivity and quality of job performance
- Tendency to make mistakes; poor judgment
- Forgetfulness and blocking
- Diminished attention to detail
- Preoccupation; daydreaming or "spacing out"
- Inability to concentrate on tasks
- Reduced creativity
- Increased use of alcohol and/or drugs
- Increased smoking
- Increased absenteeism and illness
- Lethargy
- Loss of interest
- Accident proneness

Physical Indications
- Elevated blood pressure
- Increased muscle tension (neck, shoulder, back)
- Elevated pulse and/or increased respiration
- "Sweaty" palms
- Cold hands and feet
- Slumped posture
- Tension headache
- Upset stomach
- Higher-pitched voice
- Change in appetite
- Urinary frequency
- Restlessness; difficulty in falling or staying asleep

Emotional Indications
- Emotional outbursts and crying
- Irritability
- Depression
- Withdrawal
- Hostile and assaultive behavior
- Tendency to blame others
- Anxiousness
- Feelings of worthlessness
- Suspiciousness

Adapted from Claus KE, Bailey JT. Living With Stress and Promoting Well-Being: A Handbook for Nurses. *St. Louis: Mosby; 1980.*

Individuality and Client Care. The dimensions of individuality discussed above are of concern to nurses whenever they are interacting with clients in a health care transaction. Nurses' and clients' perceptions determine their subjective reality at the time of the interaction. There may be differences in the two views of reality that will influence communication, acceptance of one another and ultimately whether the clients' health care needs are met. It is not uncommon for health care providers to lose sight of the focal importance of clients' perceptions in determining and achieving health care goals. To the extent that nurses and other providers view their own reality regarding definitions of health and how to achieve it as more important than clients' perceptions, neither clients' nor nurses' resources can be employed for maximal effectiveness.

IMPLICATIONS FOR NURSE–CLIENT COLLABORATION

Coping and Stress

Stress demands adaptation. Coping is the manner in which an individual responds to stress. Just as perceptions and needs are individual, patterns of coping are also individual. In a collaborative relationship, the nurse endeavors to identify the stressors experienced by the client, both by observing the client's responses to the environment and through verbal exchanges with the client. By these means, the nurse tries to help the client identify the stressors that tax energy and to identify and maintain effective coping patterns.

Clients' needs are a related and equally important consideration. Alterations in health often foster parallel, but not necessarily predictable, alterations in needs. The behaviors exhibited in response to altered needs are not always easily interpreted. A nurse who bases client care on a standardized or a personal interpretation of human needs is likely to meet with resistance and frustration. An effective nurse thoughtfully determines which needs a client perceives as most significant. For example, consider a woman who has been hospitalized because of symptoms of preterm labor. The nurse may assume that preventing a premature delivery and the associated risks to the woman and fetus is most important. The woman, however, may believe that the consequences of premature labor are not as threatening as the possible harm to her young children at home, who have no one caring for them. Her primary need is to satisfy the needs of her children for nourishment and protection. If the nurse understands this primary need accurately, other options for intervention can be reviewed, such as determining whether a relative or friend can be contacted and asked to care for the children, having a social worker make arrangements for child care, or clarifying with the client's physician whether a regimen for taking medications at home would be a safe alternative to hospitalization.

Nurses must also be sensitive to clients' individual coping style. Coping with the stress of unmet or altered needs and diminished wellness may be challenging to many clients. Successful adaptation depends upon healthy coping strategies and effective social support systems, such as family or friends. Nursing support of healthy, effective coping or suggestions for alternative coping strategies when the clients' resources seem inadequate or overwhelmed can be an important asset for clients.

Careful collaboration between nurse and client is an effective means for identification of client needs and strengths. Collaboration with appropriate family members and other individuals, including other health care professionals, is also important. When sufficient information has been obtained about how the client perceives the situation, his or her own needs, and current coping, a plan for client care can be mutually developed and implemented. This individualized plan for care should reduce client stress, use client resources, and facilitate attainment of an optimal level of wellness for the client. Chapter 22 discusses the assessment and management of stress and presents coping strategies that can be implemented by the nurse and client.

■ IDENTITY

The distinguishing character, or identity, of a person is an important component of individuality. **Identity** is the conscious sense that an individual has about personal uniqueness and general continuity of character. Although one's identity develops as a function of life experiences, there is a basic constancy that endures over time. This quality confers stability in individuals' perceptions of their environment and their behavior within it.

Self is an important aspect of identity. **Self** is used to refer to the union of elements, such as body, emotions, thoughts, and sensations, that constitute the individuality and identity of a particular person. "Self" is a reflexive term because it denotes a relationship between an entity (in this case a person) and itself. The term signifies that the attention of the individual is directed back on himself or herself in a reflective manner.

There are aspects of self that remain internal, that is, that are not shared with others. This is the private self. Internal self and subjective self are other terms used to refer to private self. Private self encompasses ideal self: impressions about what one would like to be, how one would desire to change oneself.

Individuals share some aspects of self in their interactions with others. This projection of self into social activities is called the public self. Aspects of self observable to others may also be called external self or objective self. The more comfortable one is with oneself, the more similiarity there is likely to be among one's private self, public self, and ideal self. For some individuals, however, private self, ideal self, and public self are quite disparate, a situation that produces considerable stress.

Self-concept

Self-concept is an organized pattern of beliefs about oneself. It is essentially synonymous with phenomenal self, encompassing one's collection of self-perceptions related to the multiple aspects of human experience. Self-concept is a product of life events and self-reflection. Cooley[30] referred to self-concept as "the looking-glass self." It evolves as one examines one's own responses to common, as well as extraordinary, life situations. Judging personal abilities, motivations, accomplishments, failures, conflicts, and pleasures among other attributes contributes to self-concept.

Self-concept is also influenced by considerations external to oneself. Interactions with others have significant impact, particularly those who are valued or perceived as powerful. Individuals' impressions of others' opinions about them grow out of these interactions. The impressions are then integrated into self-concept.

The ways in which an individual may describe the self are practically limitless. Descriptors such as man, woman, feminine, masculine, husband, teacher, tall, fat, aggressive, competent, clumsy, intelligent, and so on, may be part of one's mental picture of self. These characterizations relate to the various components of self-concept discussed below. They serve to differentiate self from others.

Perceptions that individuals have of themselves go beyond basic descriptors; individuals perceive themselves in terms of values as well.[2] A man does not think of himself simply as a father and a student who drives a cab, but rather as a good father, an A, B, or C student, and a successful or unsuccessful cab driver.

Although an individual's self-concept may not be congruent with objective assessments by acquaintances or professionals, it represents reality to that individual. Whether or not an individual's self-perceptions would be regarded as accurate by others, self-concept is a strong determinant of behavior.

It is possible for individuals to have concepts about themselves that are completely at variance from the ways in which they are regarded by others. A woman who considers herself a great wit may be surprised to learn that others are bored by her stories. A student who believes he is "just average" might be pleased to find that his teachers and peers judge that he is very bright. A self-concept that differs significantly from the concept that others hold can be a source of considerable distress. When the messages one receives from others diverge from inner messages to oneself, internal conflict and confusion may result. Consistent disagreement can alter self-concept.

Components of Self-concept. Body image, gender identity, self-esteem, and role performance are components of self-concept. Each of the components develops and changes as individuals gain experiences in their environment.

Body Image. **Body image** is the cluster of attitudes and beliefs one holds about one's body, including qualities such as appearance, functioning and overall wellness. It has a great impact on individuals' adaptation to their environment. Body image is shaped by physical and psychological growth and development. Cultural and societal values also influence the gradual formation of body image. Definitions of the ideal body vary considerably from culture to culture. Whereas one cultural group may value a generous build, members of another group may describe a person with such a body as excessively fat. Beliefs about body function are also culturally grounded. For example, the Chinese view body functioning as a balance between the forces of yin and yang—optimum functioning is harmony between these forces.[32] Among Americans, optimum body functioning is more likely to be considered in terms of what one is able to do or produce. This notion tends to cause Americans to devalue physical and functional evidence of aging. Youth, beauty and vitality are prized to the extent that maintaining a positive body image may be difficult for the elderly in America. By contrast, in other cultures, such as African or Chinese, evidence of aging is likely to bestow respect, for it is seen as suggestive of wisdom and knowledge.[31]

The impact of societal values can be seen by reflecting

upon adolescence in America. Experiences during adolescence have a profound impact on the development of body image, and ultimately self-concept.[2,31] Peer groups are formed and rigid standards are set for what is right or wrong and who is a good companion or group member. The need for acceptance by one's peers is very strong even though values of the peer group may differ from one's familial or cultural values. Major changes that occur in the contour and function of the body, as well as changes in hormone levels influencing the development of secondary sex characteristics, result in new feelings and drives. The combination of social and personal pressures forces the adolescent to find new means to cope with stress, resolve role confusion, and decide who he or she is within the framework of standards held by the peer group. Successful completion of these tasks will result in development of a positive body image.

Gender Identity. Identification with one's sex as male or female, or **gender identity,** is an important component of self-concept. During the first few moments after birth most parents inquire about the sex of their newborn, which is a reflection of the importance attached to sexual identity, or gender identity. Bardwick[33] hypothesized that parents reward or punish behaviors in their children beginning early in infancy according to their own definitions of sexually appropriate behavior. She also suggested that young girls tend to be less troublesome than boys of comparable ages because of parental pressures for gender identification and what is considered to be gender-appropriate behavior. In her opinion, many girls are punished more severely than boys for exhibiting certain troublesome behaviors because they are considered to be "unladylike."

Gender identity has a strong influence on how an individual is socialized. It affects how one is evaluated as a person, what opportunities become available, and what life choices are made. Social labeling and gender-related expectations are often internalized and become part of how one sees oneself as a person. Gender identity and a related concept, sexuality, are discussed in more detail in Chapter 23.

Self-esteem. **Self-esteem** is the degree to which an individual likes or dislikes the self.[2,34] It develops out of perceptions of success or failure in interacting with the environment. As individuals attempt to master social roles they are either rewarded, in the form of praise, or punished, by being ignored, blamed, or criticized. For most individuals, there is a mixture of positive and negative experiences, some having more impact, others less. To the extent that the overall impressions of the experiences are positive, high self-esteem ensues; if the opposite is true, the outcome is more likely to be low self-esteem. High self-esteem is reflected in a sense of confidence and satisfaction with oneself. Self-esteem is closely linked to the concept of **self-acceptance,** which is the ability to acknowledge and be comfortable with the various attributes one perceives about oneself.

BUILDING NURSING KNOWLEDGE

How Can the Nurse Help Maintain the Self-Esteem of Adolescents Who Are Hospitalized?

Miller SA. Promoting self-esteem in the hospitalized adolescent: Clinical interventions. *Issues Comprehen Pediatr Nurs.* 1987; 10:187–194.

The subject of this article is self-esteem among adolescents who undergo hospitalization. The author stresses that self-concept is the single most important factor affecting behavior. Moreover, adolescence is a particularly critical period during which self-concept is forming. Illness and hospitalization during adolescence can interfere with the achievement of developmental tasks, which in turn may interfere with the adolescent's ability to gain and maintain self-esteem.

Miller reviews literature on the benefits of self-esteem and the impact of hospitalization during adolescence, and derives a number of clinical approaches that may assist the nurse to care for the adolescent in the hospital. Miller highlights the fact that when the adolescent has a lengthy hospitalization, the nurse may actually become a significant other. This situation makes the development of a relationship of trust very important to preserving the adolescent's self-esteem. Maintaining strict confidentiality in the nurse–adolescent relationship is important to trust, as is respect for the adolescent's privacy and fear of embarrassment.

The adolescent may incorporate feedback from the nurse into his or her own self-concept, Miller emphasizes. Positive verbal feedback supports a positive self-image; thus, it is very important for the nurse to take time to listen responsively to the adolescent. Group activity is also very important, and self-esteem can be promoted by seeing that the adolescent attends school sessions and other group activities available in the hospital.

Miller also stresses the importance of involving the adolescent in formulating the plan of care and assuring that choices are offered. Self-monitoring tools promote involvement; techniques such as checklists, charts, and calendars help build the adolescent's sense of pride and gives the nurse opportunities for positively recognizing the adolescent's progress. The challenge to the nurse is to minimize the adoption of the sick role by the adolescent and to maximize attention to maintaining normal development during the potentially stressful period of hospitalization.

Role Performance. **Role performance** is the way an individual participates in society. It is influenced by perceptions of body image, gender identity, and self-concept. As the components of self-concept evolve, one's role performance changes. One may be an adolescent in high school, and then a professional nurse, and then a mother, and eventually a grandmother. Some roles in society are long-lasting, such as being female and possibly being a mother or a wife; others may be short-term, such as being a college student or an Olympic swimmer.

The Healthy Self

According to Maslow,[7] no one is able to attain ideal psychological health because our imperfect society forces inhibitions and restraints upon all of its members. A few exceptional people have been able to approximate total personality integration, or the meshing of mental processes with environmental demands, to establish a totally effective personality. Characteristics of the healthy self are reflected in the behaviors exhibited by individuals who have achieved a high degree of need satisfaction.[2] Such individuals feel capable of coping with life and are successful in enhancing the quality of their own lives. They are mostly positive about themselves and their own life experiences. These positive feelings enable them to cope with life openly and directly while experiencing little threat or fear. There is strong identification with humanity among such individuals.

Criteria for Emotional Health. Jahoda[34,35] developed criteria useful for assessing the state of one's emotional health. These criteria, which are described on the following pages, include attitudes toward the self; growth, development, and self-actualization; integration; autonomy; perception of reality; and environmental mastery.

Attitudes Toward the Self. Emotional health entails a healthy self-concept. This requires accessibility of the self to one's own consciousness. It implies that a person can say "I know who I am and I like myself." Allport[36] suggested that the mature personality possesses an ability for self-objectification: viewing oneself objectively, as if through the eyes of another person. Self-objectification demands temporary detachment from self, a difficult accomplishment. Self-detachment allows individuals to survey their ideals and goals in relation to their abilities, to compare their physical attributes to those of others, and to evaluate their opinion of themselves relative to others' opinions about them, as though they were making these observations of a stranger, someone not significant or important to their lives. To be truly emotionally healthy, one must have an intact sense of selfhood that includes recognition of shortcomings, which are then accepted in relation to recognized strengths. Emotionally healthy individuals find it possible to accept themselves and their nature without chagrin or complaint and without focusing unnecessarily on their shortcomings.[37] For the individual who has a large reservoir of positive life experiences to draw from, negative experiences or criticisms can be evaluated from a perspective that prevents them from becoming overwhelming.[2] In some instances these negative environmental interactions become positive learning experiences resulting in behavior changes. For example, the healthy self may acknowledge that a criticism is justified, and as a result alter behavior under similar circumstances in the future.

As discussed above, a sense of identity, which reflects the individual's ability to maintain inner sameness and continuity, is accrued from all life experiences.[38] The healthy self has a strong sense of identity due to positive experiences that have led to a considerable degree of need satisfaction and enhancement of the self.

Agreement of the objective self with the subjective self also facilitates development and maintenance of a healthy self. If one perceives that others view one much as one views oneself, there are no major inconsistencies that could become sources of emotional conflict. Feelings of dignity, integrity, and worth are allowed to develop.

Growth, Development, and Self-actualization. Growth, development, and self-actualization are important components of emotional health. Many psychologists see emotional health as an ongoing process in which individuals constantly strive to realize their own potential. This process has variously been referred to in the literature as self-actualization, self-realization, growing, or becoming. The healthy self desires to achieve this state. There is motivation to realize capacities and talents, to be devoted to a mission or a vocation, and to be active rather than resigned or lazy.[13] In pursuing one's full potential, one usually demonstrates an investment in living, which is evidenced by concern for others, issues concerning the world, and interests that are particularly significant to the individual self.

Integration. Integration of the personality refers to the relatedness of all processes and attributes within the individual.[34] **Integration** is reflected as a coherence or continuity of personality. In psychoanalytic theory, the **ego,** one of three divisions of the psyche, serves as an organized conscious mediator between the individual self and reality. The **id** is another of three divisions of the psyche. It serves as the unconscious source of psychic energy derived from instinctual drives and needs. The **superego,** the third of three divisions of the psyche, is only partly conscious and represents internalization of parental conscience and rules of society. It functions to reward or punish through a system of moral attitudes, conscience, and a sense of guilt. One aspect of integration as a criterion for emotional health, in psychoanalytic terms, is evidenced by a balance of psychic forces so that the ego can accommodate its corresponding id and superego and does not aim to eliminate or deny their demands.[39] This means that there is flexibility among the unconscious, preconscious, and conscious forces of the psyche so that one can respond to varying situations appropriately.[40]

A healthy individual may use considerable self-expression in one situation, such as a gathering of close friends, but exercise careful self-restraint in another, such as a work performance evaluation meeting with a supervisor. The healthy self is autonomous and can exercise self-control with the capability of altering behavior in varying situations when conforming to expected behaviors is seen as desirable. Lack of flexibility, or the lack of capacity to conform to a variety of expectations, suggests a personality integration problem.

A second aspect of personality integration pertains to having a unifying outlook on life. This results from an ability to incorporate self-extension (involvement in worldly activities and issues) with self-detachment (discussed above) into a personal philosophy of life.[37] Experiences are interpreted from an individual's perspective in terms of goals central to personal existence. One individual may develop an "aesthetic" philosophical approach to life, for instance, in which the quest for beauty becomes of prime importance; while another individual may develop a "religious" philosophical approach in which there is a continuous search for values and reasons underlying all things pertaining to life and death.

A final aspect of personality integration is exhibited in the ability to adapt to stress. The healthy individual is able to satisfy basic personal needs in ways that are socially acceptable. Strong feelings of self-security allow the individual to tolerate most tensions and frustrations without inner damage.

Autonomy. Autonomy connotes that the individual has a self-governing relationship with the environment. In the context of the healthy self, autonomy means that one has learned to depend upon oneself—on one's own growth, development, understanding, motivation, and potential for conscious decision-making—for need resolution. There is relative emotional independence from the impact of the physical and social environment along with inherent feelings of security and trust. The healthy self is able to maintain a high degree of serenity and happiness in the midst of circumstances that may be problematic or frustrating. Even in circumstances where conflict cannot be resolved rationally, the healthy individual is able to withstand the tension without inner damage to the state of emotional health.

Perception of Reality. Perception of reality is relatively undistorted in the healthy self, meaning that what the individual perceives corresponds well with what is actually so according to consensus. Although different individuals may view identical situations in diverse ways, there is a large degree of objectivity to these perspectives. One teacher may view a particular child as problematic while another teacher may view the same child as creative when in actuality both views may be accurate as they pertain to this particular child.

In viewing the world, the healthy self has relative freedom from need-distortion. This means that one is able to view situations one wishes were different without distorting them to fit personal wishes.[31] The healthy self does not eliminate needs and motives, but rather continually tests reality for its degree of correspondence to personal wishes. Healthy parents desiring their child to do well in school, for instance, usually seek objective evidence of success and accept evidence even if it is contrary to their hopes and expectations. Individuals who are less emotionally healthy, on the other hand, probably will not seek objective evidence. If confronted with evidence that is contrary to their wishes, individuals with compromised emotional health will often refuse to accept the evidence.

Not only do individuals possessing healthy selves experience relative freedom from distortion of their own needs, they can also arrive at conclusions about other people that are relatively free from distortion. This results in an ability to predict the behavior of others to a certain degree, a requirement for development of appropriate interpersonal relationships.

Environmental Mastery. Mastery of the environment is essential to the healthy self and is reflected in (1) the ability to love; (2) adequacy in love, work, and play; (3) adequacy in interpersonal relationships; (4) efficiency in meeting situational requirements; (5) capacity for adaptation and adjustment; and (6) efficiency in problem-solving. The healthy self is capable of developing an intimate relationship with another individual and maintaining the positive commitment inherent in such a relationship. Full integration of sexuality into the personality is considered by some authorities to be an extremely sensitive indicator of emotional health, particularly when there is sexual sensitivity and gratification with a loved partner.[38] The healthy self also exhibits proficiency in work, creativity within the limitations of personal capacities, and can experience relaxation through rest and recreation. Capacity to develop effective interpersonal relationships with others allows the healthy self to meet needs that are mutually beneficial, as well as to act for the benefit of others. With a reservoir of positive life experiences from which to draw, the healthy self is able to use problem-solving abilities efficiently so that adaptation and adjustment to new situations and changing life circumstances can take place.

Identity and Nursing Care

Identity is often threatened by actual or perceived alterations in wellness, for health alterations often engender change. The range of actual or anticipated changes that can be associated with fluctuations in wellness is extensive and usually directly related to the magnitude of the health alteration. Some changes are minor and may be considered merely inconveniences, others may compromise existence in profound ways. Even emotionally healthy individuals experience some distress when faced with illness-imposed changes, for example, in body functioning, daily routine, or level of independence. Those whose identity is more fragile may be overwhelmed by these kinds of demands on coping abilities and emotional reserves.

Although wellness promotion and health maintenance is an integral aspect of the nursing role, nurses most commonly encounter clients who are seeking health care because they perceive they may be ill. Therefore, sensitivity to the unique impact of the health care experience on aspects of identity and self-concept is a requisite for effectiveness as a nurse. This is true whether or not there has been an actual diagnosis of illness.

Communication skills, in particular listening, but also effective use of questions facilitate establishing nurse–client trust (see also Chaps. 13 and 14). The atmosphere in which communication takes place must be nonjudgmental and supportive. Individuals providing personal information must feel certain that it will be used professionally and effectively for their own benefit.

Many health care experiences involve some degree of change in role performance. Clients often find it difficult to be dependent on nurses or other health care providers for assistance with activities of daily living or basic personal care or comfort measures. Role changes of this nature may be particularly difficult for individuals who are customarily independent and self-supporting. A bank president, for example, who is responsible for large sums of money and numerous employees, may find it very stressful trying to adapt to a perceived subservient role when hospitalized for surgery. The surgical procedure itself may not be as problematic to this client as the feelings of loss of control over his own life, the imposition on his privacy due to diagnostic procedures and postsurgical care, or the distress due to perceived insensitivity to these concerns on the part of health care providers.

Role change is only one parameter of self-concept that may be altered in clients. Many clients experience changes in body image due to the effects of aging, surgery, accidents, or disfiguring diseases. Others experience threats to gender identity or self-esteem.

Nurses have a responsibility to recognize and minimize the effects of changes in health on the client's self-concept. Collaboration with the client, other individuals significant to the client, and other health care providers will enable the nurse to gain an understanding of the nature of alterations in self-concept the client is experiencing and their potential impact on wellness and well-being. Refer to Chapter 23 for a discussion of common illness-related problems with identity and self-expression, and related strategies for their collaborative assessment and management.

GROWTH AND DEVELOPMENT

The manner in which growth and development have progressed and the point in maturation attained at any given moment in time are key to the uniqueness of each individual.

Maturation is the process of progressive changes that permits functioning of the organism or cell. Learning is a relatively permanent alteration of behavior that results from life experiences, and is in part dependent on a satisfactory maturational process. As life progresses and experiences accrue, the individual self evolves and changes. Pursuit of one's potential is a lifelong process that progresses through characteristic phases in which there are typical challenges and responses.

Fertilization of the human ovum initiates a complex network of chemical and physical processes that form the basis for growth of body tissues and organs, changes in enzyme systems and metabolic activities, and adaptation to the environment. Growth and development proceed in an orderly fashion from conception until death, and during the span of a lifetime one passes through periods of growth, maintenance, and decline.

The term **growth** reflects those aspects of maturation that can be measured, such as increase in length, weight, or volume of the body as a whole or any of its parts, including organs and tissues. The term **development** represents both the quality and the magnitude of maturational changes. Development can be viewed from the psychosocial, physical, cognitive, or moral perspective (see Chap. 11).

Growth and development do not take place independently in discrete systems, but rather as a continuum of interactions between innate genetic potential and the multiple components of the environment. The degree to which full genetic potential is fulfilled by an individual depends upon the interaction of many physical, intellectual, behavioral, emotional, social, and cultural forces.

Theories of Individual Development

Several psychologists have developed theories about psychosocial development; however, no single theory is universally and unequivocally accepted. Reference to several major theories is useful for portraying the characteristic phases an individual progresses through during the process of growth and development.

Freud's Stages of Psychosexual Development. Freud[15] developed the concept of id, ego, and superego as three different levels of consciousness within the psyche. All of his work was based on the belief that sexual impulses underlie human behavior. His perception was that symptoms of psychological abnormality could always be traced to an erotic urge or to a sexual wish that had been repressed because of potential threat to the moral component of the psyche.

Freud proposed five stages for psychosexual development, as outlined in Table 10–4. He acknowledged that development does not always proceed smoothly through each of these five stages because anxiety, threat, or frustration block the process of maturation. Such blocking is termed **fixation.** Fixation is intimately related to subsequent episodes of **regression,** or a return to earlier forms of impulse gratification. Symptoms of regression are particularly common during periods of severe stress such as illness or hospitalization.

Erikson's Stages of Psychosocial Development. Erikson[41,42] refined Freud's notions of personality development with particular emphasis on child development. His focus was on development of the "healthy personality." Rather than a psychosexual focus in which the stages of man develop in a predictable sequence, Erikson proposed a psychosocial developmental process. Each age, or stage, is dependent upon the completion of tasks dictated by the previous stage, and each focuses on a central problem envisioned as a conflict between opposite characteristics. The eight stages of development proposed by Erikson are detailed in Table 10–5.

Buhler's Concept of Life Goals. Buhler[43] views life as a process characterized by an intent toward fulfillment. The phases of this intent or self-determination are outlined in Table 10–6. After reading several biographies of individuals considered to be exceptionally successful, Buhler noted that an inner coherence due to some unifying or integrating principle was common to most of these individuals. This suggested to her that life is lived under certain directives, toward fulfilling certain long-range goals.

Fulfillment is defined by Buhler as an overall feeling of satisfaction, accomplishment, or success at the period in life

TABLE 10–4. FREUD'S STAGES OF PSYCHOSEXUAL DEVELOPMENT

Stage	Age	Characteristic
Stage 1: Oral period	0–1 year	Pleasurable activities center on activities of the mouth such as sucking or biting.
Stage 2: Anal period	2–3 years	Critical developments during this period involve selective retention and expulsion of feces, as well as learning self-mastery.
Stage 3: Infantile genital period	3–4 years	During the first phase of this stage, called the phallic stage, the child discovers erotic pleasure in fondling the genitals and in masturbation. The child associates the genitals with a love object with whom he or she wishes to have sexual relations. A boy views his mother as the desired object yet recognizes that he cannot have her to himself because his father is a powerful competitor for her affections. This conflict is referred to as the Oedipus complex. A girl similarly desires her father as the love object, referred to as the Electra complex. The superego evolves in an effort to control unacceptable erotic urges.
Stage 4: Latency period	4 or 5 years to puberty	The child's sexual interests and impulses lie dormant.
Stage 5: Mature genital period	14 or 15 years to 18 or to 21 years	Interest in the opposite sex and adult sexuality develop.

Adapted from Freud S. An Outline of Psychoanalysis. *London: Hogarth; 1973.*

TABLE 10–5. ERIKSON'S STAGES OF PSYCHOSOCIAL DEVELOPMENT

Stage	Age	Characteristic
Stage 1: Trust vs mistrust	0–1 year	Children's fundamental attitudes about the dependability of the world are built primarily on the relationship with the mother or mother substitute during infancy. Needs for nurturing, security, and a feeling of continuity are paramount.
Stage 2: Autonomy vs shame and doubt	1–3 years	Development of a sense of self-control without loss of self-esteem should occur. Parental firmness is important. It lets children know that they are in a trustworthy world that will prevent them from overstepping their boundaries. Parental flexibility and patience that allow children to gain self-control over increasing motor skills are also important.
Stage 3: Initiative vs guilt	3–6 years	During this exploratory phase of development, children learn from playing games and asking questions. There is more evidence of being guided by a conscience in dealing with the effort to achieve a balance between daring and caution. Fears and phobias are common.
Stage 4: Industry vs inferiority	6–12 years	The need to do something worthwhile and earn recognition for it becomes important. Social conditioning is more directly related to development of male and female roles.
Stage 5: Identity vs identity diffusion	12–18 years	In the transition between childhood and adulthood, adolescents must accept a new body image and perform certain tasks relevant to establishing a sexual role, selecting an occupation, becoming independent of the family, and acquiring a social rather than egocentric response to persons and society. Without successful mastery of these tasks, individuals will develop identity confusion and will not know "who they are" or "where they are going."
Stage 6: Intimacy vs isolation	Early adulthood	Once a sense of identity has developed, individuals can move toward intimate relationships in the form of friendship, sexual intimacy, and parent–child interactions and responsibilities. Without a sense of freedom to love and be loved, individuals may develop a sense of isolation and alienation from the family, friends, and society.
Stage 7: Generativity vs self-absorption	Middle adulthood	The major focus is on creating the next generation and providing the necessary nurturing and caretaking inherent in this responsibility. Development of a sense of balance between commitment to self and commitment to others leads to a sense of productiveness and fulfillment.
Stage 8: Ego integrity vs despair	Old age	Emphasis is on maintaining productivity and involvement in the welfare of others. As limitations are imposed on physical and mental functioning, prevention of despair has much to do with wisdom and a sense of satisfaction with what has been accomplished.

Adapted from Erikson EH. Childhood and Society. *2nd ed. New York: Norton; 1963.*

TABLE 10–6. BUHLER'S PHASES OF SELF-DETERMINATION TOWARD LIFE GOALS

Phase	Age	Characteristic
1	0–15 years	Self-determination is prepared and built up. Different types of behavior develop that prepare one for goal-setting.
2	15–25 years	Life goals are set experimentally and programmatically. First thoughts develop about life belonging to oneself. Beginning goals may include the search for fulfillment. The focus of the search may be a partner to love or a God to believe in or both.
3	23–50 years	Life goals become specific and definite.
4	45–65 years	Success and failure are assessed. This is seen as a crisis period in life because many individuals are forced to reorient themselves due to retirement, drastic reductions in income, less opportunity to interact with colleagues, reduced abilities, or the beginning of severe illness.
5	60+ years	Rest or continuation of striving with a closure experience of fulfillment or unfulfillment, resignation, or despair.

Adapted from Buhler C. The course of human life as a psychological problem. Hum Develop. *1968; 11:184–200.*

when an individual begins to experience closure. Each individual anticipates or visualizes fulfillment differently; however, it is the anticipation peculiar to an individual that provides the direction necessary for unifying lifetime endeavors in order to meet long-range goals.

According to Buhler, the manner in which individuals experience the present is based on past experiences, while their outlook on the future is greatly influenced by the way the present is being experienced. Healthy individuals, therefore, are able to view the future with some meaningful continuity to the present.

Havighurst's Developmental Tasks. Havighurst[44] promoted the concept of developmental tasks and, as a result, developed six stages of these tasks, outlined in Table 10–7, to describe the process of growth and development. A **developmental task** was defined by Havighurst as a task that arises at or about a certain period in the life of an individual. According to Havighurst, each task must be accomplished with success in order for the individual to achieve happiness, as well as success in accomplishing future tasks. Failure to accomplish a task successfully will lead to unhappiness, disapproval by members of society, and difficulty in accomplishing more advanced tasks. It is Havighurst's opinion that once a task is learned it has been mastered for life. Mastering a task can be likened to learning a game. Once a child has learned to play baseball, for example, he or she will always understand how to play the game.

Piaget's Theory of Cognitive Development. Piaget[45,46] developed a theory of cognitive development consisting of five childhood phases, as summarized in Table 10–8. He used the term "cognitive development" to refer to the manner in which an individual learns to think and reason. According to Piaget, cognitive development evolves in an orderly and sequential process. This process consists of phases and is somewhat influenced by an individual's intelligence, ability to perceive, and ability to process information. A progression of mental abilities should become apparent as individuals progress through the phases of cognitive development. Capacity for logical rather than illogical thinking, complex as opposed to simple problem-solving, and understanding abstract concepts in addition to simple ideas should eventually be attained. While progressing through the phases of cognitive development proposed by Piaget, individuals must assimilate available information, accommodate to new information by learning, and adapt to changing circumstances.

Kohlberg's Theory of Moral Development. Kohlberg[47,48] proposed six stages of development within three levels of reasoning that individuals go through when making moral decisions (Table 10–9). Moral decisions are decisions related to right and wrong. When individuals make moral decisions those decisions are based on their perception of whether or not the decision will facilitate successful interaction within the environment. In other words, the decision is related to its impact on the ability to live successfully in society.

According to Kohlberg, development through the levels of reasoning requires exposure to a situation posing problems, or contradictions with one's current moral structure, leading to dissatisfaction at the current level and an atmosphere of interchange and dialogue that allows one to evaluate conflicting moral views in an open manner. It is Kohlberg's contention that development of moral values can occur randomly, meaning that this development is not necessarily age-specific, and that development of moral values can be learned in social institutions, such as schools, where principles of successful living in society are taught.

Levinson's Stages of Life Structure. **Life structure,** the basic pattern or design of a person's life at a given moment,[49] changes and evolves as an individual passes from one phase of growth and development to another. It is the configuration of life circumstances that results from an individual's important personal choices. Understanding the present life structure of an individual is one mechanism for determining the state of development for that individual. When an individual's life structure fails to change as per-

TABLE 10–7. HAVIGHURST'S DEVELOPMENTAL TASKS

Age Period	Developmental Tasks
Infancy and early childhood	Learning to walk Learning to eat solid foods Learning to talk Learning to control the elimination of body wastes Learning sex differences and sexual modesty Achieving psychological stability Forming simple concepts of social and physical reality Learning to relate emotionally to parents, siblings, and other people Learning to distinguish right from wrong and develop a conscience
Middle childhood	Learning physical skills necessary for ordinary games Building wholesome attitudes toward oneself as a growing organism Learning to get along with peers Learning an appropriate masculine or feminine social role Developing fundamental skills in reading, writing, and calculating Developing concepts necessary for everyday living Developing conscience, morality, and a scale of values Achieving personal independence Developing attitudes toward social groups and institutions
Adolescence	Achieving new and more mature relationships with peers of both sexes Achieving a masculine or feminine social role Accepting one's physique and using the body effectively Achieving emotional independence from parents and other adults Achieving assurance of economic independence Selecting and preparing for an occupation Preparing for marriage and family life Developing intellectual skills and concepts necessary for civic competence Desiring and achieving socially responsible behavior Acquiring a set of values and an ethical system as a guide to behavior
Early adulthood	Selecting a mate Learning to live with a partner Starting a family Rearing children Managing a home Getting started in an occupation Taking on civic responsibility Finding a congenial social group
Middle age	Achieving adult civic and social responsibility Establishing and maintaining an economic standard of living Assisting teenage children to become responsible and happy adults Developing adult leisure-time activities Relating to one's spouse as a person Accepting and adjusting to the physiological changes of middle age Adjusting to aging parents
Later maturity	Adjusting to decreasing physical strength and health Adjusting to retirement and a reduced income Adjusting to death of a spouse Establishing an explicit affiliation with one's age group Meeting social and civic obligations Establishing satisfactory physical living arrangements

Adapted from Havighurst RJ. Developmental Tasks and Education. *3rd ed. New York: David McKay; 1972.*

TABLE 10–8. PIAGET'S PHASES OF COGNITIVE DEVELOPMENT

Phase	Age	Significant Behaviors
Sensorimotor	0–2 years	Most action is reflexive.
Stage 1: Use of reflexes	0–1 month	Perception of events is centered on the body.
Stage 2: Primary circular reaction	1–4 months	Objects are perceived as extensions of the self.
Stage 3: Secondary circular reaction	4–8 months	Acknowledgment of the external environment. Actively makes change in the environment.
Stage 4: Coordination of secondary schemata	8–12 months	Distinguishes a goal from a means of attaining it.
Stage 5: Tertiary circular reaction	12–18 months	Tries and discovers new goals and ways to attain goals. Rituals are important.
Stage 6: Inventions of new means	18–24 months	Interprets the environment by mental image. Uses make-believe and pretend play.
Preconceptual	2–4 years	Uses an egocentric approach to accommodate to environmental demands. Everything is significant and related to "me." Explores the environment. Language development is rapid. Associates words with objects.
Cognitive thought	4–7 years	Egocentric thinking diminishes. Thinks of one idea at a time. Includes others in the environment. Uses words to express thoughts.
Concrete operations	7–11 years	Solves concrete problems. Begins to understand relationships such as size. Understands right and left. Cognizant of viewpoints.
Formal operations	11–15 years	Uses rational thinking. Reasoning is deductive and futuristic.

Adapted from Piaget J. The Origin of Intelligence in Children. *New York: Norton; 1963.*

TABLE 10–9. KOHLBERG'S LEVELS OF REASONING AND STAGES OF MORAL DEVELOPMENT

Level of Reasoning	Stage	Characteristics
Preconventional	1: Punishment and obedience orientation	The physical consequences of an action determine whether it was good or bad. If punished, the activity was wrong, but if not punished the activity was right. Avoidance of punishment and unquestioning deference to power are valued.
	2: Instrumental relativist orientation	Actions are taken to satisfy an individual's own needs. Loyalty, gratitude, or justice are not taken into account.
Conventional	3: Interpersonal concordance orientation	Good behavior is that which is approved by others. One earns approval by being "nice" to others.
	4: Law-and-order orientation	Making a right decision means doing one's duty, showing respect for authority, and maintaining the given social order for its own sake.
Postconventional	5: Social contract, legalistic orientation	One's standard of behavior is based on adherence to laws that protect the rights and welfare of others. Personal values are recognized and one avoids violating the rights of others.
	6: Universal-ethical-principle orientation	One respects others and believes that interpersonal relationships are based on mutual trust.

Adapted from Duska R, Whalen M. Moral Development: A Guide to Piaget and Kohlberg. *New York: Paulist Press; 1975.*

sonal needs change, developmental problems result. The life structure is then in conflict with the individual's personal needs, which prohibits those needs from being met. It is within the context of life structure that individuals meet or fail to meet their needs, and achieve or fail to achieve their personal goals. Life structure is a critical factor in allowing self-actualization to occur.

The concept of individual life structure was developed by Levinson and colleagues,[49] primarily as a framework for studying the character of human life and its evolution over a span of years. An individual's life structure has many components such as vocation, interpersonal relationships, relation to self, use of solitude, and a personal philosophy of life. All of these components of life structure involve relationships with individuals, groups, and institutions. Also, all of these components are influenced by and influence an individual's personality. Levinson and colleagues felt that once the character of human life was identified and better understood through use of the concept of life structure, it would then be possible to study changes in personality, marital and occupational commitments, and other parts of human life in more detail.

In examining relationships between the individual self and the rest of an individual's world, Levinson and associates determined that the primary components of life structure are choices. Important choices in adult life have relevance for work, family, friendship, love relationships of various kinds, where to live, involvement in leisure, religious, political, or community activities, and achievement of personal goals. In characterizing each choice within the life structure, one must understand one's relationships with the choice and determine how it is connected to both the self and the environment.

Usually only one or two components, or choices, of life structure have a central place in the life of an individual. They receive the largest share of a person's time and energy. Others, although important, are more peripheral, or even marginal, and are apportioned much less time and energy. Central components of life structure are occupation, marriage–family, friendship and peer relationships, ethnicity, religion, and leisure pursuits (Fig. 10–4). Occupation and marriage–family components are usually the most central, but there are significant variations among individuals. Throughout a lifetime components may shift to the periphery from being central, or vice versa, as when an individual who has committed much time to an occupation begins detaching from it to become more involved with family.

Because life structure is a concept that is value-neutral, a life structure may be developed from choices that are not necessarily common in society. One may substitute the choice of marriage, for instance, with any of a number of arrangements to meet one's need for closeness, intimacy, and love. Such substitutes have as much potential validity within the context of a particular individual's life as the choice of a traditional marriage. The criterion for determining whether a particular life structure choice is effective is whether or not the choice and resulting activities seem to be "working" for the individual, whether or not the individual is coping well with life.

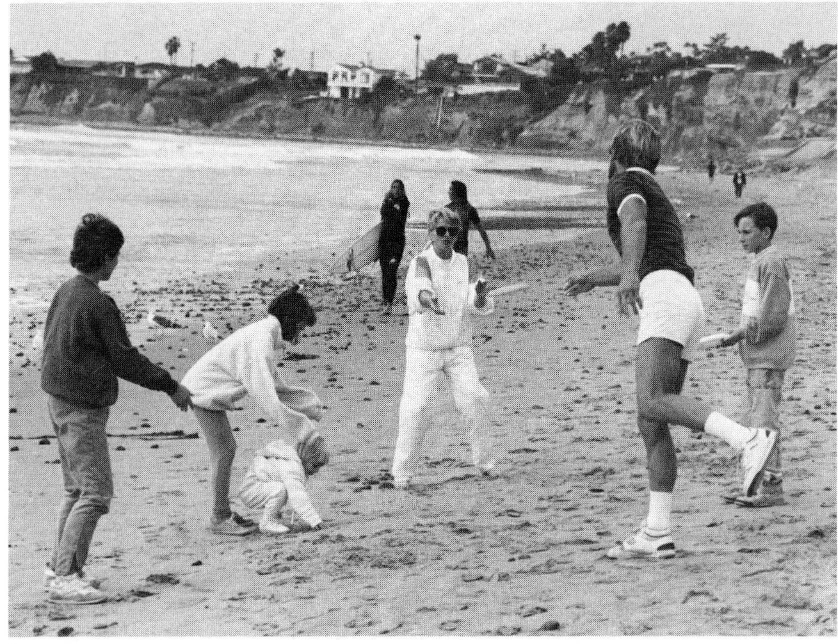

A

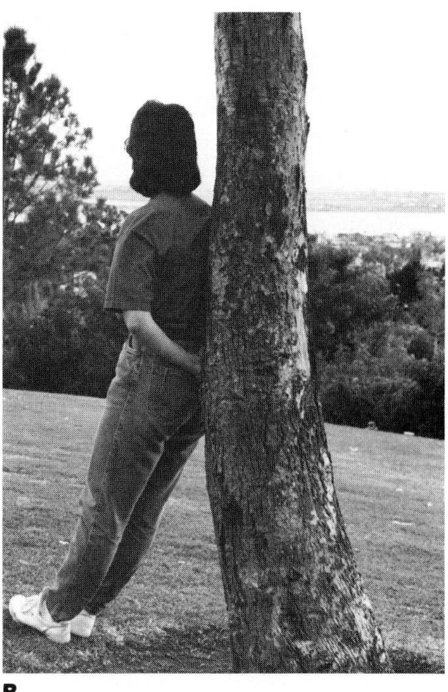

B

Figure 10–4. A. Sharing time with family is an important part of some individuals' life structure. **B.** For some, solitude is critical.

Life-style represents an individual's typical way of life, which emerges from the life structure. The personal choices that shaped the life structure affect the nature and arrangement of life activities. Life-style, therefore, reflects the quality, or character, of an individual's life choices.

The concepts of life structure and life-style are related but distinct. For example, the life structure choice to remain unemployed might result in a life-style of leisure, particularly when there is no economic necessity to earn a living and it is economically feasible that one's life activities revolve around avocational pursuits. Similarly, the life structure choice to marry might result in a family-centered life-style in which family and community relationships and activities are directed toward meeting the needs of growing children.

Levinson and co-workers found that life structure evolves through a relatively orderly sequence of eras and developmental periods during the adult years. Eras are comprised of alternating stable, or structure-building, periods and transitional, or structure-changing, periods (Fig. 10–5). These periods shape the course of psychosocial development during adulthood.

The primary task of each stable period is to build a life structure. This requires that decisions be made about certain choices. A structure is formed around these choices, and personal values and goals within the structure are pursued. During each transitional period of about 4 or 5 years, the existing life structure is partially or totally destroyed and the foundation is laid for a new one. Transitional periods are times to question and reappraise one's course in life, explore various possibilities for change, and make crucial decisions that form the basis for a new life structure in the ensuing stable period.

Success in resolution of the developmental tasks specific to each period is necessary for evolution of that period. A period begins when its major tasks become predominant in one's life and ends when these tasks lose their importance and new tasks emerge to form the beginning of a new period. A life structure is considered to be satisfactory when it is viable, or reasonable, within society and also suitable to oneself.

The following discussion of the evolution of life structure is based on the work of Levinson and colleagues and is presented in some detail to exemplify many of the parameters and relationships inherent in human growth and development. Events that occur commonly during identified periods in the life structure of an individual are summarized in Table 10–10.

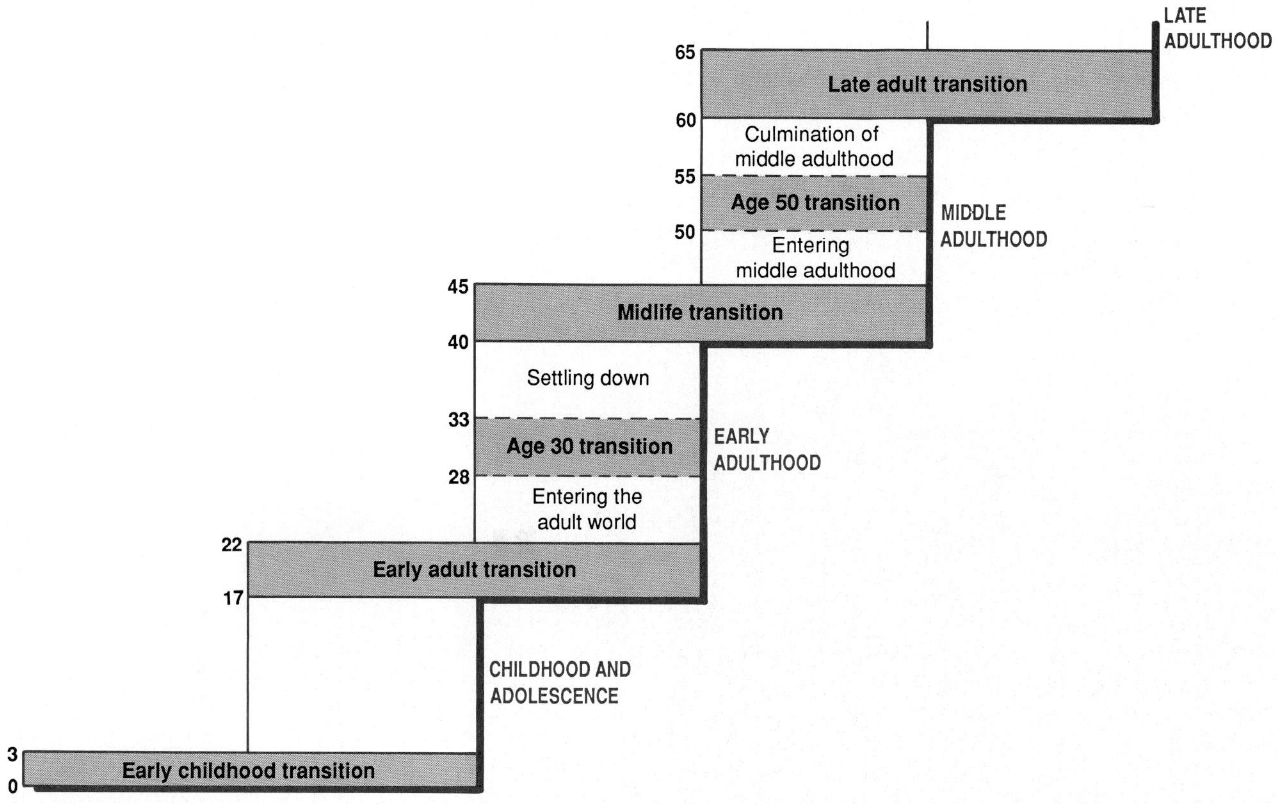

Figure 10–5. Theoretical model for life structure. (*Adapted from Levinson DJ, et al.* The Seasons of a Man's Life. *New York: Knopf; 1978. Copyright 1978 by Daniel J. Levinson. Reprinted by permission of Alfred A. Knopf, Inc.*)

TABLE 10–10. EVENTS THAT OCCUR COMMONLY DURING PERIODS IN THE LIFE STRUCTURE

Period	Events
Childhood and Adolescence	
Early childhood transition	Live with and be part of a family Be cared for and protected
Childhood	Start school Make friends who are peers Develop a sense of neighborhood Become more disciplined, industrious, and skilled
Adolescence	Experience tremendous physical and emotional changes
Early Adulthood	
Early adult transition	Move out of the family home Decrease financial dependence on parents Enter new and more autonomous relationships Enter a new role for which one is more responsible such as college, the military, or a job
Entering the adult world	Form relationships that will lead to marriage and family Begin a vocation Establish a home base Participate in religious, political, recreational, or other types of groups
Age 30 transition	Form a "dream" of one's placement in the world Establish mentor relationships Be part of a marriage Raise children Experience vocational advancement Earn an advanced degree
Settling down	Experience greater social rank, income, power, fame, quality of family life, or creativity Respond to greater social pressure and responsibility due to success
Middle Adulthood	
Midlife transition	Resolve unmet goals of adolescence Experience improved love relationships, including a greater capacity for intimacy Be more responsive as a friend Be a facilitating parent Participate in a caring relationship with own parents Serve as a mentor to young adults
Entering middle adulthood	Question the direction one's life is taking Begin to face personal mortality
Age 50 transition	Resolve important unmet needs Solidify one's personal philosophy of life Become closer to significant others
Culmination of middle adulthood	Retire from vocation Stabilize life-style
Late Adulthood	
Late adult transition	Adapt to gradual physical and mental decline Face personal mortality

Adapted from Levinson DJ, Darrow CN, Klein EB, et al. The Seasons of a Man's Life. *New York: Knopf; 1978. Copyright 1978 by Daniel J. Levinson. Reprinted by permission of Alfred A. Knopf, Inc.*

Childhood and Adolescence. Childhood and adolescence consist of the early childhood transition and pre-adulthood. During childhood and adolescence one ordinarily lives with and is part of a family, or at least an equivalent social unit. The family provides protection, opportunity for socialization, and support for growth. One is relatively dependent and vulnerable during this time while growing to become a self-sufficient member of society.

Early childhood transition, or transition into childhood, begins before birth and continues into the second or third year of life. During this time the infant learns to distinguish "me" from "not me" and develops into a separate individual. For the next 3 to 4 years the child's social world expands from the immediate family to encompass a larger sphere that includes school, friends who are peers, and a sense of neighborhood. The child also becomes more disciplined, industrious, and skilled. Usually at around the age of 12 or 13 years the child makes a transition to adolescence. This is a time of tremendous physical change, as well as psychological and psychosocial change.

Early Adulthood. Early adulthood begins in the late teens and lasts approximately 20 to 25 years. It is a time of peak physiological and intellectual functioning. One experiences maximal levels of strength, sexual capability, cardiac and respiratory capacity, and general biological vigor, as well as optimal memory, abstract thought, and ability to learn specific skills and resolve well-defined problems. This is also the period in which one encounters the most stress as personal gratification is sought but hampered by residues of childhood conflict.

Early adult transition, or transition to adulthood, most commonly takes place between the ages of about 17 and 22 years. This time serves as a bridge between pre-adulthood and early adulthood. The major developmental tasks are to terminate one's adolescent life structure, leave the pre-adult world, and initiate a life structure for early adulthood. Existing relationships with important persons and institutions need to be modified and one must separate from the family of origin.

Gradually, as one learns more about the self and the world, choices are made which form the basis for living in the adult world. One may live in the same kind of community, maintain the same ethnic and religious ties, and enter an occupation and marriage appropriate for the world in which one was raised, thereby becoming the kind of person that is consistent with the expectations of parents, family, and childhood friends. Discontinuity results when an individual's life in the late 20s turns out to be markedly different from the life that it seemed at adolescence the individual would have entered.

Entering the adult world usually takes place between the early and late 20s. The first life structure is built during these years. Two primary but contrasting tasks must be accomplished during this period. The first task is to explore the possibilities for adult living, which results in testing a variety of initial choices regarding a vocation, interpersonal relationships, values, and life-style (Fig. 10–6). Secondly, one must create a stable life structure. Difficulty may arise in finding a balance between these two tasks. If the first task is allowed to predominate, life may take on a transient and rootless quality, while if the second task predominates there is danger of committing oneself prematurely to a structure.

Age 30 transition takes place in the late 20s. It is a time used to resolve flaws in the initial life structure and create a basis for a more satisfactory structure in the future. Some people sense this time to be a "last chance" to change life for the better. This transitional period has been referred to as the "age 30 crisis"[50] because some people experience major emotional difficulties at this time in their lives.

Settling down takes place during the late 30s as one begins to realize youthful aspirations and goals while investing in the central components of one's own life structure, such as work, family, friendships, leisure, or community involvement. The two major tasks of this period are to establish a "niche" in society or the community, becoming a valued member, and to build a better life for oneself. One enters this period as a junior member in a world in which there is aspiration to become a senior, or expert, member.

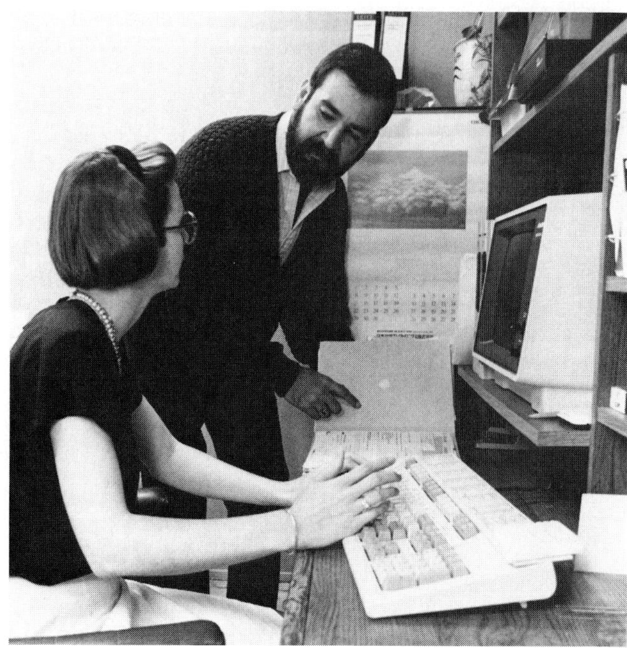

Figure 10–6. Career development is a central component of the life structure for many individuals.

Middle Adulthood. Middle adulthood begins at about 40 years of age. During the next two decades gradual changes take place in human biological and psychological functioning. If one is not severely ill or impaired and normal development has not been grossly hampered, one can maintain most activities and interests throughout middle adulthood. Physical and mental powers diminish gradually during this era and there is usually a modest decline in elemental drives such as lustful passions, capacity for anger and moral indignation, self-assertiveness, ambition, and the wish to be cared for and supported. One suffers less from the tyranny of such drives, which may foster life enrichment. Often there is a sense of freedom from petty vanities, animosities, envies, and moralisms associated with early adulthood.

Midlife transition begins somewhere around age 40 and usually takes close to 5 years to complete. One of the major tasks of this period is to terminate the era of early adulthood. This requires review and reappraisal of one's entire life. The individual must deal with the disparity between what is and what was dreamed of. Many questions are raised regardless of the outcome of youthful efforts. Also, during this period there is a sense of loss of youthful vitality, which often becomes an insult to narcissistic pride. Physical changes that begin to be noticed may be a fundamental threat to one's being. Many individuals have difficulty with this era because what has turned out to be is so different from what was hoped for. Some individuals have such serious difficulty with this transition that it has been termed the "midlife crisis."[50]

The second major task of midlife transition is to take first steps toward beginning middle adulthood. This involves modifying negative elements of the present life structure and testing new choices, which will eventually have an impact on building a new life structure for middle adulthood. One essentially must come to terms with the failures already experienced and arrive at a new set of choices around which to shape a new life. As this process is completed a person becomes more uniquely individual, acquiring a new identity with increased ability to use inner resources and pursue personal goals.

Entering middle adulthood takes place at about 45 years of age. By this time in the life cycle one has had an opportunity to question and search and is now at a point where it is necessary to begin forming a new life structure. The life structure that emerges in the middle to late 40s varies greatly from one individual to another in its suitability for the self and workability in the world. Some individuals have suffered such irreparable defeats earlier in life that they are not successful in working on the tasks of their midlife transition. They lack the internal and external resources required for creating even a minimally adequate life structure. Moreover, they are now faced with new experiences at a time of constriction and decline that requires adaptation. Other individuals start middle adulthood with a life structure that will allow special satisfactions and fulfillments as life progresses. For these individuals, middle adulthood is often the fullest and most creative era in the life cycle.

Age 50 transition usually takes place between the ages of 50 and 55 years. The functions of this period are similar to those of the age 30 transition in early adulthood. During this period an individual can continue to work on the tasks of midlife transition and further modify the life structure formed in the middle to late 40s, so that there is a more satisfactory fit with the self and the world.

Culmination of middle adulthood takes place from about 55 to 60 years of age. This period is devoted to building a second middle adulthood life structure that will facilitate completing the era. For many individuals who can rejuvenate themselves with new aspirations and activities that enrich their lives, the decade of the 50s is often a time of great fulfillment.

Late Adulthood. Late adulthood begins in the early 60s. The character of living begins to be altered as a result of numerous biological, psychological, and social changes. The reality and experience of bodily decline become more and more apparent. Continued physical and mental changes intensify the experience of one's own aging and pending mortality. Increasing frequency of death and serious illness among loved ones, friends, and colleagues are constant reminders of one's own decreasing vigor and capacity. Most individuals in their 60s have at least one major illness or impairment such as heart disease, cancer, endocrine dysfunction, defective hearing or vision, or some form of emotional distress. All of these conditions require adaptation, or changes in accustomed patterns of living, in order to accommodate to changes in bodily function.

In the United States, an individual changes generations in the 60s. One becomes "elderly" or a "senior citizen" rather than "middle-aged." These somewhat negative connotations reflect personal and cultural anxiety about aging. With more and more people living well into and beyond their 80s, the period from the early 60s to the mid-80s might more appropriately be recognized for its potential as a distinctive and potentially fulfilling period in the life cycle.

Late adult transition takes place from about 60 to 65 years of age. The tasks of this transitional period are to conclude the efforts of middle adulthood and prepare oneself for the new era to come. Late adult transition is a period of important psychological development and represents a major turning point in the life of an individual.

Individuals who survive into their 80s and beyond may suffer from a variety of infirmities and usually at least one chronic illness. The process of aging generally becomes very evident. Life structure is restricted at this point in the life cycle and typically contains only a few important relationships. For those who are ill or physically restricted, the place of residence, or even one room in that residence, may become the individual's total environment. Some experience severe personal decline and social deprivation, causing life to lose meaning. The developmental tasks during this time are to come to terms with the reality of dying and preparing for one's own death.

Other Theories of Psychosocial Development. Like other developmental theorists, Gould[51] and Sheehy[52,53] have described ages and stages in the process of growth and development at which there are predictable crises. The ages emphasized begin with the transition from adolescence to adulthood. Gould described this period as a time of turmoil when individuals begin to reject their parents' values and establish themselves as individuals in their own right. At this age one's sense of autonomy is precarious and easily eroded. Close relationships with peers are longed for but may be unstable, resulting in temporary rebound to parents for security. The 20s are seen as a time for "taking hold in the adult world" and are characterized by needs to make commitments and to explore options. Individuals at this age feel like adults and try to act like adults. This is the time when one tries to "shape a dream," which requires preparation for life's work and development of the capacity for intimacy. During the late 20s young adults begin to feel that they have achieved their independence and they seldom question the appropriateness of the commitments they have made; however, beginning in the early 30s, they begin questioning goals and the meaning of life and consider alternate courses.

Sheehy[52,53] expanded on the work of other developmental theorists in two ways. In her book *Passages*, she compared the developmental rhythms of men and women and provided a description of what she saw as predictable "passages" for couples. She found that development over time is the same for both sexes, but that men and women rarely struggle with developmental passages at the same age. Men seem to become increasingly confident during their 20s while women lose some of the assurance they had during adolescence; men seem to settle down in their 30s while women tend to become restless; and men begin to feel that their power and dreams are slipping away in their 40s while women begin to realize their full potentials.

In her book *Pathfinders,* Sheehy analyzed the second half of life, which goes beyond the work of Gould and Levinson. Her work presented a more optimistic picture of the later years of life than Levinson. She described the period beginning at age 45 as the "comeback decade." She also described the "freestyle 50s" with potential for the happiest period of life, the "selective 60s," the "thoughtful 70s," and the "proud to be 80" periods.

More recently, Whitbourne,[54] another adult development researcher, studied 94 adults over a period of five years. She found that her data failed to support the findings of Levinson and others that identity is periodically restructured over the course of adulthood. While Whitbourne had expected to find that identity developed in a more continuous process than described by other researchers, what she actually found was that the adults in her study showed an amazing constancy in identity. She found that her adult subjects had an enduring sense of identity and purpose and a persistent sense of what was important to them and what was not, usually centered around the social roles involved with family and work. Whitbourne found that among her subjects there were no regular, predictable shifts in identity. Periods of transition typified by confusion and self-doubt did not characterize the experience of her subjects. Change was a possibility for implementing identity and preserving well-being when there was the right combination of circumstances, readiness, or need on the part of the individual. Nevertheless, the basic tendency among Whitbourne's subjects was toward verifying the belief that their purpose in life was good. Thus, according to Whitbourne, most normal adults, at any given point in their lives, know the answer to the question, "Who am I?" The answer is derived from the practical context of their everyday lives and from a sense that they are loving with their families, competent in their work, and that they follow a code of ethics that gives their life purpose.

While challenging the notion that stages and crises are a necessary feature of adult development, Whitbourne does acknowledge the fact that individuals undergo identity change during adulthood. To Whitbourne, however, these changes are not predictable by a chronological timetable and must be understood from the context of the individual's own unique circumstances. Future research may ultimately be necessary to resolve the disparity between the positions of authorities on either side of this theoretical issue. The nurse, however, benefits from understanding that while certain periods of life may bring particular challenges to identity into focus, for any given individual these challenges may or may not be relevant.

Growth, Development, and Client Care

Stages of growth and development are key to the uniqueness of each individual. Nurses can use the information presented in this chapter as a guide when collaborating directly with clients, as well as other individuals significant in their lives, to determine where clients fit in the ongoing process of growth and development. Freud's stages of psychosexual development, Erikson's stages of psychosocial development, and Buhler's concept of life goals can be useful for identifying parameters of individual psychosocial development that may be threatening, or potentially threatening, to a client's level of optimal well-being. Havighurst's developmental tasks can be used to identify an individual client's stage of physical development. The nurse's understanding of the stages of cognitive development, as proposed by Piaget, and moral development, as proposed by Kohlberg, achieved by a particular client can also provide insights into the meaning of the client's behavior. Accurate information about the client's state of individual growth and development, including the nature of particular problems they encounter, will enable nurses to develop plans for care that will be effective in assisting clients to achieve a personal level of optimal well-being and wellness.

In order to be an effective nurse, one must also recognize the major components of life structure important to an individual client. Once these components have been identified, it should be possible to project how a threat, or potential threat, to optimal health or well-being may influence these aspects of a client's life. If the major component of life structure for a particular client is the family and that client is the sole source of financial support for the family, for example, the client will likely have difficulty adapting to enforced long-term hospitalization. Having identified the importance of family financial security to the client, the nurse should be able to identify appropriate resources for the client to consider. Such resources may include hospital or community-based social, financial, or psychological services. Actively addressing this concern should reduce the client's stress level and facilitate a positive response to other health care interventions provided.

Every nurse should be aware that there are multiple life-style options in contemporary society. Options chosen by a particular client may be different from those chosen by the nurse. In order for nurses to be of assistance to clients, nurses need to view these options from a client's perspective and not laden with value judgments.

HUMAN SEXUALITY

Human sexuality is a complex phenomenon that influences individuality and the life choices made by an individual. Needs for procreation, love, and intimacy are needs that must be reasonably well satisfied before an individual is capable of achieving a high level of well-being.[7,16,17] The ability to procreate is highly dependent upon healthy biological functioning. Fulfillment of love and intimacy needs requires development of reciprocal relationships between an individual and others. One can have a physical sexual relationship with another individual without much effort if it is agreeable to the other individual. Development of a loving and intimate sexual relationship, however, requires sincere interest in, as well as understanding of, the needs of the other person and willingness to honestly share oneself with that person.

Sexuality, including one's self-concept pertaining to sexuality, influences interpersonal relationships, life-style, and health status. As individuals mature, strong identification with their gender develops. **Gender** refers to sex classification, which can be biologically or behaviorally derived. Gender identity refers to the individual's perception of himself or herself as masculine or feminine, a perception that may or may not correspond to the individual's biological sex. **Gender role** is the way an individual acts as a male or female and is the primary source of a person's sense of femininity or masculinity. These concepts are also discussed in Chapter 23.

Stages of Sexual Development

Physical sexual development begins at conception and continues throughout life. Sociosexual development is initiated at birth, through interaction with others. Table 10–11 summarizes age-related changes in sexuality.

Infant, Toddler, Preschool Child. During these periods, sexual development is strongly influenced, in some cases restricted, by parental attitudes and sanctions. Genital stimulation occurs as a natural outcome of body exploration to establish body boundaries in infancy and continues into the preschool period as part of developing body awareness and mastery. Strong negative reactions to these natural behaviors by parents create confusion and conflict about sexuality that sometimes persists into adolescence and adulthood.

School-aged Child. Socialization regarding gender identity and gender roles is strong during this period. Girls

TABLE 10–11. DEVELOPMENT OF SEXUALITY

Stage of Development	Characteristics
Infant (birth to 1 year)	Biological identity as male or female Genital self-stimulation as part of exploration of body boundaries Gender role conditioning by parents begins
Toddler/preschool child (1–5 years)	Recognizes differences between males and females Beginning development of gender identity Continued body exploration and self-stimulation; beginning of sexual modesty; learning that self-stimulation is not appropriate public behavior (in most cultures) Begins learning about gender-appropriate behavior in own culture Curiosity about sexual behavior of others, about origin of babies
School-aged child (5–12 years)	Gender identity becomes stronger Internalizes gender-appropriate roles Middle childhood age group prefers same-sex friends Curiosity about other's bodies, especially of opposite sex Masturbation continues, but less common Increasing modesty, needs for privacy Sex play with peers Testing limits, eg, sex-oriented jokes, slang (especially later childhood) In later childhood, increased interest in special friend of opposite sex
Adolescence (12–18 years)	Physical sexual maturity attained Intense emotions regarding body changes, relationships with persons of opposite sex Increasing masturbation, sexual fantasies Increasing concern about own sexuality Sexual experimentation with a partner
Young adulthood (18–35 years)	Acceptance of one's sexuality Integration of biological sex, gender, roles, sexual expression Concerns about safe sex, pregnancy, sexual relationships
Middle adult (35–65 years)	Increased capacity for physical and emotional intimacy Interest in procreation as an aspect of sexuality Conflicts about gender roles, sex roles
Older adult (65+ years)	Variation in sexual desire; diminished in some, unchanged in others Health problems may interfere with sexual expression Need for physical intimacy continues

demonstrate a widespread preference for the masculine role and ambivalence about identifying with the feminine role.[55] Although most preferred friends are of the same sex, sexual curiosity about the opposite sex is strong, peaking in the preadolescent years.

Adolescence. During adolescence, both males and females become sexually mature physiologically. The gonads develop fully and secretions of androgens and estrogens are at peak levels. The capacity to respond quickly and repeatedly to sexual stimuli is common to both sexes. Adolescents often experience emotional pressure to modify their sexual desires and behaviors dramatically in order to remain in conformance with society's values.

Young Adulthood. Because one of the tasks for young adults is developing intimacy and solidarity rather than existing in isolation,[56] sexual intimacy usually occurs and intimacy issues such as learning to give and receive love, choosing whether or not to marry, and choosing a marital or sexual partner(s)[57] must be addressed. Most young adults make some commitment to a sexual relationship, whether marital or nonmarital, and usually experience social legitimization of their sexual activities for the first time. Use of contraception, exposure to sexually transmitted diseases (including AIDS), and pregnancy are concerns of men and women in this age group.

Middle Adulthood. Adulthood is the time in one's life typically devoted to parenting and consolidation of a sexual relationship[56] and the image of the "sexual self." The quality of one's self-concept during adulthood greatly affects the way in which one meets demands for gender role performance.

New opportunities for women in the marketplace often create sex role conflicts for both men and women.[56] Many women feel that they must cope with the combined responsibilities of maintaining a career and raising children while men often feel that their roles, as traditionally defined, are not supported. If adult males and females unwillingly assume responsibilities and roles that vary from those that they have been prepared by life experiences to fulfill, there may be resulting strains in sexual relationships. Honest communication of feelings and negotiation of new role definitions and functions are essential for couples in transition from the traditional world to the contemporary world.

Late Adulthood. Physiological changes have some impact on sexuality between 50 and 65 years of age. As estrogen levels decrease, women experience the transition to menopause. Depression in middle-aged women has frequently been attributed to menopause; however, data from studies over the past 20 years indicate that melancholy and depression at this time in the life cycle are probably more directly related to changes in role and loss of responsibility as children mature and leave home than to diminishing hormone levels.[32,56,58] Levels of androgen in men also decrease gradually during this period. These physiological changes and concommitant involution of sexual organs and structures cannot be equated with cessation of sexual functioning or diminution of its importance, as sexual interest has been found to remain quite consistent throughout adulthood.[56] Some individuals, both male and female, have even reported increasing sexual interest and activity as they became older.[55,59]

Attitudes Related to Sexuality

Cultural Influences. The culture of a society serves as the component of that society through which boundaries are defined between what behavior is sexual and what behavior is not sexual.[56,60] These boundaries are directly related to the internal logic and consistency of the culture. In some cultures where food is valued highly, for example, sharing food with a member of the opposite sex is considered to be a sexual act.

Many cultural opinions about sexuality are related to the state of health experienced by an individual and the effects of sexual activity on that state. In some cultures, sexual activity is believed to result in weakness or poor health, while in other cultures it is highly encouraged. Taboos against incest are common to most societies, although definitions about what constitutes an incestuous relationship vary from one society to another. The precise definition of incest within a given society is frequently based on inheritance rights or other relationships that might cause a family to incur undesirable obligations.

Sexual modesty is considered to be important in most societies. Aspects of sexual response that are influenced by cultural norms include attitudes about what is considered to be erotic, whether intercourse is restricted to marriage or a comparable relationship, lengthy versus brief precopulatory stimulation, whether the female plays an active or passive role in sexual activities, the usual positions for intercourse, and duration of the act of intercourse. The position assumed for intercourse often reflects other aspects of cultural belief and environmental conditions. A couple that values privacy for sexual intercourse but must sleep in the same room with other individuals, for example, may choose a side-to-side position because it is believed to be less noticeable to others in the room.

Religious and Ethical Influences. Religious teachings affect what an individual perceives to be ethical behavior, including ethical sexual behavior. Although the sexual drive is considered to be a divine endowment according to Judaic teachings,[61] it is to be exercised only within marriage. Protestant ethics pertaining to sexuality are predominantly concentrated on the value of human relationships.[62] Members of the Roman Catholic faith are struggling with efforts to personalize the ethics of sexuality but at the same time subscribe to the biblical image of humans.[63] The multitude of differing opinions about whether use of contraceptives is ethical behavior, for example, constitutes one of the contemporary challenges facing many Catholics.

Historical Influences. Historical concepts about sexuality have had a major impact on what parents and social institutions, including schools and churches teach about sexuality. These concepts continue to affect the development of individual attitudes about sexuality in our changing contemporary society.

The Victorian era, in the late 1800s, had a profound effect on individual understanding of sexuality.[64,65] Chastity, particularly among women, continuing even within marriage was the major emphasis of teachings, both formal and informal, about sexuality at this time. Sexual intercourse was deemed acceptable only for the purpose of procreation within marriage. Self-control resulting in denial of sexual desires and avoidance of all temptations was expected of everyone.

Partly as a result of the common attitudes about sexuality held during the Victorian era, a double standard developed that differentiated acceptable male sexual behavior from acceptable female sexual behavior.[61,66] This standard dictated that certain behaviors, particularly premarital intercourse, were acceptable for men but not for women. As a result of this double standard, both men and women have experienced psychological conflict.[61] Men were taught to require virginity in a wife but encouraged to waive this as a requirement for premarital sexual partners; women were taught that they must remain virgins until marriage but were pressured by men to participate in premarital intercourse.

Factual information about sexuality, including acceptable ways of expressing one's sexuality, is much more readily available now than it was previously; however, attitudes from the Victorian era and those resulting from the double standard for sexual behavior still influence individual perceptions about sexuality. Sexual issues confronting many individuals in contemporary society, either personally or among significant others, include premarital cohabitation, homosexuality, extramarital sexual relationships, and exposure to sexually transmitted diseases.

Human Sexuality and Nursing Care

Human sexuality is intimately linked to individuality. Self-concept, level of health, and life circumstances have a dramatic impact on an individual's success in fulfilling the basic need for sexual gratification. Nurses need an understanding of the client's sexual orientation and experience with sexuality to assist clients to find satisfactory ways to meet this need. Information gathering should include identification of the client's stage of growth and development; sexual experience or commitments (adolescent experimentation, premarital cohabitation, marriage, loss of a sexual partner, homosexuality); health status; and the client's perceptions about problems in meeting the need for sexual gratification.

In order to gain sufficient information and understanding about client sexuality, nurses must accept and understand their own sexuality. Nurses must assess clients' personal attitudes about sexuality and life experiences with sexuality without judgmentalness or imposition of their own values. Clarification of personal attitudes about sexual issues should enable nurses to address client needs in a caring but nonjudgmental manner. For example, a nurse who is opposed to homosexuality must confront personal negative feelings about caring for clients who have become infected with the HIV virus through homosexual activity. While nurses need not feel pressured to change personal values, they must remember that attitudes are conveyed openly through comments and actions, as well as subtly. Disregard for a hospitalized client's need to spend some uninterrupted time alone with a sexual partner, for example, would indicate that the nurse did not value this client need.

IMPLICATIONS FOR NURSE–CLIENT COLLABORATION

Human Sexuality

An individual's sexuality is a central factor in his or her personal choices and life structure. Thus, sexuality is a key to achieving need satisfaction and life goal attainment. An appreciation of the client's experience of sexuality, his or her sexual self-image, and how it is affected by illness is vital to the nurse's efforts to support the client's well-being. In a collaborative nurse–client relationship, the nurse is sensitive to the complex feelings the client may have about sexuality, and tries to understand how to help the client feel comfortable with himself or herself and with others while adapting to the changes of illness.

SUMMARY

Each individual is a unique being. There are no two human beings who are exactly alike because no two individuals experience identical interactions with the environment. Individuals' perceptions of self in the world and how effectively they interact in their environment are dependent upon how well their needs have been satisfied during the process of maturation. Stress results when an individual's needs have not been met satisfactorily. Stress creates potential for alterations in one's self-concept and one's perception of reality. These altered perceptions may interfere with normal growth and development and result in an inability to achieve an optimal level of well-being.

With a sound understanding of the dimensions of individuality, factors that influence the development of identity, characteristics of healthy individuals, and parameters of normal growth and development, including human sexuality, nurses are in a position to individualize nursing interventions on behalf of the client. Psychosocial development, cognitive development, moral development, life goals, and human sexuality issues must be considered when obtaining accurate data about a client. Finally, nurses need to explore the major components of life structure important to an individual client to effectively determine the potential impact of a health alteration.

A plan for nursing intervention and support can be

designed that is based on a client's unique needs. Accurate identification of client's needs amenable to nursing intervention is the result of sincere concern, as well as careful collaboration with clients and other individuals significant to them. The nurse is in a unique position to individualize client care so that it is effective in meeting the client's personal needs and ultimately facilitating the client's efforts to achieve self-actualization.

REFERENCES

1. Davis BD. The importance of human individuality for sociobiology. Perspec Biol Med. 1982; 26:1–18.
2. Rushton JP, Fulker DW, Neale MC, et al. Altruism and aggression: The heritability of individual differences. *J Personality Soc Psych.* 1986; 50:1192–1198.
3. Combs AW, Syngg D. *Individual Behavior: A Perceptual Approach to Behavior.* New York: Harper; 1959.
4. Jourard SM. *Personal Adjustment: An Approach Through the Study of Healthy Personality.* 2nd ed. New York: Macmillan; 1971.
5. Jourard SM. *The Transparent Self.* New York: Van Nostrand Reinhold; 1971.
6. Shlien JM. Phenomenology and personality. In: Wepman JW, Heine RW, eds. *Concepts of Personality.* Chicago: Aldine; 1963: 291–292.
7. Maslow AH. *Motivation and Personality.* 2nd ed. New York: Harper & Row; 1970.
8. Gatens C. Sexuality and disability. In: Woods NF, ed. *Human Sexuality in Health and Illness.* 3rd ed. St. Louis: Mosby; 1984: 370–398.
9. Pervin-Dixon L, Sexuality and the spinal cord injured. *J Psychosoc Nurs Mental Health Serv.* 1988; 26:31–35, 37.
10. Selye H. *Stress Without Distress.* New York: Signet; 1975.
11. Rogers CR. *On Becoming a Person.* London: Constable; 1977.
12. Fromm E. *Escape from Freedom.* New York: Avon; 1941.
13. Maslow A. Deficiency motivation and growth motivation. In: Jones MR, ed. *Nebraska Symposium on Motivation.* Lincoln, NB: University of Nebraska Press; 1955:1–30.
14. Allport G. *Becoming: Basic Considerations for a Psychology of Personality.* New Haven: Yale University Press; 1955.
15. Freud S. *An Outline of Psychoanalysis.* London: Hogarth; 1973.
16. Kalish RA. *The Psychology of Human Behavior.* Belmont, CA: Wadsworth; 1966.
17. Jourard SM. *Healthy Personality: An Approach from the Viewpoint of Humanistic Psychology.* New York: Macmillan; 1974.
18. Schweppe JS. *Man: A Remarkable Animal.* Chicago: Research and Education Fund; 1970.
19. Selye H. *The Stress of Life.* New York: McGraw-Hill; 1956.
20. Wolf S, Goodell H, eds. *Stress and Disease.* 2nd ed. Springfield, IL: Thomas; 1968.
21. Lazarus RS. The self-regulation of emotion. In: Levi L, ed. *Emotions: Their Parameters and Measurement.* New York: Raven; 1975:55–57.
22. Mason J. Emotions as reflected in patterns of endocrine integration. In: Levi L, ed. *Emotions: Their Parameters and Measurement.* New York: Raven; 1975:171–175.
23. Welford AT. Stress and performance. In: Welford AT, ed. *Man Under Stress.* New York: Halsted; 1974:1–2.
24. Pilowsky I. Psychiatric aspects of stress. In: Welford AT, ed. *Man Under Stress.* New York: Halsted; 1974:125–131.
25. Seyle H. *Stress.* Montreal: Acta; 1950.
26. Frankenhaeuser M. Experimental approaches to the study of catecholamines and emotions. In: Levi L, ed. *Emotions: Their Parameters and Measurement.* New York: Raven; 1975:214–216.
27. Pelletier K. *Mind As Healer, Mind As Slayer.* New York: Dell; 1977.
28. Johansson G, Gardell B. Work-health relations as mediated through stress reactions and job socialization. In Maes S, Spielberger CD, Defares PB, Sarason IG, eds: *Topics in Health Psychology.* New York: John Wiley, 1988:271–285.
29. Claus KE, Bailey JT. *Living with Stress and Promoting Well-Being: A Handbook for Nurses.* St. Louis: Mosby; 1980.
30. Cooley CH. *Human Nature and Social Order.* New York: Scribners; 1902.
31. Lidz T. *The Person: His and Her Development Throughout the Life Cycle.* 2nd ed. New York: Basic Books; 1976.
32. Spector RE. *Cultural Diversity in Health and Illness.* Norwalk, CT: Appleton & Lange; 1991.
33. Bardwick JM. *Psychology of Women: A Study of Bio-Cultural Conflicts.* New York: Harper & Row; 1971.
34. Jahoda M. *Current Concepts of Positive Mental Health.* New York: Basic Books; 1958.
35. Jahoda M. The meaning of psychological health. *Social Casework.* 1953; 34:349–354.
36. Allport GW. *Personality: A Psychological Interpretation.* New York: Henry Holt; 1937.
37. Maslow AH. A theory of human motivation. *Psychological Rev.* 1943; 50:370–396.
38. Erikson EH. Growth and crisis of the healthy personality. In: Senn MJE, ed. *Symposium on the Healthy Personality.* New York: Josiah Macy Jr Foundation; 1950:91–146.
39. Hartmann H. *Essays on Ego Psychology: Selected Problems in Psychoanalytic Theory.* New York: International Universities Press; 1964.
40. Kubie LS. The fundamental nature of the distinction between normality and neurosis. *Psychoanal Q.* 1954; 23:167–204.
41. Erikson EH. *Childhood and Society.* 2nd ed. New York: Norton; 1963.
42. Erikson EH. *Identity: Youth and Crisis.* New York: Norton; 1968.
43. Buhler C. The course of human life as a psychological problem. *Human Devel.* 1968; 11:184–200.
44. Havighurst RJ. *Developmental Tasks and Education.* 3rd ed. New York: David McKay; 1972.
45. Piaget J, Inhelder B. *The Psychology of the Child.* New York: Basic Books; 1969.
46. Piaget J. *The Origins of Intelligence in Children.* New York: Norton; 1963.
47. Kohlberg L. The cognitive–developmental approach to moral education. *Phi Delta Kappa.* 1975; 56:670–677.
48. Duska R, Whelan M. *Moral Development: A Guide to Piaget and Kohlberg.* New York: Paulist Press; 1975.
49. Levinson DJ, Darrow CN, Klein EB, et al. *The Seasons of a Man's Life.* New York: Knopf; 1978.
50. Jaques E. Death and the mid-life crisis. *Int J Psychoanal.* 1965; 46:502–514.
51. Gould RL. *Transformations: Growth and Change in Adult Life.* New York: Simon & Schuster; 1978.
52. Sheehy G. *Passages.* New York: Dutton; 1974.
53. Sheehy G. *Pathfinders.* New York: Morrow; 1981.
54. Whitbourne SK. *The Me I Know: A Study of Adult Identity.* New York: Springer-Verlag; 1986.
55. Littlefield LM. *Health Education for Women: A guide for health professionals.* Norwalk, CT: Appleton-Century-Crofts; 1986.

56. Woods NF. *Human Sexuality in Health and Illness.* 4th ed. St. Louis: Mosby; 1987:63–82.
57. Duvall EM. *Marriage and Family Development.* 5th ed. Philadelphia: Lippincott; 1977.
58. Horney K. *Feminine Psychology.* New York: Norton; 1967.
59. Kalish RA. *Late Adulthood: Perspectives on Human Development.* Monterey, CA: Brooks/Cole; 1975.
60. Davenport W. Sex in cross-cultural perspective. In: Beach FA, ed. *Human Sexuality in Four Perspectives.* Baltimore: Johns Hopkins University Press; 1977.
61. Rosenheim E. Sexual attitudes and regulations in judaism. In: Money J, Musaph H, eds. *Handbook of Sexology.* New York: Excerpta Medica; 1977:1315–1323.
62. VanGennep FO. Sexual ethics in Protestant churches. In: Money J. Musaph H, eds. *Handbook of Sexology.* New York: Excerpta Medica; 1977:1334–1338.
63. Sporken P. Marriage and sexual ethics in the Catholic church. In: Money J, Musaph H, eds. *Handbook of Sexology.* New York: Excerpta Medica; 1977:1325–1331.
64. Williams JH. *Psychology of Women.* New York: Norton; 1977.
65. Fogel CI. Sexual dysfunction. In: Fogel CI, Woods NF, eds. *Health Care of Women: A Nursing Perspective.* St. Louis: Mosby; 1981:146–170.
66. Reiss L. The double standard in premarital intercourse: A neglected concept. *Social Forces.* 1956; 34:224–230.

BIBLIOGRAPHY

Allport G. *The Person in Psychology.* Boston: Beacon; 1968.

Ansbacher H, Ansbacher R, eds. *Superiority and Social Interest: A Collection of Alfred Adler's Later Writings.* New York: Viking; 1973.

Asher CC. The impact of social support networks on adult health. *Med Care.* 1984; 22:349–359.

Baumeister RF, Shapiro JP, Tice DM. Two kinds of identity crisis. *J Personality.* 1985; 53:407–424.

Buhler C. The life cycle: Structural determinants of goalsetting. *J Humanistic Psychol.* 1966; 6:37–52.

Buhler C. Human life goals in the humanistic perspective. *J Humanistic Psychol.* 1967; 7:36–52.

Campbell JD. Similarity and uniqueness: The effects of attribute type, relevance, and individual differences in self-esteem and depression. *J Personality Soc Psychol.* 1986; 50:281–294.

Caplan G. Loss, stress and mental health. *Comm. Mental Health J.* Feb, 1990; 26:27–48.

Costa PT, McCrae RR, Zonderman AB. Environmental and dispositional influences on well-being: Longitudinal follow-up of an American national sample. *Brit J Psychol.* 1987; 78:299–306.

Dunn HL. *High Level Wellness.* Arlington: Beatty; 1961.

Erikson EH. *Life History and the Historical Moment.* New York: Norton; 1975.

Freedman RJ. Reflections on beauty as it relates to health in adolescent females. Women & Health. 1984; 9:29–45.

Fromm E. *The Heart of Man: Its Genius for Good and Evil.* New York: Harper & Row; 1964.

Janis IL, Mahl GF, Kagan J, Holt RR. *Personality: Dynamics, Development, and Assessment.* New York: Harcourt, Brace & World; 1969.

Johnson DW. *Reaching Out: Interpersonal Effectiveness and Self Actualization.* 2nd ed. Englewood Cliffs, NJ: Prentice-Hall; 1981.

Johnson JE, Lauver DR. Alternative explanations of coping with stressful experiences associated with physical illness. *Adv in Nurs Sci.* Jan, 1989; 11:39–52.

Jourard SM. *Self-Disclosure: An Experimental Analysis of the Transparent Self.* New York: Wiley; 1971.

Kalish RA. *Late Adulthood: Perspectives on Human Development.* Monterey, CA: Brooks/Cole; 1975.

Kalish RA, Reynolds DK. *Death and Ethnicity: A Psychocultural Study.* Los Angeles: University of Southern California Press; 1976.

Laing RD, Phillipson H, Lee AR. *Interpersonal Perception: A Theory and Method of Research.* New York: Springer; 1966.

Maddox GL. Aging differently. *Gerontologist.* 1987; 27:557–564.

McCracken AL. Sexuality practice by elders: The forgotten aspect of functional health. Journal of Gerontological Nursing Oct, 1988; 14:13–18

Montagu A, ed. *Culture and Human Development: Insights into Growing Human.* Englewood Cliffs, NJ: Prentice-Hall; 1974.

Montagu A. *Touching: The Human Significance of the Skin.* 2nd ed. New York: Harper & Row; 1978.

Pincus S. A sense of self. *Perspec Biol Med.* 1982; 26:30–38.

Ramsey P. *The Patient As Person.* New Haven: Yale University Press; 1970.

Rogers CR. Remarks on the future of client-centered therapy. In: Wexler DA, Rice LN, eds. *Innovations in Client-Centered Therapy.* New York: Wiley; 1974.

Rothman B, Sebastian H. Intimacy and cognitively impaired elders. *Canadian Nurse.* May, 1990; 86:32,34.

Stewart WA. *The Formation of the Early Adult Life Structure in Women.* New York: Teachers College Press; 1976.

Volden C, et al. The relationship of age, gender, and exercise practice to health life-style and self esteem. *Appl Nurs Res.* 1990; 3(1):20

CHAPTER 11

Growth and Development Across the Life Span

Behavioral Objectives

Upon completion of this chapter, the student will be able to:

1. Describe attitudes of nurses that are helpful for assisting clients in all phases of growth and development.
2. Describe the essential nature of collaboration between the nurse and client as it relates to promoting human growth.
3. Define growth and development.
4. List five major principles of growth and development.
5. Describe the expected changes in physical growth and development across the life span.
6. Summarize major points about psychosocial development for each stage of the life span.
7. Describe the focus of nurse–client collaboration for promoting/maintaining normal growth and development of individuals at each stage of the life span.
8. List two common health problems for each stage of the life span.
9. Describe responsibilities of the nurse in collaborating with clients to manage common health problems encountered in each developmental phase of the life span.

KEY TERMS

accommodation
assimilation
attachment behaviors
cephalocaudal
cognitive development
critical periods
development
fine motor control
gross motor control
growth
individuation
learning disorder
magical thinking
maturation
moral development
object permanence
parallel play
phase
proximodistal
psychosocial development
puberty
therapeutic play

Nurses' primary professional focus is on individual clients and their human responses to health problems. One of the most remarkable features of human beings is the pattern of change that occurs in body and behavior over the life span. Changes that mark the stages of life are so familiar that they are commonly taken for granted. An individual's human responses to illness are shaped significantly by these changes and the stage of life in which health problems are encountered.

To understand human responses to health problems, nurses must first know the characteristics of human coping that are natural to each phase of life and be familiar with changes brought about by simply getting older. A study of growth and development over the stages of the life cycle provides nurses with such an understanding. This knowledge helps nurses to anticipate the health needs common to a given age or stage of development.

Nurses, through the practice of nursing, endeavor to assist clients to resolve health problems. Nurses do this by interacting with clients to identify what clients' health problems are, to establish what measures might be taken to improve clients' health state, and to engage clients in taking those measures with assistance, when needed, from nurses. The collaborative approach that is the basis for this text emphasizes that the best way to help clients resolve health problems is to involve them in the health care decision-making process.

Collaboration on health decisions is a basic value of the nurse–client relationship. Collaboration involves the fundamental way in which health care decisions are made and refers to a relationship in which clients are full participants. Human beings have a basic need to control the life circumstances that affect them; collaboration addresses that need. Collaboration, as a model for client care, has certain restrictions, the most important being informed consent. Clients must be capable of understanding the consequences of a health care decision before they can take responsibility for the decision. The client's stage of growth and development is important because, to a large extent, it determines the client's capacity to take that responsibility.

Knowledge of growth and development is therefore crucial within the collaborative framework for two reasons. It helps nurses anticipate the health decisions that may be necessary and it enables nurses to foresee possibilities for clients' participation in decision making and the limitations on that participation. Principles of growth and development guide nurses in evaluating the extent to which the collaborative approach is appropriate at a particular developmental stage and assist nurses to maximize clients' participation within their developmental limits. Thus, on the basis of an understanding of growth and development, nurses are able to incorporate collaborative values into client care.

This chapter provides an overview of growth and development across the life span, with an emphasis on wellness promotion and on the common health problems experienced in each of the nine stages of development. Responsibilities of nurses for client care and opportunities for nurse–client collaboration, relative to promoting growth, development, and wellness and addressing common health problems, are also discussed. The chapter stresses the options available to nurses for incorporating collaboration as a value into client care throughout the life span.

IMPLICATIONS FOR NURSE–CLIENT COLLABORATION

Knowledge of Growth and Development

Knowledge of growth and development is crucial within the collaborative framework for two reasons. It helps nurses anticipate the health decisions that may be necessary and it enables nurses to foresee possibilities for clients' participation in decision making and the limitations on that participation.

INTEGRATING GROWTH AND DEVELOPMENT CONCEPTS IN COLLABORATIVE CARE

Nurses who use a collaborative model of care to assist clients to resolve health problems recognize that knowledge of growth and development is a critical component of that model. Nurses use their knowledge to decide when and to what extent they will involve clients in making health care decisions. In addition, because participating in decision making fosters development, nurses can make a conscious choice to use the collaborative model of care as another means of supporting clients' growth and development throughout the life span.

Attitudes and behaviors demonstrating openness and acceptance toward people of all ages are essential to maintain communication between nurses and clients. Clear and open communication offers a better opportunity for clients' health and developmental needs to be assessed accurately and for an appropriate plan of care to be developed. It also increases the likelihood that the plan will be implemented successfully.

For example, nurses who care for children may not always agree with the values, ideas, and behaviors demonstrated by parents' childrearing practices; however, judging parents is not helpful and can disrupt the collaborative relationship. Thus, nurses need to determine whether the parents' attitudes, values, and behaviors could result in harm to their children. At the same time, nurses must convey to the parents that they respect them and their right to make decisions about childbearing and childrearing practices. Nursing intervention is appropriate if parents need information about child development or assistance with parenting skills, or if the child is likely to be or has been physically or emotionally harmed by the parents. In all situations, accepting parents, remembering their rights as parents, and listening to their concerns and viewpoints increase their receptivity to proposed nursing interventions and their willingness to collaborate in health care decisions affecting their children.

Communication skills are a critical aspect of collaboration throughout the life span. Chapters 13 and 14 focus on communication in the nurse–client relationship. Although the skills outlined there are appropriate for clients of all ages, nurses working with children often find a need to use a special communication technique: therapeutic play. This technique is especially useful with toddlers and preschool children, whose language skills may not be sufficiently developed to express the fears and concerns that usually accompany illness, and in particular, hospitalization. Moreover, because developmental regression is a common phenomenon among clients of all ages when ill, play therapy is often effective with school-aged children as well.[1]

Therapeutic play is a means of enabling children to accept their health problems and treatments by engaging them in specially designed play activities that help them express fears, conflicts, and other feelings. It is meant to be healing for children who are attempting to cope with or master feelings associated with the experiences associated with illness or trauma. It is a natural means of communicating with children, for they often use play to express themselves in learning and in socializing. Play has been described as the work of children.

Therapeutic play is useful in introducing children to hospital routines, in helping them to cope with separation from parents and other loved ones, in promoting normal socialization during hospitalization and in reducing fear of injections, surgery and other painful procedures.

For example, prior to giving a child an injection, a nurse might help the child to gain control over this potentially fearful situation by having the child play nurse and give a doll a shot with a water-filled syringe. The nurse might also encourage the child to express emotional feelings by helping the child to talk to the doll. The nurse might supply phrases like: "This will feel like a sting," "this will hurt a little," and "you held very still—what a big boy!" These techniques must be performed according to scientific principles and used purposefully with an understanding of clients' growth, development, and health needs. Detailed instruction of therapeutic play skills is beyond the scope of this chapter. The reader can learn these skills through focused study and supervised experiences with therapeutic play during clinical assignments.

In addition to using therapeutic play with children, nurses interact with clients of all ages, using verbal and nonverbal communication. The application of verbal communication skills varies with clients' age and developmental level. Nurses use knowledge of growth and development to guide their choice of words and amount of detail when communicating with clients, whether they are interviewing, teaching, assessing learning, planning care, assisting with problem solving, or developing interpersonal relationships.

Interactions with clients that are based on sound developmental rationale, such as addressing adults by their full names or calling children by their nicknames, demonstrate nurses' understanding of the social formalities appropriate to clients' developmental level. Nonverbal communication, such as posture, intonation, and facial expression, is as important as verbal communication and can reflect respect and caring to clients of all ages. Attention to such concerns is helpful in establishing positive rapport.

The ability of nurses to make crucial decisions about the appropriateness and timing of specific approaches with clients is not merely intuitive, but is the result of both knowledge about and experience with persons of all ages. Needs and capacity of individuals to speak and to make decisions about health are greatly affected by development. Nurses who understand growth and development know that although some clients may have reached the stage of development at which they would ordinarily make health care decisions, they may nevertheless be limited in their ability to participate fully in decision making. Limitations emanate from impaired mental capacity and reduced consciousness and from youth itself. Even so, nurses who value collaboration ensure that clients are appropriately informed and involved to the fullest extent possible in making health care decisions.

Ultimately, the implementation of caregiving requires clients' consent and cooperation. When adult clients have had major surgery, for example, they usually are instructed, as part of their postoperative care, to cough and deep breathe to prevent the pneumonia that results from a pooling of secretions in the lungs. Nurses can explain the rationale and benefits of coughing and the consequences of not coughing and make painstaking efforts to influence clients and gain their cooperation. Clients, however, ultimately choose whether or not to follow these instructions, implying informed consent if they follow through. Children, too, decide whether or not they will cooperate, but the techniques employed to gain their cooperation must be tailored to their age and development. Thus, the judgments involved in assessing clients' capacity to decide and in selecting nursing approaches appropriate to gaining clients' participation require integrating knowledge of growth and development.

DEFINITIONS OF GROWTH AND DEVELOPMENT

Although it is true that human development generally follows certain predictable patterns, it is exciting to consider growth and development as a dynamic process and each human being as infinitely complex and uniquely different from all others. The terms *growth* and *development* are frequently used synonymously to describe a particular set of changes, but growth and development are actually very different processes.

Growth

Growth is a quantitative term used to describe a physical change, such as an increase in size, height, or weight. Growth begins at conception and is measured in pounds (or kilograms) and inches (or centimeters). Individual growth depends primarily on inherited genetic traits. Although the potential for growth is dependent on nature, growth and development patterns are also affected by environment, especially those nurturing influences that help to promote consistent health.[2] Significant trauma, for example malnutrition or emotional or physical abuse, has been shown to negatively influence or arrest growth. Because a specific chronological age comparison is somewhat arbitrary and physical growth parameters are so broad, individual children are better assessed by comparing their physical growth with age group norms.[3] Most physical growth is completed by late adolescence at about 18 years of age, as is illustrated in Table 11–1.

Development

Development, in contrast to growth, is a qualitative term used to describe changes in psychosocial, cognitive, or moral functioning. For example, the change of a child's social interest from the family to the world outside the family reflects development. Development is more difficult to measure than growth because it is complex and abstract.

Maturation is another term used to describe qualitative changes; however, the terms *maturation* and *development,* although closely related, are not synonymous. Development describes a gradual change or expansion of a person's capabilities; **maturation** describes a differentiation or increasing complexity of those capabilities that may come with age.

Psychosocial Development. Erik Erikson's classic research described the emotional and social development of the healthy personality.[4] **Psychosocial development** is a term used to describe the personality changes that occur as a result of interactions between people. Human values such as trust, independence, self-esteem, and maturity develop as people experience positive and consistent interactions with influential role models.

TABLE 11–1. EXPECTED PHYSICAL GROWTH BY CHRONOLOGICAL AGE

Age	Stage	Physical Growth
Birth–4 weeks	Neonate	*Weight gain:* 140–200 g (5–7 oz)/week *Height:* 1 in. in first 4 weeks *Vital signs:* Pulse 100–180 Respirations 35–70 Systolic BP 64–94
1–12 months	Infant	*Weight gain:* 85–200 g (3–7 oz)/week (Birth weight doubles in 4–6 months and triples by the end of the first year.) *Height:* approximately 1.25 cm (½ in.)/month (Birth length increases by about 50% by the end of the first year.) *Vital signs:* Pulse 100–120 Respirations 30–40 Systolic BP 76–86
1–3 years	Toddler	*Weight gain:* 2–3 kg (4.5–6.5 lb)/year (Birth weight quadruples by age 2½.) *Height:* at 1–2 years, 12 cm (4.5 in.) (Height at 2 years is approximately 50% of eventual adult height.) at 2–3 years, 6–8 cm (2.75–3.25 in.) *Vital signs:* Pulse 70–120 Respirations 20–35 Systolic BP 80–96
3–5 years	Preschooler Early Childhood	*Weight gain:* 2–3 kg (4.5–6.5 lb)/year *Height:* 5–7.5 cm (2–3 in.)/year (Birth length doubles by 4 years of age.) *Vital signs:* Pulse 70–100 Respirations 20–30 BP 80–110/40–65
6–12 years	School Age Middle childhood, Preadolescence	*Weight gain:* 2–3 kg (4.5–6.5 lbs)/year *Height:* 5 cm (2 in.)/year (Birth length triples by 13 years of age.) *Vital Signs:* Pulse 70–100 Respirations 20–30 BP 80–120/45–70
13–18 years	Adolescent	*Weight gain:* variable Females: range 7–25 kg (15–25 lb) mean 17.5 kg (38 lb) Males: range 7–30 kg (16–65 lb) mean 24 kg (52 lb) Height: variable Females: range 5–25 cm (2–10 in.) mean 20.5 cm (8.25 in.) (95% of mature height at menarche) Males: range 10–30 cm (4–12 in.) mean: 27.5 cm (11 in.) (95% of mature height at 15 years of age) *Vital signs:* During adolescence the pulse rate decreases slightly and systolic BP increases slightly compared with school-age children. This pattern continues into adulthood.

Adapted from Tanner JM, Davies PSW. Clinical longitudinal standards for height and weight velocity of North American children. J Pediatr. *1985; 107:317–329.*

Erikson's theory of personality development is helpful to nurses because it describes expected emotional health from birth through later adulthood (refer to Chapter 10 for an extensive discussion of developmental theories).

Cognitive Development. Jean Piaget[5] defined **cognitive development** as the ability of the individual to think and reason in a logical manner. Piaget's primary hypothesis was that intellectual development is an adaptive process occurring as a regulatory function of both physiological and intellectual growth.[5] Adaptation occurs through both **assimilation,** learning from new experience, and **accommodation,** modifying old ways of thinking to fit new situations.

Piaget acknowledges that all persons are born with an inherited predisposition for intellectual development that can meets its potential only through adequate stimulation. In early childhood, parents and siblings are the primary source of intellectual stimulation, but when the child enters school, teachers and friends also influence cognitive development.

Moral Development. Kohlberg's theory of moral development, outlined in Chapter 10, is closely related to cognitive development.[6] **Moral development** is the term used to describe development of internal beliefs and attitudes of fairness, social justice, respect, and loyalty. Structured religious or spiritual beliefs and rules are also a part of moral development. Changes in psychosocial, cognitive, and moral development are dependent on one another and together describe the processes occurring as the body and mind develop.

PRINCIPLES OF GROWTH AND DEVELOPMENT

Some general expectations, or principles, can be stated about growth and development. All persons follow certain patterns of growth and development that are predictable, continuous, and with expected sequences.

Growth and development proceed in an orderly and regular neuromuscular direction following cephalocaudal and proximodistal patterns. **Cephalocaudal** is a term used to describe the pattern of acquisition of skills occurring along the vertical axis of the body, from head to tail. For example, infants achieve control of the head first, then the shoulders, and next the trunk, before learning to sit or walk. The term **proximodistal** is used to describe the development of skills from the midline to the outside of the body. Infants, as an example, first begin to move both arms bilaterally and then to use their hands together before using each arm separately or beginning to use the fingers to manipulate objects.

Both cephalocaudal and proximodistal growth and development patterns reflect the sequence of nervous system maturation. Children who are growing and maturing normally thus crawl before they walk and walk before they run, for example, in relationship to the sequence of changes in the nervous system needed to support motor development. Each new skill developed depends on the successful achievement of a less sophisticated, or less developed, skill.

The rate of growth and development varies greatly from child to child. This is especially evident during times of rapid growth, such as adolescence. Box 11–1 summarizes these principles.

BOX 11–1. PRINCIPLES OF GROWTH AND DEVELOPMENT

1. Human growth and development follow a predictable, continuous, and sequential pattern.
2. Neuromuscular growth and development follow both cephalocaudal and proximodistal patterns.
3. Each stage of development is dependent on adequate completion of the previous stage, and is itself the foundation for the development of new skills.
4. Growth or development may temporarily be stalled or regress during critical periods.
5. Individual variations in growth and development patterns depend on genetics, environment, and positive or negative factors that are present or absent during critical periods.

STAGES OF GROWTH AND DEVELOPMENT

Like the principles of growth and development, each stage of development builds on the preceding stage in which skills or tasks were learned. Growth and development occur in phases. A **phase** is a particular period in a cycle of changes. During each phase, growth and/or development progress.

The timing of developmental changes is predictable and correlated with defined age periods such as infancy (ages 1 to 12 months) and toddlerhood (ages 1 to 3 years). After a period of developmental progression, advances may temporarily stall, or even regress, and then progress again.

Certain developmental phases have critical periods. **Critical periods** of development are those periods during which the person is more vulnerable to physical, chemical, psychological, or environmental influences.[7] Although critical periods often manifest in certain stages of growth and development, they are not specifically related to a given stage and may show up in any phase; however, the person is probably most vulnerable to environmental, physiological, or interpersonal stimulation or deprivation during times of most rapid structural change and growth. The embryonic phase of prenatal development can be looked upon as a critical period. It is a period of especially rapid cell growth in which normal tissue development is strongly influenced by factors such as maternal health. Interruption of nutrition or exposure to toxins during this period can result in irreversible congenital anomalies. Critical periods of development might also include those times during the preschool and school-age phases when children demonstrate cognitive, psychosocial, and neurological readiness to learn. Stimulation during these periods promotes the acquisition of new skills, while a lack of stimulation may result in a significant slow-down in development. An understanding of critical periods influences nurses' assessments and interventions with clients at all points in the life span. Nurses must be cognizant of influences that may stall development. What types of nutrition are most needed during times of accelerated growth? What changes in nutrition are necessary during adulthood? What experiences can a parent provide to best prepare a child to begin school? Such questions must be addressed if nurses wish to facilitate a client's development.

ASSESSMENT OF GROWTH AND DEVELOPMENT

Growth and development are evaluated by comparing an individual's characteristics with the characteristics that are expected for a person of the same age group. For example, the average 11-year-old boy measures about 55 in. in height, but normal variations for boys of that age will range from 52 to 58 in. Such standards, or normal variations, enable comparison. They provide "yardsticks" for evaluating an individual's features and capacities and for assessing an individual's health.

Assessment of the physical, cognitive, and psychosocial capabilities expected on the basis of a client's age is a basic responsibility of nurses. Moreover, by repeatedly comparing a norm or standard with clients' actual abilities on certain tasks, nurses gain an appreciation of what to expect and of the normal variations that occur.

Growth is relatively easy to assess: clients are measured and weighed, and comparisons are made with standardized height and weight charts.

Development is more difficult to measure. Maturational changes in children and adults are best measured by combining observations with standardized developmental tests. Examples of standardized tests include the Denver Developmental Screening Test (DDST), and the Vineland Social Maturity Scale. The Denver Developmental Screening Test is used to assess the level of developmental maturity in infants and young children. The Vineland Social Maturity Scale is used to assess adaptive behaviors and social readiness in school-age children.

Nurses, with appropriate study, can administer such tests to gather data about developmental levels of children. These data are an important part of the assessment base needed to plan nursing interventions. This information, when combined with that gathered by psychometrists (test interpreters), developmentalists, or psychologists who are skilled in cognitive or neuromotor assessment, provides a measure of development.

Nursing students can best use developmental theory by first identifying a client's chronological age, and then comparing the chronological age with expected norms or standards that are demonstrated for that age group. For example, nursing students working for the first time with school-age children and their families can identify expected physical growth norms, ways that school-age children think (Piaget), and expected social skills (Erikson). Nurses with little previous experience with children can use this comparative information to complete a quick assessment of school-age children. For example, they should have a blood pressure of 120/80 (see Table 11–1); they are learning to follow rules (will remain NPO before blood is drawn); they are influenced by teachers and friends (will probably cooperate with nurses); they are able to problem solve (can understand an explanation of a procedure); and they derive feelings of competence from tasks completed (may proudly describe participation in the experience to a sibling).

Nursing students can validate specific behaviors observed in clients with those described in the sections for each age group within this chapter. In this way, the concepts of growth and development become real, dynamic, and useful to students in the practice of nursing. The application of principles and concepts of growth and development truly becomes a foundation for the process of nursing.

■ GROWTH AND DEVELOPMENT BEFORE BIRTH

All study of human growth and development begins at conception. The antepartal time is considered to be a critical period in the development of family roles and structure. It is a time of *family* growth and development.

The importance of both parents' involvement in a pregnancy is apparent if this period is recognized as the time during which individuals become parents by beginning to learn new roles in their interdependent relationship to each other and their expected child. Not only the mother is pregnant; the couple is pregnant in the sense that both parents are preparing for the child and adapting to their new situation. The father is an integral part of the pregnant couple during both pregnancy and the birth process, contributing emotional support and assistance in preparing for the delivery itself.

Positive attitudes toward pregnancy and childbirth are directly related to pregnant couples' prior experiences with relatives' and friends' pregnancies. Cultural expectations, maternal and paternal age and stage of maturity, maternal health status, family planning and desire for children, and presence of a secure marital relationship influence whether or not the pregnant couple can integrate the significant emotional and physiological changes of childbearing into their lives in a secure manner.

Prenatal Development

Embryonic Phase. The embryonic phase begins at the moment of conception as the sperm enters the cell membrane of the ovum and ends at about 8 weeks of gestation when all major organ systems are in early stages of development. The embryonic phase is a critical period of development. During this phase, massive cell proliferation occurs, during which all organs and sensory systems are rapidly developing and are sensitive to any traumatic influences such as infection, ingestion or inhalation of toxic chemicals, and radiation.

Fetal Phase. The fetal phase begins at about 8 weeks of gestation and lasts until birth occurs, generally at about 40 weeks of gestation. The fetal phase is a period of rapid cellular growth. During the first trimester (conception through the 12th week of pregnancy), fetal organ systems differentiate and begin to function. Late in the second trimester (the 13th week through the 24th week of pregnancy), the fetus moves with enough force that its movements can be felt by the mother. The major organ systems are now completely formed, but organ growth and tissue growth continue throughout the entire prenatal period. During the third trimester (the 25th week until the end of pregnancy), significant brain development occurs and the fetus gains most of its body weight. Subcutaneous fat is deposited, the skin becomes smooth, and moderate amounts of scalp hair cover the head.

Influences on Growth and Development Before Birth. Many influences contribute to the healthy growth and development of the fetus. These influences can be grouped into two primary categories, genetic and environmental. Factors in either category act alone and in combination to support both the formation and rapid enlargement of vital organs and the development of physiological systems to coordinate organ function. Normal healthy genes provide basic structural normality, and individual variations in traits such as hair, skin, and eye color. Unhealthy or damaged genes result in a wide range of structural and functional abnormalities, some of which are incompatible with life.

Environmental influences originate first in the woman carrying the child, for she is, in fact, the fetus' environment. Overall health at the time of conception and life-style choices throughout pregnancy strongly influence fetal well-being. Every environmental element to which the pregnant woman is exposed has the potential to affect the fetus. Positive elements, such as sound nutrition, moderate exercise, and minimal stress, support optimal fetal development. Conversely, exposure to infections (particularly viral infections), radiation, and chemicals may damage organs' structure and alter their function. "Chemical" is a broad ranging term. Although it includes environmental pollutants such as smog or pesticides, the chemicals that have the most significant capacity to cause fetal damage are those intentionally ingested by pregnant women. Alcohol, nicotine and all drugs, whether prescription medications or "street drugs" such as cocaine, marijuana, and methamphetamines, can alter fetal development. Many of the alterations are so significant that normal life is never possible for a fetus that is exposed. Moreover, even small amounts of these chemicals can cause significant damage. Experts emphasize that there is no such thing as a safe level of intake for nicotine, alcohol, cocaine and other such drugs during pregnancy.[8]

Prenatal Health Care

Prenatal health care is important to the health of both the fetus and its parents. Diseases from genetic and environmental causes or the consequences of these diseases may often be minimized by good prenatal care. Prevention, screening, early treatment, and the psychosocial support that are part of prenatal care may make a critical difference, not only to the health of parents and babies, but to the integrity of the family as well. Although experts unanimously agree on the importance of prenatal care, it is not uniformly available to all pregnant women in the United States. There are not enough programs for women without health insurance, and they are not always readily accessible to those in need. This is a public policy that nurses can actively work to change (see Chapter 4).

Community outreach programs and education in high schools emphasizing the importance of prenatal care to positive pregnancy outcomes are part of the health promotion role of nurses. If more women become aware of the importance of prenatal care and are motivated to seek it, society as a whole benefits.

Components of Prenatal Health Care. Ideally, prenatal care begins before pregnancy. Young women of childbearing age should be encouraged to begin a relationship with a primary health care provider to establish a trusting relationship conducive to health promotion. A health assessment conducted before pregnancy or early in pregnancy identifies potential hazards to the mother and fetus and provides the basis for health education to avoid or minimize associated risks.

Regular prenatal care should continue throughout pregnancy. It involves continuing risk assessment, health promotion, and health education. Experts advise evaluating fetal and maternal well-being approximately monthly until the last month of gestation, when they recommend weekly visits. Women experiencing any complications of pregnancy should visit their physician or midwife more frequently. These women often require additional screening for both maternal and fetal health problems and benefit from further supportive care.

Health teaching is ongoing throughout prenatal care. Although all health care providers share responsibility for health teaching, nurses are often able to recognize special needs for teaching and provide needed information or resources. Nurses and others also encourage women to seek preparation for childbirth classes. These classes provide basic information about normal physical and emotional changes during pregnancy, labor and delivery. Most also emphasize techniques to cope with labor pain. This kind of preparation alleviates considerable anxiety and facilitates couples' active participation in pregnancy and the birthing process.

Comprehensive prenatal care and education are important factors in healthy growth and development of the fetus, mother, couple, and family.

■ THE NEONATE (BIRTH TO 4 WEEKS OF AGE)

Physical Growth and Development

The typical healthy neonate has certain characteristics that are evident to physicians and nurses when they perform physical assessments of neonates as a basis for their respective plans of care. Characteristically, neonates, in adjusting to life outside the uterus, cry lustily, breathe rapidly and irregularly, have a fast pulse rate, have strong muscle tone so that when an extremity is moved away from the body it springs back to the flexed position, and withdraw from imposed stimulation. They have an even, pink color that varies somewhat with ethnic background.

The head of neonates appears large in relation to the rest of the body, the face is round with fat pads in the cheeks, and the lower jaw or mandible is small. The chest is cylindrical in shape, the abdomen is rounded and protuberant, and the extremities appear short in relation to the body (Fig. 11–1). Weight, length, and vital signs are important indicators of general well-being (see Table 11–1) as is head circumference, which averages 33–35 cm (13–14 in.) at

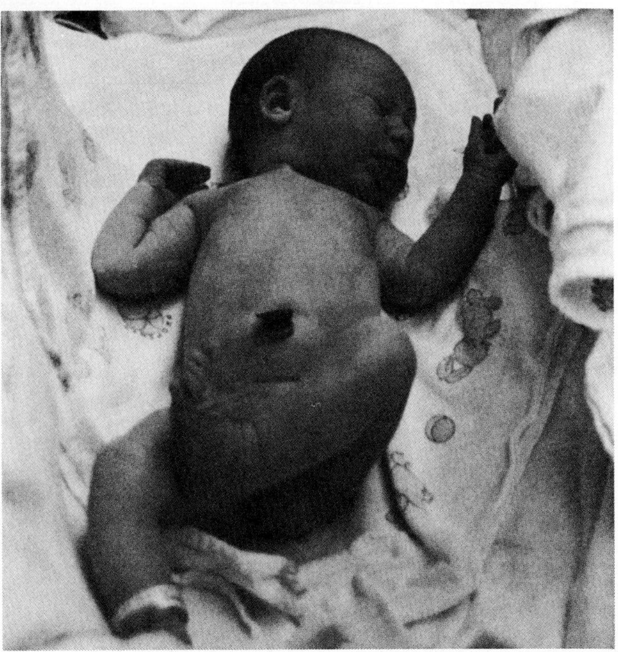

Figure 11–1. Physical characteristics of neonates. (*From Sherwen LN, Scoloveno MA, Weingarten CT.* Nursing Care of the Childbearing Family. *Norwalk, CT: Appleton & Lange; 1991.*)

birth.[9] Head-to-toe assessment for intact and symmetrical structures and functions, maturity level, and sensory motor evaluations is completed while protecting neonates from heat loss, which is a significant stressor and potential cause of pathology. Parents frequently ask for results of this examination and for an interpretation of the results. Nurses incorporate the results into a plan of care for the neonate and into the teaching plan for parents so they learn about and provide care for their neonates.

During the first 4 weeks of life, the neonate typically gains 5 to 7 oz each week and grows about 1 in. in length from the newborn measurement.

Psychosocial Development

It is not uncommon for parents to describe neonates as dependent and helpless. At the same time, they may comment on neonates' alertness, responsiveness to their voices, and strength in sucking and grasping. These comments indicate that parents recognize certain needs and capabilities within neonates. Nurses find such comments helpful in planning teaching for parents about care and development of their neonates.

Psychosocial Characteristics. Although each neonate is indeed unique, it is possible to describe the basic psychosocial characteristics of neonates. Neonates are vulnerable because they rely on others to meet their basic needs for nourishment, warmth, shelter, clothing, hygiene, and protection. The psychosocial behavior of neonates is partly a reflection of their growth and development. For example, they have little intentional control over their movements during the first weeks of life, and although they have the capacity to use their senses, their ability to differentiate stimuli is still limited.

Although neonates' communication modes are basic and generalized, neonates can be powerful communicators with others. Their primary means of expression include crying, looking, quieting, listening, and reflex activities such as grasping the finger of another person. Adults respond to these means of expression in positive ways that typically involve smiling, cuddling, soothing, and other caring behaviors.

As neonates rely on others to meet their needs, they also depend on others to interpret their expressions of these needs. Although it is true that neonates are vulnerable and dependent, they are also equipped to interact with others who can care for and nurture them so that they can grow and develop. Typically, near the end of the neonatal period, neonates are awake and alert for longer intervals of time during which they more intensely concentrate on caregivers. This maturation enhances the neonate and caregiver communication patterns. In addition, although adults must provide care for them, neonates are increasingly responsive and thus able ideally to receive and thrive on the care given. Though it is apparent that neonates depend on their parents or caregivers to meet their basic needs, the reverse is also true in that neonates increasingly reinforce nurturing behaviors of parents. An example is when parents soothe, through holding and talking, diapering, or feeding, a crying neonate who in turn quiets and visibly relaxes. Clearly, an interdependence exists between neonates and parents that serves to promote both the growth and development of neonates and the parents' development in the role of parent.

It should be noted that a change has occurred in the use of the term *parent*.[10] Once it was used only as a noun, meaning that people viewed themselves as being parents; today, it is used increasingly as a verb and people concentrate on learning to parent. Accepting the idea that parenting is a learned behavior means that nurturing activities do not automatically occur simply because people become parents, which is an idea that parents may find helpful to discuss. In addition, parents may need to learn that a healthy parent–neonate relationship is basic to healthy growth and development of neonates. Finally, parents may require assistance to understand that this relationship cannot remain static but, of necessity, will change and develop over time.

Neonate–Parent Attachment Behaviors. Attachment behaviors have been studied as part of psychosocial development for many years by researchers, beginning with Bowlby, a developmental psychologist.[11] **Attachment behaviors** are mutually responsive reactions and interactions between parents and child that indicate that the cues, that is, the behavioral requests to have needs met, given by one person are accurately interpreted and acted on by the other person.

Attachment is affected by health status of neonates and parents, by neonates' sensorimotor capabilities and responses, by sociocultural expectations, by parents' expectations and their economic and health resources, and by parents' abilities and willingness to determine the needs and cues of neonates.

Attachment is apparent when neonates and parents provide cues that stimulate appropriate responses from the other (Fig. 11–2). Nurses can assess attachment. For example, nurses can readily assess whether parents hold the neonate so that they have direct and sustained eye contact. Nurses then observe if the neonate responds by quieting and attending to parents' verbal and nonverbal communications.

Nurses should be knowledgeable about results from research conducted on attachment and the related areas of parenting. Some researchers assert that in the United States there is a focus on mother–infant attachment reflective of a cultural rather than a scientific theory of development that may restrict women in their choices of mothering styles.[12] Women receive many conflicting and cultural messages about the correct way to be mothers. Often, these messages do not correlate with the experiences of reality that women have.[13] There are many faces of motherhood and ways to be a mother that are affected by multiple forces such as the woman's personal history, social position, economic and social forces in her culture, health, quality of relationships with family and friends, and her children's characteristics.[14]

Cognitive Development. Emotional development is only one aspect of neonatal psychosocial development. According to Piaget, neonates' cognitive development is primarily sensorimotor.[15] That is, neonates are active participants in learning through their senses and through motor activities, which progress from reflexive behaviors such as sucking and grasping to purposeful activities fairly rapidly. These cognitive processes are discussed more fully in the section on the infant.

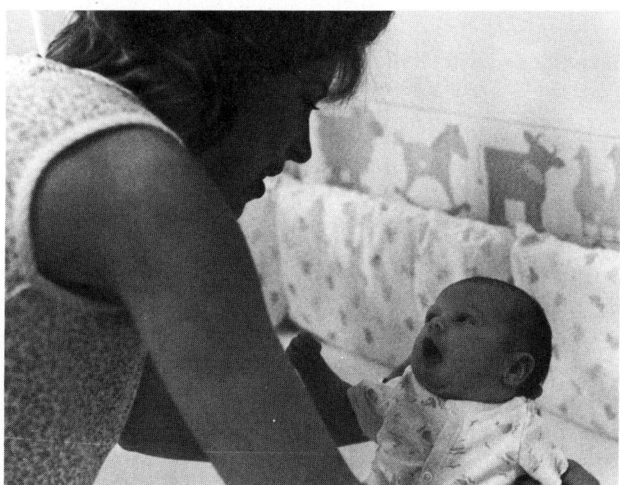

Figure 11–2. Parent–neonate attachment. (*From Sherwen LN, Scoloveno MA, Weingarten CT:* Nursing Care of the Childbearing Family. *Norwalk, CT: Appleton and Lange; 1991.*)

Wellness Promotion

Nurses have many opportunities to teach and guide parents in promoting wellness and health in their neonates. The Committee on Practice and Ambulatory Medicine in consultation with the American Academy of Pediatrics (1988)[16] recommends that children be given regular and comprehensive care beginning with a prenatal visit and continuing after birth of the neonates. Assessments include health history; length, weight, and head circumference; screening of vision and hearing; developmental and physical assessment; metabolic screening (dictated by state laws); and parental counseling.

Common Health Problems and Responses of Neonates to Illness

Health problems that commonly affect neonates include colic, diaper rash, and thrush. Regurgitation of feedings may also occur.

Colic. Approximately 10 to 20 percent of neonates will experience colic, beginning in the first 2 to 3 weeks of life.[17] Parents may express concern about their neonates having a fussy period without reason every day. Colic is characterized by periods of extreme fussiness, irritability, and crying. The occurrence of colic may be associated with gastrointestinal abnormalities or food allergies, but is rarely associated with a specific cause.

Nurses need to learn how parents define the situation, what they have tried to alleviate the problem, the factors that aggravate it, and the advice they have received from their physician or primary care provider. Parents may need assistance with feeding and calming techniques. Episodes of colic decrease as the neonate grows older and this problem rarely demands specific medical treatment.

Diaper Rash. Diaper rash, an irritation and breakdown of the skin caused by wetness, urine, or stool in the diaper, is another common health problem of neonates. It is important to know how cloth diapers are washed or, if disposable diapers are used, whether different brands seem to make a difference. Keeping the diaper area clean and as dry as possible is important, and exposing the area to air is also helpful. Also, ointments or creams, such as zinc oxide and vitamin A and D ointment, are sometimes useful. If these measures are not successful, parents should seek consultation with their health care provider, as cases lasting longer than 4 days are usually caused by *Candida albicans*.[18]

Thrush. Some neonates develop thrush, a fungal infection caused by the *Candida albicans* organism, which can affect the oral mucosa or the diaper area. In the mouth, thrush manifests as white patchy lesions and has the appearance of milk coating the mucous membranes and tongue. In the diaper area, the anus and surrounding skin develop beefy red lesions, which may bleed as the skin continues to break down.[18] Thrush requires medical treatment.

Regurgitation. Parents may comment that the neonate seems to "spit up" after feedings. It is important to obtain an accurate description of the type, amount, timing, and duration of this problem. In addition, nurses should assess for the pattern of weight gain by the neonate and the feeding methods used, including when and how the parents burp the neonate and with what success. Depending on the outcome of this assessment, nurses may be able to teach or guide the parents in feeding and burping, or may find it necessary to refer the parents to their primary health care provider.

Responses of Neonates to Illness. Parents need to learn that neonates show a generalized rather than a specific reaction to illness because their development is immature. They may express illness either by being quieter and less responsive than usual or by being more irritable. Responses depend in part on the specific illness.

Responsibilities for Client Care

Care of neonates includes performing ongoing assessments, collaborating with parents in making decisions about care of the neonates, meeting basic needs of neonates, and evaluating effectiveness of actions taken.

Assess Parents' Knowledge and Skills. When collaborating with parents of neonates, nurses first need to assess parents' knowledge, skill, and capacity to understand neonatal behaviors. Nurses can include parents in the assessment of their neonates by pointing out expected physical characteristics and psychosocial behaviors, clarifying and interpreting information about the assessment, supporting them in learning how to understand and meet the needs of their neonates, and facilitating parent–infant attachment and their development as parents (Fig. 11–3). To accomplish these responsibilities nurses can use specific activities such as demonstrating care techniques, discussing expected developmental milestones, encouraging parents to ask questions, and reassuring parents that their child care skills are progressing well.

Review Neonatal Physical Characteristics With Parents. Parents may benefit by reviewing the following points about neonates:

- Neonates tend to lose 5 to 10 percent of their body weight in the first days after birth, but typically regain it by 10 to 14 days of life. They usually need to be fed every 2 to 4 hours in the first days of life.
- Neonates need regular daily care schedules such as sleep and feeding schedules.
- The urine initially eliminated is dilute because neonates cannot concentrate urine well for the first 2 weeks, and only gradually develop that ability during the first year of life. Diapers may have a pink stain related to the urates in the urine.
- Bowel elimination usually begins within the first 24 hours of birth. The first stool is black-green and consists of amniotic fluid, cells, and intestinal juices.[9]

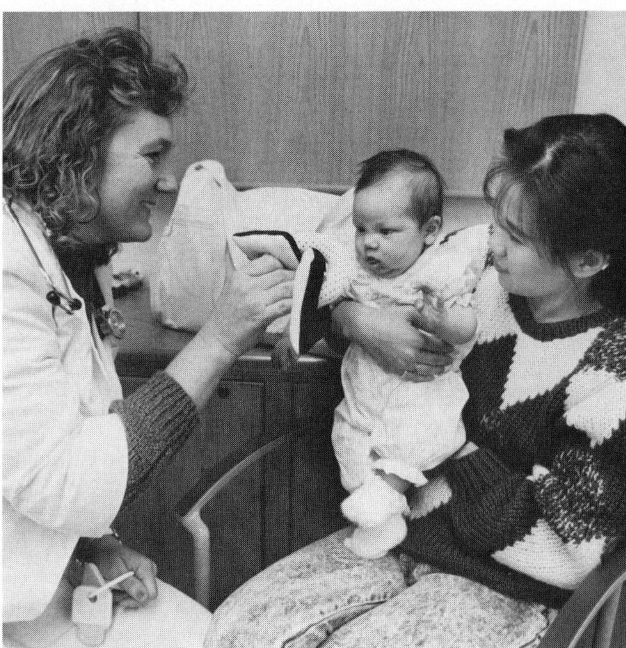

Figure 11–3. Nurse interacting with parents and neonates.

- Breast-fed neonates tend to have stools more frequently than those who are bottle-fed. Neonates often eliminate stools after their feedings, but not all neonates have daily stools. Stool color and consistency can vary, depending on many factors. Foul-smelling, greasy, bulky, or mucus-containing stools should not be considered normal.
- Neonates have characteristic "soft spots" or fontanelles on their skulls. Parents may ask questions about these places where the cranial bones have not yet fused. The anterior fontanelle usually closes by 18 months and the posterior fontanelle closes by 2 to 4 months. In some newborns, the posterior fontanelle may be only the size of a fingertip. Parents should be encouraged to touch the fontanelle so that they are comfortable in washing the neonate's scalp during the bath.

Finally, nurses can respond to parents' concerns about whether their neonates are healthy and normal.

Teach Parents About Neonates' Basic Needs. Teaching and guiding parents to meet basic needs of neonates focuses on feeding neonates when they are hungry; rocking, singing, and talking gently to soothe and quiet them; protecting them from infections; maintaining body temperature within normal ranges; providing a balance between stimulation and quiet time; accepting neonates as unique beings with specific sleep, eating, elimination, and communication patterns; and promoting safety.

Teach Hygiene and Safety Skills. Nurses should teach parents to prevent infection in neonates by using good handwashing techniques and by performing correct hygiene for eyes, umbilical cord, skin, scalp, and anal-genital areas. Nurses can teach parents to promote safety by instructing them to use correct temperatures for bathing, to prevent chilling during and after bathing, to use firm, supportive mattresses, to avoid placing a pacifier on a cord around the neonate's neck, to use only approved pacifiers, to place a hand on neonates whenever they are on an elevated surface without siderails, to use siderails in the crib, to keep the nares clear of mucus, to cover neonates so that blankets do not interfere with breathing, to maintain body temperature, and to position neonates on the right side after feedings.

Reinforce Parenting Skills. Many parents may express concern about whether they are good parents. Nurses need to assess how parents define the phrase "good parent" and then help them set realistic expectations for themselves and their neonates. Nurses can also validate when parents function in the expected and desired manner.

Nurses should suggest that the parents help and encourage one another as they are learning and becoming comfortable with their parental responsibilities. Eventually parents should perceive responses from the neonates that help them feel confident in their ability to care for their neonate. Parents should be encouraged to enjoy their neonates in addition to taking seriously their responsibility to care for them, because it can be a challenge to achieve and maintain a balanced perspective on the responsibilities of being parents.

THE INFANT (1 TO 12 MONTHS OF AGE)

Physical Growth and Development

Physical growth and development continue to be of major importance during infancy and, in fact, progress more rapidly during this period than at any other time. Nurses find that parents of infants are receptive to learning about the rapidly changing physical growth and development (see Table 11–1, and Figs. 11–4 through 11–7) and appreciate having these complex relationships pointed out.

Many parents find comfort in knowing that their infant's physical development is within normal limits. Nurses can share with them the following characteristics of an infant.

During the first year, infants develop increasingly greater motor control that follows a cephalocaudal and proximodistal pattern. They gain head control by 3 months, trunk control by 6 months, and leg control by 9 months. They achieve eye–hand coordination so that they can reach for and hold objects by approximately 6 months of age. They roll over from prone to supine then supine to prone positions at 6 months. By 7 months they sit alone, and by 12 months gradually learn to walk. The ability to control the large muscle groups necessary for these movements is referred to as **gross motor control.**

Fine motor control refers to coordination of small mus-

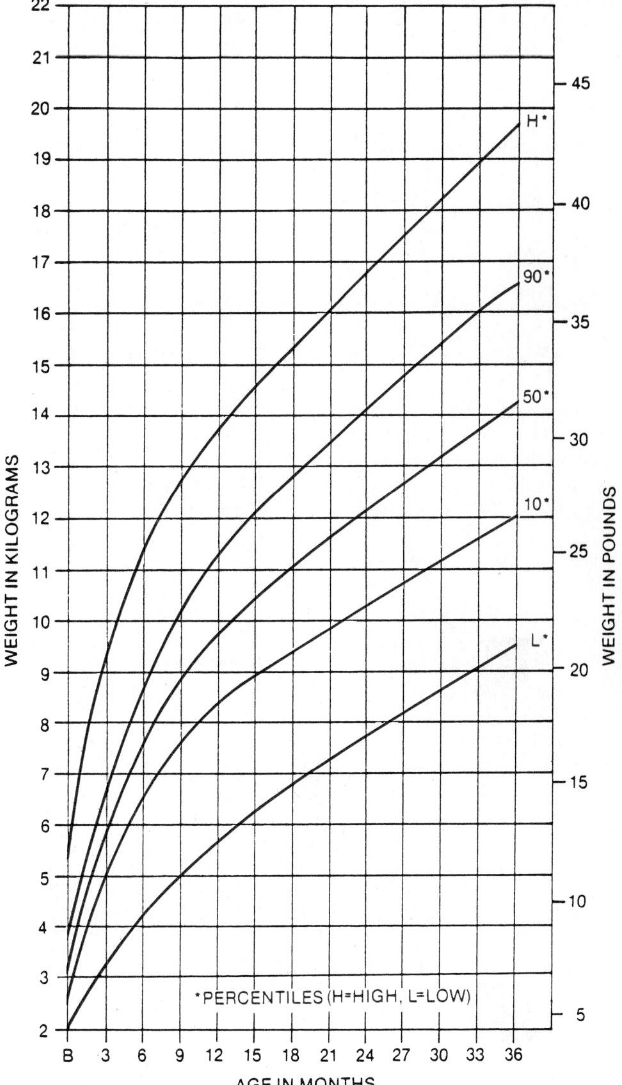

Figure 11–4. Weight-by-age percentiles for girls, ages birth to 36 months, including highest and lowest values at each age. (*From Pomerance HH.* Growth Standards in Children. *New York: Harper and Row; 1979:26.*)

cle groups so that delicate, subtle, and precise motor activities are possible. Eye–hand coordination and fine motor control permit infants to gradually refine arm, hand, and finger movements. This enables infants, by approximately 9 months, to use their thumbs and index fingers in a pincer grasp to pick up small objects such as pieces of cereal.

Psychosocial Development

Psychosocial development in infants involves all of the major aspects of development vital to maturation in later stages: emotional, cognitive, moral.

Emotional and Social Development. Emotional development involves the continuation of establishing trust versus mistrust that was begun in the neonatal period.

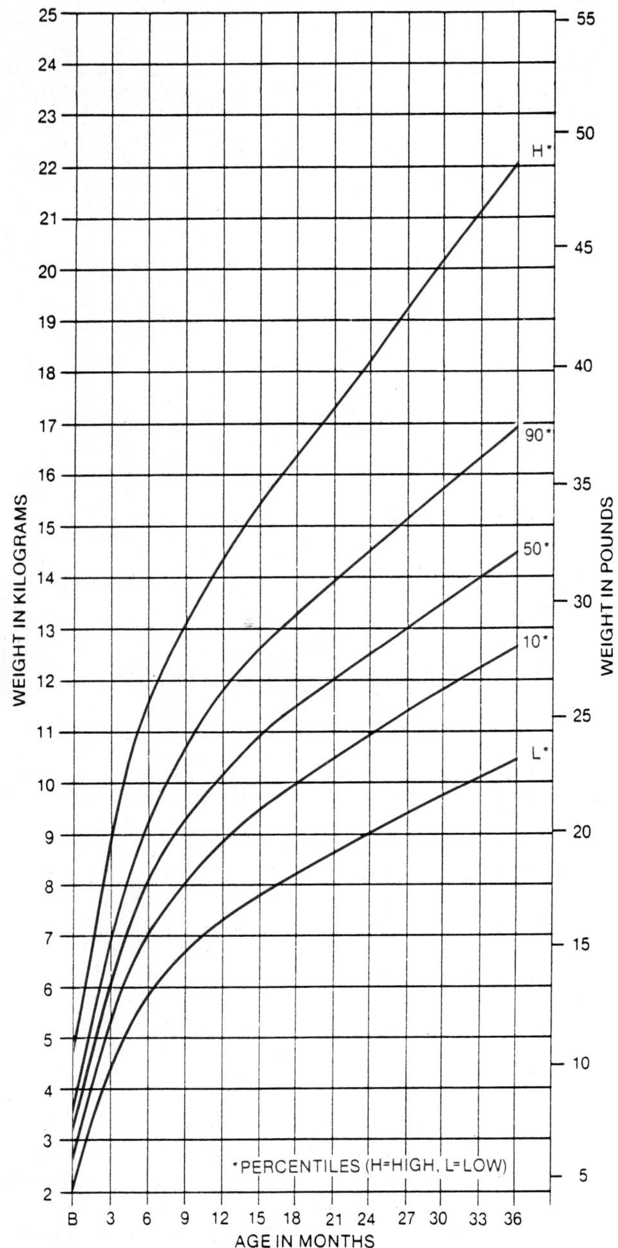

Figure 11–5. Weight-by-age percentiles for boys, ages birth to 36 months, including highest and lowest values at each age. (*From Pomerance HH.* Growth Standards in Children. *New York: Harper and Row; 1979: 25.*)

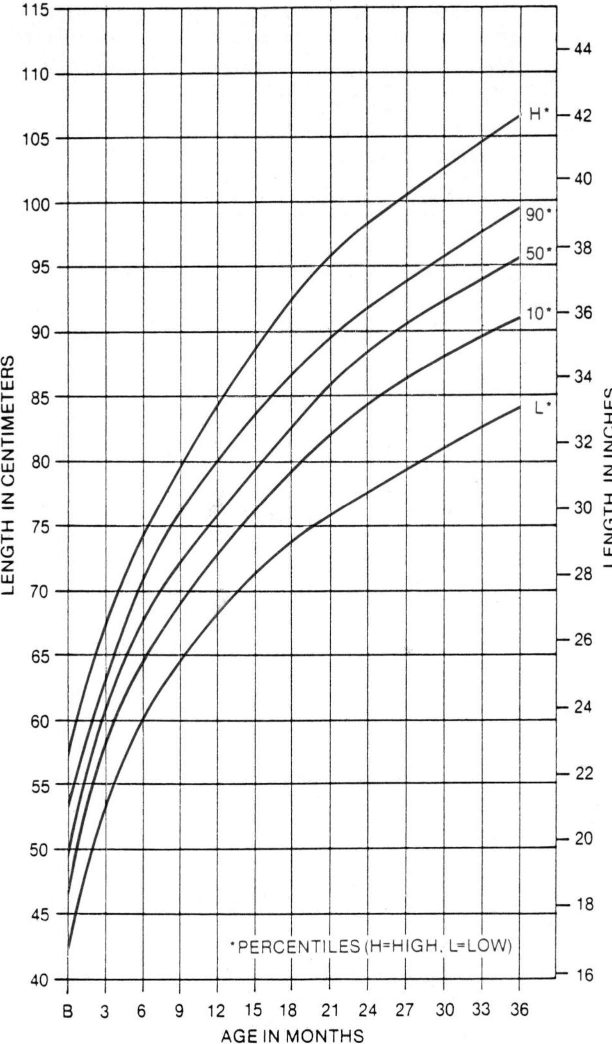

Figure 11–6. Length-by-age percentiles for girls, ages birth to 36 months, including highest and lowest values at each age. (*From Pomerance HH.* Growth Standards in Children. *New York: Harper and Row; 1979:30.*)

Infants who develop a pattern of trust will sleep, play, or become quiet after their needs are met in a timely manner. Such infants seem to "relax" as if to say, "I know that my parents take good care of me." Infants thrive on this care and the parents thrive on the infants' responses to them and the care they give. Parents learn to trust that their infants will express their needs and then respond in a predictable way once the needs are met.

Erikson suggests that it is desirable for infants to develop a pattern of trust versus mistrust, and that both trust and mistrust can serve a protective function.[4] For example, parents do not allow strangers to provide care for their infant until they learn that they can trust the person to provide care. One way of thinking about mistrust is that it *can* indicate that the individual is making thoughtful judgments about people and situations that might represent danger.

Another major concept in emotional development of infants is sexuality and body image. Infants are aware of their bodies as evidenced by apparent enjoyment in sucking their thumb, fingers, hands, or toes. They also play with their hands, feet, and genitalia. They smile at their image in a mirror and they put everything into their

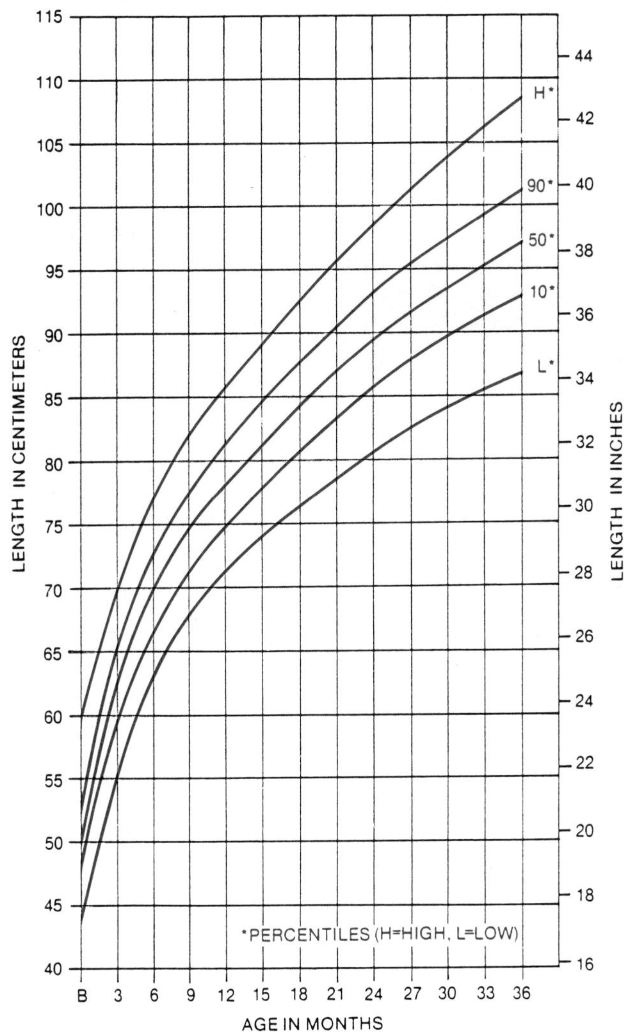

Figure 11–7. Length-by-age percentiles for boys, ages birth to 36 months, including highest and lowest values at each age. (*From Pomerance HH.* Growth Standards in Children. *New York: Harper and Row; 1979:29.*)

mouths. Parents may need to be informed that all of these actions are normal aspects of development and the beginning of self-concept.

Social interactions are another important aspect of emotional development. Infants play games with others such as peek-a-boo and patty cake (Fig. 11–8). They begin to babble and coo at approximately 1 month of age and progress to speaking words such as "da da," "ma ma," and "bye bye," which are ways in which they can interact with others. Smiling, laughing, waving, and reaching out to others are methods by which they interact in a purposeful way. They respond to and sometimes verbalize the word "no." They respond to adults' emotions, and may hug or kiss on command. They imitate sounds, facial expressions, and actions of others. By 7 to 9 months, infants have a greater awareness of self as separate from mother or father. This is called **individuation.** They may cry when separated from them or when approached by "strangers." Self-esteem is developed through both physical activities and the reactions that others have toward infants.

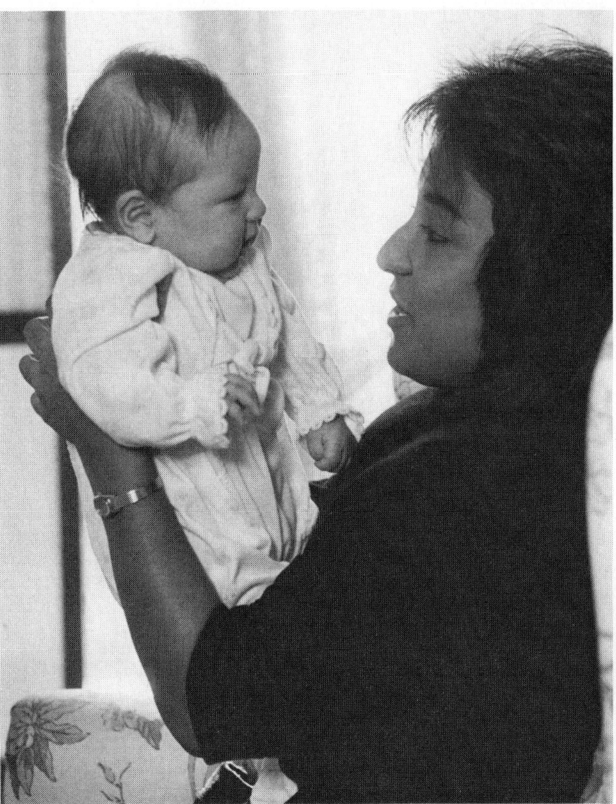

Figure 11–8. As part of their emotional and social development, infants interact with others in many ways.

Cognitive Development. Cognitive abilities continue to develop as infants grow and are exhibited in an increasing ability to concentrate and to recognize and respond to a friendly person or familiar environment. Infants learn about their world through their senses. They can anticipate feedings and going "bye bye" and may become excited when they see their parents, their bottle, or outdoor clothing. They may show fear of strangers, which is related to both cognitive and emotional development. They begin to learn **object permanence** (the awareness that unseen objects do not disappear) as evidenced by searching for objects even when they are out of sight. They demonstrate understanding of the words, behaviors, and expressions of others by their response. Their play activities are an important way of developing their cognitive, emotional, and physical capabilities, all of which give them increasing control over their environment.

Moral Development. Moral development, according to Kohlberg, is not evident until 2 years of age[6]; however, even an infant learns that some actions are approved by adults and others are not permitted.

Wellness Promotion

Wellness promotion guidelines are provided for infants by the Committee on Practice and Ambulatory Medicine and the American Academy of Pediatrics (1988)[16] (Fig. 11–9), who recommend history, physical, length, weight, head circumference, developmental/behavioral assessment, vision and hearing screening, anticipatory guidance of parents, and immunizations at 2, 4, and 6 months. Urinalysis is conducted at 6 months, and hemoglobin and hematocrit are assessed at 9 months, although there is some question about the need to run these tests more often. Tuberculin testing is recommended at 12 months.

Immunization schedules are published by the American Academy of Pediatrics[16] and are generally used as the standard recommendation. Parents need to understand the necessity of having their infants immunized fully (refer to Table 11–2).

Common Health Problems and Responses of Infants to Illness

Factors Causing Infant Illness. Whether infants die or are at risk for further health problems is related to specific factors. Factors that cause illness in infants include, but are not limited to, low birth weight, lack of prenatal care, teenage pregnancy, and poverty.[19, 20]

Infection and Communicable Disease. Infants may experience a variety of infections of the ears, upper respiratory tract, and gastrointestinal tract. Infants who do not receive immunizations or who are incompletely immunized are at risk for the acute illnesses and long-term complications from the health problems the immunizations are intended to prevent.

Accidents. Accidental deaths occur more often in infants than in any other age group.[20] Accidental injuries occur from falls, especially those involving infants who roll off surfaces without rails or sides. The National Safety Council reported that one of the four main causes of non-motor vehicle deaths in 1986 was falls.[21] Aspiration of small objects, including defective pacifiers, and crib rails that permit an infant's head to become wedged are other potential problems.

Anemia. Iron deficiency anemia is considered one of the most common nutritional problems of infancy, especially for infants living in poverty, according to data from the National Health and Nutrition Examination Survey, 1976–1980.[20] There is some evidence, however, that the incidence of iron deficiency anemia is decreasing. This may be due, in part, to improvement in feeding iron-fortified formula to infants who are not breast-fed and who are enrolled in the Special Supplemental Food Program for Women, Infants, and Children (WIC).[22]

Responses of Infants to Illness. Infants may well change their movement or activity level when ill. For example, infants may lie very quietly or may show greater activity when they have an elevated temperature, or they may protect ("splint") a body part that causes pain. Infants often give a generalized body response to illness, sometimes because they cannot yet localize the source of the illness. For example, infants with an infection either of the respiratory tract or of the urinary tract may change their feeding behaviors in response to pain and feeling of tiredness.

Infants also show generalized responses to illness because they lack the capacity to completely comfort (cure) themselves and so cry and fuss in an effort to receive attention and care. In this way infants indicate to parents or caregivers that they are needy, and also, as they quiet when appropriate care is rendered, that parental interventions were effective.

Responsibilities for Client Care

Nurses are in an excellent position to collaborate with parents of infants who have any of the common infant health problems. For instance, nurses can assist parents to learn to take cues from their infants so they begin to include *them* in the process. Even though infants have limited ability to participate because of immature development and lack of life experiences, nonetheless they can and do give cues to caregivers about their needs.

Nurses should assess what parents know and if they correctly understand the particular knowledge about infant growth and development that they will need to care for their infant. In doing this, nurses determine what the parents consider to be priority issues or topics to address during their interactions.

Provide Nutritional Information. Parents may be told that infants vary in the amount and number of feedings needed, but as a general rule of thumb, they consume 4+ oz. six times a day at 1 month, gradually increasing to 6 or 7 oz. four times a day at 5 months. Solid foods may be started at about 6 months, beginning with single-grain infant cereals and then slowly adding strained or pureed infant foods one at a time, avoiding foods that tend to cause allergic responses until later. It is wise for parents to seek specific guidance from qualified professionals on the subject of infant feeding.

Promote Parents' Understanding of Feeding Behavior. Teaching parents about infants, rooting, sucking, swallowing, and extrusion reflexes and their effects on feeding is important. The rooting reflex, the reflex by which infants turn their head toward a sensory stimulus to the cheek, enables infants to "search" for the nipple. Sucking and swallowing reflexes enable infants to safely ingest fluids from breast or bottle. Parents may feel less concerned about infants pushing the spoon of cereal out of their mouths, a manifestation of the extrusion reflex, if they understand that the tongue functions in a reflex manner and infants do not necessarily do this on purpose.

RECOMMENDATIONS FOR PREVENTIVE PEDIATRIC HEALTH CARE

Committee on Practice and Ambulatory Medicine

Each child and family is unique: therefore these Recommendations for Preventive Pediatric Health Care are designed for the care of children who are receiving competent parenting, have no manifestations of any important health problems, and are growing and developing in satisfactory fashion. Additional visits may become necessary if circumstances suggest variations from normal. These guidelines represent a consensus by the Committee on Practice and Ambulatory Medicine in consultation with the membership of the American Academy of Pediatrics through the Chapter Presidents. The Committee emphasizes the great importance of continuity of care in comprehensive health supervision and the need to avoid fragmentation of care.

A prenatal visit by the parents for anticipatory guidance and pertinent medical history is strongly recommended.

Health supervision should begin with medical care of the newborn in the hospital.

	INFANCY						EARLY CHILDHOOD					LATE CHILDHOOD					ADOLESCENCE[1]			
AGE[2]	By 1 mo	2 mos	4 mos	6 mos	9 mos	12 mos	15 mos	18 mos	24 mos	3 yrs.	4 yrs.	5 yrs.	6 yrs.	8 yrs.	10 yrs.	12 yrs.	14 yrs.	16 yrs.	18 yrs.	20+ yrs.
HISTORY Initial/Interval	•	•	•	•	•	•	•	•	•	•	•	•	•	•	•	•	•	•	•	•
MEASUREMENTS Height and Weight	•	•	•	•	•	•	•	•	•	•	•	•	•	•	•	•	•	•	•	•
Head Circumference	•	•	•	•	•	•														
Blood Pressure										•	•	•	•	•	•	•	•	•	•	•
SENSORY SCREENING Vision	S	S	S	S	S	S	S	S	S	S	O	O	O	O	S	O	O	S	O	O
Hearing	S	S	S	S	S	S	S	S	S	S	O	O	S[3]	S[3]	S[3]	O	S	S	O	S
DEVEL./BEHAV.[4] ASSESSMENT	•	•	•	•	•	•	•	•	•	•	•	•	•	•	•	•	•	•	•	•
PHYSICAL EXAMINATION[5]	•	•	•	•	•	•	•	•	•	•	•	•	•	•	•	•	•	•	•	•
PROCEDURES[6] Hered./Metabolic[7] Screening	•																			
Immunization[8]		•	•	•			•	•	•			•					•			
Tuberculin Test[9]	←					•→	←		•		→						←		•	→
Hematocrit or Hemoglobin[10]	←				•	→	←		•		→	←		•		→	←		•	→
Urinalysis[11]	←			•		→	←		•		→	←		•		→	←		•	→
ANTICIPATORY[12] GUIDANCE	•	•	•	•	•	•	•	•	•	•	•	•	•	•	•	•	•	•	•	•
INITIAL DENTAL[13] REFERRAL										•										

1. Adolescent related issues (e.g., psychosocial, emotional, substance usage, and reproductive health) may necessitate more frequent health supervision.
2. If a child comes under care for the first time at any point on the schedule, or if any items are not accomplished at the suggested age, the schedule should be brought up to date at the earliest possible time.
3. At these points, history may suffice: if problem suggested, a standard testing method should be employed.
4. By history and appropriate physical examination: if suspicious, by specific objective developmental testing.
5. At each visit, a complete physical examination is essential, with infant totally unclothed, older child undressed and suitably draped.
6. These may be modified, depending upon entry point into schedule and individual need.
7. Metabolic screening (e.g., thyroid, PKU, galactosemia) should be done according to state law.
8. Schedule(s) per Report of Committee on Infectious Disease, *1986 Red Book.*
9. For low risk groups, the Committee on Infectious Disease recommends the following options: ① no routine testing or ② testing at three times—infancy, preschool, and adolescence. For high risk groups, annual TB skin testing is recommended.
10. Present medical evidence suggests the need for reevaluation of the frequency and timing of hemoglobin or hematocrit tests. One determination is therefore suggested during each time period. Performance of additional tests is left to the individual practice experience.
11. Present medical evidence suggests the need for reevaluation of the frequency and timing of urinalyses. One determination is therefore suggested during each time period. Performance of additional tests is left to the individual practice experience.
12. Appropriate discussion and counseling should be an integral part of each visit for care.
13. Subsequent examinations as prescribed by dentist.

N.B.: Special chemical, immunologic, and endocrine testing are usually carried out upon specific indications. Testing other than newborn (e.g., inborn errors of metabolism, sickle disease, lead) are discretionary with the physician.

Key: • = to be performed: S = subjective, by history: O = objective, by a standard testing method.

Figure 11–9. Wellness promotion guidelines. (*From Committee on Practice and Ambulatory Medicine. Recommendations for preventive pediatric health care.* Pediatrics. *March 1988; 81(3.)*

TABLE 11–2. RECOMMENDED SCHEDULE FOR IMMUNIZATION OF HEALTHY INFANTS AND CHILDREN[a]

Recommended Age[b]	Immunizations[c]	Comments
2 months	DTP, HbCV,[d] OPV	DTP and OPV can be initiated as early as 4 weeks after birth in areas of high endemicity or during epidemics
4 months	DTP, HbCV,[d] OPV	2-month interval (minimum of 6 weeks) desired for OPV to avoid interference from previous dose
6 months	DTP, HbCV[d]	Third dose of OPV is not indicated in the U.S. but is desirable in other geographic areas where polio is endemic
15 months	MMR,[e] HbCV[f]	Tuberculin testing may be done at the same visit
15–18 months	DTP,[g,h] OPV[i]	(See footnotes)
4–6 years	DTP,[j] OPV	At or before school entry
11–12 years	MMR	At entry to middle school or junior high school unless second dose previously given
14–16 years	Td	Repeat every 10 years throughout life

[a] For all products used, consult manufacturer's package insert for instructions for storage, handling, dosage, and administration. Biologics prepared by different manufacturers may vary, and package inserts of the same manufacturer may change from time to time. Therefore, the physician should be aware of the contents of the current package insert.
[b] These recommended ages should not be construed as absolute. For example, 2 months can be 6 to 10 weeks. However, MMR usually should not be given to children younger than 12 months. (If measles vaccination is indicated, monovalent measles vaccine is recommended, and MMR should be given subsequently, at 15 months.)
[c] DTP = diphtheria and tetanus toxoids with pertussis vaccine; HbCV = *Haemophilus* b conjugate vaccine; OPV = oral poliovirus vaccine containing attenuated poliovirus types 1, 2, and 3; MMR = live measles, mumps, and rubella viruses in a combined vaccine; Td = adult tetanus toxoid (full dose) and diphtheria toxoid (reduced dose) for adult use.
[d] As of October 1990, only one HbCV (HbOC) is approved for use in children younger than 15 months.
[e] May be given at 12 months of age in areas with recurrent measles transmission.
[f] Any licensed *Haemophilus* b conjugate vaccine may be given.
[g] Should be given 6 to 12 months after the third dose.
[h] May be given simultaneously with MMR at 15 months.
[i] May be given simultaneously with MMR and HbCV at 15 months or at any time between 12 and 24 months; priority should be given to administering MMR at the recommended age.
[j] Can be given up to the seventh birthday.
Reprinted with permission from the Academy of Pediatrics, Committee on Infectious Diseases. Report of the Committee on Infectious Diseases, 1991. *22nd ed. Elk Grove Village, IL: American Academy of Pediatrics; 1991; 17.*

Infants actually have to learn to eat food, whereas normally they can coordinate sucking and swallowing as they drink fluids.

Some parents are concerned about colic in infants. The approaches identified in the earlier discussion of neonatal colic are effective until colic is outgrown, usually around age 3 months.[9]

Assist Parents to Cope with Infants' Growing Independence. By the end of infancy, infants demonstrate beginning signs of autonomous behavior that parents find challenging. Nurses can assist them to view this behavior as a positive sign of normal development and to find ways to cope successfully with it such as creating a safe play area in which infants can be free to explore freely while still under close visual supervision.

Provide Safety Information. Safety promotion and accident prevention are important in care of infants. Teaching should be based on the physical capabilities of the infant, always anticipating that infants will rapidly acquire new skills. Infants are most at risk for accidents from falls once they can roll over. Thus, parents should develop the habit of always placing one hand on their infant to prevent the infant from rolling when it is being dressed or diapered. Safety during bath time is another area for teaching, in relation to possible drowning, hot water burns, chills, or falls. When infants begin to walk, actions to child-proof the house, such as removing breakables from low tables, securing stairs with safety gates, installing latching devices on cabinets, and plugging unused outlets become increasingly important.

Encourage Parents to Promote Play. Preparing for the changing stimulation and play needs of infants and for their planned quiet time are other topics that parents may wish to discuss. Parents can be assisted to promote normal development of their infants by their choice of play materials and activities and their planned interactions with them. A variety of visual, auditory, tactile, and kinesthetic stimulation in early infancy promotes optimal development.

Assist Parents to Cope With Ill Infants' Needs. Nurses can assist parents to learn how to interpret the various cries of infants—cries that express hunger, tiredness, excessive heat or excessive cold, overstimulation, and discomfort or pain. Parents can learn to also observe the movements of infants and to note that these too are related to feeling states and that infants will show a change in their activity level when ill. Parents, with the assistance of nurses, can learn the significance of behavior as well as behavior changes in their infants.

Nurses can teach parents a systematic problem-solving method to use to gather information about their infants' health. Parents should be taught to consider infants' current behaviors; specific symptoms; severity and duration of symptoms; measures implemented and their outcomes; allergies; factors that aggravate or alleviate the condition; and infants' behaviors in this illness compared with behaviors during wellness. Parents' observations can be written and then shared logically and quickly with a primary health care provider. In teaching parents how to use this problem-solving approach, nurses provide them with a concrete, positive, and systematic way to respond to illness or injury of infants. If parents apply this method at the first sign of illness or injury, they will have a greater sense of control over the situation. In addition, nurses can guide them to understand that infants often develop signs and symptoms of illnesses quickly. Parents should therefore be counseled to act calmly and systematically to observe and then to communicate promptly facts and impressions they have of their ill infant.

Anticipatory guidance can be used with parents to help

them share feelings of fear, worry, inadequacy, and guilt about the illness of an infant. It is constructive for parents to express these feelings to one another as a way of coping, because infants frequently respond not only to the sensations associated with illness but also to their parents' expressions of their feelings. It is not helpful to an ill infant to have parents who cannot cope.

Nurses can use other areas of specialized knowledge to assist parents in responding to their ill infant. As infants may experience separation anxiety, it is helpful for one of the parents to stay with the ill infant, if hospitalization is required. Infants prefer the comfort and security of familiar people and objects, so parents should be prepared to offer them a favorite toy to hold rather than purchase a new toy. Spending additional time with infants during illness can be important to parents as they implement and observe the response to prescribed treatment. It can be a challenge for parents to get an infant to take medicines and parents may appreciate nursing assistance or teaching. (The reader should refer to a pediatric nursing textbook for suggested approaches.)

Parents need to understand the effects of the prescribed treatment and the information about their infant's illness so that they can fully participate in giving care to the infant, especially when hospitalization is not required. Parents also need to know when to seek additional assistance from their health care provider. Parents may notice that ill infants seem to lose some of their recently learned skills, and may seem to regress developmentally. Both of these responses to illness are normal, and generally will pass once the infant recovers and again has energy and interest, and is able to return to daily activities.

Finally, when the parents successfully cope with their infant's illness, they should evaluate how and why they were successful in coping so that they provide their own positive reinforcement. This process encourages them to develop a sense of themselves as competent parents. In turn, when parents trust themselves as being competent in meeting their infant's needs in illness and in wellness, the infant's sense of trust in them is increased.

■ THE TODDLER (1 TO 3 YEARS OF AGE)

Physical Growth and Development

Toddlers leave the relative dependence of infancy and move toward the increasing independence of childhood. Their major tasks during this stage are to further develop and refine skills learned during the first year of life, such as walking and talking and feeding themselves. These skills make it possible for toddlers to achieve an increasing independence.

The term *toddler* is an appropriate descriptive term that characterizes the pattern of locomotion of children in this age group. They tend to toddle with their feet planted several inches apart and their arms held out to help maintain balance. Being able to walk is an important milestone for toddlers because it enhances their autonomy by underscoring the sense of being a unique person who is separate from mother and father. Toddling is adaptive. By toddling, and later by walking, it becomes possible for children to explore the immediate environment without having to rely solely on someone else to bring objects, people, and experiences to them. The act of walking and exploring enhances cognitive development because toddlers can experiment with and manipulate their environment. There is an obvious interdependence among their physical and psychosocial growth and development.

The physical appearance of toddlers is quite different from that of infants. Infants have a relatively long body trunk and shorter extremities, whereas toddlers' legs begin to lengthen and often appear to be bowed (Fig. 11–10). Toddlers' head circumference increases by about 2 cm per year (average at 1 year is 46 cm.)[9] The chest and head circumferences are nearly equal. The abdomen continues to be prominent as it was in infancy, but toddlers' appetite changes and their weight gain slows (see Table 11–1, and Figs. 11–4 through 11–7).

Near the end of the second year, but frequently not until the end of the third year, toddlers learn bowel and bladder

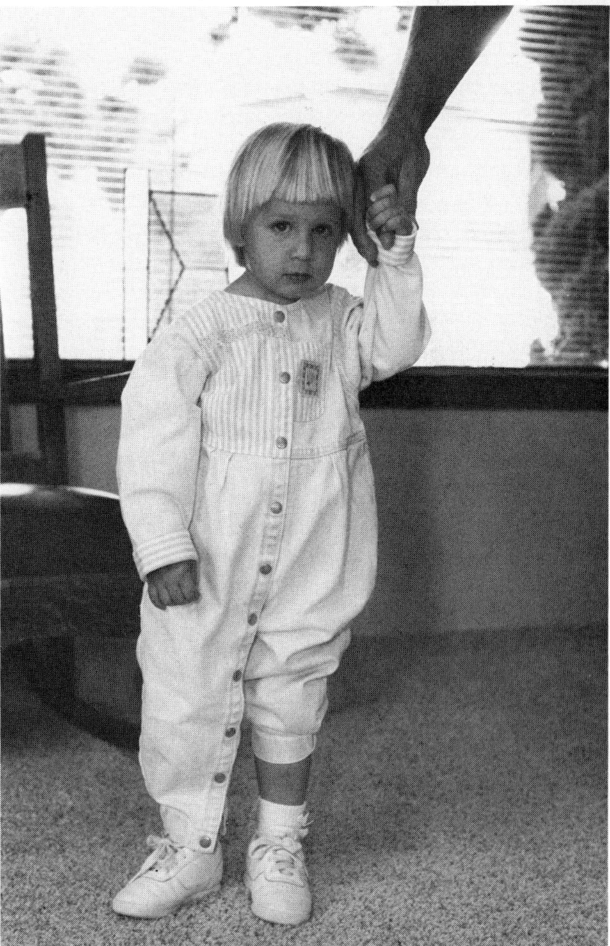

Figure 11–10. Physical characteristics of toddlers.

control. Two-year-olds can walk alone, run, climb up and down stairs, jump, throw a ball overhand, assist with dressing by removing clothing and dressing with assistance, build a four- to eight-cube tower, scribble, and dump objects from a container.[23] Both eyes work well together, hearing is well developed, and speech is telegraphic (meaning that they use two or three words together such as "me do").

It is important for toddlers to be allowed to use their newly developed motor skills as they attempt to drink from a cup and begin using a spoon to feed themselves; however, they also enjoy eating finger foods, which supports their developing autonomy and practice of motor skills.

Psychosocial Development

Emotional and Social Development. Erikson describes the work of the toddler as developing a pattern of autonomy versus shame and doubt.[4] In this effort, toddlers imitate the behaviors of persons who are significant in their lives. Good role models are important as they develop in this area and gradually learn self-control and will power. Because it is essential that toddlers have the freedom to explore on their own within safe limits, it is necessary that their role models have a flexibility and self-confidence that allow this behavior.

The fact that objects have permanence takes on greater meaning as the child moves from infancy into the toddler stage. Toddlers can tolerate their parents being out of sight, but are braver around strangers when their parents are present. Separation anxiety is a significant concern, but toddlers are influenced by their parents' responses to separation. As their parents prepare to leave for the evening, toddlers, about to be left at home with a baby-sitter, frequently protest. If the parents then vacillate about leaving, and return to offer one more hug, toddlers typically respond by wailing and clinging to the parents. Toddlers who observe their parents showing calm, firm responses, may cry briefly on seeing them go out the door, but usually gradually quiet when baby-sitters provide comfort by hugging and playing with them.

Play is a natural way for toddlers to enhance their physical and psychosocial development. Toddlers enjoy playing near others, but are frequently unable to share objects or engage in interactive activities. In **parallel play,** toddlers play "beside" but not "with" their playmates although by age 3, they are likely to participate in an interactive game like tag. Their attention span is limited to minutes because they are so delighted by activity and exploration. The types of play activities that appeal to toddlers are those that allow them to use large muscles, those that include rhythmic and repetitive motions, and those involving language because they are learning to communicate with words and behaviors.

Toddlers have the ability to tolerate frustration to some extent, but temper tantrums are common and expected. They find it difficult to make choices between activities. For example, toddlers will want to please their parents by putting aside toys and accompanying them on an errand, but they also want to continue playing with their toys and so demonstrate their frustration with the two choices by protesting.

Another aspect of psychosocial development involves self-concept and body image. Toddlers express a desire to please parents and to feel grown up by becoming toilet trained. They continue developing their sense of self-esteem not only through others' responses to them but also through the activities their bodies are capable of achieving. Although value judgments should be used cautiously, typically toddlers identify with words and phrases such as good boy, good girl (or bad boy/girl), me, and mine. They respond to adult verbal and nonverbal communications as a way of integrating who they are becoming as individuals. Interactions with others, therefore, make a major contribution to toddler development.

Sexuality is another aspect of psychosocial development at this age. Toddlers begin to develop some gender-based expectations and beliefs in response to parental behavior modeling. During the second year of life toddlers begin to describe themselves as a girl or a boy, and can accurately apply gender labels such as mommy, daddy, brother, or sister to those around them.

Toddlers do identify with parents of the same sex and imitate their behaviors such as playing house, being a mommy, going to work, and disciplining the children. There is considerable confusion among toddlers about the social role aspect of sexuality primarily because toddlers think in very concrete ways. For example, a young toddler has difficulty understanding why parents sleep together in the same bed and desire privacy, rather than sharing their bed with their toddler as well. Children learn most about the social roles of men and women by observing their parents interact with one another.

Cognitive Development. Toddlers show curiosity about themselves, their surroundings, other children, and adults. Their primary way of learning is through their sensory and motor interactions but begin preconceptual activities, simple problem solving and symbolic thought around age 2. They are egocentric and intuitive, and much of their learning occurs as a result of their perspective on how the environment and others relate to themselves. They may begin to make associations between activities or ideas, but cannot generalize or use deductive reasoning.[5] For example, toddlers will associate outdoor clothing with going somewhere, but going somewhere has a limited meaning related narrowly to their past experiences.

Rituals provide security for toddlers, language is becoming well developed, and they begin to understand the concept of time as evidenced by their responding appropriately to the request to "wait." Cause and effect have little meaning unless the situation is made specific and immediate. For example, when a toddler is cautioned not to pull the tail of the family cat, but pulls it anyway, a frequent consequence is that the child is scratched by the cat. The toddler may still require assistance to see the relationship between this action and the subsequent outcome. Moreover, the toddler may need assistance to learn that it is acceptable to pull on certain things but not others.

Toddlers can be thought of as travelers and explorers; they climb onto counters, open drawers, investigate contents of purses, and attempt to explore outside the house. They continue to use their mouth to test taste, texture, size, and shape as they did during infancy. All of these modes act to enhance cognitive development but raise safety concerns as well.

Moral Development. Kohlberg describes the moral development of toddlers as being external to the individual; that is, the toddlers' sense of right versus wrong is decided primarily by their parents or others significant in their life.[6] Toddlers can understand morality in terms of good or bad, right or wrong, and attempt to obey parents to receive their approval and avoid punishment for misdeeds.

The morality of young children has its beginnings in their ability to see themselves in relation to others.[24] The two dimensions of morality in this stage of development are inequality and attachment. The former contributes to morality as a sense of justice. The young child is less powerful than others because of size, but this diminishes as the child grows and develops. The latter dimension, attachment, provides a definition of morality as love or care. It is based on reciprocal relationships and focuses on a broader definition that includes all of the qualities of pure love such as respect and justice. Hence, the toddler's concept of morality relies heavily on their real relationships with others. Moreover, toddlers become egocentric if they do not have relationships with others.

Wellness Promotion

Preventive care recommended for toddlers by the Committee on Practice and Ambulatory Medicine in consultation with the American Academy of Pediatrics in 1988 includes a complete health history and physical examination with height and weight; vision and hearing by history; developmental and behavioral examination; immunizations at 15, 18, and 24 months; tuberculosis skin testing once between 15 months and 4 years, and annual routine testing for members of high-risk groups; hemoglobin, hematocrit, and urinalysis once between 15 months and 4 years, with additional tests at the discretion of the primary care providers; and anticipatory guidance and counseling.[16]

Common Health Problems and Responses of Toddlers to Illness

Toddlers commonly have health problems related to their increasing mobility, their immature immune system, their curiosity, and their inability to make judgments about the safety of activities. They are at risk for accidental injury and death and also accidental poisoning.

Abuse and Neglect. Nonaccidental injury, or child abuse and neglect, are threats to children at all ages, and toddlers, by challenging parents through their increasing demands for autonomy, increase their vulnerability. The Centers for Disease Control estimates that 1.6 million children are abused or neglected annually.[25]

AIDS and Other Infections. AIDS is a disease that affects infants and toddlers, as well as adult clients. Initially, children contracted the virus from infected blood products, but increasingly infants are infected by being born to infected mothers and fathers. The Centers for Disease Control has reported that between 1981 and 1990, 1141 children under age 5 have died from AIDS.[26] In some locations, HIV infection has become the leading cause of death among young children. For example, in New York state in 1988, AIDS was the leading cause of death among Hispanic children aged 1 to 4 years and the second leading cause of death among black children aged 1 to 4.[26] Although these figures do not make this a common health problem for toddlers, nurses need to be aware that it is an increasing health problem for this age group.

Infections of the ears, the respiratory tract, and the gastrointestinal tract are common among toddlers. For toddlers who have repeated ear infections, it is especially important to provide health teaching and to test their hearing. Families whose toddlers have repeated respiratory infections may need to check for pollution as one source of the problem.

Lead Poisoning. Lead poisoning is again being described as a health threat to many children in the United States. In 1988, the US Department of Health and Human Services reported that an estimated three to four million children under 6 years of age had elevated blood lead levels.[27] This health problem is especially important in toddlers because they put objects into their mouth that are not meant to be ingested and because of the negative effects that lead has on the developing nervous system.

Sleep Disturbances. Toddlers may experience sleep disturbances in the form of night terrors or nightmares. Sleep disturbances need to be treated on an individual basis and parents should be counseled to do a a problem-solving assessment similar to that described in the section on infants. Sleep disturbances can have a variety of causes and there is no one answer or method of addressing this problem. Generally, parents find that toddlers quickly acquire or regain skill over problematic behaviors, such as nightmares, given comforting and patient assistance from their parents (see also Chapter 28).

Dental Caries. Parents may or may not be aware of dental caries as a health threat, or they may believe that because the "baby teeth" or deciduous teeth will be shed, they need not be overly concerned with caries. Health teaching can assist parents to appreciate that healthy deciduous teeth influence the formation of healthy gums and permanent teeth, decrease the potential for oral and gastrointestinal illness, and have a potential influence on self-esteem, as reflected in a pleasing facial appearance.

IMPLICATIONS FOR NURSE–CLIENT COLLABORATION

Collaborating with the Toddler

The developmental characteristics of toddler behavior define the possibilities and limits for collaboration during that stage of development. For example, toddlers are explorers and their natural curiosity about the environment serves to enhance their cognitive, social, and physical development. They are beginning to understand the concept of time and can respond appropriately to the nurse's request to "wait." To the toddler, however, cause-and-effect still have little meaning. Warnings, even about specific dangers often go unheeded because the toddler does not associate the consequences of actions with personal behavior. Aware of these characteristics, the nurse is able to make appropriate decisions about how to structure a safe but interesting space for the toddler that invites an investigation of the surroundings while protecting the toddler from danger.

Responses of Toddlers to Illness. Although toddlers want to assert their independence under normal conditions, they often need support for relinquishing it during illness. It is helpful for parents to communicate to toddlers that they are willing to do activities for the toddlers until they feel well enough to perform the activities themselves. This approach allows toddlers to know that their dependence is only temporary and that they will be well cared for by their parents.

Separation anxiety, a concern when toddlers are well, is even more of a concern during illness; therefore, they may be unable to tolerate having their parents out of sight. Parents who are unable to stay with a toddler may try leaving some personal item or belonging of theirs with the toddler as a reminder that they will return.

Toddlers value their newly acquired mobility and may be reluctant to relinquish it even when they are ill; therefore, a physician's order for "bed rest" has little meaning in their care without proper support. Parents can promote rest, however, by introducing stories, songs, and games with the theme of mobility and provide these as a substitute. Toddlers benefit when rituals are maintained and realistic choices continue to be offered to them, as establishment of routines and development of autonomy are developmental achievements during this age. During illness, toddlers may seem negative, but refusing medicines or treatments can be seen as an attempt to regain some control. As with infants, the parents' reactions, not only to the illness but also to toddlers' behaviors, will influences toddlers' responses.

Responsibilities for Client Care

Nurses work with both parents and toddlers in collaborative activities designed to promote normal growth and development. Nurses collaborate with toddlers by playing with them as a way of easing into physical assessment activities, in the process gaining their trust and cooperation. Play in the form of modified role playing or "pretend" is also a means of preparing toddlers for new life experiences with a sense of confidence. For example, children preparing for a brief hospitalization can "practice" by playing out admission procedures or putting on a hospital gown. Parents also can prepare children by continuing the "pretend" process.

Nurses can modify many of the techniques used with neonates and infants in promoting wellness and health in toddlers. Modifications in approaches are based on recognition of their increasing ability to be involved in activities and in making decisions as well as acknowledging parents as being more experienced in the parental role.

BUILDING NURSING KNOWLEDGE

How Do Toddlers Deal with the Crisis of Sudden Illness and Hospitalization?

Reynolds EA, Ramenofsky ML. The emotional impact of trauma on toddlers. *MCN.* 1988; 13(2):106–109.

Reynolds and Ramenofsky analyze the impact of hospitalization from a toddler's point of view and discuss ideas for helping toddlers during illness. The toddler's security comes from a sense of reliable accessibility to the parent. When separated, they are likely to look for and cry for their parents; however, stress from the situation can alter parents' usual responses to the toddler, causing the child further distress. Children may perceive parents as having given up their role as protectors by allowing strangers to perform painful procedures.

The authors argue that nurses can implement several actions to alleviate the effects of hospitalization on toddlers. They recommend that parents be included in toddlers' treatment, but caution that parents need support to be able to participate in their child's care. Providing adequate information and answering questions about treatment procedures and outcomes can help parents to cope. If toddlers must undergo painful procedures, the authors emphasize that parents should be prepared for this possibility ahead of time. This helps them manage their own anxiety so that they can be ready to help their toddler later.

Nurses can observe children for signs of pain such as crying, guarding (protecting a part of the body by not moving it), or grimacing, and take appropriate action to alleviate the pain or prevent it when possible. Nurses can also help offset the impact of immobility by wheeling the child's bed to a playroom or patio. Such interventions cannot undo the event, but can help reduce the physical and emotional stresses of toddlers.

Assess Toddlers' Health and Development. Toddlers are best assessed during play (Fig. 11–11). Toddlers readily provide assessment cues to nurses in such situations. Nurses can then discuss their assessment with the parents and determine similarities and differences between parents' and nurses' observations. Parents can be especially helpful in sharing whether or not these are typical behaviors of their toddlers. Together, nurses and parents can determine what

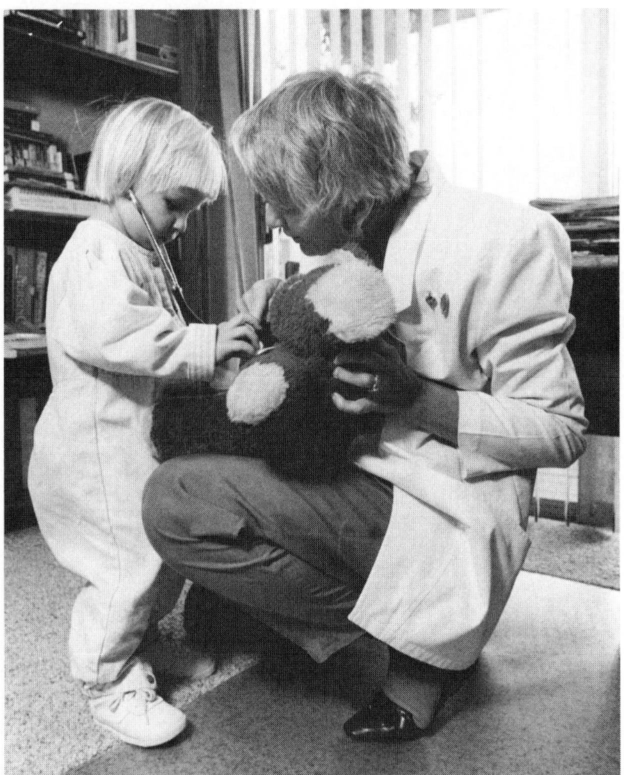

Figure 11–11. Assessment of a toddler's health is best done while playing with the child.

growth and development needs the toddlers have, which strategies that parents already use should be continued, and the need to develop additional strategies or modify those currently used.

Help Parents to Support Toddlers' Independence. Specifically, nurses should emphasize the importance of supporting toddlers in their future development of new skills and refinement of skills already learned. As toddlers move toward exercising autonomy, parents can encourage that movement by allowing them to make choices within safe limits. Parents should be aware of their own values on limit setting and discipline. Both parents should agree on the approaches that they will use, and then consistently reinforce these limits until they need to be modified or deleted.

It can be a challenge for parents to keep up with and anticipate activities of toddlers; however, they should avoid unnecessary restrictions on the toddlers' physical activities. Parent–toddler relationships will become strained if parents cannot permit toddlers sufficient space and time to test newly acquired gross and fine motor skills without interruptions.

While assessing toddlers, nurses can point out to parents that their child is changing rapidly and so parents will have to modify their expectations. Whereas parents were once able to do everything for an infant, they find that their toddler increasingly wants to do things as independently as possible and comes to parents primarily for approval or assistance.

Toddlers usually demonstrate an ability to participate with parents in making decisions that ultimately affect their growth and development; however, parents may need to have this capacity of the toddler pointed out to them. For example, toddlers often want to help brush their teeth or dress themselves and are able to perform a certain part of these activities. They need their parents' approval and recognition for what they can do; at the same time, they usually require the assistance from their parents to successfully complete the tasks. Nurses can assist parents to foster competence in their toddlers by discussing approaches that foster independence. Parents sometimes become so child-focused that they feel guilty if they acknowledge that they, as well as the toddler, have needs and rights. They can be tempted to perform activities themselves because of the greater amount of time required when toddlers perform the activities. Parents need to reach a balance, hopefully in consensus with their toddlers, to the extent possible.

Assist Toddlers and Parents to Adjust to Separation. Adjusting to separation is another area wherein nurses can assist parents. Discussing approaches that promote toddler independence aids parents to deal with separation. Parents may also appreciate assistance from nurses about how to keep toddlers safe while at the same time promoting their explorations and "travels."

Anticipatory teaching can be a major contribution in helping parents prepare for, manage, and enjoy development of toddlers. If parents are willing to consider toddlers as partners in the growth and development process who will give cues and responses to parents, if parents can learn to trust themselves and one another as capable parents, and if parents can maintain a sense of perspective and humor, it becomes easier to appreciate the "traveling, exploring toddler."

Review the Immunization Schedule with Parents. Nurses may need to reinforce with parents the importance of having toddlers properly immunized. Although the incidence of communicable diseases has been diminishing because of effective immunization programs, the only way this trend can continue is with the perseverance of universal immunizations. News reports of childhood deaths attributable to measles in Pennsylvania in 1991 are testimony to the importance of vigilance in health teaching about the importance of immunizations. The incidence of mumps has also been increasing in recent years.[28]

Reassure Parents About Toddler Behavior During Illness. The restrictions on toddlers' mobility and autonomy during illness sometimes stimulate intense behavioral reactions. Toddlers express their frustration with illness-imposed limitations by resisting treatments, angry outbursts, crying, and even tantrums. These behaviors may be stressful and embarrassing for parents. They may perceive that other adults view their child as spoiled and unmanageable, and them as ineffective parents.

Nurses can help parents accept that these behaviors are not unique to their child and do not reflect on their parenting skills, but are instead an expected developmental response to illness. Encourage parents to continue to give their toddler affection and warmth, while remaining firm in enforcing the limits that are necessary to promote recovery. Enlist their guidance in maintaining routines and rituals that are important to their child. Effective nurse–parent collaboration enhances toddlers' security and facilitates their coping with the stress of illness and restriction.

■ PRESCHOOL-AGE CHILD (3 TO 5 YEARS OF AGE)

Physical Growth and Development

Preschool-age children have mastered many gross motor skills and some fine motor skills, and have developed the ability to communicate both verbally and nonverbally. During the preschool years, they continue to refine these skills and learn additional ones in preparation for taking their place in the broader world of neighborhood and school.

Children between the ages of 3 and 5 years are taller and slimmer than toddlers (see Table 11–1, and Figs. 11–12 through 11–15). Their legs begin to straighten and eruption of the deciduous teeth ends.

Motor development of preschool-age children is concentrated on fine motor development, in contrast to toddlers who are developing gross motor skills. Most children display noticeably more precisely controlled and graceful movements than they demonstrated as toddlers. This characteristic is important. Preschool-age children are learning to take initiative in situations, which is easier to accomplish if they are able to control their bodies. Moreover, the ability to keep up with their peers and to participate successfully in games and other physical activities enhances preschoolers' self-esteem. Development of fine motor skills assumes particular importance in creative play such as using pencils, crayons, or paints. This development of motor skills makes interactive play more likely, as children with well-developed skills are in a better position to participate fully in these activities with peers. In addition, it is through interactive, social play that social and physical skills are enhanced.

Psychosocial Development

Emotional and Social Development. The sense of trust and autonomy that most children develop during the first 2 years of life continues to consolidate during the preschool years. When preschool children have a firm foundation in these two aspects of development they are in a strong position to develop a pattern of initiative versus guilt, which, according to Erikson,[4] is the developmental task at this age. Children cannot develop initiative in isolation, but must have a foundation of psychosocial security based on appropriate interactions with their parents so that they can then reach out and explore their expanding world.

Preschool-age children have a sense of curiosity, adventure, an intensified desire to explore, an interest in gender role play, and an involvement in creative play with others. Whereas toddlers learn to assert their beginning autonomy, often expressing it through gross motor activities and the word "no," preschoolers learn to show initiative through creative, social play using fine motor and gross motor skills and with the characteristic question that expresses their curiosity: "why?" Preschoolers tend to be more confident of their ability to tolerate separation from parents. Parents, generally feeling greater confidence in their ability as parents, find that they enjoy this more socialized child who seems to have developed more stable moods and more social skills.

Some of the social skills develop through practice in successfully completing self-care activities related to eating, dressing, toileting, and sleeping. Additionally, play is a major factor in socialization of preschool children. Children at this age develop an ability to play *with* others rather than alongside them, as they did during the toddler stage. Children who feel trusting and autonomous are able to express themselves more fully in play activities with other children than are children who are mistrusting and doubtful of their competence.

Children in this age group find dress-up play appealing to their creativity and imagination. This type of play is a good outlet for expressing feelings and ideas that they cannot understand in an abstract or conceptual form. They may need assistance to interpret the meaning of some events and situations because they use magical thinking and are unable to manage abstract ideas. **Magical thinking** is the belief that an event happens because of one's thoughts. For example, a child who wishes that someone in the family would "go away" or "leave me alone" may think that wishing made the event occur if that family member subsequently becomes ill and is hospitalized.

Preschool-age children are unable to differentiate between reality and fantasy in all situations. This point becomes especially important if they misbehave, as they need assurance that although parents do not like the misbehavior they still love them. Otherwise, preschoolers may decide incorrectly that because they did something "bad," they are "bad," and because parents do not like "bad" children they will not like them. Therapeutic play can help them in coping and in determining what is real and what is fantasy.

Social interactions play an important role in psychosocial development of children in the preschool stage. They have a sense of conscience in relation to others. They are able to work, play, and talk with others in an interactive manner. They are increasingly aware of gender differences and cultural norms in their interactions. They tend to identify with the parent of the same sex and their play activities may have a sexual exploratory focus. They still fear intrusion into their bodies, and to some extent even into their

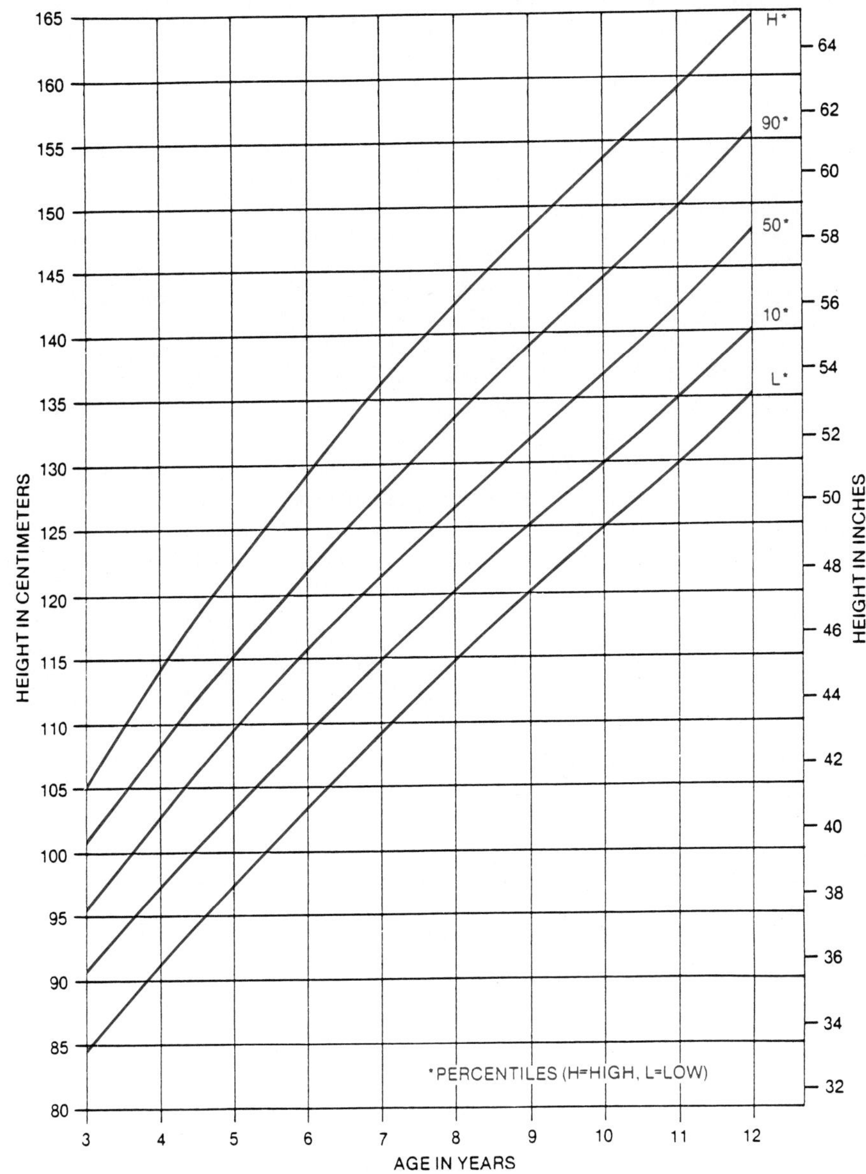

Figure 11–12. Stature-by-age percentiles for girls, ages 3 to 12 years, including lowest and highest values at each age. (*From Pomerance HH.* Growth Standards in Children. *New York: Harper and Row; 1979:32.*)

personal space. They continue to benefit from positive reinforcement about their appearance and their competence expressed in behaviors as a part of continuing development of sexuality and body image.

Cognitive Development. The cognitive ability of preschool children reflects both magical thinking and a concrete way of thinking. For instance, when 4-year-old children play with blocks, they can build a castle and pretend that there are alligators in the moat. At the same time, they are able to state, very matter-of-factly, that "these are really pretend alligators, just for fun." The growing ability to think opens a new world of fantasy, worry, and thought.

Preschoolers also display a continuation of the egocentric thinking demonstrated by toddlers. Preschool-age children exhibit this egocentric thinking by believing that everyone around them is aware of their thoughts. They are increasingly able to see relationships between some ideas but consider primarily one idea at a time. Their ability to judge size, shape, volume, mass, age, and time is still limited.[5]

Moral Development. Preschoolers' moral development proceeds to a point where they begin to understand fair and just behavior in a limited manner. They repeat behaviors that satisfy them and their significant others. Preschool-age children are less dependent on parents to set external limits on their behaviors. They assume a more active role in this regard. Loyalty and fairness are concepts that are not yet fully understood.[6]

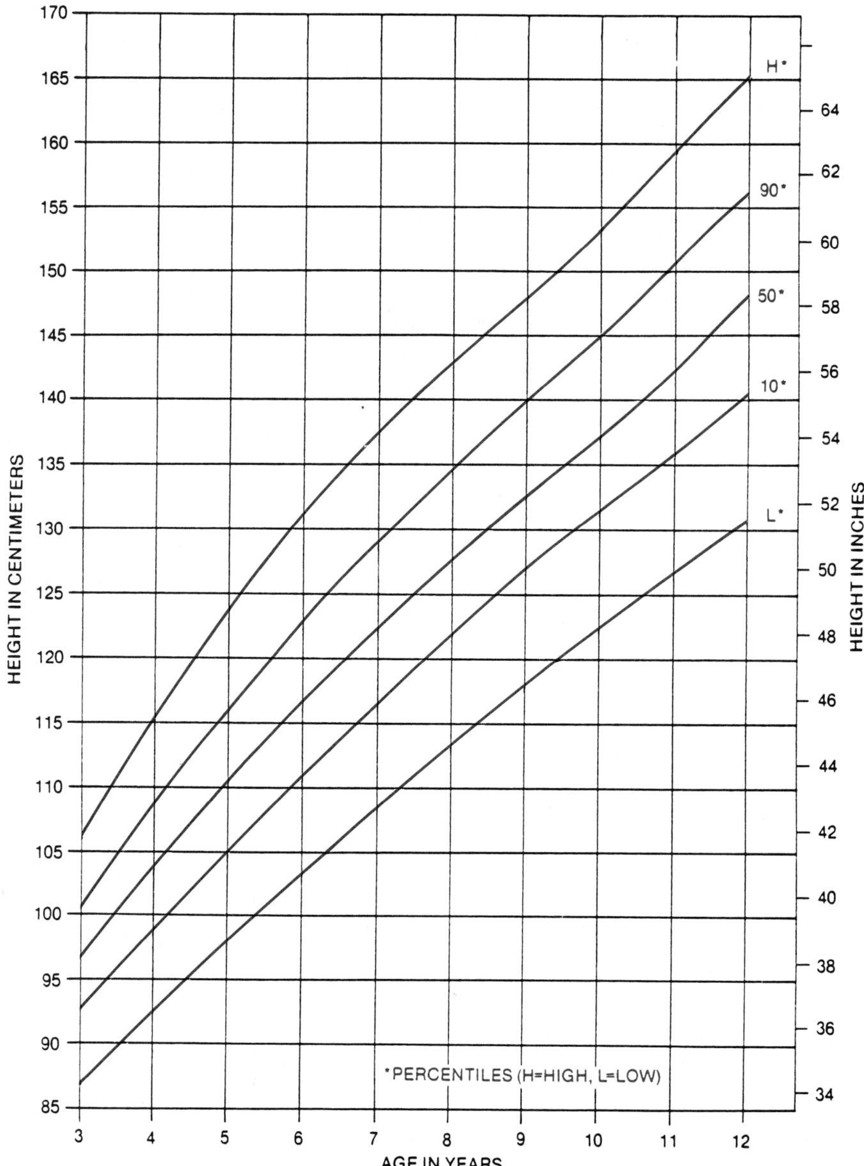

Figure 11–13. Stature-by-age percentiles for boys, ages 3 to 12 years. (*From Pomerance HH.* Growth Standards in Children. *New York: Harper and Row; 1979:32.*)

Wellness Promotion

Preschool-age children have the same need for health promotion and disease prevention as toddlers. The recommendations made by the Committee on Practice and Ambulatory Medicine in concert with the American Academy of Pediatrics are the same as those for toddlers except for the following: blood pressure is monitored yearly; vision and hearing are monitored by objective rather than subjective examination beginning at age 4 years; immunizations are required only at age 5; and the initial dental referral is made at age 3 years.[16]

Common Health Problems and Responses of Preschoolers to Illness

Infections. Because preschool-age children are still developing their immunity, they are likely to contract infections of the ear, nose, throat, skin, and urinary tract. Urinary tract infections can be avoided by good hygiene practices such as having children wash their hands both before and after toileting. Teaching girls to wipe from front to back after toileting, which keeps fecal organisms away from the urethra, and avoiding bubble baths, which cause irritation and dryness of genito-urinary mucosa also protects girls from urinary tract infections. Children who are completely immunized will be protected against the communicable diseases for which immunization is available.

Accidents. Preschool-age children are at risk for accidental injury and death. Accidents include burns, falls, drowning, and fires. Other sources of accidental injury or death are poisonings, including lead poisoning, and motor vehicle–related causes. Adults have a responsibility to provide a

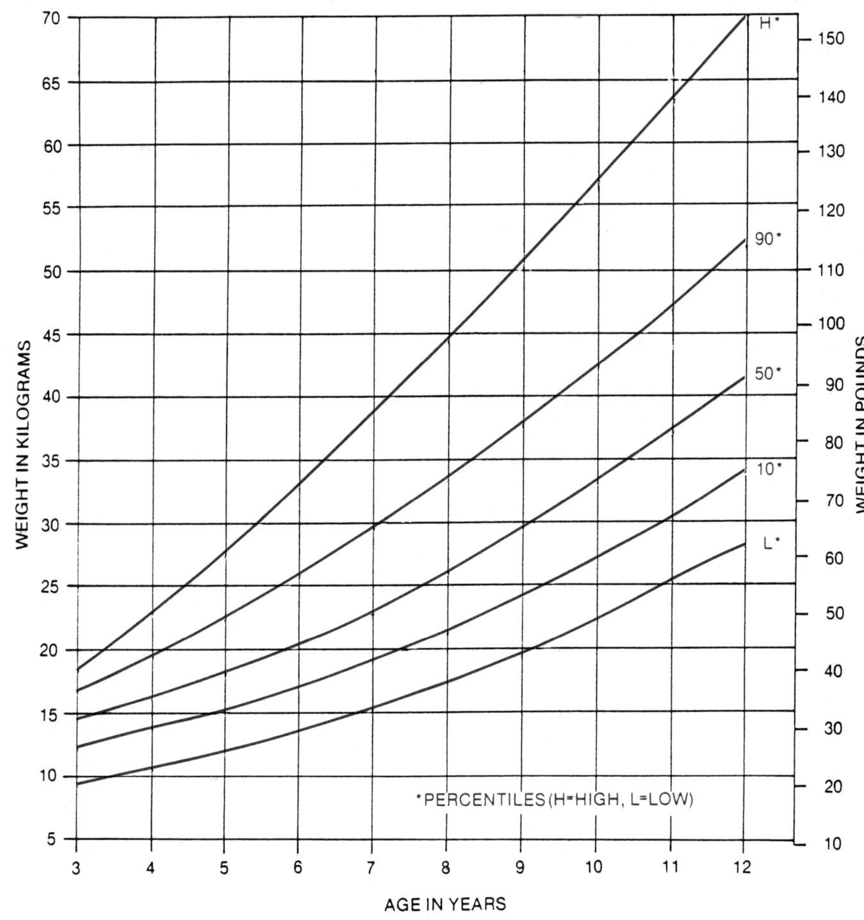

Figure 11–14. Weight-by-age percentiles for girls, ages 3 to 12 years. (*From Pomerance HH.* Growth Standards in Children. *New York: Harper and Row; 1979;32.*)

safe environment for children and to protect them from injury and death.

Abuse and Neglect. Abuse and neglect are all too common in the preschool period. Emotional, sexual, and physical abuse are frequent, but overprotection or unnecessary restriction of children is also a form of abuse. Parents are often the abusers, but relatives, neighbors, baby-sitters, day-care providers, and others in contact with preschoolers may also be responsible. Although children are dependent on adults for their nurturance and safety, even preschool-age children can be taught how to protect themselves from strangers or from others who touch them in inappropriate ways.[29]

Obesity and Malnutrition. Obesity is one of the most common preventable health problems of children in the United States today.[30] Approximately 25 percent of US children are obese, and children of two obese parents have about an 80 percent incidence of obesity.[31] Obesity often becomes apparent in preschool years when children fail to become slimmer as they grow taller.

Although too complex a topic to discuss in this chapter, obesity is considered to have both physiological and emotional etiologies and consequences. That is, obesity appears to be influenced both by genetics and by dietary patterns. In addition, obesity also has physical and emotional outcomes leading to high blood pressure and heart disease in later years and to decreased self-esteem as obesity becomes a factor in the child's social adaptation.

A sometimes overlooked nutritional and health problem of children in the United States is that of chronic hunger and malnutrition. Malnutrition can occur either from inadequate intake of quantity of food or quality of nutrients. About 20 million people in the United States, 12 million of whom are under the age of 16, are considered to be malnourished.[32] This constitutes almost 10 percent of the US population.

Responses of Preschoolers to Illness. Ill preschoolers experience an intensification of their fear of real and imagined threats to their body integrity. Preschoolers have only recently begun to achieve a sense of control over their body and some parts of their environment, such as knowing where their house is located and where their toys are kept in their room.

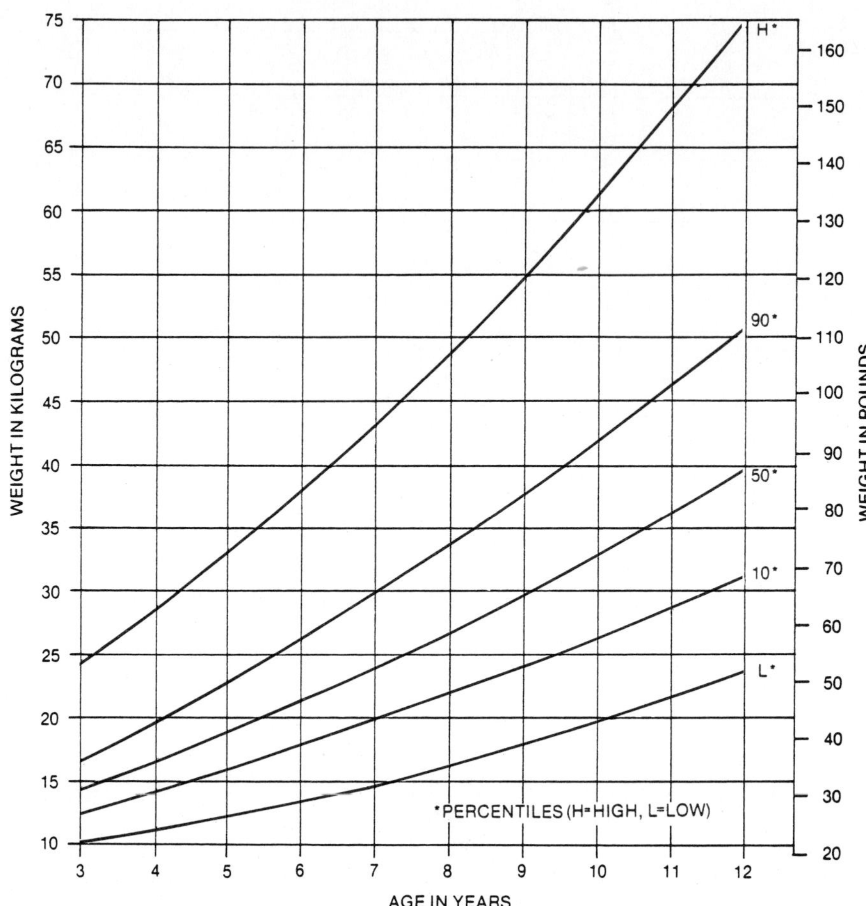

Figure 11–15. Weight by age percentiles for boys, ages 3 to 12 years. (*From Pomerance HH.* Growth Standards in Children. *New York: Harper and Row; 1979:32.*)

Illness shakes preschoolers' sense of security and feelings of control. Preschoolers who are hospitalized, even for relatively minor surgical procedures, are faced with an unfamiliar environment, with persons they have never seen before, changes in usual home routines, threats of procedures that could be painful or even mutilating, and a sense that there is a possibility of being abandoned by their parents.

Nurses must be aware that ill or hospitalized preschoolers are most likely to be frightened and have difficulty coping with fears, even when this may not be obvious in their behavior. Nurses can provide security by giving clear explanations in advance of treatments, by setting a consistent routine when possible, by working through fears by using play in a therapeutic way, and by including familiar persons such as parents in care routines (Fig. 11–16).

Responsibilities for Client Care

Conduct a Developmental Assessment. Nurses have many opportunities to promote normal growth and development of preschool-age children through collaborative efforts with children and their parents. With consideration for a child's development, nurses can expect that most children will find it appealing to be considered as "helpers" in achieving and maintaining normal growth and development.

Preschoolers who enjoy being praised for following directions can cooperate with nurses during health and developmental assessments. Preschoolers enjoy answering questions and demonstrating their skills and accomplishments.

Include Preschoolers in Decision Making. Nutrition, dental hygiene, sleep and rest, handwashing, toileting, dressing, and socialization activities are some of the daily decisions in which nurses can include children, enabling them to participate in making choices. There are limits to decision making by preschool children, however, because they lack the judgment and ability to consistently determine consequences of choices. Moreover, offering too many choices may be stressful to the child.

Nurses, in cooperation with parents, can use games, stories, drawings, and similar methods that are concrete, simple, and action oriented to elicit from children an assessment of their like s, dislikes, knowledge, and motivation to participate in any of these daily decisions. Nurses

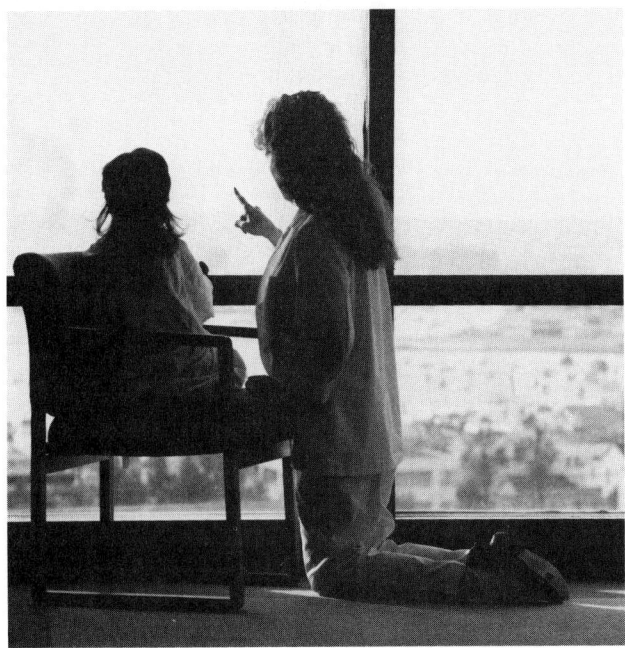

Figure 11–16. Developing a relationship with hospitalized preschoolers is a way to decrease their fears.

then can assess parents' need and willingness to respond to teaching and guidance about supporting development of decision-making in their children. Ideally parents, nurses, and children together should determine the aspects of health behavior on which they will focus their efforts.

Encourage Play. Preschoolers express their feelings, both positive and negative, through play, because they have not yet developed the sophisticated verbal skills needed to describe them. The play of preschoolers is therefore considered to be very productive and can be used by nurses as a way of interacting with and assessing the child. Using fantasy and therapeutic play, nurses can assess, develop, implement, and evaluate a teaching plan in an effort to address the issues surrounding wellness and health promotion of preschool-age children.

IMPLICATIONS FOR NURSE–CLIENT COLLABORATION

Collaborating with the Preschooler

Although preschoolers lack the judgment to determine the consequences of poor choices and may be confused by too many choices, they nevertheless find it appealing to be considered as "helpers" in the activities of normal growth and development and can participate in many of the daily decisions that are part of those activities. Some of the areas in which preschoolers can truly become a part of the collaborative effort are nutrition, hygiene, sleep and rest, and socialization. Simple, clear choices support preschoolers' growing independence within defined limits, choices such as what flavor of toothpaste to use in toothbrushing, whether to take crackers or fruit when snacks are passed out, what toy to nap with, or whether to sing a song or have a book read at bedtime. These are all health-promoting decisions that preschoolers can make.

Promote Protection. Preschool children are in a transition period. Their world is expanding, both in reality and in their active imaginations. Their impulsive desires to explore and master their environment expose them to safety risks. Their developing cognitive capacity makes the time right for teaching important safety rules like using seat belts in automobiles, crossing streets only with adult supervision, and not communicating with strangers; however, their immaturity makes surveillance and reinforcement from parents a continuing need. Preschoolers are also vulnerable to fears and concerns that grow out of their magical thinking and fantasies. Graphic television programs, an argument between parents, or a news story about a disaster, for example, may stress and confuse them. Parents can protect preschoolers from these worries by helping them to interpret events in their environment.

Caregiving gives nurses an ideal opportunity for teaching preschoolers about ways they can protect themselves through good health and safety habits, as well.

Assist Ill Preschoolers' Coping. Nurses can support ill or injured preschool-age children in their efforts to cope with illness or injury, through the use of therapeutic play. Therapeutic play differs from play therapy used by psychologists and psychiatrists. Even so, only experienced nurses should use therapeutic play. Common themes of this play are coping with fears of bodily intrusion and mutilation, learning that thoughts cannot cause illness and injury, and adjusting to separation from parents. Children who are ill need an understanding caregiver who will allow them to regress when they need to during the illness or injury but also encourage them to continue showing initiative during illness or injury when they can. This kind of sensitive support strengthens and fosters feelings of success and competence in working through health problems.

■ THE SCHOOL-AGE CHILD (5 TO 12 YEARS OF AGE)

School-age children have developed inner strength and sufficient maturity to reach outside themselves and their families. The major developmental tasks during this period are cultivation of appropriate interactions with peers and others; enhancement of intellectual skills, primarily in school; refinement of fine motor skills; and expansion of gross motor skills.

Physical Growth and Development

The physical growth and development of children during the school-age years continues at a relatively steady pace until the prepubescent stage at 10 to 12 years, when growth begins to accelerate (see Table 11–1 and Figs. 11–12 through 11–15). Facial shape changes because facial bones grow faster than does the skull. School-age children become slimmer, their legs lengthen noticeably, their neuromotor coordination is well developed, they lose deciduous teeth, and they experience eruption of the permanent teeth. They can effectively ride a bicycle and manipulate the fine motor skills needed in playing musical instruments or board games, writing, coloring, and drawing; they have the physical coordination and psychosocial skills needed for team sports and activities; and they are able to manage all aspects of self-care and activities of daily living.

Psychosocial Development

Emotional and Social Development. To accomplish the tasks necessary for emotional and social development, school-age children need opportunities to learn about and to apply rules for interacting with people outside their families. These opportunities have a direct and an indirect effect on their development of competence in physical and psychosocial activities.

During the school-age years, children usually learn that not all families interact in the same manner, that families have different norms of acceptable behaviors for children, and that cultural or ethnic background may affect family expectations of children. These factors affect both the interactions that children have outside their families and the development of their skills. To be effective in relating to others, children need to develop an awareness and an appreciation for differences among families (Fig. 11–17).

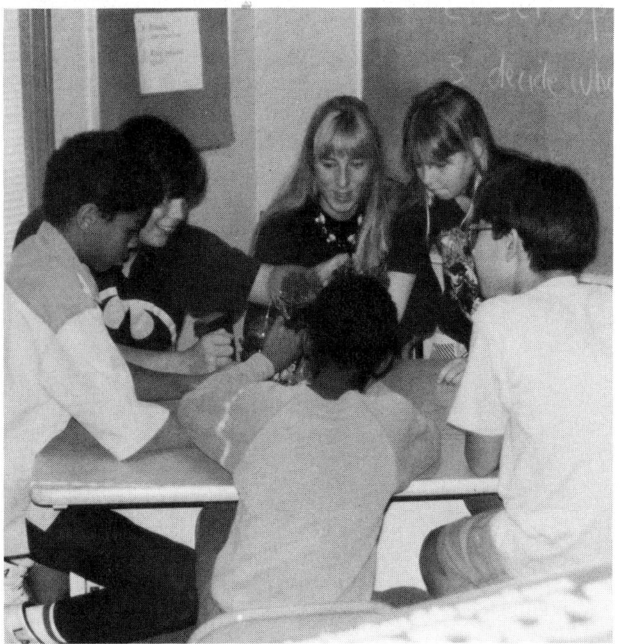

Figure 11–17. Children can develop an awareness and appreciation for differences if exposed to a variety of peers.

Erikson describes the psychosocial task of school-age children as that of developing a pattern of industry versus inferiority.[4] Rules are learned and projects are undertaken and completed (Fig. 11–18). Teachers and peers become influential role models in this stage. Children establish realistic standards of behavior and achievement that lead them to feel competent and in control of their behaviors. This stage is pivotal for growing children who must learn to compete and collaborate with persons outside their families.

Parents can assist school-age children in these efforts by encouraging their industriousness and by supporting them as they reach out to other adult role models. Parents who are unable or unwilling to be supportive of their school-age children may subconsciously want their children to remain dependent on them. There may be other reasons, however, for not supporting school-age children such as the lack of knowledge about what to do, how to show support, or even why it is important to provide support. Because parents have needs and rights as well as responsibilities, it is important for nurses to learn more about their attitudes or behaviors when assessing family interaction. Only then can a collaborative relationship be established among nurse, parents, and child. School-age children need to take responsibility for and control of their attitudes, behaviors, and values with the guidance and support of parents and other significant adults.

School-age children's sexuality and body image development are related not only to physiology but also to feelings of competence, acceptance, and recognition. Children rely to a large extent on others' responses to them for verification that they are worthwhile. Being able to contribute, feeling one's accomplishments are worthwhile, and learning about how their bodies function and how they are changing are important to developing self-acceptance.

School-age children tend to be members of groups of

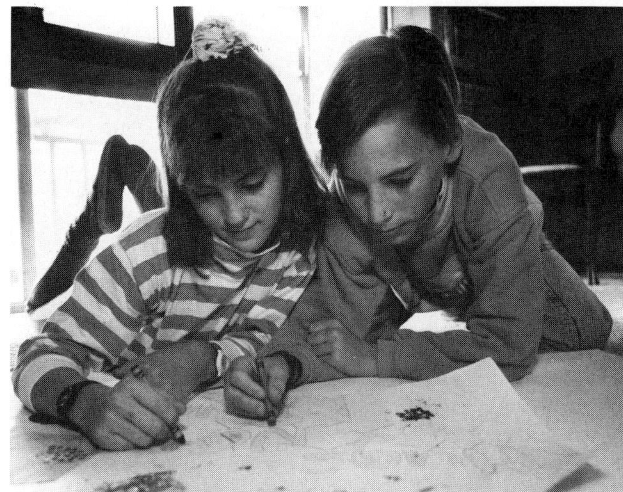

Figure 11–18. School-age children demonstrate their industriousness by working together on projects.

the same sex and have same-sex best friends. At about age 11 they begin to show an interest in members of the opposite sex.

School-age children develop understanding of certain concepts about gender. These elements include general stability, that all boys grow up to be men and all girls grow up to be women; general constancy, that even though girls dress in boys' clothes, they remain girls, and though boys dress in girls' clothes, they remain boys; and a genital basis to gender, that is, the sex organs of boys and girls differ.[33]

Cognitive Development. Cognitively, school-age children are able to apply reasoning skills to understand ideas or concepts. For example, they manipulate numbers in math and they can discuss social issues, such as homelessness, at a basic level. They learn the alphabet, then put the letters together in various combinations as they learn to read and write. They can draw relationships between concepts of time and space. They are able to memorize, are no longer bound by magical thinking, and like to categorize and organize collections in many different ways (by size, shape, or color, for example).

School-age children can make judgments after considering a number of factors, but they need to handle or manipulate objects concretely to understand concepts. Piaget refers to this as the concrete operational stage. These children become increasingly logical and capable of complex reasoning as they near the end of the school-age period. They begin to problem solve, reverse concepts, tell time, and draw conclusions. Because they are becoming more socialized and decentralized, they consider the opinions of others in their thinking.[5]

Moral Development. Moral development of school-age children, according to Kohlberg, is shaped by social behaviors especially in the context of family and cultural expectations.[6] School-age children begin to understand rules that are specific to defining appropriate behavior for specific settings or situations such as the home or school. Children conform with norms to gain approval of significant others. They learn that it is important to follow school, family, and religious rules and to respect authority figures such as parents and teachers for both their disciplinary roles and their intrinsic and human qualities.

Wellness Promotion

Many school-age children are healthy; however, a large number of children in this age group live in poverty and do not receive preventive medical and dental care. A National Health Interview Survey found that 52.2 percent of children in the United States between the ages of 5 and 17 were in excellent health. Given the value that is placed on health and fitness, more needs to be done to improve the health of children in the United States.

During the school-age years, children need preventive health care as much as they did when they were younger. The Committee on Practice and Ambulatory Medicine in concert with the American Academy of Pediatrics recommends a schedule similar to that for preschool-age children with the following exceptions: tuberculin tests are not recommended; dental examination schedules are set by the child's dentist; a subjective report on vision is acceptable at age ten; and an objective hearing examination is recommended once at age 12 unless otherwise indicated.

School-age children need specific attention given to anticipatory guidance on the topics of sexuality, substance abuse, accident prevention, stress, fears, and tension. These are subjects that are especially relevant because increasing numbers of school-age children are exposed to them through the mass media, in their peer interactions, at home, and elsewhere. Related problems are largely preventable, which makes these topics even more relevant in counseling for health promotion.

Common Health Problems and Responses of School-age Children to Illness

Nutritional Problems and Obesity. School-age children are at risk for nutritional problems, whether they have an excessive, inadequate, or poor-quality nutritional intake. They can be greatly influenced by peers, media advertisements, or poor nutrition habits to consume foods that are high in sugar, fats, and cholesterol and deficient in vitamins and minerals. Although the school-age child may begin to gain excessive weight during the prepubertal time partially because of hormonal influences, the primary cause of obesity remains excessive food intake coupled with inadequate exercise. Poor nutritional habits can lead to long-term or chronic health problems for school-age children.

Dental Health Problems. Poor nutrition and poor dental hygiene contribute to dental caries and other dental problems in school-age children. All permanent teeth except the third molars (wisdom teeth) erupt during the school-age years. School-age children with malocclusion of the teeth may be referred for orthodontia during the school-age period, with aggressive interventions usually initiated as dentition becomes complete.

IMPLICATIONS FOR NURSE–CLIENT COLLABORATION

Collaborating with the School-age Child

The moral development typical of the school-age period makes it possible for school-age children to participate in an expanded scope of health-related decisions. School-age children begin to understand the rules that define appropriate behavior in specific settings and situations in the realms of family, church, and school. School-age children conform with those norms for behavior to gain approval from significant others, and they are able to associate their own behavior with the consequences of that behavior. Thus, school-age children often are able to make decisions independently that are consistent with the limitations they learn for given situations.

Accidents. Accidents are a leading cause of injury and death in school-age children. The American Automobile Association Traffic Safety Department reports that 75 percent of all disabling bicycle injuries and 75 to 80 percent of all bicycle fatalities are associated with head injuries.[34] The report continues with the information that 42 percent of fatalities and 55 percent of injuries in bicycle and motor vehicle accidents involve children under the age of 15 years.[34] Other causes of accidental injury or death are drowning, burns, and firearms. Burns are a major health threat to children, with children less than 9 years of age accounting for 73 percent of all burn deaths in children.[35]

Visual and Hearing Deficits. Children of school age frequently have visual and hearing deficits that often account for poor academic performance, behavior difficulties, and other physical problems such as headaches. Ideally, these sensory problems should be diagnosed during the preschool years, as hearing and vision problems are the fourth and fifth most common health problems in children.[36] Nearly one third of school-age children have some degree of visual deficit.[36] Nurses can refer these children for diagnosis and possible treatment if an initial screening reveals a problem or if parents or children request it based on their observations and experience.

Learning Disorders. The term **learning disorder** describes all of those behaviors that indicate impaired neurological or intellectual processing problems. Learning disorders, such as dyslexia and attention deficit disorder (ADD) occur in about 10 to 20 percent of all children[37] and often predispose children to behavior and school problems.

Nurses should be informed if children have any of these problems, how they are being treated, and what effect these conditions and their treatment may have on childrens' health care needs. For example, some children have difficulty reading, writing, or calculating figures. If these children are also confronted with a chronic illness such as juvenile diabetes, they may be frustrated by the complexities of taking insulin and adjusting insulin dosages.

Although school-age children receive assistance from adults when they are younger, they are expected to assume more responsibility for their care as they mature. As a result, learning problems often become apparent during the school-age years. Nurses can discuss with children and their parents modifications that can be made in health care practices, based on strengths rather than limitations of the children. For example, pictures of diabetic meal plans showing numbers of daily allowances per food group may be more easily understood than printed food lists.

Communicable Disease. School-age children are at risk for infections of the skin, respiratory tract, and gastrointestinal tract as well as for the common communicable diseases of childhood. These infections are a common health problem for younger children because they come into contact with other children at a time when they are still developing immunity. In addition, handwashing practices may not be followed adequately, children may come to school even though they are ill, or they may become ill while at school. All of these factors put school-age children at risk for contracting communicable diseases.

The high incidence of communicable disease in this age group makes missing school a common occurrence. Missing school can create problems for children; if it happens too often, they can fall behind in their school work and feel overwhelmed, thus affecting their sense of competence and self-esteem. Children who are well nourished and rested, who receive appropriate preventive health care, and who exercise regularly, however, will usually recover quickly after treatment for communicable diseases.

Chronic Illness. Although many US children are in excellent health, 10 to 15 percent have chronic illnesses such as diabetes mellitus, asthma, or cystic fibrosis. Furthermore, 1 out of 20 children with a disability or chronic illness experiences impaired functioning on a daily basis.[19]

Chronic illnesses have a special impact on children, their families, schools, and the health care system. These children and their families face multiple problems such as economic strain, possible social rejection, family and marital stress, fatigue during times of acute exacerbation, and emotional frustration.

Responses of School-age Children to Illness. School-age children, although more mature than preschoolers, still carry over some of the fears and fantasies from the earlier stage. These fears may become evident during periods of stress, such as during a serious illness or hospitalization. School-age children are very concerned about their bodies, especially as puberty nears. When an illness occurs, these normal concerns may be intensified to the degree that children lose their ability to reason logically about their situation. Nurses can recognize that school-age children may look far more calm and accepting than they actually feel. Nurses can provide reassurance to children by providing consistency in their schedules and environment, for example, by assigning the same staff each day. In addition, nurses can encourage expression of feelings by spending time with children and conveying an accepting and nonjudgmental attitude.

Responsibilities for Client Care

Nurses can interact and collaborate with school-age children to a greater extent than was possible with younger children. Although parents are very much a part of assessment of needs and health teaching, school-age children can accept more responsibility for their healthy development. Nurses can appeal to their sense of industry, their desire to be competitive in reaching goals, and their perceptions of themselves as competent and capable people as a realistic way to interest and involve them in activities to promote healthy development.

Approach School-age Children as Clients. School-age children are generally capable of and interested in sharing responsibility for their health or wellness. Nurses can invite them and their parents to share their individual perceptions, ideas, questions, and concerns about wellness or health promotion.

School-age children have both the knowledge and the capacity to begin making health choices for themselves. They can be separated from their parents to preserve privacy during examinations and can participate in all phases of collaboration, as partners in preventing many health problems and as active participants in the recovery process when illness or injury occur. At this age, children also can begin to participate in some aspects of their health care separately from their parents.

Much of the child's motivation to participate may be based on past experiences in exercising self-care, self-control, initiative in setting goals, and a sense of industry in meeting goals. Children who believe that they share control and responsibility for their health with parents and health care providers, will likely function more fully in collaborative efforts than will children who believe that someone or something else is responsible and in control. Attitudes of parents and health care providers also have an effect on childrens' desire to participate in collaborative efforts.

Facilitate Sex Education. Wellness promotion for school-age children should address sexuality, with special attention given to pregnancy. Nurses should provide concrete information, but should do so with sensitivity and respect. Although school-age children may be able to cite facts about pregnancy and its relationship to sexuality, they often lack an accurate understanding of the reasons why school-age children become pregnant. Parents may be uncomfortable discussing this topic with their children, so nurses must assess parents' needs as well.

Promote Drug Awareness. Substance abuse is recognized as a national health threat. School-age children need to learn strategies that give them control over the temptation to use substances that can harm them. They need to be given better reasons to avoid substance use than others may present to encourage use. Reinforcement of drug avoidance strategies will be necessary, as will encouragement of positive activities that will keep children healthy.

Promote Accident Prevention. Accident prevention is another area in which school-age children must learn to share responsibility with their parents. Health promotion activities are designed to inform them about types of accidental injury and death for which they are vulnerable, how to reduce the likelihood of such accidents, and how to become safety conscious.

Assist School-age Children to Cope with Illness. School-age children who are ill benefit from a caring approach and brief, honest information about the illness. School-age children may act brave even when they do not feel brave. It is helpful for nurses to remember that school-age children are poised between childhood and adolescence. More advanced physical growth and development may tempt adults to expect greater psychosocial and intellectual maturity than the growing child actually possesses. Nurses can use strategies to promote positive self-concept in school-age children, which is especially important to ill children. For example, one strategy is to have children create a collage of themselves or make a commercial for themselves.[38] For children who have mental, emotional, or physical deficits, it is important to assess their capacities and to use art materials that are safe and appropriate for their conditions.[39]

School-age children, their parents, and nurses have many opportunities to collaborate in addressing the common health problems. School-age is a time of preparation for the transition to adolescence and for development of inner strength and maturity that will enable developing an identity as unique and capable individuals.

■ THE ADOLESCENT (12 TO 18 YEARS OF AGE)

The transition from late childhood, often termed *preadolescence* or prepuberty, into adolescence is marked by considerable variation among individuals. This transition may begin as early as 9 years of age, and terminates at puberty, the period during which children become physically capable of sexual reproduction. Puberty begins between 9 and 14 years of age in girls and between 12 and 16 years of age in boys. Its onset is influenced by heredity, culture, nutritional status, and state of health. Physiological maturation of male and female sex organs occurs over a 3- to 4-year period.[3] This individual variation in the physiological maturation process is a serious concern in preadolescents, who often feel awkward or embarrassed if they differ from their peers in appearance.

Adolescence, the period of life that begins at puberty and extends for approximately 5 to 8 years, is generally thought of as a time of transition into physical and psychosocial maturity. It is difficult to determine the point at which adolescence ends and young adulthood begins. Rather than trying to set arbitrary dividing lines, it is useful to consider this a time of "becoming." This perspective makes the developmental tasks of adolescence easier to understand.

Physical Growth and Development

The physiological and structural growth that occurs during adolescence has been described by Tanner and Davies.[3] Most of the linear growth in adolescents occurs in a very short period of 18 to 36 months, and is completed during the pubertal period. Girls may gain 5 to 20 cm (2 to 8 in.) in height and 7 to 25 kg (15 to 55 lb) in weight during this time. Although boys experience their growth spurt about 2 years later than girls, their physical changes are dramatic. The average boy may grow 10 to 30 cm (4 to 12 in.) in height and gain 7 to 30 kg (15 to 65 lb) in weight during this time.[3]

Hormonal influences in puberty and adolescence cause changes in the skin and sweat glands. In girls, estrogen production makes the texture of the skin softer, thicker, and more vascular. In boys, the skin becomes thicker as a result of androgen production.

The sebaceous, eccrine, and apocrine glands become very active during this time. The increased sebaceous gland activity contributes to the development of acne in adolescents. The eccrine glands are fully functional and secrete perspiration during exercise or during emotional stimulation. Apocrine glands, also fully functional, are distributed in limited areas of the body in conjunction with hair follicles. The apocrine glands produce a thick secretion that has a strong and unpleasant odor when acted on by skin bacteria.

Gender takes on specific importance because females mature biologically about 2 years earlier than males.[3] The physical changes that occur as hormones act on target receptors in the body include not only the rapid increase in body size and corresponding increase in muscle and bone mass discussed above, but also changes in body composition and shape, rapid development of the gonads, and development of secondary sex characteristics. Reproductive growth is complete in most teenagers by age 17.

Adolescents have increasing manual dexterity, physical strength, and endurance that allow them to perform the physical actions required for health maintenance and health promotion; however, integration of these physical capabilities with the emotional maturity or motivation to make healthy choices is a challenge for the typical adolescent.

Psychosocial Development

Emotional and Social Development. The peer group is the primary influence in an adolescent's life. Teenagers become more independent from their families, often to the confusion of their parents. The psychosocial tasks of adolescence include establishing a group identity, developing a consistent sense of personal identity including an irreversible sexual identity, and forming close personal relationships with both male and female friends.

Erikson termed the psychosocial task that adolescents face as the problem of "identity versus identity confusion."[4] Sometimes this conflict is described as group identity versus alienation.[40] Adolescents are preoccupied with questions about the meaning of life and with development of goals for the future. This process of developing a personal identity is a complex phenomenon. It reflects adolescents' heritage and family values, their past life experiences, beliefs and hopes for the future, and their perception of the demands and expectations of other significant persons in their lives.

In this process of self-discovery, traditional cultural or societal values that were accepted during childhood are often questioned. Adolescents may experience periods of preoccupation, confusion, and discouragement. Experimenting with adult roles helps adolescents to form an adult identity. Dating, leaving home to attend school, taking a job, and babysitting are activities that enable adolescents to examine adult responsibilities and roles. Parents can assist adolescents with this process by helping them to consider alternatives and encouraging logical problem solving.

Cognitive Development. As adolescents leave childhood behind, they begin to think in different ways. The conceptual skills of adolescence are described as the stage of formal operations.[5] Adolescents now are able to think about things changing in the future, such as expecting some differences in their relationships with their parents. They also are able to anticipate the logical consequences of their behaviors, and are able to see abstract relationships between themselves and their environment.

Adolescents are frequently biased and egocentric mostly as a result of a lack of life experiences. Although adolescents still demonstrate impatient or impulsive behaviors, they are becoming more flexible and able to delay gratification for long-term rewards.

Even though adolescents are capable of abstract reasoning, they remain idealistic and feel omnipotent when considering their long-term health needs. Adolescents rarely take seriously the notion that they might die at a young age, and although they frequently express somatic concerns, they may consider disease and illness to be concerns of the elderly. In some respects, adolescents believe they will live forever, and are unwilling to see a relationship between personal behaviors and ill health, except in the most superficial ways.

Practice in dealing with difficult decisions together with encouragement from significant friends or family will motivate adolescents to become less impulsive and self-centered when problem solving.

Moral Development. The change from conventional to postconventional morality begins in adolescence but is not well integrated in an individual's value system until adulthood.[6] During this transitional time adolescents begin to challenge traditional values in much the same way that they examine their identity. Younger adolescents (under age 15) still accept traditional family and social values for the most part; however, older adolescents are able to see distinctions between moral behavior and social convention, and begin to interpret these values in a very personal way.

Many older adolescents develop a value system that allows them to consider several alternatives before making decisions. This value system enables older adolescents to consider others in relationship to self. For example, older adolescents, although still influenced by their peers, tend to be more consistent in the ability to look beyond solely personal interests when making behavior choices.

Wellness Promotion

Adolescence is generally considered to be a time of good health. Health promotion centers primarily on teaching and guidance. Adolescents are eager learners and are anxious to learn about their own bodies and their emotional reactions to life.

Parents are involved in a different and more distant way in health decisions regarding their teenagers. It is im-

BUILDING NURSING KNOWLEDGE

Does Adolescent Behavior Increase Their Risk for Heart Disease?

Pebler MA, Hester NO, Connor K. A cardiovascular risk assessment of high school sophomores. *Issues Compr Pediatr Nurs.* 1987; 10:331–341.

In this study, the investigators explore adolescents' health needs to determine if strategies are needed to promote lifestyles that enhance fitness. They randomly selected 100 high school sophomores in a western US city to be subjects in this study. Subjects were asked to complete a questionnaire that dealt with six risk factors of heart disease: (1) family history of heart disease, (2) smoking, (3) lack of exercise, (4) elevated blood pressure, (5) obesity, and (6) stress. All of these factors except family history are associated with increased risk of heart disease and can be modified.

The findings were that 31 percent of the subjects had a family history of heart attack, 24 percent had a family history of stroke, and 51 percent had a family history of high blood pressure. Fifteen percent of the subjects reported smoking sometime and four subjects reported smoking as many as 20 cigarettes per day. Thirty-nine percent of subjects reported that their parents smoked. Most subjects reported that they exercised regularly; only six subjects reported that they did not exercise. The length of exercise sessions varied with gender, females exercising for shorter periods.

The researchers found that nine subjects, all male, had high blood pressure (systolic blood pressures greater than 140 mm Hg or diastolic blood pressures greater than 90 mm Hg). Of the male subjects, 13 were determined to be obese according to Metropolitan Life Insurance charts; 17 females were also found to be obese. Stress resulting in physical symptoms such as headache, irritability, or sleeplessness was reported by 51 percent of the subjects. The authors concluded that their study demonstrated that adolescents participate to various degrees in health behaviors that are not conducive to fitness.

portant to reassure teenagers that information shared during health counseling sessions will be kept confidential and will not be shared with parents without the teenager's consent.

Common Health Problems and Responses of Adolescents to Illness

Motor vehicle accidents, suicides and homicides, drownings, and burns are the major causes of mortality and morbidity in adolescents.[35] Adolescents' strong need to conform and to look like their peers may lead to concern about their state of health. Adolescents frequently have physical complaints in instances where no illness or disability exists, and can usually be helped to feel less anxious with information and reassurance.

Accidents. Behavior that results in adolescent health problems is often the same behavior that complicates adolescent social development. The most frequent causes of death in adolescents include motor vehicle accidents; accidents of other types, including drug and alcohol abuse; and suicide. In fact, for white males (ages 15 to 24 years) in the United States, motor vehicles, suicide, and homicide are the leading causes of death, whereas homicide is the main cause in young black males of these ages.[41]

Alcohol and Drug Use. Negative health behaviors such as alcohol and drug consumption can, in and of themselves, be detrimental to adolescents. In addition, these health behaviors can lead to associated problems including homicide, motor vehicle accidents, and drowning. It was estimated that in males 15 to 19 years of age, 40 to 50 percent of deaths by drowning in 1986 were related to alcohol consumption.[35]

Nutritional Deficits and Obesity. Nutritional deficits, including excessive and insufficient food intake, are additional negative health behaviors that place adolescents at risk for poor health in adulthood. Nutrition intake, both over and under necessary amounts, may be linked to inadequate daily exercise patterns. Excessive intake of "fast foods" may be another factor associated with nutritional deficits in adolescents.

Teen Pregnancy. Adolescent pregnancy is both a physical and a socioemotional problem. In addition to the physical risks encountered by all pregnant women, adolescents are at additional risk for premature births, fetal or maternal death, hemorrhage, infection, and infants with low birth weight.[19] As adolescents are growing rapidly themselves, they may not be adequately nourished to sustain both themselves and the rapid growth of their unborn children. Additionally, pregnant adolescents experience an interruption in the development of their identity. They may experience identity diffusion when they become parents before attaining their full psychosocial development. Furthermore, relationships with peers and family members, educational and career goals, and the establishment of independence from parents are interrupted by pregnancy.

Sexually Transmitted Disease. Sexually transmitted diseases such as chlamydia, herpes, gonorrhea, and syphilis are additional risks for sexually active adolescents. HIV infection is a threat as well. Discussion of these topics is beyond the scope of this chapter; the reader is referred to texts that provide full discussion of these subjects.

Nurses should offer anticipatory guidance in the areas of contraception and safe sex. Also, support for adolescents who do not engage in sexual activity and who may need reassurance that their behavior is normal and healthy is another form of guidance that can be very helpful.

Responses of Adolescents to Illness. When actual illness or injury occurs, adolescents may assume an overconfident attitude that hides their real fears. Adolescents are fearful of losing control and may need to be reassured that nurses and physicians can be more helpful to them when they

IMPLICATIONS FOR NURSE–CLIENT COLLABORATION

Collaborating with Adolescents

Collaboration with adolescents is greatly facilitated by nurses' acceptance and understanding of individuals' experience in this stage of life. Adolescents are preoccupied with questions about the meaning of life and with development of goals for the future, which are a part of an emerging personal identity. During self-discovery, adolescents may experience periods of preoccupation, confusion, and discouragement. Traditional cultural and societal values often are questioned and role experimentation is common. Nurses can assist adolescents during this period by helping them consider healthy alternatives and by encouraging them to do logical problem solving.

accurately describe their symptoms, including intensity of pain. Adolescents also need support in discussing their fear of illness, loss of control, and loss of privacy often associated with illness.

Sometimes, concerns about confidentiality cause teenagers to conceal their real concerns. A girl may present with a complaint like a sore throat or an upset stomach when she is really afraid she may be pregnant.

Responsibilities for Client Care

Nurses must be well acquainted with growth and development theory if they are to be effective in working with adolescents and in counseling and reassuring parents. The inherent ambivalence that adolescents face in all areas of development is less confusing when parents have provided consistent support and secure boundaries from early childhood.

Approach Adolescents as Clients. Collaboration with adolescents is an active, challenging, and rewarding experience for nurses. Parents are less directly involved in decision making about their teenagers' social and health issues, but are still essential to teenagers' well-being and security. The role of parents is to provide a supportive environment in which teenagers can mature and learn. Nurses working with teenagers must be aware of the important role parents play in motivating their adolescent to make healthy choices; therefore, nurses frequently find it beneficial to include parents in the collaborative process with adolescent clients.

Collaboration with teenagers begins during the initial psychosocial or physical assessment in which a trusting relationship begins to develop between teenager and nurse. Nurses should assess teenagers' developmental level and maturity level so that a comfortable rapport can be initiated. Teenagers who feel respected often feel less threatened by a health history and examination procedures.

Be an Active, Available Listener. Adolescents desperately require a willingness on the part of nurses to listen to their concerns and to take their problems seriously. Nurses must assure teenagers that whatever is said in confidence will not be reported to their parents; however, nurses must also caution adolescents that there may be occasions during which permission to share confidential information with parents or others may be requested of them.

Nurses convey a genuine respect to teenage clients by encouraging them to talk and by reassuring them that their concerns are real and are shared by other adolescents of the same age. Adolescents can be asked their opinion about health issues or can be asked to write their own health goals or health care plan.

Build Trust. Collaboration with parents of adolescents usually takes the form of facilitating a trusting relationship and clear communication between parents and teenager. Parents also need encouragement to know that they are doing well in their parenting role, and teenagers need positive reinforcement when they verbalize praise for their parents' guidance.

In maintaining the trusting relationship, nurses must be cautious to remain a facilitator, not taking sides with either the parent or the teenager when decisions are made but, rather, assisting them to reach either consensus or compromise.

Encourage Adolescents' Expression of Health Concerns. Because adolescents may anticipate censure or rejection, they are reluctant to describe negative health behaviors such as drug use, alcohol consumption, or unprotected sexual activity. Nurses can encourage accurate sharing of information by remaining relaxed and asking pertinent history information in a confident and direct manner.

Myths about health behaviors and illness can be corrected through clear and concise health teaching (Fig. 11–19). Adolescents should be encouraged and supported as they begin to take more responsibility for achieving and maintaining positive health habits.

Educate Parents About Expected Adolescent Behavior. Parents may need to hear that adolescents' beginning separation from them is not synonymous with decreasing love and affection for them. They may resist the increasing influence of others on their teenager, and may need to be guided to see that this process is necessary to developing an adult level of maturity and self-confidence. Nurses who are supportive and nonjudgmental with parents are likely to be perceived as helpers in the development of a healthy and happy adolescent rather than as a threat to parental authority.

Teaching parents what to expect from their teenager, what behaviors are "normal," and how to provide secure limits and rules is often helpful. Parents may need support to problem solve rationally and to be able to set reasonable limits. Nurses can also coach parents regarding nonthreatening ways to approach their teenagers to discuss emotionally charged topics such as sexuality and substance abuse.

Encourage Regular Health Checkups. The adolescent years provide nurses with multiple opportunities to pro-

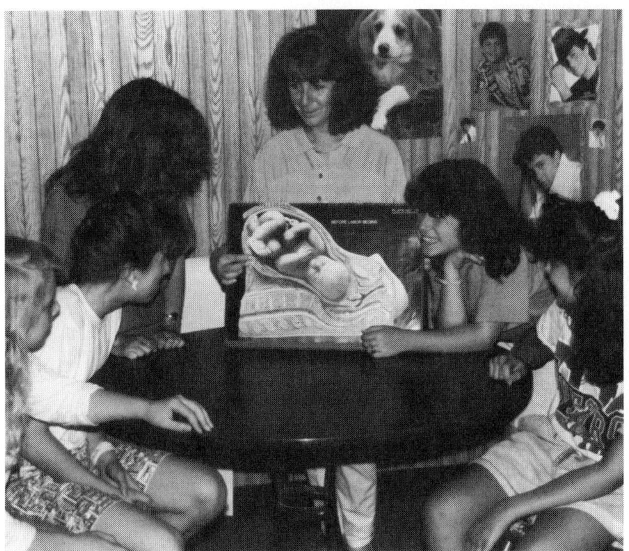

Figure 11–19. Nurses should encourage adolescents to discuss health concerns and provide teaching for the issues that are important to this age group. (Courtesy of Mary Ann Scoloveno.)

mote wellness. In addition, nurses are often in a unique position to influence others in contact with adolescents, such as teachers or guidance counselors, to promote wellness.

The American Academy of Pediatrics recommends that teenagers have a health examination at least every 2 years. Parents should not be present during these examinations. Routine immunization boosters of tetanus toxoid and diphtheria toxoid (Td) should be administered between the ages of 10 and 14 years[16] (see Table 11–2).

Adolescents may require health teaching in the areas of nutrition, dental and personal hygiene, sexual activity, sexually transmitted diseases including AIDS, and contraception. Nurses, who use a nonjudgmental approach with adolescents, encourage them to discuss health issues and concerns. This kind of discussion facilitates informed choices about health and behavior.

Nurses are also available to parents to provide similar anticipatory guidance and health education in areas of wellness promotion and injury prevention.

■ THE YOUNG ADULT (18 TO 35 YEARS OF AGE)

Physical Growth and Development

The significance of young adulthood, the period of life between 18 and 35 years of age, is not as much related to chronological age and physical growth as it is to psychosocial maturation. Young adulthood is a time of rapid personal and social change. Typically, emancipation from parents is achieved during this time, and new social groups are formed. Whether adults marry and establish a family, or remain unmarried with or without a "significant other," they begin an identification in a personal way with other adults. Generally, by age 18, physical growth is complete.

Most persons have achieved their final height but weight will vary throughout adulthood as a result of genetic and cultural influences and life-style behaviors such as nutritional intake, activity level, state of health, and personal values.

The most recent actuarial information (health, morbidity, and mortality statistics) about adult height and weight from life insurance companies in the United States and Canada is listed in Table 11–3. The insurance companies have made an attempt to relate weight by age to the lowest mortality rates for that age, thus indicating, in a quasi-scientific way, desirable weights for men and women during young and middle adulthood.

Psychosocial Development

Emotional and Social Development. Successful mastery of the developmental tasks during adolescence prepares young adults to meet the responsibilities and tasks of young adulthood in a confident way. The foremost developmental tasks of young adults are choosing a career path and building close, personal relationships (Fig. 11–20). Sometimes these tasks conflict with one another. Young adults with high goals for career achievement may forego personal relationships to pursue education or work experiences they consider critical to goal attainment. Others may invest energy in personal relationships at the expense of career achievements. The key to healthy development is balance.

Effective relationship skills are an asset in personal life and one's career. Learning them is an interactive process. In healthy relationships, individuals achieve a balanced perspective of their own needs and the needs of those close to them so both the individuals and the relationship can develop fully. Achievement of this balance depends on mature and mutual interactions with other persons.[4]

Young adults who learn to trust themselves and others in intimate relationships experience growing self-confidence and self-esteem that persist, even in times of personal adversity. They continue to learn from social and occupational experiences rather than becoming threatened or discouraged.

Young adults who fail to accomplish this task are isolated from peers, remain inward-focused and are unable to be close or spontaneous with another young adult. They become insecure, or even withdrawn and distrustful. They engage in successive, superficial relationships that are devoid of real reciprocity, intimacy, or closeness.

Self-esteem and positive social relationships influence other aspects of young adults lives, including academic, occupational, and life-style choices. The role of self-esteem and quality social relationships as a motivator for positive health behaviors is significant, and conversely, there is evidence linking low self-esteem to poor state of health.[42–44]

Cognitive Development. Like the older adolescent, thinking and reasoning skills in young adults are well developed

TABLE 11–3. HEIGHT-WEIGHT COMPARISON NORMS

Men					Women				
Height (in shoes)[a]		Weight in Pounds (in indoor clothing)[b]			Height (in shoes)[a]		Weight in Pounds (in indoor clothing)[b]		
ft.	in.	Small Frame	Medium Frame	Large Frame	ft.	in.	Small Frame	Medium Frame	Large Frame
5	2	128–134	131–141	138–150	4	10	102–111	109–121	118–131
5	3	130–136	133–143	140–153	4	11	103–113	111–123	120–134
5	4	132–138	135–145	142–156	5	0	104–115	113–126	122–137
5	5	134–140	137–148	144–160	5	1	106–118	115–129	125–140
5	6	136–142	139–151	146–164	5	2	108–121	118–132	128–143
5	7	138–145	142–154	149–168	5	3	111–124	121–135	131–147
5	8	140–148	145–157	152–172	5	4	114–127	124–138	134–151
5	9	142–151	148–160	155–176	5	5	117–130	127–141	137–155
5	10	144–154	151–163	158–180	5	6	120–133	130–144	140–159
5	11	146–157	154–166	161–184	5	7	123–136	133–147	143–163
6	0	149–160	157–170	164–188	5	8	126–139	136–150	146–167
6	1	152–164	160–174	168–192	5	9	129–142	139–153	149–170
6	2	155–168	164–178	172–197	5	10	132–145	142–156	152–173
6	3	158–172	167–182	176–202	5	11	135–148	145–159	155–176
6	4	162–176	171–187	181–207	6	0	138–151	148–162	158–179

[a] Shoes with 1-in. heels.
[b] Indoor clothing weighing 5 pounds for men and 3 pounds for women.
Source of basic data: Build Study, 1979, *Society of Actuaries and Association of Life Insurance Medical Directors of America, 1980.*

and include both concrete and abstract problem-solving capabilities; however, the quality of reasoning and judgment differs in adults as compared with adolescents. Most adults are more objective and less egocentric with problem solving than they were as teenagers.[5] For example, adults can more often separate feelings from facts in a situation. They are better able to listen to others' ideas and feelings on a topic. They may still wish to have their way, but are increasingly able to consider another's logic and feelings and to perhaps be influenced by them.

Adults learn both in formal educational or vocational programs, and in informal ways from their co-workers or friends.

Moral Development. Kohlberg[6] and other developmentalists[45] believe that capacity for moral development is established by late adolescence. In general, the young adult has internalized beliefs, values, and attitudes that guide behavior and influence personal decision making.

Principles of social justice, ethical values, religious beliefs, and personal responsibility are integrated into the young adult's social relationships with family, friends, and colleagues. Although beliefs and values are well developed, they can still be influenced by life experiences and, therefore, be changed or modified. The person reaching adulthood with a poorly defined sense of social responsibility is

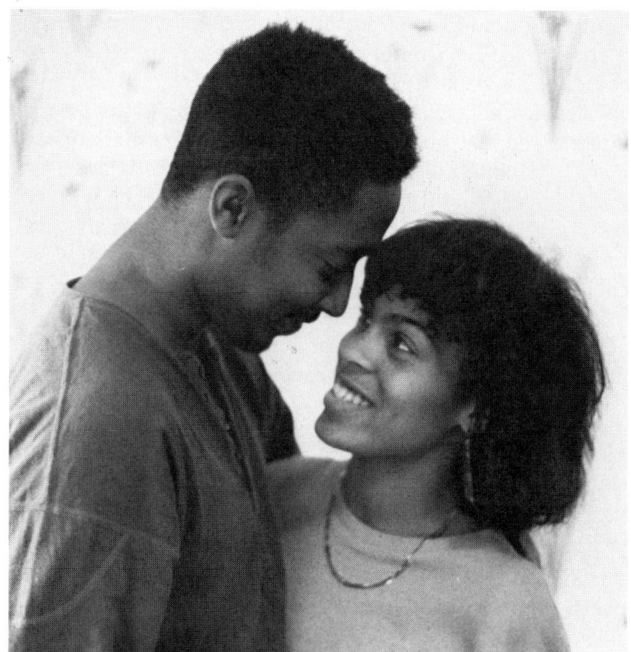

Figure 11–20. The principal developmental task of young adults is the formation of close relationships with significant others. (Courtesy of Carol Weingarten.)

less able to make consistent moral decisions than is the person with well-defined social values.

Wellness Promotion

Young adulthood is generally a time of wellness and physical stability; however, young adults should be encouraged to establish a relationship with a health care provider who will meet their needs for both routine wellness care and episodic (illness) care.

Young adults should seek a health assessment on a regular basis. Many times they receive health assessments during preemployment physicals or during routine (annual or semiannual) occupational health examinations. Frequently, young adults are required to establish a relationship with a health care professional when purchasing life or health insurance.

Young women should begin receiving routine gynecological care, including breast examination and cervical testing for cancer (Pap smear), at least by age 18 or as soon as sexual activity begins. Young men should receive routine care, including testicular examination for cancer, when physical growth is complete, at about 18 to 20 years of age. Men must learn to perform testicular examination on themselves much the same as women learn to perform breast self-examination.

Baseline diagnostic data can be collected early in adulthood. Recommended health screening includes a routine urinalysis, hemoglobin and hematocrit, lipid profile (low-density and high-density cholesterol and triglycerides), blood pressure, vision and hearing examinations, and venereal disease screening if sexually active. An ECG (electrocardiogram) may be recommended for persons with a strong family history of heart disease or hypertension. A routine tuberculosis tine test and a tetanus toxoid should be updated every 10 years.

Common Health Problems and Responses of Young Adults to Illness

Accidents. Accidents are the leading cause of death in young adults, with motor vehicle accidents producing the most deaths in both sexes.[46] Accidental injuries also include industrial accidents, drownings, and traumatic injuries incurred in violent attacks or in athletic or recreational activities.

Stress. Stress reactions culminating in maladaptive coping behaviors may be seen in young adults who are unable to cope with the responsibilities of adulthood. Stress can precipitate either physical illnesses, emotional illnesses, or combinations of both. Stress-related physical symptoms may include fatigue, interrupted sleep, headache, physical pain, overeating, anorexia, gastrointestinal pain and bleeding, and respiratory illnesses.

Obesity. Obesity has become a health problem that is frequently seen in young adults. Although the physiology of obesity is not yet completely understood, it has long been acknowledged by health care providers that social learning is a contributing factor. Individuals learn to overeat, just as they choose or make decisions about exercising. Therefore, positive life-styles can also be learned. Nurses can teach changes in diet and exercise and can encourage spouses and family members to support each other's desire to reduce weight and increase fitness.

Substance Abuse. Substance abuse in young adults contributes significantly to poor health states as well as to accidental or violent deaths. It is a major social and interpersonal problem that affects individuals from all economic groups. Alcohol, cocaine, methamphetamines, and heroin, for example, produce temporary feelings of well-being that make their use a common maladaptive coping behavior among individuals who are stressed or unable to find meaning in their lives. Barbiturates and antidepressant type drugs are also frequently abused. The "war on drugs" has become a national concern. Politicians, health care professionals, educators, and law enforcement agencies are among the many groups working to curb this growing problem. Nurses can play a role in health education to prevent substance abuse and also provide counseling and support for individuals trying to free themselves from addiction; however, the complex causes of substance abuse make it a challenging problem to solve.

Chronic Health Problems. Hypertension and early coronary artery diseases have also become health problems for young adults. These health problems are related primarily to an unhealthy life-style, particularly a high-fat diet and smoking.[47] There is evidence that use of nicotine is decreasing in all age groups, but high school seniors and college students still smoke in significant numbers. Nearly 20 percent of high school seniors smoke a half pack or more daily.[48] In this age group, cigarette smoking appears to be a social behavior that is often influenced by family and friends. According to a recent study, lung cancer is still a major cause of death and a change in this trend depends in large part on smoking cessation.[47]

Responses of Young Adults to Illness. In the young adult, as in the adolescent, illness is a threat to self-esteem. Any bodily change associated with aging, loss of function, or change in physical appearance carries with it the potential for feelings of inferiority.

Most adults cope well with minor illnesses and are able to seek appropriate intervention, initiate, and carry out health treatments. Even young adults begin to understand that death can occur at any age as they see close friends die from accidents, malignancies, or cardiac disease. Thus, young adults may become very anxious when ill, seemingly out of proportion to the problem presented. This may lead to a dependency on parents, spouses, or friends until the anxiety is diminished. Typical worries of young adults in response to illness include worries about job security, financial resources and costs, and security in social relationships. Additionally, young adults may have little experience with life crises.

Nurses caring for hospitalized or ill young adults must recognize anxiety and actively intervene to decrease fear and agitation. Supportive interventions by nurses or family members can often provide clients with the strength necessary to cope with a situational crisis.

Responsibilities for Client Care

Facilitate Consolidation of Life Goals. A priority for nurses working with young adults is to develop a mutual, trusting relationship with clients. Nurses must quickly assess young adults' developmental level, expressing respect for clients by soliciting their concerns.

Young adult clients have the physical and emotional capacity to identify life goals and to initiate a course of action to achieve these goals; however, many young adults are ambivalent and filled with misgivings when faced with the responsibility of making important decisions by themselves.

As discussed above, career selection is a major developmental task of young adulthood. One of the primary ways in which personal identity and self-esteem are expressed is through commitment to an occupation. Career choice is influenced by gender, parental occupation, ability, and previous quality of education. Young adults who are unable to make a career choice may have difficulty defining personal interests or strengths and making decisions or commitments.

Nurses working with young adults must be aware of the difficulty and distress some persons experience when making life choices. Nurses are often in a position to recognize anxiety behaviors precipitated by this stressor, and may be able to help clients increase awareness of their stress. A supportive approach and the ability to be an attentive listener can enhance clients' ability to recognize and work through these decisions in a successful way.

Nurses are frequently influential in helping clients to clarify their ideas and goals and to encourage their attempts at problem solving. Nurses can counsel and listen to clients' concerns, assist in the examination of alternatives, and praise and positively reinforce decisions to take action.

Encourage Good Health Practices. Because young adults feel well, they may develop a nonchalant attitude about health care. This period has a very important influence on later stages of adult health. It is during times of good health that nurses can offer positive reinforcement of healthy behaviors and assist clients to recognize behaviors that may precipitate poor health in the future. Nurses should inform young adults of the long-term and short-term dangers of poor life style choices to encourage them not to smoke, to drink only in moderation, to eat nutritionally sound foods, to exercise, and to learn appropriate ways of managing stress.

Assist Young Adults to Develop Coping Skills. Nurses recognize that symptoms in young adults may be stress related, that is, the result of overwork, lack of sleep, poor dietary practices, or unhealthy health habits such as alcohol and substance abuse. Clients can begin to eliminate or modify poor health habits only when they become aware that their physiological symptoms are precipitated by or intensified by inadequate coping.

Nurses can educate and work with young adults to establish more effective coping skills. Clients need to hear that anxiety-precipitated symptoms commonly occur and can be effectively dealt with by making life-style changes. Nurses can reassure clients that they are not mentally ill, but are actually in a position to recognize danger signs and to modify behavior in positive ways.

Recognize the Right of Young Adults to Make Personal Choices. Because some adults prefer to make decisions based on personal study, nurses may find it helpful to provide health information in book, pamphlet, or list format. Support groups can also be of benefit to young adults.

Nurses sometimes feel frustrated when working with clients who are unwilling to take responsibility for their own health. Long-held beliefs and values are the basis for health behaviors. Changes in life-style require changes in values, a process that takes time, reinforcement and repeated exposure to new ideas. Nurses who have a positive, but realistic attitude and convey information without trying to control clients' decisions build trust. This approach is more effective in developing a collaborative nurse–client relationship.

The nurse–client collaborative interaction continues even when the client is very dependent and appears powerless in regard to meeting personal health requirements. Nurses can reinforce that they will be available for support and education and that they recognize that the process of behavior change is a difficult one. This attitude conveys that they have confidence that change is possible and that the client will not always be dependent on them.

■ THE MIDDLE ADULT (35 TO 65 YEARS OF AGE)

Physical Growth and Development

More than 80 million people in the United States, one third of the population, are considered to be middle-aged.[49] This section focuses on both early middle and late middle adulthood.

Chronologically, middle adulthood covers the years from 35 to 65 years of age, but as with other stages of human development, middle adulthood is a time of wide physiological and psychosocial variation. The physiological aging process is influenced by many variables, among them heredity, patterns of physical activity, states of physical and emotional health, nutrition, environment, stressful life experiences, and financial status.

During the middle years of life, physical changes (some

degenerative) occur as part of the aging process, but the onset is extremely variable and depends on health state, inherited tendencies, nutritional status, attitude, and regularity of activity and exercise. With the increased focus on health and fitness in US society, many adults in the middle years of their lives learn new physical skills or maintain proficiencies developed during their youth. Others may focus on developing and maintaining strength and stamina as well as exploring hobbies and recreational activities that also support physical fitness. There are those, however, who do not pursue physical activities either because they are not motivated or because they lack resources (ie, financial) to pursue physical fitness, and whose health may consequently suffer.

In general, body weight redistributes around the waist, hips, and abdomen during middle adulthood. Also, skin changes resulting from decreased turgor and elasticity and decreased muscle tone may be evident especially in overweight, less active individuals. The skin becomes coarser and wrinkled, and facial hair may appear in women. Loss of bone calcium may predispose adults to skeletal and small bone changes to the point in older adulthood where several inches in height may be lost. Near the end of middle adulthood, both males and females experience hormonal changes. In women, menopause indicates the end of reproductive ability. Reproductive ability in the female ceases in the fifth decade of life and reduced hormonal production may contribute to a change in sexual function in both males and females. Coping with the realization that the ability to bear children is gone may be difficult for some women; other women welcome this change. The physiological changes accompanying menopause can be an uncomfortable reminder of aging in some women, but can often be lessened in intensity by hormone replacement therapy. In some men, reduced testosterone production may decrease sexual function and reproductive ability, but ordinarily sexual function remains intact in men and women.

Psychosocial Development

Emotional and Social Development. From a psychosocial perspective, aging is a function of cognition. The old adage "you are only as old as you feel" can be applied to the time of middle adulthood. Because of improved health care and medical technology, control of disease, emphasis on healthy life style choices and the shift in responsibility for good health from health care providers to individuals, the functional life span has been extended by several decades. Correspondingly, persons now expect to live in a productive and vigorous fashion well into late adulthood.

The primary psychosocial task of middle adulthood is to show caring for others in active and satisfying ways.[4] Middle adulthood is the time of life in which the new generation is nurtured. Adults become more outwardly focused than in young adulthood, committing themselves to their spouse, to children, to others, or to creative projects (Fig. 11–21). This is often a richly satisfying period in life, a time when people can relinquish competitiveness and comparisons to others. Healthy middle adults are able to live comfortably with their successes without brooding about their failures.

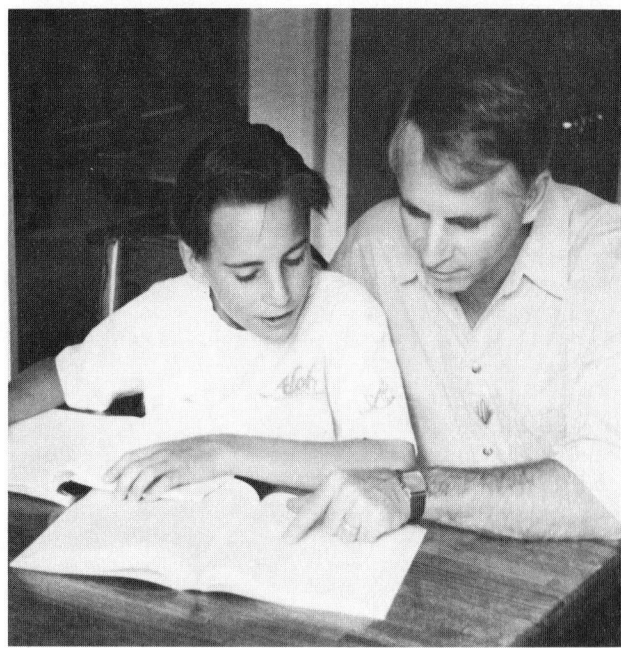

Figure 11–21. People in middle adulthood commit themselves to the nurturing of their children.

Adults who fail to direct their energy outward become self-indulgent and rigid. Self-absorbed adults experience an overwhelming sense of stagnation and an acute sense of loss over "what might have been."

Middle adults with careers often reach their peak of productivity and effectiveness during this life stage. This is affirming and gratifying. As they near the end of the middle adult years, retirement plans become a focus and many adults look forward to having more time to spend with loved ones, on hobbies, or other leisure pursuits.

For those who have not met their personal or career aspirations, "midlife crisis" ensues. This is a period of reexamination of what is important and meaningful in life. Some adults in midlife crisis feel a sense of urgency and despair and may engage in self-destructive behaviors. Some respond by returning to school or seeking a second career. When individuals confront midlife crisis with constructive re-evaluation and responses, life is rejuvenating, rather than defeating.

Cognitive Development. The capacity for cognitive or intellectual growth during middle adulthood, in the absence of neurological disease, remains active. Learning is characterized by adults in their middle years as both purposeful and enjoyable. The significant cognitive capacity of persons in middle adulthood is reflected in the peak occupational performance discussed above and in individuals who enroll in college during middle adult years. Some individuals seek an education that prepares them for a new career or contributes to career advancement.

Moral Development. Most middle adults remain concerned about justice and fairness. They strive to live in such a way that they do not infringe on others choices. Some function as mentors: knowledgeable, experienced individuals who serve as guides for someone younger. Other middle adults demonstrate greater altruism and compassion for others by actively working to protect the rights of disadvantaged populations. They may become involved with charitable organizations and devote considerable energy to causes outside the sphere of personal needs.

Wellness Promotion

Adults experience varying degrees of physical aging during middle adulthood. Organ systems and body parts age at different rates in different individuals; however, physiological changes are inevitable. The emotional feeling of "being old" may surface during this time of development, largely related to attitude, self-esteem, or the absence of significant supportive persons. Feelings of depression in middle-aged adults are often related to loss: loss of children or friends, loss of body integrity, loss of youthful appearance, and loss of the dreams established at a younger age. Some middle adults also notice changes in sleep patterns, sexual function, and energy level. It is therefore essential that persons in middle adulthood seek regular health screening and make deliberate decisions about how they will respond to these feelings and changes.

Differences between active, energetic adults and prematurely debilitated adults are a function of genetics, learning, healthy life-style, and personal attitudes. Clients may need to learn information and strategies that are useful in maintaining health well into old age. As with other stages of life, elimination of unhealthy life behaviors assists adults to feel well, to look younger, and to maintain a higher level of energy.

Adequate nutrition, regular aerobic exercise such as walking or swimming, continued social interaction and recreation, adequate amounts of rest and solitude, and purposeful life goals are health behaviors to be promoted with clients in this age group (Fig. 11–22). Nurses are in a position to reinforce healthy behaviors and interpret undesirable behaviors as having serious long-term health effects.

Common Health Problems and Responses of Middle Adults to Illness

Obesity. Obesity continues to be a health problem for some persons in middle adulthood, most often as a result of diets high in fat and carbohydrates, compounded by inadequate amounts of physical exercise. The basal metabolic rate (BMR) decreases by about 20 percent from age 40 to age 65, which also increases the potential for weight gain.[50] Obesity predisposes clients to health problems such as coronary artery disease, diabetes mellitus, hypertension, and orthopedic problems. Adults who are depressed or isolated may turn to food or alcohol for comfort, which may contribute to unwanted weight gain.

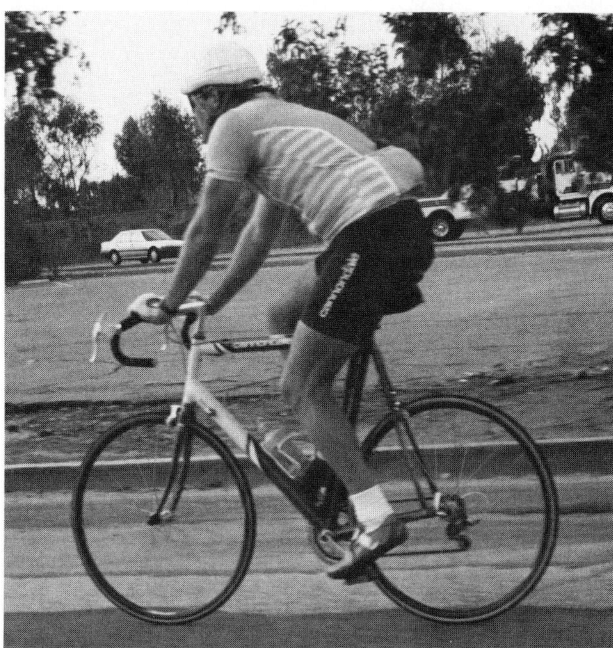

Figure 11–22. Adults should be encouraged to participate in healthy behaviors such as exercising.

Dental, Auditory, and Visual Problems. Dental health problems can develop as aging continues but can be largely prevented by good hygiene, including gum massage to stimulate circulation. Presbyopia, the farsightedness of middle age, develops and glasses are usually needed for reading, sewing, or other activities that require visual acuity at close range. Auditory reaction time slows and sound discrimination decreases. Sensory changes precipitate body image concerns particularly if appliances, such as canes and hearing aids, become necessary. Sensory changes may predispose individuals to accidental injuries in the home or when driving the car.

Accidents. The incidence of disabling accidents increases in this age group. Motor vehicle accidents resulting from alcohol use, impaired vision, or decreased response time are the most common types of accidental injury in men. Both men and women suffer other accidental injuries including lacerations and falls at work and in the home, especially from ladders and steps. Additional causes of accidental injury include exposure to cold (hypothermia)[51] and drowning.[52] Alcohol and drug abuse continue as a cause of illness and accidental injury for persons in middle adulthood.

Chronic Respiratory Problems. Chronic illnesses resulting from unhealthy life-styles can be a frequent source of lost work days in middle-aged adults. Respiratory and pulmonary illnesses such as asthma, obstructive lung disease, and cancers of the respiratory tract may develop after years of cigarette smoking or environmental or occupational pollution.

The incidence of cardiovascular disease increases in the latter part of middle adulthood. Hypertension, coronary artery disease, and stroke are more prevalent among individuals over 55 years old.[53] Although some of the heightened risk is a factor of age-related loss of elasticity in blood vessel walls, and is therefore unavoidable, most of the factors that contribute to cardiovascular disease are under individuals' control.

Cigarette smoking, high blood cholesterol levels, obesity, physical inactivity, high sodium intake, and stress significantly increase individuals' chances of developing cardiovascular disease. Individuals can modify or eliminate all of them by personal choices. In fact, age-adjusted death rates for major cardiovascular disease have steadily declined since 1978, and this is due, at least in part, to healthier life-styles.[53]

Degenerative Musculoskeletal Disease. Muscles lose tone and strength in the later years of middle adulthood, particularly among inactive individuals. With appropriate exercise, rest and nutrition, middle adults can maintain or even improve muscle tone and strength, despite aging. Osteoporosis, loss of bone density, is associated with advancing age and is especially likely in postmenopausal women. Regular activity can also mitigate the occurrence of osteoporosis.

Cancer. Although great progress has been made in early detection, treatment, survival, and quality of life for persons with cancer, it remains as the second leading cause of death in the United States. Men have a high incidence of bladder and lung cancer; for women, breast, colon-rectal, and uterine cancers are most common.[54]

Responses of Middle Adults to Illness. Most adults adjust gradually to the aging process. Many are motivated to take excellent care of themselves so that their strength and energy are maintained and the physiological processes of aging are controlled. Middle-aged adults have highly individualized responses to illness. Since many of them are active in careers, concern about lost productivity or job status may be a primary concern. For others inability to maintain family responsibilities creates considerable stress. Most middle-aged adults are uncomfortable with illness-associated dependency on others and may find life-style restrictions burdensome; however, illness forces many to confront the reality of diminishing vitality and motivates them to change unhealthful habits.

Since most adults in this age group have experienced serious illness and death of loved ones, they often consider their own death as a plausible outcome of illness, even when the illness is not life threatening. Nurses who appreciate that the experience of illness for this age group is complex and individualized can effectively facilitate positive adaptation.

Responsibilities for Client Care

Establish Mutuality in Communications. Whether nurses encounter middle-aged adults in acute care, rehabilitation, or wellness-oriented settings, showing respect for clients' autonomy and individuality is crucial. Most adults wish to be informed and consulted about procedures and treatment options whether they are undergoing routine screening or seeking help for a serious health alteration. A man who is worried about the effects of progressive age-related hair loss needs a supportive and sensitive approach as much as another man facing the burden of surgery. Nurses who demonstrate by a warm and caring manner their awareness that all health problems cause some degree of threat earn clients' trust. This is the basis for effective communication and collaboration.

Adults throughout the period of middle adulthood may have health concerns and fears of future disability or inability to function autonomously. Nurses can acknowledge these concerns, find out what clients are willing and able to do to modify the situation, and discuss or demonstrate strategies that can be used to accomplish client goals.

It is important for nurses to listen to concerns about aging, life transition, and goals for the future. Nurses can assist individuals to develop a realistic understanding of the physiological and social life changes that they are experiencing, and encourage a positive attitude toward healthy life practices. If clients wish, their spouses or another family member can be included in the health assessment and care planning activities.

Encourage Clients to Modify Unhealthy Habits. Most adults wish to maintain good health and independence, and are motivated to seek health care and change some life-style behaviors. Others may not make those choices; however, nurses can continue to provide support for the actions these clients do take to maintain health.

Nurses can reinforce positive health behaviors that help minimize the effects of changes resulting from aging. Individuals who maintain a nutritious diet and a balance between activity and rest, who have time for socializing and for being alone, and who maintain a positive attitude are frequently the same individuals who are interested in and willing to collaborate with nurses so that they successfully manage health and illness.

Encourage Clients to Seek Preventive Health Care. Clients are encouraged to seek regular, preventive health care including complete diagnostic and laboratory data when indicated. Some experts recommend complete yearly physical examinations. Clients who prefer or can afford only selected screening should have hearing and vision tests, blood pressure checks, and dental care annually. Because of the morbidity and mortality associated with cancer in this age group, it is also recommended that women have yearly mammograms after age 40, pelvic examinations with Pap testing, and examinations of stool specimens for occult blood. Men should have annual occult blood testing and testicular and prostate examinations. Nurses have a responsibility to teach clients how to perform self breast and testicular examinations, to recognize the signs and symptoms of cancer, and to seek health care if they experience these or other unusual symptoms.

Reinforce Positive Self-image. Many adults begin to notice signs of aging in their skin, muscle tone, and energy level as they experience middle adulthood. Recognition of physical aging can be moderately or significantly threatening to self-esteem and body image especially to those who equate their personal worth with external (physical) appearance.

This same realization that physical aging changes are beginning to occur can be a motivating factor in health behavior. Persons who wish to maintain or improve their appearance, stamina, or overall feelings of good health may be motivated to eat and exercise properly, get adequate amounts of rest and relaxation, and avoid health hazards, such as smoking, alcohol, excessive sun exposure, and overeating, that may accelerate the aging process.

Nurses can support clients' enthusiasm for physical fitness by positively reinforcing healthy decision making, by praising the client who has made progress toward personal health goals (such as a steady weight loss), and by offering information or correcting misperceptions so that the client can be more effective in meeting goals.

THE OLDER ADULT (65+ YEARS)

Physical Growth and Development

In the United States, nearly 35 million people are considered older adults. That number is projected to increase to 59 million by 2020, including more than 6 million who are 85 years and older, and 266,000 who are 100 years and older.[49]

Age-related physiological changes generally become more evident as chronological age increases. The same factors that influence the aging process in middle adulthood also apply to older adults, with degeneration being especially apparent in those over age 80.

Many of the physiological changes described for the middle-aged adult apply to the older adult as well. The older adult must adapt to a relative decline in physical development. For example, many older adults experience less keen memory, hearing, vision, taste, and smell. They may experience a slower reaction time than previously, which requires adjustments in activities, such as driving a motor vehicle, that demand rapid decision making and reactions. Changes in appetite, food intake, sleep patterns, exercise, and elimination patterns may require adaptations or adjustments. Some older adults find that they adjust by eating smaller portions of blander food, that they have a decrease in appetite, or that they prefer to eat many small meals daily rather than three large ones. Many older adults will describe a greater sensitivity to temperature of food and beverage.

It is important, however, to avoid viewing older adults only as declining in health and vigor. Many adults can and do retain vitality and zest for life well into this development stage, as evidenced by those who compete in the Senior Olympics, who participate in worldwide travel, who continue in the work force, and who are productive in scientific and academic areas. Although there are older adults who are frail rather than vigorous, this is also true of people in the other developmental groups. Aging is not synonymous with debilitation and dependency.

Psychosocial Development

Emotional and Social Development. The psychosocial task of older adults is to develop a satisfying sense of the past and of their accomplishments and to reconcile these with wishes for what might have been.[4] Older adults are able to develop a perspective on life, based on experience, and desire to pass on this wisdom to others. Erikson suggests that older adults are developing a pattern of ego integrity versus despair.[4] Ego integrity implies that older adults have a sense of trust in themselves and others, permitting them to function both autonomously and interdependently. They now begin to bring those unique dimensions together into an integrated whole, which contributes to a sense of overall well-being. Their goal is to develop a wise perspective of the past and integrate it into a present way of living that is not overly concerned with death.

Psychosocial development encompasses sexuality and body image, which may be affected by aging particularly because it causes some structural changes including loss of muscle strength and tone. Conversely, adults who are comfortable with themselves, with their image of themselves, and with their bodies will incorporate changes related to aging into their body image, which can continue to be positive. The capacity to maintain an intimate relationship continues for many older adults.

Frequently nurses encounter older adults who have outlived their spouses, children, or friends. Although they have life experiences to rely on in managing these losses, they too may benefit from a supportive approach in this effort. It is helpful to assess whether or not older adults have developed effective coping strategies for managing losses of loved ones. Ideally, older adults have developed the capacity to accept their approaching death. Nurses can be supportive of these individuals and facilitate this adaptation among those who have not prepared themselves emotionally for death.

Cognitive Development. Many of the points made about cognitive functioning in middle-aged adults apply to older adults. Abilities vary depending on how well developed they are and how well they are exercised. Adults who valued and developed the ability to express ideas may continue to seek opportunities to remain intellectually active, for example, in professions such as science, education, and law, in entertainment, and in human rights endeavors.

BUILDING NURSING KNOWLEDGE

How Important Is Social Support to Health Promotion Among Older Adults?

Ryan MC, Austin AG. Social supports and social networks in the aged. *Image:* J Nurs Scholarship. 1989;21(3):176–180.

In this article, Ryan and Austin are concerned about the role of the social environment, and especially of social support, in health promotion and health maintenance. Social support is the degree to which a person's basic social needs are gratified through interaction with others. These needs include affection, esteem, approval, belonging, identity, and security and are provided through one's social network, the social relationships that make others accessible.

The authors reviewed research on the subject of social support among older adults. They noted that recent research shows that social support has direct effects on health and well-being. To be healthy, older adults must achieve a fit between their own needs and abilities and the resources and demands of the environment.

Research data summarized by Ryan and Austin suggest that social support is related to illness among older adults. For example, the availability of social networks influences how quickly an elderly person is hospitalized following the onset of illness. Social support conceivably may reduce the likelihood of the onset of physical and mental illness. There is also evidence of an association between lack of social ties and increased incidence of death among older adults. Social support apparently mediates the health effects of major life events.

Moral Development. Older adults build on their previous moral development. Although moral development is usually completed in the early adult years, older adults have the capacity to modify their values and beliefs. Adults who have experienced a satisfying life as a result of their values and beliefs will generally retain these values and beliefs. Their moral legacy may be reflected in some older adults' final estate planning, which may include donations to institutions or entities that are consistent with their values.

Wellness Promotion

Older adults often cope well with changes in their lives, seek preventive health care on a regular basis, and engage in a wide range of healthy self-care practices. Many experience vigor and well-being to the extent that they require only support and validation for what they are doing to maintain health.

As in middle adulthood, older adults need to exercise self-care activities such as maintaining appropriate nutrition, sleep, exercise (Fig. 11–23), socialization, and recreational activities and seeking regular health care including immunizations and health screening. Maintaining hydration is also an important part of wellness for older adults. They require 2½ quarts of water daily. They should obtain at least 1½ quarts from beverages and the rest from food sources.

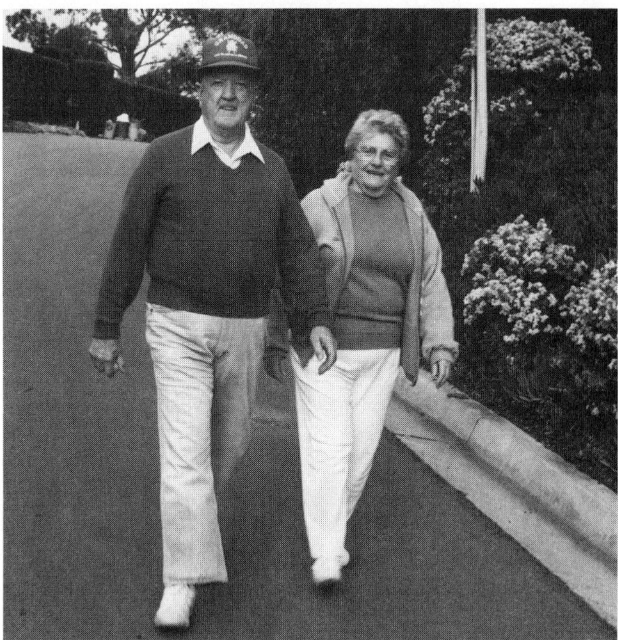

Figure 11–23. Older adults can help to maintain health and prevent illness by participating in regular exercise.

Common Health Problems and Responses of Older Adults to Illness

As organs and organ system aging occurs, many changes become apparent that render them generally less able to function well. Such organ stress can also result in disease. Tissue and cellular aging contributes to the organ degeneration as do heredity and an unhealthy life-style. For some older adults these processes and factors result in chronic illness or disability that may make it difficult for them to independently care for themselves. Approximately 1.5 million persons are currently in 20,000 long-term-care facilities in this country, according to Katz, who predicts that the number will increase to 4.5 million in 10 years.[55]

Cardiovascular, respiratory, and musculoskeletal diseases cause major physiological impairments that often result in psychosocial deficits as well. These common health problems were described earlier in the section on middle age.

In addition, suicide, infections, arthritis, and diabetes are common in older adults. Cancer in persons aged 65 and older is the second leading cause of death.[56]

Sleep Disturbances. Older adults often express concerns about disruptions in their sleep patterns. It is important to conduct an assessment to learn more about the factors contributing to this problem, rather than simply suggesting remedies to alleviate the sleep pattern disruption.[57]

Sensory Deficits. Many older adults experience a decline in sensory abilities including a decrease in visual, hearing, and taste acuity. These changes require modifications in life-style to prevent injury and perhaps strengthen remaining abilities. This may involve cooking with different flavorings, adjusting lighting or other safety features, or providing assistive devices, such as eyeglasses.

Accidents. Accidents, especially from falls, are common in older adults. It is possible to predict individuals who are most at risk for falls.[58] Another common health problem is the large number and types of medications that some older adults consume, often without knowledge of the possible interactions and effects. This occurrence can be considered a source of accidental injury and should always be considered in client assessments.

Depression. Depression is a common psychiatric disorder among the elderly; some maintain that it is the most common disorder.[55] Behavioral and psychological deficits are common health problems for many older adults.[56] Etiology varies, and for some of these problems there may be multiple causes or contributing factors. Depression, substance abuse, abuse of older adults (especially females over age 75), and Alzheimer's disease all have behavioral and emotional components and manifestations.

The loss of a spouse triggers a combination of physical and emotional responses. It is often a threat to self-concept and sense of wholeness. It disrupts personal routines and social activities. After years of identity as part of a couple, being alone can be intensely difficult. One study, however, showed that the transition from being a spouse to being a widow or widower is not always unwelcome.[59] If approached correctly, older adults can use this transition as a time to determine their strengths and identify contributions that they might yet make to society.

Dementia. Dementia is a global decline in intellectual functioning. It is usually progressive and irreversible and frequently causes significant interference with social functioning. Although only 5 percent of 65 to 74 year olds have dementia, it is a more common problem after age 80, when 30 percent are effected.[60] Alzheimer's disease is responsible for 60 to 70 percent of dementia.[60] Alzheimer's disease is a significant problem for many families, because many of those affected are cared for at home—usually by wives or daughters.[61,62]

IMPLICATIONS FOR NURSE–CLIENT COLLABORATION

Collaborating With Older Adults

To collaborate successfully with older adults, nurses must see the value of wellness promotion for this age group. Sharing perspectives and reaching a consensus with older individuals may lead to goals that seem so small as to be insignificant, but may in actuality represent a portion of wellness that proves to be very important to the client. For example, older clients may decide to work on a hobby that once was interesting and that might continue to stimulate their mind and body in ways that enhance self-esteem. Helping older clients to find or resume such outlets makes a substantial contribution to their health.

Responses of Older Adults to Illness. Responses to illness vary with the individual. They are affected by past experiences, coping skills, attitudes, beliefs, values, knowledge, and physical condition. Older adults who are ill have concerns similar to those of middle adults, discussed earlier.

Responsibilities for Client Care

Provide Knowledge for Illness Prevention. Some older adults lack the knowledge, capacity, or motivation to maintain or attain their optimal level of wellness. Depression, chronic illness, disability, and overreliance on multiple medications create a need for assistance in developing a greater focus on wellness in their lives. Older adults also may need assistance in managing accident prevention and safety promotion activities. Maintaining or improving diet is often a challenge, especially for older adults who are below or near the poverty level or who live alone.

Regular exercise is as necessary for older adults as for younger people (see Fig. 11–23). To many older adults, however, exercise may seem to be an overwhelming challenge or may not seem to be a priority. Nurses can support and reinforce the need for health- and wellness-focused activities that older adults are performing. For example, older adults who enjoyed a certain hobby at one time can be encouraged to continue with these creative activities. Nurses also have a responsibility to discuss with older adults both potentially harmful and potentially helpful activities.

Express the Value of Health Promotion. To successfully collaborate with older adults, nurses must see the value in wellness promotion for these clients and must see them as contributors to the process of collaboration. Sharing perspectives and reaching a consensus with clients can lead to the achievement of goals that, however small, may prove to be very important to a client. Nurses should also encourage socialization through community-based activity groups, for example, hot lunch programs, hobby and craft groups, and recreational groups where older adults gather to pursue interests and socialization.

Assist with Relocation. Having to move from one's home is a common experience during late adulthood. The reason for the move may be deteriorating health, loss of a spouse, financial problems, or fear of crime, among others. Older adults may relocate to another independent housing situation such as a small apartment, but more commonly the move is to a family member's home, retirement facility, long-term care facility or nursing home. These moves are almost universally stressful, and in some cases may be life threatening.[1] Nurses can help older clients and families anticipating this problem to prepare for it. The most important consideration is involving the older adult in the decision about the move. Discussing available alternatives, their benefits and disadvantages, and the timing and circumstances of the move will enable clients to retain feelings of control. Moreover, when family members share their feelings, even negative feelings, about the move, share collaborative problem solving, and achieve resolution of associated conflicts, stress for all is reduced.

Older adults and their families need continued support and assistance after the move. Older adults experience loneliness and loss of dignity and personal integrity. Families feel grief, guilt, and uncertainty about the decision. Frequent visits from family, socialization with other members of the new "community," recreational activities, personal space, and opportunities to reminisce about the past with attentive listeners facilitate elders' adaptation. If they are able to adapt successfully, their family members can better accept the new living arrangements as well.

Assist Older Adults with Transitional Adjustment. Nurses can collaborate with older adults in discussing their concerns regarding health, illness, injury, self-care, death, and needed resources. Possible effective strategies include engaging clients in a life review or reminiscence,[1,56] exploring alternate ways of adapting and coping with the health problems, and discussing economics of their health care that are frequently overwhelming to adults on fixed incomes.

Nurses can also learn from older clients, which requires an open, accepting attitude toward them and toward aging. Listening to clients' personal perspectives on age-related needs also provides an opportunity to gather assessment data. After nurses share their professional perspective, they can work toward a consensus and develop a plan to meet clients' expressed needs.

Although collaboration is generally appropriate and effective with older adults, in some situations clients may be unable to participate in this process. For example, clients with some chronic illnesses lack the capacity to express a perspective pertaining to the health problem. In this situation, nurses may need to meet with family members or rely on past discussions in which clients shared their preference for action in the event that they became incapacitated (Chapter 3). Clients may even have left written instructions in anticipation of this occurrence. Older adults may, temporarily or over an extended period, need to rely on other family members to act in their best interest in discussions with nurses, not unlike the time when the older adults acted on behalf of their infants and young children.

Nurses can support older clients in making transitions needed to maintain or achieve healthy life practices. Nurses can encourage older adults to express feelings about loss of loved ones, their family home, or career and then assist them to resolve these feelings with beneficial actions. In some cases nurses may determine that a referral is needed to help the clients cope with these feelings of loss.

Be Available to Discuss Issues Surrounding Death and Dying with Older Clients and Family. Nurses who have a collaborative relationship with older adults may be in a position to discuss death, dying, and a living will with older adults. Murray and Zentner stress that dying, which announces the finality of life, can be a final growth experience for the aged and the culmination of a purposeful life if it is acknowledged and dealt with openly and meaningfully.[1] This statement implies that mutual interaction is necessary even near the end of life.

SUMMARY

The assessment of clients' stage of growth and development is the beginning point of the process of nursing. All human beings grow and develop in predictable and continuous patterns, even though variations in rate and capability vary from person to person.

Because growth and development occur in an orderly fashion beginning at conception, these human phenomena become an appropriate structure for the classification of the nurse–client collaboration necessary for wellness. Nurses who are knowledgeable about expected developmental behavior and abilities are able to approach clients with confidence and interact with them in ways appropriate to their level of understanding.

Collaboration between nurses and clients is an important component in the process of assisting clients of all ages to achieve their optimal growth, development, health, and wellness. Nurses also use the collaborative approach when they involve clients across the life span in decision making in an attempt to resolve health problems.

Use of the collaborative model is predicated on a commitment to consider clients as participants, to the fullest extent possible, in creating a health care contract. This model requires that nurses understand human responses to wellness, health, illness, and trauma in each of the life stages. Knowledge of growth and development across the life cycle, integrated with other specialized nursing knowledge, skills, and attitudes that are based in the arts and sciences, creates a framework within which collaboration can occur.

Nurses who use the collaborative model recognize limitations imposed when clients cannot understand consequences of a health care decision or cannot take responsibility for the decision. The sources of these limitations can be the level of growth and development and the client's health–illness state. In the collaborative model nurses focus on clients and their responses to health and illness.

REFERENCES

1. Murray RB, Zentner JP. *Nursing Assessment and Health Promotion Strategies Through the Life Span.* Norwalk, CT: Appleton & Lange; 1989.
2. Hagerman RJ. Growth and development. In: Hathaway WE, Groothuis JR, Hay WW, Paisley JW, eds. *Current Pediatric Diagnosis and Treatment.* Norwalk, CT: Appleton and Lange; 1991.
3. Tanner JM, Davies PSW. Clinical longitudinal standards for height and weight velocity of North American children. *J Pediatr.* 1985;107:317–329.
4. Erikson E. *Childhood and Society,* 2nd ed. New York: WW Norton; 1963.

5. Piaget J. *The Theory of Stages in Cognitive Development.* New York: McGraw-Hill; 1969.
6. Kohlberg L. The cognitive-developmental approach to moral education. *Phi Delta Kappa.* 1975;56:670–677.
7. Colombo J. The critical period concept: Research, methodology and theoretical issues. *Psychol Bull.* 1982;81:260–275.
8. Chasnoff I, Jones KL. Presentations at Drug Victims × 3: Mothers, Babies and Society, A Conference on Perinatal Substance Abuse, San Diego, Jan 26, 1990.
9. Sherwen LN, Scoloveno MA, Weingarten CT. *Nursing Care of the Childbearing Family.* Norwalk, CT: Appleton & Lange; 1991.
10. Caldwell B. Education of families for parenting. In: Youngman M, Brazelton T, eds. *In Support of Families.* Cambridge, MA: Harvard University Press; 1986:229.
11. Bowlby J. *Attachment and Loss.* New York: Basic Books; 1969: vol 1.
12. McCartney K, Phillips D. Motherhood and child care. In Birn B, Hays D, eds. *The Different Faces of Motherhood.* New York: Plenum Press; 1988:157–183.
13. Willard A. Cultural scripts for mothering. In: Gilligan C, Ward J, Taylor J, Bardige B, eds. *Mapping the Moral Domain.* Cambridge, MA: Harvard University Press; 1988:225–243.
14. Birns B, Hays D, eds. *The Different Faces of Motherhood.* New York: Plenum Press; 1988.
15. Ginsberg H, Opper S. *Piaget's Theory of Intellectual Development: An Introduction.* Englewood Cliffs, NJ: Prentice-Hall; 1969.
16. Committee on Practice and Ambulatory Medicine. Recommendations for preventive pediatric health care. *Pediatrics.* 1988; 81(3).
17. Foye H, Sulkes S. Developmental and behavioral pediatrics. In: Behrman R, Vaughan V, eds. *Nelson Essentials of Pediatrics.* Philadelphia: WB Saunders; 1990:32–33.
18. Weston WL. Skin. In: Hathaway WE, Groothuis JR, Hay WW, Paisley JW, eds. *Current Pediatric Diagnosis and Treatment.* Norwalk, CT: Appleton & Lange; 1991.
19. Hughes D, Johnson K, Rosenbaum S, Liu J. *The Health of America's Children: Maternal and Child Health Data Book.* Washington, DC: Adolescent Pregnancy Prevention: Prenatal Campaign/ Children's Defense Fund; 1989.
20. Miller C, Fine A, Adams-Taylor S. *Monitoring Children's Health: Key Indicators,* 2nd ed. Washington, DC: American Public Health Association; 1989.
21. National Safety Council. *Accident Facts, 1987 Edition.* Chicago: National Safety Council; 1987.
22. Vazquez-Seoane P., Widom R, Pearson HA. Disappearance of iron deficiency in a high risk infant population given supplemental iron. *N Engl J Med.* 1985;313:1239–1240.
23. Frankenberg WK. *Denver Developmental Screening Test.* Revised. Boulder, CO: University of Colorado Medical Center; 1978.
24. Gilligan C, Wiggins G. The origins of early morality in early childhood relationships. In: Gilligan C, Ward J, Taylor J, Bardige B. *Mapping the Moral Domain.* Cambridge, MA: Harvard University Press; 1986:111–138.
25. Centers for Disease Control. Fatal injuries to children—United States, 1986. *MMWR.* 1991; 39:442–450.
26. Centers for Disease Control. Morbidity attributable to HIV infections/AIDS—United States, 1981–1990. *MMWR.* 1991; 40: 41–44.
27. US Department of Health and Human Services Agency for Toxic Substances and Disease Registry. *The Nature and Extent of Lead Poisoning in Children in the States: A Report to Congress.* Atlanta, GA: Public Health Service; July 1988.
28. Centers for Disease Control. Mumps—United States, 1985–1986. *MMWR.* 1987;36:151–155.
29. Lewin L. Establishing a therapeutic relationship with an abused child. *Pediatr Nurs.* 1990;16(3):263–264.
30. Kaplan DW, Mammel KA. Adolescence. In: Hathaway WE, Groothuis JR, Hay WW, Paisley JW, eds. *Current Pediatric Diagnosis and Treatment.* Norwalk, CT: Appleton & Lange; 1991.
31. Wilson MH. Obesity. In: Hockleman RA, et al. *Primary Pediatric Care.* St. Louis, MO: CV Mosby; 1987.
32. Brown JL. Hunger in the United States. *Sci Am.* 1987;256(2): 37–41.
33. Littlefield VM. A developmental perspective: What? In: Littlefield VM, ed. *Health Education for Women: A Guide for Nurses and Other Professionals.* Norwalk, CT: Appleton & Lange; 1986.
34. American Automobile Association Traffic Safety Departments. *Teacher's Guide to Bicycle Safety: Kindergarten–Grade 8.* Washington, DC: American Automobile Association; 1988:3.
35. Centers for Disease Control. Fatal injuries to children—United States, 1986. Leads From The Morbidity and Mortality Weekly Report. *JAMA.* 1990;264(8):952–953.
36. Sullivan L. How effective is preschool vision, hearing and developmental screening? *Pediatr Nurs.* 1988;14(3).
37. Rogers M. Early identification and intervention of children with learning problems. *Pediatr Nurs.* 1986;12:21–26.
38. Winkelstein M. Fostering positive self-concept in the school-age child. *Pediatr Nurs.* 1989;15(3):229–233.
39. Rollins J. Art materials: Recommendations for children under 12. *Pediatr Nurs.* 1988;14(3):251–252.
40. Newman B, Newman PR. *Development Through Life: A Psychosocial Approach.* Chicago: Dorsey Press; 1987.
41. Fingerhut L, Kleinman J. International and interstate comparisons of homicide among young males. *JAMA.* 1990;263(24): 3292–3295.
42. House J, Landis K, Umberson D. Social relationships and Health. *Sci.* 1988;241:540–545.
43. Hallol JC. The relationship of health beliefs, health locus of control and self-concept to the practice of breast self-exam in adult women. *Nurs Res.* 1988;31:137–142.
44. Baker AW. *Relationships Among Perceptions of Health State, Level of Self-Esteem, and Self-Reported Health Behaviors in Adolescent High School Students.* (unpublished dissertation) Ann Arbor, MI: Dissertation Abstracts International; August 1986.
45. Chally PA. Theory derivation in moral development. *Nurs Health Care.* 1989;11(6):302–306.
46. Centers for Disease Control. Years of potential life lost before ages 65 and 85—United States, 1987 and 1988. *MMWR.* 1990; 39:20–22.
47. Ockene J, Kuller L. Svendsen K, Meilahn E. The relationship of smoking cessation to coronary heart disease and lung cancer in the multiple risk factor intervention trial (MRFIT). *Am J Public Health.* 1990;80(8):954–958.
48. National Institute on Drug Abuse: Unpublished data 1990. In: Statistical Update on Lung Disease. American Lung Association; 1991.
49. US Department of Commerce. Projections of the population of the United States by Age, Sex, and Race, 1988–2080. *Population Estimates and Projections Series,* 1989;25:1018.
50. Tucker L, Friedman G. Walking and serum cholesterol in adults. *Am J Public Health.* 1990;80(9):1111–1113.
51. Petersdorf R. Hypothermia and hyperthermia. In: Wilson J, et al, eds. *Harrison's Principles of Internal Medicine,* 12th ed. New York: McGraw-Hill; 1991:2198.
52. Wallace J. Drowning and near-drowning. In: Wilson J, et al,

eds. *Harrison's Principles of Internal Medicine*, 12th ed. New York: McGraw-Hill; 1991:2200.

53. American Heart Association. *1991 Heart and Stroke Facts*. Dallas: American Heart Association; 1991.
54. Mendelsohn J. Principles of neoplasia. In: Wilson J, et al, eds. *Harrison's Principles of Internal Medicine*, 12th ed. New York: McGraw-Hill; 1991:1576.
55. Katz I. In: Tarini P. Elderly's unmet need: Geriatric psychiatry. *AMA News*. Chicago: AMA 1990:vol 11, pp. 13–14.
56. Yurik AG, Spier BE, Robb SS, Ebert NJ. *The Aged Person and the Nursing Process*. Norwalk, CT: Appleton & Lange; 1989.
57. Prinz P, Vitiello M, Raskind M, Thorpy M. Geriatrics: Sleep disorders and aging. *N Engl J Med*. 1990;323(8):520–526.
58. Tinetti M, Speechley M, Ginter S. Risk falls among elderly persons living in the community. *N Engl J Med*. 1988;319(26): 1701–1707.
59. Aldersberg M, Thorne S. Emerging from the chrysalis: Older widows in transition. *J Gerontol Nurs*. 1990;16(1):4–8.
60. Rowe J, Besdine R. *Geratric Medicine*, 2nd ed. Boston: Little, Brown; 1988.
61. Burggraf V, Stanley M. *Nursing the Elderly: A Care Plan Approach*. Philadelphia: Lippincott, 1989.
62. Pallet PJ. A conceptual framework for studying family caregiver burden in Alzheimer's-type dementia. *Image*. 1990;22:52–58.

BIBLIOGRAPHY

Andresen GP. A fresh look at assessing the elderly. *RN*. 1989;52: 28–40.

Castiglia PT, Glenister AM, Haughey BP, Kanski GW. Influences on children's attitudes toward alcohol consumption. *Ped Nurs*. 1989;15:263–268.

DiFranza JR, Tye JB. Who profits from tobacco sales to children? *JAMA*. 1990;20:2784.

Duffy M. Determinants of health promotion in midlife women. *Nurs Res*. 1988:358–362.

Erikson EH. *The Life Cycle Completed: A Review*. New York: WW Norton; 1985.

Gilligan C. *In a Different Voice: Psychological Theory and Women's Development*. Cambridge, MA: Harvard University Press; 1982.

Gillis A. Promoting health among teenagers. *Int Nurs Rev*. 1988;35: 10–12.

Haretsell M. New products. *J Pediatr Nurs*. 1990;5:50–60.

Hegeman K. A care plan for the family of a brain trauma client. *Rehabil Nurs*. 1988;13:254–258.

Mason JO. From the Assistant Secretary for Health-Infant mortality. *JAMA*. 1989;16:2202.

Peck R. Psychological development in the second half of life. In: Neugarten BL, ed. *Middle Age and Aging*. Chicago: University of Chicago Press; 1968.

Strong R, Wood WB, Burke WJ, eds. *Central Nervous System Disorders of Aging*. New York: Raven Press; 1988.

Thomas B. Self-esteem and life satisfaction. *J Gerontol Nurs*. 1988; 14:25–30.

Thompson RS, et al. A case-control study of the effectiveness of bicycle safety helmets. *N Engl J Med*. 1989;320:1361–1367.

Trice LB. Meaningful life experience to the elderly. *Image*. 1990;22: 248–251.

Trocchio J. Life as a bell-shaped curve. *Ger Nurs*. 1989;10:71.

US Department of Health and Human Services. *Annual Immunization: Recommendations of the Immunization Practices Advisory Committee*. Atlanta, GA: Public Health Service, Centers for Disease Control; 1986.

Weinstein L, Abrams R, Ayers C. Increasing awareness of sugar ingestion among children. *Pediatr Nurs*. 1988;14:277–279.

Williamson J. Mutual interaction: A model for nursing practice. *Nurs Outlook*. February 1981:104–107.

Winkelstein ML. Fostering positive self-concept in the school-age child. *Ped Nurs*. 1989:229–232.

CHAPTER 12

Becoming a Client

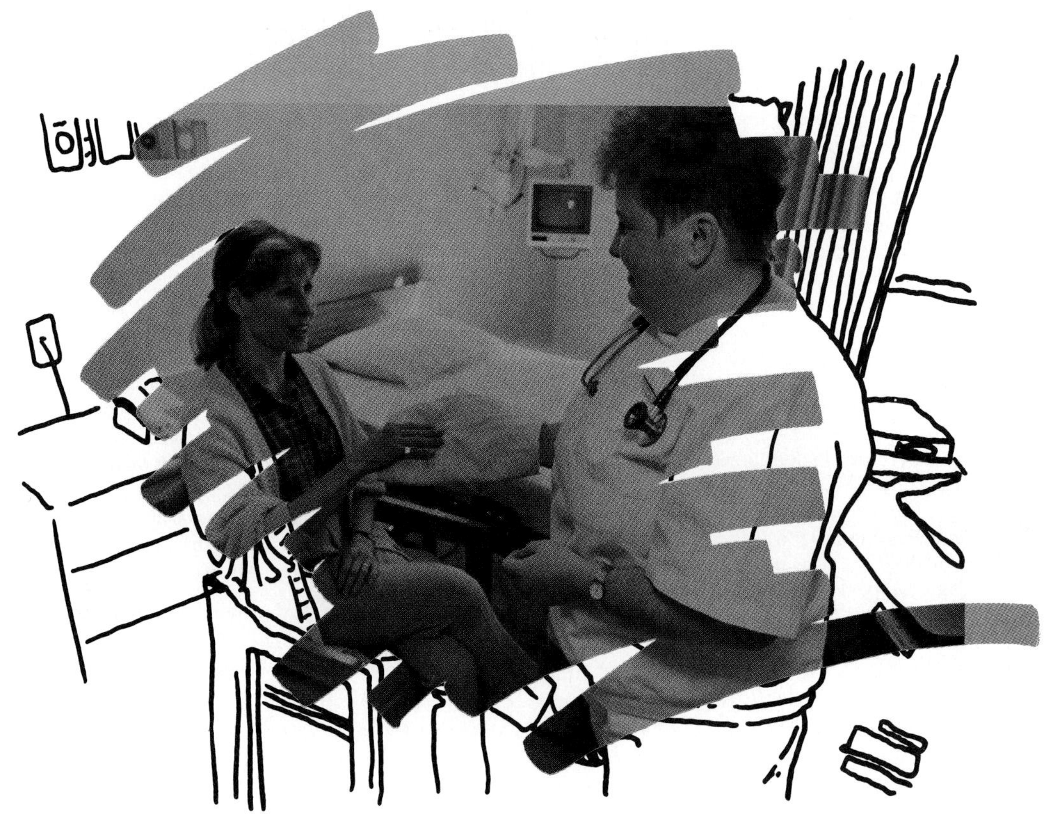

Behavioral Objectives

Upon completion of this chapter, the student will be able to:

1. Describe the holistic perspective of health.
2. Identify variables affecting popular definitions of health.
3. Identify variables to health-seeking behavior in illness.
4. Define "sick role."
5. List two rights and two obligations inherent to the sick role.
6. Discuss the implication of the Szasz-Hollander model for client care.
7. Describe the three stages of illness and state key client problems in each stage.
8. Outline stress-provoking features of the hospital experience.
9. Describe several psychological responses to the hospital stay.
10. Discuss the importance of social class, ethnicity, and other cultural variables for nurse–client collaboration.

KEY TERMS

acute illness
bias
body image
chronic illness
denial
holism
illness behavior
locus of control
primary socialization
regression
role
secondary socialization
self-care
sick role
social network
social support
socialization

The author wishes to acknowledge Victoria Moore, BA, MA, for her contributions to this chapter.

> I wish I knew what you mean about being sick. Sometimes I've felt so bad I could curl up and die, but had to go on because the kids had to be taken care of, and besides, we didn't have the money to spend for the doctor—how could I be sick? . . . How do you know when you're sick anyway?[1]

Definitions of health and illness vary widely with individual perceptions. Clinical evaluations of health and illness stress the identification and management of objective symptoms, such as body temperature, blood pressure, and white blood cell counts. In contrast, clients evaluate their own health status in relative terms that are rooted in the subjective, functional, everyday experiences of life. Health is not always clearly distinguishable from disease; it is a dynamic phenomenon that may vary from moment to moment, even in a single individual.

There are many different ways of examining the meaning of health. One way is to explore the complex relationship of health to social behavior. For instance, many diseases and their progression are inherently social in nature. Social variables are important determinants of the likelihood that an individual will contract an illness.[2] Unhealthful living conditions and stressful life-styles increase susceptibility to many diseases, such as heart disease, high blood pressure, diabetes, and cancer. Even deciding who is sick and who is well is a process that is sensitive to social influences. Thus, some clients are more frequently labeled as sick because of their socioeconomic status, ethnicity, or gender.[3–5] For example, a study done by The American Psychological Association in 1985 found that "women receive 73 percent of all prescriptions written for mood-altering, psychotropic drugs."[6] A woman describing symptoms such as insomnia, anxiety, or nervousness may be offered a prescription for Valium, while a man with similar complaints may receive counseling on ways to reduce stress. The woman in this case is defined as ill and in need of medical intervention, while the man is viewed as basically healthy and consequently is offered advice on how to remain so.

One of the most powerful influences on human behavior, and thus health, is provided by being a member of a social group such as a family, student body, working unit, religious organization, or ethnic group. Groups have shared views, values, norms, and meanings. One's group memberships therefore can be expected to exert significant influence on one's point of view regarding health, illness, and health-seeking behaviors, and can determine response to diagnosis, treatment, and recovery. Persons of different groups often have differing perspectives about many spheres of life, so it is always possible that the nurse and client may not share a similar view of the client's situation. It is precisely because of this expected disparity between views and opinions that the collaborative approach, which acknowledges the fundamental right of persons to differ, is so important in nursing practice. In fact, research suggests that the quality of provider–client interaction largely determines the outcome in health care,[7–11] and that collaboration between client and provider is conducive to a positive treatment outcome.[12]

This chapter emphasizes the experience of illness as it is perceived by the client. A summary of relevant theoretical perspectives and research on the subjective experience of illness is presented, with the focus on the social-psychological aspects of becoming, being, feeling, and being viewed as ill, as well as participating in self-care and making the transition back to wellness. Information in the chapter should enable nursing students to better understand, communicate with, treat, and be an advocate for their clients.

CONCEPTS OF HEALTH AND ILLNESS

Health as a Subjective Concept

Health is an abstract concept that is difficult to describe and measure (see Chap. 5). The concept of health has changed over time, and differs from culture to culture and from individual to individual.[13] The discipline of medicine historically has defined health merely as the absence of disease. Other definitions include objective parameters that indicate a norm or standard of health (eg, body temperature of 98.6F or blood pressure reading of 120/80). As mentioned in Chapter 5, the World Health Organization defines health as "a state of complete physical, mental, and social well-being and not merely the absence of disease."[14]

The holistic perspective on health that has become increasingly accepted in nursing is one that acknowledges an individual's adaptation to the environment. Blattner, an expert on holistic health, contends that **holism** is "a philosophical and biological concept which implies wholeness, relationships, processes, interactions, freedom, and creativity in viewing living and even nonliving entities."[15] The holistic approach emphasizes egalitarian (or equal) relationships between the nurse and client, collaboration, health maintenance, education, and the treatment of the entire person (as opposed to specialization and simple relief of symptoms).[16] The nurse attempts to understand, assess, and care for clients in light of their health potential as it exists within the scope of their individual social, economic, occupational, physical, and emotional environment. Any nursing assessment of health, then, can only be made with the view that people are complex beings who exist in relation to a complex world.

Because nurses can expect to interact with a diverse client population, it is crucial that they acquire information and skills that will sharpen their ability to communicate with a variety of clients. One important difference between the nurse and the client is the clinical training and socialization the nurse receives. It is useful, then, to gain an understanding of the subjective perception of individuals who may or may not define themselves as ill. On what basis does the average person define and evaluate his or her own health status? How does the individual determine that he or she is ill? What moves a person to seek help from a health care professional? What factors act as deterrents to health-seeking?

Before nurses can begin to comprehend the point of view of another, in this case the client, it is necessary to first understand their own outlook. Only in this way can personal philosophy be separated from the client's point of view, an important step in arriving at an empathetic understanding of the client's health beliefs.

Personal Definitions of Health

People define health in accordance with personal and familial experience and through an implicit understanding of societal expectations. These personal, family, and societal influences coalesce into an integrated belief system about health and health behavior and form the basis for personal actions in pursuit of health. Baumann suggests that individuals use a three-component set of criteria to determine health status. She found that clients measure (1) their sense of well-being, (2) the presence or absence of symptoms, and (3) their ability to carry on with day-to-day responsibilities.[17] Other experts argue that the ability to perform everyday activities far outweighs the presence or absence of symptoms. That is, for the client, attendance to symptoms is dependent on the extent to which those symptoms interfere with life.[18,19]

Thus, it may be primarily the social consequence rather than the physiological state that influences individuals to define themselves as healthy or sick. The presence or absence of symptoms alone may not constitute a perception of oneself as healthy or ill. Social interaction, the ability to work, and relationships with significant others who communicate their feelings about health and illness often override the presence or absence of symptoms. It is not uncommon for people to depend on a referral network consisting of spouses, other family members, and friends for health and illness information. Many health care professionals, physicians and nurses included, admit that they themselves tolerate and deny many symptoms of illness until they are no longer able to get up out of bed and report to work. The definition of health is inextricably intertwined with people's perception of themselves as active members of the community in which they interact: Health, therefore, is a subjective state.

Personal Definitions of Illness

Deviation from a perception of oneself as healthy begins the redefinition of oneself as sick. The definition and experience of illness reflect interpretations based on ethnic background, religious affiliation, race, gender, occupation, and status in society, among other factors. Personal values and beliefs about illness are significantly affected by relationships with parents, teachers, and friends, whose definitions of illness may either vary from or reinforce one's own. This, then, is the social basis of variation in response to signs of illness.

That individuals report a wide diversity of responses to a similar set of symptoms has been widely documented.[20–23] For example, two individuals may respond differently to the symptoms of the "common cold." One person may manage the symptoms by taking decongestants and aspirin while continuing with routine activities. Another individual may feel unable to report to work and will require bed rest and a visit to the physician. Moreover, if a symptom is statistically common or considered "inevitable" it is less likely to be perceived as a sign of ill health. For instance, forgetfulness and fatigue, seen as natural consequences of the aging process, are less likely to be perceived as signs of disease in an older person. Conversely, as Denton notes, when a society or group values working, then the inability to work may become an indicator of illness.[24]

What specific factors influence the perception and experience of illness? Tagliacozzo and Ima's work suggests that the more information and experience an individual has with illness, coupled with a motivation to be well, the more likely the individual is to identify a state of illness and to seek help.[25] These ideas have been supported by recent research.[26,27] Several researchers have substantiated the fact that individuals with higher levels of education and higher socioeconomic status are more likely to initiate and engage in effective communication with health care workers.[28,29] Clients who typically have the least amount of objective information available to them—that is, members of the lower-middle, working, and lower classes—may be more susceptible to illness, and are the least likely to access the health care system. Clients who are the least skilled in communicating about their health status are often in most need of empathetic intervention on the part of the nursing staff.

Variables Affecting Illness Behavior

Rosenstock's Health Belief Model. In the 1950s, Rosenstock developed a health belief model[30] that offers one framework for understanding illness behavior (Fig. 12–1). The health belief model was an attempt to predict how individuals would act with regard to their health based on their beliefs about health. Essentially, the health belief model proposes that an individual's readiness to take action on a health problem depends on the perception of the health threat and on health motivation. The four main variables of the model are:

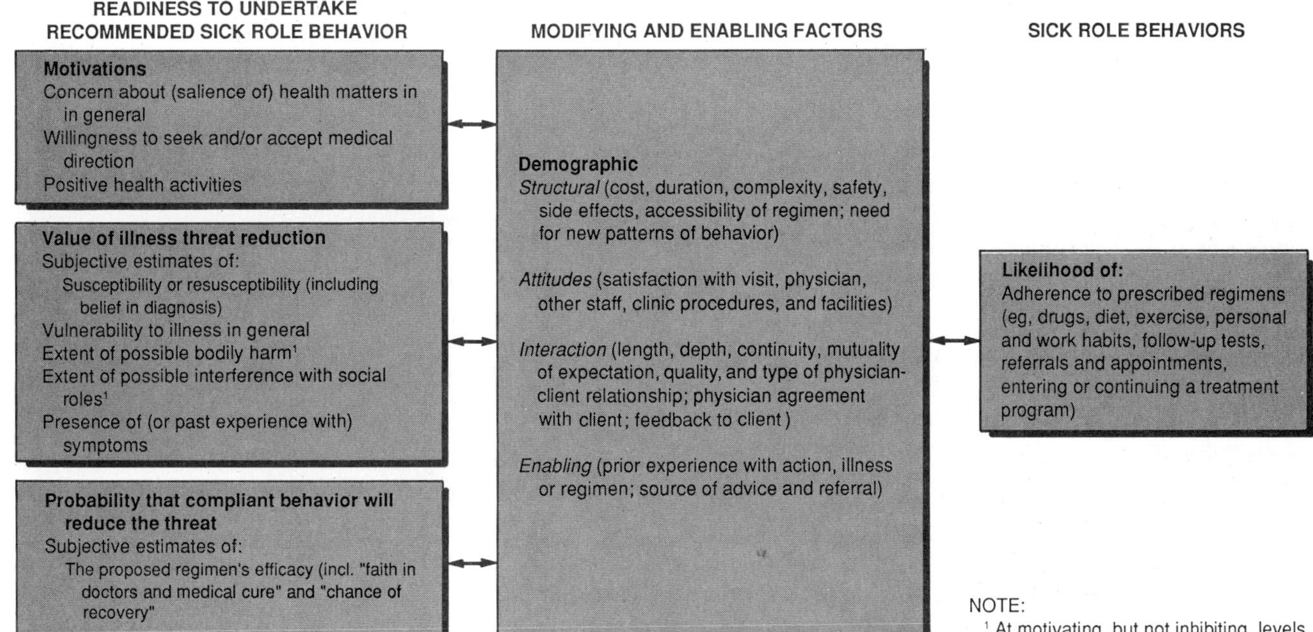

Figure 12–1. Rosenstock's health belief model adapted to the explanation of sick-role behavior. (*Source: Freeman HE, Levine S, Reeder LG.* Handbook of Medical Sociology. *Englewood Cliffs, NJ: Prentice-Hall; 1979: 266.*)

1. *Perceived susceptibility.* This refers to individuals' acknowledgment or acceptance of the possibility of illness, and may vary from complete denial to an open expression of fear regarding their perceived vulnerability to illness.
2. *Perceived seriousness.* Like perceived susceptibility, the degree of perceived seriousness can vary, depending on individuals' understanding of the negative health consequences of the condition and the effects of the condition on family, employment, and social obligations.
3. *Perceived benefits of taking action and barriers to taking action.* The acceptance of susceptibility to illness and recognition of its severity prompts individuals to take action and seek treatment. However, a conflict arises if a given treatment, although necessary to reduce the threat of illness, is seen by a client as being inconvenient, expensive, unpleasant, painful or upsetting. These conflicts can become barriers to effective treatment.
4. *Cues to action.* This last variable refers to the necessity of a stimulus (internal or external) to trigger the individual to take action. These cues can be specific, such as a notice from the dentist to schedule a check-up, or abstract, such as a radio announcement about a free hearing screening.

Rosenstock's model is based on the belief that individuals have both an emotional and an analytical response to a perceived threat of illness, and that action taken in response to this threat is based both on individual motivation and on internal or external cues.

Mechanic's Variables. Another health belief model is offered by Mechanic, who argues that the individual relies on and is influenced by 10 significant variables that explain the diversity of responses to signs of illness.[31] He developed his theory of illness behavior and help-seeking with an emphasis on the subjective perception of symptoms and the ability of the individual to cope with the perceived symptoms and illness situation. Mechanic's central theme is that **illness behavior** is a culturally and socially learned response pattern. Mechanic's 10 variables are listed in Box 12–1. Life experiences that may influence diversity in the impact of some of the variables, and related research, are discussed below.

BOX 12–1. MECHANIC'S 10 VARIABLES OF ILLNESS BEHAVIOR

1. Visibility or recognizability of symptoms by the individual.
2. The frequency, persistence, or recurrence of symptoms.
3. Perceived seriousness of symptoms by the individual.
4. Functional interference: the extent to which symptoms disrupt the individual's family, work, or other social activities.
5. The individual's level of information, knowledge, and cultural understanding relative to the symptoms.
6. The degree of tolerance toward symptoms expressed by others exposed to the individual.
7. The extent to which the psychological aspects of the illness interfere with the individual's basic needs.
8. The degree to which other needs compete with the illness response.
9. The possible alternative interpretations of symptoms considered by the individual.
10. The availability, physical proximity, financial cost, and psychological cost of treatment.

From Mechanic D. Medical Sociology. *New York: Free Press; 1978.*

Recognition of Signs and Symptoms. To what extent does the individual recognize that he or she is ill? Although fever or inflammation may be easily identified as symptoms of ill health, it is significantly more difficult to detect the presence of a breast lump, unless one is familiar with and practices routine breast self-examination. Overt, recognizable symptoms and particularly visible signs will generally cue the individual to seek diagnostic help, whereas subjective or subtle symptoms, such as gastric upset or fatigue, may not. Conversely, a person may experience a potentially life-threatening disorder such as high blood pressure, without being aware of any symptoms at all.

Number and Duration of Symptoms. An individual may be able to ignore the symptoms of the common cold, but may find it difficult to ignore a combination of symptoms such as a cold accompanied by a cough, chest pain, and fever. It becomes increasingly more difficult to ignore symptoms when they increase in number and persist over time.

Seriousness of Symptoms. The perceived seriousness of symptoms is an important factor in one's definition of oneself as ill. Many people deny, ignore, or remain unaware of sets of symptoms even when these symptoms are known by them to be signs of serious disease. For example, many people are aware that acute chest pain with accompanying difficulty in breathing and pain in the left arm may denote serious heart disease, but continue to misinterpret and ignore such symptoms. When asked, many clients report that they had indeed experienced warning signs of an impending heart attack, but interpreted the symptoms as inconsequential—the results of poor eating habits, stress, or gas.

Functional Interference. Symptoms that interfere with activities of daily living or result in absence from work or school tend to be viewed as serious and usually lead to a perception of oneself as ill and to help-seeking behavior. The woman who is no longer able to meet her responsibilities as a corporate executive because she is experiencing intermittent chest pain will be more likely to see her physician than her counterpart who is experiencing a slight gastric upset that does not interfere with job attendance.

Cultural and Socioeconomic Class Interpretation of Symptoms. Cultural and societal expectations greatly influence the acknowledgment and experience of illness. Zborowski, in a classic study of pain responses, found that Italian Catholic, Jewish, and Anglo-Saxon Protestant men responded very differently to symptoms of pain.[20] The onset of pain was important to the men in each group, but emerged as the most important indication of illness for the Italian Catholic men. In contrast, the Anglo-Saxon Protestant men felt most constrained by any interference in their life-style and activities, while the Jewish men exhibited considerable concern about the disease itself and the predictions for cure. These three very different examples of responses to signs of illness are grounded in cultural, familial, ethnic, and religious influences.

Differences were also noted in the men's responses to the hospitalization experience. The Anglo-Saxon Protestants tended to express their pain privately and were very concerned about adopting a "good client" role—that is, being cooperative with the health care professionals. The Italian Catholic men, whose cultural imperatives dictated a more dominant role in the home situation and less affective expression, became highly emotional in the hospital, openly expressing pain, anxiety, and fear. The Jewish men were more emotional overall, were more likely to express their feelings and fears, but at the same time refused extra pain medication, were concerned about drug dependency, and consistently questioned the hospital staff about their health status. The Italian Catholic and the Jewish men demonstrated similar behavior in the hospital, but their behaviors were based on a different set of values, beliefs, and meanings.

Cultural factors may also explain variations in health behavior between men and women. Women tend to report more bouts with illness and the presence of more symptoms than do their male counterparts. Nathanson suggests that it may be culturally more acceptable for women to acknowledge and report symptoms because it is more in keeping with the stereotypic female role in society.[33] Likewise, men's social roles may prevent any signs of "weakness," such as illness, thus limiting the number and types of symptoms reported. However, the nature of one's responsibilities may also be a factor here. Marcus and Seeman, researchers on illness and gender roles, reported that women who have "fixed role obligations," that is, jobs with relatively inflexible schedules, have lower morbidity rates than women with flexible role obligations. They hypothesize that individuals with less flexible work schedules may be less inclined to define themselves as ill or to permit themselves to stay home from work when ill, and state that this has formerly been more characteristic of men.[34] As more women have entered the labor force, studies reveal, as might be expected, that their susceptibility to the more serious (and often stress-related) illnesses has also increased.[35,36] A study of female clerical workers found that employees who were both married and parents were at twice the risk for heart disease as other working women or homemakers.[6] However, in a study on the effects of stress, it was noted that contrary to current belief, "top-level, high-paid, successful women and men live longer than anyone else."[6] A possible reason for this finding may be a variable called person–environment fit. MacBridge asserts that good person–environment fit contributes to good mental and physical health and self-esteem, and relieves work-related stresses.[37] This theory was supported in a study on work-related stress among female nurse educators.[38] Other variables related to diminished work stress are autonomy and opportunities for personal goal-setting.[35,36] Thus, as women's roles become more complex and varied, their risk for stress-related illness may increase, but this negative consequence can be minimized by factors such as these.

The cultural context of male and female relationships may also affect our interpretation of the health of women. Considerable evidence exists in support of the idea that women are frequently labeled as ill by a health care profession that is dominated by men, at the level of the physician. For example, processes that are normal physiological events in the life of a woman have been defined as pathological and in need of medical or surgical intervention. Menstruation, pregnancy, childbirth, and menopause are the most frequently cited examples of misinterpreted natural phenomena.[39–41] Phyllis Chesler and other feminist psychologists and psychiatrists also argue that women are more likely to be labeled as mentally ill than are men, even when male and female clients are evaluated for identical symptoms. That is, a female client is more likely to be diagnosed as neurotic than is a male client with the identical complaint of diffuse (not specific to a situation) anxiety.[42–44] Further research is needed to explore both the innate and culturally defined perceptions of health status differences between men and women. However, it must also be recognized and accepted that men and women are biologically more similar than different, and that gender differences, exaggerated by cultural and social expectations, affect the type and quality of health care men and women receive.

Social network and social support are other sociocultural variables that have been shown to influence illness and illness behavior. These terms have sometimes been used interchangeably in the literature, yet have slightly different meanings. Hall and Wellmann characterize **social network** as a weblike structure comprising one's relationships.[45] It has neither a positive nor a negative connotation. **Social support** is the positive, need gratifying consequences of interpersonal relationships, including affection, approval, belonging, identity, and security. Cohen and Syme clarify the distinction between social network and social support by stating that social network represents the structure of a relationship and social support, the function.[46]

Studies addressing social support and illness have consistently shown that there is increased health risk for persons with low quantity or quality of interpersonal relationships.[47] Social relationships have been shown to positively influence resistance to infection and to some cancers.[48] Although the mechanism through which social support is health protective has not been consistently explained, there is considerable research that indicates that social support has a positive impact on health, behavior during illness, and recovery from illness.[47,49–54]

Health, illness, and illness behavior are also influenced

by socioeconomic class. The conditions associated with poverty such as nutritional deprivation, poor sanitation, inadequate housing, and resultant chronic fatigue negatively affect health. Poverty increases life stresses and therefore increases susceptibility to disease.[55] Moreover, the poor have limited access to health care due to geographical isolation, lack of transportation, lack of money, and lack of health insurance.[56–64] Health education and primary preventative care is also less available to the working-class poor.[62,65] Because of these constraints, the poor tend to disregard symptoms of chronic illness and symptoms that are not immediately disabling although potentially life-threatening, and instead rely on self-care and systems of peer referral.

There is growing evidence that increasing numbers of the middle-class are also experiencing limited access to care because of lack of health insurance.[60,66] Wilensky reports that at least one third of the uninsured are members of families whose income is twice the poverty line, and about half of the uninsured are employed all or part of the year.[60] Clearly, the problem of paying for health care in today's society is a complicated issue, with more elements than socioeconomic class playing a role. However, equally clearly, those at the lower end of the economic spectrum are most severely affected presently.

In conclusion, many factors influence clients' perceived experience with illness (Fig. 12–2). A subjective assessment of health status—in terms of the presence, number, severity, and type of symptoms—coupled with clients' cultural background, affect ability and inclination to recognize or define illness and seek appropriate health care. As Leininger notes[67]

> Individuals from different cultures perceive and classify their health problems in specific ways and have certain expectations about the way they should be helped. To ignore such cultural differences may seriously interfere with the patient's progress toward his culturally defined health state. Moreover, what may seem to the nurse to be resistance or uncooperativeness of the patient to nursing or medical help could well be traced to the cultural background differences between the patient and the nurse.

When nurses incorporate a holistic definition of health and illness into their care plans, they take into account clients' perceptions of health and illness. The variables discussed are client factors to be assessed by nurses in order to help identify the beliefs, values, and cultural differences that may be affecting the responses of a particular client. As much as possible, nurses must become conscious of the personalized meaning they attach to health and illness in order to refrain from biasing or interfering with objective assessment of a client's experience.

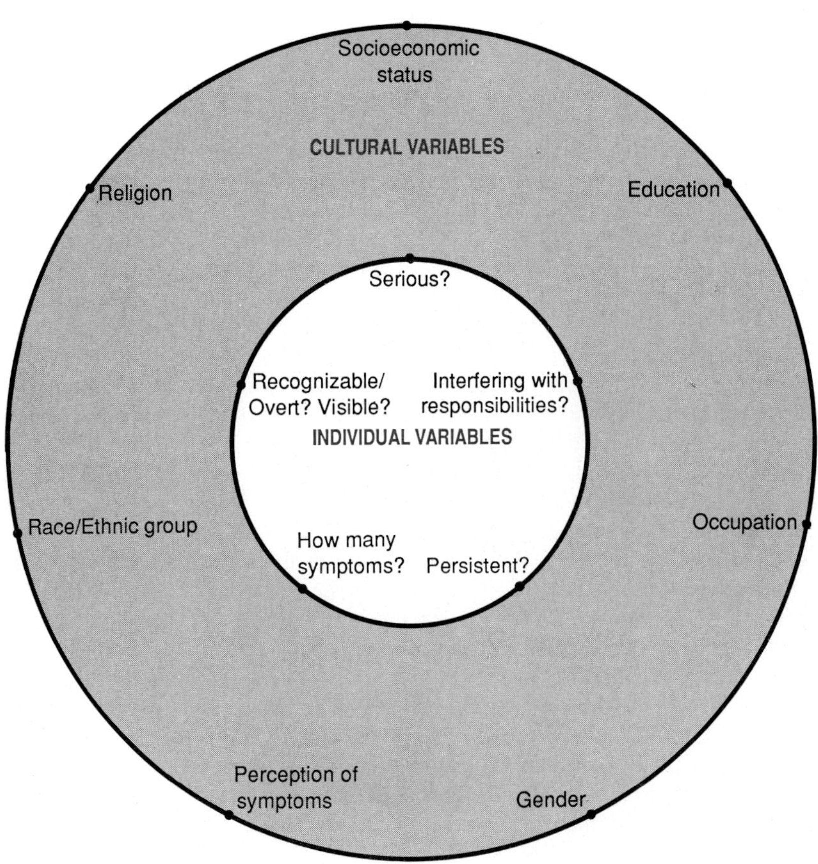

Figure 12–2. Variables influencing the client's perceived experience with illness.

The Decision to Seek Health Care

The decision to seek health care, upon recognizing or defining oneself as ill, is likewise based on cultural influences and situationally specific circumstances. That is, people may or may not seek treatment depending on their anticipated ability to gain access to the health care system. Commonly, people first seek the help and advice of their spouses, family, and friends before making contact with a health professional.

The concept of **self-care,** in which the client is encouraged to "create his own reality, his own health, and is considered to be the best resource for achieving his own level of optimal wellness,"[15] is becoming increasingly popular as costs of health care and insurance premiums continue to rise.[68,69] Examples of this trend can be seen in the increased availability of self-help books and over-the-counter self-diagnostic kits such as pregnancy tests and tests for hidden intestinal bleeding. According to Blattner, more than 70 percent of visits to a physician are unnecessary.[15] Clients who practice self-care are encouraged to view their health from a holistic perspective. That is, they consider the mind and the spirit as well as the body when defining wellness or illness. Becoming in tune with one's physical, psychological, and spiritual self is something that takes practice. Because self-care depends on intuition regarding one's own health status, some people practice meditative techniques that enhance their ability to self-assess and diagnose symptoms. The nurse's role in client self-care can be seen as "an extension of the client and his needs."[15] Thus, rather than a medical emphasis on the illness status of a client, the focus of self-care is on the client's health status, integrating body, mind, and spirit. (For additional discussions of self-care, see Chaps. 5, 22, 32, 33, and 37.)

The individual's perception of symptoms, in combination with the disruptive nature of the symptoms, and the interaction between the individual and significant others who recognize the presence of symptoms and encourage either self-care or health-seeking behavior, are all factors that may lead the individual to make contact with the system of health care delivery.[23,70] Factors that delay this process include fear, lack of information, worries about cost, and the higher priority of other role obligations.

Once the individual does move toward health-seeking behavior and is defined as ill by a health care professional, the individual assumes what is called the "sick role."

THE SICK ROLE

The Concept of Role

A **role** is a system of norms, functions, and values that provides a set of rules for behavior for members of certain social categories. Each social category is associated with different behavioral expectations and different roles. Individuals typically assume several societal roles simultaneously: one can be a daughter, a sister, a mother, a wife, and a nurse. However, each of these roles embodies different symbolic meanings, values, and expectations.

> **BUILDING NURSING KNOWLEDGE**
>
> **Who Do Older Adults Hold Responsible for Their Health?**
>
> Schafer SL. An aggressive approach to promoting health responsibility. *J Gerontol Nurs.* 1989; 15:22–27.
>
> Noting the trend to self-care and the documented relationship between health practices and decreases in illness and death, Schafer designed a study to explore the self-care attitudes of older adults living in the community. It looked at the plans older people have for making changes in their health habits and their perceptions about who is responsible for personal health and who or what could assist them to make habit changes.
>
> Schafer interviewed 319 participants in a health screening program. The average age of participants was 70 years. A large proportion of participants (65 percent) viewed themselves as being most responsible for their own health; 14 percent felt the physician was most responsible; 13 percent suggested the responsibility was a partnership between self and others, such as between themselves, the physician, and their spouses or children.
>
> Most participants engaged in healthy life-style practices. Seventy percent engaged in physical activity routinely. Sixty-nine percent reported eating breakfast routinely. Seventy-five percent reported routinely feeling rested on awakening. Eighty-six percent reported that they did not smoke. Fifty-three percent reported visiting a physician one to four times a year.
>
> Forty-eight percent of participants indicated they planned changes in their health habits. Of these, 40 percent indicated that self-reliance was important and 15 percent indicated health care professionals of various types could assist. Nurses were not mentioned as a category of professionals to help. The investigator concluded that nurses need to be more visible and aggressive in assisting people with life-style practices.

Individuals demonstrate qualities of both uniqueness and conformity in filling their role responsibilities. That is, each individual approaches and enacts his or her roles (such as parent, spouse, nurse) as an individual, demonstrating creativity and originality. However, the meanings and definitions assigned to these roles reflect shared group standards.

Roles are acquired through a process of **socialization,** which is defined by Lott[6] as "the process of learning those behaviors that are appropriate for members of a particular status group." The child's interaction within the family is called **primary socialization.** The socialization that older children, young adults, and adults receive as they progress through school, interact with others, and observe others who share a similar role is called **secondary socialization.** Socialization is a lifelong process that transmits cultural expectations from one member to another, from group to group, and from generation to generation.[71]

Nurses, too, learn appropriate professional role behavior through the secondary socialization of formal education in a school of nursing and by observing experienced nurses in a clinical setting. In school, nursing students not only acquire technical skills but learn how to *behave like nurses.* The learning involves information about at least four interrelated roles in the health care setting: that of the nurse, physician, client, and client's family. The behavior of one individual in a given setting will influence the others. Changes in role expectations for any one group (eg, nurses or clients) will affect and change roles of members from the other groups.[72,73] Therefore, it can be said that related roles form a system, and that these roles are reciprocal in the sense that changes in any one role effect changes in the others. This fact has important implications for individuals who become clients.

Parsons' Sick Role Theory

The **sick role** is a social role that embodies a set of norms and values about health and illness behavior. It is the role that individuals take on when they define themselves as ill. Talcott Parsons, a renowned medical sociologist, developed a theory about the role of a sick person that revolutionized theories about health and illness behavior. Parsons drew an analogy between social life and biological organisms in his discussion of illness in society. He postulated that the structure of society is similar to the anatomy of a biological organism, and that the function of society can be compared to the physiology of an organism. A biological organism cannot exist without the successful functioning of the heart and its component parts; society cannot exist without the institution of the health care system and the coordination of its many members in a systematic and orderly fashion.[74]

According to Parsons, society depends on the effective and interdependent functioning of each part, much as does the human body. The survival of society is dependent on the interaction and cooperation between healthy, functioning members. When illness strikes, the usual functioning of an individual is threatened. Illness, then, is dysfunctional not only for the individual but for the larger group. While today we acknowledge that illness, although usually considered a negative event, can be a precipitating factor toward a period of positive growth and change, Parsons felt that illness is an undesirable yet inevitable consequence of human life that society must legitimize for those members who fall ill. Society empowers certain individuals with the right and responsibility for defining societal members as ill. The health care system acts as the gatekeeper to the sick role. In this way society carefully monitors entrance into the realm of the legitimately ill. Thus, Parsons developed the idea that individuals in society must assume a new role when they become ill, the sick role, in order to acquire care and to legitimize "sick" behavior.

Characteristics of the Sick Role

According to Parsons, the sick role is not static and is not acquired in the same way by all clients. The role is learned—through feeling sick and interaction with one's family, community, and culture—and is acquired largely on an unconscious level. The sick role is unfamiliar to most people. It is not assumed with ease, and involves feelings and behaviors that reflect fears and anxiety about health status and mortality. Specifically, the sick role consists of two obligations or responsibilities, and two rights or privileges. Upon entrance into the sick role, the client is expected to (1) seek professional help in order to overcome the disease and (2) articulate the desire to get well. In return for meeting these obligations, the client is afforded two rights: the right to be exempt from daily responsibilities and the right to be absolved of any responsibility for the illness state.[75]

Traditional Client–Provider Relationship

Parsons believed that the aim of the health care system should be to maintain the ongoing and productive functioning of society. The health care professional was viewed as the expert who was charged with legitimizing disease, preventing malingering, and managing the client's care.

According to Parsons, men and women, as health care professionals, take on separate but complimentary roles. He assigned the more active role, or what he called the functional or instrumental role, to the physician, who he assumed would be male. Parsons assigned women to what he called the expressive or affective role, assuming that they would fill the role of the nurse. As an agent of the physician, the nurse was expected to exhibit supportive, nurturant behaviors, but in no way to interfere with the physician nor to encourage malingering by behaving in an overly empathetic or sensitive manner with the client. Parsons also characterized client behavior. He described appropriate client behaviors as those that are passive in nature, childlike, compliant, and cooperative. Thus, Parsons viewed the relationship between physician, nurse, and client as symmetrical and balanced.

Many health care professionals still agree with Parsons' expectations for physician, nurse, and client roles. Professionals who received their training in years past may be particularly in agreement with his model. In recent years, however, the Parsonian model has been subject to a great deal of scholarly analysis, and criticism of the model and its implications has been voiced by health care professionals and consumers alike.

Limitations of Parsons' Model

Although Parsons was one of the first to attempt a model for health and illness, outlining specific roles for health professionals and clients, he does not adequately describe the role of the client in the contemporary system of health care delivery. His model places too much emphasis on the active involvement of the health care professional, specifically the physician; not enough emphasis on the active involvement of the client; and fails to acknowledge the important interactional and shared aspects of the provider–client relationship. These omissions severely limit today's applications of his theory in light of the ideal of collaborative health care. Nevertheless, Parsons can be considered a pioneer in the development of sick-role theories, and his model, while dated, provided a foundation from which other theories have been developed.

Twaddle, for example, found that a good deal of sick role variation exists. He interviewed approximately 600 married couples who lived in Rhode Island, in which the male partner was between the ages of 60 and 64.[19] He was interested in discovering how individuals determine health status, how they define illness, and what kinds of behaviors were exhibited by clients when they were defined as ill. Twaddle observed that individuals respond to the sick role differently, partly in terms of the status and role of the legitimizing agent. This means that the attitude and demeanor of the health care professional affected how individual clients responded to their illnesses. Subjective feelings and perceptions of symptoms also affected individuals. These were related to the nature and severity of the disease, and to the nature of the individuals' well-role responsibilities.

Twaddle concluded that the sick role is more complex than Parsons decribed it, and is more dependent on situationally specific and culturally bound processes not addressed by Parsons. He also found little support for Parsons' contention that individuals are absolved from their daily responsibilities and that clients will tend to malinger if not monitored. Twaddle and other researchers have documented statistically that clients tend to maintain their normal well-roles, even when defined as sick, and are more likely to resume responsibilities in the home and the workplace before it is medically indicated rather than malingering in the sick role as Parsons feared they might.

Another criticism of Parsons' model concerns its professionalist bias. Parsons assumed that physicians legitimately exert control over their clients and expected that all physicians would be neutral, unbiased, objective, and fair in these interactions. Reeder argues that relationships between physicians and their clients are not innately fair and objective. Quite to the contrary, "the client may be treated as an object; he may receive little information concerning the treatment processes and the possible outcomes. The professional's conception of his relation to his client determines such communication failures."[76] Recent changes in the health care delivery system, including the growth of the medical bureaucracy and a general move toward health maintenance and disease prevention, have resulted in a move toward increasing client control over health care interaction.

Locus of Control: A Shift Toward Increased Client Participation

Psychologists have long acknowledged that people who feel they have some degree of control in their lives are less likely to perceive themselves as helpless when faced with a crisis.[77] While the Parsonian model advocated that the client relinquish control to the health care professional—namely the physician—current health care models promote increased participation by clients in their own health care. Thus, the **locus of control,** which can be defined as the perceived measure of control an individual has in a given situation, which formerly resided with the health care professional, shifts to the client. This shift in locus of control promotes clients' increased participation and control over their health and encourages clients to take a more active role in their own health care.[77] Today, clients are expected and encouraged to ask questions, get second opinions, and make decisions based on the information they receive. Clients who participate in their own health maintenance and illness prevention are less likely to become depressed and apathetic when ill and are more likely to accept the responsibility for their recovery from illness.[77] Thus, when clients retain a level of control over their health care, they change their position from a passive and helpless stance to a more active and collaborative one.

> **IMPLICATIONS FOR NURSE–CLIENT COLLABORATION**
>
> **Locus of Control**
>
> While traditional health models emphasized client passivity, current health models promote increased participation by clients in their own health care. This new perspective implies an important change in the way health care professionals and clients relate. Nurses who have adopted the contemporary outlook endeavor to support the client's locus of control by inviting the client to participate in the health care decision-making process and by acknowledging the client's fundamental right to differ.

A Collaborative Model for Provider–Client Interaction

Nurses interested in establishing collaborative interactions with their clients need a model of interaction that examines behavior as a function of an entire set of role obligations. This ideal model would regard both client and nurse as active participants in the provider–client relationship. Szasz and Hollender refined Parsons' model into a trimodel scheme that incorporated the client in the decision-making process.[78] This model acknowledges the variation that exists in provider–client interaction and categorizes the variations (Table 12–1).

Szasz and Hollender contend that an appropriate client role is an active one that exercises some degree of power in the provider–client relationship. Thus, the collaboration between individuals is paramount in the caring process; the nurse–client relationship is viewed as reciprocal. Szasz and Hollender call this relationship mutual participation. Nurses are both instrumental (functional) and expressive (caring) toward clients. In turn, clients are given, and take, responsibility and an active role in the care process. Note that Szasz and Hollender suggest that the future relationship between client and professional might be weighted toward the client, who may call on a health care provider as an expert consultant.[78] This model provides a fuller view and a healthier characterization of the role the client should have the option to assume.

TABLE 12–1. THE SZASZ-HOLLENDER TYPOLOGY OF PROVIDER–CLIENT INTERACTION

Types of Provider–Client Relationships	Provider Role	Client Role	Clinical Application
Active/passive	Does something to client	Unable to respond	Anesthesia, coma, delirium
Guidance/cooperation	Tells client what to do	Cooperates or obeys	Acute health problems: severe infectious processes, life-threatening organ failure
Mutual participation	Helps client help self	Partner, participant (uses expert help)	Less severe acute and chronic health problems

Adapted from Szasz TS, Hollender MH. A contribution to the philosophy of medicine. Arch Intern Med. *1956; 97:585–592.*

THE EXPERIENCE OF ILLNESS

The experience of illness is a complex socio-psychological event. Responses to acute illness are very different from responses to chronic disease. Taking on the sick role usually involves a move from independence to dependence. "Forced dependency as a consequence of illness adds another dimension to the complexity of the sick role."[79] Many individuals are reluctant to become dependent on others, while some clients have strong needs for dependency. Nurses can help clients accept an appropriate level of dependency within the context of respect and collaboration.

Information about medications, side effects, diagnosis, treatment, and prognosis should be shared with clients as they are ready. Nurses can elicit ideas about how much information is desired from clients. While clients have a right to information about their care, they also have the right not to know, as they desire. Although this type of subtle interaction between nurse and client takes skill, with time and experience a sensitive nurse can learn to ascertain what clients want to know through informal yet focused discussion. It is important to mention that structural barriers exist in many health care organizations that work to prevent nurses from providing all the information necessary about health and illness status to the client. For instance, physicians' orders, hospital policy, departmental regulations, and sometimes state or federal legislation may dictate the type and amount of information that a nurse may share with a client. Consumer groups and nursing organizations are involved in minimizing these barriers to collaboration.

Stages of Illness

Lederer describes three stages of the illness experience, which exist on a continuum with considerable overlap (Fig. 12–3). Clients do not move uniformly from one stage to another in discrete steps. The three stages are:

1. A transition from a perception of the self as healthy to a perception of the self as ill.
2. The illness-acceptance stage and help-seeking process.
3. The convalescence stage, beginning with a move toward wellness and a transition out of the sick role.[80]

A client's smooth progression through the stages of illness depends in part on the nature and severity of the disease itself. An **acute illness,** one that can be recognized by a severe, rapid onset of pronounced symptoms of usually short duration, allows little time for a smooth transition from a well role to a sick role. A **chronic illness**—characterized by its long duration, frequent recurrence, or

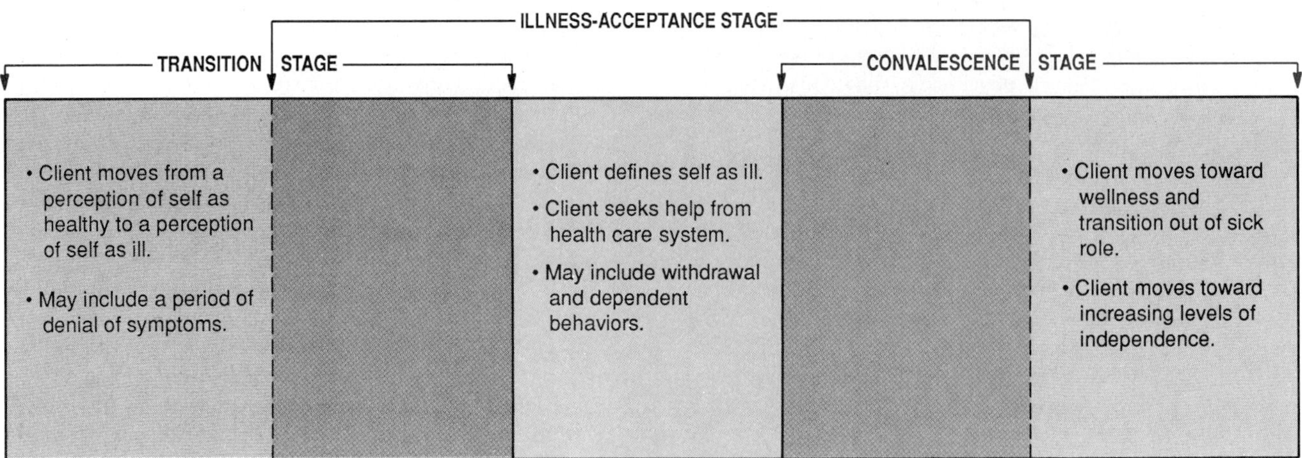

Figure 12–3. Lederer's stages of the illness experience as a continuum.

fluctuations between acute and chronic symptoms—may allow the client more time for adjustment to the sick role.

The Transition Stage. This stage is often very unpleasant for an individual. It involves changes in self-perception and development of fear and anxiety. Clients may undergo a period of **denial,** in which symptoms are ignored or minimized. Sometimes this leads to behavior that is seen as uncooperative or problematic by nurses. A client who has just been diagnosed with diabetes may refuse to follow the recommended diet, and instead continue to eat foods known to be unhealthful for diabetics. This type of denial is used by a client as a coping mechanism to help minimize the threat to well-being that a newly diagnosed disease brings.

For some clients, the denial becomes a primary mode of adaptation and no transition is made into the illness role—at least until the disease becomes incapacitating and forces dependency. Usually, however, as symptoms persist or become viewed as incapacitating, anxiety increases and clients indeed experience illness. At this point clients may begin to withdraw from routine responsibilities and to attend more clearly to the body and its functions.[80] Occasionally concern about bodily functioning becomes all-encompassing, and "minor variations in temperature, digestion, pulse, and elimination take on significant importance."[80] This behavior is also a coping response that clients use to maintain a level of control in a threatening situation. Monitoring external or physical responses to illness may help clients to come to terms with the internal or psychological aspects of an illness.

Individuals have many fears about entering the sick role, as it is an unfamiliar role laden with unfamiliar expectations for behavior. It typically involves a change in body functioning and body image, and may involve a degree of loss of control over one's physical self. This loss of control may be seen by clients as a kind of "betrayal" by the body. Routine functions such as breathing, eating, and elimination may be disrupted by the onset of illness and become cause for invasive medical procedures in a health care institution. When individuals seek health care attention, the role of nurses is crucial. Clients need to receive information in understandable terms, given with empathy, understanding, and a clear set of expectations. In this setting nurses act as liaisons between clients and an environment in which unfamiliar and often frightening procedures may be performed.

The Acceptance Stage. As individuals define themselves as ill and make contact with the health care system, they may temporarily withdraw or regress as control is transferred to professionals. **Regression** is used by clients as a mode of adjustment to a perceived threatening situation. Characterized by a return to a level of behavior appropriate for an earlier age or level of development, this coping mechanism may cause mature adults to react to their increased dependence by behaving in an often childish manner. Wu states that dependent behaviors can be classified into three categories of behavioral response: (1) cooperation and compliance with the directions and requests of health care personnel; (2) the need for actual physical assistance in the performance of daily activities; and (3) the need for effective support such as acknowledgment of feelings, approval, reassurance, physical embrace, and protection. Other possible responses to the sick role include anger and egocentricity.[79] Because so many routine activities are suspended when clients enter the sick role, it is understandable that they become very concerned with the characteristics of the illness and its management. Clients may begin to feel that their world revolves around their illness, the progression of their disease, the dosages of medication, and the like.[80]

The Convalescent Stage. This stage is analogous to the stage of adolescence. During adolescence, the young adult is neither a child nor an adult; during convalescence, the client is neither ill nor healthy, but rather is in a state of transition. A client is typically regaining strength and moving toward increasing levels of independence. Many clients are hesitant to leave the sick role, not because of dependency needs or malingering, but because of fears about relapse and the health consequences of resuming their regular set of role obligations. They require sensitive caring and psychological support to gain the strength necessary to relinquish the sick role and assume the well role. Exchanges of information about the well-role requirements should include answers to questions clients may have about the resumption of activities, work, leisure, diet, sexual activity, and stress management. Guidelines for follow-up care and appropriate referrals may be provided at this time. Open and honest communication between nurse and client during this stage can help make the client's transition from the sick role to the well role a positive experience.

IMPLICATIONS FOR NURSE–CLIENT COLLABORATION

Stages of Illness and the Sick Role

Clients' needs change as they progress through the stages of illness and again when they make the return to wellness. Difficulties may arise in either accepting or relinquishing the sick role. Depending on many physical, emotional, and social factors, a client's need for dependency on the nurse may be increased during the transition to illness, particularly when illness interferes with the ability for self-care. The client's capacity to fully collaborate in decision-making may be limited for a time both by physical condition and by personal attitudes about illness. Nevertheless, opportunities should be created for the client to communicate personal expectations for health care, because such expressions may ease the acceptance of illness and because cooperation with health instructions is more likely when the plan of care is compatible with the individual's health concerns and beliefs. Such opportunities are equally important during convalescence, and may also ease the transition to wellness and movement toward increasing levels of independence.

Movement Through the Stages of Illness. Not all clients move predictably from sickness to health; there is wide variety in the rapidity and means by which clients make the transition back to wellness. Some people identify illness quickly, seek help, and recover rapidly. Others, consistent with Mechanic's analysis, have difficulty defining themselves as ill. Still others move slowly from one phase to the next. Some clients expect to relinquish the sick role rapidly but are unable to do so because of the nature of their disease or their lack of resources. This is particularly true of clients with chronic illnesses. Some clients are cured at the end of an acute bout with illness; others will never be cured. A client's perception of the process and experience of illness affects movement through the stages of illness in profound ways. Those clients who must permanently adopt a new role, as in chronic illness, need special help both from the health care provider and the client's family and friends. (See Chap. 8 for a complete discussion of the role of the family in health and illness.) Such clients must often undergo an entire resocialization process as they readapt to former roles and adjust to new ones.

The client's participation is an important part of this process. Clients are more likely to follow instructions when they understand the reasons for a particular therapeutic regimen. It is difficult for clients to comply with a client care plan if it conflicts with their cultural experience or health beliefs. When a client does not accept the therapeutic plan, nurses can encourage collaboration by attempting to identify and respond to clients' concerns. Nurse–client collaboration can also be enhanced if expectations of both nurse and client are clearly stated. Supporting clients as they move through such dramatic life changes is the subject of many advanced and continuing education courses for nurses.

The Hospital Experience

Although the experience of illness from the perspective of clients can be understood by examining a bout with a cold or a visit to the physician's office, the experience is illustrated even more dramatically by an episode of hospitalization. It is here that clients are thrust into the sick role and come face to face with a large, unfamiliar, technological institution that is organized around a routine completely different from the one they are accustomed to. Communication takes place in a language clients often do not understand, and information about process and procedure is often monopolized by caregivers. Little, if any, preparation exists for the hospital experience. Some hospitals have community awareness programs that encourage and sometimes even sponsor tours of the hospital. Others offer pamphlets and instructional booklets to help a client prepare for a planned procedure. Still, it is not uncommon for an individual to enter the hospital unexpectedly, with little time to make the psychological transition from home to hospital. Hence, clients may experience many fears and anxieties about entering the hospital, and may be unskilled in negotiating their way through the hospital system.

The Admission Procedure. A hospital is comprised of clients and nonclients. For clients who arrive at the hospital other than in an emergency situation, the initial introduction to the institution occurs during the admission process. Personal questions are asked about financial status, insurance, and nearest kin. Clients may become exceptionally anxious at this juncture. They may hesitate to reveal information about employment status and salary, and are often stunned when asked about the names and addresses of nearest relatives "in case of an emergency." Mortality is no longer a vague, obscure possibility for the future—it becomes instead a stark potential reality for the present.

Introduction to the Room. Clients often share a room with one or two other clients who are complete strangers. The hospital room lacks personal belongings. Unisex pajamas are issued, clothing that is, according to Woods, neither male nor female, but neuter.[81] The style of hospital garb typically fails to protect privacy; the gown opens at the back and hangs shapelessly away from the body. Personal effects are usually removed to another location for safekeeping. The client is issued a wrist tag that is identified by a hospital number. There are no locks on the door and privacy is at a premium. Schuster contends that privacy becomes increasingly important to persons when they are threatened with all these affronts to individual identity. She found that clients experience threats to personal sense of privacy when[82]:

1. *They cannot meet expectations (their own or others');* for example, when a client is unable to comply with the respiratory therapist's instructions for ventilation treatment.
2. *They cannot make sense of what is happening;* for example, when laboratory tests or other procedures are performed with little or no explanation.
3. *They are unable to understand the language of the health personnel* and find diagnostic terms misleading and unclear.
4. *They perceive themselves as unacceptable to others;* for example, if the diagnosed disorder carries a negative social stigma (eg, HIV infection, alcohol-related disease, mental health disorders).
5. *They experience perceived role conflict;* for example, when a client expects nurse–client collaboration but instead is presented with an authoritative nurse who insists on client compliance and passivity.
6. *They are subject to persistent unexplained or unwelcomed presence of others;* for example, when nurses, doctors, laboratory personnel, and others enter the room without knocking and without introducing themselves, or when visitors stay too long.

These are all threatening situations in which withdrawal to one's own defined space might be a typical coping response. Ironically, in the hospital no such space exists. Nurses, however, can create a situation that is conducive to client dignity by minimizing the factors that intrude upon the client's perception of privacy. Schuster reports that clients can feel more self-confident and can experience a true sense of well-being when[81]:

1. They are able to make sense of the situation around them.
2. They are able to exchange information with caregivers.
3. Information is supplied clearly and at appropriate times.
4. Nurses and other caregivers are available when the client feels needy.
5. Encouragement and other overt caring messages are received.
6. They feel that the staff is competent and acts professionally.

In the hospital setting, clients often desire to "stake out a territory" they can call their own. That is, clients feel more comfortable in the hospital room when there is space to place personal belongings on the bedside table or on the bed itself. Personal belongings such as a bed jacket, pillow, pictures, or books help the client adjust to the hospital and illness experience by reducing the realm of the unfamiliar (Fig. 12–4).

Client–client and client–provider interactions strongly influence a client's sense of personal privacy. For example, clients who are hospitalized in the same room may establish a degree of camaraderie that can reduce fear and anxiety. Conversely, some client roommates may find that they have little in common and may engage in conflict.

Interaction with nurses (and other health care providers) can be positive or negative. These possible interactions have been discussed throughout the chapter. Schuster cited the following example that depicts the negative ramifications that can result when nurses respond insensitively to clients:

> We were having a conversation about normal life and were talking calmly and everything. Then she [the nurse] asked me what my husband did for a living and I said, "Well, right now, he's not working. We're living on welfare." And she said, "You mean we're floating you?" And that just didn't hit me right at the time. It just made me feel like two cents when she said that. And she came back later to see if I needed anything and I just said, "No, I don't need anything," and I turned my back just to avoid talking to her. And she probably didn't mean what she said. It just didn't hit me right; I felt bad about being on welfare right now and to have somebody come up with "Well we're paying . . . supporting you." Well, it made me feel worse.[81]

The experience of hospitalization limits clients' ability to control their environment, and thus has consequences for personal privacy, dignity, and self-esteem. Nurses who acknowledge this important aspect of the experience of illness in a hospital can help the client exercise some control over both the physical and psychological space of the environment.

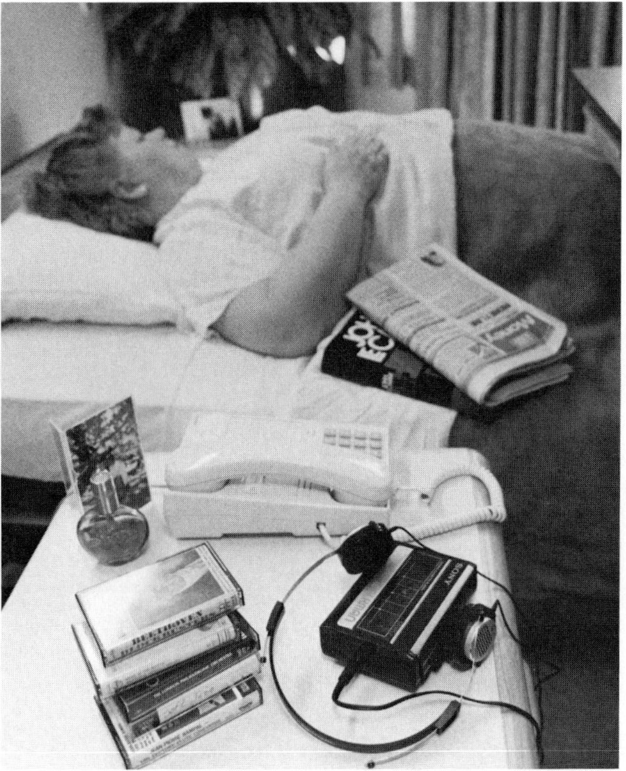

Figure 12–4. Space for personal belongings helps clients feel more comfortable in the hospital setting.

Personal Functions. Upon admission, clients are asked to discuss personal, medical, and social data with strangers. Processes normally not publicly discussed are now openly probed, measured, and charted. Even more problematic is the fact that the same or similar questions are asked repeatedly by different members of the health care team. Clients are often embarrassed to be asked as well as to answer questions about personal habits, urine output, and the regularity and timing of bowel movements. Clients may be uncomfortable complying with a request for sputum, urine, or stool samples. Questions about the date of the last menstrual period, number of pregnancies, abortions, alcohol and drug use, sexual activities, and diet can be disconcerting and embarrassing to clients. Clients fear that their answers will elicit value and moral judgments or that their disclosures will not be kept confidential. It is often unclear to clients why certain questions are being asked at all, which leads to more uncertainty. If and when hospital staff assist clients with excretory functions or hygiene, clients may be further embarrassed and may have feelings of complete loss of control over physical self and functioning.

Nurses can assist clients to understand the rationale behind the taking of a complete medical, health, and social history. For example, a woman who is preparing to undergo a mammogram to screen for breast cancer may hesitate to answer questions about her menstrual periods, number of pregnancies, age at which she first became pregnant, and her current method of contraception. Nurses can reduce anxiety by prefacing questions with a brief explanation of how the answers to these questions will provide valuable information to assist with proper diagnosis and treatment. Clients may feel freer to provide detailed information when the information is placed within the context of a collaborative assessment and when efforts to collaborate are acknowledged, accepted, and encouraged.

The Hospital Staff. Clients see a world of white- and pastel-uniformed individuals. It is often extremely difficult for clients to distinguish roles and functions of staff members. For example, most clients experience difficulty in differentiating registered nurses, licensed or practical nurses, and nurse aides. In addition, because staffing of hospital shifts often varies, clients cannot predict which nurses will appear on a given shift unless this information is explicitly shared with them. Questions a client saves for a specific nurse may never get asked if that nurse's assignment or hours change. This lack of continuity, caused by staffing irregularities or concerns with cost-effective staffing, can create added anxiety for a client who may look to the nurse as a constant in this strange environment of variables.

Clients often have unrealistic expectations about their relationship with the nursing staff at the hospital. The image of nurses as it is portrayed in childhood stories, on television, and in the movies is very different from that of real nurses in a real hospital. Clients discover all too quickly that nurses are responsible for duties that frequently preclude prolonged interaction with them. When clients notice that nurses are rushed, they usually tend to refrain from "bothering" them. Most clients want to be viewed as cooperative and don't want to risk offending nurses by making too many demands. Clients may be simultaneously desperate for understanding and empathy and acutely sensitive to signs of disapproval, rejection, or lack of interest.

The hospitalized client is separated from family and friends for long periods of time. Clients who feel understood and cared for by nurses will likely feel less alone. Nurses may embody for the client both the real and the symbolic aspects of the experience of illness and the world of the sick. That is, nurses not only care for and interact with clients, but also represent images and feelings clients may have about illness, caring, and recovery. These images may be positive or negative. Nurses who can recognize and identify these client expectations can better understand their clients' perspective and make appropriate adjustments in the care they provide. Generally, collaboration between nurse and client leads to a more positive hospitalization experience.

Medical Language. The technical terms associated with diagnosis and treatment are especially confusing to many clients. Physicians, nurses, and other health care personnel communicate with one another, in the presence of the client, in unfamiliar jargon. The client's usual vocabulary often includes words, phrases, and abbreviations that are also used in the hospital with completely different meanings. SOB may be used to describe shortness of breath. Similarly acronyms, including BS for bowel sounds, CABBAGE for coronary artery bypass graft, and CAT scan for computed axial tomography, exemplify the extent to which medical communication can be misunderstood by the client.

While the language is undoubtedly confusing, Denton notes that the hospital staff often underestimates the ability of clients to understand health care information and thus is reluctant to make an effort to explain procedures and treatment.[24] Without clear explanations, clients understand just enough to be frightened and not enough to gain a clear and accurate picture of the situation. Some nurses and physicians believe that divulging information to the client causes tension and anxiety for the client. This assumption, usually incorrect, permits health care providers to avoid collaborative interaction with the client. This is a serious omission when one considers that there is increasing evidence that nurse–client interaction is *essential* to the positive recovery of the client.[83] Studies on nurse–client interaction and communication reveal that the more information nurses provide, the less anxiety clients experience. Further, less tension results when specific details are provided. According to Lowenberg, "a healing partnership and expressive nurturance are crucial elements of the [nurse–client] relationship."[83]

Psychological Responses to the Hospital Stay

People respond in various ways to the hospital experience. (See Chap. 6 for a complete discussion of adaptation and coping strategies.) While fear and anxiety are typical emotions, they are expressed in a wide variety of ways. Some individuals will adopt what they interpret to be an "ideal client" image, and will work toward achieving approval from the nursing and medical staff. This approval-seeking behavior often conceals a client's true feelings. An outward appearance of control and stability may mask underlying feelings of uncertainty, fear, and anxiety. One client described such a situation by stating, "Maybe our appearance of being strong hid the fact that we needed help."[84] Clients who apear to be adapting well to their hospital stay are often in need of as much attention as clients who express their fears and worries openly.

In marked contrast, other individuals may act out their feelings of emotional conflict, expressing their anxiety or hostility through behavior that is seen as destructive or socially inappropriate. In an attempt to gain some degree of control over their hospital experience, some clients may openly violate hospital regulations. Some clients act out in nonaggressive ways, such as refusing to adhere to visiting hours or to take prescribed medications, ignoring smoking regulations or dietary restrictions, or simply not cooperating with nursing care. Others will act out with rage and anger at the staff: "People told me that when I escaped, threw tantrums, or tried not to show up for dialysis, that was my way of saying how I felt."[84] Still other clients will withdraw and exhibit signs of depression. A wide variety of psychological responses to hospitalization exists. Nurses need to recognize seemingly inexplicable behavior such as crying, giggling, laughing uncontrollably, refusing to cooperate, screaming, and physically abusing the staff by hitting, scratching, biting, or kicking as possible responses to stress. Once nurses understand these signs of ill-adjustment to the experience of illness and hospitaliza-

BUILDING NURSING KNOWLEDGE

What Kinds of Personal Control Are Important to Hospitalized Clients?

Dennis KE. Dimensions of client control. *Nurs Res.* 1987; 36:151–156.

Although hospitals are generally viewed as places where the ill receive proper care, Dennis notes that clients who are hospitalized face many unknowns and often have a stressful experience. Dennis argues that loss of personal control can be an important aspect of that stress. Studies reviewed on the subject indicated that promoting responsibility and choice (both of which enhance control) has a significant impact on well-being. However for some individuals, taking control is stress-inducing.

Dennis designed a study to identify activities that give clients a sense of control. Seventy clients hospitalized for various medical and surgical conditions were studied by a Q-sort technique, a method of ranking attitudes and judgments for statistical analysis. The aim was to determine the relative importance that clients attached to controlling hospital events. Dennis also interviewed the clients to ascertain factors that influenced their attitudes.

Results showed that having information was very important to clients, particularly information about their condition and whether it was improving or deteriorating. Understanding what their diagnosis meant to their way of life in general, and what activities would be restricted, was also important.

Clients differed, however, on how actively involved they wanted to be in decision-making about diagnostic tests and treatments. Some clients desired an active role in the major decisions such as the selection of method of therapy, treatments, and medicines, but were less concerned about having control over self-care or deciding when things were done, or such aspects as wearing their own apparel. Other clients were more concerned about their role as client and knowing what was expected of them, but did not have a desire to participate in decisions about diagnostic tests or treatments. Still others placed emphasis on independence and maintaining self-integrity. These clients wanted to do things for themselves, perform their own procedures, and set their own schedules. They indicated little concern for knowing about hospital schedules and routines. Dennis concluded that while clients wanted control, the marked differences in manner of attaining it underscore the importance of individualized plans of care.

tion, they can begin to intervene in appropriate and helpful ways.

From the perspective of clients, then, the experience of hospitalization can be described as a move from the familiar to the unfamiliar in almost every regard. Clients awaken in a strange room, in an institution filled with strangers. Clients are subject to questions that are at once embarrassing and frightening. Procedures are performed without careful explanation and often involve a degree of discomfort. Private bodily functions become topics of open discussion and concern by strangers. Even the language used by health care providers is unfamiliar, technical, and confusing. All of these factors can contribute to clients' lack of adjustment to the hospital experience. Chapter 22 presents further information on assessment and management of stress related to the hospital experience.

Aspects of Illness and the Hospital Experience

Body Image Changes. Every individual develops a self-concept while moving through the life cycle. One's view of one's physical body is an important part of this self-concept. As discussed in Chapter 10, **body image** can be defined as "the mental picture one holds of one's own body." Young children and infants often feel quite comfortable with their physical selves; they don't typically suffer from a sense of self-consciousness about their bodies. However, as individuals mature into pre-adolescence and adolescence, they become increasingly self-conscious about their physical selves. Particular parts of the body take on meanings that are associated with maturity, masculinity, femininity, and sexuality.

Hospitalization and illness typically alter the body image, at least temporarily. Although normal changes in body image occur during adolescence, adulthood, pregnancy, and aging, these changes can be anticipated and shared with others. During illness and hospitalization, however, body image change is often unanticipated. Common hospital procedures such as catheterization, medication, and surgery all affect body image. In the hospital the body becomes more visible, not only to physicians and nurses but to all who enter the room. Hospital gowns restrict clients' ability to conceal their bodies. This forced exposure may cause clients to feel that their bodies are not important or not deserving of respect and privacy. To avoid embarrassment caused by this exposure, clients often attempt to dissociate themselves from what is happening to their bodies. Combined with a tendency by health care providers to focus on parts of the body instead of the whole person, this dissociation can lead to a sense of the body as an object rather than an integral part of the self.

Clients who lose a part of their body suffer not only the physical loss of tissue, but also must face an altered body image. Because certain body parts are associated with notions about masculinity and femininity, the loss of a testicle or a breast may cause distortions in sexual identity.[79] Woods suggests that any surgery that removes a part of the body, including internal organs that are unseen by the client, has a significant meaning, and thus also has a potential for negatively altering body image.[81] Assessment and management of body image and body image changes are discussed in Chapter 23.

Pain. Pain is a complex experience that is not easily communicated from one person to another. Because clients have difficulty in describing their pain, nurses may misjudge the amount or type of pain a client is having. Nurses and clients may undergo what Graffam calls "mutual withdrawal."[85] The client realizes that he or she is unable to express the experience of pain to the nurse, and the nurse decides that the client is no longer complaining because the pain was not as severe as originally reported.[85] Because the client is usually dependent on the nurse for pain relief, interaction between nurse and client involves issues of control. A collaborative nurse–client relationship is crucial in determining the type and intensity of pain a client is experiencing. Responses to pain vary widely; some clients tolerate pain far longer than do others. Because each client experiences pain differently, it is important for nurses to assess each report of pain as a unique event.

Graffam studied 100 clients and 51 nurses in an attempt to identify the components of nurse–client interaction surrounding pain. She found that nurses and clients tended to agree about the occurrence of pain and its severity *except* in the cases of severe pain. Severe pain, as reported by clients, was judged to be less severe by the nurses. The effort to assess pain was minimal by the nurses in Graffam's study; in fact, the nurses expected that clients would self-disclose their pain experience. Nurses tended to assess pain in terms of the client's appearance, behavior, level of agitation, and by inference. Although nurses often did not ask the clients to describe their pain, when they did, it was difficult for clients to provide accurate and meaningful descriptions of their pain.[85]

Benoliel and Crowley cite the case of a client who was asked to "tell me about your pain" by a nursing instructor. The client responded to the question by saying, "It's interesting that you ask, because no one ever has. . . . What kind of pain are you interested in? Are you interested in the pain that is racking my body right now and from which I will never recover? Are you asking about the pain of my life when I lost my daughter? Are you talking about the pain of my loneliness because I have no one who cares?"[86]

Pain, then, is a subjective state that is difficult to interpret and express. An open and honest dialogue between nurse and client is essential in determining the amount and degree of the client's pain because correct interpretation and expression are crucial to achieving pain control. The nurse's response to a client's expression of pain should include not only a physical assessment, but also a thorough evaluation of what the client *says* about the pain.[87] The correct interpretation of both the objective and the subjective data will help the nurse determine an appropriate response to the client's pain. A discussion of the physiological and psychological aspects of pain, pain assessment and pain management is presented in Chapter 29.

■ COLLABORATION: EASING THE TRANSITION TO THE SICK ROLE

Many factors inhibit clients from making a smooth transition into the sick role. It is important that nurses be aware of this and be prepared to assess and intervene in a potentially problematic transition.

Nurses can assist clients in the sick-role experience, both in the hospital setting and elsewhere, by participating with them in therapeutic interaction (Fig. 12–5). However, social class, ethnicity, and other cultural variables often interfere with effective communication between nurse and client. The first step toward overcoming these barriers is sensitivity to the possibility of a problem. Second, nurses must be aware of biases they bring to the health care setting and must attempt to deal with them in a rational and constructive way. Likewise, nurses should endeavor to understand clients' biases. **Biases** are subjective feelings that reflect a particular point of reference or point of view. Biases have many origins, but regardless of their source can interfere with effective collaboration. Client behavior based on a particular social background may conflict with a nurse's idea of what is appropriate in a health care situation. Similarly, a nurse's behavior may conflict with clients' concepts of appropriateness. Collaborative communication within the nurse–client relationship is based on mutual acceptance

IMPLICATIONS FOR NURSE–CLIENT COLLABORATION

Biases

Biases are subjective feelings that reflect a personal and often unreasoned point of view on something. Biases are brought to the nurse–client relationship by both nurse and client and can complicate or interfere with caregiving. The exchanges of opinions, values, and information in a collaborative relationship increases the nurse's opportunities to identify the social differences between the nurse and client and thus to minimize the potential impact of biases while maximizing empathy and caring.

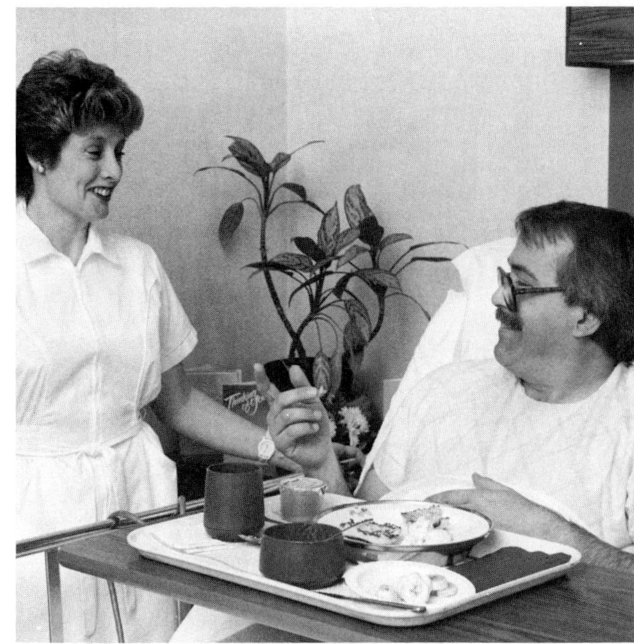

Figure 12–5. Therapeutic interaction assists clients to adapt to the sick role.

BOX 12–2. PROVIDERS' SELF-EVALUATION

- Have I really listened?
- Am I sure I understand my client's questions?
- Did I jump too quickly to my own conclusions?
- Did I identify a surface problem or the underlying cause?
- Have I shared my impressions with the client to ensure that my perceptions are an accurate reflection of his or her feelings?

of differences between nurses and clients and mutual recognition of common goals. Chapters 13 and 14 elaborate on communication and the nurse–client relationship.

Collaboration requires that nurses acknowledge the need for active client participation in the health care experience and deliberately facilitate it. Effective nurses use many different approaches to promote collaboration, but consistently demonstrate caring and respect for clients' needs, feelings and concerns. Listening, teaching, negotiating, and exchanging ideas are fundamental to success.

The notion of self-critique on the part of nurses is a crucial one. Rosenberg suggests that health care professionals should routinely perform self-evaluations when reviewing or anticipating interaction with clients (Box 12–2). He suggests that professionals ask themselves a set of questions, the answers to which will illuminate both the strengths and weaknesses of the provider–client interaction. Rosenberg contends that "We can all give something valuable to someone who is ill by being willing to see and willing to hear. Then perhaps we can begin to understand more fully what the experience of illness can mean."[84]

SUMMARY

Becoming a client compels individuals to confront challenges to their individuality and their identity. There are many determinants of health and illness behavior. Rosenstock's health belief model and Mechanic's theory of illness behavior present overlapping points of view about the variables that influence becoming a client.

Sick role theory is another approach to understanding the experience of being a health care client. The Parsons, Twaddle, and Szaz-Hollender theories of sick role behavior and provider–client relationships provide varying perspectives. In contemporary health care, the shift in locus of control suggested by Szaz and Hollender is preferable. This collaborative approach recognizes clients' rights to take responsibility for informed health care decision making.

It has frequently been assumed that when an individual enters the sick role, the transition will be unproblematic and routine. Clients are often expected to assume a posture of passivity, dependency, and compliance. It is similarly assumed that health care professionals will take the active role in assessing, diagnosing, and prescribing a treatment regimen on behalf of clients. This chapter has described the extent to which these assumptions about nurse–client interactions are inadequate.

Even when clients actively participate in health and illness care, however, the experience of illness is difficult for most. Moving through the stages of illness raises questions about one's ability to function effectively in the roles that give life meaning. Therefore, threats to self-concept and body image are part of the illness experience for many clients; for some, there are actual alterations that entail coping and adaptation. If illness involves becoming a hospital client, the threats and stresses are often multiplied. New routines, loss of privacy and personal space and a foreign environment are among the many difficulties clients encounter as part of the hospital experience.

Effective nurse–client interaction may be hindered by the many social, cultural, institutional, and psychological barriers between the two participants. The experience of illness and entrance into the sick role embody a complex set of processes that differ from one client to the next. Nurses must acquire skills that will enable them to become aware of the many meanings that clients ascribe to the experience of illness. By acquiring a comprehensive understanding of the variables that affect the subjective client experience with illness, nurses can attempt to engage clients in a collaborative effort toward wellness. Nurses promote the integrity of clients by acknowledging each client as an individual who deserves attention, care, information, understanding, and respect.

REFERENCES

1. Koos EA. *The Health of Regionville.* New York: Columbia University Press; 1954.
2. Knowles JH, ed. *Doing Better and Feeling Worse.* New York: Norton; 1977.
3. Weaver JL. *National Health Policy and the Underserved.* St. Louis: Mosby; 1976.
4. Ehrenreich J, ed. *The Cultural Crisis of Modern Medicine.* New York: Monthly Review Press; 1978.
5. Corea G. *The Hidden Malpractice.* New York: Morrow; 1977.
6. Lott B. *Women's Lives: Themes and Variations in Gender Learning.* Belmont, CA: Brooks/Cole; 1987.
7. Cleary PD, Mechanic D, Weiss N. The effect of interviewer characteristics on responses to a mental health interview. *J Health Soc Behav.* 1981; 22:183–193.
8. Wolinsky FD, Wolinsky, SR. Expecting sick role legitimation and getting it. *J Health Soc Behav.* 1981; 22:229–242.
9. Ross CE, Wheaton B, Duff RS. Client satisfaction and the organization of medical practice: Why time counts. *J Health Soc Behav.* 1981; 22:243–255.
10. Hall JA, Roter DL, Rand CS. Communication of affect between patient and physician. *J Health Soc Behav.* 1981; 22:18–30.
11. Pritchard P. Stress and anxiety in physical illness: The role of the general nurse. *Nursing Times.* 1981; 22:162–164.
12. Levinson DT, Merrifeld J, Berg K. Becoming a patient. *Arch Gen Psychiatry.* 1967; 17:385–406.
13. Wilson RN. *The Sociology of Health.* New York: Random House; 1970.

14. World Health Organization Convention, Geneva, 1960.
15. Blattner B. *Holistic Nursing*. Englewood Cliffs, NJ: Prentice-Hall; 1981: 16–18, 63, 82.
16. Lowenberg JS. Holistic health and the social movements of the sixties: Strands of continuity. Unpublished manuscript; 1980.
17. Baumann B. Diversities in conception of health and physical fitness. In: Skipper JK, Leonard RC, eds. *Social Interaction and Patient Care*. Philadelphia: Lippincott; 1965.
18. Colontino A. Lay concepts of health. *Health Values*. 1988; 12:3–7.
19. Twaddle AC. Health decisions and sick role variations: An exploration. In: Schwartz HD, Kart GS, eds. *Dominant Issues in Medical Sociology*. Reading, MA: Addison-Wesley; 1978:5–15.
20. Zborowski M. Cultural components in responses to pain. *J Soc Issues*. 1952; 8:16–30.
21. Shelp EE, Perl M. Denial in clinical medicine: A reexamination of the concept and its clinical significance. *Arch Int Med*. 1985; 145:697–699.
22. Lowery BJ. Psychological stress, denial, and myocardial infarction outcome. *Image*. 1991; 23(1):51–55.
23. Germain CP, Nemchick RM. Diabetes self management and hospitalization. *Image*. 1988; 20:74–78.
24. Denton J. *Medical Sociology*. Boston: Houghton-Mifflin; 1978.
25. Tagliacozzo DM, Ima K. Knowledge of illness as a predictor of patient behavior. In: Schwartz HD, Kart GS, eds. *Dominant Issues in Medical Sociology*. Reading, MA: Addison-Wesley; 1978: 125–133.
26. Garo LC. Explaining high blood pressure: Variation in knowledge about illness. *Am Ethnol*. 1988; 1:98–119.
27. Turk DC, Rudy TE, Salovey P. Implicit models of illness. *J Behav Med*. 1986; 9:453–474.
28. Duff RS. Patient care, the poor, and medical education. In: Kosa J, Zola K, eds. *Poverty and Health*. Cambridge, MA: Harvard University Press; 1975:335–350.
29. Hollingshead AB, Redlich FC. *Social Class and Mental Illness*. New York: Wiley; 1958.
30. Rosenstock IM. Historical origins of the health belief model. In Becker MH, ed. *The Health Belief Model and Personal Health Behavior*. Thorofare, NJ: Slack; 1974.
31. Mechanic D. *Medical Sociology*. New York: Free Press; 1978.
32. Wolinsky FD. *The Sociology of Health*. Boston: Little, Brown; 1980.
33. Nathanson C. Illness and the feminine role. In: Schwartz HD, Kart GS, eds. *Dominant Issues in Medical Sociology*. Reading, MA: Addison-Wesley; 1978:23, 31.
34. Marcus AC, Seeman TE. Sex differences in reports of illness and disability. In *J Health Soc Behav*. 1981; 22:174–182.
35. Johansson G, Gardell B. Work–health relations as mediated through stress reactions and job socialization. In: Maes S, Spielberger CD, Defares PB, Sarason IG, eds. *Topics in Health Psychology*. New York: John Wiley; 1988:271–285.
36. Cox T, Cox S. Working women: Occupational health and safety. In: Maes S, Spielberger CD, Defares PB, Sarason IG, eds. *Topics in Health Psychology*. New York: John Wiley; 1988: 287–294.
37. MacBridge A. *On-the-job Stress: A Review of the Literature*. Toronto: Clark Institutes of Psychiatry; 1982.
38. Langemo DK. Impact of work stress on female nurse educators. *Image*. 1990; 22:159–162.
39. Haire D. The cultural warping of childbirth. In: Ehrenreich J, ed. *The Cultural Crisis of Modern Medicine*. New York: Monthly Review Press; 1978:185–200.
40. Marieskind HI. *Women in the Health System*. St. Louis: Mosby; 1980.
41. Sandelowski M. *Women, Health and Choice*. Englewood Cliffs, NJ: Prentice-Hall; 1981.
42. Rusek SB. *The Women's Health Movement*. New York: Praeger; 1979.
43. Navarro V. Women in health care. In: Albrecht GL, Higgins PC, eds. *Health, Illness and Medicine*. Chicago: Rand McNally; 1981:327–337.
44. Chesler P. *Women and Madness*. New York: Avon; 1972.
45. Hall A, Wellman B. Social networks and social support. In: Cohen S, Syme SL, eds. *Social Support and Health*. New York: Academic Press; 1985:23–41.
46. Cohen S, Syme SL. Issues in the study of social support. In: Cohen S, Syme SL, eds. *Social Support and Health*. New York: Academic Press; 1985:3–20.
47. House J, Landis K, Umberson D. Social relationships in health. *Science*. 1988; 241:540–545.
48. Pilisuk M, Parks SH. *The Healing Web: Social Networks and Human Survival*. Hanover: University Press of New England; 1986.
49. Kessler RC, McLeod JD. Social support and disease etiology. In: Cohen S, Syme SL, eds. *Social Support and Health*. New York: Academic Press; 1985:219–238.
50. Ryan MC, Austin AG. Social supports and social networks in the aged. *Image*. 1989; 21:176–179.
51. Caplan G. Support systems. In: Caplan G, ed. *Support Systems and Community Mental Health*. New York: Basic Books; 1974.
52. Wortman CB, Conway TL. The role of social support in adaptation from physical illness. In: Cohen S, Syme SL, eds. *Social Support and Health*. New York: Academic Press; 1985:285–298.
53. Mishel MH. Uncertainty in illness. *Image*. 1988; 20:225–231.
54. Ellison E. Social support and the constructive–developmental model. *West J Nurs Res*. 1987; 9:19–28.
55. Kosa J. Nature of poverty. In: Kosa J, Zola K, eds. *Poverty and Health*. Cambridge, MA: Harvard University Press; 1975:335–350.
56. Callahan D. Meeting needs and rationing care. *Law, Med Health Care*. 1988; 16:261–266.
57. Blendon RJ, Donelan K. The public and the emerging debate over national health insurance. *N Engl J Med*. 1990; 323:208–212.
58. Syme LS, Berkman LF. Social class, susceptibility, and sickness. In: Schwartz HD, Kart CS, eds. *Dominant Issues in Medical Sociology*. Reading, MA: Addison-Wesley; 1978:400–402.
59. Wilensky GR. Viable strategies for dealing with the uninsured. *Health Affairs*. 1987; 6:33–46.
60. Wilensky GR. Filling the gaps in health insurance. *Health Affairs*. 1988; 7:133–149.
61. United States Congress: Congressional Budget Office. Rising Health Care Costs: Causes, Implications and Strategies. Washington, DC: Congressional Budget Office, 1991.
62. Popp RP. Health care for the poor: Where has all the money gone? In: Lindeman CA, McAthie M, eds. *Nursing Trends and Issues*. Springhouse, PA: Springhouse; 1990:420–425.
63. Brecht MC. Nursing's role in assuring access to care. *Nurs Outlook*. 1990; 38:6–7.
64. Fuchs VR. The competition revolution in health care. *Health Affairs*. 1988; 7:5–24.
65. McKinley JB. The help-seeking behavior of the poor. In: Kosa J, Zola K, eds. *Poverty and Health*. Cambridge, MA: Harvard University Press; 1975.
66. Huey FL. How nurses would change U.S. health care. In: Lindeman CA, McAthie M, eds. *Nursing Trends and Issues*. Springhouse, PA: Springhouse; 1990:319–331.
67. Leininger N. The culture concept and its relevance to nursing. *J Nurs Ed*. 1967; 6:27–37.

68. Steiger NJ, Lipson JG. *Self-Care Nursing: Theory and Practice.* Bowie, MD: Brady; 1985.
69. Hill L, Smith N. *Self-Care Nursing.* 2nd ed. Norwalk: Appleton & Lange; 1990.
70. Sundeen SJ, Stuart GW, Rankin ED, Cohen SA. *Nurse–Client Interaction.* 4th ed. St. Louis: Mosby; 1989.
71. Lewis GF. Socialization and social roles in life cycle perspective. In: Folta JR, Deck ES, eds. *A Sociological Framework for Patient Care.* New York: Wiley; 1979.
72. Schulman S. Mother-surrogate after a decade. In: Jaco EG, ed. *Patients, Physicians, and Illness.* New York: Free Press; 1979.
73. Stein LI, Watts DT, Howell T. The doctor–nurse game revisited. *N Engl J Med.* 1990; 322:546–549.
74. Parsons T. Definitions of health and illness in light of American values and social structure. In: Jaco EG, ed. *Patients, Physicians, and Illness.* New York: Free Press; 1979:120.
75. Parsons T. Family, illness therapy and the modern urban American family. *J Soc Issues.* 1952; 8:31–34.
76. Reeder LG. The patient client as a consumer. In: Schwartz HD, Kart GS, eds. *Dominant Issues in Medical Sociology.* Reading, MA: Addison-Wesley; 1978:111–117.
77. Mischel W. *Introduction to Personality.* New York: Holt, Rinehart & Winston; 1986:169–170.
78. Szasz T, Hollender MH. The basic models of the doctor–patient relationship. In: Schwartz HD, Kart GS, eds. *Dominant Issues in Medical Sociology.* Reading, MA: Addison-Wesley; 1978:100–107.
79. Wu R. *Illness and Behavior.* Englewood Cliffs, NJ: Prentice-Hall; 1973.
80. Lederer HD. How the sick view their world. In: Meyers ME, ed. *Nursing Fundamentals.* Dubuque, IA: Brown; 1967:155–167.
81. Woods NF. *Sexuality in Health and Illness.* 4th ed. St. Louis: Mosby; 1987.
82. Schuster EA. Privacy, the patient and hospitalization. In: Folta JR, Deck ES, eds. *A Sociological Framework for Patient Care.* New York: Wiley; 1979.

    (this reference has no number.) Van Kaam AL. Nurse in the patient's world. In: Meyers ME, ed. *Nursing Fundamentals.* Dubuque, IA: Brown; 1967.
83. Lowenberg JS. *Caring and Responsibility: The Crossroads of Holistic Practice and Traditional Medicine.* Philadelphia: University of Pennsylvania Press; 1989.
84. Rosenberg ML. *Patients: The Experience of Illness.* Philadelphia: Saunders; 1980.
85. Graffam S. Congruence of nurse–patient expectations regarding nursing intervention in pain. *Nurs Leadership.* 1981; 1:12–15.
86. Benoliel JQ, Crowley DM. The patient in pain. In: Folta JR, Deck ES, eds. *A Sociological Framework for Patient Care.* New York: Wiley; 1979:363–378.
87. Feldman HR. Pain. In: Patrick ML, Woods SL, Craven RF, et al. *Medical-Surgical Nursing: Pathophysiological Concepts.* Philadelphia: Lippincott; 1991.

BIBLIOGRAPHY

Baum A, Taylor SE, Singer JE, eds. *Handbook of Psychology and Health.* Vol. 4, *Social Psychological Aspects of Health.* Hillsdale, NJ: Erlbaum; 1984.

Becker MH. The health belief model and sick role behavior. In: Becker MH, ed. *The Health Belief Model and Personal Health Behavior.* Thorofare, NJ: Slack; 1974.

Bond J, Bond S. *Sociology and Health Care: An Introduction for Nurses and Other Health Care Professionals.* New York: Churchill Livingstone; 1986.

Brown NJ, Muhlenkamp AF, Fox LM, Osborn M. The relationship among health beliefs, health values and health promotion activity. *West J Nurs Res.* 1983; 5:155–163.

Ehrenreich B, English D. *Complaints and Disorders: The Sexual Politics of Sickness.* Old Westbury, NY: Feminist Press; 1973.

Faulkner A. *Nursing: A Creative Approach.* East Sussex, England: Bailliere Tidell; 1985.

Folta J. The humanization of services and the use of technology in patient care. In: Folta J, Deck E, eds. *A Sociological Framework for Patient Care.* New York: Wiley; 1979.

Gow KM. *How Nurses' Emotions Affect Patient Care: Self-studies by Nurses.* New York: Springer; 1982.

Grasska MA, McFarlane T. Overcoming the language barrier: Problems and solutions. *Am J Nurs.* 1982; 89:1376–1379.

Haddon R. Tri-care: A new concept in health care. *Nurs Health Care.* 1989; 10:197–201.

Hover-Kramer D. Creating a context for self-healing: The transpersonal perspective. *Holistic Nurs Pract.* 1989; 3:27–34.

Kirscht J. The health belief model and illness behavior. In: Becker MH, ed. *The Health Belief Model and Personal Health Behavior.* Thorofare, NJ: Slack; 1974.

Leininger MM. *Reference Sources for Transcultural Health and Nursing: For Teaching, Curriculum, Research, and Clinical-Field Practice.* Thorofare, NJ: Slack; 1984.

Lipkin GB, Cohen RG. *Effective Approaches to Patient's Behavior.* New York: Springer; 1980.

MacElveen-Hoehn P. The cooperation model for care in health and illness. In: Chaska NL, ed. *The Nursing Profession: A Time to Speak.* New York: McGraw-Hill; 1983.

McEwan PJM, ed. Health self-care. *Soc Sci Med.* special edition. 1989; 2:117–264.

Molzahn AE, Northcott HC. The social bases of discrepancies in health/illness perceptions. *J Adv Nurs.* 1989; 2:132–140.

Morley P, ed. *Developing, Teaching and Practicing Transcultural Nursing.* Salt Lake City: University of Utah College of Nursing; 1981.

Murray RB, Zentner JP. *Nursing Concepts for Health Promotion.* Englewood Cliffs, NJ: Prentice-Hall; 1979.

Pender NJ, Pender AR. Attitudes, subjective norms and intentions to engage in health behaviors. *Nurs Res.* 1986; 35:15–18.

Rosenstock IM. Why people use health services. *Milbank Memorial Fund Q.* 1966; 44:94–125.

Schaeffer MH. Environmental stress and individual decision-making: Implications for the patient. *Patient Ed Counsel.* 1989; 13:221–235.

Schuster EA. Privacy, the patient and hospitalization. In: Folta J, Deck E, eds. *A Sociological Framework for Patient Care.* New York: Wiley; 1979.

Shillinger FL. Locus of control: Implications for clinical nursing practice. *Image.* 1983; 15:58–63.

Smith JA. *The Idea of Health.* New York: Teachers College Press; 1983.

Spiegal AD, Backhaut BH. *Curing and Caring: A Review of the Factors Affecting the Quality and Acceptability of Health Care.* Jamaica, NJ: Spectrum; 1980.

Szasz TS, Hollender MH. A contribution to the philosophy of medicine. *Arch Inter Med.* 1956; 97:585–592.

Wallston BS, Wallston KA. Social psychological models of health behavior: An examination and integration. In: Baum A, Taylor S, Singer JE, eds. *Handbook of Psychology and Health.* Vol 4, *Social Psychological Aspects of Health.* Hillsdale, NJ: Erlbaum; 1984.

Woods NF, et al. Being Healthy: Women's Images. *Adv in Nsg Sci.* 1988; 11:36.

UNIT FOUR
Nurse–Client Collaboration

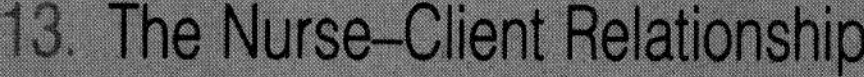

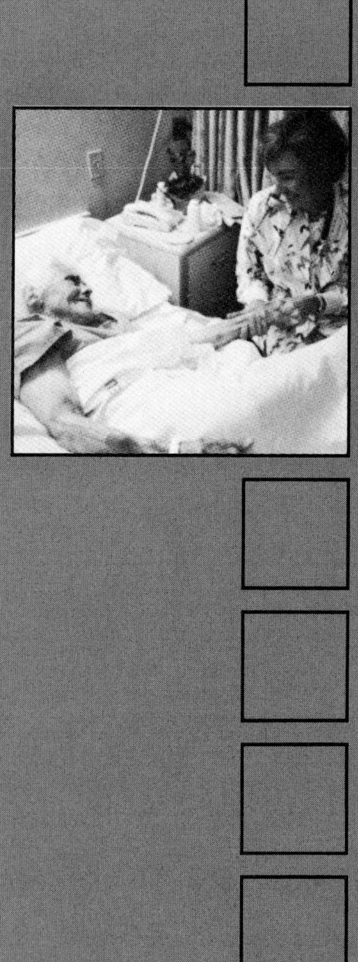

CHAPTER 13

The Nurse–Client Relationship

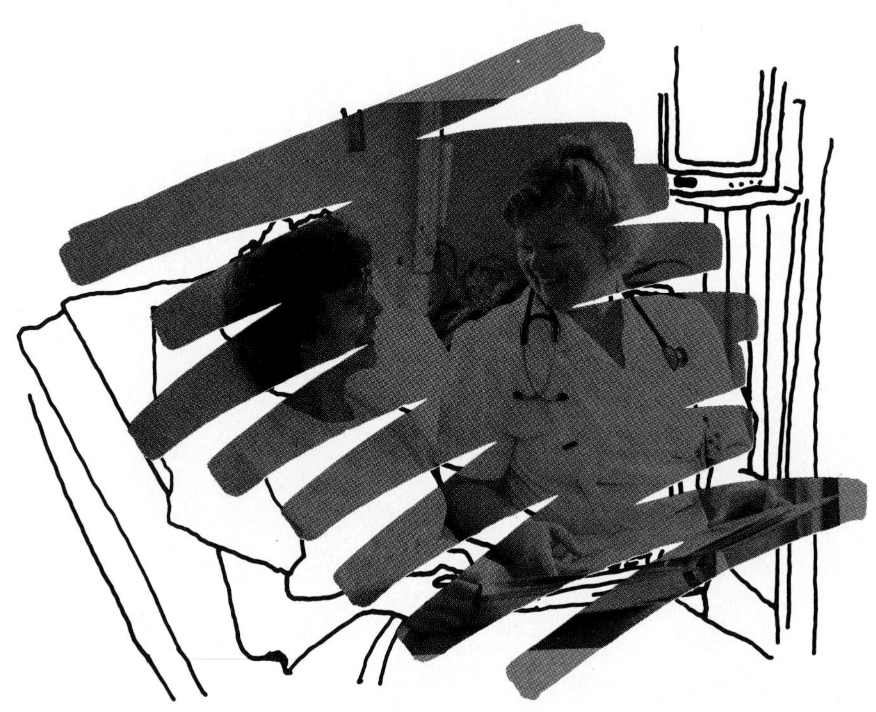

Behavioral Objectives

Upon completion of this chapter, the student will be able to:

1. Discuss the characteristics of the following types of relationships: human to nonhuman, human to ideology, human to deity, and human to human.
2. Compare and contrast the professional and nonprofessional interpersonal (social) relationship.
3. Describe the characteristics of an effective helper.
4. Identify the three phases of the helping relationship as defined by Gazda and associates.
5. Explain the following concepts: empathy, respect, warmth, concreteness, genuineness, self-disclosure, confrontation, immediacy, trust, autonomy, and mutuality.
6. Identify at least one task of each of the four phases of the helping relationship as defined by Sundeen and associates.
7. Describe how collaboration occurs in each phase of the nurse–client relationship.

KEY TERMS

action phase
autonomy
concreteness
confrontation
contract
empathy
facilitation phase
genuineness
helping relationship
immediacy
interpersonal relationship
intrapersonal relationship
manipulation
mutuality
nurse–client relationship
orientation phase
preinteraction phase
respect
self-disclosure
sympathy
termination phase
therapeutic use of self
transition phase
value clarification
warmth
working phase

The nurse–client relationship is at the core of every nursing role—teaching, advocating, caring, curing, counseling, and administrating. Imogene King[1] has defined the **nurse–client relationship** as a shared learning experience between the nurse and the client in which a health problem is explored, and attempts are made to resolve or adapt to the situation. The relationship allows a sense of connectedness to develop between the nurse and the client. Without this sense of connectedness, little sharing and exploration can occur.

Some relationships can be helpful; they are growth producing and vital to all concerned. Frequently such positive relationships are also collaborative; both individuals share responsibility not only for the maintenance of the relationship, but also for the attainment of mutually established goals. Collaboration allows both participants to participate at a level appropriate to their individual capabilities. On the other hand, there are relationships that do not reflect collaboration but rather reflect control. Such relationships can leave the participants feeling uncared for and manipulated. These relationships have no place in nursing. It behooves the nurse to have a clear understanding of what comprises a positive, collaborative relationship, and to strive for this type of relationship with all clients. This chapter covers the various types of human relationships, focusing on that form most important to nurses and clients—the helping relationship.

■ TYPES OF RELATIONSHIPS

Human to Nonhuman

Individuals can feel related to many things that are not human. For instance, it is not uncommon for people to develop very intense feelings of relatedness to pets. The expression "a dog is a man's best friend" conveys this idea. A pet can help to relieve loneliness and isolation and provide an individual with an outlet for nurturant needs. A study reported by Cain[2] explores the role a pet can play in the interaction of the family system. Pets have also been used effectively in nursing homes to provide elderly clients with something to care for and to love.

Because of their symbolic significance, objects such as wedding rings, photo albums, and souvenirs also can be a source of relatedness to an individual. Frequently people who have lost everything in a natural disaster grieve deeply for what might seem to others to be meaningless trinkets. But these kinds of objects carry with them memories and links to important times in individuals' lives. The worth of such objects cannot be measured by their material value but only by their personal significance to the owner.

Activities such as sports or work can also be a source of relatedness for people. The "football widow" can readily attest to her husband's devotion to the sport. Perhaps the sport provides the individual an opportunity for an exciting, though vicarious, experience not readily available in everyday activities. The computer hobbyist is similarly devoted to computer work. Certainly work, for many people, offers a challenge and provides an outlet for creativity. Many individuals derive their sense of value and purpose from their work accomplishments. This is evident in some of the interviews reported in Terkel's book entitled *Working*.[3]

Human to Ideology

Ideological beliefs can also be a source of relatedness for individuals. A person might devote a whole life to the furthering of one particular belief or cause. Others may embrace the same cause with less dedication, yet still devote considerable energy and time to its fruition. There are many examples of people who exemplify this type of relatedness to an ideology. For instance, in the 1984 Presidential election, Reverend Jesse Jackson represented what he called the Rainbow Coalition. His stated goal was to obtain political power for members of US society such as blacks, the poor, and other minority groups who feel disenfranchised within the mainstream of American politics. Mother Teresa, who devotes her life to serving the poor and homeless, is an example of an individual who has dedicated her life to an ideology of love and service to her fellow human beings. Whether or not the ideology is a popular one, some individuals dedicate themselves to ideology as a prime source of connectedness and gratification.

Human to Deity

Any discussion of relationships would be incomplete without mention of the relationship many individuals have with whatever they conceive to be their deity. This relationship will vary from individual to individual along a continuum from an absence of concern about spiritual entities to a strong sense of and need for faith.

Human to Human

The human relationship can be either intrapersonal or interpersonal. The **intrapersonal relationship**, or the relationship individuals have with themselves, is essential for growth and change. It is only from examining one's feelings and thoughts that one can come to understand and accept oneself. Travelbee[4] believes that self-acceptance and self-love are the precursors to developing positive relationships with others.

The **interpersonal relationship** is a social relationship—that is, it occurs among people within a social context such as marriage, family, friendship, school, business, church, or health care setting. There is, however, a difference between the nonprofessional social relationship developed between friends and the professional social relationship developed between a health care provider and a client. In a nonprofessional relationship, participants are usually on a fairly equal footing from the start and share responsibility for the progress of the relationship as long as it goes on. There is generally a mutual expectation that each will respond to the other with help and understanding. Each participant shares problems. Neither the duration of the relationship, nor the time and frequency of meetings, is predetermined. Occasionally there may be a formal ending of the relationship, but that is not always the case.[5]

Contrast this type of relationship with the professional relationship, also called the **helping relationship**, which has an explicit contract and predetermined meetings. In the beginning of the helping relationship the nurse assumes the predominant responsibility for the relationship, but as the relationship progresses, the balance of responsibility shifts toward the client. The change occurs as the client becomes increasingly aware of the parameters of informed consent and self-participation. This shifting of power and responsibility from the nurse to the shared domain of both nurse and client is the essence of collaboration. Both client and nurse share the task of keeping the relationship goal-directed and continually assessing progress made toward accomplishing mutually determined goals. The client and the nurse both assume active roles in a collaborative effort directed to meeting the health needs of the client; therefore, it is inappropriate for the nurse to use the client to resolve

IMPLICATIONS FOR NURSE–CLIENT COLLABORATION

Social and Professional Relationships

Social relationships are varied in their nature and character. The professional relationship is a special kind of social relationship, differing from other kinds of social relationships in that it is goal directed. Some professional relationships are collaborative. Collaborative relationships between nurse and client are quite different from professional relationships that are not collaborative. The foundations of collaboration rest on certain essential values of human interaction: egalitarianism, the value of equality among humans; self-determination; and respect. In a collaborative relationship, power and responsibility for goal attainment are the shared domain of nurse and client. In professional relationships that are not collaborative, responsibility for goal attainment rests largely with the professional.

personal needs and problems. Nurses must learn not to personalize client behavior as rejection, nor to expect gratification and praise from all clients. Table 13–1 compares professional and nonprofessional social relationships.

The rest of this chapter will discuss the helping relationship as characterized by the nurse–client relationship. Joyce Travelbee[4] describes this relationship as one in which a nurse therapeutically uses self to work with clients—individuals, families, or communities—to meet identified nursing needs.

Travelbee does not specify what the nursing needs are that are met within the context of the relationship, but she does specify the therapeutic use of self as the modality by which these needs can be met. The **therapeutic use of self** refers to the nurse's ability to use personality characteristics consciously and in full awareness in order to form a relationship and to structure nursing interventions. This goal is an idealistic one in that no one is ever totally aware of unconscious motivations that influence behavior. Yet, it is a worthy goal for nurses to integrate into their personal and professional development. An example of this would be a nurse who possesses the gift of humor. Using self therapeutically suggests that humor be used appropriately and not in a situation where a more thoughtful response would be in order.

Carl Rogers,[6] a noted humanistic psychotherapist, has also contributed to the understanding of helping relationships. Rogers defines a helping relationship as one "in which at least one of the parties has the interest of promoting the growth, development, maturity, improved functioning and improved coping with life." Another view of the helping relationship offered by Gazda and associates[7] is that the relationship facilitates personal growth and problem-solving through communication.

These definitions are similar, yet each provides a unique contribution to the understanding of the helping relationship. Travelbee provides a broad definition specifying who the client can be, whether individual, family, or community. She also identifies the concept of the therapeutic use of self as a way to meet nursing needs. Rogers is specific about what the needs are. Gazda introduces the important concept of communication as a vehicle to meeting the needs with which the client presents.

■ CHARACTERISTICS OF AN EFFECTIVE HELPER

Although there is no single personality type that has been identified as an effective helper, there are certain character-

TABLE 13–1. COMPARISON OF PROFESSIONAL AND NONPROFESSIONAL RELATIONSHIPS

Professional	Nonprofessional
One person takes the *responsibility of helping* while the other seeks help.	Neither person is in a position of having responsibility for helping the other.
There is a specific *purpose* to the relationship.	A specific purpose is not necessary.
Goal directed.	Not necessarily goal directed.
Focus of the relationship is on the needs of the helpee.	Each person seeks to have own needs met as well as to meet needs of the other.
Behaviors based on persons taking roles of professional and client.	People in social roles—certain social behavior is expected.
Relationship entered through necessity.	Relationship entered by choice.
Choice of whom to enter relationship with usually not available to either party.	People can choose with whom they care to become involved.
Behavior on part of helper reflects a balance between spontaneity and purposeful planned interventions.	Behavior on part of participants is spontaneous.
Helper focuses on discovering client characteristics that engender respect and caring in helper.	Feelings of liking, fondness, or love for the other are usually involved.
Helper does not judge the client as a person but does confront maladaptive client behavior and challenge client to change.	People may be judgmental in attitude.
Self-disclosure on part of helper is used as a strategy to facilitate the relationship.	Mutual sharing of such intimacies.
Empathic feelings for the helpee translated into helpful action.	Sympathetic feelings for the other may preclude or prevent helpful action.
Control is shared between helper and client. The client chooses to remain in the relationship and retains the right to decline or accept the helper's services.	Control is more evenly shared.
There is usually a definite and anticipated *ending* to the relationship, ideally when the goals of the relationship have been accomplished.	Relationships may continue indefinitely; ending usually is not anticipated.

BOX 13–1. CHARACTERISTICS OF AN EFFECTIVE HELPER

- Friendly, understanding, and well adjusted emotionally
- Aware of personal values
- Aware of personal motives and goals
- Aware of personal feelings
- Aware of personal strengths and weaknesses
- Has a sense of purpose in life
- Able to use a collaborative approach

IMPLICATIONS FOR NURSE–CLIENT COLLABORATION

Awareness of Client Values

Clients vary greatly in the values they hold for health care. The discovery of client values is known to aid nurses in planning care that is appropriate to clients' individual needs. One of the advantages of the mutual interaction model of client care discussed in Chapter 37 and throughout the text is that it acknowledges the rights of clients to participate in decisions vital to their health. Clients have authority derived from expertise, an expertise based on their special understanding of their own values. As the nurse interacts with a client in a collaborative relationship, the client is drawn into the decision-making process and reveals personal values to the nurse. The nurse's awareness of these values and sensitivity to them provides the essential foundation for planning care.

istics that helpers must possess (Box 13–1). It would seem to be basic that helpers must be friendly, understanding, and well adjusted emotionally. However, more than this is required of the helper. Gazda identifies the necessity for helpers to become as aware as possible of their own values, motives, feelings, strengths, weaknesses, and purpose in life. In addition, the ability to use a collaborative approach increases effectiveness as a helper. These factors enable one to use oneself effectively in the therapeutic manner suggested by Travelbee.[4]

BUILDING NURSING KNOWLEDGE

What Is the Effect on the Helping Relationship of Nurses' Attitudes Toward the Client?

Moss AR. Determinants of patient care: Nursing process or nursing attitudes? *J Adv Nurs.* 1988; 13:615–620.

Personal attitudes are related to personal values and nurses as well as clients bring attitudes to the helping relationship. Moss argues that too often caregiving is influenced by the attitudes of nurses who, on the basis of first impressions, categorize clients into types.

Moss reviewed a number of studies demonstrating the negative effects of categorizing clients. One study indicated that nurses associated negative traits with clients with specific problems. It compared nurses' responses to a client labeled as "alcoholic" with their responses when the client was described as someone who had been hospitalized for 4 days. Nurses viewed the client more favorably when not designated an alcoholic.

Another study examined nurses' attitudes about gender by having them describe a socially competent man, woman, and an adult of unspecified sex. The findings were that the attributes of the competent man and adult were similar, but the feminine traits were less positive and included dependence, submissiveness, and emotional excitability.

Moss emphasizes that when nurses categorize clients, there is a danger of initiating a self-fulfilling prophecy. Clients may come to view themselves as the nurses view them. Nurses may behave toward clients in such a way that clients will respond with the predicted behavior. For example, if a nurse believes a certain type of client is demanding, the nurse may respond slowly or begrudgingly to the client's requests. The client in turn may cope by being more adamant, thus becoming the demanding person the nurse expected to encounter. Moss concludes that it is vital for the profession to identify the factors that influence nurses' attitudes in order to take steps to assure that nurses deal with individual clients rather than types of people, behavior, or illnesses.

Awareness of Personal Values

If nurse helpers are to be able to value and appreciate clients as people, nurses need keen awareness of their own values. Nurses must recognize what issues have personal importance and what principles guide personal life decisions. Tripp-Reimer and co-workers[8] suggest that a nurse's lack of awareness regarding personal values can be a major source of nurse–client misunderstandings. On the other hand, awareness of one's own values permits greater acceptance of different values in others.

The process of increasing one's awareness of personal values is referred to as **values clarification.** (For further discussion of personal and professional values and values clarification, see Chap. 34.) There are so many value-laden issues with which nurses are confronted that it is essential to incorporate ongoing personal values clarification into nursing practice. Simon[9] identifies three stages in values clarification. First, the individual freely chooses a belief after carefully examining all the alternatives and identifying the consequences of such a belief. Second, the individual publicly affirms the chosen belief. Third, the individual makes life decisions and takes actions based on this belief. This process allows nurses to be clear regarding values about such issues as client rights versus nurse responsibilities, quality of life, euthanasia, abortion, surrogate motherhood, and honesty.

Likewise, a client's right to value and to believe in things that are quite different or even in opposition to nurses' views must be accepted and respected.[10] However, maladaptive or disruptive behaviors of clients do not have to be accepted; these need to be confronted and clients helped to change. Using a values clarification approach with clients can prove beneficial in assisting them to identify what is really important, what is not, and which behaviors are in conflict with stated values. The principle that guides nurses is that it is the behavior resulting from a value that is rejected, not the client. The following example illustrates a nurse's acceptance of clients, despite differences in their values.

Cynthia Brown is a nurse in an obstetrical unit where a large number of second-trimester abortions are performed. Ms. Brown, a devout Catholic, is personally opposed to abortion and is clear about her own values on this issue. She is also aware that many other people do not share her beliefs about abortion and she is able to accept value judgments that are different from her own. This acceptance guides her care of clients who have abortions performed. She is able to focus on the physical and emotional distress of clients without a need to judge them. Occasionally a client asks Ms. Brown if she would ever consider having an abortion. She states her own position in a way that acknowledges the difference between the client's values and her own but in no way implies condemnation of the other person.

Awareness of Personal Motives and Goals

The motives and goals of helpers also need close scrutiny. Nurses' efforts should be directed to facilitating the growth of clients. This does not mean that in the course of helping relationships, nurses will not experience self-growth, be challenged to change, or feel satisfaction that their role has been a facilitative one. In fact, a helping relationship has the potential to provide all of these things for nurses. But the primary motivation should be directed toward clients' well-being, and the goals of the relationship are mutually derived with clients for the purpose of benefiting them. For instance, if the goal of a nurse is to exercise power, then he or she may use manipulation or coercion to achieve client compliance with the *nurse's* goals. Note that nurses seeking power would probably not derive goals *with* clients but rather *for* clients. Likewise, nurses may be motivated to build their own self-esteem within the relationship and be a friend to clients rather than a helper. Such nurses might hesitate to confront a client about maladaptive behavior for fear of disrupting the relationship and causing the client to reject them, as the following example illustrates.

Nurse Rodriguez had been working with Mrs. Malnner for several months. Mrs. Malnner was 50 pounds overweight and had uncontrolled diabetes. When Mrs. Malnner came into the clinic she frequently brought her lunch, which usually consisted of a sandwich, potato chips, cookies, and a regular soda. Ms. Rodriguez had observed Mrs. Malnner with her brown bag lunch on several occasions.

Mrs. Malnner's examinations revealed no progress in weight reduction and a consistently high serum glucose level. Ms. Rodriguez asked Mrs. Malnner, "What do you think the problem is?" Mrs. Malnner lowered her eyes and said, "I don't know. I try so hard to follow the diet you gave me. I think it's my metabolism." Ms. Rodriguez replied, "I know how hard it is to stick to the diet and that you are trying your best." Mrs. Malnner said, "You are the only one who understands me. The doctor only yells at me."

Nurse Rodriguez should have confronted Mrs. Malnner about the lunchtime behavior that had been frequently observed. Instead, she offered a sympathetic response that the client liked but that did not facilitate the client's growth. Perhaps the nurse's motives were to meet her own needs—to feel liked, to be seen as kind and understanding. Her motives in this interaction were not geared toward Mrs. Malnner's well-being.

> **BUILDING NURSING KNOWLEDGE**
>
> **How Important Is Understanding the Client's Perspective to the Helping Relationship?**
>
> Kasch CR, Dine J. Person-centered communication and social perspective-taking. *West J Nurs Res.* 1988; 10:317–326.
>
> Kasch and Dine contend that the ability to use person-centered communication is the foundation of a nurse's ability to help clients. In person-centered communication, the beliefs, intentions, or role of the other person are addressed in every interpersonal encounter.
>
> Kasch and Dine focus on the factors that account for the ability to communicate in a person-centered way. One important factor is "perspective-taking." Perspective-taking refers to the range of capacities that allow one person to understand the viewpoint of another. For instance, the ability to make inferences concerning others' attitudes and the causes and motivations for their actions is important, as is the ability to understand the rights, obligations, and expectations associated with their social roles. Perspective-taking involves the capacity to recognize the multiple viewpoints that the people in a situation might have.
>
> Kasch and Dine argue that perspective-taking is important because it allows nurses to encounter clients as unique individuals who are responding to the pressures of the social roles they occupy. They contend, however, that nurses show considerable variation in their perspective-taking capability, and conclude that research is needed to provide a better understanding of how communication can be used to facilitate important nursing goals.

Awareness of Personal Feelings

An awareness of personal feelings is also an essential prerequisite for nurse helpers. Unrecognized feelings can result in behaviors that are not facilitative to clients, and can in fact confuse clients about their standing in the helping relationship. Nurses need to be able to pull back from an interaction and ask the following questions:

1. What am I feeling about/towards this client?
2. Do my feelings seem appropriate for the content of our communication?

3. Does the client remind me of someone else in my life? If so, are my feelings influenced either positively or negatively by the similarities I see?
4. What effect do my feelings have on my behavior with the client?
5. Are these feelings something that should be dealt with in the context of the relationship, or should I deal with these feelings by myself or with help?

Answering these questions is a way for nurses to recognize that their emotions influence their behavior in the nurse–client relationship. Even when the feelings are not related to the nurse–client relationship, it may seem to clients that they are. Clients may then feel rejected, misunderstood, or even angry. Not all personal feelings are appropriate for nurses to share with clients, but nurses' selective self-disclosure can help clients to realize that they need not interpret all of the nurses' behaviors personally.

Sometimes, nurses' feelings are reflections of the reciprocal nature of relationships. For example, a nurse may become aware of feeling discouraged whenever talking with a certain client. Rather than indicating negative feelings towards the client, these feelings may be a result of the client's disheartened emotional state influencing the nurse. The client may not have shared these feelings directly, and may even be unaware of them. Recognizing this possibility enables the nurse to address the client's feelings, and his or her own as well, to their mutual benefit.

Awareness of Personal Strengths and Weaknesses

Nurses also need to have an awareness of their strengths and weaknesses to be effective helpers. It is impossible for every nurse to be effective with every client or even to like each one. It is difficult for a nurse to be effective with clients who have a problem that is similar to an unresolved problem in the nurse's own life. In situations such as these, once nurses become aware that they are identifying with a client's situation in a nonhelpful way, the best course of action is to refer the client to someone else. The following example illustrates such a situation.

> Nurse Johnson's daughter died of leukemia at the age of 3 years. He has been unable to resolve his feelings of anger toward God. Whenever he assesses a spiritual need in a client, he refers the client to the hospital chaplain or to another nurse. His awareness that this is an area of weakness allows him to be an effective helper in other areas of client need.

Sense of Purpose

Nurses need to have a sense of purpose in life. This sense of purpose is communicated effectively to clients as caring, concern, and interest. When nurses experience enjoyment in living, satisfaction with career choice, confidence in their ability to make a difference in the lives of others, and enthusiasm for activities of daily living, it is obvious to others that they are aware of a clear purpose for living. Nurses who are able to present such positive attributes can be a source of hope to clients as the relationship progresses. Clients can see in the nurse a sense of purpose and direction that perhaps are momentarily absent from their own life due to the demands of illness.

Ability to Use a Collaborative Approach

A helping relationship is by its very nature a collaborative one. In fact, according to Williamson,[11] initiating the relationship is the first step toward collaboration. Together, nurse and client, both active and responsible, develop, implement, and evaluate the goals of the relationship. Collaboration ensures that the relationship moves in a direction that best meets clients' needs, rather than in a direction assumed by nurses to be in the clients' best interest. As active rather than passive participants, clients have a greater stake in the success of the relationship and the success of the mutually established goals. Collaboration removes nurses from an authoritarian role and clients from a subservient role and places them both in partnership roles.

CONCEPTUAL MODELS AND THE HELPING RELATIONSHIP

There are many ways of conceptualizing the process of the helping relationship. Two models are presented in this chapter. The first was developed by Carkhuff and coworkers.[12–14] Gazda and associates[7] have taken the Carkhuff model and applied the principles to specific professional fields such as health care and education. An advantage of using the Carkhuff model is that the concepts have been operationalized. This facilitates the application of the concepts to specific nursing situations and the phases of the helping relationship. Carkhuff also identifies levels of responses, which can serve as a basis for progression of learning experiences for nursing students. Beginning students will probably only be comfortable functioning within the first and second phases of the model, whereas students who have progressed within nursing education will be able to use all three phases of the Gazda model.

The second model, described by Sundeen and coworkers,[5] is designed specifically for nursing practice. This model contributes a perspective that is somewhat different from the Carkhuff model. However, the concepts have not been operationalized with the specificity of those in the Carkhuff model and may be more difficult for the beginning student to apply.

Gazda's Application of the Carkhuff Model

Gazda and associates[7] identify three phases of the helping relationship: the facilitation, transition, and action phases. There are communication techniques specific to each phase (Table 13–2) which demonstrate qualities that Gazda refers to as facilitative, transition, and action dimensions. These dimensions interact to accomplish the goals of each phase. Each of the techniques and dimensions is defined in this

TABLE 13–2. KEY CONCEPTS OF A HELPING RELATIONSHIP ACCORDING TO GAZDA AND ASSOCIATES

Facilitation Phase	Transition Phase	Action Phase
Helpee describes symptoms. Helper suspends acting on evaluations. Helpers' tenderness emphasized; helper "earns the right" to be judgmental later in the process.	Helpee defines problem and accepts responsibility for its change. Helper gently presses the helpee toward recognizing helper's role. Helper cautiously and tentatively becomes more evaluative.	Helpee takes appropriate actions to solve problem. Helper may be judgmental. Helper's self-confidence and knowledge are emphasized.
Procedural goals: Self-exploration.	Procedural goals: Better self-understanding and commitment to change.	Procedural goals: More appropriate action or direction
Facilitation Dimensions[a]	**Transition Dimensions**[a]	**Action Dimensions**[a]
Empathy (depth of understanding).	Concreteness (ability to be specific).	Confrontation (pointing out discrepancies).
Respect (belief in).	Genuineness (honesty, realness).	Immediacy (helper and helpee telling it like it is in the "here and now").
Warmth (caring, love; nonverbal).	Self-disclosure (ability to convey appropriately "I've been there too").	

[a] Each of the dimensions involves the act of perceiving (becoming aware of) and responding (acting on awareness).

From Gazda G, Asbury FS, Balzer FJ, et al. Human Relations Development. *4th ed. Boston: Allyn & Bacon; 1991.*

chapter and applied in Chapter 14. Table 13–2 outlines the key concepts of a helping relationship according to Gazda and co-workers.

Facilitation Phase. The first phase is the **facilitation phase,** in which clients describe the symptoms of their problem. Nurses make no judgment during this phase but encourage clients to continue with self-exploration. This goal is facilitated through the use of empathy, respect, and warmth.

Empathy. When helpers are able to both understand clients' feelings and to express that understanding in words, the helper is said to convey **empathy.** Empathy is the key to establishing a helping relationship with another person. In order to be empathic, nurses must first listen carefully to what clients say when describing feelings and problems. Secondly, nurses must think of words that accurately represent a client's feelings and situation. Third, nurses must express these words in order to convey to clients that they are attempting to understand the clients' position.[15]

It is essential to differentiate empathy from sympathy. **Sympathy** means to feel the same feelings that the other has, not just to understand the feelings. When a nurse feels the same as the client, then objectivity is lost and the nurse is unable to help the client. Empathy includes objectivity, which allows nurses to help clients to look at alternatives to their present situation.

Respect. Belief in a client's ability to solve his or her own problems is a key element of **respect.** Respect is developed as a nurse comes to learn about a client's uniqueness and capabilities. A nurse demonstrates respect by communicating a belief that clients can help themselves; by supporting clients' efforts to solve problems rather than taking over tasks in which they can be self-sufficient; and by fully attending to the client (attending behaviors will be discussed in Chap. 14).

Warmth. The nurse's ability to communicate caring to the client is expressed as **warmth.** When empathy and respect are present, warmth is also communicated. Warmth is communicated primarily through nonverbal behaviors such as gesture, tone of voice, touch, and facial expression.[16] Sometimes, however, words are very effective in communicating that a nurse is really concerned about a client.

Transition Phase. During the **transition phase** of a helping relationship, nurses work with clients to define the problem. Sometimes a client may have a very clear idea of the problem. At other times, a client may require a nurse's assistance to clarify the problem in the midst of a confusing array of facts. At still other times a client may rely completely on a nurse to define the problem. Once the problem is defined, nurse and client work towards goal collaboration and defining their mutual responsibility to achieve the goals. Nurses help clients to understand how a nurse can help them to reach the goals, and clarify the client's personal role in this same process. For instance, a client who is working on learning more effective communication skills with his wife may need the input of a nurse's professional knowledge about communication and interpersonal relationships in order to know how to change. The client's role may involve practicing the skills shared by the nurse and keeping a diary of daily interactions so that he and the nurse can evaluate his progress.

During the transition phase nurses sensitively help clients to recognize their own role in the problem and in its solution. This involves cautiously sharing an evaluation of the effectiveness of the clients' behavior. Because the relationship is still fragile, nurses must be careful to balance any evaluation of client behavior with ample use of warmth, respect, and empathy. The transition dimensions that facilitate goal achievement during the transition phase are concreteness, genuineness, and self-disclosure.

Concreteness. **Concreteness** is being specific when discussing a problem rather than being vague and ambiguous. The nurse who uses concreteness in a helping relationship responds directly to specific concerns expressed by clients and requests clarification of vague or abstract statements.[17] Nurses assist clients to enumerate clear and definite alternatives to deal with the problem situation.

Genuineness. The ability to communicate who one really is, is called **genuineness.** Helpers are genuine when they are consciously aware of feelings and appropriately match verbal and nonverbal behaviors to those feelings. Helpers who are genuine mean what they say and do so in a constructive way. Clients know where they "stand" with such a helper.

Self-disclosure. Self-disclosure is a powerful tool to convey that a nurse has "been there too." **Self-disclosure** is sharing aspects of one's inner self or personal experiences. If self-disclosure is appropriate or relevant to a client's situation, it can lead to greater closeness between nurse and client. If a nurse has had a similar problem and has found a solution to the problem, this can be reassuring to a client. However, if self-disclosure is premature or irrelevant, it may confuse and take the focus away from clients.[18] In addition, it is not appropriate to use self-disclosure in an effort to solve nurses' personal problems.

Action Phase. The **action phase** is where the hard work of the relationship is undertaken. In this phase, nurse and client collaborate on developing a plan to deal with the present problem and at the same time devise a method to deal with future problems. In the instance of the client needing to improve his communication skills with his wife, the client and nurse might first identify a need to practice listening skills. The plan might include specific exercises in which the client practices listening and then validates what he heard. Other techniques would be built into this plan so that perhaps on a weekly basis the client would be adding to his repertoire of communication skills.

In planning for the future, the nurse and client could identify specific situations that might arise that would interfere with his ability to communicate with his spouse. Together, nurse and client would examine and perhaps even role-play ways in which the client could handle these situations with increased effectiveness.

During the action phase nurses share specific evaluations of clients' behaviors and plans. These evaluations let a client know a nurse's perspective about which behaviors are maladaptive and contributing to the problem, and which are adaptive behaviors. Nurses also let clients know whether or not the plans for change seem appropriate. The action dimensions relevant to this phase are confrontation and immediacy.

Confrontation. After a strong relationship has been developed with the client a nurse may move on to the use of confrontation. **Confrontation** is the process of informing a client of the discrepancy between what the client has said and what the client has been doing. Confrontation can be extremely threatening and should be used only in a relationship in which mutual caring exists.

Immediacy. The concept of **immediacy** refers to the communication between the nurse and the client about their relationship as it exists at that moment in time.[7] Because immediacy may produce anxiety in either nurses or clients, it is essential that a strong base relationship be present before this technique is used. It is difficult to talk about things that are presently happening with the people that are involved. It is always easier to talk about people who are not present, or about things from the past. However, immediacy allows nurses and clients to resolve obstacles in the relationship that stand in the way of problem resolutions.

Sundeen, Stuart, Rankin, and Cohen Model

The second model of the helping relationship, developed by Sundeen and others,[5] looks at interactive concepts separate from the phases of the nurse–client relationship. In this model all the concepts operate to some degree in the three interactive phases of the relationship. The interactive concepts are trust, empathy, caring, autonomy, and mutuality. The phases of the relationship are the pre-interaction, orientation, working, and termination phases. The interactive concepts are described here first. Table 13–3 correlates the interactive concepts with the phases of the relationship.

Interactive Concepts

Trust. Trust is confidence that another will accept one for who one is and will respond genuinely. An individual develops an attitude of trust based on past experiences. The first experiences of trust stem from the parent–child relationship, in which the parent could be depended on to meet the child's needs for love, food, and comfort. Trust develops over time and can vary with each interpersonal relationship. Trust is reciprocal and must be developed in each nurse–client relationship (Fig. 13–1).[15]

Thomas[19] has identified a number of characteristics present in the trusting individual. This person is comfortable with increasing self-awareness and is able to share this awareness with others. The trusting individual is open to differences in people and does not feel a need to change others. New experiences are welcomed. Generally this individual displays congruence between words and actions over time. Lastly, this individual is future oriented and can postpone gratification of immediate need for larger goals. The individual who is distrustful tends to display the opposite characteristics. Nurses can use these behaviors to assess trust in clients as well as in self.

Trust can be enhanced within the helping relationship when nurses are honest and consistent with clients. With-

TABLE 13–3. CORRELATION OF INTERACTIVE CONCEPTS WITH PHASES OF THE NURSE–CLIENT RELATIONSHIP ACCORDING TO SUNDEEN AND ASSOCIATES

Interactive Concept	Orientation Phase	Working Phase	Termination Phase
Trust	Limited. Based on past experience. Begins to grow as contract is established.	Grows as commitment to relationship is tested and validated. Demonstrations of concern are facilitating.	Falters as termination becomes a reality but reasserted if well established during working phase. Tendency to be trusting in similar future situations.
Empathy	Difficult because of lack of awareness of the person as an individual.	Occurs more frequently as participants communicate more openly and learn to interpret nonverbal cues.	Helps toward successful termination, since feelings can be shared and understood more easily. Allows more accurate expression of feelings.
Caring	Expressed as an initial positive feeling toward another person—not specific to the individual. Relatively superficial.	Grows steadily as participants gain in appreciation of each other and share meaningful experiences together.	If termination is successful, feeling of caring will be shared by participants as part of termination process.
Autonomy	Both individuals essentially autonomous. Little data about contributions that each could make to the relationship.	Some autonomy given up by each participant in favor of area of expertise of other person. Sharing becomes important.	Both participants resume earlier autonomy as relationship is given up. Autonomous behavior of each is enhanced by behaviors learned during the relationship.
Mutuality	Limited. Tentative beginnings of sharing at an information level. Need for careful validation.	High level. Sharing of information and feelings. Deep appreciation of the uniqueness of the person. Teamwork. Interdependence.	Given up as each participant returns to more independent functioning.

From Sundeen S, Stuart S, Rankin E, Cohen S. Nurse–Client Interaction: Implementing the Nursing Process. *4th ed. St. Louis: Mosby; 1989.*

out trust the helping relationship is not able to progress beyond the most preliminary level. In the mutual interaction model it is essential that trust flows mutually between client and nurse.

A simple example of trust occurs when a nurse keeps the commitments made to a client. Such commitments may involve returning promptly with needed pain medication, calling the physician or the chaplain, or checking on a diet order as promised.

Indication of a deeper level of trust occurs in the following example, in which the nurse accepts a client's sharing of self without judgment.

> Mrs. Laker had been in labor for 16 hours. She was exhausted but she also seemed to be afraid of something. Ms. Mitchell had been her nurse for the last 6 hours and had developed a positive relationship with Mrs. Laker. Ms. Mitchell said, "I can see you are exhausted; you have worked so hard today, but there seems to be something else bothering you. If there is, perhaps it is something that I could help you with." Mrs. Laker began to sob softly and said "I wanted to abort this baby at 23 weeks but the doctor wouldn't do it. Now I'm so afraid that the baby will die or there will be something wrong with the baby—you know, it'll be a punishment from God because I wanted to get rid of the baby. But now I really want the baby and I'm scared." Ms. Mitchell took Mrs. Laker's hand in hers, touched Mrs. Laker's forehead gently, and said "What an awful feeling to carry around—that God would punish you in such a way."

Empathy. Sundeen and co-workers[5] define empathy in similar fashion to the Gazda definition. The inclusion of this concept in both models supports the importance of empathy to the helping relationship.

Caring. According to Erich Fromm,[20] caring includes an interest in what happens to another, respect for another's individuality, a feeling of involvement in another's well-being, and a knowledge of the other's needs. It is difficult to imagine a helping relationship in which a nurse "cared for" but did not "care about" the client. The presence of caring contributes to the development of trust and empathy.

Caring is demonstrated in the same manner as warmth is demonstrated in the Gazda model—that is, by being kind, gentle, and attentive to clients. Nurses also show caring by taking time to discuss the purpose and expected benefits of procedures that clients find painful but are in their best interest. Caring is communicated in a nurse's attitude while working with clients. Through a gentle and attentive approach a nurse is saying that a client is worthy of care (Fig. 13–2).

Autonomy and Mutuality. The capacity for self-direction is defined as **autonomy.** It is characterized by independence, openness to new experiences, the ability to make decisions and take responsibility for the consequences, and a tolerance of others who are different from self. **Mutuality** is concerned with the process of sharing with another person.

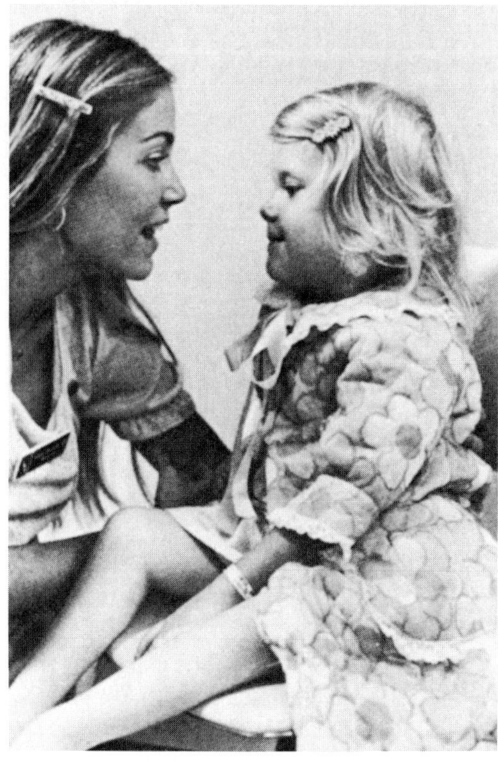

Figure 13–1. Establishing trust is important for clients of all ages. (*From Fritz PA, Russell CG, Wilcox EM, Shirk FI.* Interpersonal Communication in Nursing: An Interactionist Approach. *Norwalk, CT: Appleton-Century-Crofts; 1984: 143. Courtesy of Suzanne Edwards, Children's Memorial Hospital, Chicago, Illinois.*)

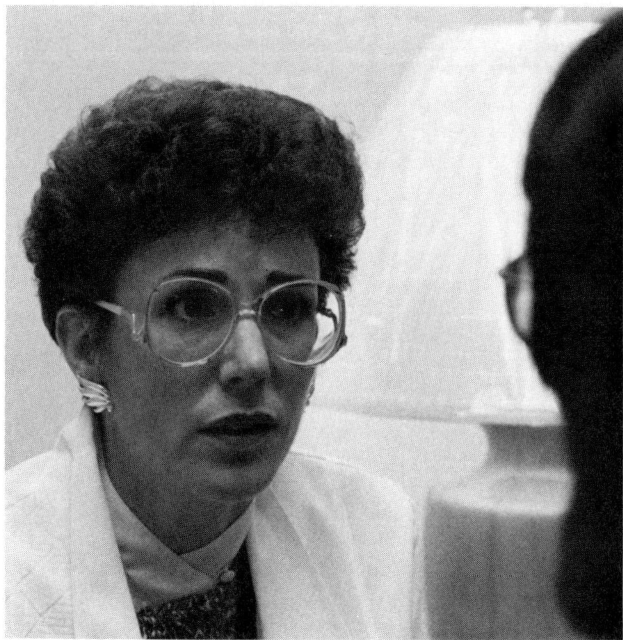

Figure 13–2. The nurse communicates warmth and caring to the client.

It is helpful to examine these two concepts as they occur on a continuum and also as they interact in a relationship.[5]

When clients initially seek health care, there are areas in which they may choose to relinquish their autonomy and allow health professionals to be in control. In fact, in the beginning of a helping relationship, clients may seem to be in a dependent role in relationship to nurses. Yet nurses must be aware that clients have *chosen* this dependence and may just as easily choose to reject this role. The ultimate control rests with clients, who can either choose to accept or to decline the helping relationship as an inalienable right.

As the relationship progresses, clients may choose and/or nurses may encourage increasing client autonomy and control. The balance of power, control, and decision-making moves toward client and away from nurse. The degree to which this shift of power occurs is an individual matter. Some clients believe their health status is under their own control and will want to exert a great deal of power. These individuals are referred to as "internals" in the locus of control theory.[21] Other clients operate with the belief that their health is controlled by outside forces, and will probably be willing to let nurses be in charge. Such individuals are referred to as "externals," and will require more encouragement from the nurses to join in a collaborative effort. (See Chaps. 12 and 23 for additional information on the locus of control theory.)

The issue of control is an important one for nurses to be clear about. Nurses might be tempted to usurp control and decision-making from an "external" client who seems passive and dependent. This would be an inappropriate nursing response. Ultimately clients must be able to manage their health needs without the direct continual assistance of nurses. Therefore, a nurse's goal is to encourage greater participation and independence in health-related matters.[22] On the other hand, complete self-direction by clients is not usually fully successful either. The ideal, then, is to arrive at an appropriate level of autonomy that encourages collaboration appropriate to clients' condition and circumstances.

According to Sundeen and others[5] "the process by which clients assume an appropriate level of autonomy without blocking the provision of necessary health care services is mutuality." The helping relationship is most effective when nurse and client each contribute their unique strengths to meet clients' needs. Nurses contribute theoretical knowledge that allows identification of problems and possible solutions. Clients contribute a knowledge of self that may influence their response to nursing interventions. The following interaction illustrates the presence of autonomy and mutuality in a relationship.

> Mrs. Garcia had given birth to her first child, a son, 2 days ago and was suffering from an anesthesia-induced spinal headache. The nursery nurse who brought Mrs.

BUILDING NURSING KNOWLEDGE

How Important Is Reciprocal Trust and What Factors Promote It?

Thorne SE, Robinson C. Reciprocal trust in health care relationships. *J Adv Nurs.* 1988; 13:782–789.

Thorne and Robinson note that trust is one of the most important ingredients of the health care relationship. They argue, however, that it must be reciprocal, especially in chronic illness. According to these authors, current knowledge reflects an understanding of trust from the point of view of health care professionals rather than the meaning it has for clients. This article discusses the findings from a study that looked at trust from the client's perspective. The study included 77 chronically ill clients and employed an interview approach to explore clients' perceptions of their relationships with their caregivers.

Clients described relationships that evolved in a predictable pattern. In the initial stage, clients had absolute trust in their caregivers. This was based on the naive assumption that solutions to their health problems would be found. Because the health problems were chronic, easy remedies did not exist. Thus, a loss of initial trust was inevitable. A stage of "shattered trust" ensued. This stage was accompanied by marked distress in clients, including feelings of anger, suspicion, and intense vulnerability. It did not last long, however, because clients recognized their ongoing need for health care. The final stage was a stage of "guarded alliance" in which trust was more selective and based on an informed rather than a naive perspective of the skills of professional care. Clients felt that blind faith was no longer possible once they had knowledge about the realities of professional care.

During the course of prolonged illness, clients also developed their own skills in illness management, including aspects in the domain of professional expertise. Clients participated in health care decision-making. Many found that it was as important to be trusted by their health care professionals as it was to have trust in them. Experiencing trust from the caregiver seemed to validate the client's ability to make competent health decisions, and contributed to the client's self-esteem and satisfaction with the relationship. The authors conclude that there are significant advantages when reciprocal trust is achieved. To facilitate it, they argue that health care professionals need to become sensitive to the client's perspective by listening and soliciting the client's ideas.

Garcia's baby to her could see that Mrs. Garcia was unable to care for her baby independently.

Nurse: Would you like me to take the baby back to the nursery, or could I help position the baby so that you can feed him?

Mrs. Garcia: This headache is killing me, but I want to hold my baby. Do you think I can safely feed him if I don't sit up?

Nurse: Why don't I position the baby next to you so that you can feed him and I'll come back in ten minutes to burp him for you. Then you can finish feeding him. (Mutuality—sharing the care.)

IMPLICATIONS FOR NURSE–CLIENT COLLABORATION

Caring, Autonomy, and Mutuality

The nature of a collaborative relationship is to recognize, acknowledge, and respect the individual's right to be autonomous or self-determined, to make their own choices. Dignity is based on self-determination. Caring is reflected in nurses' efforts to protect the client's dignity. Thus a collaborative relationship is a caring relationship.

Phases of the Nurse–Client Relationship. The following discussion focuses on four phases of the helping relationship described by Sundeen and associates: the preinteraction, orientation, working, and termination phases.[5]

Preinteraction Phase. In the **preinteraction phase** a nurse becomes aware of personal thoughts, feelings, and preconceptions about a client. This is the only phase in which clients are excluded as active participants. Perhaps a nurse has heard from others that a client is difficult and demanding. It is essential that nurses be aware of their reactions to such a report in order to be objective and to avoid communicating rejection to clients. On the other hand, a nurse may have received information suggesting that a client is experiencing certain needs. Armed with such data, a nurse will be attuned to client behaviors that validate or invalidate the presence of specific needs.

At this time, nurses also conceptualize what should be accomplished with a client. For instance, in the case of the client who has been described as difficult, a nurse might decide to focus attention on gathering data about the reason for the client's behavior. Goals would encourage the client to express thoughts and feelings freely and to help the client identify problem areas.

Orientation Phase. The **orientation phase** is the first phase of the relationship in which nurse and client interact with one another. Communication may be somewhat tentative, with each participant "feeling the other out." Orientation involves getting to know one another, sharing expectations for the relationship, and establishing mutual goals.

Introduction. It is courteous and professional for nurses to begin the interaction by telling clients their name. Nothing is more depersonalizing than to have a health care professional enter a client's room to perform a procedure on the client without introduction or explanation.

Nurses should also explain the nursing role, especially in relation to the client. Telling a client, "I'm Mary Jones, your nursery nurse for the day" provides a client with some information and direction about the purpose of this helping relationship.

Asking a client's name is a sign of respect. Many clients wish to be addressed by their first name; however, that needs to be confirmed. The nurse should not presume such familiarity without clients' permission.

Sharing Expectations. Another important task of the orientation phase is the establishment of mutual expectations, sometimes referred to as a **contract** (See also Chaps. 3 and 37). This is not to be confused with a legally binding document. In fact, this contract is not established in a businesslike manner but instead a warm and informal approach is used. A nurse–client contract is a verbal agreement that addresses mutual expectations regarding length, frequency, and location of meetings; the overall purpose of the relationship; the duration of the relationship; and the manner in which confidential material will be handled. The following interaction illustrates the establishment of a contract.

Nurse Jason: Mr. Tate I will be working with you during your five-day stay to help you practice insulin injections and to review your new diet. I'm wondering if we could find a time of the day that is good for both of us.

Mr. Tate: I'm not an early morning person, so anytime after 11 o'clock would be good. It takes me that long to wake up, and can we meet every day? I'm afraid I'll be a slow learner when it comes to the injections.

Nurse Jason: What about 1:00 P.M.? That's usually a good time for me and we could spend time together before visiting hours started. I think I can meet every day.

Mr. Tate: That sounds fine. About the diet, I have very definite likes and dislikes when it comes to food. Am I going to have to eat certain foods or will I have some flexibility?

Nurse Jason: I think we can work in enough of your preferences to make this a diet you can live with. In fact, why don't you give me a list of your likes and dislikes and I will consult with the dietician about how to include your preferences and still come up with a good diet.

Mr. Tate: That sounds good.

Nurse Jason: Perhaps at the end of the week we can plan some time to see how well we have accomplished our goals and what you can do when you are at home. There's one more thing, sometimes as I work with clients and we get to know each other they share confidential information with me. I want you to know that I respect that, and if for any reason I had to share our conversation, I would first let you know my reason.

Mr. Tate: Okay—when do we start?

Nurse Jason: How about one o'clock today?

In the above interaction the nurse and client have mutually arrived at the frequency and the schedule of meetings. In addition, both client and nurse have had input into the establishment of goals. This contract negotiation is not limited to the orientation phase, but as a client's or nurse's situation changes, the contract may need renegotiation at any point during the relationship.

Nurses begin to assess clients by gathering data. Through this process nurses begin to view clients as unique persons. Clients, likewise, are formulating ideas about nurses and comparing new perceptions to ideas previously held and to previous experiences. Clients are attuned to nurses' demonstrations of caring and trustworthiness during this phase. It is not uncommon for clients to test nurses in an effort to gauge their sincerity and interest. This testing behavior may be in the form of rudeness, or clients may wait some place other than the agreed-upon meeting place to see if a nurse cares enough to look for them.

Mutual Goal Setting. When both client and nurse begin to see each other as unique individuals, they are ready to establish more specific goals for the relationship. Trust begins to develop as both nurse and client perceive a mutual commitment to the relationship. By agreeing on the terms and goals of the relationship, two autonomous individuals have developed a degree of mutuality. Caring develops out of an appreciation of each other's uniqueness, and with caring comes a greater capacity for empathy. Nurse and client have clarified their roles within the relationship. All of these things are signals that the relationship is entering the working phase.

Working Phase. During the **working phase** nurse and client engage in active problem-solving. The process is very intense, and is characterized by periods of growth and resistance to growth. Clients are encouraged to share deep feelings and to examine reactions and coping responses to situations.

Many feelings are shared in the course of a helping relationship. This sharing challenges a nurse's ability to respond effectively. Feelings such as vulnerability, anger, hostility, sadness, and affection are all feelings that commonly arise and must be dealt with by nurses.

Feelings. Sometimes clients reveal so much of themselves that they feel vulnerable and exposed. They may respond to needs for security by pulling back from nurses and distancing themselves, perceiving "if I can again cover my feelings, I'll be safe." Clients may fear that nurses will betray their trust and somehow use their shared feelings and experiences in such a way as to hurt them. Nurses responding to such situations need to validate clients' feelings of vulnerability and communicate understanding and trustworthiness. The following example illustrates this point.

> Mr. Crowley was getting ready to be discharged to a nursing home. Mr. Saunders, his nurse, noted how saddened Mr. Crowley seemed whenever the topic of the nursing home came up. Mr. Saunders asked Mr. Crowley what he was feeling, and Mr. Crowley discussed his feelings of anger, depression, and rejection that his family was putting him into a nursing home. After their discussion Mr. Crowley said he felt better because he got his feelings out in the open. However, later in the day when Mr. Saunders returned to the room, Mr. Crowley was very curt in his communication. Mr. Saunders wondered if Mr. Crowley was now feeling vulnerable, and so he asked Mr. Crowley, "Do you feel uncomfortable with me since you shared how you felt about the nursing home? If you do, I can understand, but I want to reas-

sure you that I respect what you shared with me and I will use what you told me only to help you."

Anger is another feeling that often arises in the working phase that needs to be confronted. Anger can be seen as a frightening emotion because it carries with it the potential to harm oneself or others.[23] People learn various ways of coping with anger as a part of their normal development. Some people displace their anger to someone who is less threatening or less meaningful to them. For instance, a client who is angry at a physician for not coming to see her for 2 days may snap at a nurse who comes into her room to take her vital signs. The client is releasing some of her anger by snapping at the nurse, and this avoids a confrontation with the physician.

Some people handle angry feelings through silent behavior. Silence can be used to control or to mask anger that a client feels. Still others turn their anger inward and blame themselves for misfortune or punish themselves by overeating, drinking, or other excessive self-destructive behaviors.

Because anger can be expressed in different ways nurses need to validate that a client is indeed angry. This exploration may be helpful to clients because by confirming clients' anger, nurses are also communicating acceptance of angry feelings. Nurses also must help clients to identify the source of the angry feelings and the circumstances that have given rise to the anger. The anger may have originated from a source and circumstances outside of the nurse–client relationship and clients may displace feelings toward nurses. Or, the anger may stem from the nurse–client relationship itself. A client may perceive a nurse as having moved in too close, and anger may be used as a distancing maneuver. Perhaps a client resents the dependency that illness causes; again, the client may vent anger toward the nurse. Sometimes anger stems from a breach of trust between nurse and client. Whatever the cause of the anger, the only way to deal with it constructively is to discuss it objectively and to examine alternative ways of dealing with the feelings.

Hostility is another feeling that may arise within a nurse–client relationship. Sometimes people use hostility as a protective mechanism because it keeps others at a distance.[24] This is a self-defeating behavior. Clients who approach nurses in a hostile manner may be rejected. Clients then feel increasingly hostile and feel the need for greater self-protection from the "uncaring" health care system. Hostility does not usually occur in a trusting relationship unless clients perceive nurses have let them down or violated their trust in some way. In situations in which clients show hostility, it is important for nurses to be aware of personal feelings and express them to clients in a nonhostile manner. The following example is indicative of this type of a response toward a hostile client:

> Mr. Brown, it is very difficult for me to keep coming into your room when you speak to me in that way. I don't like it. But I care about you and I would like to be able to talk with you about what the problem is.

A client who has grown to trust a nurse may also feel comfortable in sharing memories of loss or past hurt or experiences in which the client felt ashamed or embarrassed. A nurse who is privy to this knowledge has been given a gift of self by the client and therefore the nurse should handle such revelations with absolute respect. Frequently when talking about such incidents the client feels sad and may feel the urge to cry. In such situations nurses should assure clients that these feelings are normal and that crying itself is not only acceptable, but often healing. Tears can "wash away" some of the pain and give clients a feeling of renewal in having expressed emotions that have then been accepted by a nurse.

Feelings of sadness frequently generate a similar response in nurses. It is unlikely that a truly compassionate nurse would be unmoved by some of the difficulties and tragedies that clients share. At times like this, it is appropriate and illustrates genuineness on the part of a nurse to say "When I listen to all that you have had to deal with, it makes me very sad." On the other hand some nurses may feel very uneasy when a client cries. Nurses may know that tears are beneficial; however, that doesn't guarantee that nurses will feel comfortable when clients cry.[23] This is another situation in which awareness of personal feelings allows nurses to respond appropriately to clients.

It is quite natural for feelings of mutual affection to develop occasionally between nurses and clients as the helping relationship progresses. These feelings of affection may transcend the boundaries of the professional relationship and nurses must set limits in this area. Nurses may also have feelings of affection that are inappropriate to the role as a helper. Nurses who realize, for example, that their own objectivity is being lost, that they are becoming angry at people who set limits on the client, or that they are delaying nursing evaluation of goal achievement should consider that the relationship may be veering away from its professional limitations. In these instances nurses benefit greatly from collaboration with another professional such as a nurse peer, a supervisor, or a counselor/social worker. By discussing personal feelings with an objective yet informed listener, nurses are better able to understand the basis for their reactions and also to identify ways of channeling these feelings so that nursing care is not adversely affected.

Behaviors. In addition to feelings that arise within the relationship, there are also some troublesome client behaviors that pose challenges for nurses. These behaviors include manipulation, overdependent or demanding behavior, and silence.

Manipulation occurs when clients try to use nurses to meet their own needs. Some clients may manipulate through lack of honesty or by playing one staff member against another. The result is the same—nurses feel used or manipulated and may respond with anger. It is essential that nurses examine these feelings of discomfort and identify their source. Nurses need to stand firm against being manipulated by clients because the result can be destructive to nurse, client, and their relationship.

Overdependency, a demanding behavior, occurs when clients fear that needs will not be met. Fear or insecurity causes clients to increase calls for help. Some clients do this by putting on their call light frequently or making many requests for assistance in areas where they should be independent. Again, a nurse's reaction is critical to effective care.[25] The natural spontaneous reaction is usually anger. Yet if nurses feel angry and withdraw, this will only increase clients' fears of being alone and abandoned. The following example illustrates an effective nursing response to demanding behavior.

> Mrs. Smith, a 52-year-old client recovering from a recent myocardial infarction, put her call light on for the seventh time in an hour. Nurse Wu had responded to each of Mrs. Smith's requests with increasing irritation. When the call light went on for the seventh time, Nurse Wu said to herself that something was obviously wrong; that perhaps Mrs. Smith's requests were not expressing her real needs. Nurse Wu went into the room, sat down next to Mrs. Smith's bed, and said, "Mrs. Smith, you have put your light on seven times in the last hour. At first I felt irritated, but then I realized there is probably something else bothering you that I haven't really taken care of. Why don't we talk for a few minutes?" Mrs. Smith looked down and said, "I know I've been a nuisance . . . but you know last night I had chest pain right at this time. I think I just want to know that you are close by in case I need you."

Silence is another behavior that may trouble nurses. Sometimes silence is comfortable and reflects the degree of trust and caring between two individuals that allows them to sit quietly together without words. At other times, nurses may deliberately use the technique of silence to enable clients to focus completely on what has transpired between them. However, in other situations in which silence occurs, both nurses and clients may feel anxious. The problem with silence is that neither party knows what the other is feeling or thinking. Silence can mean a client is angry, or sad, or even too frightened to talk. Nurses may have a clue as to the meaning of silence from clients' nonverbal behavior, but without verbal confirmation from clients, nurses cannot be certain about what clients are experiencing.[23] Nurses may then react with a strong desire to leave the situation to reduce their own anxiety. This reaction will probably not benefit clients. It would be more effective for a nurse to say to the client, "When we have these long periods of quiet, I wonder what you are feeling and thinking. I'm uncomfortable because I'm not sure how to reach you." This type of response is not only genuine but also communicates that the nurse cares about the client and is willing to "stick it out" in the situation even though it doesn't feel good to do so.

When dealing with any of these troublesome behaviors nurses must strive to remain aware of personal feelings and reactions. It is natural for nurses to want to withdraw, retaliate, or respond with anger or hostility when these behaviors are directed at them. It is essential to recognize that reacting with anger or withdrawal merely reinforces clients' maladaptive responses and diminishes therapeutic effectiveness. Nurses need to be aware of their own feelings, discuss them with a peer or a supervisor if necessary, and plan a response that will assist clients to deal with their feelings constructively rather than to reinforce unhealthy patterns. Nurses who act as helpers can be a vital influence in changing lifelong patterns of unhealthy behavior by increasing self-awareness of feelings and preventing them from dictating behavior. Table 13–4 summarizes nurse responses to difficult client feelings and behaviors (see also the discussion on "Blocks to Empowering Communication" in Chap. 14).

As the working phase continues, nurse and client explore alternatives to identified problems and work toward accomplishment of mutually determined goals. Both nurse and the client share responsibility for keeping the relationship goal-directed. When the goals have been accomplished or when nurses and clients find that circumstances prevent their continuing to meet, the relationship enters into the final phase of termination.

Termination Phase. The **termination phase** represents the formal ending of the helping relationship. Ideally, clients will have been prepared for termination from the moment the contract was established. It is helpful for nurses to remind clients periodically throughout the relationship that there will be an ending.

When a positive helping relationship ends, it is usually with feelings of ambivalence. There is satisfaction that mutually established goals were met, but there is also sadness about the impending loss of a significant other. Because of these conflicting feelings, termination can be very painful. Though difficult, termination can be a positive learning experience for nurse and client. It offers an opportunity to review the course of the relationship and to be aware of its deep meaning. A review of goal accomplishment can lead to feelings of satisfaction for both nurse and client. Feelings about termination also need to be shared. Clients will react to termination in much the same way that they have dealt with previous losses; feelings of anger, rejection, fear, and sadness are common. The exploration of these feelings can be beneficial and growth producing for both nurses and clients.[5]

Factors such as sufficient time and appropriate settings in which to develop the helping relationship, and the health condition of a client, impinge on the development of the nurse–client relationship. Some nurses will be able to relate to clients on a long-term basis and will readily see the applicability of the concepts related to the helping relationship. Other nurses may be in contact with clients for very limited periods of time and may not be able to develop deep relationships, but will see the phases of the relationship condensed into a brief interaction. Whatever the situation, the goal of the helping relationship is the same: to get to know a client in order to support the client's growth.

TABLE 13–4. SUMMARY OF NURSE RESPONSES TO DIFFICULT CLIENT FEELINGS AND BEHAVIORS

Client's Feelings	Nurse's Response
Anger in the form of silence, self-denigration, or hostility	1. Validate that the feelings are anger. 2. Let clients know that it is appropriate to express anger. 3. Explore the source of the anger. If the source is outside of the nurse–client relationship, assist clients to develop a plan to deal with anger appropriately and with the appropriate individual. If the source of the anger is the nurse–client relationship, assist clients to discuss the reasons for anger towards a nurse and to identify ways of handling it. 4. Examine clients' usual ways of handling anger. 5. Assist clients to evaluate effectiveness of coping methods. 6. Continue to assess one's own reaction to prevent withdrawal or angry reprisals toward clients.
Vulnerability: Client has shared personal information then reacts by withdrawing from nurse	1. Validate clients' feelings. 2. Accept clients' feelings. 3. Continue to respond to clients with patience. 4. Avoid pressing clients to share deep personal feelings. Clients need time to feel "safe" again. 5. Continue to demonstrate trustworthiness to clients. 6. Continue to assess own reactions to prevent mutual withdrawal.
Sadness	1. Acknowledge the normalcy of sad feelings in light of what client has shared. 2. Verbally and nonverbally convey understanding of acceptance of feelings. 3. Encourage continued expression of feelings—both verbally and through crying if appropriate. 4. Examine own reactions to crying. Nurses' uneasiness and desire to withdraw from the situation may communicate rejection to clients.
Affection: Inappropriate to boundaries of nurse–client relationship	1. Firmly and clearly set limits on the expression of affection that transcends professional boundaries. 2. Firmly set limits on sexual advances made by clients. 3. Reiterate goals of relationship. 4. Analyze own feelings toward client. If nurses feel affection that is inappropriate to the relationship, they may lose objectivity towards clients and be ineffective helpers.
Client Behaviors	**Nurse's Response**
Manipulation	1. Be firm with client. 2. Do not allow self to be manipulated. 3. Be aware of angry feelings and desire to withdraw from client.
Overdependency/demanding behavior	1. Identify source of client's insecurity. 2. Attempt to plan interventions mutually to meet client's real needs. 3. Be aware of inclination to avoid client and thus increasing the demanding behavior.
Silence	1. Communicate to client that silence may be unsettling or be constructive. 2. Communicate interest in what client is feeling. 3. Communicate desire to be with client even though silence may feel uneasy. 4. Be aware of desire to run away from client.

■ COLLABORATION WITHIN EACH MODEL OF THE HELPING RELATIONSHIP

Whether the Gazda model or the Sundeen model is applied to the helping relationship, collaboration is an activity that guides each model. Implicit in each model is the idea of working *with* a client and facilitating the client's growth—not doing *for* a client or in any way usurping the client's autonomy.

The names of the phases in the Gazda model clearly identify this as a collaborative approach. The first phase, facilitation, is designed to help clients to self-explore and to identify problems with the assistance of nurses. As clients progress through the transition phase to the action phase, nurses' intent is to support clients' problem-solving. This support takes the form of acceptance of clients, assistance in problem identification, and exploration of solutions and alternatives. But in the end, it is important that clients take action to deal with their own situations.

In the Sundeen model, the concepts of autonomy and mutuality are also consistent with a collaborative approach. The attitude of respect for clients' desires to be self-sufficient, while at the same time offering to share in helping, exemplifies collaboration. In the preinteraction phase, clients are excluded from active participation. However, in the orientation, working, and termination phases clients are active participants in goal establishment, goal achievement, and goal evaluation.

SUMMARY

The collaborative helping relationship is essential to all aspects of nursing practice. The helping relationship is the most important tool available to nurses in assisting clients to meet health needs. When the relationship is developed in a collaborative manner with clients, the best that nurse and client have to offer is brought to bear on clients' health problems. Nurses share theoretical expertise and knowledge of possible solutions, and clients share expertise regarding self. Combining these different but essential perspectives assures nursing care that is individualized to a specific client.

Gazda, Sundeen, and their associates offer two models of helping relationships. Gazda's model identifies three phases of the helping relationship: the facilitative, transition, and action phases. Gazda also identifies qualities that facilitate the goal achievement of each phase, including empathy, respect, warmth, concreteness, genuineness, self-disclosure, confrontation, and immediacy. These concepts are examined in more depth in Chapter 14.

Sundeen's model of the helping relationship identifies the interactive concepts of trust, empathy, caring, autonomy, and mutuality. These concepts are present in the four phases of a relationship—the preinteraction, orientation, working, and termination phases.

The thread of collaboration runs through both models. Clients are active participants with nurses in developing and maintaining the relationship. This shared responsibility, power, and decision-making ensures better health care.

REFERENCES

1. King I. *Toward a Theory for Nursing*. New York: Wiley; 1971: 98.
2. Cain A. A study of pets in the family system. In: Katcher A, Beck A, eds. *New Perspectives on Our Lives With Companion Animals*. Philadelphia: University of Pennsylvania Press; 1983.
3. Terkel S. *Working*. New York: Pantheon; 1974.
4. Travelbee J. *Interpersonal Aspects of Nursing*. 2nd ed. Philadelphia; Davis; 1971.
5. Sundeen S., Stuart G., Rankin E, Cohen S. *Nurse–Client Interaction Implementing the Nursing Process*. 4th ed. St. Louis: Mosby; 1989.
6. Rogers C. *On Becoming a Person*. Boston: Houghton-Mifflin; 1961.
7. Gazda GM, Asbury FR, Balzer FJ, et al. *Human Relations Development*. 4th ed. Boston: Allyn & Bacon; 1984.
8. Tripp-Reimer T, Brink P, Saunders L. Cultural assessment: Content and process. *Nurs Outlook*. 1984; 23:78–82.
9. Simon S. *Values Clarification: A Handbook of Practical Strategies for Teachers and Students*. Hart, NY: Leland Howe & Howard Kirschenbaum; 1972.
10. Wilberding JZ. Values clarification. In: Bulechek GM, McCloskey JC, eds. *Nursing Interventions: Treatments for Nursing Diagnoses*. Philadelphia: Saunders; 1985: 173–184.
11. Williamson JA. Mutual interaction: A model of nursing practice. *Nurs Outlook*. 1981; 29:2.
12. Carkhuff RR. *Helping and Human Relations: A Primer for Lay and Professional Helpers*. Vol 2, *Practice and Research*. New York: Holt, Rinehart & Winston; 1969.
13. Berenson BG, Carkhuff RR. *Sources of Gain in Counseling and Psychotherapy: Readings and Commentary*. New York: Holt, Rinehart & Winston; 1967.
14. Truax CB, Carkhuff RR. *Toward Effective Counseling and Psychotherapy: Training and Practice*. New York: Holt, Rinehart & Winston; 1967.
15. Norton BA, Miller AM. *Skills for Professional Nursing Practice*. Norwalk, CT: Appleton-Century-Crofts; 1986.
16. Tomlinson A. The use of experiential methods in teaching interpersonal skills to nurses. In: Kagan CM, ed. *Interpersonal Skills in Nursing*. Dover, NH: Croom Helm; 1985.
17. Wilson HS, Kneisel CR. *Psychiatric Nursing*. 3rd ed. Menlo Park, CA: Addison-Wesley; 1988.
18. Stuart G., Sundeen S. *Principles and Practice of Psychiatric Nursing*. 4th ed. St. Louis: Mosby; 1990.
19. Thomas M. Trust in the nurse–patient relationship. In: Carlsen C, ed. *Behavioral Concepts in Nursing Intervention*. Philadelphia: Lippincott; 1970.
20. Fromm E. *The Art of Loving*. New York: Harper & Row; 1956.
21. Shillinger FL. Locus of control: implications for clinical nursing practice. *Image*. 1983; 25:58–63.
22. Lewis FM. Experienced personal control and quality of life in late-stage cancer patients. *Nurs Res*. 1982; 31:113.
23. Podrasky DL, Sexton DL. Nurses' reactions to difficult patients. *Image*. 1988; 20:16–21.
24. Tedesco-Carreras P. Communicating with difficult patients. *Imprint*. 1986; 33:36–38.

25. Kasch CR. Toward a theory of nursing action: Skills and competency in nurse–patient interaction. *Nurs Res.* 1986; 35:226–230.

BIBLIOGRAPHY

Arnold E, Boggs K. *Interpersonal Relationships: Professional Communication Skills for Nurses.* Philadelphia: Saunders; 1989

Benner P, Wrubel J. Caring comes first. *Am J Nurs.* 1988; 88:1072–1075.

Benner P, Wrubel J. *The Primacy of Caring.* Menlo Park: Addison-Wesley; 1989.

Cannon M. To Sharon with love. *Am J Nurse.* 1979; 79:692.

Carlson E. *Behavioral Concepts in Nursing Intervention.* Philadelphia: Lippincott; 1976.

Clay M. Development of an empathetic interaction skills schedule in a nursing context. *J Adv Nurs.* 1984; 9:343.

Cooper M. Convenantal relationships: Grounding for the nursing ethic. *Adv Nurs Sci.* 1988; 10:48–59.

Gadza G, Asbury FS, Balzer FJ, et al. *Human Relations Development.* Boston: Allyn & Bacon; 1984.

Gordon S. *Prisoners of Men's Dreams: Striking Out for a New Feminine Future.* Boston: Little, Brown & Co, 1991.

Hofling K, Leninger M, Bregg E. *Basic Psychiatric Concepts in Nursing.* Philadelphia: Lippincott; 1976.

Larson D. Helper secrets. *J Psychosoc Nurs.* 1987; 25:20–27.

Travelbee J. *Interpersonal Aspects of Nursing.* Philadelphia: Davis; 1971.

Watson J. Nursing of the caring edge: Metaphoricae vignettes. *Adv Nurs Sci.* 1987; 10:10–18.

CHAPTER 14

Communication As a Collaborative Process

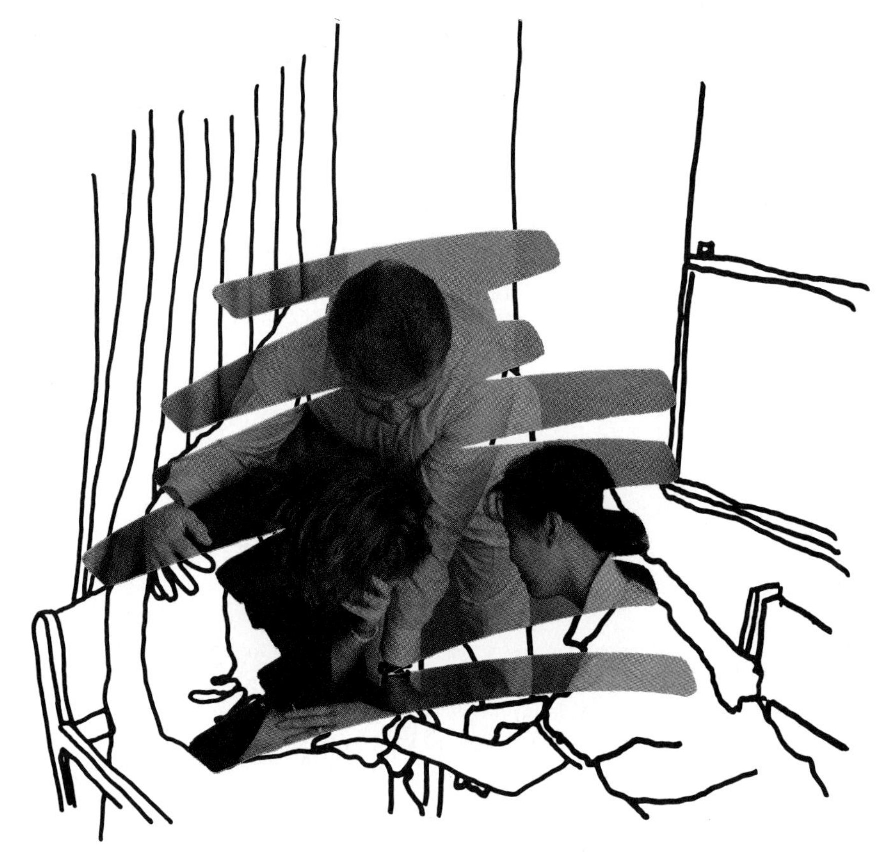

BEHAVIORAL OBJECTIVES

Upon completion of this chapter, the student will be able to:

1. Define communication.
2. Identify five components of the communication process.
3. Discuss three processes necessary for the sharing of information.
4. Describe three major modes of communication.
5. State five goals of communication in nursing.
6. Explain the role of listening in the process of communication.
7. Identify and explain at least four approaches that support and six approaches that hinder collaborative communication.
8. Demonstrate empathy, warmth, respect, genuineness, concreteness, confrontation, and immediacy in actual or simulated nurse–client relationships.
9. Discuss variations in communication techniques that can be used with special populations such as the elderly, children, and clients of different cultural backgrounds.
10. Identify two types of interviews and describe situations in which each type would be most appropriate and effective.
11. Describe at least five approaches or guidelines for effective interviewing.
12. Describe the relationship of communication to the collaborative process.

KEY TERMS

assertive communication
attending behavior
body language
communication
connotative meaning
context
denotative meaning
direct question
empowering response
evaluation
feedback
incongruent communication
intergroup communication
internal feedback
interpersonal communication
interview
intimate distance
intrapersonal communication
language
message
metacommunication
nonverbal communication
open-ended question
perception
personal distance
person-to-group communication
receiver
response time
sender
social distance
transmission
verbal communication

Communication occurs whenever people interact. In fact, it is impossible *not* to communicate. Even when we say nothing we can communicate a myriad of ideas, feelings, and expressions through a glance, a touch, or even our posture. Communication is essential to all aspects of our lives and permeates all phases of the collaborative nurse–client relationship. In Chapter 13, establishing the relationship was identified as the first step in the collaborative process. Communication is the tool for establishing and maintaining the relationship.

Most of us probably believe that we communicate well, and yet everyone has been frustrated on occasion at not being really "heard" or at not being able to really "hear" another. Sometimes there is too much talking and very little communication occurring. This is a painful situation commonly encountered by clients trying to make wants and feelings known to the health care system. Nurses need to know how to communicate to build successful collaborative nurse–client relationships, what occurs when communication is ineffective, and what to do to communicate therapeutically.

Communication is a complex process that involves more than just talking, although talking is a vital part of communication. For important communication to occur, the listener must show the speaker that the listener has correctly interpreted what the speaker has said. If the listener has not heard or interpreted the message correctly, then the speaker can move to clarify the message and thus keep channels of communication open. In the Watergate era, President Nixon's advisors coined a phrase "communication gap" to describe the problems the government experienced sending messages that could be easily and correctly interpreted. That same phrase is often used to describe miscommunications that can occur between spouses, parents and children, teachers and students, and nurses and clients. The results of such miscommunication can range from the absurd to tragic. An example from Virginia Satir's book *Peoplemaking*[1] in which she describes a husband and wife that she is seeing in therapy illustrates this point.

> In the course of the sessions the husband reveals that one of his pet peeves is the fact that his wife serves spinach, a vegetable which he hates, several times a week. The wife is shocked by her husband's revelation as she reveals that she *also* hates spinach. She serves it because years earlier when they were first married she overheard her husband extol the virtues of spinach to a young nephew. The wife assumed that her husband loved spinach and began to include it as a regular part of their meals. The wife had never validated her assumption with her spouse and he in turn had never communicated his feelings about eating spinach.

Nurses need to be aware of how the gaps in communication occur, what can be done to prevent them, and how to recover the relationship when miscommunications occur. This chapter addresses the interrelationship between communication and collaboration. Definitions of communication are given, and goals of communication in nursing, levels of communication, how the components of the communication process interact, and factors that facilitate and hinder collaborative communication are addressed. Application of the facilitative, transition, and action dimensions of Gazda's human relations model (described in Chap. 13), and the nurse's role in interviewing, are discussed to emphasize the critical role of effective communication in collaboration.

■ DEFINITIONS OF COMMUNICATION

Communication has been defined by many theorists in a variety of ways. The definitions of Lewis, Travelbee, and Ruesch and Bateson synthesize the importance and purposes of communication.

Garland Lewis[2] defines communication as "all the processes by which people influence each other" (p. 2). Lewis portrays interpersonal communication as a dynamic process in which there is an attempt "to understand the other person's point of view, from his frame of reference which includes his feelings about the situation" (p. 70).

Joyce Travelbee[3] sees communication as a "process of sharing or transmitting thoughts and feelings. . . . It is a dynamic force capable of profoundly influencing and affecting the degree of interpersonal closeness" (p. 68).

Ruesch and Bateson[4] define communication as "all of the procedures by which one mind may affect another's" (p. 6). These broad definitions encompass not only written and oral speech but also music, the pictorial and performing arts, and in fact all human behaviors.

■ IMPORTANCE OF COMMUNICATION

From the preceding definitions it is clear that communication is essential to all human endeavors. Without the ability to communicate individuals are very much alone. Since communication is so inextricably woven into the pattern of our lives, it is difficult to imagine life without communication. To appreciate the significance of communication it is helpful to reflect on situations in which communication is limited. Think of being alone in a foreign country without the necessary language skills; how frightening and frustrating to be unable to communicate basic needs. Or, imagine being in a coma and having no way to understand or ask about what was being done for you or to you. Reflect on the frustration experienced by very young children as they try to communicate wants and needs with inadequate language skills.

Communication allows individuals to understand and to be understood by other persons. It is the basis for all social relationships. An individual's first experiences with communication occur within the social relationship between self and parent.[5] It is in this relationship that the individual learns through verbal and nonverbal communication how the world (typified by the parent) will respond to needs for love, comfort, and security. If these first experiences with communication are positive ones, a foundation for a sense of self-value and belonging is developed that influences all subsequent communications.

IMPLICATIONS FOR NURSE–CLIENT COLLABORATION

Definition of Communication

Communication in professional relationships is a collaborative function. Communication refers to an exchange of messages, while collaboration involves communication that is directed toward identifying common goals and plans. The essence of both is mutuality (sharing)—exchanges of ideas, opinions, values, feelings, and energy—between nurse and client as they jointly participate in making health care decisions.

■ THE PROCESS OF COMMUNICATION

Components of Communication

In order to examine the process of communication it is necessary to interrupt the process—thus artificially giving it a beginning and an ending. By punctuating communication in this manner, what is really a complex and ongoing process appears to be much simpler than it really is. For the purpose of study, an interaction may be isolated from the total communication, as the following interaction illustrates:

A. Nurse: Do you mean that you were awake the entire night?

B. Client: No . . . it just seemed that way. The last time I looked at the clock it was about two A.M. I probably dozed off after that, but I just couldn't stop thinking.

A. Nurse: What were you thinking about?

In this interaction, *A* sends a message to *B:* "Do you mean that you were awake the entire night?" *B* receives the

BUILDING NURSING KNOWLEDGE

How Important Is Communication in Nursing?

Sarvimaki A. Nursing care as a moral, practical, communicative and creative activity. *J Adv Nurs.* 1988; 13:462–467.

Sarvimaki holds that nursing is "communicative interaction," an idea clearly allied to the collaborative view set out in this text. The author develops the idea that the very foundation of nursing lies in its value of reaching understanding between nurse and client. Communicative interaction is distinguished by the fact that participants have no preconceived ideas of how the other should act. This, according to the author, contrasts with "success-oriented action" in which one person tries to influence or control the other. Communicative interaction is not oriented towards success, but towards reaching understanding.

In Sarvimaki's view, not all verbal acts represent communication, particularly when they are intended to control another's behavior. Communication involves a special "communicative attitude," which manifests itself in striving for mutual understanding, coordination, and co-action rather than striving to control.

The view of nursing as communicative interaction emphasizes that the client's mind, interpretation, and experience of the situation play an active part in the process of caregiving. Changes in the client's health are looked upon not as the results of nurse's actions, but of the client's own activity and of the client's experiences in the interaction with caregivers. Nursing is thus creative co-action. Nurses cannot confer health and well-being but can assist others to these states. The nurses and client join efforts, wills, capacities, knowledge, and understanding to reach a common goal: the best possible health for the client.

message and returns a message to *A*: "No . . . it just seemed that way." *A* receives this message and sends another: "What were you thinking about?" This provides a simple way to analyze the interaction. However, analysis increases in complexity when *A* is viewed not only as sending a message to *B* ("Do you mean that you were awake the entire night?") but also of simultaneously receiving nonverbal messages *from B*. *B* may be looking downcast, fidgeting with the bed covers, or staring out the window, for example. While receiving a verbal message from *A*, *B* is also sending nonverbal messages and receiving *A*'s nonverbal messages. So, simply to identify *A* as the sender and *B* as the receiver, when both are simultaneously sending and receiving messages, is artificial, but useful for learning purposes. In reality, the process is a much more dynamic and complex one than the study model indicates.[6]

For the purpose of study it is appropriate to identify five functional components of the communication process in an interaction. Figure 14–1 depicts the interaction of the components.

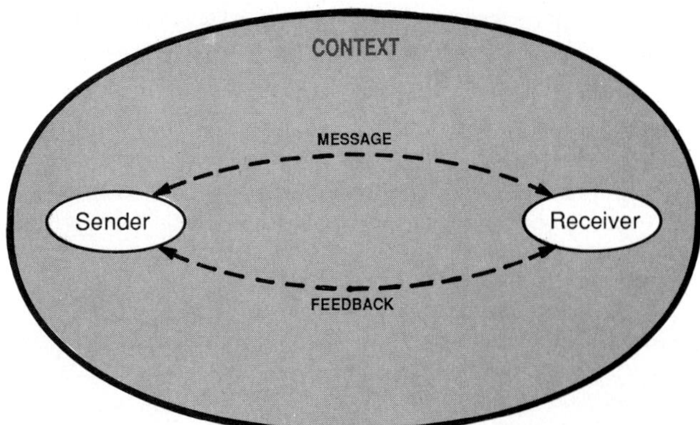

Figure 14–1. Components of the communication process.

Context. The first component is that of the **context,** which refers to the setting and circumstances in which the interaction occurs. This important factor in each interaction includes not only the physical setting but also the dimension of time and the individual qualities of each participant within the interaction.[6] What happens in the here and now is unique and can never duplicate what is past or be duplicated in the future.

Sender. The **sender** is the second component of the communication process, and refers to the individual who is sending the message. All the anatomical structures and physiological processes necessary for thinking and speech, and the body parts involved in the communication of nonverbal messages, are part of the sender.

Message. The **message** is the third component. It includes verbal and nonverbal behaviors and the total impact conveyed by these behaviors. The words used, the tone of voice, and the body language are all parts of the message that is sent. These concepts are detailed in Modes of Communication later in the chapter.

Receiver. The fourth component, the **receiver,** refers to the person who receives the message and includes all the senses that are used in this process.

Feedback. The fifth component is **feedback,** which refers to the message that the receiver returns to the sender in response to the sender's message. In the earlier example, *B* qualifies the connotative meaning of the word "entire" by saying: "No . . . it just seemed that way." However, while *B* is sending *A* feedback, *A* in turn is sending feedback to *B*. *A* may be nodding her head in agreement, indicating understanding of *B*'s qualifying statement; or *A* could have a furrowed brow, indicating the need for additional information. In addition to the feedback *A* and *B* provide each other, they each also receive internal feedback.

Internal feedback implies more than just the sense of hearing. It also includes the physiological messages that the

IMPLICATIONS FOR NURSE–CLIENT COLLABORATION

Feedback

Feedback is a very important tool available to the nurse who wishes to initiate and maintain a collaborative relationship with a client. Giving feedback enables the nurse to share a developing understanding of the client's needs, to clarify meanings, and to request confirmation from clients about the accuracy of the nurse's understanding. Receiving feedback provides nurses with essential information about the client's experience that can be useful in planning and evaluating client care. Feedback is important in nurse–client communication because collaboration depends on shared meanings; feedback is the mechanism for establishing shared meanings.

body sends to itself. These messages, which arise within both the sender and the receiver, include things such as fatigue, hunger, restlessness, anxiety, and boredom. Such internal feedback can greatly affect how an interaction is interpreted. For instance, if during the interaction between *A* and *B*, *A*'s stomach begins to rumble and growl, *A* may feel embarrassed. In embarrassment *A* no longer focuses attention on *B*, but is distracted. *B* may then interpret *A*'s behavior to mean that *A* is not really concerned about *B*.

Subprocesses in Communication

In addition to considering the components of the communication process it is also important to examine how information is shared. Ruesch[7] identifies three processes that are necessary for the sharing of information. They can be considered subprocesses within the overall communication process. These subprocesses include perception, evaluation, and transmission.[8]

Perception. Gazda and co-workers define **perception** as "the process whereby one person discerns both the overt and covert, or disguised, behavior of another" (p. 24). In order to be an effective communicator and helper, nurses must develop skills for interpreting the behavior of others. The ability to do this is affected by the needs, values, past experiences, expectations, and prejudices operating in a nurse as well as in a client. Clients whose past experiences with health care professionals have been negative, may perceive a nurse's offer to talk with them as useless or insincere. Moment to moment, perceptions are affected by past experiences. Clients may be blocking a meaningful interaction with a caring nurse because of misperceived messages. Most interpersonal difficulties result from faulty perceptions.

If information is to be accurately exchanged between a sender and a receiver, the receiver must perceive the message as the sender intended. This is no easy task. Nurses can facilitate the communication process by sharing perceptions, asking clients for feedback concerning their perceptions, comparing perceptions, and arriving at a mutual understanding, as the following example shows.

Nurse Jones: When Dr. Clinton left your room today, I noticed you seemed concerned. Your face looked so serious. I wondered what was troubling you.

Mrs. Mannel: Did I look worried? I had a lot on my mind, but actually Dr. Clinton gave me good news. He said the tests came back negative, and I could go home tomorrow. I don't know why I should look worried—although I am very tired. The hospital routine doesn't allow for much rest.

Nurse Jones: Perhaps I misinterpreted what I saw. Maybe we could arrange for some uninterrupted rest time for you this afternoon—and if you are going home tomorrow, there is no reason to wake you up at night to take your vital signs. I'll let the other staff know.

Evaluation. The second process identified by Ruesch,[7] **evaluation,** involves the ability to analyze the message that has been sent. The process of evaluation allows the individuals to interpret the message that is received. Evaluation involves many of the same factors that influence perception. An individual may evaluate a situation differently depending on the prevailing circumstances. The change in circumstances can be either internal, such as a shift in mood, or external. For example, a nurse may be able to respond to the demands of clients more effectively when well rested than when tired. Lack of sleep may lead to interpreting a client's demands as a personal burden. When rested, looking beyond the demand to determine the meaning of clients' behavior is possible.

Transmission. The third process needed for the sharing of information is the **transmission** or the actual expression of the message from the sender to receiver. Transmission depends on an adequate channel sending the message. For instance, if the sender has a speech impediment, this would certainly affect the clarity of a message. If a nurse chooses to transmit a message to a client through an intercom system that is functioning poorly, the client may have difficulty evaluating the message because of other noise that is transmitted. When the primary language of the sender and receiver differs, transmission of clear messages is a challenge.

LEVELS OF COMMUNICATION

Communication occurs on several levels: intrapersonal, interpersonal, person to group, and intergroup.

Intrapersonal Communication

The intrapersonal level was discussed in Chapter 13, as it concerns the relationship an individual has with self. **Intrapersonal communication** is the way in which persons converse with themselves and gives an indication of the level of self-esteem and self-worth felt by an individual.[9] Some individuals engage in very negative self-talk that reflects a low self-esteem and low self-worth. They tend to ruminate on their failures and repeatedly tell themselves that they can't do something and that they are not worthy. Sometimes students similarly allow a low test grade or an instructor's critical comment to affect self-esteem and motivation unduly. Negative self-talk is destructive behavior to whoever engages in it. Nurses need to develop a positive relationship to self and need to orient their thoughts and internal dialogue realistically. If they find that their thoughts are consistently of a negative, self-deprecating nature, then they need to take stock of what is occurring in their lives to cause this. The consequence of such negative internal dialogue is very powerful. Nurses can inadvertently communicate lack of confidence to clients, which in turn undermines clients' hope and strength. Nurses need to develop a self-accepting, open, and honest communication pattern with self to be able to be aware of successes as well as failures and to learn from both.

Interpersonal Communication

The second level on which communication occurs is the interpersonal. **Interpersonal communication** refers to communication with another person. Most of the remainder of the chapter will focus on this level of communication.

Person-to-Group Communication

The third level is **person-to-group communication.** Nurses are frequently involved in teaching classes to other professionals or to the public. For instance, CPR (cardiopulmonary resuscitation) certification classes are frequently conducted by nurses; much of prepared childbirth education is provided by nurses; nurses present scholarly papers at large professional gatherings; and frequently, nurses conduct small group sessions for educational or counseling purposes.

Intergroup Communication

Communication that occurs at the cultural or societal level, or group to group, is termed **intergroup communication.** An example of this is the lobbying action of the American Nurses' Association to persuade Congress to increase support for nursing education.

Another example of intergroup communication is the legislative lobbying efforts of nurse practitioner groups to receive third-party reimbursement for services provided to clients.

■ MODES OF COMMUNICATION

Various modes of communication are available to the nurse. Several may be employed at the same time. Effectiveness is enhanced when the nurse is skilled in more than one mode and can suit the mode to the situation. The two major modes of communication are verbal and nonverbal communication; however, these major modes comprise several modes (or channels) within them. Metacommunication (discussed later in this chapter) is also considered a communication mode.

Verbal Communication

Verbal communication primarily involves the physiological and cognitive mechanisms necessary for speech production and reception. Although the verbal mode is most commonly associated with the term "communication," the spoken word represents only a small segment of total communication.

Verbal communication involves the use of word symbols that are organized into a formal structured system to convey thoughts and feelings. This structured system is called **language.** Even the most primitive human cultures have developed a language system. Susan Langer,[10] a philosopher, has said that without language there can be no articulate conceptual thinking. Our language is the tool by which our thoughts can be organized into meaningful symbols.

Hayakawa[11] states that "cooperation through the use of language is the fundamental mechanism of human survival" (p. 22). Language can be used in such a way as to create peace and harmony or to create arguments and conflict. Because of the power inherent in the use of language, nurses need to be aware of how they use language to communicate.

Because language is comprised of word symbols, and symbols can have different meanings determined by culture, experience, age, sex, and other variables, it is important to examine the meaning of words. Words can have both a denotative or a connotative meaning.

Denotative meaning refers to the relationship that exists between an object in the physical world and the word that stands for that object. For instance, the denotative meaning of the word "tree" could be "a woody perennial plant having a single main axis or stem (trunk) commonly exceeding 10 feet in height" (*Webster's New World Dictionary*). Although most people probably have a similar thought picture for the word "tree," the **connotative meaning,** or the personalized meaning, might be quite different. For instance, to one person the word "tree" might conjure up an image of the old oak tree where she had a tree house as a child. To another individual the word "tree" might bring a memory of the tree that fell into the house during a lightning storm. The connotative meaning varies with past experiences, present frame of reference, and other variables.[6]

Frequently in verbal exchanges, the participants assume, often erroneously, that words have the same meaning for all people. Because words are only symbols, they can never create exactly the same meaning to all people. The meaning of words becomes even less distinct with words that are more abstract. Ask 10 people for definitions of abstractions such as justice, love, freedom, and pain, and the result will be at least 10 different definitions for each word.[6]

Nurses need to be aware that their words can be interpreted far differently than intended, and that one's interpretation of meaning may be influenced by many factors including educational level and life experiences. Keeping this in mind, nurses need to make sure that communication is as clear as possible and is appropriate to a client's level of understanding. For instance, in explaining perineal care to a 14-year-old postpartum mother, the nurse may need to use other terms besides "labia" and "perineal care" to describe the procedure. This might not be necessary for someone more mature or more widely read. The key is to match words and explanations to the level of clients' understanding.

Nurses first need to establish that they really understand clients' use of words. Nurses are unable to assess accurately or problem-solve without a base of knowledge provided by communication. Therefore, any ambiguities need to be clarified as they occur so that nurses have a clear sense of what clients are communicating.

Nonverbal Communication

The second mode of communication is nonverbal. **Nonverbal communication** includes all forms of communication that do not involve words. Probably 60 to 70 percent of all communication occurs through this mode. Nonverbal behavior can be fascinating but sometimes frustrating because the process of interpreting the meaning of nonverbal cues lacks precision. Frequent validation of nurses' interpretation of nonverbal communication is therefore essential. Perceptive nurses will be aware of nonverbal behavior or cues to assess threads in communication, intensity of feelings, conflicts, and motives. Frequently these are communicated nonverbally even if clients do not express them in words.[8]

Categories of Nonverbal Communication. Ruesch and Keys[12] describe three categories of nonverbal communication: sign, action, and object.

Sign nonverbal communication involves all gestures from the simple raised thumb of the hitchhiker to the complex system of sign language used by the deaf. Sign nonverbal communication is perceived primarily through the sense of sight.

Action nonverbal communication involves all body movements that are not specific signals. This would include for example running, dancing, and exercising. Action nonverbal communication is perceived through sight, hearing, and touch.

Object nonverbal communication includes the use of material things. The way people decorate their homes, or the kind of clothes they wear, gives nonverbal messages to others. All the senses are involved in perceiving object nonverbal communication.

Characteristics of Nonverbal Communication. Gazda and co-workers[8] analyze nonverbal communication using a number of general characteristics.

Multiple Channels. The first characteristic is that nonverbal communication can be transmitted and received through multiple channels, including response time, body, voice, and environment.

Response Time. **Response time** refers to the promptness with which a speaker's presence or words are acknowledged. For example, say that a family member approaches the nurse's station for a status report about a loved one. The family member stands for 5 minutes before any nurse in the nurse's station looks up or greets the person. Through interpretation of response time, the family member probably receives a negative nonverbal message about the courtesy and concern of the nurses.

Body. Another channel for the communication of nonverbal behaviors is the body. In fact, the body is so communicative that it is said to convey **body language.** Body language is conveyed through physical appearance, posture and gait, facial expression and eye contact, hand gestures, and touch (Fig. 14–2).

- *Physical appearance.* One of our first impressions of a person is his or her physical appearance. The way the person dresses, grooming, and choice of accessories are clues to

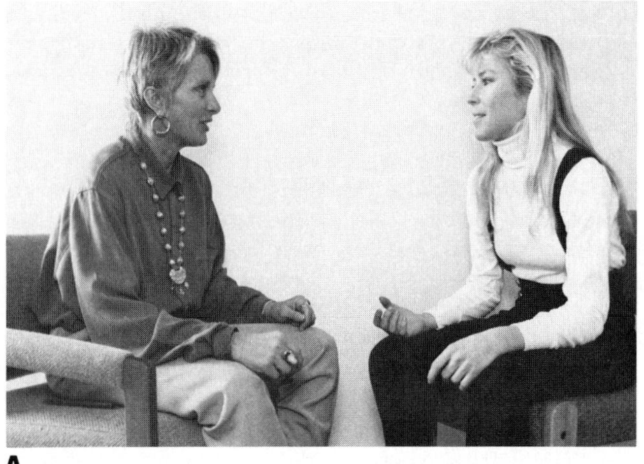

A

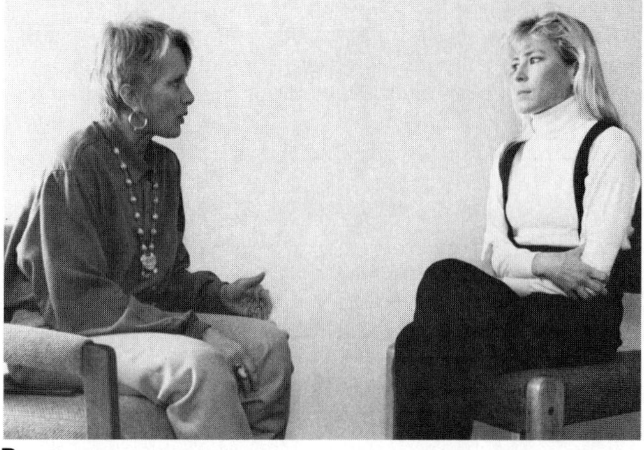

B

Figure 14–2. Nonverbal communication sometimes conveys meaning more effectively than words. **A.** The posture of these people indicates openness to communication. **B.** The listener's posture suggests resistance to communication.

social status, physical well-being, marital status, occupation, culture, self-esteem, and even religion.

- *Posture and gait.* The way people stand and move reflects emotions, physical well-being, and self-concept. Stooped shoulders and a slow gait may indicate a sense of despair or physical discomfort, whereas a straight posture with a quick purposeful gait communicates a sense of well-being.
- *Facial expression and eye contact.* Facial expression is probably the richest expression of body language and the most difficult to interpret. The face may reveal genuine emotions or contradict actual feelings. Frequently, individuals are unaware of their facial expressions and the messages being communicated via their faces. Eye contact is an important aspect of facial expression. Making eye contact with another often signals the desire to communicate. Averting the eyes may communicate discomfort and signal a desire to end the interaction. Generally, maintaining eye contact is beneficial to the conduct of an interaction. Also, the level at which eye contact occurs is significant. A nurse who looks down on the client may appear controlling. Sitting across from a client at the same eye level communicates equality and respect.
- *Hand gestures.* Gestures may be used to emphasize, punctuate, or clarify the verbal message. Sometimes the gesture combined with other nonverbal behaviors takes the place of the verbal message. For instance, when a police officer gestures to a motorist to pull over, there is usually little doubt about the police officer's message. Similarly, when a client grimaces and clutches his chest with his hand, the nurse is probably correct to interpret this message to mean the client is in pain.
- *Touch.* Much of nursing involves touch, which is a powerful tool for communicating caring, concern, and competence (Fig. 14–3).

Nurse Johnson enters Mrs. Hoya's room and pulls the curtain around the bed. The nurse pulls up a chair next to the bed and, smiling at Mrs. Hoya and putting her hand on Mrs. Hoya's arm, says, "I promised I'd come back."

By touching Mrs. Hoya's arm and making eye contact, Nurse Johnson communicates the message, "Why don't we have that talk that got interrupted this morning:" However, touch can also have other meanings determined by social and cultural conventions, and therefore must be used purposefully and with discrimination. Some clients feel that touch violates their privacy, others only interpret touch as a sexual expression. Nurses must be sensitive to a client's reaction to being touched. If a client pulls away from a nurse's touch, it may be that the client is uncomfortable with being touched and this should be respected. In addition, nurses should explain when touching is an essential aspect of an intervention.

Voice. Nonverbal communication also occurs through the channel of the voice. The tone of voice, rate of speech, loudness of voice, and diction all convey messages about the speaker.

Mrs. Miller: Did the doctor tell you the results of my liver biopsy yet?

Nurse Robert: Well (pause) no (longer pause), but I'm sure he will be in later to talk to you. Let's get on with your treatment (at faster speed).

The use of pauses and a change in the rate of speech may give a variety of negative nonverbal messages including the message that the speaker is being less than truthful with the listener.

Environment. The environment can also be a channel for nonverbal communication. The distance one stands from another sends out many messages. In normal social interactions people consciously maintain a distance between themselves. Hall[13] describes **intimate distance** as 18 inches

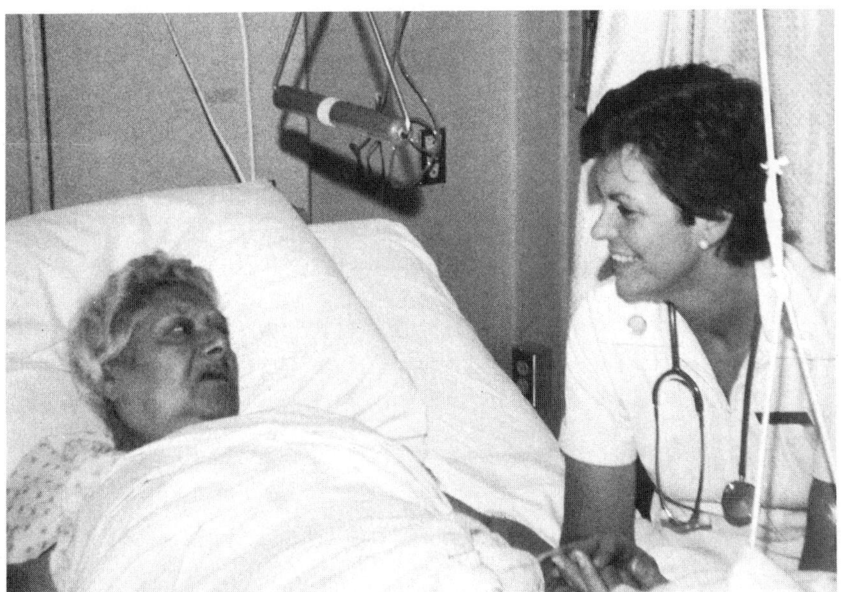

Figure 14–3. Nonverbal communication and touch can be effective in establishing a nurse–client relationship. (*Source: Hames CC, Joseph DH.* Basic Concepts of Helping: A Holistic Approach. *2nd ed. Norwalk, CT: Appleton-Century-Crofts; 1986; 93. Photo by Dayle Joseph.*)

or less, **personal distance** as 18 inches to 4 feet, and **social distance** as 4 to 12 feet (Fig. 4–4).

Nurses need to be aware that many of the physical ministrations that they provide are an invasion of clients' intimate space. Such an invasion may cause clients a certain degree of discomfort. Both nurses and clients usually feel more at ease when nursing measures are conducted within the personal space. This provides a level of closeness needed in a helping relationship but does not impose a level of intimacy. The social distance is appropriate for nurses working with groups. At this distance, a nurse is present but without physical contact. Communication is usually less threatening because personal sharing of feelings and thoughts is usually not required.

Arrangement of furniture and personal belongings is another way the environment can be a channel for nonverbal messages.

> Mr. Johnson, an 82-year-old client admitted for congestive heart failure, is very particular about how his personal belongings are placed at the bedside. He insists that his eyeglasses be placed in the upper drawer of the nightstand. His toiletries must be kept right alongside of his glasses. On his bedside stand is a clock and a stack of newspapers. Any attempt to rearrange his belongings results in an outburst of anger.

In this example, Mr. Johnson is sending nonverbal messages through his arrangement of personal effects in the environment. Some nurses may interpret his behavior to mean that he has a rigid personality. Others realize his nonverbal behavior is a way of ordering his environment and maintaining some semblance of control over what happens to him.

Multiple Functions. The second general characteristic of nonverbal communication is that it can serve various purposes. For instance, it can make a complete statement, as when a coach uses signals to convey a message to athletes. Sometimes it can be used to accentuate verbal behavior, as when a child stamps his feet while yelling "No!" At other times nonverbal communication can be used to illustrate verbal behavior, as when a fisherman gestures to describe the size of his catch. Sometimes individuals use nonverbal communication to regulate an interaction. For example, a nurse glancing at his or her wristwatch sends a clear message that it is time for the interaction to end.

Unconscious. Although at times nonverbal behavior is consciously chosen for purposes such as these, more commonly this behavior is unconscious. This is true of habitual gestures, which may not convey significant meaning, and of nonverbal communication related to underlying emotions. Unconscious behavior is the third general characteristic of nonverbal behavior.

Emotional Expression. A fourth characteristic is that it is a means of expressing emotion. Nonverbal channels are the primary means by which a person communicates feelings. Body language and voice tones that accompany verbalizations frequently give emphasis or expand the meaning of the words selected. In some cases, individuals' bodies convey emotions before they have become aware of the feelings or feel comfortable talking about them. For example, a student in a sex education class may blush and fidget in her seat during an explanation of fertilization of an ovum. Later, she requests your assistance because she fears she is pregnant.

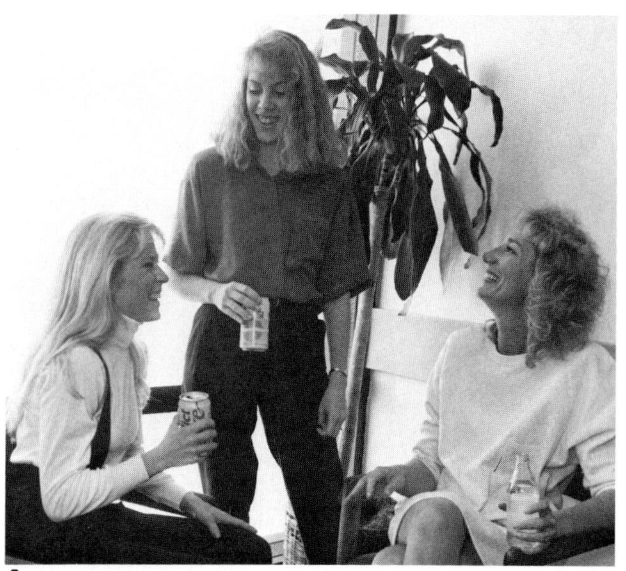

A

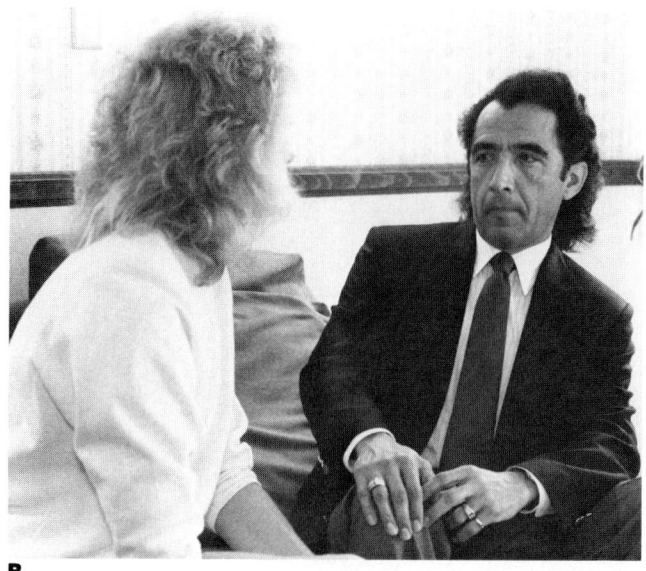

B

Figure 14–4. Personal space influences communication in social and professional interactions. **A.** Each of the individuals in this group of friends is comfortable interacting within each other's personal space. **B.** Encroachment into another individual's personal space creates tension.

IMPLICATIONS FOR NURSE–CLIENT COLLABORATION

Nonverbal Communication

Because nonverbal communication is often unconscious, it provides nurses with a valuable source of messages about a client's personal experience; it can substantially enhance the understanding nurses derive from clients' verbalizations. Observations of expressive behaviors such as body language, facial expressions, and even patterns of movement communicate much about clients' needs and values. Sometimes nonverbal messages portray clients' feelings more accurately than verbal accounts. Sensitivity to clients' nonverbal communication can thus increase nurses' understanding of clients and facilitate their collaboration on health care decisions.

Genuineness. The fact that nonverbal behavior is often unconscious and associated with emotion causes many communication experts to believe that this behavior is more genuine than words, which are more subject to conscious control. In situations in which the verbal and nonverbal messages are incongruent—that is, conveying different or even contradictory meanings—it is likely that the nonverbal is the more accurate indicator of the speaker's true feelings. For example, if a client says "everything is fine," but his lips are pinched tightly together and his hands firmly clasped, a nurse would be correct in inferring that the verbal message is not completely accurate.

Multiple Meanings. A sixth general characteristic of nonverbal communication is that a given behavior can have multiple meanings. For example, silence may be one person's characteristic way of expressing anger, whereas this behavior from another individual may have another meaning such as indifference or embarrassment. Some persons cry easily, even when the precipitating event does not have great significance to them, whereas for others tears are a rare occurrence and suggest intense feeling. There is even variability in the meaning of a given nonverbal message displayed by one individual under different circumstances. A person may frown when displeased, but show a similar facial expression when concentrating deeply. An observer must take in the entire context in which the behavior is occurring before making specific inferences about its meaning.

Cultural Variability. Finally, nonverbal behavior varies culturally. In Italy, kissing is a common greeting, even among friends of the same sex. In the United States, that behavior is not generally accepted. Individuals of Hispanic heritage often show respect by casting their eyes downward, a gesture many Anglos would interpret as deceitful. Applying one's own cultural norms when interpreting nonverbal communication displayed by persons from another culture can result in errors.

Despite the complexity of nonverbal communication and the pitfalls associated with casual interpretation of nonverbal messages, certain characteristic meanings of common nonverbal behaviors can be recognized. Table 14–1 identifies nonverbal behaviors frequently associated with four emotional states. The helper is cautioned, however, to interpret nonverbal behavior carefully and to consider the context of the entire interaction when ascribing meaning to nonverbal behavior.

Metacommunication

Virginia Satir[14] uses the term **metacommunication** to describe the total impact of the verbal and nonverbal mes-

TABLE 14–1. NONVERBAL BEHAVIORS FREQUENTLY ASSOCIATED WITH FOUR EMOTIONAL STATES

	Depression	Anxiety	Anger	Low Self-worth
Head	Down	Stiff movement; chin down	Forward or tilted upward	Downward
Face	Frown	Flushed; pale	Angry frown (eyebrows down at center)	Half-smiles; quickly follows your expressions
Mouth	Down-turned; tightness	Tightness; clenching teeth	Lips tensed; pushed forward	Quivering; halting speech
Eye contact	Little or none	Darting glances; vigilant	Excessive; defiant	Low; peeking
Hands	Rubbing; clutching	Tightness; gripping; sweaty palms	Clenching; fist thumping (symbolic hitting)	Restless
Posture	Hunches while sitting	Frequent movement; crouching; hunches shoulders	Edge of chair	Way back as if to be invisible, or on edge as if to run; protective
Position	Moves away	Angled away; protective		
Distance	More than usual	Moderately away	Moves into others' space	More than usual or, if they trust you, extra close
Energy	Low	May be high	High	Low
General	Lack of interest in people or activities	Jerky movements; tics; guards "territory"	Acting out, such as slamming door, jerking or shoving objects, extra noisy	Watching for signs of approval or disapproval from others

Source: Gazda GM. Group Counseling: A Developmental Approach. *2nd ed. Boston: Allyn & Bacon; 1978.*

sages individuals send. She calls metacommunication "a message about a message" (p. 76). It can be considered to be a clarification of the literal (verbal) message as well as a reflection on the nature of the relationship between the individuals communicating. Nonverbal metacommunication occurs in any of the channels described above. Verbal metacommunication can be an attempt to explain message-sending. For example, a person may label a message, saying "It was just a joke," or explain why the message was sent: "I thought you were down—I wanted to cheer you up a little" or "I was trying to get you to offer to help me."

Because metacommunication can involve quite an assortment of messages, interpretation can be challenging. This is especially true if literal communication and metacommunication do not jibe. This lack of agreement is called a double message or **incongruent communication.** Selecting an appropriate response when one has received an incongruent communication is difficult. To be a sensitive listener often means "hearing" what the speaker is not saying, which may be more significant in some cases than what is said. Effective communicators strive to send congruent messages to avoid misunderstandings or even mistrust on the part of the receiver. Techniques for responding to incongruent communication are described later in this chapter.

■ GOALS OF COMMUNICATION IN NURSING

The primary purpose of communication is to transfer meaning; that is, to impart a message (an idea, a feeling, opinion, information) to another person or people in such a way that both sender and receiver(s) share a common perception of the content and intent of the message. Accurate transfer of meaning between client and nurse and among health care providers is critical to collaboration in health care.

Nurses use communication skills to transfer meaning in varied situations; for example, when teaching, facilitating expression of feelings, alleviating anxiety, and promoting client problem-solving. Often professional communication also requires assertiveness as a means of transferring meaning.

In each of these situations, nurses need to communicate in a manner that is collaborative rather than controlling or manipulative. The choice of a collaborative communication style reflects a nurse's belief that clients can and should participate in their own health care. The following discussion expands on transfer of meaning in the nurse–client relationship. Specific techniques for collaborative communication follow later in the chapter.

Teaching

Nurses are frequently involved in formal or informal teaching of clients about their health care. The following examples illustrate collaborative communication in a teaching situation.

- I'm Jeff Smith, one of the nurses from the nursery. I invited all of you new mothers together so you could share your concerns about caring for your infants. We'll all have a chance to exchange ideas with each other. You may also want to ask me questions and I'll also demonstrate various ways of bathing and dressing babies for those of you who would find that helpful.
- Mrs. Nguyen, let's practice together the breathing techniques you learned in your Lamaze class. That will help us to work together more effectively later when your labor is stronger.
- Mr. Swanson, why don't we take a few minutes to review those leg exercises on the exercise plan you and the physical therapist developed to help us decide whether you need any assistance from me to do them correctly.

Collaborative communication in teaching is discussed in greater detail in Chapter 20.

Facilitating Expression of Feelings

Facilitating expression of feelings is a powerful skill in the nurse–client relationship. Expressing feelings is an effective means of defusing one's emotions and preparing for problem-solving. Sharing oneself via expression of feelings provides opportunities for personal growth. Such openness, however, is perceived as a risk by some individuals. Clients may believe that exposing personal feelings will cause nurses to perceive them as weak or unworthy. Fearing rejection, they may withhold expressing their concerns. Nurses who are able to effectively communicate empathy, respect, and caring will create a climate of trust in which open expression of feelings is more likely to occur. The following example illustrates this.

Nurse Reed: I notice you seem to be apprehensive today. Is something on your mind you'd like to talk about?

Ms. Javcob: Dr. Smith said I could go home today and . . . well . . . I'm not sure that's such a good idea.

Nurse Reed: The thought of being discharged is making you uneasy? . . . Could you tell me a bit more about that?

Ms. Javcob: It's difficult to talk about . . . but since the mastectomy, I don't feel like myself. Maybe I lost more than a breast in surgery.

Nurse Reed: The idea of returning to your home roles—being a wife and mother—seems a little overwhelming?

Ms. Javcob: I . . . a little I guess. . . . Somehow I'm feeling rather inadequate.

Helping clients to get in touch with and to express their feelings increases self-awareness. It is a beginning point for dealing with the feelings.

Alleviating Anxiety and Fear

Anxiety is frequently associated with alterations in health status. Nurses are often called upon to clarify information clients have received about their health or illness and to assist clients with common anxiety-producing situations such as preparing for surgery or diagnostic tests. In this example, the nurse invites collaborative exploration of a client's fears about anesthesia.

Mr. Gagne: The thing that scares me most about surgery is the spinal anesthesia. I'm afraid it'll leave me paralyzed.

Nurse Mendoza: Paralysis is a frightening thought. Let's talk about spinal anesthesia. Maybe our discussion will put your mind at ease.

An opportunity to identify and discuss fears or anxiety is often sufficient to alleviate or even eliminate them. Chapter 22 provides more information about common health care experiences that produce anxiety in many clients.

Promoting Problem-solving

As discussed in Chapter 13, the transition and action phases of the nurse–client relationship involve the client's identifying a problem, making a commitment to action to solve the problem, and acting on the commitment. Collaborative communication during these phases of the relationship often provides the impetus for clients to make a decision and act upon it. Nurses facilitate client exploration of personal values, particularly values that may conflict with one another. This may require that nurses press clients for more concreteness or specificity—which may be more threatening to clients. To prevent this, it is important that a sufficient level of trust be developed before using more confrontational communication.

Ms. Catalfa: I'm really confused. Dr. Li says my stomach problem may be helped by medicine, but that often surgery is necessary. I can't decide whether to try the medicine for a while—or just get it over with and have the operation now.

Nurse Kohn: I get the feeling you are uneasy about the surgery, but unwilling to go through too much more of the kinds of symptoms you've been experiencing.

Ms. Catalfa: Yes, the pain and the nausea, and now this bleeding has been really awful—I mean, it was really scary to see blood when I vomited last week. But the idea of surgery—I'd be laid up for a while . . . I'd have pain. . . .

Nurse Kohn: You have to choose between two alternatives, neither of which looks desirable. It's not an easy situation, but that seems to be the reality right now.

Ms. Catalfa: You're right. There's no getting around it. I might as well stop feeling sorry for myself and get some more information. Can you tell me anything about that drug Dr. Li mentioned? I can't even remember the name of it.

In helping clients to recognize attitudes or behaviors that are not conducive to problem-solving, nurses facilitate clients' making alternative choices.

Asserting a Point of View

Assertive communication involves presenting facts and feelings in a rational emphatic way, but not in a way that devalues the listener. This differs from aggressive communication, which is more forceful and often hurtful or degrading to the person being addressed. Assertive communication is particularly effective in situations in which there is potential for conflict. Whereas aggressive communication often promotes defensiveness during disagreements, assertiveness enhances mutual and self-respect.

Palmer and Deck[15] identified six assertive behaviors that often need reinforcing among nursing students:

1. Using "I" statements.
2. Using "I think" to express a thought and "I feel" to express a feeling.
3. Developing awareness of self-devaluing statements.
4. Using stronger words to accurately identify the here-and-now feeling.
5. Assuming an assertive posture (being aware of nonverbal behaviors) while speaking.
6. Using slow, deliberate speech.

■ APPROACHES THAT FACILITATE OR HINDER COMMUNICATION

Nurses need to be aware of communication approaches that empower others and encourage collaboration, and those that diminish others and block the collaborative approach. Before discussing specific approaches it is helpful first to discuss general concepts of empowering communication.

Empowering Responses

An **empowering response** is one that acknowledges clients' verbal and nonverbal communication in a way that communicates acceptance.

Important elements of an empowering response are empathy, respect, and warmth. An empowering response accurately reflects both the content and the feelings underlying what a client has said. It also involves active listening and the creation of a nonthreatening atmosphere in which clients are free to express themselves. Through the use of empowering responses, nurses define their role as helping individuals and assist clients to perceive themselves in an accurate way. Empowering responses demonstrate that the nurse is sincere in trying to understand and is interested in the client.

Several types of empowering techniques can be used to facilitate communication in the collaborative relationship. Among these are the art of listening; the use of attending behaviors; and the use of Gazda's facilitative, transition, and action dimensions (described in Chap. 13).

Listening. It would seem to be a given that effective communication requires listening. However, listening is so critical to collaborative communication, and such a highly professional skill, that it deserves separate discussion.

Listening is an active process, as contrasted with hearing, which is a passive process. Listening is also an art that involves not only the use of the auditory senses but the use of a "third ear," so to speak, that allows the listener to be aware of verbal and nonverbal behavior, the concurrent metacommunication, the context, and the effects of internal perception. This is no easy task, and no one is able to do this all of the time; however, *awareness* that listening is a crucial ingredient to successful communication is the first step to being an effective listener. Certainly everyone has been involved in interactions in which the listener seemed distracted or disinterested. The effect on the speaker can be devastating. However, when the listener really focuses on the speaker and responds appropriately to the speaker's message, the effect of being truly heard can be quite uplifting.

Attending Behaviors. Gazda and associates[8] define **attending behaviors** as those physical acts that the listener uses to communicate interest in the speaker. Effective use of attending behaviors is fundamental to collaborative nurse–client communication. As emphasized earlier, nonverbal and metacommunication significantly affect communication. A listener using attending behaviors is consciously selecting nonverbal behaviors with the intent of encouraging the speaker to continue. Being given the benefit of another's time, energy, and attention enhances the speaker's self-respect and encourages self-exploration. As Table 14–2 shows, a given nonverbal modality can also communicate inattentiveness and thereby block further communication. Inattentiveness connotes rejection, which is injurious to trust and communication in a collaborative relationship.

Facilitative Dimensions. In Chapter 13 the facilitative techniques—empathy, respect, and warmth—were discussed in terms of their impact on the development of helping relationships. Here, these techniques are operationalized so that they can be readily applied in nurse–client interactions.

Gazda has developed a four-level scale to assess the effectiveness of responses in the helping relationship. This scale is used to rate sample responses in the following discussion. In global terms, level 1 and 2 responses are not considered effective and may even be hurtful; level 3 responses are facilitative, but minimally helpful in the transition and action phases of a helping relationship; and level 4 responses demonstrate significant helper involvement and are most constructive in promoting helper problem-solving. Level 3 and especially level 4 responses require skill and practice to use effectively. They are particularly useful in collaborative nurse–client relationships.

It is important to note that no one can be completely effective in communicating all of the time. Beginning nursing students frequently become discouraged when attempts to apply new knowledge about communication are not completely satisfactory. Most clients are not rebuffed by an occasional nontherapeutic remark or behavior if they sense that a nurse is genuinely interested and accepting.

Empathy. When a nurse is empathic, true understanding is communicated to a client.[16] Empathy is not typified by such overused expressions as "I know just how you feel" or

TABLE 14–2. HOW NONVERBAL MODALITIES COMMUNICATE ATTENTIVENESS OR INATTENTIVENESS

Nonverbal Modality	Inattentiveness	Attentiveness
	These behaviors are likely to close off or slow down the conversation.	These behaviors encourage communication because they show acceptance and respect for the other person.
Space	Distant/very close	Approximately arm's length
Movement	Away	Toward
Posture	Slouching; rigid; seated leaning away	Relaxed, but attentive; seated leaning slightly toward other person
Eye Contact	Absent; defiant; jittery	Regular
Time	Continue with present action before responding; in a hurry	Respond to first opportunity; share time with helpee
Feet and legs (in sitting)	Used to keep distance between the persons	Unobtrusive
Furniture	Used as a barrier	Used to draw persons together
Facial Expression	Does not match feelings; scowl; blank look	Matches own or other's feelings; smile
Gestures	Compete for attention with words	Highlight own words; unobtrusive smooth
Mannerisms	Obvious; distracting	None, or unobtrusive
Voice; volume	Very loud or very soft	Clearly audible
Voice; rate	Impatient or staccato; very slow or hesitant	Average, or a bit slower
Energy level	Apathetic; sleepy; jumpy; pushy	Alert; stays alert throughout a long conversation

From Walters RP. Amity Friendship in Action, Part I. *Copyright © 1980, Richard P Walters. Boulder, CO: Christian Helpers, Inc.*

"I understand." Instead, the empathic response attempts to identify or name a client's feelings and enhance a client's perception that the listener wants to understand the client's situation.

Empathic responses may be assessed using Gazda's four-level scale, as follows:

- Level 1 essentially does not communicate empathy; it is hurtful and irrelevant.
- Level 2 only partially communicates an awareness of the surface feelings of the client.
- Level 3 provides an accurate reflection of surface feelings.
- Level 4 identifies underlying feelings and conveys that a client is understood beyond his or her own level of immediate awareness.

The following examples illustrate the four levels of empathic responses made by a nurse to a client's statement.

Example 1

Client: The harder I try to get along with my son, the more I feel he just wants to be left alone.

Nurse's Response

Level 1: He's making it plain how he feels. Why not just accept that? (Hurtful response.)

Level 2: That's a shame. (Communicates a partial awareness of surface feelings only.)

Level 3: It must be hard for you to reach out and have him reject you. (Surface feelings accurately reflected.)

Level 4: It is upsetting not to get the response you want. It sounds like you take rejection pretty hard. (Underlying feelings identified—helper adds content to add deeper meaning.)

Example 2

Client: I'm really worried about that CAT scan. Is it painful?

Nurse

Level 1: It's as easy as one, two, three. (Doesn't deal with feelings at all.)

Level 2: Yes, it can be scary. (Partially acknowledges surface feelings.)

Level 3: It is kind of scary having a test that you know nothing about. (Accurately acknowledges surface feelings.)

Level 4: Having tests you don't know anything about can be upsetting. I wonder if it's even more worrisome thinking about the possible outcome. (Acknowledges underlying feelings.)

Respect. Respect communicates a belief in the client and is assessed on the four-level response scale as follows:

- Level 1 imposes the nurse's values or opinions on the client. This kind of response devalues the client as an individual.
- Level 2 indicates that a nurse is withholding himself or herself from involvement with a client. This can be communicated by declining to enter into a relationship, by ignoring a client's statements, or by responding in a casual or mechanical manner.
- Level 3 indicates that a nurse is open to the development of a helping relationship and a client is perceived as a person of worth, capable of thinking and acting responsibly.
- Level 4 indicates that a nurse is willing to expend personal energy for a client in order to further the helping relationship. This communicates that the client is indeed a valued individual.

The following examples illustrate the four levels of respect responses made by a nurse to a client's statement.

Example 1

Client: The staff really treats me like I'm a child. Everyone tells me what to do—no one ever asks me my opinion. After all, it is my body.

Nurse

Level 1: Well, you are sick. Don't you think you should let us take care of you? (Imposes nurse's opinion on client.)

Level 2: I don't think that I can help you with this. This is a personal matter between you and the staff. (Declines entering into relationship.)

Level 3: It makes you angry not to be included in your health care decisions. Let's talk about what we might be able to do. (Communicates openness to developing a relationship with client.)

Level 4: It bothers you a lot not to be recognized for your own abilities to handle your life. I'll certainly do what I can to help and I'll discuss this with the rest of the staff so that everyone is aware of the need to involve you in the planning. (Communicates acceptance of client as a person of worth and willingness of nurse to make extra effort to help.)

Example 2

Client: When that nurse came in this morning she just about took my head off. She never even said good morning—just "turn over so I can give you your shot."

Nurse

Level 1: You should have given her a piece of your mind. (Imposes nurse's opinion on client.)

Level 2: The nurse actually did that to you? (Casual remark, declines involvement.)

Level 3: It really upset you to be treated like that. I'm here if you want to discuss it. (Open to a helping relationship with client.)

Level 4: It hurts to be treated like an object. Would you like to talk about ways that you can deal with situations like this? Also I'm willing to talk to the nurse, if that would make you feel better. (Shows involvement and commitment on part of nurse.)

Note the similarity between the level 3 empathy responses and the level 3 respect responses. When a listener is nonjudgmental in responding, the response combines both respect and empathy.

Warmth. Through warmth the nurse conveys genuine caring (Fig. 14–5). Warmth is communicated primarily through the use of nonverbal behaviors. Also, words such as "You're really in pain, let me do what I can to help," convey caring. The four levels of warmth are delineated by Gazda and associates[8] as follows:

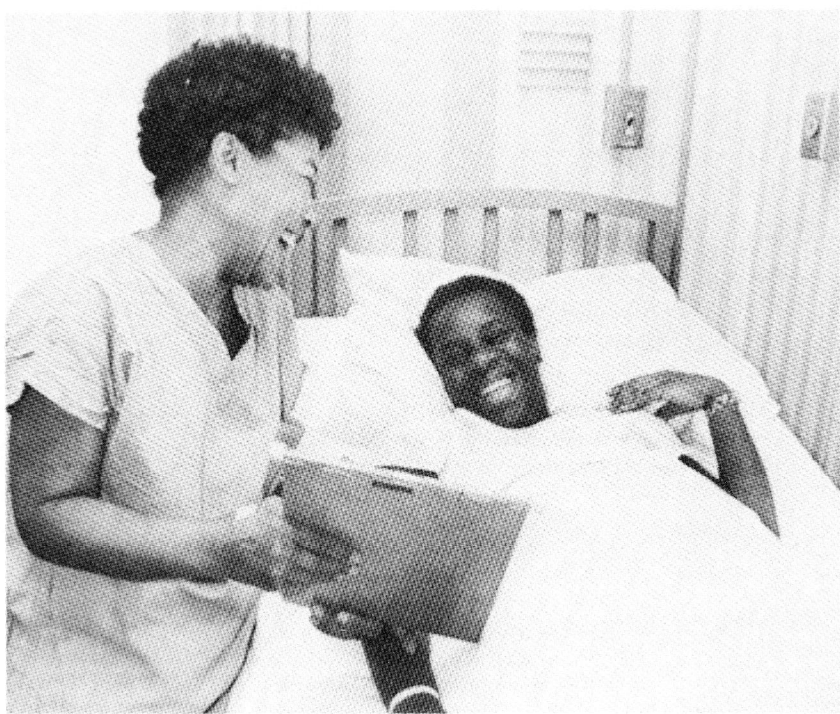

Figure 14–5. The nurse uses warmth in the delivery of basic nursing care. (*Source: Fritz PA, Russell CG, Wilcox EM, Shirk FI.* Interpersonal Communication in Nursing: An Interactionist Approach. *Norwalk, CT: Appleton-Century-Crofts; 1984; 143. Courtesy of Dennis Cryier, Evangelical Hospital Association, Oak Brook, Illinois.*)

- Level 1 displays visible disapproval or disinterest.
- Level 2 is characterized by neutral or absent gestures and responses that sound mechanical.
- Level 3 clearly shows attention and interest.
- Level 4 indicates that a nurse is intensely involved and attentive to the interaction. The client feels accepted and valued.

The following example illustrates these levels of warmth in a nurse's response to a client's statement.

Client: I just want to get out of here. (Urgent voice tone, tense facial muscles.)

Nurse

Level 1: Oh? So do I! (Goes on with tasks.)

Level 2: Looks at client, but does not change affect. Says without expression, "That's too bad." (Mechanical expression.)

Level 3: Sits down next to the client, shows concern on face, offers to talk about situation. (Clear nonverbal response.)

Level 4: Uses most effective attending behaviors. Demonstrates positive affect. Appears alert. Voice tones are appropriate to the seriousness of the interaction. Vocal quality seems relaxed, serious, and concerned. Maintains eye contact. Closer proximity than level 3 and may make physical contact such as a touch on the arm or shoulder. (Intense nonverbal communication.)

Sometimes a nurse can be very empathic and respectful but still not be perceived as a warm individual. In this situation, the nurse may find it takes longer to build a solid base for a helping relationship. On the other hand, a nurse may display high levels of warmth and low levels of empathy and respect. This occurs when a nurse doesn't really care about a client or seeks to manipulate a client. Insincerity can usually be detected by clients.

Transition Dimensions. After a nurse has developed a solid basis for a relationship through the consistent use of empathy, respect, and warmth, the relationship is ready to move on to the use of the transition dimensions of concreteness, genuineness, and self-disclosure. The nurse tentatively begins to evaluate the client's words and behaviors.

Concreteness. A nurse who displays concreteness is specific in communication and tries to elicit specificity from the client. The four levels of concreteness[8] include:

- Level 1: A response that is vague or hurtful.
- Level 2: A response that is general or intellectual. A nurse may ask for specificity but with behavior that does not model it.
- Level 3: A clear, specific, and concrete response. A nurse accepts abstractions from a client but models specificity.
- Level 4: A very specific response that actively solicits specificity from a client.

The following examples illustrate these levels of concrete responses from a nurse to a client's statement.

Example 1

Client: All of these hospital procedures make me uneasy.

Nurse

Level 1: We all have things that really unnerve us in our lives. (A vague response.)

Level 2: Having things done to you can be scary, but I find that if I let myself be open to new experiences I often profit from them. (An intellectual response.)

Level 3: Having things done to you that you do not understand is frightening. (A specific response.)

Level 4: When things are done to you that you do not understand, you feel frightened. I wonder if we could talk about what it is that frightens you. (Nurse responds specifically and elicits a specific response from client.)

Example 2

Client: The nurses here all seem too busy to talk to me.

Nurse

Level 1: Being busy is a way of life here. (A hurtful response.)

Level 2: Did you talk to any of the nurses about this? (A general response.)

Level 3: You'd like to have someone to spend some time with you and show they are interested in you. (A specific response.)

Level 4: You're feeling neglected and ignored. Why don't we talk about these feelings and ways for you to get the kind of care you need. (The nurse responds specifically and elicits specific client responses.)

Genuineness. A genuine person is one who "has it all together," a congruent person. The four levels of the genuineness scale[8] include:

- Level 1: A nurse is defensive, punitive, or deceitful to the client.
- Level 2: A nurse gives incongruent verbal and nonverbal messages.
- Level 3: A nurse's responses are congruent; however, the nurse refrains from displaying feelings.
- Level 4: A nurse's responses are not only congruent but also spontaneous. Whether the reason is positive or negative the nurse is real. When the response is negative the nurse conveys it in a manner that is constructive to a client and opens up new areas for exploration.

The following examples illustrate the levels of genuineness in a nurse's response to a client's statement.

Example 1

Client: My baby is being kept in the nursery. I'm really worried about him. I'm also worried that the separation will interfere with breast feeding.

Nurse

Level 1: Well, that's not my territory—you'll have to deal with the nursery staff about that problem. (Defensive response.)

Level 2: As a nurse on this unit, I can assure you that we will do all we can to help you. (No nonverbal display of interest or wonder.) (Incongruent verbal and nonverbal behavior.)

Level 3: I can see you're upset about this, but to be honest with you, I'm a new nurse here and I'm not sure how I can help you. (Congruent verbal and nonverbal response.)

Level 4: I can see this is a problem for you. I'm a little shaky about dealing with it because of my newness on this unit. But I will go to the nursery and see if I can get some answers for you. (Shows concern and willingness to help nonverbally.)

Example 2

Client: Does it ever bother you to give injections and to see all the blood and gore? (Client asks as nurse changes a dressing.)

Nurse

Level 1: Why should those things bother me? (Nurse is flip with client.)

Level 2: In my line of work, you learn to get used to everything. (Face shows disgust.) (Incongruent verbal and nonverbal behavior.)

Level 3: Yes, sometimes it bothers me a lot. (Congruent verbal and nonverbal behavior.)

Level 4: Yes, sometimes I really feel bothered by what I see. I realize that some unpleasant things are temporary in the process of getting well. It's very satisfying to be part of that. (Congruent verbal and nonverbal behavior and expression of feelings.)

Self-disclosure. In order for clients to get the most out of a relationship they eventually have to get to know nurses so that they can relate to them more fully. This knowledge comes through a nurse's appropriate use of self-disclosure. The four levels of self-disclosure are:

- Level 1: A nurse withholds all personal information.
- Level 2: A nurse may answer some direct personal questions, but does not volunteer information.
- Level 3: A nurse reveals personal ideas, attitudes and experiences relevant to a client's situation, but in a general fashion.
- Level 4: A nurse freely and spontaneously shares personal information that is relevant to a client's interests and concerns.

The following examples illustrate the four levels of self-disclosure used by a nurse in responding to a client situation.

Example 1

Client: I just can't seem to get the knack of giving myself an insulin injection. Did you ever have trouble when you were learning?

Nurse

Level 1: Oh, you'll get it soon. (Shares no personal information.)

Level 2: Yes, it was hard, but my situation as a nurse is different from yours. (Answers direct question; does not volunteer information.)

Level 3: Oh yes. I remember it was very difficult for me to give injections. (Reveals personal reaction in a general way.)

Level 4: Gosh yes. I can remember before my first "real" injection I practiced what I would say, how I would give the injection, and I injected dozens of willing oranges. (Freely shares specific personal information.)

Example 2

Client: I've been in the hospital so long I'm afraid that this will become a permanent condition. Have you ever been hospitalized?

Nurse

Level 1: It's more important that we talk about you. (Refuses to answer personal question.)

Level 2: Once when I had my son. (Answers question but volunteers no information.)

Level 3: I was hospitalized once and I found it uncomfortable. (Answers personal question in a general way.)

Level 4: I remember when I had my son I felt homesick and uneasy. I missed all my familiar things. It gave me a greater appreciation for how difficult it is to be in the hospital. (Freely shares specific personal information in response to question.)

Action Dimensions. The last two dimensions that Gazda and associates[8] identify are confrontation and immediacy. Confrontation and immediacy involve being evaluative; that is, nurses make judgments about what clients are saying and doing. These dimensions are referred to as action dimensions because it is through the expeditious use of confrontation and immediacy that clients are able to take action toward problem resolution. It is unlikely that beginning nursing students will have the opportunity to apply these concepts unless clinical experiences allow for time and continuity to develop a long-term relationship. However, the dimensions are certainly requisite in a professional nursing career. Both client relationships and peer relationships present situations in which professional nurses must be able to use confrontation and immediacy.

Confrontation. Confrontation involves informing a client about discrepancies between what the client has been saying and doing. In order for confrontation to be effective, a client must be able to work with what is said. Thus, the confrontation should not be so abrupt or threatening that a client becomes defensive and cannot hear the feedback, nor should the confrontation be so weak that a client misses the point. Gazda and associates[8] identify a number of helpful techniques to increase or decrease the intensity of a confrontational comment. These techniques are summarized in Table 14–3.

The four levels of confrontation move from a denial or acceptance of discrepancies to a firm identification of discrepant behavior.

- A level 1 confrontation means that a nurse accepts discrepancies expressed by a client, ignores the discrepancies, or gives premature advice that closes off fruitful exploration.
- A level 2 confrontation means that a nurse does not overtly accept or deny discrepancies in a client's behavior, but does not point them out to the client either.
- A level 3 confrontation involves a nurse's tentative acknowledgment of discrepancies in a client's behavior.
- A level 4 confrontation involves a nurse's firm acknowledgment of discrepancies in a client's behavior and the specific consequences of the discrepancies. This enables clients to deal with problematic areas of which they were either completely or partially unaware.

The following examples illustrate the four levels of confrontation used by nurses.

Example 1

Nurse Johnson has been seeing Mr. Murtz in the medical clinic to help him deal with his diabetes. They have worked together for several months with only limited success at lowering Mr. Murtz's blood sugar levels. This morning Mr. Murtz's blood sugar level was 350. While he was sitting in the waiting room, Nurse Johnson observed him eating a chocolate candy bar. Yet when he met with Nurse Johnson, he acted surprised about his high blood sugar level. He stated he was following his diabetic diet.

Nurse

Level 1: I . . . uh . . . well, I'm so glad you came to the clinic today. It shows you're willing to really work on this problem of controlling your diabetes. (Ignores discrepancy entirely.)

Level 2: We have to really look at your diet so you can control this diabetes. (Does not refer to discrepancy.)

Level 3: With such a high blood sugar level I wonder if you are having difficulty with your diet. (Tentative acknowledgment of discrepancy.)

Level 4: When I saw you munching on that candy bar and then I saw what your blood glucose level was, I recognized that you are having a problem. Can we talk about what you can do to stick to this diet? I'm really worried about what will happen if the diabetes is not controlled. (Firm directional statement about discrepancy.)

Example 2

Miss Sloan had surgery 5 days ago and wheezes when she breathes. She has been instructed to use an incentive spirometer to help loosen secretions. Nurse Goa enters

TABLE 14–3. TECHNIQUES THAT CHANGE THE INTENSITY OF CONFRONTATION

Decrease Intensity	Increase Intensity
Establish a relationship of trust and caring.	Personalize the confrontation.
Talk about people in general instead of the client specifically.	Be very specific about events.
Use words such as "sometimes," "maybe," "once in a while," "often." These words give the client loopholes and make the confrontation sound less accusatory.	Deal with issues that are recent.
Use humor.	Confront actions, not just words.
Give confrontation in a positive, caring way.	Use what the client has said or done earlier to contradict what the client is saying or doing now.

Miss Sloan's room to remind her that it is time to use the incentive spirometer. Miss Sloan agrees and begins the treatment. However, as soon as Nurse Goa leaves, Miss Sloan stops the treatment and lights up a cigarette. Five minutes later Nurse Goa returns to check on Miss Sloan's progress. Nurse Goa finds Miss Sloan sitting across the room from the incentive spirometer and notices the cigarette smoke in the room. Miss Sloan says "I just stopped using it, that treatment really helps me breathe."

Nurse

Level 1: Great, you finished your treatment, I'll be back later to tell you when it's time for another. (Ignores the discrepancy entirely.)

Level 2: You can really tell a difference after you have used the incentive spirometer. (Does not refer to discrepancy.)

Level 3: The treatment is really important. There's a smell of cigarette smoke in here. (Points out discrepancy in a tentative manner.)

Level 4: Miss Sloan, the treatment should take a full 5 minutes—but I think you even managed a cigarette break in there. Let's talk about what has happened here. (Firm directional statement about discrepancy.)

Immediacy. In the helping relationship, immediacy refers to communication exchanged between nurse and client about their relationship at a particular moment in time.[8] Because the communication can involve both positive and negative information, immediacy can increase the anxiety level of both nurse and client.

To be comfortable with the dimension of immediacy, nurses must be comfortable with their own self-image. If a nurse is threatened by what a client says about the value of the relationship, it may indicate that the nurse is in the relationship to meet personal rather than client needs.

Nurses should be continually evaluating the strengths and deficiencies of a nurse–client relationship and should be aware of cues from clients that indicate that obstacles in the relationship are blocking effective problem-solving. Nurses need to deal with these obstacles and resolve them if the relationship is to help clients deal with important problems.

The levels of immediacy range from a nurse's ignoring all cues from clients about the relationship, to a nurse's concise discussion of what is occurring in the nurse–client relationship.

- A level 1 response either ignores all cues from a client that there is a problem in the relationship, or uses a client's feelings in a destructive way.
- A level 2 response may give superficial acknowledgment about the interpersonal issue but does not discuss it.
- A level 3 response is characterized by the nurse's acknowledgment of the interpersonal difficulty followed by a general rather than a personal discussion.
- A level 4 response makes a precise interpretation about the nurse–client relationship and discusses the issue in a direct, personal, and explicit manner.

The following examples illustrate the four levels of immediacy used by a nurse in responding in a client situation.

BUILDING NURSING KNOWLEDGE

What is the Meaning of Reassurance?

Teasdale K. The concept of reassurance in nursing. *J Adv Nurs.* 1989; 14:444–450.

Some authorities do not agree that reassurance has value for clients. They argue that it may be a way of dismissing clients' concerns with stereotyped responses or trite expressions that do not relate to the clients' needs. Others feel that reassurance helps clients attain a sense of psychological well-being. Teasdale points out that the phase "reassure the client" is one of the most commonly used in nursing, yet little is known about it and little analysis is given to what the phrase really means.

Teasdale reasoned that reassurance might have several different meanings, and argued that without precise meanings for the term, it is difficult to conduct research to establish the benefits or risks. Teasdale designed a study employing the content analysis technique to identify the usage of the term within a popular nursing journal over a 6-month time period.

Three distinct uses of the term were identified: (1) reassurance as a state of mind, (2) reassurance as a deliberate attempt to restore confidence, and (3) reassurance as an optimistic expression. Reassurance as a state of mind was characterized by journal descriptions of clients who expressed feelings of threat or anxiety and then reported increased confidence gained from a new interpretation of their situation. Clients achieved new interpretations by chance, by deliberately seeking information, or when another person took deliberate, effective action to restore their confidence.

Reassurance as a purposeful attempt to restore confidence was characterized by journal descriptions of nurses who made observations that the clients looked anxious and worried, and then took action to produce a state of calmness in clients. The range of actions included verbal assurances, information-giving, use of touch, use of other people, or other sources of data.

Reassurance construed as an optimistic expression was characterized by journal descriptions of nurses who made observations that clients were anxious and worried, but who then confined the plan of action to verbal assurances, repeated pledges or promises intended to improve clients' feeling state. These findings are important, Teasdale argues, because understanding the uses that the term "reassurance" has in nursing may facilitate future research on the effectiveness of the various actions used by nurses to reassure clients.

Example 1

Mrs. Crowley is an oncology client who has just been readmitted for the fourth time in a year. All of the nursing staff know her well and really like her. Nurse Blake has been her primary nurse.

Mrs. Crowley seems very upset when Nurse Blake enters the room. Nurse Blake says, "You really seem worried, can I help in any way?" Mrs. Crowley says "What do you care? You get paid to be nice. It's part of your job."

Nurse Blake

Level 1: If I wasn't paid to be here you can bet I'd be someplace else. (Destructive.)

Level 2: You seem angry with me—we can talk about that later . . . but right now I have to take you to X-ray. (Gives token acknowledgment to expression of immediacy and then postpones discussing it.)

Level 3: You seem uneasy about our relationship. I wonder what is bothering you. (Reflects the client's feelings about the relationship in a general way.)

Level 4: I'm sorry to see that you doubt my positive feelings for you. I wonder if you are afraid of getting close to me. (Current and specific interpretation of the behavior.)

Example 2

Mr. Collins has been seeing Mrs. Kidwell, a psychiatric liaison nurse in the clinic, for 6 months. Mr. Collins has been recently unemployed and is experiencing a moderate degree of depression. Mrs. Kidwell had to cancel their last appointment. This week Mr. Collins refuses to look at her and answers her in monosyllables and shrugs of his shoulders.

Mrs. Kidwell

Level 1: If you don't care to talk today, Mr. Collins, that's fine with me. I'm quite busy. (Destructive and ignores the issue between nurse and client.)

Level 2: You seem bothered today, but I'd like to know what happened with the job interviews you went on last week. (Gives token recognition to expressions of immediacy and then changes the subject.)

Level 3: You seem upset today. Can I help? (Reflects feelings of immediacy, and then shows openness to sharing responsibility for improving the relationship.)

Level 4: You seem angry. I wonder if when I cancelled our appointment last week, you thought I was deserting you. (Explicit and specific interpretation of immediacy.)

The foregoing discussion has emphasized the use of verbal communication in each phase of the helping relationship. Communication of each of the dimensions discussed above is enhanced with the use of appropriate nonverbal behavior. Table 14–4 provides examples of ineffective and effective nonverbal behaviors that are frequently associated with high or low levels of each dimension.

Other Techniques. In addition to the communication dimensions identified by Gazda and associates,[8] Sundeen and others[6] identify other techniques that are helpful to nurses in communicating with clients and that work well within the Gazda model. These techniques are summarized in Table 14–5.

Blocks to Empowering Communication

Sundeen and co-workers[6] identify failure to listen as the primary block to effective communication. Nurses who fail

TABLE 14–4. EXAMPLES OF INEFFECTIVE AND EFFECTIVE NONVERBAL BEHAVIORS

	Ineffective Behaviors	Effective Behaviors
	Helper nonverbal behaviors likely to communicate low levels of the dimension	Helper nonverbal behaviors likely to communicate high levels of the dimension
Empathy	Frown resulting from lack of understanding.	Positive head nods; facial expression congruent with content of conversation.
Respect	Mumbling; patronizing tone of voice; engages in doodling or self-stimulating behavior to the point of appearing more involved in that than with the client.	Spends time with client; fully attentive.
Warmth	Apathy; delay in responding to approach of client; insincere effusiveness; fidgeting; signs of wanting to leave (e.g., remains standing some distance from client).	Smile; physical contact; proximity.
Concreteness	Shrugs shoulders when helpee is vague instead of asking for clarification; vague gestures used as a substitute for gestures or words that carry specific meaning.	Draws diagram to clarify an abstract point; clear enunciation.
Genuineness	Low or evasive eye contact; lack of congruence between verbal and nonverbal behavior; less frequent movement; excessive smiling.	Congruence between verbal and nonverbal behavior.
Self-disclosure	Bragging gestures; points to self; covers eyes or mouth saying, "It was no big deal."	Gestures that keep references to self low-key—eg, a shrug accompanying the words when talking about a personal incident.
Confrontation	Points finger or shakes fist at helpee; tone of voice that communicates blame or condemnation; loudness of voice may intimidate some. Wavering voice; unsure of self.	Natural tone of voice.
Immediacy	Turns away or moves back when immediacy enters the conversation.	Enthusiasm.

From Gazda G, Asbury FS, Balzer FJ, et al. Human Relations Development. *Boston: Allyn & Bacon, 1984.*

TABLE 14–5. ADDITIONAL EMPOWERING COMMUNICATION TECHNIQUES

Technique	Definition	Therapeutic Value
Silence	Periods of no verbal communication among participants.	Nonverbally communicates nurse's acceptance of client.
Establishing guidelines	Statements regarding roles, purpose, and limitations for a particular interaction.	Helps client to know what is expected.
Giving broad openings	General comments asking the client to determine the direction the interaction should take.	Enables client to decide what material to discuss and encourages continuation of the interaction.
Reducing distance	Diminishing physical space between the nurse and client.	Nonverbally communicates that nurse wants to be involved with client.
Acknowledgment	Recognition given to a client for contribution to an interaction.	Demonstrates the importance of client's role within the relationship.
Restating	Repeating to the client what the nurse believes is the main thought or idea expressed.	Asks for validation of nurse's interpretation of the message.
Reflecting	Directing back the client's ideas, feelings, questions, or content.	Attempts to show client the importance of client's own feelings, and interpretations.
Seeking clarification	Asking for additional input to understand the message received.	Demonstrates nurse's desire to understand client's communication.
Seeking consensual validation	Attempts to reach a mutual denotative and connotative meaning of specific words.	Demonstrates nurse's desire to understand client's communication.
Focusing	Questions or statements to help the client develop or expand an idea.	Directs conversation toward topics of importance.
Summarizing	Statement of main areas discussed during interaction.	Helps client to separate relevant from irrelevant material; serves as a review and closing for the interaction.
Planning	Mutual decision-making regarding the goals, direction, and so on, of future interactions.	Reiterates client's role within relationship.

From Sundeen S, Stuart G, Rankin E, Cohen S. Nurse–Client Interaction: Implementing the Nursing Process. *St. Louis: Mosby; 1989.*

to listen to the client communicate that the client is not important. Other blocks to effective communication include failure to probe, failure to explore the client's meaning, following standard forms too closely, being judgmental, using false reassurance, defending, giving advice, stereotyped responses, and changing topics. Each of these is discussed individually.

Failure to Listen. There are three common barriers to effective listening. The first block is lack of attentiveness. When nurses make eye contact with clients and display appropriate nonverbal and verbal behaviors in response to clients, the nurses are being attentive listeners. By contrast, nurses who repeatedly glance at the clock or allow other concerns to flood their thoughts are not attending to the speaker, and this will be communicated to clients loudly and clearly.

The second barrier to effective listening is responding to content instead of meaning. If a client tells a nurse that he is tired because he lies awake all night and worries about his diagnosis, and the nurse responds that she will get him sleeping medication, then the nurse has missed the whole point of the client's communication.

Effective listening is also blocked when nurses' responses are subjective—that is, when nurses respond to clients from a personal feeling state.

Subjective response:

Client: My son hasn't been to see me at all during this hospitalization.

Nurse: Well, that is certainly a selfish way to treat you. Doesn't he know that you need him?

Empowering response:

Client: My son hasn't been to see me at all during this hospitalization.

Nurse: Sounds like that hurts.

Failure to Probe. Although probe is sometimes given a negative connotation, its meaning is to explore thoroughly, a positive action in therapeutic communication. Probing is a way of achieving mutual understanding. Effective probes clarify or pinpoint clients' statements, giving a nurse a richer understanding of client perspective. When clients' statements are general or vague, failure to probe can result in communication remaining on a superficial level, which trivializes client concerns. Inviting elaboration, on the other hand, is a gift of oneself that enables clients to reveal more significant feelings if they desire.

Failure to Examine Clients' Meaning. There are many occasions in human communication when words or messages are ambiguous—that is, may convey several meanings. Sometimes the context or the topic of conversation is sufficient to suggest intent, but assuming what is meant by a speaker is usually unwise. It is quite possible that the listener's interpretation and the intent of the speaker will differ. The differences in interpretation can be the basis for further miscommunication, which may have a harmful effect on the interaction—even on the relationship itself.

In a nurse–client relationship, failure to verify a client's meaning can lead to inappropriate nursing care. For example, a new mother may say to a nurse: "It really hurts me to breast feed. I think I should wean my baby." If the nurse does not seek clarification about what the client means by "it really hurts me," the nurse may come to the wrong conclusion about the kind of support to provide. The "hurt" may be related to the development of mastitis, an infection that should be treated; it may be an emotional, not a physical, pain; or the hurt may be the result of the baby sucking incorrectly. Each of these meanings would require a different nursing response.

Following Standard Forms too Closely. Using standard forms to obtain health information provides valuable information in a brief period of time. However, relying on such forms entirely cuts off exploration of clients' feelings and perceptions about their situation and relegates clients to the role of objects. If pressed for time, nurses can note areas of further concern for future follow-up and can promise to return later to discuss them.

Being Judgmental. This is different than the technique of confrontation, which is sharing of objective evaluation. Being judgmental essentially communicates to clients that they should think and feel as the nurse does. Statements such as "That's good," "that's bad," "you shouldn't do . . . ," or "you should do . . ." are judgmental and place nurses' values, beliefs, and perceptions above those of clients.

False Reassurance. Comments such as "Everything will be fine" attempt to wipe away the pain of a client's situation. Such remarks deny or block clients' expressions of feelings. They are meaningless and insulting. False reassurance is often used when nurses are uncomfortable with the topic or emotions a client is sharing. Clients feel genuine reassurance when they feel accepted and secure as a result of other effective communication with a nurse.

Defending. When nurses feel the need to protect others, they may block a client's discussion of feelings or opinions. For instance, if a client says "That nurse Sara Blackwell is so rough; I hate it when she comes on the three to eleven shift," and a nurse responds by defending Sara Blackwell, the nurse is rejecting the client's opinion. Defending statements convey the message to clients that "You do not have the right to have feelings or to complain."

Giving Advice. Offering solutions to clients' problems implies that they are unable to be self-directed and make decisions. It often results from a helper's personal need to feel needed by others. This differs from supplying additional information, which is a collaborative approach to problem-solving. Giving clients information supplements their knowledge with additional facts so they are better equipped to make their own decisions.

Stereotyped Responses. These include platitudes, cliches, and other trite expressions that deny the uniqueness of each client. For instance, if a nurse responds to a client's statement of pain by telling the client to "Keep a stiff upper lip," the nurse has implied that the client is being weak and that the nurse is unwilling to help.

Changing Topics. This is a nonempowering technique because it puts nurses in charge of the material discussed. It sends a message to clients that a nurse is not listening or that "We will talk about what I decide is important." Changing the subject may serve to protect nurses from possible anxiety, or may result from failure to hear the significance of what the client is saying.

Responding to Incongruent Communication

When messages are incongruent it is difficult to know to which message to respond. In trying to decide how to respond, it is helpful to consider the phase of the nurse–client relationship (as discussed in Chapter 13) in which the communication takes place.

If the relationship is in the facilitative[8] or orientation phase,[6] then nurses should probably respond to the nonverbal message. If a client is uncomfortable with a nurse's response, the nurse can explain that even though the client said one thing, the nurse picked up a different feeling from the client.

In the action[8] or working phase[6] of the relationship, nurses can confront clients in a direct fashion about the dilemma caused by two conflicting messages.

The issue of congruency is also important to nurses' communication. The concept of genuineness described in Chapter 13 refers to congruency. For instance, if a nurse has a family member seriously ill and hospitalized, it would be incongruent for the nurse to be smiling all day. This is not to suggest that a nurse should share personal problems with clients, but an acknowledgment that "this is not one of my better days" would be sufficient for clients to know that any nonverbal messages of uneasiness are not directed at or caused by them.

■ COMMUNICATING IN SPECIAL SITUATIONS

There are nurse–client situations in which special skills are required on the part of nurses because the verbal channel of communication is not present or is inadequate. Some examples are clients who speak a language different from nurses', aphasic clients, noncommunicative clients, and children. In these situations, the importance of nonverbal communication is magnified.

Differing Primary Language

When nurse and client speak different languages, interpreters are often used to overcome this barrier to communication. Many hospitals keep a list of volunteers or employees who speak another language and could serve as an interpreter for clients. Sometimes there is a family member who speaks English and can facilitate communication with the client. However, the use of translators is not always without problems. Frequently translators lack sufficient knowledge of health care terminology to communicate nurses' ideas to clients. Furthermore, there are regional differences within languages. For example, Spanish spoken in the Southwestern United States is different from Puerto Rican Spanish.[17] There also are many dialects among Southeast Asian immigrants.

Thus, special care must be taken in the training of interpreters so that they can converse in regional dialects and know various cultural health practices. In addition, nurses must avoid the use of medical jargon with clients and must be very attuned to nonverbal communication. Whenever possible nurses should attempt to communicate using clients' language. No matter how limited nurses' expertise, attempts to use a client's language communicate a high level of caring.

Aphasic Client

Aphasia is a term that refers to impairment or loss of the ability to communicate using language (see also Chap. 29). The impairment may be expressive, receptive, or total. Clients with expressive aphasia know what ideas they wish to communicate, but cannot select the correct words to do so. Receptive aphasia refers to the inability to decode incoming messages. In total aphasia, verbal messages can neither be formulated nor interpreted. Communicating with aphasic clients requires the nurse to be particularly sensitive to personal nonverbal communication and to client nonverbal behaviors. It is also important to demonstrate patience and acceptance as a client struggles for words. The use of signs, signal systems, or pictures of common objects can be utilized to facilitate communication.

Nonverbal Client

Clients who do not communicate verbally present a special challenge to nurses. Nurses may need to just sit quietly with nonverbal clients and accept that silence is all that they can handle at the time.[18] Nurses' physical presence and the ability to allow clients to be silent communicates acceptance.

Elderly Client

Age-related changes in cognitive perceptual functioning often influence communication patterns in the elderly.[19] Hearing loss is common. Some older adults experience attention deficits, distractibility, and loss of short-term memory capacity. These problems create difficulty with word finding and increased use of vague terms.[20] Maintaining the topic of conversation is harder and interruptions are likely. Changes in the shape of the oral cavity, loss of teeth or poorly fitting dentures interfere with articulation, so elders' speech may be harder for others to understand.

These barriers make careful listening even more important for this age group than for clients in general. Observing nonverbal behaviors closely to glean clues to meaning averts misunderstanding. Touch is a sensory pathway that tends to remain intact through the aging process, so incorporating more touch in interactions with older clients is an effective way to convey interest and concern.[19] Box 14–1 summarizes additional approaches to increase communication effectiveness with clients who are older.

BOX 14–1. APPROACHES TO FACILITATE COMMUNICATION WITH OLDER CLIENTS

- Repeat a message in a different way if it is not understood at first, rather than speaking more loudly.
- Eliminate competing noise, such as television, radio.
- Face clients with hearing deficits and speak distinctly, without shouting.
- Use gestures or objects to augment your words as well as to assist clients to express themselves.
- Carefully attend to clients' nonverbal behaviors.
- Allow clients time for composing a verbal response before prompting or repeating your question.
- Do not pretend to understand when you do not, but avoid frequent requests for clients to repeat statements.
- Note signs of fatigue. Clients with hearing problems understand less when they are tired.
- When possible, choose areas for communication that have sound-absorbing characteristics, such as carpets, upholstered furniture, and drapes, rather than hard floors and exposed windows. The latter tend to exaggerate background noise and increase distraction.
- Use touch liberally unless clients indicate touch is not acceptable.

From Yurik AG, Spier BE, Robb SS, and Ebert NJ. *The Aged Person and the Nursing Process.* Norwalk, CT: Appleton & Lange; 1989.

Children

The last example of special communication problems concerns nurse–client interactions that involve children. In order to facilitate communication with children the nurse needs to (1) know and apply concepts of child development and (2) be versatile in use of alternative communication modes such as the use of play and art. Play offers children a constructive outlet to express feelings and fears. Art can be a way for children to communicate to nurses what they are not able to verbalize or express in any other way.

Table 14–6 summarizes thought processes, typical communication patterns, and general techniques for communicating with children of various developmental levels. While such generalizations are very useful, they cannot be applied without judgment. No two children will respond in exactly the same way to a situation. Even the same child may react to the same stimulus differently at different times. Illness is especially likely to alter children's communication

TABLE 14–6. TECHNIQUES FOR COMMUNICATING WITH CHILDREN

Developmental Level	Thought Processes, Typical Communication Patterns	Recommended Communication Techniques
Newborn (birth to 1 mo)	Mouthing, rooting, sucking. Attends to stimulation with eye movements, staring, facial and body movement (eg, reaching). Demands relief from discomfort by crying. If overstimulated looks away, arches back, rapidly moves arms and legs, cries.	Use high-pitched voice, make eye contact about 8 inches from the face. To calm crying newborn, hold while making soothing sounds, patting newborn, moving in rocking fashion.
Infant (1 mo to 1 yr)	Signals by smiling, cooing, blowing, laughing. Delay in gratification of needs is threatening. Few words (mama, dada) by late in first year. Imitates facial and body gestures at 1 to 2 months, initiates nonverbal behaviors (reaching to be held, pushing objects away, shaking head) around 6 months. Fear of strangers begins around 6 months.	Make contact slowly, respect personal space, mimic parents' tone and behavior. Interact with or through parents to prove one is a "safe" person, keep parent in view during interaction. Respond to needs promptly.
Toddler (1 to 3 yr)	Vocabulary increases, but not consistently verbal. Children are egocentric, believe that others know what they know, so may refuse to be verbal when prompted. Can effectively use gestures—pointing, pushing, pulling adult, shaking head.	Focus on child. Set concrete limits and abide by them consistently. Allow child to explore new environment (eg, equipment used for health assessment). Use concrete explanations, short sentences, incorporate child's words when possible.
Preschool (3 to 5 yr)	Talks for the fun of it, engages others in conversation. Vocabulary limited, each word has only one meaning. Can answer direct questions about self, feelings. Still egocentric. Ascribes human feelings, needs, and motives to objects, believes most events are controlled by adults. Views events in cause–effect terms with cause near in time to effect; feel they can cause events by own thoughts.	Use direct concrete questions, explanations; avoid analogies (shot is a "little stick in the arm" may evoke image of a stick from a tree poked into the arm; better to say "needle stick"). Prepare for new experiences (eg, medical treatment) by allowing manipulation of objects involved or viewing, then participating as procedure is carried out on a doll. Using play to reenact the event after it is over will also reduce feelings of powerlessness.
School Age (5 to 12 yr)	Thinking is still concrete, but can reason logically, to understand cause and effect. Grasps that body has internal parts that perform functions. Can make choices between alternatives, even if all are undesirable. Can grasp that something can hurt and still be good for them. Able to mentally rehearse to prepare for a difficult event. Is open and candid if trust is established—can precisely express concerns and needs for help.	Show interest in child's point of view. Listen actively. Provide information and support to prepare for new experiences. Use actual objects or pictures (eg, of internal organs, operating room) for explanations of illness or procedure. Give choices whenever possible. Involve child directly in activities or procedures—give opportunity to perform task or assume key role.
Adolescent (12 to 18 yr)	Ability to think abstractly begins around age 11 and develops throughout this period. Fluctuations between adult and childlike thinking and behavior are common. Group identity is important; is evidenced by appearance, selection of activities, modes of verbal expression.	Convey acceptance, respect. Listen actively. Use conversational tone when questioning to avoid impression that the "right" answer is expected. If possible, spend time when no demands are made. Focus questions on essential information versus global inquiries, especially with younger adolescents. If dealing with intimate or private concerns, assure confidentiality.

and response patterns. Commonly, regression to earlier behavior patterns is noted during illness.

■ INTERVIEWING

Up to this point the focus has been on the use of communication in a helping relationship. Another situation in which communication skills are important is gathering information in an interview. An **interview** is a structured conversation with a specific purpose.

Students frequently experience difficulties with the interviewing process. Their foremost concern is the lack of comfort they feel when they ask personal questions. Many students believe that "it's none of their business" to inquire about such personal topics as bowel habits and sexual activity. That perception is true in a social relationship; it is not true, however, in a professional relationship. Nurses depend on an accurate and comprehensive data base in order to develop an effective care plan with a client. Nurses need to know what information is important and to explain the reason for seeking such data to clients. *All* information is not relevant *all* of the time. For instance, if a client is admitted to the emergency room with a broken arm, it would probably not be pertinent to ask about bowel habits. Most likely that information will not affect the plan of care. However, in a postpartum unit it would be negligent of a nurse to fail to make the same inquiry, because constipation is a frequent concern of new mothers. If nurses are clear about why certain information is needed and can state the purpose to clients, most clients are willing to provide the requested data.

Students also feel discomfort when asking personal questions because of the newness of and unfamiliarity with their professional role. With time and experience, the role "fits" better and it becomes more natural to ask questions that once caused embarrassment.

The other aspect of interviewing that causes students difficulty is not knowing what to ask, how to ask it, and how to organize what is asked. These concerns are dealt with under *Types of Interviews*.

Purpose of an Interview

The primary purpose of an interview is to collect data. The data may be used as part of a research study, to admit a client to the health care system, or (most frequently) to complete a nursing data base for collaborative care planning (Fig. 14–6). Interviewing is an essential tool in the nursing process. Without interviewing it is difficult if not impossible to obtain a complete data base from which the nursing diagnoses and the plan of care are derived.

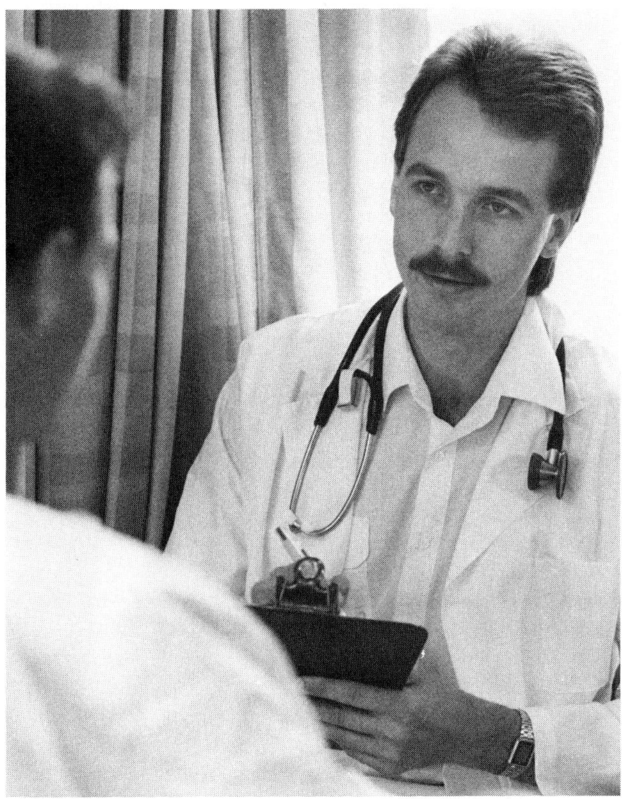

Figure 14–6. A formal interview is conducted to obtain a comprehensive data base.

The data sought by nurses are different from data sought by the medical staff. The latter seek specific factual information about a disease or illness. Nurses, on the other hand, are interested in clients' *total response* to disease or illness. The nursing interview may be organized around nursing problems, body systems, basic needs, or any other framework that guides nursing practice.

Types of Interviews

The interview can be either informal or formal. Both informal and formal interviews seek information about (1) clients' past health history, (2) current concerns, (3) level of understanding about health and current problems, and (4) care and assistance desired.

Informal Interview. The informal interview may be conducted in a variety of settings; for example, the waiting room of a clinic, the school nurse's office, or a client's home. The informal interview is usually direct and seeks to obtain expeditiously the most important data. The following example illustrates a nurse's informal interview.

Seeking information about current concern and past health history

Nurse: What brings you to the hospital today?

Client: My arthritis is really acting up. I can barely cope with the pain.

Nurse: Is this a long-standing problem? Tell me more about it.

Client: I've had it for several years. I've been taking a drug called Clinoril, but I ran out about a week ago.

Asking about understanding of current problem

Nurse: Without the drug your arthritis is much worse?

Client: I don't know if it's worse, but I don't cope with it as well.

Asking about assistance client needs

Nurse: What would you like us to do for you today?

Client: Well, I would like to get another prescription for Clinoril. But I heard that relaxation techniques are effective with arthritis pain. I would like to talk about this with you or the doctor.

In the above example, the nurse is using both open-ended and direct questions to obtain the necessary information. Both types of questions are useful. However, they each seek different types of information. **Open-ended questions** do not restrict responses to a specific topic or theme. However, they can be used to seek elaboration from clients on a particular topic. They encourage client involvement and self-exploration because they elicit responses that are more than one or two words in length. In answering this type of question, clients provide their thoughts, perceptions, and feelings regarding the issue under discussion. For instance, in the above example when the nurse asks the open-ended question "What brings you to the hospital today?", the client provides an explanation for the present hospital visit.

On the other hand, **direct questions** usually seek yes, no, or other short responses from clients. In the above example, "Is this a long standing problem?" is a direct question, followed by an open-ended statement, "Tell me more about it."

It is important that nurses match the appropriate type of question to the type of information that is sought. In some situations, it is essential to obtain factual information quickly so that clients' problems can be expeditiously handled. At other times, it is more important to understand the clients' perceptions of their problem. Usually, however, a mix of open-ended and direct questions is most effective.

In addition to the use of open-ended and direct questions, the empowering communication techniques presented earlier in the chapter are useful tools within the interview situation. Additional general suggestions for inquiring about health history, current health status, and nursing care and assistance needed appear in Table 14–7. The reader will also find sample questions pertinent to specific alterations in functioning in the Assessment sections in Chapter 16 and each of the chapters in Unit 6.

Formal Interview. The formal interview is usually longer and more structured than the informal interview. Frequently nurses use a printed form, checklist, or outline that may consist of topic headings or questions. This approach seeks to guarantee a complete and comprehensive data collection. Box 14–2 summarizes suggestions for effective interviewing.

BOX 14–2. SUGGESTIONS FOR EFFECTIVE INTERVIEWING

1. Establish a verbal contract with clients. This includes giving clients the interviewer's name, title, role, or position. The purpose for the interview, which is usually to form the basis for planning or evaluating care, is also explained. The client is informed of the approximate length of the interview and whether the nurse will be taking notes. The issue of confidentiality is also discussed.
2. Sit at client's level.
3. Make the setting as private and as free from distractions as possible.
4. Attend to clients' immediate physical needs before expecting that they can focus on the interview.
5. Vary the approach and format to meet the clients' needs. For instance, a client who is deaf, unable to talk, or easily fatigued will necessitate a modification in a nurse's approach.
6. Use both direct and open-ended questions, depending on the type of information sought. An effective interviewer balances the use of these two approaches.
7. Collect only data that are not available elsewhere. It is a waste of both clients' and nurses' time to seek information that is readily available on the chart.
8. Collect only information that is relevant to client care.
9. Respect the clients' rights to refuse to provide all requested data.
10. As the interview draws to a close, inform clients that the process is almost complete. A statement such as "I only have two more questions" helps clients to focus on the interview without wondering how much longer it will last. This also gives clients an opportunity to raise any final questions before the interview is over.
11. Summarize the data acquired through the interview process. This provides a mechanism to validate data with clients and to assure that nurses' perceptions are correct.

TABLE 14–7. SUGGESTED QUESTIONS FOR CLIENT INTERVIEW

I. Past health history, level of general health knowledge	1. Tell me about yourself, your family and your past health problems. 2. What kind of things have you found helpful in maintaining your health? 3. Describe the things in your life that make it difficult to stay healthy. 4. How do you usually react when you feel sick? 5. When you feel sick, what do you need from the people around you to help you feel better?
II. Current concern and level of understanding	1. Tell me the symptoms of the problem you are experiencing. 2. Describe how you handled this health problem when you first noticed it. 3. Does anything make you feel better? 4. How do you feel now? 5. What do you know about your illness? 6. What have you been told about the treatments or tests that are planned for you? 7. What do you expect to result from your treatment? 8. Who has provided you with this information?
III. Assistance desired	1. Is there anything that requires further explanation? 2. As you think about this situation, what do you anticipate will be the hardest part of it? 3. Illness frequently disrupts a person's daily routine. Do you anticipate any specific problems? 4. How do you think your illness/condition will affect your family? 5. What do you think would assist you in feeling more comfortable? 6. Who is available to help you?

SUMMARY

Communication encompasses the process of interacting with others. Its main purpose is the transference of meaning. This purpose has many implications for nurses in teaching, facilitating others' expressions of feelings, relieving anxiety, promoting problem-solving, and asserting self. The collaborative approach is inherent in each of these aspects. Communication can be collaborative, when clients' thoughts and feelings are valued and sought after. Or it can be controlling, as when nurses limit or block clients' input. To provide effective care, nurses must understand the importance of collaborative, empowering communication and the techniques that facilitate as well as hinder this process.

Communication occurs through verbal and nonverbal modes. The nonverbal mode—which involves the use of response time, body, voice, and environment—comprises the majority of communication. Nonverbal communication presents a greater challenge to nurses in making the correct interpretation and most appropriate response. Metacommunication, which refers to the meaning behind the verbal and nonverbal modes, is another important element in understanding the communication process.

Empowering communication, which is essential to collaboration, responds to clients' verbal and nonverbal messages and communicates acceptance. Specific techniques of empowering communication include the use of listening, attending behaviors, and the techniques of warmth, empathy, respect, concreteness, genuineness, self-disclosure, confrontation, and immediacy.

Several listener behaviors can serve as barriers to empowering communication. The most important block is failure to listen to what clients are really saying. The other blocks include failure to probe, failure to examine clients' meaning, following standard forms too closely, being judgmental, using false reassurance, rejecting and defending statements, giving advice, making stereotyped responses, and changing the topic.

The interview is presented as an example of a structured conversation with a specific purpose—to gather information. Interviews can be informal or formal; different techniques are appropriate to each type. Interviewing is a necessary nursing activity which serves to collect data for research, admission to a health care unit, and planning collaborative client care. Effective communication skills on the part of nurses are integral to the interview process.

REFERENCES

1. Satir V. *Peoplemaking*. Palo Alto, CA: Science and Behavior Books; 1972.
2. Lewis GK. *Nurse–Patient Communication*. 2nd ed. Dubuque, IA: William C. Brown; 1973.
3. Travelbee J. *Interpersonal Aspects of Nursing*. Philadelphia: Davis; 1971.
4. Ruesch J, Bateson G. *Communication: The Social Matrix of Psychiatry*. 2nd ed. New York: Norton; 1968.
5. Erikson EH. *Childhood and Society*. New York: Norton; 1963.
6. Sundeen S, Stuart G, Rankin E, Cohen S. *Nurse–Client Interaction: Implementing the Nursing Process*. 4th ed. St. Louis: Mosby; 1989.
7. Ruesch J. *Disturbed Communication: The Clinical Assessment of Normal and Pathological Communicative Behavior*. New York: Norton; 1972.
8. Gazda G, Asbury FS, Balzer FJ, et al. 4th ed. *Human Relations Development*. Boston: Allyn & Bacon; 1991.
9. Wilson HS, Skodol CR. *Psychiatric Nursing*. 3rd ed. Menlo Park, CA: Addison-Wesley; 1988.
10. Langer S. *Philosophy in a New Key*. New York; New American Library; 1951.
11. Hayakawa SI. *Language Meaning and Maturity*. New York: Harper & Row; 1954.
12. Ruesch J, Keys W. *Non-verbal Communication*. Los Angeles: University of California Press; 1968.
13. Hall ET. *The Hidden Dimension*. Garden City, NY: Doubleday; 1969.
14. Satir V. *Conjoint Family Therapy*. 3rd ed. Palo Alto, CA: Science and Behavior Books; 1983.
15. Palmer ME, Deck ES. Teaching assertiveness to seniors. *Nurs Outlook*. 1981; 29:305.
16. Rogers C. Empathic: An unappreciated way of being. *Counseling Psychologist*. 1975; 5:2.
17. Wilson D. Working with translators. *Calif Nurse*. 1987; 83:8.
18. Quinn M. Whose turn to break the silence? . . . Nurses when they are unable to communicate with patients. *Nurs Times*. 1986; 82:47.
19. Yurick AG. Communication: Hearing and speech of the elderly person and the nursing process. In: Yurick AG, Spier BE, Robb SS, Ebert NJ, eds. *The Aged Person and the Nursing Process*. Norwalk, CT: Appleton & Lange; 1989: 516–558.
20. Peach RK. Language functioning in communication disorders in aging. In: Mueller HG, Geoffrey VC, eds: *Communication Disorders in Aging*. Washington, DC: Gallaudet University Press; 1987.

BIBLIOGRAPHY

Arnold E, Boggs K. *Interpersonal Relationships Professional Skills for Nurses*. Philadelphia: Saunders; 1989.

Bebb R. Care to talk? . . . Communication a very important issue. *Nurs Times*. 1987;83:40–41.

Burgoon J, Buller D, Hale J, Deturk M. Relational messages associated with nonverbal behaviors. *Human Communic Res*. 1984;10: 354.

Burnard D. Meaningful dialogue. *Nurs Times*. 1987;83:43–45.

Kasch C. Interpersonal competence and communication in the delivery of nursing care. *Adv Nurs Sci*. 1984;71.

Nimocks MJA. Communication and the terminally ill: A theoretical model. *Death Studies*. 1988;11:323–344.

Phillips A. Alternative systems of communication. *Geriatr Nurs*. 1987;7:25–27.

UNIT FIVE
The Nursing Process as Collaboration

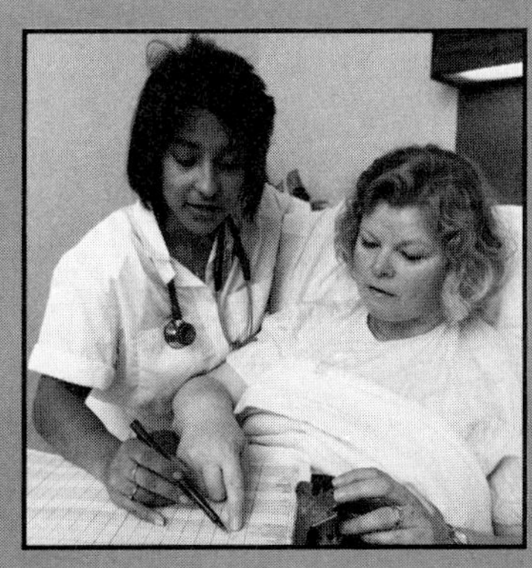

CHAPTER 15

Professional Decision Making and the Nursing Process

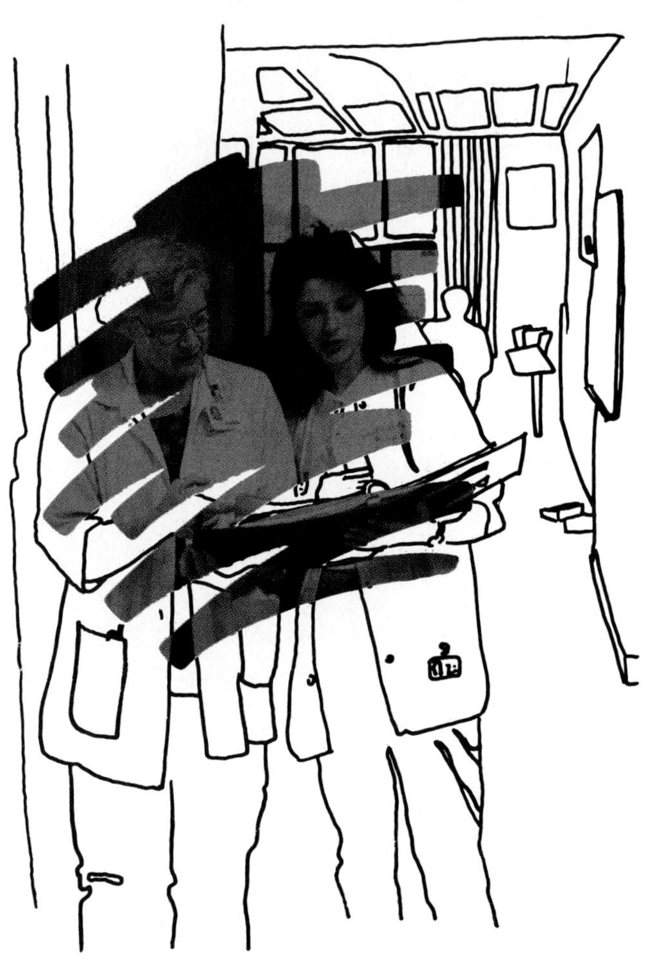

Behavioral Objectives

Upon completion of this chapter, the student will be able to:

1. Define professional decision making.
2. Describe the advantages of a systematic, deliberative process such as the nursing process.
3. Discuss the use of nonsystematic approaches to decision making.
4. Compare the formats of the four nursing process models.
5. Describe the phases and steps of the Berger–Williams model.
6. Describe inductive and deductive reasoning processes for data collection.
7. Identify data evaluation strategies for improving data analysis.
8. Identify the factors in the decision environment that influence the complexity and uncertainty of professional decision making.
9. Describe three decision analysis methods for enhancing decision making.
10. Describe the characteristics of the decision maker that influence decision making.
11. Discuss the collaborative role of clients in health care decisions.

KEY TERMS

assessment phase
data analysis
data collection
decision analysis methods
decision environment
deductive reasoning
evaluation
heuristics
hypothesis
implementation
inductive reasoning
management phase
maximizing strategy
nursing diagnosis
nursing process
optimizing strategy
planning
preventive care
professional decision making
rehabilitative care
restorative care
satisficing
supportive care

Professional nurses make decisions constantly in the course of their daily routines. Decisions about a client's state of health and appropriate actions to take are the foundation of professional nursing practice. These decisions are made within the context of the nursing process, a logical, systematic, and deliberative framework for decision making that enables nurses to make rational and effective decisions.

Professional decision making is a methodical, systematic way of acquiring and combining information to make choices from among a set of alternatives.[1] Decision making can be characterized as *rational* when knowledge of the relevant data, alternatives, choices, and their possible outcomes is thorough and when the alternative chosen is the best one possible for achieving the desired goal.[2] In health care, few decisions are truly rational because (1) not all information is known; (2) some information is unreliable (that is, it varies or changes from one situation to the next); and (3) characteristics of the decision maker and variables in the decision environment sometimes influence the decision process and outcomes. Hogarth[3] states that health care professionals' decision making can be labeled "bounded rationality." Bounded rationality means that given a lack of complete information, decision makers still aim for the best possible outcomes using the most accurate and complete data available.

In this chapter, the term *rational decision making* implies that decision making is "bounded" and not purely rational.

The nursing profession, as other professions, subscribes to the values of science—control, precision, systematic procedures, scrutiny, and deliberation. Thus, professional nurses value the systematic approach to decision making. Systematic decisions, those based on methodical analyses, professional knowledge, and scientific facts, are viewed as more rational, more carefully considered, and thus more likely to be appropriate to the client care problems nurses encounter.

This chapter discusses the relationship of professional decision making to client care. An overview of several common nonsystematic approaches to decision making is provided. The nursing process, a deliberative systematic model for making decisions, is described in terms of its organizational structure, content, and steps. The factors that influence decision making and contribute to the complexity of health care decision making are then discussed. The nature of the decision task, the decision environment, and the characteristics of the decision maker that may influence decision making are described. Several decision analysis methods that enhance decision making are presented. Finally, a philosophy of professional decision making, the collaborative philosophy, which has particular value for contemporary nursing, is discussed.

APPROACHES TO DECISION MAKING

Professional nurses are characterized, in part, by self-directing behaviors, by decision making based on a well-defined body of knowledge, and by accountability for the actions and outcomes of their decision making. The approaches nurses use to make health care decisions should reflect these professional behaviors. There are several approaches to decision making. Some approaches are more systematic, reliable, and trustworthy than others and should be used by professional nurses when appropriate.

Systematic Approaches

A systematic approach uses a structured, organized method to analyze situations and gain understanding concerning the rational choice to make. Using a systematic approach, professional nurses actively identify, evaluate, and select essential information for making decisions. The current decision situation is compared with prior knowledge and experiences to gain insight about the decisions that must be made. If previous knowledge is not available, nurses seek out appropriate resources to assist in the decision process. Thus, systematic decision making is an organized, deliberative, and directed process. The nursing process, described later in the chapter, is an example of a systematic approach to decision making.

Nonsystematic Approaches

Other approaches to decision making are less systematic and may lead to an incorrect understanding of the situation and errors in judgment. There may be little analysis and deliberation during the decision-making process when nonsystematic approaches are used. Information and solutions may be selected with little consideration of the appropriateness for the current situation. Nonsystematic approaches were used frequently in the past by nurses because of the state of nursing practice at that time. Nurses did not have the responsibility and accountability for the decisions that today's professional nurses view as routine practice. Although there are some benefits to these nonsystematic approaches, especially when combined with a more systematic approach, nurses must be cautious not to rely on a nonsystematic approach when a more reliable, rational, and deliberative approach is available. In this section, nonsystematic approaches to decision making are described.

In the past, nurses commonly relied on four nonsystematic decision approaches: tradition, authority, trial and error, and habit. These methods evolved because early nursing training and practice occurred in religious, military, and physician-controlled hospitals.[4] Thus, authority and tradition models were the primary basis for decision making. In addition, education in academic institutions, with the subsequent knowledge and skills in scholarly inquiry, are recent additions to nurses' education. Therefore, nurses relied on an approach such as trial and error to make decisions, as it was the only approach available.

Tradition. Tradition is an approach based on beliefs, values, customs, or norms that have been handed down over time. Most traditions are not based on scientific knowledge; however, they often are held as "truth" by those who ascribe to them. Many nursing practices are based on tradition passed from nurse to nurse. For example, the time of day when vital signs are monitored often is not based on the best time to capture important data related to a client's physical condition. Usually, this practice is based on the "tradition" that vital signs are taken at a set time each day, frequently the beginning of each shift.

Many times, traditions are difficult to change especially if those in authority support the "old ways." Even in situations where changes in practice are recommended on the basis of research findings, those who support the traditional approach may block or hinder the change with the explanation, "That's how we always perform this procedure." Others may deny accountability and justify their decisions by using the same explanation, "This is the way it's always been done."

Some traditions have had a positive influence on practice because they are based on important values, such as caring. Some traditions also have been the impetus for new discoveries and changes in practice. For example, Nightingale's guidelines for maintaining a clean, safe environment for clients led to the evolution of the current principles of hygiene and aseptic techniques. Nurses continue the tradition of maintaining a clean, safe environment for clients. Today, however, nurses' decision making goes beyond the reliance on traditional practices. Decision making is more deliberative and less passively accepting of directives. For example, good handwashing is a tradition. Professional nurses not only practice good handwashing but also examine the hygiene situation specific to a client. Nurses assess clients' risk for nosocomial infections and develop specific plans for preventing these infections in clients.

Although traditions in nursing often are important, some lack the scientific evidence to support their continued practice. Therefore, nurses should examine decisions based on traditional practices for their effectiveness in meeting clients' needs.

Authority. Authority, as an approach to decision making, means that information and direction come from other individuals who are respected, powerful, or revered,[4,5] or from an established policy or regulation. Nurses' early image as "handmaidens" evolved from the practice of acting on the basis of decisions of the administrative matron, physician, or military officer. In most situations, decision making was not considered the responsibility of nurses. Nurses today experience a range of decision-making responsibilities from independent nursing judgments to interdependent judgments in collaboration with other health care professionals.

There are situations in which authority is an accepted and appropriate decision-making approach. For example, in an emergency situation, a leader is usually selected to direct the actions of others as there is limited time for discussion or deliberation. Also, institutional policies often direct how practice is implemented. In both cases, an authority directs decision making and serves to protect consumers.

Although decision making by authority may be appropriate in some situations, it should not be used as a substitute for discretion and rational decision making when the latter is appropriate. Also, authorities can be wrong. For example, policies often need to be changed or updated so as to be consistent with current knowledge. Professional nurses, therefore, question, examine, and systematically challenge practices based on authority to ensure that the directive is consistent with accurate, effective, and optimal decision making.

Trial and Error. Trial-and-error decision making connotes that one or more interventions are tried until something succeeds in improving the situation. Trial-and-error decision making was common in the past. Nurses did not have the knowledge base or the research skills to study clinical problems systematically.

There are many disadvantages to the trial-and-error method of decision making. First, this approach may be time-consuming. The time lost searching for a solution may produce negative consequences for clients who require immediate, successful interventions. In addition, there may not be a clear relationship between the client situation, the choice of intervention, and the client outcome. Implementation of unsafe or inappropriate nursing actions may result.[5] Without explicit documentation of the decision-making process and subsequent outcomes, it is difficult to replicate the decisions in new situations, share knowledge about the decision making with other nurses, and document the quality of care delivered to clients.[5]

When essential information is not available, particularly in very complex or unusual situations, then the judicious use of trial-and-error decision making may be necessary. The process, however, should be as systematic as possible, with alternatives sequentially narrowed by trying approaches one by one and observing and documenting clients' responses to each approach.

Trial-and-error decision making should not be used when more systematic and deliberative processes are available. For example, in treating pressure sores nurses used to try different interventions until something worked. Today, however, nurses use research-based knowledge to evaluate the efficacy of different interventions for achieving specific outcomes for clients with these problems. Nurses no longer rely on trial-and-error methods to diagnose and treat pressure sores.

Habit. Habit, also called tenacity, means that nurses use prior decision behaviors to make choices for current client situations without deliberating on their appropriateness for new situations. Although in some cases habitual strategies can be a starting point for identifying decision options, nurses who rely on habit may not systematically consider new information. In addition, contradictory information often is blocked as it does not support the habitual decision.[4] For example, Johnson reported that nurses frequently selected an intervention to relieve pain before assessing the client and did not alter their choices even when information about the client was available.[6] In other words, the nurses implemented pain interventions they had always used in the past, and did not deliberate about the appropriate use of the interventions for the new client.

As with other nonsystematic approaches, habitual practices are not always wrong to use, but they should not be used in place of a more systematic decision-making process. Williamson suggested that practices based on habit should be investigated for effectiveness.[4] Further, nurses should not blindly implement a practice without considering the scientific basis of the practice and the appropriateness for clients.

In summary, several nonsystematic approaches to decision making may be used by nurses. Although nonsystematic approaches can be useful in guiding practice and stimulating further systematic deliberation, these approaches may be unreliable and may result in errors in judgment. Professional nurses rely more heavily on systematic and deliberative approaches to decision making.

IMPLICATIONS FOR PROFESSIONAL COLLABORATION

Authority

When nurses use authority as a basis for their decision making, they are directed by others who are respected, powerful, or revered. Nurses' early image as handmaidens evolved from their practice of basing professional decisions on the directives of a matron, physician, or military officer. In the past, authority for decision making rested in one's position. Today, nurses make a wide range of independent professional decisions and participate in an equally broad range of collaborative decisions, decisions that represent the consensus of health care professionals from various disciplines working together. Collaboration is characterized by the sharing of authority for decision making, and authority rests not with one's position, but with one's expertise.

Nurses should seek the best information and knowledge available in making decisions. They should evaluate, and not passively accept, rules, regulations, and physicians' orders. Professional nurses today also have greater responsibility and accountability for their decisions. They must justify their decisions on the basis of methodical analyses, professional knowledge, and scientific facts.

■ THE NURSING PROCESS: A SYSTEMATIC MODEL FOR MAKING PROFESSIONAL DECISIONS

The **nursing process** is a deliberative systematic approach for making decisions about a client's health state and improvements that can be achieved through nursing therapies, the specific nursing implementation to accomplish these changes, and the effectiveness of the implementation. Although there are several systematic nursing process models, in this chapter the Berger–Williams collaborative two-phase model is used as an example of the structure and content of the nursing process.[7] Approaches and strategies for processing information and making effective and efficient decisions through the use of the nursing process are described.

Model Variations

Nursing literature has not emphasized nursing process as an important aspect of nursing practice until relatively recently. Although offering comfort and supportive care to clients has long been a dominant theme in descriptions of nursing, emphasis on using a systematic process to identify approaches to care was not apparent until the 1950s. Several nursing process models with varying numbers of steps have evolved to help nurses organize client care. The American Nurses' Association described a five-phase model for nursing process in their 1973 document, *Standards for Nursing Practice*.[8] As seen in Table 15–1, there are differences in the steps and terms used in the two-, three-, four-, and five-phase models, but in general the processes are similar.

In each nursing process model, some steps help nurses assess the health state of clients, and other steps organize the actions to be performed to assist clients. Models usually include assessment data, a nursing diagnosis, desired outcomes, implementation, and evaluation data. Thus, nursing process models focus on several types of decisions that nurses make concerning clients: the health problem amenable to nursing treatment, called the nursing diagnosis; the desired nature of change in health status; what should be done to achieve that change; and what to do if the desired change is not accomplished as a result of actions taken.

In describing the steps, different authors emphasize different phases. For example, in the five-phase model, particular importance is placed on determining the nursing diagnosis. In the four-phase model, nursing diagnosis is incorporated into the assessment phase. Authors also may vary the terminology used in the models. For example, authors use the terms *implementation, intervention, action,* and *treatment* to describe the step of carrying out the plan of care. The terms *outcomes, goals,* and *objectives* are used interchangeably, with *outcome* being the currently preferred term. Although the variation in the models may initially be confusing, as nurses work with different nursing process terminology used in various health care settings, transitions to different models are easily made.

Regardless of model, the steps of the nursing process, from assessment to evaluation, are not necessarily distinct and sequential. Several steps may be considered concurrently. For example, nurses consider client information that is important for formulating the nursing diagnosis and for deciding on the appropriate actions to take. Or, in selecting an action, nurses consider the nursing diagnosis, the desired outcomes, and other possible approaches and consequences. The nursing process is both systematic, that is, organized and deliberative, and dynamic, that is, changing to meet the needs of clients. As new information is available, or clients' needs change, or the plan is not as effective as first conceived, nurses can initiate changes in all or part of the steps in the nursing process to improve the plan of care.

Decision Making in the Nursing Process

The Berger–Williams model[7] is a two-phase, six-step nursing process model (see Table 15–1). This model illustrates the organizational structure of the nursing process and the decision making that occurs in a deliberative nursing process model. The chapters in Unit VI provide examples of application of this model.

TABLE 15–1. COMPARISON OF NURSING PROCESS FORMATS

Two-Phase Model	Three-Phase Model	Four-Phase Model	Five-Phase Model
1. Assessment a. Data collection b. Data analysis c. Nursing diagnosis	1. Assessment	1. Assessment	1. Assessment 2. Nursing diagnosis
2. Management a. Planning b. Implementation c. Evaluation	2. Decision 3. Action	2. Planning 3. Intervention 4. Evaluation	3. Planning 4. Intervention 5. Evaluation

Assessment. Assessment is the first step of the Berger–Williams nursing process model.[7] The purpose of the **assessment phase** is to obtain information and to formulate a decision about a client's health status. The assessment phase consists of three steps: data collection, data analysis, and developing nursing diagnoses.

Data Collection. During **data collection,** nurses systematically identify, evaluate, and select information. Nurses use a variety of sources, such as clients, families, health records, physicians, nurses, and other health care professionals, to gather accurate, relevant, and high-quality information. Nurses also use well-developed sensory-perceptual skills, such as listening, touching, and observing, to assess clients and gather information.

Nurses usually categorize the information they collect according to the type of data, for example, historical, physical, or diagnostic. This structure provides order to the data collection procedures, helps identify missing data, and assists nurses in managing the large amount of information collected. Chapter 16 discusses the client history, physical examination in depth.

There are two approaches for collecting data for making decisions about the client health state: a deductive reasoning process and an inductive reasoning process.[5] The difference between approaches is based on whether data collection is guided by a hypothesis or concludes with a hypothesis. A **hypothesis** is a tentative assumption.

In **deductive reasoning,** thinking moves from general principles, for example, the hypothesized nursing diagnosis, to the collection of specific data that confirm or negate the nursing diagnosis. Hypotheses are based on scientific knowledge; however, they still require careful evaluation and verification.

Physicians frequently use a hypothesis-driven, deductive data collection approach. Within the first few minutes of interaction with clients, physicians generate three to five hypotheses about the client health state, that is, the medical diagnoses. Next, information is gathered to confirm the hypotheses. New hypotheses are formed if the data fail to confirm or negate the original hypotheses. This deductive reasoning process is used to more efficiently manage large amounts of data when making decisions.

The second approach to collecting data during the assessment phase is an inductive reasoning approach.[5] In **inductive reasoning,** thinking moves from particular facts to a general principle. In terms of decision making, inductive reasoning means that nurses collect information first and then make a hypothesis (nursing diagnosis) concerning a client's health state.

Inductive processes are used frequently in nursing because, until recently, nursing diagnoses were not well developed and verified. Nurses could not place as much confidence in their hypotheses as physicians did; therefore, they did not use them to narrow and focus their data collection. Instead, nurses collected information and then made decisions about the health state of clients.

Although an inductive process can be useful in some situations, there is a serious limitation to this data collection approach. Nurses are very susceptible to information overload because of the large amount of data they collect. Information overload is the inability of the short-term memory to process information in large quantities. The short-term memory is limited in capacity and duration.[9,10] Only five to nine chunks of information can be processed by short-term memory at any one time. In addition, short-term memory of data lasts only about 30 seconds without repeated rehearsal of the information. Because of these biological limits, inductive approaches often produce large amounts of data that cannot be completely and accurately processed. To compensate for memory processing limitations, people often simplify and generalize information. As a result, important data may not be processed correctly or adequately, and errors in judgment may result.[11]

Researchers and practitioners have observed difficulties in data collection and decision making related to information overload in nursing.[10] According to several researchers, nurses gather too much data, have difficulty with the identification of essential data, do not discriminate between the usefulness of data items, and do not base their confidence in the decision on the value of the information collected.[12–14] In addition, large amounts of data often are used to bolster confidence in the decision even though the data do not increase diagnostic accuracy and may hamper the decision process as a result of information overload.[11,12,14,15] Therefore, improvements in data collection and decision making may occur if nurses used deductive reasoning strategies more frequently when making decisions about the client's health state.

To illustrate a hypothesis-driven deductive data collection approach, consider a nurse whose new client is an elderly woman. From the nurse's knowledge about elderly people, the nurse identifies several hypotheses concerning the client's health state. One possible nursing diagnosis could be functional incontinence as this is a frequent problem for the elderly. The nurse then focuses data collection on information that would confirm or negate this hypothesized diagnosis. Because of this focused data collection technique, the nurse is less likely to experience information overload and the subsequent errors in judgment.

Data Analysis. Once the data concerning the client health state have been collected, the next step in the assessment phase of the nursing process is **data analysis,** the process of analyzing and interpreting the data. This step leads to the decision on the nursing diagnosis (see Table 15–1).

As in the data collection step, nursing process models assist in the analysis of client data. For example, in the Berger–Williams model,[7] nurses use a matrix (see Chap. 17) to help identify information that is relevant and important to consider. A nursing process matrix is a rectangular arrangement of rows and columns into which specific data concerning a client's functioning are recorded. The matrix also helps to alert nurses to data that are irrelevant, redundant, or noncontributory so that this information can be eliminated from the analysis and thus decrease information overload.

There are several data evaluation strategies to help nurses identify and use the best quality data for data analysis. A strategy is a plan or guide for effectively and efficiently accomplishing a task.

Importance of the Data. Determining the importance of the data used in the decision-making process is the first strategy. Data items are evaluated on importance based on whether the information is essential, contributory, or noncontributory for making the nursing diagnosis.

ESSENTIAL DATA. Essential data are pieces of information that are highly relevant, discriminate one nursing diagnosis from another, and are definitive in making a decision.[10] Essential data are necessary to recognize and consider for formulating an accurate nursing diagnosis. Essential data are observed when the diagnosis is formulated and are not observed when the diagnosis is absent. Without these characteristics, the information is of little value in discriminating between several nursing diagnoses.

CONTRIBUTORY DATA. A second type of important data is contributory data. Contributory data are data that are helpful in making a decision but are not essential for making the decision.[10] For example, information such as "change in client's sleep pattern" may contribute to or help establish the nursing diagnosis of Chronic Pain but it is not essential for making the diagnosis; nor does it discriminate between several other nursing diagnoses.

NONCONTRIBUTORY DATA. Noncontributory data are irrelevant, redundant, conflicting, or nondiscriminatory pieces of information.[10] They are not important for making the nursing diagnosis and, in fact, may be harmful. Collecting noncontributory information often overloads nurses with information and may produce errors in judgment.[10]

Type of Measurement. Another strategy for data analysis is evaluation of the type of measurement used in collecting the information. Whenever possible, a quantitative or numerical measurement should be used to obtain data. Nurses can accurately assess and document comparisons and changes in clients' status when numerical scales are used. An observation that a client "slept well" does not convey as much useful information as the number of hours of sleep or the number of interruptions of sleep. Clients' perceptions of their health also can be quantified, for example, asking a client with chest pain to rate the pain on a scale of 1 to 10 ("1" being the lowest level of pain and "10" being the greatest degree of pain). During the next pain episode, a comparison in the intensity of pain can be made and documented.

Nurses also use qualitative data to accurately measure phenomena. Qualitative scales use descriptive words such as very hot, hot, warm, cold, and very cold instead of numbers. Qualitative words often are not as precise as quantitative measures but still can be useful for comparisons.

A common error made by nurses and other health care professionals is recording a judgment about an observation, rather than the actual quantitative or qualitative measurement, and considering this the qualitative data. For example, a client may be described as having "normal blood pressure." "Normal," however, is a judgment, not data. Likewise, nurses often erroneously record interpretations of behavior such as "the client is depressed" or "the client is anxious" as qualitative data. A more accurate communication would be one that describes the *behavior* a client exhibited to cause the *interpretations* of "depressed" or "anxious." This is not to imply that nurses' interpretations are not important. Nurses' judgments or interpretations are a necessary part of data analysis. Nurses interpret data to make diagnoses and to evaluate care, but these interpretations must be about the *meaning* of the data, and not be mistakenly considered data in themselves.

Source of Information. During data analysis, the source of information also should be evaluated for appropriateness and accuracy in providing information. The source of information refers to who or what provided the data. Generally, clients and health care professionals are the best sources of data; however, in some situations, family members or friends are able to remember or make observations that others have missed. If a client's status permits, for example, he or she is not unconscious or confused, data should be verified with the client for accuracy.

Nursing Diagnosis. In the last step of the assessment phase, nurses make nursing diagnoses. One definition of a **nursing diagnosis** is "a clinical judgment about an individual, family, or community that is derived through a deliberate, systematic process of data collection and analysis. It provides the basis for prescriptions for definitive therapy for which the nurse is accountable. It is expressed concisely and includes the etiology of the condition when known" (p. 109).[16] Chapter 17 provides other recognized definitions of nursing diagnosis.

Most often, nursing diagnoses are statements of actual or potential problems. An actual problem is one that a client presently is experiencing, for example, "Severe Activity Intolerance." A potential problem denotes that a client may be at risk for developing a health problem, for example, "Potential for Mild Activity Intolerance." Judgments concerning wellness or health also are nursing diagnoses; however, these wellness diagnoses currently are not as well developed as problem-oriented nursing diagnoses. A wellness diagnosis might be "Excellent Exercise Tolerance." Although wellness diagnoses are not as well established as problem-oriented diagnoses, client strengths that support a healthful life-style should be assessed and documented. Further description of nursing diagnosis development and the numerous nursing diagnoses included in the taxonomy of nursing diagnoses are described in Chapter 17 and Unit VI.

Although nursing diagnosis often is considered a step in the nursing process, it is difficult to separate it from the data analysis step. It is the result of the data analysis and is the label or name given to the condition determined to be present in the analysis step. Analysis of client data results in nursing diagnoses, etiologies, and supporting data. The etiology is the cause of the health state or the factors related to the health state. The supporting data are the essential and contributory information (signs and symptoms) that corroborate or confirm that the diagnosis is appropriate. Supporting data also are called cues (according to the cognitive science perspective) or defining characteristics (according to the North American Nursing Diagnosis Association framework).

In making a nursing diagnosis, nurses judge the likelihood of a diagnosis being present as each data cue is added to the data base. Essential data are the most useful for estimating likelihoods because these cues have greater discriminating power. In nursing, however, making predictions often is difficult because the essential data have not been identified and verified for all nursing diagnoses. Until essential cues for diagnoses are available, nurses must make the best diagnostic judgments possible based on available knowledge and clinical experience. In contrast to nurses, physicians have identified many of the essential cues for their diagnoses and can estimate the likelihoods of diseases (medical diagnoses) based on those essential cues. Because of the availability of data, physicians often use a decision analysis method called Bayes' theorem to help them estimate the likelihood of a diagnosis given certain cues. A description of Bayes' theorem as an aid for improving decision making is presented later in this chapter.

Management. Once the decision has been made as to the nature of a client's health state, that is, the nursing diagnoses, a second phase of decision making in the nursing process begins (see Table 15–1). The **management phase** involves planning, implementation of the plan, and evaluation of the results.

Planning. **Planning** incorporates specifying desired outcomes, selecting nursing implementation, and determining evaluation criteria. Making these choices is difficult as the decision process is complex. There must be consistency between the management decisions and the decisions made in the assessment phase. The relationships among parts of the nursing process sound simple; that is, nurses make nursing diagnoses, determine desired outcomes, and then select appropriate implementation. In reality, however, these choices are not made sequentially nor are they independent of each other.

Desired outcomes are anticipated changes in the client health state. Implementation describes the actions, activities, or treatments that are used to achieve desired outcomes. Implementation approaches are selected because of the consequences (outcomes) they either produce or avoid. Thus, desired outcomes and implementation must be analyzed together to select the best option(s) for addressing the factors causing the client health state.

Nurses use standards to guide their choice of desired outcomes, nursing implementation, and evaluation criteria for inclusion in the care plan. Effective choices are relevant, realistic, and desirable.

Relevance of desired outcomes, implementation strategies, and evaluation criteria pertains to their relationship to the nursing diagnosis and etiology. Nursing students and novice nurses sometimes have difficulty clearly showing these relationships in their assessment and management decisions.

Nurses' decision making should reflect a consistent relationship among the diagnostic statement (including the etiology and defining characteristics), the desired outcomes, and the evaluation criteria. Similarly, there should be a clear relationship among the diagnostic statement, the desired outcomes, and the nursing implementation. These relationships are discussed in greater detail in Chapter 18. They are illustrated in Figure 15–1, using decision making about the nursing diagnosis Activity Intolerance as an example.

Another characteristic of each of the elements of a care plan is that they are realistic. Realistic desired outcomes and evaluation criteria are based on clients' capabilities, desires, and general health goals. Realistic nursing implementation strategies address a client's current health state and aim to facilitate attaining the desired outcomes. Nursing implementation encompasses four levels of care: preventive, supportive, restorative, and rehabilitative.[7,17]

Preventive care is the type of care clients diagnosed as "healthy" would require. Clients and nurses work together to develop desired outcomes and approaches that focus on (1) promoting and maintaining a healthy state, (2) identifying risk factors that predispose clients to future illnesses, and/or (3) developing a preventive care plan to avoid potential problems. For example, a relevant and realistic plan of preventive care can be developed for a client related to nutritional education to reduce risk factors for colon cancer.

Supportive care is concerned with clients who have early stages of alterations in their health state. In general, these clients are able to carry out activities of daily living independently, although nurses may provide some assistance. During supportive care, the extent of the problem is assessed, and desired outcomes and implementation approaches are developed with the focus on managing the existing problem and preventing further disruption. Clients requiring this level of care may need follow-up to manage the care plan over time. An example of this type of problem would be a client with severe sunburn. The associated nursing diagnosis of High Risk for Impaired Skin Integrity is made because of the reported risk factor of frequent sun exposure without sunscreen. A nurse and client would develop a plan of relevant desired outcomes and approaches to support the resolution of the sunburn and reduce the risk for the more serious problem.

Restorative care focuses on the management of acute health problems of a more severe nature. These problems are more critical and multidimensional in nature and require complex nursing implementation. During restorative care, a client's health state is monitored closely. If the client's responses to illness are not immediately addressed, severe consequences may result. Clients with problems such as altered mobility and altered nutrition often need restorative care to improve their current level of functioning and avoid permanent loss of function.

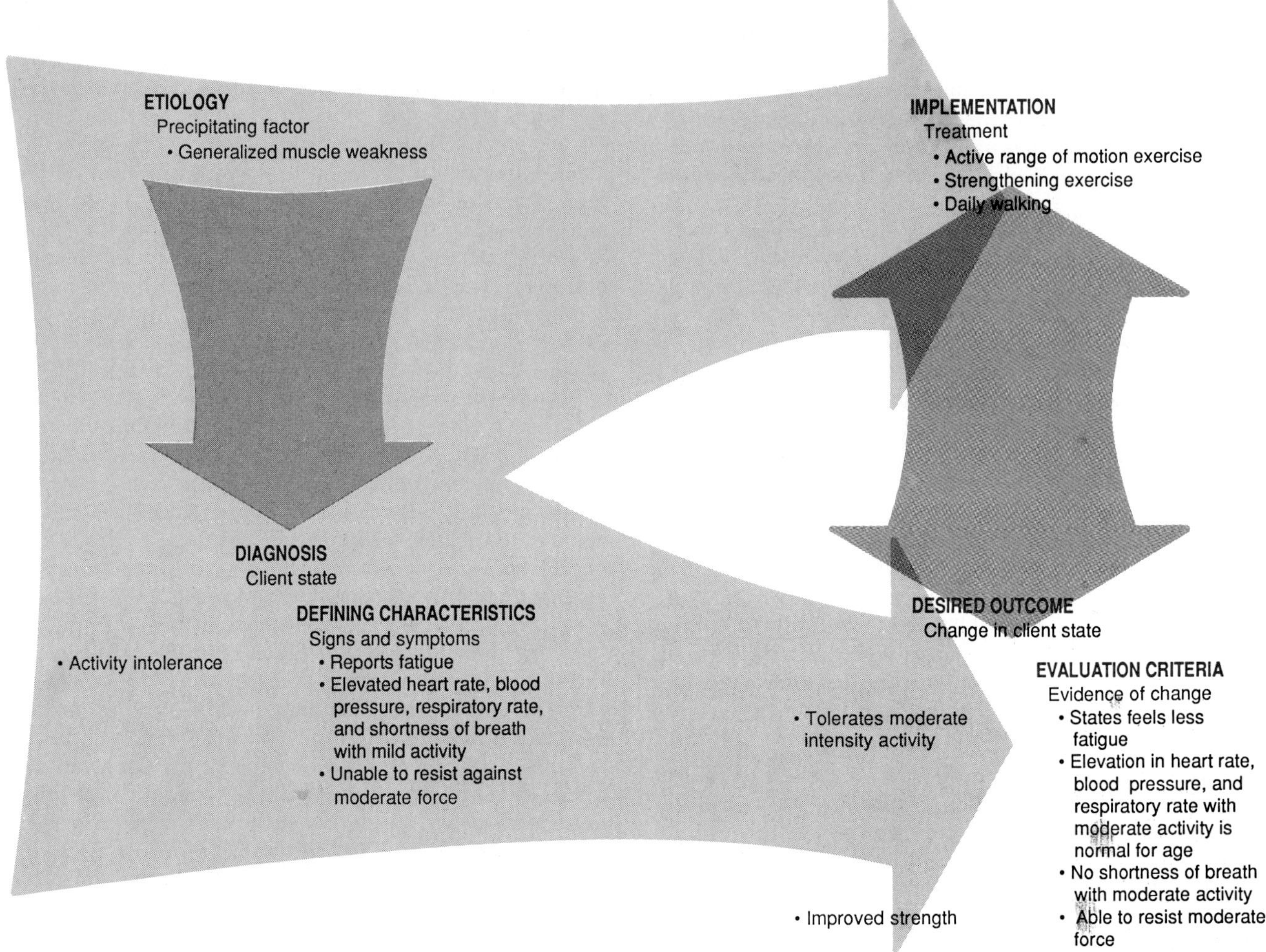

Figure 15–1. Interrelated decisions in the nursing process using as an example Activity Intolerance.

Rehabilitative care requires a management plan that assists clients to return to optimal health after an illness. In some cases, rehabilitative care helps clients achieve new self-definitions and acceptance of permanently altered states of being. Frequently, this level of care is required after severe illness or with multiple health problems; thus, there may be a long period during which nurses and clients work together to achieve desired outcomes. The process of rehabilitative care may be both time-consuming and complex, requiring an extensive understanding of human adaptation and behavior modification. A realistic management plan for rehabilitative care, for example, might focus on teaching a client how to manage activities of daily living after a severe hip fracture.

Desired outcomes, implementation strategies, and evaluation criteria also are selected on the basis of their relative desirability. Relative desirability is the value decision makers assign to the possible outcomes, strategies, and criteria.

Relative desirability also is based on the nature of the outcome desired by a decision maker. If a "perfect solution" is desired, the decision maker would search for the best solution for the problem. This type of desirability is referred to as a **maximizing** or **optimizing strategy.** To achieve an optimal decision, each alternative is evaluated against the others for achieving the outcomes. Maximizing strategies, however, often require valuable time, resources, and expertise. In some situations, like an emergency situation, they may not be practical.

A second strategy for determining the desirability of desired outcomes and proposed implementation is called satisficing. The term **satisficing** is a neologue, a new word derived from the terms *satisfy* and *suffice.* In satisficing, a decision maker searches for a solution only long enough to find one that works and meets the needs of the situation.[18] Certainly, the best decision-making strategy for clients is a maximizing strategy if the time, resources, and information are available. In many instances, however, every alternative solution cannot be considered so nurses may need to be satisfied with a choice that is adequate or suffices for the situation.

Implementation. **Implementation** is giving nursing care. It is activating the plan; that is, carrying out the proposed implementation strategies. Although there are many specific examples of nursing implementation, each of them fits into one of four general categories: therapeutic, teaching, monitoring, and referral.[19]

Therapeutic Implementation. Therapeutic nursing implementation is the most direct form of nursing care. It encompasses treatments and procedures such as skin care, applying sterile dressings, administering medications, and therapeutic communication.

Teaching. Teaching clients is another major category of nursing implementation. Teaching, that is, providing clients with the information they need to care for their health and well-being, is an important aspect of nurse–client collaboration. Nurses' role in health teaching is discussed in Chapter 20.

Monitoring. Another type of nursing action is monitoring; that is, observing and gathering information about a client's current condition and noting any changes in status. Much of this information is used in nursing decision making; however, nurses also "monitor" for other health care professionals. Compared with other providers, nurses spend more time with clients, so they are able to gather information that is useful to physicians, chaplains, social workers, and dietitians, among others.

Referral. The final category of nursing action, referral is also collaborative. Nurses refer clients to other health care professionals to provide continuity of care. Referral may include coordinating the activities of several health care professionals or departments within the health care facility or in the community to provide services to clients. An example of a referral would be a nurse contacting a social worker to provide community services to a client after hospital discharge.

Evaluation. **Evaluation** is a critical step in the nursing process. It is the process of determining the accuracy, significance, and value of assessment and management. It involves comparing outcomes of care to the desired outcomes stated in the plan. If decisions and outcomes are not evaluated, then there is no way of knowing whether the care rendered was appropriate and effective. Evaluation, therefore, is an important aspect of professional decision-making approaches.

An important function of evaluation is to build into the nursing process an element of correction and adjustment. Adjustment means that nurses make modifications to correct any errors and unsuitable decisions, and to better achieve the desired health care goals. As few health care plans are perfect and health care situations change frequently, adjustments and revisions of client care plans are essential to outcome achievement.

Evaluation activities are ongoing throughout the nursing process. Evaluation is done by periodically monitoring progress and responses to the activities specified by the care plan. The differences between desired outcomes and achieved outcomes determine whether the plan should be continued, modified, or stopped. Final evaluation occurs when client care is completed. During terminal evaluation, all phases and steps of decision making during the nursing process are critiqued. Chapter 18 discusses evaluation in detail.

■ NATURE OF DECISIONS IN HEALTH CARE

Decision making in the nursing process is influenced by the interaction between the decision task and the decision environment. Factors associated with the task and the environment contribute to the complexity and uncertainty of decision making in health care.

Decision Task

In the previous section, the process of making diagnostic and treatment decisions is described as a complex and deliberative process because of the many factors associated with the decision task. These factors include the amount and relevance of data, the number of possible client health states, the numerous potential desired outcomes and implementation, the type of reasoning process used, the level of desired care, and the dynamic nature of decision making in the nursing process. The use of a nursing process model and related decision-making strategies is suggested as a way to help organize and systematically structure decision making and reduce some of the complexity and cognitive strain of the decision task.

Decision Environment

The decision environment also influences the complexity of decision making. The **decision environment** is the context—that is, the circumstances, conditions, and setting—in which decisions are made.[20]

Open and Closed Systems. A decision environment is considered a closed system or an open system depending on the availability and certainty of information. In a closed system, there is complete knowledge of relevant variables, values, alternatives, and outcomes.[2] Alternatives can be accurately weighed against each other and an optimal choice made. In other words, rational decision making in its purest form can occur in a closed system. A closed system of decision making, however, is rare in the health care environment. In contrast, an open system[2] of decision making is one in which there is incomplete knowledge of relevant factors, multiple alternative actions and outcomes, and limited information about the likelihood of achieving desired outcomes and the expected values of actions.

Uncertainty and Complexity of Health Care Decisions

Because health care decision making is done in an open system, there is considerable uncertainty and a high degree of complexity in the process. Uncertainty means that all information about a situation is not known beyond doubt. The best that health care professionals can do is state the probability that their decisions are accurate. Thus, decision making in the health care environment is labeled probabilistic. That is, it is not possible to predict precisely or with certainty the outcomes of decisions[20]; only the probability or likelihood of success can be estimated. The uncertainty and probabilistic nature of the health care environment is a reason why people make reasonable and purposeful decisions,[3] but do not make purely rational decisions. As described earlier in the chapter, health care decision making is labeled bounded rationality[3] because of these limitations in available knowledge.

Some health care professionals, including nurses, have difficulty making decisions because they wish to think and act as if health care decisions are made in a purely rational, certain, and closed system. As a result, some professionals experience anxiety, frustration, and decreased confidence in their decision making when the desired decision environment does not match the actual environment. Accepting the probabilistic nature of the health care environment and learning to make decisions in this open system help health care professionals develop better decision-making skills and experience greater satisfaction with decision-making behaviors.

Reasons for Uncertainty and Complexity. An understanding of the reasons for the uncertainty and complexity of health care decision making helps health care professionals manage these difficult situations in a successful manner. Keeney[20] suggested that illuminating the issues related to making probabilistic judgments promotes insight and creativity in making decisions in an open and uncertain decision environment. Keeney[20] described several reasons for the uncertainty and complexity of health care decision making: (1) little or no data are available; (2) some data are available but too expensive or time-consuming to collect; (3) decisions change over time and are sequential in nature; and (4) the behavior of other influential individuals or the effect of external factors—that is, other health care professionals, family, governmental bodies, consumer groups, and administrators—may not be predictable.

IMPLICATIONS FOR PROFESSIONAL COLLABORATION

Uncertainty

Decision makers in health care are forced to make decisions without the benefit of complete information and, thus, are frequently faced with uncertainty. The likelihood that decisions are accurate can only be estimated; outcomes cannot be precisely predicted. Decisions made on this basis are said to have bounded rationality in that they are decisions aimed at the best possible outcome given the information available. One way to help reduce uncertainty and to increase the probability that outcomes are reached is to collaborate with professional peers on decisions for which data are limited. Sometimes, another point of view can identify an additional and important aspect for consideration that contributes to the overall precision of decision making.

Limited Data. In nursing, a consistent problem in decision making is the issue of little or no data on which to base nursing decisions. Knowledge about previous diagnostic and treatment decisions is limited as clinical research concerning decision making by nurses is only about 20 years old. This area of research in nursing is at a seminal level. Nurses currently are studying the relationships between cues and client health states, etiologies and health states, and treatments and subsequent client outcomes. New hospital accreditation policies also are stimulating research and clinical efforts to develop more accurate measures of client outcomes. Although the nature of health care decision making will always be uncertain, nursing research is helping to reduce some of the unnecessary complexity and uncertainty by providing more and better information on which to base nurses' client care decisions.

Costs of Collection. During the past decade, the costs of sophisticated technology and laboratory testing were a major concern for consumers, hospital administrators, insurance companies, nurses, and physicians. In response to this financial crisis, researchers began studying medical decision making to determine if the amount of diagnostic testing and information could be reduced and still produce accurate decisions. There also was concern that young physicians were not developing their diagnostic and treatment skills. Large amounts of unnecessary and redundant information were being used to bolster confidence about their decisions, a practice that was far too expensive and time-consuming. Current medical decision-making research focuses on identifying factors that predict outcomes so that treatment choices can be made wisely and resources used appropriately.

For nursing, the major cost consideration is time. Comprehensive data collection is time-consuming. Increasingly complex nursing care is a fact of life in most health care facilities. Often, immediate care demands compel nurses to make a choice between action and continued data collection, although they may feel considerable uncertainty about what the best action would be.

Changes Over Time. Decisions and outcomes of decision making are influenced by time. Often the consequences (ie, outcomes) cannot be evaluated until a future time. For example, a client may be discharged from an acute care facility with desired outcomes that will not be achieved until some future date. The nurse developing the care plan must therefore consider the long-term implications of the alternatives in the decision-making process.[20] As "long-term horizons"[20] are uncertain, the complexity of the decision process is increased.

Time is also a factor in the sequential nature of decisions. Choices that are made today often affect the availability and desirability of alternatives in the future.[20] The current choice of one nursing implementation strategy may prevent the use of another strategy later.

Priorities of care change over time, adding another element of uncertainty to the decision process. It is often difficult to predict how clients will respond to treatment; therefore, changes in priorities of care might be difficult to anticipate. For example, a client requiring supportive care may experience complications that necessitate a change to a restorative plan of care. Anticipating changes over time adds to the complexity of health care decision making.

Influence of Others. Another characteristic of the complexity of decision making is the influence of others on the decision-making process. Many people, in addition to clients, may be affected by care decisions.[20] For example, the decision to discharge a client with Alzheimer's disease to a nursing home may have significant financial and emotional consequences for the family members.

Other health care professionals' decision making also may be affected by the decisions nurses make with clients. For example, decisions made by nurses may affect the options available to a dietitian or physician. These professionals' choices, in turn, have an impact on nurses' decision making. Considering other health care professionals' treatment plans adds complexity to the decision-making process.

Other factors and entities also influence the decision-making process. Some of these include governmental policies and regulations, accrediting boards, professional regulations, laws, ethical and moral principles, hospital policies and procedures, and the influence of informed consumers.[20] Intangibles such as the good will of clients, workload allocation, reputation of the institution, work satisfaction, and esthetics also may be factors that are important to consider in the decision-making process.[20]

The Use of Decision Analysis Methods to Limit Uncertainty and Complexity

Several systematic and deliberative techniques help health professionals analyze problems in the uncertain, complex, and open system of health care decision making. These techniques are referred to as **decision analysis methods.** Four decision analysis methods that aid decision making are Bayes' theorem, decision trees, and decision analysis matrices and networks. These decision analysis techniques break problems into manageable pieces to improve the accuracy of decision making. Keeney[20] described decision analysis as "a formalization of common sense for decision problems which are too complex for informal use of common sense" (p. 806). Decision analysis methods combine the subjective judgments of the decision maker with objective mathematical data.

Advantages of Decision Analysis. There are many advantages to using a decision analysis method. First, decision analysis methods increase judgmental accuracy by guiding the decision maker in identifying relevant and essential information, and in weighing the value of the information. Decision analysis methods also help identify important but missing data. By logically diagramming decision problems, the decision maker also is better able to analyze the situation and predict the potential outcomes for a client. In addition, the process and rationale for decision making are made explicit. Thus, hidden extraneous variables influencing the decision-making process are recognized. Decision analysis techniques also help decision makers assess the value and costs of acquiring additional information.

Limitations of Decision Analysis. Despite its advantages, decision analysis in health care situations has limitations. According to Baumann and Deber, several factors preclude the routine use of decision analysis in disciplines such as nursing that use process-oriented approaches.[21] These factors include unexpected events that make the problem hard to define, a lack of standardized alternative solutions, the fact that nursing implementations are not mutually exclusive, and the related difficulty in separating the effects of a large number of interdependent actions.

The decision analysis methods that follow are more appropriately used to make institution-wide decisions, for example about policies and procedures. This does not negate the need for a systematic process for many nursing decisions, particularly in developing client care plans, but implies that lengthy decision analyses are impractical for routine care decisions.

Bayes' Theorem. Bayes' theorem is a statistical method used for making clinical diagnostic judgments. Bayes' theorem assists decision makers in estimating the probability of the presence of a diagnosis given the presence of clinical cues and in revising the probability of the diagnosis with the appearance of any new cue. Bayes' theorem combines information about the rate of incidence of the diagnosis, the probability of the cue occurring, and the probability of a cue given a certain diagnosis.[22–25] Consider the example of a nurse who is estimating the likelihood of activity intolerance after observing an increase in a client's systolic blood pressure during bathing. To use Bayes' theorem, the nurse would need to know (1) the incidence of activity intolerance, (2) the probability of an increase in systolic blood pressure regardless of diagnosis, and (3) the frequency of occurrence of an increase in systolic blood pressure with activity intolerance.

The common use of Bayes' theorem in nursing is unlikely in the near future given the current limited knowledge about the probability of clinical cues and their association with nursing diagnoses. Abraham[24] nevertheless argues that the logic underlying Bayes' theorem is important for nursing practice. Nurses need to consider base rate information—that is, the incidence or rate of occurrence in the population of various clinical cues—when making diagnostic judgments and estimating the likelihood of successful outcomes.

Decision Trees. A decision analysis technique that can be used fairly easily by nurses and clients is a decision tree. A decision tree[22,25] is a branching diagram, like a tree, representing various alternative choices and outcomes. Trees can be used for both diagnostic and implementation decisions.

In nursing, decision trees have been used to estimate the likelihood of potential diagnoses given certain data. Jones,[26] for example, developed a decision tree for estimating the risk of pressure sores given client data such as age, mobility, nutrition, pain, and hydration. Decision trees have a variety of formats. Jones'[21] is set up in a yes–no structure. With each question about the presence or absence of a cue (eg, incontinence), the nurse responds "yes" or "no." With each response, the probability of the risk for pressure sores is given. (Probabilities are based on results of clinical research, ideally, or can be estimated from clinical experience.) The nurse continues responding "yes" or "no" as new data (branches) are added to the tree and new probabilities are given. After considering all of the risk factors, the nurse can estimate the risk of pressure sore development in the client.

Decision trees also help nurses identify the value of alternative implementations for achieving specific outcomes. For example, there are several possible alternatives for intervening when the nursing diagnosis is High Risk for Medication Noncompliance related to health beliefs. Figure 15–2 illustrates three implementations that might alter health beliefs and reverse the risk for noncompliant behavior. These implementations include a medication log, a teaching program, and administration of the medication by the daughter. The desired outcome is compliance with the medication regimen.

The decision tree in Figure 15–2 uses a format different from the one described above. In the figure, the shaded box or decision node represents the management decision to be made for the nursing diagnosis. Three branches from the decision node represent the possible approaches to accomplish the desired outcome. This decision tree is a fairly simple decision problem. For more complex decisions, additional branches (ie, implementations) may be added to the tree if needed. For each branch, there is a chance node (diagrammed as a circle) representing the possible outcomes for that implementation. In Figure 15–2, the outcomes are compliance (C) and noncompliance (NC). The estimated probability (p) of the implementation strategy achieving the outcome is given. At the tips of the branches are rectangular boxes representing the final outcomes and the probabilities for achieving these outcomes. By comparing the data in each box, the best and worst outcomes can be estimated. In Figure 15–2, the best outcome for the diagnosis would be achieved by a teaching program in which family members are included in the instruction (compliance, $p = 0.80$). The worst outcome is achieved when the daughter administers the medication (noncompliance, $p = 0.90$). This is reasonable because there is less impact on the client's health beliefs, the causative factor, when the daughter administers the medications; therefore, there is a lower probability of self-adherence to the medication regimen.

BUILDING NURSING KNOWLEDGE

What Models of Decision Making Do Nurses Use in Making Diagnostic Decisions?

Jones JA. Clinical reasoning in nursing. *J Adv Nurs.* 1988; 13:185–192.

To show how nurses approach the diagnosis of client problems, Jones reviews the three models of decision making currently in use: the hypothesis/generation testing model, the decision analysis model, and the information processing model.

Under the hypothesis generation/testing model, nurses pick up cues from clients. Conscious and subconscious decisions are made about which cues are relevant and which are not. This process, called "narrowing the field," reduces cognitive strain but can lead to inaccurate inferences. Early in the diagnostic task, a nurse sets up a tentative hypothesis about the health problem. Preliminary information is organized into crude clusters. When a cluster matches a diagnostic pattern, a hypothesis results. Increased respiratory rate and effort, bluish discoloration around the lips, and noisy breathing might lead to the hypothesis "difficulty in breathing." The nurse then finds evidence to prove or disprove this "hunch," and accepts, refines, or rejects the hypothesis. This model has been criticized for the errors of omission and commission that result from the early narrowing of possibilities.

The decision analysis model reduces intuition-based approaches. This model views decision making as taking place over time and encompassing a series of decision events, the outcomes of which determine the subsequent path the decision-making process takes. This model takes the form of a decision tree, the branches of which are created by "yes–no" questions. At each branching point, a decision has to be made and the consequences of the decision evaluated. The diagnosis of risk of pressure sores would begin with a question about whether the client had experienced previous immobility. If "no," decision makers would then query whether clients were currently confined to bed. Under this model, each branch is followed to evaluate the need for further assessment and the probability of competing diagnoses. This model requires a great deal of high-quality information, which Jones points out is often unavailable in real clinical situations.

The information processing model uses "if–then" inference statements called production rules. For example, a rule for the diagnosis of pressure sores might be "if a client is frail, then the client's mobility level will be decreased." Information about frailty leads to an inference about mobility. This statement may trigger another related rule. Problem solvers operate by using a larger number of rules derived from past learning and experience. According to Jones, this model has the advantage of making decision-making logic easy to comprehend, lends itself to computer simulation programs, and is helpful to beginning clinical decision makers.

Decision Matrix. Another decision aid for reducing the uncertainty and complexity of decision making is a decision matrix. As in a decision tree, the data in a decision matrix are pictorially organized to help the decision maker identify and analyze the alternative choices.

Matrices, like decision trees, can be used for diagnosis or implementation decisions. The use of the Berger–

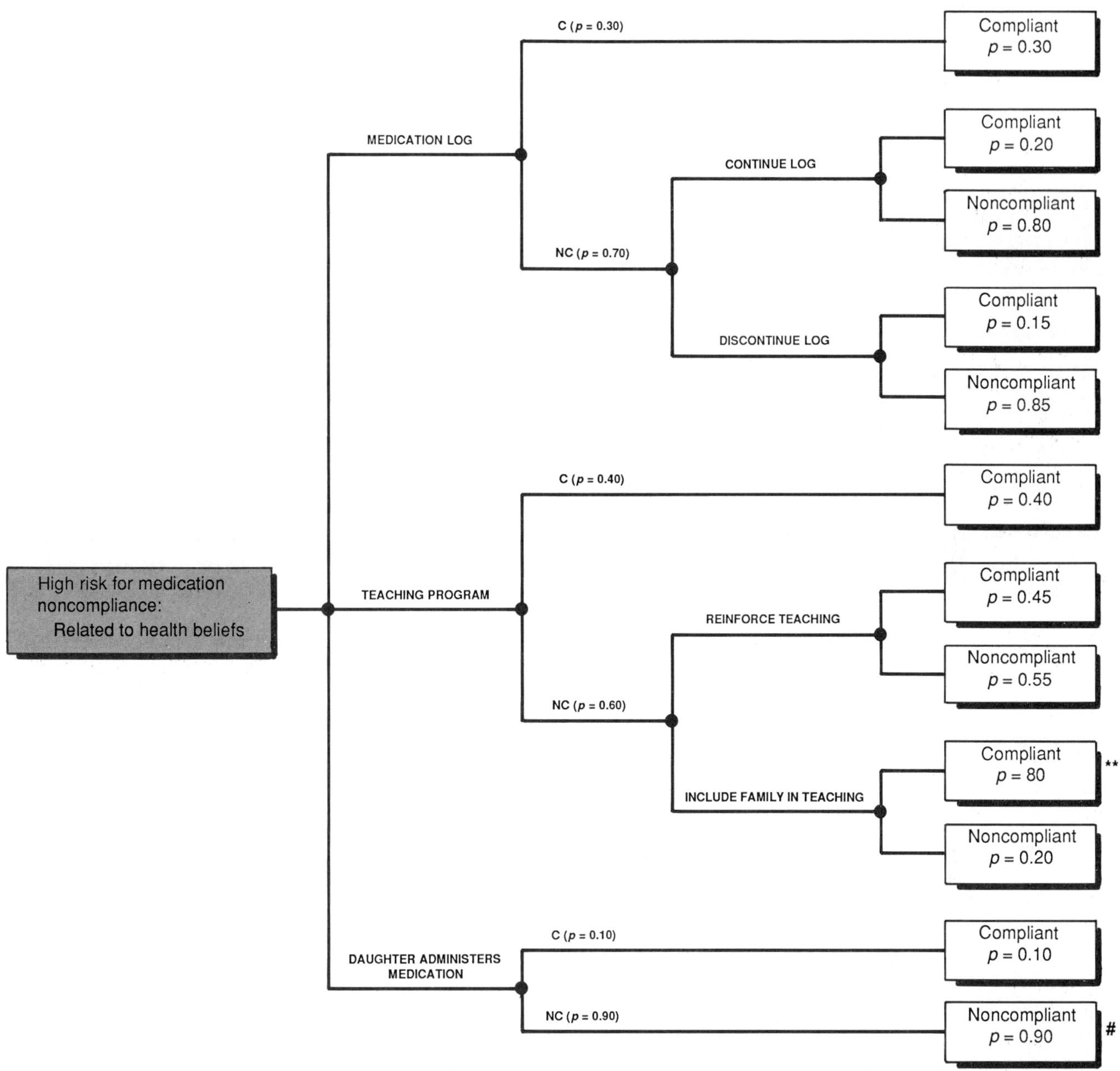

Figure 15–2. Decision tree: alternatives and outcomes for High Risk of Medication Noncompliance Related to Health Beliefs. ** = best outcome (family members are included in the instruction), # = worst outcome (less impact on the client's health beliefs).

Williams matrix for diagnostic decisions was discussed above. The same structure can be applied to implementation decisions. A matrix is developed in which implementations are organized in rows and outcomes are displayed in columns; probabilities are then analyzed. Once the procedure for completing a decision matrix is learned, this decision aid is fairly simple to use in the clinical setting.

Decision matrices can be used for a wide variety of clinical situations. Maclean[27] demonstrated the use of a decision matrix for choosing an implementation by which elderly clients can improve their tolerance to activity. The implementations analyzed were active range of motion, progressive walking, an aerobics class, and dance therapy. These alternatives were evaluated for their usefulness in achieving the desired outcomes of safety, socialization, increased physical conditioning, increased energy, and increased autonomy. A decision matrix of numerical probabilities and utilities was developed, which enabled the selection of the best option and greatly simplified the decision process.

Determining Implementations and Outcomes. An example of a decision matrix is shown in Figure 15–3. Once the client health state is diagnosed, three to five possible implementations and three to five desired outcomes are identified. Implementations and outcomes are selected following the criteria described previously in the nursing process section of this chapter. Although matrices can be designed to accommodate up to 10 implementations and outcomes, limiting the number to three to five each more clearly focuses on the critical aspects of the problem, decreases the processing time, and prevents information overload that can occur when a large number of items are simultaneously analyzed.

Determining Probabilities. After the implementations and outcomes are selected, the estimated probability for each implementation is determined. A number is assigned that reflects the estimated likelihood that the implementation will be effective for a given outcome. Each implementation is assigned a probability separately; however, the probabilities across the various outcomes must add up to exactly 100. This deliberative process of weighing implementations and outcomes helps assure that a rational choice is made.

Making the Decision. Once probabilities are assigned, the decision maker decides which outcomes are the most important and ranks them. Overall totals are determined by multiplying the probability in each cell by the rank assigned to the outcome of the cell.

The final step is to compare the total from each alternative implementation. The implementation with the greatest total is considered the preferred or rational choice.

Networks: The Critical Path Method. One of the greatest sources of complexity in clinical decision making has to do with the numbers of professionals, procedures, and tasks that may be involved in the care of a single client, particularly when the client is hospitalized with a serious illness. Necessary tasks are frequently varied in nature, require different time frames and personnel for completion. Too often, this leads to coordination problems, bottlenecks, and inefficiency. Inefficiency increases costs.

In the current climate of health care, in which cost-effectiveness is essential, providers have turned to decision aids to improve efficiency and reduce costs without sacrificing the quality of care. Networks or project analysis methods (methods designed to streamline decision making in complex undertakings) have thus generated considerable interest among health care professionals. They are increasingly being employed in the clinical settings that care for clients with complex problems.[28]

One such method is the critical path method. This method provides a way of formalizing care planning using time as the critical analytic factor. The critical path method assumes that any care plan entails jobs or tasks that must be completed by a certain time in order for a client to progress within the overall time frame (days of hospitalization) allotted for his or her condition. Institutions that use the critical path method develop typical critical paths for the common diagnosis-related groups treated (see Chap. 35 for more on diagnosis-related groups). Critical paths are similar to standard care plans with the addition of a timeline.

To employ the critical path method, a diagram is made of all of the tasks to be performed in the course of care for a client with a given problem. Tasks are identified that must be completed before other actions can be undertaken. For example, if a client with pneumonia is admitted, prompt initiation of antibiotic therapy is usually critical to the client's improvement and progress. However, it is usually necessary to obtain a sputum specimen before antibiotic therapy can be initiated. To be able to produce the specimen, the client may need to breathe humidified air for a period of time; this requires procuring and installing a humidifier. The critical path for such a client identifies not only the order in which these tasks are to be performed, but also the time frame for their completion.[28,29] It also identi-

Nursing Diagnosis: Activity intolerance R/T sedentary lifestyle

	Outcome A Increased exercise R = 3	Outcome B Reduced fatigue R = 1	Outcome C Increased socialization R = 2	Total Score
Implementation 1: Active range of motion	p = 40	p = 30	p = 30	120 + 30 + 60 = 210
Implementation 2: Progressive walking	p = 50	p = 25	p = 25	150 + 25 + 50 = 225
Implementation 3: Dance therapy	p = 40	p = 20	p = 50	120 + 20 + 100 = 240

p = the estimate of probability that an implementation will achieve an outcome; probabilities are assigned on a scale of 0 to 100; probabilities for each implementation must add up to 100.

R = the rank or value assigned to an outcome; largest number equals the most desired or important outcome.

Total score is computed by multiplying the rank times the probability for each implementation and adding the totals by row. The rational choice is the implementation with the largest total score. In the example above, dance therapy is the rational choice.

Figure 15–3. Decision matrix for selecting implementations and outcomes.

fies those tasks that can be delayed without impeding the overall progress of the plan.

The critical path method is integral to case management nursing, described in Chapter 2. Undoubtedly, the critical path method will become more widely used as greater numbers of institutions turn to managed care (see Chap. 35) to cope with constraints on their financial resources. The critical path method not only simplifies and streamlines decision making, it has the added advantage of focusing the attention of the health care team, the client, and the client's family on the desired outcomes of care.[29]

Although decision analysis techniques are fairly simple to use, additional reading and some practice may be needed by the beginning practitioner. Further information on the use of decision analysis techniques can be found in Grier[2]; Keeney[20]; Balla, Elstein, and Christensen[22]; Tanner[23]; Abraham[24]; Jones[26]; MacLean[27]; and Bailey and Claus.[30]

■ THE INFLUENCE OF DECISION MAKER CHARACTERISTICS ON DECISION MAKING

The process of making clinical decisions was described in the previous section as complex and uncertain because of the many factors associated with health care decision tasks and the health care decision environment. Decision making also is influenced by the personal characteristics of the decision maker. How a person processes information to make both optimal and less than optimal decisions may be affected by characteristics such as level of knowledge, experience, and expertise; the use of techniques to aid in learning and the influence of cognitive biases; values, attitudes, and beliefs; risk-taking behaviors; and other factors such as communication skills and comfort level. In this section, the characteristics of decision makers that positively and negatively influence decision-making behaviors are described. As stated earlier, illuminating the complexity of health care decision making should promote insight and skill for making accurate, effective, and rational decisions.

Expertise

Over time, nurses gain expertise in clinical decision making through the acquisition of knowledge about nursing, clients, and health care. Knowledge is based on education and experience. Benner[31] described five levels of proficiency in nursing: novice, advanced beginner, competent, proficient, and expert. As nurses develop expertise, Benner suggests, they rely more on experience than abstract principles, perceive the situation more as a whole and less as equally relevant parts, and engage more actively in the situation. Thus, expert nurses rely less on rules, observe meaningful patterns, discriminate between relevant and irrelevant data and alternatives, and intuitively grasp the situation as a whole.[31] Because of these perceptual and processing abilities, expert nurses use better decision-making strategies and achieve more effective outcomes than nurses with less knowledge and experience.

BUILDING NURSING KNOWLEDGE

What Role Does Experience Play in Clinical Decision Making?

Holden GW, Klingner AM. Learning from experience: Differences in how novice vs. expert nurses diagnose why an infant is crying. *J Nurs Educ.* 1988; 27(1):23–29.

Holden and Klingner sought to determine whether theory versus skill acquisition based on practical experience influences clinical decision making and particularly nursing diagnosis. They chose the problem of diagnosing why an infant is crying, because of its prevalence and because of the multiple possible competing causes.

Two groups of subjects were selected. The first group consisted of 70 baccalaureate nursing students, 26 of whom were in their first semester of nursing school, 29 of whom were in their final semester of nursing school, and 15 of whom were also parents. The second group consisted of 30 experienced, practicing pediatric nurses from a hospital in a large midwestern city.

Subjects were exposed to a computer program for diagnosing the cause of an infant's crying by searching for relevant facts from among available information. Subjects determined the single correct hypothesis from among several possibilities. Information was related to the infant (age, how often usually cries, general health, etc), the parents (breast feeding, experienced, how they usually respond to a cry, etc), the situation (what infant was doing, noise level and temperature in the room, etc), and the time (time since the last feeding, time since diapers changed, hours infant slept, etc). The nine competing hypotheses were hungry, teething, sick, startled, wet diapers, too hot or cold, wants to play, tired, and in pain.

The experienced nurses and parents differed from both of the student groups on various measures. Pediatric nurses were the most efficient in diagnosing and quickly identified the relevant information units. The parents were the most accurate and made no diagnostic errors.

Contrary to expectations, there were few differences between junior and senior students; both took more trials to come up with the relevant information than the pediatric nurses and the parents. Holden and Klingner emphasize that this in no way deprecates the education the students were receiving, but is evidence of the subtle but important cognitive changes that occur with clinical experience.

Several researchers documented differences in information processing and decision making among novice and expert nursing decision makers.[31–38] Superior problem solving of some nurses was based on their superior knowledge base, a wide range of experiences, and a realistic perception of the probabilistic nature of health care decision tasks.[32] Experts also are able to process larger amounts of information than nonexperts.[9,33,34] This processing advantage may be due to experts' ability to rapidly organize information.[9] Thus, experts are better able to code and organize information in memory for easier storage, search, and retrieval, and with less cognitive strain from information overload.

Experts also are able to match the appropriate cognitive strategy to the decision task. Hammond and colleagues[38] examined intuition and analytic reasoning and noted that there was not a single cognitive strategy, but a continuum of cognitive activity in relation to the complexity of the task. Using judgments from expert highway engineers on nine tasks, Hammond and associates[38] demonstrated that intuitive cognition was most commonly used in situations of low certainty, brief time, and with large numbers of perceptually measured cues. Analytic cognition was used when more time was available and situations were less complex relative to numbers, depth, and high certainty of cues. As judgmental accuracy was related to the correct match between cognitive strategy and task complexity, it is possible that in certain situations intuitive cognition is best and, in others, an analytic strategy is best. The use of intuition and analytic models in making judgments is controversial. As noted by Hammond and associates,[38] "Good intuition is often said to be the mark of a true expert, yet intuition often is despised as mere guesswork hiding behind analytical laziness. Good analytical ability is often praised as high competence, yet often dismissed as nothing more than slavish 'going by the book' " (p. 754). Currently, little is known about the analytic and intuitive strategies used by nurses during decision making. More research focused on this important area is needed so that decision makers can achieve the best possible decisions.

Heuristics and Cognitive Biases

Although experience is certainly necessary for building clinical expertise, inappropriate use of past experience can lead to poor decision making. Few people realize that their retrieval of past events and the use of recalled information can be biased.

Heuristics. All people use heuristics to help solve problems. **Heuristics** are easy-to-use cognitive strategies, "rules of thumb," or procedures that simplify cognitive processing of information[39]; however, heuristics can lead to severe, persistent errors when other information is not used to clarify and verify the situation.[11,39]

Tversky and Kahneman[39] stated that heuristics help people assess the probability of an uncertain event and predict values of uncertain quantities. For example, people judge the distance of an object, in part, by the clarity of the object. The heuristic "the clearer the object, the closer it is" makes solving a distance problem almost an unconscious process. Distances, however, are underestimated when visibility is good and overestimated when visibility is poor because the contours and clarity of the object change.[39] Thus, reliance on clarity alone can lead to systematic errors in judgment. Other factors that influence the judgment of probable distance should be considered.[39]

Heuristics are used by nurses to solve problems. They help simplify the search for information and experiences stored in the memory. Like most people, nurses may not be aware that they use heuristics and that, although helpful in retrieving information, heuristics can produce judgments based on data with little validity.[39]

Cognitive Biases. Even experts are susceptible to cognitive biases when not using a systematic deliberative process of decision making.[39] Examining cognitive biases or errors in subjective assessments of probability that people experience when making judgments can help nurses be more aware of and avoid weak decision strategies.

On the basis of extensive research findings, Tversky and Kahneman[39] described many common cognitive biases to which people are susceptible. Representativeness, small sample biases, availability, and salience are four of these cognitive biases that may be problematic for health care professionals.

Representativeness. Nurses may be influenced by the perceived likeness or similarity to something well known.[39] For example, a new decision situation occurs and a nurse recalls a similar situation from the past. This information should be a starting point for making hypotheses and systematically assessing the new situation; however, people often exhibit the same behaviors they used in the recalled instance because the new situation seems the same. For example, Aspinall[40] asked a nurse in a decision task why she diagnosed a client with renal failure when there were no criteria or data demonstrating renal failure. The nurse responded that in her experience clients with hepatic disease often had renal failure. The nurse subject demonstrates the cognitive bias of representativeness—if it looks similar, it must be similar. Clearly, other information was available to the nurse to disconfirm the hypothesis of renal failure, but the nurse ignored the information because the situations seemed the same. The more a new situation resembles a previous situation, the more likely it is that other information will be ignored.

There are other flaws in relying on representativeness of information. Generally, base rate information is ignored if an object seems representative. Tversky and Kahneman[39] described this cognitive bias as insensitivity to prior probability of outcomes. The probability of an event, for example, a diagnosis or outcome, should be based on the frequency or base rate of that occurrence in a population.[24] If it is a rare event, it is less likely to be the same as the recalled or representative event. As mentioned previously, nurses' decision-making accuracy can be improved when more deliberative processes are used.[24] For example, Bayes' theorem uses data on incidence and frequency of occurrence of cues and diagnoses to estimate the likelihood of a specific diagnosis.[24,25] This deliberative process helps control the influence of the representativeness bias on decision making.

Small Sample Biases. Representativeness is also influenced by a small sample bias.[39] One experience is considered equally representative as many experiences; that is, small samples are considered highly representative of the population. As described in the following section on the availability bias, single experiences often are more easily recalled and exert a disproportionate influence on judgment. Single or small samples, statistically, do not represent populations well; therefore, errors in judgment are more likely to occur. Thus, for several reasons, people are likely to make errors when judging the representativeness or similarity of one situation with another.

Availability. Availability is also a cognitive bias that limits the search for other information on which to base decisions. As with representativeness, data of little validity often influence judgment.[39] Availability is the ease in which experiences are recalled.[11,39] Experiences that are more clearly and easily remembered may have undue influence on what is understood about a current decision situation. More relevant, accurate, and essential information might not be recalled or might be ignored.

Availability is also influenced by the recency of events. More recent events are recalled more easily than past events.[39] If expertise is developed over time through the storage of multiple experiences, the use of only recent events for decision making is contradictory to the advantages of expert decision making. Although information processing of long-term memory may be more difficult for past events, a deliberative search may reveal experiences more relevant to the current situation.

Salience. Salience is a cognitive bias that makes some information more available in memory than other information. Salience is defined as the attention-getting quality of information.[39] Experiences that are very positive or very negative usually are more salient and more easily recalled. Because they are processed easily, there is a greater probability that these salient variables will influence current decision making. For example, a rare but shocking death of a client will be easily remembered compared with the large number of clients that survive in the same situation. Thus, decision making can be influenced by the shocking quality or salience and not by the rarity of occurrence in the current decision situation. Salient situations, therefore, not only are readily available, but further lead to a small sample bias as well.

Values, Attitudes, and Beliefs

The values, attitudes, and beliefs of the decision maker strongly influence the type of information used in the decision-making process and the desirability of options.[11] Values are the qualities or entities that people have affective regard for or perceive to be important; for example, intelligence, freedom, or family. Attitudes reflect the character, disposition, or temperament of a person; independence, patience, and sensitivity are examples. Beliefs are the opinions or convictions of a person; for example, thoughts about what people should and should not do. In clinical decision making, nurses' values, attitudes, and beliefs influence the information that is considered essential and important to collect, the diagnostic label assigned to clients' health states, and the perceived desirability and selection of outcomes and implementation.

When the values, attitudes, and beliefs of nurses and clients are the same, then similarities in client care planning preferences are likely. When they are different, however, which is the more likely case, whose values, attitudes, and beliefs govern what and how decisions are made?

In some situations, nurses' beliefs, for example, "eating a healthy diet to prevent heart disease," may be better for clients than their own value of "eating everything on the plate." If, however, nurses develop a plan of care based on only their own beliefs, the plan is unlikely to produce successful client outcomes. Instead, nurses' systematic assessment of clients' value systems and collaborative development of outcomes and implementations acceptable to client and nurse are more likely to be appropriate and successful.

Sometimes decision makers may not be aware that personal values, attitudes, and beliefs are influencing decision making. For example, MacLean[11] described a commonly held belief, called ageism, that elderly people are dependent, rigid, weak, incapable of change or learning, often confused, need protection, and cannot manage their own lives. Decision makers who believe this stereotype of the elderly would be unlikely to consider implementation strategies that promote independence, humor, autonomy, or life-style changes. Therefore, decision makers must examine the legitimacy of their own beliefs, attitudes, and values before including them as factors influencing decision making concerning other people.

There are other decision situations in which the values, beliefs, and attitudes of other parties must be considered, for example, family and society. Lynn[41] described several conflicts of interest concerning others during health care decision making; for example, the conflict within a client who values the best care possible but does not want to burden family members with medical bills, or the ethical dilemma faced by the physician concerning a client's desire to continue driving a car when that conflicts with society's right to protection from drivers with poor vision.[41] Lynn also described the dilemma between the value American society places on providing quality health care to all people and the value society places on controlling health care costs.[41] Does care or cost influence the decisions that are made?

There are no correct or easy answers in decision situations involving values, attitudes, and beliefs; however, a systematic, deliberative assessment of these factors can identify the influence and impact of these decision maker characteristics on the decisions being considered. The only incorrect strategy is to ignore the influence of decision maker characteristics in making decisions.

Risk-taking Behaviors

Another type of attitude that affects decision making is the risk-taking attitude of decision makers. Risk is defined by von Winterfeldt, John, and Borcherding[42] as the "probabilistic estimate of uncertain events and the losses that can result from an activity" (p. 277). A risk assessment is an estimate of the likelihood of an event and the consequences if the event occurs. For example, the assessment of risk for developing a pressure sore is based on how likely it is that a sore will occur and the losses if one should occur.

Risk assessments by people, however, often do not adhere to the technical formula for assessing risk.[42] Intuitive or quasi-rational processes of risk assessment are common and often result in misunderstanding and judgmental errors.[42,43] These errors in judgment occur because perceptions of risk are influenced by the biases and attitudes of decision makers toward risk taking.

Von Winterfeldt, John, and Borcherding[42] examined the risk ratings of laypeople related to accidents with highly variable probabilities of occurrence. They found that risk was evaluated from the perspective of personal risk to the subject and to the likelihood of a relatively high disaster. Information concerning the probability of the accident was not used in the judgment of risk.

While investigating nurses' propensity to risk, Grier and Schnitzler[44] found that risk-taking behaviors depended on nurses' education and the situation. Students in a master's degree program accepted greater risk than nurses in less advanced degree programs in both chance and nursing skill situations. Nurses with associate degrees or diploma degrees used similar risk-taking strategies regardless of whether outcomes depended on nursing knowledge or chance. Better educated nurses appeared to use knowledge more than chance to assess decision risk.

Kahneman and Tversky[45] demonstrated that risk preference varies depending on whether the decision results in loss or gain. Generally, decisions involving losses are associated with risk-taking behaviors and those associated with gains are risk aversive.[11,39,45] Nightingale[46] and Nightingale and Grant[47] reported similar findings when examining risk preference and admitting rates of emergency room physicians and decision making in critical care situations. In both studies, physicians used significantly more risk-taking behaviors when choices were framed in terms of loss instead of gain. A mediating factor that several investigators of risk-taking behaviors have identified is the concept of regret.[47,48] Willingness to take risks may be judged on how much "regret" the individual would feel: the greater the potential regret, the greater the risk behavior.[48]

In nursing, risk preference behaviors are demonstrated in client care plans that focus on preventing problems such as falls (loss) but fail to develop related plans for maximizing benefits (gains) such as increased mobility for the same clients. As a nurse would feel more "regret" if a client fell than if a client was not able to be up walking several times a day, decision making may be driven more by avoiding losses than in achieving gains. If a client with the same risk for falling developed atelectasis, the nurse might take greater risks in mobilizing the client because of the "loss" associated with atelectasis.

Other Decision Maker Characteristics

Other decision maker characteristics such as confidence, communication skills, feelings of stress, self-direction, power and control, and comfort level may influence decision making.[49–52] For example, DeWolf reported that nurses making ethical decisions were influenced primarily by their personal degree of comfort in the situation and not by ethical or decision-making principles.[49] Similarly, the communication skills of nurses appear to influence the accuracy of decision making in emergency situations.[50,51] For example, difficulty obtaining information in a triage environment from intoxicated, hysterical, very young, confused, non-English-speaking, or frightened clients may decrease the accuracy of diagnostic and management decisions.[50,51] Nurses with better communication skills may be able to acquire relevant and essential information more readily than those nurses with less developed skills.

■ THE COLLABORATIVE MODEL OF PROFESSIONAL DECISION MAKING

For a number of reasons, there has been a shift in the locus (or center) of decision making from the traditional model of

BUILDING NURSING KNOWLEDGE

Is Locus of Control a Factor in Clinical Decision Making?

Neaves JJ. The relationship of locus of control to decision making in nursing students. *J Nurs Educ.* 1989; 28(1): 12–17.

Neaves contends that the success of efforts to improve nursing practice relies on recognition of nursing as an autonomous profession. In turn, this requires that rank and file nurses develop professional skills and attitudes. Literature shows, however, that not all nurses are interested in independent practice; many prefer to relinquish control to others, perhaps to the detriment of quality care. Studies indicate that nursing students score higher than other women in altruism, nurturance, deference and submission, and philanthropic service to others, and lower in values related to theoretical acquisition, independence, and leadership.

To gain insight into this problem, Neaves investigated the role of internal locus of control in decision making. Internal locus of control was defined as the belief that rewards are contingent on one's own behavior. Literature suggests that people with high internal locus of control tend to be independent, decisive, and self-directive. Neaves hypothesized that her subjects would show this pattern.

Two groups of subjects were selected: one group of 51 seniors in a diploma program, and another group of 49 seniors in a baccalaureate program. Each subject was given two questionnaires, one on locus of control measured by Rotter's scale and one on decision making, a forced-choice scale entitled the Medication Administration Questionnaire. This scale has general statements and hypothetical situations involving decision actions and choices accompanied by independent and dependent options for action.

The findings supported Neaves' hypothesis. Those people with higher internal locus of control tended to select independent responses on the decision-making scale. Those with a higher external locus of control (the belief that reward is the result of luck, chance, or the actions of powerful others) tended to select dependent responses. Responses were not significantly associated with the type of nursing education program in which the subject was enrolled. Neaves concluded that external locus of control may interfere with full development for professional practice.

control by the health care professional to that of client-centered control.[53] Within the traditional model, health care professionals (usually the physician) make decisions for clients. The traditional decision-making model also has been called paternalism, meaning that the locus of decision making is external to clients. Currently, there is a shift away from the traditional model toward a more participatory or collaborative relationship between clients and health care professionals. In the collaborative team model,[54] clients are active team members who are involved in all aspects of the decision-making process. The shift from health care professionals from different disciplines separately interacting with clients to a collaborative team approach has increased collegiality, respect, and communication among professionals to more effectively meet the complex needs of clients.

The Collaborative Role of Clients in Health Care Decisions

The participation of clients in decision-making steps in the nursing process is inherent in the collaborative model. The collaborative model states that clients bring essential expertise to the decision-making process—expertise about their own needs, outcomes, values, and past experiences. Clients should be involved in identifying important data during the assessment phase and working with nurses to make decisions concerning their own health state. In the management of the nursing process, clients should be actively involved in developing care plans and participating in the implementation of appropriate strategies. Clients also should share in the evaluation process by identifying those aspects of the plan that are successful and those that require modification. Use of a collaborative model increases the likelihood that a feasible, appropriate, satisfying, and successful plan of care is developed, implemented, and evaluated.

Benefits of Collaborative Decision Making

With mutual planning, clients take an active role in their care; therefore, clients' needs and preferences are more likely to be considered in the decision-making process. Also, clients are more likely, able, and willing to carry out the plan of care. Thus, client satisfaction with care should be high.

IMPLICATIONS FOR NURSE–CLIENT COLLABORATION

Clients as Decision Makers

The collaborative model holds that clients bring essential expertise to the decision-making process—expertise about their own needs, values, and experiences. Client should be involved in assessment and in arriving at the decisions that will affect their health. Clients should also be involved in generating the management plan and in the evaluation process. A collaborative model, one that includes clients in decision making, helps ensure that a feasible, appropriate, and ultimately successful plan emerges.

In the collaborative view, it is only through acknowledging and facilitating clients' roles and participation in decision making that effective client care decisions are reached. Thus, professional decision making in nursing is not only a systematic deliberative process, but a shared participative process between nurses and clients.

SUMMARY

Decision making concerning client health care occurs in an increasingly complex, dynamic, and uncertain decision environment. The many factors associated with the decision task and the decision maker add to the complexity and uncertainty of professional nurses' decision making.

To make the best possible decisions in this complex and uncertain health care environment, professional nurses use the nursing process, a systematic, deliberative approach to achieve the best possible client outcomes using the most accurate, essential, and complete data available. Strategies to enhance data collection and diagnostic reasoning are used within the nursing process to enhance decision making. In addition, decision aids such as decision trees, decision matrices, and critical paths, help nurses improve their decision behaviors.

Researchers continue to investigate nurses' professional decision making to understand the processes that nurses use, the decisions that nurses make, the outcomes that are achieved, and the variables that influence rational decision making. Knowledge concerning decision making enables nurses to routinely make decisions with a high probability of being effective. Decision making is the foundation of professional nursing practice.

REFERENCES

1. Janis IL, Mann L. *Decision Making: Psychological Analysis of Conflict, Choice, and Commitment.* New York: Free Press, Macmillan; 1977.
2. Grier MR. Decision making about patient care. *Nurs Res.* 1976; 25(2):105–110.
3. Hogarth R. *Judgement and Choice.* New York: Wiley; 1987.
4. Williamson YM. *Research Method and Its Application to Nursing.* New York: Wiley; 1981.
5. Burns N, Grove S. *The Practice of Nursing Research.* Philadelphia: Saunders; 1987.
6. Johnson J. *Nurse's Use of the Decision Making Process in Patients With Short Term and Long Term Pain.* Chicago: University of Illinois; 1974. Master's thesis.
7. Berger K. *Berger–Williams Model of the Nursing Process.* 1990. Personal communication.
8. *ANA Standards for Nursing Practice.* Kansas City, MO: American Nurses' Association; 1973.
9. Klatzky R. *Human Memory,* 2nd ed. San Francisco: Freeman; 1980.
10. MacLean S. *Amounts and Relevance of Patient Data Gathered by Nursing Students.* Chicago: University of Illinois; 1983. Master's thesis.

11. MacLean SL. The decision-making process in critical care of the aged. *Crit Care Nurs Quart.* 1989;12(1):74–81.
12. Gordon M. Predictive strategies in diagnostic tasks. *Nurs Res.* 1980;29(1):39–45.
13. Gordon M. The diagnostic process (1980). In: Kim M, Moritz D, eds. *Classification of Nursing Diagnosis: Proceedings of the Third and Fourth National Conferences.* New York: McGraw-Hill; 1982: 46–53.
14. Hammond K, Kelly K, Schneider R, Vancini M. Clinical inference in nursing: Analyzing cognitive tasks representative of nursing problems. *Nurs Res.* 1966;15(2):134–138.
15. Elstein A. Clinical judgment: Psychological research and medical practice. *Science.* 1976;194:696–700.
16. Shoemaker JK. Essential features of a nursing diagnosis. In: Kim MJ, McFarland GK, McLane AM, eds. *Classification of Nursing Diagnoses: Proceedings of the Fifth National Conference.* St. Louis, MO: Mosby; 1984:104–115.
17. Jones DA, Dunbar CF, Jhirovic MM. *Medical-Surgical Nursing: A Conceptual Approach.* New York: McGraw-Hill; 1982.
18. Simon H. *Administrative Behavior.* 2nd ed. N.Y. McMillan, 1957.
19. Rezler A, Stevens B. *The Nursing Evaluator in Education and Service.* New York: McGraw-Hill; 1978.
20. Keeney RL. Decision analysis: An overview. *Operations Res.* 1982;30(5):803–838.
21. Baumann A, Deber R. The limits of decision analysis for rapid decision making in ICU nursing. *Image.* 1989;21(2):69–71.
22. Balla JI, Elstein AS, Christensen C. Obstacles to acceptance of clinical decision analysis. *Br Med J.* 1989;298:579–582.
23. Tanner CA. Research on clinical judgment. In: Holzemer WL, ed. *Review of Research in Nursing Education.* Thorofare, NJ: Slack; 1983:1–32.
24. Abraham IL. Diagnostic discrepancy and clinical inference: A social-cognitive analysis. *Genet Social Gen Psychol Monogr.* 1986; 112(1):41–102.
25. Winkler RL. Judgmental and Bayesian forecasting. In: Makridakis S, Wheelwright SC, eds. *The Handbook of Forecasting: A Manager's Guide,* 2nd ed. New York: Wiley; 1987.
26. Jones J. Clinical reasoning in nursing. *J Adv Nurs.* 1988;13:185–192.
27. MacLean SL. Activity intolerance. In: Maas M, Buckwalter K, eds. *Nursing Diagnosis and Interventions for the Elderly.* Redwood City, CA: Addison-Wesley; 1991.
28. Dunston J. How managed care can work for you. *Nursing 90.* 1989;20(10):56–59.
29. Zander K. Nursing case management: Strategic management of cost and quality outcomes. *J Nurs Adm.* 1988;18(5):23–30.
30. Bailey JT, Claus KE. *Decision Making in Nursing: Tool for Change.* St. Louis, MO: Mosby; 1975.
31. Benner P. *From Novice to Expert.* Menlo Park, CA: Addison-Wesley; 1984.
32. Carnevali D, Mitchell P, Woods N, Tanner C. *Diagnostic Reasoning in Nursing.* Philadelphia: Lippincott; 1984.
33. Shanteau J, Phelps R. Judgement and swine: Approaches and issues in applied judgement analysis. In: Kaplan M, Schwartz S, eds. *Human Judgement and Decision Processes in Applied Settings.* New York: Academic Press; 1977.
34. Chase WG, Simon HA. Perception on chess. *Cog Psychol.* 1973; 4:55–81.
35. Corcoran S. Planning by expert and novice nurses in cases of varying complexity. *Res Nurs Health.* 1986;9:155–162.
36. Westfall V, Tanner C, Putzier D, Padrick K. Activating clinical inferences: A component of diagnostic reasoning in nursing. *Res Nurs Health.* 1986;9:269–277.
37. Hammond K. Toward a unified approach to the study of expert judgement. In: Manpower JL, Phillips KD, Renn O, Uppuluri VR, eds. *Expert Judgement and Expert Systems.* Berlin: Springer-Verlag; 1987:vol. 35, pp. 1–16.
38. Hammond K, Hamm R, Grassia J, Pearson T. Direct comparison of the efficacy of intuitive and analytical cognition in expert judgement. *IEEE Trans Syst Man Cybernet.* 1987;SMC-17(5):752–770.
39. Tversky A, Kahneman D. Judgment under uncertainty: Heuristics and biases. *Science.* 1974;18:1124–1131.
40. Aspinall MS. Use of a decision tree to improve accuracy of diagnosis. *Nurs Res.* 1979;28(3):182–185.
41. Lynn J. Conflicts of interest in medical decision-making. *J Am Geriat Soc.* 1988;36:945–950.
42. von Winterfeldt D, John RS, Borcherding K. Cognitive components of risk ratings. *Risk Anal.* 1981;1(4):277–287.
43. Hammond K, Anderson K, Sutherland J, Marvin B. Improving scientists' judgments of risk. *Risk Analy.* 1984;4(1):69–78.
44. Grier M, Schnitzler C. Nurses' propensity to risk. *Nurs Res.* 1979;28(3):186–191.
45. Kahneman D, Tversky A. Choices, values and frames. In: Arkes H, Hammond K, eds. *Judgement and Decision Making.* Cambridge: Cambridge University Press; 1986:194–210.
46. Nightingale S. Risk preference and admitting rates of emergency room physicians. *Med Care.* 1988;26(1):84–87.
47. Nightingale S, Grant M. Risk preference and decision making in critical care situations. *Chest.* 1988;93(4):684–687.
48. Feinstein AR. The "chagrin factor" and qualitative decision analysis. *Arch Intern Med.* 1985;145:1257.
49. DeWolf MS. *Clinical Ethical Decision Making: A Grounded Theory Method.* Chicago: Rush University; 1989. Doctoral dissertation.
50. Budassi-Sheehy S, Barber J. Triage in emergency care. In: *Emergency Nursing Principles and Practice,* 2nd ed. St. Louis, MO: Mosby; 1985:86–91.
51. Willis D. A study of nursing triage. *Emerg Nurs.* 1979; November/December:8–11.
52. Cianfrani K. The influence of amounts and relevance of data on identifying health problems. In: Kim M, McFarland G, McLane A, eds. *Classification of Nursing Diagnoses.* St. Louis, MO: Mosby; 1984:150–161.
53. Billie D. Locus of decision making in patient and family education: Its effects on promoting wellness. *Nurs Administration Quart.* 1987;11(3):62–65.
54. Duncanis AJ, Golin AK. *The Interdisciplinary Health Care Team.* Germantown, MD: Aspen; 1979.

BIBLIOGRAPHY

Bailey JT, Hendricks DE. Decisions made easy. *Nursing 90.* 1990; 20(1):120–122.

Benner P, Tanner C. Clinical judgment: How expert nurses use intuition. *Am J Nurs.* 1987;87:23–31.

Christensen PJ, Kenney JW. *Nursing Process: Application of Conceptual Models.* 3rd ed. St. Louis: Mosby; 1990.

Corcoran-Perry S, Graves J. Supplemental-information seeking behavior of cardiovascular nurses. *Res Nurs Health.* 1990;13:119–127.

Gorzeman J, Bowdoin C. *Decision Making in Medical-Surgical Nursing.* Toronto: BC Decker; 1990.

Grobe SJ, Drew JA, Fonteyn ME. A descriptive analysis of experienced nurses' clinical reasoning during a planning task. *Res Nurs Health.* 1991;14(4):305–314.

Hughes KK, Young WB. The relationship between task complexity and decision-making consistency. *Res Nurs Health*. 1990;13:189–197.

Husted G, Husted J. *Ethical Decision Making in Nursing*. St. Louis: Mosby-Year Book; 1991.

Itano JK. A comparison of clinical judgment process in experienced registered nurses and student nurses. *J Nurs Educ*. 1989;28(3):120–126.

Iyer PW, Tapitch PJ, Bernocchi-Losey D. *Nursing Process and Nursing Diagnosis*. 2nd ed. Philadelphia: Saunders; 1991.

Johnson S, et al. Students' stereotypes of patients as barriers to clinical decision making. *J Med Educ*. 1986;61:727–735.

Kassirer JP, Kopelman RI. *Learning Clinical Reasoning*. Baltimore: Williams & Wilkins; 1991.

Malek C. A model for teaching critical thinking. *Nurse Educator*. 1986;11:20–23.

Miers M. Developing skills in decision making. *Nursing Times*. 1990;86(30):32–33.

Pyles S, Stern P. Discovery of nursing gestalt in critical care nursing. *Image*. 1983;15:51–57.

Rew L, Barrow E. Nurses' intuition: Can it co-exist with the nursing process? *AORN J*. 1989;50:353–358.

Shamian J. Effect of teaching decision analysis on student nurses' clinical intervention decision making. *Res Nurs Health*. 1991;14:59–66.

Short L, et al. Medicating the postoperative elderly: How do nurses make their decisions? *J Gerontol Nurs*. 1990;16:12–17.

Thiele J, et al. An investigation of decision theory: What are the effects of teaching cue recognition? *J Nurs Educ*. 1986;25:319–324.

Waterworth S, Luker KA. Reluctant collaborators: Do patients want to be involved in decisions concerning care? *J Adv Nurs*. 1990;15(8):971–976.

Yates JF. *Judgment and Decision Making*. Englewood Cliffs, NJ: Prentice-Hall; 1990.

CHAPTER 16

Client History and Health Examination

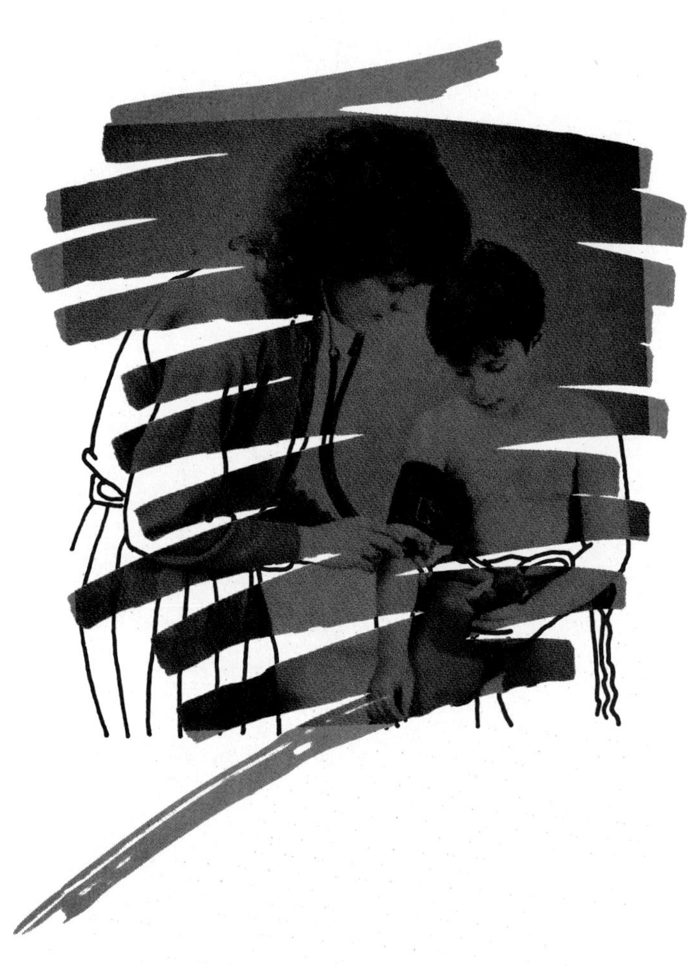

SECTION 2. HEAD-TO-TOE ASSESSMENT

Behavioral Objectives

Upon completing this chapter the reader will be able to

1. List the elements of the data base for health assessment.
2. Differentiate subjective from objective data.
3. Define the health history and health examination and state their purposes; define subjective and objective manifestations.
4. Outline the elements of the health history and describe their contents.
5. Identify interview techniques that are appropriate to each phase of the health history.
6. Describe the procedure for height, weight, and other body measurements.
7. Define body temperature, describe factors that regulate and alter it, outline the procedure for measuring oral, rectal, and axillary temperatures, and discuss the expected findings.
8. Define respiration, describe factors that regulate and alter it, outline the procedure for measuring respiration, and discuss the expected findings.
9. Define pulse, describe factors that regulate and alter it, outline the procedure for measuring apical and peripheral pulses, and discuss the expected findings.
10. Define blood pressure, describe factors that regulate and alter it, outline the procedure for measuring blood pressure by auscultation, palpation, and flush methods, and discuss the expected findings.
11. Outline the order of the head-to-toe examination.
12. Define inspection, palpation, percussion, and auscultation.
13. List several observations for each body area and system included in the health examination and identify the method of observation appropriate for each.
14. Relate observations of the head-to-toe examination to the nurse's role.
15. State the purpose of health assessment by nurses and describe the nurse's focus in doing a health assessment.
16. Discuss the importance of collaboration in the health history and examination.

KEY TERMS

auscultation
basal metabolic rate
blood pressure
body temperature
chest vibration
conduction
convection
data base
diastolic blood pressure
evaporation
health assessment
health examination
health history
inspection
Korotkoff sounds
medical data base
nursing data base
objective data
ophthalmoscope
otoscope
palpation
percussion
point of maximal impulse
precordium
pulse
pulse pressure
pulse rate
pulse rhythm
pulse symmetry
pulse volume
radiation
respiration
respiratory depth
respiratory rate
respiratory rhythm
respiratory quality
sphygmomanometer
subjective data
systolic blood pressure
turgor

Assessment is a critical phase of the nursing process. All plans for the client's care derive primarily from assessments of the client's health. Decisions on implementation are possible only after the client's needs, problems, and capacity for self-care become clear.

This chapter comprehensively covers the many important techniques and skills involved in health assessment and includes major blocks of content on the health history and examination. History-taking and examination skills are, without doubt, some of the most basic and fundamental skills taught within the nursing curriculum. That is because they are both applicable to virtually every client encounter and useful in just about every setting for nursing practice. Skill in these aspects requires time and effort on the student's part, but once the investment is made, it reaps rewards over the entire course of one's professional career.

Although this chapter emphasizes the process and techniques of health assessment, it also goes beyond the practical aspects of assessment to integrate a particular philosophy of approach—the philosophy of nurse–client collaboration. Nurse–client collaboration proposes that client self-determination should be a central value in caregiving. Further, it asserts that client self-determination is maximized when clients are involved in their care and when they actively participate in health care decisions.

The assumptions of collaboration are uniquely appropriate to health care in the 1990s because they are consistent with both the changing patterns of health and illness in society and the changing patterns of professional practice as an outgrowth.[1] Movement toward a more health-oriented delivery system—one that recognizes the influence of life-style on health—clearly highlights the importance of clients' active participation in the decisions that ultimately affect their lives and their health.

Mutual interaction is the nursing model that embodies the collaborative philosophy. It conceptualizes the nurse–client relationship as a series of interpersonal exchanges that evolve in character as caregiving progresses.[2] It thus has implications for all phases of the nursing process, foremost among them, health assessment.

During health assessment, collaboration centers on information sharing.[2] Nurses and clients trade observations, opinions, and facts in a mutual effort to pinpoint the clients' health needs and problems. The sharing process begins with the health history and continues through the health examination and laboratory diagnostic phase as more specific data accumulate. Throughout, the nurse and client are partners, first exchanging and sharing information for assessment, then negotiating a consensus on priorities for the client's care (see Chaps. 18 and 37 for more detail). It seems logical to expect that when clients sense early in the process that they are welcomed as partners in decision making, they will understand and actively join in the nurse's effort to identify relevant information.

Collaboration during the assessment has a special meaning, however, because the character of the interaction during this phase sets the interpersonal tone, not only for the initial encounter, but for the remainder of the nurse–client relationship as well. Thus, the patterns initiated during assessment go a long way to shape the process of care. A give-and-take relationship at this point in caregiving is important for two reasons: (1) it helps nurse and client to accumulate the information necessary to reveal the client's needs; (2) it establishes their agreement on the nature and goals of the relationship to follow. On reading this chapter the student will achieve not only a basic understanding of the skills of health assessment, but also a recognition of the role that collaboration plays in assessment and in nursing.

Section 1. General Concepts of Health Assessment and Vital Sign Measurement

ORIENTATION TO HEALTH ASSESSMENT

Basic Health Assessment Concepts

Health assessment can be looked on as a holistic process because it evolves from interaction, which will be discussed below, and because it is focused on an entire range of physical and psychosocial factors that are part of getting to know the client as an individual.

Nurses are interested in clients as whole, functioning individuals. Consequently, during health assessment, nurses take all of the factors that act to facilitate or impede a client's health into consideration. These encompass biological, psychological, social, familial, vocational, recreational, cultural, and spiritual considerations. To acquire information over such a wide range of dimensions, the nurse engages the client in a relationship that is structured initially around the health history and examination. On the basis of the data that accumulate, the nurse, in collaboration with the client, establishes a comprehensive and individualized plan for the client's care.

Definition of Health Assessment. **Health assessment** is the first phase of the nursing process. It refers to the data-gathering process that is conducted for the purpose of identifying, describing, and analyzing the client's health needs and problems. To identify the current health status of the client, the nurse employs the tools of health interviewing, observation, and laboratory diagnostics to develop a complete and accurate body of health information from which to make an appraisal.

Purpose of Health Assessment. In addition to identifying the current health status of the client, the nurse undertakes health assessment as the essential first step at arriving at an appropriately individualized plan of care for the client. Planning client care on the basis of thorough client assessment lies at the very foundation of contemporary nursing practice. The vast number of articles on assessment in the nursing literature gives testimony to that fact. Without client assessment, only standardized care can be rendered, and it has long been recognized that standard care, based on statistics and norms rather than a person's clinical manifestations of need, may or may not be appropriate to the problems of the individual client.

Health Assessment as Part of the Nurse's Role. Health assessment in the comprehensive and formal sense has not always been an acknowledged part of the nurse's role. Until about 25 years ago, nurses were expected only to obtain specimens for laboratory analysis and to monitor clients' vital signs in addition to the other traditional nurses' duties. Although nurses generally watched for and recognized changes in their clients' conditions, they had little training in health assessment to prepare them for that responsibility. As health care grew increasingly more complex and specialized, and technology more prevalent, demands were placed on nurses to make greater and more sophisticated contributions to client health assessment. At about the same time these changes became apparent, nurses were looking for professional autonomy. They showed themselves capable of a larger role by defining a systematic method for professional decision making known as the nursing process and by building a science of nursing. As a consequence, health assessment skills are now considered essential to the role of the nurse and are part of the fundamental content of the nursing curriculum.

Today, more than ever before, nurses are using their assessment skills with self-assurance in whatever setting they care for clients. Nurses routinely do health histories and health examinations as part of client care and use data from laboratory and other diagnostic testing to derive definitive statements, called nursing diagnoses, that describe the client's state of health.

The nursing process, as Chapter 15 established, is the logical framework around which the nurse's professional contributions to client care are organized. Health assessment, as the initial phase in the nursing process, includes all activities employed by the nurse to gain information about the client during the initial encounter and every subsequent encounter. A client's state of health can change very quickly; thus, in any setting, the nurse must always be focused on the client's immediate mental and physical status and the transformations they might be undergoing.

Health assessment is therefore an ongoing activity for the nurse. Each time a nurse encounters a client, whether in an examining room, at the bedside, or in the client's home, he or she undertakes to formally or informally assess the client's health. Health assessment by expert nurses (whose knowledge and skills are so well integrated as to be automatic) is frequently a process of intuitive interpretation.[3] No matter what the focus of the nurse's attention, however, at another level the nurse is always alert to how well the client is responding and coping, physically, mentally, and socially. It is therefore clear that health assessment skills have the broadest applicability to clinical practice and that, just as clearly, they are fundamental to any nurse's performance as a health care professional.

Health Assessment Data

The Data Base. The information that emerges from the health history and examination and the subsequent diagnostic testing is collectively referred to as the **data base.** The initial data base is established when the client enters the health care setting. As indicated earlier, it covers just about any facts about client habits or patterns of living that might be pertinent to the health problem. The initial data base is important not only because it is used to pinpoint the health problem, but also because it becomes the yardstick or standard, also referred to as the "baseline," against which all future changes in the client's condition, positive or negative, will be compared.

Focus of the Data Base. Although the basic components remain the same, it should be noted that the data base for a well person varies somewhat from that for an ill person. The data base of a well person (the adult or child who undergoes a routine and, ideally, regular evaluation of personal health) has a different emphasis. Generally, the well person has no signs or symptoms of disease. Thus, well-person assessment endeavors to establish the client's concept of health and the client's level of satisfaction with his or her own personal health, as well as to identify the client's immediate state of health. The well-client data base also thoroughly covers the client's life-style and health practices, which have an important bearing on the client's current and future state of health.

Unlike the well client, the ill client, by definition, has certain subjective and objective manifestations of disease. The data base for the ill client thus centers around those manifestations, the client's concerns about them, and the facts of the onset and progress of the client's illness. Although questions of life-style may be relevant to the client's health state, generally they are focused in reference to the client's current illness episode.

Although the best data bases are comprehensive, not all information that the caregiver might collect will be relevant. The goal is to construct a *defined data base,* a data base that contains a comprehensive range of relevant information.

To construct a defined data base the nurse first considers whether the client is well or ill. In the former case, the nurse asks about the client's previous health state and its relationship to the present; in the latter case the nurse begins with the nature of the presenting problem and the immediate subjective and objective manifestations of illness. The setting and the service rendered by the agency or institution or unit in which the nurse works is also a determining factor. Specialized units usually have a predefined data base that caregivers are expected to obtain. Such data bases generally exclude information that is not immediately pertinent. Clients who enter the intensive care unit for treatment of heart failure, for instance, are not expected to answer questions about a family history of breast or ovarian cancer. Thus, judgment is used in constructing a defined data base. It is important to focus and limit the data base by looking at the most obvious features first. The nurse must consider, "Who are my typical clients and what are their problems?" "What do I need to know to provide good care to clients with those kinds of needs?" "What is unnecessary for me to know?" The data base can always be expanded as needed.

Components of the Data Base. Nurses need a thorough familiarity with each of the components of the data base.

The Health History. The **health history** is an organized body of information comprising the clients' verbal reports about their own health state. The health history may be the most important part of the data base, not only because it is the first aspect and thus serves to define and focus the other aspects, but also because it may produce as much as 85 percent of the relevant information in the health assessment.[4]

The health history guides the assessment process. The client's presenting problems, the problems that bring the client to seek help, are elicited by the health history. They determine the focus of the health examination, the techniques of observation, and even the laboratory tests that will be used to collect information on the client's signs of health or illness.

The health history is also a teaching tool. It is a time when the nurse and client jointly review the client's health patterns and have an opportunity to exchange ideas. During the health history, they can address the positive aspects of the client's health practices, as well as habit changes that might be helpful for the future. For example, if the nurse discovers that a client maintains her body weight by eating a healthy diet but fails to perform regular breast self-examinations, praise for the former may enhance the client's self-esteem, and instruction about the latter, along with a careful consideration of the barriers the client experiences, may serve to change the client's habits.

The Health Examination. The **health examination** is the hands-on portion of health assessment, the phase in which caregivers use their observation skills to identify the physical signs of health and illness. The health examination verifies, supplements, or calls into question the findings from the health history. It identifies the client's state of physical integrity or abnormality as well as functional abilities and disabilities. For accurate health examinations to result, the nurse must have both observational skill, which depends on well-trained and acute sensory perception, and a methodical cognitive process served by a well-organized body of knowledge about health and illness.

Laboratory and Diagnostic Tests. Laboratory and diagnostic tests provide another source of data that amplify and validate the data of the health history and health examination. In recent years the technology of medical diagnosis has developed to such a stage that many aspects of health that lie outside the clinical perception of the caregiver can be measured. Internal body processes can be evaluated with a high degree of accuracy. A client's complaint of cough and chest pain during the health history, for example, may lead the caregiver to suspect pneumonia. When this suspicion is reinforced by the caregiver's examination finding of abnormal breath sounds over the chest, a definitive diagnosis can be confirmed or ruled out by a chest x-ray. Diagnostic tests can also bring to light abnormalities that had not been suspected by the caregiver. This is the function of a "screening test," a diagnostic test employed when there is no immediate sign of illness.

The results of laboratory and diagnostic tests are used not only to establish the client's medical diagnosis, but also to monitor and evaluate the effectiveness of nursing implementation once it is under way. For example, the nurse caring for the client who receives a diagnosis of pneumonia will be interested in the client's subsequent chest x-rays as a way of determining whether the actions taken during caregiving have been effective.

Types of Data Bases. Two types of data bases are used by nurses: the nursing data base and the medical data base.

Nursing Data Base. The **nursing data base** is the body of information collected by the nurse. It focuses on how adaptive are the client's health habits and how illness and health care are affecting the client. The nursing data base contains information that is necessary to design a plan for nurse–client management.

The focus of the nursing data base is a reflection of the nature and scope of nursing practice as outlined in the American Nurses' Association's *Social Policy Statement.*[5] That document defines the domain of nursing as the "diagnosis and treatment of human responses to actual or potential health problems" (p. 9). To fulfill this responsibility nurses must be able to identify (1) the client's current health status, (2) the effect of the client's life-style on the current state of health, (3) past patterns of wellness and illness, (4) the client's responses to episodes of illness, (5) the client's current risk factors for future illness episodes, (6) past and present social and cultural factors that may affect health and health care, (7) immediate stressors and coping mechanisms, (8) the effect of the client's illness on his or her self-care capacity, and (9) available resources.

The nurse uses the information obtained in these areas to make nursing diagnoses and, with the client, to establish a plan of treatment (care) that further maximizes health where it is present and minimizes the disruption to the client's life and health that is caused by illness.

Medical Data Base. The **medical data base** is the body of information collected by physicians, nurse practitioners, physician's assistants, and nurses. It is generally focused on the client's disease process and the objective of its construction is to determine appropriate medical management. The medical data base contains the client's presenting problems, the chronological time line of their development, an examination of the client's body systems, and a battery of laboratory and diagnostic test results. The result is a medical diagnosis that labels the client's pathophysiological process and defines the direction of medical therapy.

Comparison of Data Bases. It is clear from the above descriptions that the medical data base and nursing data base are different in their orientations; the medical data base is oriented to the client's disease; the nursing data base is oriented to its impact. Both of these types of data bases are highly relevant to the practice of nursing. Nurses have an independent role as the ANA's statement has established, for which the nursing data base is highly relevant. Nurses also participate in the client's medical management, and for that role, the medical data base is particularly pertinent.

The Data. Data are pieces of information that are collected and collated by caregivers to help them carry out the responsibilities of clinical practice.

Types of Data. Two general kinds of data are found in medical and nursing data bases: subjective data and objective data.

BUILDING NURSING KNOWLEDGE

What Data Does the Nurse Need to Do a Client Assessment?

Carnevali DL. Daily living and functional health status: A perspective for nursing diagnosis and treatment. *Arch Psychiatr Nurs.* 1988;11(6):330–333.

Carnevali notes that nurses must be clear about what differentiates nursing from other health disciplines as they perform client assessments. She states that nurses always deal with medical information in assessing; however, they use this information in a supportive fashion as physicists depend on mathematics to solve problems in physics. Thus, the focus of nurses differs from the focus of physicians and other health care professionals.

According to Carnevali, two categories of data are especially important to nurses: data on daily living and data on functional health status. The interrelationships between these two categories are also important. For example, nurses are interested in how the client's functional health status balances with the requirements of daily living.

The daily living category has important subcategories. Activities, which include anything the client does, is one. Activities, in turn, are affected by the client's presenting health situation. Nurses are also interested in how past activities have contributed to the client's present condition, and how the client's present condition affects his or her ability to perform current and future activities.

Events and demands in daily living, environment for daily living, and values and beliefs are other important subcategories. Events are anniversaries, holidays, travel, medical treatments, and other important occurrences that generate a positive or negative response in the client. These responses, such as motivation, fear, and dread, in turn affect participation in health care.

Demands are expectations of self and others that influence behavior and generate an emotional response. Nurses are interested in whether the client's functional health resources are sufficient to meet demands. The environment creates demands. Nurses are interested in the drain of physical, microbial, and interpersonal factors on the client's functional health status. Values and beliefs, especially regarding health and health care, and an individual's priorities in life also can be crucial elements in a client's participation in health care.

To assess the client's functional health status, nurses consider the client's age, stage of development, and achievement of developmental tasks. Functional health status is greatly affected by pathology; therefore, nurses are also interested in the medical diagnosis and treatment activities as they assess health. The focus, however, is on how these affect the client's ability to meet daily living requirements.

Subjective Data. **Subjective data** is the name given to the information that the client verbally reports. The health history, therefore, comprises subjective data. Anything that the client recalls and says about his or her health is considered subjective data. The client's statements about current feelings and problems, reports of signs and symptoms of illness, personal evaluations of the cause and effects of illness, and recall of past history and events are all considered subjective. Subjective data represent the client's world from the client's point of view as the client experiences it. They are perceptible only to the client and can be verified only indirectly through others' observations. Subjective data related to unusual body sensations are referred to as symptoms in the medical data base, but as subjective manifestations in the nursing data base.

Objective Data. **Objective data** is the term used for all other data. Objective data are the data derived from clinical observation and testing. They are detected by the caregiver's senses—smell, touch, hearing, and vision—and they are detected through the use of tools of measurement such as a thermometer, a urinometer, and a sphygmomanometer. Posture, facial expression, skin color and condition, body proportions, and movement are all observable and their observation contributes objective data. Likewise, blood pressure, body temperature, respiratory rate, pulse, height, and weight are measurable as are blood hemoglobin and hematocrit, blood and urine glucose, and myriad other aspects of the body's physiochemistry. Their measurement also contributes objective data. Objective data related to the unusual appearance, smell, sound, or feel of the body are referred to as signs in the medical data base, but as objective manifestations in the nursing data base (Box 16–1).

Sources of Data. Data sources for health assessment are of two types: primary and secondary. *Primary data* come directly from the client. *Secondary data* come from all other sources including the client's family and friends, other health professionals and personnel, medical and nursing records and reports, and the health science literature that is pertinent to the client's problems and needs.

The Client. The client is usually the most appropriate source for obtaining health data, particularly subjective data. Only the client can provide a complete, thorough, accurate description about inner symptoms and experiences. Usually the self-responsible adolescent or adult client is able to discuss episodes of illness and describe health practices, current health status, and medication regimen in considerable detail. Sometimes it is unfeasible for the client

BOX 16–1. CHARACTERISTICS OF SUBJECTIVE AND OBJECTIVE DATA

Subjective Data	Objective Data
Must rely on client's verbal reports; information only indirectly verifiable	Verifiable by tools
Apparent only to client	Apparent to examiner
Called symptoms in medical data base	Called signs in medical data base
Called subjective manifestations in nursing data base	Called objective manifestations in nursing data base

to provide reliable data, especially when the individual is very young or mentally disabled. Clients who are confused or unconscious or unable to talk for physical reasons may not be able to provide the information necessary.

Family/Significant Others. Data may also be obtained from the family/significant others. Talking with the family is a good means of validating the information provided by the client. Family members frequently have valuable insights and information about the client, the client's condition, and the client's responses to illness. Family members are often able to identify additional specific and special client needs. Sometimes the family member or significant other is the only source of information, particularly when the client is critically ill, incoherent, intellectually impaired, or unconscious. In these situations, the nurse must rely on data provided by the family and other secondary sources.

Nursing and Medical Records. Any record containing health-related information can be of assistance in establishing a data base. The nursing and medical records originate from various sources. Records often are available from prior hospitalization(s) or can be transferred from other community health settings. Other sources of records include outpatient clinic records, physician's office records, public health agency records, or home health service records. Records may also be available from nurse clinicians in private practice who have cared for the client. Health care records from facets of the client's life such as military or school can provide useful information about the client's health. In the hospital, information from the physician's admitting history and physical examination can also be helpful. Indeed, this is one of the most common secondary sources used by the nurse in the hospital setting.

Professional Peers. Data obtained by professional peers (social workers, occupational and physical therapists) after the client is admitted often are helpful to the nurse. These data can be used to confirm or disconfirm health information obtained by the nurse to provide a clearer or more complete picture of the client's status.

Health Science Literature. Current health science literature provides information that can assist the nurse in compiling a comprehensive client data base. Information obtained from printed sources can also aid the nurse (and client) in developing creative nursing interventions and is helpful in planning individualized care. Printed material can provide a review that refreshes the nurse's fund of information in the areas of specific etiology, causative factors, pathophysiology, treatment, and expected outcomes for the client's health problem.

Data Collection as a Collaborative Process

Using the collaborative approach to data collection means that there is free exchange of information between the nurse and the client. The client and the nurse work jointly as partners in producing the data. Their roles in this process are complementary. The nurse's role is to facilitate, encourage, and guide the client's participation in assessment. The client's role is to respond openly and to provide thorough, accurate self-reports.

Client Concerns About Data Collection. The client often has significant concerns about the assessment process. These result from prior experiences and shape the client's expectations for the current experience. The client's concerns usually include but may not be limited to the important issues of privacy and control. The client's level of pain or discomfort, physical and psychological, also influences attitudes toward and expectations about health assessment.

Loss of Privacy. Privacy is an important concern for clients who undergo health assessment. There are generally two aspects to a client's concern about privacy: protection of confidentiality and protection of modesty.

Clients are often uncomfortable or embarrassed about answering the personal questions that are part of the health history. Frequently they are reluctant or hesitant to reveal details even about their past or present illnesses. The nurse must be sensitive to this reluctance. Sometimes the client feels the information requested is of such a personal nature that he or she is being asked to divulge the most private of inner secrets. The client, moreover, may be unaware of the nurse's commitment to professional confidentiality and may fear that the nurse will transmit those secrets to others. Generally, the nurse will be successful in alleviating those fears by:

- assuring the client about the confidential nature of the communication
- stating the reason for asking
- conveying the purpose served by the client's answers

The client's concerns about confidentiality often constitute one of the first problems to arise within the nurse–client relationship. How the issue is resolved may have a significant bearing on the relationship to follow. Sensitivity to the client's concerns about confidentiality sends the client an important message about the nurse's trustworthiness.

Clients also worry that their bodies will be immodestly exposed during health examination. Although this may not be an overriding concern for some individuals, for others it is the source of considerable worry. Personal modesty is therefore an important aspect for the nurse to address as the examination phase of health assessment begins. The nurse can protect the client's modesty by:

- conducting the examination in a private area
- being careful to use a screen or close the door to the examination area
- providing the client with an examination gown or sheet prior to beginning the examination
- reassuring the client that every effort will be made to cover the parts of the client's body that are not being examined
- covering each body part immediately after finishing that portion of the examination

Taking these measures to protect the client's modesty not only will reduce the client's worries about body exposure, it will convey to the client that the nurse is aware of and concerned about the client's personal feelings.

Loss of Control. Clients who have severe illnesses or chronic conditions often feel powerless because they sense that they cannot control their bodies and because, no matter what they do, they will be unable to change their situation significantly.[6] The sense of powerlessness is closely related to feelings of helplessness. Clients with a sense of powerlessness not only feel that they are unable to help themselves, they also may fear that others will be unable to help them.

There are times when feelings of powerlessness and helplessness can be overwhelming. When clients become overwhelmed and are unable to cope with these inner feelings, their capacity to participate in health assessment frequently diminishes. It is important to note, moreover, that questioning and examining may contribute to a client's underlying sense of powerlessness; the client may feel obliged by his or her dependency to surrender control to health professionals. These feelings may further diminish the client's morale and manifest in a tense and upset appearance.

When such feelings and attitudes block communication, the nurse can assist by accepting the client's feelings and by striving to understand the meaning of the client's behavior. Looking at the situation from the client's point of view helps the nurse to understand how frightening it is to experience a loss of control.[7] Usually the state of being overwhelmed is temporary. With the support of the nurse, other health care professionals, and family members, the client eventually regains composure and the ability to cope; however, while the client remains distraught, the nurse may have to rely on family members, significant others, or other secondary sources for health information.

Pain/Discomfort. Clients frequently fear they will experience pain or other forms of discomfort, particularly during the examination phase of health assessment. Children are often fearful; adults are less often so although they too may anticipate pain. Anticipation of pain is not exclusive to clients who are ill; those clients who are undergoing a routine health evaluation, well children or well adults, may also fear discomfort. Anticipation of pain and discomfort may interfere generally with the client's ability to participate in an open and spontaneous manner during the health assessment process. This is one of the purposes for collaborative exchanges during health assessment. By providing the client with descriptions of what is to be done, what the client will experience, and why the various maneuvers are important, the nurse may be able to alleviate the client's fears and facilitate the client's relaxation.

Many clients, it should be noted, are already experiencing pain and discomfort when they seek assistance. They may have concerns about examining procedures and fear that these procedures will worsen the pain or cause them to feel even more uncomfortable. When the nurse senses that the client is in immediate discomfort, it often facilitates assessment to address the problem of pain before beginning the health assessment process. Often there are measures the nurse can take to alleviate the client's discomfort before going on.

Collaborative Values. Although collaborative values are germane to all phases of the nurse–client relationship and to each step of the nursing process, their application to assessment is especially important because of the foundation it sets for the interactions to come. The values of collaboration are communicated to the client from the very opening of the assessment process and are made apparent in the way the nurse approaches the client. The most important collaborative values that are conveyed during assessment are:

- mutual participation in decision making
- informed consent
- informed dissent

Mutual Participation in Decision Making. From the beginning, the nurse invites the client to participate in a joint exploration of the client's situation and to come to a mutual assessment of the client's state of health. The nurse seeks information but is also interested in encouraging the client to explore and come to a better understanding of his or her own situation. The interaction during assessment involves dialogue, sharing, negotiation, and the development of a nurse–client consensus on decisions about the client's care. This contrasts with the more traditional health care interaction that is directed by the professional and centers on interrogation and prescription giving. Interaction during assessment goes beyond the surface level. At a deeper level, the client gains an understanding about the kind of relationship that is developing with the nurse and forms an opinion about his or her own influence in the relationship. When the value of mutual participation is operating, the client learns that control in the relationship is shared with the nurse, and that the nurse and client are partners in making the health care decisions.

Informed Consent. Clients have the right to control their bodies. That principle has been well established in law (*Schloendorff v. Society of New York Hospitals,* 221 N.Y. 125 N.E. 92 (1914)). More specifically, every adult client of sound mind has the right to consent to health procedures performed on his or her body. Although this principle derives from the law, it is also one of the central values of collaboration and is applicable to health assessment as well as to the other phases of the client's care. Thus, the nurse is always careful to remind the client that he or she has the right to consent. Moreover, it is part of the nurse's role to provide the client with a description of what health assessment will entail and to describe generally the benefits and risks of the procedures that will be performed. Clients often have questions about health assessment and the purpose of the various maneuvers. The nurse answers the client's questions in language the client can understand, and ensures that the client understands the possible consequences of declining to undergo assessment. There may be instances in which the nurse directs these explanations to the client's family members or to others acting on behalf of the client; these situations generally involve parents or guardians of children, or guardians of the mentally ill or mentally retarded, or relatives of individuals who are semiconscious or unconscious. (See also Chaps. 3 and 34).

Informed Dissent. The client may choose to decline proposed treatments or procedures or to reject health recommendations. Although the nurse has an obligation to use all constructive means to influence the client to accept health care (see Chap. 37), the client ultimately bears responsibility for his or her own health care decisions. The nurse's role is to ensure that the client's decisions are indeed informed decisions.

Exchanges Between Nurse and Client During Data Collection. During the data collection process, the nurse explains what is being done, why it is being done, and what the client will experience, and then shares findings. The nurse acts as the client's guide and interpreter during the health care experience. The nurse always explains what is to occur next, emphasizing why the procedure is important and how the procedure relates to the client's overall care.

During assessment the client is always treated with the utmost respect. Indeed, acts of mutual exchange are inherently respectful acts. The nurse lays personal feelings aside and accepts the client and his or her beliefs. In doing this the nurse directly and indirectly communicates caring and concern for the client and the client's health. Listening to the client and hearing what the client has to say are important in themselves and also convey to the client an implicit message that the nurse cares about what the client is experiencing. Empathy is important in relating and understanding the client's feelings. The fact that the developing relationship is collaborative is a signal to the client that the nurse is empathic and views the client as an individual.[8]

Exchanges of Information and Observations. As the nurse obtains health information, the nurse shares the findings with the client. The nurse also ensures that the client has opportunities to raise concerns and request clarification of information. The nurse does this by frequently asking such questions as "Is there anything else you wish to know?" and "Do you have any questions or concerns about the items we've just discussed?" The nurse also facilitates complete disclosure by asking such questions as "Is there anything else I should know about this problem?" Additional client input provides an opportunity for the nurse to identify the client's current knowledge level and sources of information. The nurse can then tailor explanations to the client's need for information and the client's level of understanding. This can lay the foundation for mutual understanding, trust, and agreement on a plan of action. It may also help to further clarify the client's responsibilities for self-care and health maintenance. The nurse discusses each issue from the standpoint of giving any and all information relevant to the client's concern.[9] The sharing of information and observations provides opportunities for clarifying the plan of action and for reviewing the nurse's expectations of the client and the client's expectations of the nurse.

Techniques for Promoting Client Collaboration in Data Collection. Collaboration can be facilitated by various means. By using the approaches described above and those that follow, the nurse is generally able to establish trust and to influence the client to become involved in the health assessment process.

- *Stress the benefits of health assessment.* The major benefit of health assessment is that the information enables the development of a comprehensive and individualized plan of care for the client. Care can be tailored to the client's personal needs and values.
- *Link benefits to client's goals and values.* The client is more likely to participate freely in health assessment once he or she understands how participation helps the attainment of personal goals. The nurse can invite the client to share what he or she is hoping to achieve by seeking health care assistance. With this information, the nurse may be able to "link" or to establish the relevance of assessment procedures to the client's own objectives. This is particularly important when the client is unfamiliar with health procedures.
- *Reassure the client of confidentiality and privacy.* The nurse should reassure the client that the information being collected for the data base will be held in the strictest confidence and will be available only to those directly engaged in the client's care. By reassuring the client in regard to confidentiality, the client may be more forthcoming with information and willing to participate in the health assessment process.
- *Promote physical and emotional comfort during data collection.* The nurse must be attuned to the client's level of comfort throughout the entire health assessment process. Physical comfort measures are instituted as indicated. This may include conducting the health assessment in small components rather than in its entirety at one time. Or assessment may be resumed after the client is experiencing less pain or stress. Physical comfort measures are provided; for example, a pillow on which the client can rest his or her head. An important emotional comfort measure for the client is the knowledge that he or she is in control of the situation.
- *Limit the demands on the client for data collection.* If the client is hospitalized in settings where health care providers are trained, there is potential for repeated requests for health history information. These requests may originate with the admitting physician, service resident, interns, medical students, staff nurses, nursing students, or dietitian. The nurse works with the client to determine which of these interviews should be "granted." This is important to conserve the client's energy. Once these decisions are made by the client, the nurse acts as the client's advocate in upholding the decision.

Consulting With Professional Peers for Data Collection. In the process of completing the nursing assessment, the nurse may choose to consult formally or informally with fellow professionals to verify or acquire additional information, gain insight, or obtain a different perspective (Box 16–2). Frequently nurses consult with each other when they are unsure about some aspect of the client's care or if there is a need to verify information. In some instances, it may be prudent to elicit the assistance of a nurse clinician who can provide specialized information. At other times the physician may be the appropriate peer with whom to consult. Consultation with other ancillary care providers, such as respiratory therapists and dietitians, can often provide a clearer picture of the total client and his or her health care practices and activities.

Making the Decision to Consult. The nurse must become comfortable in consulting with peers, whether on a formal or an informal basis. Whenever there is need for verification, clarification, or additional information, the nurse should use all available resources.

THE HEALTH HISTORY

Basic History-taking Concepts

The health history can be looked on as the client's story about his or her state of health and how it developed. The client's story is important to nurses not only because of the facts about the client's body and state of mind it provides, but also because of the insight it gives into the client's expectations for health care and the ideas he or she holds for what the outcome will be. Almost all clients have their own agenda for health care.[10,11] They come with ideas about the nature, causes, and severity of their problems and with preferences regarding the kind, conditions, and goals of care, which they will usually share if invited.[12] They even come with preferences for the way they wish to work with the caregiver, some welcoming the opportunity for a collaborative relationship and some preferring a more traditional approach.[13]

Effective caregiving requires that caregivers understand clients' agendas. As Chapter 37 describes, caregivers and clients often hold different points of view on caregiving.[14–18] Differences in outlook influence the caregiving process, sometimes impeding goal attainment. Caregivers are therefore wise to work with clients toward developing a consensus about the strategies and priorities of care and the kind of relationship they are to have.[19] (See Chap. 37 for information on how to establish consensus.) This requires a consideration of the client's agenda as history taking proceeds. Although caregivers are not obligated to follow the client's preferences, they are obligated to negotiate differences in the service of an agreement. Give-and-take is a key aspect of establishing a workable care plan. It begins with the health history as clients are invited to tell their story.

BOX 16–2. PROCESS OF CONSULTATION

Prior to Requesting Consultation

- Clearly identify the problem and all its facets.
- Compile complete data concerning the problem at hand.
- Obtain the client's permission before consulting with a source not involved in the current care.

Selecting the Consultant

- Choose the consultant with the appropriate skill or knowledge in the area.

Discussion With the Consultant

- Outline the problem and its issues.
- Discuss and analyze the consultant's recommendations.

Action

- Record consultant's recommendations in the client's chart.
- Implement and evaluate the effectiveness of the recommended activities.

IMPLICATIONS FOR NURSE–CLIENT COLLABORATION

History Taking and Caring

History taking is the initial context for the communication of caring. Clients have a need for their caregivers to understand their concerns. They also have a need for information about their health. One of the ways that a nurse communicates caring is to invite clients to tell their story in their own way during history taking and to encourage this process through appropriate acknowledgments of what they say. This not only communicates caring; it also initiates the client's involvement in assessment. Another way to communicate caring during history taking is to invite clients to ask questions related to their health concerns and to offer information in response.

Purpose of the Health History. The primary purpose of the health history is to collect subjective data. As established above, another purpose is to initiate a relationship with the client. The nurse endeavors to develop a rapport during history taking that will lead to mutual trust and understanding. The nurse also uses the health history introduction to discuss the client's role in a collaborative assessment process and to convey to the client that he or she is to be a partner in decision making.

The History-taking Process. To compile a history, the nurse conducts a health interview, which is an interview focused on the client's health information. The nurse does the interview in phases and employs various interview techniques to elicit the client's self-reports. (See Chap. 14 for more about interview phases and techniques.) Table 16–1 lists helpful interviewing techniques and the purposes they serve.

During the health interview, clients are invited to dis-

TABLE 16–1. INTERVIEWING TECHNIQUES FOR THE HEALTH INTERVIEW

Technique	Example	Application
Open-ended question	What brings you here today?	Allows client to discuss openly and without restraint.
Closed or direct question	How long have you had this pain?	Used to obtain very specific details or in an emergency situation.
Facilitating	Go on, what do you mean by indigestion?	Purposely encouraging client to continue talking to provide additional information.
Reflecting	You say the lump just appeared?	Clarifies and expands information.
Listening	(Silently nodding the head)	Indicates to client that you are attentive and continue to be interested.
Suggesting leads	Tell me about your family.	Directs conversation to a specific area.
Requesting clarification	Do you mean you have blood in your urine *each* time you urinate?	Clarifies informational point and ensures accuracy of data.
Restating	I see, you get the pain each time after eating fried foods.	Validates nurse's perception of the information.
Verbal observation	The expression on your face seems to indicate you are uncomfortable. Are you having pain?	Provides feedback to validate or deny observation perception.
Focusing	Oh yes, we were discussing how you felt when your wife had to go back into the work force.	Brings client back to the point at hand when the conversation has wandered.
Using silence	(There is no conversation from either the client or the nurse.)	Permits client to recall events, organize thoughts, or move to another area.
Summarizing	You said the pain always occurs at night when you lie on your left side after you have been bowling and have drunk three or four cans of beer.	Provides a composite review of data for the client to confirm or correct.

cuss their health concerns and to convey their personal understanding of the health problem. Clients generally find this process reinforcing.[10] The opportunity to tell their story in their own words without interruption, which Stiles and associates have referred to as "patient exposition," conveys to the client that the caregiver is interested and concerned.[10] Stiles and associates studied approaches to the health interview and found that on reviewing (with the caregiver) the symptoms, circumstances, and feelings associated with their problem, clients were more likely to be affectively satisfied with the health interview.[10]

Once the client has had the opportunity for exposition, another type of exchange becomes appropriate. The caregiver is able to follow up with pertinent questions, reflect the information obtained to check its accuracy, clarify relationships, and fill in gaps. Periodically during this phase of the interview, the caregiver interjects information or observations calculated to promote collaboration with the client, to help bring out the information necessary to crystallize the client's health problems, and to define their mutual understanding of the client's needs for direct care. Clients want information about their condition and about treatment, and appreciate feedback.[10] Indeed, clients' cognitive satisfaction with the health interview may depend on the quantity and quality of information obtained in feedback exchanges during this phase.[10] For example, on learning that a client has a history of breast masses but has never been taught the technique for breast self-examination, the interviewer might take the opportunity to mention the importance of self-monitoring and a goal for care might be skill in self-examination.

The concluding segment of the health interview is used for summarizing a mutual understanding of the client's problem. The caregiver gives a verbal overview of the findings and their implications for care, and also may discuss resources available to assist the client and nursing support the client can expect during the period of caregiving.

Approaches to the Interview. The health interview begins by introducing oneself to the client. The caregiver discusses purpose, process, roles, and time required for the interview, describing what will happen and addressing the client's specific concerns, if any, about the impending process of health assessment.

During the first phase of the interview, the caregiver's approach is unstructured, informal, and open-ended; the caregiver encourages the client to speak freely. It is important to begin with topics that are unlikely to threaten the client. The interviewer frequently asks a question such as "What prompted you to seek health care today?" The open-ended approach invites clients to answer in the way they choose and in a manner that supports their sense of composure in the situation. It gives clients an opportunity to become comfortable with the interviewer and the situation. Once the client begins to relax it is easier to discuss topics that may be more personal or sensitive. Clients can be encouraged to share by asking such questions as "What do you think has caused your problem?" and, "What do you think the course of your illness will be?" Ultimately, the client's cooperation determines the extent and detail of the data obtained.

Generally clients are a little nervous as the interview begins. When the caregiver senses that a client is especially anxious, the client may be helped by an acknowledgment of those feelings and by reassurance that they are common. The caregiver can also reassure the client that he or she need not answer every question. Usually, this will reinforce the client's sense of control and facilitate cooperation in the health interview.

Although several content areas are important to cover in the health interview, as long as the client spontaneously provides the caregiver with relevant information, direction of the interview is unnecessary. Enlow and Swisher, experts on history taking, state that "Facts are not sought, rather they are permitted to emerge."[20] Caregivers encourage elaboration on relevant aspects by using such open-ended utterances as "Tell me more about that" and "How did you feel about that?" They avoid direct questions and questions seeking yes/no answers except for those instances in which information about specific signs and symptoms is necessary. Again, such approaches prompt additional information while encouraging the client's participation and control of the interview process.

Although the caregiver's approach need not be directive, neither is it laissez-faire. A balance is sought between relinquishing and retaining complete control. To protect client autonomy, caregivers seek to avoid an interrogating style in which rapid-fire questions are thrown at the client[21]; instead they emphasize techniques that encourage the client to spontaneously discuss the health problem, giving the client freedom to move from topic to topic according to his or her personal priorities. Nevertheless, clients sometimes fail to spontaneously give important information, and when that happens, caregivers appropriately use direct but sensitively worded questions, exerting control to pinpoint a time line, clarify a sequence of events, or fill in a gap.

One aspect that may not always come out is the client's agenda.[22] For a variety of reasons generally having to do with their beliefs about who controls the relationship and whose goals will be dominant, clients may not tell caregivers about their expectations or preferences. When clients fail to reveal this information, it is appropriate to ask them for it. Generally, this is done during the concluding segment with such questions as "What do you hope will be done for you?" and "What do you hope the outcome will be?"[23]

Preparation for the Health Interview. Conducting a good health interview requires preparation before the interview begins. That preparation includes three aspects: (1) reviewing the health information that is available from other sources, (2) selecting the time and preparing the setting, and (3) preparing the client.

Review of Health Records. Prior to interviewing the client, the caregiver reviews all data from previous medical and nursing records. On the basis of this information, the caregiver may also elect to consult relevant texts and authoritative journals for the latest information relevant to the client's past health problems. This is especially important when the client's health problem is chronic and likely to influence the current needs and when the caregiver has had little experience with it.

Selection of Place and Time. The caregiver also gives attention to the setting and the timing of the interview. The setting should be private and well lighted and have a comfortable air flow and air temperature. The caregiver times the interview so as to provide an uninterrupted period that is sufficient to cover the relevant topics.

Timing is important. Before beginning a health history, the caregiver considers the client's probable state of mind. If the client is severely ill, it may be necessary to postpone the health history or to interview a family member instead. This may also hold true if the client has just received distressing news of some sort and is emotionally upset.

Preparing the Adult Client. Adults may or may not prefer to have a relative present and should be consulted. Other aspects of preparing adults have been addressed above.

Preparing the Child. Preparing children usually requires that the caregiver consider their age. Children under 7 years may be limited in their ability to understand and answer health-related questions and may have difficulty producing the information required. Younger children are often reassured when their parent is present and are more relaxed and responsive to the interviewer. For children in this age group, the parent may take responsibility for providing a significant portion of the information. The younger the child, the more the parent will be involved in the health interview. The caregiver takes advantage of this opportunity to observe parent and child interact, which may prove helpful in establishing a nursing diagnosis.

The caregiver addresses opening instructions and explanations to parent and child, taking care to use language the child can comprehend. Children of preschool age or younger may feel more comfortable if allowed to explore the examination area briefly; many children have questions about the objects they see and are more at ease when they have the opportunity to satisfy their curiosity and allay their concerns. Older children and especially adolescents may prefer that the parent is not present and their preference should be established. Opening instructions and explanations for teenagers follow the pattern used for the adult client with special attention to the aspect of confidentiality, as this is often an important concern for clients in this age group.

Preparing the Elderly Client. The elderly also have special needs. Timing, for instance, may be especially important. Some elderly clients become fatigued, confused, or disoriented late in the day; thus, their capacity for clear thinking is diminished, a reason to schedule interviews early. The caregiver should also be careful to allow sufficient time for the interview, as the elderly client's past health history may be long, and to provide enough time so that the atmosphere is unhurried. Special attention should be paid to the client's comfort during the interview. Arthritis and other musculoskeletal problems are common in this age group and can make sitting for long periods difficult. Hearing and vision loss may complicate history taking. The caregiver should be careful to sit close to the client, within the client's field of vision, and to speak in a clear, low-pitched voice, using a slow, distinct speech pattern. Elderly clients may also prefer to have a relative or a friend present as a source of support.

Recording the Health History. A great deal of information accumulates during the health history, and for the beginning interviewer there is a tendency to want to record information as the client speaks. Copious note taking during the interview, however, diverts the interviewer's attention from what the client is saying, potentially resulting in a loss of important data, and frequently interferes with the spontaneity of the client's answers. The interviewer should have a small pad and pencil available to jot very brief details, but note taking during history taking is kept to a minimum.

The caregiver uses the period *immediately following* the interview to digest the information that the client has provided, put it in logical order, and organize it into the proper format for recording. The health history is generally recorded on a special form devised for that purpose by the institution in which the caregiver is employed (Fig. 16–1). The form may be placed in the client's medical record, in the care plan Kardex along with the client's care plan, or on a clipboard at the client's bedside, depending on institutional procedure. Sometimes the history is entered directly into the computer, and the computer history format designates specific information to obtain and its recorded order.

Format of the Health History. Just as there are two complementary data bases in health care, there are also two corresponding orientations toward the health history: nursing and medical. Much attention has been paid by nurses to the nature of the nursing history. There is agreement that the nursing history should reflect the domain of nursing; however, no similar consensus has been reached on the nursing history format or its definitive content. Indeed, the orientation and format may be unrelated to diagnostic appropriateness and accuracy. One study showed that whether the data base was nursing or medical made little difference to the number and quality of the nursing diagnoses subjects generated from history data.[24]

Because nursing as a profession has not yet reached a consensus, nursing history forms differ from institution to institution, varying considerably in the sequence and organization of data and even in the specific information required. Institutions even vary in the place where nursing history data are stored and in the policies for disposition of these data after the client's discharge. Some hospitals keep nursing histories with the medical record, and some do not. Practicing nurses thus gear their history taking to the conventions of the institution.

This text views health assessment as a collaborative process in which information is exchanged by the various professionals who each have a role in the client's care. Professional exchanges promote teamwork and a comprehensive mode of care that benefits the client. The written record, of which the health history is a significant part, provides an important avenue for the collaborative exchange of information in institutional settings. To do a health assessment, nurses must be familiar not only with the nursing data base but also with the medical data base, because some of the information that nurses use to formulate nursing diagnoses may well come from the record of the physician's history and examination. Likewise, some of the information that other health professionals use may be obtained from the nursing history. To promote information exchange, the format for history recording proposed in this text reflects nursing's domain, yet has structural similarities and logical relationships to the medical record. A common format promotes ease of information exchange; this, in turn, promotes the sharing of information and interprofessional communication.

Content of the Health History. The nursing and medical histories can be looked on as two complementary aspects of the health history. Each addresses its respective practice, yet each alone provides insufficient information for caregiving. Only when these two aspects are taken together is the picture of the health of the client complete. Thus, nurses and physicians both contribute significantly to the collection of historical information and need a working understanding of one another's respective contributions. The sections that follow highlight the contributions of the nurse, describing the subjective data for which the nurse is responsible, but also outline the contributions of the physician, pointing out their value to the nurse. Table 16–2 lists the major content areas of the health history, distinguishing nursing and medical elements.

Elements of the Health History

Biographical Data. The health interview generally begins with the collection of *biographical data.* Important information commonly includes name and address, telephone number, sex, date of birth, marital status, nationality, religion, occupation, and the source of the information. When this information is already available in the client's record, the interviewer need only verify its accuracy.

During this part of the interview, the interviewer forms an initial impression of the client's ability to give reliable information. If the client's apparent mental state causes the interviewer to question the accuracy or validity of information, family members or significant others are also interviewed.

Primary Concern/Chief Complaint. The first elements of the health history establish the client's health concern(s) and reason(s) for seeking health care. These will vary ac-

NURSING ASSESSMENT—ADMISSION INFORMATION

ADMISSION

DATE ______ TIME ______ ID Band Checked ______
ARRIVED: WALKING ______ W/C ______ GURNEY ______
FROM: HOME ______ ER ______ MD OFFICE ______ OP AREA ______
OTHER HOSP (NAME) ______
ECF (NAME) ______
VITAL STATISTICS: T ______ P ______ R ______
BP ______ HT ______ WT ______

ORIENT TO: CALL LIGHTS ____ BED ____ SIDE RAILS ____ BATHROOM ____ ROOM LIGHTS ____
TV ____ MEALS ____ SMOKING POLICY ____ VISITING HRS/RULES RE: CHILDREN ____
SIGNATURE ______ RN/LVN/NA

VALUABLES

DENTURES: UPPER ______ LOWER ______ PARTIALS ______ OTHER ______
DEVICES: CANE ______ CRUTCHES ______ WALKER ______ W/C ______ GLASSES ______
CONTACTS ______ HEARING AID L ______ R ______ PROSTHESIS ______
OTHER VALUABLES: DESCRIPTION DISPOSITION

CHECK HERE IF NO OTHER VALUABLES: ____ SEE PATIENT BELONGINGS FORM ☐ INITIAL

PSYCHOSOCIAL/CULTURAL

OCCUPATION ______ EDUCATION ______
RELIGION ______ PASTORAL CARE DESIRED ______
MARITAL STATUS ______ NAME PREFERRED ______
CULTURAL PRACTICES ______
LANGUAGE SPOKEN ______ LANGUAGE UNDERSTOOD ______
APPEARANCE DURING INTERVIEW: RELAXED ____ ANXIOUS ____ OTHER ______
COMMENT: ______
CONTACT: ______ PHONE ______

SLEEP/REST/COMFORT

PAIN: DENIES ____ YES ____ LOCATION ______ DURATION ______
QUALITY: SHARP ____ DULL ____ PRESSURE ____ OTHER ______
PRECIPITATED BY ______
RELIEVED BY ______
SLEEP ROUTINE ______
SLEEPING AIDS ______
COMMENTS ______ INITIAL

GENERAL INFORMATION

PT EXPRESSED REASON FOR HOSP ______
SYMPTOMS ______
DURATION ______ INITIAL

GENERAL INFORMATION

PAST (MAJOR) ILLNESSES / SURGERIES / SHUNTS: YEAR:

CHRONIC ILLNESSES: DIABETES ______ HEART PROB ______ GASTRITIS / ULCERS ______
↑ BP ____ CANCER ____ SEIZURES ____ LUNG DISEASE ______ LIVER ______
COMMENTS ______
ANY BLOOD TRANSFUSIONS ____ YEAR ____ REACTIONS ______
MEDS CURRENTLY USING (Rx & NON-Rx): DOSE: REASON:

MEDS TAKEN IN LAST 24 HRS (INCLUDE TIME) ______

DISP. OF MEDS: HOME ____ TO PHARMACY c̄ RECEIPT ____ RECEIPT TO CHART ____ NONE ____
ALLERGIES: MEDICATION ______ REACTION ______
MEDICATION ______ REACTION ______
FOOD ______ REACTION ______
OTHER ______ REACTION ______
NO KNOWN ALLERGIES ______
PREFERRED DIET: ______
LAST MEAL: ______
SMOKING PPD ______ YEARS ______ STOPPED ______ NONE ______
ETOH USE ______
HAVE YOU HAD A DRINK IN THE LAST 24 HRS? ______
HAS ALCOHOL EVER CAUSED YOU A PROBLEM? ______
HAVE OTHER PEOPLE VERBALIZED CONCERN ABOUT YOUR DRINKING? ______
HAVE YOU EVER THOUGHT ABOUT CUTTING DOWN? ______
DO YOU EVER TAKE A PILL FOR NERVES, PAIN, SLEEP? ______
WHAT KIND ______ DOSE ______ HOW OFTEN? ______
WHAT OTHER DRUGS HAVE YOU USED? (e.g. POT, CRYSTAL, COCAINE) ______
HAVE DRUGS EVER CAUSED YOU A PROBLEM? ______
EXERCISE ______ X WEEK ______ X MINUTES ______
FORM ______
INFORMATION RECEIVED FROM: PT ______ SO ______ OLD CHART ______
MD ______ OTHER ______ INITIAL

2640-33 (12-89)

Figure 16–1. Example of a health history form (*continued*) (*Courtesy Sharp Cabrillo Hospital, San Diego, CA.*)

SUBJECTIVE

SENSORY

VISION: NO DIFF___ GLAUCOMA___ CATARACTS___ BLIND___ OTHER___

HEARING: NO DIFFICULTY___ IMPAIRED___ COMMENTS ___ INITIAL

CIRCULATION

NO DIFFICULTY___ PACEMAKER___ AICD___

CHANGE IN SENSATION/EXTREMITIES___ DESCRIBE ___

Hx OF BLEEDING___ LOCATION___ DURATION___ COLOR___

COMMENTS ___ INITIAL

VENTILATION

NO DIFFICULTY___ SOB___ WHEN ___

COUGH___ NON-PRODUCTIVE___ PRODUCTIVE___ DESCRIBE ___

HOME OXYGEN___ WHY ___

COMMENTS ___ INITIAL

NUTRITION

NO DIFFICULTY___ CHANGE IN APPETITE___ WHEN___ WT CHNG?___

NAUSEA/VOMITING ___ DIFFICULTY SWALLOWING/CHEWING___

COMMENTS ___ INITIAL

ELIMINATION

BOWELS: LAST BM___ BM FREQUENCY___ DIARRHEA___ CONSTIPATION___

RECENT CHNG___ LAXATIVES___ ENEMAS___ DESCRIBE STOOL ___

BLADDER: NO DIFFICULTY___ URINE DESCRIPTION ___

FREQ/URGENCY___ PAIN/BURNING___ INCONTINENCE___ RETENTION___

COMMENTS ___ INITIAL

SKIN

NO DIFFICULTY___ ITCHING___ BRUISING___ RASHES___

OTHER ___

COMMENTS ___ INITIAL

MOBILITY

INDEPENDENT___ ASSIST DEVICE___ NEEDS ASSIST___

ACTIVITY PATTERN ___

FRACTURES ___ PARALYSIS___ UNABLE ___

COMMENTS ___ INITIAL

REPRODUCTIVE

MALE: PROSTATE PROBLEMS___ DESCRIBE ___

PENILE DISCHARGE___ DESCRIBE ___

FEMALE: CHNG IN MENSTRUAL CYCLE___ LMP___ MENOPAUSE___ LAST PAP___

VAGINAL DISCHARGE___ DESCRIBE ___ LAST BREAST EXAM___

NO DIFFICULTY ___

COMMENTS ___ INITIAL

SIGNATURES	DATE/TIME	UNIT

OBJECTIVE

NEURO.

ORIENTATION: PERSON __ PLACE __ TIME __ SPEECH: CLEAR __ IMPAIRED __ NO RESPONSE __

LOC: AWAKE/ALERT___ DROWSY___ RESP TO PAIN ONLY___ NO RESPONSE___

COMMENTS ___ INITIAL

CARDIAC

APICAL PULSE___ REG __ IRREG __ COLOR: PALE __ PINK __ FLUSHED __ CYANOTIC __

U EXTREMITIES: RADIAL P(R)___ (L)___ BRACHIAL P(R)___ (L)___ CLUBBING___

L EXTREMITIES: TEMP (R)___ (L)___ COLOR(R)___ (L)___ EDEMA(R)___ (L)___

PULSES: PEDAL(R)___ (L)___ POST TIBIAL(R)___ (L)___ POPLITEAL(R)___ (L)___

COMMENTS ___ INITIAL

RESPIRATORY

BREATH SOUNDS: CLEAR___ CRACKLES___ RHONCHI___ WHEEZES___

LOCATION ___

COMMENTS ___ INITIAL

G.I.

ABDOMEN: APPEARANCE ___ GIRTH___ BOWEL SOUNDS___

MOUTH/GUMS/TEETH: INTACT___ BLEEDING___

COMMENTS ___ INITIAL

ELIMINATION

ENTEROSTOMY ___

STOOL APPEARANCE ___

CATHETER ___

URINE APPEARANCE ___

COMMENTS ___ INITIAL

SKIN

COLOR ___ TEMP ___ TURGOR ___

SKIN DESCRIPTION ___

DECUBITUS ULCER___ FLOW SHEET INITIATED___ ADMISSION PICTURE___

DESCRIPTION ___

COMMENTS ___ INITIAL

MOBILITY

EXTREMITY STRENGTH: RUE ___ LUE ___ RLE ___ LLE ___

LIMITED ROM ___ CONTRACTURE ___

JOINT SWELLING/DEFORMITY ___

ABNORMAL EXTREMITY ___

COMMENTS ___ INITIAL

INFECTION CONTROL NEEDS NO☐ YES☐ DESC.

SAFETY NEEDS: NO☐ YES☐ DESC.

Figure 16–1. (*continued*).

SHARP
CABRILLO HOSPITAL

PATIENT HISTORY SHEET

DATE INITIATED	PATIENT PROBLEM LIST	DATE RESOLVED	CURRENT HOSPITAL HISTORY	DISCHARGE / ENVIRONMENTAL
				LIVES ALONE WITH SPOUSE FAMILY OTHER
				HOME APARTMENT STAIRS
				IF ALONE: ANY OUTSIDE HELP
				TRANSPORTATION AVAILABLE
				DISCH. DESTINATION
				PT / FAMILY SERVICES NEEDED
				NOTIFIED
				OTHER NEEDS
				TEACHING NEEDS
				COMMENTS
			DIAGNOSTIC STUDIES W/RESULTS	
				PATIENT IDENTIFICATION

Figure 16–1. (*continued*).

TABLE 16–2. ELEMENTS OF THE HEALTH HISTORY

Nursing History	The Medical History
Biographical data	Biographical data
Primary concern	Chief complaint
Current understanding	History of present illness
Past health problems/ experiences	Past medical history
Personal, family, and social history	Family history Personal and social history
Subjective manifestations	Review of systems

cording to the nature of the situation and the type of health assessment—well person or ill person—required.

The *primary concern* is that aspect of the client's condition or problem about which he or she is most concerned. To bring out the client's primary concern, the caregiver repeats the client's reason for seeking help and asks, "What about your condition bothers you the most?" The primary concern may be the same as the reason for seeking help or some related aspect. For example, the client may seek help for a problem of leg weakness. The primary concern may be the weakness itself, the physical threat it may represent (paralysis, disability), or a functional effect of the weakness, such as the inability to work or pursue valued activities. The primary concern is of considerable interest to the nurse because it provides clues to the client's awareness of the health problem and the client's priorities in relation to it. The nurse's effectiveness in assisting the client may stem from an understanding of the client's primary concern.

The specific reason or problem for which the client is seeking help is referred to as the *chief complaint* (commonly abbreviated on the medical record as CC). In some situations, it is up to the nurse to establish the chief complaint. The chief complaint is elicited by asking the client, "What brought you here today?" The client may be seeking a routine examination. More commonly, the chief complaint will identify some sign or symptom of illness. For example, the client may state, "I've had a headache and blurred vision for the last 2 days." The chief complaint is *not* a diagnosis, but a list of the main symptoms the client has noted and their duration. Knowledge of the chief complaint is essential to the caregiver because it designates the problem for which the client usually expects treatment, and because it provides the focus for the primary concern.

Current Understanding/History of Present Illness. The *current understanding* deals with the client's understanding of the causes and consequences of the current condition and level of health knowledge. The ill client is asked to outline his or her personal understanding of the symptom needing attention, its relationship to present and future health, personal ideas on the cause of the symptom, including aggravating and alleviating factors, and effects the symptom is having on self-care and daily activities. As the well person usually has no symptoms, the caregiver asks the client about his or her usual state of health and the factors that have contributed to it.

Knowing how the client perceives his or her health assists the nurse in establishing nursing diagnoses. To elicit the current understanding, the interviewer might request clients to "describe your current state of health" or to "identify the factors you feel have affected your health." The caregiver also asks, "Do your current symptoms keep you from doing what you want to do?"

The current understanding also emerges from the *history of the present illness* (HPI). The history of the present illness is the client's narrative or chronological story about the problem for which she or he seeks attention. When the medical record is available, it may be unnecessary for the interviewer to elicit this element of the health history; however, to elicit the HPI, the caregiver asks the client to "Tell me all you can about your problem."

Four major aspects should emerge in the client's story: (1) details of the onset of the illness, (2) character of the problem, (3) progress of the problem, and (4) current status of the problem. Each of these aspects incorporates important specific pieces of information that are helpful in establishing a medical diagnosis, but that may also assist the nurse in formulating nursing diagnoses. Box 16–3 gives suggestions on how to elicit specific elements of the current understanding and history of present illness.

Past Health Problems/Experiences, Past Medical History. *Past health problems/experiences* emphasizes the client's responses to past health problems and treatment and inventories important health care experiences such as hospitalizations and the client's attitudes toward them. Information in this category provides nurses with a description of factors that may shape clients' expectations for their current experience and outcomes. Sometimes these have a positive influence on care and sometimes they interfere with clients' progress toward health care goals. By understanding the client's past history, the caregiver is prepared to anticipate the client's responses, to help clarify the client's understanding of the current situation, and perhaps even to resolve conflicts between the client's understanding and that of the health care team.

This aspect relates closely to the *past medical history*, the elements of which are questions about childhood and infectious diseases, immunizations, accidents, surgical procedures, allergies, and current medications (Box 16–4). The past medical history is important to determining medical treatment, may suggest the client's medical prognosis, and is helpful to nurses because it directs the interview about the client's past responses to illness and treatment. When this information is available in the medical record, it is important that the caregiver familiarizes himself or herself with it before interviewing the client.

Personal, Family, and Social History. The *personal, family, and social history* provides the caregiver with an important body of information about the client as an individual and,

BOX 16–3. ELEMENTS OF THE CURRENT UNDERSTANDING AND HISTORY OF PRESENT ILLNESS

Onset of Health Problem	
Time of onset	First date noticed?
Mode of onset	Sudden? Gradual?
Situation	What was client doing at the time?
Precipitating events	What seemed to bring the problem on?
Character of Problem	
Location of symptom/sign	
Quality of symptom	Description of sensation/feeling
Severity of symptom	Mild? Moderate? Severe?
Duration of symptom	How long did it last?
Associated symptoms	What other symptoms accompanied the problem?
Relief	What did client do for relief?
Relation to habits	Was symptom related to anything client usually does?
Progress of Problem	
Sequence of symptom development	In what order did symptoms come on?
Persistence	How long did symptoms last?
Recurrence	Did the problem come back?
Changes	Has the symptom changed in severity or character?
Situation change	How did change in situation affect problem?
Current Status of Problem	
Current symptoms	Which symptoms are bothering the client now?
Location	Where are they located?
Severity	How severe are the current symptoms?

particularly, insight into the client's well-being and self-expression patterns (see Chaps. 22 and 23). Effective nursing requires that the caregiver know more about the client than facts related to physical health. It is during this segment of the health history that the caregiver comes to know the client as a whole, functioning person.

The personal, family, and social history of the adult contains the range of information outlined in Table 16–3. The general areas of inquiry include the client's vocation, family and social relationships, leisure activities, cultural and spiritual factors, sexual factors, health habits, and psychological factors, including stress and coping patterns, self-image, and sick role behavior. In addition to the specific categories, the interviewer tries to gain an understanding of the priority that each of these various elements has in the client's life. That is, the caregiver strives to understand the client's life structure (see Chaps. 10 and 23 for more about life structure). Personal, family, and social histories are also done for children, in which case the focus is on the client's relationships with the parents, the living conditions, peer relationships, school adjustment, activities, and diet.

BOX 16–4. ELEMENTS OF THE PAST HEALTH PROBLEMS/EXPERIENCES, PAST MEDICAL HISTORY

Immunizations

Names and dates of vaccinations received (measles, mumps, rubella, tetanus, polio, pertussis, etc)

Accidents

History of all major accidents (apart from illness) and the injuries suffered, particularly ones that might have required treatment in an emergency department

Surgeries

Major illnesses that resulted in a need for surgery, the date and type of surgery received (these are listed chronologically in the medical record.)

Allergies

A list of allergic reactions and their dates, causes, and precipitating circumstances

Current Medications

A list of all medications, including over-the-counter medications, the client is currently taking and the conditions for which they were prescribed or are used

Probably one of the most important aspects of the personal, family, and social history for nurses is the summary it provides of the client's activities of daily living. This aspect is elicited by asking the client to describe his or her activities in the course of a normal day. Information about the client's usual activities helps the caregiver decide on the kind of teaching and counseling the client may need to cope with illness.

Another very important part of the personal, family, and social history is the sexual history. This segment includes questions about the client's sexual orientation and patterns. This is important to nurses because sexuality is such an important aspect of social interaction and because many illnesses not only have a serious effect on clients' self-image and therefore their feelings about their personal attractiveness to others, but also interfere physically with clients' capacity to have and maintain sexual relationships.

The sexual history may be uncomfortable for client and nurse. A factor that helps ensure that the client remains comfortable in the interview is the nurse's own comfort in asking sexual questions. The caregiver's uneasiness is usually conveyed to the client and is contagious. Nurses are generally comfortable with this area when they understand its vital importance to clients and the comfort and relief clients experience given an opportunity to share sexual concerns. A sexual history is appropriate, moreover, not only

TABLE 16–3. ELEMENTS OF THE ADULT PERSONAL, FAMILY, AND SOCIAL HISTORY

A. **Vocational/Educational/Financial**
 1. Type of work
 2. Type and amount of education
 3. Financial well-being
 4. Impact of illness

B. **Home and Family**
 1. Household roster
 2. Locale of family members
 3. Living arrangements
 4. Marital status
 5. Role responsibilities
 6. Impact of illness

C. **Social, Leisure, Spiritual, and Cultural**
 1. Description of social life
 2. Leisure interests
 3. Ethnic rituals/practices
 4. Religious beliefs/practices
 5. Impact of illness

D. **Sexual**
 1. Orientation/pattern
 2. Satisfaction
 3. Education/information
 4. Impact of illness

E. **Activities of Daily Living**
 1. Description of daily activity pattern
 2. Impact of illness

F. **Health Habits**
 1. Tobacco, alcohol, and other drug use
 2. Diet/description of daily intake
 3. Exercise pattern
 4. Sleep pattern
 5. Hygiene practices

G. **Psychological**
 1. Stressors/coping patterns
 2. Self-concept
 3. Health beliefs/sick role pattern

TABLE 16–4. SEXUAL HISTORY QUESTIONS FOR VARIOUS AGE GROUPS

Preschool: Questions are directed to parent or guardian.

- Have you begun providing sex education for your child?
- Have you talked to your child about sexual abuse, how to avoid it, and what to do if it occurs?
- Do you maintain bedroom and bathroom privacy in your home?

School Age: Questions are directed to the child.

- Tell me what you know about having babies.
- Tell me what you know about menstruation or having periods.
- Are you careful not to let anyone touch your (vagina, penis)?
- Have you and your family or your teachers talked about the kinds of touching that are not right? Parts of your body that other people should not touch?

Adolescence: Questions are directed to the adolescent.

- Tell me what you know about pregnancy.
- Tell me what you know about birth control.
- Tell me what you know about sexually transmitted disease.
- When did you begin to mature sexually?
- Girl: Are you menstruating? When did your menstrual period begin?
- Boy: When did you first notice your body changing?
- Are your friends sexually active?
- Are you sexually active? Describe your sexual pattern.
- What precautions do you take against pregnancy and sexually transmitted diseases?
- Tell me what you know about sexual abuse. Have you experienced sexual abuse?

Young Adult

- Are you sexually active?
- Describe your sexual pattern.
- What precautions do you take against pregnancy or sexually transmitted diseases?
- Are you satisfied with your sexual relationship(s)?

Middle and Older Adult

- Are you sexually active?
- Describe your sexual pattern.
- Have you experienced any changes in your sexual function?
- Are you satisfied with your sexual relationship(s)?

for adults but also for children and adolescents. Table 16–4 covers sexually focused questions that might be appropriate for various age groups. The guidelines for obtaining a sexual history are outlined here:

- *Begin with other areas of the history.* The nurse should delay the sexual history until there has been time to establish an initial rapport with the client. Explain why the sexual history is important and the types of questions that will be asked.
- *Provide privacy.* Interview the client in a quiet room. Direct questions to parents if the child is a preschooler. Otherwise direct questions to the client. For adolescent clients, interview the client without parents, siblings, peers, or roommates.
- *Maintain eye contact.* Making eye contact assists the nurse in evaluating the client's expressions, which may provide significant information about the client's attitudes. Avoid the tendency to look away or to gaze at notes. Clients may conclude that the nurse is uncomfortable with the topic of sex.
- *Avoid expressions of personal attitude.* Offer no opinions or advice. Maintain a neutral facial expression. Be matter of fact in addressing clients' questions. Give the client time to respond. Do not challenge the client's responses, even

if it is suspected that the client may be disclosing incomplete information.

- *Use correct anatomical terms.* Avoid using euphemisms for identifying the genitalia. Use correct anatomical terms.

Because the range of information in a complete personal family and social history is so vast, the caregiver must exercise judgment in collecting data. Discretion must be used about what questions to ask. Generally this is guided by the nature of the client's presenting problem. If the client, for example, has entered the hospital for treatment of an illness or injury that may cause temporary disability, it is appropriate to inquire about the client's arrangements for meeting job and home responsibilities in order to evaluate the need for social service intervention. If the disability might persist beyond discharge, it is also appropriate to ask the client about his or her place of residence and its characteristics (room arrangement, stairs, etc), which could present barriers to postdischarge care. By considering the nature of the client's problem, the caregiver is able to tailor the personal, family, and social history to the situation.

It should be noted that the family history accompanying the medical data base is oriented differently from the one nurses compile. The medical family history is a brief medical history of the client's family elicited to define familial patterns of disease. It is recorded in a branching diagram called a genogram that covers three generations of the client's family. The age and major medical problems are identified for each living family member, and the age and cause of death are listed for each deceased family member (Fig. 16–2). This information is helpful to nurses when there is a family illness pattern that has implications for the client's self-care. Nurses are vitally interested in teaching clients self-monitoring procedures for diseases that have a familial pattern, such as breast cancer and heart disease.[25]

Subjective Manifestations/Review of Systems. These two aspects of health assessment are identical in their orientation. They are both a review of the major systems of the body for the purpose of identifying the *subjective manifestations* that are present, the cardinal signs and symptoms of illness as reported by the client. Because the list is long, the caregiver generally works from a prepared list that serves as a memory cue. When going over such a list, it is important that the caregiver translate items into language that the client can understand. The client may not understand a question about diaphoresis, for example, but probably will understand one about sweating or perspiration. The list of questions that are appropriate for each organ system appears in Section 2. The major content areas include general questions and questions about the integument, head, ears, eyes, nose, throat, breasts, chest and cardiovascular, gastrointestinal, genitourinary, musculoskeletal, and neurological systems. Understanding the client's subjective manifestations enables nurses to tailor caregiving to the specific physical needs of the client. Moreover, nurses are then able to explore the consequences of these manifestations for the client's activities of daily living.

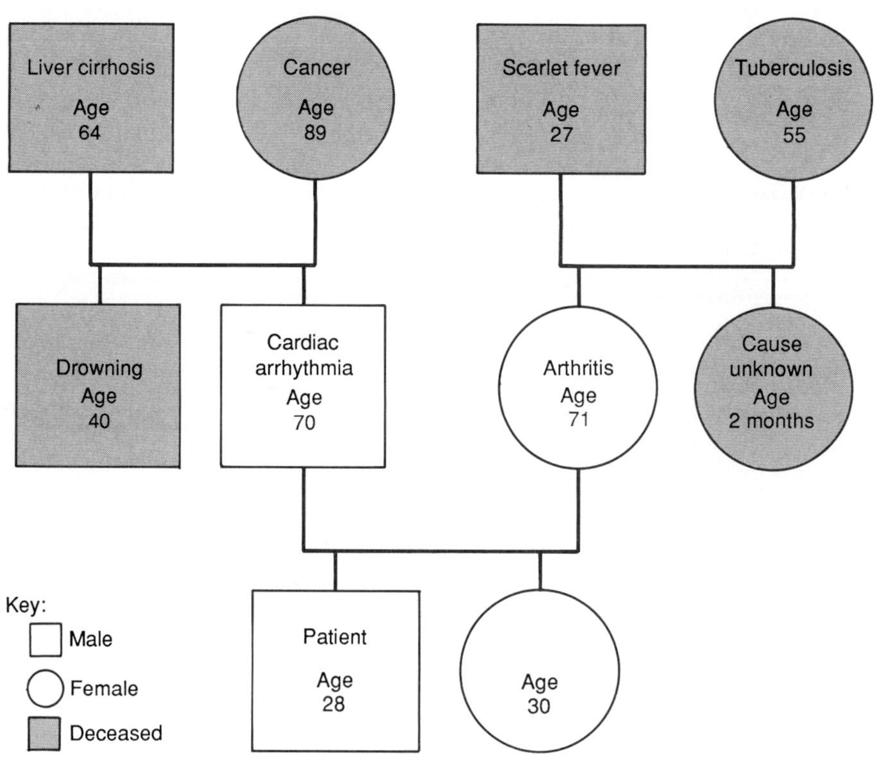

Figure 16–2. Genogram.

Types of Health Histories

There are three types of health histories: comprehensive, limited, and self-administered. The type of health history the caregiver conducts depends on the client's need or problem, the situation, and the health care setting.

Comprehensive. When the client undergoes a thorough well-person assessment or enters an acute care facility for the first time, a comprehensive health history is obtained. A comprehensive health history is one in which all of the elements of the history are thoroughly addressed.

Limited. A limited history is appropriate when the client has a specific need or an urgent health care problem. A limited history is one that addresses only the information needed to make decisions about the client's immediate problem. Thus, only those aspects of the past history, personal, family, and social history, and subjective manifestations that are relevant to the current situation are elicited. For example, a limited history might be done for a child admitted to an ambulatory surgery center for a tonsillectomy.

Self-administered. Self-administered histories are prepared histories in the form of questionnaires that clients read and fill out themselves. They are frequently used in outpatient and ambulatory care settings, and can be either comprehensive or limited in their scope. There are many different formats for self-administered health histories.

Self-administered histories are helpful because they save professionals time, freeing them for other responsibilities. Some clients prefer them because they can respond to them at their own pace; however, self-administered questionnaires have the disadvantage of being impersonal and of limiting the amount of detail that can be acquired. Unless a special effort is made, self-administered histories provide no opportunity for discussion or exploration with the client and no opportunity for the client to gain the reinforcement that goes with a chance to tell his or her story. When self-administered histories are used, they should always be preceded by thorough directions for use and followed up at their completion with a discussion of the client's answers with the client. Person-to-person exchanges centered on the content of the self-administered form diminish the inherent disadvantages of this approach.

THE HEALTH EXAMINATION

The health examination is that phase of health assessment in which the caregiver uses vision and other sensory modes to gain objective data about the client's health state.

Basic Health Examination Concepts

Purpose of the Health Examination. The purpose of the health examination is to collect objective data. The nurse assesses the client's current overall health status to establish a baseline against which future examination findings can be compared.

Phases of the Health Examination. There are five phases to the health examination: (1) preparing the examination room or area, the equipment, and the client; (2) obtaining measurements and vital signs; (3) collecting laboratory specimens as indicated; (4) conducting the head-to-toe examination, and (5) recording the examination data.

Preparation. The first phase is preparation. The examination room or area should be clean and well lit and arranged conveniently. The tools to be used should be available, easily accessible, and in good operating condition. Box 16–5 lists the tools and supplies commonly used during the health examination. Figure 16–3 depicts some of the tools that are used during the examination.

Preparation also requires that clients are given information about the purpose of the examination and what they can expect and might experience. Client preparation for the health examination encompasses two areas: physical preparation and psychological preparation.

Physical Preparation. One aspect of preparing the client for the examination is to have the client urinate or "void" before the health examination begins. If a urine specimen is required, it can be obtained at this time.

Another aspect of preparing the client for physical examination is removal of the client's clothing. If a complete health examination is done, ask the client to undress completely and don an examination gown. If a limited examination is planned, that is, an examination of only one or two body systems or areas, the client needs only to remove the clothing from that specific area. It may be necessary to

BOX 16–5. TOOLS AND SUPPLIES COMMONLY USED DURING THE HEALTH EXAMINATION

- Sphygmomanometer
- Stethoscope
- Thermometer
- Percussion hammer
- Tape measure
- Tuning fork
- Nasal speculum
- Tongue depressors
- Otoscope
- Ophthalmoscope attachment
- Penlight
- Lubricant
- Disposable gloves
- Vaginal speculum
- Safety pin
- Cotton or small cotton-tipped swab
- Watch with seconds calibration
- Disposable pads
- Drapes

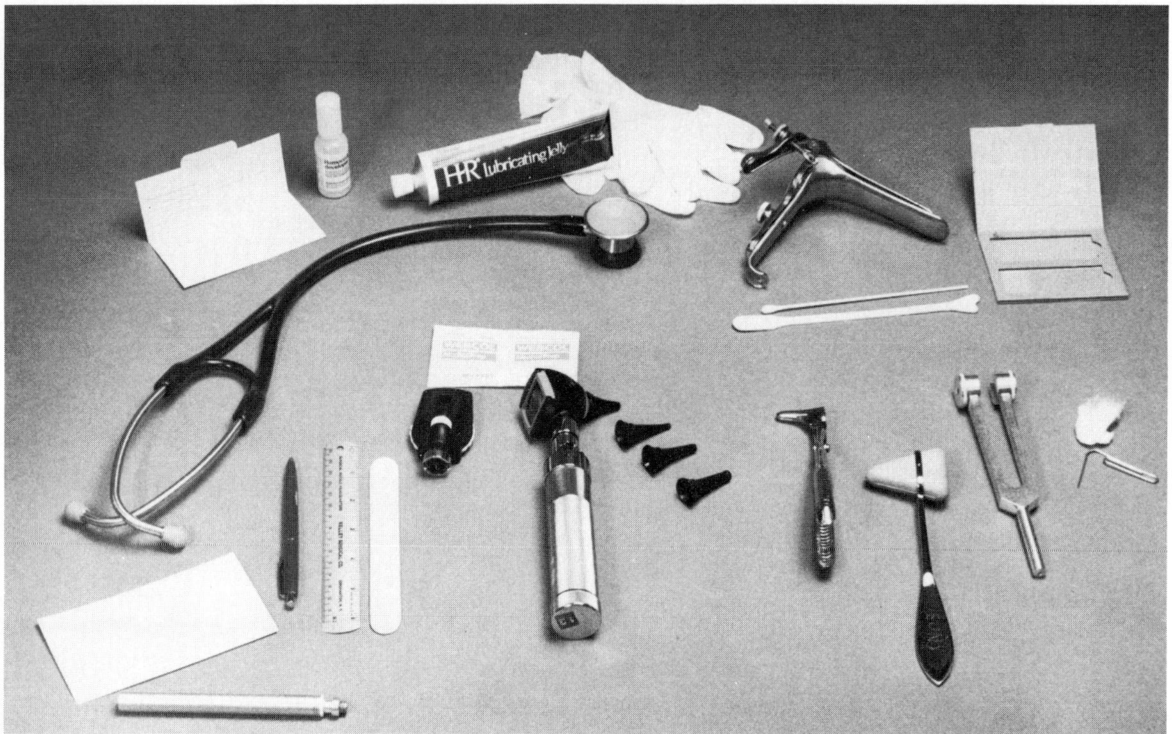

Figure 16–3. Tools that are used during the health examination. (Source: *Block GJ, Nolan JW.* Health Assessment for Professional Nursing: A Developmental Approach. *2nd ed. Norwalk, CT: Appleton-Century-Crofts; 1986.*)

cover the client with a blanket to prevent chilling during the examination, particularly if the room temperature is cool or the client is older or very ill.

The physical examination requires that the client assume various positions during the process. This facilitates the examination by providing access and visibility to the body area being examined. The positions that are most useful are the recumbent position, the dorsal recumbent position, the knee-chest position, the lithotomy position, and Sims' position. Table 16–5 shows these positions and lists their purposes.

As the client assumes the various positions the nurse must ensure that the client's privacy is maintained. This is done by draping the client's body with a sheet or one or more disposable drapes. In addition to privacy, drapes also provide warmth. Table 16–5 shows the most effective way to apply a drape for each of the examination positions.

Psychological Preparation. To prepare the client psychologically, explain the examination procedure to the client. Invite the client's questions and endeavor to answer them as fully as possible. This approach should help to alleviate anxiety. Show the equipment that will be used and outline its use especially to very young clients. This usually enhances the client's sense of control in the situation.

During this early phase of the examination, the nurse focuses on continued development of rapport with the client and takes the opportunity to reinforce the collaborative values initiated at the time of the health history. During the health examination, the client confirms or disconfirms initial impressions of the caregiver. The client may require additional assurances that the caregiver will take the necessary measures to assist the client to feel comfortable during the examination. As the examination proceeds, nurse and client discuss the findings, adding to the exchanges begun in the health history. This process facilitates later exchanges during which the nurse and client review and verify findings as the examination draws to a close. Collaborative give-and-take during the examination provides additional opportunities for the client to expand on his or her health problems or health status from a personal perspective.

Measurements and Vital Signs. Height, weight, head and limb circumferences, limb length measurements, temperature, pulse, respiration, and blood pressure are taken as the second step in the health examination process. These measurements are discussed in detail below.

Laboratory Specimen Collection. Various specimens are collected for laboratory analysis that provide additional objective data to be used in arriving at definitive diagnoses. Usually specimens are collected after measurements are taken and before the head-to-toe examination begins. Diagnostic test results are an essential component of the health examination. Procedures for collecting laboratory specimens appear in Unit VI in the respective chapters on human functional dimensions to which they are related.

TABLE 16–5. CLIENT POSITIONS AND DRAPING FOR THE PHYSICAL EXAMINATION

Position	Purpose
Recumbent	Head and neck, anterior thorax and lungs, breasts, axillae, heart
Dorsal recumbent	Pelvis, vaginal
Knee-chest	Rectum
Lithotomy	Vaginal, pelvis
Sims'	Rectum for nonambulatory males and for females receiving a rectal but not a vaginal examination

From Flynn JBM, Hackel R. Technological Foundations in Nursing. *Norwalk, CT: Appleton & Lange; 1990.*

Head-to-Toe Examination. One systematic method of examining is to begin at the head and work toward the feet. This is the so-called *head-to-toe examination* (Box 16–6). It is the fourth phase of the health examination.

The head-to-toe examination is the orderly review by the caregiver of the client's body parts and body systems. It literally begins at the client's head and proceeds in an observational sequence to the neck, the trunk and upper limbs, and finally the lower limbs. Observations of body areas are combined with the nurse's focus on specific body systems. For example, the examination of the head combines observations of the anatomical features of the head with an assessment of the neurosensory functions of vision, hearing, taste, and smell.

The advantage of the head-to-toe examination is that it applies a pattern of organization that helps ensure that all aspects of the health examination are completed and none are inadvertently ignored.

BOX 16–6. HEAD-TO-TOE ORDER OF EXAMINATION AREAS

- Skin
- Hair
- Nails
- Head
- Face
- Ears
- Eyes
- Nose
- Sinuses
- Mouth
- Throat
- Neck
- Breasts and axillae
- Thorax/back
- Heart and peripheral vessels
- Upper extremities
- Abdomen
- Anus and rectum
- Genitalia
- Lower extremities

Recording. The final phase of the health examination is recording of findings. The objective data are organized according to body systems (respiratory, cardiovascular, gastrointestinal, etc) and compiled into a written record. The order in which systems are recorded corresponds to the order of the head-to-toe examination. Naturally, all information recorded must be factual and devoid of the caregiver's interpretations.

Recording health information accomplishes several objectives. The recording format organizes the data and this organization process assists the caregiver in formulating the nursing diagnosis and aids the development of the plan of care. Putting the data into written form ensures that the data are available to all caregivers working with the client and that they can be used for future reference. Lastly, recording the data creates a legal record that can be used as evidence when there is controversy about some aspect of the client's care or treatment. Prompt recording is advisable to ensure accuracy and completeness of the record.

Methods for Examining. There are four classical methods or techniques of examining: inspection, palpation, percussion, and auscultation.

Inspection. To inspect means to visually look at, to observe, and to examine. All body parts are subjected to **inspection** during the health examination. Because the body is symmetrical, each body part is compared for similarities and differences with its counterpart on the opposite side of the body. This identifies variances in size, shape, position, form, or color that may suggest abnormality.

Technique. Your eyes are the tools of inspection. During inspection, visually observe the client. Instruments are frequently employed to enhance the examiner's vision. Some instruments provide illumination (otoscopes, penlights, or adjustable-neck examination lamps). Other instruments give magnification as well as illumination (ophthalmoscopes). Instruments are helpful to observe hard-to-visualize areas. Still other tools assist inspection by removing barriers to observation. Tongue depressors, for example, aid visualization of the back of the throat by depressing the tongue so that the structures behind it can be seen.

Palpation. To palpate means to feel. Clinically, the term **palpation** means to examine by use of touch. Many body parts are examined by palpation during the health examination. The caregiver places his or her hands on the client to feel characteristics of the underlying tissue that cannot be visualized. Through palpation, it is possible to identify such features as size, shape, and position of underlying masses, texture and temperature of the skin, or movement, vibration, or pulsation of internal structures. It is also possible to demonstrate tenderness. Touching tender areas usually causes recoil from the painful stimulus.

The examiner's hands are the tools of palpation. Using various parts of the hand—sometimes only the tips of two fingers, sometimes all of the fingers, sometimes the fingers and the palm of the hand—the examiner systematically touches areas of the body such as the chest, abdomen, lymph nodes, breasts, and even the face.

There are three types of palpation: light palpation, deep palpation, and ballottement.

Light palpation is the use of gentle touch to palpate tissue. During light palpation, an indentation in the tissue of about ½ in. (1 cm) is made (Fig. 16–4A). Light palpation is helpful to identify areas of tenderness and superficial masses. Light palpation is accomplished using the procedure outlined below.

Light palpation is generally not helpful for sensing deep structures. To assess deep structures, such as the major organs of the abdomen, deep palpation is necessary. During deep palpation, an indentation of about 1 in. (2 cm) is made in the tissue (see Fig. 16–4B). Deep palpation can be done using one or two hands. When two hands are used, the top hand provides the pressure for the inward movement and the lower hand is used to detect sensations. Caution should be used when performing this technique, as the pressure can result in internal injury if not done correctly.

Ballottement is a type of palpation that has a specific and limited use. It detects masses of tissue that are floating within a fluid in the body, such as the fetus that floats in the amniotic fluid of the pregnant uterus. The mechanism of this technique is that a floating tissue mass can be made to move upward in the fluid by gently tapping the surround-

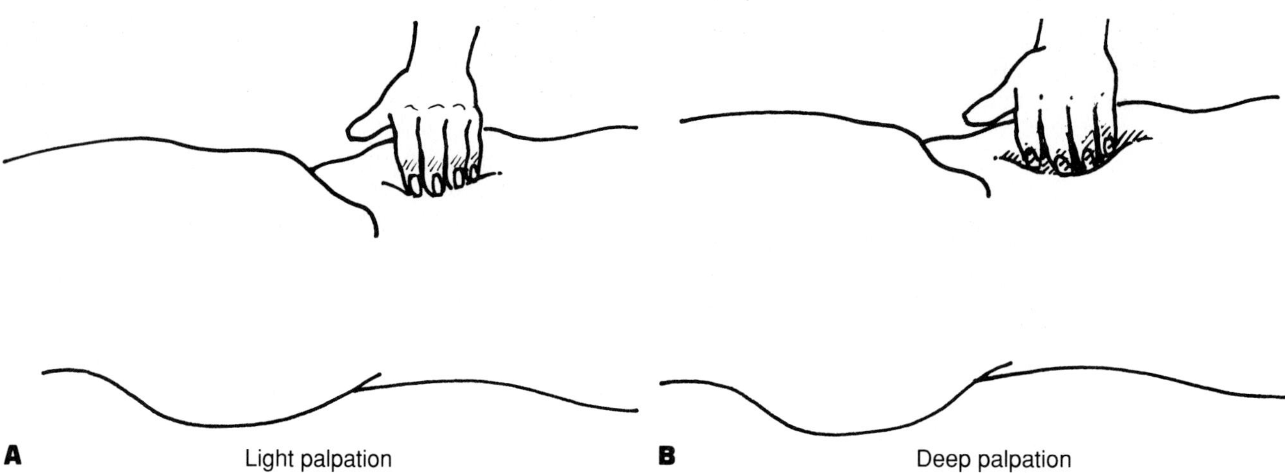

Figure 16–4. Light and deep palpation.

ing tissue. As the floating mass sinks back to its original position, a rebounding tap is felt by the examiner's fingers. This technique is also used to detect the presence of fluid accumulation within the abdomen (ascites).

Palpation, particularly of such areas as the abdomen, is easier when the client is relaxed. Often clients are afraid that palpation will cause pain. They become tense even before the examiner begins. Reassuring the client that discomfort is usually minimal and that palpation will be stopped if the client experiences pain usually helps clients to relax during the procedure. Sometimes the presenting problem of the client involves pain. It is helpful to know the areas of the body in which the client is experiencing pain before beginning palpation. With that information, the caregiver can approach those areas with special care.

Technique. Place your fingers at a 45-degree angle to the skin. Gently push downward. Simultaneously move the palpating hand in a circular motion. This enables the perception of density and mobility of the underlying tissue. Instruct the client to indicate whenever he or she feels a tender spot or painful area. Observe the client for nonverbal expressions of pain.

Percussion. **Percussion** is the technique of tapping the skin surface with the fingers or with an instrument to produce sounds. The characteristics of the sounds that result vary with the density of the underlying tissue. Disease may alter tissue density and thus change the sounds tissue provides when tapped.

Percussion is used to assess the condition of tissue that lies beneath the surface of the skin by the sound emitted. In addition, various internal structures can be located, size determined, boundaries outlined, and density identified. Percussion can also identify, by the sound emitted, whether the area is filled with fluid, is filled with air, or is solid. The sounds are evaluated by the examiner according to their intensity (amplitude), pitch (number of vibrations per second), duration (length of sound), and quality (resonance).

Generally the examiner's fingers are the tools used for percussing. There are two techniques for percussing, direct and indirect. In the direct method, one or two fingertips of the examiner's hand are used to tap directly on the client's body surface. A percussion hammer or a fist can also be used for direct percussion. In the indirect method, the examiner uses the fingers of one hand to tap the finger of the other hand, which is placed on the client's skin (Fig. 16–5). Indirect percussion is the hands-on technique most people think of in reference to the health examination.

The five categories of percussion sound are flatness, dullness, resonance, tympany, and hyperresonance (Table 16–6). The sound elicited is described as tympany if it is high-pitched and drumlike, and dull if it is thudlike. A hollow organ such as the stomach will produce a musical, high-pitched tympanic sound, whereas the sound heard from percussing a dense solid organ such as the liver will be dull, which is a short, soft thud in quality. Resonance is similar to the sound obtained when talking through a cardboard tube. It has a clear, moderately low-pitched quality and is the sound obtained when palpating air-filled lungs. Hyperresonance is a deep rebounding sound, much like that which occurs when talking inside a cave or cavern. It has a booming quality, is abnormal, and is heard over a fluid-filled emphysemic lung. Flatness lacks rebound vibration from the underlying area. This response to palpation is received over very dense tissue such as muscle and bone.

Technique. Place the palmar surface of the finger (referred to as the pleximeter) of one hand firmly on the client's skin. Use the first or second finger of the other hand (referred to as the plexor), applying wrist action, to tap on the knuckle

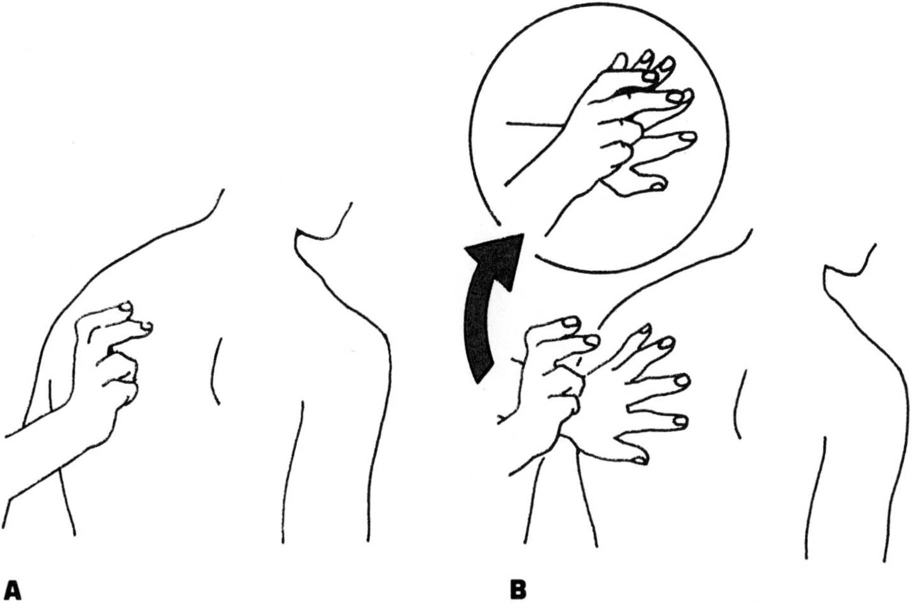

Figure 16–5. Percussion technique. Percussion can be done either **(A)** with one hand (direct) or **(B)** with both hands (indirect).

TABLE 16–6. SUMMARY OF PERCUSSION SOUNDS

Type	Sound	Example
Flatness	Lacks rebound vibration	Very dense tissue, eg, muscle and bone
Dullness	Blunt	Solid organ, eg, liver
Resonance	Hollow	Air-filled area, eg, air-filled lung
Tympany	High-pitched, drumlike	Hollow organ, eg, lung or stomach
Hyperresonance	Rebounding, booming	Abnormal sound, eg, area filled with much fluid, as with an emphysemic lung

of the positioned finger. Listen for the sounds produced. The resounding vibrations and sounds are translated and interpreted as physical findings.

Auscultation. **Auscultation** employs the sense of hearing to assess naturally occurring body sounds. The examiner listens to the sounds originating internally to assess the functioning status of a particular organ or structure. Categories of sound assessment include frequency, volume, quality, and duration. Sounds are auscultated in the cardiovascular, respiratory, and gastrointestinal systems.

The Stethoscope. Auscultation can be done by placing an ear directly on the client's body surfaces. Usually, however, an *acoustical stethoscope* is used to amplify body sounds. It detects surface vibrations that are a continuation of visceral vibrations generated inside the body, and magnifies the sounds emitted so they are audible to the examiner. There are times and situations, however, in which an acoustical stethoscope cannot magnify the sound sufficiently so that it can be heard. In these instances, an ultrasound stethoscope is often employed. Ultrasound stethoscopes are discussed later in the chapter.

An acoustical stethoscope has several standard components. These are the chestpiece, flexible plastic tubing, approximately 12–18 in. in length, connecting to rigid tubes called binaurals, and earpieces made of plastic or hard rubber (Fig. 16–6). The chestpiece itself usually has two components, a diaphragm and a bell; however, some models have only the diaphragm. The diaphragm is the flat disk-shaped piece of plastic that is affixed to the chestpiece. It is used for detecting higher-pitched sounds such as bowel sounds. The bell is the cone-shaped device attached to the back of the diaphragm. It is used for lower-pitched sounds such as heart sounds.

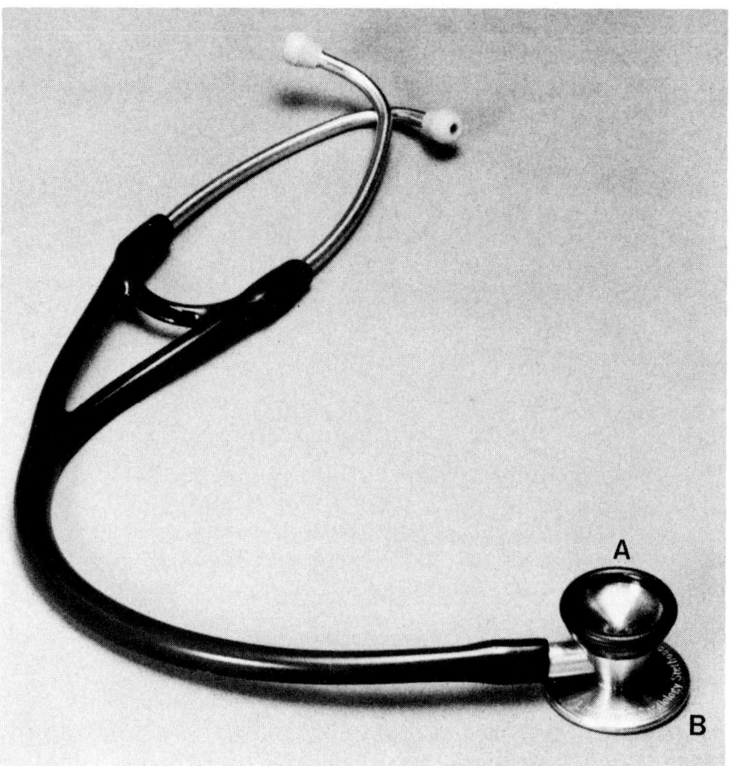

Figure 16–6. Acoustical stethoscope. **A.** Bell. **B.** Diaphragm. (Source: *Block GJ, Nolan JW.* Health Assessment for Professional Nursing: A Developmental Approach. *2nd ed. Norwalk, CT: Appleton-Century-Crofts; 1986.*)

The chestpiece picks up the surface vibrations and transmits them through the tubing, binaurals, and earpieces into the user's ears, where they are translated into sound. As the stethoscope is a closed system, most of the vibration is prevented from dissipating into the surrounding air. The earpieces are positioned slightly forward to facilitate hearing as this is the same approximate position as the ear canal. Excess pressure applied when using the bell or insufficient pressure applied when using the diaphragm results in inadequate transmission of vibrations.

When using a stethoscope that has a chestpiece with both a diaphragm and a bell, the examiner is careful to position the chestpiece properly when rotating from one mode to the other or before each use. A distinct "click" can be felt when the chestpiece locks into position. Failure to appropriately position the chestpiece will obliterate the sounds.

Technique. Position the earpieces in the ears. Lock the diaphragm or bell, whichever is to be used, into position and test for sound by tapping. Apply the diaphragm or bell to the skin surface. Hold the diaphragm firmly against the skin. Apply the bell lightly to the skin surface.

Organizing the Examination. There are several approaches the nurse can use when determining the organization or sequence in which the health examination is conducted. The examination can be conducted by body system or body region, or a combination of the two can be used. These formats all ultimately result in a complete health examination.

Body Systems. When using the body system approach to the health examination, the nurse examines all areas and structures connected with that particular system. For example, if the gastrointestinal system were being examined, the nurse would begin the examination with the mouth, continue to the abdomen, and end with the rectum. Although this approach provides data, it is inefficient. It can be taxing, particularly for a debilitated client, as the client is asked to sit up for the oral examination, lie down for the stomach, liver, and intestine examination, and change positions yet a third time for the rectal examination. Under the systems approach, when the examiner completes the revision of one system, she or he moves to the next.

Body Regions. The body region approach to the health examination is to examine all systems and structures in a particular area. For example, if the upper extremities were being examined, the nurse would collect data about the skin, muscle, bone and joint movement, circulation, and neurological function present in this area. When the examination of one body part is completed, the examiner moves to another. This approach also provides health assessment data and is more efficient; it requires less energy expenditure by the client, who can remain in one position. It does require that the examiner consider several examination facets simultaneously and remember and carry them out in order to end with a comprehensive examination.

Mixed. The mixed approach, as the word implies, is a combination of the body system and body region approaches. An example of this health examination approach is to use the body region method to conduct the health examination but to omit the neurological system and visual testing assessments until the end of the examination. As was stated earlier, the type of health examination that is done depends on the client's condition and needs and the nurse's intuition about other body involvements.

Measurements and Vital Signs

Height Measurement. *Height* measurement is the length of the individual or the vertical distance measured from the top of the head to the heels. Height is an indicator of health status and is used to assist with identification of genetic disease, organ/system dysfunction, and hormonal disturbances. For example, the child whose growth rate falls outside the standardized growth parameters for the child's age could have inadequate pituitary function.

Equipment. A vertical measuring tool, typically one combined with a scale for weight measurement, is required to obtain a height measurement. Cloth, metal, paper, plastic or wooden measurement devices that are attached to a wall surface are also acceptable devices. Weight scales that have an attached height measurement bar provide an efficient way to measure the height of young children or adults. Infants are measured with a tape measure or horizontal ruler.

Technique. Ask the client to remove shoes or slippers. Heel height will increase the measured height and obscure the client's actual measurement. Encourage the client to stand erect. Make a written note of the height so it can be accurately recorded later in the client's chart.

When measuring the height of a child who cannot stand alone, place the child in the supine position, extend the legs, and measure from the heels to the top of the head. Be sure the legs are fully extended to obtain an accurate measurement.

Norms and Expected Findings. The norms and expected height–weight ratios for adults are listed in Table 16–7. The reader is referred to Chapter 11 for values for children. It is a fact that people gradually decrease in height as they age. There is an inverse relationship between age and height. This decrease occurs as a result of the osteoporosis (decreased bone density) and kyphosis (thoracic spinal curvature) that occur with aging. The aging process may cause a decrease in height of as much as 1 to 3 in.

Special Considerations, Precautions, Sources of Error. It is important to have the client stand as straight as possible during height measurement. Older adults with skeletal malformations or poor posture may require some assistance to stand straight.

Height is usually obtained in inches but charted in feet and inches. The nurse can convert inches into feet and inches by dividing the number of inches of height by 12.

Some facilities use the metric system for obtaining and

TABLE 16–7. HEIGHT–WEIGHT COMPARISON NORMS

Men					Women				
Height (in shoes)[a]		Weight in Pounds (in indoor clothing)[b]			Height (in shoes)[a]		Weight in Pounds (in indoor clothing)[b]		
ft	in.	Small Frame	Medium Frame	Large Frame	ft	in.	Small Frame	Medium Frame	Large Frame
5	2	128–134	131–141	138–150	4	10	102–111	109–121	118–131
5	3	130–136	133–143	140–153	4	11	103–113	111–123	120–134
5	4	132–138	135–145	142–156	5	0	104–115	113–126	122–137
5	5	134–140	137–148	144–160	5	1	106–118	115–129	125–140
5	6	136–142	139–151	146–164	5	2	108–121	118–132	128–143
5	7	138–145	142–154	149–168	5	3	111–124	121–135	131–147
5	8	140–148	145–157	152–172	5	4	114–127	124–138	134–151
5	9	142–151	148–160	155–176	5	5	117–130	127–141	137–155
5	10	144–154	151–163	158–180	5	6	120–133	130–144	140–159
5	11	146–157	154–166	161–184	5	7	123–136	133–147	143–163
6	0	149–160	157–170	164–188	5	8	126–139	136–150	146–167
6	1	152–164	160–174	168–192	5	9	129–142	139–153	149–170
6	2	155–168	164–178	172–197	5	10	132–145	142–156	152–173
6	3	158–172	167–182	176–202	5	11	135–148	145–159	155–176
6	4	162–176	171–187	181–207	6	0	138–151	148–162	158–179

[a] Shoes with 1-in. heels.
[b] Indoor clothing weighing 5 pounds for men and 3 pounds for women.
Source of basic data: Build Study, 1979, *Society of Actuaries and Association of Life Insurance Medical Directors of America, 1980.*
Copyright 1983 Metropolitan Life Insurance Company.

recording height. Boxes 16–7 and 16–8 show metric equivalents.

Recording. The client's height is recorded on the vital signs graphic or designated flowsheet. Accuracy is important. Height, weight, and body surface area data are used by other departments to calculate laboratory test results, drug dosages, anesthetic agent doses, nutritional supplements, and amount of radiation required by individual clients for specific radiologic procedures.

Weight Measurement. *Weight* is defined as the measurement of quantity or mass as determined by a scale. Frequently weight and height are plotted together on a standardized height/weight chart that compares the two measurements. An overall assessment of the ratio of height to weight provides valuable clues about the client's current health and nutritional status. If a client's weight is excessive for the measured height, it may indicate excessive food intake or retention of fluid. If weight is insufficient for height, it may be indicative of inadequate food intake, gastrointestinal malfunction or disease, or the presence of other disease processes.

Equipment. Two types of scales for weight measurement are available today: mechanical and electronic. The mechanical scale indicates weight on a gauge or by use of a balance lever; the electronic scale provides a digital readout of the weight.

There are various models of weight measurement devices designed specifically to meet the needs of the client who is unable to stand on a conventional scale. In addition to the scale models that clients stand on, there are stretcher and bed scales that provide tables on which clients can lie if they are unable to stand unassisted (Fig. 16–7). Still another model provides a built-in chair on which clients sit while being weighed (Fig. 16–8). These types of special-

BOX 16–7. CONVERSION FORMULA FOR METERS AND INCHES

1 m = 39.4 in.
To convert meters to inches:
meter(s) × 39.4 = inches
To convert inches to meters:
inches ÷ 39.4 = meters

BOX 16–8. MEASUREMENT EQUIVALENTS

1 in. = 2.5 cm
1 ft = 0.3 m
1 ft = 30.5 cm
1 cm = 0.4 in.
1 m = 39.4 in.
1 m = 3.28 ft

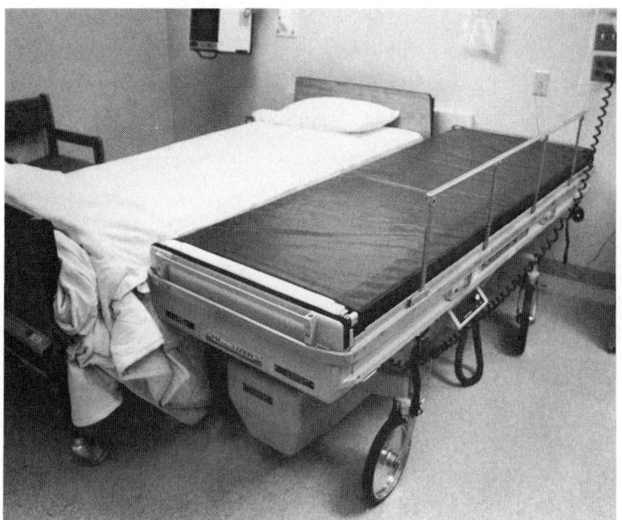

Figure 16–7. Bed scale.

purpose scales have casters and can be transported to the bedside. Infant scales vary from adult scales in that, before recording the infant's weight measurement, the weight of the protective scale platform covering must be subtracted from the infant's weight reading (Fig. 16–9).

Technique. Obtain the client's weight by using the scale model appropriate to the client's condition and functional abilities. Follow the procedure recommended for the scale model used.

To ensure that an accurate weight is obtained, weigh the client before breakfast. Ask the client to void prior to obtaining the weight reading. Remove all nonessential clothing such as shoes, slippers, robe, and jacket (Box 16–9). This ensures that the measurement obtained is free of extraneous sources of additional weight. Be sure to place a paper towel on the scale platform as both an infection control and sanitary measure.

When using a bar balance scale, slide the counterweight until the bar balances at the indicated mark. When using the gauge or digital readout scale, simply make a notation of the reading so it can be recorded accurately later in the client's chart. For further instructions on how to use the available scale model, refer to the accompanying instruction manual.

When using the stretcher table or chair model scale, always use the same type and amount of linens while weighing the client or weigh the linens before or after the client transfers to the scale stretcher platform or chair. Subtract the weight of the linens from the weight reading obtained.

While weighing the client, observe the client's appearance and make a judgment about whether the client's weight appears appropriate to height. This is an important step in evaluating nutrition.

Place a disposable scale paper, cloth diaper, or paper towel on the scale platform as a sanitary measure before weighing an infant. Infants frequently urinate in response to the stimulation of the procedure and may defecate. Completely undress the infant and remove the diaper. Place the infant on the covered scale platform. Be aware of the infant's safety needs and potential for falling. After obtaining the weight measurement, which is measured in grams, redress the infant and wrap in a blanket to minimize heat loss or cold stress.

Similarly to the adult, weigh the infant at the same time each day before being fed to exclude extraneous factors such as weight of the formula just ingested and obtain as true a weight as is possible.

Norms and Expected Findings. Insurance companies have devoted a great deal of research to determine height-to-weight averages, which are used as a standard for comparison. These averages are compiled into actuarial tables and are accepted as normal ranges by the medical profession. Actuarial tables indicate height–weight ratios for various body build types and sex (see Table 16–7).

Special Considerations, Precautions, Sources of Error. The accuracy of the weight measurement depends on the precision of the scale used, the conditions under which the weight measurement is obtained, and the accuracy of the nurse's technique and recording. Clients may try to balance themselves on the scale by holding onto someone or something else. The nurse should ensure that the client does not inadvertently lean against a wall or hold onto the scale,

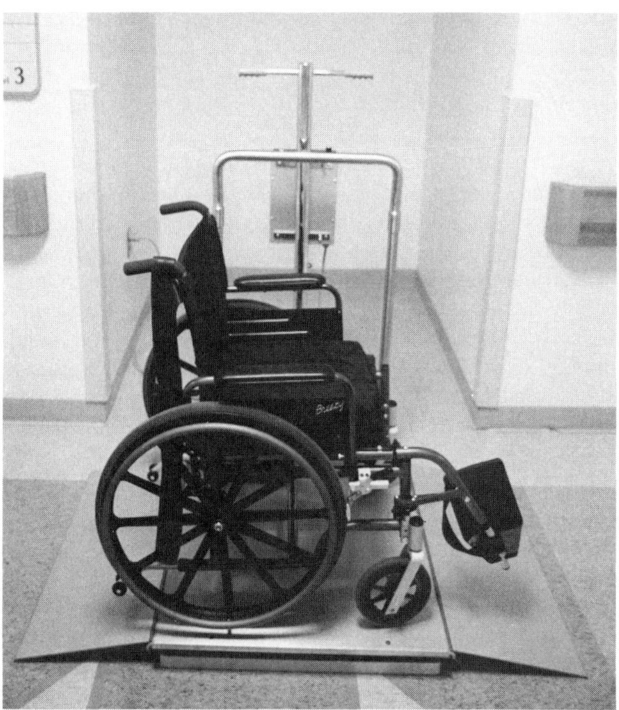

Figure 16–8. Chair scale.

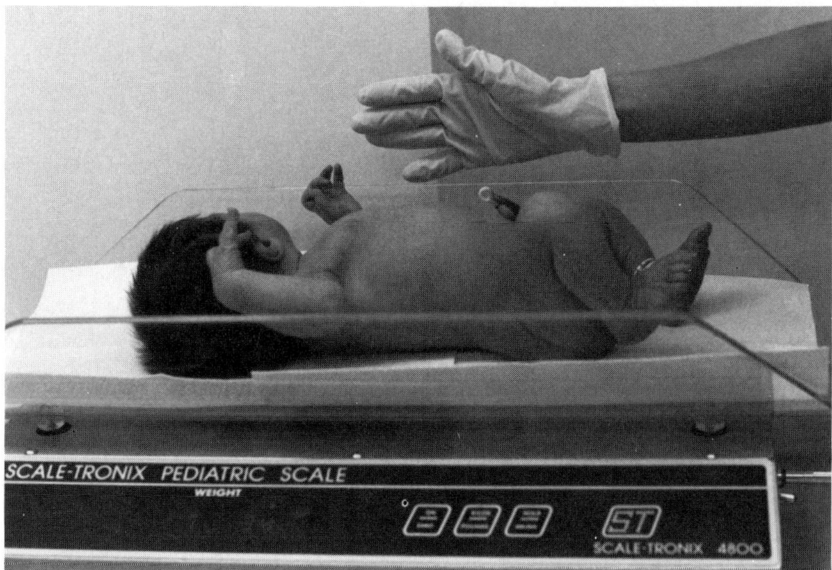

Figure 16–9. Weighing an infant. (Source: *Sherwen LN, Scoloveno MA, Weingarten CT.* Nursing Care of the Childbearing Family. *Norwalk, CT: Appleton & Lange; 1991.*)

because this will give an inaccurate reading. Assistance from others may also inadvertently contribute to measurement errors. Those assisting need to be reminded to avoid putting pressure on the stretcher table or bed frame, which will falsely increase the client's weight reading.

The nurse should ask the client if he or she has had a recent unexplained weight increase or decrease. Gain or loss of 10 or more pounds in one month could indicate dysfunction or disease. If the client has experienced a weight change, the nurse should inquire about the presence of other signs or symptoms, such as nervousness, decreased energy, and frequent urination. Such symptoms may be associated with and may provide clues to the etiology. Also, the nurse should inquire about the regularity of mealtimes and quantity of food intake.

Recording. The client's weight is recorded on the vital signs graph or designated flowsheet. As with height recording, the accuracy of this information is important. It provides valuable medical data and is also used by other departments.

Some facilities use the metric system for weight measurement and record the weight in kilograms as the unit of measure (Box 16–10).

BOX 16–9. PROCEDURE CONSIDERATIONS THAT ENSURE OBTAINING ACCURATE WEIGHT

The client should:

1. Void before being weighed.
2. Be weighed at the same time each day, preferably on awaking and before breakfast. A weight obtained in this manner is called a "metabolic weight."
3. Wear the same type of clothing, for example, with or without a robe, with or without slippers.

Head Circumference, Limb Length, Limb Circumference. *Head circumference* is the measurement of the head at the level of its greatest diameter. Head circumference measurement is usually done for infants and children as an indirect indicator of brain growth. It is performed routinely on children until the age of 2 years. Head circumference measurement would, however, be an appropriate adult measurement if indicated. Such client statements as "My head seems to have grown because my hat is too small now" and "I have these terrible headaches and my head seems like it's getting larger" suggest a need to measure head circumference. An increase in the measurement may indicate cerebrospinal fluid accumulation with corresponding abnormal growth of the skull.

Limb circumference is the distance around a specific area on the arms or legs. *Limb length* is the measurement between two specific bony landmarks or other anatomically identified areas.

Arm and leg length and circumference measurements usually are obtained only if a growth abnormality is suspected on admission to the health agency during the initial physical examination; however, these measurements may be obtained more frequently following surgery, for example, or if edema of the extremity is present or suspected.

BOX 16–10. CONVERSION FORMULA FOR KILOGRAMS AND POUNDS

1 kg = 2.2 lb
1 lb = 0.45 kg
To convert kilograms to pounds:
kilograms × 2.2 = pounds
To convert pounds to kilograms:
pounds ÷ 2.2 = kilograms

Equipment. A flexible tape measure is needed for head circumference, limb length, or limb circumference measurement.

Technique

Head Circumference. When measuring the head, place the measuring device, usually a paper or cloth tape, just above the eyebrows (the supraorbital ridge) anteriorly and across the area of greatest protrusion of the occipital bone posteriorly. It is important that the client remain still for the measurement.

Limb Length. For limb length, the exact points of measurement must be indicated. The area to be measured is determined by the nature of the client's problem. For example, if a bone graft has been inserted into the tibia, the measurement is made between the patella and the malleolus.

Limb Circumference. Limb circumference is measured bilaterally and the measurements are compared. To ensure accuracy, measurements should be taken at the same level on both limbs. The purpose for the measurement determines the point at which the measurement is taken. For example, if muscle atrophy of the leg is suspected, then thigh or calf measurement would be indicated. The most common points for leg measurement are the midthighs and calves. Arm circumference measurement is less common, and the level for measurement is determined by the purpose of the procedure. Note the exact level or place where the circumference is measured on the Kardex or work sheet. This helps to ensure procedural consistency by all caregivers. If limb circumference is done frequently, use an indelible marker to indicate on the skin surface the exact placement of the measuring tape. Place the measuring tape snugly but not tightly around the area being measured. If there is a tissue indentation, the tape measure has been too tightly applied.

Norms and Expected Findings. The norms and expected findings for head circumference and height and weight measurements for ages birth to 18 years appear on the inside back cover. Similar to height and weight, head circumference is evaluated by comparing the measured value to a chart of standard values. Measurements should neither increase nor decrease from day to day. Findings other than this are abnormal and the nurse should consult with the physician about such findings.

Limb length and circumference should also be stable from day to day and should be symmetrical. Limbs may differ a small amount in length normally.

Special Considerations, Precautions, Sources of Error. The limb length or circumference measurement reading will be inaccurate if it is not obtained at the same points on both the right and left limbs.

Head circumference measurements may vary if the client moves during measurement or if tape measure placement varies from one time to the next.

Recording. The information obtained from these measurements is recorded in the client's chart on the vital signs graph or flowsheet. Measurement can be recorded in either centimeters or inches (see Box 16–8).

Body Temperature Measurement. One of the most common and important activities of the nurse is to measure body temperature. Body temperature, one of the body's vital signs, is considered to be a cardinal indicator of health status.

Basic Concepts About Body Temperature. Body temperature is the balance maintained between the amount of heat produced in the body and the amount of heat lost. Ordinarily, heat production and heat loss are balanced to maintain a relatively constant body temperature. Heat balance is a manifestation of physiological homeostasis. Body temperature is an excellent indicator of health or illness because temperature changes accompany many diseases and indicate an alteration in condition that may be otherwise unobservable. Thus body temperature is measured to monitor body functioning.

Definition. **Body temperature** is the level of hotness or coldness of the body measured in heat units called degrees. There are two types of body temperature: surface temperature and core temperature. Surface temperature is the temperature of the skin and outer tissue layers and increases or decreases in direct relation to the environmental temperature. The surface temperature can vary from 68F to 104F (20C to 40C) without causing damage to the body for the reason that the skin, subcutaneous tissue, and fat provide insulation against heat loss and protect the body from high environmental temperatures.

Core temperature is the temperature of the deep structures such as the heart and liver. It remains relatively constant within 1 degree of 98.6F (37C). When the client's temperature is assessed, the core temperature is measured in the mouth (oral), rectum, or axillae.

Body Temperature Regulation. The hypothalamus, the skin and deep body thermoreceptors, and the major body organs all participate in the regulation of body temperature.

The hypothalamus, located deep in the brain between the cerebral hemispheres, acts as the body's thermostat and is stimulated by an increased or decreased temperature of its blood flow. Receptors in the hypothalamus along with thermoreceptors in the skin monitor and control the balance between heat production and heat loss.

The temperature receptors located in the skin of the body are very important to the control of body temperature and the initiation of heat conservation mechanisms. The skin is endowed with both cold and warmth receptors; however, there are 10 times more cold than warmth receptors. Thus, peripheral temperature detection is the detection of mainly cool rather than warm temperatures.[26] When the skin is chilled over the entire body, receptor reflexes act to (1) provide a stimulus for shivering, (2) inhibit the process of sweating, and (3) promote vasoconstriction.[26]

Deep body thermoreceptors assist the skin receptors in controlling body temperature. Although skin receptors are found wherever there is skin, deep body thermoreceptors are found only in certain areas, mainly in the spinal cord, in the abdominal viscera, and in and around the great veins.[26] Deep body thermoreceptors function differently from skin receptors because they are exposed to the core temperature, whereas skin receptors are exposed to surface temperature. Like skin receptors, however, they detect mainly cold rather than warmth and are probably involved in preventing low body temperatures.[26]

Effector organs also contribute to temperature balance. Body organs under the stimulus of nerve impulses and increases in norepinephrine and epinephrine circulating in the blood are able to augment their rate of cellular oxidation. This is known as *chemical thermogenesis* and results in heat production. The rate of heat production can be increased by as much as 10 to 15 percent by this means.[26] Endocrine glands also participate in this process. Cooling of the thermostat cells in the hypothalamus increases its output of a hormone that stimulates the output of thyroxine by the thyroid gland. Increases in thyroxine also increase the rate of cellular metabolism. Female reproductive hormones also augment metabolic rate to support the body's needs during ovulation and pregnancy.

Body temperature varies somewhat with exercise and with extremes of environmental temperature, because the temperature regulatory mechanisms are not 100 percent effective.[26] Moreover, the ability of the body to regulate temperature is lost or impaired at 106F (41.4C) or above, or below 83F (28.3C) (Fig. 16–10).[26]

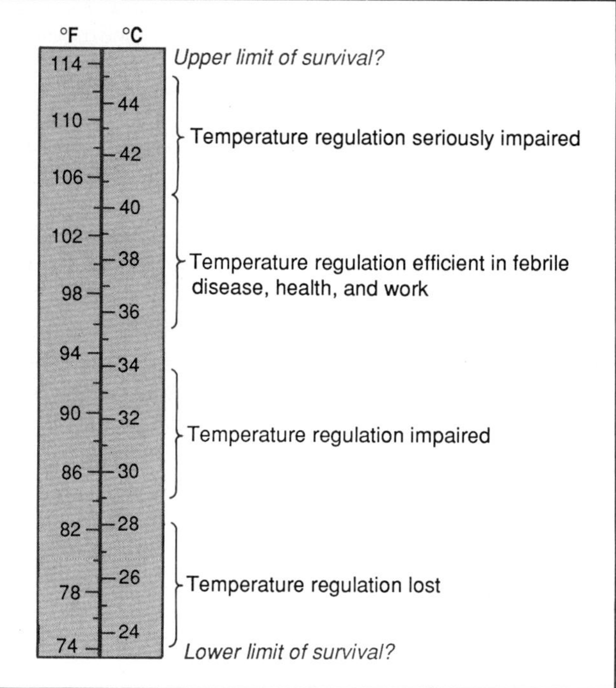

Figure 16–10. Extreme ranges of body temperature at which the body's ability to regulate temperature is impaired or lost. (Source: *DuBois EF. Fever and the regulation of body temperature.* American Lecture Series, *Pub. No. 13, 1948. Courtesy of Charles C Thomas, Springfield, IL.*)

HEAT PRODUCTION AND CONSERVATION. Four factors influence the production of body heat: (1) basal metabolic rate, (2) muscle activity, (3) hormone secretion, and (4) circadian rhythm. (For further information about circadian rhythm, see *Factors Affecting Body Temperature,* later in this chapter.)

The body constantly produces heat as a result of cell metabolism. All people have an individual minimum rate at which their body cells oxidize nutrients to produce energy. That rate is referred to as the **basal metabolic rate** (BMR). The BMR is the rate at which heat is produced hourly by the body's cells when they are under basal conditions. Thus, to measure the BMR, the individual must be subjected to such conditions. The individual must not have eaten within 12 hours of BMR measurement, must have just awakened from a restful night's sleep, must have performed no strenuous exercise, must be experiencing no psychological or physical stress, and must be surrounded by an ambient (room) temperature between 68F and 80F.[26]

Because the BMR is measured under basal conditions, it directly reflects the metabolic efficiency of the body. When the basal metabolic rate increases, body heat production also increases, and when heat production exceeds heat loss, body temperature increases. Temperature increases above expected norms constitute fever.

Conversely, when the basal metabolic rate falls, body heat production drops and, in turn, body temperature falls. Temperatures below expected norms result in hypothermia. All factors associated with alterations of body temperature (daily cycles, exercise, stress, environmental factors; see below) are associated with increases or decreases in the BMR.

The basal metabolic rate reflects the chemical breakdown of high-energy phosphate bonds in adenosine triphosphate, which liberate energy in the body's cells. Each bond releases 12,000 calories of energy per mole of adenosine triphosphate (ATP) under the physical conditions of the body.[26] Metabolism is calculated in kilocalories per square meter of body surface area. A 20-year-old male requires approximately 38.5 kilocalories per square meter per hour.[26]

Muscle activity also contributes to heat production. See the discussion of exercise below. During periods of muscle inactivity heat production comes from the body's core. During periods of muscle activity, however, muscle cells produce most of the body's heat.

The body has several mechanisms for preventing excessive cooling. Muscle activity and chemical thermogenesis were mentioned earlier. Vasoconstriction and shivering also act to prevent excessive cooling. When the core temperature drops below normal, that is, less than 98.6F (37C), the hypothalamus initiates the mechanisms described above, but also initiates heat-conserving mechanisms. *Vasoconstriction,* the shunting of blood from the extremities to the vital core organs, acts to conserve body heat. During vasoconstriction, blood is shunted from the large arteries to the large veins, bypassing the capillaries and peripheral capillary constriction. The observable sign of blood shunting is the blanching of the peripheral nail beds; nail beds become pale or bluish in color.

Shivering is a supplementary heat-producing mechanism that occurs when vasoconstriction is unable to conserve sufficient heat. Shivering produces heat by causing intense involuntary activity in large skeletal muscles. Heat production can be increased to four to five times its usual rate by this means.[26] *Piloerection*, erection of hair caused by contraction of muscle around a hair follicle, usually accompanies shivering.

HEAT LOSS. There is a constant loss of body heat to the environment. Eighty-five percent of the heat produced by the body is lost through the skin, the remainder through perspiration, excrement (urine and feces), and water vapor exhaled from the lungs during respiration.

Heat is lost through four mechanisms: (1) conduction, (2) convection, (3) radiation, and (4) evaporation (Fig. 16–11).

Conduction is heat loss from a warmer area or object to a cooler area or object, for example, from the body to objects in the environment such as the bed and chair. For conduction to occur, the warmer and cooler objects must be in direct contact. Only a minute amount of heat is lost from the body by direct conduction from the skin to things in the environment (see Fig. 16–11).[26]

Convection is loss of heat to surrounding air or fluid. Again, the surrounding air or fluid must be cooler in temperature than the source of heat for convection to occur. For the body to lose heat by convection, heat must first be conducted to the body surface. It is then dissipated from the body when the individual sits in a cool area. Air currents carry the heat away from the body (see Fig. 16–11).

Radiation is the transfer of heat from one object to another without the necessity of contact between those objects. It involves the radiation of infrared heat rays, a type of electromagnetic wave.[26] The human body radiates heat rays in all directions. So do all objects in the environment that have a temperature above absolute zero. When body temperature is greater than the temperature of environmental objects, there is a net transfer of heat to those objects. Loss of heat by radiation accounts for approximately 60 percent of the heat loss from an undressed individual at normal room temperature (see Fig. 16–11).[26]

Evaporation is the conversion of a liquid to a gaseous form. The conversion of water to steam provides a commonplace example of evaporation.

Radiation and conduction are the most important means of heat loss as long as body temperature exceeds the temperature of the environment; however, when the temperature of the environment surpasses body temperature, evaporation becomes the most important means of heat loss.[26] Evaporation of perspiration exemplifies this mechanism. Increased body temperature causes the sweat glands to produce sweat. As the sweat evaporates, it promotes heat loss in an attempt to lower the body temperature. When water evaporates from the body surface, 0.58 calorie (kilocalorie) of heat is lost for each gram of water that evaporates (see Fig. 16–11).[26]

When the body overheats, it relies on evaporation for heat loss. The hypothalamus activates the sweat mechanism and initiates an autonomic response that causes the skin's superficial blood vessels to dilate (*vasodilation*). As perspiration evaporates heat is released and the body is cooled.

Factors Affecting Body Temperature. Many factors affect body temperature, some of which already have been touched on. Those factors all have an effect on metabolic rate. They include diurnal cycles, exercise habits, hormones, stress, and age as well as changes in environmental temperature and humidity.

DIURNAL VARIATIONS. The body has a 24-hour cycle of temperature change that is predictable in well individuals. A 24-hour pattern is referred to as a *diurnal cycle.* Body temperature shows a 24-hour pattern to its fluctuation (Fig. 16–12). Body temperature is higher in the late after-

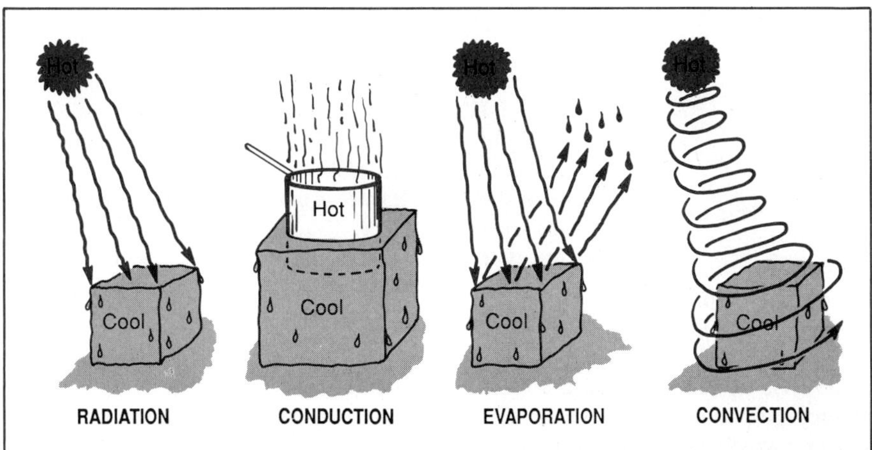

Figure 16–11. Methods of heat transfer.

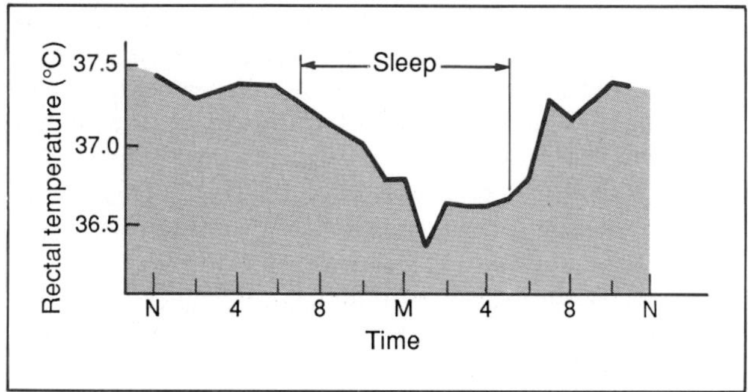

Figure 16–12. Diurnal cycle temperature variations.

noon and early evening than it is in the morning before one awakes. The highest temperature during this daily pattern occurs at about 1300 hours (1 PM), gradually decreases until it reaches its lowest ebb at about 0100 hours (1 AM), then slowly begins to increase with a sharp increase occurring about 0600 hours (6 AM). The temperature variation during this cycle can range from 1.0F to 1.5F (0.5C to 0.8C) (see Fig. 16–12); however, diurnal cycles differ for individuals who work during the night and sleep during the day. These people often experience a reversed temperature fluctuation cycle.

EXERCISE. As described above, muscle activity patterns influence body temperature fluctuations. Exercise produces large quantities of body heat that act to increase body temperature. Vigorous exercise can raise body temperature to as much as 101F to 104F (38.3C to 40C). When the individual is a well-trained athlete, the amount of heat produced during exercise may increase as much as 20 times over that produced under basal resting conditions.[26]

HORMONES. Hormones have a strong effect on body temperature fluctuation. Several hormones including sex hormones have their own daily or monthly cycles, which, in turn, influence body temperature changes. The body temperature of men remains fairly constant during a month; that of women has greater variance. This variance is directly related to the female hormonal changes that occur during the menstrual cycle. As the progesterone level increases and decreases, so does female body temperature. When the progesterone level is low, the temperature decreases 2F to 3F (3.6C to 5.4C) below baseline and remains at this level until midcycle, when the progesterone level increases and ovulation occurs. When ovulation occurs, the temperature increases 0.5F to 1.0F (0.3C to 0.6C). This increase in progesterone level increases the body temperature. The elevated body temperature continues until the onset of menstruation. This hormonal-related temperature change is the basis for the basal body temperature method of birth control.

Normal fluctuation in thyroid secretion also affects body temperature changes as established above. Thyroid secretion normally fluctuates on a diurnal cycle, which, in turn, contributes to the daily cycles of body temperature. Disease of the thyroid, however, acts to disrupt the normal pattern.[27]

STRESS. Stress, both physical and psychological, may cause the body temperature to fluctuate. The body responds to stress by secreting additional epinephrine and norepinephrine, which initiate chemical thermogenesis, producing additional heat. When stress abates, circulating epinephrine and norepinephrine diminish and cellular metabolism returns to its previous rate.[26]

AGE. Age also plays a role in temperature regulation. Temperature variations are common in both infants and the elderly. The normal newborn rectal temperature is 96F to 99.5F (35.5C to 37.5C),[28] whereas the temperature of an elderly person often is below 96.8F (36C). In addition, these two age groups experience difficulty maintaining adequate temperature control, but for different reasons. An infant's thermoregulatory mechanism is not fully developed, nor is an infant able to shiver. Moreover, an infant's large surface area relative to mass causes more rapid heat loss when exposed to a cool environment. In the elderly, advancing age brings deterioration in thermoregulation. This is the result of less subcutaneous tissue to insulate and conserve body heat, coupled with decreases in sweat gland activity, in arterial blood flow as a result of arterial changes, and in the body's metabolic rate. Aging also changes the extent of the diurnal temperature peak and trough. The temperature highs and lows become less extreme as one ages.[29] Both of these age groups are at risk for hypothermia.

ENVIRONMENTAL TEMPERATURE. The temperature of the external environment also affects body temperature. By the process of radiation, elevated environmental temperature causes the temperature of the blood to increase. This elevated blood temperature signals the hypothalamus to activate cooling mechanisms. The hypothalamus, through its effect on the sympathetic nervous system, in turn activates sweat glands to produce perspiration, which causes a cooling of the skin via evaporation.[26]

The level of humidity influences the rate of body heat lost through evaporation. Increased humidity causes the perspiration to evaporate more slowly.

Decreased environmental temperature also affects body temperature. Body temperature in the early morning during exposure to winter environment temperature can be 96F (35.5C). When the skin temperature drops to 95F (35C), the client shivers uncontrollably. This occurs because the body shunts the warm blood from the surface to the core organs. If skin temperature is below 90F (32.2C), the body's heat loss mechanisms are lost.[30] This shunting of blood is also the reason the client may experience severe muscle cramps with movement (see *Thermal Abnormalities* and *Norms and Expected Findings* for additional information).

Thermal Abnormalities. Disorders of thermoregulation include hyperthermic conditions such as heat stroke, heat exhaustion, heat cramps, and fever, as well as hypothermic conditions such as generalized hypothermia and frostbite.

HYPERTHERMIA. *Hyperthermia* (fever) is, by definition, a core body temperature above 102.2F (39C) and is usually the result of brain or spinal cord injury or trauma such as head injury and stroke.

Fever. *Fever* is an elevated body temperature above 100F (38C). Although not an illness in and of itself, fever is an indicator or sign of the presence of disease. Fever signifies that there is disequilibrium between the amount of heat produced and the amount of heat lost. Fever frequently accompanies infection; however, it can also be caused by noninfectious processes such as brain or spinal cord trauma or tumor, dehydration, and hyperthyroidism.

When an individual becomes ill with an infection the body's metabolic rate increases, resulting in an increased body temperature. The resultant hyperthermia (fever) is sometimes called pyrexia.

The physiological process that leads to fever involves toxic protein breakdown products called *pyrogens* that act on the hypothalamus to alter its thermostatic control. The hypothalamic thermostat is "turned up" in effect. Pyrogens are secreted by toxic bacteria or are produced within the body by the breakdown of degenerating tissue. The alteration in thermostatic control brings all mechanisms for raising body temperature into play, including heat production and heat conservation.[26] Vasoconstriction, shivering, and piloerection occur. Shivering causes the production of additional body heat, even though body temperature is already elevated. Heat production continues as heat loss diminishes, resulting in fever. As the client's metabolic rate climbs, heart and respiratory rate increase to meet the new demands for oxygen to support cellular oxidation. The client has chills and complains of feeling cold. The client's skin feels hot and dry.

Many bacterial pyrogens act directly on the hypothalamus; others, especially the endotoxins from gram-negative bacteria, cause severe fever by acting in an indirect manner. Bacteria or their breakdown products act indirectly by causing the release of a substance called leukocyte pyrogen into the blood after they are phagocytized by the blood leukocytes and macrophages.[26]

As the client begins to recover and thermostatic feedback is restored, heat-dissipating mechanisms begin to operate. The client will usually sweat profusely. This is referred to as *diaphoresis.* The skin becomes flushed and cool to the touch. The sensation of chills abates and the client begins to feel warm again. In lay terminology, this process is referred to as "the fever breaking."

Fever is a serious condition that, if left untreated, will result in potentially severe complications. These complications are related to increased metabolic rate and manifest themselves in increased heart and respiration rate, depletion of energy reserves, and dehydration, all of which occur in direct relation to the body's heightened rate of oxygen consumption. Oxygen requirements increase 7 percent for every 1F or 12 percent for every 1C of temperature elevation.[26]

If the increased temperature is prolonged, dehydration can result if there is not adequate fluid replacement. Dehydration occurs because the body's increased metabolic rate demands the use of additional water. Dehydration is discussed in detail in Chapter 31. Signs and symptoms of dehydration are flushed skin that is dry to the touch and muscle cramping. Fever above 108F (42.2C) can cause unconsciousness.[31] If untreated, prolonged high temperature (above 105F or 40.5C) can result in irreversible brain damage or death. Ventricle fibrillation, a potentially fatal cardiac arrhythmia, may occur when the core temperature reaches 88F to 90F (31.1C to 32.2C).

Heat Stroke. *Heat stroke* is a life-threatening situation that occurs when body temperature rises to dangerous levels and reaches 106F to 108F (41.1C to 42.2C). Unfortunately, there is a limit to the rate at which the body is able to lose heat through maximal sweating. When this limit is reached heat stroke occurs. Heat stroke results because the body is unable to dissipate any additional heat. This can happen as a result of thermoregulation inadequacy or failure (refer to Fig. 16–10). In addition, the hypothalamic temperature regulation function is severely compromised because of the high body temperature.

Predisposing factors include very hot environmental temperature accompanied by high humidity, excessive exercise, age, and chronic illnesses such as cardiac disorders that interfere with the ability to adapt to environmental or physical stress. Obesity is another predisposing factor. Some drugs also promote this condition by causing vasodilation (such as diazoxide and hydralazine), by reducing the capacity to sweat (such as atropine and methantheline), or by increasing the basal metabolic rate (such as levothyroxine sodium) (Box 16–11).

Clinical signs and symptoms of heat stroke include dizziness, visual disturbances, abdominal cramping, confusion, and loss of consciousness. The skin feels hot and dry to the touch; convulsions can occur. The client's respirations and pulse are increased as the body attempts to release heat via exhaled air and increased cardiac output. Blood flow to the skin and muscles is increased in an attempt to dissipate heat via radiation.

HEAT EXHAUSTION. *Heat exhaustion* occurs when the client's temperature reaches 102.2F to 104F (39C to 40C) and results in depletion of the body's water and sodium through sweating. This, in turn, creates electrolyte imbalances and decreased blood volume. Heat exhaustion is likely when perspiration is very profuse and when the individual fails to ingest oral replacement fluid.

Signs and symptoms of heat exhaustion include hypotension, tachycardia, pale skin that feels cold and clammy to the touch, and client complaints of headache, thirst, nausea, dizziness, or weakness. There is an increase in pulse rate and postural hypotension.

HEAT CRAMPS. *Heat cramps* are intermittent skeletal muscle spasms associated with elevated body temperature. Heat cramps are very painful and result from the rapid sodium and water depletion that occurs during vigorous exercise,

BOX 16–11. DRUGS RELATED TO DEVELOPMENT OF HYPERTHERMIA

Anticholinergics
Phenothiazines
Tricyclic depressants
Monoaxinoxide inhibitors
Glutethimide
LSD
Amphetamines

From Budassi S, Barber J. Emergency Nursing Principles and Practices. *St. Louis, MO: CV Mosby; 1986.*

particularly when the client is not acclimated to a high level of activity. The occurrence of heat cramps is rather common in hot climates.

HYPOTHERMIA. Hypothermia may be accidental, as in prolonged exposure to cold, or may be intentional or induced, as in preparation for heart or brain surgery. Circulation can be stopped for relatively long periods in hypothermic clients because cellular oxygen needs are greatly reduced. There are no permanent ill effects from controlled induced hypothermia.

Hypothermia occurs when the rate of heat loss surpasses the rate of heat production. By definition, hypothermia is low core body temperature between 77F and 95F (25C and 35C). It is a life-threatening condition. Infants and the aged are prone to hypothermia.

Hypothermia can be either generalized or regional. Generalized hypothermia is a very serious body condition. Early clinical signs and symptoms of hypothermia include confusion, memory loss, decreased level of consciousness, difficulty standing and speaking, and pupil dilation. If the condition continues, the pulse and respiration rate decrease and blood pressure begins to decrease. This is followed by cardiac dysrhythmias and loss of consciousness. The automatic body response of shivering may fail to occur when the body temperature drops to about 86F (30C).[32] Also, at this point muscle rigidity occurs.

When cardiac dysrhythmias occur, the client's condition has reached a critical state. Atrial fibrillation is the most common hypothermia-related cardiac dysrhythmia. The core rewarming must increase slowly at the rate of 1 to 2 degrees an hour and must increase at the same rate as the external temperature to inhibit ventricular fibrillation.

When hypothermia is present, the nurse monitors laboratory data for complete blood count (CBC), blood urea nitrogen (BUN), electrolytes, serum amylase and glucose levels, coagulation studies, and arterial blood gases (ABG). Intake and output are recorded every 15 to 30 minutes. Neurological status checks are done at least hourly. Usually a 6-second recording of cardiovascular function is also done hourly. External and core temperature is monitored hourly and adjustments are made accordingly.

A decrease in sodium and water absorption with a resulting fluid shift into the extracellular spaces occurs in hypothermia. This fluid shift can cause hemoconcentration and hypovolemia. The client is at risk for hyperglycemia because the hypothalamus inhibits the release of insulin from the pancreas. [30]

When hypothermia occurs in a specific body area it is called *frostbite.* Ice crystals form and expand in extracellular spaces causing cell membranes to rupture.[33] Although this causes damage to body tissue, it is not life threatening. Affected areas are usually the fingers, toes, nose, cheeks, or ears.

The external cold temperature induces vasoconstriction, which causes the blood flow to the area to decrease as a heat-conserving mechanism. Decreased blood flow, in turn, causes vessel occlusion and results in ischemia of the area. Factors that increase the risk for frostbite include moisture, malnutrition, and disease, especially diabetes, arteriosclerosis,[30] and other disorders that affect circulation.

Superficial frostbite appears as a shallow blanched wheal and disappears on rewarming, but the affected area becomes reddened. The client complains of burning, tingling, and numbness in the affected area.

Equipment. Clinical thermometers are used to measure body temperature.

Types of Thermometers. The several types of thermometers available for clinical use—glass, electronic, and disposable—are all capable of accurately measuring body temperature.

MERCURY-IN-GLASS THERMOMETERS. A glass thermometer is composed of a hollow core glass tube, usually containing mercury, that is marked with a graduated scale of units. When the hollow tube contains mercury the device is referred to as a mercury-in-glass thermometer. It works by the following method. Heat from the body is transferred to the mercury inside the tube, causing its temperature to increase. As its temperature increases, the mercury expands and rises in the hollow tube. Once the column stabilizes at its new height, temperature is registered, and the column will not reposition itself unless the tube is snapped or shaken vigorously. The unit scale on the side of the tube is marked with either Fahrenheit or centigrade calibrations (Fig. 16–13).

Glass thermometers are specifically designed for oral and axillary use or for rectal use. The two types are differentiated by the shape of the mercury-containing bulb (see Fig. 16–13). The oral thermometer has a long, thin bulb, which permits a greater surface area between the thermometer and the body tissue. The rectal thermometer has a short, wide bulb, which makes insertion into the rectum safe and easy. Some glass thermometers are color coded on the top end, red signifying rectal use and blue signifying oral use.

Glass thermometers have certain advantages over other types. They are durable, inexpensive, easy to obtain, and accurate; however, they also have certain disadvantages, one being that glass thermometers require a relatively long period of time to obtain a reading (3 to 5 minutes) and another being that they are breakable.

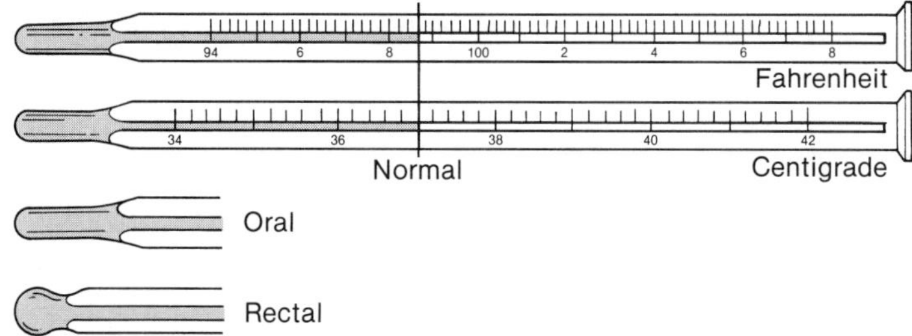

Figure 16–13. Mercury-in-glass thermometers calibrated in Fahrenheit and centigrade units. (Source: *Smith S, Duell D.* Clinical Nursing Skills. *2nd ed. Norwalk, CT: Appleton & Lange; 1989.*)

ELECTRONIC THERMOMETERS. Electronic thermometers (Fig. 16–14), which use batteries as a power source, are also available and widely used. Electronic thermometers consist of an attached heat-sensitive probe, a digital display unit for indicating the temperature reading, and a thin wire connecting the two. Digital displays are available in either the Fahrenheit or centigrade scale. With some electronic thermometers different heat-sensitive probes are available for oral and rectal use. With other units, a single probe provides for all uses. Disposable covers for the heat-sensitive probe are provided as a sanitation and infection control measure. After the disposable cover is attached, the probe is inserted and left in place until the electronic thermometer registers a temperature that it signals by an audible or visible cue. The time required for the electronic thermometer to register is about 10 to 15 seconds. Electronic thermometer readings are said to be accurate to within plus or minus 0.2 degrees of the body's actual temperature. Baker[34] found that even though insertion lengths vary, the difference between readings obtained using an electronic and a glass thermometer are not clinically significant.

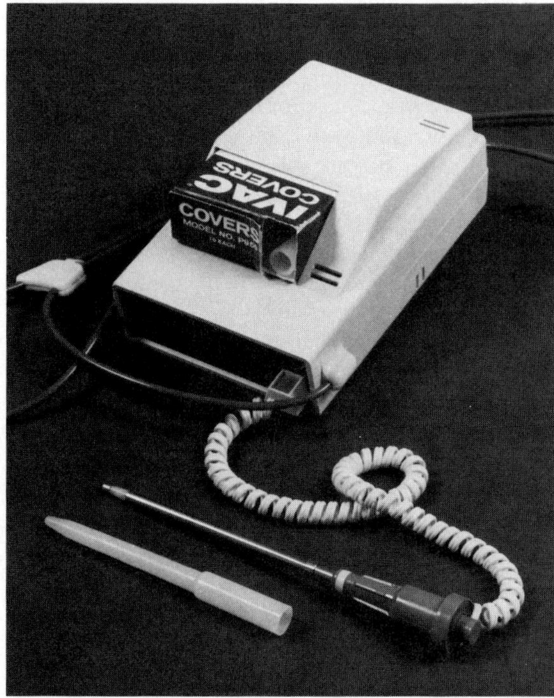

Figure 16–14. Electronic thermometer. (Source: *Smith S, Duell D.* Clinical Nursing Skills. *2nd ed. Norwalk, CT: Appleton & Lange; 1989.*)

With electronic thermometers, readings are quickly obtained and displayed in large, easy-to-read numbers. The disadvantages of electronic thermometers are the initial purchase expense, which is relatively high, the continuing expense of purchasing disposable probe covers, and the environmental pollution caused by the disposal of single-use plastic covers.

DISPOSABLE THERMOMETERS. A relative newcomer to clinical use is the disposable, single-use thermometer. It is employed in the same manner as a glass thermometer. It uses a chemically impregnated plastic strip that responds to heat by changing color (Fig. 16–15). A temperature reading can be obtained in 45 to 60 seconds with this type of thermometer. The strip is discarded after use.

Chemical disposable thermometers have the advantage of being simple to use, easy to read, and accurate. Their disadvantages include expensive purchase price and the environmental pollution caused by disposing of single-use items.

Temperature Scales. Body temperature is measured in heat units called degrees. Two scales of measurement are used to indicate degrees of temperature: the Celsius scale and the Fahrenheit scale. Box 16–12 provides a formula that is used to convert temperature measurement from one scale to the other.

Thermometer temperature scales are calibrated in either Fahrenheit or Celsius (centigrade) units. Each long line on the Fahrenheit and Celsius scales delineates one temperature degree; however, the scales differ in their designation of units assigned to shorter lines. The shorter lines on the Fahrenheit scale indicate 0.2-degree increments, but each of the short lines on the Celsius scale indicates 0.1 degree (refer to Fig. 16–13).

Technique. Proper technique helps ensure that nurses' temperature measurements are accurate. As is apparent from the discussion of equipment above, body temperature can be measured at any of three sites: in the oral cavity under the tongue (sublingual area), in the rectal canal, or in the axillae. Temperature is best measured, however, in a

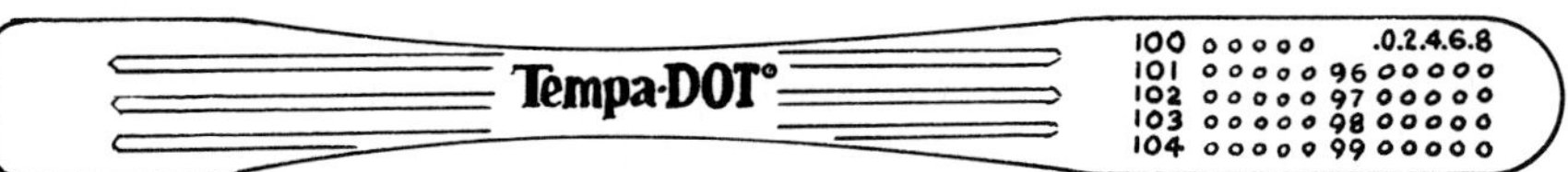

Figure 16–15. Single-use, disposable thermometer.

closed orifice with abundant vascularization. Blood vessels act as outlets for body heat and, in large numbers, serve to localize heat at the measurement site. When that site is a closed orifice, the influence of environmental temperature on the measurement is minimized. The sublingual areas of the oral cavity and rectal canal are both appropriate by these criteria. Both are closed orifices and both have heavily vascularized mucosal membranes. The axillae, on the other hand, meet neither criterion. The axillae, however, provide an acceptable alternative site for use when other sites are unavailable or unsafe for some reason. A fourth potential site for measuring temperature, the tympanic membrane of the ear, is thought to accurately reflect core body temperature. Like the hypothalamus, the tympanic membrane is served by the internal carotid artery, a large artery that carries blood directly away from the core.[35,36] Nevertheless, measurement of tympanic temperature requires the insertion of a speculum into the ear canal, which increases the complexity of temperature taking; thus, this site is not in wide clinical use.

Regardless of the site for temperature measurement, some general guidelines should be followed for temperature measurement:

- Discuss the procedure with the client before beginning and, to the extent possible, involve the client in decision making regarding the procedure.
- Select the most appropriate site using the considerations discussed above and below.
- Collect and assemble all necessary equipment including the thermometer, thermometer sleeves for electronic thermometer probes, gloves and lubricant for rectal use, cleansing tissue, pen, and recording sheet.
- Cleanse your hands using good medical asepsis; be sure to warm your hands during this procedure if you anticipate touching the client's skin.
- Position the client appropriately for the site and method of temperature measurement you are going to use.

Selecting the Oral Site. Each area for measuring temperature has advantages and disadvantages. Oral temperatures are convenient and easily obtained, but they require that the client is alert, able to follow directions, and cooperative. Oral readings, moreover, are influenced by a number of conditions that may render them inaccurate. Factors that affect the environment of the mouth have the potential to alter oral temperature. Neff and associates, for example, examined the effect of mouth breathing on sublingual temperatures. They found that open mouth breathing reduces measurements by an average of 0.82F (0.31C).[37] Mouth breathing is sometimes associated with rapid breathing. Under such conditions a rectal temperature is preferable.[38] Other factors also alter the environment of the mouth; for example, smoking or ingesting hot or cold liquids within 15 minutes of temperature measurement may alter oral temperature.

Selection of a measurement site should be made on the basis of a consideration of these factors. If the client meets the requirements for an oral temperature (alert, cooperative, able to follow directions), then the oral site is generally appropriate. Even children who fulfill the criteria may have their temperature measured orally. The oral route is inappropriate for very young children, however, or for clients who are confused or comatose or who are being supervised for seizures. The danger of accidental injury from biting or otherwise breaking an oral thermometer is substantial for all of these groups. Painful mouth lesions, oral surgery, and the presence of head, neck, or facial dressings that act as a barrier to the oral route are additional factors that make the oral route inappropriate. Still another factor is the use of oxygen by face mask. Humidified, cooled oxygen may lower the reading when a glass thermometer is used. Moreover, even temporary removal of the mask places a seriously ill client at risk for reduction of arterial oxygen levels (hypoxia).[39] Oral temperatures are not contraindicated when oxygen is being delivered by cannula or catheter, however, provided that the other client criteria are met. Additionally, the oral site is inappropriate for clients who have nasogastric or endotracheal tubes in place, which make it difficult for clients to keep their mouths closed for temperature measurement.

BOX 16–12. CENTIGRADE AND FAHRENHEIT CONVERSION FORMULAS

To convert centigrade to Fahrenheit:
F = (C × 9/5) + 32
To convert Fahreneheit to centigrade:
C = (F − 32) × 5/9

TECHNIQUE FOR ORAL TEMPERATURE MEASUREMENT. The technique for oral temperature measurement is outlined in Procedure 16–1. Also, explain the reasons for the site selection you have made, or if the situation permits, invite the client to participate in the selection of the site. Emphasize the importance of retaining the thermometer bulb or tip directly under the tongue while at the same time depressing the tongue gently over it and closing the lips. This

(Text continues on page 457.)

PROCEDURE 16–1. ASSESSING BODY TEMPERATURE

PURPOSE: To Identify elevations in temperature requiring treatment

EQUIPMENT: Oral or rectal thermometer, tissue paper wipes, disposable gloves, lubricant for rectal temperature

ACTION	RATIONALE
1. Wash your hands.	1. Removes transient organisms that may be pathogens, preventing transmission to the client.
2. Discuss the procedure and its expected benefits with the client.	2. Active participation is more likely if the client understands the expected behaviors and anticipated benefits.
3. Prepare the client.	
a. For oral route: Inquire if client has recently smoked, eaten food, or had oral fluids. If so, wait 15 minutes before taking oral temperature.	a. Hot and cold substances, as well as smoking, alter temperature of oral cavity.
NOTE: An oral thermometer, especially the glass variety, should never be used if there is any potential that the client could break the thermometer by biting it.	
b. For axillary route: Pull curtains around bed; expose axilla; pat dry with tissue if damp.	b. Privacy reduces embarrassment or distress associated with body exposure.
c. For rectal route: Pull curtains around bed. Request or assist client to Sims' position (lateral position with upper leg flexed) and drape with bed linens.	c. Privacy reduces embarrassment or distress associated with body exposure. Position facilitates access to rectum. Draping keeps client warm and prevents unnecessary exposure.
4. If the thermometer has been stored in disinfectant, rinse with cool water before using. Dry with tissue or paper towel.	4. Removes irritating disinfectant. Hot water may cause bulb to break.
5. Hold thermometer with fingertips at end opposite bulb and read mercury level, holding thermometer at eye level. If mercury level is above 35.5C (96F), grasp thermometer securely, stand away from solid objects, and sharply flick thermometer downward until the mercury reading is below 35.5C (96F).	5. Mercury should be below 35.5C (96F) before taking temperature. Shaking thermometer lowers mercury level. Standing in an open area prevents breakage of thermometer.
NOTE: Electronic thermometer discussed below.	

(continued)

PROCEDURE 16–1. (continued)

6. Take the temperature.

   a. Oral:

      (1) Ask client to open mouth and gently insert thermometer under the tongue into the posterior sublingual pocket.

      (1) Heat from superficial blood vessels in posterior sublingual pocket reflects body core temperature.

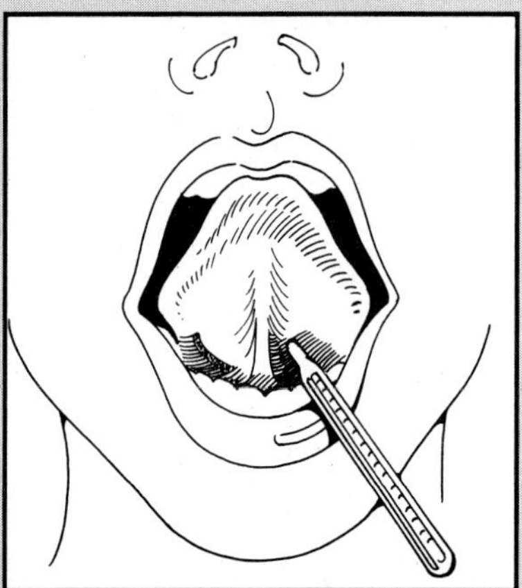

      (2) Request that the client keep thermometer in place by closing lips, not teeth, around thermometer.

      (2) Proper thermometer position is needed to obtain accurate reading. Biting the thermometer can cause injury from broken glass or mercury poisoning if ingested.

      (3) Leave the thermometer in place for 3 to 5 minutes or as directed by agency policy.

      (3) Allows sufficient time for accurate reflection of body temperature.

   b. Axillary:

      (1) Place thermometer bulb in center of axilla, lower arm over thermometer, and place arm close to the body, then across chest.

      (1) Maintains position of thermometer against superficial blood vessels in axilla to measure skin temperature. Reading is 1F or .5C lower than oral temperature.

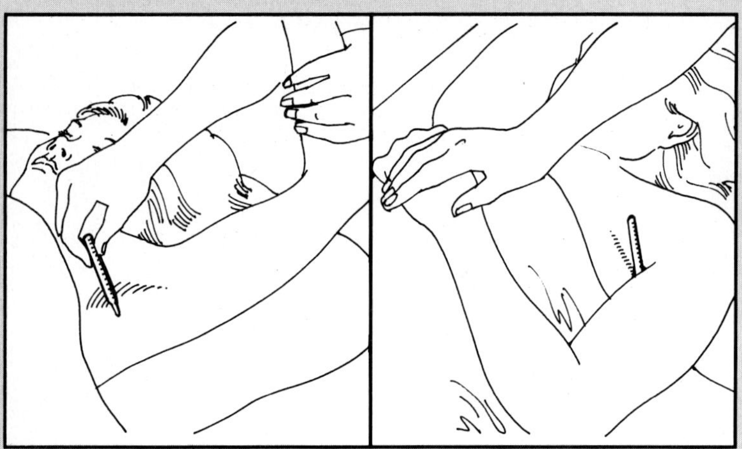

(continued)

PROCEDURE 16–1. (continued)

(2) Request client to hold thermometer in place 5 to 10 minutes or as directed by agency policy.

(2) Five to ten minutes allows sufficient time to obtain accurate reflection of body temperature.

(3) If a client is a child or a confused adult, hold thermometer in place.

(3) Client may injure self on thermometer. Movement will result in inaccurate reading.

c. Rectal:

(1) Don clean disposable gloves.

(1) Fecal material may contain pathogenic organisms. Gloves prevent skin contamination by direct contact.

(2) Place a liberal amount of lubricant on thermometer, covering bulb end and 2.5 to 3.5 cm (1 to 1½ in.) of thermometer shaft.

(2) Lubrication facilitates thermometer insertion and minimizes trauma to rectal mucosa by reducing friction.

(3) Separate client's buttocks with nondominant hand.

(3) Exposes the anus.

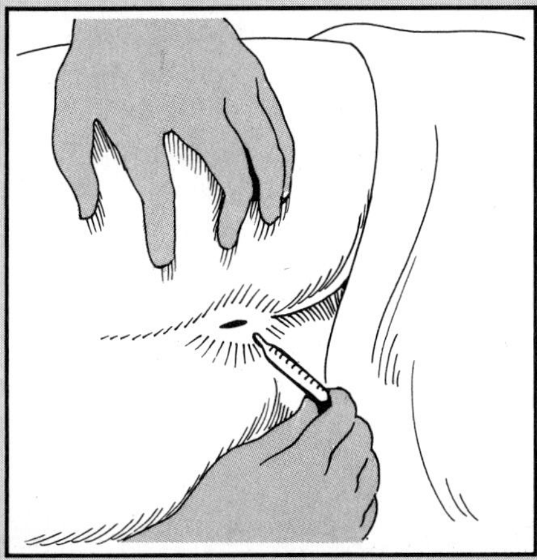

(4) Ask client to take a deep breath and blow it out. Insert thermometer into anus with bulb pointing toward umbilicus as client inhales. Insert thermometer 3.5 cm to 4 cm (1½ in.) for adult, 2.5 cm (1 in.) for a child, and 1.5 to 2.5 cm (½ to 1 in.) for infant.

(4) Taking a deep breath helps to relax the anal sphincter. Pointing bulb toward the umbilicus follows the contour of the rectum, minimizing the risk of trauma to rectal wall or mucosa. Rectal cavity reflects body core temperature.

(continued)

PROCEDURE 16–1. (continued)

(5) Hold thermometer in place 2 to 4 minutes or as directed by agency policy.	(5) Holding the thermometer reduces risk of accidental injury to client. Two to four minutes allows sufficient time to obtain accurate reflection of body temperature. Reading will be 1F or .5C higher than oral temperature.
7. Carefully remove thermometer and wipe off any adhering matter with the tissue. Wipe down in a rotating fashion from tip to bulb. Dispose of tissue.	7. Wipe from area of least contamination (shaft) to area of greatest contamination (bulb).
8. Hold thermometer at eye level; rotate until mercury column is visible. The end of the mercury column nearest your hand indicates the client's temperature.	8. Refraction of light will distort reading if mercury column is not read at eye level.
NOTE: On a Fahrenheit thermometer, each long line on the scale represents 1 degree, each short line represents 0.2 degree. On a Celsius (centigrade) thermometer, each long line represents 0.5 degree, each short line represents 0.1 degree (see Fig. 16–13).	
9. If temperature was taken rectally, clean client's anal area to remove remaining lubricant or feces. Dispose of tissue in container marked "Organic Waste" or "Infectious Waste."	9. Maintains client comfort. Prevents transmission of microorganisms to environment or other clients.
10. Remove gloves by pulling them off at wrist and turning them inside out. Dispose of gloves in same receptacle as tissue.	10. Prevents transmission of microorganisms to another client or to the environment.
11. Assist client to a comfortable position, if needed.	11. Maintains client comfort.
12. Wash thermometer in lukewarm soapy water; rinse in cool water and dry.	12. Removes organic materials that could harbor and support growth of microorganisms.
13. Record temperature reading on client's vital signs flowsheet or medical record according to agency policy. Usually, axillary readings are designated by placing an "A" next to the value. Rectal readings are designated by placing an "R" next to the value.	13. Temperature reflects client's health status. Noting consecutive readings on a flowsheet facilitates comparison of values and shows trends.
14. Discuss temperature value with client and actions client can take to reduce it if elevated, for example, increase fluid intake (see Chap. 31), breathing exercises (see Chap. 27).	14. Client needs accurate information about health status to be actively involved in self-care.

(continued)

PROCEDURE 16–1. (continued)

15. Shake down the mercury in the column and store thermometer in its container.

15. Provides clean storage and protects from breakage.

16. If temperature is significantly elevated, report to appropriate RN or physician. Repeat assessment in 30 minutes to 1 hour. Take nursing or medically ordered measures to reduce elevated temperature or according to agency policy.

16. Elevations in temperature frequently indicate an infectious process, which could become serious if not treated. Reducing temperature promotes client safety and comfort.

VARIATIONS WHEN USING ELECTRONIC THERMOMETER

1. Remove thermometer from charging unit. Select blue probe for oral or axillary routes, red probe for rectal route.

1. Charging unit must remain connected to power source. Separate probes for oral or axillary and rectal routes prevent cross-contamination.

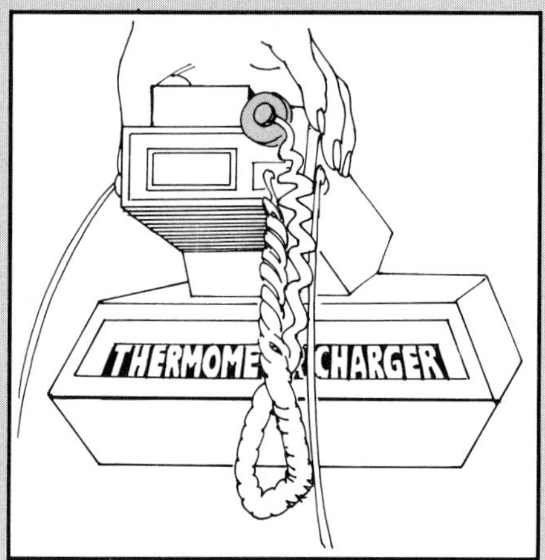

2. Proceed as above, steps 1 to 3.

3. Grasp probe as illustrated and insert it into one of the disposable probe covers until it locks into place. Do not touch button end of probe; it is for ejection of probe.

3. Disposable probe cover is a barrier, preventing transfer of microorganisms from client to probe and then to another client.

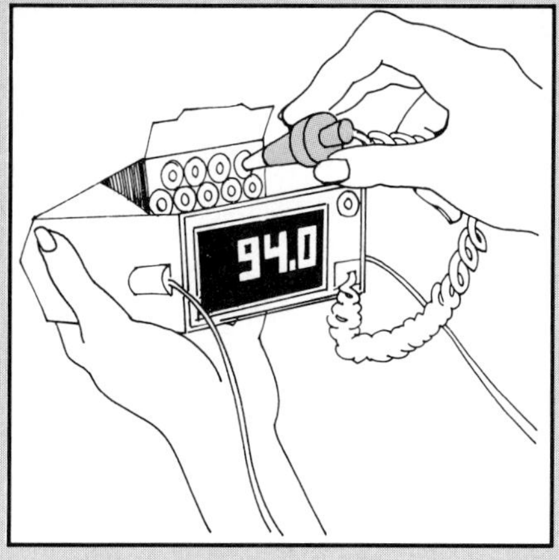

(continued)

PROCEDURE 16–1. (continued)

4. Prepare and place probe for desired route as described in step 6 above. Hold probe in place until an audible or visual signal alerts you that the maximum temperature has been reached. The time is considerably shorter than required with a mercury thermometer. Read temperature on face of thermometer unit.

4. The same contact points are required to register an accurate reading as with a mercury thermometer, but it is computerized to generate a reading more rapidly. Reading on display disappears when probe is replaced to ready unit for next use.

5. Eject probe into appropriate trash receptacle by pushing ejection button while holding probe over trash can. Probes used for rectal temperatures are usually disposed of in infectious waste containers.

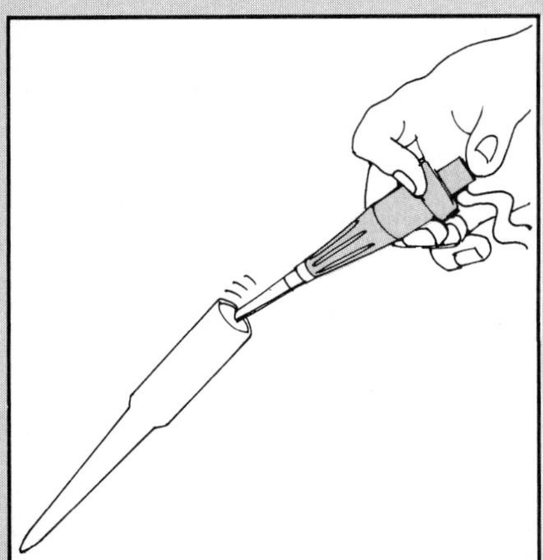

5. Ejection device prevents contact with probe. As there is potential for mucosal damage with rectal temperature, blood may be present on probe after use. Universal precautions require disposal in infectious waste containers.

(continued)

PROCEDURE 16–1. (continued)

6. Replace probe in storage well. Continue with steps 13–16 above; return temperature unit to charging unit.

6. Battery will wear down if not being charged when not in use.

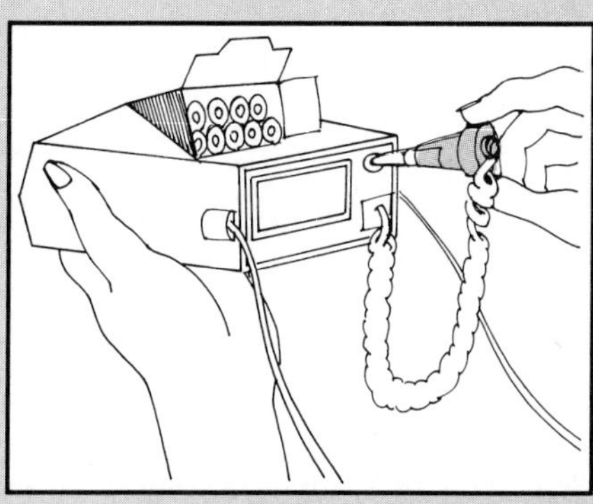

RECORDING: See step 13 above. Some health care agencies stipulate recording of vital signs in other locations besides client's flowsheet.

ensures that the oral cavity is closed during the procedure and that the thermometer is in contact with the heat source. Stress to the client that he or she should breathe nasally during the procedure. Be sure to remind the client of the time it will take for the thermometer to register (full 3 minutes or longer for a glass thermometer, 10 to 15 seconds for an electronic thermometer). Before inserting the thermometer, remember to shake down the mercury column in a mercury-in-glass thermometer and to position the disposable sleeve of an electronic thermometer probe.

Selecting the Rectal Site. Rectal temperatures have the advantage of accuracy because the thermometer comes into contact with the densely vascularized intestinal membrane and because the influence of ambient temperature on the reading is minimal. Rectal temperatures have the disadvantage, however, of being more invasive than either oral or axillary temperature measurement. Clients may fear pain when this method is used. Indeed the rectal site may be inappropriate for clients who have large, inflamed, external or internal hemorrhoids. Clients may also fear embarrassment, and nurses must take measures to ensure the client's privacy. Moreover, although using the rectal site does not require that clients are fully alert and cooperative, they must be closely supervised to prevent position changes that might result in accidental mucosal perforation by a rectal probe. Rectal temperatures are preferred for infants and young children who are unable to cooperate for the oral procedure; however, rectal temperatures are generally not used for newborns because of the higher risk within this group of accidental damage to the rectal mucosa. Rectal temperature generally registers 0.1F or more higher than oral temperature (Box 16–13).

In the past, authorities felt that the rectal site was inadvisable for clients who had sustained a coronary occlusion (heart attack), reasoning that stimulation of rectal mucosa induced a reflex slowing of heart rate by the vagus nerve. Indeed, many hospitals required that temperature be measured using the oral or axillary routes for all post-coronary clients. The efficacy of such policies was called into question, however, when it was demonstrated that vagus nerve stimulation failed to correlate with rectal temperature measurement.[40] Such policies are therefore no longer in use.

TECHNIQUE FOR RECTAL TEMPERATURE MEASUREMENT. Procedure 16–1 reviews the technique for rectal temperature measurement. As with the oral method, discuss the procedure with the client, assuring him or her that privacy will be protected. Assist the client into Sims' position. Be sure to ask the client about rectal tenderness and examine the rectal area closely for lesions before placing a rectal probe. If desired, use an adjustable neck lamp to illuminate the rectal area for visualization. Supervise the client during the procedure, making sure that the client remains still.

BOX 16–13. COMPARISON OF TEMPERATURES FOR ORAL, RECTAL, AND AXILLARY MEASUREMENTS OF BODY TEMPERATURE

Area	Average Reading		Time Required to Obtain (min)	Variance
	F	C		
Oral	98.6	37	3–8	None
Rectal	99.6	37.5	2–4	1 F higher
Axilla	97.6	36.4	10	1 F lower

Selecting the Axillary Site. Temperatures measured at the axillary site are generally regarded as the safest but the least accurate; however, research done by Ecoff and Joyce, who studied children, suggests that the measurement differences between axillary and other sites may be clinically insignificant.[41] Axillary temperature measurement is preferred for newborns and young infants because insertion of a rectal thermometer risks mucosal damage and stimulates defecation. Axillary temperatures are unlikely to cause client embarrassment. On the other hand, they take significantly longer to register and the nurse must hold the thermometer in place. Axillary temperatures are inappropriate for any client who has had surgery involving the axilla or is receiving any other treatment to that area. Axillary temperatures usually register 1F (0.6C) lower than oral temperatures (see Box 16–13).

TECHNIQUE FOR AXILLARY TEMPERATURE MEASUREMENT. Discuss the procedure with the client, reminding the client that the thermometer must be left in place for a full 10 minutes. Electronic thermometers register in 1 minute or less. Explain that you will be holding the thermometer in place to prevent shifting of the probe. Hold the thermometer in place as it is registering, and gently hold the arm in position if the client is a child.

Norms and Expected Findings. It is important for the reader to understand the terms that apply to body temperature.

Normothermia is a term applied to body temperatures that fall within the range of normal. Although there are individual variations, the usual range for an oral temperature of a resting adult is 97F to 100F (36C to 37.8C). Rectal temperature is usually 1F higher (98F to 101F) than the temperature taken orally. The axillary temperature is usually 1F lower (96F to 99F) than the oral temperature (Box 16–13).

Special Considerations, Precautions, Sources of Error. As has been discussed earlier in this section, the nurse assists the client in selecting the route to be used for the temperature measurement if possible. If this is not realistic, the nurse selects the route of temperature measurement that is appropriate to the client's condition and health status.

The nurse should return to the bedside to remove the oral thermometer of a responsible adult in a timely manner within the required time for measurement, as clients become irritated when the thermometer is left in the mouth longer than the required time.

The nurse must be gentle and cautious when inserting a rectal thermometer, as poor technique, carelessness, or inattention could result in injury to the rectum. Because of the risk of rectal perforation, the rectal route is avoided with neonates.

It is important not to leave the side of a client when a rectal thermometer or probe is in place. In addition, children should be observed very closely while the temperature reading is being obtained to ensure their safety.

It should be noted that many thermometers do not register hypothermic temperatures so a special low-registering type with a scale that extends to 80F (27C) must be used.

The axilla should be dry before taking an axillary temperature as the moisture can interfere with the transfer of body heat from the area to the thermometer bulb.

Most facilities have a policy of routinely taking the temperature of all clients twice every 24 hours. If the client's temperature is elevated, it should be monitored by the nurse at least every 4 hours or more frequently if indicated or ordered by the physician.

Each facility will have a policy that states the point at which a temperature elevation is to be reported to the physician. In most facilities, the client's physician is to be notified of a temperature of 100F (37.7C) or greater.

Recording. Each temperature reading obtained is recorded on a flowsheet in the client's chart. The site at which the temperature was obtained is always identified if it is axillary or rectal. The rectal temperature is noted as such on the flowsheet by placing an "R" above the plot; an "A" above the plotted temperature reading identifies an axillary temperature. No site notation is required for a temperature reading obtained orally (Fig. 16–16).

When the client has a temperature elevation, a nurse's note is written that contains the nursing process initiated in response to the elevated temperature. Also, the nurse documents that the client's physician was notified of this finding.

Measurement of Respiration. Oxygen is vital to the cellular metabolism. During respiration, oxygen is taken into the body to resupply the cells so they can continue metabolic activity and carbon dioxide waste is discharged with each breath.

Basic Concepts of Respiration. The terms *respiration* and *oxygenation* are used interchangeably. Clinical measurement of respiration is actually a matter of observing and counting the client's respiratory cycles.

Definition. **Respiration** is the exchange of oxygen and carbon dioxide in the lungs. It consists of three phases: ventilation, which is the movement of air into and out of the lungs; diffusion, the mechanism by which gases cross the alveolar-capillary membrane; and perfusion, the exchange of cellular gases to and from the blood. See Chapter 27 for more detail on the physiochemistry of respiration.

Respiratory Cycle. Respiration comprises a two-part cycle: *inspiration* (inhaling), the taking of oxygen-rich air into the lungs through the nose, trachea, and bronchi, and *expiration* (exhaling), or removal of carbon dioxide waste containing gases from the lungs out the respiratory passages into the air. Ventilation results from the differences in air pressure between the lungs and the atmosphere that occur with the movement and changing size of the thorax.

Normal respiration has an even, regular pattern, is quiet, and occurs without effort. The number of breaths taken by the client per minute is referred to as the respiratory rate.

Vital Sign Record

BLOOD PRESSURE RECORD

Date																				
Time																				
>200 -200																				
-190																				
·180																				
-170																				
-160																				
-150																				
-140																				
-130																				
-120																				
-110																				
-100																				
- 90																				
- 80																				
- 70																				
- 60																				
- 50 <50																				

f° c° **TEMPERATURE RECORD**

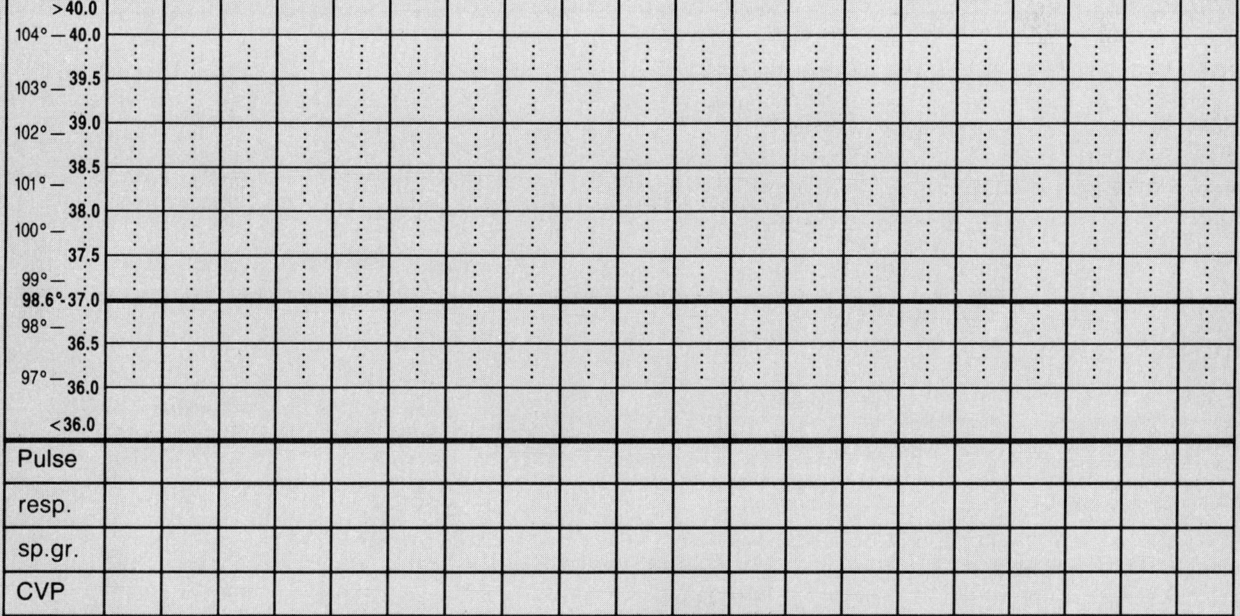
>40.0
104° — 40.0
103° — 39.5
102° — 39.0
38.5
101° —
38.0
100° —
37.5
99° —
98.6° 37.0
98° —
36.5
97° — 36.0
<36.0
Pulse
resp.
sp.gr.
CVP

N 4.08 Rev. 7/89
12605

Figure 16–16. Example of a temperature, pulse, and respiration (TPR) graphic recording form. (*Courtesy of St. Louis University Hospital, St. Louis University Medical Center, St. Louis, MO.*)

Mechanics of Breathing. Movement of the thorax is controlled by the central nervous system. Impulses from the brain's respiratory center pass over the phrenic nerve, which stimulates the diaphragm to contract and move downward into the abdomen from its resting position (Fig. 16–17). This enlarges the intrathoracic space. The abdominal organs move down and forward into the abdomen, and the rib cage lifts upward and expands outward to create more room for lung expansion. Increased intrathoracic space causes a decrease in the pressure inside the lung (intrapulmonic pressure), which becomes lower than the atmospheric pressure. When the pressure inside the lung is less than atmospheric pressure, air flows into the lungs and the inhalation phase of the respiratory cycle occurs (see Fig. 16–17).

The diaphragm then relaxes and returns to its original position; the ribs move downward and inward. This maneuver decreases the intrathoracic space. The decrease in intrathoracic volume results in an increase in the pressure in the lungs. When the lung pressure becomes greater than the atmospheric pressure, air flows out through the nose and mouth; this is exhalation. Thoracic size changes as a result of contraction and relaxation of the thoracic muscles. Pressure changes in the lungs are created by the increasing and decreasing size of the thoracic cavity.

The muscles that normally assist with inspiration are the scaleni, levatores costorum, sternocleidomastoideus, pectoralis major, platysma myoides, and serratus posterior superior. They elevate the ribs and sternum, and raise the ribs to create additional space for the lungs to expand. Accessory muscles also assist with expiration to move the diaphragm up to its original position. These are the rectus abdominis, external and internal obliques, and transverse abdominis. In addition, other muscles depress the ribs. These are the internal intercostals, serratus posterior inferior, and quadratus lumborum.

When a disease of the heart or lungs is present, respiratory rate often increases. This frequently places an extra burden on the respiratory system. Respiratory mechanics under these conditions often require assistance from muscles called the accessory muscles of respiration. Use of these muscles is a sign of respiratory distress.

Control of Respiration. Respiration is controlled primarily by the respiratory center of the central nervous system, which is excited by feedback signals initiated by changes in the chemical composition of the blood.[26] Signals from other parts of the nervous system also have a significant influence on the respiratory center during exercise.[26]

The respiratory center is composed of three major groups of neurons that ensure continuation of involuntary automatic respiration. The dorsal portion of the medulla controls mainly inspiration. The ventral group, located in the ventrolateral part of the medulla, causes inspiration and expiration, depending on which neurons in the group are stimulated.[26] The third group comprises the neurons of the pneumotaxic center located in the dorsal superior portion of the pons. The pneumotaxic center controls rate and pattern of breathing.[26] Output from this center ensures adaptation of respiratory rate and rhythm to meet the body's needs. Voluntary control of respiration is mediated by the cerebral cortex and permits conscious, willful acts such as holding one's breath and deliberate overbreathing.

The objective of respiration is to maintain the proper concentrations of oxygen, carbon dioxide, and hydrogen

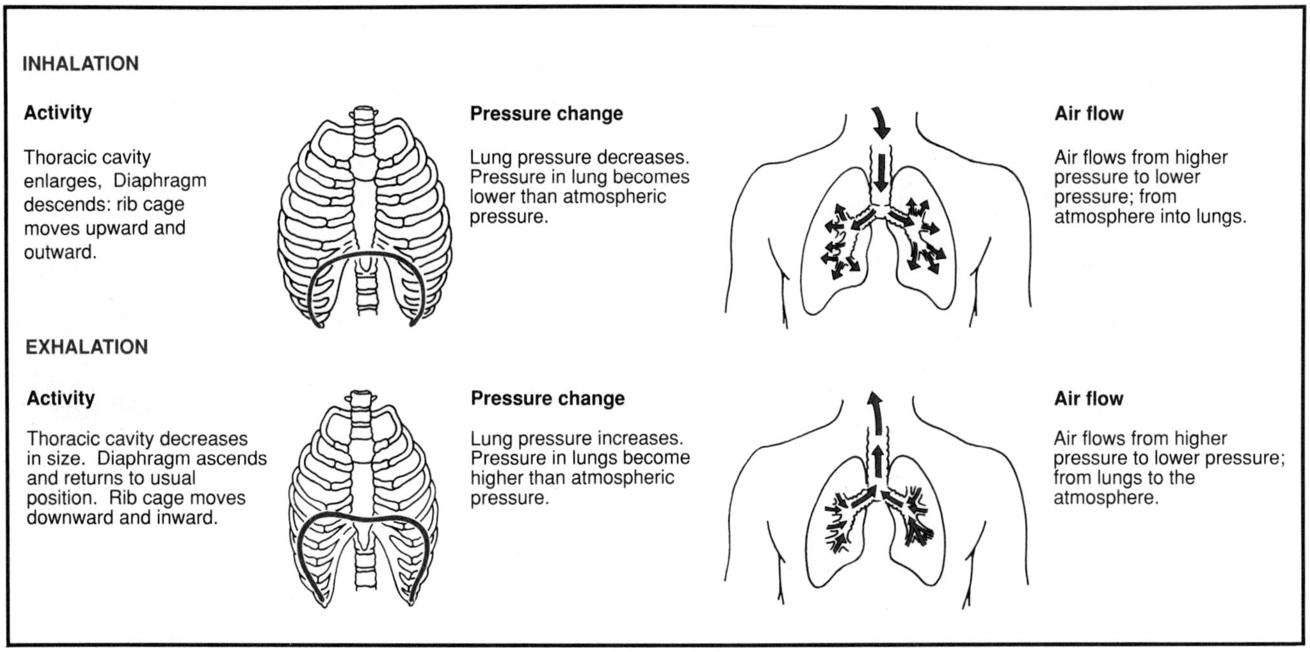

Figure 16–17. Movement of the diaphragm increases and decreases thoracic cavity space which, in turn, affects the pressure in the lung. Pressure changes in the lungs cause inspiration and expiration.

ions in body fluid. Excess carbon dioxide and hydrogen ions have an excitatory effect on the respiratory center that results in a stimulation of ventilation. Chemosensitive neurons in the respiratory center are activated primarily by accumulation of carbonic acid in the blood. Carbon dioxide itself has little direct effect on these neurons, but has a potent indirect effect by its ability to combine with water and form carbonic acid. Carbonic acid, in turn, dissociates into hydrogen and bicarbonate ions. Hydrogen ions, through their potent stimulating effect on the respiratory center, cause an increase in the rate and depth of ventilation and, thus, in the volume of air inhaled and exhaled per unit of time, the effect of which is a reduction in the partial pressure of carbon dioxide in the blood.[26]

Unlike hydrogen ions, oxygen has no significant direct effect on the respiratory center in controlling respiration. It does, however, participate in respiratory control through its ability to act on the peripheral chemoreceptors located in the carotid and aortic bodies, which, in turn, transmit signals to the respiratory center.[26] In addition, respiratory rate is affected by body temperature. Increases in body temperature have a direct stimulating effect on the respiratory center. They also have an indirect effect; they act to increase cellular metabolism throughout the body which augments the chemical stimuli for increased respiration.[26]

Factors Affecting Respiration. Anatomic, metabolic, environmental, and other factors have the potential to influence respiratory rate, depth, rhythm, volume, and quality. It is important that nurses understand the relationship of these factors to respiration.

Age and Gender. As the thorax grows, intrathoracic space expands and thus the area available for lung inflation increases. Because the male thoracic cavity is structurally larger on average than the female thoracic cavity, the total lung capacity of men is usually greater than that of women of the same age group. The average vital capacity of a young adult man is about 4.6 L, whereas in the young adult woman, it is 3.1 L.[26] Likewise, vital capacity is usually greater in tall individuals because of their relatively larger thoracic dimensions.

There are gender differences, moreover, in type (quality) of breathing. Female respirations are costal, which means they are accomplished primarily through the use of the costal muscles. Male respirations, on the other hand, are diaphragmatic, which means they occur primarily through depression of the diaphragm.

Age is another factor. Clearly, the vital capacities of children increase as they grow. Chest circumference increases from 33 cm at birth to 44.6 cm at age 5 years. Respiratory rate also varies inversely with age until adulthood, decreasing from 30 beats per minute at birth to 25 beats per minute at age 5 years and 18 beats per minute at age 10 years[42] (Box 16–14).

BOX 16–14. VARIATIONS IN RESPIRATORY RATE BASED ON AGE

Age	Rate
Infant	30+
Child	22–28
Adolescent	18–22
Adult	14–20

Growing older also affects respiration. The elderly experience a loss of lung capacity with age for two reasons: (1) skeletal changes in the thorax that reduce intrathoracic volume, and (2) loss of lung compliance. Because the compliance (elasticity) of lung tissue diminishes with age, the lung capacity of elderly individuals is frequently less than that of younger individuals of comparable size. Loss of lung compliance is accompanied by a reduction in the vital capacity.[26]

Disease. Disease alters respiration. Paralysis of the respiratory muscles, for example, drastically diminishes vital capacity. This situation sometimes develops when clients contract poliomyelitis, or following spinal cord injuries. The vital capacity, normally about 4600 mL, may be reduced to as little as 500 to 1000 mL.[26] Any disease that reduces pulmonary compliance will also reduce vital capacity. Tuberculosis, chronic asthma, lung cancer, and chronic bronchitis all reduce the pulmonary compliance and thus vital capacity. Another factor that also reduces pulmonary compliance is the congestion of the lungs accompanying increased pulmonary blood pressure that develops when the left ventricle of the heart fails.[26] The lungs become stiff and lose expansibility; vital capacity is correspondingly diminished.

Metabolism. Any activity, for example, exercise or digestion, increases the respiratory rate and depth in a compensatory mechanism to increase blood flow and oxygen to the cells to meet demand. During periods of rest, the respiratory rate decreases.

Fever, which reflects an increased rate of metabolism, also results in increased respiratory rate. During fever, body cells require a greater supply of oxygen to fuel metabolic increases. The increased oxygen need that results is provided for by an increase in the number of respirations per minute. Stimulation of the respiratory center to increase respiratory rate is a direct result of the effect of body temperature on the center and an indirect result of increases of carbon dioxide in the blood from metabolic rate increases.[26]

Stress. Stress and emotions such as anger, fear, and anxiety cause an increase in the respiratory rate. This happens as epinephrine and norepinephrine are released by the adrenal glands in response to the perception of threat. Pain causes stimulation of the sympathetic nervous system which, in turn, also increases the rate and depth of respiration.

Medications. Side effects of various medications alter respiratory rate. Drugs such as thyroid hormone supplements, amphetamines, and cocaine increase respiratory rate; barbiturates and narcotics decrease respiratory rate (Box 16–15).

BOX 16–15. DRUGS THAT ALTER RESPIRATORY RATE

Increase Rate	Decrease Rate
Thyroid hormone supplement	Anesthetics
Epinephrine	Narcotics
Progesterone	Sedatives
Salicylate	Atropine
Digitalis	
Amphetamines	
Cocaine	

Environment. Environmental factors such as altitude, air pollution, and environmental temperature affect respiration.

There is an inverse relationship between altitude and oxygen content of air. As altitude increases, the oxygen content of air decreases, which results in compensatory increases in respiratory rate. The respiratory center of the brain detects a decreased oxygen level and accelerates the respiratory rate and depth.

Air pollution has basically the same effect as altitude, resulting in a decreased oxygen content per unit of air. Pollution molecules take up "space" in the air that normally would be occupied by oxygen. Oxygen can also combine with various pollutant molecules, rendering it more difficult to dissolve in the blood.

Environmental temperature is another factor. During periods of excessive environmental temperature, the body attempts to compensate by initiating heat loss mechanisms, one component of which is an increased cardiac output which, in turn, requires a corresponding increase in respirations.

Characteristics of Respiration. Respirations are described in terms of rate, depth, rhythm, quality, chest vibration, and breath sounds.

Rate. **Respiratory rate** is the number of respiratory cycles that occur in one minute. Although respiratory rates vary from person to person, the average rate ranges between 12 and 20 per minute for an adult (see Box 16–14). Respiratory rate is directly linked to the body's constantly changing demand for oxygen and is affected by many factors discussed earlier. A constant ratio is maintained between respiratory and heart rates. The usual ratio is one respiration for each four beats of the heart. Alteration of this ratio can reflect insufficient oxygenation.

Fever increases the rate by about four breaths per minute for every 1F (0.3C) of temperature elevation. Increased cranial pressure decreases respiratory rate as brain function is depressed.

The usual adult respiratory rate of 12 to 20 is referred to as *eupnea*. If the respiratory rate is above 24 respirations per minute, the condition is considered to be abnormal and is called *tachypnea*. This pattern can result from increased cellular activity such as during exercise or anxiety. Pregnancy and fever also cause tachypnea because of increases in metabolic cellular demands. *Hyperventilation* refers to a pattern of increased rate and depth. Causes of hyperventilation include central nervous system lesions, meningitis, encephalitis, cerebral hemorrhage, cerebral trauma, tumors, hyperthyroidism, acidosis caused by metabolic imbalance, hypotension, and pain.

If the respiratory rate is below 10 per minute, the state is called *bradypnea*. Bradypnea can result from central nervous system depression or dysfunction. Drug overdose can result in central nervous system depression. Anesthetic agents also cause bradypnea, as can cerebral tumor and increased intracranial pressure. Skeletal deformities such as arthritis and conditions that impair thoracic movement such as tumors can also contribute to bradypnea as can pneumothorax and atelectasis.

Apnea is the temporary interruption or prolonged but nonpersistent absence of respirations. Prolonged apnea is a respiratory arrest.

Depth. **Respiratory depth** refers to the volume of air that is inhaled and exhaled. Depth varies and is described as deep, normal, or shallow.

Respiratory depth is assessed by observing the range and symmetry of the chest movement during inspiration and expiration. The symmetry of chest expansion is noted when assessing respiration depth. Both sides of the chest should expand equally. If chest expansion is asymmetrical, a condition known as *atelectasis* may exist. This is partial or complete collapse of a lung. Atelectasis is a very serious condition and the nurse who suspects it should consult with the physician immediately.

Hypoventilation is a state in which the intake of air is in insufficient quantity to meet metabolic demand. Both rate and depth of respiration may be decreased. Insufficient oxygen is taken in and insufficient carbon dioxide is exhaled. As carbon dioxide is retained, the pH of the blood drops below 7.2 and the client becomes acidotic. Acidosis is a serious and potentially life-threatening condition. (See Chap. 31 for more on acidosis.)

Gravity has an effect on ventilatory depth. One of the reasons that clients are encouraged to ambulate as early as possible after surgery is to counteract the biomechanics of gravity. Gravity constantly exerts a force against the outward excursion of the thorax, which can impede ventilation when the client is in a weakened state. Reduced ventilation results in the pooling of secretions in the lungs, a predisposing factor in the development of pneumonia.

Rhythm. **Respiratory rhythm** refers to the cadence or pattern of respiration. Respiratory rhythm is described as being either regular or irregular. Respirations should be regular, smooth, and evenly spaced. The inspiratory phase is slightly longer than the expiratory phase. Irregular respirations are unevenly spaced and have no pattern. Irregular respirations in a newborn are a normal and expected finding; however, irregular respirations in an adult client are abnormal. One irregular respiratory rhythm that is frequently observed in very seriously ill clients is *Cheyne-Stokes respirations*. This pattern consists of a period of hyperventilation followed by a period of apnea. This pattern is repeated until finally the client's condition deteriorates and death occurs. Clearly, Cheyne-Stokes respirations signify a respiratory emergency that requires immediate and intensive medical treatment.

Quality. **Respiratory quality** refers to the distinctive traits or characteristics of respiration. Respirations should be effortless and quiet. The chest under normal conditions moves only slightly, and the movement that does occur is symmetrical. Any observations other than these indicate a decrease in the quality of the respirations. "Diaphragmatic" breathing means that ventilation occurs through depression of the diaphragm.

Dyspnea is the term used to describe difficult or labored breathing. Pronounced physical effort is exerted to breathe and the use of the accessory muscles is required to carry out respiration. Clients who are dyspneic experience a shortness of breath on exertion. A small amount of exercise leads to a disproportionately large increase in ventilation. The clients often have an unpleasant sensation of breathlessness. They may be aware of the increased effort needed to expand and contract the chest wall, may sense fatigue in the respiratory muscles, and may have the uncomfortable sensation that they urgently need to breathe again before expiration is completed, a condition referred to as "air hunger." Some clients also experience a sense of "tightness in the chest." Clients with this condition often feel severely apprehensive. Labored breathing is apparent to the observer through the anxious appearance of the client, by the client's use of the accessory muscles of respiration, and by the flaring of the nostrils on inspiration, which is another sign of respiratory distress. Because dyspnea signifies that there is insufficient oxygen in the bloodstream to meet body demands, any client who becomes dyspneic requires immediate medical attention to correct the condition. Clients who have chronic respiratory disease often have oxygen or medication available to treat their condition; they should be assisted to use available modalities. If they fail to respond to treatment promptly, however, they too will require immediate medical attention. (See also Chap. 27.)

Orthopnea is the inability to breathe adequately while lying down. Under normal conditions, the volume of air in the lungs changes as body position changes. The air volume in the lungs decreases when the individual lies down and increases when the person is standing. This is because the diaphragm is pressed upward by the abdominal contents when the individual is lying down and also because the pulmonary blood volume increases, leaving less space available for air.[26]

When orthopnea occurs, it is readily observable. The client can breathe adequately only while sitting, standing, or lying propped up by several pillows. The assessment of this condition includes identifying the number of pillows that are required to position the client, so that he or she can inhale an adequate amount of air.

Chest Vibration. **Chest vibration** is another characteristic of respiration. It refers to the vibrations that are felt over the chest wall when the client speaks. For information concerning chest vibration, refer to the section *Thorax and Lungs,* later in this chapter.

Breath Sounds. When respirations are not quiet, audible sounds are apparent, sometimes to the unaided ear, but always by stethoscope. These sounds can be assessed by the nurse and include wheezing, stridor, crackles (rales) and gurgles or rumbles (rhonchi).

Equipment. The equipment needed to assess respirations includes a watch with the capability to indicate seconds and a stethoscope if breath sounds are to be assessed. (See *Thorax and Lungs* for more about assessing breath sounds).

Technique. Place the client's arm across the chest and proceed to take the pulse. After counting the pulse, continue holding the client's wrist, observing the rise and fall of the chest that occur with each respiration. This method of counting improves accuracy in measurement. The client can consciously or unconsciously modify his or her breathing while being observed; this method avoids making the client self-conscious.

Usually, counting the number of respirations that occurs in 15 seconds and multiplying by 4 provides an accurate respiratory rate; however, if the respiratory pattern is in any way unusual, for example, rate, rhythm, depth, or sounds of respiration are altered, the respirations should be counted for one full minute (Procedure 16–2).

Norms and Expected Findings. Respirations are automatic and should be quiet and require no exertion. The expected rate is 12 to 20 cycles per minute. Respiratory rhythm should show regular cycles. The depth of respirations should be even and appropriate to activity. Occasional sighs are expected. Respiratory quality should be nonlabored without flaring of the nostrils or use of the accessory muscles of respiration. No abdominal muscle retraction should occur.

Special Considerations, Precautions, Sources of Error. As discussed earlier, the nurse should obtain the respiratory rate assessment without the client's awareness that it is being done. The recommended method decreases the potential that the rate count will be inaccurate.

The nurse should wait 5 to 10 minutes after the client has been active or received treatment before assessing respirations. Activity or stress increases the metabolic rate, thereby increasing cell oxygen consumption which, in turn, increases the respiratory rate.

If the client has a respiratory rate above 30 or below 12 cycles per minute, the nurse should proceed to monitor respirations every 15 minutes. If the pattern persists longer than 30 minutes or if the client has additional signs of respiratory distress such as dyspnea or use of the accessory muscles, the client may require medical intervention and the nurse should confer immediately with the physician.

A potential source of error in respiration measurement involves failure to position the stethoscope chestpieces correctly (see the discussion about the technique of using the stethoscope earlier in this chapter).

Recording. Both normal respirations and deviations from the expected findings are recorded in the client's chart. Deviations are discussed with the physician and the time the physician was notified is included.

PROCEDURE 16–2. ASSESSING RESPIRATIONS

☐ **PURPOSE:** To determine general information of client's respiratory function

☐ **EQUIPMENT:** Watch with second hand or digital display of seconds

ACTION

1. Observe client for signs of acute stress, pain, or recent activity, such as flushed face, rapid audible respirations, extraneous movements, guarding posture, clenched jaw, and tears. Defer assessment if signs are present; initiate intervention as appropriate.
   NOTE: Discussion of procedure is deferred for this assessment, as clients' awareness that respiratory rate is being assessed may cause them to be overly conscious of their breathing, which may alter rate.
2. Observe the rise and fall of the chest. Assess regularity of respirations by noting intervals between breaths.
3. If movement is regular, count for 15 seconds and multiply by 4; if irregular, count for 1 minute.
4. Note amount of chest movement with each breath to determine depth of respirations. Chest excursion may be assessed (see Fig. 16–51) for more definitive data about depth of respirations.
5. Note whether respirations are noisy or silent, effortless or labored. If noisy or labored, auscultate breath sounds. (See discussion later in this chapter.)
6. Discuss results with client. Initiate teaching as appropriate.

☐ **RECORDING:** Note respiratory rate on client's vital signs flowsheet. Note changes in rhythm, depth, or quality of respirations on progress notes. Discuss atypical findings for client with client's physician.

A nurse's note for normal respirations might appear as follows: respiratory rate 12; shallow; regular; no chest vibrations present; lungs clear to auscultation.

The following nurse's note describes abnormal respirations: respiratory rate 32; shallow; irregular; respirations labored with apparent abdominal retraction; chest vibrations felt over anterior and posterior chest wall; wheezing heard on inspiration and expiration without use of stethoscope.

Pulse Measurement. Pulse is another cardinal sign that has been used by nurses to assess clients' immediate health.

Basic Concepts About Pulse. Pulse assessment is an important tool for evaluating the functions of the cardiovascular system and its capacity to respond to peripheral oxygen demands.

Definition. **Pulse** is defined as the elastic expansion and recoil of an artery in response to pressure waves created by the beating of the heart.

Arterial wall elasticity enables the arteries to respond in a dynamic way to the conditions created by the pressure wave, expanding as pressure increases (systole) and recoiling as it diminishes (diastole).

A wave of pressure begins in the aorta as the volume of blood ejected by the heart (stroke volume) passes through the aortic valve into the aorta during ventricular systole. It quickly overcomes the inertia of blood in the central aorta and continues farther and farther out into the arterial tree. The blood ejected into the aorta travels much more slowly than the pressure wave itself. Therefore, the pulse that is palpated in a peripheral artery is the result of the propagation of the pressure pulse but is unrelated to the actual flow of blood.[43] As arteries branch, the pulse wave diminishes substantially, and by the time it reaches the capillaries, the pulse wave is almost absent.[26]

The pulse reflects many features of cardiovascular function. In addition to heart rate and cardiac output, pulse reflects arterial compliance, blood volume, and the general resistance of the vascular bed. One of the most common reasons for measuring the pulse, however, is to gain information on the rate at which the heart is beating. Pulses can be felt over peripheral arteries as they pass over bony prominences. Counting a pulse by palpating a superficial artery is a common nursing procedure. The most accurate method for counting the pulse, however, is not by palpation, but rather by auscultation of the heart itself. Certain pathological circumstances sometimes cause imperceptible weak pulses to occur.[26] Although their corresponding heartbeats may be audible, weak pulses palpated at a peripheral site may go uncounted, resulting in an underestimation of heart rate.

Pulse Regulation. Pulse rate and volume are regulated under normal conditions by nervous reflexes that initiate negative feedback signals for the constant adjustment of the circulation (see Chap. 6 for more information on negative feedback mechanisms). Those reflexes, the baroreceptor and chemoreceptor reflexes and the central nervous system ischemic response, act to maintain an optimal relationship among arterial pressure, cardiac output, and total peripheral resistance, all of which are reflected in pulse rate and volume.[26] Any factor that disturbs the balance is counteracted by these reflexes.

The baroreceptor mechanism relies on pressure-sensitive cells located in the walls of the large systemic arteries. A rise in arterial pressure stretches the baroreceptors and causes them to rapidly transmit signals to the central nervous system, inhibiting the vasomotor center of the medulla and exciting the vagal center. Feedback signals are then sent back through the parasympathetic branch of the autonomic nervous system to the circulation to adjust arterial pressure downward.[26] The net effect is a decrease in heart rate and strength of contraction and vasodilation throughout the peripheral circulation. Arterial pressure drops as cardiac output and peripheral resistance decrease; however, **pulse pressure,** the difference between the systolic and diastolic pressure (see *Blood Pressure Measurement,* later in this chapter), is maintained because the reduction in peripheral resistance results in a greater venous return to the heart, increasing the volume ejected (stroke volume) with each heartbeat.[26] Thus pulse volume (strength) remains relatively constant under normal conditions.

The chemoreceptor reflex involves chemosensitive cells that are located in the carotid bodies, one of which lies in the bifurcation of each common carotid artery, and in several aortic bodies adjacent to the aorta. Diminished blood flow through these structures stimulates the chemoreceptors, which are sensitive to a reduction in available oxygen and an increase in carbon dioxide and hydrogen ion concentration.[26] The vasomotor center becomes excited and acts to elevate arterial pressure by initiating vasoconstriction and by increasing heart rate and contractility, thus adjusting the arterial pressure upward when it becomes too low.[26] Pulse rate increases correspondingly.

The central nervous system ischemic response acts directly on the vasomotor center of the brain. When blood flow to the lower brain stem is insufficient, ischemia results. *Ischemia* is defined as a local oxygen deficiency and carbon dioxide buildup. The ischemic response activates only when arterial blood pressure falls below 60 mm Hg.[26] Under these abnormal conditions the neurons of the vasomotor center become strongly excited, causing a rise in arterial blood pressure in the same manner as the chemoreceptor reflex. This mechanism causes strong vasoconstriction as well as an increase in heart rate and contractility[26]; however, because stroke volume decreases in inverse proportion to the increase in heart rate, and because strong vasoconstriction greatly increases peripheral resistance, the pulse pressure narrows, and the pulse weakens correspondingly.[26,27]

Heart rate varies continuously in response to demand but constantly maintains a rate that supports adequate circulation. A pulse rate that is insufficient to meet demand indicates circulatory pathophysiology.

Pulse Characteristics. When the nurse palpates the client's pulse, specific pulse characteristics are assessed. They include rate, rhythm, volume, and symmetry.

PULSE RATE. **Pulse rate** is the number of ventricle contractions or heartbeats that occur in one minute and indirectly reflects cardiac output. An adult pulse rate below 60 beats per minute is called *bradycardia;* a rate above 100 beats per minute is called *tachycardia.*

PULSE RHYTHM. **Pulse rhythm** is the cadence or pattern of the pulse. Pulse rhythm is either regular or irregular. The usual pulse rhythm is regular and evenly spaced. If the rhythm is irregular, the nurse determines if the irregularity is a regular-irregular or irregular-irregular pattern. A *regular-irregular pulse* is one that is indeed irregular but has a regular, predictable pattern to the irregularity. An *irregular–irregular pulse* is one in which there is no pulse pattern whatever; the pulse occurs at random. An irregular pulse is a sign of cardiac pathology. A pulse with an irregular rhythm is referred to as an *arrhythmia.*

PULSE VOLUME/AMPLITUDE. **Pulse volume,** also referred to as the strength or quality of the pulse, results from the force and intensity of the left ventricle contraction, which creates the wave of pressure felt at peripheral points as a pulse. It is sometimes referred to as the amplitude of the beat. Words used to describe pulse volume include strong, "bounding," which indicates effective ventricle contraction, and weak or "thready," which indicates decreased cardiac output and inefficient cardiac function. A pulse of adequate amplitude cannot be easily eliminated when pressure from the fingers gently pushes the artery against the underlying bone.

Ordinarily, the arteries have elasticity and expand with each volume output; however, when the arteries become hardened, as they do in arteriosclerosis, they lose their capacity to expand; the pulse quality changes, becoming "weak," and can be difficult to palpate. When the pulse volume is weak, the heart rate increases as the body's homeostatic mechanisms attempt to counterbalance the decreased cardiac output by increasing the heart rate.

PULSE SYMMETRY. **Pulse symmetry** refers to the fact that in normal circumstances, peripheral pulses are equal on both sides of the body, sometimes referred to as bilateral equality. For example, the popliteal pulses of both legs should have the same rate, rhythm, and volume. Lack of symmetry reflects the perfusion status of the area with the weaker pulse.[26]

Factors Affecting Pulse Characteristics. Pulse rate is a direct reflection of metabolic rate. A body demand for an increase in the metabolic rate results in a corresponding increase in the heart rate to supply the cells with the additional blood and oxygen. The accelerated metabolic process is required to meet the increased demand for energy. Factors that increase or decrease body demand include age, sex, activity, stress (both physical and psychological) and emotions, disease, and medications.

AGE. As age increases, the body's metabolic rate decreases. Age therefore is associated with a decreased demand for oxygenated blood supplied to the cells. Moreover, the heart muscle, like other body muscles, becomes less effective, efficient, and forceful in its contractions as it ages. There is an inverse relationship between age and pulse; as age increases, the pulse rate decreases (Box 16–16).

Another factor associated with aging is loss of arterial vessel wall elasticity, as described previously. This occurs in *arteriosclerosis,* a pathological process of the arteries that causes hardening of the vessel wall. Arterial expansion is decreased in arteriosclerosis as the artery walls lose some or most of their elasticity and are unable to "give" or expand to accommodate the bolus of blood that passes through with each ventricular contraction. When the arterial vessel wall cannot expand and recoil, the pulse is more difficult to palpate.

BOX 16–16. EXPECTED PULSE RATE BY AGE GROUP

Age Group	Range	Average
Infant	100–160	120
Child	80–90	85
Adult	50–90	80
Elderly	60–90	70

SEX. Pulse rate and strength are influenced by factors associated with sex. The pulse rate of the adult female is ordinarily 7 to 10 beats higher than the pulse rate of the adult male. This difference reflects female hormonal effects on cellular metabolism. Likewise, pregnancy has an important effect on the pulse. Cardiac output rises 30 to 50 percent by the twelfth week of pregnancy.[44] Elevation in cardiac output is accompanied by a rise in pulse rate of 8 to 10 beats per minute above nonpregnant levels.

ACTIVITY. Physical exertion increases the cells' demand for blood so they can continue to meet the increased metabolic oxygen demand. Acceleration in metabolic rate causes the pulse rate to increase; however, the long-term effect of consistent regular exercise results in a very efficient cardiovascular system. Overall pulse rate slows to under 60 beats per minute, a condition known as athletic bradycardia, and the heart readily meets an increased demand with only a slight increase in pulse rate. (See also Chap. 30.)

Body position affects pulse rate. Less energy is required for muscle activity while lying quietly than while standing. Hence pulse rate is lower in recumbent individuals than in those who are standing.

STRESS AND EMOTIONS. Emotions that are frequently accompanied by an increase in pulse rate include anxiety, excitement, fear, and anger. Epinephrine and norepinephrine, both of which raise the basal metabolic rate, are secreted in response to physical and psychological stress; they cause an increase in the heart rate. Pain as a form of stress also causes an increase in pulse rate. Grief and depression, on the other hand, are accompanied by an output of acetylcholine, which decreases the heart rate.

DISEASE. Diseases that alter metabolic rate, either increasing it or decreasing it, are accompanied by a corresponding change in heart rate. Hyperthyroidism, a condition discussed earlier in which excessive thyroid hormone is secreted, is associated with increased heart rate; hypothyroidism is associated with decreased heart rate. Infection accompanied by fever, which signals a rise in metabolism, also increases pulse rate. For every 0.5C (0.9F) of temperature elevation, the heart rate is increased by 7 to 10 beats per minute.

Pulse changes also accompany changes in cardiac valve and muscle function and alterations in the electrical conduction of the heart. Valvular diseases cause a variety of alterations in pulse strength and rhythm. Narrowing (stenosis) and insufficient closure (regurgitation) of the aortic valve are associated, for example, with a weak pulse.[44] A severely diseased heart muscle, on the other hand, may be associated with alternating strong and weak pulse waves known as *pulsus alternans.*[26] Pulsus alternans results from a mechanical oscillation that alternately augments and reduces stroke volume. It signifies severe dysfunction of the left ventricle of the heart.[27] Electrical conduction disturbances in the heart, by their effect on heart rate and rhythm, also alter pulse rate and rhythm. Irregular heartbeats may be insufficiently strong to eject enough blood to create a strong pressure wave, or may be so fast as to allow insufficient time for adequate ventricular filling. In either case a *pulse deficit,* pulses that can be heard over the apex of the heart but are imperceptible to the touch, may result. The greater the pulse deficit, the more serious is the underlying problem.[26]

HEMORRHAGE. Hemorrhage decreases venous return to the heart and thus reduces cardiac output. Approximately 10 percent of the total volume of blood can be lost with no significant effect on arterial pressure or cardiac output.[26] Loss of more than this reduces cardiac output at first and then arterial pressure. Hemorrhage initiates the powerful autonomic reflexes described above and causes a profound vasoconstriction and a marked increase in heart activity, both of which result in a rapid, weak pulse. The pulse rate may rise from 70 to 200 beats per minute.

POSITION CHANGES. When an individual changes from a lying or sitting position to a standing position, blood may momentarily pool in the dependent extremities. This reduces venous return to the heart and activates the autonomic reflexes described above. The body responds with an increase in heart rate and vasoconstriction.

MEDICATIONS. Drugs that are central nervous system depressants such as hypnotics and sedatives decrease heart rate. Cardiac drugs have specific functions and can either slow or strengthen the heartbeat (eg, digitalis), increase the heart rate (eg, atropine, epinephrine), or improve electrical conduction (eg, propranolol hydrochloride, procainamide hydrochloride) to enhance pulse. Drugs that affect the basal metabolic rate also increase or decrease the heart rate (eg, levothyroxine sodium, methimazole).

Equipment. To assess the client's pulse, the nurse needs a watch that indicates seconds and an acoustical stethoscope for auscultating the apical pulse or a Doppler stethoscope in the event that apical sounds are inaudible.

Doppler ultrasound stethoscopes are used when peripheral pulses are impalpable and the apical pulse is inaudible with an acoustical stethoscope. Rather than amplify sounds, the Doppler ultrasound stethoscope detects the movement of underlying tissue or blood cells by the use of sound waves. A battery-operated probe containing a volume-controlled audio unit and a transducer gives off sound waves of high ultrasonic frequency that are directed into the body. These waves are reflected off of red cells as they course through blood vessels. As the red cells move in relation to the stationary instrument, the frequency of reflected waves shifts slightly, producing an audible sound—an effect known as the Doppler shift—which is detected by the transducer and transmitted into the Doppler head set attached by a long cord. Dopplers can detect the movement of blood cells to a depth of 5 cm,[45] but are unable to detect movement in deep vessels or in underlying bone such as in the chest or abdomen. Thus the use of the Doppler for pulse detection is reserved for peripheral pulse sites. Doppler stethoscopes are also used in the indirect measurement of blood pressure.

Technique. The technique of pulse assessment follows from the nurse's decisions about the site and method to be used. The sites available are the apical area, which is assessed using an acoustical stethoscope, and the peripheral pulse sites, which are assessed by palpation or with the use of a Doppler ultrasound stethoscope. Regardless of the method or site used, the client should be resting and relaxed for pulse assessment. Clients who have been active should be allowed to rest for 5 to 10 minutes before beginning.

Selecting the Apical Site. The apical pulse site is preferable whenever the client has or is suspected to have a cardiac arrhythmia (an irregular cardiac rhythm). The apical site is advantageous because it provides clear, audible sounds for rate counting and rhythm assessment. Apical pulses are required when the client is taking certain heart medications, particularly those of the digitalis family. Digitalis causes slowing of the heart and is usually contraindicated when the heart rate falls below 60 beats per minute. Thus an accurate pulse count prior to administration of the drug is essential. Undercounting the heart rate may result in unnecessary withholding of the drug. Thus, the apical site is preferred.

The apical site is also used to detect a pulse deficit when a client is known or suspected to have a cardiac arrhythmia. The procedure for assessing pulse deficit requires two nurses for its performance. One nurse counts the radial or other peripheral pulse as the other nurse counts the apical pulse. The apical pulse will be either the same as or greater than the peripheral pulse count. A difference between the two counts constitutes a pulse deficit. Pulse deficits usually signify cardiac dysfunction and, when detected, indicate the need for an immediate consultation with the physician. A peripheral pulse count that is higher than the apical count signifies a counting error.

LOCATING THE APICAL AREA. The apical site is located on the anterior surface of the chest directly over the **point of maximal impulse** (PMI). This is the small area (generally less than 2 cm in diameter) where the apex of the heart is in closest proximity to the chest wall. The site is found lying over or just inside of the midclavicular line at the fifth intercostal space in adults; the midclavicular line is an imaginary line that passes vertically from the midpoint of the clavicle. The PMI may be found at the fourth intercostal space in children under 7 years of age, and may lie slightly to the left of the midclavicular line. The impulse of the heart beating is palpable in about 50 percent of the adult population. Sometimes the apical impulse is actually visible (Fig. 16–18).

TECHNIQUE FOR APICAL PULSE MEASUREMENT. Procedure 16–3 outlines the technique for apical pulse measurement. Before beginning, locate the PMI and place the bell or diaphragm of the acoustical stethoscope over the apical site. Remember to check the earpieces of the stethoscope for debris that might impede sound transmission and to lock the chestpiece into position before beginning your count.

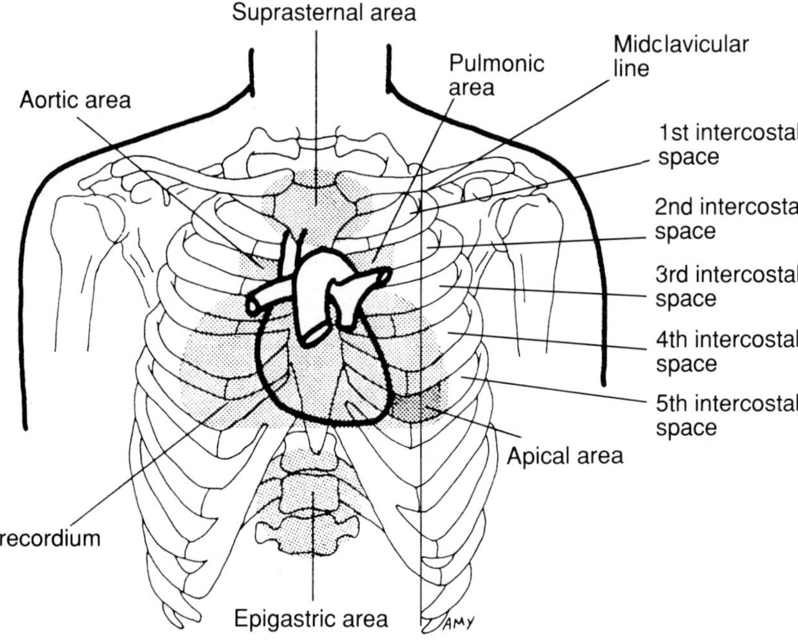

Figure 16–18. Physical landmarks for locating the apical area. (Source: *Berger KJ, Fields WL.* Pocket Guide to Health Assessment. *Reston, VA: Reston Publishing Co.; 1980.*)

PROCEDURE 16–3. ASSESSING APICAL PULSE

PURPOSE: To directly assess pumping action of the heart in clients with dysrhythmias, certain diseases, or who are taking certain medications.

EQUIPMENT: Stethoscope, watch with second hand or digital display of seconds.

ACTION	RATIONALE
1. Discuss the procedure, desired client participation, and anticipated benefits with the client.	1. Active participation is more likely if the client understands expectations and benefits.
2. Wash your hands.	2. Removes transient organisms from your hands that could be pathogens, preventing transmission to the client.
3. Observe the client for indicators of acute stress, pain, or recent activity, such as flushed face, rapid audible respirations, guarding posture, extraneous movements, clenched jaw, and tears. Defer assessment of pulse rate if signs are present; intervene as appropriate.	3. Emotional and physical stress (pain, exercise, etc) can elevate pulse temporarily. Value obtained may not reflect the general cardiac status of client.
4. Request or assist client to assume supine position, with head slightly elevated. Sitting position is also satisfactory.	4. Promotes comfort and access to PMI (point of maximal impulse).
5. Screen client; expose chest.	5. Prevents embarrassment or discomfort from body exposure.
6. Locate PMI while holding diaphragm of stethoscope in your other hand (see also Fig. 16–18).	6. Pulse will be most readily auscultated at this location. Diaphragm of stethoscope will be warm, which is more comfortable to the client.

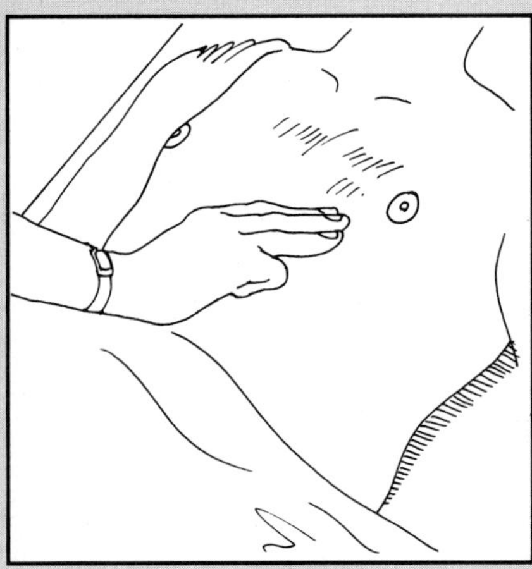

(continued)

PROCEDURE 16–3. (continued)

7. Place the diaphragm of the stethoscope over the PMI and listen for normal heart sounds: S_1 (lubb) and S_2 (dupp). Assess rhythm by noting interval between beats.

7. Reflects closing of atrioventricular valves (S_1) and semilunar valves (S_2). Regularity of beats determines time of counting.

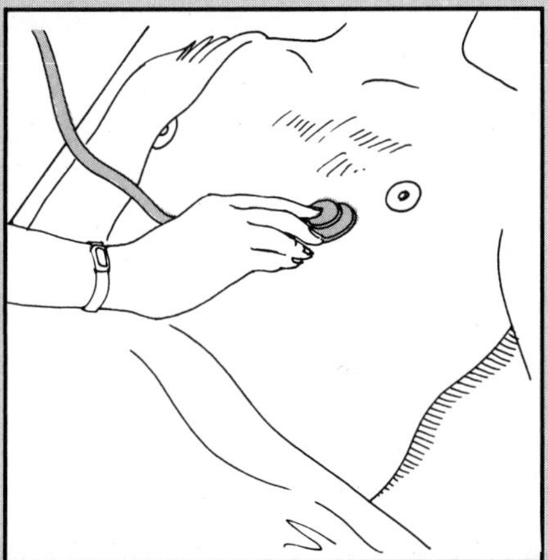

8. If heart beat is regular, count for 30 seconds and multiply by 2; if irregular, count for 1 full minute.

8. Minute rate of irregular heartbeat can be determined only by counting for 1 full minute.

9. Note loudness of sounds to determine strength of heartbeat.

9. Weak sounds suggest poor cardiac function. Loud sounds indicate strong heart action; very loud sounds may reflect cardiac enlargement.

10. Discuss results of assessment with client. Initiate teaching as appropriate.

10. An informed client can be a more active participant in health care and self-care.

11. Assist client to replace gown or clothing and bed covers, if needed. Open curtain, if desired.

11. Promotes well-being.

VARIATION: APICAL–RADIAL PULSE

NOTE: This assessment is rarely done because most clients with cardiac pathology that causes pulse deficit (apical pulse greater than radial pulse) will have continuous electronic cardiac monitoring.

1. Discuss reason for simultaneous assessment by two nurses with client.

1. Allays anxiety client may feel because of unusual assessment.

2. One nurse auscultates apical pulse while second palpates radial pulse.

2. Both values are necessary to determine whether pulse deficit is present.

3. One nurse holds watch so both can see it, gives signal to start counting and to stop after 1 minute.

3. Counting must be simultaneous.

(continued)

PROCEDURE 16–3. (continued)

4. Nurses compare rates, strength, and rhythm of pulses. — 4. Defines magnitude of deficit, if present.

RECORDING: Record apical pulse on client's vital signs flowsheet or medical record. On flowsheets, apical pulse is designated with "A" next to entry. Note changes in rate, rhythm, or strength or pulse deficit in progress notes. Discuss atypical findings for client with client's physician.

Warm your hands and the chestpiece to be used before placing it on the client's chest. The sounds of the heart beating can be heard as an audible lubb-dupp, which are S_1, the first heart sound, and S_2, the second heart sound, respectively. S_1 and S_2 together represent one beat of the heart. Count the number of beats. (The section on the *Cardiovascular System* later in this chapter goes into more detail on the cardiac cycle and heart sounds.)

Note the regularity of the apical rhythm. Regularity is characterized by an equal duration of the time lapses between beats. Irregularity is characterized by unequal intervals between each beat. On detecting an arrhythmia, describe it as either a regular-irregular pattern, as noted earlier, or an irregular-irregular pattern. Detection of an arrhythmia is another indication for an immediate consultation with the physician, who may wish to evaluate the arrhythmia further by ordering an electrocardiogram (see Chap. 27.)

Selecting the Peripheral Site. The peripheral pulse sites all lie distal to the heart and are used frequently for pulse measurement. The radial site is readily accessible and is the site for routine pulse assessment. Other pulse sites may be selected when the radial is unavailable or impalpable or when additional information is needed. For example, the carotid and femoral arteries are used when other pulses at other peripheral sites become impalpable or when the client is a child. Likewise, the carotid artery may be used when information about circulation to the brain is needed, or the femoral site may be used when information about circulation to the leg is needed. The popliteal pulse reflects circulation to the lower leg; the dorsalis pedis reflects circulation to the foot. Thus the site selected depends on the situation, the age of the client, and the information needed.

LOCATING THE PERIPHERAL SITES. Table 16–8 lists the peripheral pulse sites and reviews their uses. After selecting the site for pulse measurement, palpate the area over the artery. Exerting moderate pressure, place the distal pads of the middle two fingers over the arterial site. Move your palpating fingers over the site until a pulse is detected. If you feel no pulse or only a weak pulse, modify the pressure of your palpating fingers. Excessive pressure will obliterate the pulse; insufficient pressure may make the pulse undetectable. (See Fig. 16–57.)

TECHNIQUE FOR PERIPHERAL PULSE MEASUREMENT. Procedure 16–4 outlines the procedure for taking a peripheral pulse, both by palpation and with the use of a Doppler ultrasound stethoscope.

Once the peripheral pulse is located evaluate it for rate, rhythm, and volume. Pulse volume refers to the strength or quality of force created by each pulse. Pulse volume is usually the only variable assessed for lower extremity pulses. Pulse volume ranges from absent (no pulse) to bounding

TABLE 16–8. SUMMARY OF PERIPHERAL PULSE SITES

Site	Use
Temporal: superior and lateral to the eye	Easily accessible; used primarily in infants and children
Carotid: below angle of jaw at edge of sternocleidomastoid muscle	Frequently used during crisis; palpable after peripheral sites are not
Brachial: antecubital fossa between biceps and triceps muscles	Used when radial site is not available; used for blood pressure auscultation
Radial: thumb side, inner aspect of wrist	Most frequently used site; convenient and accessible
Femoral: next to inguinal ligament	Used when radial site is not available; evaluates circulation status of lower extremity; evaluates arterial perfusion during CPR
Popliteal: popliteal fossa behind knee	Located deep in tissue; site less readily available and more difficult to locate; evaluates lower extremity circulation
Posterior tibial: medial ankle below malleous	Evaluates circulation status of lower extremities
Pedal: top of foot	Must be palpated gently; this artery is absent in about 10% of the population.

(an unusually full pulse). The expected finding is a pulse that is easily felt with moderate pressure and is obliterated only by the application of additional pressure. Weak pulses, sometimes referred to as "thready" pulses because of their characteristic feel, may be obliterated using even moderate pressure. Bounding pulses, on the other hand, are difficult to obliterate even with strong pressure. Pulse volume is described and recorded using a numerical scale (Box 16–17).

Pulses should be detected in distal extremities. If pulses at the radial, dorsalis pedis, or posterior tibial sites are undetectable, palpate the femoral and carotid sites. Diminished pulses at these sites indicate poor perfusion and shock. A palpable radial pulse generally signifies a systolic blood pressure of at least 80 mm Hg.

Assess pulse symmetry by comparing pulses bilaterally for their volume. Pulses are said to be symmetrical when those on either side of the body, both radial pulses and both femoral pulses, for example, show equal pulse volume.

When using the Doppler ultrasound stethoscope, turn on the battery-powered unit. Apply conductive gel to the probe. Do not use any gel other than the conductive gel. Place the earpieces in your ears. Place the probe over the artery and adjust the volume. The sounds over an artery have a pulsating and pumping quality, whereas those over a vein are softer and may vary with respiration. Be sure to wipe the remaining gel off of the probe and return the instrument to the battery recharging unit when finished.

COUNTING PULSES. Counting procedure is an important factor in obtaining an accurate pulse measurement. The traditional method of counting pulses is to label the first beat counted as 1; the remainder follow in series as 2, 3, 4, and so on. Hargest, however, encourages a counting procedure that labels the first beat as 0, analogous to the time of birth as indicating 0 months of age.[46] The rationale is that the interval between two beats is a single pulse sequence. Therefore, by beginning with 0, the caregiver avoids overestimating heart rate. The traditional counting method, on the other hand, can result in an error of 4 beats per minute when the pulse is counted for 15 seconds and multiplied by 4.

The duration of the interval for counting is another issue. There is controversy about whether the pulse should be counted for 15-, 30-, or 60-second intervals. Some authors advocate counting for 30 seconds and multiplying by 2[47,48]; others advocate counting for a full 60 seconds for all clients[49]; still others advocate counting for 60-second intervals only for clients who have a slow or rapid pulse[50] or an irregular pulse,[51,52] and counting for 15-second intervals and multiplying by 4 when the pulse rate is normal and regular.[50]

It is clear that judgment is needed in the selection of a counting interval. The 15-second interval is commonly used because it is time-saving, but it may result in inaccuracy. For the most accurate count, using the 30-second interval and multiplying by 2 is preferable. When the client's heart rate is unusually slow, rapid, or irregular, or if there is any doubt as to the accuracy of the pulse, count the pulse for a full 60-second interval.

BOX 16–17. PULSE VOLUME DESCRIPTION SCALE

Scale	Description
0	Absent
1 +	Thready, weak, easily obliterated
2+	Normal, easily palpated
3+	Strong, forceful
4+	Bounding, difficult to obliterate

Norms and Expected Findings. Although there is great individual variance, the usual pulse rate range for an adult according to the American Heart Association is 50 to 100 beats per minute, with the average considered to be 72 beats per minute. The pulse rate of an infant spans 100 to 160 beats per minute and that rate decreases until adolescence, when the usual pulse rate is 60 to 100 beats per minute. The average rate remains unchanged until older adulthood, when the pulse further decreases to 60 to 90 beats per minute.

The rhythm should be regular; however, occasional premature beats in a healthy client are not significant. The pulse amplitude should be symmetrical and vary with the size of the artery.

There should be no variation in amplitude of a single artery beat-to-beat. The pulse character should be neither bounding nor thready.

Special Considerations, Precautions, Sources of Error. When taking a pulse in the carotid artery, palpation should be gentle so as to avoid compression of the artery. Compression can cause vagus nerve stimulation, which can result in reflex bradycardia. Both carotids should never be palpated simultaneously because under this condition, even partial compression can decrease blood flow to the brain or result in reflex bradycardia.

The nurse should never use the thumb to assess the client's pulse. The thumb has an artery near its ventral surface. Palpating with the thumb may result in the nurse's mistaking his or her own pulse for that of the client.

If an irregular pulse is found, the nurse should then assess the rate and rhythm apically.

Recording. All components of the pulse assessment are recorded in the client's chart. In some facilities, the information is noted on a vital signs graphic sheet in the chart and in others on a flowsheet at the bedside. Specific findings concerning rate, rhythm, and volume are also to be recorded in the client's chart in the nurse's notes. In addition, any abnormal findings are recorded along with the nursing interventions initiated in response to these abnormal findings. Abnormal pulse assessment findings are to be reported to and discussed with the physician and so noted in the client's chart. An example of a nurse's note for abnormal pulse is: pulse 122, irregular, volume 1+, peripheral pulses symmetrical.

Blood Pressure Measurement. Blood pressure is an important component in the assessment of the client's health status and cardiovascular system. It yields data about ventricular contraction force and cardiac output and the status of the arterial and circulatory systems. Blood pressure is measured in millimeters of mercury (mm Hg).

Basic Concepts About Blood Pressure. It is possible to measure both arterial and venous blood pressures, although the measurement of arterial blood pressure is much more common.

Arterial blood pressure is measured by two general means: direct and indirect. The direct method, which is impractical in nonhospitalized clients, involves cannulating an artery for the purpose of measuring arterial pressure with a calibrated pressure transducer. The indirect method, the more common method used in homes and hospitals, employs a sphygmomanometer that operates on the basis of the occluding auscultatory technique. In this technique, sounds are detected over an artery after the flow of blood is temporarily occluded. To fully understand blood pressure measurement, nurses need a good understanding of what blood pressure is and what it reflects about the body's physiology.

Definition. **Blood pressure** is the pressure of the blood within the systemic arteries that is maintained by the contractile force of the left ventricle, the peripheral resistance to blood flow created by arterioles and capillaries, the elasticity of the arterial walls, and the viscosity and volume of the blood.

Blood Pressure Physiology. Arterial blood pressure readings provide a measure of the adequacy of the interplay of these factors in maintaining sufficient circulation to the body's tissues.

CARDIAC CONTRACTILITY. Blood pressure is created by the the pumping action of the heart in the closed circulation system of the arteries and veins. The contractile strength of the heart muscle is an important factor in determining the volume of blood the ventricles eject and, thus, in maintaining a cardiac output sufficient to meet the body's needs. The contractile strength of the heart is dependent on autonomic reflexes and the integrity of the cardiac muscle and electrical conduction system. Sympathetic nervous stimulation increases the contractile strength of the heart muscle; parasympathetic stimulation reduces it. Any factor that reduces sympathetic reflex activity, damages the myocardium, or interferes with the conduction of electrical impulses to the heart muscle will reduce cardiac contractility. When the degree of the cardiac dysfunction that results exceeds the ability of circulation to adapt, arterial blood pressure will drop as well.

PERIPHERAL VASCULAR RESISTANCE. *Peripheral vascular resistance* is the friction created between the blood flowing and the elastic walls of the arteries and arterioles. Three factors contribute to peripheral resistance: (1) arterial diameter, (2) compliance of arteries, and (3) viscosity of the blood.

There is a direct relationship between vascular resistance and arterial blood pressure. When vascular resistance increases, the blood pressure also increases as long as the volume of blood remains constant. There is an inverse relationship between vessel lumen size and peripheral resistance; the smaller the lumen, the greater the peripheral resistance. A small lumen creates increased peripheral resistance and results in an increase in blood pressure. When vasodilation occurs, the peripheral vascular resistance decreases and the blood pressure also decreases.

The diameter of arterioles plays a very important role in an individual's blood pressure. The resistance of the arterioles accounts for about 50 percent of the resistance in the entire systemic circulation.[26] Arterioles constrict and relax independently of each other. Their diameter changes as needed to meet the body's needs and demands and to maintain an adequate amount of blood in the circulation.

The compliance of arteries also plays a role in blood pressure maintenance. As previously established, blood vessel wall elasticity permits expansion (distention or dilation) and contraction to accommodate the varying blood pressure forces exerted against it. When blood vessel walls lose their elasticity, as happens in arteriosclerosis, the walls are unable to dilate or enlarge to accommodate the flow pressure increases.[26] The unyielding wall contributes to an increase in both systolic and diastolic blood pressure.

The blood's thickness or *viscosity* is determined by the amount of protein molecules and the number of red blood cells (*hematocrit*) present. The higher the hematocrit, the thicker or more viscous the blood. Increased viscosity causes flow resistance. Thicker blood flows more slowly through the vessels just as syrup flows more slowly than water. "Thick" blood has more difficulty flowing through smaller vessels particularly, as the thickness is a cause of the resistance. There is a direct relationship between blood viscosity and blood pressure. When viscosity increases, so does the blood pressure; likewise, when viscosity decreases, blood pressure decreases.

VENOUS RETURN AND BLOOD VOLUME. *Venous return* is the quantity of blood flowing from the systemic veins into the right atrium of the heart each minute. It is also plays an important role in blood pressure maintenance. For blood pressure to remain stable the venous return must be equal to *cardiac output,* the quantity of blood pumped into the aorta each minute. Under normal conditions the amount of venous return is determined by blood volume, arterial pressure, and total peripheral resistance. Any factor that alters these variables will cause a corresponding fluctuation in venous return.

Blood volume by its effect on venous return is a significant factor in the maintenance of arterial blood pressure. As established above, hemorrhage that exceeds 10 percent of the total blood volume is eventually accompanied by a fall in arterial blood pressure. Circulatory shock is a state in which cardiac output is inadequate to supply local tissues with nutrition. Individuals can be in shock as a result of hemorrhage, however, and yet have a normal blood pressure because of the strong vasoconstrictive reflexes that operate in hemorrhage. Despite vasoconstriction, once 35 to 40 percent of the total blood volume is lost, venous return becomes insufficient to maintain cardiac output, and arterial pressure falls to zero.[26]

Blood Pressure Characteristics. Arterial blood pressure has two phases: systolic and diastolic.

Systolic Blood Pressure. **Systolic blood pressure** is the pressure exerted against the arterial wall as the left ventricle contracts and forces blood into the aorta. It is the maximum pressure that is exerted against the vessel wall. This force creates characteristic sounds after flow through an artery has been temporarily occluded. These are known as **Korotkoff sounds.** During arterial blood pressure measurement, the artery is auscultated and the examiner hears these sounds. They follow a pattern (described below) the beginner soon learns to recognize.

Diastolic Blood Pressure. **Diastolic blood pressure** is the arterial pressure that is measured as the left ventricle relaxes and the heart is at rest. This is the minimal constant arterial wall pressure. During the diastolic phase, the examiner hears a change in the sound that gradually decreases until it becomes inaudible. Phase IV muffled sounds correspond to diastole in children; the disappearance of sound in phase V corresponds to diastole in adults.[53]

Pulse Pressure. Pulse pressure was defined above as the difference between systolic and diastolic pressures. It is obtained when the systolic reading is subtracted from the diastolic reading. For example, if the blood pressure reading is 140/80, the pulse pressure is 60 (140 − 80 = 60). Pulse pressure varies with arterial elasticity. When the difference between the high and low pressures is greater than 30 to 40 mm Hg, the arteries have lost some of their elasticity.

Pulse pressure also varies with the volume of blood the left ventricle puts out with each beat. As established above, this volume changes with the rate and strength of the heartbeat and with the rate of venous return to the heart. A rapid transfusion may increase pulse pressure, whereas hemorrhage will decrease it. Moreover, increased heart rate leaves less time for ventricular filling, which can result in decreased pulse pressure.

Blood Pressure Regulation. Blood pressure is regulated both by circulatory responses, which act to make immediate corrections, and by kidney function, which acts to make long-term adjustments. The circulatory responses mediated by the baroreceptors and chemoreceptors have been previously discussed (see *Pulse Measurement*). Kidney function also plays a role in blood pressure adaptation by regulating circulating blood volume; together with the circulatory responses described above, arterial blood pressure is maintained within homeostatic limits.

Because the circulatory reflexes adapt over time and lose their ability to initiate further change, long-term blood pressure adjustment depends on renal processes. Whenever the blood pressure falls very low, the juxtaglomerular cells located adjacent to the glomeruli secrete the enzyme renin into the blood. The rate of this secretion is also augmented by sympathetic nervous signals. Renin acts on a plasma protein to produce angiotensin I, which is converted by an enzyme into a potent vasoconstrictor substance known as angiotensin II. This substance acts on the blood vessels to immediately raise arterial pressure, but also has longer-term effects. Angiotensin II acts directly on the kidneys to decrease the excretion of salt and water. It also stimulates the adrenal cortex to secrete aldosterone, which has the same effect.[26] The net effect is an elevation in blood volume and ultimately arterial pressure.[26]

Factors Affecting Blood Pressure. The client's blood pressure varies continually as it responds to the body's demands. It is affected by age, sex, race, physical activity, central nervous system response to emotions such as fear, anxiety, and stress, circadian rhythm, body position, body size, and medications (Table 16–9).

AGE. Age is an important factor affecting blood pressure. Blood pressure increases gradually during childhood and then stabilizes in early adulthood. The arteries of many older adults lose their compliance. Loss of arterial elasticity is associated with increased systolic blood pressure (Box 16–18).

TABLE 16–9. FACTORS THAT INFLUENCE BLOOD PRESSURE

Factor	Blood Pressure Response	Reason
Age	Increases as age increases	Vessel wall elasticity is reduced.
Sex	Higher in males than females under age 50	Male cardiac output is greater than that of females.
Race	Hypertension more frequent in blacks	Unknown
Physical activity	Increases with increased activity	Increased activity increases cellular demand for increased oxygen supply.
Emotions/stress	Increases	Central nervous system response releases epinephrine, which causes cardiac acceleration.
Diurnal cycle	Varies with time of day and biorhythm	Unknown
Position	Lying to standing increases; standing to lying decreases	Gravity exerts effects on circulatory system.
Medication	Increases or decreases depending on action	Medications cause vasodilation or vasoconstriction, affect cardiac output, and affect blood volume.

BOX 16–18. BLOOD PRESSURE CHANGES THAT OCCUR WITH AGING

Age	Usual Blood Pressure
Infant	63 mean
Toddler	96/30
Preschool-age child	96/60
School-age child	105/60
Adolescent	120/75
Young adult	130/85
Middle adulthood	160/95
Older adulthood	170/95

SEX. Sex also plays a role in affecting blood pressure. Blood pressure of women under 50 years of age is lower than in men of the same age. This variance is thought to be due to the influence of female hormones on blood pressure.

RACE. Race may also be a factor in blood pressure. There continues to be disagreement as to the cause of blood pressure differences between blacks and Caucasians. Some authorities feel the differences are the result of genetic factors; others associate environmental factors such as diet, stress, and socioeconomic status.

PHYSICAL ACTIVITY. Physical activity increases the body's metabolic rate and the heart pumps faster to supply the cells with blood and carry away wastes. Cardiac output increases, which, in turn, increases the peripheral vascular resistance and the blood pressure. The client should therefore be encouraged to relax before the blood pressure reading is obtained. The reading should be delayed for 30 minutes after exercising.

EMOTIONS AND STRESS. Emotions and stress can cause an elevated blood pressure reading. Stress induces a response by the sympathetic nervous system. This response increases the heart rate which, in turn, increases cardiac output, resulting in a higher level of peripheral resistance.

BODY RHYTHM. Blood pressure has a diurnal cycle. It is highest in the late afternoon and early evening and lowest in the early morning.

BODY POSITION AND POSTURE. Moving from a lying to a standing position affects blood pressure readings. The lying systolic pressure is about 10 mm Hg lower and the lying diastolic pressure is 5 mm Hg lower than the standing readings. This difference is due to the effect of gravity. A blood pressure difference of 30 mm Hg or greater between the lying and standing readings could be a symptom of hypovolemia.

BODY WEIGHT. There is a direct relationship between weight and blood pressure. As weight increases, both systolic and diastolic blood pressures increase.

MEDICATIONS. Medications are specific for either increasing or decreasing blood pressure. This is accomplished by the medication's effect on blood vessel walls or on cardiac output. Specific medications can cause vasodilation to occur; other medications are specific for causing vasoconstriction. In addition a third category of medications act on cardiac output and affect blood volume.

Equipment. The most common method of measuring arterial blood pressure is by the indirect method, a method that requires no direct catheterization of the artery. A **sphygmomanometer** comprises an inflatable bladder enclosed in an unyielding cuff, an inflation bulb or other device to increase pressure in the bladder, a manometer filled with mercury or an aneroid gauge or digital readout unit to register the pressure applied, and a valve on the inflation bulb to control deflation of the bladder. The cuff is wrapped around the client's limb generally at the upper arm, but sometimes around the thigh or leg.[53]

Types and Components of Sphygmomanometers. Three types of sphygmomanometers are available that are differentiated by their method of display pressure values: mercury manometers, aneroid gauges, and electronic models with digital display units.

All three types have a compression cuff linked to a single air pump. The cuff consists of an inflatable rubber bladder covered by a fabric cuff. A bulb pumps air into the bladder and there is a valve to regulate air escape during decompression.

MERCURY MANOMETERS. The mercury manometer model has a mercury reservoir connected to a hollow glass tube that is graduated and calibrated in units. As pressure in the bladder rises during inflation, a column of mercury rises correspondingly in the tube from a reservoir. The pressure is indicated at the level of the meniscus of mercury once it stops rising. To avoid distorted readings, the meniscus must be read at eye level. On release of the valve, air moves out of the bladder, pressure decreases, and the level of mercury in the manometer falls (Fig. 16–19).

ANEROID GAUGES. The aneroid gauge models have a circular dial with calibrations and a needle that points to the calibrations. These models contain an internal bellows. Movement in the bellows is created by increases and decreases in bladder pressure which, in turn, cause the indicator valve to move. The aneroid gauge model is more portable and thus more convenient but also less accurate than the mercury manometer model (see Fig. 16–19).

ELECTRONIC SPHYGMOMANOMETERS. Some institutions have electronic models with digital readout displays. An acoustical stethoscope is unnecessary with these models. A light flashes on the display unit to indicate systolic and diastolic pressures. These models are accurate and convenient to use but are expensive to purchase (Fig. 16–20).

Selecting Cuff Size. The width of the blood pressure cuff is very important and can greatly affect a blood pressure reading. The cuff should be 20 percent wider than the diameter of the limb on which it is used. The upper two thirds of the arm should be covered by the cuff. A cuff that is not wide

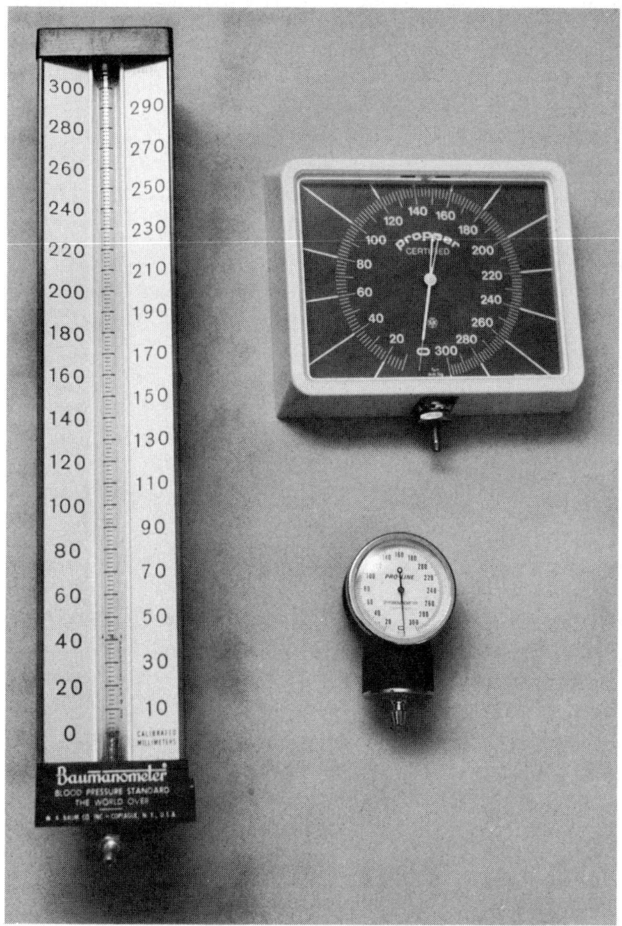

Figure 16–19. Two types of sphygmomanometers: mercury manometer and two aneroid gauges.

enough will give an incorrect (usually higher) reading as it is insufficient in size to compress the artery. Using a cuff that is too wide can give a false low reading. See Table 16–10 for appropriate bladder dimensions.

Blood pressure cuffs are available in six different widths. Most facilities, however, use only three sizes: the regular adult cuff, a small size for children, and the wide cuff, which is used for obese clients, particularly those with large muscular upper arms, or for obtaining blood pressure in the thigh (Fig. 16–21).

Other Equipment. When measuring blood pressure with a sphygmomanometer an acoustical stethoscope is also necessary. The stethoscope amplifies the sound of the pulse. Other equipment, such as ultrasound stethoscopes and arterial catheters, is also sometimes used.

ULTRASOUND STETHOSCOPES. There may be times when the pulse cannot be auscultated or palpated. Conditions such as artery obstruction, decreased blood volume, and obesity interfere with blood pressure measurement by these means. When such conditions exist, the ultrasound (Doppler) stethoscope can be used (see Procedure 16–4) to obtain the measurement.

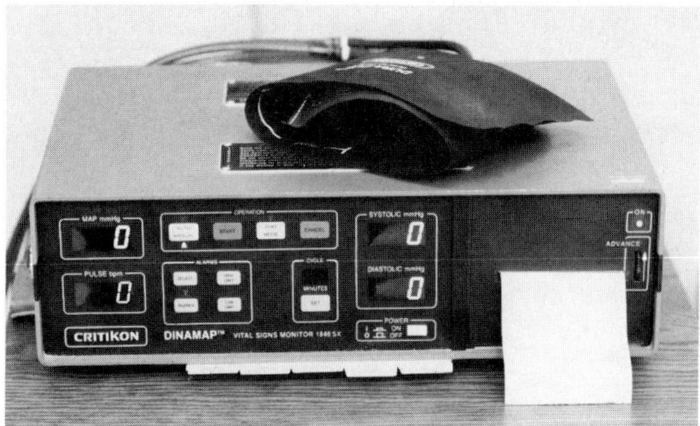

Figure 16–20. Electronic sphygmomanometer.

The Doppler translates blood cell movement into sounds. When the nurse hears the sound using the Doppler, it indicates that the cuff pressure is equal to the blood pressure in the vessel and that the blood is once again flowing and is no longer occluded by the pressure in the cuff. This sound denotes the systolic blood pressure reading.

ARTERIAL CATHETERS. A direct blood pressure measurement that is usually done in intensive care settings can be obtained with a pressure-sensitive catheter that is inserted into a major artery. When there is a need to record rapid blood pressure changes, an electronic transducer is used. The blood pressure is displayed on an electronic recording device. This piece of equipment prints the blood pressure readings on a paper graph.

TABLE 16–10. RECOMMENDED BLADDER DIMENSIONS FOR BLOOD PRESSURE CUFFS

Arm Circumference at Midpoint[a] (cm)	Cuff Name	Bladder Width (cm)	Bladder Length (cm)
5–7.5	Newborn	3	5
7.5–13	Infant	5	8
13–20	Child	8	13
24–32	Adult	13	24
32–42	Wide adult	17	32
42–50[b]	Thigh	20	42

[a] Midpoint of arm is defined as half the distance from acromion to olecranon. Use nonstretchable metal tape.

[b] In persons with very large limbs, indirect blood pressure should be measured in leg or forearm.

From Frohlich ED. Recommendations for Human Blood Pressure Determination by Sphygmomanometer. *Dallas, TX: American Heart Association; 1987: p. 21, with permission.*

PROCEDURE 16–4. ASSESSING PERIPHERAL PULSE

PURPOSE: To obtain general information about client's cardiac function and adequacy of peripheral circulation

EQUIPMENT: Watch with second hand or digital display of seconds; Doppler ultrasound unit (DUS) may be used for peripheral pulses too faint to be palpated; ultrasound conducting gel

ACTION	RATIONALE
1. Discuss procedure with the client, including desired client participation and anticipated benefits.	1. Active participation is more likely if client understands expected behavior and anticipated benefits.
2. Wash your hands.	2. Removes transient organisms that could be pathogens, preventing transmission to the client.
3. Observe client for indicators of acute stress, pain, or recent activity, such as flushed face, rapid audible respirations, extraneous movements, guarding posture, clenched jaw, and tears. Defer assessment of pulse rate if these signs are present; intervene as appropriate.	3. Emotional and physical stress (pain, exercise) can elevate pulse temporarily. Value obtained may not reflect general cardiac status of client.
4. Screen client if body exposure is likely.	4. Prevents embarrassment or discomfort associated with exposure.
5. Request or assist client to position that provides access to the pulse site desired.	5. Optimum positioning conserves client and nurse energy.
6. Support arm if assessing radial pulse. 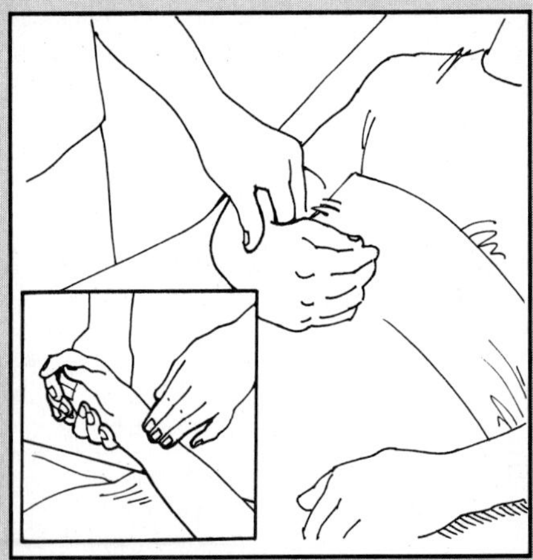	6. Conserves client energy, comfort.
7. Place tips of first two fingers on skin over artery at desired pulse site (see Fig. 16–57).	7. Fingertips are most sensitive to arterial pulsation. Thumb is contraindicated because it has a pulse.

(continued)

PROCEDURE 16–4. (continued)

Action	Rationale
8. Place two fingers over pulse site to obliterate pulse initially and then relax pressure so pulse becomes palpable.	8. Pulse is more accurately assessed with moderate pressure. Too much pressure impairs blood flow and results in inaccurate assessment.
9. When pulse is felt, assess rhythm by noting intervals between beats. If intervals are equal, begin count with 0, then 1, and so on. When the estimated pulse rate is less than 100 beats per minute, count for 15 seconds and multiply total by 4.	9. Pulse must be located before rate is determined. Timing should begin with count of 0. 1 is the second beat after timing begins. Rates of 100 beats per minute or less can be accurately and efficiently assessed in 15 seconds when rhythm is regular.
10. If pulse is irregular, count for 1 minute. NOTE: Irregular pulse may require assessment of apical pulse. If arrhythmia is a new finding, confer with client's physician.	10. Accuracy of count cannot be assessed by multiplying 15-second rate when pulse is irregular.
11. Assess strength of pulse by noting the sensation of vessel fullness as it contacts fingers.	11. Strength reflects volume of blood ejected against arterial wall with each contraction.
12. Compare strength of pulse on opposite extremity. NOTE: When assessing pulses of the leg and foot, rate is usually omitted; strength of pulsation is the major focus.	12. A primary reason for assessing peripheral pulses other than radial pulse is to determine condition of peripheral circulation. Comparison of pulses bilaterally provides a more complete picture.
13. Assess the elasticity of the arterial wall by running your fingertips along the artery.	13. Reflects the general integrity of the peripheral circulation. Particularly important in assessment of foot and leg pulses.
14. Assist client to a comfortable position if necessary.	14. Promotes well-being.
15. Discuss results of assessment with client; initiate teaching if appropriate (see Chap. 27).	15. An informed client can be a more active participant in health care and self-care.
16. Wash your hands.	16. See step 2.

VARIATION: PULSE ASSESSMENT WITH DOPPLER

Action	Rationale
1. Begin as above, steps 1 to 5.	1. See steps 1 to 5 above.

(continued)

PROCEDURE 16–4. (continued)

2. Plug headset and/or speaker into jack next to volume control.

2. Headset transmits sound to nurse; speaker transmits sound to room so client can hear if desired. Speaker option not available on all models.

3. Apply conducting gel to skin over pulse location or on narrow end of transducer housing.

3. Air interferes with optimum transmission of ultrasound waves. Gel creates an air-free connection between transducer and client's skin.

4. Turn on the Doppler and place the narrow end of the housing over the expected pulse location, using light pressure. Turn dial at top to adjust volume.

4. Skin transducer interface via gel transmits sound of cells flowing through artery. Sound has a pulsating, whooshing quality.

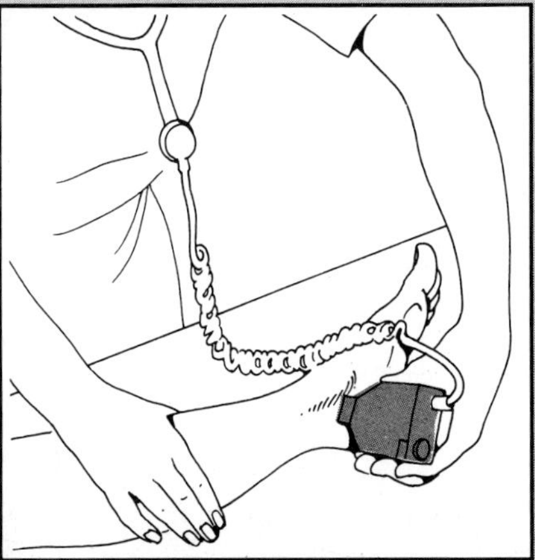

NOTE: Intermittent sounds with a windy quality may be heard as well. These are venous sounds, heard because of proximity of major veins and arteries. Only pulsating sounds indicate intact arterial circulation.

5. Reposition probe as needed until pulse is heard or you are certain pulse is not obtainable.

5. Pulse sites are approximate and vary slightly from person to person.

6. Remove gel from client's skin and Doppler. Complete procedure as in steps 12 to 15 above.

6. Promotes comfort; protects equipment. Dried-on gel interferes with transmission of signal.

NOTE: Alcohol should not be used to clean transducer face because it causes corrosion. Use dry or damp paper towel only.

RECORDING: Record radial pulse on client's vital signs flowsheet. Note changes in rhythm or strength in progress notes. A separate flowsheet is often used to record data about peripheral circulation; if not available, record method of assessment and strength and regularity of pulse in progress notes. Discuss findings atypical for client with client's physician.

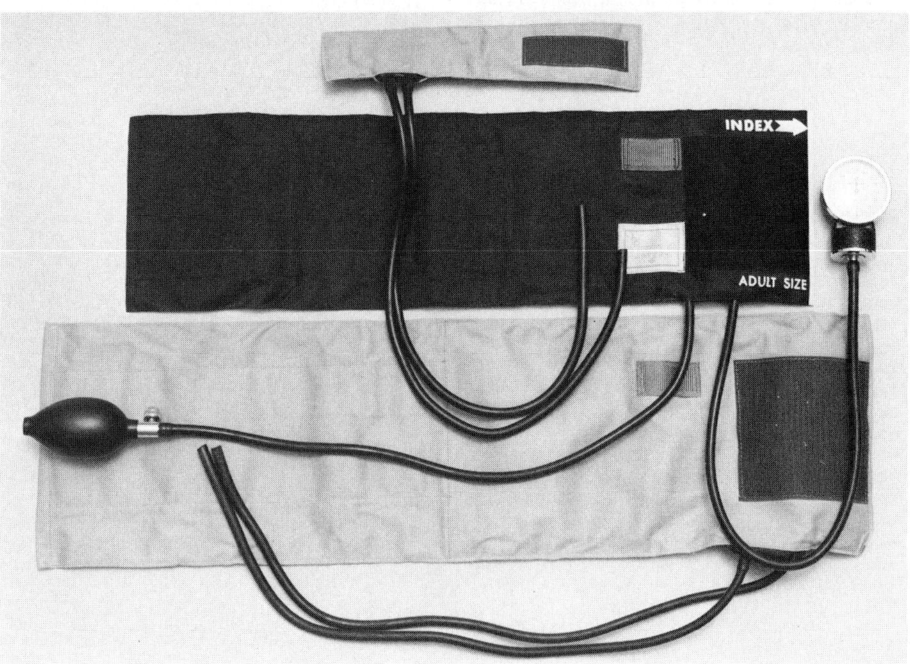

Figure 16–21. Blood pressure cuff sizes: small size for children, regular adult cuff, and wide cuff for obese clients or for obtaining blood pressure in the thigh.

As insertion of an arterial catheter is an invasive procedure, it is used only for clients who are critically ill and require direct frequent blood pressure monitoring.

Technique. The indirect method of obtaining an arterial blood pressure is commonly used. The basic process of obtaining a blood pressure reading consists of three steps: (1) attaching the blood pressure cuff, (2) inflating the cuff and occluding the artery, (3) deflating the cuff and simultaneously listening for the return of pulse sounds as the artery refills with blood. Three techniques can be used to obtain a blood pressure reading: auscultation, palpation, and flushing.

Auscultory Technique. An auscultory blood pressure is one in which the examiner, using a stethoscope, listens to the sounds created as blood courses through an artery. The blood pressure registers on the manometer or gauge. The principle of the auscultory method is that cuff pressure occludes blood flow through the artery. As the cuff is deflated, blood once again begins to flow through the artery, creating a distinct pattern of sounds referred to earlier as Korotkoff sounds. These are summarized in Box 16–19. Phases I, IV, and V are particularly significant. Phase I is characterized by the regular tapping of the pulse sounds, which gradually becomes louder. This phase designates the systolic blood pressure reading (Fig. 16–22). As phase IV begins, the pulse sounds suddenly become muffled and less clear. This is the diastolic reading for children. At phase

BOX 16–19. PHASES OF KOROTKOFF SOUNDS

Korotkoff sounds are named after the Russian physician Nikdai S. Korotkoff, who first noted them. These sounds occur in phases that correspond to the arterial pressure changes created by the cardiac cycle and, thus, can be used to measure arterial pressure indirectly.

When an artery has been occluded (as when a sphygmomanometer cuff is applied to a limb and the bladder inflated), blood will begin to flow again as the occluding force is released. The level at which the flow begins is the level at which the peak pressure created by left ventricular contraction overtakes the occluding force. The flow produces sharp, rhythmic, knocking sounds that correspond to the heartbeat. As pressure over the artery is gradually released, these sounds change in character and intensity through a series of phases and finally disappear. Korotkoff sounds occur in five phases:

- *Phase I:* The pressure level at which the first faint, clear tapping sounds are heard. The sounds gradually increase in intensity as the cuff is deflated.
- *Phase II:* That time during cuff deflation when a murmur or swishing sounds are heard.
- *Phase III:* The period during which sounds are crisper and increase in intensity.
- *Phase IV:* That time when a distinct, abrupt muffling of sound (usually of a soft, blowing quality) is heard.
- *Phase V:* That pressure level when the last sound is heard and after which all sound disappears.

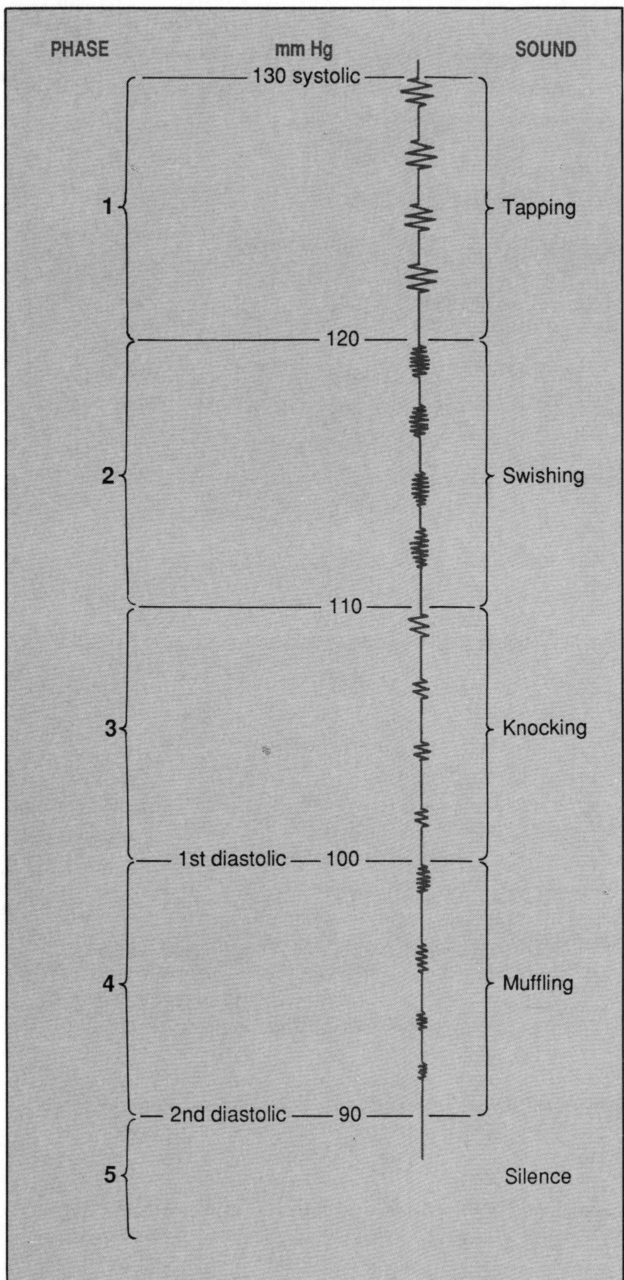

Figure 16–22. Visualization of pulse sounds heard when auscultating blood pressure.

V, the pulse sounds become inaudible. At this point, the pressure in the cuff is lower than the minimum pressure in the artery. This is the diastolic blood pressure reading for adults.

Procedure 16–5 outlines the technique for assessment of blood pressure. To obtain an auscultory blood pressure reading, place the stethoscope chestpiece over the area where the brachial artery pulse is palpated prior to cuff inflation. To auscultate the blood pressure, close the pressure control valve and inflate the cuff. When the cuff pressure reaches the point where it exceeds the systolic pressure in the vessel, it compresses the artery and occludes blood flow. Slowly open the pressure release valve to deflate the cuff.

Measuring the blood pressure in the thigh requires that the client be prone (lying on the abdomen) and that a wide cuff be used. When the client is unable to assume a prone position, the side-lying position with the knee slightly flexed can be used. Place the cuff at the midthigh above the knee, with the cuff bladder positioned over the posterior aspect. Palpate the pulse and place the stethoscope over the popliteal artery.

The systolic reading obtained on the thigh will be 5 to 15 mm Hg higher than the brachial artery reading. The diastolic reading will be lower.

When measuring the blood pressure in the leg, the client can be either lying down or sitting for the procedure. Place the cuff on the leg with the lower cuff edge at the malleolus. Palpate the pulse and place the stethoscope over the posterior tibial or dorsal pedis artery. The process is then the same as when taking a brachial blood pressure.

Palpatory Technique. There are instances when the blood pressure is inaudible with an acoustical stethoscope, but can be palpated. Obtaining a blood pressure reading by palpation is usually done only in emergency situations when cardiac output is decreased and does not produce sounds loud enough to be heard through a stethoscope.

To palpate the blood pressure, inflate the cuff to the point at which the pulse can no longer be felt. Continue to inflate the cuff 30 mm Hg more and then, using the pressure control valve, slowly decrease the cuff pressure. As the mercury falls, watch the manometer or gauge for the reading when the pulse is first felt again; this is the systolic reading. The diastolic reading is not obtained using this method.

Flush Technique. When the pulse is impalpable and Korotkoff sounds are inaudible, and when electronic equipment is unavailable, the flush technique can be used. It uses skin color change as an indicator of blood pressure and is employed primarily for measuring blood pressure of infants.

Apply the blood pressure cuff to the infant's arm as usual.

Bandage the limb, beginning distally and working proximally; this forces venous blood out of the extremity while reducing arterial inflow. Inflate the cuff to approximately 150 mm Hg and release the bandage. Slowly release the pressure in the cuff until you see a vascular flush; the pale limb will become suddenly reddened. The reading at the flush point is the mean blood pressure reading—the midpoint between systolic and diastolic blood pressures.

PROCEDURE 16–5. ASSESSING BLOOD PRESSURE

PURPOSE: To assess pressure within the circulatory system during the phases of the cardiac cycle: systole and diastole

EQUIPMENT: Sphygmomanometer, blood pressure cuff of appropriate size, stethoscope

ACTION	RATIONALE
1. Situate the client in a quiet environment and put him or her at ease. Make sure the room temperature is comfortable.	1. Environmental factors influence the accuracy of readings.
2. Assess the client for signs of acute stress, pain, or recent activity, such as flushed face, rapid audible respirations, extraneous movement, guarding, clenched jaw, and tears. Defer BP assessment if signs are present; intervene as appropriate. Ask if client has smoked or ingested caffeine within past 30 minutes.	2. Emotional and physical stress (pain, exercise), caffeine, and nicotine* can elevate blood pressure temporarily. Value obtained may not reflect general cardiovascular status.
3. Wash your hands.	3. Removes transient organisms from your hands that could be pathogens, preventing transmission to the client.
4. Check equipment to see that valve opens and closes freely, bladder has no residual air, tubing connections are air tight, and gauge reads zero. Grasp rolled cuff, turn valve clockwise, inflate bladder—gauge should indicate pressure; release valve—gauge should return to zero.	4. Faulty equipment compromises accuracy of reading.
5. Check cuff width as illustrated. 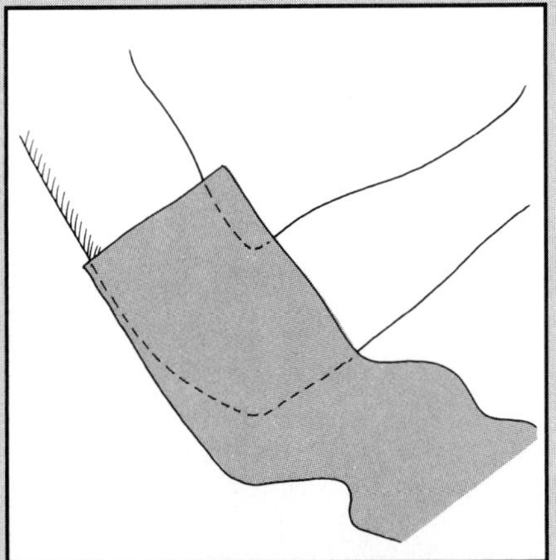	5. Cuff should be 20 percent wider than the diameter of the arm to compress an adequate portion of the brachial artery to achieve an accurate reading. The length of the bladder within the cuff should be at least 80 percent of arm circumference.
6. Discuss the procedure, desired client participation, and anticipated benefits with the client.	6. Active participation is more likely if the client understands expectations and benefits.

(continued)

PROCEDURE 16–5. (continued)

7. Request or assist the client to assume a sitting or low Fowler's position, with the forearm slightly flexed and supported at heart level with palm of hand turned up. You and client should be within 5 ft of manometer, which should be at your eye level.

7. Position of the arm and/or the body can significantly alter blood pressure. If position is other than described, note this in progress notes. If client is too far from manometer, you will be unable to read it; if it is not at eye level, parallax will distort reading, especially on vertical gauge.

8. Expose upper arm. Locate the center of the bladder inside the blood pressure cuff and center it over the brachial artery.

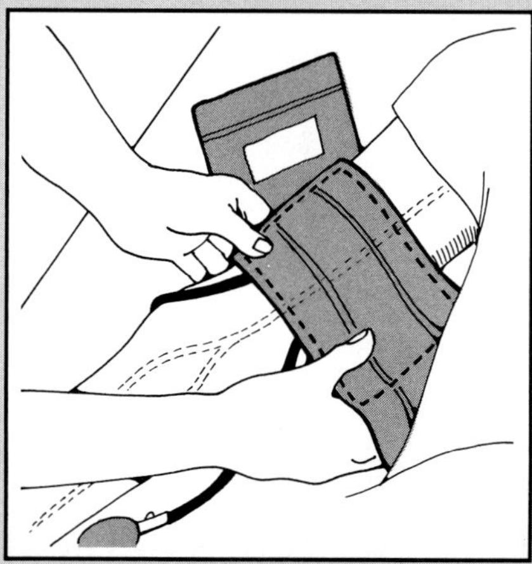

8. Removing clothing and centering bladder promote even compression of artery, which is necessary for accurate reading.

9. Wrap the fully deflated cuff evenly and snugly around the client's arm, so bottom edge of cuff is 1 in. above antecubital space. No more than two of your fingers should fit under cuff.

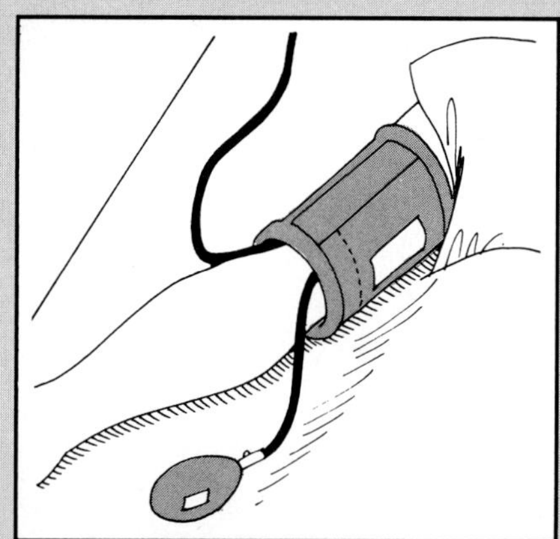

9. Loose cuff allows significant inflation of bladder before artery is compressed, resulting in falsely high readings. If cuff is too close to antecubital space, cuff edge will interfere with auscultation.

(continued)

PROCEDURE 16–5. (continued)

10. Place stethoscope earpieces in your ears. Palpate brachial artery in the medial aspect of upper arm above the antecubital space. Place the stethoscope diaphragm over the artery.

10. Facilitates accurate placement of stethoscope for optimal transmission of Korotkoff sounds.

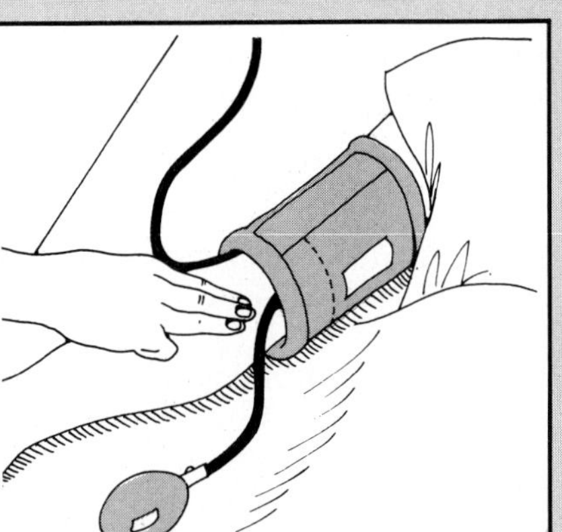

11. If no recent previous readings are recorded, and client is unaware of usual BP, close inflatable bulb valve and inflate bladder while palpating artery until pulse is obliterated. Open valve and deflate bladder.

NOTE: Some hypertensive clients have an auscultatory gap: a band of about 40 mm Hg on which no sounds are heard. To avoid recording an erroneously low reading, pump the cuff to 30 mm Hg above the highest recent reading when assessing clients with a history of hypertension.

11. Indicates artery is occluded, an approximate indication of systolic pressure. Maximum inflation for auscultatory assessment is 20 to 30 mm Hg above this level or above client's usual range. Greater inflation is unnecessary and causes discomfort.

12. After 15 seconds, place stethoscope bell or diaphragm over artery and reinflate cuff to pressure determined in step 11. Open valve partially. Release pressure at a rate of 2 to 3 mm Hg per second.

12. Slower rate of deflation is uncomfortable for client; faster rate results in inability to note precise pressure at which Korotkoff sounds change.

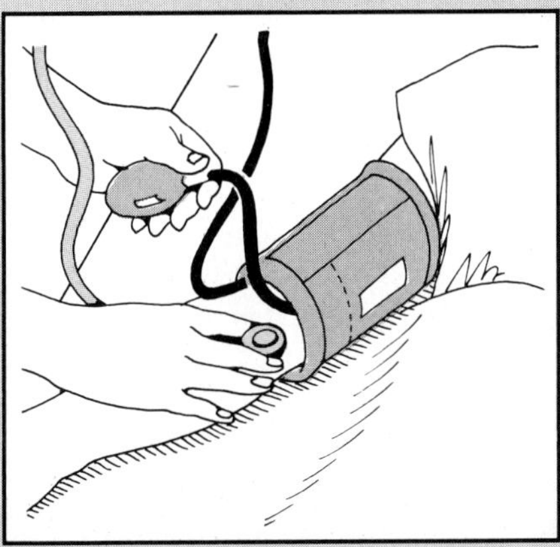

13. Note pressure at which first of a series of faint rhythmic tapping sounds is heard (Korotkoff phase I). This is the systolic reading.

NOTE: If sounds are heard immediately upon releasing the valve, quickly deflate bladder, allow 15 to 20 seconds of rest (may elevate arm above heart level to decrease venous congestion from repeated occlusion of veins, which can alter reading). Reinflate 20 mm Hg above previous reading to assure detection of first sound.

13. The first Korotkoff sound begins when the artery has opened just enough to allow spurts of blood to flow through, representative of systole (contraction).

(continued)

PROCEDURE 16–5. (continued)

14. Note pressure at which sounds become muffled with a soft blowing quality (Korotkoff phase IV) and at which sounds disappear (Korotkoff phase V); then deflate cuff rapidly and completely before removing.

14. The disappearance of sound (phase V) occurs when the artery is completely open and there is no more turbulence to create sound. This is considered the diastolic reading in adults. The muffling of sound (phase IV) is recorded as diastole in children.

15. If there is a need to repeat the procedure, wait 1 to 2 minutes.

15. Permits blood sequestered in veins to begin flowing.

NOTE: Some agencies require that both phases IV and V of the Korotkoff sounds be recorded.

16. Remove cuff; replace in storage area. Assist client, if needed, to a comfortable position.

16. Promotes well-being.

17. Discuss results of assessment with client. Initiate teaching as appropriate.

17. An informed client can be a more active participant in health care and self-care.

VARIATION: THIGH BLOOD PRESSURE

Complete procedure as above, except assist the client into prone or sidelying position. Popliteal pulse is used (see Fig. 16–57). Wrap cuff as illustrated; usually a large, adult-sized cuff is needed. With client recumbant, BP in thigh is about 3 mm Hg higher than in the brachial artery at heart level.[a]

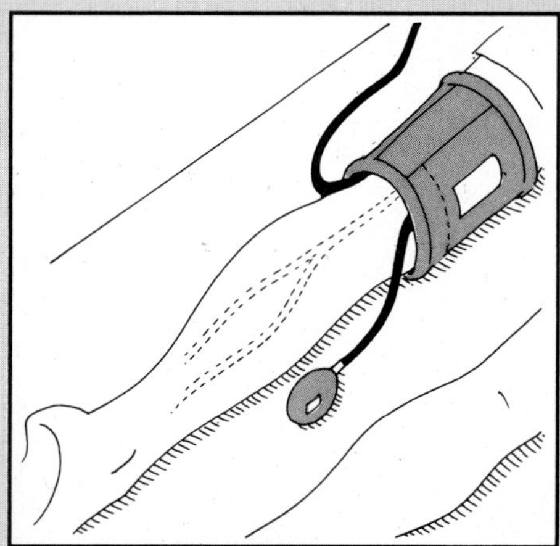

RECORDING: Record systolic and diastolic readings on client's vital signs flowsheet or medical record. If variations in position or technique were necessary, note variation and reason in progress notes. Discuss atypical values with client's physician.

[a] Ganong WF. *Review of Medical Physiology,* 15th ed. Norwalk, CT: Appleton & Lange; 1991.

Sites for Arterial Blood Pressure Measurement. Blood pressure measurements can be obtained over several sites.

UPPER ARM. Blood pressure readings are commonly obtained over the brachial artery in the upper arm or the antecubital fossa. These sites are usually convenient for both the nurse and the client.

The blood pressure cuff should cover about the upper two thirds of the arm. The cuff is applied securely to the arm approximately 1 to 2 in. above the antecubital fossa.

THIGH. The blood pressure measurement obtained using the thigh assesses the pressure in the popliteal artery that is located behind the knee in the popliteal space.

LEG. Blood pressure obtained in the lower leg assesses the pressure in the posterior tibial or dorsalis pedis artery.

Selecting a Procedure. It has been recognized for some time that direct blood pressure measurements, the standard by which other methods are evaluated, do not correlate perfectly with indirect blood pressure measurements. Investigators have found, for example, that indirect systolic pressures are generally lower than direct systolic pressure readings taken simultaneously, and that indirect diastolic pressure readings are generally greater than simultaneous direct diastolic readings.[54,55] As the indirect auscultory method is so commonly used, these differences have raised questions about indirect measurement technique.

Researchers have recommended that the diaphragm over the upper arm brachial artery technique be used whenever small variations in blood pressure are significant as they often are in critical care settings.[56] Nevertheless, use of the diaphragm at the antecubital fossa may be easier for some people and may be an acceptable alternative when small errors are unimportant.

VENOUS BLOOD PRESSURE MEASUREMENT. Venous blood pressure is the continuous pressure that is exerted against the vein walls at all times by the circulating blood.

To obtain an accurate venous pressure, a central venous catheter is inserted into a major vein and threaded through the superior vena cava into the right atrium. The catheter, when connected to a manometer, provides a relatively accurate pulmonary venous pressure reading.

Norms and Expected Findings. There is a great variance in blood pressure readings that is considered within the range of normal. Blood pressure continually changes.

Normotensive Blood Pressure. The term *normotensive blood pressure* is applied to individuals whose arterial blood pressure is within the parameters specified as normal for that individual's age group. The expected reading in a healthy adult is 100 to 140 mm Hg systolic and 60 to 90 mm Hg diastolic. A pulse pressure of 40 mm Hg or less is a typical finding. The normal range for an older adult is higher, as blood pressure increases with age because of the loss of vessel wall elasticity (see Box 16–18).

As there is a slight difference in the blood pressure in each arm, when taking the client's blood pressure for the first time, it is important to take it in both arms. In this way, the difference in the readings between the two arms can be determined. A difference of 5 to 10 mm Hg is expected. A difference between the two readings of more than 15 mm Hg may indicate the presence of cardiac disease, such as a narrowing of the aorta or some other type of arterial obstruction.

Blood pressure readings change with body position and will vary according to whether the client is lying down, sitting, or standing. If, however, on sitting or standing there is a decrease of 20 mm Hg or more, the client may complain of dizziness. This decrease is called *orthostatic hypotension* and is caused by a sudden decrease in blood volume, side effects of medications, or extended period of bed rest.

Abnormal Findings. Blood pressure can either be too high or too low and in either case may lead to serious consequences.

Hypertensive Blood Pressure. The American Heart Association defines *hypertension* as a blood pressure that is above 140 mm Hg systolic and 90 mm Hg diastolic.[53] The primary causes of hypertension include loss of vessel wall elasticity. It results from the increased peripheral resistance that occurs because of narrowing of peripheral blood vessels (vasoconstriction) (see *Peripheral Vascular Resistance* earlier in the chapter). Any arterial pressure increase of more than 20 mm Hg over the client's usual baseline when there are no extenuating circumstances (such as recent exercise or activity) can be considered hypertension.

The diagnosis of hypertension is made by formulating the average of readings that are taken on at least two subsequent visits. The causative factors of hypertension are seldom identified, and usually the symptoms are treated rather than the cause. Often, hypertension indicates that there is an underlying disease frequently of the kidneys. It is estimated that one third of the North American population has hypertension.[57] As hypertension often presents no symptoms, it has been estimated that 50 percent of the people who have hypertension are not aware of their problem. This is why it is called the "silent killer."

For some yet unknown reason, hypertension occurs twice as frequently in blacks as Caucasians. Some theorists feel the racial difference could be genetic or environmental in origin. Hypertension affects twice as many women as men.

Hypertension is a major health problem that puts the client at risk for stroke and heart attack. It can cause damage in the heart, kidneys, eyes, and brain. Congestive heart failure occurs from hypertension-caused heart damage. Kidney damage is often reflected by the presence of protein in the urine. Changes in blood vessels that occur because of hypertension can be seen in the retinal eye grounds. Cardiovascular accident (CVA) is the result of hypertensive vessel damage in the brain.

Symptoms that cause clients to seek medical attention and that ultimately identify hypertension include blurred vision, severe headaches sometimes in association with nausea and vomiting.

Hypotensive Blood Pressure. *Hypotension* is defined as a blood pressure that is below 95 mm Hg systolic and 60 mm Hg diastolic. Causes of hypotension include hypovolemia and cardiac disease.

Hypotension is a relative status and is defined in terms of the individual's baseline blood pressure. If the baseline blood pressure is hypertensive, this realigns the definition of hypotension for that individual.

Client symptoms that prompt medical attention frequently include dizziness and blurred vision, confusion, and skin that feels cold and clammy to the touch. Another usual client complaint is orthostatic hypotension.

SHOCK. Hypotension can also be a sudden crisis resulting from circulatory collapse. It is a life-threatening condition that, if untreated, can cause death. Symptoms include a sudden fall in blood pressure, increased heart rate, and apprehension. The skin feels cold and clammy to the touch.

Shock is extreme hypotension that occurs because an adequate amount of blood is not reaching vital organs. If not treated, shock can result in cellular destruction, decreased organ function, and ultimately death.

During an episode of shock, the skin feels cold. The client perspires because the autonomic nervous system is stimulated. Pulse becomes rapid and thready as cardiac output decreases. Respirations are fast and shallow to compensate for a change in acid–base balance (metabolic acidosis) that develops. Temperature decreases because the reduced oxygen supply to the cells interferes with cellular metabolism and the production of heat.

Causes of shock include excessive blood loss, severe edema as a result of capillary damage, weeping wound(s) or burn(s), excessive fluid loss during sweating, vomiting, or diarrhea, fluid and electrolyte imbalance, and capillary engorgement that reduces blood volume.

Special Considerations, Precautions, Sources of Error. When taking the blood pressure with a mercury gauge manometer, the gauge should always be vertical and at eye level. This is important to avoid a parallax reflux, an error caused by the angle from which the fluid meniscus is viewed.

If the blood pressure cuff is applied loosely or is not an appropriate size, it will not provide an accurate reading. If the cuff is deflated too slowly or is reinflated without waiting 30 seconds, venous congestion occurs and results in an inaccurate reading.

To get an accurate blood pressure reading, the stethoscope diaphragm must be firmly in contact with the skin over the area of the artery. This is accomplished by ensuring the client's limb is fully extended and there is no clothing covering the area on which the stereoscope is to be placed. Also, the stethoscope must fit properly in the nurse's ears to clearly hear the various blood pressure sounds.

There may be a silent period between the systolic and diastolic sounds (usually occurs between the first and second Korotkoff sounds) during which pulse sounds are not heard. This is called an auscultory gap. This phenomenon occurs in clients with "venous congestion" or hypertension. Even though there are no audible pulse sounds, the radial pulse is still palpable during the auscultory gap.

If there is question as to the accuracy of the reading, always recheck the blood pressure. When it becomes necessary to repeat the blood pressure procedure, the cuff bladder must be completely deflated for at least 30 seconds before beginning the procedure again. If there is no recovery period between the two readings, a false reading is possible because of the venous congestion that develops.

Recording. The blood pressure readings are charted on a vital signs graph or flowsheet. The blood pressure is recorded by placing the systolic reading over the diastolic reading with a line or slash separating the two:

$$\frac{\text{systolic}}{\text{diastolic}}$$

When an *auscultory gap* (period in which no sound is heard) occurs, it is recorded indicating the area of the gap, for example, auscultory gap from 190 to 150. When blood pressure is monitored more frequently than every 4 hours, a separate blood pressure graph is used in most facilities.

The American Heart Association recommends that three blood pressure values (Korotkoff sounds) be recorded, the tapping systolic reading, the muffled sounds, and the point of absence of sound.[53] An example of this method of recording would be 130/80/60; however, individual facility policy will indicate whether this method of recording is to be used or if only the systolic and diastolic measurements are to be recorded.

Whenever there is an abnormal or unusual blood pressure reading or related symptom(s), a nurse's note is written indicating the findings, identifying any possible cause for the deviation, and stating whether the physician was notified. Nursing interventions initiated are also recorded.

Objective Manifestations Overview

The *objective manifestations overview* refers to the head-to-toe examination of the body, the aspect of health assessment in which each body area and system is observed using the four modalities of observation—inspection, palpation, percussion, and auscultation. The objective manifestations overview is conducted for the purpose of confirming information obtained in the health history and to identify health problems the client may not have reported. In approaching this overview, nurses are interested in clients' physical find-

IMPLICATIONS FOR PROFESSIONAL COLLABORATION

Sharing Data on Subjective and Objective Manifestations

A review of the subjective manifestations (symptoms) and objective manifestations (signs) of illness provides the nurse with detailed information on the client's immediate state of health. It enables the formulation of nursing diagnoses that are more specific and precise than are possible when such data are unavailable; however, data collection can be tedious and time consuming, for nurses and clients alike. Demands on the client are minimized and professional efficiency is increased by sharing data on signs and symptoms through the medical record. Information sharing reduces unnecessary repetition of effort and is an important part of collaboration.

ings, but they are also interested in clients' social and psychological responses to those findings.

The content of the objective manifestations overview is outlined in detail in the next section of this chapter. During the examination nurses not only make observations; they also ask specific questions about the body area or system being examined—questions about the subjective manifestations that may correspond to the physical findings. Generally, direct questions are used to elicit specific information about subjective manifestations during this phase. The sections on the head-to-toe assessment that follow outline these questions and how they might be worded.

Types of Health Examinations

The objective manifestations overview can be a complete, thorough examination inclusive of all body areas and systems, or it can be a partial examination tailored to the client's primary concern and chief complaint. Self-examinations are also a form of health examination.

Complete. The complete health examination is usually done when the client is admitted to a hospital or during the initial visit to an outpatient setting or doctor's office. A complete picture of the client's health and physical findings, coping mechanisms, and impact on daily living are compiled in an initial client data base. This data base can be used as a basis for identifying present health care needs and for making future comparisons.

Partial. A partial health examination is carried out during subsequent return visits, for example, to the outpatient setting or as follow-up examination in a hospital. A partial examination is done to identify changes that have occurred during the interval since the initial examination or previous examination. Partial health examinations focus directly on the client's specific problem area(s) rather than on the client's overall state of health.

Self-Examination. Often, as part of the expectation that clients will take control of their health care, they are taught how to do self-examinations of those body parts that are accessible and constitute a special risk for disease or abnormality. Examples of self-examination are breast self-examination for women and a scrotal self-examination for men. The client is taught how to do the procedure and is instructed about findings that could indicate the presence of a problem. The client is instructed to consult with his or her health care provider when abnormalities are detected. Self-examination is a very important part of health education. Teaching self-examination techniques is also an important responsibility of the nurse. Techniques for breast and scrotal self-examination are described later in the chapter.

Section 2. Head-to-Toe Assessment

■ GENERAL ASSESSMENT

Overview

General assessment refers to a broad overview of the physical appearance and demeanor of the client. General assessment consists of the nurse's overall impressions of the client's state of health, mental status, speech, body development (height and weight) and posture, movement, gait, and energy level. Inspection is the examination technique used to conduct a general assessment. To accompany the nurse's observations, there is a list of important history questions that apply to the client's overall state of health and appear in Table 16–11. In this text, the list includes requests for information about the endocrine and hematologic systems, which are vital to overall health and which have manifestations that can be observed as part of a general assessment.

Conducting the General Assessment

The general assessment consists of observations of the client while he or she is walking, sitting, and lying down. It begins at the first encounter with the client, usually on entering the client's room, whether in the hospital, clinic, or home, to conduct the health history. It continues throughout the interview and the health examination. As the client is interviewed, certain key observations are made that help in formulating an overall assessment of the client's health. Measurements of the client's height and weight and vital signs taken early in the health examination often confirm the impressions of the general health of the client.

Preparation. No special preparation is necessary for the general assessment. Initial observations can be made as you encounter the client, whether he or she is sitting, standing, or lying. Usually the client assumes a sitting position for the

TABLE 16–11. SAMPLE CLIENT HISTORY QUESTIONS FOR SUBJECTIVE MANIFESTATIONS: GENERAL ASSESSMENT

1. How would you rate your overall health? Are you generally healthy? Or are you frequently or chronically ill?
2. Have you recently gained or lost weight?
3. Are you always hungry (*polyphagia*) or do you have a poor appetite (*anorexia*)?
4. Do you feel energetic most of the time? Or are you frequently fatigued?
5. Do you exercise?
6. Do you have difficulty falling asleep or staying asleep (*insomnia*)?
7. Do you have fevers or night sweats?
8. Have your hands or feet enlarged in size recently (*acromegaly*)?
9. Does change in weather bother you (temperature intolerance)?
10. Do you feel excessively thirsty (*polydipsia*)?
11. Do you have frequent infections?
12. Have you ever been told you were anemic?
13. Have you ever had a blood transfusion? Why was this necessary and when did it occur?
14. Does _____ (subjective manifestation) interfere with your usual daily activities? How?

health history, remains seated for the examination of the head, neck, and thorax, lies down for the examination of the breasts and abdomen and for much of the neuromuscular examination, and stands for evaluation of posture, gait, and balance. Thus, as the examination progresses, there is ample opportunity to make general observations while the client is in each position. Many times the client's overall status is evaluated during the course of giving care. General observations can be made while giving the client a bed bath, changing a dressing, or watching the client ambulate to the bathroom. To obtain measurements, the following equipment is needed: scale with a measuring arm to collect height and weight data, a sphygmomanometer to measure blood pressure, a stethoscope, and a watch with a second hand to measure pulse and respirations.

IMPLICATIONS FOR NURSE–CLIENT COLLABORATION

General Assessment

Collaboration and general assessment go hand in hand, and both commence when the health interview begins. Here the initial trust the nurse works to establish is very important. General assessment is enhanced by the client's spontaneity in the health interview. In turn, a good general assessment (especially observations of the client's mental status) enables the nurse to make an initial evaluation of the client's capacity for collaborating and to assess the potential limitations created by the client's state of health.

Inspection. Begin the observation with the client's mental status, speech, and appearance and then progress to observations of body development and proportions, movement, and energy level. These observations can be made as you take the client's history, measure the client's vital signs, or carry out the activities that are part of caring for the client.

Mental Status. The mental status examination that accompanies general assessment is informal in comparison to the more detailed one done as part of the evaluation of the neurological system (discussed later in the chapter). It encompasses the initial impressions of the client's level of consciousness, orientation, behavior, and mood.

Level of consciousness is the client's alertness and awareness of the surroundings. At first glance, note whether the client is fully alert, lethargic, or unresponsive. A fully alert individual is awake, knows who he or she is (person), where he or she is (place), what the situation is, and what the date and time are.

Levels of consciousness other than alertness include *confusion, lethargy, delirium, stupor,* and *coma.* Box 16–20 lists definitions of these terms. If the client appears to be sleeping, note whether he or she can be aroused to a fully alert state. Does the client become more alert when gentle touch

BOX 16–20. LEVELS OF CONSCIOUSNESS

Alertness	Client is awake, attentive, appropriately responsive to stimuli, and oriented to person, place, situation, and date.
Confusion	Client's attention drifts; client is easily distracted, has decreased memory, is disoriented, has difficulty giving clear, appropriate answers to questions.
Lethargy	Client is drowsy, falls asleep easily, but arouses easily to sound of voice.
Delirium	Client is severely confused and has disordered perceptions (may hear sounds and see images that others do not see—hallucinations), reacts inappropriately to stimuli, shows marked anxiety and motor and sensory excitement (agitation).
Stupor	Client is only intermittently awake and then is arousable only for short periods; requires loud noise or tactile or painful stimuli for arousal; has limited awareness during response; responds only with movement and moaning.
Coma	Client is unarousable; moves involuntarily and assumes intermittent or fixed decerebrate posture in response to painful stimuli. In the decerebrate posture, the body is rigidly extended, neck is arched, and wrists, fingers, and feet are flexed.

From Seidel HM, Ball JW, Dains JE, Benedict GW. Mosby's Guide to Physical Examination. *St. Louis, MO: CV Mosby; 1991.*

is applied? If the client fails to respond to touch, does a painful stimulus such as a gentle pinch elicit a response?

If the client is awake, but does not seem fully alert, make a judgment about the client's level of alertness. The information to be considered in arriving at this judgment might include the flow of the client's speech, the quality of the client's voice, the clearness of the client's articulation, and the clarity and organization of the client's thoughts. Note how promptly the client responds to questions and whether the client's attention drifts, or whether it is necessary to touch the client to gain his or her attention. Assess the client's orientation by asking the client, "What is your name?" "Where are you?" "What day is this?" Remember that it is common for people who are in an unfamiliar environment for any period to lose track of the exact date; however, they should be able to give a generally correct response. Clients who are moved from room to room in the hospital may not remember their room number, but they should know that they are in the hospital. Time disorientation can reflect anxiety or emotional depression.

Note also whether the client's behavior is appropriate to the situation. Clients who become disoriented or confused may behave in a manner that is inappropriate to the situation. Confusion refers to a variety of behaviors including decreased concentration and attention span, inappropriate response to questions, recent or remote memory loss, or inappropriate behavior.

In addition to the client's level of consciousness, be aware of the client's mood as you interact. Mood is the quality or character of a client's emotional expression. Does the client seem fearful or anxious, angry or hostile, happy or sad? Mood is apparent in the client's posture, facial expressions, and other nonverbal behavior. Note whether the client's emotional expressions match the thoughts he or she communicates. Severe stress may be manifested when the client's mood does not match the content of his or her verbalizations.

Speech. When the client is awake and during a conversation, form an immediate impression about the client's speech and use of language. Observe the fluency, spontaneity, and clarity of speech. Note the quality of the client's voice. The ability to speak without hoarseness or difficulty in articulating reflects the function of cranial nerve X—the vagus nerve. The ability to produce certain sounds such as "B," "M," and "W" and rounded vowels reflects the function of cranial nerve VII, the facial nerve; the ability to articulate "L," "T," and "N" sounds reflects the function of cranial nerve XII, the hypoglossal nerve.

Although observation of the client's speech is part of assessing the level of consciousness, there are also expressive aspects to be assessed. Note the delivery of the speech—whether the client speaks hesitantly, uses rapid-fire delivery, or stutters. Note whether the client presents ideas in an orderly fashion. Note whether the client uses words in an unusual way or substitutes words that do not seem to fit the message. Difficulty using language may signify cerebral dysfunction and is referred to as *aphasia,* the inability to express oneself through speech. These are all important observations that reflect the client's cognitive and emotional state. When the client speaks in a foreign language, assessing expression may be difficult. A rough evaluation can be made by observing the client as he or she communicates with friends and significant others in the native language. Compare the client's speech with that of the other speakers.

Appearance. The client's appearance comprises a combination of features that include dress, facial expressions, manner, apparent age, race, and gender. Note whether the client's clothes are neat, clean, and appropriate to the situation. Observe the client's dress for its character and style and for what it might reveal about the client's social identity. Such information can be helpful during caregiving.

Observe the apparent care given to aspects of personal hygiene such as hair and skin, and note the presence of body odors. In illness, self-care can be neglected. Observe female clients for the manner in which makeup is applied, a feature that may reflect on the client's self-concept. Note whether the client appears older or younger than the stated age. This can provide clues to the client's overall state of health or illness.

Manner applies to the characteristics of the client's actions, whether spontaneous and communicative, outgoing, withdrawn, polite, or abrupt. Observe for involuntary signs of emotion such as a sweaty brow, underarms, or palms. Note whether the client appears overtly anxious. Does the client laugh inappropriately, wring his or her hands, or appear overly excited? Note the presence of signs of emotional depression, which may include apathy, inertia, confusion, anger, and disorientation.

Nutrition. Nutrition is very important to evaluate. Note whether the client appears obese or undernourished and the degree of the obesity or undernourishment. Confirm the observations by taking height and weight measurements and by asking relevant questions during the health history. From this information, compare the client's usual and actual weight with the desired weight for the client's height. A history of weight gain or loss indicates the need to obtain a detailed diet history and assess for specific nutrient deficiencies during the health history and examination.

Body Development and Proportions. Body development reflects growth, maturation, and sex (see inside back cover). Bone length and muscle mass increase from birth to about age 20. Secondary sex characteristics should become apparent during early adolescence. Stature also reflects advancing age. Sex and age interact to cause a loss of stature from bone demineralization in old age, particularly in older women.[58] Muscle mass also decreases during later adulthood, and the ratio of body fat to lean body mass increases.[59] Thus, body development changes not only in childhood, but throughout the life-span.

Genetic heritage is another important factor in body development and proportions. Both an unusually short stature with short limbs (dwarfism) and an unusually tall stature with long limbs (Marfan's syndrome) have a genetic basis. Ethnicity is related to genetic heritage and also affects body development and proportions. Stockiness, for example, the relation of body mass to an individual's height, has been shown to be related to ethnicity.[60] Racial differences in bones have been documented by research; blacks register greater bone mass and density than other groups.[61,62] The ratio of arm span to height is also different. Steele and Mattox have reported that the arm span of black females is 6.5 cm longer in relation to height, on average, than that of white females.[63] Height and weight, moreover, are greater on average in black and white males than in Hispanic and Asian males.[64] Moreover, black males and females are leaner on average than white males and females; blacks have also been found to carry a greater proportion of their subcutaneous fat on their upper rather than their lower trunks than do whites.[64,65] Although there are demonstrable racial differences in physique and body proportions, there is also a considerable overlap among racial groups, and this overlap is important to keep in mind when evaluating individual clients.[66]

During the general assessment, observe the overall development of the body and note the relationship between height and weight and whether body development is appropriate for the client's age. For children 2 years of age or older, height and weight can be obtained using a standing scale. Observe the muscle mass and shape of each body part and observe the two sides of the body for symmetry. Next, look for any obvious malformations, and note obvious disproportions. Does the client's head appear too large for the rest of his or her body? Are the client's limbs symmetrically disproportionate or uncommonly long or short in relationship to the trunk?

Posture, Movement, and Gait. On first encountering the client, note the client's posture. Some postural variations are a feature of individuality or personality; others signify the presence of illness. Posture often gives clues to inner feelings and particularly emotions. A slumped posture, for example, may be a manifestation of emotional depression. Posture can also indicate the presence of fatigue in that slumping may express the intense feeling of heaviness that people feel in their backs and limbs when fatigued. Posture also manifests pain. Clients who are experiencing pain, particularly over the abdomen, sometimes assume a protective posture to guard the painful area.

Movement is another important observation in the general assessment. Throughout the examination, note whether the client's movements are fluid and coordinated or awkward and jerky. Observe if the client's movements seem involuntary, that is, if the client is unable to control his or her movement. Twitches, tics, and tremors are examples of involuntary movement.

Note the client's gait. Gait assessment is broken into two phases, the stance phase and the swing phase. The stance phase has three parts, heel-strike, midstance, and pushoff. The heel strikes the floor, moves to full contact with the floor, and finally pushes off. The swing phase also consists of three parts: acceleration, swing-through, and deceleration. As weight begins to shift from the weight-bearing foot, the swing of the free leg accelerates; the free foot then moves ahead of the weight-bearing foot and slows down in preparation for heel strike. Abnormality in either phase of the client's gait results in an awkward and uncoordinated appearing gait. This type of gait does not have the expected characteristic of smoothness.

Observe the position of the body during the gait. The head and shoulders should be erect and positioned over the pelvis. There should be a minimum of shifting of the pelvis and trunk during walking. The heels should be placed from 2 to 4 in. apart, and a wider stance, which is expected in toddlers, should be noted as a possible sign of abnormality in older children and adults. Observe foot dragging, shuffling, or limping as the client walks. Note whether the client has obvious difficulty with balance. Balance reflects the functioning of the balance mechanism of the inner ear and the cerebellum. Clients experiencing balance problems associated with an uncoordinated gait may tend to watch their feet while walking.

Energy Level. Energy level reflects the integrated functions of several body systems and is a good indicator of healthy nutrition, oxygenation, mobility, neurosensory function, and mental status. Observe the client for obvious signs of fatigue such as slumped posture or slow or little movement. Fatigue may signify a loss of sleep. It may also signify interference with energy metabolism or diminished circulation. If these seem to be possibilities, observe for associated signs, such as a pallorous or flushed skin color or noisy or labored respirations. The client's speech may be broken into short phrases with apparent intermittent shortness of breath. These are signs of cardiovascular and respiratory distress. Musculoskeletal weakness can also give the picture of a reduced energy level. Weakness is detected during the examination of the musculoskeletal system as each muscle group is checked for strength.

Special Considerations, Precautions, and Sources of Error

The general assessment is formed in stages, beginning as the nurse enters the client's presence. As first impressions are formed, the nurse must always keep in mind that the examination of the body systems to follow will produce data that either confirm or negate initial impressions; it is thus very important that the nurse be prepared to revise these initial impressions. The variations of general assessment findings throughout the life cycle are contained in Table 16–12.

Recording

The general assessment is recorded at the beginning of the health examination. It is an objective statement expressing the nurse's impression of the physical health and mental and emotional status of the client during the nurse's assessment. It is not intended to include speculation about how the client might appear and the client's behavior when out

TABLE 16–12. OBJECTIVE MANIFESTATION FINDINGS AND LIFE-CYCLE VARIATIONS: GENERAL ASSESSMENT

Examination Technique	Expected Findings	Common Life-Cycle Variations
INSPECTION		
Mental Status		
Level of consciousness	Fully alert on arousal, normal sleep–wake pattern, no lethargy, confusion or fluctuation in level of consciousness.	
Orientation	Unhesitatingly states person, place, date, and situation.	
Mood and behavior	Attentive to examiner. Affect and behavior appropriate to age, status, background, and situation.	
Speech	Fluent, well-articulated speech; speech pattern appropriate to age. No hoarseness apparent—cranial nerve X—the vagus.	Speech development begins at age 3–4 months with babblings, cooing, laughing. Imitative vocalization apparent by age 9 months and word formation appears by age 1 year. Loss of dentition and ill-fitting dentures, as well as loss of speech discrimination capacity with advanced age, may alter speech or increase response time in later years.
Appearance	Appropriate attire; no obvious signs of distress; adequate hygiene.	
Nutrition	Weight appropriate to height, age, and dietary intake. No obesity or emaciation. See height–weight tables, Table 16–7.	Body fat decreases from age 1–6 years in both sexes followed by a period of body fat accumulation and then an early adolescent growth spurt.
Body development	Appropriate to age; consistent with genetic heritage.	Secondary sex characteristics should be apparent by age 13 in girls and age 14 in boys.
Body proportions	Symmetrical development; limbs in proportion to trunk. Proportions consistent with genetic heritage.	Infant head is large relative to body size. From age 1 to 5 years head decreases in proportion to size. Loss of height with advanced age by as much as three inches (7.5 cm) from adult peak. Neck and trunk shorten; arm span increases relative to height.
Posture	Erect; flexible, appropriate to activity and situation.	Newborn posture is one of partial flexion changing by age 4 months to a symmetrical position. Slumped posture in teens. Stooped posture with age.
Movement	Appropriate to activity; no involuntary movements.	Slower mobility with old age.
Gait	Fluid, balanced, coordinated; no staggering, lurching, dragging of feet or watching feet while walking.	Children aged 12–18 months show wide-stanced gait, little balance, but most progress to ability to run by age 18 months. Many elderly show slowing of gait and some have specific gait abnormalities associated with neuromuscular conditions.
Energy level	Activity appropriate to situation without apparent fatigue, faltering, or difficulty in self-restraint.	

From References 4, 42, and 59.

of the nurse's presence; only the immediate observations of the client are included. Information regarding overall health is obtained from the client during the interview and is recorded in the health history as subjective data. Box 16–21 contains examples of subjective and objective general assessment findings. Before attempting to record a general assessment or any other aspect of the health examination, review the list of abbreviations in Box 16–22. The use of standard abbreviations increases the nurse's efficiency in recording.

Role of the Nurse and the General Assessment

The general assessment is an important nursing skill. It is the process of making an initial assessment from immediate, holistic observations of the client. The ability to rapidly

BOX 16–21. RECORDING THE GENERAL ASSESSMENT

Subjective Manifestations

General health. The client rates his overall health as good. Weight has not fluctuated more than 5 pounds during adulthood. Sleeps 7 hours a night, feels energetic, and exercises daily by walking 4 miles at a moderate pace. Denies polyphagia, anorexia, insomnia, fevers, or infections. Has never had a blood transfusion or been told he was anemic.

Objective Manifestations

Appearance. Healthy appearing and alert; oriented to person, place, situation.
Mobility. Moves easily and has erect posture; no uncoordination or involuntary movement.
Speech and manner. Responds in a pleasant, cooperative, unhurried, confident manner; no hoarseness or difficulty articulating.
Energy level. No apparent fatigue.

assess a client's status is learned through practicing and gaining knowledge. Rapid evaluation is imperative when the nurse is presented with a client who is in acute distress and in need of immediate nursing care or referral. The ability to accomplish an accurate initial assessment may give the nurse immediate clues to the client's health problems and needs. The general assessment is the only aspect of the client evaluation that gives a broad overview of each client as an individual. It thus personalizes the health record. It is important to note that the nurse employs general assessment skills in every encounter with a client, not only the first encounter. Thus general assessment is as much a part of monitoring the client's health as it is of making an initial evaluation. Monitoring is assessment that is carried out after the nursing diagnoses are made, during the course of caregiving.

■ INTEGUMENT

Overview

The assessment of the integument includes the inspection and palpation of the skin, mucosa, hair, and nails. Percussion and auscultation are not generally used as modes of skin observation. The history questions relating to this assessment are summarized in Table 16–13.

Topographical Anatomy

The skin is the largest organ system of the body and has protective, sensory, and regulatory functions. The skin protects the body from hazards in the external environment and assists in the maintenance of the internal structures. It contributes to the regulation of body temperature and absorbs external sensory stimulation that is experienced as pain, heat, cold, and touch. The skin has three layers: the *epidermis*, the *dermis*, and the *subcutaneous layer*. The mucosa lining the nasal, oral, and other body cavities is considered an extension of the skin because it communicates with the air and is susceptible to external temperature changes as well as internal physiological changes such as anemia (which causes pallor) and hepatitis (which causes jaundice).

The most superficial of the three layers of the skin is the *epidermis*. The outer layer of the epidermis is composed of dead keratinized cells that are continually shed as underlying layers are renewed. These keratinized, or cornified, cells are the major components of the hair and nails. Melanocytes in the second (basal) level of the epidermis determine skin and hair color and protect the body from harmful ultraviolet radiation by increasing the pigmentation of the skin. The underlying *dermis* supplies the skin with blood vessels, sensory nerve endings, sebaceous glands, eccrine and apocrine sweat glands, and connective tissue (collagen and elastin), and also provides for the storage of fluids and electrolytes. The third level of the integument is the *subcutaneous layer*, a repository for fat cells that contribute to the important functions of temperature regulation and protection, or cushioning, of the body from traumatic assaults from the environment.

Conducting an Examination of the Integument

The inspection and palpation of the skin and mucosa begin with the examination of the head and neck and continue throughout the physical assessment as each body part is exposed to view.

Preparation. A thorough examination of the skin is possible only if the client is undressed (but draped) and the trunk and extremities are exposed in turn for inspection. Bright lighting that does not cast shadows on the skin is essential to accurately determine color changes. A glove is needed to palpate rashes and other lesions that might be infectious. A small transparent ruler is useful to correctly document the size of skin lesions; a hand-held magnifying glass can aid in the identification of lesions. As noted above, the skin assessment is incorporated throughout the physical examination and the client is seated part of the time, lying down part of the time, and may even be standing as the skin is assessed.

Inspection and Palpation. Inspection and palpation are the techniques used for skin assessment. Good observational skills elicit information about skin color, moisture, texture, temperature, vascularity, edema, masses, and lesions, as well as mucosal color and moisture; nail color, shape, and condition; and hair color, pattern, texture, and cleanliness.

Skin. Inspect the client's skin color. Skin color varies from individual to individual and from region to region over the surface of the body. Shades and tones range from pale ivory to deep brown according to the client's genetic heritage, exposure to the sun, and state of health. Note any changes in skin color, particularly *flushing*, a rosy appearance to the skin that occurs with fever, certain emotional states, and sexual arousal; *pallor*, unnatural paleness; *cyanosis*, a bluish discoloration of the skin; and *jaundice*, a yellow discoloration of the skin caused by faulty bile metabolism or excre-

BOX 16–22. ABBREVIATIONS USED FOR RECORDING THE HEALTH HISTORY AND HEALTH EXAMINATION

A	aortic
AAL	anterior axillary line
AC	air conduction
ADL	activities of daily living
AGE	angle of greatest extension
AGF	angle of greatest flexion
A-P diam	anterior-posterior diameter
ARDS	adult respiratory distress syndrome
ausc	auscultation
A-V	arteriovenous
A&W	alive and well
BC	bone conduction
BP	blood pressure
CC	chief complaint
cm	centimeter
CN	cranial nerve
CV	cardiovascular
CVA	costovertebral angle
dx	diagnosis
DPT	diphtheria, pertussis, tetanus
EENT	eyes, ears, nose, and throat
EOM	extraocular movements
F	father
FH	family history
Gen	general
GEO	geographic
GI	gastrointestinal
gm	gram
GU	genitourinary
HEENT	head, eyes, ears, nose, and throat
H&P	history and physical
HPI	history of present illness
ht	height
Hx	history
ICS	intercostal space
ID	identifying data
insp	inspection
kg	kilogram
Ⓛ	left
LAAL	left anterior axillary line
LBCD	left border cardiac dullness
LICS	left intercostal space
LLQ	left lower quadrant
LLSB	lower left sternal border
LMP	last menstrual period
LOC	level of consciousness
LRSB	lower right sternal border
LSB	left sternal border
LUQ	left upper quadrant
M	mother, mitral
marit	marital
MAL	midaxillary line
MCL	midclavicular line
mg	milligram
MIL	midinguinal line
mm	millimeter
MMR	measles, mumps, rubella
MS	musculoskeletal
MSL	midsternal line, midscapular line
nl, NL	normal
NP	neuropsychiatric
N&V	nausea and vomiting
OB	obstetrical
O.D.	right eye
O.S.	left eye
O.U.	both eyes
P	pulmonic
PAL	posterior axillary line
palp	palpation
Pap	Pap smear
perc	percussion
PERRLA	pupils equal, round, reactive to light, and accommodation
PMH	past medical history
PMI	point of maximal impulse or intensity
P/SH	personal and social history
Psych	psychiatric
pt	patient
Ⓡ	right
RAAL	right anterior axillary line
RICS	right intercostal space
RLQ	right lower quadrant
ROM	range of motion
ROS	review of systems
RSB	right sternal border
RUQ	right upper quadrant
Rx	treatment
S_1	first heart sound
S_2	second heart sound
S_3	third heart sound
S_4	fourth heart sound
SH	social history
SOB	shortness of breath
T	tricuspid
TB	tuberculosis
TM	tympanic membrane
TOPV	trivalent oral polio vaccine
TPR	temperature, pulse, respiration
ULSB	upper left sternal border
URI	upper respiratory infection
URSB	upper right sternal border
WNL	within normal limits
wt	weight

From Berger KJ, Fields WL. Pocket Guide to Health Assessment. *Reston, VA: Reston Publishing Co.; 1980.*

tion. These changes are apparent by comparing the skin over one body region with the skin over another, or by comparing an unnatural skin color with the normal skin color.

Generalized skin color changes are difficult to assess in darkly pigmented individuals. Because of this difficulty, it is necessary to develop special skills for observing pigmented skin. Flushing is difficult to see in brown- or black-skinned individuals. It can sometimes be observed by looking at the tips of the ears. Pallor and cyanosis are important signs of physical distress. In individuals with naturally brown skin, pallor may appear as a yellow-brown skin tone

TABLE 16–13. SAMPLE CLIENT HISTORY QUESTIONS FOR SUBJECTIVE MANIFESTATIONS: INTEGUMENT

1. Is your skin itchy (*pruritic*) or painful in any areas?
2. Do you have any rashes? How long have they been apparent?
3. Do you have any bug bites? Have you been exposed to contagious skin conditions such as scabies, lice, and impetigo?
4. Has your skin felt unusually oily (*seborrhea*), dry (*xerosis*), or rough (scaly or crusted)?
5. Have you noted a change in skin color, either loss of pigmentation (*vitiligo*) or increased coloration (*hyperpigmentation*); a change in color, size, or sensitivity of a mole; or an incidence of increased bruising?
6. Do you have a family tendency toward skin cancers or other skin problems?
7. Has there been a recent change in the texture of your hair or the condition of your scalp? Have you had unusual hair loss (*alopecia*) or hair growth (*hirsutism*)?
8. Have you noticed changes in the shape, color, or brittleness of your nails?
9. Does _____ (subjective manifestation) interfere with any of your usual daily activities? How?

change; in those with black skin, an ashen gray tone may appear. Generally these changes can be confirmed by the appearance of the nail beds, the *palpebral conjunctiva* (mucosa of the eyelids), and the mucosa of the inner surfaces of the mouth, known as the *buccal mucosa*. All of these areas may appear pale or ashen when discoloration is unapparent over the skin itself. Jaundice also may be difficult to see, and is best observed over the sclera (whites) of the eyes in dark-skinned individuals.

Next, note skin moisture. Observe the client for the presence of perspiration. Sweat is commonly found over the brow and in the axilla and the skin folds. Note the absence of perspiration, which may suggest dehydration. Dehydration is particularly likely when the client's lips are also cracked. Observe the skin for the roughness or smoothness of its texture. People with disorders of the thyroid gland may have uncommonly smooth, soft skin (overactive gland) or dry, flaky skin (underactive gland). After inspecting, palpate the skin to further assess smoothness, moisture, skin temperature, and apparent edema. Palpation confirms the findings of inspection and is the only way to determine skin temperature, whether overly warm (as in fever) or overly cool (as when the circulation to the skin is diminished).

After making these observations, inspect and palpate the skin for lesions (see Tables 16–14 and 16–15). Primary skin lesions are those that first appear on previously healthy skin. Secondary skin lesions represent alterations of primary lesions.

Lesions, in particular macular (flat) lesions, are difficult to evaluate by inspection when the skin is darkly pigmented. Apparent discolorations that might suggest the presence of lesions may be nothing more than normal variants of pigmentation pattern.[67] Moreover, black skin has

BUILDING NURSING KNOWLEDGE

How Do Nurses Form Their Initial Assessments of Clients?

Price B. First impressions: Paradigms for patient assessment. *J Adv Nurs.* 1987;12:699–705.

Price notes that an initial assessment of the client usually comprises both formal and informal elements. The nurse makes baseline observations, takes a health history, and makes other clinical measurements. In addition, however, the nurse also informally appraises the client "as a person." This aspect of personal appraisal, according to Price, has not been given sufficient acknowledgment for its importance to caregiving.

This study explored the criteria that nurses use to make this informal appraisal. Past studies have focused on how nurses, lacking the prestige of physicians, have had to enter into open negotiations of role and status with the client. These studies documented how stressful these negotiations are to nurses whose personal feelings of insecurity, control, and reward during the initial assessment also influence the future professional relationship with the client.

Price interviewed nursing students, observing them as they conducted initial assessments with clients, and also studied client records to identify informal assessment categories. Price found that the nursing students in his sample, in fact, used informal categories of assessment.

One of the most significant categories related to the clarity of the "hospital career" of the client. Hospital career refers to the series of events that the client is likely to experience in the hospital. The career for a client who is admitted to have surgery is more clear than that of a client who is admitted for an unknown diagnosis. Nursing students welcomed clients with clear careers and enjoyed briefing them on what they might expect during their stays. Such interviews were strongly structured around giving information and protocols. Nursing students were less enthusiastic about interviews with clients who faced an unclear career. The sequence of such interviews was much more variable. Information was given more hesitantly. In many instances, students sought to keep the assessment at a very simple level, in contrast to the more detailed questions asked of clients with clear careers.

Age was another important informal category. Although the nursing students often favored elderly clients, those elders whose moods were surly or critical had shorter interviews and were asked more closed questions. This resulted in a more formal and mechanical style of interview. With young adults, an important issue during the interview was whether they would adhere to the health care plan. Because they were similar in age, the students sought to establish a professional distance between themselves and their young adult clients. When the professional distancing appeared to be resented or not totally respected by the client, the students often suspected the client would not adhere to client role expectations. Those clients were sometimes labeled as "uncontrollable," "immature," or "lacking in insight" by the students.

Price concluded that nurses cannot expect to exclude informal variables from assessment and that nurses' own feelings should be given more account. Nursing educators should make it a goal to help students become more aware of social factors in action and to deal with them to the client's benefit.

TABLE 16–14. PRIMARY LESIONS

Illustration	Name and Characteristics	Examples
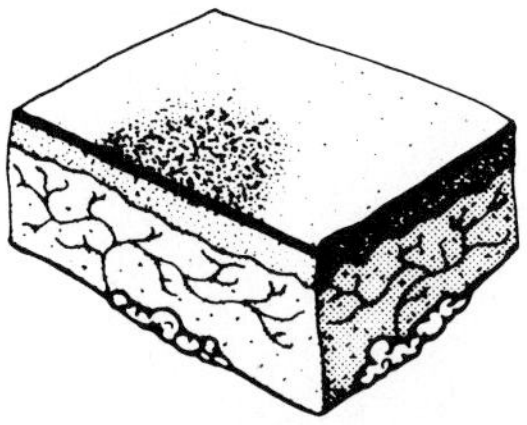	*Macule:* Flat, nonpalpable colored spot up to 1 cm in diameter.	Freckle, vitiligo, petechia
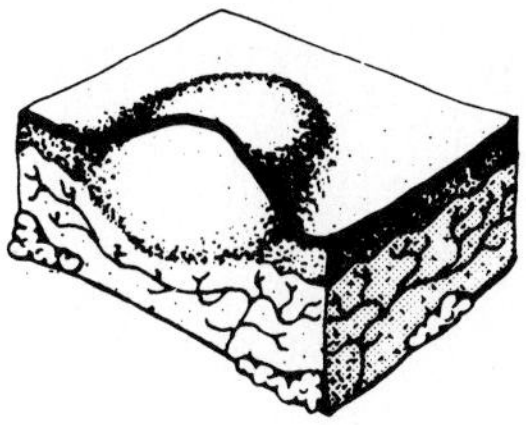	*Papule:* Solid, elevated circumscribed lesion, up to 1 cm in diameter.	Acne, measles
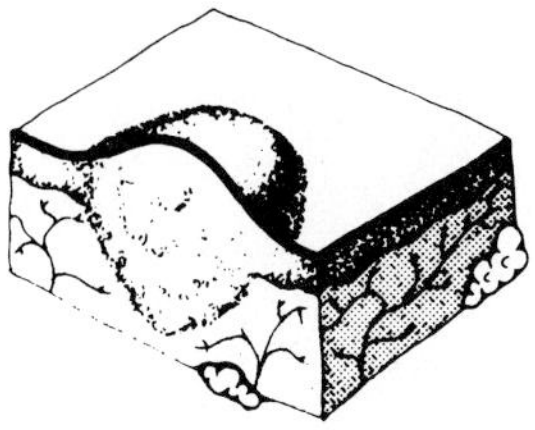	*Nodule:* Solid, elevated circumscribed lesion 0.5–2 cm in diameter.	Wart, basal cell carcinoma
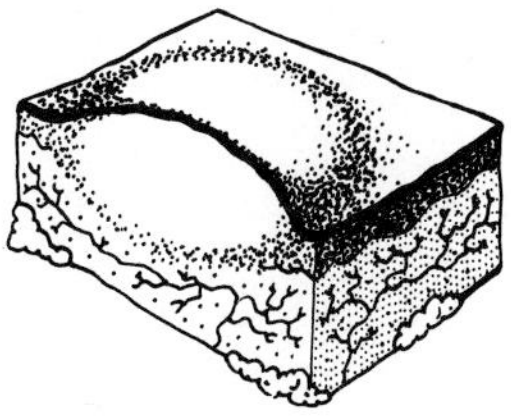	*Plaque:* Raised patch on skin or mucous membrane, 2–3 cm in diameter.	Psoriasis, thrush
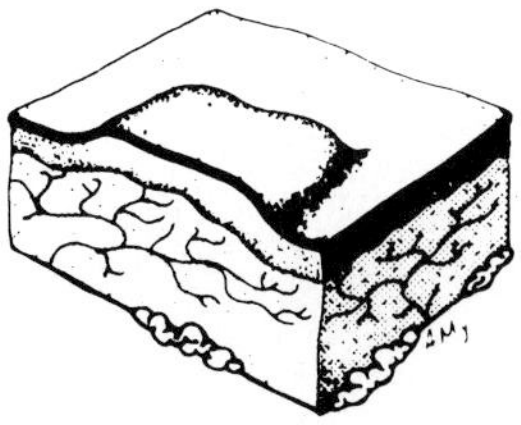	*Wheal:* Transient elevation of skin, white in center with red periphery, 5–10 cm in diameter.	Hives, urticaria, insect bite
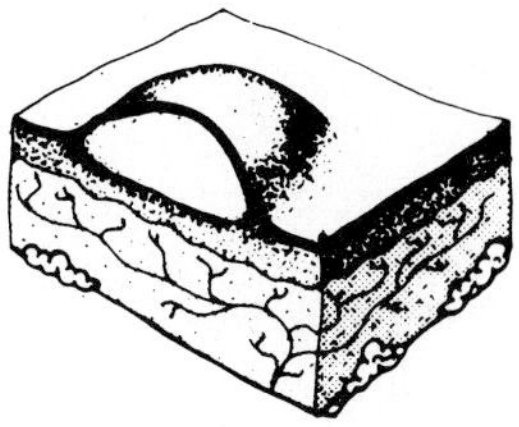	*Vesicle:* Circumscribed skin elevation filled with serous fluid, up to 1 cm in diameter.	Herpes simplex, chickenpox
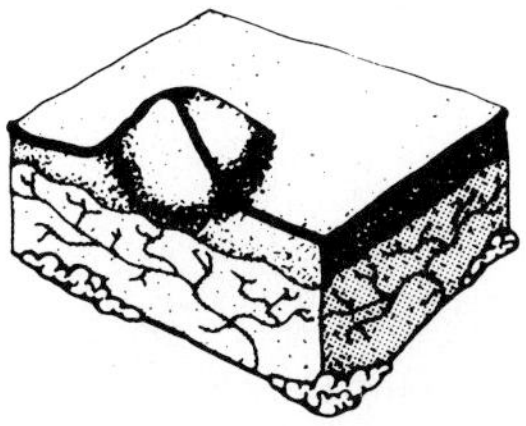	*Pustule:* Pus-filled, elevated, circumscribed lesion of variable size.	Acne vulgaris, impetigo

(*continued*)

TABLE 16–14. (continued)

Illustration	Name and Characteristics	Examples
	Cyst: Encapsulated fluid-filled mass.	Epidermoid cyst
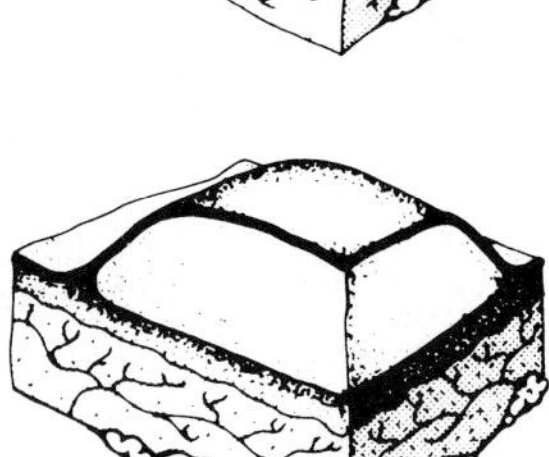	*Bulla:* Elevated, circumscribed lesion >0.5 cm in diameter, filled with serous fluid.	Pemphigus, second-degree burn
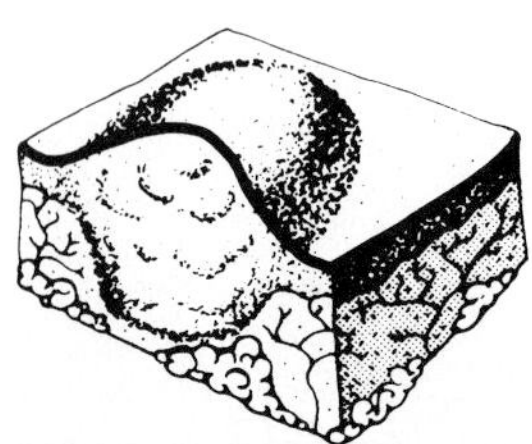	*Tumor:* Solid elevated mass > 1 cm in diameter.	Cavernous hemangioma

All illustrations, except plaque, reproduced from Berger KJ, Fields WL. Pocket Guide to Health Assessment. *Reston, VA: Reston Publishing Co.; 1980.*

TABLE 16–15. SECONDARY LESIONS

Illustration	Lesion/Description	Examples
	Scale: Dried, thin epithelial flake.	Dandruff, psoriasis
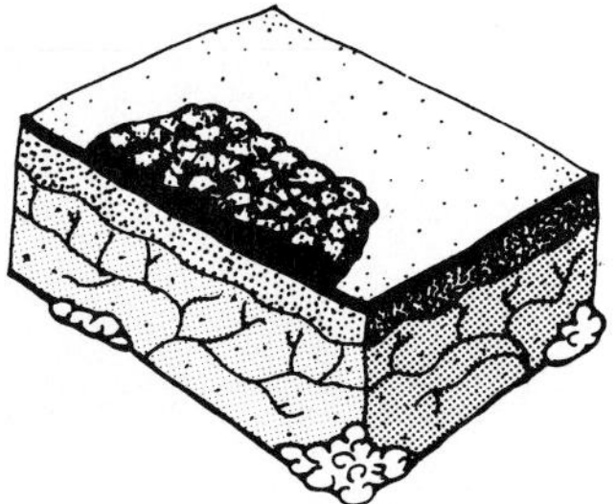	*Crust:* Dried exudate.	Impetigo, eczema

TABLE 16–15. SECONDARY LESIONS (continued)

Illustration	Lesion/Description	Examples
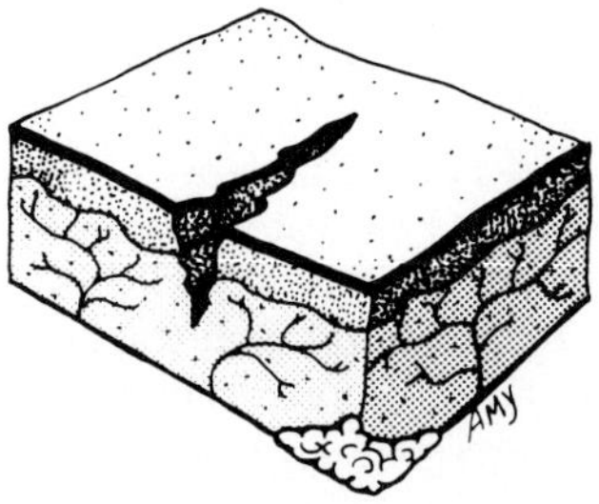	*Fissure:* Linear crack in skin, usually extending through epidermis.	Chapping, allergic dermatitis
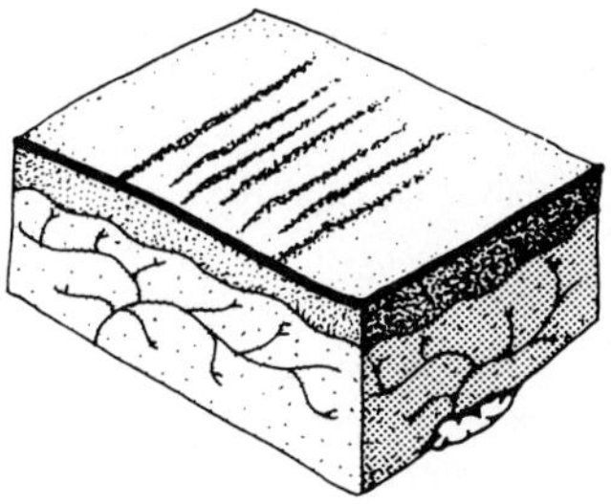	*Excoriation:* Traumatized area; abrasion, scratch marks.	Eczema, chickenpox
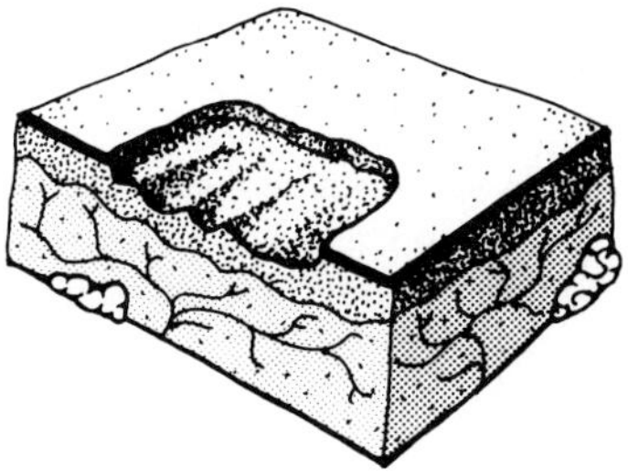	*Ulcer:* Circumscribed area of destroyed epidermis; may extend into corium and subcutaneous tissue.	Stasis ulcer, secondary to varicose veins, chancre
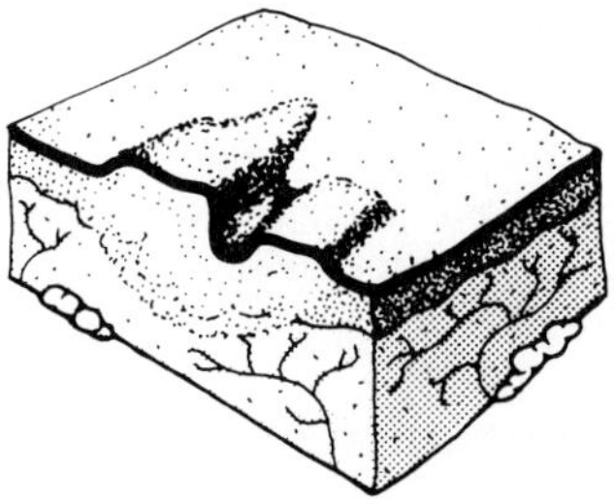	*Scar:* Fibrotic area of dermis caused by destruction of dermis and/or subcutaneous layers.	Healed surgical incision
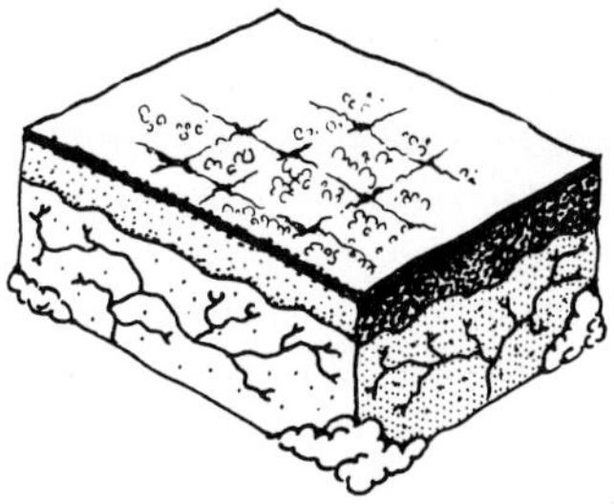	*Lichenification:* Crustlike, thickened, rough, scaly, area, often related to chronic irritation.	Psoriasis

All illustrations, except lichenification, reproduced from Berger KJ, Fields WL. Pocket Guide to Health Assessment. *Reston, VA: Reston Publishing Co.; 1980.*

been documented to react differently than other skin types to common skin conditions.[67] Thus, skills to aid inspection are helpful. By gently stretching the skin, you may be able to better visualize a suspected lesion on darkly pigmented skin. To differentiate a simple variation of color from a lesion, it may be necessary to gather additional data by asking the client whether the discolorations observed are old or new, and whether any unusual subjective manifestation such as itching and pain is associated with it.

Palpation is particularly useful for evaluating skin lesions and masses over skin of any color. Skin lesions are flat (macular) or raised (papular). Some lesions have depth and others are fluid-filled. These characteristics can be determined only by feeling the surface of the skin. Palpate the client's skin by touching it with your fingers and running them over any apparent lesions or rashes to confirm whether these are flat or raised. You may want to glove your hands before palpating skin lesions.

After identifying the presence of lesions, describe them according to their type (primary or secondary), location, number and distribution, and color. Skin changes may appear as a single unit or in a collection. A grouping of lesions may occur if there are more than one, and a pattern may be apparent in their relation to one another. Describe the pattern of grouping. Common terms used to describe grouping include "clustered" (grouped together), "diffuse" (widespread over the skin surface), "linear" (in a straight line), "circular" (in a circle), and "confluent" (blending together or impinging on one another). Finally, note the presence of discharge from any lesions that are present and describe the discharge for color and amount. Masses, collections of subcutaneous tissue that may represent enlarged lymph nodes or tumors, are defined by location, size, contour, consistency (whether the mass is hard or soft), tenderness, and mobility (whether the mass moves or is fixed over underlying tissue).

Skin turgor is another important observation that is done by palpation, with the aid of inspection. **Turgor** is the term used to describe the skin's elasticity. Test turgor by gently pinching an area of skin such as over the wrist or abdomen. Note how quickly the skin returns to its former contour. The skin should recoil promptly. Turgor is decreased when the skin is slow to recede.

Nails. Nails should be translucent and smooth. The convex contour of the nail plate should not be marred by splitting, clubbing, or separation from the underlying nail bed. Abnormal findings are often attributable to systemic diseases. Spoon nails, for instance, nails that are concave instead of convex in shape, may indicate severe anemia or infections of the nail bed. *Clubbing*, an exaggerated convexity associated with enlargement of the tips of the fingers, accompanies severe, long-standing oxygenation dysfunction.

After inspecting, palpate the nails. Compression of the nails elicits information about flexibility of the nail plate and tenderness of the nail bed.

Hair. Observe the hair of the scalp for color, pattern of hair distribution or loss, texture, and cleanliness. Thorough inspection of the hair requires that the hair be moved so that the underlying scalp can be viewed. Note if there are any lesions, bald spots (alopecia), or parasites on the scalp or hair shafts. Head lice (pediculosis) and ringworm (tinea capitis) are frequently found when inspecting and palpating the hair. It is best to glove your hands for palpating the hair and scalp.

There is a wide variation in normal patterns of hair growth, particularly in childhood and adolescence, a factor that should be kept in mind in evaluating the hair.[68] Hair texture, a reflection of the structure and protein composition of the hair, varies with race.[69] Mongoloid hair is straight, and hair shafts are round; negroid hair is curly, and hair shafts are flat; caucasoid hair is wavy, and hair shafts are elliptical.

The many variations of normal skin characteristics are outlined by life cycle phases in Table 16–16.

Special Considerations, Precautions, and Sources of Error

Thoroughness is the key to effective examination of the skin, mucosa, nails, and hair. The integument can reflect systemic changes (disease processes in other parts of the body), and a nurse with keenly developed observational skills can identify these subtle changes, such as a slight jaundice of the skin caused by liver disease. The nurse must take care to examine the entire body surface and not just the area, or areas, of concern to the client. The client may be unaware of skin lesions on body surfaces, such as the back, where they are less noticeable. Gloves should be worn during palpation of skin lesions and rashes to avoid contamination of the nurse's hands and subsequent spread of infection.

Recording

A carefully written record communicates examination findings to other members of the health care team. The subjective manifestations of the integument are recorded in the health history; objective skin manifestations are grouped with the rest of the physical findings. Skin lesions are described according to their distribution, configuration, color, and type (primary or secondary). Examples of a written record are presented in Box 16–23.

Role of the Nurse and the Assessment of the Integument

Physiological changes such as hypoxia can initially manifest as subtle changes in skin color. Nurses in hospitals, clinics, and community settings are frequently the first members of the health care team to observe these variations and decide on the follow-up care required by the client. The nurse may also be the first professional to notice malignant changes in a mole or other lesion and to make an appropriate early referral. Hospital nurses take special note of erythematous (red) skin color changes on the buttocks or over bony prominences so they can initiate early precautions to prevent skin breakdown. The evaluation and referral of skin lesions by community health nurses and school nurses can alert public health officials to communicable disease outbreaks in schools or communities.

TABLE 16–16. OBJECTIVE MANIFESTATION FINDINGS AND LIFE CYCLE VARIATIONS: INTEGUMENT

Examination Technique	Expected Findings	Common Life-Cycle Variations
INSPECTION		
Skin		
Color	Uniform and consistent with ethnicity; no jaundice, pallor, erythema.	Pigmentation appears over face, nipples, areolae, axillae, and vulva during pregnancy. Irregular pigmentation with age and weathering.
Vascularity	Absence of enlarged or dilated blood vessels.	Peripheral vasodilation apparent during pregnancy. Vessels appear more prominent with age as skin becomes thinner and vascular lesions proliferate as the skin becomes more friable.
Lesions	With the exception of scattered freckles and moles the normal skin is free of lesions.	Acne and comedones (blackheads) occur with puberty. Sun exposure contributes to an increased number of lesions with aging.
Consistency/texture	Moist appearing, smooth; pores barely visible; not oily, dry, scaly, or crusty.	Skin of infants and children appears smoother than that of adults. Peeling of skin may be apparent in newborns.
Mucosa		
Moisture	Shiny and moist.	Increased sweating in adolescence and pregnancy. Dull and dry with aging; sweat gland activity reduced.
Color	Pink with some variation among racial groups.	
Hair		
Quantity	Appropriate for age.	Both men and women experience scalp hair thinning with age and women may note increased facial hair.
Distribution	Appropriate to age and sex.	Coarse hair appears in axillae and pubic areas during adolescence. Recession of scalp hair often occurs with aging and leg and axillary hair may become scanty.
Texture	Not brittle or dull.	
Color	Consistent with genetic heritage; lustrous.	Graying with age.
Nails		
Color	Translucent with color variation by ethnicity and no staining or discoloration.	
Shape	Smooth convex surface with firm adherence to nail bed.	
Lesions	None.	
Nail base	Intact with no redness or swelling.	
Consistency	Smooth.	
PALPATION		
Skin		
Moisture	Dry but not scaly.	Oiliness with puberty, increased dryness with age and weathering.
Temperature	Warm to the touch.	Digits increasingly cool with age.
Texture	Smooth.	Thins with age.
Elasticity	Mobile and recoils immediately on pinching skinfold.	Laxness with age. Loss of turgor from reduced elasticity and subcutaneous fat.
Lesions		Rashes and growths occur throughout the life-span.
Hair		
Texture	Flexible.	
Nails		
Quality	Flexible and not brittle or dry.	More brittleness and slower growth with age; loss of luster; toenails may thicken.

From References 4, 42, and 59.

BOX 16–23. RECORDING THE ASSESSMENT OF THE INTEGUMENT

Subjective Manifestations

Integument. Reports no rashes, lumps, itching, dryness, or color changes of the skin and mucous membranes. No brittleness or lesions of nails. No recent change in color, texture, or quantity of hair. No family or personal history of skin cancer.

Objective Manifestations

Skin. Pink, smooth, warm, moist with good turgor. Scattered nevi on trunk and upper arms but no rashes, abnormal pigmentation, or masses. One solitary circular erythematous lesion on right upper arm with raised vesicular border.
Mucosa. Pink, moist, and without lesions.
Nails. Strong, flexible, and pink without clubbing or lesions.
Hair. Thick and normally distributed with temporal graying. Recession of scalp hair consistent with male balding pattern.

TABLE 16–17. SAMPLE CLIENT HISTORY QUESTIONS FOR SUBJECTIVE MANIFESTATIONS: HEAD, FACE, AND NOSE

1. Have you had any accidents or injuries to your head, face, or nose? Are there any painful areas or lumps?
2. Do you have headaches?
3. Have you noticed any rashes or sores on your scalp? Do you have itching of your scalp? Have you noticed any bugs on your scalp or hair?
4. Do you have a history of sinus pain (*sinusitis*) or a sensation of pressure in your sinuses?
5. Do you have a nasal discharge (*rhinorrhea*) or congestion (*rhinitis*)? Is this symptom related to seasons of the year? Do you have an adequate sense of smell?
6. Do you have nosebleeds (*epistaxis*)?
7. Does ______ (subjective manifestation) interfere with any of your usual daily activities? How?

Nurses with effective assessment skills and a clear understanding of skin health and disease are in an advantageous position to increase client awareness of environmental hazards. Chemicals and insecticides, for instance, are dangerous solutions that contaminate unprotected skin. Even soaps and perfumes can cause rashes on sensitive skin. Health education should become a routine aspect of any skin assessment, with particular stress on the dangers of excessive sun exposure and the role of weathering in the formation of potential skin cancers.

■ HEAD, EAR, EYE, NOSE, AND THROAT

Head, Face, and Nose

Overview. Assessment of the head, face, and nose combines the description of the symptoms elicited from the client during the health history interview and the examination techniques of inspection and palpation. Table 16–17 suggests questions the nurse can ask to obtain significant and pertinent information about this critical area of the body.

Topographical Anatomy. An understanding of the anatomy of the head and associated structures is essential to both thorough assessment and accurate description of physical findings. The skull, or cranium, is the hard protective covering for the vital brain tissues and has four anatomical divisions: the frontal, temporal, parietal, and occipital bones (Fig. 16–23). The skeletal portions of the face consist of the nasal bones, the zygomatic arches, the maxilla, and the large mandibular bone that forms the movable jaw (Fig. 16–24). The paranasal sinuses are cavities in the cranial and facial bones (Fig. 16–25). They are lined with ciliated mucous membrane and, with the nose, aid in warming, humidifying, and filtering inspired air. The sinuses closest to the facial surface are the frontal, maxillary, and anterior ethmoidal. The posterior ethmoidal and sphenoidal sinuses lie deeper in the cranial cavity. The sinuses drain into the nasal cavities.

The scalp that covers the cranium is composed of five layers: skin, subcutaneous tissue, the muscular epicranius, a fatty layer, and the pericranium, which extends into the suture lines that bind the cranial bones together. Situated beneath the mandible are the submandibular salivary glands. The other two pairs of salivary glands are the parotids, located laterally on the jawbone just below the ears, and the sublingual glands beneath the tongue. The ducts of these three pairs of glands open into the mouth and are evaluated during assessment of the oral cavity.

The external nose is supported by bone posteriorly and by cartilage anteriorly. The interior nose consists of two nares divided by the nasal septum, which is also composed of bone and cartilage (Fig. 16–26). Three turbinate bones (inferior, middle, and superior) protrude from the lateral surfaces of the nares into the nasal cavities. The highly vascular mucous membrane covering the turbinates acts in conjunction with the rest of the nasal mucosa to warm and filter atmospheric air. This vascular cover has the capacity to swell when inflamed and occlude the nasal cavity. Near the tip of the septum is another vascular area (Kiesselbach's plexus) that is associated with nosebleeds (epistaxis). The nose is also the sensory organ for smell.

Conducting an Examination of the Head, Face, and Nose. Aspects of the examination to be covered here are inspection of the head, face, nose, and sinuses and palpation of the head and sinuses. Visualization of the internal nose is accomplished by the use of a light source and occasionally a nasal speculum. Transillumination of the frontal and maxillary sinuses requires a penlight but is beyond the scope of this text. The areas examined are inspected and palpated

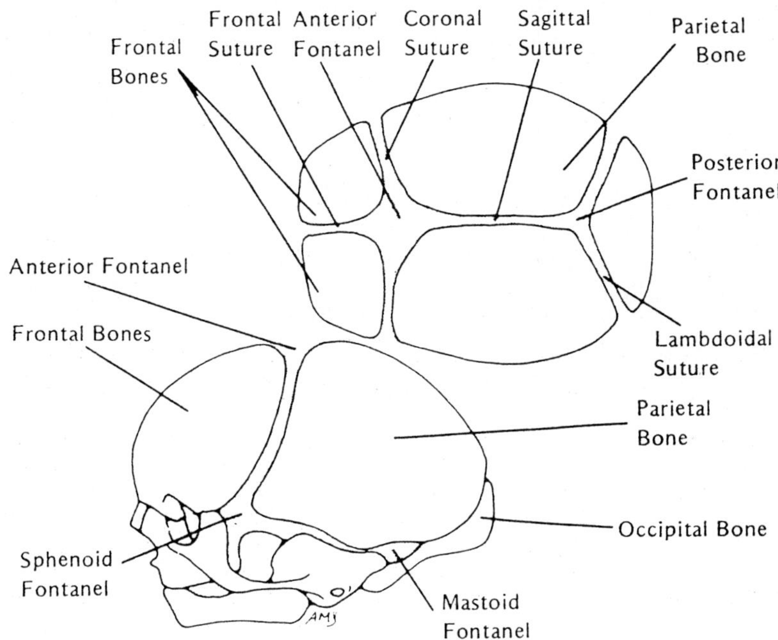

Figure 16–23. Infant skull showing skull bones and fontanels. Fontanels close by 18 months of age. (Source: *Berger KJ, Fields WL.* Pocket Guide to Health Assessment. *Reston, VA: Reston Publishing Co.; 1980.*)

simultaneously. Assessing smell requires an available source of familiar odors.

Preparation. The client sits facing you at eye level during this examination. You should have near at hand a light source, such as a penlight or otoscope, and a nasal speculum.

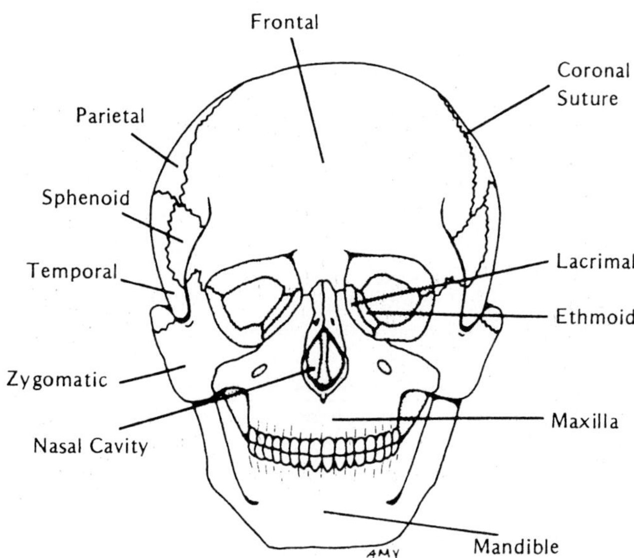

Figure 16–24. Facial bones. (Source: *Berger KJ, Fields WL.* Pocket Guide to Health Assessment. *Reston, VA: Reston Publishing Co.; 1980.*)

Inspection and Palpation. Inspect and palpate each area, head, face, and nose, in turn.

Head. Inspect the head for size, contour, position, and condition of the scalp. When the client is a child under the age of 2 years, measure the circumference of his or her head. This procedure is easier if the parent holds the child's head to stabilize it. Norms for head size vary with race; for example, the average head circumference of Asian newborns is slightly smaller than that of Caucasian or black newborns.[70] (See inside back cover for head circumference norms.) While inspecting the head, examine the scalp for

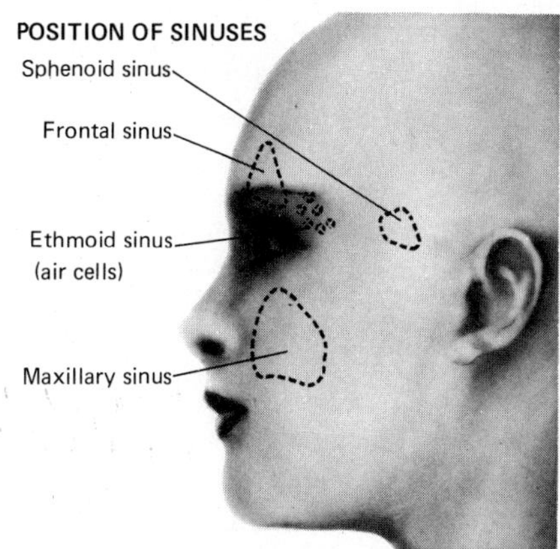

Figure 16–25. Position of sinuses. (Source: *Block GJ, Nolan JW.* Health Assessment for Professional Nursing: A Developmental Approach. *2nd ed. Norwalk, CT: Appleton-Century-Crofts; 1986.*)

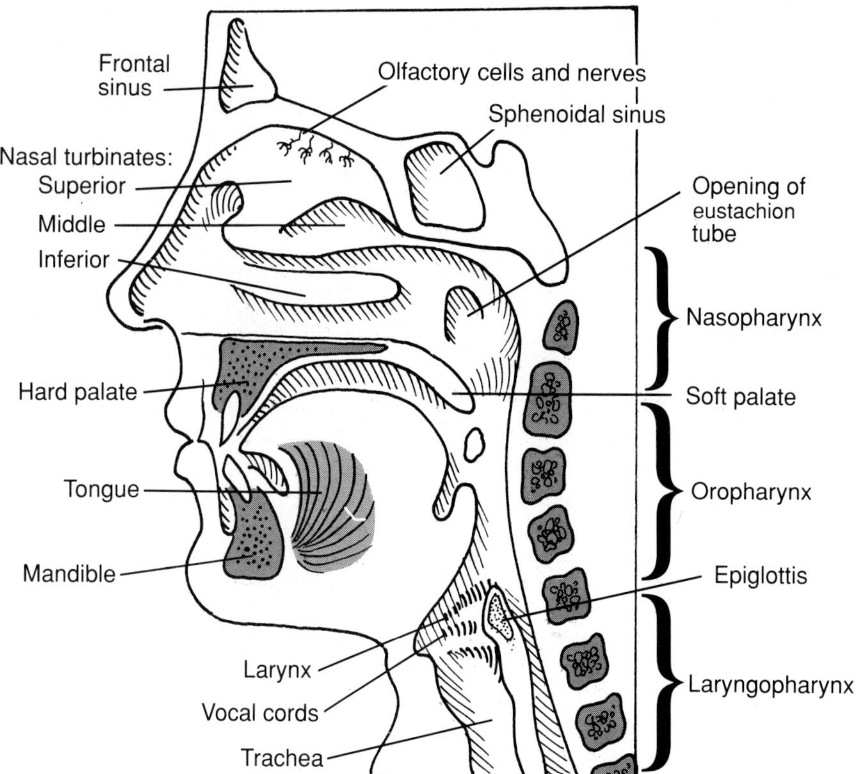

Figure 16–26. Structure of the nose in relation to the pharynx.

scaliness and seborrhea (greasy, scaly patches), and for rashes, lesions, and infestations (lice). This is done by separating the hair at intermittent locations over the scalp. Palpate the skull and scalp for masses and tenderness.

Face. Observe the face for proportion, contour symmetry, edema, masses, and skin condition. Note carefully the facial expression and particularly the symmetry of facial muscle movement. Facial muscle movement reflects the function of cranial nerve VII, the facial nerve. Damage to a facial nerve causes facial muscle paralysis. Jaw movement reflects the function of cranial nerve V, the trigeminal nerve, and is checked by asking the client to clench the teeth. Sensation over the face also reflects the function of cranial nerve V. Palpate the areas over the paranasal sinuses and note any tenderness. Lastly, if there is a mass on the face, palpate it for size, contour, consistency, tenderness, induration, mobility, and boundaries.

Nose. Evaluate the external nose for deformity, discharge, and the presence of lesions around the nostrils. Look for obvious deviation of the nose which appears as nasal asymmetry. Note any edema or discoloration that might indicate recent trauma. Ask the client to tip his or her head slightly backward and shine a light into the nasal cavity. You may need to stabilize the client's head with your hand. The inferior turbinates and nasal septum will be visible. Check the nasal passages for patency. Evaluate the integrity and color of the mucosa. The septum is observed for deviation and perforation.

Smell. The sense of smell is important to one's ability to enjoy food, and when diminished may contribute to poor nutrition.

The sense of smell reflects the function of cranial nerve I, the olfactory nerve. The easiest way to assess the client's sense of smell is to be aware of the client's reaction to odors that are present in the environment. Failure to react to an obvious odor may suggest a diminished sense of smell, a common problem associated with nasal congestion. A simple way to check smell is to ask the client to identify the familiar odors of items on the meal tray or of items that might be in the client's cupboard or refrigerator. Coffee and orange juice are good examples. Ask the client to close his or her eyes before presenting the stimulus, first to one nostril and then to the other.

The physical manifestations expected to be noted during head, face, and nose assessment are described in Table 16–18.

Special Considerations, Precautions, and Sources of Error. Palpation of the head is an intimate procedure regarded by some clients as an infringement of personal space. Careful explanation of the necessity for cranial palpation may alleviate client anxiety about this procedure. Children in particular may react negatively to strangers touching their heads without taking time to develop a friendly and trusting relationship.

Careful explanation before each procedure is performed alleviates client concern. As children can be espe-

TABLE 16–18. OBJECTIVE MANIFESTATION FINDINGS AND LIFE CYCLE VARIATIONS

Examination Technique	Expected Findings	Common Life Cycle Variations
INSPECTION		
Head		
Size	In proportion to body size.	Head circumference measures 13–14 inches at birth in the average size neonate (7 lbs). Head size changes in dimension and proportion until adolescence, and reaches 90% of final size by age 6. Bone suture lines may be overriding at birth, but generally flatten by age 6 months. Anterior fontanelles close by 19 months, posterior by 1–2 months.
Contour	Symmetrical.	Irregularities can be normal, especially at the back part of skull.
Position	Straight and midline; no sustained tilting.	
Scalp	Color of skin, free of lesions, and covered with hair.	Balding with age.
Face		
Proportion	Spacing of sensory organs symmetrical.	Variations with genetic inheritance. Nose and jawbones grow at an accelerated rate during adolescence, particularly in males. In advanced age loss of skin elasticity and subcutaneous fat lead to apparent prominence of orbital and facial bones and sagging of facial features. Nose elongates with age. Loss of teeth; jaw bone resorption results in noticeable shrinkage of lower face.
Skin condition	Clear and color consistent with rest of skin.	Variation in skin color by ethnicity.
Color, pigmentation		With age, loss of skin capillaries leads to graying of facial skin.
Movement	Symmetrical, able to clench teeth, move jaw side to side. Able to purse lips, wrinkle forehead.	
Expression	Alert with smooth expressive movement.	
Edema	None.	
Lesions/Masses	None.	
Nose		
Septum	Intact and midline.	Nonobstructive deviation frequent and normal occurrence.
Mucosa	Moist and pink; not red or gray; no crusting, edema, lesions.	
PALPATION		
Head		
Masses	None.	
Tenderness	None.	
Sinuses		
Tenderness	None.	
ASSESSMENT OF SMELL	Able to differentiate familiar odors.	Some loss of smell acuity with advanced age.

From References 4, 42, and 59.

cially anxious during a head and neck examination, it is usually best to initiate this assessment by examining a less threatening body system first. Some aspects of the neurosensory examination, for instance, coordination tests and evaluation of deep tendon reflexes, can distract and relax children and permit them to gradually adjust to both the nurse and the new environment.

During the head and face assessment, the nurse readily observes paired facial features such as eyes and ears and bilateral sides of the nose and mouth and notices that all individuals have some degree of asymmetry of their head, face, and features. Learning the acceptable range of normal variation among these features requires diligent practice and verification of findings by the student's instructor.

Recording. Box 16–24 demonstrates the recording of the subjective and objective findings of the evaluation of the head, face, and nose.

Role of the Nurse and the Assessment of the Head, Face, and Nose. Placing clients at ease and ensuring their comfort are major criteria for successful physical assessment of the head and associated structures. Palpation of the head creates an appropriate opportunity for the nurse to teach safety measures that prevent cranial injuries, such as the consistent use of seat belts in the car and of helmets when riding bicycles and motorcycles.

Observation of inappropriate facial expressions (depression, rage, fear, or hostility) can alert the nurse to previously undetected psychiatric or mood disturbances, as well as clues to body self-image. These clues can prompt the nurse to initiate discussions that guide clients to express concerns they may have in this area.

Ear

Overview. The assessment of the ear includes inspection and palpation of the external structures, palpation of the mastoid bone, which lies behind the ear, and testing of auditory acuity (hearing function). Table 16–19 lists questions useful in obtaining subjective information from the client about the health of the ear.

Topographical Anatomy. The ear is divided into three anatomical areas: the external, middle, and inner ear. Only the external ear and tympanic membrane, the window to the middle ear, can be observed. The *auricle,* or *pinna,* and the auditory canal constitute the external ear. The air-filled middle ear contains the bony ossicular chain, and the inner ear is the site of the sensory functions of hearing and equilibrium (Fig. 16–27).

The cartilaginous auricle, also referred to as the pinna (Fig. 16–28), is covered with skin. It has a lower fleshy portion called the lobule (ear lobe). The lobule is susceptible to infection because it is the site of ear piercing. Wide individual variations occur in the size and shape of the external ear. The auditory canal is composed of cartilage laterally and bone medially and is lined with skin, hair, and ceruminous glands. The glands secrete wax (*cerumen*) that, together with the hair, traps foreign particles and prevents them from reaching the tympanic membrane. Poor drainage of cerumen can cause occlusion of the canal and impede hearing. The tragus, the small projection anterior to the entrance of the ear canal, is contiguous with the cartilage that forms the lateral portion of the auditory canal.

The internal structures of the ear are not visible from the surface of the ear and must be observed through a special instrument called the otoscope (Fig. 16–29). The structures of the ear that can be observed with the use of the **otoscope** include the external ear canal and the tympanic membrane and its landmarks. The tympanic membrane forms the border between the environment and the middle ear. The middle ear contains the ossicles (malleus, incus, and stapes), the three tiny bones that transmit sound waves to the internal ear and make hearing possible (see Fig. 16–27). The ossicles form the landmarks of the tympanic membrane that are visible with the otoscope (Fig. 16–30). Other landmarks of the

TABLE 16–19. SAMPLE CLIENT HISTORY QUESTIONS FOR SUBJECTIVE MANIFESTATIONS: EAR

1. Do you have a history of ear pain or injury (trauma) to your ears?
2. Have you ever had ear infections? If so, how frequently do they occur?
3. Have you noticed drainage from your ear canals? What does it look like? *Pus* (purulent discharge)? Blood? Clear fluid? Do you have a history of inflammation in your ear canal (swimmer's ear or otitis externa)? Do your ear canals itch?
4. Do you hear buzzing (*tinnitus*) in your head or your ears? Do you experience popping sounds in your ears when you swallow? When you speak, does your voice reverberate in your head (*autophonia*)?
5. Have you had dizziness, a spinning sensation (vertigo), or nausea associated with your ear discomfort or hearing problem?
6. Do you have difficulty hearing others? Do you need to turn up the radio or television to hear adequately?
7. Do you have speech problems?
8. Does ______ (subjective manifestation) interfere with any of your usual activities? How?

BOX 16–24. RECORDING THE ASSESSMENT OF THE HEAD, FACE, AND NOSE

Subjective Manifestations

Head. Occasional tension headache. No history of head injury.
Face. No complaints of facial pain, involuntary movements, or masses.
Nose and sinuses. One or two colds yearly. Recent onset of nasal congestion with copious clear discharge. No epistaxis or sinusitis.

Objective Manifestations

Head. Erect and midline. No lesions, masses, or tenderness. Scalp clear and free of parasites.
Face. Appropriately expressive with symmetrical movements and clear skin. Able to clench teeth and move jaw from side to side.
Nose and sinuses. Straight and symmetrical. Mucosa pink, with clear discharge. Septum intact and slightly deviated to the right. Nasal cavities barely patent. Frontal and maxillary sinuses nontender.
Smell. Correctly identifies odor of coffee.

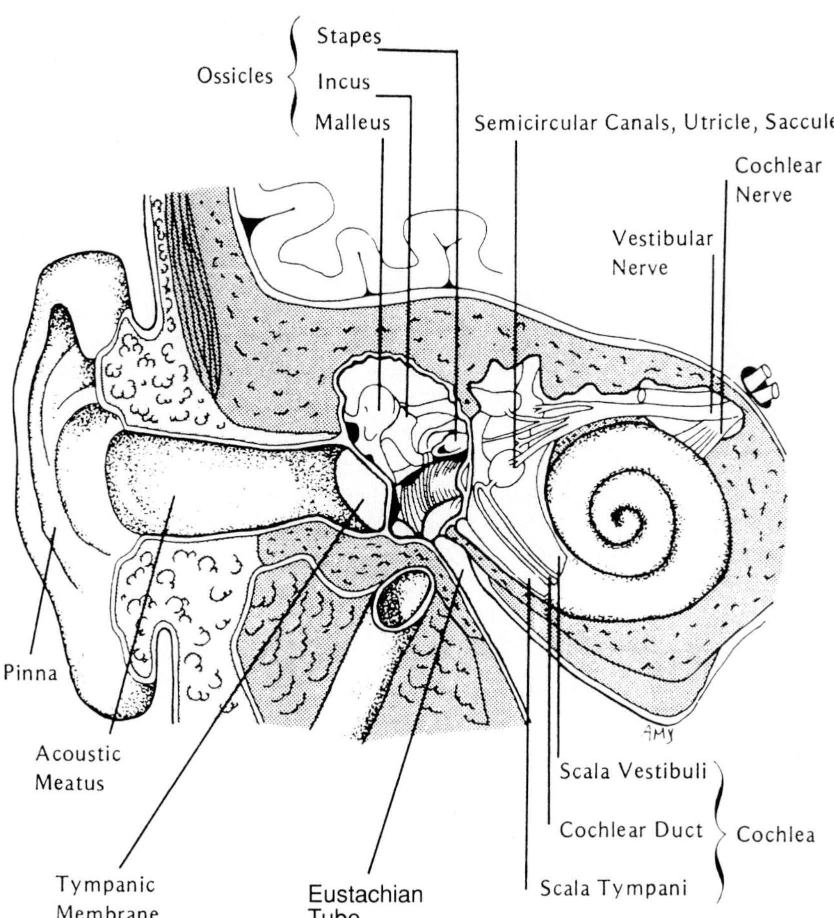

Figure 16–27. Anatomy of the external, middle, and inner ear. (Source: *Berger KJ, Fields, WL.* Pocket Guide to Health Assessment. *Reston, VA: Reston Publishing Co.; 1980.*)

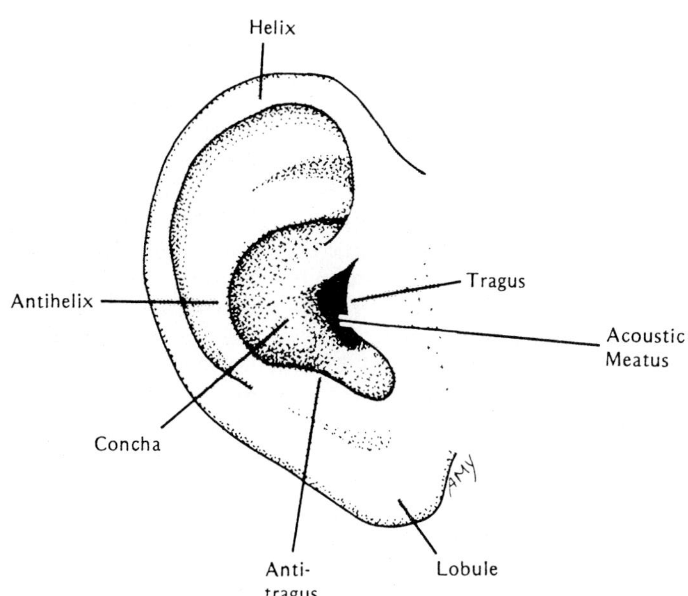

Figure 16–28. The pinna. (Source: *Berger KJ, Fields WL.* Pocket Guide to Health Assessment. *Reston, VA: Reston Publishing Co.; 1980.*)

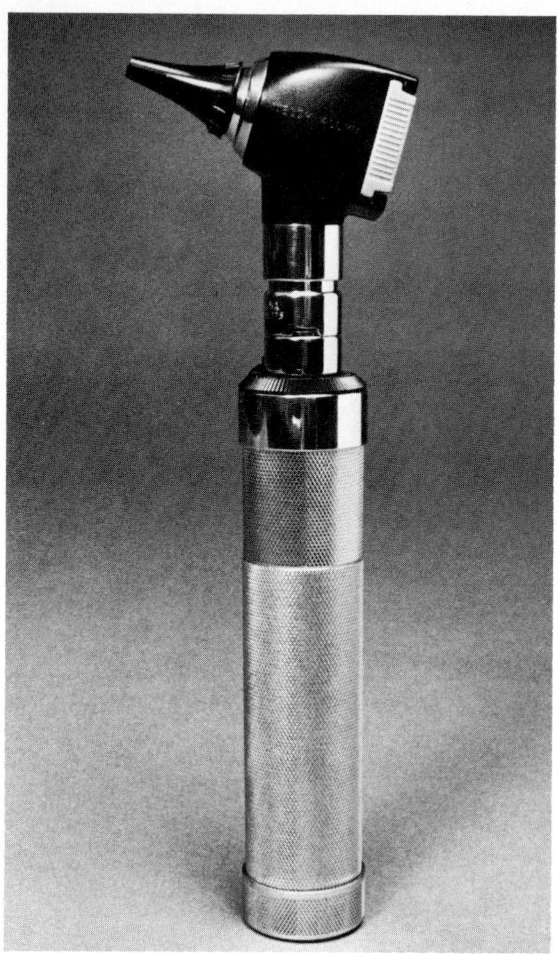

Figure 16–29. Otoscope. (Source: *Block GJ, Nolan JW.* Health Assessment for Professional Nursing: A Developmental Approach. *2nd ed. Norwalk, CT: Appleton-Century-Crofts; 1986.*)

tympanic membrane are the annulus, a fibrotic ring holding the membrane in place, the cone of light (a reflection of the otoscope light on the taut pars tensa), and the malleolar folds that anatomically separate the superior pars flaccida from the inferior pars tensa.

Observation of the tympanic membrane is an advanced technique taught later in the nursing curriculum. (For a discussion of the evaluation of the internal ear and the use of the otoscope, the reader is referred to a textbook of physical assessment.)

The mastoid process behind the ear is the lower portion of the temporal bone and has air-filled spaces that communicate with the middle ear. Infections in the middle ear can spread into the mastoid cells and cause a serious inflammation called mastoiditis. The eustachian tube connects the middle ear with the throat (pharynx) and equalizes the pressure between the middle ear and the environmental air in the auditory canal. When inflammations of the middle ear (*otitis media*) or throat (pharyngitis) disrupt this equilibrium and allow fluid to enter the middle ear, the client experiences pain and sometimes hearing loss. The ossicles articulate with one another to transmit and amplify sound to the internal ear, the site of the auditory nerve (cranial nerve VIII). Beyond the middle ear is the inner ear, which contains the cochlea, the end organ receptors of hearing and balance. Dysfunction in the inner ear structures (cochlea, vestibular apparatus, and the neural end organ for cranial nerve VIII) can cause vertigo, dizziness, and tinnitus as well as sensorineural hearing loss.

Conducting an Examination of the Ear. The examination of the ear incorporates inspection and palpation of the external ear (auricle, tragus, and mastoid process) and assessment of auditory acuity. The simple hearing tests presented here are for screening purposes and do not replace audiometric testing.

Preparation. Seat the client facing you at eye level for the assessment of the ears and hearing. A tuning fork (512 Hz is considered adequate for these tests) is needed to complete the examination. Have children sit on their parents' laps during the ear assessment to allay their fears about this examination.

Inspection. Inspect the auricle for size, shape, and position in relation to the head and eyes. Check to see that the auricles are level with one another. Examine the skin surrounding the ear, particularly the portion behind the ear and overlying the mastoid bone, for scaling, flaking, redness, lesions, and masses. Note any apparent discharge from the ear. Look for lesions and foreign objects in the portions of the ear canal visible to the eye.

Palpation. Gently compress the auricle between the thumb and the first finger, beginning at the top and working toward the lobule. This maneuver elicits the subjective symptom, tenderness, and detects growths and masses. Pressing the index finger against the tragus will cause discomfort when the auditory canal is inflamed.

Hearing. There are two types of hearing loss: conductive and sensorineural. *Conductive hearing loss* results when air vibrations to the inner ear are mechanically disrupted by occlusion of the auditory canal with a foreign body, cerumen, or swelling; fluid formation in the normally air-contained middle ear (inflammation); or fusion of the ossicular bones (otosclerosis). *Sensorineural hearing loss* occurs when aging or disease processes interfere with the transmission of sound to the brain by way of cranial nerve VIII.

Several easily performed tests can effectively screen clients for hearing dysfunction. Most readily available is the whisper test. To perform this test, stand behind the ear to be tested and occlude the other ear by covering it with one hand. In this way, the client cannot read the examiner's lips and it is assured that only one ear is being tested at a time. Softly whisper a word toward the uncovered ear and ask the client to repeat what he or she heard. The whispered word should be audible from a distance of 2 ft. The watch tick test, performed in the same manner, is largely unfeasible because modern watches rarely tick.

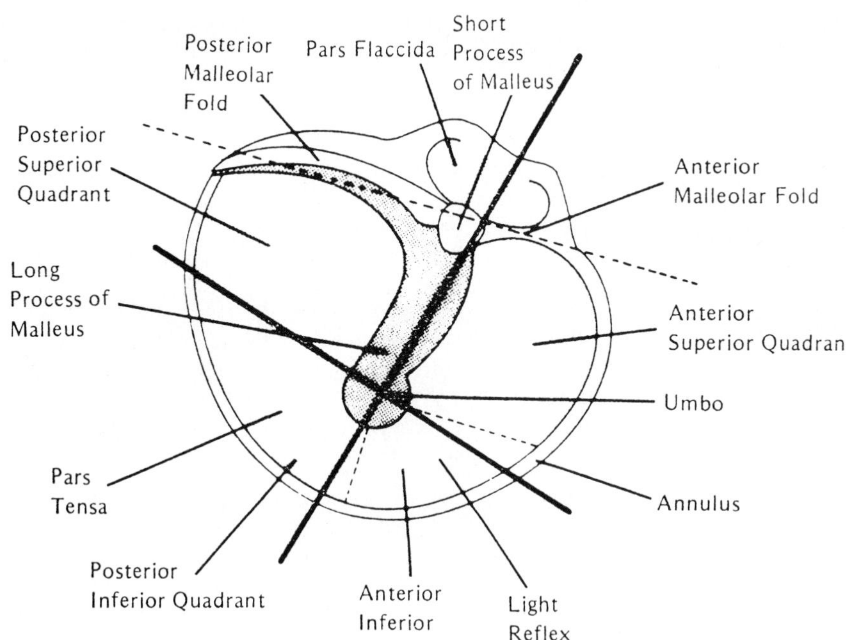

Figure 16–30. Landmarks of the tympanic membrane. (Source: *Berger KJ, Fields WL.* Pocket Guide to Health Assessment. *Reston, VA: Reston Publishing Co.; 1980.*)

Two tuning fork tests are also used to evaluate hearing. They are helpful in differentiating conductive from sensorineural hearing loss. They depend on the conduction of vibrations through air and bone. These tests require that the fork vibrates adequately and that the client understands the tests and the responses. To set the fork vibrating, hold it by the stem and tap it against the fleshy part of your palm. Perform the *Weber test* by placing the vibrating tuning fork in the center of the client's head (Fig. 16–31). Instruct the client to tell you if the sound is heard in one or both ears. The desired response is "both ears." If the sound is heard better in one ear than the other, the client may have either a conductive or a sensorineural hearing loss in one ear. In conductive hearing loss, the sound lateralizes to the poor ear because environmental noise is not getting through. In sensorineural hearing loss, the sound lateralizes to the good ear because that ear does not have nerve damage.

The *Rinne test* compares air conduction with bone conduction. Normally, sound conducted by air is heard twice as long as bone-conducted sound. To perform the test, first place the vibrating tuning fork behind the client's ear directly on the mastoid process and ask the client to tell you when the sound is no longer heard. When this occurs, remove the tuning fork from the mastoid bone and hold it a few inches from the external ear where the client again hears the sound if air conduction is not impeded (Fig. 16–32). Diminished air conduction occurs when the auditory canal is impacted or occluded with cerumen or the middle ear is filled with fluid.

Pure tone audiometry confirms the diagnosis of hearing loss detected by the previously described tests (the whisper test and the tuning fork tests). Referral for audiometric testing is essential for prompt treatment and possible correction of hearing dysfunction.

The expected objective manifestations associated with inspection and palpation of the external ear and the mastoid process are found in Table 16–20. Life cycle variations, including changes in hearing, are described as well.

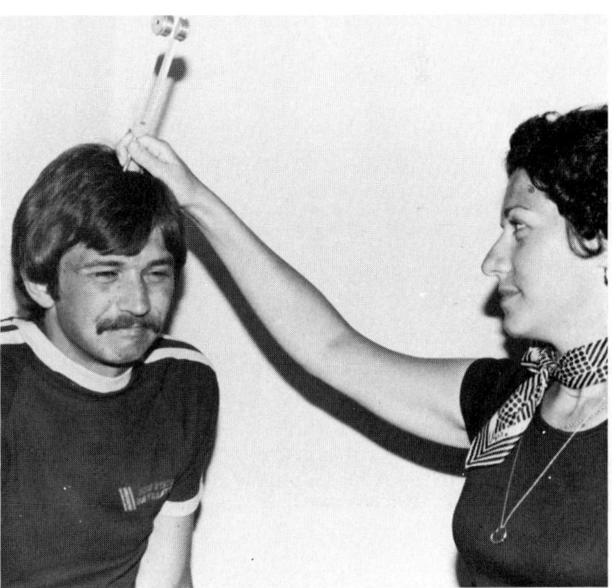

Figure 16–31. Performing the Weber test. (Source: *Block GJ, Nolan JW.* Health Assessment for Professional Nursing: A Developmental Approach. *2nd ed. Norwalk, CT: Appleton-Century-Crofts; 1986.*)

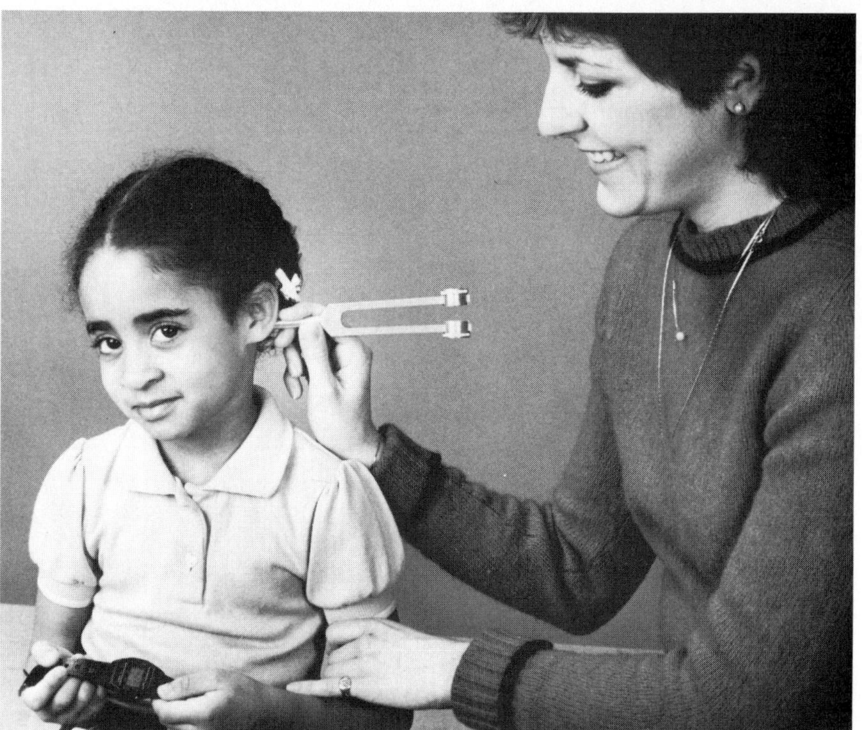

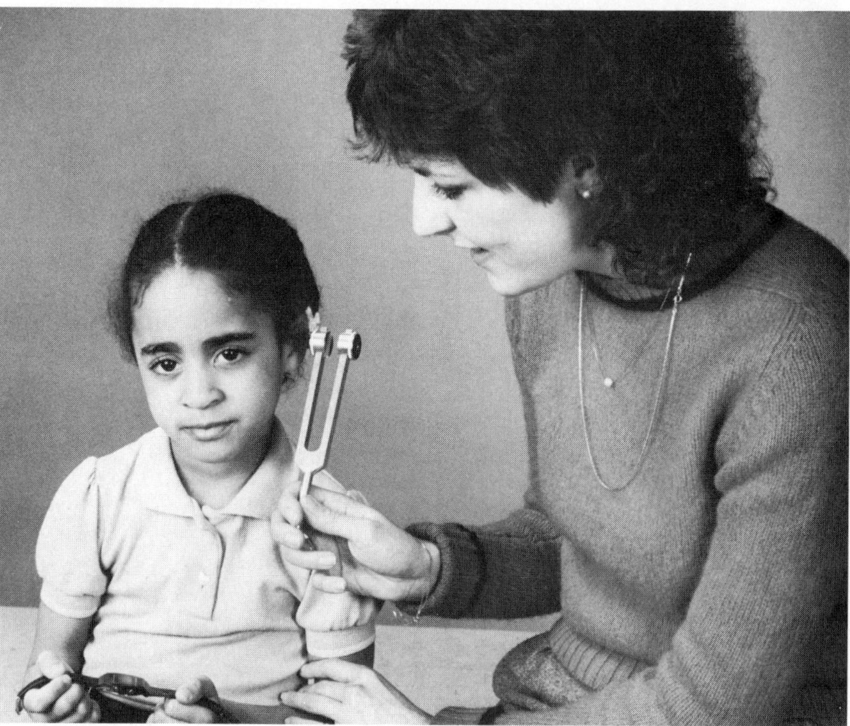

Figure 16–32. Performing the Rinne test. (Source: *Block GJ, Nolan JW.* Health Assessment for Professional Nursing: A Developmental Approach. *2nd ed. Norwalk, CT: Appleton-Century-Crofts; 1986.*)

Special Considerations, Precautions, and Sources of Error. Pain elicited by pressure on the tragus can alert the nurse to inflammation in the auditory canal (otitis externa). This is a clue to refer the client for further evaluation. The hearing tests described here are only screening tests and are not definitive tests for the diagnosis of hearing loss. Referral for audiometric testing and follow-up is essential.

Unsteady stance and unstable gait can be associated with dysequilibrium caused by inner ear disease, as can tinnitus (ringing in the ears), nausea, and vomiting. Signs

TABLE 16–20. OBJECTIVE MANIFESTATION FINDINGS AND LIFE CYCLE VARIATIONS: EAR

Examination Technique	Expected Findings	Common Life Cycle Variations
INSPECTION		
Auricle		
Size	Between 4 and 10 cm in vertical span.	Auricle grows in proportion to the head.
Shape	No deformities, gnarling, or thickening.	Shape of the auricle is often familial. The ear lobule may elongate with aging and creases form in a linear pattern.
Position	Bilaterally symmetrical with top of ear horizontal to the corner of the eye.	
Lesions	None.	
Masses	None present on or behind the ear.	
Mastoid Process	No swelling, redness, or skin lesions.	
PALPATION		
Auricle		
Lesions	None.	
Masses	None.	
Tenderness	None, especially with palpation of tragus.	
Mastoid Process	No tenderness or masses.	
HEARING TESTING		
Voice	Soft whisper heard from a distance of 2 feet with opposite ear occluded.	Hearing is acute in infancy as manifested by alertness to noise stimuli. A brisk Moro reflex (abduction, extension of all four extremities) should follow loud sudden noises. Head turns to source of sound by 4–6 months of age. In childhood, hearing is manifested by attentive, responsive behavior and normal progress in social and educational spheres. Speech development reflects hearing acuteness and by 7th year all sounds should be phonetically correct. Engorged capillaries in eustacian tubes may cause a sense of fullness in the ears during pregnancy. With advanced age, speech reception and discrimination may be reduced.
Weber test	Tuning fork vibrations heard equally loud in each ear, do not lateralize to either.	
Rinne test	Tuning fork heard approximately twice as long by air conduction as by bone conduction.	
Pure tone audiometry	All frequencies within the normal speech range (300–3000) heard at 0–20 decibels.	Gradual sensorineural hearing loss frequently accompanies aging. Auditory reaction time increases.

From References 4, 42, and 59.

indicative of ear difficulties include not only degree of deafness and problems associated with balance but subjective symptoms like ear pain, dizziness, tinnitus, and vertigo. Little children who are unusually irritable and exhibit diminished appetite, disturbed sleep pattern, and diarrhea may be showing systemic signs of middle ear infection.

Recording. Box 16–25 describes a pattern for adequately recording the subjective and objective findings of the examination of the external ear and the evaluation of hearing acuity.

Role of the Nurse and the Assessment of the Ear. The sensory functions of the ear, hearing and equilibrium, account for many client complaints. Hearing difficulties may be brought to the nurse's attention by family members who notice the client has become inattentive and withdrawn. The nurse may detect hearing dysfunction while obtaining the client's health history or giving care. The client may fail to respond to stimuli or misunderstand when others speak or ask questions. A client with hearing loss is often unaware of the disabling effects of progressive deafness on his or her personal relationships. Young children may manifest

BOX 16–25. RECORDING THE ASSESSMENT OF THE EAR

Subjective Manifestations

Ears. Hearing is adequate. No tinnitus, vertigo, earaches, or history of infection. No drainage from the ear canal.

Objective Manifestations

Ears. Top of ears positioned even with the corner of the eyes. Right and left ears without tenderness, discharge, lesions, or deformities. Ear lobes show creasing and elongation consistent with aging. No foreign bodies or cerumen visible in outlet of auditory canal.
Hearing. Hears whisper at 2 ft. No lateralization with Weber test, AC > BC with Rinne test (AC = air conduction, BC = bone conduction).

TABLE 16–21. SAMPLE CLIENT HISTORY QUESTIONS FOR SUBJECTIVE MANIFESTATIONS: EYE

1. What was the date of your last vision test? What were the results? Who tested you?
2. Do you wear glasses? Do you wear contact lenses? When was the last time you had your prescription changed? What type of correction do you have?
3. Do you have any difficulty seeing? Is your vision ever blurred? Do you ever see double (*diplopia*)?
4. Do you have pain around your eyes? Do your eyes itch or tear excessively? Do you ever have pinkeye?
5. Are your eyelids ever swollen (*edema*)?
6. Have you had trouble with crossed eyes (*strabismus*)? Do you suffer from eye fatigue?
7. Have you ever noticed blind spots (*scotomata*)?
8. Do you have pain in the eyes? Do you have eye pain in bright light (*photophobia*)? Have you been tested for glaucoma? What were the results?
9. Does _____ (subjective manifestation) interfere with your usual daily activities? How?

hearing loss by speech delay or school learning difficulties, observations that prompt the school nurse to do a thorough ear assessment.

The nurse may be able to take steps to improve the client's hearing as an outcome of having performed an ear assessment. A thorough assessment of the external ear using the techniques of inspection and palpation, complemented by a hearing evaluation, will yield significant information about the health of the external, middle, and inner ears.

Eye

Overview. The assessment of the eye comprises that part of the client history in which clients are asked about the subjective manifestations associated with their eyes and vision and the eye examination, in which the eyes are observed for the objective manifestations of eye tissue integrity, eye movement, and acuity of vision. Questions for subjective manifestations are summarized in Table 16–21.

Topographical Anatomy. For the purposes of examination, the structures of the eye can be divided into two groups: the external structures and the internal structures.

External Structures. The external structures of the eye include the orbit, eyebrow, eyelid, eyelashes, conjunctiva, sclera, cornea, iris, pupil, nasolacrimal (tear) duct, and extraocular muscles, which control the movements of the eye (Fig. 16–33).

The *orbit* is the opening in the skull in which the eye is located; it provides protection for the eye as do the eyebrows, eyelids, and eyelashes. The inner and outer *canthi,* ordinarily referred to as the corners of the eye, are the points at which the eyelids meet. The *sclera,* or white of the eye, is one of the layers of eyeball tissue; part of the sclera is readily visible from the surface of the eye. The *extraocular muscles,* which are not visible from the surface, attach to the sclera and align and move the eyes in the various fields of gaze. The *conjunctiva* is the colorless membrane that covers the inside of the eyelid and the surface of the eyeball up to the junction of the cornea. The *cornea* is a transparent tissue layer covering the iris, the pigmented band surrounding the pupil, and the *pupil* itself or opening of the eye, which dilates and constricts to modify the amount of light entering the eye. To drain the tears that constantly wash across the eye, the *tear duct* sits in the inner canthus of the eye and leads internally into the nose.

Internal Structures. The internal structures of the eye (Fig. 16–34) are not visible from the surface of the eye and must be observed through a special instrument called the **ophthalmoscope** (Fig. 16–35). The structures of the eye that can be observed with the ophthalmoscope include the lens, the vitreous, the macula, the optic disc, and the tiny blood vessels, arterioles and venules, that serve the internal lin-

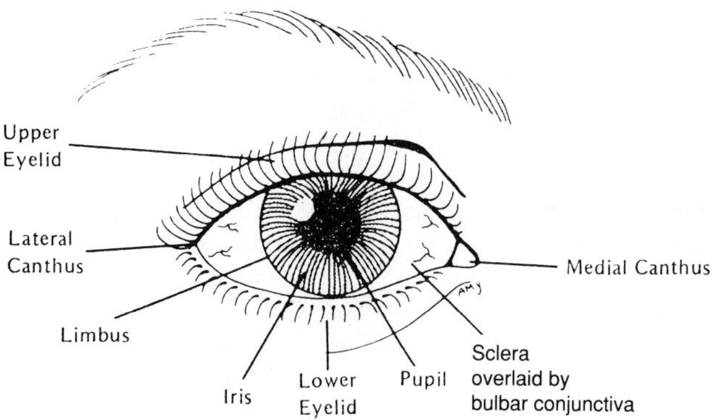

Figure 16–33. External structures of the eye. (Source: *Berger KJ, Fields WL.* Pocket Guide to Health Assessment. *Reston, VA: Reston Publishing Co.; 1980.)*

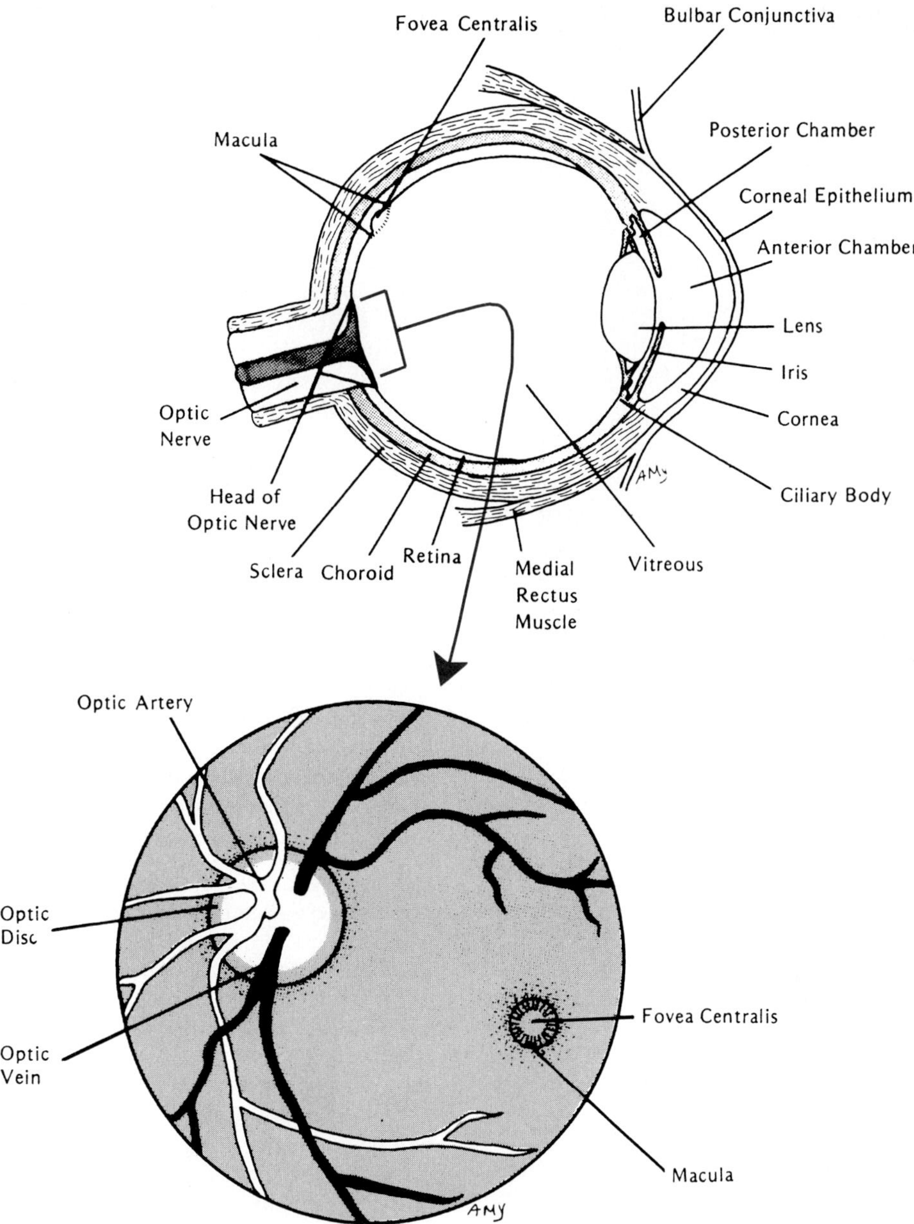

Figure 16–34. Internal structures of the eye. (Source: *Berger KJ, Fields WL.* Pocket Guide to Health Assessment. *Reston, VA: Reston Publishing Co.; 1980.*)

ing of the eye, the retina. These structures are very important to vision. Significant abnormalities can severely impair the client's ability to see or may in some cases even result in blindness. Observation of the internal eye is an advanced technique taught later in the nursing curriculum. The student, however, may observe nurses and physicians conducting ophthalmoscopic examinations and should be aware that the purpose is to observe the structures of the internal eye. (For a discussion of the evaluation of internal eye structures, the reader is referred to a textbook of physical assessment.)

Conducting an Examination of the Eye. Two aspects of examination of the eye are covered in this text: inspection and palpation of the external structures and vision testing. These examination techniques aid the nurse in assessing the overall integrity of the tissue of the eye and the basic adequacy of vision function.

Preparation. For most aspects of the examination of the eye, the client should be in a sitting position facing you at eye level. You will need a penlight and a Snellen chart or newspaper for the eye examination.

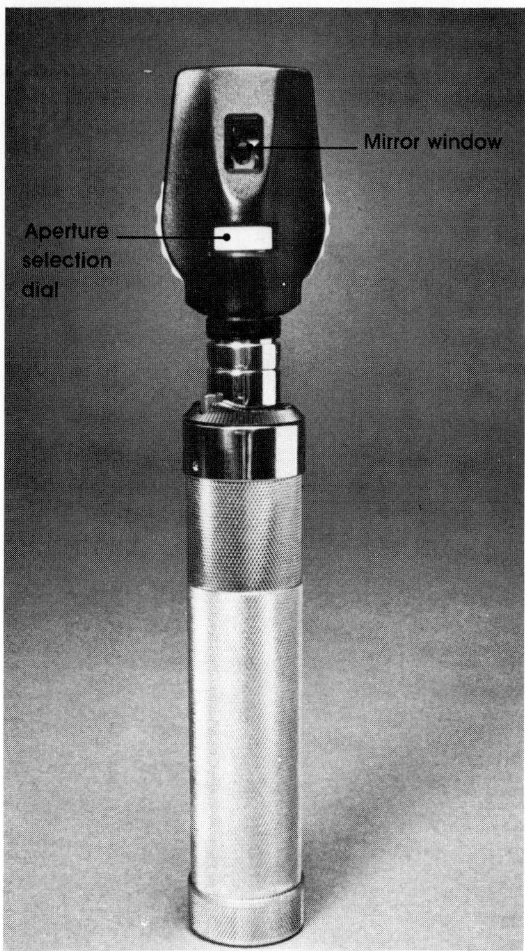

Figure 16–35. Ophthalmoscope. (Source: *Block GJ, Nolan JW.* Health Assessment for Professional Nursing: A Developmental Approach. *2nd ed. Norwalk, CT: Appleton-Century-Crofts; 1986.*)

Inspection. In general, the inspection of the eye involves assessing the characteristic features of the eye structures and eye movement. When inspecting the eyes, it is important to check the color, texture, size, shape, position, and movement of eye structures. The eyes should also be inspected for abnormalities of ocular tissue. Abnormalities are commonly manifested in swelling, pain or tenderness, fluid discharge or pus (exudate), sores, bumps or rashes (lesions), discolorations, changes in contour, or absent or uncoordinated movements of those structures that are expected to move.

Eyebrows, Eyelashes, Eyelids, and Tear Ducts. To assess the external eye structures, note the eyebrows and eyelashes for hair texture, quantity, and distribution. Observe the eyebrows for movement and the eyelids for blinking, drooping, and adequacy of closure. Movement of the eyelids reflects the function of cranial nerve III, the oculomotor nerve, which, when paralyzed, results in the inability to raise the eyelid completely. This abnormality is called *ptosis.* It is also important to assess the characteristics of the surface of the eyelids and observe the nasolacrimal duct for apparent abnormalities.

Conjunctiva. Inspection of the conjunctiva involves observing both the bulbar and palpebral portions. To inspect the *bulbar conjunctiva,* the conjunctiva covering the eyeball itself, retract the client's eyelids using the thumb and index finger, placing pressure on the upper and lower rim of the orbit. Observe the color, texture, and integrity of the conjunctiva.

To observe the palpebral conjunctiva, the portion that lines the inner surface of the eyelid, the client must direct his or her gaze upward as the lower lid is retracted. Upper lid eversion is necessary for full evaluation of the palpebral conjunctiva, but this is an advanced technique and is done only if the client is having symptoms that make upper lid conjunctival inspection essential. (For a discussion of this technique the reader is referred to a textbook of physical assessment.)

Sclerae. Inspect the sclera for color and particularly color change. Normally white, the sclera becomes yellow-tinged when the client is jaundiced, a condition associated with liver disease in which the skin, eyes, mucous membranes, and body fluids turn yellow from the deposit of bile pigment. In African-American individuals, however, yellowish deposits do not necessarily indicate abnormality.

Cornea. Next, examine the cornea with a light. Ask the client to look straight ahead while holding a penlight at an oblique angle to the eye and move it slowly across the corneal surface. Look for clarity, discolorations, and deviations of the contour of the cornea.

The check for corneal sensitivity involves touching the cornea with a wisp of cotton. This usually causes pain in the eye and reflects the function of cranial nerve V, the trigeminal nerve. Testing for corneal sensitivity is an advanced technique taught later in the nursing curriculum. (Refer to a textbook of physical assessment for a description of this technique.)

Iris. Inspect the iris for its color and shape. The color reflects family and genetic heritage. Color is usually present and consistent in both eyes; the shape is round and symmetrical.

Pupil. Observe the pupils for degree of dilation or constriction. Estimate the diameter in millimeters. After noting the size of each pupil, inspect them as a pair for symmetry.

Next, check the pupils for reactivity to light. To evaluate the ability of the pupil to react to light, darken the environment to the extent possible and shine a bright light such as a penlight into each pupil. Ask the client to avoid looking at the light, and bring the light rapidly into the field of vision from the outer corner of the eye to prevent the client from looking at the light as it approaches. Watch for constriction of the pupil into which the light is shined (Fig. 16–36). This is called a *direct reaction to light*. The pupil is also expected to constrict, although to a lesser degree, when the light is shined in the other eye. This is called a *consensual reaction to light*. Assess it in the same way; only watch for a reaction in the eye opposite to the one in which the light is shining. The response of the pupils to light reflects the function of cranial nerves III (oculomotor nerve), IV (trochlear nerve), and VI (abducens nerve).

The pupils are also expected to change in size to accommodate for near and distant vision, dilating to bring in more light when looking at a distant object. To assess *accommodation*, hold a finger 15 cm (6 in.) in front of the client and ask the client to look at it. Observe the pupil response as the client looks first at the finger and then at a distant object.

Eye Alignment. Eye alignment is important for vision. Faulty eye alignment is known technically as *strabismus*, but commonly referred to as crossed eyes. To inspect the alignment of the eyes, observe the reflection of light on the cornea. After darkening the room, have the client look straight ahead and direct a penlight to the bridge of the client's nose. When the eyes are in alignment, the light reflects from the same part of the cornea in each eye. This is called the *Hirchberg test*.

Extraocular Movements. Although the extraocular muscles themselves cannot be visualized, the adequacy of their function can be assessed by checking eye position and movement. To inspect the extraocular movements, check the eyes first for their position at rest. Observe the symmetry of eye position.

Next, look at the eyes in motion. Watch the eyes as they move through the *six cardinal fields of gaze* (Fig. 16–37). Have the client moves his or her eyes to follow the movement of a penlight. Ask the client to hold his or her head in a fixed position facing you while following the light with eyes only. Trace a large letter "H" form in the air with the penlight, moving first to the extreme right and moving the light up and down on that side. Then repeat the procedure on the left. Observe the eyes for their ability to follow the penlight with balanced, smooth, symmetrical movement. The position and movement of the eyes reflect the innervation of cranial nerves III, IV, and VI.

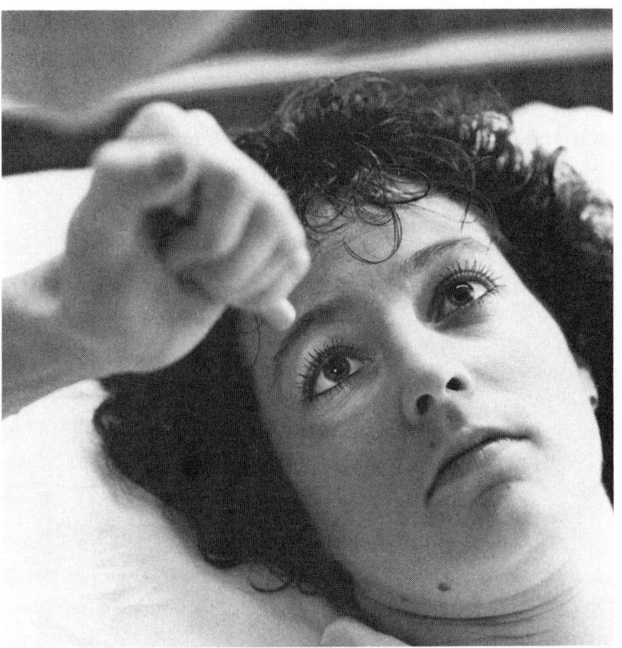

Figure 16–36. Assessment of direct and consensual reactions to light.

Palpation. The eye examination relies mainly on inspection; however, it also includes an important observation that requires the technique of palpation.

Ocular Tension. Palpation of the eyeball is done to assess ocular tension, the hardness or softness of the eyeball. This technique can be helpful in diagnosing the client's state of hydration, because in a condition of dehydration the eyeball can become unexpectedly soft. Some diseases such as glaucoma, a serious chronic disease of the eye that can lead to blindness, result in increased ocular tension, and the eyeball feels harder to the touch.

To palpate for ocular tension, ask the client to look downward. Place both index fingers on the upper eyelid. Apply gentle pressure (ballottement) to the eyelid with one finger and then withdraw the finger. Keep the other finger in place to feel for the degree of hardness or softness of the eyeball tissue as it rebounds against the finger.

Vision. Basic vision testing is a useful technique to identify whether impaired vision might interfere with the client's ability to cope or might place the client at risk for accidents. Vision reflects the function of cranial nerve II, the optic nerve.

A very basic check of functional ability is done simply by shining a penlight from a lateral position toward the client's eye. While doing this, turn the penlight on and off and ask the client to identify when the light is on or off.

Another basic check involves moving a hand in front of the client's face at a distance of 30 cm (1 ft). Periodically stop the movement, and ask the client to identify when the hand movement has stopped. Still another easy check for vision, particularly near vision, is simply to have the client read. After ascertaining that the client is literate and proficient in the language of the copy presented, ask the client to read a portion of newsprint at normal reading distance, 30 to 36 cm (12 to 14 in.). The client should be able to read the copy.

The formal screening test for vision involves the use of the Snellen chart or another standardized eye assessment

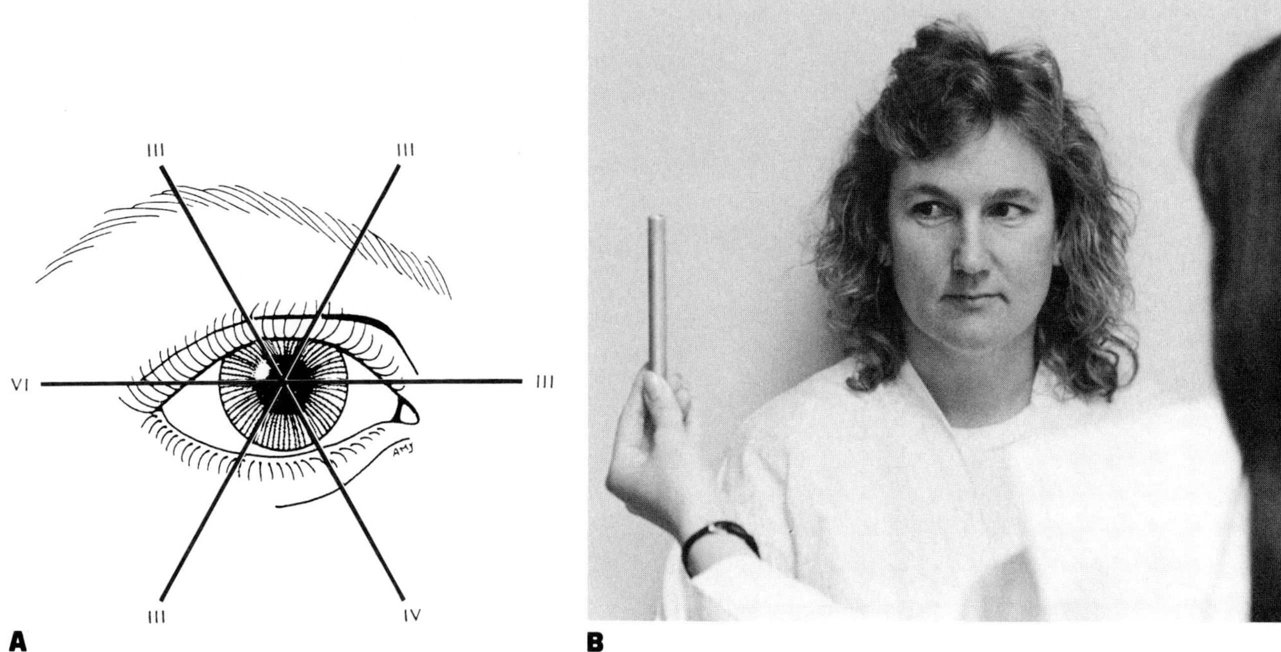

Figure 16–37. Extraocular movements. Roman numerals refer to cranial nerve controlling direction of gaze. (**A** from *Berger KJ, Fields WL.* Pocket Guide to Health Assessment. *Reston, VA: Reston Publishing Co.; 1980.*)

chart (Fig. 16–38). Ask the client to stand or sit 6 m (20 ft) from the chart, wearing corrective eyeglasses if these are necessary for distant vision. Test each eye separately, covering the eye that is not being tested. Ask the client to read the letters on the chart, starting with the larger letters. The lines of letters are graded according to the degree of visual acuity they represent.

Color vision is checked by asking the client to differentiate the red and green lines on the Snellen chart. Request the client to "read the letters over the green line." The green line is line 6 on the chart. Likewise, ask the client to "read the letters over the red line." Line 8 is the red line.

Peripheral vision is also important to the client's ability to cope with the environment. Peripheral vision includes the images in the visual field that surround those in central focus.

In checking peripheral vision, it is important to check the client's vision in four peripheral fields: (1) the nasal field, which is the inner or proximal field; (2) the temporal field, which is the lateral field; (3) the upward field; and (4) the downward field. Peripheral vision is tested simply by comparing the client's visual fields with those of the examiner. It is assumed that the examiner has good peripheral vision.

To conduct the check, the examiner stands directly in front of the client so that their eyes are at the same level. Looking at the client's nose, ask the client to look directly at your nose. Check each eye separately. Cover the client's left eye when the client's right eye is checked. Reverse the order for your own eyes, covering the right eye (Fig. 16–39). To check the nasal field of vision of the client's right eye, extend your right arm; raise the index finger and slowly bring the finger to a midline position between examiner and client. Ask the client to state when your finger comes into view. Note whether you can also see the finger. Also note the point of the client's visualization as the degrees (of a circle) it is distant from the central point of vision (the nose). Repeat for the temporal field, this time extending the left arm to the side, bringing in the raised index finger from the left. Again, compare the point at which you can see the finger with the point at which the client states he or she sees it and note it as the number of degrees from the point of central vision.

After checking the nasal and temporal fields, conduct the procedure again for upward and downward fields. To check the upward field, move the arm and raised index finger in from the lower periphery. To check the downward field, move the arm in from the upper periphery.

When all fields are checked in one eye, repeat the entire process for the other eye. This procedure is referred to as *gross confrontation*.

The expected findings for the various external structures of the eye and for vision and some of the common variations of findings that occur with the phases of the life cycle are outlined in Table 16–22.

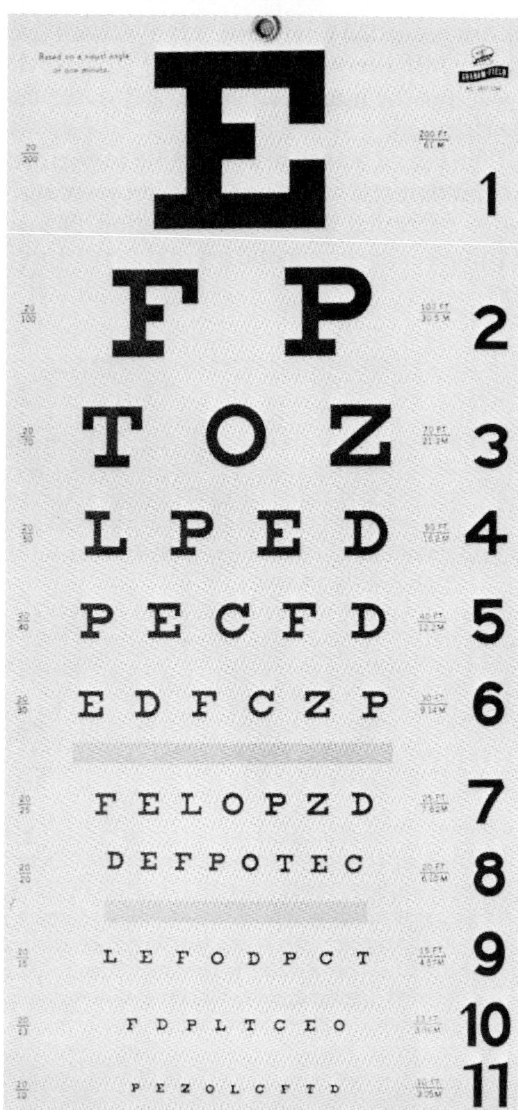

Figure 16–38. Snellen chart. (Source: *Block GJ, Nolan JW.* Health Assessment for Professional Nursing: A Developmental Approach. *2nd ed. Norwalk, CT: Appleton-Century-Crofts; 1986.*)

Special Considerations, Precautions, and Sources of Error. Because of the importance of the eye and its structures and of the function of vision, it is necessary that the examiner use gentle technique in carrying out the examining procedures, particularly on such procedures as retracting the eyelids. The surface of the eye is delicate. Not only is it vulnerable to abrasions and bruises, but it is also very sensitive to pain. Careful technique prevents client discomfort. Instruments such as penlights should be used with great caution in the area of the eye, and to minimize the risk of nosocomial infection, the examiner should make sure that gloves are donned before conducting the parts of the examination that involve touching the eye.

Recording. The final step in the assessment of the eye is to record the findings. The subjective manifestations are recorded as part of the health history (Box 16–26).

Role of the Nurse and the Assessment of the Eye. Understanding what are the expected characteristics of the healthy eye enables the nurse to quickly assess apparent abnormalities, to alert the client to the need to get further evaluation, or, if necessary, to make a referral for medical treatment.

Nurse generalists in the hospital may find that clients who are there for other reasons develop eye problems while in the hospital that require assessment. Moreover, loss of visual acuity is a very common difficulty experienced by clients. When the loss of vision is severe, it may interfere with important functional dimensions such as mobility. A plan of client care that involves ambulation to preserve mobility may require that the nurse first assess the client's vision to determine if it is sufficient to support safe ambulation.

Nurses who work in community health and advanced practice settings frequently are faced with situations in which eye assessment skills are important. Often the nurse is the first health care professional to see a family member

BOX 16–26. RECORDING THE ASSESSMENT OF THE EYE

Subjective Manifestations

Eyes. Last vision test, 3/27/88. Vision R—20/40, L—20/20. Tested by Dr. Leventhal. Does not require corrective lenses. Reports no difficulty seeing; denies blurred or double vision; denies pain around eyes; reports pinkeye in right eye for last 24 hours, itching of right eye, swelling of right eyelid; no itching or swelling of left eye; denies strabismus or eye fatigue; no scotomata, no pain in eyes, no photophobia. Tested for glaucoma, 2/12/85; reports results were normal.

Objective Manifestations

Eyes

- *Lids.* Right—tearing, green crusting on lower lid; no edema; left—no tearing, crusting, or edema. No ptosis.
- *Conjunctiva.* Right—reddened (erythematous); left—no erythema.
- *Cornea.* No clouding bilaterally.
- *Sclera.* White, bilaterally.
- *Iris.* Brown, round bilaterally.
- *Pupil.* PERRLA.
- *Nasolacrimal duct.* No discharge from inner canthus.
- *Alignment.* Light reflex symmetrical.
- *Extraocular movement.* No strabismus.
- *Vision.* Snellen: OD 20/40; OS 20/20. Visual fields: 60 degrees nasally, 50 degrees upward, 90 degrees temporally, 70 degrees downward by confrontation.

TABLE 16–22. OBJECTIVE MANIFESTATION FINDINGS AND LIFE CYCLE VARIATIONS: EYE

Examination Technique	Expected Findings	Common Life Cycle Variations
INSPECTION		
Eyebrow/eyelashes		
Color/texture	Consistent with age and family heritage	Graying is observed with advanced age.
Condition	Shiny, flexible hair shafts, not broken or dry; no tenderness, redness, or swelling of the hair follicles	
Quantity	Present in moderate to dense thickness; thinning or absence may suggest illness	Thinning may be the result of plucking in young women but also occurs with advanced age.
Distribution	Thick, short eyebrow hairs along arched bone prominence above orbit; eyelash hairs long or short, extending from edges of eyelids in double or triple rows	
Eyelids		
Color	Consistent with body skin color; appropriate to family heritage	
Shape	Consistent with family heritage; no turning outward (ectropian) or turning inward (entropian) of the edges; no extra fold of skin covering the inner corner of the eye (epicanthal folds)	Epicanthal folds are commonly found in Asian children. They are present in 20 percent of Caucasian children but should disappear by age 10. Ectropian and entropian are found more often in older adults.
Position	Able to open eyes fully on request; no drooping; white of eye not visible on eye closure; no squinting in the absence of high light intensity	Gradual loss of lid elasticity leads to drooping of the eyelids in the elderly.
Movement	6–12 blinks per minute; no staring or twitching	
Swelling	None	
Lesions	None	
Discharge	No crusting	
Nasolacrimal duct		
Color	Pink, no redness in the area of the opening (punctum)	
Tearing	No spilling of tears in the absence of a stimulus (crying, foreign body); no absence of tears	Tearing is not common before 3 months of age.
Swelling	No distention of the duct	Occasionally the opening (punctum) of the duct is imperforate in the neonate (a condition that requires surgery) and the duct may become distended. Lacrimal gland function may change during pregnancy and pregnant women may complain of dry eyes.
Discharge	None	
Eyeball and orbit		
Eyeball size	Symmetrical	
Orbital contour	Smoothly arched	
Position in socket	Symmetrical depth; no recession of eyeball into the orbit (enophthalamus) or protrusion of the eyeball from the orbit (exophthalamus)	
Spacing of orbits	No unexpected width (hypertelorism) or narrowing (hypotelorism) between the eyes	
Conjunctiva		
Color	Transparent; palpebral pink, bulbar white; no pallor of palpebral conjunctiva; no red, yellow, or brown discoloration	Pink or red discoloration of the conjunctiva representing inflammation (pinkeye or conjunctivitis) occurs frequently in children, is often associated with discharge, and may accompany a cold or other illness. Patches (plaques) and infiltration of discoloring substances (degenerative infiltrates) accompanying advanced age may appear on the conjunctiva of the elderly.
Moisture	Glistening; moist appearance; no dullness	
Lesions	None	
Swelling	None	
Discharge	No drainage or pus	

(continued)

TABLE 16–22. (continued)

Examination Technique	Expected Findings	Common Life Cycle Variations
Sclera		
Color	White to light brown varying with genetic heritage; no yellow discoloration in light-skinned individuals	The sclerae of newborns may be slightly bluish, which fades as the infant ages.
Contour	Smoothly rounded; no irregularities	
Cornea		
Color	Transparent, not cloudy or pigmented; no gray discoloration around the outer edge (limbus)	Elderly persons sometimes acquire an arc or circle of gray-colored degenerative material (arcus senilis) around the limbus of the cornea. This does not interfere with vision.
Contour	Smoothly rounded; no bulging; no abrasions, ulcerations, or swellings	
Iris		
Color	Symmetrical and consistent with family and racial heritage; no absence or dulling of color	
Pupil		
Size	3 to 6 mm, symmetrical; neither widely dilated or narrowly constricted (pinpoint); small size difference (0.5 mm) not significant	Pupils of infants are frequently slightly smaller. Pupils may also be slightly smaller in the aged.
Shape	Perfectly round	
Reactivity	Prompt constriction in response to direct and consensual light stimulus and accommodation for near vision; no sluggishness or absence of reactivity	
Eye alignment	Corneal light reflex symmetrical	Strabismus is a congenital condition found in 3–5 percent of children. When eyes are not aligned, double images (diplopia) are passed to the brain. Gradually the child learns not to use the deviating eye. Early detection can prevent this situation. Intermittent strabismus in which eyes converge toward a common point is not abnormal before 3 months of age.
Extraocular movement	Smooth, symmetrical movements through all six cardinal positions of gaze—no divergence in any position	Short periods of constant jerky movements of the eyeball (nystagmus) may be seen in infants who are not yet focusing, usually before 6 weeks of age.
PALPATION		
Ocular tension	Prompt rebound of indented sclera when examining finger is withdrawn; no spongy or hard consistency	Glaucoma, a condition of increased intraocular pressure, occurs in 1.5 percent of the middle-aged population and is the most common cause of blindness in that group.
VISION TESTING		
Visual acuity	Able to accurately call out letters in the 20/20 test line of Snellen chart or other eye testing chart from a distance of 6 m (20 ft)	Peripheral vision fully developed at birth in term newborns. From birth until age 4–5, children are myopic. 20/20 visual acuity is reached by age 5. Because vision is so important to learning, visual screening is a very important aspect of the health care of children. In middle age, the lens of the eye loses elasticity and fails to accommodate to near vision. Farsightedness again results (presbyopia) and reading glasses become necessary.
Color vision	Able to differentiate between green and red lines on Snellen chart	
Near vision	Able to read newsprint at a distance of 30 cm (1 ft)	
Visual field integrity	Able to identify object from angle of 60 degrees nasally, 50 degrees upward, 90 degrees temporally, and 70 degrees downward	Because peripheral vision is most often affected by glaucoma, gross confrontation is an important part of the screening examination of middle-aged adults.

From References 4, 42, and 59.

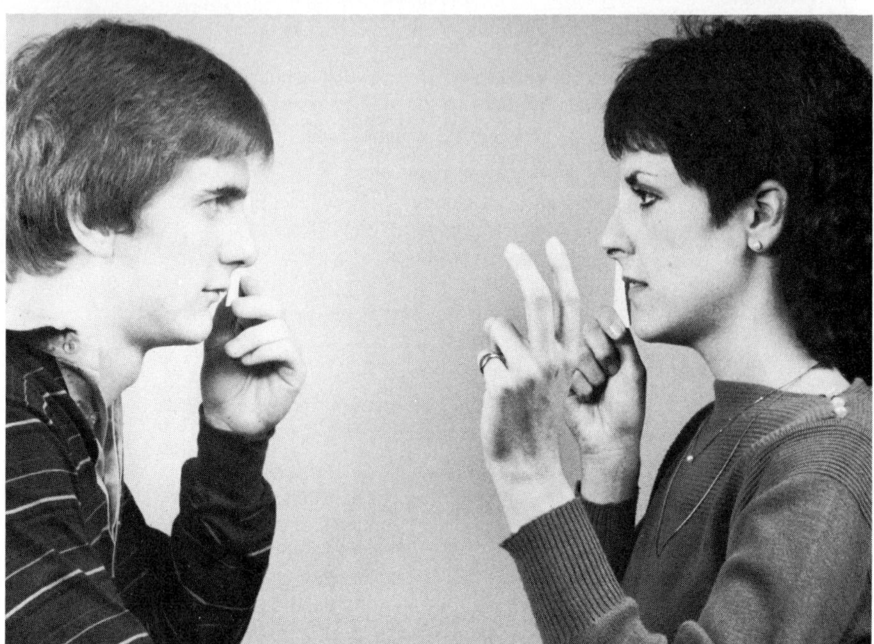

Figure 16–39. Testing the right nasal field of vision. (Source: *Block GJ, Nolan JW.* Health Assessment for Professional Nursing: A Developmental Approach. *2nd ed. Norwalk, CT: Appleton-Century-Crofts; 1986.*)

who has developed an eye abnormality. The school nurse, for instance, uses eye assessment skills to do vision screening on the population of children in the school and with children who get foreign objects in their eyes or who may have abrasions or infections in the eye. Nurse practitioners are frequently called on to perform complete eye examinations in clinic settings. These are only a few of the many applications of the assessment of the eye in nursing practice that make it a valuable skill for the student to develop.

Mouth and Throat

Overview. Physical assessment of the mouth and throat consists primarily of inspection and occasionally of palpation. The purpose is to examine the oral cavity, the teeth and gums, and to visualize the oropharynx. The subjective questions relating to the health of the mouth and throat are found in Table 16–23.

Topographical Anatomy. The structures of the oral cavity are the lips, the teeth and gums, the tongue, the buccal mucosa that lines the cheeks, the hard and soft palates that form the roof of the mouth, and the oropharynx or back of the throat (Fig. 16–40). The *oropharynx* consists of the anterior and posterior pillars that produce the fauces for the tonsils, if the tonsils have not been surgically removed. The posterior pharynx is covered with mucous membranes and lymphoid tissue, similar to the tonsils. The buccal mucosa lines the inside of the cheeks and lips. The ducts from the salivary glands open into the oral cavity and are visible as small openings in the mucosa. The parotid duct opens opposite the second upper molars and the mandibular ducts are located in the mucous membranes beneath the tongue. The fleshy connection between the underside of the tongue and the floor of the mouth is the *frenulum.* The bony roof of the mouth is called the *hard palate* and its posterior portion is the *soft palate.* The *uvula* is an extension of the soft palate and is the soft, pendulous tag of tissue seen hanging from the roof of the mouth. The average adult has 32 teeth. The number of teeth in children varies by developmental stage and age.

Conducting an Examination of the Mouth and Throat. Assessment of the mouth and throat begins with inspection of the lips and progresses to visualization of the internal structures. Sometimes it is necessary to palpate the buccal mucosa, the tongue, and the gums.

Preparation. The client sits facing you at eye level. You will need a penlight and a tongue blade to adequately visualize the mouth and throat and gloves to protect your hands while palpating oral structures. Assessment of taste requires a source of flavors—salty, sweet, sour, and bitter.

Inspection. Inspect the lips and the oral cavity including the teeth, gums, buccal mucosa, tongue, hard and soft palate, and anterior and posterior pharynx.

Look closely at the client's lips for color, lesions, and dryness before asking her or him to open the mouth. Dry weather and constant lip licking can cause cracking and fissures. Anemia may make normally pink lips appear pale and lack of oxygenation can cause them to appear bluish. Ask the client to open the mouth and direct inspection from the front to the back of the oral cavity. Holding the penlight in one hand and the tongue blade in the other, observe the teeth and gums. The appropriate number of teeth should all be present and free of decay.

TABLE 16–23. SAMPLE CLIENT HISTORY QUESTIONS FOR SUBJECTIVE MANIFESTATIONS: MOUTH AND THROAT

1. When was your last dental examination?
2. Do you wear dentures?
3. Do you have toothaches or sensitive teeth?
4. Do you have broken teeth or teeth with cavities (*caries*)?
5. Do you grind your teeth (*bruxism*)?
6. Are there any sores in your mouth?
7. Do your gums bleed (*gingivitis*)?
8. Do you experience sore throats (*pharyngitis*) or difficulty swallowing (*dysphagia*)?
9. Do you have persistent hoarseness?
10. Does _____ (subjective manifestation) interfere with any of your usual daily activities? How?

The gums should not be swollen or show evidence of bleeding and they should adhere closely to the teeth. Touch the tongue blade gently to the gums to determine their texture. Healthy gums are firm and not spongy and do not bleed because they are inflamed (gingivitis). To check alignment, instruct the client to lightly close the upper and lower teeth together. Ask the client who wears dentures or a partial plate to remove these; then note if there are any lesions on the gums caused by ill-fitting dental appliances.

Inspect the tongue by asking the client to protrude it from the mouth and move it from side to side to permit its assessment for movement and alignment, surface texture, color, and coating. Movement of the tongue reflects the function of cranial nerve XII, the hypoglossal nerve. Note any involuntary tremors that might be indicative of neurological dysfunction. Ask the client to curl the tongue backward by pressing the tip against the hard palate; this permits observation of the underside for lesions and also of the floor of the mouth. Find the openings of the submandibular salivary glands and note if they are inflamed or swollen. Blood vessels visible on the floor of the mouth are frequently enlarged in adults and are a normal finding.

Use the tongue blade to retract the sides of the mouth and assess the buccal mucosa for color and lesions. Place the tongue blade on top of the client's tongue, hold it down, and ask the client to say "ahh" to facilitate visualization of the back of the throat (Fig. 16–41). The uvula and soft palate should rise symmetrically during this maneuver and not deviate to one side or the other. The movement of the uvula and soft palate reflects the function of cranial nerve IX, the glossopharyngeal nerve, and cranial nerve X, the vagus nerve. This maneuver may elicit the gag reflex, which also reflects the function of cranial nerves IX and X.

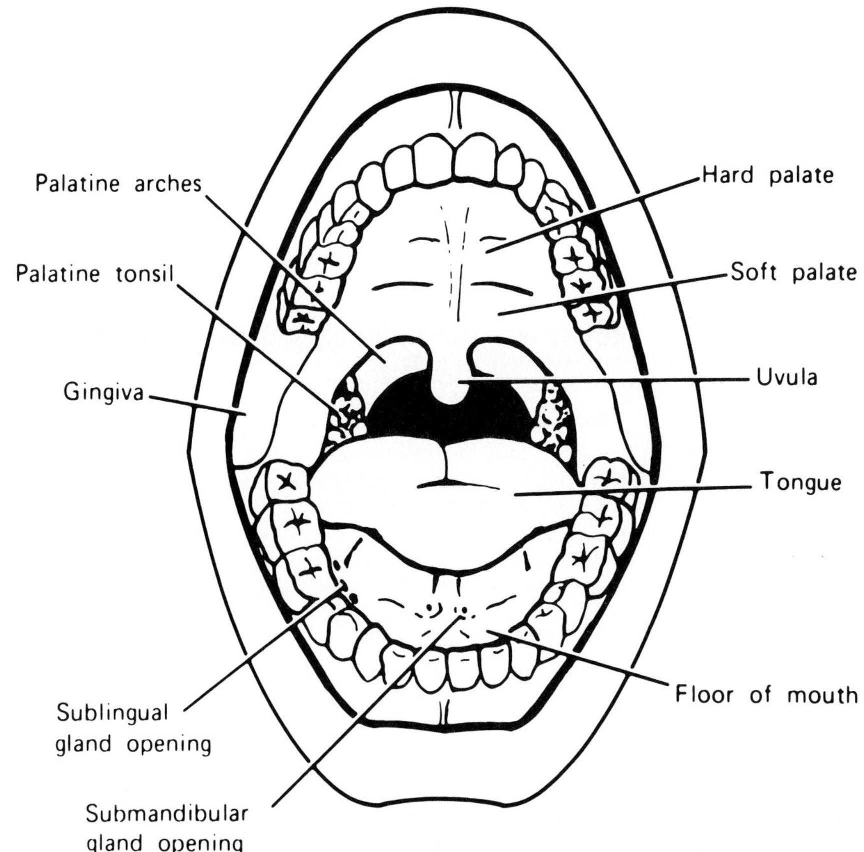

Figure 16–40. Oral cavity. (Source: *Fields WL, McGinn-Campbell KM.* Introduction to Health Assessment. *Reston, VA: Reston Publishing Co.; 1983.*)

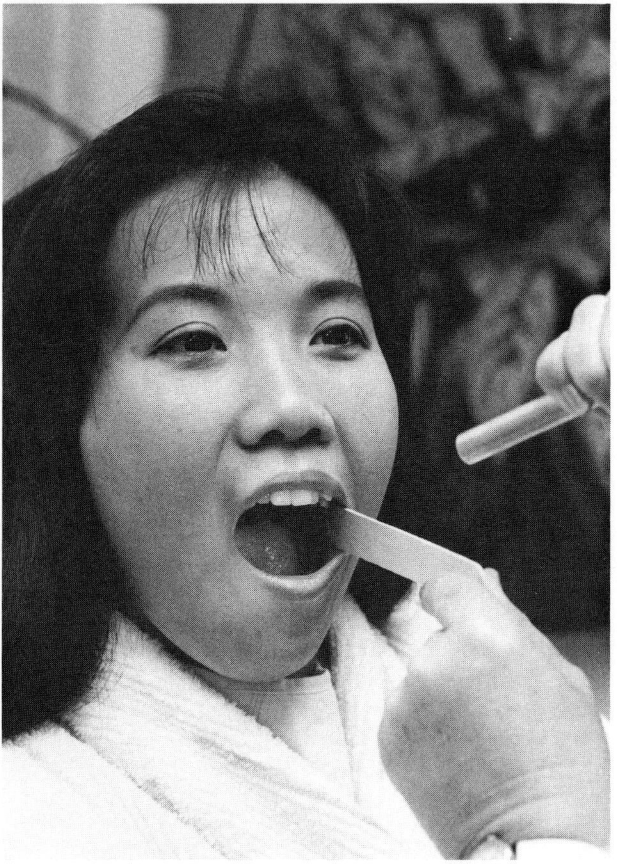

Figure 16–41. Assessing the buccal mucosa.

The mucous membranes of the oropharynx are usually the same color as the lining of the mouth. When the tonsils are red and swollen, the client may have tonsillitis. Sometimes, inflamed tonsils have pus (exudate) on the outer surfaces. The posterior pharynx contains patches of lymphoid tissue similar to the tonsils and this tissue can also become swollen and exude discharge (pharyngitis). Complete the inspection of the mouth and throat by lightly touching the tongue blade to the oropharynx in the area of the tonsils to elicit the gag reflex.

Palpation. Put on a glove before running your index finger along the inside of the cheeks to assess the buccal mucosa for tenderness or nodules. Use gloved hands to pull the lower lip outward to improve the view of the mucosa. It is sometimes necessary to grasp the client's tongue to determine its consistency and check for swellings or masses.

Taste. The sense of taste, which diminishes with age, reflects the function of cranial nerve VII, the facial nerve, and cranial nerve IX, the glossopharyngeal nerve. If there is reason to suspect that the client's sense of taste is diminished, it can be assessed easily as the client eats a meal by simply asking the client to close his or her eyes, protrude the tongue, and identify the various foods presented on the tip of a spoon. When possible, the flavors presented should include salty, sweet, sour, and bitter tastes.

Table 16–24 describes the expected findings of the head and neck examination as well as the normal variations.

Special Considerations, Precautions, and Sources of Error. The oral cavity contains several structures (teeth and gums, buccal mucosa, tongue, and oropharynx), each of which needs thorough evaluation. A systematic plan carefully adhered to with each assessment helps the nurse to avoid omissions. For example, it is systematic to start from the front, first inspecting the lips and then proceeding to the assessment of the gums and teeth, the buccal mucosa, the tongue, and finally the oropharynx. Nurses sometimes tend to focus most carefully on the pharynx and the tonsils and forget how significant dental caries, gum disease, and oral lesions are to the general good health of the client. Use of a penlight and tongue blade is indispensable to the completeness of the examination.

Recording. The data elicited from the client relating to the health of teeth, gums, oral mucosa, tongue, and pharynx are recorded in the health history along with the rest of the information he or she relates about the head and sensory organs. Objective findings are also recorded as part of the head and neck examination. Examples of a written record containing your findings are in Box 16–27.

Role of the Nurse and the Assessment of the Mouth and Throat. The oral cavity is the site of many pathological conditions, such as cancer, gum disease, tooth decay, and inflammation of the mucosa and tonsillar tissue from allergy or infection. Sometimes cancers go undetected because they are painless and difficult to see, lying under a client's dentures or tongue where the client is unable to observe them. The nurse who carefully observes the mouth for lesions can help prevent the development of a serious condition.

BOX 16–27. RECORDING THE ASSESSMENT OF THE MOUTH AND THROAT

Subjective Manifestations

Dental exam. Last dental exam Oct. 14, 1990.
Teeth. No dentures, missing teeth, or caries. Denies bruxism, sensitive teeth, or gum disease.
Mouth. No oral lesions.
Throat. Rarely has sore throat. Denies dysphagia and persistent hoarseness.

Objective Manifestations

Lips. Moist, pink, and without lesions.
Mucosa. Buccal mucosa intact, pink and moist.
Teeth. Clean, aligned, and no visible caries. Numerous fillings.
Tongue. Mobile, midline, and extends without tremors.
Throat. Tonsils are small, no redness or exudate. Uvula is midline and elevates with phonation.
Taste. Able to distinguish sweet from sour flavors.

TABLE 16–24. OBJECTIVE MANIFESTATION FINDINGS AND LIFE CYCLE VARIATIONS: MOUTH AND THROAT

Examination Technique	Expected Findings	Common Life Cycle Variations
INSPECTION		
Lips		
Shape and Position	Symmetrical; consistent with genetic heritage.	
Movement	Symmetrical for all facial expressions.	
Condition	Moist without dryness, cracks, or fissures.	
Color	Pink to brown depending on genetic heritage; no cyanosis, pallor.	
Lesions	None.	
Teeth		
Alignment	No malocclusion.	Newborn is edentulous but may show small bumps on gum ridges which disappear in 4–8 weeks. Deciduous teeth erupt at approximately 6 months of age. Permanent teeth begin to appear in around 6th year. Final molars appear between 17 and 25 years of age. Children and some adults may wear braces. Teeth become progressively worn with advancing age and may be lost due to aging and poor care.
Presence	The average adult has 32 teeth.	Children will have various stages of tooth development.
Caries	None.	Incidence less frequent after age 20.
Dentures	Well-fitted; no slipping or audible clicking sounds when talking or chewing.	Some adults will have missing teeth and will be using dentures or partial plates.
Gums		
Color	Pink; not retracted, inflamed, bleeding.	Mottled in dark-skinned people. Increased vascularity and growth of connective tissue of gums may occur during pregnancy. Gum tissue becomes less elastic and more vulnerable to trauma with advancing age.
Lesions	No bleeding, swelling, or sores.	Ill-fitting dentures will cause sores on gums.
Tongue		
Color	Pink like the oral mucosa; not red.	
Texture	Irregular lingual papillae; no denuding or smooth appearance.	In advanced age, taste buds may appear atrophic.
Mobility	Moves freely, without tremor or deviation.	
Undersurface	No lesions or swelling; easily visible venous pattern when tongue raised.	Sublingual varicosities not uncommon with aging.
Buccal Mucosa		
Color	Pink; no plaques or angiomas.	
Texture	Smooth, moist, shiny.	
Lesions	None.	
Salivary ducts	Visible opposite the second upper molar and under the tongue.	
Palate/Uvula		
Color	Soft palate pink, hard palate whiter.	
Contour	Smooth and symmetrically arched; no visible cleft in palate. Uvula free hanging—pear shaped.	Bony prominence on hard palate not uncommon.
Movement	Uvular and palate rise symmetrically and midline with palpation (cranial nerve IX, glossopharyngeal; cranial nerve X, vagus).	
Lesions	None.	

(continued)

TABLE 16–24. (continued)

Examination Technique	Expected Findings	Common Life Cycle Variations
Pharynx		
Tonsils		
Size	Small or flat; symmetrical scale for recording tonsillor size: 1+ Tonsil edges barely visible 2+ Tonsil edges midway between tonsillor pillars and uvula 3+ Tonsil edges touching uvula 4+ Tonsil edges meet midline	Often chronically enlarged in childhood or may be surgically absent.
Color	Same pink as oral mucosa.	
Discharge	None.	
Lesions	None.	
Posterior pharyngeal wall		
Color	Pink; small amount of redness not significant.	
Edema	None.	
Discharge	None.	
Lesions	None.	
Movement	Intact gag reflex; midline elevation uvula; able to swallow (cranial nerve IX, glossopharyngeal; cranial nerve X, vagus).	
PALPATION		
Mouth		
Floor	Nontender; no swellings, masses, plaques, or lesions.	
Walls	Soft; compressible; nontender; no lesions, tumors, or plaques.	
Soft palate	No submucous cleft.	
Salivary ducts	Nontender; no swelling or calculi.	
Tongue	Soft, uniformly compressible, nontender tissue; no swelling or masses.	
ASSESSMENT OF TASTE	Differentiates sweet, sour, bitter, and salty tastes (cranial nerve VII, facial; cranial nerve IX, glossopharyngeal).	Some deterioration of taste discrimination may occur with advanced age.
ASSESSMENT OF VOICE, PHONATION	Pitch consistent with sex, age, and genetic heritage; no hoarseness (cranial nerve X, vagus).	Male voice pitch lower at puberty; female voice pitch may lower after menopause.

From References 4, 42, and 59.

Examining the mouth is also important because the condition of the mouth manifests and provides clues to the causes of generalized illness. Paleness of lips and buccal mucosa may indicate anemia or other oxygenation problems. Signs and symptoms of pharyngitis, on the other hand, may explain the cause of a client's fever. A dry mouth may indicate dehydration.

Evaluating the state of the teeth is a traditional and particularly important nursing function. The condition of the teeth may determine whether or not the client is able to eat a house diet while in the hospital or whether he or she may require specially prepared food—a soft diet. Moreover, the state of the teeth and the client's dental hygiene can be indicative of the client's level of self-esteem. School nurses sometimes find that inattentive children suffer from toothaches caused by dental decay.

The ability of the client to swallow and thus to eat depends on the coordinated movement of the tongue and palate. By observing this movement, the nurse is able to judge the client's ability to handle liquids and solid foods.

Neck

Overview. During the assessment of the neck the nurse inspects and palpates simultaneously. Evaluation of the neck includes observation of the skin and underlying structures, palpation of the cervical lymph nodes and neck vessels, and determination of neck muscle strength. Palpation of the thyroid gland, normally part of the head and neck assessment, is an advanced technique and is not included in this text. The health history questions related to evaluation of the neck are included in Table 16–25.

Topographical Anatomy. The neck is bounded by the lower jaw (the mandible) above and the clavicle bones below. The major muscle masses are the sternocleidomastoid muscles visible on both sides of the neck when the head is turned to the side and the powerful trapezius muscle that attaches at the base of the skull and runs downward to attach at the sternum and clavicles. The trachea is midline over the suprasternal notch and the lobes of the thyroid gland lie on either side of the trachea and partially under the sternomastoid muscle. The carotid artery runs anterior to the muscle and its pulsations are observed low in the neck. The facial-cervical lymph nodes surround the ears and extend along the chin line and on either side of the sternomastoid muscles (Fig. 16–42). Lymph nodes are flat or nonpalpable if they are not inflamed.

Conducting an Examination of the Neck. The assessment of the neck encompasses inspection to detect symmetry of the neck structures (muscles, trachea, thyroid, and carotid pulsations) and palpation to uncover enlargement or tenderness of the facial-cervical lymph nodes (*lymphadenopathy*). Palpation of the carotid artery is necessary to determine the rate and rhythm of the carotid pulse. Ordinarily, the examination of the neck also includes the palpation of the thyroid gland; however, this is an advanced technique that is taught later in the nursing curriculum. It is therefore not covered in this text. The client participates in the neck assessment by actively bending the head and neck so you can assess range of motion (ROM) and by pressing the head against resistance to determine muscle strength.

Preparation. The client sits facing the examiner at eye level for the neck examination. No special equipment is needed for this assessment.

Inspection. Begin by asking the client to raise the chin and tilt the head backward. This makes visualization significantly easier. Begin the neck assessment by inspecting the musculature from the front and from each side. The neck should have no significant asymmetry such as unilaterally (one-sided) overdeveloped sternomastoid muscles or underlying masses that cause the muscles to bulge. Ask the client to bend the head forward to touch the chin to the sternum (flexion) and then raise the chin toward the ceiling so the back of the head (occiput) is pointing toward the feet (hyperextension). Next have the client bend the neck so each ear in turn is pointing toward the shoulder (lateral bending) and, then, to rotate the head so he or she is looking over the shoulder. Finally, ask the client to move his or her head against the resistance you apply, and return it to the midline position, against this resistance. Muscle strength should be symmetrical, and the client should be able to strongly oppose resistance to midline rotation. This reflects the function of cranial nerve XI, the accessory nerve. The range of motion should be smooth and the flexibility symmetrical.

The skin of the neck is inspected for scars, discolorations, and masses. Enlarged lymph nodes (lymphadenopathy) or thyroid nodules may be visible as masses just under the skin and musculature. Pulsations of the carotid arteries and venous pulsations of the jugular vessels are often detected in the base of the neck (just above the clavicle bones) in the seated client. The jugular veins should be flat (not distended or full) when the client is seated at an angle of 40 degrees or greater.

Palpation. Palpate the neck to determine the consistency and strength of the trapezius muscles. Place your hands on the client's shoulders and ask the client to shrug the shoulders while you press downward to determine the strength of the trapezius muscle.

Next palpate the facial-cervical lymph node chains starting behind the ears (postauricular nodes) and moving in front of the ears (preauricular nodes), the back of the head (occipital nodes), under the jawline (submandibular and submental nodes), and along both sides of the sternomastoid muscles (anterior and posterior cervical nodes). These lymph nodes are frequently not palpable but if they are felt they must be evaluated for precise location, size, shape, mobility, consistency, and tenderness. Determination of location helps you to distinguish between lymphadenopathy and masses on the neck muscles or on the lobes of the thyroid gland.

Glands are evaluated in the same manner as lesions and masses. Size is estimated in millimeters or centimeters. Shape is the determination of outline (discrete or matted together); mobility refers to the ability of the node to move over the underlying tissue as opposed to being fixed (stuck) to the underlying tissue. Consistency is the degree of hardness or softness characteristic of the enlarged node, and tenderness is the client's subjective response to palpation of the affected node.

The carotid pulses are palpated approximately midneck and anterior (medial) to the sternomastoid muscles. The rate and rhythm of the carotid pulses should be equal (the same on both sides).

Objective manifestations of the expected findings of the neck assessment are found in Table 16–26.

Special Considerations, Precautions, and Sources of Error. Care must be taken to avoid undue pressure while palpating the neck vessels and assessing the carotid pulse.

TABLE 16–25. SAMPLE CLIENT HISTORY QUESTIONS FOR SUBJECTIVE MANIFESTATIONS: NECK

1. Have you experienced neck stiffness?
2. Do you have neck pain?
3. Has your neck been injured in an accident?
4. Are there any lumps in your neck? Are they painful?
5. Does _____ (subjective manifestation) interfere with any of your usual daily activities? How?

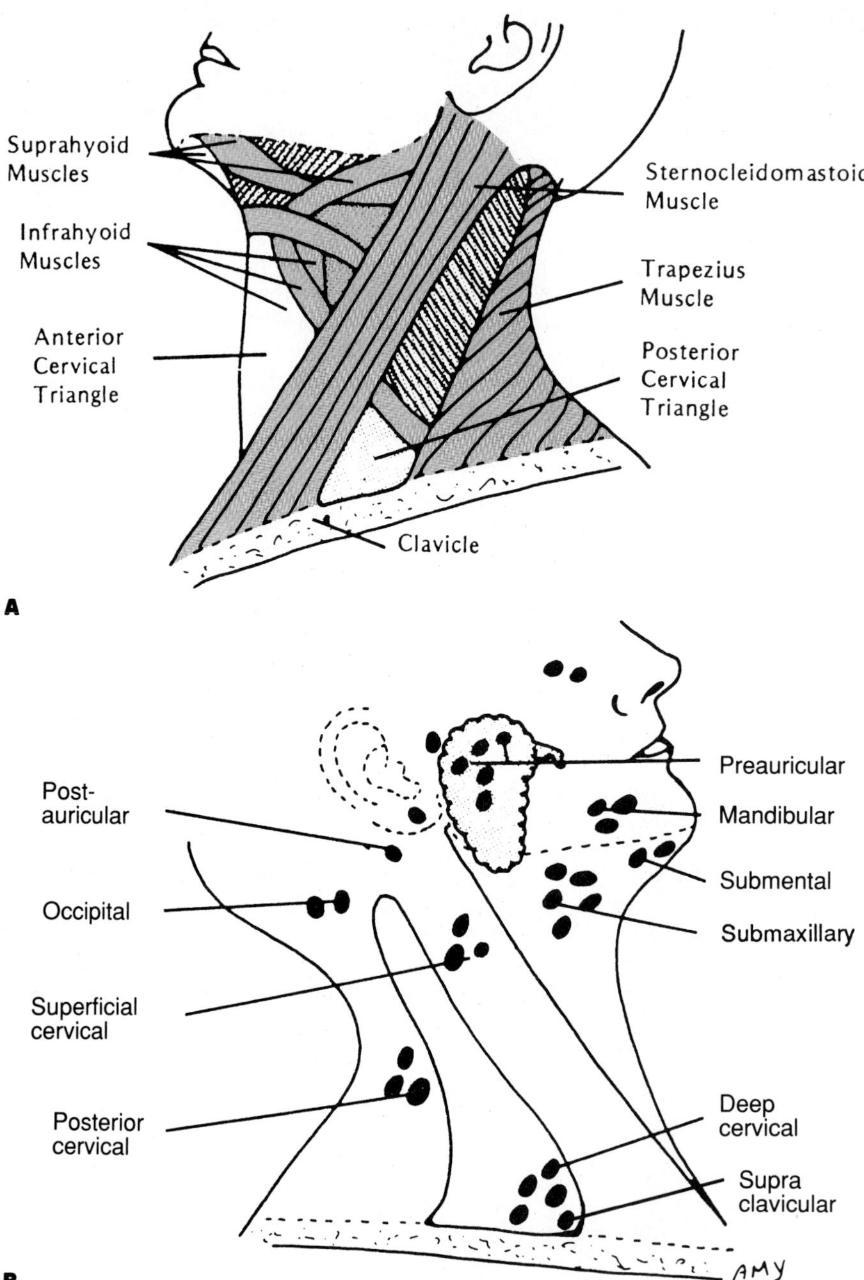

Figure 16–42. Muscles of the neck **(A)** and lymph nodes (muscles, trachea, thyroid, and lymph glands) **(B)**. (Source: *Berger KJ, Fields WL.* Pocket Guide to Health Assessment. *Reston, VA: Reston Publishing Co.; 1980.*)

Palpation should be limited to one side at a time to prevent occlusion of the artery or precipitation of bradycardia (slowing of the pulse). As abnormal growths, enlarged lymph nodes, and thyroid nodules may all be visible or palpated in the neck region care must be taken to differentiate between these masses. A clear understanding of the neck anatomy or location of neck structures is the most effective safeguard against error.

Recording. Recording the assessment of the neck requires a notation about each structure evaluated (musculature for strength and flexibility, the carotid pulse for rate and rhythm, and the facial-cervical nodes for location, size, shape, mobility, and tenderness). The presence or absence of masses, scars, or skin lesions constitutes part of the neck writeup. The objective data from your physical examination, as well as the client's subjective symptoms, are presented in Box 16–28.

Role of the Nurse and the Assessment of the Neck. Important indications of health, especially head and neck infections, can often be confirmed by a careful neck examination. Swelling of the lymph nodes occurs with such diverse conditions as ear inflammations, throat infections, and tooth

TABLE 16–26. OBJECTIVE MANIFESTATION FINDINGS AND LIFE CYCLE VARIATIONS: NECK

Examination Technique	Expected Findings	Common Life Cycle Variations
INSPECTION		
Symmetry	No masses or bulging; angles of the jaw equidistant from respective shoulders.	Neck diameter and length small in relationship to head size in infancy and early childhood. Gradual increase in proportionate size of neck during childhood. Head control evident in infant beginning at 3 months of age.
Head movement	Smooth, coordinated; no involuntary movement.	
Range of motion	Flexion: normal is 45 degrees, able to touch chin to sternum. Hyperextension: normal is 55 degrees. Lateral bending: normal is 40 degrees, ear nearly touching shoulder. Rotation: normal is 70 degrees.	With age or injury, neck flexibility diminishes.
Curvature	Cervical concavity present.	In advanced age, shortening of neck parallels shrinking of spine.
Pulsation	Diffuse undulent pulse may be visible at base of neck.	
Venous distension	Neck veins flat at 45-degree angle or higher in sitting position.	Loss of skin elasticity and muscle tone results in a more evident appearance of neck arteries and veins in advanced age.
Thyroid	Small and symmetrical; no enlargement or masses.	Transient diffuse enlargement of the thyroid is common in pregnancy.
Lymphadenopathy	None.	
Skin	Clear; no masses, swelling, scars, discoloration, or rashes.	
PALPATION		
Lymph nodes	Nonpalpable and nontender.	Commonly enlarged but nontender in healthy children.
Pulsations	Carotid artery with symmetrical amplitude, smooth upstroke, and gradual descent.	
Masses	None.	
Muscle strength	Sternomastoid and trapezius muscles strong against resistance.	Less strength in very old age.

From References 4, 42, and 59.

and gum diseases. Lymphadenopathy is a warning signal to the nurse to extend the assessment to the head and sensory organs to detect the sites of infection. Lumps in the neck need to be referred for a thorough evaluation of masses growing on the musculature or the lobes of the thyroid gland. Stiffness or pain in the neck occurs from hyperextension of the neck in motor vehicle accidents (whiplash), increasing osteoporosis (demineralization of bone) in the elderly, sports injuries, and meningitis in children, to name a few causes of discomfort associated with the neck. All of these conditions require that the nurse assess and refer the client for further evaluation as expeditiously as possible.

BOX 16–28. RECORDING THE ASSESSMENT OF THE NECK

Subjective Manifestations

Neck. No stiffness or pain of neck muscles. No history of traumatic injury. No masses or lumps noted in the neck area.

Objective Manifestations

Neck. Supple with full range of movement. No masses. Muscles strong against resistance. No muscle atrophy. No deformity.
Nodes. No facial-cervical lymphadenopathy.
Vessels. Jugular veins flat at 40 degrees. Carotid arteries with regular rate and rhythm.

■ BREASTS AND AXILLAE

Overview

The breasts of all men, women, and children need to be examined by the two physical assessment modes of inspection and palpation. Furthermore, the breast examination should be used by the nurse as an opportunity to teach breast self-examination to female clients. Self-examination is the most effective method for early detection of malignancies. Health history questions appropriate to the com-

TABLE 16–27. SAMPLE CLIENT HISTORY QUESTIONS FOR SUBJECTIVE MANIFESTATIONS: BREASTS AND AXILLAE

1. Do you perform monthly breast self-examination?
2. Do you have a history of breast lumps (masses)? When were they first noticed? Is their presence related to your period (menses)?
3. Do you have breast tenderness at any time during your menstrual cycle (menses)?
4. Have you noticed any swelling or enlargement of your breasts? Are you pregnant or breastfeeding?
5. Do you have discharge from your breasts? When did you first notice this? What is the color and odor of the fluid from your nipples?
6. Have you had any breast surgery?
7. Do you have axillary tenderness, lumps, or rashes?
8. Have you or anyone in your family had breast cancer?
9. Does ______ (subjective manifestation) interfere with any of your usual daily activities? How?

plete evaluation of the client's breast health are found in Table 16–27.

Topographical Anatomy

The adult female breast is composed of glandular and fibrous tissue and fat cells (Fig. 16–43). The proportions of these components vary with age and general body weight. Glandular tissue of the breast responds to the hormonal variations of pregnancy and the menstrual cycle; as a result, breast tissue undergoes changes with age and estrogen stimulation. Female children, for instance, have a small amount of glandular tissue that increases with puberty and postmenopausal women experience a loss of glandular tissue. Because breast tissue often extends to the clavicles, palpation of the supraclavicular (just above the clavicles) and infraclavicular (just below the clavicles) areas is included in the thorough breast examination. Lymph nodes that drain the breasts are located in the axillary, supraclavicular, and infraclavicular areas (Figs. 16–43 and 16–44).

The male breast is composed of a minimal amount of glandular tissue located just beneath the nipples and areola. This tissue has the capacity to enlarge in males in response to the hormones of puberty and to some medications. Enlargement of male breasts is referred to as *gynecomastia.*

For the purposes of location and description of abnormal findings the breasts are divided into quadrants (Fig. 16–45).

Conducting an Examination of the Breasts and Axillae

Preparation. At the beginning of the examination, the client is seated so you can observe the contours of the breast. Following the seated inspection ask the client to lie flat while you palpate the breast tissue. No special equipment is needed besides *warm* hands. (To assure that your hands are warm, hold them in warm water for a moment

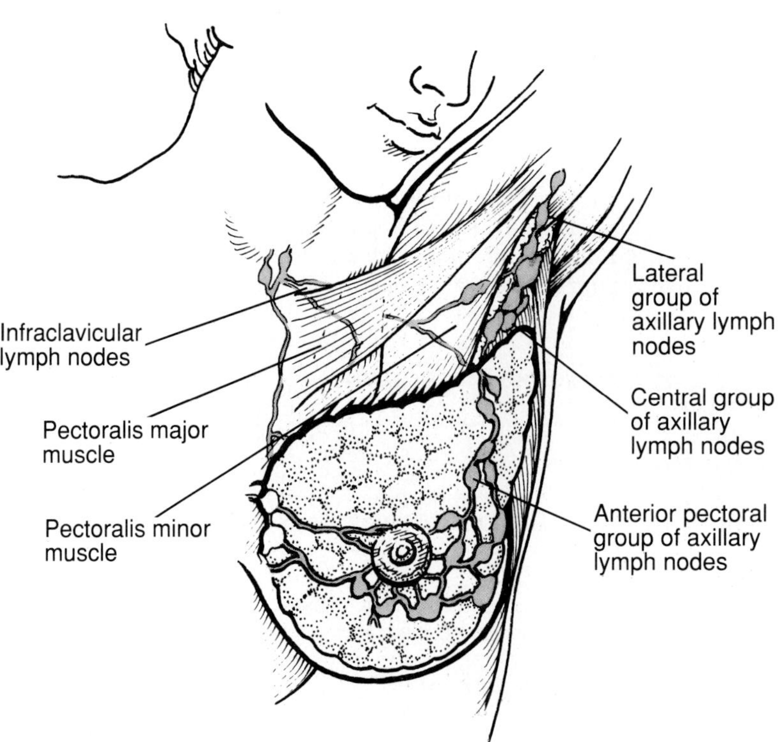

Figure 16–43. Anatomy of the female breast. (*Source: Block GJ, Nolan JW.* Health Assessment for Professional Nursing: A Developmental Approach, *2nd ed. Norwalk, CT: Appleton & Lange; 1986.*)

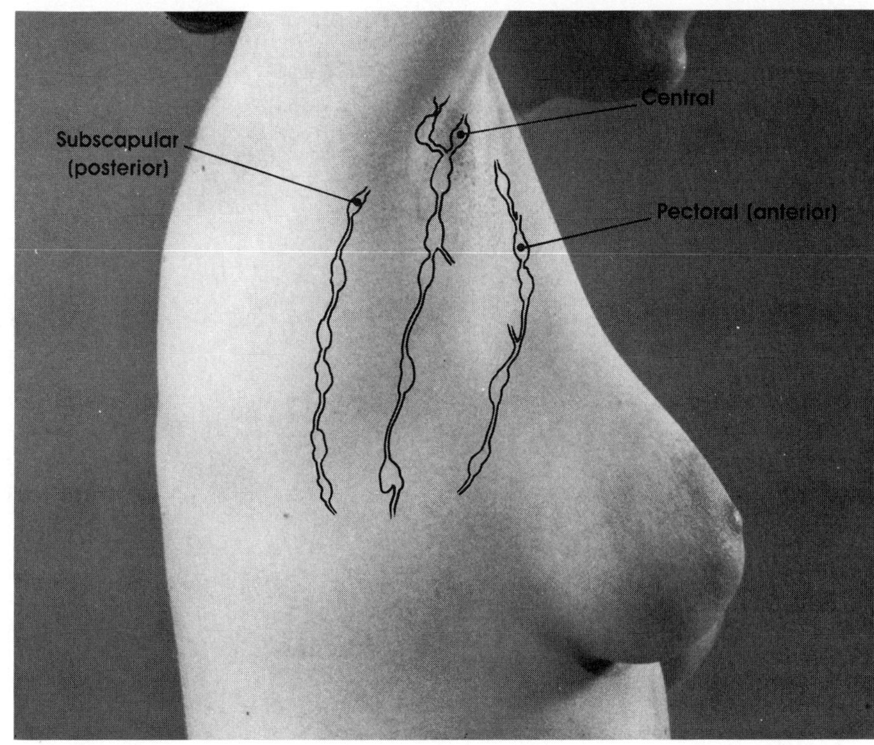

Figure 16–44. Lymph nodes of the axillary and clavicular areas. (Source: *Block GJ, Nolan JW.* Health Assessment for Professional Nursing: A Developmental Approach. *2nd ed. Norwalk, CT: Appleton-Century-Crofts; 1986.*)

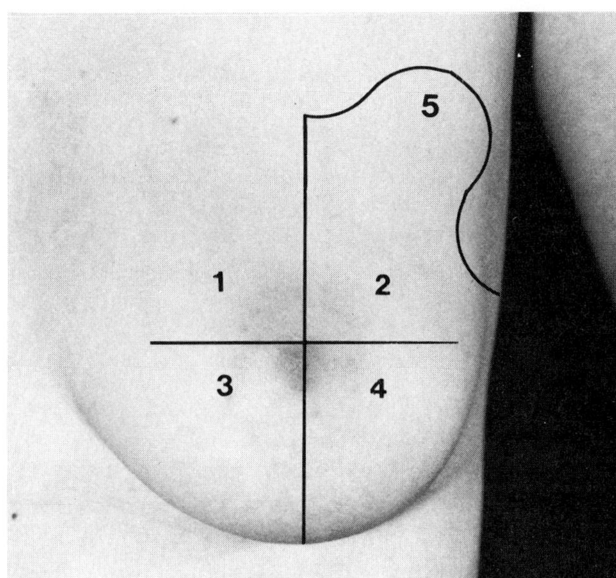

Figure 16–45. Breast quadrants. **1.** Left upper inner. **2.** Left upper outer. **3.** Left lower inner. **4.** Left lower outer. **5.** Tail of Spence. (Source: *Block GJ, Nolan JW.* Health Assessment for Professional Nursing: A Developmental Approach. *2nd ed. Norwalk, CT: Appleton-Century-Crofts; 1986.*)

and dry them just before beginning the breast examination.) The client should wear a gown over her upper body that the examiner can move as needed to fully observe and palpate the breasts without obstruction but at the same time provide adequate coverage to preserve the client's modesty.

Inspection. Inspect the axillary and clavicular areas and the breasts in females and males. Because the development of breast tissue is associated primarily with females, it is easy to forget that it is also important to examine the breasts of males.

Axillary and Clavicular Areas. Inspect the axillary and clavicular areas for swelling and lesions. Masses located either just above or just below the clavicles may be enlarged lymph nodes associated with infection, or they may be tumors. Masses in the axillae may also be enlarged lymph nodes, indicating infection in the area of the corresponding arm.

Breasts. Visually inspect the breasts while the client is seated and undraped. Observe the development, symmetry, and superficial appearance of the breasts.

Breast development is easily evaluated by applying Tanner's five stages of breast development.[71] Tanner's first stage is the stage from birth to the onset of adolescence and is called the infantile stage. The second stage is called the bud stage. In this stage the breast tissue is slightly elevated and the areolar diameter enlarges. Breast tissue further enlarges during the third stage, but there is no

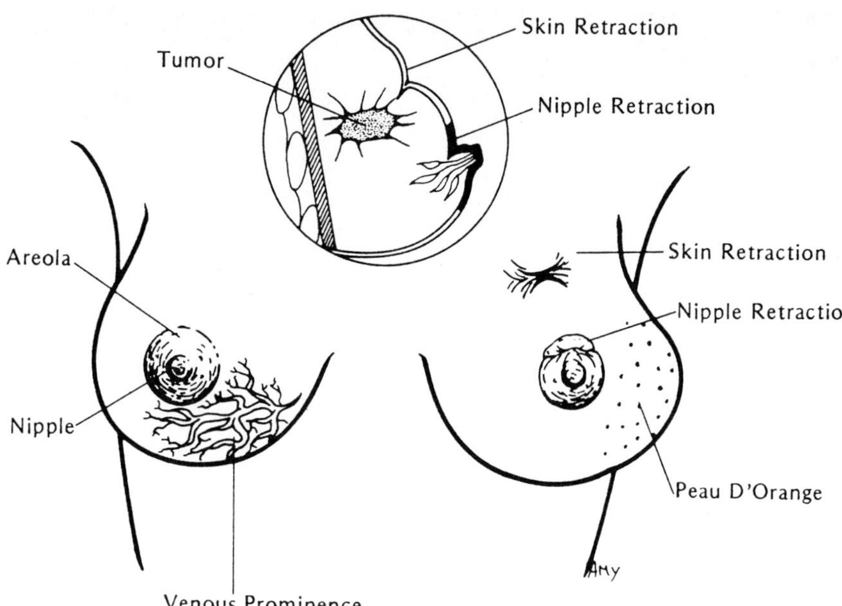

Figure 16–46. Abnormalities of the breast. (Source: *Berger KJ, Fields WL.* Pocket Guide to Health Assessment. *Reston, VA: Reston Publishing Co.; 1980.*)

change in contour between the areola and breast. In the fourth stage, the areola and papilla have a separate contour and appear as a secondary mound distinct from the breast. Such contour distinctions are best observed by viewing the client's breasts from the side or lateral vantage point. In mature breasts, the fifth stage, further enlargement of the breast tissue occurs, and the nipple projects from the areola.

To evaluate mature breasts that are especially pendulous, ask the client to lean forward. This allows the breasts to fall away from the chest wall and permits their contours to be more easily observed for smoothness and symmetry. Breasts are commonly slightly unequal in size, but recent changes in the size of one breast may signify infection or underlying tumor.

Inspect the superficial appearance of the breasts for pigmentation, lesions, rashes, masses, or redness. Edema may appear when the lymph channels from the breast become blocked by tumor cells. Edema creates the porous appearance characteristic of an orange peel, referred to as *peau d'orange* (Fig. 16–46).

Next, ask the client to raise her hands above the head. This position helps to reveal one of the most important signs of underlying masses referred to as "dimpling" (see Fig. 16–46). Requesting the client to tighten the muscles surrounding the breasts by pressing her hands on her hips may also help in visualizing superficial masses. These maneuvers are not necessary in the male client because breast tissue is small in amount and masses are more easily visible.

Nipples and Areola. Observe the nipples and areola for position. Nipple position is usually symmetrical; that is, the nipples point in the same direction, whether everted or inverted. Nipple inversion is a normal variant, but recent inversion of a previously everted nipple is referred to as "retraction." Retraction caused by subcutaneous fat loss may occur normally in elderly women, but the nipple can be manually everted when this is the case. Retraction also occurs in malignancy, and nipple position is fixed. Retraction of the nipples can be observed as the woman assumes

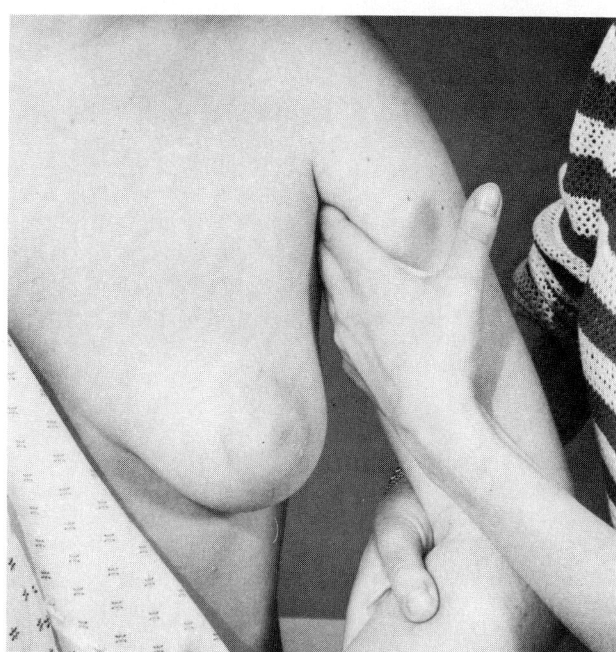

Figure 16–47. Position for palpation of axillary lymph nodes. (*Source: Block GJ, Nolan JW.* Health Assessment for Professional Nursing: A Developmental Approach. *2nd ed. Norwalk, CT: Appleton-Century-Crofts; 1986.*)

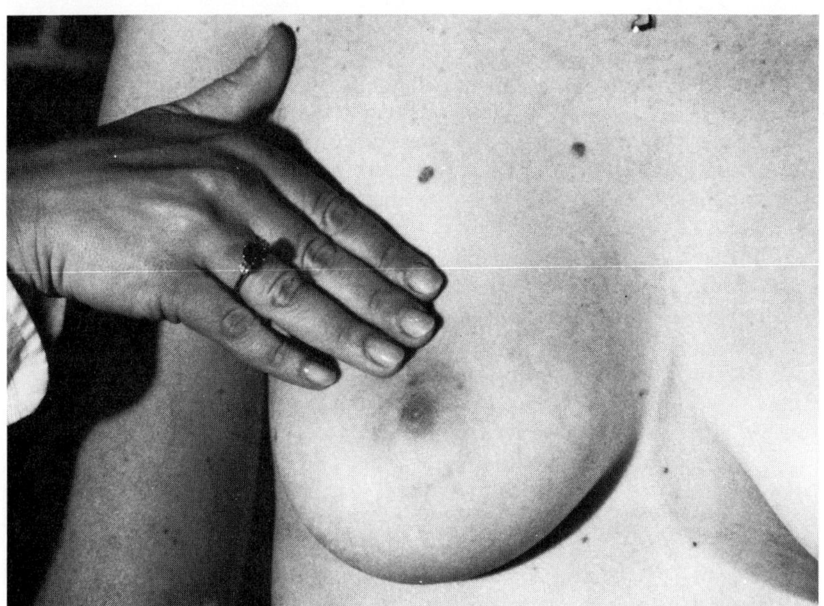

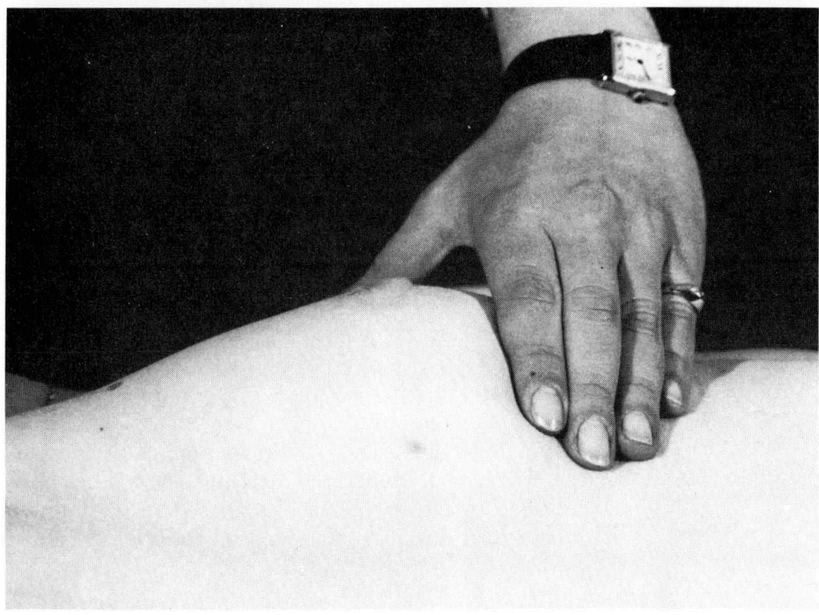

Figure 16–48. Patterns of palpation of breast tissue. (Source: *Block GJ, Nolan JW.* Health Assessment for Professional Nursing: A Developmental Approach. *2nd ed. Norwalk, CT: Appleton-Century-Crofts; 1986.*)

any of the positions recommended above for evaluating breast contour.

While observing the nipples for position, also note their color. The color of the nipples in Caucasian individuals is usually pink, but nipples and areola become brown in pregnancy. In darkly pigmented individuals, the nipple and areola are darker than the surrounding skin and become darker still in pregnancy. Inspect the nipples for discharge and the areola for ulcerations and rashes.

Palpation. Palpation includes not only the tissue of the breast, areola, and nipples, but also that of the axillary, and clavicular lymph nodes. Palpation of the male breast follows the same procedure as for the female breast.

Axillary and Clavicular Nodes. While the client is still in the sitting position, ask her to place her arms at her sides so that the muscles are relaxed. Support the client's left arm with your right arm, and palpate the axilla with your left hand. Supporting the client's arm facilitates relaxation. Palpate both the anterior and posterior axillary folds and high in the axillae for masses (Fig. 16–47). Enlargement of lymph nodes can signify infection or tumors. Then, standing in front of the client, palpate the supraclavicular and infraclavicular areas bilaterally for masses.

Breast and Nipples. When you have completed your assessment of the axillary area place the client's arm above her head to flatten the breast tissue and facilitate your ability to feel for breast masses. Gently, but firmly, palpate the breasts in a circular or a linear pattern (Fig. 16–48), evaluating the consistency of the underlying tissue. The elasticity of young breasts is apparent with palpation and the lobules of glandular tissue can be defined by the examining hand. Tenderness is noted and masses are evaluated for size, shape, consistency (degree of hardness), relationship to the surrounding tissue, and mobility. Hard, fixed (immobile) masses can be indicative of cancer. Palpate the nipple and areola for masses, tenderness, and discharge. Breasts of males and children are palpated for masses and tenderness and the axillary areas for evidence of lymphadenopathy.

Breast Self-Examination. Every breast examination should be considered a teaching examination. Clients need continual reinforcement of the correct techniques for effective self-examination. During the assessment the client can demonstrate back to you the techniques you have just taught her. Self-examination includes inspection of the breasts in a mirror and palpation of breasts and axilla. Some women palpate their breasts while lying down; others prefer palpation while bathing or showering. Literature illustrating breast self-examination is widely available and is an important adjunct to health teaching. Because the consistency and degree of tenderness of breast tissue may change following ovulation, instruct the client to palpate her breasts shortly after her menses.

In addition to reviewing the technique of breast self-examination with the client, it is also a good idea to review the guidelines proposed by the American Cancer Society for detection of breast cancer in asymptomatic women:

1. Breast self-examinations should be performed every month when a woman is 20 years of age or older.
2. Women from 20 to 40 years of age should have a physical examination of the breast at least every three years, and women over 40 years should have one every year.
3. Women between the ages of 35 and 39 should have a mammogram to serve as a baseline for future mammograms.
4. Women 40 to 49 years should have a mammogram every 1 to 2 years, depending on their risk factors and the findings of previous mammograms.
5. Any woman over 50 years of age should have a mammogram every year.[72]

Instruction in self-examination is important for all clients, but may be especially important for some women who may have less exposure to health information and who may also have less access to health care. In a review of research on the subject, Nemcek noted that that the breast is the most common site of cancer in both black and white women; however, black women have an approximately 20 percent greater mortality rate from the disease.[73] Nemcek suggests that this may be related in part to insufficient self-detection, a possibility in view of the fact that black women were found in a National Cancer Institute survey (1980) to be less aware of breast cancer symptoms than others surveyed.[74] In Nemcek's study, black women who performed breast self-examination irregularly or not at all perceived numerous barriers to carrying out the procedure, such as fear of finding a lump, concern about an inability to recognize lumps, feelings of embarrassment, and difficulty in remembering when to perform breast self-examination. Presumably, these same perceptions might interfere with regular breast self-examination among women of all ethnic groups.[73] To be effective, instruction in breast self-examination needs to address these barriers.

The expected physical findings from breast assessment, as well as the variations of normal and the changes associated with aging, are found in Table 16–28.

Special Considerations, Precautions, and Sources of Error

The breasts of all clients require physical evaluation regardless of age or gender. Children and men are often neglected because nurses and other health care providers forget that these groups can also suffer from breast diseases and cancers. Any breast masses and lesions detected during assessment require immediate referral for further evaluation. Because the consistency and degree of tenderness of the breasts of menstruating women are related to variations in the hormonal cycle, the breasts are most effectively palpated just after menses.

Recording

Box 16–29 demonstrates the recording of both subjective and objective data collected during the breast assessment.

Role of the Nurse and the Assessment of the Breasts and Axillae

Physical examination of the breast and axillary area, using the techniques of inspection and palpation, is the most effective method of detecting early breast cancer. Self-examination by clients themselves is responsible for saving many lives from progressive malignancy. The most

BOX 16–29. RECORDING THE ASSESSMENT OF THE BREASTS AND AXILLAE

Subjective Manifestations

Breasts. No family history of breast cancer. Does breast self-examination each month following her menses. Notes generalized breast tenderness prior to menses. No history of masses or swelling of the breast tissue, nipple discharge, or surgery. Denies axillary tenderness, lumps, or rashes.

Objective Manifestations

Breasts. Symmetrical contours bilaterally. No palpable masses or tenderness. Nipples are erect and without discharge or masses. Areola free of lesions. Axilla clear of rashes, enlargements, or tenderness.

TABLE 16–28. OBJECTIVE MANIFESTATION FINDINGS AND LIFE CYCLE VARIATIONS: BREASTS AND AXILLAE

Examination Technique	Expected Findings	Common Life Cycle Variations
INSPECTION		
Breasts		
Size and symmetry	Wide variation in size, one breast frequently larger than the other.	Breast budding appears after age 9 years in female. Asymmetry common in teenage girls. Breasts enlarge with pregnancy—may double or triple in size. Loss of firmness in breast tissue of women who have had more than one pregnancy. Loss of elasticity of tissue leads to flattening and drooping of breasts with advancing age. Gynecomastia frequent in teenage boys and may occur in some elderly males.
Shape	Wide variety, but should be symmetrical, no dimpling.	
Skin	Color dependent upon ethnicity, should be uniform and without lesions.	
Contour	No skin retraction, dimpling, flattening or apparent masses.	
Color	Even distribution of pigment consistent with genetic heritage.	
Areola/Nipple		
Size/Shape	Symmetrically round, and the same color.	Areola will enlarge with pregnancy.
Direction	Usually erect but can be normally inverted.	
Lesions/Masses	None.	
Retraction	None.	
Discharge	None.	Pregnant female may have leakage of colostrum and the lactating female involuntary expression of milk.
Axilla	Skin intact, no lesions or masses.	Deodorants frequently cause rashes. May appear swollen in pregnancy and lactation.
Hair distribution	Women frequently shave the underarms.	Children rarely have axillary hair until puberty.
PALPATION		
Breasts		
Consistency	Most breast tissue is glandular.	Young breasts are elastic while aging causes a stringiness to breast tissue. Breasts firm, hard in pregnancy.
Tenderness	None.	Breasts tender prior to menses.
Masses	None.	
Areola/nipple		
Masses	None.	
Tenderness	None.	
Discharge	None.	Discharge usual in lactating women.
Axilla	No tenderness, masses, or lymph node enlargement.	

From References 4, 42, and 59.

significant role of the nurse in promoting the health of women may be in teaching clients how to examine their own breasts and in motivating them to do so on a regular monthly basis. By making every breast examination a teaching exam the conscientious nurse constantly reinforces client knowledge.

■ THORAX AND LUNGS

Overview

Examination of the respiratory system uses several assessment skills: proficient interviewing technique, identification of anatomical landmarks, inspection of the skin and respiratory effort, palpation and percussion of the thorax, auscultation of the breath sounds, and astute clinical judgment. Table 16–29 lists the health history questions pertinent to evaluation of the thorax and lungs.

Topographical Anatomy and Surface Projections of the Lungs

Bony landmarks constitute the most important anatomical feature of the chest for evaluation of the lungs and thorax. One easily identifiable landmark is the *suprasternal* notch. It is visible at the base of the ventral aspect of the neck as the rounded bony depression between the clavicles. The most significant anterior chest markings, however, are the sternum and its adjacent superior portion, the manubrium. These two palpable bones are joined together at the manubriosternal junction (formerly called the sternal angle or the angle of Louis). This easily distinguished feature marks the attachment of the second rib and permits the accurate numbering of the rib spaces. The first seven ribs articulate directly with the sternum, the next three are attached to the superior costal margins. Ribs 11 and 12 are not attached to the ribs above them and are termed "floating ribs." The costal junctures join the ribs together into a protective structure for the lungs, heart, and great vessels and can also be the site of significant chest wall pain (costochondritis). The delicate clavicular bones articulate laterally from the superior surfaces of the manubrium. Reference lines are imaginary vertical lines that define anatomical areas of the chest and facilitate location and description of physical findings. Figure 16–49 shows the landmarks and location of reference lines on the anterior chest. Lines over the anterior thorax are the *midsternal, midclavicular,* and *anterior axillary lines.* Lines over the lateral thorax are *the anterior, mid-,* and *posterior axillary lines.*

TABLE 16–29. SAMPLE CLIENT HISTORY QUESTIONS FOR SUBJECTIVE MANIFESTATIONS: THORAX AND LUNGS

1. What was the date of your last chest x-ray? What were the results?
2. Do you have a cough? Do you bring up *phlegm* (productive cough)? What color is the phlegm (*sputum*)? Is there blood in the sputum (*hemoptysis*)?
3. Do you have hoarseness or change in your voice?
4. Do you experience shortness of breath (dyspnea)? Does this occur with physical activity or when sitting still?
5. Do you *wheeze* (asthmatic breath sounds)? Is the asthma related to allergies, stress, or exercise?
6. Do you have chest pain or pain when you take a deep breath?
7. Do you have a history of pneumonia or bronchitis?
8. Have you had night sweats or any contact with tuberculosis? Have you been tested for tuberculosis? Results?
9. Do you smoke or live with a smoker? How much do you smoke?
10. Does _____ (subjective manifestation) interfere with any of your usual activities of daily living? How?

Posteriorly the largest bony mass consists of the paired scapulae. These two projections are located on either side of the thoracic spine high in the upper back. Imaginary vertical reference lines pass through the midscapula (called the *midscapular lines*) as well as through the midspine (called the *spinal line*). The most prominent bony projection of the spine is C7, the seventh cervical spinous process located at the base of the neck (see Fig. 16–49 for the location of anatomical landmarks and reference lines of the posterior thorax).

While examining the thorax, the nurse visualizes the underlying anatomy to gain a clear idea of which lung fields he or she is percussing or auscultating. Anteriorly, the apices of the lungs rise slightly above the inner one third of the clavicles and the bases are at the approximate level of the sixth to eighth ribs (Fig. 16–50).

Posteriorly, the lower projection of the lungs is at the level of the tenth thoracic spinous process but may descend to the twelfth process with deep inspiration.

The left lung has two lobes; the right lung has three. The middle right lobe is located anteriorly and can be auscultated only over the anterior chest wall (see Fig. 16–50 for anterior, posterior, and right and left lateral views of the lobes of the lungs).

Conducting an Examination of the Thorax and Lungs

The thorax is examined from the front, back, and sides and requires space to maneuver around the client and a quiet environment to allow you to hear even the faintest breath sounds.

Preparation. The client should be seated facing you with the thorax exposed. You need to have a clear view of the anterior chest and must be able to move into a position that permits a full view of the back as well. The debilitated client may need assistance leaning forward and maintaining a comfortable position while you visualize the back and listen to the breath sounds over the posterior thorax.

You will need a stethoscope to auscultate the lungs and a watch with a second hand to count the respiratory rate.

Inspection. Begin your evaluation by noting the contour or shape of the thorax. This includes the anterior, posterior, and transverse dimensions of the chest. The normal healthy adult has an oval-shaped chest. The anteroposterior diameter is smaller than the transverse diameter and, in Caucasians, has a ratio of 1:2. The chest configuration may change with age or long-standing respiratory disease. Osteoporosis, usually associated with the aging process, can cause *kyphosis,* an outward hump high in the upper back, and chronic obstructive pulmonary disease (COPD) can lead to an increase in the anteroposterior chest diameter causing what is commonly called a *barrel chest.* The oval contour may also be marred by slight asymmetries that have no pathological significance. Frequently people will have a mild *scoliosis* (curvature of the spine) or a slight protrusion (*pigeon breast*) or depression of the sternum (*funnel chest*) (see Chaps. 27 and 30 for further discussion of these ab-

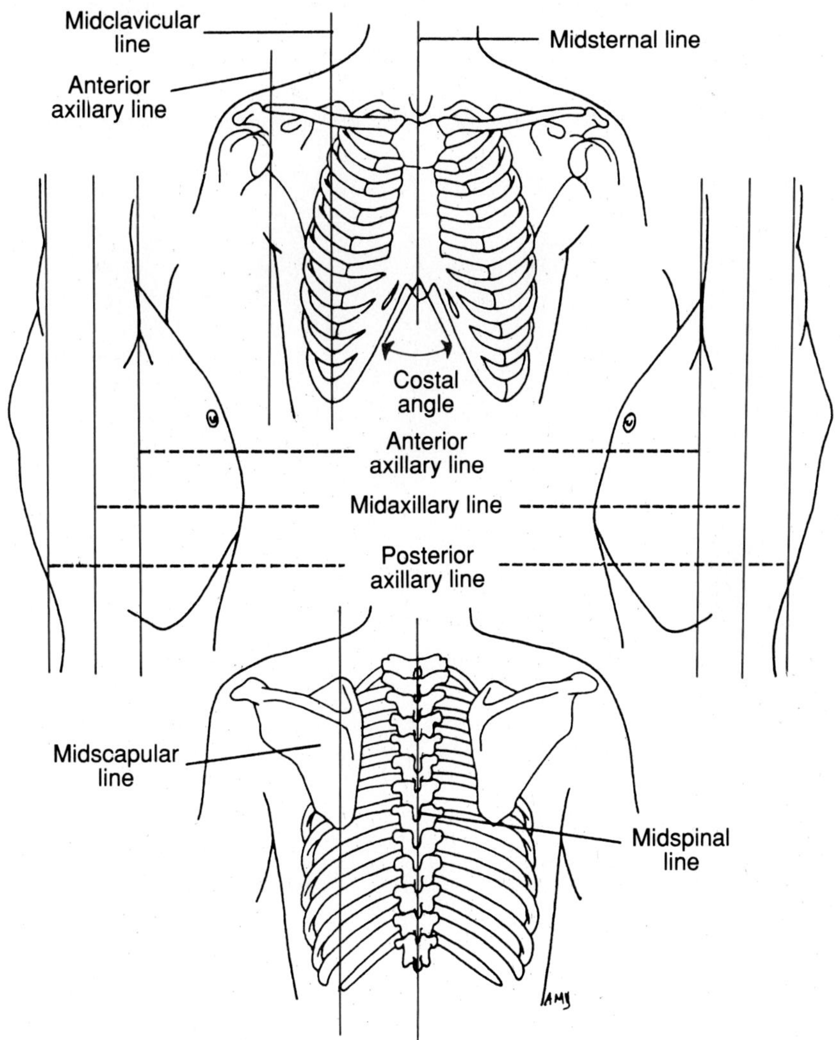

Figure 16–49. Topographical landmarks of the thorax. (Source: *Berger KJ, Fields WL: Pocket Guide to Health Assessment. Reston, VA: Reston Publishing Co.; 1980.*)

normalities). All of these asymmetries have the potential to be hazardous to health.

The respiratory movements of the healthy chest are even and symmetrical. The respiratory rate is measured by counting the number of breaths taken per minute by the resting client. The breaths should not be labored (dyspnea); that is, the client should not appear to be "working hard" to catch his or her breath. The neck muscles bulge outward, the shoulders pull upward, and the client looks worried when gasping for air. The intercostal muscles between each rib lie flat during normal effortless breathing, but can retract (pull in) or bulge outward with respiratory distress.

Palpation. After inspecting the contour or shape of the chest and assessing the rate and rhythm of respirations, place two hands on the client's back and palpate the musculature for tenderness and assess the *respiratory excursion* (Fig. 16–51). Excursion is determined by allowing the hands, placed gently and at right angles to the spine, to move with the client's inspirations and expirations. The examiner's hands should move outward and symmetrically with each deep inspiration. Muscle tenderness or pain with respirations may occur from superficial skin lesions, deeper bruises or masses, tumors, or musculoskeletal injuries such as cracked ribs, muscle strains, and inflammations.

Next, elicit vocal fremitus by instructing the client to verbalize words or numbers such as "ninety-nine" and feel for the vibrations with your hands resting lightly on his or her back. Sound increases in intensity and clarity when it passes through fluid instead of through air. When the normally air-filled lungs become fluid-filled, or consolidated, with the cellular by-products of pneumonia the vibrations of fremitus feel more pronounced to your palpating hands.

Percussion. Percuss the chest wall for resonance (the sound produced by striking the thorax over normal lung tissue). This technique calls for striking a pleximeter finger,

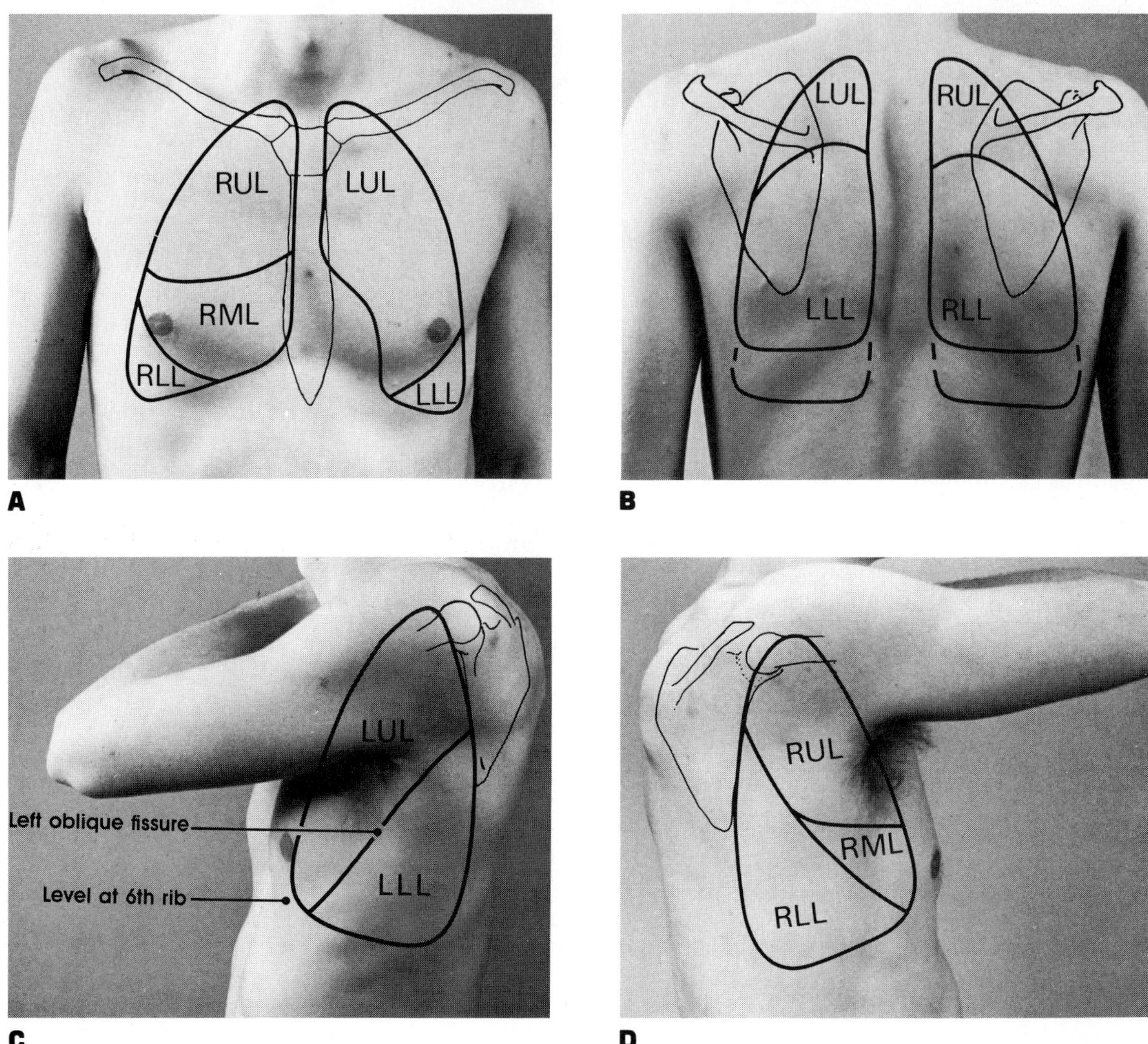

Figure 16–50. Surface projections of the lungs. **A.** Anterior view. **B.** Posterior view. **C, D.** Lateral views. (Source: *Block GJ, Nolan JW.* Health Assessment for Professional Nursing: A Developmental Approach. *2nd ed. Norwalk, CT: Appleton-Century-Crofts; 1986.*)

the one lying flat against the body surface, with the index finger of the other hand (the plexor).

Percuss the back, or posterior thorax, systematically from the upper midback to the approximate level of the diaphragm and around the lateral walls of the chest (Fig. 16–52). The air-filled lung emits a resonant percussion note and the fluid- or tumor-filled lung, a note best described as dull. Hyperresonance is the sound produced by the emphysematous or overextended lung. A flat sound is produced when the examiner's finger strikes bone.

Auscultation. Using the diaphragm of the stethoscope, listen from side to side over the posterior thorax following the pattern illustrated for percussion in Figure 16–52. Stay close to the spine to avoid the bony scapulae and ask the client to slowly and deeply inhale and exhale through her or his mouth each time you move your stethoscope. Listen especially to the bases of the lungs because fluid tends to accumulate there. Move the stethoscope slowly around the lateral walls of the chest to hear the breath sounds from the middle right lobe of the lung as they are heard only over the anterior thorax. Anteriorly auscultate the apices of the lungs (located in the supraclavicular area) and continue listening down the chest wall, staying close to the sternum.

Breath Sounds. Three breath sounds are normally heard in the lungs. *Bronchial breath sounds* are caused by turbulent air flow in the large airways (bronchi) and are heard with the stethoscope placed over the trachea. *Bronchovesicular sounds* are less coarse and are produced in the bronchioles and

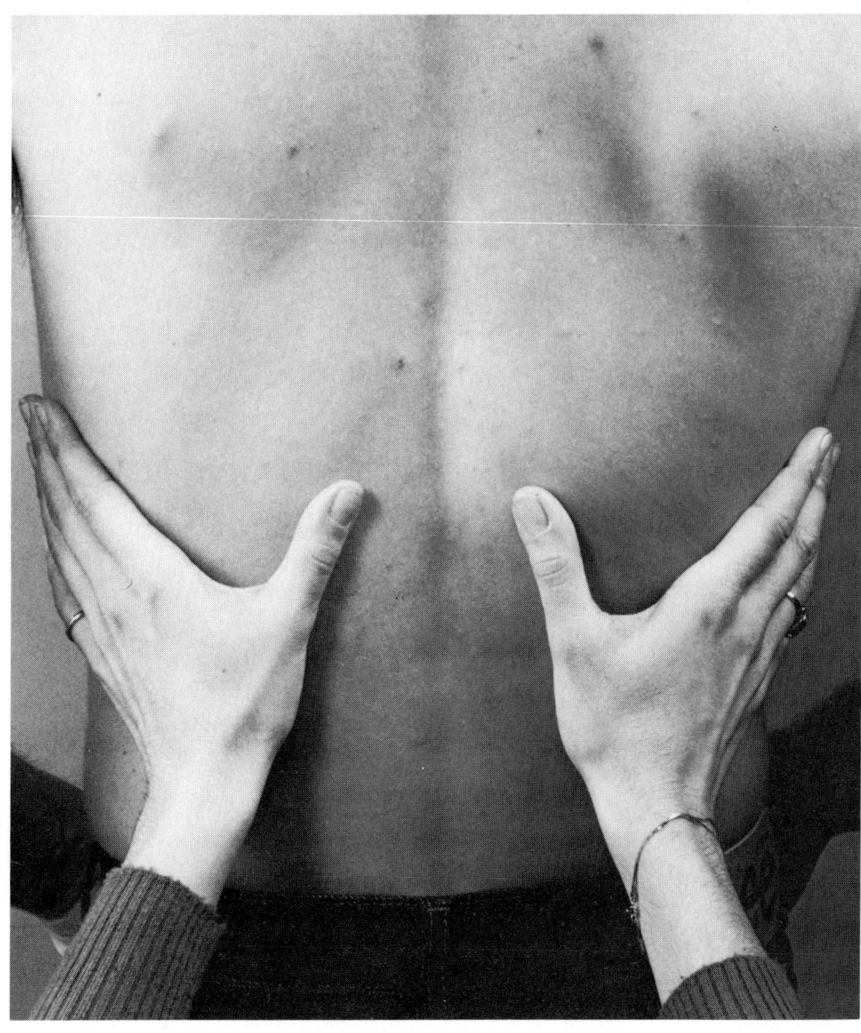

Figure 16–51. Hand placement for respiratory excursion. (Source: *Block GJ, Nolan JW.* Health Assessment for Professional Nursing: A Developmental Approach. *2nd ed. Norwalk, CT: Appleton-Century-Crofts; 1986.*)

heard best over the manubrium. The majority of breath sounds are produced by air exchange in the small air spaces (alveoli) and are known as *vesicular sounds*. Extra sounds that should not be heard are discontinuous *crackles* (formerly called *rales*), continuous rumbles or gurgles (formerly called *rhonchi*), and *wheezes*. Crackles or rales are fine sounds arising from fluid seeping into the alveoli in such conditions as congestive heart failure (CHF) and pneumonia. Wheezes are high-pitched and shrill and are characteristic of bronchial asthma. Rumbles or rhonchi have a harsh, snoring quality and are produced by the mucus and fluid of bronchitis.

Voice Sounds. As consolidation progresses, changes in vocal sounds are heard through the stethoscope as well. Normally voice sounds are faint and muffled but when transmitted through bronchial secretions they are heard loudly and clearly. Ask the client to say "ninety-nine" as you auscultate the lung fields. In the consolidated lung the words will be clearly audible. This phenomenon is called *bronchophony*. Whispered pectoriloquy is an increase in the transmission of the whispered "ninety-nine." Finally, ask the client to say "ee." If the sound you hear is "ay" instead of "ee" your client has an E-to-A change sometimes called egophony. If there is an absence of sound over an area of the lungs consider the possibility of *pneumothorax* (collapsed lung), a foreign body obstructing the flow of air through the lungs, or a mass expanding into the alveoli and preventing oxygen exchange. (See also Chap. 30.)

The expected findings and life cycle variations of the assessment are found in Table 16–30.

Special Considerations, Precautions, and Sources of Error

Following a systematic pattern during assessment of the lungs should preclude forgetting any essential portions of the respiratory examination. Haste and carelessness result in failure to note important pathological signs and symptoms. The nurse should always listen thoughtfully to each auscultatory area and move back and forth constantly comparing sides. Correlating the client's subjective symptoms with objective physical findings helps in the early detection of respiratory illness.

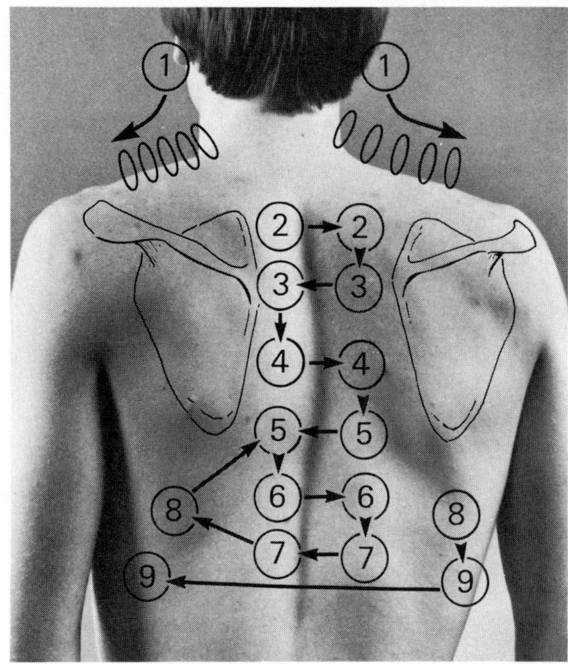

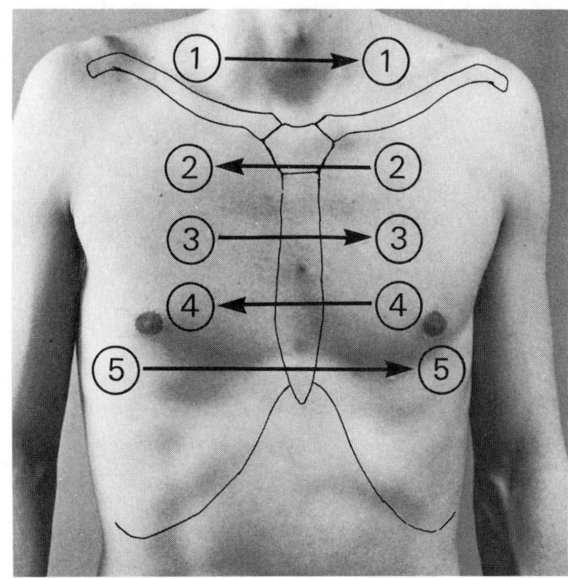

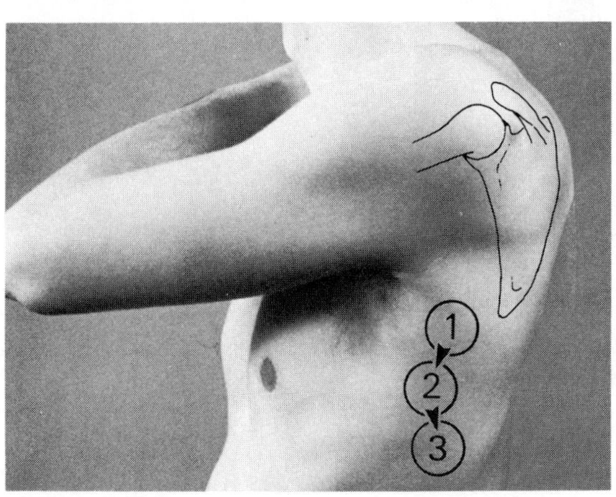

Figure 16–52. Pattern for percussion and auscultation. (Source: *Block GJ, Nolan JW:* Health Assessment for Professional Nursing: A Developmental Approach. *2nd ed. Norwalk, CT: Appleton-Century-Crofts, 1986.*)

Although it is recommended that the client be seated during assessment of the posterior thorax and auscultation of the lungs, sometimes ill and elderly clients, especially those who are hospitalized, may be unable to sit unassisted or at all. If possible ask a co-worker to hold the client in an upright position during the assessment. If even this small amount of exertion is in your judgment detrimental, complete the examination by rolling the client first to one side and then to the other so that both lungs can be heard equally well.

Recording

The recording of the respiratory assessment consists of the client's account of his or her pulmonary status and the findings from the physical examination. Box 16–30 highlights an example of a written record of the thorax and lung evaluation.

Role of the Nurse and the Assessment of the Thorax and Lungs

Pneumonia is a serious and often life-threatening complication of hospitalization, especially for clients on surgical units or elderly clients. The nurse's skillful pulmonary assessment can detect early signs of lung consolidation and prevent death and debility. Nurses in extended care facilities have a special obligation to be very vigilant in the prevention of respiratory illness in the elderly for whom they care.

Individuals of all ages are susceptible to pulmonary diseases such as bronchitis, pneumonia, and influenza and to dysfunctions like asthma and pneumothorax. The pediatric nurse and the school nurse have ample opportunities to assess the respiratory status of their child clients. In addition, pulmonary history taking and assessment provide an ideal atmosphere in which to begin talking to clients who smoke about the health risks inherent in this habit. It

TABLE 16–30. OBJECTIVE MANIFESTATION FINDINGS AND LIFE CYCLE VARIATIONS: THORAX AND LUNGS

Examination Technique	Expected Findings	Common Life Cycle Variations
INSPECTION		
Thorax		
Shape/Dimension	Anterior-posterior (A-P) diameter smaller than the transverse.	The infant thorax is round, the A–P diameter equal to the transverse. Adult proportions reached by age 6–7 years. The transverse diameter of the chest increases by 2 cm in pregnant women and the circumference by 5–7 cm. With advanced age and shrinking of thoracic spine, A-P diameter of chest expands.
Configuration/contour	Slightly convex with minor or no sternal depression or projection. Spine straight.	Benign structural anomalies common. Slight scoliosis or kyphosis with age giving barrel chest appearance.
Skin	No scars, masses, or discoloration.	Often freckles, moles, and sun damage.
Movement	Symmetrical and without retractions or bulging of the intercostal spaces; rhythmic respirations.	Loss of muscle strength over chest results in underventilation in alveoli of lower lung fields in older adults.
Respiration		
Rate	12–20 cycles per minute.	Respiratory rate 30 cycles per minute at birth; 25 cycles per minute at age 2 years, and 18 cycles per minute at age 10 years.
Rhythm	Regular cycles with inspiratory phase slightly longer than expiratory phase.	
Depth	Even; appropriate to activity, with occasional sighs.	
Ratio of respirations to heart rate	1 respiration per 4 heart beats.	
Quality	Quiet at rest, nonlabored; no flaring of nostrils, no intercostal or abdominal retraction. No tachypnea, hyperpnea.	
Type of breathing	Diaphragmatic in male; costal in female; no Cheyne-Stokes or Kussmaul breathing.	
PALPATION		
Thorax		
Tenderness	None.	
Lesions	None.	
Respiratory excursion	Equal and symmetrical.	
PERCUSSION		
Lungs		
Quality	Symmetrical and resonant, not dull or flat.	
AUSCULTATION		
Lungs		
Quality of breath sounds	Vesicular breath sounds in the lung fields; no wheezes, crackles, or rumbles.	With advanced age increased A-P diameter may result in reduced intensity of breath sounds.
Voice sounds	Vocal resonance heard as murmur through chest wall while client speaks; no bronchophony, whispered pectoriloquy; egophony.	

From References 4, 42, and 59.

BOX 16–30. RECORDING THE ASSESSMENT OF THE THORAX AND LUNGS

Subjective Manifestations

Lungs. Last chest x-ray one year ago; reports entirely normal. Denies history of bronchitis, pneumonia, cough, or hemoptysis. No vocal changes or hoarseness. No exposure to tuberculosis. Reports wheezing as a child related to seasonal allergies now controlled with antihistamines. Client does not smoke and has no contact with secondary smoke.

Objective Manifestations

Thorax. Thorax is symmetrical and without skin lesions or bony abnormalities. Respiratory rate is 16 per minute, regular, and unlabored, with full respiratory excursion.
Lungs. Resonant throughout, with vesicular breath sounds bilaterally. No wheezes or crackles present.

is also an opportune time to begin a preventive strategy with potential teenage smokers. (See also Chap. 27.)

CARDIOVASCULAR SYSTEM

Overview

Assessment of the heart includes a careful history, especially in relation to life-style patterns that affect coronary health. The physical examination consists of precordial inspection and palpation and auscultation of the heart sounds. Evaluation of the peripheral vessels in the extremities and measurement of the blood pressure complete the examination. The information necessary to elicit from the client prior to the physical examination is found in Table 16–31.

TABLE 16–31. SAMPLE CLIENT HISTORY QUESTIONS FOR SUBJECTIVE MANIFESTATIONS: CARDIOVASCULAR SYSTEM

1. Do you have high blood pressure (hypertension)? Are you on medication?
2. Do you have dizzy spells or vertigo?
3. Do you have chest pain (*angina*)? Where does the pain go (radiation)? Do you have sweating (diaphoresis), shortness of breath (dyspnea), skipping heartbeats (*palpitations*), racing heart (*tachycardia*), or nausea?
4. Does your shortness of breath come and go (intermittent)? Does it come on unexpectedly (paroxysmal)? Does it occur when lying down (recumbent)? Does it occur only at night (*paroxysmal nocturnal dyspnea*)?
5. How many pillows do you use at night?
6. Do you have a cough? At night (nocturnal)? In the daytime (diurnal)? Do you cough up blood (hemoptysis)?
7. Do your feet swell? Are your shoes tight at the end of the day?
8. Do you have leg pain? Does it occur with exercise (*claudication*)? Do your legs hurt at rest? Change in leg color (cyanosis, pigmentation)?
9. Do you have swollen leg veins (*varicosities*)?
10. Do you have numbness or tingling of the feet (*paresthesia*)?
11. Did anyone in your family die of heart disease?
12. Do you have any diseases that affect your heart, such as diabetes, obesity, or lung disease?
13. Do you smoke, drink excessive amounts of alcohol, or eat a high-fat diet?
14. Do you exercise? Are you under stress?
15. Does _____ (subjective manifestation) interfere with your usual daily activities? How?

Topographical Anatomy

The heart is located behind and to the left of the sternal bone in the anterior chest wall (Fig. 16–53). The second rib demarcates the approximate position of the great vessels as they leave (the aortic artery) or enter (the vena cava) the atria. The left and right atria constitute the base of the heart, even though they are anatomically superior to the ventricles or apex. The four-chambered heart lies at such an angle that the right ventricle makes up most of the anterior surface.

The most muscular and powerful chamber of the heart, the left ventricle, pulsates against the chest wall at approximately the fifth intercostal space (ICS) at the midclavicular line (MCL). This pulsation is called the **point of maximal impulse (PMI).**

The pulse felt at the PMI reflects the phases of the cardiac cycle described earlier in this chapter. In particular, the PMI corresponds with ventricular systole, the phase in which the heart ventricles contract and eject blood; blood flows from the right ventricle through the pulmonic valve into the pulmonary artery, and from the left ventricle through the aortic valve into the aorta. A characteristic "lubb" sound, the first heart sound referred to as S_1, accompanies the closure of the pulmonic and aortic valves. This sound corresponds to the onset of ventricular systole and the apical pulse felt over the PMI. The period between impulses represents ventricular diastole, when the atria contract to eject blood through the tricuspid (right atrium) and mitral (left atrium) valves into the ventricles. A characteristic "dupp" sound, the second heart sound referred to as S_2, accompanies the closure of the tricuspid and mitral valves. This sound corresponds to the onset of ventricular diastole (Fig. 16–54).

The sounds of the valves closing, like other body sounds, project to the surface of the body. Each valve is best heard over a specific area; these are collectively referred to as auscultatory areas, because they are the ideal areas for positioning the head of the stethoscope to hear sounds made by the valves. The closure of the tricuspid valve is heard best in the left fifth intercostal space close to the sternum. The closure of the mitral valve is best heard in the left fifth intercostal space medial to the midclavicular line. The closure of the pulmonic valve is best heard in the left second intercostal space close to the sternum, and the closure of the aortic valve is best heard in the right second intercostal space

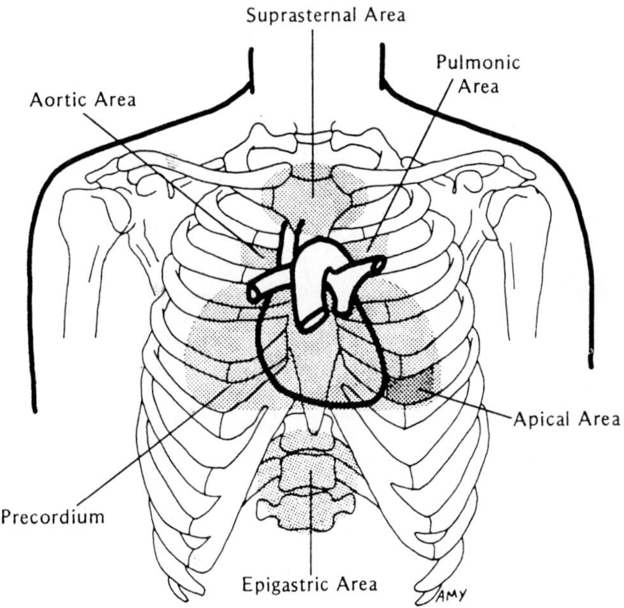

Figure 16–53. Orientation of heart and auscultatory areas. (Source: *Berger KJ, Fields WL.* Pocket Guide to Health Assessment. *Reston, VA: Reston Publishing Co.; 1980.*)

also close to the sternum (see Fig. 16–53). The area of the chest overlying the heart is referred to as the **precordium.**

Conducting an Examination of the Cardiovascular System

Preparation. The client is examined in two positions, seated and supine, and is disrobed to the waist. The equipment needed consists of a stethoscope with a bell and a diaphragm, a sphygmomanometer to take the blood pressure, and a watch with a second hand to determine heart rate.

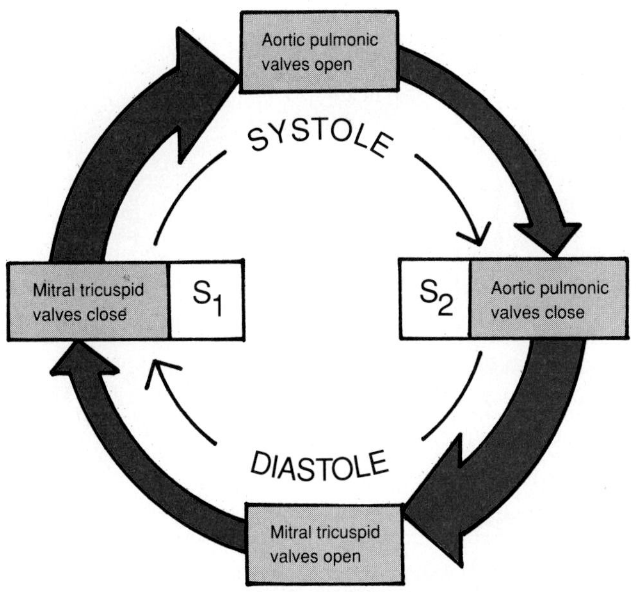

Figure 16–54. Events of the cardiac cycle.

Inspection. With the client seated and the thorax fully exposed, note the contour of the chest.

Precordium. There should be no significant abnormalities of the sternum, such as depression or protrusion, or crookedness of the thoracic spine. Carefully observe the anterior chest wall for visible pulsations and note their force and location. The only pulsation normally seen is the PMI located at the fifth ICS at the MCL; however, the PMI will not be visible in obese clients or in women with pendulous breasts. The PMI is small (2 cm or less in diameter) and has a regular rhythm. No other pulsations are usually visible in a healthy adult of average body build. Any evidence of intercostal bulging or retraction or pulsations in areas other than the PMI is not an expected finding unless the client has respiratory disease or is very thin.

Blood Vessels. The carotid arteries, supplying oxygenated blood to the brain, and the internal and external jugular veins, returning blood from the brain to the heart via the vena cava, pass just beneath the skin on both sides of the neck and are visible to the naked eye. Inspect the carotid pulse, located in the lower third of the neck just medial to the border of the sternomastoid muscle, for presence, symmetry, and rhythm (Fig. 16–55). The pulsation should be strong but not so forceful that it causes the head to bob.

Venous pulsations from the internal and external jugular veins are visible at the base of the neck (see Fig. 16–55). Tangential (oblique) lighting and elevation of the client to at least 30 degrees facilitate visibility. The external jugular vein with its diffuse and undulant (wavy) pulsation is easier to see than the internal jugular vein. Assess the venous pulsations for amplitude and the veins for distension. Prominent pulsations may be indicative of right-sided heart failure. Fullness or distension of the jugular vein into the jaw line when the client is seated to 45 degrees can indicate greatly increased pressure in the vessels from heart disease or atherosclerosis. Normally the neck vessels lie flat when the client is seated and distend only when he or she is supine. See Figure 31–6, which shows how jugular venous distension is assessed.

Observe the peripheral vessels in the extremities for the presence or absence of visible pulsations. Neither pulsations nor varicosities (distended veins) should be noticeable. The status of the skin (color and temperature) and the presence, absence, and distribution of hair on the arms and legs also indicate competency of the blood exchange and flow mechanisms of the peripheral vessels.

Palpation. Palpate the precordium with the palm of the hand in a systematic pattern at the auscultatory anatomical sites (see Fig. 16–53 for the location of the precordium).

Apex and Precordium. Generally, the PMI in the fifth ICS at the MCL is the only pulsation palpable. The PMI is felt as

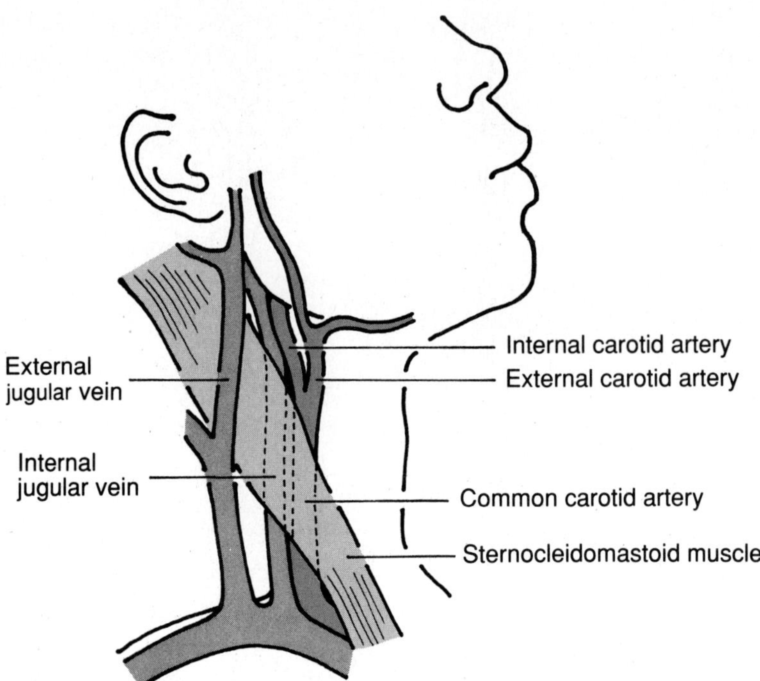

Figure 16–55. Location of the carotid artery and internal and external jugular veins.

a light tap with a diameter of about 1.5 cm and is most easily felt when the client is seated and bending slightly forward or lying on the left side. These positions bring the apex of the heart into closer proximity to the anterior chest wall. Abnormal movements of the chest wall are caused by forceful contractions of the heart musculature. They are called "lifts" or "heaves." Others, called "thrills," are murmurs associated with turbulent flow through the valves of the heart. First, place your whole hand gently on the client's anterior chest covering the second ICS on the right and left sides of the sternal border (Fig. 16–56). Next, move your hand until it covers the entire left sternal border. Finally, place your palpating hand across the chest at the fifth ICS with your fingers at the PMI to evaluate the face of the apical impulse (see Fig. 16–56).

Blood Vessels. Examine the arterial pulses by palpating them with the second and third fingers, using the distal pads. If the client's pulse is difficult to find, vary the pressure you apply with the fingers. Also vary the position of your fingers slightly, going thoroughly over the area where the pulse is usually found. The presence of fat or tissue swelling may make it difficult to perceive pulsations. Pulses are best felt over bony prominences. When you locate a pulse, make sure it is the client's pulse and not your own. You will be able to distinguish the two by checking your own apical pulse as you palpate the client's peripheral pulse. If the pulses correspond, it is likely you are palpating your own pulse.

First, palpate the carotid pulses in the neck. Be sure to palpate them one at a time to prevent occlusion of the vessels by your touch. Unilateral palpation prevents subsequent cutting off of the blood supply to the brain. The importance of following this procedure cannot be stressed too strongly. Note the amplitude (strength), rate, and rhythm of the carotid pulses.

Palpate the pulses of the upper extremities (temporal, brachials, and radials), the lower abdomen or inguinal area (femorals), and the lower extremities (popliteal, posterior tibial, and dorsalis pedis) and evaluate them for presence, rate, rhythm, and symmetry (Fig. 16–57). The peripheral pulses should be symmetrical (the same in paired extremities), reflect the cardiac rate bilaterally, and have a regular rhythm.

Pulse rate has been found to vary with race, but in

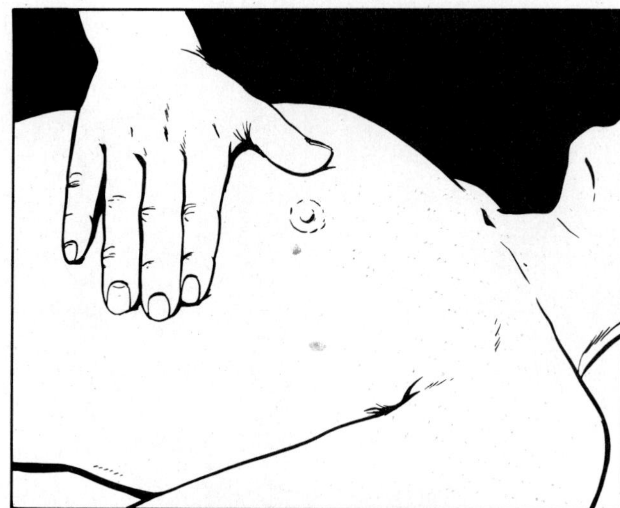

Figure 16–56. Palpating the precordium and point of maximum impulse (PMI). (Source: *Rudy EB, Gray VR.* Handbook of Health Assessment. *3rd ed. Norwalk, CT: Appleton & Lange; 1991.*)

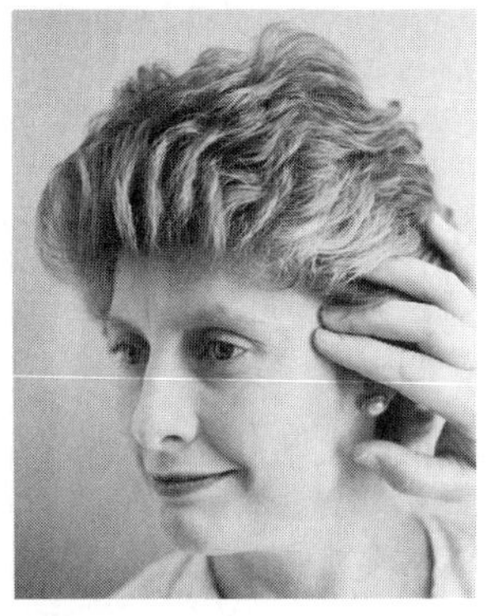
A

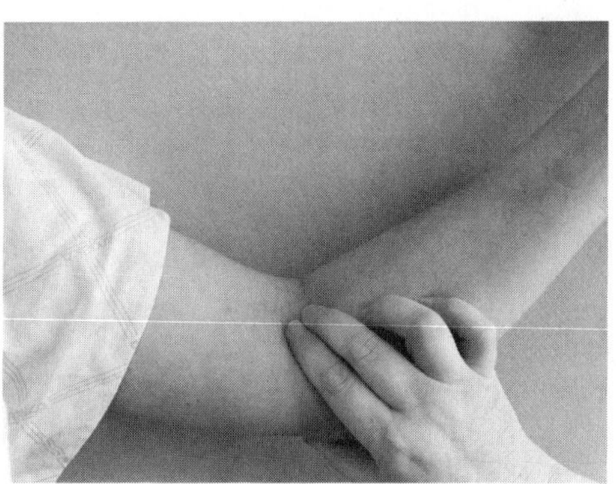
B

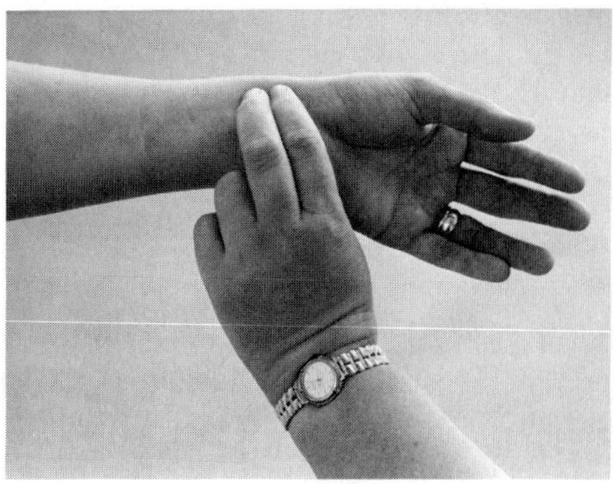
C

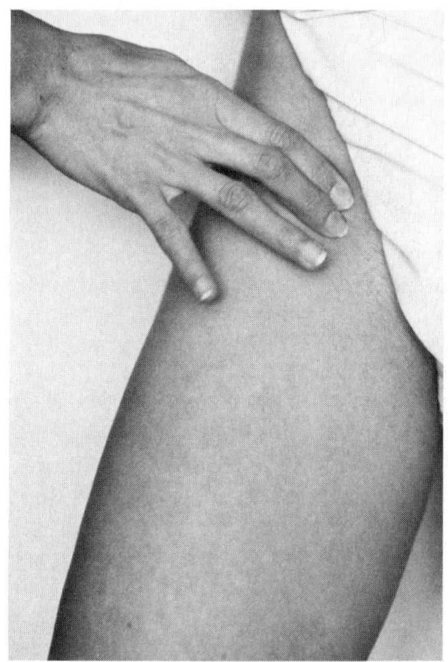
D

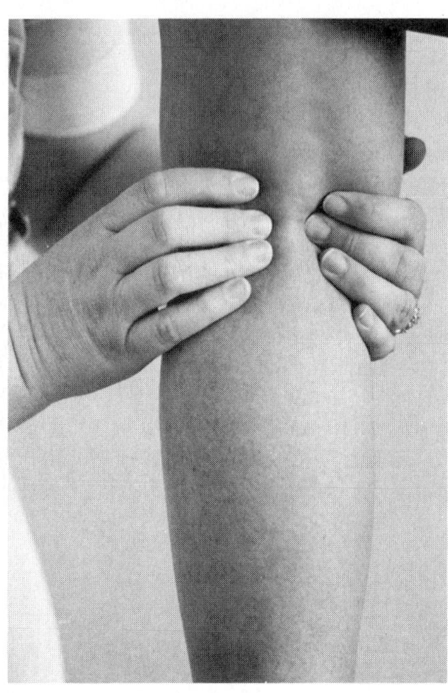
E

Figure 16–57. Palpating the peripheral arteries. **A.** Temporal. **B.** Brachial. **C.** Radial. **D.** Femoral. **E.** Popliteal. **F.** Posterior tibial. **G.** Dorsalis pedis.

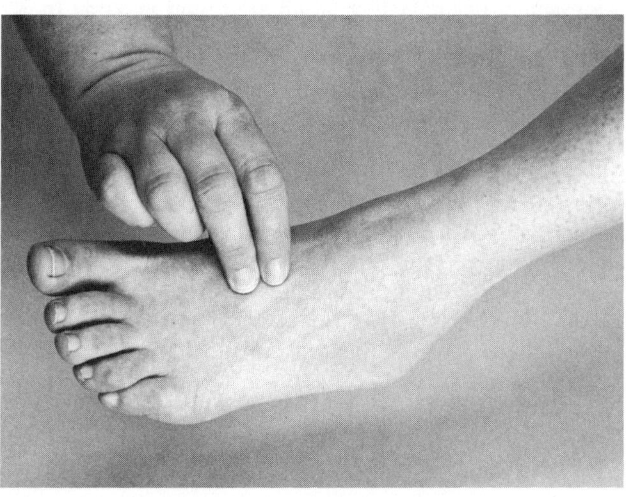
F

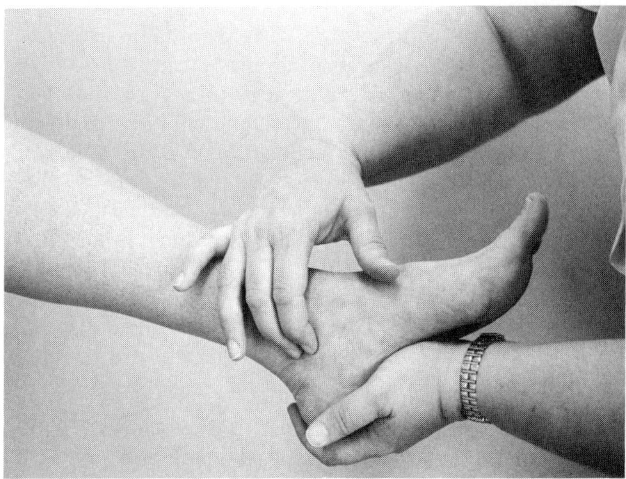
G

males only. The findings of Lui and associates indicate that the pulse rates of black male subjects are lower on average than the pulse rates of white male subjects, by as many as two to four beats per minute.[75] The same difference was not observed between black and white females, however.

Auscultation. Check Figure 16–53 to review the locations for auscultation of the precordium.

Heart Sounds. The first heart sound (S_1) is heard throughout the precordium, but the sound is more concentrated along the left sternal border and at the apex. The S_2 sound, or "dupp," is heard at the apex as well, but is louder directly over the base of the heart (right and left second ICSs at the sternal borders). Paired valves that do not close simultaneously cause a "split" heart sound. Inspiration produces a delay in closure of the pulmonic valve and creates a split S_2, which is normal in the healthy heart.

Begin auscultation of the heart by placing the diaphragm of the stethoscope at the second ICS to the right of the sternum (aortic area). Concentrate very hard on the S_2 sound, listening for splitting, rate, rhythm, and intensity of the sound. Slowly "inch" the stethoscope across the sternomanubrium junction and concentrate on the sounds of pulmonary valve closure. A sinus arrhythmia (a heart rate faster with inspiration than with expiration) is often heard in this location, especially in children. Move the stethoscope slowly down the left sternal border stopping at each ICS to carefully evaluate the heart sounds and to listen between them to systole and diastole. The sound of S_2 will increase moving toward the fifth ICS at the left sternal border (the tricuspid valvular area). Carefully "inch" the stethoscope horizontally until reaching the apical area, which generally coincides with the PMI. It may be helpful to have the client lean forward slightly to make the mitral valve sound as audible as possible, especially if the client has a thick chest wall. After completing auscultation with the diaphragm, turn the head of the stethoscope over and repeat the entire process with the bell. Placing the bell of the stethoscope very lightly on the chest facilitates the audibility of low-pitched sounds such as S_3 and S_4, as well as the sound of selected murmurs. The diaphragm accentuates the high-pitched sounds of S_1 and S_2. The third heart sound, S_3, is the sound of rapid ventricular filling and may be heard in healthy children and young adults during the resting phase of the ventricles (diastole). Other diastolic sounds are S_4, the sound of atrial contraction, and OS, the opening snap of a damaged mitral valve. Neither of these sounds is heard in the normally functioning heart. The sound of an ejection click (EJ), a clicking sound heard as blood is ejected, particularly from the left ventricle, signals a malfunctioning mitral valve. The extra heart sounds (S_3, S_4, OS, and EJ) are evaluated for timing in the cardiac cycle (systole or diastole) and location of maximal intensity.

Murmurs. *Murmurs* are the sound of turbulent blood flow through a faulty valve or an abnormal opening in the heart or great vessels. Evaluate murmurs by describing their timing in the cardiac cycle, their location (the auscultatory area best heard), radiation if any (listen to the neck and axilla for radiation of murmurs), intensity (as graded on a scale of 1 to 10), pitch (high, medium, or low), and quality (musical, rumbling, harsh, blowing, ascending, descending, or plateau).

After completing the cardiac assessment with the client seated, ask the client to lie down and repeat the entire examination. Listening to the heart in two positions is essential because some heart sounds change with positioning. The functional heart murmur of childhood for instance is classically heard better when the child is supine.

Vascular Sounds. Auscultate the carotid arteries for *bruits* (turbulence in the vessels) and the jugular veins in children for a venous hum (turbulence in the jugular). A *venous hum* is a continuous sound (heard in both systole and diastole) just above the medial third of the clavicles while the child is seated. The epigastric area (Fig. 16–53) is auscultated for bruits in the abdominal aorta, and the inguinal area is auscultated for bruits in the femoral vessels.

Blood Pressure. Evaluation of the blood pressure is an important part of a thorough cardiovascular assessment. The blood pressure is taken in both arms and while the client is sitting, standing, and supine. Sometimes the pressure is also taken in the thigh, but this procedure requires the use of a large cuff referred to as a thigh cuff (see earlier section on *Measurements and Vital Signs*). The normal range of adult blood pressure is 100/60 to 140/90. The difference between the two arms is less than 10 mm Hg. When the client rises from a seated to a standing position the orthostatic drop should not exceed 10 mm Hg. The thigh pressure is usually as much as 10 mm Hg higher than the blood pressure in the arm. It should be noted that blood pressure, like pulse rates, has been found to vary with race. Lui and associates found that in their sample black participants had a higher average systolic blood pressure than white participants for every age, sex, and education group.[75] They also tended to have a slightly higher diastolic blood pressure.

The findings expected to result from the cardiovascular assessment of the healthy adult are found in Table 16–32.

Special Considerations, Precautions, and Sources of Error

The cardiac examination should be divided into manageable components. The nurse should concentrate on one segment at a time, first carefully inspecting the precordium and the vessels and then moving on to palpation of the auscultatory areas and the peripheral pulses. After palpation, the nurse should place the stethoscope on the chest wall and listen to the heart sounds, concentrating on S_1 and S_2 and then on systole and diastole. Extra sounds between S_1 and S_2 are sometimes heard and should be timed for the points at which they occur in the cardiac cycle. Clients' vocalizing or movement will interfere with precise auscultation of heart sounds. Cardiac assessment takes time and clients should be prepared for this so that they do not become alarmed when the nurse seems to be listening to their heart for what may seem like a very long time.

TABLE 16–32. OBJECTIVE MANIFESTATION FINDINGS AND LIFE CYCLE VARIATIONS: CARDIOVASCULAR SYSTEM

Examination Technique	Expected Findings	Common Life Cycle Variations
INSPECTION		
Thorax		
Configuration	Contour symmetrical and without significant boney abnormalities of the thoracic spine and sternum.	
Precordium		
Pulsations	2 cm or less in diameter. Only the PMI should be visible in the 5th ICS at the MCL.	
Neck		
Carotid arteries	Pulsations visible and regular in the lower third of the neck alongside the sternomastoid muscle.	
Jugular veins	Diffuse, undulant pulsations visible at the base of the neck. Veins flat when seated and may distend when supine or leaning back less than 40 degrees.	
Extremities—Peripheral Vascular		
Pulsations	None visible.	
Venous distension	None.	
Hair distribution	Present—sparse to dense.	Amount decreases with age.
Skin color/temperature	Color appropriate to genetic heritage and remainder of body and warm to the touch; no cyanosis, pallor, or mottling.	
Nail shape/color	Oval nails, pale pink color; no nail thickening; no clubbing.	
PALPATION		
Precordium		Palpation of apical impulse may be difficult in adolescents as muscle mass increases in males and breast mass increases in females.
Lifts/pulsations	Only the PMI is palpable at the 5th ICS at the MCL.	Children under age 7 years have PMI at the 4th ICS; PMI reaches 5th ICS by age 7 years. Enlarged uterus shifts diaphragm upward in pregnancy altering position of heart so that apex moves laterally.
Neck and Extremities		
Pulses	(**Caution:** simultaneous bilateral palpation of carotids should not be done.) No pulse deficit. Bracheal and radial pulses in the arms; femoral in the inguinal area; popliteal, posterior tibial, and dorsalis pedis in the lower extremities all palpable and regular in rate and rhythm.	
Evaluation of pulse rate	60–100 beats per minute in adults; 70–150 in children; varies with age, physical activity, emotional status; no pulse deficit.	Pulse rate reduced as child grows and cardiac output increases.
Rhythm	Regular; occasional premature beats not significant.	
Amplitude	All pulses present, symmetrical; amplitude varies with size of artery; no variation beat to beat; neither bounding nor thready. Evaluation scale: 1 + Greatly diminished 2 + Slightly diminished 3 + Normal 4 + Bounding	With advanced age, blood vessels may lose compliance, which results in loss of pulse amplitude.

(continued)

TABLE 16–32. (continued)

Examination Technique	Expected Findings	Common Life Cycle Variations
Elasticity of arterial walls	Soft, pliable, not resistant to compression.	With advanced age, blood vessels may show resistance to compression.
AUSCULTATION		
Precordium		
Heart sounds S_1	S_1 sound loudest in the right and left 2nd ICS; S_2 loudest along the left sternal border and the apex. "Lubb" sound synchronous with carotid upstroke, louder, duller, lower pitched, and slightly longer than 2nd sound at apex. Splitting of S_1 may be heard over tricuspid area.	
S_2	"Dupp" sound synchronous with descent of carotid pulse wave, louder than first sound at base. Splitting may be heard over pulmonic area during inspiration.	Split S_2 common in children; child may have functional systolic murmur.
Extra sounds, friction rubs, murmurs	None.	
Neck and Extremities		Venous hum commonly heard in children.
Carotid bruit	None.	
Femoral bruit	None.	
Blood pressure assessment	Varies with age. Range 100/60 to 140/90. Difference between limbs should be less than 10 mm Hg. Orthostatic drop should not exceed 10 mm Hg.	Blood pressure decreases somewhat during second trimester of pregnancy and may rise thereafter, but not more than 30 mm Hg systolic or 15 mm Hg diastolic. May increase with age and with the use of oral contraceptives.

From References 4, 42, and 59.

Recording

The blood pressure and the pulse rate are often recorded along with the respiratory rate at the beginning of the physical examination writeup. The cardiac assessment, the evaluation of the neck vessels, and the assessment of the peripheral vascular vessels are recorded together. The record also includes subjective information obtained from the client during the initial interview. Box 16–31 presents an example of a record of subjective and objective findings.

Role of the Nurse and the Assessment of the Cardiovascular System

Nurses have a long tradition of participation in the clinical evaluation of the heart and circulation. The measurement of pulse rate and blood pressure for many years has been an important nursing responsibility. In recent years the scope of the nurse's evaluation of this system has expanded to include the full range of physical examination techniques. Thus the nurse has an even more important role in evaluating circulation.

For today's nurse, physical evaluation of the heart and peripheral vessels is only one aspect of the cardiovascular assessment. The nurse also is in a vital position to appraise the client's risk factors for heart and vascular disease by taking into account the health history. Clients with health risks such as smoking, a high-fat diet, obesity, sedentary life-style, and a family history of early heart disease need to be counseled about the necessity of making behavioral changes that will reduce their risk of heart disease and atherosclerosis. Nurses above all are teachers and therefore are expected to demonstrate, by their own healthy behaviors and by client education, how to replace poor habits with healthful habits.

BOX 16–31. RECORDING THE ASSESSMENT OF THE CARDIOVASCULAR SYSTEM

Subjective Manifestations

Cardiovascular. No family or personal history of heart disease or vascular disease. Maintains a low-fat diet, exercises regularly with 30-minute walks. Does not smoke, rarely consumes alcohol, and maintains a steady weight appropriate to body build. Has a history of normotensive blood pressure. Experiences no dizziness, chest pain, or dyspnea. Has noted no cough, skin color changes, palpitations, or arrhythmias. Denies pedal edema, paresthesia, or leg pain.

Objective Manifestations

Cardiovascular. BP 122/78. HR 84 and regular. Precordium without lifts or thrills. PMI 5th ICS at the MCL. S_1 and S_2 regular, no extra sounds or murmurs. Neck vessels without bruits; carotid pulse 80 and regular. Peripheral pulses present, symmetric, and regular; skin of extremities pink and warm.

■ ABDOMEN AND GASTROINTESTINAL SYSTEM

Overview

The assessment of the abdomen includes health history questions related to gastrointestinal function. Pertinent questions are listed in Table 16–33. All four of the examination modes are used in the abdominal examination, but their usual order is altered. Auscultation precedes percussion and palpation so that the nurse can hear the bowel sounds before they are disturbed by manual pressure. Percussion alters both the frequency and the intensity of bowel sounds.

Topographical Anatomy

Generally the surface of the abdomen is divided into quadrants by two intersecting reference lines. One line runs vertically from the xiphoid process through the umbilicus to the pubic symphysis and the other runs horizontally through the umbilicus (Fig. 16–58). These lines guide the examiner's hands and also allow the examiner to pinpoint and describe the physical findings. Figure 16–59 shows the underlying organs of the abdominal quadrants and Box 16–32 lists the abdominal contents (organs and intestines) located in each quadrant.

Conducting an Examination of the Abdomen and Gastrointestinal System

Preparation. The client is supine for the abdominal examination, with the head resting on a small pillow and arms straight at the sides. Knees may be flexed to relax the abdominal wall muscles. The breasts of the female client are covered and a drape is placed over the genitalia and legs of all clients. A stethoscope is needed for this examination.

Inspection. It is best to begin inspecting the client's abdomen from a seated position. This position enables the examiner to view across the surface of the client's abdomen. Observing the shadows apparent from this position aids visualization of contour deviations.

TABLE 16–33. SAMPLE CLIENT HISTORY QUESTIONS FOR SUBJECTIVE MANIFESTATIONS: ABDOMEN AND GASTROINTESTINAL SYSTEM

1. Have you had a change in appetite? What is your usual weight?
2. Do you have difficulty swallowing (dysphagia)?
3. Are there any foods you have difficulty tolerating?
4. Have you felt nauseated? Have you vomited (*emesis*)? Is there blood in your vomitus (*hematemesis*)?
5. Do you experience indigestion? Heart burn (*pyrosis*)? Belching (*eructation*)?
6. Do you use antacids and, if so, how often?
7. Does your abdomen feel bloated after eating (*distention*)?
8. Do you have abdominal pain? Is it associated with eating?
9. Have you had abdominal surgery and, if so, when and where?
10. Does _____ (subjective manifestation) interfere with any of your usual daily activities? How?

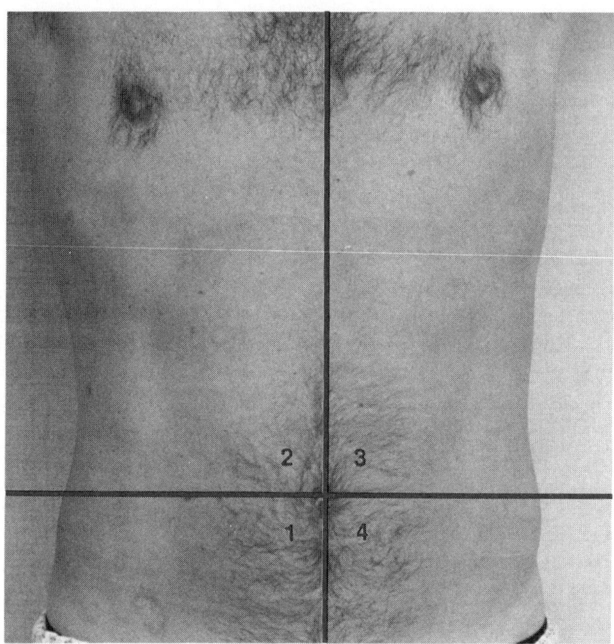

Figure 16–58. Abdominal quadrants.

Next, look at the skin over the abdomen, and note the presence of scars or discolorations. Scars may represent old surgeries. Ask the client to identify the cause of any scars found. Pigmentation may be apparent, particularly if the client has been exposed to the sun or is pregnant. Look for the presence of linear bluish-gray or silvery-gray discolorations over the abdomen and upper thighs. These are called striae and often accompany weight gain, pregnancy, or the presence of large amounts of fluid in the abdomen, known as ascites.

The contour of the abdomen is usually flat as the client lies in the recumbent position. The obese client will have a rounded, protuberant abdominal contour; the overly thin client will have a concave or scaphoid abdominal contour. Be sure to inspect for symmetry. In addition to obesity, generalized symmetrical distension also occurs in pregnancy or may represent ascites, large tumors, or the collection of gas in the abdomen. Ask the client to take a deep breath. This will lower the diaphragm, compress the organs in the abdomen, and possibly reveal previously unseen bulges or masses.

Note the location and contour of the umbilicus. It should be at the center of the abdominal quadrants, and should not be shifted upward, downward, or laterally. It may be everted, but should not be inflamed or swollen or have an obvious bulge protruding from it, suggestive of a hernia. It is particularly important to inspect the umbilicus of newborn clients. Note whether the cord is present and its condition and whether it is dry and odorless as expected, and look for signs of inflammation or herniation.

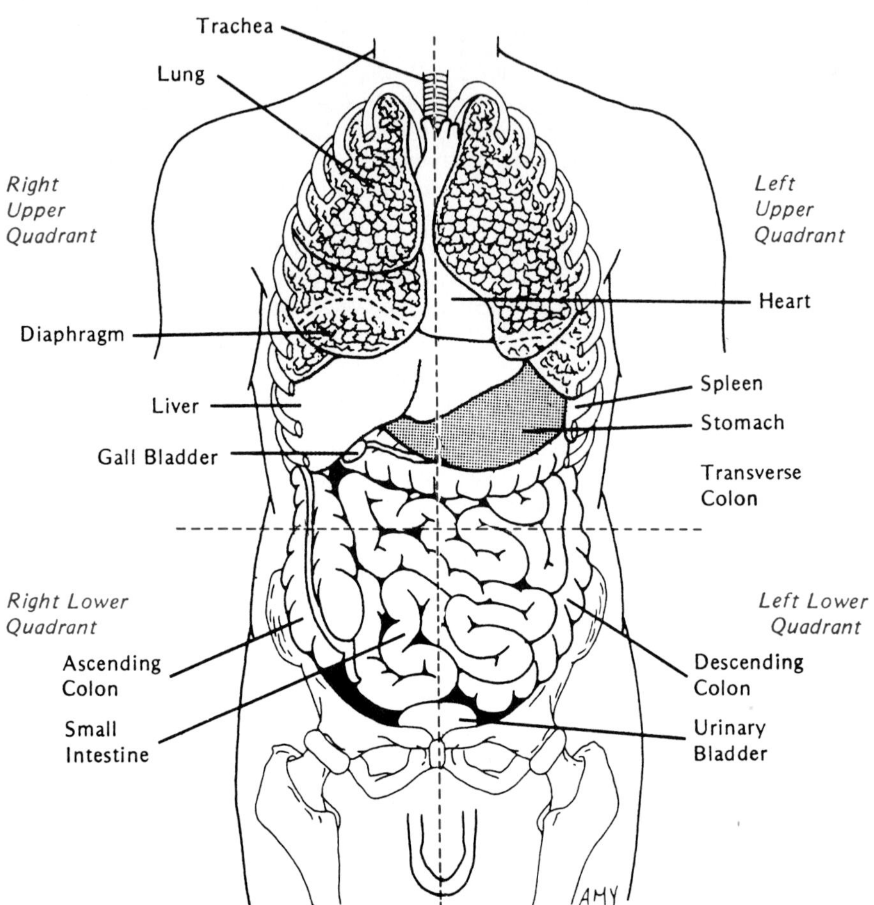

Figure 16–59. Topographical anatomy of the abdomen. (Source: *Berger KJ, Fields WL.* Pocket Guide to Health Assessment. *Reston, VA: Reston Publishing Co.; 1980.)*

Note any behavior from the client that may indicate the presence of pain. Reluctance to move, cough, or take a deep breath, called guarding, may be an important clue. Be sure to ask the client if he or she is experiencing abdominal pain. If the answer is affirmative, ask the client to locate the pain over the surface of the abdomen.

Auscultation. Following inspection, use the diaphragm of your stethoscope to listen to each quadrant of the abdomen for bowel sounds and vascular sounds. Make sure the diaphragm of your stethoscope is warm before touching it to the surface of the client's abdomen. A cold stethoscope or hands may initiate contraction of the abdominal muscles. To auscultate the abdomen, place the warm diaphragm gently on the surface of the abdominal skin and hold it in place with very light pressure. Excessive pressure will have the same effect as palpation on the bowel sounds.

With the stethoscope in place, listen for bowel sounds. Bowel sounds are an expected finding of auscultation. An absence of bowel sounds is ominous and may signify intestinal obstruction. The normal bowel produces gurgling sounds every 5 to 15 seconds. Gastrointestinal complaints associated with diarrhea induce high-pitched, loud, tinkling noises referred to as hyperactive bowel sounds.

BOX 16–32. LOCATION OF ORGANS IN ABDOMINAL QUADRANTS

Upper Right Quadrant	**Upper Left Quadrant**
Liver	Left lobe of liver
Gallbladder	Stomach
Duodenum	Spleen
Head of pancreas	Left kidney
Right adrenal gland	Body of pancreas
Right kidney	Left adrenal gland
Hepatic flexure of colon	Splenic flexure of colon
Ascending colon	Transverse colon
Transverse colon	Descending colon
Lower Right Quadrant	**Lower Left Quadrant**
Lower lobe of right kidney	Lower lobe of left kidney
Cecum	Sigmoid colon
Appendix	Descending colon
Ascending colon	Left ovary
Right ovary	Left fallopian tube
Right fallopian tube	Left ureter
Right ureter	Left spermatic cord
Right spermatic cord	

Midline

Bladder
Uterus

Percussion. Using the fingers to strike the abdomen (refer to the assessment of the thorax), percuss all four quadrants of the abdomen. As you percuss remember which organs lie beneath your fingers. Note the sound of dullness over the liver and spleen and the tympany of the air-filled organs over the stomach and intestines. Percussion of the midline in the lower abdomen may elicit the dullness of a full urinary bladder. While percussing, observe the client's face for indications of pain caused by the examination. If the client has complained of pain before the examination, percuss, and palpate, the painful area *last*.

Palpation. Begin this phase of the examination by lightly and very gently palpating each quadrant of the abdomen to localize areas of pain, superficial masses, and enlarged tender organs. Following light palpation repeat the process, but this time press deeply into the muscle wall to delineate the abdominal organs and locate any abnormal masses. Use one or both hands to accomplish deep palpation (Fig. 16–60). Identification of the borders of abdominal organs using the technique of palpation is covered later in the nursing curriculum.

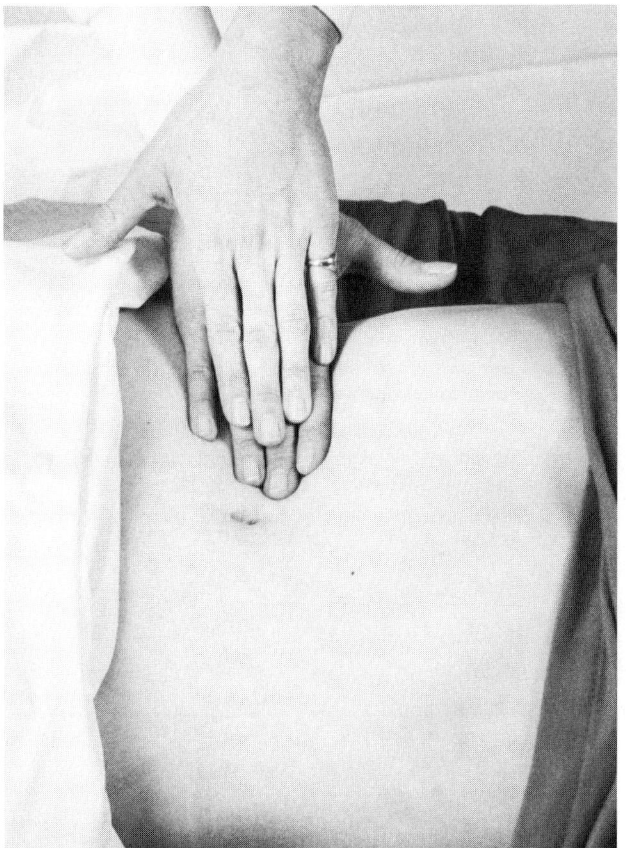

Figure 16–60. Deep palpation of the abdomen. (Source: *Block GJ, Nolan JW.* Health Assessment for Professional Nursing: A Developmental Approach. *2nd ed. Norwalk, CT: Appleton-Century-Crofts; 1986.*)

Table 16–34 describes the expected findings of the examination and life cycle variations.

Special Considerations, Precautions, and Sources of Error

Physical assessment of the abdomen is greatly enhanced by an adequate gastrointestinal review of systems. A complaint of pain, for instance, should lead the examiner to alter the examination pattern. The tender area should be percussed and then palpated gently.

Remember that the sequence of the examination modes must be altered and the abdomen auscultated prior to percussion and palpation. Changing the order of the examination avoids overstimulation of bowel activity and misleading hyperactive bowel sounds.

Recording

A sample recording of the gastrointestinal review of systems and the findings from the physical examination is found in Box 16–33.

Role of the Nurse and the Assessment of the Abdomen and Gastrointestinal System

Loss of appetite, nausea, vomiting, and abdominal pain are frequent health problems that clients experience. The physical examination of the abdomen generally confirms the problems reported by the client during the health interview. Nurses in all clinical settings encounter clients who have illnesses and distressing symptoms related to the organs of the abdomen. Because these organs play an essential role in health, accurate assessment and referral of abnormal findings is an important nursing responsibility. Nurses also have occasion to counsel clients about nutrition, weight control, and problems with elimination. Health teaching in these areas is enhanced by the ability to obtain the necessary subjective information from the client and relate it to physical examination findings.

BOX 16–33. RECORDING THE ASSESSMENT OF THE ABDOMEN AND GASTROINTESTINAL SYSTEM

Subjective Manifestations

Abdomen. Client denies weight change or loss of appetite. Usual weight is 162 pounds. Client is a vegetarian, has an adequate understanding of good nutrition, and has no food intolerances. Denies dysphagia, heartburn, indigestion, nausea, and vomiting.

Objective Manifestations

Abdomen. Flat and symmetrical, without visible pulsations or peristaltic movements. Skin clear; umbilicus without herniation or lesions. Nontender to deep palpation. Liver 2 cm below the right costal margin. Tympany over the gastric air bubble in the left upper quadrant. No evidence of abnormal masses or enlarged organs.

TABLE 16–34. OBJECTIVE MANIFESTATION FINDINGS AND LIFE CYCLE VARIATIONS: ABDOMEN AND GASTROINTESTINAL SYSTEM

Examination Technique	Expected Findings	Common Life Cycle Variations
INSPECTION		
Abdomen		
Skin	Same pigmentation as rest of body; no rashes or scars; no tight, shiny skin.	Straie may appear over pregnant abdomen. With advanced age, loss of skin elasticity leads to skin redundancy.
Contour	Symmetrical, no obvious masses, no distension.	Rounded contour in children gives pot-bellied appearance in toddler—slimming occurs by age 5 years. Abdominal wall slackens with aging.
Umbilicus	No herniation or lesions.	
Movement	Visible peristalsis in very thin individuals.	
Pulsations	Arterial pulsations may be visible in epigastrium in thin individuals.	
AUSCULTATION		
Abdomen		
Bowel sounds	High-pitched, gurgling peristaltic sounds occur every 5–15 seconds over all quadrants.	
Vascular sounds	None.	
PERCUSSION		
Abdomen		
Percussion notes	Tympany over gastric bubble and air-filled bowel. Liver dullness in RUQ.	
PALPATION		
Abdomen		
Tenderness	None.	
Masses	None.	
Organs		
Uterus		Pregnant uterus protrudes gradually. As uterine fundus rises, umbilicus flattens and may protrude.
Liver	Liver edge felt 2–3 cm below right costal margin; smooth, sharp edge; nontender.	Liver size decreases after age 50, paralleling decrease in body weight.
Spleen	Nonpalpable; nontender.	
Kidneys	Usually nonpalpable; nontender.	The kidneys enlarge during pregnancy, returning to normal 6–8 weeks following delivery.
Gallbladder	Nonpalpable; nontender.	Gallbladder may become distended during pregnancy.
Descending colon	Firmness may be felt in LLQ from collected fecal matter.	
Urinary bladder	Ordinarily nonpalpable; occasionally palpable above symphasis pubis when distended with urine.	
Pulses	Femoral pulses present, strong, and symmetrical. Aorta midline in epigastrium.	

From References 4, 42, and 59.

■ ANUS AND RECTUM

Overview

Assessment of the anus, the rectum, and the perianal region is a continuation of the abdominal evaluation. Some of the health history questions are of necessity overlapping. Table 16–35 lists the questions appropriate to the complete evaluation of the lower intestinal tract. This text covers the inspection of the anus and perianal region. The rectal examination, which requires inserting a gloved finger through the anus for the purpose of palpating the rectum, is an advanced technique taught later in the nursing curriculum.

TABLE 16–35. SAMPLE CLIENT HISTORY QUESTIONS FOR SUBJECTIVE MANIFESTATIONS: ANUS AND RECTUM

1. Do you have diarrhea? Bloody or black stools (*melena*)?
2. Is there pus or mucus in your stool?
3. Do you have hard stools? Are you constipated?
4. Do you use laxatives or enemas on a regular basis?
5. Have you experienced pain with a bowel movement (*dyschezia*)? Feel the need to pass stools frequently and without results (*tenesmus*)?
6. Do you have anal itching (*pruritis*) or painful hemorrhoids?
7. Do you lose control over your bowels (*fecal incontinence*)?
8. Does _____ (subjective manifestation) interfere with any of your usual daily activities? How?

Topographical Anatomy

The rectum and anus form the distal portion of the gastrointestinal tract. The anus, the external opening of the rectal canal, is a muscular sphincter covered with hairless integument. This sphincter is normally closed. The skin and tissue surrounding the anus is called the perianal region.

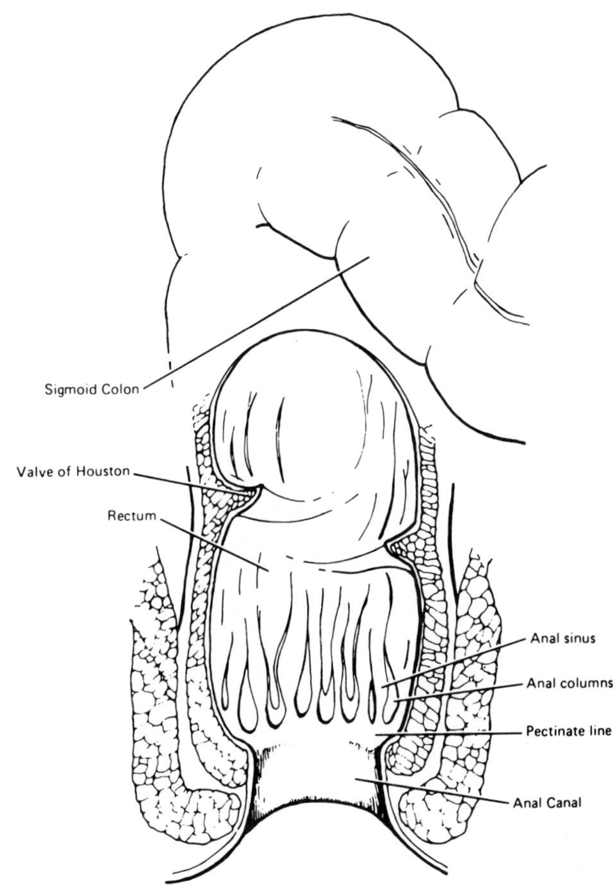

Figure 16–61. Anatomy of the rectum and anus. (Source: *Fields WL, McGinn-Campbell KM.* Introduction to Health Assessment. *Reston, VA: Reston Publishing Co.; 1983.*)

The rectum is lined with moist mucous membrane and joins with the anus at the anorectal junction (Fig. 16–61).

Conducting an Examination of the Anus and Rectum

Preparation. Position the client on the left side with the right leg flexed across the body. Arrange the drape to cover the external genitalia. Gloves and good lighting to adequately visualize the perianal area are needed. The rectum and anus of the female client are frequently assessed in conjunction with the pelvic examination.

Inspection. After placing the client in a left lateral position, spread the buttocks apart with gloved hands. Observe the skin color and texture of the perianal area and inspect the anus for rashes, fissures, excoriations from itching, and dilated veins (hemorrhoids).

The expected findings of the physical examination of the anal region are listed in Table 16–36.

Special Considerations, Precautions, and Sources of Error

Clients often react with embarrassment when discussing bowel dysfunction and anal problems. The nurse's professional attitude and skillful physical examination will dispel anxiety.

The anal area can be difficult to expose to view, especially in the obese client, and lighting is often a problem. The examining room lamp must be moved into a position that fully illuminates the perianal area.

Recording

This physical assessment of the rectum and anus is limited to inspection of the perianal area. This limitation increases the value of the health history in the detection of functional disorders. Box 16–34 is an example of the written record of the history and physical findings of a rectal and anal evaluation.

Role of the Nurse and the Assessment of the Anus and Rectum

Clients frequently complain of discomfort related to bowel function and of discomfort in the anal area. The health

BOX 16–34. RECORDING THE ASSESSMENT OF THE ANUS AND RECTUM

Subjective Manifestations

Anus. No history of diarrhea or constipation. Does not use laxatives or enemas. Denies flatulence, painful defecation, or fecal incontinence. No itching in perianal region and no history of hemorrhoids.

Objective Manifestations

Anus. Skin of perianal region without rashes. No anal fissures, hemorrhoids, or other lesions.

TABLE 16–36. OBJECTIVE MANIFESTATION FINDINGS AND LIFE CYCLE VARIATIONS: ANUS AND RECTUM

Examination Technique	Expected Findings	Common Life Cycle Variations
INSPECTION		
Anus		
Color	More pigmented than surrounding skin	
Lesions	No rashes, masses, or fissures	Hemorrhoids are often visible in pregnant females or clients with chronic constipation.
Hair	None	
Perianal skin		
Color	Same as surrounding skin	
Hair	Sparse, coarse, circumanal	Anal hairs may appear at puberty.
Lesions	No rashes or lesions	

From References 4, 42, and 59.

history and visual inspection of the perianal area should yield sufficient information for the nurse to make an accurate nursing assessment and provide for follow-up care or referral. Discussion of elimination problems frequently centers around the retention of stool. This is especially true in the geriatric population where many individuals use laxatives excessively. Teaching healthful habits like daily exercise and increased intake of dietary fiber and fluid may help clients to decrease their reliance on laxatives and enemas to combat constipation.

GENITOURINARY SYSTEM

Overview

Inspection of the external genitalia of male and female clients lies within the purview of the beginning nurse. More complex evaluations, such as the internal examination of the female pelvic organs or the digital examination of the inguinal area for herniations in the male, are left to the advanced practitioner; however, a complete health history pertinent to the reproductive and urinary systems and inspection of the external genitalia will alert the nurse to refer the client to the advanced practitioner. Table 16–37 lists questions relevant to obtaining information about genitourinary functioning in both men and women.

Topographical Anatomy

Female. The external genitalia, or vulva, of the female is depicted in Figure 16–62. The *mons pubis* is the fatty pad overlying the symphysis pubis (the junction of the pubic bones). This prominence is hair free until puberty when the advent of sparse pubic hair marks the beginning of adult reproductive functioning. The *labia majora* are symmetrical folds of adipose tissue that form the lateral border of the vulva. Contained within this protective covering are the *labia minora,* two folds of mucous membrane that enclose the vestibule. Opening onto the vestibule are the *urethral meatus,* the *vaginal introitus,* and the ducts of *Bartholin's*

TABLE 16–37. SAMPLE CLIENT HISTORY QUESTIONS FOR SUBJECTIVE MANIFESTATIONS: GENITOURINARY SYSTEM

Female

1. Have you noticed an increase in the discharge from the vagina? What is its color, odor, and consistency?
2. At what age was your first period (menarche)? Date of your last menstrual period (LMP)? What is the duration of your period (menses)? Do you have pain or cramps (*dysmenorrhea*)?
3. Have you ever been pregnant? How many living children?
4. Have you stopped having periods (*menopause*)?
5. Do you have pain with intercourse (*dyspareunia*)?
6. What is your method of contraception?
7. When was your last Pap smear? Was it normal?

Male

1. Have you had prostate trouble? A change in your urinary stream?
2. Have you noticed rashes or sores on your genitals? Discharge from your penis?
3. Do you have painful testicles? Any lumps or swellings?
4. Are you able to achieve an erection and ejaculation?
5. Do you perform regular testicular self-examination?

Female and Male

1. Do you have painful urination (*dysuria*)? A sensation that you have to urinate even when the bladder is empty (urgency)? Do you pass frequent small amounts of urine (frequency)?
2. Do you awaken at night to urinate (*nocturia*)?
3. Do you experience dribbling of urine (*incontinence*)? Do you pass urine when you cough, sneeze, or laugh (*stress incontinence*)?
4. Have you had a problem with kidney stones (*calculi*)?
5. Have you had reproductive surgery? Problems with infertility?
6. Does _____ (subjective manifestation) interfere with any of your usual daily activities? How?

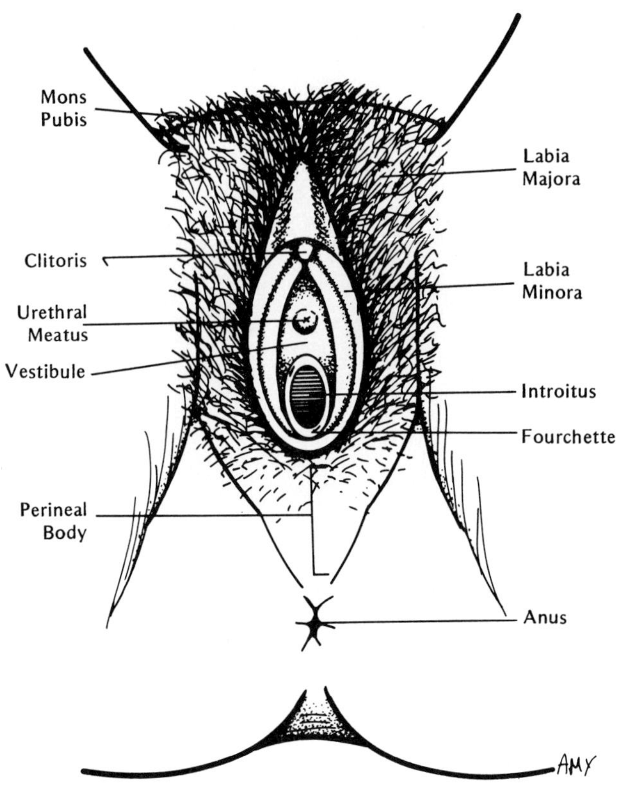

Figure 16–62. External female genitalia. (Source: *Berger KJ, Fields WL.* Pocket Guide to Health Assessment. *Reston, VA: Reston Publishing Co.; 1980.*)

glands. The *clitoris* and *prepuce* are the most anterior structures of the vulva. The perineum, located between the vagina and the anus, is frequently the site of rashes and lesions.

The internal structures of the female reproductive system are the vagina, cervix, uterus, and adenexa (the fallopian tubes and the ovaries). These structures are pictured in Figure 16–63. Examination of the internal structures calls for advanced technique taught later in the nursing curriculum. Internal examination requires a vaginal speculum (Fig. 16–64).

Male. The external male genitalia consists of the penis and *scrotum*. The pubic hair that appears at puberty is distributed in a diamond-shaped pattern above the penis. The shaft of the penis is hairless and extends to the glans. The sensitive glans is covered by the prepuce or foreskin unless it has been surgically removed (circumcision).

The urethral meatus opens centrally at the tip of the penis. The scrotum is a wrinkled pouch with two compartments, each containing a testicle. The left scrotum usually hangs somewhat lower than the right. The *testes* are oval in shape and have a smooth contour and rubbery consistency. The *epididymis* lies across the top of the testicle and extends into the *vas deferens,* a cordlike structure that extends from the seminal vesicles and which together with nerves and vessels passes into the inguinal canal as the *spermatic cord* (Fig. 16–65).

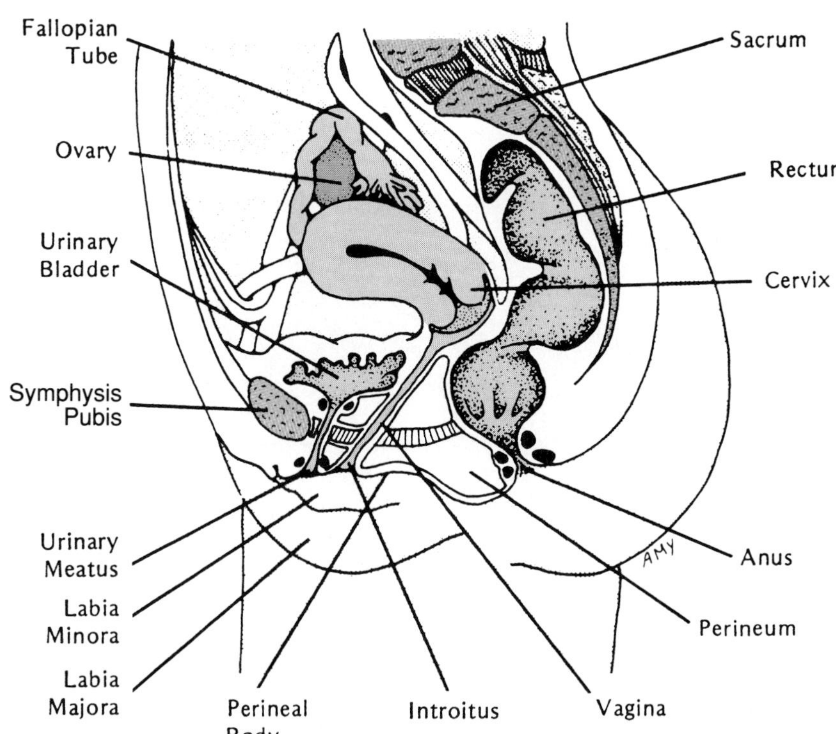

Figure 16–63. Internal female pelvic organs. (Source: *Berger KJ, Fields WL.* Pocket Guide to Health Assessment. *Reston, VA: Reston Publishing Co.; 1980.*)

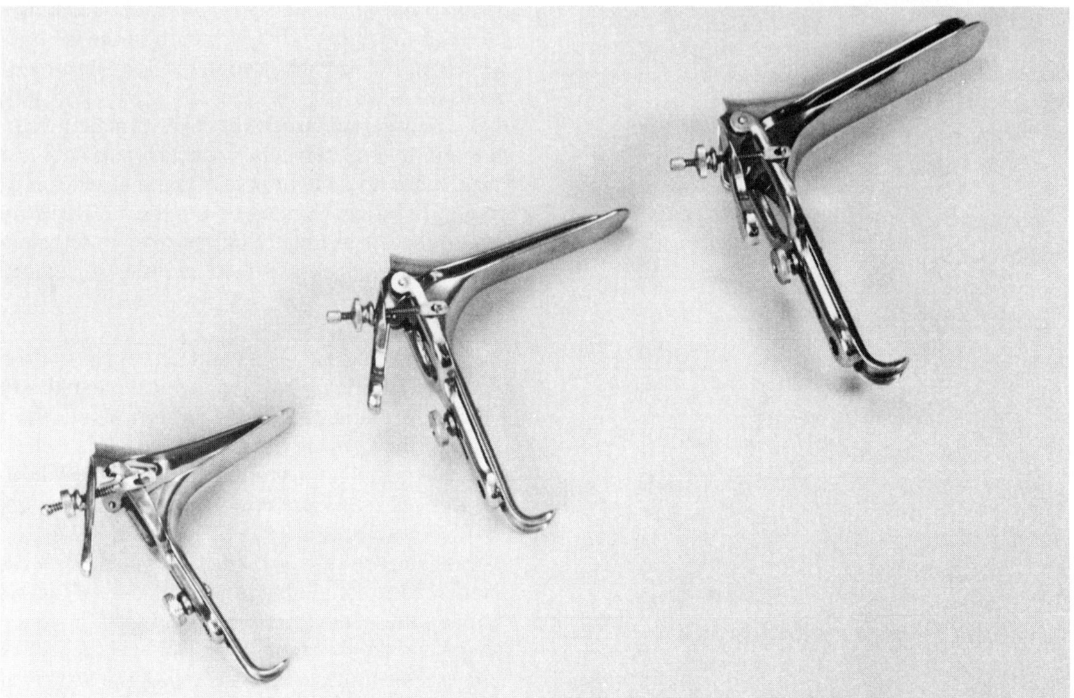

Figure 16–64. Vaginal speculums: left, small; center, medium; right, large. (*Source: Block GJ, Nolan JW.* Health Assessment for Professional Nursing: A Developmental Approach. *2nd ed. Norwalk, CT: Appleton-Century-Crofts; 1986.*)

Conducting an Examination of the Genitourinary System

Preparation. The female client lies on her back with her knees bent and her feet apart for the examination of the external genitalia. A drape is placed over her lower body and positioned so that the pelvic region is exposed.

Examine the male client either supine or standing. The standing position affords a better opportunity to observe bulging (herniation) in the groin where the spermatic cord passes through the inguinal canal.

The examiner wears gloves when palpating the penis and scrotum and spreading apart the female labia.

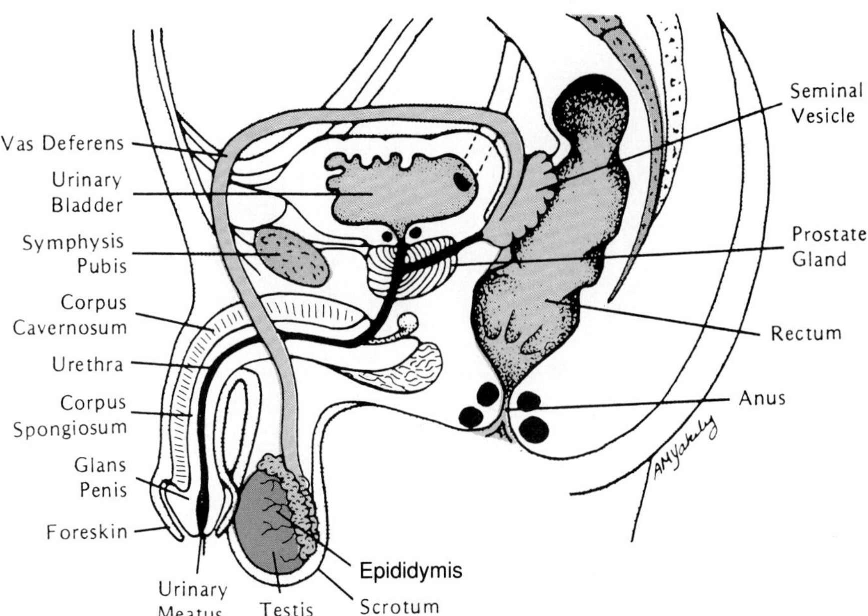

Figure 16–65. Cross-section of the male genitalia. (Source: *Berger KJ, Fields WL.* Pocket Guide to Health Assessment. *Reston, VA: Reston Publishing Co.; 1980.*)

Inspection

Female Genitalia. During childhood the female genitalia grow slowly at varying rates. At puberty they substantially increase in size and pubic hair appears. The clitoris becomes more erectile; the blood vessels of the labia minora become more apparent. The labia majora and mons pubis become more prominent. Vaginal secretions increase as the menstrual cycle begins. In older women, the labia and clitoris become flatter, and vaginal secretions are reduced.

Assess the external female genitalia for sexual maturity by noting the presence or absence of pubic hair and its distribution (inverted triangle). The hair should be free of infestations (lice) and the underlying skin should have no lesions or rashes. The labia majora are usually symmetric and may be shriveled or full in appearance. Next, separate the labia with the fingers of one gloved hand and inspect the labia minora. The labia minora are usually moist and dark pink. As you spread apart the labia assess the clitoris for size, the urethral meatus for lesions, and the vaginal introitus for swelling of the Bartholin's glands and presence of discharge. The perineum and the mucous membranes of the labia and vestibule are vulnerable to lesions and rashes.

Male Genitalia. At birth one or both testes may remain in the inguinal canal, and the final descent is accomplished in the postnatal period. At puberty, sparse hair appears at the base of the penis, and the scrotum skin reddens or darkens. The penis enlarges, and the pubic hair gradually becomes curly, dense, and coarse as adolescence progresses. With aging the scrotum becomes more pendulous.

Observe the male client for the quantity and distribution of pubic hair (diamond-shaped). Inspect the penis for lesions and rashes and the scrotum for size and shape. The penis should be proportionate to body size. If the foreskin is present ask the client to retract it so you can observe the urinary meatus for the presence of urinary discharge and lesions.

Palpation. In this text, palpation of only male genitalia is described. Gently grasp the penis between two gloved hands and palpate the shaft for masses and tenderness. Express urethral discharge by compressing the tip of the penis. Penile discharge is an abnormal finding. Feel the scrotal contents between your thumb and first two fingers delineating the testicle, epididymis, and spermatic cord on each side. Note the presence, size, shape, mobility, contour, and consistency of each testicle. Palpate the epididymis and spermatic cord for masses, swelling, and tenderness.

Testicular Self-Examination. Teach the male client to examine his penis and scrotum on a periodic basis to detect testicular cancer and penile lesions. Instruct him to place his thumb and fingers on either side of the scrotum and palpate the contents for growths, masses, and tenderness and to report any abnormalities to his physician.

Findings from the assessment of the external genitalia and expected life cycle variations are summarized in Table 16–38.

Special Considerations, Precautions, and Sources of Error

Some elderly clients may be unable to assume the position used for examining the female external genitalia.

Frequently, both the nurse and client are uncomfortable during the reproductive and sexual history interview and during the physical examination. This is especially true if the client and the nurse are of the opposite gender. The nurse's professional demeanor and thorough explanation of the benefits of the examination help allay embarrassment on the part of both.

Recording

Examples of the written record of the male and female genitourinary assessment are found in Box 16–35.

Role of the Nurse and the Assessment of the Genitourinary System

The nurse's role in genitourinary assessment is to encourage men and women to become more familiar with changes in their own urinary and reproductive systems. A woman should be aware when normal vaginal discharge increases, becomes odoriferous, or causes vulvar or perineal itching. These signs and symptoms, or the appearance of lesions on the genitalia, are an indication that she must seek medical care.

Teaching the male client the risks of testicular cancer, a disease that occurs primarily in younger men, is very important. While assessing the client's genitalia, the nurse can also use this time to demonstrate testicular self-examination and encourage its regular practice. All men should be advised to seek medical care for scrotal masses, penile lesions, and urethral discharge.

BOX 16–35. RECORDING THE ASSESSMENT OF THE GENITOURINARY SYSTEM

Subjective Manifestations

Female. Denies vaginal discharge or STD (sexually transmitted disease) contact. Menarche age 14; periods last 3 days and are without pain. Has never been pregnant; uses condoms for contraception. LMP 1/23/91. No dysuria, urgency, frequency, or history of cystitis. Last Pap 1 year ago.
Male. Denies penile discharge or STD contact. No scrotal masses, tenderness, or skin lesions. No history of prostate trouble, urinary difficulties, or sexual dysfunction.

Objective Manifestations

Female. External genitalia with normal female hair distribution. No lesions, scars, or masses on vulva. Mucous membranes moist and vaginal introitus without swelling or discharge.
Male. Normal male hair distribution. Circumcised penis without lesions; urinary meatus opens centrally at tip. Scrotum is proportionate in size; left testicle slightly lower than right. Testes smooth, firm, and nontender. Epididymis and spermatic cord without masses. No evidence of inguinal herniation when standing. Taught testicular self-examination.

TABLE 16–38. OBJECTIVE MANIFESTATION FINDINGS AND LIFE CYCLE VARIATIONS: GENITOURINARY SYSTEM

Examination Technique	Expected Findings	Common Life-Cycle Variations
INSPECTION		
Female Genitalia		
Hair pattern	Inverted triangular pattern over mons pubis; sparse hair on upper thighs may be evident.	Will appear at puberty. Decreases in amount and greys with normal aging.
Labia	No lesions or rashes.	Vasculature increases in puberty.
Vestibule	Openings of urethra and vagina. No swellings or discharge.	Normal discharge changes throughout the menstrual cycle and the life cycle, with scant discharge in the aged.
Perineum	Free of rashes, masses, lesions. Scars may be visible in multiparous women.	Healed scars from childbirth and episiotomy common.
Male Genitalia		
Hair pattern	Diamond-shaped distribution, often extends onto thighs.	Pubic hair appears about age 10. Greying and thinning of hair occurs with aging.
Penis	No lesions present. Urethral meatus centrally located. No penile discharge, inflammation, edema.	Uncircumcised male will have foreskin that is easily retracted.
Scrotum	Left lower than right; scant hair; no varicose veins; no inflammation, edema, discharge.	Slight testicular atrophy occurs in the aged.
PALPATION		
Penis	No masses, lesions, or tenderness on the shaft.	Growth of penis and scrotal sac is proportional to body size in puberty.
Urethral meatus	No expressible discharge.	
Scrotum	Mobile oval-shaped testicles present bilaterally, 4 × 3 × 2.5 cm in size; firm rubbery consistency; no masses; testes freely mobile in scrotal sac.	

From References 4, 42, and 59.

Both men and women need to be aware of the signs and symptoms of cystitis (urinary tract infection). The manifestations are dysuria, urgency, frequency, and, sometimes, hematuria. Cystitis can progress to become a kidney infection if treatment is delayed.

■ MUSCULOSKELETAL SYSTEM

Overview

Many of the general observations of the musculoskeletal system are made when the nurse first encounters the client. Recall that during the general assessment phase the nurse notes the client's body development and proportions, posture, and gait. In this part of the examination the nurse does a more in-depth review of the musculoskeletal system, observing the structure and movement of the thorax and back, the limbs, and the joints. The health history questions in Table 16–39 assist the nurse in localizing any client complaints related to specific muscle groups or the skeleton.

Topographical Anatomy

The skeletal system consists of the skull and the vertebral column with its attachments. The attachments, sometimes called the appendicular skeleton, include the ribs, the shoulder girdle, the pelvis, and the limbs (Fig. 16–66).

TABLE 16–39. SAMPLE CLIENT HISTORY QUESTIONS FOR SUBJECTIVE MANIFESTATIONS: MUSCULOSKELETAL SYSTEM

1. Do you have stiffness or weakness of muscles or joints? Which joints are involved? Is the discomfort related to activity? Does it occur at rest? At what time of day?
2. Are your joints swollen? Are they red or hot?
3. Do you have rheumatism or gout?
4. Do you have difficulty getting out of bed or up from a chair? Do you have a problem combing your hair or brushing your teeth? Can you feed yourself?
5. Have you experienced difficulty walking? Do you have pain in your hip joint? Do you limp?
6. Do you feel pain, stiffness, or cramping in your calves? Does this discomfort occur with walking or other exercise (intermittent claudication)? Do you have pain at night? Is the pain in one or both legs?
7. Have you ever broken a bone (fracture)? Have you experienced joint dislocation? Have you had any sprains or strains? Do you have any bony deviations?
8. Have you had back pain? Is it associated with numbness or tingling of the legs? When does it come on? Does it travel down your leg (radiation)?
9. Are your feet painful? Do you have corns or bunions?
10. Does _____ (subjective manifestation) interfere with any of your usual daily activities? How?

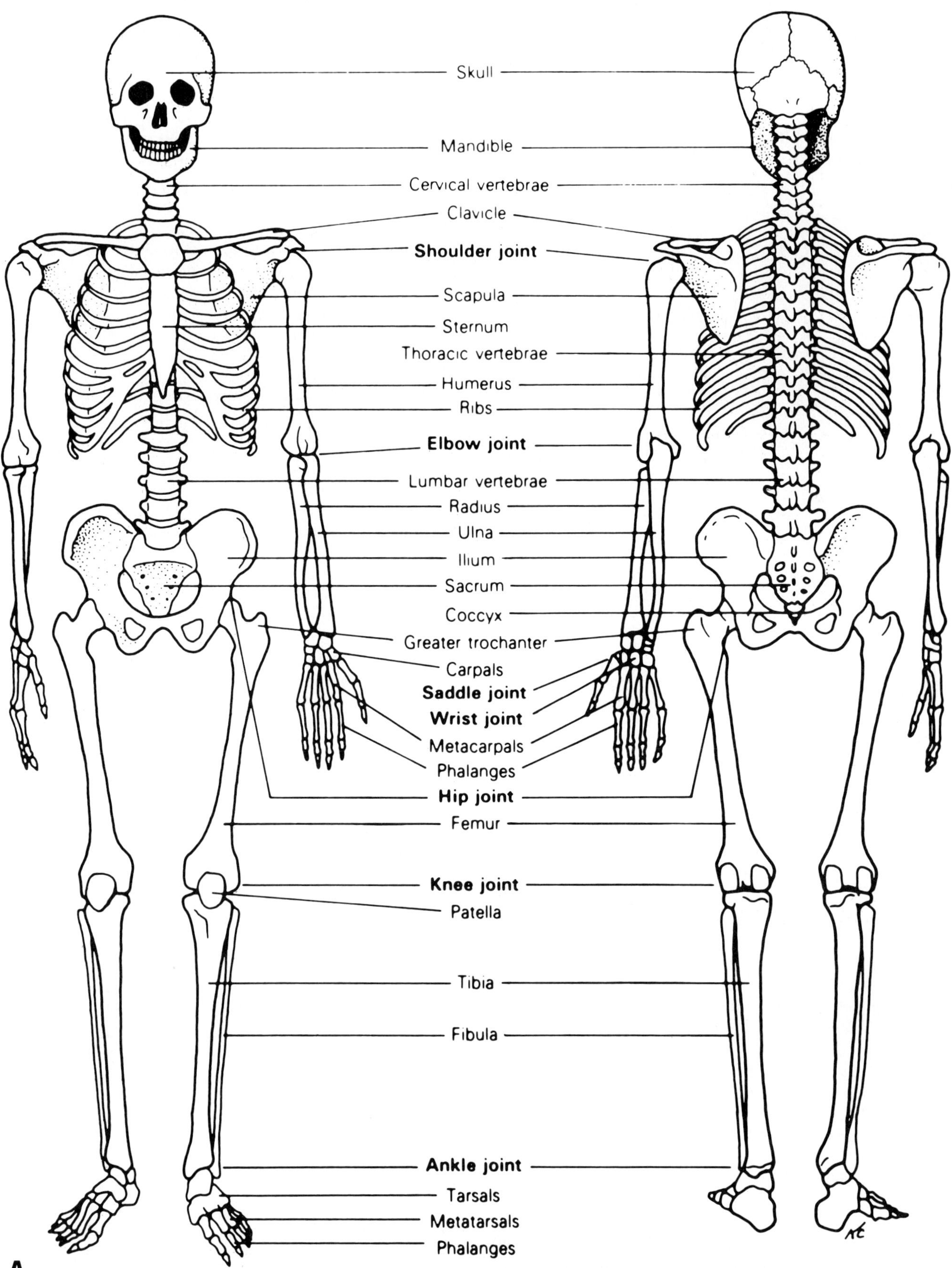

Figure 16–66. Skeletal system. **A.** Skeleton. **B.** Wrist, hand, and finger. **C.** Ankle and foot. (*continued*) (Source: *Fields WL, McGinn-Campbell KM.* Introduction to Health Assessment. *Reston, VA: Reston Publishing Co.; 1983.*)

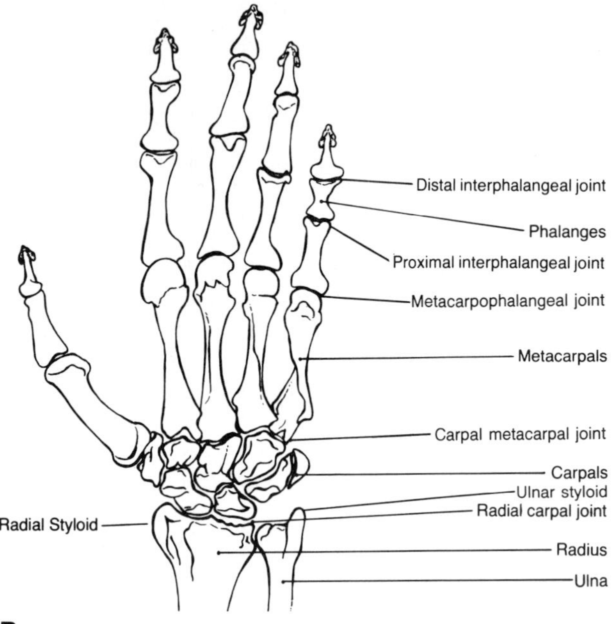

B

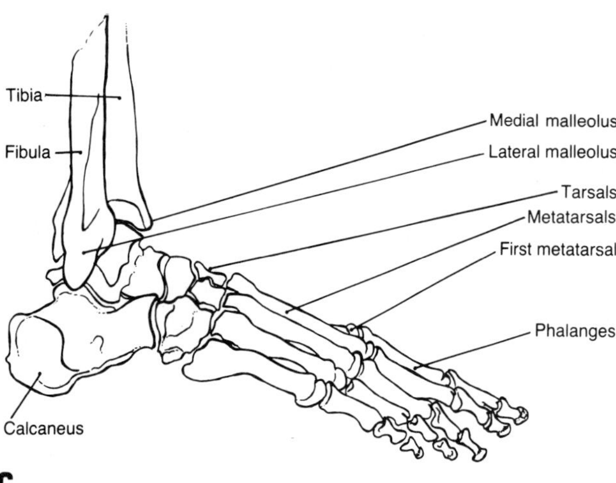

C

Figure 16–66. *(continued)*

The skull was discussed with the face and nose previously in the chapter.

The spinal column is composed of 26 vertebrae (Fig. 16–66). The cervical spine has 7 vertebrae (C1 to C7), the thoracic spine has 12 vertebrae (T1 to T12), and the lumbar spine has 5 vertebrae (L1 to L5). The remaining bones of the spine are the sacrum, composed of 5 fused vertebrae, and the coccyx, with 3 to 5 rudimentary vertebrae.

The bones of the thorax besides T1 through T12 of the spinal vertebrae are the sternum and the 12 pairs of ribs. All the ribs articulate posteriorly with the vertebral column, but only the first 7 pairs are attached directly to the sternum by the costal cartilages. Ribs 8, 9, and 10 attach to the cartilage of the seventh rib. The rib cage is depicted in Figures 16–49 and 16–53.

The appendicular skeleton consists of the bones of the upper and lower extremities, the shoulder, and the pelvis. The shoulder is made up of the scapula (shoulder blades) posteriorly, the clavicles (collar bones) anteriorly, and the head of the humerus. The long bones of the upper extremities are the humerus of the upper arm and the radius and ulna of the forearm. A notch in the ulna articulates with the hand. The bones of the hand are the carpals (wrist bones), the metacarpals (palms of the hands), and the phalanges (finger bones). (See Fig. 16–66 for the skeletal anatomy of the upper extremities.)

The lower extremities are attached to the pelvic girdle. The pelvis is composed of the paired innominate bones, which in the adult are a fusion of the ilium, ischium, and pubic bones. These bones are distinct in children and fuse as they grow. The two innominate bones, or hip bones, join at the pubic symphysis anteriorly and articulate posteriorly with the sacrum. The large heavy femur bone of the thigh articulates with the pelvis at the acetabulum, a depression on the lower lateral side of each hip. The other bones of the lower extremities are the patella or kneecap, the tibia or shin bone, and the small fibula, which is positioned laterally to the tibia. The talus, the ankle bone, articulates superiorly with the lower leg bones and inferiorly with the tarsal bones of the instep of the foot. The largest of the seven tarsal bones is the calcaneus, the bone that forms the prominence of the heel. The five metatarsals of the foot attach to the five phalanges, or toes. (See Fig. 16–66 for the anatomy of the pelvis and lower extremities.)

Three types of joints, or articulations, connect bones or cartilage together. Fixed joints occur in the skull, or cranium. The symphysis pubis is an example of a slightly movable joint; freely movable joints occur in the hips, shoulders, ankles, and wrists. Joints are frequently the site of traumatic injury or rheumatologic disorders. (See also Chap. 30.)

Muscle groups cover the bones and ligaments. Ligaments connect bones and cartilage, serving to support and strengthen joints. Tendons bind the musculoskeletal system together. These three types of connective tissue protect bones and internal organs and allow for mobility of body parts. All three tissues, as well as selected bony prominences, are palpated during the physical examination.

Conducting an Examination of the Musculoskeletal System

Preparation. The client's entire body is examined during the musculoskeletal assessment so the client must completely disrobe, except for underpants, and wear a gown. The client will need to stand, sit, and move around during the evaluation to enable assessment of gait, mobility, strength, and range of motion (ROM). No special equipment is needed for this examination.

Inspection and Palpation. It is customary to inspect and palpate each body part in turn. Before observing specific areas, take the opportunity to look once again at the client's body as a whole. Observe the symmetry of the two sides of the body, and compare the sides for evidence of masses, swellings, or deformities.

Thorax and Back. Ask the client to stand with the back of the gown open. Inspect the contour of the back. The head and shoulders should be erect and the hip bones are usually level. Observe the scapulae bilaterally. Note if they are level. Unevenness may signify an abnormal spinal curve. Abnormal curvatures of the spine include an exaggerated thoracic convexity (kyphosis), a pronounced lateral curvature (scoliosis), an exaggerated lumbar concavity (*lordosis*), and humpback (*gibbus*). (See Chap. 30.) Checking for scoliosis is particularly important in children. Early referral may prevent severe spinal deformity, surgery, and pain. Palpate the spinal processes and paravertebral muscles to assess for tenderness, noting the level at which it occurs.

Shoulders, Arms, and Hands. Examine the shoulders, arms, and hands of the client while the client is seated. Ask the client to elevate the shoulders and rotate them forward and backward. Note the presence of *atrophy* (wasting) of the muscles, deformity, or masses as the client goes through these movements. Note any behavior on the part of the client that might indicate that movement is painful. Palpate the muscles of the shoulders for tenderness and spasm.

Next, observe the muscle structure of the upper arms and forearms. Compare the two arms. Look at the elbows, and note any redness, swelling, nodules, or deformities. Then, have the client put his or her elbow through active range of motion. Make sure that the client has his or her upper arm next to the trunk (adducted) while supinating and pronating the forearm. This will prevent the shoulder from participating and inadvertently increasing forearm movement. Observe for any sign of pain or joint fixation during joint movement. (See Chap. 30 for further details on assessing range of motion of the elbow.) Check the arm for muscle tone and strength. See below for the details of the technique. Palpate the elbow for tenderness.

Inspect the wrists for shape, deformity, redness, swelling, or masses. Compare the two wrists for symmetry. Have the client move his or her wrists through active range of motion. Observe for any sign of pain during movement. Palpate the wrists for tenderness. Then, inspect and compare the hands. Look at the structure and observe for masses, swelling, and redness. Palpate the joints of the hands for tenderness. Tenderness, swelling, and deformity of the joints may reflect arthritis. You may note that the thumb muscles are more prominent on the dominant hand; this reflects their greater use. Ask the client to put his or her fingers through active range of motion and observe for signs of joint fixation, pain, and discomfort. Check the fingers for muscle tone and strength.

Hips and Pelvis. Inspect the pelvis while the client is in the sitting position. The iliac crests should be level and parallel to the floor. Palpate the iliac crests, the anterior spines, and, while the client is lying down, the symphysis pubis. Pain over any of these areas may suggest pelvic trauma. Palpate the muscles of the hips and buttocks for tenderness. Have the client perform active range of motion and check for any sign of pain on movement or joint fixation. Check for muscle tone and strength. (See Chap. 30.)

Legs and Feet. Inspect the muscles of the anterior and posterior thigh. Compare for leg length and muscle size. If there are any apparent discrepancies, measure leg length (anterior-superior spine of the pelvis to the medial malleolus of the foot) and thigh and leg circumferences. Ask the client to move his or her legs and watch for any sign of muscle spasm. Palpate the muscles for tenderness.

While the client remains in the sitting position, observe and compare the knees, noting deformities, swelling, redness, and masses. If the client is a child, ask the child to stand and observe for bowleggedness (*genu varum*), knock knees (*genu valgum*), or hyperextension (*genu recurvatum*). Palpate the bony and muscular structures and note any points of tenderness. Have the client move his or her knees through active range of motion, and note signs of pain or joint fixation. Check the legs for muscle tone and strength.

Next, look at the ankles and inspect them for swelling, redness, and deformity. Look for hallux valgus, a deformity often caused by ill-fitting shoes in which the great toe deviates toward the second toe and may overlap it. With continuous trauma, this may become painful and is referred to as a bunion. Observe the soles of the foot for flattened arches. Palpate the bony and muscular structures of the foot for tenderness. Ask the client to put his or her ankle and toe joints through active range of motion and note signs of pain or joint fixation.

Range of Motion. Range of motion is evaluated by noting the joint mobility demonstrated by the client during active and passive range of motion and comparing it with the standard of mobility expected for each joint. (See Chap. 30 for detailed coverage of range-of-motion assessment.)

Muscle Tone. Muscle tone, a function of musculoskeletal and neurological integrity, can be evaluated by moving the client's joints through passive range of motion. In passive range of motion, support the client's joints and move them through the full range of motion. The client should make no effort. This contrasts with active range of motion in which the client moves his or her own joints. While moving the client's joints, note that a level of tension is present in the muscles. A lack of tension in a muscle is referred to as *flaccidity*. Flaccid muscles are soft and flabby. Excessive tension is characteristic of *spasticity*. Spastic muscles are hard from tonic spasm, a state of continuous contraction. Either of these types of abnormal tone may accompany muscles that are paralyzed.

Muscle Strength. Muscle strength is evaluated informally by observing the client walk and move as part of general observation. This provides a gross estimate of the strength or weakness of major muscle groups. Muscle strength is also evaluated formally as part of the musculoskeletal or neurological phase of the health examination. The formal evaluation is done by having the client flex each muscle and then asking him or her to resist an opposing force applied by the examiner. Muscle strength for each muscle group is then compared bilaterally.

All muscles should be evaluated for strength during the complete examination; this can be done when checking each joint for range of motion. For example, as the client moves his or her elbow through active range of motion, ask the client to flex the biceps muscle. Then apply opposing force by

TABLE 16–40. EVALUATING SCALE FOR MUSCLE STRENGTH

Function Level	Grade	% Normal
Flaccid muscle, no evidence of contractility	0	0
Slight muscle contraction, no movement	1	10
Full passive range of motion only	2	25
Full active range of motion with gravity assisting, no resistance	3	50
Full active range of motion against gravity, some resistance	4	75
Full active range of motion, full resistance	5	100

Adapted from Malasanos L, et al. Health Assessment. 4th ed. St. Louis, MO: CV Mosby; 1989.

placing one hand on the back of the client's arm and, putting the fingers of the other hand around the client's wrist, pulling on the wrist. The client should be able to resist the force applied. Be sure that the degree of force used is appropriate to the development and age of the client; less force should be exerted in checking the strength of children and the elderly. Note any weakness. Each muscle group should be examined in this manner. Evaluate the strength of the muscles of the neck by asking the client to hold his or her head still as you attempt to turn the head, using moderate pressure, first to one side and then to the other; the client should be able to hold his or her head still. (See Chap. 30 for more details on muscle strength assessment.)

BOX 16–36. RECORDING THE ASSESSMENT OF THE MUSCULOSKELETAL SYSTEM

Subjective Manifestations

Denies stiffness, pain, or weakness of the joints or muscles. Has no history of arthritis but complains of pain in finger joints. No difficulties with activities of daily living. No hip pain, limping, difficulty with gait. Had a fractured right ankle in 1985 that healed without complication; no other bone injuries or deformities. No history of back pain or injury. Feet are without bony deformities, corns, or bunions.

Objective Manifestations

Shoulders. Full symmetrical range of motion, no pain on movement. No deformities. No muscle atrophy. Full resistance to opposing force. No masses, redness, swelling.
Elbow. Full symmetrical range of motion. Full resistance to opposing force.
Wrist. Full symmetrical range of motion.
Fingers. Swelling of distal interphalangeal joints of second and third fingers of both hands. Range of motion diminished in those joints. All other joints show full symmetrical range of motion.
Spine. Posture erect in sitting and standing positions. Full range of motion with no pain on movement.
Pelvis/hips. Iliac crest level in sitting and standing positions. No tenderness on palpation. Full active range of motion.
Knees/ankles/toes. Full active range of motion. No deformities, masses. No muscle atrophy. No tenderness, swelling, redness. Full resistance to opposing force.

The scale in Table 16–40 is helpful in evaluating muscle strength. Muscle strength of grade 3 or less represents disability.

The expected findings from inspection, palpation, range of motion, and muscle strength testing are found in Table 16–41 along with life cycle variations.

Special Considerations, Precautions, and Sources of Error

A complete musculoskeletal evaluation takes effort on the part of the nurse and the client and requires space for the client to move around so that the examiner can assess gait and range of motion. Cramped quarters and client inertia should not preclude a complete assessment.

Even if a client has been previously evaluated, a periodic reevaluation is necessary to detect new findings or changes in the musculature or the skeleton. Arthritic changes, for instance, result from aging and from injury and can appear at any time in the life span.

Recording

The record of the assessment of the musculoskeletal system encompasses health history information and physical findings from inspection, palpation, and muscle strength testing. Box 16–36 presents an example of the record of the musculoskeletal assessment.

Role of the Nurse and the Assessment of the Musculoskeletal System

A thorough musculoskeletal examination is essential to the evaluation of changes in joints, bones, and muscles. Arthritis may appear first in the small bones and digits of the hands. Early detection permits early treatment and prevention of deformities.

School health nurses are frequently called on to evaluate sports injuries and playground accidents because children often sustain fractures, sprains, and strains at school. School nurses are mandated in most states to do scoliosis screening of preadolescent children to detect spinal curvature during the growth spurt. The nurse can refer children for further evaluation and treatment if needed.

■ NEUROLOGICAL SYSTEM

Overview

The complete examination of the neurological system includes an assessment of mental status, the cranial nerves, cerebellar function, the sensory and motor systems, and a variety of reflexes. Many of the aspects of the neurological examination are checked informally while conducting the health history or while examining the various regions of the body such as the head and the limbs. By the time the musculoskeletal examination is completed, much of the neurological examination has also been completed. What remains is the formal testing of certain aspects of mental status, formal testing of balance and coordination and sensory perception, and evaluation of the tendon reflexes. Table 16–42 provides health history questions to be asked to obtain information about neurological function.

TABLE 16–41. OBJECTIVE MANIFESTATION FINDINGS AND LIFE CYCLE VARIATIONS: MUSCULOSKELETAL SYSTEM

Examination Technique	Expected Findings	Common Life Cycle Variations
INSPECTION		
Total body	Symmetry between sides; no deformities, skin lesions, swellings, or masses	Bones of infants are soft and flexible. Lumbar and sacral curves begin developing at 6–12 months of age. Bone atrophy of aging may cause loss of height.
Thorax and back	Erect posture with normal spinal curvature. Full ROM from the waist. Flexion: 70–90 degrees; extension: 30 degrees standing, 20 degrees prone; rotation: 30–45 degrees; lateral bending: 35 degrees.	Lumbar and sacral curves develop in infancy between 6 and 12 months of age. An increase in shoulder breadth occurs in males during adolescence.
Extremities	Equal limb length and diameter; muscle mass proportionate to body size. Joints without swelling, redness, discoloration, or deviation from midline. Full ROM of arms, legs, and all joints (see Table 30–5).	Legs short, bowed, feet flat before age 1; arms, fingers short in infancy. At puberty hands, feet, and extremities grow out of proportion to rest of body; muscle mass expands in males.
Movement	Fluid movement, coordinated gait, and steady balance when moving about and walking. No staggering, lurching, dragging of feet while walking. No toeing in or toeing out. No unusually short steps or wide-based walk.	Movement random and uncoordinated in infancy; muscular development proceeds cephalocaudally. Increased skill and coordination in childhood. Large muscles grow faster than smaller ones, resulting in lack of coordination in puberty.
PALPATION		
Muscles	Slight resistance to passive movement. No tenderness, masses, or involuntary movements.	
Joints	Symmetrical and without masses, swelling, or edema. Temperature the same as surrounding skin; nontender.	
Bone	Firm and without tenderness, masses, or abnormal prominences.	
Strength	Able to hold head still against resistance; able to shrug shoulders against resistance; able to maintain partially extended position of arm against pulling and pushing forces; able to straighten and flex fingers against resistance; able to raise from supine to sitting position without support; able to raise head and shoulders while lying prone; able to raise thigh and flex hip against resistance; able to maintain tight knees against pulling and pushing from side; able to rise from deep knee bend; able to extend knee against resistance; able to extend and flex feet against resistance.	Increased muscle strength during childhood, adolescence; some loss of strength with advanced age.

From References 4, 42, and 59.

Topographical Anatomy

The cells and nerve fibers of the neurological system link every part of the body and regulate and coordinate all bodily activity. The central nervous system (CNS) is made up of the brain and spinal cord. The peripheral nervous system comprises all the ganglia and nerves that lie outside the skull and vertebral column.

The brain, or cerebrum, is the location of mental processes, emotions, and consciousness and is the initiator of motor and sensory activity. The cranial nerve nuclei are situated within the brain.

The spinal cord is located in the vertebral canal and consists of 31 pairs of small nerves, each of which innervates a separate area of the body surface known as a dermatome (Fig. 16–67). The reflex arc in the spinal cord transmits impulses to and from the CNS to the periphery.

Conducting an Examination of the Neurological System

Preparation. The client wears a gown for the neurological examination. Mental status, language and speech, cranial nerve evaluation, and deep tendon reflexes (DTRs) are generally assessed in the seated position. Cerebellar function

TABLE 16–42. SAMPLE CLIENT HISTORY QUESTIONS FOR SUBJECTIVE MANIFESTATIONS: NEUROLOGICAL SYSTEM

1. Do you have headaches? Are they associated with nausea or vomiting? Have you had a head injury?
2. Do you ever experience dizziness, weakness, or vertigo?
3. Do you ever feel faint (*syncope*) or have blackouts? If so, how often? When?
4. Have you ever had convulsions (seizures, epilepsy)? How long have these been occurring? Do you take medicine?
5. Are you forgetful?
6. Do you have trouble swallowing (*dysphagia*), speaking (*dysphasia*), or talking (*dysarthria*)?
7. Do you experience numbness (*anesthesia*) or tingling (*paresthesia*) in any body part?
8. Do you have a problem moving your limbs (*paresis* or *paralysis*)? Do you have tremors?
9. Do you lose balance or feel uncoordinated?
10. Do you have a problem controlling your bowels or bladder (incontinence)?
11. Does _____ (subjective manifestation) interfere with any of your usual activities? How?

(balance and coordination) requires the client to stand and to ambulate. Motor and sensory testing is often done with the client lying supine.

The equipment used in the neurological assessment comprises the tuning fork for auditory testing and vibratory sensation, a reflex hammer to elicit deep tendon reflexes, a cotton wisp and a sterile safety pin or other sharp object for sensory assessment, and an eye chart for testing visual acuity.

Mental Status. Level of consciousness is evaluated as a part of the initial encounter of the client, as is mood, behavior, and speech. During this formal phase of the mental status examination, the nurse checks the client's general knowledge, abstract reasoning, judgment, memory, ability to do mathematical calculation, thought process and content, and ability to execute motor skills.

Knowledge. The client's knowledge and vocabulary usually become apparent during the health history. If for some reason there is some doubt about the client's cognitive functioning, ask the client certain questions to further check cognitive status. Test knowledge by requesting the client to name several past presidents or names of vegetables or

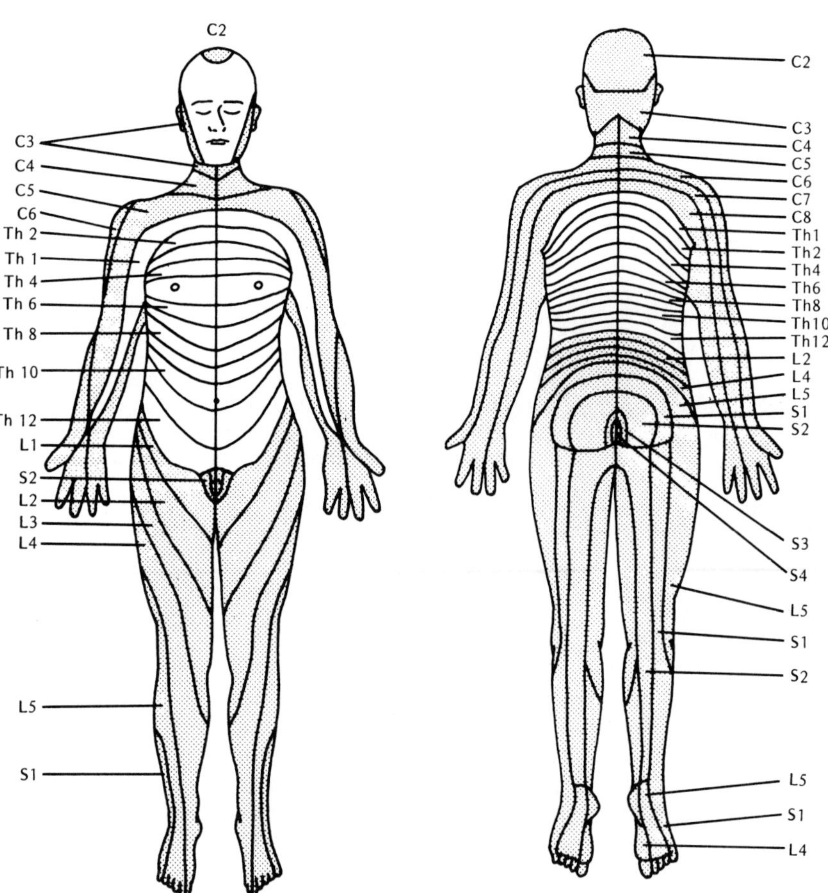

Figure 16–67. Dermatomes. (Source: *Berger KJ, Fields WL.* Pocket Guide to Health Assessment. *Reston, VA: Reston Publishing Co.; 1980.*)

examples of some class of objects that would be within the client's frame of reference. Be sure to take into account the client's age and cultural and educational background in assessing knowledge base.

Abstract Reasoning and Judgment. Generally, the social history and the information it provides about the client's daily life, level of functioning, and self-care practices will provide adequate data to evaluate abstract reasoning and judgment. If that information suggests a pattern of irresponsibility, impulsiveness, or irrational behavior implying poor judgment, a more detailed evaluation is necessary. Check abstract reasoning by asking the client to explain a fable or metaphor such as "a stitch in time saves nine" or "a rolling stone gathers no moss." Assess judgment by evaluating the client's ability to make decisions according to common sense and with appropriate thought processes. A client who is able to handle daily responsibilities of business and family is assumed to have intact judgment. If the history seems to refute this, ask the client how he or she might handle a specific situation like a family or personal crisis that you describe. The client's answer should show the ability to consider a range of options and the application of sound reason.

Memory. The health history also serves as an assessment of the client's memory of present and past events. If the client seems forgetful or has large gaps in memory, do a formal evaluation. Check immediate recall by reciting a list of items and asking the client to repeat them. The client should repeat them correctly and in the order given. Check recent memory by showing the client a few common objects and then, 10 minutes later, asking the client to recall the objects. The client should be able to list the objects. Check remote memory by asking the client about personal facts or past events that can be verified. Some items may have to be verified by family members. Ask the client for his or her mother's maiden name or the name of the college or high school he or she attended.

Calculation. Mathematical calculation is related to memory and also reveals cognitive functioning. If doubt about either exists, formally assess the client's ability to calculate. Check the client's ability to calculate by doing simple addition and subtraction problems without paper and pencil. For example, ask the client to subtract by sevens starting with 100.

Thought Process and Content. While interviewing the client during the health history, the nurse also gains an appreciation for the client's thought process and content. The client's thinking should show logic, coherence, and relevance to the topics discussed. During this phase of the neurological examination, observations of illogical or unrealistic thought process can be followed up by asking the client about obsessive thoughts related to decisions, fears, or guilt. Ask the client whether he or she has the feeling of being controlled or watched or followed by others. Ask the client about repeated thoughts and actions, such as checking and rechecking to see if something has been done. Illogical, unrealistic thinking or compulsive behavior may indicate a mental disorder.

Execution of Motor Skill. The client should be able to carry out the activities of self-care after reaching a certain age. Inability to complete a simple task because of a lack of comprehension, known as *apraxia,* is indicative of cerebral disorder. For example, ask a female client to comb her hair or put on lipstick; her inability to carry out such activities, when the motor capacity is intact, may signify apraxia.

Language and Speech. The client's speech should be clearly enunciated and easily understood. Slurring of words, unusual intonation, and extremely rapid or slow speech can be indicative of anxiety and depression as well as neurological dysfunction. The ability to answer questions requires the cognitive skills to interpret meanings and formulate responses. Individuals with auditory defects may have difficulty hearing words and processing answers. Make adjustments for people whose primary language is not English.

Cranial Nerves. The 12 pairs of cranial nerves have many vital sensory and motor functions in the human body. The cranials serve the very important senses of vision, hearing, taste, and smell. They innervate the muscles of the face and participate in facial sensation and movement (thus serving facial expression). They have a crucial role in the movement of the tongue and palate and play an essential role in mastication and swallowing. They innervate the larynx and are important to phonation and to the client's ability to communicate vocally. They innervate the muscles that move the eyes and head, carry vital sensory information necessary for balance, and serve the parasympathetic nervous system. Thus, cranial nerve function is crucial to everyday functioning, adaptation, and coping. Damage or disease can interrupt any of the functions served by the cranials, depending on which nerves are affected. Blindness, deafness, and interference with nutrition and communication are only a few of the human problems that result from cranial nerve dysfunction. All of these are dysfunctions that affect nursing care and represent problems in which nurses have a vital interest.

Formal examination of the cranial nerves is considered by some educators to be an advanced technique; therefore, a detailed summary of the traditional examination of the cranial nerves is not presented in this chapter. Several informal and simple standard checks for each of the cranial nerves have already been discussed in previous sections. It is important to note that because of the kinds of client behavior served by cranial nerve function—the movement of the eyes and head and the ability to smile or frown, to vocalize and swallow, to see, and to hear—every time a nurse encounters a client, a cranial nerve check is done. Consciously or unconsciously, the nurse compares the client's behavior with standards of health and with the client's previous appearance, and through this process, abnormal-

TABLE 16–43. SUMMARY OF CRANIAL NERVES

Nerve	Function	Expected Response
Cranial I: olfactory	Smell reception and interpretation	Eyes closed; correctly differentiates familiar odors with each nostril
Cranial II: optic	Visual acuity	Accurately calls out letters on 20/20 test line of eye chart
	Color vision	Differentiates between red and green lines on Snellen chart
	Near vision	Able to read newsprint at distance of 1 ft (30 cm)
	Peripheral vision	Identifies object 60 degrees nasalward, 50 degrees upward, 90 degrees temporally, 70 degrees downward
Cranial III: oculomotor	Pupillary reactivity, lens adaptation	Pupil size symmetrical, neither widely dilated nor pinpoint in average room light; prompt constriction in reaction to direct and consensual light stimuli
	Eyelid elevation	Able to retract eyelid fully on command
	Movement of eye upward and outward, upward, and inward, and medially	Smooth, symmetrical movements through all six cardinal positions of gaze
Cranial IV: trochlear	Movement of eye downward and inward	Smooth, symmetrical movements through all six cardinal positions of gaze
Cranial V: trigeminal	Tearing (lacrimination) sensation to eye and face	Brisk blink response to touch of cornea Eyes closed, indicates facial and oral tactile perception; correctly identifies facial pain stimulus and distinguishes hot and cold applications over three regions; forehead, cheek, and jaw
	Movement of muscles of mastication (masseter, temporalis, pterygoideus)	Symmetrical tension in muscles of clenched jaw; able to move jaw laterally against resistance
Cranial VI: abducens	Movement of eye laterally	Smooth, symmetrical movements through all six cardinal positions of gaze
Cranial VII: facial	Taste to anterior two thirds of tongue	Perceives sweet, sour, bitter, and salty tastes with each side of anterior tongue
	Secretion of sublingual and submaxillary salivary glands	
	Movement of facial muscles, scalp, ears, forehead, around eyes, lips: facial expression	Able to elevate eyebrows, frown, close eyes tightly, show teeth; with jaw closed, whistle, puff cheeks, and smile symmetrically; able to make labial speech sounds (B, M, W)
Cranial VIII: acoustic	Hearing	With opposite ear masked, hears whispered voice from 2 ft (60 cm) and correctly repeats words whispered
		With opposite ear masked, hears ticking watch from same distance at which examiner is just able to hear it
		Weber: no lateralization
		Rinne: air conduction longer than bone conduction
	Balance	Able to tandem walk, stand with feet together without postural deviation; able to appose finger to nose or finger to finger without past pointing

(*continued*)

TABLE 16–43. (continued)

Nerve	Function	Expected Response
Cranial IX: glossopharyngeal	Position of palate and uvula	Uvula elevates midline[a]
	Sensation of mucosa of pharnyx and palatine tonsils; taste to posterior one third of tongue	Perceives touch stimulus on pharyngeal mucosa[a]
	Secretion of parotid salivary gland	Salivation in response to spicy food
	Movement of pharynx Swallowing phonation	Gag reflex intact[a]
Cranial X: vagus	Movement of palate, pharynx, and larynx Phonation	Able to phonate without hoarseness or articulation difficulty
	Swallowing	Able to swallow without regurgitating and breathe with ease
Cranial XI: accessory	Movement of trapezius and sternocleidomastoid muscles	Able to raise shoulders against resistance; able to turn head side to side
		Able to strongly oppose resistance to attempt to return chin to midline
Cranial XII: hypoglossal	Movement of the tongue	Tongue protrudes to midline No tremors, fasciculations, atrophy
		Able to oppose resistance
		Pronunciation of "R" words intact (eg, rugged, ragged, third, riding); also L, T, and N sounds

[a] Nerves IX and X both participate in this response.
From Berger and Fields.[42]

ities become apparent. Table 16–43, a summary of the functions of each pair of cranial nerves, is provided for easy review.

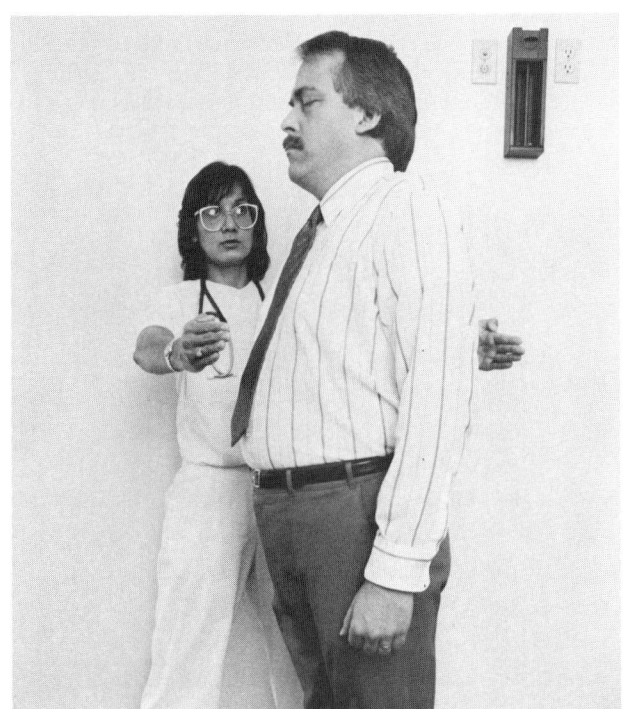

Figure 16–68. Romberg test.

Cerebellar Assessment. Cerebellar assessment is the evaluation of balance and coordination. Position yourself so that you have a full view of the standing client. Ask the client to walk across the room using his or her normal gait pattern. Evaluate the client's gait, including arm swing, for smoothness and coordination. Next, ask the client to walk in a straight line with the heel of the front foot coming down directly in front of the toes of the back foot. The client should accomplish this test, called the tandem walk, without a severe loss of balance, although some individuals will experience swaying and may have to move their arms to maintain an upright position. There should be no reeling, lurching, or falling in the normal client.

Ask the client to stand still with feet together, arms at sides, and both eyes closed. Observe for swaying or other signs of imbalance. This test is known as the *Romberg test* (Fig. 16–68). If the client loses his or her balance, the test is called a positive Romberg sign.

Fine motor coordination and position sense of the extremities can be evaluated by point-to-point testing and rapid alternating movement tests. It is usual for the client to be seated while testing the upper extremities and lying down while testing coordination of the lower extremities. Ask the client, with his or her eyes open, to alternately touch the index finger of one hand first to his or her own nose and then to your finger. Move your finger around so

TABLE 16–44. GRADING SCALE FOR REFLEXES

Grade	Reflex Response
0	No response
1+	Diminished or sluggish
2+	Active, expected response
3+	Brisker than expected, slightly hyperactive
4+	Brisk, hyperactive, showing intermittent clonus (involuntary contractions)

that the client has to extend the arm and reach toward you to complete the cycle. Test both hands and observe the movement for ease and accuracy.

Alternating hand movements are a second test of upper extremity coordination. Ask the seated client to alternately supinate and pronate the hands on his or her knees, gradually moving them as rapidly as possible. Observe this motion for speed and fluidity of movement.

Ask the client to lie down to complete the assessment of coordination and position sense. Have the client place one heel on the knee of the other leg and run the heel all the way down the shin to the great toe. Have the client repeat this procedure with the heel on the other leg.

Ask the client to repeat the heel-to-shin test with the eyes closed to enable you to evaluate position sense. Test the alternating movement skill of the lower extremities by asking the client to tap his or her feet against the palms of your hands.

Motor Assessment. Neurological assessment of the motor system consists of evaluation of the muscles for size, symmetry, tone, and strength. The muscles should be symmetrical and well developed on both sides of the body. There should be no wasting of muscle tissue or unusual bulk. (See Musculoskeletal system, earlier in this chapter, and Chap. 30 for evaluation of muscle tone, strength, and movement.) Observe closely for involuntary muscle movements such as tics, fasciculations, tremors, and twitches. Notice if these movements are generalized or localized, continuous or intermittent, and whether they occur with activity or relaxation. Unusual or involuntary muscle movement can be indicative of neurological disease.

Sensory Assessment. Sensory testing is generally performed with the client in the supine position with the eyes closed. The sensory system is assessed for response to the stimuli of light touch, superficial pain, vibration, discrimination, and sometimes temperature. Test light touch by stroking the client's skin with a wisp of cotton following the pattern of dermatomes (Fig. 16–67). It is not necessary to test each dermatome, but testing should be done symmetrically on both sides of the body and on enough skin surface of each extremity and the face to make a valid determination that sensation to light touch is intact. As you systematically touch three areas on each side of the face (forehead, cheek, and chin bilaterally) and three or more different areas of the arms and legs, ask the client to tell you when he or she feels your touch. If sensory loss is suspected attempt to detect the boundaries of loss by testing more specific dermatomes. The client states whether there is no sensation (*anesthesia*), decreased sensation (*hypesthesia*), or increased sensation (*hyperesthesia*).

Following approximately the same dermatome pattern and again instructing the client to close the eyes use a sterile safety pin to assess for response to pain. Alternate the sharp and dull (head) ends of the pin as a test of discrimination and accuracy.

Temperature is tested with two test tubes, one filled with warm and the other with cool water. Alternately place each tube against the client's skin. Temperature testing is not usually done if pain sensation is normal because the nerve pathways of pain and temperature are the same.

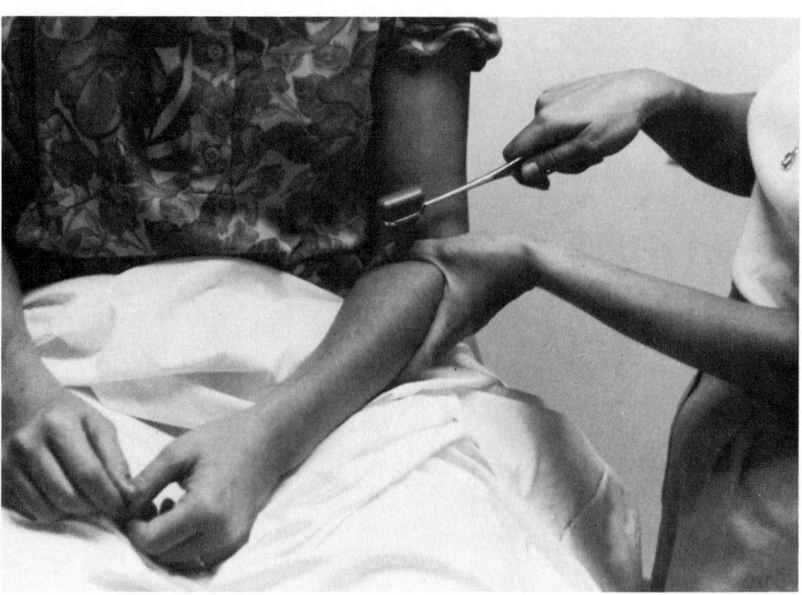

Figure 16–69. Biceps reflex. (Source: *Block GJ, Nolan JW.* Health Assessment for Professional Nursing: A Developmental Approach. *2nd ed. Norwalk, CT: Appleton-Century-Crofts; 1986.*)

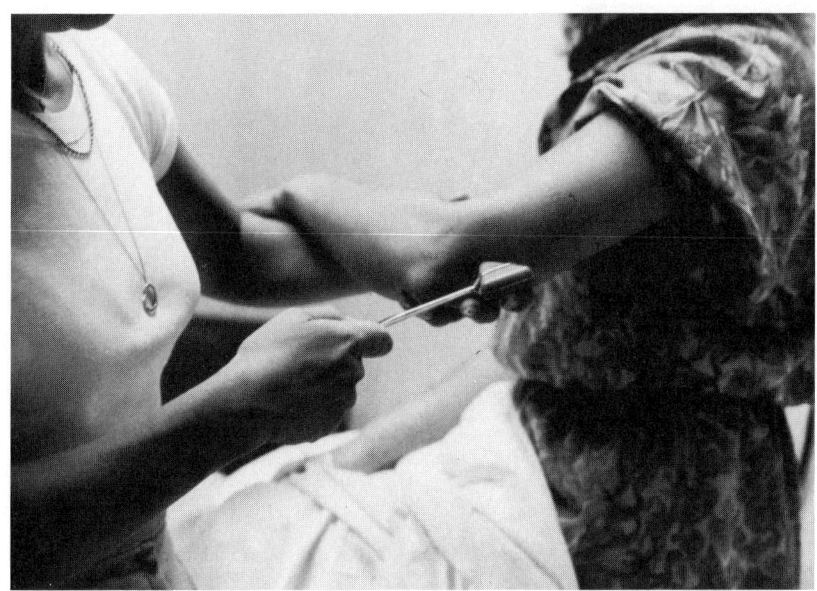

Figure 16–70. Triceps reflex. (Source: *Block GJ, Nolan JW:* Health Assessment for Professional Nursing: A Developmental Approach. *2nd ed. Norwalk, CT: Appleton-Century-Crofts; 1986.*)

Vibratory sensation is a test for peripheral neuropathy. Set a low-pitched tuning fork (128–256 Hz) vibrating and place it on a distal bony prominence (interphalangeal joint of the left or right great toe and a distal interphalangeal joint of each hand). If the client indicates perception of this sensation, stop testing. If the client is uncertain, then proceed to place the vibrating tuning fork on more proximal joints (wrist or elbow of upper extremities, ankle or knee of lower extremities).

The discrimination tests (two-point discrimination and point localization) assess the integrity of the nervous system. Touch the client lightly with your fingertip and ask him to state where he or she felt your touch. Test two-point discrimination by touching the client with the sides of two sharp objects (pins or opened paper clips) and asking the client to state whether he or she felt one or two points.

Reflexes. The deep tendon reflexes are tested with a reflex hammer, and the superficial reflexes, with the tip of the hammer handle or a tongue blade torn longitudinally. When testing reflexes it is imperative that the client is fully relaxed so an adequate response is elicited when the tendon is struck with the reflex hammer. Hold the hammer lightly and strike using a brisk movement from your wrist. Reflexes are graded on a scale of 0 to 4+ (Table 16–44).

The deep tendon reflexes commonly tested are the biceps, triceps, and brachioradialis reflexes of the upper extremities and the ankle and knee reflexes of the lower extremities. Most frequently the client is seated during deep tendon reflex testing but these reflexes can be elicited with the client supine as well.

Biceps Reflex. To test the biceps reflex ask the client to rest his or her arm on the lap with the elbow slightly flexed and the palm facing downward. Place your thumb or index finger on the biceps tendon, which should be palpable in the antecubital space (Fig. 16–69). Strike your finger with the pointed end of the hammer to elicit the reflex. If you are successful the elbow will flex slightly and the biceps muscle will contract.

Triceps Reflex. Pull the client's arm across the chest or hold the arm outward with the hand hanging down (Fig. 16–70). Strike directly on the triceps tendon, which is located just above the olecranon process (elbow). Watch for contraction of the triceps muscle and slight extension of the arm.

Brachioradialis Reflex. The brachioradialis tendon is located just above the wrist bone on the thumb side of the forearm (Fig. 16–71). Ask the client to rest his or her hand on the leg or knee and strike the tendon with the flat side of the reflex hammer to elicit flexion of the forearm and slight supination of the hand.

Patellar Reflex. It is most convenient to elicit the two reflexes of the lower extremities if the client is seated on the edge of the examination table or bed. With the client's knees over the table and the legs very relaxed, strike the reflex hammer just below the knee, the site of the patellar tendon (Fig. 16–72). As the tendon causes the quadriceps muscle to contract, extension of the lower leg should be observed.

Achilles Tendon Reflex. The ankle reflex is elicited by dorsiflexing the client's foot with your hand and striking the Achilles tendon at the back of the ankle (Fig. 16–73). You will observe and feel a downward movement (plantar flexion) of the foot.

Abdominal and Plantar Reflexes. Two sets of superficial reflexes are considered in this text: the abdominal reflexes and the plantar reflex. The client must be lying supine to test the abdominal reflexes. The abdominal reflexes are elicited when the abdomen is stroked above and below the umbilicus. The stroke, with a tongue blade or the end of the reflex hammer, will cause the abdominal muscles to con-

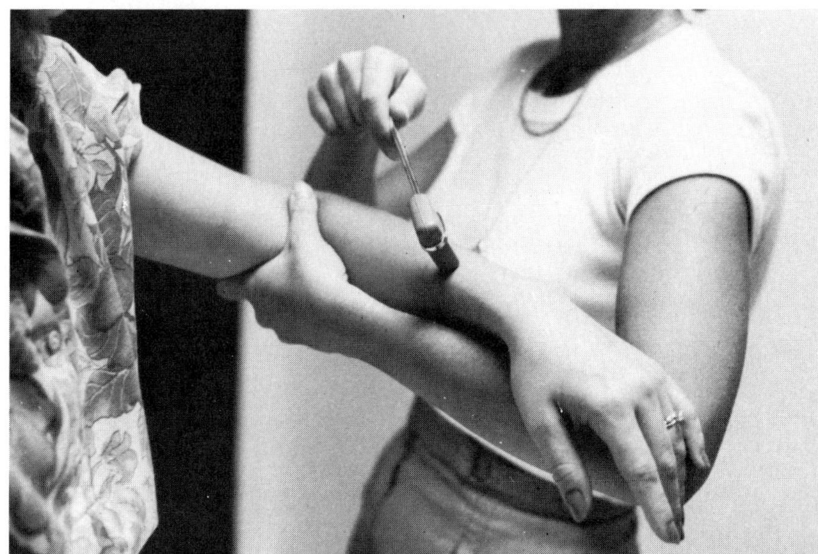

Figure 16–71. Brachioradialis reflex. (Source: *Block GJ, Nolan JW.* Health Assessment for Professional Nursing: A Developmental Approach. *2nd ed. Norwalk, CT: Appleton-Century-Crofts; 1986.*)

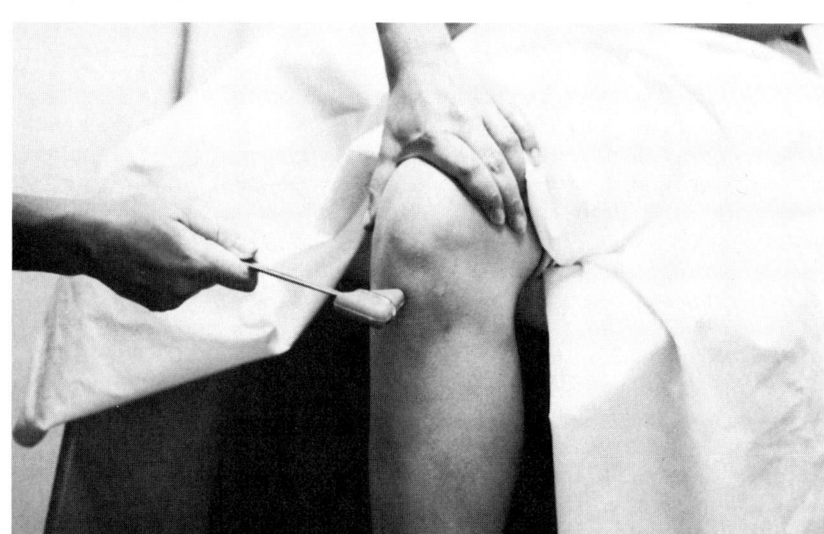

Figure 16–72. Patellar reflex. (Source: *Block GJ, Nolan JW.* Health Assessment for Professional Nursing: A Developmental Approach. *2nd ed. Norwalk, CT: Appleton-Century-Crofts; 1986.*)

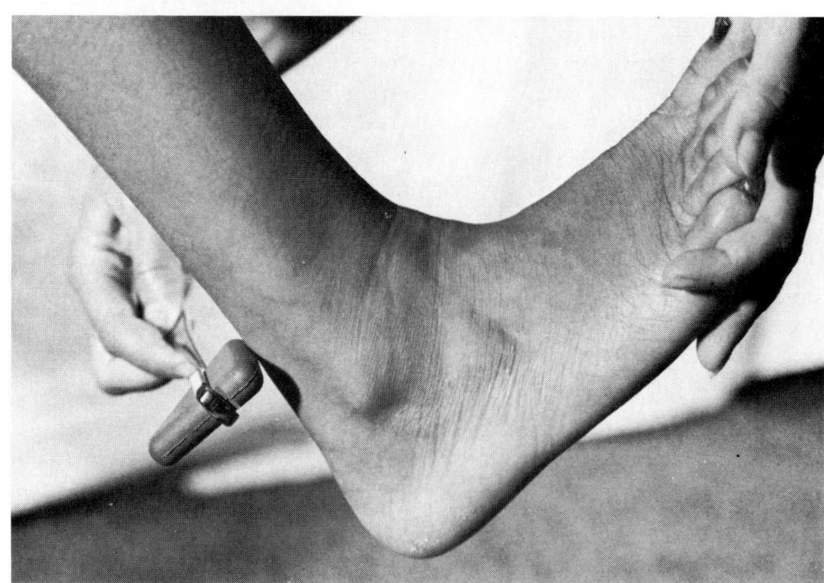

Figure 16–73. Achilles tendon reflex. (Source: *Block GJ, Nolan JW.* Health Assessment for Professional Nursing: A Developmental Approach. *2nd ed. Norwalk, CT: Appleton-Century-Crofts; 1986.*)

tract and the umbilicus to move toward the stimuli.

The plantar reflex is elicited by drawing a dull object like the handle of the reflex hammer or tongue blade across the sole of the foot from the heel to the toe. Avoid drawing the object up the center of the foot as some clients will find this ticklish. In the normal adult the toes will flex or curl downward in response to this stimulation. Dorsiflexion of the great toe and spreading out or fanning of the other toes constitute the Babinski response and indicate significant neurological disease.

Objective findings and life cycle variations for the neurological system are found in Table 16–45.

Special Considerations, Precautions, and Sources of Error

If sensory deficits are suspected, withhold judgment of cognitive functioning until further evaluation can been done. An impairment such as vision or hearing loss may make clients susceptible to the suspicion that they have diminished mental functioning. The nurse must be certain the clients have the necessary sensory organ functioning to permit them to hear, see, and process the information given them.

Many well-functioning people forget names, dates, and other information because they are distracted or stressed. Simple forgetfulness should not be confused with dementia or organic brain disease.

Knowledge and vocabulary can be related to social status and not necessarily to intellectual functioning.

The cultural background and circumstances of the client must be included in any mental status assessment. Immigrants, for instance, may possess extensive knowledge and information but their limited English language skills may prevent them from responding appropriately to questions and requests.

Recording

A sample recording of both the subjective information obtained from the client and the objective findings from the physical assessment is found in Box 16–37.

Role of the Nurse and the Assessment of the Neurological System

Nurses in virtually every setting in which nursing is practiced find neurological assessment skills, formal and informal, essential for evaluating the health and functional capacities of their clients. Nurses in occupational and recreational settings, schools, hospitals, clinics, and in the home setting all use neurological assessment to evaluate and monitor their clients' conditions. Regardless of work setting, prudent nurses acknowledge the importance of having thorough initial data on the client's nervous system function for use as comparison standards for later assessments.

A less thorough, abbreviated form of neurological assessment is also practiced frequently by nurses in many settings. Brief but formalized "neuro checks," for example, are a very important nursing responsibility in caring for clients whose central nervous system function must be closely monitored. Neuro checks are also used to track the progress of clients who have a primary disease of the central nervous system or who have a severe disease of some other body system that has secondary effects on the nervous system. See Chapter 29 for further discussion of neuro checks.

Informal neurological assessment also has an important place in nursing. It is important to point out that nurses, educated to be aware of the signs of health and illness, habitually, automatically, and often subliminally conduct informal follow-up examinations whenever they encounter clients, subconsciously comparing the client's immediate level of consciousness, expression, behavior, and movement to observations made during previous en-

BOX 16–37. RECORDING THE ASSESSMENT OF THE NEUROLOGICAL SYSTEM

Subjective Manifestations

Denies headaches or head injury. Has no dizziness, faintness, or blackouts. No history of seizures or forgetfulness. Has never experienced dysphagia, dysphasia, or dysarthria. Has no problem with balance or coordination.

Objective Manifestations

Mental status. Alert, oriented to time, place, and person with full cognitive functioning. Behavior appropriate.
Language and speech. Fluent and coherent and well enunciated.
Cranial nerves. See Head, Ears, Eye, Nose and Throat examination.
Cerebellar function. Stance and gait steady, Romberg negative. Well-coordinated point-to-point testing and rapid alternating movements.
Motor. No atrophy, fasciculations, or tremors. Muscle mass, tone, and strength appropriate for age and sex.
Sensory. Intact to pain, vibration, and light touch.
Reflexes. Superficial reflexes: plantar and abdominal present bilaterally. Deep tendon reflexes: all intact; 2+ and symmetrical; no right or left ankle clonus.

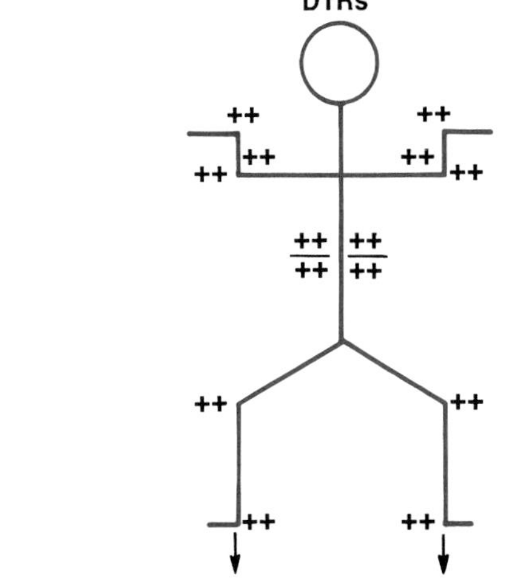

TABLE 16–44. OBJECTIVE MANIFESTATION FINDINGS AND LIFE CYCLE VARIATIONS: NEUROLOGICAL SYSTEM

Examination Technique	Expected Findings	Common Life Cycle Variations
MENTAL STATUS		
Knowledge and vocabulary	Appropriate to age, education, cultural background, and life experiences.	
Judgment and abstraction	Able to discern abstract meaning from a proverb or plot a rational course of action.	
Memory	Adequate recall of present, recent, and past memory.	Forgetfulness is common with distraction.
Calculation	Able to subtract serial 3s or do other simple math exercises.	Level of education may mediate math ability.
LANGUAGE AND SPEECH		
Speech	Clearly articulated and enunciated; speech pattern appropriate to age; no hoarseness, nasality, dysarthria, or voice weakness.	See general survey.
Language	Able to use and interpret language with ease, taking into account primary language. No difficulty sending or receiving verbal, written, or gestural messages.	
CRANIAL NERVES		
HEENT examination	See Table 16–41 for expected cranial nerve functions.	Hearing, taste, and smell sometimes decrease with age. Vision changes throughout the life span.
CEREBELLAR ASSESSMENT		
Balance	Gait coordinated and smooth. No wavering or loss of balance while performing Romberg test.	
Coordination	Able to perform coordination tests smoothly and accurately; steady tandem walk. Finger-to-nose test shows no past-pointing. Heel-to-shin test shows smooth, accurate movements. Alternating motion test shows smooth forearm supination and pronation. Tandem walking test shows no lurching, reeling, or widening steps.	Dominant hands and feet are often more skillful than nondominant. Less agility with age.
MOTOR ASSESSMENT		
Muscles	Symmetrical development with good tone and full strength.	Strength and development may diminish with age.
Size	Full development; no wasting or flabby hypertrophy; symmetrical.	
Tone	No spasticity, rigidity, excessive firmness, or flabbiness.	
Strength	Able to resist opposing force appropriately with all muscle groups.	
Movement	No involuntary movements such as tics, fasciculations, tremors, or twitches.	

TABLE 16–45 (continued)

Examination Technique	Expected Findings	Common Life-Cycle Variations
SENSORY ASSESSMENT		
Light touch, pain, temperature, position, and vibration	Responses present and symmetrical over all dermatomes tested.	Thresholds to touch, pain, and temperature higher in infancy than in childhood. Diminished sensory function in advanced age due to loss of brain cells and increased peripheral nerve conduction time.
REFLEXES		
Deep tendon reflexes (DTRs)	Biceps, triceps, brachioradials, patellar, and Achilles reflexes all present and symmetrical.	
Superficial reflexes	Abdominal and plantar reflexes bilaterally intact.	Babinski response is expected in infancy.

From References 4, 42, and 59.

counters. The importance of these "informal" assessments should not be underestimated because they are sometimes the first step in undertaking life-saving professional action.

SUMMARY

This chapter has covered all of the basic concepts and skills that enable a nurse to carry out a complete health assessment, including the essential competencies of health history taking and the health examination. In addition to stressing the practical aspects of health assessment, this chapter has examined the process of health assessment from the standpoint of nurse–client collaboration, a philosophical perspective that stresses the importance of client self-determination through participative decision making.

The health history, as presented in this chapter, is focused on the domain of nursing and is oriented to the client's responses to illness. The essential elements of the health history that nurses compile include the client's primary concern; current understanding; past health care experiences; personal, family, and social history; and subjective manifestations. Each of these elements is described and suggestions given for how the nurse might obtain the corresponding client information.

The health examination performed by nurses incorporates all of the basic physical measurements, including height, weight, and other body dimensions, as well as measurement of vital signs (temperature, pulse, respiration, and blood pressure). The health examination also incorporates a complete head-to-toe orderly observation of body regions and systems using the classical techniques of examination: inspection, palpation, percussion, and auscultation. The purpose of the head-to-toe assessment is to identify the client's objective manifestations of health and illness. Thus, the parameters of normal that are manifested in expected findings also have been identified in the interest of aiding the student to differentiate healthy findings from those that suggest the presence of illness.

Equipped with the knowledge presented in this chapter, students will be well prepared to begin the process of developing their clinical skill in health assessment. Mastery takes time and effort; it does not happen overnight, or even in the course of a single semester. Students therefore must be dedicated to the objective of learning and honing their assessment skills throughout their time in nursing school. With time, the skills practiced by students will gradually become automatic, freeing them to concentrate on the client's responses rather than on how to do a particular procedure. Health assessment is intrinsic to the nurse's role and a fundamental nursing responsibility. Thus, the time and effort taken to master assessment is well spent.

REFERENCES

1. Kasch CR. Establishing a collaborative nurse–patient relationship: A distinct focus of nursing action in primary care. *Image: J Nurs Scholarship.* 1986;18(2):44–47.
2. Williamson JA. Mutual-interaction: A model of nursing practice. *Nurs Outlook.* 1981;29(2):104–107.
3. Benner P. *From Novice to Expert: Excellence and Power in Clinical Nursing Practice.* Menlo Park, CA: Addison-Wesley; 1984.
4. Block GJ, Nolan JW. *Health Assessment for Professional Nursing: A Developmental Approach.* Norwalk, CT: Appleton-Century-Crofts; 1986.
5. American Nurses' Association, Congress for Nursing Practice. *Nursing: A Social Policy Statement.* Kansas City, MO: American Nurses' Association; 1980.
6. Thorne SE, Robinson CA. Guarded alliance: Health care relationships in chronic illness. *Image: J Nurs Scholarship.* 1989;23(3): 153–157.
7. Kasch CR, Dine J. Person-centered communication and social perspective taking. *West J Nurs Res.* 1988;10(3):317–326.
8. Wheeler K. A nursing science approach to understanding em-

pathy. *Arch Psychiatr Nurs.* 1988;2(2):95–102.

9. Hogue E. (1985). *Nursing and Informed Consent.* Owings Mills, MD: National Health Publishing (a division of Rynd Corp.).
10. Stiles WB, Putnam SM, Wold MG, James SA. Interaction exchange structure and patient satisfaction with medical interviews. *Med Care.* 1979;17(6):667–678.
11. Molde S. Understanding patients' agendas. *Image: J Nurs Scholarship.* 1986;18(4):145–147.
12. Eisenthal S, Emery R, Lazare A. "Adherence" and the negotiated approach to patienthood. *Arch Gen Psychiatry.* 1979;36: 393–398.
13. Morse JM. Negotiating commitment and involvement in the nurse–patient relationship. *J Adv Nurs.* 1991;16:455–468.
14. Scheff TJ. Negotiating reality: Notes on power in the assessment of responsibility. *Social Problems.* 1963;16:3–17.
15. Bloom SW, Wilson RN. Patient–practitioner relationships. In Freeman HE, Levine S, Reeder LG, eds. *Handbook of Medical Sociology.* Englewood Cliffs, NJ: Prentice-Hall; 1972.
16. Lazare A, Eisenthal S. A negotiated approach to the clinical encounter: Attending to the patient's perspective. In Lazare A, ed. *Outpatient Psychiatry.* Baltimore, MD: Williams & Wilkins; 1979.
17. Anderson WT, Helm DT. The physician–patient encounter: A process of reality negotiation. In Jaco EG, ed. *Patients, Physicians, and Illness.* New York: Free Press; 1979.
18. Lazare A, Eisenthal S, Frank A. A negotiated approach to the clinical encounter: Conflict and negotiation. In Lazare A, ed. *Outpatient Psychiatry.* Baltimore, MD: Williams & Wilkins; 1979.
19. Roberts SJ, Krouse HJ. Enhancing self-care through active negotiation. *Nurse Practitioner.* 1988;13(8):44–52.
20. Enlow AJ, Swisher SN. *Interviewing and Patient Care.* New York: Oxford University Press; 1986.
21. Barsky AJ, Kazis LE, Freiden RB, Goroll AH, Hatem CJ, Lawrence RS. Evaluating the interview in primary care medicine. *Social Science Med.* 1980;14A:653–658.
22. Eisenthal S, Lazare A. Evaluation of the initial interview in a walk-in clinic. *J Nerv Ment Dis.* 1976;162(3):169–176.
23. Kleinman A, Eisenberg L, Good B. Culture, illness, and care: Clinical lessons from anthropologic and cross-cultural research. *Ann Intern Med.* 1978;88:251–258.
24. Andersen JE, Briggs LL. Nursing diagnosis: A study of quality and supportive evidence. *Image: J Nurs Scholarship.* 20(3):141–144.
25. Keller ML, Ward S, Baumann LF. Processes of self-care: Monitoring sensations and symptoms. *Adv Nurs Sci.* 1989;12(1): 54–66.
26. Guyton AC. *Textbook of Medical Physiology.* 8th ed. Philadelphia: WB Saunders; 1990.
27. Wilson JD, Braunwald E, Isselbacher KJ, et al. *Harrison's Principles of Internal Medicine.* 12th ed. New York: McGraw-Hill; 1991.
28. Whaley LJ, Wong DL. *Nursing Care of Infants and Children.* 4th ed. St. Louis, MO: CV Mosby; 1991.
29. Mason DJ. Circadian rhythms of body temperature and activation and the well-being of older women. *Nurs Res.* 1988;37(5): 276–281.
30. LaVoy K. Dealing with hypothermia and frostbite. *RN.* 1985; 48(1):53–56.
31. Lohman M. Fever: Different types, different causes. *Nursing 88.* 1988;18(4):98–101.
32. Birdsall C. How do you handle heat loss? *Am J Nurs.* 1985; 85:367.
33. Budassi S, Barber J. *Emergency Nursing Principles.* St. Louis, MO: CV Mosby; 1986.
34. Baker NC. The effect of type of thermometer and length of time inserted on oral temperature measurements of afebrile subjects. *Nurs Res.* 1984;33:109.
35. Wilson R, Knapp C, Traber D, Priano L. Tympanic thermography, a clinical and research evaluation of a new technique. *South Med J.* 1971;64:1452–1455.
36. Holdcroft A, Hall G. Heat loss during anesthesia. *Br J Anaesth.* 1978;50:157–164.
37. Neff J, Ayoub J, Longman A, Noyes A. Effect of respiratory rate, respiratory depth, and open versus closed mouth breathing on sublingual temperature. *Res Nurs Health.* 1989;12: 195–202.
38. Durham M, Swanson B, Paulford N. Effect of tachypnea on oral temperature measurement estimation. *Nurs Res.* 1986;36: 211–214.
39. Felton CL. Hypoxemia and oral temperatures. *Am J Nurs.* 1978; 78:57.
40. Creative Care Unit. Turnabout: Rectal temperatures for postcoronary patients. *Am J Nurs.* 1977;77:997.
41. Ecoff M, Joyce B. Temperature measurement in children. *Am J Nurs.* 1981;81:1010–1011.
42. Berger KJ, Fields W. *Pocket Guide to Health Assessment.* Reston, VA: Reston Publishing Co.; 1980.
43. Henneman EA, Henneman PL. Intricacies of blood pressure measurement: Reexamining the rituals. *Heart Lung.* 1989;18(3): 263–271.
44. Sherwen LN, Scoloveno MA, Weingarten CT. *Nursing Care of the Childbearing Family.* Norwalk, CT: Appleton & Lange; 1991.
45. Hudson B. Sharpen your vascular skills with the Doppler ultrasound stethoscope. *Nursing 83.* 1983;13:55–57.
46. Hargest TS. Start your count with zero. *Am J Nurs.* 1974;74:887.
47. Smith S, Duell D. *Clinical Nursing Skills.* Los Altos, CA: National Nursing Review; 1985.
48. Bellack JP, Bamford PA. *Nursing Assessment: A Multidisciplinary Approach.* Monterey, CA: Wadsworth Health Sciences Division; 1984.
49. Billings DM, Stokes LG. *Medical Surgical Nursing.* St. Louis, MO: CV Mosby; 1987.
50. Bates B. *A Guide to the Physical Examination.* 4th ed. Philadelphia: JB Lippincott; 1987.
51. Wieck L, King EM, Dyer M. *Illustrated Manual of Nursing Techniques.* 3rd ed. Philadelphia: JB Lippincott; 1986.
52. Hollerbach AD, Sneed NV. Accuracy of radial pulse assessment by length of counting interval. *Heart Lung.* 1990;19(3): 258–264.
53. Frohlich ED. (chairman). *Recommendations for Human Blood Pressure Determination by Sphygmomanometers.* Dallas, TX: American Heart Association; 1987.
54. London SB, London RE. Comparison of indirect pressure measurement (Korotkoff with simultaneous direct brachial artery pressure distal to the cuff. *Adv Intern Med.* 1967;13:127–142.
55. Raftery EB, Ward AP. The indirect method of recording blood pressure. *Cardiovasc Res.* 1968;2:210–218.
56. Byra-Cook CJ, Dracup KA, Lazik AJ. Direct and indirect blood pressure in critical care patients. *Nurs Res.* 1990;39(5):285–288.
57. National Institutes of Health. The 1988 *Report of the Joint National Committee on Detection, Evaluation, and Treatment of High Blood Pressure.* NIH Publication No. 88-1088. Bethesda, MD: US Government Printing Office; 1990.
58. Judd HL. Menopause and postmenopause. In Pernoll ML (ed):

Current Obstetric and Gynecologic Diagnosis and Treatment. Norwalk, CT: Appleton & Lange; 1991.
59. Seidel HM, Ball JW, Dains JE, Benedict GW. *Mosby's Guide to Physical Examination*. St. Louis, MO: CV Mosby; 1991.
60. Meredith HV. Variation in body stockiness among and within ethnic groups at ages from birth to adulthood. *Adv Child Dev Behav*. 1987;20:1–60.
61. Nelson DA, Kleerekoper M, Parfitt AM. Bone mass, skin color and body size among black and white women. *Bone Mineral*. 1988;4:257–264.
62. Politzer WS, Anderson JB. Ethnic and genetic differences in bone mass: A review of the hereditary vs. environmental perspective. *Am J Clin Nutr*. 1989;50:1244–1259.
63. Steele MF, Mattox JW. Correlation of arm-span and height in young women of two races. *Ann Hum Biol*. 1987;14(5):445–447.
64. Maguire MS, Meredith HV, Spurgeon JH. Comparison of body size and form among ethnic groups of active duty United States Army men and women referred to a weight control program. *Hum Biol*. 1988;60(4):579–585.
65. Zillikens MC, Conway JM. Anthropometry in blacks: Applicability of generalized skinfold equations and differences in fat patterning between blacks and whites. *Am J Clin Nutr*. 1990; 52:45–51.
66. Himes JH. Racial variation in physique and body composition. *Can J Sports Sci*. 1988;13(2):117–126.
67. McLaurin CI. Cutaneous reaction patterns in blacks. *Dermatol Clin*. 1988;6(3):353–362.
68. Barth JH. Normal hair growth in children. *Pediatr Dermatol*. 1987;4(3):173–184.
69. Dekio S, Jidoi J. Amounts of fibrous proteins and matrix substances in hairs of different races. *J Dermatol*. 1990;17:62–64.
70. Alvear J, Brooke O. Fetal growth in different racial groups. *Arch Dis Child*. 1978;53:27–32.
71. Tanner JM. *Growth at Adolescence*. 2nd ed. Oxford: Blackwell Scientific; 1962.
72. American Cancer Society. *1985 Cancer Facts and Figures*. New York: American Cancer Society; 1985.
73. Nemcek MA. Health beliefs and breast self-examination among black women. *Health Values*. 1990;14(5):41–52.
74. National Cancer Institute. *Breast Cancer: A Measure of Progress in Public Understanding*. Washington, DC: Department of Health and Human Services; 1980. Technical Report Publication No. 81-2291.
75. Liu K, Ballew C, Jacobs DR Jr, and the CARDIA Study Group. Ethnic differences in blood pressure, pulse rate, and related characteristics in young adults. *Hypertension*. 1989;14(2): 218–225.

BIBLIOGRAPHY

Bernstein L, Bernstein RS. *Interviewing: A Guide for Health Professionals*. 4th ed. Norwalk, CT: Appleton-Century-Crofts; 1985.

Cassell EJ. Talking With Patients. Cambridge, MA: MIT Press; 1985

Coulehan JL, Block MR. *The Medical Interview: A Primer for Students of the Art*. Philadelphia: FA Davis; 1987.

Muscari ME. Obtaining the adolescent sexual history. *Pediatr Nurs*. 1987;13(5):307–309.

Northouse PG. *Health Communication: A Handbook for Health Professionals*. Englewood Cliffs, NJ: Prentice-Hall; 1985.

CHAPTER 17

Nursing Diagnosis

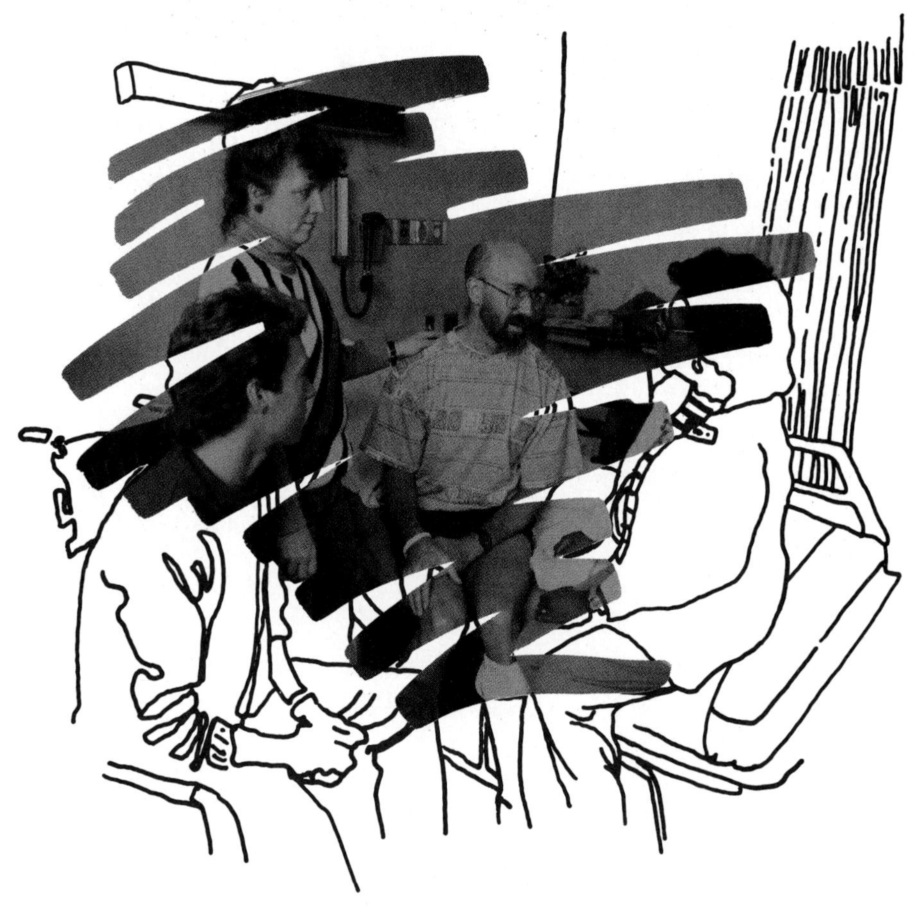

Behavioral Objectives

Upon completion of this chapter, the student will be able to:

1. Define nursing diagnosis and differentiate it from medical diagnosis.
2. Identify the relationship of nursing diagnosis to nursing process.
3. Trace the historical development of nursing diagnosis.
4. Define taxonomy.
5. Summarize the progress to date and future directions in the development of nursing's diagnostic taxonomy.
6. Identify the components of a nursing diagnosis statement.
7. Formulate nursing diagnosis statements from the list of approved diagnoses, their etiologies, and defining characteristics.
8. Differentiate the methods of stating actual and potential nursing diagnoses.
9. Outline the process of diagnostic reasoning.
10. Describe the most common type of diagnostic error and its sources.
11. Correlate several common sources of diagnostic error with the novice and the expert.
12. Identify six advantages of nursing diagnosis to nursing practice.

KEY TERMS

category label
contributing factor
cue
defining characteristic
diagnostic label
diagnostic reasoning
etiology
inference
inferential leap
manifestation
nursing diagnosis
organizational framework
PES format
potential diagnosis
problem
related factor
risk factor
taxonomy

Nursing diagnosis, a process whereby nurses interpret assessment data and apply standardized labels to health problems they identify and anticipate treating, is evolving rapidly in clinical and educational settings. Not coincidentally, this evolution parallels the overall process of professionalization of nursing.

Traditionally, nurses have relied on the language and therapeutics of other sciences. This has inhibited the establishment of nursing as a free-standing profession. Efforts by nurses to identify and name the conditions that they study and treat, on the other hand, foster nursing's professional identity by clarifying its distinct services to society and by providing a vehicle for the building of its science.

This chapter reviews the historical development of nursing diagnosis, establishes definition of its terms and concepts, and offers guidelines for formulating actual and potential diagnostic statements from the North American Nursing Diagnosis Association's list of approved diagnoses. The process of diagnostic reasoning and sources of diagnostic error are explored, to assist the student in beginning efforts to enhance diagnostic accuracy. Finally, several exercises are included at the end of the chapter to provide the student practice in identifying and stating nursing diagnoses.

■ HISTORICAL DEVELOPMENT OF NURSING DIAGNOSIS

Preconference Era

Diagnosis by nurses of health problems amenable to their treatment is not really new. In fact, throughout history nurses have diagnosed problems and intervened in their care. During the Crimean War, Florence Nightingale identified and treated such health problems as alterations in comfort and nutrition; and fear, anxiety, and potential for injury. In fact, Nightingale, by her writings, teachings, and example, set the precedent for the scrupulous data collection and goal-directed planning of care that today so characterizes the practice of nursing.

The term nursing "diagnosis" first appeared in the nursing literature in the 1950s.[1,2] At this time, a fundamental change began to occur in the process whereby nurses moved from data collection to care planning.[3] Nurses began to include a step in the process for data analysis and grouping and identification of the health issue at stake prior to care planning (Fig. 17–1). Nursing diagnosis encompasses the analysis and grouping of data. It is now universally accepted as an essential aspect of the professional decision-making process used by nurses: the nursing process. See Chapter 15.

Historically, nursing interventions tended to be disjointed and episodic. Nurses often looked upon each piece of assessment data as a separate, discrete entity, neither seeking nor perceiving relationships among groups of symptoms. Intervention strategies were planned and carried out in relation to what were considered to be a series of independent findings. For example, if soft tissue swelling, frequent infections, and delayed healing were observed in a client, nurses would likely have interpreted and managed each symptom separately. Some interventions would have been used to reduce swelling, some to avoid or control infection, and others to promote healing.

Consider the gains if nurses instead ponder the possibility of a relationship among these symptoms, uncover a cause, and organize a treatment plan corresponding to the diagnosis, Altered Nutrition: Less Than Body Protein Requirements. With nursing diagnosis as a component of decision-making methods, nurses necessarily become more systematic in the collection and interpretation of data, and effect a change in the basis of their clinical operations, from symptom management to problem-solving.

Conference Era

Prompted initially by a perceived need to clarify the nurse's role and to distinguish it from that of other health professionals' in their own practice setting, two faculty members at St. Louis University, Kristine Gebbie and Mary Ann Lavin, called together the First National Conference on the Classification of Nursing Diagnosis in 1973. The group organized around the task of identifying, standardizing, and classifying health problems treatable by nurses. This conference heralded a now-international professional movement, the ninth conference of which was held in 1990. The task force, now known as the North American Nursing Diagnosis Association (NANDA), consists of nurse theorists, nurse researchers, nurse educators, and nurse clinicians.

The impetus for the work of NANDA and its national conference groups derives from the need to establish a vocabulary that specifically reflects the treatment domain of nursing practice. In addition to being requisite to nursing's status as a profession, such a vocabulary serves to coordinate communication among nurses in relation to the health problems they are observing and treating, and is as much for purposes of social policy as it is, says Carpenito,[4] to "clarify nursing for nurses" (p. 11).

Approved nursing diagnoses are listed in Box 17–1. Though not included in the box, accompanying each diagnosis are possible contributing factors (etiologies), as well as the signs and symptoms of the health problem (defining characteristics). These are used by nurses to help formulate the diagnostic statement and tailor it to the individual client characteristics and circumstances.

An "approved" nursing diagnosis is one accepted by NANDA as having been refined to the point of clinical usefulness, and approved for beginning clinical validation through formal research methods. Practitioners using approved nursing diagnoses, etiologies, and defining characteristics are in fact participating in the preliminary testing of the health problems described by the diagnostic labels.

IMPLICATIONS FOR PROFESSIONAL COLLABORATION

History of Nursing Diagnosis

The development of nursing diagnosis has been one of the most important collaborative efforts in the history of the nursing profession. The First National Conference on the Classification of Nursing Diagnosis in 1973 heralded what is now an international movement in nursing. One result of the initial conference was the development of the North American Nursing Diagnosis Association (NANDA). This group of nurse theorists, nurse researchers, nurse educators, and nurse clinicians collaborates on issues related to nursing diagnosis in their efforts to develop a diagnostic vocabulary that reflects the treatment domain of nursing practice.

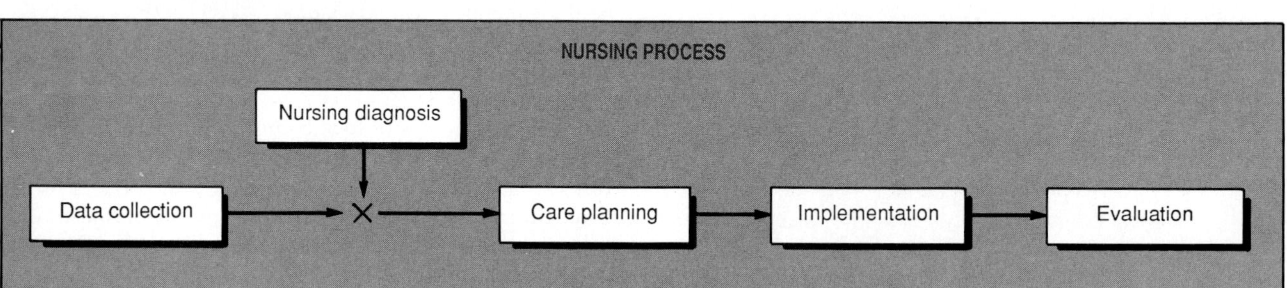

Figure 17–1. Nursing diagnosis as a separate step in nursing process.

BOX 17–1. NANDA-APPROVED NURSING DIAGNOSES ORGANIZED UNDER THE NINE HUMAN RESPONSE PATTERNS OF TAXONOMY 1 (REVISED 1990)

Pattern 1:	**Exchanging**
1.1.2.1	Altered Nutrition: More than body requirements
1.1.2.2	Altered Nutrition: Less than body requirements
1.1.2.3	Altered Nutrition: Potential for more than body requirements
1.2.1.1	Potential for Infection
1.2.2.1	Potential Altered Body Temperature
1.2.2.2[b]	Hypothermia
1.2.2.3	Hyperthermia
1.2.2.4	Ineffective Thermoregulation
1.2.3.1[a]	Dysreflexia
1.3.1.1[c]	Constipation
1.3.1.1.1[a]	Perceived Constipation
1.3.1.1.2[a]	Colonic Constipation
1.3.1.2[c]	Diarrhea
1.3.1.3[c]	Bowel Incontinence
1.3.2	Altered Urinary Elimination
1.3.2.1.1	Stress Incontinence
1.3.2.1.2	Reflex Incontinence
1.3.2.1.3	Urge Incontinence
1.3.2.1.4	Functional Incontinence
1.3.2.1.5	Total Incontinence
1.3.2.2	Urinary Retention
1.4.1.1[c]	Altered (specify type) Tissue Perfusion (renal, cerebral, cardiopulmonary, gastrointestinal, peripheral)
1.4.1.2.1	Fluid Volume Excess
1.4.1.2.2.1	Fluid Volume Deficit
1.4.1.2.2.2	Potential Fluid Volume Deficit
1.4.2.1[c]	Decreased Cardiac Output
1.5.1.1	Impaired Gas Exchange
1.5.1.2	Ineffective Airway Clearance
1.5.1.3	Ineffective Breathing Pattern
1.6.1	Potential for Injury
1.6.1.1	Potential for Suffocation
1.6.1.2	Potential for Poisoning
1.6.1.3	Potential for Trauma
1.6.1.4[a]	Potential for Aspiration
1.6.1.5[a]	Potential for Disuse Syndrome
1.6.2[d]	Altered Protection
1.6.2.1	Impaired Tissue Integrity
1.6.2.1.1[c]	Altered Oral Mucous Membrane
1.6.2.1.2.1	Impaired Skin Integrity
1.6.2.1.2.2	Potential Impaired Skin Integrity

Pattern 2:	**Communicating**
2.1.1.1	Impaired Verbal Communication

Pattern 3:	**Relating**
3.1.1	Impaired Social Interaction
3.1.2	Social Isolation
3.2.1[c]	Altered Role Performance
3.2.1.1.1	Altered Parenting
3.2.1.1.2	Potential Altered Parenting
3.2.1.2.1	Sexual Dysfunction
3.2.2	Altered Family Processes
3.2.3.1[a]	Parental Role Conflict
3.3	Altered Sexuality Patterns

Pattern 4:	**Valuing**
4.1.1	Spiritual Distress (distress of the human spirit)

Pattern 5:	**Choosing**
5.1.1.1	Ineffective Individual Coping
5.1.1.1.1	Impaired Adjustment
5.1.1.1.2	Defensive Coping
5.1.1.1.3[a]	Ineffective Denial
5.1.2.1.1	Ineffective Family Coping: Disabling
5.1.2.1.2	Ineffective Family Coping: Compromised
5.1.2.2.2	Family Coping: Potential for Growth
5.2.1.1	Noncompliance (specify)
5.3.1.1[a]	Decisional Conflict (specify)
5.4	Health-seeking Behaviors (specify)

Pattern 6:	**Moving**
6.1.1.1	Impaired Physical Mobility
6.1.1.2	Activity Intolerance
6.1.1.2.1[a]	Fatigue
6.1.1.3	Potential Activity Intolerance
6.2.1	Sleep Pattern Disturbance
6.3.1.1	Diversional Activity Deficit
6.4.1.1	Impaired Home Maintenance Management
6.4.2	Altered Health Maintenance
6.5.1[c]	Feeding Self-care Deficit
6.5.1.1	Impaired Swallowing
6.5.1.2[a]	Ineffective Breastfeeding
6.5.1.1.3[d]	Effective Breastfeeding
6.5.2[c]	Bathing/Hygiene Self-care Deficit
6.5.3[c]	Dressing/Grooming Self-care Deficit
6.5.4[c]	Toileting Self-care Deficit
6.6	Altered Growth and Development

Pattern 7:	**Perceiving**
7.1.1[c]	Body Image Disturbance
7.1.2[b,c]	Self-esteem Disturbance
7.1.2.1[a]	Chronic Low Self-esteem
7.1.2.2[a]	Situational Low Self-esteem
7.1.3[c]	Personal Identity Disturbance
7.2	Sensory/Perceptual Alterations (specify) (visual, auditory, kinesthetic, gustatory, tactile, olfactory)
7.2.1.1	Unilateral Neglect
7.3.1	Hopelessness
7.3.2	Powerlessness

Pattern 8:	**Knowing**
8.1.1	Knowledge Deficit (specify)
8.3	Altered Thought Processes

Pattern 9:	**Feeling**
9.1.1[c]	Pain
9.1.1.1	Chronic Pain
9.2.1.1	Dysfunctional Grieving
9.2.1.2	Anticipatory Grieving
9.2.2	Potential for Violence: Self-directed or directed at others
9.2.3	Posttrauma Response
9.2.3.1	Rape-trauma Syndrome
9.2.3.1.1	Rape-trauma Syndrome: Compound reaction
9.2.3.1.2	Rape-trauma Syndrome: Silence reaction
9.3.1	Anxiety
9.3.2	Fear

[a] New diagnostic categories approved 1988; [b] Revised diagnostic categories approved 1988; [c] Categories with modified label terminology; [d] New diagnostic categories approved 1990.

North American Nursing Diagnosis Association. NANDA nursing diagnosis taxonomy II. *St. Louis: North American Nursing Diagnosis Association, St. Louis University School of Nursing, 1990.*

NANDA actively seeks input from practicing nurses regarding the development and refinement of nursing diagnoses. The association publishes guidelines for submitting new diagnoses to its Diagnosis Review Committee. Direct input into the proceedings of the national conferences is possible through membership and participation in NANDA and any of its regional associations.

The goals of NANDA include:

- Further validation and refinement of existing diagnoses and their etiologies and defining characteristics.
- Generation of new diagnoses.
- Incorporation of approved nursing diagnoses into the 10th revision of the World Health Organization's *International Classification of Diseases*.
- Development of a category of wellness diagnoses describing clients' strengths and potential for growth.
- Refinement of the taxonomy initially endorsed at NANDA's seventh conference (this taxonomy replaces the alphabetized listing of diagnoses used previously).

BUILDING NURSING KNOWLEDGE

How Are Nursing Diagnoses Developed?

Levin RF, Krainovitch BC, Bahrenburg E, Mitchell CA. Diagnostic content validity of nursing diagnoses. *Image.* 1989; 21:40–44.

When NANDA's review committee reviews diagnoses, some clinical testing has already been done. But the diagnoses, as Levin and associates note, remain in an early state of development and additional research is necessary to develop them for clinical use. This report describes a study to validate the defining characteristics for six common nursing diagnoses: Impaired Physical Mobility; Pain; Self-care Deficit: Feeding, Dressing, or Bathing; Impaired Skin Integrity; Anxiety; and Knowledge Deficit.

A random sample of 600 registered nurses was asked to complete a questionnaire using a five-point scale to rate the relevance of defining characteristics for the six diagnostic labels. These scores were used to establish which defining characteristics were critical, which supporting, and which irrelevant.

Of the questionnaires returned, 148 were usable, most from nurses who worked in staff nursing positions. One hundred twenty four respondents (88.6%) indicated that they used nursing diagnosis in their practice. The diagnosis with the highest rating score was Impaired Skin Integrity; this was followed by Self-care Deficit. Thus for these diagnoses the defining characteristics were found to have high validity.

Two common diagnoses, (1) Anxiety, and (2) Pain, received the lowest overall rating scores. A previous study confirmed this finding, but also found that two of the specific defining characteristics for the diagnosis of Pain received high rating scores. Those characteristics were the verbalization of pain and a facial expression of pain. The investigators recommended that NANDA certify the two defining characteristics as critical to the diagnosis of Pain.

A **taxonomy** is a classification system that organizes known phenomena into a hierarchical structure and helps direct the discovery of new phenomena. An example of a taxonomic system from zoology is the familiar division into kingdom, phylum, class, order, family, genus, and species. Strictly speaking, the alphabetized list of approved nursing diagnoses constitutes a nomenclature, or system of names. The specification of a nomenclature and its successor, a taxonomy, are important preliminary steps in building nursing theory and science.

DEFINITIONS OF NURSING DIAGNOSIS

No single definition of nursing diagnosis is sufficiently comprehensive to convey its identity as a concept, a skill, and an international professional movement. Yet a definition of nursing diagnosis is needed to permit understanding of the multifaceted thing it is, and to separate it from things that it is not. Basic to any definition is the recognition that nursing diagnosis exists both as part of a process (the nursing process, consisting of data collection, nursing diagnosis, planning, implementation, and evaluation), and as a process unto itself (the diagnostic reasoning process).

Several of the most enduring definitions of nursing diagnosis are found in Box 17–2. Key words and terms emerging from these definitions are judgment, conclusion, inference, person's response, and actual or potential health problem.

A nursing diagnosis is a *conclusion* a nurse reaches after collecting and analyzing data relative to a client's holistic health status. It is a professional *judgment* in that, in addition to the collection and analysis of data, nurses make

BOX 17–2. DEFINITIONS OF NURSING DIAGNOSIS

Gebbie and Lavin: The judgment or conclusion that occurs as a result of nursing assessment.[6]

Mundinger and Jauron: A statement of a person's response to a situation or illness which is actually or potentially unhealthful and which nursing intervention can change in the direction of health.[7]

Aspinall: A process of clinical inference from observed changes in the patient's physical or psychological condition.[8]

Gordon: Actual or potential health problems that nurses, by virtue of their education and experience, are capable and licensed to treat.[3]

Shoemaker: A clinical judgment about an individual, family or community which is derived through a deliberate, systematic process of data collection and analysis. It provides the basis for prescriptions for definitive therapy for which the nurse is accountable. It is expressed concisely and it includes the etiology of the condition when known.[9]

North American Nursing Diagnosis Association: A clinical judgment about individual, family, or community responses to actual or potential health processes/life processes.[10]

IMPLICATIONS FOR PROFESSIONAL COLLABORATION

Diagnostic Vocabulary

Nursing diagnoses are professional judgments that are made by nurses about the meaning of assessment data gathered from clients. Nursing diagnoses are also labels given to the problems that nurses address; such labels provide a vocabulary that serves to coordinate communication among nurses in relation to the health problems they observe in practice. By identifying the health conditions that are primarily resolved by nursing interventions or therapies, a diagnostic vocabulary serves to define the professional domain of nursing. Thus, the development of nursing diagnoses, a collaborative activity in itself, not only serves to enhance communication among nurses but also unifies their efforts in the service of clients' health problems.

interpretations as to the meaning and significance of these findings both individually and collectively. This conclusion, this judgment, forms the basis for nursing action: treatment.

The term *inference* is useful in defining nursing diagnosis because it emphasizes the tentative and assumptive nature of diagnoses. *Webster's Collegiate Dictionary* describes inference as "a conclusion arriv[ed] at by reasoning from evidence," and warns that "if the evidence is slight the term comes close to *surmise*."[5] In recognizing that elements of both judgment and inference are part of nursing diagnoses, one can appreciate the need to limit or control the influences of bias and subjectivity on the part of the diagnostician and in the act of diagnosing, so that the diagnostic conclusion reached is as logical and factually based as possible. Inference in the context of diagnostic reasoning is discussed in greater detail later in this chapter.

A *person's response* to health and illness situations constitutes the focus, or phenomenon of concern, to nurses and is the object of nurses' diagnostic activities. In 1980, the American Nurses' Association (ANA) issued *Nursing: A Social Policy Statement*,[11] which defined the nature and scope of the profession in this way: "Nursing is diagnosis and treatment of human responses to actual or potential health problems" (p. 9). *Actual or potential health problems* to which nurses direct their diagnosis and treatment, then, are human responses—to the health challenges encountered in birth, illness, wellness, growth and development, and death.

The most essential and distinguishing feature of any nursing diagnosis is that it describes a health condition *primarily resolved by nursing interventions or therapies*.[11] There is, however, some difficulty in applying this criterion to the broad spectrum of health problems that nurses have historically, do currently, and will in the future identify and treat. The boundaries of nursing practice, particularly those that are shared with other health care professions, are dynamic and not easily delineated.

To assist in clarifying the boundaries of nursing, as well as to provide a framework for the development and classification of nursing diagnoses, the ANA[10] outlines the following categories of health problems, the treatment of which lies within the profession's domain:

1. Self-care limitations.
2. Impaired functioning in areas such as rest, sleep, ventilation, circulation, activity, nutrition, elimination, skin, and sexuality.
3. Pain and discomfort.
4. Emotional problems related to illness and treatment, life-threatening events, or daily life experiences, such as anxiety, loss, loneliness, and grief.
5. Distortion of symbolic functions, reflected in interpersonal and intellectual processes, such as hallucinations.
6. Deficiencies in decision-making and ability to make personal choices.
7. Self-image changes required by health status.
8. Dysfunctional perceptual orientations to health.
9. Strains related to life processes, such as birth, growth and development, and death.
10. Problematic affiliative relationships (p. 10).

Although the above categories are not in themselves nursing diagnoses, standardization of diagnostic labels developed from within this framework helps to ensure a discipline-specific perspective for the intervention activities of professional nurses.

FORMULATING NURSING DIAGNOSIS STATEMENTS: PES FORMAT

When communicating nursing diagnoses, either verbally or in writing, it is customary to use a format; that is, a general plan of arrangement or organization. Formats are important because they streamline communication by specifying the important information and how to present it. Formats are also important because they are used in common by the group adopting them and thus they unify a group's approach to communication around shared understanding and expectations.

The conventional format for documenting nursing diagnoses is the **PES format,** which indicates the direction of the relationship between the health problem (P), its etiologic factors (E), and defining characteristics, or signs and symptoms (S).

- *P = Problem.* This is a concise statement of the client's actual or potential health problem or health state. The **problem** statement, also called a **diagnostic label** or **category label,** comes from the list of approved nursing diagnoses (Box 17–1). An example is Impaired Skin Integrity.
- *E = Etiology.* This specifies source(s) from which the health problem is thought to arise, also called **related** or **contributing factors.** The **etiology** of a problem is its cause (to the extent that cause and effect can be known, or shown). A nursing diagnosis can, and often does, have several etiologies as its probable cause. These factors—whether biological, environmental, circumstantial, or

interpersonal—interact to produce the health problem. Each diagnostic label describing an actual problem has accompanying listings of possible causative factors. Examples of etiologies for the diagnosis Impaired Skin Integrity are *shearing forces, physical immobilization,* and *nutritional deficit.*

- *S = Signs and Symptoms.* These are observed, reported, or measured findings that serve as supporting evidence of the diagnosis, also called the **defining characteristics** or **manifestations.** As with etiology, each diagnostic label has a corresponding list of possible signs and symptoms. Examples of defining characteristics for the diagnostic label Impaired Skin Integrity are *disruption of skin surface* and *destruction of skin layers.*

Table 17–1 illustrates the PES components for several nursing diagnoses.

When communicating nursing diagnoses, either verbally or in writing, it is customary to link the PES components with words that indicate the direction of the relationship between the problem, its etiologic factors, and defining characteristics. The problem and etiology are linked with the indicator *related to;* the defining characteristics are linked by the indicator *as evidenced by.* Using the first diagnosis from Table 17–1 to illustrate documenting diagnostic statements in this way, the diagnosis for the client experiencing pain would be written:

> Pain related to surgical incision as evidenced by client statements: "it hurts when I move," "sharp knifelike pain," guarding behaviors, tightened brow, elevated heart rate.

Additionally, it is common practice to abbreviate related to and as evidenced by as *R/T* and *AEB,* respectively. Using the second diagnosis from Table 17–1 to illustrate these abbreviations, the diagnosis for the client experiencing constipation would be written:

> Constipation R/T immobility, fluid volume deficit, and use of narcotic analgesics AEB no BM × 5 days, hypoactive bowel sounds, straining at stool.

GUIDELINES FOR USE OF THE TAXONOMY OF NURSING DIAGNOSES

It is important to recognize that classification of the phenomena to which a profession addresses itself is a sizable and ongoing task. The development and refinement of nursing's nomenclature of health problems is in its earliest stages and subject to much revision based upon the research and clinical reports presented and reviewed at each of NANDA's conferences and by the Diagnosis Review Committee. Work on existing diagnoses is incomplete: several have etiologies and defining characteristics "to be developed," making clinical use difficult and frustrating. Other diagnoses are observed to "come and go" from the approved list from conference to conference. This apparent state of flux is both necessary and usual in the process of taxonomy development. One has only to look at the system of names describing health problems treatable by physicians not many years ago (eg, chilblains, consumption, dropsy) to appreciate our own progress to date, as well as the enormity of the overall task before us.

Guidelines for Problems (P)

Definitions of Health Problems. Many diagnoses have accompanying definitions to help clarify for nurses just what the health problem is conceptualized to be. These definitions are important for the student of nursing diagnosis to consider because they clarify more about the problem than is apparent from the label alone. For example, the definitions accompanying the diagnoses Fear and Anxiety draw a

TABLE 17–1. SAMPLE NURSING DIAGNOSES IN PES FORMAT

Problem	Etiology	Defining Characteristics
Pain	Surgical incision	"It hurts when I move" "Sharp, knifelike pain" Guarding behaviors Tightened brow Elevated heart rate
Constipation	Immobility Fluid volume deficit Narcotic analgesics	No BM × 5 days Hypoactive bowel sounds Straining at stool
Activity intolerance	Hypoxemia	Subjective breathlessness during AM self-care Heart rate elevation of 30 bpm over baseline upon ambulating to bathroom Pallor
Self-esteem disturbance	Recent divorce Physical incapacity to resume occupation	"What's the use?" "Who would care?" "Just another cripple" "I'd leave me too" Inability to accept positive reinforcement Nonparticipation in therapy

particularly useful distinction between the two problems: Fear is an emotion that has an identifiable source or object that the client validates, while anxiety is an emotion whose source is nonspecific or unknown to the client. Other good examples of such definitions accompany the diagnoses Social Isolation, Powerlessness, Altered Parenting, and Ineffective Family Coping.

Until definitions accompany all approved diagnoses, it will be important for nurses collaborating in care to establish consensus regarding the meaning and scope of the health problems stated.

Making Diagnostic Labels Specific. Some nursing diagnoses need to be accompanied by qualifiers or specifiers based on the characteristics of the health problem as it manifests itself in a particular client. For example, the diagnosis Fear needs to be specified as to the object of a client's particular fear (eg, death, pain, disfigurement, malignancy). Similarly, the diagnosis Knowledge Deficit needs to be specified regarding the content of the deficiency (eg, use of incentive spirometer, counting the pulse rate, respiratory muscle strengthening exercises).

Following are several nursing diagnoses needing specification, with examples of qualifying client circumstance in italic typeface.

- Fear: *Postoperative Pain*
- Knowledge Deficit: *Self-monitoring of Oral Anticoagulation Therapy*
- Altered *Peripheral* Tissue Perfusion
- Altered Nutrition: Less Than Body *Potassium* Requirements
- Altered Nutrition: More Than Body *Calorie* Requirements
- Self-Care Deficit: *Bathing and Feeding*
- Noncompliance: *Prescribed Activity Restrictions*

Guidelines for Etiologies (E)

Making Etiologies Specific. Etiologies cited for nursing diagnoses are often broad categories or examples—again, needing to be made specific based on characteristics of the problem and the client being treated. For example, one of several possible etiologies listed for the diagnosis Fluid Volume Excess is compromised regulatory mechanism. Considering this to be the cause of the fluid excess in a particular client, the nurse would need to specify which regulatory mechanism and in what way compromised (eg, inappropriate ADH secretion by the neurohypophysis) before the diagnosis could be formally stated (leaving aside the question as to whether this problem is independently treatable by nurses or would need referral).

Several etiologies needing to be made specific are listed below, along with examples of such specification in parentheses:

- Situational crisis (recent diagnosis of terminal illness)
- Psychological injuring agent (hurtful relationship, verbal abuse)
- Developmental factors (developmental arrest, extremes of age)

Nursing Diagnosis as Etiologies. Nursing diagnostic labels may rightfully serve as etiologies for other diagnoses. Examples are Anxiety related to knowledge deficit, and Activity Intolerance related to decreased cardiac output.

Etiologies as the Focus of Treatment. The treatment plan formulated for a given diagnosis must include interventions aimed at resolution or management of the etiologic factors as well as at the health problem itself. In fact, in some instances nursing treatment will be directed almost exclusively at the etiology of a problem, with the logical expectation that if the causative factors are reduced in influence, the problem should begin to resolve. This will be especially true in instances where a nursing diagnosis has as its etiology another nursing diagnosis. Consider treatment approaches to the diagnosis Ineffective Breathing Pattern related to high abdominal incision pain. Predictably little effectiveness would be shown were the interventions to be focused solely on reviewing the rationale for slow, deep, symmetrical breathing, demonstrating the technique, and encouraging the client in its performance, without some plan for alleviating the client's pain.

Medical Diagnoses as Etiologies. Because, as mentioned, the etiology of a nursing diagnosis becomes a focus of intervention in the treatment of the overall problem, citing a medical condition or diagnosis as the etiology is conceptually inadvisable if the problem statement is to retain its identity as a health problem primarily resolved by nursing therapies. And yet many problems of concern to nurses and amenable to their treatment *are* consequent to medical conditions. Examples are Ineffective Airway Clearance that results from chronic obstructive pulmonary disease (COPD), and Sensory-Perceptual Alterations resulting from open heart surgery. In these instances nurses should isolate those aspects of the contributing pathological state that are *modifiable by nursing intervention,* and cite these factors as etiologic. Problem statements might include Ineffective Airway Clearance related to thick tracheobronchial secretions, Knowledge Deficit: Effective Cough and Hydration Techniques and Respiratory Muscle Weakness; and Sensory-Perceptual Alterations related to sensory overload, sensory deprivation, and sleep pattern disturbance. These problem statements are more clearly worded, and provide a much sharper focus for nursing intervention.[12]

Guidelines for Defining Characteristics/Signs and Symptoms (S)

Making Defining Characteristics Specific. As with problem statements and statements of etiology, the list of defining characteristics (signs and symptoms) cited for each diagnosis often describe a nonspecific symptom category and need to be modified to reflect the particular situation presented by the client being diagnosed. For example, one of the possible defining characteristics for the diagnosis Impaired Gas Exchange is *abnormal blood gases.* In formulating this diagnostic statement for clinical use, the specific blood gas value used to diagnose the problem should be cited in the statement (eg, Po_2: 54 mmHg and/or Pco_2: 50 mmHg) rather than the nonspecific symptom category, abnormal blood gases.

Several defining characteristics are cited below in nonspecific form as they appear in the taxonomy, followed in parentheses by examples of proper specification:

- Respiratory Depth Changes (shallow breathing)
- Blood Pressure Changes (hypotension)
- Autonomic Responses (dilated pupils, increased heart rate)
- Altered Electrolytes (hypokalemia)
- Change in Mental State (confusion, lethargy, apprehension)

Major or Critical Defining Characteristics. Major (also called critical) defining characteristics are designated signs and/or symptoms that must be present for the health problem to be considered present. These major defining characteristics must be present in a client data base profile in order to diagnose the corresponding health problem with any degree of certainty. For example, the diagnosis Altered Parenting has as its critical defining characteristics *inattentive to infant/child needs,* and *inappropriate caretaking behaviors.* It is essential that these characteristics be present in the client's situation (in addition, perhaps, to several other noncritical signs) for the diagnosis of this problem.

The assignment of major or critical status to a defining characteristic is based upon research and/or extensive clinical experience in which the signs and symptoms of a health problem are tested for their ability to predict most reliably the presence of the diagnosis, and can therefore be used with confidence by the nurse diagnostician. Presently, NANDA has not designated major defining characteristics for all of the approved nursing diagnoses, although nurse clinicians and scholars have done considerable research to accomplish this goal.[13–17] It is incumbent upon the Diagnostic Review Committee and the general membership of NANDA to continue efforts to identify the defining characteristics that are critical for each nursing diagnosis.

GUIDELINES FOR DIAGNOSING HIGH-RISK STATES AND POTENTIAL HEALTH PROBLEMS

Determining a Risk State for Diagnosis

Predicting a potential health problem in a client involves an estimation of probability. The potential for an event, or pattern of response, to occur can truly be said to exist in almost any situation. Consider the potential health problems facing the postoperative client. This risk state includes Potential for Body Image Disturbance, Potential for Sleep Pattern Disturbance, Potential for Ineffective Airway Clearance, Potential for Constipation, and Potential for Aspiration, to name only a few. To include each of these diagnoses in the client's treatment plan without regard for probabilities, and formulate expected client outcomes and interventions for each, would be pointless.

What is needed is an appraisal of clients' health status and the identification of **risk factors** that place them at higher risk for the health problem than the general population. For example, all persons recovering from abdominal surgery have a potential for constipation owing to the effects of general anesthesia and narcotic analgesics, manipulation of abdominal viscera, and postoperative immobility. There is a tacit understanding of this risk among all nurses, and monitoring and intervention are carried out to avert the problem as part of routine nursing care; hence there is no need to state the problem on an individualized nursing care plan. (However, this potential problem should be on record in a Standards of Care Manual or Standardized Care Plans. See Chapter 18.) A client is at higher risk than the general population of postoperative clients if, for example, the history reveals dependence on laxatives or the client demonstrates fluid volume deficit, prolonged immobility, or noncompliance with nursing prescription for ambulation. The diagnosis indicating this potential and its risk factors would then be stated so that additional or more intensified interventions, beyond those which are routine, could be planned.

Stating Potential or High-Risk Diagnoses

Several of the approved diagnoses in Box 17–1 address potential dysfunctional states. These **potential diagnoses** identify the presence of risk factors, but not the actual health problem. Examples of such high risk diagnoses are:

- Altered Nutrition: Potential for More Than Body Requirements
- Potential for Aspiration
- Potential for Infection
- Potential for Impaired Skin Integrity
- Potential for Injury
- Potential for Poisoning
- Potential for Suffocation
- Potential for Violence

Although these diagnoses are listed formally as potential problems, rightfully any diagnosis from the approved list can be stated as a potential problem by simply adding the modifiers "potential" or "high risk" to the label. For example, Self-esteem Disturbance is written Potential for Self-esteem Disturbance, and Impaired Gas Exchange becomes Potential for Impaired Gas Exchange.

Potential nursing diagnoses cite defining characteristics as risk factors. The diagnostic statement includes only two parts: the health problem at risk and the risk factors; for example, Potential for Ineffective Individual Coping, Risk Factors: malignant biopsy results, absence of interpersonal support system, and history of alcohol abuse.

Table 17–2 provides guidelines for formulating nursing diagnosis statements.

TABLE 17–2. GUIDELINES FOR FORMULATING NURSING DIAGNOSIS STATEMENTS

Guideline	Correct Example	Incorrect Example
1. Use definitions accompanying diagnoses to clarify meaning of the label and accurately diagnose the client health problem.	1. Anxiety R/T threatened change in health status AEB "I'm feeling nervous," "Just wish my operation were over," frequent fidgeting with sheets, rearranging personal articles, and tense shoulder and jaw muscles.	1. Anxiety: *pain due to surgery* R/T threatened change in health status AEB "I'm feeling nervous," "Just wish my operation were over," frequent fidgeting with sheets, rearranging personal articles, tense shoulder and jaw muscles (anxiety has no known source, if source is known, fear is more accurate).
2. Make diagnostic labels specific to manifestations exhibited by the client.	2. Knowledge deficit: *dietary sources of protein* R/T lack of exposure AEB "What should I eat to get protein?" "I never learned about what we get from foods," "Is fruit high in protein?"	2. Knowledge deficit: *protein* R/T lack of exposure AEB "What should I eat to get protein?" "I never learned about what we get from foods," "Is fruit high in protein?"
3. Make etiologies specific to manifestations exhibited by the client.	3. Sleep pattern disturbance R/T *awakening to feed newborn* AEB "I'm always tired," "I never feel rested when I get up in the AM," "The baby wakes me up every couple of hours all night long." or Potential for infection, R.F. *Diabetes, gangrenous toe and incision, L. leg.*	3. Sleep pattern disturbance R/T *social cues* AEB "I'm always tired," I never feel rested when I get up in the AM," "The baby wakes me up every couple of hours all night long." or Potential for infection, Risk Factors: *Chronic disease, tissue destruction.*
4. Make defining characteristics specific to manifestations exhibited by the client.	4. Pain R/T uterine contractions AEB *fixed stare, jaw clenched, moaning, rolling from side to side, arms rigid, fists clenched during contractions.*	4. Pain R/T uterine contractions AEB *Facial mask of pain, distraction behavior, alteration in muscle tone.*
5. Be sure the etiology does not restate the diagnosis.	5. Impaired skin integrity R/T *pressure on skin over boney prominence, shearing force.*	5. Impaired skin integrity R/T *pressure sore, L. hip.*
6. Avoid medical diagnoses as etiologies; instead, identify aspects of the disease that can be modified by nursing intervention.	6. Impaired physical mobility R/T *pain and muscle weakness, L. leg.*	6. Impaired physical mobility R/T *arthritis.*
7. Do not confuse etiology with specification of the diagnostic statement.	7. Knowledge Deficit: *breast feeding* R/T lack of exposure to information.	7. Knowledge Deficit R/T *breast feeding.*
8. Use the taxonomy to guide identification of the etiology.	8. Anxiety R/T *change in role: motherhood:*	8. Anxiety R/T birth of newborn child.

Diagnosing the Potential for a Medical Problem

Nurses were speaking the language of prevention long before it became economically imperative to do so. Today, many of the activities that make up the professional nursing role involve the promotion of health and prevention of illness and complications. Hence, the prevention of some medical conditions is logically and justifiably within the domain of nursing. Potential for Atelectasis, Potential for Joint Contractures, and Potential for Thrombophlebitis, though not so designated within NANDA's list of approved diagnoses, are examples of health problems *primarily resolved by nursing interventions or therapies;* problems that nurses, as Gordon[3] states, "by virtue of their education and experience are capable and licensed to treat" (p. 2).

Scrutiny of the entire scope and context of situations in which these and other potentials for a medical condition are diagnosed is necessary, however, to determine that the problem can and will respond *primarily* to nursing intervention. Certainly there are medical conditions that are not directly preventable by nursing therapies, such as potential for asthma, potential for breast cancer, and so on. Additionally, once the potential for a medical condition becomes an *actual* problem, it loses its designation as a nursing diagnosis and is referred to a physician.

Collaborative Problems

Collaborative problem is a designation proposed by Carpenito for potential physiological complications that nurses monitor.[4,19] This term and the concept have been somewhat controversial among nursing scholars and clinicians. Although there is considerable agreement that collaboration is an important element in health care, more often it is the process of collaborative management, rather

Functional Dimensions \ Manifestation Categories	Berger-Williams Model for Holistic Assessment			
	Physical	**Cognitive**	**Emotional**	**Self-conceptual**
Wellness and Well-being				
Self-expression				
Skin and tissue integrity				
Nutrition				
Elimination				
Oxygenation	Hx COPD. RR 24, shallow. Skin cool, pale. Sits with chest supported by arms. Shoulders rise with breathing. States "I get extemely winded even walking to the phone."	"I don't know of any breathing techniques other than the ones I'm using and have used for years."	"Shortness of breath frightens me real bad." "I live in fear of losing my wind." "I just seem to panic when my breathing gets tough."	"What's the use of trying?" "I'm just a puffy old guy who's always spittin' up phlegm."
Sleep–rest patterns				
Neurosensory integration				
Mobility				
Fluid balance				

Figure 17–2. The Berger-Williams Model for holistic assessment.

Berger-Williams Model for Holistic Assessment				Identified Nursing Diagnosis
Sociocultural/ Life-structural	Developmental	Sexual	Environmental	
				Ineffective breathing pattern related to: ■ Deconditioned diaphragm: second-degree chronic lung disease. ■ Lack of knowledge: effective breathing techniques. ■ Fear. ■ Decreased self-esteem AEB: rapid, shallow breathing; pallor; activity intolerance; use of accessory respiratory muscles.

Figure 17–2 (continued).

than the stipulation of a problem as collaborative, that receives greater support.[20–26] Collaborative management involves the activities of clients, nurses, and other health care providers. It encompasses planning, implementing, and evaluating client care related to nursing diagnoses, as well as monitoring aspects of client status related to the disease process. Therefore, it is nursing, not the health problem, that is collaborative in nature. Collaborative management is achieving increasing recognition as a cost-effective and a quality affective model for health care delivery.[27] See Chapters 1, 18, and 35.

■ DIAGNOSTIC REASONING

Lest it appear from the foregoing discussion of the mechanics of nursing diagnosis statement formulation that nurses have only to select a label for a problem from an "approved list," and follow a formula for deciding upon its cause and symptoms from an "ingredients index" accompanying that list, the process of diagnostic reasoning will now be examined.

Diagnostic reasoning is the process through which nurses arrive at a nursing diagnosis. Also referred to as inferential reasoning or clinical problem-solving, it can be thought of as a mental equation: a + b + c = d. Like an equation it is orderly and systematic; unlike an equation not all of its factors and operations exist in our conscious awareness. The challenge of refining the process of diagnostic reasoning is to bring into one's conscious awareness all of the factors and operations influencing the equation, and necessary in arriving at an accurate "answer," or diagnosis.

Components

Although diagnostic reasoning is a purely mental process, reaching a diagnostic decision at its conclusion is to a large extent collaborative. When nurse and client share the appraisal of the problem that each has reached independently, the decision (diagnosis) that results may be different from one that either would have made alone. Mutual input increases the validity of the diagnosis.

Diagnostic reasoning comprises several elements, including collecting and organizing the data, clustering cues to generate inferences, and validating inferences.

Collecting and Organizing the Data Base. By virtue of nursing's unique orientation and commitment to holism, nurses collect an enormous volume of data relative to a client's health status. Consequently, in the process of assembling this data base nurses need some place to "put" the information as it is collected. Ideally, this storage device would contain compartments that could keep the data separated and organized. Such a device is called an **organizational framework.**

Organizational frameworks also serve as guides for assessment. Their compartments consist of headings corresponding to the attributes that nurses accept as comprising the nature of humans, health, illness, and nursing. In this way, the framework helps guide the deduction of diagnoses that are within the domain of nursing.

Organizational frameworks are neither new nor unique to nursing. Traditionally, nursing utilized medicine's organizational framework for the collection and organization of data. However, as nursing's own knowledge base and conceptual orientation became increasingly differentiated and complex, the biologic-mechanistic medical framework was found to be insufficiently comprehensive for use by nurses as a tool for holistic assessment. The organizational framework for generalist medical practice and three frameworks for nursing practice are compared in Table 17–3.

Figure 17–2 (*see* previous page) represents an expansion of the Berger-Williams model for Holistic Assessment found in Table 17–3. The vertical axis of the grid contains the categories of human functional dimensions typically in-

TABLE 17–3. COMPARISON OF SELECTED ORGANIZATIONAL FRAMEWORKS

Medicine	Nursing		
Body Systems	Berger-Williams Model for Holistic Assessment	NANDA Taxonomy I Revised	Functional Health Patterns
Cardiovascular	Physical	Exchanging	Health Perception-Management
Respiratory	Cognitive	Communicating	Nutritional-Metabolic
Neurological	Emotional	Relating	Elimination
Endocrine	Self-conceptual	Valuing	Activity-Exercise
Metabolic	Sociocultural/Life-structural	Choosing	Sleep-Rest
Hematoimmune	Developmental	Moving	Cognitive-Perceptual
Integumentary	Sexual	Perceiving	Self-Perception-Self-Concept
Gastrointestinal	Environmental	Feeling	Role-Relationship
Genitourinary		Knowing	Sexuality-Reproductive
Reproductive			Coping-Stress Tolerance
Psychiatric			Value-Belief

vestigated by nurses. The horizontal axis contains the manifestation categories of the Berger-Williams Model, which represent the multiple facets of individuals' holistic nature. Data are collected relative to a functional dimension category (vertical axis) and are pursued in terms of the nature of their manifestations (horizontal axis). Figure 17–2 provides an example of data collection relative to the functional dimension, oxygenation. Physical indicators related to oxygenation have been collected and documented, as well as cognitive, emotional, and self-conceptual manifestations. Upon analysis of these data a nurse can see the multiple etiologies and manifestations of the dysfunction and is thus aided in the formulation of a descriptive, comprehensive nursing diagnosis statement, as well as in the planning of comprehensive client care. (See Chapter 18.) Although oxygenation is a physical function, considering only its physical elements could not accurately identify nor effectively correct the oxygenation problem. The dual axes of the model emphasize that a unidimensional approach to client care does not acknowledge the multiple variables that underlie clients' responses to health problems.

As data collection continues and observations and findings regarding all of the functional dimensions (fluid balance, neurosensory integration, and so on) are assembled, it is typical to find factors that contribute to one problem within other functional dimension categories. An example is a nurse's identification that a client's weight is greater than that recommended for his or her age and sex (nutrition dimension). The nurse reasons that this is responsible in part for the client's discomfort and difficult breathing during activity (mobility dimension) and therefore is a likely contributing factor to his or her activity intolerance.

Organizational frameworks are necessary to structure the volume of information nurses accrue in the assessment of clients. They facilitate diagnostic reasoning by guiding data collection and organizing it into manageable parts. Organizing incoming information in this way increases its availability for retrieval and facilitates subsequent identification of relationships from among the data.

The selection of any one framework over another, so long as it is designed to organize nursing data, is an individual choice.

Clustering Cues to Generate Inferences. A **cue** is a piece of information, a raw fact. Through the senses nurses notice and seek cues regarding clients' health status and functioning. Sweaty palms, restlessness, and heart rate of 102 beats per minute are cues. A cue is inert; in itself it says nothing beyond what it represents: sweaty palms are sweaty palms, restlessness is restlessness, a heart rate of 102 is a heart rate of 102. In the process of diagnostic reasoning, cues are the units of information that are collected and recorded for later analysis. Cues are free of interpretation; they are purely objective and carry no symbolic meaning.

An **inference** is the assignment of meaning to cues. It is not until individual cues are grouped together (clustered) and interpreted collectively that they can begin to assume the identity of a phenomenon greater (or other) than what each represented individually. Sweaty palms, restlessness, and heart rate of 102, when interpreted as a cluster, can now mean anxiety, shock, fear, or pain.

Inferences are created, whereas cues exist. The process of creating inferences from cues, therefore, carries with it the risk of logical error. If the cues sweaty palms, restlessness, and heart rate of 102 were grouped and interpreted in a client who also manifested gurgling respiratory sounds and a rapid, shallow breathing pattern—and these additional cues were overlooked or ignored by the person assigning meaning to the cluster—the inferences (anxiety, shock, fear, or pain) would be erroneous (the more likely inference being, in this case, ineffective airway clearance).

Nursing diagnoses are inferences, whereas defining characteristics are cues. The process of clustering assessment cues and developing inferences as to their collective identity can be likened to playing the game of Scrabble, where the individual letters represent cues and completed words represent diagnostic inferences. As players collect the seven letters (cues) and place them on the rack, they begin to entertain possibilities for the formulation of words (diagnoses). The goal is to develop a word (diagnosis) that would include as many letters (cues) as possible. Sometimes, completed words (diagnoses) seem to formulate themselves on the letter rack; at other times a player needs to arrange and rearrange the letters (cues) on the rack in order to "see" a word (identify a diagnosis). The better or more experienced player sees words (diagnoses) others would have missed given the same selection of letters (cues). Ultimately, all words formulated on the letter rack need to be found a place on the Scrabble board, connected to the overall matrix of words. The analogy here is that a logical fit is necessary between the diagnostic inference and the total client profile. Table 17–4 illustrates cue clustering within the oxygenation functional dimension to generate a nursing diagnosis.

Validating Inferences. An inference is as much a guess as it is a hypothesis. Once a diagnostic inference is formulated, nurses develop and implement a treatment plan designed to resolve or reduce the problem represented by that inference. Erroneous inferences can have serious consequences; among them, potential client harm resulting from treatment of a nonexistent health problem, or from treatment withheld for a missed diagnosis. Consequently, it is essential to seek validation of diagnostic inferences prior to implementing treatment.

Four approaches to the validation of inferences are recommended.[28] First, consult with an authoritative source. This may be a clinical nurse specialist, nurse educator, textbook, or published research. Seek confirmation of the logical and scientific integrity of the diagnostic statement. Is it reasonable that this particular etiology is responsible for this problem in this client, and would these be the expected signs and symptoms?

Second, reexamine the cues (Fig. 17–3). Could the cues in this diagnostic statement support any other diagnosis, or

TABLE 17–4. EXAMPLE OF CLUSTERING CUES TO GENERATE INFERENCES (NURSING DIAGNOSIS) WITHIN OXYGEN FUNCTIONAL DIMENSION

Assessment Data	Cue Clustering		Nursing Diagnosis
History COPD RR: 24, shallow Skin cool, pale Sits with chest supported by arms. Shoulders rise with breathing. "I don't know any breathing techniques other than the ones I'm using and have used for years." "Shortness of breath frightens me real bad." "What's the use of trying? I'm just a puffy old guy who's always spittin' up phlegm." "I just seem to panic when breathing gets tough." "I get extremely winded even when walking to the phone." "I live in fear of losing my wind."	Sits with chest supported by arms. Shoulders rise with breathing. "I get extremely winded even when walking to the phone."	Deconditioned diaphragm and use of accessory respiratory muscles; activity intolerance	Ineffective breathing pattern R/T deconditioned diaphragm, lack of knowledge of effective breathing techniques; fear; decreased self-esteem, AEB rapid shallow breathing, pallor, activity intolerance, use of accessory respiratory muscles.
	"I don't know any breathing techniques other than the ones I'm using and have used for years."	Lack of knowledge	
	"Shortness of breath frightens me real bad." "I just seem to panic when breathing gets tough." I live in fear of losing my wind."	Fear	
	"What's the use of trying?" "I'm just a puffy old guy who's always spittin' up phlegm."	Decreased self-esteem	

only the one chosen? Consider the cues from the data base that were felt *not* to be a part of the cluster supporting this diagnosis. Is there some other cluster of which they are a part, or could several of them, together with cues from this cluster, suggest an altogether different diagnosis? (Recall from the example in the discussion of inference the ramifications of the overlooked cues of gurgling respiratory sounds and rapid, shallow breathing pattern.)

Third, validate inferences with the client. Share with the client the cluster of cues you've identified and what it is you feel they represent. Clients often have remarkable insights into what underlies their patterns of response and can be a great resource in validating nurses' conclusions. Additionally, people benefit significantly from having their situations reflected back to them. Indeed, collaborating with clients in this way is many times all the intervention that is necessary.

Fourth, seek evidence of the reliability of the diagnostic inference from within the appropriate reference group. Do most professional peers conclude the same explanation for the available cues?

The above approaches are excellent strategies for seeking validation of diagnostic inferences prior to the institution of treatment. The only way to achieve or confirm val-

IMPLICATIONS FOR PROFESSIONAL COLLABORATION

Validation

Once nurses complete the diagnostic reasoning necessary to infer a diagnosis, they share the inferences derived through diagnostic reasoning with other nurses and health care professionals. This collaboration is focused on validating the diagnosis. Nurses also collaborate with clients on the diagnosis. Sharing the diagnostic inference with clients gives them an opportunity to judge the accuracy of the diagnosis from a personal point of view. It is also the first step in reaching a consensus with clients about the nature of the health problem and the direction of the care plan.

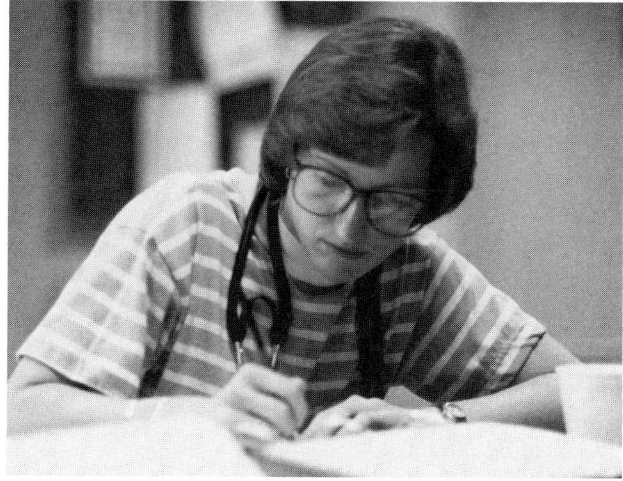

Figure 17–3. Reviewing records is part of the diagnostic process.

idation of a diagnosis, however, is to treat and evaluate it. If favorable and predicted outcomes result, strong evidence exists that the problem, its etiology, and defining characteristics were accurately inferred.

Sources of Diagnostic Error

There is much scientific curiosity within the nursing profession regarding the diagnostic reasoning process, strategies effective in increasing diagnostic accuracy, and sources of diagnostic error. Many of the principles identified through research thus far have come from studying differences in the diagnostic strategies employed by experts and novices.[29–32] The following discussion focuses only on the most common type of diagnostic error, the inferential leap, and several of its sources.

As the term implies, the **inferential leap** involves a jump to a conclusion, based upon premature termination of the data-gathering/data-analysis phase of the nursing process. Numerous studies have shown that this jump to an erroneous conclusion is most frequently made because not all of the variables were known or examined at the time the inference was formulated. Interestingly, the novice will often close the search for cues prematurely (insufficient data gathering) whereas the expert will terminate prematurely the analysis of cues (insufficient data analysis).[29]

The novice tends to close the search for cues prematurely because of a lack of appreciation for the scope of the problems to be diagnosed. Diagnoses such as Disturbance in Self-concept and Ineffective Individual Coping are reported to be at the highest level of abstraction among nursing diagnoses[33] and are therefore quite difficult to know fully, let alone see and discriminate from among other diagnostic possibilities. The expert has an advantage in this regard by virtue of a greater breadth of experience, both with the label and with the clinical presentation of clients demonstrating the problem.

Additionally, the novice will often halt the collection of data and conclude a diagnosis prematurely because of a discomfort with uncertainty. The novice has a tendency to move with a sense of urgency to assign a diagnosis, any diagnosis, in order to experience the comforting sense of direction that comes with having a client's "problems" labeled. The novice may mistakenly feel that reserving judgment pending greater diagnostic certainty will brand him or her as being inexpert. The expert, on the other hand, tends to enjoy uncertainty and finds stimulation in weighing and rearranging cue clusters.

The erring expert will occasionally overutilize knowledge from previous experience, which fosters a tendency to stereotype clients and their health alterations, thereby obscuring vital relationships among assessment data. Carnevali[34] cites Francis Bacon's observation that once an opinion has been made, the mind tends to "draw all things to support that judgment, ignoring the presence of contrary or ill-fitting data" (p. 41). Novices are more purist in this regard, because they have a limited experiential base from which to draw stereotypes and their objectivity is therefore freer from contaminating influences.

The above descriptions of the predispositions and tendencies of the novice and expert diagnostician should not be used to characterize a nurse in terms of relative expertise. Nor should they be interpreted as a sequence of developmental tasks to be accomplished in the evolution of novice to expert.

They are offered, instead, to ground firmly in reality the process of developing diagnostic skill by acknowledging that errors are inherent in this process, and to stimulate

IMPLICATIONS FOR PROFESSIONAL COLLABORATION

Diagnostic Error

Sharing the diagnostic inference with expert nurses or other health care professionals who have an interest in a client's care is an important collaborative activity that has the benefit of preventing or minimizing diagnostic error. As points of view are shared and factors considered, alternative diagnoses are often considered and weighed. Collaboration to validate diagnoses thus reduces the likelihood that important variables will be overlooked and reduces the chance that the nurse will err in the diagnosis by making an inferential leap.

BUILDING NURSING KNOWLEDGE

What Factors Influence Diagnostic Reasoning?

Woolley N. Nursing diagnosis: Exploring the factors which may influence the reasoning process. *J Adv Nurs.* 1990; 15: 110–117.

According to Woolley, several ingredients are essential to accurate nursing diagnosis. These include an awareness of the central concepts of nursing, the problem-solving process, and logical thinking. Woolley identifies the factors that influence the nurse's diagnostic reasoning process as (1) the experience of the diagnostician, (2) the nature of the diagnostic task, and (3) the nature of the setting.

Woolley argues that experience has a profound effect on the reasoning process; it is what gives the expert the ability to combine and interrelate knowledge gained from theory and clinical practice to make accurate diagnoses. Experience is linked to being able to accurately assess the probability that a given diagnosis applies. Biases also have a profound effect on diagnostic reasoning. If unexplored, they may negatively affect standards of care. Thus nurses need to examine their own beliefs and value systems and to develop self-awareness.

Several environmental factors also influence diagnostic reasoning. Technology creates added responsibility for nurses who must master its use and employ the data in nursing diagnosis. Role responsibilities also affect diagnostic reasoning. Work pressure often creates conflicting demands for nurses, and performing physical tasks may take time from the process of formulating diagnoses. Developing effective clinical decision-making strategies is a professional responsibility. Awareness of the variables that can influence the process facilitates gaining diagnostic skill.

in the diagnostician a quest for the attainment of higher levels of skill.

PROFESSIONAL ADVANTAGES OF NURSING DIAGNOSIS

Nursing diagnosis has many advantages for professional practice. A review of the nursing literature by Baer[35] revealed, among other benefits, that nursing diagnosis

- Assists in organizing, defining, and developing nursing knowledge.
- Aids in identifying and describing the domain and scope of nursing practice.
- Focuses nursing care on the (client's) response to problems.
- Prescribes diagnosis-specific nursing interventions that should increase the effectiveness of nursing care.
- Facilitates the evaluation of nursing practice.
- Provides a framework for testing the validity of nursing interventions.
- Provides a standardized vocabulary to enhance intra- and interprofessional communication.
- Prescribes the content of nursing curricula.
- Provides a framework for developing a system to direct third-party reimbursements for nursing services.
- Indicates specific rationales for (client) care based on nursing assessment.
- Leads to more comprehensive and individualized (client) care (p. 92).

These advantages underscore the value of the development and application of the taxonomy of nursing diagnoses to individual nurses and the profession at large. Two additional benefits deserve emphasis: support of the independent role of nurses and promotion of collaboration.

Chapter 2 discusses the importance to nursing of being recognized as a profession by other health care providers and the public. Autonomy, control, and accountability in practice were among the characteristics of a profession delineated there. A universally accepted classification system: the taxonomy of nursing diagnoses, that clearly specifies the domain of nursing practice confers a measure of autonomy and simultaneously provides a vehicle through which to demonstrate accountability. Chapter 18 further clarifies this concept.

The philosophy on which this text is based stresses the importance of collaborative decision making. Consistent naming of client conditions treated by nurses enhances awareness among health care providers and clients of the role nurses can play in supporting clients' efforts to achieve and maintain optimal health. This awareness enhances communication, mutual goal setting, and working together toward goal attainment.

SUMMARY

Nursing diagnoses are standardized labels that represent clinical judgments made by professional nurses, and describe health problems primarily resolved by nursing therapies. Nursing diagnosis focuses nursing assessment and intervention on the human response to altered health states, thus constituting a unique, distinct, and imperative component to comprehensive health care. No longer a clinical luxury, nor even an option, nursing diagnosis is mandated as part of competent registered nurse criteria by many state Nurse Practice Acts, as well as constituting the very core of the ANA's formal definition of nursing.

Developing actual or potential nursing diagnosis statements from the North American Nursing Diagnosis Association's approved diagnoses consists of specifying a problem statement (P), probable risk factors or etiologies (E), and the signs and symptoms (S) of the problem. Clinically, nursing diagnoses are formulated through the process of diagnostic reasoning, which in this chapter includes collecting and organizing the data base, clustering cues, generating diagnostic inferences, and seeking validation of inferences prior to treatment. Diagnostic skill is learned and enhanced both cognitively and experientially.[36]

Identification, standardization, and classification of health problems treatable by nurses is a continuing task; one that the discipline of nursing has commenced relatively recently. Because of its present embryonic state of development, the clinical nurse often finds the approved list of diagnoses clumsy, incomplete, and inelegant. It is. And yet it is only through repeated and persistent clinical application that nursing diagnosis finds promise of evolving and emerging as clinically pertinent, useful, and accurately descriptive. Additionally, amidst the process of developing a diagnostic taxonomy nurses find a stimulus and mechanism for the advancement of nursing theory and science, and a maximized potential for the delivery of high-quality, reliable, professional health care.

REFERENCES

1. Fry VS. The creative approach to nursing. *Am J Nurs.* 1953;53: 301–302.
2. Hornung GJ. Nursing diagnosis: An exercise in judgment. *Nurs Outlook.* 1956;4:29–30.
3. Gordon M. *Nursing Diagnosis: Process and Application.* 2nd ed. New York: McGraw-Hill; 1987.
4. Carpenito LJ. *Nursing Diagnosis: Application to Clinical Practice.* 3rd ed. Philadelphia: Lippincott; 1989.
5. *Webster's New Collegiate Dictionary.* 9th ed. Springfield, MA: Merriam; 1986.
6. Gebbie KM, Lavin MA. *Classification of Nursing Diagnoses: Proceedings of the First National Conference.* St. Louis: Mosby; 1975.
7. Mundinger MD, Jauron DG. Developing a nursing diagnosis. *Nurs Outlook.* 1975;23:94–98.
8. Aspinall MJ. Nursing diagnosis: The weak link. *Nurs Outlook.* 1976;24:433.
9. Shoemaker J. Essential features of nursing diagnosis. In: Kim MJ, McFarland GK, McLane AM, eds. *Classification of Nursing Diagnoses: Proceedings of the Fifth National Conference.* St. Louis: Mosby; 1984.

10. North American Nursing Diagnosis Association. *Classification of Nursing Diagnoses: Proceedings of the Ninth National Conference.* Philadelphia: Lippincott, 1991.
11. American Nurses' Association. *Nursing: A Social Policy Statement.* Kansas City, MO: ANA; 1980.
12. Davie JK. Medical diagnoses as etiologic-related factors to nursing diagnoses. *Newsletter South Cal Nurs Diagnosis A.* 1989;6:3.
13. Levin RF. *Yesterday, today and tomorrow: Nursing diagnosis research.* Paper presented at the First Mid-Atlantic Regional Conference on Nursing Diagnosis. Philadelphia: June, 1984.
14. Metzger KL, Hiltunen E. *Diagnostic content validation of ten frequently reported nursing diagnoses.* Paper presented at the meeting of the North American Nursing Diagnosis Association. St. Louis: March, 1986.
15. Silver SM, Halfmann TM, McShane RE. The identification of clinically recorded nursing diagnoses and indicators. In Kim MJ, McFarland GK, McLane AM, eds. *A Classification of Nursing Diagnoses: Proceedings of the Fifth National Conference.* St. Louis: Mosby, 1984.
16. Levin RF, Krainovitch BC, Bahrenburg E, Mitchell CA. Diagnostic content validity of nursing diagnoses. *Image.* 1989;21:40–44.
17. Fehring RJ. Validating diagnostic labels: Standardized methodology. In Hurley M, ed. *Classification of Nursing Diagnoses: Proceedings of the Fifth National Conference.* St. Louis: Mobsy; 1986.
18. Woodtli AO. Validation of defining characteristics: Clinical design. *J Neurosci Nurs.* 1988;29:324–326.
19. Carpenito LJ. *Nursing Care Plans and Documentation: Nursing Diagnoses and Collaborative Problems.* New York: Lippincott, 1991.
20. Davie, JK. Independent and Interdependent/Collaborative Nursing Practice, *Newsletter of the Southern California Nursing Diagnosis Association.* 1989;5:3, 24:433.
21. Moccia P. 1989: Shaping a human agenda for the nineties. *Nursing and Health Care.* 1989;10:15–17.
22. Chavigny KH. Coalition building between medicine and nursing. *Nursing Economics.* 1988;6:179–183, 204.
23. Aiken LH. Charting the future for hospital nursing. *Image.* 1990;22:72–78.
24. Atkinson LD, Murray ME. *Understanding the Nursing Process: Fundamentals of Care Planning.* New York: Pergamon, 1990.
25. Mitchell PM. Components of nursing practice. In Patrick ML, Woods SL, Craven RF, Rokosky JS, Bruno PM, eds. *Medical-Surgical Nursing.* New York: Lippincott, 1991.
26. Craft CA. Issues pertinent to implementation of nursing diagnosis. In Carlson JH, Craft CA, McGuire AD, Popkiss-Vawter S. *Nursing Diagnosis: A Case Study Approach.* Philadelphia: Saunders, 1991.
27. Zander K. Nursing case management: Strategic management of cost and quality outcomes. *J Nurs Adm.* 1988;18:23–30.
28. Iyer PW, Taptich BJ, Bernocchi-Losey D. *Nursing Process and Nursing Diagnosis.* 2nd ed. Philadelphia: Saunders, 1991.
29. Benner P. *From Novice to Expert: Excellence and Power in Clinical Nursing Practice.* Menlo Park, CA: Addison-Wesley; 1984.
30. Tanner CA. Toward the development of diagnostic reasoning skills. In: Carnevali DL, Mitchell PM, Woods NF, Tanner CA, eds. *Diagnostic Reasoning in Nursing.* Philadelphia: Lippincott; 1984.
31. Tanner CA, Padrick KP, Westfall UE, Putzier DJ. Diagnostic reasoning strategies of nurses and nursing students. *Nurs Res.* 1987;36:358–363.
32. Woodley N. Nursing diagnosis: Exploring the factors which may influence the reasoning process. *J Adv Nurs.* 1990;15:110–117.
33. Kritek PB. Current nomenclature and classification systems: Pertinent issues. In: Kim MJ, McFarland GK, McLane AM, eds. *Classification of Nursing Diagnoses: Proceedings of the Fifth National Conference.* St. Louis: Mosby; 1984.
34. Carnevali DL. The diagnostic reasoning process. In: Carnevali DL, Mitchell PH, Woods NF, Tanner CA, eds. *Diagnostic Reasoning in Nursing.* Philadelphia: Lippincott; 1984.
35. Baer CL. A futuristic process for nursing practice. *Topics in Clinical Nursing. Nursing Diagnosis.* 1984;5:89.
36. Carroll-Johnson RM, ed. *Classification of Nursing Diagnoses: Proceedings of the Eighth Conference.* Philadelphia: Lippincott; 1989.

BIBLIOGRAPHY

Bulecheck GM, McCloskey J. *Nursing Interventions: Treatments for Nursing Diagnoses.* Philadelphia: Saunders; 1985.

Burke L, Murphy J. *Charting by Exception.* New York: Wiley; 1988.

Carpenito LJ. *Nursing Diagnosis: Application to Clinical Practice.* 2nd ed. Philadelphia: Lippincott; 1987.

Carpenito LJ. Nursing diagnosis in critical care: Impact on practice. *Heart Lung.* 1987;16:595–600.

Christensen PJ, Kenney JW. *Nursing Process: Application of Theories, Frameworks, and Models.* 3rd ed. St. Louis: Mosby, 1990.

Carroll-Johnson R. *Classification of Nursing Diagnoses: Proceedings of the Eighth Conference.* Philadelphia: Lippincott; 1989.

Gordon M. *Manual of Nursing Diagnosis, 1991–1992.* St. Louis: Mosby, 1990.

Gordon M. Nursing implementation of nursing diagnosis: An overview. *Nurs Clin North Am.* 1987;22:875–879.

Hannah KJ, Reimer M, Mills WC, Letourneau S, eds. *Clinical Judgement and Decision Making: The Future With Nursing Diagnosis.* New York: Wiley; 1987.

Kim MJ, Moritz D. *Classification of Nursing Diagnosis: Proceedings of the Third and Fourth National Conferences.* New York: McGraw-Hill; 1982.

Kim MJ, McFarland G, McLane AM. *Classification of Nursing Diagnoses: Proceedings of the Fifth National Conference.* St. Louis: Mosby; 1984.

Kritek P. Nursing diagnosis in perspective: Response to a critique. *Image.* 1985;17:3–8.

McLane A, ed. *Classification of Nursing Diagnoses: Proceedings of the Seventh National Conference.* St. Louis: Mosby; 1987.

McLane A. Measurement and validation of diagnostic concepts: A decade of progress. *Heart Lung.* 1987;16:616–624.

Miller E. *Diagnosis Based Nursing Practice.* Norwalk, CT: Appleton & Lange, 1990.

Pocket Guide to Nursing Diagnoses. St. Louis, MO: Mosby; 1990.

Thelan L, Davie J, Urden L. *Textbook of Critical Care Nursing: Diagnosis and Management.* St. Louis: Mosby; 1990.

CHAPTER 18

Making, Writing, and Evaluating Client Care Plans

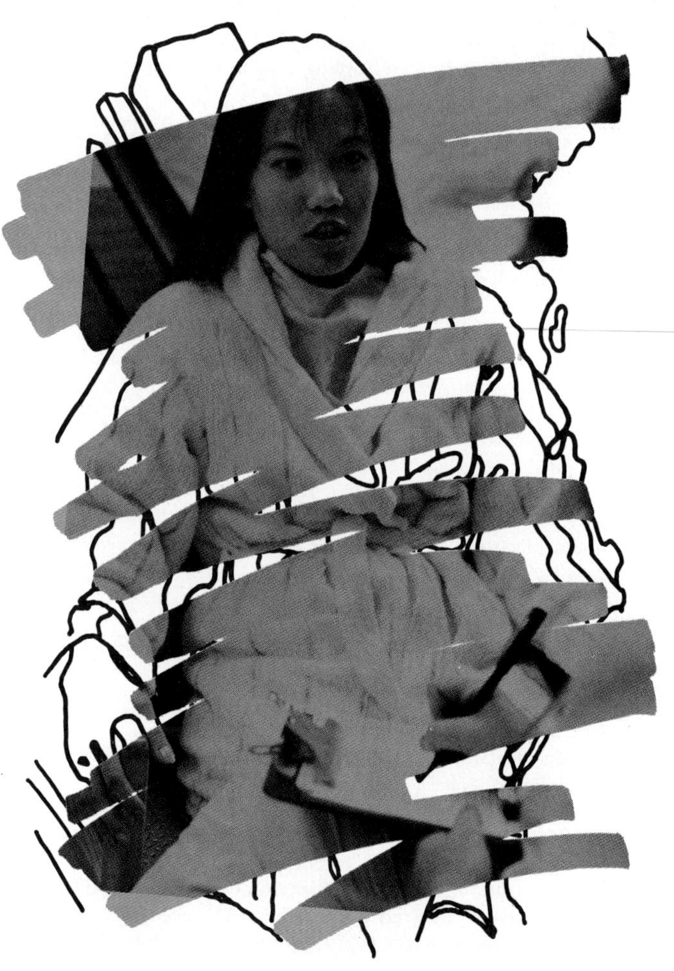

Behavioral Objectives

Upon completion of this chapter, the student will be able to:

1. Define the terms desired outcome, nursing implementation, evaluation criteria, and evaluation.
2. List the benefits of the individualized client care plan.
3. Identify criteria for priority setting.
4. List elements to be considered when establishing deadlines for desired outcomes.
5. Formulate desired outcome statements that are specific, client oriented, and measurable.
6. State the major differences between long-term and short-term outcomes.
7. Describe the proper format for a nursing implementation statement.
8. Describe possible differences and similarities between evaluation criteria and desired outcome statements.
9. Describe four activities involved in the evaluation phase of the nursing process.
10. State the difference between situational and structured reporting.
11. Identify the characteristics of effective reporting.
12. State guidelines for recording information on the client's chart.
13. State the benefits of collaborative planning for the client and the nurse.
14. Identify two types of evaluation used to determine the quality of client care.
15. Describe the purpose and steps of a quality assurance evaluation.

KEY TERMS

audit
client care plan
client record
collaborative functions
dependent functions
desired outcome
discharge planning
evaluation
evaluation criterion
formative evaluation
independent functions
interdependent functions
Kardex
long-term outcome
monitoring
nursing implementation
nursing order
priority setting
problem-oriented record
quality assurance program
retrospective evaluation
short-term outcome
source-oriented record
standard care plan
standard of care
summative evaluation

Making, writing, and evaluating a plan for individualized client care is a professional responsibility of all nurses. Constructing a unique plan to guide the delivery of nursing care to every client requires a wide range of knowledge and skills. A clear understanding of the nursing process and well-grounded decision-making skills are essential. Proficiency in assessment of health status and the ability to carry out diagnostic reasoning are required. Knowledge of effective implementation for resolving health problems is important as well.

It is common in nursing literature and in many clinical practice settings to refer to the plan for resolution of client health problems as a *nursing* care plan. This text uses the term *client* care plan, because this term more accurately communicates the concept of a collaborative approach to planning—that is, planning undertaken by client and nurse together. The collaborative approach emphasizes that nurse and client share responsibility for client health and recognizes clients' power in decision making regarding health and health care. Collaborative planning reflects clients' beliefs and values, as well as nurses' knowledge; it is essential to the delivery of individualized care.

Writing the care plan that client and nurse have developed is a nursing responsibility. The selection of concise language that accurately and completely conveys the intent of the planners is critical, not only to enable the plan to be used as a guide by all nurses caring for a client, but to facilitate evaluation of the plan's effectiveness.

This chapter describes the process of collaborative planning and provides specific instructions for writing client care plans efficiently and effectively. It delineates processes for evaluating client care plans of individual clients, as well as institutional evaluation procedures. Reporting and recording as vehicles for communicating evaluation are emphasized and guidelines for both are included.

■ THE CLIENT CARE PLAN

A **client care plan** is a blueprint for assisting a client to resolve the health problems that client and nurse have identified as a result of their collaboration. As discussed in Chapter 17, nursing diagnoses are judgments or conclusions about a client's health-related problems that can be resolved primarily by nursing remedies. Nursing diagnoses, in turn, direct nurses' professional decisions about recommendations for alleviating these client problems (see also Chap. 15). A client care plan, however, embodies not only nurses' conclusions about courses of action to take, but clients' conclusions as well. Thus, a client care plan is a document that reflects collaborative exchanges and clients' informed consent.

A client care plan has four components: (1) diagnostic statement, (2) desired outcome statement, (3) nursing implementation, and (4) evaluation criteria. The development of the nursing diagnoses and the process of writing clear and complete diagnostic statements are discussed in Chapter 17. The clearly stated nursing diagnosis is the basis for each of the other elements in the plan.

The **desired outcome** statement describes the expected client status when a nursing diagnosis has been resolved. It indicates what nurse and client wish to accomplish as a result of nursing implementation. Desired outcome statements are analogous to behavioral objectives such as those provided at the beginning of this chapter. Whereas behavioral objectives for a chapter or course specify expectations for learning identified by the author or teacher, desired outcome statements on a client care plan specify expectations for improved health status identified by nurse–client collaboration. In some clinical practice settings and nursing process literature, the terms *objective* or *goal* are used instead of desired outcome. Increasingly, however, outcome is the preferred term. This is because it is consistent with nursing audit and quality assurance terminology and also because it cues the writer of the plan to formulate statements that describe client behavior.[1–3] In fact, the term, *outcome,* is gaining wider use throughout the health care system in recent years, particularly in health care institutions using case management. Case management is a model of health care delivery that emphasizes collaborative development of institutional protocols (standards) for client care. The collaborators include clients, nurses, physicians, and other members of the health care team. The protocols use health outcomes as a core concept. Outcomes as related to quality assurance and case management are discussed in a later section of this chapter.

Nursing implementation describes the collective activities of nurse and client that they select to correct or alleviate the health problem identified in the nursing diagnosis statement. Although the terms *nursing intervention, nursing order,* and *nursing action* are used in place of implementation in some settings, these terms connote activities "done to" or "done on" a client, rather than a balanced problem-solving approach involving nurse and client. In this text, the term *nursing implementation* is used throughout to emphasize a more collaborative nurse–client relationship.

Evaluation criteria are statements that describe acceptable evidence that outcomes have been achieved. Evaluation criteria are used to determine whether desired outcomes have been met as a result of the nursing implementation. If actual client status matches that described in the criteria, this signifies that the desired outcomes have been attained.

Each of these elements of the client care plan relate to one another and to the stated nursing diagnosis. The processes for developing each of the components and for selecting language to effectively communicate them on a written client care plan are discussed in detail in the sections that follow.

■ NATURE OF COLLABORATIVE CLIENT CARE PLANS

Each client responds differently to the challenge of achieving and maintaining health. As discussed in Chapters 5 and 12, even the definition of health varies from individual to individual. Several clients facing the same health problem may desire or be capable of achieving health-related outcomes that are quite different, but valid within each person's value system and life circumstances. The methods that each client would find acceptable for attaining the desired outcomes would also be likely to differ.

Recognizing these realities, nurses have long believed in the importance of individualized care plans. A collaborative care plan is inherently an individualized plan. In a collaborative process for deriving care plans, an individual client's values about health, concerns about health, and capacities for achieving health are essential to the exchange. The process of shared decision-making empowers clients. It enhances trust, demonstrates respect for clients, and communicates caring. All aspects of the plan—diagnoses, desired outcomes, nursing implementation, and evaluation criteria—are developed as a direct result of nurses' collaboration with clients.[4]

From the foregoing discussion, it can be seen that collaborative client care plans have several distinct benefits:

- They embody clients' as well as nurses' concepts of health and values for health.
- They address clients' primary concerns.
- They draw from clients' own resources and capabilities.
- They are the outcome of a shared decision-making process that empowers clients and communicates nurses' respect for clients' individuality.
- They reflect clients' informed consent.
- They enhance clients' motivation to carry out the plan.

- They are efficient and effective because they reflect clients' values.

A collaborative client care plan is an essential component of all levels of nursing care. Nurses who interact with clients primarily in a health assessment capacity can assist clients with health promotion by facilitating identification of life-style factors, health beliefs, and behaviors or knowledge deficits that may be interfering with maintenance of optimal health. A collaborative care plan focused on illness prevention and promotion of well-being can be the result. Nursing approaches identified as *preventive* client care throughout this text are most commonly used in such plans.

Planning for health promotion and illness prevention is also appropriate in acute care and rehabilitation settings, although the initial emphasis in such settings may be on health restoration. Client care plans to facilitate restoration of health for clients who are acutely ill are perhaps the most widely used types of care plans. Here, *supportive* and *restorative* approaches are most useful.

In a rehabilitation setting, facilitating adjustment to long-term or permanent alterations in health is the primary goal of client care plans. This focus also applies when nurses collaborate with clients being discharged from acute care settings while still needing supportive care. Involving family and community resources becomes especially important in such situations. Nursing approaches identified as "rehabilitative" are most appropriate for these clients.

Collaborative planning with clients facing terminal illness is yet another function of professional nurses. Because of the intensity and complexity of responses to terminal illness by both clients and their loved ones, constructing care plans for terminally ill clients is one of the most challenging aspects of practice.

MAKING CLIENT CARE PLANS

Processes of Collaborative Care Planning

Collaborative care planning involves three distinct processes: (1) the nurse's application of professional knowledge; (2) the interaction between client and nurse through which agreement and consent are achieved (making the plan); and (3) documentation of the results of the interactive planning process (writing the plan).

The Nurse's Application of Professional Knowledge. Nurses make assessments and diagnoses, and identify possible implementation and evaluation strategies to recommend to clients. Many resources can be called upon to support this process. They are discussed later in the chapter.

Making the Plan. This is the interaction between client and nurse through which agreement and consent are achieved. Nurses share professional recommendations with clients. Nurse and client discuss the health problems both have identified to determine which ones both agree need to be addressed. They discuss the level of wellness that each realistically believes the client can achieve. These ideas are the focus for the diagnoses and desired outcomes in the client care plan. The focus for strategies to achieve the outcomes (implementation), and for criteria to evaluate progress toward the desired outcomes (evaluation criteria), are also mutually developed by client and nurse. Additionally, collaborative prioritizing of client problems, desired outcomes, and nursing implementation is part of this interactive process. A detailed discussion of each phase of making the plan follows in the next sections.

Documenting the Results of the Interactive Planning Process. The collaboratively developed plan must be recorded according to the format of the institution so that it can be used as a central information source for all caregivers. A detailed discussion of this process is given in Writing Client Care Plans, later in the chapter.

Resources for Planning

The development of a powerful client care plan can be facilitated by employing resources that support individual nurses' knowledge base (Fig. 18–1).

Clients. Active participation by clients in the development of a care plan is a necessary condition if the plan is to meet individual needs. Clients are the best source of information about their needs, which are unique and may change as their health status changes. Likewise, client values and beliefs cannot be overlooked when planning care. A client could not be expected to participate in activities that are in conflict with personal principles, no matter how appropriate these activities might seem to nurses. When nurses actively seek client participation, emphasizing that mutual contributions result in a plan specifically tailored to reflect clients' unique needs, preferences, values, and resources, client motivation is reinforced.

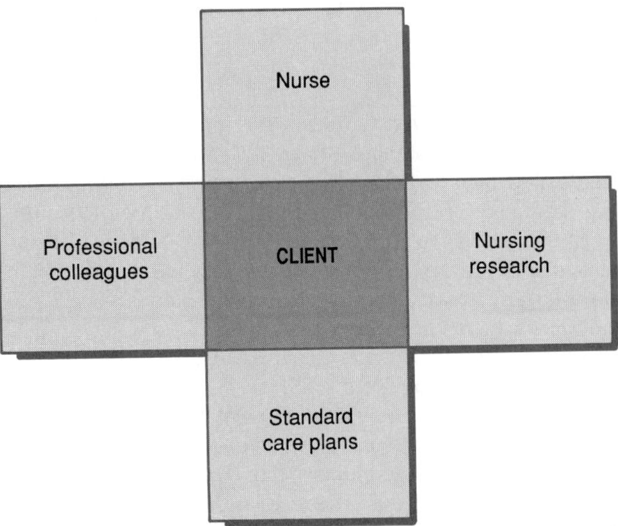

Figure 18–1. Resources for client care planning.

Colleagues. Other members of the health care team can be excellent resources for developing a client care plan. For example, social workers and discharge coordinators are usually aware of available community services. Physicians may have data from previous contacts with a client and also can provide information about the current medical plan for care. Specialists such as physical therapists, dietitians, enterostomal therapists, and others can contribute information from their respective fields. Clinical nurse specialists (see Chap. 1) are excellent resources, as are experienced staff nurses. Sharing of information and ideas about nursing care commonly occurs on an ongoing basis among staff nurses who are fellow members of a particular unit.

Using professional colleagues as resources when making care plans gives each client the benefit of the collective expertise of the entire team. Client care conferences, in which the caregivers involved in the care of a client or group of clients meet to develop or update care plans, are held regularly in many health care facilities. Informal sharing on a one-to-one basis is also effective.

Nursing Research. Nursing scholars and practitioners are becoming increasingly more involved in research to improve nursing practice. Results of nursing research can be applied in collaborative care planning. Nursing research may have many different foci. It may be directed at identification or refinement of nursing diagnoses to more clearly delineate those health problems amenable to nursing treatment. The focus may be to characterize effective nursing implementation for specific health problems or in certain situations or conditions. The impact of health problems on various aspects of an individual's life is also a frequent research topic. Differences in response to illness, or preferred care approaches related to social, economic, and cultural variables, are other nursing research foci. The results of nursing research are reported in nursing and related professional journals, as well as in nursing textbooks. Indexes are available to locate studies that may be relevant to a specific client situation. Chapter 32 describes in detail the role of nursing research in improving the quality of nursing care.

Standard Care Plans. Standard care plans are another resource for collaborative planning. A **standard care plan** is a preprinted plan that focuses on commonly recurring nursing diagnoses and provides general directions for desired outcomes and client care related to each diagnosis. Therefore, standard care plans can be used as a basis from which to build an individualized collaborative plan.[1] Samples of standard client care plans are included in Chapters 22 through 31 of this text. Examples are also provided later in this chapter (see pages 607–608).

Standard care plans are often developed by nurses at a particular health care facility and kept on file for reference. An advantage of these plans is that they reflect that facility's standards of care and may relate more specifically to the resources that are available in that setting.[5]

Earlier forms of standard care plans were commonly written for specific medical diagnosis, such as gastric ulcers, diabetes mellitus, or arthritis. Some facilities continue to use standard plans based on medical diagnoses, but these are usually not useful as a basis for collaborative client care plans. Standardized guidelines for care related to medical diagnoses are useful, in that they identify important aspects of client care for all clients having the medical diagnosis in question, but they are more accurately called **standards of care,** not client care plans.

> **IMPLICATIONS FOR PROFESSIONAL COLLABORATION**
>
> **Standard Care Plans**
>
> Used appropriately, standard care plans increase efficiency by reducing the time and effort (and sometimes a duplication of effort!) needed to generate the collaborative plan. Standard plans cannot be used without individualized alterations, however, and nurses must always judge which aspects of a standard plan are appropriate to a client's problem.

The appropriate use for standard client care plans is as a resource for developing collaborative plans, not as a replacement for them. Used appropriately, standard care plans increase efficiency by reducing the time and effort needed to generate care plans and avoiding duplication of effort. However, standard care plans have significant limitations that must be emphasized. The standard care plan cannot serve as a complete care plan for any client. Many clients have several nursing diagnoses arising from a disease or its treatment and manifestations of the problem that are peculiar to them and their unique situations. The use of standard plans without individualized alterations also excludes client participation in the planning process. This lack of collaboration can significantly reduce the effectiveness of the plan. Not only might client acceptance of the standard outcomes and approaches be reduced, but also, some of these outcomes and approaches might actually be inappropriate for the client in question. Additionally, if standardized plans are used as a shortcut too early in the assessment phase of the nursing process, insufficient data may be gathered to accurately identify the most relevant nursing diagnoses.

In some institutions, standard care plans are stored in a computer memory. Like other care plans, computerized care plans provide nurses with a number of alternatives for desired outcomes and implementation for a given nursing diagnosis, as well as the option of entering individualized statements. In this way, maximum benefits of both the standard plans and the collaborative plan can be obtained. Refer to Chapter 21 for a detailed discussion of this and other computer applications to nursing care.

Setting Priorities

The Nature of Priority Setting. When nurse and client collaborate to develop a client care plan, one of their tasks is to

BUILDING NURSING KNOWLEDGE

What Are the Influences on the Nurse's Priority Setting?

Hendrickson G, Doddato TM. Setting priorities during the shortage. *Nurs Outlook.* 1989; 37:280–284.

The current shortage of nurses means that fewer nurses have responsibility for more tasks. The investigators in this study examined how nurses pick and choose among their competing tasks to set priorities under these conditions. Using a questionnaire, 206 nurses who worked on several types of nursing units in a very large hospital were asked about their perceptions on the choices they were required to make.

The general finding was that the availability of nursing personnel is just as influential as client needs in the setting of priorities for care. The nurses indicated that the most important professional tasks were documentation of care, preparing and giving medications, and administering treatments. When they were overburdened, nurses gave priority to activities that needed immediate attention and were often unable to practice their role as they envisioned it.

Thus functional activities—tasks such as turning clients in bed, giving coughing and deep breathing therapy, monitoring and adjusting intravenous infusions, taking vital signs, giving bed baths, ambulating clients, and answering client call bells—received more attention than collaborative tasks. When nurses were forced to choose among competing tasks, the collaborative category—defined by the investigators as participating in medical rounds, attending inservice training, doing client teaching, and giving the client and family psychosocial care—and developing care plans received less attention. This was despite the fact that many nurses believed collaborative activities to be central to their nursing role.

set priorities. **Priority setting** is a decision-making process that is used to rank the urgency or relative importance of nursing diagnoses, desired outcomes, and/or nursing implementation. Effective priority setting is a collaborative process involving a client, nurses, and other health care team members. The mutually determined priorities are then communicated in the written client care plan.

IMPLICATIONS FOR PROFESSIONAL COLLABORATION

Priority Setting

Priority setting refers to decisions that rank the urgency or relative importance of a client's nursing diagnoses. Effective priority setting is a collaborative process involving a client, nurse, and other health care team members. Priorities change as the client's condition or situation changes. Priority setting is facilitated by the use of professional criteria and guidelines and standards of care, and by consulting colleagues for their special expertise and skill in clinical judgment. Priority setting is also enhanced by consulting with clients and their families about their concerns and preferences when ranking diagnoses.

Successful priority setting requires a high level of clinical judgment and sensitivity to nuances in client communication. Nurses not only use assessment data collected from a specific client, but also draw from past experiences and knowledge.[6] Experienced nurses recognize priorities readily because they are able to mentally scan the vast amount of information they have gained through past education and through long experience. They can anticipate problems and draw conclusions relevant to a given client situation. The process used by expert nurses has often been described as intuitive.[7] Novice nurses lack situational experience and therefore make judgments within the context of textbook knowledge, which is valid but less encompassing. Skill in setting priorities grows and develops as a nurse's level of knowledge and experience expands.[6]

Priorities assigned to a problem or desired outcome do not remain constant. They change as a client's condition or situation changes or as problems are resolved as a result of nursing implementation. In addition, several problems may be considered high priority simultaneously. As high-priority problems are partially resolved, attention is directed at those of lower priority. The dynamic nature of priority setting makes it a challenging and continuous process.

Reasons for Priority Setting. Priority setting improves the quality and efficiency of nursing care. Any situation in which resources for problem-solving are not infinite requires decisions about how to best use available resources. Ranking client health problems, desired outcomes, or nursing implementation is a way of allocating resources—of client, nurse, and institution. When thoughtful mutual consideration by nurse and client is given to identifying the problems most needing resolution, these problems can receive maximum focus. In contrast, if arbitrary or indiscriminate choices about delivering care are made, some important problems may be ignored.

Client satisfaction is also enhanced when care delivery is organized according to a ranking of problems that has been mutually developed. Trust in health care providers is increased when there is concrete evidence that the providers value client input and concerns. Clients achieve more gratification in achieving outcomes they have helped to develop; they are more likely to participate actively in care activities to meet the outcomes when the expected benefits are clear.

Factors in Priority Setting. Although setting priorities is a complex process, use of criteria or guidelines is helpful.

Frameworks such as Maslow's hierarchy of needs (Chaps. 6 and 10) are used by some nurses to rank the relative urgency of problems, or the seriousness of the consequences if a problem is not resolved. Typically, the highest priority is assigned to physiological needs, such as oxygen, fluids, and food, which are considered more basic to life. Needs that Maslow characterized as secondary (or higher-level) needs—such as safety and security, love and belonging, and self-esteem—would be assigned a lower level of priority by nurses using Maslow's hierarchy. Nurses who effectively use Maslow's hierarchy of needs or other structured systems to aid their efforts at prioritizing realize that rigidly applying such systems to all situations is inappropriate. Such systems can only be considered guides. Other factors, such as knowledge from the physical and social sciences, nurses' understanding of disease processes, and other factors to be discussed below, also enhance accurate interpretation of the urgency of problems. However, nurses' determination of the urgency of problems provides only part of the picture. Clients' perceptions of urgency also play a role in the final ranking.

Clients' beliefs, values, and desires affect their perception of the urgency of problems. Moreover, their perceptions may differ from nurses' perceptions. For example, a nurse may feel that instructing a client about the special diet that has been prescribed for her should be given a high priority. The client, however, may be more concerned about communicating with professional colleagues about an important project nearing deadline and may be unwilling or unable to focus attention on diet teaching until her concerns about her professional responsibilities are resolved. Clients may also want to consult with family members or other significant support persons before making decisions about treatment options. As nurses and clients collaborate to prioritize problems, nurses are responsible to ensure that clients have all the information necessary to make informed decisions and that strong consideration is given to their input.

Resources available to nurses and clients may also influence the ordering of priorities. If a service desired by a client is not offered in the health care setting in which care is being given, then the problem may be given a lower priority, at least temporarily. Nurses can try to locate a referral source for the service, to contact when circumstances permit. Client resources, such as finances or home environment, also play a role in the setting of priorities.

Situational variables, such as special procedures or diagnostic tests, may take temporary precedence over the ranking of priorities established by client and nurse. These events involve considerations about efficient use of resources for an entire client population. When possible, however, established priorities should be considered when scheduling routine therapies and care activities.

When considering the process of ranking the urgency of problems, it is useful to recognize that client care plans are not developed for life-threatening emergencies. Priorities in such situations are determined by protocols (written guidelines for action in specified situations) or standards of care, which supersede priorities on a care plan. However, emergencies allow the purest application of a need hierarchy. For example, when the most basic need, oxygenation, is in serious jeopardy, as in massive hemorrhage or cardiac arrest, all efforts are focused on restoring oxygenation. No one questions whether other needs may also require attention until the oxygenation problem has been resolved.

Developing Desired Outcomes

Definition and Purpose of Desired Outcomes. As noted previously, a desired outcome is a projection of client condition or status when the health problem identified in the nursing diagnosis has been resolved to the extent possible, given a client's overall health status. It describes the expected influence of nursing implementation. Desired outcomes may refer to biological, psychological, sociocultural, and spiritual aspects of health, as well as to related knowledge and skills.[8] They may relate to maintenance or restoration of health as well as to prevention of complications and future illness. Desired outcomes do not describe nursing care measures. Their purpose is to provide direction for the planning of specific nursing implementation and to form the framework for the evaluation phase of the nursing process.[9]

Determining the Focus of Desired Outcomes. Because the desired outcome represents an improvement in or an absence of the problem identified in the nursing diagnosis, nurses develop desired outcomes by reviewing the problem component of the nursing diagnosis statement (see Fig. 15–1). They then convert the problem component to a description of a *desired* health condition that would exist were the problem absent. The health condition is the focus of the desired outcome. Determining the converse of the problem is the first step. For example, suppose a client had a nursing diagnosis of Constipation. The converse of "constipation" is "no constipation." A health condition corresponding to "no constipation" would be "a healthy bowel elimination pattern." Therefore one possible focus for the desired outcome for the nursing diagnosis of constipation would be: healthy bowel elimination pattern. The desired outcome focus is the basis for the written desired outcome statement that nurses write on the care plan document, as will be seen in the later section on writing desired outcome statements.

Desired outcomes are also derived from the etiology component of the problem statement, because eliminating the etiology is often the most effective way to correct a problem. Suppose the etiology of the above client's constipation were "a diet lacking in fiber and a sedentary lifestyle." Using the process described above of identifying the converse of the diagnosis statement component and describing a corresponding health condition yield desired outcomes such as "greater intake of dietary fiber" and "increased exercise." As can be seen from this discussion, it is not unusual to have several desired outcomes that relate to one nursing diagnosis.

Long-term and Short-term Outcomes. The projected time period for achieving desired outcomes is used to differentiate types of outcomes. **Long-term outcomes** describe complete resolution of a problem, often characterizing desired client status in broad, global terms. In the example above, the outcome focus "healthy bowel elimination pattern," derived from the problem component of the diagnosis, represents a long-term outcome, as it describes complete resolution of the problem. Depending on the magnitude of the changes needed in dietary and exercise habits, these outcomes may also be considered long term.

Nurses frequently use long-term outcomes in discharge planning. **Discharge planning** is a process that attempts to project client health status and needs for continuing care at the time of discharge from the health care agency. Discharge outcomes describe the general level of functioning to be demonstrated by clients at the time client care is terminated. Discharge planning is important because it acknowledges the relatively short-term nature of the care relationship in the acute care setting and emphasizes the importance of facilitating clients' transition to self-care in their own environment. Discharge planning is discussed further in Chapter 7.

Short-term outcomes are more precise, relate to more immediate changes in client status, and often represent steps toward long-term outcomes. Short-term outcomes may focus on behavior changes that would contribute to the desired health condition described in long-term outcomes or to the knowledge and skills needed to achieve long-term outcomes. Clients who are striving to achieve a healthy bowel elimination pattern by changing eating and exercise habits may need to gain specific knowledge about types of exercise, foods high in fiber, and how exercise and fiber relate to bowel functioning before being ready to make a commitment to these life-style changes. Short-term outcomes relating to clients' level of knowledge of these topics would thus be logical steps toward the long-term outcomes.

Selecting Realistic Deadlines. Deadlines provide a specific time frame for projected achievement of both long- and short-term outcomes. They represent target dates for evaluation of progress toward or attainment of desired outcomes. The nature of the problem and the available resources influence deadlines. It is important that clients' resources—such as personal strengths, support persons, environment, and finances—as well as deficits in levels of functioning be considered.

Realistic deadlines give both client and nurse a sense of achievement. Unrealistic deadlines can lead to frustration with the entire health care experience. Setting appropriate deadlines requires clinical judgment. As with priority setting, proficiency comes with experience. It is important for novice nurses to recognize, however, that in some situations, projecting outcome achievement may be somewhat arbitrary, even for expert nurses. It may not be possible to predict, for example, what time period will be required for a given client to achieve a given improvement in activity tolerance. The importance of setting deadlines, then, lies not so much in their absolute accuracy as in the fact that a specific target date for reassessment has been designated. Evaluating outcome achievement at designated intervals prevents problems from persisting beyond acceptable time periods without modification of treatment approach.[10]

Nurse–Client Collaboration in Outcome Development. Nurse and client collaborate to identify outcomes that correlate to each of the client's nursing diagnoses. This is another opportunity for nurses and clients to discuss priorities. Clients with multiple nursing diagnoses may have a considerable number of desired outcomes. Attention needs to be given to clients' preferences, resources, and deficits in both the selection and the ranking of these outcomes. Nurse and client need to identify and consider physiological, emotional, intellectual, spiritual, financial, and environmental factors that could hinder or enhance attainment of the desired outcomes when making the plan.

Professional Collaboration in Outcome Development. Health care team members in facilities using the case management model develop collaborative health outcomes. In these settings, outcomes for nursing implementation may be integrated into the interdisciplinary case management plan. This system strongly emphasizes accountability and mutuality in outcome achievement. Although the ultimate responsibility for specific outcomes is assigned to one group of providers (eg, nurses, physicians), the collaborative nature of the plan encourages everyone on the health care team to contribute to overall outcome achievement.

Establishing Nursing Implementation

Definition and Purpose of Nursing Implementation. Nursing implementation encompasses all of the collective client and nurse activities that facilitate a client's achievement of the desired outcomes. It includes assessing, communicating, performing technical skills, teaching and counseling, among other activities. In some cases, the appropriate nursing implementation may even be to do nothing. For example, some clients are able to resolve problems identified through collaborative assessment without nursing assistance. Other clients may be unwilling to accept assistance that nurses feel is in the clients' best interests to accept. Because a collaborative nurse–client relationship encourages a stronger client role than do some of the more traditional approaches to nurse–client relationships, in situations in which an informed client refuses nursing care, nurses would respect these wishes. The intensity of nursing involvement in nursing implementation, therefore, like other aspects of the client care plan, is influenced by clients as well as nurses.

The definition of nursing implementation is further clarified by many state Nurse Practice Acts (see also Chap. 3) as being independent or dependent. **Dependent functions** are prescribed by physicians but carried out by nurses. **Independent functions** refer to care that nurses themselves are licensed to plan and carry out. As discussed in Chapter 17, the American Nurses' Association's *Social Policy Statement* and the ongoing work of the North American Nursing Diagnosis Association (NANDA) have clarified and expanded the definition of nursing's unique domain of practice and hence the definition of independent nursing implementation. A third category, **interdependent** or **collaborative functions,** describes activities that are performed jointly with other members of the health care team. In this text, the client is seen as a key member of the health care team; hence collaborative activities include those carried out by nurse and client as well as by nurse and other caregivers.

Independent and collaborative implementation are key components of a client care plan, whereas dependent implementation appropriate for a given client situation is found in agency standards of care or noted in physicians' orders.

Determining the Focus of Nursing Implementation

Desired Outcomes/Etiology. A review of the desired outcomes gives nurses specific direction in selecting the appropriate focus for nursing implementation to alleviate a client problem (see Fig. 15–1). Recall the example of the client with constipation. The desired outcomes related to the etiology "greater fiber intake" and "increased exercise" suggest implementation such as exploring ways to increase fiber intake, assisting the client with meal planning that includes high-fiber foods, and discussing various exercise programs to find one that interests the client. The short-term outcomes that relate to knowledge and skills needed to attain the long-term outcomes suggest several more areas of focus for implementation: for example, teaching about causes of constipation and about the role of dietary fiber and exercise in promoting bowel function. Even when the problem component of two diagnoses is the same, different etiologies suggest different foci for implementation, as illustrated in Table 18–1. Were a client's constipation related to suppression of defecation because of lack of privacy for elimination, a nurse would approach the situation differently. In the latter case, the primary implementation focus would be to make environmental changes to create privacy. In these examples, the relationship between the content focus of the outcome and that of the implementation is quite direct. In some cases, more theory application will be necessary to determine the appropriate focus. For example, were the desired outcome "increased muscle strength," a nurse would need to know what components contribute to muscle strength in order to select related implementation foci.

Defining Characteristics. The defining characteristics (the signs and symptoms of the diagnosis) that a client exhibits may further refine the focus for nursing implementation. If the client whose constipation was related to a sedentary life-style evidenced this etiology by statements such as "I can't find time to exercise because of my work" and "I'm too busy to take a walk," a nurse would approach the problem differently than if "I hate exercise" and "Exercise is so boring" were the defining characteristics. In both cases, the general focus would be increased exercise, but the specific strategies nurse and client would employ to achieve this result would differ with the individual situation. In one case, time management may be a focus; in the other attitude change or exploration of a variety of different types of exercise may be more effective.

Using the defining characteristics a specific client demonstrates also makes the nursing implementation appropriate to clients' level of wellness. If the sedentary client in the previous example were not ambulatory, but rather acutely

TABLE 18–1. COMPARISON OF NURSING IMPLEMENTATION FOCUS FOR NURSING DIAGNOSES WITH THE SAME PROBLEM COMPONENT BUT DIFFERENT ETIOLOGIES

Nursing Diagnosis/Etiology	Examples of Nursing Implementation Focus
Altered Nutrition: less than body requirements for protein R/T *insufficient income to purchase food*	Teach about low-cost food sources of protein. Obtain social service consult to determine eligibility for food stamps.
Altered Nutrition: less than body requirements for protein R/T *perception of being overweight*	Inform clients about low-calorie foods high in protein and how to reduce calories per serving (remove visible fat from meat, remove skin from chicken). If actual weight is appropriate for height, obtain psychological consult to rule out/treat anorexia nervosa or bulimia.
Impaired Skin Integrity R/T *shearing force* (friction on skin from sliding movement)	Teach clients to avoid putting head of bed higher than 30 degrees (prevents sliding to foot of bed) and to change positions after 30 minutes. Obtain footboard so client will not slide down in bed.
Impaired Skin Integrity R/T *altered sensation*	Assist clients to devise a turning schedule to prevent remaining in one position for greater than 2 hours. Obtain special bed to reduce pressure, if needed.
Sleep Pattern Disturbance R/T *psychological stress*	Provide active listening to promote resolution of stress. Encourage daily vigorous exercise. Teach relaxation techniques.
Sleep Pattern Disturbance R/T *pain*	Provide back massage at bedtime. Assist to comfortable position, using pillow supports as needed.

ill and immobilized in bed, these factors would be reflected in the defining characteristics. The nursing implementation for such a situation would have to be directed at assisting elimination without increasing exercise, because the client's condition precludes participating in exercise. Table 18–2 contains additional examples.

Nurse–Client Collaboration. Collaboration with the client in the selection of nursing implementation is just as important as in other aspects of care plan development. Although nursing knowledge and experience is an important factor in identifying safe and effective implementation, consideration of clients' values, beliefs, and desires will increase the likelihood of the implementation being successful.[4] Implementation that is unacceptable to a client may result in client stress, resistance, and distrust.

Institutional Resources and Limitations. Institutional resources and limitations are another consideration in the identification of nursing implementation. In some cases, this may mean that a strategy that both nurse and client favor as a way to alleviate a given problem may have to be modified or replaced by another. Suggesting implementation that is unrealistic for the setting, is against agency policy, or requires materials or personnel that are unavailable invites frustration for both nurse and client.

A related concern is that the proposed nursing implementation be congruent with other therapies a client is receiving or that are planned by other members of the health care team. Health care professionals represent a significant institutional resource. Optimum results are achieved when the involved health care professionals coordinate their efforts and expertise.

Developing Evaluation Criteria

Definition and Purpose of Evaluation Criteria. Evaluation criteria are statements that describe specific evidence that desired outcomes have been attained. They represent standards or measures that are used by client and nurse to gauge progress toward desired outcomes in the course of giving care (formative evaluation) and outcome achievement at the termination of care (summative evaluation). A more detailed discussion of these types of evaluation is presented later in this chapter.

Evaluation criteria are developed when making the plan. That is, as nurse and client collaborate to identify the focus of desired outcomes and for nursing implementation, they also identify the type of client behavior, level of functioning, or health status that would demonstrate that the implementation is resulting in progress toward and/or attainment of the desired outcomes. Evaluation criteria are then expressed succinctly by nurses when writing the plan and, finally, applied as part of mutual evaluation. The term *outcome criteria* is also used to refer to a standard used for evaluation.

Determining the Focus of Evaluation Criteria. The focus of evaluation criteria is often similar to that of the desired outcomes, because the evaluation criteria describe evidence that the outcomes have been achieved.

Client Status or Functioning. Evaluation criteria are developed by examining the client status or functioning implied by each desired outcome and asking the questions: "How would an observer know whether this status had been achieved?" or "What would be evidence of this functioning?" Recall the example from the earlier discussion of developing outcomes, in which the desired client status was that of having a healthy bowel elimination pattern. Listing characteristics of a healthy bowel elimination pattern would be a way to begin generating possible evaluation criteria to correspond to that desired outcome.

Defining Characteristics. The defining characteristics stated in the nursing diagnosis statement help individual-

TABLE 18–2. COMPARISON OF NURSING IMPLEMENTATION FOCUS FOR NURSING DIAGNOSES WITH THE SAME ETIOLOGIES BUT DIFFERENT DEFINING CHARACTERISTICS

Diagnosis/Etiology/Defining Characteristics	Examples of Nursing Implementation Focus
Altered Nutrition: more than body requirements for calories R/T excessive intake relative to metabolic need AEB *weight 10% over ideal for height/frame, "I never exercise," "I love desserts."*	Discuss alternative desserts low in fat. Discuss value of exercise, alternative types of exercise.
Altered Nutrition: more than body requirements for calories R/T excessive intake relative to metabolic need AEB *weight 10% over ideal for height/frame, reports eating/drinking at restaurants once or twice a week for business, work responsibilities cause late dinners most nights.*	Discuss substituting mineral water for alcohol. Discuss selection of lower-calorie entrees—eg, broiled versus breaded or fried, avoiding cream sauces. Discuss late afternoon nutritious snack and light evening meal instead of heavy dinner late in the evening.
Constipation R/T inadequate fluid intake AEB *decreased frequency, hard dry stool, "I never drink water during the day—too busy."*	Teach relationship between fluid intake and healthy elimination. Problem-solve with client ways to make fluid intake part of daily routine—eg, substituting water for coffee at work breaks, keeping pitcher of water or fruit juice on desk at all times.
Constipation R/T inadequate fluid intake AEB *decreased frequency, hard dry stool, "I only drink at meals, I never think of drinking during the day—I'm a little forgetful."* (Client is elderly, lives alone.)	Teach relationship between fluid intake and healthy elimination. Discuss reminders client can integrate into daily routine—eg, getting a glass of liquid at every TV commercial or setting a timer.

ize evaluation criteria. Because the defining characteristics portion of the diagnostic statement lists the signs and symptoms exhibited by a particular client that indicate the problem is present, it follows that the converse or absence of these characteristics would indicate that the problem has been resolved. The earlier example of the client with constipation can again be used for illustration. Suppose the client exhibited defining characteristics of constipation that included decreased frequency of bowel movements; abdominal distension; and hard, dry stools. Stating the converse of these conditions—"increased frequency of bowel movements," "absent or diminished abdominal distension," and "soft, moist stools" would provide a starting point, a focus from which to derive more precise evaluation criteria.

Client Strengths, Deficits, and Preferences. Individual client strengths, deficits, and preferences also influence the focus of evaluation criteria. Recall that two possible etiology-related outcomes were suggested for the client with constipation: greater fiber intake and increased exercise. When client and nurse discuss the evaluation criteria related to each of these outcomes, they will consider the type of changes in diet and exercise that *this particular* client is willing to make. Thus, even though two clients may have similar or even identical desired outcomes, the criteria that set the expectations for how each client will exhibit that outcome may be quite different.

Characteristics of Evaluation Criteria. Useful evaluation criteria have the following characteristics. They:

- *Relate to client outcomes.* As stated above, evaluation criteria represent evidence of outcome achievement.
- *Specify client behavior or status.* Evaluation criteria are client centered, not nurse centered. A common error when developing evaluation criteria is to address whether or not nursing implementation was carried out. Although evaluation seeks to determine whether nursing implementation was effective, this is done by examining *client* status. If the desired change in client status occurred, it is assumed the implementation was instrumental in bringing about that change. The particular client behavior that is specified in the evaluation criteria is determined by an individual client's situation, as discussed above.
- *Describe measurable or observable behavior.* Evaluation criteria that identify measurable or observable client behaviors indicating attainment of outcomes minimize ambiguity and inconsistency in evaluation. This is particularly challenging when abstract concepts such as knowledge or comfort are the focus of desired outcomes. Different evaluators may not agree on client attainment of the desired level of knowledge or comfort unless more measurable or observable behaviors are specified in evaluation criteria. For example, behavioral evidence of knowledge may be correct verbalization of specific facts or correct performance of a skill.
- *Contain only one behavior per criterion.* Sometimes more than one client behavior must be demonstrated for an evaluator to consider that a desired outcome has been met. In this case, several criteria are written, each describing one behavior. The evaluator can then more easily determine which criteria have been met and which require continued attention.
- *Are realistic.* The behaviors specified in evaluation criteria must be attainable by the individual client for whom they are written and within the time frame specified by the deadline date for evaluation. Individual strengths and limitations influence the level of wellness that may be attained by each person. These strengths and limitations must be considered when developing evaluation criteria.

WRITING CLIENT CARE PLANS

The care plan that has been generated through the collaborative process discussed thus far (determining the focus of desired outcomes, nursing implementation, and evaluation criteria for each of the clients' nursing diagnoses) requires further refining to be useful as a guideline for nursing care. In a sense, the plan at this stage can be considered a draft or worksheet that must be strengthened by the selection of precise language and recorded on the care plan forms used by the health care agency. The resulting client care plan is then a useful document to guide the nursing care of a particular client.

Client care plans are usually written in a column format, which facilitates both recording and use of the plan for reference during care. The columns correspond to the phases of the nursing process, although there is considerable variation among health care agencies in the number of columns used and in the column headings. A three-column format with the headings Nursing Diagnosis, Desired Outcome, and Nursing Implementation is probably the most commonly used. As noted previously, synonyms such as "problem" instead of diagnosis, "goal" instead of outcome, and "nursing order" or "nursing intervention" instead of implementation are possible variations. Additional columns entitled Evaluation, Evaluation Criteria or Outcome Criteria, Deadline Date, Resolution Date, and Nurse's Signature are sometimes added and, rarely, an Assessment column is present. Usually baseline assessment and ongoing data appear on flowsheets or progress notes that are separate from the care plan.

Writing the nursing diagnosis statement was discussed in Chapter 17. The sections that follow discuss how to write clear and succinct statements for each of the remaining columns of a client care plan. Because the plan is used by many nurses besides the nurse who collaborated with the client to make the plan, clarity of expression is very important.

Formulating Clear and Succinct Desired Outcome Statements

Recall that the desired outcome is a description of favorable client status achieved when the nursing diagnosis has been resolved. When writing the care plan, nurses construct at least one desired outcome statement for each of the clients' nursing diagnoses. Often, several desired outcomes, in-

BOX 18–1. GUIDELINES FOR WRITING OUTCOME STATEMENTS

- Describe client behavior, status, functioning, or condition.
- Use positive terms.
- Relate each desired outcome statement to only one nursing diagnosis.
- Specify the expected time frame for outcome attainment.

cluding short-term and long-term outcomes, are written for each diagnosis. The focus of each desired outcome collaboratively identified by client and nurse is the basis for the desired outcome statements the nurse writes on the care plan form. The guidelines in Box 18–1 apply to transforming the more general outcome focus to a concise written desired outcome statement. These guidelines are examined in greater detail below.

Describe Client Behavior, Status, Functioning, or Condition. Client behavior refers to what the client will do, how the client will look, or what the client will say. Status, functioning, or condition may be an attribute such as strength, knowledge, or mental status; or a body function such as respiratory rate, urine output, or as in the previous example, bowel elimination pattern. To emphasize the client-centered nature of desired outcome statements and distinguish them from nursing activities, the words "The client will . . ." or "The client will demonstrate . . ." may be used as the first phrase of the written outcome statement. The outcome focus is added to complete the statement.

Recall the example in the discussion above about identifying the focus of desired outcomes. Several were suggested: (1) "healthy bowel elimination," (2) "greater fiber intake," (3) "increased exercise," (4) "knowledge about foods high in fiber," and (5) "understanding of the role of fiber-rich foods and exercise in bowel elimination." Desired outcome statements generated from these foci might include:

1. "The client will demonstrate a healthy bowel elimination pattern."
2. "The client will eat fiber-rich foods."
3. "The client will increase exercise."
4. "The client will learn dietary sources of fiber."
5. "The client will learn how fiber and exercise promote bowel elimination."

Use Positive Terms. Stating outcomes in terms of what one desires to see, rather than listing undesirable conditions that a client should not exhibit, is the preferred format for desired outcome statements. Positive desired outcome statements provide a better foundation for clearly stated evaluation criteria, as will be seen below.

Relate Each Desired Outcome to Only One Nursing Diagnosis. Combining seemingly related behaviors or conditions that actually relate to two separate diagnoses in one outcome statement creates confusion. An outcome statement such as "The client will experience maximal comfort and demonstrate functional grieving during terminal stage of illness" is actually derived from two diagnoses: Alteration in comfort related to physical effects of terminal illness and Dysfunctional grieving related to impending death. An outcome statement derived from more than one nursing diagnosis does not as readily facilitate selection of related nursing implementation or evaluation of outcome attainment.

Specify the Expected Time Frame for Outcome Attainment. When the outcome statements are complete for a given diagnosis, target dates can be added for each outcome, as discussed previously. Clearly written desired outcome statements (Fig. 18–2) are the basis for nursing implementation, discussed below.

Communicating Nursing Implementation Effectively

Communicating decisions on implementation to other caregivers demands the same kind of precision that is needed for other parts of the written care plan. Nursing implementation statements describe the nursing care selected to facilitate client attainment of desired outcomes. Often, several implementation statements correspond to one desired outcome. The statements should be brief and precise. They must be specific enough that any health care provider using the plan would have a clear understanding of the actions to be taken. Box 18–2 and Figure 18–3 identify components that should be included in statements of nursing implementation. Nursing implementation statements containing all of these components are called **nursing orders** by some authors.[3,5,9,11] The sections that follow clarify each of these components.

Subject. Often, nurses carry out the implementation, and so "the nurse" is an implied rather than a stated subject.

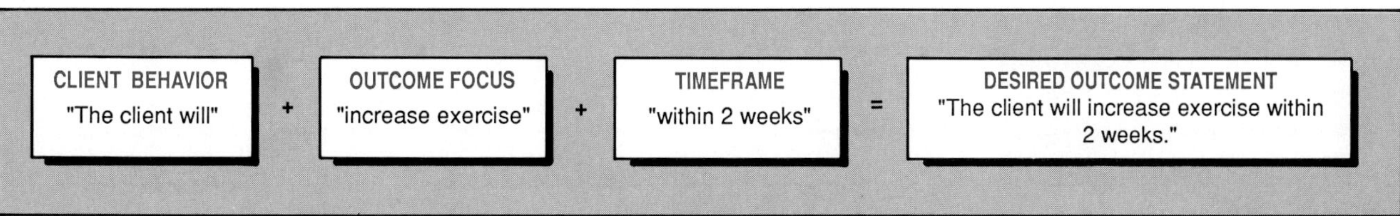
CLIENT BEHAVIOR
"The client will"
+
OUTCOME FOCUS
"increase exercise"
+
TIMEFRAME
"within 2 weeks"
=
DESIRED OUTCOME STATEMENT
"The client will increase exercise within 2 weeks."

Figure 18–2. Writing desired outcome statements.

BOX 18–2. COMPONENTS OF NURSING IMPLEMENTATION STATEMENTS

- Subject
- Focus
- Action verb
- Time
- Quantity/condition
- Date
- Signature

However, if action is to be taken by someone other than a nurse, such as a family member or another member of the health care team, the subject should be identified. In some cases, "the client" is the implied subject of nursing implementation statements. This occurs when the activity identified to achieve the desired outcome is performed by a client, but observed or verified by a nurse. For example: "Ambulate 10 minutes t.i.d. (three times a day)" or "Sit in chair at least 1 hour q (every) shift" would be carried out by a client, not a nurse, although a nurse may assist as needed.

Focus. Identifying the focus for nursing implementation is part of the process of making the plan, discussed previously. In the earlier example, reviewing the desired outcomes for the diagnosis "Constipation related to a diet lacking fiber and a sedentary life-style" produced several foci for implementation: "fiber intake," "exercise," and "knowledge about causes of constipation." Each one of these foci, when combined with the other components identified in Box 18–2, would make a complete nursing implementation statement.

In some situations, the nurse may need to clarify the focus originally identified when making the plan. A more specific focus will result in a more precise implementation statement. For example, consider a nurse who is collaborating to make a care plan with a client scheduled for surgery. The nurse and client may agree that the client needs assistance with "expression of feelings" (general implementation focus). The nurse realizes that "Facilitate expression of feelings" does not provide adequate direction for other nurses who may use the client care plan. To produce an implementation statement that is more precise, the nurse might consider the following questions: How would one facilitate this client's expression of feelings? What feelings are relevant? Using knowledge of communication and knowledge about the client to answer these considerations, the nurse writes a more precise statement, such as "Provide opportunities to talk about concerns regarding the outcome of surgery."

Action Verb. Because nursing implementation statements describe action, a precise action verb is critical. The verb selected should relate to the implementation focus as well as to specific clients' needs. Actions related to fiber intake for the earlier diagnosis of constipation could include: *serve* foods high in fiber, *provide* a list of high-fiber foods, *explore* the client's food preferences that contain fiber, or *develop* a menu plan containing high-fiber foods. The selection would depend on the individual client situation. Possibly, all would be appropriate. Often several different types of nursing implementation are needed to facilitate the achievement of each desired outcome.

Time. Time includes frequency, duration, and/or the specific hour of the day the action is to be implemented. Phrases such as "t.i.d." (three times a day), "q4h" (every 4 hours), or "at 0800, 1400, and 2000" can be added when appropriate. The action "Serve foods high in fiber," for example, would be more precise with the phrase "at least two meals qday (every day)." However, not all implementation is time dependent. The other implementation examples in the preceding paragraph would not need to be carried out at specific times of the day, and so would have no time designations.

Quantity/Condition. Modifiers specifying quantity (such as number, distance, or volume) or conditions under which an activity should be carried out (such as "ambulate *at least 20 feet using a walker*" or "assist client to transfer to a chair *using a hydraulic lift*" or "irrigate wound *aseptically*") improve the clarity of nursing implementation statements.

Date. In some facilities, the date on which the implementation is first entered on the care plan, as well as the dates of any revisions, are recorded on the plan. A target date for completion of the activity is also helpful. For example, "Develop a menu plan containing high-fiber foods" may have phrases such as "within 3 days" or "by October 1" added. These date specifications facilitate timely execution of implementation.

Signature. In some practice settings, the nurse who writes a nursing implementation statement is required to sign it.

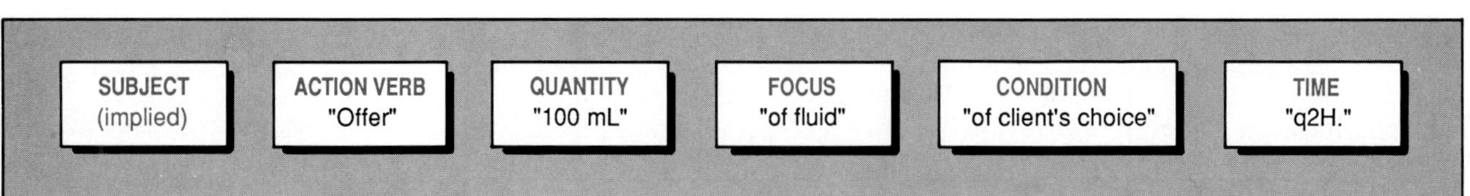

Figure 18–3. Identifying components of a nursing implementation statement.

Similarly, if the implementation is revised, the nurse making the revision so indicates by signing the revision.

In keeping with the value placed on brevity in written care plans, nursing approach statements are not usually written as complete sentences, and modifiers such as adverbs and adjectives are kept to a minimum. Articles, such as "a/an" and "the," are also customarily omitted. Medical terminology and abbreviations that have been approved by the facility are used when possible. Thus, one might write: "Apply warm sterile soaks to LUE b.i.d." rather than "Apply warm sterile soaks to the client's left upper extremity twice a day"; or "Husband to assist with tub bath qAM" rather than "Have husband help client with bath every morning." Table 18–3 includes several examples of correct implementation statements. (A list of symbols and abbreviations that are commonly used in writing care plans is included in Box 18–7, later in this chapter.)

Writing Evaluation Criteria

Evaluation criteria describe specific behaviors (including aspects of physiological functioning) that indicate that the desired outcomes have been achieved. Nurses write the criteria in the evaluation column of the care plan at the same time as the rest of the elements of the plan. Then on the designated deadline date for outcome achievement, nurse and client compare actual client behavior to the criteria. They may also use evaluation criteria prior to the final target date to gauge progress. When actual behavior matches the criteria, the desired outcome is considered to have been met. If the client is unable to demonstrate the behavior specified in the criteria, a judgment must be made about whether to continue with the plan or alter it in some way. Types of evaluation and evaluation activities are discussed in greater detail later in this chapter.

TABLE 18–3. COMPARISON OF CORRECT AND INCORRECT NURSING IMPLEMENTATION STATEMENTS

Correct	Incorrect
Offer 100 mL of fluid of client's choice qh (every hour).	Encourage fluids.[a]
Assist client to ambulate 10 minutes t.i.d. (three times a day).	Ambulate t.i.d. (three times a day).[b]
Observe independent ambulation around perimeter of nurse's station b.i.d. (twice a day).	Encourage ambulation.[c]
Turn side, back, side q2h (every 2 hours) odd hours.	Turn q2h (every two hours).[d]
Up in chair 20 min. 2x q (twice per) shift.	Up in chair q.i.d. (four times a day).[e]

[a] Omits quantity and frequency.
[b] Omits quantity and condition.
[c] Omits time, quantity, and condition.
[d] Omits condition.
[e] Omits time and quantity.

Like desired outcome statements, evaluation criteria are stated in positive terms for clarity. "No respiratory wheezes," for example, is not as precise as "Breath sounds clear on auscultation." A client with "no wheezes" could have other abnormal breath sounds. It is easier to explicitly describe a desirable condition that would indicate outcome achievement than to generate an exhaustive list of undesirable conditions, the absence of which would indicate outcome achievement.

The components of evaluation criteria statements are identified in Figure 18–4 and discussed below.

Focus. The collaboratively identified focus for each evaluation criterion is incorporated in the written statement. The focus may be stated as one of the elements below, or may be combined with one or more of them to make a clear, complete statement.

Subject. As with the desired outcome statements to which evaluation criteria relate, the implied subject of the criteria statement is often the client. However, as discussed previously, the foci of evaluation criteria frequently are client attributes or functions such as respiratory rate, muscle strength, facial expression, and the like, which are considered evidence of a given desired health state described in the desired outcome statement. In this case, the attribute or function may be the subject of the criteria statement. For example, evaluation criteria relating to the desired outcome "Client will demonstrate an effective breathing pattern" might include "Regular and unlabored respirations at rest: 16 to 20 per minute."

The evaluation focus itself also may be the subject of evaluation criteria statements. For example, one evaluation focus for the client with constipation related to a diet lacking in fiber and a sedentary life-style, discussed previously, was "absent or diminished abdominal distension." An evaluation criteria statement based on this focus might be "Soft, nondistended abdomen."

Action Verb. Verbs used in evaluation criteria statements should describe observable behaviors or, when possible, measurable conditions that would verify the achievement of the corresponding desired outcome. Verbs describing overt action are most readily evaluated. Conversely, verbs like "understand," "feel," or "cope" that may be found in desired outcome statements, are not acceptable in evaluation criteria, because such verbs do not describe behavior that is observable. An inference would be necessary to evaluate whether understanding, for example, had been achieved. To facilitate consistent evaluation, more specific actions that are observable and that nurse and client agree would indicate understanding or coping or other abstract behaviors are used in criteria statements. "States," "verbalizes," "lists," and "describes" are examples of verbs that can be used to evaluate understanding, feeling or coping.

Often, "is (will be)" or "has (will have)" are implied verbs in evaluation criteria statements. They are omitted for the sake of brevity. This was the case in the earlier example

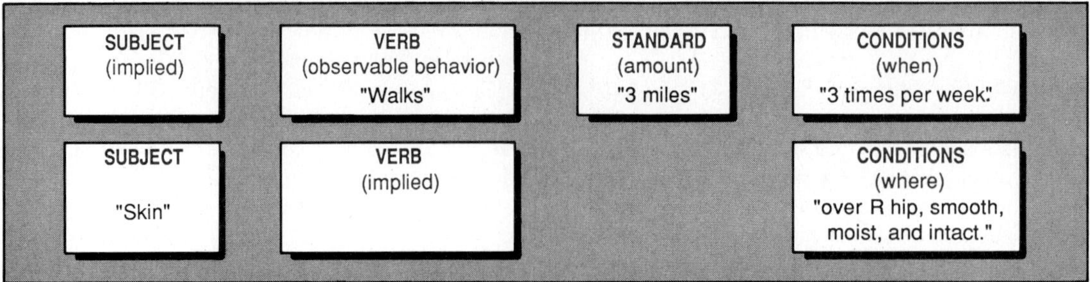

Figure 18–4. Identifying components of evaluation criteria statements.

regarding abdominal distension. The statement could have read: "The client will have a soft, nondistended abdomen" or "Abdomen will be soft and nondistended." However, the meaning of the statement is evident without including the verb, and the resulting statement is more concise.

Standard or Measure. Standard or measure specifies such quantities as time, distance, frequency, or amount. Recall the sample desired outcome statement: "The client will increase exercise." A corresponding evaluation criterion might be "The client will exercise for *30 minutes three times a week.*" The level of expected performance specified by the standards, in this case, 30 minutes and three times a week, depends on the individual client situation.

Conditions. Conditions refer to specific circumstances under which the behavior is to be performed—for example how, when, where. The statement above, "The client will exercise for 30 minutes three times a week," could be modified to read "The client will perform *aerobic* exercise for at least 30 minutes three times a week." This modification adds another condition, "how"; "aerobic" specifies a type of exercise. "When" conditions include such phrases as "30 minutes before bedtime," "with every meal," "during social events," or "when aware of symptoms of anxiety." "Where" conditions might be "at home," "at work," and so on. These additional descriptive elements may be selected on the basis of nurses' professional knowledge and expertise or clients' resources and preferences.

Desired Outcome Statements as Evaluation Criteria. Some client care plan forms do not have a column for evaluation criteria. In this case, desired outcome statements are modified so that they may be used as substitutes for evaluation criteria. This situation creates a need for more precise desired outcome statements. When evaluation criteria are not part of the written plan, desired outcome statements should be expanded to include the components of evaluation criteria described above. A simple way to do this is to add the phrase "as evidenced by" (abbreviated "AEB") to the desired outcome statement, followed by components that would ordinarily be part of the evaluation criteria. When evaluating outcome achievement, nurses look for the evidence specified. Box 18–3 illustrates this.

The complete written care plan stating all of the client's nursing diagnoses with corresponding statements of desired outcome, nursing implementation, and evaluation criteria is a comprehensive guide for the care of the client. The written plan should be shared with the client so that both nurse and client can verify that it communicates their mutual intent. The plan may be kept at the client's bedside, in the client's chart, or in a central file in the nurses' station. Some agencies have the capacity to store care plans in a computer system. In any case, the plan must be readily accessible to all personnel caring for the client.

The Client Care Plan for Mrs. Mildred Stone, on pages 606–608 shows a sample client care plan with two problems; a partial data base precedes the plan. This plan can be compared to the standard care plans that appear on pages 607–608. (Copy in italic print shows how the standard care plans can be modified for a particular client.)

■ CARE PLANS WRITTEN BY STUDENTS

The practice of professional nursing is built on a knowledge base of theories, models, and scientific principles from the

BOX 18–3. DESIRED OUTCOME STATEMENTS AS EVALUATION CRITERIA

Desired Outcome

Client will attain a healthy bowel elimination pattern.

Evaluation Criteria

One soft, formed BM qd (every day).
Abdomen soft, nondistended.

Modified Desired Outcome Statement

Client will demonstrate a healthy bowel elimination pattern AEB one soft, formed BM qd (every day) and soft, nondistended abdomen.

IMPLICATIONS FOR NURSE–CLIENT COLLABORATION

Written Care Plan

Sharing the written care plan with clients enables nurse and client to verify that it communicates their mutual intent. This is another act that reflects the interdependency of the collaborative approach. The written plan is often kept at a client's bedside where it is readily accessible to all personnel who act as caregivers to the client. Access to the plan promotes continuity, facilitates evaluation, and invites ongoing collaboration among members of the health care team.

behavioral and natural sciences and the humanities. Learning to apply this knowledge to construct effective individualized care plans is a major part of nursing education. Students preparing for professional nursing practice are required to develop and use comprehensive care plans for clients in a variety of health care settings. Writing client care plans not only assists students to assimilate information, but also provides a vehicle for communicating students' knowledge to an instructor. A client care plan written by a student reflects the student's ability to apply theory, to think critically and logically, to use reference materials, and to communicate with the client.

Components of Student Care Plans

Student care plans include all of the elements of a collaborative client care plan discussed earlier, plus several additional components (Box 18–4).

Comprehensive Data Base. It is common for student plans to include a detailed comprehensive data base, organized according to a specific conceptual framework. By reviewing all of the data a student used to identify the nursing diagnoses, and the organization of the data, the evaluator of the care plan gains insight about the student's diagnostic reasoning ability. Such an evaluation can confirm that the student recognizes what data are relevant to collect and can effectively apply diagnostic reasoning skills to analyze the data. Conversely, problems with which the student needs further assistance, such as faulty data clustering or premature closure of the assessment phase, may also be inferred.

BOX 18–4. COMPONENTS OF STUDENT CARE PLANS

- Comprehensive data base
- Nursing diagnosis statements
- Scientific basis for nursing diagnoses
- Desired outcome statements
- Nursing implementation statements
- Standard care related to medical diagnoses
- Scientific rationale for nursing implementation
- Evaluation Criteria
- Validation of outcome attainment
- Recommendations for alterations in the plan

Scientific Basis for the Nursing Diagnosis. A column discussing the scientific basis for the nursing diagnosis is another adjunct often found on student plans. Students may be expected to use basic science facts to interpret how the identified etiologic factors bring about the problem named in the diagnostic statement and how the specific defining characteristics exhibited by the client are produced. For the nursing diagnosis "Constipation related to a diet lacking in fiber and a sedentary life-style, as evidenced by decreased frequency of bowel movements and abdominal distension," used as an example in the sections above, a student might be expected to explain normal bowel physiology, with emphasis on the role of fiber and regular exercise, and to discuss how this physiology is altered, producing abdominal distension and decreased frequency of bowel movements, when adequate fiber and exercise are lacking. An analysis such as this evidences the depth and breadth of the student's knowledge as well as the ability to apply that knowledge appropriately.

Scientific Rationale for Nursing Implementation. In a similar way, a column in which the student explains the scientific rationale for nursing implementation provides important information for the instructor and valuable learning for the student. As the column title implies, students are expected to set forth the rationale for the nursing implementation they have selected, using facts and theories from the physical and social sciences. This explanation demonstrates students' understanding of how and/or why the approach selected will facilitate a client's achievement of the desired outcomes and therefore resolve the nursing diagnosis. Requiring science-based explanations of nursing diagnoses and implementation encourages students to use reference materials to enhance their knowledge and facilitates integration of theory and practice concepts.

Validation of Desired Outcome Achievement. Student care plans may also include more detailed validation of desired outcome achievement than is common on clinical plans. In the clinical setting, client behavior that demonstrates progress toward outcome achievement is recorded in the client chart rather than on the care plan. (See later discussion of Written Communication: Recording.) Requiring documentation of client progress toward desired outcomes on the care plan emphasizes the importance of the evaluation step in the nursing process and encourages students to incorporate evaluation strategies in their nursing care.

Recommendations for Alterations in the Plan. Recommendations for alterations in the plan if outcomes are not met may also be required on student care plans. In the clinical setting, the client care plan is considered a fluid document and such changes would be made in the course of day-to-day nursing care. Nurses and clients may discuss altering a desired outcome, for example, or consider a

CLIENT CARE PLAN FOR MRS. MILDRED STONE

Relevant Data Base (4/15/92)

Subjective

C/O abdominal distension and rectal pressure. Usual bowel elimination pattern: 1 soft formed stool after breakfast qd. Usually drinks a cup of hot lemon water at breakfast to stimulate a BM; prefers plain water to drink during day. Likes cooked fruit and vegetables or soft ripe fruit. Can't chew crisp fruits or vegetables—becomes SOB. Also likes whole wheat bread, bran flakes softened with milk. Does not exercise much due to SOB, but sometimes took short walks in the afternoon PTA. C/O fatigue when OOB since admitted.

Objective

Abdomen firm and distended; hypoactive bowel sounds × 4 quadrants; one small, dry, hard BM in last 3 days. Fluid intake 600 mL/day last 3 days. Consumes less than ½ of food on trays (soft diet). Using BSC, up in chair ×2 qd, no ambulation since admitted two days ago. HR ↑ 30 bpm, RR ↑ 10/min. p̄ transfer to chair or BSC.

Nursing Diagnosis	Desired Outcome	Nursing Implementation	Evaluation Criteria
Constipation R/T limited physical activity, inadequate fluids and decreased dietary fiber AEB 1 hard, dry BM in 3 days, distended abdomen, hypoactive bowel sounds.	1. Reestablish normal elimination pattern by 4/20.	1a. Assist to BSC within 20 min of finishing breakfast. 1b. Do not schedule tests or treatments until 40 min p̄ breakfast.	1. 1 soft formed BM q AM.
	2. Increase daily fluid intake by 4/16.	2a. Offer 300 mL hot lemon water c̄ breakfast qd. 2b. Increase fluids on meal trays to 400 mL. 2c. At least q2h, remind client to take frequent sips of water 2d. Keep water pitcher within reach at all times.	2. Fluid intake at least 1600 mL qd: Day shift: 1000 mL PM shift: 500 mL Night shift: 100 mL
	3. Increase fiber intake by 4/17.	3a. Request at least 1 cooked fruit and vegetable on each tray. 3b. Request bran flakes or whole wheat bread on breakfast tray. 3c. Request between meal snacks of soft ripe fruit 1–2 × d. 3d. If unable to eat all of food on tray, suggest fluids and high-fiber foods be consumed first. 3e. Consult with dietitian about serving 6 small meals qd if unable to eat 75% of food on meal trays.	3. Eats at least 5 servings of high-fiber foods qd (bran, whole grains, fruits, vegetables).
	4. Increase activity—see nursing diagnosis for Activity Intolerance, below.		
Activity Intolerance R/T imbalance between O_2 supply and demand and immobility AEB verbal reports of fatigue and SOB, RR and HR ↑ p̄ minimal activity.	1. Tolerates mild activity by 4/25.	1a. Assist with gradual increase in exercise qd; as SOB ↓, increase amount of exercise.	1. Able to slowly walk 20 feet s̄ SOB. RR ↑ <5/min, HR ↑ < 15 bpm.
	2. Improved O_2 supply during mild exercise by 4/20.	2a. Teach pursed lip and diaphragmatic breathing exercises. 2b. Assist to practice both exercises for 3 minutes at least 2× q shift (day and PM). 2c. Increase length of exercise sessions by 1 minute qd. 2d. Discuss how use of these breathing techniques can improve exercise tolerance; ask client to use them during transfers to chair and BSC.	2. See #1

Nursing Diagnosis	Desired Outcome	Nursing Implementation	Evaluation Criteria
	3. Improved energy level by 4/25.	3a. Schedule care to allow time for rest periods after meals, bathing and transfers to BSC and chair. 3b. When RR ↑ = <2 and HR ↑ = < 10 p̄ transfers, move chair and BSC 5 feet from bed. Reassess tolerance; gradually increase distance qd.	3. States does not feel fatigued p̄ walking 20 feet at a slow pace.

STANDARD CARE PLAN: CONSTIPATION RELATED TO LIMITED PHYSICAL ACTIVITY

Mrs. M. Stone

Desired Outcome	Implementation	Evaluation Criteria
1. Healthy bowel elimination pattern. *By 4/20.*	1. Teach relationship between exercise and bowel elimination.	1. Regular elimination of soft formed stool; frequency dependent on individual variables. *1q AM.*
2. Increased physical activity appropriate to client's health status. *By 4/25.*	2. Collaborate with client to develop a progressive aerobic exercise program appropriate to client's health status. *Transfers to chair, walks c̄ assistance.*	2. Regular participation in exercise program of choice. *Progressive ambulation: bed to chair, increasing distances, then ambulation in halls.*

STANDARD CARE PLAN: CONSTIPATION RELATED TO INADEQUATE FLUID INTAKE

Mrs. M. Stone

Desired Outcome	Implementation	Evaluation Criteria
1. Healthy bowel elimination pattern. *By 4/20.*	1. Teach role of fluids in healthy bowel elimination.	1. Regular elimination of soft, formed stool; frequency dependent on individual variables. *1 q AM.*
2. Fluid intake matches metabolic needs. *By 4/16.*	2. Plan schedule of daily fluid intake with client that incorporates personal likes/dislikes and accommodates usual daily routines. *a. Hot lemon water 300 mL q AM.* *b. Trays: 400 mL each.* *c. Offer water q2h.*	2. Daily intake of fluids matches needs as determined by calculation of body surface area. *Day shift 1000 mL.* *PM shift 500 mL.* *Night shift 100 mL.*

STANDARD CARE PLAN: CONSTIPATION RELATED TO INADEQUATE DIETARY FIBER

Mrs. M. Stone

Desired Outcome	Implementation	Evaluation Criteria
1. Healthy bowel elimination pattern. *By 4/20.*	1. Teach role of fiber in healthy bowel elimination.	1. Regular elimination of soft, formed stool; frequency dependent on individual variables. *1 q AM.*
2. Greater fiber intake. *By 4/7.*	2a. Teach food sources of fiber. 2b. Collaborate with client to make a menu plan that incorporates high-fiber foods that client likes. *1. 1 cooked fruit or veg, q tray.* *2. Bran flakes or whole wheat toast q AM.* *3. 1–2 fruit snacks (ripe/soft) qd.*	2. Daily intake of at least five servings of high-fiber food.

STANDARD CARE PLAN: ACTIVITY INTOLERANCE RELATED TO BED REST/IMMOBILITY

Mrs. M. Stone

Desired Outcome	Implementation	Evaluation Criteria
Improved activity tolerance appropriate to level of wellness. *By 4/25.*	1. Assist with exercises in bed according to client's tolerance. 2. Teach client the benefits of regular exercise in health maintenance. 3. Collaborate with client to develop a progressive aerobic exercise program to be initiated when client's condition allows. *a. Transfer to chair b.i.d.* *b. ↑ distance to chair by 5′qd p̄ can tolerate transfer (RR ↑ < 2, P ↑ <10).*	Progressive increase in activity tolerance AEB decreased complaints of fatigue, activity-related changes in P, R, BP WNL for health prognosis. *Will walk slowly 20 ft s̄ SOB.*

STANDARD CARE PLAN: ACTIVITY INTOLERANCE RELATED TO IMBALANCE BETWEEN OXYGEN SUPPLY AND DEMAND

Mrs. M. Stone

Desired Outcome	Implementation	Evaluation Criteria
Improved activity tolerance appropriate to level of wellness. *By 4/25.*	1. Teach diaphragmatic and pursed lip breathing exercises. 2. Collaborate with client to devise a schedule gradually increasing frequency of breathing exercises. *Pursed lip and diaphragmatic breathing per 3 min 2 × shift; increase by 1 min qd.* 3. Discuss the value of using these techniques during exercise. 4. Schedule rest periods between activities that cause fatigue. *Rest p̄ meals, transfers, bath.*	Progressive increase in activity tolerance AEB decreased complaints of fatigue, activity-related changes in P, R, BP WNL for health prognosis. *See above.*

change in implementation when client circumstances suggest these changes are in order. Challenging nursing students to recognize the need for changes in a care plan they have written and to identify possible alternatives is good preparation for professional practice.

Medically Ordered Implementation and Standard Nursing Care. Students may also be requested to include medically ordered implementation and standard nursing care related to clients' medical diagnoses on their care plans. As discussed earlier in the chapter, clinical client care plans usually address only those problems that are collaboratively identified by client and nurse. However, there are benefits to including routine nursing care and medically ordered care on student client care plans: (1) students become familiar with specific nursing assessments and implementation that are considered standard for clients with common medical diagnoses, knowledge that is expected of professional nurses; and (2) by identifying and discussing the scientific rationale for these nursing actions and examining relationships between medical and nursing diagnoses, students develop critical thinking and problem-solving skills that are essential for functioning in the professional role.

Common Student Problems in Writing Client Care Plans

Common sources of diagnostic error were discussed in Chapter 17. The discussion here focuses on difficulties related to writing other elements of the care plan.

Common pitfalls when writing desired outcome statements and evaluation criteria are (1) stating outcomes as nursing behaviors rather than client behaviors, (2) selecting client behaviors that are not observable or measurable, (3) failing to consider the actual resources and desires of the client. A common error in nursing implementation statements is lack of specificity.

Stating Outcomes as Nursing Behaviors Rather Than Client Behaviors. This error occurs most often when students view nursing as a task-oriented rather than a problem-solving endeavor. To write outcome statements that are client centered, keep in mind the purpose of a collaborative client care plan that was set out in the beginning of this chapter: to assist a client to resolve health problems. Focus on the meaning of "outcome"—that is, an outcome is a result, not a means to attain a result. It may be helpful to think of the plan as a map that clients and nurses develop to assist clients to reach a specified destination. The outcome is the client's destination.

Selecting Client Behaviors that are Not Observable or Measurable. As emphasized in the previous sections, desired outcome statements relating to abstract concepts like knowledge, strength, comfort, and the like require corresponding evaluation criteria (or additional "as evidenced by" clauses) that specify how an evaluator would recognize that the expected change had occurred. To avoid the error of neglecting to specify a measurable or observable behavior, ask yourself the following question: Would two nurses using the desired outcome statement and evaluation criteria that I have written to make independent evaluations of this client's progress reach the same conclusion? Have I identified what "knowledge" or "comfort" mean *for this client* relative to *this nursing diagnosis?*

Failing to Consider Client Resources and Desires. Recall that the process of developing desired outcome statements and evaluation criteria begins with stating the converse of the problem and of the signs and symptoms that evidence the problem. In other words, nurses devise a description of a desired health state representing absence of the problem. Then, through collaborative efforts clients and nurses modify this "ideal" outcome so it describes a health state that is realistic and acceptable to a client. This modification to tailor the desired outcome to the individual is a critical step, but one not always carried out by students in their initial attempts to develop client care plans. Student–client collaboration after the student has analyzed the data, while not always possible given the time constraints of student clinical laboratories, is a worthwhile standard to strive for.

Writing Statements that are Not Sufficiently Specific. Writing nursing implementation statements may also be a challenge for beginning students. The most common student error related to nursing implementation statements is writing statements that are not sufficiently specific. To return to the analogy of the map used earlier, the nursing implementation represents the route to the destination. If the directions are vague, the student and the client will get lost!

This error probably relates, at least in part, to the limited experience that students have with nursing implementation strategies. Until one is exposed to the wide range of possibilities for nursing implementation, it may be difficult to write succinctly about them. Another contributing factor is students' reliance on standard care plans as resources. Standard care plans are valid resources for care planning; the key is in knowing how to use them. By their very nature, standard care plans are very general, because they are not based on individual client data. Therefore, students must view nursing implementation statements listed in standard care plans as broad guidelines, insufficient to stand alone on a care plan written for a specific client.

To use nursing implementation recommended on a standard plan, the student must modify the broad statement according to the guidelines for writing precise nursing implementation statements provided in this chapter, using the client data base. For example, to modify the general statement "Encourage fluids," one should ask oneself, what would a nurse need to know about the client to encourage him or her to drink more fluids? Information such as what fluids the client likes, whether hot or cold fluids are preferred, and how much fluid the client needs each day (based on formulas for calculating fluid needs found in Chap. 31), would help the student write a specific prescription for this client; one that would be clear enough to be used effectively by other caregivers without necessitating additional data gathering.

A major constraint that underlies many of the problems discussed above is the fact that students often do not have the opportunity to use their client care plans to guide the care of the clients for whom they were written. Because students do not usually have regular day-to-day contact with clients, their care plans are more often a retrospective analysis, completed after having cared for the client. This situation may lead students to view making and writing care plans as an exercise rather than as a learning experience that has relevance to the "real world" of nursing. Although it may be true that the sometimes lengthy product of a student's effort to create an individualized care plan bears little resemblance to the care plans in use in clinical settings, the process of making and writing both plans is the same. The skills required—communication, clinical judgment, critical thinking, concise writing—are the same. Students who invest themselves in the care planning process with enthusiasm and commitment thus gain a proficiency that is essential to their professional future.

■ EVALUATING CLIENT CARE PLANS

Evaluation has been mentioned repeatedly throughout the foregoing discussions of making and writing client care plans. In the context of collaborative nursing process, **evaluation** is a systematic comparison of a client's health status to standards mutually developed by the client and a nurse. As such, this evaluation addresses the quality of the client care plan and the client's progress toward the desired outcomes on the plan (the mutually developed standards) and reflects the quality of nursing care. Evaluation is an integral component of professional accountability.

Considerations that relate to the quality of the plan include the accuracy of the diagnoses, the appropriateness of the desired outcomes and evaluation criteria, the effectiveness of the nursing implementation, the clarity with which each of the elements of the plan is expressed, and the currency of the plan. These considerations will be discussed in the later section on Evaluation Activities.

Types of Evaluation

Although evaluation is often called the final step in the nursing process, it is more accurately described as an aspect of the nursing process that is not only terminal, but is concurrent with other steps as well. This dual characterization is consistent with descriptions in the literature of various professions, which identify these types of evaluation processes as formative and summative. Formative evaluation refers to a concurrent or ongoing process; summative evaluation to a final or summary process. Nursing literature also uses the term *retrospective evaluation.* Box 18–5 highlights the distinctions between these types of evaluation.

Formative Evaluation. **Formative evaluation** is ongoing—that is, it is an inherent part of *making, writing,* and *implementing* the client care plan. As previously discussed, evaluation is part of the decision-making process used to identify the health problems that should be addressed on the plan and select desired outcomes, evaluation criteria, and implementation strategies. Formative evaluation during implementation of the plan gauges client progress toward the desired outcomes. If expected client progress is not evident, nurses seek to identify and correct factors contributing to the lack of progress.

Summative Evaluation. **Summative evaluation** occurs on the target dates specified in the plan and at the termination of care. Its focus is outcome achievement. Summative evaluation determines whether outcomes were *met, partially met,* or *not met.* Failure to achieve outcomes by the target date or the discharge date calls into question the quality of the plan and of the formative evaluation process. Lack of progress toward desired outcomes should have been noted during formative evaluation, and action taken as noted above.

Retrospective Evaluation. **Retrospective evaluation** occurs after the termination of care. Its focus is the overall quality of care on a given nursing unit or in the health care agency as a whole. Retrospective evaluation activities are usually applied in institutional evaluation, also called quality assurance. Retrospective evaluation processes are discussed later in this chapter.

Evaluation Activities

Evaluation activities that are applied as client care plans are being implemented including monitoring, analyzing, collaborating, and deciding. **Monitoring** is the ongoing collection of data about a client's condition. Analyzing involves comparison of client status to evaluation criteria. In collaborating, nurses discuss their analysis and perceptions with clients and obtain client feedback. Deciding is the mutual determination by client and nurse of whether to continue with, modify, or terminate the plan.

BOX 18–5. TYPES OF EVALUATION

Formative Evaluation

Ongoing part of nursing process.

Summative Evaluation

Occurs on specified target dates and at termination of care or discharge.

Retrospective Evaluation

Occurs after termination of care or discharge.

Monitoring. Monitoring is a continuous aspect of client care. It includes such activities as measuring, inspecting, examining, and listening. Some monitoring is prescribed by the client care plan or the medical orders, or is implied by clients' nursing and medical diagnoses. The time and frequency of the monitoring may be specified—for example, by a target date in the care plan or physician's orders—or it may be done at nurses' discretion. An astute nurse makes specific as well as holistic observations during every contact with a client. Subtle variations in a client's demeanor, alertness, or color, for example, may herald a significant change in status. Sometimes a specific deviation cannot be identified, but a nurse may note that "something's just not right" with a client. The nurse's perceptiveness may then prompt the gathering of additional data, increasing the frequency of monitoring, or taking corrective action.

The data obtained during monitoring are used to update the client care plan, recorded on flow sheets or client progress records, and may also be reported to other caregivers. Methods of reporting and recording are addressed later in this chapter.

Analyzing. Nurses analyze data obtained during monitoring activities to determine client achievement of or progress toward desired outcomes. In formative evaluation, nurse and client compare current data with baseline data and with desired or expected data. The baseline data, gathered during the initial client assessment, provide evidence of the existence of the problem. The desired data, stated as evaluation criteria, provide evidence of outcome achievement. If the prescribed nursing implementation is contributing to resolution of a client's problem, the current data should indicate a status somewhere between baseline and optimum. Recall, again, the previously discussed client with constipation. One sample desired outcome for this client was "The client will learn about dietary sources of fiber." Suppose that an evaluation criterion for this desired outcome was "The client will correctly identify at least three food sources of fiber," and that, on initial assessment, the client had been unable either to name any foods high in fiber or to state how fiber could assist in preventing constipation. If the client later states that she plans to add bran (a high-fiber food) to her diet to increase fiber intake, a nurse's analysis would validate that progress toward the outcome has been noted. If no progress was noted, further analysis would be needed to identify the reasons.

On outcome target dates, or at discharge or termination of care, nurse and client carry out summative evaluation. Current data are compared to desired data—the evaluation criteria—to validate outcome achievement rather than progress. If at this time the client in the example can name three or more high-fiber foods, the outcome has been met. Other possible conclusions of summative evaluation are "outcome partially met" or "outcome not met."

When formative evaluation reveals little or no progress toward a given desired outcome, or summative evaluation indicates that the outcome was not met or was only partially met, continued analysis is required to determine why the expected progress did not occur. The following questions can be used in this analysis.

Is the care plan current? A care plan that is not updated regularly is unlikely to be an effective plan. A client care plan must be considered a fluid document. Every nurse caring for the client needs to take responsibility for making changes based on data obtained during monitoring. Consistent evaluation on target dates also contributes to updating.

Was the planned nursing implementation actually carried out? Most clients' care plans contain several nursing diagnoses, each with prescribed implementation. Sometimes nursing implementation for other health problems is given priority, resulting in a lack of expected progress toward the outcome in question.

To determine whether planned care was given, nurses should check with the client, review the chart, and check with other nurses caring for the client. By participating in the initial development of the care plan, clients demonstrate willingness to accept and/or participate in the nursing implementation described on the plan. They will usually be able to state whether the planned care was implemented. In addition, nurses routinely document the date and time specific nursing care is given in the client's record (see later discussion). Therefore, if the care prescribed on the plan was given, it should be noted in the chart. Finally, discussing the unmet outcome with other nurses assigned to the client, informally or in client care conferences, should reveal the extent to which the nursing implementation in question was rendered.

If the care was not given as planned, and the client is still motivated to achieve the outcome, the care plan for that outcome can be continued as written with a new target date. However, when the analysis indicates that the prescribed care was implemented, the quality of the care plan itself must be questioned.

Is the nursing diagnosis accurate? Diagnostic errors (see Chap. 17) may result in misdiagnosis. As discussed above, all of the components of a client care plan are derived from the nursing diagnosis statement. Therefore, it follows that if the problem, its etiology, or the defining characteristics are incorrect or not clearly stated, one or more elements of the plan are likely to be faulty as well.

Are the desired outcome and evaluation criteria acceptable to the client, realistic, specific, and measurable or observable? Errors relating to the selection and manner of stating the desired outcome and related evaluation criteria are a common reason for unmet outcomes.

Outcomes and evaluation criteria unacceptable to clients typically result when nurses do not solicit or respect client input. If the desired outcome is not really desired by a client, lack of outcome attainment is a predictable result. A client is not likely to participate in achieving outcomes that are not personally meaningful and important. Likewise, if a client does not agree that the behavior specified in the evaluation criteria is reasonable, that behavior would not be a useful way to determine outcome achievement.

Unrealistic outcomes are destined to be unmet outcomes. The degree to which a client's problem can be resolved depends on factors such as age, general health, finances, and support from family or significant others. Not taking these resources or deficits into consideration when identifying expected client outcome behavior and setting target dates can result in outcomes that are unattainable.

Evaluation criteria that do not describe specific and measurable/observable client behavior related to the desired outcome do not lend themselves to consistent evaluation. In this case, the conclusion that the outcome has not been met may even be in error, a result of the evaluator's inability to interpret the criteria.

Does the nursing implementation statement provide sufficient direction to caregivers? If the nursing implementation statement is broad and general (eg, "assist with ambulation," "encourage coughing and deep breathing," "offer emotional support"), it is unlikely that the client will receive consistent care. And if each nurse is treating the client's problem differently, it is impossible to determine which approach, if any, is effective.

Does the prescribed nursing implementation designate effective therapeutic client care related to the identified problem and its etiology? This question addresses the effectiveness of the implementation. If expected progress toward desired outcomes did not occur, despite clear and appropriate desired outcomes and evaluation criteria, and clearly written and consistently performed nursing implementation, it is a logical conclusion that the implementation was not effective. Perhaps the prescribed implementation failed to address the etiology of the problem. Perhaps the frequency specified was insufficient. Perhaps the implementation was not powerful enough to support a change in the status quo. Implementation strategies such as monitoring, measuring, checking, recording, reporting, and notifying are more likely to maintain equilibrium than they are to bring about an improvement in health status.[10] Perhaps the nursing implementation was not acceptable to the client. A client could not realistically be expected to participate in activities that violate personal desires or beliefs, no matter how effective these activities might seem to a nurse. Nursing implementation is, in a sense, the "core" or "meat" of a client care plan. Identifying effective strategies requires collaboration, creativity, and persistence. The reward is clients' successful achievement of improved health status.

Collaborating. Collaboration is the essence of successful care planning. The earlier discussion of making client care plans emphasized that care plan development is a shared responsibility of nurse and client. The same is true of the evaluation of the plan. By discussing the results of the nurse's analysis, client and nurse can reach a mutual conclusion about whether further action is needed (Fig. 18–5).

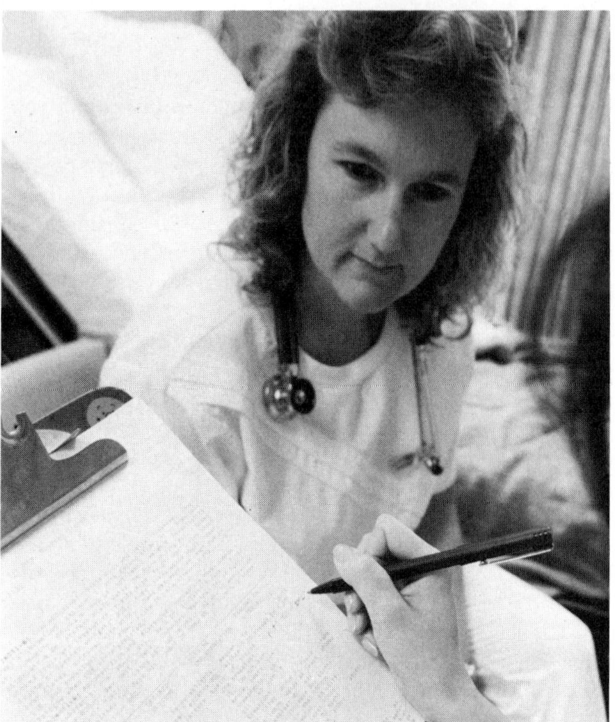

Figure 18–5. A client signs off on her client care plan after collaborative evaluation with the nurse.

Deciding. Deciding is the final outcome of the evaluation process. It is also a mutual process, based on the analysis discussed above. Together, nurse and client reach a decision to terminate, continue, or modify the plan of care.

Termination of the Plan. If the desired outcomes are achieved by the designated target date, the nursing diagnosis is considered resolved and related nursing implementation may be terminated. Nurse and client then write "Resolved" in the evaluation column for that nursing diagnosis and signs and dates the entry.

Continuation of the Plan. If partial achievement of desired outcomes is noted on the target date, a decision to continue the plan without revision may be made. The plan may also be continued when analysis determines that outcomes were not met, but that all elements of the plan are determined to be appropriate. In this instance, a nurse writes "Continue with plan" and a new target date is selected.

Modification of the Plan. Partially met or unmet outcomes may result in a decision to revise desired outcomes or nursing implementation. The method for deleting portions of the plan which no longer apply and for recording revisions depends on agency policy.

■ COMMUNICATING EVALUATION

Communicating the judgments or conclusions reached through evaluation is an essential component of collaboration. Communication between health care providers and with clients is a regular activity in any health care agency. Much of this communication occurs through structured, organized methods and vehicles, thereby enhancing effectiveness and efficiency, imperative for continuity and coordination of care. Two standard communication modes are used consistently in health care: reporting (oral communication) and recording (written communication).

Oral Communication: Reporting

The general purpose of reporting is to communicate information about a particular topic. In health care, most reports relate to clients' status or progress toward expected outcomes of care set out in the medical treatment plan and the client care plan. Reports may be exchanged between providers and clients, providers and clients' families or significant others, and among members of the health care team. Some reports are situational and informal; others are structured, following a consistent pattern, order, or format.

Situational Reporting. Situational reporting occurs regularly between clients and nurses. Sometimes situational reports occur as part of assessment or monitoring activities, but frequently they happen during nursing care activities. Often, clients spontaneously report changes in symptoms or concerns about their illness or their health care experience. Sometimes such reports are solicited by nurses. Nurses also share information about clients' current status or perceptions about progress toward goal attainment while carrying out monitoring or other nursing care.

Situational reporting between health care team members is also a common occurrence. Information such as results of laboratory or other diagnostic tests, sudden changes in a client's condition, or other unexpected events may be shared in situational reports. For example, a nurse may telephone the client's physician to report significant changes in the client's vital signs or the appearance of abnormal breath sounds.

Structured Reporting. Structured reporting between nurse and client is part of their collaborative evaluation of the client care plan on specified target dates or in preparation for termination of care. At these times, nurses report their professional opinion about the extent to which desired outcomes were achieved, and solicit client input. Nurses then record the collaborative nurse-client judgments on the care plan.

Structured reporting between health care team members is a regular component of their daily routine. A structured report is given whenever a nurse relinquishes responsibility for care to another team member, such as at change of shift or when the client is transferred to another nursing unit. Nursing students are usually expected to give a structured report to a staff nurse at the conclusion of clinical laboratory as well.

Change of Shift Reports. The change of shift report addresses all of the clients on a given nursing care unit. It is a summary of each client's current status, including the significant events and changes occurring during the previous shift. Many units develop a protocol for change of shift report to assist nurses to focus on the most relevant data to report. Generally, the following information is included: clients' priority problems, progress toward resolution of the problems, and significant changes indicating a deterioration or improvement in condition. Often nurses also mention recent diagnostic tests and their results; specific treatments such as intravenous therapy, dressing changes, or physical therapy that have been completed or that are needed; and new medical and nursing orders.

Walking Rounds. Protecting client confidentiality is an important issue when giving any report. Thus, the correct place for reporting is an area that provides privacy. In some agencies, reporting is accomplished through the use of walking rounds in which staff members walk from room to room, giving information about each client at that client's bedside. When using a walking rounds report format, clients should be included in the communication, not merely talked about.

Client Care Conferences. Structured reports among health care team members are also shared at client care conferences. These are interdisciplinary meetings held regularly in many agencies to address client health problems that may require the expertise of several disciplines. Client care conferences are discussed in more detail in Chapter 19.

Characteristics of Effective Reporting. Effective reporting promotes continuity, quality, and efficiency in client care. Time is a commodity in short supply on many nursing units. Therefore, an effective report is focused, orderly, precise, concise, and comprehensive.

- *Focused.* Identify the client being discussed by name, room number, primary physician, and admitting diagnosis. When the purpose of the report relates to specific aspects of client care or client problems, include information relevant to those aspects only.
- *Orderly.* All information that is relevant to one client or topic or aspect of the report should be given before going on to address additional clients or topics.
- *Precise.* Select terminology that clearly describes the event or situation; quantify when possible. Broad generalizations and vague statements are of little value.
- *Concise.* Only pertinent information is included in an effective report. Rambling on about extraneous details wastes time, and important information may be missed.
- *Comprehensive.* Thoroughness is not sacrificed for the sake of brevity. Include all data that are relevant and necessary to portray an accurate account of a situation or event.

Figure 18–6 provides an example of a change of shift report that meets these standards. It concerns a client, Mrs. Mildred Stone, who was admitted to the hospital because of increasing respiratory difficulty and whose partial care plan (two problems) appears on pages 606–608.

Becoming a competent and effective reporter requires considerable knowledge and experience. Students gain and practice these skills as they progress through their nursing program, and refine them as professional nurses.

BUILDING NURSING KNOWLEDGE

How Accurate Are Nurses' Intershift Reports?

Richard JA. Congruence between intershift reports and patients' actual conditions. *Image.* 1988; 20:4–6.

Richard argues that many factors in the hospital environment interfere with nurses' information processing. This may lead to the communication of inaccurate information about clients. Factors such as noise, workload demands, and the volume of information that nurses need to process may all interfere with accurate reporting.

Richard designed a study to determine the percentage of error in intershift reports, the reports by offgoing nurses to the oncoming nursing personnel. No attempt was made to determine the causes of error. The investigator observed and listened to a total of 57 intershift reports on 19 client care units in a large hospital. Reports were rated according to preestablished guidelines. The investigator then visited and checked each client to make an independent assessment of their conditions. A total of 584 clients were visited.

The overall agreement between reports and client conditions was 70 percent for the day shift, 72 percent for the evening shift, and 68 percent for the night shift. The rate of items omitted from reports was 11.76 percent. The most common omission was in the category of fluid intake and output values. This was a particular problem on the night shift.

The rate of lack of agreement between items reported and the client's condition was 12.36 percent. The most common item on which nurses erred was intravenous needle or catheter insertion sites. Of 409 IV site reports, 107 did not correspond. Another common item was intravenous infusion rates. Of 286 rate reports, 74 were off. These deviated anywhere from 10 to 50 percent of the reported rate. The mode of report had an effect on the rate of errors. Taped reports were more likely to have omissions than were face-to-face reports. Richard concludes that what is reported does not always accurately reflect a client's condition, and recommends that oncoming nurses check clients shortly after going on duty to verify the reports they receive.

Written Communication: Recording

The primary purpose of written interprofessional communication is to provide formal, legal documentation of treatment plans and progress made toward meeting clients' health care goals. Written communication is also a vehicle for coordinating client care. The client care plan, discussed previously, is one example of written interprofessional communication. Two other examples, the client's record and the Kardex, are discussed below.

The Kardex. The **Kardex** is a form that is used in hospitals and other inpatient facilities as a ready reference to communicate data about a client quickly and succinctly. In most agencies it is considered a working document rather than a

Mrs. Stone, age 64, in room 218 bed 2, a patient of Dr. Dean, admitted 5 days ago for exacerbation of her emphysema. The primary care concern during this shift should include follow-up on the nursing diagnosis of constipation related to decreased mobility. Assist Mrs. Stone to be up in a chair for dinner and continue to urge fluids 400 mL per tray plus 400 mL during each shift. Mrs. Stone also has ineffective airway clearance related to thick sputum and ineffective cough; she needs to be encouraged to cough and deep-breathe and continue to urge fluids. She coughs up dime-sized amounts of thick stringy sputum and becomes dyspneic upon exertion, requires frequent rest periods. Respiratory rate is 24 per minute at rest and 36 upon exertion. Mrs. Stone is scheduled for a pulmonary function workup tomorrow.

Figure 18-6. Change of shift report for Mrs. Mildred Stone.

legal document, so information is recorded in pencil to facilitate updating as needed. The Kardex consists of a series of cards, one for each client on the unit, that are organized in a portable file or notebook. It is kept in a central and accessible location in the nurses' station.

Each Kardex card has labeled sections to categorize data. Most individual health care institutions devise a format for Kardex cards that is specific to their needs, so the appearance of the cards varies. Information typically available in the Kardex includes the following:

1. Demographic data about a client; for example, name, room number, age, religion, and date admitted. Names of family or significant others who should be contacted in case of emergency may also be listed.
2. The physician who admitted the client, medical diagnosis, concurrent health problems, allergies, and medical or surgical procedures since admission.
3. Information about client requirements or restrictions related to activities of daily living, such as diet, fluid, activity, and elimination; as well as needs for assistive devices such as dentures, glasses, hearing aids, canes or crutches; and safety precautions such as restraints or siderails.
4. Continuing intravenous therapy orders, including type of solution, additives, rate of administration, bottle number, date, and start and finish times.
5. Other treatments ordered by the physician, such as oxygen therapy, skin care, irrigations or dressing changes, as well as nursing management of these therapies—that is, specific variations related to the client's individual needs.
6. Laboratory and diagnostic tests, including the date tests were ordered and the date tests should be performed.
7. Special services, such as physical therapy, respiratory therapy, social service, or other consultations needed on a regular or one-time-only basis. Frequency of the service, date, and/or time scheduled may also be listed.
8. List of medications and administration times. In many agencies, this information appears on a separate Kardex.

To be useful, the Kardex must be kept up to date. Generally, the ward clerk or a specific nurse is assigned the task of noting changes ordered by the physician. However, every nurse caring for the client shares in the responsibility for adding or deleting information relating to nursing management as changes occur.

Health care facilities using computerized hospital information systems (see Chap. 21) may have an option to use an automated computerized Kardex. This system greatly streamlines creating the initial document and updating it as changes occur. Although the same type of information is available in an automated Kardex, the presentation and location of information may differ from the traditional Kardex file.

The Client Record. The **client record** (also called a medical record or chart) is a permanent, legal document that is a compilation of a client's health history and current health status. It describes client progress; therapies that have been completed, are ongoing, or are planned; as well as considerations for discharge and comprehensive follow-up care. The chart should be an accurate chronological account of clients' health status, health care, and responses to care since being admitted to the facility. Records are retained by health care facilities after clients are discharged for a period of years, depending on laws in the state in which the facility is licensed.

Medical records may be used in court, as evidence in malpractice lawsuits, by insurance companies to calculate appropriate payment to providers, and by the government to determine eligibility for Medicare reimbursement. (See also Chaps. 3 and 35.) As will be seen in a later section, clients' records are also used to evaluate quality of care in health care facilities.

Because the chart is a continuous description of client health status and progress toward treatment goals, it serves as a vehicle for health care team members to communicate with each other. Physicians, nurses, dietitians, discharge planners, physical therapists, social workers, and respiratory therapists are only some of the health care professionals who use the chart as a communication tool.

There are two types of client records: source-oriented and problem-oriented records. The **source-oriented record** contains a separate section for each discipline (such as nursing, laboratory, physical therapy, dietary, medicine) to record pertinent observations, care, or response to care. The chart is generally separated into sections through the use of dividers with tabs signifying the source of the data or the name of the form on which data are recorded; for example, nurses' progress notes, physicians' progress notes, medical history, and so on. Data within each section are entered in chronological order. Although this type of record facilitates data entry and retrieval by each discipline, it has the disadvantage of fragmenting data. The user may have to peruse several sections of the chart to obtain important information about one client problem.

In the **problem-oriented record** (POR), also called the problem-oriented medical record (POMR), client data are arranged according to identified client problems rather than the data entry source. All providers contribute to a single problem list in the front of the chart that notes a client's actual or potential problems, including the nursing diagnoses, medical diagnoses, and diagnoses formulated by other health care team members (for example, social workers, dietitians, and physical therapists). Problems are listed and numbered in the order in which they are identified. Each entry on the problem list is dated (Fig. 18–7). When the problem is resolved the date of resolution is documented. A client's progress related to these problems can be readily discerned, because all disciplines also use a common form for progress notes. Entries made in the progress notes refer to the name and number of the problem on the problem list. This format fosters a collaborative approach, as any provider making relevant observations about any problem on a client's problem list may write a corresponding progress note. For example, a nurse may write a progress note on a problem originally identified by the physician or respiratory therapist. The major sections of a POMR include data base, problem list, plan of care, and progress notes. Box 18–6 describes the information found in each of these sections of the POMR.

Both source-oriented and problem-oriented records use similar record-keeping forms to organize data, although the forms may be located in different parts of the chart. Table 18–4 lists typical chart forms and describes information found on each.

Nursing Entries in the Client Record. Because nurses provide client care around the clock, many chart entries are made by nurses. Important considerations in charting these entries include content, format, and mechanics.

Content. Content refers to the actual information conveyed (that is, which events require documentation in the chart) and the choice of language used. Although there may be some institutional variation in designating relevant events to document, the following information is most commonly noted.

- *Client assessment.* Client assessment is a description of elements of a client's functioning and health status that are particularly relevant to that client's medical and nursing diagnoses. Generally, a comprehensive assessment of these elements is done at the time a nurse assumes care. Then, selected elements are reassessed as needed

BOX 18–6. LOCATION OF INFORMATION IN PROBLEM-ORIENTED MEDICAL RECORDS

Data Base

Medical and nursing history and physical forms; histories/examinations performed by other providers (eg, dietitian, social worker); diagnostic reports.

Problem List

Health problems identified by all providers, in chronological order (see Fig. 18–7).

Plan

Medical treatment plan, frequently stated in three parts: diagnostic work-up, proposed therapy, and client education; and client care plan developed by client and nurse. Plans by other disciplines may also be included.

Progress Notes

Narrative notes by all providers written in SOAP format that describes client progress related to each problem (see later discussion); discharge summary, written when care is terminated. Flowsheets, such as graphic sheet or daily care sheet, may also be found in this section.

PROBLEM LIST			
NUMBER	DATE	PROBLEM	DATE RESOLVED
#1	4/15	*Ineffective Airway Clearance*	
		R/T thick mucous	
		secretions and weak cough.	
#2	4/15	*Emphysema.*	
#3	4/15	*Constipation R/T limited*	
		physical activity, inadequate	
		fluids and ↓ dietary fiber.	
#4	4/15	*History of smoking.*	
#5	4/15	*Activity Inolerance R/T*	
		imbalance between O_2	
		supply and demand and immobility.	
#6	4/15	*Low income.*	
#7	4/15	*Isolation—lives alone.*	

Figure 18–7. Problem list for Mrs. Mildred Stone—POMR Format.

TABLE 18–4. RECORD-KEEPING FORMS USED IN CLIENT MEDICAL RECORDS

Form	Information Recorded
Admission sheet (face sheet, personal data sheet)	Legal name; address; age; sex; birthdate; marital status; occupation; employer; next of kin; person to notify in emergency; insurance information; religious preference; date, time, and reason for admission; attending physician; medical record number.
Medical history and physical form	Summary of health history and physical examination performed by physician. Initial medical treatment plan may be included.
Physician's order sheet	All directives for care written by the physician, such as medications, treatments, diagnostic tests, restrictions.
Nursing history	Results of initial nursing assessment (see Fig. 16–12).
Problem list	Used in POMR to note health problems identified by all providers, in chronological order (see Fig. 18–7).
Progress notes	Description of client response to treatment plan; significance of new data; alterations in treatment plans, if any. Source-oriented records have forms for each discipline (eg, nurse's notes).
Flowsheets	Forms to record specific observations or measurements made on a repeated basis. May have spaces for entries designated by times, dates, or both. There are many types of flowsheets. The following are examples.
Graphic	Routine vital signs; temperature, pulse, respiration, blood pressure displayed as a graph (Fig. 18–8).
Daily care/assessment	Record of routine care (eg, hygiene, skin care, safety precautions, treatments) and regular assessments (eg, intake and output, weight, activity level) (see Fig. 18–9).
Medication administration record (MAR)	Name, dosage, route, and schedule of all ordered medications; record of who administered medication and when it was given.
Other	Diagnostic reports: laboratory, x-rays, scans, sonography, other tests Operative (surgery) reports Anesthesia records Consultation reports Discharge summary Consent forms

throughout the shift. Unit VI in this text identifies and explains assessment data relevant to each major functional category: oxygenation, nutrition, fluid balance, elimination, mobility, sleep–rest cycles, skin integrity, neurosensory integration, and self-expression. Data relevant to specific medical diagnoses are addressed in later nursing courses. The assessment may be recorded on a flowsheet or on progress notes, depending on agency policy.

- *Environmental assessment.* Selected aspects of a client's environment, such as the presence and operation of technical equipment (eg, intravenous lines, drainage tubes, oxygen delivery equipment) and safety equipment (siderails, restraints) should be noted. Often, daily care flowsheets have checklists to facilitate documentation about equipment. In some cases, environmental assessment may also include notations about personal items the client displays or uses.
- *Nursing implementation.* All nursing care that is provided, whether related to a client's nursing diagnosis or ordered by a physician must be documented. In many institutions, a daily care flowsheet is used to document routine care; more detailed descriptions, if necessary, may be written on the progress notes or nurse's notes.
- *Care by other providers.* Generally, individual providers are responsible for documenting the care they provide. In some health care facilities, however, a nurse assigned to a particular client is expected to note visits and care by others, such as the physician, laboratory technician, or x-ray technician. Tests or therapy performed in other departments are also noted by the nurse caring for the client at the time the therapy or test is done.
- *Client's response to implementation.* Note both desired and unexpected responses to care that are given. Clients' perceptions about their illness and their health care experiences are also significant. If unexpected events or responses to care are noted, it is advisable to describe corrective action taken as well as the outcomes of those actions.
- *Care that is omitted.* If care that is ordered on a client care plan or by a physician is not given, the omission and the reason for it should be documented.
- *Visits by significant others.* Contact and support from loved ones is an important resource during illness. When family, significant others, or a client's clergy visit, this is usually noted in progress notes.

Language is the other aspect of content to be considered when writing in the client's record. The purpose of documentation is to convey information. Therefore, the language used in chart entries should be accurate and concise.

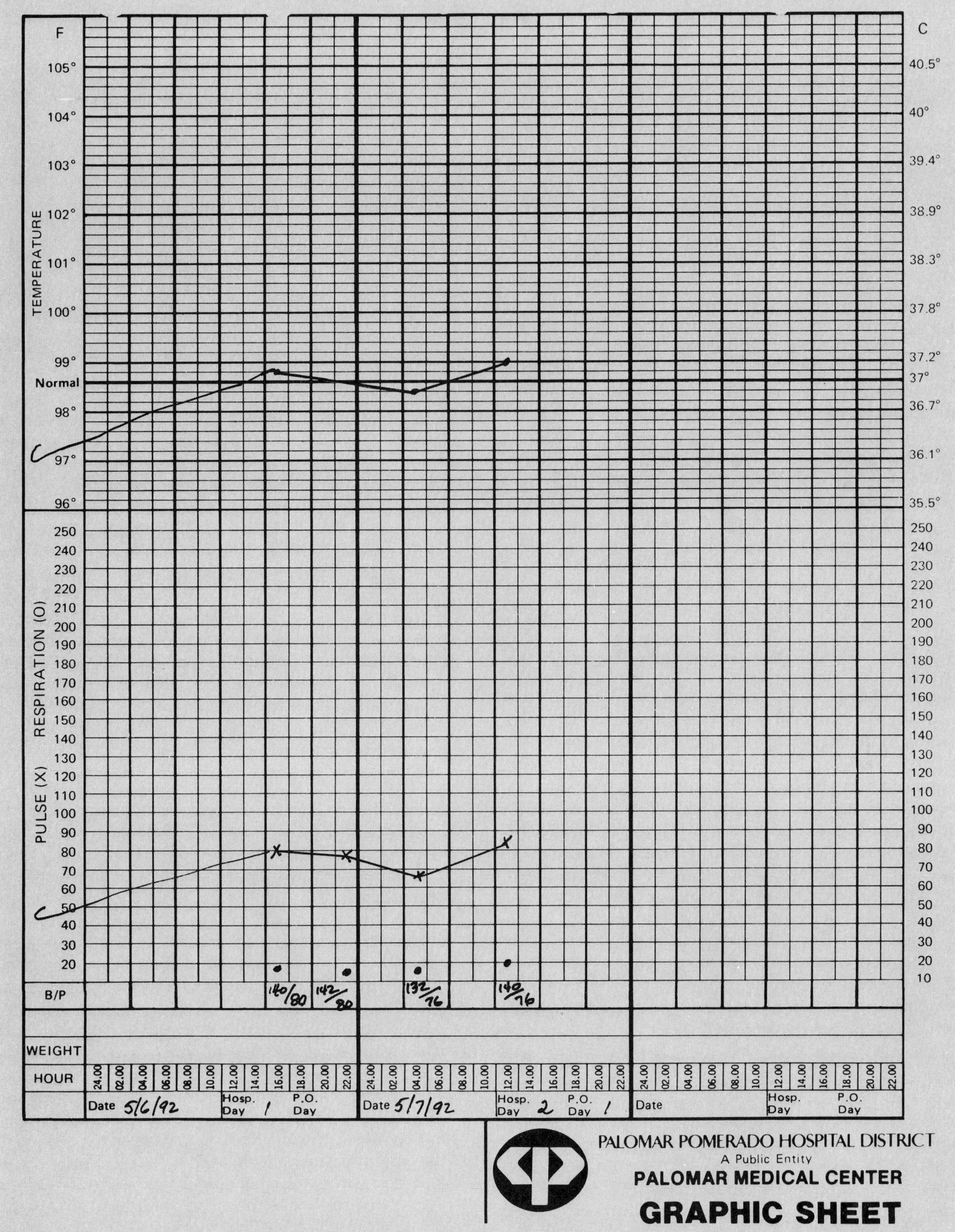

Figure 18–8. Sample graphic flowsheet. (*Source: Palomar Medical Center.*)

Descriptive notes in objective language are preferable to entries that are vague or that could be construed as value-laden or judgmental.[12] For example, state "Teeth discolored, gums receding, food debris noted" not "Poor oral hygiene"; or "Walked 10 yards without assistance, pulse increased 5 beats per minute after exercise, returned to baseline in 5 minutes" rather than "Walked 10 yards without assistance, tolerated well." The phrase "tolerated well," although frequently used, is ambiguous; its use should be avoided.

Sometimes a client's own words will convey an idea most clearly. When quoting a client directly, quotation marks should be used.

Accuracy also incorporates completeness. Record all relevant details, without sacrificing conciseness. Data that support or that may be pertinent to ruling out a particular diagnosis should be included. As noted above, learning to recognize what information is relevant to a given situation begins during basic nursing education and continues throughout professional life.

When recording assessment data, it is preferable to describe all findings, including findings considered normal, rather than to use global terms such as "normal" or "WNL" (within normal limits). A complete description lends itself to accurate interpretation of the information.

Some authorities caution against nurses' charting interpretations or judgments about the significance of data. It is this author's opinion that making and communicating professional inferences or judgments is a nursing responsibility. Nursing diagnoses are in fact professional inferences. When charting an interpretation of data, support the interpretation by documenting facts as well. In this way a more complete picture is presented.

A concise statement is one that conveys the intended meaning in as few words as possible. It is not always necessary to write complete sentences when charting. Articles (a, an, and the) may be omitted. Limit adverbs and adjectives to those necessary for accuracy and clarity. Omit "client" as the subject of sentences. It is understood that the client is the subject of the record. Write "Ate 25% of breakfast," not "Client ate 25% of breakfast." However, when action by others, such as the physician or other therapist, is documented, identify the person by name and title.

Using correct medical terminology when charting also contributes to conciseness. Often, one medical term can convey meaning that would require several words if conventional language were used. Furthermore, use of appropriate language conveys professionalism.

Format. Format is a second consideration when charting. The format of an entry on a client record refers to the way the information is presented. It includes the manner in which chart entries are organized as well as elements that must be included in each entry. The date, time, and signature of the writer are essential elements of every chart entry, including entries on flowsheets or checklists.

Date and Time. This refers to the date and time of the assessment or care described in the note. Generally, there are designated spaces on chart forms for these entries. In some cases, a new form (such as a daily care flowsheet) is used each day. In this case, the date is stamped or entered only once, when the first chart notation is made.

Signature. The signature identifies the caregiver writing the entry on the chart form. In most cases, this is the person who gave the care or made the observation described. The signature must include the signer's first name or initial, last name, and title (RN, SN, LVN). Because the format of checklists or flowsheets does not lend itself to signing each entry, such forms usually have a designated space on the form for signatures. In addition to signing in that space, it is recommended that providers documenting care or assessments on a flowsheet initial every entry.[12] To conform with legal standards for documentation, there must be a corresponding signature for every set of initials that appears on a flowsheet (Fig. 18–9).

Organization. Organization of descriptive entries, such as progress notes, is necessary for clarity. As the discussion of source-oriented and problem-oriented records noted, these records use different modes of organizing information. POMR progress notes are organized according to client problems. All entries require a standard systematic format. The format originally proposed for POMR notes is "SOAP," which is an acronym for *s*ubjective data, *o*bjective data, *a*ssessment, and *p*lan. Some agencies add IE for *i*mplementation and *e*valuation; others add R for *r*evision. A condensed version, APIE, in which *a*ssessment combines subjective data, objective data, and interpretation, is also used. In some facilities, a further condensation, PIE, is preferred.

A complete progress note names a problem from the problem list, and describes current progress in the form of a SOAP note. The appropriate content for each of these elements is discussed below. (A sample POMR progress note appears in Fig. 18–11).

- **S:** *Subjective* data are what a client states about the problem. Data may be recorded as a direct quote, or longer statements or discussions can be paraphrased. Subjective data may be omitted if no relevant client statement has been elicited.
- **O:** *Objective* data are information gathered by health care team members through observation. Physical assessment data, laboratory test results, and client behavior such as crying, shouting, or fidgeting with the sheets are examples of objective data.
- **A:** *Assessment* refers to the interpretation or inference made from the subjective and objective data. It is an estimation of a client's progress toward previously identified desired outcomes related to the problem being addressed in the note, or may identify changes in status relative to the problem that suggest a need for revision of the current desired outcomes.
- **P:** *Plan* is a brief statement describing the intended action to be taken relative to the above assessment—for example, to provide specific care, continue monitoring, or notify the physician. Some agencies specify that the plan

should specify therapeutic, diagnostic, and educational actions related to the problem.

- **I:** *Implementation* is a description of the actual action taken. It is preferable that this entry elaborate on the plan, not repeat it.
- **E:** *Evaluation* is the documentation of a client's response to the implementation. It should indicate the extent of resolution of the problem identified in the assessment entry.
- **R:** *Revision* describes changes in the implementation that are planned. Revisions may be recommended when satisfactory resolution of the problem has not occurred as a result of the plan recorded above.

In contrast to problem-oriented records, the overall organizational pattern of notes within each section of source-oriented records is time-related. Therefore, nurses write narrative style progress notes in chronological order in the Nurse's Notes section of the chart. Although there is no mandated format for narrative notes that corresponds to the SOAP format in POMR, each narrative entry should be organized logically to facilitate a reader's comprehension and interpretation of the note. Several organizational approaches are commonly used:

- Charting may be organized to reflect an application of the nursing process. This approach is similar to the SOAP format, in that assessment data are recorded first, followed by a reference to the nursing diagnosis, if appropriate; then implementation and client's response are noted. No headings are used to separate or distinguish each of the elements, but the order is clear.
- Body systems is another common organizational strategy for ordering narrative nurse's notes. In this case, assessment data are listed system by system, often in "head-to-toe" order. Sometimes the body system being addressed is named to further categorize the information. For example, a nurse may write: "Neurological: alert, oriented ×3, PERRLA. Cardiovascular: color pale, P = 80, strong, regular; pedal pulses strong and equal bilaterally . . ." The note would continue until relevant aspects of all body systems had been addressed.
- Functional categories, such as nutrition, oxygenation, self-expression, and others listed above, may also be used to organize narrative entries. For clarity, the function being discussed should be identified. For example: "Nutrition: States appetite still poor. Consumed only 10% of food on breakfast tray. Weight loss since admission 5 lbs. Will consult with family about possibility of bringing favorite dishes from home."

The choice of organizational approaches may be determined by agency policy, or by individual nurse preference. It is recommended that students practice writing both SOAP and narrative-style notes, and experiment with several different ways to organize narrative progress notes.

Mechanics. A third charting consideration is mechanics. Mechanics refers to aspects of actually writing the note. It includes legibility, spelling, grammar, timing of entries, and specifications regarding errors, use of space on forms, abbreviations, and writing in ink.

Legibility, Spelling, and Grammar. Legibility and correct spelling and grammar are necessary for clear communication among health care team members. Charting that is unreadable because of illegible handwriting, misspellings, and poor grammar contributes to misunderstandings about client status.[13] Such errors also connote carelessness and lack of professionalism and so reflect negatively on the quality of care given. Were a chart with these kinds of errors presented as evidence in a court of law, a jury might form an unfavorable opinion about the care a client received.[12]

Timing. Timing relates to frequency and sequence of entries. Some institutions require that notations be made at a specified frequency, such as every 2 hours, to demonstrate vigilance and continuity of care.

Whether or not frequency of charting is specified by agency standards, it is advisable to chart assessment data and client care at the time they occur. If it is not practical to make chart entries as events happen, personal working notes should be kept. Then, when making official entries into a client's chart, the working notes will provide detailed and accurate information so that a complete and orderly sequence of events is communicated.[13] Some practitioners attempt to streamline charting by writing entries that include references to procedures or care not yet completed, in anticipation of doing them later. This is a dangerous practice that could be construed as deliberate falsification of records, an illegal and unethical activity.

Although charting in source-oriented records is expected to be a chronological account of events, occasionally circumstances require what is called a "late entry."[12] For example, suppose the nurse caring for a client provides the ordered care at 8:00 AM but is unable to chart it at that time. Then suppose another nurse completes a treatment at 9:00 AM and charts it immediately. When the first nurse returns to chart the 8:00 care, a routine chronological entry is impossible, because there is no space between the 7:00 and 9:00 entries. Therefore, a late entry is required. The nurse would write: "Late Entry 10 AM. 8 AM Wound care completed. Incision clean, dry and intact."

Space. Space is another aspect of the mechanics of charting. Blank lines should never be left between narrative entries. This includes parts of lines remaining at the end of an entry. Instead, a line is drawn to the right-hand margin (Fig. 18–10). Also, information must not be inserted into a space that has already been filled, such as one might do when editing a paper or letter. Such an alteration may be interpreted as an attempt to falsify a record. Use of the late entry (discussed above) or the error designation (discussed below) is preferred.

Errors. When an error is made in recording in a client's chart, a straight line should be drawn through the mistake so it remains legible. In some health care facilities, the word "error" is written above the lined out portion and the line-out is initialed or signed. Then the entry should be rewrit-

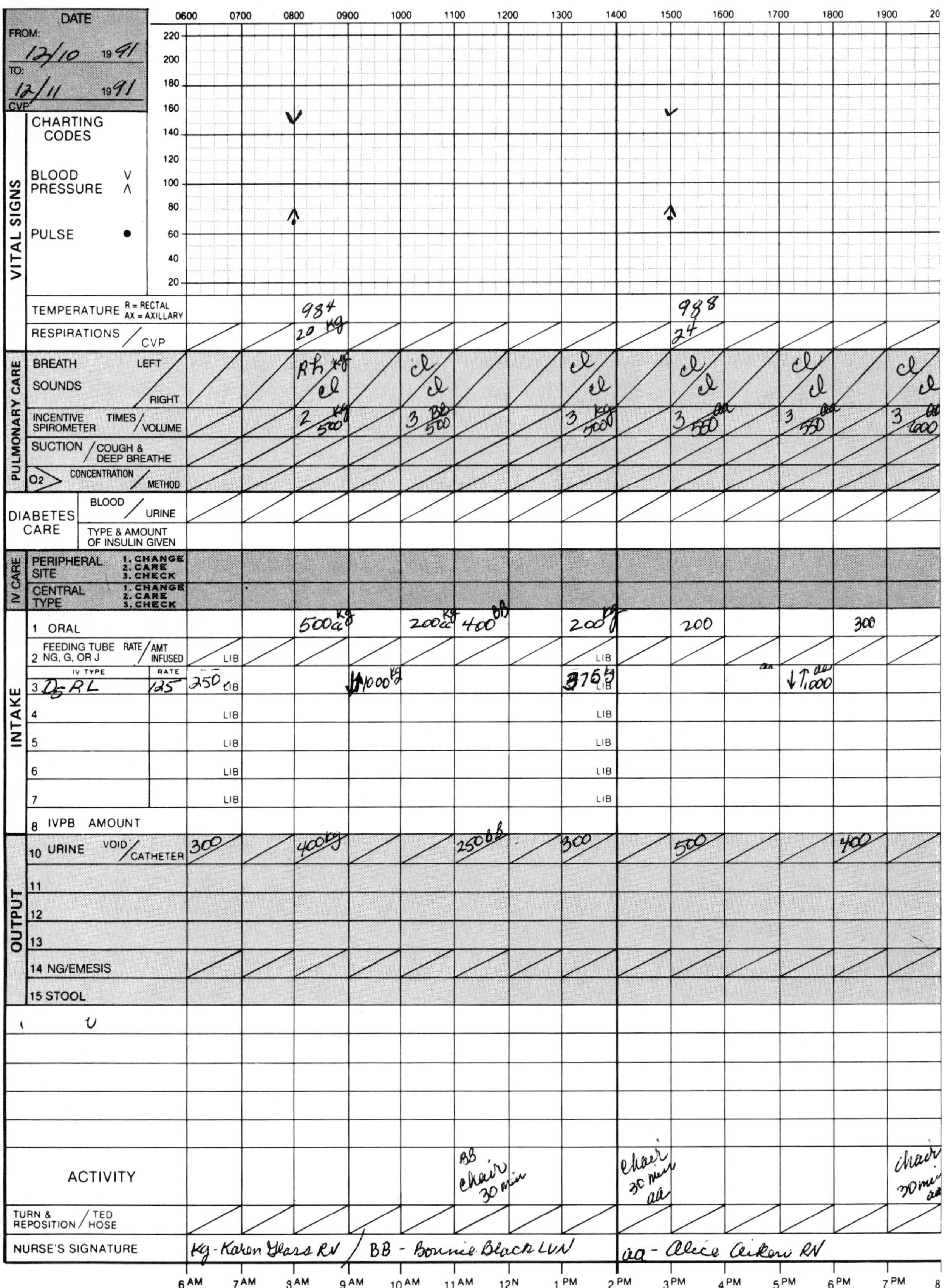

DATE FROM: 12/10 1991 TO: 12/11 1991

	0600	0700	0800	0900	1000	1100	1200	1300	1400	1500	1600	1700	1800	1900
VITAL SIGNS — CVP; CHARTING CODES: BLOOD PRESSURE V Λ; PULSE ● (scale 220–20)			V / Λ							V / Λ				
TEMPERATURE R = RECTAL AX = AXILLARY			98⁴							98⁸				
RESPIRATIONS / CVP			20 KG							24				
PULMONARY CARE — BREATH SOUNDS LEFT / RIGHT			Rh KG / cl		cl / cl			cl / cl		cl / cl		cl / cl		cl / cl
INCENTIVE SPIROMETER TIMES / VOLUME			2 KG / 500		3 BB / 500			3 KG / 500		3 aa / 550		3 aa / 550		3 aa / 600
SUCTION / COUGH & DEEP BREATHE														
O2 CONCENTRATION / METHOD														
DIABETES CARE — BLOOD / URINE														
TYPE & AMOUNT OF INSULIN GIVEN														
IV CARE — PERIPHERAL SITE 1. CHANGE 2. CARE 3. CHECK														
CENTRAL TYPE 1. CHANGE 2. CARE 3. CHECK														
INTAKE — 1 ORAL			500cc KG		200cc KG	400 BB		200 KG		200			300	
2 FEEDING TUBE NG, G, OR J RATE / AMT INFUSED		LIB						LIB						
3 IV TYPE D5RL, RATE 125	250	LIB		↓1000 KG				375 KG LIB				↓↑1,000 aa		
4		LIB						LIB						
5		LIB						LIB						
6		LIB						LIB						
7		LIB						LIB						
8 IVPB AMOUNT														
OUTPUT — 10 URINE VOID / CATHETER	300		400 KG			250 BB		300		500			400	
11														
12														
13														
14 NG/EMESIS														
15 STOOL														
ACTIVITY						BB chair 30 min			chair 30 min aa					chair 30 min aa
TURN & REPOSITION / TED HOSE														
NURSE'S SIGNATURE	KG - Karen Glass RN / BB - Bonnie Black LVN								aa - Alice Aiken RN					
	6 AM	7 AM	8 AM	9 AM	10 AM	11 AM	12 N	1 PM	2 PM	3 PM	4 PM	5 PM	6 PM	7 PM

Figure 18–9. Flowsheet with sample charting. (*Source: form courtesy of Mercy Hospital and Medical Center, San Diego.*)

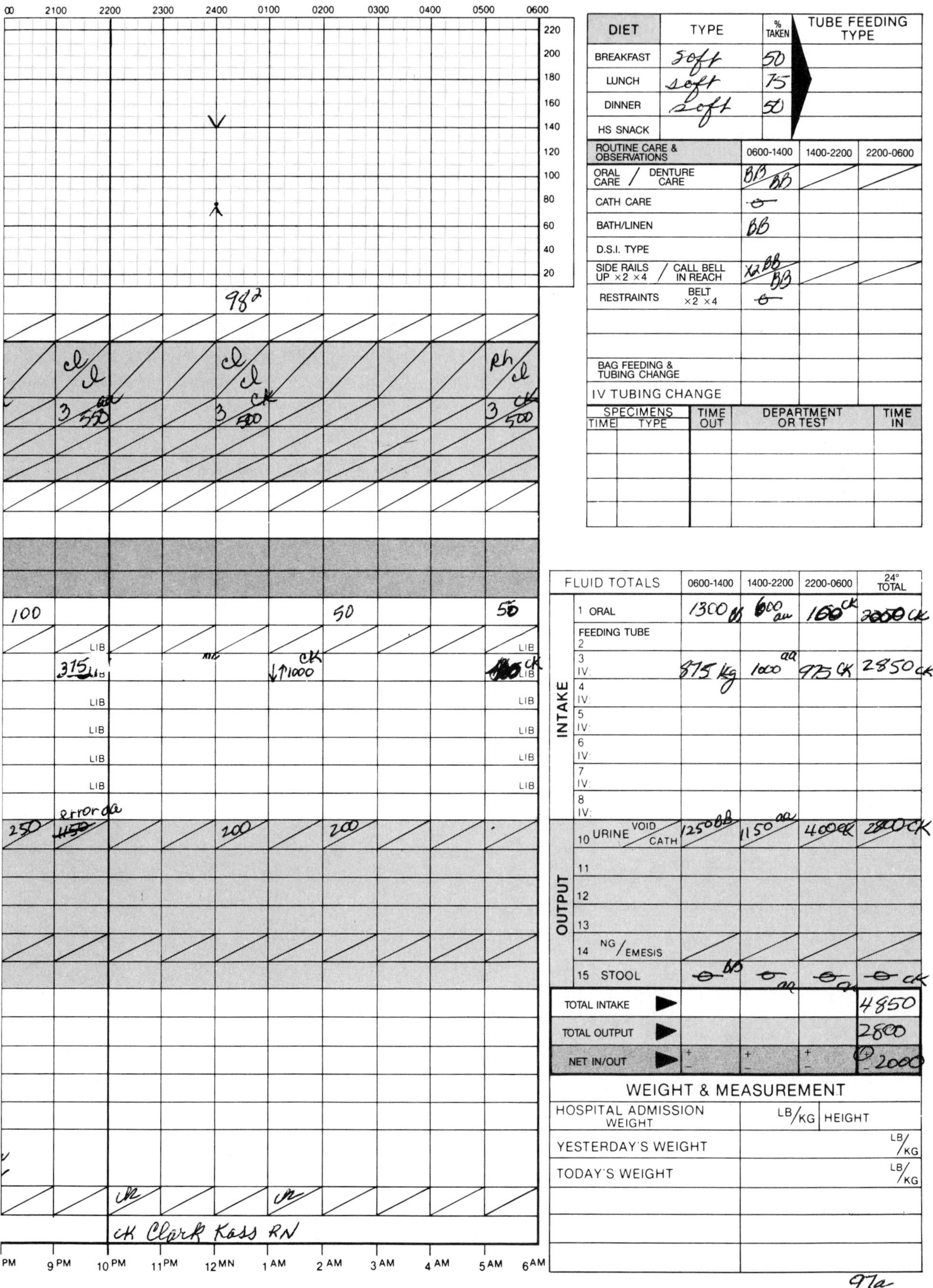

DIET	TYPE	% TAKEN	TUBE FEEDING TYPE
BREAKFAST	soft	50	
LUNCH	soft	75	
DINNER	soft	50	
HS SNACK			

ROUTINE CARE & OBSERVATIONS	0600-1400	1400-2200	2200-0600
ORAL CARE / DENTURE CARE	BB / BB		
CATH CARE	-0-		
BATH/LINEN	BB		
D.S.I. TYPE			
SIDE RAILS UP ×2 ×4 / CALL BELL IN REACH	x2 BB / BB		
RESTRAINTS BELT ×2 ×4	-0-		
BAG FEEDING & TUBING CHANGE			
IV TUBING CHANGE			

SPECIMENS TIME	TYPE	TIME OUT	DEPARTMENT OR TEST	TIME IN

	FLUID TOTALS	0600-1400	1400-2200	2200-0600	24° TOTAL
INTAKE	1 ORAL	1300 BB	600 aa	160 CK	~~2050~~ CK
	FEEDING TUBE 2				
	3 IV:	875 Kg	1000 aa	975 CK	2850 CK
	4 IV:				
	5 IV:				
	6 IV:				
	7 IV:				
	8 IV:				
OUTPUT	10 URINE VOID / CATH	1250 BB	1150 aa	400 CK	2800 CK
	11				
	12				
	13				
	14 NG/EMESIS				
	15 STOOL	-0- BB	-0- aa	-0- CK	-0- CK
	TOTAL INTAKE				4850
	TOTAL OUTPUT				2800
	NET IN/OUT	+ –	+ –	+ –	2000

WEIGHT & MEASUREMENT		
HOSPITAL ADMISSION WEIGHT	LB/KG	HEIGHT
YESTERDAY'S WEIGHT	LB/KG	
TODAY'S WEIGHT	LB/KG	

97a

Figure 18–9 (continued).

MERCY HOSPITAL AND MEDICAL CENTER
SAN DIEGO, CALIFORNIA 92103-2180

PATIENT CARE AND ACTIVITY RECORD

PATIENT ADDRESSOGRAPH

SURGERY OR PROCEDURE DATE

DATE FROM 12 / 10 / 1991 TO 12 / 11 / 1991

0800 Awake and alert, oriented x3. Lungs: Rhonchi LLL, right lung clear. No SOB. Abd firm and distended; says feels bloated. — Karen Glass RN —
~~0900 c/o abd pain~~ error KG (wrong chart) K Glass RN —

RESPIRATORY
O – ORAL
NT – NASAL TRACHEAL
NP – NASAL PRONGS
BB – BLOW BY
T – TRACHEOSTOMY
ET – ENDOTRACHEAL
MM – MIST MASK
RB – REBREATHER

LUNG SOUNDS
CL – CLEAR
RH – RHONCHI
W – WHEEZES

TUBINGS
CT – CHEST TUBE
NG – NASOGASTRIC
JP – JACKSON PRATT
G – GASTROSTOMY
J – JEJUNSTOMY

DIABETES CARE
L – LAB (if in this column)
G – GLUCOSCAN
CS – CHEMSTRIP
A – ACCUCHECK II

DRESSINGS / TREATMENTS
CDI – DRY & INTACT
DSD – DRY STERILE DRESSING
SS – STERISTRIPS
S – STAPLES
IBI – INTERMITTENT BLADDER IRRIGATION
CBI – CONTINUOUS BLADDER IRRIGATION
HEME + or – = HEMETEST POSITIVE OR NEGATIVE

OTHER
Abd – ABDOMEN
LOC – LEVEL OF CONSCIOUSNESS
A & OX – ALERT & ORIENTED TIMES
Δ – CHANGE
DC – DISCONTINUE
BSC – BEDSIDE COMMODE
S – SUPINE
P – PRONE
R – RIGHT
L – LEFT
DSI – DISEASE SPECIFIC ISOLATION
HOB – HEAD OF BED
SM – SMALL
MOD – MODERATE
LG – LARGE

IV CARE
RA – RIGHT ARM
LA – LEFT ARM
HL – HEP LOCK
A – RED/SORE
B – EDEMA
C – ROUTINE
D – ACCIDENTAL D/C
E – LEAKING
F – CLOTTED
LIB – LEFT IN BOTTLE
↑ – BOTTLE/BAG HUNG
↓ – BOTTLE/BAG DISCONTINUED

LAB DATA

FORM NO. 3135 (REV. 1/87)

SEE BACK FOR ADDITIONAL NOTES

Figure 18–10. Nurse's progress notes. (*Form courtesy of Mercy Hospital and Medical Center, San Diego.*)

ten correctly. Never erase or obliterate the mistake with ink or correction fluid. This could be interpreted as an attempt to tamper with the record. Some agency policies specify that if the nature of the error is not immediately recognizable, an additional explanatory note be written, such as "Charted for wrong client" (Fig. 18–10).

Abbreviations. Abbreviations can cause confusion and inaccurate interpretation of chart entries. Each institution has a set of approved standard abbreviations, symbols, and terms that can be used in charting. Approved standard abbreviations are generally listed in the hospital policy manual. When there is a doubt about whether an abbreviation is acceptable or when it is so similar to another abbreviation that the two may be confused with one another, nurses should not use it.[12–14] See Box 18–7 for a partial listing of generally accepted abbreviations.

Ink. Because a client's chart is a permanent legal record, all recording in it should be written in ink. Some institutions require nurses to write progress notes in different colored ink to signify the shift recording the note. For example, day shift may record in blue or black ink, the evening shift in green ink, and the night shift in red ink.

Figure 18–11 illustrates two samples of charting about Mrs. Stone, the client who was described earlier in Figure 18–5. One entry is a narrative note appropriate for a source-oriented record, and the other is in SOAP format as would be found in a problem-oriented record. Box 18–8 lists general guidelines for recording in the client record.

Computerized Charting. Computerized hospital information systems, discussed in detail in Chapter 21, can greatly simplify record keeping in health care facilities. Order entry systems that automatically enter new orders in the Kardex and pertinent portions of the chart, such as the client care plan or the medication administration record; print appropriate requisitions; and notify affected departments; save time and improve accuracy.

Hospital information systems can also be programmed to streamline progress note entries. A series of commonly used statements used to describe assessments, functions, or client activities, categorized according to the desired organizational format, is entered into the system. The phrase or phrases desired can then be retrieved and recorded as desired on a given client's progress or nurse's notes. Additional notes can be entered using a keyboard.

■ INSTITUTIONAL EVALUATION: QUALITY ASSURANCE

Institutional evaluation expands the focus of evaluation from one client's achievement of desired outcomes to the quality of health services provided throughout an entire health care agency. As discussed in Chapter 35, health care is regulated at the federal and state level by government agencies and by private sector organizations such as the Joint Commission on Accreditation of Healthcare Organizations (JCAHO) and the American Nurses' Association (ANA). Institutional evaluation initially resulted from 1972 federal legislation enacted to monitor cost and quality of care delivered to Medicare, Medicaid, and maternal-child health program recipients.[15] It has since expanded to include all recipients of health care as well as all aspects of institutional health care service. Moreover, new standards emphasize a more active process, which not only identifies deficiencies but also introduces changes to rectify the problems identified.[16]

The basis of both governmental and private sector institutional evaluation processes is peer review. That is, members of the profession being evaluated develop the standards and carry out the evaluation.[17] Then, individual departmental evaluations are coordinated so that systemwide corrections result.[15]

These systematic, comprehensive institutional evaluation programs are called **quality assurance programs** or **audits.** According to the JCAHO, the following activities should be included in quality assurance:

- Medical staff monitoring and evaluation.
- Monitoring and evaluation in other departments providing direct or indirect client care services (nursing is part of this category).
- Organization-wide functions, such as infection control, utilization review, and safety programs and issues.[1]

Types of Evaluation

Quality assurance programs may look at structure, process, or outcome.

Structure. The evaluation of structure focuses on the environment or context in which care is implemented. It includes physical facilities, equipment, staffing, administration, qualifications of personnel, inservice education, policies, and procedures. Client safety is the primary concern.

Process. Evaluation of process focuses on health care delivery. Process evaluation in a nursing quality assurance program, therefore, addresses the activities of nurses as the steps of the nursing process are implemented. Nurses' behaviors are measured against defined standards of practice.

Outcome. The third type of evaluation focuses on outcome. Outcomes are client characteristics or behaviors that are the end product of health care. The reader will recognize that this definition is consistent with that used in client care planning.

Outcome-based evaluation is a central concept in the case management model of health care delivery. In case managed care, "quality is prescribed in written detail, managed concurrently, and evaluated collaboratively" (p. 25).[18] Case management is being heralded as a possible answer to problems of health care cost containment and quality of care. This model also emphasizes the professional role of

BOX 18–7. COMMON ABBREVIATIONS USED IN RECORDING

ā	before
abd	abdomen
a.c.	before meals
ADL	activities of daily living
ad lib	as desired
AEB	as evidenced by
AMA	against medical orders
AM	morning
amb	ambulatory
amt	amount
as tol	as tolerated
BE	barium enema
b.i.d.	twice a day
BM	bowel movement
BP	blood pressure
BRP	bathroom privileges
BSC	bedside commode
c̄	with
C	Celsius (centigrade)
C&S	culture and sensitivity
CBC	complete blood count
CBR	complete bed rest
CC	chief complaint
cc	cubic centimeter
cl	clear
C/O	complains of
CPR	cardiopulmonary resuscitation
DAT	diet as tolerated
D/C	discontinue
DOE	dyspnea on exertion
dx	diagnosis
ECG (EKG)	electrocardiogram
F	Fahrenheit
GI	gastrointestinal
gtt	drop
GU	genitourinary
h	hour
HOB	head of bed
HR	heart rate
H_2O	water
HPI	history of present illness
hs	hour of sleep; bedtime
ht	height
Hx	history (of)
I&O	intake and output
IM	intramuscular
IV	intravenous
L	left
lg	large
lytes	electrolytes
meds	medications
mL	milliliter
mod	moderate
NG	nasogastric (tube)
neg	negative
no.	number
noc	night
n.p.o.	nothing by mouth
NS (NIS)	normal saline
OOB	out of bed
O.D.	right eye
O.S.	left eye
os	mouth
OT	occupational therapy
O_2	oxygen
p̄	after
p	pulse
pc	after meals
PE	physical examination
per	by
PERRLA	pupils equal, round, reactive to light, and accommodation
PM	afternoon
PMH	past medical history
PO	by mouth
postop	postoperative(ly)
preop	preoperative(ly)
prep	preparation
prn	as needed
PT	physical therapy
pt	patient
PTA	prior to admission
q	every
qd	every day
qh	every hour
qhs	every night at bedtime
q.i.d.	four times a day
qs	quantity sufficient
q2h (q3h, q4h, etc)	every 2 hours, every 3 hours, etc
R	respirations
R	right
RBC	red blood cells
R/O	rule out
ROM	range of motion
ROS	review of systems
RR	respiratory rate
R/T	related to
Rx	treatment
s̄	without
sm	small
SOB	short of breath
spec	specimen
stat	immediately; now
Sx	symptoms
T	temperature
t.i.d.	three times a day
TO	telephone order
TPR	temperature, pulse, respirations
UA	urinalysis
UGI	upper gastrointestinal
VO	verbal order
VS (vs)	vital signs
WBC	white blood cell
WNL	within normal limits
wt	weight
x	times

Symbols

Symbol	Meaning
<	less than
>	greater than
↑	increase
↗	increasing
↓	decrease
↘	decreasing
°	degree
2^0	secondary to
=	equal
=	unequal
0	none
♂	male
♀	female

SOAP Progress Note	*Narrative Nurse's Note*
#3 Constipation related to decreased mobility. *S: "I feel like my abdomen is full and there's pressure in my rectum. I haven't had a BM in 3 days. At home I take hot lemon water at breakfast."* *O: Abdomen firm and distended; hypoactive bowel sounds all 4 quadrants; took 300 mL from breakfast tray; drank 240 mL hot lemon water at 0930; passed one 2" piece dark brown hard, dry stool.* *A: Still constipated. Had only one 2" piece hard, dry, stool.* *P: Continue nursing care plan #3. Dietary notified re: client request. Add 240 mL hot lemon water to breakfast tray.* *P. Schmidt, RN*	*0830 Abdomen firm and distended, hypoactive bowel sounds all 4 quadrants; states "feels full" and has a feeling of "pressure in rectum." Hasn't had BM for 3 days. Encouraged to drink fluids on breakfast tray, but took only 300 mL. Refused to sit in chair for meal. Says feels too short of breath and tired. Turned to R side.* *0930 States at home she takes hot lemon water to stimulate BM. Dietary notified re: client request. Given 240 mL hot water c̄ lemon. Assisted to bedside commode. Passed one 2" piece dark brown, hard, dry stool.* *P. Schmidt, RN*

Figure 18–11. SOAP progress note and narrative nurse's note.

nurse clinicians. (See Chapters 1, 35, and 36 for further discussion.)

Steps in the Quality Assurance Process

The steps of the quality assurance process provide for an organized problem-solving approach. These steps, which are discussed in greater detail below, include (1) selecting the topic, (2) identifying standards and criteria, (3) collecting data, (4) interpreting data, (5) selecting and implementing solutions, and (6) reevaluating.

Select the Topic. The first step in an audit is selection of the topic or focus. The topic can vary greatly, depending on the agency, department, and scope of the audit. For example, an audit could focus on a medical diagnosis, a nursing diagnosis, a particular procedure performed frequently in a given department, or a recurrent client complaint. Nursing service areas often targeted for study are those that are high risk, high volume, or are problem prone.[19]

BOX 18–8. GENERAL GUIDELINES FOR RECORDING IN THE CLIENT RECORD

- Record assessment data, nursing implementation, and client response to care. Include client's words as appropriate.
- Record all relevant data concisely.
- Write descriptive notes in objective language. Avoid judgmental or global terms. Support interpretations with data.
- Organize information in progress notes according to hospital policy or a consistent organizational format of your preference.
- Record events at the time they occur.
- Include time, date, and signature in all entries.
- Write legibly in ink.
- Use correct grammar and spelling in all entries.
- Use only approved abbreviations, terms, and symbols.
- Do not leave blank lines in nurse's or progress notes. Draw a single line through blank lines or parts of lines.
- Correct errors promptly, using a single strike-out line, "error," and initials. Do not erase or obliterate entries.

BUILDING NURSING KNOWLEDGE

What is Quality Assurance?

New NA. Quality measurement: Quick, easy and unit-based. *Nurs Manag.* 1989; 20:50–51.

In this article, the author discusses what quality assurance is and why it is important. The author notes that systems of quality measurement are evolving to meet the demands for data created by regulatory bodies, consumers, insurance companies, and hospital managers. Each institution communicates its standards of care through policies, procedures, and standard care plans. New contends that measuring quality is an important tool for assessing compliance with standards and plays a role in many aspects of the problem-solving process. Recognizing that compliance with standards is low helps identify problems, and the use of data makes problem-solving more systematic. Quality measures can indicate the success or failure of a solution to a problem. The ultimate reason for quality measures is to improve care.

The quality measures proposed by New include the use of "screening criteria," criteria to detect problems in quality; and "problem-oriented criteria," application of standards of care to specific problems. New reports on one institution's efforts at quality assurance. Each month personnel select five criteria for study. Two are chosen by nursing administrators and three others are chosen by nursing staff members. These are then used to evaluate unit care. For example, one criterion selected was "Each client on the unit wears an identification bracelet." Data are collected, scores tallied, and results shared with the staff. If results do not meet the institution's goal, unit nurses are involved in the problem-solving that follows.

Determination of the target population is part of the topic selection process. Audits can be of a general nature, including, for example, all surgical clients or all clients with the nursing diagnosis, pain. They can also focus on clients within a specific group, such as cholecystectomy clients or surgical clients who develop ineffective airway clearance.

Identify Standards and Criteria. Once a topic or problem is selected for evaluation, specific standards must be identified. Standards define the ideal. They are used as a basis to which evaluators compare the structure, process, or outcomes being evaluated. Sources for the development of standards include research findings, professional literature, professional organizations, and legal decisions.

Nursing standards describe nursing practice ideals for a particular institution or agency. The ANA has developed standards for practice that have subsequently become a baseline for determining client care standards in many health care agencies.[2] Besides being used to evaluate the quality and appropriateness of client care, the defining of nursing standards provides for the defense of client care practices should the need arise and promotes research to improve nursing practice.[5]

Standards are broad statements. Criteria quantify the standard; they are measurable characteristics related to the standards. The process of developing criteria from standards for quality assurance is the same as that used in the planning phase of the client process when evaluation criteria are derived from desired outcomes. Without measurable characteristics that can be used to interpret standards, the quality assurance program cannot be consistently applied.

The audit criteria and standards are made even more specific by determining expected compliance levels. An expected compliance level defines the desired degree of attainment of criteria and standards. It can be expressed as the percentage of the time that the criterion could be expected to be met.[15] For example, a 100-percent compliance level might be expected for the criterion "postsurgical clients being discharged from the hospital can verbalize symptoms indicating a need to call the physician." A lower compliance level may be deemed appropriate for other criteria.

Collect Data. Data collection is fundamental to the quality assurance process. Important questions to consider regarding data collection are: Who will be responsible for gathering the data? When will data be collected? What tools will be used?

As stated earlier, peer review is the basis for the quality assurance process. Therefore, the people gathering data for each department within the agency are expected to be practitioners of the profession being evaluated. Auditors may be employees of the agency, people familiar with the agency, people who are not at all associated with it, or a combination of these. The type of group deemed most effective depends on the type of audit and the entity conducting it.

The timing of the data collection may be concurrent—that is, while a client is under the care of an agency—or retrospective, after a client has been discharged. In the early history of mandated quality assurance programs, most audits were retrospective. This type of audit has proved to be less than satisfactory as a sole method of evaluating care. The JCAHO, in particular, has shifted its emphasis in recent years to concurrent monitoring.[15] Whether a concurrent or retrospective audit is deemed appropriate will affect the choice of tools to gather data.

Data may be gathered through direct observation, questionnaires, client interviews, and chart reviews. Direct observation is one of the most reliable methods of data collection for concurrent evaluation of structure and process. Questionnaires and interviews also are useful tools for process evaluation and are useful for outcome evaluation, as well. Either could be used for concurrent or retrospective audits, but interviews are usually limited to concurrent audits because of cost constraints. Chart reviews (which include evaluation of client care plans) can be used to evaluate structure, process, or outcome. Chart review was the method of choice for retrospective evaluation for many years and can also be used in concurrent audits. It is particularly useful when data are gathered from a large number of clients.[15] Several processes for performing a chart review to evaluate quality of nursing practice have been developed, including those by Phaneuf, Jelink, and Wandelt and Ager. The advent of the Medicare Prospective Payment System (PPS) and Diagnostic Related Groups (DRGs) has resulted in the development of new instruments as well.[20]

The most recent innovation for chart review involves the use of computers. Agencies using some hospital information systems can build subroutines into the system that will audit client care plans and documentation of care.[21]

Interpret Data. After data collection has been completed, the information that has been gathered is analyzed. Data are compared to the preselected standards. If discrepancies exist between the data and the measurement criteria related to the evaluation standards, then variables influencing the discrepancy must be identified. In a nursing audit, for example, staffing levels, method of care delivery, availability of equipment and materials, as well as competency of individual nurses are among the possible factors contributing to an unsatisfactory audit. The analysis of data concludes with proposals for action to correct the identified discrepancies.

Select and Implement Solutions. Because quality assurance implies not only evaluating health care but also taking corrective action, implementing change to correct the discrepancies or eliminate the factors that hinder the rendering of quality client care is an important next step. Choosing the best approach may be difficult, as the possible contributing variables are usually complex. In addition, cost–benefit ratios are a major factor to consider when selecting solutions.

Reevaluate. The last step in quality assurance is a reevaluation to determine the effectiveness of the change or changes that were made. Effective quality assurance programs coordinate the detection and resolution of problems and result in efficient, quality care.

The parallels between evaluation processes at the individual client level and at the institutional level should be clear from the above discussion. In both cases, participants use similar evaluation activities and strive for comparable goals, knowing that determined successful efforts will affect not only the client's welfare but that of health care facilities.

SUMMARY

Client care plans illustrate the nursing process in action. They are vital to promoting continuity, efficiency, and quality of client care. Making the care plan is a collaborative process in which nurse and client identify the focus of each component of the plan: outcomes, nursing implementation, and evaluation criteria. Writing the care plan involves selection of precise language for communicating the plan. A variety of resources, including colleagues, nursing research, and standard care plans, are available to assist nurses in developing an individualized client care plan.

Making and writing a client care plan involves setting priorities based on the urgency of the problem, client desires, situational variables, and resources available to client and nurse. Desired outcomes need to be developed after priorities have been determined. Desired outcomes can be long- or short-term. They describe the hoped-for client status as a result of the nursing care rendered. The selection of appropriate nursing implementation is the next step in the care planning process. Implementation encompasses all the nursing activities that assist the client to achieve the desired outcomes.

Evaluating care plans is a critical aspect of the nursing process that plays a role in the planning portion, when evaluation criteria are established, as well as being a separate step in the nursing process. The evaluation phase of the nursing process involves monitoring, analyzing, deciding, and collaborating with the client. Evaluation can be formative, summative, or retrospective.

Reporting and recording are ways of communicating evaluation at the individual client level. Reporting is oral communication whose purpose is to share information about a client's progress. It can be situational or structured. Recording is written communication conveyed through a client's record, which is also called the chart.

Evaluation at the institutional level occurs through the quality assurance program, or audit. This is a planned and systematic evaluation of the care given to a group of clients. It can focus on structure, process, or outcomes of care. Regardless of whether evaluation occurs at the individual client level or at the institutional level, the result is quality client care and an increased commitment of nurses to the outcomes of their practice.

Collaboration is essential to individualized care planning. Collaborative planning emphasizes shared responsibility for client health and recognizes clients' power in decision-making related to health and health care. It enhances trust, demonstrates respect for clients, and communicates caring. Collaborative planning reflects clients' beliefs and values, as well as the knowledge and ethics of nurses.

REFERENCES

1. *The Joint Commission Guide to Quality Assurance.* Chicago: Joint Commission on Accreditation of Healthcare Organizations; 1988.
2. *ANA Standards for Nursing Practice.* Kansas City, MO: American Nurses' Association; 1973.
3. Mayers MG. *A Systematic Approach to the Nursing Care Plan.* Norwalk, CT: Appleton-Century-Crofts; 1983.
4. Williamson J. Mutual interaction: A model of nursing practice. *Nurs Outlook.* 1981;29:104–107.
5. Patterson C. Standards of patient care: The Joint Commission focus on nursing quality assurance. *Nurs Clin North Am.* 1988; 23:625–637.
6. Benner P. *From Novice to Expert: Excellence and Power in Clinical Nursing Practice.* Menlo Park, CA: Addison-Wesley; 1986.
7. Itano J. A comparison of the clinical judgment process in experienced registered nurses and student nurses. *J Nurs Ed.* 1989;28:120–125.
8. McFarland GK, McFarlane EA. *Nursing Diagnosis and Intervention.* St. Louis: Mosby; 1989.
9. Allen CV. *Comprehending the Nursing Process.* Norwalk, CT: Appleton & Lange, 1991.
10. Thelen LA, Davie JK, Urden LD. *Critical Care Nursing: Diagnosis and Management.* St. Louis: Mosby; 1990.
11. Carpenito L. *Nursing Diagnosis: Application to Clinical Practice.* 3rd ed. Philadelphia: Lippincott; 1989.
12. Byer E. Charting: The RN's best courtroom defense. *Calif Nurs Rev.* 1990;40–45.
13. Bergerson S. More about charting with a jury in mind. *Nursing 88.* 1988;51–56.
14. Cohen MR. Play it safe: Don't use those abbreviations. *Nursing 87.* 1987;46–47.
15. Iyer P, Taptich B, Bernocchi-Losey D. *Nursing Process and Nursing Diagnosis.* 2nd ed. Philadelphia: Saunders; 1991.
16. Maciorowski LF, Larson E, Keane A. Quality assurance, evaluate thyself. *J Nurs Admin.* 1985;15:38–40.
17. Gordon M. *Nursing Diagnosis: Process and Application.* New York: McGraw-Hill; 1985.
18. Zander K. Nursing case management: Strategic management of cost and quality outcomes. *J Nurs Adm.* 1988;18:23–30.
19. Peters DA, Pearlson J. Clinical evaluation: Research or quality assurance? *J Nurs Qual Assur.* 1989;3:1–6.
20. Yura H, Walsh M. *The Nursing Process.* 5th ed. Norwalk, CT: Appleton & Lange; 1988.
21. Ozbolt J, Abraham IL, Schultz S. Nursing information systems. In: Shortliffe EM, Perrault LE, eds. *Medical Informatics: Computer Applications in Health Care.* Reading, MA: Addison-Wesley; 1990.

BIBLIOGRAPHY

Alfaro R. *Application of Nursing Process: A Step by Step Guide.* Philadelphia: Lippincott; 1986.

American Association of Critical Care Nurses. *Outcome Standards for Nursing Care of the Critically Ill.* Laguna Niguel, CA: AACN; 1990.

Botsford J. Implementing outcome standards: A planning strategy. *AORN J.* 1984;40:572–575.

Brucker M, Reedy N. Quality assurance—An overview. *J Obstet Gynecol Neonatal Nurs.* 1977;9–13.

Cassidy DA, Friesen M. QA: Applying JCAHO's generic model. *Nurs Manag.* 1990;21:22–27.

Cushing M. The legal side: Failure to communicate. *Am J Nurs.* 1982;82:1597.

Fredette S. Common diagnostic errors. *Nurse Ed.* 1988;13:31–35.

Green E, Katz J. A quality assurance tool that works overtime. *RN.* 1989;52:30–31.

Hodges LC, Icenhour ML. Measuring the quality of nursing care. In: McCloskey JC, Grace HK, eds. *Current Issues in Nursing.* St. Louis: Mosby; 1990:242–248.

Jones J. Clinical reasoning in nursing. *J Adv Nurs.* 1987;13:185–192.

Klaassens E. Improving teaching for thinking. *Nurse Ed.* 1988;13: 15–19.

Krenz M. Linking nursing diagnosis, quality assurance, and nursing standards. *J Adv Med-Surg Nurs.* 1989;1:53–61.

Krenz M, Karlick B, Kiniry S. A nursing diagnosis based model: Guiding nursing practice. *J Nurs Adm.* 1989;19:32–36.

Krevitz L. A quality assurance model for nursing. *Nurs Manag.* 1987;18:82–84.

Lovett R. Clinical practice evaluation in an oncology setting. *J Nurs Qual Assur.* 1989;3:24–35.

McElroy D, Herbelin K. Writing a better patient care plan. *Nursing 88.* 1988;50–51.

Miller V, Rew L. Analysis and intuition: The need for both in nursing education. *J Nurs Ed.* 1989;28:84–86.

Moriconi D. Quality assurance in diagnosis-based nursing practice. In: Miller E, ed. *How to Make Nursing Diagnosis Work: Administrative and Clinical Strategies.* Norwalk, CT: Appleton & Lange; 1989: 175–194.

Pardue S. Decision-making skills and critical thinking ability among associate degree, diploma, baccalaureate, and master's prepared nurses. *J Nurs Ed.* 1987;26:354–360.

Phaneuf M. *The Nursing Audit and Self-Regulation in Nursing Practice.* New York: Appleton-Century-Crofts; 1976.

Polaski A, Vitron S, Carrier B, Carlson D. A multidimensional teaching-learning strategy for the nursing process. *Nurse Ed.* 1988;13:19–23.

Short NM, Bair L. Standards of care: Practicing what we preach. *Nurs Manag.* 1990;21:32–39.

Smith-Marker CG. The marker model: A hierarchy for nursing standards. *J Nurs Qual Assur.* 1987;1:7–20.

Smith-Marker CG. The marker umbrella model for quality assurance: Monitoring and evaluating professional practice. *J Nurs Qual Assur.* 1987;1:52–63.

Tappen R. Critical thinking. In: Tappen RM, ed. *Nursing Leadership and Management: Concepts and Practice.* 2nd ed. Philadelphia: Davis; 1988:125–133.

Tennenhouse D. *Risk Prevention Skills.* Danville, CA: Contemporary Forums; 1988

Tonges MC, Bradley MJ, Brett JL. Implementing the ten-step monitoring and evaluating process in nursing practice. *Qual Rev Bull.* 1990;16:264–269.

Tribulski J. Nursing diagnosis: Waste of time or valued tool? *RN.* 1988;51:30–34.

Wyszewianski L. Quality of care: Past achievements and future challenges. *Inquiry.* 1988;25:13–22.

CHAPTER 19

Collaborating with the Health Care Team

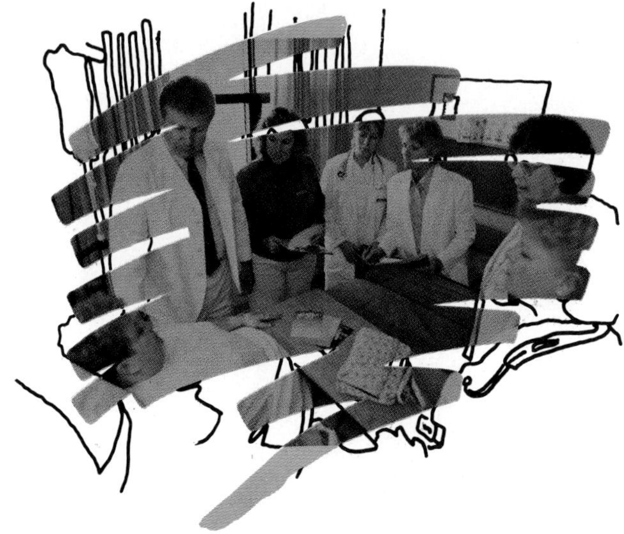

Behavioral Objectives

Upon completion of this chapter, the student will be able to:

1. Describe the components of a team.
2. Describe the three stages of group development and outline several principles of group dynamics.
3. Outline the role and complementary functions of members of the health care team.
4. Discuss the need for collaboration among health care professionals.
5. Identify the aims of collaboration within the health care team.
6. Describe the complementary nature of medical and nursing diagnoses.
7. Discuss two factors that determine the nature of a collaborative professional relationship.
8. List modes of collaboration seen in health care settings.
9. Compare the roles of the initiator and maintainer in relation to group dynamics.
10. Explain how nurses can take on the role of initiator and maintainer in the health care team.
11. List four behaviors that nurses can use to facilitate collaboration of team members and participation of clients in the decision-making process.
12. Describe the importance of clients' participation as a member of the health care team.
13. Identify potential obstacles to collaboration among health care team members.
14. Discuss intrinsic and extrinsic factors that facilitate collaboration among team members.
15. Describe potential ethical issues related to collaboration.

KEY TERMS

accountability
advocacy
assertiveness
authoritarian
autocratic
autonomy
cohesiveness
collaboration
consolidated client record
consultation
democratic
detente
group dynamics
health care team conference
laissez-faire
risk taking
team
territoriality

For many years, health care professionals from many disciplines have worked side-by-side in a team approach to health care. A health care team is a group of professionals with clearly defined roles and different kinds of expertise who work together on common goals while providing client care. Collaboration is the highest form of the team approach. A collaborative health care team considers clients as central members of the team and integrates the contributions of all team members to provide the best possible care.

A collaborative relationship requires communication and mutual respect among team members. Collaboration among health care team members facilitates effective client care by encouraging information sharing, efficient and comprehensive care planning, and continuity of client care. Collaboration is a model for communication that promotes joint problem solving by health team members. A collaborative relationship develops when each team member recognizes and accepts the unique contributions the others make in planning and providing care.

This chapter explores the nature of teamwork in health care, the process of team building, and collaboration as the essence of teamwork in health care settings. It examines the special characteristics of collaborative teamwork, modes of collaboration in health care settings, and factors that influence the development and maintenance of collaborative relationships in health care.

WHAT IS A TEAM?

A **team** is defined by *Webster's New Collegiate Dictionary* as "a number of persons associated together in work or activity."

Richardson, an authority on team building, notes that the term *team* often describes a group of individuals with a particular goal toward which they strive.[1] This is in contrast to a *group,* which is defined simply as a number of persons or things gathered or classified together.

Most of the literature on the subject of teamwork conveys that a team is an identifiable unit with clear separation of roles and responsibilities among its members. The team is expected to have decision-making capabilities and a system of communication.

Characteristics of a team include:

1. a composition of two or more members
2. an interplay between members
3. common objectives
4. common rules
5. specific roles and responsibilities of members
6. a sense of cohesion among members[2]

This generic view of a team is a helpful starting point in understanding how a team approach may be applied to the health care setting.

The concept of team is common to many aspects of life.[3] For instance, in various sports, individual athletes function as a team. Family members often function as a team when working on home maintenance tasks. Each member may have a different role to play, but all work toward a mutual goal. Striving to achieve their aim is what draws individual members closer. Each member's contribution to the team is looked on with equal importance. The underlying feeling of solidarity is often characterized by the term *team spirit.*

Nature of a Collaborative Team

In a collaborative team, decision making is shared among all team members. In a collaborative health care team, for example, the group leader takes a democratic approach, including the contributions of the client and other health care professionals as part of the dynamics of the team. The members of a collaborative team work interdependently to achieve goals and make decisions. In noncollaborative teams, leaders make decisions. This is referred to as an autocratic style of leadership. The autocratic leader discourages creative thought and collaboration among team members.

> **IMPLICATIONS FOR PROFESSIONAL COLLABORATION**
>
> **Collaborative Teamwork**
>
> In any endeavor, a team is a group of people with clearly defined goals and different expertise who are focused on a common activity. In the health professions, that activity is client care. The collaborative team is the highest form of team approach, in health care as well as in other pursuits. The collaborative team interacts in a collegial manner to share decision-making and planning activities. This contrasts with the traditional view of the team in which the leader makes all the decisions. The decisions that emerge from shared decision making are different from those that any single member might have made, but reflect the collective knowledge and various points of view of group members.

Group Dynamics

To understand how a team develops and functions, it is important to examine the concepts of group dynamics, group development, and styles of group leadership. Each of these affects the others and the group: the nature of group dynamics influences and is influenced by group leadership; the stage of group development has an effect on group dynamics and is affected by group dynamics; and so on. Because a team is one kind of group, the processes that characterize group development and functioning also underlie team building, discussed in a later section.

Group dynamics (or group process) refers to the patterns and activities of interaction and communication among group members. Individuals work and interact differently when they are alone than when they are in a group. Behavioral scientists have found that group work tends to increase motivation and stimulate creative problem solving.[4]

In one particular example, a hospital was having difficulty in facilitating timely discharge of clients from medical care units because individual health care professionals were not communicating discharge plans among themselves or to the clients. To find a solution, a representative team of health care professionals was formed. Members shared their perspectives of the problem and agreed to work collaboratively on a solution. The team's common goal was timely preparation of clients for discharge. By collaborating in the problem-solving process, the team members felt they had all contributed toward the solution and were thus more motivated to support the program implementation.

A factor that significantly influences the dynamics of a group is climate. Climate is the perceived mood among group members. In the positive climate of a collaborative group, mutual trust and support are enhanced. Cohesiveness, or the degree of commitment to common goals, grows in a supportive group environment. Such a climate enhances both individual contributions to the group and group productivity.

Activities such as relating, facilitating, influencing, and deciding are part of group dynamics. Group members may demonstrate each activity in a variety of ways, some of which are listed in Box 19–1.

- Relating refers to the use of modes of communication, both verbal and nonverbal. Health care team members use communication techniques such as questioning, interviewing, and reflecting on pertinent client information. Relating is also important in developing and maintaining the relationships among group members.
- Facilitating fosters relationships in the group and supports the group in accomplishing its tasks. A health care team facilitates productivity of team members by improv-

BOX 19–1. GROUP ACTIVITIES AND BEHAVIORS

Relating
- Demonstrate ability to interact effectively with other group members.
- Impart knowledge and information.
- Discuss and share goals and expectations.
- Explain group rules and norms.
- Elicit information from other group members.

Facilitating
- Intervene to improve communication.
- Initiate and support contacts with group members.
- Be sensitive to the impact of control on group behavior.
- Support roles of group members.
- Foster positive relationships within the group.

Influencing
- Understand the meaning and effects of power within the group.
- Express self clearly and logically.
- Support effective communication among group members.
- Modify behavior of self and group members.
- Negotiate with group members.

Deciding
- Use a variety of resources to gather information.
- Use effective problem-solving techniques.
- Apply decision-making models.
- Predict potential consequences of actions.
- Include all group members in decision making.

ing group communication or supporting members' roles.

- Influencing means that group members use their understanding of such concepts as power and control and their effects on group dynamics. For instance, members of the health care team may use behaviors such as negotiating, delegating, and bargaining to influence the actions and decisions of the team.
- Deciding is the use of problem-solving methods to reach a group decision. For example, health care team members gather information from various sources and then make informed decisions about a client care plan.

Factors Influencing Group Dynamics. Several factors influence group dynamics (Fig. 19–1): type of group, stage of group development, power and authority, rules and norms, cohesiveness, decision-making method, and style of group leadership. The influence of each factor varies in different groups. In one group, the balance of power may be an important issue, whereas in another group, the development of rules and norms may be the most influential factor.

Type of Group. Groups are usually categorized as primary or secondary. Primary groups are those that form an individual's informal social support network, including family and friends. Usually, primary groups are long-lasting and members have strong affiliations with one another. Secondary groups, which are more formal in structure and purpose, develop to perform a specific task. The health care team is a secondary group.

Group Development. Groups develop through a succession of stages, just as individuals pass through life stages. In groups, as in people, the rate of development varies. In one group, some stages may occur simultaneously; in another, development may move backward. A three-stage process of group development is illustrated in Figure 19–2.

In the first stage, dependence, members get to know each other. At this time, members may have individual agendas, because group cohesion has not yet occurred. Communication also is being established and may be tenuous until trusting relationships are developed. For instance, health care professionals form individual views of clients' needs in this stage of a health care team's development. Similarly, clients may find it difficult to question a decision made by health care professionals without their participation.

The second stage, independence, is characterized by the development of a group identity, group structure, and roles of members. At this point, care providers begin to understand clients' priorities and include clients in interactions. Thus learning to know clients facilitates other team members' recognition of them as important members of the health care team.

During the final stage, interdependence, the group moves toward its goals, thereby stimulating productivity. In this stage, the health care team acts to meet clients' needs

BUILDING NURSING KNOWLEDGE

What is an Interdisciplinary Team?

Mariano C. The case for interdisciplinary collaboration. *Nurs Outlook.* 1989; 37(6):285–288.

The importance of interdisciplinary collaboration has been widely expounded, but little emphasis has been placed on interdisciplinary education. This may reflect a lack of understanding of what interdisciplinary teamwork is. Mariano endeavors to describe interdisciplinary teamwork and how it can be facilitated.

After reviewing a wide range of literature on the subject, Mariano notes that an interdisciplinary team is more than a collection of people. It has structure, direction, an identification, and "group energy." Clear, specific goals, member consensus regarding priorities, and agreement on the action to be taken all enhance interdisciplinary teamwork; goal conflict interferes with it. Goal conflict arises out of value differences that create disagreement about objectives or how to achieve them.

Role conflict, fostered by overlapping competencies and role preconceptions, is another problem. A thorough knowledge of one's own discipline is essential to see how that discipline contributes to the whole. Team members who feel secure and competent professionally can communicate their discipline's strengths, limitations, and contributions. Interdisciplinary decision making requires an explicit definition of the problem, clarity of member roles, generation of options and alternatives, and commitment to action with specified responsibilities.

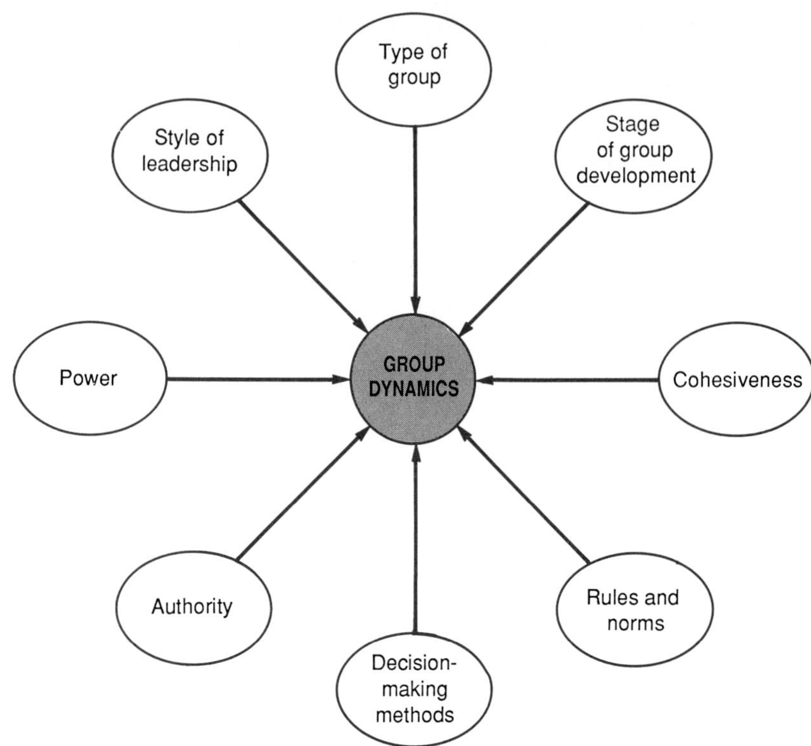

Figure 19–1. Factors influencing group dynamics.

and actively seeks client participation in decision making. Clients benefit from the collaborative efforts and mutual goal setting of the health care team at this stage.

Power and Authority. Power and authority are two factors that influence group dynamics. Power is the ability to influence the actions or behavior of others. In many cases, power is achieved by virtue of one's position. An individual in a position of leadership usually carries authority, the right to command and make decisions.[5] Power and authority are not the same, although they are related. Authority connotes an individual's right or responsibility to take charge; power relates to an individual's ability to move the group toward its goals. One member of a group may be the designated authority figure, but this person may not have the power to influence the group's decisions.

Power may also be conferred on an individual whom the group views as an expert. In such cases, knowledge is thought of as equal to power. Some power is obtained through coercion. Coercion may move a group toward its goals, but often at the cost of negative feelings among group members.

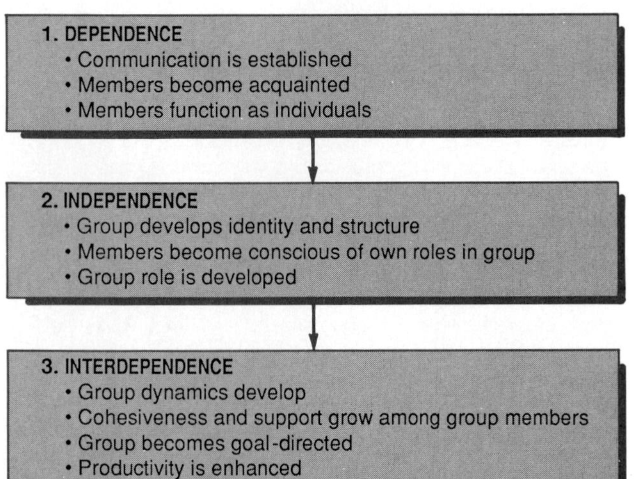

Figure 19–2. Stages of group development.

Rules and Norms. Rules and norms are sets of standards that affect the behavior and attitudes of the group. Rules are usually formal statements of appropriate and inappropriate behavior for group members. For example, standards of practice are rules that guide health care professionals as they carry out their duties and responsibilities in providing prudent client care. In contrast, norms are usually unwritten rules developed by a group to facilitate conformity among its members. For the health care team, norms may focus on such things as acceptable relationships among health care professionals or the way to address clients. Rules and norms differ from one group to another, so individuals who move from one group to another often have to learn new standards.

Norms may be explicit or implicit. Explicit norms may be presented to new members verbally or in writing when they join a group. Implicit norms are often less clear and may not be expressed until there is a violation of the norm. For instance, a nurse may be accustomed to taking a lunch

IMPLICATIONS FOR PROFESSIONAL COLLABORATION

Interdependence

A collaborative health care team is unique because it recognizes clients as participating members of the team. All teams go through several phases of development: dependence, independence, and interdependence. Interdependence is the final stage in which the team moves toward its goals. In becoming interdependent, the collaborative health care team is unusual because clients, as members of the team, are included in the decisions made. This aspect of interdependence is particularly important because clients' participation is often helpful in clarifying the team's objectives and because clients benefit from the opportunity to influence the decisions that affect their health.

break at 12:30 each day. She goes to work on a new unit, where the group members have an understanding that breaks are to be scheduled around client meals and care. This was never explicitly stated to the new nurse, but she gradually learns through other members' behavior that she must conform to the group's norms. One way to avoid confrontations on such issues is for group members to ask questions to elicit information about norms.

Cohesiveness. **Cohesiveness** refers to the degree of togetherness or bonding among group members. Cohesiveness is directly related to the members' level of satisfaction with the group and the group's goals, actions, and outcomes. In turn, cohesiveness influences group process and productivity. Cohesiveness is enhanced when members feel they are an important part of the group, that their contributions are valued, and that the group's work is purposeful.

Decision-making Methods. Decision-making methods differ among groups. In general, decision making involves the evaluation of several possible alternatives. Groups make decisions in several ways. For example, one group may use the process of consensus in reaching decisions. That is, members present various sides of an issue and discuss the alternatives until agreement is reached. All members support the final decision because they feel that their ideas were appreciated and their suggestions taken into account. Collaborative teams usually reach decisions by consensus. Additional information on decision making is presented in Chapter 15.

Styles of Group Leadership. Another important consideration in examining group process and development is leadership. Lippitt[6] suggested that a leader's function is to help the group members:

- decide on goals
- focus on effective goal-centered modes of group process
- use resources efficiently
- evaluate productivity
- think creatively
- learn from past experiences

A leader also should be able to delegate some responsibilities to other group members as appropriate.

One of the most widely described categorization systems of leadership styles was developed by White and Lippitt.[7] They described three general styles of leadership: autocratic, democratic, and laissez-faire. Characteristics of groups under various styles of leadership are summarized in Table 19–1.

In general, the **autocratic** leader makes all the decisions for the group; group members are kept "in the dark." In some situations, leaders may elicit suggestions from group members, but autocratic leaders use little or none of this input in making decisions. Autocratic leaders usually set the rules and norms for the group and hold all the power.

Under an autocratic leader, a group's level of cohesiveness and morale are low. Scapegoating of one member, that is, blaming the group's failure or poor morale unjustly on one individual, is common. The group's productivity may be high with close supervision by the leader. A health care example of autocratic leadership is a physician or another health care professional who views clients paternalistically. If health care professionals identify goals and make decisions for clients, clients may not choose to follow the treatment regimen. For example, a physician may prescribe an antihypertensive medication for a client, informing the client that he must take the drug twice daily. The client experiences dizziness, nausea, and dry mouth after 2 days on

TABLE 19–1. CHARACTERISTICS OF GROUPS UNDER VARIOUS STYLES OF LEADERSHIP

	Leadership Style		
Members' Characteristics	**Autocratic**	**Democratic**	**Laissez-Faire**
Level of cohesiveness	Low	High	Low
Level of morale	Low	High	Low
Productivity level	May be high	High	Low
Level of satisfaction	Low	High	Low
Level of independence	Low	High	Varies
Level of participation in decision making	Low	High	Low
Responsibility	Leader-centered	Member-centered	Noncentered

the drug. He avoids contacting the physician regarding these side effects, because he believes the physician to be an authority but may stop taking the drug because of the discomfort. Because the physician is directing his care, the client is unwilling to question her decisions.

The **democratic** leader supports group members' active participation in decision making. Because all members' ideas and opinions are included, creative thinking is stimulated. Individual members feel a high level of cohesiveness and morale. Members' satisfaction is also high, which has a positive effect on productivity. Democratic leadership in health care involves mutual client-practitioner goal setting and decision making about strategies to meet goals. With this approach, adherence to the treatment plan is likely, because clients have invested energy in developing the plan. Moreover, they are more inclined to confer with providers about difficulties they experience with the treatment, because their previous input was valued. A physician using democratic leadership would explain potential side effects of the antihypertensive medication to the client and elicit his or her concerns regarding the treatment regimen. After experiencing an episode of dizziness and nausea, the client would probably communicate with the physician, who might then consult a pharmacist to determine an alternative drug with fewer side effects.

In the **laissez-faire** leadership style, neither the leader nor the group takes responsibility for decisions or actions because the leader feels comfortable in allowing things to develop on their own. Group work tends to remain undone because the group members are unclear about the group's purpose and goals. Members feel a lack of cohesiveness and experience low morale. Because they do not understand what is expected of them, they may feel unsatisfied and express frustration. The leader and group members may become apathetic, and decision making may disintegrate. Productivity is low. This form of leadership may occur when a health care team cannot focus on mutual client goals because of lack of direction by a determined team leader or when individuals' workloads prohibit effective group dynamics and leadership.

Factors that Interfere with Successful Group Dynamics. Factors that hamper a group may be categorized as intrapersonal, intragroup, and interpersonal. These factors can influence the group at any point in its development.

Intrapersonal factors include factors peculiar to one member that affect the entire group. For example, a member may have personal problems that hamper the individual's ability to participate in the group. A member may also hold personal beliefs that conflict with the group's goals. In addition, any change in the group's composition, such as addition or loss of members, may alter the group's dynamics.

Intragroup factors are those that relate to group dynamics. For example, as a result of a struggle for power by group members, the group may become divided. Emphasis may be placed on the power struggle, rather than on the work at hand, thus hindering the development of a collaborative environment.

Interpersonal factors relate to communication among group members and include personality conflicts, prejudices, and ineffective communication.

Team Building

Team building is the development of a group of individuals into a cohesive, effective team that can accomplish specific goals.[8] It is important to understand that not all groups are teams. Not all characteristics of a team apply to a group. For example, a group may not have formalized specific roles and responsibilities for its members and may lack the sense of cohesiveness characteristic of teams. Team building requires the development of trust and a team identity, productive growth, clearly determined goals, and mutual decision making among all team members.

The stages of team building are essentially the same as those of group development, although specific activities in each stage may differ because of the differences between teams and groups. Farley and Stoner propose a four-step model of team building in which the second and third stages correspond to the independence stage of group development, discussed earlier.[9] Table 19–2 identifies typical member behaviors and tasks, as well as team tasks and ideal outcomes for each of the four stages of team building.

A Team Approach to Health Care Delivery

The main purpose of a health care team is to establish an effective process to achieve specific goals related to health care delivery. Goals may include providing comprehensive client care, teaching, implementing a program of education or research, or developing a model of clinical practice.

Londey describes three types of health care teams.[10] The first type has a specific set of rules equally applied to all members, as well as a common goal. By this definition, the hospital as a whole may be considered a team. The goal of the hospital is to provide quality health care to all clients. All employees must follow certain hospital policies to meet that standard. A second kind of team is formed in circumstances in which management of a group is more productive than managing individuals. This type of group is often used in instructional situations, such as a classroom or a clinical rotation for nursing students.

The third type of team is formed to enhance the efficiency of the team members. The health care team is an example of this type of team. When the team approach is used in health care delivery, the team's common goal is to meet the client's needs. In the process of building a team, a sense of cohesion develops among team members. In a collaborative health care team, the client is considered an integral member who actively participates in decision making.

The team approach to health care delivery has been advocated by medicine and nursing. In 1980, the American College of Physicians approved the Institute of Medicine's recommendation that the team approach to health care delivery be taught in medical schools.[11] In the same year, the

TABLE 19–2. STAGES OF TEAM BUILDING

Stage	Behaviors	Member Tasks	Team Tasks	Ideal Outcomes
Orientation	Caution with opinions Politeness Ambiguous relations Lack of focus	Learn expectations of self Make social comparisons Question belonging to group	Develop trust in others Define boundaries	Develop acquaintances Identities begin to form Little productivity
Adaptation	Develop social mechanisms to differentiate members Team identity beginning	Discovering roles of self	Structure and climate conducive to team work developing Team identity beginning	Group roles developing Developing common language
Emergence	Bargaining Form alliances Power struggles Disagreement Defend opinions	Finding identity as team member Able to confront and collaborate	Determine who is in control Determine how control is exercised Rules and norms	More comfortable with differences "We" identity
Working	Complementary relationships	Honest disclosure Individual decisions and solutions negotiated	Decision making Planning Productivity	Cohesiveness among members Acceptance of feedback

Adapted from Farley MJ, Stoner MH. The nurse executive and interdisciplinary team building. Nurs Admin Quart. *1989; 13(2):24–30, 26.*

American Nurses' Association (ANA) described the ideal approach to the development of teamwork between nurses and physicians as a "collegial, collaborative joint practice."[12] In recent years, a considerable body of literature on teamwork and collaboration has developed, as discussed below.

■ WHAT IS COLLABORATIVE TEAMWORK IN HEALTH CARE?

The essence of teamwork in health care settings is collaboration among health care professionals and between health care professionals and clients. The ANA's *Social Policy Statement* stresses the importance of partnership as a segment of collaboration "with recognition and acceptance of separate and combined spheres of activity" (p. 7).[12] The roles of health care team members may differ, but each member shares in the responsibility of meeting clients' health care needs.

Styles describes collaboration as "a potent force to achieve . . . professional aims."[13] As the basis of teamwork, collaboration encourages:

- information sharing
- efficient care planning
- comprehensive care planning
- prevention of complications
- continuity of care

By definition, collaborative teamwork develops from collegial interactions in which decision making is shared among team members to achieve a common purpose. In some health care teams, decision making may be reserved for one or two key members and may not include client participation. Thus, not all health care teams are collaborative.

Types of Working Relationships in Health Care Teams

The ANA's *Social Policy Statement* addresses three types of working relationships among health professionals (Fig. 19–3). In the first type of relationship, **authoritarian,** the individual in the position of authority or power gives direction and makes all decisions for others. This is similar to the autocratic leadership style described earlier in this chapter. Clients have little or no participation in decision making, passively accepting directions from health care providers. Communication tends to be fragmented and the quality of care is potentially jeopardized.

In the second type of relationship, **detente,** there is an accepted balance of authority between individuals with some degree of mutuality regarding goals (Fig. 19–3B). The mutual goal of the health care professionals is to meet the client's needs. Each professional accepts and recognizes the others' roles and responsibilities. Each is governed by his or her own practice realm within accepted standards of practice of each profession. Detente is similar to the paternalistic or traditional model, in that the client's participation in decision making is still not recognized by the caregivers. Detente may be considered a precursor to a collaborative relationship.

Collaboration, the third type of relationship, stems from a recognition of the unique contributions of each member in a working relationship. Collaboration means working together toward common goals in a cooperative manner and sharing responsibility for problem solving and decision making. Clients are equal members of the collaborative health care team (Fig. 19–3C). All members of the team interact, so that communication is encouraged. This facilitates comprehensive, integrated care. All team members share responsibilities for decision making.

In reality, no working relationship is purely of one

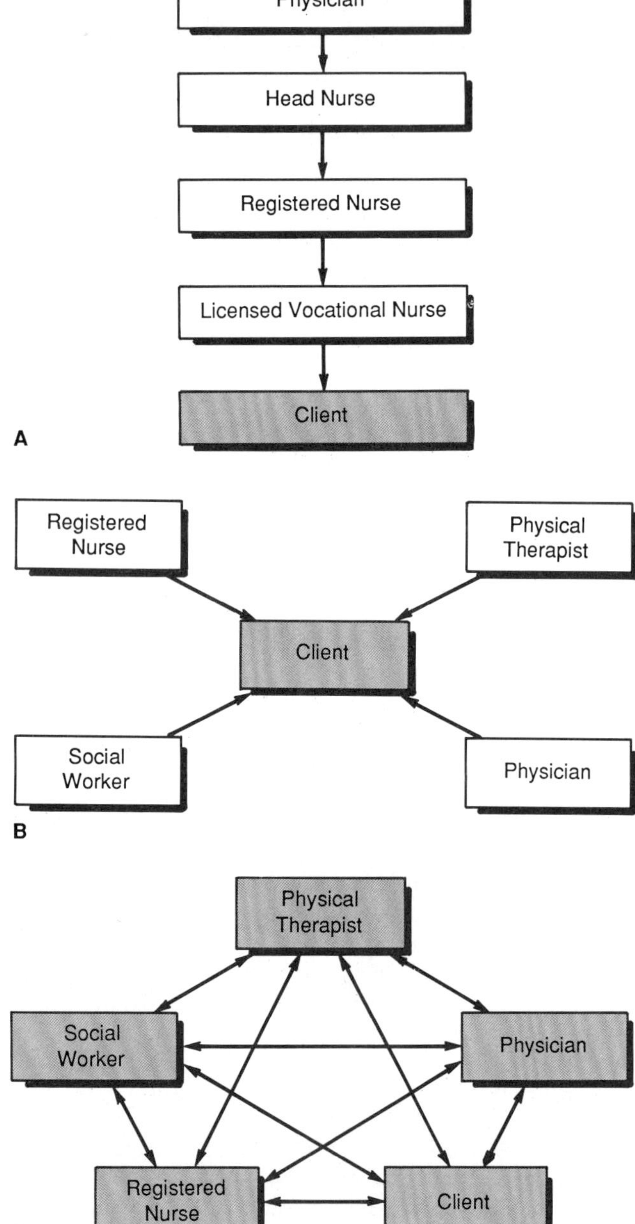

Figure 19–3. Three types of working relationships among health care professionals. **A.** Authoritarian relationship. **B.** Detente relationship. **C.** Collaborative relationship.

type. Rather, working relationships tend to exhibit characteristics of all three types, most commonly of the latter two. It is important for nurses to be able to assess working relationships with their clients and other health team members to facilitate collegial interactions and effective goal attainment.

■ THE NEED FOR COLLABORATIVE TEAMWORK

The need for a team approach to health care delivery is rooted in the complexities of the health care system and current health care trends. Over the past 30 years, changes in health care such as technological developments, the growth of specialization, and shortages of health care professionals have been the impetus for the advancement of teamwork.

Advances in Technology

Technology is an extremely important factor in the evolution of the health care system. Advances in technology have enabled the health care team to better diagnose, treat, and rehabilitate clients with various forms of illness. With the developments in technology, there is a corresponding increase in specialization. As knowledge becomes more fragmented, there is a greater need for communication and collaboration among health care team members. For example, today's health care team relies on expert technicians to interpret various diagnostic findings. Consultation with specialists for diagnostic and treatment plans is common.

Specialization of Professionals

The continuing growth of specialization within the health care professions is a direct result of the increases in medical knowledge and in the complexity of client problems. A collaborative team approach facilitates coordination of care by health care professionals. Pluckhan remarks that "the alternative to working together is working alone, which is totally unrealistic in today's society."[14] If health care professionals and clients do not work together as a team, client care suffers.

Often, it is a health care professional who makes the decision to consult with one or more specialists to strengthen treatment decisions and who takes responsibility for coordinating a team approach to care. However, it is equally likely that a client makes the choice to seek care from several specialists for different health problems. For example, a client may see a cardiologist for a heart problem, a urologist for a prostate problem, and a nurse practitioner or family physician for minor ailments. In this case, the client is the key member on this team. Unless the client informs each of the providers about the care he or she gets from others, overlapping or contradictory treatment plans may be developed by each. If providers emphasize a collaborative approach to health care with individual clients, the clients are more likely to recognize the importance of their own active involvement as decision makers and communicators.

Shortages of Health Care Professionals

Shortages of health care professionals in some areas have also influenced the development of collaborative teamwork. A collaborative approach is efficient as well as effective for guiding use of scarce health care resources because it eliminates duplication of effort, averts inappropriate services or treatments that may be considered when there are no clear, mutually defined treatment goals, and fosters each team member's contributing to team goals according to his or her specific professional preparation and role on the team.

MEMBERS OF THE HEALTH CARE TEAM

Each member of the health care team differs in role, experience, and educational preparation. The following section describes how the client and various health care professionals function as collaborative team members.

The Client

The overall goal of the health team is to facilitate clients' achievement of optimal health. With a collaborative philosophy, this can be accomplished only when clients are central members of the health care team. Clients bring a particular expertise and life experiences to the interaction with health care professionals. The ANA *Social Policy Statement* identifies the importance of clients' participation in health care:

> What is equally important is the growing realization that individuals, families, and groups have considerable responsibility for their personal health and for development of their potentials for achieving it. A public increasingly knowledgeable about health and health care systems is becoming more and more involved in related public and political decisions.[12]

In other words, clients have the right to participate in decisions related to their own well-being. Just as it is imperative for health care team members to exchange information, clients should also participate in information exchange throughout their care.[15] Ethically, each individual has a right to self-determination. That is, each client has the right to accept or reject health care, as well as to be a part of the decision-making process as a member of the health care team.

Clients vary in the degree to which they participate in health care decision making. Many consumers now question their physicians, nurses, and pharmacists freely regarding treatment and may choose not to follow directives. Researchers once labeled this behavior "noncompliance,"[16–18] but more recently, it has been deemed a form of "self-regulation" by which clients attempt to retain control of their own lives.[19] This definition is also in keeping with that used in the North American Nursing Diagnosis Association (NANDA) definition of noncompliance: a person's informed decision not to adhere to a health care recommendation. It is the responsibility of health care professionals to provide clients with information based on their distinct areas of expertise, so that clients are sufficiently well informed to participate in decision making.

IMPLICATIONS FOR PROFESSIONAL COLLABORATION

The Client as Team Member

The health care team is formed to enhance the efficiency and effectiveness of the members of the group. The team's common goals are focused on meeting the client's health care needs. Principles of group dynamics indicate that group structure is a factor in a group's ability to realize its objectives. Thus, in team health care delivery, and particularly in collaborative teamwork, the client is an integral member of the team. The client's participation in decision making serves to increase the efficiency of team communication and to enhance the likelihood that the plans that emerge will be effective within the context of the health supports and constraints the client faces in daily life.

The Physician

Physicians have traditionally been considered to have the most critical role in the health care system. The primary role of physicians is to diagnose, treat, and prevent disease. To accomplish this, physicians use treatment modalities such as medication and surgery, as well as make referrals for therapies provided by other professionals, such as respiratory therapists, physical therapists, and others.

Although the traditional perspective of the physician as leader of the health care team prevails in some places, it is becoming more common for physicians and other health care providers to participate as equals, each with different and important contributions to client health.

In 1970, the American Medical Association included a conceptual difference between the primary roles of physicians and nurses in its policy statement, *Medicine and Nursing in the 1970's*.[20] The physician's role was described as that of curing whereas the nurse's role was that of caring for clients. Although the same distinction is often made in statements written by nurses and is also a commonly held lay perception of physician and nurse roles, neither role is mutually exclusive in a collaborative relationship. "Caring" and "curing" are not opposite ends of a continuum nor mutually exclusive. Rather, physicians' and nurses' roles encompass both processes, but to differing degrees.

The Registered Nurse

In 1859, Florence Nightingale defined nursing as having "charge of the personal health of somebody. . ." and the nursing responsibility ". . . to put the patient in the best condition for nature to act upon him."[21] The promotion of clients' well-being is at the core of nursing care. Historically, a nurse's primary role has been regarded as providing consolation and assistance. The ANA's definition of nursing in its *Social Policy Statement* incorporates both the historical and contemporary conceptions of nursing: "Nursing is the diagnosis and treatment of human responses to actual or potential health problems."[12] Nursing diagnosis is a relatively contemporary concept (see Chap. 17). It is a means of identifying a client's particular response to illness, which reflects a broad range of physiological and psychological reactions. Nursing diagnoses form the basis for the nursing actions undertaken jointly with clients to alleviate problems.

Nursing has changed over the course of its history and it is continuing to change. Currently, nurses practice as generalists or specialists. Nurses in either role function collaboratively with other members of the health care team. Most nurses are generalists, providing comprehensive care to clients in hospitals, nursing homes, ambulatory care settings, industries, hospices, and private practice (see Chap. 1).

Nurse specialists provide care to clients who have specific care needs. Specialists have refined their expertise through advanced education and clinical experience. The additional knowledge base and expertise of nurse specialists facilitates collaboration. One way that nurse specialists collaborate is by sharing their knowledge and experience (Fig. 19–4).

The Physical and Occupational Therapists

Physical and occupational therapists assist clients to attain optimum musculoskeletal functioning after injury, illness, or surgery. Physical therapists prescribe specific exercises and therapies to strengthen muscles and prevent further loss of function. Occupational therapists help clients attain independence in activities of daily living. For example, an occupational therapist may help a client learn the use of special appliances for the home to enable the client to perform personal hygiene, dressing, or home maintenance chores.

Physical and occupational therapists work in hospitals, rehabilitation centers, long-term-care facilities, ambulatory care settings, and private practices. Many clients receive therapy in their homes. Physical and occupational therapists collaborate with the health care team by assessing client needs for rehabilitation, recommending exercises, specialized equipment, or environmental modifications, providing treatments, and evaluating client progress (Fig. 19–5).

BUILDING NURSING KNOWLEDGE

What is the Definition of Physician–Nurse Collaboration?

Baggs JG, Schmitt MH. Collaboration between nurses and physicians. *Image: J Nurs Scholarship.* 1988; 20(3):145–149.

Baggs and Schmitt review a wide variety of literature on the subject of collaboration. Their survey indicates that interdisciplinary health care teams who interact collegially and collaboratively are more efficient and effective and achieve improved client outcomes.

Baggs and Schmitt look at collaboration as nurses and physicians working cooperatively together, sharing responsibility for solving problems and making planning decisions. Key elements of collaboration are coordination, cooperation, and sharing. Cooperation implies planning and working together in a helpful way; however, being cooperative does not mean being unassertive. In fact, assertiveness is necessary for making the compromises that are part of collaboration.

Sharing is an important part of collaboration, goal setting, planning, problem solving, decision making, and responsibility. Consultation is a form of sharing, but it is different from the sharing involved in collaboration because it is limited to only the planning phase of client care.

BUILDING NURSING KNOWLEDGE

How Do Physicians View Nurses' Authority?

Katzman EM. Nurses' and physicians' perceptions of nursing authority. *J Professional Nurs.* 1989; 5(4):208–214.

Collaboration rests on the ability of health care team members to influence one another as they make decisions. Mutual influence generally implies a balance of power and authority in a relationship. Katzman notes that over the last several decades scholars have examined the power or lack of power of nurses to implement changes in their roles, particularly as those roles interface with the roles of physician co-workers. This study endeavors to identify whether there is consensus or conflict between nurses and physicians regarding the decision-making authority of nurses.

A survey, called the Authority in Nursing Roles Inventory, was completed by a sample of 110 mostly female nurses (98%) and 53 mostly male physicians (79%), all of whom were between 33 and 49 years of age. Items on the survey concerned nurses' authority to take responsibility for certain actions such as changing an inappropriate client diet, questioning inappropriate physician orders, deciding the frequency of vital sign measurements, teaching clients about health promotion, or answering clients' questions about medical treatment regimens.

Katzman found a significant difference between nurses and physicians on all items with respect to their perceptions of both current nursing practice and of ideal nursing practice. Nurses generally perceived themselves to have more authority to initiate health assessments, answer clients' questions about medical regimens and change clients' diets than did physicians, suggesting that many nurses do not seek discussion or recognition from physician co-workers before performing these roles. The two groups also disagreed about the amount of authority nurses should have in health policy making, client care decision making, and establishing standards of nursing care. Nurses were generally more dissatisfied with the status quo than were physicians.

The researchers concluded that there is a need for closer communication and greater consensus regarding the scope of nursing practice, and programs are necessary to aid all health care professionals to understand the link between quality, cost-effective health care, and the authority of nurses to function fully within their legal scope of practice.

The Social Worker

Social workers focus primarily on discharge planning, referrals to community agencies, and client and family counseling. At the initial contact with a client, a social worker

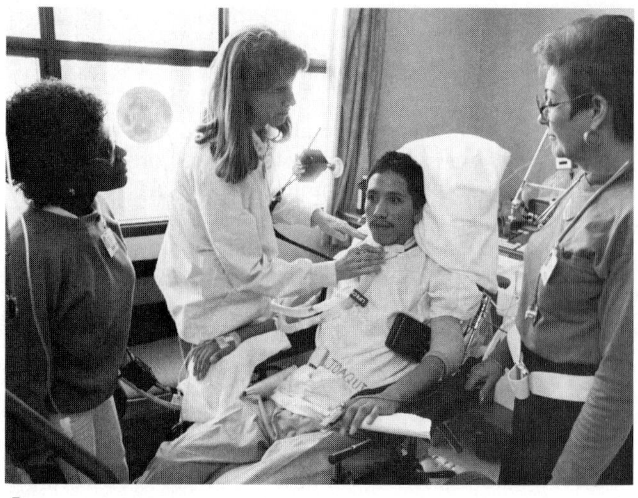

A

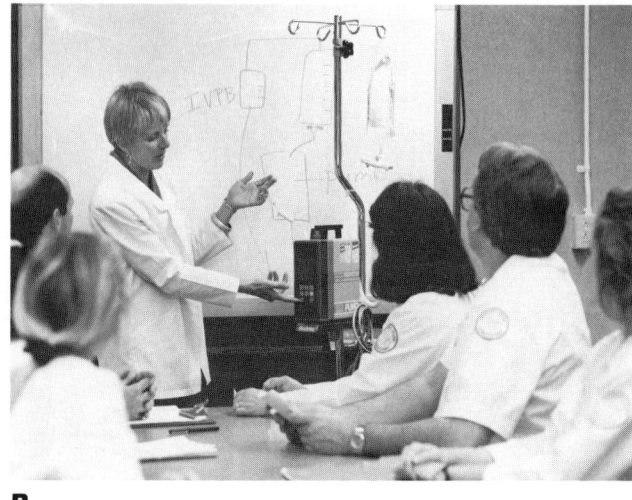

B

Figure 19–4. A. Clinical nurse specialist with staff nurse and client. **B.** Clinical nurse specialist as educator.

may assess such factors as work history, family and social supports, emotional status, general health habits, substance abuse, and discharge planning needs. Social workers are knowledgeable about organizations that provide free or low-cost supplies or equipment and collaborate with other members of the health care team, such as community health nurses, to share such information and make recommendations for referrals.

Social workers practice in hospitals, nursing homes, health care clinics, health departments, and private practice. Over the past decade, the social worker's role has been refined and expanded into that of a primary caregiver and client advocate who helps clients cope with emotional and environmental problems. For instance, in a hospice, the social worker collaborates with nurses and clients to obtain resources for clients and families such as homemaking services and visiting nurses, as well as providing emotional support.

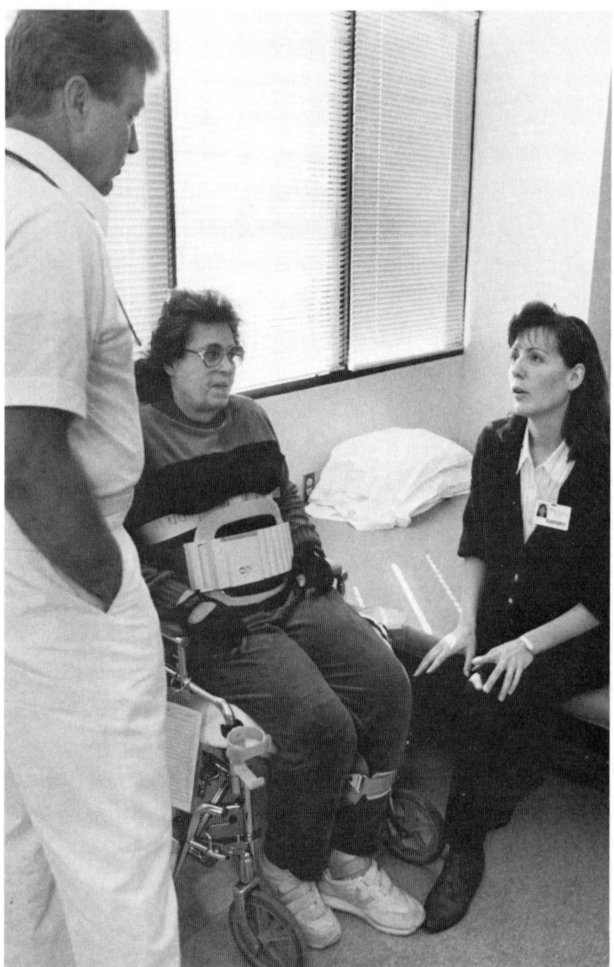

Figure 19–5. Physical therapists often work with nurses and clients to promote optimum musculoskeletal functioning.

The Registered Dietitian

Registered dietitians provide nutritional counseling and therapy. In hospitals, long-term-care facilities, and ambulatory care centers, dietitians assess clients' nutritional status and make recommendations for dietary therapy (Fig. 19–6). Dietitians take into account such factors as clients' cultural background, ethnicity, and socioeconomic status, all of which influence dietary habits. They prepare an individualized nutritional plan for each client based on such variables and communicate these recommendations to the health care team.

The Chaplain

Chaplains assist clients and families in meeting their spiritual needs. Clients, family members, or health care professionals may request chaplain services. In a hospital, a chaplain may be asked to provide spiritual counseling, rites (such as communion), or prayer. Some chaplaincy services

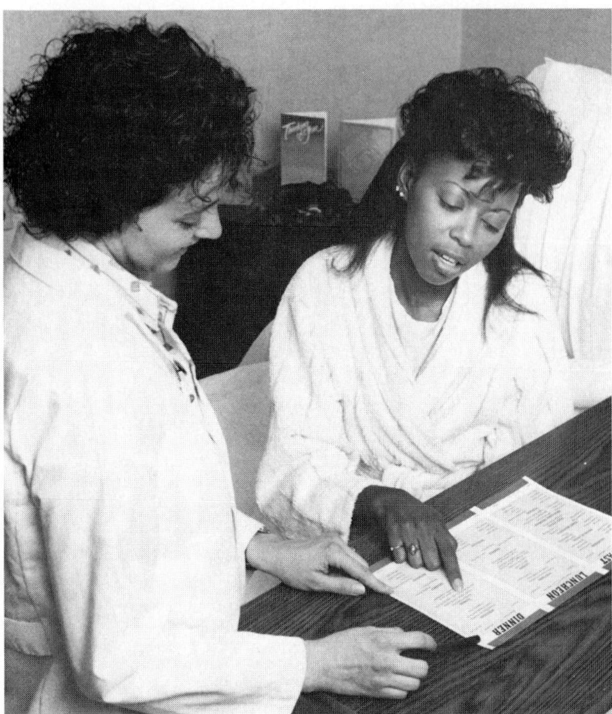

Figure 19–6. Dietitian planning menu with hospitalized client.

have developed programs to help other health care professionals address ethical and moral issues surrounding such topics as life-sustaining measures, living wills, and death and dying. For example, the health care team may find it difficult to deal with a terminally ill client who refuses all treatment. A chaplain can facilitate discussion of health care professionals' concerns while providing insight into clients' wishes.

The Discharge Planning Coordinator

Discharge planning coordinators are relatively new members of the health care team. A discharge planning coordinator is usually a nurse or social worker who arranges placement and services to maximize clients' quality of life after discharge from a health care facility. Discharge planning coordinators provide information and alternatives to the health care team regarding clients' discharge placement. To support the goals of the health care team, discharge planning coordinators may arrange for adult care or meals-on-wheels, obtain homemakers or visiting nurses, assist with long-term-care placement, or help clients and families obtain information about living with a particular illness. In a hospital, a discharge planning coordinator often begins a relationship with a client and family on the day of admission. The discharge planning coordinator collaborates with community health nurses in arranging nursing care measures for the client in the community. (Refer to Chap. 7 regarding the role of the community health nurse.)

The Pharmacist

Pharmacists dispense medications prescribed by qualified professionals, including physicians, psychiatrists, dentists, and nurse practitioners. Pharmacists collaborate with members of the health care team about indications for specific drugs, drug interactions with other drugs or foods, drug side effects, and over-the-counter medications. In prescribing the proper medication and dosage, a prescriber may confer with the pharmacist for recommendations about the lowest-cost drug, the most rapidly acting drug, or the drug with the fewest side effects, for example. In filling prescriptions, pharmacists provide important information to clients, such as written material about a medication and instructions for its use.

Collaboration between nurses and pharmacists is of paramount importance. Pharmacists recommend and dispense medications, and nurses administer them. Nurses may collaborate with pharmacists for several important reasons related to client care. For instance, pharmacists can provide information to nurses about drug interactions, optimum administration schedules, or drug compatibility with intravenous solutions.

Other Members of the Health Care Team

Other important members of the health care team help meet the needs of particular clients. Each of these professionals makes important contributions to a collaborative health care team.

The Dentist. The role of dentists is limited to the diagnosis and treatment of dental abnormalities and disease. Dentists may prescribe certain medications within their realm of practice. Dentists also contribute important preventive education to clients and families regarding oral diseases and oral hygiene.

Clients often contact dentists for preventive care as well as for dental problems. Some dental problems may result in systemic diseases or altered nutrition if untreated. Nurses or other health care professionals may recommend that clients seek the services of a dentist.

The Ophthalmologist and Optometrist. Both ophthalmologists and optometrists treat visual disorders. Clients often seek their services on the recommendation of another health care team member. Ophthalmologic nurses, who specialize in the care of clients with visual disorders, work closely with ophthalmologists and optometrists in the assessment, planning, and management of client needs.

The Chiropractor. Chiropractors focus on improving the function of the nervous system through various treatment modalities. Chiropractors use treatments such as spinal manipulation, diet, exercise, and massage.

The Licensed Vocational Nurse. Licensed vocational nurses (LVNs) or licensed practical nurses (LPNs) perform specific nursing care functions under the supervision of registered nurses or physicians in long-term-care facilities, hospitals, health clinics, and physicians' offices. LVNs collaborate with other members of the health care team about client care needs and the effectiveness of care. For example, while giving a bed bath, an LVN may observe that an elderly client on bed rest is developing skin breakdown. The LVN communicates the assessment of the problem to other health care team members, who develop a plan of skin care.

The Respiratory Therapist. Respiratory therapists assess and treat clients with respiratory problems. In some health care settings, respiratory therapists and nurses collaborate to plan and provide clients' treatments. For example, a nurse and respiratory therapist may perform postural drainage for a client with chronic lung disease, monitoring the effectiveness on a flowsheet to facilitate communication among health care team members. Respiratory therapists may also administer medications in respiratory devices as ordered by a physician. Both respiratory therapists and nurses evaluate the effectiveness of such treatments and communicate their findings to the other members of the health care team.

Future Directions in the Health Care Professions

To provide more efficient and effective care to clients, health care professionals must periodically examine their own procedures. Some professions, for instance, may experience a shortage of professionals in a particular specialty or geographic area. In response to the current shortage of registered nurses, Chicago's Rush-Presbyterian-St. Luke's Medical Center has created a new worker called a "nurse extender."[22] Because of the close working relationship between a nurse extender and a registered nurse, this model is called a practice partnership.[23] Under the direction of a nurse, nurse extenders assist clients in daily living activities such as bathing, transferring, or dressing. Nurse extenders also perform many tasks considered outside the realm of nursing but still vital to client care, such as transporting, taking phone messages, obtaining and inventorying equipment, and making beds. This enables nurses to spend more time with clients. Thus far, the nurse extender position has been implemented only in hospitals, but there could be wide application of such a role in other settings.

In 1988, another ancillary health worker, the registered care technician (RCT), was proposed by the American Medical Association (AMA). The AMA proposal called for RCTs to be trained to perform basic bedside care under the supervision of a physician. After generating controversy and opposition from nurses and nursing organizations, the RCT proposal was quietly withdrawn by the AMA in 1990.

Notwithstanding this controversial proposal, the use of ancillary health caregivers, who function under the direction of a professional, is intended to facilitate effective client care management. Such positions support a collaborative environment by enabling health care professionals to carry out professional level care activities.

■ THE BASIS FOR TEAMWORK

Improving or maintaining optimal health is the foundation for teamwork among health care professionals. Over the past 20 years, the focus of client care has changed from being solely disease-oriented to the current focus on health promotion and disease prevention. The health care team assists clients both in times of illness and in wellness. Members of a collaborative health care team establish a common focus in order to provide for clients' health needs. That common focus is expressed by mutual goal setting by the health care team. The following situation shows how the health care team works to meet the needs of a client by mutual goal setting.

> The client, Mr. Lane, has been receiving chemotherapy and radiation treatments for colon cancer and was to be discharged from the hospital shortly. Mr. Lane was scheduled to receive therapy at home to manage his pain with the use of a patient-controlled analgesic (PCA) pump. Recent changes in the economics of health care and technological developments, such as the PCA pump, have increased the responsibilities of the client and family in providing care in the home, as in Mr. Lane's case.
>
> Before discharge, members of the health care team, including Mr. Lane's physician, a nurse, a social worker, and a discharge planner, met with Mr. and Mrs. Lane. Although Mr. Lane had lived with cancer for the past year, he was unaware of the community resources available to him. As Mr. Lane had become more dependent in daily living activities over the past 2 months, Mrs. Lane had reduced her work hours to help her husband at home. Mrs. Lane felt anxious at the prospect of the PCA pump in the home, stating, "What if the pump fails to work? What if the medication runs out?" After Mr. and Mrs. Lane expressed their concerns, the health care team helped the Lanes sort out the cognitive and emotional needs they perceived as most important.
>
> Three major needs were identified, and the health care team concurred that goals would be developed in order to meet these needs. The Lanes' primary need was for direction about pain management at home. They also needed guidance about Mr. Lane's personal care. Finally, they needed financial assistance information.
>
> The health care team determined that the overall goal was to develop and implement a home program that would provide the Lanes with information and resources to meet Mr. Lane's daily care needs. Each health care team member's contributions would focus on helping Mr. and Mrs. Lane adapt to changes necessitated by Mr. Lane's treatment and functional status. The physician prescribed the medical plan of care, including the medication regimen, follow-up diagnostic tests, and activity schedule. The nurse focused on Mr. and Mrs. Lane's responses to Mr. Lane's illness, the performance of daily living activities, and education about pain management. The discharge planner recommended home health nurses. The social worker addressed financial concerns and identified community resources, such as cancer support groups, to help the Lanes cope with Mr. Lane's physical and psychological changes.

Collaboration among health care team members means that a relationship is established with clients and that professionals work together to meet clients' needs. Shared goals enable health care team members to have a clearer understanding of each member's role and responsibility. Health care team members must also be willing to share and communicate with each other to develop mutual goals. Care may become fragmented if health care team members have different goals or if the client is not considered a team member in goal development.

Medical and nursing diagnoses provide another avenue for teamwork. Diagnosis has long been considered the purview of physicians; nurses have long been crucial contributors to resolving medical diagnoses. Supporting the medical treatment plan continues to be an important nursing responsibility.

The term *diagnosis* is gaining wider use in health and other professions. For example, an auto mechanic may "diagnose" a car's problem. Within the health professions, physicians historically have centered their practice on diagnosing diseases, social workers use the term *casework diagnosis* to describe social problems experienced by clients, and nurses use the term *nursing diagnosis* to denote clients' responses to health problems. Although medical and nursing diagnoses differ in their area of focus, in collaborative practice, medical and nursing diagnoses complement one another to promote mutual goal setting.

Nursing and medicine also use similar steps in the diagnostic process. Information is first collected from clients and other sources, such as family members and past health records. Nursing and medicine use some similar techniques for gathering information, such as interviewing, observing, and examining. Both analyze and synthesize data in order to arrive at a diagnosis.

Diagnosis as a means of communication is an important aspect of a collaborative team effort in health care delivery. Communication and sharing of information among health care team members should occur throughout the process of diagnosis and care. While most health care team members are familiar with medical diagnostic terms, nursing diagnosis is new to many health care professionals. Part of a nurse's collaborative role as the NANDA taxonomy is further developed and refined is to educate other team members about the meaning of nursing diagnosis terminology and the ways in which their expertise can contribute to collaborative resolution of nursing diagnoses. There are several modes through which health care team members facilitate collaborative communication with each other; these will be discussed later in the chapter.

Advocacy and Accountability

Advocacy and accountability are two aspects of professional behavior that affect teamwork. **Advocacy** refers to health care professionals' focus on protecting clients' interests. Providers recognize the need for client advocacy when they determine that a client has needs that are not being met, or is in jeopardy of having rights violated, but is unable to take individual responsibility to change the situation. They demonstrate advocacy by speaking or acting in the client's behalf to meet the need or to prevent the potential violation of rights. All members of the team, including nurses, share in the responsibility to act as client advocates. Nursing has paid particular attention to advocacy as a part of the nurse's role, and nurses function as client advocates in virtually every setting in which nursing is practiced.

As part of a team, each member is responsible for his or her own performance. **Accountability** refers to the health care professional's acceptance of this responsibility. Although each member of the health care team is accountable for his or her professional contributions, collaborative decision making is necessary by virtue of the responsibilities derived from a common focus on the well-being of the client. Team members also are accountable to one another, as well as to the client in this regard.

Consider the example of an elderly nursing home resident who will be returning home in a week after recovering from a fractured hip. As client advocate, the social worker focuses on the client's ability to obtain and use resources effectively in the home and to adapt to a role change as someone else performs household tasks, as well as the impact of the client's social support network on her adaptation to changes at home. In the role of client advocate, the nurse has to consider, among other factors, the client's need for information about medications and treatments, the client's ability to maintain functional independence, and safety precautions in the home. The social worker and nurse rely on each other to help the client in meeting her needs in the home environment.

Suppose, for example, that this client confides to the nurse that she has never had a stranger working in her house before and that she is afraid to have the homemaker assistant that the social worker has arranged come into her home. The client also adds that she did not express her feelings to the social worker because she was afraid that if she did, she

IMPLICATIONS FOR PROFESSIONAL COLLABORATION

Diagnosis as a Means of Communication

Diagnosis is an important aspect of a collaborative team effort. The process of diagnosis promotes information sharing. Information sharing, in turn, enhances diagnostic accuracy, expands planning options, and facilitates group consensus.

Diagnosis is also important because it is the process of labeling client health problems. These labels provide the common language by which health care team members are able to talk about clients' needs and share ideas on the nature of clients' health problems. As precise statements of client problems, diagnoses provide a specific basis for the team's goal with each client; thus, diagnoses serve to unify the efforts of team members. Although medical and nursing diagnoses differ in their focus, medical diagnoses being oriented largely to the nature of clients' disease and nursing diagnoses to clients' responses to illness, both are concerned with clients' health status and are indispensable and frequently interdependent components of client care.

would not be allowed to go home. Acting as an advocate for the client, the nurse first explores the client's ideas for alternatives to a homemaker assistant or ways to make the use of this helper more acceptable, then promises to communicate the client's concerns to the social worker for collaborative problem solving. The nurse's actions demonstrate client advocacy as well as professional accountability.

THE NATURE OF COLLABORATIVE PROFESSIONAL RELATIONSHIPS

Collaboration among health care team members is essential to teamwork. The nature of collaborative professional relationships is determined by two factors, communication and mutual respect.

Communication

Communication is the first step toward developing a collaborative relationship (see Chap. 14). Health care team members exchange information, observations, judgments, and recommendations regarding client care. Informal communication is ongoing as team members carry out client care responsibilities in a shared working space. Physical proximity among health care team members facilitates interdisciplinary functioning and communication.[24] Each individual has a unique style of communication. In some cases, health care team members may need to alter their style if the communication behavior inhibits teamwork. Some questions that can help health care team members evaluate their communication style are:

- Am I open to the ideas of others and willing to share my ideas?
- Are my verbal and nonverbal communications consistent?
- Do I express my ideas freely in a group or only to certain individuals?
- Do I assume that everyone knows what I am attempting to communicate?
- Do I include listening as a component of my communication style?

Through awareness of communication strengths and deficits, health care team members can enhance their effectiveness in expressing themselves in groups. Although disagreements occur in most groups at times, open communication facilitates problem solving and helps the team reach consensus. Further information regarding collaborative modes of communication may be found in Chapter 14.

IMPLICATIONS FOR PROFESSIONAL COLLABORATION

Communication

Communication is essential to the development of a collaborative relationship. Style of communicating influences communication and may inhibit or enhance team relationships. Qualities that enhance communication are openness, consistency, avoidance of assumptions about others' understanding, and careful listening to others' messages. Good communication provides a basis for mutual respect.

IMPLICATIONS FOR PROFESSIONAL COLLABORATION

Mutual Respect

Good communication supports an atmosphere of mutual respect and mutual respect promotes good communication. Mutual respect means that health care team members appreciate and support the distinct yet complementary expertise of each other, that they have a collegial relationship with each other. Under conditions of collegiality, status differences are minimized, efficiency and effectiveness are highlighted, ideas are received with objectivity, the contributions of others are accepted, and responsibility is assumed by all.

Mutual Respect

The second characteristic of a collaborative relationship is mutual respect. Mutual respect exists when each team member appreciates and supports the distinct yet complementary expertise of other team members. Mutual respect is also referred to as collegiality.

Styles emphasize the significance of mutual respect when she states the following benefits of collegiality:

1. It minimizes professional status distinctions.
2. It centers on one's efficiency and effectiveness.
3. It supports information sharing among colleagues.
4. It encourages objectivity in listening to all ideas.
5. It accepts the contributions of others.
6. It advocates critical evaluation of performance.
7. It facilitates mutual decision making.
8. It allows responsibility taking rather than abdicating.[25]

Mutual respect among health care team members contributes to the aims of teamwork. When health care team members respect each other, "individual endeavor is potentiated, not pooled—respect then follows, with the acknowledgment and encouragement of the contribution that others make to our mutual task" (p. 143).[25] Without effective communication skills and mutual respect among health care team members collaborative relationships cannot develop.

MODES OF COLLABORATION IN HEALTH CARE SETTINGS

Collaboration takes many forms, some formal, others informal. With formal modes of collaboration, the communication process has a clear purpose and acknowledged structure. For example, formal means of collaboration include the health care team conference, consultation, and consolidated client records. Informal collaboration usually occurs in one-to-one interactions between health care professionals, such as in the spontaneous discussion of a client's

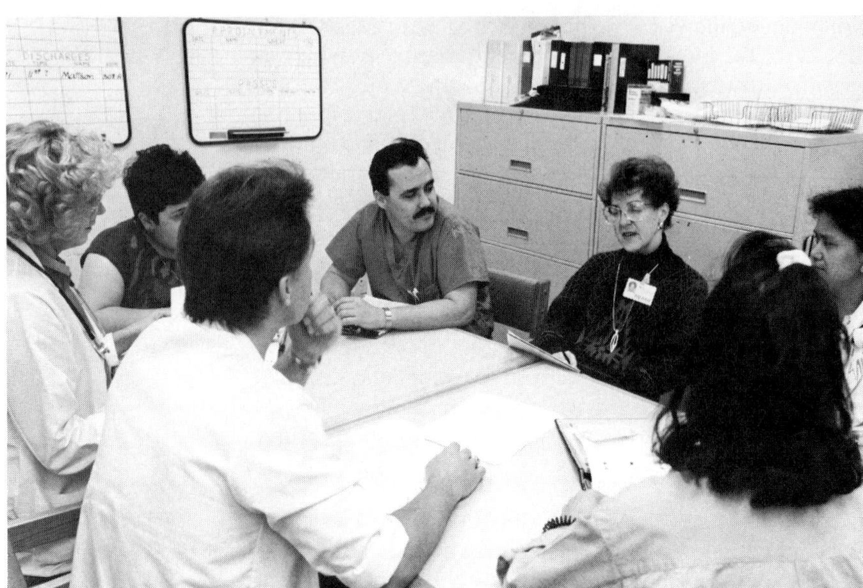

Figure 19–7. Members of the health care team in a team meeting.

health problems. Informal collaboration is seldom structured and may relate to only one specific aspect of client care.

Health Care Team Conference

To foster a unified effort in care planning, **health care team conferences** usually have a stated purpose, focus on client problems and coordinated care, and meet regularly (Fig. 19–7). For example, a conference may be organized to help resolve a complex client problem current therapy is not resolving. Several different professional perspectives often are needed to address complex problems.

The health care team conference usually follows a format that is dictated by its purpose. Box 19–2 outlines a typical presentation by the health care team in a hospital setting. Through collaboration, the health care team clarifies and redefines actual and potential client problems, formulates objectives, plans interventions, and evaluates the effectiveness of therapeutic measures.

The conference begins with a client profile, including the reason for seeking health care assistance and a description of the client's personal, social, and health history.

Ideally, the course of the hospitalization is described from the viewpoint of all health care disciplines. For instance, the physician may explain diagnostic test results and the effectiveness of a medication regimen. The nurse may describe the client's physical and psychosocial responses to illness. The physical therapist may describe the client's activity tolerance in ambulating and balance. A collaborative care plan is then developed. Desired outcomes and interventions may be reconsidered at future conferences and revised as necessary.

Consultation

Another formal mode of collaboration is consultation. **Consultation** occurs when one or more health care team members contact an expert to help solve problems.[26] The expert, or consultant, is usually a specialist who has knowledge and experience related to the particular situation. The consultant usually does not make decisions, but provides the health care team with possible alternatives to solve the problem. The health care team decides whether to use or discard any or all of the consultant's proposals.

Making Referrals. The procedure of requesting a consultation is referred to as making a referral. Consultation may be either formal or informal, but a referral commonly means a formal course of action.

Health care settings may have a consultation form,

BOX 19–2. TYPICAL FORMAT OF THE HEALTH CARE TEAM CONFERENCE

1. Client profile
2. Family/significant other(s)
3. General health/social history
4. Present diagnoses
   - Medical problems
   - Nursing problems
   - Collaborative problems
5. Course of present illness
   - Tests/procedures
   - Medical therapeutic measures
   - Nursing therapeutic measures
   - Consultations with other team members
6. Presentation of care plan
   - Client/team goals
   - Evaluation of interventions
7. Course of decision making
   - What is the team's course of action?

which is a written document of interdisciplinary communication. There are usually two sections to the form. The first part is completed by the health care team member initiating the referral, and includes a brief overview of the client and reason for the referral. The consultant receives the referral, assesses the client's situation, and recommends a plan of action on the second half of the form. The completed referral form then becomes part of the client's permanent record. As such, all members of the health care team have access to the consultation record to facilitate coordination of care.

Types of Consultation. Consultations generally are divided into two major categories: intradisciplinary and interdisciplinary. Intradisciplinary consultation occurs within a particular discipline. Nurse-to-nurse consultation is becoming more common as part of the expanding role of the nurse. In many settings, a nurse generalist may consult and collaborate with a nurse specialist. Interdisciplinary consultation occurs when different disciplines collaborate. A nurse requesting a consultation with a dietitian is an example.

Consolidated Client Records

Health care team members document the care they provide and clients' responses to care to indicate progress toward desired outcomes. In some health care facilities, each health care profession has its own system of recording client information. Each professional writes in a different area in the client record. For example, nurses do not document care in the same section of the client's chart as physicians. This unconsolidated system does not facilitate communication among health care providers.

Consolidated client records are a means of communicating client responses and progress that encourages collaboration. A **consolidated client record** is a record in which written communication by health team members is documented on one common form rather than in several areas of the client record. This system facilitates communication because it integrates the contributions of the entire health care team.

Different health care settings consolidate different segments of the client record. The client problem list, progress notes, and clinical protocols are most commonly consolidated. The problem-oriented medical record (POMR) is used by professionals in many health care settings today as a format for consolidating client problem lists and progress notes. The problem list is a cumulative record of actual and potential client problems documented by health care team members. Integrated progress notes enable all disciplines to contribute to and document the plan of care in one place in the chart.[27] All team members can easily read each other's documentation.

Integrated progress notes serve several important purposes. First, replication of efforts may be reduced. Second, each discipline's plan of care is enhanced in a collaborative environment in which team members' knowledge and suggestions have equal importance in affecting the client's care. The POMR is discussed further in Chapter 18.

■ CONCEPTUAL DEFINITIONS OF COLLABORATIVE ROLES

To meet clients' needs, each team member performs two categories of activities: task functions and maintenance functions. The two types of activities complement each other in teamwork. Task functions include behaviors that help identify and meet goals. Maintenance functions are activities that keep the team working together in a cohesive manner.

Role of Initiator

The role of initiator is primarily task oriented. The initiator can be either the leader, who coordinates the team's efforts, or a member, who facilitates the team's efforts. The functions of the initiator include:

- Introducing or proposing objectives; identifying a client problem; suggesting alternative solutions to a problem. *For example,* "We will first discuss Mrs. Crane's adjustment to the nursing home."
- Requesting information; asking for suggestions; stimulating discussion. *For example,* "What interventions have we implemented thus far?"
- Giving information; presenting ideas or facts; giving suggestions. *For example,* "Involving Mrs. Crane's daughter in her care would help her adjustment."
- Clarifying information; restating ideas; expanding on discussion. *For example,* "What you are telling me is that we should focus on. . . ."
- Synthesizing information; pulling ideas together to summarize. *For example,* "So far, we have discussed. . . ."
- Focusing the group onto the task at hand. *For example,* "That is a good point, but perhaps you could develop it after we finish discussing Mrs. Crane's adjustment."
- Reacting constructively to ideas of others. *For example,* "That's a very good suggestion and sounds realistic."

Role of Maintainer

The role of maintainer is to foster good group dynamics, so that group work may move along in a positive direction. The maintainer and initiator roles are compared and summarized in Box 19–3. Some of the functions of the maintainer role include:

- Encouraging other team members; recognizing their contributions to the team. *For example,* "Thank you for your input."
- Harmonizing among team members to appease differences in viewpoints. *For example,* "We haven't reached any decision on this matter. Perhaps we should table the discussion."
- Sensitizing others in the group to feelings; sharing perceptions, attitudes, opinions, and emotions. *For example,* "It concerns me that you seem upset. . . ."
- Compromising one's own stance to facilitate group cohesiveness. *For example,* "We've made two good points here. Is there a middle ground where we could agree?"

BOX 19–3. FUNCTIONS OF THE INITIATOR AND MAINTAINER ROLES

Role of Initiator
- Introduce ideas
- Request information, ideas
- Give information
- Clarify information, ideas
- Synthesize ideas
- Focus group
- React to ideas

Role of Maintainer
- Encourage members
- Harmonize members
- Sensitize members
- To facilitate compromise
- Encourage participation
- Propose goals

- Encouraging the participation of all team members; keeping open lines of communication. *For example,* "What do you think about. . . ."
- Proposing goals for group function and dynamics. *For example,* "In today's meeting, let's try to keep the discussion centered on the issues."

THE NURSE'S ROLE IN COLLABORATION

Nurses serve as initiators and maintainers in the health care team. In the role of initiator, a nurse takes on a leadership role in planning and implementing client care measures. As maintainer, a nurse takes on roles that complement and support the roles of other health care team members.

The Nurse as Initiator

In the role of initiator, nurses perform key tasks as team members: they assess needs, identify goals, make referrals, and request consultations. Nurses take a leadership role and ask for team members' input in identifying client needs and goals. As initiator, a nurse may propose new ideas or help to pull information together, clarify team discussion to refocus on goals, and evaluate the effectiveness of the plan of care. Nurses also recommend referrals to other health disciplines. For example, a nurse discusses his or her assessment findings with the team regarding a diabetic client's need for foot care. In interviewing the client, the nurse finds that the client has never been told of the importance of good foot care. The nurse examines the client's feet during a bed bath and finds the client's nails are long and dirty, with a possible infection between two toes of the right foot. As part of the care plan, the nurse recommends a referral to a podiatrist for further assessment and treatment.

The Nurse as Maintainer

In the role of maintainer, nurses support collaborative relationships within the health care team. The maintainer role includes team conference leader or participant, consultant, and discharge planner. Taking notice of communication problems within the group, calling members' attention to nonproductive communication in a nonthreatening way, and involving all members in group process are ways nurses can maintain collaborative teamwork.

In all of these roles, nurses facilitate communication among disciplines. Setting an example to other professionals and being cordial and receptive are positive ways in which a nurse may be a team advocate.

Collaboration and Alternative Models of Client Care Delivery

The current focus on collaboration has extended the scope of nursing practice and expanded nurses' roles. The expanded scope of nursing practice has resulted in greater independence in decision making in some health care settings.[28,29] The status of nurse–physician collaboration was the focus of studies in 1972 by the ANA and the AMA. The two organizations formed a committee, the National Joint Practice Commission (NJPC), which significantly contributed to improving nurse–physician collaboration. The NJPC identified several models of client care delivery that support nurse–physician collaboration, including primary nursing, case management, expanded nursing roles, and practice partnerships. Primary nursing has formed the basis for new models of nursing practice that further support a collaborative environment.

Primary Nursing. Although several new models of care delivery are in use across the nation, primary nursing remains one of the most widely practiced models. The NJPC defined primary nursing as "the performance of clinical nursing functions by professional nurses with minimal or no delegation of nursing tasks to others."[30] Primary nursing enables a nurse to develop a depth of understanding of a client's health care needs. Thus, the nurse is better able to function in a collaborative role. The clinical credibility of nurses is more frequently recognized in a primary system. Physicians are more supportive of primary nurses' expanded responsibilities as they observe nurses performing detailed assessments, making nursing diagnoses, and planning successful comprehensive therapeutic measures. Additionally, primary nursing has been a major factor in retaining nurses in many health care settings as nurses experience a higher degree of job satisfaction.

Case Management. Case management is an innovative system of nursing care delivery in which a nurse (case manager) plans the nursing care for clients and delegates aspects of care to other nursing personnel. Case management is an extension of primary nursing in that one nurse plans the client's care but other caregivers provide care. Case managers have collaborative relationships with all members of the health care team, in particular with physicians. The clients' needs and the level of skill of the nursing personnel determine how a case manager delegates the work.

Overall responsibilities of the case manager include the following:

- Evaluation of outcomes of nursing care
- Promotion of collaborative relationships
- Allocation of resources to provide care
- Development of the discharge plans
- Evaluation of cost-effective nursing care[31]

On admission, a case manager assesses a client's needs and identifies initial goals with the client and family. The case manager then collaborates with the health care team to determine the completeness of the plan. Thus, in a case management system, mutual goal setting between the client and health care team is promoted.

Important Qualities of Nurses in Collaborative Roles

In a collaborative environment, nurses' expanded roles complement roles of other team members. Along with the expanded role, nurses can use certain behaviors to bolster collaborative relationships. These behaviors include assertiveness, accountability, risk taking, and autonomy.[32]

Assertiveness is the expression of confidence and self-assurance that one's ideas and rights are important and should be recognized. An assertive nurse works collaboratively with the health care team, sharing information, offering constructive suggestions, and requesting information. There is a difference between assertiveness and aggressiveness. Aggressive behavior usually tramples on another's rights, which leads to conflict and impairs the collaborative relationship.

Accountability is the assumption of responsibility for one's actions and decisions. (See the discussion earlier in this chapter.)

Risk taking means taking action or stating a value that is outside of the prevailing group norm. For example, a nurse may recommend alternative forms of pain relief, such as acupuncture, to the health care team for a client who is not responding to traditional therapies.

Autonomy is independence or freedom to choose one's actions. Professional autonomy implies control of professional roles and self-directed practice. However, being autonomous does not signify isolation as an individual practitioner. Responsible exercise of autonomy requires accountability to one's profession and shared responsibility for meeting clients' needs.[33]

■ FACTORS THAT FACILITATE COLLABORATION

Several factors are essential to maintaining collaborative relationships. Some of these factors have been discussed in detail in this chapter. They are now summarized and presented as a framework for collaboration.

As shown in Figure 19–8, factors that influence collaboration may be intrinsic or extrinsic to the members of the health care team. Professionals must demonstrate personal maturity and self-confidence. Nurses who know the facts and can state them confidently will be held in high regard by other professionals. Team members must be accountable for their own actions and be willing to take on responsibility if they want to be treated as colleagues. Clinical credibility is built on clinical competence. Individual team members should use their expertise to the maximum. Finally, professionals must be willing to accept the changes that collaborative relationships entail.

External factors, interactions between health team members that foster collaboration, include mutual respect which develops out of the contributions each member makes to team functioning. Clearly defined roles and responsibilities lead to clear understanding of what is expected of each team member. Open lines of communication encourage all team members to participate in problem solving. Finally, joint educational and clinical experiences should be part of the education of all health care professionals.[24] Collaboration will then be expected by all those involved in health care delivery.

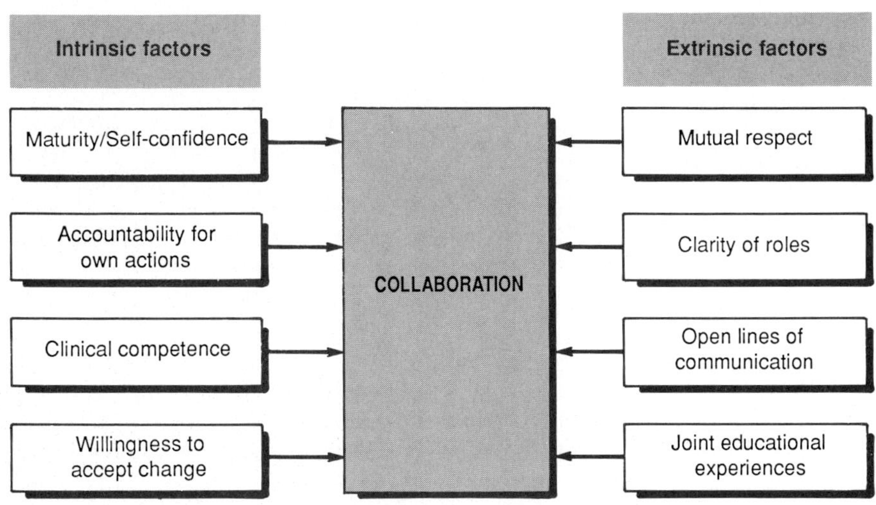

Figure 19–8. Factors that facilitate collaboration among members of the health care team.

■ OBSTACLES TO COLLABORATION AMONG HEALTH CARE TEAM MEMBERS

Many of the obstacles to collaborative relationships can be traced to traditional role relationships of the past. By understanding the factors that hinder collaboration, nurses and other health care team members will be able to help overcome them.

Traditional Role Relationships

In the traditional model of care, there is a hierarchy with the physician at the apex and the client at the base. Communication flows downward from the physician to the client; there is little upward communication. Most communication from the physician takes the form of orders, with little exchange of ideas or alternatives. Care is fragmented, because individual care providers focus on their own goals for clients and their own perceptions of clients' needs.

Territoriality

As applied to human behavior, **territoriality** is the innate need to claim control and to dominate various facets of one's existence.[14] Territoriality can be seen in the demarcation of work roles in the health care system. Some physicians may perceive the expanding role of nurses as a threat to their professional territory. Barriers to communication often develop in response to this threat. Territoriality, however, is not limited to nurse–physician relationships. Overlapping work roles among other health care disciplines also cause territorial responses. Differences in each discipline's understanding of others' roles may result in poor collaboration. Thus, territoriality may prevent the health care team from working together for clients' health.

Interprofessional Communication Problems

Several researchers have identified potential problems in interprofessional communication. In a study of interactions between nurses and physicians, McLain observed that the degree to which communication is open among health professionals is directly related to the level of collaboration.[34] Lynaugh and Bates, authorities on interpersonal communication, consider that a lack of communication between nurses and physicians is related to separate education.[35] It has also been suggested that communication problems are related to differences in the ways nurses and physicians structure their work.[36]

Another factor influencing collaboration is the use of language. In the past, physicians and nurses have used similar medical terminology. With the development of a taxonomy of nursing diagnoses, physicians may find some nurses' language confusing. In addition, nursing diagnosis may alarm some physicians, who feel that "diagnosing" is within their exclusive realm. Nurses who use new terms

BUILDING NURSING KNOWLEDGE

Is Nurse–Physician Communication Collaborative?

Katzman EM, Roberts JI. Nurse–physician conflicts as barriers to the enactment of nursing roles. *West J Nurs Res.* 1988; 10(5):576–590.

Katzman and Roberts note that interprofessional conflicts between nurses and physicians have been a part of nursing history since Florence Nightingale. They designed a study to assess the current impact of sex-role behavior on professional communication between female nurses and male physicians and to determine the themes that characterize that communication. The research method they employed was participant observation. The researchers observed 14 female nurses in traditional roles and 11 female nurse practitioners as they interacted with their male physician colleagues in a 350 bed nonprofit, nonsectarian northeastern U.S. hospital.

The researchers found several themes in their observational data. The first was that nurses subordinated their own professional judgment about client care to the decision-making power of the physician. For example, when a physician informed a client she could leave the hospital, but then failed to write an order for the client's discharge, the nurse tried to contact the physician, who did not return her call. The nurse noted that the client was depressed about the situation, but said, "There is nothing we can do about it." The researchers also found that nurses were unaware of the effect of their powerlessness on client's well-being, blaming instead the client–physician relationship.

Another theme was stereotypical sex role behaviors. For example, while discussing a drug policy about which they disagreed, a female nurse practitioner stood while the male physician sat. The physician repeatedly interrupted her as she was writing a note in a client's chart, in order to continue the debate. Although the nurse practitioner's behavior indicated her obvious exasperation, the male physician, nevertheless, talked in a calm, deliberate manner, periodically picking up the phone to make calls unrelated to the discussion. The researchers noted that women in the United States are raised to behave in ways that make men feel superior, and a passive demeanor is experienced by women as more congruent with sex-role expectations.

A final theme was lack of interaction between nurses and physicians, a surprising finding in view of the demands client care make for regular communication. During one morning's observation, for example, 9 of 18 physicians came and left the unit without interacting with a single nurse. Physicians conducted weekly conferences on the units. Nurses were invited; however, because of client care responsibilities, only a few could attend. Interactions were most infrequent when new or part-time nurses outnumbered the regular, seasoned staff. Nurses often cited lack of medical knowledge as a barrier to communication with physicians. Noting this sense of inferiority, the researchers drew parallels between the nurse–physician relationship and the wife–husband relationship. They concluded that programs are necessary to bring nursing and medical students together to find solutions to this age-old dilemma.

must explain their use clearly to other professionals. Health care professionals should also avoid the use of jargon or confusing language. Open communication among team members is facilitated if all members make efforts to integrate and clarify terminology that is unique to a particular discipline.

Ambiguity of Expectations

Weiss, an authority on health care professional roles, examined interaction patterns among physicians, nurses, and clients. She found that all three groups held different expectations about collaboration and its effects.[37] For example, clients' beliefs were more in keeping with a traditional rather than a collaborative model of practice. They acknowledged nurses' roles in health care, but they felt that physicians had higher levels of responsibility. Weiss also found some attitudes and behaviors of nurses that potentially hamper collaboration. Some nurses in her study had difficulty identifying themselves as professionals or recognizing their unique expertise, and some felt uncomfortable taking on responsibility.

Differences in Education

Health care professionals from different disciplines generally share little or no coursework or clinical experiences during their preparation for practice.[38] Members of any one discipline thus may have little direct knowledge of the clinical knowledge and skills of other health team members.

There is evidence that collaboration may be enhanced through educational activities. Woodman and Sherwood report that nurses and physicians who experience collaborative working conditions during their training tend to develop knowledge, skills, and attitudes that facilitate successful collaboration later in their practice.[38]

Resource Allocation and Reward System Differences

Differences in resource allocation and reward mechanisms among professionals on the health care team foster frustration and resentment. For example, there is a large difference in the average earnings of physicians and the average earnings of most other health care professionals. Although differences in education can account for some of the discrepancy, historical patterns of economic discrimination against women play a significant role. The magnitude of the variance has caused considerable ill feeling among health care professionals, which is a deterrent to effective collaboration. Bruce identified differences in social status or a lack of what he called social proximity as a critical determinant of different disciplines' abilities to work collaboratively.[39]

■ COMPARING COLLABORATIVE AND NONCOLLABORATIVE BEHAVIORS

What is the difference between the behavior of team members who are acting collaboratively and the behavior of those who are not? How can nurses and other health care team members support collaborative interactions? First, they can apply the following examples of collaborative and noncollaborative situations to daily practice. The following are examples of collaborative interactions:

1. In initially addressing clients and colleagues, follow institutional or personal preferences. Ask clients their preferred method of address. For colleagues, respect personal preferences as well, unless institutional policy specifies address.
2. Be prepared to discuss your client with other members of the health care team. Know the current plan and goals.
3. Ask questions to clarify information from other health care team members. For instance, ask the pharmacist, "We will be administering this experimental drug to clients. Could you give the team information about its action and potential side effects?"
4. Initiate consultation with other members of the health care team in conferences and rounds. For example, ask the social worker, "What alternatives are available for Mr. Jones when he returns home, as his wife feels she needs help with his daily care?"
5. Demonstrate responsibility for your own actions within the realm of professional practice. This means being accountable to clients, to other health professionals, as well as to yourself.
6. Encourage shared educational experiences among health care team members. For instance, bedside client care rounds may be an opportunity to learn and use assessment skills.

The following are examples of noncollaborative interactions:

1. Be closed-minded about change: maintain the attitude "that's how I learned it" or "that's how we've always done it."
2. Do not try to be current on your client's condition and response to treatment; "I don't know, I've been off for a few days."
3. Avoid asking other members of the health care team to clarify orders or issues that affect your client care.
4. Avoid responsibility and accountability for your actions. Take the attitude "That's what was ordered" in response to questions from health care team members.
5. Do not seek educational experiences that may promote collaboration and maintain clinical competence.

■ ETHICAL ISSUES IN COLLABORATION

This chapter has emphasized the importance of joint efforts on behalf of clients by all members of the health care team. Most of the literature on professional ethics in health care focuses on the moral commitment of individual practitioners to clients.[40] Little has been written on the ethical responsibilities of the health care team as a whole.[41] Pellegrino and Thomasma state that "there is not as yet any fully developed ethical theory to define the obligations of a group of individuals (the team) making decisions which affect the well-being of another person (the client)."[42] With the growth of technology and the increasing ability to prolong life, the health care team faces many ethical decisions.

What if an individual professional's values conflict with the decisions of the health care team? If an error is made, who is responsible—the individual practitioner or the group? Are the moral obligations of individual practitioners the same as those of the group? There are no simple answers to these questions.

Another potential problem is the changing nature of today's health care delivery system. One example is the impact of the shorter length of hospitalization as a result of the federal prospective payment system. A coordinated effort by the health care team is required to meet more acute client needs in a shorter period of time. Meeting the needs of greater numbers of clients who have serious health problems with dwindling economic resources poses another challenge. Whose needs shall be met; whose excluded?

Some guidelines are available to help the team address ethical conflicts. First, the team is guided by ethical principles and theories (see Chap. 34). Clients' rights are primary and must be respected. Second, team members should have a common understanding of value-laden terms such as "accountability," "autonomy," and "quality of care." Achieving a common understanding requires time and commitment. Third, team members should openly communicate their concerns about moral issues. The team should discuss, rather than ignore, ethical perspectives and issues. Discussing ethical issues also facilitates achievement of a common understanding. Finally, the team should consult with an ethics committee in complex ethical dilemmas.

■ EVALUATING THE EFFECTIVENESS OF THE COLLABORATIVE HEALTH CARE TEAM

Evaluation determines whether the care plan and implementation have met identified outcomes. (See discussion in Chap. 18.) This final section addresses the importance of evaluating the effectiveness of the collaborative health care team in terms of outcomes of care. Specific strategies for this evaluation are still being developed.

The NJPC recommended the formation of a formal evaluative group in each health care setting, a **joint practice committee,** to monitor health care team relationships and quality of care issues and to make recommendations that would promote collaboration. The committee should comprise members of several different health care disciplines.

The nurse–pharmacist therapeutics committee is one example of a joint practice committee. In one institution, a health care team was concerned about the apparent lack of communication between nurses and pharmacists. After reviewing the situation, the institution's nurse–pharmacist therapeutics committee decided that pharmacists should function on specific units. Satellite pharmacies were opened on units so that pharmacists were directly available to nurses. Pharmacists also began to participate in client rounds, fostering the collaborative model. In 1990, the NJPC revised nursing standards to focus on clients as the center of care. It is anticipated that these changes will affect other health care providers' evaluation of client care.[43]

Another approach to evaluating the effectiveness of collaboration is examining both subjective and objective outcomes. In evaluating subjective outcomes of using a collaborative model in a hospice setting, Dobratz reports positive responses from health care team members as well as from clients. Nurses felt more of a challenge in their expanded role, and physicians revealed more acceptance of nurses' participation in decision making. Clients felt more caring and support from the health care team along with an increase in communication.[44]

Evaluations of objective outcomes might take the form of documenting comparative costs of collaborative and noncollaborative models of client care. Possible factors for comparison would be length of hospital stay for clients with identical health problems, and retention of professional staff under collaborative and noncollaborative models.

SUMMARY

Providers from many diverse disciplines make up a health care team. Many factors, such as power and authority, stage of group development, and cohesiveness, influence how teams function.

Effective collaborative health care teams facilitate the delivery of quality client care. Health care professionals become colleagues in the health care setting, each recognizing the unique contributions of other members. Teams that incorporate clients as members of the team can plan and implement efficient and comprehensive care through information sharing and shared decision making. For clients who participate in a coordinated team effort, the result is integrated, personalized care. The need for a team approach is apparent from the complexities of today's health care system and current health care trends.

Collaboration may take several forms in health care settings. Formal modes of collaboration include interdisciplinary team conferences, client care rounds, and problem-oriented documentation. Informal collaboration usually occurs in the form of discussion of client health problems and concerns.

In a collaborative environment, health care team members may take on several roles, depending on such factors as the health care setting, client problems and needs, and health care team members' experience. In a collaborative model, roles of health care professionals may be distinct in several areas and overlap in others.

Collaboration has promoted the expansion of the nurse's role. Nurses today function interdependently with other health professionals. Several new models of nursing practice, including case management and practice partnerships, are being implemented to meet the changing client needs and facilitate collaboration in the health care team.

Several factors can either promote or hinder collaboration among health care team members. Factors that enhance collaboration include accountability for one's own actions, demonstration of clinical competence, willingness to accept change, mutual respect among colleagues, and open lines of communication. Collaboration may be hindered by traditional models of care, professional territoriality, interprofessional communication problems, ambiguity of expectations, differences in education, organizational or bureaucratic problems, and resource allocation and reward system differences.

Today's health care team faces many ethical problems and ethical dilemmas. Collaboration among health care team members facilitates coordinated efforts in ethical decision making. Collaboration among the health care team is an important model for communication, focusing efforts on meeting clients' needs in a caring, efficient, and comprehensive manner.

REFERENCES

1. Richard AT. Nurses interfacing with other members of the team. In: England D, ed. *Collaboration in Nursing*. Rockville, MD: Aspen Systems Corp; 1986:163–185.
2. Dincanis AJ, Golin AK. *The Interdisciplinary Health Care Team*. Germantown, MD: Aspen Systems Corp; 1979.
3. Smith AE. Nurses, physicians and hospitals are a team. *Am Nurse*. 1989;21–31:4.
4. Reese B, Brandt R. *Effective Human Relations in Business*. Boston: Houghton Mifflin; 1981.
5. Davis RC. *The Fundamentals of Top Management*. New York: Harper and Row; 1951.
6. Lippitt R. How to get results from a group. In: Bradford LP, ed. *Group Development*. Washington, DC: National Training Labs, National Education Association; 1961.
7. White R, Lippitt R. Leader behavior and member reaction in three social climates. In: Zander E, ed. *Group Dynamics: Research and Theory*. 2nd ed. New York: Harper and Row; 1960.
8. Blechert TF, Christiansen MF, Kari N. Intraprofessional team building. *Am J Occup Ther*. 1987;41(9):576–582.
9. Farley MJ, Stoner MH. The nurse executive and interdisciplinary team building. *Nurs Admin Quart*. 1989;13(2):24–30.
10. Londey D. On the action of teams. *Inquiry*. 1978;12:213–218.
11. American College of Physicians. The Institute of Medicine Report: A manpower policy for primary health care. *Ann Intern Med*. 1980;92:843.
12. American Nurses' Association. *Nursing: A Social Policy Statement*. Kansas City, MO: ANA; 1980.
13. Styles M. Reflections on collaboration and unification. *Image*. Winter 1984, pp. 21–23.
14. Pluckhan ML. Professional territoriality: A problem affecting the delivery of health care. *Nurs Forum*. 1972;11(3):300–310.
15. Engstrom B. Communication and decision-making in a study of a multidisciplinary team conference with the registered nurse as conference chairman. *Int J Nurs Stud*. 1986;23(4):299–314.
16. Blackwell J. Patient compliance. *Med Intel*. 1973;289(5):249–252.
17. Eraker, SA, Kirscht JP, Becker MH. Understanding and improving patient compliance. *Ann Intern Med*. 1984;100(2):258–268.
18. Ryan P, Falco SM. A pilot study to validate the etiologies and defining characteristics of the nursing diagnosis of noncompliance. *Nurs Clin North Am*. 1985;20(4):685–695.
19. Conrad P. The meaning of medications: Another look at compliance. *Soc Sci Med*. 1985;20(1):29–37.
20. Mechanic D, Aiken L. A cooperative agenda for medicine and nursing. *N Engl J Med*. 1982;307:747–750.
21. Nightingale F. *Notes on Nursing: What It Is and What It Is Not*. London: Harrison and Sons; 1859. (Facsimile edition: JB Lippincott; 1946.)
22. Donovan M, Slack J, Robertson S, Andreoli K. The unit assistant: A nurse extender. *Nurs Manage*. 1988;19(10):70–78.
23. Manthey M. Practice partnership. The newest concept in care delivery. *JONA*. 1989;19(2):33–35.
24. Mariano C. The case for interdisciplinary collaboration. *Nurs Outlook*. 1989;37(6):285–288.
25. Styles MM. On nursing: Toward a new endowment. St. Louis, MO: CV Mosby; 1982.
26. MacKay BJ. Nurses interfacing with the community. In: England DA, ed. *Collaboration in Nursing*. Rockville, MD: Aspen Systems Corp; 1986:187–209.
27. Weed LL. *Medical Records, Medical Education, and Patient Care*. Chicago: Yearbook Medical Publishers; 1969.
28. Reifsteck SW. Physician, nurse relationships. *Top Health Care Finances*. 1990;16(3):12–21.
29. McLain BR. Collaborative practice: A critical theory perspective. *Res Nurse Health*. 1988;11(6):391–398.
30. The National Joint Practice Commission. *Guidelines for Establishing Joint or Collaborative Practice in Hospitals*. Chicago: Neely Printing Co; 1981:4.
31. Cronin C, Maklebust J. Case-managed care: Capitalizing on the CNS. *Nurs Manage*. 1989;20(3):38–47.
32. Mauksch IG. Nurse–physician collaboration: A changing relationship. *JONA*. June 1981;35–38.
33. McKay PS. Interdependent decision making: Redefining professional autonomy. *Nurs Admin Quart*. 1983;7(4):21–29.
34. McLain BR. Collaborative practice: A critical theory perspective. *Res Nurse Health*. 1988;11(6):391–398.
35. Lynaugh JE, Bates B. The two languages of nursing and medicine. *Am J Nurs*. 1973;73:66–69.
36. Stein LI, Watts DT, Howell T. The doctor and nurse game revisited. *N Engl J Med*. 1990;322(8):546–549.
37. Weiss SJ. The influence of discourse on collaboration among nurses, physicians, and consumers. *Res Nurs Health*. 1985;8:49–59.
38. Woodman R, Sherwood J. Effects of team development intervention: A field experiment. *J Appl Behav Sci*. 1980;16:214–227.
39. Bruce N. *Teamwork for Preventive Care*. Chichester, UK: Research Studies Press (John Wiley & Sons); 1980.
40. Abramson M. Collective responsibility in interdisciplinary collaboration: An ethical perspective for social workers. *Social Work Health Care*. 1984;10(1):35–43.
41. Newton LH. Collective responsibility in health care. *J Med Philos*. 1982;7(1):11–21.
42. Pellegrino ED, Thomasma DC. *A Philosophical Basis of Medical Practice*. New York: Oxford University Press; 1981:245.

43. Eubanks, P. Nursing restructuring renews focus on patient centered care. *Hospitals.* 1990;64(8):60–62.
44. Dobratz MC. Hospice nursing. Present perspective and future directives. *Cancer Nurs.* 1990;13(2):116–122.

BIBLIOGRAPHY

Baggs JG. Intensive care unit use and collaboration between nurse and physicians. *Heart Lung.* 1989;18(4):332–338.

Baggs JG, Schmitt MH. Collaboration between nurses and physicians. *Image Journal of Nursing Scholarship.* 1988;20(3):145–149.

Cartlidge A, Bond J, Gregson B. Interprofessional collaboration in primary health care. *Nursing Times.* 1987;83(46):45–48.

Friedman H, DiMatteo M, eds. *Interpersonal Issues in Health Care.* New York: Academic Press; 1982.

Iles PA, Auluck R. From organizational to interorganizational development in nursing practice: Improving the effectiveness of interdisciplinary teamwork and interagency collaboration. *J Adv Nurs.* 1990;15(1):50–58.

Moulder P, Staal A, Grant M. Making the interdisciplinary team approach work. *Rehabilitation Nursing.* 1988;13(6):338–339.

Murphy TG. Improving nurse/doctor communications. *Nursing 90.* 1990;20(8):114–118.

Pickard MR, Barbato HL. Strategies for collaboration. *Nursing Management.* 1990;21(9):44–45.

Raines C. Personal value systems: How they affect teamwork. *AORN J.* 1988;48(2):324, 326, 328–330.

Smith A. Nurses, physicians, and hospitals are a team. *American Nurse.* 1989;21(2):4.

White S, Rainey T. Collaboration benefits critically ill patients. *Focus Critical Care.* 1989;16(4):325–326.

Wodarski L, Bundschuh E, Forbus W. Interdisciplinary case management: A model for intervention. *J Am Diet Assoc.* 1988; 88(3):332–335.

CHAPTER 20

Teaching and Learning as Collaboration

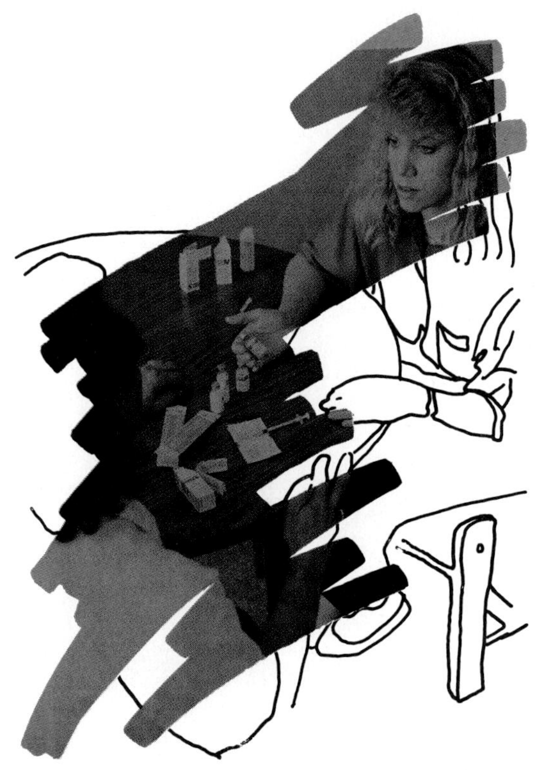

Behavioral Objectives

Upon completion of this chapter, the student will be able to:

1. Define teaching and learning.
2. Describe how each of the steps in the teaching–learning process is carried out collaboratively.
3. Discuss social and professional factors that support client teaching as an integral aspect of client health care.
4. Compare and contrast the definitions of learning and the premises about how learning occurs in behaviorism and the Gestalt-field theory.
5. Describe the types of behaviors that are characteristic of each of the three domains of learning.
6. Discuss the mental operations that are necessary to acquire and process information.
7. List and discuss factors that contribute to an individual's readiness, ability, and learning style.
8. Identify components of the standard health assessment that produce data relevant to health teaching.
9. Identify elements of a client's support system that may influence learning and/or application of health-related knowledge in daily activities. Discuss how these elements may be assessed and incorporated in the teaching–learning process.
10. Discuss at least four etiologies of the Knowledge Deficit nursing diagnosis, explaining how each contributes to a knowledge deficit.
11. Name and describe the components of a teaching–learning plan and form behavioral objectives for such a plan.
12. Compare and contrast informal and structured health teaching and describe situations in which each is appropriate.
13. Discuss the advantages and disadvantages of individual and group teaching approaches and describe situations in which each would be more appropriate.
14. Describe teaching approaches and teaching aids that are appropriate for health teaching.
15. Describe three ways in which client learning may be validated.

KEY TERMS

behavior
behavioral objective
cognitive style
conditioned response
conditioned stimulus
conditioning
feedback
field
Gestalt
knowledge deficit
learning
learning domain
learning objective
literacy
negative reinforcement
positive reinforcement
primary reinforcement
prime
prompt
readiness
response
return demonstration
secondary reinforcement
simultaneous mutual interaction
stimulus
teaching

Recognition of individuals' responsibility for their health and respect for their right to participate actively in health care decisions are primary values in contemporary health care delivery. Information is a critical component of both rights and responsibilities. It follows, then, that if clients are to be full participants in health care decisions, they must have an opportunity to obtain information. Health care providers are an obvious resource for clients needing to learn more about their health and health care.

Even before client education became a point of emphasis in health promotion and health care delivery, nurses perceived teaching as part of their caring role. Nurse Practice Acts in many states mandate client teaching as a component of nursing care. Today, changes in the client population and in health care delivery make meeting clients' needs for health education more critical, yet more challenging. To confront these challenges, nurses need knowledge and skills relevant to teaching and promoting learning.

This chapter presents a collaborative view of teaching and learning that is in keeping with trends in client–provider relationships in health care. **Learning,** defined as the modification of a behavioral tendency by experience, is viewed as an ongoing process. It occurs whether or not there are concerted efforts by others to teach. However,

teaching, or deliberately influencing learning towards specific goals, can have a powerful impact. A teaching–learning interaction is a special form of communication, a process that in many ways parallels the nursing process as discussed in Chapter 18. When all participants in the teaching–learning process perceive the roles of teacher and learner as shared, as is implied by the concept that teaching and learning are collaboration, all participants benefit. To help beginning nursing students participate in collaborative teaching–learning interactions, this chapter introduces basic concepts from major learning theories. Domains of learning and mental operations supporting learning and memory are addressed, with emphasis on application of these concepts to planning and executing health teaching.

This chapter emphasizes the individual characteristics that influence clients' participation in a teaching–learning process. Guidelines are provided for assessing these and other related attributes for the purpose of diagnosing and planning to meet health-related learning needs. Finally, the chapter describes elements of the teaching–learning plan (objectives, content, teaching methods, and evaluation approaches) as well as practical strategies for implementing teaching–learning plans and documenting client teaching.

■ FACTORS SUPPORTING THE NEED FOR CLIENT TEACHING

Social Factors

Patient Bill of Rights. In the early 1970s the American Hospital Association (AHA) published the Patient Bill of Rights.[1] This document acknowledges the rights of clients to receive understandable information about their diagnosis, treatment, and prognosis so they can make informed decisions about available treatment options. It also recognizes clients' rights to obtain health-related information so they can be active, informed participants in their own care. Health care options and treatment modalities are becoming increasingly complex, making straightforward communication from providers even more critical to informed client decisions. The Patient Bill of Rights, while not a legal document in all states, serves as a guideline for providing services in many hospitals. Some states have recognized specific patient rights by law.[2]

IMPLICATIONS FOR NURSE–CLIENT COLLABORATION

Importance of the Nurse as Teacher

The collaborative philosophy holds that clients retain a significant measure of responsibility for their own health, and that health care outcomes are enhanced by nurses' respect for clients' right to actively participate in health care decisions. For clients to be competent participants in health care decisions, they must have an opportunity to obtain relevant information. The nurse is often one of the client's most important information sources. As a teacher of health concepts and facts, nurses can be significant influences on clients and an important support to clients' collaboration in decision making.

Informed Consent. The doctrine of informed consent reinforces clients' rights to knowledge about their health and autonomy in making decisions about health matters. Legally, informed consent principles specify that clients must be given information about their diagnosis; the purpose, probable success and risks of proposed treatment; treatment alternatives; and the consequences of not receiving the proposed treatment.[3] The quality of information given is an important consideration, because information must be provided in a manner that clients can understand.[4] Health care terminology can be confusing and unintelligible to clients. Although statutes regulating informed consent vary from state to state, informed consent always requires that information be provided in everyday terms. Informed consent provides opportunities for clients and health care professionals to share information and participate in the decision-making process so that client autonomy in health-related matters is preserved. More detailed information about ethical responsibilities associated with informed consent is presented in Chapter 34; further discussion of laws relating to health care is found in Chapter 3.

The Consumer Movement. The consumer movement has helped make client education an integral part of health services.[5] Many consumers have become dissatisfied with the dependency that has traditionally characterized their relationships with health care providers. They not only seek information about health and health care as individuals but also have formed groups that lobby for changes in health care policy, including more emphasis on health education programs. Consumer awareness, therefore, has fostered a more active client role in health care as well as promoted the consumer education that supports such a role. Consumerism and its impact on health care are discussed further in Chapter 37.

Increase in Chronic Illness. At the present time, chronic illnesses such as diabetes, emphysema, and hypertension account for a significant portion of health care services sought by clients. This is at least partially attributable to the increasing numbers of elderly persons in our population. As the average life expectancy continues to increase, incidence of chronic illness is expected to increase as well. Moreover, with current changes in health care payment systems (discussed below), more care must be provided in outpatient settings, and more responsibility for care and early recognition of illness falls to clients themselves. Increased health knowledge can help people prevent, control, or limit the effects of chronic disease.[6] For many chronically ill clients, therefore, effective health teaching may be crucial to their quality of life.

Emphasis on Health Promotion. Levin suggested that client education has often been too narrowly focused on providing specific illness-related information after a disease has been diagnosed.[7] With the emerging emphasis on health promotion and disease prevention, there is a growing need for client education related to self-care and wellness. Some self-care education programs are now available to consumers. These programs are holistic in that they emphasize supporting and improving physical, emotional, and social well-being. Examples include stress management, nutritional counseling, childbirth preparation classes, and exercise and physical fitness classes. Nurses can participate in the wellness self-care movement by being positive role models and by routinely including identification of needs for information about health promotion and self-care in their client assessments. Health promotion strategies can then be integrated into client health education plans.

Health Care Payment Systems. The implementation of prospective payment for Medicare patients and limitations on length of stay being imposed by government and third-party insurance companies (discussed in Chap. 35) have stimulated some health care delivery institutions to view client education as one way of promoting early discharge. However, shorter hospital stays reduce the time available for client education, and hospital nurses may be faced with the dilemma of teaching clients whose needs for information are greater than ever, while their readiness to learn is hampered by the acuteness of their illness.

At the least, these changes require that nurses facilitate client learning earlier and more efficiently.[8] Determining learning priorities, developing a teaching–learning plan, and covering various portions of the plan as the client moves between different types of service settings will be an increasingly important part of the nursing process. Written documentation of the client education plan will also be crucial to coordinate the client learning that has been accomplished in various settings.

Professional Factors

Professional Standards. Various professional groups have endorsed the responsibility of professional health care providers to provide client education (see Chap. 2). In 1975, the American Nurses' Association (ANA) published a document entitled *The Professional Nurse and Health Education* that affirmed the nurse's responsibility to teach clients and families about their health needs and the behavioral changes recommended to achieve and maintain a healthy state.[9] Specific responsibilities in various client care settings were described. During hospitalization, for example, nursing responsibilities include assessing clients' knowledge levels about their condition, preparing the client for surgery and other procedures, and making plans for discharge teaching and continuing care after discharge.

In 1976, the Joint Commission on Accreditation of Hospitals, now called the Joint Commission on Accreditation of Healthcare Organizations (JCAHO), began to include standards for patient education as part of the criteria for accrediting health care organizations.[4] These standards require that client learning opportunities be provided as an integral part of all health care services. Because nurses constitute the largest group of health care professionals and have the skills needed to facilitate collaborative teaching and learning, they often provide these client services.

Nurse Practice Acts. Many state Nurse Practice Acts explicitly include client teaching as part of the role of the professional nurse.[2] Although the legal role of the nurse in client education has been generally mandated, specific standards of practice regarding nursing implementation of the teaching–learning process have not been consistently outlined. Today, professional nurses facilitate client learning as one of many practice activities. In almost all health care settings nurses have the most consistent, ongoing contact with clients. Often these contacts include informal, spontaneous teaching as well as planned, formal, organized teaching–learning sessions. Mutual collaboration and information sharing between client and nurse about learning needs and goals can facilitate learning of both client and nurse during nurse–client contacts.

Professional Literature. Cohen's review of literature about client learning described the impact of client education on health status.[10] The nonresearch literature that he reviewed stressed the general importance of client education and described steps in the teaching–learning process that need to be implemented in health teaching. The review of research literature revealed the importance of assessment to individualize teaching approaches and objectives. It also indicated concrete benefits of planned structured teaching, such as shorter hospital stays and in some instances fewer complications. An analysis of research in the area of client preoperative instruction concluded that preoperative teaching results in impressive cost savings and improved client physical and psychosocial well-being.[11] However, while the nurses in the studies recognized the need to provide preoperative education, the amount of time and the comprehensiveness of instruction they provided was far below what the research evidence suggested was needed. Reasons given included lack of time and lack of overt support for nurse-delivered client education.

Wilson-Barnett and Osborne[12] provide additional explanations for nurses omitting teaching. Some of the reasons these authors cited were nurses' perceived lack of time, lack of awareness of clients' needs for information, and lack of confidence and knowledge about how to carry out teaching activities.

The information presented in this chapter is intended to provide a foundation for the knowledge nurses need to do successful health teaching.

■ CONCEPTS RELATED TO LEARNING

Learning Theories

A learning theory is a systematic way of describing the process by which individuals relate to their environment in order to use themselves and their environment more effectively. Since the 17th century, psychologists have developed learning theories supported by experimentation. From these theories, several different schools of thought regarding learning evolved during the 19th and 20th centuries. None of these theories proves conclusively that learning occurs only in one particular way. Contemporary research and discourse about learning continue to refine earlier concepts. However, even as learning theories are crystallized or modified, they provide useful bases for developing educational programs.

Because nurses assume pivotal responsibility for providing health education to clients, they need a basic understanding of major learning theories. This knowledge is necessary to plan and conduct effective client teaching. Two broad families of learning theories are discussed here: behaviorism and the Gestalt-field theories. These theories have generated significant scientific interest and inquiry in recent decades.

Behaviorism. Behaviorists define learning as a "change in observable behavior that occurs as a result of stimuli and responses becoming related according to mechanistic principles."[13] Several key words in this definition require further explanation. First, behavior. To a behaviorist, a **behavior** is "publicly observable activity of muscles or glands of external secretion as manifested, for example, by movements of parts of the body, or the appearance of sweat, tears or saliva."[14] The physiological, especially the neural, basis for the "observable activity" is regarded as the basis for changes in behavior (learning). Mental activities, because they are not observable, are not considered relevant to the learning process. Some behaviorists do, however, acknowledge mental reaction (thinking), considering it a symbolic movement, and therefore a symbolic response, that takes place as an intermediate step between the overt stimulus and the overt response. In this view, thought is not a covert, mysterious process that causes behavior, but is the behavior itself.[13]

Stimuli and responses are also key concepts in the behaviorist definition of learning. A **stimulus** is the cause of learning. Stimuli are events or agents in the environment that act upon the organism. The environment consists of an individual's physical and social surroundings, described in objective terms. Because of the objective, physical nature of environment, anyone can see, hear, feel, smell, or taste the environment of anyone else. A **response** is an organism's overt physical reaction to stimulation from the environment.

Behaviorists describe stimuli and responses as mechanistically related because they believe that humans have innate needs (or drives) and reflexes which are "built in." Therefore, responses are preprogrammed and automatic. A specific stimulus always elicits the same response, unless changes in the environment modify the automatic response. Humans, like machines, passively wait for environmental activity, and then react in a predictable fashion.

Behavior, then, is controlled solely by its consequences. Because the consequences depend on the environment (which includes the teacher), learning is dependent on the teacher; the learner is passive. To change behavior (that is, to produce learning) a teacher must create new relationships or associations between stimuli and responses. This process is called **conditioning.** There are two basic types of conditioning: classical and instrumental.

Classical Conditioning. Classical conditioning relies on stimulus substitution. Early classical conditioning experiments were done on animals by the Russian physiologist, Ivan Pavlov. Others who contributed to classical conditioning theory include J. B. Watson and the more contemporary E. R. Guthrie.

In classical conditioning, a stimulus related to a given drive, called an adequate stimulus, is presented, eliciting the expected response. Then a second, neutral, stimulus is presented at the same time as the adequate stimulus. The repeated pairing of the adequate and the neutral stimuli causes the organism to associate the two stimuli. Eventually, the organism learns to respond to the neutral stimulus in the same way as to the adequate stimulus, even in the absence of the adequate stimulus (Fig. 20–1). The new (formerly neutral) stimulus is called a **conditioned stimulus;** the response to that stimulus, a **conditioned response.**

The following example uses classical conditioning techniques to describe how you teach a dog to come to you when you call its name. First, present a piece of meat at some distance from the dog, but within its sight and smell. The meat is an adequate stimulus—the dog will approach it. As the dog approaches, present the neutral stimulus as well: Call the dog's name. With repetition of the combined stimuli, the dog will soon come in response to the calling alone, having learned to respond to the conditioned stimulus in the same way it instinctively responded to the original stimulus.

A conditioned response tends to be extinguished—that is, to become weaker and disappear over time—as the association between the adequate and neutral stimuli fades. Giving the organism a reward, or reinforcement, when it demonstrates the conditioned response will strengthen and maintain the response. The reinforcement is not needed to establish the conditioned response, only to maintain it over time. In order to maintain the conditioned response in the above example (coming when called), you must reward

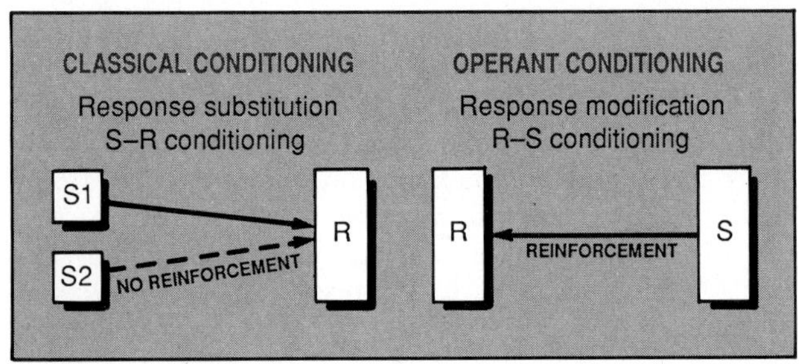

Figure 20–1. Types of conditioning.

the dog in some way when it comes to you, at least some of the time. Reinforcement is discussed further below.

Classical conditioning is the basis for the Lamaze method of prepared childbirth. It is used to replace the unconditioned response to pain (muscle tension) with a conditioned response of muscle relaxation. After teaching the woman to relax her muscles in response to a specific stimulus (the command "relax"), the teacher or the woman's partner presents the command at the same time as a painful stimulus. After successive pairing of these two stimuli, the painful stimulus will elicit the relaxation response. Other responses, such as patterned breathing, may be conditioned in the same way. The woman will then respond to the pain of labor by relaxing her muscles and initiating a specific breathing pattern. In this case the reward that strengthens and maintains the response does not come from the environment, as with the example of the dog. Instead, it is internal—a feeling of mastery over a potentially stressful life event: labor and childbirth.

Instrumental Conditioning. Instrumental conditioning is based on the work of E. L. Thorndike in the early 1900s. Contemporary theorists C. L. Hull, B. F. Skinner, R. M. Gagne, and Albert Bandura also employed instrumental conditioning (sometimes called operant conditioning) concepts in their learning theories. Rather than presenting a stimulus to elicit a response from a learner, as in classical conditioning, a teacher using instrumental conditioning offers a feedback stimulus (reinforcement) after the learner displays a given response. In other words, the response precedes the stimulus (see Fig. 20–1). Each time an organism displays the desired behavior (response), whether spontaneously or with guidance, the reinforcing stimulus is presented. For example, a parent might use instrumental conditioning to teach a child appropriate social behavior by praising the child each time he or she remembers to use good manners. Therefore, the desired response is instrumental in bringing about the reinforcing stimulus, but the stimulus that prompted the desired response in the first place is not central to the learning process. Instrumental conditioning involves a response that accomplishes something. After multiple presentations of a reward for a given behavioral response, the learner actively selects and displays that behavior to obtain the reinforcement.

The reinforcement is selected because it satisfies a need of the organism. The experience of need satisfaction when a certain behavior occurs increases the likelihood that the behavior will be repeated in the future. To be most effective, reinforcement must be closely associated in time with the desired behavior. If future repetitions of the behavior are followed by similar reinforcement, the behavior will become stronger, eventually becoming a habit. Irregular reinforcement (that is, providing reinforcement for most but not all occurrences of the desired behavior) has been found to be most effective in strengthening behaviors.

Reinforcement is further categorized in operant conditioning theory. **Positive reinforcement** is a stimulus whose presence strengthens the response. **Negative reinforcement** is a stimulus whose withdrawal strengthens the response. Negative reinforcement, therefore, is seen as psychologically different from punishment. Both positive and negative reinforcement can be primary or secondary. **Primary reinforcement** strengthens a certain behavior because it satisfies a basic or biological need of the organism. **Secondary reinforcement,** or higher-order reinforcement, is effective because it has acquired value indirectly through learning and hence strengthens behavior as a primary reinforcer would. Money and praise are examples of secondary reinforcers for humans.

Operant conditioning is used more often than classical conditioning in human learning. Behavior modification programs that promote weight loss or attempt to eradicate addictions (cigarettes, alcohol) rely on operant conditioning, as do biofeedback techniques. Many teachers use principles of operant conditioning in school settings. In a sense, the grading systems used by most schools can be viewed as operant conditioning systems, in that students who display desired behaviors are rewarded with good grades.

Gestalt-field Theories. Gestalt-field psychology originated in Germany in the early 20th century. Its major premises almost directly contradict the mechanistic, physiologically based ideas that underlie behaviorism. The basis for Gestalt psychology was Max Wertheimer's assertions, in 1912, that an organized whole is more than the sum of its parts. Gestaltists consider the whole organism, rather than just its nervous system, as having a significant role in learning. Gestalt learning theories have been developed by German psychologists Wolfgang Kohler and Kurt Lewin and American psychologists Rollo May and Gordon Allport, among others.

Gestalt-field theorists define learning as a process of gaining or changing insights, outlooks, expectations, or thought patterns that provides a potential guide for future behavior.[13] A gain or change in insight or thought patterns implies a new way of looking at one's environment or the elements within it. Thus, for Gestaltists, learning is not observable behavior but rather a change in experience—a mental or psychological process unique to each individual. A change in behavior may be evidence of learning, but it is not learning itself. In fact, one may have a change of behavior without learning, or learning without a change of behavior.

The concept of *Gestalt,* a German noun, is not easily translated into English; therefore, the term has been carried over into English psychological literature. **Gestalt** refers to an organized configuration or pattern, including all that the pattern is composed of. The term **field,** as used by Gestaltists, encompasses a person, the person's environment, and the interaction between the two. The Gestalt-field, the complex organized entity of individual and environment, influences learning.

Environment is not construed to be simply one's surroundings, but rather what one makes of one's surroundings: one's perceptions. Environment is, therefore, time- and situation-dependent. One may perceive the same external surroundings quite differently at different times or under different circumstances. Similarly, two individuals in identical physical surroundings might have different perceptions and therefore different fields.

Gaining or changing insights, or learning, occurs through a process of **simultaneous mutual interaction** within the person's field—that is, between individual and environment. Each affects the other. The individual is not mechanistically dependent upon the environment as postulated in behavioral learning theory, but may also influence the environment. Simultaneous mutual interaction implies that at any time during learning, the individual's behavior may alter the environment and vice versa. Moreover, each person's reality—what he or she perceives in a given situation—influences learning in that situation.

Therefore, what an individual learns in any given situation depends on the environment, on the individual, and on the interaction between them. Environmental factors include how the stimuli are presented (visual, tactile, auditory, and so forth), how many stimuli there are, and whether the stimuli enhance or interfere with other stimuli. Individual factors include how and whether the stimuli are received; how they are perceived, which is influenced by past experiences and memory; and how the individual reacts to stimuli and uses them for goal achievement. Simultaneous mutual interactions are continuous individual–environment exchanges that occur throughout the stimuli presentation and stimuli reception-perception-utilization processes. The stimuli may be objects, facts, ideas, processes, or other individuals' behavior. Moreover, since individuals' perceptions are part of their environment, the stimuli may originate from an individual's own mind. Figure 20–2 represents learning from a Gestalt-field point of view.

From a perspective of a Gestaltist, the tension that motivates learning is a sense of purpose, an attempt to find meaning in the environment or use the environment advantageously. Learning involves gaining understanding of phenomena in the perceptual field, appreciating relationships among them, and developing abilities to use the environment effectively or in new creative ways. This implies

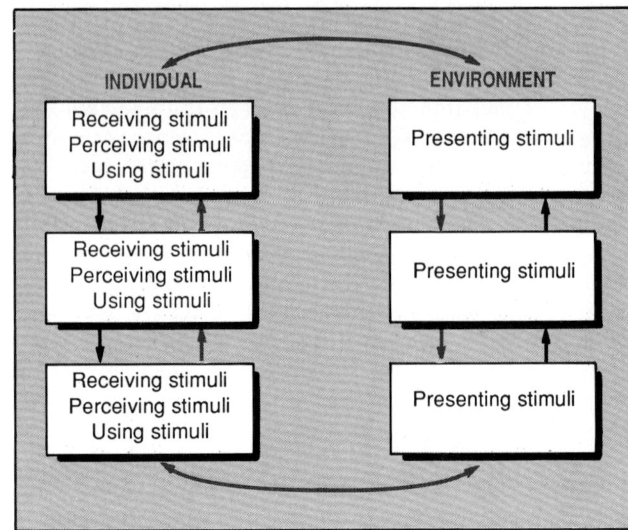

Figure 20–2. Gestalt-field view of learning.

that personal involvement is necessary to the learning process.

The learning experience is an interactive event between individual and environment in which, through acting and seeing what happens, a person learns the consequences of the action. This insight can then influence future behavior. In contrast, behaviorists contend that simply being exposed to the environment in which the appropriate stimuli are presented is sufficient to bring about learning.

Gestalt-field theory has particular relevance in a collaborative approach to teaching and learning. The concept of simultaneous mutual interaction implies that, in effect, the roles of teacher and learner merge. Each is influenced by the other; therefore, each is both a teacher and a learner simultaneously. Moreover, the demeanor, approach, communication style, and a myriad of other variables related to both participants can be expected to influence the teaching–learning interaction.

IMPLICATIONS FOR NURSE–CLIENT COLLABORATION

Gestalt-field Theory

According to Gestalt-field theory, learning occurs through a process of simultaneous mutual interaction between the individual and the environment. In building a collaborative relationship, the nurse and client share experience. Each becomes an important aspect of the other's environment, interacting mutually, and through interaction, gaining insight into themselves as persons and into their role as partners in the process of moving toward optimal health for the client. Under Gestalt-field theory, teaching and learning can be shared, and for each participant, personal change is a possibility.

Humanistic Learning Theories. Gestalt-field theory is the basis for various humanistic learning theories, which include theories of motivation and behavior, such as those of Abraham Maslow and Carl Rogers. In humanistic learning theories, the impact of emotions and culture on perceptions, and therefore on learning, is given particular importance. The need to attain a feeling of personal adequacy is seen as a major factor that drives learning. Taking responsibility for one's own learning through self-evaluation and self-feedback is one way to foster feelings of personal adequacy.[15] Therefore, teaching–learning plans based on humanistic learning theory often incorporate opportunities for learner self-evaluation.

Albert Bandura's social learning theory blends concepts of behaviorism, Gestalt-field, and humanistic learning theory. Bandura contends that imitation, the act of copying a model or example, is the basis of learning. Imitation, or modeling, is most likely to occur when the learner identifies with the individual being modeled. Identification, a concept derived from psychoanalytic literature, is a process in which individuals take on beliefs, attitudes, and values of another and incorporate them as part of their own personality. For example, young children commonly identify with their parents. Later, other role models such as teachers and peers may become objects of identification.

According to social learning theory, reinforcement also has a role in learning. Behaviors that are rewarded are more likely to become permanent or habitual. Both modeling and reinforcement occur in a social context; that is, in group interaction. Group membership and social dynamics influence modeling and the impact of reinforcement. For example, Bandura states that individuals are most likely to imitate those with high prestige, and reinforcement of behavior given by high-prestige individuals is most powerful. Furthermore, group pressure increases the likelihood that a given behavior will occur, as does observing others receive rewards for the behavior.[16]

Both major learning theories, behaviorism and Gestalt-field theory, as well as humanistic and social learning theories, have useful applications for nurses. Important concepts from each of these learning theories, with implications for collaboration, appear in Table 20–4 at the end of the chapter.

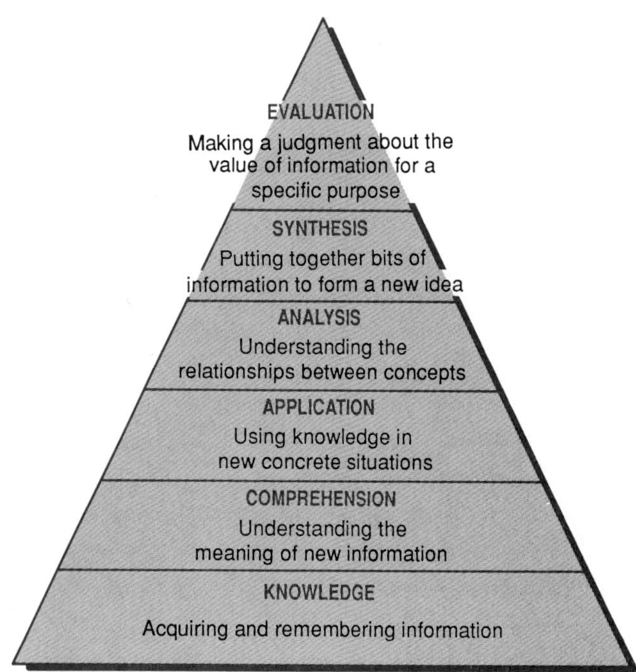

Figure 20–3. Taxonomy of the cognitive domain.

Domains of Learning

Benjamin Bloom described three domains of learning: cognitive, affective, and psychomotor.[17] A **learning domain** is a particular category, or class, of learning in which learning behaviors or abilities are defined and organized according to their relative complexity or difficulty. The domains are not mutually exclusive. Most learning situations require skills from more than one domain. Identifying the learning domains and skills applicable in a learning situation helps the teacher to sequence instruction and select teaching approaches.

Cognitive Domain. The cognitive domain comprises intellectual skills. Bloom[14] identified six levels of cognitive behaviors:

1. *Knowledge:* acquiring and remembering information.
2. *Comprehension:* understanding the meaning of new information; that is, ability to restate information in one's own words.
3. *Application:* using knowledge in new concrete situations.
4. *Analysis:* understanding the relationships between concepts.
5. *Synthesis:* putting together bits of information to form a new idea.
6. *Evaluation:* making a judgment about the value of information for a specific purpose.

Higher-level cognitive learning is based on previous learning of lower-level skills (Fig. 20–3). For example, before learners can use information or knowledge in their daily lives (level 3), they must be able to remember (level 1) and restate (level 2) that information. Before learners can compare or describe relationships between concepts (level 4), they must remember (level 1), restate in their own words (level 2), and use the information in concrete situations (level 3). In most health teaching situations, the minimum level of cognitive learning desired of clients is application: using knowledge to improve health. For example, clients with high blood pressure need to know and understand their medication regimen in order to use this information to help monitor their responses to the medication.

Affective Domain. The affective domain involves learning that deals with feelings and emotions, including beliefs, values, and interests (Fig. 20–4). Learning about ethics and moral behavior is also included in the affective domain. Krathwohl, Bloom, and Masia[18] identified five levels of behavior in the affective domain:

1. *Receiving:* attending to phenomenon, to another's expression of ideas or beliefs.
2. *Responding:* reacting verbally and nonverbally to phenomenon, to another's expression of ideas or beliefs.
3. *Valuing:* attaching worth to an object or belief; exhibiting commitment.
4. *Organizing:* building a consistent value system by bringing together different values and resolving conflicts among them.
5. *Characterizing:* acting and responding in ways that reflect a consistent value system.

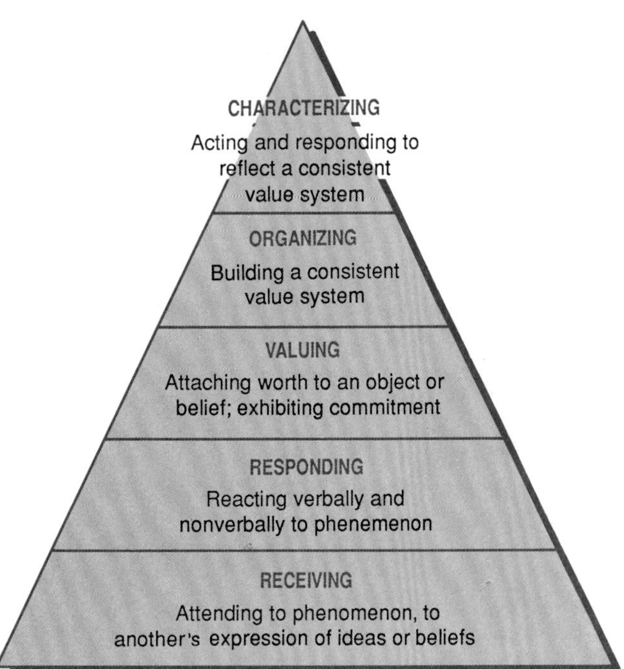

Figure 20–4. Taxonomy of the affective domain.

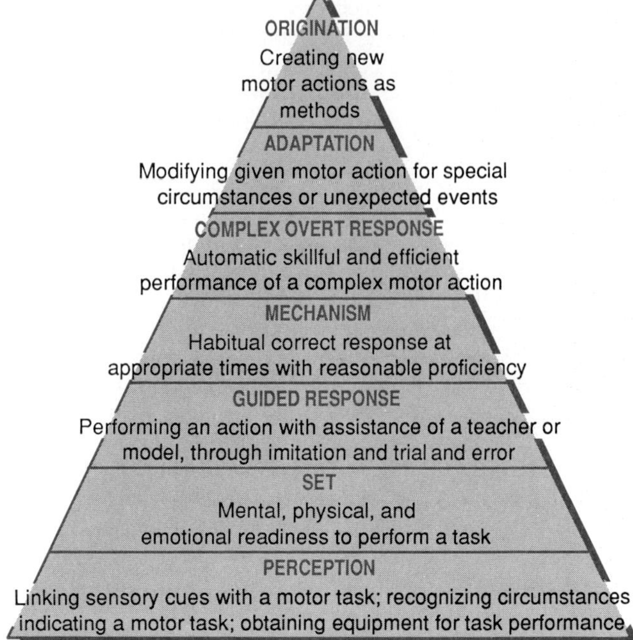

Figure 20–5. Taxonomy of the psychomotor domain.

Nurses can be sensitive to affective aspects of learning by observing clues about clients' feelings toward learning new health competencies. For example, a client must be willing to look at his colostomy stoma site (receiving) before he can be expected to recognize the importance of colostomy self-care (valuing).

Clients are not likely to be motivated to learn health practices that conflict with their strongly held cultural or religious beliefs. For example, helping a client with high blood pressure learn to control this disease often involves teaching about following a prescribed medication regimen, limiting the amount of sodium in the diet, and using stress management strategies. A particular client may value learning about managing stress and taking prescribed medications safely but resist learning about low-sodium diets because of cultural food preferences for foods high in sodium. To be effective, the teaching plan should focus on the knowledge the client is motivated to apply. The nurse might present information about the risks of a high-sodium diet and alternative methods of seasoning foods but place greater emphasis on the other strategies that the client valued more.

Psychomotor Domain. The psychomotor domain involves skills that require integration of mental and motor activity (Fig. 20–5). The classification model devised by Simpson[19] has seven levels of behavior:

1. *Perception:* linking sensory cues with a specific motor task. Recognizing circumstances under which a given motor task is indicated; obtaining appropriate equipment if needed for task performance.
2. *Set:* readiness to take a particular action. Includes:
   - Mental set: mentally focusing on the action to be performed.
   - Physical set: assuming the correct body position to initiate the action.
   - Emotional set: willingness to perform the action.
3. *Guided response:* performing an action with assistance of a teacher or model through imitation and trial and error.
4. *Mechanism:* habitual correct response at appropriate times with reasonable proficiency.
5. *Complex overt response:* automatic skillful and efficient performance of a complex motor action.
6. *Adaptation:* modifying given motor action for special circumstances or when unexpected events occur.
7. *Origination:* creating new motor actions as methods.

Psychomotor learning illustrates the overlap between the domains. For example, for a client who is learning to give a self-injection, cognitive knowledge about the equipment and the drug and affective learning about the value of the injection will influence the learning of the motor actions of preparing the syringe and administering the injection.

Mental Operations in Learning

Learning involves acquiring, processing, and using information, endeavors that are different from one another but that may occur simultaneously. Performing them entails several mental operations, or cognitive processes. The level of proficiency with which individuals perform these operations is directly related to their ability to learn and also seems to be related to overall intelligence.

Acquiring Information. Acquiring information includes both sensory reception and discrimination.

Sensory Reception. Sensory reception is a function of neurosensory integration; sense organs receive signals, which are transmitted via the nervous system to the brain. Sensory reception is not always a conscious process, and it is more or less continuous.

Discrimination. Discrimination involves the ability to distinguish figure from background; that is, recognizing which stimuli within the perceptual field are relevant in a given situation or context. Stimuli may be objects, actions, ideas, facts, or processes. They may be external or internal. Discrimination is more difficult when the field contains many simultaneous stimuli, particularly if they are complex.

Processing Information. Processing of information involves ascribing meaning to that information through association, generalization and concept formation.

Association. Association refers to the ability to link ideas or objects. At the simplest level, association involves pairing ideas, but clustering of multiple related ideas is also association. The latter, however, also requires generalization (discussed below). Naming objects is an example of simple verbal association: A visual stimulus (the object) is associated with a verbal response (the name). Association involves recall, or the ability to retrieve the correct response from memory. It may also involve stimulus coding, or mentally transforming a stimulus into a different type of symbol. Because language is a significant element in human learning, individuals often use verbal coding, such as forming acronyms, labels, or other word associations, to facilitate learning. Visually oriented learners may, instead, transform words into mental images. (See the discussion of learning styles later in the chapter.)

Sometimes associations are formed gradually, sometimes instantaneously. Individuals can make both forward and backward associations. In a forward association, one recalls the response when the stimulus is presented. For example, a teacher holds up a syringe, and the student recalls the name: syringe. In a backward association, when given the response, one recalls the associated stimulus: given the cue "syringe," the student selects the correct object. Linking ideas or linking ideas and objects is easier when the information is meaningful to the learner. Then stimuli can be organized or clustered. This involves processes called generalization and concept formation, both of which also depend upon recall.

Generalization. Generalization means perceiving similarities among stimuli. One may generalize among current stimuli or among current stimuli and those in memory. A young child learning names of objects in the environment learns that small furry objects with four legs are called cats. When encountering a puppy or a gopher the child is likely to call it a cat. The child has noted the more obvious similarities in the animals and generalized that all such objects are cats.

Concept Formation. Concept formation means classifying or organizing stimuli that have some elements or attributes in common. When older, a child will appreciate that although all of the small four-legged objects are different, they share common attributes which link them—they are all animals. The child has now grasped the concept of animal and would most likely be able to recognize that a new stimulus, for example a lion, having attributes in common with other familiar animals, belonged to the same category. Categorizing or conceptualizing relationships often requires abstraction—that is, appreciating qualities or characteristics that are not material, do not exist in concrete form. Therefore, although verbal processes play a role in concept formation, it is not an entirely verbal process. Concept formation permits an individual to use an object or idea in many different situations.

Using Information. Using information refers to its application in cognitive, affective, and psychomotor activities in daily life. Generally, the higher-level behaviors in each of the learning domains are related to using information. For example, application, analysis, and synthesis are cognitive behaviors related to using information in life situations; valuing, organizing, and characterizing are affective behaviors requiring ability to use values; mechanism, complex overt responses, adaptation, and origination are psychomotor behaviors involving application of psychomotor skills to daily life.

The greater one's ability to grasp sophisticated, complex concepts, the more effectively one can function in one's environment. The ability to formulate and link concepts is essential for the critical thinking skills needed to recognize and understand basic rules or principles underlying natural phenomena—such as the laws of physics, human physiology, or the functioning of a simple machine. Creative thinking and problem-solving skills that facilitate adaptation to new situations depend upon concept learning as well. In one way or another, all that we do depends upon our ability to perform the mental operations involved in acquiring and processing information, whether we perform mundane and routine tasks or make complex and innovative attempts to find new meaning and new ways to use our environment.

Collaborative View of Learning

Discussions of learning are often accompanied by parallel discussions of teaching. Although teaching and learning are in fact complementary processes, learning occurs at all times, whether or not there is intentional teaching. Individuals learn from all experiences. When two individuals interact, they learn about one another and from one another. This is true regardless of the relationship between them: whether they are parent and child, teacher and student, client and nurse, or shopkeeper and customer. What is learned is influenced by the attitudes of the individuals and their approach to the interaction. For example, a directive, critical parent teaches children that they cannot solve their own problems, but must remain dependent. An unfriendly, discourteous shopkeeper teaches customers to shop elsewhere. Authoritative, insensitive nurses teach clients not to trust them.

A collaborative view of learning, like the mutual interaction model of nursing practice, emphasizes the importance of dialogue between individuals—that is, a mutually respectful exchange of ideas. A collaborative approach to all interactions with clients teaches clients that nurses can be trusted. The resulting climate of openness provides opportunities for nurses to learn much about clients, which facilitates selection of appropriate formal teaching topics and approaches. Figure 20–6 illustrates exchanges of messages and responses between teacher and learner, characteristics of individuals that influence learning (discussed below), and the influence of the environment.

CHARACTERISTICS OF LEARNERS THAT INFLUENCE LEARNING

Characteristics of learners are personal qualities or attributes that determine whether a person can learn and predict which teaching approaches are likely to be effective. Certain characteristics may also suggest which topics are appropriate. Some of the characteristics are innate and relatively permanent; others are time- and situation-dependent. Nurses need to understand these characteristics and their influence on learning and recognize their manifestations in a given client. Three major characteristics discussed here are readiness, ability, and learning style.

Readiness

Readiness is willingness to take action or to participate in a teaching–learning interaction. Several factors—including motivation, past experiences with learning (especially health related), current physical condition, and developmental stage—determine a client's readiness for health teaching.

> **IMPLICATIONS FOR NURSE–CLIENT COLLABORATION**
>
> **Teaching and Learning in a Collaborative Relationship**
>
> Learning is the modification of a behavioral tendency by experience—a human process that occurs whether or not there has been an effort to teach. Teaching refers to the deliberate acts of people to influence the learning of others toward specific goals. In any collaborative relationship, including the one between nurse and client, teaching and learning merge. The nurse is both a teacher and a learner and so is the client. Nurses learn about clients and teach them things that make health an easier goal to achieve. Clients teach nurses about themselves and about the supports and constraints that bear on their achievement of health, and, in turn, learn how to use their supports and work around their constraints in order to become healthier.

Motivation. Motivation is the force or drive that generates behavior. An individual's current situation (or field, to use a term from Gestalt learning theory), including internal as well as environmental phenomena, creates a desire for change. An unmet need, whether biological, emotional, or social, or any event that causes disequilibrium in the individual, may motivate a person to seek new information or be open to it when it is offered. Havighurst calls such sensitive periods in which individuals are particularly ready and able to learn "teachable moments."[20] An effective teacher recognizes teachable moments and enhances them using knowledge about the learner and learning theory.

Health Beliefs. Motivation to learn about health and health care relates to a person's health beliefs. Rosenstock's Health Belief Model, discussed in Chapter 12, postulates that several independent variables—including perceived susceptibility, severity, benefits/costs, and barriers—help explain an individual's health behavior. Recently, Rosenstock, in collaboration with Strecher and Becker, incorporated self-efficacy as an additional significant variable to be included in the Health Belief Model.[21] The concept of self-efficacy, the conviction that one can successfully execute behaviors required to produce certain outcomes, was first identified by Bandura as part of his social learning theory.[16] Individuals' health beliefs are influenced by their present knowledge about health and illness and their cultural heritage.

Present Knowledge about Health and Illness. Present knowledge about health and illness directly influences an individual's beliefs about personal susceptibility to illness in general and about the severity—the physical and social consequences—of a given disease. The more individuals know about health and illness, the more realistic are their beliefs about personal susceptibility and the potential impact of disease. Recognizing that one is personally at risk for illness because of age, occupation, or life-style, for example, motivates interest in learning about prevention, whereas believing one is not susceptible decreases motivation.

Knowledge may also affect beliefs about self-efficacy. Lack of certain information or skills may cause individuals to believe they lack ability to carry out necessary self-care. Therefore, their interest in learning about self-care may be diminished, even though they are aware of personal risk of a health problem or have been diagnosed with a specific illness. When clients are knowledgeable about their disease but do not seem motivated to participate in self-care practices, assessment of their attitudes and beliefs using the health belief model can provide the nurse with insights to individualize teaching about self-care.

Some health problems present confusing cost versus benefits pictures to clients, because the immediate detect-

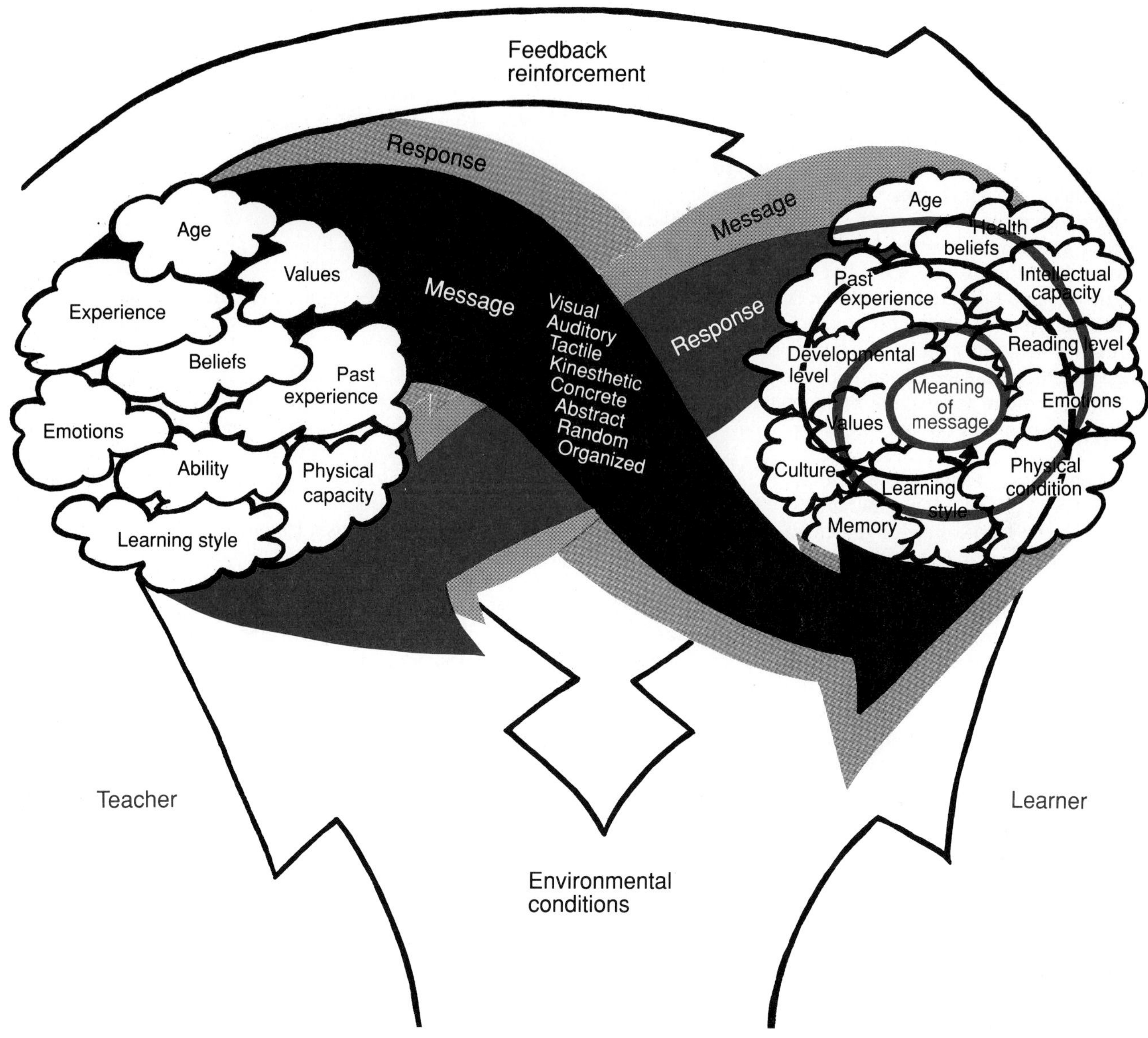

Figure 20–6. Collaborative view of teaching–learning.

able effects do not seem severe, and the treatment causes discomfort, pain, or interference with life-style. For example, high blood pressure has been called the "silent killer" because a client can have this disease for years without experiencing symptoms or obvious effects of the disease. Furthermore, clients who are treated with antihypertensive drugs often experience side effects, such as weakness, lethargy, and impotence, that are more bothersome than the disease itself. These clients may discontinue treatment, because they felt better before they took the medication. The cost (inconvenience, discomfort) of the treatment seems to outweigh its benefits.

Many preventive health care practices, such as losing weight or stopping smoking, require clients to modify or give up behaviors that are pleasurable and gratifying. It may be difficult for people to give up something that is pleasurable when they are presently feeling good or the behavior meets a need. Again, careful assessment of attitudes through soliciting client health beliefs can provide the nurse with information that can be used to modify the teaching plan to make it more acceptable to the client.

Cultural Heritage. Cultural heritage can also have a significant impact on health beliefs. According to Redman people of various ethnic backgrounds may (1) differ in their knowledge about disease, (2) classify disease symptoms into categories that differ from those of the current medical system, and (3) have a variety of ideas about the causes of disease.[22] Additionally, culture influences the way people interact with authority figures and express feelings or requests for assistance. Sensitive questions can determine the degree to which clients have integrated beliefs considered typical of their cultural group.[23] Nurses can gain insight about clients' cultural health beliefs, values, and practices by asking questions that elicit their ideas about (1) what caused a health problem and why it started; (2) what will happen to them as a result of the disease; (3) what treatment they desire and the results they expect to obtain from treatment; and (4) the fears they have about their illness. Showing respect for clients' cultural beliefs while providing scientifically based health information requires sensitivity and understanding. For more detailed information about cultural variability in response to disease, see Chapter 9.

Past Learning Experiences. Readiness to learn is also influenced by past learning experiences. Negative associations with the learner role or the client role will interfere with readiness; conversely, positive feelings tend to promote an open attitude toward learning.

A client's willingness to participate in teaching–learning may also be affected by past encounters with health care providers. Studies have shown that clients are satisfied with health care when (1) their expectations are fulfilled, (2) their concerns are respected and they receive feedback about their condition, and (3) their relationship with a health care provider is warm and sincere.[24] (See also Chap. 12.) Clients who have had unsatisfactory past experiences with providers may be wary of any nurse, including one who attempts to engage them in teaching–learning.

Additionally, past prevailing social attitudes toward health care have been oriented toward rapid cure and the client as a passive recipient of care—people follow directions, take a pill, and they get well. Most people have had experiences with providers that reinforced the passive recipient role. A teaching–learning interaction requires a more active participant role, which some clients may initially be reluctant to assume. Understanding and acceptance by the nurse fosters the client's trust and willingness to pursue teaching–learning. Assessing past experiences may supply information that will enhance nurse–client collaboration during development and implementation of a teaching–learning plan.

Emotional Status. Emotions can enhance or interfere with readiness to participate in teaching–learning. The role of emotion in learning has been addressed by proponents of all the major learning theories. Behaviorists describe emotions or emotional needs as one type of internal drive that stimulates behavior. Gestalt-field theorists emphasize the significance of an individual's field—the psychological forces, including emotions, that are occurring in any given situation. Proponents of humanistic learning theory and social learning theory address the impact of intensity of emotion. Bandura and Walters stress that states of moderate emotional arousal are most conducive to learning.[25] Lack of emotion, or extremely intense emotion, prevents a person from learning, because it produces either lack of arousal or too much arousal. In health teaching situations, anxiety, fear, and panic may accompany health alterations and their treatment. Some clients respond to a serious illness by using psychological coping mechanisms such as anger, denial, or hostility. Generally, these emotional reactions precede a client's acceptance of an altered health state. Health teaching is not likely to be effective until a client accepts the reality of an illness. The nurse should attempt to identify the client's coping mechanisms and facilitate expression of emotions before initiating a teaching–learning interaction.

Physical Condition. A personal health crisis may stimulate clients to be open to learning and amenable to change even if their ability to participate is somewhat limited. Some clients' readiness to participate can best be determined by whether they ask questions about their condition and the type of questions they ask. However, even if clients express interest, an unstable health state, fatigue, or pain will limit attention span. Limited teaching that centers on clients' expressed concerns is appropriate whenever clients' physical condition permits participation. Although extensive teaching–learning contacts should be delayed until the client's condition improves, it is important to begin teaching while the client's attention is heightened as a result of a recent health crisis.

Developmental Stage. A person's learning capabilities and interests change throughout life. Teaching plans should be developed with clients' developmental level in mind. Developmental concepts are presented in Chapter 11; refer to that chapter for a detailed description of developmental stages. Table 14–6, on communicating with children, is another resource. The following discussion covers specific factors for nurses to consider when designing teaching–learning plans for clients of various age groups.

Infants. Infants (birth to 1 year) learn primarily through imitation and sensorimotor activity. Imitation of facial expressions and gestures begins as early as 1 to 2 months of age. Spontaneous purposeful motor responses involving objects in the immediate environment begin at around 6 months. The primary caregiver (parent or a substitute) plays a key role in the infant's life. Health teaching is directed toward helping parents understand and implement health care practices to promote or restore their child's health as well as recognize when to seek assistance from a health care provider.

Toddlers. Toddlers (ages 1 to 3) learn through observing what others around them do. Since the toddler's environment may be expanded beyond the home setting, other role models besides the parents may influence their behavior. Toddlers are capable of learning some simple self-care practices, such as brushing teeth and washing hands, and may be quite interested in acquiring these skills to assert their independence. Although vocabulary expands considerably during toddlerhood, toddlers are not consistently verbal when prompted to speak, nor do they process information verbally. Therefore, they need pictures to illustrate concepts or activities to be learned or objects to manipulate and practice with. Health teaching for parents is also appropriate.

Preschool Children. Preschool children (ages 3 to 5) gradually become more social in their activities. Thinking beyond the immediate surroundings begins; preschoolers can remember past events and imagine the future. This is the beginning of learning by concept formation, which is critical to later development of logical thinking. During this stage, children can exert increasing control over their emotions and learn to assume greater independence in self-care and grooming. Modesty becomes important to children during this period. Play activities can be an important way of teaching about health needs. The nurse should answer the child's questions in simple, easily understood words. Nurses may need to negotiate with preschool children by offering positive rewards for following recommended health care practices. Including parents in health teaching will enable them to reinforce good health practices with their children.

School-age Children. School-age children (ages 5 to 12) are generally interested in learning about their daily lives and forming relationships with peers. Learning rules is important at this age. School-age children can understand cause-and-effect relationships and begin to develop logical reasoning skills that contribute to problem-solving. They can learn positive health care practices but may have difficulty sticking with these practices over time. A parent (or a substitute) should learn health care information as well and reinforce the child's behavior. Nurses can enhance learning by incorporating the child's activities of daily living in the teaching plan. Important concepts to be explored during this period include death and sexuality.

Adolescents. Adolescents (ages 12 to 18) become increasingly adept at logical reasoning and abstract thinking skills. These skills promote the ability to reason hypothetically—that is, to construct possible explanations for events and then logically evaluate the hypotheses. Physical appearance, peer identity, and being like one's friends are important during this period. Adolescents therefore have great difficulty following health care practices that make them feel isolated or different from their friends. Health teaching that emphasizes the immediate benefits of following recommended practices is more effective than threats of negative outcomes if the care practices are ignored.

Adolescents are concerned with establishing their own identity separate from their immediate family. Independence and autonomy are important to adolescents. Legally, the age of informed consent in most states is 18; however, from an ethical and developmental standpoint it may be appropriate for adolescents to be encouraged to make some informed decisions about their own health care by the age of 13 or 14. Parents and adolescents may disagree about the merit of certain recommended health care practices. Disagreement can create conflicts that nurses must consider in making or implementing the teaching–learning plan.

Young Adults. Young adults (ages 18 to 30) are at their prime physically and mentally. Maturation is essentially complete, although drives for self-improvement are strong. Establishing careers, earning a living, forming new relationships with a marriage partner or a significant other, and possibly becoming parents are important pursuits for young adults. They may neglect their own health care needs because they feel "too busy" because of the many obligations they have undertaken or because they are more focused on providing for the health needs of other family members.

Young adults need information about risks to their health and about life-style adjustments they can make to promote health, as well as assistance to deal with fears and problems adapting to illness. If they have previously been generally healthy, they may have a hard time accepting an illness or recommended changes in health care practices. Some may fear they will lose their job if their employer finds out that they have a health problem.

Middle-aged Adults. Middle-aged adults (ages 30 to 65) often experience their first major episode with a chronic disease. Common health problems in this age group include depression, obesity, and cardiovascular disease. Concerns about health often center on the ability to maintain a career or usual life-style in spite of health deficits or alterations in body functioning. Health care practices designed to retard disease or promote health—such as rest, regular exercise, a prudent diet, and stress reduction—are of particular benefit to the middle-aged adult; however, these practices may require major life-style adjustments. Some adults in this age range can adapt to such changes, but change is often threatening to middle-aged adults. If adults can see personal meaning and relevance in proposed health promotion or treatment regimens, they are more likely to participate in them.[26,27]

Older Adults. While it is not true that aging is synonymous with declining, older adults (age 65 and over) experience age-related physiological changes that influence learning modes and learning pace.[28] Diminished sensory acuity, especially hearing and vision, and difficulties with thinking and remembering related to altered blood flow to the brain, are common. Despite these changes, older adults are quite capable of learning. In fact, the rate of loss of mental power can be decreased by continued stimulation.

Learning is facilitated when information is presented and organized to minimize skills or modalities that have been altered by aging or disease and to enhance present level of functioning. For example, pacing of learning activities is especially important for older adults. They work best

BUILDING NURSING KNOWLEDGE

Can You Teach the Elderly?

Weinrich SP, Boyd M, Nussbaum J. Continuing education: Adapting strategies to teach the elderly. *J Gerontol Nurs.* 1989; 15:17–21.

This report is concerned with teaching and learning among the elderly. The elderly already account for 31 percent of all hospital stays, and most elderly people have at least one chronic health problem; many have multiple problems. These problems require knowledge and information to support self-care which, considering the high cost of health care, could prove to be cost-effective.

Weinrich and colleagues inventory the various physical changes of aging that can interfere with learning, which they acknowledge create barriers to learning. They also stress that learning is not impossible, so long as teaching strategies are geared to the elders' special needs. Some of the changes that interfere include sensory losses (sight, hearing, touch, taste, and smell). Teaching strategies that compensate for sensory losses enhance learning. For example, the use of visual aids to reinforce auditory input often improves learning among the hearing impaired.

Most research supports the premise that the ability of older adults to learn and remember is virtually as good as ever; nevertheless, cognitive changes occasionally occur. These include slowed cognitive functioning, decreased short-term memory, and increased reaction time. Where such barriers exist, learning may be enhanced by slowing the pace of presentation or repeating information frequently.

Overall educational level of elderly persons is frequently lower than that of the population as a whole. Elders were raised in an era when consumerism and health education were nonexistent. This group may not feel comfortable in teaching–learning situations. Promoting attitude and self-image changes may be a necessary step to achieving learning objectives.

at their own pace; success decreases when activities are timed or they feel rushed.

Because remembering isolated facts is difficult, highly organized material is important. Repeat important ideas, eliminate extraneous concepts, and use pictures to clarify abstract ideas and brochures or posters with large print to facilitate learning. Also, individuals over the age of 65 have diminished ability to ignore environmental distractions, and so a quiet, controlled environment is important.[29]

Older adults, like middle-aged adults, often resist change; therefore, collaborative development of teaching–learning goals that the clients find meaningful is especially important for successful health teaching.

Ability

Ability to learn is influenced by intellectual capacity, reading comprehension, physical capacity, and age. Individualizing the teaching plan according to the learner's ability promotes success and enhances motivation to participate in teaching–learning.

Intellectual Capacity. Intellectual capacity, or intelligence, refers to a person's capacity for reasoning, comprehension, and other mental activities. It relates to aptitude rather than level of performance on a specific mental task. Intelligence is believed to be an innate characteristic; that is, it is not enhanced or lost as a result of life experiences or aging. Intellectual capacity is often inferred from verbal and calculation skills, but such inferences must be made with caution. For example, an intelligent person may be illiterate, because of lack of exposure to written language. Also, people sometimes underestimate the intelligence of persons whose primary language is different from theirs.

Matching teaching and learning activities with learners' intellectual capacity is important. Concepts, materials, and teaching approaches that are too easy or difficult are likely to be boring or frustrating and therefore not supportive of effective learning.

Reading Comprehension. Estimates indicate that approximately 27 million adults in the United States are functionally illiterate; that is, they cannot cope with the minimal reading requirements of everyday life.[30] Educational background, such as high school graduation, may not correlate with literacy skills. The median reading level of US adults is about 10th grade; this means that about one-half of adults read at or below this grade level.

Literacy encompasses the ability to recognize words as well as comprehend their meaning in context. Reading comprehension is an important determinant of what the client is able to understand in teaching–learning situations. Some people can sound out words but have limited understanding of what they have read. Therefore, it is important for a health educator to assess a client's reading comprehension before using written handouts as a teaching tool.

Often, adults who have limited reading and comprehension skills are embarrassed and hide their lack of skill. Some behavioral cues that a client is unable to read include unusual menu selections, inability to use mechanical devices that have clearly marked written operating instructions, inattention to printed materials, questions about procedures that have been described on written instruction sheets, and mouthing or pointing to words when attempting to read.[31] Clients with reading difficulties sometimes admit that "the words get mixed up" or blame their difficulty on poor eyesight or glasses that are not strong enough. If the nurse suspects the client has limited reading and comprehension skills, alternative teaching materials can be used, such as drawings and diagrams that illustrate important concepts, or tape-recorded instructions.

Physical Capacity. Neurosensory and neuromuscular functioning create the physical capacity for learning. The functioning of sense organs influences whether environmental stimuli are received accurately, are distorted, or are not received at all. A person needs a fully functional nervous system for effective transmission and interpretation of impulses and response to stimuli. The nature of the response is determined to some degree by motor capacity—

the ability to move in a purposeful manner. Coordinated motor responses are particularly important in psychomotor learning.

Neurosensory or neuromuscular deficits may limit what an individual can learn or may dictate modification of teaching approaches. Moreover, an individual's emotional responses to these deficits may further compromise learning. Teaching and learning under such circumstances are challenging, but success can be particularly rewarding. A collaboratively developed teaching–learning plan is a first step to successful learning.

Age. As detailed in the earlier section on developmental stages, physical, mental, and emotional capacity to learn develop gradually. Therefore, children's learning is limited by their age level. Once maturity in each of these capacities has been attained, age ceases to be an influencing factor on learning until late adulthood. After the age of 60, learning capacity gradually deteriorates, although the rate and amount of loss vary considerably.

Learning Style

Learning style refers to a learner's preference for particular sensory-perceptual, environmental, and social factors in a teaching–learning situation.

Sensory-perceptual Factors. Sensory-perceptual factors relate to the sensory channel through which stimuli are received and retained in memory. Auditory, visual, and kinesthetic (body awareness, body position in space) channels are the major modalities relevant to teaching–learning situations. It is believed that heredity and environment influence development of modality strength, the particular sensory modality through which an individual most efficiently accomplishes a learning task. School-aged children typically demonstrate a dominant modality, but they gradually learn cognitive strategies to transfer information from one modality to another. Therefore, in adulthood, identification of modality strength by observation or testing is more difficult. Planning educational experiences to match a learner's modality strengths may enhance learning potential; therefore, researchers are attempting to find ways to identify modality strengths in adults. Relying on modality preference is an alternative way of individualizing learning approaches although preference does not determine modality strength.

Cognitive style refers to thought processes and ways an individual ascribes meaning to symbols. Cognitive style has been defined as the psychological dimensions that represent consistencies in an individual's manner of acquiring, storing, processing, and using information.[32] How individuals ascribe meaning to information is influenced by their tendencies toward abstract versus concrete thinking, as well as by their predominant processing mode. Some individuals are primarily verbal; they use verbal symbols (words) to conceptualize and categorize. For others visual processing, imagery, predominates. These modalities are also involved in storing (remembering) information and in using information in daily life.

Cognitive style mapping is a process of identifying an individual's ways of acquiring, processing, storing, and using information to devise approaches to instruction that capitalize on cognitive style. For example, people with poorly developed verbal discrimination skills will have difficulty learning unless the teacher identifies, defines, and organizes important concepts. In contrast, those with a high level of discrimination ability may find it stimulating to discover these concepts on their own. Concrete thinkers may have to manipulate objects to understand their function, whereas abstract thinkers may infer function from an abstract approach.

Environmental Factors. Environmental aspects of learning style refer to conditions such as temperature, noise, lighting, and clutter. Some people are easily distracted by extraneous stimuli such as an uncomfortable chair, noise, or the movement of others and therefore prefer a quiet, secluded learning setting. Others can concentrate amidst chaos, and may even prefer extra stimulation during learning activities.

Social Factors. Social factors refer to the kinds of learning interactions learners prefer. Some learners need teacher-dominated modes of instruction; others need independent activities or group interaction, such as discussion or role-playing. Whereas most learners have definite preferences for particular modes of learning, the relationship of these preferences to achievement has not been determined. Providing opportunities for different learning modes is likely to stimulate learners' active participation.

■ CONCEPTS RELATED TO TEACHING

Teaching is by nature an interactive process. Communication skill is therefore a major factor in the effectiveness of teaching efforts. The communication skills discussed in Chapters 13 and 14 are critical to the establishment of a trusting nurse–client relationship, which is the basis for health teaching by the nurse.

Health teaching is generally focused on knowledge that will help clients assume greater responsibility for their own care or adapt to health alterations. Because of the nature of the nurse–client relationship, health teaching is often informal and spontaneous, occurring in the context of nursing care without specific planning. In contrast, structured teaching is based on an organized plan. Both approaches are most effective when based on learning theory and consideration of individual client characteristics.

Informal Teaching

Nurses are often asked for advice, because they are respected as resources by family, friends, and clients. Often the most important assistance a nurse can give is to recognize the true nature of the need being expressed. People often ask for information and advice when they are confused and uncertain. They ask questions to make contact with a resource, not to obtain an answer to the specific question. Therefore, even when a question may seem like a clear-cut opportunity for teaching, exploration may be the most effective response.

Taking an exploratory approach using active listening (see Chap. 14), rather than giving advice, will clarify the person's need. Ultimately, exploration may lead to a discussion that is in fact an informal teaching session. However, in some situations the context of a question may show that providing information without further exploration is appropriate. Moreover, observant nurses often recognize a client's need and readiness for information during routine nursing care. For example, postoperative clients are encouraged to turn from side to side every 2 hours. However, turning is painful, so many clients feel a conflict: They wish to avoid complications, but also wish to avoid pain. Demonstrating techniques to minimize pain while clients are trying to turn is effective. The reinforcing effect of moving with a minimum of pain increases the likelihood that they will continue to turn regularly.

Such "teachable moments" are most productive when they provide a link between the clients' present knowledge and future problem-solving.[33] Reviewing the comprehensive data base obtained upon admission prior to providing care will help the nurse create such a link. However, even when nurses lack such client assessment data, sensitive observation and communication can promote client learning. For example, a client who says, "I know I should exercise more, but I can never find the time" is giving a nurse an opportunity to explore current knowledge level and address future strategies for healthy life-style adaptations.

Structured Teaching

Structured teaching involves the use of formal, planned teaching–learning programs. In structured teaching programs, the content and methods of delivery are often predetermined. Some health educators feel that a consistent teaching approach assures that all clients receive all the information they need. Lindeman and Van Aerman's research on preoperative teaching supports this belief. They found that a systematic, structured program of preoperative instruction was more effective in improving clients' postoperative experience than informal preoperative teaching.[34] The same result was found by Marshall and colleagues in their study of clients undergoing coronary artery bypass surgery.[35] Those with structured teaching gained more knowledge than those receiving unstructured teaching, but the former approach was more expensive in staff time and resources. Future research is needed to determine if the extra cost is justified by the greater client benefits.

Although the focus of structured programs is the cognitive and psychomotor domains, they can provide opportunities for addressing emotional concerns as well. Nurses may do structured health teaching to individuals or groups.

Group Teaching. Structured group teaching programs are often developed based on common teaching–learning needs of a health care agency's clients. Obesity, hypertension, diabetes, cancer, childbirth preparation, basic infant care, and recovering from addictions are some examples of topics covered (Fig. 20–7).

Group teaching is an effective way to enhance learning, because group members can become resources for one another. Group members often motivate one another to make changes in life-style or even belief systems. The exchange of ideas is often more stimulating in a group than in one-to-one discussions. Group members also provide support for one another. It is particularly helpful if some members of the group have successfully adapted to an alteration in health that other members have recently encountered. They can offer invaluable practical tips and encouragement through their example of successful adaptation.

Individual Teaching. Structured programs can also be effective for individual teaching. Individual teaching, rather than a group format, may be used because of the complexity of the information, the immediacy of the client's need, individual learning problems, or simple logistics. For example, in acute care settings, most teaching is provided on a one-to-one basis, because clients are usually at different stages of convalescence, making effective group teaching difficult. Moreover, short hospital stays frequently dictate that nurses integrate teaching with other care activities or risk losing the opportunity to teach at all.

A major disadvantage of structured programs is that nurses may fail to recognize individual client concerns and learning needs. Therefore, it is important to acknowledge clients' feelings and individualize instruction based on a client's readiness and willingness to learn. Often this can be accomplished by describing the structured program, then asking clients to decide when, if, and how much of the information they wish to learn.

An individualized structured teaching plan is generated collaboratively by a nurse and a client. The process for creating an individualized structured teaching plan paral-

IMPLICATIONS FOR NURSE–CLIENT COLLABORATION

Advice and Teachable Moments

People often ask for information and advice when they are confused and uncertain, and nurses, because they are respected as resources, frequently receive their questions. Sometimes, behind a request for information, is another, deeper, more urgent concern. A collaborative approach, one that invites clients to express themselves fully, may help clarify the nature of clients' needs. Active listening is essential. The nurse may feel a temptation to offer advice, but this may shut off clients' communication before the nurse can be certain of their needs. By ascertaining the client's need before responding, however, the nurse is able to take advantage of "teachable moments" by initiating an informal teaching plan geared to a client's real concern.

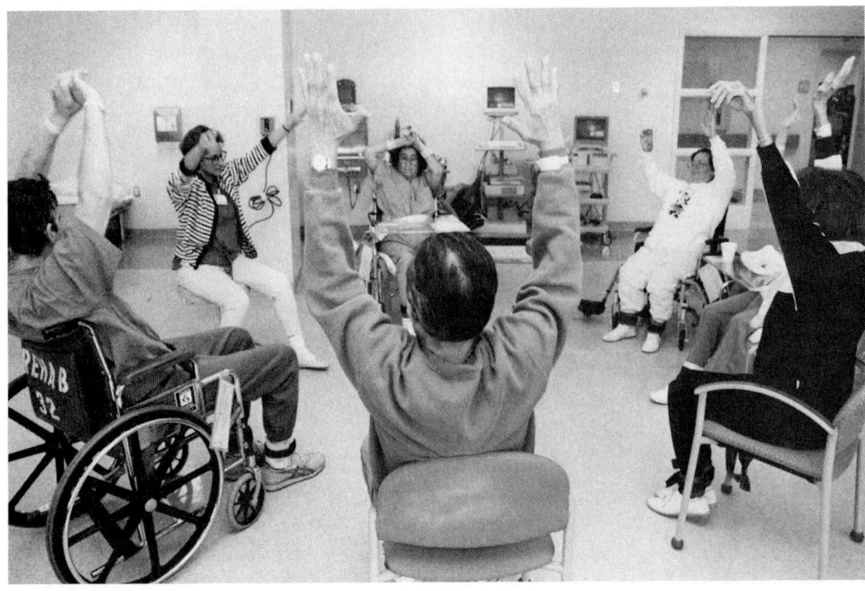

Figure 20–7. Group teaching in a rehabilitation facility of exercises to improve oxygenation.

lels that for developing individualized client care plans (see Chap. 18). It is detailed later in this chapter.

COLLABORATION IN THE TEACHING–LEARNING PROCESS

Collaborating with Clients

The nurse and client share responsibility for implementation of the teaching–learning process. The ultimate goal is to enhance clients' self-care competencies so they can achieve and maintain optimal health. Active participation in a mutual exchange of information promotes learning. In a collaborative teaching–learning process, both client and nurse are active learners and teachers. Clients assume the role of learner when acquiring new self-care competencies and the role of teacher when communicating their personal perspective of health. Nurses assume the role of learner as they strive to understand the beliefs, motivations, and desires of clients and the role of teacher when providing information.

In the past, clients were often expected to comply with providers' health care recommendations passively.[4] (See also Chap. 12.) Health care professionals considered themselves qualified to decide what knowledge and skills clients needed to improve their health; however, clients are the experts about their personal perceptions, beliefs about health, and desires for learning. Moreover, because of the consumer movement and public media, clients are informed and involved in their own care. Studies have documented that clients want to know about their health and health care.[10,11,36,37] A collaborative approach to health teaching effectively meets clients' needs for information and for participation.[38,39] Through shared responsibility, client and nurse can set learning goals and objectives. (See also Chap. 37.)

IMPLICATIONS FOR NURSE–CLIENT COLLABORATION

Is Group Teaching a Good Method for Client Health Education?

Sultemeier A. An innovative approach to teaching prenatal nutrition. *J Com Health Nurs.* 1988; 5:247–254.

Sultemeier observed that despite costly individual teaching about nutrition, many prenatal clients develop anemia, excessive weight gain, and have inadequate diets. This report describes an experiment with group teaching to see if it improved client follow-through.

One concern was to find teaching aids that used terminology that could be understood by the average client and that were sensitive to cultural preferences and limited financial resources. Sultemeier put together a slide presentation featuring a community health nurse who stressed the staff's concern for each client's well-being. The accompanying narration introduced the topic of nutrition, addressed the four basic food groups, and dealt with items that should be omitted from clients' prenatal diet. Sultemeier also prepared a teaching guide for use by the community health nurses who would lead the class discussions.

A 2-month clinical trial of group teaching was conducted. The experimental group had 18 subjects. The control group of 20 subjects received individualized teaching. Evaluation was based on the subjects' recall of dietary intake over a 48-hour period and on a nutritional questionnaire.

Sultemeier found that 6 of the 20 clients in the control group showed an appropriate weight gain after one month, and 2 showed an improved dietary intake; on the other hand, 7 of the 18 clients in the experimental group showed an appropriate weight gain and 9 showed improved dietary intake. Sultemeier concluded that the group method was more effective than the individual method for teaching prenatal nutrition to pregnant women.

Clients and providers sometimes have divergent ideas or competing goals.[39,40,41] Negotiation is an effective way to bridge these differences.[4,40,42,43] Negotiation implies mutual recognition of the validity of another's viewpoint and commitment to reaching mutually acceptable outcomes. Negotiation often involves compromise by both participants. For example, hypertensive clients are often advised to limit their sodium intake. In discussing sodium intake with a hypertensive client, a nurse may discover that the client is unwilling to give up certain high-sodium foods. Rather than trying to impose limitations the client finds unacceptable, the nurse might negotiate with the client some alternative ways for limiting sodium consumption, such as eliminating other high-sodium foods that are less important to the client and using herbs or lemon juice for seasoning. The alternatives may result in a higher-than-ideal sodium intake, but effectively reduce former levels of sodium intake.

Collaborating with Other Health Care Professionals

Frequently, several health care professionals are involved in teaching–learning with clients. For continuity and reinforcement, it is important that each professional communicate with the others about content, progress, and approaches being used. When providers collaborate, they reinforce each others' teaching. This not only facilitates clients' learning and retention but also promotes client trust in the providers. Furthermore, if the client moves rapidly through various health care settings, communication between agencies is essential to effective coordination of teaching and learning. For example, a client may first visit a clinic or office setting, and then be admitted to a hospital, transferred to an extended care facility, and finally discharged with orders for a home care or community health nurse follow-up. Sharing the teaching plan and reporting progress each time the client moves to a new facility contributes to progress toward the client's learning goals.

■ OVERVIEW OF THE TEACHING–LEARNING PROCESS

The teaching–learning process includes phases that are similar to those of the nursing process.[22] (See Chap. 15.) Both include assessment, diagnosis, planning, implementation, and evaluation. The nurse can collect data for the purpose of assessing client learning needs as part of the general health assessment. Assessment of learning needs is described in greater detail in the next section of this chapter.

The nursing diagnosis established in the teaching–learning process is a summary statement about a specific learning need, or Knowledge Deficit. It represents a judgment mutually agreed upon between the client and nurse.

The teaching–learning plan is also developed collaboratively. It defines the behavioral objectives (client behaviors that show that learning has taken place), as well as the teaching–learning strategies that client and nurse will use to meet these objectives. Client and nurse then collaboratively implement the plan. Evaluation determines whether each learning objective has been met. During evaluation, the nurse and client determine if the teaching and learning activities were effective in promoting progress toward the learning objectives.

■ ASSESSMENT OF LEARNING NEEDS

Data Collection

During the assessment phase of the teaching–learning process, clients and nurses collaborate through mutual interaction to determine clients' learning needs. Nurses make informal observations of clients' abilities to perform self-care activities as part of routine nursing care. However, relying only on informal, unfocused observation may cause important information to be missed. Only comprehensive assessment can accurately assess learning needs. This assessment should incorporate data from the basic health assessment, address individual learner characteristics that may influence learning, and consider the client's support system.

Basic Health Assessment. Several elements of the standard health history and physical assessment provide important clues to client learning needs (see Chap. 16). The sections of the health history covering primary concern; current understanding; past health problems; personal, family, and social history; and subjective manifestations are particularly relevant, as are the general observation, musculoskeletal, and neurosensory assessments in the physical examination.

Health History. When discussing a client's primary concern, nurses explore the health concern that the client considers most important at present. Past health problems are health deviations that occurred before this contact with a health care provider. Clients' manner of speaking about their health concerns, particularly the vocabulary used, is a useful clue to learning needs. Nurses gain additional information when surveying clients' perceptions about what makes their symptoms worse, or alleviates them. For example, consider a client whose primary concern is several days of frequent urination accompanied by burning. The client states that she has had similar complaints in the recent past and believes that limiting fluid intake improves her symptoms. A nurse would recognize that this client needs health teaching to help her identify symptoms requiring assistance and to understand the importance of ample fluid intake. Further discussion about other past health problems may reveal more learning needs.

Personal, family, and social history is a rich source of relevant data. Particulars about a client's occupation, lifestyle, habits, family structure, social activities, and usual coping strategies reveal overall health knowledge and the degree to which the client applies that knowledge to daily life.

As discussed in Chapter 16, the overview of subjective manifestations is a means of determining whether clients have been experiencing symptoms that they have not reported. Clients often fail to report symptoms because they do not know the symptoms are significant. An astute nurse can identify potential topics for client teaching when discussing subjective manifestations.

Physical Examination. The general observation portion of the physical examination provides initial impressions about mental status, nutrition, mobility, energy level, and coordination, which can be indicators of clients' learning needs and physical capacity to learn or perform self-care skills.

Some self-care activities require stamina and strength. A musculoskeletal examination, including assessments of range of motion, muscle strength, and activity tolerance, assists nurses to make judgments about clients' capacity to perform such activities.

Additional essential information about clients' capacity to learn is obtained from the neurosensory examination. Here, data about memory, use of language, judgment and abstraction abilities, coordination, and visual and auditory acuity are particularly relevant to selection of content and teaching approaches.

Learner Characteristics Influencing Learning. In addition to the data obtained in the basic health assessment, other factors, such as health beliefs, reading comprehension, and learning style also need to be assessed for planning teaching–learning activities. Table 20–1 presents assessment considerations and sample questions for these general learner characteristics. Some health care facilities use assessment forms specifically related to a particular health problem (for example, diabetes or hypertension) to collect detailed, relevant information.[44]

Assessing the Client's Support System. People who are learning new health practices are often influenced greatly by their immediate family and friends. Nurses should therefore determine who else besides the client should be included in the teaching–learning process.

Parents are usually included in teaching–learning activities for children, because of parents' responsibility for their children's health supervision. Frequently, teaching parents has multiple benefits. Besides providing information to promote family health, it reduces the anxiety of both children and parents.[45] For adults, particularly those who need help with activities of daily living, it may also be helpful to include family members in the teaching activities. Rankin and Duffy believe that the family system should be included in the assessment process, because without family support the client may have difficulty adopting new behavior.[46] For example, a hypertensive client will be better able to maintain a low-sodium diet if his spouse, who does the food shopping and cooking, is involved in discussions about preparing flavorful low-sodium meals.

A client's support system can affect motivation to learn health behaviors. Champion found that social influence (encouragement from significant family members or friends) had a positive influence on women's intent to learn breast self-examination.[47]

Sometimes the client's social network has a negative influence on learning or application of learning. Although it is not possible to include all significant others in health teaching, it is valuable to obtain clients' impressions of how family or friends, or even work associates, may influence new health behaviors. For example, a client who sets a goal of reducing calorie intake but who regularly eats lunch at restaurants with work associates may find ordering low-calorie dishes difficult when others select high-calorie foods. If anticipatory guidance, including strategies to handle such situations, is part of the health teaching, the client will be more likely to achieve the goal.

Nursing Diagnosis of Learning Needs

A nursing diagnosis related to health education acknowledges that a client lacks information needed to be an active, informed participant in his or her health care.[48] It is a summary statement that identifies a client's specific health-related learning needs (knowledge deficits) and the conditions or circumstances that are causing or contributing to the client's lack of knowledge. The Knowledge Deficit diagnosis is derived through analysis of the data obtained in the client assessments and is the basis for a collaboratively developed teaching–learning plan. Redman states that nursing diagnosis statements related to teaching–learning needs help to focus the teaching–learning process by summarizing a knowledge and/or skill deficit; emotional reactions, attitudes, and beliefs that interfere with learning; and environmental or social conditions that influence learning behavior.[49]

Knowledge Deficit. Knowledge deficit is the inability to state or explain information or demonstrate a required skill related to disease management procedures, or the inability to explain or use self-care practices recommended to restore health or maintain wellness.[50,51] A diagnosis of Knowledge Deficit is incomplete without specification of the knowledge or skills the client needs. (See also Box 20–1.)

Etiologies of Knowledge Deficit. The North American Nursing Diagnosis Association (NANDA) has approved six possible etiologies for the Knowledge Deficit diagnosis: lack of exposure, lack of recall, information misinterpretation, cognitive limitation, lack of interest in learning, and unfamiliarity with information resources.

Lack of Exposure. Lack of exposure implies that a client has not had opportunities to obtain knowledge needed to improve level of wellness or self-care skills. Recall the previous discussion of concepts related to learning. Both major learning theories, behaviorism and Gestalt-field theory, emphasize the importance of the environment in learning. Unless learners are exposed to relevant stimuli (behaviorism) or have an opportunity to gain needed insight through in-

TABLE 20–1. ASSESSING LEARNER CHARACTERISTICS TO IDENTIFY LEARNING NEEDS AND GUIDE APPROACHES FOR HEALTH TEACHING

Observations and Sample Questions

READINESS

Does the client demonstrate an intention to learn?

Motivation: How interested is the client in matters that affect health, in general? How interested in learning particular new health care practices?

Health beliefs/present knowledge:

- How would you describe your health?
- What kinds of things do you do regularly to keep yourself healthy? (Eg, exercise, watch diet, avoid alcohol, meditate.)
- Where did you learn about these things? (Eg, family, friends, books, magazines.)
- Are there changes you think would improve your overall health that you have not been willing or able to make?
- What do you think keeps you from making these changes? (Eg, time, cost, family needs.)
- What kinds of things do you do to get better when you don't feel well?
- Do you have any health problems at present?
- What are your concerns about (current health problem[s])?
- I notice you are being treated for (problem). Have you felt better since starting treatment?
- Have the (treatments, medicines, restrictions) caused any difficulties for you? (Eg, discomfort, cost, inconvenience.)
- What about having (problem) is the hardest? (Eg, how you feel, what you can't do because of disease, what you can't do because of treatments, cost.)
- Do you think there's anything you can do to minimize that difficulty?
- Do you ever worry that (problem) will get worse?
- If (problem) gets worse, how do you think it will affect you? (Eg, how you feel, what you can do.)
- Do you think there's anything you can do to keep (problem) from getting worse? How hard would those things be for you to do?
- Are there health problems you are aware of that you may be at risk for? (Eg, because of age, diet, occupation, habits [smoking, alcohol, lack of exercise], family history.)
- (If yes to above) Do you feel the (identified risk[s]) is/are a serious problem?
- What do you think keeps you from changing circumstances that increase your risk?

Cultural heritage:

- Do you use any treatments or medicines (eg, herbs or poultices) that you believe are used most often by persons from your cultural group?
- Does your doctor know that you use them?
- Have you ever felt that advice or a prescription you were given by a doctor or nurse was contrary to values or beliefs that you consider important?
- If so, what did you do?

(See also Chap. 9 for additional information about the impact of culture on health beliefs.)

Past experiences with health care/health teaching: How might the client's past health care experiences influence motivation to participate in health teaching now?

- Have you used other health care facilities in the past?
- What is your general feeling about that (those) experience(s)? Did you like your doctor? Nurses? Did you feel that they gave good care? Cared about you?
- Do you remember anyone teaching you anything about what was wrong with you? How to help yourself get better? How to keep from getting sick again?
- (If yes to above) Did you like having more information about your health? Was it helpful? Could you use the information in your daily life?
- (If no) Do you wish someone had told you more about any of those things?
- Would you like more information about (current problem)?

Emotional status: Is the client's emotional status optimum for learning? Emotional status is not assessed via direct questions about emotions. Nurses can make inferences about client's emotional status by observing nonverbal behaviors and noting relevant statements about emotions, worries, and concerns. (See also Chaps. 13 and 14.)

Considerations:

- Does the client exhibit extremes of emotion (very intense or lacking emotion)?
- Is the client using coping strategies (eg, anger, denial) that must be attended to before new health care practices can be learned?

Physical condition: Might the client's health status interfere with learning? Use data from general health assessment.

Considerations:

- Is the client able to participate in learning activities?
- Is the client's physical state of health stable enough so attention can be directed toward meeting learning needs?
- Are there inhibiting factors such as pain present?

Developmental stage: Does developmental level suggest particular content or teaching approach? Determine by noting chronological age and observing client's behavior. (See also Chap. 11.)

ABILITY

What are the client's strengths and limitations related to learning capacity?

Intellectual capacity: Does the client possess the cognitive skills needed to understand how new information and/or skills can affect his or her health status? Infer from conversation, vocabulary, and clarity of expression. Use data from mental status assessment. Note whether English is client's primary language.

Reading comprehension: Will reading problems limit client's grasp of written information?

- Do you enjoy reading?
- Does reading help you to learn or remember?
- Do you find it easy to learn something by reading about it?

(continued)

TABLE 20–1. (continued)

Observations and Sample Questions

Also, observe client behavior when given written material. Does the client read newspaper, magazines, or instruction pamphlets? Does the client follow written instructions?

Physical capacity: Does the client have the physical capacity to learn self-care skills? Use data from general health assessment.

Considerations:

- Does the client have any limitations in sensory perception skills (eg, seeing, hearing, touch) that affect learning ability and suggest modifications in teaching approach?
- Does the client demonstrate the motor and coordination skills needed for self-care?

Age: See Developmental stage, above.

LEARNING STYLE

Does the client have a preferred way of learning?

Sensory-perceptual factors:

- Do you find it easier to learn new things by talking about them? Reading about them?
- If you are learning how to use equipment, do you prefer that someone demonstrate how it works? Help you make it work? Would you rather experiment and figure it out for yourself?
- Do you tend to picture how things work in your mind? Talk to yourself about how things work?

Environmental factors: What environmental conditions does the client prefer when learning?

- When you are trying to learn new things, are you bothered by noise, clutter, or the activity of other people around you?
- Do you find you can easily ignore what's going on around you when you are really interested in learning something?

Social factors: What social conditions does the client prefer when learning?

- Do you like to learn on your own? To learn with a group?
- Do you like the teacher to decide on what things about a subject are more important to learn? Do you think the teacher should decide the best way to learn how to do something, and then tell you how?

CLIENT SUPPORT SYSTEM

To what extent might significant others enhance learning? Use data from personal, family, and social history in basic health assessment.

- Would it help you to learn abut the things you need to do to take care of yourself if your (husband, wife, friend, daughter, son) learned with you?
- Do you think (significant other, family member) would be interested in learning about that? Would he or she help you do it at home?

Additional considerations:

- Does the client have family or friends who may support and/or assist with learning and maintaining health behaviors?
- Might significant others interfere with this?

teraction with the environment (Gestalt-field), there can be no learning. Once there is exposure to information, mental operations for acquiring that information—sensory reception and discrimination—come into play. Processing the information—that is, making associations and generalizations and forming concepts—then enables the learner to remember and use the information.

Lack of Recall. Lack of recall implies that a learner has been exposed to relevant information but is unable to recall and apply it to the current situation. Lack of recall can result from ineffective processing of information: inability to make associations and generalizations or form concepts at the time the information was presented. Often ineffective processing relates to teaching approaches. Learners are better able to make associations if teachers illustrate relationships in the teaching process. Lack of recall may also occur when a learner has not used information regularly. In this situation, new associations—that is, new learning—interferes with recall.

Information Misinterpretation. Information misinterpretation is also a problem of receiving or processing information. If a learner is unable to receive stimuli, whether because of neurosensory deficits or environmental interference (such as noise), the stimuli cannot be effectively processed into meaningful ideas. As with lack of recall, the teaching approach can influence a learner's interpretation of material. If the concepts are not clearly presented, are not meaningful to the learner, or seem unrelated to past learning, the learner will be less able to understand them.

Cognitive Limitation. Intelligence level determines learning ability. Some health care concepts may be impossible for a person of below-average intelligence to grasp. The learner must be able to make associations and generalizations and record them in memory to understand most health and self-care concepts. In some cases, simplifying the ideas or carefully organizing them in sequence may help clients understand. Presenting concrete examples can also help correct a knowledge deficit related to cognitive limitations.

Lack of Interest in Learning. Lack of interest in learning means that a nurse believes a client needs information but is unwilling to participate in teaching–learning. Without client interest, attempts to teach are futile (see also Table 20–1). Before abandoning efforts to carry out teaching, however, the nurse should further explore underlying causes for lack of motivation. As emphasized above in the section on learner characteristics, several factors may cause a person to seem disinterested in learning. Perhaps the client believes the proposed information is unrelated to current needs, or feels too sick to participate. Perhaps the client's cultural beliefs or anxiety are interfering. Nurse–client communication and negotiation may eliminate the barriers to teaching–learning.

Unfamiliarity with Information Resources. Unfamiliarity with information resources suggests that there is no lack of ability or interest, but that the learner is not aware of sources to obtain desired information. Like lack of exposure, unfamiliarity with information resources eliminates the environmental stimulus or interaction that is a requisite for learning. Expanding learners' awareness of resources for health information will not only assist in the current situation but also help them be more informed health care consumers in the future.

Stating the Knowledge Deficit Diagnosis. A complete Knowledge Deficit diagnosis specifies the knowledge or skill that a client lacks, identifies the etiology, and lists the signs and symptoms that are evidence of the deficit. Two aspects of the diagnostic statement for Knowledge Deficit, specification and defining characteristics, are worthy of emphasis.

In order for health teaching to be appropriately focused, nurse and client must mutually determine the specific information or skill the client needs. The more precise the identification of the knowledge deficit, the more likely it is that the teaching will be effective. This is because the specification of the knowledge deficit not only determines what nurses will teach but also guides the selection of teaching approaches.

Note that the specification of the deficit is different from the etiology. As discussed in Chapter 17, the phrase "related to" (R/T) is used to designate etiology, and a colon (:) is used to designate specification of a diagnostic label. However, it is a common error to state the knowledge deficit as follows: "Knowledge Deficit related to breastfeeding." This implies that breastfeeding is the cause of the knowledge deficit, when in fact breastfeeding is the subject or content area needing attention. As written, there is no etiology for the knowledge deficit. A nurse would need to reexamine the data base and or communicate further with a client to determine the factor contributing to the knowledge deficit about breastfeeding, and then restate the diagnosis. A correct statement might be: "Knowledge Deficit: breastfeeding related to lack of exposure to information about breastfeeding techniques as evidenced by. . . ."

A second important point related to the Knowledge Deficit diagnosis is including defining characteristics in the diagnostic statement. Although defining characteristics are considered a necessary part of any diagnostic statement, they are particularly important for Knowledge Deficit. Defining characteristics clarify whether the lack of knowledge is the problem or the etiology of another problem. This suggests the importance of validating the diagnosis and of fully exploring related signs and symptoms, whether nurses infer a knowledge deficit from observed behaviors or from a direct client statement. Box 20–1 provides examples of correctly stated Knowledge Deficit diagnoses. The nursing diagnosis table on page 679 presents a general overview of the Knowledge Deficit nursing diagnosis, with examples of defining characteristics that present with each etiology.

BOX 20–1. SAMPLE STATEMENTS OF KNOWLEDGE DEFICIT DIAGNOSIS

1. **Specified Deficit:** Knowledge Deficit: Correct use and side effects of antihypertensive drugs.

   Etiology: R/T misinterpretation of information.

   Defining Characteristics: AEB continued blood pressure elevations after 2 weeks on prescribed medication, "I took only half the dose after a few days, because the pills made me feel funny," and "I didn't think taking the pills twice a day was so important."

   Complete Statement:
   Knowledge Deficit: Correct use and side effects of antihypertensive drugs R/T misinterpretation of information AEB continued blood pressure elevations after 1 week on prescribed medication, "I took only half the dose after a few days, because the pills made me feel funny," and "I didn't think taking the pills twice a day was so important."

2. **Specified Deficit:** Knowledge Deficit: Risks associated with exercise in pregnancy.

   Etiology: R/T lack of exposure to information.

   Defining Characteristics: AEB recent diagnosis of first pregnancy, "I don't know much about what to expect about being pregnant," "I'm a competitive runner, I need to keep up my workouts," and "I know I'll have the discipline to stick to my workout schedule even though I may feel tired."

   Complete Statement:
   Knowledge Deficit: Risks associated with exercise in pregnancy R/T lack of exposure to information AEB recent diagnosis of first pregnancy, "I don't know much about what to expect about being pregnant," "I'm a competitive runner, I need to keep up my workouts," and "I know I'll have the discipline to stick to my workout schedule even though I may feel tired."

NURSING DIAGNOSIS: KNOWLEDGE DEFICIT			
	Assessment		
	Defining Characteristics/Manifestations		
Nursing Diagnosis	**Subjective Data**	**Objective Data**	**Etiology**
A. Knowledge Deficit (specify) *8.1.1.*	Verbalizes a need for specific health-related information. Verbalizes insufficient health care information. Makes a direct request for specific information. Verbalizes lack of prior experience with this health problem.	Incorrect performance of skill related to health or health care. Unable to answer questions about specific health problem or related self-care.	Lack of exposure
B. Knowledge Deficit (specify) *8.1.1.*	Verbalizes a need for specific health-related information. Verbalizes insufficient health care information. Makes a direct request for specific information. Verbalizes forgetting information previously provided.	Incorrect performance of skill related to health or health care. Unable to answer questions about specific health problem or related self-care. Inaccurate follow-through of previous instructions.	Lack of recall
C. Knowledge Deficit (specify) *8.1.1.*	Expresses an inaccurate perception about information previously given.	Incorrect performance of skill related to health or health care. Unable to answer questions about specific health problem or relates self-care. Inaccurate follow-through of previous instruction.	Information misinterpretation
D. Knowledge Deficit (specify) *8.1.1.*	Makes a direct request for specific information. Verbalizes forgetting information previously provided. Expresses an inaccurate perception about information previously given. States is confused about information previously given. Reports inability to concentrate.	Incorrect performance of skill related to health or health care. Unable to answer questions about specific health problem or related self-care. Inaccurate follow-through of previous instruction. Simple vocabulary for age level. Difficulty recognizing common symbols. When given several items belonging to a category, unable to name the category Unable to explain a simple proverb. Unable to perform simple math exercises. Unable to repeat 7 digits forward or 4 backward.	Cognitive limitation
E. Knowledge Deficit (specify) *8.1.1.*	States doesn't see need to know about self-care or health condition: "I'm not really that sick." States doesn't feel well enough to learn. Expresses dislike for school-type situations. States it will be too hard to make lifestyle changes related to health condition. States prefers to use health treatments typical of own cultural group.	Incorrect performance of skill related to health or health care. Unable to answer questions about specific health problem or related self-care. Inaccurate follow-through of previous instruction. Inappropriate or exaggerated behaviors (eg, hysterical, hostile, agitated, or apathetic.)	Lack of interest in learning
F. Knowledge Deficit (specify) *8.1.1.*	Verbalizes a need for specific health-related information. Verbalizes insufficient health care information. Makes a direct request for specific information. Verbalizes lack of prior experience with this health problem. States doesn't know how to get information about health state or self-care.	Incorrect performance of skill related to health or health care. Unable to answer questions about specific health problem or related self-care.	Lack of familiarity with information resources

CLIENT–NURSE MANAGEMENT OF TEACHING–LEARNING

Nursing management encompasses planning, implementing the plan, and evaluating its effectiveness. The table on pages 680–681 presents general approaches to alleviate knowledge deficits for the etiologies discussed above. These general approaches can serve as guidelines when developing specific teaching–learning plans for individual clients or for groups.

Planning

The planning step of the teaching–learning process is a continuation of the collaborative nurse–client relationship established during the assessment. It includes developing objectives, identifying relevant content, and selecting teaching methods and learning activities. Choosing an appropriate environment, scheduling teaching–learning sessions, and determining criteria and timing for evaluation are also part of planning.

For effective collaborative planning, client preferences about involvement should be considered. For example, some clients are willing to leave the decision about subject matter and teaching method to the nurse. Other clients clearly state what they want to learn and how they prefer to learn. Sometimes, clients who are initially reticent become more active as the teaching–learning process progresses.

Providing a written teaching–learning plan that lists possible behavioral objectives, subject matter to be covered at each teaching session, and proposed methods of evaluation is an effective means of collaborating in planning for meeting teaching–learning needs. The nurse can then make revisions based on the client's input.

After a general plan has been agreed upon, many

CLIENT–NURSE MANAGEMENT OF TEACHING–LEARNING

Nursing Diagnosis	Desired Outcomes	Implementation	Evaluation
A. Knowledge Deficit R/T lack of exposure to information. *8.1.1.*	1. Gains knowledge needed for self-care. 2. Adheres to proposed health care practices.	1. Institute individualized teaching program based on areas of knowledge and/or skill deficit and characteristics of learner. 2. Incorporate teaching aids as appropriate.	1. Correctly verbalizes relevant health related information. 2. Self-care at level desired by client.
B. Knowledge Deficit R/T lack of recall. *8.1.1.*	1. Gains knowledge needed for self-care. 2. Adheres to proposed health care practices.	1. Determine reason for lack of recall and correct if feasible. 2. Institute individualized teaching program that includes the reteaching of prior information and/or skills. 3. Supplement teaching with use of aids that foster recall (eg, written instructions or audiotape of instructions). 4. Collaborate with client to schedule intermittent access to health care providers to reinforce learning. 5. Include family member/significant other in teaching–learning activities if feasible.	1. Correctly verbalizes relevant health related information. 2. Self-care at level desired by client.
C. Knowledge Deficit R/T information misinterpretation. *8.1.1.*	1. Gains knowledge needed for self-care. 2. Adheres to proposed health care practices.	1. Determine possible source(s) of misinterpretation (eg, influence of family, friends, media; personal characteristics such as health beliefs, ability, language barrier, learning style). 2. Modify previously implemented teaching plan to address source of misinterpretation. 3. Supplement teaching with written materials and other media appropriate to intellectual ability and learning style.	1. Correctly verbalizes relevant health-related information. 2. Self-care at level desired by client.
D. Knowledge Deficit R/T cognitive limitation. *8.1.1.*	1. Gains knowledge needed for self-care. 2. Adheres to proposed health care practices.	1. Institute individualized teaching program within ability of client. 2. Supplement teaching with use of aids that foster recall (eg, written instru-	1. Verbalizes relevant health care information within own intellectual ability.

nurses make a more detailed teaching plan that lists the specific points to be covered in order of presentation. This kind of plan is a useful aid for beginning nurses. It promotes efficiency and decreases the likelihood of omitting important concepts. The written plan is even more useful if it specifies the teaching methods and materials to be used. The following sections describe how to prepare a teaching–learning plan.

Defining Objectives. A **learning objective** is a statement that describes the behavior a learner should be able to demonstrate after completing a learning experience.[52] Because objectives describe learner behavior, the term **behavioral objective** is sometimes used in educational literature. Note the similarity between the definition of behavioral objectives and desired outcome statements, as discussed in Chapter 18. Objectives have the same role in a teaching–learning plan as desired outcomes have in a client care plan; the term "objective" is used here to conform with terminology in educational literature. A behavioral objective must include:

1. Specific observable learner behavior
2. The conditions under which the behavior will be demonstrated
3. The criteria that indicate acceptable level of performance[52]

Box 20–2 illustrates these three critical components of a behavioral objective. As the box illustrates, there may be more than one condition in a single objective. Criteria may specify a standard ("at least three") or a time ("within 2 days").

Preparing sound behavioral objectives requires considerable practice. Objectives, like desired outcome state-

Nursing Diagnosis	Desired Outcomes	Implementation	Evaluation
	3. Receives assistance/support from family or significant others as needed.	mentations or audiotape of instructions. 3. Include family member/significant other in teaching–learning activities if feasible. 4. Supplement teaching with written materials and other media appropriate to intellectual ability and learning style.	2. Self-care at level of client's capability. 3. Uses support systems as needed to assist in carrying out own health care practices.
E. Knowledge Deficit R/T lack of interest. *8.1.1.*	1. Identifies types of information or skills, is interested in learning. 2. Gains knowledge needed for self-care. 3. Adheres to proposed health care practices.	1. Use active listening to explore reason for lack of interest with client and/or family/significant others. 2. Explore client's level of understanding about specific health problem. 3. Therapeutic communication to assist client to achieve acceptance of health state (see Chaps. 13 and 14). 4. Supply information regarding benefits of health-related knowledge to client. 5. Secure assistance from family/significant others to interest client in learning. 6. Negotiate with client to develop teaching plan that addresses client's interests. 7. Use alternative sensory modalities to stimulate interest in learning. 8. Include family member/significant other in teaching–learning activities if feasible.	1. Accurately verbalizes description of health problem, its seriousness, and ways he or she can improve health status. 2. Verbalizes interest in learning about specific health care practices. 3. Uses support systems as needed to facilitate self-care. See also A1 and 2, above.
F. Knowledge Deficit related to unfamiliarity with information resources. *8.1.1.*	1. Gains knowledge of information resources needed for self-care. See also A1 and 2, above.	1. Provide a list of other information sources such as health care agencies, community agencies, support groups, and/or other health care professionals. 2. Explain types of information and services available from each source. 3. Role-play contact with agency of choice. 4. Provide referral to agency of choice if needed.	1. Explains purpose and availability of relevant information resources. 2. Prepares a list of phone numbers and/or addresses of above resources.

IMPLICATIONS FOR NURSE–CLIENT COLLABORATION

Can a Collaborative Approach to Client Teaching Improve Health Education Outcomes?

Clark JM, Haverty S, Kendall S. Helping people to stop smoking: A study of the nurse's role. *J Adv Nurs.* 1990; 16:357–363.

Clark and colleagues were concerned about the slow decline of smoking among women. To explore whether or not teaching by nurses helps women stop smoking, they devised a new approach, one that included the client in the planning. The framework was based partly on the health belief model and partly on the nursing process. It consisted of assessing the smoker's motivation, beliefs, fears, and worries about continuing or giving up smoking. Then a course of action was planned *with* the smoker, not *for* the smoker. During the implementation phase the nurse played a supportive and encouraging role.

Of the 68 clients in the study, 54 were followed up at 6 months, and 42 at 1 year. At 1 year after the teaching interaction, seven clients had stopped smoking, five had cut down substantially, 13 had made at least one attempt to give up smoking, and 17 had made no change in behavior. There was a significant correlation between motivation to stop and concern about health consequences.

Analysis of the tape-recorded interactions showed that nurses were generally able to make a detailed assessment of clients; however, they had some difficulty eliciting clients' true level of motivation. The nurses had a difficult time engaging clients to participate in working out a cessation strategy. Two clients with strong motivation participated fully; but in general, the nurses tended to fall back on prescriptive advice and telling the clients what was "best," not focusing on the client's needs or allowing the client to think about what would work best. In the successful interventions (those in which the client stopped or reduced smoking), there was clear evidence of client involvement in the planning process and the clients did more of the talking.

The researchers concluded that the findings indicate that attempts to help people are unlikely to be successful unless the individual's real concerns are addressed.

ments, should be specific and observable or measurable so the client and the nurse can readily determine whether they have been achieved. Mager cautions against using vague or loaded words, such as "know" or "understand" (see also Box 20–3).[52] These words could be interpreted differently by different observers. Box 20–4 lists samples of effective words to describe client behavior, arranged according to the learning domains described earlier in this chapter. The table is not meant to be an exhaustive list, but rather to provide examples for guidance. Because the affective domain deals with emotions and attitudes, which are abstract, selecting relevant observable behaviors is most challenging for that domain.

Objectives should also be mutually acceptable and attainable. If they are unrealistically high, clients may become frustrated and give up. It is also advisable to sequence objectives so that learning begins with the most basic concepts, and then builds on basic concepts to more complex content. Nurses use the cues in the data base to develop objectives that are observable, relevant, and attainable to share with clients. Then nurse and client confer to modify these objectives and make final selections for the teaching–learning plan. When there are many objectives related to several different subjects, nurse and client may choose to prioritize them to facilitate implementing the plan.

BOX 20–2. COMPONENTS OF BEHAVIORAL OBJECTIVES

The client will *correctly identify* (behavior)
at least *three side effects* (criterion) of atenolol
from a *list of common side effects of antihypertensive drugs* (condition).

Within 2 days (criterion)
the client *will demonstrate* (behavior)
three ways to hold her newborn for breastfeeding (criteria)
that *promote maternal comfort* (condition)
and facilitate correct latching of the newborn (condition).

Identifying Content. Content is the general topic or subject to be addressed in a teaching–learning plan. The content to be taught is implied by the nursing diagnosis statement, which specifies the subject of the knowledge deficit. Also, the list of defining characteristics may include examples of specific misconceptions or errors that the client has exhibited.

Two additional content considerations should be addressed during planning: depth and organization. The nurse determines the amount of detail for a particular teaching–learning situation from the data base and the collaboratively developed objectives. Client interest and ability are major determinants of depth of content to be presented. For example, one client who is learning to give self-injections of insulin may want to know the mechanics of a safe injection but not the reasons for each aspect of the procedure. A second client may want to know the under-

BOX 20–3. WORDS TO AVOID WHEN STATING BEHAVIORAL OBJECTIVES

- Know
- Learn
- Understand
- Comprehend
- Grasp meaning of
- Appreciate
- Interpret
- Integrate
- Evaluate
- Value
- Feel

BOX 20–4. EFFECTIVE WORDS FOR BEHAVIORAL OBJECTIVES RELATED TO DOMAINS OF LEARNING

Cognitive Domain[a]

Knowledge
- state
- write
- recite
- identify
- select
- recognize
- list
- name
- verbalize

Comprehension
- define terms
- describe
- explain
- summarize main points
- discuss main ideas

Application
- use
- exercise
- consume foods
- take medication
- drink
- seek health care
- perform personal hygiene (behavior related to content taught)

Analysis
- compare
- contrast
- differentiate
- classify
- distinguish
- identify relationships

Synthesis
- make a plan
- discuss relationships

Evaluate
- apply standards
- evaluate using standards

Affective Domain[b]

Receiving
- listen
- pay attention

Responding
- participate
- interact

Valuing
- state commitment
- identify personal values

Organizing
- identify others' values
- compare values

Characterizing
- consistently act on stated commitment

Psychomotor Domain[c]

Perception
- identify equipment
- observe skill
- state when skill appropriate

Set
- describe skill
- state steps of skill

Guided Response
- imitate steps
- perform with prompts

Mechanism
- demonstrate skill
- execute skill

Complex Overt Response
- demonstrate skill in various circumstances

Adaptation
- modify skill for specified circumstances
- modify skill in unexpected circumstances

[a] Adapted from Bloom BS. *Taxonomy of Educational Objectives. 1. Cognitive Domain.* New York: Longman; 1956.
[b] Adapted from Krathwohl DR, Bloom BS, Masia BB. *Taxonomy of Educational Objectives. 2. Affective Domain.* New York: Longman; 1964.
[c] Adapted from Simpson EJ. *The Psychomotor Domain.* Washington, DC: Gryphon; 1972; 3.

lying principles in order to remember correct execution of the mechanics.

Organization of content refers to the order in which concepts are presented. Ordering ideas from simple to complex, familiar to unfamiliar, or concrete to abstract facilitates understanding. However, when trying to master a procedure, most people find that learning the steps from beginning to end is best.

Robert Gagne[53] proposed a four-level hierarchy to sequence information:

1. Establish a factual foundation: Present terminology and basic facts.
2. Develop conceptual understanding: Show relationships between facts and link facts to form concepts.
3. Use principles and rules: Show relationships between two concepts and among two or more concepts.
4. Engage in problem solving: Infer cause and effect, predict consequences, and apply principles to real situations.

This organization seems particularly relevant to health teaching, since the information provided is usually intended for application in daily life. Box 20–5 shows how this hierarchy may be used to teach a client about the importance of following a prescribed medication schedule.

BOX 20–5. SEQUENCING CONTENT FOLLOWING GAGNE'S HIERARCHY

TOPIC: Teaching clients the importance of following a prescribed schedule for time and dose of medication.

Facts

1. Medications are prescribed for a specific desired effect in the body.
2. To be effective medication must be at a certain concentration in the body.
3. Drugs are used up by the body at a fairly predictable rate.
4. Sometimes a medication has other effects besides the effect it is given for.

Concepts

1. Therapeutic level: the concentration of medication in the body needed for the drug to do its work. Achieved when the amount taken in replaces the amount used up.
2. Side Effects: effects that are not harmful, but may be uncomfortable, that medications may produce when therapeutic level is achieved.
3. Toxic Effects: dangerous effects that may happen if too much medication is in the body at any one time.

Principles

1. To keep the therapeutic level, drug must be taken as scheduled.
2. "More is better" does not apply to medicines. Taking more than is prescribed, or taking doses too close together, may cause toxic effects, because some of the previous dose may not yet be used up.
3. Sometimes side effects must be accepted in order to have the medication do what it is supposed to in the body.

Problem-solving

1. What will happen if you take only half the prescribed dose? Will the medication be able to do its job?
2. You are told to take your pills in the morning and before bed. What will happen if you forget to take the medication in the morning? Could you take it at noon?
3. If you realize that you forgot your morning pill at bedtime, should you take them both together?
4. If you sometimes skip pills to get rid of side effects, can the pills you do take do the job they are supposed to?

Selecting Teaching Methods and Learning Activities. Experienced health care providers develop preferred styles of teaching. Sometimes, however, their styles reflect the common misconception that teaching is simply supplying information. Like most people, health care providers tend to repeat behaviors that are comfortable and that have been successful in the past. However, nurses need to develop skill in a variety of teaching methods to be effective in different situations.

The learning domain implied by the behavioral objective is one guideline for selecting teaching approaches. Cognitive learning can be facilitated by strategies and aids such as lecture, reading material, or films. Affective learning demands more personal interaction between teacher and learner; discussion techniques are one way of facilitating this type of learning. Learning psychomotor skills requires the use of performance strategies such as demonstration and return demonstration. When choosing teaching methods, nurses should also consider client characteristics documented in the data base: readiness, ability, and learning style.

A given teaching method typically implies corresponding learning activities. Collaborating with clients to select learning activities that are meaningful and stimulating enhances motivation and facilitates learning. The following discussion describes teaching methods and learning activities that are effective for health education. Combining several strategies in a teaching session keeps the learner's interest and promotes learning in more than one domain.

Explanation or Lecture. The most common method of providing information is explanation or lecture. It is particularly efficient for teaching groups but can also be used effectively with individuals. It consists of one-way transmission of verbal messages from teacher to learner. Because the teacher controls the presentation, content can be effectively organized and important concepts appropriately emphasized. This format has two limitations: It uses only one sensory modality and provides minimal opportunity for learner participation or reinforcement. Both contribute to learner inattention. These limitations can be mitigated by using visual aids such as posters or transparencies and by combining lectures with discussion.

Discussion. Discussion is the verbal exchange of ideas between two or more persons. Discussion encourages learner participation and is therefore particularly useful in a collaborative teaching–learning model. Discussion provides ongoing opportunities for teachers to discover learners' ideas, determine their level of understanding, and provide feedback and reinforcement. Effective use of discussion questions encourages learners to expand their thinking.

Generally, the teacher guides or facilitates discussions, but the give-and-take between participants creates unpredictable sequencing of information. This may be an advantage for some learners but is confusing to others. Moreover, because the teacher must exercise considerable patience and skill to resist the urge to control the flow of ideas, discussion is a difficult method for inexperienced teachers to use. Even the most proficient facilitator may be unable to maintain all learners' interest and active participation in a group discussion. However, learners who do actively participate often gain greater depth of understanding than could be expected with an explanatory approach.

Role-playing. Role-playing is an effective, interactive teaching strategy that involves emotions, attitudes and values. It is useful in health teaching because clients' emotional concerns often are paramount in health related situations. If these concerns are not addressed before the nurse makes any attempts to convey information or teach self-care skills, learning will be compromised.

In role-playing, each participant is assigned a role in a scenario based on a real-life situation. Often, the teacher also takes a role, which provides an opportunity to teach by means of modeling, or providing examples of behavior that participants may imitate.

Role-playing involves the scenario itself and the follow-up discussion in which participants examine the feelings evoked and relate them to the situation. The aim of the discussion is to help participants find meaning in the experience that they can apply to their own circumstances. A teacher facilitating role-play needs sensitivity, self-awareness, and communication skills to help participants overcome self-consciousness and promote their personal growth.

Behavior Rehearsal. Behavior rehearsal is similar to role-playing, but instead of taking on roles, learners play themselves in imagined situations. It is best used in one-on-one interactions; often the teacher takes on the role of a participant's significant other. Behavior rehearsal is especially useful to help clients prepare for anxiety-provoking future events. The simulation enables participants to try various behaviors, realize their consequences, and confront feelings without the intense negative effects they fear in the actual situation. The teacher's responsibility in behavior rehearsal is to suggest the simulation, suggest closure at an appropriate point, and initiate discussion after each scenario. As with role-playing, a high level of interpersonal skill is required to help participants develop awareness of feelings and insight into consequences of behavior.

Demonstration-coaching. Demonstration-coaching is used to teach psychomotor skills. It is useful for teaching clients and families self-care procedures. Rordan states that demonstration-coaching requires sequential steps or levels to help learners achieve progressively higher levels of proficiency:

1. The teacher explains and demonstrates the entire procedure.
2. The teacher demonstrates individual steps in the procedure while explaining each action and why it is done in that way.
3. The teacher performs the procedure while the learner describes each action, and then coaches the teacher on the next step.
4. The learner handles the equipment, tries parts of the procedure that involve new skills, and practices these skills with teacher guidance.
5. The learner performs all the steps of the procedure with the teacher's coaching.
6. The learner performs the entire procedure while explaining each action and the reason for it.
7. With teacher coaching, the learner demonstrates how to deal with errors or unexpected situational variations.[33]

This paradigm is applicable to teaching any type of motor skill. Each successive level builds on the competency gained in previous levels, but certain steps may be repeated, merged with other steps, or eliminated to accommodate individual learners' abilities. The steps in levels 1 and 2 could be presented on film or video to permit repeated viewing by the learner without additional teacher time. The procedure or equipment used can be modified to accommodate a client's home or work situation or other life-style needs.

The exchange of roles (observer, performer, coach) in levels 3–7, maintains learner involvement. However, teachers should schedule additional practice time for mastery of most skills after the formal teaching session. Research suggests that short practice periods interspersed with other activities are more effective for skill learning than one long practice period.[54]

Teaching Aids. Teaching aids are important adjuncts to effective teaching. Teaching aids help gain and maintain learners' attention by enhancing a presentation. Most involve visual or tactile modalities. Examples include written materials, pictures and diagrams, models, audiovisual programs, and self-paced learning programs, some of which are computer assisted.

Written Materials. Written materials, such as pamphlets, books, instruction sheets, and outlines, can be used before a teaching session to help learners prepare, to supplement or reinforce information during a teaching session, or as a review at the end of a teaching session. Written materials also serve as a reference for learners when they no longer have access to the teacher.

Written materials must be of a suitable reading level to be useful. Many adults in America have limited reading ability or are are unable to read at all. Written materials used for health teaching should be written at the sixth- to eighth-grade level. Materials that use simple sentence structure, avoid words with three or more syllables, and include concrete examples are most likely to be effective. Many professional organizations, government agencies, and non-profit organizations such as the American Heart Association distribute free or low-cost printed educational materials to health care professionals or consumers.

Pictures and Diagrams. Pictures and diagrams are useful for communicating concepts and complex relationships. Because pictures tend to be remembered more readily than words, they are potent reinforcers of verbal teaching techniques. Pictures and diagrams are available for purchase in many forms, such as flipcharts, posters, photographs, transparencies, and slides. They are also easy for teachers to prepare on their own. The most effective pictorial aids are simple and uncluttered, contain words as well as pictures, and use color for emphasis. Realism does not necessarily make pictures more powerful: in fact, the excessive detail in realistic pictures may detract from the intended message.

Models. Models are similar to pictures, but add the dimensions of tactile stimulation and perspective. Anatomical models can be invaluable in teaching people the location and structure of their internal organs, which helps them understand the meaning of their symptoms or recommended self-care strategies (Fig. 20–8). Models also help teach psychomotor skills.

Audiovisual Programs. Film, audiotapes, and videotapes can be used to present content, teach skills, or stimulate learning of attitudes and values. The realistic action in film and videotapes makes them engrossing and involves learners intellectually and emotionally. These media are therefore powerful means of portraying affective responses to health care problems or stimulating group discussions or nurse–client interactions. For example, the film "From the Other Side of the Stethoscope" portrays the emotional responses and coping strategies of a young physician who becomes ill with cancer. Because the responses illustrated are common to many people with cancer, but exhibited by an individual perceived by many to be powerful and strong, the film gives permission to express and examine feelings many clients tend to hide.

Many health care agencies use closed-circuit television to present information to clients. Often, a variety of programs are available, including descriptions of common health problems, self-care strategies, and diagnostic tests. The value of such programs is enhanced if clients can discuss them with a health care provider after viewing.

Videotaping also enhances teaching of motor skills. Not only is a videotape a useful way of presenting skills, but videotaping practice sessions enables teacher and learner to critique the performance simultaneously or separately. Viewing one's actions on videotape often helps improve technique. Moreover, the teacher's feedback will be more precise if it refers to a concrete example of the action or the error.

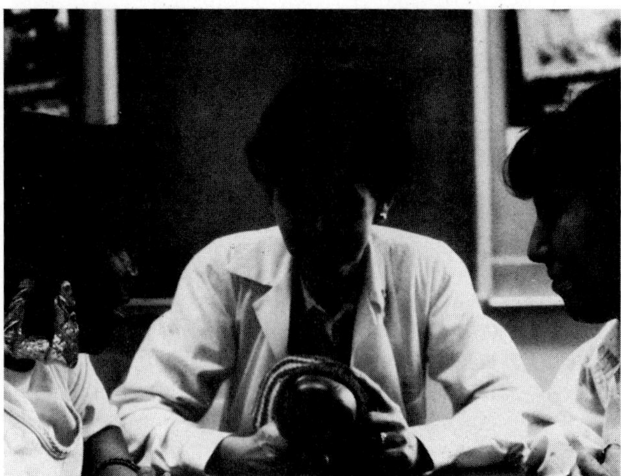

Figure 20–8. Using a model to teach body structure and function. (*From Sherwen LN, Scoloveno MA, Weingarten CT.* Nursing Care of the Childbearing Family. *Norwalk, CT: Appleton & Lange; 1991.*)

Audiotapes can be used to augment or repeat content explained in individual or group teaching sessions. Although tapes are no more effective in conveying information than live lectures, the learner can stop and start the tape and repeat all or part of it as needed. A possible health care teaching application of audiotapes is to record discharge instructions on an audio cassette for clients to take home. As more and more families obtain VCRs, health care professionals may begin to prepare videotaped discharge instructions, which would reinforce self-care skills and operation of equipment.

Self-paced Learning Programs. Also called autotutorial or programmed instruction, self-paced learning programs present information in small segments and require learners to answer frequent questions. In this way, learners are given immediate feedback and can work at their own pace. Programmed instruction requires that learners take individual responsibility for learning, as no teacher–learner interaction occurs. Nevertheless, research has demonstrated significantly higher learning results from programmed instruction than from typical explanatory presentations of the same content. Equal amounts of information are learned in far less time.[55]

With the introduction of computers into most aspects of our lives has come CAI, or computer-assisted instruction. CAI is a form of self-paced autotutorial instruction. Because of sophisticated branching techniques possible with computers, learners' answers determine the type of subsequent prompt that they receive from the computer. High-technology interactive video systems, which combine the capabilities of the video and computer media, are capable of even more realistic and individualized feedback.

CAI simulations are highly effective for teaching psychomotor skills as well as conveying direct information. Not only does CAI take less time to complete than traditional teaching strategies, but greater transfer of learning results.[55] Chapter 21 provides more information about health teaching applications of computer technology.

Evaluation Strategies. Many teaching–learning plans incorporate evaluation strategies and schedules in addition to objectives, content, and teaching–learning activities. (See sample teaching plan, Table 20–3.) This helps make evaluation a mutual responsibility. Collaborative evaluation is detailed in a later section.

Choosing an Environment Conducive to Learning. Environment shapes learning. Because space is often at a premium in health care facilities, securing an appropriate location for teaching–learning activities may be challenging, but should be considered a priority. Although environmental conditions are not completely under nurses' control, obtaining appropriate space and teaching aids is a necessary part of planning for teaching–learning. The nurse may have to alter the physical environment to make it supportive of learning and free of distractions. Individual preferences for learning environment should be accommodated when possible. The following general considerations are relevant in most teaching–learning situations.

Environmental conditions that affect sensory-perceptual proficiency, such as lighting and noise level, have a significant impact on learning. Poor lighting and extraneous noise interfere with reception and discrimination of stimuli. If learners are unable to see or hear well, they are likely to become frustrated and disinterested.

Conditions related to physical comfort should also be considered. Discomfort is distracting. Poor ventilation, extremes of temperature, uncomfortable chairs, or a too-crowded room contribute to inattention.

Physical environment also includes equipment to support presentation of material. Having all teaching aids and any related equipment in working order and accessible saves time. Arranging chairs so all learners can see audiovisual materials or participate in group interaction enhances effectiveness.

Privacy may also be a concern for some clients. If the subject matter is sensitive, or if self-care skills involve body exposure, most learners prefer private one-on-one teaching.

Scheduling Teaching–Learning Sessions. Mutual scheduling of teaching–learning sessions fosters learning. When possible, plan teaching–learning activities in 15- to 20-minute segments.[56] Although adults can maintain concentration for as long as an hour under optimum conditions, optimum conditions cannot be ensured for health teaching. Frequently, clients' physical and emotional condition limits attention span. Certain medications may also interfere with cognitive functioning. Moreover, treatments or therapies may contribute to fatigue.

Clients may prefer a particular time of day for teaching–learning. For example, some people feel most alert early in the morning; others prefer the late afternoon. Clients' other nursing care needs and nurses' other responsibilities must also be considered.

As stated earlier, nurses perceive that time limitations are the most common reason for omitting health teaching. Scheduling health teaching as an integral part of nursing care is one way to demonstrate its value to nurses and clients alike.

Using Teaching–Learning Contracts. A teaching–learning contract is a verbal or written agreement between client and nurse. It is somewhat different from a teaching–learning plan (described in the next section). Typically, teaching–learning contracts outline mutually acceptable learning objectives, a time frame, as well as clients' and nurses' responsibilities in achieving the specified objectives. Reinforcers or rewards a client will receive for accomplishing objectives may be specified. The contract may also describe a structured means for evaluating learning progress. Development and implementation of the contract require collaboration and negotiation between client and nurse. The contract is often signed by both parties to signify the mutual commitment it implies.

The Written Teaching–Learning Plan. The activities of defining objectives, identifying content, selecting teaching and evaluation methods, choosing the setting, and scheduling the teaching sessions culminate in a written teaching–learning plan. The components of these plans vary depending on agency policy. Two slightly different samples appear in Tables 20–2 and 20–3. Table 20–2 is a discharge teaching plan for parents of newborns at risk for sudden infant death syndrome (SIDS). Table 20–3 is a partial plan for hypertension education for clients at risk. The complete hypertension education teaching plan is part of a funded research study to determine the effectiveness of churches in black communities in reaching high-risk groups for anticipatory teaching about hypertension.

Implementing the Teaching–Learning Plan

A comprehensive, collaboratively developed teaching–learning plan is the foundation for client teaching activities. Implementing the plan effectively depends upon an individual nurse's sensitivity and communication skills. However, successful implementation of a teaching plan requires consistent awareness of several additional considerations. They are discussed below.

Facilitative Teaching Behaviors. Most people respond positively to warm, friendly health care providers who demonstrate a willingness to listen to their concerns and recognize their rights to autonomy and self-determination. A collaboratively developed teaching–learning plan is consistent with this approach. Maintaining a climate of mutual responsibility and flexibility as the plan is implemented fosters clients' self-confidence and openness, thereby making a successful outcome likely. Even with a strong commitment to change, change is difficult. Therefore, support and respect from nurses as clients attempt change are important contributing factors to continued motivation. Box 20–6 summarizes facilitative teaching behaviors, appropriate when implementing a teaching–learning plan.

Giving Feedback. Feedback is information about the quality and accuracy of a response. It is most helpful if it is given immediately or shortly after the response. Feedback can be positive (validating correct responses) or negative (telling a learner the response was incorrect). Negative feedback is more valuable if it clearly specifies what the error was, why the response was wrong, and the criteria for correct performance. Learners then need an opportunity to correct the error and reach their objectives. Involving learners in identifying ways to correct errors increases their motivation and enhances their feelings of accomplishment.

Although feedback is appropriate for all types of learn-

TABLE 20–2. TEACHING–LEARNING PLAN FOR USE OF PEDIATRIC APNEA MONITOR

Objectives	Strategy	Evaluation
Parents will:		During return demonstration, parents will:
1. Visually identify parts of the monitor and explain the function of each part of the monitor.	1. One-to-one discussion with use of pamphlet and instruction sheet for apnea monitor.	1. Point out the 3 critical parts of the apnea monitor and explain the function of each.
2. Correctly apply monitor leads and turn on the monitor.	2. Viewing and listening to videotape or film showing correct use of apnea monitor in the home.	2. Securely apply monitor leads in correct location and turn on the monitor.
3. List, in order of priority, the steps to be taken when alarm sounds.	3. One-to-one discussion of monitor use.	3. Write a list of the actions to take when the alarm sounds in order of priority, and save for future reference.
4. Demonstrate actions to be taken when alarm sounds.	4. Demonstration of steps to be taken when alarm sounds.	4. When alarm sounds, exhibit correct actions.
5. Discuss when the monitor should be used and describe situations in which it is safe not to use it.	5. Several return demonstrations with immediate feedback and reinforcement.	5. Describe indicators for use of the monitor and situations in which it is safe to leave the child off the monitor.
	6. Daily phone calls to the home following client discharge, decreasing in frequency as family becomes more independent.	
	7. Share teaching with home-care nurse assigned to family.	

Adapted from Van Hoozer HL, Bratton BD, Weinholtz D, et al. *The Teaching Process: Theory and Practice in Nursing.* Norwalk, CT: Appleton & Lange; 1987; 224.

ing, it is especially important for learning psychomotor skills. Learners generally require frequent, detailed feedback during initial practice sessions. As learners progress, they need less teacher feedback and can be encouraged to provide their own feedback or compare their performance to a standard.

Giving Positive Reinforcement. As discussed in the sections on learning theory earlier in the chapter, reinforcement shapes learner behavior. It is a necessary condition for learning. Positive reinforcement in health teaching usually takes the form of verbal praise or encouragement from health care providers. Nurses should reinforce efforts to meet objectives as well as actual achievement of objectives. Sometimes more tangible positive reinforcement, such as a chart on which teacher and learner can record progress, is effective.

Success is reinforcing in itself. If the teaching plan provides for content and methods that facilitate progress toward objectives and provides sufficient challenge, the learner's personal satisfaction provides intrinsic positive reinforcement.

Using Prompts and Primes. Primes and prompts are stimuli that elicit recall. They enhance progress and provide opportunities for positive reinforcement.

A **prime** is a teacher stimulus that tells the learner the exact response that is desired. For example, the teacher may state a word or phrase and ask learners to restate or write exactly what was said. Demonstrating the steps of a skill and requesting the learner to imitate each step is another example of a prime.

A **prompt** is a hint or clue that helps the learner think of the correct response. The clue may be a word, a picture, or a question. Research has shown that primes and prompts stimulate learner interest and enthusiasm, but that constant repetition of the same type of cue is likely to produce boredom.[57]

Using Practice and Repetition. Educational researchers have found that repeated practice is essential for learning and retention. Practice and repetition, or overlearning, are beneficial for cognitive, psychomotor, and social behaviors. As noted previously, several short practice sessions lead to better performance than one long session. Giving feedback during practice ensures that the behaviors repeated are not erroneous. Periodic review of previous learning is another way to use repetition to link new concepts and skills with past learning.

Even with adequate practice, studies of long-term retention show that within 1 year people forget 50 percent of what they learn, unless the information or skills are used frequently. This suggests that health teaching should focus on information and skills that have immediate application to clients' self-care.

Facilitating Transfer of Learning. Transfer of learning refers to learners' ability to use knowledge in more than one setting or situation. Clients participate in teaching–learning interactions to be able to take responsibility for their health and self-care. Therefore, they must be able to relate what they learn to their own life situations.

For example, it may be relatively easy for a client with high blood pressure to select low-sodium foods in a con-

TABLE 20–3. SAMPLE HYPERTENSION EDUCATION TEACHING PLAN

Session 1: Understanding Risk Factors in Hypertension
Time: 20–30 minutes
General Objective: To provide an overview of strategies for managing risk factors associated with hypertension

Objectives	Content	Teaching–Learning Activities/Aids
Identify at least two characteristics of high blood pressure.	Understanding high blood pressure A. What kind of disease is high blood pressure (HBP)? 1. HBP is a potentially dangerous disease that is frequently called "the silent killer" because there are no symptoms in the early stages of the disease.	Prior to beginning teaching, ask class participants, "What do you think HBP is?"
	2. HBP is also called hypertension (refer to booklet). 3. It is one of the most serious diseases in the United States; 55 million Americans have HBP.	Distribute booklet *High Blood Pressure and What You Can Do About It* by Marvin Moser.
	4. Anyone can get HBP. All races, ages, sexes, and socioeconomic groups have HPB. 5. Blacks have HBP more frequently than whites: a. One out of every four black adults has high blood pressure. b. High blood pressure is the leading cause of death among blacks. c. High blood pressure often develops early in life and is especially severe in blacks.	Ask group: "Is there an ethnic group that is more prone to get HPB than another?" "Which ethnic group?"
Describe what blood pressure is and how it is measured.	B. What is blood pressure? 1. Blood pressure is the force with which your heart pumps blood through the body. It involves blood flowing through heart and blood vessels. Compare to faucet.	Show poster of heart and blood vessels. Explain how the heart works in pumping blood through the body. Have learners turn to p. 7 in booklet for comparison of heart and blood vessels with a faucet, and p. 6 for picture of BP equipment.
	2. Measuring BP is done with a BP instrument called sphygmomanometer: a. Systolic b. Diastolic	Hold up large and small sphygmomanometers and stethoscope. Pass around group. Ask for volunteer to have BP measured.
Differentiate between (1) systolic and diastolic blood pressure recording, and (2) normal and abnormal blood pressure. State the ranges for normal and high blood pressure.	3. Normal BP a. Systolic (SBP) 140 or less b. Diastolic (DBP) 89 or less 4. Occasional increases in blood pressure levels are not unusual; however, if your blood pressure reaches abnormally high levels and stays high, then you are considered to have high blood pressure (HBP). High blood pressure is also called hypertension. Hypertension is: a. SBP = greater than 140 and/or b. DBP = 90 or higher	Refer to booklet for sample of how BP is recorded on chart.
Identify at least three risk factors associated with high blood pressure.	C. What are the causes of HBP? Although the exact causes for high blood pressure are not known in 90% of cases, certain risk factors or associations usually are present. 1. *Hereditary factors.* High blood pressure tends to run in families. This suggests that some inherited factor predisposes certain people to developing this disease. 2. *Race.* High blood pressure occurs one-and-a-half to two times more frequently among blacks than among whites. It develops, on the average, five to ten years earlier; is generally more severe with higher blood pressure levels; and progresses more rapidly with earlier complications. 3. *Environmental and life-style factors.* In many cases, your environment and/or life-style may determine whether you develop high blood pressure. These factors include where you live, salt intake, weight, stress, alcohol consumption, lack of exercise, and many other less proven factors.	Ask the group: "What are some things that cause HBP?" Which of these factors can be changed? Answer: ■ Smoking ■ Obesity ■ Dietary Na^{+} and cholesterol intake ■ Exercise ■ Stress Which of these cannot be changed? Answer: ■ Age ■ Sex ■ Race ■ Family

From Eva Smith, unpublished material.

BOX 20–6. FACILITATIVE TEACHING BEHAVIORS

1. Acknowledge that coping strategies are used by clients to protect them from real or imaginary threats.
2. Realize that a variety of personal attributes, past learning experiences, and the present situation affect clients' reactions to their health status and to the changes in behavior recommended for clients.
3. Recognize that clients with the same condition react and adapt differently; use different teaching approaches based on the needs of individual clients.
4. Conduct a careful assessment of the beliefs, reactions, and situation of each client, and make decisions about teaching based on facts, not assumptions.
5. Initiate teaching according to the clients' readiness to learn; establish rapport before suggesting changes in client's behavior.
6. Use empathy and understanding to lay the groundwork for effective teaching.
7. Understand and accept clients' reactions such as fear and frustration.
8. Use support to acknowledge client stress and efforts to cope.
9. When clients use coping strategies, such as denial, that are detrimental to teaching, gradually introduce them to reality.
10. Refrain from reinforcing negative opinions and inaccurate ideas expressed by clients.
11. When the coping strategies used by clients do not hinder their condition or treatment, do not try to interfere with the strategies being used.

Source: Merritt, SL. Patient self-efficacy: A framework for designing patient education. *Focus Crit Care.* 1989; 16:68–73.

trolled hospital environment. However, typical contemporary American dietary practices, such as consuming prepared foods containing preservatives and eating in fast food restaurants, may make it difficult to limit sodium intake outside the hospital. To enhance transfer of learning about sodium intake to a client's daily routine, a nurse might suggest that the client modify several of his or her typical daily menus to comply with the prescribed sodium restrictions.

Strategies to facilitate transfer of learning should be a focus of most health teaching. Practice exercises that demand increasing levels of independent decision making are an effective way to help clients apply learning to their everyday life experiences.

Collaborative Evaluation

Evaluation, like each of the previous steps in the teaching–learning process, is a collaborative activity. It includes validating learning and modifying the teaching–learning plan, if desired learning has not occurred. As discussed in Chapter 18, evaluation is an ongoing as well as a terminal process. Nurses and clients evaluate progress toward objectives during teaching–learning activities and may modify strategies or objectives as a result. Feedback, discussed above, is an example of ongoing evaluation. At the conclusion of the teaching–learning sessions, client and nurse execute a more formal evaluation using predetermined evaluation methods or tools. This is also the time when teachers elicit feedback from learners about the effectiveness of their teaching. This may be done verbally or by providing a written form.

Validating Learning. Several methods may be used to determine to what degree learners have attained the knowledge, attitudes, and skills specified in the objectives. They include verbal, written, and observational techniques.[33,58]

Verbal evaluation techniques may take the form of a self-report of learning by clients; more often, however, the teacher asks the learner questions about the learning experience. Although verbal questioning is stressful for some individuals, a sensitive low-key approach can make the evaluation a natural extension of teaching–learning activities. Observation of clients' nonverbal behavior during questioning provides additional clues to their level of confidence about the material being tested. (Refer to Chap. 14 for a discussion of nonverbal behavior.)

For verbal questioning to be an effective evaluation tool, the questions must be carefully planned. Questions should follow a logical order and relate to the level of learning specified in the teaching–learning objectives. For example, to evaluate the first level of learning in the cognitive domain, knowledge, a nurse might ask a client "Can you name three foods you should avoid on a sodium-restricted diet?" To evaluate application, a third-level cognitive behavior, a question such as "Let's see how you would decide whether a sample menu for one day's meals had too much sodium" would be appropriate.

Written evaluation techniques include tests and questionnaires. The former are usually used to determine knowledge level, the latter to evaluate attitude changes resulting from the teaching–learning interaction. Written examinations are challenging to construct, but they do provide a useful record of client performance. Because they are closely associated with classroom situations and performance expectations, some individuals become anxious when confronted with written tests. Using practice tests as part of the teaching–learning experience may alleviate anxiety. If teachers and learners score the test together and discuss clients' answers, nurses will obtain more detailed information about what clients have learned.

Observation is used to evaluate performance of motor behaviors, such as self-care skills. Ideally, nurses would observe clients performing self-care under realistic circumstances. Often, however, a return demonstration in a simulated setting must suffice. In a **return demonstration,** the client performs a skill without coaching (Fig. 20–9). Many nurses use checklists or rating scales to evaluate client performance of motor skills. Checklists identify desired behaviors, often in a specified sequence; rating scales describe several levels of performance for each behavior. Rating scales are useful for successive evaluations. Clients may then note their progress to higher levels of proficiency.

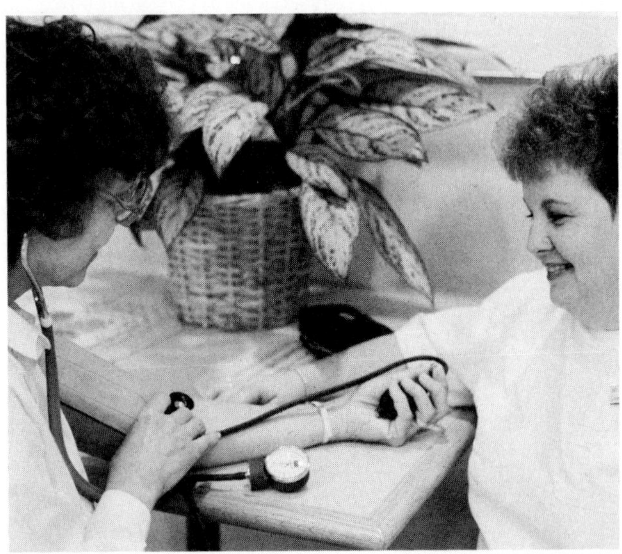

Figure 20–9. Formal individual teaching. The nurse observes a client's return demonstration of blood pressure assessment.

Sample items for a checklist and a rating scale for evaluating preparation of medication for self-injection appear in Figure 20–10.

Videotaping clients as they perform self-care skills is another way to evaluate skills. This method enables teachers to provide concrete feedback and provides an opportunity for collaborative evaluation.

Modifying the Teaching–Learning Plan. When evaluation indicates that teaching–learning objectives were not met or were only partially met, nurse and client must decide on possible reasons for the unsatisfactory outcome and try to correct it. As discussed above, nurse and client usually become aware of a need to modify the plan during the teaching–learning activities; however, sometimes it is not until the final formal evaluation phase that the need for modification becomes apparent.

Failure to meet objectives may be related to learner characteristics and behaviors, the complexity of the material, teaching–learning approaches, environmental conditions, the amount of time available, or a combination of these. After client and nurse systematically appraise the role of each factor, they can reach collaborative decisions about solutions. Sometimes, setting more realistic objectives is the answer; scheduling more frequent teaching–learning sessions, changing teaching approaches, or providing more practice time may also be considered. A strong mutual commitment to achieving the overall goal of enhancing client ability to take responsibility for self-care enhances the likelihood of successful resolution of teaching–learning problems.

Documenting Teaching–Learning. As Chapter 18 showed, documentation of client care is a crucial nursing responsi-

CHECKLIST:

_____ 1. Draws accurate amount of medication into syringe with correct aseptic technique.
_____ 2. Identifies appropriate site for injection.
_____ 3. Cleanses skin at site.

RATING SCALE:

Rating	Levels of Functioning
3	_____ a. Firmly wipes top of vial with alcohol swab
	_____ b. Removes needle cover without difficulty
	_____ c. Smoothly draws up desired amount of medication without contaminating medication or equipment
2	_____ a. Wipes top of vial with alcohol swab
	_____ b. Removes needle cover
	_____ c. Draws up desired amount of medication without contaminating medication or equipment
1	_____ a. Does not cleanse top of vial
	_____ b. Removes needle with needle cover or contaminates needle as cap is removed
	_____ c. Obtains air bubbles as withdraws medication and has difficulty expelling air or obtains incorrect dosage of medication

Note: A rating of at least 2 is required for each behavior for performance to be considered acceptable.

Figure 20–10. Sample checklist and rating scale items.

GROSSMONT HOSPITAL WOMEN'S HEALTH CENTER
DOCUMENTATION OF PATIENT/FAMILY EDUCATION

PATIENT ASSESSMENT			EDUCATION
	I would like to have my nurse discuss or show me. (Pt. initial)	I feel comfortable doing. (Pt. initial)	Discussed, demonstrated or observed. (Nurse sig.)
FEEDING-BREAST			
Proper positioning and latch on			
Maintaining infant airway & breaking suction			
Reason for frequent feedings			
Frequency & positions for burping			
Appearance of colostrum & milk			
Reason for supplemental feedings			
Indications of adequate feedings			
Storage of breast milk			
FEEDING-BOTTLE			
Proper position for burping			
Frequency & positions for burping			
Frequency & amount of feedings			
Indications of adequate feedings			
DIAPER CHANGE			
Number of expected wet diapers			
Number of expected stools			
Normal variations in BM			
BABY CARE			
Bathing			
Cord Care			
Foreskin/Circumcision Care			
Cleansing Genitals (boys/girls)			
Bulb Syringe			
Wrapping & dressing infant			
Use of Thermometer			
When to call Pediatrician			
Infant safety & infant car seat			
SELF CARE			
Changes of Vaginal Discharge			
Appropriate activity level			
Peri-care & sitz bath			
Incision Care, C-Section			
Bowel & bladder changes			
Breast Care			
Diet & Fluids			
Postpartum Blues			
Administration of Rhogam and/or Rubella Vaccine			

OTHER ______

I have received instructions and/or demonstrations as indicated. I understand that this information is not necessarily complete and definitive, therefore, I have been instructed to contact my physician regarding additional questions.

SIGNED: ______ WITNESS: ______

DATE: ______ ADDRESSOGRAPH

GHF-N-78 (Rev. 3-90)

Figure 20–11. Sample documentation of teaching. (*Courtesy of Grossmont Hospital Women's Health Center, San Diego.*)

bility. The client record serves as a means of communication among health care providers and as legal validation of the care provided. All of the characteristics of effective recording discussed in Chapter 18 apply to charting about client teaching. Often, however, documentation of health teaching is incomplete or omitted, particularly when teaching is done informally.

When client and nurse develop a formal teaching–learning plan, it serves as documentation of the teaching–learning objectives and accomplishments. Or, if a nurse incorporates teaching–learning objectives into the overall client care plan, then progress relevant to those objectives can be routinely charted. In some health care facilities, client teaching is documented on a separate client education sheet (Fig. 20–11). Such a document is useful when all clients on the unit have similar educational needs. To provide consistency in teaching and streamline documentation, the agency that uses the form shown in Figure 20–11 provides a handbook for clients and staff that outlines specific content related to each of the topics on the form. This form also emphasizes collaborative responsibility for identification of learning needs by providing a space for clients to identify the topics they wish to focus on. A nurse who verifies client demonstration of a particular topic or skill documents that the content related to that topic has been learned, and the client also signs to verify her participation.

When there is neither a formal teaching–learning plan nor a specific teaching protocol, nurses must take responsibility for clearly documenting their client teaching. Barron suggests that progress note entries about client teaching include information about content, method, and evaluation.[59] The description of content should be specific and concise. Although the actual information conveyed may be too lengthy, the topic must be clearly identified. In describing the teaching method, indicate, for example, whether explanation, discussion, or demonstration was done and note handouts or other resources that were provided.

Evaluation data should include evidence of client learning, such as a correct return demonstration or correct verbalization of specific facts. Effective documentation verifies that nurses have met their responsibilities for client education and facilitates continuity if clients are transferred to another unit or another health care facility or are discharged with home health care follow-up.

SUMMARY

Health education is part of all health care providers' responsibility to their clients. Although nurses have long recognized this responsibility and endeavored to meet it, they have not consistently achieved optimum results. Often, perceived time constraints and lack of confidence about teaching ability impair nurses' effectiveness as teachers.

Nurses can become more competent health teachers by consistently assessing client characteristics that influence learning and recognizing the importance of a collaborative approach to clients' learning needs (Table 20–4). Nurses who are vigilant about diagnosing clients' learning needs, who consider clients' needs, abilities, and preferences when selecting teaching approaches, and who incorporate teaching aids to enhance verbal presentations, are effective teachers.

A formal teaching–learning plan is an effective way to organize and document client teaching, but informal teaching is also appropriate in many situations. Group teaching for clients with similar needs is another possible approach.

If health education is given a priority in all health care facilities, clients' abilities to take responsibility for health promotion and self-care will be greatly strengthened. This will not only empower health care consumers but also enhance providers' sense of professional accomplishment and improve the efficiency of health care delivery.

REFERENCES

1. American Hospital Association. *A Patient's Bill of Rights.* Chicago: AHA; 1973.
2. Rothman DL, Rothman NL. The legal basis for patient education practice in nursing. In: Redman BK, ed. *Issues and Concepts in Patient Education.* New York: Appleton-Century-Crofts; 1981: 104–117.
3. Roach WH. The patient's right to know. In: Bille DA, ed. *Practical Approaches to Patient Teaching.* Boston: Little, Brown; 1981: 35–52.
4. Falvo DR. *Effective Patient Education.* Rockville, MD: Aspen Systems; 1985.
5. Stanton MP. Patient education in the hospital health-care setting. *Patient Ed Counsel.* 1983;5:14–22.
6. Pender N. *Health Promotion in Nursing Practice.* 2nd ed. Norwalk, CT: Appleton-Century-Crofts; 1987.
7. Levin LS. Patient education and self-care: How do they differ? *Nurs Outlook.* 1978;26:170–175.
8. Kernaghan SG. Preadmission preoperative teaching: A promising option, but easier said than done. *Promoting Health.* 1985; 5:26–28.
9. American Nurses' Association. *The Professional Nurse and Health Education.* Kansas City: ANA; 1975.
10. Cohen SA. Patient education: A review of the literature. *J Adv Nurs.* 1981;6:11–18.
11. Cook TD. Major research analysis provides proof: Patient education *does* make difference. *Promoting Health.* 1984;4:18–22.
12. Wilson-Barnett J, Osborne J. Studies evaluating patient teaching: Implication for practice. *Int J Nurs Stud.* 1983;20:33–44.
13. Bigge L. *Learning Theories for Teachers.* New York: Harper & Row; 1982.
14. Hebb DO. *A Textbook of Psychology.* Philadelphia: Saunders; 1958.
15. Rogers C. *Freedom to Learn.* Columbus: Merrill; 1969.
16. Bandura A. *Social Learning Theory.* Englewood Cliffs, NJ: Prentice-Hall; 1979.
17. Bloom BS, ed. *Taxonomy of Educational Objectives. 1. Cognitive Domain.* New York: Longman; 1956.

TABLE 20–4. LEARNING CONCEPTS AND THEIR IMPLICATIONS FOR COLLABORATION

Theory/Concept	Implications for Collaboration
■ Behavior that is rewarded is more likely to be repeated. Rewards must immediately follow desired behavior to have reinforcing effect.	■ Learn from the client what reward is meaningful; provide this reward consistently and immediately during practice.
■ Cognitive feedback confirms accurate responses and corrects errors.	■ Give direct verbal feedback that explains errors and affirms correct responses, so errors are not inadvertently rewarded with correct aspects of the behavior.
■ Behavior is more likely to be retained if it is repeated.	■ Provide many opportunities to practice desired behaviors.
■ Once a behavior has been learned, intermittent reinforcement maintains behavior most effectively.	■ When mastery of a desired behavior has been demonstrated, reward the behavior some of the time, but not every time.
■ An individual's past experiences and current perceptions affect a given learning situation.	■ Assess clients' beliefs relative to the topic(s) being considered for teaching. Find out about clients' past experiences with learning. Provide concrete evidence to refute erroneous perceptions that interfere with learning.
■ The person–environment interaction influences learning. Environment can enhance or interfere with learning.	■ Assess current status (eg, interest, motivation, internal distractions such as pain or fear) and external environment. Correct environmental conditions that could cause distraction or interference.
■ Learning is goal directed. It is deeply influenced by the learner's personal goals.	■ Plan teaching and learning in collaboration with the client, with emphasis on the learner's goals and desired paths to reach them.
■ New learning is built on past learning.	■ Find out what a client knows about a topic before beginning teaching. Link new information to past information.
■ Learning is a total (holistic) experience. The perceptual features of a learning situation are important influences.	■ Use multiple sensory modalities (touch, sight, movement) to enhance learning.
■ Some learners have specific modality preferences for learning.	■ Ask individuals how they feel they learn best, then use their preferred modality whenever possible.
■ Attaining mastery/success: achieving new insight or successfully manipulating the environment (eg, equipment) is self-reinforcing and encourages further learning.	■ Structure learning experiences to match abilities of the learner, so a challenge is perceived, but success is achievable.
■ Humans have a natural potential for learning. Subject matter seen as having personal relevance is more readily learned.	■ Learn as much as possible from clients about themselves and their lives. Provide links between what is being taught and clients' life experiences. Show how content has application in a client's life.
■ Human behavior is directed toward increasing feelings of personal adequacy.	■ Enhance learners' feelings of personal adequacy by being nonjudgmental and demonstrating acceptance and caring.
■ Needs perceived as immediate receive a person's attention before actual or potential future problems.	■ Deal with current needs and concerns that clients define before trying to direct clients' attention to learning about subjects that the provider identifies as important.
■ Learning that involves a change in one's perception of oneself is threatening and tends to be resisted.	■ Provide nonthreatening learning environment with pace of learning/change determined by the learner, particularly when learning involves significant change by the learner.
■ All learners are not motivated by the same learning situation. Preferred learning style influences receptivity to material presented.	■ Tailor the learning environment to the needs, preferences, and abilities of the learner.
■ Anxiety and stress influence learning. Low to moderate stress enhances learning, whereas high stress interferes with learning.	■ Assess client's stress level before attempting teaching. If stress level is high, assist with stress-reduction techniques before attempting teaching.
■ Taking responsibility for one's own learning through self-evaluation and self-feedback fosters development of feelings of personal adequacy.	■ Collaborate with the client to devise self-evaluation instruments that the client can use to evaluate learning.
■ People with high expectations about their ability to engage in or execute a behavior achieve better behavioral outcomes than those who have less confidence.	■ Give encouragement and support during teaching, emphasizing evidence that the client has the ability to learn the behavior being taught.
■ Imitation of models is more likely if models are perceived to be similar to oneself.	■ Use language and nonverbal communication that are similar to the client's when possible. Call attention to similarities between yourself and client.
■ Culture is an important variable in observational learning. Imitation is less likely if models are of a different culture than oneself.	■ When possible, assign caregivers from a cultural background similar to a client's.

TABLE 20–4. (continued)

Theory/Concept	Implications for Collaboration
■ Identification (change that becomes an enduring part of a person's behavior) is more likely when the model is seen as warm, empathic, and willing to explain.	■ Establish client trust by a consistent warm and open approach.
■ Continued imitation of a behavior is more likely when that behavior has been rewarded.	■ When desired behavior is imitated, praise or give other positive acknowledgement for the behavior.
■ Imitation is more likely if models are perceived as having high prestige.	■ Health care providers are often held in high regard by clients, so providers exhibiting healthy behaviors or evidence of healthy life-style choices (such as not smoking, being of optimum weight for height, appearing physically fit) can positively influence clients' choices.
■ Imitation of a number of different behaviors of models besides the specific behavior intended or rewarded is likely.	■ Unhealthy behaviors by role models may be imitated even without contingent rewards.
■ Group pressure to perform any behavior makes it more likely to occur.	■ Using a group setting for teaching can facilitate adoption of desired behaviors, because group members who embrace the new behaviors can influence those who are less willing to change.
■ Forgetting occurs because new associations interfere with previously acquired associations.	■ Provide opportunities to review prior learning if that knowledge is necessary to grasp new material.
■ Discrimination is a requisite for learning.	■ Assess functioning of sensory organs prior to teaching; do not rely on modalities in which client has deficits (eg, hearing, vision).
■ Discrimination is more difficult for most learners when many complex stimuli are presented.	■ Keep extraneous environmental stimuli to a minimum; present essential learning stimuli in appropriate sequence for the topic/concept.
■ Discrimination and verbal association are prerequisites for generalization and concept formation.	■ See above. Before presenting concepts, provide opportunities to learn vocabulary needed to understand the concepts. Organize presentation of information from simple to complex; concrete to abstract. Present complex or abstract concepts after simple and concrete concepts are learned.

18. Krathwohl DR, Bloom BS, Masia BB. *Taxonomy of Educational Objectives. 2. Affective Domain.* New York: Longman; 1964.
19. Simpson E. The classification of educational objectives in the psychomotor domain. In: *Contributions of Behavioral Science to Instructional Technology: The Psychomotor Domain.* Washington DC: Gryphon; 1972.
20. Havighurst RJ. *Developmental Tasks and Education.* New York: McCay; 1976.
21. Rosenstock IM, Strecher VJ, Becker MH. Social learning theory and the health belief model. *Health Ed Q.* 1988;15:175–183.
22. Redman BK. *The Process of Patient Education.* St. Louis: Mosby; 1988.
23. Tripp-Reimer T. Cross-cultural perspectives on patient teaching. *Nurs Clin North Am.* 1989;24:613–619.
24. Becker MH. Understanding compliance: The contributions of attitudes and other psychosocial factors. In: Cohen SJ, ed. *New Directions in Patient Compliance.* Lexington, MA: Heath; 1979.
25. Bandura A, Walters R. *Social Learning and Personality Development.* New York: Holt, Rinehart & Winston; 1963.
26. Armstrong MI. Orchestrating the process of patient education: Methods and approaches. *Nurs Clin North Am.* 1989;24:597–604.
27. Johnson EA, Jackson JE. Teaching the home care client. *Nurs Clin North Am.* 1989;24:589–595.
28. Spier BE. The nursing process as applied to the cognitive aspects of aging. In: Yurik AG, Spier BE, Robb SS, Ebert NJ. *The Aged Person and the Nursing Process.* Norwalk, CT: Appleton & Lange, 1989.
29. Kick E. Patient teaching for elders. *Nurs Clin North Am.* 1989;24:681–687.
30. Personal communication, Literacy Volunteers of America, Syracuse, New York, January 1992.
31. Loughrey L. Dealing with the illiterate patient . . . You can't read him like a book. *Nursing '83.* 1983;13:65–67.
32. Ausburn LJ, Ausburn FB. Cognitive styles: Some information and implications for instructional design. *Ed Commun Technol.* 1978;26:337–354.
33. Rordan JW. *Nurses As Health Teachers: A Practical Guide.* Philadelphia: Saunders; 1987.
34. Lindeman CA, Van Aerman BH. Nursing intervention with the presurgical patient: The effects of structured and unstructured preoperative teaching. *Nurs Res.* 1971;20:319–332.
35. Marshall J, Penckofer S, Llewellyn J. Structured postoperative teaching and knowledge and compliance of patients who had coronary artery bypass surgery. *Heart Lung.* 1986;15:76–79.
36. Barrett N, Schwartz MD. What patients really want to know. *Am J Nurs.* 1981;81:1642.
37. Barsevick AM, Lauver D. Women's informational needs about colposcopy. *Image.* 1990;22:23–27.
38. Roter D. An exploration of health education's responsibility for a partnership model of client–provider relations. *Patient Ed Counsel.* 1987;9:25.
39. Williamson JA. Mutual interaction: A model of nursing practice. *Nurs Outlook.* 1981;29:104–107.
40. Eisenthal S, Emery R, Lazare A, Udin H. Adherence and the

negotiated approach to patienthood. *Arch Gen Psychiatry*. 1979; 36:393–398.

41. Kim HS. Collaborative decision-making in nursing practice: A theoretical framework. In: Chin PL, ed. *Advances in Nursing Theory Development*. London: Aspen; 1983.
42. Kasch CK. Establishing a collaborative nurse–patient relationship: A distinct focus of nursing action in primary care. *Image*. 1986;18:44–47.
43. Kasch CK. Toward a theory of nursing action: Skills and competency in nurse–patient interaction. *Nurs Res*. 1986;35:226–230.
44. Hill MN, McCombs NJ, eds. Hypertension. *Nurs Clin North Am*. 1981;16:299–376.
45. Vulcan BM, Nikulich-Barrett M. The effect of selected information on mothers' anxiety levels during their children's hospitalizations. *Journal of Pediatric Nursing*. 1988;3(2):97–100.
46. Rankin SH, Duffy KL. *Patient Education: Issues, Principles and Guidelines*. Philadelphia: Lippincott; 1983.
47. Champion VL. Effect of knowledge, teaching method, confidence and social influence on breast self-examination behavior. *Image*. 1989;21:76–80.
48. Pokorny BE. Validating a diagnostic label: Knowledge Deficit. *Nurs Clin North Am*. 1985;20:641–655.
49. Redman BK. *The Process of Patient Education*. St. Louis: Mosby; 1984.
50. Gordon M. *Manual of Nursing Diagnoses, 1991–92*. St. Louis: Mosby; 1990.
51. McFarland GK, Mcfarlane EA. *Nursing Diagnoses and Intervention*. St. Louis: Mosby; 1989.
52. Mager RF. *Preparing Instructional Objectives*. 2nd ed. Belmont, CA: Fearon; 1975.
53. Gagne R. *The Conditions of Learning*. New York: Holt, Rinehart & Winston; 1970.
54. Van Hoozer HL, Bratton BD, Ostmoe PM, et al. *The Teaching Process: Theory and Practice in Nursing*. Norwalk, CT: Appleton-Century-Crofts; 1987.
55. Van Hoozer HL. Determining strategies for teaching. In: Van Hoozer HL, Bratton BD, Ostmoe PM, et al. *The Teaching Process: Theory and Practice in Nursing*. Norwalk, CT: Appleton-Century-Crofts; 1987.
56. Craft MJ. Selecting and using teaching strategies, resources and materials for client education. In: Van Hoozer HL, Bratton BD, Ostmoe PM, et al. *The Teaching Process: Theory and Practice in Nursing*. Norwalk, CT: Appleton-Century-Crofts; 1987.
57. Dwyer FM. Behavioral approach to visual communications. Association for Educational Communications and Technology: *Instructional Communications and Technology Research Report*. 1980;11:21–25.
58. Albanese MA, Gjerde CL. Evaluation. In: Van Hoozer HL, Bratton BD, Ostmoe PM, et al. *The Teaching Process: Theory and Practice in Nursing*. Norwalk, CT: Appleton-Century-Crofts; 1987.
59. Barron S. Documentation of patient education. *Patient Ed Counsel*. 1987;9:81–85.

BIBLIOGRAPHY

Becker MH, ed. *The Health Belief Model and Personal Health Behavior*. Thorofare, NJ: Slack; 1974.

Benner P. *From Novice to Expert: Excellence and Power in Clinical Nursing Practice*. Menlo Park, CA: Addison-Wesley; 1984.

Bille DA, ed. *Practical Approaches to Patient Teaching*. Boston: Little, Brown; 1981.

Dennison PD, Keeling AW. Clinical support for eliminating the nursing diagnosis of knowledge deficit. *Image*. 1989;21(3):142–144.

DeTornay R, Thompson MA. *Strategies for Teaching Nursing*. 2nd ed. New York: Wiley; 1982.

Devine EC, Cook TD. A meta-analytic analysis of effects of psychoeducational interventions on length of postsurgical hospital stay. *Nurs Res*. 1983;32:267–273.

Doak L, Doak C. *Teaching Patients With Low Literacy Skills*. Philadelphia: Lippincott; 1985.

Doak L, Doak C. Lowering the silent barriers to compliance for patients with low literacy skills. *Promoting Health*. 1987;86–88.

Filbeck R. *Systems in Teaching and Learning*. Lincoln, NE: Professional Educators Publications; 1974.

Fortin F, Kirovac S. A randomized controlled trial of preoperative patient education. *Int J Nurs Stud*. 1976;13:11–24.

Gazda GM, Corsini RJ, eds. *Theories of Learning: A Comparative Approach*. Itasca, IL: Peacock; 1980.

Geffner BA, Armstrong ML, eds. Patient teaching. *Nurs Clin North Am*. 1989; 24(3):580–693

Gilliland MM. What patients can teach you about your patient teaching. *Nursing '81*. 1981;11:52–53.

Herje PA. Hows and whys of patient contracting. *Nurs Educator*. 1980;5:30–34.

Hyman RT. *Ways of Teaching*. 2nd ed. Philadelphia: Lippincott; 1974.

Jenny J. Humanistic strategy for patient teaching. *Health Values*. 1979;3.

Jenny J. Knowledge deficit, not a nursing diagnosis. *Image*. 1987; 19(4):184–185.

Keefe JW, ed. *Student Learning Styles*. Reston, VA: National Association of Secondary School Principals; 1979.

Kim MJ, McFarland GK, McLane AM. *Pocket Guide to Nursing Diagnosis*. St. Louis: Mosby; 1990.

Langford T. Establishing a nursing contract. *Nurs Outlook*. 1978;26: 386–388.

Lauer P, Murphy SP, Powers MJ. Learning needs of cancer patients: A comparison of nurse and patient perceptions. *Nurs Res*. 1982; 31:11–16.

Littlefield VM. *Health Education for Women: A Guide for Nurses and Other Health Professionals*. Norwalk, CT: Appleton & Lange; 1986.

McFarland GK, McFarlane EA. *Nursing Diagnosis and Intervention*. St. Louis: Mosby; 1989.

McKeachie WJ. *Teaching Tips*. 7th ed. Lexington, MA: Heath; 1978.

Megenity JS, Megenity J. *Patient Teaching: Theories, Techniques and Strategies*. Bowie, MD: Brady; 1982.

Pohl M. *The Teaching Function of the Nursing Practitioner*. 2nd ed. Dubuque, IA: Brown; 1973.

Reilly DE. *Behavioral Objectives—Evaluation in Nursing*. New York: Appleton-Century-Crofts; 1980.

Reynolds MA, Bingle JD. *Structured Preoperative Teaching*. CURN Project, Michigan Nurses' Association. New York: Grune & Stratton; 1981.

Rogers C. *On Becoming a Person.* Columbus: Merrill; 1969.

Smith CE, ed. *Patient education: Nurses in partnership with other health care professionals.* Orlando: Grune & Stratton; 1987.

Smoyak SA. Teaching as coaching. *Nurs Outlook.* 1978;26:361–363.

Steckel SB, Swain MA. Contracting with patients to improve compliance. *Hospitals.* 1977;51:81–84.

Streiff LD. Can clients really understand our instructions? *Image.* 1986;18:48–52.

Swain MA, Steckel SB. Influencing adherence among hypertensives. *Res Nurs Health.* 1981;4:213–222.

Walsh PL. Design considerations for adult patient education. *Patient Counsel Health Ed.* 1982;4:84–88.

Whitman NI, Graham BA, Gleit CJ, Boyd MD. *Teaching in Nursing Practice: A Professional Module.* Norwalk, CT: Appleton-Century-Crofts; 1986.

Woldrum KM, Ryan-Morrell V, Towson MC, et al. *Patient Education: Foundations of Practice.* Rockville, MD: Aspen; 1985.

CHAPTER 21

Computers as an Aid to Collaboration

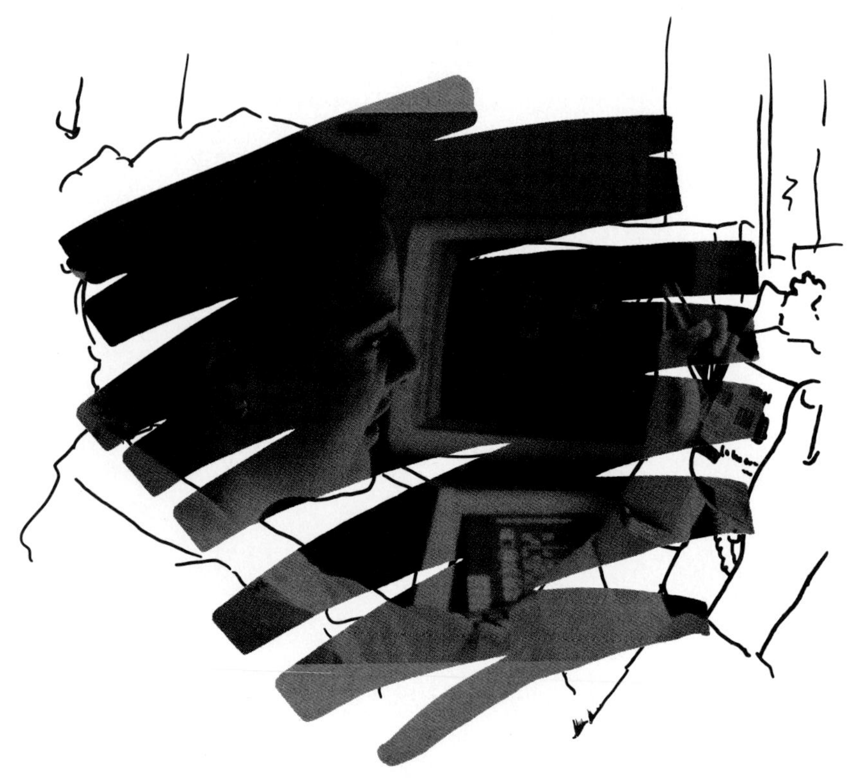

Behavioral Objectives

Upon completion of this chapter, the student will be able to:

1. Differentiate between computer hardware and computer software and describe the function of the various parts of the computer.
2. Describe five applications of computers in clinical practice.
3. Identify four advantages of computer use by nurses in clinical practice.
4. Identify three disadvantages of computer use by nurses in clinical practice.
5. Discuss the issues of privacy, confidentiality, and security as they relate to computer use by nurses.
6. Describe four types of computer-assisted instruction.
7. Discuss how computer-assisted instruction can be used in nursing education.
8. Discuss how computer-assisted instruction can be used in client education.
9. List three ways computers can assist nurses in conducting research.
10. List four computer applications used by nursing administrators.
11. Describe three types of general applications software.
12. Discuss how computers aid in collaboration among health care professionals in nursing practice, nursing education, nursing research, and nursing administration.

KEY TERMS

arithmetic/logical unit
assembly language
bit
byte
central processing unit
computer
computer-assisted instruction
control unit
hardware
high-level language
hospital information systems
machine language
microchip
microprocessor
primary memory
programs
random-access memory
read-only memory
secondary memory
software

In our society computers are found at supermarket checkout counters, banks, airports, hospitals, clinics, and physicians' offices. Computers are used for many purposes in health care, including financial management and billing. Computers perform a wide range of activities that save time and help nurses provide quality nursing care. Nurses use computers in clinical practice, education, research, and administration, and computer use by nurses is growing rapidly.

Computers are a powerful aid to professional collaboration. For example, the availability of computerized care plans and reference materials developed by expert nurses allows all nurses with access to a computer to benefit by indirect collaboration with these experts. In the future, as health care facilities expand their computer capabilities and more nurses become computer literate, computers will play an even greater role in aiding in collaboration than they do today.

Although computers have been used in health care since the 1960s, computer use by nurses has increased rapidly in recent years. Nurses need to be familiar with computers because computer use by nurses will continue to grow in the years ahead. Advances in computer technology are making computers smaller, faster, and more powerful. New and improved uses for computers in health care are being developed. Nurses must have a basic understanding of computers if they are to play an active role in deciding how they want computers to work for them.

Computers are important tools in nursing practice, nursing education, nursing research, and nursing administration. There are many advantages to the use of computers by nurses in clinical care. For example, computers can save nurses time in documentation and make documentation more complete and legible. Yet the issues of client privacy and the confidentiality and security of data are concerns associated with computer use in clinical practice.

Computers are also used in education. Computer-assisted instruction (a method of teaching in which the computer takes the role of the teacher) is used by nursing students and nurses, as well as by clients.

Computerized literature searches help researchers and students find information on the topic they are studying. Researchers also use computers to assist them in data collection, data analysis, and results reporting. Telecommunications technology makes it possible for nurses from different areas of the country to collaborate on joint research projects.

A number of computer programs assist nursing administrators to best use the nurses working for them and to maintain records. Computers can calculate daily the number of nurses needed on each unit based on how ill clients are on the individual units. Nursing administrators may also use a computer to schedule nurses' days off so that an optimal number of nurses are working at any one time.

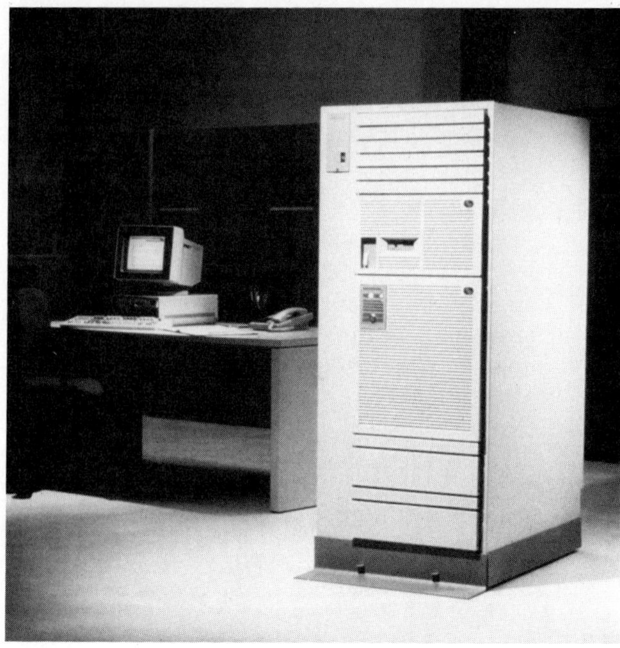

Figure 21–1. Mainframe computer. (*Courtesy of IBM.*)

■ WHAT IS A COMPUTER?

A **computer** in its complete form is a machine that accepts input; stores, retrieves, and processes information; and generates output. Humans also do these things; however, the computer performs calculations with greater speed and reliability, can store larger amounts of data, and responds more precisely and predictably. Although there are different types of computers, they work on similar principles. The main components of the computer are the central processing unit (CPU), the memory, input devices, and output devices. These physical components of the computer are called **hardware.** For the computer to work it must have instructions, or **programs.** Computer programs are sets of instructions and are referred to as **software.**

Types of Computers

There are three basic types of computers: mainframe computers, minicomputers, and microcomputers. The three types vary not only in their physical size but also in the amount of data each can process and store and the speed with which the data can be processed. The mainframe computer (Fig. 21–1) is the largest of the three and has the most memory, power, and speed. A minicomputer is a medium-sized computer. A microcomputer (Fig. 21–2) is the smallest type of computer. Personal computers used in homes, elementary and secondary schools, and small businesses are generally microcomputers. Laptop computers and notebook computers so small that they fit into a pocket are also microcomputers. Today the distinction between the three types of computers is somewhat blurred because new technology has made microcomputers as powerful and speedy as the minicomputers of a few years ago.

Computer Hardware

The main components of a computer are the CPU, memory, and input and output devices. This section briefly describes each of these components.

Central Processing Unit. The **central processing unit** (CPU) controls a computer's operations and performs all of its calculations. The CPU is composed of two parts: a control unit and an arithmetic/logical unit. The **control unit** determines the sequence of operations and routes data be-

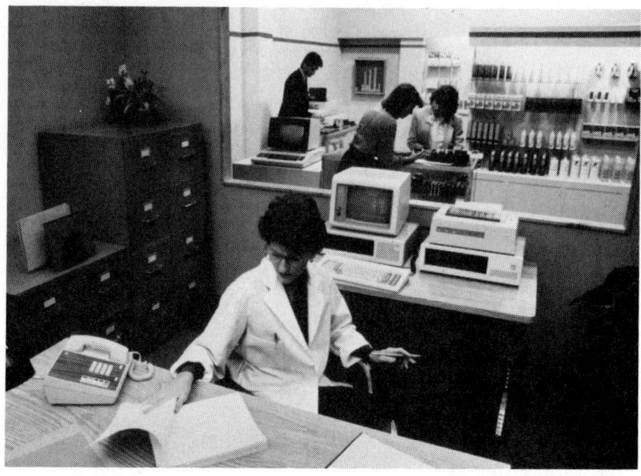

Figure 21–2. Microcomputer. (*Courtesy of IBM.*)

tween the different parts of the computer. The **arithmetic/ logical unit** performs the actual operations, such as addition, subtraction, and comparison of data. The CPU, however, can do nothing without the instructions provided by a computer program. Computer programs are discussed later in the chapter.

Memory. The computer stores data in specific numbered "locations" and retrieves the data later by specifying that the contents of a location should be retrieved. A series of on/off switches leads an electrical current to the particular location, and the data are moved between the CPU and its memory banks by electronic pathways called registers.

Data are represented in computer memory as groups of *bi*nary digi*ts*, or **bits.** Bits contain only two values, 0 and 1. By use of seven bits, all the letters of the alphabet in uppercase and lowercase, numbers, punctuation marks, and a number of special characters can be represented. The American Standard Code for Information Interchange (ASCII) is a commonly used binary code. Table 21–1 shows some of the bit strings in ASCII code and the characters they represent. An eighth bit is often added as a check for errors.

A group of eight bits is called a **byte.** Each byte represents one letter or character. A typed double-spaced page of 250 words contains approximately 2000 bytes.

The advantage of using binary numbers and coding systems for representing data in a computer is that the values can be represented inside the computer by switches that can be on or off. For example, 1 might equal switch or power on, and 0 might equal switch or power off. As discussed above, there are a series of on/off switches called registers that control the movement of data within the computer.

People often describe their computers as having 640 K of memory or a 20-megabyte hard drive. K represents kilobytes, or approximately 1000 bytes (1024 bytes to be precise). Therefore, 640 K memory means the computer can store approximately 640,000 bytes of data (approximately 320 pages of typed double-spaced text) at once. A megabyte contains 1 million bytes. Therefore, a 20-megabyte hard drive can store 20 million bytes (approximately 3600 double-spaced typed pages) of data.

There are two types of computer memory: primary and secondary (see Box 21–1). Primary memory is used to run the computer. Secondary memory is used primarily for long-term storage of data.

Primary Memory. **Primary memory** is the space within a computer that allows for immediate access. Two types of primary memory are stored within the computer: read-only memory and random-access memory.

Read-only memory (ROM) is permanently imprinted in a computer, and can be read from but cannot be changed or written onto. People operating the computer have no control over ROM, because ROM is meant to be read only by the computer itself. The computer uses ROM to tell it how to start itself up when it is turned on and how to process electronic data from the keyboard to the CPU and from the CPU to the printer and screen. The programs used by the control unit of the CPU to oversee the computer's functions are called firmware. ROM also contains decoders that translate data entered as letters and numbers on a keyboard into binary digits.

Random-access memory (RAM) is the main memory of

TABLE 21–1. ASCII CODES FOR SELECTED CHARACTERS

Character	Binary Code	Character	Binary Code
A	100 0001	0	011 000
B	100 0010	1	011 0001
C	100 0011	2	011 0010
D	100 0100	3	011 0011
E	100 0101	4	011 0100
F	100 0110	5	011 0101
G	100 0111	6	011 0110
H	100 1000	7	011 0111
I	100 1001	8	011 1000
J	100 1010	9	011 1001
K	100 1011		
L	100 1100		
M	100 1101	blank	010 0000
N	100 1110	$	010 0100
O	100 1111	(	010 1000
P	101 0000	)	010 1001
Q	101 0001	•	010 1010
R	101 0010	+	010 1011
S	101 0011	′	010 1100
T	101 0100	-	010 1101
U	101 0101	•	010 1110
V	101 0110	/	010 1111
W	101 0111	=	011 1101
X	101 1000		
Y	101 1001		
Z	101 1010		

BOX 21–1. TYPES OF MEMORY AND STORAGE DEVICES

Primary Memory

(memory within a computer available for immediate access)

ROM (Read-Only Memory)	***RAM (Random-Access Memory)***
Tells computer how to start up and process data between the keyboard and the CPU	Where programs and information are temporarily stored while computer is in use
ROM cannot be changed by computer user	Information in RAM is lost when computer is turned off unless saved in secondary memory

Secondary Memory

(where large amounts of information can be stored on a long-term basis in storage devices; access to secondary memory is slower than access to primary memory)

Storage Devices

Floppy disks	Hard disks	Magnetic tapes and disks

IMPLICATIONS FOR PROFESSIONAL COLLABORATION

Understanding Computer Components

Effective client care in the future demands that nurses understand the use of computers in the clinical setting. The results of a nurse's collaboration with a client can be implemented only if these results are communicated to others who have a role in care giving. Computers maximize efficiency in professional communication and help ensure that the benefits of clients' participation in health care decision making are realized.

most computers. When a computer is described as having 640 K of memory, the memory referred to is random-access memory. It is called "random access" because data stored any place in the memory can be accessed randomly in an equal amount of time. A very important point to remember is that information in RAM is lost when the computer is turned off or power is lost, unless the information has been saved in secondary storage (to be discussed below). A person using the computer controls RAM. The computer user reads or writes instructions and data to RAM and stores information there temporarily while completing a particular job or task. Because software applications are stored in RAM while in use, it is necessary before buying software to know how much RAM memory is required to run the software and to compare that amount with how much RAM the computer has.

Secondary (Peripheral or Auxiliary) Memory. **Secondary memory** is a place where information can be stored on a long-term basis. It is where information from RAM is stored before a user turns off the computer. Secondary memory can provide large amounts of storage at less cost than ROM or RAM; however, accessing the information takes longer. Because of limited space, data in secondary memory are stored on a device, such as a floppy disk or diskette, hard disk, or magnetic disk or tape.

Floppy disks or diskettes are used with microcomputers. They are flexible plastic disks thinly covered with magnetic material and then encased in an envelope of heavier plastic. The rigidity of the outer envelope varies with the type of disk. Floppy disks come in different sizes (8-, 5¼-, 3¼-, and 3-inch squares, for example) and different formats (single or double sided, single or double density, and high capacity). The type of computer generally determines the type of floppy disk used. The type of floppy disk determines how much data can be sorted. For example, a double-sided, double-density 5¼-inch disk can store 360 kilobytes or approximately 180 typed double-spaced pages of material. Floppy disks have many advantages. They are portable, relatively inexpensive, and can be carried from home to job or school in a small carrying case.

Floppy disks, however, are relatively fragile. Mistreatment of floppy disks can result in loss of the information on the disk. These disks should always be stored in their protective paper jackets. The parts of the disk visible in the openings in the protective plastic cover should never be touched. Writing on the label on a disk with anything other than a felt-tip pen, exposing the disk to excessive heat or cold, bending the disk, or getting liquid, dirt, or smoke on the disk may damage it. Exposing the disk to a magnet or electromagnet can also damage it. Placing a disk on top of a computer terminal may damage the disk because the terminal uses large electromagnets to operate.

Hard disks, introduced by IBM in 1973, are used in many microcomputers and minicomputers. They are hard, metal, recordlike platters, generally encased in a nonremovable sealed container built into the computer. Hard disks come in different sizes, identified by the number of megabytes of data they can hold. The storage capacity of a hard disk (eg, 20, 30, 40, 60, or more megabytes) is much greater than the storage capacity of a floppy disk, and access to data on a hard disk is also much quicker. A 10-megabyte hard disk can store the same amount of material as approximately thirty 5¼-inch double-sided, double-density diskettes. Data can be copied from the hard disk to a floppy disk when the user wishes to transfer information from one place or computer to another.

Magnetic disks and magnetic tapes are used as secondary storage devices in mainframe computers and minicomputers. Both allow for the storage of large amounts of data at a relatively low cost.

Input Devices. To be processed by a computer, data must be entered into the computer with an input device. There are many types of input devices, including (1) a keyboard, which looks like a typewriter keyboard; (2) a joystick, which is used in many computer games; (3) a light pen, with which a user makes selections by aiming at a desired spot on the computer screen and pressing a button on the pen; (4) a touch screen, on which a user makes selections by touching the computer screen in the appropriate spot; and (5) a mouse, which is a hand-held pointing device. Data can also be entered using a universal product code (bar code). Universal product code readers are commonly seen at supermarket checkout counters but are also used to read the bar codes on medical supplies for billing and inventory purposes. Optical scanning is another method of entering data into a computer. Test answer sheets are frequently scanned to enter students' answers in a computer so that the computer can analyze and grade the tests. This is done with the National Council Licensure Examination (NCLEX-RN).

Floppy disks or diskettes, hard disks, and magnetic disks and tapes can be input devices as well as storage devices. Voice-recognition systems also exist. Although voice-recognition technology is still at a beginning level, it offers great promise, particularly for handicapped users. Rather than typing at a keyboard, users direct the computer by spoken command.

Output Devices and Media. Once data have been entered into the computer and processed, the user needs to be able to retrieve the information in usable form. The two most common output devices are the printer, which provides the output typed on a piece of paper, referred to as hard copy, and the computer terminal, which temporarily displays output on a monitor screen that looks like a small television screen. A computer terminal may also be referred to as a CRT (cathode-ray tube terminal) or a VDT (video display terminal).

Other output devices or media include the secondary storage devices already discussed (floppy disk, hard disk, and magnetic disk and tape). Plotters can be used to make hard copy of graphs and other visual images. Output may also be in the form of microfilm or microfiche, voice or musical output, or photographic material.

Computer Software

The programs or sets of instructions that control computer hardware and make a computer run are called computer software. There are two types of software: systems programs and applications programs. Systems programs control the function of the computer itself. The disk operating system (DOS) is a systems program. Applications programs perform a specific function or task. For example, word processing software allows a user to prepare and edit text. Computer games, billing systems, nurse scheduling systems, and grocery store inventory systems are other examples of applications software.

Systems programs are generally written by manufacturers and supplied with the computer hardware. The systems program must be loaded in the computer before applications software can be used. Applications programs can be written by or for users or purchased as preprogrammed software packages.

Computer programs are written in various programming languages. There are three levels of computer programming language: (1) machine language, (2) assembly language, and (3) high-level languages.

Machine Language. **Machine language** is the only language the computer understands directly and consists of the binary numbers 0 and 1, representing on and off electronic impulses. Each type of computer has its own machine language. Programming, or writing sets of instructions for a computer, in machine language is very complex and time-consuming. Because of the difficulties of communicating in low-level languages like machine language, high-level languages were developed.

Assembly Language. **Assembly language** uses abbreviations or mnemonic codes rather than binary code. Assembly language is still considered a low-level language. A device called an assembler translates assembly language into machine language so the computer can understand the program.

High-level Languages. **High-level languages** were created to simplify computer programming. High-level languages closely resemble English. There are a number of high-level languages. BASIC (Beginners All Purpose Symbolic Instruction Code) is probably the most widely used microcomputer language. It is considered to be easy to learn because it is the programming language closest to English. Other common programming languages include FORTRAN (Formula Translator), COBOL (Common Business Oriented Language), and PASCAL (named after the 17th-century French mathematician Blaise Pascal). FORTRAN is used primarily for medical, scientific, and technical applications. COBOL, as the name implies, is oriented to business and accounting applications. PASCAL is used for both business and scientific applications and is popular with microcomputer users. A device called a compiler translates high-level languages into machine languages.

■ HISTORICAL OVERVIEW: COMPUTERS IN HEALTH CARE

Landmarks in Computer Technology

Computers have changed radically since they were introduced just over 40 years ago. A review of landmarks in the historical development of computer technology provides perspective for understanding how computers are used in health care today.

First-generation Computers. In 1951, the UNIVAC I was the first electronic computer to become commercially available. The UNIVAC covered a floor area of about 220 square feet. Its CPU was about 8 feet high and 15 feet long and weighed about 5 tons. The 5000 vacuum tubes it used required a great deal of electrical power and generated a great deal of heat, thus necessitating air conditioning. First-generation computers using vacuum tubes, although commercially available, never became widely used because of their very large size and the unreliability of the vacuum tubes.

Second-generation Computers. The transistor, invented in 1947, served the same purpose as the vacuum tube but was much smaller, was more reliable, and used less energy. Second-generation computers, which used transistors, were therefore faster and smaller, and used less energy than first-generation computers. These computers prevailed from approximately 1958 until 1964.

Third-generation Computers. In the late 1950s new technology made it possible to place thousands of miniature transistors on a small piece of silicon called a **microchip,** or an integrated circuit. The work of thousands of vacuum tubes could be done by one chip; however, it was not until 1964 that IBM introduced a computer using this newer technology, thus making it feasible for businesses and hospitals to begin using computers in their day-to-day operations. The microchips lasted longer, cost less, used less power, generated less heat, and were smaller and faster than transistors. The introduction of integrated circuits marked the beginning of the third generation of computers.

Fourth-generation Computers. In 1969, M. E. Hoff of Intel Corporation built an entire CPU on a single chip. The miniaturized CPU on a chip is called a **microprocessor.** The development of these microminiaturized circuits on a chip led to the start of the fourth generation of computers in 1975, when the microprocessor on a chip was refined. With this new technology, computers became even faster, smaller, more reliable, more durable, and able to store more information.

Microcomputers are part of this fourth generation of computers. In 1977, one of the first fully assembled, programmable microcomputers, the Apple II, appeared on the market. In late 1981, IBM entered the microcomputer market with the IBM-PC.

Fifth-generation Computers. Computer technology has changed rapidly over the last 20 years and continues to change as ways to process larger amounts of data more rapidly are discovered. The fifth generation of computers is currently being designed with new hardware architecture and new software.

History of Computers in Health Care

The early focus of health care computing was on the financial and business aspects of health care. During the 1960s, hardware and software became available that enabled hospitals and other health care agencies to use computers for the business and financial aspects of their operation. The development of software for client care and health care administration followed. As late as 1973, no hospitals in the United States or Europe had successfully completed a total hospital computer system,[1,2] although a number of hospitals had begun to implement such systems. In 1983, Fedorowicz[3] reported that "of the nation's 4800 short-term care hospitals over 50 beds in size, 98 percent had computerized business and financial systems in hospital or shared" (p. 36); however, only about 20 percent had a hospital information system that included client care information (see the next section). Since that time there has been a rapid increase in computer use in health care agencies.

In the late 1970s and early 1980s, a number of companies developed prototype hospital information systems. These prototype systems were then marketed to other health care facilities and adapted as required. El Camino Hospital in Mountain View, California, had one of the first computer systems to include nursing documentation. This system was developed in the 1970s. IBM, HBO, Burroughs, and Shared Medical Systems were other companies that developed early hospital information systems.

The use of bedside computers by nurses is a relatively new development in health care computing. Bedside computers make it possible for nurses to record client data at the bedside as the data are collected and to check the client care plan or record without returning to the nurses' station. According to Hammond and Stead, "the idea of bedside terminals has been around for many years. [However,] only recently, with advances in networking technology and cheaper hardware, have bedside terminals become economically feasible" (p. 5).[4] Soontit[5] describes the design and installation of a bedside nursing computer system, MedTake, which she believes is "the first use of computers by nursing at the bedside—possibly the only *operational* bedside system in the country" (p. 23). MedTake is now in use in 32 facilities in the United States.[6] In 1988, Hughes[7] described another bedside computer, CliniCare, which had just completed initial installation.

■ CLINICAL NURSING PRACTICE

Most nurses in the United States who use computers in their professional practice work in hospitals. Therefore, this section focuses primarily on health care computing in hospitals.

Hospital Information Systems

Hospital information systems are automated information systems that facilitate communication of relevant client care and administrative information within a hospital. A hospital information system may be as simple as a computer that keeps track of admissions, discharges, and transfers and makes that information available to nursing units and ancillary departments throughout a hospital. A complex hospital information system may store the majority of clients' records and relay most communications between departments. Hospital information systems have also been called medical information systems, patient care information systems, and patient data management systems.

Types of Hospital Information Systems. Hospital information systems vary widely in their configuration (the combination of hardware and systems software being used) and scope (number and type of applications software available). A hospital information system may be anything from a relatively small computer system designed to meet the needs of a single department, such as nursing, pharmacy, laboratory, or dietary, to a large system that integrates the use of microcomputers with a minicomputer or a mainframe computer to meet the needs of a whole institution.

Health care institutions have several options when they decide to acquire a computer system. They may decide to purchase or lease a computer and hire computer programmers to develop a hospital information system designed specifically to meet their needs. Another alternative is to buy a hospital information system that has been developed and tested by someone else. There are numerous commercial hospital information systems. When a system is purchased, a number of factors can be individualized, such as the way the computer screens are set up and the terminology used for specific tests. As a result of this customization and the ability to purchase different applications packages, computer systems vary from hospital to hospital even when the hospital information system was purchased from the same vendor.

Applications of Hospital Information Systems. Some of the common applications nursing departments use are (1) admission, discharge, and transfer; (2) order entry; (3) various nursing documentation applications; (4) client teaching guides; (5) clinical reference manuals; and (6) results reporting.

Admission, Discharge, and Transfer. Admission, discharge, and transfer (ADT) are usually some of the first functions automated because they are integrated with the billing applications. ADT systems allow nurses to obtain basic biographical information on clients before they arrive on the unit. When a discharge or transfer is entered in the computer, all the appropriate departments (eg, dietary, housekeeping, pharmacy, admitting) are automatically notified, thus saving nurses many phone calls. Information about beds available and a client's location on the unit is also readily available.

Order Entry. Order-entry systems allow orders to be entered at a terminal on the unit. The orders are automatically sent to the appropriate department and requisitions are printed out in the department. For example, a physician orders a blood test. When the order is entered in the computer, it is automatically noted on the computerized Kardex, and the requisition slip and labels for the test tubes are printed in the laboratory. Figure 21–3 shows a sample computer-generated Kardex or client care summary. This process saves nurses time because they do not have to record the order in the Kardex, make out a requisition slip, stamp the requisition slip and labels with the client's addressograph card, and call the laboratory to tell them the test has been ordered. This not only saves telephone time but decreases the chances of lost or delayed requisition slips. In some hospitals, up to 80 percent of physicians enter their own orders at the computer terminal, almost eliminating order transcription as a nursing function. Order-entry systems are usually programmed to accept only complete orders, which forces physicians and nurses to be thorough in their entries.

Many order-entry systems are part of fully integrated hospital information systems in which all departments are connected to the computer, and information entered in one place is automatically recorded in all appropriate places in a client's record. Therefore, orders are automatically sent to any department needing the information, printed on the unit, and entered in the appropriate place in the medical or nursing care plan or in the Kardex. For example, if a physician changes a client's diet order, the order is automatically sent to the dietary department and the change is made on the Kardex. Any new orders that are entered are also printed on the unit to alert nurses that a new order has been written. The hospital information system can also be programmed so that if a test or procedure requiring a special preparation from the pharmacy is ordered, not only is the test scheduled but the preparation is automatically ordered from the pharmacy and added to the client's bill as well.

Nursing Documentation. Computerized nursing documentation applications are less widely used than ADT and order-entry systems; however, the use of nursing documentation systems is increasing. Nursing assessments, client care plans, medication administration records, nursing notes, and discharge plans are some of the forms of nursing documentation that have been computerized. Computerized documentation has many advantages. It is typed and therefore legible. The computer can be programmed to identify the date and time of all entries as well as the initials or name of the person making the entry.

Nursing Assessments. Nursing assessments completed on a computer tend to be more complete than handwritten nursing histories, because the computer is often preprogrammed so that certain questions must be answered. A nurse cannot move ahead until required questions are answered.

Client Care Plans. Client care plans can be developed on some hospital information systems. The computer helps nurses develop care plans in several ways. The computer can store standard care plans in a format determined by the institution, to be used by nurses as the basis for developing individualized client care plans. Computer-assisted care planning can therefore help novice nurses formulate care plans and remind experienced nurses to be more complete. Standard care plans usually have a number of options from which to choose. In addition to choosing from the list of options presented, nurses may type in their own desired outcomes, evaluation criteria, and implementation strategies. The nurses using these systems create care plans by choosing options from the standard care plan menus at the terminal with a light pen, a touch screen, or by cursor movement. Figure 21–4 shows a nurse using a light pen to create a care plan, and Figure 21–5 a sample of a plan that might be created in this way. A care plan can be developed quickly when selections are made from a menu.

Albany Medical Center in Albany, New York, uses Protouch, an integrated information system that includes an electronic patient record. A unique feature of the system is a collaborative approach, in which physicians' orders and nursing care plans are placed in the same document.[8] Nurses generate care plans on the computer in language similar to that used in the NANDA taxonomy.

Other, standalone systems that are not part of a hospital information system can help nurses create client-specific care plans. Standalone systems run on a microcomputer. Two examples of programs that can be used as standalone systems to create client care plans are RN ACT care plan generator and COMMES Protocol Consultant CareLink, and ULTICARE.[9,10]

Medication Administration Records. Medication administration records have been computerized on some hospital information systems. The computer is often programmed to automatically print a list of medications to be administered at predetermined times during the day. A nurse, using the printout for a particular client, administers the medication and then charts it on the computer. If the medication is not charted and given within a specified time after the scheduled time due, the computer prints a reminder that the medication is overdue. For injections, the computer may require nurses to specify the injection site before it will document that the medications were given. Some computer

```
18  -0516      TECHNICON  DEMONSTRATION  HOSPITAL
09/04/91  12:00  NN      (QABSSP)                                    PAGE 001
- - - - - - - - - - - - - - - - - - - - - -
DEMPSEY, ELIZABETH          F   49
MR#: 10003259     ACCT#: 50060281                            PATIENT CARE SUMMARY
SERV: MEDI        1S          104B
MD: JONES, ROBERT    ADM: 09/04/91
DX: ANEMIA
- - - - - - - - - - - - - - - - - - - - - -

SUMMARY: 09/04  07:00 AM TO 03:00 PM

PATIENT INFORMATION:
   09/04    DRUG/SUBSTANCE ALLERGY: ASPIRIN
   09/04    DIETARY ALLERGY: EGGS
   09/04    ADMIT DX: ANEMIA

ALL CURRENT MEDICAL ORDERS:

DOCTOR TO NURSE ORDERS:
   09/04 6.ACTIVITY, UP AD LIB W/ASSIST, (BC).
   09/04 7.T-P-R-BP BID, (BC).
   09/04 8.CHECK URINE FOR GLUCOSE AND ACETONE AC & HS, (BC).

DIET:
   09/04 5.DIET: REGULAR, NO CAFFEINE, START WITH DIN TODAY,(BC).

MEDICATIONS
 * 09/04 9.LASIX FUROSEMIDE TAB 20 MG, # 1, PO, DAILY AT, 8 AM,
         STARTING TOMORROW, (09/05/91 08 AM-..), ( BC ).
 * 09/04 10.VALIUM DIAZEPAM TAB 5 MG, #1, PO, TID, (09/04/91 01 PM-..),(BC).
   09/04 11.NEMBUTAL PENTOBARBITAL CAPS 100 MG, #1, PO, PRN SLEEP,BC).
         R= TIME TO RENEW
         *= SCHEDULED MED

LABORATORY:
   09/04 1.CBC, TOMORROW, (09/05/91), (BC).
   09/04 2.URINALYSIS, TOMORROW, (09/05/91), (BC).
   09/04 3.GLUCOSE, RAND, TODAY, COLLECTED, (09/04/91), (BC).

RADIOLOGY:
   09/04 4.(IN PROGRESS) X-RAY: CHEST, AP SUPINE, INDICATIONS:
         COUGH, SCHEDULE: TODAY, HANDLING: WHEELCHAIR, (BC).
ANCILLARY:
   09/04 12.CARDIOLOGY ECG 12-LEAD, INDICATIONS: CHEST PAIN, TODAY, (BC).
   09/04 13.RESPIRATORY THERAPY. IPPB, DURATION: 5 MIN, PRESSURE LIMIT: 20
         CM H2O, SALINE 0.45%, QID, (BC).

                              LAST PAGE
```

Figure 21–3. Sample computer-generated Kardex. (*Courtesy of TDS Healthcare Systems Corporation, Atlanta, Georgia.*)

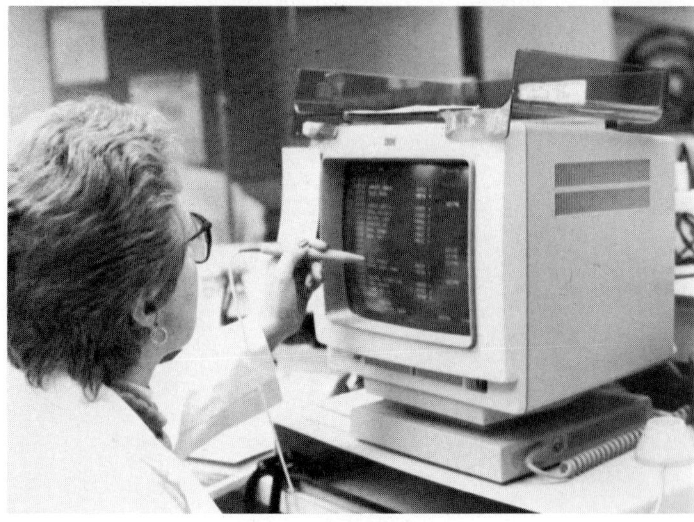

Figure 21–4. A nurse using a light pen to create a nursing care plan for a client. (*Courtesy of Carol Weingarten.*)

systems also have reference materials on drugs and drug compatibilities, which nurses can easily review. The computer can perform drug dosage calculations faster and more accurately than nurses can. Computer support for medication administration can save considerable nursing time and significantly reduce medication errors.

Nurses' Notes. Nurses' notes can be entered quickly by choosing statements appropriate for a particular client from multiple preprogrammed choices. For example, if a nurse wished to chart something about a client's activity level, the computer might have preprogrammed the following statements:

- Ambulating ad lib
- Ambulated length of hall _____ times
- Ambulated in room with assistance of one person
- Up in chair _____ hours
- Uses cane
- Uses walker
- Uses crutches
- Uses one crutch
- Other __________

A nurse would choose one or more of the preprogrammed statements, filling in the blank if required, or choose "other" and type in whatever was necessary. Nurses' notes may also be entered by typing entries on the keyboard; however, this is tedious for nontypists. The output of computerized charting is typewritten, making it more legible than handwritten notes and, therefore, more likely to be read by other health care providers. Moreover, there is a considerable reduction in time spent on documentation when computer systems are used, especially with bedside units. Computerized charting at the bedside has been estimated to save about 1 hour per shift.[11]

Discharge Planning. Discharge planning has also been computerized at some hospitals. Romano describes the computerized approach to discharge care planning at the National Institutes of Health (NIH).[12] The computer system facilitates the discharge planning process by providing structured nursing and multidisciplinary assessment forms, by improving communication between health care providers, and by providing comprehensive multidisciplinary outcome summaries that are legible and well organized. The computer system as described by Romano clearly aids in collaboration among health care providers.

Client Teaching Guides. In 1988, one California hospital added a client teaching application to its hospital information system. System planners hoped that by making it easy for nurses to structure a comprehensive teaching plan for a client and by providing clear documentation of what had been taught and the client's response to teaching, the system would provide for continuity of client teaching from shift to shift. The ability to print a comprehensive teaching plan with minimal effort from a hospital information system encourages nurses to conduct effective client teaching and allows nurses to review the entire proposed plan with clients before it is implemented, thus promoting collaboration between client and nurse.

Clinical Reference Materials. The computer can store many types of reference materials that nurses can retrieve and print as desired. For example, a nurse can use a computer to retrieve and print information about an unfamiliar procedure or laboratory test. Such information can greatly enhance nurses' ability to provide clients with accurate, up-to-date information before tests or procedures.

Results Reporting. The hospital information system may include a laboratory subsystem that not only analyzes data, but also reports the results. The laboratory computer can, for example, calculate the complete blood count (CBC) and white blood count (WBC) on a blood specimen and record the result in the appropriate client's record. The results can be printed out on the nursing unit or, if a printer is not

```
IN-B -0396     TECHNICON  DEMONSTRATION  HOSPITAL
12/16/91  12:12PM          PAGE 001             NURSING CARE PLAN
AVERETT GREGORY                         M  62  221B  SERV:MEDI
   10003408  ADM:10/15/91  ASTEN, THOMAS            07:00 AM 12/16/91

==================================================================

RESP. NURSE:                            ALT. NURSE:
DX: COPD  603.5 ...OSTEOARTHRITIS ...                  **:      PAS:

REAL OR POTENTIAL PROBLEM:                                   ENTRY  COMP
                                                               BY:  DATE:

12/13 PROBLEM--AIR EXCHANGE IMPAIRED: R/T SOB                  DD
  EXPECTED OUTCOMES                            C/P:   D/L:
    12/13  GOAL--NO DYSPNEA                    Q4H    DISCH DD
    12/13  GOAL--LUNG SOUNDS CLEAR BILATERALLY
             (COMPLETED)                       QSH    12/16 DD      12/16
    NURSING INTERVENTIONS
    12/13  --ASSESS RATE, DEPTH, CHARACTER OF
           RESP--BID                                        DD
    12/13  --ASSESS FOR APPREHENSION,
           RESTLESSNESS, COMFORT, AND CYANOSIS              DD
    12/13  --PROVIDE O2--3L PRN (COMPLETED)                 DD      12/16
    12/13  --PROVIDE PILLOW FOR SLPINT WHEN
           COUGHING                                         DD
    12/13  --PATIENT POSITION--HOB ELEVATED                 DD

REAL OR POTENTIAL PROBLEM:                                 ENTRY  COMP
                                                             BY:  DATE:
    12/13  PROBLEM--SKIN IMPAIRMENT  DECUBUTI  :R/T--OPEN AREA:
           LOCATION--COCCYX                                 DD
    EXPECTED OUTCOMES                                    C/P:  D/L:
    12/13  GOAL--HEALED AREA/INCISION                    DAILY DISCH DD
    12/13  GOAL--NO ENLARGEMENT OF AREA                  DAILY DISCH DD
    NURSING INTERVENTIONS
    12/13  --OBSV AREA FOR REDNESS, SWELLING,
           DRAINAGE, ODOR, AND TENDERNESS                            DD
    12/13  --MAINTAIN ADEQUATE HYDRATION/FLUIDS--
           -3000CC/DAILY                                             DD
    12/13  --EMPLOY PREVENTATIVE/COMFORT
           MEASURES--SHEEPSKIN                                       DD
    12/13  --KEEP AREA CLEAN AND DRY                                 DD
    12/13  --HEAT LAMP FOR 15 MINS QID                               DD

                                LAST PAGE
```

Figure 21–5. A client care plan generated on a computer. Most computer systems accommodate some customizing for consistency with hospital philosophy. This plan reflects terminology and approach that is somewhat different from that used in this text. (*Courtesy of TDS Healthcare Systems Corporation, Atlanta, Georgia.*)

available, may be visible at the computer terminal only. The results are available to nurses and physicians quickly, as there is no need to telephone the laboratory for results. The computer not only reports the results but also identifies any values that are outside the normal range, making it less likely that abnormal values will be overlooked.

Bedside Computers

How bedside computer terminals are used varies with the type of computer system and the applications available. At a minimum, nurses should be able to enter data routinely collected at a client's bedside, including vital signs, intake and output, admission history, treatment and therapy administrations, and specimen collection. Bedside terminals can also be used to verify medication orders and record medication administration. Other forms of nursing documentation, such as nurses' notes and client care plans, can be entered and checked at the bedside.

Bedside computer systems may be designed as standalone systems or to interface (communicate) with a hospital information system. Standalone systems do not communicate with other computers in the hospital, such as the pharmacy or laboratory computer, and, as a result, nurses cannot check the results of a lab test from the bedside. A bedside computer that interfaces with a hospital information system allows nurses to have access to the information available in the hospital information system and to communicate with other areas of the hospital, such as the pharmacy or the laboratory. MedTake and CliniCare, two of the bedside computer systems currently on the market, are sold as standalone systems or integrated systems depending on the buyer's preference.

The input devices used by bedside computer systems vary. One system, CliniCare, uses a touch screen monitor and an optional hand-held terminal.[7] Figure 21–6 shows the CliniCare system. Another system, MedTake, uses small terminals with simplified keyboards. The keyboards have a numeric keypad for entering temperatures, blood pressures, and heart and respiratory rates, and function keys labeled with common client care activities (eg, Temp, I&O, Diet, Meds).[13] Figure 21–7 shows a MedTake bedside terminal. Both systems are designed to be user friendly (easy to use with minimal instruction). Data can also be entered from a terminal with a full keyboard located at the nurses' station or other location. The IBM 7690 clinical workstation uses a touchscreen system. The system is designed for use by physicians and other caregivers, as well as nurses.[11]

Advantages. Bedside computer terminals offer nurses a number of advantages. Recording nursing assessments and interventions at the bedside as they are performed results in more thorough and accurate documentation. Documenting care as it is provided rather than at the end of the shift provides other health care providers with more timely data on which to base decisions. While at a client's bedside, a physician can review a nurse's most recent observations of the client and make decisions based on the most up-to-date information.

The ability to check clients' care plans or medication administration records at the bedside can save time and increase accuracy. For example, a nurse does not have to make repeated trips to the nurses' station to check a client's Kardex or to determine when the last dose of pain medication was administered. When medications are given with the CliniCare system, the bar code reader in the hand-held

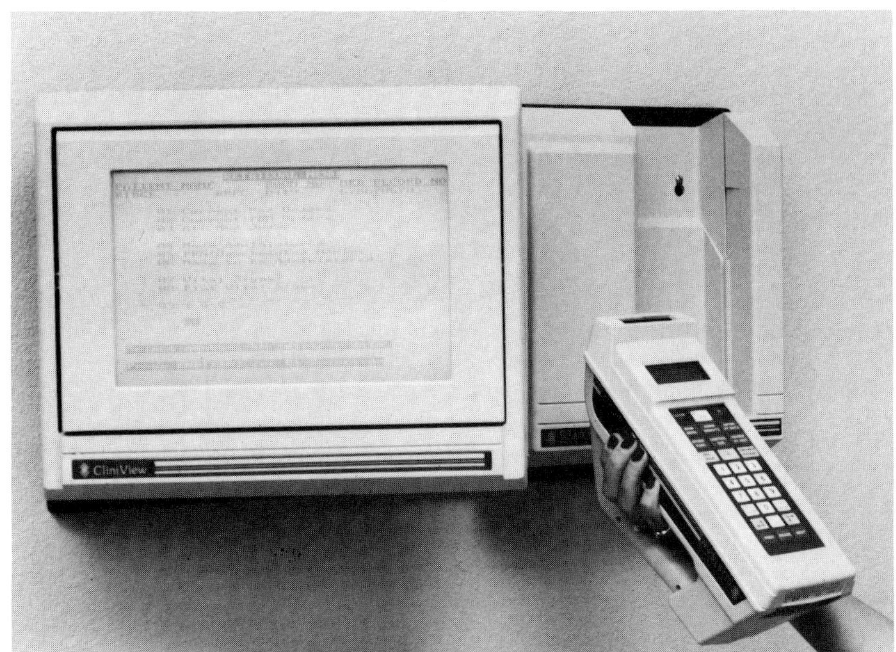

Figure 21—6. A small hand-held computer and touch screen can be used at a client's bedside. (*Courtesy of CliniCom, Inc., Boulder, Colorado.*)

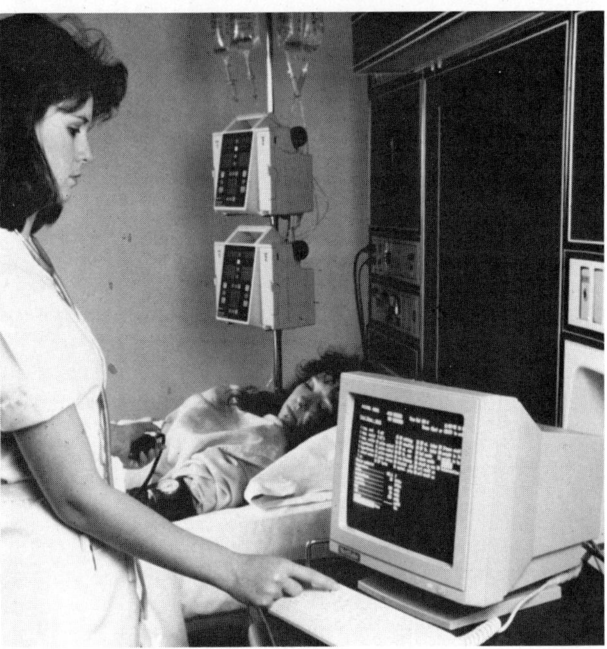

Figure 21–7. Bedside computer terminal. (*Courtesy of Micro Healthsystems, Inc., West Orange, New Jersey.*)

unit checks the client's identification band and the bar code on the unit dose of medication, then verifies the order. If client, medication, dosage, and time are correct, the green status light on the hand-held terminal is illuminated. If there is any discrepancy, the red status light is illuminated and a message such as "incorrect dosage" is displayed on the screen.[7]

Clients' vital signs are recorded once on the bedside terminal and are automatically added to the graphic chart, which can be printed on demand. This process saves time by eliminating multiple recordings in different locations.

Printed shift reports, assessments, and care plans are more legible than handwritten reports and therefore more frequently read by other health care providers. As entries are made at the bedside, the computer automatically notes the date and time and the person making the entry. Most states do not legally recognize computer signatures, so nurses must sign their notes at the end of the shift. Thus nurses have the opportunity to review what was charted during the day for each client and to make any corrections.

Disadvantages. The major disadvantages of bedside computers relate to the privacy and security of client information. Bedside computer systems include security systems to protect the system from unauthorized access. With one commonly used type of security system, each employee authorized to use the bedside terminal is given a security code number. The code number must be entered each time the employee wishes to use the computer. Security codes are similar to signatures, and it is very important that nurses not give other people their code numbers to use. A person who learns a nurse's security code could enter the computer system and not only gain access to client data but also alter or destroy the data. It is also possible for unauthorized persons to view client data visible on the computer terminal or display screen when a health care provider is entering or reviewing data.

Client Monitoring Systems

Physiological monitoring is an important aspect of client care. Computers aid this process.

As with hospital information systems and bedside computer systems, physiological monitoring systems vary from institution to institution in their setup and capabilities. Cardiac arrhythmia monitoring systems are used extensively in intensive care units (ICUs), emergency rooms (ERs), and operating rooms (ORs) to monitor for irregularities in cardiac rhythm. Figure 21–8 shows an ICU with monitoring systems at a client's bedside. There are two types of arrhythmia systems. One is a detection surveillance system, which alerts a nurse when an arrhythmia occurs. The second type of arrhythmia system interprets the electrocardiogram (ECG).

Computerized monitoring systems are also available to monitor vital signs, oxygen saturation, pulmonary artery pressure, and central venous pressure. A number of special-purpose systems are used in critical care areas. For example, there are computer-assisted ventilators, blood gas analyzers, pulmonary function systems, intracranial pressure monitoring systems, and drug infusion pumps.[3]

Client monitoring systems, particularly of the surveillance type, are used widely in critical care areas. Monitoring systems that diagnose, particularly EKG systems, are also quite common. In a growing number of treatment intervention systems, the microprocessor not only interprets what is happening but changes the setting on equipment. For example, in response to changes in a client's condition, the computer can alter the ventilator setting. These automated approaches to client monitoring free nurses from the technician role of watching machinery and permit them to focus attention on clients, clients' families, and the nursing process.

Special-Purpose Computer Systems and Software

An increasing number of special-purpose software programs for microcomputers aid health care professionals in providing quality health care. There are programs to analyze the nutrient content of recipes, meals, and diets, to analyze blood gas values, or to provide health care professionals with guidelines for weaning clients from a ventilator. Medical imaging such as computerized axial tomography, clinical laboratory, operating room, pharmacy, blood bank, clinic appointment scheduling, and infection control systems are other examples of special-purpose computer systems.

Many of these special software programs can be used

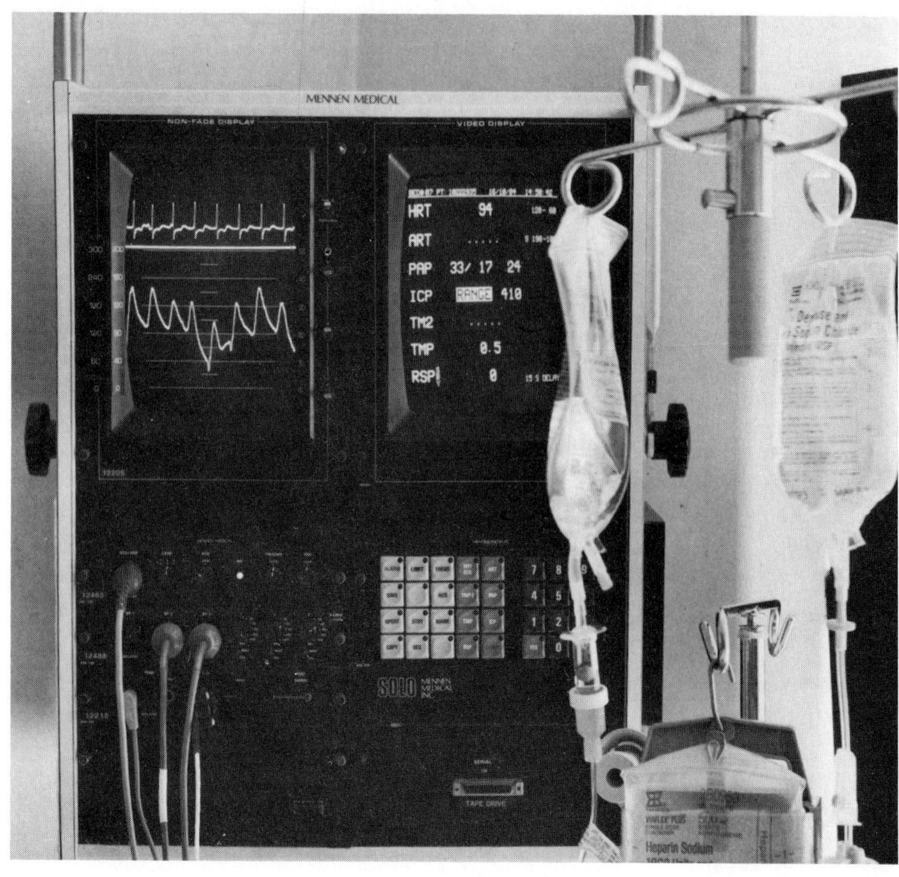

Figure 21–8. Monitoring systems at a client's bedside in an intensive care unit. (*From DeGroot KD, Damato MB.* Critical Care Skills. *Norwalk, CT: Appleton & Lange; 1987.*)

to assist in client teaching. For example, programs that provide clients with a fitness profile or risk factor analysis after they answer a series of questions can form the basis for further dialogue between clients and nurses.

The number of special-purpose computer systems and computer software programs available prohibits mentioning them all here. The reader is referred to the *Computers in Nursing* "Annual Software Exchange," published yearly as a special supplemental issue in March/April. This information lists software by general categories, such as education, management, and practice. Within each category are a number of subcategories. Listings for each software program includes title, the computer system for which it is written, the population to which the program is targeted, a synopsis of the program, the cost, and where to obtain the program.[14]

Decision Support Systems

Computerized decision support systems assist professional decision making. For example, they alert nurses whenever clients have an abnormal value on a laboratory test or whenever medications are ordered that might be contraindicated because of a client's condition or past history or because of incompatibility with other medications the client is currently taking. Programs are being developed that will allow the computer to analyze a nursing history and generate a list of nursing diagnoses and a care plan for each nursing diagnosis.

Decision support systems, or expert systems as they are sometimes called, can be viewed on a continuum. Systems that assist in decision making are at one end of the continuum and systems that actually make decisions are at the other end.[15] Three examples of decision support systems that vary in their role in decision making are described here: the HELP System, COMMES, and the ULTICARE system.

The HELP (Health Evaluation Through Logical Processing) System assists in decision making by providing nurses with interpretations, warning alerts, and treatment protocols. The HELP System also looks at the interrelationship between medications and laboratory results. For example, a warning alert is printed if a client receiving oral potassium supplements has an elevated potassium level. Although the HELP system assists in decision making, it does not actually make decisions.

COMMES (Creighton On-Line Multiple Modular Expert System) is another example of a decision support system. COMMES was originally run on a mainframe computer; however, it is now available for use with a microcomputer. The system is designed to simulate the input provided by professional consultants in several different areas. Staff nurses can use COMMES to help construct client care plans; to identify nursing diagnoses supported by client assessments; or to assess their own learning needs, develop a tutorial, and earn continuing education units.[9]

The HELP System and COMMES have been used for many years. New decision support systems are also being developed to assist nurses in many different areas. The ULTICARE system is designed to allow custom tailoring to adapt to many different types of hospital systems. It incorporates nursing assessment, diagnosis, care planning, and documentation of care. It also has the advantage of providing feedback to nurses about their diagnostic inferences, placing it on the opposite end of the decision support continuum from the HELP System. It can also integrate data from other services such as laboratory and pharmacy, creating a comprehensive electronic medical record. Some of the new systems are being developed for microcomputers, which will make them less expensive to purchase and therefore more widely available to nurses. One such system is CareLink. It can be programmed to serve as an institution-specific reference and provide patient-specific decision support for care planning. It also can assist with teaching plans, discharge planning, and can interface with other hospital information systems.[10]

BUILDING NURSING KNOWLEDGE

What Is the Value of Computerized Client Assessment?

Halloran EJ. Computerized nurse assessments. *Nurs Health Care.* 1988;9:497–499.

Cost cutting is one of the most important trends in health care. Efforts to cut costs until now have been directed toward the medical aspect of illness. Dependency on nursing services has not received the attention it needs, considering that nursing constitutes 20 to 30 percent of hospital expense. Better use of nursing manpower is therefore an important economic concern. Halloran feels that a computerized nursing data base may aid delivery of cost-effective care.

In developing a data base, Halloran states that four factors are important: (1) nursing goes on 24 hours a day; (2) client conditions may change drastically and frequently; (3) nurses perform several activities simultaneously (eg, combining the bed bath with client teaching); and (4) clients are viewed by nurses as individual and unique. However, there are common patterns of a need for care within hospitals.

Halloran describes a computerized classification system that was put into practice by one acute care hospital. The system included 61 nursing diagnoses derived from the clinical characteristics of clients requiring varying levels of care. Nurses gathered information on each client in their nursing unit by identifying the appropriate diagnostic descriptors once daily and entered the data by use of a hand-held computer terminal. Scanner bar codes developed for each nurse's social security number were used to enter data for each client. Findings showed that level of nursing care was determined by nurses' judgments about clients' actual need for nursing rather than the medical diagnosis. Halloran concludes that computerized nursing assessment using nursing diagnosis may promote more efficient and economical health care delivery.

BUILDING NURSING KNOWLEDGE

How Do Nurses Feel About the Use of Computers to Assist Client Care?

Bongartz C. Computer-oriented patient care. *Comput Nurs.* 1989;6(5):204–210.

Bongartz observes that the computer revolution is making an impact. More and more hospitals are incorporating computers into nurses' working environments. Some nurses, however, are reluctant to accept the change to computerization. Bongartz designed a study to survey the attitudes of professional nurses toward computerization and to gain insight into how nurses perceive the influence of computers on the nurses' role.

A questionnaire was used by the investigator to elicit subjects' attitudes toward computers. It was completed by 440 nurses who worked in a hospital that used computers and 277 nurses who worked in a hospital that did not use computers to support client care.

Out of 100 possible points, 100 being the most positive or favorable score, the user group average score was 70.05; for the nonuser group, it was 72.22. The difference was statistically significant since the nonuser group had a more favorable attitude. Both groups were more favorable than unfavorable toward using computers to support client care. The nonuser group, however, perceived the use of the computer as a greater possible threat to job security, but felt more positively that the computer would give nurses more time for direct client care. The nonuser group also felt more positively that the computer would cut time needed to handle information and reduce paperwork. There were no differences between the groups about legal ramifications of the use of computers, nurses' willingness to use them, or the benefit of computers to the institution.

Issues Associated With Computer Use in Clinical Practice

Nurses' Attitudes. Some of the early studies on health care personnels' attitudes toward computers[16–19] found nurses to have negative attitudes toward computers. More recent studies[20,21] and studies conducted at hospitals where nurses viewed the hospital information systems as being of direct benefit to them[22,23] have found nurses to have more positive attitudes toward computers. As the number of nursing documentation applications increases, nurses' attitudes will no doubt continue to become more positive.

Time Saving and Error Reduction. Some of the advantages of computer use by nurses in clinical practice have already been mentioned. For example, computer systems have been shown to decrease the amount of time required for charting. In addition, charted information is more legible, because computer output is typewritten. Documenta-

BUILDING NURSING KNOWLEDGE

What Is Computer Anxiety and How Does It Affect Nurses?

Jacobson SF, Holder ME, Dearner JF. Computer anxiety among nursing students, educators, staff, and administrators. *Comput Nurs.* 1989;7(6):266–272.

Jacobson and associates observe that most nurses have had little involvement in either the hospital or educational computer revolutions, and many nurses are reticent to acquire computer skills. Reasons offered for this include lack of opportunity to learn, demands of client care, and alienation between the perspectives of computer professionals and nurses. A final factor is computer anxiety.

Computer anxiety is analogous to math anxiety and test anxiety. In fact, computer anxiety correlates positively with math anxiety, being female, and taking a health professional major. Nurses may be particularly prone to computer anxiety because they are predominantly female (whereas the computer culture is overwhelmingly male), but also because they often perceive automation as dehumanizing.

This article reports a study of 129 undergraduate nursing students, 68 nurse graduate students, 256 staff nurses, 104 nurse managers, and 71 nurse educators. The investigators presented each subject with a questionnaire designed to measure computer anxiety, the Oetting Computer Anxiety Scale.

The average scores for all groups except the graduate students were in the "mild anxiety" range. The graduate students were in the "comfort range," that is, they were not bothered by computer anxiety. More graduate students and nurse educators had computer education. Twenty percent of the sample had no experience with computers, 16 percent had computers at home, and 49 percent reported that they were not currently expected to use computers in their jobs. Those with computers at home showed lower computer anxiety. Nurses with less education had more computer anxiety than nurses with more education.

Jacobson and colleagues concluded that the fact that having a computer at home was associated with lower anxiety suggests that some sort of desensitization may take place, and nurses may benefit from having computer equipment brought into the work setting well in advance of instruction. Other studies have shown that nurses value computer knowledge highly. This factor, together with the finding that nurses' computer anxiety is in the mild range, bode well for nurses' ultimate acceptance of computers, according to the investigators.

tion is not only legible but also complete. With bedside computer terminals, client data are entered in a more timely fashion. Computer systems that help nurses develop care plans also save time. Medication administration systems have been shown to reduce error and to save charting time.

Privacy, Confidentiality, and Security. Among the major disadvantages nurses have cited of computer use in nursing practice are the impersonal nature of the computer and the lack of privacy or security.[24,25]

The issues of privacy, confidentiality, and security are very important. In any health care setting, clients must disclose a certain amount of information about themselves if health care providers are to be able to work with them; in other words, clients must give up a certain amount of privacy. Clients, however, have a right to expect that information disclosed is held in confidence and is shared only with those health care professionals who need the information to provide them with care.

With traditional paper records, people must review the record itself and only one person at a time may have access to it. Computers have drastically changed the accessibility of client records. With some hospital information systems, the record can be accessed from any terminal in the hospital or even from a physician's office, whether or not the person accessing the information is providing care for a particular client. The ethical behavior of health care workers becomes very important in protecting clients' rights. For example, a nurse could obtain access to the medical records of hospitalized co-workers without ever physically going to the unit where a co-worker is hospitalized. This behavior is highly unethical. Clients have also been able to gain access to their records by reading what is on the computer screen or by using someone's security code to enter the system. Clients or other persons can learn nurses' security codes by observing nurses entering their security codes or by overhearing nurses tell someone their security codes.

Security involves the physical security of the hardware and software as well as protection of data from destruction or modification (either deliberate or accidental). Physical security includes measures such as appropriate fire extinguishers (fire sprinklers would ruin the computer), locked doors, limited access, and even closed-circuit television monitoring of the main computer. Data security includes measures such as backing up (making a duplicate copy of) the information on the computer system at least daily and storing the backup copy in a separate, physically secure location. Controlling access to the computer system with passwords, codes, or badges is another data security measure. Different levels of access codes are built into some hospital information systems, so that a staff nurse's code, for example, would allow the nurse to perform different activities than a nurse's aide or a physician. Some hospital information systems automatically record all users and transactions performed on the computer system, including the type of transaction, when it was made, and the location of the terminal where the transaction was made, thus providing a record that can be used to identify the source of any altered, lost, or incorrectly used data.

Downtime, Response Time, and Lack of Availability of a Computer Terminal. Nurses have also cited some very practical disadvantages of using computers in clinical practice, such as downtime (time when the computer is not available to perform its usual activities) and lack of access to a computer terminal.[24] With technological advances, unscheduled downtime and response time (the time it take for the computer to do something) have both decreased. The cost of computer terminals has also decreased, making it possible to purchase more terminals for the same number of dollars.

EDUCATION

Computer-Assisted Instruction

Computer-assisted instruction (CAI) is a method of teaching that involves interaction between the learner and the computer. The computer takes on the role of the teacher. CAI has been shown to be at least as effective as traditional forms of education.[26] CAI can be used by students and nurses as a means of self-teaching, thus offering the potential for all nurses to have access to high-quality education anywhere in the country, at any stage in their careers. Most CAI software today is written for use on a microcomputer. As microcomputers have decreased in price, their use has become more widespread. Many colleges and universities and some hospitals have microcomputer laboratories where students or nurses can use CAI software.

There are different types of CAI programs.

Drill-and-Practice. Drill-and-practice CAI is the most common and least complex type of CAI presently in use. A learner is presented with a series of questions or problems about material that has already been learned and has the opportunity to master the topic through repeated practice.[27] Drug dosage calculations, intravenous drip rate calculations, and medical terminology and abbreviations are some of the topics that drill-and-practice CAI is well suited for.

Tutorial Programs. Tutorial programs present new material and are similar to programmed instruction; however, CAI generally requires learners to be more active. Tutorials generally present information, ask a learner to answer questions about the information, and provide the learner with feedback. Color and graphics are used to increase interest and help hold learners' attention.

Simulations. Simulations present learners with "real-life" situations and are designed to assist learners in developing problem-solving and decision-making skills in a safe environment. In this way, students can make decisions and receive feedback about the effects of those decisions. The feedback often includes the scientific reason for the effects of the decision.

Interactive Video Instruction. Interactive video (IAV) instruction can provide learners with "true-to-life" simulations. IAV combines CAI with a videotape or videodisc player so that video pictures as well as graphics can be incorporated into the design of the software. Interactive videodisc technology is still relatively expensive but no doubt will decrease in cost as microcomputers and videotape players have done in recent years.

In conjunction with the American Heart Association (AHA), Actronics, Inc. developed an interactive videodisc system to teach the American Heart Association CPR/ACLS (cardiopulmonary resuscitation/advanced cardiac life support) Learning System. Figure 21–9 shows a nurse using this system, which was originally designed to teach CPR to the lay public. Edwards and Hannah[28] found no significant difference in learning between a control group of laypersons who received traditional CPR instruction and an experimental group who learned CPR with the interactive videodisc system. The system now includes advanced life support (ALS) instruction and has been approved by the AHA for ALS certification. The interactive videodisc learning system allows nurses to learn at their own rate and to review the content as often as desired, and allows quality CPR instruction to be available in areas where there is limited access to traditional CPR courses.

The *American Journal of Nursing* (AJN) Company has produced IAV programs on nursing care of the elderly client with chronic obstructive pulmonary disease and acute cardiac disorders. An IAV program on ethical dilemmas and legal issues in caring for the elderly is also available. There are also an increasing number of other companies producing IAV programs. The Fuld Institute of Technology in Nursing Education offers workshops, serves as a clearinghouse for current information, including reviews of software and hardware, and develops IAV programs.

Computer-Assisted Instruction in Nursing Education

Computer-assisted instruction software related to nursing is marketed by many companies. Depending on the vendor, software goes through an extensive review process

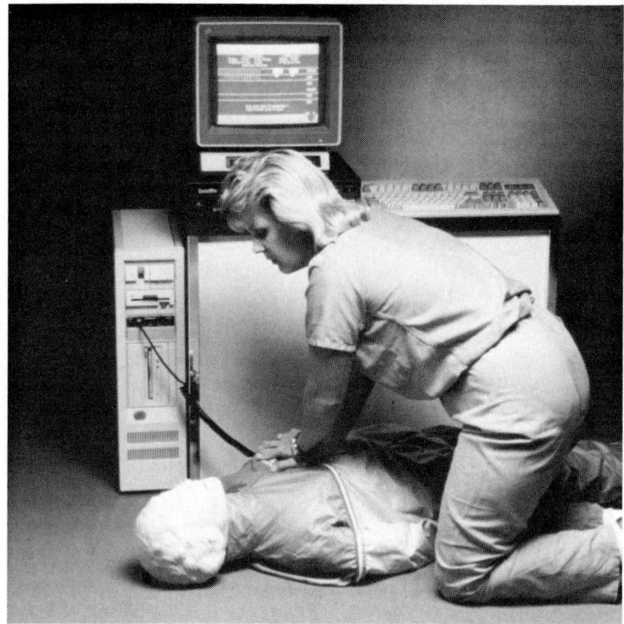

Figure 21–9. A nurse using an interactive videodisc system to learn cardiopulmonary resuscitation. (*Courtesy of Actronics, Pittsburgh, Pennsylvania.*)

before it is placed on the market. As a result, users benefit from the collaborative efforts of many experts. One can also purchase authoring systems to create CAI lessons tailored to meet a specific need.

The National League for Nursing (NLN) publishes an annual *Directory of Educational Software for Nursing* edited by Bolwell.[29] The directory contains descriptions, evaluations, and purchasing information for many software programs of interest to people in nursing education. Each program included in the directory has been rated by a pool of health care professionals for its ease of use, use of microcomputer attributes, ability to stimulate interest, and the overall impression it made on the reviewers. Use of microcomputer attributes refers to qualities that make the CAI program different from traditional methods of instruction, such as the use of graphics or animation, interactivity, provision of immediate feedback, and ability to perform rapid calculations.

The journal *Computers in Nursing* publishes an annual software exchange as a special supplement to the March/April issue. The software listed covers general practice as well as specialty areas and includes software other than educational software, such as management software packages. Unlike the NLN directory of educational software, the *Computers in Nursing* software exchange does not review and rate the programs.

One of the big advantages of CAI is that it allows for individualized, independent learning that is at least as effective as traditional classroom instruction. CAI can be used not only in formal undergraduate and graduate nursing education but also in staff development and continuing education.

Computer-Assisted Instruction in Client Education

The use of computers in client education promotes collaboration between clients and nurses. Nurse and client can decide together which CAI program or which parts of a CAI program are most appropriate. After a client completes an interactive CAI program, a nurse can follow up the lesson with individualized discussion. Clients can also ask more specific and sophisticated questions because of what they learned in the CAI program. Nurses' time is better spent answering any questions clients have after the CAI program and reinforcing and individualizing the content. Because it is a tedious and time-consuming task to teach the same material repeatedly, each client may not receive the same quality of presentation. Nurses believe client education is important; however, there is not always enough staff to allow nurses to spend long periods with individual clients. The use of CAI in client education can help make this process more individualized and productive.

Numerous client education software packages are currently available on topics such as diabetes, cataracts, weight control, hypertension, risk factors in coronary artery disease, arthritis, and allergies. CAI software for client education is based on the same principles as CAI software for nursing education. As with nursing education CAI, many CAI programs that are not known to the general nursing community have been developed and are available in individual institutions.

Many software programs are available that run on standard IBM or Apple microcomputers. Some features, however, are common to any quality CAI program. CAI programs should be interactive to involve clients in their own learning. The program should provide clients with positive reinforcement and feedback. The content presented should be factually correct. Programs should be reviewed by a nurse for quality before clients are asked to use them. CAI allows clients to work at their own pace and to repeat the program as many times as they like.

A typical CAI lesson may start with tutorial or drill-and-practice interactions and lead up to a game or simulation. The programs should be interactive and should require a response from clients. Because clients do not interact with filmstrips, videotapes, or other media that are often used in client education, it is easy for them to become bored. The interactive nature of CAI keeps clients involved in their own learning.

Clients are given feedback and reinforcement after each choice. After a correct choice, clients may be told "good choice" or "very good"; the content is summarized briefly as additional reinforcement. If an incorrect choice is selected, clients are not told "incorrect," which might be viewed as a reprimand. Instead, the program may state "not really" or "try again" and may give information to help select the correct answer. Clients then have the opportunity to choose again.

Many programs attempt to individualize the presentation by including "lifestyle" or "personal" questions. For example, clients may be asked how much they smoke or how much they weigh. A glaucoma program might contain content on several potential treatment regimens. Clients are instructed to review the treatment plan prescribed by their physician, thus individualizing the program specifically to them.

Some programs can also produce a printout to document clients' completion of the program. A printout has two potential benefits. Clients can keep a copy as a reference and further reinforcement of the content. Another copy can be placed in the medical record as documentation that the teaching took place. The Joint Commission on Accreditation of Healthcare Organizations (JCAHO) requires that documentation of client teaching and learning out-

IMPLICATIONS FOR NURSE–CLIENT COLLABORATION

Computerized Client Teaching

The goal of computerized client teaching plans is to improve continuity in client teaching. Increased availability of computerized teaching plans encourages nurses to conduct more client teaching. These plans invite collaboration as nurse and client review the plan together before the client begins and as the nurse assesses and documents the client's response to teaching. Computerized teaching plans are beneficial not only because they increase nurses' efficiency but, more importantly, because they free nurses to concentrate on clients' learning.

comes be included in the client record.[30] Computer printouts tend to be more complete and legible than handwritten documentation because of the time involved in writing a lengthy summary of a client teaching session.

CAI has great potential in client education. It can be used in a variety of settings. Bell points out that microcomputers may be placed in waiting rooms or designated teaching rooms in ambulatory care centers or transported to the bedside of inpatients on a movable cart.[31] If clients have compatible computers at home, they may borrow the floppy disks containing the program for use at home. Clients may also gain access to educational programs from home via a modem (a device that allows computers to communicate with one another via the telephone).

In summary, CAI offers many benefits in client education and can be used in a variety of settings. Consumers are becoming more aware of the importance of good health and demanding accurate and complete information from health care professionals. CAI allows health care professionals to meet consumers' challenge in a cost-effective way.[31]

NURSING RESEARCH

Computers facilitate the research process in a number of ways. Computerized literature searches are a particular advantage to researchers because they save time and can increase the scope of the search and the number of data bases that can be searched. The computer can also help researchers collect and analyze data, prepare research reports, and disseminate research findings.

Computerized Literature Searches

The sharing of ideas in scientific literature is an especially important form of professional collaboration in nursing and other disciplines. The number of nursing and related journals has increased dramatically in recent years, making a thorough manual literature search very time-consuming and tedious. Many data bases (collections of related information) can be accessed by computer. The National Library of Medicine MEDLARS (Medical Literature Analysis and Retrieval Systems) contains at least 20 data bases that can be searched on-line. MEDLINE (Medical Literature Analysis and Retrieval System On-Line) is one of the world's largest bibliographic data bases of medical information.[32] The listings found in the *International Nursing Index*, the *Index Medicus*, and the *Index to Dental Literature* are contained in the MEDLINE data base and can be searched simultaneously. This process takes much less time than manually searching several indexes. The citations found in the *Cumulative Index to Nursing and Allied Health Literature* (CINAHL) can also be searched on-line by subscribers. CINAHL includes some journals and magazines not referenced in the *International Nursing Index*.

To perform an on-line search of these data bases, one needs a computer terminal or microcomputer with a modem, telecommunications software (software that permits two computers with modems to communicate with one another over telephone lines), a telephone line, and a printer (if a hard copy of the search results is desired). Telecommunications technology allows subscribers anywhere in the world to access the data bases. Many people with microcomputers can conduct literature searches from their homes or offices. Telecommunications will be discussed further in a later section.

There is generally a charge for on-line literature searches, which varies with the data base being searched. A beginning researcher may need the help of a librarian. In addition to searching a data base, a researcher can print the citations that appear applicable to a project and, in some cases, abstracts of articles as well.

Another option in computerized literature searches is a relatively new technology, CD-ROM (compact-disk read-only memory). With CD-ROM systems, the data base is stored on a compact disk (CD) and a microcomputer searches the data base on the compact disk drive. There is an annual subscription fee of close to $1000 for the MEDLINE or CINAHL data bases rather than a charge per search. The high cost of the hardware and the annual subscription fee make CD-ROM systems too expensive for most individuals. Some libraries, however, are installing CD-ROM systems that make it possible for users to conduct literature searches without a charge.

Computerized literature searches make it easier for students and nurses to find current articles relevant to client care. This process allows practicing nurses to collaborate indirectly with experts in many areas of nursing. At Beth Israel Hospital and Brigham and Women's Hospital in Boston, nurses can execute a literature search from the computer terminal on their client care unit using a program called PaperChase. PaperChase was developed at these institutions and is now available to other institutions and individuals for a fee. Using this program, nurses at one of these hospitals can search the literature for relevant research relating to care of their clients; for example, new research on the treatment of decubitus ulcers.

IMPLICATIONS FOR PROFESSIONAL COLLABORATION

The Computer as an Aid to Nursing Research

Computers vastly increase nurses' access to the world of nursing information. Computer literature searches place nurses in instantaneous contact with research findings on virtually any topic relevant to client care. Computers also aid in the process of conducting nursing research by making data collection, data analysis, and results reporting much more efficient. Computers thus support the development of nursing knowledge and the ability of nurses to share that knowledge in service of the goal of effective client care.

Computers as an Aid in Conducting Nursing Research

Data Collection. Computers can also help researchers to collect data. Cox, Harsanyi, and Dean describe how computers can facilitate data collection when used in developing and sorting mailing lists and randomizing subjects.[33] Many nursing organizations and nursing journals maintain mailing lists on a computer so that names can be added and deleted without retyping the lists. In addition to names and addresses, these lists often include information about nurses' clinical specialty, practice location (eg, hospital, nursing home, or school of nursing), and educational level. A nurse researcher who wants to study nurses with an associate degree who work in critical care units might purchase such a mailing list and use the computer not only to identify nurses who meet these criteria but also to print mailing labels. The computer also can be used to randomly select the nurses that will be studied, saving the researcher time and eliminating potential bias in subject selection.

Computer simulations can be used to collect data in nursing research.[33] A researcher could use simulations similar to those used in CAI or an IAV program to present subjects with a situation so that the subjects' reactions or skills in the particular situation could be studied. For example, it might be difficult to study nurses' decision-making skills during an actual cardiac arrest. With an IAV program that simulates a cardiac arrest situation, however, the researcher can study many nurses making decisions in exactly the same situation. Even if it were feasible to study nurses' decision making during a real cardiac arrest, it would be impossible to find two that were exactly the same. As another example, in studies involving physiological variables, the computer monitoring systems described earlier can greatly assist in data collection.

Data Analysis. Computers offer researchers a tremendous advantage when analyzing data. There are many preprogrammed statistical packages for use on a mainframe computer or a microcomputer. Some of the most widely used statistical packages are SPSS, SAS, and Minitab. The computer increases not only the speed with which data can be analyzed but also the accuracy of the calculations.

Results Reporting. Once research is complete, the results must be reported if the findings are to have an impact on nursing practice. The word processing capabilities of the computer greatly aid researchers in writing reports of their research. Many different word processing software packages are available. With word processing, it is easy to change or move words, sentences, or paragraphs, making revisions simple. Many word processing software packages include features such as spelling checkers and a thesaurus. The computer also makes it easy for several people to collaborate on a report. Each person can write a separate section or piece of a section and the final draft can be put together on the computer. Reports do not need to be fully retyped each time a change is made. The revisions are simply made on the computer and the new version is printed.

Telecommunications. Access to many of the computerized bibliographic data bases, as mentioned earlier, requires telecommunications technology. Telecommunications technology also enables people from all over the country to collaborate on research projects. People can send raw data as well as reports to each other instantly, without waiting several days for materials to arrive by mail.

There are computer bulletin boards to which researchers gain access via their telephones with the same hardware and software needed to access the bibliographic data bases. Bulletin boards are often aimed at people with similar interests, thus allowing researchers to identify and communicate with others who have similar research interests.

For two computers to talk with one another, each computer must be connected to a piece of hardware called a modem, have a telecommunications software package, and be connected to a telephone line. A modem may be internal (installed inside the computer itself) or external (a piece of equipment that connects to the computer). Modems make the signals produced by computers compatible with telephone equipment. When a message is sent, the modem converts the computer signal so it can be transmitted over the telephone wires. The other person's modem then converts the telephone signal back to a signal the computer can understand.

NURSING ADMINISTRATION

The computer's abilities to sort information, to present information in various configurations, to summarize data, to do mathematical calculations quickly and accurately, and to transmit information to multiple locations all contribute to its usefulness to the nursing administrator. Many applications programs perform functions specific to nursing administration. There are systems for mainframes that can be purchased as part of an integrated hospital information system or independently. There are also many microcomputer-based systems. Selected administrative computer applications are described briefly below.

Patient Classification Systems

Both manual and computerized patient classification systems can be used to assign nursing staff based on how severely ill clients are. With any patient classification system, clients are assessed on a number of criteria, and their abilities or need for nursing care are rated. A client's total rating score, or acuity, indicates how much nursing care the client requires. Ideally, a fully integrated hospital information system would automatically calculate a client's acuity

IMPLICATIONS FOR PROFESSIONAL COLLABORATION

Computers as an Aid to Nursing Administration

Computers substantially ease the task of ensuring adequate services and supplies. Computers release nurses from the repetitive and time-consuming tasks that keep them from direct interaction with clients. To the extent that computers make the administration of client care more efficient, they support collaboration with other health care professionals and with clients.

by searching the client's records for the specific criteria. In most cases, however, nurses must rate clients on each criterion. Depending on the system, this process may be done on-line, on forms that are optically scanned in a central location, or on forms that are then tallied by hand or manually entered in the computer. Obviously, the greatest amount of time is saved when the acuity data can be entered on-line, making the data immediately available for analysis and use.

Unit Staffing Based on Client Acuity

Computerized patient classification systems can be integrated with staffing systems that allow nursing administrators to optimize the use of staff while minimizing the cost. Most computerized staffing systems can also generate various types of reports of staff usage and client acuity by unit over time. This information is helpful to administrators when planning budgets, forecasting future needs, and identifying trends.

Scheduling Systems

Computer scheduling systems help nurse managers produce staff schedules that best use their personnel resources while still considering individual needs. Computerized scheduling systems create schedules that automatically incorporate work preferences, special requests, patient acuity levels, and compute nursing costs.[34] These systems objectively formulate schedules, reducing any staff concerns regarding favoritism. It takes much less time to prepare a schedule with a computerized scheduling system than it does to perform the same task manually, thus saving nurse managers time on a tedious, repetitive task and freeing them to work more closely with staff on client care issues.

Inventory Systems

Computerized inventory systems keep track of supplies received and disbursed; they also can be integrated with the client billing system, keep track of expiration dates of dated supplies, and provide summary reports of supplies used and available on the nursing unit at any given time. The bedside computer by CliniCare described earlier has a bar code reader. If a hospital has a computerized inventory system, nurses charge supplies to each client by scanning the client's identification bracelet and then scanning the bar codes of the supplies as they are used. The system bills the clients and orders more supplies for the unit. This eliminates the need for charge slips and charge stickers and decreases the number of lost charges.

Quality Assurance

Quality assurance programs evaluate the quality of the care provided in an institution. The Joint Commission on Accreditation of Healthcare Organizations requires that hospitals have quality assurance programs; however, there is no requirement that they be computerized. Ideally, a computerized quality assurance program would compile the data for the quality assurance reports as part of the hospital information system.[35] In most institutions, however, nurses must audit the charts manually. Even so, once the audits are completed, the computer not only organizes the data better, but also calculates the data and produces the report faster.[33] The timeliness of the reports allows for early identification of problems. Nurses can then collaborate with other health care professionals to develop and implement needed changes before the problem can be magnified by time.

Personnel Files

Personnel files can be maintained using a data base management system, as noted earlier; however, information systems designed specifically for maintaining nursing personnel files eliminate the time needed to create and organize a data base from scratch. Nursing administrators purchase the information system and have only to input the required data.

GENERAL COMPUTER APPLICATIONS SOFTWARE

There are three major applications areas for which many preprogrammed software packages have been written. These general-purpose computer applications are not specific to nursing or to the health care field; however, they are particularly helpful for nursing administrators, nursing researchers, nursing educators, and nursing students. These applications areas are word processing, electronic spreadsheets, and data base management systems.

Word Processing

Nursing administrators and managers benefit from word processing as do nursing researchers, nursing educators, and nursing students. Word processing makes the preparation of reports and mailings easier. Policy and procedure manuals are easier to update and change when they have been created initially with a word processor.

Students who want to learn one computer skill that would benefit them for years to come should learn word processing. Although there are numerous word processing software packages, once a nurse has learned how to use one, it is easy to learn others, because there are certain tasks all word processors do even if different commands are needed to perform the task.

Electronic Spreadsheets

Spreadsheets have been used by accountants and bookkeepers for years to organize their work. On spreadsheets, numbers are organized in rows (horizontal) and columns (vertical). Electronic or computerized spreadsheets perform mathematical calculations on these columns and rows of numbers. The computer can perform mathematical functions more quickly and accurately than a person could, even with a calculator or adding machine. Many spreadsheet software programs are available. Lotus 1-2-3 is one that is widely used.

Electronic spreadsheets can help nursing administrators in the budgeting process. For example, a nursing administrator could use an electronic spreadsheet to figure out what the difference in cost would be between giving the nurses in the institution a 2 percent, 3 percent, or 4 percent raise. If all nurses' salaries were on a spreadsheet, it would be easy to write a formula that would calculate the raise for each nurse and then total them. The computer would complete the calculations quickly and accurately. Spreadsheets thus allow nursing administrators to do "what if?" speculations when preparing budgets.

Nursing researchers use electronic spreadsheets to analyze data. Nursing educators use them to compute students' grades quickly and accurately.

Data Base Management Systems

A data base management system is a software program designed to allow users to create their own computerized filing systems. With a data base management system, users can create a data base, add and delete data, sort data, and find and extract pieces of data that meet specifications. A nursing administrator might have all nursing employees' records in a data base. If license expiration dates were a part of the employee record, the administrator could use the data base management system to identify and print a list of all employees who needed to renew their licenses in the next month. Nursing educators and researchers also use data base management systems in much the same way nursing administrators do to organize student records or research data.

SUMMARY

Computer use in health care settings is becoming more and more commonplace. Initially, computers were used in health care settings primarily for billing and accounting. Today, nurses use computers in clinical practice for many purposes.

Nurses use computers in clinical practice to document nursing care; communicate physicians' orders; receive and send information about admissions, discharges, and transfers; monitor clients; and receive clients' laboratory and test results. Decision support systems may assist nurses in professional decision making by alerting them to abnormal laboratory results or changes in a client's vital signs or by helping a nurse create a care plan for a particular client. Bedside computers offer a number of advantages. Because nursing assessments are recorded as they are performed, they are not only more timely, but also more thorough and accurate. Errors are reduced when a client's care plan and medication record can be checked right at the bedside. Nurses have a responsibility to protect the confidentiality and maintain security of the clients' information, whether a computer is located at the nurses' station or at the bedside.

Computers are useful tools in education because they allow for individual, self-paced learning. The interactive nature of CAI helps maintain learners' interest, whether learners are students, nurses, or clients.

Researchers use computers to conduct literature searches, collect and analyze data, and report the results of their research. Nurse researchers can collaborate with one another via computer using telecommunications technology.

Computers are also useful tools for nursing administrators. A number of computer programs are designed to assist nursing administrators with staffing based on client acuity and scheduling. General computer applications software such as word processing, electronic spreadsheets, and data base management systems help nursing administrators as well as other nurses to prepare reports and letters, create budgets, and maintain personnel records and mailing lists.

REFERENCES

1. Collins MF, ed. *Hospital Computer Systems.* New York: Wiley; 1974.
2. Deland EC, Waxman BD. Review of hospital information systems. In: Bekey GA, Schwartz MD, eds. *Hospital Information Systems.* New York: Marcel Dekker; 1972.
3. Fedorowicz J. Hospital information systems: Are we ready for case mix applications? *Health Care Management Rev.* 1983;8(9):36.
4. Hammond NE, Stead WW. Bedside terminals: An overview. *MD Comput.* 1988:5(1):5.
5. Soontit E. Installing the first operational bedside nursing computer system. *Nurs Management.* 1988;18(7):23.
6. Murphy R. Micro Healthsystems, Inc., personnel communication; August 1991.
7. Hughes S. Bedside terminals: CliniCom. *MD Comput.* 1988; 5(1):22–28.
8. Booker, E. Piecing together a distributed system at Albany Medical Center. *Comput Healthcare.* 1989;10(11):20–22.
9. Ozbolt J, Abraham IL, Schultz S. Nursing information systems. In: Shortliffe EM, Perreault LE, eds. *Medical Informatics.* Menlo Park, CA: Addison-Wesley; 1990.
10. New products. *Comput Healthcare.* 1990;11(3):62.
11. New products. *Comput Healthcare.* 1990;11(4):43.
12. Romano CA. A computerized approach to discharge care planning. *Nurs Outlook.* 1984;32(1):23–25.
13. Pesce J. Bedside terminals: MedTake. *MD Comput.* 1988;5(1):16–21.
14. Annual Software Exchange. *Comput Nurs.* 1991;7(2):Suppl.
15. Ronald JS, Skiba DJ. *Guidelines for Basic Computer Education in Nursing,* Publ. No. 41-2177. New York: National League for Nursing; 1987.
16. Melhorn JM, Iegler WK, Clark GM. Current attitudes of medical personnel toward computers. *Comput Biomed Res.* 1979;12:327–334.
17. Reznikoff M, Holland CH, Stroebel CF. Attitudes toward computers among employees of a psychiatric hospital. *Mental Hyg.* 1967;51:419–425.
18. Rosenberg M, Reznikoff M, Stroebel CF. Attitudes of nursing students toward computers. *Nurs Outlook.* 1967;15:44–46.
19. Startsman TS, Robinson RE. The attitudes of medical and para-

medical personnel toward computers. *Comput Biomed Res.* 1972; 5:218–227.

20. Merrow SL. Nurse educators' and nursing service personnel's knowledge of and attitudes toward computer use in nursing practice. In: Ackerman MJ, ed. *Proceedings of the ninth annual symposium on computer application in medical care.* Los Angeles: IEFE Computer Society; 1985.
21. Bongartz C. Computer-oriented patient care. *Comput Nurs.* 1989;6(5):204–210.
22. Giebink GA, Hurst LL. *Computer Projects in Health Care.* Reading, MA: Addison-Wesley; 1975.
23. Hodge MH. *Medical Information Systems.* Germantown, MD: Aspen Systems Corp; 1977.
24. Merrow SL. *Nursing Educators' and Nursing Service Personnel's Knowledge of and Attitudes Toward Computer Use in Nursing Practice.* Doctoral dissertation, Northeastern University; 1984.
25. Pollock E. Applications: How far have we come? Part II. *Comput Healthcare.* 1990; 11(4):24–26.
26. Belfry MJ, Winne PH. A review of the effectiveness of computer assisted instruction in nursing education. *Comput Nurs.* 1988;6(2):77–85.
27. DeTornyay R, Thompson M. *Strategies for Teaching Nursing.* New York: Wiley; 1987:279.
28. Edwards MJ, Hannah KJ. An examination of the use of interactive videodisc cardiopulmonary resuscitation instruction for the lay community. *Comput Nurs.* 1985;3(6):250–252.
29. Bolwell C. 4th ed. *Directory of Educational Software for Nursing,* New York: National League for Nursing; 1991.
30. Patterson CH. Standards of patient care: The Joint Commission focus on nursing quality assurance. *Nurs Clin North Am.* 1988; 23(3):625–638.
31. Bell JA. The role of microcomputers in patient education. *Comput Nurs.* 1986;4(6):255–258.
32. National Library of Medicine. *Medlars: The World at Your Fingertips,* NIH Publ. No. 86-1286. Washington, DC: US Govt Printing Office; October 1986.
33. Cox HC, Harsanyi B, Dean LC. *Computers and Nursing: Applications to Practice, Education and Research.* Norwalk, CT: Appleton & Lange; 1987.
34. Products. *Comput Healthcare.* 1989;10(10):54.
35. Mikuleky MP, Ledford C. *Computers in Nursing: Hospital and Clinical Applications.* Menlo Park, CA: Addison-Wesley; 1987.

BIBLIOGRAPHY

Albrecht C. Hours of direct nursing care: Assessing baseline data for an automated system. *Comput Nurs.* 1987;5(2):46–49.

Arnold JM, Bauer CA. Meeting the needs of the computer age in continuing education. *Comput Nurs.* 1988;6(2):66–76.

Ball MJ, Hannah KJ, Gerdin-Jelger V, Peterson H, eds. *Nursing Informatics: Where Care and Technology Meet.* New York: Springer-Verlag; 1988.

Barhyte D. Ethical issues in automating nursing personnel data. *Comput Nurs.* 1987;5(5):171–174.

Bloom KC, Leinter JE, Solano JL. Development of an expert system prototype to generate nursing care plans based on nursing diagnoses. *Comput Nurs.* 1987;5(4):140–145.

Bratt EM, Vockell EL. Using the microcomputer to give student personalized feedback on preparing patient health histories. *Comput Nurs.* 1987;5(4):146–151.

Brodt A, Stronge J. Nurses' attitudes toward computerization in a midwestern community hospital. *Comput Nurs.* 1986;4(2):82–86.

Brudenell I, et al. Adult learning styles and attitudes toward computer assisted instruction. *J Nurs. Educ.* 1990;29(2):79–83.

Chase SK. Knowledge representation in expert systems: Nursing diagnosis applications. *Comput Nurs.* 1988;6(2):58–64.

Curl L, Hoehn J, Theile JR. Computer applications in nursing: A new course in the curriculum. *Comput Nurs.* 1988;6(6):263–268.

Dobberstein K. Computer-assisted patient ed. *Am J Nurs.* 1987; 87(5):697.

Fitzpatrick T, Farrell L, Richter-Zeunik M. An automated staff scheduling system that minimizes payroll costs and maximizes nurse satisfaction. *Comput Nurs.* 1987;5(1):10–14.

Gerber RM, Atwood JR, Hinshaw AS, Erickson JR. Optical scanning and computer technology in nursing research. *Comput Nurs.* 1986;4(6):241–245.

Graves JR. Personal library management. *Comput Nurs.* 1987;5(6): 225–230.

Greipp ME. CAI made a difference. *Comput Nurs.* 1988;6(6):231, 243.

Grobe SJ, Ronald J, Tymchyshyn P. *Computers in Nursing Education.* Kansas City, MO: American Nurses' Association; 1987.

Hebda T. A profile of the use of computer assisted instruction within the baccalaureate nursing education. *Comput Nurs.* 1988; 6(1):22–29.

Hodson KE, Manis J, Thayer M, Webb S, Hunnicutt C, Hoogenloom A. Computerized management program for the skills laboratory of a school of nursing. *Comput Nurs.* 1988;6(5):215–221.

Holzemer WL, et al. The development of a computer-based tutorial for an introductory course on nursing research. *Comput Nurs.* 1989;7(6):258–265.

Howard EP. Use of a computer simulation for the continuing education of registered nurses. *Comput Nurs.* 1987;5(6):208–213.

Johnson D. Decisions and dilemmas in the development of a nursing information system. *Comput Nurs.* 1987;5(3):94–98.

Koch EW, et al. Nursing students' preferences in the use of computer assisted learning. *J Nurs. Educ.* 1990;29(3):122–126.

Kosidlak J, Kerpelman K. Managing community health nursing: A personal computer tool for assessing, monitoring, and planning the distribution of public health nursing resources at the community level. *Comput Nurs.* 1987;5(5):175–180.

Larson C. Use of the microcomputer as a tool for subjective grading. *Comput Nurs.* 1987;5(5):186–191.

MacDonald F. Computer applications in diabetes management and education. *Comput Nurs.* 1987;5(5):181–185.

Mark B, Lange L. Spreadsheets in nursing administration: Not as easy as 123. *Comput Nurs.* 1987;5(6):214–218.

Masten Y, et al. Automated continuing education and patient education. *Comput Nurs..* 1990;8(4):144–150.

McNeal GJ. Designing a test bank computer program. *Comput Nurs.* 1989;7(1):29–34.

Meade CD, Wittbrot R. Computerized readability analysis of written materials. *Comput Nurs.* 1988;6(1):30–36.

Nicoll L. The microcomputer: An alternative for data analysis. *Nurs. Res.* 1987;36(5):320–323.

Paganelli BE. Criteria for the selection of a bedside information system for acute care units. *Comput Nurs..* 1989;7(5):214–221.

Peterson HE, Gerdin-Jelger V. *Preparing Nurses for Using Information Systems: Recommended Informatics Competencies.* New York: National League for Nursing; 1988.

Plummer CA, Warnock-Matheron A. Training nursing staff in the use of a computerized hospital information system. *Comput Nurs.* 1987;5(1):6–9.

Rizzolo MA. Guidelines for creating test question banks. *Comput Nurs*. 1987;5(2):65–69.

Rizzolo MA. What's new in interactive video. *Am J Nurs*. 1989; 89(3):407–408.

Romano CA. Privacy, confidentiality, and security of computerized systems. *Comput Nurs*. 1987;5(3):99–104.

Romano CA, Damrisch SP, Heller BR, Parks PL. Levels of computer education for professional nursing. *Comput Nurs*. 1989;7(1): 21–28.

Schodt D, Jackson B, Borup P, Balliram N, Swan W. Implementation of a hospital information system: The use of a nursing task force. *Nurs. Management*. 1987;18(7):23–25.

Soja ME, Lentz KE. Development of a hospital-based computer users' course for student nurses. *Comput Nurs*. 1987;5(1):15–19.

van Bemmel JH. Computer assisted care in nursing: Computers at the bedside. *Comput Nurs*. 1987;5(4):132–139.

Van Ort S. Evaluating audio-visual and computer programs for classroom use. *Nurse Educator*. 1989;14(1):16–18.

UNIT SIX
Fundamental Nursing Assessment and Management

CHAPTER 22

Wellness and Well-being

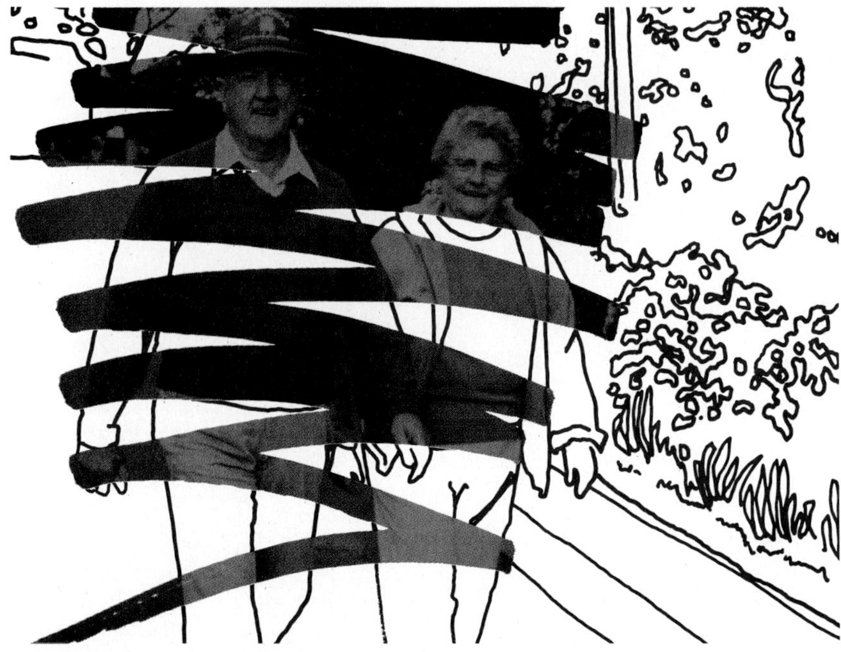

Behavioral Objectives

Upon completion of this chapter, the student will be able to:

1. Define the concepts of health, wellness, and well-being.
2. Discuss the development of the wellness movement in the United States.
3. Discuss the relationship between the health of the individual and life-style practices.
4. Describe the basic elements of a wellness life-style.
5. Describe the objective and subjective manifestations of wellness and altered wellness.
6. Identify several factors that enhance or alter wellness.
7. Identify the wellness tasks related to various developmental stages.
8. Describe the impact of illness on wellness.
9. Discuss elements of health care experiences that can influence an individual's level of wellness.
10. Outline the elements of the health history that are pertinent to assessing wellness and well-being.
11. Discuss the implications of selected objective manifestations for assessing wellness and well-being.
12. Discuss the role of diagnostic tests in assessing wellness.
13. List the nursing diagnoses that are most commonly associated with altered wellness and well-being.
14. Describe preventive care measures for wellness and well-being.
15. State the relevance of self-management techniques for making life-style changes.
16. Describe supportive, restorative, and rehabilitative care measures available to assist clients with altered wellness or well-being.
17. List the nurse's responsibilities for admission of the client to the hospital.
18. Define medical and surgical asepsis and describe nursing procedures aimed at preventing nosocomial infection.
19. Discuss ways nurses can support and enhance the wellness and well-being of clients who are receiving treatment for health alterations.
20. Discuss the nurse's role in assisting the client with stress and describe several stress management techniques.
21. Discuss the nurse's role in reducing environmental hazards and reducing accidents.
22. Outline the nurse's role in managing fever.
23. Outline the principles of safe medication administration.
24. Describe the procedures for giving medication by the oral, subcutaneous, intramuscular, intravenous, rectal, and vaginal routes.
25. Describe the procedures for eye and ear instillations.
26. Describe three systems of measurement in current use for prescribing drugs.
27. State the formula for medication dosage calculation.
28. Outline the key aspects of the care of the client prior to, during, and after surgery.

KEY TERMS

absorption
ampule
anaphylaxis
chemical name
distribution
drug
drug tolerance
excretion
fitness
generic name
hardiness
intradermal
intramuscular
intravenous
locus of control
medical asepsis
medication
metabolism
nosocomial infection
official name
patient-controlled analgesia
perioperative nursing
potentiation
privacy
prn order
proprietary name
relaxation response
resilience
self-efficacy
side effect
stat order
sterile technique
subcutaneous
surgical asepsis
therapeutic effect
toxic effect
trade name
universal precautions
vial
well-being
wellness

Although the traditional image of nursing is one of caring for the sick or incapacitated, the scope of nursing practice extends far beyond the care of physiological conditions of the body or the nurturing of the disabled. In recent decades, changing patterns of morbidity and mortality, coupled with the skyrocketing costs of medical care, have focused increasing attention on measures that serve to promote health and prevent disease and disability. The major threats to health no longer come from disease-producing bacterial or viral agents but rather from chronic conditions produced and fostered by life-style factors or environmental hazards.[1] Increasingly the scope of health care reaches beyond the acute-care setting to encompass not only the physiological but the psychological, social, and environmental factors that influence and determine an individual's level of health.

The concepts of wellness and well-being are integral to a focus on health promotion and disease prevention. Promotion of health and maintenance of a sense of well-being is the ultimate goal of all nursing actions; however, the foundation of the wellness framework is the concept of active self-responsibility, personal action to protect and promote one's own health. Within this context, individuals are active participants and determinants of their own level of wellness rather than just passive recipients of health-related care. The goal of high-level wellness is achieved through a collaborative effort between individuals and nurses or other health care providers. Barbara Blattner, author of *Holistic Nursing*,[2] writes:

> Both the nurse and the client have within themselves the knowledge, tools, material, and energy to maintain health. What clients may lack in factual or technical expertise, they make up for in "inside" information about themselves. This contribution is respected and encouraged by the nurse, for without it and the client's participation, none of the lifestyle changes will occur or be maintained for any length of time. (p 175)

When the client is a full participant in health care decision-making, the role of the nurse becomes that of educator and facilitator. Nursing practice focuses on the cultivation of "self-care," the education of clients in the maintenance and promotion of health, the motivation of clients for active application of this knowledge, and the development of life-styles and behaviors by clients that are conducive to health and yet reflective of clients' needs and preferences.[3]

For individuals faced with illness or disability, nurses provide those aspects of care that clients cannot accomplish for themselves; however, the ultimate goal is still the empowerment of clients for self-determination and self-management so that they will be able to attain their own level of optimal health and well-being.[1]

Because the concepts of wellness and well-being are integral to all aspects of nursing practice and are the foundation for the development of a collaborative approach to client care, this chapter serves as an introduction to the fundamentals of wellness and related client assessment and management. Basic concepts related to an understanding of the promotion and maintenance of optimal wellness will be presented in this chapter. In subsequent chapters, these concepts will be expanded to focus on specific aspects of fundamental nursing care.

Section 1. Understanding Wellness

This section is designed to develop readers' understanding of wellness and its implications for nursing practice. Incorporation of the concepts of wellness and well-being into daily nursing practice begins with an application of the evolution of the basic definitions and the principles that constitute the wellness framework. Additionally, theories from nursing, the social sciences, and a variety of related fields are presented to facilitate an understanding of human needs and behaviors and how these contribute to each person's experience of health and well-being throughout the life cycle. This section also examines alterations in wellness that occur in the course of daily living and within the context of the health care experience. This material is presented to assist nurses in identifying actual or potential alterations in wellness in clients encountered in daily nursing practice.

■ OPTIMUM WELLNESS

Evolution of the Wellness Movement

The current emphasis on wellness is a relatively new movement which began in the late 1970s. The focus of the movement has been the development of a wellness-oriented life-style that includes not only physical fitness but also nutritional awareness, stress management, self-development, positive human relations, and environmental sensitivity. Although a complete discussion of the wellness movement is beyond the scope of this chapter, a brief description of its evolution and leaders is included.

Halbert L. Dunn is considered by many as the father of the wellness movement. As a retired public health service physician, he began lecturing and writing articles in the 1950s about the concept of "high-level wellness," which he defined as "an integrated method of functioning which is oriented toward maximizing the potential of which the individual is capable, within the environment where he is functioning."[4] His classic text, *High Level Wellness*,[5] provided a theoretical framework for wellness. The major points of emphasis within Dunn's framework included the need for maximizing each individual's potential, the importance of mind-body-spirit connections, and the idea of purposeful direction toward a higher level of functioning. He believed there was no single level of optimal wellness, but rather within each individual the potential for moving forward to a personal level of wellness.[6] Although Dunn's work was not widely acknowledged at the time it was published, it greatly influenced many of the health care professionals who were instrumental in the development of the wellness movement years later.

Although a variety of factors influenced the growth of the wellness movement in the 1970s, a major impetus was the publication of several landmark works. In 1974 the Canadian Ministry of Health and Welfare released a document entitled *A New Perspective on the Health of Canadians*.[7] This was the first major work that presented epidemiological evidence on the significance of life-style and environmental factors on health and illness. It proposed a number of national health-promotion strategies and called for Canadians to assume more responsibility for their own health. Although largely ignored in Canada, it strongly influenced many medical leaders in the United States.

In 1977 the Senate Select Committee on Nutrition and Human Needs published a report on dietary goals for the United States.[8] This document disclosed the links between diet and disease and called for sweeping changes in American food consumption patterns. Closely following *Dietary Goals for the United States* was a document entitled *Healthy People* released by the Department of Health, Education, and Welfare in 1979.[9] Basically an American version of the earlier Canadian document, this report called for a shift away from high technology and hospital-centered medical treatment in favor of health-promoting and disease-preventing life-style and environmental strategies.

One of the major leaders of the wellness movement in the 1970s was John W. Travis, a physician who chose not to practice traditional medicine with its focus on the treatment of disease. Together with Regina Ryan, he founded the Wellness Resource Center in Mill Valley, California, and focused his practice on assisting clients and health care professionals to develop and maintain wellness-oriented life-styles.

Travis uses a continuum to illustrate his concept of wellness (Fig. 22–1). Moving from the center point of the continuum to the right indicates increasing levels of health and well-being, while moving to the left of center shows a progressively worsening state of health. The figure also demonstrates the difference between the treatment model (traditional medicine), which stops after curing evidence of disease, and the wellness model, which begins at any point on the continuum with the goal of helping a person move as far to the right as he or she is willing or capable of going. Central to this model is the principle of self-responsibility. According to Travis, each individual is responsible not only for caring for the physical self, but also for using the mind constructively, channeling stress energies positively, expressing emotions effectively, becoming creatively involved with others, and staying in touch with the environment.[10]

This central theme of self-responsibility was echoed by other leaders of the wellness movement such as Donald B. Ardell, Ph.D., a wellness consultant and author. In Ardell's view, high-level wellness is a life-style-focused approach that individuals develop in the pursuit of the highest level of health within their capability. Ardell believes that high-level wellness can be achieved only through the development of a personal life-style that focuses attention on the areas of self-responsibility, nutritional awareness, environmental sensitivity, physical fitness, and stress awareness and management. To be effective, this life-style must also be dynamic and ever-changing as the individual matures and evolves through the life span.[11]

The impact of the concepts generated by wellness movement can be seen in many aspects of everyday life. The recent explosion of weight-loss clinics, smoking cessation classes, fitness centers, employee wellness programs, and the similar health-oriented services can be attributed in part to the wellness movement. The significance of this movement can also be seen in the multitude of books, articles, and conferences currently available on the subjects of health promotion, stress management, and life-style modification.

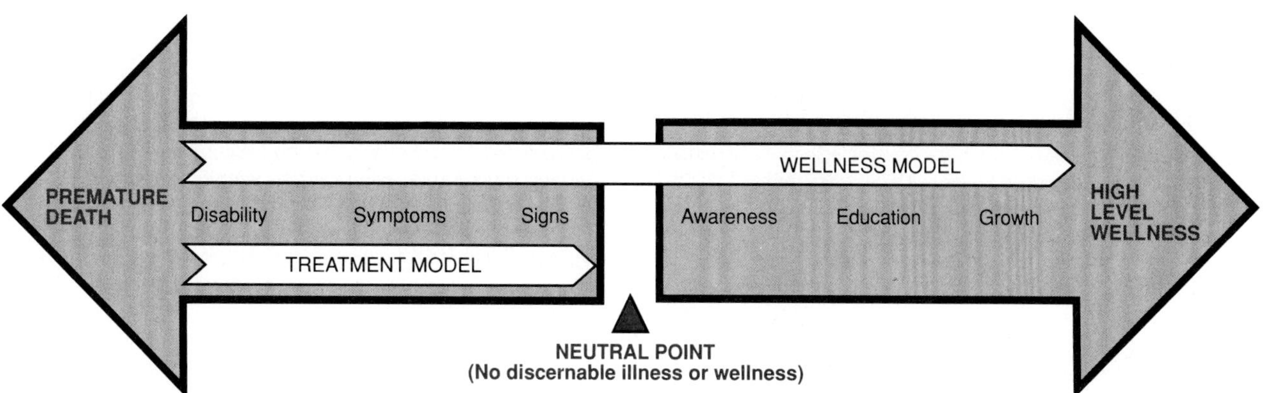

Figure 22–1. This illness–wellness continuum emphasizes going beyond the treatment model of wellness to high-level wellness. (*From Ryan RS, Travis JW. The Wellness Workbook. Berkeley: Ten Speed Press; 1988.*)

Wellness and Nursing

The focus of nursing on promoting and maximizing an individual's health began with Florence Nightingale, who defined nursing as "that care that puts a person in the best possible condition for nature to either restore or preserve health."[12] As nursing evolved, its focus became more directed on prevention and cure of disease and rehabilitation; however, nurses have always identified health promotion as the component of care that differentiates their profession from that of other health care professionals.[6]

With the advent of the wellness movement, nursing reemphasized its focus on health promotion and the holistic care of the individual. In 1974, Cynthia Oelbaum identified those behaviors that characterize optimal wellness in the adult (Box 22–1). Although stated in somewhat dated terminology, this list of individual criteria illustrates the broad scope of nursing's concept of wellness. Wellness extends far beyond physiological functions of the body to include psychological, social, spiritual, and environmental aspects of daily life. Oelbaum emphasizes that no one behavior or function is necessarily more important than another, and that a balanced and integrated approach is necessary for optimal health and well-being.[13]

Nursing has traditionally adopted a holistic perspective, viewing the client as a balance of mind, body, and spirit. These parts cannot be separated, and each dimension—mind, body, and spirit—affects and is affected by the others. Barbara Blattner has developed a holistic nursing model that incorporates the concepts of high-level wellness. Her model focuses on nine life processes that can be used to reach wellness: self-responsibility, caring, stress, life-styling, human development, problem-solving, communication, teaching–learning, and leadership and change. Her book, *Holistic Nursing*, presents theories and methodologies that can be used by nurses to facilitate clients' achievement of their maximum potential or highest level of wellness.[2]

Another model of health promotion for nursing has been developed by Nola Pender. Although it does not address the concept of wellness directly, Pender's model focuses on those factors that influence an individual's decision to engage in activities that sustain or increase level of

IMPLICATIONS FOR NURSE–CLIENT COLLABORATION

Self-responsibility

Self-responsibility has been a central theme in the wellness movement as it has evolved in both the United States and Canada. It is also a key value of the collaborative philosophy of client care. In a collaborative relationship, the nurse and client jointly make health care decisions. This fosters the client's self-responsibility even while the client's capacity for self-care (the ability to carry out the activities of daily living independently) may be diminished.

BOX 22–1. AN ADULT IN OPTIMAL HEALTH

A. Performs Activities of daily living.
B. Has a stable Body image perceived as being socially acceptable.
C. Provides for his own Comfort and relaxation (psychological and physical).
D. Efficiently Disposes of metabolic wastes.
E. Obtains and maintains an Environment conducive to well-being.
F. Has an appropriate intake and healthy distribution or excretion of Fluids and electrolytes.
G. Guards himself against overwhelming changes. Regulatory and defense systems intact and helpful.
H. Maintains good Hygiene.
I. Builds and maintains meaningful Interpersonal relationships. Is comfortable with Interdependence.
J. Juxtaposes the tasks of his various life roles with minimal conflict while keeping in touch with his own needs.
K. Accumulates Knowledge and skills that bring him success in his chosen life roles and self-esteem.
L. Holds expectations and makes decisions reflecting understanding of his own Limitations and situational realities.
M. Maintains optimal Motor function (strength, range of motion, locomotion, gross and fine coordination).
N. Obtains, digests, and metabolizes appropriate amounts of food that promote good Nutrition.
O. Efficiently uses Oxygen.
P. Demonstrates Personality growth and creative expression appropriate to his developmental level and prized by his culture.
Q. Demonstrates high Quality cerebral functioning (to remember, think abstractly, transfer knowledge, concentrate, and solve problems).
R. Mobilizes Resources to meet his needs (internal, significant others, community). Begins by expressing his needs freely to an appropriate person.
S. Receives and recognizes Sensory input (the five senses, balance, proprioception, and body scheme).
T. Is a Team member of his own prevention/rehabilitation team. Has sufficient understanding, initiative, self-control, and financial resources to maintain health.
U. Recognizes and cherishes the Uniqueness of his own identity and the Uniqueness of each other person.
V. Demonstrates functional Verbal and nonverbal communication.
W. Attains healthful balance of productive Work and rest.
X. Humanistically eXpresses his love and respect for all life and the quality of that life.
Y. May have symptoms, but they are Yielding to prescribed therapy. Uses therapies to help him carry out his wellness work.
Z. Demonstrate a Zeal for living.

From Oelbaum CH. Hallmarks of adult wellness. Am J Nurs. *1974;74:1623.*

well-being, self-actualization, and personal fulfillment. Understanding the factors that motivate clients to engage in health-promoting activities is an important part of nursing care and is a central component of Pender's model.[1] A discussion of motivation as a factor influencing wellness can be found later in this chapter.

Carolyn Chambers Clark has described the concept of "wellness nursing," a collaborative nurse–client relationship in which the nurse functions as role model and facilitator. Clark views clients as experts in their own wellness, and believes the purpose of nursing practice is to assist clients to be independent and able to provide self-care measures that enhance wellness.[14] The actual concept of wellness is examined through six areas of activities that generally promote high-level wellness: eating well, being fit, feeling good, caring for self and others, fitting in, and being responsible.[15] These dimensions of wellness and the concept of the collaborative nurse–client relationship are the foundations upon which this and subsequent chapters are based.

Defining Health, Wellness, and Well-being

Although the concepts of health, wellness, and well-being are often used interchangeably in the literature, some distinctions are necessary for clarification. As discussed in Chapter 5, the concept of health is a relative and highly individualistic term. Individuals' definitions of health are unique and are influenced by their developmental status, social and cultural background, personal experiences, self-concept, and value system. Smith[3] has proposed four models of health: role performance, clinical, adaptive, and eudaemonistic. Box 22–2 provides a brief summary of each model; a discussion and clinical descriptions can be found in Chapter 5. These four models encompass the wide variation of beliefs and meanings attributed to the concept of health. Recent studies by Laffrey[16] and Woods and associates[17] have verified the wide variation in personal definitions of health reported by individuals.

Wellness is a function of the eudaemonistic model of health.[3] In this model, health is regarded as the full expression of a person's physical, emotional, social, and spiritual potential. This view of health is the one used in much of nursing literature today because it focuses on the complex nature of human beings rather than just the treatment or prevention of disease. Increasingly, the eudaemonistic view of health is being accepted and expressed by the public as well. A study by Woods and co-workers[17] of women's images of health reflected a strong emphasis on concepts such as healthy life-styles, a positive body image, a positive emotional state, satisfying social relationships, and a sense of harmony, all components of the eudaemonistic model.

Wellness, then, is a process or life-style that is oriented toward attaining an individual optimal level of physical fitness and physical–emotional harmony that supports a sustained zest or joy of living and provides maximum resistance to disease.[18] It is a unique and individualized state for each person that is strongly influenced by physical makeup, life circumstances, and personal choices. Individuals engaged in wellness activities are constantly striving to move toward their highest level of ability or potential in an effort to create a more satisfying and productive life.[19]

BOX 22–2. MODELS OF HEALTH

- **Role Performance Model:** Prime indicator of health is the ability of the individual to carry out expected functions.
- **Clinical Model:** Health is the absence of signs and symptoms of disease.
- **Adaptive Model:** Health is the ability of the individual to successfully respond to stimuli in the environment.
- **Eudaemonistic Model:** Health is the full expression of a person's physical, emotional, social, and spiritual potential.

Well-being, although closely related to wellness, can be differentiated as individuals' subjective perception of their current level of functioning and satisfaction with life. It is an integral but intangible component of wellness—that aspect that is focused on "feeling good." A substantial portion of nursing care is directed toward fostering and sustaining well-being in clients.

A positive sense of well-being expressed by an individual does not necessarily indicate a high level of health or the absence of disease. A person can be handicapped, in pain, elderly, or chronically ill and yet still sustain well-being. A study of individuals with severe chronic obstructive pulmonary disease (COPD) by Parson[20] indicated that many of these individuals maintained a moderately high sense of well-being despite the severe physical limitations imposed by their illness. Conversely, low levels of well-being may be found in "healthy" physically fit individuals who are experiencing excessive stress and anxiety in their daily lives due to occupational, interpersonal, or environmental factors.

Dimensions of Wellness

Personal Behavior and Health. Increasingly it is being acknowledged that many of the fundamental causes of poor health in contemporary society are the result of personal behavior, life-style, and environmental factors, and fall within the realm of individual personal responsibility. Two now-classic studies that have demonstrated the significant affects of personal behavior on health are the Framingham Heart Study and the Alameda County Study.

The Framingham Heart Study was begun in 1949 and has followed over 5000 residents of a small town in Massachusetts for the past 40 years. The purpose of the study was to identify factors that contributed to the development of coronary heart disease and high blood pressure. The results of the study have indicated that heart disease is more prevalent among individuals with high blood pressure, high cholesterol levels, and low levels of exercise, and among those who smoke. Obesity was also identified as a significant contributor to hypertension and elevated cholesterol levels.

The Alameda County Study examined the relationship of personal habits to the individual health of 7000 adults in Alameda County, California. The results of the study correlated both physical well-being and life expectancy to the adherence to seven basic practices:

1. Sleeping 7 to 8 hours each night.
2. Eating three meals a day at regular intervals with little snacking.
3. Eating breakfast every day.
4. Maintaining desirable body weight.
5. Avoiding excessive alcohol consumption.
6. Getting regular exercise.
7. Not smoking.

The physical health of subjects who followed all seven good health practices was consistently about the same as subjects who were 30 years younger but followed few or none of these practices.[21] Subsequent follow-ups of this study sample have continued to support the relationship between cigarette smoking, alcohol consumption, physical exercise, hours of sleep, and maintaining ideal weight and mortality. Social factors were also identified as having an important influence on health. It was found that the strength of an individual's social networks (eg, marriage, contact with close friends and relatives, church membership, and ties with formal or informal groups) was inversely related to life expectancy.[22] Other studies have shown that social support contributes to increased positive health behaviors[23,24] and to psychological well-being.[25]

Elements of a Wellness Life-style. As these studies have indicated, the development of a personal life-style that focuses on achieving high-level wellness can have a significant impact on an individual's level of health. The following discussion elaborates on Clark's[15] concept of an integrated wellness life-style and the six elements listed earlier in the chapter.

Eating Well. Eating well means selecting and ingesting foods that provide appropriate nourishment and satisfaction. Adequate nutrition plays a vital role in the maintenance and promotion of well-being. Not only does good nutrition provide the essential nutrients needed for normal growth and development, it also contributes to maintaining the alertness and energy that is needed for full and productive living.[1]

Making good food choices has important health implications. Although the role of diet in diseases such as heart disease, adult-onset diabetes, hypertension, dental caries, and cancer is not always clear, certain relationships, such as the role of excessive fat intake in the development of cardiovascular disease, have been identified. Choosing healthy foods begins with a basic understanding of the composition and use of various nutrients in the body.[26]

The process of eating provides far more than daily nutrient requirements, however. Many psychological, emotional, and social needs are met in the act of eating. People engage in eating for the pleasurable sensations and esthetic enjoyment. Many people equate eating with social interaction. Ethnic and cultural backgrounds have important influences on eating behavior. In every society, food and eating behaviors are accompanied by many rituals, customs, and beliefs.[27] Eating well includes an understanding of how and what one eats and why, including the meaning that food has for each particular individual.

Many authorities believe that nutrition represents an area with a great deal of potential for enhancing wellness. In 1980, the federal government issued an abbreviated set of dietary guidelines for Americans. This set of guidelines has been revised twice since then. The most recent revision in 1990 adds specific suggestions to some of the seven guidelines, which have remained essentially the same since the first edition. The guidelines are:

1. Eat a variety of foods.
2. Maintain a healthy weight.
3. Choose a diet low in fat, saturated fat, and cholesterol.
4. Choose a diet with plenty of vegetables, fruits, and grain products.
5. Use sugar only in moderation.
6. Use salt and sodium only in moderation.
7. If you drink alcohol, do so in moderation.[28]

Although no guidelines can guarantee optimal health or well-being, these general statements can assist individuals in evaluating their dietary habits and moving toward general improvements. Basic eating habits based on moderation, variety, and sound nutritional practices can be an important part of an integrated wellness life-style. A detailed discussion of nutrition and the 1990 *Dietary Guidelines for Americans* can be found in Chapter 25.

Being Fit. **Fitness** is a state in which body systems function optimally. One of the most significant factors affecting physical wellness is the type and amount of exercise that the body receives. A wide variety of positive physiological benefits result from a combination of sound nutritional practices and a regular exercise program, including improved cardiovascular endurance; increased muscle strength and endurance; reduced blood pressure, pulse rate, and percentage of body fat; and reduced blood cholesterol and triglyceride levels. Exercise is also known to improve digestion, nutrient use, and elimination.[29]

In addition to physiological benefits, regular exercise also provides a wide range of beneficial effects that significantly contribute to a positive sense of well-being. These include:

1. Increased energy.
2. Reduced fatigue.
3. Fewer bodily aches and pains.
4. Fewer colds and increased resistance to disease.
5. Improved self-esteem and self-regard.
6. Improved sleep.
7. Increased self-confidence and assertiveness.
8. Increased libido and enhanced sexual vitality.[18]

Regular exercise has also been shown to be an effective stress reduction technique in addition to maintaining strength, coordination, and endurance.[30]

Although the traditional view of "being fit" focuses on cardiac fitness, a wellness perspective is more comprehensive and includes four areas of physical fitness: (1) muscle strength and endurance, (2) flexibility, (3) cardiorespiratory fitness, and (4) body composition.[31] An exercise program that enhances fitness in all four areas is desirable. Fitness and the benefits of exercise are discussed further in Chapter 30.

Feeling Good. Feeling good evolves from functioning with a sense of purpose, successfully meeting life's challenges, and maintaining a sense of personal control over life circumstances. It relates to an individual's ability to reduce or manage stress, to rest and relax, and to maintain a positive outlook on life in general. For some people, the concept of feeling good refers primarily to *physical* wellness. They enthusiastically focus their attention on exercising regularly and eating properly, but often disregard the holistic nature of wellness. The concept of holistic wellness refers to the interrelationship of the physical, mental, emotional, spiritual, and social dimensions within each individual. Optimal health and wellness are achieved only when a stable balance or sense of harmony exists between all the parts of the whole.

The spiritual dimension of life, therefore, is a vital force in determining an individual's overall well-being. It is a unifying force that integrates all other dimensions of human beings—physical, mental, psychological, and social.[32] Spirit gives meaning and direction to an individual's life, and is the basis for a sense of satisfaction or dissatisfaction with living. Important signs of spiritual health include a sense of inner tranquility and feelings of being at peace with nature, fellow humans, and for some, with God.

Feeling good as an aspect of wellness also encompasses a balanced response to stress. Stress is an integral part of modern-day life. Chapter 6 introduces the concept of stress and describes Selye's General Adaptation Syndrome (GAS)—the uniform set of physiological changes that occur within the body in response to various stressors.

In Western industrialized society today, exposure to stress comes not so much from physical threats as from the by-products of modern civilization. These include physical factors such as noise, polluted air and water, and rushed schedules; emotional stressors such as financial worries, frustrations at work, marital strife, and sexual dysfunctions; and spiritual problems such as inner emptiness, chronic boredom, and lack of fulfillment. Noise, urgency, frustration, and worry are the constant companions of most people today. These pressures of modern-day life can cause prolonged, excessive stress—not necessarily at extremely high levels, but enough to cause physical consequences that accelerate the aging process, sap vitality, and increase susceptibility to disease.[18] The emotional consequences of excessive stress are as harmful as the physiological ones.[33] In reality they may be even more detrimental because they inhibit effective coping practices and reinforce the initial stress response.

Individuals who maintain well-being or a sense of feeling good develop stress-reduction and stress-management strategies that meet their unique needs and life-style. Many different techniques for stress management are recommended including both active and passive types of relaxation. Active methods include a variety of physical activities ranging from walking, jogging, and swimming, to yoga and dancing. Active relaxation can also occur on a psychological level in the form of activities such as reading or needlework. Passive relaxation can be achieved through the use of mechanisms such as massage or spas that directly relax the muscles as well as the mind, or through the use of a multitude of psychological relaxation techniques.[34] A discussion of various relaxation techniques can be found in Section 3 of this chapter.

Caring for Self and Others. Self-care refers to those activities an individual performs in order to achieve, maintain, or promote maximum health. Caring for others includes an ability to nurture and support, to relate well, and to communicate effectively. Conceptually, self-care includes much more than an ability to carry out activities of daily living and basic health practices. It includes caring for self in the sense of liking oneself. Maintaining adequate sleep and rest patterns, engaging in recreational activities, and sustaining an ability to laugh and enjoy life are critical components of physical and psychological wellness, but self-care also includes individual actions directed toward self-nurturance, self-improvement, and personal growth.[1] In a collaborative model, nurses serve as educators and consultants in assisting clients to recognize the importance of all of these aspects of self-care.

Although a wellness perspective emphasizes the importance and potential of the individual, it is critical to recognize that one cannot attain wellness without positive relationships with others. Numerous studies have indicated that the presence of a confidant, friend, or social support system is important for both physical and emotional health.[25,35–38] A social support system is the set of interpersonal relationships through which the individual maintains a social identity; receives emotional support, material aid, and information; and makes new social contacts. It evolves throughout a person's life span and plays a significant role in maintaining psychological and physical integrity of the individual over time. Developing and nurturing social relationships is an important component of wellness.

Social wellness requires a balance between receiving support from others to meet one's own needs and being able to offer support and assistance to others. Individuals who spend all of their time and energy meeting the needs of others often fail to adequately meet their own basic needs. Conversely, those who focus primarily on themselves may neglect or ignore their responsibilities to others. Maintaining a balance between one's own needs and the needs of others requires an ability to say no when others' demands exceed one's capabilities, and to assertively seek assistance when needed.

Fitting In. Fitting in refers to an individual's ability to adapt and function and live in harmony with the surrounding environment. In recent years increased attention has been focused on the effects of environmental factors such as smog, water pollution, noise, and overcrowding on the health and well-being of individuals, as well as on the consequences of human life-styles and choices on the environment. Although many of these problems may seem too monumental or pervasive for personal action, there are techniques people can employ to decrease environmental destruction and to modify their personal and community environmental spaces to enhance wellness.

Ardell[11] differentiates the concept of environment into three aspects—the physical, the social, and the personal. Physical environment refers to the air, water, and other natural or physical components that surround us. Social environment is a reflection of the economic, governmental, and cultural influences in our lives. The personal component of environment refers to an individual's immediate surroundings or "space" and all the stimuli or forces that influence the person at any particular time. Although there are limitations to the extent that people can alter their physical and social environments, the personal environment is under greater individual control.[11]

Increasing one's sensitivity to the impact that personal choices have on the environment, and becoming more aware of the influences the multiple stimuli in one's home, work, and social surroundings have on oneself, are important steps toward creating positive environmental conditions. "Fitting in" includes taking responsibility for protecting the environment and protecting oneself from harmful environmental elements. Personal actions such as conserving precious natural resources, reducing consumption, recycling, and proper disposal of trash and other wastes are protective of the physical environment.

Choosing to live and work in smoke-free areas; following basic safety practices; minimizing exposure to known pollutants, infectious agents, carcinogens, and excessive noise; and providing for personal space and privacy for self and family are ways of enhancing one's personal environment to protect health and promote wellness.

Optimal well-being also requires attention to the emotional and spiritual elements in the environment. Although more difficult to identify and isolate, these aspects of daily living have a profound impact on an individual's level of wellness. Social interaction with others—family, friends, co-workers—creates unique emotional climates. If these climates are highly stressful, individuals may expend a great deal of physical and emotional energy attempting to adapt, leaving them continually exhausted and irritable. Studies have shown that stressful, anxiety-filled work environments may increase the incidence of psychosomatic illness, accidents, and interpersonal conflicts, just as angry, unloving home environments can produce emotional distress and various destructive behaviors among family members.[18]

BUILDING NURSING KNOWLEDGE

What Determines the Actions People Take on Behalf of Their Own Well-being?

Keller ML, Ward S, Baumann LJ. Processes of self-care: Monitoring sensations and symptoms. *Adv Nurs Sci.* 1989; 12:54–66.

Self-care is defined as the activities that people personally engage in to maintain life and health. The authors note that Orem's theory stipulates that nursing involves helping people to engage in effective self-care. According to the authors, a large number of studies on self-care indicate such behavior is the product of subjective perceptions—what people believe and how they feel.

This article reviews research based on the Common Sense Model of self-care, a model that assumes people are problem-solvers whose behavior is guided by their personal definitions of health threats. The model holds that individuals construct meanings for body sensations based on (1) the bodily experience, (2) information from the environment, and (3) past experiences with illness. The process of self-care occurs in three stages: representation, coping, and appraisal.

Representation is the stage in which individuals organize, analyze, and interpret information from their inner and outer environment. Coping, the selecting and executing of responses, depends on the representation formed. For example, if a woman interprets headache as due to flu, she will probably take different coping actions (self-medicate with aspirin, go to bed) than if she interprets it as due to food poisoning (call doctor immediately). Appraisal involves the individual's evaluation of the effectiveness of coping.

Research on the process of representation formation shows it is affected by personality factors, and particularly by the tendency to repression. Some individuals tend to avoid negative emotion more than others. Research shows these individuals report fewer side effects from medical treatments because they are less aware of incoming stimuli. Research also shows that people form representations based on associations of symptoms with disease labels and that these associations are learned early in life. Coping actions are related to associations. Identity is also a factor and is a link between representation and coping. Subjects related a large number of physical changes and symptoms to "aging," and did not report using health care providers as a strategy to cope with such changes.

In each case self-care is influenced. People who do not experience sensations may fail to initiate self-care activities. Those who believe their sensations are due to a specific cause may monitor only those sensations that they associate with that cause, and may ignore others that are also important. Those who attribute sensations to old age may conclude that the best strategy is acceptance of the sensation. The authors conclude that it is paramount for nurses to assess their client's representations if they are to assist them with self-care.

Conversely, a work or home environment that allows opportunities for continued self-development and expression, provides frequent positive "rewards" and support for accomplishments, and allows people to fulfill meaningful roles contributes to individuals' psychological and emotional well-being. Individuals who recognize that their home or work environments are stress filled can initiate change. First, they can examine the extent to which their own behavior or their responses to the behavior of others contributes to the problem; then they can make a conscious effort to discontinue those actions. Often one person's efforts can be a catalyst for others to make positive changes as well.

Being Responsible. Self-responsibility is the key element in the development and practice of a wellness life-style. Each of the dimensions of wellness depends on individuals accepting personal accountability for the use of their inner resources and decision-making skills. Being responsible requires self-awareness—an ability to recognize one's limitations as well as one's strengths. It also demands that individuals become active, knowledgeable, and informed participants in matters related to health and well-being.

Many of the determinants of poor health lie within the realm of personal responsibility. Research has linked the conditions most often causing death in contemporary society—heart disease, cancer, and stroke—to unhealthy personal habits such as excessive alcohol intake, smoking, overeating, excessive stress, and a sedentary life-style. These common patterns of life all lie outside the realm of traditional health care but within the scope of individual personal choice.

Active self-responsibility does not eliminate or discount the need for intervention or treatment by health care professionals. Rather, in seeking the assistance of a physician or nurse, individuals are exercising responsibility for their health by entering into a client relationship with a professional. The extent to which individuals are able to meet their health needs should determine the extent of the assistance from the professional. The goal of professional intervention should be to maintain, restore, or increase the ability of individuals to provide their own self-care. Nurses can best facilitate self-responsibility through education of clients and through mutual goal setting and decision-making. Increased knowledge promotes self-confidence, self-reliance, and motivation—all important determinants of an individual's exercise of self-care behaviors.

The Experience and Manifestations of Wellness

What does it feel like to experience wellness? How can one recognize wellness in other individuals? Because the concept of wellness is multifaceted and encompasses all aspects of human existence, a description of the characteristics of wellness covers a variety of areas.

Self-esteem/Self-acceptance. Individuals who have attained a high level of wellness like themselves and their accomplishments. They have a high level of self-awareness. They are aware of their feelings and conflicts; they understand their personalities and motivations and are able to deal with difficult situations and learn from them. They are able to identify their strengths and limitations and accept both aspects of themselves. They exhibit a sense of confidence and self-worth that is evident to those around them.

Closely tied to self-esteem is a positive body image. Well individuals feel good about their bodies and the way they look. This positive sense of self is evident in the way they dress, their posture, and the way they express themselves. They are comfortable with touching and being touched by others.

Satisfying Interpersonal Relationships. Individuals who like themselves are able to establish mutually satisfying relationships with others. They are able to share personal feelings, and maintain long-standing relationships based on mutual trust, loyalty, and caring. Well individuals are generally outgoing, well liked by others, and interesting to be with. They are focused on meeting the needs of others as well as meeting their own needs.

Fitness and Energy. Individuals experiencing high-level wellness are physically fit, active, and energetic. They have the stamina to engage in daily activities with zeal and enthusiasm and seem indefatigable. They are able to sleep well and awake feeling refreshed and energized.

Positive Outlook. The manifestation of wellness that is generally most apparent to others is a continued sense of optimism and happiness. Well individuals feel good—about themselves, their relationships with others, and life in general. They do not dwell on past mistakes, or what might have or should have been, but rather look forward to the future with enthusiasm and positive expectations. They have a healthy sense of humor and a strong sense of self-control and self-confidence.

Inner Harmony. High-level wellness also manifests itself through an internal sense of harmony or peace. Individuals experiencing high-level wellness often report a sense of deep inner happiness or joy. This sense of inner satisfaction comes from discovering who one really is and finding one's unique place in the universe. This internal tranquility increases one's ability to love and trust and is often manifested as an abiding sense of peace, hope, and faith.

Focus and Sense of Purpose. People also demonstrate wellness through a clear sense of purpose in life. Knowing themselves and having global ideas of what they wish to accomplish enables well individuals to set reasonable life goals and remain focused as they pursue them. The sense of purpose is not characterized by rigidity, but rather by determination and flexibility. Well individuals deterred from achieving a particular aim would be more likely to explore alternative paths or new choices rather than become discouraged or give up.

■ FACTORS AFFECTING WELLNESS

There are many determinants of wellness. The discussion here addresses values, philosophy, and spirituality; life-style; locus of control, self-efficacy, and self-concept; hardiness and resilience; culture and socioeconomic status; and age-related variables.

Values, Philosophy, and Spirituality

Values are those beliefs one holds as to how one ought to behave and which goals or end states are personally or socially preferable. Values provide the basis for making decisions or choices and largely determine how individuals react to various internal or external environmental stimuli. Values are shaped by family and life experiences, and they evolve and change as a result of maturation, interpersonal relations, and social circumstances.[1]

Closely related to values are the concepts of spirituality and personal philosophy. Personal philosophy represents a value system; that is, it is the way in which an individual's personal values relate to one another, guide personal choices, and shape that individual's concept of how to live. Spirituality emanates from an individual's sense of values and is the quality that gives meaning and direction to life. It provides a vital, deepening, and unifying force within each person, and is the integrating factor that determines an individual's overall well-being.

Often, values, personal philosophy, and spirituality are embodied in an individual's religious preference. Active involvement in one's church and church activities are a central aspect of living for many. For others, spirituality is experienced through the process of self-actualization and the development of a personal connection to a greater reality in the form of nature, history, or whatever has particular meaning for an individual.

Life-style

An individual's choice of life-style directly reflects personal values. Life-style is an individual's unique way of living. It encompasses everything from communications styles and self-expression to career choices, recreational activities, and interpersonal relationships. Life-style choices compatible with the dimensions of wellness discussed above (eating well, exercising regularly, and so on) promote wellness. Conversely, many life-style options are health defeating. Pender[33] emphasizes this by characterizing life-style patterns as "expressions of health" (p. 118). She further suggests that members of health care disciplines broaden their perspectives by researching life-style patterns.

Locus of Control, Self-efficacy, and Self-concept

An individual's personal sense of mastery and control in large part determines the extent to which he or she engages in wellness behaviors. **Locus of control** refers to the extent to which individuals believe that events in their lives are self-controlled (an internal orientation), or are determined by forces outside themselves such as fate, luck, or chance (an external orientation).[39] Studies indicate that individuals who believe they have little personal control over events that happen to them do not engage in health promotion activities.[40] Conversely, internally controlled individuals are thought to be more self-directed, more assertive in seeking assistance and information, and more likely to change behavior patterns. Although it is not an absolute indicator, various research studies have indicated that internally directed individuals are more apt to wear automobile seat belts, schedule preventive dental care, take prescribed medications, use contraception, and have positive attitudes

BUILDING NURSING KNOWLEDGE

Is Religion Important to the Health of Elders?

Mull CS, Cos CL, Sullivan JA. Religion's role in the health and well-being of well elders. *Pub Health Nurs.* 1987;4:151–159.

The investigators note that while nursing emphasizes holism, which includes the spiritual dimension, few studies have examined religiosity as a factor in health. Their study looked at the relationships between religious activities, beliefs, and perceived health status.

The authors noted varying definitions of religiosity in the literature ranging from a narrow definition (attendance at formal religious services) to a broad, dimensional definition (religiosity as ideological, ritualistic, experiential, intellectual, and consequential). Their literature review showed that religiosity is related to demographic variables: Women are more religious than men. Religion is linked to health behavior: Mormons show a 30 percent lower incidence of most types of cancer. People who are uncertain of their religious beliefs have more headaches, loneliness, worry, and anxiety. A belief in life after death is a predictor of an individual's world view; religion has been shown to be positively related to happiness, well-being, good adjustment, and life satisfaction.

The investigators interviewed 380 predominantly female, well elderly subjects living in senior housing in a midwestern city. Health was measured by a self-rating system, and by interviewing subjects about common symptoms. Self-management was assessed by a survey about activities of daily living. Well-being and religiosity were measured by questionnaires.

Attendance at religious services was positively associated with health and functional capacity. Prayer, meditation, and watching or listening to religious programs were negatively correlated with the same variables, suggesting that as health declines, these activities become more important. The number of diagnosed health problems was positively correlated with frequency of prayer and belief in life after death. The number and intensity of symptoms were correlated positively with all religious activities.

The investigators concluded that when functional ability is compromised, or symptomatology increases, the nurse should be alert to the availability of alternatives to church/synagogue attendance. Identifying appropriate religious services on radio and TV, providing religious reading material, and engaging in-house visiting clergy should become part of the plan of care for the elderly.

IMPLICATIONS FOR NURSE–CLIENT COLLABORATION

Self-efficacy and Self-confidence

Self-efficacy, a personal belief that one can do something, is closely allied to one's sense of self-confidence. Self-confidence is a consciousness of one's own power. A collaborative nurse–client relationship facilitates both self-efficacy and self-confidence through an endorsement of the client's participation as a full partner in decision-making. A decision-making partnership provides an implicit acknowledgement of the client's personal strengths and knowledge and creates opportunities for the explicit reinforcement of the client's skills.

about physical exercise, cardiovascular fitness, and certain other preventive and health promotion behaviors.[41,42]

Locus of control is a measurable concept. The Health Locus of Control (HLC) scale developed by Wallston and associates[43] can be used to measure individuals' locus orientation and possibly predict or explain their health-related behaviors. Self-efficacy theory provides another perspective on the reasons that some people act to promote or improve their health and others do not. **Self-efficacy** refers to an individual's perceived belief that he or she can successfully execute a required behavior necessary to produce a desired result.[44] The theory is based on the interactive model of human behavior that is the basis for Bandura's social learning theory (discussed in Chap. 20).[45] Self-efficacy theory assumes that information from sources such as personal experience with the task or activity, observing another person perform the task, and verbal persuasion, influences individuals' beliefs about their own ability to successfully execute the requirement.[46]

Many studies have found efficacy expectation a primary factor in the health decisions individuals make. When faced with difficult situations, people who have serious doubts about their capabilities often decrease their efforts and give up, while those with a strong sense of efficacy exert greater effort to master the problem.[44] Nursing interventions that promote self-efficacy can assist clients in initiating or maintaining health promoting behaviors.

Self-concept is directly related to an individual's locus of control and sense of self-efficacy. It refers to an individual's unique perception of his or her own body (appearance and functions) and nonbody (spiritual, emotional, and intellectual makeup) images. The self-concept forms the foundation for a person's perception and interpretation of daily events and stressors. As such it largely determines attitudes, levels of aspiration, and motivation. It has a direct impact on a person's participation in self-care activities and on overall sense of well-being. Individuals with poor self-concepts are likely to feel they have little personal control over life events and low self-efficacy. Often they will neglect illness prevention or health-promotion activities, saying to themselves "Why bother? I'm not worth the effort. I couldn't do it anyway." Discussions of self-concept and self-expression can be found in Chapters 10 and 23.

Hardiness and Resilience

As discussed earlier, ineffective responses to stress negatively influence wellness. Hardiness and resilience are personality characteristics that researchers have found to influence individuals' responses to stress in their lives in a positive way.[47–51] **Hardiness,** as defined by Kobasa and colleagues, encompasses control (a belief that one can influence life events), commitment (a sense of purpose that promotes a desire to be actively involved in life events), and challenge (a belief that change is to be expected in life and provides opportunities for growth).[49] **Resilience** is the ability to restore balance by integrating difficult life events into life experience.[51] It involves courage, flexibility, self-reliance, and the ability to find continued meaning and purpose in life.

Individuals having these qualities do not necessarily experience less stress or illness than others, but their response to these or other misfortunes modifies their risk. Hardy, resilient individuals use more effective coping strategies; thus, loss and change are less likely to overwhelm them.

Nurses can make inferences about hardiness and resiliency from verbalizations, expressions of emotion, and evidence of generalized psychological responses to stress. Some researchers have suggested that a hardiness training program that teaches strategies to develop control over one's life, to become more committed to oneself, and to choose to perceive unexpected events as a challenge, could help vulnerable individuals develop increased resistance to stress.[52,53] This kind of teaching may benefit all individuals facing long-term stressors such as chronic disease.

Culture and Socioeconomic Status

Socioeconomic status profoundly affects an individual's lifestyle, health practices, and, therefore, his or her level of wellness. In general, poor people get sick more often and stay sick longer because of inadequate health maintenance, lack of prevention, poor nutrition, and limited access to adequate personal health services. The poor are more vulnerable to disease and less able to cope with it than those in higher socioeconomic populations.[54] There is also evidence that low-income groups are less likely to have effective social networks to call upon for support during illness.[37]

Poverty may also exert a negative influence on an individual's motivation to engage in health-promoting activities. More pressing needs for physiological essentials, such as food, shelter, and safety, must be met before individuals can devote energy to activities that have less immediate impact on survival. Focusing on such a basic need level has tremendous psychosocial implications and inhibits any attempts to meet security, belonging, self-esteem, and other higher-order needs that are related to high-level wellness.

Cultural background strongly influences health beliefs and, consequently, participation in activities related to wellness. Health values, attitudes, and behaviors are learned within the context of the family beginning at an early age. Every cultural group has its own health culture and defines the traditional ways its members cope with illness and

BUILDING NURSING KNOWLEDGE

Is Hardiness Related to Well-being?

Lambert VA, Lamberrt CE, Klipple GL, Mewshaw EA. *Image.* 1989;21:128–131.

The purpose of this study was to determine whether or not social support and a personality characteristic, hardiness, would predict well-being in women with rheumatoid arthritis, a type of joint inflammation that is painful, chronic, progressive, and can cause severe deformity. The authors note that the conditions created by the disease, the need to deal with symptoms, manage complex health care regimens, deal with alterations in body appearance, and face uncertainty, can be overwhelming.

A sample of 122 mostly Caucasian women, 21 to 81 years of age, seen in a clinic on the East Coast was used in the study. Well-being was measured by a standardized questionnaire. Social support was measured by another questionnaire on the number of supports available and the individual's satisfaction with the supports. Hardiness was measured by Kobasa and Associates' hardiness scale. Severity of illness was measured by a test of three important parameters of rheumatoid arthritis: duration of morning joint stiffness, blood sedimentation rate, and joint function of limbs and spine.

Length of morning stiffness was negatively correlated with psychological well-being: Greater stiffness resulted in reduced well-being. Both satisfaction with available social support and hardiness were significant predictors of well-being, when the severity of disease as a variable was controlled. The investigators concluded that psychosocial care should include plans for fostering and facilitating use of the client's social support system regardless of the severity of illness. Caregivers should find out whether clients are satisfied with the quality of the social support provided. When few supports exist, caregivers should link clients with support systems. Caregivers should also identify those clients who are less hardy, since they are at risk for less effective coping. Hardiness is manifested in a desire to be actively involved in ongoing life events and in believing and acting as if one has influence over the course of life events.

maintain well-being.[55] These include attitudes toward wellness and illness, health practices (diet, relaxation, exercise), familial and community support systems, and healing rituals. Collaborating with clients to establish a plan of care that respects cultural differences and is consistent with their values and belief systems is essential if nurses are to effectively assist individuals or families to develop optimal health behaviors.[55,56] (For further discussion of sociocultural influences on health, see Chapter 9.)

Age

An adequate understanding of the process of human development is crucial for nurses who are focused on maintaining and fostering wellness behaviors in clients. Sound knowledge and application of various developmental theories enable nurses to anticipate age-specific areas of expected growth in clients as well as prevent potential stage-related hazards to wellness. Chapter 11 presents a detailed discussion of the principles and theories of growth and development. Only a brief application of those concepts to the wellness process is presented here.

As previously stated, an individual's level of health and well-being is largely determined by life-style and personal health habits, most of which are learned through the developmental process. The family plays a critical role in the development and practice of health-promoting and protective behaviors. Health-related decisions regarding diet, location and quality of residence, use of professional health care services, and leisure time activities affect all family members. The health practices of children and adolescents are greatly influenced by the examples set by adults within the family. Those behaviors that are most satisfying to the individual are retained and reinforced, and largely determine their potential for experiencing wellness. Likewise, inappropriate health habits such as overeating, lack of exercise, use of alcohol and tobacco, and ineffective coping patterns are often established in early childhood and adolescence and carried into adulthood. As the primary source of socialization, the family must assume responsibility for fostering and supporting the healthy self-care activities of all family members.[57]

Bruhn and associates[58] integrated the wellness process with developmental theories by proposing specific health tasks for the individual to accomplish at each developmental phase of the life cycle. Table 22–1 outlines the developmental stages and tasks proposed by Erickson and Havinghurst, and provides examples of basic wellness tasks that must be mastered for each of these developmental stages. The maximal potential for wellness at each developmental level is dependent upon satisfactory completion of the various wellness tasks in previous stages of development. A range of tasks is appropriate at each stage, but certain basic tasks need to be completed at each stage so that a person may progress.[58]

Infants. High-level wellness for the infant actually begins before birth with proper prenatal care, adequate maternal nutrition, and maternal avoidance of environmental hazards such as smoking, alcohol or drug ingestion, certain medications, toxic substances, and radiation. After birth the single most important factor affecting the infant's physical, emotional, and cognitive development and health is parental influence.[29]

The development of a healthy personality and psychological wellness is a lifelong process that begins in infancy. Emotionally healthy parents and stable families provide a sound environment and support system for growing children. Psychological wellness begins when the infant first learns to trust that the world is a safe and secure place. Consistent and predictable love from parents contributes significantly to the development of self-esteem and self-love.[27,48]

Other important wellness tasks related to infancy include adequate nutrition to meet the needs related to rapid growth and metabolism, and periodic health supervision by health care professionals to monitor growth and development and administer routine immunizations. Safety measures become increasingly important as the infant develops

TABLE 22–1. RELATIONSHIP BETWEEN DEVELOPMENTAL TASKS AND WELLNESS TASKS FOR EACH STAGE OF THE LIFE CYCLE

Erickson's Eight Stages of Man	Havinghurst's Developmental Tasks	Examples of Minimal Wellness Tasks for Each Developmental Stage
I. Infancy (trust vs mistrust)	I. Infancy and early childhood ■ Learning to walk. ■ Learning to take solid foods. ■ Learning to talk. ■ Learning to control elimination of body wastes. ■ Learning sex difference and sexual modesty. ■ Achieving physiological stability. ■ Forming simple concepts of social physical reality.	■ Ability to perform psychomotor skills. ■ Learning functional definition of health. ■ Learning social and emotional responsiveness to others and to the physical environment.
II. Early childhood (autonomy vs shame and doubt)	■ Learning to relate oneself emotionally to parents, siblings, and other people. ■ Learning to distinguish right and wrong and developing a conscience.	■ Learning about proper foods, exercise, and sleep. ■ Learning dental hygiene.
III. Late childhood (initiative vs guilt)	II. Middle childhood ■ Learning physical skills necessary for ordinary games. ■ Building wholesome attitudes toward oneself as a growing organism. ■ Learning to get along with mates.	■ Refining psychomotor and cognitive skills. ■ Developing self-concept. ■ Learning attitudes of competition and cooperation with others. ■ Learning of social, ethical, and moral differences and responsibilities.
IV. Early adolescence (industry vs inferiority)	■ Learning an appropriate masculine or feminine role. ■ Developing fundamental skills in reading, writing, and calculating. ■ Developing concepts ncessary for everyday living. ■ Achieving personal independence. ■ Developing attitudes toward social groups and institutions.	■ Learning that health is an important value. ■ Learning the self-regulation of basic physiological needs—sleep, rest, food, drink, and exercise. ■ Learning risk-taking and its consequences.
V. Adolescence (identity vs role confusion)	III. Adolescence ■ Achieving new and more mature relations with age mates of both sexes. ■ Achieving a masculine or feminine social role. ■ Accepting one's physique and using the body effectively. ■ Achieving emotional independence of parents and other adults. ■ Achieving assurance of economic independence. ■ Selecting and preparing for an occupation. ■ Preparing for marriage and family life. ■ Developing skills and concepts necessary for civic competence. ■ Desiring and achieving socially responsible behavior. ■ Acquiring a set of values and an ethical system as a guide to behavior.	■ Learning economic responsibility. ■ Learning social responsibility for self and others. ■ Experiencing social, emotional, and ethical commitments to others. ■ Accepting oneself and one's physical development. ■ Reconciling discrepancies between personal health concepts and observed health behavior of others. ■ Learning to cope with life events and problems. ■ Consideration of life goals and career plans and acquiring necessary skills to reach the goals. ■ Learning the importance of time to self and the world. ■ Experiencing degrees of structure or flexibility in social institution and interpersonal relationships.

(*continued*)

TABLE 22–1. (continued)

Erickson's Eight Stages of Man	Havinghurst's Developmental Tasks	Examples of Minimal Wellness Tasks for Each Developmental Stage
VI. Early adulthood (intimacy vs isolation)	VI. Early adulthood ■ Selecting a mate. ■ Learning to live with a marriage partner. ■ Starting a family. ■ Rearing children. ■ Managing a home. ■ Getting started in an occupation. ■ Taking on civic responsibility. ■ Finding a congenial social group.	■ Commitment to marriage partner and assumption of long-term responsibilities for family. ■ Selecting a career. ■ Commitment to membership in social gruops and organizations. ■ Incorporating health habits and practices into life-style. ■ Learning the importance and place of noncommitment.
VII. Middle adulthood (generativity vs stagnation)	VII. Middle age ■ Achieving adult civic and social responsibility. ■ Assisting teenage children to become responsible and happy adults. ■ Establishing and maintaining an economic standard of living. ■ Developing adult leisure time activities. ■ Relating oneself to one's spouse as a person. ■ Accepting and adjusting to the physiological changes of middle age. ■ Adjusting to aging parents.	
VIII. Maturity (ego integrity vs despair)	VIII. Later maturity ■ Adjusting to decreasing physical strength and health. ■ Adjusting to retirement and reduced income. ■ Adjusting to death of spouse. ■ Establishing an explicit affiliation with one's age group. ■ Establishing satisfactory physical living arrangements.	■ Becoming aware of risks to health and adjusting life-style and habits to cope with risks. ■ Adjusting to loss of job, income, and family and friends through death. ■ Redefining self-concept. ■ Adjusting to changes in personal time and new physical environments. ■ Adjusting of previous health habits to current physical and mental capabilities.

From Bruhn JG, Cordova FD, Williams JA, Fuentes RG. The wellness process. Community Health. *1977;2:209–221.*

motor skills and hand-to-mouth activity. The majority of accidents for this age group occur in the home, with falls, burns, and aspirations of foreign objects as the most common.

Toddler. During the second year of life a child's personality comes into its own. The individuality of the child becomes more apparent as the toddler faces the task of developing a sense of autonomy versus one of shame or doubt. This task is accomplished as toddlers begin to assert their independence and to explore the world. Toddlers quickly learn that their behaviors have an impact on their environment and the people within that world.[54] This knowledge forms the initial foundation for the development of an individual's sense of control and self-efficacy.

Wellness tasks for this age include an increased focus on safety as the toddler's inquisitive nature and rapidly developing motor skills increase safety risks. The health goal for toddlers focuses primarily on the provision of opportunities for maximal growth and development while maintaining a healthy and safe environment.

Preschool. The preschool period (ages 3 to 5 years) is considered an ideal time to teach wellness behaviors because it is when parental influences have the greatest impact on the child.[57] Healthy families can promote a healthful family lifestyle by encouraging an appropriate balance of activity and rest, fostering nutritionally sound dietary practices, and promoting regular exercise. Parents need to be aware that they are probably most influential when they "practice what they preach." Parents who say that sensible eating and exercise are important but do the opposite are usually less successful in establishing wellness behaviors in their children.[58]

An important component of psychological development occurring during the preschool years is the emergence of self-concept. The family functions to give the child a sense of social and personal identity. Like a mirror, the family reflects back to the child a picture of who they are and how valuable they are to others. Positive reflections provide the child with a sense of satisfaction and worth. The development of a favorable self-concept and sense of autonomy is thought to have a positive influence on health practices.[57]

School-age. For many children, the school-age years are the healthiest time of their lives. Energy levels are high and seemingly endless, and the ability to recover from illness or injury is rapid and relatively complete. School-age children exhibit increasing physical and emotional independence from parents and are exposed to new ideas, attitudes, perspectives, and behaviors as contact with the world outside the family expands.

Safety behaviors are an important consideration for this age group. An important element in safety promotion involves education regarding risk-taking behavior. Parents can promote safety by helping children to identify and avoid potentially hazardous situations. Increasing cognitive maturity, including the ability to learn from past experiences and to anticipate probable outcomes from contemplated actions, enables school-age children to take an active part in accident prevention, to make decisions about risk-taking behaviors and their consequences, and to develop personal values related to health.

An important wellness-related developmental task for school-age children is learning to cope effectively with stress. Although many people tend to view childhood as relatively carefree, school-age children confront many problems related to change, competition, frustration, and failures that must be confronted and adequately dealt with. Many of the health problems encountered in adolescence and young adulthood (reckless driving, suicide, alcohol and drug abuse, obesity, and so on) are related to stress and inadequate coping skills. Families of school-age children can play an important role in promoting mental and emotional health by equipping children with the skills necessary to cope with the outside world, thus potentially preventing future health problems in adolescence and adulthood.[57]

Adolescent. Adolescence has long been considered a critical period in human development. Throughout the teenage years, adolescents experience many complex changes physically, emotionally, cognitively, and socially. Rapid and significant developmental adjustments create a variety of stresses and problems that affect adolescent well-being. The overwhelming physical changes of puberty may seem inconsequential when compared to the social and psychological changes that take place during adolescence.

By the time individuals reach adolescence, a substantial part of their health-related behavior has already been established. As adolescents spend increasing amounts of time away from home, parental influence over dietary and health habits diminishes and the influence of peer pressure takes on added significance. Adolescents may engage in many destructive health behaviors because of peer pressure, such as unhealthy dietary habits, smoking, alcohol and drug abuse, reckless driving, and indiscriminate sexual practices. Adequate educational programs and a supportive home environment can assist adolescents to resist negative peer pressure, to make positive health-related decisions, and to be positive role models for peers.

One of the central developmental tasks of adolescence is the establishment of a sense of identity or self-concept. Self-image and self-esteem are very much tied to body image. Adolescents who perceive their bodies as less than ideal often have low self-confidence and may spend months or years rejecting their bodies and attempting to alter themselves beyond recognition. Inadequate self-esteem can have significant consequences for future adult health behaviors.

Young Adult. Young adults enter new roles of responsibility in relation to work, home, and self. Acceptance of responsibility for self-care during this period is of paramount importance for future health. Independent health behaviors practiced as a young adult with respect to nutrition, exercise, sexual practices, alcohol, smoking, drug use, and family life will largely determine the quality of life in the later years.

Stress plays an integral part in young adults' lives. Newly acquired responsibilities related to college, partner selection, marriage, childbearing, job demands, and social expectations can produce overwhelming stresses. Internal pressures to succeed and excel contribute to the potential risks to health. Assisting young adults to identify and reduce stress-producing behaviors or situations can be effective in preventing future health problems. Initiation of programs for exercise or nutritional improvement can boost the ability to cope with high levels of stress. The incorporation of stress-reduction techniques into the young adult's lifestyle can also be extremely effective.[57]

Middle Adult. Middle adulthood is a period of social, psychological, and biological change. For many, this extended period after the children leave home is a time of maximum economic productivity and marital satisfaction. For others, the transition into middle life is as critical as adolescence and in some ways more difficult. It is a period of reexamination and reevaluation of life goals and adult roles.[27]

Wellness tasks for middle-aged adults focus on guarding against the onset of preventable chronic diseases through continued healthy habits and regular practice of established methods of early detection and treatment. Many of the basic health practices identified by Belloc and Breslow,[21] such as maintaining ideal weight, participating in regular moderate exercise, and abstaining from smoking or excessive alcohol consumption, take on added significance at this stage of life.

Middle and later adulthood often presents a midlife crisis in relation to body image for many men and women as the inevitable signs of aging and gradual decline become impossible to ignore. In our contemporary society, all physical signs of aging are considered to be negative, so even an older person with a healthy body image may face problems.[2] Learning to accept aging in self and others is a basic developmental task for the middle adult.

Older Adult. Wellness behaviors take on added significance with the elderly population. Although today's elderly are healthier than in the past, studies indicate that 85 percent of older Americans suffer from at least one chronic disease.[59] Considering that the average life expectancy for those who reach the age of 65 is an additional 16.9 years,[60] the importance of wellness measures that work to maintain or improve functional ability and limit the effects of disabling conditions cannot be overstated. Small gains in health promotion or even slight reductions in the rate of decline can make a significant difference in the quality of life and the degree of independence of the elderly person.[57]

Health-promotion activities for the elderly focus on adequate nutrition, safety measures, exercise, stimulating social and leisure activities, and fostering independence.[29,59] Alterations in visual and auditory perception are common with advancing age and are a major contributor to safety problems encountered by the elderly client. A safety assessment should include an examination of the physical environment as well as an evaluation of the functional capacity of the elderly individual.[59]

Exercise and physical activity play a key role in the maintenance and promotion of a sense of positive wellbeing for the elderly. The value of exercise in maintaining strength, endurance, flexibility, and cardiovascular fitness has long been acknowledged. Recent research has also linked physical activity with psychological and emotional well-being. A study by Horgan found that frequency of physical activity was the leading behavior related to a positive self-perception of health by elderly subjects.[61]

One of the major tasks of the elderly is a continual adaptation to the multitude of physical, psychological, and social changes that accompany aging. The health of older adults, to a great extent, is dependent on their ability to cope with the multiple stress-producing life events they encounter. Adjustment to retirement, loss of loved ones, moving to retirement homes or care facilities, and changes in health and physical appearance are some of the major adjustments of later life. Adaptation to retirement includes not only adjusting to a new leisure life-style, but also coping with profound changes in role, status, and income. The inevitable loss of spouse and close friends alters lifelong roles and relationships and may contribute to problems of loneliness and social isolation. Physical limitations resulting from chronic illness may restrict mobility or independence and have a devastating effect on self-esteem. Although many of the adjustments of old age cannot be avoided, many of the negative effects can be diminished through anticipatory guidance. Planning for expected stressful events such as retirement or relocation can offset many potential problems.[57]

ALTERATIONS IN WELLNESS

Dimensions of Altered Wellness

As discussed earlier, the level of wellness that individuals experience is largely determined by the life-style and personal choices that are made throughout life. Each person adapts and reacts to the stresses and demands of daily life in a unique way. As a result, each individual life-style is a collection of the conscious and unconscious behaviors that meet perceived needs. Although personal actions can do much to facilitate the achievement of wellness, there are many daily activities and personal habits that diminish wellness and contribute to the development of serious health problems. These unhealthy behaviors can be examined in terms of the dimensions of wellness described earlier in this chapter. Many of these problems are discussed in detail in subsequent chapters, and so will only be addressed briefly here.

Eating Poorly. Adequate nutrients and healthy dietary patterns are an integral part of a wellness-oriented life-style. Unfortunately, for many Americans unhealthy nutrition is a way of life. Forty-five percent of the American food dollar is spent on eating in restaurants; 8 percent of meals are eaten in the car. Typically, meals eaten out are high in fat, sugar, salt, and calories, and low in complex carbohydrates.[62] Meals prepared at home are increasingly comprised of "convenience" foods that are highly refined, processed, colored, preserved, and artificially sweetened.

In the United States, obesity is the most frequent nutritional disorder among children and adults.[62] The prevalence of obesity increases with increasing age until age 64, then declines. Over 29 percent of 50- to 64-year-olds are overweight; the median percentage of adults who are overweight is 20.9 percent.[63] The typical American diet is comprised of excessive amounts of saturated fats, cholesterol, sugar, and salt. The overconsumption of these nutrients has been linked to a number of chronic diseases including cardiovascular disorders, hypertension, diabetes, and breast and colon cancers. The Surgeon General has documented that two thirds of all deaths in the United States are related to diseases whose incidence has been linked to dietary factors.[64] A detailed discussion of problems resulting from poor nutrition can be found in Chapter 25.

Lack of Fitness. Coupled with unhealthy nutritional habits is a basically sedentary life-style for many Americans. Present estimates indicate that 58 percent of adults are sedentary, and only one third of all adults participate in some form of exercise on a weekly basis.[63] These figures are distressing, not only because the benefits of exercise are well-documented, but also because adults set the life-style models that greatly determine the health practices of succeeding generations.

Inactivity is a serious health hazard that has been linked to conditions such as hypertension, chronic fatigue, premature aging, poor musculature, and inadequate flexibility. These conditions, in turn, are major contributors to lower back pain, injury, tension, obesity, and coronary heart disease.[29] A sedentary life-style may also encourage the development of other harmful life-style practices such as overeating, smoking, and alcohol ingestion, and has serious implications for emotional and psychological well-being. Additional information related to physical fitness can be found in Chapter 30.

Feeling Stressed. Stress is an unavoidable element in modern society. Stress affects both sexes and all ages, and over time can produce health-damaging effects. The relationship of excessive stress to physical illness is well documented. Stress-linked diseases or conditions have been identified that affect every body system. Peptic ulcers, irritable bowel syndrome, asthma, arthritis, coronary artery disease, hypertension, diabetes, alcoholism, insomnia, cancer, migraine headaches, and a variety of sexual dysfunctions are examples of disorders whose origins are linked to varying degrees of stress.[65,66] Hypertension alone affects more than 61 million Americans and predisposes its victims to other lethal consequences such as arteriosclerosis, congestive heart failure, and stroke.[67]

There are so many pressures and stressors inherent in contemporary life that very few people can avoid stress-related disease. However, research has indicated that certain types of individuals are more prone to stress-related disorders. Drs. M. Friedman and R. Rosenmann concluded that individuals with "striving personalities" (Type A) are prime candidates for heart disease, hypertension, and other physical ailments.[68] Type A behavior is a life-style or general orientation to life where high-level stress is an integral part of everyday life. These individuals live their lives according to the calendar and the clock—they do everything rapidly including eating, working, walking, driving, and speaking. Type A individuals are extremely competitive and are classic "workaholics." Even when the job is done they are unable to unwind and feel guilty for "doing nothing."[69] According to Friedman and Rosenmann, over 90 percent of the males under age 60 who have heart attacks display Type A behavior.

Although Type A personality is certainly a potent risk factor for the development of stress-related disorders, it is the individual's inability to cope with the high levels of stress that results in altered wellness. For many Type A individuals, the drive to compete and excel may produce feelings of personal satisfaction and may earn the person community respect.[70] Ineffective coping leaves anyone, regardless of personality type, "feeling stressed." Many unhealthy personal habits, such as smoking, overeating, and drug or alcohol abuse, are related to ineffective coping.

Ceasing to Care for Self or Others. Competent self-care is vital for the maintenance of health and well-being. Individuals may choose, consciously or unconsciously, not to participate in self-care activities for a variety of reasons. Lack of knowledge, poor motivation, lack of financial resources, or poor self-concept may influence an individual's choices. Nonparticipation in basic preventative and health maintenance activities can have serious negative effects on wellness. For the well individual, failure to engage in regular dental care or screening procedures such as breast self-examination may lead to diseases reaching an advanced state before medical treatment is sought. Lack of prenatal care during pregnancy produces increased incidence of poor pregnancy outcomes, such as premature labor and delivery and low-birth-weight infants. Individuals with diagnosed but treatable conditions, such as hypertension or diabetes, may suffer irreversible damage if self-care practices are not routinely performed.

Caring for others means recognizing the inherent value in all individuals and being respectful of others' needs and rights. Sometimes caring for others requires taking responsibility for their health and well-being; often, it means acknowledging their needs to take care of themselves, to make their own choices. Failure to care for others thereby produces unhealthy relationships in which one member attempts to control the other, or situations of neglect in which needed nurturing and support is not given. In some cases, inability to care for others is manifested in violence: child, spouse, or elder abuse.

Difficulty Fitting With the Environment. Environmental interaction includes minimizing one's own negative impact on the environment as well as recognizing all external factors that influence a person's biological, psychological, spiritual, and social functioning. A multitude of stressors, most created by human civilization in the external environment, can have a negative influence on wellness. Individuals whose approach to the environment is to exploit it are in fact contributing to the stressors that detract from wellness. Accidents related to environmental factors are a major health hazard for all age groups but especially for the young and the elderly. For infants and young children, the majority of accidents occur in the home environment—mostly falls, burns, and aspirations of foreign objects. As children mature, their environment expands to include the use of bicycles, skateboards, and of course, automobiles. Accidents of all kinds are the leading cause of death among children and adolescents under age 19, and almost half of the fatalities are the result of motor vehicle accidents.[71] Mortality statistics only illustrate a portion of the health impact of accidents for adolescents. For every youth killed in an automobile or other accident, hundreds more are injured, maimed, or incapacitated.

For the elderly, environmental hazards represent an important health threat. Alterations in visual and auditory acuity and tactile sensation are common with advancing age. Visual impairment and decreased mobility and coordination increase the likelihood of falls, a major problem with the elderly. Other sensory impairments also decrease the elderly person's awareness of environmental hazards and may lead to unintentional injury.

Lack of Self-responsibility. The ability to assume responsibility for one's actions, decisions, and health status is a trait that is learned as an individual matures and develops.

The fact that not all people develop an adequate sense of self-responsibility is evident from the large number of individuals who engage in nonhealthful activities. Many health-damaging behaviors such as smoking, drug and alcohol abuse, and unsafe sexual practices are utilized by individuals attempting to cope with excessive stress, disappointments, or lack of meaning and purpose in their lives. Initiation of these behaviors often begins in adolescence and continues throughout adulthood.

Smoking. Smoking is recognized to be the single most preventable cause of death in the United States. There is extensive evidence linking tobacco use with disease, disability, and premature death; for example an estimated 434,000 Americans died of diseases attributable to smoking in 1988. Current male smokers over 35 are 22 times more likely to die prematurely of lung cancer than nonsmoking males; for female smokers in the same age group, the risk of premature death due to lung cancer is 12 times greater than for nonsmokers.[72] Cigarette smoking is responsible not only for cancer of the lung and bronchus, but also for cancers of the larynx, pharynx, mouth, esophagus, bladder, and stomach. It is also a well-known contributing factor in the development of heart and blood vessel disease, chronic bronchitis and emphysema, and peptic and gastric ulcers.[72]

Although there has been a dramatic shift in the smoking behavior of Americans over the past 20 years, roughly 30 percent of adult Americans continue to smoke.[73] Recent public awareness of the hazards of "secondhand" smoke to children, unborn fetuses, and others in the immediate environment has facilitated the development of smoke-free areas and encouraged the development of smoking-cessation programs; however, smoking remains a serious health concern.

Alcohol and Drug Abuse. Alcohol and drug abuse are other behaviors with major implications for adolescent and adult health. Alcohol is a factor in more than 5 percent of all deaths in the United States and 42 percent of all highway fatalities.[74] Alcohol abuse is also directly related to cirrhosis of the liver, cerebrovascular disease, and various cancers.

Experimentation with drugs such as marijuana, cocaine, hallucinogens, or prescription medications also poses great risks for individuals. Drug use reportedly produces feelings of physical and psychological well-being that many individuals desire; however, the effect is temporary and continued drug use may lead to physical and psychological dependency. Drug use also leads to many physical, mental, and social problems for the individual, family, and community at large.

Unsafe Sexual Activity. Sexual activity is a natural form of self-expression throughout all stages of human development. Indiscriminate or unsafe sexual practices, however, have serious implications for wellness. The primary health hazards related to sexual activity are unplanned pregnancies and transmission of sexually transmitted diseases (STDs), problems that carry with them physical as well as psychological and social ramifications. Indiscriminate sexual practices may also lead to feelings of lowered self-esteem and self-worth. Additional information related to unsafe sexual practices can be found in Chapter 23.

The Experience and Manifestations of Altered Wellness

A variety of objective and subjective signs may be indicative of altered wellness. Although many of these conditions are normal reactions to everyday events, repeated or persistent manifestations of these characteristics are generally problematic.

Anxiety and Fear. Individuals faced with unfamiliar or threatening situations or conditions often experience anxiety and fear. Although these two concepts are often interrelated, anxiety refers to an unpleasant feeling of dread of the unknown while fear is related to a specific known threat in the environment.[75]

Individuals experiencing anxiety and fear often display a wide variety of signs, symptoms, or behaviors. Physiological signs and symptoms include increased heart rate, respirations, and blood pressure; insomnia; trembling; and anorexia. Intellectually individuals may be unable to concentrate or solve problems. Emotionally they may appear agitated, withdrawn, or distraught.[76]

Depression. Depression is a common reaction that can be maladaptive if it is prolonged or severe. Depression is usually exhibited in changes in feelings and thought content. Depression is often caused by loss of self-esteem related to the loss of a valued person or object.[75]

The observable feelings that a depressed person exhibits are sadness, apathy, and a lack of energy. There may also be a noticeable withdrawal from social contacts with other people. Depressed individuals often express feelings of failure and lack of a sense of personal worth or value to others.[75]

Physical Signs and Symptoms of Stress. Although the nonspecific generalized stress response described by Selye is evident in everyone experiencing stressful events, each individual's specific response to stress is unique. The interplay of factors such as genetic potential, personality, organ vulnerability, and general state of health and fitness, as well as previous experience with stress, creates a highly personalized response. Manifestations of stress cover a wide range of behaviors. Some of the most common include overeating or lack of appetite; excessive smoking or drinking; irritability; sleep disorders; fatigue; depression; sweating; muscle tension; and numerous physical complaints, for example, headaches, palpitations, and altered elimination.

Pain. Pain is the number one symptom or complaint that causes an individual to seek health care. It influences quality of life and sense of well-being more than any other health-related problem. A description of the clinical manifestations of pain is difficult because of the private and individualistic nature of each person's pain experience. Persons with acute pain often exhibit pronounced physiological responses such as tachycardia, tachypnea, elevated blood pressure, and diaphoresis. Because of adaptive changes over time, these manifestations may not be present in an individual who is suffering with chronic pain. Body movements associated with acute pain include holding affected body parts, grimacing, or lying listlessly because one is afraid to move. Many people also exhibit affective behaviors such as crying or moaning.

Fatigue. Individuals who are experiencing any form of altered wellness often exhibit symptoms of fatigue. Physical signs of fatigue include dark circles under the eyes, frequent yawning, ptosis (drooping) of the eyelids, and an expressionless face. If the fatigue is significant, changes in behavior and performance will be present, such as increasing irritability, disorientation, listlessness, and an inability to concentrate or think clearly.

Powerlessness. Powerlessness is an individual's perceived lack of control over a current situation. It is often associated with illness or may be the result of unsatisfactory interpersonal or social relationships. People experiencing powerlessness feel that any action that they take will have no significant effect on the outcome of the present situation.

Manifestations of powerlessness are difficult to predict. Individuals may appear passive or apathetic. They may express dissatisfaction or frustration over their inability to act, or may express doubt regarding their role performance. Feelings of powerlessness may lead to depression, and result in many of the manifestations discussed in that earlier section.

Loneliness. The significance of social relationships to wellness is reflected in Holmes and Rahe's Social Readjustment Rating Scale[77] (see also Chap. 6, Fig. 6–4). The death of a spouse ranks highest on the scale, reflecting the amount of disruption associated with the event. Three of the other most disruptive life events on the scale are also related to changes in social relationships: divorce, marital separation, and death of a close family member.

Loneliness is an emotional response resulting from a lack of intimacy or human contact. Although usually associated with an individual who is isolated because of illness or unfamiliar surroundings, loneliness can occur even when one is surrounded by familiar objects and friends.

Manifestations of loneliness may be difficult to identify as it is commonly hidden or disguised by the individual. Often it is expressed through withdrawal, depression, or a profound sense of hopelessness. Others, however, may complain of vague physical symptoms such as headache, or may display hostility or anger toward those around them.[76]

Internal Conflict and Dissatisfaction. Altered states of wellness are often characterized by the presence of internal conflicts and personal dissatisfaction with the current situation or with life in general. Prolonged internal conflicts may manifest themselves through the use of inappropriate coping mechanisms such as overeating, excessive drinking or smoking, use of recreational drugs, or other self-destructive behaviors.

Factors That May Alter Wellness

Life Change and Crisis. Chapter 6 introduces the concepts of change, stress, and crisis and outlines the physiological and psychological responses that occur as a result of stress. Stress is produced by any kind of change—negative or positive. Research by Holmes and Rahe resulted in the development of the Social Readjustment Rating Scale (see Chap. 6, Fig. 6–4), which quantifies the amount of change in a person's life over a given period of time.[77] Their research revealed a marked correlation between high amounts of change in an individual's life and an abrupt and serious change in their emotional and/or physical health. Although the Social Readjustment Rating Scale measures predominately major life events over a 1-year period, further research by Holmes and Rahe indicated that even a few days of stress and change can result in minor illnesses such as headaches, stomachaches, and colds.[78]

Crisis is an acute variation of stress that is so severe that the individual reaches a state of social and psychological disorganization in which the ability to function deteriorates. Crises can be described as developmental (maturational) or situational (see Chaps. 6 and 8). Developmental crises are periods of transition that every person experiences during life that are accompanied by changes in thoughts, feelings, and abilities (eg, adolescence, middle age). Situational crises are external events that may occur suddenly or unexpectedly (eg, natural disasters, death of parent or spouse). The essential factor influencing the occurrence of a state of crisis is the individual's inability to resolve the problem through normal coping methods.

Crisis carries with it a profound sense of helplessness and powerlessness. Individuals feel they are faced with an insurmountable problem that they cannot master or control. Disorganization of all aspects of life may occur in response to the acute level of emotional and psychological distress. Although crisis is characteristically of relatively short duration, the impact on well-being is devastating. Additional information related to crisis can be found in Chapter 6.

Illness. The concept of illness was introduced in Chapter 5. Although the terms illness and disease are often used interchangeably, illness is a much broader concept. Disease generally refers to a biomedical condition that results in a malfunction of a body organ or system. Illness is the perception and reaction of individuals and those around them to a state of not being well. Although the concept of illness does include disturbances caused by biological and psychological changes, it also includes personal, social, and cultural reactions to disease. Illness involves the whole person and is unique for each individual. Often changes in self-concept, social relationships, and coping patterns accompany illness.

Change in Self-concept. Altered self-concept may occur as individuals experiencing illness are faced with changes in their physical condition and their ability to function normally. Illness often forces one to regress to a state of dependency on others. For many people, this loss of control is regarded as a threat. Alterations in individuals' perceptions of themselves, their bodies, or their worth have a profound effect on their satisfaction with life and overall well-being. Disturbances in self-concept have been linked with conditions such as obesity, anorexia and bulimia, and alcoholism. Chronic illness or disability can produce varying degrees of feelings of low self-esteem and powerlessness. Individuals may look different because of disability or may feel different because of the limitations imposed by the disease. They may also feel that they can no longer affect personal destiny, which undermines decision-making abilities and self-efficacy. Feeling different and inferior to others can lead to a desire to retreat from all interactions or social activities and can seriously impair social and spiritual health.[32] A detailed discussion of self-concept can be found in Chapters 10 and 23.

Change in Social Relationships. Altered relationships with family and friends often accompany illness. The type of effect depends on the severity of the illness, family sociocultural beliefs and practices, and the roles normally performed by the ill person.

The severity of the illness dictates to a large extent the degree of dependency that a person must assume during the illness. Critical illness may leave individuals totally dependent on others for even the maintenance of simple bodily functions. Less severe illness may allow individuals to continue to perform some aspects of self-care, but often assistance from family members or health care providers is still necessary. Many clients may experience difficulty in relinquishing control and allowing others to care for them.

A family's sociocultural beliefs influence not only how a client perceives illness but also from whom assistance is sought and what types of treatment will be considered most advantageous. Many cultures may advocate the use of folk medicine or lay remedies prior to seeking professional medical care and may prescribe caregiving roles within the family.

The daily roles the ill person normally performed have a profound effect on the degree of change that occurs in family and social relationships. Each family member is affected differently depending on which member of the family is ill. The degree of change is generally related to how dependent each family member is on the ill person.

Change in Coping Patterns. Often altered coping occurs with the development of illness. Personal illness may seriously impair an individual's ability to use normal coping mechanisms. Physical stressors related to illness, such as pain, fatigue, or the effects of medications, may seriously impair problem-solving skills and decision-making. Increased dependency may foster the use of immature and less effective coping mechanisms. Normal outlets for tension release, such as physical activity, may not be possible due to illness.

Coexistence of Wellness and Illness. Because wellness and illness are conditions that exist as part of a continuum, they are not mutually exclusive concepts. An illness does not always disrupt physical, emotional, and social functioning. Moreover, the nature of an individual's response to illness is a significant variable influencing the degree to which the illness interrupts wellness. Many individuals cope with illness in such a way that their physical and emotional harmony, self-concept, zest for living, and usual healthy life-style choices are basically unchanged. For them, illness and wellness coexist. On the other hand, when the actual or perceived interference with one's life routine brought on by illness is significant, the illness may be all-consuming. The change to an illness orientation may be temporary and self-limited, or the illness-related deviations may be so great that individuals must reframe their former definition of wellness.

Health Care Experiences. As Chapter 12 emphasizes, there is considerable variation in the ways individuals experience the stages of illness and the process of becoming a client.

Becoming a Client. Recognition that something is, or may be, wrong can take considerable time. Once individuals accept that symptoms are present, they may still take no action. A "wait and see" attitude, with the hope that symptoms will improve or disappear, is common. At some point in the transition from wellness to illness, action specific to the symptoms is taken. Individuals may try self-care remedies, consult with family or friends about the symptoms, or contact a health care professional.

Contact with a health care professional is made in order to validate the reality of the illness as well as to seek advice on a treatment plan. Individuals often experience varying degrees of anxiety related to the decision to seek professional help. Even minor symptoms may be construed to be early signs of a serious condition.

When an actual diagnosis of illness is validated by a health care professional, the transition to the client role begins. Often, becoming a client involves actual or perceived loss of control. Most people experience ambivalence related to relinquishing control to a health care provider; however, they may view the provider's recommendations as the only solution for attaining the desired goal of cure. Although some individuals are able to accept a degree of dependency upon the health care system, many will attempt to retain varying degrees of control over the situation through information-seeking and self-care. In a collaborative provider–client relationship, this client involvement is fostered and encouraged.

Any experience with physical illness is stress producing and represents a potential threat to an individual's well-being. Even a minor illness, such as a cold, saps vitality, alters daily routines, and interferes with normal social interactions. When the illness requires intervention by health care professionals and/or hospitalization, another variable is added. For some, the health care experience has a profound impact on well-being. Chapter 12 discusses ways that assuming the client role and entering the health care system can be stressful. The discussion here focuses on the implications these stressors have for client well-being.

Admission to the Hospital. Hospital admission has been compared to the culture shock that is experienced by individuals arriving in a foreign country. There is a different mode of dress, food, daily routines, and language. In a very real sense, a hospital is a separate and unique community. Individuals are thrust into an unfamiliar environment and surrounded by strangers who expect conformity to their established way of life. Culture shock for healthy individuals is disorienting and stressful, particularly during the initial period of adaptation. For seriously ill individuals, the stress of entering the hospital environment only compounds already high stress levels. Anxiety and fear are common emotions experienced with hospitalization. Nurses can work with clients to relieve anxiety and fear related to the hospital experience through adequate orientation and preparation, and the maintenance of a warm, supportive, collaborative relationship. The following discussion addresses the impact on wellness of common experiences associated with hospitalization, including loss of autonomy, loss of privacy, sensory overload and deprivation, social isolation, exposure to risk, pain, threat to body image, and worry about the future.

Loss of Autonomy. Loss of autonomy is frequently associated with hospitalization. Autonomy refers to independence and freedom to choose actions. For most adults, autonomy is part of feeling good and taking responsibility, two elements of a wellness life-style discussed previously. In fact, without autonomy, responsibility is a relatively meaningless term. Admission to the hospital usually involves loss of personal choice—for example, regarding what one wears, where personal possessions are kept, and decisions about a daily schedule. There are often established rules and schedules as to when one must eat, sleep, bathe, urinate, and when one may or may not have pain medication or visitors. The ill adult is often considered incompetent to engage in self-care activities and must follow "doctor's orders." Nursing care is often focused on the completion of physical and medical tasks (baths, medications, dressings) rather than on individual needs, making clients feel as if they are a piece of equipment or machinery that needs to be worked on. This loss of control and individuality is often very difficult to accept and may lead to decreased self-esteem, a sense of powerlessness, and a generalized feeling of altered wellness.[74] Nurses can humanize the hospital experience and minimize loss of autonomy by responding to clients as individuals and encouraging clients to collaborate in their own care.

Loss of Privacy. Loss of privacy is another aspect of hospitalization that is closely related to loss of autonomy. **Privacy** can be defined as "the right of the individual to decide what information about himself should be communicated to others and under what conditions" (p. 223).[79] People need varying degrees of privacy based on their personalities and social and cultural backgrounds. Intrusion into privacy leaves one feeling invaded and uncomfortable.

The hospital environment invades all aspects of privacy. The physical surface of the body, including intimate parts, is examined, pushed, washed, rubbed, and excised by caregivers who are total strangers. Questions are asked about all aspects of life, including bodily functions. Personal information is recorded in a chart that many people read. Modesty is often difficult to maintain with hospital gowns that open down the back and only thin curtains separating one patient from another. Nurses can show respect for an individual's privacy by knocking before entering the room, asking permission before opening or disturbing personal articles, taking care to avoid unnecessary exposure of clients during procedures, and refraining from discussing clients or their care in public places such as hallways, elevators, or the hospital cafeteria.

Sensory Overload or Deprivation. Optimum stimulation contributes to wellness. It is a way of connecting with one's environment. Often, clients experience excessive or insufficient stimulation during hospitalization. Sensory overload occurs when the individual receives more sensory stimulation stimulation than can be tolerated. Bright lights, noise, unfamiliar machinery, pain, visitors, and a disturbed sleep–wake cycle all combine to overwhelm the hospitalized client. Seriously ill individuals, often restricted in movement, can do little to control the incoming stimuli. Intensive care units are especially prone to producing sensory overload.

Sensory deprivation, the opposite of sensory overload, occurs when the level of sensory input is too low to permit normal functioning. Sensory deprivation can be the result of a restricted environment, reduced sensory input, or elimination of order and meaning from sensory input.[80] Elderly clients are particularly prone to sensory deprivation. Many of these individuals have reduced visual, auditory, taste, and tactile sensations, and wear eyeglasses, hearing aids, and dentures to compensate for their sensory deficits. It is not uncommon to find these prosthetic devices in a bedside drawer out of the hospitalized person's reach. Elderly clients depend on these devices in order to communicate with

IMPLICATIONS FOR NURSE–CLIENT COLLABORATION

Loss of Autonomy

Whenever an individual is hospitalized, an automatic loss of autonomy occurs. Just by entering the hospital—a world characterized by formal rules, policies, and informal behavior norms that are the creation of others—the client gives up an aspect of personal autonomy. A collaborative nurse–client relationship is particularly beneficial in this context because it promotes the preservation of the client's self-determination by encouraging the client's active participation in health care decision-making.

the sensory environment; without them their sensory input is severely impaired.[80]

Both sensory overload and sensory deprivation result in marked physical, psychological, and emotional reactions. Individuals may appear fatigued, withdrawn, confused, agitated, and disoriented to time and place. Severe sensory alterations can lead to disturbed thought patterns, illusions, sensory distortions, and hallucinations. Nurses need to increase their awareness of clients' sensory environment and its effect on clients. Additional information related to sensory deprivation and overload can be found in Chapter 29.

Social Isolation. Relationships with family members and significant others meet individuals' needs for affection, closeness, belonging, and understanding. These feelings are an essential aspect of wellness. Moreover, illness threatens security, so it often intensifies the need for love and belonging. Hospitalization separates clients from their usual sources of social support at a time when their needs are the greatest. Although clients may be surrounded by people (nurses, physicians, roommates) within the hospital environment, interactions with them do not usually serve to meet intimacy and belonging needs. If clients require isolation techniques because of an infection, the sense of abandonment and loneliness increases dramatically.

The separation and loss of intimacy caused by illness and hospitalization significantly affects the well-being of family members as well as clients. Medical crisis can modify patterns of social interaction within families and mutual needs and expectations for intimacy often are not met.[81] A study by Gilliss of family stress levels related to coronary bypass surgery found that spouses actually experienced higher levels of subjective stress than the clients.[82] Family members reported high levels of frustration with their inability to comfort or care for the client. Feelings of insecurity and fear may actually cause family members to withdraw emotionally, further increasing the client's sense of social isolation.

Exposure to Risks. Risks threaten wellness because of their potential for harm and because of the stress associated with threat. Risks common to hospitalized clients include physical injury, exposure to nosocomial infections, potential negative effects of medications, and risks associated with surgical procedures.

PHYSICAL INJURY. Several types of physical injuries can occur in hospitals. Acutely ill or physically debilitated clients are prone to injury from falls or improper transfers. The increasing use of advanced technology and equipment may expose clients to the dangers of electrical shock or improper radiation exposure. A detailed discussion of nursing measures related to providing a physically safe environment for hospitalized clients can be found in Section 3.

EXPOSURE TO NOSOCOMIAL INFECTIONS. Exposure to nosocomial infections represents a major threat to client well-being. **Nosocomial infections** are hospital acquired, which means they develop *after* hospital admission. They include infections clients acquire during their hospitalization or that they manifest after discharge. A hospital is one of the most likely places to acquire an infection as it harbors a high concentration of microorganisms that may be antibiotic resistant and more virulent than microorganisms normally found in the community. Hospital-acquired infections affect over 2 million patients each year in the United States or approximately 6 percent of all people admitted to acute care facilities.[83] Surgical patients have the highest incidence of infection. Nearly 70 percent of all nosocomial infections develop in postoperative patients.[84]

Factors that predispose an individual to acquiring an infection include age, the degree to which body defenses have been compromised by illness or drugs, the type and number of invasive procedures performed, and the length of hospitalization. The major sites affected by nosocomial infections are the urinary tract, surgical wounds, respiratory system, and the bloodstream.[83] A detailed discussion of epidemiology and the chain of transmission of infection can be found in Chapter 7. A discussion of infection control measures is included later in Section 3.

EFFECTS OF MEDICATIONS. One common treatment used in acute care settings that exposes the client to substantial risk is receiving multiple medications. A **medication** is any substance that is used therapeutically in the diagnosis, treatment, or prevention of disease. The safe and accurate administration of medications is a major component of nursing care in acute care settings. Proper use of medications can promote a sense of well-being in the client through intended therapeutic actions. For example, analgesics can help ease the pain of a surgical incision, antibiotics can combat infection, and vitamin supplements can supply needed nutrients and enhance nutritional status.

Unfortunately, medications have both desirable and undesirable effects on the body. Most drugs in addition to their intended therapeutic action also produce unintended side effects, which may be harmless or potentially harmful. For example, some analgesics, such as morphine, are effective in relieving pain but may also produce nausea and diffuse itching. Many times the side effects are tolerated in order to receive the beneficial action of the drug. An antibiotic, such as penicillin, may be effective in fighting an infection, but can also cause a severe and potentially fatal anaphylactic reaction in susceptible persons.

Some people are concerned about ingesting medications because they view them as undesirable chemicals. They feel that using what they consider unnatural substances carries inherent risks of disrupting balance and function within the body. Another concern that makes some people hesitant about taking pain medications is the fear of becoming addicted. Providing accurate information about drugs and their effects, while being sensitive to client concerns, can reduce the stress associated with fears such as these. Fear of pain or distress related to invasion of body boundaries from medications administered via injection or intravenously is another common stressor related to receiving medications, even among adult clients.

Nurses are sometimes insensitive to these kinds of concerns, feeling that they are juvenile or insignificant in light of the overall disease process or its therapy. Also, because administering medications is so much a part of nurses' daily routines, they may forget having had similar feelings themselves. These kinds of responses are not helpful to clients. Accepting the genuineness and intensity of whatever concerns clients may have about receiving medications and empathically working with them to resolve their feelings are more effective and caring approaches.

Any medication has the potential to harm a client if administered improperly. It is the responsibility of the nurse to ensure that clients receive safe and therapeutic doses of prescribed medications. Medication errors can be avoided through the practice of basic principles of medication administration and sound nursing judgment. Nurses must understand an ordered drug's action, administer it properly, and monitor the client's response. In addition, knowledge of the client's condition and previous responses assists the nurse in determining whether a particular drug or dosage is appropriate and should be given. The principles of safe medication administration are presented later in this chapter.

SURGICAL PROCEDURES. Surgical procedures alter all aspects of an individual's well-being. Physiologically the integrity of skin, blood vessels, major organs, and other body tissues are compromised. Psychologically, surgery represents a major threat to life itself, as well as altering body image, self-esteem, and self-control. Socially, surgery produces significant changes in family dynamics, role performance, and life-style. Table 22–2 outlines the major alterations in well-being related to surgical procedures. Basic pre- and postoperative nursing care is discussed in Section 3 of this chapter.

Exposure to Pain and Discomfort. For most clients, the hospital experience includes undergoing a variety of therapeutic treatments, diagnostic testing, and invasive procedures. Although these measures are implemented to facilitate diagnosis, promote healing, and prevent complications and/or disability, they often subject clients to varying degrees of pain and discomfort.

The experience of pain is a subjective phenomenon that can significantly alter wellness. Pain is a direct barrier to usual activities that most individuals consider part of being well. Margo McCaffery, a recognized authority in the nursing care of clients in pain, states that "pain is whatever the person experiencing it says it is and [it] exists whenever he says it does."[85] Pain is comprised of two components: physiological alterations or stimuli and psychological reactions. The integration of these two components produces a unique pain experience for each individual. Although all individuals have the some basic physiological makeup, there are differences that make some people more or less susceptible to pain than others. Individuals' psychological responses to pain are influenced by the degree of powerlessness they experience, the presence and attitudes of other people, the amount of information they are given, the degree of threat the pain imposes, personal and past experiences with pain, cognitive level, and the extent to which they have used pain for secondary gains.[85] (Secondary gains are advantages such as attention or other desired responses that some people derive from illness or its symptoms.)

How individuals react to or express pain is largely determined by what the pain means to them and their previous experiences with pain (including cultural and social influences). Clients undergoing an acutely painful experience may withstand the pain surprisingly well if they view the experience as beneficial. Examples include a woman giving birth to a healthy infant or an individual who has undergone restorative surgery. Conversely, clients who view the pain as serving no useful purpose or as a threat to body image or life-style, may experience anxiety, fear, and depression, which serve to exacerbate the pain sensation.

Adequate pain management is vital to client well-being. Unrelieved pain taxes clients' coping abilities both physically and emotionally. It directs clients' attention inward and drains emotional and physical energy. Clients may feel powerless and controlled by the pain and may react with depression, irritability, withdrawal, or hostility. Nurses can use a wide variety of pain control measures to assist clients in maintaining an acceptable level of comfort. The relaxation techniques presented later in this chapter are often effective pain relief measures. A detailed discussion of pain and other pain control measures is presented in Chapter 29.

Disturbance of Body Image and Self-esteem. In addition to physiological threats, the hospital environment also poses many psychological threats to the client. As was discussed earlier, admission to the hospital often involves a loss of privacy and personal control. Additional psychological threats include a disturbance of body image due to invasive and/or surgical procedures and high levels of emotional stress related to fear and anxiety.

Emotional adjustment to many of the therapeutic treatments used in the hospital setting may be a difficult task for clients. Some treatments such as traction, although designed to promote healing of damaged skeletal tissue, may have negative consequences on client well-being due to complications related to immobility, sensory deprivation, and extended hospitalization. Renal dialysis or diabetic dietary restrictions, although physiological life-saving therapies, require profound psychosocial and emotional adjustment on the part of clients and family members. Nurses can assist clients in adapting to therapeutic treatments through continued client education and support, and through encouraging their active involvement in the therapeutic regimen. Careful attention to each client's unique needs and responses enables individuals to receive maximum benefits from the treatments while minimizing stressful effects.

Invasive procedures and tubes are an integral part of today's high-tech acute care settings. Chemical dyes, radioactive substances, and a host of other materials may be injected into the body for diagnostic purposes. Tubes and

TABLE 22–2. ALTERATIONS IN WELL-BEING RELATED TO SURGICAL PROCEDURES

Alteration	Associated Stressors
Disruption of skin integrity	Potential infection of surgical incision Potential wound dehiscence or evisceration Change in body image/self-esteem
Disruption of circulatory system	Possible postoperative hemorrhage Excessive fluid losses Problems related to venous stasis (thrombus, thrombophlebitis) Potential infection/inflammation at IV site
Alteration of respiratory function	Potential respiratory depression related to use of anesthetics and narcotics Pooling of respiratory secretions in lungs/alveoli Decreased lung expansion related to immobility and pain Potential trauma to larnyx during intubation/extubation
Alteration in nutrition	Potential negative nitrogen balance Problems with postoperative nausea and vomiting
Activation of the stress response	Increased risk of infection Increased fluid retention/potential fluid overload
Alteration in elimination	Decreased peristalsis Potential problems with paralytic ileus Abdominal distension Constipation Postoperative urinary retention Potential urinary tract infection related to catheterization
Decreased physical mobility	Increased risk of venous stasis Pooling of respiratory secretions Potential problems with skin breakdown Decreased muscle strength/joint mobility
Alteration in body temperature	Increased vasodilation from anesthetic agents Exposure of internal organs to cold operating room (OR) environment Infusion of cool IV fluids Fever related to infectious process
Sleep pattern disturbance	Alteration of normal biorhythms Use of narcotics/anesthetics Round-the-clock monitoring/assessment Postoperative pain
Alteration in comfort	Postoperative pain Irritation from tubes/drains Muscular soreness related to OR positioning
Fluid and electrolyte imbalance	Excessive fluid losses Restricted oral intake Potential fluid overload from IV fluid administration Increased aldosterone and antidiuretic hormone secretion
Alteration in sensory perception	Loss of consciousness Decreased sensation/orientation related to use of narcotics Sensory overload or deprivation
Alteration in body image	Loss of body part or function Permanent incisional scar Invasion of body by tubes, equipment Possible alteration in sexual expression
Alteration in role performance	Changes in family relationships Possible financial difficulties Permanent life-style alterations
Self-care deficit	Forced to assume dependent role Change in normal hygiene routines Sense of powerlessness Invasion of privacy Loss of self-esteem
Fear/anxiety	Decreased attention span Inability to learn Disturbance of sleep/rest Increased conflict in interpersonal relationships

other devices may be inserted through the skin or any number of natural or surgical openings in the body. Aside from the obvious physiological hazards these procedures may present, invasive procedures can significantly affect an individual's sense of control and personal space. The distinction between where the body begins and the environment ends becomes blurred, especially in areas such as an intensive care unit where the many invasive tubes are connected to elaborate monitoring devices. Even "common" tubes such as intravenous lines, urinary catheters, or nasogastric tubes may be viewed as threatening by clients.

Any invasive procedure alters one's sense of body boundary. Even minor surgery that leaves little or no visible incisional scar may entail removal or manipulation of internal organs, leave individuals feeling invaded, and alter body image. Major surgical procedures that result in visible physical changes or functioning may require extensive psychological adjustment. Impairment of sexual functioning or role performance due to surgical intervention can lead to sustained problems with self-expression and self-esteem, and may significantly alter individuals' relationships with significant others (see Chap. 23).

Fear and Anxiety. Diagnostic testing procedures are a frightening experience to many people. Clients may fear the pain or discomfort involved with the procedure, the results of the procedure and their implications, or possible complications resulting from the procedure itself. Not knowing what to expect only adds to the sense of dread.

Fear is a natural response to the experience of surgery. The threat of undergoing anesthesia and literally placing one's life in the hands of strangers may elicit powerful reactions of fear and anxiety. Fear of never waking up, or of the development of serious complications, are universal whether expressed or not. If the surgery is exploratory in nature or involves a biopsy, the fear that a malignant tumor may be discovered or that parts of the body will be removed while anesthetized can be very disturbing. Preparation of clients for diagnostic testing and/or surgery and providing necessary emotional support are critical nursing interventions that will be discussed later in this chapter.

The concepts of wellness and well-being are integral components of professional nursing practice. Using a collaborative approach, the ultimate goal of nursing is to facilitate each client's progress toward his or her own level of optimal wellness. The following sections provide a guide for assessment of clients and management of problems related to alterations in wellness, as well as approaches to maintain or enhance well-being when health is compromised.

Section 2. Assessment of Wellness and Well-being

■ WELLNESS AND WELL-BEING DATA COLLECTION

The assessment guide presented on the following pages focuses on the data necessary for assessing wellness and well-being. It concentrates on the general elements of wellness, especially the personal, social, and stress and coping elements. The details of assessing more specific aspects of wellness are found in other chapters in Unit VI. For instance, a detailed guide for assessing self-expression is located in Section 2 of Chapter 23; a guide for assessing nutrition appears in Section 2 of Chapter 25; a guide for assessing cardiovascular function appears in Section 2 of Chapter 27; one for neurosensory integration appears in Section 2 of Chapter 29; one for assessing sleep and rest appears in Section 2 of Chapter 28; and one for assessing musculoskeletal fitness appears in Section 2 of Chapter 30. The reader is referred to those chapters for in-depth coverage.

Wellness and well-being assessment are important because they provide an overall understanding of a client as a person and an understanding of how clients' health problems are influenced by the pattern of their lives. Wellness and well-being assessments contribute a description of the context in which clients' health problems have evolved and in which they will be resolved. Client strengths and resources are as important a part of wellness assessment as are the factors that are creating health problems. It is through the overall understanding that emerges from a wellness assessment and the appreciation of how the various pieces of a client's situation fit together that an appropriate plan of client care can be devised.

Wellness assessment is an ongoing process, but it is an especially important priority at the beginning of a nurse–client relationship. Thorough and accurate wellness assessments depend on full, open exchanges between nurses and clients during the health history and examination. The level of rapport a nurse establishes with a client in the opening moments of the health interview is usually a significant factor in putting a client at ease and may enhance or detract from the interaction that occurs thereafter. Given that the assessment of wellness and well-being often involves issues that are of a personal nature, such as life-style and coping patterns, skill in enlisting client's cooperation and collaboration is of paramount importance. Generally clients will respond to a nurse once they sense the nurse's caring and concern and once they experience the nurse's spontaneity and openness. The nurse's invitation to the client to become a partner in the decision-making process is also an extremely important factor. It supports clients' sense of control in the situation and conveys to clients that they are not alone, a message that builds trust.

Wellness and Well-being History

Much of the data on which a wellness assessment is based cannot be measured or directly verified for the following reasons:

1. Psychological and emotional functioning is difficult to quantify and measure and thus assessment of these aspects is heavily reliant on a client's self-report.
2. Clients' assessment of their own functioning is subjective. Individuals may feel that they are coping well when in fact others, including health care professionals, would not agree.
3. Assessment by family members is subjective. Although they may have more intimate knowledge of a client than nurses, they are only reporting their perceptions of a client's well-being.
4. Nurses' perceptions and assessment of clients is also subjective, and may be influenced by personal values, experiences, and psychological state.
5. Dissimilar perceptions resulting from different values and cultural beliefs held by clients and nurses may contribute to a misinterpretation of assessment data.[75]

Thus, while clients' self-reports are vital to a wellness and well-being assessment, validation of the messages conveyed in these reports is necessary to ensure that nurses understand clients' and family members' points of view. (For more on this subject, see Chapter 14.) Nurses verbalize their understanding of clients' statements, especially those that can be interpreted in various ways, and ask clients to provide clarifying feedback.

Further, self-report data must be augmented by nurses' observations, and for this nurses need skill in "reading between the lines." Because so much of the data in a wellness and well-being assessment come from the health history, it is necessary for nurses to evaluate whether clients' self-reports correspond to their behavior. Does a client report feeling good but look dejected, sad, or depressed? Does a client state that "things are under control" but show outbursts of irritability? Such inconsistencies are an important part of the wellness and well-being assessment.

Still another important point is that value differences between nurses and clients may interfere with both data collection and data interpretation, and may skew the nurse's assessment. (For more about values in health care see Chaps. 9 and 34.) Thus, it is important for nurses to evaluate the tone, that is, the quality or character, of the communication during history taking. In everyday social exchanges, there are sometimes awkward moments when the tension level rises inexplicably. These also occur between nurses and clients as they are getting to know one another. Nurses should look upon these moments as signals and as important clues. Sometimes they signal that a client has underlying feelings about the topic. When such moments occur, a nurse makes mental notes to follow up either immediately or later in order to determine their significance to the client. Establishing their meaning may help a nurse to better understand a client's subjective experience.

Primary Concern. History taking should begin by focusing on a client's primary concern, the aspect of the health problem about which the client is most concerned. Life-style and health habits are frequently factors in illness, and illness generally interferes with clients' well-being. Thus, a client's primary concern is important because it is a direct reflection of a client's well-being and is an indicator of how illness is impinging on well-being.

Clients differ in their awareness of the links between their life situation and their health problems. Some clients will recognize that their health problem is related to life stressors, life-style, or health habits. Some clients may actually identify being "overstressed" as their primary concern. History taking should focus on how the client's present situation influences well-being. Nurses can obtain that data by asking "What about your problem bothers you the most?" Clients with the same chief complaint (reason for seeking health care) can have very different primary concerns. Such differences can have an important impact on the selection of caregiving strategies. For example, a client may come into the health care agency with a chief complaint of back pain. The client's primary concern may be the pain itself, the pathological significance of the pain, or some consequence of the back pain such as an inability to work. This is illustrated by the two examples presented below. Care strategies would differ in each case. In any event, the primary concern represents a threat to client well-being and provides valuable information for developing strategies to enhance wellness.

- Brian Berry is a 36-year-old single man admitted to the hospital for back pain. When asked, "What about this problem bothers you the most?" Brian responds "I've never had pain like this before. I'm not sure if I can stand it much longer." Brian's primary concern is his ability to tolerate severe pain.

  Melissa Landon, on the other hand, a 25-year-old single woman, is also admitted with back pain. When asked the same question, she responds "Well, the pain is terrible, but the thing is that I've already missed too much work, and my boss said that if I miss any more, he'd fire me. I've got a brand new condo with payments to make!"

  While the chief complaint for both Brian and Melissa is back pain, their primary concerns differ. Melissa's primary concern is the potential threat her illness poses to her financial security and life-style.

Current Understanding. A client's interpretation of the present problem has an important affect on the actions taken to achieve and maintain well-being. The client's interpretation is influenced by the perceived causes of the problem and the impact of the problem on daily living. The perceived cause of the problem will affect the client's perception of self-efficacy and confidence in his or her personal ability to change the problem. Often, the impact of the problem on a client's daily living is a key factor influencing a motivation for change. The following example demonstrates the nurse's use of current understanding data.

- Mr. Jones has had a cough and hoarseness for the past three months. Mr. Jones has smoked for 10 years and recently increased his smoking from one to two packs a day. When asked about the cause of his cough, Mr. Jones links it to his increased smoking, which he says is because of stress at work. Knowing this, the nurse is able to direct the assessment to the reasons for stress at work.

Past Health Problems/Experiences. Information about the client's response to past illness and previous health care experiences enables the nurse to identify experiences the client has had that may shape responses to the present situation and especially to caregiving. Some clients bring fears and anxieties with them that they formed during previous hospitalizations. Consequently, they may approach the current situation with a lack of confidence in themselves and others. Other clients have successfully weathered intense pain and other effects of illness or had other adverse experiences related to illness and health care and have grown from them. Eliciting a history of past health problems can help nurses identify potential health problems as well as client strengths, as the following example illustrates.

- Mrs. Bertini is admitted to the hospital for an appendectomy. While obtaining the history of her health problem, the nurse asks about previous surgeries and finds out Mrs. Bertini had an operation as a child. Mrs. Bertini volunteers that she remembers having had unbearable pain and is worried about repeating that negative experience. The nurse notes this information and Mrs. Bertini's apparent need for preoperative teaching regarding patient-controlled pain relief measures.

Personal, Family, and Social History. The personal, family, and social history is one of the most important elements of the wellness/well-being assessment. This is the part of the history that deals with many of the particulars of wellness and well-being—information about life-style and habits, social and leisure life, spiritual and cultural values, and significantly, the client's sense of control over his or her life and personal satisfaction with life circumstances.

The personal, family, and social history is a process of real exchange between client and nurse. It is the part of the history in which nurses come to know a great deal about clients as individuals, the part in which clients share their goals and desires as well as life difficulties and problems. Moreover, in this part of the history nurses gain further knowledge about clients' overall health and their understanding of the factors that affect it. The personal, family, and social history involves two-way communication and presents an opportunity for nurse and client not only to identify, but also to discuss, possible factors that could lead to future health problems. Table 22–3 contains suggested questions for obtaining personal, family, and social history information relevant to client wellness and well-being. The following example illustrates the importance of a client's personal, family, and social history.

- Mr. Dodd is admitted to the hospital with a diagnosis of possible peptic ulcer disease after vomiting blood. The nurse pays special attention to his personal, family, and social history because of the association of stress with this disease. Mr. Dodd reports he was an executive in a major corporation but has been unemployed for the past 5 months. He has been looking for a job, but has found nothing satisfactory. He reports frequent arguments about money with his wife who recently returned to work as a legal secretary. Mr. Dodd said he had stopped smoking several years ago but started again 2 months ago. To get a clearer picture about Mr. Dodd's coping ability, the nurse asks Mr. Dodd about his understanding of the effects of stress on health, whether he exercises regularly, and what he does to relax. This initial sharing shows Mr. Dodd that the nurse is genuinely concerned, and provides the nurse with a clearer picture of what kind of assistance to offer Mr. Dodd.

Subjective Manifestations. Nurses' inquiries regarding subjective manifestations of well-being are essential to gain a comprehensive perspective on clients' symptoms. Table 22–4 reviews several areas that are important in a total assessment of well-being.

Wellness and Well-being Examination

The wellness examination produces a great deal of information about the client's level of fitness, nutrition, stress, and general health. This information is the basis for establishing wellness goals and provides the baseline for evaluating progress once implementation of approaches begins. Areas of particular importance when conducting a wellness examination are clients' vital signs, body weight, and general appearance. These are very important general indicators of wellness status.

Measurements

Vital Signs. Measurements of vital signs including pulse, respiration, and blood pressure and body weight are often affected by excessive stress or emotional reactions. Rapid heart rate; shortness of breath with rapid, shallow respirations; and elevated blood pressure may indicate severe anxiety, fear, or pain. Clients exhibiting these signs should be assessed carefully to determine the underlying cause.

Body Weight. Weight is used to assess the nutritional status of a client. Body weight should be compared to standardized norms and deviations greater than 10 percent should be assessed further with clients. Also, recent

TABLE 22–3. WELLNESS AND WELL-BEING HISTORY: PERSONAL, FAMILY, AND SOCIAL HISTORY QUESTIONS

A. **Vocational**
1. What type of work do you do?
2. Have you changed jobs recently?
3. How do you feel about your work?
4. Are you satisfied with your work?
5. What stresses are associated with your work? How do you handle them?
6. How do your family members feel about your work?
7. Are you optimistic about your prospects for the future?
8. Does your work bring you into contact with pesticides, solvents, x-rays, or other harmful agents?

B. **Home and Family**
1. Who are the members of your family who are most significant to you? What family members live with you? What are their relationships with you?
2. Where do you live? What type of residence is it?
3. How long have you lived at your current address?
4. Have there been any changes in your family group recently? Births? Deaths? Have you recently married, separated, divorced?
5. Are you financially responsible for any family members?
6. Do any of your family members have a chronic illness or serious disability?
7. Who acts as caretaker for him or her?
8. Are you satisfied with your family life?
9. What family problems most concern you?
10. Do you keep pesticides, solvents, or other potentially harmful substances in your home? How do you store them?
11. What precautions do you take to prevent fire and accidents in your home?
12. Do your family members wear seatbelts when driving?

C. **Social, Leisure, Spiritual, and Cultural**
1. What community groups are you a member of?
2. What do you do to relax?
3. Do you enjoy occasional solitude?
4. What hobbies do you enjoy?
5. Are you satisfied with your social relationships?
6. Do you enjoy your neighbors?
7. Do you have a circle of good friends?
8. Do you enjoy new people and getting to know them?
9. Do you feel your life has purpose?
10. Are there any routines or practices based on your ethnic origins that are important in your daily life?
11. Do you practice a religion? Which one?
12. Are there any special religious practices that are part of your daily routine?
13. Do you attend religious services? How often? Would you like to attend religious services or see the clergy while you are in the hospital?

D. **Sexual**
1. Are you satisfied with yourself in your role as a man or woman?
2. Have you had changes in your sex life recently? Have you noticed a change in your desire for sex?
3. Are you satisfied with your sex life?
4. What precautions do you take to prevent unwanted pregnancies? Sexually transmitted diseases?

E. **Habits**

Exercise
1. Do you engage in regular exercise? What type? How often?
2. Do you engage in recreational sports?
3. Do you do yoga, limbering, or stretching exercises?
4. Do you feel you are fit? Are you satisfied with your fitness program?
5. Have your exercise habits changed recently?

Sleep
1. How much sleep do you average a day?
2. Do you wake up feeling fresh and relaxed?
3. Do you fall asleep easily at night?
4. Do you sleep on a firm mattress?
5. Are you satisfied with the amount of rest you get?
6. Have your sleep habits changed recently?

Diet
1. What is your concept of the foods to include in a healthful diet?
2. Do you sometimes skip meals? Eat more than you should? Eat between-meal snacks?
3. Do you pay attention to the ingredients in the food you eat? Vitamins and minerals? Roughage and fiber? Saturated fats, cholesterol, salt, or processed sugar?
4. Do you read the labels for nutrients in packaged foods?
5. What guidelines do you follow for planning meals?
6. Have you changed your diet habits recently? For what reason?
7. Are you satisfied with your diet? With your weight? With your nutritional state?
8. Do you avoid any foods for health reasons? What foods? Are you aware of foods suspected to increase the risk of cancer and heart disease?
9. What problems do you encounter in providing a healthful diet for yourself and your family?

Beverages
1. Do you drink coffee, tea, and cola? How much do you drink per day?
2. Do you drink beer, wine, or other alcoholic beverages? How much do you drink a day?
3. Do you drink and drive?

Tobacco Use
1. Do you use tobacco? Do you know about the effects of tobacco on health?
2. Do you permit smoking in your house?

Other Substances
1. Do you use drugs to feel good? Get high? Relax? Reduce pain? What drugs do you use?
2. Have your substance use habits changed recently?
3. Do you use aerosol sprays?
4. Are there products that you avoid for health reasons? Which ones?

Hygiene
1. What are your regular personal hygiene habits?
2. Have you changed your habits recently?
3. Do you brush your teeth and floss regularly?
4. What do you do in your home to prevent the spread of illness in your family?

TABLE 22–3. (continued)

Health Assessment

1. Do you pay attention to the way your body looks and feels?
2. Do you know the seven early danger signs of cancer?
3. (If male) Do you know how to do a testicular self-examination? Do you do testicular self-examinations regularly?
4. (If female) Do you have a pap smear regularly? Do you know how to do a breast self-examination? Do you do breast self-examinations regularly?
5. Do you take your own pulse or blood pressure? What is your usual pulse? What is your usual blood pressure? Do you know what they should be?

F. **Psychological**

Stressors

1. Are you aware of any stress factors in your life? What are they?
2. What is your understanding of the effects of stress on health?
3. Do you feel happy, relaxed most of the time?
4. Have you had any big changes in your life recently? What were the effects on you, overall?
5. Are you accident prone?

Coping

1. What helps you most when you feel stressed?
2. Do you ever pamper yourself?
3. Do you meditate or use any relaxation methods regularly?
4. Have you attended classes to learn relaxation skills?
5. What outlets do you have for your emotions?
6. Do you consider it acceptable to cry, feel sad, angry, or afraid?
7. Are there people close to you with whom you can share problems?
8. Are you able to forget your problems when solutions are not possible?
9. Do you read articles or books about promoting health?
10. Do you find each day interesting and challenging?
11. Do you look forward to the future?
12. Do you try to keep yourself open to new experiences?
13. Are you able to laugh at yourself or laugh with others over something funny?
14. Do you tend to be shy or sensitive?

Sick Role/Health Beliefs

1. Do you believe that there are things you can do to make yourself well?
2. Does it seem to you that your health is affected by accidental happenings or luck?
3. Do you feel that your health depends on how well you take care of yourself?
4. Do you feel that you are to blame when you get sick?
5. Have you ever attended classes on personal health?
6. Who do you consult when you do not feel well?
7. Do you feel that it is important to consult health care professionals to maintain your health?
8. Do you have regular contact with your physician and dentist?
9. Do you ever question your health care professional or seek a second opinion when you do not agree with the recommended care or treatment?
10. Do your financial resources enable you to maintain routine, preventative health care?

changes in body weight may indicate need for further assessment. Unintentional weight loss or gain may signal physical illness or an emotional disturbance. For a detailed description of nutritional assessment, see Chapter 25.

Objective Manifestations

General Observations. General observations are an important aspect of a wellness examination. Wellness and well-being are reflected in facial expressions, eye movements, motor behavior and gestures, grooming and dress, and mood.

Facial Expression. Facial expression can indicate feelings of gladness, excitement, anger, strength, weakness, depression, or powerlessness. These expressions can be intentional or unintentional. Client feelings also are demonstrated by speech. Client speech can be described as calm, clear, articulate, slow, drawn out, excited, trembling, or garbled. Nurses should note facial expressions and verbal statements that do not seem to correspond. These require further assessment.

Eye Movement. Eye movement can indicate clients' emotions and well-being. Nurses should assess clients' use of eye contact during interaction. Too much eye contact may indicate anger or lack of trust in the nurse–client relationship. Too little eye contact can indicate anger or withdrawal. Poor eye contact can also result from a sense of hopelessness. Cultural factors, too, influence client eye contact.

Motor Behavior. Motor behavior reflects client wellness and relates to posture and kinetics (the nature of body movement). The manner in which individuals carry themselves indicates how they feel about themselves. An erect standing and sitting posture reflects wellness, while slouched posture and slumped positioning in a chair may reflect physical illness or emotional distress. Body movements and gestures also reveal feelings about self. Anxiety can be indicated by many behaviors such as toe tapping, constant, nonpurposeful hand movements, nail or lip biting, picking on hair, or trembling. In contrast, wellness is indicated by relaxed purposeful movements.

Grooming and Dress. Grooming and dress also express clients' feelings about themselves (see Chap. 23, Section 2 for more on this topic). The hygiene of the skin, hair, nails, and teeth are indicators of self-esteem. Inadequate hygiene can be related to low socioeconomic status or a sign of depres-

TABLE 22–4. SUBJECTIVE MANIFESTATIONS QUESTIONS RELATED TO WELLNESS AND WELL-BEING

A. **General**
   1. Do you generally feel healthy and energetic?
   2. Do you have any aches, pains, or other symptoms that bother you?
   3. Do you ever become angry or agitated over little things?
   4. Are you frequently nervous?

B. **Integumentary**
   1. What do you do to protect your skin from the sun?
   2. Do you sweat profusely when it is not hot?

C. **HEENT (head, eyes, ears, nose, and throat)**
   1. Are you bothered by frequent colds? Allergies?
   2. Does your mouth ever feel dry when you are not thirsty?
   3. Do you have trouble with your eyesight? Hearing?

D. **Chest, cardiovascular**
   1. Do you ever have difficulty breathing?
   2. Does your heart ever seem to pound?

E. **Gastrointestinal**
   1. Do you have difficulty digesting your food?
   2. Are you bothered by an upset or acid stomach?
   3. Do you have a soft, formed bowel movement regularly without discomfort?

F. **Musculoskeletal**
   1. Do your joints hurt when you move?
   2. Do you experience neck stiffness or muscle tension?
   3. Do you suffer from muscle twitches?

G. **Neurological**
   1. Do you have difficulty with balance?
   2. Do you ever stutter or stammer when you speak?
   3. Are you bothered by headaches?
   4. Do you ever feel lightheaded or faint?

sion or hopelessness. Moreover, hygiene (or the lack of it) has a bearing on well-being and wellness. Poor hygiene increases clients' exposure to potential infectious organisms. Cleanliness promotes wellness by supporting the body's natural defense mechanisms and thereby reducing a client's risk for infection. Dress is related to hygiene. Clothes are also a defense against illness and injury, and therefore should be appropriate to the season.

Mood. Mood registers the inner experience of an individual. It is a subjective overall impression of how an individual feels. Assess affect in the context of the other general observations reviewed. Does the client display feelings of anxiety or fear such as irritability, nervous laughter, or general nervousness? Demonstrate depression or hopelessness by a flat affect or withdrawal from social contact? Portray a "genuineness"? Does the client share "true feelings"?

Integument. Assess the overall condition of the skin. Intact skin is an important first line of defense against infection. Note skin color, temperature, and moisture. Healthy skin is dry, warm, and neither pale nor flushed. Is there excess perspiration? Skin pallor and clamminess can occur in response to stress. Sympathetic stimuli, common in anxiety, cause vasoconstriction with pallor and coolness of the skin. Conversely, physical and emotional stress may increase body metabolism and raise body temperature. The body responds with vasodilation and increased sweat production to promote heat loss by evaporation. Sweat glands are most numerous on the palms of the hands and soles of the feet, so sweaty palms and feet may indicate a stress response.

HEENT (Head, Eyes, Ears, Nose, and Throat). Assess the eyes and mucous membranes of the mouth for signs of a stress response. Fatigue, tiredness, apprehension, or fear can often be noted in a client's eyes. The sympathetic nervous system stimulates contraction of the radial muscle of the iris, producing pupil dilatation and increased visual acuity, while decreasing saliva producing mouth dryness.

Chest. As noted earlier, respiratory rate may increase in response to stress. Hyperventilation, when extreme, can result in loss of consciousness. In most instances, clients will experience paresthesia (an abnormal sensation such as numbness or tingling), faintness, or impaired consciousness, but will not actually lose consciousness. Respiratory signs can also provide clues to relaxation. The smooth muscles of the respiratory passages relax in response to sympathetic stimulation, resulting in bronchodilation. This is to improve oxygenation during "fight-or-flight". (For more information on the fight-or-flight response see Chap. 6.) During relaxation, however, parasympathetic stimulus produces bronchoconstriction. Noisy breathing heard when someone dozes or sleeps is the result of parasympathetic-induced bronchoconstriction. Thus noisy breathing can signify relaxation.

Cardiovascular. As noted earlier, cardiovascular changes occur in response to stress-induced sympathetic stimulus. Increased pulse rate and cardiac contractility increase cardiac output. Anxiety and stress can increase the heart rate to over 100 beats per minute, called sinus tachycardia. Most clients will not experience symptoms but some may describe palpitations (a sensation of pounding of the heart). Increased sympathetic tone can also trigger a cardiac arrhythmia such as premature heart contractions. Clients usually are unaware of this change in heart rate and rhythm, but those having numerous premature beats may experience palpitations or a "missed beat" and notice an irregular heart rhythm. These clients need further evaluation (see Chap. 27). Medical treatment may be required and is focused on correcting the underlying cause.

Stress also produces blood pressure elevations as a result of several factors, including constriction of blood vessels in the skin, kidneys, and abdominal organs; elevated levels of norepinephrine; and increased blood volume, as in response to increased renin and mineralocorticoid secretion. Vessels in the heart and skeletal muscles dilate with sympathetic stimulation to provide oxygen and nutrients for action. Collaboration in stress management is an important nursing intervention for clients who have stress-related cardiovascular symptoms. Relaxation, a parasympathetic response, slows metabolism, producing a corresponding decrease in heart rate and blood pressure.

Abdomen. Assess the abdomen for gastric and abdominal discomfort. Loss of appetite, indigestion, nausea and/or vomiting, abdominal cramping or pain, diarrhea, constipation, bloating, or flatus may be stress related. Gastric motility, blood supply, and acid secretion are increased by anxiety and decreased by depression. The sympathetic nervous system triggers constriction of duodenal blood vessels, making its mucosa vulnerable to trauma from gastric acid. Ulcers in the duodenum—that is, open lesions in the mucous membrane of that part of the intestine—are a common result of chronic stress.

What are the client's bowel habits? Assess for abdominal distension and auscultate bowel sounds. Peristalsis is decreased and anal sphincters contract in response to sympathetic stimulus, predisposing individuals to constipation, bloating, and flatus. Parasympathetic dominance, which may result from chronic stress, may cause irritable bowel syndrome with alternating diarrhea and constipation. Chapters 16 and 26 address the gastrointestinal assessment in greater detail.

Genitourinary. Assess the client's urinary output. Stress triggers increased aldosterone production, promoting sodium and water reabsorption by the kidneys and decreased urine output (for more on this subject, see Chaps. 26 and 31). Sympathetic stimulus activates relaxation of the detrusor muscle (bladder) and contraction of the urinary sphincter, also reducing urinary output. Relaxation promotes parasympathetic stimulation that facilitates urination by contraction of the bladder muscle and relaxation of the urinary sphincter. Parasympathetic dominance with chronic stress can cause urinary frequency.

Musculoskeletal. Note muscle strength and tone, range of motion, and activity tolerance. Anxiety-induced sympathetic stimulation produces increased muscle tension to bolster motor activity in the "fight-or-flight" response. Excessive tension can lead to muscle twitching, stiffness, fatigue, and general body aches and pains, especially in the chest, back, and neck. Parasympathetic stimulation results in loss of skeletal muscle tone. See Chapter 30 for a full mobility assessment.

Functional mobility is a critical element of well-being and wellness. Exercise increases skeletal muscle flexibility and efficiency, cardiac efficiency, and peripheral blood flow. It improves coordination, respiratory functioning, sleep, and vitality because fatigue is reduced. Activity in the form of exercise slows the effects of aging by preventing osteoporosis. Exercise promotes general well-being and enhances muscle tone, strength, and general fitness (see Chap. 30).

Neurological. Assess for headaches, hyperattentiveness, restlessness, irritability, inability to concentrate or relax, and insomnia. Examine mental status to determine whether client is experiencing abnormalities in thinking, feeling, or behaving. These observations can be made while providing routine client care. A baseline mental status assessment (discussed in Chap. 16) is essential. See also Chapter 29 for a complete discussion of neurosensory integration. Any mental dysfunction noted during care can be compared to the baseline assessment. Sympathetic nervous stimulation increases mental alertness and mental activity. Sustained stimulation produces the symptoms of anxiety but eventually causes lethargy, fatigue, lack of initiative, inactivity, and withdrawal due to exhaustion and parasympathetic dominance. Signs of altered mental status such as increased confusion, memory loss, and change in emotional response may be the result of disease processes, medication side effects, sensory overload or deprivation, depression, or hopelessness. These changes in mental status can be related to chronic stress, illness, or hospitalization. Elderly clients are especially susceptible to confusion as a result of a sudden change in their environment such as a move to an extended care facility or hospital. Existing sensory deficits need to be noted. Visual and auditory deficits occur with aging. If the loss occurred gradually over a number of years, elderly clients may have adapted in their home environment and be unaware of the loss. A new, strange environment may accentuate these sensory deficits. Collaborative client care is required to deal with these needs.

Diagnostic Tests

Every diagnostic test bears in some way on clients' wellness. Some tests reveal information on nutritional health (found in Chap. 25), while some reveal information about cardiovascular status (Chap. 27), musculoskeletal fitness (Chap. 30), or neurosensory integration (Chap. 29). The reader is referred to those chapters for information on those diagnostic tests. The discussion in this section focuses specifically on tests that reveal data about the physical changes related to stress.

Several laboratory tests and the electrocardiogram can detect a possible stress response and yield valuable information for assessing well-being. Client preparation for these tests is important because physical and emotional stress often alters results. Nurses should review clients' understanding of diagnostic tests and prepare clients or educate them for self-preparation. Although the diagnostic tests discussed in this section reflect something about clients' stress response, they are not usually ordered by the physician for that general reason. Rather, they are ordered to pinpoint a specific pathophysiological problem or to assist in narrowing the differential diagnosis. Nurses, however, can incorporate test results to establish nursing diagnoses and should examine clients' medical records for completed tests that reflect fitness, nutrition, and stress level.

Laboratory Tests. Blood and urine tests that may reflect physiological response to stress include blood glucose levels, free fatty acid levels, and 24-hour urine tests for vanillylmandelic acid (VMA).

Blood glucose is regulated primarily by the hormones insulin and glucagon. Other hormones that contribute to glucose metabolism include adrenocorticotropic hormone (ACTH), epinephrine, and adrenocorticosteroids. Secretion of these hormones is increased by stress-induced stimulation of the sympathetic nervous system. Increased amounts of these hormones and gluconeogenesis causes elevated blood sugar (hyperglycemia). Therefore, acute stress may cause elevations of blood sugar in otherwise healthy individuals. Fasting blood sugar (FBS) is used to assess altered glucose metabolism. The client must not eat for at least 4 hours prior to the test, but may drink water. Adult reference values for fasting serum are 70 to 110 mg/dL.[86]

Free fatty acids are formed in the body by the breakdown of triglycerides and lipoproteins. Anxiety and the "fight-or-flight" response increases free fatty acid levels. Excessive fatty acids are associated with elevated levels of very-low-density lipoproteins. These lipoproteins are atherogenic; that is, they promote atherosclerosis, the fatty degeneration and thickening of blood vessel walls. High levels increase the client's risk of coronary artery disease. The free fatty acid test requires a fasting venous blood sample. Adult reference values are 8 to 20 mg/dL.[86]

Urine studies are used to assess adrenal function. The adrenal medulla secretes two hormones, epinephrine and norepinephrine, called catecholamines. These hormones are used by the body in its "fight-or-flight" response to stress. Vanillylmandelic acid (VMA), a major product of catecholamine breakdown, is used as a screening test.

All catecholamine metabolite urine tests require a 24-hour urine specimen (see Chap. 26). It is important that all urine be saved for 24 hours and that the specimen be kept cold to reduce bacterial growth. Certain foods such as coffee, tea, chocolate, carbonated beverages, bananas, avocados, and vanilla extract must be restricted because they interfere with test results. However, the client should not fast, as fasting increases catecholamine levels. Ideally, clients should stop taking any drugs that act on the sympathetic nervous system 3 to 7 days before the test, for accurate results. An acid preservative may need to be added to the urine collection bottle. Blood pressure, height, and weight should be recorded on the lab slip, along with the date and time the collection started and ended. Adult reference value for the VMA test is 0.7 to 6.8 mg/24 hours.[86] If it is abnormal, other catecholamine metabolite urine tests will be done.

Electrocardiogram. A discussion of the electrocardiogram (ECG) and the nurse's role can be found in Section 2 of Chapter 27. Relevant portions of an ECG tracing, along with an interpretation of their significance, are frequently found in the medical record. The ECG tracing reveals electrographic evidence of tachycardia, arrhythmias, and premature beats, all of which can be stress related. These findings have particular significance as a stress response when the physician finds no other evidence of pathology.

NURSING DIAGNOSIS OF WELLNESS AND WELL-BEING STATUS

The assessment phase culminates in the formulation of diagnostic statements that identify actual or potential client problems that require nursing implementation. The formulation of nursing diagnoses involves the analysis and interpretation of assessment data that have been collected and validated. Conclusions are drawn regarding client concerns, responses, needs, and problems.

Accurate identification of appropriate nursing diagnoses is the most important and difficult step of the nursing process. It requires an ability to integrate data, using critical thinking skills and sound clinical judgments (see Chap. 17). Client collaboration is essential because self-responsibility is enhanced when clients participate actively in the identification of nursing diagnoses. For the diagnostic statement to be useful, it must label the problem and contain a description of the etiology or probable cause of the problem. Inclusion of the etiology individualizes the diagnostic statement and forms the foundation for the development of an individualized plan of care.

Because of the holistic nature of well-being and wellness, all approved nursing diagnoses reflect an alteration in well-being and wellness in one form or another. A discussion of some of the most significant diagnoses related to well-being and wellness, including defining characteristics (subjective and objective data) and the established etiologies for each of these diagnoses, are presented in this chapter. Additional diagnoses that reflect well-being and wellness are presented in later chapters of Unit VI.

Health-seeking Behaviors

Health-seeking behavior is defined as a situation in which a client, while in stable health, actively seeks ways to change life-style, health habits, and/or the environment in order to achieve a higher level of well-being and wellness. Unlike the majority of nursing diagnoses, this diagnostic statement reflects a positive condition in which an individual is striving for high-level wellness. The key defining characteristic is the client's desire for information to promote health.

Specific etiologic factors have not been identified for this diagnosis. However, it can be appropriately applied to clients who are actively seeking knowledge about health and how to achieve it, who are expressing an interest in increased exercise or self-care, or who are expressing concerns regarding the impact of environmental factors on their health status. More detailed defining characteristics are provided in the table Sample Nursing Diagnoses for Wellness and Well-being on pages 757–758.

SAMPLE NURSING DIAGNOSES: WELLNESS AND WELL-BEING

Nursing Diagnosis	Defining Characteristics/Manifestations: Subjective Data	Defining Characteristics/Manifestations: Objective Data	Etiology
Health-seeking Behaviors: Seeks out and participates in weight-loss program 5.4	Asks questions regarding healthy weight loss methods. Verbalizes concern about weight. Verbalizes concern regarding family health history/personal risk for developing disease due to excess weight. Verbalizes desire to alter dietary habits.	Actively participates in prescribed dietary/activity program Joins support group to reinforce lifestyle change.	*Cognitive:* Exposure to information regarding health risks associated with obesity
Altered Health Maintenance: Substance abuse 6.4.2	Reports frequent feelings of being overwhelmed. States is worried about using "too much booze and pills." Verbalizes difficulty managing stressors without drugs/alcohol.	Smell of alcohol detected during visit. Displays flat affect (eg, does not participate in care, initiate interaction). Speaks in monotone. Limited eye contact with nurse.	*Emotional:* Ineffective individual coping.
Anxiety 9.3.1	"I feel so wound up." My stomach feels like it's tied in knots." "I am so afraid of what they might find."	Heart rate 80. Trembling. Restlessness. Unable to remember instructions given to prepare for diagnostic test. Poor eye contact when speaking. Awake most of previous night.	*Physical:* Threat to health status: Uncertainty about result of diagnostic tests.
Fear of pain 9.3.2	Reports of distress. States feelings of dread or apprehension: "I'm afraid of severe pain." "I can't handle it." Verbal reports of insomnia, nausea, palpitations. Many questions about upcoming surgery. "I've never had surgery. I don't know what to expect."	Pulse increased above baseline. Respiratory rate increased above baseline. Drawn expression when discussing surgery. Refuses meals.	*Cognitive:* Knowledge deficit: Pain associated with surgery.
Powerlessness 7.3.2	"It doesn't matter what I want—I can't do it anyway." "There's nothing I can do—they make the rules." "What do I know about any of this?"	Lack of participation in treatments or daily regimen. Refuses to participate in decision making (eg, when to bathe or get out of bed).	*Environmental:* Illness-related regimen.
Hopelessness 7.3.1	"I don't have any energy—it doesn't make sense. I don't do anything. They won't let me." "I may as well give up—all I can do is lay here." "Why bother."	Infrequent eye contact. Excessive sleep (more than 12 hours/day). Withdraws from social contact. Passively allows care. Refuses to participate in self-care.	*Environmental:* Prolonged activity restrictions.
	Verbal expressions of profound despair: "I'm never going to get better." "Don't waste your time on me." "I don't want to live like this." "Nothing I do will help."	Excessive sleep (more than 12 hours/day). Withdraws from social contact. Passively allows care. Refuses to participate in self-care. Eating less than 50% of diet. Decreased verbalization.	*Physical:* Deteriorating physiological condition: AIDS.
Spiritual Distress 4.1.1	"I need my priest to give me communion." "God seems so far away since I can't go to mass." "I don't understand why God let this happen to me."	Personal clergy unable to visit due to distance.	*Self-Conceptual:* Separation from religious ties.

(continued)

SAMPLE NURSING DIAGNOSES: WELLNESS AND WELL-BEING (continued)

Nursing Diagnosis	Risk Factors
Potential for Infection *1.2.1.1*	Physical Invasive procedures: Foley catheter. Peripheral IV fluids while n.p.o. Central line for parenteral nutrition. Decreased WBCs.
Potential for Infection *1.2.1.1*	Receiving chemotherapy. Tissue destruction: Excoriation from fecal incontinence. Raw perianal area associated with urinary incontinence. Red open area on sacrum. "My bottom sure is sore."

Alteration in Health Maintenance

Alteration in health maintenance describes a client at risk for illness or disease because of an inability to identify, manage, or explore options to maintain wellness. The presence of unhealthy life-style behaviors is a major defining characteristic of this nursing diagnosis. Etiologic factors include alterations in communication skills; perceptual–cognitive impairments such as confusion; ineffective individual or family coping; unachieved developmental tasks; and lack of material resources.

Etiology: Alterations in Communication Skills. Communication profoundly affects an individual's ability to maintain or promote health. Impaired verbal skills or language differences prevent a client from expressing health needs or communicating effectively with health care professionals. A client's inability to provide a nurse or physician with accurate assessment data may result in erroneous or ineffective treatment of illness or disease. Language differences also may impair the effectiveness of health education or discharge teaching.

Etiology: Perceptual–Cognitive Impairments. Perceptual–cognitive function is the ability to gather information through the senses and process that information through intellectual skills such as understanding and reasoning. Perceptual–cognitive impairments include limitation of the senses such as blindness or deafness, or brain dysfunction such as memory loss or confusion. These impairments may reduce the level of knowledge an individual acquires about a health condition or prescribed treatment. A lack of ability to make deliberate and thoughtful judgments can create a delay in seeking professional assistance. Signs and symptoms of disease may be ignored or disregarded as irrelevant. Health education or discharge instructions may be misinterpreted, not assimilated and remembered, or not followed, resulting in inadequate health maintenance or an exacerbation of disease.

Etiology: Ineffective Individual or Family Coping. Strategies that enable a person to deal with life difficulties are coping mechanisms. They may be personal behaviors such as working out to reduce tension, or crying, or family-based behaviors such as turning to a parent for love and support. Ineffective coping occurs when an individual or family uses strategies such as avoidance of a problem that prevent reduction of stress in a healthy manner. Ineffective coping can lead to altered health maintenance in several ways. Health practices may suffer because of preoccupation with individual or family problems. Or, individuals may develop unhealthful coping habits such as smoking, alcohol or drug abuse, or eating disorders. Inability to cope effectively with life stressors can actually increase clients' needs for health maintenance by predisposing them to stress disorders and lowering their resistance to disease.

Etiology: Unachieved Developmental Tasks. Unachieved developmental tasks implies an individual's failure to meet a developmental goal that is appropriate to his or her age. For instance, a 30-year-old man who states he continues living at home so his mother can cook, clean, and do his laundry for him has not achieved the level of independence expected for adults. An individual's potential level of wellness can be significantly altered by unachieved developmental tasks. Lack of education about nutrition, safety, fitness, or health-protecting practices during childhood or adolescence can have a significant impact on adult health. An inability to meet basic needs for safety and security, or love and belonging, at various developmental stages, may result in the development of a distorted value system or a lack of motivation for self-care.

Etiology: Lack of Material Resources. Lack of material resources results most commonly from inadequate financial resources for the essentials of daily life, such as food, clothing, and access to health care. It is a major barrier to health maintenance. Increasing numbers of people in the United

States lack financial resources and access to adequate health services. Many rural and inner-city areas have a severe shortage of qualified physicians and other health care professionals. The overwhelming cost of health care services prohibits many individuals from seeking health assistance. Financial barriers are not limited to unemployed or lower-class clients. Many middle-class families are unable to afford adequate health insurance and may avoid seeking medical care until health problems interfere significantly with their lives. Preventive and health-promoting services such as mammograms for women and immunizations for infants and children are often not reimbursed by standard health insurance policies and may be unaffordable luxuries for many individuals. (See Chap. 35 for further discussion of health care delivery.)

Diversional Activity Deficit

Diversional activity deficit describes a state in which clients experience reduced stimulation from or interest in recreational activities. The major defining characteristic is an observed or stated boredom caused by inactivity. Etiologic factors include lack of diversional activity in the environment, long-term hospitalization, and frequent or lengthy treatments.

Etiology: Lack of Diversional Activity in the Environment; Long-term Hospitalization. Reduced diversional activity is often experienced by immobilized clients and may result in boredom or depression. Even clients who initially were able to cope effectively with hospitalization may begin to experience diversional activity problems when their confinement becomes prolonged.

Standard hospital diversions such as television or radio may be meaningless to someone who is not interested in typical commercial television programs or for someone with severe hearing or visual problems. Also, these diversions are not as meaningful for clients experiencing pain or emotional upset. Unable to participate in their usual hobbies or recreational activities and confined to a monotonous environment, clients often begin to display emotional hostility or apathy in response to their situation.

These same symptoms may also be found in individuals who are adapting to major life changes. When children leave home or individuals retire, many routine daily activities are eliminated. This may leave individuals feeling "lost" and not knowing quite what to do. Elderly clients who experience sensory losses are also vulnerable to inadequate diversional activity. Severe apathy and depression are characteristic of many of the residents of long-term care facilities.

Etiology: Frequent or Lengthy Treatments. Long-term care can seriously affect client well-being. For example, clients who must spend long hours each week attached to renal dialysis machines often become frustrated and angry at their confinement and inability to perform normal activities. Clients undergoing chemotherapy or radiation therapy also are often required to spend countless hours in health care facilities without the benefit of diversional or recreational activities.

Anxiety

Anxiety is defined as a vague feeling of uneasiness or apprehension that clients cannot relate to an identifiable source or threat. Anxiety is associated with future, anticipated events. Any change or threat of change in an individual's life situation can create stress and anxiety. A degree of anxiety is healthy because it motivates growth. Severe anxiety interferes with normal activity and is detrimental to wellness and well-being. Etiologic factors include threat to or change in health status and threat to or change in environment.

Etiology: Threat to or Change in Health Status. Illness and treatment of illness, whether as outpatient or inpatient, cause stress and anxiety. Illness frequently requires individuals to change routines and habits. Change in behavior pattern or habits often creates stress. Habits develop because they meet some basic need. Changes in health status may also cause changes in one's body structure and function. This may threaten identity and therefore well-being. These threats may be so severe or so obscure that clients may be unable to identify the source of the threat but, nevertheless, experience apprehension. Client anxiety regarding change or threat to health status sometimes serves as the motivation for developing new wellness behaviors.

Etiology: Threat to or Change in Environment. The environment a person chooses as part of the life structure reveals many things about that person and about what he or she considers important. Environment generally includes the person's home, work milieu, area for activities, and area for interpersonal contact; however, it can include a hospital bed that a client identifies as his or her own. Environment can be the basis for a sense of security. Thus, a disruption or change in environment can lead to anxiety.

Fear

Fear is defined as a feeling of apprehension that clients can validate and relate to an identifiable source. It often engenders feelings of powerlessness or loss of control. The sensations associated with fear characterize the absence of well-being. Fear is related closely to anxiety and elicits many of the same physiological and emotional responses. As discussed earlier, fear differs from anxiety in that with fear individuals can identify the actual threat, whereas with anxiety the source of discomfort is unknown. Because the source of fear can be identified, the actual threat should be named in the diagnostic statement (eg, fear of pain, fear of mutilation, or fear of death). Fear can occur in response to a variety of health situations or problems. Some etiologic factors include environmental stimuli, lack of knowledge, and separation from one's support system in a potentially threatening situation.

Etiology: Environmental Stimuli. Clients are often threatened by environmental stimuli. Loud noises, darkness, strangers, and heights are fears shared by many people. Health care environments include many unfamiliar sounds, smells, and people and can be very frightening places, especially for children. Children may also fear strange equipment or machines, needles, and diagnostic or therapeutic procedures. Adults more often fear the discomfort that equipment like needles or procedures can cause. Fear triggered by environmental stimuli may seriously threaten well-being.

Etiology: Knowledge Deficit. Unfamiliarity with a situation leaves individuals especially vulnerable to fear. Fear of the unknown is particularly stressful. Imagination can compound fear as individuals attempt to envision potential outcomes. In the Hospital Stress Rating Scale developed by Volicer and Bohannon, seven of the ten most stressful items noted are related to fear of the unknown (eg, thinking you might lose your sight, thinking you might have cancer, not being told what your diagnosis is, not knowing the results or reasons for treatment, and so on.[86] Lack of knowledge contributes to a fear of loss of control. Knowledge of what to expect in a given situation promotes a sense of control. Nurses can decrease much of the stress and fear encountered by clients through meaningful and accurate communication. Adequate preparation of clients for tests and procedures can eliminate unnecessary stress.

Etiology: Separation from Support Systems. The fear response is exacerbated during potentially threatening situations by separation from support systems. Although this reaction may be most pronounced in children who are separated from parents, it is a universal experience. Clients faced with threatening situations such as hospitalization, invasive diagnostic procedures, or surgery, need the support and comfort of their significant others. Having to face such frightening situations alone may be overwhelming.

Powerlessness

Powerlessness is defined as a client's perceived lack of control over a current situation, immediate event, or future outcome. The key defining characteristic is an expressed inability to control. This is in conflict with well-being, which requires a perception of control over life events and a sense of satisfaction with life circumstances. In powerlessness, individuals have the expectation that the outcome of their behaviors is not determined by what they do (internal control) but rather by the influence of outside forces (external control). Major etiologic factors include the health care environment, an illness-related regimen, and interpersonal interactions.

Etiology: Health Care Environment. The impact of the health care environment on an individual's sense of control was discussed earlier in this chapter and in Chapter 12. Lack of privacy, altered personal territory, and the forced dependent status often found in acute care settings dramatically alter an individual's sense of control. Generally, clients who exhibit an orientation toward internal control will experience greater distress in an acute health care environment than clients with an external control orientation because the former are more self-directed.

Etiology: Illness-related Regimen. Medical care can create a sense of powerlessness, especially when all treatment choices seem undesirable. The illness removes power to make choices because clients face deteriorating health if they do not participate in the treatment regimen. Nurses can promote clients' feelings of control and power in these situations with empathetic listening and by helping clients to define what power they have within the prescribed regimen. Nurses can then support clients in seizing that power.

Etiology: Interpersonal Interaction. Interaction between clients and health care professionals profoundly affects clients' sense of control. Lack of explanations from caregivers or a lack of collaboration with clients regarding health care decisions increases clients' sense of powerlessness. To promote clients' sense of personal power, nurses need to make an effort to involve clients in mutual planning about their care. Collaborative care is characterized by the avoidance of paternalism, the philosophy that the health care professional "knows best." Even clients who are debilitated, are still able to make some choices and decisions. Retaining a sense of power and control enhances clients' self-esteem and gives meaning to life. Prolonged states of powerlessness ultimately lead to hopelessness.

Hopelessness

Hopelessness is a subjective state in which clients feel that alternatives or personal choices are limited or nonexistent. This results in inability to mobilize energy for solving health problems. Hopelessness is the absence of optimism that is such an important part of well-being. Like powerlessness, hopelessness represents personal loss of control. The major defining characteristic of hopelessness is passivity, which is manifested by decreased verbalization and/or decreased affect. Etiologic factors include prolonged activity restriction, deteriorating physiological conditions, long-term stress, and loss of spiritual belief or belief in individual transcendent values.

Etiology: Prolonged Activity Restrictions. Functional mobility is a vital component of well-being because mobility confers independence. Prolonged activity restrictions create feelings of isolation and helplessness. Limitations on activity, therefore, can have a devastating effect on an individual's self-esteem and sense of purpose in life. Clients may exhibit signs of profound depression or apathy and may show little interest in participating in the limited activities available to them.

Etiology: Deteriorating Physiological Conditions. Although clients can experience wellness and well-being without every body system functioning optimally, generalized deterioration signifies impending cessation of function. This implies dependence and, eventually, death.

Heart disease, kidney disorders, respiratory failure, cancer, and AIDS are examples of progressive conditions in which clients experience increasing pain, discomfort, or weakness. Although many people are able to cope successfully with long-term chronic diseases for many years, prolonged treatments with no positive results or the development of new or unexpected symptoms may leave individuals feeling that all the effort has been futile and that no solution is possible.

Etiology: Long-term Stress. As discussed in Section 1, stress is a direct threat to well-being, particularly when it is long term. Stress associated with failure to achieve valued life goals (marriage, children, financial success) despite prolonged effort may leave individuals feeling exhausted and without options. Extended caretaking responsibilities for a disabled or ill child, spouse, or parent also saps strength and may eventually overwhelm the caretaker.

Hopelessness that develops from the effects of long-term stress is not necessarily the result of a catastrophic event. The cumulative effect of daily pressures, environmental stressors, and normal developmental life changes may deplete energy reserves and coping resources. If an additional, unexpected stressor such as hospitalization or illness occurs, vulnerable individuals may feel completely overwhelmed.

Etiology: Loss of Spiritual Beliefs or Belief in Individual Transcendent Values. Hope is often closely linked with spiritual well-being. It arises from an individual's faith, life goals, relationships with others, feeling needed, and having something to accomplish. Crisis events in individuals' lives such as the loss of someone or something valued (spouse, child, friend, financial security, health, job) may be accompanied by a loss of individual spiritual beliefs or belief in transcendent values. Such a loss can leave individuals feeling that there is no purpose in life. Religious individuals may feel that God has deserted them and may question their most fundamental values. Such profound spiritual distress may render individuals more susceptible to physical or mental deterioration. See also the following nursing diagnosis, Spiritual distress.

Spiritual Distress

Spiritual distress describes clients experiencing a disturbance in their value and belief system: those principles that integrate and give meaning to their lives. As discussed above, spiritual values and beliefs that give life meaning and purpose are essential to well-being. The major defining characteristics of this diagnosis are behaviors that suggest disruption in values and beliefs such as questioning the meaning of life, death, and suffering. Etiologic factors include separation from religious or cultural ties and change in beliefs or value system.

Etiology: Separation from Religious or Cultural Ties. Beliefs and values are formed by many factors including religion and culture. These factors shape a client's concept of well-being. Beliefs and values based on religious and cultural ties provide some clients with a frame of reference used to organize information and are a powerful resource for adapting to stress. Therefore, separation from religious and cultural ties because of illness or hospitalization can significantly threaten clients' well-being.

Etiology: Challenged Belief or Value System. Beliefs and values are an integral part of life. They frequently assume increased importance during a time of stress such as illness or hospitalization. New situations and experiences can force individuals to face aspects of reality they have not considered or ever imagined could occur. For example, treatment of severe health problems such as organ failure (heart, liver, kidney, lung) may challenge a client's or family member's definition of life and death. When events challenge the core values that formerly guided a client's decision-making, the sense of uncertainty and isolation that ensues is often profound.

Potential for Infection

Potential for infection is the state in which clients are at an increased risk for attack by pathogenic organisms. As discussed in Section 1, illness and hospitalization greatly increase an individual's potential for infection because of compromised body defenses and a high concentration of organisms within the physical environment. Environmental exposure, invasive procedures, tissue destruction, malnutrition, and the effects of pharmaceutical agents are all risk factors because they affect the body's primary and secondary defenses against infection. As discussed in Chapter 17, multiple risk factors must be present for a client to be diagnosed as having Potential for infection.

Risk Factor: Environmental Exposure. Minimizing the number and kinds of organisms to which clients are exposed promotes wellness by reducing the risk of infection. Potential for infection is reduced by eliminating reservoirs of organisms, controlling portals of exit and entry into the potential host, and controlling the transmission of organisms. See Chapter 7 for more about environmental exposure and health. Environmental exposure is controlled by use of proper handwashing and sterile technique for invasive procedures, discussed in Chapter 24.

Risk Factor: Tissue Destruction/Invasive Procedures. Normal body defense mechanisms are threatened by all invasive procedures, diagnostic or therapeutic. Skin and mucous membranes provide a first line of defense, physically and chemically. Sweat glands prevent overgrowth of bacteria. The skin's acid pH prevents pathogenic organisms from growing on the skin. Traumatic opening of the skin, whether therapeutic, such as an intravenous line, or accidental, increases the client's risk for infection (see also Chap. 24). Any procedure involving invasion of body boundaries or entering body cavities with instruments or devices carries with it the risk of introducing pathogenic organisms or providing a vehicle for access. For example, invasion of the bladder by a catheter is a common risk factor for infection in hospitalized clients.

Risk Factor: Malnutrition. Nutrition influences primary and secondary defense mechanisms. Adequate protein, carbohydrate, fat, and vitamin and mineral intake is needed to maintain tissue integrity and promote wound healing. Good nutrition promotes protein synthesis necessary for production of leukocytes for phagocytosis of invading pathogens. Malnutrition slows healing and compromises defenses, increasing the body's vulnerability to infection. See Chapter 25 for more about the role of nutrition in health.

Risk Factor: Effects of Pharmaceutical Agents. Some drugs pose a threat to secondary lines of defense. For example, corticosteroid therapy and chemotherapy are immunosuppressives, meaning they interfere with the body mechanisms that identify and destroy pathogens. Antibiotics are used to inhibit growth or kill pathogens. Although given to destroy disease-producing organisms, they may also destroy normal flora that are part of the body's natural defense against infection. Chemotherapy is effective against cancer cells because they are rapidly dividing cells. Areas in the body in which normal cells undergo rapid mitotic division, such as bone marrow (where leukocytes are produced), are also affected by chemotherapeutic agents. Bone marrow suppression results in decreased numbers of leukocytes, leaving the individual vulnerable to infection.

Stating the Wellness and Well-being Diagnosis

A nursing diagnosis of the client's wellness and well-being status is the basis for mutual planning. An effective diagnostic statement identifies the problem, a specific etiology, and the defining characteristics exhibited by the client.

The taxonomy of nursing diagnoses lists general etiologies for nursing diagnoses related to altered wellness and well-being. These etiologies have been discussed. General etiologies or contributing factors can be made more specific with assessment of the individual client. Specific contributing factors are important because they direct nursing implementation. Client care is often based on the etiology of an identified problem.

The taxonomy also lists many signs and symptoms called defining characteristics that are associated with each nursing diagnosis. No individual client experiences all of these signs and symptoms at one time. Including clients' signs and symptoms in the diagnostic statements facilitates development and evaluation of desired outcomes. The following are examples of complete statements of a wellness and well-being nursing diagnosis.

> Fear of dying related to first hospitalization as evidenced by "I have never been in the hospital before," "I'm afraid of it because my mother died in the hospital 15 years ago"; pulse rate of 100; respirations 32, clinging to overnight bag while sitting in chair; and tense erect posture while in bed.
>
> Hopelessness related to long-term stress of caring for house-bound husband for the past 8 months as evidenced by "I can't take any more of this—I feel like I don't have a life"; "I used to get out of the house, but I don't want anyone to visit"; "I don't know what to do"; no eye contact made during history taking.
>
> Potential for infection; risk factors: 75-year-old client with chronic lung disease admitted to hospital for abdominal surgery; indwelling Foley catheter and intravenous line; client reports poor appetite, eats only one meal a day.

Assessment of wellness and well-being is the process of collecting data for identification of actual or potential client care problems. Assessment is not only the first step in the nursing process, but an ongoing component of all other steps in the process. Analysis of that data in collaboration with clients leads to identification of problem areas and the formulation of individualized nursing diagnoses and a client care plan.

Section 3. Nurse–Client Management of Wellness and Well-being

Management of wellness and well-being encompasses planning, implementing, and evaluating client care related to promoting, maintaining, or improving wellness and well-being. Nurses and clients collaborate in planning desired outcomes of care, based on assessment data. An individual's ability to meet his or her own health needs determines the nature and extent of nursing implementation. A primary goal of nursing management is to maintain, restore, or increase individuals' capacity for self-care.

Much of the content in this section deals with clinical procedures and approaches aimed at preserving clients' current level of wellness and promoting well-being even though illness is present. This reflects the philosophy of the authors that wellness practices do not emphasize healthy living to the exclusion of treatment of disease, but rather, encompass recognition of the elements of health and wellness that even ill clients possess and the promotion of wellness-oriented behaviors in the face of disease as much as in a state of health.

PLANNING FOR OPTIMUM WELLNESS AND WELL-BEING

Planning for optimum wellness begins with setting priorities and determining desired outcomes. Client assessment and the formulation of nursing diagnoses identifies client needs and actual or potential problems that affect client wellness and well-being. In the collaborative approach, this information is shared with clients and a variety of alternatives are identified and explored by nurse and client. The nurse–client interaction involves sharing, discussion, and exploration of options because both parties are active participants in the process.

Every effort should be made to address needs that clients feel are most important. For example, a young woman admitted to the hospital for treatment of injuries sustained in a motor vehicle accident may have many obvious nursing problems including severe pain, impaired mobility, and potential for infection. Upon assessment of this client, however, a nurse may discover that her greatest concern is an unfinished project at work. Facilitating communication with a co-worker who is able to make arrangements for completion of the project during the client's hospitalization will allay much of the client's distress and enable her to focus her energy and attention on recovering from her injuries.

Based on the individualized nursing diagnoses and the mutually determined priorities, nurses collaborate with clients and family members to plan desired client outcomes or goals. These outcomes should reflect the highest level of wellness and independent functioning possible. The individualized nursing diagnosis and outcomes are the basis for nursing implementation.

NURSING IMPLEMENTATION TO PROMOTE WELLNESS AND WELL-BEING

The final step in the planning phase of the nursing process is the collaborative selection of a course of action that will best meet the client's needs. The goal of nursing actions is to assist and support clients in achieving effective self-care. For this reason, it is imperative that clients have an active role in the decision-making process. Clients' feelings and opinions have a great effect on their participation in the therapeutic regimen. Encouraging clients to express feelings, to participate in self-care, and to make informed decisions affirms clients' self-worth and promotes self-responsibility, one element of wellness.

The table of Nurse–Client Management of Wellness and Well-being, on pages 764–766, presents appropriate outcomes, implementation, and evaluation criteria for nurse–client management of the nursing diagnoses related to wellness and well-being that are presented in this chapter. These are provided as examples only. Individualized plans of care should be developed for all clients based on their own particular needs and situation.

Preventive Care

Preventive care focuses on the healthy, disease-free client. Its goal is assisting clients to obtain a high level of wellness through health maintenance or improvement and disease prevention. Nursing actions directed toward health protection focus primarily on health education, immunizations, and screening. Table 22–5 summarizes health-protective approaches for clients at each developmental stage. Nurses can also help clients to develop a self-management program to change unhealthy behaviors.

Health Education. Health education is a major focus of preventive client care. The goal of health education is to provide individuals with the knowledge necessary to incorporate health-promoting and health protective behaviors into their life-style. Health education empowers individuals to make responsible informed life-style choices.

Nurses educate clients regarding the elements of a wellness life-style discussed in the first section of the chapter: eating well, being fit, feeling good, caring for self and others, fitting in, and being responsible.[15] Education related to principles of nutrition, fitness, and stress reduction assists clients to develop an individualized program of high-level wellness. Client education about the negative effects of habits such as smoking, consumption of excessive alcohol and drugs, irresponsible sexual activity, unbalanced nutrition, lack of exercise, and prolonged stress on wellness and well-being enables clients to recognize and eliminate habits that are detrimental to wellness. Teaching clients about the importance of immunizations, basic health maintenance, and principles of safety, sanitation, and hygiene is also part of health protection. Avoiding hyperthermia and hypothermia is an example of a topic for health education that is related to safety and fitting in with the environment. Maintaining body temperature is important to health and well-being. Generally, heat production and loss are balanced to maintain a relatively constant body temperature; however, body temperature is affected by the external environment (see Chap. 16). Cold winter temperatures can lower body temperature (hypothermia), whereas elevated summer temperatures cause increased body temperature (hyperthermia). Preventive education regarding hypothermia and hyperthermia promotes client health and well-being. Boxes 22–3 and 22–4 provide client education for avoiding hypothermia and hyperthermia.

Vehicles for Health Education. Printed material is an important vehicle for education in health promotion and illness prevention behaviors. Many health care professionals use printed material in the form of pamphlets for health education. Health-related articles found in general interest and consumer health magazines are a new and different form of client health education. Consumer interest in health information has resulted in the proliferation of magazines and articles that target health-seeking individuals of all ages and life-styles. Consumers consider magazines a valid source of information and they use them to meet their health education needs.[87] The advantage of these materials is that they are written for the general public rather than health care professionals. Nurses can use consumer health articles as a basis for client health education, after evaluating them for accuracy. Misinformation can be clarified for clients while accurate information can be reinforced.

Another vehicle for health education is radio and television. This media facilitates education of clients who are unable to read. It also has value as a vehicle for getting health promotion information to individuals with limited access to health care services because of inadequate financial resources or limited availability of health services. Videotape or closed circuit systems enable use of television for small group and individual health education. Radio, video, and printed health information must be available in varied languages to be most effective.

Immunization. Immunization is a means of protecting individuals from certain infectious diseases. Stimulation of immunity by vaccines has greatly reduced the incidence and severity of many infectious diseases around the world.

NURSE–CLIENT MANAGEMENT OF WELLNESS AND WELL-BEING

Nursing Diagnosis	Desired Outcome	Implementation	Evaluation Criteria
Health-seeking behavior: Participation in weight loss program R/T exposure to information regarding health risks associated with obesity *5.4*	1. Verbalizes understanding of factors that contribute to current physical condition.	1a. Assess current nutritional patterns (see Chap. 25). 1b. Assess factors that influence eating patterns (stress, boredom, cultural practices/beliefs). 1c. Assess activity patterns (see Chap. 30). 1d. Assess client's knowledge of basic nutrition/caloric value of favorite foods. 1e. Review diet diary (see Chap. 25) with client to identify factors that contribute to increased intake.	1a. Client identifies personal eating patterns that contribute to weight gain. 1b. Client accurately describes role of exercise in weight control.
	2. Adopts life-style changes necessary for attainment of weight-loss goals.	2a. Collaborate with client to plan a balanced, acceptable diet that considers cultural and personal preferences. 2b. Assist client in setting realistic weight-loss goals. 2c. Discuss ways to manage stress and deal with emotions instead of eating. 2d. Involve significant others in treatment plan as much as possible. 2e. Explore alternative exercise programs with client. 2f. Support selection of exercise program that fits client's preferences and daily routines. 2g. Provide positive reinforcement for verbal and behavioral indicators of healthy changes in eating and exercise.	2a. Client reports ability to successfully follow prescribed dietary plan. 2b. Client reports/describes participation in exercise regimen. 2c. Client reports weight loss of 1–2 lb/wk.
Altered health maintenance: Substance abuse R/T ineffective individual coping *6.4.2*	1. Cessation of excessive use of alcohol or other drugs.	1a. Assess client's history of abuse and possible past attempts at reducing substance use. 1b. Discuss effects of drugs and alcohol on health.	1. Client reports cessation of alcohol and drug use.
	2. Effective stress management.	2a. Assess client's other coping skills. 2b. Assist client in identifying other methods for coping with stress (eg, exercise or relaxation technique). 2c. Be supportive of functional coping behaviors such as use of progressive relaxation. 2d. Assist client to identify personal strengths and set realistic goals for change. 2e. Explore available resources and support systems with client. 2f. Refer to a community support group for individuals who are recovering from substance abuse.	2a. Client reports uses exercise and meditation to manage stress. 2b. Client participates regularly in a community support group.
Anxiety R/T threat to health status: Uncertainty about results of diagnostic tests *9.3.1*	1. Decreased anxiety.	1a. Encourage client to discuss feelings. 1b. Engage in active listening at least twice a shift. 1c. Encourage client to explore possible factors contributing to anxious feelings. 1d. Provide clear, concise information about all client care activities. 1e. Reduce as many stressful environmental stimuli as possible. 1f. Remain with client during severe anxiety. 1g. Provide opportunities to discuss test results when available.	1a. Client identifies factors that trigger anxiety. 1b. Decreased anxiety AEB: decreased trembling and restlessness ("I feel calmer now, my stomach isn't so upset"); improved eye contact when speaking; sleeps throughout night.

Nursing Diagnosis	Desired Outcome	Implementation	Evaluation Criteria
	2. Uses relaxation techniques as needed.	2a. Assess client's knowledge and experience with relaxation techniques. 2b. Teach a relaxation technique such as guided imagery or meditation.	2. Performs progressive relaxation technique several times a day.
Fear of pain R/T knowledge deficit: Pain associated with a surgical procedure *9.3.2*	1. Reduction in fear.	1a. Encourage client to discuss feelings. 1b. Engage in active listening at least twice a shift. 1c. Assess client's knowledge and experience with relaxation techniques. 1d. Teach a relaxation technique such as guided imagery or meditation.	1. Reduced fear AEB: "I can see now that there's not so much to be afraid of," relaxed expression, pulse and respiratory rate at client's usual baseline.
	2. Verbalizes accurate knowledge of procedures and methods to control pain.	2a. Provide information regarding techniques to control pain. 2b. Encourage questions. 2c. Discuss procedures within client's level of understanding.	2a. Client verbalizes understanding of techniques to control pain. 2b. Client is able to describe expected sensations and what he or she can do to minimize unpleasant sensations.
Powerlessness R/T illness-related regimen *7.3.2*	1. Reduction in feelings of powerlessness. 2. Recognition of aspects of situation client can control.	1a. Facilitate verbalization through active listening. 1b. Discuss aspects of treatment regimen that are most difficult for client; explore possibilities for changes with other health care team members. 1c. Facilitate client's identifying factors under own control. 1d. Ask client how he or she prefers to participate in care. 1e. Discuss all treatments and procedures with client. 1f. Acknowledge the importance of client's space. 1g. Keep personal effects within reach.	1. Reduced sense of powerlessness AEB: describes changes in environment that give feelings of control, participates in decisions related to care, participates in self-care activities.
Hopelessness R/T prolonged activity restrictions *7.3.1*	1. Reduction in feelings of hopelessness.	1a. Facilitate expression of feelings through active listening, open-ended questions, nonverbal acceptance. 1b. Encourage client to explore and verbalize feelings related to physical condition/activity restriction. 1c. Acknowledge reality of situation; recognize both abilities and deficits. 1d. Assist client to set realistic goals for progress/future. 1e. Accept negative emotions and avoid false reassurances.	1. Reduced feelings of hopelessness AEB: identifies realistic goals for coping with activity restrictions, demonstrates interest in appearance and personal hygiene, participates in at least one group activity daily, active participation in self-care activities.

(continued)

NURSE–CLIENT MANAGEMENT OF WELLNESS AND WELL-BEING (continued)

Nursing Diagnosis	Desired Outcome	Implementation	Evaluation Criteria
	2. Identifies personal/ social resources to facilitate coping with changes in function.	2a. Assist client in identifying activities that can be performed independently. 2b. Assist client in identifying personal strengths and sources of support. 2c. Collaborate with client in planning schedule of daily activities; respect client preferences as much as possible. 2d. Provide opportunities for social interaction/ diversional activities. 2e. Encourage visits by significant others. 2f. Provide positive reinforcement for behaviors that demonstrate initiative (eg, self-care, increased appetite, increased interaction). 2g. Inform client of agency and community resources available to assist. 2h. Introduce client to other individuals who have coped successfully with a similar situation.	2a. Verbalizes feelings of confidence and self-worth. 2b. Lists agencies to contact for assistance prior to discharge.
Hopelessness R/T deteriorating physical condition (AIDS) *7.3.1*	1. Reduction in feelings of hopelessness.	1. See 1a, 1c, 1d, 1e, above.	1. Reduced feelings of hopelessness AEB: participation in self-care, initiation of interactions with others, reduction in negative remarks about self and situation.
	2. Identifies personal/ social resources to facilitate coping with changes in function.	2. See 2a–2h, above.	2. See 2a and 2b, above.
	3. Participates in decision-making for the future.	3. Facilitate client's identifying factors under own control.	3. Identifies realistic alternatives for future.
Spiritual distress R/T separation from religious ties *4.1.1*	1. Feelings of spiritual comfort.	1a. Acknowledge client's spiritual concerns. 1b. Encourage client to express thoughts and feelings. 1c. Offer to arrange visits by clergy, provide privacy during visit. 1d. Provide client privacy for religious practices during hospitalization. 1e. Arrange to have objects that provide spiritual comfort at bedside.	1a. Verbalizes has achieved restored closeness to God, sense of peace during prayers and after receiving communion from local priest. 1b. Specifies what spiritual assistance is needed.
Potential for infection R/F: Invasive procedures, decreased WBCs, receiving chemotherapy 1.2.1.1	1. Client remains free of infection throughout treatment regimen.	1a. Monitor vital signs every 4 hours. 1b. Monitor urine for altered color and odor. 1c. Wash hands before client contact. 1d. Encourage or assist with daily hygiene. 1e. Discontinue invasive procedures as soon as possible. 1f. Strict aseptic technique for all invasive procedures and IV site care. 1g. Prevent client exposure to infective visitors. 1h. Teach client and family techniques to prevent infection.	1a. Client will remain afebrile 1b. IV sites free of signs of infection: redness, swelling, heat, purulent drainage. 1c. Urine remains free of bacteria. 1d. Client will verbalize knowledge of techniques to prevent infection.

TABLE 22–5. HEALTH-PROTECTIVE BEHAVIORS THROUGHOUT THE LIFE SPAN

Developmental Level	Immunizations	Screening Procedures	Health Education
Infants (0–1 year)	DPT and oral polio at 2, 4, and 6 months of age.	At birth: PKU, hypothyroidism, congenital hip dysplasia, developmental assessment, instillation of silver nitrate drops or erythromycin ointment in eyes, injection of 1 mg vitamin K to prevent hemorrhagic disease. Complete physical examination every 2–3 months.	Parent education: normal growth and development, breastfeeding, nutrition practices, safety measures, management of common childhood illnesses, importance of regular helath supervision (well baby checks).
Toddlers and preschool children (1–5 years)	MMR at 15 months of age. DPT and oral polio at 18 months of age.	Complete physical examination every 3 months to age 2; every 6 months to age 3; and annually to age 5. Vision and hearing screening. Developmental assessment. TB testing at age 3.	Parent education: dental development, discipline measures, accident prevention, nutritional practices, normal growth and development. Child education: dental self-care, feeding self-care, dressing, basic hygiene practices.
School-age children (5–12 years)	DPT and oral polio boosters at age 5 or 6. Tetanus booster at age 10. Girls should receive rubella vaccine before puberty if not previously immunized.	Complete physical examination annually. TB test every 3 years. Vision and hearing screening. Dental check-ups every 6 months.	Healthy diet habits. Accident prevention and safety measures. Preparation for physical changes of puberty. Substance abuse education.
Adolescents (12–18 years)	Oral polio at 12–14 years. Tetanus booster, if needed.	Complete physical examination at puberty, including blood pressure, cholesterol, CBC, UA. BSE (female). TSE (male). Pap smear and pelvic examination for females, if sexually active. TB test at 12 years. Dental check-ups every 6 months.	Proper nutritional practices. Sex education/methods of birth control. Sexually transmitted diseases. Safe driving skills. Substance abuse counseling. Safety practices. Preparation for adult roles. Methods for monthly BSE or TSE.
Young adults (18–30 years)	Tetanus at age 20 and every 10 years. Hepatitis B for high-risk populations/occupations. Rubella for females if serum test negative.	Complete physical examination at age 20 and every 5 years. Monthly BSE (female). Monthly TSE (male). Pap smear and pelvic examination every 2 years for healthy females; every year for high-risk groups. Blood pressure screening. VDRL. Regular dental check-ups.	Sexual counseling on birth control, sexually transmitted disease. Life-style counseling: Stress management, nutrition, physical fitness, parenting skills, environmental health.
Middle-aged adults (30–65 years)	Tetanus booster every 10 years. Influenza for high-risk individuals annually.	Complete physical examination every 5 years. Montly BSE (female). Monthly TSE (male). Pap smear and pelvic examination every 2 years; annually after age 40. Baseline mammogram at age 35; annually after age 40. Stool guaiac at age 50 and annually after. Sigmoidoscopy at age 50.	Warning signs of serious illness. Cancer detection. Continuation of life-style counseling. Anticipatory guidance for retirement/"empty nest."

(*continued*)

TABLE 22–5. (continued)

Developmental Level	Immunizations	Screening Procedures	Health Education
		Glaucoma testing routinely after age 40. Blood pressure screening.	
Older adults (65+ years)	Annual influenza. Tetanus booster every 10 years. One-time pneumococcal.	Complete physical examination every 2 years. Blood pressure annually. Monthly BSE (female). Monthly TSE (male). Annual mammogram (female). Annual stool guaiac. Glaucoma screening every 3–5 years. Pap smear and pelvic examination annually. Regular vision and hearing screening.	Home safety. Life-style counseling: Nutritional changes, retirement/relocation, adjustment to changes related to aging, cancer detection.

DPT = diphtheria, pertussis, tetanus; MMR = measles, mumps, rubella; PKU = phenylketonuria (an inborn error of metabolism that causes mental retardation); TB = tuberculosis; CBC = complete blood count; UA = urinalysis; VDRL = Venereal Disease Research Laboratory (test for syphilis); BSE = breast self-examination; TSE = testicular self-examination.

For example, smallpox has been eliminated as a health threat in many countries through immunization. Although most immunizations are given to children, a variety of immunizations are available for disease prevention throughout the life span. For example, the tetanus toxoid booster is required every 10 years throughout life, and older adults should receive an annual flu shot to prevent influenza.

Client education is an important part of immunization. Individuals need to know about the importance of obtaining immunizations. Concern about possible adverse reactions leads some individuals to refuse immunization, but in most cases with careful history and assessment, the consequences of acquiring the disease are more serious than complications from immunizations.

Immunizations prescribed by primary care providers are administered by nurses. Obtaining a thorough history including allergies before administering a vaccine and carefully observing clients receiving an immunization is an important nursing responsibility. It is not possible to deter-

BOX 22–3. CLIENT EDUCATION FOR AVOIDING HYPOTHERMIA

Action	Rationale
1. Wear mittens rather than gloves	1. Fingers adjacent to each other give off heat that keeps the other fingers warm.
2. Keep dry.	2. Wetness and moisture help transfer cold to the body surface.
3. Avoid tight-fitting shoes or boots.	3. Tightness interferes with circulation and therefore heat distribution.
4. Do not drink alcohol.	4. Causes vasodilation and adds to rate of heat loss.
5. Keep active.	5. Muscle activity generates heat.
6. Eat high-calorie foods.	6. Calories supply energy that the body converts to heat.
7. Do not smoke.	7. Nicotine constricts blood vessels and reduces blood flow to the extremities.
8. Avoid exposure to wind.	8. Wind in addition to cold environmental temperatures enhances heat loss by convection, which creates an even colder chill factor.
9. Wear several thin layers of clothing rather than thick layer of outerwear.	9. Traps warmed air between layers.
10. Wear a hat.	10. The head is very vascular with minimal insulating fat. If head is uncovered, loss of body heat is significant.

(Adapted from Budassi SA, Barber J. Emergency Nursing Principles and Practice. *St. Louis: Mosby; 1986.*

BOX 22–4. CLIENT EDUCATION FOR AVOIDING HYPERTHERMIA

Action	Rationale
1. Avoid strenuous activity or exercise during hot weather.	1. Activity increases the amount of body heat produced.
2. Drink three quarts of fluid on a hot day.	2. Replaces body fluid lost in increased perspiration.
3. Wear loose-fitting clothing.	3. Provides for body heat dissipation via evaporation and convection.
4. Ventilate living areas well.	4. Circulation of air removes air warmed by radiation.
5. Wear light hat with good ventilation when outdoors.	5. Provides skin protection from sun and environmental heat.

mine before administration whether a client will have an adverse reaction. Nurses should inform clients of possible adverse effects and how to deal with them and question clients about their occurrence on return visits for health care. Finally, it is important for individuals to maintain an accurate record of when they received immunizations. Usually, health care providers record immunizations in clients' health records, but giving clients a record to keep for personal reference promotes self-responsibility. Table 22–5 lists the immunizations that are recommended at each developmental stage.

Screening. Screening procedures are used to identify individuals at risk or in the early stages of disease development. Early diagnosis and prompt treatment of health problems can often halt the pathological process and prevent disability. A growing number of people are interested in learning more about health, illness, and medicine to be able to self-screen with more accuracy. Many people keep a *Physician's Desk Reference* or other drug reference at home to inform themselves about prescribed medications and facilitate self-responsibility in taking prescription medication. Also, many screening procedures can be performed independently by individuals. Examples include a monthly breast or testicular self-examination, use of home kits for the detection of pregnancy or occult blood in stools, checking pulse before and after activity, monitoring weight, and frequent self-assessment for the seven warning signs of cancer. Box 22–5 lists these warning signs. Some screening such as blood pressure checks for hypertension are easier if done with the assistance of a family member or significant other. Nurses often teach clients and families correct techniques and how to select equipment that will produce accurate results. Other screening programs such as annual Pap smear, mammogram, and testing for diabetes, elevated cholesterol, and glaucoma require the services of a health care professional. To be effective, screening requires health education. Individuals need to know about the importance of screening procedures for early detection and treatment of health problems. Clients need information about procedures that they can perform independently and those requiring professional assessment. Increased knowledge enables clients to exercise self-care behaviors. Refer to Table 22–5 for screening procedures that are recommended for each developmental stage.

Preventive client care is provided in a variety of settings including physicians' offices, nurse practitioner clinics, industrial health clinics, and community care facilities. Nurses in all of these settings use education, immunization, and screening for health protection and promotion. Frequently long waiting periods in preventive care settings result in feelings of boredom and lethargy, or anger and frustration, which diminish a client's sense of well-being and may increase stress levels. Stocking the waiting room in a health care facility with educational materials and presentations about wellness and health maintenance makes possible productive use of client waiting time (Fig. 22–2). Educational pamphlets and videotape presentations can provide clients with important wellness and health maintenance information. Nurses who solicit clients' questions about information presented in the waiting area while assisting them to prepare for the health examination enhance the effectiveness of the educational materials and reinforce their use.

BOX 22–5. SEVEN WARNING SIGNS OF CANCER

- Change in bowel or bladder habits
- A sore that does not heal
- Unusual bleeding or discharge
- Thickening or lump in breast or elsewhere
- Indigestion or difficulty swallowing
- Obvious change in wart or mole
- Nagging cough or hoarseness

IMPLICATIONS FOR NURSE–CLIENT COLLABORATION

Self-care

The collaborative philosophy, centered as it is on self-responsibility, acknowledges the client's capacity for self-care and endorses the client's active participation in therapeutic routines, both in the hospital and at home.

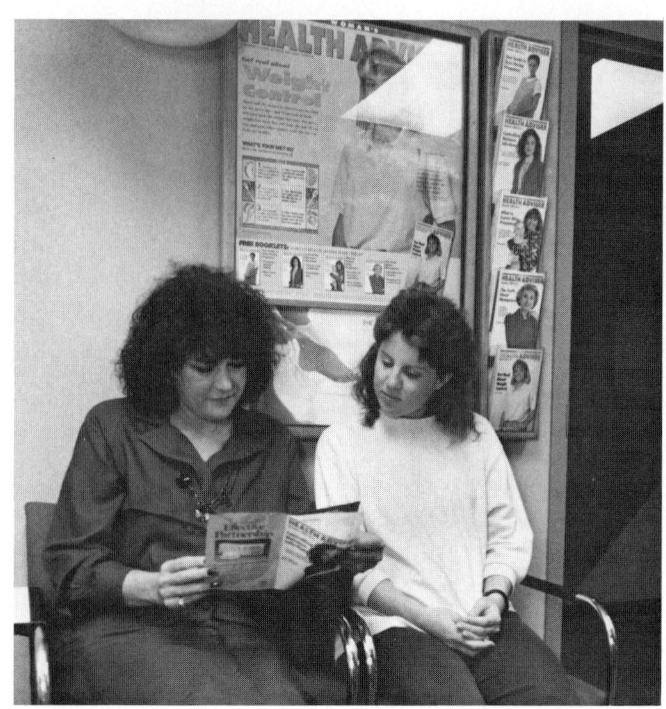

Figure 22–2. A waiting room with educational materials makes positive use of time clients spend waiting to see a health care provider.

Industrial health clinics employ nurses who promote employee health. They screen for health problems such as hypertension or obesity and assess for work-related hazards such as exposure to chemicals. Screening programs also provide an opportunity to educate employees about elements of a wellness life-style. In some communities, mobile facilities run by nurses are available to companies for employee health promotion and screening (Fig. 22–3).

Community health includes a variety of settings such as schools, home health, and public health clinics. Preventive care in these settings involves health education and screening for age-appropriate threats to health. Use of printed material, video, and small group presentations on threats to health and elements of a wellness life-style is effective in these settings.

In all of these client care settings, clients are active participants in health care decision-making. Nurses are facilitators and educators. First-level nursing practice focuses on promotion of self-care through education, motivation, and development of life-style and behaviors conducive to health. Pender[1] has proposed a health promotion model that incorporates ideas from Rosenstock's Health Belief Model (see Chaps. 5 and 12) and Bandura's Social Learning Theory. The model lists factors that influence and determine individuals' participation in health-promoting behaviors (Fig. 22–4). This model can be useful to nurses in assessing and planning with clients for health promotion.

Self-management. Self-management is a method of personal change that can be used by anyone, adolescent or adult, who has a health goal to achieve. Self-management stresses that self-knowledge and self-belief, an understanding of the environmental events that reinforce behavior, and systematic planning are all important to success in changing oneself. Motivation and will power alone are usually insufficient conditions; changing oneself usually requires more than simply wanting to change or deciding to change; it also requires rational strategies. Self-management is useful in

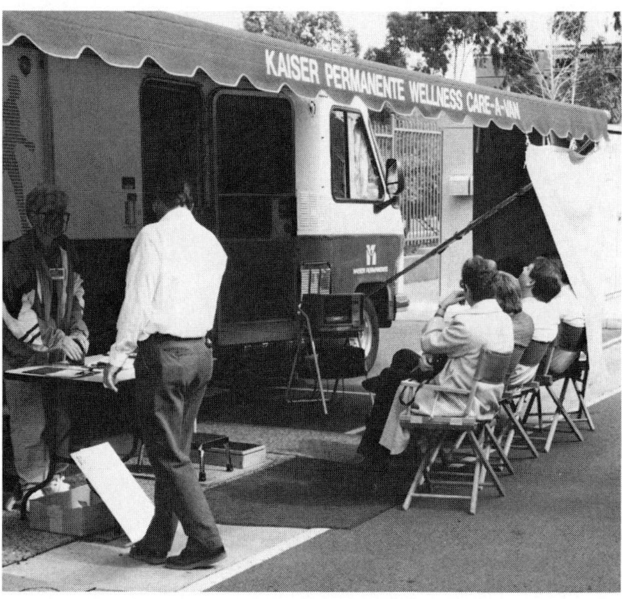

Figure 22–3. This mobile Wellness Care-A-Van travels to work sites to provide wellness checks for employees.

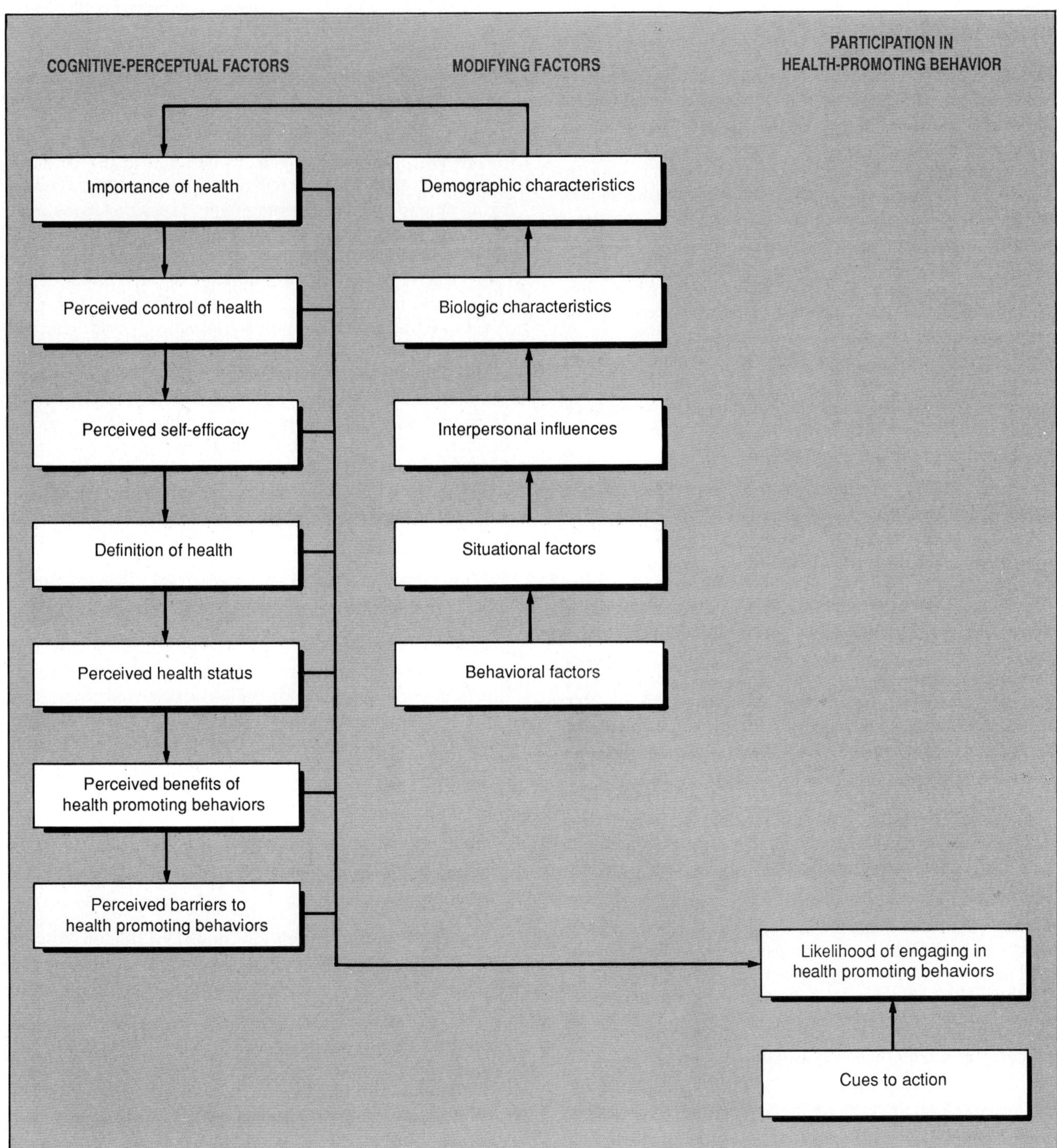

Figure 22–4. Nurses can use Pender's Health Promotion Model to assess factors that may influence clients' willingness to participate in health-promoting activities. (*From Pender NJ.* Health Promotion in Nursing Practice. *2nd ed. Norwalk, CT: Appleton & Lange; 1987.*)

nursing because it provides strategies that nurses can teach to clients, many of whom desire to make changes in their lives.

A summary of self-management philosophy and techniques is included under preventative care because self-management can be used for developing new, health-enhancing habits. Adding an exercise program to one's daily activities, for example, is a common new pattern that can be achieved through self-management. Self-management can also be used, however, as a way to change long-established, health-endangering habits. Smoking, overeating, and stress are common patterns in the lives of those who develop chronic health problems. Correspondingly, smoking cessation, weight reduction, and stress management are preventative health goals for which self-management can be employed. The method can be used just as effectively to achieve rehabilitative health goals, however, once a health problem has developed. Nurses can make significant contributions to clients' well-being by teaching self-management techniques; and by using these techniques themselves, nurses can enhance their own health and well-being.

Learning Theory, Personal Outlook, and Self-management. Self-management helps individuals to gain control over their behavior. As a method for personal change, it draws principles from several theories of learning, incorporating cognitive and perceptual learning, but also leans heavily on behaviorism.[88] (See Chap. 20 for more information on theories of learning.) The foundation of self-management is that change involves learning—learning about oneself and learning about one's environment.

Self-management emphasizes the importance of internal locus of control and high self-efficacy to success in personal change.[88] People may want to change but lack the belief that they can change themselves or that they have the knowledge, skills, or resources needed to change. Self-management proposes that both internal locus of control and greater self-efficacy can be gained through a methodical process of self-assessment and selection of the right self-control strategies.[88]

Process of Self-management. The process of self-management entails three systematic steps: (1) self-assessment and goal-selection, (2) development of an action plan, and (3) progress measurement and improvement maintenance.

Self-assessment and Goal Selection. Self-assessment is the first step in the method and leads to goal selection.

ASSESSING OUTLOOK. The process of self-management begins with an identification of where an individual's locus of control lies. Change in a person's beliefs about who or what controls behavior often comes slowly.[87] Nurses can assist clients by helping them to assess their own locus of control. Figure 22–5 shows a simple scale that can be used for that purpose. By completing the scale, an individual can determine whether he or she has an internal or an external locus of control. Clients who have an internal locus of control generally have an easier time achieving success in personal change. Research shows that self-management is an effective instrument for shifting locus of control from external to internal.[89] By employing self-management people learn that they can achieve greater control over their environments. However, clients who are initially externally oriented may require more self-management trials to achieve ultimate success.

ASSESSING BEHAVIOR. The next step is to identify the behavior that is to be changed. In addition to the patterns mentioned above, that behavior might be related to managing time, developing or maintaining social relationships, changing personal feelings, or even to achieving personal fulfillment. Taking inventory of one's patterns is easier when a self-assessment questionnaire of the type shown in Figure 22–6 is employed.

Once the self-description is completed, a basic concept to keep in mind for interpreting the results is that wellness and well-being are represented by balance. Balance is represented by the scores across the four self-management areas—work, social, health, leisure. Williams and Long recommend that the person taking the inventory look for areas in which scores are minimal or negative, because negative scores indicate areas where change might be desirable, and suggest that scores should be on the positive side in all areas.[88]

SETTING PRIORITIES. The next step is to set priorities. There are any number of changes that an individual might make, but time and other constraints usually make only a few realistic. The object is to decide on which goals have the greatest personal importance. The process of priority setting is undertaken by making a list of behavior changes in order of their importance. The individual decides which are really essential. For example, a personal list might look like this:

1. Overcoming feelings of depression
2. Stopping smoking
3. Starting an exercise program
4. Becoming more self-directive
5. Making new friends

In this list, changing personal feelings has the top priority for the individual, and self-management might be concentrated on that priority at first. A priority list becomes the basis for goal-setting.

ASSESSING PERSONAL RESOURCES. Many changes require resources for their accomplishment. Where does one find, or help another to find, resources? Reviewing personal assets by focusing on personal abilities or reviewing personal successes can help to place individuals in touch with their inner resources. Another way is to go over those things that generally elicit others' compliments. Compliments from others serve to highlight personal resources that an individual may have come to take for granted.[88] Remembering the compliments that one has gained while wearing a certain outfit, for example, may serve as a resource of inner strength during weight reduction.

The influence of the environment also needs to be as-

Using the scale −3, −2, −1, +1, +2, +3, indicate the extent to which you agree or disagree with each of the following items. Let −3 represent complete disagreement and +3 complete agreement. Put the number representing the degree of your agreement or disagreement by each item. Directions for scoring your responses are given at the conclusion of the inventory.

1. Whether or not I get to be a leader depends mostly on my ability.
2. To a great extent my life is controlled by accidental happenings.
3. I feel like what happens in my life is mostly determined by powerful people.
4. Whether or not I get into a car accident depends mostly on how good a driver I am.
5. When I make plans, I am almost certain to make them work.
6. Often there is no chance of protecting my personal interest from bad-luck happenings.
7. When I get what I want, it's usually because I'm lucky.
8. Although I might have good ability, I will not be given leadership responsibility without appealing to those in positions of power.
9. How many friends I have depends on how nice a person I am.
10. I have often found that what is going to happen will happen.
11. My life is chiefly controlled by powerful others.
12. Whether or not I get into a car accident is mostly a matter of luck.
13. People like myself have very little chance of protecting our personal interests when they conflict with those of strong pressure groups.
14. It's not always wise for me to plan too far ahead because many things turn out to be a matter of good or bad fortune.
15. Getting what I want requires pleasing those people above me.
16. Whether or not I get to be a leader depends on whether I'm lucky enough to be in the right place at the right time.
17. If important people were to decide they didn't like me, I probably wouldn't make many friends.
18. I can pretty much determine what will happen in my life.
19. I am usually able to protect my personal interests.
20. Whether or not I get into a car accident depends mostly on the other driver.
21. When I get what I want, it's usually because I worked hard for it.
22. In order to have my plans work, I make sure that they fit in with the desires of people who have power over me.
23. My life is determined by my own actions.
24. It's chiefly a matter of fate whether or not I have a few friends or many friends.

Scoring procedures for the I, P, and C scales

There are three separate scales used to measure one's locus of control: Internal scale, Powerful Others scale, and Chance scale. There are eight items on each of the three scales. To score each scale add up your answers to the items appropriate for that scale. (These items are listed below.) Add to this sum +24. (This removes the possibility of negative scores.) The possible range on each scale is from 0 to 48. Theoretically, a person could score high or low on all three dimensions. The higher the score on a scale, the more inclined the individual is to believe in that particular form of control.

Scale	Items
Internal scale	(1, 4, 5, 9, 18, 19, 21, 23)
Powerful Others scale	(3, 8, 11, 13, 15, 17, 20, 22)
Chance scale	(2, 6, 7, 10, 12, 14, 16, 24)

Figure 22–5. Levenson locus of control scale. (*From Levenson H. Activism and powerful others: Distinction within the concept of internal–external control. J Personality Assess. 1974;38:381–382.*)

sessed. Environmental events strongly affect behavior. One object of self-management is to make social influences and external physical events work together with one's inner resources rather than in opposition to them.[88] Identifying setting events, that is, events that set the stage for a particular response, is helpful. For example, an individual might notice that he or she eats more when eating alone than when eating with friends. Eating with friends or eating alone are different setting events for eating behavior. Awareness of such patterns can help in devising an action plan to avoid overeating. The consequences of behavior are also important. An important step in self-management is to arrange for immediate consequences that reinforce good habits. For example, eating with friends may reinforce eating less by substituting social conviviality for the feeling of immediate psychological comfort that overeating creates for some people.

BASELINE ASSESSMENT. To judge progress in behavior change, it is also necessary to quantify behavior that helps and interferes with goal attainment, and to do so over a period of time. This requires a framework for record-keeping, and data to provide a yardstick for evaluating progress.

The initial appraisal acts as the baseline assessment. For several days or a week, the individual keeps track of a certain behavior, referred to as the target behavior. Recording for a week allows an individual to see cycles in personal behavior. The individual simply counts how many times a behavior is repeated or how long a behavior is performed in the course of a day. By recording what happens immediately before or after a target behavior occurs, an individual also can establish the setting events and consequences of that behavior. For example, an individual who wishes to cease smoking would count the number of cigarettes smoked over a period of several days, but would also note the conditions surrounding smoking. Was he or she conversing with others, drinking coffee, or working at the computer while smoking? Fre-

Your life is probably characterized by many different behaviors. To learn how you spend your time, indicate how frequently you engage in each of the behaviors listed in the inventory, using the following time distinctions:

Never: Under no circumstances do you ever engage in the behavior.
Rarely: You engage in the behavior a few times a year.
Periodically: You engage in the behavior a few times a month.
Regularly: You engage in the behavior several times a week.
Always: You engage in the behavior every time an opportunity presents itself.

Rate your response in the right column with the answer that *best* corresponds to your level of participation in each behavior by using the following points: 0 = never; 1 = rarely; 2 = periodically; 3 = regularly; and 4 = always.

Behavior	Rate
1. Filing work materials	_____
2. Rambling in conversation	_____
3. Flossing my teeth	_____
4. Creating art objects	_____
5. Overextending myself in work commitments	_____
6. Keeping my word	_____
7. Using hard drugs	_____
8. Attending art and cultural exhibits	_____
9. Attaining work goals	_____
10. Criticizing others behind their backs	_____
11. Getting adequate rest at night	_____
12. Playing a musical instrument	_____
13. Jumping from one task to another	_____
14. Initiating conversation	_____
15. Eating excessively	_____
16. Attending concerts	_____
17. Completing work assignments on time	_____
18. Interrupting others during conversation	_____
19. Participating in vigorous physical activity	_____
20. Writing creatively (e.g., poetry, short stories)	_____
21. Putting off unpleasant, but necessary, tasks	_____

Behavior	Rate
22. Listening closely to others' comments	_____
23. Smoking cigarettes	_____
24. Reading leisurely (e.g., poetry, fiction, magazines)	_____
25. Setting working goals	_____
26. Dominating conversation	_____
27. Drinking water	_____
28. Gardening/working in the yard	_____
29. Losing work-related materials	_____
30. Encouraging others	_____
31. Eating junk food	_____
32. Engaging in outdoor nature activities	_____
33. Reading course/professionally related materials	_____
34. Reprimanding others	_____
35. Doing stretching exercises	_____
36. Engaging in a hobby not otherwise listed in questionnaire	_____
37. Failing to meet deadlines	_____
38. Showing affection toward others	_____
39. Gulping meals	_____
40. Dancing	_____

Scoring Instructions: Give yourself 0 to 4 points credit for never-to-always responses to the positive items, and subtract 0 to 4 points for never-to-always responses to the negative items. Total your scores within each of the four areas outlined below. If you gave very few never or always responses, don't be alarmed. We consider the other categories more realistic alternatives for most individuals.

Work				**Social**			
+Items	*Positive credit*	*−Items*	*Subtraction points*	*+Items*	*Positive credit*	*−Items*	*Subtraction points*
1	_____	5	_____	6	_____	2	_____
9	_____	13	_____	14	_____	10	_____
17	_____	21	_____	22	_____	18	_____
25	_____	29	_____	30	_____	26	_____
33	_____	37	_____	38	_____	34	_____
Total A	_____	Total B	_____	Total A	_____	Total B	_____

Subtract B from A to get your work self-management score.

Subtract B from A to get your social self-management score.

Health				**Leisure activities**			
+Items	*Positive credit*	*−Items*	*Subtraction points*	*All + items*			
3	_____	7	_____	4	_____	24	_____
11	_____	15	_____	8	_____	28	_____
19	_____	23	_____	12	_____	32	_____
27	_____	31	_____	16	_____	36	_____
35	_____	39	_____	20	_____	40	_____
Total A	_____	Total B	_____	Total A	_____	Total B	_____

Subtract B from A to get your health self-management score.

Add A and B to get your leisure activities score. Because this subscale contains only positive items, one can score twice as high in this area. For comparison with other subscales, we suggest that you divide by 2 your leisure activities' total.

Figure 22–6. Self-description form. (*From Williams RL, Long JD.* Toward a Self-Managed Life Style. *3rd ed. Boston: Houghton Mifflin; 1983. Adapted from a presentation by Sandra Thomas, Damaris Olsen, and Robert Williams on "The Development of a Naturalistic Self-management Inventory" at the American Education Research Association, New York, 1982.*)

quencies of all of these items would be monitored and recorded for analysis later.

WRITTEN GOALS. Self-management experts advocate written goal lists. Successful people have been found to be more likely to use "to-do" lists than unsuccessful people.[90] Goals are related to one's priorities, as discussed above, and thus should be related to genuine desires for change. Goals break down overall priorities on a weekly and daily basis into manageable, accomplishable objectives. For example, if physical fitness is a long-term priority, the daily objective list would contain some kind of physical activity.

Goals established must be measurable. Some goals can be difficult to quantify. Reducing anxiety is such a goal. One must question, what constitutes anxiety? An accelerated heart rate? Butterflies in the stomach? If becoming less anxious is the goal, then to quantify such a goal, individuals might ask themselves in what ways anxiety is expressed or what things anxiety prevents them from doing. For example, anxiety might prevent a person from speaking up in a group. Knowing this, a corresponding daily objective could be to make one comment per day in a group setting.

Goals established should be achievable, but they should also provide a challenge. When goals are set too high, they are likely to be dropped; when they are set too low, they provide no stimulation.[88] What represents a challenge varies from individual to individual. Williams and Long suggest that when an individual consistently meets a goal, the level of expectation can be increased.[88]

Developing an Action Plan. In addition to establishing goals, some analysis of behavior is necessary to develop a workable action plan. That process is called task analysis. For example, the task of speaking up in a group setting may require that the individual analyze how to prepare for speaking up. It may be easier for an individual to speak at the beginning of a group session than later. Or an individual might make mental notes of appropriate comments to make in the group.

After tasks are analyzed, they must be scheduled. Activities can be grouped and sequenced in such a way as to make them easier to accomplish. Factors to consider are the number of activities and personal energy level.

ARRANGING ENVIRONMENTAL SUPPORT. The next aspect is to arrange environmental support—physical, social, and internal. Physical environment refers to the places the individual is most productive; social environment refers to the people who provide direction, feedback, and encouragement; the internal environment refers to personal thoughts that help a person change. Certain tasks can be readily accomplished in one setting but not another. For example, the goal of increased studying is made easier to accomplish when a quiet place is available for study. The goal of eating less may be aided by seeking an environment where food temptation is minimized and pleasure from sources other than food is available.

ARRANGING HELPFUL CONSEQUENCES. Target behaviors are examined for intrinsic reinforcers, that is the natural reinforcement they offer. When these are insufficient, external reinforcers are also sought. Pairing enjoyable activities with the target behavior, for example, increases the likelihood of repeating the behavior.[88] Joggers wear headsets so that they can listen to music, which makes the activity of jogging more enjoyable.

Evaluating Progress and Maintaining Improvements. Along with implementing the action plan, record-keeping is important because it lets individuals see what they have accomplished each day and also what remains to be accomplished. There are various methods of recording, but with any method, the most important consideration is accuracy. Records that are made several hours after a behavior are likely to be inaccurate. On the other hand some behaviors do not lend themselves to on-the-spot recording. Having a paper and pencil ready may be impossible, but sometimes a wrist counter can be worn. It may be unnecessary to record some infrequent behaviors immediately, but if the individual has difficulty remembering the count, chances are there will be inaccuracy in behavioral evaluation.

RECORD-KEEPING. Record-keeping generally relies on frequency counting. This involves counting a target behavior and totaling the count for a day. For example, the number of blocks jogged may be counted and totaled for each day. Each day's count can then be plotted on a graph and the lines connected to show progress. Visual display of the counts provides a sense of progress, which is a form of reinforcement.

Another record-keeping method is product assessment. The target behavior may involve producing a product of some sort; for example, a person who wishes to improve job performance might keep track of tasks, jobs, or projects completed each day to evaluate output increases. Product output can also be graphed cumulatively to show an individual that he or she is accomplishing change goals.

Williams and Long emphasize that long-term success of any self-management program requires that one learn to shift from artificial support to natural support.[88] This needs to be done gradually. The first task is to analyze whether any of the strategies of the action plan should become a permanent part of one's daily routine. For an individual with a tendency to overeat, it may be important to eliminate the cookie jar altogether. Another strategy is to find substitutions for artificial rewards. Self-approval statements can be substituted for frequency counts and graph recording. Once self-management has been applied successfully in one life area, most people have no trouble applying the method to other areas of their lives as they decide to make changes.

Supportive Care

Supportive care focuses on clients who are exhibiting early changes in health status. Physiological alterations (for example, diminishing eyesight due to a cataract) and psychological alterations (such as fear of blindness) are evident; however, clients are coping with the changes and continue to function in a fairly independent manner. Typically, these clients are seen in a physician's office, outpatient clinic, or possibly the hospital setting if admitted for diagnostic testing such as tumor biopsy or minor surgery such as a cataract extraction. The goals of supportive care are to assess the problem, select appropriate implementation, and help prevent more serious disruptions or alterations in the client's health. Supportive care occurs in some of the same settings as preventive care, but with a different focus. Minor alterations in health often serve to motivate clients to develop life-style and behaviors more conducive to health. Supportive care includes promoting client self-responsibility, preparing clients for health care experiences, preventing infection, and supporting well-being.

Promoting Self-responsibility. Entry into the health care system, whether as an outpatient or inpatient, typically forces clients to assume a passive dependent role. Although clients often are able to function in an independent manner, many of their daily routines may be prescribed or dictated by physicians' orders or organizational policy. The effects of the loss of independence and autonomy on client well-being include anxiety, fear, and physical signs and symptoms of stress such as irritability, altered appetite, sleep disturbance, and muscle tension.

To promote client well-being, nurses support self-responsibility. Nursing care, therefore, includes interventions that promote clients' abilities to maintain, restore, or increase involvement in self-care. Mullin[91] suggests that nurses ask themselves two questions before performing client care: (1) Why am I doing this (activity)? and (2) How is this (activity) assisting the individual to be his or her own self-care agent? If the answer to the first question is "because the physician ordered it" or "because this is the way we always do it," an assessment of actual client needs may be in order, to ensure that unnecessary care is not provided. If the answer to the first question is "because the client does not know how to do it," a more appropriate nursing action might be to provide the client with the necessary knowledge to independently meet care needs.

The second question helps nurses to focus on the importance of active client participation in all facets of care. The role of nurses becomes one of "client advocate," assisting clients to obtain the necessary care while maintaining maximal independence, dignity, and self-esteem. Ambulatory hospitalized clients who have an established routine for taking prescribed medications at home, for example, should be encouraged to continue with the established schedule provided it is not pharmacologically harmful or contraindicated. Altering client medication schedules to fit set hospital administration times may alter the serum levels of the drug, confuse clients, and result in medication errors after discharge. The second question also emphasizes the importance of continued client education. Enhancing client understanding of the condition and prescribed treatments can decrease anxiety and/or fear, and promote self-confidence and feelings of self-efficacy—all important components of subjective well-being. Clients who are used to caring for themselves and others may experience difficulty accepting assistance for themselves. (See Chap. 12 for additional discussion.)

Nursing measures directed at assisting self-care should also include family members. The most compelling problem identified by families is a lack of knowledge about their loved one's condition and care.[92] Providing explanations and instruction for family members is an essential component of basic nursing care. A family that is knowledgeable about a client's condition and care requirements will be more willing and able to participate in client care. The participation of family members not only aids clients' recovery but also helps family members to feel productive and increases their feelings of self-worth. Increasing family understanding and involvement also fosters the development of a supportive home environment that enhances client wellness and participation in prescribed therapeutic regimens after discharge. By including the family, nurses promote caring for self and others. The balance and reciprocity in this dimension of wellness is important not only for client well-being, but also for family well-being. An elderly client who needs assistance with bathing and range of motion is one example of a situation in which family member involvement with an intervention is directed at assisting self-care. The family can be educated regarding the importance of range of motion, how it can be incorporated in the bath, and how the client can actively participate. Family members' sense of woth is enhanced as they participate in the client's recovery.

Preparing Clients for Health Care Experiences. Anxiety and fear are common reactions to many health care experiences. Admission to a health care facility, diagnostic testing, and surgical procedures can be stressful events for clients and family members. Clients' sense of "feeling good" is enhanced as stress is reduced through preparation for health care experiences. Preparing clients for various procedures or treatments is an important part of nursing care that promotes well-being.

Admitting the Client to the Health Care Facility. Nurses play an important role in ensuring that clients' basic needs are met during admission to the health care facility. Generally, except for emergency admissions, preliminary information is gathered by the admitting office prior to the actual admission to the nursing unit. Information collected includes personal data (name, date of birth, next of kin, address, religion) as well as information related to the reason for admission, physician's name, and health insurance or financial arrangements. Clients are also asked to sign a general consent to treatment form, which permits the health care facility to provide routine care.

Nurses are responsible for preparing the room and admitting clients to the nursing unit. The following activities should be carried out prior to the client's arrival:

- *Positioning and Preparing the Bed.* In most cases the bed should be adjusted to its lowest position to make it easier and safer for ambulatory clients to get into bed. The bed should be opened with the bedspread, blanket, and top sheet folded to the foot of the bed. If a client is arriving by stretcher, the bed should be placed in high position, and furniture in the room should be arranged to allow easy access to the bed.

- *Assembling Necessary Supplies and Equipment.* Basic supplies including bath basin, water pitcher, bedpan or urinal, emesis basin, and towels should be on hand. A hospital gown should be available, although clients may prefer to wear personal clothing. Basic equipment such as bed controls, overbed lighting, and call bell should be checked to ensure that they are in good functioning order.
- *Assembling Specialized Equipment.* Some clients may require the use of specialized equipment or supplies such as oxygen equipment, suctioning apparatus, cardiac monitoring intravenous poles, or an overhead trapeze. These items should be available and ready for client use upon arrival.

A friendly supportive attitude that conveys interest and concern for the client's needs helps to allay anxiety and fear experienced by the client and family members. Inquiring about and prompt attention to any immediate concerns that clients or family members express facilitates the development of a sense of security that needs will be met and initiates a trusting nurse–client relationship. For many clients, entering the hospital is like entering another world. Moreover, worries about the seriousness of their health problem and the kinds of treatment that may be required intensify feelings of alienation. Nurses' sensitivity to the personal significance of the transition to the sick role can be a major support (see also Chap. 12). Guidelines for basic nursing actions related to admission of the client can be found in Box 22–6.

BOX 22–6. GUIDELINES FOR CLIENT ADMISSION TO THE HEALTH CARE FACILITY

1. Introduce yourself to the client and significant others who are present. Introduce the client to other clients in the room and to any staff members encountered. Even though the client cannot be expected to remember all the names, no one should be in the client's immediate environment without being introduced.
2. Explain and demonstrate the use of the equipment within the client's area—for example, use of call system, overhead lighting, bed controls, overbed table, and television controls (if applicable). Show location of bathroom and showers, and available closet or storage space.
3. Place an identification bracelet on the client's wrist (if not already done) and explain its purpose.
4. Provide information about the agency and normal daily routines to the client and family members. Inform the client about meal hours, visiting hours and restrictions, and smoking regulations. Describe other areas of the facility that the client or family members may use, such as the cafeteria, lounges, chapel, or gift shops. Explain how the client may obtain a television or radio (if applicable).
5. Inform the client of agency policies regarding valuables and personal articles. Treat personal articles with respect and store valuables such as money, jewelry, and keys in a secure manner following agency procedures.
6. Obtain and record the client's vital signs, height, and weight. Collect specimens as needed.
7. Obtain a basic nursing and health history. Document information obtained so that the client does not have to repeat the same information to other caregivers. Ensure that allergy alerts are posted in appropriate places if needed.
8. Encourage the client and family members to ask questions and clarify needed information.
9. Encourage the client to adjust the environment within the limits of comfort, safety, and therapeutic effectiveness.
10. Begin implementation of physician's admitting orders.

Preparing for Diagnostic Tests. Client preparation for diagnostic tests should include both physical and psychological dimensions of care. Although the measures required for physical preparation are usually dictated by agency policy or physician preference, psychological preparation is based on nurses' assessment of individuals' specific needs. Both physical and psychological needs must be met in order to secure reliable test results and maintain client well-being.

Physical Preparation. The extent of physical preparation depends on the specific diagnostic test ordered. Some tests, such as a routine chest x-ray, require only a simple explanation to the client; however, many studies require more extensive preparation measures such as dietary restrictions, bowel preparation, or sedation. Many diagnostic procedures are performed on an outpatient basis, which means that clients are responsible for some aspects of self-preparation. Nurses must verify that clients are adequately informed of the purpose and rationale of the ordered preparation. Written instructions are beneficial and help to avoid misunderstandings. It is important for nurses to determine whether clients have followed preparation instructions properly before the test is begun to avoid invalid or inaccurate results.

Psychological Preparation. Diagnostic tests are frightening experiences for many people. Individuals may fear the pain or discomfort associated with the test, or experience anxiety about what the results may show. Fear of the unknown increases the stressful nature of the procedure. Clients and family members need accurate explanations of what the test entails and why it is necessary. The explanations should take into account the client's current level of understanding and how much the client needs or wants to know.

Studies have indicated that sensory information—how something looks, feels, sounds, and so on—is most useful in preparing clients for specialized procedures.[93] Basic guidelines for preparing clients include the following.

- Describe physical sensations, but do not evaluate them. Tell clients that they will feel a burning or stinging sensation, but not that it will be "awful" or "unbearable."
- Explain the causes of the sensations to clients. Knowing what to expect and what causes it will reduce problems of misinterpretation or clients fearing that something has gone wrong.
- Only prepare clients for those aspects of the experience that are noted by most clients. Over preparation may only serve to increase fear and anxiety.
- Objective information such as where the test will take place, who will do it, how long it will last, and when the results will be available is also helpful in assisting clients to develop realistic expectations for the experience.

Preparing for Surgery. Preparing clients for surgery involves many of the same principles and guidelines used in preparing clients for diagnostic procedures. As discussed earlier in this chapter, surgical procedures have a profound impact on every aspect of client well-being. Although many of the effects of anesthesia and surgery are unavoidable, studies have indicated that increased education and preparation of clients preoperatively can significantly increase the rate of recovery from surgery and reduce the incidence of postoperative complications.[94,95] In addition to preparing clients psychologically by providing objective and subjective sensory information, nurses are responsible for preoperative education of the client and family members in effective measures to manage pain, and the physical activities necessary to decrease postoperative complications and facilitate recovery. Preoperative teaching enables clients to become active participants in postoperative care and enhances individual well-being by fostering personal control.

Pain Management. Adequate management of postoperative pain is essential to client well-being. In most cases, postoperative pain management relies predominately on the use of narcotic medications; however, postoperative pain management begins preoperatively with the client teaching that is done. Without this teaching, the postoperative measures in all likelihood will not be as effective. Preoperative client teaching should focus on how narcotics can be used effectively along with relaxation techniques (deep breathing or guided imagery) to facilitate pain management during postoperative recovery.

McCaffery and Beebe[85] have identified four important elements regarding postoperative pain management that should be included in preoperative client teaching:

- Pain medications are generally ordered on a PRN (as needed) basis. Instruct clients to ask for medication before the pain becomes severe and unbearable. Pain medications are most effective if administered at regular intervals around the clock. Emphasize that clients should not assume nurses will automatically bring the pain medication, or that nurses will know when they are in pain.
- A 2- to 4-hour time restriction is generally ordered between medication doses to prevent oversedation. If the prescribed pain medication is not adequately controlling the pain during that time period, different medications or dosages can be ordered. Clients need to be encouraged to verbalize problems with inadequate pain management so that the medication and/or dosage can be adjusted until they are comfortable.
- There is very little danger of addiction to medications when used in the management of postoperative pain. Clients should not "suffer in silence" or hold off in asking for medication in the days after surgery because of fear of addiction.
- Effective pain management facilitates client participation in the activities and exercises necessary for recovery and prevention of complications.

Pain management is enhanced through client control of therapy. **Patient-controlled analgesia** (PCA) is a drug delivery system that enables clients to administer pain medication as they need it. The device is an intravenous infusion pump that administers a small preprogrammed dose of analgesic when the client pushes a button. This device is used in some institutions for pain management. Its use is not limited to clients with terminal illness. PCA has the advantage of giving clients control over their pain management. Client anxiety and feelings of powerlessness are reduced because they are in charge of their own medication administration. This enhances pain relief. Additional information related to pain control can be found in Chapter 29.

Deep-breathing Exercises. Deep-breathing exercises are taught preoperatively to hyperventilate the alveoli, expand the lungs, and facilitate oxygenation of tissues, thus preventing many of the respiratory complications of surgery.

Coughing Exercises. Coughing facilitates the removal of accumulated mucous in the respiratory tract and prevents pulmonary postoperative complication. Clients should be taught coughing exercises preoperatively to facilitate postoperative implementation. It is much harder to teach the necessary concepts or to gain clients' cooperation when they are in acute pain or drowsy from pain medication, both of which make it much more difficult for clients to focus mentally. Chapter 27 contains procedures for effective breathing and coughing exercises that are taught as part of preoperative client preparation.

Leg Exercises. Frequent movement of the extremities promotes return of blood through the venous circulation to the heart. This helps to prevent postoperative complications, such as inflammation of a vein with formation of a blood clot that can move to the lungs as a pulmonary embolus. As with other postoperative measure, leg exercises need to be learned during preoperative education to facilitate successful implementation during the client's postoperative recovery. Additional information related to leg exercises can be found in Chapter 27.

Frequent Turning. Frequent turning in bed and early ambulation promote circulation, enhance healing, and help to prevent problems associated with immobility. Before surgery, clients should be instructed that they will need to turn side to side at least every 2 hours postoperatively. Use of the siderails to facilitate turning is helpful. The importance of other mobilizing technique such as sitting at the edge of the bed and progressive ambulation should be reviewed with clients prior to surgery. These techniques are described in detail in Chapter 30.

Preventing Client Infections. A safe environment is an important component of health and well-being. Microorganisms are naturally present everywhere in the environment, both in the client's home community and in the hospital community. The hospital environment generally has a larger population of microorganisms than other environments. Most are harmless and some are even beneficial at times. An *infection* is the invasion of body tissues by microorganisms capable of producing disease. *Disease* is said to be present if the proliferation of the microorganisms produces an alteration in tissue function.

Microorganisms vary in their ability to produce disease, in the severity of the diseases they produce, and in their communicability. No organism is pathogenic—that is, disease-producing—all of the time; however, many naturally harmless microorganisms can cause disease in susceptible individuals. Infection control measures, which control or eliminate the source and transmission of infectious agents, help protect clients from disease. Control of infection is an important aspect of all nursing actions.

Supporting Normal Body Defenses. Individuals have many natural defense mechanisms that protect against invading organisms. Although many body systems, such as skin, respiratory tract, and gastrointestinal tract, are easily accessible to pathogens, each body system has unique protective physiological mechanisms.

The body's first line of defense is the mechanical barrier provided by intact skin and mucous membranes. Although bacteria and fungi can live and multiply on the skin and mucosal membranes, they cannot invade the body unless the skin or mucosa are cracked or broken. Normal physiological processes such as the constant shedding of skin cells, the ciliary action of the nasal mucosa, and the production of stomach acids also function to prevent the entrance of microorganisms. Client and nursing actions that facilitate and support normal defense mechanisms serve to enhance health and decrease disease susceptibility. Table 22–6 outlines the major physiological barriers to microorgan-

TABLE 22–6. NATURAL BODY DEFENSE MECHANISMS

Body System	Defense Mechanisms	Actions to Enhance Defense
Integumentary	Intact surface impenetrable by microorganisms. Constant shedding removes organisms adhering to outer layer. Secretion of sebum, a fatty acid, kills some bacteria. Slightly acidic pH of skin inhibits bacterial growth.	Avoidance of trauma or abrasions, which disrupt skin surface. Regular bathing to remove dead cells and excess organisms. Use of lotions or creams to prevent excessive dryness and cracking of skin.
Digestive	Regular shedding of epithelial cells rids mouth of colonizing bacteria. Intact mucosal layer provides a protective barrier. Saliva flow washes away organisms. Saliva contains microbial inhibitors such as lysozyme and lactoferrin. High acidity of stomach contents inhibits bacterial growth. Rapid peristalsis of small intestine prevents colonization of bacteria. Normal flora of large intestines kills or inhibits bacterial growth.	Regular oral hygiene to promote healthy teeth and mucosa. Maintenance of adequate hydration to facilitate saliva production and mucosa integrity. Assure that meats and fish are properly refrigerated and adequately cooked before eating. Avoidance of excessive use of antacids, which neutralize stomach acid. Ingestion of adequate amounts of fiber and fluids to promote peristalsis and prevent constipation. Adequate exercise to promote intestinal motility. Wash hands after using bathroom.
Respiratory	Cilia and moist mucous membranes lining nose and throat trap inhaled organisms. Coughing and sneezing mechanisms remove trapped organisms. Macrophages in lungs ingest foreign particles.	Avoidance of smoking, air pollution, and other factors that alter cilia and mucous membranes. Adequate hydration to maintain mucosal integrity.
Genitourinary	Low pH of vaginal secretions (after puberty) inhibits growth of many microorganisms. Presence of normal flora (lactobacilli) in vagina inhibits bacterial growth. Intact epithelium lining provides protective barrier. Flushing action of urine flow washes away microorganisms found in urethra and bladder. Intact epithelium lining urethra provides protective barrier.	Avoidance of excessive douching, which alters normal pH. Use of cotton underclothes to absorb excessive moisture and retard bacterial growth. Adequate fluid intake to promote normal urination. Frequent urination to prevent bladder distension and urine. Practice effective perianal hygiene. Urinate after intercourse.

isms and actions that support them. Additional information on natural defenses can be found in Chapters 7 and 24.

If the body's natural barrier mechanisms fail, other secondary defense mechanisms help to protect individuals, such as inflammation, increased production of white blood cells, and production of antibodies to counter disease-producing microorganisms that invade the body (see also Chap. 24). A healthy life-style, adequate nutrition, and effective stress management help to enhance these body mechanisms. Other measures such as routine immunization programs also help to prevent the development of infectious diseases.

Identifying Clients at Risk. Many factors increase clients' susceptibility to infection. Assessment of these factors assists nurses in identifying those individuals who are at risk.

Age. The risk of infection is greatest in newborn infants and the elderly. At birth, newborns are protected only by antibodies received from their mothers. Their immune system is immature and incapable of producing the needed immunoglobulins and white blood cells. As infants grow, their immune systems mature but they remain susceptible to many infectious agents.

The aging process decreases the effectiveness of the immune system. There is a progressive loss of cellular regulation in the body and an increased susceptibility to disease. Aging also alters the structural integrity of the skin and mucous membranes, which increases elderly individuals' exposure to pathogens.

Stress. As discussed earlier in the chapter, exposure to excessive levels of stress decreases individuals' resistance to infection or disease. Continued high levels of adrenocorticosteroids decrease anti-inflammatory responses, deplete energy stores, and lead to a stage of exhaustion. Thus, clients encountering hospitalization or surgery are particularly prone to the development of infections, not only because of the exposure to invasive organisms, but also because of the high levels of physiological and emotional stress that many experience.

Heredity. Some individuals have a genetic susceptibility to the development of infections. Familial tendencies for immune abnormalities affect the production of antibodies and alter immune responses, resulting in increased risk of infection.

Nutritional Status. Adequate nutrient intake is essential for the maintenance of normal body defenses and adequate tissue repair. Negative nitrogen balance, often experienced as a result of illness or injury, decreases individuals' ability to fight or resist infection. (See also Chap. 25.)

Existing Disease. Any disease that alters the body's defense mechanisms places clients at risk of infection. Diseases that directly affect the immune system, such as AIDS or leukemia, are particularly perilous. However, chronic conditions such as diabetes or emphysema also deplete individuals' energy and nutritional reserves and leave them vulnerable to infection.

Medical Therapy. Some drugs and medical therapies compromise clients' immune responses and increase susceptibility to infection. Antineoplastic drugs and radiation therapy, which are used in treating cancer, also destroy normal cells and lower the body's resistance to infection. Steroid medications suppress the inflammatory process and increase protein breakdown. Some antibiotics administered to combat infections can have adverse effects. Antibiotic therapy often destroys the normal flora of the intestines or vagina, thus allowing the proliferation of bacteria that would usually be inhibited.

Diagnostic procedures can also predispose clients to infection. Many of these procedures involve a disruption of skin barriers or an invasion of internal body cavities. Although these procedures may be performed under sterile conditions and not directly introduce pathogens into the body, the trauma sustained by skin or mucous membranes may leave the client vulnerable to subsequent infection.

Client Environment. A client's environment is a potential risk factor for infection. Some environments harbor agents of infection to a greater extent than others. People are the most common source of infection to others and to themselves. This means that individuals with close contact with large numbers of people, such as those of low socioeconomic status, are at increased risk of infection. Poverty profoundly affects an individual's life-style and health practices. Inadequate health practices and poor nutrition often associated with poverty increase clients' susceptibility to infection. As previously discussed, the hospital community also has characteristics that increase infection risk.

Applying Principles of Medical Asepsis. The presence of microorganisms does not necessary mean that an infection can or will occur. The development of an infection requires a cyclical six-step process commonly known as "the chain of infection" (see Chap. 7). Elements of the infectious process include the infectious agent, the reservoir (or source), a portal of exit from the source, a mode (method) of transmission, a portal of entry, and a new, susceptible host. Infection is prevented or controlled by "breaking" or interrupting the chain of infection.

Medical asepsis refers to all measures that limit the growth and/or spread of microorganisms. Surgical asepsis is the method by which all microorganisms are eliminated, and is described later in the chapter under Restorative Care. With medical asepsis, objects are identified as clean or dirty. Clean objects harbor microorganisms, but none that are considered infectious. Dirty objects are soiled with potential disease-producing microorganisms. Basic household sanitation is a form of medical asepsis. Additional procedures are used in the hospital community because hospital microbe populations are larger and often more virulent and because clients who are ill have increased susceptibility to infection.

Traditionally, infection precautions have focused on preventing the spread of microorganisms from individuals who were exhibiting manifestations of infection. More re-

BUILDING NURSING KNOWLEDGE

Do Current Handwashing Procedures Take a Toll on Nurses' Skin?

Seitz JC, Newman JL. Factors affecting skin condition in two nursing populations: Implications for current handwashing protocols. *Am J Infect Control.* 1988;16:46–53.

The investigators note that handwashing has undeniable importance as a procedure for preventing nosocomial infection. Yet in their view, current practices are based largely on untested traditions and beliefs, and some practices may actually compromise the natural ability of the skin to protect against microbes. Their objective was to document the effects of frequent handwashing on nurses' skin.

In this study, two populations of nurses were studied to examine the effects of daily handwashing and certain environmental variables. Nurses' scores were compared to those of housewives and female office workers, who experienced seasonsal dry skin but were not subjected to high-frequency handwashing.

Ninety-seven nurses, ages 20 to 65, were selected from two hospitals, one in Wisconsin and one in Arizona. These nurses continued their routine handwashing procedures during the study. Those prone to dry skin or who had skin diseases on the hands were eliminated from the sample. The sample of housewives and secretaries was taken from another ongoing study.

For both groups of nurses, photos of the backs of hands were taken in July and August and again in January and February. Prior to the study, scores on a scale of 0 to 10 were given each subject for erythema, scaling, and cracking. Graders had no knowledge of subject group assignment or season of the year. Scores were grouped according to age, locale, work area, and handwashing frequency. Summer to winter differences in scores were analyzed.

Wintertime hand erythema, scaling, and cracking scores for Wisconsin nurses were significantly higher than those for the Arizona nurses or those of housewives and secretaries prone to dry skin. Summertime scaling scores for Wisconsin nurses were also higher.

There was no difference in Wisconsin nurses' scores when sorted by frequency of handwashing or work area. Older age was associated with higher scaling and cracking scores in the summertime. Wintertime scores were higher than summertime scores. Wintertime cracking scores were higher for nurses working in general and maternity areas. Arizona nurses experienced no significant differences in scaling, cracking, or erythema associated with frequency of handwashing or work area; however, older age was associated with greater scaling.

The most profound variable in the study was winter season climate. The investigators linked this to low indoor humidity, which fluctuates dramatically with outdoor temperature. They reasoned that the range of the skin's tolerance for temperature and humidity changes is low, and when exceeded, the skin can no longer replace its surface moisture. In the winter climate even moderate handwashing frequency (one to two times per hour) compromised the integrity of the skin, which the investigators concluded suggests the need for reevaluating guidelines for handwashing protocols with specific interventions to alleviate the symptoms of dry skin. They proposed substituting milder cleansers and using hand lotion treatment.

cently, it has become increasingly apparent that infectious pathogens are transmitted not only from symptomatic individuals but from asymptomatic individuals whose body substances (blood, wound drainage, feces, urine, airway secretions) contain the infectious agents. As a result, the value and effectiveness of some of the traditional infection control measures such as isolation and double bagging soiled items are now being questioned.

Handwashing. Handwashing is the single most important means of preventing the spread of infection. Handwashing should be practiced by everyone in the health care community including clients, visitors, nurses, and other health care providers. The purpose of handwashing is to remove microorganisms that might be transmitted to a new susceptible host. The Centers for Disease Control (CDC)[96] recommend that caregivers wash their hands:

- On arrival at the hospital
- Before meals
- After toileting
- Before contact with clients who are susceptible to infection
- After caring for infected clients
- After touching any body substance (even if gloves were worn)
- Before and after contact with wounds
- Before and after invasive procedures (injections, suctioning, catheterization)
- After handling contaminated equipment
- Between giving care to different clients
- Before leaving the unit for the day

Differences of opinion exist about the appropriate choice of cleansing agents, the necessary length of time, and the ideal frequency of washing. Friction, not soap, is the most effective component of handwashing. It is generally accepted that handwashing is the most valuable method of infection control and that it is not done frequently enough. Recent studies have indicated that fewer than half of all client contacts by health care personnel were preceded or followed by handwashing even when the clients were known to have infectious diseases.[97]

Various products are available for handwashing. The CDC recommends the use of plain soap for most general care and for instances where the sole purpose of handwashing is to remove soil and transient organisms. Plain soap, however, only *removes* organisms—it does not kill them. Therefore, in dealing with high-risk clients or in areas where exposure to many virulent pathogens is likely, washing with a product that contains an antimicrobial ingredient is recommended.[97]

The basic techniques for adequate handwashing are presented in Procedure 22–1. These techniques are intended for use with medical asepsis. Techniques for cleansing the hands prior to sterile procedures, such as surgical operations or delivering an infant can be found in a text dealing with operating room procedures. Some authorities advocate the removal of rings prior to handwashing; total bacteria counts on the hands, especially of gram-negative

BUILDING NURSING KNOWLEDGE

Is the Amount of Soap Used in Handwashing Important?

Larson EL, Eke PI, Wilder, MP, Laughon BE. Quantity of soap as a variable in handwashing. *Infect Control.* 1987;8:371–375.

The investigators note that there are a number of influences on the effectiveness of handwashing: the agent used, amount of friction applied, and frequency of washing. Yet little is known about the importance of the amount of soap used. Official guidelines fail to specify a recommendation for amount of plain or antimicrobial soap. Many institutions are changing from bar to liquid soap for hygienic and practical reasons. Some soap dispensers are set to dispense a standard amount. This study compared the antimicrobial effects of four products when used in two different amounts, 1 or 3 mL, per handwash.

Forty adult subjects with no skin diseases who were receiving no antibiotic medications were chosen for the study. They were randomly assigned to one of four handwashing agents, ten subjects per group. One group used an antiseptic agent with 4 percent chlorhexidine gluconate (Hibiclens); two groups used alcohol-based handrinses (Calstat and Hibistat); and one group used a liquid nonantimicrobial soap (Safe'n Sure). Within each product group, subjects were randomly assigned to use 1 or 3 mL of product per wash.

Following an initial handwash with control soap, a baseline culture was obtained for each subject. Subjects washed their hands with their assigned product 15 times a day under supervision for 5 days using a standardized handwashing procedure. Hand cultures were obtained after the first and last handwash on days 1 and 5.

Significant differences were found among product groups on day 1. After 15 washes on day 5, however, bacterial counts were the lowest of any test period, and there were no differences in reductions of bacterial counts associated with antiseptic products. With antiseptic products, there was a statistically significant dose-related response. Subjects using 3-mL doses had fewer bacterial counts than those using 1-mL doses, on both days 1 and 5. Reductions in bacterial counts with antiseptic products were greater when large quantities of soap were used, whereas counts in subjects using control soap were the same or higher when more soap was used. The investigators concluded that in clinical areas where there are high-risk clients, and where personnel perform tasks where hand hygiene is important (handling newborns, doing invasive procedures, caring for clients with open wounds, etc), the use of antiseptic soap in amounts of 3 to 5 mL per handwash is indicated to reduce bacteria.

organisms, are significantly higher when rings are worn. Rings also interfere with handwashing and the donning of gloves. Studies have indicated, however, that thorough handwashing reduces the bacterial count in ring wearers to that of non-ring wearers.[97] Generally the removal of all rings except a plain wedding band is considered effective.

Use of Gloves. Use of gloves is an important component of medical and surgical asepsis. Donning of gloves for surgical asepsis will be discussed later in this chapter under *Restorative Care.* With medical asepsis, gloves reduce the possibility that health care workers will be infected with organisms from clients, reduce the likelihood of caregivers transferring their own organisms to the client, and reduce the possibility that caregivers will transfer organisms from one client to another.

Clean, nonsterile gloves are indicated in many health care situations. Nurses should use clean gloves whenever there is the risk of contact with damaged or broken skin, contaminated material, mucous membranes, and any body fluids including blood, urine, feces, sputum. Also, all health care providers with chapped skin or cuts should wear clean gloves for their own protection. Disposable, nonsterile gloves are made of either latex or vinyl. Latex gloves are a natural material that is more flexible and durable than vinyl (which is a synthetic rubber), so they should be used for tasks that are likely to stress the gloves. Health care worker allergy to latex or the powder used in latex gloves necessitates the use of vinyl in all situations.[98] Often special efforts to obtain these gloves is necessary. Disposable, nonsterile gloves are easily applied and are designed to fit either hand. Keeping a box of disposable gloves at every bedside encourages their frequent use (see Fig. 22–7).

Gloves should be changed after direct contact with a client's excretions or secretions, even if care has not been completed. While a special technique is not needed to re-

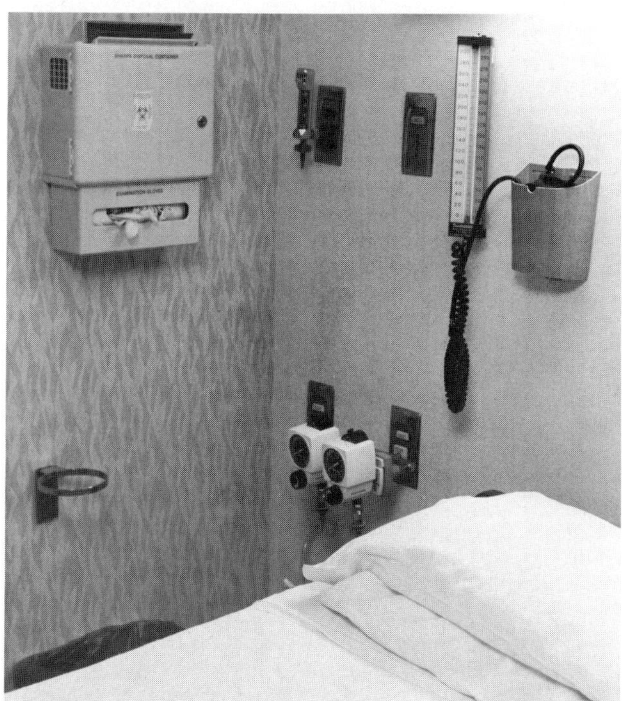

Figure 22–7. A dispenser for clean disposable gloves and a container for disposal of used syringes in each client's room facilitates carrying out universal precautions.

PROCEDURE 22–1. HANDWASHING

PURPOSE: To remove soil and transient organisms from the hands, thereby preventing transmission of pathogens from one client to another.

EQUIPMENT: Liquid or bar soap, warm running water, and paper towels.

ACTION	RATIONALE
1. Remove and store all jewelry except watch and plain wedding band. Push watch and long sleeves above the wrists.	1. Jewelry harbors microorganisms that are difficult to remove with normal handwashing technique. These organisms may be transferred to the client.
2. Adjust water flow so no splashing occurs; adjust water temperature to lukewarm. Avoid contacting sink with hands or uniform as you wash.	2. The sink is a reservoir of microorganisms. Contact and/or splashed water will transfer organisms to you, which could then be transmitted to clients. Hot water depletes protective skin oils, increasing risk of chapping and breaks in the skin. Chapped or broken skin provides a portal of entry for organisms, increasing infection risk to nurses.
3. Wet hands and wrists, keeping hands lower than elbows.	3. The hands have a greater microbial population than forearms. Gravity causes water and suspended microorganisms to flow downward and off the hands. If hands are higher than elbows, wrists and forearms will be contaminated by microbes from hands.
4. Apply soap and rub hands and wrists to create a generous amount of lather. NOTE: Bar soaps harbor microbes. If used, rinse bar thoroughly to remove them.	4. Lather suspends transient microorganisms so they can be flushed from the hands.

(continued)

PROCEDURE 22–1. (continued)

5. Wash for 10 to 30 seconds, cleaning all surfaces of hands and fingers, with firm, brisk rubbing motions.

5. Firm rubbing creates friction, which dislodges transient microbes.

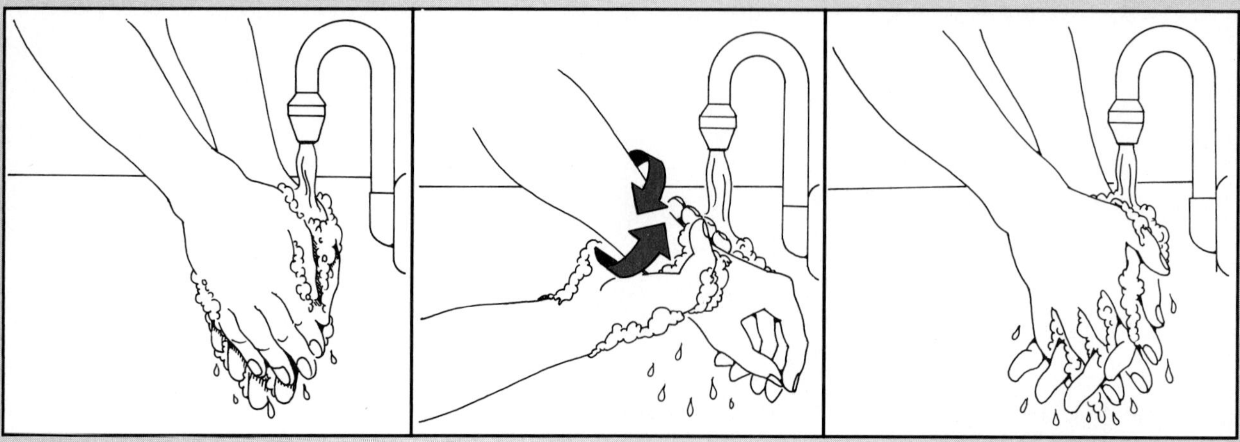

6. Clean under nails and around nailbeds with fingertips and nails from opposite hand.

6. Microbes lodge under and around nails. Transient microbes may become resident flora and colonize if not removed. Short nails are less likely to harbor microbes.

7. Thoroughly rinse each hand, holding fingertips downward.

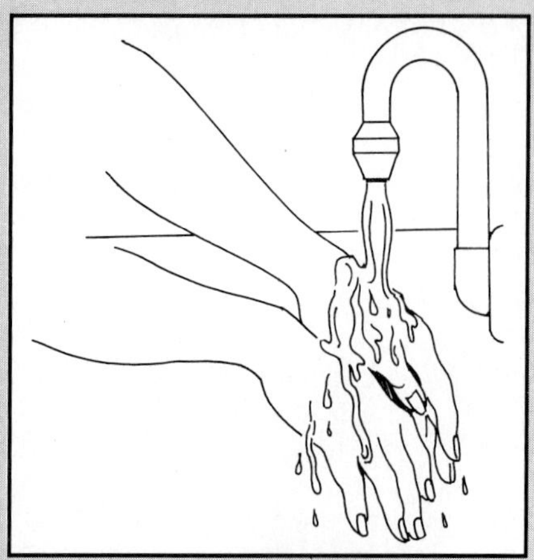

7. Rinsing removes lather with suspended microbes. See also step 3, above.

8. Repeat steps 4 to 7, if hands were grossly contaminated.

8. No studies support a specific length of time for effective washing; however, it is generally accepted that length of washing should correspond to degree of contamination.

9. Dry hands thoroughly with paper towels.

9. Drying well prevents chapping (which would create a portal of entry for organisms).

(continued)

PROCEDURE 22–1. (continued)

10. If faucet is hand regulated, protect your hand with the paper towel when turning off the water.

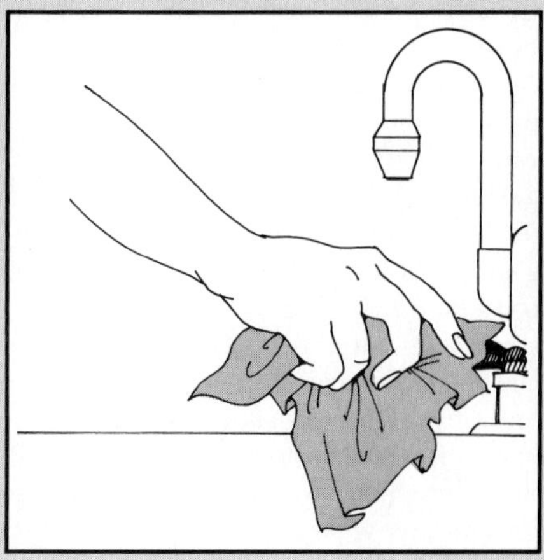

10. The faucet handle is contaminated. The paper towel creates a barrier, preventing transfer of microbes to your hands.

11. Apply lotion to hands if desired.

11. Hand lotions contain emollients, which replace skin moisture lost during handwashing, thereby preventing cracking and chapping.

RECORDING: No recording is necessary.

move gloves, there is no reason to soil one's hands while removing gloves. Removing nonsterile gloves as one does sterile gloves, described in Procedure 22–4 steps 7 and 8, prevents bare hand contact with dirty gloves. Used gloves should be discarded into a waste receptable marked "infectious waste." If nursing actions do not require additional contact with body substances, additional gloving is not necessary. It is important to note that the use of gloves does not eliminate the need for effective handwashing after client care is completed. Nonsterile gloves have been found to be prone to tiny, invisible tears, allowing organisms to enter and contaminate hands.[99] Moreover, organisms on the hands multiply rapidly inside the warm, moist environment of the glove even when external contamination does not occur. Handwashing is thus essential after gloves are removed.

Use of Gowns. Gowns are used primarily to prevent routine soiling of caregivers' clothing when providing client care. Gowns are not necessary for most client care; however, they are indicated when clothes are likely to be soiled with infective secretions or excretions such as when changing the bed of a client with infectious diarrhea or holding an infant with a respiratory infection.

Gowns are long to cover all outer clothing. They open in the back and are secured with ties at the waist and neck. Long sleeves with tight-fitting cuffs provide added protection. When gowns are indicated, they should be worn only once and then discarded. Those made of cloth can be laundered for reuse while paper gowns are disposable. In some situations plastic aprons are worn over gowns, because isolation gowns are not impervious to moisture.

There is no special technique for donning a clean gown as long as it is fastened securely at the waist and the neck with an overlap of the gown at the back to ensure coverage of the clothing; however, the gown should be removed carefully to minimize contamination of hands and clothing. To remove a gown, first loosen the waist ties, and then the neck ties. Slip your hands inside the gown sleeves without touching the outside of the gown. Then pull the gown off the shoulders without turning the sleeves inside out. Hold the gown at the shoulders and fold the outside surfaces together to reduce contact with the soiled gown. Discard the gown into a receptable for soiled linen or trash and wash hands (Fig. 22–8).

Use of Masks. Wearing a mask and protective eyewear (goggles or glasses) may be necessary when caregiving measures create a risk for client body substances splattering the caregiver's eyes, nose, or mouth. Masks also protect caregivers from inhaling microorganisms transmitted through the air from infected clients (respiratory isolation)

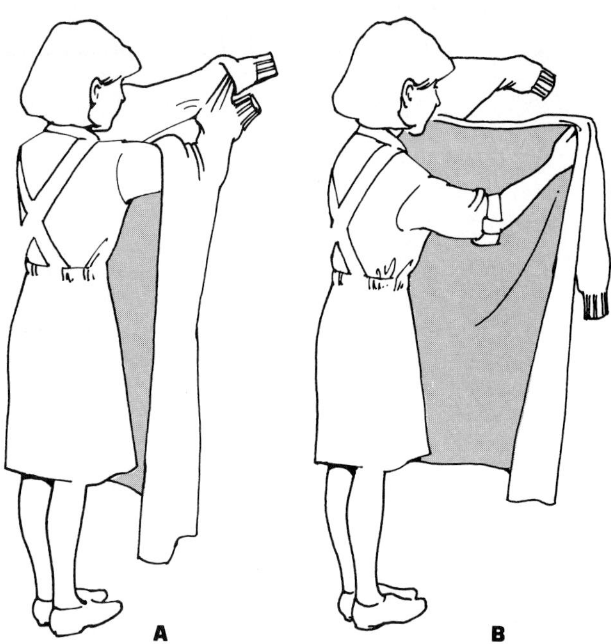

Figure 22–8. A nurse protects herself from contact with organisms when removing an isolation gown by **(A)** slipping her hands out of the sleeves without touching the outside of the gown; and **(B)** pulling the gown off her shoulders and folding it inside out for disposal.

and prevent contamination of clients having limited resistance from organisms in the caregiver's respiratory tract (reverse isolation). Masks are worn by caregivers, visitors, or clients based on the needs of the situation. When entering a client's room to administer care or visit, caregivers or visitors wear masks. If clients with a contagious respiratory infection or compromised immune function must leave their rooms, they should wear a mask.

A mask is applied by holding the top strings. Position the mask over the bridge of your nose, bring the ties above your ears, and tie the upper strings at the top back of the head. If you wear glasses, the top edge of the mask should fit under your glasses to reduce fogging of the glasses as you exhale. Pull the lower edge of the mask so that it fits under your chin. Tie the lower strings at the nape of the neck (Fig. 22–9). Most masks have a flexible metal strip to secure them over the bridge of the nose.

A properly applied mask should fit snugly over the nose and mouth so pathogens cannot enter or escape from the sides. Talking should be kept to a minimum when wearing masks. Masks that become moist are ineffective and should be discarded. Before removing a mask, wash your hands. Begin removing mask by loosening the lower strings. Dispose of the used mask in a waste receptable marked "infectious waste." A mask should never be lowered around the neck and reused.

Use of Private Rooms. The CDC suggests that in general private rooms can reduce the transmission of infectious organisms by separating infected or colonized clients from susceptible individuals. It is also suggested that the use of private rooms may encourage the practice of handwashing by personnel before leaving the room and contacting other clients, especially if a sink is available at the door. Nevertheless a private room is not necessary to prevent the spread of many infections.[96]

The CDC recommends the use of a private room for individuals with infections that are highly contagious or especially virulent. Additionally, a private room is suggested for infected individuals with ineffective hygiene habits. When it is unavoidable that infected individuals share a room, it is important that they be placed with appropriate roommates. Generally, infected clients should not share a room with a highly susceptible individual or one for whom the consequences of infection could be quite severe. When an infected person shares a room with an uninfected person, it is important for both clients and health care personnel to practice good personal hygiene and medical asepsis. Individuals with the same infectious disease may share a room.

Care of Contaminated Equipment. Used articles usually need to be enclosed in an impervious bag and sealed before they are removed from the client area. This practice is used to protect personnel in the health care facility who may come in contact with the soiled equipment or supplies. Bagging items used in client care is also necessary to protect other clients from cross-infection. CDC guidelines indicate that bagging is necessary only if the articles are contaminated with infectious material.

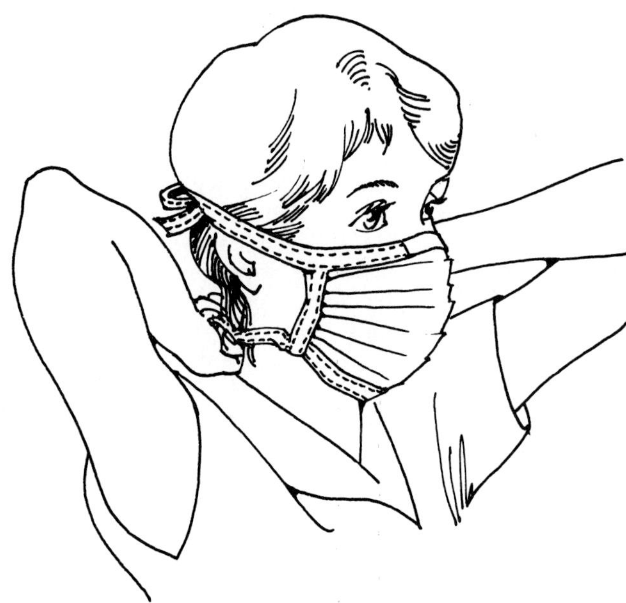

Figure 22–9. Apply a disposable mask so the top ties go over your ears and tie at the back of your head and the lower ties tie at the base of the neck. Adjust the mask to fit over your nose by bending the metal strip at the top of the mask.

Double bagging of infected materials is used in some hospitals to prevent contamination of the bag's outer surface. The procedure requires the nurse in the client's room to close the first bag tightly. That nurse then places the first bag into a second, clean bag. The second bag is held outside the client's room by a second "clean nurse" or a self-supporting hamper. The second bag is closed securely. Double bagging, although common in the past, is unnecessary as long as the single bag is impervious and not easily penetrated, and the articles can be placed in the bag without soiling the outside. With either method, the outer bag must be specially labeled or colored to indicate it contains infectious material.

Much of the equipment and supplies in health care facilities today is designed for single use only and should be disposed of after one use. Some items are reusable. Individual facilities may have specific guidelines for the handling and care of reusable equipment. Nurses need to become familiar with the standard policies of the agency in which they work.

Isolation Precautions. Since 1983, the CDC has recommended two major forms of isolation precautions: disease-specific and category-specific precautions. The rationale behind these precautions is to interrupt transmission of organisms by placing barriers (gloves, gowns, masks) between the infective substances and health care providers. With disease-specific precautions, certain isolation practices are recommended for each infectious disease. This is the least costly and time-consuming method and ensures that clients are not "overisolated" with unnecessary precautions. The category-specific precautions (Table 22–7) are used more commonly and include isolation precautions for eight categories of diseases based on mode of transmission. When category-specific isolation is used, a cart stocked with all the items needed (eg, gowns, masks, gloves, bags) is parked in the hallway outside the client's room to facilitate adhering to correct precautions (Fig. 22–10).

In 1987, due to the increasing prevalence of the human immunodeficiency virus (HIV) which causes acquired immunodeficiency disease (AIDS), the CDC recommended that the Universal Blood and Body Fluids Precautions be expanded and applied to *all* clients, especially those in emergency care areas where the exposure to blood is increased and the infection status of clients is unknown. Under these **universal precautions** the blood and certain body fluids of all clients are considered potentially infectious with HIV and other blood-borne organisms, and strict adherence to infection control measures for minimizing the risk of exposure to blood and body fluids is vital. Careful disposal of items contaminated with blood and body fluids is also critical. However, it is equally important that items that have not contacted blood and body fluids be disposed of in conventional trash containers. All trash placed in waste containers marked "infectious waste" must receive special treatment.

Box 22–7 outlines the specific guidelines for universal precautions. It is important for health care professionals to realize that the risk of HIV infection through client contact is very small and can be all but eliminated through the careful use of universal precautions. Of the thousands of documented accidental exposures of health care workers to HIV-infected body substances, less than half a dozen workers have been infected. Over 40 percent of these exposures were classified as preventable. The majority of the accidents were related to recapping needles or the improper disposal of needles and sharp instruments.[100]

Caring for Psychosocial Needs of Isolated Clients. Ambulatory clients in a hospital often express feelings of being "trapped" or "caged." Surrounded by unfamiliar and sometimes threatening sights and sounds, with few distractions to redirect their attention, hospitalized clients are constantly reminded of the fragility of health. The implementation of infection control measures can have even more profound psychosocial implications for individuals being isolated. Strict confinement to a private room can be devastating, especially for children. Clients may feel unclean, undesirable, and rejected. Friends and relatives as well as health care workers may spend less time with isolated clients due to fear of contracting the disease or the inconvenience of dealing with the prescribed isolation procedures. The resulting social isolation and sensory deprivation can have a profound effect on client well-being.

Education of clients and significant others about the epidemiological aspects of their condition and the proper procedures for the specified isolation procedures can help to allay unnecessary fears and help to prevent the spread of infection. Visitors and health care workers need to be particularly sensitive to clients' feelings of loneliness or undesirability. Health care providers should spend time with clients to listen and talk about their feelings regarding isolation. Care should be taken to ensure that clients are not "overisolated" with unnecessary precautions.

Although beneficial for all clients confined to the hospital for an extended period of time, diversional activities are an especially important part of care for isolated clients. Varying the daily routine and physical environment may help relieve monotony. Clients can be involved in scheduling times for pesonal care or treatments around visitors or favorite television shows. Providing space for clients to display cards, family pictures, or posters in the room creates a pleasant, cheerful environment as well as providing informal validation of social supports. Displaying religious articles, providing opportunities for clients to participate in religious rituals, or arranging for visits with appropriate clergy are important activities that should not be overlooked or ignored. For some clients, access to daily newspapers, magazines, or library books are pleasant diversions. Discussing clients' usual hobbies or recreational activities may also provide ideas for other activities.

Supporting Client Well-being. Many nursing interventions support or enhance client well-being. Although most of these interventions are not complex or highly technical, they are a vital component of good nursing care and do much to facilitate clients' achievement of optimal health.

TABLE 22–7. CATEGORY-SPECIFIC ISOLATION PRECAUTIONS

Isolation Category	Purpose	Room	Gowns	Masks	Gloves	Handwashing	Care of Contaminated Articles
Strict Isolation Diphtheria, smallpox, varicella (chickenpox)	Designed to prevent transmission of highly contagious or virulent infections that may be spread by both air and contact.	Private room is indicated. Door should be kept closed. In general, people infected with same organism may share a room.	Indicated for all persons entering the room.	Indicated for all persons entering the room.	Indicated for all persons entering the room.	Hands must be washed after touching the client or potentially contaminated articles and before taking care of another client.	Contaminated articles should be discarded or bagged and labeled before being sent for decontamination and reprocessing.
Contact Isolation Acute respiratory infection in children, conjunctivitis, herpes simplex, influenza, rubella, viral pneumonia	Designed to prevent transmission of highly transmissable or epidemiologically important infections that do not warrant strict isolation.	Same as strict isolation.	Indicated if soiling is likely.	Indicated for those who come close to the client.	Indicated if touching infective material.	Same as strict isolation.	Same as strict isolation.
Respiratory Isolation Measles, meningitis, mumps, pneumonia, pertussis	Designed to prevent transmission of infectious diseases primarily over short distances through the air (droplet transmission).	Same as strict isolation.	Not indicated.	Indicated for those who come close to the client.	Not indicated.	Same as strict isolation.	Same as strict isolation.
Tuberculosis Isolation (AFB Isolation) Pulmonary and laryngeal tuberculosis	Designed to prevent the spread of acid-fast bacilli (AFB).	Private room with special ventilation is indicated. Door should be kept closed. In general, people infected with the same organism may share a room.	Indicated only if needed to prevent gross contamination of clothing.	Indicated only if the client is coughing and does not reliably cover the mouth.	Not indicated.	Same as strict isolation.	Articles are rarely involved in transmission of tuberculosis. Articles should be thoroughly cleaned and disinfected or discarded.

TABLE 22–7. (continued)

Isolation Category	Purpose	Room	Gowns	Masks	Gloves	Handwashing	Care of Contaminated Articles
Enteric Precautions Amebic dysentery, cholera, diarrhea, gastroenteritis, viral meningitis, polio	Designed to prevent infections that are transmitted by direct or indirect contact with feces.	Private room is indicated if client hygiene is poor.	Indicated if soiling is likely.	Not indicated.	Indicated if toucing infective material.	Same as strict isolation.	Same as strict isolation.
Drainage/ Secretion Precautions Minor or limited abscesses, burns, decubitus ulcers, skin infection, wound infection	Designed to prevent infections that are transmitted by direct or indirect contact with purulent material or drainage from and infected body site.	Not indicated.	Indicated if soiling is likely.	Not indicated.	Indicated if touching infective material.	Same as strict isolation.	Same as strict isolation.
Blood/Body Fluid Precautions AIDS, hepatitis B, malaria, syphilis	Designed to prevent infections that are transmitted by direct or indirect contact with infective blood or body fluids.	Private room is indicated if client hygiene is poor. In general, people infected with same organism may share a room.	Indicated if soiling of clothing with blood or body fluids is likely.	Not indicated.	Indicated if touching blood or body fluids.	Hands must be washed immediately if they are potentially contaminated with blood or body fluids and before taking care of another client.	Same as strict isolation. Used needles must be placed in puncture-proof container for disposal.

Managing Stress. Effective stress management is an integral component of individual well-being. It promotes the sense of "feeling good," which is essential to well-being. The nurse's role in stress management extends beyond controlling sources of biological and environmental stressors in the acute care setting. It also includes assisting clients to assess their current stress levels, evaluate the adequacy of their coping mechanisms, and develop competence in using various stress management techniques. Pender[1] identifies three areas of intervention in stress management: (1) minimizing the frequency of stress-inducing situations, (2) psychological preparation to increase resistance to stress, and (3) counterconditioning to avoid psychological arousal resulting from stress.

Reducing Exposure to Stressful Situations. Attempting to eliminate all stressors is unrealistic and virtually impossible; however, clients can learn to reduce and control many of the stressful situations they encounter. Assisting clients to become aware of their current stress levels and identifying stressors that are amenable to change is an important nursing function.

Nurses can assist clients to reduce or control sources of stress in the environment using techniques such as avoiding unnecessary change, time management, and environmental modification.[1,101,102]

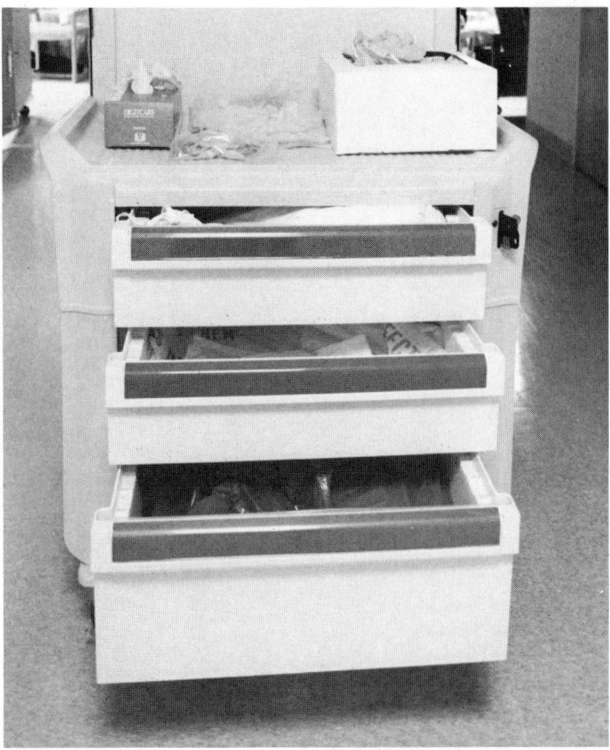

Figure 22–10. An isolation cart outside a client's room contains all the supplies needed to carry out category-specific isolation procedures.

AVOIDANCE OF UNNECESSARY CHANGE. Clients who are already experiencing stress should be encouraged to avoid any unnecessary changes during this time, such as taking on new responsibilities at work or moving to a new residence. By controlling planned change, individuals can prevent additional stress that could lead to exhaustion and illness.

TIME MANAGEMENT. The inability to accomplish personal goals due to lack of time is expressed frequently by most people. This lack of time to care for oneself is stressful and promotes ill health. For example, individuals may be unable to follow a prescribed diet or treatment regimen because their time is devoted to caring for family, helping friends, or volunteering in the community. The following time management techniques help to minimize stress through the analysis and restructuring of daily life according to a plan based on an individual's values and personal goals.

- *Identify values and personal goals.* Clients must identify what it is they value most: family, religious beliefs, health, happiness, honesty, and so on. This information will help them to decide upon their own personal goals, and to prioritize these goals as to which is the most and least important. A person may value providing care for her sick mother. She may also desire to follow a low-salt diet and exercise regimen prescribed to treat her own heart disease. Ordering the priority of the goals will determine how she plans her time.
- *Identify time that is wasted.* This activity follows from the clarification of values and personal goals. Encourage clients to regularly schedule a block of time to analyze and reflect on their progress toward achieving these personal goals. Have them describe a typical day or week in their lives, and analyze this time with their personal goals in mind. At this point it is important to focus on time that is wasted on activities unrelated to these goals. An individual may have unrealistic expectations of himself and be overcommitted to family and community projects. Overcommitment of one's time can lead to frustration, inability to meet one's own and others' expectations, and stress.
- *Restructure time.* When time-wasting activities and valued pursuits have been identified, nurses work with individuals to plan daily activities with personal goals in mind. The focus is using time efficiently and effectively to achieve these goals with the least stress, while still allowing time for relaxing and restorative pursuits when time pressures are not a factor. Clients learn to "say no" to commitments that are low on the priority list, to delegate responsibility to others, and to seek assistance when necessary. Nurses can encourage clients to break tasks down into smaller parts and recognize the value in the accomplishment of each part to enhance self-esteem and minimize frustration. Clients also need to learn to recognize and avoid procrastination. Procrastination leads to stressful feelings of urgency as deadlines or due dates draw

BOX 22–7. CDC GUIDELINES FOR UNIVERSAL PRECAUTIONS

1. Universal precautions apply to blood and other body fluids containing visible blood. BLOOD IS THE SINGLE MOST IMPORTANT SOURCE OF HIV, HBV, AND OTHER BLOODBORNE PATHOGENS IN THE OCCUPATIONAL SETTING.
2. Universal precautions also apply to semen and vaginal secretions, tissues, and the following fluids: cerebrospinal fluid, pleural fluid, synovial fluid, peritoneal fluid, pericardial fluid, and amniotic fluid.
3. Universal precautions do not apply to feces, nasal secretions, sputum, sweat, tears, urine, and vomitus unless they contain visible blood.
4. Universal precautions do not apply to saliva. Gloves need not be worn when feeding clients and when wiping saliva from skin.
5. All health care workers should routinely use appropriate barrier precautions to prevent skin and mucous membrane exposure when contact with blood or other body fluids of any client is anticipated. Gloves should be worn for touching blood and body fluids, mucous membranes, or non-intact skin of all clients, for handling items or surfaces soiled with blood or body fluids, and for performing venipuncture and other vascular access procedures. Masks and protective eyewear or face shields should be worn during procedures that are likely to generate droplets of blood or other body fluids. Gowns or aprons should be worn during procedures that are likely to generate splashes of blood or other body fluids.
6. Universal precautions are intended to supplement rather than replace recommendations for routine infection control, such as handwashing and using gloves to prevent gross microbial contamination of hands.
7. Hands and other skin surfaces should be washed immediately and thoroughly if contaminated with blood or body fluids. Hands should be washed immediately after gloves are removed.
8. All health care workers should take precautions to prevent injuries caused by needles, scalpels, and other sharp instruments or devices during procedures, when cleaning used instruments during disposal of used needles, and when handling sharp instruments after procedures.
9. Do not recap used needles by hand; do not remove used needles from disposable syringes by hand; do not bend or break or otherwise manipulate used needles by hand. Place used disposable syringes and needles, scalpel blades, and other sharp items in puncture-resistant containers for disposal. Locate the puncture-resistant containers as close to the use area as is practical.
10. Use sterile gloves for procedures involving contact with normally sterile areas of the body. Use examination gloves for procedures involving contact with mucous membranes unless otherwise indicated and for other client care or diagnostic procedures that do not require the use of sterile gloves. Gloves should be changed after contact with each client. Do not wash or disinfect surgical or examination gloves for reuse. Use general-purpose utility gloves (eg, rubber household gloves) for housekeeping chores involving potential blood contact and for instrument cleaning and decontamination procedures.
11. Health-care workers who have exudative lesions or weeping dermatitis should refrain from all client care and from handling client care equipment until the condition resolves.
12. Although saliva has not been implicated in HIV transmission, to minimize the need for emergency mouth-to-mouth resuscitation, mouthpieces, resuscitation bags, and other ventilation devices should be available in area where the need for emergency mouth-to-mouth resuscitation is predictable.
13. Handle soiled linens as little as possible and minimize shaking or other agitation to diminish contamination of air and personnel. Wet linen soiled with bloody fluids must be placed in leak resistant bags in the room in which it was used.
14. Put all specimens of blood and listed body fluids in well-constructed containers with secure lids to avoid leakage during transport. Avoid contaminating outside of container when collecting specimen.
15. Follow agency policies for the disposal of infective waste, both when disposing of and when decontaminating materials. Excretions containing blood should be poured down drains that are connected to a sanitary sewer.

U.S. Department of Health and Human Services, Public Health Service. Update: Universal precautions for prevention of transmission of human immunodeficiency virus, hepatitis B virus, and other bloodborne pathogens in health care settings. MMWR *1988; 37:1–7; and 1989; 38:9–18.*

near and a task is not yet finished. Finally, nurses can assist clients in planning wise use of free time.

ENVIRONMENTAL MODIFICATION. Environmental modification is another way of reducing exposure to stress. It involves identifying aspects of the environment that are stressful and avoiding them, decreasing contact with them, or changing them if possible. This includes minimizing stressful contact with other people and changing the physical environment to minimize stress.

The hospital setting is one in which exposure to stressful situations, altered time management, and environmental stressors are present. Often there is complete disruption of individuals' usual patterns of living. Measures by health care personnel that support or encourage normal routines can reduce stress and foster a sense of individual control. For hospitalized clients, this may mean rearranging the surroundings, moving to another room, changing roommates, changing the times of certain activities, or even changing nurses. Other measures related to altering one's personal environment to reduce stress were discussed in Section 1.

Providing Psychological Preparation. The use of anticipatory guidance to prepare clients for unfamiliar or frighten-

IMPLICATIONS FOR NURSE–CLIENT COLLABORATION

Stress Management

Interaction between nurse and client that accomplishes a reduction in client stress is a true example of successful collaboration. To assist relaxation implies a high level of mutual understanding and trust—a real partnership characterized by easy give and take. Not only must the nurse understand the sources of the client's stress and the appropriate measures to take, but the client must trust in the nurse's understanding and recognize their common goals.

ing experiences is an important stress-management activity of nurses. Orientation to the hospital environment and preparation measures for health care experiences were discussed earlier in this section.

Decreasing Physiological Responses to Stress. As discussed in Section 1, individuals' life-style practices and general physical condition greatly influence their perceptions and reactions to stressful events. The importance of adequate nutrition, rest, regular exercise, and relaxation in the prevention of stress-related disorders and the promotion of physical and mental well-being is well documented.

Clients can also moderate their physiological response to stressors through the mind modulation that links the cognitive appraisal of stress to the physical response. Controlling the body through the mind involves bringing the autonomic nervous system under conscious control and balancing sympathetic nervous system activity with the effects of parasympathetic stimulation; that is, balancing muscle tension with relaxation, and anxiety and fear with calmness. Individuals can also learn to control the release of endorphins, the neuropeptides that modulate pain control and immune function. Techniques that reduce or control the physiological responses to stress are receiving increasing attention within the health care community. These stress management techniques have been shown to be extremely useful in managing the pain of childbirth, controlling hypertension, and alleviating anxiety-related symptoms such as tension headaches, insomnia, and chronic muscle tension.[103] The relaxation response, biofeedback, and exercise are effective means of moderating the physiological stress response.

RELAXATION RESPONSE. The relaxation response first described by Dr. Herbert Benson, a Harvard researcher, is a physiological response that is the opposite of the fight-or-flight response.[104] It can be elicited by psychological means. The **relaxation response** is a state of heightened parasympathetic stimulation leading to decreased anxiety, tension, and pain, and an increased feeling of well-being. There is a corresponding reduction in sympathetic stimulation, so metabolism is slowed, heart rate and blood pressure are decreased, and breathing is slowed. In addition, the brain releases endorphins, which increase well-being, control pain and discomfort, and promote healthy immune function. The relaxation response is not the same as sleeping. Individuals achieve relaxation through the conscious control of muscle tension. The actual techniques do not require any special equipment or physician's order and may be done in a variety of settings. This conscious control requires discipline and self-responsibility to practice the technique and incorporate it into daily life. Relaxation can be induced through controlled breathing exercises, progressive muscle relaxation, guided imagery, meditation, and thought stopping.

Before learning to relax, individuals first must become aware of the tension in their bodies, such as tightness in jaw or neck muscles, tension headaches, or feelings of tightness in the chest and back. Nurses should encourage clients to "scan" their bodies for these signs periodically throughout the day. Clients then learn a variety of relaxation techniques that can be used in different situations. The only necessary components for eliciting a relaxation response are: (1) a quiet environment that is free of external distractions, (2) a comfortable position (usually sitting or reclining) that individuals can maintain for at least 20 minutes, (3) a passive attitude that is gained by emptying all thoughts and distractions form the mind, and (4) an object, phrase, sound, or image to dwell upon.[103]

Relaxation techniques can only be effective if clients are interested and participate willingly. Nurses can describe the steps of the various techniques and the sensations that clients can expect to experience; however, as with any skill, commitment and practice are needed to develop proficiency. The ultimate goal is for clients to be able to recognize signs of tension in themselves and to independently initiate relaxation methods of their choice as needed to effectively reduce the effects of stress. The following techniques can be used to evoke the relaxation response. Client instructions for eliciting the relaxation response are summarized in Box 22–8.

- *Controlled breathing.* Individuals are usually not conscious of breathing because it is automatically controlled by the respiratory center in the brain. During controlled breathing exercises, individuals concentrate on taking deep breaths that make full use of the lungs to maximize oxygenation and elimination of carbon dioxide and other waste products. Conscious control of breathing slows the respiratory rate, counteracting the effects of sympathetic stimulation.
- *Progressive relaxation.* Edmund Jacobson, a physician, first described progressive relaxation as an antidote to stress. Progressive relaxation works by progressively tensing and relaxing major muscle groups in systematic fashion until they are all in a state of relaxation. Clients focus on the feelings associated with relaxation such as heaviness and warmth. With practice, individuals are able to achieve deeper and deeper relaxation.[1,101] Procedure 22–2 describes how to teach clients progressive relaxation. Box 22–8 contains a shortened method that clients can do by themselves.

BOX 22–8. INSTRUCTIONS FOR ELICITING THE RELAXATION RESPONSE

Deep Breathing Exercises

1. Scan your body for tension.
2. Place one hand on your abdomen and one on your chest.
3. Inhale slowly and deeply through your nose into your abdomen to push up your hand as much as feels comfortable. Your chest should move only a little and only with your abdomen.
4. When you feel at ease with step 3, smile slightly, inhale through your nose and exhale through your mouth, making a quiet, relaxing, whooshing sound like the wind as you blow gently out. Your mouth, tongue, and jaw will be relaxed. Take long, slow, deep breaths which raise and lower your abdomen. Focus on the sound and feeling of breathing as you become more and more relaxed.
5. Continue deep breathing for about 5 or 10 minutes at a time, once or twice a day, for a couple of weeks. Then, if you like, extend this period to 20 minutes.
6. At the end of each deep-breathing session, take a little time to once again scan your body for tension. Compare the tension you feel at the conclusion of the exercise with that which you experienced when you began.
7. When you become at ease with deep breathing, practice it whenever you feel like it during the day when you are sitting or standing. Concentrate on your abdomen moving up and down, the air moving in and out of your lungs, and the feeling of relaxation that deep breathing gives you.

Progressive Relaxation

(Often more effective if preceded by breathing exercises above.)

The following is a procedure for achieving deep muscle relaxation quickly. Whole muscle groups are simultaneously tensed and then relaxed. Repeat each procedure at least once, tensing each muscle group from 5 to 7 seconds and then relaxing from 20 to 30 seconds. You may want to make a tape of the basic procedure to facilitate your relaxation. Remember to notice the contrast between the sensations of tension and relaxation.

1. Curl both fists, tightening biceps and forearms (Charles Atlas pose). Relax.
2. Wrinkle up your forehead. At the same time, press your head as far back as possible, roll it clockwise in a complete circle, reverse. Now wrinkle up the muscles of your face like a walnut: frowning, eyes squinted, lips pursed, tongue pressing the roof of your mouth, and shoulders hunched. Relax.
3. Arch back as you take a deep breath into the chest. Hold. Relax. Curl toes simultaneously tightening calves, thighs, and buttocks. Relax.

Guided Imagery

1. Close your eyes, take a deep breath, and let it out slowly. As you take in another breath, you are concentrating your thoughts on a happy, relaxing day at the beach.
2. Let your breath out, and feel yourself relax and become more comfortable. It is warm and the sun is bright as you lie on the warm beach. The sun feels good on your skin, and you feel the pleasant, cool breezes from the ocean.
3. As you lie there peacefully, you hear the rhythmic lapping of the water against the shore, and it quietly echoes the sounds of the beach.
4. With each breath, you are more relaxed, comfortable, and sleepy. Your body relaxes in the sun and you feel well.
5. Pause for 5 to 10 minutes.
6. You are feeling comfortable, and you slowly open your eyes.
7. You are awake, alert, refreshed, and feel calmly active and actively calm.

Breathing exercises and progressive relaxation from Davis M, Eschelman ER, McKay M. The Relaxation and Stress Reduction Workbook. *3rd ed. Oakland, CA: New Harbinger; 1988.*

Guided imagery reprinted with permission from Kandzari JH, Howard JR. The Well Family: A Developmental Approach to Assessment. *Boston: Little, Brown; 1981:105.*

- *Guided imagery.* This technique quiets the sympathetic nervous system as individuals focus on an image that they create in their minds. The focus is on the feelings that accompany the image rather than the clarity of the image. Commercially prepared written exercises or tape recordings that describe various images are available; however, to be effective the focused image must be one that the individual finds personally relaxing or soothing. If no prepared exercise is available nurses can ask clients to describe and focus on a scene or experience that they find particularly peaceful or happy. In a quiet soothing voice, nurses can then "guide" clients through the image—asking questions to stimulate client imaginations and further their involvement in the projected image (Fig. 22–11). A guided imagery exercise is found in Box 22–8.
- *Meditation.* This technique was demonstrated as effective treatment of high blood presure in a classic study by Herbert Benson.[104] Clients allay their anxiety by learning to concentrate on one thing and blocking out other thoughts. Clients are taught to focus their thoughts by (1) chanting a mantra (a simple word or sound that they chant over and over) aloud or silently; (2) counting or repeating a phrase as they inhale and exhale with each breath; or (3) fixing their gaze on a particular object.
- *Thought stopping.* This technique allays anxiety by interrupting stress-producing thoughts that lead to negative emotions. Clients may experience stress from obsessive thoughts or worries that are repetitive, intrusive, unrealistic, irrational, or unproductive. Clients, through disciplined practice, learn to concentrate unwanted thoughts and then stop and empty their mind.[101]

BIOFEEDBACK. Biofeedback is a mechanical process in which physiological information related to internal body functioning is "fed back" to the individual. Research with biofeedback has demonstrated that many autonomic ner-

PROCEDURE 22–2. TEACHING PROGRESSIVE RELAXATION

PURPOSE: To achieve a relaxed state; can be used to promote sleep.

EQUIPMENT: Copy of relaxation technique to be read until the client learns the technique; and special equipment as needed, eg, radio, tape recorder, phonograph.

ACTION	RATIONALE
1. Discuss the purpose and expected benefits of the technique with the client. NOTE: Use easily understood language. Some individuals find soft music or a picture of a serene setting useful aids in relaxation.	1. Client will be more likely to participate if the purpose and benefit of relaxation is understood.
2. Reduce environmental stimulation, including lights, noise tactile irritants.	2. The reticular activating system (RAS) is aroused by all types of sensory stimuli. Activating the RAS produces alertness.
3. Assist client to assume a comfortable position—either lying or sitting. NOTE: Correct alignment enhances comfort. If relaxation is being used to promote sleep, lying in bed is recommended.	3. Physical discomfort activates the RAS, and frequently promotes muscle tension.
4. Instruct client to inhale slowly and deeply, hold breath for several seconds, and then to exhale slowly and deeply. Repeat two or three times. NOTE: Speak in a soothing and slow tone of voice throughout procedure.	4. Breathing is a significant variable in the stress (autonomic nervous system) response. Controlling breathing reduces stress response. Focusing on the rhythm of breathing diminishes thought patterns (cerebral cortex) that would stimulate the RAS.
5. Beginning with the facial muscles, instruct the client to alternately contract (or tense) and relax each muscle group three times. For example, ask the client to frown then relax the face. Each exercise should end with the muscle group in a relaxed position. Ask the client to notice the difference in the way the muscle group feels when it is tense and when it is relaxed. NOTE: Continue deep, slow breathing as needed to aid in relaxation. Suggesting the client let the muscle or body part feel heavy is helpful to many clients. When the client learns the technique, repeated tensing and relaxation is unnecessary.	5. Recognizing the difference in the feeling of a tense and relaxed muscle is necessary to achieve a relaxed state. Many individuals are not aware of the difference.

(continued)

PROCEDURE 22–2. (continued)

6. Progress through each muscle group of the body from head to toe, as described above. As you progress, alternate sides of the body as appropriate (first tense and relax the right shoulder muscles, then the left, etc).	6. Focusing on one muscle group at a time enhances client's awareness of how a relaxed state feels. Ultimately all skeletal muscles should be simultaneously relaxed.
7. To end the procedure, ask the client to say "I feel relaxed."	7. Emphasizes client's control. Clients' belief in their ability to relax enhances effectiveness of techniques.
8. If relaxation is being used to promote sleep, provide adequate covers, leave bed in low position with siderails up, and call light within reach. Turn lights low or off.	8. Comfort and security reduce cortical activity (see step 4), which would stimulate the RAS.

RECORDING: Note technique taught, level of mastery demonstrated by client, and level of relaxation reported by client. If used to promote sleep, note whether sleep achieved or delayed.

vous system functions can be brought under conscious control if individuals receive information about the ongoing processes. Pender[1] describes the four basic operations of biofeedback as:

1. Detection and amplification of the bioelectrical potentials.
2. Conversion of bioelectrical signals to easy-to-process information.
3. Feedback of information to the client.
4. Voluntary control of target response through learning based on feedback.

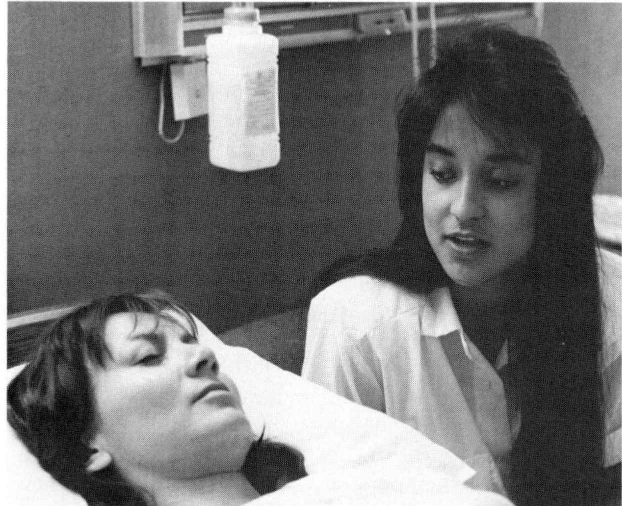

Figure 22–11. Nurse assisting client to perform guided imagery.

For example, clients are taught to monitor muscle tension, skin temperature, brain waves, or heart rate as early indicators of stress through feedback from a machine that is connected to their bodies, and converting body signals to visual or auditory signals. This feedback enables them to detect subtle internal changes and take measures to counteract the response before it becomes severe or prolonged. Biofeedback alerts individuals to sources of stress and provides information on the effectiveness of the techniques used to decrease the stress. The ultimate goal of biofeedback is the achievement of a generalized state of relaxation without information being fed back to clients by a machine. Biofeedback training is a long-term process. It is currently used to treat stress-linked conditions such as tension or migraine headaches, hypertension, muscle spasms, insomnia, and asthma.

EXERCISE. Regular exercise is known to improve general health and to reduce strain and nervous tension brought about by stress. In addition, individuals who exercise regularly often experience feelings of euphoria. This benefit is thought to be related to the exercise-induced release of neuropeptide endorphins. Pender[1] describes the following as characteristics of good exercise:

- It should be enjoyable.
- It should be vigorous enough to make use of a minimum of 400 calories.

- It should sustain the heart rate at 70 to 85 percent of maximum potential for 20 to 30 minutes (approximately 120 to 150 beats per minute for most people).
- It should produce rhythmical movements, with muscles alternatively contracting and relaxing.
- It should be repeated for 30 to 60 minutes, 4 to 5 days per week.
- It should be systematically integrated into the individual's life-style.

Reducing Mild Pain. Adequate pain control contributes significantly to clients' physical and emotional well-being. Mild pain, although not debilitating or overwhelming, can limit activities, interfere with rest and sleep, and make individuals feel irritable and unpleasant. Although pharmacological measures are frequently associated with pain management, a number of other measures can be used to promote client comfort.

The nurse's main objective in management of mild pain is to assist clients to reduce their own pain. Nurses support self-responsibility in management of mild pain by educating clients regarding measures they can use independently to promote comfort. Nurses facilitate client well-being by supporting use of the various noninvasive techniques available for pain management. The relaxation and guided imagery techniques discussed earlier are effective pain control techniques. Relaxation not only reduces muscle tension and anxiety but also draws the individual's attention from the pain and provides a sense of personal control. Other effective mild pain control measures include the use of distraction and cutaneous stimulation. These measures as well as a detailed discussion of moderate and severe pain can be found in Chapter 29.

Promoting Comfort. Closely related to relaxation and mild pain control are a variety of nursing functions that serve to enhance client comfort. Adequate rest and relaxation is necessary for well-being and high-level wellness. Nursing measures that promote physical and psychological comfort eliminate unnecessary stressors and facilitate the recuperative process.

Physical Comfort. The importance of physical comfort in determining clients' sense of well-being cannot be overstated. The nurse's role in supportive care is encouragement of client self-care through informing clients of basic measures that will promote their physical comfort.

Positioning is an effective comfort measure. Some individuals, such as clients who are in labor or recovering from uncomplicated surgery, may need to be reminded to change positions every hour or so. These clients often believe that movement will enhance pain and are pleasantly surprised that a change of position promotes comfort instead. Encouraging correct anatomical alignment and providing extra pillows if needed to support joints and extremities reduces potential sources of irritation or discomfort. Maintaining clean, dry, smooth surfaces under extremities protects skin integrity while promoting physical comfort. These and other nursing measures to promote client comfort are described in more detail in Chapters 24 and 30.

Hygiene measures greatly contribute to a sense of physical comfort. Besides their cleansing effect, bathing, shampooing hair, shaving, and oral care enhance individual self-esteem, stimulate circulation, and promote feeling refreshed and relaxed.

Supporting normal bowel functioning through the use of fluids, diet, and exercise enhances well-being and helps clients avoid discomfort from abdominal distension or cramping. Nurses must be sensitive to each individual's personal hygiene and elimination needs. Many of these practices are determined by cultural and familial influences and are integral components of client well-being. A detailed discussion of nursing measures that promote hygiene and elimination can be found in Chapters 24 and 26.

Maintaining Client Safety. Maintaining client safety is also part of promoting comfort. Client safety is influenced by personal safety awareness. Clients who are capable of self-care may need to be oriented to the potential hazards and safety features of an unfamiliar environment or unfamiliar treatments. Client and family orientation to a new environment such as a hospital, physician's office, or outpatient clinic is an important nursing intervention to promote client safety. Individuals receiving supportive care in the home environment may need education regarding potential hazards in that environment, particularly if there has been a recent change in health status. Clients can self-manage treatments such as application or heat or cold, for example, but the treatments may pose hazards that nurses should call to clients' attention.

Clients with mobility, sensory, or communication impairments who are capable of self-care have special safety needs. Clients with impaired mobility are at risk because they often need assistive devices or support from another person to facilitate their movement. Clients with sensory impairments, whether visual or auditory, are at greater risk of injury because of inability to perceive a potential danger, especially in a new environment. Clients with communication impairments are at risk because they may be unable to express needs for assistance. Nurses need to be aware of the special safety needs of clients with mobility, sensory, or communication impairments and take steps to reduce these hazards. These clients also benefit from education regarding their special safety needs to facilitate safe self-care.

Psychological Comfort. Psychological comfort is also a critical element of high-level wellness. Adequate rest and relaxation and joy in living can only be achieved if clients feel secure and well cared for. Many sources of discomfort have emotional as well as physical aspects. Meeting an individual's physical comfort needs promotes psychological comfort; however, many other nursing actions are necessary to reduce anxiety and foster peace of mind.

Actively listening to clients' personal concerns and alleviating them when possible, making provisions for client privacy, fostering social support systems, and demonstrating acceptance of clients as individuals all serve to promote self-esteem and personal security. Incorporating family members in an individual's care, personalizing clients' hospital space, and preserving normal routines when possible fosters familiarity and may decrease anxiety levels and promote well-being.

Many of the client preparation measures discussed earlier in this chapter help reduce fear and anxiety that clients experience in the health care environment. Nurses who answer questions honestly and offer explanations about procedures and agency policies or routines eliminate much of the fear of the unknown and help clients to feel more at ease.

Caring is the essence of nursing practice. One way of communicating caring is therapeutic use of self. Therapeutic use of self involves use of interpersonal communication techniques to convey warmth and acceptance. Effective communication contributes greatly to individuals' psychological comfort and overall sense of well-being. Communication and human relationship skills are used to facilitate clients' active involvement in the solution of their problems. (See also Chaps. 13 and 14.)

Restorative Care

Restorative care focuses on individuals with acute health problems that require more complex nursing implementations. Clients requiring restorative care in the hospital or home environment often are faced with a multitude of physiological and psychological disruptions that threaten individual well-being; however, nurses can support their wellness through promotion of the dimensions of a wellness life-style discussed in Section 1. Accurate nursing assessment and prompt goal-oriented implementation are necessary to return individuals to optimal functioning.

The role of the nurse at this level of care is much more action oriented. Although teaching and other facilitating measures are part of restorative care, clients needing acute care are ill enough to require assistance from nurses with many activities of daily living that they are unable to perform independently. Nurses can support individual clients' sense of control by cooperative planning of care.

Nursing interventions that promote the clients' beliefs in their own capability to master a current health problem will assist clients to initiate or maintain health-promoting behaviors. Nurses can facilitate self-responsibility through education and mutual goal-setting and decision-making. Although nursing implementation is more direct in restorative care, nurses should focus on empowering clients for as much self-management as they are capable of.

Promoting Safety Measures. Maintaining a physically safe environment for acutely ill or debilitated clients is an important nursing responsibility. Physical safety promotes client well-being by supporting individuals' sense of "feeling good." When clients feel physically safe, they are able to relax and rest while focusing energy on getting well. Physical safety measures related to the prevention of fires, falls, electrical shock, and radiation exposure must be incorporated into daily nursing care.

Fire. The hospital and home environments are always at risk for fires. The most common causes of institutional and home fires are careless smoking in bed and faulty electrical equipment. Smoking regulations should be clearly explained to all hospitalized clients and family members, and should be strictly enforced. Today, smoking is not permitted in many health care facilities, except in a few designated areas. If smoking is allowed, disoriented clients should be permitted to smoke only under direct supervision. Providing adequate ashtrays in smoking areas and the proper disposal of ashes and used matches can help to prevent trash can fires.

Special fire safety precautions are needed when oxygen therapy is used in client care. Oxygen is highly combustible. Nurses promote client safety when oxygen is used by posting no smoking signs and checking that all electrical equipment is functioning correctly and is grounded properly. See Chapter 27 for more information on oxygen safety measures.

In the event of an institutional fire, nurses have three priorities: (1) to notify authorities of the existence and location of the fire; (2) to protect clients from injury; and (3) to attempt to contain the fire if it poses no immediate threat to clients or self. Most health care agencies have established procedures to be followed in emergency situations. Nurses should become familiar with the fire and evacuation policies of their employing institutions and participate in agency fire drills.

Clients cared for in the home have similar fire safety needs. Clients should not smoke in bed and disoriented individuals need direct supervision when smoking. Smoke detectors should be installed throughout the home. The family should have a plan of escape in case of fire and practice that plan on a regular basis. Use of oxygen therapy and electrical equipment in the home demand caregiver awareness of the safety hazards inherent in their use. Use of electrical equipment in the home creates special hazards because of the potential for old or inadequate wiring. Outlet circuit breakers may be needed to prevent electrical overload and risk of fire.

Falls. Falls are the most common threat to physical safety for elderly or debilitated clients. Altered body function and disorientation associated with serious illness increases the likelihood of falls for clients in home care settings. The unfamiliar environment of the acute care setting increases the risk of falls among all hospitalized clients. Broken bones due to falls are more common in older clients, whose bones have lost density.

Prevention of falls begins with the identification of those clients considered to be at risk for falling. Examples of individuals who are at increased risk for falls include those with:

- A known fall before or after admission.
- Altered mental status (confusion, disorientation, uncontrolled restlessness, sedation).
- A seizure disorder.
- Limited mobility or abnormal gait.
- Severely limited hearing or vision.
- A recent escape from restraints or a history of crawling out of bed.

- Unwillingness or inability to call for help with ambulation.
- A recent history of dizziness or syncope.
- New medications or taking medications that cause dizziness, confusion, or hypotension.
- Equipment to assist ambulation that is new to them (eg, crutches or walkers).
- Elimination problems such as incontinence, urgency, or catheters.[105,106]

In addition, caution should be exercised with clients who are experiencing severe pain, who have been confined in bed for a few days or longer, or who recently underwent a surgical procedure.

Nursing measures that help to prevent falls are outlined in Box 22–9. Confused or disoriented clients may require the additional use of restraints and/or mechanical bed alarms for protection from falls. Restraints must be used with great caution. Often they cause more injuries than they prevent, and they cause significant loss of well-being and self-esteem.[107] A detailed discussion of the correct use and application of various restraint mechanisms can be found in Chapter 30.

Electrical Shock. Much of the equipment used in client care is electrical. Everyone involved in direct client care must be familiar with the safe use of electricity and be aware of the potential hazards for electrical injury to clients. Particular care must be exercised when multiple pieces of equipment are in use for a single client and when working with clients especially vulnerable to electrical injury, such as those with indwelling catheters or wet dressings.

The body's natural defense against electrical shock is dry intact skin. All electrical equipment emits a low-level leakage current, which normally is undetectable by individuals in contact with the equipment. However, the natural defense mechanism of the skin is decreased in the presence of moisture including sweat, urine, or wet dressings or when the skin surface is broken by abrasions or invasive instruments. Under these conditions even minor leakage current can produce substantial electrical injury.

Electrical injury is prevented through use of properly grounded equipment. Grounded equipment has a three-pronged electrical plug. The two short prongs transmit power to the equipment while the longer third plug serves as the grounding device to carry stray current or electrical shorts to the ground and away from the equipment operator. The grounding plug is required on all medical equipment.

Despite the use of properly grounded equipment, leakage currents can flow through clients if the equipment is grounded at two different points. For this reason all electrically operated equipment for one client should be plugged into the same cluster of wall outlets.[108] Additional safety measures related to electrical hazards are listed in Box 22–10.

Radiation Exposure. Unnecessary or excessive exposure to ionized radiation in the acute care setting is a health concern for both clients and health care workers. Exposure results primarily from the radioactive materials used in therapeutic procedures and diagnostic testing such as x-rays, fluoroscopy, and nuclear medicine tests.

Clients are exposed to excessive radiation when diagnostic tests are ordered indiscriminately or unnecessarily, when tests are repeated, or when too many views are re-

BOX 22–9. NURSING MEASURES TO PREVENT FALLS

- Assign high-risk clients to rooms near the nursing station for close observation.
- Alert all health care providers to client's "at risk" status (eg, Kardex and chart notations; signs over bed, outside clients' room, or near intercom console at nurses' station).
- Keep client's bed in low position except while giving care.
- Keep siderails raised at all times if client is confused or disoriented.
- Emphasize to client and family members the importance of seeking assistance for ambulation or transfers.
- Make sure call light or bell is within easy reach and remind client where it is before leaving the room.
- Answer all calls promptly and courteously.
- Place all personal items, TV controls, etc, within easy reach.
- Observe client frequently.
- Provide client with well-fitting nonskid footwear.
- Schedule frequent toileting or provide a bedside commode.
- Place a nightlight in client's rom.
- Arrange furniture and equipment to allow clear walkways free of obstacles to the bathroom or door.
- Instruct client in the correct use of ambulatory aids such as canes, crutches, or walkers.
- Teach client to change positions slowly and carefully.
- Provide frequent comfort measures (position changes, pain relief).
- Provide psychosocial stimulation (companionship recreational activities).

BOX 22–10. SAFETY MEASURES TO REDUCE ELECTRICAL HAZARDS

- Keep clients as dry as possible.
- Use only grounded electrical devices.
- Check cords for fraying or other signs of damage before using. Do not use if damage is evident.
- Always pull a plug from the wall outlet by firmly grasping the plug and pulling straight out. Never pull a plug using the cord only.
- Avoid overloading outlets.
- Do not touch the bed, client, or any device attached to the client when plugging in electrical equipment.
- Report loose or broken receptacles to the engineering department.
- Report any shocks experienced while using equipment.
- Do not use extension cords.
- Check all clients' personal electrical applicances through engineering department for safe functioning.

quested. Improper physical preparation of clients may also result in unnecessary radiation exposure as when clients are given inadeqauate bowel preparation prior to a barium enema, or when dye tablets are not given at the proper time.

Exposure of health care workers to radiation is limited through the use of protective shields—lead aprons, gloves, and drapes. Exposure to radiation should be kept to a minimum and monitored with film badges. Special precautions are necessary for pregnant caregivers, as they are at special risk. Special precautions are also necessary when working with clients who have radioactive isotopes placed inside the body for diagnostic or treatment procedures. Rubber gloves must be worn when handling specimens or body wastes and exposure to these clients should be limited.

Important considerations when caring for a person with implanted radioactive substances or receiving x-rays are time and duration of exposure, distance from the source, and shielding. Radiation exposure is decreased by limiting the time of exposure and increasing the distance from the source of radiation. Shielding by the use of lead-lined gloves and/or an apron also reduces exposure. Therefore, health care providers can reduce their radiation exposure by carefully tallying the time spent with clients and increasing distance from clients when possible. Client care must be well planned before entering the room so that the care provider's time of exposure is kept to a minimum while maintaining safe, adequate client care. Several tasks should be implemented with each trip into the room. It is not necessary to avoid all contact with clients if these precautions are followed.

Radiation implants as a medical treatment modality prevent the wellness behavior of "fitting in." Positive social interaction with others contributes to well-being. Thus, the environmental isolation required during radiation implantation threatens clients' well-being. Teaching about the reasons for isolation helps. Client's sense of isolation can be reduced somewhat by providing a radio or television in the room.

Promoting Comfort. Comfort is often elusive for acutely ill clients. All of the comfort measures discussed under supportive care are also important as part of restorative care, but clients require more direct assistance from nurses to achieve comfort. Besides the physical discomfort associated with illness or treatments, the lack of homelike surroundings, fewer social and family contacts, inability to carry out religious rituals, and invasions of privacy are significant barriers to comfort. Nurses who are friendly, kind, and empathic can lessen the impact of these barriers. Small acts like knocking before entering a client's room to show respect for privacy, responding promptly to requests for help, or offering to arrange visits from clergy are comforting to clients. Clients also report that having the same caregiver every day is important to feelings of comfort. It is sometimes difficult for nurses in the high-intensity atmosphere of acute care settings to remember the importance of warmth and caring to well-being, but it is a critical element of care at all levels.

Maintaining Infection Control: Surgical Asepsis. Providing a safe environment for acutely ill clients includes infection control. The principles of medical asepsis were discussed earlier in this section under Supportive Care. Medical asepsis is designed to limit the growth and/or spread of pathogens in order to prevent infection. Items are considered contaminated if they are known to be, or suspected of harboring pathogens (eg, soiled dressing or linens). Some client care situations require surgical asepsis.

Surgical asepsis, also referred to as **sterile technique,** is the method by which items and specific areas in the health care setting are kept free of microorganisms. Surgical asepsis, therefore, goes beyond medical asepsis in that it requires the elimination of all microorganisms, not just pathogens. An item is either sterile or it is not; the presence of even one microorganism or spore renders an item contaminated or unsterile. Nurses working with a sterile field or object must realize that the slightest break in technique results in contamination. The practice of surgical asepsis requires extreme conscientiousness and strict attention to detail. If an item in use becomes contaminated, it must be set aside and the procedure begun again with new sterile equipment.

Surgical asepsis is routinely practiced in the operating room, labor and delivery suites, and special diagnostic areas; however, there are many common procedures performed in general care areas that also require strict sterile technique. Sterile technique should be used during any procedure that involves any sterile body part or cavity, or that results in breaking of the skin or mucous membranes. Examples of specific common procedures requiring sterile technique include:

- Bladder catheterization
- Tracheobronchial suctioning
- Administration of injections
- Insertion of intravenous catheters
- Dressing changes

but do not include:

- Vaginal douches or medications
- Nasogastric tube insertion/irrigation
- Enemas

Although sterile technique is used for procedures in the acute care setting, it may not be required in the home setting. Acute illness and exposure to a concentration of infectious agents in the acute care setting greatly increases potential for infection while hospitalized. This increased risk of infection requires the use of surgical asepsis for all invasive procedures in the acute care setting. In contrast, individuals who are recuperating and return home to an environment where there are fewer microorganisms may not need to adhere to surgical asepsis. For example, some clients who perform self-catheterization use sterile technique while hospitalized, and clean technique at home. A client's health status influences which technique is required. Potential for infection increases in proportion to the deterioration of a client's health. Therefore, visiting nurses who catheterize frail elderly clients in a home setting use sterile technique, while elderly clients able to perform self-catheterization use clean technique. However, some procedures always involve risk of serious infection; for these, sterile technique is always used. An example is insertion and care of an intravenous catheter.

Applying Principles of Surgical Asepsis. When performing a sterile procedure, nurses must observe basic guidelines to maintain surgical asepsis and protect clients from the threat of infection. These guidelines are described below. Box 22–11 presents general principles guiding the practice of surgical asepsis.

1. All objects on a sterile field must be sterile. A sterile field is a work area for assembling and handling sterile supplies. Never assume that an object is sterile. Check packages for sterility expiration dates, which should be clearly marked. Check sterilization indicators inside large packages to ensure that all contents have been exposed to the sterilization process. The outside of commercially packaged sterile items should be marked with the word "sterile." Always inspect a package containing sterile items for dryness and intactness. Any package that appears torn, open, punctured, or wet should be considered contaminated and discarded.
2. Sterile objects become contaminated when touched by an unsterile object, because microorganisms are transmitted by direct contact. For example, if any part of a nurse's sterile gloved hand touches a client's bed linen, or if the tip of intravenous tubing touches a clean disposable glove, the items are no longer sterile. Whenever the sterility of an object is questionable, the item is assumed to be unsterile and cannot be used in a sterile procedure. Sterile items that will be used on open wounds or enter sterile body cavities should only be handled with sterile forceps or sterile gloved hands.
3. Sterile items that are out of the field of vision or held below waist level are considered contaminated because undetected contact with unsterile items is possible. Likewise, turning one's back on a sterile field, or leaving it unattended, presents a risk of undetected contamination. Always keep sterile gloved hands in sight above waist level to prevent unknown contact with unsterile objects.
4. Microorganisms are transmitted by air currents. A sterile object can become contaminated through prolonged exposure to air. Nurses should avoid activities that create air currents when working with sterile equipment. Doors should be closed and traffic kept to a minimum. Avoid reaching across a sterile field. This prevents microorganisms falling on to it. Instead, reach around a sterile field. Items on a sterile field are moved as little as possible to minimize the possibility of contamination caused by air currents.
5. Microorganisms are transmitted via droplets. Laughing, sneezing, or coughing over a sterile field can contaminate it with microorganisms from the oral cavity and respiratory tract. Some nurses advocate the use of masks whenever working over a sterile field or open wound. Nurses with upper respiratory tract conditions should wear masks when working with sterile equipment.
6. Moisture is a medium by which microorganisms are transferred to a sterile object or field because of capillary action or gravity. Capillary action is movement of fluid against gravity in a tube or fiber. Care must be exercised to avoid splashing or spilling when pouring sterile liquids into containers on a cloth sterile field, because bacteria from the surface under the cloth can move through the wet, sterile field by capillary action. Sterile waterproof barriers are often used beneath sterile objects to prevent contamination from capillary action. Fluids also flow in the direction of gravity; therefore, the tips of wet forceps are always held below the level of the handles. If the tips are held up, the fluid could flow onto the handle and become contaminated by the hands. When lowered again, the contaminated fluid would again travel and contaminate the tips. For the same reason, nurses who are performing a surgical hand scrub always hold their hands higher than the elbows to prevent contaminants from the forearm from traveling to the hands.

BOX 22–11. GENERAL PRINCIPLES GUIDING THE PRACTICE OF SURGICAL ASEPSIS

- Microorganisms are present on the skin, in body cavities with an opening to the exterior of the body, in many body fluids, and on all objects in the environment not subjected to sterilization procedures.
- Intact skin prevents bacteria and viruses from entering the body; broken skin provides a portal of entry for organisms. Prolonged exposure to moisture causes maceration of skin and compromises its effectiveness as a barrier to microorganisms.
- A sterile object is free of all microorganisms.
- The skin cannot be sterilized; however, rigorous cleaning can remove transient microorganisms and some resident flora.
- All items that are not sterile are contaminated; microorganisms are present on contaminated items.
- If there is any doubt about the sterility of an item, it is considered contaminated; sterile items that are not kept within one's field of vision are considered contaminated.
- Microorganisms require a mode of transmission to move from one place to another. They can be transmitted by:
  - *direct contact* with contaminated items
  - *airborne droplets* (eg, when speaking, laughing, coughing, sneezing)
  - *air currents* (eg, via dust, lint particles, or microscopic skin flakes)
  - *fluids*
  - *gravity*
  - *capillary action* (the movement of a liquid along a fine fiber or tube against gravity)
- Microorganisms cannot penetrate dry cotton fabric, nonwoven paper, or plastic wrappers.
- A moist, dark environment promotes the growth of many microorganisms.

7. The edges of a sterile field are considered contaminated. As a general rule the outer 2.5 cm (1 in) margin of a sterile field is considered unsterile since it is in such close proximity to an unsterile surface. All objects placed on a sterile field must be inside the 2.5 cm (1 in) margin. Any object that falls onto the margin is considered contaminated.

Preparing Clients. Before starting a sterile procedure, nurses must first assess clients' knowledge or experience with sterile technique. Clients' cooperation should be enlisted to prevent inadvertent contamination of sterile items. Clients should be asked to avoid any sudden movements of body parts that may be covered with sterile drapes. It is important that clients refrain from touching any supplies and avoid talking, sneezing, or coughing over sterile areas. Anticipating clients' needs and ensuring their comfort prior to beginning a procedure also helps avoid problems with disruption.

Performing Sterile Procedures. Nurses should gather all equipment or supplies that will be needed prior to beginning a sterile procedure. Anticipating what will be needed and having a few extra supplies on hand in case of accidental contamination, prevents having to leave the unwrapped sterile items unattended. Simple procedures such as an intramuscular injection require few supplies and minimal preparation. More complex procedures, such as bladder catheterizations or dressing changes, usually require a sterile field and the use of a variety of sterile supplies. Many hospitals today have prepackaged disposable kits for these common procedures. Using these kits facilitates preparation as all supplies that are needed are included in one single package, but may be more costly.

Establishing and Maintaining a Sterile Field. A sterile field can be any size depending on the procedure and the amount of equipment needed. The inside of a sterile package can serve as a small sterile field. Larger sterile fields can be created through the use of sterile drapes. Once the field is established, a nurse adds sterile supplies by placing them directly on the field or transferring them with sterile forceps. Procedure 22–3 describes the preparation of a sterile field.

PROCEDURE 22–3. ESTABLISHING A STERILE FIELD

PURPOSE: To provide a work area for placement of sterile supplies needed to perform a sterile procedure.

EQUIPMENT: Package containing sterile drape (may be called "Barrier Towel"), and additional supplies as dictated by specific care to be given.

ACTION	RATIONALE
1. Wash your hands.	1. Removes transient microbes, thereby reducing possibility of contamination.
2. Assemble all necessary supplies. Inspect all packages for dryness, intactness, indication of sterility and expiration date. Discard any packages marked sterile that appear damp or whose wrappers are damaged.	2. A sterile field may not be left unattended to retrieve extra supplies. Because sterility cannot be assured, an unattended sterile field is considered contaminated unless covered by a sterile drape. A torn or wet wrapper permits entry of microbes.
3. Select a clean, dry work surface that is at a comfortable working height.	3. A wet surface beneath a sterile field permits transmission of microbes through the drape by capillary action, unless the drape is impervious to moisture.

(continued)

PROCEDURE 22–3. (continued)

4. Open the package containing the drape according to the guidelines in Box 22–12.

   4. These techniques prevent client infection by maintaining sterility of supplies.

5. Without touching the drape, inspect it to locate the corner that has been diagonally folded. Then grasp the corner with your thumb and forefinger.

   5. The corner is folded to facilitate holding it. The outer 2.5 cm (1 in) of a sterile field may be touched during its preparation. The entire border of the field is therefore considered contaminated and all sterile items must be placed inside this border.

6. Lift the drape from its wrapper, allowing it to unfold. Prevent contact with unsterile items by stepping away from the work surface as you lift the drape and by holding your arm well away from your body.

   6. Microorganisms are transmitted by direct contact with an unsterile object.

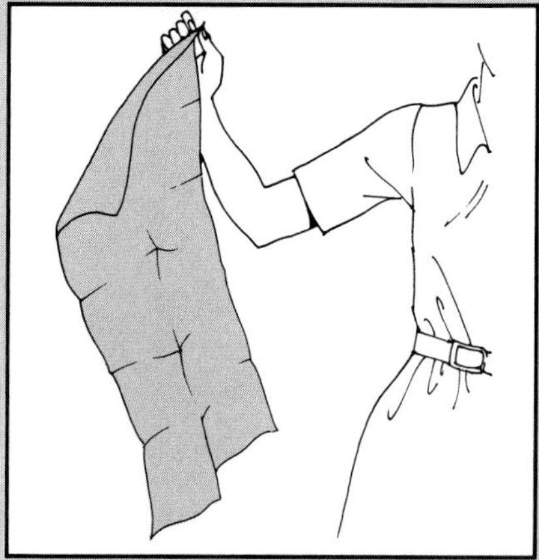

NOTE: Disposable drapes may not unfold readily. Gently shaking the drape may help, but avoid vigorous movement.

7. Grasp the adjacent corner of the drape with your other hand. Place the drape on the work surface. Either side of the drape may placed facing up. Do not lean or reach over the drape while positioning it.

   7. Leaning or reaching over the drape as it is placed on the table may contaminate it by direct contact or via air currents.

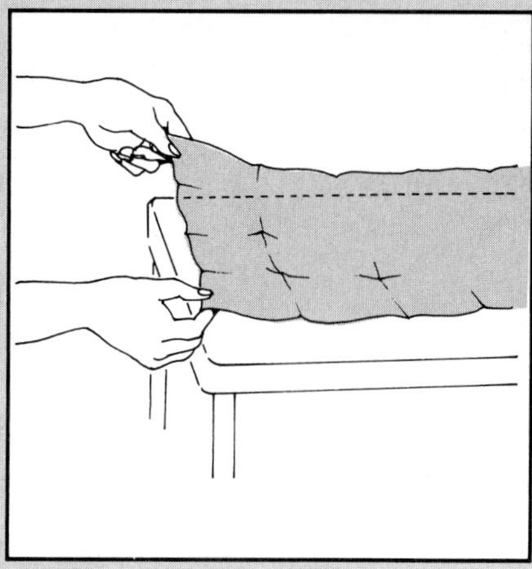

(continued)

PROCEDURE 22–3. (continued)

8. Open sterile supplies needed for the procedure as described in Box 22–12.

8. These techniques prevent client infection by maintaining sterility of supplies.

9. Minimize reaching over the sterile while adding supplies:

9. See step 7, above.

a. Drop small lightweight items on the field from a height of about 15 cm (6 in.).

a. This distance is small enough to assure accurate placement on the field and great enough to prevent wrappers from contacting and contaminating the field.

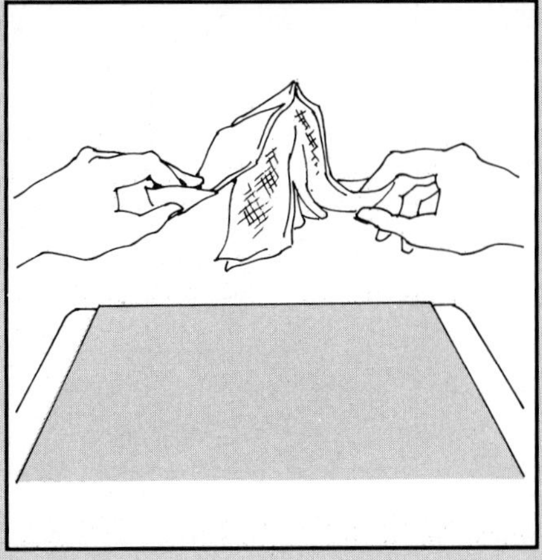

b. Place bulky items such as sterile basins near the margin (see step 5, above) of the sterile field, holding one edge of the item in its sterile wrapper as shown. See also Box 22–2.

b. Dropping bulky items could cause them to bounce or slip off the sterile field. The wrapper provides a barrier between your hand and the sterile item. See step 6, above.

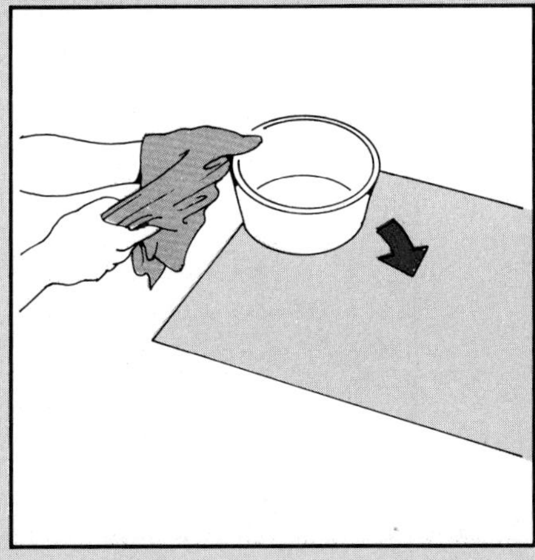

10. If sterile solution is to be used, pour according to guidelines in Box 22–13.

10. These techniques will maintain sterility of field and solution.

11. Rearrange sterile items on field if necessary after putting on sterile gloves. See Procedure 22–4.

11. See step 6, above.

RECORDING: Document procedure performed according to guidelines for that procedure. Preparation of a sterile field need not be documented separately.

BOX 22–12. GUIDELINES FOR OPENING STERILE PACKAGES

Inspect all packages for dryness, intactness, indication of sterility, and expiration date. Do not use any packages marked sterile that appear damp or whose wrappers are damaged.

Peelpacks

1. Grasp the tabs above the sealed edge as shown.

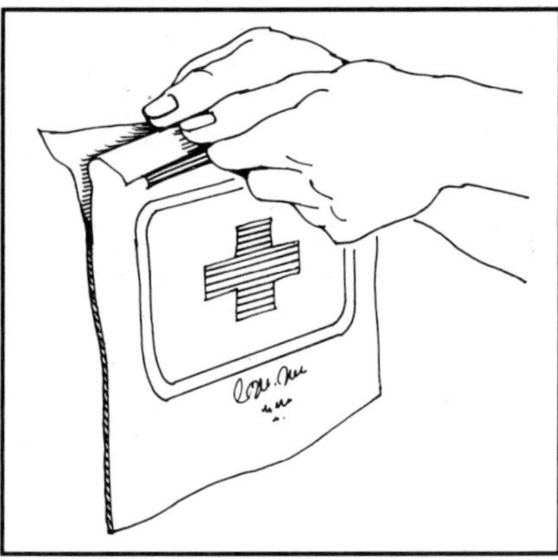

2. Peel edges apart to break seal.
3. Package may be placed on a flat surface and top wrapper removed to completely expose contents as shown, creating a small sterile field for contents of package.

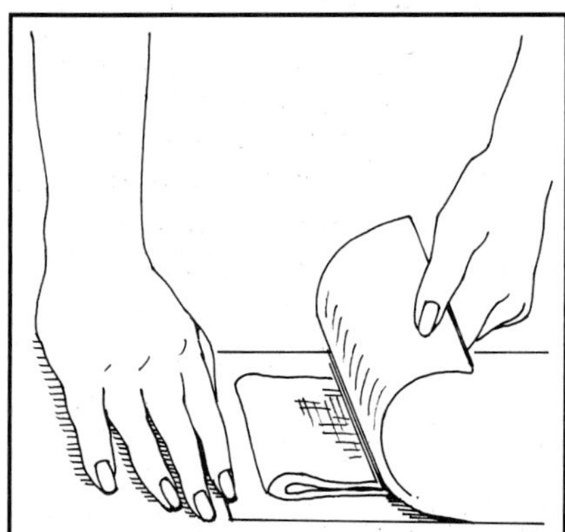

4. Contents may be dropped on another sterile field.

Peelback Containers

1. Hold the bottom of the container with one hand.
2. Grasp corner tab of peelback top; pull to remove top.

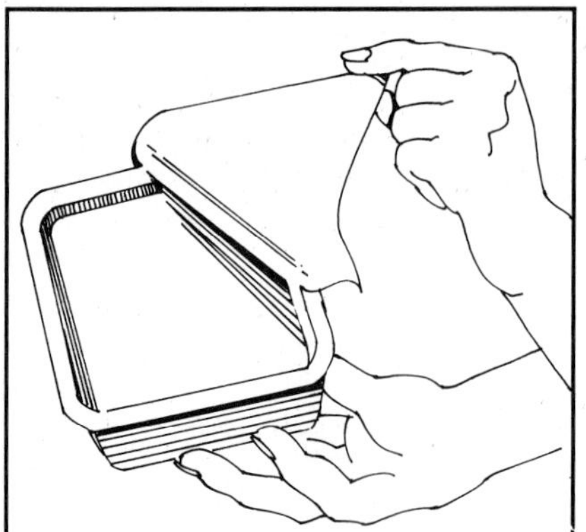

3. Container may be used as self-contained sterile field for contents.
4. Sterile solution may be added if needed, or contents may be placed on a another sterile field and container used to hold sterile solution. Refer to Box 22–13.

Envelope Wrapped Package on a Surface

1. Center the package on the work area so the outer flap of the wrapper faces away from you.
2. Reach around, not over the package and open the flap, pulling it away from you. Touch only the outside of the wrap.

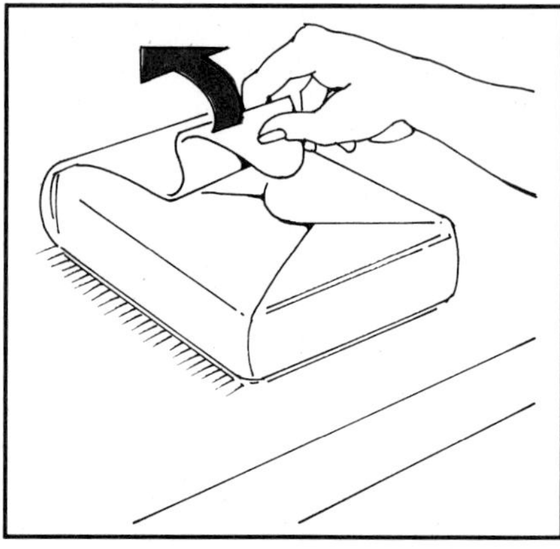

3. Open side flaps in sequence, using right hand for right flap and left hand for left flap. Touch outside surface only, as shown. Avoid reaching over package.

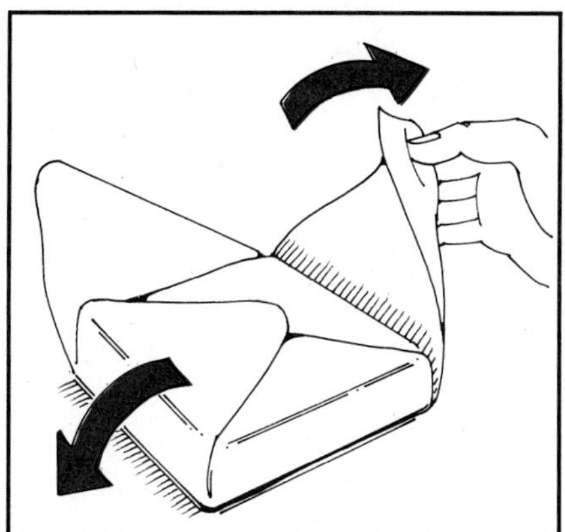

4. Open inner flap by pulling turned down corner toward you. If flap is large, step away from the table so wrapper does not contact your uniform. If inner corner is not turned down, touch outside of wrap only, as in step 3.

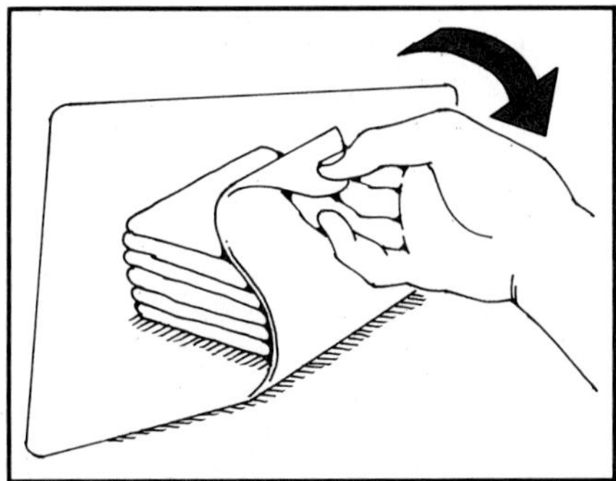

5. Wrapper may be used for sterile field. Additional items may be added as necessary. See Procedure 22–3.

Envelope Wrapped Package Held in Hand

1. Hold the package in one hand so the outer flap of the wrapper faces away from you.

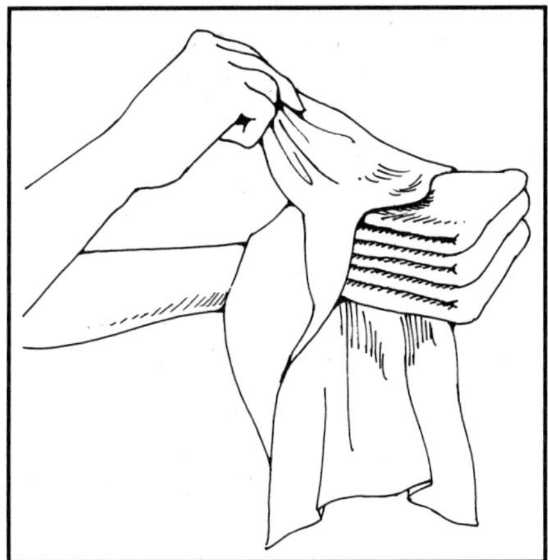

2. Open the package as in steps 2 to 4 above, pulling the flaps back toward you as you open each one.
3. Gather the opened flaps with your free hand and hold them against the opposite arm, as shown. The sterile item can now be placed on a sterile field without risk of contacting the field with the parts of the wrapper that you have touched.

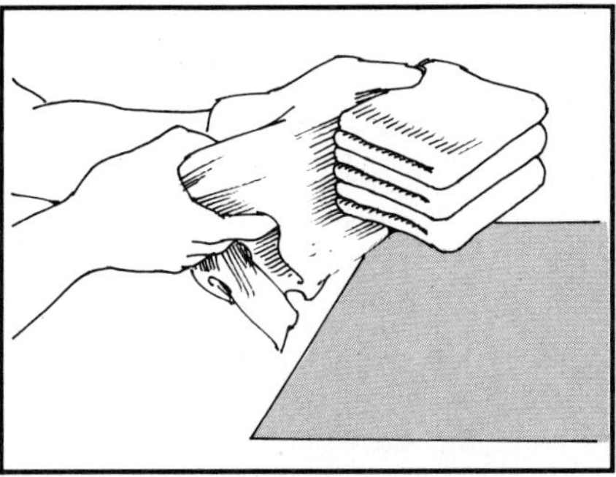

Opening Sterile Packages. Before opening a sterile package the nurse should prepare a work surface. A bedside table or countertop that is above waist level, clean, and dry provides a convenient surface on which to place the sterile items. Agency-sterilized items and large commercially prepared procedure kits are typically wrapped in muslin or paper in an "envelope style" with the four corners of the outer wrap folded around the sterile item in a uniform way. Many smaller items are packaged in "peel packs." Box 22–12 lists guidelines for opening sterile packages.

Pouring Sterile Liquids. Sterile liquids are commonly packaged in plastic or glass bottles. The inside of the bottle and its contents are considered sterile while the outside and the cap are considered clean. Guidelines for pouring sterile solutions are found in Box 22–13.

Using Sterile Forceps. A forceps is a two-bladed instrument that is used for grasping or manipulating equipment or body tissue. A variety of styles of forceps are available. Thumb forceps look like tweezers; ring forceps (sometimes called transfer forceps) have handles like scissors. The blades or tips of forceps are varied according to their intended uses. In most cases, forceps are packed with commercial kits, but may be individually packaged in some agencies. Guidelines for the use of sterile forceps are found in Box 22–14.

Donning Sterile Gloves. Sterile gloves are worn during many procedures to maintain the sterility of equipment and to protect clients. There are two gloving methods—open and closed. The open method is most frequently used outside the operating room. The closed method is practiced in the operating room and requires that the nurse wear a sterile gown. Students desiring information about the closed method are referred to an operating room text.

Sterile gloves are available in a variety of sizes. It is important to select the proper size. The glove should not stretch so tightly that it tears; however, it should fit snugly so that items can be picked up or manipulated easily. Procedure 22–4 outlines the steps of open gloving technique.

Specific procedures that require sterile technique such as wound care, venipuncture, and insertion of Foley catheters are discussed in conjunction with related care in other Unit VI chapters. Breaks in sterile technique increase a client's risk for infection. Infection produces fever. Nurses can promote the well-being of clients experiencing an infection through fever management.

Managing Fever. Body temperature is precisely regulated by physiological and behavioral mechanisms. Generally, heat production and loss are balanced to maintain a relatively constant body temperature. Normal physiological function depends on a small variation in body temperature. Central nervous system function is impaired when body temperature varies 4°C (9°F) above or below normal. Nurses use knowledge of temperature control mechanisms (see Chap. 16) to promote client temperature regulation.

Body temperature is altered as a result of changes in environmental temperature and in temperature-regulating

BOX 22–13. GUIDELINES FOR POURING STERILE SOLUTIONS

1. Check medical order to verify name and strength of solution ordered for procedure.
2. Obtain correct solution. Do not use solution from previously opened bottle unless time and date of first use are written on the label. Most agencies allow solution from an opened bottle to be used for a 24-hour period before discarding remaining contents. Some solutions may have a specific expiration date or time indicated on the label. If solution has been refrigerated, place in a basin of hot water to warm it to room temperature.
3. If using solution from an unopened bottle, write current time and date on the label where it can be readily seen.
4. Prepare sterile field and sterile container for solution as needed. See Procedure 22–3 and Box 22–12.
5. Remove the lid and place it on a nonsterile surface so the inside of the lid is facing up, to prevent contamination of inside surface of lid.
6. Grasp solution bottle with its label facing the palm of your hand to prevent solution, which may drip or run down the side of the bottle, from obliterating the label.

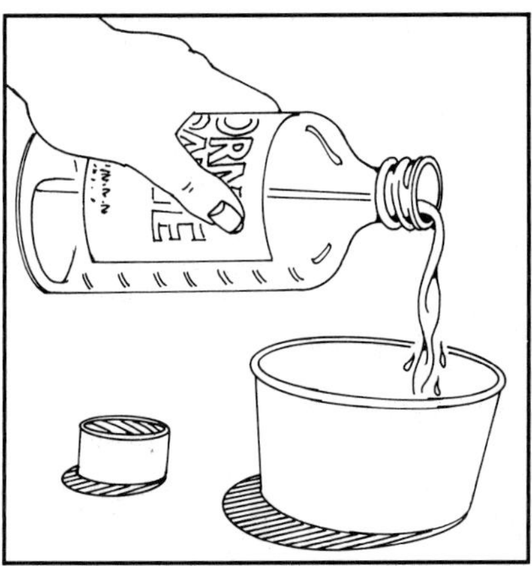

7. Hold the solution bottle about 10 cm (4 in.) above the receiving container and pour slowly to avoid splashing. Do not allow the lip of the bottle to contact the receiving container.
8. Replace lid on the bottle securely. Store according to agency policy.
9. Record specific care given, identifying type and strength of solution used.

mechanisms. Prolonged exposure to an excessively cold environment can cause hypothermia, and prolonged exposure to high temperatures causes hyperthermia (heat stroke). The best treatment for these conditions is prevention. Client education for preventing body temperature changes associated with increased or decreased environmental temperature was discussed in this section under *Preventive Care.*

Fever is an elevation in body temperature caused by disease. The hypothalmic regulator of body temperature acts as if it is set at a higher than normal level, which activates temperature-raising mechanisms and causes an elevation in body temperature. Temperature elevation usually

BOX 22–14. GUIDELINES FOR USE OF STERILE FORCEPS

1. As with all sterile items, forceps must be held above the waist and within sight at all times.
2. The handles are considered contaminated, unless held with sterile gloves.
3. Always hold the tips lower than the handle. Forceps are frequently used in conjunction with solutions. Because fluid flows downward due to gravity, raising the tips and then lowering them again to continue the procedure would allow the solution to contact the hands, become contaminated, and then flow back to the tips, contaminating them.
4. Dry, sterile forceps that have been handled with ungloved hands may be placed on the edge of a sterile field so that the tips are within the field and the handles are outside it.

produces a sensation of chilliness with shivering due to vasoconstriction. Fever stimulates sweating. Sweating is a process that transfers heat from the body through evaporation of water from the skin and mucous membranes of the respiratory tract. Water loss due to evaporation can produce dehydration with decreased skin turgor, dry mucosa, and thirst. With fever, the body's metabolic rate and rate of oxygen consumption increases. Pulse and respiratory rates increase. Confusion may result because of insufficient oxygen available for the brain. Energy reserves are depleted, causing lethargy. Fever is one of the body's defense mechanisms. Fever between 37 and 38°C (98.6 and 100.4°F) helps to activate the body's immune system by stimulating antibody production. Antibodies work best at temperatures higher than normal, and microorganism growth is inhibited. For this reason, not all fevers are treated by physicians. If treated, traditional therapy consists of fluid, antipyretics, and antibiotics when a specific organism can be identified as the cause.

Independent nursing measures can be implemented to promote heat loss during fever, enhancing clients' well-being. Nursing measures for management of fever include special assessments, dress, activity, fluids, nutrition, and bathing.

Special Assessments. Special assessments are required for a client with fever. Vital signs including temperature, pulse, and respirations should be monitored at least every 4 hours, more frequently if elevation is significant. Temperature assessment is required before and within 1 hour after administering antipyretics such as Aspirin or Tylenol prescribed by the physician. These drugs reduce body temperature by acting on the hypothalmic thermoregulating center. More frequent assessments are required if the fever does not respond to antipyretic and other independent nursing measures. Because of the loss of electrolytes in perspiration, laboratory results including sodium, potassium, and chloride must be monitored.

Dress. During chills, which may precede onset of fever, an extra blanket helps to keep clients more comfortable. Blankets should be removed when clients feel warm. Removing clothing during fever promotes heat loss through radiation and conduction. Reducing room temperature with cool cir-

PROCEDURE 22–4. PUTTING ON AND REMOVING STERILE GLOVES: OPEN GLOVING

PURPOSE: To prevent transmission of microorganisms from caregiver to client and from one client to another.

EQUIPMENT: Undamaged package of sterile gloves in caregiver's size. Additional supplies dictated by specific care to be given.

ACTION	RATIONALE
1. Wash your hands. Remove rings with stones.	1. Handwashing removes transient microbes, thereby reducing possibility of contamination. Rings increase risk of tearing gloves.
2. Assemble all necessary supplies. Inspect all packages for dryness, intactness, indication of sterility, and expiration date. Do not use any packages marked sterile that appear damp or whose wrappers are damaged.	2. A sterile field may not be left unattended to retrieve extra supplies. Because sterility cannot be assured, an unattended sterile field is considered contaminated unless covered by a sterile drape. A torn or wet wrapper permits entry of microbes, so contents are contaminated.
3. Open the outer wrapper according to guidelines in Box 22–12. Discard wrap. Place the inner package on a clean, dry work surface that is at a comfortable working height and provides enough space to unfold the glove wrapper without contacting sterile supplies already prepared. 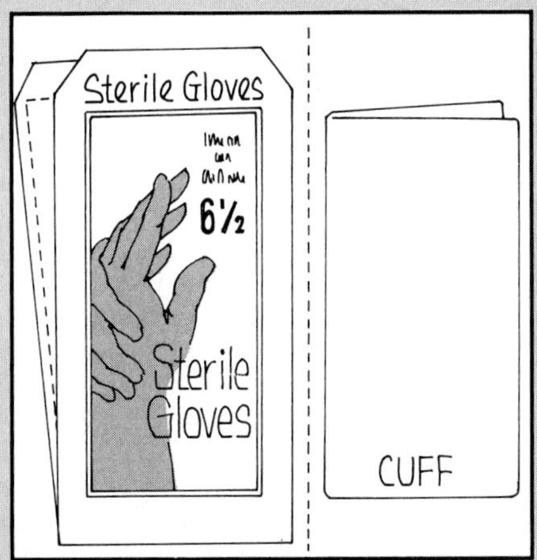	3. A wet surface beneath the package would permit transmission of microbes through the wrapper to the gloves by capillary action. Contact between the glove wrapper and the sterile field would transmit microbes to the sterile field, because the outside of the wrapper is not sterile once placed on work area.

(continued)

PROCEDURE 22–4. (continued)

4. Open inner wrapper according to directions printed on package. Illustration below is typical. Pull wrapper firmly to keep it flat, touching only exposed "cuffs" of wrapper. Gloves will be positioned next to each other, palm up, with thumbs to the outside, bottom cuffed.

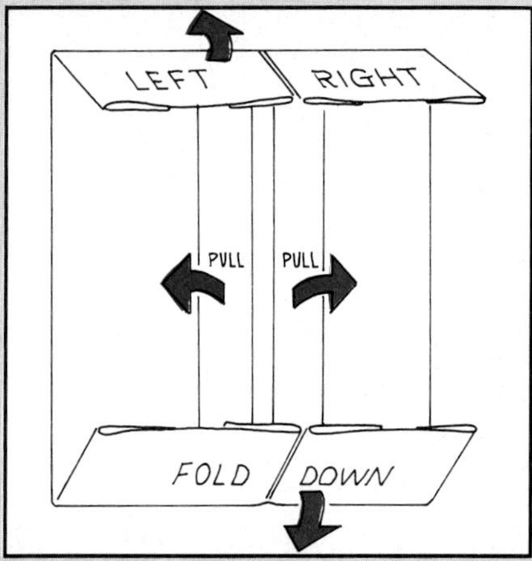

4. Correctly opening the inner wrapper creates a sterile field for the gloves. If wrapper returns to folded position after you have touched it, gloves may be contaminated by contact with wrapper.

5. Grasp the folded edge of the cuff of one glove. Lift it above the work area and away from your body. Insert your other hand into the glove and pull it on. Do not adjust the cuff or placement of fingers inside the globe. If the outside of the glove touches any unsterile object, the glove must be discarded.

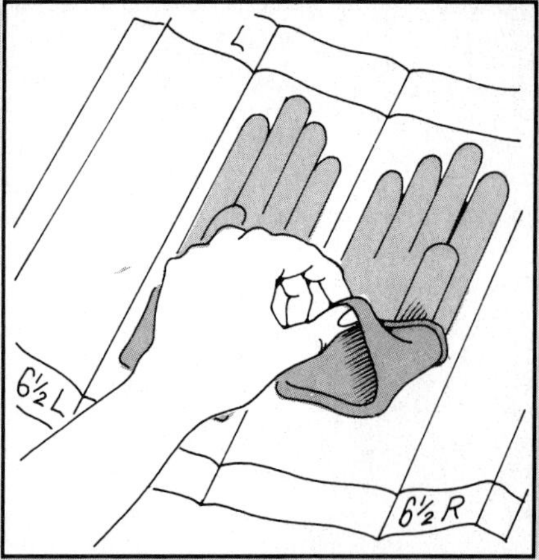

NOTE: It is usually easier to put the first glove on the nondominant hand. Incorrect finger placement can be adjusted when both gloves are on.

5. These actions prevent the outside of the globe from contacting unsterile objects such as your hand, uniform, or the work surface, which would allow transmission of microbes to the glove.

(continued)

PROCEDURE 22–4. (continued)

6. Slip your gloved hand *under* the cuff of the remaining glove, lift it up as above, and pull it on. Do not flex the wrist of the gloved hand while lifting or putting on the second glove. Hold the gloved thumb away from the opposite hand and arm.

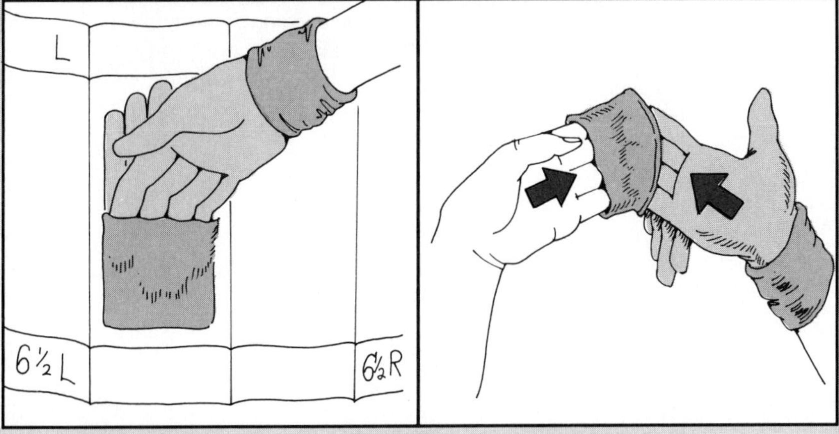

6. Holding the second glove under the cuff without flexing the wrist or adducting the thumb prevents contact between the sterile gloves and exposed skin, thereby keeping both gloves sterile.

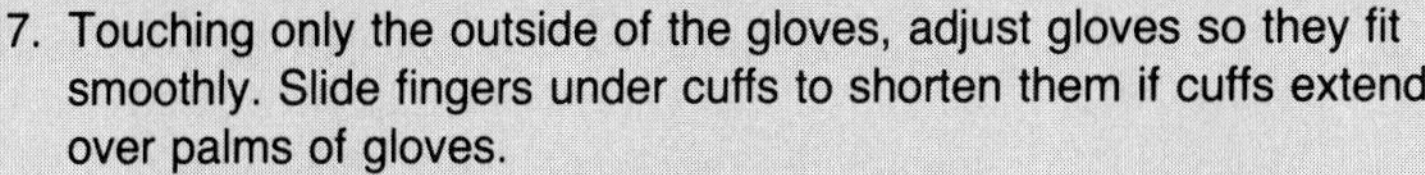

7. Touching only the outside of the gloves, adjust gloves so they fit smoothly. Slide fingers under cuffs to shorten them if cuffs extend over palms of gloves.

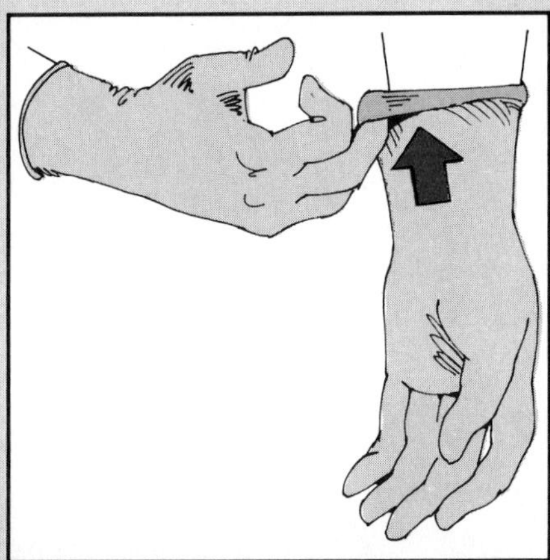

7. Contact with the unsterile inside of the gloves would transfer organisms to the outside of the gloves. Smooth fit improves dexterity during procedure.

8. Carry out sterile procedure without extraneous movement. Gloved hands must remain in sight above waist level at all times.

8. Excessive movement increases risk of contacting unsterile objects and creates air currents that could transmit organisms to client or sterile field. Keeping gloves in sight assures awareness of accidental glove contamination.

(continued)

PROCEDURE 22–4. (continued)

9. To remove gloves: a. Grasp outside of one glove near the wrist and remove it by turning it inside out. Once removed, the glove may be held in the still gloved hand or placed with used equipment from procedure.

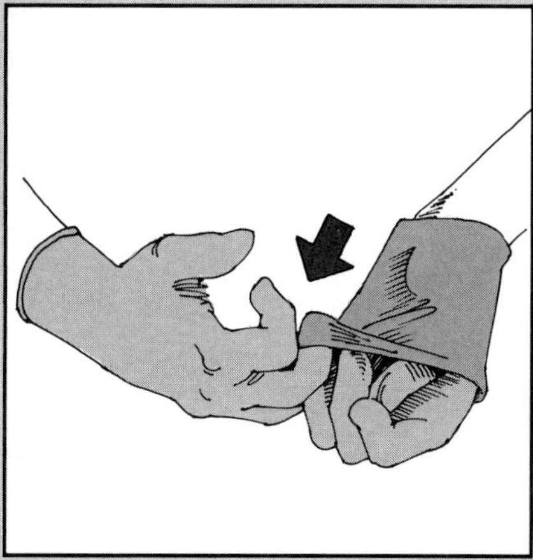

9a. During the procedure, gloves have contacted organisms from the client's skin. Touching the outside of the glove and inverting it when removing glove prevents transmitting these organisms to the nurse's hands.

b. Slip ungloved thumb or fingers inside remaining glove and remove it by turning it inside out. Do not touch outside of glove.

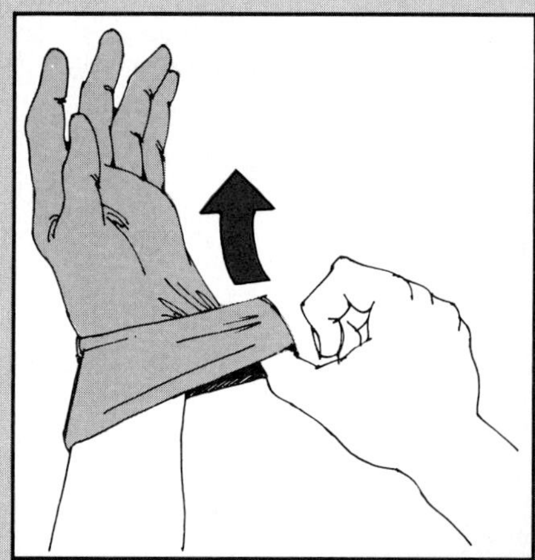

b. Prevents contamination of nurse's hand with organisms from outside of glove. If first glove was held, it will be contained inside second glove.

10. Discard gloves and other used equipment according to agency policy.

10. Equipment contacting blood or bloody secretions requires special handling according to CDC Guidelines for Universal Precautions.

11. Wash your hands. See Procedure 22–1.

11. Microorganisms flourish in moist warm environment inside gloves. Thorough washing removes most transient organisms. See Procedure 22–1.

RECORDING: Specific reference to use of sterile gloves is not usually required. Documentation of specific procedure should indicate sterile technique was used.

culating air and applying a cool washcloth to the forehead promotes comfort and cooling.

Limited Activity. Activity increases oxygen demand, so frequency of activity should be reduced. Febrile clients need frequent rest periods. Limiting physical activity also reduces the body's heat production.

Nutrition and Fluids. Fluids are important to prevent dehydration. Extra fluids are needed to replace fluids lost due to increased metabolism. A febrile client with normal cardiac and renal function should drink at least 3 liters of fluids a day to replace losses through sweating. Oral hygiene is important because oral mucosa drys with dehydration.

Nutrition is vital with the increased metabolism associated with fever. Nurses should use measures to stimulate appetite and provide well-balanced meals (see Chap. 25) to meet clients' increased needs.

Cooling Baths. Bathing clients with tepid (21.1 to 29.1°C or 70 to 85°F) water reduces the body's surface temperature. Keeping the bathed body part exposed to cool air circulating in the room enhances surface cooling through evaporation. Vital signs should be assessed prior to starting the bath to be able to evaluate effectiveness of the treatment. If antipyretic medications are prescribed, administer them before starting the bath to enhance fever reduction. An icebag applied to the head during the bath relieves headache and promotes comfort; a hot water bottle applied to the feet helps to prevent chills and shivering, which counter the desired effect of a tepid bath because they increase metabolic rate. Bathing is done in the same sequence as a bed bath. Cold wet compresses can be placed on the neck, groin, and axilla to promote cooling of large superficial blood vessels. A tepid bath should not exceed 30 minutes.

If body temperature elevates to 41°C (105°F), the rate of cellular metabolism increases so much that the body's regulatory mechanisms can no longer overcome the rate of heat production. A hypothermic (cooling) blanket is necessary to prevent brain damage. A cooling blanket contains coils through which cold water or antifreeze are circulated. Care must be taken to avoid cooling the client too rapidly or too much. Rapid cooling can cause shivering, which increases the client's metabolic rate, countering the action of the cooling blanket. Drugs to relax skeletal muscles may be prescribed to prevent shivering.

Special care is needed when using a hypothermia blanket to prevent skin damage. The hypothermia blanket is covered with a bath blanket to protect the skin. Lanolin, cold cream, or mineral oil is applied to the skin to prevent drying. The skin must be checked at least once an hour and the client should be turned at least every 2 hours to promote skin integrity. The client's temperature is monitored continuously with a rectal probe thermometer to determine the effectiveness and duration of treatment.

Administering Medications. The safe and accurate administration of medications is an important nursing responsibility, particularly in the acute care setting. A **medication** or **drug** is a chemical substance used for therapeutic purposes: diagnosis, treatment, cure, or prevention of disease. Drugs are a primary component of medical care for clients with alterations in health status.

Although medications have many therapeutic effects, they can also produce many harmful effects if administered improperly. The safe administration of medications requires that nurses: (1) understand the basic concepts of pharmacology; (2) understand the mechanism of action, specific desired effects, and common undesirable effects (side effects) of all drugs they give; (3) identify the client; (4) skillfully perform the techniques necessary for proper administration; (5) effectively assess and monitor the client's response after receiving the medication; and (6) communicate medication effects to the prescriber. Nurses are legally responsible for every drug dose they administer.

Collaborative effort is necessary for the safe and effective use of medications. Physician, nurse, and pharmacist all have important roles in ensuring that clients receive maximum benefit from prescribed medications. Nurses also collaborate with clients in assessing the effects of medications and through the sharing of drug information.

Adequate client knowledge related to medications they are taking is essential in promotion of client self-responsibility. As teachers, nurses must provide information about the drug name, expected therapeutic action, dosage amount and timing, route and technique of administration, duration of drug use, major adverse effects and ways of minimizing them, and major drug interactions. With this knowledge, clients can be active participants in their care related to medication administration.

Clients cared for in the home may have family members administering their medications. This requires that nurses teach the family how to administer medications safely and accurately. The principles presented in this discussion to guide safe medication administration by nurses are also useful for client and family education.

Basics of Pharmacology. Safe administration of medications begins with a basic understanding of names and forms of medications, mechanisms and effects of drug action, and factors influencing drug action.

Drug Names. A single drug may have as many as four different names. The **chemical name** provides an exact description of the chemical composition of the drug and is rarely used by health care providers. The **generic name** is the name given by the manufacturer who first develops the drug. Often the generic name is derived from the chemical name. The **trade** or **proprietary** (brand) **name** is the name under which a manufacturer markets a drug. Because the same drug can be manufactured by many different companies, one drug may have many trade names. For example, acetaminophen (generic name) is known by the trade names of Anacin-3, Datril, Panadol, Tempra, and Tylenol.

In 1962, federal legislation mandated that there be one **official name** for each specific drug. Many times a drug's generic name also becomes its official name. This is the name by which each drug is listed in official pharmacological publications. The *United States Pharmacopeia* (USP) and the *National Formulary* (NF) are now published as a single volume by the United States Pharmacopeial Convention. It is an official publication that provides standards for drug quality and strength in the United States. The *Physicians' Desk Reference* (PDR) is an annually revised reference readily available to hospitals, physicians, and nurses, but it is not an official reference; the information in it is provided by drug manufacturers. The *British Pharmacopoeia* (BP) sets the standards for drug quality and strength in Canada. The *Canadian Formulary* (CF) is recognized by the Canadian Food and Drug Act and has some drugs not included in the *British Pharmacopoeia*.

Classification. Drugs may be classified according to their effect on a body system (eg, cardiac drugs); the symptoms relieved (eg, decongestant), or their desired effect (eg, stool softener). Classification systems are designed to organize the vast body of information related to medications, but are by no means exact. Drugs classified together may have very different chemical or physical compositions, but similar effects. Likewise, one drug may be found in several different categories because of simultaneous effects on various body systems. Nurses must learn the general characteristics of medications in each class.

Types of Preparations. Drugs are available in a variety of forms or preparations. Some drugs may be manufactured in several types of preparations such as tablets, pediatric elixirs, capsules, and suppositories, while other drugs may be available in only one form. The form in which the drug is available determines the route of administration. It is important that the nurse administer the form specified in the medication order. Table 22–8 outlines some of the common forms of medications.

Mechanism of Drug Action. Medications are administered to produce a therapeutic effect. The study of the mechanisms of drug action is pharmacodynamics. Drugs do not introduce new responses in the body, but rather act to alter existing physiological activity. Drugs interact with the body in several different ways—by altering body fluids, altering cell membranes, and most commonly by binding or interacting with chemical receptor sites at the cellular level. Once administered, all drugs go through four stages, absorption, distribution, metabolism, and excretion. Pharmacokinetics is the study of these four drug processes. Each drug has its own unique pharmacokinetic properties.[109]

ABSORPTION. **Absorption** is the process by which a drug is transferred from its site of entry into the body to the circulatory system. This process occurs in the gastrointestinal tract, subcutaneous tissue, muscle tissue, and the skin. Drugs that are injected directly into the bloodstream are immediately absorbed.

Medications are absorbed at different rate and in different ways. The rate of absorption is influenced by the following factors:

1. *Solubility of the drug.* Drugs must be in liquid form to be absorbed; therefore, drugs that dissolve easily are absorbed more rapidly. For this reason it is important to administer oral drugs with an adequate amount of fluid, and to reconstitute and dilute drugs only with the diluent recommended by the manufacturer, so that drug solubility is enhanced.
2. *Drug pH.* pH is a measure of the degree to which a solution is acidic or alkaline. It affects the ability of an oral medication to be absorbed. Acidic drugs pass through the gastric mucosa rapidly. Drugs that are basic are not absorbed until they reach the small intestines.
3. *Route of administration.* Each route of administration has a different influence on drug absorption depending on

TABLE 22–8. COMMON FORMS OF DRUGS

Form	Description
Capsule	Powder, liquid, or oil form of medication enclosed in a gelatin shell.
Elixir	Medication in a clear liquid containing alcohol, water, sweeteners, and flavoring. Designed for oral use.
Liniment	Medication mixed with alcohol, oil, or soapy emollient, which is applied to the skin.
Lotion	Drug in liquid suspension designed for topical use.
Lozenge	Flat round preparation containing drug in a flavored or sweetened base that dissolves in the mouth to release the medication. Also known as a *troche*.
Ointment	Semisolid preparation of one or more drugs applied to the skin.
Paste	Semisolid preparation, thicker and stiffer than ointment; absorbed more slowly than ointment through the skin.
Pill	Mixture of powdered drug with cohesive material in round, oval, or oblong shape.
Powder	A drug ground into fine particles from a solid for inhalation or application to the skin.
Solution	A drug dissolved in another liquid substance. May be used orally, parenterally, or externally.
Suppository	One or more drugs mixed into a firm base, such as gelatin, designed for insertion into a body cavity. The preparation melts at body temperature, thus releasing the medication for absorption.
Suspension	Fine drug particles dispersed in a liquid medium. Must be shaken before use.
Syrup	Medication dissolved in a concentrated sugar solution to mask unpleasant taste.
Tablet	A powdered form of medication compressed into a hard small disk or cylinder. May be a variety of colors or sizes. Enteric-coated tablets are covered with a substance that is insoluble in gastric acids, thus reducing the possible gastric irritation.

the physical nature of the affected tissues. Generally, injected medications are more rapidly absorbed than oral medications. The presence or absence of food in the gastrointestinal tract may significantly alter the rate of absorption.

4. *Circulation to the site of absorption.* The amount of blood flow to the absorption site profoundly affects the absorption rate. Topical medications applied to abraded skin are absorbed rapidly, while an injection administered into an area with low blood flow will be poorly absorbed. Because muscles have a greater blood flow than subcutaneous tissue, intramuscular injections are more rapidly absorbed.
5. *Concentration of dose.* High concentrations of a medication are absorbed more quickly than low doses.

DISTRIBUTION. **Distribution** is the process by which a drug is transported from the site of absorption to the site of action. Organs having the most extensive blood supply such as the heart, brain, liver, and kidneys receive the distributing drug the most rapidly while other organs receive the drug later. The rate and extent of distribution depend on the physical and chemical properties of the medication and the physiology of the person taking the drug. Drugs that are fat-soluble tend to accumulate in adipose tissue.

Distribution may be general or selective. Water-soluble drugs, for example, cannot pass through the blood–brain barrier, and therefore are relatively ineffective on the central nervous system. A drug's binding to albumin, a protein found in the blood, also affects the drug's distribution. Most medications bind to this protein to some extent. When bound to albumin, drugs cannot exert their pharmacological effect. Drugs are in their active form when they are not bound to albumin. The distribution process is very important because the amount of drug that actually gets to the desired receptor sites determines the extent of the pharmacological activity.

METABOLISM. **Metabolism,** or biotransformation, is the process that changes the drug into an inactive form and prepares it for excretion. Most of this process takes place in the liver, where a variety of enzymes degrade and detoxify the active chemicals. For this reason, individuals with impaired liver function are at greater risk for problems with drug toxicity as the metabolism and elimination rates are decreased. Older adults often have decreased liver function and so are at greater risk for toxicity.

EXCRETION. **Excretion** is the process by which the metabolites and drugs are eliminated from the body. The kidneys are the primary organs of excretion, although some products are excreted through the intestines, respiratory tract, and sweat, salivary, and mammary glands. The efficiency of kidney function decreases with age. Elderly clients may require smaller doses of a medication due to diminished excretion rates.

Effects of Drug Action. All medications produce a variety of physiological effects in the body—some desirable and some undesirable. A **therapeutic effect** is the desired or intended physiological effect for which the drug was prescribed. For example, a narcotic is given to relieve pain.

Drugs may also act unpredictably, be harmful, or have unpleasant effects. **Side effects** are those effects that are unintended and undesirable. Side effects are often predictable, and may be harmless, mild, severe, or even lethal. Common side effects of narcotics are stupor and sleep. Side effects are often tolerated in order to achieve the drug's therapeutic effect; however, if the side effects are too severe, the physician may have to discontinue the drug or alter the dosage. Unlike side effects, idiosyncratic reactions are unpredictable. These reactions occur when an individual overreacts or underreacts to a drug or has a reaction different from normal. It is impossible to anticipate an idiosyncratic reaction because it is unpredictable.

Toxic effects are adverse reactions that result from a drug overdose, or from abnormal accumulation of the medication in the body. As mentioned above, elderly clients and those with impaired kidney or liver function are at high risk for toxic effects. Excessive amounts of a drug in the system can have lethal effects. For example, high doses of certain common potent antimicrobial drugs can cause severe, permanent auditory and kidney damage.

A drug allergy is the immunological response to a drug to which the individual has been sensitized. The allergic reaction may be mild or severe, and may occur immediately or be delayed for hours or days. Typically signs and symptoms of allergic reactions include urticaria (hives), pruritus (intense itching), wheezing, nausea or vomiting, and diarrhea. **Anaphylaxis,** a severe, life-threatening allergic reaction, results in severe respiratory distress, and may be fatal. Individuals with known drug allergies should wear an identification bracelet to alert nurses and physicians. Nurses should always check drug allergies before administering any prescribed medication.

Drug tolerance exists when an individual needs increasing dosages of a particular medication in order to maintain a given therapeutic effect. Opiates, alcohol, and barbiturates are examples of drugs that are known to cause drug tolerance.

Drug interactions occur when one drug modifies the action of another drug. Drug interactions are common among individuals who take multiple medications. A drug may potentiate (increase) or antagonize (decrease) the action of another drug. **Potentiation** or synergism means that the combined effect of two drugs is greater than the anticipated effects of each drug given alone. For example, a muscle relaxant given in combination with an analgesic produces more effective pain relief than the individual drugs would be expected to achieve. Giving codeine with aspirin allows a lower dose of the narcotic to be given. Antagonism occurs when one drug interferes with the action of another. For example, an antacid taken with tetracycline decreases the absorption of the tetracycline.

Factors Influencing Drug Action/Effects. Individual responses to drugs vary considerably. A number of factors are known to influence the action or effect of medications.

AGE. The very young and the elderly have an increased responsiveness to drugs. Infants lack many of the enzymes necessary for mature metabolism, have immature organ systems, have variations in the amount of protein circulating in the blood, and have a larger percentage of total body water and lower fat stores. Because of the many physiological changes associated with aging, the elderly also absorb, metabolize, react to, and eliminate drugs differently than younger adults. Decreased gastric motility, lower levels of circulating serum albumin, and decreased kidney and liver function all contribute to altered drug effects in older adults.[110]

BODY WEIGHT. Body weight significantly affects drug action. The greater the body weight, the higher the dosage of drug required to effect the same response. Likewise, children need proportionately smaller doses of medications. Methods sometimes used to calculate pediatric dosages based on body weight are discussed later in this chapter.

SEX. Men and women react differently to the same drugs due primarily to differences in distribution of fat and water, hormonal balance, and body size and weight. Women usually have more fat reserves while men have greater water reserves. As a result, women tend to absorb more fat-soluble drugs, while men absorb a greater percentage of water-soluble ones.

ILLNESS AND DISEASE. Any pathological condition that impairs the function of major body organs has a significant effect on drug actions and/or effects. Diseases that affect circulatory, kidney, and liver function have the most profound effects on pharmacokinetics.

GENETIC EFFECTS. Many individuals, because of genetic makeup, may metabolize or react differently to specific drugs. For example, because of genetic effects some individuals produce red blood cells that are deficient in an enzyme called glucose-6-phosphate dehydrogenase (G-6-PD). This deficiency results in the destruction of red blood cells when given certain drugs such as aspirin. Metabolic patterns are often similiar in families. Many family members may share a particular drug sensitivity or reaction.

ENVIRONMENT. Drug actions may be affected by environmental factors. Sensory deprivation or overload may affect drug responses—clients in intensive care units may not receive the full benefit of an analgesic when surrounded by overwhelming noise and stimulus. Environmental temperature also influences drug action. Warm temperature produces vasodilation and may enhance the absorption of topical drugs. Conversely, cold weather causes vasoconstriction, which reduces topical absorption.

TIME OF ADMINISTRATION. As a rule, presence of food in the stomach delays the absorption of oral medications. Some drugs are given with food to prevent gastric irritation. These factors need to be considered when planning a medication schedule.

PSYCHOLOGICAL FACTORS. A number of psychological factors influence an individual's use and response to various drugs. The meaning or significance of the drug or drug taking often determines client compliance or acceptance of a prescribed therapy. The client's expectations of the medication can also affect drug action. This is one of the reasons why nurses tell clients to expect pain relief in a certain time when administering pain medications. The placebo effect (see Chap. 29), where an inactive substance produces effective pain relief, is a classic example of the impact of client expectations on drug effect.

General Considerations in Medication Administration

Legal Aspects. The production, distribution, prescription, and administration of drugs in the United States and Canada is governed by state, federal, and provincial laws. The major federal acts controlling drugs are the Food, Drug, and Cosmetic Act (1938) and its amendments, which require proof of the safety and efficacy of a drug before it can be sold; and the Controlled Substances Act (1970), which sets strict controls on the manufacture and distribution of narcotics and other controlled substances. The Canadian Food and Drug Act was passed in 1953 with many subsequent amendments. Enforcement of the Canadian Narcotic Control Act is the responsibility of the Royal Canadian Mounted Police.[110]

At the state level, nurse practice acts define and set limits on the scope of professional nursing functions including many aspects of the administration of medications. It is important for nurses to know specific limitations in their particular state. To practice beyond the scope of defined nursing practice endangers clients and leaves nurses open to possible medical malpractice suits. In the past, only physicians prescribed medications; however, today many states have granted medication prescription rights to nurse practitioners.

The legal responsibilities associated with the preparation, administration, and evaluation of medications are immense. Under the law, nurses are accountable for their actions and judgments instituted during the performance of professional duties. Nurses are expected to know the purpose, side effects, and expected action of prescribed medications before administering them. Likewise nurses are expected to use professional judgment in assessing whether a medication order is reasonable and within the standards of normal practice. Nurses should question an order that appears unreasonable and refuse to administer the medication until the order is clarified. Not only do unclear orders raise the possibility of harm to clients, they also put nurses at risk for a lawsuit. The nurse who administers a drug according to an incorrectly written medication order will be held responsible for the error.

Systems of Measurement. Three systems of measurement are used in North America for drug therapy: metric, apothecary, and household. Because all three systems are currently being used in prescribing medications, nurses must become familiar with all three systems and be able to convert from one system to another as needed.

METRIC SYSTEM. The metric system is the most frequently used system of measurement for drug administration. It is a logically organized system based on units of 10. Multiplying or dividing by 10 forms secondary units (100, 1000, 0.1, 0.01). The basic units of measure are the meter (length), the liter (volume), and the gram (weight). Nurses use volume and weight units for doing drug calculations. Latin prefixes are used to designate subdivisions of the basic units of measure: deci- (0.1), centi- (0.01), milli- (0.001). Greek prefixes designate multiples of the basic units: deka- (10), hecto- (100), kilo- (1000). See Box 22–15. Drug doses use fractions or multiples of a basic unit. Fractions are written in decimal form: for example, one-half of a gram is written 0.5 g. A zero should always be placed in front of a decimal when writing fractions to prevent errors in interpretation.

APOTHECARY SYSTEM. The apothecary system is a much older system of measurement that was brought to the United States and Canada from England during colonial days. Although physicians and pharmacists formerly used the apothecary system extensively, it has been replaced by the metric system in most health care facilities. Many aspects of this system are familiar to most North Americans. The units of measurement in this system are easily found in the home. Fluid is measured in pints and quarts, weight is measured in pounds, and length is measured in feet and inches. The basic unit of weight is the grain (equal to the weight of a grain of wheat in colonial days), and the basic unit of volume is the minim (a volume of water equal to the same grain of wheat). The units of weight in ascending order are the grain, dram, ounce, and pound. The units of volume in ascending order are the minim, fluid dram, fluid ounce, pint, quart, and gallon.

Quantities in the apothecary system are designated by lower-case Roman numerals. The Roman numeral follows rather than precedes the unit of measure. For example, 3 grains would be written as gr. iii.

HOUSEHOLD MEASUREMENTS. Household measurements are also familiar to most people. Included in household measures are drops, teaspoons, tablespoons, cups, and glasses. Although pints and quarts are household measures, they are also used in the apothecary system. These units of measurement are quite convenient; however, household utensils are often very inaccurate and vary considerably in size. Household measurements are not frequently used because of their inaccuracy. When accuracy is not critical, it is safe to use household measures, such as with many over-the-counter drugs (antacids, cough syrups, etc).

Table 22–9 gives an example of some of the most frequently used equivalents between the three systems of measurement. It should be noted that there are discrepancies among these equivalents. These represent approximate, not exact equivalents.

Drug Dosage Calculations. All problems relating to drug dosages can be solved by the use of a proportion. The prescriber's order will supply the name of the medication, strength or dosage of the drug, method or route of administration, frequency of administration, and any other spe-

BOX 22–15. METRIC SYSTEM: RELATIONSHIPS OF UNITS FOR VOLUME AND WEIGHT

Units	0.000001	0.001	0.01	0.1	1	10	100	1000
Prefixes	Micro-	Milli-	Centi-	Deci-		Deka-	Hecto-	Kilo-
Weight	Microgram (μg)	Milligram (mg)	Centigram (cg)	Decigram (convert to grams)	Gram (g)	Dekagram (dg)	Hectogram (hg)	Kilogram (kg)
Equivalents (read across)					1000 g			1 kg
					100 g		1 hg	
					10 g	1 dg		
		1000 μg	100 cg	(10 decigrams)	1 g			0.001 kg
		100 mg	1 cg		0.1 g			0.01 kg
		10 mg			0.01 g			0.1 kg
	1000 μg	1 mg			0.001 g			
	1 μg	0.001 mg						
Capacity		Milliliter (mL)		Deciliter (dL)	Liter (L)			
Equivalents (read across)		100 mL		1 dL	0.1 L			
		1000 mL			1 L			
		1 mL			0.001 L			

TABLE 22–9. EQUIVALENTS OF MEASUREMENT

Apothecary	Metric	Household
15 or 16 minims	= 1 milliliter (mL)	= 15 drops (gtts)
1 dram (ʒ)	= 4 or 5 mL	= 1 teaspoon (tsp)
4 ʒ	= 15 mL	= 1 tablespoon (tbsp)
1 fluid ounce (℥)	= 30 mL	= 2 tbsp
1 grain (gr)	= 60 milligrams (mg)	
7½ gr	= 500 mg	
15 gr	= 30 g	
1 pound (lb)	= 454 g	
2.2 lb	= 1 kilogram (kg)	

cial instructions. The medication container or package will provide the strength of the medication on hand. Box 22–16 contains a sample drug dosage calculation.

CONVERTING BETWEEN SYSTEMS. Sometimes a medication order will be written in one system of measurement and the drug will be supplied in another. In these instances, it is necessary to convert one of the measurements so that they are both expressed in the same measurement system. Before beginning a conversion, a nurse must know the equivalents required to make the conversion (Table 22–9). Use the equivalents to set up a proportion. The known equivalent is placed on the left side of the proportion and the equivalent to be determined is placed on the right. Only two different units of measure may be used in each proportion. The units of measure must be in the same position on the right as they are on the left. Box 22–17 contains an example of a dosage calculation with a conversion among systems.

PEDIATRIC CALCULATIONS. Calculating pediatric dosage requires caution. A child's smaller size dictates that proportionately smaller dosages of medication are needed. Although physicians generally calculate the safe dosage based on the child's size, nurses must be able to check the dosage via the principles of safe pediatric dosages. Unlike standard adult drug dosages, children's dosages vary considerably. Pediatric dosages can be based on weight or body surface area.

Drug references are available that designate pediatric dosages for specific drugs in milligrams per kilogram of body weight. If the weight has been measureed in pounds, convert the weight to kilograms before calculating the correct drug dosage. Using pediatric dosage parameters specified for a particular drug rather than a standard formula is considered to be the safest method for calculating pediatric drug dosages. If no such reference is available for a given drug, a formula based on body surface area (BSA) is recommended.

BSA is determined by using a standard nomogram and plotting in the child's height and weight. A straight line is drawn between the child's height (left column) and the child's weight (right column). The point at which the line crosses the surface area column (center) is the child's estimated body surface area. A child who is 4 feet, 2 inches tall and weights 75 pounds has a body surface area of 1.05 m^2 (Fig. 22–12). The formula for calculating a child's dose of medication is a ratio of the child's BSA to the surface area of an average adult (1.7 m^2) times the normal adult dose.

$$\text{Child's dose} = \frac{\text{Surface area of child}}{1.7\ \text{m}^2} \times \text{Normal adult dose}$$

Distribution Systems. Systems and standard policies for the storage and distribution of medications vary among health care facilities. All agencies have a designated area for stocking and dispensing drugs. Many agencies have specially designed medication rooms with locked cupboards for controlled substances. Others may use mobile medication carts or individual storage units adjacent to the client's room (Fig. 22–13). All systems are designed to provide safe storage and administration of medication. Medications are de-

BOX 22–16. SAMPLE DRUG DOSAGE CALCULATION

Physician's medication order: Aspirin 650 mg q4h po prn for pain. Drug available: Aspirin 325 mg tablets.

	Known equivalent		Unknown equivalent
1. Set up proportion; units of measure same both sides of proportion.	$\frac{325\ \text{mg}}{1\ \text{tab}}$	=	$\frac{650\ \text{mg}}{X\ \text{tab}}$
2. Cross-multiply.	325X	=	650 × 1
3. Solve for X.	X	=	$\frac{650}{325} = 2$ tabs

BOX 22–17. DRUG DOSAGE CALCULATION WITH CONVERSTION BETWEEN SYSTEMS

Physician's medication order: Phenobarbital gr ¾ po bid.

Drug available: Phenobarbital elixir 20 mg per 5 mL.

Step 1: Convert measurements to same system.

	Known equivalent		Unknown equivalent
Set up proportions; units of measure same on both sides of proportion.	$\frac{1\ \text{gr}}{60\ \text{mg}}$	=	$\frac{3/4\ \text{gr}}{X\ \text{mg}}$
Cross-multiply.	1X	=	60 × ¾
Solve for X.	X	=	45 mg

Step 2: Calculate amount of drug to be given.

	Known equivalent		Unknown equivalent
Set up proportion; units of measure same on both sides of proportion.	$\frac{20\ \text{mg}}{5\text{mL}}$	=	$\frac{45\ \text{mg}}{X\text{mL}}$
Cross multiply.	20X	=	5 × 45 = 225
Solve for X.	X	=	$\frac{225}{20} = 11.25$ mL

Answer: Give 11.25 mL of available phenobarbital elixir.

livered to the nursing unit through three supply systems: stock supply, individual supply, and unit dose system.

STOCK SUPPLY. With a stock supply system, large amounts of commonly used medications (eg, aspirin) are kept available on each unit. Individual doses are taken from bulk containers and dispensed by nurses. Although this system is not used as commonly as in the past, narcotics are still usually provided in stock supply.

INDIVIDUAL CLIENT SUPPLY. This provides a separate supply of medications for each client in specially labeled drawers or storage bins. Pharmacists dispense only the amount of medication a client will use for a limited period of time and nurses are responsible for administering individual doses at the prescribed times.

UNIT DOSE SYSTEM. The unit dose system supplies medications in individual packaged and labeled doses (Fig. 22–14). The individual doses for each shift or 24-hour period are delivered to the floor from the pharmacy. The unit dose system is increasing in popularity as many believe it saves time in preparation and reduces the incidence of medication errors.

Medication Orders. No medication can be administered to a client without a medication order from a physician or some other qualified health care professional. Ideally all medication orders should be written; however, in an emergency a physician may give an order verbally or by telephone. Institutional policies vary as to who may accept a verbal order and write it on a client's chart.

A medication order is incomplete unless it contains the following essential components:

1. *The client's full name.* The full name is used to distinguish the client from others with the same last name. Most

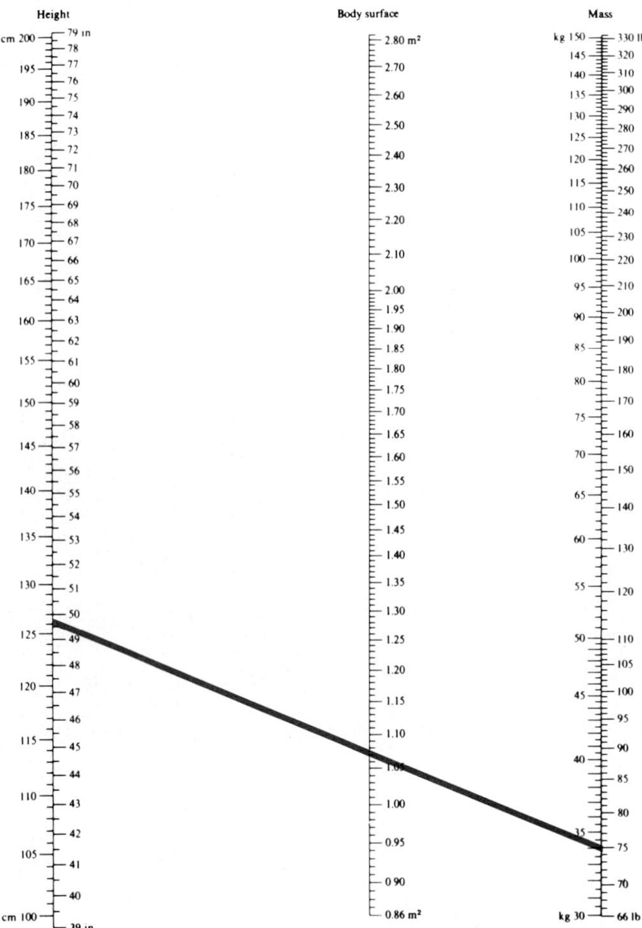

Figure 22–12. Sample nomogram to determine body surface area by plotting height and weight on the parallel axes.

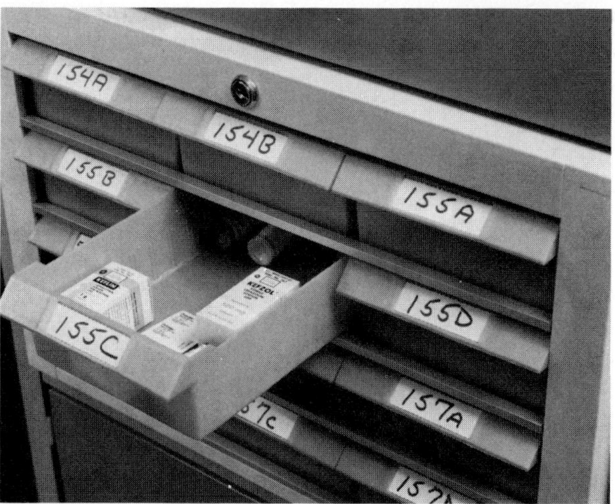

Figure 22–13. Unit dose cart. (*From Smith S, Duell D. Clinical Nursing Skills: Nursing Process Model; Basic to Advanced Skills. 3rd ed. Norwalk, CT: Appleton & Lange; 1992.*)

institutions imprint the client's name and identification number on all forms.

2. *Date.* The date should include the day, month, and year. Some agencies also require that the time of day be included to clarify exactly when certain orders should end.
3. *Drug name.* The drug name must be clearly written. Correct spelling is important, as many drugs have similar names. Prescribers may order drugs using generic or trade names.

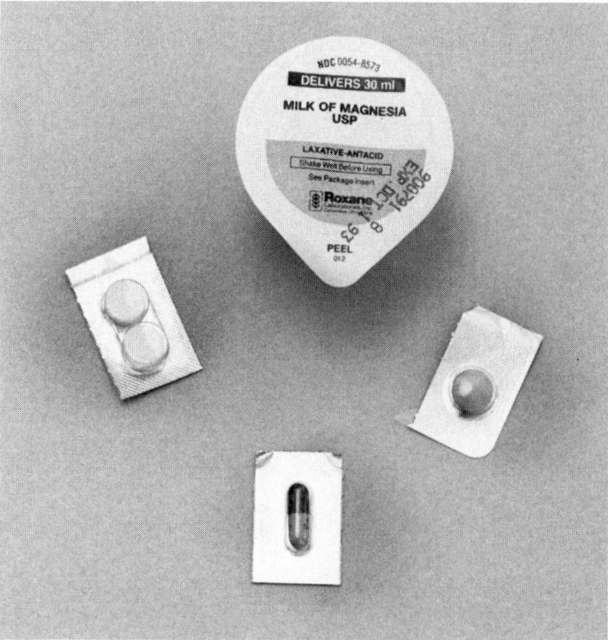

Figure 22–14. Samples of individually packaged drugs for a unit-dose system of dispensing medications.

4. *Dosage.* The dosage should include the amount and/or strength of the prescribed drug.
5. *Route of administration.* Many drugs may be administered by more than one route, so it is important that the prescribed route be clearly stated. A nurse who believes a client's condition makes the ordered route inappropriate must contact the prescriber to change the route of administration. For example, a client who is nauseated and vomiting will be unable to take oral medications and may require parenteral administration of medications until the nausea subsides. Nurses may not arbitrarily change the route of medication because the dosage may need to be changed. However, it is acceptable and appropriate for a nurse to request another form of a drug for administration by the ordered route. For example, a nurse can substitute the liquid form of an oral medication for a tablet if a client is having difficulty swallowing the tablet, so long as the ordered dosage is given.
6. *Time and frequency of administration.* Nurses need to know when to initiate drug therapy and at what intervals the medication should be given.
7. *Signature.* The signature of the prescriber makes the drug order a legal request. An unsigned order has no validity in a health care agency or in a court of law.

Medication orders often contain abbreviations. The abbreviations may be used to indicate dosage, routes of administration, and special information for nurses to follow when dispensing the drug. Table 22–10 lists abbreviations commonly used in medication orders. Some professionals believe abbreviations should be eliminated because one may be confused with another. For example, qod for every other day can be read as qid if not carefully written.

TYPES OF MEDICATION ORDERS. The four common types of medication orders are based on the frequency of medication administration. A single order is to be given only once at a specified time. Preoperative medications are frequently single orders. A **stat order** is also a single order, but is to be given immediately. Stat orders are frequently given in emergency situations or when a client's condition changes suddenly.

Routine orders are carried out at regular intervals until the prescriber cancels the order or an automatic stop order takes effect. Automatic stop orders are used in many institutions to automatically discontinue certain medication orders within a specific time.

Medications to be administered as the client needs them are called **prn orders.** This allows nurses to administer the medication based on an assessment of clients' needs. Such orders are frequently used for the administration of analgesics for pain and specify a minimum interval of time that must elapse between doses. For example: Tylenol tabs ii, q4h, prn mild pain.

VERIFYING MEDICATION ORDERS. Medication orders must be transcribed to an appropriate medication form, often called a medication administration record (MAR). Increasingly, hospitals are using computerized printouts of medications

TABLE 22–10. ABBREVIATIONS COMMONLY USED IN MEDICATION ORDERS

Abbreviation	Meaning
ac	Before meals
ad lib	Freely; as desired
bid	Twice a day
c̄	With
cap	Capsule
D/C	Discontinue
elix	Elixir
hs	At bedtime; hour of sleep
IM	Intramuscular
IV	Intravenous
IVPB	IV piggyback
OD	Right eye
OS	Left eye
OU	Both eyes
pc	After meals
po	By mouth
prn	As needed; when necessary
q	Every
qd	Every day
qh	Every hour
qid	Four times a day
qod	Every other day
qs	Sufficient quantity
s̄	Without
SC or SQ	Subcutaneous
ss̄	One-half
stat	Immediately
supp	Suppository
tid	Three times a day

administration records, which reduces the incidence of errors. Although the procedures and/or forms vary among institutions, it is critical that all transcribed orders be verified—that is, compared to the written order in a client's chart—by a registered nurse to assure accuracy and thoroughness of transcription. If the order as written in the chart seems incorrect or incomplete, a nurse then contacts the prescriber to clarify any questions.

Client Assessment. Client assessment is a vital part of nursing responsibilities associated with the administration of medications. Assessment related to medications begins at admission to the health care facility and is a continual process that extends through discharge teaching.

MEDICATION HISTORY. A medication history is an important component of a complete nursing history. A review of clients' previous and current drug practices, including the use of prescription drugs, over-the-counter medications, and recreational drugs (alcohol, marijuana, etc) is included in a medication history. Documentation of known or suspected drug allergies or adverse reactions is also important. For more detailed information about client history-taking see Chapter 16.

PHYSIOLOGICAL ASSESSMENT. Physiological assessment is an integral part of routine medication administration. Nurses must assess relevant aspects of clients' current physical or mental status prior to the administration of any medication. For example, blood pressure should be measured prior to the administration of antihypertensives. Not only does this practice enable nurses to exercise sound professional judgment in determining the appropriateness of the prescribed medication, but it also provides baseline assessment data upon which clients' response to medications can be measured. For a more detailed review of physical assessment see Chapter 16.

LEARNING NEEDS. Assessment of a client's learning needs related to medications is also an ongoing process. As stated earlier, clients should be aware of the purpose of their prescribed medications, expected side effects, and necessary administration techniques or schedule. Hospitalized clients are frequently discharged with new or altered prescribed medication regimens. Client understanding of ordered medications is necessary for safe and effective use of medications.

Principles of Safe Administration. Safety is of utmost importance when administering medications. As discussed earlier, medication errors can have harmful and even potentially lethal consequences. Nurses should follow the guidelines of the "five rights" to ensure safe drug administration: that is, right drug, right dose, right time, right route, and right client.

Right Drug. Administration of the right drug is ensured through carefully checking medications listed on the medication administration record with the physician's original written order. When preparing to administer the drug, nurses should check the label of the drug container against the confirmed medication record three times—when removing the container from storage, as the drug is removed from the container, and as the container is returned to storage. If a unit-dose medication is being used, the drug should be checked when removing it from the drawer, before placing it in the medicine cup, and once again before leaving the unit dose cart with the medication. Some nurses prefer to take the medication administration record to the bedside, completing the third check there.

Nurses should only administer medications that they have personally prepared. Drugs from an unmarked container or one with an illegible label should never be used. If the client questions a medication, nurses should withhold the medication until they can recheck the medication orders. Clients are often alert to changes in the appearance or numbers of medications, so their comments must be taken seriously. Rechecking to ensure that the change in prescribed regimen is indeed ordered prevents potential medication errors and may ease client concerns.

Right Dose. Compare the dosage printed on the unit dose package (or stock supply bottle) with that printed on the medication administration record. Sometimes the wrong dosage is supplied by the pharmacy. Although the use of the unit-dose system eliminates the need for many drug calculations, nurses must still be able to calculate dosage accurately to verify accuracy of administered amounts. Careful attention to detail when pouring liquid medications or filling syringes also ensures that the client receives the correct dose. Always doublecheck any calculations that indicate the need for multiple pills/tablets or that require the splitting of a tablet.

Right Time. Nurses should know why a medication is ordered for a certain time of day and whether that time schedule may be altered. For example, medications ordered for three times a day could be given three times during waking hours (8 AM, 2 PM, 8 PM), or could be given every 8 hours around the clock (8 AM, 4 PM, 12 MN). If the ordered medication is an IV antibiotic, the physician would probably want it administered every 8 hours, while a routine medication such as an iron supplement could be given three times during waking hours. Most institutions have a recommended time schedule for medications ordered at regular intervals, but nurses should also consider client preferences, particularly for drugs they have been taking prior to admission on a particular schedule.

When administering medications, nurses should ensure that medications are given within 30 minutes of the prescribed time. For some drugs, such as insulin given prior to a meal, the correct time is a high priority.

Right Route. Check that the drug that has been supplied is the appropriate form for the ordered route. Check the ordered route with the prescriber if there are any questions. When administering parenteral medications, proper technique must be followed to ensure that the medication is delivered exactly as ordered (eg, IM versus SQ). Nurses may never arbitrarily change the route or dosage.

Right Client. Ensuring that a medication is administered to the correct client is vital. In acute care settings, nurses are often responsible for administering medications to several clients within a short time frame. Clients often have similar names, and it may be difficult to associate names and faces accurately. The only reliable way to verify a client's identity is through checking the identification bracelet or asking a client to state his or her name; however, nurses should not rely on a client's answering when his or her name is called. Some hospitalized clients are confused or scared and may answer to the wrong name.

Narcotic Safety. In addition to the "five rights," additional safety measures must be employed when administering narcotics and other controlled substances. Narcotics are stored in a double-locked cabinet or drawer. Federal law requires that each nursing unit keep an accurate record of the administration of all narcotics. Although the actual forms and procedures may vary among institutions, narcotic records generally require the name of the client, drug dose, time, physician's name, and the signature of the nurse administering the drug. The form is filled out as the narcotic is removed from the locked cabinet. If a portion or all of a narcotic dose must be discarded or is wasted, an additional nurse's signature is generally required to corroborate the disposal of the narcotic substance. Only licensed individuals can administer narcotics. Students administering narcotics are supervised by a licensed person, who countersigns the narcotic record.

It is common practice for narcotics to be checked and the exact count verified at specified intervals—usually at the change of shift. Discrepancies in the narcotic count should be reported and investigated promptly.

Table 22–11 outlines some additional principles related to the safe administration of medications. These guidelines should be incorporated into each nurse's normal practices to ensure client safety and well-being.

Administering Oral Medications. Oral preparations (pills, tablets, capsules, elixirs) are the most commonly prescribed forms of medication. Generally unless a client is experiencing impaired gastrointestinal functioning or is unable to swallow, the oral route is the safest, cheapest, and easiest method of medication administration, especially for self-administration (Procedure 22–5).

Benefits of the oral route include reduced costs, simplified administration, and the ability to provide a systemic drug effect without violating the client's skin or mucous membrane barriers. Disadvantages of this administration route include the unpleasant taste of many drugs, harmful gastric side effects, and problems with absorption that may be encountered because of the presence or absence of food in the stomach at the time of administration.

Although most oral medications are relatively easy to administer, some clients may have difficulty with swallowing them or may find their taste objectionable. Assisting clients to a sitting or standing position and providing them with at least 60 to 100 mL of fluid often facilitates swallowing tablets or capsules. If a client must remain flat or is on a strict fluid restriction, nurses should check with the pharmacist to see if a liquid form of the medication is available. Time-released or enteric coated drugs may not be crushed.[110]

A variety of techniques can be used to mask or reduce the unpleasant taste of medications. Suggest that clients place medications further back on the tongue where there are fewer taste buds. Or, medications can be diluted with fruit juices or cold carbonated beverages. Administering medications with crushed ice numbs the taste buds and reduces unpleasant taste. Crushing and mixing the medication with soft foods such as applesauce, ice cream, or pudding may mask the taste; however, it is important to ensure that crushing a medication does not change its therapeutic properties. If medications cannot be crushed or diluted, have juices or other beverages on hand to offer immediately after administration.

Clients with nasogastric (NG) feeding tubes can receive oral preparations through the feeding tube. In most instances, liquid preparations are preferred. The guidelines for administration of oral medications via NG tube are presented in Box 22–18.

Administering Topical Medications. Topical medications are designed to be applied to the skin or mucous membranes for absorption. Although not all drugs are readily

TABLE 22–11. GUIDELINES FOR THE ADMINISTRATION OF MEDICATIONS

Action	Rationale
1. Use medical asepsis for oral medications, surgical asepsis for parenteral medications.	1. Protects clients from injury.
2. Verify medical order prior to administering drugs.	2. Promotes safety and accuracy.
3. Before administering any medication, know client's diagnosis, purpose of the medication, its therapeutic effects, secondary effects, and any pertinent nursing implications.	3. Knowledge enables nurses to make informed professional decisions regarding appropriateness of medication order.
4. Check client's allergy list before administering a medication.	4. Prevents administration of medications with potentially harmful effects.
5. Check the expiration date on the medication.	5. Outdated medications may have reduced potency or be chemically altered from original condition.
6. Do not leave medications unattended. If you must interrupt medication preparation for more urgent tasks, return the medications to their storage area before leaving. Repeat safety checks when resuming medication preparation.	6. Unattended medications may be removed by unauthorized individuals. Interruptions cause loss of concentration and possible errors. Repeating safety checks prevents errors.
7. Do not return an unused unlabeled medication to a container or transfer medications from one container to another. An unopened unit dose package may be returned to a client's medication drawer in the unit dose cart so client can be credited for unused drug.	7. Prevents inadvertent mixture of medications or placing of medication in incorrect container.
8. Identify clients prior to administering medication by checking their identiband or asking their name.	8. Prevents administering the drug to the wrong client.
9. Discuss the purpose and side effects of drugs with clients.	9. Promotes self-responsibility.
10. Observe that clients take the medication. Do not leave the medication at the bedside, assuming a client will take it.	10. Ensures correct administration of prescribed drug to the correct client.
11. Special precautions may be required for certain drugs. Most agencies require that two registered nurses doublecheck the dosages of anticoagulants, insulin, and certain intravenous medications. Check institutional policies.	11. Prevents accidental errors in dosage with potentially lethal drugs.
12. Chart a medication immediately after administering it. Some nurses initial the medication administration record before taking the medication to a client's room. If the medication is not taken, this is indicated when the drug is returned to the cart or discaded.	12. Prevents potential overdose. Failing to chart promptly may cause another nurse to repeat the dose thinking it has not been given. Initialing when leaving the cart verifies intent to administer medications and prevents repeated doses and omitted charting because of interruptions that interfere with returning to the cart to chart immediately after administering medication.

PROCEDURE 22–5. ADMINISTERING ORAL MEDICATIONS

PURPOSE: To provide medication for a specific therapeutic effect, when rapid absorption is not a major consideration.

EQUIPMENT: Medication supply, disposable medication cups, client's medication administration record (MAR), drinking water or juice, and straws.

ACTION	RATIONALE
1. Follow general guidelines for administration of medications (Table 22–11).	1. These guidelines facilitate safe, error-free preparation of medication.

(continued)

PROCEDURE 22–5. (continued)

2. Before preparing oral medications, verify that no tests or procedures are scheduled requiring the client to be n.p.o.

   Most oral medications may be safely deferred until test/procedure has been concluded. If in doubt about significance of delayed administration, consult physician.

3. Check the client's MAR to determine the medication(s) to be given.

   Oral medications are usually given at routine times on a client care unit. Frequently a client will have several medications ordered for each administration time.

4. To prepare tablets or capsules, compare the dosage ordered with the dosage available to determine how many tablets/capsules should be given.

   NOTE: Some tablets are scored to facilitate administration of ½ or ¼ tablet. Do not break capsules or unscored tablets. Consult with physician or pharmacist.

   Many medications are dispensed in several strengths corresponding to the commonly prescribed dosages, but individual client needs may require that less than 1 or more than 1 tablet be given at each administration time. This comparison of the order and drug label represents the first safety check.

5. Remove the correct number of tablets/capsules from the supply. Compare the drug name and strength on the label with the order on the MAR. Do not remove the wrapper of unit dose medications. Place packet into a medication cup.

   NOTE: Some nurses prefer to place each wrapped drug on the MAR next to the order. A third check that all medications ordered for the current time have been correctly prepared can then be done prior to placing all drugs into a medication cup.

   This is the second safety check. Intact wrapper provides positive identification of the drug at the bedside, providing opportunity for third safety check and ready identification of any drugs refused or held because of assessment data obtained at the time of administration. Unused medications can be returned safely to the supply.

6. If dispensing tablets/capsules from a stock supply, pour the required number into the bottle cap, then into the medication cup. Compare the label to the order a third time before returning the bottle to the shelf. Avoid touching medications with your fingers, if possible.

   Extra tablets poured inadvertently can be readily returned to the stock container from the cap before being mixed with other drugs in the medication cup. Third safety check at the bedside is impossible because drugs cannot be positively identified.

7. Repeat the above steps for al medications to be given at this time. Compare the number of drugs ordered for current time to the number of drugs in the cup(s) prior to leaving the preparation area.

   NOTE: Many nurses place drug(s) requiring specific assessment (eg, pulse, BP) prior to administration in separate cups to aid them in remembering to carry out the assessment prior to giving the medication.

   Following a specific routine for each drug reduces medication errors. Comparing the number of drugs ordered with the number prepared prevents omissions.

(continued)

PROCEDURE 22–5. (continued)

8. Follow the same safety checks for preparing liquid medications. If available in unit dose form, do not open lid until at the bedside. If pouring from a stock bottle, calculate the correct volume required for ordered dosage prior to pouring liquid.

8. See step 5 above. Prior calculation reduces likelihood of pouring incorrect amount.

9. To pour the correct volume, hold bottle with your palm on the label and pour liquid into a graduated medicine cup held at eye level. If cup is not marked in sufficiently small increments to measure the required amount, use a syringe to obtain the correct dose.

9. Palming the label prevents liquid that drips during pouring from obliterating the label. Using appropriately graduated container to measure dosages prevents errors related to incorrect estimation. If a meniscus is not read at eye level, parallax (the apparent displacement of objects caused by a change in the observer's position) will distort perception and result in inaccurate dosage.

10. Take medications to client's room. If supplies (such as juice, foods to mix with crushed medications) are needed, take these in with the medications.

NOTE: Some nurses also take the MAR into the client's room to match with ID bracelet and to perform third safety check. Others chart on MAR prior to leaving medication preparation area.

10. Taking all necessary supplies to complete the procedure saves nurse time and energy.

11. Identify client by reading client's ID bracelet. You may also ask clients to state their name.

NOTE: Complete special assessments before giving medications.

11. Positive identification prevents giving medications to the wrong client.

12. Match drug labels with MAR if third safety check was not previously completed. Discuss drug effects/precautions with client.

12. Informed clients are able to take greater responsibility for decisions regarding health care.

13. Remove drug wrappers. Offer medications according to client's preference for order of drugs, number taken at once, liquid/food of choice, etc. Encourage intake of additional 60 to 100 mL of fluid after medications have been swallowed.

NOTE: Placing the medications under the tongue or on the back of tongue facilitates swallowing them. Mix crushed tablets or contents of capsules with food for clients who have difficulty swallowing pills. Do not crush enteric coated tablets or granules from time-release medications.

13. Respecting client's preferences promotes trust. Extra fluid facilitates drug moving to stomach rather than remaining in the esophagus.

(continued)

PROCEDURE 22–5. (continued)

14. Remain with client until all medications have been swallowed.	14. Verification of actual ingestion of medication is necessary for documentation of administration.

RECORDING: Note name, strength, route, and time of administration according to agency policy. The MAR is the usual location for this information. Specific assessment data (P, BP) may also recorded on the MAR in some agencies. Additional information regarding client response to the medication may be placed in the nurse's notes, but generally only untoward effects are documented for routine medications.

absorbed through the outer skin layers, absorption can be facilitated by thorough cleansing of the skin with soap and water prior to application, and prolonged contact of the drug with skin. The use of solvent penetrants in combination with drugs also enhances absorption.[109]

There are a variety of different kinds of topical agents, including (1) local anesthetics, (2) emollients for moisturizing and soothing skin, (3) cleansing agents for the skin or mucous membranes, (4) antipruritics, (5) antiseptics and antibiotics, and (6) anti-inflammatory agents. Topical medications are generally applied for the local effects on the immediate area of application; however, some topical medications are absorbed through the skin or mucous membranes into the bloodstream and exert a systemic effect. Nitroglycerin paste is an example of a systemically acting topical agent.

Skin Applications. Topical medications such as creams, lotions, and ointments are frequently supplied in tubes, jars, and multiple-use containers. Nurses should remove only enough medication from the container for one application (Fig. 22–15). Unless contraindicated, the skin should always be cleansed with soap and water prior to medication application. If the skin is inflamed or irritated, the soap can be omitted but the area should be rinsed with water.

Gloves are sometimes indicated when nurses apply these preparations. Lotions or emollients may be applied directly to intact skin. A tongue blade, cotton balls, or cotton-tipped applicators may be useful in applying ointments or topical liquids. Gloves should always be worn when working with systemically acting medications, or when there is a risk of infection transmission. Sterile technique is required if the client has open, draining wounds.

Conditions that require the administration of topical medications are often a source of discomfort or embarrassment to the client. Skin lesions or rashes may be sensitive to the touch and may require extreme care in cleansing or application of lotions or ointments. Nurses need to be aware of the impact these conditions can have on clients' self-esteem or self-image, and make every effort to convey acceptance.

BOX 22–18. GUIDELINES FOR ADMINISTRATION OF MEDICATIONS THROUGH A NASOGASTRIC TUBE

1. Liquid forms of medication are most easily adminstered via NG tube. Consult with pharmacy to have all drugs that are available in liquid form to be dispensed as liquids.
2. Simple compressed tablets can always be crushed and mixed with liquid. Use a glass mortar and pestle, or crush the tablet inside the unit dose package.
3. It is preferable to dissolve a soft gelatin capsule in 20 to 30 mL of warm water rather than sticking a needle into the capsule and squeezing out the contents.
4. Capsules containing powders can be separated and the contents mixed with liquid.
5. Do not crush enteric-coated tablets or sustained-release preparations. These are intended to dissolve in the intestines, not the stomach. Consult with the physician or pharmacist for alternative forms of the drug.
6. Administer buccal or sublingual tablets as intended, if possible.
7. Clients receiving continuous tube feedings generally have residual feeding solution in the stomach, so medications that are inactivated by milk (such as tetracycline) are unlikely to be effective. Absorption of most drugs will be slowed by the presence of the tube feeding formula in the stomach. If an empty stomach is critical to a drug's absorption, consult with the physician to arrange intermittent rather than continuous feedings.
8. Verify the placement of the NG tube before administering medications. (See Procedure 22–19, step 5.)
9. Use a large syringe to administer medications. Remove the plunger and pour the medications into the barrel. Use positive pressure to instill the medications, rather than gravity. Most crushed tablets will not dissolve in liquid, and viscous liquid medications will not move through small-lumen tubes via gravity.
10. Flush the tubing with 30 to 50 mL of water to clear the tubing after administering medications to prevent their plugging the tube. (See Procedure 22–20.)
11. Record the total volume of liquid (medications and water) instilled on the intake and output (I&O) record.

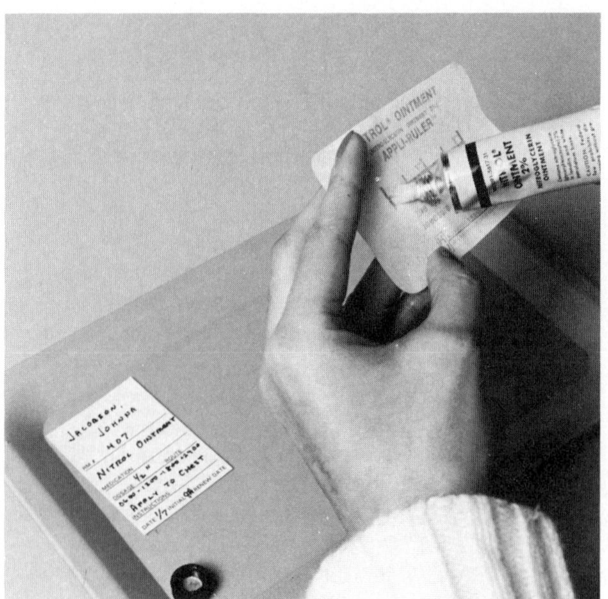

A

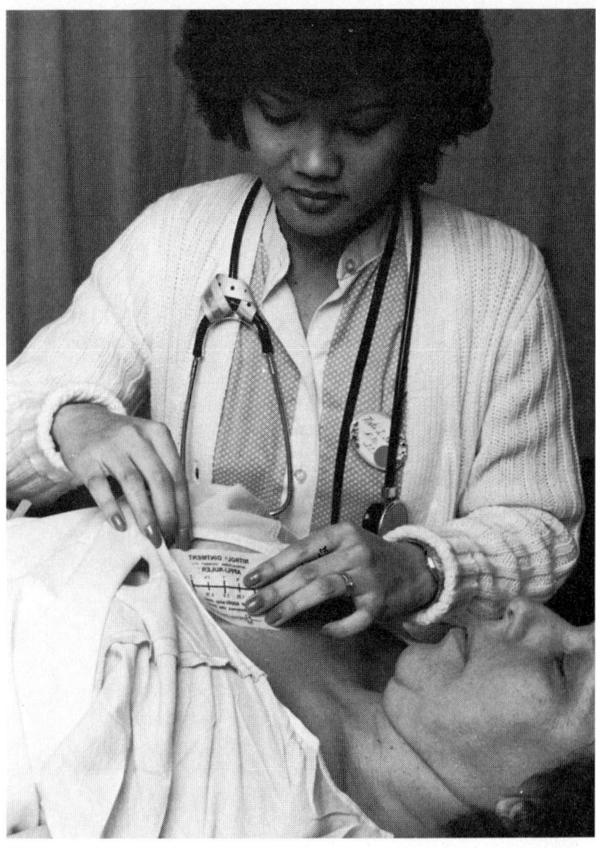

B

Figure 22–15. Application of topical medication. **A.** This topical medication is applied using special papers to measure the dosage. **B.** The paper is applied to the skin and remains in place until the next dose is given. (*From Smith S, Duell D.* Clinical Nursing Skills: Nursing Process Model; Basic to Advanced Skills. *3rd ed. Norwalk, CT: Appleton & Lange; 1992.*)

Oral Applications. Some medications are inserted directly onto the mucous membranes of the oral cavity for systemic absorption. Examples include buccal tablets, which are placed in the cheek pouch; and sublingual tablets, which are placed under the tongue. It is important that clients understand that these tablets are not to be chewed or swallowed, but must be held in the mouth until totally absorbed.

Eye Applications. The eye is an extremely delicate organ that is susceptible to injury or infection. For this reason, all procedures involving the eye require the use of sterile technique. The cornea of the eye is extremely sensitive; therefore preparations intended for use in the eye must be instilled in the lower conjunctival sac to avoid direct contact with the cornea. Typical eye preparations include artificial tears/lubricants, antibiotic drops or ointments, and medications for the treatment of glaucoma. Procedure 22–6 describes installation of medications into the eye. Information about eye irrigations can be found in Chapter 24.

Ear Instillations. The ear and the external auditory canal are not sterile organs. In general, medical aseptic technique is used to instill medications or irrigate the ear canal. If, however, there is a possibility that the tympanic membrane is ruptured or damaged, sterile technique should be used to prevent the introduction of materials into the middle or inner ear. Procedure 22–7 outlines instillation of medications into the ear. Information about ear irrigations can be found in Chapter 29.

Nasal Instillations. Like the ear, the nose is not considered a sterile cavity and medical aseptic technique is acceptable for the instillation of medications. To administer nosedrops, request clients to assume a sitting or recumbent position with the head tilted back. As with the procedure for instillation of eye or ear medications, the filled dropper should be held in the dominant hand with the heel of the hand resting against the head to prevent inadvertent injury from the dropper. The drops should be administered gently taking care not to touch the inside of the nares with the tip of the dropper. Encourage clients to keep their head tilted back for several minutes to maximize the effectiveness of therapy. Because the nasal passages drain into the back of the throat, clients may experience an unpleasant taste in their mouths from the medication. Nurses can provide a tissue for expectoration.

Nasal medications may also be administered in the form of a spray. A small atomizer is often used to disperse the medication. This method is often much easier for clients to perform independently. However, clients should be cautioned against the overuse of these preparations. Many

PROCEDURE 22–6. INSTILLING MEDICATIONS INTO THE EYE

▭ **PURPOSE:** To deliver locally acting medication to the cornea and conjunctiva.

▭ **EQUIPMENT:** Eyedrops, tissues, cotton balls or washcloth, and client's medication administration record (MAR).

ACTION

1. Follow general guidelines for administration of medications (Table 22–11).
2. Be sure the client is aware of the purpose, expected benefits, and usual sensations associated with the medication, as well as desired client participation to facilitate instillation.
3. Although the eye is not sterile, it is vulnerable to infections; therefore aspetic technique is used for eye instillations. Eye medications used for one client should not be shared with another client.
4. If encrusted secretions are present, cleanse the eyelid and lashes with soft cloth or cotton ball moistened in warm water. Wipe from inner to outer canthus. To avoid possible cross-contamination, use a separate cotton ball or a different portion of the cloth for each eye.
5. Ask or assist the client to assume a supine or a sitting position with head tilted back.
6. Rest the heel or the side of your dominant hand lightly on the client's forehead while holding the dropper or tube vertically between thumb and index finger. Gently pull downward on the lower lid with the other hand, exposing the conjunctival sac. Ask client to look upward.

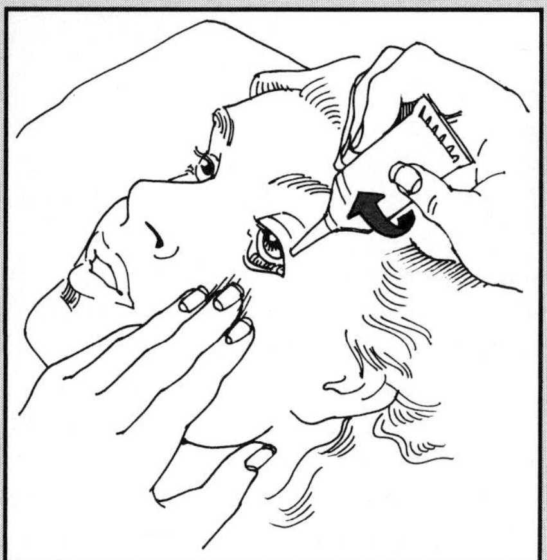

7. Squeeze gently to dispense the required number of drops into the conjunctival sac, not on the cornea. If medication is in ointment form, squeeze a ribbon of ointment from inner to outer canthus, rotating your hand toward the forehead to disconnect the ointment strip as you near the outer canthus. Do not touch the eye or surrounding tissue with the dropper or the tip of the tube. If accidental contact occurs, the dropper or tube must be discarded.
8. Ask client to close eye gently, keeping it closed for 2 to 3 minutes to spread the medication over the surface of the cornea, but not to squeeze eye tightly closed, as this will force medication out of the eye. If drops were instilled, apply gentle pressure on the lacrimal duct for 1 to 2 minutes to delay medication overflow into the duct. This action will increase local effectiveness of medication and decrease systemic absorption. Some eye medications cause systemic side effects if drained undiluted into lacrimal ducts. Some clients may prefer to apply duct pressure themselves.
9. Repeat for other eye, if ordered.
10. Excess medication may be wiped from eyelids from inner to outer canthus, using a tissue or cotton ball.

▭ **RECORDING:** Record medication administration, appearance of eye and/or drainage, and any unexpected reactions to the medication according to agency policy.

PROCEDURE 22–7. INSTILLING MEDICATIONS INTO THE EAR

PURPOSE: To deliver locally acting medication into the auditory canal.

EQUIPMENT: Medication, cotton balls, washcloth or tissue, and client's medication administration record (MAR).

ACTION

1. Follow general guidelines for administration of medications (Table 22–11).
2. Be sure the client is aware of the purpose, expected benefits, and usual sensations associated with the medication, as well as desired client participation to facilitate instillation.
3. Use medical asepsis for ear instillations unless tympanic membrane is ruptured. Then sterile technique is required.
4. The ear is sensitive to cold. Warming medication to body temperature will diminish discomfort, although this may be contraindicated for some medications. Carrying the container in your uniform pocket for 15 minutes or immersing the container in a cup filled with warm water for several minutes will warm contents.
5. Ask or assist the client to assume a side-lying position with the affected ear facing upward. Clean discharge from external ear with a soft cloth, cotton ball, or cotton-tipped applicator. Do not attempt to clean inside auditory canal.
6. Gently straighten the auditory canal to facilitate entry of medication: Pull the pinna slightly upward and backward for adults; for a child under 3, pull downward and backward. This may cause slight discomfort if the client has an ear infection. Rest the heel of your hand lightly on the client's head near the ear as you introduce the medication to prevent injury to the ear should the client move unexpectedly.
7. Direct the flow of drops against the side of the canal, as direct application on the tympanic membrane is uncomfortable. Administer the prescribed amount of medication. Gently massage the tragus (area directly anterior to the ear) to facilitate dispersing medication into the canal.

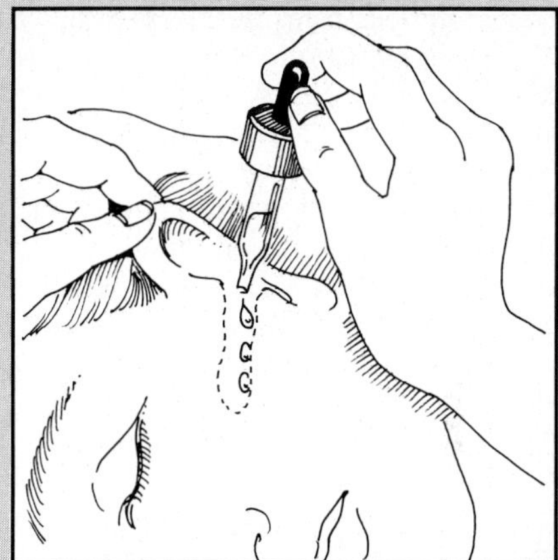

8. Inform the client of the importance of remaining on the side for 5 minutes to prevent immediate drainage of the medication out of the ear. A cotton ball may also be placed loosely in the ear to absorb drainage after the client sits up.
9. Repeat for other ear, if ordered.

RECORDING: Record medication administration, appearance of the ear and/or description of drainage, and any unexpected reactions to the medication according to agency policy.

sal medications have systemic effects with prolonged use. The use of nasal decongestants for more than 3 to 5 days also produces a rebound effect of increased nasal congestion.

Vaginal Applications. Vaginal medications are applied as creams, foam, jellies, suppositories, or irrigations (douches). Medical aseptic technique should be used unless there are open wounds present in the vagina; then sterile technique is required. An applicator that facilitates placement of the medication high into the vaginal cavity is provided with many vaginal preparations.

The administration of vaginal medication is often embarrassing for client and nurse. If a client is used to instilling vaginal medications, she will probably prefer to administer it herself. In fact, a client who is able should be encouraged to do vaginal applications herself because this promotes self-responsibility. The nurse's role is to assess a client's ability to manipulate the applicator or suppository and position herself to insert the medication, and to teach her how to do the application. Prior to instillation suggest she urinate to reduce discomfort from a full bladder during instillation and absorption.

For proper application, tell a client to lie on her back with her knees bent and legs flexed outward at the hip, spread the outer and inner labia apart with one hand, gently insert the filled applicator approximately 5 cm (2 in.) into the vagina, and then push the plunger until the applicator is empty. Vaginal suppositories can be inserted in the same manner with an applicator or gloved finger.

If assistance from a nurse is needed, every effort should be made to reduce embarrassment and to protect clients' privacy through projecting a professional, matter-of-fact attitude and minimizing exposure by draping. Open a sheet, ask the client to hold one corner, and let the adjacent corners fall over each knee. The fourth corner falls over the perineum but is folded back to visualize the perineum. Following insertion of the medications, clients should remain in a supine position for at least 10 minutes to facilitate absorption of the medication. A sanitary napkin may be needed to absorb excess drainage. Instillation of these preparations at bedtime is often recommended.

Rectal Instillations. Rectal medications are supplied in the form of rounded, bullet-shaped suppositories (Fig. 22–16). Suppositories have a lanolin, glycerin, or gelatin base that is solid at room temperatures but melts at body temperature. Usually, suppositories are administered to soften fecal matter and stimulate defecation; however, systemic effects can be achieved with rectal preparations of drugs for clients unable to tolerate medications by mouth. Drugs to reduce fever (antipyretics) and drugs to treat nausea and vomiting (antiemetics) are sometimes given rectally.

The administration of rectal medications is often embarrassing for clients and inexperienced nurses. In some instances, clients can be taught self-administration. If a nurse administers a rectal suppository, measures to protect the client's privacy and reduce embarrassment discussed above for vaginal preparations are important. Procedure 22–8 describes the technique for administration of a rectal suppository.

Administering Medications by Inhalation. Medications such as bronchodilators and decongestants are often administered by inhalation. A hand-held atomizer or nebulizer is used to dispense a specified dose of medication in the form of a fine mist (Procedure 22–9). Inhalation medications are most effective when self-administered by clients, as the ejection of the mist must coincide with deep inhalation through an open mouth. A closed mouth around the inhalator will not deliver medication deeply enough into the

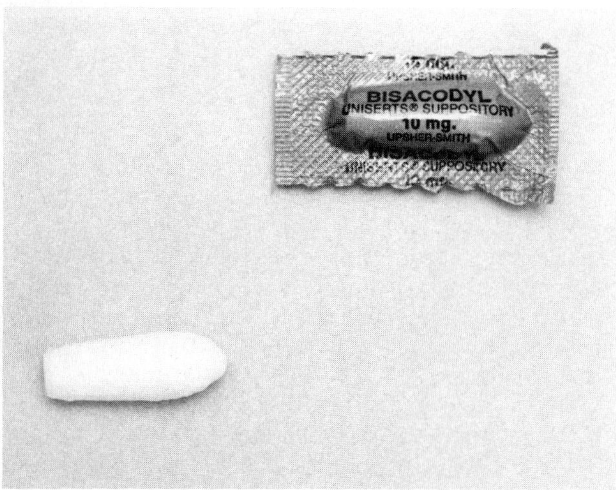

Figure 22–16. Foil-wrapped rectal suppository; unwrapped suppository; note rounded tip to facilitate insertion.

lungs. In an acute care setting, nebulized medication is also often delivered with specialized oxygen equipment or intermittent positive pressure machines.

Administering Parenteral Medications. This term refers to medications given by routes other than oral, topical, or inhalation. Nurses administer drugs parenterally by the following routes: **intradermal** (into the dermal layer of the skin), **subcutaneous** (into the subcutaneous tissue), **intramuscular** (into selected muscle tissue), and **intravenous** (into a vein). Figure 22–17 illustrates these layers of tissue. Administration by each of these routes is an invasive procedure that requires the penetration of the protective skin barrier and the placement of medication into body tissues. Injections are used for clients who cannot take medications by mouth, and to administer medications (such as insulin) that cannot be given orally. The absorption of injected medications is usually much more rapid and complete than with oral preparations. For this reason, it is the method of choice for emergency situations.

The administration of parenteral medications requires greater skill and caution than oral preparations. Meticulous aseptic technique is required to prevent infection. Because these medications are absorbed so quickly, and are irretrievable once injected, it is essential that nurses administer them carefully and precisely. Accurate location of injection sites and use of proper technique prevents tissue damage and reduces client discomfort. Clients receiving parenteral medications must be monitored closely because toxic as well as therapeutic effects develop rapidly.

Receiving medications by injection is a source of anxiety and discomfort for most clients. Aside from the actual physiological pain involved, many individuals fear needles and may avoid any medical treatment that involves injections. Nurses can reduce physical discomfort through careful choice of site, proper positioning of the client, and skillful injection technique. Apprehensive or fearful clients should be adequately prepared prior to an injection and should be encouraged to express their concerns. Box 22–19 outlines some techniques that can be used to minimize client discomfort related to injection.

Equipment. Needles and syringes come in a wide variety of sizes and types, each designed for a specific use. Nurses must use professional judgment to determine the most appropriate equipment needed to effectively deliver the medication as ordered.

SYRINGES. Syringes consist of three parts: (1) the tip, which connects to the needle; (2) the barrel or outside of the syringe, which is marked with measurement increments; and (3) the plunger, which fits inside the barrel (Fig. 22–18). Syringes vary in size to hold from 1 to 50 mL (Fig. 22–19). Generally only syringes from 1 to 3 mL in volume are used for injections. Larger syringes may be used for adding medications to IV fluid or for wound irrigations. Most syringes used today are made of plastic and are disposable. Some are prefitted with a needle; all are individually packaged in a sterile wrapper or rigid plastic container.

PROCEDURE 22–8. ADMINISTERING A RECTAL SUPPOSITORY

PURPOSE: To provide local effect on gastrointestinal tract or systemic effect when oral route is impossible or contraindicated.

EQUIPMENT: Clean gloves, water-soluble lubricant, disposable waterpoof underpad, suppository, and client's medication administration record (MAR). If laxative suppository: bedpan, commode, and toilet tissue.

ACTION

1. Follow general guidelines for administration of medications (Table 22–11).
2. Be sure the client is aware of purpose, expected benefits, and usual sensations associated with the medication, as well as desired client participation to facilitate administration.
3. Provide privacy. Ask or assist client to assume a side-lying position. Raise bed to comfortable working height. Arrange bed covers so buttocks are exposed, but client is otherwise covered. Place underpad under buttocks.
4. Unwrap suppository. Don clean glove. Lubricate tapered end of suppository and your index finger.
5. Raise client's buttock to expose anus. Ask client to take a deep breath to facilitate relaxation. Touch anal sphincter lightly with suppository, then wait several seconds. Sphincter will contract, then relax as a reflex response to being touched.
6. Gently insert suppository. Use your index finger to direct the suppository 3 to 4 inches (2 inches for children) along the rectal wall, toward the umbilicus. It must be inserted beyond the internal sphincter to prevent expulsion. Do not insert it into a fecal mass. The suppository must contact the rectal mucosa to be absorbed.

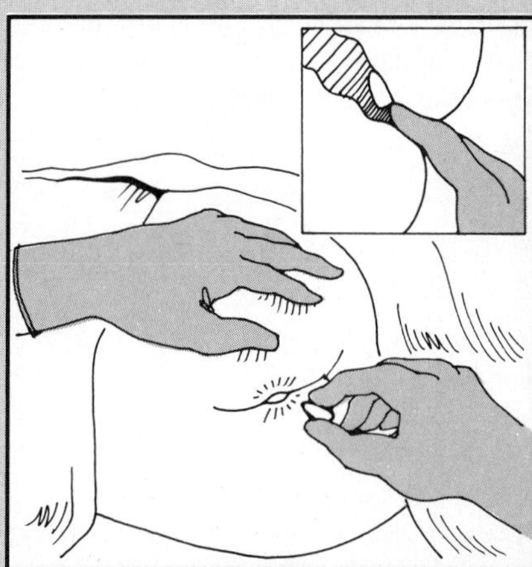

7. Withdraw your finger. Applying slight pressure over the anus with tissue or holding the buttocks together briefly will assist the client to overcome the reflex urge to defecate.
8. Turn glove inside out to remove it, and discard. Cover client. Wash hands. Inform client that remaining in side-lying position for up to 30 minutes will enhance absorption of systemic medication. If suppository is a laxative, urge to defecate may be strong within 5 to 10 minutes. Leave call bell in reach. Some clients may prefer a bedpan and toilet tissue be left in the bed to prevent soiling.

RECORDING: Record medication administration and any unexpected reactions to the medication according to agency policy.

NEEDLES. Needles also consist of three parts: (1) the hub, which attaches to the syringe; (2) the shaft, which is connected to the hub, and (3) a slanted or beveled tip (Fig. 22–18). The bevel of the needle is designed to make a narrow slit-type opening in the skin that seals easily when the needle is removed, and prevents seepage of blood or medications. When attaching a needle to a syringe, a nurse may grasp the hub of the needle to ensure a tight fit; however, the shaft and the tip must remain sterile.

Needles are manufactured in a variety of gauges and lengths. The gauge is a number referring to the diameter of the needle shaft. The lower the gauge number, the larger the needle diameter (eg, an 18-gauge needle is larger than a 25-gauge needle). The selection of gauge number of needle depends on the viscosity of the medication to be administered. Thick medications or blood transfusions require a larger-gauge needle. Needle lengths vary from ⅜ to 2 inches. Nurses select needle length based on clients' size, amount of subcutaneous fat, and the ordered route (eg, intramuscular injections require longer needles than subcutaneous injections). Box 22–20 outlines basic guidelines for the selection of appropriate needle and syringe sizes.

MEDICATION CONTAINERS. Parenteral medications may be packaged in ampules, vials, or prefilled cartridges or syringes. An **ampule** is a clear glass container with a constricted neck that holds a single dose of medication. Ampules are available in several sizes, from 1 to 10 mL. The neck of the ampule must be broken off to withdraw the medication. Use of a filter needle to withdraw medication that has been reconstituted prevents microscopic glass

PROCEDURE 22–9. ADMINISTERING MEDICATIONS BY INHALATION

▭ **PURPOSE:** To deliver medication to the respiratory tree, usually for local effect.

▭ **EQUIPMENT:** Medication cannister, metered dose inhaler (some clients may also use aerochamber), and client's medication administration record (MAR).

ACTION

1. Follow general guidelines for administration of medications (Table 22–11).
2. Be sure the client is aware of purpose, expected benefits, and usual sensations associated with the medication, as well as desired client participation to facilitate instillation.
3. If the client is unfamiliar with the inhaler, provide opportunity for the client to manipulate the equipment and ask questions.
4. Discuss the critical elements for correct use of the inhaler:
    a. Shake cannister, remove mouthpiece cover.
    b. If aerochamber will be used, attach it to inhaler, remove its mouthpiece cover.

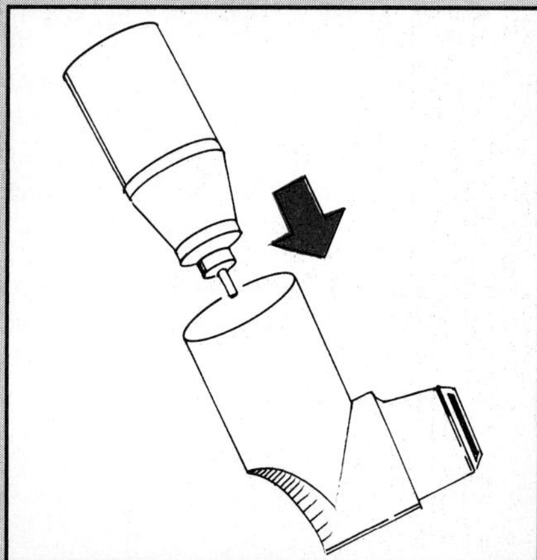

    c. Invert inhaler. Hold inhaler with three-finger grip: index and middle fingers on cannister, thumb supporting mouthpiece.
    d. Place mouthpiece into open mouth (cannister points up).
    e. Exhale fully, then place teeth and lips around mouthpiece. Aerochamber has a raised lip on mouthpiece to assist with correct placement of mouth.

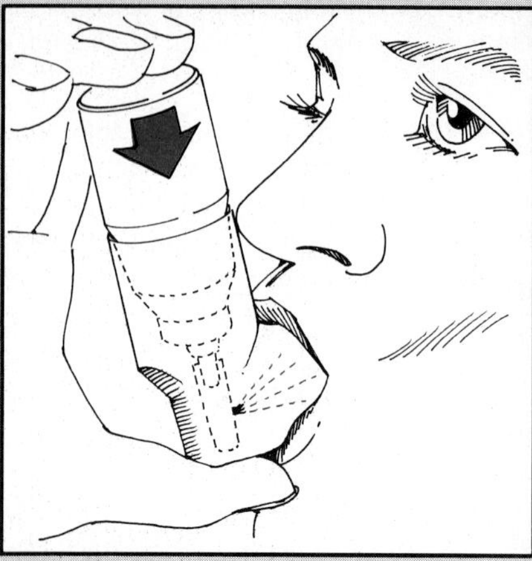

    f. While inhaling slowly and deeply through the mouth (about 5 seconds), press down on cannister to deliver measured dose of medication into airways. With aerochamber, client can inhale after depressing cannister and still obtain aerosolized medication. Some clients may find it easier to inhale through the mouth if they hold their nose. It is important that the mist be inhaled, not swallowed.
    g. Hold breath for 10 seconds to allow medication to reach deeper airways.
    h. Remove mouthpiece, exhale normally.
    i. If client is to take more than one dose at each use, wait several minutes before inhaling second dose.
    j. Caution client about the risks of overuse: development of drug tolerance and possible increased side effects.
    k. Inhaler and aerochamber can be rinsed with warm water and dried after use.
5. Request that client verbalize steps for using inhaler to assess level of understanding. Clarify misunderstandings, if any.
6. Ask client to self-administer medication with inhaler while you observe. (Nurse must observe each use if medication administration is to be charted on MAR.)

▭ **RECORDING:** Record medication administration, level of client participation, and any unexpected reactions to the medication according to agency policy.

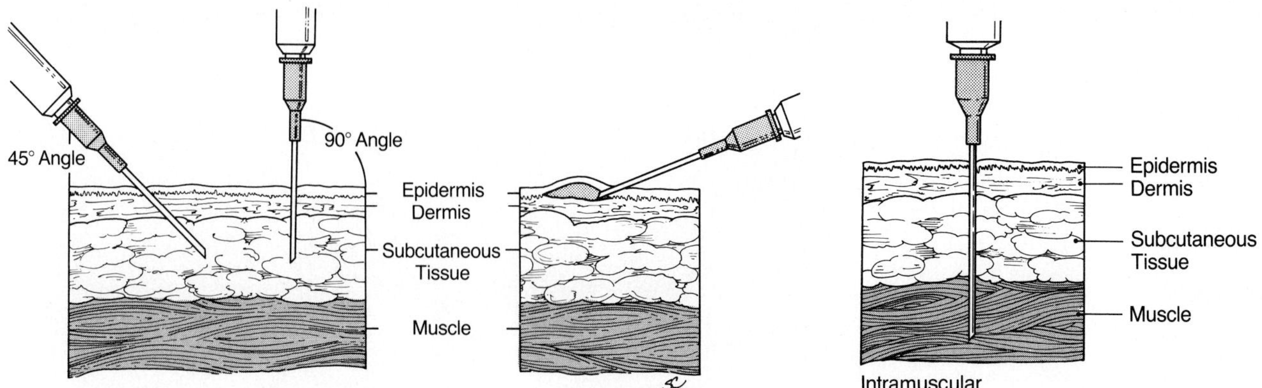

Figure 22–17. Schematic drawing of tissue layers, illustrating locations for parenteral medications. (*From Smith S, Duell D.* Clinical Nursing Skills: Nursing Process Model; Basic to Advanced Skills. *2nd ed. Norwalk, CT: Appleton & Lange; 1988:311,316.*)

shards from being injected into the client. Procedure 22–10 illustrates how to prepare medication from an ampule.

A **vial** is a glass container with a self-sealing rubber cap through which medication can be withdrawn. Vials come in a variety of sizes and may be single- or multidose containers. Unlike an ampule, a vial is a closed system and requires the injection of air to facilitate removal of the medication. Procedure 22–11 describes the preparation of medication from a vial.

Medications in vials may be in liquid or powdered form. Drugs that deteriorate when stored in liquid form are supplied as powders and must be reconstituted with a sterile diluent or solvent (generally sterile water or saline) prior to administration. Each medication has specific directions printed on the label concerning the type and amount of diluent that is required for proper reconstitution. The correct amount of diluent must be prepared following the steps outlined in Procedure 22–11, and then injected into the vial containing the powdered drug. Most medications dissolve easily; however, it may be necessary to rotate the vial to thoroughly dissolve the medication. The reconstituted solution should be clear and free of particulate matter prior to administration. Once dissolved, the medication can be withdrawn from the vial following the outlined procedure.

Many parenteral medications are available in a variety of prefilled cartridges or syringes. These systems provide a single dose of medication in a disposable syringe with attached needle, or a cartridge-needle unit that must be loaded into a reusable cartridge holder for administration. Tubex and Carpuject are two examples of these systems

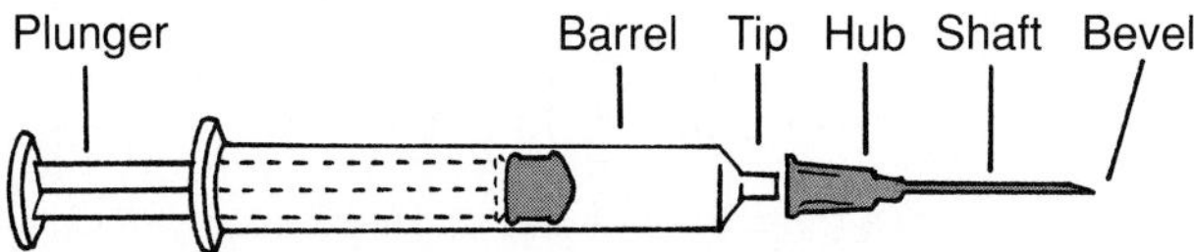

Figure 22–18. Parts of a syringe and needle.

BOX 22–19. NURSING MEASURES TO REDUCE DISCOMFORT RELATED TO INJECTIONS

1. Select a needle that is the smallest gauge appropriate for the site and solution to be administered.
2. Select a proper injection site using anatomical landmarks. Avoid sensitive areas of the body. Select a site that is healthy and nonirritated.
3. Rotate injection sites to avoid repeated trauma to tissues.
4. Applying ice to the insertion site prior to administration numbs pain receptors. (Many clients will find the ice more painful than the injection.)
5. Allow the skin to dry after cleansing with antiseptic. Antiseptic is irritating to the tissues if carried in by the needle insertion.
6. Make sure the outside of the needle is free of medication that may be irritating to the subcutaneous tissues.
7. Do not administer more fluid in one injection than is recommended for the selected site or route: No more than 0.1 to 0.5 mL intradermally; no more than 1.5 mL subcutaneously; no more than 2 mL into a small muscle or 5 mL into a large muscle. (Avoid giving large dose by dividing dose, if possible.)
8. Insert the needle into relaxed musculature. Position the client as comfortably as possible to reduce muscle tension. If injecting into the dorso- or ventrogluteal sites, have client internally rotate the leg, or flex the upper leg if in a sidelying position.
9. Use a quick dartlike motion to insert needle.
10. Hold the syringe steady while the needle is in body tissues.
11. Inject the medication slowly to allow it to spread into the tissues.
12. Divert the client's attention from the injection through conversation or relaxation techniques.
13. Apply counterpressure with a dry gauze square as needle is removed. Remove needle in quick, smooth motion.
14. Massage the area of injection after administration, unless contraindicated. Massaging helps spread the medication into the surrounding tissues and enhances absorption.

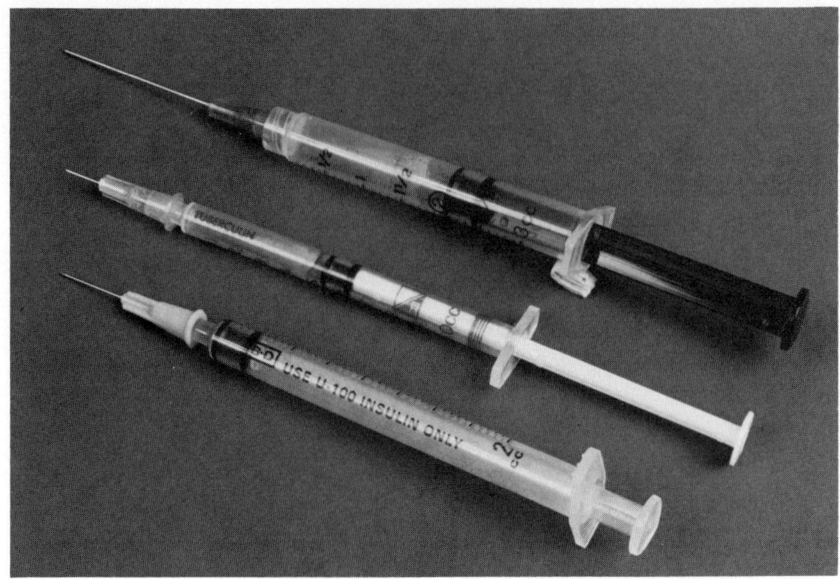

Figure 22–19. Three types of syringes. Top, 3-mL, syringe. Middle, tuberculin syringe. Bottom, insulin syringe. (*From Smith S, Duell D.* Clinical Nursing Skills: Nursing Process Model; Basic to Advanced Skills. *2nd ed. Norwalk, CT: Appleton & Lange; 1988:305.*)

that are currently available (Fig. 22–20). In settings where certain medications and dosages are used routinely, as in surgical units, these prepackaged injectable medications save time and reduce errors. Many narcotics and emergency medications are available in prefilled form.

Mixing Medications. Many times a client may require the administration of two parenteral medications at the same time. If the two drugs are compatible, it is possible to mix them in the same syringe and administer them in a single injection. Drug compatibility charts should be available on all nursing units. If there is any question about the compatibility of two medications, a pharmacist should be consulted before they are mixed.

MIXING DRUGS FROM TWO VIALS. When mixing drugs from two different vials, it is important to withdraw the correct amounts of each medication without contaminating or mixing the remaining medication in either vial (Procedure 22–12). Insulin preparations are commonly mixed in one syringe from two vials. When preparing insulin injections it is important that the correct insulin syringe be used, and that the regular (rapid-acting) insulin be aspirated into the syringe first. Because of the inherent risk of contamination when mixing drugs from two vials, the trend is toward premixed single-dose preparations, when possible.

MIXING DRUGS FROM A VIAL AND AN AMPULE. Because ampules do not require the injection of air, first withdraw the

BOX 22–20. CRITERIA FOR SELECTING NEEDLES AND SYRINGES

1. *Route of administration.* Select a needle that will deposit the medication accurately into the specified tissue. A longer needle is needed to administer medication intramuscularly (usually 1 to 1½ inches) than subcutaneously (usually 3/8 to 5/8 inches). See Figure 22–17 for cross-section of skin layers.
2. *Viscosity of medication solution.* Viscous fluids require a larger-gauge needle. The administration of blood products requires a 16- or 18-gauge needle to prevent damage to the blood cells.
3. *Amount of medication to be administered.* The larger the amount of solution, the larger the syringe needed. Care should be taken to select a syringe slightly larger than actual volume of medication (eg, 5-cc syringe used for 3 cc of medication). Syringes filled to capacity are difficult to manipulate. Check that the syringe is marked in increments that allow for accurate measurement of medication (eg, accurate delivery of 0.25 cc of medication requires a syringe marked in increments of one-hundredths of a cc).
4. *Body size.* Intramuscular medications should be deposited deep into the chosen muscle mass. Clients with large amounts of adipose tissue require longer needles to ensure that the medication is delivered to muscle tissue. Children or slender adults require shorter needles.
5. *Site of administration.* Always choose a needle that will deposit the medication deep into the chosen muscle but away from any vital structures such as bones, blood vessels, or nerves. An intramuscular injection into the deltoid muscle requires a shorter needle than an intramuscular injection into the gluteal muscle.
6. *Type of medication.* Specialized insulin syringes must be used when administering insulin injections. Extremely irritating solutions (eg, some iron preparations) require the use of longer needles to ensure that the medication is not inadvertently injected into subcutaneous tissue.
7. *Client comfort.* The narrower the needle, the more comfortable the injection. Always select the smallest-gauge needle that is appropriate for site and medication to avoid unnecessary discomfort.

PROCEDURE 22–10. PREPARING MEDICATION FROM AN AMPULE

PURPOSE: To withdraw medication contained in an ampule in preparation for parenteral administration.

EQUIPMENT: Ampule containing ordered medication, sterile syringe and needle, filter needle, alcohol swabs, and client's medication administration record (MAR).

ACTION	RATIONALE
1. Follow general guidelines for administration of medications (Table 22–11).	1. These guidelines facilitate safe, error-free preparation of medications.
2. Remove medication trapped in the neck of the ampule by holding it upright and rotating your wrist several times, by moving the ampule downward as if to trace a large circle, or by flicking the stem with your finger.	2. Circular or rotational movement creates centrifugal force; flicking creates turbulence. Both will overcome the surface tension holding the liquid in the neck and move the medication into the lower portion of the ampule.

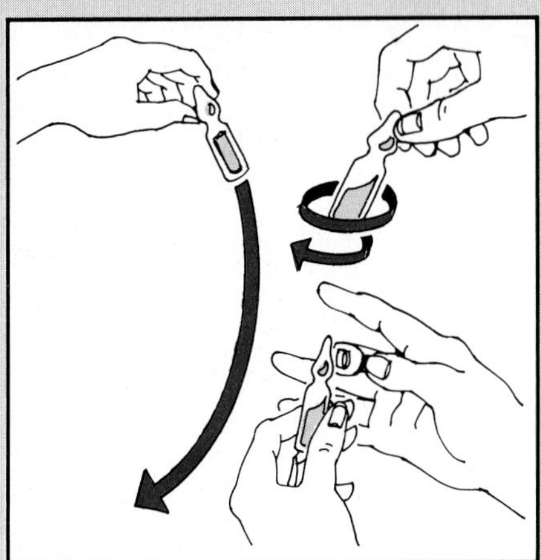

ACTION	RATIONALE
3. Place an alcohol swab around the neck of the ampule. Keeping your fingers away from the neck, break off the top of the ampule.	3. The alcohol swab protects the nurse's fingers from the sharp edges of the ampule as well as from glass fragments.

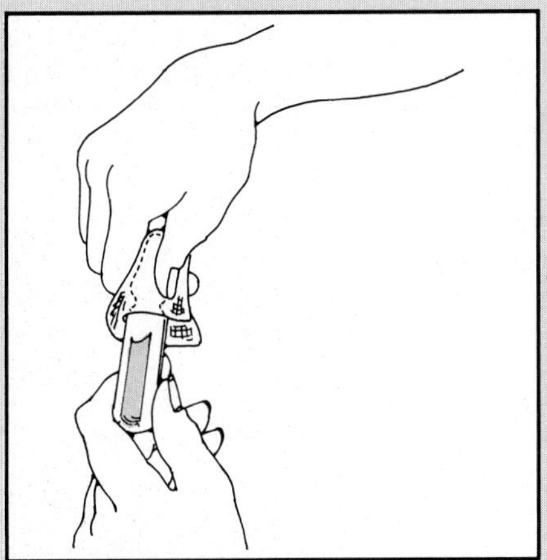

(continued)

PROCEDURE 22–10. (continued)

4. If filter needles are available in your agency, place one on the syringe without touching the needle shaft or the tip of the syringe. Use a firm twisting motion to secure needle.

4. Filter needles prevent tiny glass shards, which are deposited in the medication when the ampule is broken, from entering the syringe with the medication. Although client injury related to these glass shards has not been documented, experts recommend use of a filter needle as a precaution. Contact with the syringe tip or needle would transfer organisms to the syringe, to the medication, and subsequently to the client. Medications injected through the skin must be sterile.

5. If the syringe has a preattached needle, the needle may be reserved and reattached to give the medication. Remove the needle in its protective cap using a twisting motion and place it on a clean dry surface.

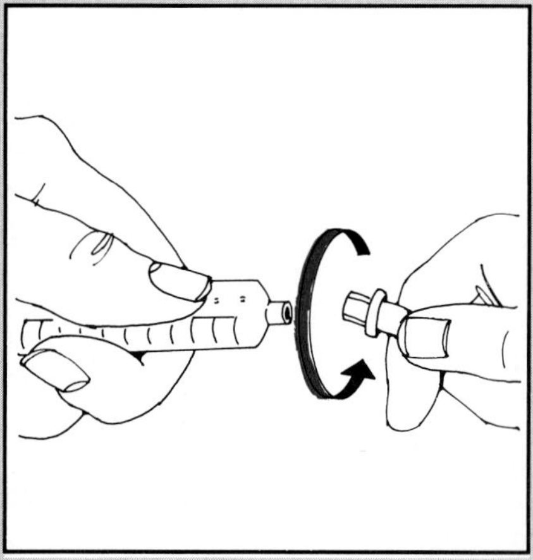

5. Filter needles may not be used to administer medications. Pulling on the needle rather than twisting will remove the needle cap rather than the needle. The reserved needle and cap will remain sterile because the flange on the needle cap prevents contact between the inside of the needle hub and the surface of the work area.

6. Pull firmly to remove filter needle cap. Insert the needle into the ampule without its touching the rim of the ampule.

6. See step 5, above. The rim of the ampule is considered contaminated. Contact would contaminate the needle and therefore, the medication, creating potential for client infection.

7. Keeping the tip of the needle below the level of fluid, pull on the plunger to withdraw the ordered amount of medication. The ampule may stand upright on a flat surface or be inverted. If inverted, the ampule and syringe should be held in the nondominant hand, as shown, and must not be tipped at an angle. The upright ampule may need to be picked up and tipped slightly to withdraw the last part of the fluid if needle is short.

7. Pulling on the plunger creates negative pressure within the syringe, causing fluid to move from the ampule into the barrel of the syringe. Air will also move into the syringe if the needle tip is not below the surface of the fluid. Surface tension will prevent the fluid in the ampule from running out when it is inverted, but unless the opening is very small, holding the inverted ampule at an angle will break the surface tension and allow the fluid to run down the needle.

(continued)

PROCEDURE 22–10. (continued)

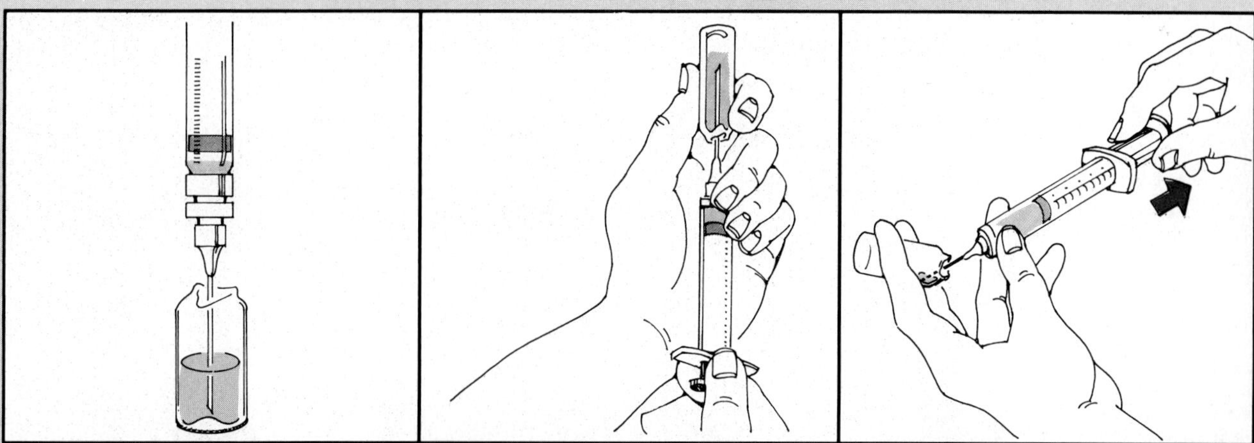

8. Recap and remove filter needle, discard in sharps disposal containers. Replace it with reserved needle or another sterile needle of appropriate length and gauge for medication administration. Do not touch the syringe tip, needle shaft, or inside of needle hub when changing needles. Use a firm twisting motion to attach the new needle.

8. Filter needle must be removed prior to expelling fluid because particles trapped in the filter needle would be expelled with the medication as fluid flows through it in the opposite direction. See also step 4, above. A twisting motion will secure needle.

9. Remove needle cap, place it on work surface. Hold syringe vertically, needle up. Tap sharply on syringe barrel to release air bubbles trapped in the liquid. Pull back slightly on plunger, then push it upward to expel air that has moved to the top of syringe.

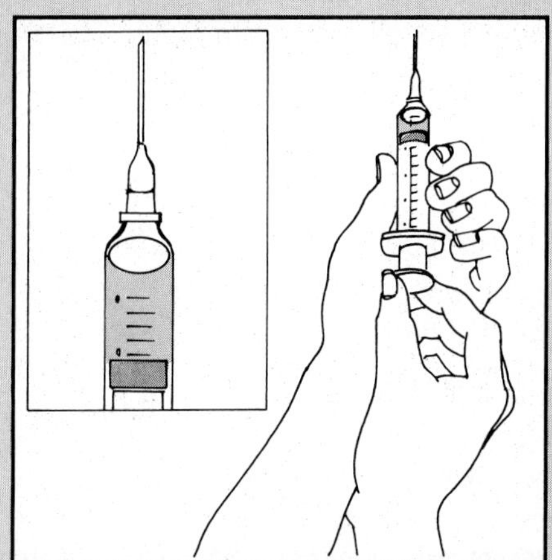

9. Cap may trap air or fluid. Air must be expelled to assess accuracy of medication dosage. Syringe position described facilitates removal because air bubbles suspended in a liquid rise. Tapping on the barrel of the syringe releases surface tension, freeing trapped bubbles. Pulling back on plunger before expelling air moves any medication still in needle into the syringe, so it is not expelled with the air.

(continued)

PROCEDURE 22–10. (continued)

10. Recheck amount of medication to assure accurate dosage. If there is excess, hold the syringe vertically, needle down over a trash container or sink and push downward on plunger until excess is expelled. Do not allow needle to contact sink or trash container.

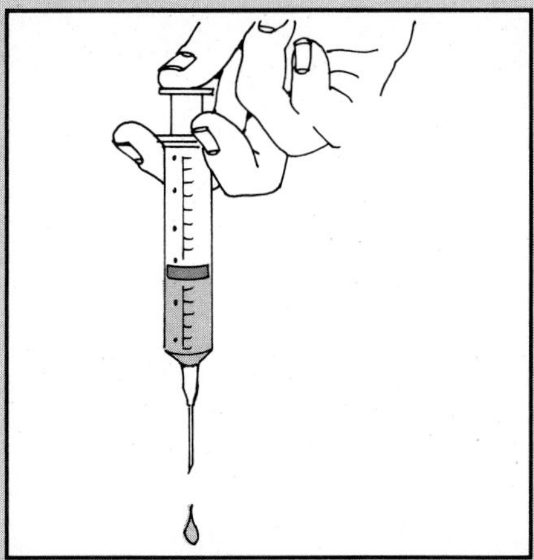

10. Accurate dosage is necessary for therapeutic effect and prevention of client injury. Excess is discarded by inverting syringe to avoid medication running down needle and syringe. Medication on outside of needle can cause tissue irritation. Vertical position allows accurate reading of amount.

11. If medication is to be administered at the bedside, recap needle, using care not to touch needle with outside of cap or your hand. Do not recap if medication is to be added to another container at the work area.

11. Recapping the needle creates potential needle stick injury to the nurse, so is not done except to maintain the sterility of the needle during transport to another area.

12. Discard ampule in sharps disposal container. Leave work area clean and dry.

12. Glass may cause injury when trash is removed, so glass items are separated from other trash.

RECORDING: Record administration of medication according to agency policy.

required amount of medication from the vial following the outlined procedure. Once the accurate dose is obtained in the syringe and any excess air has been expelled, the prescribed amount of medication can be withdrawn from the ampule using the same needle and syringe.

DISPOSAL OF EQUIPMENT. All syringes, glass vials, and ampules must be discarded in specially marked containers (often called "sharps" disposal containers) found in the medication preparation area and in all clients' rooms (Figs. 22–7 and 22–21). Used syringes are not recapped before discarding them because recapping needles is the most common cause of needle stick injuries. These containers also prevent needle stick injuries to personnel handling trash because they are impervious to penetration by needles. When full they are destroyed with infectious wastes, not emptied.

Intradermal Injections. An intradermal injection is the administration of medications into the dermal layer (below the epidermis) of the skin (see Fig. 22–17). The intradermal route has the slowest absorption rate of any of the parenteral routes. For this reason, it is commonly used for diagnostic purposes—primarily allergy and skin testing.

Intradermal injections involve very small volumes of medications (eg, 0.1 mL), and are typically administered on the inner forearm, upper chest, and upper back. Accurate skin testing requires that the site be intact and readily visible. For this reason, avoid administering intradermal injections in areas that are irritated, discolored, heavily pigmented, or extremely hairy. Procedure 22–13 outlines the steps involved in an intradermal injection.

Following the injection, the exact location and time of the injection must be recorded in the client's record. It is also helpful to mark the site of the injection with indelible ink to facilitate assessment of client reaction to the medication. Most skin tests must be "read" or evaluated within 48 to 72 hours.

PROCEDURE 22–11. PREPARING MEDICATION FROM A VIAL

PURPOSE: To withdraw medication contained in a vial in preparation for parenteral administration.

EQUIPMENT: Vial containing ordered medication, sterile syringe and needle (select length and gauge based on mode of administration and size of client), alcohol swabs, and client's medication administration record (MAR).

ACTION	RATIONALE
1. Follow general guidelines for administration of medications (Table 22–11).	1. These guidelines facilitate safe, error-free preparation of medication.
2. Remove the metal or plastic cap on top of the vial. If vial is multidose, label with current date and time. A previously used multiple dose vial will have no cap.	2. Protective cap covers rubber seal, maintaining its sterility. Most open multidose vials may be used for 24 hours before discarding contents.
3. Cleanse rubber seal of previously used vial with alcohol swab, using firm circular motion. An unused vial need not be cleansed unless seal was touched during cap removal.	3. Friction removes bacteria from surface. Although alcohol is an antiseptic, its effectiveness varies. It is not effective unless allowed to dry.
4. Obtain syringe. Pull firmly on needle cap to remove it. Pull down on plunger to draw a volume of air into syringe equal to the volume of medication to be given. NOTE: Injecting too much air will create positive pressure inside the vial. The compressed air will displace the plunger and may eject it from the barrel of the syringe.	4. The vial is a closed container, so fluid withdrawn must be replaced with air to keep the pressure inside the vial equalized. If air is not injected, negative pressure is created by withdrawal of fluid, making withdrawal of correct volume difficult.
5. Insert the needle through the stopper and inject the air into the air space in the vial to avoid creating bubbles. Some nurses prefer to invert the vial and syringe as in step 6, below, before injecting air.	5. See step 4, above. Air bubbles are to be avoided because they make withdrawing the correct amount of medication more difficult.

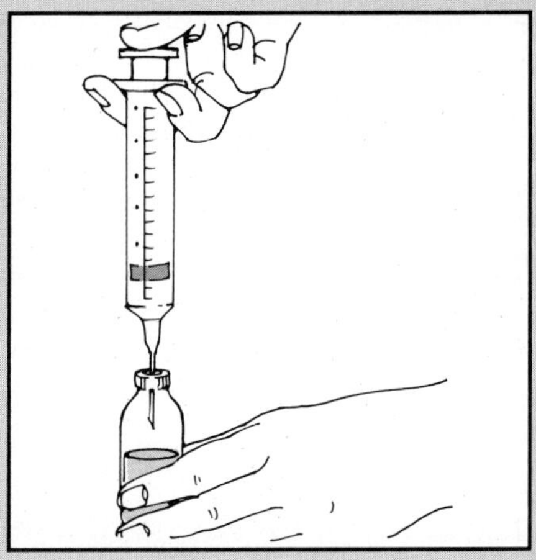

(continued)

PROCEDURE 22–11. (continued)

6. Invert the vial and syringe unit. Stabilize both syringe and needle in the nondominant hand, using one of the grips illustrated.

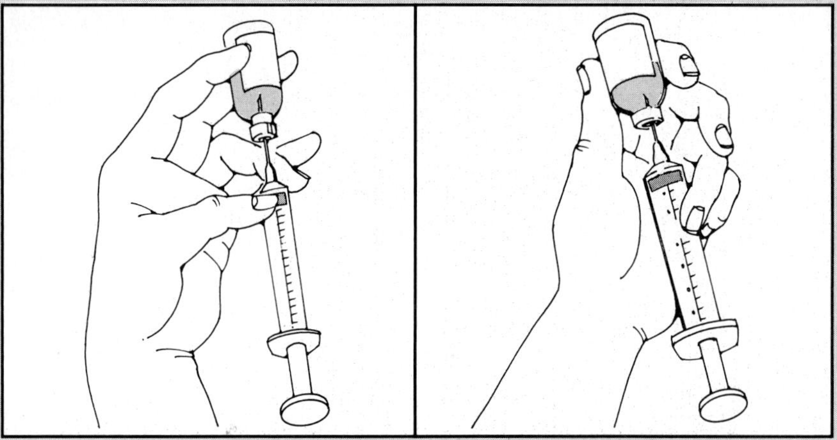

6. Either method leaves the dominant hand free to manipulate the plunger with minimal risk of inadvertently withdrawing needle from vial and contaminating it.

7. Holding syringe at eye level, with the needle below the fluid–air interface, pull down on plunger slowly to withdraw the required amount of medication.

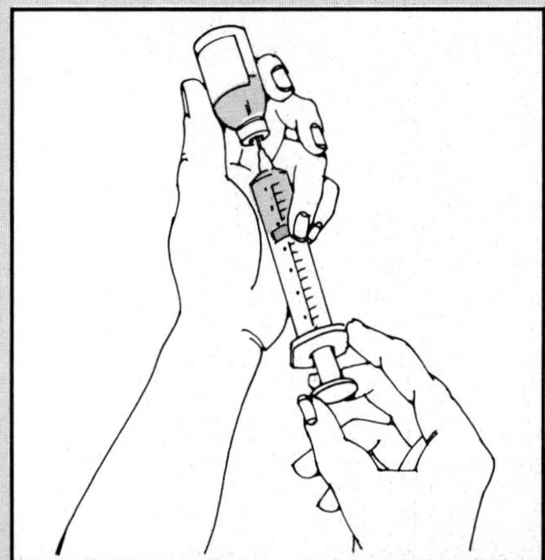

NOTE: Some experts advise withdrawing enough medication to wet the inside of the syringe, replacing it into the vial, and then removing measured amount. Wetting the syringe decreases air bubbles.

7. When a meniscus is not viewed at eye level, parallax (the apparent displacement of objects caused by a change in observer's position) will distort the nurse's perception and result in an inaccurate dosage. If the needle is in the air space, air will be drawn into the syringe. Rapidly withdrawing the medication creates turbulance with resulting air bubbles.

8. Check for air bubbles before removing needle from vial. Tap syringe barrel sharply to move air to the top of the syringe, then eject air into vial. Recheck medication volume, return excess or obtain more as needed. Remove needle from vial.

NOTE: Air bubbles which lodge in the shoulder of the syringe may be difficult to remove. Withdrawing a bolus of air from the vial will often trap the bubble so it can be expelled.

8. Tapping on the barrel of the syringe releases surface tension, freeing trapped bubbles so they can rise. Assuring accuracy of dosage before removing needle eliminates need to recleanse and repuncture stopper to obtain additional medication, thereby saving time.

(continued)

PROCEDURE 22–11. (continued)

9. If medication is to be administered at the bedside, recap needle, using care not to touch needle with outside of cap or your hand. Do not recap if it is to be added to another container at the work area.	9. Recapping the needle creates potential needle stick injury to the nurse, so is not done except to maintain the sterility of the needle during transport to another area.
10. Discard empty vial in trash container for glass items. Store vial containing medication according to agency policy. Leave work area clean and dry.	10. Glass may cause injury when trash is removed, so glass items are separated from other trash.

RECORDING: Record administration of medication according to agency policy.

Subcutaneous Injections. Subcutaneous injections involve the administration of medication into the loose subcutaneous tissues between the skin and muscle tissue (see Fig. 22–17). Because there is subcutaneous tissue all over the body, a variety of sites may be used to administer subcutaneous injections. Common sites are the lateral anterior thigh, the outer aspect of the upper arm, the scapular areas of the upper back, and the abdomen (Fig. 22–22). Absorption of subcutaneous medications is slower than intramuscular or intravenous routes; however, the entire dose is absorbed if the client's circulatory status is adequate. The subcutaneous route is used for many medications including insulin and heparin.

Equipment needed for a subcutaneous injection depends upon the prescribed drug. Insulin injections must be prepared with special insulin syringes calibrated by units rather than milliliters. Heparin may be administered with a tuberculin syringe and a 25- to 27-gauge needle. Ordinarily no more than 1 mL of solution is administered subcutaneously. Clients who require repeated subcutaneous injections (eg, diabetics) must rotate injections sites in an orderly fashion to minimize tissue damage, avoid client discomfort, and

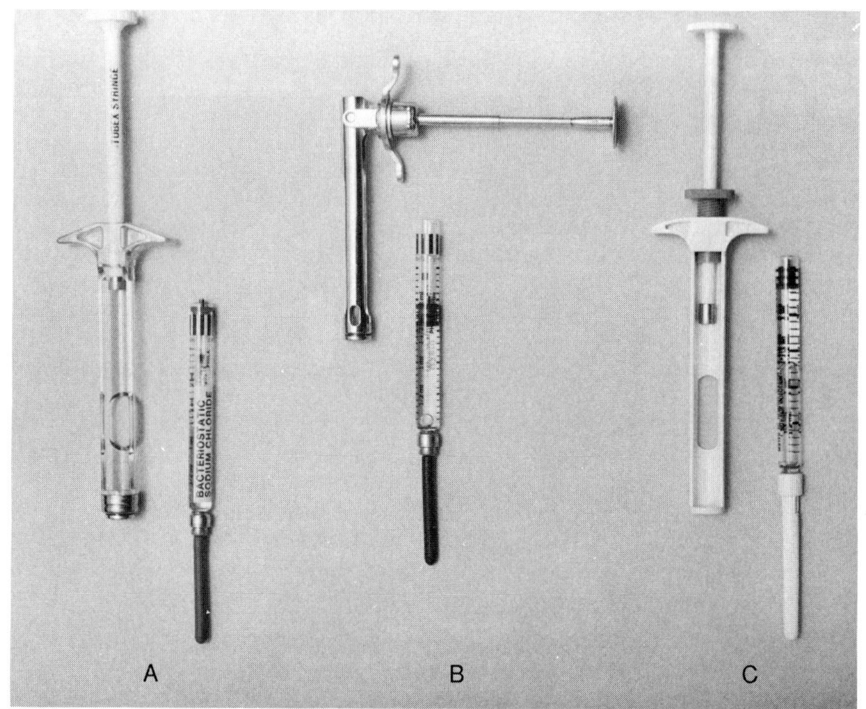

Figure 22–20. Samples of cartridge-type syringes. **A, B.** Two types of Tubex syringes. **C.** Carpuject syringe.

PROCEDURE 22–12. MIXING TWO MEDICATIONS IN ONE SYRINGE

PURPOSE: To simultaneously administer two compatible drugs via subcutaneous or intramuscular routes, thus sparing client the discomfort of two injections.

EQUIPMENT: Vials and/or ampules containing ordered medications, sterile syringe and needle (select length and gauge based on mode of administration and size of client), alcohol swabs, and client's medication administration record (MAR).

ACTION

1. Follow general guidelines for administration of medications (Table 22–11) and the techniques for preparing medications from vials and ampules (Procedures 22–10 and 22–11) to maintain accuracy and asepsis in preparation of medications.
2. Determine which drug should be withdrawn from its container first. To minimize the possibility of contaminating a multiple-dose vial and most easily obtain the correct amounts of both drugs, follow these guidelines:
   a. If one container is a single-dose vial and the other is a multiple-dose vial, withdraw from the multiple-dose vial first.
   b. If one container is a vial and the other is an ampule, withdraw from the vial first.
   c. If mixing two forms of insulin, withdraw regular insulin first.
3. If both medications are in vials, inject air into both before withdrawing either medication. This will decrease the likelihood of mixing medications when adding air. The vial containing the medication to be withdrawn first ("vial 1"), should be injected with air last.

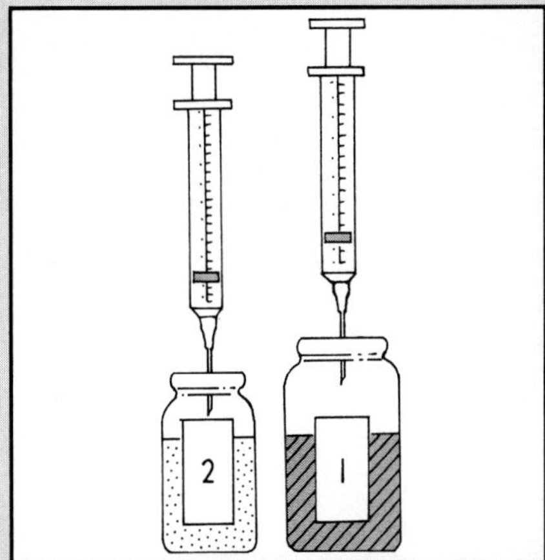

4. Withdraw medication from vial 1.

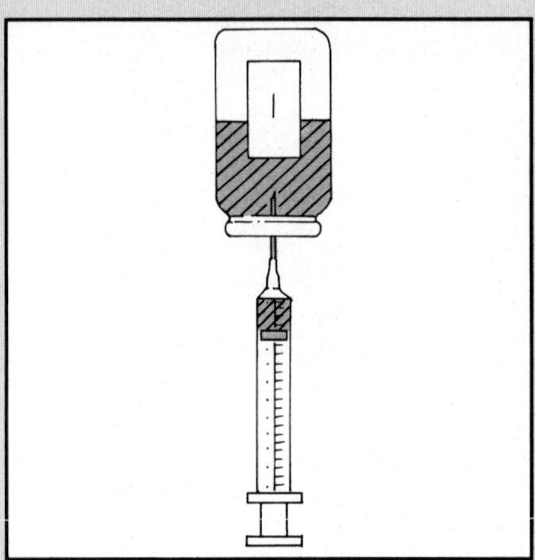

5. Withdraw medication from vial 2. Use extreme caution to withdraw only the ordered amount of medication and to avoid creating air bubbles. Excess medication cannot be returned to vial 2, because syringe now contains a mixture of two medications. If air bubbles enter the syringe, they must be expelled into the air, not into vial 2 because some fluid is likely to be expelled with the air. Some experts recommend changing needles prior to withdrawing medication from vial 2. This cannot be done when mixing insulin, as the needles on insulin syringes are not removable. The needle will not carry medication into the second vial, as withdrawing it through the rubber stopper of vial 1 will remove residual medication from the outside of the needle.

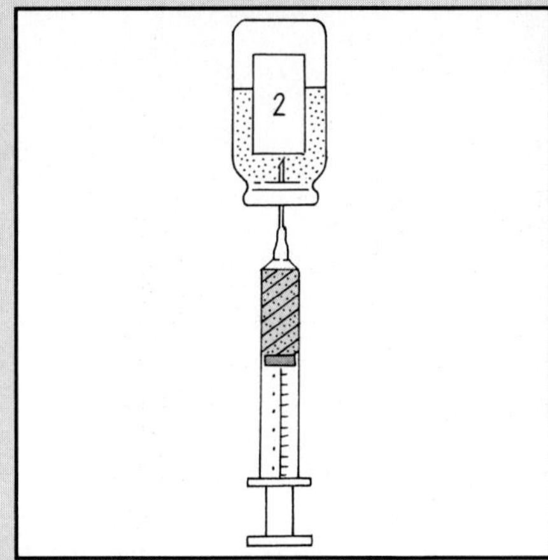

6. Medications are now ready for administration as ordered.

RECORDING: Record administration of medication according to agency policy.

PROCEDURE 22–13. ADMINISTERING AN INTRADERMAL INJECTION

PURPOSE: To inject medication into the dermal skin layer. Generally used for sensitivity testing (allergies, presence of antibodies).

EQUIPMENT: Sterile tuberculin syringe, ⅜ to ⅝ inch 26- or 27-gauge needle, alcohol swabs, medication/allergen to be administered, client's outpatient record or medication administration record (MAR), and one clean glove.

ACTION	RATIONALE
1. Follow general guidelines for administration of medications (Table 22–11).	1. These guidelines facilitate safe, error-free preparation of medication.
2. Prepare correct drug dosage from vial or ampule (see Procedures 22–10 and 22–11).	2. This method results in aseptic administration of required amount of drug.
3. Identify client by reading client's ID bracelet. You may also ask client to state name.	3. Positive identification is essential immediately before administering any drug to prevent giving drug to the wrong client.
4. Discuss reason for the procedure, usual sensations, expected client participation, and expected benefits.	4. Client will be more willing to participate if reasons and benefits are clear. Because many clients are apprehensive about procedures involving needles, extra efforts to inform and relax client are warranted.
5. Discuss possible injection sites with client. Determine client's site preference. Screen client if client desires.	5. Respecting clients' rights of choice regarding their bodies promotes trust in the nurse and diminishes clients' feelings of powerlessness.
6. Cleanse the skin at the site using a firm circular motion from center outward, not a back-and-forth motion. Alcohol and/or acetone swabs may be used depending on agency policy. Remove needle cap from syringe. 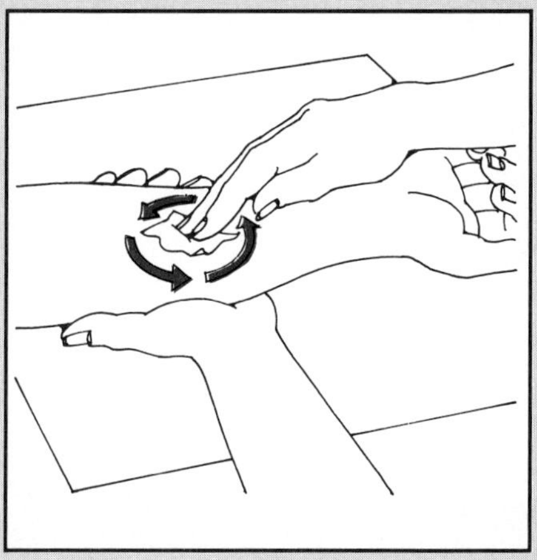	6. Alcohol and friction remove surface organisms, preventing their being transmitted through the skin via the needle. A back-and-forth motion is less effective because it moves skin flora from surrounding skin to site. Acetone removes skin oils, which may affect test results in some cases.

(continued)

PROCEDURE 22–13. (continued)

7. Wearing a clean glove, if desired, pull skin taut over injection site by spreading skin between thumb and index finger of nondominant hand. If forearm is used, skin may be stretched by grasping arm from below while it is resting on a table.

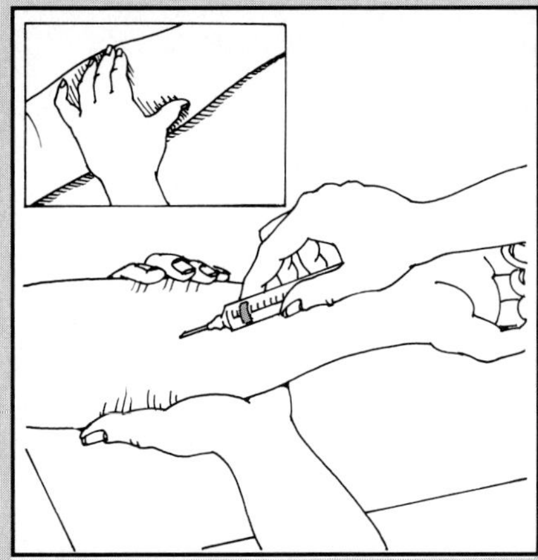

7. Taut skin is easier to pierce with needle, so client discomfort is lessened. Glove protects nurse in case of bleeding (not expected with intradermal injections).

8. Hold syringe as shown, parallel to skin with needle bevel up. Resting your fingers on client's skin helps to stabilize the syringe during insertion. Insert needle at a 15-degree angle or less. Advance needle far enough to place bevel just under the surface of epidermis. Outline of the bevel will be clearly visible under skin surface.

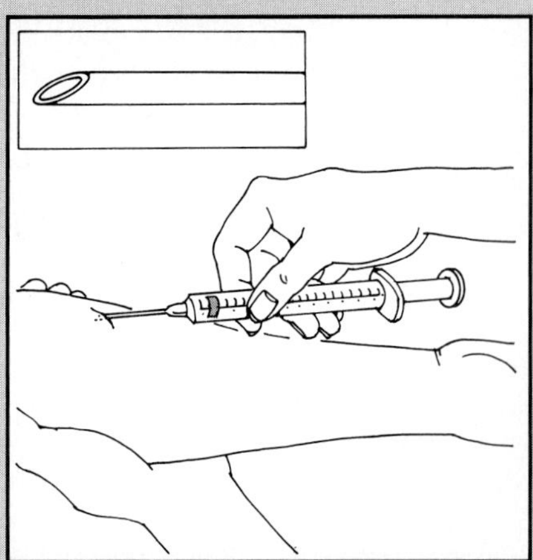

8. Insertion of the needle at a greater angle will cause needle to enter subcutaneous tissues, not dermis. When entire bevel is under skin surface, medication will be deposited between dermal layers, as desired.

(continued)

PROCEDURE 22–13. (continued)

9. Holding syringe steady with dominant hand, slowly push plunger with nondominant hand to inject medication. You should feel slight resistance as medication is injected. A wheal (small raised area like a blister) should be produced on skin surface, as fluid is injected, but no fluid should leak from wheal.

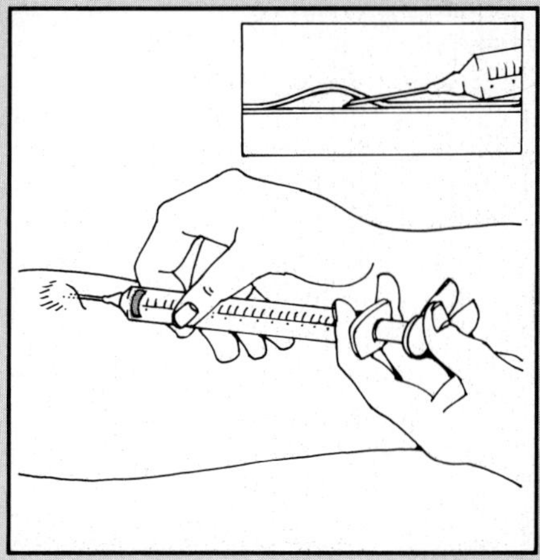

9. Syringe movement and tissue distension are sources of injection pain. Slow injection causes gradual distension and less pain. Resistance is created by skin layers. Fluid pushes a small area of epidermis upward, creating a wheal. If no wheal develops, needle insertion was too deep. Leaking indicates needle insertion was too shallow.

10. Withdraw needle at same angle it was inserted, without massaging site.

10. Minimizes discomfort. Massage may disperse medication, preventing observation of local reaction.

11. Dispose of glove, syringe, and needle in puncture-proof container, labeled for used needle disposal. Do not recap needle.

11. Recapping used needles creates a risk of needle stick injuries and subsequent infection. Labeled puncture-proof container protects other personnel from injuries.

12. Wash your hands.

12. Removes transient organisms, preventing transmission to other clients or personnel.

13. Observe site for unusual itching or redness. Provide client information about site care and reassessment for reaction. Site may be marked to aid later assessment.

13. The most common reason for intradermal injections is allergy or antibody testing. Reactions take several days to appear.

RECORDING: Note time, date, and location of injection. State name and strength of medication. Describe any immediate local or systemic client reactions.

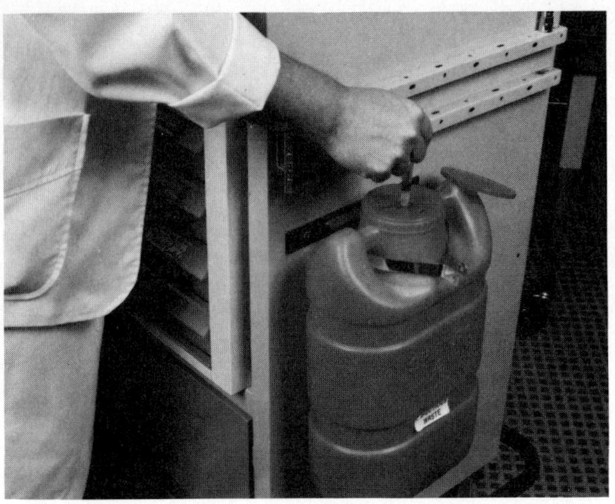

Figure 22–21. Puncture-resistant container for disposal of used syringes in medication preparation area. (*From Smith S, Duell D.* Clinical Nursing Skills: Nursing Process Model; Basic to Advanced Skills. *3rd ed. Norwalk, CT: Appleton & Lange; 1992.*)

facilitate absorption (Fig. 22–22). Procedure 22–14 describes the steps for administering a subcutaneous injection.

Intramuscular Injections. Intramuscular injections are used for medications that are irritating to subcutaneous tissue, which require larger than 1 mL of volume, or which need to be absorbed more rapidly. Because of rich vascularity of the muscle tissue, intramuscular medications are absorbed rapidly and completely; however, caution must be exercised to avoid injury to tissue, nerves, and blood vessels.

A number of sites are appropriate for intramuscular injections. Frequently used sites include the ventrogluteal, dorsogluteal, vastus lateralis, and deltoid muscles. When selecting a site, consider the condition of the tissue and suitability of the site for the type and volume of medication to be administered.

VENTROGLUTEAL SITE. This site is gaining favor for use both with children and adults. It is situated away from major blood vessels or nerves, and there are generally fewer fatty deposits than in the buttock area. It is also further away from the rectal area and tends to be less contaminated. The ventrogluteal site can be used for deep IM, Z-track, and large-volume injections, and is accessible with the client in a supine, prone, or side-lying position.

The ventrogluteal site is easily located by placing the palm of the hand over the client's greater trochanter with the fingers pointing toward the head. The right hand is used to identify landmarks on the left hip, and the left hand is used on the right hip. With the index finger on the anterior superior iliac spine, the middle finger is extended back toward the buttock until it points toward the iliac crest. The lowest point of the triangle formed by the index finger, the middle finger, and the iliac crest is the injection site (Fig. 22–23).

DORSOGLUTEAL SITE. The dorsogluteal site is commonly used for intramuscular injections; however it provides the slowest absorption rate and the greatest risk for injury to nerves and major blood vessels of all the intramuscular sites. Excessive fat accumulation in this area may make visualization of anatomical landmarks difficult and result in medication being deposited into subcutaneous rather than muscle tissue. The dorsogluteal site can be used in adults and older children; however, it is generally not appropriate for children under the age of 3 years because the muscle is not sufficiently developed until the child has been walking for several years.

To locate the injection site, palpate the posterior iliac spine and the greater trochanter. An imaginary line should be drawn between these two landmarks. The injection site is lateral and slightly superior to the imaginary line. An injection may be administered at this site with the client in a prone or side-lying position (Fig. 22–24).

VASTUS LATERALIS MUSCLE. The vastus lateralis muscle is usually well developed in both adults and children, and is located away from major nerves and blood vessels. For this reason, it is increasingly recommended as an intramuscular site, especially for infants and small children. The muscle is situated on the anteriolateral aspect of the thigh. The middle third of the muscle, one hand's breadth below the greater trochanter to one hand's breadth above the knee, is suggested as the injection site (Fig. 22–25). The rectus femoris muscle, which is situated on the midanterior thigh, can also be used for intramuscular medications; however, injections in this muscle tend to cause considerable discomfort for many clients (Fig. 22–25).

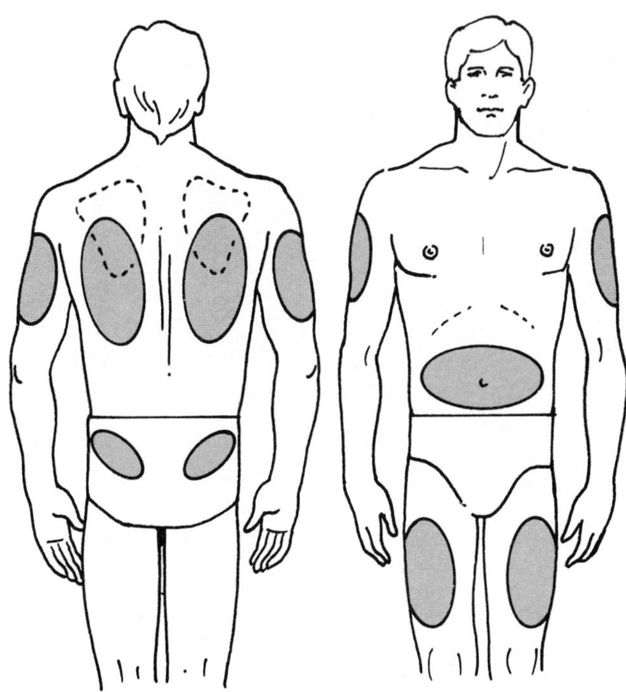

Figure 22–22. Sites for subcutaneous injections. Site rotation is important to prevent tissue damage.

PROCEDURE 22–14. ADMINISTERING A SUBCUTANEOUS INJECTION

PURPOSE: To inject medication into subcutaneous tissue. This route is preferred for nonirritating medications when sustained effect is desired.

EQUIPMENT: Sterile syringe (insulin or 2- to 3-mL size), ⅝ inch 25-gauge needle, alcohol swabs, medication to be given, client's medication administration record (MAR), and one clean glove.

ACTION	RATIONALE
1. Follow steps 1 to 5 of Procedure 22–13.	
2. Choose an area of the selected site that is free of lesions, tenderness, or inflammation.	2. Medication is more readily absorbed from healthy tissue.
3. Cleanse the skin at the site with an alcohol swab, using a firm circular motion from center outward, not a back-and-forth motion. Allow alcohol to dry before penetrating skin with needle.	3. Alcohol (if allowed to dry on the skin) and friction remove surface organisms, preventing their being transmitted through the skin via the needle. A back-and-forth motion is less effective because it moves s' flora from surrounding skin to sit

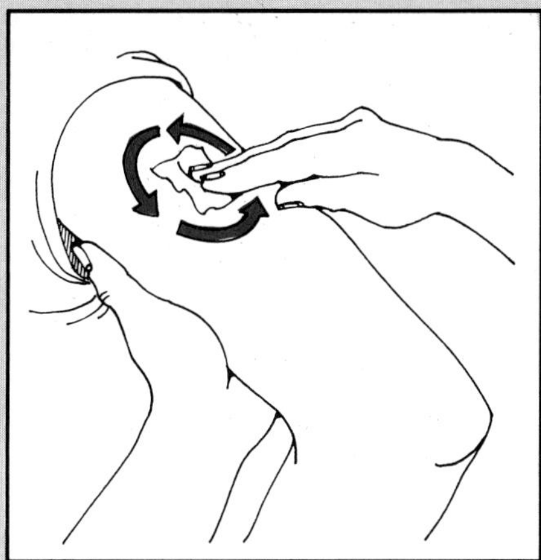

NOTE: Wearing a clean glove on the nondominant hand is recommended because needle penetration of a capillary may cause a small amount of bleeding from the injection site.

(continued)

PROCEDURE 22–14. (continued)

4. Remove needle cap from syringe. Stabilize the skin by pinching a fold of skin between thumb and index finger or spreading skin with thumb and index finger of nondominant hand.

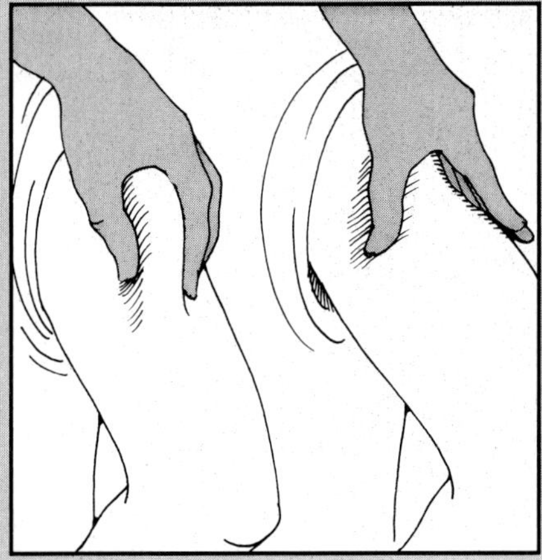

4. Spreading skin facilitates piercing of skin by needle, decreasing pain. Some experts recommend pinching a fold of skin when client is very thin to prevent injecting medication into muscle.

5. Grasp syringe with thumb and four fingers or with thumb and index finger. Stabilize your hand or wrist on the client's skin, as shown.

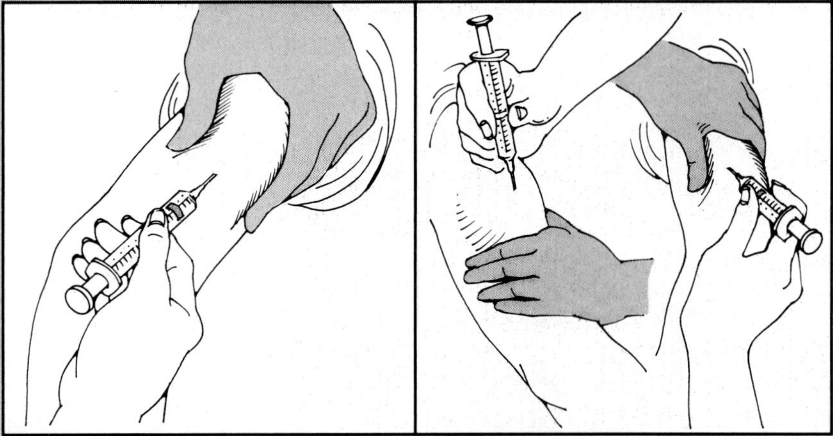

5. Either grip facilitates needle entry. Stabilizing hand helps to control the force and distance of needle insertion.

6. Quickly insert needle at a 45- to 90-degree angle, depending on the amount of subcutaneous tissue.

6. Quick needle insertion reduces stimulation of cutaneous nerves, reducing discomfort. For clients with minimal subcutaneous tissue, inserting needle at a 45-degree angle prevents injection into muscle, which may result in medication being absorbed too rapidly with decreased duration of action.

(continued)

PROCEDURE 22–14. (continued)

7. Release skin and pull back on plunger with nondominant hand while stabilizing syringe with dominant hand.

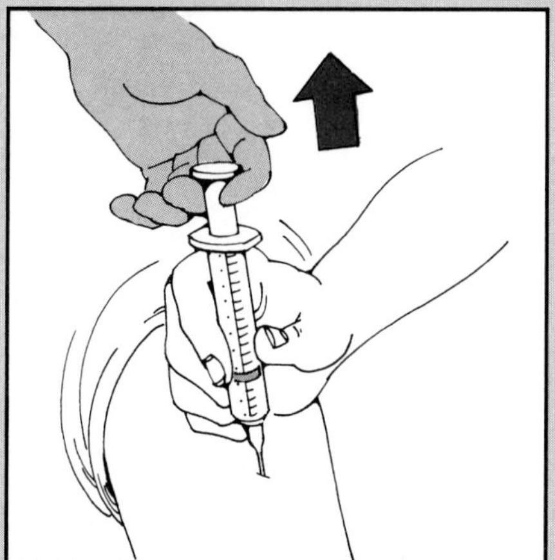

7. Stabilizing the syringe with the same hand that was used to insert needle (rather than changing hands so dominant hand aspirates) prevents syringe and needle movement, which would stimulate nerve endings, producing pain.

8. If blood enters syringe, withdraw needle and obtain new medication. If aspiration produces no blood, push slowly on plunger with nondominant hand to inject medication into subcutaneous tissue.

8. Blood indicates needle is in a blood vessel, so needle is withdrawn to prevent intravenous injection of medication, which could cause client harm. Medication is injected slowly to prevent rapid tissue distension, which would increase nerve stimulation and increase discomfort.

9. Spread skin around needle, then quickly withdraw needle.

9. Taut skin and rapid withdrawal minimize nerve stimulation, reducing pain.

10. Massage injection site with gloved hand, unless contraindicated for specific medication.

10. Massage stimulates circulation, enhancing absorption of medication.

11. Discard needle and syringe without recapping needle, in specially marked puncture-proof container. If glove contacted blood, discard in infectious waste container per CDC guidelines.

11. Recapping used needles creates a risk of needle stick injuries and subsequent infection. Labeled puncture-proof container protects other personnel from injuries.

12. Assist client, if needed, to a comfortable position; replace covers.

12. Comfort promotes well-being.

13. Wash your hands.

13. Removes transient organisms, preventing transmission to other clients or personnel.

RECORDING: Note time, date, and location of injection. State name and strength of medication. If the client is an inpatient, this recording is usually done on the MAR. Additional recording regarding client's response to the medication, including desirable and/or undesirable effects, may also be necessary. This is done on the nurse's notes.

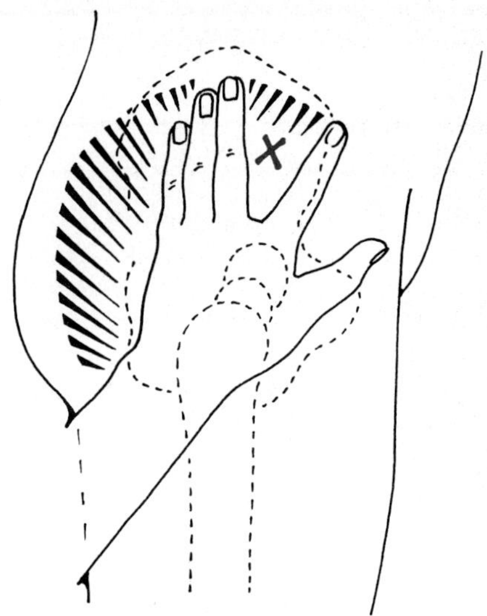

Figure 22–23. Anatomical landmarks for locating the ventrogluteal site for intramuscular injections. Give injection at the bottom of the "V" formed by the fingers. (Hand need not remain in place while injection is given.)

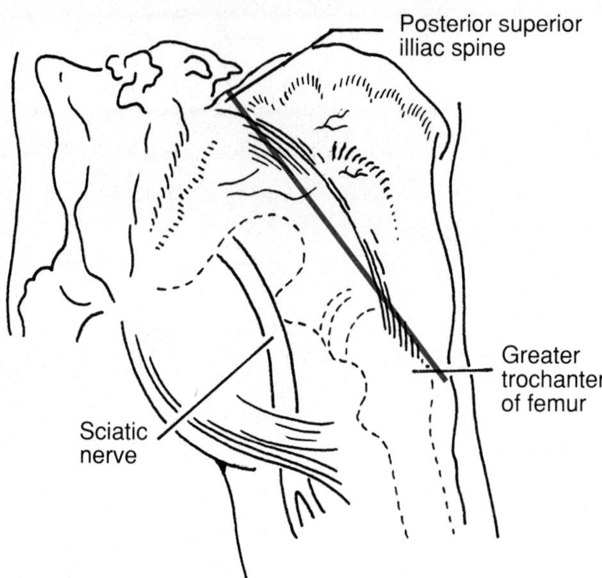

Figure 22–24. Anatomical landmarks for locating the dorsogluteal site for intramuscular injections. Place the injection above the diagonal line.

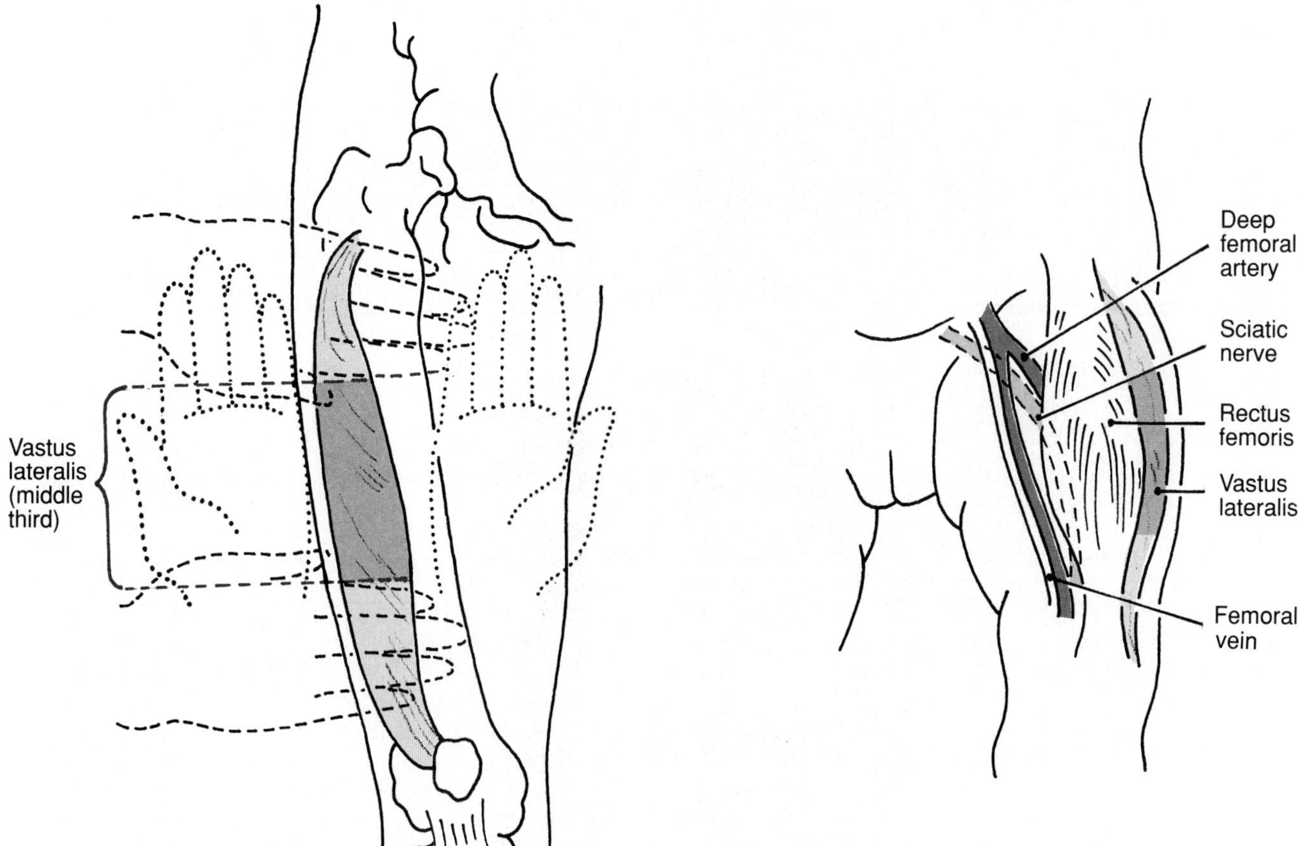

Figure 22–25. Anatomical landmarks for locating the vastus lateralis site for intramuscular injections. Give injection in the middle one-third of the muscle (rectangular space formed by hand placement).

PROCEDURE 22–15. ADMINISTERING AN INTRAMUSCULAR INJECTION

PURPOSE: To inject medication into a muscle. Provides more rapid absorption, but shorter duration of effect than subcutaneous injection.

EQUIPMENT: Sterile syringe (3mL size), 1 to 1½ inch, 22- or 23-gauge needle, alcohol swabs, medication to be given, and client's medication administration record (MAR), and one clean glove. Note: A longer needle is required for obese clients.

ACTION	RATIONALE
1. Follow steps 1 to 5 of Procedure 22–13.	
2. Determine if needle is of sufficient length to penetrate muscle at site selected by assessing the amount of subcutaneous tissue, as follows: Gently squeeze tissue over muscle with your thumb and index finger. Lift pinched tissue slightly. Estimate the distance between your thumb and finger. One half of this distance is the length of needle needed to reach, but not penetrate the muscle. Add an additional ½ inch to assure muscle penetration. Obtain new needle of appropriate length, if necessary. 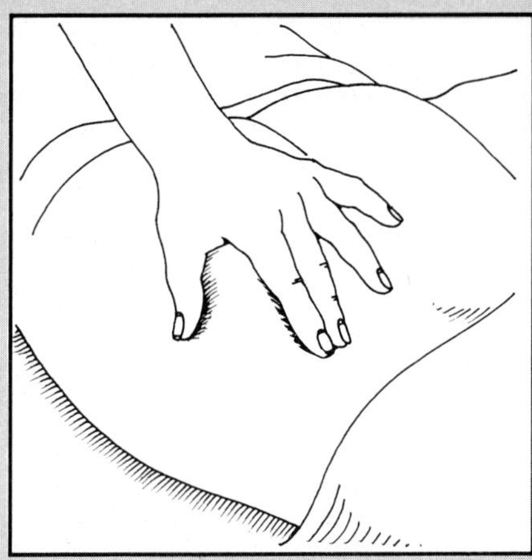	2. Subcutaneous tissue is loose and easily isolated from muscle, which has greater density. Method described raises two thicknesses of subcutaneous tissue, hence ½ the thickness represents depth of tissue above muscle. Medications given IM are usually irritating to subcutaneous tissue and if injected they may cause severe pain, sterile abscesses or tissue necrosis, so the additional ½ inch is important to prevent inadvertent subcutaneous injection. While a 1- or 1½-inch needle is sufficient for most sites in average-sized clients, obese clients may require a 3- to 6-inch needle.
3. If necessary, assist the client to assume a position that provides the nurse easy access to the selected site. Adjust covers and gown so sites can be visualized with minimal exposure of client. Use boney landmarks (Figs. 22–23 to 22–26) to precisely locate correct location for injection. Site should be free of lesions, tenderness, hardness, or inflammation.	3. Good access to site allows use of optimum body mechanics and correct injection technique. Minimizing client exposure prevents chilling and demonstrates respect for client's privacy. Use of landmarks identifies muscle region without major arteries or nerves. Avoid sites with lesions, tenderness, or inflammation, because medication is more readily absorbed from healthy tissue.

(continued)

PROCEDURE 22–15. (continued)

4. Cleanse the skin at the site with an alcohol swab, using a firm circular motion from center outward, not a back-and-forth motion. Allow alcohol to dry before penetrating skin with needle.

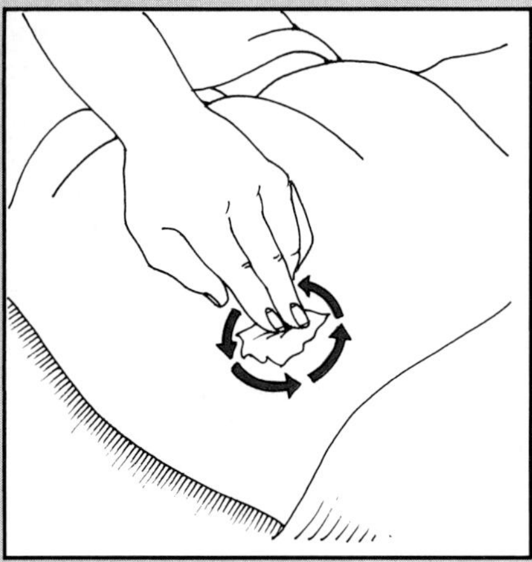

NOTE: Wearing a clean glove on the nondominant hand is recommended because needle penetration of a capillary may cause a small amount of bleeding from the injection site.

4. Alcohol (if allowed to dry on the skin) and friction remove surface organisms, preventing their being transmitted through the skin via the needle. A back-and-forth motion is less effective because it moves skin flora from surrounding skin to site.

5. Remove needle cap from syringe. Stabilize the skin by spreading skin with thumb and index finger of nondominant hand.

5. Spreading skin facilitates piercing of skin by needle, so fewer nerve endings are stimulated and pain is minimized.

6. Grasp syringe with thumb and index finger. Stabilize your hand or wrist on the client's skin, as shown.

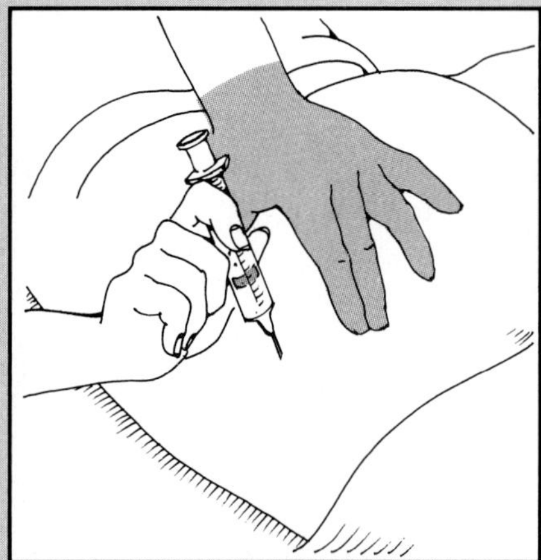

6. This grip will facilitate needle entry. Stabilizing hand helps to control the force and distance of needle insertion.

7. Quickly insert needle to the hub at a 90° angle.

7. Quick needle insertion reduces stimulation of cutaneous nerves, reducing discomfort. Inserting entire length of needle at 90-degree angle deposits medication well into muscle.

(continued)

PROCEDURE 22–15. (continued)

8. Release skin and pull back on plunger with nondominant hand while stabilizing syringe with dominant hand. Do not allow partial withdrawal of needle while aspirating.

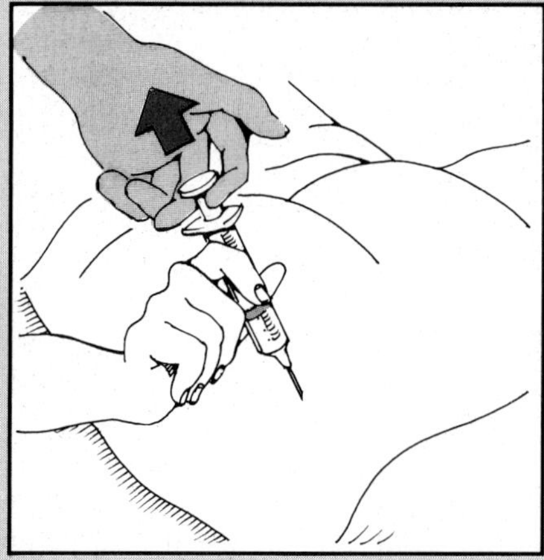

8. Stabilizing the syringe with the same hand that was used to insert needle (rather than changing hands so dominant hand aspirates) prevents syringe and needle movement, which would stimulate nerve endings, producing pain. Partial withdrawal of needle could result in subcutaneous injection.

9. If blood enters syringe, withdraw needle and obtain new medication. If aspiration produces no blood, push slowly on plunger with nondominant hand to inject medication into muscle.

9. Blood indicates needle is in a blood vessel, so needle is withdrawn to prevent intravenous injection of medication, which could cause harm to client. Medication is injected slowly to prevent rapid tissue distension, which would increase nerve stimulation and increase discomfort.

10. Spread skin taut around needle, then quickly withdraw needle.

10. Taut skin and rapid withdrawal minimize nerve stimulation, reducing pain.

11. Massage injection site with gloved hand.

11. Massage stimulates circulation, enhancing absorption of medication.

12. Discard glove, needle, and syringe without recapping needle, in specially marked puncture-proof container.

12. Recapping used needles creates a risk of needle-stick injuries and subsequent infection. Labeled puncture-proof container protects other personnel from injuries.

13. Assist client, if needed, to a comfortable position; replace covers.

13. Comfort promotes well-being.

14. Wash your hands.

14. Removes transient organisms, preventing transmission to other clients or personnel.

15. If drug was a PRN medication, return in 30 to 40 minutes to observe whether desired effects were obtained.

15. Observation is necessary to make a decision regarding subsequent administration of this drug to the client.

RECORDING: Note time, date, and location of injection. State name and strength of medication. If the client is an inpatient, this recording is usually done on the MAR. Additional recording regarding client's response to the medication, including desirable and/or undesirable effects, may also be necessary. This is done on the nurse's notes.

DELTOID MUSCLE. The deltoid muscle is located on the lateral aspect of the upper arm. It is a relatively small muscle and is close to the major nerves and artery of the arm. The major advantages of the deltoid site are its easy accessibility and rapid absorption. The deltoid is used primarily in adults for single injections of small volume (less than 2 mL but preferably 1 mL) (Fig. 22–26).

The injection site is located by imagining a line across the lateral aspect of the upper arm, even with the lower edge of the acromion process, and a second lower line even with the axilla. The injection site is in the center one third of the rectangle that is formed by these boundaries, about 1.5 to 2 inches below the acromion process (Fig. 22–26).

INJECTION TECHNIQUES. Procedure 22–15 outlines the general principles and steps for the administration of intramuscular injections. In addition to the basic injection technique, many sources advocate the use of the air lock technique and Z-track injections when administering intramuscular medications.

The air lock technique is the aspiration of a small bubble of air (0.2 mL) into the syringe after the desired amount of medication has been prepared. When the injection is administered, the air bubble clears the needle of medication and prevents leakage of medication through the subcutaneous tissues as the needle is withdrawn. This technique is recommended by drug manufacturers when administering iron dextran (Imferon) and some of the diphtheria and tetanus toxoids prepared with aluminum adjuvant, to prevent skin staining or abscess formation. Use of this technique with all intramuscular injections, however, may lead to overdose errors, as the amount of medication left in the hub and needle is not part of the syringe barrel calibration. Clearing the hub and needle of medication may actually inject the client with as much as 10 percent more medication than was actually ordered.[111]

The Z-track technique is another commonly used injection procedure that prevents leakage of medication from the muscle site into subcutaneous tissue. With the Z-track method, the skin and subcutaneous tissue overlaying the injection site are displaced 1 to 1½ inches laterally prior to insertion of the needle. The tissue must remain retracted as the needle is inserted and the medication is slowly administered. After waiting 10 seconds for the medication to disperse, simultaneously remove the needle and release the skin. This technique forms a zigzag needle path through clients' tissue (Fig. 22–27) and seals the medication into the muscle.

Intravenous Medications. Medications administered by the intravenous route are injected directly into a client's vein and have an immediate effect. Once administered, these medications cannot be removed or their action slowed. For this reason, it is critical that nurses exercise the utmost caution in the administration of intravenous medications. To prevent infection, strict adherence to the principles of surgical asepsis must be maintained during all aspects of intravenous medication administration.

Many of the client concerns related to needles and injections also apply to intravenous medications. Nursing

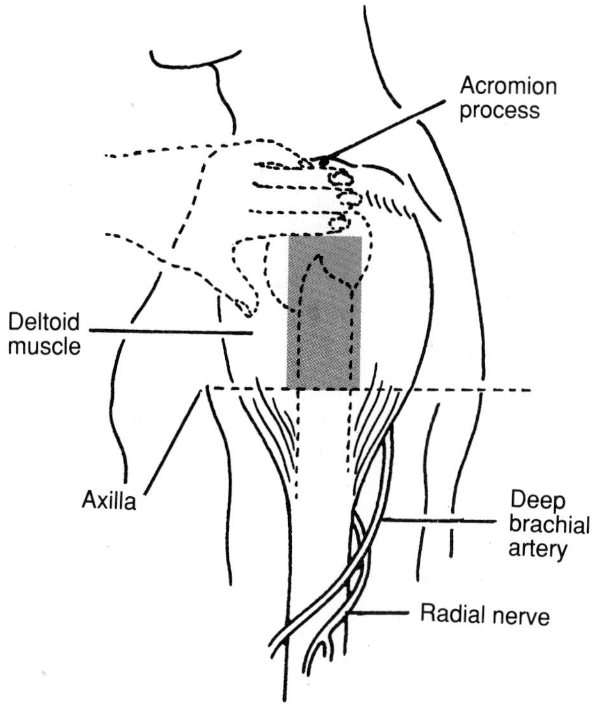

Figure 22–26. Anatomical landmarks for locating the deltoid site for intramuscular injections. Give injection in the rectangle formed by the planes of the landmarks.

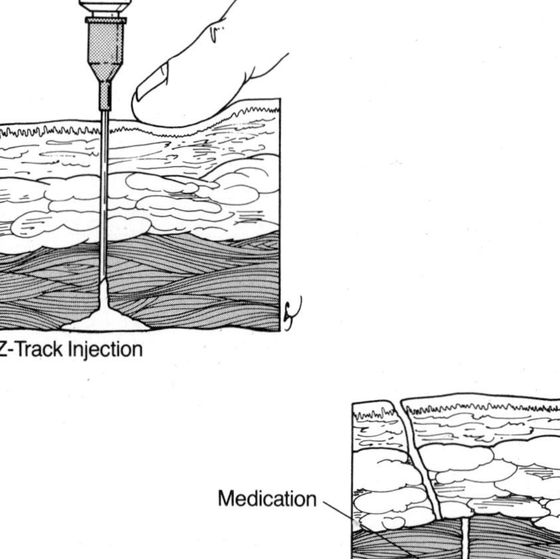

Figure 22–27. Z-track technique for intramuscular injections prevents tracking of medications to the skin. (*From Smith S, Duell D.* Clinical Nursing Skills: Nursing Process Model; Basic to Advanced Skills. *3rd ed. Norwalk, CT: Appleton & Lange; 1992.*)

measures designed to educate and prepare clients for venipuncture and continuous IV therapy can be found in Chapter 31. Because many intravenous medications are extremely irritating to body tissues, nurses should always verify placement of the IV needle prior to administration. Irritating medications such as potassium preparations or Valium must be well diluted and should be initially infused at a slow rate so nurses can assess clients' response to the particular drug. Refrigerated medications should be warmed to room temperature prior to administration to reduce venous spasm. Careful attention to the IV site and the client response throughout intravenous medication administration is necessary to maintain client comfort and to avoid potential hazards.

IV medications can be administered by one of three methods: (1) as an additive to a large-volume container of IV fluids, (2) as intermittent small-volume doses through the use of piggyback or volume-controlled infusions, and (3) through injection of a small bolus of medication directly into an existing IV line or heparin lock (IV push). In all three of these methods, the client has an existing IV infusion or site. A detailed discussion of basic IV procedures can be found in Chapter 31.

ADDING MEDICATION TO AN IV FLUID CONTAINER. Of the three methods of intravenous medication administration, the dilution of the drug in a large-volume (500 to 1000 mL) container of IV fluids is the safest and easiest. In many institutions, this procedure is performed in the pharmacy prior to the fluids being delivered to the nursing unit. Potassium chloride and multivitamin solutions are examples of two drugs commonly added to IV fluids. Medications added to large-volume containers are administered continuously over several hours. Accurate labeling of containers to which medications have been added is important to avoid inadvertent overdoses. The steps for adding medications to intravenous containers are outlined in Procedure 22–16.

SMALL-VOLUME INFUSIONS. Intravenous medications can also be administered intermittently through the use of small-volume (50 to 100 mL) infusions, also called additive sets. A drug is added to a compatible solution and administered at prescribed intervals, such as every 4 hours. Some piggybacks are prepared in the pharmacy; others by nurses. The medication in solution is introduced into the primary intravenous line through the use of a short section of tubing (secondary tubing) that is attached to the uppermost Y-port or injection site of the primary tubing. The piggyback is regulated to infuse over a 30- to 90-minute interval. When the infusion is complete, the primary IV solution must be readjusted to its prescribed rate. IV antibiotics are frequently administered by the piggyback method (Procedure 22–17).

Small-volume infusions can also be administered through the use of volume control sets. These administration sets have different names depending on the manufacturer (eg, Soluset, Buretrol, Pediatrol). They consist of a small-volume container (100 to 150 mL), which is attached directly below the primary IV bag or bottle. The container is filled with a prescribed amount of fluid from the primary IV; medication is added into the volume control set through the injection port. This type of equipment is used primarily to administer fluids and medications to children and elderly clients who require careful monitoring of fluid volume (see Chap. 31). The procedures for filling and infusing through these administration sets vary according to manufacturer's design. Package directions should be followed carefully to ensure proper functioning (see also Procedure 31–8).

IV PUSH (BOLUS). An IV push (bolus) is the administration of a concentrated dose of medication directly into the systemic circulation. This method is used in emergency situations or when a rapid response to the drug is desired. An IV push is the most dangerous method for administering drugs as the entire dose is administered in a short time. Therefore, effects are immediate and there is no way to correct errors. Administration of IV push medications is an advanced procedure. In many institutions only physicians or specially trained nurses may administer IV push medications. These medications may be administered through a direct venipuncture, through the injection port of an existing IV line, or through the use of a heparin lock. Procedure 22–18 outlines the general technique for the administration of an IV drip medication via a heparin lock.

Promoting Client Comfort and Well-being. Nursing measures that serve to enhance client well-being are an important component of any aspect of medication administration. The safe administration of medications is critical to client well-being. Safety considerations have been stressed throughout the preceding discussion. Other important elements related to client well-being include the identification of client needs and the promotion of collaborative administration.

Identification of Learning Needs. Education of clients and family members is an important aspect of medication administration. Unless clients are properly informed about the purpose of the prescribed medications and the correct methods for taking the drugs properly, they cannot be expected to maintain the prescribed regimen. In addition, clients require some basic knowledge of the anticipated effects of the drugs—both desirable and undesirable ones—as well as an understanding of the effects that will be experienced if the medication is not taken properly.

Client teaching related to medications should be an integral part of daily nursing practice and not reserved for "discharge" instructions. It is important that nurses assess clients' readiness, motivation, and current level of knowledge. Some clients' may desire a detailed description of drug action or effects, while others may only be capable of or interested in focusing on some basic facts. More information about learner assessment and teaching approaches can be found in Chapter 20.

Collaborative Administration. Closely related to client education is the concept of collaborative administration. Health care facilities vary widely in their policies related to client self-medication, but all clients can become involved in medication administration at some level. Encouraging clients to

(Text continues on page 866.)

PROCEDURE 22–16. ADDING MEDICATIONS TO AN IV SOLUTION CONTAINER

PURPOSE: To deliver intravenous medication continuously over several hours.

EQUIPMENT: IV fluid container containing ordered solution, ampule or vial containing ordered medication, sterile 5- to 20-mL syringe and 19- to 20-gauge needle (transfer needle may be used), alcohol swabs, medication label, and client's medication administration record (MAR).

ACTION	RATIONALE
1. Follow general guidelines for administration of medications (Table 22–11) and technique for preparing medication from an ampule or vial (Procedures 22–10 and 22–11).	1. These guidelines facilitate safe, error-free preparation of medication.
FOR NEW IV CONTAINER 2. Remove protective cover from injection port: *Glass bottles:* metal ring, disc (leave latex disc in place). *Plastic bottles:* screw-cap. *Plastic bags:* plastic pop-off or pull-off cap. Do not touch tip of port or top of bottle. If accidental contact occurs, cleanse with friction and alcohol swab. Let dry. NOTE: Vacuum in glass bottles causes depressions in latex disc over openings in stopper, so their location can be determined without breaking seal.	2. Cover prevents transfer of microbes from environment to port and fluid by direct contact. If contact of opened port occurs, friction and antiseptic action of alcohol will remove or kill microbes. (Alcohol must dry for antiseptic effect.)
3. Insert the needle of the syringe containing medication into medication port (pierce latex seal on glass bottle) and inject medication. Do not inject medication into air vent port on glass bottle or port for tubing insertion on plastic bag. With glass bottle, medication may be injected into triangular or larger round opening. Vacuum will draw medication into bottle.	3. Port is provided for easy addition of medications. It is self-sealing to prevent leaking. Tubing port is not self-sealing. Injection of liquid into air vent may result in spilling.

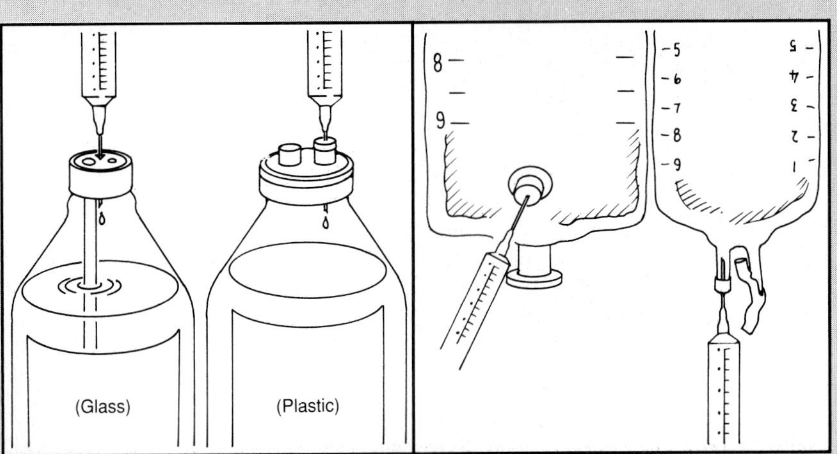

(continued)

PROCEDURE 22–16. (continued)

4. Remove and discard syringe without recapping in specially marked puncture-proof container.

   4. Recapping needles creates risk for needle stick injuries. Container prevents injury to other personnel.

5. Gently agitate container.

   5. Movement increases rate of diffusion of medication throughout container. Complete mixing of medication in IV solution assures uniform rate of administration of drug to client.

6. Fill out and affix medication label to IV container. Spike container with IV tubing (see Procedure 31–4). Set is now ready for administration (see Procedure 31–10). If client has existing IV, new tubing may be unnecessary (see Chap. 31.)

   6. Label alerts other staff to presence of medication so precautions related to the specific drug can be observed.

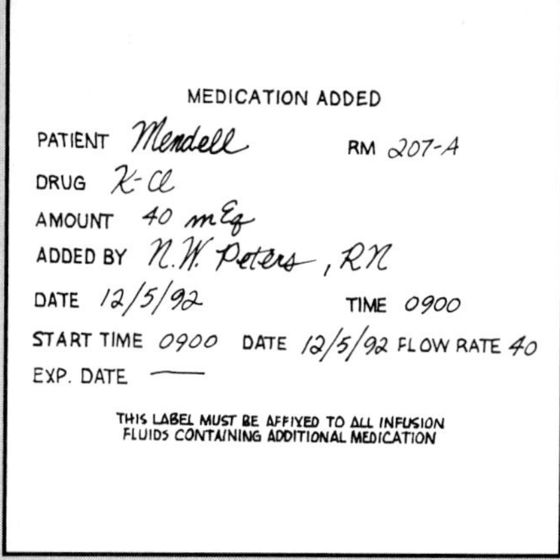

MEDICATION ADDED

PATIENT Mendell RM 207-A

DRUG K-Cl

AMOUNT 40 mEq

ADDED BY N.W. Peters, RN

DATE 12/5/92 TIME 0900

START TIME 0900 DATE 12/5/92 FLOW RATE 40

EXP. DATE —

THIS LABEL MUST BE AFFIXED TO ALL INFUSION FLUIDS CONTAINING ADDITIONAL MEDICATION

7. If medication container is a vial, and the entire amount is to be added to the IV solution container, a transfer needle may be used in lieu of a syringe:

   7. Transfer needle acts as a conduit between vial and IV container. It eliminates several steps and therefore saves time as well as potential for contamination.

   a. Remove needle cover from short end of needle, insert needle into vial.

   b. Remove needle cover from long end of needle and insert needle/vial unit through latex disc (see step 3, above). Medication will be drawn into bottle by vacuum.

      b. Negative pressure rapidly pulls the liquid from the vial to the bottle. The disc is removed before connecting the IV tubing.

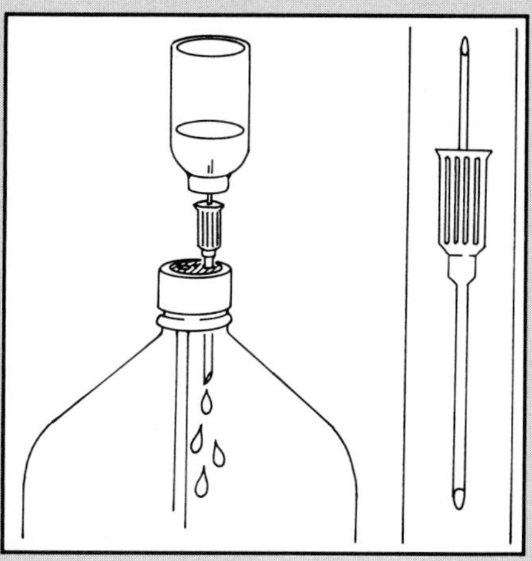

(continued)

PROCEDURE 22–16. (continued)

c. For IV bag, invert bag, then insert needle/vial unit into medication port. Squeeze and release bag until vial is empty.

c. Because the bag has no vacuum, pressure gradient must be created manually. Squeezing bag pushes air into vial which then displaces some of medication into bag. Inverting bag utilizes gravity to assist in the fluid transfer.

8. Take IV container to client's room, identify client (see step 10, below), and infuse as ordered (see Procedure 31–10).

8. See step 10 and Procedure 31–10.

FOR CURRENTLY INFUSING IV

9. Determine whether the amount of solution remaining in container is sufficient to adequately dilute drug to be added.

9. IV drugs have immediate effect. Insufficient dilution may irritate vein as well as intensify drug effect, causing potential harm to the client.

10. Discuss the reason for the medication and expected benefits with the client.

10. Client will be less anxious if reasons and benefits are clear.

11. Identify client by reading client's ID bracelet. You may also ask clients to state their name.

11. Positive client identification is necessary immediately prior to giving drug to prevent medicating the wrong client.

12. Slow IV to keep vein open (KVO) rate (see Chap. 31).

12. Medication port is near tubing insertion site. At a normal infusion rate, concentrated drug may enter tubing before adequate mixing can occur.

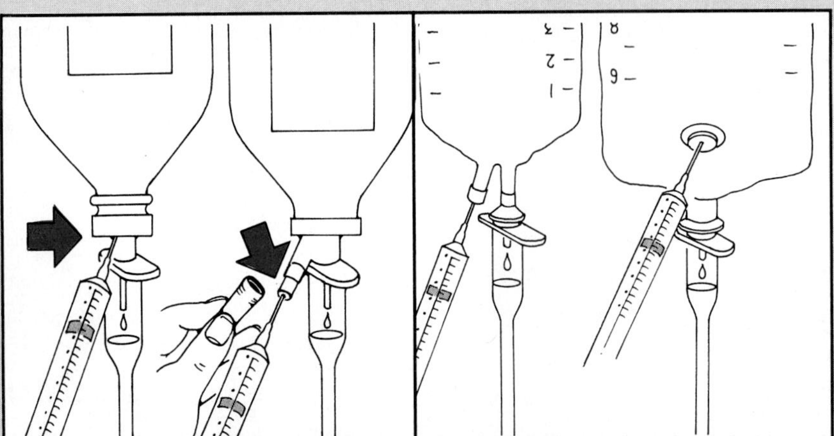

13. Cleanse medication port with alcohol swab, using firm rotational motion. Insert needle, and inject medication.

13. See steps 2 and 3, above.

14. Remove syringe, agitate container, discard syringe as above.

14. See steps 4 and 5, above.

15. Readjust IV flowrate to ordered infusion rate. Affix completed medication label as above.

15. See step 6, above.

(continued)

PROCEDURE 22–16. (continued)

16. Assess the infusion, the site and the client periodically during the infusion. Reregulate drip if necessary, or reposition limb to improve flow. If severe pain or swelling occurs at site, or other untoward effects occur, discontinue infusion and consult physician.

16. These actions promote early detection and correction of problems related to infusion mechanics and/or undesirable reactions to the medication.

RECORDING: Record IV solution and medication according to agency policy. Some agencies require entry on MAR and I&O/IV record; others indicate medication as IV additive on IV record without MAR recording.

PROCEDURE 22–17. ADMINISTERING IV DRIP MEDICATIONS VIA PIGGYBACK (ADDITIVE SET)

PURPOSE: To deliver medications by intravenous drip.

EQUIPMENT: Ordered medication in a 50- to 100-mL infusion bag, alcohol swabs, sterile 18 to 19-gauge 1-inch needle or needle-lock device, client's medication administration record (MAR), and IV secondary administration set if tubing change is needed, based on agency policy.
If medication has not been prepared by pharmacy: Vial/ampule of ordered medication, sterile syringe and needle, and 50- to 100-mL infusion bag of D_5W or 0.9% NaCl (often called "partial-fill" or "addit").
If medication is not compatible with client's IV solution: Also obtain a 250 mL container of 0.9% NaCl or D_5W and a standard IV administration set with additive ports, and an additional 18- to 19-gauge needle.

ACTION	RATIONALE
1. Follow general guidelines for administration of medications (Table 22–11). If medication has not been prepared by pharmacy, follow techniques for preparing medications from vial or ampule (see Procedures 22–10 and 22–11).	1. These guidelines facilitate safe and error-free preparation and administration of medications.
2. If ordered medication has not been prepared for IV infusion by pharmacy, inject medication into infusion bag of NaCl or D_5W, using technique for new container described in Procedure 22–16. Affix medication label.	2. This will result in aseptic preparation of correct medication for infusion readily identifiable by all personnel during infusion.
3. Check compatibility of medication and client's IV solution. If incompatible, prepare 250 mL NaCl or D_5W to use as a flush line. See Procedure 31–4.	3. Flush line prevents mixing of incompatible solutions
4. Take prepared medication to client's room. Identify client by checking ID band. You may also ask clients to state their name.	4. Positive identification is essential immediately before administering any drug to prevent giving drug to the wrong client.

(continued)

PROCEDURE 22–17. (continued)

5. Discuss the reason for the procedure, expected client participation, usual sensations, and expected benefits with the client.

5. Client will be more willing to participate and less anxious if there is an opportunity to clarify concerns and the reasons and benefits for the procedure are clear.

6. Assess IV site for redness, swelling, warmth, and tenderness. If none are present, proceed with next step.

6. These are indicators of inflammation due to vein irritation by solutions. Medications are often more irritating than standard IV solutions, so it may be advisable to consider a new venipuncture if vein is already irritated.

7. If the medication is compatible with the primary IV solution, remove and discard empty container from prior infusion and spike medication container with secondary tubing still connected to port on primary line (clamp should be closed). If using new tubing, cleanse the highest injection port on the primary line, and attach a needle or needle-lock device to secondary line and insert it into port. Back-fill secondary tubing by opening clamp and holding the container lower than the port. When drip chamber on secondary line is one-half full, hang container, leaving clamp open. If medication is not compatible with IV solution, or if several medications not compatible with each other are ordered, see steps 12 to 14.

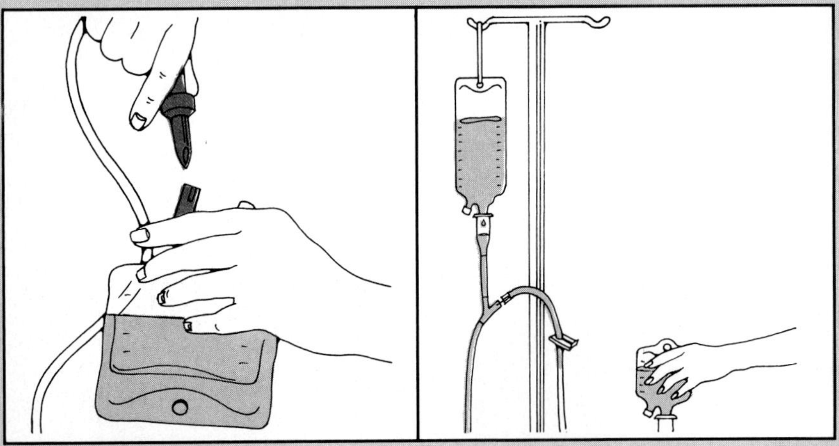

7. Setup from previous medication is usually left connected to the primary line after the medication has infused to minimize disruption of closed system (which creates possibility of contamination). Backfilling rather than priming the tubing also introduces air into the medication container. When the container is a plastic bag, adding air is necessary to prevent creation of a vacuum as medication infuses (bag will collapse). A vacuum in the bag prevents remaining medication from infusing. Backfilling is preferred, but not necessary for other types of containers or if vented secondary tubing is used.

(continued)

PROCEDURE 22–17. (continued)

NOTE: The highest port has a check valve that temporarily stops the flow of the primary infusion while the secondary infusion is running. If other ports are used, the primary infusion will continue to flow because these ports have no check valves.

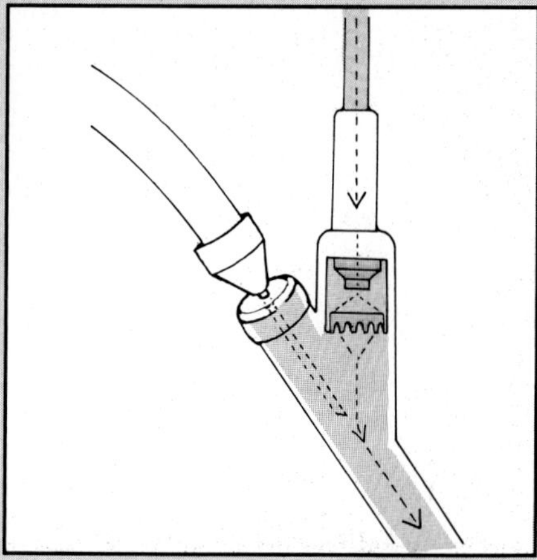

8. If using new tubing, clamp temporarily and secure secondary line with tape or needle-lock device so it cannot accidently pull out of the port; then reopen clamp. Tubing used for previous piggyback should already be taped in place.

8. Accidental separation of secondary line is one cause of needle-stick injuries to health care personnel, and would cause loss of medication to floor or client's bed.

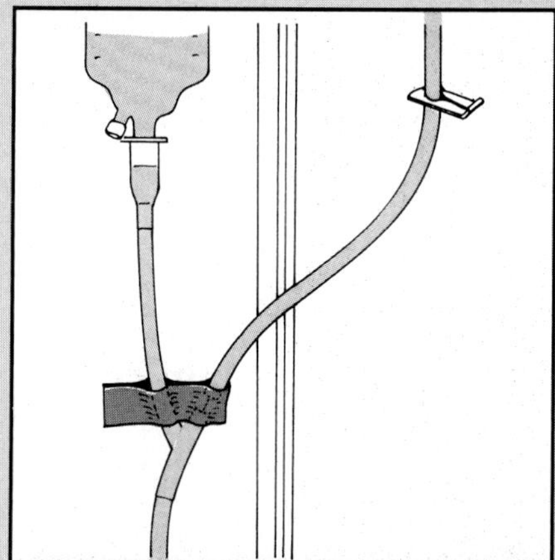

(continued)

PROCEDURE 22–17. (continued)

9. Hang the primary container so it is lower than the secondary (medication) container. If multilevel overhead IV hanger is not available, use extension hook contained in secondary administration set to lower the primary bottle. Use the clamp on the primary line to regulate flow of medication at the ordered or recommended rate. Medications may be infused over 15 to 90 minutes; 30 minutes is most common.

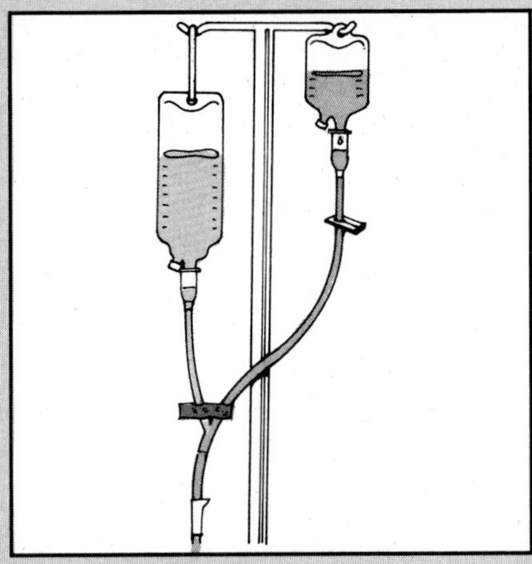

9. The greater the height of a column of liquid, the faster the flow. The faster flow from the higher secondary container will close the check valve so medication will infuse according to the setting on the primary tubing. When the level of fluid in the secondary tubing is even with the drip chamber of the primary line, the primary line will have the greater height so the check valve will open and the primary line will resume infusing.

10. Assess the infusion, the site and the client periodically during the infusion. Reregulate drip if necessary, or reposition limb to improve flow. If severe pain or swelling occurs at site, or other untoward effects occur, discontinue infusion and consult physician.

10. These actions promote early detection and correction of problems related to infusion mechanics and/or undesirable reactions to the medication.

11. When infusion is complete, close clamp on secondary line, reassess and/or reregulate primary infusion at ordered rate.

11. Promotes fluid and electrolyte balance.

NOTE: Some agency IV policies recommend pinching off primary line just above the port so medication remaining in secondary tubing will run in, then closing secondary clamp.

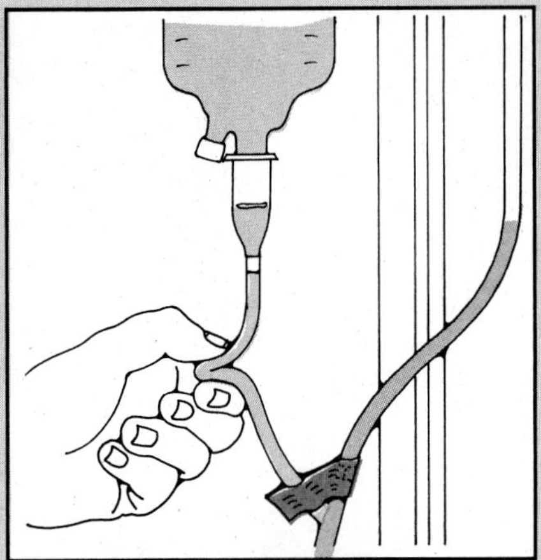

(continued)

PROCEDURE 22–17. (continued)

12. If medication previously infused is not the same as current medication, but is compatible, above procedure can be followed. If medications are not compatible, use separate secondary tubing for each medication. It is permissible to leave the secondary tubing still attached to the previous medication container hanging on IV stand for use at the next administration time, but needle guard should be securely in place and a new needle or needle-lock device used for next infusion. Connect and back-fill as for new tubing (see step 8, above).

12. Medications that are not compatible may precipitate, clogging venipuncture device, or may inactivate one another.

13. If primary solution and the medication are incompatible, prepare 0.9% NaCl or D_5W for use as flush line as you would a primary IV (see Procedure 31–4), but attach an 18- to 19-inch gauge, 1-inch needle or a needle-lock device to the needle adapter at the end of the tubing.

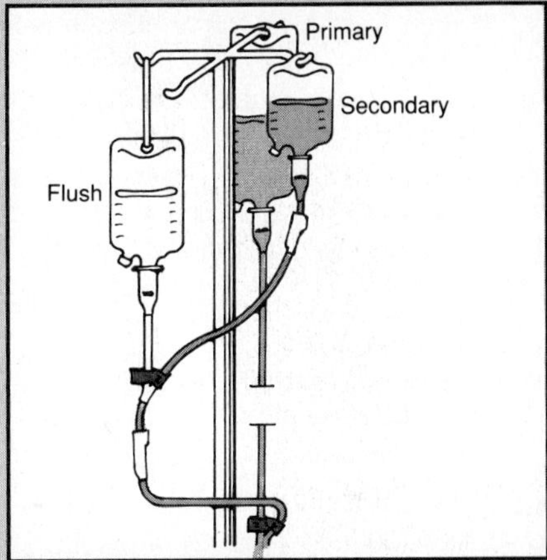

13. NaCl or D_5W will be used as a flush line, preventing primary solution and medication from mixing. Confer with physician to determine whether either of these solutions is contraindicated for client.

14. Insert the needle or needle-lock device on primed flush line into one of the lower ports on the primary tubing, secure as above. Close the clamp on the primary line and open the clamp on the flush line to keep vein open (KVO) rate.

14. Solution in flush line acts as a buffer, preventing mixing of medication and primary IV solution.

15. Connect medication to flush line as described above in steps 7 to 9 and administer medication according to steps 10 and 11. When medication container is empty, allow flush solution to flow for 5 minutes, and then separate flush line from primary line, recap or replace needle or needle-lock device, and leave in room for future use. Readjust flowrate of primary solution to ordered rate.

15. When medication has infused, the solution in flush line will flush medication into client's vein (see rationale 9, above), preventing mixing of primary solution and medication.

RECORDING: Record administration of IV medications and solutions according to agency policy. Usually recording will be necessary on both the MAR and the I&O record. Narrative recording on nurse's notes may also be expected for some medications or if unexpected reaction to medication occurs.

PROCEDURE 22–18. ADMINISTERING IV DRIP MEDICATIONS VIA A HEPARIN LOCK

PURPOSE: To deliver medications by intravenous drip to a client not receiving continuous IV fluids.

EQUIPMENT: Ordered medication in a 50- to 100-mL infusion bag, or vial/ampule of ordered medication, sterile syringe and needle, and 50- to 100-mL infusion bag of NaCl or D_5W; IV administration set; sterile syringe/needle (22 gauge, 1 in) with 1- to 2-mL sterile normal saline (2 syringes of saline if medication is incompatible with heparin); sterile syringe/needle (22 gauge, 1 in) with 1 to 2 mL heparin flush solution (100 μL/mL); alcohol swabs; sterile 18-gauge, 1-inch needle; tape; and client's medication administration record (MAR). In some agencies, "flush solution" of D_5W or NaCl with primary infusion tubing is intermittantly connected to heparin lock and medication infused as a piggyback rather than directly into heparin lock. Secondary tubing is then required for medication. If needleless system is in use: Needleless cannula with threaded lock replaces 18-gauge needle on primary line, needlelock device is used on secondary line, and prefilled (heparin and saline) needleless syringes may be used to flush heparin lock.

ACTION	RATIONALE
1. Follow general guidelines for administration of medications (Table 22–11) and techniques for preparing medications from vial or ampule (Procedures 22–10 and 22–11) to prepare syringes of heparin flush solution, sterile saline (if needed), and ordered medication (if not preprepared in IV solution by pharmacy.)	1. These guidelines facilitate safe and error-free preparation and administration of medications.
NOTE: Check agency policy for amount of heparin flush solution and saline. Saline syringe may not be necessary if flush IV setup is used.	
2. If ordered medication has not been prepared for IV infusion by pharmacy, inject medication into infusion bag of NaCl or D_5W, using technique for new container described in Procedure 22–16. Affix medication label.	2. This will result in aseptic preparation of correct medication for infusion readily identifiable by all personnel during infusion.

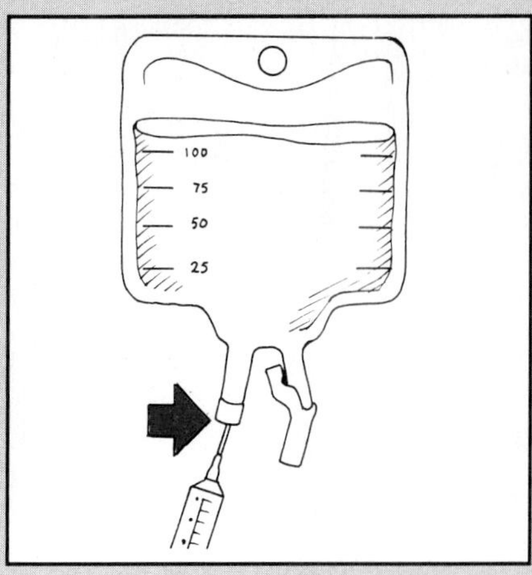

(continued)

PROCEDURE 22–18. (continued)

3. Use secondary tubing if IV flush setup is being used or primary tubing without additive ports if medication will be infused directly into heparin lock. Attach 18-gauge 1-inch needle or needle-lock device to secondary tubing, and 18-gauge 1-inch needle or needleless cannula to primary tubing. Leave protective caps on.

NOTE: IV tubing used for prior infusion of the same drug may be reused for a 48- to 72-hour period. Check agency policy.

3. Secondary tubing is of appropriate length for piggyback administration, but too short to allow client movement if medication is to be infused directly into heparin lock. Needleless system is not available for injection ports on IV tubing, but needle-lock device prevents accidental separation of secondary tubing from port.

4. Take prepared medication to client's room. Identify client by checking ID band. You may also ask client to state name.

NOTE: Some clients will answer "yes" when asked, "Are you Mr. (name), even when it is not true.

4. Positive identification is essential immediately before administering any drug to prevent giving drug to the wrong client.

5. Discuss the reason for the procedure, expected client participation, usual sensations, and expected benefits with the client.

5. Client will be more willing to participate and less anxious if there is an opportunity to clarify concerns and the reasons and benefits for the procedure are clear.

6. Assess IV site for redness, swelling, warmth, and tenderness. If none are present, proceed with next step.

6. These are indicators of inflammation. IV flow may be sluggish, even if heparin lock is patent. Insertion of new heparin lock at another site may be necessary.

7. Hold heparin lock with one hand to stabilize it. Cleanse port with alcohol swab, using firm rotational motion. Let dry.

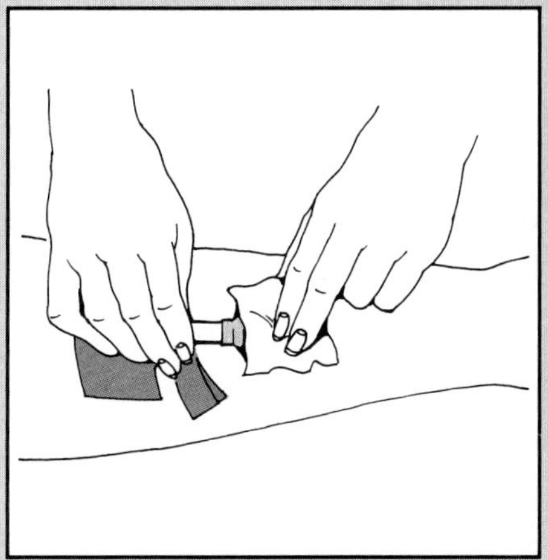

7. Stabilizing heparin lock prevents its moving, which causes discomfort and may dislodge cannula. Alcohol (if allowed to dry) and friction remove microbes, preventing their being introduced into the client's circulatory system when the needle is introduced.

(continued)

PROCEDURE 22–18. (continued)

8. To infuse medication directly into the heparin lock, first insert needle (or needleless cannula) of syringe with sterile saline. Aspirate for blood return. If there is blood return, flush IV cannula with saline and continue with next step.

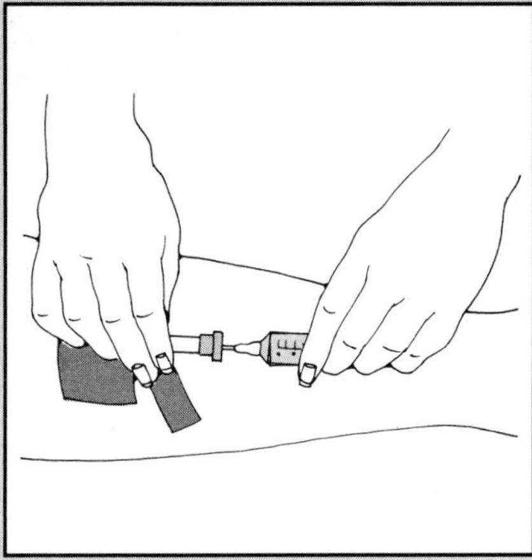

NOTE: Some agencies prescribe flushing with 1 mL of heparin flush solution, omitting aspiration and saline if medication to be infused is compatible with heparin.

8. Aspiration is a means of assessing patency of cannula. Lack of blood return suggests cannula has been dislodged from vein or is clotted. New site is required. Saline clears heparin from lock. Do not flush forcefully to dislodge clot.

9. Cleanse port as in step 7. Insert needle or needleless cannula attached to IV tubing/bag containing medication. Regulate drip rate according to medical order, your drug research, or agency policy.

9. See step 7. Optimum infusion rate is determined by type of medication, its stability, and how irritating it is to vein.

10. Secure needle/tubing to skin adjacent to port with tape (see Procedure 31–6). Needleless cannula is secured with threaded guard, but tubing should be taped.

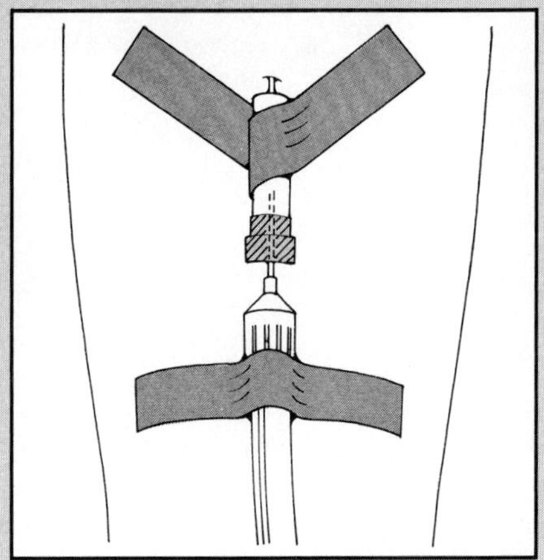

10. Taping or threaded guard prevents accidental separation of needle/tubing from heparin lock during infusion.

(continued)

PROCEDURE 22–18. (continued)

11. If a "flush" setup will be used, insert its needle (or needleless cannula) into heparin lock. Partially open the roller clamp on the flush line to infuse IV solution. If solution flows readily, insert needle (or needle-lock device) on secondary line into highest injection port on flush line and back-fill secondary tubing (see Procedure 22–17). Close roller clamp on secondary line. Secure secondary tubing with tape if needle-lock device not available.

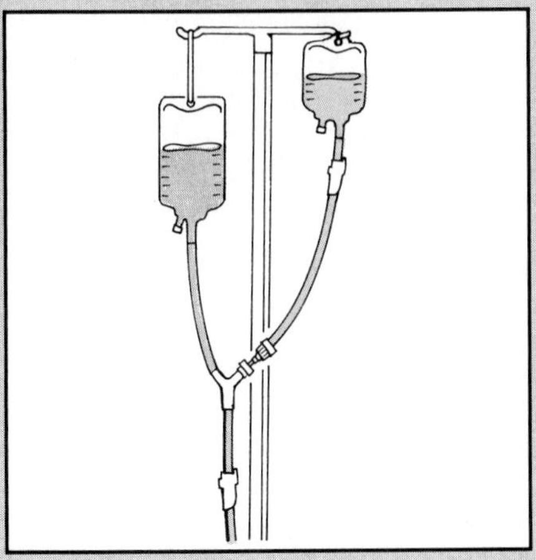

NOTE: If solution does not flow, remove needle. Obtain syringe with heparin flush solution or sterile saline and aspirate heparin lock for soft clots.

11. If solution in "flush" setup infuses readily, heparin lock is patent and drug can be infused.

12. After infusing several mL of "flush" solution, open roller clamp on secondary line. Regulate infusion with clamp on primary line (see Procedure 22–17).

12. See steps 9 to 11, above.

13. Assess the infusion, the site, and the client periodically during the infusion. Reregulate drip if necessary, or reposition limb to improve flow. If severe pain or swelling occurs at site, or other untoward effects occur, discontinue infusion and consult physician.

13. These actions promote early detection and correction of problems related to infusion mechanics and/or undesirable reactions to the medication.

14. When medication infusion is complete, allow several mL of "flush" solution to infuse. Then close roller clamp and withdraw needle/tubing. Remove and discard used needle (or needleless cannula) on flush line in specially labeled container. Replace with sterile 18-guage, 1-inch needle with cover or sterile, capped needleless cannula. Empty medication container and secondary tubing may remain connected to flush setup.

14. Flush solution clears medication from cannula. Needle is discarded rather than recapped to prevent needlestick injury to nurse. New needle maintains sterility of tubing and solution.

15. Cleanse heparin lock port as in step 7, above. Inject 1 mL of heparin flush solution into heparin lock.

15. See step 7, above. Heparin is an anticoagulant. When it fills the heparin lock and the IV cannula, clots are prevented from forming, even though no solution is flowing through the intravenous device.

16. If medication was infusing via primary tubing into heparin lock, remove needle/tubing and replace needle or needleless cannula, as in step 14, above. Then cleanse port as in step 7, and flush heparin lock using second syringe of sterile saline, followed by 1 mL of heparin flush solution.

16. See steps 7, 14, and 15, above. If medication is compatible with heparin, saline flush may be omitted.

17. If heparin lock is not used regularly for medications, heparin flush solution should be reinjected regularly according to agency policy.

17. See step 14, above.

RECORDING: Record administration of IV medications and solutions according to agency policy. Usually recording will be necessary on both the MAR and the I&O record. The heparin flush solution is also considered a medication and is recorded on the MAR. Narrative recording on nurse's notes may also be expected for some medications or if unexpected reaction to medication occurs.

become active participants in medication administration greatly facilitates their understanding and motivation, and may improve the effectiveness of the prescribed regimen.

When feasible, clients should participate in decisions regarding the scheduled times or methods of administration. Tailoring the medication regimen to clients' needs and life-style enhances self-esteem and may improve motivation to continue with the therapy. Clients also need to play an active role in the assessment of drug effects. A client who is knowledgeable about the expected therapeutic and undesirable effects of prescribed drugs may be capable of detecting subtle physiological changes or developments long before they become readily apparent to health care personnel. Collaboration with clients enables the physicians and nurses to modify or adjust a medication regimen to achieve maximum client benefit with a minimum of discomfort or undesirable effects.

Perioperative Nursing Care. Surgical intervention is often a component of the treatment of an acutely ill or injured client. Nurses play an important role enhancing well-being in all aspects of the care of surgical clients. **Perioperative nursing** is the name given to the many nursing activities performed before, during, and after surgery. The surgical experience is divided into three phases: preoperative, intraoperative, and postoperative.

Preoperative Phase. The preoperative phase begins when the decision is made that surgery is necessary, and extends until a client is safely transferred to the operating room. Nurses' primary function during the preoperative phase is to prepare clients both psychologically and physically for the surgical experience.

Preparing Clients Psychologically. Surgery can be a very frightening and stressful experience to clients and family members. They require accurate information about the purpose of the surgical procedure and what is to be expected throughout the perioperative period. Psychological preparation also includes meeting the specific learning needs of clients and family members in relation to postoperative care.

INFORMED CONSENT. Legally no invasive or surgical procedure can be performed unless clients understand the purpose of the procedure, what it involves, the expected results and possible risks, and any alternative treatments or procedures that might be available. Primary responsibility for informing clients and obtaining a consent for treatment rests with the surgeon; however, nurses often play an important supportive role in educating clients and clarifying information.

A consent form must be signed prior to the final preparations for surgery. The main purpose of obtaining an informed consent is to enable clients to become active participants in the decision-making process. With an understanding of the potential risks and benefits of the proposed surgery and any available alternatives, clients are able to make an informed decision and retain the right to control what happens to their bodies. For clients' consent to be valid, three conditions must be met: (1) clients must be capable of giving consent; (2) clients must have received sufficient information necessary to make an intelligent decision; and (3) the consent must be voluntarily given—not coerced.[102]

Although the surgeon is responsible for discussing the procedure with clients and obtaining the consent, nurses are often asked to serve as witnesses. As client advocates, nurses should assess clients' capability, understanding, and willingness to proceed with the planned surgical procedure. Nurses may clarify general information and provide support to clients; however, if a client has specific questions about the planned surgery or expresses doubts or hesitations, the surgeon should be notified. The legal and ethical considerations related to informed consent are discussed in Chapters 3 and 34.

PREOPERATIVE TEACHING. Education of clients and family members is an important preoperative nursing function. Preoperative teaching generally focuses on teaching the client effective measures to manage postoperative pain, and the physical activities that are necessary to prevent postoperative complications. Preoperative teaching allows clients to participate actively in the recovery process and enhances individual well-being by fostering a sense of personal control and accomplishment. A detailed discussion of preoperative teaching related to pain management was presented earlier in this chapter. Deep-breathing exercises, coughing exercises, leg exercises, and early ambulation are discussed in Chapter 27.

Preparing Clients Physically. The physical preparation of clients varies with the type of surgery, the surgeon's orders, and the special needs of the individual client. Certain nursing functions related to nutrition and hydration, hygiene and skin preparation, elimination, rest and sleep, care of valuables and prostheses, and preoperative assessment are appropriate for all surgical clients.

NUTRITION AND HYDRATION. Surgical clients are at risk for developing alterations in nutrition and hydration status as a result of inadequate preoperative intake or excessive intraoperative or postoperative losses. Because of the potential danger of clients vomiting and aspirating while under general anesthesia, they are generally required to fast at least 6 to 8 hours prior to surgery. Clients and family members must be informed of the importance of taking nothing by mouth (n.p.o.). Clients may rinse their mouths with water or mouthwash, and brush their teeth, as long as they do not swallow any fluids. If clients eat or drink during the fasting period, the surgeon must be notified.

HYGIENE AND SKIN PREPARATION. Adequate hygiene and skin preparation activities prior to surgery help to remove microorganisms from the skin and reduce the incidence of postoperative infection. Surgical skin preparation involves special cleansing of skin and sometimes removing hair from the areas surrounding the surgical site. The skin may be cleansed by scrubbing the operative site one or more times with an antimicrobial soap or solution. Often this can be done by clients in the shower the morning of or the evening prior to surgery.[112] Clients' nails should also be cleaned and polish from at least one nail is removed to allow circulatory assessment. Cosmetics must also be removed the day of surgery so that lips and skin are readily visible for circulatory assessment.

Removal of hair at the surgical site is no longer a standard practice. For many years, shaving the entire area surrounding the incision site was routine the evening prior to surgery. The purpose of shaving was to remove any microorganisms that resided in the body hair. Current Centers for Disease Control (CDC) guidelines recommend that unless the hair around the surgical site is so thick that it interferes with the surgical procedure, it should not be removed. The CDC also recommends that if hair removal is necessary, that it be done either by clipping or by using a depilatory cream rather than shaving.[113] Shaving, if performed at all today, is now most often done immediately prior to surgery—usually in the surgical holding area. This practice eliminates time for bacteria to grow in any small cuts that result from the shaving procedure.

ELIMINATION. Routine enemas prior to surgery are no longer prescribed, however, nurses should carefully assess clients preoperatively for needs related to elimination. Because the administration of anesthesia slows bowel activity, clients who have not had a bowel movement for several days prior to surgery may need an enema or suppository ordered preoperatively to help prevent problems with postoperative constipation.

Clients undergoing gastrointestinal or abdominal surgery always require bowel preparation. The surgeon may order cathartics and/or a series of cleansing enemas to empty the gastrointestinal tract. This prevents problems with postoperative constipation as peristalsis does not return for 24 to 48 hours after the bowel is handled. An empty bowel also reduces the risk of injury to the intestines during surgery and prevents contamination of the surgical wound if the bowel is opened or resected.

Nurses should ensure that clients empty their bladders prior to surgery. A Foley catheter is often inserted prior to surgery to prevent bladder distension and accidental injury, especially for clients having pelvic surgery. If a catheter is not ordered, clients should void just prior to the administration of preoperative medications.

REST AND SLEEP. Adequate rest and sleep are essential if clients are to cope successfully with the stress of surgery and heal properly. Nurses can promote rest by employing a variety of physical and psychological comfort and relaxation measures, many of which were discussed earlier in this chapter. Encouraging clients to express fears and concerns regarding the impending surgery, and answering questions in an honest and supportive manner, may reduce anxiety and enable clients to relax. See Chapter 28 for a discussion of nursing measures to promote sleep. Often, surgeons order a sedative the night prior to surgery to assist clients to get a good night's sleep. Preoperative medications are frequently ordered the day of surgery to sedate clients, reduce respiratory secretions, and provide analgesia. Typically these medications are administered 45 minutes to 1 hour prior to surgery.

CARE OF VALUABLES AND PROSTHESES. Prior to surgery nurses secure all valuables and prostheses and make provisions for their safe-keeping. It is preferred that valuables such as money and jewelry be given to family members; if this is not possible they should be labeled and locked in a secure place. If clients are reluctant to remove a wedding band or religious ornaments, these may be allowed if taped securely in place. However, wedding bands must be removed if there is any danger that clients will experience swelling in the hand or fingers.

All prostheses (eyeglasses, contact lenses, artificial limbs, etc) must be removed prior to surgery. These items should also be labeled and stored for safekeeping. Nurses should also check for the presence of loose teeth or removable bridgework. These can become dislodged and obstruct breathing during anesthesia procedures.

PREOPERATIVE ASSESSMENT. Prior to transfer to the operating room, nurses are responsible for complete assessment of clients. In most institutions a preoperative checklist is used to ensure that all procedures required for surgery have been completed. In addition to verifying the preparation measures that have already been discussed (removal of prosthesis, skin preparation, informed consent, npo, etc), nurses verify preoperative lab work results, obtain and record vital signs, and verify that the client's identification bracelet is correct and secure. The recorded vital signs are utilized as baseline data to which to compare client responses during and after the surgical procedure. Preoperative abnormalities in the vital signs, such as an elevated temperature, should be reported immediately. The preoperative checklist, client chart, and operative permit accompany clients to the operating room.

Intraoperative Phase. The intraoperative phase begins when the client enters the operating room and ends with admission to the postanesthesia area (recovery room). Operating room personnel function as a team to meet the needs of clients undergoing surgery. Each member of the team is responsible for specific aspects of client care. Major nursing functions include protecting clients from injury, assisting with the surgical procedure, and maintaining accurate documentation.

Protecting the Client. Anesthetized clients are highly vulnerable to injury. Because clients are unresponsive, they are totally dependent upon the operating room personnel to meet all of the basic physiological and safety needs. Protecting clients from injury during transfer and positioning for the surgical procedure is one aspect of protective nursing care. Clients are positioned to maintain optimal visualization and access for the surgeon, good airway and monitoring access for the anesthesiologist, and physiological safety for clients.

Some surgical procedures require that clients be placed in unusual positions; however, nurses must make every effort to maintain clients in correct physiological alignment and protect them from unnecessary pressure, abrasions, or other injuries. Care must be taken to avoid extending any joints beyond the limits of normal range of motion, to prevent neuromuscular impairments or damage. Anesthetized clients are so relaxed that it is relatively easy to place them in a position that they normally could not assume. Because surgical clients are often in one position for several hours, padding of bony prominences and careful alignment is critical.

All members of the surgical team including nurses protect clients through meticulous attention to sterile technique.

Assisting with Procedures. Usually there are two designated nursing roles in the operating room: the scrub nurse and the circulating nurse. The scrub nurse assists the surgeon by providing sterile instruments and supplies (Fig. 22–28). Because such a wide variety of specialized instruments are used, scrub nurses must have extensive knowledge of all instruments and their use, must be able to anticipate which instrument the surgeon requires, and must be able to pass it quickly and smoothly without disrupting the surgeon's concentration or technique. Scrub nurses are also responsible for disposing of soiled gauze sponges, needles, and instruments. Accurate counts of the number of sponges and other instruments are necessary to ensure that none are left inside a client.

The circulating nurse functions as an assistant to the scrub nurse and the surgeon. The circulating nurse's responsibilities include assisting with positioning clients and applying sterile drapes, assisting the scrub nurse and surgeon to don sterile gowns and gloves, obtaining and opening sterile supplies, adjusting operating room lights, maintaining documentation, and assisting with the counting of sponges and instruments at the end of the procedure.

Maintaining Documentation. Throughout the intraoperative period, the circulating nurse must maintain accurate documentation of procedures performed by operating room personnel. Typical documentation includes client positioning, medications administered, sponges and instrument counts, client data such as vital signs, presence of dressings or drains, and types of safety devices used. This intraoperative data is useful to other health care personnel who care for clients postoperatively.

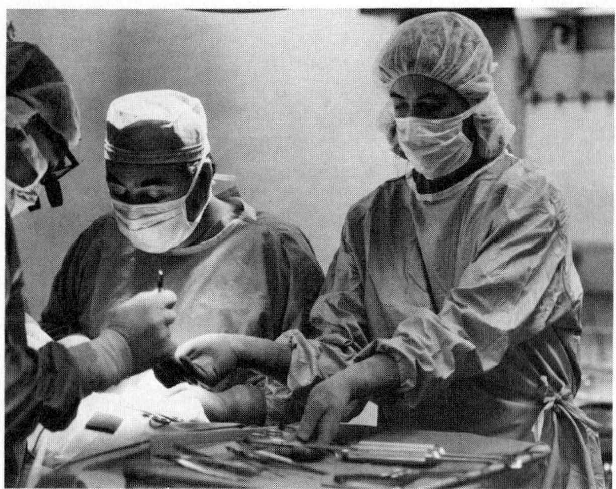

Figure 22–28. The scrub nurse assists the surgeons in the operating room.

Postoperative Phase. Postoperative nursing care is often complex because of the multitude of physiological changes that clients experience as a result of anesthesia and surgery. The focus of postoperative nursing care is maintaining physiological functioning, providing for client safety and comfort, and preventing postoperative complications. The postoperative phase is usually divided into two stages: the immediate postoperative stage and the ongoing recovery stage.

Immediate Postoperative Stage. After surgery, clients are immediately transferred to the postanesthesia room (PAR), also commonly referred to as the postanesthesia care unit (PACU) or recovery room (RR). Recovery room nurses are skilled in client assessment and monitoring. During a client's stay in the postanesthesia area, assessment is continuous (Fig. 22–29). Clients are carefully monitored until their physiological status is stabilized and they can be safely transferred to the general surgical unit. Critically ill clients are often transferred directly from the operating room to an intensive care unit. Continuous assessment of clients includes frequent assessment of respiratory status, cardiovascular status, neurological status, fluid balance, wound condition, and client comfort and safety.

ASSESSING RESPIRATORY STATUS. Recovery room nurses assess clients' respiratory rate, rhythm, and depth, as well

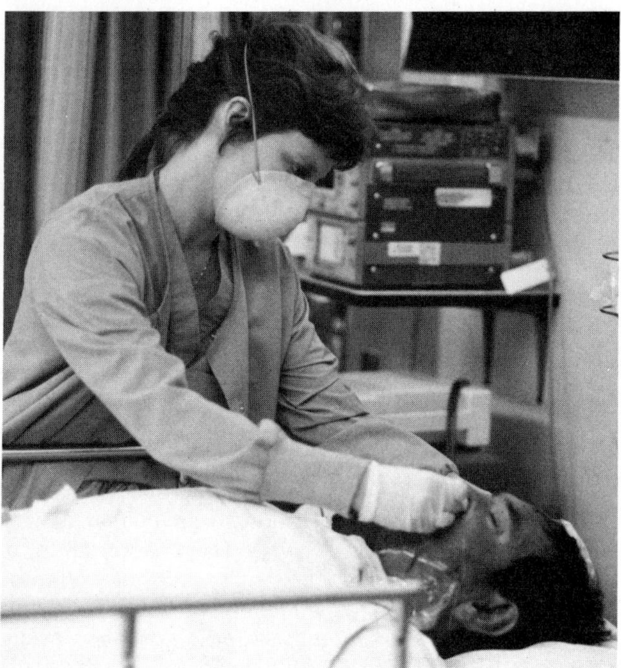

Figure 22–29. Recovery room nurse provides constant assessment and care for clients recovering from the effects of anesthesia.

as monitoring breath sounds, chest wall expansion, and color of mucous membranes. Artificial oral or nasal airways are often left in place to maintain patent air passages until normal reflexes return and the client is able to control the tongue, swallow, and cough. See Chapter 27 for a discussion of airway equipment.

Airway obstruction is the most common recovery room emergency. It may be caused by a number of conditions including accumulation of mucous secretions, obstruction by the tongue, aspiration of emesis, laryngospasm, or laryngeal edema. Nursing measures to promote airway patency include positioning clients on one side with the neck slightly extended to prevent aspiration or occlusion of the pharynx by the tongue. The administration of oxygen, suctioning of excessive secretions, and initiation of coughing and deep-breathing exercises when clients are responsive also help to promote adequate tissue oxygenation.

ASSESSING CARDIOVASCULAR STATUS. Careful assessment of the client's cardiovascular status, including the blood pressure, heart rate, and rhythm, is done at least every 15 minutes throughout the recovery period. Often electronic equipment that performs continuous assessment is used. Postoperative vital signs are compared to baseline data collected during the preoperative phase. Significant differences between baseline and postoperative readings, or changes in vital sign status, should be reported immediately.

Perfusion is assessed by examining the color of the nail beds and the skin. Pale, cyanotic, and cool skin may be a sign of circulatory problems. Peripheral pulses should be checked in clients who have had vascular surgery or who have casts or other restrictive devices on an extremity. Pulses distal to the injury or surgical area should be compared with the pulses in the unaffected extremity. A more detailed circulatory assessment can be found in Chapter 16.

Hemorrhage is a common circulatory problem in the postoperative period. Internal hemorrhage usually results in the operative site becoming tight and distended. External hemorrhage is manifested by excessive bloody drainage on dressings and bedclothes, or through surgically placed drains. Classic vital sign changes reflective of shock (increased pulse and respiratory rates, restlessness, decreased blood pressure, pallor, and cool clammy skin) are found with either type of hemorrhage. Any indicators of hemorrhage should be reported to the surgeon immediately.

ASSESSING NEUROLOGICAL STATUS. Assessment of clients' level of consciousness is an important component of post-anesthesia care. The use of general anesthetics results in a complete loss of reflexes and consciousness. As the effects of anesthesia wear off, clients demonstrate return of neurological function in the following order: (1) responds to stimuli (loud noise or touch), (2) drowsy, (3) awake but not oriented, and (4) awake and oriented. Nurses assess pupil and gag reflexes, and voluntary activty, and arouse clients by calling their names in a normal tone of voice. Clients are oriented through repeated explanations that the surgery is over and this is the recovery room. The amount of time necessary for recovery from anesthesia is determined by the kind of anesthetic agent used, the dosage, and individual client response to it.

ASSESSING FLUID BALANCE. Postsurgical clients must be monitored carefully for signs of fluid and electrolyte imbalances. Accurate measurement of intake and output helps monitor renal and circulatory status. Maintenance of ordered intravenous fluids and/or blood products provides clients with the only source of intake during the immediate postoperative period. Careful attention to IV flow rates and insertion sites prevents potential problems with fluid volume excess or deficit. All sources of client output are also carefully monitored. Nurses must assess and record the color, consistency, and amount of drainage from all tubes and suction equipment. Nurses also ensure that all tubes or drains are patent and that all equipment is functioning properly.

ASSESSING WOUND CONDITION. Most surgical wounds are covered with a sterile dressing in the operating room to protect the incision and to collect drainage. Recovery room nurses inspect the surgical dressing and note the color, consistency, and amount of any visible drainage. Large amounts of bright red drainage may be indicative of hemorrhage and should be reported immediately. If a dressing becomes saturated, drainage may ooze down the client's side and pool on the bedclothes. It is important that the nurse check under the client for such wound drainage. Wound assessment and care is discussed in Chapter 24.

ASSESSING CLIENT COMFORT AND SAFETY. Attention to clients' comfort and safety needs is an important aspect of recovery room care. As clients regain consciousness, pain is often prominent. Severe pain may make clients extremely restless and cause changes in vital signs. Because narcotics are potentiated by anesthetics, reduced dosages of narcotic analgesics are often administered in the recovery room. Clients must be assessed carefully for their response to the medication and their need for additional pain relief as the effects of anesthesia wear off.

Other measures related to physical and emotional comfort and safety are also important. Clients often complain of being cold as they awaken. Many intraoperative factors influence clients' temperature, including the cold operating room temperature, the exposure of clients' internal body surfaces, the infusion of cool IV fluids, and the effects of some anesthetics. Nurses should provide clients with warmed blankets and regularly assess their body temperatures. Frequency of assessment depends on client condition and surgeon orders. It is critical that the assessments be made as often as client condition requires. Positioning in correct alignment, turning at least every 2 hours, and the use of siderails are other means of promoting physical safety.

Ongoing Recovery: Facilitating Normal Physiological Functioning. Postoperative nursing measures after transfer from the recovery room to the general surgical unit assist clients to regain normal physiological functioning and prevent common postoperative complications. These measures include:

- *Maintaining respiratory function.* Prevention of respiratory complications requires adequate lung expansion and aggressive pulmonary hygiene measures. Clients are encouraged to do deep-breathing exercises every 1 to 2 hours while awake. Active participation by the client is essential for optimum lung expansion. If secretions accumulate coughing is added to routine care. As discussed under supportive care, adequate preoperative preparation of clients facilitates active participation. Careful attention to adequate pain relief measures also enhance client participation. Clients may also be encouraged to use incentive spirometers to facilitate lung expansion. Suctioning may be necessary for clients who are unable to mobilize and expectorate secretions. (See Chap. 27.)
- *Preventing circulatory stasis.* Frequent changes of position and early mobilization of surgical clients facilitate circulation and prevents the pooling of blood. Leg exercises and the application of antiemboli stockings may also prevent concentration of blood elements and the formation of clots (see Chap. 27).
- *Maintaining fluid balance.* Maintaining intravenous fluid intake as ordered is an important aspect of postoperative recovery. Clients receive continuous IV fluids until they can take in sufficient fluids by mouth to meet daily fluid requirements. When bowel sounds are noted, oral intake is initiated in small amounts, beginning with clear liquids.
- *Promoting adequate nutrition.* Dietary intake following surgery is dependent upon the extent of the surgery and the organs involved. Clients who have abdominal or gastrointestinal surgery may be given nothing by mouth and maintained on intravenous fluids for several days to allow peristalsis to resume. Generally these clients have a nasogastric tube in place. Other clients usually progress from a diet of clear liquids, to full liquids, to a light diet, to a regular diet within a few days. Postoperative clients benefit from liberal fluid and protein intake when normal gastrointestinal function returns. Healing is also enhanced by vitamins A and C and zinc. See also Chapters 24 and 25. Gastric intubation, the insertion of a tube into the stomach via either the nose, mouth, or a gastrostomy opening, prevents gastric distension, nausea, and vomiting associated with stasis of gastrointestinal secretions because of absent or diminished peristalsis. Nasogastric (NG) tubes remove gastric contents through direct suction, called decompression. Negative pressure may be generated via wall suction or portable suction units (Fig. 22–30). Tubes commonly used to maintain gastric decompression include the Levin tube (a single-lumen tube) and the Salem sump tube (a double-lumen tube) (Figs. 22–31 and 22–32). Procedure 22–19 describes the management of nasogastric suction. To maintain effective decompression, the nasogastric tube must be patent. Procedure 22–20 describes the technique for irrigating a nasogastric tube to maintain patency. Nasogastric tubes are required until peristalsis resumes. For most clients the tubes can be discontinued and oral intake resumed 1 to 3 days postoperatively. The initial diet is clear liquids with advancement to a regular diet as tolerated.
- *Promoting normal elimination.* The return of peristalsis is determined by the assessment of bowel sounds. Typically bowel function is slowed in the immediate postoperative period. Problems with nausea can be avoided in clients who do not have NG tubes by limiting oral intake to small sips of fluids and progressing dietary intake slowly. Early ambulation and adequate hydration facilitate normal bowel functioning and prevent problems with postoperative constipation.
- Normal urinary function may also be diminished during the immediate postoperative period. Aldosterone production increases as a response to surgery so the body conserves fluid. Moreover anesthetic and narcotic agents may reduce sensation of bladder fullness and impair bladder tone. Nurses must assess all clients for urinary retention and clients who do not have indwelling catheters for difficulties with urination. Postoperative clients who have not voided within 6 to 8 hours after surgery must be monitored closely for bladder distension. Nursing measures that facilitate urinary elimination include assisting clients into as normal a position as possible, providing privacy, and maintaining adequate hydration (see also Chap. 26). If a client has not voided within 8 hours of the surgery, bladder catheterization (also discussed in Chap. 26) may be necessary. Accurate intake and output records should be maintained on all surgical clients for at least 48 hours.

PREVENTING INFECTION. As discussed earlier in this chapter, surgical clients are at high risk for developing an infection. Common sites of infection include the bladder, lungs, and surgical wound. Many of the postoperative nursing measures already discussed protect clients against infection. Adequate hydration and the promotion of urinary elimination help to prevent bladder infections. Strict attention to sterile technique when catheterizing clients also prevents the introduction of pathogens into the body. Aggressive pulmonary hygiene through the use of hourly deep-breathing exercises, incentive spirometry, and early ambulation promote pulmonary expansion, remove pooled secretions, and prevent the development of postoperative pneumonia.

Surgical wounds generally are covered with a sterile dressing to prevent contamination and to collect drainage. Nurses are responsible for protecting the incision and promoting the healing process. Strict attention to sterile technique during dressing changes, maintaining patency of surgical drains, and frequent handwashing when caring for clients help prevent the transmission of pathogens. Frequent assessment of the surgical site is necessary for the detection of early signs and symptoms of infection. A detailed description of wound care can be found in Chapter 24.

PROMOTING COMFORT AND REST. As the effects of anesthesia wear off, clients may become increasingly uncomfortable. Incisional pain is one source of client discomfort, but tension and irritation from tubes, tight dressings, muscular aches from positioning in the operating room, and gastric discomfort all may contribute to clients' distress.

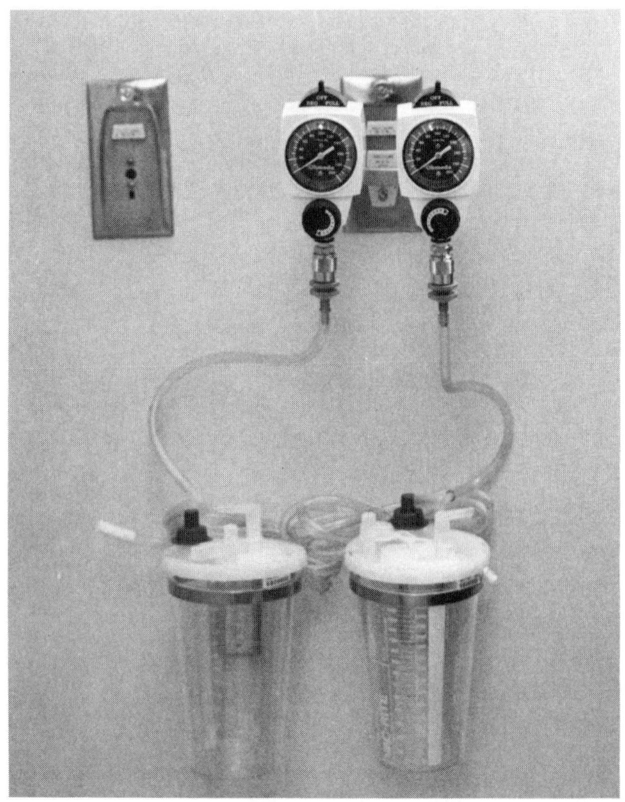

A

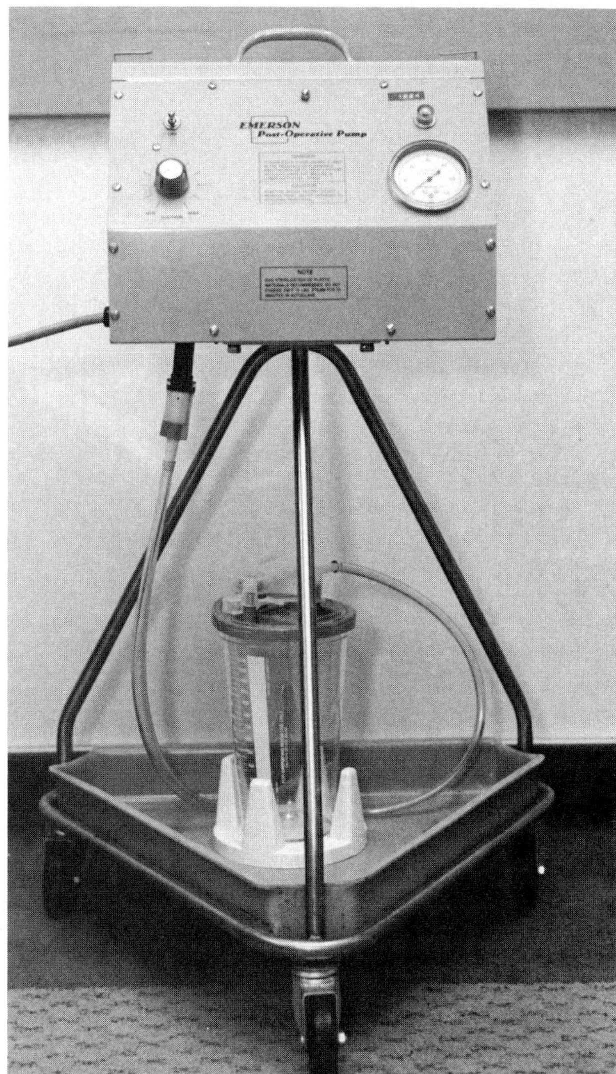

B

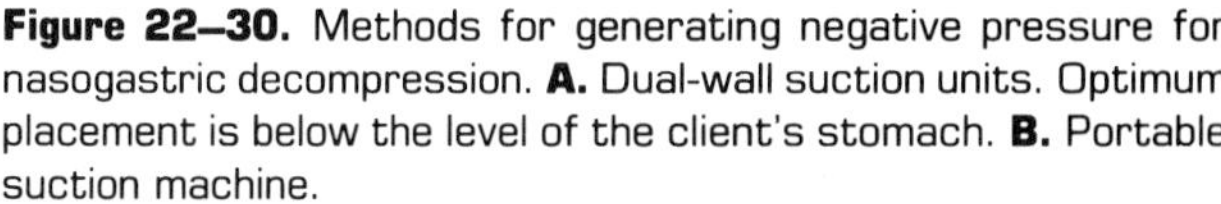

Figure 22–30. Methods for generating negative pressure for nasogastric decompression. **A.** Dual-wall suction units. Optimum placement is below the level of the client's stomach. **B.** Portable suction machine.

Nursing comfort measures such as relaxation, imagery, diversion, and administration of medications were discussed earlier in this chapter. Other interventions related to the relief of severe pain can be found in Chapter 29. Adequate pain management and the promotion of rest is a vital part of postoperative nursing care. Clients in distress will be unwilling to participate actively in the postoperative exercises and activities that are necessary for recovery.

MEETING THE PSYCHOLOGICAL NEEDS OF SURGICAL CLIENTS. As discussed earlier in this chapter, the surgical experience may have a profound effect on client self-esteem and body image. The presence of wounds, bulky dressings, multiple tubes, and visible drainage containers may be distressing for some clients. If the surgical procedure produces permanent changes in bodily appearance or functioning, both client and family members may have a difficult time adjusting.

Nurses should be alert for signs or behaviors that indicate problems with self-esteem or adjustment. Encouraging clients and/or family members to participate in nursing care activities as soon as possible enhances self-confidence and may prevent potential problems. Maintenance of hygiene practices and a pleasant environment foster client well-being. Encouraging clients to discuss feelings related to body image or role performance with nurses and family members also contributes to the maintenance of positive self-esteem and self-worth.

Rehabilitative Care

Nursing measures related to well-being extend beyond the acute care setting to include a focus on rehabilitation. Nurses assist clients to develop a long-term plan to facilitate health promotion and optimal client well-being. Support and education of clients and family members is an impor-

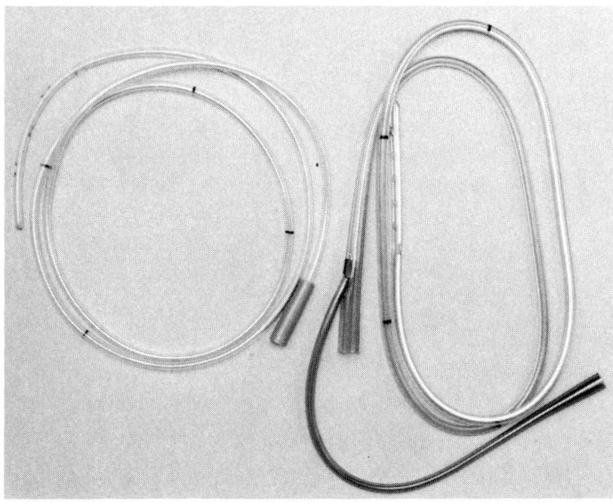

Figure 22–31. Nasogastric tubes used for gastric decompression. Left, Levin tube. Right, Salem sump tube (note "pigtail").

tant aspect of rehabilitative care. The most important ingredient in rehabilitative care is the expression of caring by the caregiver to clients.

A long-term plan of care to promote client health and well-being may include services provided in a variety of health care settings such as rehabilitation centers, adult day care, respite care, home health care, long-term care facilities, and hospice care. Rehabilitation centers are designed to assist individuals in returning to their optimal level of physical and emotional functioning. They facilitate client life-style changes needed because of loss of a body part such as amputation or loss of physical function such as occurs with a stroke. The goal of rehabilitative care is restoring individuals to their previous level of health or the maximum level that is possible for them. Rehabilitation is an educational process that promotes self-responsibility. Clients must participate actively for the process to be effective.

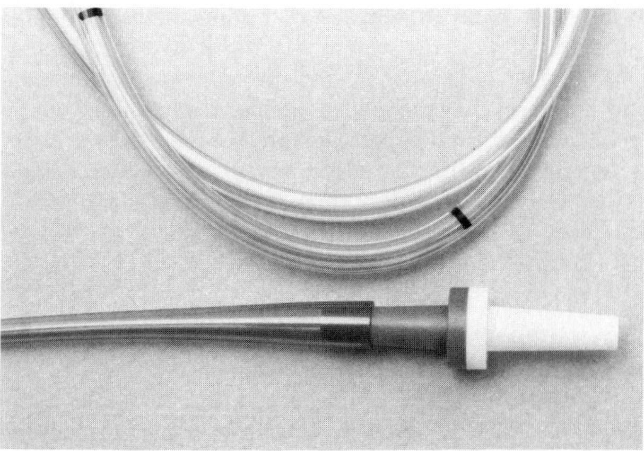

Figure 22–32. Antireflux valve for use with a Salem sump tube.

Some adults need special health care services to maintain independence. Adult day care provides an alternative to institutionalization for clients who need limited amounts of assistance in daily activities. Day care centers provide health services for clients able to remain at home at night. They are also used by families caring for clients at home while continuing their employment or other routine activities. This is an ideal setting for health education to promote wellness life-style behaviors in older adults.

Respite care refers to health services provided intermittently for a a dependent family member who is routinely cared for in the home by family. This is a frequently much needed support enabling a dependent family member to remain in the home and avoid institutionalization. Respite care enables permanent caregivers to have a rest from the daily responsibilities of caring for a dependent family member. It enables caregivers to do things that they would otherwise be unable to do like take a vacation with spouse and children. These temporary health services can be provided in clients' homes or in an institution.

Recovering adults' independence and well-being can also be supported through use of home health care and homemaker services. Home care services are used for clients who need care that family members cannot provide without assistance or additional education. It also enables client care for health problems that are not covered by insurance in the acute care setting or for clients with limited financial resources. Nurses in the home can assess client and family adaptation to long-term illness, teach self-care, counsel client and family regarding adaptation to chronic illness, and collaborate with client and family in planning and administering direct care. Homemaker services provide support for clients who need assistance with self-care and activities of daily living.

Institutionalization in a long-term care facility may be necessary for some adults with declining health and increasing dependence. These facilities provide extended care including personal and psychosocial services. A variety of levels of service are available within long-term care including independent living, intermediate care, and personal care for clients that are no longer able to care for themselves without direct skilled assistance. Whatever the level of care, these institutions become "home" for these clients. Clients and family may need support as they make the decision for institutional care.

Nurses can assist clients and families to choose a long-term facility by helping them define their options and then supporting a choice that matches clients' personality while meeting the clients' physical needs. Participation of client and family is vital to minimizing the stress of such a significant life change. Institutional care affects changes in interpersonal relationships. An important intervention during this transition is fostering clients' personal support systems. Nurses can counsel clients and family regarding the feelings of anger and guilt that underlie many family interactions as a result of the transition to long-term care. Nurses

(*Text continues on page 879.*)

PROCEDURE 22–19. MANAGING NASOGASTRIC SUCTION

PURPOSE: To maintain patency of nasogastric tube so decompression of stomach is maintained, preventing postoperative abdominal distension, nausea, and vomiting. To promote client comfort and tissue integrity while NG tube is in place.

EQUIPMENT: Regulator and gauge for wall suction or portable suction machine, connecting tubing and collection container, syringe with tip that fits tightly into lumen of NG tube (usually 50-mL size), water-soluble lubricant, cotton-tipped applicators, lemon glycerine swabs or mouthwash, 1-inch hypoallergenic adhesive tape, adhesive remover, and catheter plug for ambulatory clients.

ACTION	RATIONALE
1. Check physician's order for type, amount, and duration of suction to be maintained. NOTE: High suction is likely to damage gastric mucosa unless tube is a dougle-lumen tube with an air vent such as a Salem sump tube.	1. Maintainance of gastric decompression is not an independent nursing function. Suction orders may be for high (80 to 100 mm Hg) or low (30 to 40 mm Hg); intermittent or continuous. A specific schedule for suction may also be ordered.
2. Discuss the purpose of the suction and associated assessments and trouble-shooting, usual sensations, desired client participation, and expected benefits with the client.	2. Client will be less anxious and more willing to participate if reasons and expected benefits of procedure are clear.

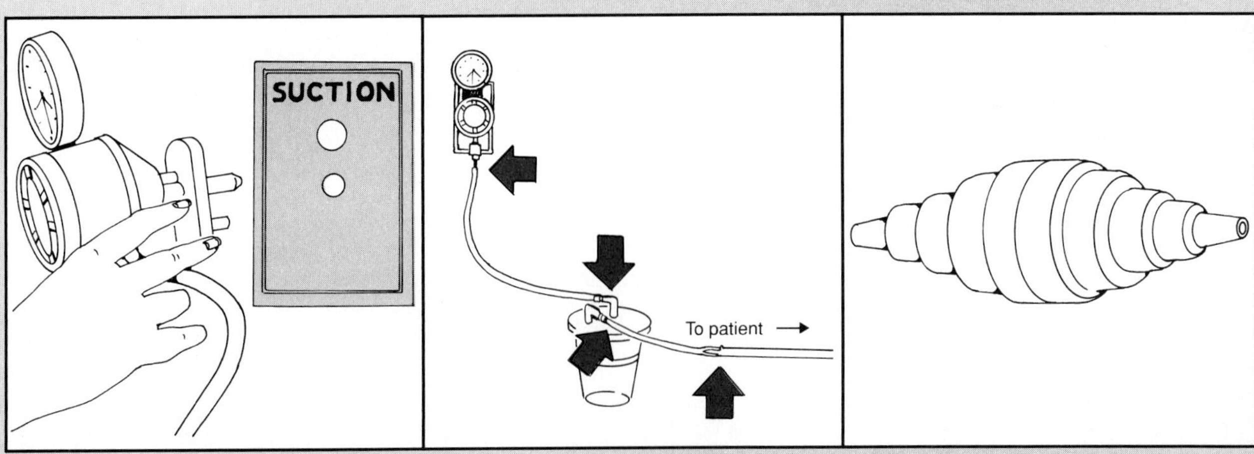

ACTION	RATIONALE
3. Attach NG tube to connecting tubing, and then attach tubing to suction container and suction source, making sure that all connections are tight. Turn on suction as ordered. A five-way adapter may be needed to join NG to connecting tubing.	3. Connecting tubing allows client to move freely in bed without pulling on the NG tube. Tight connections prevent pressure leaks, which decrease the effectiveness of the suction apparatus.
4. When system is on, assess for proper functioning at least q2h:	4. Client is receiving no benefit if system is not functioning.

(continued)

PROCEDURE 22–19. (continued)

a. Any fluid in the connecting tubing should be moving toward the suction source.

a. Lack of fluid movement suggests tube is blocked or placed incorrectly. Check for kinks in tube. See also step 5.

b. There should be no leaking of fluid at connection points or from the air vent ("pigtail") of a Salem sump tube.

b. Leaks suggest a block and ineffective connections. Reflux from pigtail has several causes; see step 6.

c. There should be no sounds of air movement, except with Salem sump, which should produce a hissing sound at the pigtail opening.

c. Air intake sounds at sites other than the pigtail decrease effectiveness of suction in the stomach. Recheck all connections.

d. If intermittent suction is ordered, suction pump should turn on and off in a cyclic fashion; cycles last several seconds.

d. Lack of cycling indicates no suction is occurring. Client will become distended, nauseous, and may vomit. Obtain new suction equipment.

5. To troubleshoot a blocked tube:
   a. Check suction equipment. Disconnect from NG tube. If liquid in tubing then moves toward collection container, suction is working. (End of tubing may be placed in a glass of water to test if no drainage is present in the tubing.) If water does not move, tighten all connections and recheck.

5a. Mechanical malfunction is relatively easy to rule out with minimal trauma to client, so it should be done first. If all connections are tight and liquid does not move when tubing is separated from the smaller lumen of the NG tube, obtain a new suction unit.

   b. If collection container is full of drainage or plastic liner is bulging with air, turn off suction and empty container. (Drainage should be measured before discarding in toilet.)

b. Overfilled collection container may decrease suction efficiency, may trigger shut off valve.

   c. With suction off, place stethoscope just below the xyphoid process, then inject 15 mL of air via pigtail (separate NG from connecting tube to inject if single-lumen tube). A whooshing or popping sound indicates tube is in the stomach. Clearing the pigtail may also restore suction.

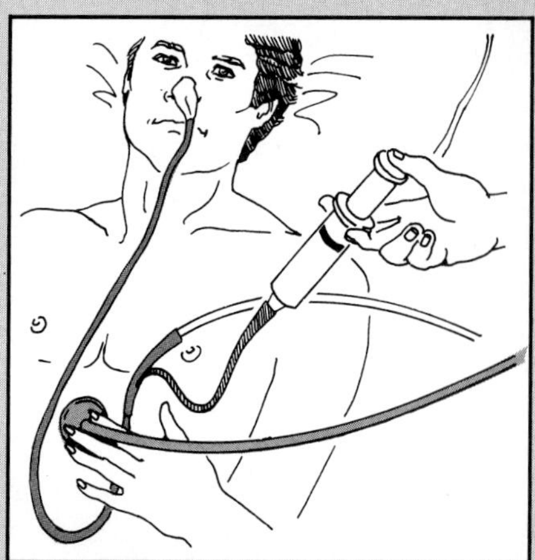

c. Sound will interfere with placement check. Air movement from the tube into the stomach can be heard with this stethoscope placement. If no sound is heard, tube is not in the stomach. Advance tube 1 to 2 inches and recheck. Pigtail prevents tube from adhering to mucous membrane because air intake via vent reduces negative pressure at inlet ports of tube. If vent is blocked, adherence to mucosa may occur, interfering with suction.

(continued)

PROCEDURE 22–19. (continued)

d. Reposition client to the opposite side, turn on suction. Reposition tube so pigtail is above level of stomach after position change (see step 6).

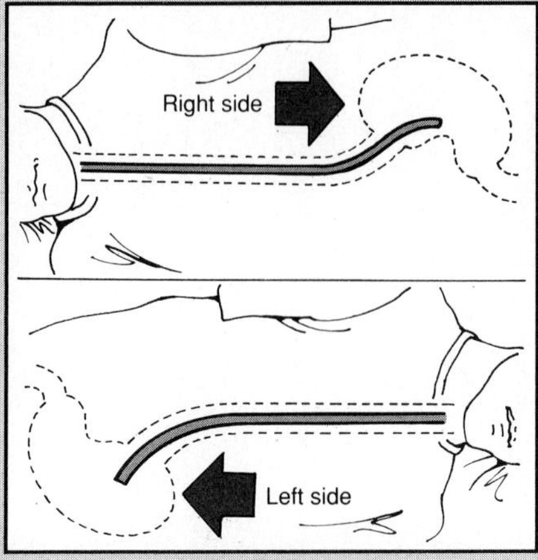

d. Client position change alters the angle/placement of tube in stomach. It may move tube away from mucosa. This is not effective if suction is on, as tube will adhere to mucosa.

e. If client has not had gastric surgery, tube may also be rotated and/or advanced or retracted 1 to 2 inches before suction is turned on. (Tape must be removed and reapplied.)

e. These measures also change the angle or position of the tube in the stomach. Movement of tube may disrupt gastric sutures; consult with surgeon before changing position of the tube.

f. Irrigate NG (see Procedure 22–20).

6. To correct reflux of gastric contents via pigtail:

6. Reflux occurs because of pressure gradients created by changes in relative heights of two fluid containers (stomach and collection containers) connected by a fluid-filled tube.

a. Pin the NG tube to the client's gown so that the air vent is above the level of the stomach—if client is side-lying, NG should be pinned to the higher, not the dependent, shoulder. Pin NG to the opposite shoulder when client turns to other side.)

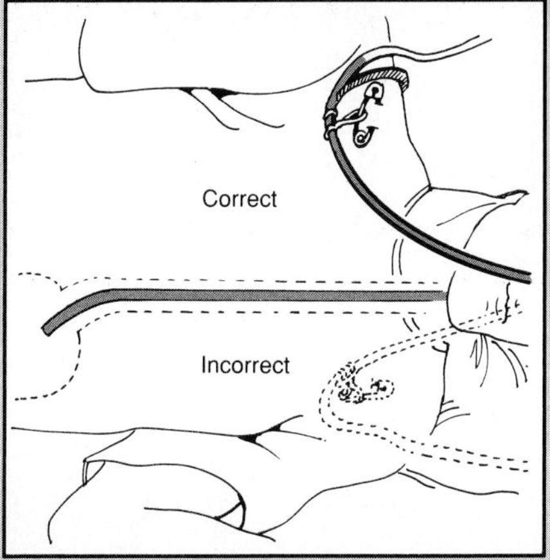

a. Gravity prevents fluid in stomach from flowing out of vent. If vent is lower than stomach, syphon effect (movement of fluids from higher to lower level without external suction) will cause reflux out of vent.

(continued)

PROCEDURE 22–19. (continued)

b. Keep the collection container below the level of the stomach. It may be necessary to obtain an extension for tubing connecting drainage container to wall suction.

b. Fluid levels in two connected containers tend to equalize. If the collection container is higher, fluid will rise in the air vent to seek the level of the container.

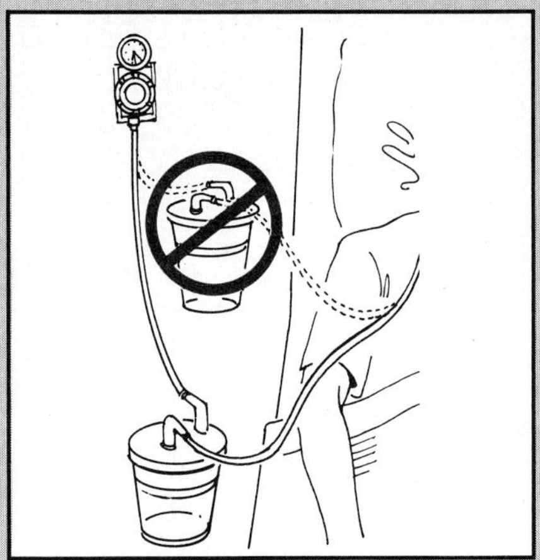

c. Maintain patency of both lumina: irrigate drainage lumen (see Procedure 22–20); inject air into air vent. Never occlude the air vent to stop reflux.

NOTE: An antireflux valve may be used to prevent spills, if available in your agency (see Fig. 22–32).

c. Blocked suction lumen will prevent air flow via vent and cause liquid to rise in vent to the level of the block. Positive pressure of air injection clears fluid from vent. If vent is occluded, mucosal damage is likely.

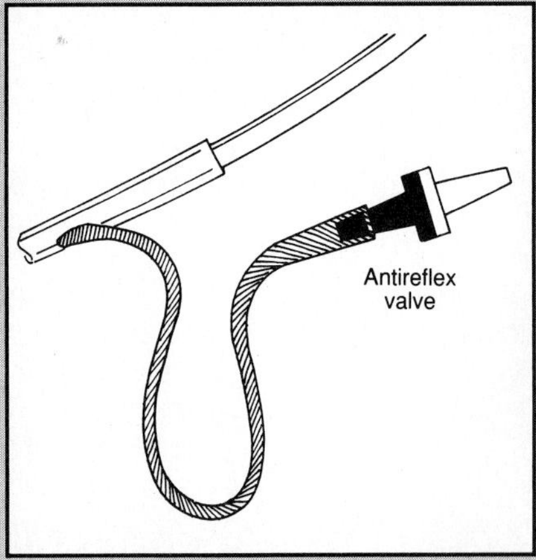

(continued)

PROCEDURE 22–19. (continued)

7. Supply clients with materials of preference for lubricating mouth: toothbrush/toothpaste, lemon glycerine swabs, NaCl gargle, iced one-half-strength mouthwash, ice chips, chewing gum, lozenges, or hard candy. Offer emollient for lips. Provide mouth care for weak or unconscious clients at least q2h (see Procedure 24–6). Check with physician to verify whether any of the lubrication techniques are contraindicated.

7. Clients with NG tubes with suction are n.p.o.; therefore, secretion of saliva is decreased, causing discomfort and cracking of lips. Tube may also irritate throat mucosa. Mouth care increases saliva production and provides supplemental lubrication to mouth, throat, and lips.

8. Assist client to clean nares with moist cotton-tipped applicators prn. Provide water-soluble lubricant for nares.

8. Mucus production in the nose is increased because the tube is an irritant. Mucosa may also be eroded because of friction caused by movement of the tube. Dried mucus around the tube increases irritation. Lubricant decreases friction. Water-soluble lubricant is preferred for the nose because it will not cause irritation if accidentlly aspirated into the lungs.

9. Retape tube to nose prn (see Procedure 25–2). Remove adhesive residue, if any, with adhesive remover. Recheck tube placement.

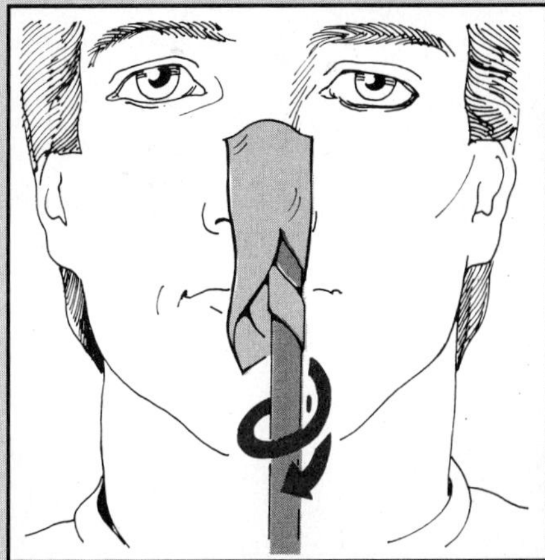

NOTE: Slight repositioning of tube in nares before retaping will change its point of contact with the nares and the throat, decreasing irritation.

9. Skin oils decrease effectiveness of adhesives and may produce a gummy residue, which is not water soluble. Cleaning and retaping promotes comfort and maintains tube placement. Manipulation of tube during care may displace tube, so placement should be rechecked.

(continued)

PROCEDURE 22–19. (continued)

10. If client is ambulatory, suction may be discontinued during ambulation. Disconnect NG from connecting tubing; plug NG with catheter plug. Turn off suction. Be sure pigtail remains above stomach level during ambulation. Resume suction as ordered when ambulation is completed.

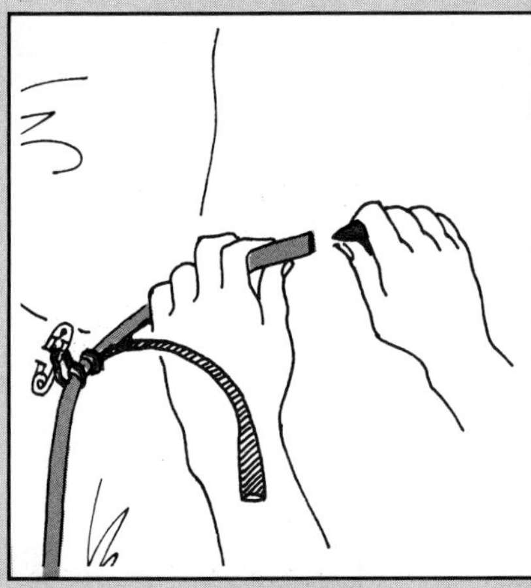

10. Short periods without decompression will not cause distension, but secretions will move from stomach out of tube via suction lumen and/or pigtail if end of tube is below level of stomach. (See step 5, above.)

11. At least q8h, assess:
    a. Abdomen for distension and bowel sounds. (Turn off suction to assess for bowel sounds.)

11a. Abdominal distension indicates build-up of gastrointestinal secretions. Suction is used to prevent this, so suction apparatus should be checked if distension occurs. Presence of bowel sounds in a postoperative client indicates suction is no longer needed, as secretions will be moved via peristalsis.

    b. Signs and symptoms of hydrogen, chloride, and potassium depletion (see Chap. 31).

b. Gastric secretions are rich in hydrogen, chloride, and potassium, which are removed by suction. Inadequate IV replacement of these electrolytes may result in deficits.

    c. Measure and assess color and consistency of drainage. Normal gastric drainage is of slightly mucoid consistency and yellow- or dark-green in color.

c. Changes in drainage may indicate complications or improvement in client's condition. Amount of secretions is expected to decrease as GI function returns.

    d. pH and/or hematest may also be ordered.

NOTE: Report presence of drainage that is frankly bloody or with coffee-ground color.

d. Occult blood may indicate damage to gastric mucosa. Some blood is expected if gastric surgery was performed.

RECORDING: Document that suction was maintained as ordered. Describe any problems encountered and action taken to correct them. Record all assessment findings and action taken, if any. Drainage is considered output and is recorded on I&O records.

PROCEDURE 22–20. IRRIGATING A NASOGASTRIC TUBE

PURPOSE: To clear nasogastric tube of obstruction, so decompression of stomach is maintained, preventing postoperative abdominal distension, nausea, and vomitting.

EQUIPMENT: Irrigation set, normal saline or tap water, and disposable waterproof underpad.

ACTION

1. Check physician's order or agency policy for type and amount of solution to be used for irrigation. Normal saline or tap water may be specified. Obtain necessary equipment. NG irrigation is a clean, not a sterile, procedure so equipment may be kept in room and reused for a 24-hour period.
2. Discuss the purpose of the irrigation, associated assessments and trouble-shooting, usual sensations, desired client participation, and expected benefits.
3. Pour solution (or obtain from tap) into reservoir. Place waterproof underpad on bed under junction of NG and connecting tubing. Check for placement. (See Procedure 22–19). If tube is in stomach proceed to next step. If not, advance tube 1 to 2 inches and check again. (Tape must be removed and reapplied).

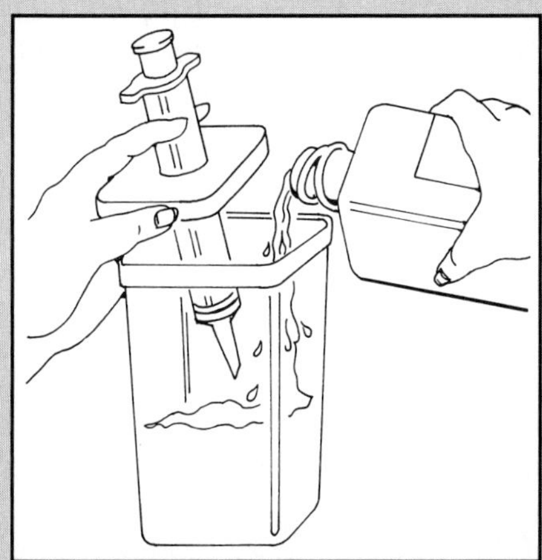

4. Draw up 30 to 50 mL in syringe and inject all of liquid into tube. If NG is a salem sump tube, keep pigtail above level of stomach during Irrigation to prevent reflux.

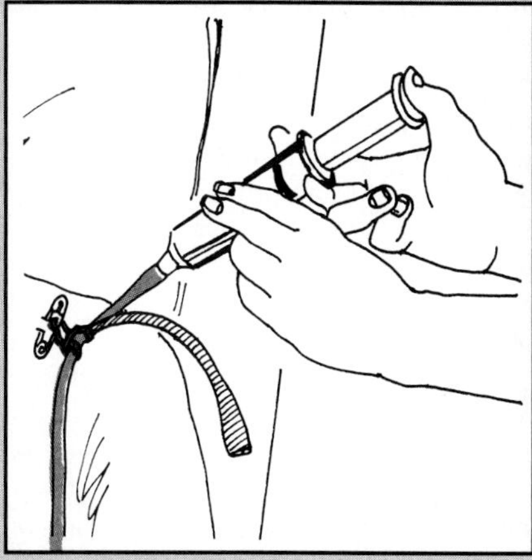

5. Reattach NG to connecting tubing. If drainage now moves toward drainage collector, check pigtail for hissing sound. Inject 10 mL of air to clear tube if no air movement can be heard.
6. Assist client to comfortable position. Store equipment at bedside for next irrigation.
7. If no return of irrigant is obtained, repeat steps 4 and 5, above. May repeat instillation a third time if second attempt is not successful. If no return is obtained after third instillation of fluid, reposition client to change angle of tubing in stomach. Tubing may be advanced 1 to 2 inches more to reach pool of liquid in stomach, if fluid still does not return.
8. If none of the above measures result in return of fluid, repeat troubleshooting measures described in Procedure 22–19. If unable to determine cause of problem, do not irrigate again, as fluid in stomach stimulates production of secretions, so is contraindicated if suction is not functioning correctly. Report status of client and equipment to charge nurse of physician.

RECORDING: Document procedure, client's response, problems, and action taken. Record total amount of fluid instilled as intake.

can facilitate communication through active listening and paraphrasing family statements. This helps family members clarify their thoughts and feelings, which enables resolution of conflicts associated with a client's move to an extended care facility.

Nurses can promote quality of life for clients living in extended care facilities by actively listening and responding to client and family needs. This enables support of individual client life-style. Personal freedom is important. Also, personal possessions such as pictures, photographs, and other items of special significance to individuals are important in promoting security by creating a homelike surrounding. Encouraging family involvement in client care enhances client well-being and family self-worth.

A community resource for care of terminally ill individuals is hospice care. It focuses on meeting the physical, psychosocial, and spiritual needs of dying clients and their families. The focal point of hospice care is improving or maintaining the quality of life prior to death. Communication, comfort, and pain relief are common needs of the terminally ill client.

Rehabilitative care, recovery, and rehabilitation can also occur outside of a health care institution in an outpatient setting. With early discharge from hospitals, more rehabilitative care is provided on an outpatient basis. For example, clients with a fractured femur have a period of hospitalization followed by the application of a cast for an extended period of time. Most of the recovery time is spent outside the health care institution, but it is an important part of rehabilitation. Optimal level of functioning returns when the cast is removed and the leg muscles are strengthened through an extended period of care on an outpatient basis.

Facilitating Life-style Changes. Acute illness or injury often necessitate an alteration of life-style, either temporary, such as care of a healing wound, or permanently, as with changes in the home environment and daily activity patterns because of loss of a body part or function. Education is important in facilitating life-style changes. See also the discussion of self-management in the earlier section on preventive care. Success often requires the inclusion of family members or significant others in a health education plan and discharge teaching. Support and acceptance by significant others largely determines the success or failure of any attempted life-style changes. Plans of care should be individualized to reflect the unique needs and situations of clients and family members. Psychological, physiological, and sociocultural variables must be considered when planning long-term care. For example, a nurse can assist a client who is a salesman to consider his frequent meals in restaurants while traveling as they plan to reduce his dietary salt and fat following a heart attack.

Discharge planning should address appropriate continuation of care after discharge from the hospital. Plans for discharge from acute care should begin on admission. Exchange of information regarding essential life-style changes throughout acute care provides opportunities for nurses to assess client understanding and reinforce what is not understood. When clients are discharged from the hospital, nurses should provide written instructions with information needed for self-care at home. Instructions should be written so clients can understand them. Clients' educational level must be considered when preparing an instruction sheet. Use words clients can understand and review the written information with clients to promote understanding. Verbal review of written instructions provides an opportunity for nurses to assess understanding of the information and reinforce what is not understood. It also provides an opportunity for nurses to make referrals to community resources if needed.

Written instructions are important because clients are being discharged from hospitals before they have fully recovered from health alterations. Hospital nurses have less time to prepare clients and families for care needed in the home. Clients often return home needing several different medications, diet and activity restrictions, and with surgical incisions that are not completely healed. The nursing diagnoses developed in collaboration with clients during hospitalization can be used to organize information clients need to know about each of their health problems. On discharge, areas that frequently require incorporation of a life-style change to promote client health and well-being include medication regimen, dietary restrictions, activity alterations, performance of special procedures, and follow-up care.

Medication administration time schedules are important in maintaining a constant, therapeutic concentration of medication in the bloodstream. A review of daily activities is important in planning a medication schedule. Nurses can use this review to help clients incorporate medication times into daily routines. For example, a drug ordered four times a day may have been given at 9 AM, 1 PM, 5 PM, and 9 PM in the hospital, but after review of the client's daily schedule may be better planned with meals (at 8 AM, 12 noon, and 5 PM) and at bedtime (11 PM) for a particular client. A schedule appropriate for the prescribed medication worked out in collaboration with clients is usually more acceptable. Clients also need information about side effects that they may experience as a result of the prescribed medication. The nurses can encourage participation in the medication regimen by discussing ways to reduce these side effects.

Clients may need to incorporate dietary changes into their lives. Clients need to understand exactly what the diet requires, what the restrictions are, and why they are needed. Dietary restrictions require inclusion of family members to facilitate incorporation of the needed life-style changes. The person planning and cooking clients' meals must be included in the teaching sessions. Some clients may need special assistance to maintain diet restrictions through help of a dietitian and/or social service. A dietitian can suggest menus, recipes, and shopping tips. Clients who are unable to shop for food or cook their meals could be assisted by a homemaker or Meals-on-Wheels arranged by social service.

Optimum recovery from some illnesses and injuries requires activity alterations: increased exercise for some, restrictions for others. Normal client activities need to be assessed to promote incorporation of these changes into individual life-style. For example, a housewife who is not to do any heavy lifting should not carry wet laundry but this is irrelevant to the client whose husband does the laundry. However, this client's normal activity patterns need to be reviewed so other activities requiring heavy lifting are not overlooked. This enables a nurse to individualize teaching to the client. If activity restrictions mean clients will be unable to care for themselves when returning home, the family may be able to provide support during this recovery. Clients who live alone may need additional help such as a home health aide. Clients with permanent changes such as an amputation or paralysis may need more extensive rehabilitation services before returning home. Clients needing to alter their life-styles by increasing exercise often need assistance to identify appropriate types of exercise and acceptable programs or schedules. Many health clubs offer help with planning exercise programs. Rehabilitation centers also sponsor exercise classes for enhancing recovery or improving well-being after specific problems such as stroke or respiratory disease.

Upon return home, some clients need to perform special procedures to maintain their health and well-being. While all new skills take time to master, some are more complicated than others. For example, consider a client who has an ulcerated area next to the stoma of his colostomy. He needs to learn special care to heal the ulceration: warm compresses to be applied three times a day. This client needs to learn how to perform the procedure at home and may need assistance with plans for incorporating the procedure into his everyday activities. For example, although compresses on open wounds are applied with sterile technique in the hospital, they can be done using a clean washcloth and clean bowl in the home. Suppose the client works from 8 AM to 5 PM. The nurse can help him select three times during the day for performing the prescribed treatments that will accommodate his work schedule and responsibilities.

Many clients discharged from a hospital need to return to their physician's office or clinic for follow-up care. Nurses need to educate clients about the importance of follow-up care. Clients with limited mobility or finances may need assistance or transportation to keep follow-up appointments. Social workers can facilitate these services.

Enhancing Self-esteem. Alterations in health threaten self-esteem. Self-esteem is related to meaning in life, feelings of competence, ability to carry out meaningful work, and opportunities for enjoyment. Any of these may be compromised by serious illness. In order to support individual efforts to regain or enhance self-esteem, nurses need to understand how clients perceive their illness experience and their current abilities to participate in meaningful life experiences. Clients' resources, coping styles, and self-efficacy are also important variables in determining the degree of threat a particular illness experience presents and the nature of nurses' approaches. Clients having self-efficacy, a strong social support network, and effective coping skills need less intensive assistance from nurses to regain self-esteem. They are often able to establish realistic rehabilitation goals and identify effective strategies to achieve them. For these clients, providing information about the specific life-style alterations that are necessary for their rehabilitation and giving positive reinforcement for progress may be sufficient assistance. They are likely to emerge from the illness experience stronger than before.

For less resilient clients, more support and active involvement from nurses is appropriate. These clients need to experience acceptance from others to rebuild acceptance of themselves. While a collaborative approach that conveys nurses' respect is ultimately valuable, they may be hesitant, even resistant to participate in planning at first. Under these circumstances, it is appropriate for nurses to take the lead in establishing rehabilitation goals to set the stage for more active client involvement later. Begin by setting small goals. Achievement builds feelings of competence. Facilitate contact with others recovering from similar problems. Interacting with those who have progressed beyond clients' current level is encouraging; being able to assist others who have to come as far creates feelings of competence and helps reestablish meaning in life. To reinforce clients' self-worth, emphasize abilities that remain, rather than limitations. Encourage exploration of alternatives for work and recreation if clients cannot return to their previous activities. Reinforce renewing contact with church, friends, or hobbies. Stress that well-being involves a balance between meaningful endeavors and play. Point out achievements and progress toward goals. Gradually shift the roles so clients become more active in generating alternatives, decision-making and recognizing progress. Although for some clients, regaining feelings of self-worth may be a long process, the rewards of participating in the process for client and nurse are great.

Promoting Adaptation to Chronic Illness. Problems associated with the effects of chronic illness, old age, and death can not be eliminated, but can be tempered through self-management. Change begins with nurses assisting clients to examine their life-style and setting priorities based on their opinion of what is most important in their health and well-being. Client priorities are the basis for goal development. Goals should present a challenge but be realistic or they will hinder adaptation. A positive attitude and positive reinforcement for change toward the goal is an important support for client adaptation. Nurses can promote adaptation to chronic illness by helping clients identify strengths to be built upon rather than focusing on the negatives and what cannot be done. This can be approached by a review of past successes. Feedback regarding progress toward established goals will assist the clients to learn new behaviors. Clear direct communication about a client's behavior helps promote change. If negative feedback must be given, be sure to balance it with some positive feedback. When identifying ineffective behavior, always include a suggestion for how it could be changed so clients can maintain a sense of control. If clients become defensive or argumentative, revert to active listening rather than threaten the trust that is essential to a meaningful nurse–client relationship. Chapters 13 and 14 elaborate on effective nurse–client communication.

Because most chronic illnesses require ongoing medical therapy or monitoring, nursing interventions often focus on assisting clients toward independent management of the disease. Client and family adaptation to the changes and restrictions resulting from the development of chronic illness can be enhanced through supportive and educative nursing actions. Incorporation of the prescribed medical regimen into customary daily activities, as discussed above, and continual self-monitoring by clients for signs or symptoms of complications or problems that require professional health services, are necessary. For example, clients with diabetes can maintain health and well-being by learning how to manage the disease. Nurses assist clients to learn how to self-administer insulin, self-monitor blood sugar, and adapt the diet, all of which are important to maintaining health and well-being. Quality of life is effected based on incorporation of these behaviors into everyday activities.

Health-promoting behaviors are also an important element of rehabilitative nursing care. Assisting chronically ill clients to incorporate exercise or activities that are designed to enhance mobility or functioning, or at least prevent degeneration of capabilities, is important for maintenance of quality of life. For example, hypertensive clients are often encouraged to incorporate regular exercise or stress-reduction techniques, such as meditation or biofeedback, into their daily schedule. Diabetic clients are taught to practice daily foot care in order to prevent future problems such as ulcers related to decreased peripheral circulation.

Referral to Support Groups/Community Resources. Support groups and community resources are often an important component of a comprehensive client care plan. There are a wide variety of community groups that function solely to provide support and encouragement to individuals with a specific health problem or need. Groups influence how their members think, feel, and act. They are a valuable resource for assisting clients in adapting to change. Often groups are sources of peer support and information gained from personal experience that may be lacking in traditional medical systems. Examples include the American Cancer Society's Reach for Recovery program for recent mastectomy clients, Weight Watchers, the United Ostomy Association, and Alcoholics Anonymous. Many groups also include significant others in their programs or meetings. Participation in self-help groups enhances self-esteem and facilitates adjustment to medical problems or conditions, because the group members are a source of encouragement and reinforcement for change.

The availability of community services such as visiting nurses, Meals-on-Wheels, or organized transportation assistance is often the critical factor in determining whether a client can independently function in the community setting during rehabilitation. Many acute care facilities now engage the services of a discharge coordinator who is able to meet the unique needs of each individual through proper referral to the appropriate agency or service.

■ EVALUATION

Evaluation of client well-being is an ongoing process that encompasses all aspects of nursing care. Evaluation of wellness and well-being is based on the desired outcomes that nurse and client developed for the client care plan. If desired outcomes are clear, specific and measurable evaluation criteria are easily identified. Nurses should be as individualized and specific as possible when selecting evaluation criteria. The nurse must continually strive to remain aware of the unique needs of each individual client. Effective evaluation requires that nurses maintain a holistic perspective. Only when all aspects of an individual's condition—including the physical, mental, emotional, and social components—are considered, can the nurse truly evaluate client well-being. Progress toward desired outcomes is monitored during the course of all levels of client care as well as on identified target dates.

SUMMARY

Wellness and well-being are broad, interrelated concepts. Wellness encompasses dimensions that relate to all aspects of individuals' lives, including eating well, being fit, feeling good, caring for self and others, self-responsibility, and fitting in with the environment. Wellness and well-being are manifested through individuals' optimism, self-confidence, energy, sense of purpose, inner peace, and overall satisfaction with their lives.

Wellness is influenced by many variables. Values, life-style, culture and socioeconomic status, self-concept, locus of control, age, and personality traits such as hardiness and resilience affect life-style choices and in turn, wellness. Wellness is altered by life experiences such as life change, crisis, and illness. Health care experiences also alter wellness. Becoming a client and, in particular, being hospitalized can threaten wellness and well-being in a profound way. Altered wellness is manifested in many different ways. Fear, anxiety, pain, stress, fatigue, depression, loneliness, powerlessness, confusion, and dissatisfaction with life circumstances are examples of how individuals experienced altered wellness.

Because wellness and well-being encompass all aspects of the individual—physical, psychosocial, and spiritual—assessment and management of wellness must focus on all aspects of a clients' life-style. Nursing diagnoses related to alterations in wellness and well-being are based on a wide variety of client problems, including those that are cognitive, physical, emotional, social, and environmental, all of which nurses need to address. An effective collaborative relationship requires mutual participation between clients and nurses during the entire process of assessment and management. Threats to well-being and wellness cannot be corrected without the clients' active participation, which is facilitated in a collaborative nurse–client relationship.

Nursing implementation to promote client wellness and well-being involves all of the four levels of client care. Client care includes screening, counseling, and/or direct physical care. Client education is important in promoting a wellness life-style and for supporting client well-being through stress management skills and facilitating self-responsibility. Preparation for health care experiences such as admission to the hospital and diagnostic and surgical procedures is vital to client well-being. Counseling is used to promote well-being, enhance self-esteem, facilitate life-style changes, and support adaptation to chronic illness. Promoting client well-being also encompasses direct physical care including preventing infection (medical and surgical asepsis), managing fever, providing comfort, protecting safety, administering medications, and perioperative care.

Although wellness and well-being are highly individualized, nurses whose approach to clients demonstrates respect and caring, and who promote client involvement and self-responsibility through collaboration, support wellness and well-being in all their clients, even those experiencing significant alterations in health.

REFERENCES

1. Pender NJ. *Health Promotion in Nursing Practice.* Norwalk, CT: Appleton & Lange; 1987.
2. Blattner B. *Holistic Nursing.* Englewood Cliffs, NJ: Prentice-Hall; 1981.
3. Smith JA. *The Idea of Health: Implications for the Nursing Professional.* New York: Teachers College Press; 1983.
4. Dunn HL. What high level wellness means. *Can J Pub Health.* 1959;50:447.
5. Dunn HL. *High Level Wellness.* Arlington: Beatty; 1961.
6. Moore PV, Williamson GC. Health promotion: Evolution of a concept. *Nurs Clin North Am.* 1984;19:195–206.
7. LaLonde M. *A New Perspective on the Health of Canadians.* Ottawa: Government of Canada; 1974.
8. US Senate Select Committee on Nutrition and Human Needs. *Dietary Goals for the United States. Washington, DC: US Government Printing Office (pub no. 052-070-03913-2);1977.*
9. US Department of Health, Education, and Welfare. *Healthy People: The Surgeon General's Report on Health Promotion and Disease Prevention.* Washington, DC: US Government Printing office; 1979.
10. Travis JW, Ryan RS. *The Wellness Workbook.* 2nd ed. Berkeley: Ten Speed Press; 1988.
11. Ardell DB. *High Level Wellness: An Alternative to Doctors, Drugs, and Disease.* Emmaus, PA: Rodale; 1977.
12. Nightingale F. *Notes on Nursing.* Philadelphia: Lippincott; 1946.
13. Oelbaum CH. Hallmarks of adult wellness. *Am J Nurs.* 1974; 74:1623–1625.
14. Clark CC. *Wellness Nursing: Concepts, Theory, Research, and Practice.* New York, Springer; 1986.
15. Clark CC. *Enhancing Wellness: A Guide for Self-care.* New York: Springer; 1981.
16. Laffrey S. Development of a health conception scale. *Res Nurs Health.* 1986;9:107–113.
17. Woods NF, Laffrey S, Duffy M, et al. Being healthy: Women's images. *Adv Nurs Sci.* 1988;11:36–46.
18. Bloomfield HH, Kory RB. *The Holistic Way to Health and Happiness: A New Approach to Complete Lifetime Wellness.* New York: Simon & Schuster, 1978.
19. Claus KE, Bailey JT. *Living With Stress and Promoting Well-Being: A Handbook for Nurses.* St Louis: Mosby; 1980.
20. Parsons EJ. Well-being: Ask the patient. *Rehab Nurs.* 1988;13: 263–264.
21. Belloc N, Breslow L. Relationship of physical health status and health practices. *Prev Med.* 1972;1:409–421.
22. Wiley JA. Life-style and future health: Evidence from the Alameda County study. *Prev Med.* 1980;9.
23. Howe HL. Enhancing the effectiveness of media messages promoting regular breast self-examination. *Public Health Rep.* 1986; 96:134–142.
24. Ellison E. Social support and the constructive-developmental model. *West J Nurs Res.* 1987;9:19–28.
25. Lambert VA, Lambert CE, Kipple GL, Mewshaw EA. Social support, hardiness, and psychological well-being in women with arthritis. *Image.* 1989;21:128–131.
26. James KS. Family nutrition and weight control. In: Bomar PJ, ed. *Nurses and Family Health Promotion: Concepts, Assessment and Interventions.* Baltimore: Williams & Wilkins; 1989:155–178.
27. Hill L, Smith N. *Self-care Nursing.* Norwalk, CT: Appleton & Lange; 1990.
28. US Department of Agriculture and US Department of Health and Human Services. *Nutrition and Your Health: Dietary Guidelines for Americans.* 3rd ed. Washington, DC: US Government Printing Office; 1990.
29. Murray RB, Zentner JP. *Nursing Assessment and Health Promotion Strategies Through the Lifespan.* Norwalk, CT: Appleton & Lange; 1989.
30. Dossey BM, Keegen L, Guzzetta CE, Kolkmedier LG. *Holistic Nursing: A Handbook for Practice.* Rockville, MD: Aspen; 1988.
31. Swinford PA. *Promoting Wellness: A Nurse's Handbook.* Rockville, MD: Aspen; 1989.
32. Carson VB. *Spiritual Dimensions of Nursing Practice.* Philadelphia: Saunders; 1989.
33. Pender NJ. Expressing health through lifestyle. *Nurs Sci Q.* 1990;3:115–122.
34. Bresler DE. Conditioned relaxation. In: Gordon JS, Jaffe DT, Bresler DE, eds. *Mind, Body, and Health: Toward an Integral Medicine.* New York: Human Sciences; 1984:19–36.
35. Grasser C. Craft BJ. The patient's approach to wellness. *Nurs. Clin North Am.* 1984;19:207–218.
36. House J, Landis K, Umberson D. Social relationships and health. *Science.* 1988;241:540–545.
37. Hammer M. "Core" and "extended" social networks in relation to health and illness. *Social Sci Med.* 1983;17:405–411.
38. Baldassare M, Rosenfeld S, Rook K. The types of social relations predicting elderly well-being. *Res Aging.* 1984;6:549–559.
39. Rotter JB. *Social Learning and Clinical Psychology.* Englewood Cliffs, NJ: Prentice-Hall; 1954.
40. Brown N. The relationship among health beliefs, health values, and health promotion activity. *West J Nurs Res.* 1983;5:155–163.
41. Hallol JC. The relationship of health beliefs, health locus of control, and self concept to the practice of breast self-exam in adult women. *Nurs Res.* 1982;31:137–142.
42. Lakin JA. Self-care, health locus of control and health value among faculty women. *Pub Health Nurs.* 1988;5:37–44.
43. Wallston B, Wallston K, Kaplan G, Maides S. Development and validation of the health locus of control (HLC) scale. *J Consult Clin Psychol.* 1976;44:580–585.
44. Jenkins LS. Self-efficacy theory: Overview and measurement of key components. *Cardiovasc Nurs.* 1988;24:36.
45. Bandura A. *Social Learning Theory.* Englewood Cliffs, NJ: Prentice-Hall; 1977.
46. Bandura A. *Social Foundations of Thought and Action: A Social Cognitive Theory.* Englewood Cliffs, NJ: Prentice-Hall; 1986.
47. Kobasa S. Stressful life events, personality and health: An inquiry into hardiness. *J Pers Soc Psychol.* 1979;37:1–11.
48. Kobasa S, Maddi S, Conn S. Hardiness and health: A prospective study. *J Pers Soc Psychol.* 1982;42:168–177.
49. Kobasa S, Maddi S, Courtington S. Personality and constitution as mediators in the stress-illness relationship. *J Health Soc Behav.* 1981;22:368–378.
50. Langemo DK. The impact of work stress on female nurse educators. *Image.* 1990;22:159–162.

51. Wagnild G, Young HM. Resilience among older women. *Image.* 1990;22:252–255.
52. Rich V, Rich A. Personality, hardiness and burnout in female staff nurses. *Image.* 1987;19:62–66.
53. Lambert C, Lambert V. Hardiness: Its development and relevance to nursing. *Image.* 1987;19:92–95.
54. Stanhope M, Lancaster J. *Community Health Nursing: Process and Practice of Promoting Health.* St. Louis: Mosby; 1988.
55. Spector RE. *Cultural Diversity in Health and Illness.* 3rd ed. Norwalk, CT: Appleton & Lange; 1991.
56. Lantz, J. Family culture and ethnicity. In: Bomar PJ, ed. *Nursing and Family Health Promotion: Concepts, Assessment, and Interventions.* Baltimore: Williams & Wilkins; 1989:47–54.
57. Szafran K. Family health protective behaviors. In: Bomar PJ, ed. *Nurses and Family Health Promotion: Concepts, Assessment, and Interventions.* Baltimore: Williams & Wilkins; 1989;258–292.
58. Bruhn JG, Cordova FD, Williams JA, Fuentes RG. The wellness process. *J Com Health.* 1977;2:209–221.
59. Yurik AG, Spier BE, Robb SS, Ebert NJ. *The Aged Person and the Nursing Process.* Norwalk, CT: Appleton & Lange; 1989.
60. Association for Retired Persons and the Administration on Aging, *A Profile of Older Americans: 1989.* Washington, DC: US Department of Health and Human Services; 1989.
61. Horgan PA. Health status perceptions affect health-related behaviors. *J Gerontol Nurs.* 1987;13:30–33.
62. Eschleman MM. *Introduction to Nutrition and Diet Therapy.* Philadelphia: Lippincott; 1991.
63. Behavioral risk factor surveillance; 1988. *MMWR.* 1990;39:1–6.
64. *Surgeon General's Report on Nutrition and Health: Summary and Recommendations.* Washington, DC: US Department of Health and Human Services, DHHS (PHS) pub no. 88-50211;1988.
65. McCance KL. Stress and disease. In: McCance KL, Huether SE. *Pathophysiology: The Biologic Basis for Disease in Adults and Children.* St. Louis: Mosby; 1990.
66. Selye H. History and present status of the stress concept. In: Monat A, Lazarus RS, eds. *Stress and Coping: An Anthology.* 2nd ed. New York: Columbia University Press; 1985.
67. American Heart Association. *1991 Heart and Stroke Facts.* Dallas: American Heart Association; 1991.
68. Friedman M, Rosenmann RH. *Type A Behavior and Your Heart.* New York: Knopf, 1974.
69. O'Flynn-Comiskey A. The type A individual. *Am J Nurs.* 1979; 79:1956–1958.
70. Cohen F. Stress and bodily illness. In: Monat A, Richard S, eds. *Stress and Coping: An Anthology.* 2nd ed. New York: Columbia University Press; 1985;40–54.
71. Fatal injuries to children—United States, 1986. *MMWR.* 1990; 39:442–450.
72. *Statistical Update on Lung Disease.* New York: American Lung Association; March 1991.
73. Smoking attributable mortality and years of potential life lost—United States, 1988. *MMWR.* 1991;40:62–71.
74. Alcohol related mortality and years of potential life lost. *MMWR.* 1990;39:173–175.
75. Barry PD. *Psychosocial Nursing Assessment and Intervention: Care of the Physically Ill Person.* Philadelphia: Lippincott; 1989.
76. Beare PG, Myers JL. *Principles and Practice of Adult Health Nursing.* St. Louis: Mosby; 1990.
77. Holmes TH, Rahe RE. The social readjustment rating scale. *J Psychosomat Res.* 1967;11:213–217.
78. Holmes TH, Rahe RE. Short-term intrusion into the life style routine. *J Psychosomat Res.* 1976;14:121–132.
79. Roberts SL. *Behavioral Concepts Throughout the Life Span.* Englewood Cliffs, NJ: Prentice-Hall; 1978.
80. Ebersole P, Hess P. *Toward Healthy Aging: Human Needs and Nursing Response.* St. Louis: Mobsy; 1990.
81. Fife BL. A model for predicting the adaptation of families to medical crises: An analysis of role integration. *Image.* 1985;17: 108–112.
82. Gilliss CL. Reducing family stress during and after coronary artery bypass surgery. *Nurs Clin North Am.* 1984;19:103–112.
83. Patrick ML, Woods SL, Craven RF, Rokosky JS, Bruno PM. *Medical-Surgical Nursing.* Philadelphia: Lippincott; 1991.
84. Garner JS. CDC guidelines for prevention and control of nosocomial infections: Guidelines for prevention and control of surgical wound infections. *Am J Infect Cont.* 1986;14:71–80.
85. McCaffery M, Beebe A. *Pain: Clinical Manual for Nursing Practice.* St Louis: Mosby; 1989.
86. Harold CE, ed. *Diagnostic Tests.* Springhouse, PA: Springhouse; 1991.
87. Jimenez SLM. Consumer journalism: A unique nursing opportunity. *Image.* 1991;23:47.
88. Williams RL, Long JD. *Toward a Self-managed Life Style.* 3rd ed. Boston: Houghton Mifflin; 1983.,
89. Pawlicki RE. Effects of self-directed behavior modification training on a measure of locus of control. *Psycholog Rep.* 1976; 39:319–322.
90. Lakein A. *How to Get Control of Your Time and Your Life.* New York: New American Library; 1973.
91. Mullin VI. Implementing the self-care concept in the acute care setting. *Nurs Clin North Am.* 1980;15:177–190.
92. Hathaway D, Boswell B, Stanford D, et al. Health promotion and disease prevention for the hospitalized patient's family. *Nurs. Admin Q.* 1987;11:1–7.
93. McHugh, NG, Christman NJ, Johnson JE. Preparatory information: What helps and why. *Am. J Nurs.* 1982;82:780–782.
94. Flaherty GG, Fitzpatrick JJ. Relaxation technique to increase comfort level of postoperative patients. *Nurs Res.* 1978;27:352–355.
95. Johnson JE, Christman NJ, Stitt C. Personal control interventions: Short- and long-term effects on surgical patients. *Res Nurs Health.* 1985;8:131–145.
96. US Centers for Disease Control. Guidelines for prevention of transmission of HIV and HIV in healthcare settings. *MMWR.* 1989;38(suppl S4):1—38.
97. Larson E. Handwashing: Its essential—even when you use gloves. *Am J Nurs.* 1989;89:934–949.
98. Jacobson G, Thiole J, McCune J, Farrell L. Handwashing, ring-wearing, and the number of microorganisms. *Nurs Res.* 1985; 34:186–187.
99. Korniewicz DM, Kirwin M, Larson E. Do your gloves fit the task? *Am J Nurs.* 1991;91:38–40.
100. US Department of Health and Human Services, Public Health Service. Update: Universal precautions for prevention of transmission of human immunodeficiency virus, hepatitis B virus, and other bloodborne pathogens in health care settings. *MMWR.* 1989;38:9–18.
101. Davis M. Eschelman ER, McKay M. *The Relaxation and Stress Reduction Workbook.* 3rd ed. Oakland: New Harbinger; 1988.
102. Dossey BM, Keegan L, Guzzetta CE, Kolkmier LG. *Holistic Nursing: A Handbook for Practice.* Rockville, MD: Aspen; 1988.
103. Richter JM, Sloan R. A relaxation technique. *Am J Nurs.* 1979; 79:1960–1964.
104. Benson H, Klipper M. *The Relaxation Response.* New York: Morrow; 1975.

105. Morton D. Five years of fewer falls. *Am J Nurs.* 1989;89:204–205.
106. Berryman E, Gaskin D. Jones A, Tolley F, MacMullen J. Point by point: Predicting elders falls. *Geriatr Nurs.* 1989;10:199–201.
107. Evans LK, Strumpf NE. Myths about elder restraints. *Image.* 1990;22:124–127.
108. Meth IM. Electrical safety in the hospital. *Am J Nurs.* 1980;80: 1344–1348.
109. Calyton BD, Stock YN. *Basic Pharmacology for Nurses.* St Louis: Mobsy; 1989.
110. McHenry LM, Salerno E. *Pharmacology in Nursing.* St. Louis: Mosby; 1989.
111. Chaplin G, Shull H, Welk PC. How safe is the air-bubble technique for I.M. injections? *Nursing 85.* 1985;15:59.
112. Association of Operating Room Nurses. Recommended practices: Preoperative skin preparation. *AORN J.* 1988;48:950.
113. Garner JS. Guidelines for prevention of surgical wound infections. Hospital Infections Program. Washington, DC: Centers for Disease Control, US Public Health Service; 1985.

BIBLIOGRAPHY

Aldane SG, Silvester LJ. The relationship of physical activity and perceived stress. *Health Values.* 1989;13:34–37.

Antonovsky A. *Unraveling the Mystery of Health: How People Manage Stress and Stay Well.* San Francisco: Jossey-Bass; 1987.

Carlson BR, Petti K. Health locus of control and participation in physical activity. *Am J Health Promotion.* 1989;3:32–37.

Connelly CE. Self-care and the chronically ill patient. *Nurs Clin North Am.* 1987, 22:621–629.

Dane JK, Sleet DA, Lam DJ, Roppel CE. Determinants of wellness in children: An exploratory study. *Health Values.* 1987;11: 13–19.

Gordon JS, Jaffe DT, Bresler DE (1984). *Mind, Body and Health: Toward an Integral Medicine.* New York: Human Sciences Press; 1984.

Greenberg JS. Health and wellness: A conceptual differentiation. *J School Health.* 1985;55:403–406.

Hastings AC, Fadiman J, Gordon JS. *Health for the Whole Person.* Boulder: Westview, 1980.

Hathaway D, Boswell B, Stanford D, Schneider S, Moncrief A. Health promotion and disease prevention for the hospitalized patient's family. *Nurs Admin Q.* 1987;11:1–7.

Johnson JE, Christman NJ, Stitt C. Personal control interventions: Short and long-term effects on surgical patients. *Res Nurs Health.* 1985;8:131–145.

Jordan-Marsh M, Neutra R. Relationship of health locus of control to lifestyle change programs. *Res Nurs Health.* 1985;8:3–11.

Mullin VI. Implementing the self-care concept in the acute care setting. *Nurs Clin North Am.* 1980;15:177–190.

Volicer BJ, Bohannon MW. A hospital stress rating scale. *Nurs Res.* 1975;24:352–359.

CHAPTER 23

Self-Expression

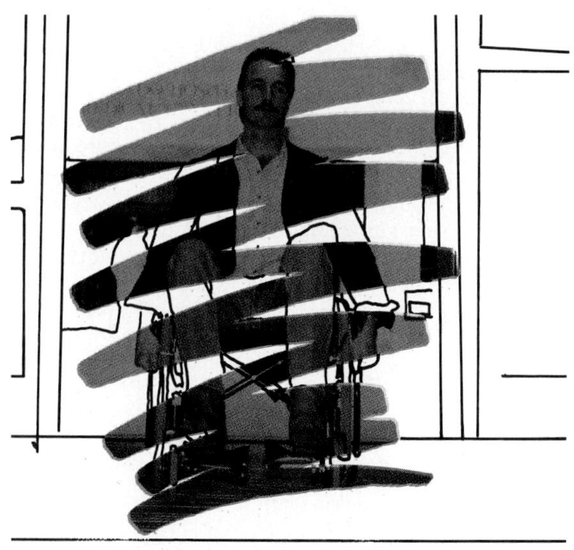

Behavioral Objectives

Upon completion of this chapter, the student will be able to:

1. Define self-expression.
2. State the importance of self-expression to health and well-being.
3. Discuss three functions of self-expression.
4. Discuss the concept of self-expression in relation to identity, self-concept, life structure, sexuality, and development.
5. Identify common modes of self-expression observed in everyday life.
6. State the importance of self-presentation and self-disclosure to self-expression.
7. State several characteristics of optimal self-expression.
8. Describe the impact of life change, illness, and loss on self-expression and state the implications for nursing practice.
9. Describe the grieving process.
10. Outline components of the client history and examination pertinent to assessing self-expression.
11. Outline nursing diagnoses related to self-expression, listing etiologies and defining characteristics.
12. Discuss nursing implementation related to self-expression for clients undergoing self-concept or body image changes, clients with concerns about sexuality, grieving clients, and dying clients.
13. Discuss the collaborative role of the nurse in assisting clients with self-expression problems.

KEY TERMS

algor mortis
ambivalence
anticipatory grief
bereavement
catharsis
denial of illness
depersonalization
distress
distress disclosure
grief
hope
insight
livor mortis
loneliness
loss
mourning
reference groups
rigor mortis
self-disclosure
self-expression
self-presentation
sex
sexuality
sexual orientation
situated identities

Human beings are expressive by nature. Indeed, the expressive character of human behavior has been counted among those features that distinguish humans from other beings. Banerjee, for example, has noted that humans are unique in their capacity to transcend the physical and biological dimensions of existence, and even the given social order, to express themselves in creative and personally satisfying ways.[1]

People express themselves through virtually every aspect of life and living, in relationships, activities, and physical behavior. Virtually any sphere of activity—physical, intellectual, cultural, or social—can be looked on as providing outlets for self-expression.

For most people, the opportunities for self-expression are discovered in a social context where they find themselves in some relationship to other human beings,[1] usually through vocational and leisure activities as well as in their family and spiritual lives.[2,3] People project themselves into the world through their roles as working person, parent, spouse, lover, friend, group member, churchgoer, artist, athlete, citizen, enthusiast, and opinion holder. All of these roles enable the individual to structure an identity and live it out in the world.

Opportunities for self-expression also present themselves in the important transitions of life, such as growing up and getting married. By participating in the rituals and traditions that surround developmental events, people express the meaning they find in life changes. Even birth and death are occasions for self-expression.[1] As Banerjee points out, the cries of a newborn and the last gasps of a dying man are highly expressive, representing that most basic motive—the desire to live. At a symbolic level, they too provide evidence of the human urge for self-expression.

In all of its many forms, self-expression is an essential dimension of human life, but its real significance lies in its embodiment of personal values and aspirations.[1] The values and aspirations embodied in self-expression give meaning to life, and acts of self-expression affirm and convey that meaning.[1,4]

The relationship between self-expression and meaning is complex. Expressive behavior does more than embody, affirm, or convey meaning, it actually gives meaning in the sense that to express oneself is intrinsically satisfying.[1] Moreover, people achieve the identity of their values in the community, to a large extent by an exchange of expression through which they form bonds to others. In relating to others, meaning is found in the love and belonging, and cooperation and sharing, that transpire. Thus, an important part of meaning in life is ultimately grounded on the mutual self-expression on which relationships are based.[1]

This textbook endorses the collaborative approach to promoting health in which nurse and client are viewed as partners in the health care experience. This approach advocates reciprocity in the holistic encounter with clients.[5–13] Reciprocity entails a give-and-take characterized not only by personal revelations from the client, but also by a sharing of self by the nurse, the ultimate result of which is an exchange of personal feeling within the context of the therapeutic relationship.[6–8,10,14] Indeed, it can be said that collaboration involves mutual self-expression between client and nurse. Empathy, warmth, genuineness, immediacy, and self-disclosure, aspects of helper–helpee interaction outlined in Chapter 13, can be looked on as forms of self-expression found in successful therapeutic interactions.[15]

Through collaboration the nurse is able to facilitate the client's coping and to foster healing.[16] Chapter 13 explores the idea that health is promoted by positive human interaction, the kind found in helping relationships. Facilitating the client's self-expression is thought to have a therapeutic or restorative value for the client. Many times this may be a primary aspect of the client's care and an essential part of the nurse's role. This chapter builds on the concepts presented in Chapters 10 through 14, relating the concepts from these chapters to a practical understanding of how the nurse acts to support and facilitate the client's self-expression.

IMPLICATIONS FOR NURSE–CLIENT COLLABORATION

Importance of Mutual Self-Expression in Caregiving

Self-expression is the process by which people share their self-understanding with others. Collaboration involves mutual self-expression between nurse and client. Sharing of self-understanding by the client helps the nurse to understand the client's needs from the client's perspective and facilitates caregiving that meets those needs. Sharing of self-understanding by the nurse is one of the most important ways that the nurse communicates empathy and caring. In turn, the nurse's sharing facilitates the client's sharing.

Section 1. Understanding Self-Expression

■ OPTIMUM SELF-EXPRESSION

Definition of Self-Expression

For much of the twentieth century, researchers in psychology and the social sciences have focused on investigating the basic constructs (identity, self, self-concept) and processes (cognition, motivation, communication) that might explain the expressive nature of human behavior. The result is a substantial body of research on human expressiveness. Studies have been undertaken on the universality of emotional expression,[17,18] the cultural rules for emotional expression,[19,20] the role expression plays in determining subjective experience,[21–26] individual differences in displaying expressions and interpreting others' expressions,[27] and the role of expression in creating impressions on others.[28–31] Nevertheless, the concept of self-expression for the most part has eluded definition.

The term *expression,* as defined by *Webster's New Collegiate Dictionary,* refers to something—an action, a gesture, or an utterance—that makes one's opinions or feelings known. *Webster's* definition emphasizes that expressions give a *true* or *vivid* impression of the personal emotions, moods, or sentiments that are aroused by objects or events in the environment and convey an accurate picture of a person's subjective reality. *Webster's* also refers to expression as being related to one's abilities and one's artistic and creative impulses.

Although dictionary definitions are helpful, they provide only a very general understanding of self-expression. Scholarly ideas add depth and precision.

A Concept of Expression. Zajonc notes that expression implies a sequence of events that at its endpoint has an "efferent process." The term *efferent* means to carry or conduct outward.[24] In the strict neurological sense, it refers to the motor contraction of any tissue or organ in response to impulses from the central nervous system. Thus, certain types of involuntary behavior, such as sweating or blushing, can be classified as expressive.[32–34] In a less restrictive sense, however, the term refers to behavior, typically facial or postural displays, but also gestures, vocalizations, laughter, and crying, that corresponds to immediate feelings.[35–37]

Expression also implies the existence of an internal state, composed of thoughts as well as feelings, that seeks externalization and thus forces itself to the surface.[24] In the classical view, cognitions and emotions seek an outlet and thus "cause" expression; however, a growing number of experts dispute this idea and argue that expression also plays a role in creating a person's experience.[23–26] Nevertheless, expression as the externalization of a person's thoughts and feelings remains the prevailing view. This concept of expression is important to nurses because it highlights the assumption on which much of nursing assessment is based—that the nurse gains important clues about the client's immediate experience from the client's behavior, involuntary and communicative.

A Concept of the Self. Self-expression is a complex concept, however, involving more than simply a behavioral display of passing thoughts or momentary moods. As Banerjee[1] points out, self-expression presupposes a self. To understand the concept of self-expression, it is therefore necessary to consider the nature of the self. Chapter 10 develops the idea of the self at length and the reader is referred to that chapter for more detail.

The Self as Subject. The self has been variously conceived by modern psychologists as the "knower"—the "I" that thinks and feels, the center of human purposes and actions that conveys a sense of self-continuity[38]; as pure "ego"—the conscious, rational aspect of the personality described by Freud[39]; or, alternately, as the "agent"—an inborn information processor that attends to, interprets, and remembers information for the purpose of constructing self theories.[40]

These ideas reflect the elusiveness of scientific formulations. Despite their elusive quality, however, these conceptions share a common vantage point, depicting the self as subjective consciousness. Psychologists have long looked on the self as a private, hidden-from-view, intrapsychic entity composed of unobservable mental events. As far back as the ancient Greeks, the self was conceived as the thinking aspect of the soul; later it was thought of as the spiritual essence of life.[41] Over the centuries, debates about the self centered around its oneness with, or separateness from, the body (see Chap. 33 for more on the question of mind–body dualism), but continued to emphasize the inwardness of the self and to represent the self as subjective consciousness.[41]

Even today, the self is looked on primarily as a separate unit of sensation and perception that is more or less isolated from the outer world.[42] Although psychologists may dispute the degree to which people are aware of their own mental events, or the precise nature of the healthy self, they agree for the most part that the locus of the self lies within the inner world of the individual.[43] Thus, they tend to emphasize the intrapsychic and intrapersonal dimensions and ascribe greater importance to these dimensions than to the social or relational context of the self.[44]

The concept of the self as an interior, private entity is extremely useful to nurses as it focuses professional attention on the inner world of the individual. Clients' responses to illness are easier to understand when nurses appreciate the importance of the inner sense of self-unity and self-continuity. Illness can then be interpreted as a threat to one's inner sense of self. Suffering, a phenomenon related to illness, also becomes easier to understand. It can be thought of as occurring whenever some crucial aspect of one's self or one's existence is endangered. It thus is a natural consequence of a threat to the self. Whether or not suffering corresponds to physical pain depends entirely on the meaning that the experience of pain has for one's sense of self.[45]

The Self as Object. The intrapsychic version of the self is by no means the only philosophical or scientific view of the self. The self as object is also an important psychological construct. This point of view focuses on the effect of social life on the inner world of the individual.

For most psychologists, the self as object is not a denial of inwardness in the strict sense, but rather an acknowledgment of the relationship between the self and the social world.[41] Cooley's formulation of the "looking glass self" best exemplifies that position. Cooley found it impossible to consider the self in isolation. He theorized that the raw material for the formation of the self came from reflections of self provided by others.[46]

Baldwin, a contemporary of Cooley's, reinforced Cooley's idea and went on to assert that the self developed as a result of its exchanges with the social world.[47] Cooley and Baldwin laid the groundwork for the later formulation of the self-concept (or phenomenal self), one of the most important formulations in modern psychology. The self-concept as defined in Chapter 10 is the organized pattern of beliefs that individuals hold about themselves.[48]

Erik Erikson, a renowned developmental psychologist, emphasized the objective, socially derived aspects of the self to an unprecedented extent. As an immigrant from Austria, Erikson became interested in the social identification problems that immigrant children experienced as they tried to adapt to their new culture. He used his personal perspective and a blending of anthropologic and psychoanalytic methods to formulate a theory of identity that stressed the importance of social as well as inner sameness.[47]

> If . . . we speak of the community's response to the young individual's need to be recognized by those around him, we mean something beyond a mere recognition of achievement; for it is of great relevance to the young individual's identity formation that he be responded to, and be given function and status as a person whose gradual growth and transformation make sense to those who begin to make sense to him.[49(p102)]

Erikson thus believed that the society strongly influenced the inner unfolding of individual identity.

Erikson's ideas had a great influence on the field of social psychology which, at about the same time, was struggling with a formulation of identity as an interactional reality.[50] Headed by G. H. Mead, sociologists at the University of Chicago were seeking to understand how people are affected by and affect each other. Like Erikson, Mead believed that the development of identity was a socially mediated process. He proposed the self to be an outgrowth of the child's adoption of the attitude of the "generalized other." By that term, Mead referred to any social group (including abstract or nonexistent groups) that gave individuals "a unity of self," that is, a consistent way of thinking about themselves.[50] In Mead's view the self did not exist apart from social interaction.

Goffman, another University of Chicago sociologist, in a lengthy essay, now a classic in social psychology, focused on the impressions that people made or tried to make on others through their behavior—an angle stressing outer image. He used the analogy of the theater, arguing that life was a stage and that social interactions were akin to "performances."[28] Goffman believed that whenever individuals confronted one another, they behaved in a fashion that was consistent with the impression they desired to make to garner social approval. Under his model, for example, honesty was not so much a quality of self as an impression strategically generated—a matter of appearing to be honest. Goffman's perspective on the self became known as the "dramaturgical perspective" and it influenced a substantial body of experimental studies on "impression management" in social interaction.[51,52]

The impact on the helping professions of these various viewpoints on the self as object cannot be overestimated. Articles in the nursing literature explore the clinical implications of the self theories just described, delineating the relationships among illness, self-concept, and social identity.[53–55] Collectively, this work has had a profound impact on the practice of nursing. Today's nurses understand that clients are more likely to follow through with health recommendations when these take the client's self-concept into account.[56] Nurses also understand that all people, themselves and clients included, have a need to affirm their self-concepts in social interaction, to modify their behavior according to their social circumstances, and to protect the images they project to others in their everyday lives.

The Unified Self. A third perspective on the self merges the self represented in inner life with the self represented in the social forum. This perspective is known as symbolic interactionism. Symbolic interactionism holds that the individual and society are inseparable and interdependent units.[41] Thus, the self does not merely exist in society; rather the self and society mutually interact and can be understood only in terms of one another.[41]

Symbolic interactionism emphasizes the symbolic meanings attached to objects, activities, and events, and suggests that people act toward the environment on the basis of the various meanings the environment holds for them.[57] The meanings of objects, activities, and events remain ambiguous until defined by the participants. People even define one another during interaction; that is, they fix the characteristics each will have (status and attributes) and the roles each will play through an implicit process of social negotiation; thus, they define the nature and context of their interaction.[57]

Identities thus derived are said to be "situated"; that is, they are fixed by one's relationship to particular other people.[41] **Situated identities** reside neither in the person nor in the environment, but rather in the relationship between the two at any point in time. A person's particular role relationships (Donny's mother, Mitch's wife, Mr. Sullivan's nurse, Laura's friend) exemplify the situated identities that someone might have in various social settings.

Symbolic interactionism also holds that people define their selves in terms of their situated identities.[57] Thus, there is a definition of "me" that corresponds to each of a person's everyday roles. For each individual, some roles have a more positive value associated with them than do others; these more highly valued roles are important to identify. An individual's self-conception comprises all of the valued "me's" an individual perceives. These "me's" are organized in a hierarchy according to the degree of positive attitude the individual holds toward them and are experienced simultaneously and holistically.[57]

Perspectives on the self that are grounded in symbolic interactionism generally reject the inner–outer metaphor for viewing the self.[47] Social psychologists who share this position prefer the terms *private self* and *public self*. The public self refers to the self that is represented to others through one's situation and manner of behavior; the private self is the way one understands oneself to be, even if unrecognized by others. This perspective allows for the merging of elements of the self. To the extent that an individual shares his or her personal self-understanding, the private self becomes public and the self is unified. According to symbolic interactionism, this process is mediated through the symbolic meanings that are shared in social transactions.

The work of Levinson, a pioneer in adult development theory, also reflects the belief that the self is to be understood in terms of its transactions with the world. Based on data from a long-term study of several individuals from differing backgrounds, Levinson and co-workers concluded that "The self is in the world, and the world is in the self."[2(p46)] By this they meant that for the individuals in their study, self and world were mutually influencing entities, bound together in enduring but changing relationships. For Levinson and his colleagues, it was the life structure—that basic design of an individual's life, apparent at any moment in an individual's choices for an occupation, group affiliation, family relationships, friendships, or even a relationship to oneself—that engaged the individual and society. Life structure can be thought of as the social framework that enables individuals to form and enact their self-concepts. Levinson et al. believed that for any individual the life structure represented an evolving pattern of the "interpenetration" of self and world.[2]

A Concept of Self-Expression. From these various perspectives, it is clear that the self is a complex and multidimensional concept that can be used to reflect alternatively on a person's inner consciousness, self-attitudes, valued social images, identities, situations, and roles. However one conceptualizes the self, the unity, continuity, and contents of the self are all of central importance to the individual, as are the individual's transactions with the environment through which unity is achieved.

The merging of an individual's private and public selves presupposes a process for connecting the self and the world; that process can be looked on generally as the process of self-expression.[1] In this text, **self-expression** is defined as the process by which a person's self-understanding is shared with others. In other words, self-expression is the process by which the private self becomes public, or at least available for others to regard.

The aspects of self that are shared in the process of self-expression vary in the importance attached to them by the individual and in the modes by which they are conveyed. In everyday social communication, an individual's verbal and nonverbal attention is frequently on the passing personal feelings, fleeting moods, momentary thoughts, and casual preferences that are part of social discourse.[31] Important social identities are usually conveyed through appearance, dress, and manner,[28] and the deepest values and commitments are revealed in the patterns of one's life.[2] In more intimate relationships, an individual may express deeply personal aspects of the self in ways that are reserved for those relationships, for example, through touch and physical closeness.[31]

The Content of Self-Expression. Levinson et al.[2] enumerated several potentially important aspects of the private self that an individual might elect to share with others. Foremost among them are a person's sharing of goals, wishes, values and ideals, modes of feeling, thought, and action. Conflicts, fears, and anxieties and ways of resolving and controlling them may be shared, as may talents, skills, and character traits. Other aspects of the private self that people often choose to express are family, ethnic, religious, social class, political, peer group, and sexual identifications.[2,57]

Modes of Self-Expression. Modes of self-expression can be thought of as parts of the person, the immediate environment, and the long-term person–environment relationship.

Many authorities[18,23,27,29] make reference to the personal communicative modes of self-expression—physical, verbal, and behavioral—that were enumerated above and in Chapter 14. Goffman classifies expressive behavior into two fundamental categories, "expressions given," by which he refers to the traditional use of words and gestures in communication, and "expressions given off."[28] Expressions given off are the messages about self that are conveyed through one's setting (place, situation) and its characteristics (decor, size, physical layout) and through one's appearance as represented in dress and personal adornment, especially the insignia of role, office, or rank.[28] For example, the practice that many physicians and nurses have adopted of wearing a stethoscope draped around the back of the neck might be looked on as a symbolization of role or status identity.

Levinson et al.[2] and Banerjee[1] both address the longer-term aspects of expression, those that deal with life patterns and the deep personal preferences and commitments that endure over time. Levinson and colleagues, for example, argue that the life-structure, as the basic design of a person's life, is itself expressive in the sense that its various components represent an individual's personal choices for life and living. Thus, as a reflection of individual preferences, the selection of vocation, avocation, personal relationships, and social and institutional identifications is an important part of self-expression. Moreover, although the choices made for one's life structure constitute expressions in themselves, life structure also contributes to self-expression in a more indirect way through the social framework it provides for the establishment of social relationships and for the building and enactment of an individual's self-concept.

Banerjee, taking a more philosophical approach, lists the many different types of potentially expressive activities that link individuals with society. For example, he mentions the expressive aspect of efforts to improve human relations through acts of personal diplomacy or through a personal study of history to gain a better understanding of others; the activities a person might undertake to control or satisfy basic needs, for self and society, such as through technological or medical discovery; and the expressive value of the creation of new ideas and novel things or aesthetic interests such as art, music, dance, literature, and poetry.[1]

The Importance of Choice. Choice making lies at the heart of self-expression because making a choice is an act of manifesting a personal preference. Preferences, in turn, are an integral aspect of inner emotions and are constituted from the interaction between an object and the internal state of the individual.[58] Because preferences are so strongly associated with emotion, a person may not always be conscious of the reasons for his or her choices.

Akin to the idea that choice making is expressive is the idea that freedom of choice is a necessary condition for expression. Banerjee stresses that without freedom of choice, an individual's actions cannot be considered expressive.[1] In his view, any behavior on the part of a person that is heavily influenced, manipulated, or forced by others reflects little about that individual's self. Thus, the music played by a child who must be forced to practice would not be classified as a reflection of the child's self; on the other hand, the child's reluctance to practice, as an exercise of freedom, might.

Choice making, however, is almost always constrained to some degree by society, usually on an ethical, legal, or economical basis. An individual's choices are thus as much determined by the resources, opportunities, and limitations of the environment as by personal preference.[2] As a consequence, some aspects of self may never be expressed during the course of a person's life, and some may have to be suppressed. Levinson et al. suggest that an individual lives out some aspects of self, while inhibiting or ignoring others, a process, moreover, that has a developmental dimension. Childhood preferences gradually evolve and ultimately may be suppressed or ignored as an individual comes to be an adult.[2]

Individual Variance in Expression. Self-expression can be viewed as a continuum that has, at one end, behavior that projects the private self into the world and ties people to others and, at the other end, behavior that shows an absence of self-projection, whose purpose seems to be to withdraw from the social world.[1] Banerjee considers both behaviors to be self-expressive. Although social withdrawal may express a negative, unhealthy denial of one's self, it is also found in the ascetic practices of yoga and other forms of meditation as an aspect of spiritual self-discipline. A withdrawal to solitude is also a way of coping with stress. Self-expression need not always be a social process. For some individuals, the most self-expressive times may be those they spend alone, away from others.

Functions of Self-Expression. Certainly a major function of self-expression is the communication of self-identity, the fixing and specifying of "who I am" in the world.[59] Schlenker argues that this function is accomplished privately through self-reflection, and publicly through the process of self-presentation and self-disclosure, discussed below. The image of self that is conveyed in any given situation represents both how an individual is and how the individual desires to be.[59]

Self-identification is a lifelong aspect of self-expression. Identity is always in a process of "becoming" in the sense that an individual's potentialities are developed and abilities actualized during the course of life.[2,60,61] Life choices are made and remade as an individual moves through the phases of development, and correspondingly, the identity one projects through self-expression also undergoes transition.

Another major function of self-expression is the establishment of interpersonal relationships. Relationships, particularly intimate ones, are a primary source of personal support. They offer a sense of closeness to others and therefore provide relief from the isolation inherent in our individual separateness. Because interpersonal relationships constitute a substantial part of the meaning most people find in living, self-expression can be viewed as essential to meeting a person's basic human needs, as classically defined by Maslow,[61] and as necessary to avoiding loneliness.

Coping is a final function of self-expression. Coping as defined in Chapter 6 is the human response to stress—that behavior by which an individual attempts to change a situation for the better. Frankl,[4] in *Man's Search for Meaning*, documents the powerful effect of self-expression as a means of coping with dire circumstances by examining the transcendent value inmates of World War II death camps derived from a search for meaning in their circumstances. *Hardiness*, the term used to refer to the personality characteristics that make a person resistant to stress, is a reflection of an individual's capacity to interpret potentially stressful situations as challenges rather than threats. A hardy person more readily perceives the opportunities for self-expression that present themselves in even the most difficult circumstances.

Clinical Relevance of a Concept of Self-Expression. A concept of self-expression is central to the philosophy of this text, which places heavy emphasis on person–environment transactions, both as they relate to an individual's experiences with health and illness and as they relate to the process by which one person is able to help another achieve health (see Chaps. 6 and 37). One might look on self-expression as mediating person–environment transactions, the outcomes of which are, alternatively, stress, illness, and decline; sameness; or growth and health. The following sections outline principles and clinical guidelines to help ensure that nurse–client transactions achieve the latter outcome.

The concept of self-expression is highly relevant and, in fact, fundamental to the clinical practice of nursing. Many nursing authorities believe that to influence health, nurse–client transactions require the context of a caring relationship.[62–64]

Caring involves self-expression. Marck argues that caring is based on equity, that is, on a process of give-and-take that incorporates the mutual sharing of self, which Marck labels "therapeutic reciprocity."[9] Examples of give-and-take include client participation in decisions about care, shared control of the professional relationship through mutual negotiation, instances of mutual self-disclosure and mutual learning, use of shared language and common terminology, exchanges of humor, and mutual accommodation of personal space. Marck stresses that reciprocity is neither inherently positive nor inherently negative, and proposes that therapeutic reciprocity, the kind that enhances health, reduces the emotional distance between nurse and client by a genuine exchange of feelings, thoughts, and experiences that are relevant to the client's care.[9]

Shared meaning and genuine exchange are influenced by the symbols used in interaction. Sarvimaki notes that the activity of nursing is loaded with symbols and meaning.[11] The words nurses use, the expressions on their faces, the tasks they perform, and how they perform them all work as symbols. A client's interpretation of what these symbols reflect about the nurse's caring ultimately influences whether the client will join with the nurse in a therapeutically reciprocal relationship.

The nurse's encounters with clients are always encounters with the clients' public selves, a seemingly self-evident idea that nevertheless bears emphasis; however, it is clients' private selves that are often deeply affected by the experience of illness. How much of their private selves clients are ultimately willing to share may depend to an important extent on the symbolism and meanings that nurses convey by their own appearance and behavior. Explicit messages that are contradicted by implicit ones can negate the communication of caring. Nurses who ask "How can I help you?" and then fail to promptly answer call lights place the client's trust at risk. If clients are not to be alone in their struggle with illness, it is paramount that all nurses develop the art of expressing caring in ways that clients can understand.

Dimensions of Self-Expression

Individual self-expression has essentially two behavioral dimensions: self-presentation and self-disclosure. Both dimensions are important in nursing, because they are the interpersonal means by which individuals communicate their self-concepts to others (Fig. 23–1).

Self-Presentation. **Self-presentation** refers to the conscious or unconscious attempts of individuals to control the images of themselves they convey to other people (immediate audiences), imagined or real, or to themselves.[65] Control implies that people make an effort to generate not just any impression, but rather a particular type of impression that is important to them.[65] Because self-presentation is involved with controlling the images or impressions one conveys, it is sometimes also referred to as the process of impression management.[30] Self-presentation is a primary means by which individuals form and maintain their self-concepts.

Strategies of Self-Presentation. A wide range of behavior is associated with self-presentation. Schneider identifies four behavioral categories: verbal, nonverbal, artifactual displays, and purposive behaviors.[66]

Verbal Self-Presentation. Almost any verbal statement can be construed as a self-presentation. Even a simple, "Hello, how are you?" which may seem uninformative, in fact suggests that the speaker has some knowledge of the normative standards of politeness. Thus, such a statement generally presents the speaker to others as a polite person. Failure to use appropriate greeting behavior in a situation, on the other hand, would present the individual as rude, distracted, or perhaps emotionally preoccupied.[66] Much verbal behavior that can be characterized as self-presentation, however, has to do with self-reports, statements that individuals make about themselves which tend to be generally positive in nature. Individuals make statements about themselves that are intended to convey social virtues such as honesty, sincerity, competence, and trustworthiness. When these statements seem to be exaggerated, people may consider the speaker to be bragging or boasting; when they seem to be minimized, people may consider the speaker to be modest.

Nonverbal Self-Presentation. Smiles, frowns, yawns, eye contact, brow knitting, head nodding, stooping, slumping, handshake firmness, and many other nonverbal behaviors have self-presentation value and are important in general person perception.[66] People who wish to gain social approval may attempt to ingratiate themselves to others through such behavior as frequent head nodding in affirmation of the opinions and ideas others express. Nonverbal behaviors are also useful for creating impressions about one's interpersonal style. They convey warmth, intensity, sincerity, modesty, shyness, aggressiveness, and many other traits. A simple "hello" conveys a social greeting, but when accompanied by a smile, eye contact, and a friendly handshake, it also communicates warmth.

Artifactual Displays. Schneider indicates that physical appearance cues, possessions, and even the situational context of behavior affect people's perceptions.[66] The fact that artifactual displays are important, Schneider notes, is confirmed by such social maxims as "dress for success" and by the frequent emphasis on the social value of status possessions.[66] Adornments, either of one's person or of one's space, are an important means of self-presentation. Associations are also an important means, if more indirect.[66] Behavior such as name dropping reflects the self-presentation value of "knowing the right people." A similar behavior is wearing apparel marked with school or organization insignias that call attention to one's affiliations. Richardson and Cialdini refer to such behavior as "basking in reflected glory."[67] Situational contexts also convey impressions. The size and placement of an administrator's office, the neighborhood in which an individual lives, the places a person goes to relax all convey messages about the type of person an individual is or wishes to be.

Purposive Behavior. Purposive behavior refers to any behavior that is designed to elicit a particular response from others. Examples of purposive behavior include favors, gifts, intimidation, expression of moral outrage, flattery, opinion, conformity, and many others. Such behaviors can be used to elicit gratitude, admiration, or fear from others. They also communicate something about the behaver as a generous, powerful, exemplary, admiring, or attractive person, and thus have self-presentation value.

Functions of Self-Presentation. Many motives have been proposed to explain why people engage in self-presentation. According to Tedeschi and Reiss, these include (1) construction of a social role, (2) maintenance of self-esteem, (3) consolidation of power and social influence, and (4) desire for social approval and avoidance of disapproval.[68] Most authorities agree, however, that a common underlying motive is the universal desire for social approval.[69]

Much behavior serves to construct and protect images that individuals associate with acceptance and admiration from others.[69] Social approval is a powerful motivator because it is a prime source of self-esteem. Hass has noted that self-esteem is a function of how people perceive themselves; therefore, anything that improves one's concept or perceptions of self generally raises self-esteem.[70] Successful self-presentation elicits social approval from others and provides information that the individual may use to shape, confirm, or alter self-perceptions.[71] Confirmation of one's impressions by others has a self-esteem–enhancing effect because it serves to bring the real self and ideal self into closer approximation.[72]

Another basic reason why people engage in self-presentation is to identify themselves to others and to de-

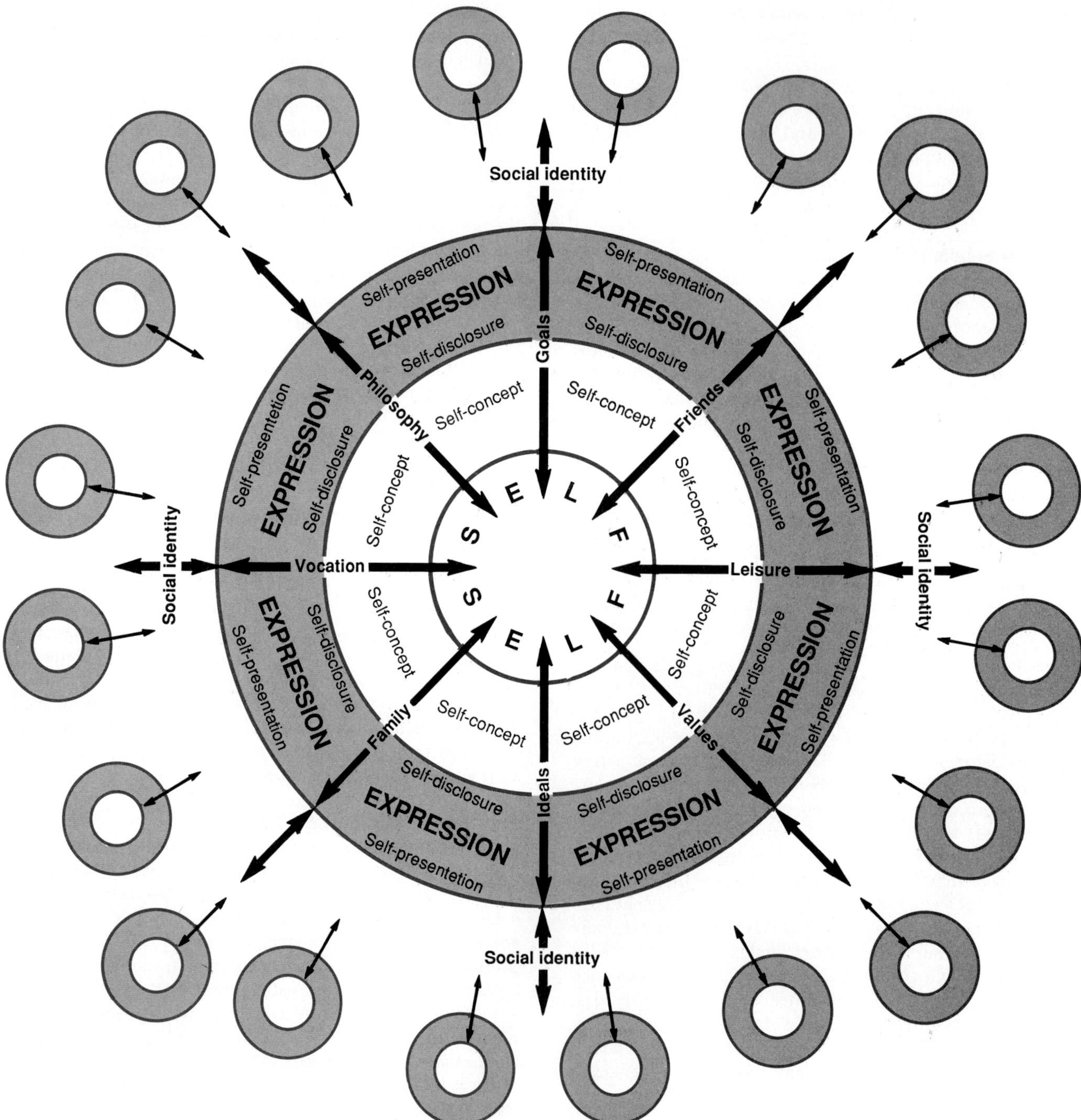

Figure 23–1. Self-expression. This diagram depicts the relationships between self-presentation and self-disclosure and the self, the self-concept and social identity. Self-presentation and self-disclosure are the interpersonal means by which individuals communicate their self-concepts to others and reinforce them to themselves. The life structure, depicted by the spokes that extend from the self into the social environment, provides the social framework for building and enacting the self-concept. Through the various aspects of the life structure, individuals are able to relate to others, and to present themselves and disclose themselves to others. The arrows depict the mutual influence between the self and the social environment.

fine themselves for others in social interaction. Through self-presentation, people call out their identity as a person through their manner, dress, and behavior. Recall that self-identification is a basic function of self-expression. Self-presentation, then, is a fundamental process for fixing identity in social situations.

Identity can be understood either from the standpoint of the individual (self-concept) or from the standpoint of others (social perception of the individual's characteristics, roles, positions). Self-presentation represents the interface between self-concept and social identity. It is a public display of self, integrating aspects of the real self with aspects of the ideal self, to which others react.[72] The reactions of others, in turn, serve to confirm or disprove the validity of persons' self-presentations and ultimately of their self-concepts.

Control is an important element of self-presentation. In striving to present themselves to others, people seek for others to regard them in a way that is consistent with their own self-concepts. When self-presentations are successful, others assign positive qualities to the individual and describe the individual in positive terms; they also behave toward the individual in a way that reinforces the individual's self-concept.[68]

Self-presentation carries risks, however. The success of a person's self-presentation is never assured, but varies with the match between the values projected and the values held by the group that acts as the audience.[59] People unfortunately make self-presentational mistakes and get caught up in incongruities regarding their social identity.[68] Thus, to a certain extent, identity is always a compromise between wishes and reality.

Self-presentation mistakes can be relatively harmless and easily correctable, such as when a person makes an uncharacteristic social blunder, for example, through inadvertently failing to greet an acquaintance. Self-presentation mistakes can also carry social consequences. One of those consequences is that others will assign negative labels to a person, labels that depict a negative social identity. Mistakes involving the presentation of aggression in social situations, for example, can result in labels of "wimp" or, alternatively, "bully."

Serious self-presentation mistakes, on the other hand, such as those exemplified in public incontinence, drunkenness, or hallucinations often result in the assignment of labels signifying social deviance, for example, "bum." Such labels are associated with varying amounts of social rejection and carry the risk of a severe loss of personal reputation. Indeed, certain types of deviance act to stigmatize an individual and lead to social ostracism.[73] Faced with the situation of coping with a spoiled identity, some individuals find it necessary to construct an entirely new identity.

Thus, most individuals strive to avoid self-presentational predicaments by projecting identities that are believable and that will be acceptable to others in their lives and adjust the identities they project somewhat to conform to their understanding of the audience they confront.[65] Generally these identities are in fairly close accord with the individual's self-understanding, and over time patterns of self-presentation become automatic and unconscious. Thus, self-presentation is strategic in the sense that it has a goal, not in the sense that it involves conscious planning or an attempt to portray a wholly inaccurate image of the self.

Clinical Importance of Self-Presentation. Self-presentation is important in any setting because all people have identities to confirm and protect. Nurses and clients are no exceptions. Human relations in general and professional relations in particular are enhanced when people understand the significance of one another's self-presentations and respond to support one another's identities.

Nevertheless, self-presentation has special significance where clients are concerned. As Chapter 12 established, clients who take on the sick role assume a new identity and relinquish aspects of a prior identity, at least for a period. Such transitions are stressful. Nurses who are able to ease identity transitions make an important contribution to the client's health.

Identity transitions are made easier by supporting the client's social presentation of self. Nurses do this in many ways, for example, by getting to know their clients as individuals, by conversing with clients about their lives, by assisting clients with their personal identity rituals (make-up, grooming, hair arrangement), by expressing interest in clients' self-reports, and by protecting clients' privacy during any activity that would be inappropriate to conduct in public. These actions and many others that will be discussed below serve to ease the identity transitions that occur between illness and wellness.

Identity transitions may be complicated by failing to support the client's social presentation of self. Although nurses generally recognize that identity transitions are an important part of illness, they are occasionally unsuccessful in helping clients to adapt to these transitions. Nurses generally accept that they are responsible for developing positive relationships with clients, but they often vary the character of their responses to clients in response to the impressions they gain from the way clients present themselves. It is well documented, for example, that nurses too often differentiate between clients who are "good" and clients who are "bad."[74–76] Good clients, as described in the literature, are cheerful, control their feelings, and are appreciative of what nurses do for them.[75] Bad clients, on the other hand, are those nurses view as highly anxious, depressed, hostile, challenging, overly dependent or independent, aggressive, impatient, unappreciative, or nonconforming, and those whose care necessitates greater energy and effort on the part of the nursing staff.[75] Although some of these clients may be manifesting long-established personality traits, many are simply reacting to the humiliating identity transition that frequently accompanies the sick role.[76]

Such client behavior may cause the nurse to feel ineffective and, as a consequence, to react defensively.[75] Too often, nurses label clients as "difficult" or "demanding" when they impede the flow of work by their complaints or fail to cooperate. These labels signal the disapproval that nurses hold and their personal perception that the client's behavior is deviant. Unfortunately, such labels serve to fix the identity of the client in the nurse's eyes, which can have negative consequences for caregiving.[77,78] As Jankin has pointed out, once nurses label clients, they no longer are able to process client data; they see only one aspect of the total person.[79] There is evidence, moreover, that nurses express personal frustration and anger by avoiding or ignoring clients labeled as difficult.[79–81]

Self-Disclosure. **Self-disclosure** is sometimes distinguished from self-presentation on the basis of being uncontrived, spontaneous, and more truly expressive of an individual's self-understanding. The goal of image control is absent or generally less important in self-disclosure. What really distinguishes self-disclosure from self-presentation is the *level* of self-understanding conveyed. Self-disclosure is not the communication of any self-understanding; rather, it is the communication of one's innermost self-understandings. As defined by Jourard, self-disclosure is the process of telling another person about oneself, sharing thoughts and feelings that may be of a deeply personal and private nature.[82]

Self-disclosure is most often a feature of close, even intimate, relationships between human beings.[31] In fact, the degree of intimacy of a relationship can be defined by the amount of self-disclosure and reciprocal sharing of self that occurs.[31] Self-disclosure involves decisions about whether to reveal one's thoughts, feelings, past experiences, and future goals to another person, to what degree, at what time, and in what place. As a feature of a relationship in which people feel free of the constraints that might serve as barriers to self-expression, self-disclosure can be considered as a correlate of interpersonal trust.[83]

Strategies of Self-Disclosure. Essentially there are two types of self-disclosure: cognitive self-disclosure, in which an individual shares self-related information, and affective self-disclosure, in which an individual shares feelings.[84] Verbal and nonverbal strategies for self-disclosure follow from the nature of the self-disclosure being made, whether cognitive or affective.

Cognitive Self-Disclosure. Cognitive self-disclosure involves the communication of personal thoughts and beliefs, and much of it is conveyed by verbal statements that begin with the words "I think" or "I believe." This type of self-disclosure characterizes the early phases of a close relationship and helps to reduce partners' uncertainty about each other's attitudes, values, and characteristics, and to develop mutual understanding. Once the partners feel that they understand one another, the exchange of factual information generally decreases.[84] Information that is conveyed in cognitive self-disclosure is related to one's own appearance, behavior, personality, or self-concept. As relationships develop, a greater range of self-references in verbal discourse emerges.[84]

Affective Self-Disclosure. Initially, in developing relationships, verbal exchanges are focused on information about the partners' selves. As the relationship progresses, that information is expanded to include statements about personal feelings. The range of emotional information also increases, and the modes of expression become more variable. The focus not only is on how partners feel about themselves, but also on how they feel about each other and the relationship.[84] Feelings may be expressed nonverbally or verbally or, for a variety of reasons, may remain unexpressed. Partners generally negotiate a relationship in which both are comfortable with the intensity of the emotion exchanged.

Even in close relationships, how and when a person expresses emotion vary.[84] It has long been recognized, for example, that the norms regulating emotional expressivity are governed by sex-role behavior. Thus, an individual's desire to protect his or her masculine or feminine identity may determine whether or not emotion is communicated and how and to what degree it is communicated.[85] Other factors include the topic of disclosure (some people have difficulty with expression of feelings on such topics as fears, weaknesses, and negative attitudes toward the other person) and the relative social status of the partners (intimate disclosure tends to flow from those low in power to those high in power).[85] Still another factor involves the consequences anticipated. Individuals tend to match the intimacy of disclosures to maintain an equal social exchange.[86] They may restrict self-disclosure to positive references and feelings about the partner in anticipation of the tension and conflict that might result from the reciprocation of an expression of negative feeling.[84]

Functions of Self-Disclosure. As with self-presentation, many motives have been identified to explain why people engage in self-disclosure, among them (1) maintenance and enhancement of relationships, (2) anticipation of rewards, and (3) reduction of anxiety.[87]

Self-disclosure is widely recognized as an important process for establishing and consolidating social relationships, particularly close or intimate social relationships.[31,88] Relationships provide the forum for self-disclosure, and self-disclosure, in turn, serves as (1) a mode for self-expression, particularly in the release of feelings; (2) a way to gain self-clarification through presenting one's ideas to another; (3) a way to obtain social validation through comparing oneself with another individual; (4) and a way to consolidate social influence through impression management during disclosure.[89]

In addition, self-disclosure supports mutuality in relationships by enabling individuals to identify their similarities in needs and skills and their shared beliefs and expectations.[89] Thus, just as self-presentation aids in self-identification, self-disclosure also contributes to the process of identity bargaining and mutual accommodation through which individuals negotiate complementary roles. When this process is successful, the role relationships that develop reinforce interdependence. In turn, interdependence provides individuals with the help they need to cope with life and living.[89] Repeated experience of mutual help, caring, and acceptance generally benefits the partners in a relationship by reducing their anxiety. Trust and a sense of confidence in each other's integrity, truthfulness, and commitment to the relationship frequently follow.[89]

Self-disclosure, like self-presentation, is not without its risks, however. Revealing personal information of a deep, secret nature makes an individual particularly vulnerable to hurt. Just as self-disclosure helps create an intimate relationship, it can also lead to negative consequences. In fact, a hallmark of self-disclosure is that it places an individual at a self-created disadvantage, which may explain the pressure for reciprocation that partners frequently experience as relationships develop.

Derlega identifies six specific risks to which individuals subject themselves through self-disclosure:

1. *Rejection.* An individual's identity may be rejected; after making a complete disclosure, individuals may find others dislike them.
2. *Embarrassment.* An individual may discover after disclosing personal interest that the other person is uninterested in a close relationship.
3. *Exploitation.* In a vulnerable moment a partner may remind the discloser of his or her weaknesses.
4. *Leaks.* One partner may share information gained through disclosure with others, only to have the disclosing partner become aware that others were told.
5. *Betrayal.* One partner may disclose information to another who then uses it against the discloser with a third party.
6. *Inequity.* One partner may disclose more than the other, causing resentment by the discloser toward the withholder.[83]

The fear of being rejected or exploited can be countered by refraining from disclosure, but the alternative is social isolation and loneliness.[83,90] Most people respond by honing their social skills for developing intimacy.[90] Others are particularly sensitive to rejection and, as a consequence, have lifelong problems in developing close relationships and are subject to considerable loneliness.

Clinical Importance of Self-Disclosure. From the client's point of view, the process of health assessment is a one-sided process of self-disclosure that often occurs in the context of a relationship with a stranger. Ordinarily such circumstances would inhibit disclosure. Nevertheless, nurses frequently request clients to disclose a significant amount of extremely personal information during the health interview. Clients are usually responsive, not because nurses are unusually successful in conveying an impression of trustworthiness, but rather because implicit in the interaction is their mutual understanding of the nurse's role, which makes it unethical for the nurse to violate the client's trust. On the other hand, clients bring the values and concerns they hold for social relationships to the health interview. As they respond to the nurse's questions, they may observe the nurse for subtle nonverbal indicators of personal attitudes and may hold an undisclosed fear that the nurse will ultimately reject them for their answers to intimate questions.

What clients may not understand is that the stakes in the developing relationship are also high for nurses. Nurse–client interaction is professional in nature, yet it shares many of the features of interaction typical of other types of close relationships, perhaps even exceeding them in the physical closeness involved in certain acts of caregiving. The personal effectiveness of nurses and, ultimately, their professional identity may depend on an ability to establish interactions based on mutual trust and acceptance and to create a climate in which clients feel comfortable to disclose bothersome thoughts and feelings that may ultimately interfere with regaining health.

Effective caregiving frequently involves client counseling, and virtually all forms of counseling emphasize the ongoing importance of self-disclosure on the part of clients.[83] Thus, nurses are concerned about the way they present themselves in the health interview because they understand that the impressions they create on the client may either enhance or hinder the development of trust and ultimately their ability to successfully counsel clients about health matters that are of concern to them. Chapter 16 discusses interview approaches available to nurses for minimizing the perceived risks of disclosure for clients and for enhancing the impressions nurses make as caring professionals.

How are close relationships with nurses potentially beneficial to clients? Not only are nurses educated to understand the psychological impact of illness and the problems associated with particular health conditions, but their bedside role gives nurses a special opportunity to get to know the client. This means that nurses are uniquely well prepared and well situated to aid clients with the distress that commonly accompanies illness. **Distress** is the state of mental or physical anguish that corresponds to stress. Clients often experience distress and need opportunities for distress disclosure.[91] There is evidence, for example, that distress disclosure has beneficial physical as well as psychological effects.[92] Nurses understand the importance of distress disclosure to clients' coping, and this benefits clients both directly and indirectly. (Distress disclosure is discussed in more detail below, under *Factors Affecting Self-Expression: Stress.*)

Self-Presentation, Self-Disclosure, and Life Activities. Life activities, particularly those that constitute life patterns and deep personal preferences and commitments, have already been identified as a mode of self-expression. They can also be examined for their value along the dimensions of self-presentation and self-disclosure.

Self-presentation occurs in face-to-face interaction, as well as in activities that communicate qualities of the self, or self-ideal, to onlookers. Such activities influence the impressions an individual makes. Consider the competitive ordinary athlete, for example. Athletic feats demand strong self-discipline and self-denial to develop and maintain the required muscle dexterity. A display of athletic skill therefore presents an individual to onlookers as a person who clearly has these personal qualities. The athlete is thus accorded the social identity of a self-disciplined person.

Self-disclosure is also possible through an individual's activities, many of which involve a deep commitment for their pursuit, perhaps at considerable personal cost. Such activities are sometimes said to reveal personal "passion." As applied to a life activity, passion reflects an intense, driving, even overwhelming motivation to be involved in and to excel in an endeavor. Life patterns that reveal a long-term devotion to an activity are therefore self-disclosing in the sense that they are indicative of a person's passions. Whereas individuals may be unable to verbalize the passionate nature of their commitments, often their passion will be apparent in the amount of time and effort they dedicate to a pursuit.

Nurses are interested in the importance of an individual's activities from the standpoint of their contribution to the person's identity. Illnesses that interrupt or make impossible the activities that are central to self-concept and social identity are likely to be especially stressful and threatening.

■ FACTORS AFFECTING SELF-EXPRESSION

Age

Age and development are important determinants not only of the modes available to an individual for self-expression and the dimensions of individual self-expression, but also of the cognitive and affective content of self-expression. Chapter 10 discusses at length the evolution of human characteristics over the life span and reviews various theories of development and age-related identity changes. The reader is referred to that chapter for comprehensive coverage of the role that age plays in self-expression.

Basic human needs and corresponding developmental tasks generally shape the character of self-expression during any given phase of development; thus, self-expression itself develops with passing time. The neonate's self-expression, for example, centers around reflex behaviors and vocalizations oriented to securing needs for food and warmth. By comparison, the infant's range is much broader and is revealed in the development of the social smile, the rudimentary beginning of social skill.

Toddlers' self-expression is centered on growing independence, curiosity about the environment, imitation of others, and use of words instead of cries to call attention to their needs, whereas preschoolers are intent on learning what their abilities are and the basic rules for playing compatibly with their peers. An overly restrictive environment during either of these stages can interfere with the child's developing sense of "who I am."

School-aged children are preoccupied with friendships, activities, and skill development, whereas adolescents devote most of their time to developing a personal and sexual identity and contemplating the future. At no time are issues of self-presentation and self-disclosure more important than during adolescence.

Young adults, on the other hand, express themselves primarily through important life choices for work, leisure, and family. Middle adulthood involves the fruition of creative goals, whereas older adulthood is a time for reflection, reminiscence, and the self-actualizing pursuits that remain within the individual's physical capacity to achieve. Thus, self-expression is clearly tied to the unique characteristics of the various phases of life and development.

Usually age and self-expression patterns correspond to one another. When an individual's self-expression patterns lag behind chronological age, the individual is said to be immature; when they go beyond chronological age, the individual is said to be precocious. Development is never complete, however, and even in adulthood, people make significant changes in their lives with the objective of finding satisfying, personally fulfilling self-expression patterns.

Personality

Personality encompasses the whole of an individual's behavioral and emotional tendencies (see Chap. 10). Personality influences how a person thinks, feels, and acts in any given situation. For any particular individual, the personality will show uniqueness, continuity, and development over time.

One of the most important aspects of the personality is the self-concept, defined previously in this chapter. Images of the self are formed and stabilized over years of personality development through repeated playing out of images in a person's imagination and through their subsequent validation in the environment by significant others.[93] The images that are most central and important to an individual form the core self-concept. These are the images that are most frequently used, most likely to be activated in the memory by social cues, to operate as salient determinants of behavior in any particular social context, and to engender stress when threatened.[93] As a determinant of behavior, self-concept is also a determinant of self-expression.

Self-concepts are generally oriented around the human qualities that people as individuals have come to value highly. Most individuals, however, perceive a gap between the self-concept (how they see themselves) and the self-ideal (how they would like to be). A wide gap between self-ideal and self-concept may be accompanied by low self-esteem, whereas a narrow gap may correspond to high self-esteem. To gain and protect self-esteem, people generally seek to merge the self-ideal and the self-concept.[65] Thus, the gap serves as a goal to motivate people to better themselves and to select self-presentations that are in line with their personal capabilities. For most people, however, the gap is never entirely closed.

Usually people hold self-ideals that are realizable; that is, they strive for those things that they have the personal or environmental resources to achieve.[65] Balance is revealed in an individual's expression of a self-assured demeanor and in the self-confident pursuit of personal goals. An imbalance of ideals and resources is also revealed in self-expression. Defensively, individuals may insist that they have achieved ideal characteristics when they have not, a tendency that may impress others as egotistical; or they may insist that they fall far short of ideal characteristics when they do not, a tendency that may impress others as revealing emotional insecurity.

When self-ideals become impossible to realize, as sometimes happens when people become seriously ill, a negative change in self-concept frequently occurs that is often reflected in an individual's self-expression. Such individuals may dwell mentally or verbally on their shortcomings, communicate a sad, dejected affect, and even withdraw from social interaction, all hallmarks of psychological depression.

Fortunately, self-concept is not a fixed entity, but rather a product of continual learning. Clients whose self-concepts are threatened by illness can learn new patterns with the help of those around them. Mastery over the most difficult circumstances can be achieved when modeling and other teaching strategies are employed to personally empower the individual to achieve change.[94] Social influences contribute to personal development by assisting in a reduction of the anxiety that often accompanies a threat to self-concept, by the interests and competencies they cultivate in the individual, and by the social networks they provide.

Neurosensory Variables

Self-expression is to a large extent a product of the neurosensory mechanisms that supply the anatomical and physiological means for communication. Although factors outside the individual act to influence self-expression, the capacity to discern those factors and to modify one's self-expression accordingly is largely a function of neurosensory information processing. The neurosensory mechanisms for communication are described in detail in Chapter 29; however, the role of the brain and sense organs is briefly outlined here to emphasize certain important features and their implications for self-expression.

The two hemispheres of the brain play distinctly different but important roles in self-expression. These roles are related to the pattern of cerebral dominance that develops in most individuals whereby certain cognitive and motor functions become progressively localized in one hemisphere or the other. The left hemisphere, for instance, is known to be adept in the functions of sequential analysis and abstraction. The right hemisphere, on the other hand, tends to organize and treat data in terms of complex wholes and works to synthesize broad meanings from fragmentary information.[95]

Researchers have firmly established the relative superiority of the left cerebral hemisphere for speech- and language-related activities.[95] For most right-handed people and the majority of left-handed people, disease or injury of the left hemisphere will result in language disorders involving the perception of verbal sensory stimuli. Such individuals, because they lose their ability to appreciate the structure of language, often have difficulty comprehending oral communications, speaking and writing clearly, and cueing the memory for the correct names for objects.[95]

In contrast to the analytic function of the left hemisphere in encoding and decoding communication, the role of the right hemisphere seems to lie in affective communication.[95] Thus, left-hemisphere disorders disturb an individual's comprehension of language and ability to speak or write, whereas right-hemisphere disorders disturb the affective aspect of speech, altering both the comprehension of emotion in others' speech and the expression of emotion in one's own.[95]

The major sense organs also play an important role in self-expression. Sensory input from vision and hearing is extremely important to communication. In fact, the loss of eyesight and hearing raises significant barriers to communication. Vision and hearing not only contribute to an individual's ability to receive the neurosensory data needed for ordinary exchange of verbal and gestural messages, they also provide the primary sensory means for an individual's experience of the environment. Loss of vision and hearing thus has an important impact on an individual's capacity for social interaction and for engagement in those expressive activities that rely on vision and hearing.

Sociocultural and Economic Variables

The place of social relationships in human self-expression has been described already, as has the societal contribution to the development of the self and the social modes by which individuals act to influence their environment in the service of self-expression. Chapter 9 discusses in detail sociocultural processes and how they affect the social experience of health and illness. The reader is referred to that chapter for an in-depth review of the ways society acts to govern and regulate patterns of individual self-expression.

The social norms for appropriate discourse in a given social context have a powerful influence on individual self-expression. Social rules for self-expression will vary with several important social factors. *Who* is in a social situation, *where* the interaction is taking place, and *what* is happening all influence the perceived meanings of interactions between individuals and the corresponding social rules that operate for individual behavior. Even nurse–client interaction is subject to social norms. Deviations from social norms are possible, but place the individual's social approval at risk, as previously noted.

Social norms are culturally determined, and cultures vary in the social behavior they approve. Thus, in pluralistic, culturally complex societies such as the United States and Canada, social groups vary in the rules they apply to regulate social situations. These differences reflect the predominant culture to which the group subscribes, whether that is the majority or any one of several minority cultures, an ethnic or religious orientation, or an upper-, middle-, or working-class distinction. Individuals learn the rules of the social groups with which they identify, and these groups exert influence on the choices of their members for self-expressive outlets and behavior.

The groups whose values and rules an individual adopts are called **reference groups.** Any group may serve as a reference group for a given person, for example, a group to which the person belongs or wishes to belong, an interaction group, a status group, a statistical category, an actual group, or a merely imaginary group. These groups exert their influence in a passive way, simply by being thought of by the individual. Reference groups influence individuals' patterns for speech and dress, their habits and rituals, their goals and attitudes, their personal philosophies, and their choices for work, family, and leisure.

Reference groups also act as yardsticks for the process of social comparison by which people evaluate themselves in relation to others.[96] People have a natural tendency to look at themselves as better off or worse off than others. Such comparisons may have positive or negative implications for an individual's self-esteem.[97] Learning that another is better off than yourself suggests that (1) you are not as well off as everyone else (negative), and (2) it is possible for you to be better (positive). On the other hand, learning that another is worse off than yourself suggests that (1) you are not as bad off as everyone else (positive), and (2) it is possible for you to get worse (negative). Thus, the effect on self-esteem will be determined by one's interpretation of the information gained. Positive interpretations should have a positive effect on self-esteem.[97]

All people, clients included, use such social reference groups to support their concept of self; to evaluate the advantages and disadvantages of their personal situation; to set their physical, social and material goals; and to appraise their own progress toward those goals. Social comparison is an important process in health and illness alike. Thus, clients may feel threatened when they are exposed to others with the same health problem but who are more ill, as sometimes happens in hospital or clinic waiting rooms.[98]

Another important social variable is the opportunity for self-expression afforded by an individual's economic resources. Any individual's self-expression can be significantly constrained by a lack of economic resources; for some individuals economics may be the deciding factor as to whether or not their personal skills and talents are developed. A child reared in poverty may have a natural musical ability, but lack the economic resources to pursue its development. A young person may be unable to attain a desired situated identity in which to express self (teacher, nurse, lawyer, social worker), if he or she is unable to pay the tuition and living expenses associated with college. Few people have the economic resources to pursue anything they wish. Thus, adaptation and adjustment are necessary, and a person's success in adapting will affect his or her well-being.

Still another sociocultural variable is access to others. Some social situations provide only a limited social network and may serve to isolate an individual from others. Living in a retirement home tends to separate the elderly from the community and their families, for example. To the extent that access to others is constrained, personal expression also may be correspondingly limited. It is difficult to sustain intimate relationships, for instance, when social contact is infrequent. Conversely, building social networks may substantially increase personal opportunities for expression and improve overall well-being by expanding one's available social resources. Nelson, for example, studied institutionalized elderly and found that those who had social networks that provided significant amounts of aid, affirmation, and affection reported less depression.[99] Thus, it is not surprising that the value of social support is widely acknowledged by nurses.[99–101]

Personal Values and Philosophy

Personal values and philosophy have an important influence on self-expression. One's world view, outlook on life, personal ethics, and spiritual framework all affect personal choices for self-expression.

Personal values and philosophy, however, reflect both individual personality and social learning. The interaction of a person's natural tendencies with environmental influences creates variability in individual self-expression. People may be socialized into any number of groups that have norms for the regulation of self-expression, and yet retain a unique perspective that represents their own personal interpretation of a group identity.

Because person and environment are mutually influencing, one can never assume that an individual's group affiliations or demographic assignments by virtue of age, sex, or ethnicity wholly determine personal self-expression patterns. For example, one individual may practice the rituals of a particular religion, but fail to accept all of the teachings of that religion for regulating self-expression, whereas another may adhere faithfully to all tenets. Those differences of personal values within a broader philosophic framework are nevertheless likely to be reflected in an individual's personal patterns of self-expression. Thus, it is important to avoid stereotypes when approaching individuals in a health care setting or any other social setting; one may become insensitive to the influence of individual value differences.

Health and Illness

Neurosensory health has a direct effect on an individual's patterns of self-expression. As long as neurosensory mechanisms operate efficiently, self-presentation and self-disclosure have the necessary biological support and will be influenced more by an individual's state of psychological and social need than by neurosensory processes. More indirectly, general health is also an important influence. Good nutrition and fitness, psychological well-being, and social satisfaction are all important ingredients for a vibrant pattern of self-expression.

Illness, on the other hand, often acts to alter self-expression, by its effect on the body (eg, body sensations such as pain and fatigue) and by its effect on neurosensory, psychological, and social processes. Especially when severe, illness can have a profound effect on the way people communicate and on the focus of their communication.

Stress

The integral relationship among health, stress, and illness was examined in Chapter 6. Stress disturbs the mind–body relationships and physiological regulatory mechanisms that are important to health. Failure to moderate stress eventually overtaxes the body's homeostatic capacity and thus contributes to the development of illness. To the extent it interferes with bodily health, stress acts as an indirect influence on self-expression.

Stress also directly influences self-expression through its effects on psychological and social processes. Psychologically, people who are distressed have a need to disclose their discomfort to others, a process sometimes referred to as **distress disclosure.** Stiles has observed that the intensity of a person's distress is related to the amount of distress disclosure made, and that disclosure helps to relieve the person's distress.[102] He depicts these relationships as analogous to the relationship of a fever to physical infection in which the fever is both a sign of disturbance and a part of the restorative process.

In distress disclosure, individuals' vocalizations, gestures, and body positions reflect their internal, phenomenological frame of reference. Distress disclosures reflect subjective experience, and convey the speaker's private awareness. They can be distinguished from other statements in that they are generally made in the first person and refer to private experience. For example, a person disclosing distress would say, "I've been very lonely," rather than, "I seldom go out on a date." The former is expressive and describes how the speaker feels; the latter is a statement of objective fact that does not make reference to a feeling state.

Upsetting or stressful events commonly generate a subjective sense of pressure that seems to derive from the feeling that strong emotions such as anger, fear, remorse, and despair are being bottled up.[102] This sense of pressure is relieved by telling others about one's private experience.

The mechanism by which distress leads to disclosure involves an increase in an individual's private self-consciousness, according to Stiles.[102] Powerful emotion forces the individual's attention to internal, subjective matters, creating a motivation for **catharsis,** the process of psychologically purging or getting rid of emotion. The process of disclosure is akin to other homeostatic self-regulating mechanisms. Once catharsis is achieved, the need to disclose is inhibited.[102]

Stiles emphasizes that the benefit of disclosure lies in the depth rather than the extent of the disclosure and in the intensity of the accompanying emotional expression.[102] Victims of stress, trauma, or bereavement are less likely to become depressed if they confide their feelings to others, and this process may prevent the physiological arousal that results in physical symptoms.[103]

Aside from stress relief, another long-term benefit of distress disclosure for the individual is self-understanding and insight. **Insight** is the mental ability to see into a situation and perceive its meanings. An increase in self-understanding constitutes psychological growth. Talk that involves the individual's internal frame of reference assists the individual to bring inconsistent feelings into awareness where they can be evaluated. The opportunity for such talk is one of the benefits of counseling.

Although there are decided benefits of distress disclosure, a prolonged need for it can take a toll on a person's social relationships. Coates and Winston refer to this as the dilemma of distress disclosure.[91] People tire of others who are unhappy and suffering.[104] Indeed, distress disclosure may even prompt rejection from others.[105] Because of the importance of social support to successful coping, the loss of this support could ultimately undermine the individual's adaptation and well-being. Nurses and other helping professionals thus have an important role to play. Their assumption of the role of listener provides the client with another outlet for distress disclosure and relieves the client's significant others from some of the burden of the client's distress.

Helpers' efforts may actually promote more than the client's psychological and social well-being. Evidence exists that by providing an opportunity for catharsis, helpers may serve to enhance the survival of those who already have a serious illness. Derogatis and associates found that clients with metastatic breast cancer (breast cancer that had spread to other organs) who readily expressed their anger and depression survived longer than those who kept their troubles to themselves.[106]

IMPLICATIONS FOR NURSE–CLIENT COLLABORATION

Self-Disclosure, Distress, Loss, and Illness

Distress is the emotional experience of stress. Distress usually requires outward expression to relieve the sense of pressure that accompanies it. Distress is part of the experience of loss. Loss, in turn, is a key aspect of identity change. Illness often brings changes in social identity and personal identity (self-concept). Illness may initiate changes in body image, role performance, sexual behavior, or future plans, all of which alter profoundly an individual's relationship to the environment. These changes are experienced as loss, the most painful aspect of which may be loss of the self-ideal. Grieving such deep losses is facilitated by opportunities for distress disclosure within the context of a caring relationship. Effective nurse–client collaboration in illness provides those opportunities.

Medication and Substance Use

Medications and drugs influence self-expression in a variety of ways. Some drugs alter mental functions, acting to change a person's mood (narcotics, cannabinoids, alcohol, antidepressants), allay anxiety (antianxiety agents, tranquilizers), stimulate or depress the mind (amphetamines, barbiturates), or alter thought processes (antipsychotic agents, hallucinogens). These agents have a dramatic effect on the mental processes and, as a result, are able to alter an individual's experience in subjectively pleasurable or disturbing ways, thus influencing self-expression. The use of these agents also has well-known social consequences. Some agents, such as the antidepressives and antipsychotics, may actually assist individuals to interact appropriately and improve their overall social functioning. Others, when abused or used inappropriately, create psychological dependence and physical addiction and may result in a life-style that fosters mental, physical, and social deterioration.

Other drugs have the ability to influence self-expression not by modifying mental processes, but by changing an individual's bodily sensations. Any of a number of drugs, for example, serve to relieve distressing symptoms that might interfere with personal comfort and thus with self-expression. Drugs that relieve pain (analgesics), reduce stomach acidity (antacids), relieve vomiting (antiemetics), reduce fever (antipyretics), relieve coughing (antitussives), relieve constipation (laxatives), or reduce edema (diuretics) indirectly improve mental outlook by relieving discomfort. The relief from symptoms that these agents provide enables individuals to divert attention from bodily symptoms and refocus on social and environmental events.

Still other drugs exert an indirect influence on self-expression by correcting the causes of distressing symptoms. Drugs that cure infection (antibiotics), improve cardiac function (cardiac glycosides, antiarrhythmics), improve metabolic homeostasis (insulin), reduce inflammation (corticosteroids), or destroy tumors (antineoplastic agents) act to improve overall health, to increase longevity, and thus to enhance the individual's opportunities for self-expression.

Sex and Sexuality

Sex and sexuality are related but distinct concepts. **Sex** relates to an individual's anatomic differentiation as male or female, and thus makes a concrete, narrow reference to the characteristics of the sex organs, and to a person's physical identity as male or female. Sex also refers to the functional characteristics that serve reproduction and to the behavioral act of engaging in sexual intercourse.

Sexuality, on the other hand, is an abstraction that refers to a pervasive characteristic of personality reflected in the totality of a person's feelings, attitudes, beliefs, and behavior related to being male or female.[107] Although sex is a narrow concept, sexuality is a broad concept that synthesizes varied aspects of an individual's expression of self.[107] Chapter 10 describes in detail the many aspects of life and living that are integrated by an individual's sexuality, including the influence of sexuality on individuality, life choices, life-style, self-concept, close and distant social relationships, roles, and health status.

Sexuality involves both gender identity, that is, the psychological identification with one's sex, and social identity, which involves others' identification of an individual with masculine or feminine traits. Sexuality also relates broadly to the desire for love, warmth, sharing, and touching between individuals that is present throughout life (Fig. 23–2). It is thus an important part of everyday human relationships and an extremely powerful motivator of human behavior. For most people, sexuality and sex correspond; that is, their psychological and social identities are heavily influenced by their biological heritage and physical identity.

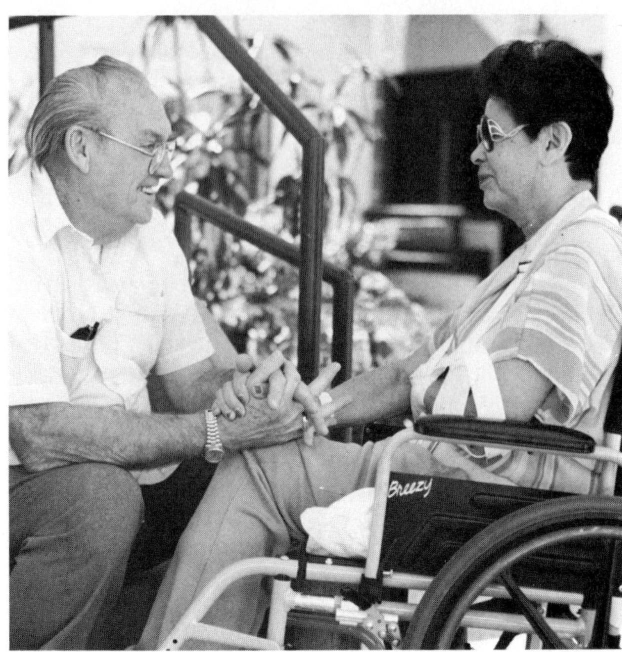

Figure 23–2. Sexuality, including the need for love and sharing, is present throughout the life span.

Sex and sexuality are extremely important factors in self-expression. The ability to express oneself by engaging in a close physical relationship with a sexual partner is of central importance to the self-esteem of most individuals. That is because the physical capacity for sex is ultimately related, for many people, to a sense of adequacy as a man or a woman. A concept of oneself as having masculine or feminine appeal may derive primary reinforcement from success in intimate relationships and sexual encounters. This concept of self as an adequate male or female is likely to carry over to other relationships where sexual activity may not be involved, but where sexuality is nevertheless a factor in interpersonal attraction.

Likewise, the capacity to conceive children is linked not only to health, but also to the psychological and social identity of many individuals. Fertility is extremely important to the enactment of male and female roles as are the physical, psychological, and social changes that accompany pregnancy and childbirth. Childbearing enables people to experience the reality of their sexuality in ways that bring personal satisfaction and social recognition; moreover, with the birth of a child, there are new roles and opportunities for self-expression that satisfy the adult need for generativity through the chance to nurture a child.

Conversely, an incapacity to engage in sexual acts is often accompanied by diminished self-esteem and even by diminished opportunities for satisfying social relationships; sexual dysfunction limits the capacity of individuals not only for reproduction, but also for social risk taking. People who suffer from a physical incapacity to have sex may be unwilling to expose themselves to the threat of embarrassment in intimate encounters and may retreat from relationships that might led to intimacy. Moreover, the loss of self-esteem that accompanies sexual dysfunction may interfere with general confidence and success in self-presentation, which may lead, in severe cases, to a loss of influence over others, to difficulty in establishing and maintaining social relationships, and to social isolation and loneliness. Thus, sex and sexuality are central to effective, satisfying self-expression; in one way or another sexuality plays a role in almost everything an individual does or does not do.

Before 1948, when Alfred Kinsey and associates published their first research in sexual behavior,[108] little information was available on sexual attitudes and practices. Kinsey's research not only provided information, it sparked the scientific legitimacy necessary for sexual behavior to become a bona fide focus of scientific inquiry and research. Since the Kinsey report, society has changed and sexuality has gained worldwide recognition as an important factor in human health. In 1975, the World Health Organization (WHO) advocated the involvement of health professionals in the education, counseling, and treatment of problems in human sexuality.[109]

During the intervening years there has been a general relaxation of the social norms pertaining to sex and sexuality. Once a taboo topic, sex is now openly discussed in social situations of all kinds and is widely covered in the media. As a result, there is a new public awareness of the importance of sexuality and sexual functioning. Nevertheless, myths and misinformation about sexual practices persist. Box 23–1 lists some of the erroneous sexual beliefs that people may hold. The importance of accurate, up-to-date information for sexual health cannot be overemphasized. The following sections therefore discuss current information on various aspects of sex and sexuality as they pertain to self-expression and health.

BOX 23–1. COMMON SEXUAL MYTHS

1. Elderly people do not want or need sexual intimacy.
2. Blacks have a greater sex drive than whites.
3. A large penis is of great importance to a woman's sexual gratification.
4. Menopause or hysterectomy terminates a woman's sex life.
5. Homosexuals are identifiable by their appearance and behavior.
6. Homosexuals are all promiscuous.
7. Contraception reduces sexual pleasure.
8. Condoms eliminate the risk of sexually transmitted disease.
9. Sexual intercourse should be avoided during pregnancy.
10. Women cannot get pregnant while they are lactating.
11. Alcohol is a sexual stimulant.
12. Masturbation causes mental illness.
13. A couple must have simultaneous orgasms to achieve sexual satisfaction or for conception to occur.
14. There is an absolutely "safe" period in a woman's sexual cycle in which coitus cannot cause impregnation.
15. Male impotency is incurable.
16. All sexually transmitted diseases can be successfully treated if caught in time.
17. AIDS is spread by kissing.
18. Contraception eliminates the risk of pregnancy.
19. AIDS is a disease of homosexuals only.
20. Sex is not important when you are sick.

All of the above are untrue statements.

Adapted from Knowlton CN. Human sexuality. *In Flynn JM, Heffron PB, eds.* Nursing: From Concept to Practice. *2nd ed. Norwalk, CT: Appleton & Lange; 1988.*

Biosexual Development. Chapters 10 and 11 introduced many of the aspects of the development of sexuality and gender identity. These concepts are examined below as they relate to self-expression.

Sexual development in the prenatal period begins at the moment of conception. Biological sex is determined by the chromosomal pattern contributed by the ovum and sperm that come together to form the zygote. The resulting pair of sex chromosomes, whether XX (female) or XY (male), is responsible for the differentiation of the embryonic gonads, the former pattern resulting in the development of ovaries and the latter, testes.[110] Sexual development after the point of conception is heavily influenced by maternal hormones that cross the placenta and by hormones produced by the fetus itself. At 4 weeks of gestation, a genital tubercle develops in both sexes and remains undifferentiated until the tenth week, when the male testes begin to secrete fetal testosterone. Under the influence of testosterone, the anterior part of the genital tubercle develops into a penis and the urethral folds fuse to form the spongy male urethra. In the absence of fetal testosterone, the female clitoris is formed from the tubercle. The urethral folds fail to fuse, resulting in the female labia. Prenatal sexual differentiation under the influence of fetal testosterone involves not only the development of both external genitalia, but also the internal genitalia and probably the brain itself.[111]

The secondary sex characteristics that distinguish male from female are under hormonal influence and develop rapidly in puberty, the period in which endocrine and gametogenic functions of the ovary first develop to the point at which reproduction can take place. The hypothalamus secretes gonadotropin-releasing factor, which stimulates the anterior pituitary to secrete the gonadotropin hormones (follicle-stimulating hormone and luteinizing hormone). Follicle-stimulating hormone stimulates the growth of the ova in the ovary and the sperm-producing cells in the testes. Cells in the ovary and testes, in turn, produce sex hormones that are responsible for secondary sex characteristics.

In males, pubertal development begins with testicular enlargement and is followed by growth of the penis and scrotum, the development of pubic, axillary, and facial hair, voice deepening, and an adolescent spurt in long bone growth and increase in bone mass. Functionally, males achieve the capacity for ejaculation, the expulsion of semen from the penis in response to intense sexual stimulation, during puberty.

In females, pubertal development begins with the appearance of breast buds and is followed by breast growth, the development of pubic and axillary hair, the appearance of vaginal secretions, hip widening, increased fat distribution to the breasts, hips, and thighs, and finally ovulation and menarche. The onset of the menstrual cycle, termed *menarche,* occurs on average at about 12.5 years of age in response to hormonal stimulation. It consists of recurrent changes in the ovaries, uterus, cervix, and vagina.

Beginning at around age 40 and lasting to approximately age 60, women undergo another reproductive transition termed the *climacteric.* The climacteric is the process through which the reproductive capacity of the woman ends. It includes both a premenopause phase and a postmenopause phase. There is no comparable process for males. Menopause, which is technically a reference to the last menstrual period, is also referred to in ordinary language as "change of life." The average age for physiological menopause is about 50 years of age; however, the actual cessation of menstrual cycles is generally preceded by a series of irregular periods. Although the menstrual cycle ceases in menopause, the capacity to experience sexual pleasure does not, and for many women, the postmenopausal period is a continuation of sexual fulfillment.

Sexual Orientation and Modes of Sexual Expression. The solidification of gender identity early in development (see Chaps. 10 and 11) and the completion of the physical changes of puberty and the sex-role learning that accompanies adolescent socialization (see Chap. 11) prepare the individual for sexual activity. At this stage, individual sexual orientation becomes apparent.

Sexual orientation refers to individuals' preferences for the sex of their partners or for the means of expression of sexual thoughts and feelings. A heterosexual orientation is one in which the individual's sexual preference is for partners of the opposite sex; a homosexual orientation is one in which the preference is for partners of the same sex; a bisexual orientation is one in which the individual accepts both same-sex and opposite-sex partners. There are also orientations in which no partners are preferred. Celibacy refers to a preference for abstaining from sexual intimacy and activity; masturbation is the practice of solitary, self-stimulation of the sexual organs.

The determinants of sexual preference are complex and are not yet well understood. Sexuality and sexual preferences probably result from the interplay of many influencing factors, inborn and learned. Concepts of masculinity and femininity and sex-role behavior are, first of all, culturally prescribed and transmitted. What constitutes appropriate, acceptable sexual behavior varies widely from one society to the next, from one social subgroup to the next, and, within a given society, from one generation to the next. A behavior that is taboo in one society or group may be accepted in another or may become accepted as that society changes. Religions also have a profound effect on sexual attitudes and practices and vary in their dispositions toward sexual activity, both inside and outside the context of marriage. Individuals who adhere to a particular religious faith may well follow its tenets relating to sexual behavior and derive their sexual attitudes from their religious beliefs.

Sexual feelings and attitudes are also influenced by early sexual attachments to one's parents and are derived from the infantile sexual pleasures that are experienced in relation to one's own body. Early childhood experiences with warm, loving relationships undoubtedly influence later feelings about closeness and intimacy. Certainly the family's influence on reinforcement of gender identity is also a powerful influence. For most individuals, gender identity is conferred at birth when they are assigned a masculine or feminine name, and it is strengthened in a myriad of ways throughout childhood and adolescence. Here again, social change is also a factor. As social attitudes about what is masculine and what is feminine evolve, family practices in reinforcing gender identity also undergo change.

Thus, it can be said that there is no universal consensus on appropriate sexual behavior and attitudes in the same way that there are no universal values and norms for what constitutes health and illness. People who are relativistic and utilitarian in their outlook will evaluate sexual actions based on their effects. On the other hand, people who are hedonistic in their outlook will espouse that pleasure is the essence of sex and will evaluate sexual acts only on the basis of whether or not they give pleasure. People who are absolutist, however, will look at reproduction as the primary purpose of sexual activity and will evaluate sexual behavior on the basis of its contribution to procreation.

Healthy, functioning people engage in a wide range of sexual behavior, and sexual arousal is achieved and expressed in a variety of ways. These modes are summarized in Box 23–2.

Sexual arousal is a very individual phenomenon and involves a variety of tactile, visual, and olfactory input and often stimulating mental images and fantasies. For some individuals, however, it is achieved only through means that may be harmful psychologically or physically to themselves or to others and, for that reason, such means are subject to social injunction. Harmful means generally involve (1) repetitive sexual activity focused on the real or simulated suffering or humiliation of oneself or one's partner (sadomasochism); or (2) sexual activity involving nonconsenting partners (rape; pedophilia, or sex with prepubertal children; sex with minors); or (3) any of a number of specific deviations including exhibitionism (exposure of the genitals to unsuspecting strangers), fetishism (use of nonliving objects, commonly clothing, to achieve excitation), voyeurism (observation of unsuspecting others who are na-

BOX 23–2. MODES OF SEXUAL EXPRESSION

Petting	Mutual kissing, caressing, stroking, massaging, genital stimulation
Coitus	Sexual intercourse with insertion of the penis into the vagina with resulting orgasm
Oral-genital contact	Fellatio (penis in partner's mouth); cunnilingus (mouth and tongue stimulation of female genitalia); anilingus (tongue stimulation of anus); mutual fellatio-cunnilingus (simultaneous, mutual oral-genital contact)
Anal intercourse	Insertion of penis into anus with resulting orgasm
Autoeroticism	Self-stimulation with or without mechanical devices

ked or in the act of disrobing), and zoophilia (sex with animals).

Human Sexual Response. The sexual response cycle is the physiological reaction, manifested by numerous body changes, to sexual arousal.[112] The physiological changes that accompany the cycle are summarized for women in Table 23–1, and for men in Table 23–2. The sexual response for both men and women is experienced in four phases: (1) excitement, in which there is a subjective sense of pleasure and accompanying physiological changes (pelvic vasoconstriction, vaginal lubrication, swelling of the breasts and external genitalia, erection of the penis, increased heart and respiratory rate and blood pressure, and perspiration); (2) plateau, in which sexual excitement reaches a peak, vaginal narrowing occurs, and the penis reaches maximum size with reflex and psychogenically stimulated erection; (3) orgasm, which is the peaking of sexual pleasure with the release of tension and rhythmic contraction of perineal and pelvic reproductive organs and the ejaculation of semen; and (4) resolution, in which there is a sense of general and muscular relaxation.

Several disturbances of the sexual response cycle can be attributed to psychophysiological difficulties and to organic factors such as diabetes, alcoholism, and other health problems. These include inhibited sexual desire (loss of interest in sex); inhibited sexual excitement, or impotence (partial or complete failure to attain or maintain erection in males) and frigidity (inability to attain or maintain genital lubrication and swelling in females); functional dyspareunia (coitus associated with genital pain in either the male or female); functional vaginismus (recurrent, persistent involuntary spasm of the musculature of the vagina during intercourse); inhibited female orgasm (failure of orgasm following sexual excitement); inhibited male orgasm (failure of ejaculation following sexual excitement); and premature ejaculation (absence of voluntary control of ejaculation).

■ CHARACTERISTICS OF HEALTHY SELF-EXPRESSION

Over the years many authorities have suggested criteria of personal health that encompass aspects of both private experience and public behavior. Their ideas are helpful for understanding what constitutes a healthy self and healthy self-expression.

Self-Awareness

Healthy self-expression promotes self-awareness.[113] Self-aware individuals are able to talk about their concepts of themselves, their self-ideals, and what they desire to do and feel they should do, without disowning any major feelings, capacities, or goals. They are aware of all of the major traits and characteristics of themselves as persons and are neither self-conscious nor uncomfortable with themselves. They see themselves realistically and objectively, both strengths and shortcomings, and do not mistake how they would like to be with how they are.[113]

Identity

When self-expression is healthy, people generally have a sense of identity that gives them a feeling of self-esteem, and they are confident in their ability to maintain their own sameness and continuity, both in their own eyes and in the eyes of others.[113] They choose self-presentations and make self-disclosures that are in keeping with their self-understanding and that communicate believable identities to others. The feelings of unreality, self-diffusion, and depersonalization characteristic of people who are undergoing profound developmental and situational changes are absent.[113] These relationships are discussed below under *Alterations in Self-Expression.*

Self-Actualization

Healthy self-expression generally leads to individual growth and self-actualization.[113] Healthy self-expression reflects a motivation for personal development and an investment in living. Self-actualizing individuals show a drive for personal development. Basic needs are met, allowing an individual to concentrate energy on vocational and avocational pursuits. Self-actualizing individuals are able to focus themselves on problems outside of themselves and express concern for the predicaments of others and balance meeting their own needs with meeting those of others.[113,114] They evoke a compassionate, warm response from others.[114]

Unifying Outlook on Life

The self-expression of healthy people displays a unifying outlook on life. People who express themselves in healthy ways generally have a philosophy that may not be articulated, but that nevertheless unifies their behavior and gives them a feeling that there is purpose and meaning to life.[113] This philosophy underlies their intentions to strive for specific accomplishments in the future, and enables them to move toward long-range goals. Through their unifying philosophy, people gain a sense of private, inner harmony.[114]

TABLE 23–1. PHYSIOLOGICAL SEXUAL RESPONSE: WOMEN

Phase	Site	Response
Excitement	Vagina	Vaginal lubrication occurs Inner two thirds of vagina lengthens and distends; color changes to dark purple Over one third of vagina fills with blood
	Labia	Labia minora enlarge, become more deeply colored Labia majora flatten and thin, move away from midline
	Uterus	Uterus elevates, pulling on vagina and making a tent or open area at inner one third of vagina
	Breasts	Breasts increase in size Nipples become erect
	Cardiovascular/respiratory	Heart rate slows early, then increases in rate Breathing may increase in rate Blood pressure increases as phase progresses
	Skin	Sex flush, measleslike rash occurs on chest or upper abdomen
Plateau	Vagina	Vaginal opening decreases in size by one third
	Labia	Sex skin reaction: labia minora change from pink to bright red in nulliparous women and from red to deep wine in multiparous women
	Clitoris	Clitorus retracts from unstimulated position to inaccessible place under clitoral hood
	Skin	Sex flush spreads to all areas of breast, chest, and abdomen
Orgasmic	Vagina	Contractions begin in outer one third of vagina; at 0.8-s intervals and recur from 3 to 15 times; time between contractions becomes longer and strength of contractions decreases
	Uterus	Uterus contracts, similar to labor
	Rectum	Rectal contractions are linked in time with vaginal contractions
	Muscular	Muscular spasm is released; some loss of voluntary control occurs, with spasms and contractions of many muscle groups
	Cardiovascular	Heart rate is two times normal Blood pressure increases by one third
	Respiratory	Breathing rate is three times normal
Resolution	Breasts	Nipple erection decreases; slower loss of breast volume Sex flush and swelling around nipples disappear
	Skin	Film of perspiration covers body
	Vagina	Within 5 to 10 seconds clitoris returns to normal position; loss of vasocongestion is slower Congestion in outer one third of vagina disappears Congestion in vaginal walls disappears in 15 minutes or more
	Labia	Labia majora return to unstimulated size Labia minora: prestimulation color returns in 15 seconds; size returns more slowly Cervix descends to unstimulated position
	Respiratory/cardiovascular	Breathing, heart rate, and blood pressure return to prestimulation condition
	Urinary	Urge to urinate is felt, particularly in nulliparous women

From Masters WH, Johnson VE. Human Sexual Response. *Boston: Little, Brown; 1966, with permission.*

Resistance to Stress

Healthy self-expression confers a resistance to stress.[113] People who are able to express themselves in healthy ways show a resilience that enables them to bounce back from adverse situations and to adapt and find new kinds of self-satisfaction when old patterns are no longer possible. They are able to laugh at themselves and discharge tension through humor.[114]

Autonomy

Healthy self-expression demonstrates autonomy, self-determination, and independence. People who express themselves in healthy ways are able to regulate their behavior from within in accordance with internalized standards.[113] They are able to balance a need for the approval of others with their own sense of self-approval, and although they consider others' opinions, they are not unduly dependent on them for their sense of self-esteem.[113] They are capable of conforming to behavioral norms, but remain free to choose whether or not to conform. Their capacity for autonomy stems from a deep private sense, derived from early childhood relationships, that they have a right to express themselves and that their fundamental personal worth makes their expressions valuable to others around them.[115]

TABLE 23–2. PHYSIOLOGICAL SEXUAL RESPONSE: MEN

Excitement	Penis	Penile erection caused by blood engorgement; penile size increases
	Scrotum/testes	Skin of scrotum tenses, becomes congested and thick Testes rise higher in scrotum, increase in size as much as 50%
	Breast	Nipples become erect and swell
	Muscular	Increasing spasm of long muscles of legs and arms and abdomen muscles occurs
	Rectum	Some voluntary contractions occur late in phase
	Respiratory	Breathing may increase late in phase
	Cardiovascular	Heart rate slows initially, then quickens
Plateau	Skin	Sex flush occurs (not as frequent as in women) over chest, neck, and face
	Muscular	Muscular tension of face, neck, abdomen, and limbs increases
	Penis	Penile glans enlarges
	Testes	Testicular size increases from 50 to 100% Elevation of testes is fully accomplished
	Blood pressure	Blood pressure increases as phase progresses
Orgasmic	Respiratory/cardiovascular	Breathing, heart rate, and blood pressure increase—generally higher than in women
	Testes	Testes, prostate gland, and seminal vesicles contract as they collect sperm and seminal fluid and expel them into the entrance of the urethra
	Muscular	Muscular spasm is released, some loss of voluntary control occurs, with spasms and contractions of many muscle groups
	Penis	Penile muscle contraction and urethral contractions result in actual ejaculation of seminal fluid out of the penis
	Rectum	Contractions are linked to genital contractions
Resolution	Penis	After ejaculation one half of erection is lost quickly; second stage is slower
	Testes/scrotum	Scrotal wall reverts to uncongested state Testes descend rapidly in most men; swelling decreases
	Skin	Skin flush disappears Perspiration is usually confined to palms and soles of feet, but sometimes is widespread
	Nipple	Nipple erection lost
	Muscular	Loss of muscle tension over a 5-minute period
	Cardiovascular/respiratory	Heart rate, breathing, and blood pressure return to prestimulation state

From Masters WH, Johnson VE. Human Sexual Response. *Boston: Little, Brown; 1966, with permission.*

Clear Perception of Reality

Healthy self-expression reveals that the individual's perception of reality is clear and relatively free from distortion.[113] People who express themselves in healthy ways do not mold their perception of events, particularly the attitudes and intentions of other people, to conform to their wishes and are able to see the implications of events even when these conflict with their inner needs. They are concerned about and show empathy for other people.[115]

Environmental Mastery

Healthy self-expression reveals two themes, success and adaptation.[113] People who express themselves in healthy ways generally have the ability to love, are competent in interpersonal relations, have the capacity to adapt and adjust, and are efficient problem solvers. They are able to establish and maintain intimate relationships and experience sexual gratification from sexual mutuality in close relationships.[113] They are able to be assertive in their relationships without alienating people with aggressiveness. They respect others' personhood as well as their own; they refrain from expressing themselves in ways that impose on the rights of others.[115] They are spontaneous and creative in their thinking and behavior.

■ ALTERATIONS IN SELF-EXPRESSION

Alterations in self-expression occur naturally over the life span, as the previous discussions of self-expression and development have established. People change in the modes and in the content of their self-expression as they grow and develop, and these changes are manifested in their self-presentations and self-disclosures. Often the changes are positive from the standpoint of the individual's self-fulfillment; however, nurses periodically encounter negative alterations in self-expression. These may be developmental in nature as, for example, when a school nurse becomes aware that a child's learning disability is taking a toll on his or her self-concept, or when an occupational health nurse learns that a young worker's angry outbursts are related to job stress. More commonly, however, nurses encounter alterations in self-expression that are situational in nature and related to illness itself.

Situational changes arise not from development, but from the interaction between individuals and their environment. Situational changes that are particularly serious or that have threatening implications are classified as crises. (Refer to Chap. 6 for detailed discussion of maturational and situational changes and their relationship to stress and coping.)

Illness is a kind of situational change that often brings crisis with it. Diseases are frequently caused by infections, toxic, and traumatic factors, all of which involve one's exposure to the environment. Illnesses caused by such agents are generally beyond the control of individuals to prevent. They can be mild or severe; they may come on slowly or suddenly, catching the person unsuspecting and unprepared. When serious illness develops, individuals usually find themselves in a personal crisis from the sudden disruption of roles and routines. This situation may also create a substantial threat to personal survival, raising the specter of permanent disability or even death. Such illnesses generally are accompanied by a temporary or long-term alteration in self-expression.

Disease may also develop as a result of patterns of individual adaptation to the environment. These illnesses frequently involve factors over which people do have control; for example, Chapter 22 documented life-style as a important factor in illness. Self-expression is directly related to individuals' choices for the structure of their lives that result in healthy or unhealthy life-styles. Thus, a complex relationship exists between self-expression and illness. Illnesses not only cause changes in self-expression, but may themselves be caused by the choices that individuals make in the interest of their self-expression. Illnesses that result from life-style factors are often of a chronic, slowly progressive nature. Nevertheless, they also represent a threat to survival and, in the periods in which they rapidly progress, are just as capable of causing personal crisis and threat.

Illness is threatening for several reasons. First, the infliction of pain or mutilation is a prominent source of psychological stress and is known to be a part of many illnesses and their treatments. People naturally seek to protect themselves from such dangers. Illness is also threatening because it places at risk not only an individual's body functions and body images, but also the self-concept in a broader sense. Social and family roles, friendships, job, avocational pursuits, future goals, ideals, and even personal possessions can be placed in jeopardy by the individual's inability to continue to pursue long-established life patterns. Often these factors have attained such a degree of psychological importance that they have become a part of the individual's personal and social identity, and thus make an indispensable contribution to the individual's psychological homeostasis. The importance that these factors assume renders the individual vulnerable to their loss or even to the threat of their loss.

Illness also frustrates people's drives to meet basic human needs. Illness interferes with the ill individual's capacity to meet needs for love, belonging, esteem, intimacy, and self-actualization. Intimate communication becomes impossible, for example, when the individual is having trouble breathing or when pain is severe. Anger and other strong emotions may have to be suppressed because the person is simply too ill to express such feelings. Needs, impulses, and desires, moreover, may have to be inhibited because the individual lacks the capacity to act on them.

Alterations in self-expression constitute one of the important ways in which people manifest the threat of illness. They communicate to others that changes are going on within the individual's private world as a result of illness. Generally, these alterations can be viewed as an indication that the individual is attempting to deal with and adapt to the impact that illness is having on the self-concept, including the individual's body image, sexuality, and/or role performance. Alterations in self-expression manifest themselves through self-presentation and self-disclosure. Individuals may suddenly or gradually show less concern about social images and indicate a greater need for self-disclosure, or they may show an increased concern for social images, avoiding those people from whom they feel a social challenge. The amount and intensity of emotion they communicate to others may change, and they may experience an urgent need to disclose mounting distress to others. Whatever the specific nature of the change, the underlying threat is to the self-concept. Thus it is important to understand the impact of illness on the self-concept.

IMPLICATIONS FOR NURSE–CLIENT COLLABORATION

Self-Presentation, Self-Ideal, Loss, and Illness

Self-presentation is the process by which individuals attempt to control the impressions they make on others to validate valued images of self. Self-presentation gives a picture of the individual's self-concept and self-ideal. It communicates individuals' understanding of how they are and how they would like to be. The sharing of the self-ideal is a very important part of self-presentation in everyday life. Illness, however, often interferes with an individual's capacity to fulfill the self-ideal, thus widening the gap between concept of self and ideal image of self. In this situation self-esteem generally diminishes. To preserve self-esteem, the ill person not only must alter his or her concept of self, but frequently must give up self-ideals that are no longer attainable. Loss of a self-ideal may be accompanied by a period of grief as adaptation takes place. Effective nurse–client collaboration provides opportunities for the client to address issues related to changing self-concept and self-ideal.

Illness, Self-Concept, and Self-expression

People everywhere cherish and protect their wholeness. Such feelings are continually reinforced and strengthened by mass media images that correspond to cultural ideals of health and beauty. With few exceptions media images focus on people who satisfy the cultural standards rather than on those who have deformities, disabilities, or other characteristics generally considered to represent misfortunes. Thus, they serve as constant reminders to the healthy and ill alike that illness is a deviation from the normative, desirable human state. Given this environment, it is clear why many individuals have difficulty adapting to body changes that are permanent in nature.

Altered Body Image. Body image is one of the most common aspects of self-concept to be affected by illness.[116,117] Illness changes the body, both structurally and functionally, and is thus related to the mental images that correspond to altered parts or functions. Body image is tied to self-esteem, of which there are two fundamental levels: basic and functional.[118] Basic self-esteem is learned early and remains relatively stable; functional self-esteem changes continuously as one's situations and relationships change and evolve. Thus, body image changes associated with illness are more likely to be of the functional type, the significance of which is that negative changes need not be permanent.

The impact of an altered body image on the self-esteem of any given individual derives from the interaction of several factors: (1) the individual's body ideal (the mental measuring stick against which the individual judges the actual body); (2) the sociocultural significance of the altered body part or process; (3) individual concept of the importance of the body part altered; (4) age, sex, and marital status. Alterations such as those associated with the breasts and reproductive organs, which affect interpersonal attractiveness, are extremely powerful in their potential to effect a negative change in body image[116]; however, the loss of a breast to a young, single, sexually active woman may well have a much different meaning than the same loss would have for an elderly widow who lives with her sister.

Illnesses That Alter Body Image. Virtually any illness can alter a person's body image. For some people, the mere fact of being ill at all may be an affront to their self-concept of strength and independence. Nevertheless, certain illnesses are particularly likely to cause temporary or permanent changes in body image that may involve a prolonged period of adjustment. Illnesses that involve the deformity, mutilation, or loss of a part of the body or that change the way people communicate, eat, eliminate body wastes, or move from place to place are likely to alter body image and diminish self-esteem, at least temporarily.

Illnesses, injuries, or surgeries that significantly alter the face, the features of which constitute a central aspect of body image, represent such a challenge and can easily alter body image. Even cosmetic surgery, which is intended to improve the appearance of the face, can negatively affect an individual's body image when the changes are unanticipated and considered undesirable by the individual.

Cardiovascular diseases frequently cause fatigue and reduce the capacity for activity, including self-care activities, thus altering body image. Treatment for cardiovascular diseases may, however, result in positive body image adjustments. For example, a pacemaker may make it possible for a previously very ill individual to resume sexual activity, which may improve the individual's self-esteem. Coronary artery bypass surgery, which is commonly performed for blockage of the coronary arteries, has been associated with diffuse positive changes in body image, including changes in individuals' perceptions of appetite, weight, energy level, breathing, elimination, and overall health.[117]

Gastrointestinal illnesses sometimes interfere with nutrition and, thus, may alter an individual's body image by altering body weight. Severe intestinal disease sometimes requires an ostomy, a surgical procedure that creates an artificial opening in the abdominal wall for the elimination of feces or urine. This radically alters not only the process of elimination but, for some individuals, also may represent a virtual assault on their body images, requiring a prolonged period of rehabilitation for the resumption of former social patterns.

Musculoskeletal and neurological diseases often compromise mobility and may also be associated with deformity. These are only a few illustrations of the ways in which illness can affect a change in body image. Although it is important to understand that certain illnesses and treatments are likely to correspond to body image alterations, negative and positive, it is also important to keep in mind that the relationship between illness and body image is highly individualistic. To predict who will and who will not face a significant adjustment, one must know a great deal about the meaning that the specific illness and its consequences have for the individual.

Altered Sexuality. The reciprocal relationship between medical illnesses and sexual functioning is widely recognized.[107] Illness may cause changes in an individual's sense of self as a man or woman, as well as a decline in the physical ability to function sexually.

Some chronic diseases are especially well known for their interference with the sexual function. Diabetes mellitus, for example, increases the incidence of impotence among male diabetics and may reduce female sexual activity through its capacity to make women vulnerable to vaginal infection.[119] Spinal cord injury results in significant changes in physical functions, including the sexual function. The erection reflex may remain intact in men, but they may lose the ability to achieve erection through mental sexual arousal.[120] This can result in severely diminished self-esteem for those afflicted.[121]

Acute illness may and often is accompanied by transient disinterest in sex or lack of desire for sexual activity

IMPLICATIONS FOR NURSE–CLIENT COLLABORATION

Sexuality

Sexuality is a very important part of individual behavior and constitutes a central aspect of self-concept. Many illnesses alter the ability to engage in sexual activity or act to change the way that individuals think about themselves as sexual beings. The experience of altered sexuality in illness can be an extremely distressing experience. Individuals who have such experiences may desperately need to disclose their distress and, in the process, to examine the nature of their problem. Nurses who are comfortable talking about sex and sexuality with clients who are distressed about altered sexuality make a significant contribution to the clients' well-being.

among individuals who are preoccupied with their symptoms.[107] Ill individuals may fear that sexual activity will aggravate their illness. Such is often the case for individuals who have suffered a myocardial infarction (heart attack), which has no direct effect on the sexual response but may nevertheless engender a fear that sexual activity will cause another attack. Thus, illness, whether acute or chronic, may result in a substantial threat to sexual identity.

Sexuality may also be constrained by admission to the hospital. Enduring diagnostic and intrusive procedures and the other identity insults that hospitalized individuals must put up with, such as being separated from significant others and having clothing, jewelry, and personal possessions removed, may dampen sexual feelings and reduce sexual desire temporarily.

On the other hand, some individuals, in the same circumstances, may react with overt sexual behavior. Individuals may use sexual behavior within the hospital setting to express a variety of needs, for instance, to reaffirm sexual identity, to express sexual feelings, to affirm an ability to function sexually, or to control the situation.[107] When nurses are confronted by or inadvertently become a witness to clients' sexual activity, their ability to respond in a helpful manner is usually challenged. Section 3 discusses attitudes and approaches that enable nurses to assist clients who have needs related to altered sexuality.

Altered Role Performance. Role performance is the component of self-concept that is directly related to life structure and the various roles it comprises. Roles involve activities that enable an individual to demonstrate personal skill and competence and are frequently tied to an individual's self-esteem. To the extent that individuals choose the roles they occupy, roles are also expressive. Roles also create situated identities, as previously discussed.

People often mutually reinforce one another in their respective roles and become important to one another's self-esteem. For the individual, each role and situated identity carries a corresponding definition of self that becomes a part of the individual's self-concept. When illness interferes significantly with an individual's physical capacity for activities, certain roles may become impossible; role relationships may be disturbed; a person's situated identities and ultimately a person's concept of self also may be threatened.

Consider a young man who sustains severe trauma to the spinal cord in a work-related accident that results in temporary, and possibly permanent, paralysis of the legs. Not only will the young man be unable to work and meet the responsibilities of bread winner, at least for several months, but paralysis will also make it impossible to do the activities associated with being a husband and father. Some of the activities and relationships from which he derived his self-esteem may be permanently lost to him, depending on the outcome of his illness. New patterns and roles will have be be learned, at least until he recovers. New ways of carrying out former roles will have to be devised, and new relationships are likely to be formed in the process.

Such pervasive life changes generally bring corresponding changes in a person's concept of self. How these influence the individual's self-esteem depends on that person's success in finding sources of reward in the new circumstances and in finding new ways to express self.

Adaptation to Self-Concept Threats. Adaptation to self-concept threats is a complex process involving the nature of the threat, its meaning to the person, its perceived outcomes and consequences, and the person's resources for coping. Adaptation generally occurs in four phases: impact, retreat, acknowledgment, and reconstruction.[122]

Impact. When a person becomes seriously ill or injured, generally there is an initial period of shock during which the person moves from little awareness that a change has occurred to at least partial awareness of what has happened. When the crisis involves something that permanently changes the appearance of the body, such as the loss of a limb, it quickly becomes apparent to everyone that the change prevents a return to previous routines and that adjustment is necessary. When the crisis does not involve changes in the appearance of the body, however, recognition of an altered state may depend on more subtle cues. Because the altered state is not readily apparent, caregivers may need to intervene to establish the significance of what has happened. When the physical foundation of the self-threat is ambiguous, realization of altered circumstances may take more time for the individual and family to integrate.

Once an awareness begins to develop, depending on the severity of the problem and its perceived consequences, the individual may express strong emotions of despair, discouragement, hostility, and anger. The despair that individuals express may be for others as well as themselves, as they realize that others' lives are also affected. Anger and hostility may also be expressed; the anger that individuals feel toward themselves for becoming ill is projected onto others.

Retreat. In the retreat phase, the individual, feeling threatened, steps back from the problem to gather energy and mourn the loss of the old self, to reflect on its meaning, and to marshal personal resources and strengths to confront patterns that must be changed. During retreat, individuals may try to reduce the perception of threat by denying that a threat exists. This is referred to as a **denial of illness.** Subtle behavior such as a refusal to take medication, inattention to symptoms, or a cheerful presentation of self that seems inappropriate in the face of reality may constitute denial of illness.

Denial is a largely unconscious mechanism; that is, there is no deliberate attempt by the individual to mislead self or others. There are, however, differences in the level of awareness at which denial operates and in the degree to which reality is denied. At the extreme level is the verbal denial of what is plainly apparent to the eyes, such as when a person who has lost a limb insists that it is still there. This is complete denial and suggests that a serious psychological disequilibrium exists. A more common form of denial is ignoring or disowning limited aspects of the problem. Still more common is minimization of aspects of the problem rather than outright denial of them. "It's not so bad!" is a statement frequently made by those who wish to deflate the importance of what has happened to them. Partial denial is common in everyday life; when it aids individuals without interfering with the activities necessary to adaptation, it is not considered unhealthy. With appropriate support, denial generally gives way to growing awareness.

Acknowledgment. During the acknowledgment phase, the individual begins to deal openly with the threat and to make the changes that are necessary. It is at this point that the person has a substantial and growing awareness that change is unavoidable, and that life roles cannot be resumed without significant modifications of patterns and arrangements for coping.

At this point individuals experience strong challenges to personal identity. They may question who they are and who they are becoming. This is a highly stressful state in which the person may have bodily symptoms of stress and unusual disturbing feelings of detachment, loss of contact, self-diffusion, and **depersonalization**, in which they feel as if they are observing what is happening to them rather than experiencing it. Individuals undergoing acknowledgment may have a strong need to talk about their feelings and the meaning of their experience and to disclose their distress to others.

Reconstruction. During the reconstruction phase, the individual repairs old concepts of self or builds what amounts to a new set of self-concepts. Individuals slowly begin to involve themselves in activities and to engage in social interaction.

This phase is fraught with risk and ambivalence. Individuals still mourn the past, fearing not only that its satisfactions are out of reach, but also that their new circumstances will fail to hold comparable satisfactions. They frequently hold conflicting emotions and opposing attitudes about their situation, an emotional state known as **ambivalence**. For example, a newly paralyzed accident victim who undergoes rehabilitation may return to sports activities as a wheelchair athlete. Although gratified by new accomplishments, the individual may nevertheless mourn the loss of previous wholeness and view the emerging self as damaged or somehow unwhole. The individual may also feel anger toward self for whatever personal responsibility he or she may have had for the accident. He or she may thus experience pride, anger, and remorse all at the same time.

These emotional polarities are energy consuming and need to be resolved as completely as possible. Part of the process of working through conflicting feelings involves disclosing them to others and examining their implications for health. Most serious illnesses are accompanied by the experience of conflicting feelings. Ambivalent individuals need the opportunity to express all aspects of their feelings in the context of a relationship that minimizes the risks of disclosure.[133] Catharsis frequently leads to insight. Yet the conditions must be right for the disclosure of strong, confusing emotions; these conditions generally include a high level of interpersonal trust, communication of empathy and caring from the helper, and the opportunity to safely put aside concerns about the impressions one is conveying to others.[13,133]

Humor is also important to resolving ambivalence. Humor allows the expression of aggressive feelings in a socially acceptable way; laughter, moreover, enables people to discharge the tension that is associated with difficult situations.[124] Humor is thus important to those in the phase of reconstruction who need to externalize the meaning of their experience in a way that will not make others uncomfortable.

Success in the phase of reconstruction depends greatly on the quality of support the individual finds in the environment, particularly from significant others. Feedback during this phase is critical, because it is on the basis of the behavior and reactions of others that the individual learns that satisfying social relationships are still possible, that social identity can be reestablished, and that self-esteem can develop again. Individuals look for indications of their worth in others' acceptance of their new identities and are sensitive to nuances in the behavior of family and friends that suggest they are regarded differently.

The lack of environmental support may have serious consequences for the individual. Reconstruction is a period of profound tension between the self-concept and the self-ideal, both of which, when illness is severe, generally must undergo substantial revision for adaptation to occur. This tension often generates feelings of shame which may focus on the basic unalterable reality that change has occurred and the fear one has that he or she may have become inadequate for the person or persons loved. Shame is a highly stressful private experience that may be communicated by a complete or partial withdrawal from visual contact; avoidance of eye contact; bowing of the head; turning of the back; autonomic skin reactions such as blushing and blanching; nervous gestures such as playing with hair or clothes, twisting fingers, hand tremors, facial tics, and

BUILDING NURSING KNOWLEDGE

Should the Nurse Use Humor With Clients?

Ruxton JP. Humor intervention deserves our attention. *Holistic Nurs Prac.* 1988;2(3):54–62.

Ruxton reviews the various reasons that humor has been ignored historically as a mode of intervention with clients. She points to the traditional discipline and regimentation of educational programs that defined humor as unprofessional. She also cites the tendency for health professionals to use in-group humor to separate themselves socially from clients and to shield themselves from the life-threatening situations to which they are constantly exposed.

In Ruxton's opinion, humor has an important therapeutic role, the value of which has not received appropriate recognition. Four functions of humor are highlighted in the article: communicative, social, psychological, and physiological. Humor is important in establishing a comfortable atmosphere and neutralizes emotionally charged events. Humor in the form of the "jocular gripe" turns individual experiences into a collective experience and can strengthen the social structure of a hospital ward. Humor also enhances persons' ability to look at situations from a new perspective, which, in turn, helps them generate new alternatives for themselves. Physically, humor provides benefits similar to those of exercise in the form of stimulation and relaxation. There also may be chemical-neurological connections involving the endorphins, the natural opiates found in the brain, which have implications for the use of humor for clients with stress-related conditions.

Ruxton reviews literature indicating that the use of humor involves certain considerations, specifically, timing, receptiveness, and content. The use of humor may be inappropriate in a time of crisis, when the caregiver is unfamiliar with the client, and when humor is at the client's expense. The use of humor is not constrained by the setting, however, and may be used in high-stress work areas. Ruxton states that humor is useful in client teaching, for children and adults with overwhelming anxieties about hospitalization or treatment, and with older adults in institutions.

showing a hesitating or vacillating manner; or by difficulty with speech articulation such as stuttering, or speaking in an especially soft, high- or low-pitched voice.[125]

Individuals who experience shame can be helped to cope by a mutual process through which others use face-saving etiquette, support the individual's facades, discharge tension with humor, respect the individual's physical and psychological privacy, and encourage the individual in special activities and accomplishments that restore pride. Feelings of worth are reinforced and restored when the individual receives encouragement and positive feedback from others, and experiences a mutual sharing of ideas for realistic problem solving, and the caring interest of those in the environment.

Dying, Grieving, and Self-Expression

Perhaps the greatest threat posed by illness is that one of its possible outcomes is always death. The fear of death is pervasive among humans, who may be unique among the species for having the capacity to contemplate their own eventuality.

Death is a biological process, yet it is one of the most social experiences an individual can have. The process of dying is symbolically the process of losing valued relationships—relationships to significant others, to valued objects such as one's home and possessions, important roles and positions at work and in the family, and the future and to personal goals—and even the relationship one has to oneself as important identities are lost.[126] Thus, the meaning of death is generally focused on profound personal losses that are highly social in nature.

Loss can be defined as the state of being deprived of or being without something one has had.[126] Loss is an integral part of the human experience and has far-reaching implications over the entire course of individual development. Birth, for example, can be looked upon as a loss of the relative security of intrauterine life.[126] Loss is also part of life and living. Most people have many experiences with loss during their lifetimes, and, paradoxically, these may be necessary for the growth of their sense of mastery over life.

Loss can be a real event or a perception derived from an individual's interpretation that endows an event with personal or symbolic meaning.[126] The more individuals have invested emotionally in a person, object, or aspect of self, the more threatened they are likely to feel as they anticipate that loss[126]; however, it is when losses are associated with significant others, the identification with whom grows out of idealization and love, that feelings of loss are likely to be accompanied by grief.

Grief and Grieving. **Grief** describes the private experience of persons who are anticipating loss or who have sustained a loss of something that is critical to their sense of well-being. It is a profound, holistic state that affects how a person thinks, eats, sleeps, and makes it through the day. Grief is a painful response that involves strong emotions such as rage, despair, and fear. It also frequently involves physical symptoms. Grieving people often show many of the signs of acute stress, among them, a feeling of choking or shortness of breath, a need for sighing, and an empty feeling in the abdomen; they may suffer from insomnia and have mental symptoms such as absentmindedness, confusion, and difficulty concentrating.[127]

Recognition of an important loss is a critical feature of the experience of a terminal illness.[128] Such a recognition is generally accompanied by grief, which is experienced by those who are being left behind and by the dying individuals themselves. Grief that is experienced before death occurs is known as **anticipatory grief**.

Bereavement is a term that is associated with grief. **Bereavement** is a role transition that survivors undergo on the death of someone close.[127] The child becomes an orphan, the spouse a widow or widower. Bereavement may or may not be accompanied by grief, depending on the closeness of the relationship involved, the circumstances of the death, and how disruptive the changes prove to be for the bereaved.

Mourning is related to both grief and bereavement. Mourning is the cultural patterning of expression of a bereaved person's grief. Cultures provide various ways for individuals to convey their grief to others through culturally sanctioned attitudes and customs. Because of the cultural plurality that exists in North America, there are many patterns of mourning found among various cultural subgroups.

The Experience of Grief. Because nurses encounter not only death, but also people who are grieving, it is important that they understand the nature of grief and how it is experienced. Carter studied 30 narrative accounts of bereaved individuals' of their experience with grieving, and found five core themes that provide an understanding of what it means to grieve[129]:

- *Being stopped* refers to the interruption that death creates in life's usual flow. Although a few individuals characterized this interruption as a pause in their activities, most experienced greater disruption related to difficulty dealing with the absolute inalterability of death, which led to feelings of being overpowered and helpless. The experience of being stopped was accompanied by sensing oneself as "falling apart" or being "unable to hold myself together."[129]
- *Hurting* is characterized by a cluster of intensely painful emotions. Feelings of sorrow and sadness, often accompanied by crying, were so strong that people described them as painful, similar to being hit, wounded, stabbed, shattered, or crushed, or as an immense heaviness or weight. Painful guilt, burning anger, and sorrowful wishing were also reported. The pain was unrelieved by anything they did, and taxed their coping capacities. As one person commented, "I can't stand it." Although pain was universal, the emotions that were associated with the pain varied.[129]
- *Missing* describes the acute awareness of what has been lost. It included wishing or yearning for the loved one's presence. The loss of the loved one was perceived as a kind of emptiness or void that left the bereaved with a sense of desolation, deprivation, abandonment, and even loneliness. Expressions of missing the loved one were simple and direct, for example, "I miss him so much."[129]
- *Holding* expresses the desire of the bereaved to preserve all that was good from the loved one's lost existence. Ways of holding included "honoring her wishes" and "carrying on his legacy." Talking about the life of the deceased in great detail was important to the bereaved. Holding was a sorting process by which the bereaved separated out the good memories and recalled them, while pushing back the painful memories.[129]
- *Seeking* describes a search for help, which takes the form of seeking comfort and meaning. Comfort was sought in rituals, prayer, staying busy, writing and reading about bereavement, and seeking out others whom the bereaved felt "really understood." The search for meaning was represented in frequent questioning ("why?") or in statements such as, "I want to use this experience to help others."[129]

For many individuals in Carter's study, the hallmark of their grieving was a sense that words were inadequate to convey their experience. The experience of grief was, in essence, inexpressible. Only those who had comparable confrontations with death were felt to provide a shared understanding, and subjects felt a special bond with people who had had similar experiences, as if they were a "secret society" into which only the same experience provided entry. Subjects also had a sense they wanted to meet the expectations they imagined others had for proper bereavement, as if there were a right way to feel or mourn or conduct oneself while bereaved. These were strong enough for some to place prescriptive impositions on themselves that they should act in a certain way, not feel as they did, or not grieve as long as they were grieving.[129]

From this picture it is clear that grief is an experience for which there may be no comparison in human experience. Cody, another researcher of the experience of grieving, also documented the pain of grief. In a study of four bereaved individuals, he found that there were both negative and positive aspects to grieving.[130] Losing someone close undoubtedly gives rise to immobilizing agony, yet the profound change in self that occurred allowed subjects to move forward with a new perspective. One subject viewed his grieving as a rite of passage through which he became more mature.[130]

By understanding the feelings of the bereaved, nurses are able to assist in this process and are provided with a direction for their efforts in caregiving: to assist in the resolution of grief. The fact that Carter's subjects sought help and gained a sense of comfort from sharing their experience with those they perceived as having been in the same situation suggests that mutuality during grieving is both possible and helpful.

The Process of Grieving. Many authorities have described models of grieving in which the grief experience proceeds in predictable stages and unfold within certain time parameters. Lindemann,[131] Engle,[132] Kubler-Ross,[133] and Bowlby[134,135] have all described patterns of grieving that have a typical sequence. These models are similar to each other, depicting stages of response not unlike those experienced by a person with an alteration in body image or self-concept. In fact, the stages of impact, retreat, acknowledgment, and reconstruction can be viewed as a model of grieving.

Although models can help to describe commonalities in grieving, manifestations of grief are highly variable and individual, and people progress and regress in unpredictable ways in their journey toward integrating loss.[136] Despite these variations, it is possible to outline clusters of experience that describe the grief reaction. These clusters should not, however, be viewed as stages with discrete boundaries.

Shock and Disbelief. The immediate response following death, regardless of whether or not the loss is anticipated, comprises shock, numbness, and often disbelief. The feeling of numbness changes to a profound sense of pain and loss, which may be associated with any of the several physical symptoms listed above. Muscular weakness, clammy sensations, feelings of exhaustion, and longing are also common. Bereaved individuals may exhibit extremes of behavior and mood or be unable to think, feel, or move.[136] They may have dreams in which the deceased is alive, and may think they have seen the deceased or have felt the deceased touch them.[136]

Yearning and Protest. Strong feelings frequently well up in bereaved individuals as numbness wears away and they begin to adapt to the loss. These feelings can last weeks or months and include anger toward the deceased for dying and leaving them, anger toward God or caregivers for allowing the death to happen, and feelings of jealousy and resentment toward others who still have their loved ones. The strength of these feelings may lead bereaved individuals to question their own mental stability; hence they may be reluctant to disclose such feelings, fearing they will be misjudged as mentally ill.[136]

Anguish, Disorganization, and Despair. As anger is exhausted and the reality and permanence of the situation are recognized, many bereaved individuals experience confusion, aimlessness, loss of motivation, and general immobility, corresponding to the sense of "being stopped," described above. At this point, the bereaved often suffer from apathy, depression, and loss of meaning to their lives; they frequently withdraw from their usual activities to solitude, but may be overcome by feelings of loneliness at the same time. Memory lapses, difficulty concentrating, and frequent loss of emotional control are characteristic. Bereaved individuals may experience anguish so intense it frightens them. They may have a strong wish and need to cry. As these feelings begin to resolve, the bereaved may have a new feeling that life is fragile. The bereaved will often seek out opportunities to reminisce and use the process of selective memory to support idealized memories of the deceased.[136]

Identification. The bereaved may adopt the behavior, admired qualities, and mannerisms of the loved one. They may take on some of the symptoms of illness that caused the loved one's death or even come to think they have the same illness.[136]

Reorganization. The process of reorganization may begin approximately 6 months after the death and may last a few years. Data from clinical studies fail to support the popular adage that grief should resolve itself in one year and, in fact, indicate a variable time schedule that may be considerably shorter or longer.[137] At this point in the adaptation process, periods of depression may be interspersed with periods of well-being. As time passes and opportunities for sharing feelings accumulate, sadness decreases and aspects of ordinary life are resumed.[136]

Elements of Griefwork. The desired outcome of grieving is that the bereaved are able to resolve the emotional pain they feel in remembering their loved one in such a way as to preserve the capacity to love and to reinvest their emotional energy in living.[136] The process of emotional resolution is stressful and has come to be associated with work, hence the term *griefwork.* Griefwork involves facing emotional pain by recognizing that what is happening is a part of life and by acknowledging and experiencing the full range of emotions associated with one's grief.[136]

There are four elements to griefwork: (1) severing the strong emotional bonds to the deceased, sometimes called *decathexis;* (2) adjusting to an altered environment; (3) developing a new social pattern and relationships; and (4) learning to live with memories of the deceased.[136] Severing emotional bonds requires that the bereaved work through the disturbances created by the loved one's death. The bereaved individual must establish a new identity or revise the former identity, and must work to fill the roles formerly assumed by the deceased, such as managing finances, cooking, and cleaning. Adjustment involves finding new ways to spend the time that the bereaved and the deceased formerly spent together and becoming comfortable with the symbols of the deceased that remain in the bereaved's daily life. Developing new relationships requires that the bereaved reenter social life and reinvest emotions in another person; it also requires an integration of the loss into the bereaved's belief system. Finally, the ability to live with memories requires that the individual in essence says goodbye, remembering the pleasures without forgetting the disappointments.[136]

When griefwork is incomplete or unsuccessful, prolonged grief occurs, making reorganization impossible for the survivor. The hallmark of prolonged grief is a sense of personal hopelessness and lack of involvement in the future.[136] Delayed grief, another outcome of incomplete griefwork, is associated with situations in which people have been unwilling to grieve, preferring to keep busy and to appear to cope well while making no reference to the loss. Symptoms and responses resembling the grieving process finally emerge after a long period of absent grief.[136] Generally the success of griefwork depends on the type of relationship lost, the nature of the death, the characteristics of the survivor, the demands of the social environment, and the quantity and quality of available social support.[136]

Dying. Advances in medical technology over the last several decades have changed the picture of mortality significantly. Deaths from many diseases are no longer automatic or, at least, are no longer quickly fatal. Some diseases that routinely caused death are now curable at least some of the time, or their progression can be substantially forestalled. Terminal diagnoses no longer mean that an individual will die now or even next month or next year. Moreover, thousands of people are treated for chronic illnesses over far longer periods than was the case in the midtwentieth century.

Technological advances are prolonging life and giving time for living, yet in a sense they are also prolonging death, thus increasing the ambiguity and uncertainty of illness. Today, people with serious illnesses often must cope with living and dying simultaneously. Periods of relative health and energy are often interspersed with periods of deterioration. Serious, seemingly terminal illnesses may respond to treatment or inexplicably remit, further compounding uncertainty. The best possible result, which for many is no further deterioration, may be impossible for health professionals to guarantee, so that the specter of death, if not quick death, remains.

Faced with this situation, individuals are forced to deal mentally with their own mortality while continuing an investment in life and living. For some people, a satisfactory adaptation may be possible. They may view their ambiguous situation as an opportunity rather than a danger.[138] For others, the ambiguity and uncertainty may be more difficult than dying itself. Both possibilities have profound implications for an individual's self-expression.

The Meaning of a Potentially Fatal Diagnosis. From the moment they receive a diagnosis of potentially fatal illness, individuals experience many losses over which they may grieve; among these are the following:

- Loss of being a healthy person functioning in society
- Loss of the ability to live without the interruption of hospitalization, clinic appointments, and painful treatments
- Loss of the ability to plan for the future, or at least the long-term future
- Eventual or sudden loss of job role
- Loss of present or future ability to care for home and family
- Loss of present or future ability to perform sexually
- Loss of present or future ability to care for one's own bodily needs and functions[139]

Individuals receiving a potentially fatal diagnosis experience these and other losses at varying points in their recognition of the implications of their illness. For some, the grieving may begin immediately; for others, it may be substantially delayed. The reaction of the person who receives the diagnosis affects significant others with varying degrees of intensity, and the reactions of significant others, in turn, have an effect on the individual. Mutually they define the situation in a way that makes it possible for them to cope.

One possibility is that they will choose not to acknowledge the possibility of death, at least at first. So long as the physical status remains uncertain, inattention to the likelihood of death may actually enhance coping by influencing ill individuals to adhere to their treatment programs[140]; however, as the physical condition deteriorates, new definitions become necessary for adaptation.

Ill individuals and their significant others who fail to acknowledge the possibility of death as the terminal phase develops, may have a need to conceal their feelings from one another, and this will affect their ability to grieve.[139] If they and their families persist in ignoring death as an outcome, using avoidance as a pattern of coping, not only will the dying person and significant others become isolated from one another, distancing themselves from their natural support systems and rendering their experience lonelier and perhaps more painful than it otherwise would be, but the long-term adjustment of the survivors may be placed at risk as well.[138]

Reactions of caregivers from prediagnosis to death and bereavement can facilitate or hinder the emotional response of the client and family as illness progresses. Caregivers who also cope by avoidance may deny the client and family an important means of support in dealing with their impending losses.[139]

The Experience of Dying. Grieving is an element of dying just as it is an element of bereavement. Kubler-Ross in the 1960 classic work *On Death and Dying,* was one of the first to investigate the experience of dying by outlining the stages of grieving through which the dying individual evolved. These included denial (of the seriousness of the condition), anger ("why me?" with rage directed at anybody and everybody), bargaining (making an arrangement with God or fate), depression (sense of loss and inevitable finality), and acceptance (an acknowledgment that if the person enters this stage, the struggle is over).[133]

Kubler-Ross awakened a generation of people to the needs of the dying person and her work has been extremely influential; however, critiques of her work have emphasized that the concept of stages ignores the complexity and depth of the dying person's experience and encourages those familiar with the theory to dismiss the dying person's reactions as a matter of developmental course, rather than to deal existentially with the content and intensity of the dying person's expressions.[141] Kastenbaum and Costa thus have emphasized the individual variability of grieving as a part of dying, just as others have emphasized the individual variability of grieving as a part of bereavement.[141] The clusters of grieving, described earlier, can be viewed as having relevance to the experience of the dying, but should not be taken as prescriptive.

It may be impossible for a living person to do justice to a description of dying. Certainly, an important part of the experience of dying derives from the social context of death. One aspect of that experience can be profound loneliness. **Loneliness** is a subjective feeling experienced in response to a deficit in social relationships and contacts that are meaningful and important.[142] It is a distressing experience that, if intense enough, can heighten the ill individual's physical symptoms. Dying frequently involves prolonged hospitalization, during which the dying person is separated from loved ones. In the course of this separation, the dying person may experience profound loneliness, mitigated to a greater or lesser extent by the perception that the separation is temporary.

Sometimes separation occurs at an emotional or social level, and this, too, can cause loneliness. Dying persons often find themselves isolated with their own grief as others seek to maintain their own composure and coping ability by ignoring the reality of the situation. The dying may even find themselves confronted with the necessity to comfort others who are unable to handle the intensity of their own emotions. Even health care professionals, who are vulnerable to becoming emotionally overwhelmed by the shear frequency of their encounters with death, are sometimes prone to defensive behavior.[143]

All of these situations in the social context reinforce the loneliness of dying. Shifts in the social context that emerge as an individual moves into the terminal stage are not always negative, however, and the extent and duration of communication changes may be mediated by factors such as pre-illness family function and communication patterns. Generally, stable relationships are less disrupted by the diagnosis and treatment of terminal illness.[116]

Another aspect of the experience of dying involves alterations in comfort and physical suffering. Pain, anorexia, nausea, vomiting, fatigue, elimination difficulty, sexual dysfunction, and breathlessness are a few of the physical problems that may accompany dying.[144] These, in turn, compound the emotional experience that often includes depression, anxiety, and fear. Terminal illness does not uniformly involve pain, but when it does, the pain is often a salient feature of the individual's experience. The pain in terminal illness is often of a chronic and progressive nature and, although it varies in intensity, often requires aggressive pharmaceutical and nonpharmaceutical interventions for control. Narcotics are often used on a regularly scheduled rather than an intermittent basis in the treatment of cancer pain.[144] Pain control is one of the most important contributions that nurses make to care of the dying.

Another important feature of the experience of dying is the emotions that are associated with dying itself, with the social situation that dying creates, and with the physical suffering of dying. Fear of the unknown is a prominent feature of the distress of many dying individuals. This fear may be so strong as to consume the limited time and energy available to the dying person. Fears and anxieties may be made more tolerable when the individual has the opportunity to disclose them to caring others. An individual's spiritual beliefs may be particularly helpful. Personal beliefs and philosophy that are relevant to the dying experience may be shared through self-disclosure and can be reinforced by caregivers as a way of expressing caring and providing comfort. Depression is often related not only to the fact of dying, but also to the physical symptoms that the individual has. Thus, relief from physical suffering may also be instrumental in bringing relief from depression.[144]

Adaptational Tasks of the Dying Person. The griefwork involved in the process of dying encompasses coping with the dying experience, hopefully moving toward acceptance, and completing a series of adaptational tasks during the course of grieving. The relative importance of each task varies with the characteristics and needs of the dying person. Humphrey has identified several adaptational tasks that the dying person may undertake.

Getting Affairs in Order. Getting one's affairs in order may be difficult given the effects of illness. If this task is delayed, the individual may lack the physical or mental capacity to participate. Denial may contribute to delay.

Coping with the Loss of Both Loved Ones and Self. The dying person may be overwhelmed by loss, not only the loss of relationships but of the world around him or her. Nevertheless, the individual must contemplate that life will go on for his or her survivors and must consider who will care for them and who will share in their lives to come. As Humphrey points out, this issue is especially poignant for the dying person.[139]

Considering Future Health Care Needs. Options for care are increasing as the hospice movement develops. Hospices are homelike institutions that specialize in the care of the dying in the terminal phase. The current lack of health care insurance facing many Americans may make hospice care unrealistic. Nevertheless, careful planning for the physical care of the dying person during the terminal phase is an issue that must be addressed in advance and is important not only to the dying person but also to the survivors.[139]

Planning for the Time Remaining. With an awareness of the limited time remaining, choices for use of that time and of remaining resources are crucial. Final acts of self-expression must be contemplated and decisions made on priorities for the days, weeks, months, or years available.

Anticipating Future Pain and Physical Losses Contributing to a Loss of Identity. The issue of pain must be realistically addressed and solutions anticipated. Changes in physical appearance and functions that interfere with self-presentation are extremely threatening, but generally unavoidable. Loss of hair, for example, is a common side effect of cancer chemotherapy. Because hair loss is such a visible change, it is a source of considerable social embarrassment for many individuals, particularly for women. It is also a constant reminder to the individual of altered identity and of approaching death. Such losses generally must be grieved, and the individual will usually require assistance to cope in a fashion that minimizes shame and guilt.[139]

Considering Being a Nonperson. Consideration of one's own nonbeing is part of the experience of dying. Humphrey notes that this existential aspect is like looking at the sun; it cannot be done for long without looking away.[139] Nevertheless, it is an issue that must be dealt with as part of the anticipatory grief process. Life review is helpful as the individual undertakes this task, and may provide a sense of fulfillment and satisfaction that will aid the dying in letting go. Religious and philosophical discussions may also be helpful to the dying who fear the transition into death.

Deciding to Speed Up or Slow Down the Dying Process. In losing one's life, one loses ultimate control. Nevertheless, it is helpful for the dying to know that individuals do retain some control over the death trajectory. At an emotional level, individuals decide to fight or give up, and this has consequences for the length of their survival. Once a person lets go, death often quickly follows.[138] Moreover, individuals have the right to refuse life-prolonging treatment, which gives them some control over the temporal aspect of death. More controversial, socially, morally, ethically, and legally, is whether they have the right to assist or be assisted in their own death.

Hope. **Hope** is an attitude that is characterized by a confident, yet uncertain, expectation of achieving a future good, which to the hoping person is realistically possible and personally significant.[145] Hall pinpoints the dilemma of hope for the terminally ill by asking, "If hope is future oriented, and if the dying supposedly have no future, are they engaging in wishful thinking and denial when they have hope?"[146(p180)] One viewpoint holds that hope is appropriate only if it is realistic. The other holds that hope is an emotion whose purpose is to maintain emotional well-being in the face of both everyday occurrences and extremely unusual dire circumstances, and thus is always valuable.[147] This latter view comes from the work Erick Fromm entitled *The Revolution of Hope*, which proposed that hope is a shared human experience that is essential to life.[148]

Hall stresses that hope is integral to humanness, and that loss of hope can be equated with loss of life itself. In a study of 11 individuals who tested positive for the human immunodeficiency virus (HIV), Hall found that all of her subjects had mechanisms for maintaining a positive outlook and that these were essential to their sense of well-being. One individual, for example, declined to join an AIDS support group because the members' constant talk of death scared him. Other individuals refused to change their activities just for the sake of preventing illnesses that might prove to be terminal. Still others looked at their survival predictions as a challenge, Hall believed, to maintain hope.[146] It was also important to Hall's subjects that they retain a future orientation.

Hall emphasizes that nurses have an important role to play in helping terminal clients maintain hope, and that trust is enhanced when nurses relate to the terminally ill in the same future-oriented way in which they relate to anyone else. Although nursing care that stimulates discussion by the dying about the meaning and quality of their lives often eases the passage from life, whether or not to talk about death must be the dying individual's choice.[146]

IMPLICATIONS FOR NURSE–CLIENT COLLABORATION

Uncertainty in Illness, Denial of Illness, and Hope

The outcome of illness is often uncertain. Many illnesses are said to be terminal in nature; that is, they rapidly accelerate the process of dying. Survival statistics enable health professionals to predict the likely timetable for any given illness. Nevertheless, individual variability makes it impossible to predict with certainty what the timetable will be in a specific case. Hope enables people to cope with difficult situations, illness included, in our future-oriented society. Denial of illness, at least the denial of certainty of death at any specific time, may be a part of maintaining hope in the face of overwhelming circumstances, and may aid individuals to deal with their situation in a way that preserves their dignity. Nurses are in a position to assist ill individuals to preserve their dignity by supporting hope.

Other Spiritual Needs. The approach of death is commonly accompanied by an inward journey to consider the meaning of one's life. The dying often have urgent spiritual needs related to a search for meaning, forgiveness, and love.[149] The search for meaning represents a need to make death significant, less fearful, and more tolerable; to deal with the frustration that dying causes; and to affirm the value of life.[149] For some individuals the answers lie in their religious beliefs, and for others, in their ability to articulate their own meaning of death.

The dying may seek relief from feelings of guilt as they review their lives and consider the unfulfilled expectations they had for themselves.[149] Forgiveness from God or from particular individuals may become extremely important. Many dying individuals find comfort in spiritual counseling from their clergy as they experience these feelings, and may have a need to express these feelings to others as they strive to identify and deal with the source of their discomfort.

The love of God and the love of others also take on new meaning. Family and friends are important sources of love, but may need assistance to express their feelings as they struggle to deal with the needs of their dying loved one and their own as well. Professional caregivers are also a source of love, especially when family and friends are unavailable or nonexistent.

Interdisciplinary teamwork to meet the spiritual needs of the dying is important. People vary in their ability to balance involvement and objectivity in the care of the dying, and members of the team can assist each other to both help the dying and maintain their own ability to carry on.

Definition of Death. Death is a very familiar word, one whose definition might appear to be self-evident. Many people assume that physical characteristics of death represent an absolute certainty apart from any variations in individual and social meaning. Nevertheless, the physical nature of death is a subject of substantial scientific, social, and public policy controversy.

The proliferation of the technology of organ donorship and transplant has brought the issue of what constitutes death to the forefront of bioethical and medical concern. Nurses who work in hospitals, particularly those in critical care settings, are frequently confronted by the human problems that surround the definition of death. This is perhaps one of the most wrenching social, ethical, and legal issues of our times and, given the expense of technologically sophisticated care, one of the most difficult economic questions as well. It is a question that bioethicists, clergy, policymakers, nurses and physicians are currently debating, one that may not soon be resolved, but in which all of us have a vital interest.

In the past, a person was considered dead when the vital functions such as heartbeat and respirations ceased, when the individual was unarousable, with no nervous reflexes, speech, or movement. Today technology has changed that picture significantly, making traditional approaches to the diagnosis of death inadequate. Is a person dead when, mechanically supported, the heart still beats, the chest rises and falls, the lungs exchange gases, and the nervous reflexes are intact and easily elicited, even though the person is unable to give any signs of cognitive functioning?

Kastenbaum has identified several ways of being dead, all of which occur in health care settings[127]:

- The *person* is dead. The individual fails to respond, shows a prolonged inability to express thoughts or feelings by any means, and generally shows none of the characteristics associated with being distinctly human. The vital processes have ceased, and the individual is functioning on a vegetative level; however, the cessation is not necessarily permanent.
- The same situation exists; however, the vital processes have returned and continue to function *with* the use of an elaborate life-support system.
- The same situation exists; however, the vital functions continue *without* an elaborate life-support system.
- The *body* is dead. All vital functions have permanently ceased.

One question that arises in relation to these various ways of being dead, and that has been subject to ethical and legal debate, is how important is the distinction between the cessation of bodily processes and the loss of a person as a person? There are also other questions. What difference, if any, is there between a body that continues to function on a vegetative level with a life-support system and a body that functions on the same level without a life-support system? How long are people obliged to continue to make elaborate life-support systems available to those who are in a vegetative state and what criteria are applicable to the cessation of life support? What means of support are people obliged to provide, and for how long, when a body in a vegetative state sustains its vital functions without elaborate mechanical devices? These questions all have practical significance to health professionals.

Medical Definition. For the past 40 years, the health care and legal communities have attempted to answer these difficult questions as well as the more basic question of what death is. By 1959, the impact of technology had manifested itself in the recognition of the concept of brain death in a pioneering report from two French physiologists, Mollaret and Boulon.[150] They documented the existence of a physiological state "beyond coma" in which there was no detectable electrophysiological activity from the brain in some comatose individuals whose breathing was maintained with a ventilator. A decade later a committee of Harvard Medical School faculty formulated the Harvard Criteria for determination of a permanently nonfunctioning brain.[151] These criteria included the following:

1. *Unreceptive and unresponsive.* There is no awareness of external stimuli (including stimuli that ordinarily would be extremely painful) or inner need.
2. *No movements and no breathing.* There is a complete absence of spontaneous respirations and all other spontaneous muscular movement.
3. *No reflexes.* The usual reflexes elicited in a neurological examination, including pupillary constriction to a light stimulus, are absent.
4. *A flat electroencephalogram for 24 hours.* Electrodes attached to the scalp fail to elicit a printout of electrical activity as obtained from living brain. The stylus records an essentially flat line indicating a lack of electrophysiological activity instead of the usual peaks and valleys of brain waves.
5. *No circulation to or within the brain for 24 hours.* Sophisticated procedures (such as the use of Doppler ultrasound) fail to detect the flow of blood in the brain, the loss of which is accompanied by death of the brain cells.

Generally the first three criteria are enough to establish a diagnosis of death, and the others are reserved for situations in which traditional criteria are inadequate. In situations where the final two criteria are applied, the Harvard committee recommended that tests be repeated 24 hours later.

The Harvard guidelines have received widespread application. Indeed, they are still used today, although procedures have been and are still being refined. During the intervening years, controversies have appeared about the extent of the loss of brain activity that constitutes brain death: whether the whole brain, that is, the cortex (upper brain) and the brainstem (lower brain), must cease to function, or whether the cessation of cortical function alone is sufficient while brainstem and vegetative functions persist. The current medical and legal standard requires that all brain functions cease, including the activity of the brainstem and higher structures.[152]

Legal Dilemmas. Despite widespread medical use of these criteria, legal dilemmas are presented to those who find themselves confronted with social questions surrounding the definition of death. Right-to-die cases have raised questions about the rights of individuals who find themselves coping with problems stemming from the failure of social policy to keep pace with technology, and these cases are gradually providing answers to questions about the withdrawal of support from those who meet the medical criteria of death. Answers, in fact, began to emerge with the case of Karen Ann Quinlan in 1976 and continued to evolve with the relatively recent case of Nancy Cruzan in 1990. Karen Ann Quinlan was a young woman in a persistent vegetative state following two periods of anoxia; her parents sought court authorization to remove her from the ventilator that sustained her respiration. The New Jersey Supreme Court in a landmark, unanimous decision authorized removal on the basis of Quinlan's constitutional rights of privacy, which the Court concluded would be lost unless the parents were given the authority to exercise it on her behalf.[153] The Quinlan case established that individuals who could not speak for themselves nevertheless could exercise their right to decline extraordinary medical treatment.

On the other hand, Nancy Cruzan, a young woman in a persistent vegetative state as a result of a 1983 automobile accident, required only tube feeding to continue to survive. Her parents firmly believed that Nancy would not have wanted treatment continued in these circumstances, in part on the basis of her own statement that she would not want to live if she could not be "at least halfway normal."[153] The trial judge authorized her parents to have their daughter's tube feeding discontinued; however, the Missouri Supreme Court reversed the decision. Nancy's parents appealed to the US Supreme Court, which characterized the case as involving both the right to die and the right to cause death. The majority opinion in the five-to-four decision stated that the Court assumed the US Constitution would grant a competent person the protected right to refuse lifesaving hydration and nutrition. Nevertheless, the Court allowed that states could restrict the right of surrogate decision makers to act on behalf of previously competent individuals by requiring clear and convincing evidence of the person's expressed decision while competent.[153]

Undoubtedly more issues will find legal resolution as the state courts take positions on similar and different cases. One issue currently before the courts is whether physicians should have the authority to stop life support in hopeless cases when the incompetent individual's surrogates desire that support be continued. Future decisions on this and other issues undoubtedly will continue to refine the legal requirements for acknowledging death in cases where technology prolongs life artificially. On the basis of the Cruzan case it is clear, however, that even in death, a person's self-expression retains a powerful influence over personal fate and the behavior of others.

Section 2. Assessment of Self-Expression

The holistic view of human behavior described in Section 1 offers a framework for assessing self-expression. Because self-expression merges subjective and objective aspects of the self, both internal (private) and external (public) aspects are of equal importance in assessment of self-expression. Access to the client's inner world of feelings, thoughts, and perceptions helps nurses understand the client's illness experience. Setting the climate for such self-disclosure facilitates a more thorough assessment by the nurse.

Assessment focuses on both the content and the process of self-expression. The content of self-expression refers to all the verbal expressions of feelings and thoughts and all observable actions or behaviors in a person that symbolize important meaning for that person. History taking elucidates the process, that is, the meaning clients place on these behaviors, enabling nurses to understand the "how" and "why" of clients' behavior: What does the behavior say about what is important to this client, at this time? What is the client experiencing and feeling, what does it mean to the client, and what is its significance now?

Assessment provides data about the client's overall state of wellness, goals, perceptions of illness, and expectations about recovery, care, and future well-being. Specific aspects of self-expression such as self-concept, body image, role performance, life structure, and sexuality are revealed through the client's self-presentation and self-disclosure, and contribute to a holistic view of the client that provides the basis for effective planning and management of care. The information the nurse elicits from the client regarding self-concept, body image, self-ideal, and life choices and goals will highlight the impact of illness on each of these areas. This information is gained through history taking, examination, and ongoing observation of the client's behavior in the nurse–client relationship and the client's relationships with significant other persons. Table 23–3 provides an overview of the components of assessment and the aspects of self-expression that are evaluated for each component.

■ SELF-EXPRESSION DATA COLLECTION

Self-Expression History

History taking allows nurses to discern themes, patterns, and priorities of the client's life. A detailed history of present and past health problems and of the client's life course assists nurses to make formulations about the client's self-concept, coping ability, current stressors, adaptation, and experiences with health care providers.

The nurse's approach to history taking is extremely important to assessing self-expression. History taking can be viewed as a formalized process of self-disclosure. By asking questions about the client's life, the nurse communicates interest in the client as a person. These expressions of interest are one of the ways that the nurse lets the client know that caregiving is a process of sharing. Such expressions of interest also encourage the client to share the information necessary for care planning. In taking a history, the nurse avoids adhering strictly to an outline, as people generally do not talk about themselves in outline form (see Chap. 16). The client's spontaneity is promoted by avoiding a set format and by inviting the client to tell his or her own story as he or she knows it, without interruption.

History taking may be complicated by the fact that the client views the nurse with a set of attitudes and expectations derived from previous experiences with other nurturers and helpers. The relationship to the nurse influences to a large extent clients' motivation to disclose the nature of their problems and their possible sources. It is not customary for most persons to discuss openly their intimate relations, thoughts, and feelings with strangers in the first

TABLE 23–3. OVERVIEW OF COMPONENTS OF SELF-EXPRESSION ASSESSMENT

Components	Aspects of Self-Expression Evaluated
History	Perception of illness, life structure, self-presentation styles, self-concept, problems, goals, preferences
Primary concern/current understanding	Self-disclosure related to immediate concern, perception of event
Past health problems/experiences	Health practices, life-style choices, body image, interaction patterns
Personal, family, social history	Sexuality, self-concept, vocational choices, life structure, activity patterns, values, social distance/closeness, beliefs, public and private self, interpersonal relationships, role performance, sense of meaning, self-esteem, reference group, life satisfaction
Subjective manifestations	Self-presentation, self-concept, body image
Examination	Body image, self-concept, self-esteem
Measurements	Body image
Objective manifestations	Self-presentation, posture, facial expression, speech, dress, manner, grooming

meeting. Self-disclosure requires courage[82] and a secure and reciprocal relationship based on mutual trust.[102]

In addition to identifying potential problems in self-expression brought on by illness, history taking is essential to identifying client strengths, resources, and resourcefulness. Effective coping is an important strength. How clients are currently coping with the illness and methods they have used for coping in the past provide data that assist the nurse in planning care. Emotional support provided by the client's interpersonal network, creative outlets, leisure pursuits, and behaviors that enhance self-esteem are other areas that may reveal client strengths.

Primary Concern. The primary concern reflects the client's most important reason for seeking help at this time. This portion of the history focuses on what about the current health problems bothers the client most and why the client is seeking help now. When the client's health problem involves the dimension of self-expression, this concern often has an impact on self-concept or the client's ability to perform meaningful activities. For example, the client may be recently widowed after a long marriage and struggling with the subsequent loss of identity. The nurse also assesses clients' expectations for the caregiving process. Clients may wonder whether they will be able to return to work or an important activity on discharge or may fear that a treatment will change their ability to have intimate relationships. The relevance of the primary concern for self-expression data collection is illustrated by the following case example and Table 23–4.

- Mr. Foster is a 62-year-old clerical worker, hospitalized for abdominal pain of 2 weeks' duration. He recently lost his wife of 30 years to an unexpected cardiac illness. Mr. Foster states that he expects his hospital stay to be short; however, his physician suspects he is suffering from an obstruction of the intestines that may require surgery. The nurse's assessment will focus on Mr. Foster's previous experiences with surgery, potential alterations in body image due to anticipated surgery, and expected changes in vocation and leisure pursuits. The recent death of Mr. Foster's wife also cues the nurse to assess life satisfaction, grieving state, and the social demands of his current interpersonal network.

IMPLICATIONS FOR NURSE–CLIENT COLLABORATION

Self-Disclosure and History Taking

History taking is a formalized process of client self-disclosure. Ordinarily, self-disclosure is reserved for close, trusting relationships in which the risks of self-disclosure are minimized, but during health assessment clients are asked to disclose intimate details about their lives to people who are virtual strangers. Although clients generally understand the nurse's fiduciary role and accord an automatic trust to the nurse, it is nevertheless important for the nurse to protect the client's privacy in regard to potentially sensitive subjects by using open-ended interview approaches, such as, "Tell me about your problem at work." Open-ended approaches leave decisions about what to disclose and how much to disclose to the client, and give the client the freedom to share the details he or she is comfortable giving.

Current Understanding. Determining the client's perspective about the health problem as it relates to self-expression requires some judgment about what may have precipitated his or her distress. For example, a client may have had repeated admissions over several years for joint pain in the knee and may currently fear the prospect of surgery and prolonged mobility limitations. As the client has had no restrictions on mobility prior to this, the loss of mobility is a new and potentially difficult challenge. The client now faces body image changes, possible loss of self-esteem, and loss of enjoyment obtained from certain activities. Thus, exploration of how health problems hamper the client's life at present and what consequences the client fears in the future is helpful.

The nurse should ask the client about the present prob-

TABLE 23–4. EXAMPLES OF PRIMARY CONCERN STATEMENTS

Primary Concern as Expressed by Client	Aspect of Self-Expression Potentially Affected
"I can't manage at home anymore." "I have been getting more and more depressed."	Self-esteem, leisure pursuits, social relationships, sexuality, life satisfaction, self-presentation
"My test results show I'm going to need a mastectomy."	Body image, sexuality, self-presentation, self-esteem, self-concept, self-disclosure
"I haven't been able to walk as well."	Self-presentation, body image, leisure pursuits, social relationships, life satisfaction
"I can't cope with taking care of my new baby."	Role performance, self-esteem, self-presentation, psychosocial development, life satisfaction, self-awareness
"My breathing has been getting worse."	Body image, self-concept, leisure pursuits, self-disclosure, social relationships
"My heart condition is worse and my doctor thinks I can't work anymore."	Vocation, role performance, body image, self-presentation, life satisfaction
"My wife passed away and I haven't been able to eat since."	Self-esteem, self-concept, self-disclosure, role performance, self-presentation, grieving and loss

lem as the client sees it, and should note changes that the client anticipates, focusing on self-esteem, interpersonal relationships, or impairment in work. Any factors that may have contributed to the present crisis and methods the client is using to adapt to the crisis should be noted.

In determining problems in self-concept/body image, it is helpful to evaluate the client's highest level of functioning before the illness occurred. Nurses can elicit this information by asking several questions: "When did you feel the best about yourself?" "What were you doing at the time?" "What helps you have a positive view of yourself?" "How did you see yourself functioning during that period?"

Reviewing clients' expectations about how the illness will affect their life patterns is also essential. Clients' accounts should include how they view the illness affecting their mood, interest in activities, involvement with others, and future choices. Understanding how the client's day-to-day life is affected by the illness helps the nurse determine areas for possible intervention.

Modifications in dress, grooming, and personal habits related to the illness also provide information about the client's self-presentation. The client may describe these changes during history taking or the nurse may observe them during the course of working with the client. Clients with mood changes from illness may be less interested in how they present themselves to the world. Clients with changes in energy level from the illness may also pay less attention to grooming and hygiene.

Clients who are coping with a loss through death or divorce may manifest health changes that have been caused or aggravated by loss. For example, weight changes, headaches, or pain are examples of symptoms that may be related to loss. A careful description of the social circumstances in which the symptoms evolved should be obtained. Exploring with the client whether there have been deaths, separations, conflicts, or losses of significant others is extremely helpful in assessing problems in self-expression.

Clients' attitudes toward the illness and their expectations of care provide important data. Some clients may be angry about past health care and have expectations of being frustrated again. Other clients may feel helpless in coping with the illness, which will affect their ability to engage in problem solving. Client expectations may not always be realistic and may need revision through education or sensitive counseling by nurses. Both client and nurse have an important role in identifying concerns to be addressed or goals to be obtained.[154]

Past Health Problems/Experiences. It is important to review the impact of past health problems on the client's self-expression. The psychological meaning of the illness can be explored in terms of the client's feelings about injury to body parts, effects on body image, and effects on self-concept and self-esteem, particularly in relation to loss. For instance, a client who has undergone drug treatment for cancer and experiences subsequent hair loss may be angry or depressed, may have lowered self-esteem related to body image changes, or may withdraw socially because of concerns about self-presentation.

Clients' motivation for and capacity to assist in recovery, and the coping mechanisms they have employed, provide information for current implementation and for assessment of problems in self-expression. Support systems and interpersonal contacts that the client has used to aid recovery in the past provide important data for current management.

The nurse should ask about chronic physical conditions to which the client has had to adapt. These data can also provide useful information about clients' coping abilities, resources, limitations, and residual problems in self-expression or sexual expression (eg, social isolation because of a body image problem).

As important as the factual data of the client's past health problems is the client's perception and response to the illness. The nurse should explore the meaning of the illness to the client and how the illness has affected self-expression by asking questions such as "How did you feel about yourself after your surgery last year?" "Did you view your body differently when you received the diagnosis of . . . ?" "Did you have negative feelings about yourself during the last episode of . . . ?" "Do you think any different about yourself after . . . ?" "Do you think others view you differently since . . . ?" The following example illustrates the importance of these data.

- Mr. Morton is a 64-year-old client, hospitalized for cardiac surgery. He suffered a stroke in the past that left him with a mild paralysis of the left side of his face. He has also been previously diagnosed with sensory loss and numbness of the lower extremities, which has limited his mobility. Mr. Morton is quite anxious about facing major surgery, but is most concerned about chronic sensory loss in his legs. In exploring Mr. Morton's response to the past problem, it is clear that he is most upset about his restricted ability to dance and the effect of this limitation on his relationship with his girlfriend. The nurse decides to explore body image changes with Mr. Morton as well as self-esteem changes, interpersonal relationships, leisure pursuits, life satisfaction, and role performance changes.

Personal, Family, and Social History. Through the personal, family, and social history, many of the dimensions of the client's self-expression are discovered. As described in Section 1, the self has many aspects. One important aspect is the social self, through which meaningful links to the world are created. Exploration of the personal, family, and social history can also provide information about how a client views self in relation to others.

Another aspect of the self is the sense of personal uniqueness derived from one's experiences with others. This feeling of individuality or distinctness from others is communicated through one's choices and experiences in personal, family, and social arenas and helps the person answer questions such as "How am I special?" "How am I different than others?" "What makes me unique?" Table 23–5 provides examples of personal, family, and social history questions.

Vocation/Occupation. The vocation/occupation component of the personal, family, and social history provides important clues about the client's life structure as well as data about formal and informal educational pursuits. The job history can provide information about the client's strengths, functional level, goals, life satisfaction, self-esteem, and self-presentation. Vocation/occupation choices demonstrate how one expresses oneself through work (Fig. 23–3). Work roles affect one's perceptions of self. Work often provides a sense of importance, productivity, mastery, and usefulness for an individual. Work relationships often have a powerful influence, positive or negative, on self-esteem. Exploring the meaning of work to the client also aids in understanding self-concept. Is work the central focus of the client's life? Does it merely provide a livelihood? Is it balanced with other areas of importance such as family? How does work affect the client's view of self and how the self is presented to the world?

Social and Leisure Activities. A review of social and leisure activities gives clues about what provides a sense of meaning and life satisfaction to the client as well as areas that may have impairments. An absence of leisure pursuits may demonstrate a lack of adequate stress-reducing mechanisms or simply may indicate that the client is focused on other areas of life.

Leisure activities can contribute to positive feelings about the self, a sense of uniqueness and mastery. They provide an expressive outlet for clients; thus, a disruption in leisure activities may result in further crisis for the client. For example, an illness that leaves a client unable to exercise may deprive the client of his or her usual outlet for coping with day-to-day stress.

Sexual History. The sexual history provides important information about the client's sexual orientation, sexual satisfaction, and possible sexual dysfunction. Sexual patterns are a significant form of self-expression. Sexual expression is affected by body image, self-concept and self-esteem, life satisfaction, and close interpersonal relationships. A review of each of these areas helps to identify problems in sexual self-expression.

Sexual history taking can often be woven into questions related to significant relationships or health problems. For instance, the nurse might ask "How do you and your spouse get along?" "Are there problems in your relationship?" "Do you feel you can talk about most things with your spouse?" "Are there areas you would like to see changed in your relationship?" "Do you think your heart condition has affected other areas of your life?" More direct questions also are required.

Psychological State. The client's mood and affect are important indicators of psychological state. How clients describe themselves and their strengths and achievements also can reflect self-esteem, a component of self-concept. The client's ability to adapt to and cope with illness in the past assists in determining the effectiveness of coping behaviors. Does the client have skill deficits that need attention or faulty problem-solving skills that need intervention?

Subjective Manifestations. A thorough assessment of problems in self-expression should include questions related to each body system. Of particular relevance are the neurological and genitourinary/reproductive systems.

Neurological aspects of the history are often of great significance, especially in clients with intellectual deficits or disturbances of memory and attention. The client may report a change in these functions during history taking. Mental status testing during the examination can reveal further data. (Examination is discussed in detail below.) Intellectual deficits, such as the inability to recall and mobilize previous experience in adapting to new situations, can create problems in self-expression. Reasoning, judgment, and problem solving may be affected by illness. Self-expression

TABLE 23–5. SELF-EXPRESSION HISTORY: PERSONAL, FAMILY, AND SOCIAL HISTORY QUESTIONS

A. **Vocational**
1. What kind of work do you do?
2. What kind of training/schooling did that require?
3. How long have you been doing this kind of work?
4. Have you changed jobs recently? What made you change?
5. What kind of experience did you have in the military? (Include combat experience.)
6. Does your work provide satisfaction?
7. What are your career goals?
8. How close do you feel toward your career ideals?
9. How does your work make you feel good about yourself?
10. How has your work affected your health?

B. **Home and Family**
1. Do you live alone or with someone?
2. Tell me about your family/spouse. (Include ages, children, duration of marriage.)
3. How is your family or spouse reacting to your illness?
4. What is a typical day like in your home?
5. What roles and responsibilities do you have in your family?
6. Does your family do things together?
7. Have you lost any family members recently?
8. Are you currently having family or marriage problems?
9. How does your family or spouse solve problems with you?
10. Would you describe your family as close?
11. How has your health problem affected your family relationships?

C. **Social and Leisure**
1. What do you do to relax, have fun?
2. Are you involved in activities outside work or your home?
3. Are you involved in church/synagogue/community activities?
4. What helps you feel good about yourself besides work and family?
5. Are you involved in sports or exercise on a regular basis?
6. Do you have friends you see on a regular basis?
7. Are there things you feel strongly about or are active in?
8. How do you feel around other people?
9. Are there groups you belong to or are active with?
10. How has your health affected your involvement with friends or activities?

D. **Sexual**
1. Are you single? Married? Divorced? Seeing someone?
2. Do you have a sexual preference (eg, heterosexual, homosexual)?
3. Are you concerned about sexually transmitted diseases?
4. Are you worried about sex?
5. Are there areas about sex that you would like more information about (eg, effects of medication on impotence)?
6. Are you satisfied with your current sexual relationship?
7. Has your health affected your sex life?
8. Are there emotional concerns/issues that have affected your sex life?

E. **Habits**

Exercise
1. Do you get regular exercise?
2. What type of exercise do you do? How often? For how long?

Diet
1. Are you on a special diet?
2. What do you pay most attention to in the foods you eat (eg, fat content, salt, calories)?
3. Has your health affected your interest in or intake of food?

Sleep
1. Do you have problems sleeping, falling asleep, or staying asleep?
2. Has your health affected your sleep patterns?

Substance Use
1. Do you smoke? How much? How long have you smoked? Are you concerned about its effects on your health?
2. Do you drink alcoholic beverages? How much and how often?
3. Do you use drugs? What kind and how often? How long have you used them?

(continued)

TABLE 23–5. (continued)

F. **Psychological**
1. How would you describe yourself?
2. What do you like best about yourself? Least?
3. What accomplishments are you proud of?
4. Has your appearance changed because of your illness? If so, how has that affected you?
5. What do your friends, family, co-workers say about you?
6. Would you describe yourself as a private person? A loner? Social?
7. Do you think people see the real you?
8. Do you feel depressed or anxious?
9. How do you cope with stress? What helps the most?
10. Are you anxious or self-conscious around people?
11. Do you have certain fears that upset you?
12. Do you ever feel hopeless or that you don't want to go on?
13. Do you feel sad for prolonged periods?
14. Do you feel discouraged? About anything in particular?
15. Have any changes (eg, death or loss) affected your mood?

can be impaired if a client has memory deficits; the data that are presented to the nurse will also be affected. Clients with aphasia (loss of previous ability to communicate words), for example, have unique problems in self-expression.

The genitourinary and reproductive system questions may reveal problems related to sexual expression. For example, past health problems of chronic urinary tract infections may have residual effects on sexual functioning. Chapter 16 provides sample questions for subjective manifestations related to these systems.

Self-Expression Examination

A thorough assessment includes data obtained from observation and physical examination of the client. Observation is especially important in assessment of self-expression, as many aspects of self-expression are communicated indirectly, subtly, or nonverbally.

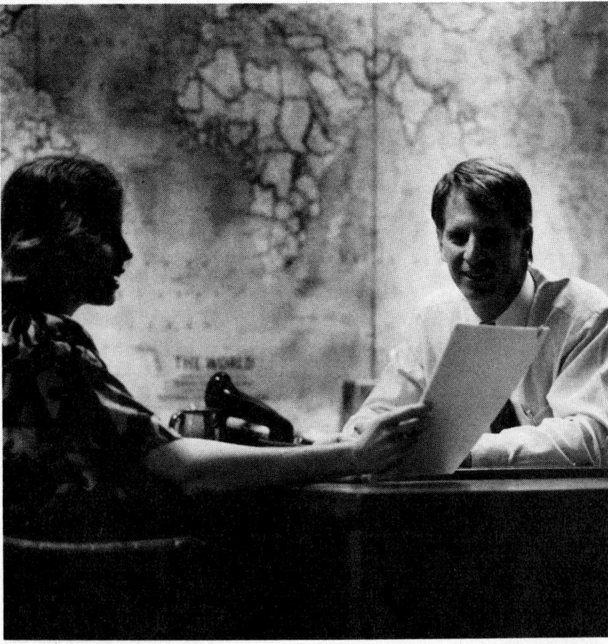

Figure 23–3. Career is an important aspect of self-expression for many people.

Measurements. Measurements of height and weight are obtained and recorded. These measurements can reveal information about the client's body image and self-esteem. Particularly important is how the client views these findings. Statements such as "I should lose some weight" and "I have always been too tall and skinny" may reflect self-concept and self-esteem issues.

Objective Manifestations. Changes from illness that affect body image, such as loss of a limb, scarring, loss of hearing or vision, and speech impairments, will affect self-expression and the modes of self-presentation a client chooses. Changes in spatial-perceptual abilities (such as lack of awareness of affected extremities) can affect how clients care for themselves, how they express themselves through activities, and how they adapt to their environment following these changes.

General Observations. The client's general appearance, sex, age, nutritional status, gait, energy level, speech, color, eye contact, gestures, and motor behavior can provide a wealth of information about self-expression.

General Appearance. Characteristics of dress and grooming should be noted as should facial expressions and gestures that may be related to self-presentation (eg, poor eye contact, stooped posture). Grooming is an important indicator of clients' ability and/or willingness to care for themselves. Manner of dress can reveal clues about reference group identification, self-concept, and level of self-esteem. Unkempt clothing may reflect a negative attitude toward self. Note any changes in dress or grooming, as well as when the changes occurred. Note how the client expresses himself or herself during the interview. Is the client restless, agitated, tense, open, or relaxed? It is also important to note personal hygiene, as this is a form of self-expression.

Posture and Mannerism. Posture and mannerisms can reflect self-presentation styles. Motor activity can also communicate data about self-expression. Note whether the client is pacing, slowed down, animated, anxious, or seems comfortable. Posture or motor behavior can be expressive of many mood states such as depression, anxiety, agitation, and fear. A client who has a self-concept or self-esteem problem may express reticent or retiring feelings in body posture, demonstrated by slumped posture, hesitation to sit down, or difficulty making eye contact with the nurse. A client who is experiencing depression with concomitant low self-esteem may be slowed in behavior or speech or present in a withdrawn fashion.

Speech. The characteristics of speech can reveal self-presentation and self-expression data. Note whether the speech is rapid or slow, hesitant, loud, or slurred. Speech that is pressured or rapid may reflect anxiety. Speech that is slowed or hesitant may reflect an inner state of mistrust, fear, or depression. Observe the self-presentation of the client and explore its meaning to the client by asking further questions.

The content and the manner of expression also can be useful in assessing self-disclosure and self-presentation. Note the quality and the quantity of speech. Is conversation coherent or disorganized? Is the client open in describing himself or herself? A withholding or guardedness of the client may reflect problems in self-disclosure. Conversely, a client who speaks freely and openly about his or her background may not have problems in self-disclosure, but may have a need for pleasing others or overcompliance.

Affect. Affect is recognized from general appearance and also from information the client directly shares. Does the client appear happy, calm, at ease with self? Does the client appear angry or depressed? Anxious, tense, or nervous? Sad? Irritable? Is the affect congruent with the content of the client's conversation? An example of inappropriate affect would be smiling when describing the death of a loved one.

Thoughts and Perceptions. Thoughts and perceptions refer to the client's ability to communicate thinking in an organized and coherent manner and to perceive reality accurately. Ask yourself if the client's thinking is presented in a clear, logical way. The content of thought can provide possible clues to the client's inner world. What is the client preoccupied with? Do the thoughts express the client's ambitions or dreams? Are the thoughts confused? Does the confusion reflect an inner emotional state, a stress response, or an organic cause (such as metabolic imbalance)? Can the content of thought be followed? Or is it confused? Is the client oriented? Does the client represent facts accurately? Sometimes this can only be determined through concurrent history from family and significant others. Is the client's self-perception congruent with reality? Does the client claim powers or skills he or she clearly does not possess?

Social Interaction Pattern. The overall way in which the client relates to the nurse may give clues to the way the client relates to other strangers. Does the client relate in a way that communicates boasting or bragging? Does the client seem uncomfortable or shy interpersonally? Does the shyness reflect an inner feeling of low self-esteem or problems in self-concept? The process or manner in which a client relates indicates how the client views himself or herself and how the client engages with the world. Is there a confidence and assertiveness about the client that communicates a positive self-concept? Does the client engage in the process of self-disclosing information? Does the client demonstrate eye contact during the interview? Does the client seem guarded in the kinds of information she or he shares or the details of that information?

Integument. Particular attention is required in examining skin for changes that may affect self-concept and body image, such as disfiguring scars, anomalies, and facial trauma/scars.

HEENT. Note any loss of function that affects self-expression, such as blindness, hearing loss, and speech difficulty. Any of these may interfere with communication of self-expression.

Breasts. Observe for changes, scarring, or other abnormalities that potentially affect body image and sexual expression.

Cardiovascular. Changes such as rapid heart rate, increased respiratory rate, and elevated blood pressure may indicate certain emotional states (fear, anxiety, shock) that reflect alterations in self-expression.

Genitourinary. Examine for structural changes that may affect sexual functioning and/or sexual satisfaction.

Musculoskeletal. Examine for areas that affect body image/self-concept such as paralysis, amputation, and limited movement or mobility. Loss of a body part such as an arm, leg, or breast, in particular, usually involves a change in body image.

Neurological. The mental status examination can confirm with greater precision changes that the client describes during history taking. For example, a client's report of memory changes can be further refined on examination to identify problems with immediate recall, recent memory, or remote memory. The following areas are examined (see Chap. 16 for techniques):

- *Immediate recall.* Ask the client to repeat seven digits forward and seven digits backward.
- *Recent memory.* Ask the client to repeat three of three objects within 5 minutes.
- *Remote memory.* Ask the client to name the past five presidents of the United States.
- *Orientation.* Ask the client for his or her full name, the place, and the current date.
- *Concentration.* Ask the client to subtract serial sevens beginning with 100. If unable to perform this test, ask the client to subtract serial threes beginning with 50.

- *Knowledge and Vocabulary.* Ask the client to name the five largest cities in the Unites States. Ask the client to compare how certain objects are similar (eg, apple and orange, table and chair, mountain and lake).
- *Judgment and Abstraction.* Ask the client to interpret a proverb, eg, "a rolling stone gathers no moss" or "people who live in glass houses shouldn't throw stones." Ask the client what he or she would do if lost in a strange city. Ask the client what he or she would do on finding a lost, stamped letter.
- *Behavior.* Is the client cooperative, restless, agitated, or demonstrating excessive motor behavior?
- *Mood.* Is the client sad, depressed, angry, hostile, agitated, euphoric, or withdrawn?
- *Thoughts.* Are the client's thoughts organized, coherent, and logical? Are there areas the client is preoccupied with or having obsessive thoughts about? Are there signs of unreality in the client such as delusions or paranoid thinking?

In addition to the mental status component of the neurological examination, the nurse assesses for problems in coordination, muscle function and movement, and balance, which may affect self-expression.

NURSING DIAGNOSIS OF SELF-EXPRESSION STATUS

The final step in assessment of self-expression is analyzing the subjective and objective findings from the history and examination to generate nursing diagnoses. To determine whether nursing intervention based on these diagnoses is indicated, the nurse must assess the degree to which the client's problems in self-expression interfere with functioning in important areas of the client's life. If the problems do not interfere, or interfere in an area of functioning not currently important to the client, intervention may not be indicated.

The following section discusses nursing diagnoses related to self-expression that have been approved by the North American Nursing Diagnosis Association (NANDA). Diagnoses are grouped according to four categories: diagnoses related to self-concept/coping, life structure, sexuality, and death and dying. Examples of subjective and objective data (defining characteristics) and established or suggested etiologies for several of the diagnoses in these categories are presented below and in tables of sample nursing diagnoses for each category. Other nursing diagnoses that may be associated with altered self-expression are listed in Box 23–3. These diagnoses may contribute to self-expression problems or result from altered self-expression.

BOX 23–3. OTHER NURSING DIAGNOSES RELATED TO SELF-EXPRESSION

Physical

- Fatigue
- Impaired Physical Mobility
- Impaired Verbal Communication
- Sensory Perceptual Alterations
- Pain
- Altered Nutrition, Less than Body Requirements
- Altered Nutrition, More than Body Requirements

Cognitive

- Altered Thought Processes
- Impaired Verbal Communication

Emotional

- Powerlessness
- Fear
- Hopelessness
- Altered Health Maintenance
- High Risk for Violence
- Spiritual Distress
- Noncompliance
- Self-Care Deficits: Bathing, Hygiene, Grooming, Dress

Self-Conceptual

- Chronic Low Self-Esteem
- Situational Low Self-Esteem
- Decisional Conflict
- Defensive Coping
- Ineffective Individual Coping

Sociocultural/Life-Structural

- Impaired Home Maintenance
- Diversional Activity Deficit
- Social Isolation
- Altered Family Processes
- Altered Parenting
- Parental Role Conflict

Developmental

- Altered Growth and Development
- Developmental Lag Related to Illness/Hospitalization

Sexual

- Rape/Trauma Syndrome

Environmental

- Impaired Adjustment
- Health-Seeking Behavior

Diagnoses Related to Self-Concept/Coping

Nursing diagnoses related to self-concept/coping include disturbances in self-esteem, body image, and personal identity; anxiety; ineffective individual coping; and impaired adjustment. Etiologies and defining criteria for these diagnoses are discussed below and included in the table Sample Nursing Diagnoses: Self-Expression Problems Related to Self-Concept/Coping on page 927.

Coping includes behavioral and cognitive patterns used by individuals in the face of difficult or problematic situations.[155] As illness can be viewed at least as difficult or

SAMPLE NURSING DIAGNOSES: SELF-EXPRESSION PROBLEMS RELATED TO SELF-CONCEPT/COPING			
	Defining Characteristics/Manifestations		
Nursing Diagnoses	Subjective Data	Objective Data	Etiology
Body Image Disturbance *7.1.1*	Reports self-deprecating thoughts Makes self-critical remarks "I'm no good any more. I can't do anything since I've been so sick." "Having other people take care of me makes me feel worthless." Rejects positive feedback	Makes poor eye contact Has low voice volume Refuses to try new things/situations	*Social/Life-Structural:* Loss of independence secondary to chronic disease
Self-Esteem Disturbance *7.1.2*	Verbal response to change in structure and/or function: "I can't believe I no longer have part of my bowel and I have to go to the bathroom through this bag." States nonacceptance of body change Verbalizes fears of rejection by others	Bowel elimination via colostomy Surgery 10 days ago Stoma healing well Does not look at stoma Does not participate in colostomy care	*Physical:* Change in body structure and function: colostomy
Impaired adjustment *5.1.1.1.1*	Family members and client verbalize unrealistic goals Refusal to discuss/acknowledge change in health status: "I'm not really that sick. I don't need to do all that."	Family visits infrequently Spouse repeatedly makes negative comments about client's prescribed diet restrictions Client has been admitted to health care facility several times with symptoms suggesting diet restrictions have not been followed	*Social:* Inadequate support systems
Ineffective individual coping *5.1.1.1*	Verbalizes inability to cope: "This is too much for me. I don't know what to do." "I'm supposed to take this medicine, but what difference will it make? I'll just skip it."	Demonstrates difficulty meeting basic needs: awakens frequently during night, eats less than 50% of food at mealtime, refuses to participate in ambulation Shows impaired judgment or problem-solving: unable to make a decision regarding which treatment option to select	*Physical:* Situational crisis: serious illness

problematic, and most likely, as a crisis, coping patterns and coping pattern deficiencies are important areas for assessment and diagnosis.

According to Wylie,[156] self-report seems to be the most appropriate way to measure self-concept. The history and client's self-report provide assessment data, which the client and nurse review together to identify deficiencies in self-concept. Self-concept is defined as the individual's unique set of perceptions, ideas, and attitudes about himself or herself. Self-concept determines aspects of self-expression in various situations.

Self-esteem is an important component of self-concept that is expressed in many ways by the client. Self-esteem may be presented both publicly and privately. For example, a client's presentation of herself may include a confident, assertive manner when interacting with others. The client may also share or self-disclose her sense of self-worth as being high, and acknowledge her competent areas. Another client may present himself in a hesitant, avoidant manner (poor eye contact, low voice volume) and express self-devaluing remarks.

Self-Esteem Disturbance. Self-Esteem Disturbance is a negative self-evaluation about self or self capabilities and may be expressed directly or indirectly. A disturbance in self-esteem can have many sources. If a client does not have a sense of belonging, a sense of competence, or a sense of worth, problems in self-esteem are likely.

Defining characteristics of Self-Esteem Disturbance include self-negating verbalizations and expressions of shame or guilt. A client with self-esteem disturbance is also likely to rationalize or reject positive feedback or reinforcement from others and exaggerate negative feedback about self. The client may demonstrate a hesitancy to try new situations or a lack of follow-through on stated plans. Clients with self-esteem disturbance are likely to project blame or responsibility for their problems onto others. Personal failures may be rationalized or clients may see themselves as unable to deal with events. Others in the client's interpersonal network may see obvious problems that the client denies. The client's self-presentation may include poor eye contact or lack of attention to grooming and dress. Self-destructive behavior, such as substance abuse, may be evident, or indirect, such as nonparticipation in therapy. Clients may present themselves in a grandiose (overinflated) way. Hypersensitivity to criticism may be present. Many of these characteristics are revealed to the nurse only through the client's self-disclosure.

No official etiologies are currently specified for Self-Esteem Disturbance; however, many situations that affect the client or the client's self-expression are possible etiologies. Illness, surgery, or accidents that change a person's life patterns may decrease feelings of self-worth. Chronic illness that interferes with a person's ability to engage in activities or relationships can lead to self-esteem disturbance. Conditions that lead to a loss of independence may also affect self-esteem. Repeated criticism or lack of positive feedback from others in the client's interpersonal network may contribute to loss of self-esteem. Situations or stressors that interfere with clients pursuing life choices or repeated failures in fulfilling those choices may create self-esteem disturbance. Loss of significant others may create a profound disturbance in self-esteem.

Body Image Disturbance. Body Image Disturbance is a disruption in the way an individual perceives his or her body. Body image disturbance may come from many sources. Defining characteristics include either a verbal or nonverbal response to actual or perceived changes in structure or function. Over the past decade, many studies have demonstrated the relationship between self-esteem and body image. In fact, Austin, Champion, and Tzeng[157] concluded from their cross-cultural study on the relationship between self-concept and body image that the strong interrelationship of these two components suggests that clients who have poor self-concepts are also at risk for poor body image and vice versa.

Etiology: Biophysical. A person's biological makeup comprises many characteristics that affect body image, including height, weight, skin color, attractiveness, body build, and physical features such as hair and eyes. Body image can be affected by acute or chronic illness, trauma, or surgery. Physical changes from aging can also affect body image. Loss of a body part or function may disrupt the body image permanently or temporarily, until the change is incorporated. Burns, amputations, breast removal, and facial trauma are all examples of significant changes in body structure and appearance that affect body image.

Etiology: Cognitive-Perceptual. How the client perceives the change in his or her body will also determine the degree of body image disturbance. A fear of rejection or of reaction by others may be present. The client's cognitive appraisal of body image may not agree with the somatic reality of body dimensions. For example, the client may state, "I think I'm too fat" (cognitive appraisal), when the actual somatic dimensions of body weight are within normal limits. Distortion can lead to problems in body image and thus problems in self-esteem.

Etiology: Psychosocial. Each individual's personal and emotional experience contributes to an internalized view of his or her body (body image) and may result in potential problems in body image. For a client whose body image centers on being athletic, immobility may create changes not only in mobility status, but also in the client's view of himself or herself based on past experiences and choices. Reactions of parents, significant others, and society to the individual also contribute to body image and can create problems. For example, if disfigurement or scarring is viewed by significant others as unattractive, this may contribute to the client's body image disturbance.

Etiology: Cultural or Spiritual. The culture in which a person lives often creates a cultural ideal for body image, which may be unobtainable by the person or in conflict with the person's own ideal. Either of these conditions can lead to a body image disturbance. Furthermore, one's culture affects feelings about body and body image and influences choices that will, in turn, influence body image.

Personal Identity Disturbance. Personal Identity Disturbance is defined as confusion over the distinctions between self and nonself. A disturbance in personal identity can be manifested by dissociation or depersonalization. Defining characteristics include vague self-image, feelings of depersonalization, the inability to separate one's own needs from those of others and failure to complete the task of the separation/individuation stage of development.[158]

No official etiologies are specified for Personal Identity Disturbance. Possible etiologies include a severe level of anxiety, threat to physical integrity, and threat to self-concept.

Anxiety. Anxiety is defined as a vague, uneasy feeling, the source of which is often nonspecific or unknown to the individual. Anxiety can serve as a signal that something is not right. However, when the intensity of the feeling is too strong, it can interfere with constructive action.

The concept of threat is important in understanding anxiety and a client's possible problems in self-expression related to anxiety. Anxiety results from an individual's internal (private) perception of threat. Each person perceives threat differently and responds with varying levels of anxiety. Exploring clients' feelings to discover the general nature of the perceived threat, its meaning, and its effect on self-expression clarifies the diagnosis and guides the selection of implementation.

Etiologies of anxiety presented here include threat to or change in health status, threat to or change in socioeconomic status, threat to self-concept, threat to or change in interaction pattern, threat to or change in role functioning, threat of death, maturational crises, and situational crises.

Defining characteristics include subjective manifestations such as apprehension, increased tension, persistent helplessness, uncertainty, fearfulness, feelings of inadequacy, shakiness, fear of unspecific consequences, and expressed concern about change in life events. Defining characteristics that are objective in nature include glancing about, poor eye contact, trembling hands, extraneous foot or hand movements, facial tension, voice quivering, a focus on self, increased wariness, and increased perspiration or sympathetic changes (pupil dilation, rapid heart rate, rapid breathing, vasoconstriction).

Etiology: Threat to or Change in Health Status. Any change or potential change in health may present a threat to a client that leads to anxiety. The actual degree of impending change may not be in proportion to the level of anxiety present. For example, a client who is admitted to the hospital for removal of a skin lesion that is not cancerous may experience a high degree of anxiety related to possible changes in health status, such as inability to walk afterward or a disfiguring scar. It is important to identify the client's concerns. Nurses should not confuse their own ideas about what they might feel under a similar threat or try to minimize the client's response.

Etiology: Threat to or Change in Socioeconomic Status. Illness can affect many areas of a client's life, particularly the ability to perform at work and earn a living. The duration of illness and the length of hospitalization and recovery can affect work and, thus, economic status and possible future life choices of the client. The cost of illness and treatment can also affect economic status. The potential loss or change in income, resources, and socioeconomic status poses a real threat that can lead to anxiety.

Etiology: Threat to Self-concept. Any threat to self-concept can lead to varying degrees of anxiety. The threat to self-concept may be related to self-esteem, role function, personal identity, or body image, or to a combination of these factors. Many life experiences have potential to threaten individuals' views of themselves as competent, whole, respected by peers, and loved by significant others. Because the self-concept is an integral part of the self, a threat to self-concept can cause significant disruption in functioning.

Etiology: Threat to or Change in Interaction Pattern. Because of the significant role of social relationships in affirming self-worth, anxiety can result from a client's perceived threat of disruption in interpersonal relationships. The interpersonal network may include family and significant others, co-workers, members of groups to which the client belongs, friends, acquaintances, and colleagues. Again the threat may be real or perceived; what is important is how the client views the threat. For example, a client may receive a great deal of support from daily interaction with co-workers. Illness may reduce or temporarily suspend that support by altering the client's mobility and limiting ability to continue with group memberships (clubs, organizations, church) that are important in the client's life structure.

Etiology: Threat to or Change in Role Functioning. Anxiety may be aroused by any change or anticipated change in role functioning. Most clients enact multiple roles through which situated identities are conferred—worker, mother, daughter, friend, professional, volunteer—and illness can affect one or more of these roles. Some roles are more critical to a person's self-expression, sense of meaning, and self-concept than others. Particular roles may be more demanding in terms of time, energy, and resources than others. A client's perception of and involvement in his or her differing roles will affect the level of anxiety experienced when these roles are threatened.

Etiology: Threat of Death. The person who is confronted with death can experience intense anxiety when the expectation of death is imminent. A person who has difficulty accepting the reality of impending death or has "death anxiety" may be experiencing denial.

Threat of loss of one's life is perhaps the ultimate threat. In health care, this threat is most often experienced in the form of a life-threatening illness, such as cancer, or through experiencing near death with the possibility of recurrence, for example, as a result of a cardiac arrest. Even for those with strong religious beliefs in a hereafter, the transition to another state of existence brings uncertainty and alarm. Those who view death as the cessation of existence may find coping with life-threatening illness even more difficult.

Etiology: Maturational Crises. Maturational crises can arouse a state of anxiety because of the unfamiliarity and unknowns of the change. Adaptation usually requires changes in thoughts, feelings, and abilities, which can also provoke a state of anxiety.

Etiology: Situational Crises. Often situational crises are sudden and unexpected and evoke uncertainty and anxiety. Anxiety will be particularly high if maturational and situational crises occur at the same time, for example, birth of a new infant with complications of an illness.

Ineffective Individual Coping. Individuals with ineffective individual coping have impaired adaptive behaviors and problem-solving abilities for meeting life's demands and roles. Any of the examples discussed above under the nursing diagnosis, Anxiety, present challenges to individuals' ability to cope, that is to adapt effectively so that the anxiety-producing event does not disrupt day-to-day functioning and the ability to meet usual role responsibilities. When the challenge is too great and coping attempts are unsuccessful, the diagnosis Ineffective Individual Coping applies.

Defining characteristics include verbalizing one's inability to cope or ask for help, inability to problem-solve, inability to meet role functions, inability to meet basic needs, altered social participation, destructive behavior toward self or others, inappropriate use of defense mechanisms, change in usual communication patterns, verbal manipulation, and high illness or accident rate. The first two examples listed are considered critical defining characteristics; that is, evidence of these behaviors is necessary to validate the presence of the diagnosis.

Etiologies for this diagnosis include maturational crises, situational crises, and personal vulnerability. Maturational and situational crises were discussed above under Anxiety; personal vulnerability will be discussed here.

Etiology: Personal Vulnerability. A condition of personal vulnerability exists when an individual lacks a repertoire of effective adaptive responses. Examples include persons with intellectual deficits who lack the capacity to learn problem-solving, individuals with psychological disorders that interfere with optimum cognitive functioning, and individuals who have not had opportunities to learn effective problem-solving because of life circumstances. Young adults experiencing the transition to adulthood, but lacking opportunities to make independent decisions as part of growing up are personally vulnerable to the challenges presented by independent living. Similarly, women who have remained dependent on a spouse to make major decisions often find they lack skills to manage independently when the relationship ends through death or divorce.

Impaired Adjustment. Impaired Adjustment is defined as the state in which an individual is unable to modify his or her life-style or behavior in a manner consistent with changes in health status. The processes normally used to maintain a satisfactory equilibrium with the environment are compromised in some way in these clients. For example, a client may be unable to use effective problem-solving techniques or self-esteem–enhancing behaviors in adapting to illness. Support systems that would normally aid a client's adjustment may be inadequate. Defining characteristics include verbalization of nonacceptance of health status change; nonexistent or unsuccessful ability to be involved in problem solving or goal setting; lack of movement toward independence; extended period of shock or disbelief; and lack of future-oriented thinking.

Etiology: Disability Requiring Change in Life-style. This may include any kind of physical illness that mandates a change in the client's present style of living. For example, a construction worker who is disabled from excessive physical labor will have to undergo a vocational change, possible job retraining, possible change in socioeconomic status, or a period of lost income. Clients with impaired adjustment are not able to meet the demand of required changes and may experience significant impact on their life structure.

Etiology: Inadequate Support Systems. Clients with inadequate support systems to assist in coping with the stress of illness often have compromised adjustment. Crisis theory stresses the importance of a support network to help restore clients' equilibrium following a stressor or crisis.[159] Clients without adequate support are likely to experience other problems in addition to compromised adjustment, such as anxiety, loneliness, and depression, which can affect self-expression.

Etiology: Impaired Cognition. Impaired cognition may result from physical or psychological causes. The client with impaired cognition is not as equipped to use the problem-solving process effectively. Problem solving is essential in adapting to changes from illness, exploring new options, and managing adjustment.

Etiology: Assault to Self-Esteem. Various factors or events can result in an assault to self-esteem that compromises client adjustment. These events may be related to body image, such as loss of a body part or function or disfigurement. They may be related to interpersonal changes, such as death, divorce, sexual changes, and loss of contact or involvement. Role changes, such as job loss or change, retirement, and birth, can also be an assault to self-esteem that leads to impaired adjustment.

Diagnoses Related to Life Structure

Life structure, as previously described, is a way of looking at the choices individuals make throughout adult life that structure life and the involvement and participation of individuals in the social environment. The diagnoses of Role Performance, which can include both occupational and social roles, and Impaired Social Interaction, which can include both close family relationships and other social relationships, are addressed here. Etiologies and defining characteristics for these diagnoses are presented in the table Sample Nursing Diagnoses: Self-Expression Problems Related to Life Structure on page 931.

Impaired Social Interaction. Impaired Social Interaction is defined as the state in which an individual participates in an insufficient or excessive quantity or ineffective quality of social exchange. When a client is unable or unwilling to maintain relationships with significant others and casual acquaintances, isolation results. This isolation can lead to further problems such as ineffective coping, changes in self-esteem, and depression. Some clients exhibit excessive dependency as a pattern of behavior. This can lead caretakers and family members to withdraw from the client, resulting in isolation.

Defining characteristics include verbalized or observed discomfort in social situations; verbalized or observed inability to receive or communicate a satisfying sense of belonging, caring, or interest; observed use of unsuccessful social interactions with peers, family, and/or others; or a reported change in any of these areas by family.

Etiology: Knowledge/Skill Deficit About Ways to Enhance Mutuality. Mutuality is required to develop and maintain satisfactory relationships. Mutuality involves a two-way process of concern, interest, caring, and involvement with another. Involvement with another in a close relationship is one of the most important forms of self-expression. Meaningful interactions require effective communication and mutuality. Therefore, if individuals lack knowledge and skills to communicate feelings or are unaware of the kinds of exchanges and behaviors that strengthen relationships, their efforts to interact with others may discourage rather than enhance relationships. Their social interactions are likely to be ineffective and unsatisfying.

SAMPLE NURSING DIAGNOSES: SELF-EXPRESSION PROBLEMS RELATED TO LIFE STRUCTURE			
	Defining Characteristics/Manifestations		
Nursing Diagnoses	**Subjective Data**	**Objective Data**	**Etiology**
Impaired Social Interaction *3.1.1*	Verbalizes discomfort in social situations: "It's different being with friends now." Verbalizes inability to participate in satisfying relationships: "I just can't get around to see my friends."	Confined to wheelchair	*Physical;* Change in physical mobility due to health
Altered Role Performance *3.2.1*	Verbalizes inability to perform role-related activities	Physical change that interferes with role: no longer able to work Verbalizes conflict in performing roles: "I can't see myself staying at home looking after the house. My work was my whole life."	*Physical:* Loss of function due to illness: cardiac illness resulting in premature retirement

Etiology: Communication Barriers. Several factors can establish barriers to effective communication that lead to impaired social interaction. Language barriers, speech barriers, culturally determined communication barriers, listening barriers, and emotional barriers can all influence the effectiveness of communication and create impairments in social interaction. (See Chap. 14 for a full discussion of effective communication.)

Etiology: Self-Concept Disturbance. Self-concept is one of the most important determinants of the involvement individuals have with one another. How one views oneself determines many aspects of self-expression, particularly how one engages with others. An individual with a poor self-concept often displays inappropriate modes of self-presentation and interpersonal communication, which are not conducive to social interaction. Others are not attracted to interact with individuals who have low self-esteem; the individuals themselves may lack the confidence to initiate interaction. Also, individuals with a self-concept disturbance often find self-disclosure threatening, so interactions that do occur remain superficial and unsatisfying. Furthermore, limited or unsatisfying interactions reinforce negative feelings about self, making resolution of both the self-concept and the relationship problems challenging.

Etiology: Absence of Available Significant Others or Peers. Absence of significant others may be a self-imposed condition resulting from the fact that the individual has chosen an isolated life-style or a temporary state resulting from a current stressor or life situation. For example, hospitalization or recovery, especially if prolonged, can interrupt a client's social network and lead to impaired social interaction. Other examples are the loss of a significant relationship and a move to an unfamiliar environment. Mood states such as severe depression or anxiety can also create withdrawal and, thus, absence of adequate contact with significant others.

Etiology: Limited Physical Mobility. Limited physical mobility, usually created by illness or trauma, can create a state of isolation and reduce the amount or frequency of social interaction. When social relationships are interrupted, the nature and quality of the relationships can also be adversely affected. The reduced frequency of contact with close friends can create a potential state of withdrawal in those friends (from perceived neglect of friendship), resulting in insufficient interpersonal contact for the client.

Etiology: Sociocultural Dissonance. Lack of familiarity or comfort in certain sociocultural settings can impair social interaction. For example, a Hispanic client who speaks little English may react to hospitalization by withdrawing from social interaction in situations that stimulate his anxiety. (See Chap. 9 for more on how sociocultural factors influence health care delivery.)

Altered Role Performance. Altered Role Performance is defined as a disruption in the way one perceives one's role performance. Defining characteristics often include a change in self-perception of the role or denial of the role. There may also be a conflict of roles or a change in others' perceptions of the role, a change in usual patterns or responsibilities or a change in the person's physical capacity to undertake the role, or a lack of knowledge about the role.

No official etiologies are specified in the taxonomy for this diagnosis; however, several conditions or situations may lead to altered role performance. Altered role performance may result when an individual and significant others have differing expectations for role performance. Role conflicts can also lead to altered role performance. This occurs when clients find that the various roles in their life structures contain incompatible elements. For example, being a busy corporate executive may be incompatible with some elements of being an available nurturing father.

Role overload or role strain is created when a person is unable to fulfill the demands of a role because of lack of time, energy, or resources.[160] Role overload can lead to altered role performance. Role ambiguity, which occurs when role expectations are unclear, can also lead to altered role performance.

Diagnoses Related to Sexuality

Sexuality is a central issue in life and individual identity. Lack of satisfactory sexual relations and lack of ability to express oneself through sexuality can contribute to problems in self-expression. Two diagnoses related to sexuality, Sexual Dysfunction and Altered Sexuality Patterns, are therefore discussed below and presented in the table Sample Nursing Diagnoses: Self-Expression Problems Related to Sexuality below.

Sexual Dysfunction. Sexual Dysfunction is defined as the state in which an individual experiences a change in sexual function that is viewed as unsatisfactory, unrewarding, or inadequate. Sexual problems may be a manifestation of a physical or emotional illness, but also commonly occur in persons who function well in other areas. (Sexual dysfunction is defined by NANDA somewhat more broadly than in the literature on sex/marital therapy, which usually refers to medical diagnoses such as premature ejaculation, orgasmic dysfunction, impotence, and vaginismus.)

Defining characteristics include verbalizations of problems, alterations in achieving perceived sex role, actual or perceived limitation imposed by disease and/or therapy, conflicts involving values, alteration in achieving sexual satisfaction, seeking of confirmation of desirability, alteration in relationship with significant other, and change of interest in self or others.

Etiology: Biopsychosocial Alteration of Sexuality Related to Ineffective or Absent Role Models. For most children learning, identification, and cognitive organization all contribute to the development of sex roles, gender identity, and a sense of masculinity or femininity. Restrictive upbringing is a common source of sexual conflict. For example, parents who are uncomfortable with their own sexuality may be unable to discuss sexuality openly with a child and may unintentionally communicate shame or embarrassment about sexuality. The lack of effective role models both in childhood and as adults can also affect sexual identity, sexual comfort, and the ability to engage in sexually appropriate behavior.

Etiology: Misinformation or Lack of Information. A person's sexual information may contain many fallacies that influence sexuality and sexual functioning. Examples of such fallacies are the belief that alcohol enhances sexual performance and that the elderly are sexually inactive. Sexual dysfunction may occur when individuals base their behavior on erroneous assumptions and beliefs. As sexuality is often a difficult or uncomfortable topic, clients may be hesitant to ask for information or clarification or to self-disclose information about their sexuality.

Etiology: Values Conflict. Because many negative societal influences and values are communicated about sex and sexuality, an individual may experience conflict in trying to reconcile sexual behavior with such values. For example, a client's belief that sexual pleasure is sinful or that sex is only for procreation may interfere with sexual satisfaction or sexual expression. Early messages in childhood about sexual expression can also lead to conflict and guilt in adult relationships.

Etiology: Lack of Privacy. For most people, privacy is an essential requirement for maintaining comfort in sexual be-

SAMPLE NURSING DIAGNOSES: SELF-EXPRESSION PROBLEMS RELATED TO SEXUALITY

	Defining Characteristics/Manifestations		
Nursing Diagnoses	**Subjective Data**	**Objective Data**	**Etiology**
Sexual Dysfunction *3.2.1.2.1*	Verbalizes problem: conflict involving values: "My priest taught us that sex was for reproduction. Now that I've had my uterus removed I don't know what to do." Alteration in achieving perceived sex role: "I don't feel as feminine as I used to since the hysterectomy." Alteration in relationship with significant other: "I seem to withdraw from my husband sexually even though I know he's interested." Seeking confirmation of desirability: "I'm constantly asking my husband how I look since the surgery."	Recent hysterectomy	*Physical:* Altered reproductive system in structure or function: hysterectomy
Altered Sexuality Patterns *3.3*	Reports difficulties: "Ever since my abortion I'm not that interested in sex." Verbalizes change in sexual behavior or attitudes	Actual limitations: "I don't know what to do since I can't afford birth control pills."	*Cognitive:* Knowledge deficit: contraception alternatives

BUILDING NURSING KNOWLEDGE

Is Sexuality Important in the Later Years of Life?

McCracken AL. Sexual practice by elders: The forgotten aspect of functional health. *J Gerontol Nurs.* 1988;14(10): 13–17.

There are many reasons for reduced sexual practice in old age: chronic illness, lack of a partner (especially for women who tend to outlive men), the societal myth that older people do not engage in sex, and, for the present older generation, a general deficit of instruction in how to give pleasure to themselves and partners through sexual expression. McCracken reviews literature confirming that although sexual interest varies from individual to individual and declines with old age, with reasonable health and a partner, sexual relations are possible into the seventh, eighth, and ninth decades of life.

McCracken stresses the importance of asking sexual questions as part of history taking with older clients. Physical aspects of the sexual response do change with age. Many elderly do not understand these changes (slower erection and ejaculation for men; fewer vaginal secretions and narrower, shorter vagina for women) and may draw incorrect conclusions about their capacity for sex. Moreover, many elderly, according to McCracken, do not understand sexual anatomy or the sexual response cycle.

Chronic illness can reduce sexual function. Many elderly are afraid to exert themselves following a heart attack; however, sexual activity is equivalent in strain to climbing a flight of stairs and may be resumed when comparable activities are resumed, according to McCracken. Diabetes is sometimes accompanied by neuropathy and cardiovascular changes that can produce impotence. The joint pain of arthritis may inhibit sexual expression. On the other hand, McCracken points out that production of adrenal cortisone tends to increase with regular sexual activity, which can help rheumatoid arthritis. The medications that are used to treat hypertension tend to reduce sexual interest. Prostate surgery sometimes causes impotence. Understanding these factors, the nurse is in a position to provide counseling and referrals to elderly who might benefit.

Many elders reside in nursing homes. Yet McCracken reviews literature indicating that staff have more difficulty with sexual expression by elderly persons than do the residents themselves. In 1974, federal regulation established that skilled nursing facilities should provide privacy for conjugal visits for married residents or for nonmarried residents who choose to associate. Unfortunately, many in long-term care facilities remain deprived of human intimacy because of lack of privacy. Change has been slow probably because of administrative concerns about liability issues and family influence. McCracken emphasizes that promoting healthy sexual function is an important part of gerontological nursing and that this situation requires remedy.

havior, especially sexual intercourse. Thus, a setting that does not allow for adequate privacy can inhibit sexual expression.

Etiology: Lack of Significant Other. Many factors can contribute to a situation in which an individual cannot fulfill one's sexual needs with a significant other. Physical and psychological separation can interfere with sexual functioning. Loss of a significant other through divorce, illness, hospitalization, or death may all affect sexual expression.

Etiology: Altered Body Structure or Function. The effects of physical illness on sexual expression can be general or specific. A person who feels ill or is in pain may not be interested in pursuing sexual activity. Many illnesses, such as diabetes, high blood pressure, and cardiovascular, pulmonary, or renal problems, have a direct effect on erectile function or libido. Damage to the genitalia or nervous system can also interfere with sexual performance and sensations. Infections of the bladder and ureters may cause discomfort and loss of interest in sex. Surgery to the reproductive system or other areas of the body can also affect sexual ability or perceptions about sexual ability. Injury to the pelvic area can temporarily or permanently alter sexual functioning. Interest and ability to engage in sexual activity may also be affected by pregnancy.

Altered Sexuality Patterns. Altered Sexuality Patterns is defined as the state in which an individual expresses concern regarding his or her sexuality. Sexuality is often a common source of anxiety and conflict. Adequate sexual behavior and expression require not only a healthy reproductive system but absence of factors that affect sexual functioning.

Defining characteristics include reported difficulties or limitations and changes in sexual behavior or attitude.

Etiology: Knowledge/Skill Deficit About Alternative Responses to Health-Related Transitions. Concerns about sexuality or problems with sexuality are often the result of inadequate information. Clients may lack information about the normal range of human sexuality and behavior, effective sexual techniques, or necessary adjustments in sexual behavior following an illness. For example, clients with a heart condition often erroneously believe that they can no longer engage in sexual activities; women who are pregnant may think that they must abstain from sexual activity throughout pregnancy.

Etiology: Altered Body Function or Structure. Successful and satisfactory sexual activity depends on the physical integrity of the sexual organs and their supporting vascular, neurological, and endocrine systems. Many illnesses and medications can interfere with sexual functioning, causing or contributing to problems in sexual expression. Disfiguring surgery can also affect an individual's sense of attractiveness or desirability.

Etiology: Conflicts With Sexual Orientation or Variant Preference. Society dictates what is considered normal sexual behavior and orientation. In the United States, for example, monogamous behavior and heterosexual orientation are considered norms. This norm of sexual orientation may, however, be inconsistent with an individual's personal orientation. This can result in conflict and feelings of guilt, shame, and ambivalence. These individuals may experience difficulty with sexual expression related to the conflicting emotional feelings about their orientation.

Etiology: Fear of Acquiring a Sexually Transmitted Disease (or Fear of Pregnancy). Problems in sexual satisfaction or sexual functioning can result from a variety of fears. Fear of rejection or abandonment by one's partner, fear of penetration, fear of punishment, fear of failure, and fear of pregnancy are only a few. Common today is a fear of acquiring a sexually transmitted disease like herpes, gonorrhea, or AIDS. All of these fears can present a threat to self in the individual and inhibit or negatively affect sexual expression. Often these fears are based on inadequate information or misconceptions about sex. The nurse's role in understanding the specific fear and the origin of that fear is important in planning appropriate intervention.

Diagnoses Related to Death and Dying

The death of a significant other is recognized as one of the most severe psychological stresses a person can experience.[137] Any individual's ability to cope with this loss is influenced by many factors, including the significance of the person lost, the conditions under which the loss occurred (sudden death or death after a prolonged illness), and the relationship to the person lost. Death can affect many areas of self-expression. The threat to self-concept and self-esteem is enormous.

The taxonomy includes two nursing diagnoses, Anticipatory Grieving and Dysfunctional Grieving, that are relevant to self-expression. Examples of subjective and objective data, defining characteristics, and established or suggested etiologies for these diagnoses are described below and presented in the table Sample Nursing Diagnoses: Self-Expression Problems Related to Death and Dying below.

Anticipatory Grieving. Anticipatory Grieving is defined as the phenomenon encompassing the processes of mourning: coping, planning, and the psychosocial reorganization that occurs when a person discovers that he or she is about to lose a loved one.[161]

Defining characteristics include the potential loss of the significant other and expression of distress at this loss. Individuals undergoing anticipatory grieving may experience many emotions, including denial, guilt, anger, and sorrow. Behavioral manifestations may include changes in eating habits, alterations in sleep patterns, alterations in activity level, and/or alterations in communication patterns. Sexual energy and libido are often affected.

There are no official etiologies for this diagnosis in the approved taxonomy, but any threat of death or separation can lead to anticipatory grieving. In fact, Rando[161] suggests that the dying person also experiences a kind of anticipatory grief. The chronic nature of many terminal illnesses can create conditions that evoke and affect the response of anticipatory grieving. Many terminal illnesses include periods of exacerbation and remission that affect both the client and significant others. Each phase of exacerbation and remission will have concomitant emotional reactions that affect the anticipatory grieving response.

Dysfunctional Grieving. Dysfunctional grieving is defined as grieving that is unusually prolonged or unresolved. There are varying degrees and manifestations of unresolved grief that can be described as dysfunctional. Grief can be unanticipated, conflicted, or chronic.[127]

SAMPLE NURSING DIAGNOSES: SELF-EXPRESSION PROBLEMS RELATED TO DEATH AND DYING

	Defining Characteristics/Manifestations		
Nursing Diagnoses	**Subjective Data**	**Objective Data**	**Etiology**
Anticipatory Grieving *9.2.1.2*	Reports change in sleep pattern and eating patterns States feels depressed mood Reports changes in activity patterns: "I don't go to church or the club anymore." Expresses guilt, anger, sorrow Reports change in libido Reports change in communication pattern	Displays sad expression Experiences mood swings: sometimes angry responses to nurses Withdraws and is not interactive	*Emotional:* Significant other diagnosed with terminal illness
Dysfunctional Grieving *9.2.1.1*	Reports verbal expression of distress: "I still miss her very much." "Every day I look for her at breakfast—wait for her to come home from school." Reports alteration in eating habits Reports alteration in sleeping habits Expresses guilt: "I should never have let her go out that night." "If only I'd made her stay home."	Cries frequently Demonstrates poor problem solving Has minimal social interaction Unable to maintain focus on conversation	*Cognitive:* Perceived significant loss: daughter killed in accident 3 years ago

Defining characteristics include verbal expressions of distress at a loss. Emotional responses, including denial, anger, sadness, guilt, crying, and anxiety, may all be present. The client may have difficulty in expressing the loss or may express unresolved issues related to the loss. Behavioral manifestations may include sleep and appetite disturbance, altered sexual patterns, and altered activity patterns. The lost person may be idealized. Daily functioning and social involvement may be affected. The client may regress psychologically to an earlier stage of development/ maturation or demonstrate alterations in concentration or cognitive functioning.

Etiology: Actual or Perceived Object Loss (Including Possessions, Job, Status, Home, Ideals, Part or Processes of the Body). This etiology, which encompasses more than just the loss of an object or significant other, reflects emphasis on the life structure, values, and areas that give a sense of meaning to the client. Thus, grieving is viewed similarly whether the loss is related to a person or a significant attachment.

Stating the Self-Expression Diagnosis

The nursing diagnosis is a specific statement about the problems identified via assessment and data analysis. An effective diagnosis statement includes three components: problem, etiology, and signs and symptoms or defining characteristics. Making the etiology and defining characteristics as specific to the individual client as possible makes the diagnostic statement more effective as a basis for planning and evaluating client care. Many of the nursing diagnoses related to self-expression have general etiologies and defining characteristics. While these are sufficient to explain the diagnosis conceptually, they do not provide enough clarity to guide care planning unless made explicit to individual clients.

For example, several diagnoses related to self-expression have etiologies of situational or maturational crises. To plan effective care, identifying the nature of the crisis underlying the diagnosis and the unique way a particular client is demonstrating the problem is needed. For example, the nursing diagnosis for a new diabetic who reacts to this situational crisis by self-destructive behavior and poor problem solving should identify the problematic behaviors so they can be addressed. Ineffective Individual Coping related to newly diagnosed diabetes, as evidenced by eating binges and skipping meals, missing medical appointments, and erratic testing of blood sugar, is a complete diagnostic statement that gives clear guidance for treatment.

Another example of a self-expression diagnosis with general etiologies is Body Image Disturbance. In this case, the basis for the diagnosis may be biophysical, cognitive-perceptual, psychosocial, or cultural. However, explicitly identifying the nature of the etiology and defining characteristics is important. An example is Disturbed Body Image related to body contour changes associated with pregnancy, as evidenced by "I hate being so lumpy," "I can't see how some women feel beautiful when they're pregnant—I feel like a blob," "I don't even want my husband to look at me," and "I can't wait until I can go on a diet to get my body back." This kind of diagnostic statement provides insight for effective nursing implementation.

Section 3. Nurse–Client Management of Self-Expression Problems

Management of problems related to self-expression includes not only addressing current problems, but also focusing on optimizing a client's potential for handling future problems and preventing further problems whenever possible. Nurse–client management includes collaborative planning of desired outcomes, nursing implementation of the plan, and evaluation of the effectiveness of the plan in meeting desired outcomes.

■ PLANNING FOR OPTIMUM SELF-EXPRESSION

Self-expression problems usually involve personal and very private aspects of the client's world. Identification of self-expression problems most often requires self-disclosure on the part of the client. The client's as well as the nurse's perception of the problem is important to planning care. A collaborative approach that solicits client input and promotes self-disclosure is particularly important in planning care for self-expression problems.

Planning requires establishing priorities with the client, determining the client's goals, identifying desired outcomes, and developing a client care plan. Prioritizing the nursing diagnoses requires the client's participation, evaluation of available resources, and a consideration of time limitations or restrictions.

The nursing diagnoses facilitate the development of both short-term and long-term outcomes. The outcomes are individualized to meet the client's current and future self-expression needs and may address preventive, supportive, restorative, or rehabilitative aspects of care. The individualized outcome statements describe a specific client behavior and establish a period within which the outcome should be attained. In this way, nurse and client can measure and document progress toward outcome attainment.

■ NURSING IMPLEMENTATION TO PROMOTE SELF-EXPRESSION

Nursing implementation is a collaborative process through which nurse and client identify nursing approaches that promote self-expression. It is important that clients participate, agree, and cooperate in this process. Because self-expression involves both the private self and the public self, the client's participation is essential to allow the nurse access to the more private self. Nurses can establish a climate that encourages client self-disclosure through the behaviors and feelings they communicate to clients. Facilitative behaviors include empathy, respect, and warmth. Therapeutic self-disclosure is sometimes helpful in communicating empathy and a genuineness to clients.[14] Sharing a similar experience or feeling with a client may promote further self-disclosure in the client.

Specific nursing approaches to assist clients with an alteration in self-expression are described below and summarized in the tables Nurse–Client Management of Self-Expression Problems on pages 937–940. These tables are organized according to the four categories used in Section 2: self-concept/coping, life structure, sexuality, and death and dying.

Preventive Care

Preventive care is directed toward clients who currently are experiencing no change in self-expression but who may be at risk for developing a problem. Individuals who are at risk for developing problems in self-expression are identified at this phase with the hope of preventing the problem by reducing or eliminating the risk factors.

Clients who are experiencing one or multiple stressors may be at risk for problems in coping, adjustment, or social interaction. Clients who are experiencing relationship changes such as separation, birth, children leaving home, and marital conflict may be at risk for problems with loss and self-concept changes. Such situational and maturational crises may place the client at risk but may not necessarily become a problem when the client receives preventive care.

Conditions That Create Risk

Situational Crises. Many events may constitute potential situational crises for clients, and suggest a need for preventive care. Changes such as starting a new job, being promoted, forming a new relationship, losing an old relationship, pregnancy and childbirth, and geographic relocation can have an impact on self-concept, coping, adaptation, and self-expression. Rahe and Holmes' classic work on the Schedule of Recent Experiences (SRE) also suggests that stressful events can have a marked effect on the illness individuals experience in the 6 months following these life events.[162] Thus, any client who has an important life change or anticipates one should be viewed as being at risk for problems in self-expression.

Clients facing a major life change often require intervention to prevent changes in self-esteem or self-concept, life structure (particularly interpersonal networks), and coping behaviors (such as leisure and emotional expression). Examples of life changes that result in situational crises are presented in Table 23–6, along with nursing approaches to address these crisis situations. According to Aguilera and Messick, crisis situations develop when one or more balancing factors are absent. These balancing factors include the client's perception of the event, available situational supports, and coping mechanisms. Crisis intervention involves working with clients to identify the balancing factors that are weak or absent and intervening to strengthen these factors.[163]

Maturational Crises. The normal process of growth and development creates changes that sometimes lead to problems in self-expression (see Chap. 11). When maturational tasks are perceived by the client as crises, intervention is necessary. Examples of maturational changes that can result in crises are presented in Table 23–7, along with nursing approaches to address these crises.

Health Education. Health education is particularly important as a means of preventing problems in self-expression. It is important for the nurse to understand the client as a total person when determining the client's need for teach-

TABLE 23–6. SITUATIONAL CRISES AFFECTING SELF-EXPRESSION

Situational Event/Stressor	Crisis	Nursing Approaches
Birth of new infant	1. Inadequate sense of self-esteem in mothering role 2. Inadequate support in family 3. Lack of knowledge in child care	1. Encourage verbalization of inadequate feelings 2. Encourage family intervention to strengthen support base 3. Provide health teaching/parent class to increase knowledge base
Loss of job	1. Self-esteem changes resulting from loss of role 2. Inadequate problem-solving skills 3. Loss of social support system	1. Promote self-esteem–building activities 2. Explore resources with client for job search and/or training, eg, vocational rehabilitation counselor, job retraining seminar
Diagnosis of physical illness	1. Body image changes 2. Temporary loss of leisure pursuits 3. Interruption of interpersonal network	1. Assist client to work through feelings associated with body image changes 2. Promote realistic adaptation and assist client in exploring substitute activities 3. Provide support to client and encourage continued contact with significant others

NURSE–CLIENT MANAGEMENT OF SELF-EXPRESSION PROBLEMS RELATED TO SELF-CONCEPT/COPING

Nursing Diagnosis	Desired Outcomes	Implementation	Evaluation
Self-esteem disturbance R/T loss of independence secondary to chronic disease *7.1.2*	1. Recognition of personal strengths	1a. Accept expressions of negative emotions regarding present condition 1b. Provide opportunities to discuss specific concerns about changes in levels of independence 1c. Encourage client to identify current aspects of independent functioning.	1. Makes realistic positive statements about abilities
	2. Participation in developing plan to maximize abilities and use supportive resources appropriately	2a. Discuss aspects of daily living in which independence is most important; problem-solve strategies to maintain self-responsibility for these areas. 2b. Engage client in discussions of realistic alternatives for coping 2c. Refer to mental health professional	2a. Engages in collaborative problem-solving with nurse. 2b. Identifies some daily activities in which independence is possible 2c. Identifies acceptable assistance when independence is not possible
Body image disturbance R/T change in body structure and function: colostomy *7.1.1*	1. Recognition and acceptance of change in body appearance and function	1a. Accept expressions of negative emotions regarding body changes 1b. Provide opportunities to discuss specific concerns about change in appearance and function 1c. Engage client in discussions of realistic alternatives for coping 1d. Encourage viewing ostomy, then progressing to participating in care as client demonstrates readiness 1e. Provide contacts with local self-help group for clients with ostomies 1f. Positively reinforce attempts at self-care, grooming, and other behaviors that suggest progress toward acceptance of body change	1a. Client statements about colostomy are descriptive and factual rather than negative 1b. Participates in care of colostomy
	2. Recognition of aspects of appearance and physical capacities are are intact and positive		2a. Maintains usual grooming and hygiene activities 2b. Positive statements about appearance, abilities to carry on usual daily activities
Impaired adjustment R/T inadequate support system *5.1.1.1.1*	1. Recognition of change in health status	1a. Discuss changes in health status 1b. Facilitate expression of feelings about changes in health status through active listening	1. Acknowledges change in health status
	2. Modification of lifestyle in response to change in health status	2a. Discuss specific problems client and spouse are having with prescribed diet 2b. Identify options for menus and recipes that meet diet prescriptions 2c. Confer with other members of the health care team about possibility for less restrictive diet 2d. Explore alternate support systems, including other clients with same diagnosis and diet 2e. Refer to appropriate community resources	2a. Verbalizes intent to adhere to modified diet 2b. Indicates talking to others with same problem is helpful and plans to continue relationship

NURSE–CLIENT MANAGEMENT OF SELF-EXPRESSION PROBLEMS RELATED TO SELF-CONCEPT/COPING (continued)

Nursing Diagnosis	Desired Outcomes	Implementation	Evaluation
Ineffective individual coping R/T situational crisis: severe illness *5.1.1.1*	1. Use of problem-solving strategies to deal with current crisis	1a. Accept expressions of negative emotions regarding illness 1b. Provide opportunities to discuss current situation; focus on identifying specific problems 1c. Discuss past problems and past coping to resolve them 1d. Engage client in discussions of realistic alternatives for coping with current illness 1e. Involve family in problem-solving discussions 1f. Provide a list of relevant community resources	1a. Identifies problems needing immediate attention 1b. Identifies past successful coping strategies 1c. Participates in planning to cope with current situation
	2. Recognition and effective use of available support		2a. Identifies resources is willing to use 2b. Initiates involvement with resources (family, community)

ing. The nurse's view of the total person is important in helping a client reach his or her maximum health potential and avoid problems in self-expression. The client's culture, religion, environment, life structure choices, developmental stage, roles, ability for self-disclosure, and self-concept are all variables that will affect the client's understanding and the nurse's subsequent teaching.

A sense of appropriate timing is essential in teaching. It is important to determine the client's level of receptivity to teaching. What does the client want to learn? What does

NURSE–CLIENT MANAGEMENT OF SELF-EXPRESSION PROBLEMS RELATED TO LIFE STRUCTURE

Nursing Diagnosis	Desired Outcomes	Implementation	Evaluation
Impaired social interaction R/T change in physical mobility related to health *3.1.1*	1. Improvement in quality and quantity of social interactions	1a. Discuss perceived barriers to social interaction 1b. Explore ways client has altered communication/interaction after change in mobility 1c. Identify communication approaches client can use to initiate contact with friends 1d. Discuss alternatives available for transportation to meet with friends 1e. Provide a list of community resources for social activities appropriate to health condition	1a. Reports improved social interactions: initiates contact with friends when interaction desired; has joined community group that sponsors social events; uses varied modes of transportation including friends, public transportation
Altered role performance R/T loss of function secondary to illness resulting in premature retirement *3.2.1*	1. Adaptation to new role/alternative role definition	1a. Accept expressions of negative emotions regarding present condition 1b. Explore possible positive outcomes of role change 1c. Engage client in discussions of realistic coping 1d. Involve family in problem-solving discussions 1e. Refer to mental health professional or community resources	1a. Actively participates in exploration of alternative role definition/role activities 1b. Positive statements about changed life-style, life activities 1c. Active involvement in new/changed role

NURSE–CLIENT MANAGEMENT OF SELF EXPRESSION PROBLEMS RELATED TO SEXUALITY

Nursing Diagnosis	Desired Outcomes	Implementation	Evaluation
Sexual dysfunction R/T altered reproductive system structure and function: hysterectomy *3.2.1.2*	1. Satisfying sexual relationship	1a. Provide opportunities to discuss specific concerns about change in appearance and function 1b. Provide opportunities for further discussion about values conflict regarding sexual expression, now that procreation is impossible 1c. Provide factual information about physical sexual functioning after hysterectomy 1d. Involve partner in discussions, if client and partner are willing 1e. Refer to mental health professional if unable to resolve conflicts	1. Reports able to discuss concerns with her partner; able to enjoy satisfying sexual relationship with partner
Altered sexuality patterns R/T knowledge deficit about contraception alternatives *3.3*	1. Concerns regarding sexuality resolved	1a. Explore concerns about loss of interest in sexual expression 1b. Determine what client knows about contraception 1c. Correct misconceptions, if any, and provide factual information about contraceptive techniques in which client is interested; include information on correct use, effectiveness, risks, and necessary associated health assessment and care	1a. Reports able to enjoy satisfying sexual relationship 1b. Selects affordable contraception; reports satisfaction with selected method

the client know about risk factors? What are the best methods to teach this client? How can the client be motivated to learn about health practices related to self-expression?

The focuses for health teaching for a client at risk for problems in self-expression are described below.

Developmental Milestones. Each stage of development with its concomitant developmental tasks provides not only an opportunity for potential change or growth but also a potential crisis. Education provided by nurses about the normal stages of development can assist clients in prepar-

TABLE 23–7. MATURATIONAL CRISES AFFECTING SELF-EXPRESSION

Stage of Maturation or Development	Crisis	Nursing Approaches
Infancy and early childhood	Inadequate preparation for parenting role	Provide health teaching on normal growth and development, infant care, and age-appropriate tasks
Young child	Inability to tolerate motor and verbal development of child, promoting excessive dependency	Provide health education on developmental tasks of preschool- and school-age children Explore resources for coping with separation behavior of child, eg, parents' support group Encourage allowing autonomy in child
Adolescence	Development of secondary sex characteristics leading to body image changes	Encourage verbalization of feelings of private self related to body changes Provide education about sexuality and normal secondary sex characteristics
Adult/middle age	Retirement with loss of role and self-esteem	Discourage withdrawal Explore alternative activities that bring life satisfaction and build self-esteem, eg, volunteer work
Late adulthood	Isolation and loneliness as a result of chronic illness	Explore resources to decrease withdrawal, eg, senior centers, church, volunteer work, support groups Encourage contact with significant others, building new social network

NURSE–CLIENT MANAGEMENT OF SELF EXPRESSION PROBLEMS RELATED TO DEATH AND DYING

Nursing Diagnosis	Desired Outcomes	Implementation	Evaluation
Anticipatory grieving R/T significant other diagnosed with terminal illness *9.2.1.2*	1. Expression of grief	1a. Provide opportunities to talk about anticipated loss 1b. Encourage grieving person to share feelings with spouse, other family members 1c. Provide anticipatory guidance about grieving: physiological, emotional responses; typical pattern of progression, regression, resolution 1d. Provide information about community resources, support groups	1. Verbal and emotional expressions of grieving
	2. Recognition of importance of experiencing the present as well as preparing for the future	2a. Encourage collaborative decision-making with spouse regarding care, treatment, amount of personal involvement desired 2b. Encourage life review with spouse 2c. Encourage taking time for sharing special experiences as spouse's health allows 2d. Provide opportunities to discuss life after loss	2a. Participates with spouse in day-to-day decisions related to current illness 2b. Describes special time shared with spouse 2c. Makes realistic statements about personal needs after spouse is gone
Dysfunctional grieving R/T loss of daughter in accident 3 years ago *9.2.1.1*	1. Resolution of grief, allowing resumption of productive personal life	1a. Accept, then confront, expressions of loss, grief, guilt 1b. Provide health teaching about healthy grieving process 1c. Encourage identification of realistic choices for personal growth and fulfillment 1d. Encourage removal and appropriate disposition of daughter's personal effects 1e. Refer to mental health professional	1a. Resumes active involvement in career/home responsibilities 1b. Resumes social interaction with peers 1c. Reports return to regular eating and sleeping habits

ing for and coping with these changes. Parents, in particular, need to appreciate the different stages of development to help their children learn and express themselves in satisfying and healthy ways.

Nurses can assist clients by providing education about age-appropriate behaviors and tasks. Chapters 10 and 11 describe these behaviors and tasks in detail. Examples include the following.

- During infancy, newborns have no separate sense of self apart from the mother, but have the capacity for expression.
- Toddlers begin to learn that their identity is separate from others and begin to learn patterns of self-expression.
- Adolescents must deal with body image changes as secondary sex characteristics develop. Teaching parents that adolescents will experience conflicts about body image as their bodies change can assist parents to provide the appropriate support during this period. During adolescence, self-esteem and self-concept continue to be molded outside the home through the influence of teachers and peers.
- Adults must deal with building of a life structure and making important choices related to education, vocation, family, meaningful activities, leisure pursuits, and fulfillment of sexual needs.
- Older adults are often faced with role changes, losses, and self-esteem and body image changes related to aging.

Healthy Self-Expression. Most people have a general awareness of what healthy self-expression means, at least in the sense that they know there are social norms and laws that prescribe appropriate social behavior. Nevertheless, many individuals lack a clear understanding of the characteristics of a healthy self and the relationship of these characteristics to self-expression. Thus, it is often beneficial for the nurse to review these characteristics with clients, particularly when the client is an individual who may be at risk for developing a problem in self-expression. Characteristics of healthy self-expression were described in Section 1 and are summarized below.

- Individuals with healthy self-expressive behaviors exhibit a clear sense of self. They acknowledge their emotions and have energy available to bring meaning to life. These individuals have a realistic view of others and an ability to relate to them in a satisfying relationship.

- Individuals with healthy self-expression can cope effectively with the realities and problems of life.
- Individuals with healthy self-expression demonstrate realistic dimensions of self-concept, among them, a positive body image, adequate self-esteem, and competent and satisfying role performance.

Sexual Patterns and Practices. Many clients can benefit from information on sexual self-expression. Despite a greater openness today regarding discussion of sex and sexuality, many individuals lack specific information that might enable them to limit the risks encountered in sexual activity. Age-appropriate education by nurses can be instrumental in preventing problems in sexual expression.

For example, nurses who work with adolescent clients who are just beginning to develop secondary sex characteristics can allay anxiety or prevent self-concept or body image disturbances in these clients by describing the normal physiological changes that occur during this period. Clients' needs for information will vary. Other content areas that might be covered include normal anatomy and physiology of sexuality, normal stages of sexual development, effects on sexuality of various illnesses, relationship of sexual practices to contraction of sexually transmitted diseases (STDs), and contraception (Fig. 23–4). Encouraging adolescent clients to ask questions and discuss concerns related to sexuality is a significant nursing intervention.

Clients whose behavior puts them at risk for contracting sexually transmitted diseases can benefit greatly from preventive care by the nurse. Clients often take risks because they lack information about safe sex practices. Nurses can provide current, accurate information about STD incidence and transmission and help clients to identify behaviors that place them at risk for contracting STDs. This is particularly important in light of the increasing incidence of acquired immunodeficiency syndrome (AIDS), syphilis, gonorrhea, and other STDs. Educating clients about the importance of limiting the number of sexual partners and using "safe sex" practices (particularly use of latex condoms and avoidance of anal intercourse) if they are sexually active can help clients to reduce their risks of contracting STDs. Common signs of sexually transmitted diseases for which clients should seek treatment are presented in Table 23–8. Guidelines for preventing AIDS transmission are presented in Box 23–4.

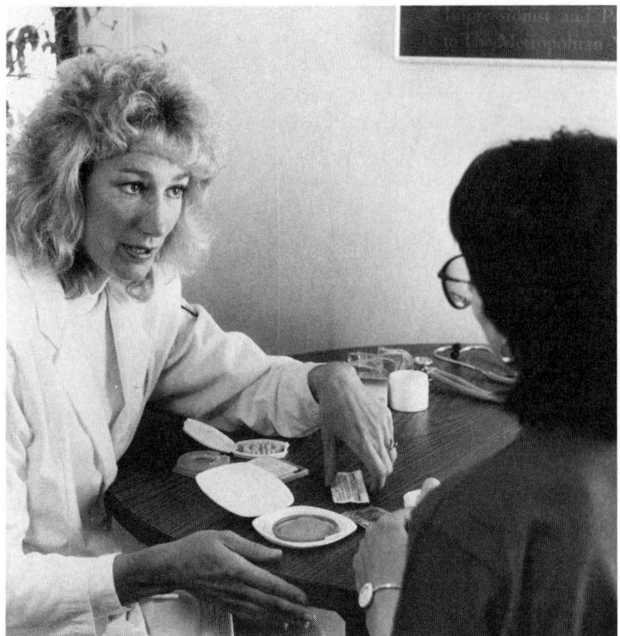

Figure 23–4. Contraceptive counseling is one way that nurses can aid clients' concerns about sexuality.

Impact of Crises/Illness. Illness is a crisis state to which individuals respond as they respond to other stressors. Educating clients about normal response patterns to stress may prevent complications and residual disability and assist clients to develop new coping patterns. Teaching a client about normal human response to stress and adaptation to crises can prevent illness and complications of illness. For instance, a client experiencing severe loss may experience anxiety and disruptions of sleep or eating patterns. The client may fail to associate these symptoms with the stress or crisis he or she is experiencing. This may further aggravate the client's anxiety. Assisting clients to recognize normal responses to grief and loss can help prevent clients from feeling overwhelmed by these physiological responses to stress.

Psychological vulnerability is greatest during the beginning of a crisis; therefore, intervention through education is particularly useful at that time. Part of coping with a crisis such as illness involves identifying and verbalizing the accompanying emotions or feelings that are experienced. Nurses can be instrumental in encouraging client self-disclosure and supporting current coping abilities. Educating clients about feelings they may experience, and communicating that such feelings are normal, can reduce clients' inner sense of turmoil and encourage further verbalization and self-disclosure.

Community Support Systems. Clients who may be at risk for alterations in self-expression may benefit from information about community support systems. Community support systems include the network of people and agencies or groups with which clients may already be familiar (such as church or support groups, or clubs). These community systems frequently have services that may be helpful to clients and assist their coping. For example, a client who is suddenly widowed may find a great deal of support and assistance in a church group or a self-help group like "Suddenly Alone" that helps clients cope with the initial stages of grief and assists them in rebuilding their lives and social networks. Similarly, a client faced with parenting a toddler may find parent teaching classes useful in coping with the stress of this stage of childhood development. A client cop-

TABLE 23–8. SIGNS AND SYMPTOMS OF SEXUALLY TRANSMITTED DISEASES

Disease	Signs and Symptoms
Acquired immunodeficiency syndrome (AIDS)	The range of symptoms associated with HIV infection may extend from minimal to the full clinical syndrome of AIDS. Clients with the clinical syndrome of HIV infection often give a history of nonspecific symptoms for months prior to diagnosis. Symptoms may include easy fatigue, poor appetite, weight loss, swollen lymph glands, diarrhea, fever, and night sweats. Other symptoms specific to opportunistic diseases occur in clients with HIV infection, such as purple to bluish skin lesions associated with Kaposi's sarcoma or shortness of breath and nonproductive cough resulting from *Pneumocystis carinii* pneumonia.
Candida albicans	Female partner: itching and redness of the vaginal and vulvar tissues; thick, curdlike discharge.
	Male partner: itching, inflammation, or cutaneous lesions on the penis.
Chlamydial urethritis	Female partner: vaginal discharge, itching; may have chlamydial endocervicitis.
	Male partner: dysuria, frequency, and mucoid to purulent urethral discharge. Some men are asymptomatic.
Gonorrhea	Female partner: mucopurulent endocervical discharge, abnormal menses, dysuria. Some women are asymptomatic.
	Male partner: dysuria, urinary frequency, and purulent urethral discharge.
Herpes genitalis	Single or multiple vesicles anywhere on the genitalia. Vesicles spontaneously rupture to form shallow ulcers, which may be very painful. They resolve spontaneously without scarring. The first occurrence (initial infection) lasts approximately 12 days; subsequent recurrences are usually milder and of shorter duration (4 to 5 days). Virus shedding occurs intermittently during latent periods between recurrences.
Syphilis	Chancre is located at the site of exposure, which heals in 4 to 6 weeks. Secondary symptoms include skin rash, mucous patches, condylomata lata, and swollen lymph glands. Clients with latent syphilis are asymptomatic, demonstrating serologic evidence of untreated syphilis without clinical signs.
Trichomonas vaginalis	Female partner: itching and redness of vulva; copious, watery, malodorous discharge.
	Male partner: itching, edema of external genitalia. Some men are asymptomatic.

Adapted from Sherwen LN, Scoloveno MA, Weingarten CW. Nursing Care of the Childbearing Family. *Norwalk, CT: Appleton & Lange; 1991.*

ing with facing a role change such as retirement may find she can preserve her self-esteem through volunteering her expertise in a business advisors' group like SCORE.

Screening. Screening for risks to self-expression may occur individually during history taking or through group-oriented screening programs targeted to identify the needs of a specific population.

Clients reveal a great deal of information about themselves during history taking and examination. In reviewing the personal, family, and social history with clients, nurses can identify areas of potential risk that require early intervention.

How clients present themselves may provide clues about potential risks to self-expression. For example, a client who presents with poor eye contact, low voice volume, or unkempt appearance may have self-esteem or body image problems. Early signs of coping problems can reveal themselves in many areas of self-expression. Clients may begin to withdraw from social interaction or forgo once meaningful activities. Clients may begin to function less effectively in their various roles and may withdraw sexually.

Group-oriented screening is carried out in programs designed for wellness and prevention. Breast cancer screening programs are an example. Frequently, as nurses interact with clients in these programs, clients will reveal information about themselves that suggests a self-expression problem. Use of standard wellness inventories for knowledge assessment in a particular area may also elicit data about risk factors for self-expression.

Risk factors can be physical, developmental, environmental, age related, familial, or life-style related. Physical risks include hospitalization, onset of severe or chronic illness, and threats to body image. Environmental risks include loss of social contact, roles changes, and changes in support systems. Life-style risks include loss of ability to engage in leisure pursuits, relationship changes, loss of meaningful activities, and socioeconomic changes that threaten self-concept. Developmental risks include the normal developmental milestones or tasks that may provoke crises, such as marriage, career choice, childbirth, and retirement.

Familial risk factors pertain to family relationships. Families at risk for crisis may include those in which parents are overcontrolling (not allowing children's moves to-

BOX 23–4. PREVENTION STRATEGIES FOR AIDS

- Avoid sexual contact with persons *known* to have AIDS.
- Avoid sexual contact with persons *suspected* to have AIDS.
- Practice "safe sex" (no exchange of body fluids including semen, urine, saliva, feces, or blood; no contact of body fluids with mucous membranes). Wear a latex condom during intercourse as a barrier to transmission of body fluids and blood.
- Avoid unnecessary transfusions of blood or blood products.
- Encourage autologous transfusions for elective surgery whenever possible.
- Administer only heat-treated coagulation factor to hemophiliacs.
- Screen all potential blood donors carefully.
- Encourage AIDS clients and persons at high risk not to donate blood, plasma, organs for transplantation or semen for artificial insemination.
- Advise parenteral drug users to use only clean, disposable needles and syringes and not to share drug equipment.
- Recommend that seropositive women delay pregnancy.
- Provide educational programs on AIDS for the public and schoolchildren.
- Use appropriate blood and body fluid precautions with known or suspected AIDS clients (see Chap. 22 for CDC guidelines for universal precautions).

Adapted from Ames SW, Kneisl CR. Essentials of Adult Health Nursing. *Menlo Park, CA: Addison-Wesley; 1988.*

ward independence); parents have difficulty with consistent limit setting; parents' own self-concepts are threatened by the normal childhood and adolescent separation behavior; and parents do not promote increased responsibility and choices in the young child or adolescent.

Age-related risk factors pertain to development. Adolescents at risk for problems in self-expression include individuals with prior problems in developmental task achievement or excessive dependency on parents; lack of opportunities for expressing independence; lack of privacy; lack of significant involvement with peer group; inability to consolidate secondary sex characteristics into a positive body image; or inability to tolerate inner emotional turmoil consistent with this stage of development.

Age-Related Approaches. Implementation to prevent possible problems in self-expression is appropriate throughout the life cycle. Preventive approaches include an emphasis on anticipatory teaching directed at promoting healthy self-expression. Examples of age-appropriate approaches are presented in Table 23–9 and described below.

Infants and Toddlers. Parent or caretaker education is particularly important during the stages of early development. It is widely accepted that the infant's relationship with parents, particularly the mother, is essential to development of self-concept and self-esteem. Consistent, sensitive, loving care by the mother or caretaker lays the foundation of trust and is essential to a healthy self-image. Nurses can teach parents about the importance of self-esteem and self-concept and the conditions that promote healthy self-concept.

A healthy relationship with the caretaker also enables the infant to begin the process of separation from the caretaker. By helping parents to understand the developmental tasks of this period, nurses may help avert a crisis at this stage. Anticipatory teaching also focuses on the physical and emotional needs of infants and toddlers.

Children. The child's sense of self continues to develop during preschool and school years. In fact, the first 5 years are believed to be the most formative period in terms of self-concept development. New mastery of physical skills and body coordination affect the young child's body image during this period.

Parents need to understand the importance of creating a stable environment, which is essential to the development of their child's self-esteem and self-concept. Adequate parental attention, affection, and promotion of autonomy in the young child, along with consistent and firm rules, reinforcement of positive behavior, and positive appraisals, all contribute to the creation of a stable environment for the young child. A parental dyad that is free from excessive tension or conflict also encourages a stable environment. The child's role in the family and relationship to siblings are being formed during this phase, which contributes to opportunities for self-expression. Providing information about family roles and normal family conflicts (ie, sibling rivalry) can help with parenting skills.

The child's exploration, testing, and attempts to master aspects of the environment must be encouraged by parents to support healthy self-concept development and the beginnings of separation. Encounters with teachers that are accepting, facilitative, and supportive of the need for mastery and growth also contribute to a healthy self-concept.

Nurses working with parents can provide teaching about the normal developmental tasks of the young child. Teaching parents about the need for environmental stimulation, mastery, and safety will encourage parents to set the conditions for healthy self-concept formation.

Nurses working with young children must promote autonomy when appropriate by offering choices and allowing as much independent behavior as is safe. Nurses can encourage self-expression in young children through the use of play activities and motor activity. Nurses can encourage parents to stay with a hospitalized child as much as possible to reduce the threat of separation.

Adolescents. The rapid changes and growth during adolescence create fluctuations in body image, self-esteem, and self-concept. As adolescents become more independent, they are confronted with life choices involving leisure activities, school curriculum, peers and friends, and sexual choices.

TABLE 23–9. PREVENTIVE NURSING IMPLEMENTATION ACROSS THE LIFE SPAN

Developmental Stage	Nursing Approach
Infant/toddler	Educate parents about needs of infant or toddler: establishing trust and a nurturing environment and promoting normal developmental tasks
Child	Provide health teaching to parents about body image, beginning separation, self-expression needs, socialization needs, and self-concept formation Educate about need for physical mastery and health and safety maintenance
Adolescent	Provide health teaching to adolescents and parents about continued growth of self-concept, identity formation, and body image integration Educate about sex role, sexuality, need for leisure pursuits, and continued development of interpersonal relationships Educate about drug and alcohol use, fertility, and contraception
Young and middle-aged adults	Provide health teaching about role acquisition and changes, normal sexual expression, and intimacy needs Educate about life structure, choices, and decisions (eg, work, marriage)
Older adult	Provide health teaching about changing life structure, body image changes, role changes, response to losses, grieving, and self-esteem changes

The need for individuality in self-expression and self-presentation is great during this stage. Nurses can be particularly helpful in assisting parents and families to understand the developmental tasks of adolescence that can lead to often disruptive behavior. As the need for personal identity becomes greater during these years, rejection of parental values and beliefs can lead to role conflicts and family adjustment problems. Anticipatory teaching can help to prevent family crises at this stage.

Nurses may be in the position to set appropriate limits for adolescents (in the hospital setting, for example) or may teach the parents the importance of appropriate and consistent limit setting. Nurses can also assist adolescents to make appropriate choices for themselves and exercise independence, which promotes a sense of personal identity.

Teaching both adolescents and their parents about the normal physiological changes occurring during this period reduces anxiety and promotes adaptation. Understanding that secondary sex characteristics are a normal part of development at this stage can reduce the threat to body image. Nurses can teach adolescents about healthy sex practices and provide information about birth control and sexually transmitted diseases, particularly AIDS. Nurses can also provide information about problems associated with drug and alcohol abuse.

Young and Middle-Aged Adults. During early adulthood, individuals continue to experience changes in self-concept, role acquisition, and life structure. Rossan suggests that many changes in identity may result from changes in social settings and reflected appraisals from others.[164]

The developmental tasks of early adulthood include choosing a career, choosing a partner, starting a family, and building additional meaningful activities; all are areas for potential risks to self-expression. Even the process of decision making in building a life structure may present a risk to some clients. For example, ambivalence about career choice or educational paths can create a threat to self-esteem for some individuals.

Counseling clients who are faced with overwhelming life decisions can help prevent problems in self-expression. The necessity to make an important life choice can provoke a state of anxiety and confusion that may constitute a risk to future self-expression and well-being. Nurses often encounter individuals who are making life choices. The anxiety surrounding decision-making sometimes provokes a state of emotional crisis that can interfere with carrying out the decision. Nurses are in a position to identify such problems, to provide clients with opportunities to disclose and examine confusing feelings, and to refer clients for further counseling, if appropriate.

Career changes as well as other role changes are often part of midlife transition for adults. Self-concept changes and reevaluation of life choices take place during this transition. Clients facing midlife changes may be at risk for self-expression problems in many areas, including losses, adjustment, and role ambiguity. Levinson suggests that an "inner reintegration" needs to occur during the midlife transition, which requires many modifications or changes to the life structure that was built during the young adult phase.[2]

Nurses can teach clients experiencing midlife changes about normal anxieties and concerns and help clients identify appropriate choices that are consistent with their value system and changing needs. Discussion with others is frequently a source of clarification, assisting individuals to examine choices and explore meanings. Often the process of describing an inner conflict to someone else enables the client to achieve a level of self-understanding for taking action. Self-disclosure often enables clients to develop increased self-awareness.

Older Adults. Late adulthood is a potential time for change and growth in many areas. Often this stage of development also includes multiple losses. Retirement, the "empty nest" syndrome as children grow up and leave home, death of family and friends, and economic changes may occur. During this stage, clients are at risk for developing problems in interpersonal changes, adjustment, loss of self-esteem, loss of roles, loss of significant meaningful activities, possible losses related to health changes, and grieving.

The existential issues of meaninglessness may be particularly salient during this stage. Erikson suggests that despair about time running out can be predominant during this stage, as multiple roles and meaningful activities are lost.[165] Loss of parenting functions, work roles, and economic provider role (with a corresponding loss of a sense of productivity) may place clients at risk for unsuccessful adaptation. Nurses can assist clients in redefining meaning and restructuring significant activities during this period.

Approaching older clients with respect communicates that clients are viewed as adults who are capable of making their own choices and providing self-care. Nurses can promote a positive self-concept and sense of individuality in hospitalized older clients by allowing as many choices as possible, respecting the need for privacy, and encouraging the adornment of space with personal, meaningful belongings. The nurse's role also includes assisting older clients to adapt to the changes occurring at this stage of life and to rebuild a satisfactory life structure.

Making Referrals to Community Agencies. Clients whom the nurse identifies as being at risk may require special, ongoing assistance. It may be necessary to refer the client to an agency of professionals who deal with the client's area of difficulty. There are a variety of community agencies that may provide support to clients experiencing an alteration in self-expression. Clients may be referred to another provider (such as physician or therapist), a hospital, a community-based agency, a voluntary agency, a self-help organization, or a governmental agency.

Community-based agencies include home health care services, crisis intervention centers, drug or alcohol centers, family planning agencies, and day-care agencies. Voluntary agencies include the American Cancer Society, American Lung Association, Arthritis Foundation, Hospice Association, and local parent teaching classes. Self-help organizations include Alcoholics Anonymous, Cocaine Anonymous, Overeaters Anonymous, Codependents Anonymous, Suddenly Alone, Parents Without Partners, and single parents groups. Governmental agencies include unemployment agencies, vocational rehabilitation services, Social Security, and the public health service.

Nurse–client collaboration to mutually identify needs and risks can facilitate the client's acceptance of the referral. Nurse and client must also identify possible impediments to following through with the referral. For example, a client with transportation problems is unlikely to attend a weekly self-help group if this need is not addressed.

Supportive Care

Supportive care focuses on clients whose situation places them at risk for developing self-expression problems. Clients entering the hospital for an illness, clients receiving a diagnosis of a serious disease, clients recently experiencing a death (or other loss), clients undergoing an exacerbation of a chronic illness, and clients facing body-altering surgery, trauma or death are all examples of clients requiring supportive care.

Supportive care is also directed toward clients who demonstrate early changes in self-expression. At this stage, problems may be alleviated or their impact reduced through early intervention. Nursing implementation for clients experiencing early changes in health status focuses on preventing further disruption or minimizing the impact of these early changes on self-expression.

Not all clients who demonstrate problems will experience a severe crisis as a result. Some clients with appropriate supportive care will recover quickly and go on to cope with their situation. For example, a client with body changes due to illness will cope adequately and may have already sought out appropriate resources (such as a support group for diabetics) and be using effective problem-solving skills to overcome the crisis. The nurse needs not only to make an adequate assessment of the client's problems, needs, and risk factors related to self-expression but to assess the client's strengths and resources in coping effectively.

Caring for Clients With a Self-Esteem Problem. Nursing care of clients with a self-esteem problem necessitates a nurse–client relationship that is collaborative, caring, warm, genuine and respectful. Clients with self-esteem problems require interventions directed toward achieving a realistic appraisal of self.

Nurses can assist these clients to acknowledge positive, not just negative, attributes. They can also be instrumental in assisting clients to own and accept tasks or accomplishments that deserve positive feedback. Nurses contribute to building positive self-esteem and self-concept by honestly pointing out clients' strengths and successes. Nurses can provide a model for clients by accepting compliments and positive appraisals of their own behaviors and actions without minimizing or devaluing them.

Body image, a central component of self-concept, can be altered by a variety of physical, psychosocial, and cultural factors. (See the discussion of Body Image Disturbance in Section 2.) Clients with physical body changes such as ostomies often need assistance to develop a realistic perception of their body image. Management includes providing understanding and support as clients explore feelings about body image. Nurses can help clients identify strengths and activities that promote a positive body image, as well as actions that assist clients to cope with altered body functions. Nurses should support client behaviors that suggest a positive adaptation to altered body image (eg, interest in self-preservation, interest in interpersonal relationships). Clients often benefit from the additional support provided by groups of other individuals with the same body changes (eg, ostomy groups, amputee groups).

Caring for Clients With a Social Interaction Problem. Several etiologies, as previously noted, can contribute to an insufficient or excessive social exchange in clients. A collaborative nurse–client relationship that uses effective interpersonal communication, conveys characteristics of the helping relationship (genuineness, empathy, and warmth), and promotes trust and self-disclosure, is an important component of care for clients with a social interaction problem. The nurse's role also includes promoting appropriate social contact with others.

In a study of the institutionalized elderly, Nelson identifies categories of social support networks, among them, spouses, relatives, friends, neighbors, health care providers, counselors, and ministers.[99] These categories apply to the interpersonal sphere of most clients and provide a basis for assisting clients to establish or reestablish adequate social interaction and social support. Through the personal, family, and social history, the nurse gathers information about the client's family, family relationships, and social network. Based on this information, nurse and client together plan ways to increase or modify the client's social interaction. Guidelines for promoting increased social interaction include the following.

- Plan with the client times at which visiting can occur.
- Encourage contact via phone or letter with important persons.
- Help the client identify barriers to initiating contact with others.
- Assist the client to initiate new contacts for support when appropriate (eg, contacting clergy).
- Encourage self-disclosure in areas that might interfere with making contact with support systems (eg, embarrassment, humiliation, fears of rejection, feelings of being a burden).
- Educate the client about the need for support systems to assist in coping with crisis and promoting self-esteem.
- Encourage contact with other clients, when appropriate, to reduce isolation or loneliness.

Caring for Clients With Concerns About Sexuality. Care of clients who express concerns about sexuality includes understanding specific reasons or etiologies for these concerns as well as manifestations of changes or impairments in sexual patterns.

Nursing management of self-expression problems related to sexuality begins with nurses examining their own attitudes and beliefs about sexuality. Unsain et al suggest the following guidelines for nurses who care for clients with concerns about sexuality.

- Work toward developing comfort in discussing sexuality with clients.
- Develop a nonjudgmental, caring, and supportive attitude.
- Avoid imposing your own values and beliefs concerning sexuality on clients.
- Develop sufficient knowledge to understand the effects of disease on sexuality and sexual functioning.
- Become familiar with the language used by clients to express sexuality and sexual functioning.
- Develop experience in interviewing clients regarding sexual matters.
- Provide a private, quiet, and relaxed atmosphere for discussion.
- Include the client's significant other, whenever possible.
- Prevent premature disclosure, and overwhelming or rushing the client (p.391).[119]

The PLISSIT Model. The PLISSIT model, described by Annon in 1976, provides a useful framework for care of clients with concerns about sexuality.[166] The model describes four levels of intervention: permission, limited information, specific suggestions, and intensive therapy. Generally, nursing care involves only the first three levels of intervention. Nurses must recognize the scope of their knowledge, comfort, and expertise in handling problems in sexuality, and know when to refer the client to the appropriate professional.

Permission. Often giving clients permission for current behavior or beliefs is sufficient to resolve concerns and prevent the development of problems (see the discussion of Health Education, under *Preventive Care*). Clients may feel that certain feelings, thoughts, or behaviors about sexuality are abnormal; hearing that these are both acceptable and normal can provide great relief.

Limited Information. Information about normal anatomy, physiology, and the effects of certain medications or diseases on sexual functioning can assist clients to change behaviors and attitudes about sexuality or accept certain limitations. For instance, diabetes may affect a male client's ability to have an erection, but not his ability to achieve orgasm.

Specific Suggestions. Nurses may be able to suggest specific courses of action to improve clients' sexual functioning or sexual satisfaction, or to enable clients to reach identified goals. Referral to a support group may be appropriate; for example, for clients with spinal cord injury that affects sexuality. Referral to a sex therapist may also be indicated.

Intensive Therapy. Referral to an appropriate professional is indicated when the preceding interventions are not helpful or have not met clients' goals. Marital therapy might be appropriate, sex therapy, or urological/gynecological intervention.

Management of clients with concerns about sexuality thus includes promoting self-disclosure and providing education, permission, suggestions, and possible referral. Because self-esteem and body image are integral aspects of sexuality, clients with illnesses that affect these areas often require interventions to support healthy sexual functioning.

Caring for Clients Who Are Having Difficulty Coping. Coping with stressors, illness, or life changes necessitates resourcefulness and the ability to problem-solve. Assessment of clients' responses to stressors or crisis helps determine whether clients' coping behaviors are effective, and guides nurse and client in strengthening existing coping behaviors or identifying a need for more effective patterns of coping. Clients must be active participants in defining coping mechanisms. Nurses can be instrumental, however, in developing with clients guidelines for actions, alternatives, and a mechanism for evaluating whether new or added coping behaviors are effective. For example, a client who is coping with prolonged work stress by excessive drinking may be encouraged to attend an Alcoholics Anonymous meeting. Nurse and client can then review the client's response to the meeting, what was learned, what support was gained, and what alternatives others use for coping with similar stresses. Nurses can also assist clients to use previously learned coping behaviors that are not being used.

Clients experiencing extreme anxiety are usually unable to problem-solve effectively. Often nurses must intervene to help manage the anxiety before these clients can proceed to effective coping and problem-solving. Clients can be taught how to recognize anxiety and ways to reduce the anxiety to a manageable level through exercise, relaxation or meditation techniques, verbalization, or cognitive intervention.

Caring for Clients With a Role Performance Problem. Clients experiencing a change in health status usually have some degree of interruption in performance of their roles. The personal, family, and social history provides the nurse with information about the roles the client is engaged in, the responsibilities involved in those roles, the importance of the roles to the client, and the contribution the roles play to the client's self-concept and life satisfaction.

Illness, either chronic or acute, necessitates adjustments on the part of individuals as they redefine roles and attempt to accommodate to necessary changes. Changes in role structure created by illness magnify the potential for individual and/or family stress. Nurses can be instrumental in teaching clients how to adapt to and cope with role changes that occur as a result of illness. Situational crises, such as divorce or unemployment, and maturational crises, such as childbirth or retirement, also require adjustment to new roles.

Role performance problems include role stress, role conflict, role overload, and role ambiguity. Assisting clients with role performance problems often includes intervention with family members or significant others. Nurses can teach clients the concepts of role sharing and role negotiation to reduce the stress.[167] Once the specific disabilities or limitations related to role expectations are identified, nurses can help clients define realistic role expectations that are congruent with the changes caused by illness, situational crises, or maturational crises. Encouraging input from family members can increase the cooperation and collaboration necessary in redefining role structures. At times, referral to a family therapist or other professional is necessary to assist families in adjusting to a family member's altered role performance.

Caring for Clients Who Are Faced With a Difficult Life Choice. Levinson describes the importance of life choices in building an individual's life structure.[2] Aspects of the self are lived out through an individual's life choices and define how the individual engages with the world. Areas in adult life that involve major choices include occupation/vocation, marriage/family, and friendship/peer relationships.

The process of making major life choices involves change, which is often stressful. Clients experiencing life transitions may be in a state of crisis as they deal with the implications of their choices. Inner emotions may include ambivalence, uncertainty, fear, sadness, depression, or anger.

Making the choices that build one's life structure also involves loss (eg, choosing to leave a job to return to school; choosing to leave a marriage; choosing to move to a more economically thriving community), and may precipitate mild or severe responses as a result. Even a planned change that is desired and is expected to improve aspects of one's life may evoke an emotional crisis in dealing with the loss.

Making a choice to pursue a certain pathway to fulfillment of goals involves giving up something. The ambivalence involved in the choice can be distressing. For example, a woman who is considering leaving an unhappy marriage may live through a period of ambivalence lasting months or even years. This state of ambivalence can create problems itself in coping (eg, sleep disruption, poor concentration, social withdrawal).

Nurses can assist clients facing a difficult life choice by promoting client self-disclosure. Assisting clients to verbalize the emotions involved in making a decision can be therapeutic and often helps clients clarify their feelings. Clients gain a perspective on what is important to them in the choice. Verbalization also assists clients to identify values and beliefs that influence their decisions. Values can be clarified through the process of self-disclosure.

The nurse's role is not to suggest a course of action for the client but to prepare the client to make his or her own choice. Nurses can assist clients with the problem-solving process by raising questions and exploring with clients areas that they may have overlooked. For example, a client considering moving to a new location to obtain a job may not have considered all of the ramifications of the choice. The nurse can ask questions that will aid the client to examine these factors, such as, "How long do you think your finances will last while you're looking for work?" or "What might happen if you don't find work and have to move back?" Self-disclosure assists clients to express, cope with, and examine emotional states associated with life change, choices, and building a new life structure. Assisting clients in the process of problem-solving and decision making—without making the decisions for the client—can be enormously helpful in assisting clients who are making a difficult life choice.

Caring for Newly Hospitalized Clients. Hospitalization has the potential to disrupt many dimensions of the client's life—physical, social, intellectual, sexual, and psychological. Nurses can help to reduce the negative effects of hospitalization by individualizing client care as much as possible. Providing time and opportunity for client self-disclosure about the threats to self-expression caused by hospitalization can also help clients adjust to the crisis. For some clients, the loss of control of their daily routine is the most disruptive aspect of hospitalization. Other clients may perceive the loss of privacy, the loss of contact with significant others, or the loss of valued roles as more disruptive.

Nurses must understand the impact of hospitalization for the individual client to plan approaches that minimize the negative effects of this experience. Clients' anxiety often can be reduced by explaining hospital routines, procedures, and tests, and whenever possible by allowing clients a choice in the management of their care. Box 23–5 presents guidelines for supporting clients' self-expression during hospitalization.

Caring for Clients Who Receive a Diagnosis of Serious Illness. Clients who have recently been diagnosed with a serious illness often experience many threats to self-expression; among these are shock and anxiety.

Shock is the numbing emotional response that often accompanies traumatic news such as the loss of a loved one or a diagnosis of serious or life-threatening illness. This response may be momentary or last for several days. Clients experiencing shock may appear to be carrying out normal activities but if asked to describe their state use phrases such as "I was in a fog," "I couldn't think clearly," "All my emotions were numb." The following guidelines can assist nurses who care for clients experiencing shock in response to traumatic news.

- Do not rush the client through this stage; allow the client time to integrate the information.
- Offer the client support and comfort, both physical and emotional.
- Stay with the client; this communicates nonverbal support.
- Provide the client an opportunity to describe what he or she is experiencing.
- Assist the client to define areas in which he or she needs assistance (eg, contacting a family member).

Clients who receive a diagnosis of serious illness usually experience a period of anxiety that can progress in intensity. They may deny the threatening information and fail to recognize its implications. They may experience fear of dying or worry that they will endure suffering and pain. Clients may also react negatively to being in a dependent role.

Because client responses to the news of illness are varied, nurses must explore each client's responses and the meaning of the diagnosis to that client. This is achieved by promoting self-disclosure. Nurses can help to establish conditions that facilitate self-disclosure by the following approaches.

- Provide a private, comfortable, unhurried environment.
- Convey a warm, concerned, interested, and permissive attitude.
- Demonstrate empathy by accurately reflecting back to clients what nurse and client have discussed and the associated feelings.

BOX 23–5. GUIDELINES FOR SUPPORTING SELF-EXPRESSION DURING HOSPITALIZATION

- Address the client by name. Ask the client how he or she prefers to be addressed.
- Express interest in the information the client reveals during history taking. Take the opportunity to share a few items about yourself that communicate who you are as a person and that might be likely to create a social bridge to the client.
- Invite the client to continue wearing his or her own clothing if the client is not acutely ill and no immediate diagnostic or therapeutic procedures are to be performed.
- Invite the client to display personal artifacts (photos, greeting cards, small figurines, and so on) at the bedside.
- Ensure that the client and the client's significant others understand visiting policies and know about facilities for visitors such as parking, cafeterias, and rooming-in arrangements. Provide space for client and family interaction (Fig. 23–5).
- Discuss daily schedules with the client so that he or she will have a mental framework of the day's activities and can make appropriate arrangements for support from significant others as well as prepare himself or herself mentally.
- Make an effort to identify the client's identity reference groups and express interest in the role identities from which the client gains self-esteem.
- Protect the client's physical privacy by closing the door and by providing and using screens or drapes during all diagnostic, therapeutic, or caregiving procedures.
- Protect the client's psychological privacy by allowing the client to reveal aspects of self and personal situation at his or her own pace.
- Communicate warmth and empathy while providing the client with opportunities for self-disclosure.
- Offer to assist (eg, to comb the client's hair, shave the client, put on makeup) if the client has difficulty with self-care activities.
- Inform the client about in-hospital church services or clergy available for spiritual counseling.
- Use humor when possible to relieve the tension associated with the embarrassments of hospitalization.

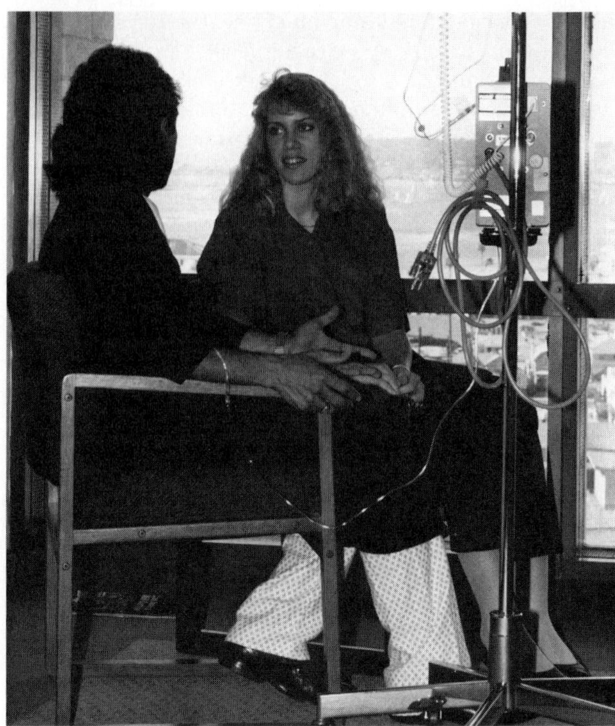

Figure 23–5. Providing space for client and family interaction during hospitalization is important to support self-expression.

- Listen to the client's concerns, beliefs, and attitudes regarding his illness. Use open-ended verbal techniques and encourage clients to expand.
- Recognize symptoms of anxiety that interfere with self-disclosure.
- Communicate in an unobtrusive way to the client, and without interrupting the flow of the client's own disclosure, personal experiences with the client's problem. It is not necessary to volunteer what the specific experience was. Clients who desire to know will respond with their own inquiries about your experience.

Clients coping with the uncertainty of an illness use various coping mechanisms, among them, information seeking and emotion control.[138] In fact, Mischel suggests that managing the uncertainty associated with an illness and its treatment may be an essential task of adapting to illness.[138] Nurses should be available to assist clients to cope with uncertainty by providing information about the illness and its course and treatment.

Other nursing approaches for clients experiencing a newly diagnosed illness include the following.

- Encourage verbalization of feelings and responses to the information.
- Give clients permission to experience the normal emotions, such as shock, fear, denial, and sadness, associated with a diagnosis of illness. (These emotions are discussed in more detail under *Restorative Care,* below.)
- Encourage self-disclosure about the client's expectations for the outcome of the illness.
- Provide clarification, education, and health teaching as necessary about the specifics of the client's illness (usual symptoms, most frequently used treatment, frequency of hospitalizations or clinic visits).
- Talk to the client about the resources and support networks available.
- Explore the client's need for additional support (eg, from clergy, nurses, support groups, therapist).
- Assist the client in developing coping patterns to deal with possible role changes or other life-structural changes (eg, a mother of a toddler diagnosed with musculoskeletal disease that severely limits mobility may need help planning for additional child care).
- Talk to the client about future needs. This will also aid the problem-solving process in coping with a future crisis. (For example, if this mother needs to be rehospitalized in the future, how can she plan for her absence with the family?)

Caring for Clients Who Anticipate Body-Altering Surgery. A change in body image as a result of surgery is a potentially profound threat to clients' self-concept.

The nurse needs to understand the client's body image and self-concept to anticipate the impact of surgery on the client. Nurses may ask clients what they currently think of their body, what they like best about their body, and what aspect of their body makes them feel the best about themselves. They can also ask clients to describe what they think will be different after surgery, what abilities related to their body they expect to change, what limitations they imagine living with after surgery, and what kind of scarring or disfigurement they expect.

Assisting the client to verbalize emotional responses to the anticipated changes communicates support and understanding. Folz describes several useful strategies in working with clients at risk for body image changes. One important strategy is client-to-client visitation programs (eg, a visit from a woman who has had a breast removed can be enormously helpful to a client anticipating this surgery). Another strategy is to employ progressive relaxation (use of breathing and visualization exercises) and desensitizing techniques (gradually becoming used to the aversive stimuli, such as gradually allowing the client to look at and care for his or her ostomy wound).[116]

Sexual functioning may also be affected by body image changes that lower self-esteem. Particular sensitivity is required to assist clients' disclosures regarding sexuality and sexual functioning. Clients may also require referral to other health care professionals or sex therapists.

Caring for Clients Who Receive a Terminal Diagnosis. Perhaps no threat to self-expression is greater than that presented to clients who receive a diagnosis of a terminal illness. Leming and Dickinson emphasize that several factors must be taken into account when working with terminally ill clients[168]: the client's perspective of time and of

BUILDING NURSING KNOWLEDGE

What Can the Nurse Do to Rebuild Clients' Self-Esteem?

McGlashan R. Strategies for rebuilding self-esteem for the cardiac patient. *Dimensions Crit Care Nurs.* 1988;7(1): 28–38.

McGlashan explores the nurse's role in dealing with the lowered self-esteem that sometimes results from the challenge of serious illness. The author defines self-esteem as the judgments—positive, negative, or neutral—that one places on one's self-concept. McGlashan contends that individuals with high self-esteem perceive themselves as worthwhile and equal to others. They are more self-confident, less anxious, and more effective in meeting demands. They recognize their limitations and expect to improve. Those with low self-esteem feel worthless, experience self-dissatisfaction, lack self-respect, and feel incapable of controlling their lives.

The diagnosis of a serious disease (such as cardiac disease) challenges a client to modify life-style, alter roles, and restructure the environment. Depending on the meaning this has for the client, the client may change his or her perception of self, sometimes in a negative way.

McGlashan points out that each client has his or her own way of dealing with lowered self-esteem. Some clients reveal their feelings, whereas others conceal them. The author stresses that special skills are needed to differentiate the client who outwardly expresses self-doubt from the client who is outwardly assured but inwardly feels incompetent. A history of past accomplishments and feelings of esteem are important in determining whether the pattern is a longstanding one or a temporary reaction.

Signs of lowered self-esteem, according to McGlashan, include verbalization of self-reproach, disinterest in appearance, lack of eye contact, and changes in gait and facial expression. Withdrawal from family and friends, low energy level, persistent comments of "I'm tired!" in later stages of rehabilitation, excessive anxiety, and reluctance to accept more self-responsibility as the condition improves are also signs of lowered self-esteem.

McGlashan identifies eight strategies that nurses can use to help rebuild self-esteem. Establishing the client's trust is paramount; this is done by creating a climate that says, "You can count on me to help you." Inspiring hope is also vital. Hope, according to McGlashan, is a powerful way to combat despair. The key to hope is to establish goals. Another strategy is to promote self-care; there is a strong relationship between self-esteem and self-control in McGlashan's view. Displaying nonverbal reassurance is another approach; positive nonverbal messages conveyed by the nurse's warmth and interest build self-esteem.

Enhancing the client's knowledge and skills is another way. Teaching and, particularly, supporting the client in what he or she already knows promote positive health behavior. The long-term nature of heart disease makes teaching more significant. Positive feedback is important. Clients want to know, "How am I doing?" Promoting support systems and, particularly, relationships that give the client a sense of belonging build self-esteem. Finally, humor is a powerful factor in coping, and laughter is an important means for retaining humanness in a difficult situation.

time running out is an individual one; the confinement of the client to a specific space (eg, intensive care unit, oncology ward) contributes to loss of personal power; the role disengagement that often follows a terminal diagnosis can have many consequences; the value meanings (including spiritual) that dying holds for a client can be positive or negative; the client's view of himself and his relationship to the world undergoes enormous changes; the client's definition of the social situation (eg, the hospital as a safe place or a foreign environment) also has an impact on the dying process.

Dying clients not only are anxious themselves but may elicit a response of anxiety in others, including health care providers and family. The nurse's role involves helping clients to identify, express, and cope with the normal feelings of anxiety associated with a terminal illness. The nurse also has a role in assisting family members to do the same. Encouraging family members to visit, allowing extended visiting hours to accommodate the family, and ordering meals for the family so they can dine with the client all communicate to family members that the nurse also has time for them and that their concerns are important. Because dying may arouse anxieties in nurses, they must also find outlets for expression of their own anxiety and helplessness in working with dying clients.

Dying clients often seek opportunities to review their lives, recall and share important memories, and review decisions and choices they have made during their lives. The therapeutic value of this "life review" cannot be underestimated. This reevaluation enables clients to begin their own grieving process and to put their affairs in order. Nurses can provide support to clients by listening as they plan for the future and review decisions and choices that must be made.

Clients facing death often experience a sense of isolation, shock, loneliness, loss of control, and abandonment. Nurses can play a role in assisting clients to cope with these painful feelings. (See the discussion of *Restorative Care,* following.) The client's family and significant others experience similar emotional distress, frustration, anger, and shock at the news of terminal illness. Anger or blaming may be directed at the nurses or physicians caring for the dying client. The nurse's role encompasses supporting the family and encouraging anticipatory grieving and, when indicated, bereavement counseling.

Caring for Clients Who Are Grieving a Loss. Clients who are grieving a loss, whether that loss is of a body part, an aspect of personal identity, a treasured object, or a loved one, will generally experience a variety of intense emotions during the course of their adaptation. The major feelings they must cope with are guilt, sorrow, depression, anger, hostility, and anxiety.[169]

Guilt. During a period of adaptation to loss many people experience some amount of guilt. Usually this sense of guilt is associated with other strong feelings related to the loss. For example, guilt may accompany the awareness of feelings of anger that are felt toward the deceased for having died, or be experienced in relation to a sense of responsibility for the loss, whatever its nature.

Nurses need to recognize that guilt is an emotion commonly experienced in relation to loss and look for signs that clients are experiencing guilt. Often these are revealed in self-disparaging statements such as "I should have gone to the doctor sooner," or "If only I had been there when he got sick."

The significance of guilt feelings often eludes those who are grieving. Clients may not understand, for example, that dwelling on the negative is a way of severing the ties with the object of the loss, and thus is an important part of adaptation. Nurses can be helpful by pointing this out.

Moreover, people who experience guilt may be unaware of its relationship to other emotions. Thus, when a client begins to express strong emotions such as anger in relation to the loss, it can be helpful to encourage such expressions, and then to reassure the client that feelings of ambivalence are normal in life crises and illness and represent normal human reactions to a stressful situation. Educating the client about the relationship between feelings of guilt and feelings of anger is often helpful.[169]

Clients who feel guilty also often have unrealistic self-expectations. Grieving clients may expect that they should maintain their usual productivity or work level and may feel guilty when they cannot. It may also be helpful, therefore, to help clients identify the self-expectations they hold that are unrealistic or irrational, and to search for goals that are appropriate under the circumstances.

Many times people around those who are grieving a loss do not understand what the grieving person experiences. Nurses can be helpful by assisting the family member or significant other to understand the nature of grief and the grieving process. Helping significant others to understand increases the likelihood that they will be able to support the client.[169] Significant others may also need to be educated about the meaning of ambivalence.

Sorrow. Feelings of sorrow, sadness, pain, and anguish are commonly associated with the experience of loss. Many individuals who experience sorrow fear that they will be overwhelmed by their mental suffering and thus distance themselves from others; others may overcompensate for this fear by becoming aggressive or demanding, behaviors that hide their true vulnerability.[169] Nurses are helpful when they identify and legitimize these feelings of sorrow for clients. Clients may be helped by understanding that emotional release and catharsis are an important part of adaptation, and that it is important to express feelings as a part of working them through. It also may be helpful to point out to clients that the hurt they experience is related to their loss and the love they have for the object of their loss. Clients may also be helped by knowing that, with time, feelings of hurt and sorrow diminish.[169]

Nurses should be mindful of the limits that clients have for the experience and expression of strong emotion. Self-control is an important value for most adults, and clients frequently need help to express emotions at a pace and with the degree of intensity that is consistent with their self-esteem. Sometimes, for example, a client may require assistance toward gentle closure of an emotion-laden conversation so as not to become overwhelmed. Noting that a client is on the verge of losing control in a situation where that might prove embarrassing to the client, the nurse can modify the situation to maximize the client's ability to cope with feelings of emotion until a time when those feelings can be more appropriately released.[169]

Depression. Depression, a subjective state that arises when the functioning interaction ceases between oneself and one's world, is a common element of loss of relationships. It is an anticipated aspect of the grieving process and is usually associated with some degree of behavioral disorganization.[161] Depression is a complex cognitive, emotional, and physical condition that produces many symptoms. These are summarized on Box 23–6. Depression may develop at any time during the process of grieving a loss; it may be short-lived or prolonged; it may remit, only to reoccur. Although painful, depression is adaptive if it facilitates the breaking down of old patterns of behavior to make way for new patterns that are necessary for the future.

Throughout the course of the client's grieving, the nurse should be aware of the likelihood of depression and monitor the client for its signs and symptoms. Helpful implementation focuses on encouraging the expression of feelings associated with the loss that is being grieved, while continuing to facilitate the client's involvement in living.[169] The client should be encouraged to talk about not only the tangible aspects of his or her loss, but also the symbolic and psychosocial aspects such as associated losses of status, roles, relationships, meaning, beliefs, dreams, hopes, and expectations.[169] Assisting the client to identify and label the specific emotions he or she experiences can be helpful; this prevents the accumulation of emotions in an undifferentiated mass of painful stimuli.[169] When emotions accumulate, it is likely that the client will fail to clearly understand the experience, will be unable to problem-solve and to deal with specific components, and will tend to feel overwhelmed by the sheer mass of feelings.[169]

Anger. Anger is a natural response whenever a person feels deprived of someone or something valued. Indeed, anger signifies an innate predisposition to attempt to find and recover what has been lost. Thus, failure to recoup what has been lost frequently results in feelings of anger. Anger also derives, however, from an unsuccessful attempt to find meaning in a loss. The quest for meaning frequently leads the grieving person to ask "Why me?" Failure to find an acceptable answer often leads to a profound sense of injustice and disillusionment.[169] The grieving person may begin to question values and beliefs that were formerly comforting.

Anger, hostility, and frustration—related emotions—can be expressed in a variety of ways. Some of the more common manifestations include: negative verbalizations, aggressive behavior, sarcasm, negativity, irritability, ten-

BOX 23–6. SUBJECTIVE AND OBJECTIVE MANIFESTATIONS OF DEPRESSION

Physical

- Weight loss or gain
- Sleep difficulties
- Decreased energy, fatigue
- Loss of interest in sex
- Anorexia

Social

- Social withdrawal
- Regression
- Dependency on others

Behavioral

- Apathy
- Lack of initiative, motivation
- Restlessness
- Agitation
- Irritability

Cognitive

- Confusion
- Depersonalization
- Disorganization
- Poor concentration
- Feels overwhelmed
- Difficulty with decision-making

Emotional

- Feels out-of-control
- Feels sense of meaninglessness
- Self-reproach
- Loneliness
- Sadness
- Tension/anxiety
- Anguish
- Despair
- Yearns for what was lost
- Shame
- Guilt
- Ambivalence
- Feels hopeless
- Feels abandoned
- Tearful/crying

sion, anxiety, withdrawal, jealousy, and stinginess. Anger may be directed at the object of the loss, at the self, or at other people.

Anger is an emotion that is poorly dealt with in our society; in general, people do not welcome the expression of anger by others. Anger that is directed at others may provide emotional release, but also may have the consequence of damaging the grieving person's interpersonal relationships. Grieving people, understanding this, often fear alienating others by expressing the bitterness and disappointment they feel. Thus it is not uncommon for grieving people to find themselves isolated with their feelings of anger. Instead of expressing their anger to others, they direct it inward, internalizing it. Internalized anger frequently results in depression and guilt.

Dealing with anger is thus a very important part of the care of the grieving. Indeed, one of the most important contributions nurses can make is to assist grieving persons with their feelings of anger. Giving clients permission, implicitly or explicitly, to ventilate their anger in the context of interaction provides an important psychosocial outlet. Expressing anger to the caregiver carries no risk to the client's relationships with significant others.

Encouraging physical outlets for anger, in addition to psychosocial expression, can also be helpful. Exercise and sports help to siphon off emotional energy that otherwise might prompt inappropriate aggressive expressions.[169] Activities such as hitting a punching bag or pounding a pillow can help to discharge feelings of anger and provide emotional release. Nurses should remember, however, that individuals will vary in their manifestations of anger and avoid communicating preset expectations for types of feeling manifestations.[169]

It is also important to help significant others to understand the client's anger. Just as they may fail to understand a grieving client's guilt, significant others may also fail to understand feelings of anger. Thus, the nurse can be helpful by assisting significant others to understand the role of anger in the adaptation process.

Anxiety. Anxiety represents a threat to a value that an individual holds as central to his or her existence. In situations of loss, anxiety is a predictable experience, as the loss itself represents a value threat.

As previously discussed, anxiety is also a normal accompaniment of the uncertainty of serious or terminal illness, which are common causes of anticipatory grief. Thus, when clients are grieving a loss of self through illness, anxiety is likely to be a feature of their experience.

Another source of anxiety is unexpressed emotions and thoughts that well up during grieving. A sense of vulnerability associated with the loss, a frightening sense of helplessness, distressing memories, heightened emotional and physical arousal, are all sources of anxiety. One of the greatest stimulators of anxiety, however, is the intrapsychic and intrafamilial disorganization with which many grieving clients must cope.[169] The need to change thought and behavior patterns, roles, and responsibilities is an important source of anxiety.

To help the client with anxiety, the nurse encourages the client to break down the anxiety into component parts, and to identify specific concerns that can then be addressed through problem-solving. Global feelings are more terrifying than are explicit, specified fears; coping with specific fears, when well defined, is easier than coping with undifferentiated feelings.[161] Individuals vary in the unique combination of specific fears they hold. Thus, the nurse's goal is to work with the client to ascertain which specific fears and issues are of concern to him or her and to assist the client to confront them. Examples of the kinds of fears people may have include: the unknown, loneliness, loss of identity, not knowing how to accept others' sympathy, being overwhelmed by sorrow, economic problems, guilt for previous actions, loss of social status, or the inability to cope with practical matters.[169]

Providing grieving clients with information can be very helpful in alleviating anxiety. Information eases uncertainty of the unknown. Clarifying information previously acquired can also be helpful, particularly when that information is erroneous and a source of concern to clients. Individuals vary in their capacity to cope with information; some people require it in smaller pieces and at a slower pace. By reviewing information concerning the loss that clients have acquired elsewhere, nurses can help clients to identify and accept its significance to their current situation.

Caring for Clients Who Are Chronically Ill. Chronically ill clients are clients who have illnesses that are generally incurable and thus last longer than several months. These clients have special needs and are often faced with many losses in addition to loss of health, among them, body image changes, loss of self-esteem, changes in relationships and roles, changes in life-style activities and leisure pursuits, changes in sexual functioning, and loss of income or financial stressors. Independence and a sense of control or mastery over their environment may be affected.

Chronically ill clients also face major disruptions in life-style that are often stressful, time consuming, fatiguing and frustrating. Disruptions include frequent clinic or physician visits, regular laboratory or other tests, medication trials and adjustments, and possible rehospitalizations for exacerbations of the illness. Chronically ill clients often suffer from chronic fatigue related to the illness and emotional exhaustion from coping with exacerbations and remissions. All of these variables have the potential to affect self-expression.

Encouraging clients to verbalize feelings about the illness can assist clients to deal with these feelings and aid nurses to plan appropriate implementation. Similar to clients who are grieving a loss, chronically ill clients must cope with a variety of emotional responses. These include feelings of anger, depression, anxiety, and hopelessness.

Nurses' realistic assessment of clients' health status and function can help to provide a sense of hope, as clients recognize activities and aspects of self-expression that are unaffected or minimally impaired by illness. Often clients with chronic illness, especially the aged, suffer from loneliness and isolation. Nurses should work with these clients in establishing a plan to reduce isolation and increase social contact.

Nurses may provide support to chronically ill clients by facilitating expression of spiritual beliefs. Nurses can also assist clients' expression of spiritual beliefs by enlisting the support of a pastoral care representative; for example, asking a priest, rabbi, or minister to visit a client.

Clients with chronic illness often have difficulty pacing their activity and conserving energy. A client with chronic lung disease, for example, may overexert himself by climbing stairs too quickly, bringing on an episode of difficult breathing. A client with chronic pain may engage in too strenuous a physical activity, aggravating the pain. Teaching clients the concept of pacing and what is appropriate to their level of limitation can facilitate clients' self-expression through physical activity.

Assisting clients to plan for and engage in activities that promote self-esteem can assist them in coping with chronic illness. Helping clients identify ways in which they can preserve autonomy and control can reduce the sense of dependency these clients often experience. Clients who are coping with a chronic illness may withdraw from activities that provide a sense of meaning in their lives because of embarrassment, lack of energy, or lack of resources. Nurses can assist clients to minimize withdrawal from meaningful activities by emphasizing the importance of such activities to self-concept, and, as necessary, helping clients reengage or define alternate forms of meaningful activities.

Clients with chronic illness often have an ongoing need for support both during times of exacerbation and remission of the illness. Referral of clients to additional appropriate resources such as a support group can meet this need. Support groups such as Better Breather, for clients with chronic lung disease, provide ongoing support for clients with this illness.

Caring for Dying Clients. As discussed previously, clients who are faced with terminal illness experience perhaps the greatest threat to self-expression. Clients and their families experience many emotions in assimilating the diagnosis of terminal illness. (See the discussion of the client with a terminal diagnosis, above.) Nursing care involves providing various types of informational, familial, and social support.[139]

Humphrey offers several general guidelines for nurses who care for dying clients.

- Perceive the dying person holistically.
- Provide information using language the client can understand.
- Facilitate meaningful discussions by assisting the client to review what meant the most during his or her life.
- Be aware of the client's values and your own.
- Do not take over for the dying person or the family.
- Assist the client in developing support networks and in maintaining important relationships.
- Spend adequate time with the client.
- Monitor your own feelings.
- Surround the client with empathic support.[139]

Humphrey also suggests the following guidelines for working with family members of dying clients.

- Maintain the relationship between the dying client and family by encouraging open communication (to the extent family style allows).
- Support family members' unique identities and their own capabilities in differentiating their own legitimate needs from those of the dying person (eg, need for a break or period of solitude away from the client).

- Assist and support family members to cooperatively assume new roles.
- Encourage family members' expressions of emotions and support them in sharing their emotions.
- Continue reality testing and planning to assist family members to understand pertinent information about the illness and its treatment.
- Assist family members to recognize that the end is near.[139]

Acknowledging Clients' Feelings. Dying clients are faced with multiple losses and experience a grieving state over these losses, which include loss of health, plans for the future, ability to care for self, ability to perform roles, self-esteem, positive body image, and eventual loss of significant others. Enormous and varied emotional responses may accompany this sense of loss. Clients often become aware of death and face these losses in a staccato fashion—experiencing brief moments of awareness and terror, denial, internal processing, and then preparedness for more information.[170]

Nurses working with dying clients have a unique opportunity to provide an empathic response to the varied shared emotions of these clients. Tyner suggests that empathy must include a communication by the nurse of attitudes and behavior that indicate a genuine effort to understand the unique meaning of the life experience, past and present, of the dying client.[171] She further suggests that nonverbal behaviors have a powerful effect of communicating empathy.

1. The face of the nurse must be used with skill to convey the message of focused attention, interest, and concern for the dying client; this includes eye contact that suggests caring and regard.
2. Body posture and gestures express empathy. For example, sitting down, being relaxed and facing others express interest and a desire to understand.
3. Hand movements by the nurse can be expressive or comforting.
4. Tactile stimulation or touching can communicate an empathic sensitivity.
5. A voice that is softly modulated and slightly low in tone is best received by an ill client.[171]

Emotions experienced by dying clients may include shock and disbelief, fear, loneliness, anger, sadness and depression, and hope.

Shock and Disbelief. Shock and disbelief are usually the first responses to a terminal diagnosis (see earlier discussion). Clients numbed with this news may appear dazed, sit motionless, cry, or demonstrate extreme behavior or mood changes. Nurses can provide support by remaining with clients, allowing for privacy, or assisting clients to contact family members during this emotional response.

Fear. The implications of death are so enormous that often clients' life energy is taken up in the denial of mortality. Dying clients are forced to face the reality of their own mortality, with all the accompanying fears: fear of pain, fear of procedures, fear of surgery, and fears regarding loss. Nurses who care for dying clients should encourage verbalization of these fears and, where possible, assist clients to cope with their fears by providing support and education.

Loneliness. Dying clients often experience loneliness, both from an existential perspective in facing death and from the isolation from significant others. Zack proposes several approaches in working with clients experiencing loneliness.

- Teach significant others about the client's needs for closeness and belonging.
- Use empathic skills, such as listening attentively and allowing the expression of feeling.
- Suggest and/or carry out measures that conserve the client's energy or relieve symptoms to enable the client to meet needs for closeness and social interaction.
- Explore use of nonsocial, creative/solitary pursuits, when indicated.
- Model and teach the skills needed for social interactions.[142]

In addition to the approaches described above, nurses can encourage contact with significant others via telephone and face-to-face visits, and provide a sense of connection to others through photographs placed at the bedside and contact with the outside world (eg, TV, radio, newspaper).

Anger. As previously discussed, anger is a normal emotional response of seriously ill and dying clients. Clients should be encouraged to verbalize the anger and assisted to understand the normalcy of this response. (See the earlier discussion of Caring for Clients Who Are Grieving a Loss.)

Sadness and Depression. Dying clients experience sadness and depressed feelings related not only to losses that have already occurred (such as the loss of a breast, loss of a job, or loss of home life), but also to losses that are impending (such as inability to function in role of mother and wife, loss of involvement in the outside world, or loss of relationships to significant others). Sadness and depression must be recognized as normal responses. Conveying a sense of caring by silently sitting with the client or by touching the client can communicate that these feelings are normal and acceptable.

Hope. Most of the literature on care of the dying client emphasizes the importance of hope as a coping mechanism. Assisting clients to maintain hope in the face of a terminal diagnosis requires sensitivity on the part of nurses. The nurse must understand the client's emotional state, knowledge of the illness and the diagnosis, and what helps the client feel hopeful. By understanding the experience of dying for the individual client, the nurse is able to identify areas of hope that can be fostered or strengthened. For example, does the client need to feel hopeful that he or she will not be alone during his or her final hours? Does the client need to feel hopeful about a pain-free death? Does the client need to feel hopeful that clergy will be available? Does the client need to feel hopeful that all interventions are being used? Does the client need to feel hopeful that he or she is still cared about? Understanding the dimensions of hope that are important to the client enables the nurse to assist the client with maintenance of hope.

Promoting Independence. Allowing dying clients to remain independent for as long as they are able enables clients to maintain a sense of dignity. Encouraging clients' participation in decision-making about care reinforces independence and a sense of control.

Maintaining Physical and Spiritual Comfort. Dying clients have many physical needs for comfort. Alleviation of pain is particularly important. Nurses must be particularly attentive to clients' needs related to skin care, breathing, movement, nutrition, elimination, pain relief, and personal hygiene. For example, clients whose mobility is limited are at risk for pressure ulcers and compromised respirations. Vigilant nursing care is required to ensure comfort and optimal physiological functioning for these clients.

Providing clients with spiritual comfort requires that nurses have an understanding of clients' belief systems and religious affiliation (see Chap. 9). Nurses who work with seriously ill or dying clients must also understand their own spiritual beliefs and values. Facilitating contact with clergy can assist clients to meet spiritual needs. Encouraging client self-disclosure about the meaning of death, belief in afterlife, and feelings associated with dying are also helpful. Prayers, Bible readings, meditation, and spiritual counseling are other ways that clients meet needs for spiritual comfort.

Hospice Care. Hospice care provides a change in focus from hospital-based curative care to palliative/supportive care. Hospice care helps terminally ill clients continue their lives with minimal disruptions. Care is provided in a homelike setting by a team of health care professionals and support staff.

Nurses should be informed about local hospice services, as there is a wide variety in the scope of these services. Nurses can be helpful to clients and families by explaining the option of hospice care.

Caring for the Body After Death. The nurse who has cared for a client while the client was alive often cares for the body after death and can be most sensitive to the requests of family and the client's prior expressed wishes regarding body care. Care of the body should occur relatively rapidly after death, as the body subsequently undergoes several physical changes. **Rigor mortis** develops within 2 to 4 hours, causing stiffening of the body. **Algor mortis**, which occurs gradually after death, causes a reduction of the body temperature and loss of skin elasticity. **Liver mortis** causes a purple discoloration of the skin in the lowermost portions of the body as red blood cells begin to break down.

To prepare the body for viewing, the nurse positions the body in the supine position, with the hands at the side or crossed on the abdomen, and closes the eyes and mouth. A pillow may be placed under the head to present a natural appearance and to prevent pooling of blood in the face. If the client wore dentures, these are placed in the mouth.

The nurse will also need to prepare the family for the experience of seeing the body. Offering a quiet, private area for viewing is most important. If family members were not present when the client died, the experience of seeing the body may be an especially emotional one. Nurses can demonstrate respect for the family's grief at this time by treating the body carefully and with respect.

After viewing by the family, identification tags are applied to the body at the ankle and wrist and the body is wrapped in a shroud. An additional identification tag is placed on the outside of the shroud.

Caring for Clients Who Express Strong Emotion. Clients who are undergoing the stress of an illness often cope with this state by expressing strong emotional reactions (either verbally or nonverbally) such as anger, hostility, sadness, or fear. Clients' expression of intense emotional states is sometimes viewed by nurses as negative or difficult behavior and can elicit nontherapeutic responses such as criticizing or withdrawal. Nurses who understand that such expressions are a form of coping behavior are less likely to label clients as difficult and more likely to respond therapeutically or in a helpful, caring manner. In their study of nurses' responses to difficult clients, Podrasky and Sexton found anger and frustration to be the two most common responses.[172] Nurses may legitimately feel anger and frustration in caring for some clients, but the expression of those emotions to the client is rarely beneficial. It is more helpful to work toward understanding the reasons for the emotional expression and assist clients to handle these emotions.

Anger. Anger is a common and normal response during the stress of grief, loss, or illness. Clients may not be fully aware of how angry they are; nurses can help them "get in touch" with the anger by providing feedback about how clients are presenting themselves to others. Nurses can point out behaviors such as rising voice volume, clenching of fists, or sarcastic comments. Other signs of anger, and nursing approaches for dealing with angry clients, were described earlier under Caring for Clients Who Are Grieving a Loss. Additional guidelines for assisting clients to cope with the expression of anger include the following.

- Give the client permission to express the anger.
- Point out to the client that anger is a normal response to the situation.
- Help the client identify signs of anger, such as hand waving, loud voice, furrowed brow, racing heart, or rapid breathing.
- Explore with the client reasons for the anger (avoid the use of "why" questions).
- Help the client distinguish appropriate anger expression from aggressive behavior.
- Give the client time to verbalize and describe the anger.
- Assist the client to identify additional sources for anger expression other than verbalization, ie, exercise or other physical release activities (use of punching bag, pillow).
- Do not use a counter response of anger toward the client.

Hostility. Hostility arises from a sense of conflict, frustration, or antagonism. Hostility may be expressed openly or may be oblique and subtle. Anger that has been denied or suppressed for a long period is often expressed as a subtle form of hostility. For example, a husband angry at his wife for routinely failing to be on time, may express hostility by remarks such as "You're always disorganized" or "Can't you get a watch?" A more direct expression of the anger about this conflict such as "I'm angry with you for keeping me waiting" may avoid the pent up anger that leads to indirect hostile expression.

Sometimes the hostility expressed by clients is related to past experiences, either in childhood or in similar situations involving other health care providers. Nurses can assist clients who cope with illness by the use of hostility in the following ways.

- Recognize the client's behavioral response with a statement that conveys concern and willingness to help (eg, "I sense that you are feeling troubled about something").
- Encourage the client to identify and express the underlying anger or conflict that leads to the hostile response.
- Give permission for expression of negative emotions by acknowledging what you perceive to be the client's feelings. Assist the client to be more direct in expression (eg, "You seem upset or angry that I kept you waiting so long").
- Do not counter with a response of hostility.
- Encourage clients who have difficulty expressing anger to test it out in the safety and context of the nurse–client relationship.
- Demonstrate empathy with the client's emotional state by paraphrasing what was said and what emotions are communicated.

Sadness. Sadness is one of the principal responses of clients who are grieving a loss. Sadness is often expressed through crying, but can also be expressed through other behaviors such as a downward cast of the eyes, a blank stare, a monotone voice or low voice volume, or a slumped posture. Nurses working with clients experiencing the emotion of sadness may find the following approaches helpful.

- Encourage the client to put into words the feeling of sadness.
- Explore with the client the sources of the sadness.
- Encourage the client to express the sadness through crying, even if it makes the nurse uncomfortable.
- Provide or make time to be with the client.
- Observe for clues in the client or ask the client if he or she would rather be alone for a while. Some clients want the comfort of another person while crying and others want solitude during this period.

Fear. The physiological responses of fear are similar to those of anxiety. However, fear differs from anxiety by the fact that fear has an identifiable source. Clients may experience fear because of a threat to physical integrity or a threat to self-concept. Nurses may find the following guidelines helpful in working with fearful clients.

- Explore with the client his or her perception of the threat.
- Identify aspects of the problem that the client controls or that can be changed; this can often help reduce fear.
- Provide time for self-disclosure to allow the client to verbalize the fears.
- Clarify or educate, as needed, regarding areas of misinformation that may unnecessarily magnify the fears.
- Educate the client that certain fears are usual and expected when undergoing surgery.

Restorative Care

Restorative care focuses on implementation for clients with a severe self-expression problem. Restorative care for clients with self-expression problems may occur in the home, clinic, or hospital setting. Clients with severe health problems can have many diagnoses that affect self-expression. The nurse's role includes approaches to treat existing problems as well as to reduce a progression of problems that are detrimental to the client.

Caring for Clients Who Grieve Dysfunctionally. Dysfunctional grief is another term for unresolved grief, that is, grief that takes atypical forms and that continues for a prolonged period to interfere with an individual's adaptation to living and coping with loss. Ordinarily grief is self-limited and resolves with time. Dysfunctional or unresolved grief, however, is similar to a wound that fails to heal properly.

Causes of Unresolved Grief. Unresolved grief results from a variety of social and psychological factors that interfere with the client's ability to complete the process of grieving. These are summarized in Box 23–7. Causes include the following.

- *Social negation of loss.* Ordinarily members of a person's social network are supportive following losses, especially losses due to death. The loss of a parent or child, for example, is generally understood by others. Some losses may not be as well recognized by society, but nevertheless are accompanied by grief. These include abortions,

BOX 23–7. CAUSES OF UNRESOLVED GRIEF

Social Factors

- Social negation of loss
- Losses deemed inappropriate for social acknowledgment
- Social isolation
- Lack of opportunity to grieve
- Uncertainty over loss

Psychological Factors

- Guilt
- Fear of a loss of self
- Reawakening of an old loss
- Multiple losses
- Individual resistance to grieving

Adapted from Lazare A. Unresolved grief. In Lazare A, ed. Outpatient Psychiatry. *Baltimore, MD: Williams & Wilkins; 1979.*

miscarriages, the death of parent or child surrogates (substitutes), or the death of a person who has achieved a position of emotional closeness in one's life. Because such losses may not be recognized as losses, others may not offer the social support they otherwise would.

- *Losses deemed inappropriate for social acknowledgment.* Some losses may be acknowledged as losses, but are of such a nature that the bereaved and others in the environment feel they are inappropriate to discuss.[173] These include the death of lovers (homosexual or heterosexual), deaths caused by the bereaved either intentionally or accidentally, and death by suicide. Such deaths leave the bereaved feeling embarrassed, shamed, or humiliated and are commonly avoided as topics in social conversation.[173]
- *Social isolation.* Social isolation, which has many causes, can interfere with an individual's ability to find the social support necessary for griefwork. Many elderly, for example, are confined to nursing homes and without relatives in the community. The lack of a social network thus limits their social resources in a time of need. The diminished importance of religious institutions, formerly an important source of support to bereaved individuals, further diminishes social resources in bereavement.
- *Lack of opportunity to grieve.* Under ideal conditions the bereaved are permitted to relinquish some of their usual responsibilities of daily living in order to take time to grieve. Neighbors and relatives assist them in necessary tasks so that they will be able to do the work of grieving. Many of the social situations that contribute to social isolation also make it necessary for some individuals to continue in their usual roles without any outside assistance. Forced to "be strong" and carry the burdens of everyday living in addition to dealing with grief, some individuals simply fail to grieve.[173]
- *Uncertainty over loss.* In some situations, it is unclear whether a person has actually died (kidnapped children, soldiers missing in action, comatose individuals on long-term life support); thus it is difficult for relatives to begin the process of grieving until the uncertainty is removed.
- *Guilt.* People who by virtue of their personality are prone to guilt or who feel intensely ambivalent toward the deceased individual may have difficulty grieving. Such people may unconsciously anticipate an experience of enormous guilt should the process of grieving begin. Often individuals who fail to grieve feel a sense of responsibility for the death through something they did or failed to do.[173]
- *Fear of a loss of self.* Some people have difficulty grieving because they perceive the deceased as a part of or an extension of their selves. For example, a woman might refer to her dead mother as "half of myself."[173] Thus the death of the loved one also represents the death of a part of self. Such individuals may feel they can never be the same or whole again.[173]
- *Reawakening of an old loss.* Some people are unable to grieve a current loss because they have a previous unresolved loss with which they have not dealt. At some level of awareness, they fear that acknowledging a current loss will reawaken the conflicts surrounding the old loss.[173]
- *Multiple losses.* Individuals who experience multiple losses simultaneously or close in time, as when several family members die in a single accident, may have difficulty grieving. Such experiences are psychologically overwhelming.
- *Individual resistance to grieving.* Some individuals resist grieving. Reasons for this resistance vary. Some view grieving as a sign of weakness. Some are concerned their grief will hurt other people. Others profoundly fear the loss of emotional self-control. For still others, the expression of the emotions of grief, such as through crying, engenders a feeling of guilt they wish to avoid.[172]

Types of Unresolved Grief. There are essentially three types of unresolved grief: chronic grief, absent grief, or delayed grief.[136]

In chronic grief, the bereaved continues to experience intense feelings characteristic of early grief long beyond the period expected. While authorities generally agree that timetables for grieving are erroneous in the consideration of individual cases, chronic grief can nevertheless be viewed as acute grief that persists beyond the expected 6 month to 1 year period of bereavement.[173] Manifestations of this type of grief include hopelessness about the future as well as extreme feelings of anger, self-blame, and depression.[136]

Absent grief occurs when survivors continue their usual activities as if nothing had happened and, at a superficial level, appear to be coping well. Underlying the outward appearance, however, they may feel depressed and have various manifestations of depression.[136]

Delayed grief is grief that is experienced minimally at the time of the loss and then resurfaces late in the form of a depression or affective disorder.[136]

Identifying Clients With Unresolved Grief. Lazare identifies several characteristics by which persons with unresolved grief can be identified.

1. Manifestations of depression.
2. Experience of prolonged grief in the past.
3. Expressions of guilt, self-reproach; panic attacks; physical symptoms such as choking sensations, breathing attacks.
4. Physical symptoms that are the same as those manifested by the dead person—often those manifested during the terminal illness (identification).
5. Feelings of pressure in the chest or under the sternum.
6. Searching behavior—looking for something that cannot be found.
7. Difficulty with specific dates that are important anniversaries in the life of the deceased.
8. Statements that the death occurred yesterday, even though it may have been months or years ago.
9. Unwillingness to remove the material possessions of the deceased—refusal to give away or pack the deceased's clothes.
10. Social relationships that seem to favor those who seem to replace the dead person (such as a dead person's sibling).

11. Diminished participation in religious and other ceremonial activities (attendance at church, visits to the grave, participation in memorial services).
12. Inability to discuss the deceased without crying.
13. Conversations marked by themes of loss.[173]

Clients who suffer from unresolved grief rarely identify their problem as grief, and may instead complain of depression or difficulty with interpersonal relationships. Nurses must be alert to the possibility of unresolved grief and attempt to confirm or disconfirm that possibility through the health history.

Implementation for Unresolved Grief. The goal of the nurse is to help clients with unresolved grief to accomplish the griefwork that they previously had been unable to complete. In many clinical settings, nurses may identify unresolved grief or suspect it exists, but have insufficient time to address the problem. Therefore, one of the nurse's most important contributions is to encourage the client to seek support in the form of counseling or a community support group. If the client is hospitalized or is making regular visits to an outpatient clinic, a mental health referral may be appropriate.

The process of getting the client into a situation of appropriate support may be complicated by the fact that many clients who experience unresolved grief fail to recognize it as such. It may be necessary to negotiate a disagreement on the nature of the problem before any action can be taken on the client's behalf. Often clients with unresolved grief attribute their distress to depression or to interpersonal problems. They may need to experience some of the grief before they are able to recognize the need for grieving. Sometimes this is facilitated by their recalling the deceased and remembering the time they spent together. Such recollections can be followed by an offer of referral.

In settings where there is time to assist clients with grief work, it is very important that nurse and client establish a solid therapeutic alliance—a trust relationship. Once the relationship is well established, there are several ways in which the nurse can be helpful. One of the most important is to act as the client's support system. This means encouraging the client to express painful emotions when they appear. The client can be encouraged to recollect the deceased through speaking about the deceased, reviewing photos and other memorabilia, and so on. It is acceptable for the nurse to inquire about the deceased and to ask questions that enable the client to recall details about the deceased. "What kind of a person was your husband?" "What did he look like?" "How long was he ill?" "When did he die?" The purpose of such questions is to encourage recall so that the accompanying emotions can be expressed and emotional release and catharsis achieved.[173]

Similar to clients whose grief follows the more typical course to resolution, many clients who experience unresolved grief have difficulty with ambivalent feelings. Once the client begins grieving, he or she may share feelings of anger with the nurse. The nurse need not—and should not—encourage the client to release a mass of negative feelings; this might well be overwhelming to the client; however, once the client begins to express anger, it is acceptable and desirable to acknowledge the feeling and to put it into context for the client, much as the nurse would for any client who is grieving a loss. Teaching the client about ambivalence may be helpful. The nurse's choice of language in these discussions is important. The client will be unlikely to open up if the nurse makes reference to anger, hate, or hostility, but may be willing to discuss feelings of disappointment, irritation, or annoyance. The use of softer words can make the difference between success and failure in such discussions.[173]

Once clients have grieved their losses, they generally experience a change in their feelings, as indicated by the following.[173]

1. Time will seem to pass again.
2. The experience of sadness may change from bitter and negative to sweet and nostalgic.
3. The client is able to discuss the deceased without losing control.
4. Holidays and other occasions become enjoyable again.
5. Searching behavior ceases.
6. Relationships to other survivors becomes more realistic.
7. The deceased is remembered more positively.

It is never too late to grieve a loss. Anderson has described a case of unresolved grief that was grieved over four decades after the death occurred.[174] Thus, the sharing of pain long suppressed can still have therapeutic effects for the individuals involved.

Helping Clients Who Are at High Risk for Unresolved Grief. The current AIDS epidemic in the United States and elsewhere is significant not only for the number of lives it is taking, but also for the number of bereavements it is creating. Because of the conditions surrounding AIDS deaths, many of these bereaved may be at high-risk for unresolved grief.

Because of the stigma attached to AIDS, many bereaved will experience complications that may interfere with their grieving process. Gay men who have not socially acknowledged their sexual orientation may view the admission of the loss of a friend as a threat to their status in the social world.[175] If the deceased was a lover, the bereaved may fear he will be shunned by others for admitting it. Many of the social rituals of bereavement, moreover, are reserved for widows and widowers. Thus, the survivors may well be excluded from those mechanisms of social support. Funerals and memorials, for example, may create awkward social circumstances for the bereaved.[175] People may not engage the bereaved in conversations about the deceased and may fail to acknowledge the loss at all. For high-risk individuals, other forms of bereavement support are thus critical. Nurses who care for clients who are dying of AIDS may be in the best position to offer support to their significant others. Nurses can provide assistance by being available to those anticipating bereavement and by helping them to express their grief at their own pace and in their own way. Such support may be a significant factor in preventing unresolved grief.[175]

Caring for Clients Who Deny Illness. Denial is not the same as maintaining hope in the face of serious or life-threatening illness. Denial involves the inability to accurately integrate and use information about one's health status. Denial serves a useful coping function in the early stages of illness but can be detrimental as the illness progresses. For example, an elderly client who denies the seriousness of symptoms may not seek treatment that, if provided early, could speed or ensure recovery.

Nurses should work with clients to gently break down the denial, facilitating acceptance. The first step is to encourage self-disclosure by the client. This enables the nurse to understand what the illness experience means to the client. Some clients may need more information about the illness to understand the implications of the diagnosis. Other clients may need help in working through fears about the illness or exploring the impact of the illness on various aspects of their lives.

Caring for Clients Who Are Unable to Accept Body Changes. Many illnesses and their treatments create profound changes in body functions and appearances. Cancer, for example, has the potential to affect many body functions; its treatment may require medication that temporarily alters a person's appearance or surgery that permanently changes body structure and function. Sometimes the results are unsightly from a cosmetic standpoint, even though the treatment itself may be life-saving. Degenerative and traumatic neurosensory conditions also sometimes result in body function changes; for example, paralysis may permanently alter an individual's ability to move and to be mobile, to eat and eliminate waste, or even to breathe.

Such changes represent a virtual assault, not only on the body, but also psychologically on the person's body image and self-concept. The person, once whole, suddenly has fewer body parts, or in the case of ostomy surgery (relocation of the ureters or large bowel opening to the abdominal wall) has a new part—the stoma. Because of trauma or illness, the person may be unable to accomplish even the most basic functions. In our society, with its emphasis on wholeness, such changes are often difficult to accept. For some individuals, however, the experience can be overwhelming and may culminate in the inability to accept the reality of the changes that have taken place.

Coping with changes that so vastly alter normal modes of adaptation is difficult for individuals under the best of circumstances. Such changes create a wide variety of needs that must be addressed—physical, psychological, and social. When needs go unmet, or when intervening variables make it impossible for needs to be met, there is always a risk of adaptation failure.

Preventive care for individuals at risk is very important. Preventive care begins right after diagnosis and before any treatment measures are taken as the client is given information about the disease and what to expect from its treatment. Preventive care continues during the treatment phase, preoperatively and postoperatively, as the client is assisted physically and psychologically through the ordeal of surgery and its aftermath.

Unfortunately, there are often gaps in the psychological preventive care that is given to clients before treatment. Clients often have questions about their disease or surgery that go unanswered.[176–178] Frequently these questions concern the potential for normal functioning after treatment and involve issues of their sexuality and how they will function as a social person.[176,179] Many clients having body-altering surgery do not understand the nature of the changes that they will undergo.[178] In Deeny's study of clients having ostomy surgery, all of the clients expressed a desire for more information about their procedure preoperatively. Several of the clients did not realize, for example, that creating an ostomy meant that the rectum and anus would be removed.[178]

Caregiving for clients undergoing major surgery is intense in the immediate postoperative period. Often, however, this care is oriented around the client's immediate physical needs. As the client's condition improves and the client gradually becomes aware of the profound differences in his or her body, the staff has usually redirected its energies to others who are more acutely ill, leaving the client to cope more or less independently with the shock of the new reality.[177] In the recovery phase, while the client remains hospitalized, the client may experience an overwhelming mix of feelings that he or she may not understand and may be unable to express. Because clients are often unable to communicate their confusion or dilemmas, busy staff may simply assume they are coping well.

Postdischarge care may also fail to address clients' psychological needs. Cancer and ostomy clients often experience periods of depression after discharge and require ongoing assistance to deal with problems of body image and self-concept.[180] Because care after discharge also may be fragmented, the postdischarge psychological state of the client may go unnoticed. Moreover, preparation for the postdischarge phase is often inadequate in regard to instruction on the psychological realities confronting clients. Oberst and Scott studied individuals undergoing ostomy surgery and found that while predischarge teaching covered the behavioral aspects of self-care thoroughly, most often it ignored psychological aspects such as providing clients with information about the temporal patterns of recovery.[179] This contributes to clients' vulnerability to problems in adaptation. Clients require not only information about what their physical and psychological symptoms are going to be, but also a timeframe against which to measure their progress. These components are too often missing from the client's preventive care.

Identifying Clients Who Are at Risk. Nurses make an important contribution by identifying individuals who are at risk for an adaptation problem and by taking preventive steps to avoid such a problem, before and immediately after treatment and in the posthospitalization phase. Denial is a common response in the phase leading up to treatment, and may not signify impending adaptation problems. Nevertheless, clients who seem to be unable to absorb information provided to them or who seem completely unaware of the reality of their situation should be monitored closely for signs of adaptation problems following treatment.

One of the most important signs of an impending problem is the client's reaction to the altered body part. Some clients, for example, completely ignore the altered area, declining to look at or touch the body part. They may act as if nothing were different. The client who becomes paralyzed on one side of the body, for example, may act as though that region simply no longer exists, failing to wash or care for the affected arm or leg. While such behavior may be adaptive in the acute phase of recovery, persistent inability to acknowledge a change should be regarded as problematic.

Many clients who undergo body-altering surgery likewise have difficulty looking at their incisions, particularly when these are associated with mutilating changes. Northouse studied women undergoing mastectomy (breast removal) and found that clients' reactions to their incisions varied considerably.[181] Nearly one half (46 percent) reported looking at their incision in the hospital approximately 1 to 3 days after surgery. Another one third (32 percent) viewed their incisions within the first 2 weeks after returning home; the remaining women (22 percent) looked at their incision between 2 and 4 weeks later. All of the women had seen the incision by 1 month after surgery.[181]

Adaptation to the reality of a body change takes time. Persistent inability to look at, touch, or handle the care of the affected body part, however, is a sign of an adaptation failure and an indication that the client is suffering from an unmet need. Oberst and Scott found in their study of clients with ostomies that the crisis period is not resolved in the 6 to 8 weeks predicted by models of acute crisis, and, in fact, is generally not resolved until 3 to 6 months postdischarge. Thus, there is a prolonged period of adaptation in which individuals will progress on varied timetables. With the proper supportive care, most clients adapt within several months of surgery. Persistent denial and resistance to acknowledging the change beyond this period should be regarded as an indicator that the client needs additional professional assistance.

Assisting Clients to Accept a Body Change. Readiness is a factor in a client's progression toward health. Readiness to look at the altered body part, for example, was found to be a factor in the timing of clients' viewing of their incisions in Northouse's study.[181] Some women in Northouse's sample were reluctant to look at their incisions even though they had the opportunity, describing a need to "work up the nerve" to do it.[181] One said, "I didn't want to look." Another said, "I was scared and didn't know what to expect." Others wished they had been forewarned about the appearance of the incision. Many were concerned about what their husbands' reactions would be, and were afraid that their husbands would be hesitant to look at the incision. Husbands in the study also reported being unprepared for what to expect.[181]

Readiness can be encouraged by helping clients to progress through the grieving process associated with important body changes. Encouraging clients to express feelings immediately before, during, and after treatment can facilitate the grieving process. Often catharsis will help the individual prepare for acknowledgement of deficits that are real and permanent.

Nurses also can be helpful by teaching clients about what they should expect from their altered body part. This teaching should be paced according to the individual's ability to integrate the information. Nurses can begin by presenting small pieces of information. Nurses can begin by presenting small pieces of information, and then gradually build a foundation. Clients who are able to handle information at a faster pace will generally respond with questions for clarification or make requests for still more information. It is also important to clarify information that clients have previously received. Sometimes this information contains significant misunderstandings that may inhibit a client's readiness to progress.

Nurses also can assist clients by gently encouraging them to consider their affected body part. Clients who become paralyzed, for example, may benefit from information that helps them interpret their confusing sensory input and understand how their injury or disease is affecting various body functions.[182] Such discussions may represent initial steps toward incorporating body changes into a renewed body image. Clients can be gently encouraged to care for the affected region of the body. This is facilitated by developing realistic short-term goals, beginning with a small, simple activity and gradually progressing to more complex aspects. Short-term goals provide realistic challenges that are important in coming to terms with self-loss.[182]

Inviting and encouraging the client to participate in the decision-making process also encourages the client to become involved in care. Making contracts with clients who are reticent to join in caregiving activities can be helpful. (See Chap. 37 for more on client contracts.)

Another approach that is often helpful is to involve family members in decision-making and care planning. Information is helpful, not only for clients, but also for family members. Family members also need to be encouraged to express their feelings. Sometimes this may mean interacting privately with spouses and other close relatives in order to assist them in coming to terms with their own feelings.

Clients can also be encouraged to interact with others who have had similar illnesses and undergone similar treatments. Clients often derive strength from seeing others who have adapted successfully to what they themselves are experiencing. Many subjects in Northouse's study, for example, took particular comfort in the support they received from other women who had undergone mastectomies. Conversations with such women helped clients feel less isolated and alone.[181]

Clients are often worried about their attractiveness to others and their social acceptability following a profound body change.[176,183] They may worry about how others will regard them sexually and have questions about their own sexual functioning. Nurses can be particularly helpful by being sensitive to these issues, by gently acknowledging their importance, and by implicitly or explicitly inviting clients to ask questions on these topics and to express their feelings. Often there are practical barriers to sexual activity that will preoccupy clients. By having the opportunity to address the issues involved, clients may be helped to adapt and come to deal with their bodies.

Finally, ongoing counseling can significantly aid the integration of difficult body image and self-concept changes. Clients who have a profound body change can benefit from regular ongoing group or individual counseling during the course of recovery. Whenever possible, such support should be encouraged and provided.

Caring for Clients With a Sexual Dysfunction. Care of clients with a sexual dysfunction builds on the approaches outlined in the earlier discussion of clients with concerns about sexuality. The etiology of the sexual dysfunction will determine appropriate nursing approaches to improve, enhance, or foster adaptation to sexual functioning. As noted in the earlier discussion of etiologies of sexual dysfunction, childhood development, lack of role modeling, and religious and values conflicts may influence an individual's sexual functioning.

Care of clients with a sexual dysfunction often necessitates referral to other providers, such as sex therapists. If a sexual dysfunction is suspected or identified, a thorough sexual history is warranted to identify a long-term or situational problem. The information gathered through the history enables the nurse to determine whether referral is appropriate. The discussion that follows outlines general approaches for the client with a sexual dysfunction.

Nurses should identify the obstacles to satisfactory sexual functioning—whether a result of illness, psychological conflicts, loss of physiological function, anxiety, communication problems in a relationship, partner rejection, or sexual fears. Depending on the source of the problem, tasks can be identified to facilitate improved sexual functioning; these include communication exercises with one's spouse, alternate coital positions or sexual techniques, substitute behaviors such as fondling or caressing, and relaxation exercises. Clients with sexual dysfunction can be advised to focus on sensual pleasure and reduce the demand they place on themselves for coitus and orgasm.

Management of sexual dysfunction is a sensitive and often difficult endeavor, as clients are often embarrassed to collaborate in discussions of intimate sexual functions. Nurses who demonstrate concern and professionalism can help build clients' trust and comfort, facilitating management of sexual needs and functioning.

Rehabilitative Care

Clients who have undergone an acute change in health status may have short-term or long-term needs during the rehabilitative phase. Rehabilitative care often focuses on reconstruction—that is, integrating the positive aspects of the changes in self-expression clients have undergone as a result of health changes. This focus necessarily includes working toward developing new life patterns as clients adjust to the changes. A new self-concept emerges with the potential for greater opportunity and risk-taking. Clients often need a great deal of support during this period, both from significant others and from health care professionals. Regaining a sense of self-esteem is critical. Nurses can be instrumental in providing feedback and encouragement to clients attempting to reenter a social world after changes in self-expression.

Supporting Life-Structural and Role Pattern Changes. Clients who are recovering from an acute health alteration may require support to reenter or reestablish former aspects of life structure and role patterns. Clients may also require assistance to initiate changes in previous patterns necessitated by health alterations.

Counseling. Counseling is frequently a component of rehabilitative care for clients with self-expression problems. Clients experiencing an alteration in self-esteem or body image often experience a prolonged period of adjustment and coping. Referral for appropriate counseling is thus an important component of care for these clients.

Referral to Support Groups. Clients with body changes as a result of illness or surgery may find support groups particularly helpful in adjusting to long-term implications of these changes. Many community support groups are available to aid coping with various health problems, as well as aspects of grief and loss.

■ EVALUATION

Evaluation of client care related to self-expression is the final component of nurse–client management of self-expression. Nurse and client together evaluate progress toward the desired outcomes and the influence of management approaches on current self-expression status. Reassessment and replanning may be necessary to achieve outcomes consistent with clients' expectations. Criteria for evaluation should be as specific and individualized as possible to facilitate evaluation.

Progress toward goals is monitored during the course of care and on the dates specified in the goals. As outcomes are met, they are recorded in the client's chart. Outcomes that are not met, along with reassessment data and additional plans, are also recorded.

SUMMARY

Self-expression, the process by which individuals share their self-understanding with those around them, is vital in both health and illness. It is the process by which people find meaning in their lives, come to know themselves and to be known by others, establish and maintain relationships, and communicate what is important to them to others. Through self-presentation, people work to place an image of themselves before those around them that will strengthen the bonds of human relationship and reinforce their own identity. Through self-disclosure people share the deepest aspects of themselves with those to whom they are close in order to further strengthen the bonds and to gain a sense of togetherness. The life structure provides the social framework through which individuals interact with others to express themselves and through which they build and enact their self-concepts.

Illness interrupts the flow of events in everyday life, and often creates conditions that inevitably alter not only the person, but the person's capacity to pursue activities. This situation often creates a crisis as the individual is faced with undeniable and permanent change. Change in one's body often creates a change in personal and social identity that is manifested by changes in self-presentation. These changes affect relationships of all kinds, but most particularly close, intimate relationships where the capacity to function in important roles, including one's sexual roles, may also be affected. Such changes are usually experienced as a loss and are accompanied by great distress. As a consequence, they initiate a process of grieving through which the individual must go in order to adapt. Grieving an important loss generally requires repeated opportunities for distress disclosure for a resolution of emotions to occur.

Sometimes death is the outcome of illness. In anticipation of death and bereavement, people grieve. At the same time they experience the intense distress that is usually associated with dying, they not only must work to adjust themselves, but to mutually help one another. During the process of dying, the dying and the bereaved deal with urgent issues of identity change and with overwhelming emotions associated with loss. At no time is the distress in an individual's life likely to be greater. Nurses are in an important position to come to the aid of those who are confronting death, to assist them with the threat they inevitably experience to their identity, and to meet their needs for distress disclosure as they attempt to adapt to profound loss.

REFERENCES

1. Banerjee SP. Dimensions of self-expression: Freedom and constraints. In Banerjee SP, Moitra S, eds. *Communication, Identity, and Self-Expression.* Delhi: Oxford University Press; 1984.
2. Levinson DJ, Darrow CN, Klein EB, Levinson MH, McKee B. *The Seasons of a Man's Life.* New York: Ballantine Books; 1978.
3. Whitbourne SK. *The Me I Know: A Study of Adult Identity.* New York: Springer-Verlag; 1986.
4. Frankl VE. *Man's Search for Meaning.* Boston: Beacon Press; 1962.
5. Kasch CR. Establishing a collaborative nurse–patient relationship: A distinct focus of nursing action in primary care. *Image: J Nurs Scholarship.* 1986;18(2);44–47.
6. Morse J. Reciprocity in care: Gift giving and the patient–nurse relationship. *Can J Nurs Res.* 1989;21(1):33–45.
7. Cooper MJ. Covenantal relationships: Grounding for the nursing ethic. *Adv Nurs Sci.* 1988;10(4):48–59.
8. Davies MD. An ode to being human. *Nurs Clin North Am.* 1971;6(4):695–701.
9. Marck P. Therapeutic reciprocity: A caring phenomenon. *Adv Nurs Sci.* 1990;13(1):49–59.
10. Paterson JG, Zderad LT. *Humanistic Nursing.* New York: John Wiley & Sons; 1976.
11. Sarvimaki A. Nursing care as a moral, practical, communicative and creative activity. *J Adv Nurs.* 1988;13:462–467.
12. Thorne SE, Robinson CA. Reciprocal trust in health care relationships. *J Adv Nurs.* 1988;13:782–789.
13. Yuen FKH. The nurse–client relationship: A mutual learning experience. *J Adv Nurs.* 1986;11:529–533.
14. Young JC. Rationale for clinician self-disclosure and research agenda. *Image: J Nurs Scholarship.* 1988;20(4):196–199.
15. Gazda GM, Asbury FS, Balzer FJ, Childers WC, Walters RP. *Human Relations Development.* 4th ed. Boston: Allyn & Bacon; 1991.
16. Frankl VE. Self-transcendence as a human phenomenon. *J Human Psychol.* 1966;6:97–106.
17. Ekman P, Sorenson ER, Friesen WV. Pancultural elements in facial displays of emotion. *Science.* 1969;164:86–88.
18. Ekman P, Oster H. Facial expressions of emotion. *Annu Rev Psychol.* 1979;30:527–554.
19. Ekman P, Friesen WV. Origins, usage and coding of nonverbal behavior. In Vernon E, ed. *Communication Theory and Linguistic Models in the Social Sciences.* Buenos Aires: DiTella; 1968.
20. Ekman P. Universal and cultural differences in facial expressions of emotion. In Cole J, ed. *Nebraska Symposium on Motivation.* Lincoln: University of Nebraska Press; 1972.
21. Cupchik GC, Leventhal H. Consistency between expressive behavior and the evaluation of humorous stimuli. *J Pers Soc Behav.* 1974;30(3):429–442.
22. Zuckerman M, Klorman R, Larrance DT, Spiegel NH. Facial, autonomic, and subjective components of emotion: The facial feedback hypothesis versus the externalizer–internalizer distinction. *J Pers Soc Behav.* 1981;41(5):929–944.
23. Riskind JH. They stoop to conquer: Guiding and self-regulatory functions of physical posture after success and failure. *J Pers Soc Psychol.* 1984;47(3):479–493.
24. Zajonc RB. Emotion and facial efference: A theory reclaimed. *Science.* 1985;228:15–21.
25. Winton WM. The role of facial response in self-reports of emotion: A critique of Laird. *J Pers Soc Behav.* 1986;50(4):808–812.
26. Izard CE. Facial expressions and the regulation of emotions. *J Pers Soc Behav.* 1990;58(3):487–498.
27. Rosenthal R. *Skill in Nonverbal Communication: Individual Differences.* Cambridge, MA: Oelgeschlager, Gunn, & Hain; 1979.
28. Goffman E. *The Presentation of Self in Everyday Life.* Garden City, NY: Doubleday Anchor Books; 1959.
29. Schneider DJ, Hastorf AH, Ellsworth PC. *Person Perception.* 2nd ed. Reading, MA: Addison-Wesley; 1979.
30. Tedeschi JT, ed. *Impression Management Theory and Social Psychological Research.* New York: Academic Press; 1981.
31. Derlega VJ. *Communication, Intimacy, and Close Relationships.* Orlando, FL: Academic Press; 1984.

32. Notarius CI, Levenson RW. Expressive tendencies and physiologic responses to stress. *J Personality Social Psychol.* 1979;37:1204–1210.
33. Ekman P, Levenson RW, Friesen WV. Autonomic nervous system activity distinguishes among emotions. *Science.* 1983;221:1208–1210.
34. McBride G, King M, James JW. Social proximity effects of galvanic skin responses in adult humans. *J Psychol.* 1965;61:153–157.
35. James WT. A study of the expression of bodily posture. *J Gen Psychol.* 1932;7:405–437.
36. Ekman P, Friesen WV. The repertoire of nonverbal behavior: Categories, origins, usage and codings. *Semiotica.* 1969;1:49–97.
37. Chelune GJ, ed. *Self-Disclosure: Origins, Patterns and Implications of Openness in Interpersonal Relationships.* San Francisco: Jossey-Bass; 1979.
38. James W. *The Principles of Psychology.* New York: Henry Holt & Co; 1890.
39. Allport GW. The ego in contemporary psychology. *Psychol Rev.* 1941;50:451–478.
40. Greenwald AG. The totalitarian ego: Fabrication and revision of personal history. *Am Psychologist.* 1980;35:603–613.
41. Schlenker BR. Introduction: Foundations of the self in social life. In Schlenker BR, ed. *The self and social life.* New York: McGraw-Hill.
42. Baumeister RF, ed. *Public Self and Private Self.* New York: Springer-Verlag; 1986.
43. Kreitler S, Kreitler H. The psychosemantic aspects of the self. In Honess T, Yardley K, eds. *The Self and Identity.* London: Routledge & Kegan/Paul; 1987.
44. Hall CS, Lindsey G. *Theories of Personality.* New York: Wiley; 1970.
45. Kahn DL. The experience of suffering: Conceptual clarification and theoretical definition. *J Adv Nurs.* 1986;11(6):623–631.
46. Cooley CH. *Human Nature and Social Order.* New York: Scribners; 1902.
47. Baldwin JM. *Social and Ethical Interpretations.* New York: Macmillan; 1897.
48. Combs AW, Snygg D. *Individual Behavior: A Perceptual Approach to Behavior.* New York: Harper & Brothers; 1959.
49. Erikson E. *Identity and the Life Cycle: A Reissue.* New York: WW Norton; 1959/1980.
50. Strauss A. *The Social Psychology of George Herbert Mead.* Chicago: University of Chicago Press; 1956.
51. Scheibe KE. Historical perspectives on the presented self. In Schlenker BR, ed. *The Self and Social Life.* New York: McGraw-Hill; 1985.
52. Tetlock PE, Manstead ASR. Impression management versus intrapsychic explanations in social psychology: A useful dichotomy? *Psychol Rev.* 1985;92(1):59–77.
53. Muhlenkamp AF, Sayles JA. Self-esteem, social support, and positive health practices. *Nurs Res.* 1986;35(6):334–338.
54. Antonucci TC, Jackson JS. Physical health and self-esteem. *Fam Community Health.* 1983;6(2):1–9.
55. Norris CM. The professional nurse and body image. In Carlson CE, ed. *Behavioral Concepts & Nursing Intervention.* Philadelphia: JB Lippincott; 1970.
56. Bonham PA, Cheney AM. Concept of self: A framework for nursing assessment. In Chinn PL, ed. *Advances in Nursing Theory Development.* Rockville, MD: Aspen; 1983.
57. Rose A. *Human Behavior and Social Processes.* Boston: Houghton Mifflin; 1962.
58. Zajonc RB. Feeling and thinking: Preferences need no inferences. *Am Psychol.* 1980;35(2):151–175.
59. Schlenker BR, ed. *The Self and Social Life.* New York: McGraw-Hill; 1985.
60. Bonner H. *On Being Mindful of Man: Essay Toward a Proactive Psychology.* Boston: Houghton Mifflin; 1965.
61. Maslow AH. *Toward a Psychology of Being.* Princeton, NJ: Van Nostrand; 1962.
62. Gadow SA. Nurse and patient: The caring relationship. In Bishop AH, Scuder JR Jr., eds. *Caring, Curing, Coping: Nurse, Physician, Patient Relationships.* Tuscaloosa, AL: University of Alabama Press; 1985.
63. Benner P, Wrubel J. *The Primacy of Caring: Stress and Coping in Health and Illness.* Toronto: Addison-Wesley; 1988.
64. Watson MJ. New dimensions of human caring theory. *Nurs Sci Q.* 1988;1:175–181.
65. Schlenker BR. Identities, identifications, and relationships. In Derlega VJ, ed. *Communication, Intimacy, and Close Relationships.* Orlando, FL: Academic Press; 1984.
66. Schneider DJ. Tactical self-presentations: Toward a broader conception. In Tedeschi JT, ed. *Impression Management Theory and Social Psychological Research.* New York: Academic Press; 1981.
67. Richardson KD, Cialdini RB. Basking and blasting: Tactics of indirect self-presentation. In Tedeschi JT, ed. *Impression Management Theory and Social Psychological Research.* New York: Academic Press; 1981.
68. Tedeschi JT, Riess M. Identities, the phenomenal self, and laboratory research. In Tedeschi JT, ed. *Impression Management Theory and Social Psychological Research.* New York: Academic Press; 1981.
69. Arkin RM. Self-presentational styles. In Tedeschi JT, ed. *Impression Management Theory and Social Psychological Research.* New York: Academic Press; 1981.
70. Hass RG. Presentational strategies and the social expression of attitudes. In Tedeschi JT, ed. *Impression Management Theory and Social Psychological Research.* New York: Academic Press; 1981.
71. Tedeschi JT. Private and public experiences and the self. In Baumeister RF, ed. *Public Self and Private Self.* New York: Springer-Verlag; 1986.
72. Tedeschi JT, Norman N. Social power, self-presentation, and the self. In Schlenker BR, ed. *The Self and Social Life.* New York: McGraw-Hill; 1985.
73. Goffman E. *Relations in Public.* New York: Basic Books; 1971.
74. Podrasky DL, Sexton DL. Nurse's reactions to difficult patients. *Image: J Nurs Scholarship.* 1988;20(1):16–21.
75. Sarosi GM. A critical theory: The nurse as a fully human person. *Nurs Forum.* 1968;7(4):349–363.
76. McGregor FC. Uncooperative patients: Some cultural interpretations. *Am J Nurs.* 1967;67(1):88–91.
77. Larson PA. Nurse perceptions of patient characteristics. *Nurs Res.* 1977;26(5):416–421.
78. Ruiz MJ. Open-closed mindedness, intolerance of ambiguity and nursing faculty attitudes toward culturally different patients. *Nurs Res.* 1981;30(3):177–181.
79. Jankin JK. The nurse in crisis. *Nurs Clin North Am.* 1974;9(1):17–26.
80. Flaskerud JH, Halloran EJ, Janken J, Lund M, Zetterland J. Avoidance and distancing: A descriptive view of nursing. *Nurs Forum.* 1979;18(2):158–174.
81. Williams F. The crisis of hospitalization. *Nurs Clin North Am.* 1974;9(1):37–45.
82. Jourard S. *The Transparent Self.* Princeton, NJ: Van Nostrand-Reinhold; 1964.

83. Derlega VJ. Self-disclosure and intimate relationships. In Derlega VJ, ed. *Communication, Intimacy, and Close Relationships.* Orlando, FL: Academic Press; 1984.
84. Fitzpatrick MA. Marriage and verbal intimacy. In Derlega VJ, Berg JH, eds. *Self-Disclosure: Theory, Research, and Therapy.* New York: Plenum Press; 1987.
85. Hill CT, Stull DE. Gender and self-disclosure: Strategies for exploring the issues. In Derlega VJ, Berg JH, eds. *Self-Disclosure: Theory, Research, and Therapy.* New York: Plenum Press; 1987.
86. Berg J. Responsiveness and self-disclosure. In Derlega VJ, Berg JH, eds. *Self-Disclosure: Theory, Research, and Therapy.* New York: Plenum Press; 1987.
87. Carpenter BN. The relationship between psychopathology and self-disclosure. In Derlega VJ, Berg JH, eds. *Self-Disclosure: Theory, Research, and Therapy.* New York: Plenum Press; 1987.
88. Derlega VJ, Berg JH. *Self-Disclosure: Theory, Research, and Therapy.* New York: Plenum Press; 1987.
89. Chelune GJ, Robison JT, Kommor MJ. A cognitive interactional model of intimate relationships. In Derlega VJ, ed. *Communication, Intimacy, and Close Relationships.* Orlando, FL: Academic Press; 1984.
90. Stokes JP. The relation of loneliness and self-disclosure. In Derlega VJ, ed. *Self-Disclosure: Theory, Research, and Therapy.* New York: Plenum Press; 1987.
91. Coates D, Winston T. The dilemma of distress disclosure. In Derlega VJ, Berg JH, eds. *Self-Disclosure: Theory, Research, and Therapy.* New York: Plenum Press; 1987.
92. Locke S, Colligan D. *The New Medicine of Mind and Body.* New York: Dutton; 1986.
93. Schlenker BR. Self-identification: Toward an integration of the private and public self. In Baumeister RF, ed. *Public Self and Private Self.* New York: Springer-Verlag; 1986.
94. Ozer EM, Bandura A. Mechanisms governing empowerment effects: A self-efficacy analysis. *J Pers Soc Psychol.* 1990;58(3): 472–486.
95. Chelune GJ. A neuropsychological perspective of interpersonal communication. In Derlega VJ, Berg JH, eds. *Self-Disclosure: Theory, Research, and Therapy.* New York: Plenum Press; 1987.
96. Schachter S. *The Psychology of Affiliation.* Stanford, CA: Stanford University Press; 1959.
97. Buunk BP, Collins RL, Taylor SE, VanYperen NW, Dakof GA. The affective consequences of social comparison: Either direction has its ups and downs. *J Pers Soc Psychol.* 1990;59(6): 1238–1249.
98. Wood JV, Taylor SE, Lichtman RR. Social comparison in adjustment to breast cancer. *J Pers Soc Psychol.* 1985;49:1169–1183.
99. Nelson PB. Social support, self-esteem, and depression in the institutionalized elderly. *Issues Ment Health Nurs.* 1989;10:55–68.
100. Muhlenkamp AF, Sayles JA. Self-esteem, social support, and positive health practices. *Nurs Res.* 1986;35(6):334–338.
101. Lambert VA, Lambert CE Jr, Klipple GL, Mewshaw EA. Social support, hardiness and psychological well-being in women with arthritis. *Image: J Nurs Scholarship.* 1989;21(3):128–131.
102. Stiles WB. "I have to talk to somebody," A fever model of disclosure. In Derlega VJ, Berg JH, eds. *Self-Disclosure: Theory, Research, and Therapy.* New York: Plenum Press; 1987.
103. Pennebacker JW, O'Heeron RC. Confiding in others and illness rates among spouses of suicide and accidental death. *J Abnorm Psychol.* 1984;93:473–476.
104. Winer DL, Bonner TO, Blaney PH, Murray EJ. Depression and social attraction. *Motivation Emotion.* 1981;5:153–166.
105. Peters-Golden H. Breast cancer: Varied perceptions of social support in the illness experience. *Soc Sci Med.* 1982;16:483–491.
106. Derogatis LR, Abeloff MD, Melisaratos N. Psychological coping mechanisms and survival time in metastatic breast cancer. *JAMA.* 1979;242:1504–1508.
107. Knowlton CN. Human sexuality. In Flynn JM, Heffron PB, eds. *Nursing: From Concept to Practice.* 2nd ed. Norwalk, CT: Appleton & Lange; 1988.
108. Kinsey A, Pomeroy W, Martin C, Gebhard P. *Sexual Behavior in the Human Male.* Philadelphia: WB Saunders; 1948.
109. World Health Organization. *Education & Treatment in Human Sexuality: The Training of Health Professionals.* Geneva: World Health Organization; 1975: Technical Report Series No. 572.
110. Moore KL. *The Developing Human: Clinically Oriented Embryology.* 4th ed. Philadelphia: WB Saunders; 1988.
111. Masters W, Johnson V, Kolodny R. *Human Sexuality.* 2nd ed. Boston: Little, Brown; 1985.
112. Masters WH, Johnson VE. *Human Sexual Response.* Boston: Little, Brown; 1966.
113. Jahoda M. *Current Concepts of Positive Mental Health.* New York: Basic Books; 1958.
114. Jourard SM. *Personal Adjustment.* New York: Macmillan; 1963.
115. Price GM. Empathic relating and the structure of self. In Honess T, Yardely K, eds. *Self and Identity: Perspectives Across the Lifespan.* London: Routledge & Kegan Paul; 1987.
116. Folz AT. The influence of cancer on self-concept and life quality. *Semin Oncol Nurs.* 1987;3(4):303–312.
117. Wright JE. Self-perception alterations with coronary artery bypass surgery. *Heart Lung.* 1987;16(5):483–490.
118. Crouch M, Straub V. Enhancement of self-esteem in adults. *Fam Community Health.* 1983;6:76–78.
119. Unsain IC, Goodwin MH, Schuster EA. Diabetes and sexual functioning. *Nurs Clin North Am.* 1982;17(3):387–393.
120. Goddard LR. Sexuality and spinal cord injury. *J Neurosci Nurs.* 1988;20(4):240–244.
121. Chicano LA. Humanistic aspects of sexuality as related to spinal cord injury. *J Neurosci Nurs.* 1989;21(6):366–369.
122. Lee JM. Emotional reaction to trauma. *Nurs Clin North Am.* 1970;5(4):577–587.
123. Young JC. Rationale for clinician self-disclosure and research agenda. *Image: J Nurs Scholarship.* 1988;20(4):196–199.
124. Ruxton JP. Humor intervention deserves our attention. *Holistic Nurs Pract.* 1988;293:54–62.
125. Lange S. Shame. In Carlson C, ed. *Behavioral Concepts & Nursing Intervention.* Philadelphia: JB Lippincott; 1970.
126. Peretz D. Development, object relationships, and loss. In Schoenberg B, Carr AC, Peretz D, Kutscher AH, eds. *Loss and Grief: Psychological Management in Medical Practice.* New York: Columbia University Press; 1970.
127. Kastenbaum RJ. *Death, Society, and Human Experience.* 3rd ed. Columbus, OH: Charles E. Merrill; 1986.
128. Benoliel JQ. Loss and terminal illness. *Nurs Clin North Am.* 1985;20(2):439–449.
129. Carter SL. Themes of grief. *Nurs Res.* 1989;38(6):354–358.
130. Cody WK. Grieving a personal loss. *Nurs Sci Q.* 1991;4(2):61–68.
131. Lindemann E. Symptomatology and management of acute grief. *Am J Psychiatry.* 1944;101:141–149.
132. Engle GL. Grief and grieving. *Am J Nurs.* 1964;64:93–98.
133. Kubler-Ross E. *On Death and Dying.* New York: Macmillan; 1969.
134. Bowlby J. *Attachment and Loss: Separation.* New York: Basic Books; 1973.

135. Bowlby J. *Attachment and Loss: Loss.* New York: Basic Books; 1980.
136. Martocchio BC. Grief through bereavement: Healing through hurt. *Nurs Clin North Am.* 1985;20(2):327–341.
137. Sowell RL, Bramlett MH, Gueldner SH, Gritzmacher D, Martin G. The lived experience of survival and bereavement following the death of a lover from AIDS. *Image: J Nurs Scholarship.* 1991;23(2):89–94.
138. Mischel MH. Uncertainty in illness. *Image: J Nurs Scholarship.* 1988;20(4):225–232.
139. Humphrey MA. Effects of anticipatory grief for the patient, family member, and caregiver. In Rando TA, ed. *Loss and Anticipatory Grief.* Lexington, MA: Lexington Books; 1986.
140. Capritto K. *The Effect of Perceived Ambiguity on Adherence to the Dietary Regime in Chronic Hemodialysis.* Unpublished master's thesis, California State University, Los Angeles.
141. Kastenbaum R, Costa PT. Psychological perspectives on death. *Annu Rev Psychol.* 1977;28:225–249.
142. Zack MV. Loneliness: A concept relevant to the care of dying persons. *Nurs Clin North Am.* 1985;20(2):403–413.
143. Glaser BG, Strauss AL. *Awareness of Dying.* Chicago: Aldine; 1965.
144. Moseley JR. Alterations in comfort. *Nurs Clin North Am.* 1985; 29(2):427–438.
145. Dufault K, Martocchio BC. Hope: Its spheres and dimensions. *Nurs Clin North Am.* 1985;20(2):379–391.
146. Hall BA. The struggle of the diagnosed terminally ill person to maintain hope. *Nurs. Sci Q.* 1990;3(4):177–184.
147. Stoner M. Measuring hope. In Frank-Stromberg M, ed. *Instruments for Clinical Nursing Research.* Norwalk, CT: Appleton & Lange; 1988.
148. Fromm E. *The Revolution of Hope.* New York: Harper & Row; 1968.
149. Conrad NL. Spiritual support for the dying. *Nurs Clin North Am.* 1985;20(2):415–425.
150. Korein J. The problem of brain death: Development and history. *Ann NY Acad Sci.* 1978;315:1–10.
151. Ad Hoc Committee of the Harvard Medical School to Examine the Definition of Brain Death. A definition of irreversible coma. *JAMA.* 1968;205:337–340.
152. Youngner SJ, Landefeld CS, Coulton CJ, Juknialis BW, Leary M. Brain death and organ retrieval: A cross-sectional survey of knowledge and concepts among health professionals. *JAMA.* 1989;261:2205–2210.
153. Annas GJ. Nancy Cruzan and the right to die. *N Eng J Med.* 1990;323(10):670–673.
154. Williamson J. Mutual interaction and model of practice. *Nurs Outlook.* 1981;2:104–107.
155. Rohde P, Tilson M, Lewinsohn P, Seeley J. Dimensionality of coping and its relation to depression. *J Pers Soc Psychol.* 1990; 153:499–511.
156. Wylie RC. *Measures of Self-Concept.* Lincoln, NB/London: University of Nebraska Press; 1989.
157. Austin JK, Champion V, Tzeng O. Cross-cultural relationships between self-concept and body image in high school age boys. *Arch Psychiatr Nurs.* 1986;3(4):234–240.
158. Townsend MC. Nursing diagnoses in psychiatric nursing: *A Pocket Guide for Care Plan Constriction.* Philadelphia: Davis; 1991.
159. Wooley N. Crisis theory: A paradigm of effective intervention with families of critically ill people. *J Adv Nurs.* 1990;15:1402–1408.
160. Heiss J. Social roles. In Rosenberg M, Turner R. *Social Psychology: Sociological Perspectives.* New York: Basic Books; 1981.
161. Rando TA. A comprehensive analysis of anticipatory grief: Perspectives, processes, promises, and problems. In Rando TA, ed. *Loss and Anticipatory Grief.* Lexington, MA: Lexington Books; 1986.
162. Sheehan DV, Hackett TP. Psychosomatic disorders. In Nicholi AM, Jr. *The Harvard Guide to Modern Psychiatry.* Cambridge, MA/London: Belknap Press of Harvard University Press; 1978: 319–353.
163. Aguilera D, Messick J. *Crisis Intervention: Theory and Methodology.* 5th ed. St. Louis, MO: CV Mosby; 1986.
164. Rossan S. Identity: Its development in adulthood. In Honess T, Yardley K. *Self and Identity: Perspectives Across the Lifespan.* London/New York: Routledge and Kegan Paul; 1987.
165. Erikson E. *Childhood and Society.* New York: WW Norton; 1963.
166. Annon JS. *The Behavioral Treatment of Sexual Problems: Brief Therapy.* New York: Harper & Row; 1976.
167. Winston K: Family roles. In Bomar P, ed. *Nurses and Family Health Promotion: Concepts, Assessment and Interventions.* Baltimore, MD: Williams & Wilkins; 1989:55–66.
168. Leming MR, Dickinson GE. *Understanding Dying, Death and Bereavement.* New York: Holt, Rinehart and Winston; 1985.
169. Rando TA. Understanding and facilitating anticipatory grief in the loved ones of the dying. In Rando TA, ed. *Loss and Anticipatory Grief.* Lexington, MA: Lexington Books; 1986.
170. Yalom I. Death and psychopathology. In Yalom I, ed. *Existential Psychotherapy.* New York: Basic Books; 1980:110–158.
171. Tyner R. Elements of empathic care for dying patients and their families. *Nurs Clin North Am.* 1985;20:393–401.
172. Podrasky D, Sexton DL. Nurses' reactions to difficult patients. *Image: J Nurs Scholarship.* 1988;20:16–21.
173. Lazare A. Unresolved grief. In Lazare A, ed. *Outpatient Psychiatry.* Baltimore, MD: Williams & Wilkens; 1979.
174. Anderson DB. Never too late: Resolving the grief of a suicide. *J Psychosoc Nurs.* 1991;29(3):29–31.
175. Houseman C, Pheifer WG. Potential for unresolved grief in survivors of persons with AIDS. *Arch Psych Nurs.* 1988;2(5): 296–301.
176. Gloekner MR. Perceptions of sexual attractiveness following ostomy surgery. *Res Nurs Health.* 1984;7:87–92.
177. Kelly MP. Loss and grief and responses to surgery. *J Adv Nurs.* 1985;10:517–525.
178. Deeny P, McCrea H. Stoma care: The patient's perspective. *J Adv Nurs.* 1991;16:39–46.
179. Oberst MT, Scott DW. Postdischarge distress in surgically treated cancer patients and their spouses. *Res Nurs Health.* 1988;11:223–233.
180. Watson PG. The effects of short-term postoperative counseling on cancer/ostomy patients. *Cancer Nurs.* 1983;6:21–29.
181. Northouse LL. The impact of breast cancer on patients and their husbands. *Cancer Nurs.* 1989;12(5):276–284.
182. Richmond TS, Metcalf JA. Psychosocial responses to spinal cord injury. *J Neuroscience Nurs.* 1986;18(4):183–187.
183. Simmons KN. Sexuality and the female ostomate. *Am J Nurs.* 1983;83:409–411.

BIBLIOGRAPHY

Allan JD, Hall BA. Between diagnosis and death: The case for studying grief before death. *Arch Psychiatr Nurs.* 1988;2(1):191–199.

Christman NJ, McConnell EA, Pfieffer C, Webster KK, Scmitt M, Ries J. Uncertainty, coping, and distress following infarction: Transition from hospital to home. *Res Nurs Health.* 1988;11:71–82.

DeFeo DJ. Change: A central concern of nursing. *Nurs Sci Q.* 1990; 3(2):88–94.

Demi AS, Miles MS. Bereavement. *Annu Rev. Nurs Res.* 1986;4:105–123.

Doka KJ. Silent sorrow: Grief and the loss of significant others. *Death Studies.* 1987;11:455–469.

Englebardt SP, Evans ML. Meeting consumer needs: Successful collaboration between an interdisciplinary health care team and bereaved parents. *Nurs Connect.* 1988;1(1):57–63.

Hinds P. Adolescent hopefulness in illness and health. *Adv Nurs Sci.* 1988;10(3):79–80.

Janelli LM. The impact of health status on body image in older women. *Rehab Nurs.* 1988;13(4)178–180.

Lambert VA, Lambert JP. *Psychosocial Care of the Physically Ill.* 2nd ed. Englewood Cliffs, NJ: Prentice-Hall; 1985.

Legal Advisors Committee, Concern for Dying. The right to refuse treatment: A model act. *Am J Public Health.* 1983;73:918–921.

McGlashan R. Strategies for rebuilding self-esteem for the cardiac patient. *Dimensions Crit Care Nurs.* 1988;7(1):28–38.

McKerracher B. How to lend support in a crisis. *Nursing 90.* Nov 1990:62–64.

Miller JF. *Coping With Chronic Illness: Overcoming Powerlessness.* Philadelphia: Davis; 1983.

Miller JF. Hope-inspiring strategies of the critically ill. *Appl Nurs Res.* 1989;2(1):23–29.

Mischel MH, Braden CJ. Uncertainty: A mediator between support and adjustment. *West J Nurs Res.* 1987;9:43–57.

Mischel MH, Braden CJ. Finding meaning: Antecedents of uncertainty. *Nurs Res.* 1988;37:98–103.

Mischel MH, Murdaugh C. Family experiences with heart transplantation: Redesigning the dream. *Nurs Res.* 1987;36:332–338.

Mitchell GJ. The lived experience of taking life day-by-day in later life. *Nurs Sci Q.* 1990;3:29–36.

Nelson PB. Social support, self-esteem, and depression in the institutionalized elderly. *Issues Ment Health Nurs.* 1989;10:55–68.

Pfeifer WG, Houseman C. Bereavement and AIDS. *J Psychosoc Nurs.* 1988;26(10):21–26.

Rowat KM, Knaff KA. Living with chronic pain: The spouse's perspective. *Pain.* 1985;23:259–271.

Sanders CM. *Grief: The Mourning After.* New York: John Wiley & Sons; 1989.

Schneider J. *Stress, Loss, and Grief.* Baltimore, MD: University Park Press; 1984.

Sowell RL, Bramlett MH, Gueldner SH, Gritzmacher D, Martin G. *Image: J Nurs Scholarship.* 1991;23(2):89–94.

Travis SS. Older adults' sexuality and remarriage. *J Gerontol Nurs.* 1987;13(6):9–14.

Watson J. *Nursing: Human Science and Human Care, a Theory of Nursing.* Norwalk, CT: Appleton-Century-Crofts; 1985.

Zisook S, DeVaul RA. Grief, unresolved and depression. *Psychosomatics.* 1983;24:247–256.

CHAPTER 24

Skin and Tissue Integrity

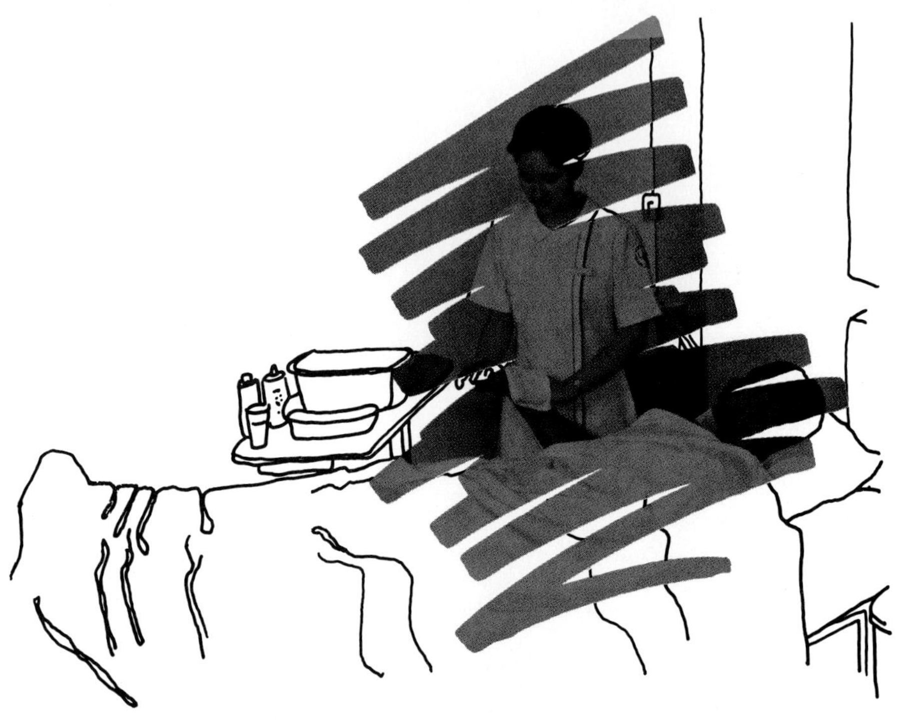

Objectives

Upon completion of this chapter, the student will be able to:

1. Discuss at least three functions of skin and mucosa.
2. Name at least four factors that influence skin and tissue integrity and describe their effects.
3. Discuss three examples of altered skin and mucosal integrity.
4. Describe the difference between primary and secondary skin lesions and list three examples of each.
5. Describe four types of wounds.
6. Discuss two processes in each of the phases of wound healing.
7. Compare and contrast healing by primary and secondary intention.
8. Discuss a collaborative approach to a health history specific to skin and tissue.
9. Describe the main elements of a skin and tissue examination.
10. State five examples of etiologies of impaired skin and tissue integrity according to the taxonomy of nursing diagnoses.
11. Discuss three examples of nursing implementation for impaired skin and tissue integrity for each of the following levels of care: preventive, supportive, restorative, and rehabilitative.
12. Discuss the importance of collaborative nurse–client management of skin and tissue integrity.
13. Discuss four general nursing approaches to enhance wound healing.

KEY TERMS

buccal mucosa
caries
collagen
conjunctiva
contusion
cornea
cyanosis
debride
dehiscence
dermatitis
dermis
ecchymosis
emollient
epidermis
epithelialization
erythema
eschar
exudate
fibroblast
gingiva
gingivitis
granulation tissue
hematoma
hemorrhage
incision
inflammation
ischemia
laceration
lesion
macrophage
normal flora
phagocytosis
pharyngitis
pilomotor activity
plaque
pressure ulcer
primary intention healing
primary lesion
rhinitis
sclera
secondary intention healing
secondary lesion
shearing
stomatitis
subcutaneous fat
tartar
thrombus
urethritis
vaginitis
wound

Skin covers all the surfaces of the body. The integument—including skin, hair, nails, and mucous membranes—comprises the body's largest organ. The integument has several purposes, including protective, excretory, secretory, sensory, and metabolic functions.

People often describe skin in terms of its appearance: firm and youthful, smooth and tan, wrinkled and leathery. We often base our first impressions of others on the appearance of skin, hair, and teeth. The appearance of skin affects the way people feel about themselves. Many individuals moisturize and apply cosmetics to their skin, color their hair, and paint their nails in an effort to improve their appearance. Applying cosmetics to enhance appearance dates back to prehistoric times. Both men and women painted their faces and bodies to attract as well as repel others.

Body odors also affect peoples' responses to others. The glands of the skin release odors that act to attract people to each other and are part of our sexuality. Various cultures have differing ideas as to which body odors are pleasant and which odors are repulsive.

Many variables affect skin, including age, exposure to sun, nutrition, ethnic background, and occupation. Some of these factors cause disruptions in skin and tissue integrity. Typical disruptions in integrity have been documented for thousands of years. Ancient cliff writings and Egyptian hieroglyphics contain references to syphilitic lesions, leprosy, and wounds. The Bible describes types of lesions and their healing. Early medical texts described the care of wounds. Many primitive cultures had "folk methods" of dealing with wounds and rashes, using a variety of mud and floral poultices. Because many alterations in health status alter skin, the assessment and care of the skin is a primary nursing concern.

This chapter addresses the anatomy and physiology of the various integumentary structures and common disruptions for which nurses may give care. Assessment for integument problems, nursing diagnoses related to skin and tissue integrity, and nursing implementation for prevention and management of integumentary problems are also discussed.

Section 1. Understanding Skin and Tissue Integrity

■ OPTIMUM SKIN AND TISSUE INTEGRITY

Intact skin and mucous membranes are part of the human body's primary defenses against a pervasive and potentially dangerous adversary: microorganisms. Integrity of skin and mucosa, therefore, protects tissue integrity throughout the body. Conversely, skin and mucosal changes often reflect changes in internal tissue integrity. Understanding the structure and function of skin and mucous membranes contributes to effective nursing assessment and management of overall health, as well as integumentary health.

Anatomy of Skin and Mucosa

Skin. To accomplish its function of protecting the body's internal environment, the skin adapts in thickness and character according to which area it covers. The soft covering of the palms of the hands differs from the soles of the feet because of their different functional needs. The skin of the eyelids has no subcutaneous fat. (Fig. 24–1) Some areas are devoid of any hair, whereas thick hair grows on the scalp and softer hair on the trunk and limbs.

The skin owes its adaptability to its three anatomical regions: the epidermis, the dermis, and the subcutaneous fat. Each region has unique functions and components while sharing specialized cells that give the skin its general properties.

Epidermis. The **epidermis** is the outer surface of the skin. Its chief function is protection of deeper tissue from the external environment. The epidermis is composed of four layers. The innermost layer is the only layer that actually produces skin cells. These cells, called basal keratinocyte cells, move up through the other epidermal layers to replenish the skin surface. This process, which normally takes 30 days, is shortened in wound healing and in aberrant conditions such as basal cell skin cancer and psoriasis, in which overproliferation of skin cells is the basis of the pathology.

The two middle epidermal layers are very active metabolically and contain a variety of cell types. Melanocytes are found here; they produce melanin, the substance that determines skin pigment and filters ultraviolet radiation from the sun. Other specialized epidermal cells provide cell-to-cell adhesion, participate in the initial identification of antigens, function as touch receptors, and give each epidermal layer its characteristic appearance.

Layers of large cornified, flattened, polyhedral cells compose the surface layer of the epidermis. The cells overlap at the margins and form interlocking ridges. This layer varies in thickness from 15 cells on the face to 100 cells on the plantar surfaces. This layer possesses properties of physical toughness, strength, flexibility, elastic return, and electrical impedance, and has a dry surface that resists moisture and microorganism growth.

Appendages. Epidermal appendages include hair, the nail unit, sebaceous glands, eccrine sweat glands, and apocrine sweat glands.

Hair. Humans have hair over the entire body surface except for the soles of the feet, palms of the hands, fingertips, glans penis, and mucocutaneous junctions (parts of the integument in which skin and mucosa merge, such as the lips). Hair develops from follicles that arise from the dermis. Follicles are present after the fifth month of fetal development; no new follicles develop after birth. Free nerve endings and arterioles and venules surround each follicle, nourishing and stimulating it. Autonomic nerve action causes hair to "stand on end" due to pilomotor stimulation.

The first hair formed in utero is called lanugo. It is a very fine, downy type hair. Most of it sloughs off before birth, but infants' hair growth continues from the same follicles. Children and adults have two types of hair: soft hair that covers the body, and longer, more coarse hair that grows on the scalp, eyebrows, and eyelashes. After puberty it also appears in the axillary and pubic areas.

Individual hairs may be straight, spiral, or wavy. Straight hair is due to straight vertical hair follicles and is typical in orientals. Spiral hair, seen in blacks, arises from curved follicles having the lower portion of the follicle horizontal to the skin surface. The white race has a combination of all three types. Generally, whites have the most body hair among racial groups, and orientals the least.

Hair has five important functions. It is a sexually attractive body element, acts to filter irritants in the nasal passages, protects the scalp and skin, serves as a shield for the eyes from sun and sweat droplets, and aids in tactile perception.

Nail Unit. The nail unit consists of the nail plate and the tissue surrounding it. The nail plate is hard, convex, rectangular, and translucent. Nail growth is continuous. Fingernails grow at a rate of about 1 mm per week; toenails grow more slowly. The fingernails and toenails protect the terminal phalanges, participate in tactile stimulation, scratch, and allow humans to grasp minute objects.

Sebaceous Glands. The sebaceous glands produce sebum, a lipid substance. They are usually associated with hair follicles. Sebum regulates skin absorption of fluid and chemicals, lubricates the hair and skin surface, carries out antibacterial and antifungal activity, and is a vitamin D precursor.

Eccrine Sweat Glands. The eccrine sweat glands are the true sweat glands, and are present all over the body. Their primary function is to produce sweat during periods of internal or external heat stress to cool the body through evaporation.

Sweating also can occur during periods of emotional stress. The palms, soles, axilla, and forehead have sweat glands that react to emotions. Sweaty palms or beads of perspiration on the brow are often indicators of fear or anxiety.

Contact Dermatitis. Contact dermatitis, a skin irritation that results from exposure to a noxious substance, may be a result of sweating. Sweat can cause salts to leak from jewelry or clothing (such as wool) and the resulting mixture of these salts and sweat produces a skin reaction.

Apocrine Sweat Glands. The apocrine sweat glands are distributed primarily in the axillae, anogenital area, abdomen, face, and scalp. Specialized apocrine glands produce cerumen (wax) in the external ear canal. Apocrine secretion occurs in response to both physical and emotional stress. In lower animals, apocrine secretions allow species identification.

Dermis. The **dermis** lies directly below the epidermis and contains the specialized capillaries, nerve ends, and lymph channels of the skin.

The dermis is composed mostly of noncellular connective tissue, including collagen, elastin fibers, and ground substance. It is divided into two layers, a thin zone that interfaces with the epidermis in wavelike projections called papillae, and a thicker layer that contains a variety of specialized cells.

The components of the dermis have specific functions in addition to giving structure to the dermis. **Collagen** is essential for wound healing and scar formation; it gives the healing wound tensile strength. Elastin fibers give the skin its ability to return to its original shape after stretching. Ground substance promotes cell migration in wound healing, acts as a glue to hold skin surfaces together while healing occurs, and influences the skin's osmotic properties be-

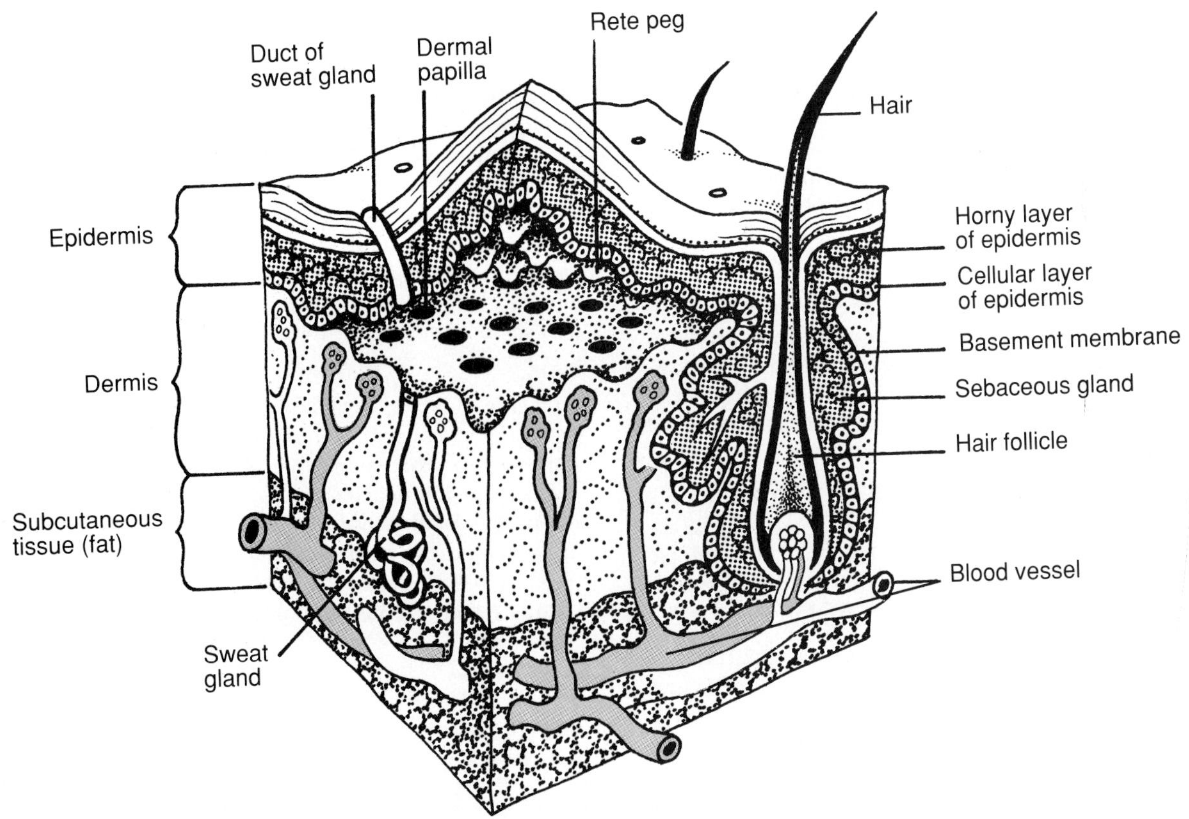

Figure 24–1. Skin cross-section.

cause of its ability to retain water (up to 1000 times its own weight).

Fibroblasts, macrophages, and mast cells are the primary functioning cells within the dermis. **Fibroblasts** act in the building and rebuilding of connective tissue. They are active in wound healing. **Macrophages** are phagocytes; they are particularly important in the inflammatory process. Mast cells are highly specialized cells that also play a role in inflammation.

Subcutaneous Fat. A lipid layer lying below the dermis, **subcutaneous fat** contains major vascular networks, the lymphatics, and nerve fibers. Its thickness varies: It is absent in the eyelids, penis, and scrotum, but prominent on hips, thighs, and buttocks. Women generally have more subcutaneous fat than men, but there is considerable variation in amounts among individuals of both sexes.

Subcutaneous fat serves several protective functions. It acts as an insulator, preventing loss of body heat in cold environments. The body retains heat because fat is a poor conductor of heat. Fat protects internal organs from impact trauma, acting as a shock absorber. It is also a storage form of energy that can be mobilized when nutritional intake is diminished.

Dermal–Epidermal Junction. This area between the dermis and epidermis is also called the basement membrane zone. The basement membrane appears to play an integral role in the inflammatory process (discussed later in the chapter) and also acts as a filter barrier that regulates the passage of molecules into the dermis.

Mucosa and Related Structures. Mucosa lines many organs that communicate with the outside of the body.

Oral Cavity. The hard and soft palate form the roof of the oral cavity. The mouth contains several types of mucosa, as well as mucosal appendages: the tongue, salivary glands, and the teeth.

Oral Mucosa. The oral mucous membranes form a continuous covering extending from the lips to the oral pharynx. The fibrous tissue covering the alveolar surfaces of the jawbone and surrounding the teeth is called the **gingiva,** or gums. The membrane covering the interior surface of the cheeks is called the **buccal mucosa.**

Tongue. The tongue is a highly specialized organ. Its primary functions are taste, speech, mastication, and sensation. The tongue has a rough, rosy texture due to the papillae on its dorsal surface. The ventral surface is smooth and delicate.

Salivary Glands. The salivary glands are located under the tongue, at the base of the jaw, and beneath the ear. Saliva—a clear, odorless, tasteless, and somewhat viscid (sticky) liquid—lubricates the oral cavity, facilitating chewing and swallowing of food, and initiates the digestion of starches. Saliva also acts as a solvent for waste excretion and assists in the regulation of water balance. The presence of food in the mouth stimulates the salivary glands; even seeing or smelling food can cause salivation because of a conditioned reflex. The dry mouth that occurs during stress is due to adrenergic (sympathetic) nervous system suppression of salivation. Saliva becomes ropey and more viscid when a person becomes dehydrated, breathes through the mouth, or ingests drugs like atropine or antihistamines.

Teeth. The teeth are suspended in the gums by periodontal ligaments. Children have 20 deciduous teeth that begin to erupt at about 6 months of age, and are lost during the early school-age period. Thirty-two permanent teeth gradually replace them. The teeth are living structures with a circulatory and nerve supply that is contained in the inner core of the tooth, called the pulp. Dentin, the primary tissue of the tooth, surrounds the pulp. Enamel, a hard substance, covers the exposed portion of the tooth, called the crown. The primary functions of teeth are to bite and masticate (chew) food.

Eyes. Fibrous membranes called the sclera and the cornea cover the eye. The **sclera,** white and opaque, extends from the optic nerve to the cornea. The **cornea** is continuous with the sclera, but is transparent and colorless. The cornea plays a role in refraction. The mucous membrane that lines the eyelids is called the **conjunctiva;** it is attached to the sclera (see Figs. 16–33 and 16–34). Tears, secreted by the lacrimal glands, keep the conjunctiva, sclera, and cornea moist. Tears cleanse the eye and protect it from contamination by pollutants.

Nose and Pharynx. The mucous membranes and accessory structures in the nose filter, warm, and moisturize incoming air. Nasal hairs screen out larger particles, while cilia on the mucosa remove smaller particles. The mucus-producing goblet cells lining the nasal passages moisturize incoming air. The abundant blood vessels in nasal mucosa also warm the air as it passes to the lower respiratory tract.

The pharyngeal (throat) mucosa is continuous with nasal mucosa and extends to the base of the larynx. It is similar to the mucosa of the respiratory tract, and contains lymphoid tissue, which makes up the tonsils. A dry sensation in the pharyngeal mucosa is part of the mechanism that stimulates thirst.

Genitalia. Glandular vaginal epithelium, which lies in folds called rugae, covers the smooth-muscle walls of the vagina. This mucosa produces a continuous flow of fluid that serves to maintain vaginal cleanliness. The vestibule (the area between the labia majora in females) contains the vaginal opening and the urinary meatus. It is covered with very thin, almost mucosal skin. Bartholin's and Skene's glands, both of which produce mucus, especially during sexual excitement, also open into the vestibule.

Mucosal tissue also lines the urethra in the male reproductive tract. The bulbourethral glands open into the urethra and produce a rather viscid secretion that lubricates the urethra.

Anus and Rectum. Mucous membranes also line the rectum and anus. The rectal mucosa lies in transverse folds that contain rectal smooth muscle. In the upper third of the anal canal, the mucosa forms vertical folds containing arteries and veins. The mucous membrane merges into skin in the distal third of the anal canal.

Functions of Skin and Mucosa

Protection. The outer layer of the epidermis is a relatively impermeable layer of interlocking cells that provides a mechanical barrier to protect underlying tissue from the environment. The epidermis resists penetration by mechanical forces as well as bacteria. The epidermis is also moisture resistant: the multilayered epidermis and the presence of sebum minimize the loss of body fluids or absorption of liquids on the surface of the skin. This ability to control diffusion affects the efficacy of topical medicines and the intensity of hypersensitivity allergic responses. The dry surface of the epidermis also serves to impede electrical current from low-voltage sources. Keratin and the melanocytes in the inner epidermal layers act to filter ultraviolet light.

Antimicrobial action is another form of protection afforded by the skin and mucosa. Even when a break occurs in the skin, the basement membrane of the dermal–epidermal junction acts as an effective filter to limit invasion of foreign substances. The cells of the dermis marshal the body's defenses if microbes do gain entrance, initiating the inflammatory response and, in some cases, a specific immunological response. The skin also hosts a variety of nonpathogenic organisms known as **normal flora.** These organisms provide further protection against invasion by pathogenic bacteria. Normal flora create a biological niche for themselves, thereby effectively competing with other bacterial strains for nutrients and space.

Mucous membranes also afford protection. When intact, mucous membranes are impermeable to bacteria, although viruses are able to penetrate them. The most effective protection afforded by mucosa is related to the secretion of mucus, which traps microbes and other foreign materials so they can be more readily disposed of, for example, by coughing. Mucus secretions also contain antimicrobial enzymes that are lethal to many invading bacteria.

Temperature Regulation. The hypothalamus and receptors in the dermis regulate body temperature. When skin receptors sense a change in environmental temperature, specific responses to conserve heat or to prevent an increase in core temperature occur.

When an individual is exposed to cold, constriction of blood vessels in the skin and subcutaneous tissue minimizes the amount of heat energy carried by the blood from the interior to the surface of the body. **Pilomotor activity,** or "gooseflesh," also appears, trapping a layer of warm air next to the surface of the body, which acts as an insulator against heat loss.

An increase in environmental or core body temperature, on the other hand, stimulates vasodilation, facilitating heat transfer from the body to the environment. Sweating occurs, enhancing heat loss by evaporation. More than 80 percent of the body heat loss occurs via the skin by radiation, conduction, convection, and/or evaporation (Table 24–1). The effectiveness of each of these processes depends on the relative differences in skin and environmental temperature and on humidity.

Sensation. Skin is an important organ of sensation. A person's ability to discriminate touch, pressure, pain, and temperature is due to a complex network of nerve fibers in the dermis. Specialized receptors as well as free nerve endings transmit the varied impulses that communicate information about the immediate environment as well as initiate important reflexes that are important in adapting to the environment. These receptors react to different thresholds of stimulation and sensation depending on the region of the body in which they occur.

Excretion. Although the skin is not a major excretory organ, excretion of varied amounts of water, salts, and urea occurs via the skin. Under certain abnormal conditions water loss via the skin can be substantial enough to cause fluid imbalance.

Lubrication. Lubrication is primarily a function of mucosa. When mucosa are irritated by chemical or mechanical stimuli, mucus is produced. The mucus protects the usually fragile membranes from damage that could result from such

TABLE 24–1. PROCESSES OF HEAT TRANSFER

Process and Definition	Application to Temperature Regulation
Radiation: Transfer of infrared rays through space.	When in proximity to, but not touching, cold objects in the environment body heat is lost. Proximity to warm objects causes a local increase in temperature.
Conduction: Transfer of heat between two objects of different temperature through molecular vibration.	When placed in contact with cold objects or immersed in a cold liquid, body heat is lost. Contact with warm objects causes a local increase in temperature. Cooling of the body by moving air (eg, wind or a fan).
Convection: Transfer of heat between objects/areas by circulating liquid or gas.	Transfer of heat from body interior to surface via blood and exhaled air.
Evaporation: Transformation from liquid to gaseous state.	Body heat is absorbed by the environment with insensible perspiration and in greater amounts with sweating, cooling the skin surface.

stimuli. Mucus also provides needed lubrication for bodily functions such as bowel elimination and sexual activity.

FACTORS AFFECTING SKIN AND TISSUE INTEGRITY

Age

Infants. A protective substance called vernix caseosa, a whitish creamy secretion produced by the sebaceous glands, usually covers a newborn's skin at birth. It is usually absorbed by the skin or removed during the infant's first bath. Lanugo, the precursor to body hair, may also be present, particularly over the shoulders and back. Newborns' skin feels soft and smooth. It is particularly vulnerable to environmental irritants, which may produce rashes. Other common skin variations include milia (small white papules caused by plugged sebaceous glands) over the bridge of the nose and forehead; acrocyanosis (bluish tinged hands and feet, related to uncoordinated vasomotor responses to temperature changes and oxygen demands); petechiae (red pinpoint capillary hemorrhages) over the head and face; and mongolian spots (area of darker pigmentation over the lower back and buttocks due to uneven melanocyte distribution in dark-skinned babies). Some newborns have birthmarks such as capillary hemangiomas (dilated capillaries), which usually disappear by the age of 1 year; or permanent birthmarks such as strawberry marks, nevus flammeus, and port wine stains.

Many newborns develop physiological jaundice at 24 to 48 hours of age. This is because the number of red blood cells needed for oxygenation in utero is greater than that needed after the transition to extrauterine life, so unneeded red blood cells are destroyed after birth, producing jaundice. Desquamation (peeling or sloughing of the outer epidermal layer) is also common during the first several weeks of life.

Infant integument problems that may require treatment include diaper rash, cradle cap, and thrush (an oral cavity yeast infection).

Toddlers Through School Age. During this time period the skin takes on the appearance and most of the functions of adult skin. It is more resistant to injury, irritation, and infection than during infancy. Nevertheless, abrasions and lacerations associated with play activities, and allergic or infectious forms of **dermatitis** (inflammation of the skin characterized by redness and itchiness), do occur.

Adolescents. Adolescents experience several skin changes associated with physical maturation. The sebaceous glands begin to produce sebum, a complex mixture of cholesterol, fatty acids, and waxy alcohols, several years prior to puberty because of stimulation by sex hormones. The larger glands of the face and scalp are particularly sensitive to androgens (male sex hormones produced by testis, adrenal glands, and ovaries), giving rise to acne and other skin eruptions. Apocrine glands become active at the onset of puberty and secrete a substance that exudes odor in the presence of bacteria. Body hair changes in character and distribution. Both boys and girls develop pubic and axillary hair and body hair becomes thicker and more noticeable. Boys also begin growing facial hair. In girls, there are increases in subcutaneous fat deposits over the hips, thighs, and breasts.

Middle-aged and Older Adults. There are few age-related skin problems affecting middle-aged adults. The next age-related integumentary changes occur later in life, although there is considerable variation in the age of onset and the rate of progress of changes. The skin of older people loses elasticity, appearing more wrinkled, with deeper folds because of collagen changes and loss of subcutaneous fat. The fingerlike projections that attach the epidermis to the dermis flatten with aging, weakening the attachment. This increases vulnerability to epidermal tears, which occur as a result of even minimal friction or shearing.[1] Blood vessels are more fragile and less protected because of collagen tissue changes, and so even minor trauma results in purpura (localized hemorrhages into the skin, initially having a red to purplish appearance, and then fading to yellowish-brown before disappearing). This is called senile purpura, because of its relationship to the aging process. The bleeding beneath the epidermis makes epidermal detachment easier, and so skin tears are a frequent complication of purpura.

Pigmentation changes related to altered melanocyte activity—such as mottling, darkened spots ("age" or "liver" spots), particularly on the face and back of hands—and gray hair are common. Sebum production diminishes after menopause in women, and in the late 70s in men; the loss of lubrication causes dry, flaky skin and dry hair. Some hair follicles cease to function, so scalp hair is thinner, but women sometimes experience an increase in facial hair because estrogen is depleted and no longer balances the influence of androgen. Nails become thicker and more brittle because of overgrowth of keratin, grow more slowly, and may appear yellow due to deposition of calcium. The skin of older adults is a less effective barrier against infection, and immune function is somewhat diminished. As a result, susceptibility to fungal, bacterial, and viral infections increases. Vascular insufficiency is more common among older adults; shiny, hairless skin and stasis ulcers are manifestations of this.

Exposure to Sun

Sun exposure is damaging to skin. Premature development of skin changes associated with aging occurs in individuals who experience frequent and regular exposure to sun without use of protective skin preparations. Sunburn is even more serious. It damages deeper skin layers and its destructive effects are cumulative. Repeated overexposure to the sun's ultraviolet rays significantly increases the risk of basal cell carcinoma, a skin cancer characterized by excessive and uncontrolled production of basal epithelial cells that invade the dermis rather than migrate upward to the skin's surface.[2] This means that children and adolescents who suffer frequent sunburn are in significantly greater jeopardy for developing this form of cancer; although sun exposure, particularly sunburn, at any age increases risk.

Nutritional Status

The integument is particularly vulnerable to deficiencies in essential nutrients, because of the rapid turnover of its cells. Protein and vitamin deficiencies in particular result in diminished maintenance of skin integrity and poor wound healing. Vitamin deficiency diseases typically produce skin manifestations such as dermatitis (vitamin B_6, niacin, riboflavin); cracks in the corners of the mouth (vitamin B_6, riboflavin); and edema (thiamin). Deficiency of vitamin C causes petechiae and bleeding gingivae. Insufficient vitamin A results in epithelial cells becoming plugged with excess keratin, forming unsightly bumps on the skin. Hyperkeratinization interferes with mucus production as well, so mucosa throughout the body becomes dry and hardened.

Personal Hygiene

Variations in personal hygiene practices impair or enhance skin and mucosal integrity. Skin, hair, and mucosa that are well cared for—cleaned regularly with mild soap and moisturized with emollients—remain in optimal condition.

Poor hygiene makes the integument vulnerable to insult and can even cause breakdown and deterioration. For example, inadequate oral hygiene promotes dental caries and permits buildup of excessive amounts of dental plaque, which eventually causes severe periodontal disease and loss of teeth.

Infrequent bathing causes skin irritation from accumulated oil, dead skin cells, perspiration, and bacteria. Skin folds are particularly vulnerable; skin in these areas may break down. Genital and anal–rectal mucosa may become excoriated from residue of urine and fecal matter. Conversely, excessive bathing, or bathing with harsh soaps, hinders the protective actions of sebum, producing dryness and compromised antibacterial action.

Health Status

The integument reflects overall health state. A healthy person generally has healthy integument: skin, teeth, nails, hair, and mucous membranes. Ill health may alter the integument.

Acute Conditions. Some acute illnesses cause temporary changes in skin and mucosal status. For example, any condition in which there is abnormal body fluid loss, such as vomiting or diarrhea, will eventually produce dry skin and mucosa, and thickened or diminished secretions (mucus, tears, saliva). Dehydration also precipitates loss of skin turgor (elasticity), so skin appears loose and flabby. The effects of dehydration are discussed in greater detail in Chapter 31.

Many minor infectious diseases have skin rashes as one manifestation. In some of these the skin is the target organ of the infectious agent; in others the skin manifestations are secondary. Dermatitis is a common response to environmental allergens; inflammation of nasal, pharyngeal, and respiratory mucosa also may occur because of allergens. Some acute illnesses such as upper respiratory infections or vaginal infections cause mucosal irritation, resulting in increased mucus production. Continuous drainage of mucosal discharge also may irritate surrounding skin.

Pressure ulcers are another example of skin changes related to health status. **Pressure ulcers** are areas of cellular necrosis that develop when soft tissue is pressed between a bony prominence and a firm surface.[3] They are often associated with periods of immobility related to illness. Pressure ulcers are discussed in greater detail later in this chapter.

Integument alterations associated with acute conditions are usually self-limiting, that is, they heal spontaneously when the causative agent is no longer present.

IMPLICATIONS FOR NURSE–CLIENT COLLABORATION

Life-style

Life-style is a frequent cause of skin problems. Personal choices regarding hygiene, diet, and sun exposure, for example, may be causal, contributing, or exacerbating conditions. A collaborative approach to dealing with skin problems involves the nurse's recognition of the importance of a client's personal preferences. Sensitive information sharing is likely to result in trust and effective problem resolution.

Chronic Conditions. Many chronic diseases generate integumentary manifestations. Some of these are diseases in which the primary pathology involves the skin. The specific type of skin change or lesion depends on the specific disease. In other cases, the effects on the skin are secondary to pathology in other organs. For example, skin is particularly vulnerable to circulatory disorders. Interference with circulation causes a wide range of skin changes. Milder manifestations include thinning of skin layers, decreased sebum production, and loss of hair. More pronounced disruption of circulation produces stasis ulcers and tissue death. Diabetes mellitus is one cause of poor peripheral circulation. Some individuals with respiratory conditions suffer similar skin changes because of low oxygen concentration in the blood, even though circulation to the skin is intact.

■ ALTERATIONS IN SKIN AND MUCOSAL INTEGRITY

Skin Pigmentation Changes

Hyperpigmentation. Some variations in the skin are the result of an increase in pigmentation. Normal color variation between races is a result of the increase in the number and size of melanocytes and the rate at which melanin is produced. An increased production of melanin produces hyperpigmentation. A suntan is one example of hyperpigmentation. Sunlight activates increased production of melanin. The ability to tan varies among individuals. Light-skinned, blue- or green-eyed individuals produce pigment more slowly than those whose skin is normally darker. Sunburn results when sun exposure exceeds an individual's ability to produce melanin. The result is redness and tenderness, often appearing several hours after the sun exposure.

Hyperpigmentation also occurs in freckles, skin changes in pregnancy (chloasma and linea nigra), aging (age spots on upper body and face), and certain drug and allergic reactions (silver nitrate, perfumes, and the antimalarials).

Hypopigmentation. Decreased or absent melanin production is quite rare. It results in a decrease in pigmentation. Albinism is a congenital lack of pigmentation that may be total or partial. Vitiligo, in which areas of normal coloring surround patchy areas without pigmentation, is an acquired condition that is thought to be due to decreased cholinesterase activity in the skin or to an autoimmune process.

Color Changes. The skin changes in color in response to a variety of internal conditions. A decrease in capillary flow or in blood components will be visible on the skin surface, causing **pallor** (pale skin). **Erythema** is a generalized area of redness that blanches when palpated. It is due to dilation of superficial capillaries. **Cyanosis,** a bluish-gray skin color, occurs when oxygen content of the intravascular hemoglobin is diminished or when blood flow rate is slowed, for example, when a person is chilled. Increased serum bilirubin level will cause the skin to have a yellowish cast, called **jaundice**.

Skin Lesions

A **lesion** is a circumscribed area of pathologically altered tissue. Skin lesions may be primary or secondary.

Primary Lesions. Primary lesions appear in previously healthy skin. They are classified according to their size, shape, and contents. Primary lesions may be flat or raised, circular or lobulated. They may be filled with clear fluid, pus, or solid matter. There are many causes of primary lesions, including trauma, allergens, infectious agents, and cancer. Advise clients to bring persistent skin lesions to the attention of a health care provider to determine cause and appropriate treatment. The terms used when describing primary lesions, with accompanying illustrations and definitions, appear in Table 16–4.

Secondary Lesions. Secondary lesions are alterations in primary lesions, such as erosion of deeper skin layers or cracking of skin surrounding a primary lesion. Scars are also considered secondary lesions because they represent dermal changes following a primary lesion. Table 16–5 provides definitions and descriptions of common secondary lesions.

Mucosal Disruptions

Oral Mucosa. Oral mucosal lesions include mechanical trauma, stomatitis, tooth and gum problems, and malignant changes.

Mechanical Trauma. Mechanical trauma to oral cavity structures is due to accidental occurrences or chronic irritants. The resultant lesion may be erosion of oral mucosa, puncture wounds, lacerations, or burns.

Examples of accidental causes of trauma include overly vigorous tooth brushing, chewing on sharp objects, biting oneself, and ingesting very hot foods or beverages. Chronic irritation develops from orthodontic braces, loose-fitting dentures, and cigarette and pipe smoking. Some treatment modalities used in health care facilities, such as oral airways and nasotrachial or orogastric tubes, also cause irritation to the oral cavity.

Stomatitis. **Stomatitis** is inflammation of the mouth. Causative factors include pathogens (bacteria, fungus, yeast, or viruses); chemical substances (ingredients in mouth-care products, medications, especially cancer chemotherapy); systemic infections (measles, syphilis); and vitamin deficiency.

Typically, stomatitis presents with numerous small vesicles on the cheeks, palate, gums, or oral pharynx. Sometimes there are also lesions on the tongue (glossitis). The vesicles soon break and leave shallow ulcers with reddened edges. The lesions are uncomfortable, and may make eating difficult. Some causative agents of stomatitis produce agent-specific lesions; for example, thrush (a yeast infection) produces white plaque-like lesions; measles produce small red spots with blue-white centers.

Tooth and Gum Problems. The most common tooth and gum problems are associated with the accumulation of dental plaque because of ineffective or infrequent oral hygiene. **Plaque** is a mixture of saliva, bacteria, and sloughed epithelial cells. Sugary foods tend to make plaque more adherent to teeth. The presence of plaque on the tooth can cause demineralization of the tooth enamel. As the enamel wears away, bacteria enter the dentin of the tooth and cause **caries** (tooth decay or "cavities"). Bacteria present in the plaque are often odor producing, causing halitosis.

Plaque is also an irritant to the gingiva. When plaque is not removed from the teeth by regular oral hygiene, plaque is transformed into **tartar,** a hard yellowish substance that forms along the gum line. Prolonged contact of the gingiva with tartar causes inflammation and bleeding of the gums, called **gingivitis.** Chronic gingivitis often progresses to periodontal disease, in which the supporting structures of the teeth degenerate, resulting in loosening and loss of teeth.

Other gum problems include hyperplasia (overgrowth of epithelial tissue), most frequently secondary to use of certain anticonvulsant medications, and sordes, a crustlike accumulation of dead cells, food debris, and microorganisms.

Malignant Lesions. Malignant lesions in the oral cavity occur on the tongue, gums, and associated bony processes. The original lesions may be whitish-gray plaques, lumps, or small ulcerations. As the disease extends, the ulcerations become more extensive and may cause numbness. Early treatment is often curative, but extensive lesions usually require radical surgical dissection. For this reason, persistent mouth sores or mouth pain should be investigated to determine their origin.

Corneal Mucosa. Disruptions of corneal mucosa result from foreign bodies or chemical injury. Foreign bodies are often small airborne particles such as dust that blow into the eye. They are easily removed and usually do little harm, although they may cause considerable discomfort because the cornea is very sensitive. When a foreign body penetrates the sclera or cornea, damage to the eye may result. This kind of injury is considered a medical emergency and must be treated immediately.

Contact lens wearers may experience corneal abrasions because of poorly fitting lenses or foreign bodies being trapped under the lens. These problems are more common with hard contact lenses.

Many chemicals are toxic to the conjunctival mucosa, sclera, and cornea. They create a burn or ulcer. Immediately flushing the eye with water for 5 minutes or more may remove the chemical before damage results. If irritation persists after flushing, medical assistance is advisable.

Nasal and Throat Mucosa. **Rhinitis** (inflammation of nasal mucosa) and **pharyngitis** (inflammation of throat mucosa) are common minor illnesses. The usual cause of acute inflammation is viral or bacterial invasion of the tissues. Mucosa become reddened and painful and mucus production increases. With bacterial infection, discharge is often purulent. Smoking causes a chronically irritated, reddened throat and a characteristic "smoker's cough" from frequent need to clear the airways of accumulated mucus.

Genital Mucosa. Disruptions of genital mucosa include **vaginitis** (inflammation of vaginal mucosa) and **urethritis** (inflammation of the urethra). Infection by bacteria, viruses, protozoa, or yeast is the most common cause of genital mucosal disruptions. The infectious agent may be sexually transmitted or be transmitted from the anal area because of incorrect wiping of the perineum in women. Occasionally, yeast infections result from disruptions in normal vaginal flora after a course of systemic antibiotic therapy. Neoplasms (tumors), foreign bodies such as a retained tampon, or chemical irritation from strong douches are other causes of vaginitis.

Symptoms include discharge that is sometimes malodorous, pruritus (itching) of the vulva and perineum, and painful urination. The vaginal mucosa appears red and may have superficial ulcerations; the urethra in males is not visualized to diagnose this condition.

Atrophic vaginitis frequently occurs in postmenopausal women, or women experiencing disruption of estrogen production for other reasons. The vaginal mucosa becomes thinner and vaginal mucus secretion declines. Some women experience pruritus with this condition. Painful intercourse is sometimes associated with atrophic vaginitis, because lubrication is diminished.

Anal and Rectal Mucosa. Hemorrhoids (enlarged veins in the mucosa of the anal canal) and anorectal fissures (cracklike lesions) are common problems of anal and rectal mucosa. Hemorrhoids have varied causes; frequently straining at stool is a contributing factor (see also Chap. 26). Anal fissures are often trauma related, resulting, for example, from passage of extremely hard stool or anal intercourse. Local pain, particularly upon defecation, and itching are symptoms of both problems.

Wounds

A **wound** is an injury to tissue that disrupts normal cellular processes. It may involve a break in the integrity of the skin or mucous membranes and/or damage to deeper tissue. Wounds may result from mechanical, thermal, chemical, or radiation trauma, or from invasion by pathogens. Surgical incisions, accidental scrapes and cuts, and pressure ulcers are examples of wounds.

Types of Wounds. Several overlapping descriptive categories including severity, cause, and contamination may be used to classify wounds.

Severity. Severity relates to type and amount of tissue damage. For example, in reference to skin integrity, closed wounds are wounds in which skin remains intact, but there is damage to soft tissue or deeper structures, and open wounds are those in which skin or mucosa is damaged. Wounds are also described in terms of extent of injury. Superficial or partial-thickness wounds involve only the epidermis and/or part of the dermis. Tissue-loss wounds are deeper wounds, with damage or destruction of subcutaneous fat, muscle, bone, or other structures.

Cause. Wounds may also be described according to how they were acquired. In an abrasion, all or part of the skin or mucosa is scraped away. Skinned knees and dermabrasions (a cosmetic skin procedure) are examples. Burns are injuries due to heat, radiation, chemicals, or electricity. Thermal and electrical burns are classified by degrees, depending on the depth of tissue injury. First-degree burns are minor, injuring only the outer epidermis; second-degree burns extend into the dermis, causing blisters; third-degree burns destroy epidermis and dermis and damage underlying tissue as well. Tissue may be charred or coagulated.

A **contusion** is a blow from a blunt object that entails soft tissue damage, but no break in the skin. Often bleeding is associated with contusions. Diffuse bleeding into surrounding tissue is called an **ecchymosis** (bruise); encapsulated bleeding is known as a **hematoma.** **Lacerations** are tears of tissue having uneven edges and often contaminated with dirt, grass, or other debris. Lacerations can involve skin and muscle layers.

A puncture wound is a wound made by a sharp pointed instrument that penetrates the dermal layer. Stepping on a nail or getting a splinter are examples of minor puncture wounds. Puncture wounds are prone to become infected because they bleed little and are difficult to cleanse. A foreign object entering deeper tissue or a body cavity such as the chest or abdomen causes a penetrating wound. If the foreign object enters and then exits an internal organ, the wound is called a perforating wound. An incision is a clean-edged cut made with a sharp instrument. Most incisions are intentional surgical wounds.

A pressure ulcer is a wound caused by lack of perfu-

TABLE 24–2. STAGES OF PRESSURE ULCERS

Stage	Illustration	Description
Stage 1	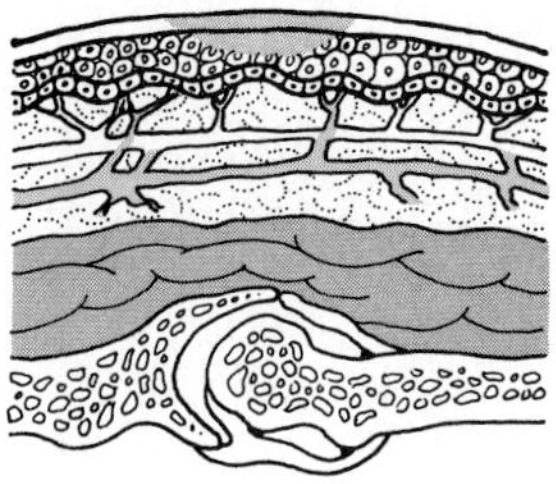	Involves epidermis only. Ranges from swollen pinkish-red mottled skin that does not return to normal color after pressure is relieved, to a moist, superficial, irregular ulceration that exposes the dermis and resembles an abrasion.
Stage 2	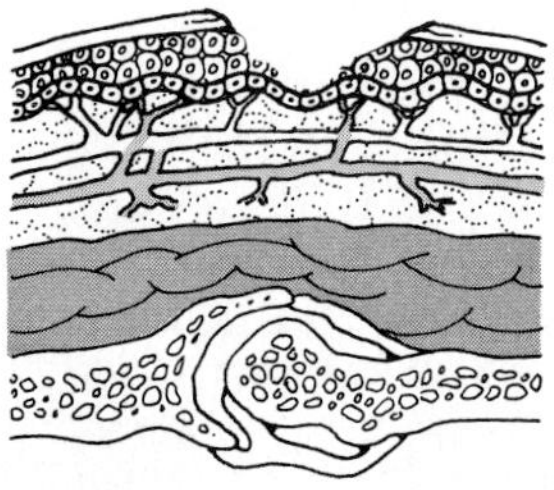	A full-thickness ulcer that extends through the dermis to subcutaneous fat.
Stage 3	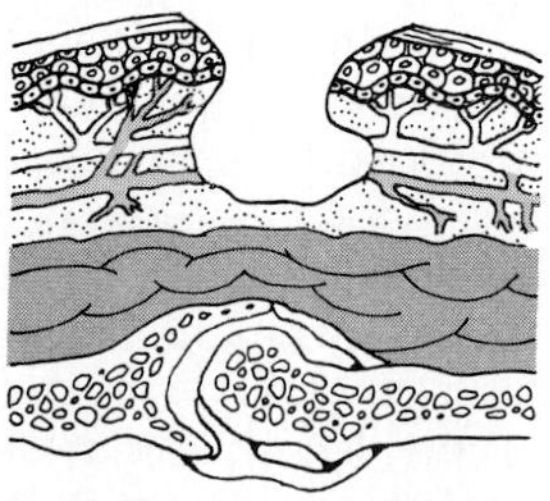	Ulceration involves deeper tissue, invading subcutaneous fat where extensive undermining can occur, because deep fascia limits the depth of penetration of necrosis.
Stage 4	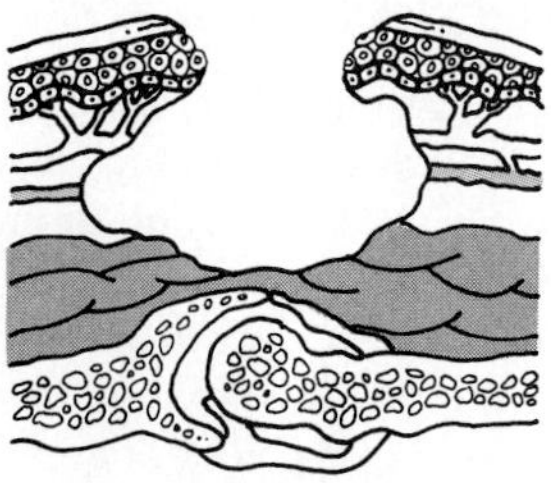	Ulcer penetrates deep fascia and muscle, and may expose bone.
Stage 5	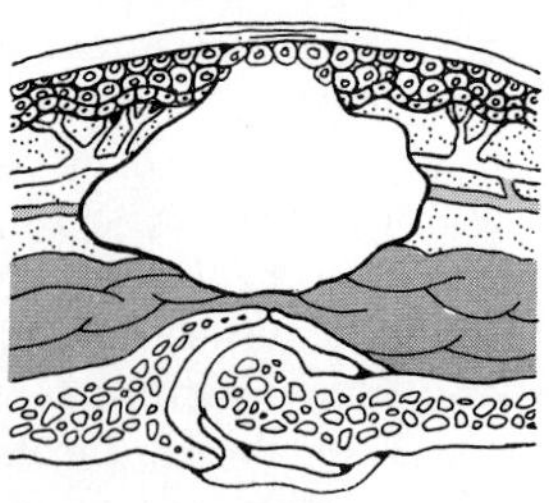	Closed-surface epidermis or draining skin defect with underlying cavity.

From Shea J. Pressure sores: Classification and management. Clin Orthopedics. *1975; 112:89–100.*

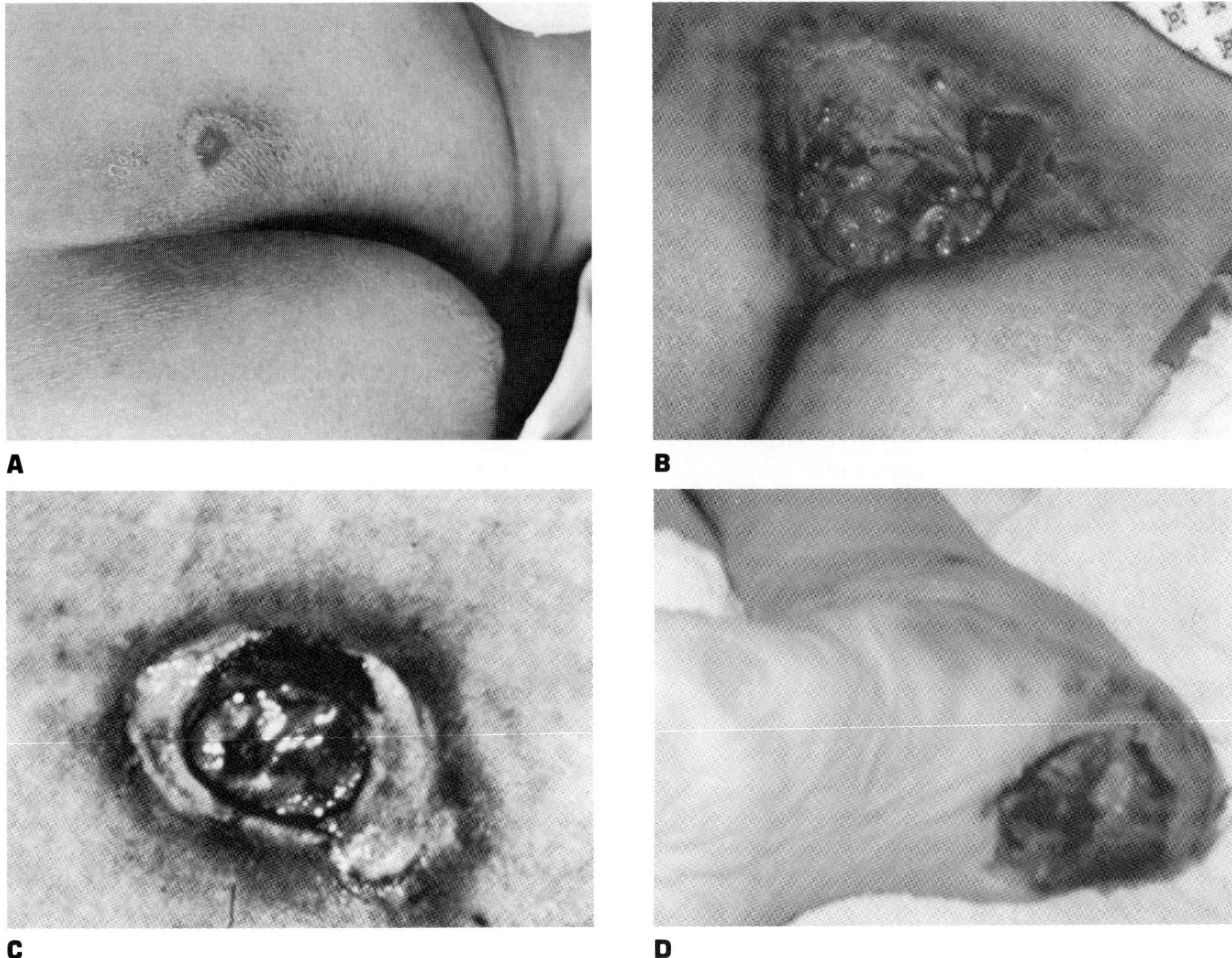

Figure 24–2. Stages of pressure ulcers. **A.** Stage 1 ulcer. **B.** Stage 2 ulcer. **C.** Stage 3 ulcer. **D.** Stage 4 ulcer. (*B–D from Smith S, Duell D.* Clinical Nursing Skills: Nursing Process Model; Basic to Advanced Skills, *3rd ed. Norwalk, CT: Appleton & Lange; 1992.*)

sion to tissue because external pressure compromises capillary circulation. Pressure ulcers are graded from stage 1 to stage 4, according to the extent of tissue damage. The stages are summarized in Table 24–2 and illustrated in Figure 24–2.

Contamination. The American College of Surgeons has classified wounds on the basis of actual or potential contamination. Contaminants are agents in the wound that may cause infection, render a surgical site less clean, or interfere with healing. Examples of contaminating agents are bacteria, fecal material, soil, and gravel particles. There are four levels in the classification:

- *Clean wound.* Wound makes no contact with body cavities having bacterial populations (normal flora). Occurs in tissue that is not infected. Example: breast surgery.
- *Clean-contaminated wound.* Wound enters an organ that has normal flora or that connects with an organ having normal flora. Example: lung surgery.
- *Contaminated wound.* Open accidental wounds; surgery with a break in sterile technique or in which gastrointestinal drainage or drainage from an infected area contacts the wound. Example: ruptured appendix.
- *Infected wound.* Wound in which microorganisms are multiplying and producing injurious effects. Example: drainage of an abscess.

WOUND HEALING

Wound healing is a spontaneous restorative process that is initiated immediately after a wound is inflicted. There are two stages of healing: inflammation and repair. The nature of repair and the length of each stage varies with the type of wound as well as with local and systemic host factors. The following sections will provide an overview of the processes in wound healing and the factors that influence healing.

Process of Wound Healing

The healing process consists of three overlapping phases: inflammation, proliferation, and maturation.

Inflammation. **Inflammation** is a nonspecific defensive response to injury. It is initiated by the release of intracellular chemicals from injured tissues. Inflammation serves to control bleeding, protect from bacterial invasion, remove debris from tissue injury, and prepare for repair.[4] Several physiological mechanisms work together to achieve these ends.

Mechanisms in Inflammation. Immediate vasoconstriction at the site of an injury and the accumulation of platelets along damaged blood vessel walls accomplish the goal of controlling bleeding. The clotting mechanism, involving a complex series of interactions among coagulation factors, produces a platelet and fibrin plug called a clot or **thrombus** to seal off the site of the injury from further blood loss.

Protection from bacterial invasion results from **phagocytosis** (ingestion and digestion of foreign cells and debris) and **epithelialization** (migration of epithelial cells to close the wound site), which occur simultaneously. Phagocytosis also accomplishes removal of debris and preparation for repair.

Phagocytosis. Vascular changes support initiation of phagocytosis. Immediately after the initial vasoconstriction, arterioles, venules, and capillaries dilate. Vasodilation increases vascular permeability, allowing cells, plasma proteins, and fluid to flow into the injured tissues from blood vessels surrounding the injury. These responses underlie formation of inflammatory exudate and produce some of the signs and symptoms characteristic of inflammation, discussed below.

Leukocytes (white blood cells) are the cells that migrate to the site of injury to carry out phagocytosis. Neutrophils are the primary leukocyte in the initial phase of the inflammation. Macrophages (reticuloendothelial cells whose primary function is phagocytosis) present in loose connective tissue are also active. As neutrophils die, monocytes become the dominant leukocyte. The monocytes are transformed into macrophages to replace those consumed in the process of clearing the wound site of debris that would interfere with the next phase of healing.

Epithelialization. Epithelialization begins with the reproduction and migration of cells from the edge of the wound toward its center. New epithelial cells continue to form, until they cover the surface of the injury, and the epidermis is as thick as before. In sutured incised wounds, a layer of epithelial cells usually covers the wound surface within 24 hours.

Inflammatory Exudate. The fluid that accumulates around the site of an injury is called an **exudate.** The characteristics of exudates depend on the type of injured tissue, cause of the injury, and duration of the inflammatory response. Serous exudate, the liquid component of blood, is produced in mild to moderate injuries. The fluid that collects inside a blister is a familiar example. Other types of exudates are described in Box 24–1. Large amounts of exudate significantly delay healing. The circulatory system must reabsorb the exudates before healing can progress.

BOX 24–1. INFLAMMATORY EXUDATES

- *Serous:* Clear exudate that accumulates in interstitial tissue in mild to moderate injuries, and is produced with injury to serous membranes such as peritoneum or pleura.
- *Serosanguineous:* Reddish, pink exudate containing red blood cells with serous drainage produced when an injury involves blood vessel damage.
- *Catarrhal:* Exudate produced with mucosal irritation such as in a cold; appears as clear liquid with strands of mucus.
- *Fibrinous:* Sticky exudate produced in severe injury or prolonged inflammation. Increased capillary permeability permits escape of fibrin molecules into interstitial space. This promotes adherence of membranes to one another, causing, for example, intestinal adhesions (sticking together of sections of intestine) or pleural friction rubs (sound made when inflamed pleura rub together). May appear as grayish, opaque membrane over tissue-loss wounds.
- *Purulent:* Thick exudate containing dead bacteria and leukocytes produced when an infection is present at the site of an injury. Color varies with causative organism; yellowish, grayish, green most common. Collection of purulent drainage is called an abscess.

Signs and Symptoms of Inflammation. Inflammation produces redness, heat, swelling, pain, and loss of function. These local manifestations are often called the cardinal signs and symptoms of inflammation. They are a direct result of the processes discussed above, as summarized in Box 24–2. If inflammation is severe or prolonged, systemic manifestations, such as weakness, malaise, and a low-grade fever, are noticeable as well. White blood cell counts show elevations in neutrophils in the acute phase of inflammation, with increased monocytes in the recovery phase.

BOX 24–2. CARDINAL SIGNS AND SYMPTOMS OF INFLAMMATION

Manifestation	Produced By
Redness	Increased blood flow to site of injury. Capillary dilation produces reddened skin.
Heat	Increased blood flow transfers body heat to site of vasodilation.
Swelling	Exudate distends interstitial tissue.
Pain	Stimulation of nerve endings by tissue distension, and by chemicals released by injured tissues.
Loss of function	Death of cells, limited mobility because of swelling and pain.

Duration of Inflammation. Inflammation overlaps with the next phase of healing, proliferation. Usually, acute inflammation peaks 24 to 48 hours after an injury, and then subsides. Inflammation is prolonged when the response is insufficient to accomplish preparation of the site for healing, as with individuals with compromised nutritional status or other physiological stressors.

Proliferation. The proliferation of several types of cells that form new tissue and, when possible, restore the function of the injured area initiates tissue reconstruction. The new tissue may be identical to the injured tissue, or be connective (scar) tissue. The amount of connective tissue required for reconstruction varies with the extent and location of the injury. In some tissue, such as muscles and nerves, minimal regeneration is possible, so considerable scarring results if the injury is extensive.

Cellular Migration. Within a few hours of an injury healthy cells at the wound margins migrate toward the center of the wound. Migrating cells include epithelium, as discussed above, and parenchymal cells. Parenchymal cells are the functional cells of internal organs—that is, those cells that actually carry out the functions of the organ, rather than giving it structure. Cellular migration continues until the cells migrating from all of the wound edges meet one another. In an incised sutured wound, the surgeon approximates all tissue layers, so cellular migration is relatively rapid. In a large tissue-loss wound, granulation tissue replaces both parenchymal cells and epithelial cells (see Capillary Budding, below). Epithelial cells eventually cover the wound surface. The process of epithelialization is faster and more economical of energy when the wound surface remains moist.[5–7] To cover a scabbed wound, epithelial cells must migrate under the thick layer of dried protein and dead cells, called **eschar.** Fifty percent of their metabolic energy is expended in secreting enzymes to dissolve the eschar, which greatly prolongs the process.[6]

Fibroplasia. Connective tissue cells called fibroblasts appear at the wound site about 2 days after an injury. These cells are the precursors of collagen, the protein molecule that makes up most connective tissue in the body. Over the course of wound reconstruction, the fibroblasts produce collagen fibers of increasing size that cross-link and overlap. Collagen supports the junction of migrating cells and gives scar tissue tensile strength.

Capillary Budding. At the same time that collagen production is progressing, blood vessels adjacent to the wound site produce capillary buds. These capillary branches eventually create a network that bridges the wound space, providing ample oxygen and nutrients to support the growth of new tissue. The new tissue that fills a large wound space or bridges the small gap between margins of a sutured wound is called **granulation tissue.** It is made up primarily of collagen, new capillaries, macrophages, and fibroblasts. Granulation tissue is pink to red because it is highly vascular. It is quite fragile and bleeds easily if traumatized.

Contraction. Myofibroblasts, cells with contractile properties similar to cardiac muscle, begin to gather around the wound edges in this phase of healing. As these cells contract in unison, they significantly reduce the surface area of the wound, facilitating epithelial coverage.[6]

The proliferative phase lasts for 2 or more weeks after an injury. An extended proliferative phase is necessary to heal large tissue-loss wounds.

Maturation. Maturation involves reorganization and remodeling of the scar. It involves continued production and alignment of collagen, balanced by selective collagen reabsorption and continued contraction. Contraction shrinks the scar. Extra blood vessels are reabsorbed and compressed as maturation proceeds, so the scar becomes pale in color like surrounding skin. Eventually, the collagen fibers become interwoven with the fibers of original tissue surrounding the wound and with each other, resulting in a serviceable scar that is nearly as strong as the original tissue. Maturation lasts several months in sutured surgical incisions and takes considerably longer in tissue-loss wounds. Table 24–3 summarizes the major events in wound healing.

Factors Affecting Wound Healing

Type of Wound. Although healing proceeds through the same phases regardless of the type of wound, the length of healing time and the appearance of the scar differ with the type of wound. These differences are summarized by the terms primary and secondary intention.

Healing by Primary Intention. **Primary intention healing** refers to the healing of a wound in which there is no tissue loss. An incised surgical wound is an example. The approximation and securing of the corresponding tissue layers enhances cellular migration and facilitates healing by primary intention (Fig. 24–3). In surgical incisions, this is accomplished when the surgeon sutures the wound edges together.

In primary intention, the phases of healing proceed relatively quickly. Inflammation is minimal, because damage is not extensive. Epithelialization is rapid, and so infection risk is slight. Little or no granulation tissue forms, because migration of matching tissue types from the wound margins facilitates tissue regeneration. A small scar is typical.

Healing by Secondary Intention. **Secondary intention healing** is the process by which tissue-loss wounds heal (Fig. 24–3). In secondary intention, all phases of healing are prolonged. Inflammation may be significant. Often there is more debris and necrotic tissue in tissue-loss wounds, extending the period of phagocytosis. Infection risk is greater. These wounds need more fibroblasts to provide a framework for granulation tissue. Moreover, considerable granulation tissue is often needed to fill the wound cavity. Often epithelial cells cannot close the tissue defect, and eschar covers the wound surface. Parenchymal migration may also be impossible, resulting in more scar tissue. Deformities are common with contraction of the large scar.

TABLE 24–3. THE PROCESS OF WOUND HEALING

INFLAMMATION

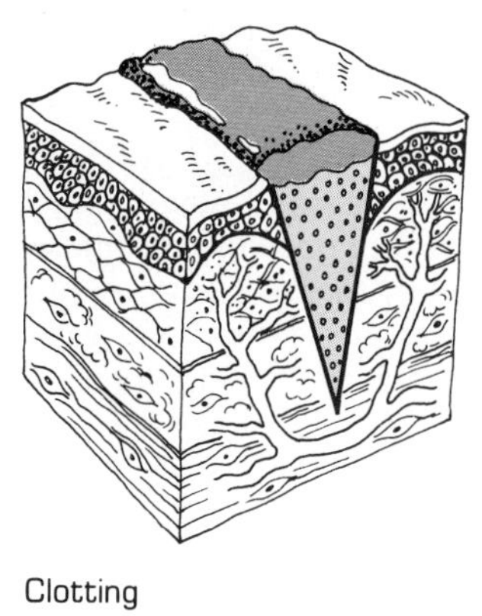

Clotting

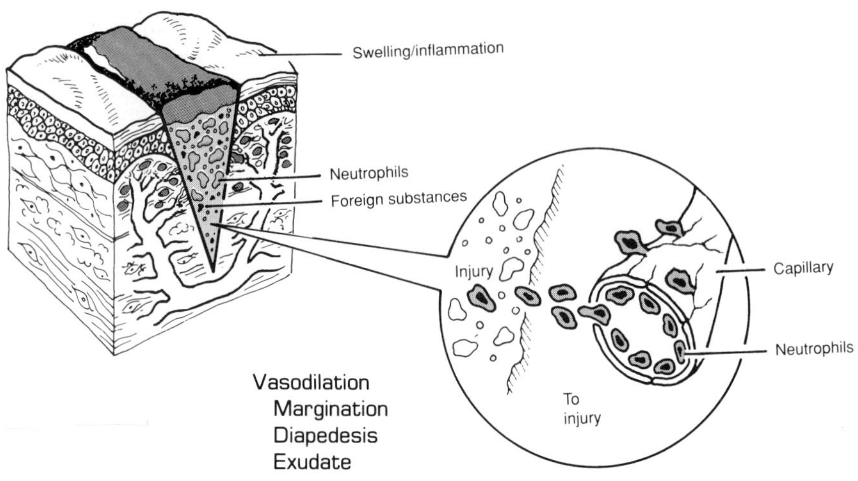

Vasodilation
Margination
Diapedesis
Exudate

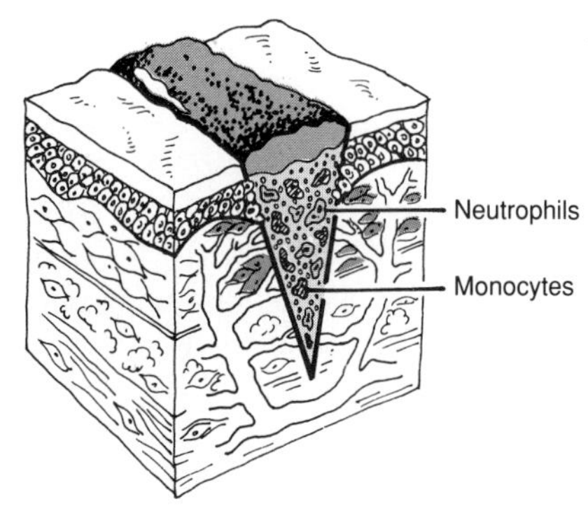

Phagocytosis

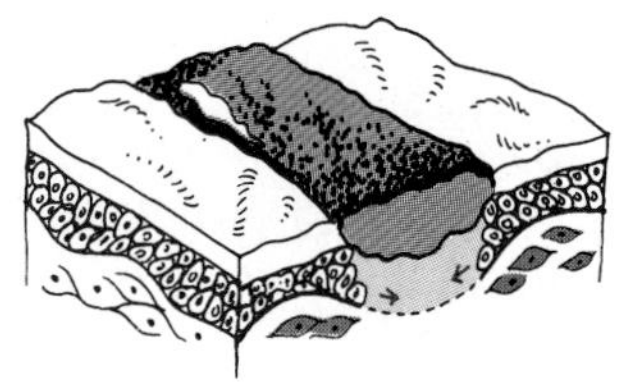

Epithelialization

PROLIFERATION

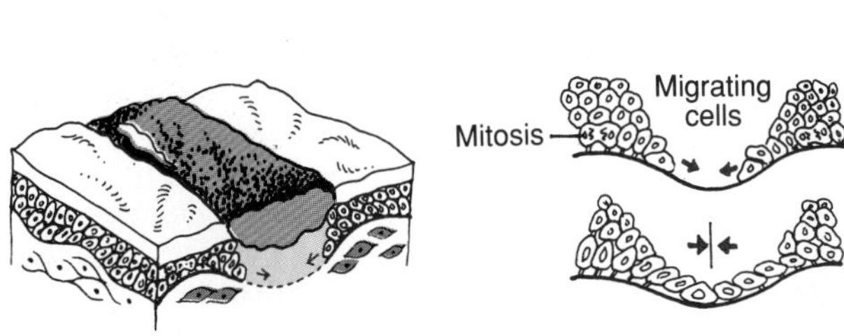

Epithelialization

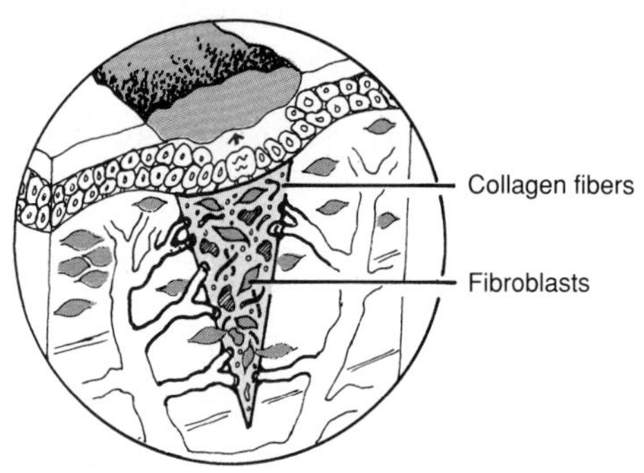

Fibroblast migration
Capillary budding

TABLE 24–3. (continued)

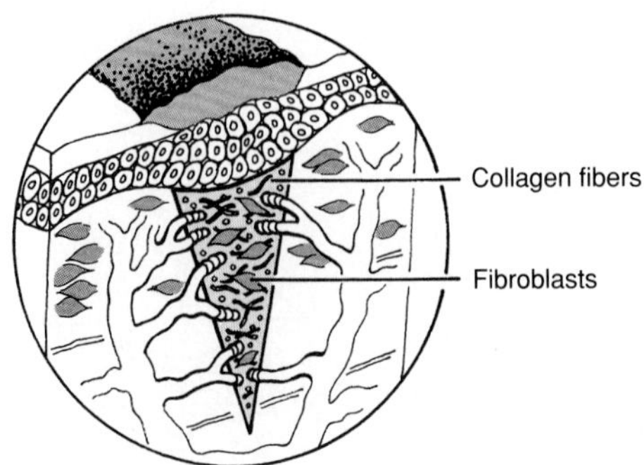

Collagen synthesis

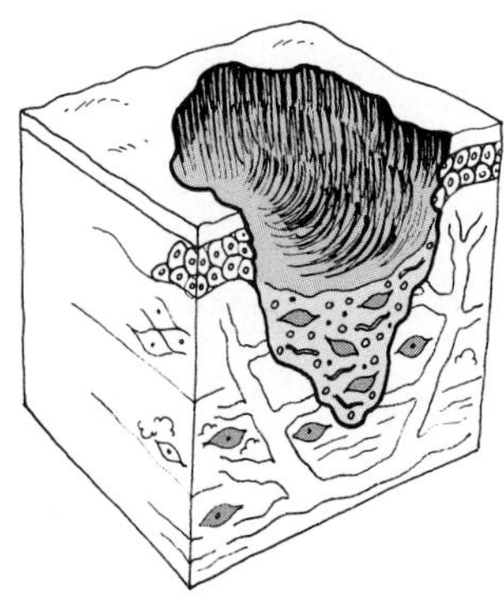
Granulation (in unsutured wounds)

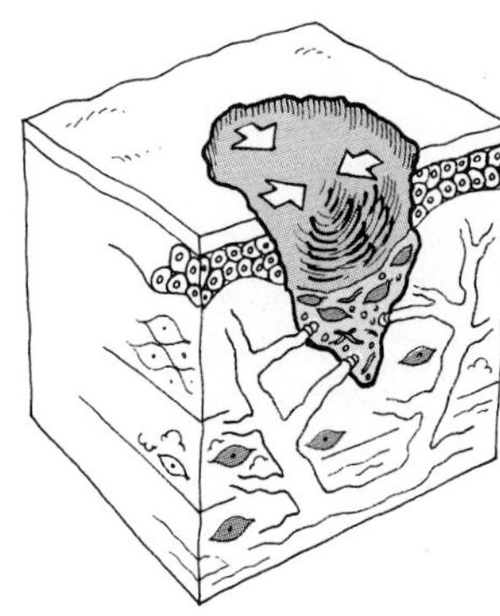
Contraction

MATURATION

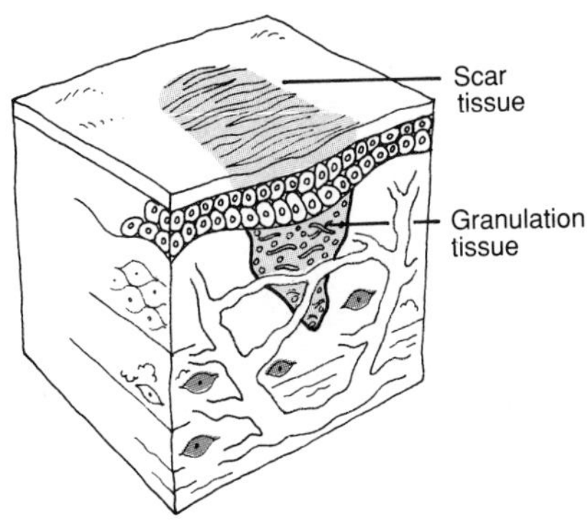

Remodeling

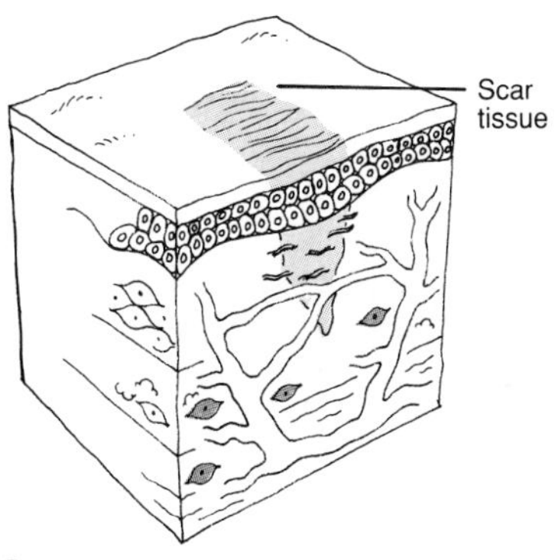

Contraction

Delayed Primary Closure. Delayed primary closure refers to a wound that is not sutured because of infection or high risk for infection. If the wound were sutured, growth of microorganisms in the wound's deeper layers would compromise healing there, while epithelial tissue on the surface of the wound would heal normally. Serious complications could occur as a result. When this type of wound is leftopen and granulation tissue development is promoted by special wound care while simultaneously treating the infection, more satisfactory healing occurs. After a time, the wound can often be closed to allow healing to conclude by primary intention.

Age. Generally, extremes of age compromise wound healing. Several physiological variables affect healing in neonates and premature infants.[8] They are prone to develop respiratory compromise and therefore decreased tissue perfusion. The defense mechanisms of phagocytosis and cellular immunity are ineffective. Because of rapid metabolism, growth, and limited nutrient reserves, basal energy needs are high. Wound healing increases energy needs, and it is therefore often a challenge to provide sufficient calories for both.[8]

Older adults are also at risk for delayed healing. Age-related changes in immune function and circulatory effi-

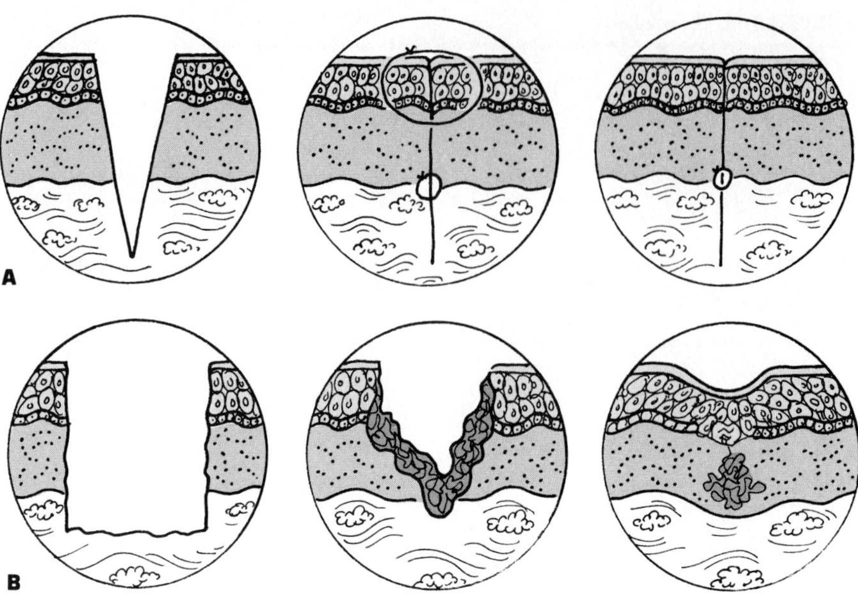

Figure 24–3. Wound healing by **(A)** primary intention and **(B)** secondary intention.

ciency delay onset of inflammation and prolong its phases. Cellular migration, replication, and maturation slow with age, extending reconstruction.[9] Moreover, diminished amounts of slow-wave sleep (see Chap. 28) reduce production of growth hormone, contributing to slower anabolic processes.[4] Nutritional deficits are relatively common among elderly individuals, an added risk factor, as discussed in the next section.

Nutritional Status. Healing is a significant energy demand. Because most clients with serious wounds are unable to ingest foods by mouth in the immediate treatment phase, those with poor nutritional status at the time of injury or surgery are at risk for complications.

Rebuilding tissue at the site of injury requires protein, which individuals can synthesize only if they take in sufficient amounts of essential amino acids. Carbohydrate and fat calories are also important. Average-sized individuals must ingest about 2800 kilocalories a day before they can use protein for tissue repair rather than for basal metabolic activity.[10] Vitamin C is also essential for effective healing. It is required for collagen synthesis, capillary formation, and capillary stability.[10,11] Vitamin A, also important for collagen synthesis, enhances epithelialization.[7,10,11] Zinc deficiency has adverse effects on healing as well. It retards epithelialization and the rate of gain of collagen strength.[12,13] Clients experiencing catabolic stressors (such as surgery and injury), or excessive gastrointestinal drainage (common with postoperative gastric suctioning) excrete large amounts of zinc and so may need supplements.[10,11,14]

Even well-nourished clients who must remain on nothing-by-mouth status for several days, and then on a clear liquid diet for more than a day, are at risk for developing deficiency states that can delay healing. Standard dextrose and electrolyte solutions deliver less than 1000 calories per day. This marginal calorie intake depletes carbohydrate reserves within 1 to 2 days, making gluconeogenesis (formation of glycogen from noncarbohydrate sources, such as amino acids) necessary and therefore depleting amino acids available for tissue replacement.[10,11]

State of the Tissue. Variables such as the general condition of the wounded tissue, tissue perfusion, surgical dead space, and microorganism population influence the healing process.

General Condition. Healthy tissue heals best. A surgical wound made in otherwise undamaged tissue is likely to heal rapidly and without complication. On the other hand, a traumatic wound that damages a large area of tissue and disrupts surrounding circulation takes longer to heal. Tissue compromised in other ways, such as by radiation (often part of therapy for cancer), or tissue exposed to extremes of heat or cold, heals slowly. Radiation also threatens the immune system, because of its interference with the production of fibroblasts.[14]

Tissue Perfusion. The vascular system is a primary factor in initiating and maintaining tissue repair. Many of the cells responsible for phagocytosis and the immune response are blood components. Phagocytosis and cell migration, cell replication, and protein and collagen synthesis also require a good oxygen supply.[7] Highly vascular tissue, such as in the head and face, heals more rapidly than less vascular tissue. Early mobility after surgery or injury improves overall circulation, and so enhances healing. Any condition that compromises circulation—such as obesity, anemia, vascular occlusion, or smoking—interferes with healing. Obesity increases the amount of adipose tissue, which is not highly vascular. Anemia reduces the amount of oxygen that is transported to healing tissue.[14] Smoking reduces hemoglobin's oxygen-carrying capacity (see Chap. 27). It is the most common cause of wound hypoxia.[6] Wound oxygen tensions have been measured at 0 for 20 minutes after smoking

BUILDING NURSING KNOWLEDGE

Do Children's Wounds Heal Differently?

Garvin G. Wound healing in pediatrics. *Nurs Clin North Am.* 1990; 25:181–193.

This article examines how wound healing in childhood differs from that in adulthood. Garvin notes that although the same physiological responses are involved, immature organ function creates some differences, especially in early infancy. While children have greater capacity for tissue repair than adults, children lack reserves and hence are more vulnerable to electrolyte imbalance, body temperature fluctuation, and rapid spread of infection, all of which affect wound healing.

Infants are vulnerable to circulatory changes, and anything that compromises circulation can reduce wound healing. Infants are also prone to develop irregular breathing patterns due to immaturity of the central nervous system. Garvin stresses that this can reduce tissue oxygen. The lining of the respiratory tract is delicate and mucous membranes do not offer the protection against infectious organisms that develops later in life. The phagocytic action needed for wound healing and cellular immunity for resistance to infection provided in later life by the white blood cells are also incompetent in the neonate. Thermoregulatory mechanisms are immature and hypothermia leads to metabolic conditions that interfere with wound healing.

Nutrition is another area of difference. Malnutrition slows healing. Infants are born with minimal energy stores; this creates a nutritional challenge for the nurse, because infants, especially those with wounds, have high energy requirements. Amino acids are needed for all aspects of wound healing. Hypoproteinemia delays collagen synthesis and wound remodeling. Oral protein intake for infants should be on the high side of published guidelines, according to Garvin. An optimal protein-to-nonprotein calorie ratio also must exist. The infant's diet should contain at least 25 to 32 nonprotein calories per gram of protein. Garvin points out that carbohydrates are needed as an energy source for white blood cell function. Clinical assessment of caloric adequacy is done by monitoring weight gain, which should be 15 to 20 g/kg per day in the young infant. Vitamin C is essential for wound healing. Infants need 35 mg per day. The mineral zinc is also important, and infants require 100 μg/kg per day.

1 cigarette.[15] Hypoxia and ischemia can also be caused by excessive tension on sutures.[13]

Dead Space. Dead space refers to areas within a sutured wound in which tissue layers on opposite sides of the wound are not aligned and in contact with one another. Dead space is inevitable when surgery involves removal of a large amount of tissue, but dead space disrupts healing because it interferes with cellular migration and tissue perfusion. Exudates that collect in or around a wound increase dead space and distort tissue because of increased tension on the wound.[16] Studies have shown that a large amount of wound fluid decreases oxygen availability in the wound.[7,14] Therefore, whenever surgeons expect a significant amount of inflammatory exudate to form after surgery, they place a drainage system adjacent to the wound to facilitate fluid removal from the incision site. Surgical drainage systems are discussed in Section 3 of this chapter.

Microorganism Population. The presence of microorganisms in a wound site increases the chance of wound infection and delayed healing. Accidental wounds are contaminated wounds and carry a greater risk of infection than wounds that occur under surgically aseptic conditions. Surgical wounds that enter body cavities having a normal bacterial population are more likely to become infected than those in which only sterile organs or cavities are entered. If drainage from a nonsterile body cavity, such as the bowel, contaminates the wound site, the infection rate is greater still.

General Health Status. Good health is predictive of good wound healing. Conversely, health-related factors such as stress and many chronic diseases are detrimental to healing.

Acute stress triggers the release of catecholamines that constrict blood vessels and reduce perfusion of injured tissue.[17] Many sensations that accompany surgery or injury create stress of this type.[18] Chronic stress inhibits healing because of the deleterious effect excessive amounts of adrenocortical hormones have on fibroblast formation. Lower cortisol levels, on the other hand, are associated with improved healing.[19]

Many disease states, such as diabetes mellitus, cancer, and hypothyroidism, compromise immune function and therefore jeopardize healing.[14] Clients with rheumatoid arthritis, alcoholism, and malabsorption syndromes are at risk for deficiencies of nutrients needed for healing, and therefore often experience delayed healing.[6] Certain therapeutic regimens are also known to hinder immune functioning as well. Steroid therapy markedly inhibits the inflammatory response and interferes with collagen synthesis.[20] Clients receiving cancer chemotherapy frequently experience diminished wound tensile strength.[14] Radiation, as discussed above, also compromises immunity.

Type of Wound Care. The materials used to dress and cleanse wounds can support or inhibit healing. If the selection of wound antiseptic is inappropriate, tissue irritation, and even destruction of granulation tissue, is possible.[21,22] Vigorous cleaning of wounds destroys developing granulation tissue even when using mild solutions. Dry gauze or wet to dry dressings adhere to healing tissue and remove viable tissue when they are removed.[23] Wound care that enhances drying of the wound surface retards epithelial regeneration, as noted above.

Complications of Wound Healing

Hemorrhage. **Hemorrhage** is excessive loss of blood. Traumatic wounds hemorrhage if damaged blood vessels are not effectively compressed. Hemorrhage in surgical wounds results when severed blood vessels are not completely sealed by suturing or cautery, or when sutures are disrupted. Unchecked hemorrhage is life threatening. Hem-

BUILDING NURSING KNOWLEDGE

Do Wounds Heal Differently in Elders?

Jones PL, Millman A. Wound healing and the aged patient. *Nurs Clin North Am.* 1990; 25:263–277.

Jones and Millman note that despite the changes of aging, most aged clients heal well. Though the aged often heal more slowly, overall they follow the same healing process. There is extreme variability in the extent to which aged adults exhibit the changes of aging, the authors point out. Because of this, two people of age 80 may have quite different wound healing times because one has had more rapid aging of tissues critical to healing. The slow healer may have lower myocardial output, or fewer alveolar–capillary units for gas exchange in the lungs, resulting in lower tissue oxygen.

Jones and Millman cite some differences in aged wound healing. Response rates for inflammation, cell migration, proliferation, and maturation are slowed in later years. Epithelialization and contraction of open wounds are delayed. There may be age-related decreases in functional efficiency and reserve capacity that may not be apparent until the individual tries to adapt to a stress such as wound healing. Compromises in cellular responsiveness may be greater when an individual is confronted with multiple stressors at once.

Nurses can promote healing by attention to energy conservation. Postoperative fatigue—a sense of muscle weakness, impaired mental acuity, and reduced psychomotor skills—is common among the aged. Little is understood about it, but it may be due to anesthesia, bedrest, lack of food, or altered sleep. Nursing care that provides time for rest and sleep and a comfortable environment is important, the authors emphasize. Disrupted sleep can lead to mental disorientation that, along with decreases in neurosensory perception of pressure, touch, pain, and temperature, reduces the aged person's awareness of danger and increases the risk of trauma.

Thermoregulation also is less efficient in the aged. The energy required to regain normal body temperature after the hypothermia of surgery may increase the risk of inadequate perfusion to the wound. Thus nursing care, Jones and Millman stress, must concern itself with the environmental temperature. Another concern is over- or underhydration, which can reduce cardiac output. Thus the authors stress that nursing must include continuous assessment of the aged client's hydration status during wound healing. Psychosocial stress is another form of energy depletion, particularly when the aged are unprepared for hospitalization. Such stress can be detrimental to wound healing and places clients at risk. Preparation for the unknown, and timely exploration of attitudes related to care and aging, can help the aged person expand awareness and gain control of situations, thus reducing the risk of stress.

orrhage from closed surgical wounds may be visible as an accumulation of bright red drainage on wound dressings or occult if bleeding is internal. Other symptoms of hemorrhage include rapid, irregular, thready pulse; pallor; and cool, moist skin. Postoperative wound hemorrhage is most common within the first 48 hours after surgery, but late hemorrhage also occurs. Late hemorrhage is often secondary to infection and typically happens on the sixth to the tenth postoperative day.

Wound Infection. Wound infections are the result of microbial contamination at the time a wound occurs, or during the healing process. Microorganisms can enter a wound at any time prior to completion of epithelialization. When microorganisms multiply and cause injurious effects, the wound is considered infected. A well-functioning immune system usually effectively contains and destroys small numbers of microorganisms. With highly virulent organisms or grossly contaminated wounds, however, bacteria multiply faster than the body's defenses can destroy them. Other risk factors, such as malnutrition, poor perfusion, extremes of age, chronic diseases, and a history of steroid therapy, predispose clients to wound infections.[7,10,11] Environmental factors such as breaks in asepsis during wound care, a lengthy surgical procedure, or delayed treatment of contaminated wounds, also contribute to infection risk.[24,25]

Signs and symptoms of wound infection include local heat, redness, edema, pain, high-grade fever, elevated white blood count, and purulent wound drainage. Clinical signs of infection become apparent within 2 to 7 days of surgery.

Wound Separation. Several degrees of wound separation may occur in surgical wounds. Superficial separation refers to separation of approximated skin on the wound surface. This usually occurs in small spaces between sutures or skin staples, but may involve larger portions of the incision. Usually, superficial separation is minor and presents no risks other than possible widening of the scar at the point of separation. **Dehiscence** is separation of the wound edges. It may be complete, involving all tissue layers, or partial. It is a more serious complication and requires immediate correction. Evisceration, that is, the spilling out of the abdominal contents, may accompany dehiscence of abdominal incisions. In some cases, partial dehiscence is occult, involving the muscle and fascia layers only. This often leads to incisional hernia. Dehiscence is not a common complication, but is two to three times more frequent in clients over the age of 60 than in younger clients.[9] It is also more common in individuals with diabetes, immunocompromise, cancer, and obesity, and with those receiving steroid therapy.[26]

Keloids. A keloid is a raised, firm, thickened scar that results from deposition of abnormal amounts of collagen into the tissue surrounding a wound. The excess collagen is not lysed during the maturation stage of healing, allowing the disproportionate tissue to continue to grow for some time after wound closure. This complication is more common among blacks.

Contracture. Wound contracture is the pathological shrinking of a scar causing loss of mobility. It should not be confused with contraction, which is a normal part of wound healing. Contractures sometimes need surgical correction.

Section 2. Assessment of Skin and Tissue Integrity

SKIN AND TISSUE DATA COLLECTION

Skin and tissue alterations often affect an individual's appearance and threaten self-concept, so some clients may be sensitive about discussing or exposing skin or tissue lesions. Discomfort related to itching or irritation may also be a feature of integumentary problems. Keeping these points in mind when gathering data about skin and tissue guides the nurse's approach to data collection. The assessment incorporates the skin, and the mucosa of the eye, nose, oral cavity and pharynx, and genital–rectal area. Particular attention is paid to any wounds or lesions in these structures.

Skin and Tissue History

The focus of the history is to obtain clients' perceptions of their integumentary problems, and the effects these problems have on their usual daily activity.

Primary Concern. A primary concern related to the integument may relate to the appearance of a lesion, its interference with activities, its cause, or other features, such as whether it is contagious or likely to recur. The nature of the client's distress guides the data-collection process as well as treatment approaches. Some skin problems may imply a need for a more comprehensive data collection, because the skin and mucosa reflect general health and provide clues to problems in other functional areas. Conversely, a skin and tissue assessment may be appropriate with other kinds of primary concerns, such as dietary or elimination problems. The following example demonstrates a nurse's use of primary concern data.

- Brenda Thomasen seeks help for a recurring rash on her face. Although this is the first time she has sought health care for this problem, she recalls two previous occurrences of this rash in the same location. Her son has a history of herpes skin lesions and she is concerned that her rash may have the same etiology. Although her son has not required treatment, she is worried that she will be unable to work if her lesions are not treated, because she has just started a job in a newborn nursery, and she realizes that newborns are highly susceptible to this infection. The nurse assures her that if the diagnosis is positive for herpes simplex type 1, medication to prevent or limit the duration of future outbreaks is available.

IMPLICATIONS FOR NURSE–CLIENT COLLABORATION

Skin and Tissue Healing

Nurse–client collaboration during the skin and tissue history is an effective means of assuring accurate determination of client concerns. Skin problems often have broad impact on client well-being; psychosocial as well as physical. Nurses who effectively solicit client participation in the assessment process are able to gain a more comprehensive understanding of the distress a client is feeling and how a skin problem affects that client's general functioning.

Current Understanding. Skin and mucosal wounds and lesions can have many possible causes. It is helpful to determine what a client believes may have precipitated the problem, what makes it worse or better, and what has been tried as a home remedy. Because skin and tissue alterations can result from injuries, infectious diseases, topical contact with an irritant or toxin, or food ingestion, it is worthwhile to explore environmental factors thoroughly with clients. Sometimes the appearance of a lesion implies its cause and helps to focus nurses' assessment questions. Other appropriate inquiries about the current eruption or exacerbation include, for example: When did the eruption appear? Have there been previous episodes? Are there other problems associated with the lesion such as itching, cold-type symptoms, localized swelling, warmth, redness, bleeding or oozing of fluid, or odor? Has the skin around the lesion changed in texture, color, or turgor? Has there been any change due to the treatment? The following is an example of current understanding.

- Anita, age 13 years, reports to a clinic with bilateral redness and swelling of the conjunctiva. She reports she has been bothered by these symptoms for 3 days, but has never had them before. She reports that she has tried rinsing her eyes with warm water, but has gotten no relief. In discussing Anita's usual skin care, the nurse learns that Anita and her friends have been trying out new makeup. The nurse suggests that discontinuing the makeup until the irritation clears and then using hypoallergenic products may solve the problem.

Past Health Problems/Experiences. This section of the history may reveal that the current alteration is a recurrence of a previous problem. Many skin conditions are chronic or recurring. Medications or treatments for other medical conditions may underlie skin or mucosal symptoms, or they may be sequelae or complications of other health problems. An example of nurses' use of past health problem data follows.

- Salvador Lopes is admitted to Ward B for treatment of leg ulcers on his lower left leg. He has a history of diabetes mellitus and reports difficulty following his dietary and skin care assessment regimen. Nurse Cataldo notices irregular scars on both legs, and asks about their cause. He states that they were the same kind of sores, but "I just can't seem to keep them from happening." Nurse Cataldo makes a mental note to explore what barriers prevent Mr. Lopes from engaging in preventive practices and seeking early care when symptoms first appear.

Personal, Family, and Social History. Life-style influences environmental exposure and ingestion of substances that may cause skin and tissue alterations. For example, hygiene habits affect oral cavity and skin health. Sun exposure for leisure or because of work increases risk for skin cancers. Occupational exposure to chemicals is a frequent cause of mucosal and skin lesions. Stress may precipitate skin rashes. A client who smokes or who has poor nutrition habits may have difficulties with healing. Smokers are also more susceptible to oral cancers. Skin and integumentary alterations are the primary manifestations of many nutritional deficiencies. Pets in the home may cause allergic lesions.

Personal history related to coping and stress level should not be overlooked. A client's sense of well-being in response to skin disruptions varies according to his or her perception of the alteration. When a client views it as temporary, and unlikely to cause scarring, the alteration is often seen as no more than an irritant. The irritant can be an enormous bother but bearable or may be viewed as only a minor problem. However, when the alteration is chronic or results in scarring, many clients grieve over the change in body image. They experience feelings of denial, depression, guilt, embarrassment, disgust, anxiety, fear, or rejection. The level of stress is highly individualized. Sensitive nurses recognize the potential significance of skin and tissue alterations and include assessment of verbal and nonverbal behavior through active listening as a focal part of their skin and tissue assessment (see also Chap. 14).

The following example illustrates a nurse's use of data from a client's personal, family, and social history. Table 24–4 provides sample questions to elicit relevant information about personal, family, and social influences on integumentary health.

- Sam Carruthers seeks health care for a small red lesion on his forehead that has been present for several weeks. The nurse notices that he also has a sunburn, and so asks about his usual leisure and occupational activities. He indicates that although his office job keeps him indoors most of the time, he participates in sailing and golf every weekend. He admits "I'm a little lazy about the sunscreen—I don't get all the SPS, SPX stuff and I keep forgetting to take it with me." The nurse realizes that Mr. Carruthers is at risk for skin cancer, and resolves to problem-solve strategies with him to help integrate sun protection into his regular habits.

Subjective Manifestations. The last part of the skin and tissue history is subjective manifestations. As discussed in Chapter 16, this portion of the history is a general overview of common symptoms that serves as a means of assuring that no relevant symptoms go unreported. Chapter 16 provides sample questions relevant to skin and tissue.

Skin and Tissue Examination

The primary modalities in the skin and tissue examination are inspection and palpation. Measurements are occasionally used.

Measurements. Measurements usually are not relevant except when lesions are present. Health care providers sometimes measure lesions to diagnose the type and evaluate progression or remission.

Assessment of weight and weight changes is important for postsurgical clients, or other clients with skin and tissue disruptions who do not have good oral intake. A 6 percent weight loss has been found to be an indicator of risk for nutrition-associated complications of surgery, such as infection and wound dehiscence.[27]

Objective Manifestations. General observations, integument, eye, ear, nose, mouth, throat, breast, cardiovascular, genitourinary, and anal–rectal examinations provide information that contributes to assessment and diagnosis of skin and tissue problems. Chapter 16 summarizes normal findings relevant to skin and tissue integrity. The following discussion addresses alterations.

General Observations. A client's overall appearance suggests actual or potential problems, as well as healthy functioning. Note whether the skin appearance is congruent with the stated age. Note facial skin color. Changes, such as pallor or jaundice, usually are visible first in the face. Body odors, and general cleanliness of the hair, body, and apparel, give clues about hygiene practices. Clients with poor oral or general hygiene habits are likely to have poor skin and mucosal health. Extensive lesions are also noticeable upon general inspection, but will need more meticulous examination in the integumentary examination. Guarding or scratching suggest lesions in unexposed areas that should be inspected later in the examination.

Integument. Examination of the integument should address skin (including lesions and wounds), skin appendages, and mucosa over all body areas. For the sake of efficiency and convenience, the integument assessment is not conducted all at once, but is integrated into the head-to-toe observations of other organs and functions. Chapter 16 describes the integument findings expected in healthy individuals. Selected indicators of problems are addressed here.

When inspecting the skin and mucosa, dryness (including tenacious mucus), flakiness, poor turgor, redness, swelling, and delayed capillary filling time suggest actual or potential skin problems. Often, skin changes such as these reflect alterations in nutritional or fluid status (see Chaps. 25 and 31). Be alert for lesions on the face and neck that are characteristic of premalignant or malignant changes. Scaly papules with underlying redness (actinic keratoses), small papules with waxy translucent borders (basal cell carcinoma), and small hard conical nodules accompanied by ulcers

TABLE 24–4. SKIN AND TISSUE HISTORY: PERSONAL, FAMILY, AND SOCIAL HISTORY QUESTIONS

A. **Vocational**
1. What type of work do you do?
2. How long have you had this job?
3. Where did you work previously?
4. Does your current or prior work involve contact with chemicals, dyes, or fibers?
5. What precautions or safety measures do you take when handling these materials?
6. Have you ever had a rash or sore that seemed related to contact with these materials?
7. Does your job involve frequent or prolonged exposure to the sun?

B. **Home and Family**
1. What are your usual home activities?
2. Do you live in an urban neighborhood? Rural?
3. Are there many kinds of plants growing around your neighborhood? Do you notice many insects around your home?
4. Does your family have pets? What kind? Who cares for the pets?

C. **Social, Leisure, Spiritual, and Cultural**
1. What are your favorite leisure activities?
2. Do you spend a lot of time in outdoor recreation?
3. Do you often get sunburned? How often do you use sunscreen?
4. Has your skin problem ever interfered with participation in social or leisure activities?

D. **Sexual**
1. Are you sexually active?
2. How do you protect yourself against sexually transmitted diseases?
3. Have you ever been treated for a sexually transmitted disease?
4. Has your skin problem ever interfered with sexual expression?

E. **Habits**

Sleep
1. Have your skin problems ever interfered with getting a good night's sleep?

Nutrition
1. What foods do you eat daily?
2. Are you allergic to any foods? What foods? What symptoms do you experience?
3. What kinds of snack foods do you prefer? Do you eat them often?

Beverages
1. How often do you drink sugared beverages, such as Coke, sweetened iced tea, or coffee?
2. How much water do you drink each day?
3. Do you drink alcoholic beverages? How often? How much?

Tobacco Use
1. Do you smoke? Cigarettes, cigar, pipe?
2. How much do you smoke each day?

Other Substances
1. How often do you take nonprescription medications, such as aspirin?
2. Do you take any prescription medications? Any that you apply to your skin?
3. Are you allergic to any medications?

F. **Psychological/Coping**
1. Do you ever feel nervous or stressed? How often does this happen?
2. Do you notice flare-ups of your skin problem when you feel nervous?
3. Is there anything about your skin problem that worries you?
4. Has having this skin problem changed the way you feel about yourself? Your body?
5. Has your skin problem caused you to miss activities or events that are important to you? Do you ever avoid going out when it flares up?
6. How do you deal with your skin problem?

IMPLICATIONS FOR NURSE–CLIENT COLLABORATION

Planning

Planning is a collaborative nurse–client function. Mutual development of outcomes and implementation is appropriate for client problems of all types. Skin problems often present a challenge, because the outcome most clients see as ideal—complete healing without scarring—is not always achievable. Moreover, nursing implementation necessary to achieve the best possible outcomes is sometimes painful and long term. Clients may become discouraged and withdrawn. Accepting clients' feelings while encouraging their continued participation in planning and in care requires empathy and skill.

with irregular borders are examples. Note the distribution of moles on the face, trunk, and extremities. Ask clients if they have noted any changes in any moles, such as increased elevation, increased pigmentation, or bleeding. These changes are characteristic of malignant melanoma. Scattered purplish macular lesions suggest Karposi's sarcoma, associated with HIV infection (AIDS). Skin tears on the arms, hands, and sacrum are common among elderly bedridden clients.[1,4]

Palpation provides information about tissue temperature and perfusion. Palpation is also important for identifying lesions. By touching lesions, the examiner distinguishes the texture and consistency of each lesion. Is skin globally warm, hot with fever, locally cool, or cold and clammy from shock? Is the area around the lesion warmer than other areas? Are there pulses distal or proximal to the lesion on the extremities? It is advisable to wear gloves when palpating open lesions.

Skin Lesions. Characteristic primary and secondary lesions are described in Tables 16–4 and 16–5. It is useful to compare lesions to intact skin areas. When describing lesions, include distribution, size, shape, color, and configuration.

DISTRIBUTION. Distribution refers to the location and symmetry of lesion placement. Symmetrical distribution means that lesions appear on corresponding body parts on opposite sides of the body—for example on both arms or both feet. Asymmetrical distribution means that only one side of the body is affected. Skin folds are an important area to scrutinize when assessing for the distribution of lesions, as this is a common location for lesions.

SIZE. Size is a familiar concept. Measure lesion size for precise diagnosis. If many lesions of varying sizes are present, describe the range of sizes found or the size of a typical lesion. It may be useful to compare the size of lesions to familiar objects, such as "dime-sized."

SHAPE. Lesions may be regular or irregular in shape. In some cases, a characteristic shape may be diagnostic of a specific lesion, for example, ringworm presents in an annular or ringlike formation.

COLOR. Lesions may be red, purple, yellow, white, or black. Some lesions are of mixed color. Note whether the color is uniform and widely distributed throughout the lesions (diffuse) or limited to the edges (circumscribed).

CONFIGURATION. Configuration refers to the general arrangement of lesions. Lesions may be singular or grouped. Grouped lesions may cluster in regular patterns, such as linear or annular, may follow the course of a cutaneous nerve, or may cluster randomly with no particular pattern.

It is also appropriate to note whether all of the lesions are similar in appearance, of if there are lesions at differing stages. If the lesions are not uniform in appearance, ask the client to point out which of the lesions represents the initial stage. Note the appearance of the skin around the lesions as well as the healed skin.

Wounds. The wounds that nurses encounter most frequently are traumatic wounds, surgical wounds, and pressure ulcers.

TRAUMATIC WOUNDS. Initial assessment of traumatic wounds should include location, type, size, and the amount of bleeding or other drainage. When clients have experienced trauma, it is important to assess their overall condition, including adequacy of breathing, pulse, and the presence of other injuries. Initially hemostasis of all bleeding wounds and maintenance of cardiorespiratory function are critical. When clients' cardiorespiratory status is stable, examine the wound for the presence of foreign bodies such as particles of dirt, clothing, or glass and note changes in drainage or appearance since the initial assessment. Many traumatic wounds need suturing or surgical repair. After treatment, assessment should be the same as for any other wound. Box 24–3 summarizes the elements in a routine wound assessment.

SURGICAL WOUNDS. It is common practice to cover surgical wounds with dressings. The type of dressing varies with the kind of procedure, complications (if any), and provider's preference. It is important to assess both the dressing and the wound regularly. If a dressing has fresh bloody drainage, assess for additional drainage in the bed. When a wound is hemorrhaging, blood flow is often too rapid for the dressing to absorb it; instead it flows into the bed under the client due to gravity. If you suspect hemorrhage, assess vital signs and notify the physician or charge nurse.

Surgeons often place devices to evacuate and contain drainage in surgical wounds (Fig. 24–4). If one or more is present, assess them also. The frequency depends on factors such as the type and location of the incision, stage of healing, and presence of complications, if any.

PRESSURE ULCERS. Pressure ulcers are preventable wounds. Preventive measures are imperative, including frequent position changes, assessment of the bony prominences of all clients at risk, and implementation to relieve pressure at the first sign of a stage-one ulcer (see Chap. 30 and Table 24–2). Once an ulcer has advanced beyond stage one, the appearance of the wound guides the selection of treatment approaches.[23] It is important to note the color of the wound and the nature of the drainage. This will help

BOX 24–3. ROUTINE ASSESSMENT OF WOUNDS

Wounds Healing by Primary Intention

- Inspect Dressing
  Note **drainage:** Amount (diameter of drainage, number of gauze pads soaked)? Color? Odor?
  Note whether dressing is secure.
- Inspect Incision
  Note **appearance:** Wound edges approximated? Separated? Healing (moderate swelling, redness)? Possible infection (wound edges red, puffy, surrounding tissue taut)?
  Note **drainage:** Amount, color, odor, consistency.
- Inspect Drainage Devices
  Note **functioning:** Intact? Functioning correctly? Needing emptying and recompression?
  Note **drainage** as above.
- Palpate Incision Edges and Surrounding Skin
  Note **tension:** Taut? Moderately swollen?
  Note **healing:** Healing ridge (1 cm wide ridge around wound) present by 7 days postsurgery?[a]
  Note **heat:** Wound area warmer than rest of body?
- Assess Pain
  Note **location:** Incisional? Deep pain? Other than incision?
  Note **intensity:** How severe on 1–10 scale? More or less severe than before? Building in intensity?
  Note **onset/duration:** Sudden? Gradual?
  Note **character:** Sharp? Dull? Knifelike? Pressure? Constant? Intermittent?
  Note **exacerbating factors:** Specific event? Specific type of movement? Movement in general?

Wounds Healing by Secondary Intention

- Assess Dressing, Drainage, and Pain as Above
- Inspect Wound
  Note **appearance:** Color of tissue—red, yellow, black? Texture of tissue—velvety, rigid, fibrotic, dry, crusted?
  Note **size, shape:** Depth of injury (stage, if pressure ulcer)? Diameter? Size changing?
- Inspect Surrounding Skin
  Note **appearance:** Healthy? Compromised? Extent of involvement.
  Note **edges:** Poorly defined? Well defined? Rolled toward base? Undermined?

[a] *Hunt TK, Goodson WH. Wound healing. In: Way LW, ed.* Current Surgical Diagnosis and Treatment. *Norwalk, CT: Appleton & Lange; 1991.*

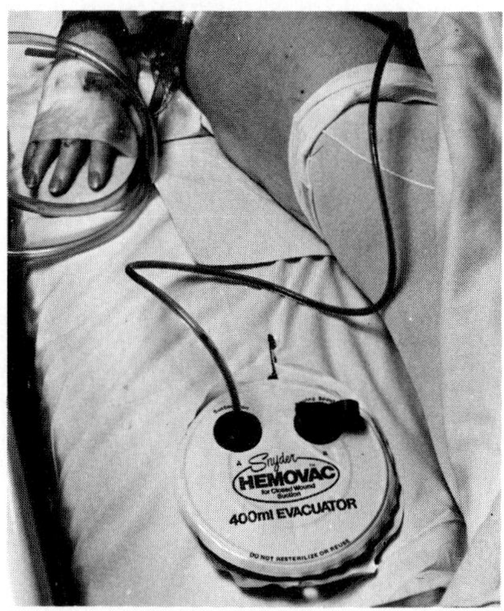

Figure 24–4. Hemovac drainage evacuation device for surgical wounds. (*From Smith S, Duell D.* Clinical Nursing Skills: Nursing Process Model; Basic to Advanced Skills, *2nd ed. Norwalk, CT: Appleton & Lange; 1988:586.*)

identify healing tissue and necrotic areas and will suggest the presence of infection (Box 24–3).

Skin Appendages. Changes in the nails and hair often accompany skin diseases and nutritional deficiencies. If nails are brittle, dry, and cracked, or hair is dull and brittle, look for other signs of nutritional deficiencies (see Chap. 25).

Alopecia (hair loss) is sometimes a side effect of cancer chemotherapy. Hair that grows after therapy is discontinued is often sparse and of fine texture. Spotty areas of alopecia may indicate disease, and warrant further investigation. One possible cause is ringworm. If there are scalp lesions, look for lice infestation (pediculosis). When checking for lice, a flashlight is useful. Eggs (nits) on the hair shaft have a pearlized appearance in the light.

Mucosa. Examine the mucosa of the eye, nose, mouth and throat, and perineal–rectal area for color changes, hydration, discharge, and evidence of disruptions. Common problems specific to each body area are discussed below in the corresponding examination sections. Table 24–5 summarizes causes of mucosal disruptions.

HEENT. The aspect of the head, eyes, ears, nose, and throat (HEENT) assessment that is most germane to skin and tissue assessment is mucosal assessment.

Eye. Note the presence of inflammation, manifested by redness (erythema) of the conjunctiva and eyelids, swelling, excess tearing or other discharge, pain, or pruritus. Trauma, allergy, or infection may be the underlying cause.

Ear. Redness, itching, scaling, pain, and discharge suggest infection in the external or middle ear. Odor may indicate infection or presence of a foreign body. Excessive ear wax (cerumen) is a concern to some clients, causing discomfort or diminished hearing acuity. Cerumen is visible in the external ear, but requires otoscopic examination to determine whether it is excessive.

Nose. Evaluate the nasal mucosa for color, lesions, discharge, swelling, or evidence of bleeding. With allergies, the nasal mucosa appears pale with a clear discharge. Infections produce reddened mucosa. Discharge may be watery or purulent. Discharge limited to one nostril is typical of a foreign body in the nose. Lesions can result from internal or external sources (Table 24–5).

Mouth and Throat. Chapter 16 addresses the expected appearance of gingivae, buccal, and pharyngeal membranes,

TABLE 24–5. CAUSES OF MUCOSAL DISRUPTIONS

Location	Internal/Biological	External/Mechanical
Eye (conjunctiva)	Infection: bacterial, viral Allergy	Abrasions (eg, from contact lenses) Chemical burns Foreign bodies
Mouth/pharynx	Infection: bacterial, viral, fungal Dehydration Mouth breathing Emesis Plaque Cancer Cancer chemotherapy	Poorly aligned teeth Trauma: braces, toothbrushes, toothpicks, biting self, hot liquids Oral airways Ortracheal tubes
Nose	Upper respiratory infections	Foreign body Manual extraction of secretions Chemicals: cocaine, caustic gas Nasogastric tube Nasotracheal tube
Vaginal/perineal	Infection: bacterial, fungal, viral, protozoa Age-related atrophy Irritation: poor hygiene, obesity	Trauma: sexual abuse Foreign body: retained tampon Chemical irritation: soaps, contraceptive foams, creams, sponges; douches
Penile/perineal	Infection: bacterial, fungal, viral, protozoa Irritation: Poor hygiene, obesity	Foley catheter Condom catheter Sexual abuse
Rectal	Infection: bacterial, viral, parasitic Trauma: hard stools Irritation: diarrhea, medications, poor hygiene, obesity Cancer	Foreign body Sexual abuse

and the tongue and teeth; Section 1 of the present chapter describes their typical lesions. Open, draining, painful lesions of the mouth and throat should be cultured to rule out infectious origin. For clients receiving care in a hospital, n.p.o. status and mouth breathing are common causes of altered oral and throat membranes. The teeth and tongue may appear coated, and saliva sticky. Without frequent mouth care, open lesions can develop. Oral mucous membranes quickly reflect fluctuations in hydration status and also suggest changes in nutritional health. For this reason assessment of oral mucous membranes should be part of nurses' routine head-to-toe assessment every shift.

Cardiovascular. The elements of the cardiovascular examination that are important to skin and tissue assessment relate to perfusion. Palpate peripheral pulses, particularly in the lower extremities, and note coolness, pallor, and mottling of the skin of the legs, indicative of acute arterial occlusion. Chronic arterial occlusion results in hairlessness, thinning skin, and color changes related to gravity: redness when dependent, pallor when elevated. Ankle edema, with shiny bluish or brownish thin skin, or open ulcers on the lower leg suggest chronic venous insufficiency.

Genitalia, Anus, and Rectum. The mucosa of the genital and anal–rectal region is vulnerable to fissures; infectious lesions, such as jock itch (tinea cruris), herpes, or venereal warts; infestations, such as scabies or lice; and irritation from accumulated secretions or excretions, warts, or hemorrhoids. When clients remain in bed for treatment of illness, nurses need to conduct perineal assessment and provide perineal hygiene several times a day. Increased perspiration, indwelling urinary catheters, and diminished ability for self-care increase clients' vulnerability to skin and mucosal disruptions.

Diagnostic Tests

There are few diagnostic tests related to skin and mucosal functioning. Culture and sensitivity, erythrocyte sedimentation rate, C-reactive protein, antibody titers, and skin testing for sensitivity to specific antigens provide information about infectious and inflammatory processes.

Culture and Sensitivity. Cultures identify causative organisms of infections. Caregivers commonly obtain culture samples from wounds with suspicious drainage and skin or mucosal lesions of unknown origin. Throat cultures are a familiar example. Sensitivity testing is a means of determining the antibiotics to which the causative organism of an infection is sensitive. Nurses sometimes obtain specimens for culture and sensitivity (C & S) testing, particularly of wounds. Specific techniques for this procedure are discussed later in this chapter.

Erythrocyte Sedimentation Rate. The erythrocyte sedimentation rate (ESR) test is a general test for an acute inflammatory process. It is a measure of the rate at which red blood cells settle to the bottom of a test tube in unclotted blood. Inflammation tends to increase the protein content of plasma, so the sedimentation rate increases when inflammation is present. The ESR does not identify the location of the inflammation. There are no food or fluid restrictions for this test. The normal range is 0 to 7 or 0 to 10 mm/h for males and 0 to 15 or 0 to 20 mm/h for females, depending on the method used.

C-reactive Protein. C-reactive protein appears in the blood about 6 to 10 hours after the onset of an acute inflammatory process, peaking in 48 to 72 hours. It is not present in viral infections, but bacterial infections and tissue destruction produce the protein. It is not specific to location, but is useful in determining if a bacterial infection is the cause of an inflammatory response. Clients must remain n.p.o. for 8 to 12 hours before the test. Normally the protein is not present (negative); a titer of greater than 1:2 is positive.

Antibody Titers. Antibody titers measure the presence or concentration of antibodies. Some are specific to particular antigens (a foreign substance that initiates formation of antibodies); others detect the presence of a general type of antibody, but do not conclusively identify the antigen. The presence of a high concentration of a particular antibody implies the presence in the body of the organism or substance that it attacks. There is no preparation for antibody titer tests. Diagnostic titers vary with the specific antibody.

Skin Sensitivity Tests. Skin sensitivity tests identify allergens, often the cause of skin and mucosal symptoms. Small amounts of the allergens commonly responsible for the type of symptoms an individual is experiencing are injected into the dermis. The sites of the injections are examined after a period of time (usually 48 to 72 hours). Local inflammation is indicative of sensitivity to the antigen.

NURSING DIAGNOSIS OF SKIN AND TISSUE INTEGRITY

Data analysis and data clustering assist nurses to determine whether a client has any skin and tissue problems that nursing therapies can address. Five nursing diagnoses apply specifically to skin and tissue. Four are discussed here. They are Impaired Tissue Integrity, Impaired Skin Integrity, Potential for Impaired Skin Integrity, and Altered Oral Mucous Membranes. The latter three diagnoses are subcategories of the first. The last, Impaired Tissue Perfusion, is discussed in Chapter 27. Refer also to the Sample Nursing Diagnoses of Skin and Tissue Problems table on page 994. Diagnoses that may accompany, result from, or produce skin and tissue problems are listed in Box 24–4.

Impaired Tissue Integrity

Impaired Tissue Integrity is the state in which an individual experiences damage to mucous membrane, corneal, integumentary, or subcutaneous tissue.

BOX 24–4. OTHER NURSING DIAGNOSES RELATED TO SKIN AND TISSUE INTEGRITY

Physical

Altered Nutrition: More Than Body Requirements
Altered Nutrition: Less Than Body Requirements
Potential for Infection
Hypothermia
Hyperthermia
Diarrhea
Bowel Incontinence
Urinary Incontinence
Fluid Volume Excess
Fluid Volume Deficit
Decreased Cardiac Output
Impaired Gas Exchange
Potential for Disuse Syndrome
Altered Protection
Impaired Physical Mobility
Activity Intolerance
Fatigue
Sleep Pattern Disturbance
Impaired Swallowing
Unilateral Neglect
Pain

Cognitive

Sensory–perceptual Alterations
Knowledge Deficit
Altered Thought Processes
Health-seeking Behaviors

Emotional

Hopelessness
Powerlessness
Dysfunctional Grieving
Anxiety
Ineffective Coping
Impaired Adjustment

Self-conceptual

Body Image Disturbance
Self-esteem Disturbance

Sociocultural/Life Structural

Impaired Social Interaction
Social Isolation
Altered Role Performance
Sexual Dysfunction
Altered Sexuality Patterns

Developmental

Feeding Self-care Deficit
Bathing Self-care Deficit
Toileting Self-care Deficit

Environmental

Potential for Injury
Potential for Trauma

SAMPLE NURSING DIAGNOSES OF SKIN AND TISSUE PROBLEMS

Nursing Diagnosis	Defining Characteristics/Manifestations: Subjective Data	Defining Characteristics/Manifestations: Objective Data	Etiology
Impaired Tissue Integrity 1.6.1.2.1	"It's harder to breathe lying on my side, I need to sit up—but my tailbone hurts too."	1-inch diameter sacral ulceration extending through dermis. Selects semi-Fowler's position unless reminded to change positions. Frequently slips down in bed.	*Physical:* Pressure and shearing from continuous use of semi-Fowler's position.
Altered Oral Mucous Membranes 1.6.2.1.1	"My mouth feels like cotton." "It's really sore at the edge of my tongue."	Xerostomia. Coated tongue. Reddened area on lateral surface of tongue. Saliva sticky, ropey. Halitosis.	*Physical:* Dehydration.
Impaired Skin Integrity 1.6.2.1.2.1	"I feel so weak." "It hurts on my left hip." "I just can't turn myself, it's too hard."	Reddened area over left greater trochanter, does not disappear after 1 hour in supine position.	*Physical:* Generalized muscle weakness and physical immobilization.
Nursing Diagnosis	**Risk Factors**		
Potential for Impaired Skin Integrity. 1.6.2.1.2.2	Altered sensation: "I notice a sore or a bruise, but I never remember getting it, and it doesn't hurt." Does not recoil and is unable to describe sensation when lightly pricked with a sterile needle while eyes are closed.		

Etiology: Altered Circulation. Interference with circulation to body tissue, **ischemia,** prevents the adequate transport to and from cells of oxygen and nutrients, cellular waste products, or both. Ischemia rapidly produces hypoxia, and eventually cellular death or necrosis. Altered circulation can result from diseases such as diabetes, arterial insufficiency, and internal blockage of vessels by plaque or clots, and from external pressure. Immobility is a factor in pathological clotting as well as a major cause of external pressure. Poor perfusion also delays wound healing. Although nurses cannot independently treat medical diagnoses as etiologies of altered tissue integrity, teaching and preventive measures to eliminate additional contributing problems, such as pressure, friction, and shearing, are important.

Etiology: Nutritional Deficit. Deficiencies in essential nutrients, particularly vitamins, produce lesions in tissues with rapid cell turnover, such as mucosa and skin. Nutrient deficits also impair wound healing, as discussed in Section 1. Overweight or underweight clients are at additional risk for pressure sores.[28] Ischemia is likely when clients with excessive adipose tissue are immobile, because fatty tissue is not highly vascular and becomes less resilient when it is dense. Conversely, muscle and a moderate amount of subcutaneous fat provide a cushioning effect against pressure that is lacking in underweight clients. In fact, two nursing studies identified underweight as the most effective predictor of skin breakdown.[28,29]

Etiology: Fluid Deficit or Excess. Dehydration produces shrinking of cells and resultant dysfunction. To maintain life-sustaining functions, fluid shifts to the intravascular space occur when total body water diminishes. Therefore, skin and mucosal changes are among the first clinical signs of dehydration. Secretions, such as tears and mucus decrease, with resultant tissue damage due to friction and irritants. Tears and mucus normally provide tissue lubrication and play a primary role in ridding tissue of irritants.

Localized fluid excess, edema, is an abnormal expansion of the interstitial space. This increases the distance between the cells and the capillaries that deliver oxygen, compromising local cellular profusion.

Etiology: Knowledge Deficit. Lack of knowledge may result in behaviors that result in skin, mucosal, corneal, or deeper tissue lesions. Examples of knowledge deficits that can lead to impaired tissue integrity include nutrition, optimal hygiene, appropriate skin care, effective use of sunscreen, correct contact lens care, and the risks associated with immobility.

Etiology: Impaired Physical Mobility. Individuals with intact musculoskeletal and neurological function relieve pressure on body parts through spontaneous movement, prompted by discomfort. Shifting in one's seat during a long lecture is a familiar example. Compromised sensory perception and capacity for independent movement, altered level of consciousness, and muscle weakness impair mobility. Impaired mobility exposes clients to pressure sore risks from altered circulation (discussed above) and mechanical forces (discussed below). Other debilitating effects of immobility that may interact to further increase pressure sore risk are discussed in Chapter 30.

Etiology: Chemical Irritants. Many chemicals destroy superficial skin layers, resulting in an injury that is similar to a burn. Caustic alkalies often produce gelatinization of tissue.

Body excretions are a source of irritating chemicals. Urine and feces contain urea and intestinal enzymes that are destructive to skin. Moreover, *Candida albicans,* a component of intestinal flora, often colonizes in fecal matter left on the skin, causing painful excoriation. Body secretions such as blood and mucus also serve as growth media for microorganisms that subsequently cause skin irritation and breakdown.

Etiology: Thermal (Temperature Extremes). Hyperthermia results in burn injuries of varying severity. Mild burns characterized by local erythema involve only the epidermis and cause minor tissue damage. More serious burns damage dermis or even deeper layers. Full-thickness burns destroy all elements of the epithelium, therefore allowing no possibility of skin regeneration. Hypothermia damages skin by causing cellular dehydration.[29] Ice crystals form between cells, pulling intracellular fluid to them as they grow. Milder forms involve transient blanching and numbness. These injuries can occur through unsafe use of heat or cold as a treatment for other injuries.

Etiology: Mechanical. Pressure, friction, and shearing are the mechanical forces responsible for disruptions in tissue integrity. Pressure is force exerted against a surface. Pressure is created on body tissue when it is compressed between a bony prominence and a firm surface. When the pressure exceeds mean capillary pressure (approximately 25 mm Hg), capillaries collapse. The tissue appears blanched and pale. Upon release of pressure, reactive hyperemia occurs, giving the skin a flushed appearance.[28–30] This compensatory vasodilation disappears if pressure is not so great or of such long duration as to cause irreversible tissue damage. When the redness does not disappear, tissue damage has occurred. This is a stage 1 (or grade 1) pressure ulcer.

Tissue tolerance for pressure is also influenced by intrinsic factors, such as nutritional status, age, and circulatory status; and extrinsic factors, such as moisture, friction, and shearing.[31] Each of the intrinsic factors was discussed previously. Moisture weakens the natural protective barrier provided by intact epidermis. The effects of friction and shearing are discussed below. The amount of pressure and the length of time the pressure is exerted are also factors. Studies designed to define the lowest amount of pressure over a particular time period that would cause tissue injury have not produced uniform results. Minimum pressures as low as 35 mm Hg to as high as 350 mm Hg have been reported, with usual time periods of 1 to 2 hours.[32–35]

Friction is the rubbing together of two surfaces. It weakens epithelium by removing cells from the epidermis, making breakdown more likely. A common source of friction is nurses' pulling clients across bed sheets when moving and repositioning them. Friction on heels, elbows, and sacrum also occurs with self-repositioning, in particular when clients move themselves toward the slightly elevated head of the bed.

In mechanics, **shearing** is the stress created from the sliding of one load against another. As this concept applies to clients in bed, one load is a client's weight, and the other is the bed. Shearing occurs most often when a client in a semi-sitting (semi-Fowler's) position slips toward the foot of the bed. Because of friction, the skin surface in contact with the sheets moves less than the deeper tissues attached to the skeleton. As illustrated in Figure 24–5, the shearing occurs where the deeper and more superficial tissue layers meet, often damaging capillaries and compromising circulation, besides damaging other cells.

Etiology: Radiation. Radiation can produce multilayered tissue destruction similar to that caused by burns. The destruction in radiation depends on the level of radiation, length of exposure, and area of the body exposed. Radiation burns occur in people undergoing radiation therapy for malignancies, as well as in those accidentally exposed. Usually side effects from radiation therapy range from mild erythema and dryness to a more severe skin loss that appears raw and moist with clear exudate. Sometimes there is scarring accompanied by loss of skin appendages, such as hair follicles, sebaceous glands, and sweat glands, and residual hyper- or hypopigmentation.[36] Although newer supervoltage radiation machines are less destructive of skin than those used in the past, areas of the body with skin folds are vulnerable to more serious damage. Although nurses do not independently treat lesions caused by radiation, nurses treat responses to the lesions, such as discomfort and body image changes, and take measures to prevent secondary lesions or infection.

Impaired Skin Integrity

Impaired Skin Integrity is a state in which an individual's skin is adversely altered, including disruption of the skin surface and/or deeper layers. External (environmental) factors or internal (somatic) factors cause impaired skin integrity. Many of the etiologic factors for this diagnosis are the same or similar to those discussed above for Impaired Tissue Integrity. Two additional factors are discussed here.

Etiology: Mechanical Factors, Restraint. Caregivers use restraints to restrict the mobility of clients who are at risk for injury or who may harm others if mobility is not restricted. Restraints also are used to prevent clients from dislodging treatment modalities, such as nasogastric tubes or intravenous lines (see Chap. 30). Often clients are restrained because they are confused, or are too young to understand the

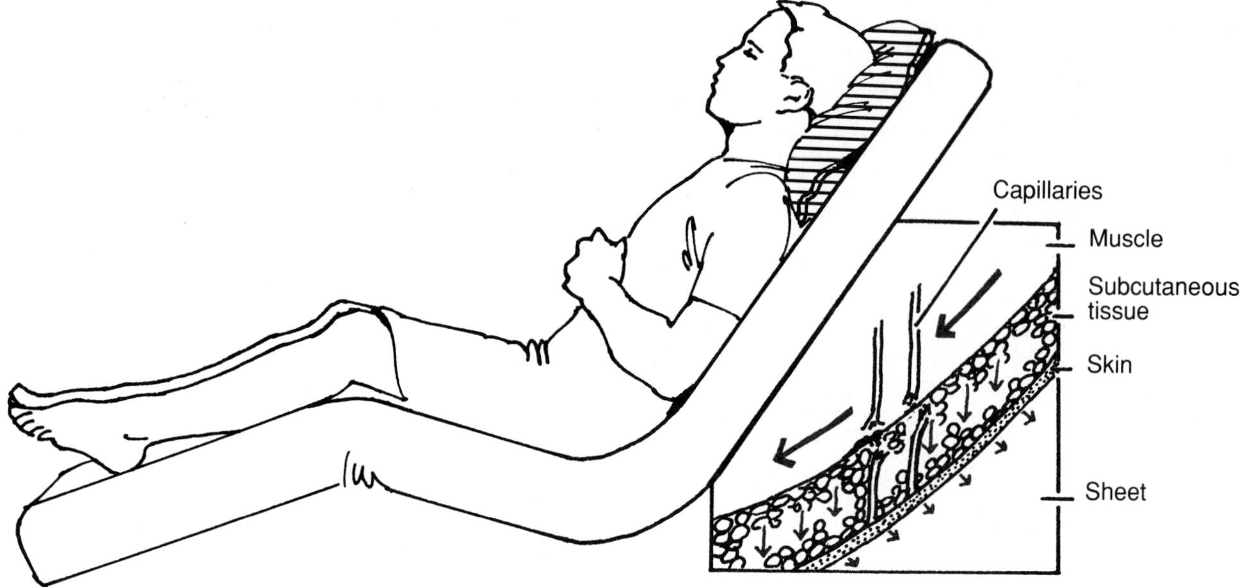

Figure 24–5. Shearing force.

importance of remaining at rest. In both cases, clients pull against restraints in an effort to move or free themselves. Even restraints that are applied correctly can cause skin damage from the pressure and friction this resistance generates. The elderly are particularly vulnerable.

Etiology: Developmental Factors. Diaper dermatitis is a skin alteration that is common among newborns and infants. The cause is prolonged skin exposure to urine and feces, which contain urea and intestinal organisms. The use of rubber pants, which prevent evaporation of moisture and therefore enhance absorption of the irritants by the skin, aggravates the rash. The perineal skin appears reddened and thickened. In 80 percent of cases lasting more than 4 days, *Candida albicans* can be cultured from the lesions.[37]

Another example of a developmental skin alteration is epidermal skin tears in older adults, discussed in Section 1.

Potential Impaired Skin Integrity

Potential Impaired Skin Integrity refers to a state in which an individual's skin is at risk of being adversely altered. The risk factors for this diagnosis are the same as the etiologies for Actual Impaired Skin Integrity. Nurses can spare a client at risk from actual skin damage by taking appropriate preventive actions.

Altered Oral Mucous Membrane

This is the state in which an individual experiences disruptions in the tissue layers of the oral cavity. Etiologies may be chemical or mechanical, or related to hydration or radiation. Mechanical and chemical etiologies of oral mucosa lesions are discussed in Section 1. The section on Impaired tissue integrity addresses changes related to hydration.

Head and neck exposure to radiation decreases saliva production, with a resulting dry mouth (xerostomia). Erythematous lesions progressing to ulceration can occur. Radiation also may affect mucosal appendages including taste buds and dental structures.[38] As with radiation injuries to the skin, nurses do not independently treat these lesions.

Stating the Skin and Tissue Diagnosis

The most useful diagnostic statements are precise descriptions of the way a particular client manifests a nursing diagnosis. For example, although damaged or destroyed tissue is the only defining characteristic for the diagnosis of Impaired Tissue Integrity, including information about the size, depth, and location of the damaged tissue provides more guidance for developing desired outcomes, evaluation criteria, and nursing implementation. Similarly, definitive statements of etiology help focus implementation effectively.

Clients with skin and tissue disruptions commonly experience more than one of the related factors listed on the taxonomy. For example, a debilitated client who develops a pressure ulcer may have a protein–calorie nutritional deficiency that makes her weak and therefore impairs her mobility. As a result of this, pressure over a bony prominence alters circulation, which finally results in the ulcer. To guide corrective nursing action effectively, the diagnostic statement should include the related factors most basic to the problem. For example: Impaired Tissue Integrity related to protein–calorie malnutrition, weakness, and physical immobility as evidenced by stage 2 pressure ulcer, ½ inch diameter, on left hip. In this case, the unique related factors are lack of adequate calories and protein and weakness that impairs mobility. Pressure and impaired circulation are, by definition, the cause of pressure ulcers, so need not be included in the diagnostic statement when there are other more significant contributing factors.

The same guidelines apply to the other skin and tissue diagnoses. Make etiologies and defining characteristics as precise as possible. For example, "Impaired Skin Integrity related to altered circulation as evidenced by disruption of skin surface on left ankle" is not as clear as "Impaired Skin Integrity related to arterial insufficiency and pressure as evidenced by ulcer, ⅛ inch deep and ½ inch in diameter with pale base and necrotic edges over left lateral malleolus." The basis for an effective client care plan is a clearly stated nursing diagnosis.

Section 3. Nurse–Client Management of Skin and Tissue Integrity

Management of skin and tissue integrity involves collaborative planning, nursing implementation, and evaluation. Refer to the Nurse–Client Management of Skin and Tissue Problems table on page 1000 for sample standard care plans with desired outcomes, evaluation criteria, and nursing implementation for clients with selected nursing diagnoses related to skin and tissue.

■ PLANNING FOR OPTIMUM SKIN AND TISSUE INTEGRITY

A client care plan for skin and tissue integrity describes expected changes in skin and tissue, criteria for evaluating the achievement of desired changes, and nursing implementation to bring about the improvements in skin and tissue condition. The statements of desired outcomes (expected changes in skin condition) and the related evaluation criteria should reflect client and nurse input. For most skin and tissue problems, the desired outcome is healing of the wound or lesion. Evaluation criteria specify the expected indications of progressive healing for the particular type of wound or lesion a client is experiencing. Sometimes, clients may have unrealistic expectations about how the skin will look after a deep lesion heals. A pleasing appearance is important to body image, and scarring may be difficult to accept. While healing of lesions is primary, nurses need to be sensitive to client concerns about disfiguring scars when developing collaborative outcomes and evaluation criteria.

Implementation must also be acceptable to clients. Because a variety of etiologies generate skin problems, implementation must incorporate multiple approaches. The example given earlier of the client whose pressure sore was related to protein–calorie malnutrition and weakness would need nursing implementation to increase intake of protein and calories, improve strength, and facilitate healing. Although nurses would have more information about approaches related to healing, clients may have considerable valuable input about dietary choices and the preferred regimen to promote strength.

Just as clearly stated nursing diagnoses are the basis for effective client care plans, collaborative plans are the basis for productive implementation.

■ NURSING IMPLEMENTATION TO PROMOTE OPTIMUM SKIN AND TISSUE INTEGRITY

Preventive Care

Preventive care related to skin and tissue integrity includes health teaching about topics such as basic hygiene, prevention and treatment of minor skin injuries, and sun protection; and screening for clients at risk for skin and tissue injury.

Health Education. Nurses provide preventive health education about skin and skin care in locations such as schools, occupational sites, clinics, wellness centers, private practice settings, and as part of home care. Often group presentations are effective, such as teaching oral hygiene to school children or protective measures against common toxic materials encountered in a particular job setting.

Teaching Basic Hygiene. Personal hygiene is influenced by advertising, cultural background, socioeconomic status, and personal preferences. Although most individuals value basic cleanliness, poverty and crowded living conditions may make adhering to hygienic practices difficult for some. A sensitive and nonjudgmental approach is essential.

School and community health nurses often teach hygiene practices, such as washing hands before eating and after toileting, brushing teeth after meals, and the importance of regular bathing and hair washing. Changes in hygiene needs corresponding to growth and development, such as use of deodorants, menstrual hygiene, and the need for more frequent facial cleansing, bathing, and shampooing during puberty are other topics that school, public health, and clinic nurses address. Teaching new mothers about postpartum hygiene and their newborns' hygiene needs is another example.

Many people are poorly informed about proper oral hygiene. Although most people brush their teeth at least daily, incorrect brushing technique, selecting an inappropriate toothbrush, and failure to include flossing are common errors. Teaching about effective oral hygiene is appropriate whenever oral assessment implies ineffective hygiene practices. Procedure 24–1 provides guidelines.

PROCEDURE 24–1. TEACHING ORAL HYGIENE

PURPOSE: To promote oral health in clients of all ages.

EQUIPMENT: Toothbrush, dental floss, and model teeth (optional).

ACTION

1. Discuss the importance of regular oral hygiene: Oral care helps prevent tooth decay and plaque, stimulates the gingiva (gum tissue), prevents halitosis, and maintains moisture of oral mucosa.
2. Discuss oral care supplies that are most effective for maintaining a healthy mouth:
   Toothbrush: A lightweight toothbrush with soft straight bristles of equal length is most effective. Hard bristles damage gum tissue. Replace a toothbrush when bristles no longer maintain the original shape of the brush. Electric or battery-operated toothbrushes are easy to use and are as effective as manual brushing in removing food particles and plaque.
   Toothpaste: Toothpaste is not required to clean teeth, prevent decay, or remove plaque. Water is sufficient to accomplish this. Sodium bicarbonate is an inexpensive product that is effective in removing stains from the teeth. Most people prefer the refreshing aftertaste that commercial toothpastes provide. Toothpastes with fluoride provide more protection against cavities than nonfluoridated products, and are especially recommended for children (but should not be swallowed). Current claims that new toothpastes prevent plaque have not been consistently substantiated.
   Dental Floss: Use of dental floss is an important means of removing food particles between the teeth, which promote plaque. It is available waxed, unwaxed, and flavored; all are equally effective if used correctly.
   Mouthwash: Mouthwash is not essential to oral health. Recent claims that it is effective in preventing plaque have not been substantiated, but it is refreshing.
   Mechanical Irrigation Devices: These devices generate an intermittent steam of water that, when directed against teeth and interdental spaces, is effective in removing debris and organisms as well as stimulating the gums. It cannot remove existing plaque, but is effective in preventing it.
   Toothpicks: Round or beveled-edge toothpicks have been found to be effective for cleaning interdental spaces and preventing plaque and gum disease.
3. Describe and demonstrate correct brushing technique, using model teeth and brush, or brush only:
   a. Hold the brush against the teeth at a 45-degree angle, so the bristles are pointing at the gumline. This allows the bristles to clean under the gum margin.
   b. Move the brush back and forth lightly over 2 to 3 teeth at a time, to the count of 10. Repeat until all of the inner and outer surfaces of all the teeth have been brushed. Following a regular order (eg, all outer surfaces of upper teeth, then all outer surfaces of lower teeth, then all inner surfaces) will facilitate reaching all teeth. Using the brush as shown will make cleaning the front teeth easier.

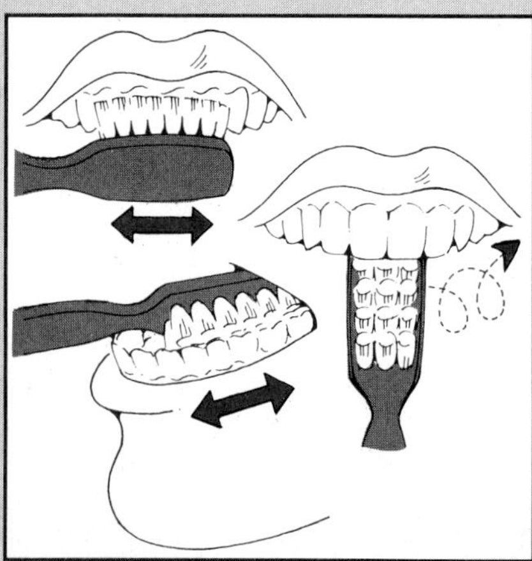

   c. Brush the chewing surfaces by placing the brush flush against the teeth and using short back-and-forth strokes. Long strokes tend to contact only the highest points of the teeth.
   d. The tongue may be brushed, if desired.
   e. Rinse the mouth as needed, moving water vigorously around the teeth and tongue so additional particles are loosened.
   f. Experts recommend brushing for 5 minutes to adequately remove plaque and food particles. It is better to brush thoroughly once a day than ineffectively several times.
4. Describe or demonstrate on model teeth the correct flossing technique:
   a. Remove a 12- to 15-inch length of floss; wrap one end around index or middle finger of each hand until the length of floss between your fingers is 1½ inches.
   b. Hold floss taut and slip it between two teeth with a gentle sawing motion, moving the floss downward toward the gums. Curve the floss around the edge of the tooth like a "C," then move the floss below the gumline until resistance is felt.

(continued)

PROCEDURE 24–1. (continued)

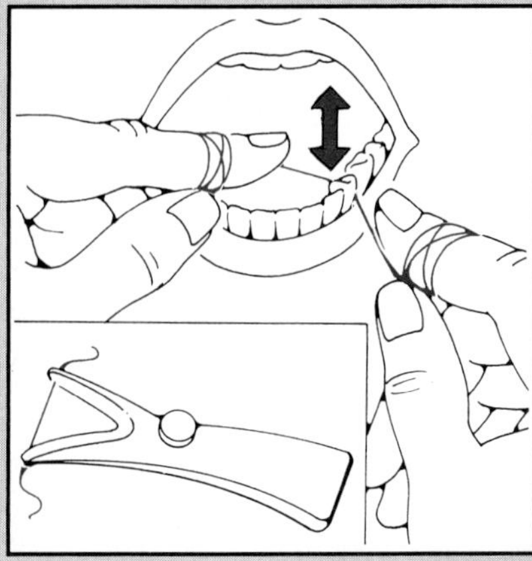

c. Move the floss up and down along the edge of the tooth from gumline to crown several times. Repeat between all teeth. It is helpful to follow a regular pattern (eg, starting at the center, then working toward the back teeth on each side of the mouth, repeating for lower teeth, or starting at the back of one side of the mouth and working toward the other side). When floss becomes frayed expose a new length by unwinding a portion from around one finger.
d. Floss handles are available and are especially useful for clients who lack dexterity needed for the above technique (see Figure above).
e. Rinse vigorously after flossing to remove loosened particles. Bleeding may indicate flossing was too vigorous or that gums are inflamed (gingivitis) because of plaque.
f. Flossing should be done at least once a day.

5. Provide additional information for parents to promote dental health in children:
   a. Avoid putting infants to bed with a bottle of milk or juice as both promote tooth decay. If a bottle is needed, use water.
   b. Fluoride treatments or vitamins with fluoride significantly decrease tooth decay in both erupted and unerupted teeth.
   c. By the time children are 2 years old, they have all their deciduous (baby) teeth; these teeth should be brushed by parents and teaching of self-brushing should begin as soon as the child can control a toothbrush.
   d. Assisting children to establish a habit of brushing teeth after every meal will significantly reduce cavities.
   e. Two to three servings of milk or dairy products per day provides calcium needed for strong teeth.
   f. Sweets and soft foods adhere to the teeth and promote tooth decay. Limit ingestion of these foods and encourage brushing or at least rinsing with water after sweet snacks.
6. Emphasize the importance of regular dental checkups every 6 to 12 months for adults and children, beginning at age 2½ to 3 years.

Prevention and Treatment of Minor Skin Injuries. Parents of young children benefit from information about protecting their youngsters from accidental injury. Bath water that is too hot is a common cause of burns and scalds. Children's natural curiosity and exploration of the environment also contribute to burn accidents. Keeping containers of hot liquids, such as beverage cups, out of reach, turning the handles of cooking pans inward, testing bath water with the wrist or elbow while filling the tub and before putting a child in it, and recognizing that toddlers' mobility expands rapidly, are simple but effective ways to prevent burns, falls, and other accidents.

All children experience cuts and scrapes as part of growing up; however, supervising their use of sharp tools and setting good examples for their safe use is a way of avoiding potentially serious injuries.

Basic first aid for minor injuries, such as gentle cleansing of cuts and scrapes with mild antiseptics, application of antibacterial ointment, and covering with a Band-Aid to keep the wound surface moist and clean, aids healing and prevents infections. Minor burns need not be covered, but application of antiseptics or topical anesthetics is soothing.

Protection from Sun Exposure. Teaching about the hazards of ultraviolet (UV) rays is an important means of preventing skin cancer. Recent evidence suggests that sun damage is cumulative, and that damage during childhood and adolescence is particularly harmful. This means that avoiding sunburn by using effective sunscreens throughout one's life must start in childhood and continue through adulthood. Even though children do not develop skin cancer, individuals that have been sunburned during the first 20 years of their lives are at greater risk of developing skin cancers as adults. To understand how to protect themselves from the harmful effects of sun exposure, individuals must grasp the meaning of SPF, or sun protection factor, that indicates the degree of protection a sunscreen provides. SPF indicates the length of time a person can stay in the sun without burning while using the sunscreen, compared to the time of sun exposure that would cause a burn on unprotected skin. Therefore, a person who would get sunburned in 15 minutes with no sun protection, using a sunscreen with an SPF of 4 could stay in the sun four times longer—in this case, for an hour—before burning. If that same person used a sunscreen with a 25 SPF, he or she would not burn in 6 hours of exposure. Reapplications are not as effective as initial applications, so that person could not expect 6 more hours of sun protection from the second application of 25 SPF sunscreen. Also, most products require application at least 30 minutes before sun exposure and reapplication after swimming for maximum effectiveness.

NURSE–CLIENT MANAGEMENT OF SKIN AND TISSUE PROBLEMS

Nursing Diagnosis	Desired Outcomes	Implementation	Evaluation Criteria
Impaired tissue integrity R/T pressure and shearing from continuous use of semi-Fowler's position *1.6.2.1*	1. Intact skin over sacrum.	1a. Establish a turning schedule that is acceptable to client and that avoids pressure on sacrum. 1b. Collaborate with physician to obtain pressure relief bed, mattress, or overlay. 1c. Maintain clean, dry, and wrinkle-free bed linen. 1d. Discuss the value of leg exercises and other movements in promoting circulation and therefore healing. Encourage use of exercises with each position change. 1e. Apply hydrocolloid dressings over ulcer. Assess dressing q shift, change according to manufacturer's directions. 1f. Clean or irrigate wound with isotonic solution such as normal saline or Ringer's lactate.	1. Progressive healing of sacral ulcer AEB: ■ Decreased depth and diameter. ■ Pale pink wound margins. ■ Presence of pink granulation tissue at base of wound, gradually filling in cavity.
	2. Avoidance of semi-Fowler's position until ulcer is healed.	2a. Discuss with client how shearing and pressure caused sacral ulcer. 2b. Obtain foam or other supports to assist client to maintain correct alignment in a side-lying position with HOB sufficiently elevated to facilitate breathing without difficulty. 2c. Obtain footboard if needed to prevent shearing in above position.	2. Client maintains turning schedule, is observed to avoid semi-Fowler's position.
Altered oral mucous membranes R/T dehydration *1.6.2.1.1*	1. Intact oral mucosa.	1a. Assist as needed with mouth care after meals and prn. Use foam toothettes instead of toothbrush if gums inflamed. 1b. Provide emollient for lips prn. 1c. If npo, assist to rinse mouth q1–2 hours. Use ¼-strength H_2O_2, normal saline, or ½-strength low alcohol mouthwash. Discuss irritating effect of alcohol, tobacco, acidic foods.	1. Absence of lesions in oral cavity AEB tongue uniformly pink.

NURSE–CLIENT MANAGEMENT OF SKIN AND TISSUE PROBLEMS (continued)

Nursing Diagnosis	Desired Outcomes	Implementation	Evaluation Criteria
	2. Healthy fluid balance.	2a. Provide oral fluids, if allowed, to compensate for losses and meet basal requirements (see Chap. 31). 2b. Maintain intravenous fluids as ordered.	Oral mucosa pink, shiny, Saliva of watery consistency, Breath fresh smelling.
Impaired skin integrity R/T generalized muscle weakness and immobilization *1.6.2.1.2.1*	1. Intact skin over left greater trochanter.	1a. See *1.6.2.1*, 1a–1d, except avoid trochanter pressure in turning schedule.	1. Skin over trochanter without redness or ulceration.
	2. Increased muscle strength appropriate to client's age, sex, and health status.	2. Provide progressive strengthening exercises to client's tolerance twice daily.	2. Serial testing of muscle strength shows progressive improvement.
	3. Improved mobility, appropriate to age and health status.	3a. Discuss relationship between mobility and healing and mobility and prevention of pressure ulcers. 3b. Collaboratively develop and use progressive ambulation regimen to client's ability.	3. Progressive increase in mobility without fatigue.
Potential for impaired skin integrity *1.6.2.1.2.2*	Skin will remain free of lesions or wounds.	Establish preventive measures in keeping with client's mobility status. Eg, if mobile reduce or eliminate environmental hazards; if bedridden, establish and maintain a regular turning schedule and exercises to stimulate circulation.	

Screening. Screening for skin changes that suggest actual or potential skin problems is part of the nurse's responsibility in preventive care, even when a skin problem is not a client's primary concern. Of particular concern are lesions that suggest malignancy, described on page 977. Other skin alterations that indicate a need for follow-up are unusual dryness, scratch marks, edema, atypical color, unhealed lesions, and thin, shiny, hairless skin. Each of these could signal problems, as discussed in Alterations in Skin and Mucosal Integrity earlier in the chapter.

Supportive Care

Nurses provide supportive skin and tissue care for clients with mild skin problems that are acute or self-limiting. One common problem for which nurses often provide supportive care is pruritus. **Pruritus** is an irritating itching sensation that individuals commonly attempt to relieve by scratching. Although this brings temporary relief, the increased blood flow caused by scratching enhances the itchy sensation, causing more scratching—setting up a continuous cycle. Pruritus may be a manifestation of a skin or systemic disease, a reaction to drugs or allergens, or a result of dry skin. Supportive care focuses on increasing comfort, protecting the skin from injury, alleviating causal factors when possible, and teaching clients strategies for prevention.

Therapeutic Baths. Although frequent bathing exacerbates pruritus, preparations such as the colloidal oatmeal preparation, Aveeno, or oils such as Alpha-Keri or Lubath are often soothing. Bran, starch, and gelatin added in a proportion of 1 or 2 ounces to a gallon of water also can be used to relieve itching.[39]

Emollients. **Emollients** are fatty or oily substances that soothe or soften dry skin or mucous membranes. Petroleum jelly, lanolin, vitamin A and D ointment, and vitamin E are examples. There are also many water-based lotions available that eliminate staining of clothing. Clients should apply emollients several times a day and especially after bathing as a preventive measure against dry skin, often a precursor to pruritus.

Topical Antipruritics. Antipruritic agents are available in the form of ointments, pastes, and lotions. For localized itching, cool compresses using normal saline, potassium permanganate, aluminum acetate (Burow's solution), or boric acid are effective (Procedure 24–2). Calamine lotion and 0.5 to 1 percent hydrocortisone ointment provide good relief as well.

PROCEDURE 24–2. APPLYING WARM OR COOL COMPRESSES

PURPOSE: To promote circulation and enhance healing, to promote suppuration, to soften dried wound exudate, and to apply medicated solution (eg, to relieve pruritus).

EQUIPMENT: Material for compress: gauze 4 × 4s or 2 × 2s, eyepads, combipads, washcloths, or towels, depending on the size and location of the application; container to moisten compresses; prescribed solution. For warm compresses: petroleum jelly, cotton-tipped applicators or tongue blades, insulating material: plastic, towels, or dry dressing materials; waterproof underpad; gauze strips or tape. External heat source such as aquathermia pad may also be used. If compresses are used on open wounds, sterile supplies, including sterile gloves and a moistureproof bag will be needed. Prepackaged sterile wet dressings are often used in this case.

ACTION	RATIONALE
1. Verify medical order for solution, location, and duration of heat therapy. Gather supplies.	1. In most health care agencies, heat therapy is not an independent nursing implementation.
2. Discuss the procedure with the client, including the expected benefits, usual sensations, and desired participation.	2. The client will be less anxious and more likely to participate if this information is shared.
3. Wash your hands.	3. Removes transient microorganisms, therefore preventing their transfer by direct contact.
4. If order is for warm compresses, warm prescribed solution or place prepackaged sterile wet dressings in dressing heater. For clean compresses, place pads/towels, etc in a basin of hot water. Preheat aquathermia pad. Sterile solution may be warmed by placing its container in a basin of very hot water.	4. Heat transfer takes time. Remaining preparation can be carried out while these materials are warming.
5. Screen client, assist with positioning, drape if necessary. Place waterproof underpad under or adjacent to body part to which compresses are to be applied.	5. Shows respect for client's needs for privacy and comfort.
6. Assess for skin integrity: general condition of skin and tissue (eg, lesions, edema); and for sensory or circulatory impairment: response to light touch, pinprick, unilateral coolness of extremity.	6. Assessment provides baseline for evaluation of effectiveness of compresses. Clients with sensory or circulatory impairment or thin/damaged skin are at greater risk for thermal injury; extreme caution is required when applying heat therapy.

NOTE: Caution is also necessary when using heat therapy with elderly, very young or unresponsive clients.

(continued)

PROCEDURE 24–2. (continued)

7. If compress is for wound, don gloves and remove existing dressing (see Procedure 24–16). Discard in moistureproof bag. Assess condition of wound and drainage.

NOTE: Inner dressing must be removed with sterile gloves. See Procedure 24–16.

7. Gloves and bag are barriers preventing transmission of organisms to nurse or environment. Assessment provides baseline to evaluate effectiveness of moist heat therapy.

8. Apply petroleum jelly to skin to be covered by warm compress. If treating an open wound, clean wound as ordered (see Procedure 24–15), then apply petroleum jelly to surrounding skin with sterile applicator or tongue blade. Skin protection is not needed for cool (room temperature) compresses to treat pruritus.

8. Provides a barrier, protecting skin from burns, maceration, or irritation, while allowing heat to penetrate deeper tissue layers.

9. Quickly wring out compress material so it is damp, but not dripping. Test temperature with your inner wrist. If too hot, cool by exposing to air. If available, a thermometer can be used. 40–45.5C or 104–114F is generally recommended for warm compresses.

9. Excess moisture will damage skin and leak from compress. Skin on inner wrist is sensitive to temperature. If this area can tolerate temperature of compress, it is likely to be tolerable to client as well.

10. Place compress lightly on prescribed area. If tolerable to client for several seconds, mold compress closely to skin surface and apply adequate compresses to cover prescribed area with 2 to 4 layers of material.

10. Skin is sensitive to sudden change in temperature, so evidence of intolerance will be prompt. Molding excludes air, which is a poor conductor of heat. Extra layers will prolong heat retention and penetration.

11. If compress is to be applied to a wound, aseptically place sterile gauze pads in a sterile basin (see Procedure 22–3), then pour warm sterile solution to cover gauze. Don sterile gloves (see Procedure 22–4) to prepare and apply compresses as above. If prepackaged sterile wet dressings are used, follow manufacturer's directions.

11. Sterile supplies prevent transfer of microorganisms from environment to wound.

12. Apply insulating layer such as plastic or dry towels over compresses. Use a sterile barrier towel over sterile compresses before additional insulating material is used. When applying compresses to an extremity, maximum insulation is achieved by wrapping insulating layer around extremity.

12. Insulation delays heat transfer to environment by convection and conduction. Moistureproof material is preferred to keep bed linens dry. Sterile barrier towel is moistureproof, so prevents contamination of wound by capillary action.

13. External heating device such as an aquathermia pad may be wrapped around or placed under insulating layer to extend the therapeutic effect of the compresses.

NOTE: Replace warm compresses every 5 minutes if no external heat source is used.

13. Warm compresses become too cold to be therapeutic within 5–10 minutes without an external heat source because heat is lost to the environment by conduction and convection.

(continued)

PROCEDURE 24–2. (continued)

14. Secure compresses, aquathermia pad, and insulating layer with tape or ties.	14. If client movement dislodges compresses, heat will no longer be directed to affected area.
15. Explain to the client that within a few minutes, the compress will feel cooler, because the body's heat receptors adapt to new temperatures rapidly, but that the compress will not actually have cooled significantly in this time period.	15. This explanation will prevent the perception that the compress is too cool to be therapeutic and the request for a hotter compress, which could cause a burn.
16. Assess client in 10–15 minutes for generalized vasodilation. If the client feels warm, provide ventilation or remove some covers. If in distress, remove the compress. NOTE: This response may cause a drop in blood pressure in clients with circulatory, pulmonary or cardiac problems.	16. Vasodilation in untreated areas of the body (consensual response) is a reflex response. It is more likely when heat therapy is applied to a large area.
17. Discontinue compress in 20 to 30 minutes. NOTE: If compress was applied to a wound, use aseptic technique for removing and disposing of compress.	17. Maximum increase in skin circulation occurs after 20–30 minutes of heat therapy. Prolonged heat (30–45 min) results in tissue congestion, followed by vasoconstriction, which prevents heat dissipation.
18. Assess the condition of the skin and/or wound. Report signs of burns or deteriorating skin condition to the physician.	18. Assessment needed to document therapeutic effect.
19. Wipe off remaining petroleum jelly, apply wound dressing if needed (see Procedure 24–16). Assist client to comfortable position; dispose, store materials according to hospital policy.	19. Shows respect for client needs for comfort and safety.

RECORDING: Note length and type of application; condition of skin before and after therapy; and systemic reaction or other problems, if any, and action taken to correct problems.

Measures to Prevent Pruritus. Eliminating the use of harsh, highly alkaline soaps is one way to prevent or minimize pruritus. Decreasing the frequency of bathing, or avoiding all soap except on the face, axilla, and perineal area, is also helpful. Thorough rinsing is important regardless of the type of soap used.

Some pruritus is the result of sensitivity to cosmetics, deodorants, or laundry products. Avoiding highly perfumed lotions and soaps and experimenting with different laundry products often eliminates itching. Sometimes extra rinsing of bed linens is helpful. Some people are sensitive to fibers used in clothing, particularly wool. Often these people can wear wool garments as long as they avoid direct contact between the wool and skin. Anyone with a sensitivity to wool also should avoid products with lanolin.

Maintaining hydration by increasing daily fluid intake to 3000 mL and raising environmental humidity via room humidifiers also improves pruritus that is secondary to dry skin.

Topical Antifungals. Nurses can offer supportive care to clients experiencing fungal skin and mucosal infections, such as vaginal candidiasis and athletes' foot. These infections often flare up in hot weather or under conditions that increase perspiration.[40] More frequent bathing, thorough drying, and loose-fitting clothing that allows air circulation can prevent flare-ups of fungal infections.

Candida albicans is a common cause of vaginitis. It produces a curdy white, cottage-cheese-like discharge, itching, and vaginal erythema. Vaginal application of nystatin is the most common treatment. It is now available over the counter. Nurses recommending its use should caution clients to seek additional care if symptoms do not disappear after the recommended course of the drug. Some clients may prefer alternative treatments such as vinegar douches (1 tsp in a pint of water) or boric acid powder in a size 0 gelatin capsule, inserted into the vagina nightly for 1 to 2 weeks.[41] Inform clients that drying labial skin folds thoroughly after bathing or showering (a hair dryer works well), wearing cotton underwear, and avoiding tight-fitting pants are effective preventive measures and promote treatment of active infections.

Athletes' foot responds to topical applications of preparations such as Tinactin, Enzactin, or Desinex in ointment, powder, or spray form. Clients should wash the affected area with mild soap and water and dry well before applying medication. Wearing sandals or leather shoes with absorbent cotton socks enhances evaporation of perspiration. Clients should avoid vinyl or plastic shoes because they trap moisture.

Sitz Bath. Sitz baths (Procedure 24–3) are soothing for clients with hemorrhoids and perineal wounds, such as episiotomies. They enhance healing by cleansing action and promoting circulation. Clients can use their bathtubs for self-administered sitz baths at home.

PROCEDURE 24–3. TAKING A SITZ BATH

PURPOSE: Application of local heat to the perineal/rectal area to reduce inflammation, enhance suppuration, and soften and remove exudates, thereby promoting healing and comfort.

EQUIPMENT: Portable sitz bath, disposable sitz bath kit or permanently installed sitz bath, towels, and bath blanket (optional).

ACTION	RATIONALE
1. Review medical order.	1. Heat application is not an independent nursing action in some health-care facilities.
2. Discuss the procedure with the client, including the expected benefits, usual sensations, and desired participation.	2. Clients will be more likely to participate and less anxious if this information is shared.
3. Fill the sitz bath ⅓–½ full of warm water, depending on the size of the tub and the size of the client. 105–115F (40.5–46C) is preferred if a thermometer is available. If a portable unit is used, fill the bag as well, then clamp the tubing. Most clients find permanent or portable sitz baths more comfortable if a towel is placed in the bottom of the tub.	3. When the client sits in the tub, water will be displaced so the water level will rise. Because portable units are small, the water cools more quickly. The bag provides a reservoir of warm water to replace the cooled water in the tub.

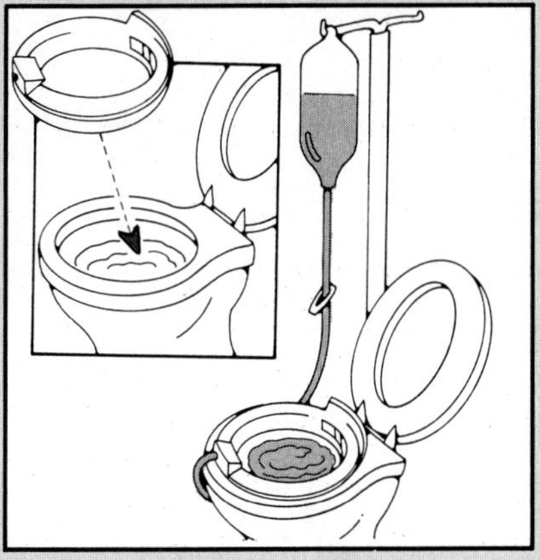

(continued)

PROCEDURE 24–3. (continued)

4. Assist client to bathroom or tub area, if necessary, or provide privacy for portable unit in client's room. Most alert mobile clients need no further assistance for sitz bath if clear explanation is given.

4. Bathing and related activities are considered private in most cultures.

5. If perineal dressings are present, don gloves to remove and discard in waterproof bag.

5. Heat is most effective if applied directly to the skin. Dressings would have an insulating effect.

6. Assess affected area for swelling, redness, drainage.

6. Assessment provides baseline for evaluating effectiveness of treatment.

7. Provide level of assistance client requires to sit in the tub, show client how to use clamp to control flow of warm water from the bag.

NOTE: Clients with cardiac, respiratory or circulatory problems should not be left unattended during heat therapy. See step 9.

7. Client safety is a primary concern, but most clients who are able prefer to perform bathing-related activities independently.

8. Provide bath blankets to drape over shoulders and legs if client desires.

8. Some clients may feel chilled when part of the body is warmed by heat therapy.

9. Show client location of nurse call button. Return to assess client response to therapy within 5 minutes. Assess for weakness, vertigo, pallor, tachycardia or shortness of breath.

9. These indicate inability to tolerate sitz bath. This is an unusual response in otherwise healthy clients, but assessment of all clients is prudent to prevent injury.

10. Return in 15–20 minutes to discontinue treatment. Alert mobile clients are able to independently discontinue treatment.

10. Maximum increase in skin circulation occurs after 20–30 minutes of heat therapy. Prolonged heat (30–45 min) results in tissue congestion, followed by vasoconstriction, which prevents heat dissipation.

11. Assess affected area as in step 6. Replace dressings if ordered (see Procedure 24–16).

11. Evaluation of effectiveness of treatments is a nursing responsibility.

12. Clean/disinfect portable or permanent sitz bath according to agency policy. Disposable units can be washed and reused by client as needed.

12. Cleaning/disinfecting removes and kills microorganisms, preventing transfer to other clients.

RECORDING: Note completion of treatment; condition of affected area before and after treatment; client's response; and problems, if any, and action taken to correct them.

IMPLICATIONS FOR NURSE–CLIENT COLLABORATION

Assisting Clients With Personal Hygiene

Many clients perceive that accepting help for personal care such as oral hygiene, bathing, or perineal care is demeaning. A nurse's ability to offer this help while demonstrating respect and seeking client input to the extent that clients are capable of giving it enables clients to retain a sense of dignity and self-respect. This kind of caring approach is the essence of collaboration.

Eye Irrigation. Although tears naturally cleanse the eyes, occasionally irritants such as debris or chemicals require removal by irrigation, as described in Procedure 24–4. Lubricants or artificial tears provide protection when tear production is diminished, or to reduce irritation from dust or contact lenses.

Ear Irrigation. Some individuals produce excessive cerumen, which may collect in amounts sufficient to interfere with hearing. Irrigating the ear (as discussed in Chap. 29) is a safe means of removing built-up wax. Caution clients against attempting to remove ear wax with cotton-tipped applicators, as they can damage organs of the middle ear.

Restorative Care

Clients with wounds, skin diseases, or health problems that interfere with the ability to perform self-hygiene and skin care need restorative skin and tissue care. Restorative skin and tissue care includes general hygiene: oral hygiene, bathing (including eye, ear, hair, nail, and perineal care), and care of lesions and wounds. Box 24–5 presents general guidelines for assisting clients with hygiene. Each of the individual elements of restorative skin and tissue care is discussed below. Health care facilities that provide inpatient care have routine times for providing hygiene related to usual daily activities. Early morning care, morning care, and hour of sleep care are the most common.

Early morning care is offered at the time of awakening. It enhances well-being and readies clients for breakfast. Early morning care consists of offering a bedpan or urinal (see Chap. 26) or helping clients to the bathroom or bedside commode and helping or providing materials for clients to wash their hands and face, perform oral hygiene, and comb or brush their hair. Clients who need glasses or hearing aids usually desire to put them on after washing their face. If these aids need cleaning (see Chap. 29), it may be done now or later with the bath. Some clients also desire to shave and apply cosmetics or makeup at this time.

Morning care (AM care) is given sometime after breakfast. It includes assistance with elimination, oral care, shower or bath, linen change, and shaving and hair care if not previously done. Often, range of motion and other in-bed exercises or ambulation (see Chap. 30), are considered part of morning care. Hour of sleep (HS) care readies clients for sleep. It encompasses helping with elimination, washing hands and face, oral care, skin care, and straightening or freshening bed linens. Chapter 28 discusses HS care in greater detail.

BOX 24–5. GENERAL GUIDELINES FOR ASSISTING CLIENTS WITH PERSONAL HYGIENE

1. Encourage independence in personal care to the extent possible considering client's physical condition and necessary restrictions related to medical and nursing treatment plans. Self-care promotes self-esteem and reduces feelings of dependence and powerlessness. Large muscle activity during self-care activities stimulates circulation and maintains muscle tone and joint mobility.
2. Adhere as closely as possible to clients' usual hygiene routines, in terms of timing, techniques, and special toilet articles or products used. Loss of control over personal routines is a significant stressor associated with illness and hospitalization.
3. Collaborate with client and physician to select the least restrictive modification given client's condition (eg, cover incision and IV site with plastic so ambulatory postsurgical client can take a shower rather than a sponge bath, use a shower chair for an alert but slightly weak client).
4. Protect client's safety during independent hygiene activities by using "occupied" signs rather than locks on showers or tub rooms, instructing client on the location and use of the call light, and checking on client at least every 5 minutes. For some clients, remaining outside the door or curtain is advisable.
5. When assisting with hygiene procedures, maintain privacy at all times: close door, pull curtains around bed, and keep all parts of body covered except part being cleaned. Hygiene activities are considered private in most cultures. Body exposure is threatening and demeaning to most individuals and also causes discomfort because of chilling.
6. Wash your hands before and after assisting with hygiene to avoid transfer of microorganisms among clients, nurse, and environment. Gloves may be indicated for some procedures (see specific procedures).
7. Apply principles of body mechanics such as raising the bed to your waist level and moving client close to the side of the bed on which you are working when assisting clients with hygiene. Refer to Chapter 30 for more information about body mechanics.

Oral Hygiene. Most clients prefer to perform oral self-care, even if they cannot get out of bed. If clients need assistance, follow the guidelines in Procedure 24–1. Bring toothbrush, toothpaste, curved basin (also called a kidney or emesis basin), dental floss, water for rinsing, and a disposable waterproof underpad. Some nurses prefer to wear clean latex gloves when doing oral care, but the Centers for Disease Control recommend wearing gloves only if there is obvious bleeding of oral mucosa (see Chap. 22).

Hospitalized clients who have dentures often require help to clean them. Procedure 24–5 outlines denture care.

Oral care is especially important for unconscious clients. They are often mouth breathers, which promotes drying of the oral mucosa and tenacious oral secretions that accumulate on the tongue and teeth. Procedure 24–6 details

PROCEDURE 24–4. IRRIGATING EYES

☐ **PURPOSE:** To cleanse eye of irritants or discharge.

☐ **EQUIPMENT:** Sterile irrigating solution (normal saline is most common; IV solution, container, and tubing may be used); sterile irrigation set (or sterile basin and toomey syringe); curved (emesis) basin; waterproof pad; and sterile gauze pad (4 × 4).

ACTION

1. Review the medical order. Wash your hands. Discuss the procedure with the client, including the usual sensations, and desired participation.
2. Request or assist the client to a sidelying position with the affected eye lowest. Place the waterproof pad so pillow, sheet, and clothing are protected. Place an emesis basin with the concave curve against the cheek to collect returned solution. The client may wish to hold the basin for closer contact.
3. If using an irrigation set, fill the syringe with sterile irrigant at room temperature. If using an infusion set, attach and fill the tubing (no needle is used). Do not allow anything unsterile to contact the tip of the syringe or tubing.
4. With your nondominant hand, retract the upper and lower lids of the affected eye to expose conjunctival sac. Administer solution so it flows from the inner canthus to the outer canthus to prevent fluid from flowing into the unaffected eye or the nasolactimal duct of the affected eye. Flush the cornea and conjunctival sac. Fifteen minutes of flushing is needed for some chemicals. Avoid contacting the cornea with the syringe or tubing tip as this will injure the cornea.

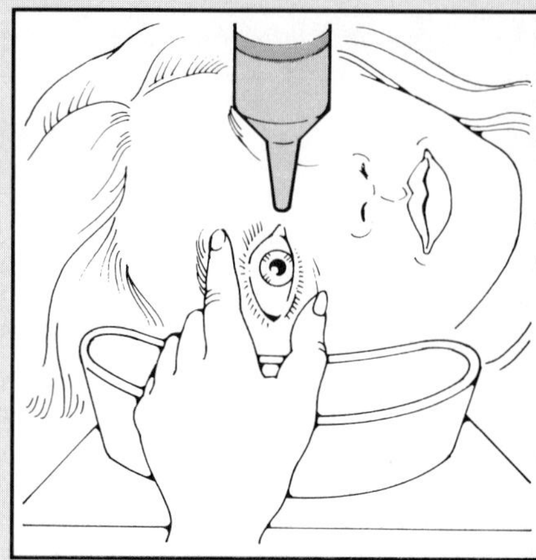

5. When the prescribed amount of irrigant has been administered, or the returned solution is clear, gently blot the eye from inner to outer canthus with a sterile 4 × 4 and dry the client's cheek. Remove and discard used equipment according to agency policy.

☐ **RECORDING:** Note the appearance of the sclera, conjunctiva, and surrounding tissue. Describe discharge, if any. Note the amount and type of irrigant and the client's response to the procedure.

oral care for unconscious clients. Many unconscious clients need oral care every 2 hours.

Hair Care. Hair care includes shaving, beard and mustache care, and combing and shampooing scalp hair. Facial hair requires daily care. Most men are uncomfortable if they are unshaven, and some may need to shave twice a day to maintain a desired appearance. Usually men prefer to shave themselves, but if they are unable, shaving is part of daily nursing care. Refer to Procedure 24–7.

Hair care is another aspect of hygiene that most clients prefer to do independently. However, clean, combed hair contributes to well-being and positive feelings about self-presentation, so clients who are unable to manage it usually appreciate help. Refer to Procedures 24–8 and 24–9. In acute care settings, time constraints may preclude shampooing a client's hair; however, any client confined to bed for several days benefits from a shampoo.

Bathing Clients. A daily bath or shower is part of most individuals' hygiene habits. Although some may feel that their relative lack of activity when in a hospital makes daily bathing unnecessary, in fact being in bed under covers increases perspiration. Bathing removes accumulated perspiration, skin oils, dead skin cells, and bacteria, and prevents body odor. It also enhances circulation and promotes relaxation and feelings of well-being. Bathing a client provides a nurse with an excellent opportunity to assess skin condition thoroughly and initiate early treatment of any lesions related to bed rest. Procedure 24–10 describes how to give a bed bath. Some clients, particularly older clients, require special care to prevent dry skin, such as use of moisturizing soap, emollients, or using soap sparingly. Foot and nail care (Procedure 24–11) and perineal and Foley catheter care (Procedure 24–12) are part of the bath, and are repeated as necessary throughout the day.

(*Text continues on page 1026.*)

PROCEDURE 24–5. CARING FOR DENTURES

▭ **PURPOSE:** To remove trapped food particles from dentures and oral cavity, to maintain oral mucosal integrity, and to promote comfort and a sense of well-being.

▭ **EQUIPMENT:** Denture brush, soft brush or toothette, denture cup or emesis basin, gauze or paper towels, cleaning agent of client's preference, and washcloth or towel.

ACTION

1. Discuss client's preferences for denture care. Most clients prefer to care for dentures independently and many are embarrassed to be seen by others without dentures in place. If assistance is necessary, encourage clients to direct the process as much as possible.
2. Wash your hands. Assemble equipment at the bedside. Ask the client to remove dentures. If client is unable to do so, use gauze or a paper towel to prevent slipping when grasping the denture to remove it. Some nurses prefer to wear gloves for denture care, but this is not required according to universal precautions. Grasp the front of the lower plate, lift it, and tip it slightly, using care not to bump it on the upper plate as you take it from the mouth. Place it in the denture cup or emesis basin. Grasp the front of the upper plate, rock it gently from side to side to break the vacuum seal, and then tip it downward slightly to pull it out of the mouth. Put it in the cup or basin.

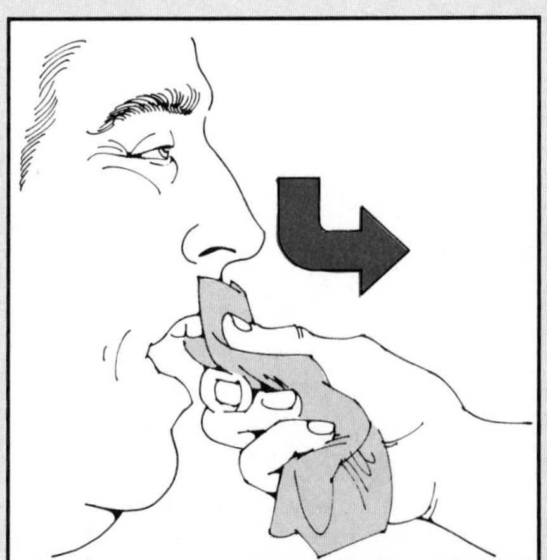

3. Brush all surfaces of both plates at the sink, using a stiff denture brush and cleaning agent of client's choice. Placing a washcloth or several paper towels in the sink will prevent chipping the dentures if they are dropped during cleaning. Rinse dentures thoroughly with running water. Do not use hot water because this may warp the dentures. Stained dentures may be soaked in denture cleaner or a solution of 5–10 mL of vinegar in 240 mL of water.
4. Clean client's tongue and gums with a soft toothbrush, inspecting gums and palate for signs of irrtation from the dentures. Offer water or mouthwash to rinse mouth and a towel or cloth to wipe mouth.
5. Give dentures to client for reinsertion. Some clients use denture adhesive, which is applied in a thin layer on the undersurface of each plate. If assistance is needed, insert the plates one at a time, upper and then lower, exerting slight pressure to facilitate adherence to the gums. If dentures are not reinserted, they should be stored in liquid in a marked denture cup.
6. Store client's oral hygiene materials as client desires.

▭ **RECORDING:** Not usually required. May be noted on checklist. If mucosal lesions are noted, describe lesions and action taken.

PROCEDURE 24–6. PROVIDING MOUTH CARE FOR AN UNCONSCIOUS CLIENT

PURPOSE: Cleansing oral cavity, maintaining integrity and hydration of oral mucosa, and preventing oral infections and lesions.

EQUIPMENT: Gauze-padded tongue blade or bite block; soft toothbrush; toothette or lemon-glycerine swabs; cleaning agent: ½-strength hydrogen peroxide, baking soda, or mouthwash; water; 50-mL syringe; emesis basin; suction apparatus with tonsil suction tip; waterproof pad; and emollient such as petroleum jelly, A & D ointment, or commercial lip balm. Gloves recommended.

ACTION	RATIONALE
1. Discuss the procedure with the client, including the expected benefits, usual sensations, and desired participation.	1. The client will be less anxious and more likely to participate if this information is shared. Even apparently unresponsive clients may be able to hear and understand.
2. Gather equipment at bedside, close door or pull bedside curtains.	2. Personal care is considered a private activity in most cultures. Unconscious clients are deserving of the same respect as alert clients.
3. Position client on the side, with head on the edge of the pillow, a curved basin below the mouth, and a waterproof pad under the head and basin. 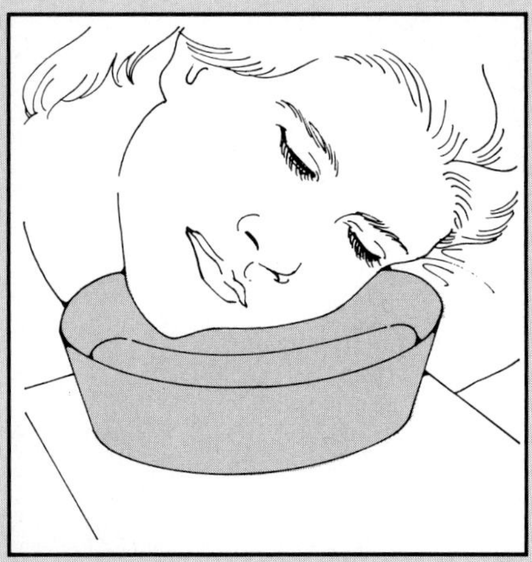	3. Unconscious clients often lack a gag reflex, so are at risk for aspiration. This position facilitates flow of liquid out of the mouth by gravity. Basin and pad protect bed linen.

(continued)

PROCEDURE 24–6. (continued)

4. Place a padded tongue blade edgewise between the back molars on one side of the mouth. A bite block may also be used.

4. Keeps the mouth open so oral care and assessment can be carried out.

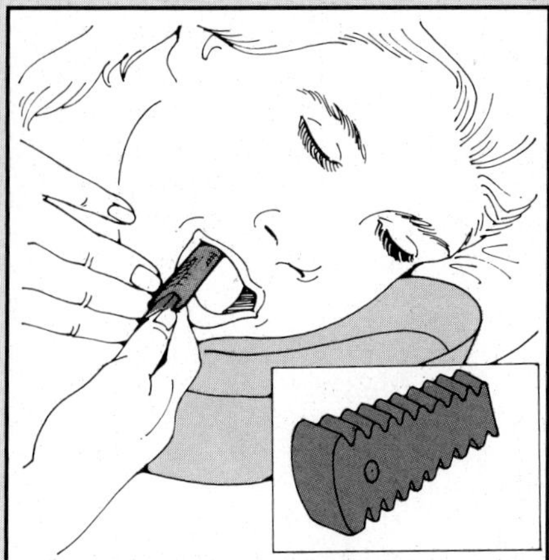

NOTE: Some unconscious clients bite reflexively when an object is placed in their mouths. Do not try to force the mouth open or place your fingers in the mouth.

5. Turn the suction unit on to low suction. Be sure tonsil suction device is attached.

5. Tonsil suction apparatus can be used to quickly remove cleaning solution or saliva, which may flow into the throat if client suddenly changes positions.

6. Moisten the toothbrush with dilute H_2O_2 or mouthwash. Do not use regular toothpaste, as it is hard to rinse. Brush all surfaces of the client's teeth and tongue as described in Procedure 24–1. Assess the condition of oral mucous membranes as you brush. Dentures of unconscious clients should not remain in their mouths as they can be aspirated; however, oral hygiene is still needed.

NOTE: Lemon-glycerine swabs or toothettes may be used as short-term substitute for brushing, but are not as effective in removing debris.

6. Unconscious clients are often mouth breathers, which contributes to drying of mucosa and formation of crusts, both of which may promote mouth lesions. H_2O_2 is particularly effective in removing organic matter and is antibacterial, so it promotes healing.

(continued)

PROCEDURE 24–6. (continued)

7. Rinse the mouth thoroughly with water from the syringe. Direct the water toward the sides, not the back, of the mouth. Use suction to remove any liquid that does not flow into the basin. Reassess mouth.

7. Rinsing in this manner reduces risk of aspiration while removing loosened debris.

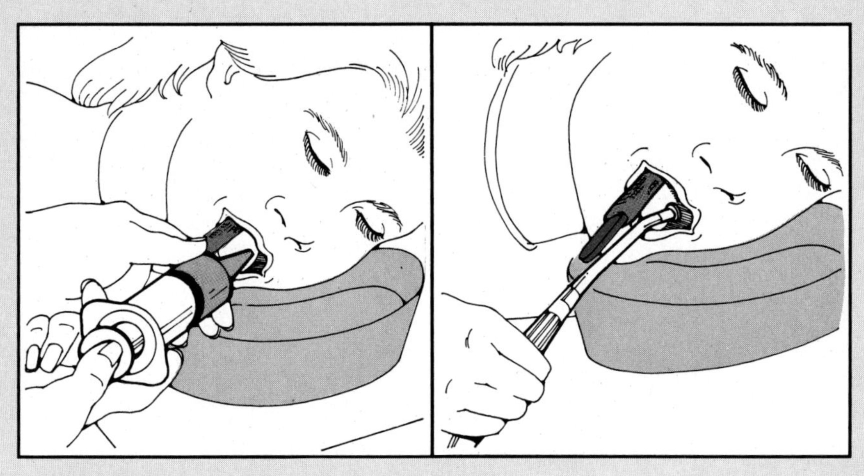

8. Dry client's face. Apply emollient to lips.

8. Emollients minimize loss of moisture from tissues and contain additional moisturizing agents.

9. Reposition client. Raise siderails. Remove equipment; clean and store according to agency policy.

9. Promotes client comfort and safety.

10. Repeat every 1–2 hours.

10. Buildup of dried secretions in the oral cavity occurs rapidly in unconscious clients because of mouth breathing and the lack of activities such as chewing and swallowing, which ordinarily contribute to oral hygiene.

RECORDING: Note procedure; condition of oral cavity before and after; problems, if any, and action taken in response.

PROCEDURE 24–7. SHAVING AND BEARD CARE

PURPOSE: Removal of facial hair to promote comfort and improve appearance.

EQUIPMENT: Razor with sharp blade, shaving cream, basin, washcloth, towel, and clean gloves (if desired). Aftershave lotion (optional). Comb for beard or mustache, scissors if trim is desired. Mirror if desired by client. Electric shaver preferred by some clients.

ACTION

1. Discuss client's preferences for time and type of shave. Some clients may prefer family member to assist. Some black clients cannot tolerate shaving because it causes skin irritation and/or ingrown hairs; often dipilatory preparations are used instead. Use of an electric shaver is recommended for clients on anticoagulant therapy, taking high doses of aspirin, or with bleeding disorders.
2. Assemble equipment and prepare area: raise bed to nurse's waist height with client in Fowler's position, place towel over client's chest to collect drips and hair. Provide privacy if client desires.
3. *If using a razor:* Soften the beard by applying a moist, warm washcloth to the face and neck for several minutes. Apply an even layer of shaving cream to face and neck. Don gloves, if desired. Holding the razor at a 45-degree angle, use firm short strokes in the direction of hair growth to remove facial and neck hair. Pulling skin taut with your other hand in opposite direction to strokes will reduce the likelihood of accidental cuts. Rinse razor frequently in basin of warm water. Some prefer to shave against the direction of hair growth—this results in a closer shave, but is more likely to cause skin irritation. When shave is complete, wipe excess lather with warm, damp cloth; dry face and neck.

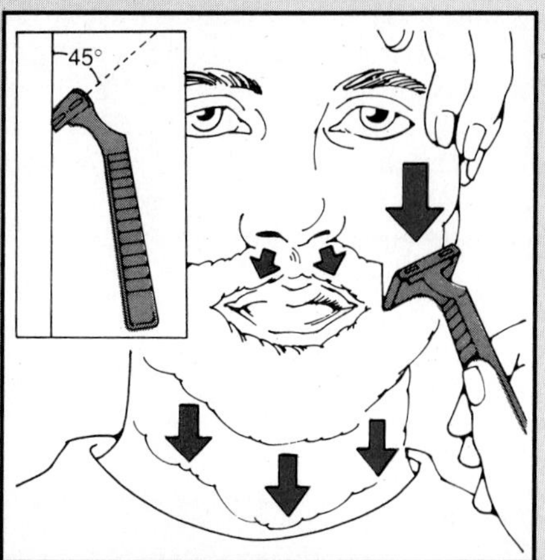

4. *If using an electric shaver:* No lather or gloves are needed. If shaver has a flat straight head, use short up-and-down strokes on face, and strokes in the direction of hair growth on sensitive areas (eg, neck). Rotary head shavers work best if circular strokes are used. Hold skin taut while shaving as with razor.
5. Use sharp scissors with blunt tips to trim beards and mustaches if client desires. Beards and mustaches should be combed daily and washed several times per week using facial soap, rinsed well and dried.
6. Provide aftershave lotion if desired, remove soiled linen, store personal items according to client preference. Clean accumulated hair from electric shaver before storing, discard disposable razor in sharps container. Razor, linen, or gloves soiled with blood require special precautions. See agency policy.

RECORDING: Not usually necessary unless problems occur (eg, excessive bleeding). Then note problem and action taken.

PROCEDURE 24–8. CARING FOR HAIR

PURPOSE: To maintain integrity of hair and scalp and promote sense of well-being.

EQUIPMENT: Comb or brush, and special products desired by client. For hair matted with blood or excessively tangled: hydrogen peroxide, alcohol, or oil. Gloves if blood is present.

ACTION

1. Discuss client's preferences for nature and timing of hair care. Most clients prefer to carry out these activities independently, but may be unable due to illness or activity restrictions.

   Daily Care: Bush or comb hair at least once per day, working from scalp to ends. Style according to client's preference. Long hair may be more easily managed if parted and groomed in sections; braiding prevents tangling. While caring for hair, assess the scalp for flaking, sores, irritated areas, or areas of hair loss; and note hair luster, texture, thickness, dryness, oiliness, or unusual loss of hair with combing.

   Special Hair Care for Black Clients: Black clients commonly have thick, curly hair that is more fragile than straight hair; scalp and hair tend to be dry. A comb with widely spaced teeth is recommended. Comb from the scalp outward with a lifting, fluffing motion. Hair-lubricating products are preferred by most black clients. Mineral oil or petroleum jelly may be used for this, if commercial products are not available. If hair is braided in cornrows, these need not be unbraided, even for shampooing.

   Tangled or Matted Hair: Tangles may be loosened by applying a small amount of oil, petroleum jelly, or alcohol. Comb out tangles in a small section of hair toward the scalp. Stabilize a short length of hair with your hand to avoid scalp trauma and comb toward the ends of the hair. If hair is matted with organic substances such as blood, wiping matted areas with gauze or cotton soaked in hydrogen peroxide is effective to clean and untangle hair strands. It is recommended that gloves be worn if blood is present. Badly tangled or matted hair is more likely to be infested with lice, so careful inspection for lice and nits (usually found near the root of the hair shaft at the nape of the neck or behind the ears) is indicated. If lice or nits are present, combing with a fine-tooth comb and a shampoo with products containing gamma-benzene-hexachloride is indicated (see Procedure 24–9). Removing tangles can be a difficult and painful process, so may need to be completed in several short sessions rather than all at once.

RECORDING: Describe special care given, noting condition of scalp and hair before and after care. Routine daily care is generally not documented, but may be noted on a daily care checklist.

PROCEDURE 24–9. SHAMPOOING

PURPOSE: To remove oil, dirt, or other substances, or to apply medicated solutions to hair and scalp.

EQUIPMENT: Shampoo, special preparations desired by client, towels, and hair dryer (optional). If bed shampoo: shampoo trough or bath blanket and waterproof sheet, extra towels, two basins, and pitcher or graduate (an irrigating bag, such as an enema bag, suspended from an IV pole may be used instead).

ACTION

1. Discuss client's preferences for location and timing of shampoo. Most clients prefer to carry out this activity independently, but may be unable due to illness or activity restrictions. Options for location of shampoo include the bed, sink, tub, or shower. A chair or gurney may be used, depending on space limitations. Dry shampoo is available if conditions prevent a wet shampoo. In some agencies, a medical order is required for a wet shampoo.

(continued)

PROCEDURE 24–9. (continued)

Shower Shampoo: This is most feasible if the shower is equipped with a hand-held device. The client can sit in a shower chair or, if space permits, lie on a gurney protected with a waterproof sheet (if a sheet is unavailable, one or more large trash bags work well for this, or make protector described below for bed shampoo).

Tub Shampoo: If the client is able to sit in a bathtub, the hair can be washed and rinsed as part of the tub bath. The shampoo must be done rapidly, however, to avoid chilling the client.

Sink Shampoo: This is easiest if the client is seated in a chair, with the back to the sink (if a chair of suitable height is not available, a bedside commode may be substituted). The head rests on the edge of the sink, which is padded with a towel. A pitcher, graduate, or irrigating bag may be needed to wet and rinse the hair. A bath blanket can be placed over the client to prevent chilling. It is possible to perform a sink shampoo with the client lying on a gurney if space permits.

Bed Shampoo: If the above locations are too difficult for the client, the bed can be protected with a plastic shampoo trough or an improvised device to channel and collect the water. To make an improvised trough: fold a bath blanket into quarters lengthwise, then form into a long roll; place the roll on the edge of a plastic sheet (or several overlapping trash bags, if no sheet is available), continue rolling the blanket tube several turns into the plastic; curve the plastic-covered tube into a horseshoe shape and position it under the client's head so the remaining plastic can be gathered into a trough and draped into a basin to catch the water.

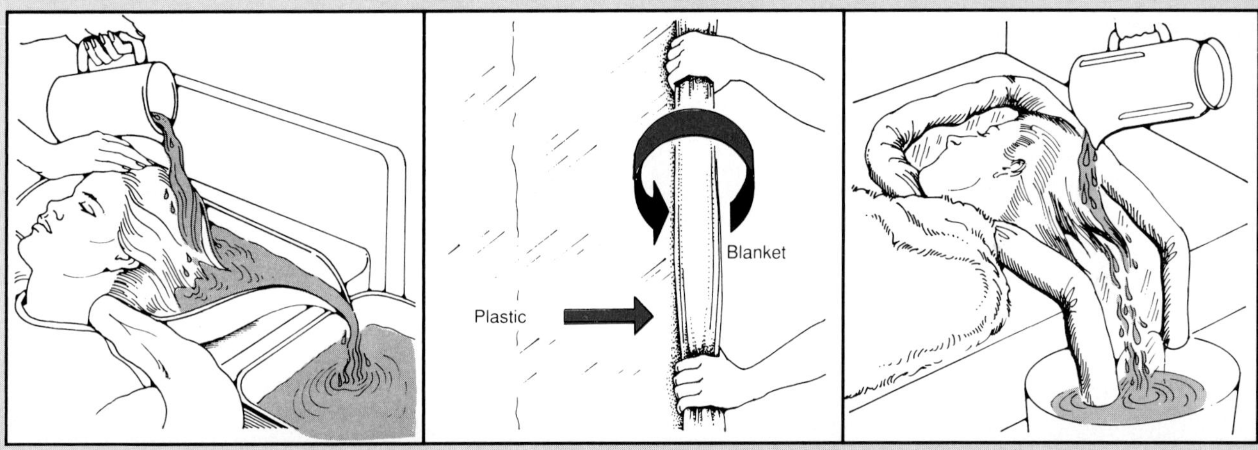

2. Position client and bed, chair, or gurney, so nurse's access to client's hair is optimal. Place a rolled towel around the client's neck and another around the shoulders. Many clients also desire to hold a small towel or washcloth over their eyes and to be covered with a bath blanket. Position protector for bed or gurney as described above.
3. Gather equipment at location selected for shampoo. For bedside shampoo, fill a large basin with warm water (105–110F, 40–41C, or warm to the inner wrist) and obtain a smaller container to pour water; or fill irrigating container with attached tubing, clamp tubing, and hang container from an IV pole at bedside. If running water is used, adjust water temperature as above before directing water over client's hair.
4. Wet hair completely. Cover client's ear with your free hand to avoid water flowing into ears. Apply a small amount of shampoo and work into a lather with both

(continued)

PROCEDURE 24–9. (continued)

hands. Massage the scalp with pads of your fingers. Rinse thoroughly with clear water. Repeat lather and rinse if necessary. Apply conditioner if desired and rinse again. Squeeze excess moisture from hair.

5. Wrap the client's head with a dry towel. Reposition if necessary so bed protector can be removed. Blot the hair dry with the towel, comb as described in Procedure 24–8. Apply special products as desired by client and blow dry hair if situation permits.
6. Assist client as necessary to comfortable bed position. Pillow and clients shoulders may be covered with a towel if hair is not completely dry.
7. Clean and store equipment according to agency policy.

RECORDING: Note condition of hair and scalp before and after shampoo; client's response; and problems, if any, and action taken in response.

PROCEDURE 24–10. GIVING A BED BATH

PURPOSE: To clean the skin, promote circulation, relax muscles, and promote comfort and well-being. Provides good opportunity for complete integumentary assessment.

EQUIPMENT: Basin, soap in soap dish, washcloth, 2 or 3 towels, bath blanket, deodorant (if client desires), lotion, clean linen and gown, and linen hamper.

ACTION	RATIONALE
1. Mutually select the optimum time for bath and associated hygiene. Typically, clients prefer to wash their face, shave, brush their teeth, and comb their hair before breakfast, and bathe at a later time. Refer to Box 24–5 for general guidelines for hygiene and Procedures 24–1 and 25–5 through 25–9 for shaving, oral and hair care. Client may prefer that a family member assist.	1. Mutual decision making communicates respect for the client. Rigid conforming to schedules is often condoned in institutions, for the sake of efficiency, but it is not always most efficient or effective to do so.
2. Discuss the procedure with the client, including the expected benefits, usual sensations, and desired participations.	2. The client will be more likely to participate and less anxious if this information is shared.
3. Assemble equipment. Screen client, raise bed. Lower siderail on near side of bed. Remove positioning aids, pillows except for pillow under head. HOB can be flat or slightly raised.	3. Conserves nurse's energy, promotes body mechanics. See Chap. 30.

NOTE: If client has been incontinent, clean thoroughly before beginning bath. If bath basin is used for this, disinfect it before using it for bath.

(continued)

PROCEDURE 24–10. (continued)

4. Remove and fold bedspread. Cover top linen with a bath blanket. Ask client to hold top of bath blanket, then pull top sheet out without exposing client. If top sheet is to be reused, fold and place on chair. Place soiled linen in hamper. Top sheet may be left in place if no bath blanket is available. Place an additional blanket on top if client is cold.

4. Bathing promotes evaporation of moisture from the skin, which lowers skin temperature. Flannel bath blanket absorbs more moisture and is warmer than a sheet.

5. Remove gown with minimal exposure of client. If client has an IV, remove opposite sleeve first, then sleeve on arm with IV. Take the IV container off the pole and slip sleeve over tubing and container, rehang, and check flowrate. If an IV controller or pump is in use, adjust screwclamp, remove tubing from machine, remove gown as above, replace tubing in machine.

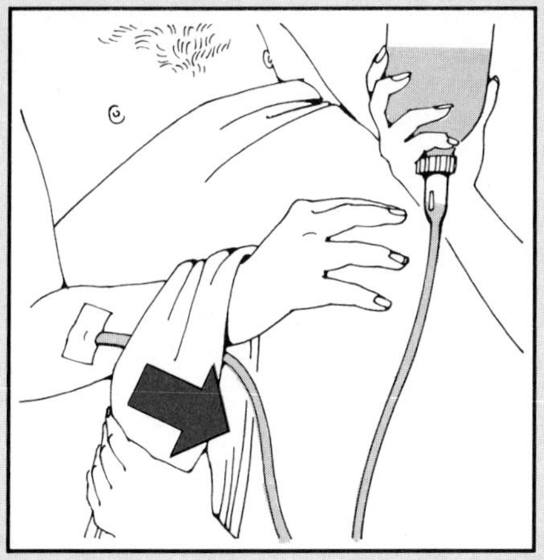

5. Removal of gown feels very invasive and generates feelings of vulnerability. Keeping exposure to a minimum shows empathy for these feelings and promotes trust.

NOTE: Never separate IV tubing to remove the gown. Disruption of this closed system could allow microorganisms to enter the bloodstream and cause serious infection.

6. Obtain water in basin. 110–115F (43–46C) is preferred. If there is no thermometer, use water as hot as is comfortable for your hands. Use slightly cooler water for very young or elderly clients. Test client's tolerance by lightly touching cheek with washcloth dampened in the water and wrung out. Water should be changed whenever it is cool or soapy.

6. Water in open basin cools rapidly by convection, conduction, and evaporation. If too cool at the start, bath will be uncomfortably cold. Elderly clients have thinner skin and diminished sensory perception, so are at greater risk for thermal injury. Testing clients' tolerance will prevent discomfort or burns.

(continued)

PROCEDURE 24–10. (continued)

7. Place a towel under the client's head. Wring out cloth and make a mitt as shown. This "mitt" technique is used throughout the bath. The towel will be used to protect bed throughout bath. Use a second towel to dry client.

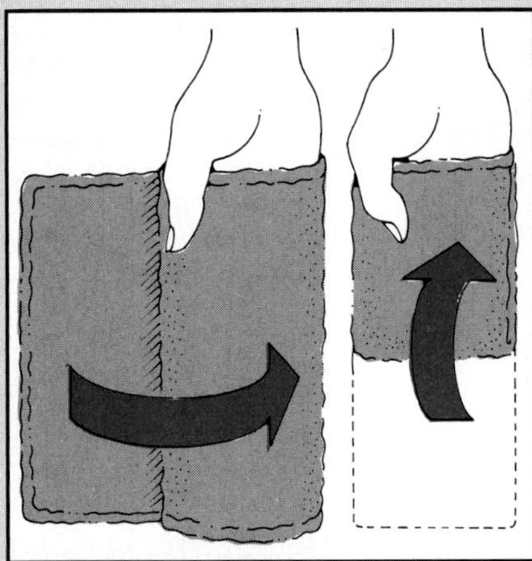

7. Towel is used to absorb moisture, protect bed linen. Mitt prevents edges of the cloth from brushing against the client's skin. This may produce a tickling sensation and may feel cool.

8. Using no soap, clean client's eyes, washing from inner to outer canthus, and shifting the cloth so you use a fresh part with each wipe. Rinse cloth before cleaning second eye. If lids are caked with discharge, let the warm cloth rest on the lid for a few seconds to soften exudate.

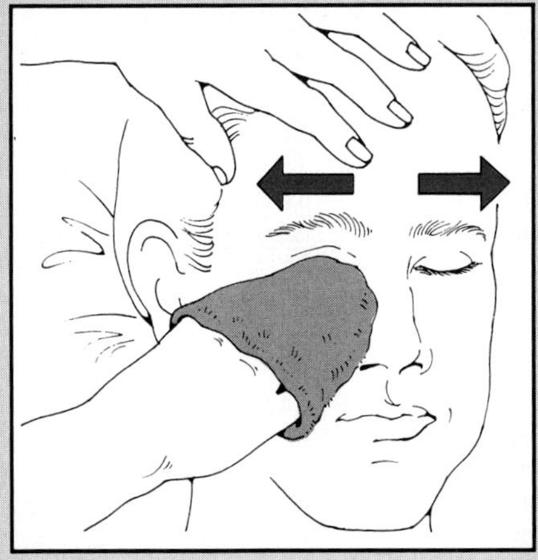

8. Soap is irritating to the eyes. Considerable discharge may be present on the eyelids, because the cleansing action of blinking ceases during sleep. Cloth is rinsed to avoid transferring organisms from one eye to the other.

(continued)

PROCEDURE 24–10. (continued)

9. Clean face, neck, and ears. Use little or no soap depending on skin condition and client's preference. Some clients use special soaps or cleansers on the face.

9. Facial skin may range from very oily to very dry. Oily skin is cleaned more effectively with soap because soap acts to reduce surface tension in water droplets and emulsifies oils; soap makes dry skin drier.

10. If soap is used, do not leave soap in basin between uses. Rub a small amount on the cloth and return soap to soap dish.

10. Adequate rinsing is difficult when giving a bed bath. Soapy water compounds the problem.

11. Rinse as needed. Dry thoroughly with second towel. Use special care in skin folds (eg, on the neck).

11. Soap residue is irritating and drying to skin and may alter the skin pH. If skin is not dried, evaporation will result in chilling. Moisture in skin folds causes maceration and possible breakdown and infection.

12. Uncover one arm. Move protective towel under the arm. Using soap, wash hand, arm, shoulder, and axilla with firm long strokes from distal to proximal. If skin is dry or thin, use gentler strokes. Pay particular attention to hands and axilla. Rinse, repeat as necessary. Dry thoroughly. Provide nail care, if needed (see Procedure 24–11). Repeat for other arm. Some nurses soak client's hands in the basin to facilitate cleaning nails. Nail care may be deferred until after bath.

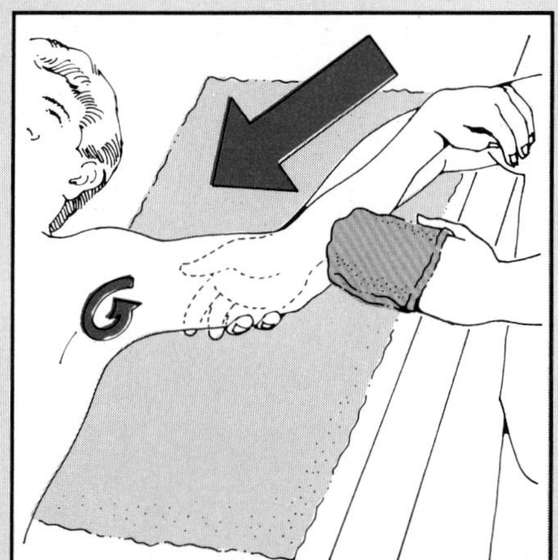

12. Firm strokes create friction, which removes bacteria, dead skin cells, and other substances; excessive friction can damage skin. Axilla and hands generally have more bacteria. Distal to proximal strokes stimulate circulation, facilitating venous return to the heart.

(continued)

PROCEDURE 24–10. (continued)

13. Expose one side of a female client's chest and wash it. Lift the breast to clean underlying skin. Note condition of skin under breast. Rinse well and dry. Repeat for other side of chest. For a male client fold down the bath blanket to expose the chest and abdomen at the same time. Wash, rinse, and dry.

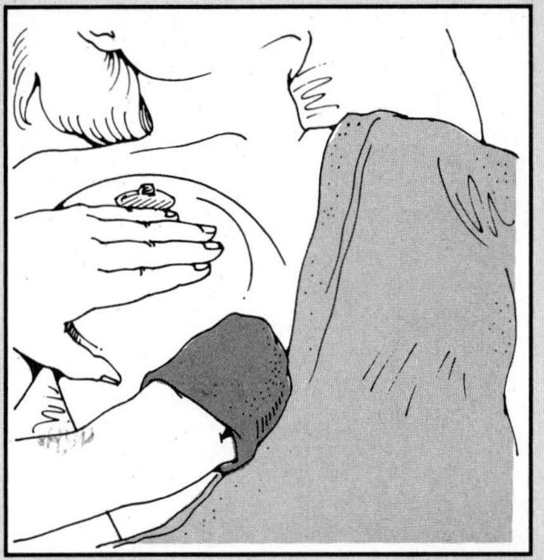

13. Most women feel uncomfortable when breasts are exposed. Exposing only the area being cleaned is less threatening. Skin fold under heavy breasts is vulnerable to excoration, especially if client perspires a lot.

14. Cover the breasts with the towel, then pull down the bath blanket to expose the abdomen. Keep the pubic hair covered. Wash, rinse, and dry the abdomen as above. Cover the chest, arms, and abdomen with the bath blanket.

14. See step 13.

15. Expose one leg; place towel under it, leaving leg flexed. Keep perineum covered. Wash foot, leg, and groin, using firm long, distal to proximal strokes. Rinse and dry. Repeat for other leg. Lotion may be applied if skin is dry, but vigorous massage should be avoided.

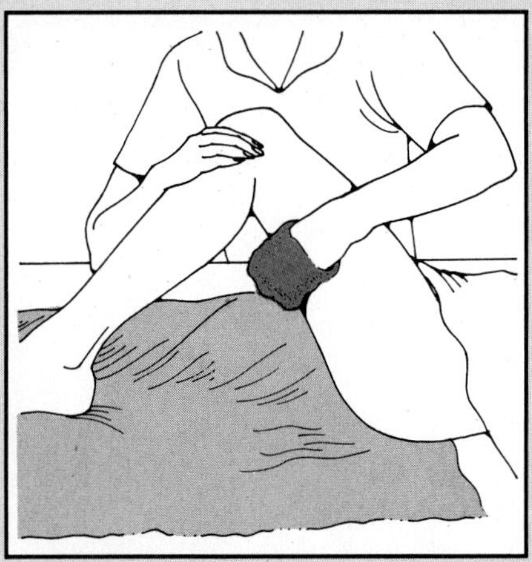

15. See step 12. Perineum is cleaned at the end of the bath. Vigorous leg massage is thought to increase the risk of freeing venous clots (emboli). Because debilitated clients on bed rest have increased risk of pathological clotting in the legs, caution is advised, even when no diagnosis of thrombophlebitis has been made.

NOTE: Foot may be soaked in basin, if desired. Client may prefer to soak feet while seated in a chair as nurse makes the bed.

(continued)

PROCEDURE 24–10. (continued)

16. Cover legs. Roll client so back is toward you. Expose back and buttocks. Place towel next to back. Wash, rinse, and dry neck, back, and buttocks as above, excluding perianal area. Apply lotion, massaging skin over bony prominences. If reddened areas or broken skin is noted, institute appropriate decubitus care in collaboration with the physician. If entire back cannot be exposed when client turns away, clean exposed part, and then turn client toward you to expose and clean remaining part.

16. Many clients spend most of their time in bed on their backs. The back has many potential pressure areas. Massage stimulates circulation, so prevents skin breakdown. If skin integrity is already disrupted, more aggressive measures are needed.

17. Return client to back. Offer option of independent cleansing of genitals. It is important that the client understand what is being asked. Use commonly understood terms like "private parts" or "between your legs."

17. Genitalia are considered the most personal parts of one's body. Genital exposure is embarrassing to most people. Having one's genitals cleaned by another makes many clients feel like they are being treated like small children.

18. If client has a Foley catheter, is confused, or lacks mobility or strength, perineal cleaning must be done by the nurse (see Procedure 24–12).

NOTE: Clients having had rectal or vaginal surgery or childbirth, or who are incontinent, are at greater risk for infection and irritation. Frequent perineal care is needed.

18. The perineal area tends to be dark, warm, and moist. Because of normal secretions, skin folds, and the bacterial population in the vaginal and anal area, odors, skin breakdown, and infection are likely if the perineum is not thoroughly cleaned. A Foley catheter provides a direct route for bacteria to enter the bladder; therefore, meticulous cleaning is essential.

19. Provide clean gown, assist client as needed to put it on. IV container and tubing should be slipped into the sleeve of the gown before the hand and arm. Reassess IV flowrate. Make occupied or unoccupied bed, as appropriate for client's activity level (see Procedures 24–13 and 24–14). Dispose of soiled linen in hamper, clean and store bath equipment and personal hygiene items, rearrange client's personal effects as desired. Place call bell in reach. Raise siderail.

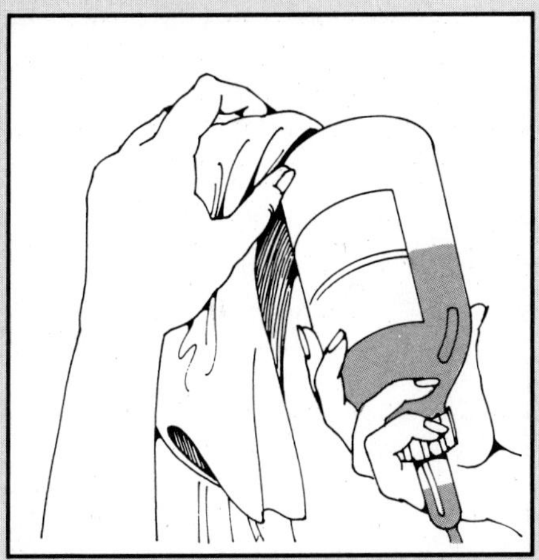

19. See step 5. Clean gown and linen, and orderly environment, promote relaxation and well-being. Personal belongings, arranged according to client's wishes, promote a feeling of personal territory. In an unfamiliar environment such as a hospital, even a small amount of personal territory diminishes feelings of alienation.

☐ **RECORDING:** Routine bathing may be recorded on a checklist, or may not be recorded unless problems are encountered. Skin or mucosal lesions noted during bath should be described, including appearance, size, location, and drainage, if any. Document nursing action taken. Note any other problems and action taken.

PROCEDURE 24–11. CARING FOR FEET AND NAILS

PURPOSE: To maintain cleanliness and integrity of nails and surrounding tissue, to promote comfort.

EQUIPMENT: Basin, towel, washcloth, moistureproof pad, nail clippers or scissors, orange stick, and lotion or other emollient.

ACTION

1. Discuss previous foot and nail problems with the client, usual foot and nail care and preferences for assistance. Some clients may prefer that a family member provide nail care. Assess condition of feet and nails.
2. Determine whether a medical order is needed to cut nails. (This policy is common because of risks associated with accidental cuts in clients with diabetes or circulatory disorders.) Assemble equipment. Foot and nail care is usually done as part of the bath, but may be done separately as needed. Screen client.
3. *Fingernails:* If dirt or other debris is trapped under nails, soaking hands in a basin of warm water for 5–10 minutes will facilitate cleaning. A soft nailbrush may be needed to loosen impacted soil. For routine care, soaking of fingernails is not usually needed, although unusually thick nails will be easier to cut if softened by soaking. If nails are long, obtain client's consent to cut them. Use a nail clipper, cutting straight across the nail, even with the tops of the fingers. If one is available, use an orange stick to clean under the nails. Apply or provide lotion to moisturize skin and cuticles. Cuticles may be pushed back with orange stick.
4. *Feet.* Feet commonly require more care because they are subject to trauma from ill-fitting shoes and they are more likely to be poorly perfused or edematous due to circulatory impairment secondary to disease or aging. Clients with diminished vision or flexibility may find self-care difficult, even though they are alert and oriented. Elderly clients' toenails are often thick and difficult to cut without soaking. Feet may be soaked with the client seated in a chair or by placing a basin in the bed (see Procedure 24–10). Dry feet thoroughly, especially between the toes to prevent maceration or fungal infections. When cutting toenails, use special care to cut straight across the nail to prevent ingrown toenails and to avoid cutting cuticles. A toenail clipper is best for this as it has a larger cutting surface. Do not cut corns or calluses. Clean under nails and apply lotion as in step 3. If any breaks in the skin, corns, ingrown nails or other lesions are noted, notify the client's physician.

RECORDING: Routine nail care is not recorded in all agencies. May be noted on a checklist. If lesions are noted or problems are encountered, describe condition and action taken.

PROCEDURE 24–12. CARING FOR PERINEAL AREA AND FOLEY CATHETER ("PERICARE")

PURPOSE: To promote cleanliness and comfort, and prevent odors, skin irritation, and infection. Perineal care is always part of the daily bath; however, it is done more frequently for clients who are incontinent, who have had rectal or vaginal surgery, and after childbirth.

EQUIPMENT: Basin, soap in a dish, washcloths, towel, disposable gloves, bath blanket, and waterproof pad. Irrigation container and bedpan may be used when giving perineal care to a woman.

ACTION	RATIONALE
1. Discuss the procedure with the client, including the expected benefits, usual sensations, and desired participation.	1. The client will be more likely to participate and less anxious if this information is shared.
NOTE: A calm, matter-of-fact approach during the explanation and the care will reduce the discomfiture of client and nurse about perineal care. The nurse must strive to view the genitals simply as body organs, mentally deemphasizing their sexual function (which is usually the root of the nurse's anxiety), but remain sensitive to client's feelings of embarrassment.	
2. Assemble equipment. Fill basin with warm water. Screen client, raise bed. Lower siderail on near side of bed. Remove positioning aids, pillows except for pillow under head. HOB can be flat or slightly raised.	2. See Box 24–5. Also, conserves nurse's energy, promotes body mechanics. See Chap. 30.
3. Cover client's torso with a bath blanket. Fold top covers down to waist. Place a towel or waterproof underpad under client's buttocks. Ask client to spread legs. Female client should also flex thighs (dorsal recumbent position). Pull top covers down to expose genitalia, drape bath blanket over lower abdomen. For a female, bath blanket should cover flexed legs, top covers cover feet only. If doing pericare as part of the bath (top covers removed) drape the male client by lowering bath blanket below genitalia and covering chest and abdomen with a towel.	3. Receiving such personal care from another often causes feelings of dependency, vulnerability, and embarrassment. These feelings are diminished somewhat by exposing only the part of the body which is to be cleaned.

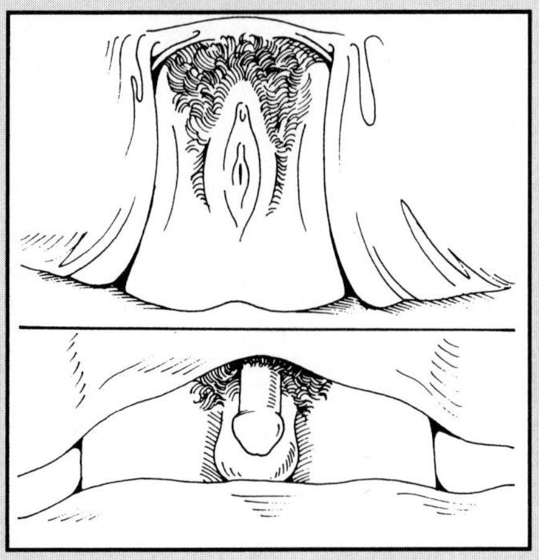

(continued)

PROCEDURE 24–12. (continued)

4. Don gloves. Wash perineum using a small amount of soap and a washcloth as follows.
   Female client: Spread labia majora. Wash from the mons pubis, downward over the urethral and vaginal openings to the base of the labia. Using a different portion of the cloth, wash folds of labia minora and majora on one side, then the other. Rinse and repeat as necessary to remove visible secretions. Rinse all remaining soap, dry well. If desired, client can be placed on a bedpan and the perineum rinsed by pouring warm water over it. This technique may be ordered after vaginal surgery.

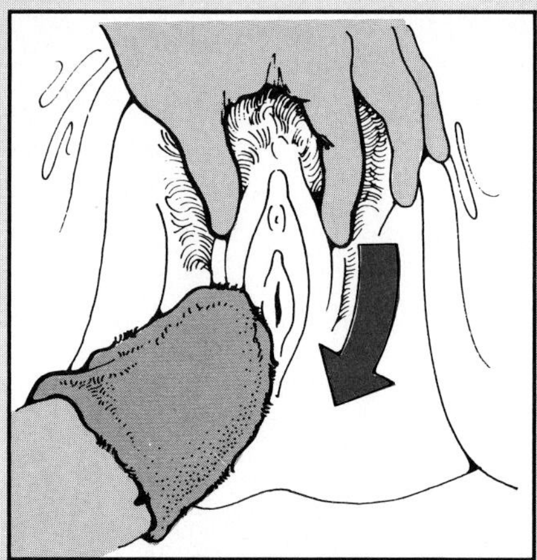

   Male client: Holding the penis by the shaft, wash the glans with a circular motion. If client is uncircumcised, retract foreskin, clean glans, then replace foreskin. Clean the penile shaft and anterior scrotum with downward strokes. Cup the scrotum gently in your hand to clean lateral and posterior surfaces. Rinse and repeat as necessary. Dry well. An erection during pericare is uncommon (see Note), but if it should occur, acknowledge that it has happened and ask the client if he prefers that you complete the care or give him a moment of privacy.

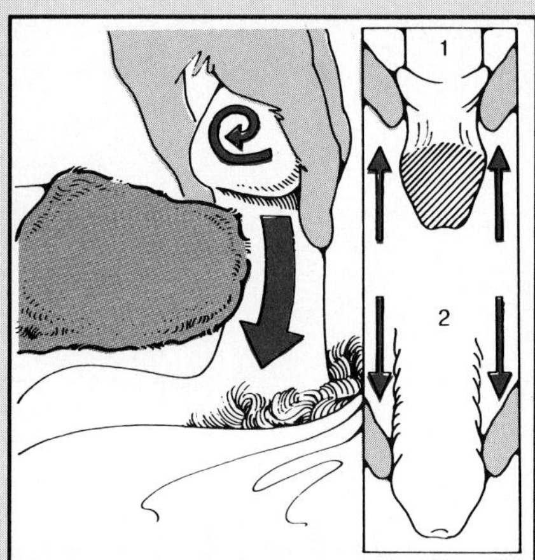

4. Gloves act as a barrier, preventing transmission of organisms from client to nurse. Gloves are optional unless known pathogens are present; however, most nurses prefer to use them. Washing genitalia as described proceeds from cleanest area to area with largest numbers of organisms, thereby minimizing transfer of organisms to cleaner area. Whitish secretions called smegma are normal in labial folds and under glans, but should be removed to decrease likelihood of growth of pathogens. Soap residue irritates skin and mucous membranes, causing itching and excoriation. Moisture, especially between labia and thighs or scrotum and thighs, promotes maceration, skin breakdown, and fungal infections. Scrotum is handled gently to avoid pressure on sensitive testicles. Ignoring an erection, should it occur, belittles the client and is likely to increase, rather than decrease, client and nurse embarrassment. Providing the client with an option for dealing with the situation shows respect.

(continued)

PROCEDURE 24–12. (continued)

NOTE: Many beginning nurses are personally embarrassed to give perineal care. For many, this is related to concerns about sexual connotations associated with handling the genitals (see step 1) and especially, the fear that a male client will have an erection during care. This is highly unlikely. Most clients feel embarrassment, which suppresses psychic stimuli needed for an erection. Composure on the part of the nurse will increase client's comfort.

5. If client has an indwelling catheter, clean the portion of the catheter just distal to the urinary meatus after completing step 4. Use the same washcloth and a small amount of soap. Hold the catheter steady to prevent its moving back and forth into the urethra as you clean it. Spread the labia of a female so the catheter can be thoroughly cleaned. Use a firm twisting motion, wiping from the meatus outward, 1–2 inches. Rinse well.

5. The catheter acts as a mucosal irritant; therefore, mucus frequently collects around the portion of the tube that exits the meatus. This mucus can be a medium for bacterial growth, increasing the risk of a urinary tract infection. Friction physically removes mucus and bacteria.

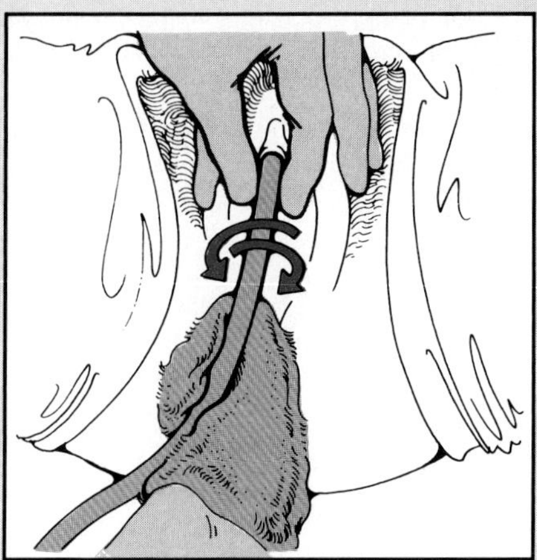

NOTE: Formerly, antibacterial soaps and ointments such as povidone iodine, and sterile catheter care kits, were recommended for Foley care. Studies have shown soap and water are equally effective, as well as cheaper and less irritating to mucosa.

(continued)

PROCEDURE 24–12. (continued)

6. Ask the client to turn to the side, facing away from you. Rearrange the bath blanket so only buttocks are exposed. Raise the top buttock and clean the anal area, starting near the genitalia and washing backward. Rinse and repeat as necessary; remove all soap residue and dry well.

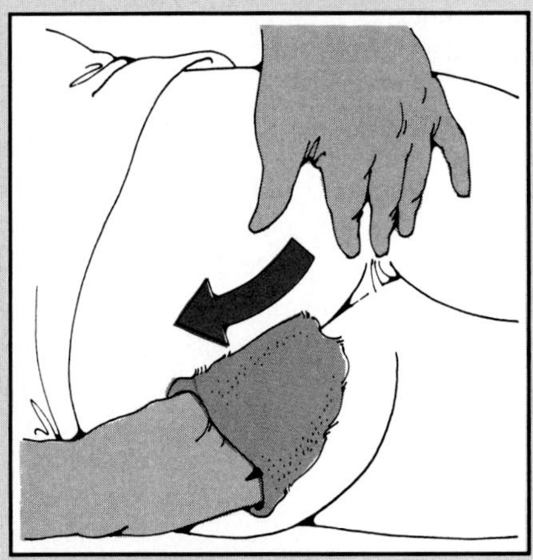

6. The anal area contains organisms such as *Escherichia coli,* which can cause vaginal or urinary tract infections. Cleaning from cleanest area to area with most organisms reduces this possibility.

7. Remove gloves, discard in waterproof receptacle. Remove underpad and drape, reposition and cover client, return bed to low position. Dispose of linen, clean and store equipment according to agency policy; or continue with bath.

7. Promotes client comfort and safety.

RECORDING: Routine perineal care may be documented on a checklist or in narrative charting. In some agencies it is not specifically charted unless problems are encountered. A narrative entry is necessary to document perineal lesions or unusual discharge and describe nursing action taken.

Shower. When possible, most clients prefer to shower. Even clients receiving intravenous fluids or with surgical incisions can shower as long as they can stand independently. Usually, nurses can cover dressings or venipuncture sites with plastic wrap taped on all edges. This prevents wetting the dressing as long as water does not flow directly on the tape. Confer with the client's surgeon to be sure there are no contraindications to showering. It is a good idea to remain outside the shower area for a short time to be sure clients are not experiencing problems and to check on them periodically. Inform clients of the location of the call light.

A shower chair is a good choice for clients able to tolerate being out of bed but unable to stand safely in a shower. They receive the benefit and enjoyment of a shower without risking accidents.

Assisted Bath. Many clients confined to bed are able to wash themselves if provided with a basin of warm water, soap, and towels. Offer to change the water as necessary and wash their backs, feet, or other areas they find hard to reach. Clients with indwelling urinary catheters may need assistance to cleanse around the catheter adequately.

Sink Bath. For ambulatory clients unable to shower, a sink bath is often preferable to a sponge bath in bed. They will need help with their backs and feet.

Tub Bath. Some health care facilities have tubs available as another alternative for hygiene. Washing and rinsing are easier in a tub than with a bed bath and many clients prefer a tub bath to a sponge bath or shower. Special precautions are necessary to prevent injury getting in and out of the tub.

Linen Change. Having a clean wrinkle-free bed in which to rest makes a significant contribution to clients' well-being, particularly with clients whose activity is limited. Procedures 24–13 and 24–14 contain detailed instructions for changing linen. The decision to make an occupied or unoccupied bed may rest with client and nurse, or medical orders may specify one or the other. Although many nurses believe that making an occupied bed conserves clients' energy, studies have shown that getting clients out of bed for bedmaking results in minimal energy cost and cardiac stress for clients.[42–44] Because early mobilization is beneficial to most clients' recovery, encourage clients who are able to get out of bed and sit in a chair during bedmaking. Elevate the lower legs of postoperative clients to avoid popliteral pressure venous stasis, decreasing the risk of pathological clotting (see Chap. 27).

(*Text continues on page 1035.*)

PROCEDURE 24–13. MAKING AN UNOCCUPIED BED

PURPOSE: To promote client comfort and relaxation.

EQUIPMENT: Top and bottom sheet, pillowcases, drawsheet (optional), waterproof underpads (optional), mattress pad, blanket and bedspread (change only if soiled), and linen hamper (varies with agency policy). Clean gloves if linen has fresh bloody drainage.

ACTION

1. Discuss need and timing of procedure with client. Linen is usually changed while clients are showering/bathing, after a bed bath, or when a client is off the unit for treatments or tests.
2. Obtain clean linen as needed. In some facilities, top sheet is reused if it is not soiled. Drawsheet and waterproof pads are needed for clients who are incontinent, have draining wounds, and/or who receive treatments such as wet compresses or wet-to-dry dressings. A pull sheet (folded drawsheet) is recommended for clients who need assistance with position changes. The minimum amount of foundation linen necessary to protect the bed should be used when special foam "eggcrate" mattresses are in use (see Chap. 30).
3. Lower head of bed, raise the bed to your waist level. Remove call bell, if attached to linen. To strip the bed of soiled linen:
   a. Don gloves if linen is soiled with bloody drainage. Loosen linen and lower siderails all around the bed.
   b. If spread is clean, fold it before removing it from the bed: fold the top edge so it's even with the bottom edge, grasp at the center of the fold and the doubled bottom edge and raise the spread from the bed, creating a second fold. Continue to fold until it can be easily hung on bedside chair without touching the floor. Fold and remove the blanket in the same manner. Fold top sheet in same manner if it is to be reused.

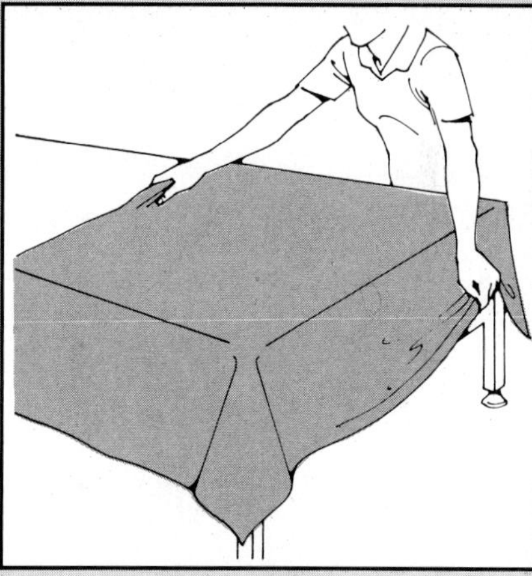

   c. Remove all pillowcases; place pillows on chair.
   d. Remove disposable waterproof underpads and dispose in waterproof trash receptacle. Gather remaining linen into a ball, rolling edges toward the center, and place in portable hamper, taking care to avoid contacting your uniform with soiled linen. If a central hamper is used, soiled dry linen can be rolled toward the foot of the bed and tucked between the end of the mattress and the footboard until you have finished making the bed. Do not place soiled linen on the floor, as it is grossly contaminated with organisms. It is likely you would contaminate your uniform when retrieving the bundle of linen from the floor for disposal in the central chute.
   e. Remove gloves.

(continued)

PROCEDURE 24–13. (continued)

4. Place foundation linen as follows:
   a. If a mattress pad is on the bed, align it on the mattress and smooth wrinkles. Replace if soiled.
   b. Place bottom sheet in the center of the bed with folded edge facing the central long axis of the bed. Unfold the sheet toward the head and foot of the bed, allowing the sheet to extend about 1 inch (2.5 cm) over the bottom edge of the mattress, hem down, and the remaining length to extend over the top edge of the mattress. Unfold the sheet toward each side of the bed and smooth wrinkles on the side nearest you. The linen on the far side of the bed can remain partially folded until the first side of the bed is made. Bed linen is unfolded in this way to minimize air currents created if linen is unfolded by waving it in the air. Air currents facilitate spread of microorganisms.

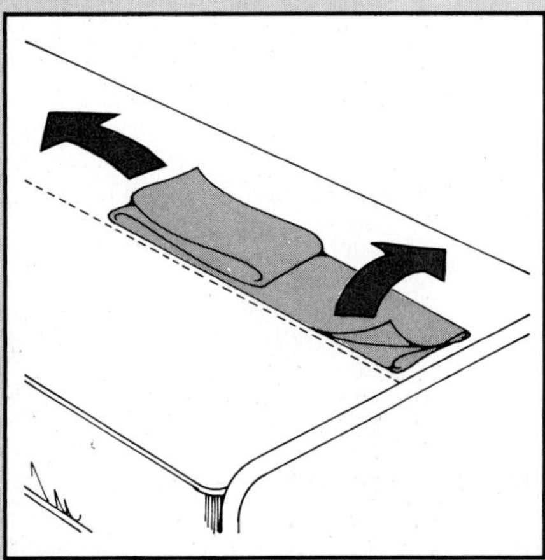

   c. Tuck the sheet under the top end of the mattress, pulling the entire length of the tucked portion well under the mattress to firmly secure it. Extra length is needed at the head of the bed to keep the sheet in place when the head of the bed is raised.

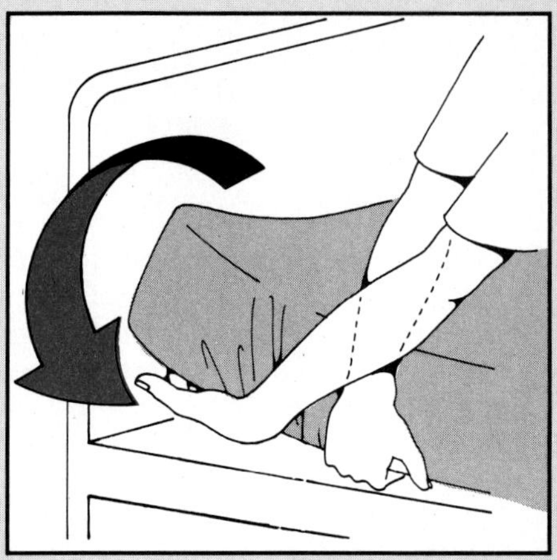

5. Miter the corner as follows:
   a. Lift the sheet (i) to form a right triangle on the mattress (ii). The triangle's base is along the side edge of the mattress; the side forming the right angle is parallel to the top edge of the bed. Place your other hand as shown to keep the sheet smooth as you form the triangle. The sheet should look like (iii.)

(continued)

PROCEDURE 24–13. (continued)

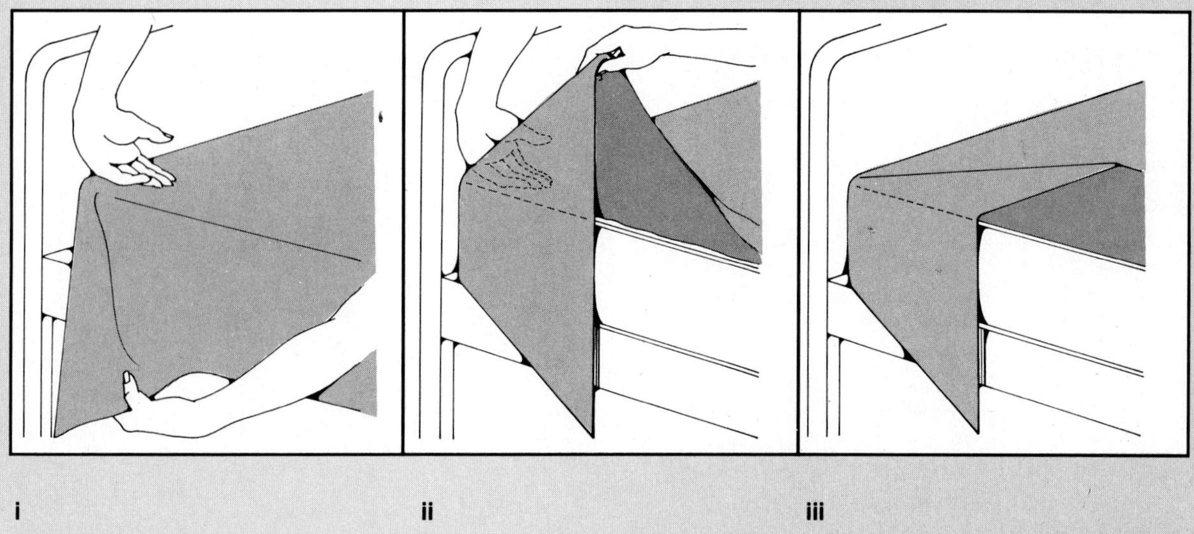

b. Tuck the lower portion of the sheet securely under the side of the mattress without disturbing the triangular fold.

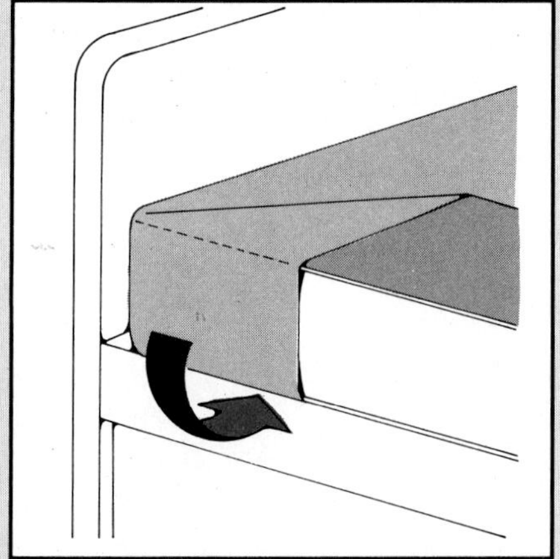

c. Hold the sheet secure at the edge of the mattress with one hand while bringing the tip of the traingle over your hand, then tucking it securely under the mattress.

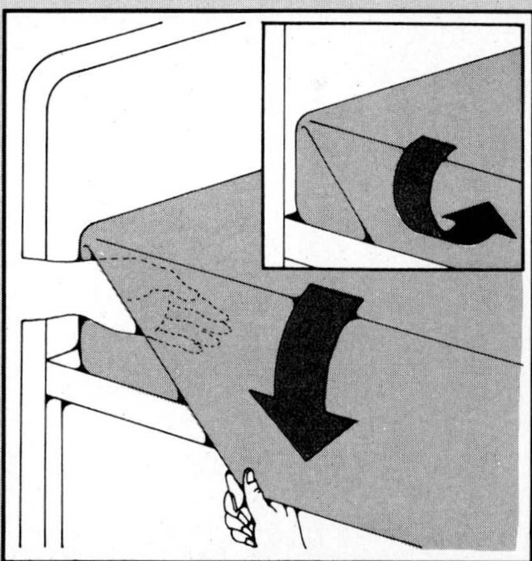

d. Secure the rest of the sheet by tucking it well under the mattress. If not securely tucked, it will pull out when the other side of the bed is made, or when the client moves in bed.

(continued)

PROCEDURE 24–13. (continued)

6. If a drawsheet is used, place it so the center fold lies along the center of the mattress. The top edge should be 12–15 inches (30–17 cm) from the head of the bed. Unfold toward each side as with the bottom sheet. Tuck in the excess draw-sheet so it extends as far under the mattress as possible (see step 5d).
7. Place the top linen as follows:
   a. Align the sheet with the fold along the center of the bed and unfold, as with foundation linen. The top edge of the sheet should be even with the top edge of the mattress, hem facing up. Smooth wrinkles.
   b. Place the blanket (if used), then the spread over the top sheet, centering, unfolding and smoothing as above, with the top edges about 6 in (15 cm) from the head of the bed. Fold the top sheet down to make a cuff over the blanket and spread.
   c. Tuck all of the top linen under the foot of the bed at one time. Make a mitered corner using all layers of linen, as in step 5, except do not tuck the tip of the triangle under the mattress.

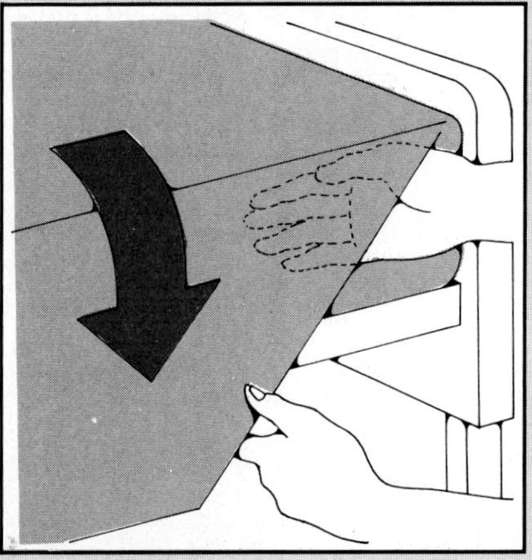

8. Move to the opposite side and finish the bed as follows:
   a. Fold or roll the top linen away from you to expose the foundation linen.

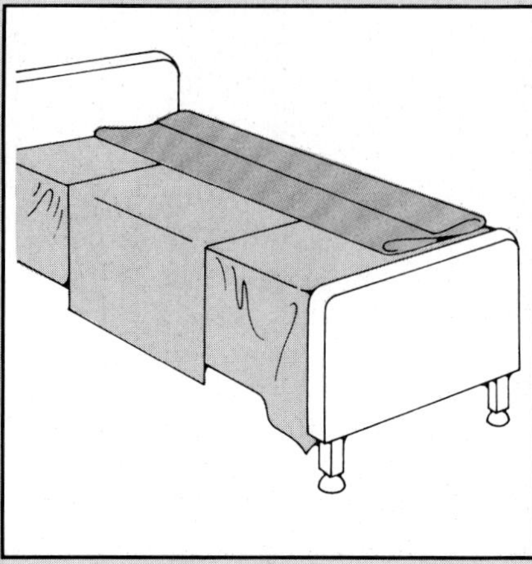

   b. Smooth the bottom sheet and tuck it in at the head of the bed, mitering the corner as in step 5. Tuck in the rest of the sheet in sections, pulling each section firmly with both hands, so the sheet is taut and secure.

(continued)

PROCEDURE 24–13. (continued)

c. Smooth the drawsheet, pull the center section tightly with both hands, then tuck it securely as far under the mattress as you can. It may be helpful to brace your knee against the bedframe for more leverage or shift your weight backwards as you pull. Tuck in the top and bottom sections the same way. The foundation should now be tight and free of wrinkles. Adjust any loose areas as necessary. Wrinkled or loose foundation linen causes client discomfort and creates pressure areas.

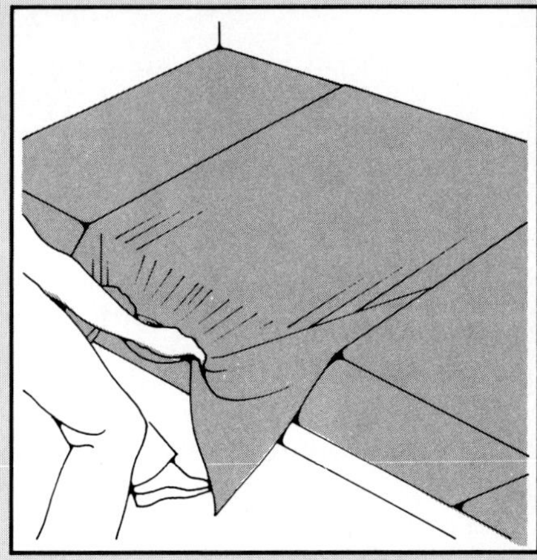

d. Smooth the top sheet, blanket, and spread, one at a time, then tuck in at the foot of the bed and miter as a unit, as in step 7. Adjust cuff at head of bed, if necessary.

e. Make a toe pleat in the top linen to prevent pressure on the client's feet: stand at the foot of the bed, reach over the bedframe, and grasp the top linen as a unit about 6 inches (15 cm) from the foot of the bed, and lift the linen toward you—creating a fold across the entire width of the bed.

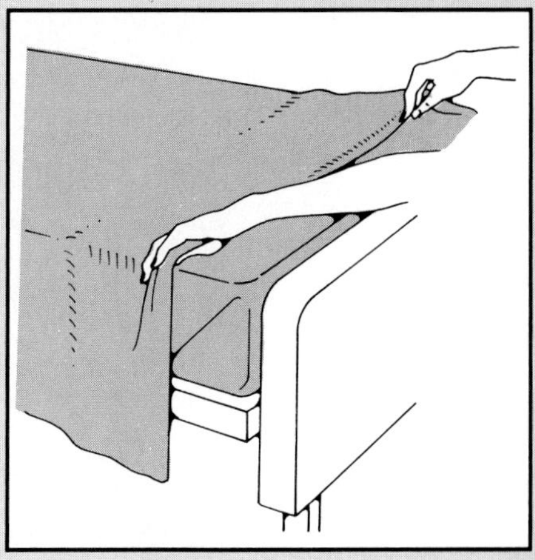

9. Replace the pillowcases:
   a. With one hand, hold the pillowcase in the center of the closed end.

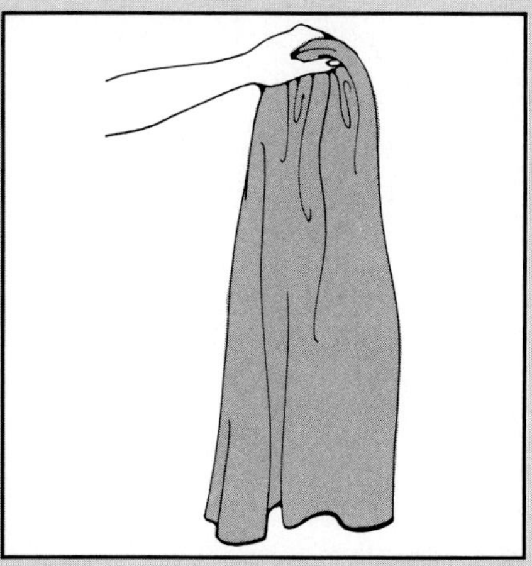

   b. With your other hand, gather up the case and invert it over the first hand and forearm.

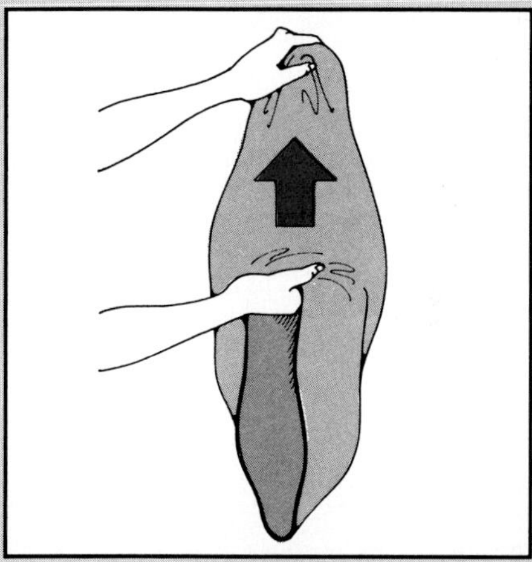

(continued)

PROCEDURE 24–13. (continued)

c. Still holding the pillowcase, grasp the center of one end of the pillow with the first hand.

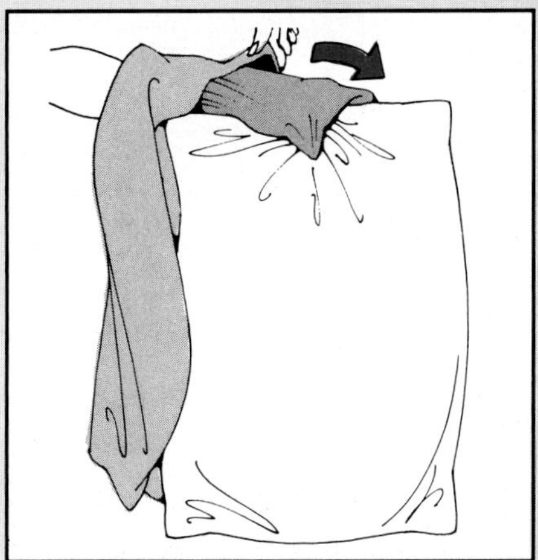

d. Pull the pillowcase over the pillow, aligning corners of case and pillow.

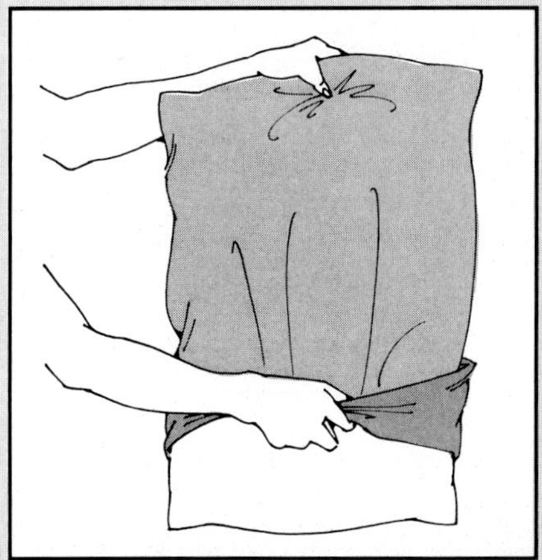

e. Place pillows on the bed according to client's preference.

10. Prepare the bed for the client:
    a. Fanfold top linen to the foot of the bed.
    b. Place waterproof pad(s) as needed over the drawsheet.
    c. Attach the call light so the client can reach it when in bed.
    d. Raise siderail on one side of the bed.
    e. Return bed to lower position unless client will return to bed via a gurney.
    f. Rearrange furniture and personal items according to client's preference.

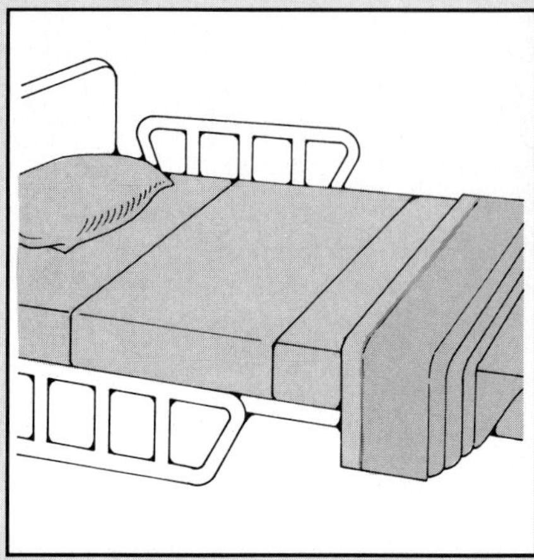

11. Assist client into bed as needed, remove soiled linen and discard in central chute or remove portable hamper. Use care to avoid contacting your uniform while carrying soiled linen. Contact transfers microorganisms.

☐ **RECORDING:** May be noted on a checklist. In some agencies bedmaking is not documented.

PROCEDURE 24–14. MAKING AN OCCUPIED BED

☐ **PURPOSE:** To promote client comfort and relaxation for clients whose condition or treatment plan precludes their getting out of bed.

☐ **EQUIPMENT:** Top and bottom sheet, pillowcases, drawsheet (optional), waterproof underpads (optional), mattress pad, blanket and bedspread (change only if soiled), and linen hamper (varies with agency policy). Two pair of clean gloves if linen has fresh bloody drainage. Because linen change is usually done after the bed bath, equipment for both procedures can be gathered at the same time.

ACTION

1. Obtain equipment. Discuss need and timing of procedure and the desired client participation with client. Linen is usually changed immediately after a bed bath, but some clients may prefer a brief rest period prior to changing the linen. A complete linen change may also be necessary after spills, emesis, excessive diaphoresis or incontinence.
2. Screen the client, close door, if desired. Raise bed to your waist height. With far siderail up, ask or assist client (see Procedure 30–11) to roll as close to the opposite edge of the bed as possible facing away from you. Remove all pillows, except one under the head; move it to the opposite side of the bed. This provides space to change the foundation linen on the near half of the bed.
3. Lower near siderail. Don gloves to handle linen soiled with fresh bloody drainage. If linen change is done immediately after the bath, client will be covered with a bath blanket, which can remain in place until the foundation linen has been changed. If top linen is in place, remove and refold spread and blanket as in Procedure 24–13, step 3b, if both are clean. If soiled, place in hamper or roll to foot of the bed and leave between end of mattress and footboard. Top sheet may be used to cover client while foundation linen is changed unless it is wet or very soiled, in which case it should be replaced with a bath blanket as in Procedure 24–10, step 4. Loosen foundation linen at the head and sides of the bed. Remove soiled disposable underpads and discard in waterproof trash container. If pads are under client, roll them with soiled foundation linen into a tight roll that extends the length of the bed. Push the roll of soiled linen as close to the client's back as possible to allow room for the clean foundation linen. Remove gloves. Discard in waterproof trash receptacle.

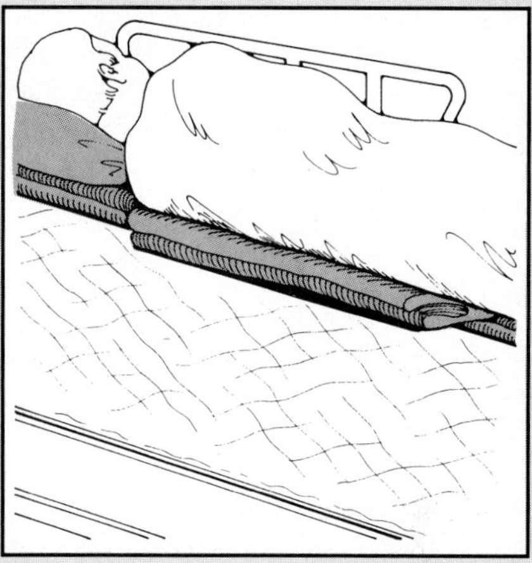

4. Replace foundation linen:
   a. Smooth the mattress pad, if clean. Replace if necessary: with pad folded in half lengthwise, align it over the mattress on the near side of the bed, then fanfold or roll the excess toward the client, pushing the roll as close to the rolled soiled linen as possible.

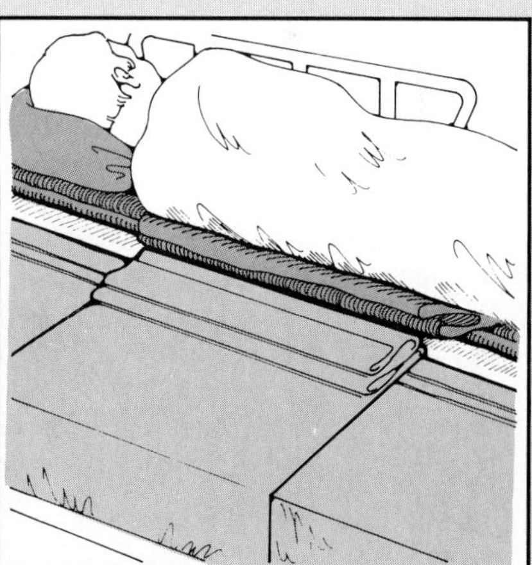

(continued)

PROCEDURE 24–14. (continued)

b. Place the clean bottom sheet in the center of the bed and unfold as in Procedure 24–13, step 4b. Roll or gather the excess as above and tuck it next to the rolled foundation linen. Miter corner at the head of the bed and tuck in the sides as in Procedure 24–13, step 5.

c. If a drawsheet is needed, position it as in Procedure 24–13, step 6. Tuck in the near side, roll or gather the excess as above. If disposable underpads are needed, place them over the drawsheet in the same way.

5. Remove the pillow under the client's head and change the pillowcase as in Procedure 24–13, step 9. Place the freshly changed pillow on the clean foundation linen. If the client cannot tolerate having no head support, replace the case on another pillow and place it on the clean side of the bed.

6. Ask the client to roll toward you, over the rolled linen. Assist if necessary (see Procedure 30–11). The client should now be facing you, lying on his or her side on the clean foundation linen. Raise the near siderail.

7. Move the chair with the clean top linen to the opposite side of the bed. Linen may also be stacked on the clean foundation, near the client's feet. This will save steps, allowing you to complete the foundation, then replace top linen without repeated walking around the bed.

8. Complete the foundation:
   a. Don clean gloves, if needed. Loosen soiled linen. Roll it into a ball toward the center of the bed. Place in hamper, or at the foot of the bed, as described above, avoiding contacting your uniform.
   b. Unroll and smooth clean linen, one layer at a time. If client is large, part of the roll may be under the client, but can usually be pulled free without difficulty. In some cases, it may be necessary to have a second nurse assist by holding the client as close to the opposite side of the bed as possible, while you free the linen.
   c. Securely tuck in the bottom sheet and drawsheet as in Procedure 24–13, steps 8a–8c. It is usually necessary to brace your knee on the bedframe for leverage or shift your weight backwards as you pull the sheets to eliminate wrinkles and achieve a taut foundation (see Procedure 24–13, step 8c).
   d. Ask or assist the client to return to a supine position in the center of the bed.

9. If extra pillows have been in use, change the pillowcases as above. Reposition client, if necessary (see Chap. 30).

10. Replace top linen:
    a. Place the clean top sheet over the bath blanket covering the client. Unfold as in Procedure 24–13, step 7a. Ask the client to hold the top edge of the sheet as you pull the bath blanket toward the foot of the bed. It may be folded for reuse or put with the soiled linen.
    b. Place the blanket, if desired, and the spread over the sheet, unfolding, aligning, and smoothing as in Procedure 24–13, step 7a. Make a cuff over the top edge of the blanket and spread with the top sheet.
    c. Tuck in and miter the corner of the top linen as a unit at the foot of the bed, as in Procedure 24–13, step 7c. Raise siderail.
    d. Repeat on other side of the bed.
    e. Make toe pleat as in Procedure 24–13, step 8e.

11. Lower the bed, rearrange furniture and personal belongings according to the client's preference. Remove soiled linen and other supplies; store or discard according to agency policy.

▭ **RECORDING:** May be recorded on a checklist. In some agencies linen change is not routinely recorded unless unusual events occur during the procedure. Rarely, a narrative entry describing the procedure and client's response is required, even for a routine linen change.

BOX 24–6. GENERAL GUIDELINES FOR CLEANSING SURGICAL WOUNDS

1. Not all surgical wounds are routinely cleansed with every dressing change. Agency policy and surgeon preference may vary.
2. Various solutions may be used to cleanse surgical wounds. Hospitals or individual surgeons frequently have specific solution preferences. Refer to the agency policy manual or physician's order sheet in the client's chart.
3. All equipment used to clean surgical wounds must be sterile, even if the wound is infected.
4. Most solutions must be poured into sterile containers (sterile specimen cups are an inexpensive and conveniently sized choice for most wounds). See also Box 22–13. The solution is applied to the wound and surrounding skin with pledgets made from gauze 2 × 2s or 4 × 4s. Pledgets may be held in a sterile-gloved hand, or with a sterile thumb forceps or a hemostat. Large cotton-tipped applicators (swabs) in foil packets containing antiseptic are available in some agencies.
5. Wounds must be cleansed from the cleanest area to the least clean area to avoid transfer of microorganisms. The following facts apply:
   - The incision line or wound has fewer endogenous organisms than the skin surrounding the incision.
   - In a vertical incision, especially one that is draining, the highest end of the incision is drier and therefore has fewer endogenous organisms.
   - A localized area of purulent drainage (eg, oozing from a small part of the incision) contains many organisms.
   - A drain site separate from the incision has more organisms than the incision and the peri-incisional skin.
6. Refer to Procedure 24–15, which describes and illustrates several cleansing methods.
7. Wound cleansing should be recorded on a checklist or in a narrative note. Describe the location, size, and appearance of the wound, the solution used to clean it, whether a dressing was applied, and the client's response to the procedure.

Wound Care. Wound care includes cleaning and dressing wounds, managing drainage systems, obtaining wound cultures, and special procedures such as wound irrigation, wet to dry dressings, and application of proteolytic enzymes. Although care of uncomplicated surgical incisions is straightforward, wounds that do not heal optimally can present many nursing care challenges. Moreover, wounds are difficult for most clients—not only are they painful, but they are sometimes disfiguring and debilitating. Nurses' recognition that having a wound represents a potential threat to clients' perceptions of their wholeness, ability to function, and physical appearance is an important factor in determining the effectiveness of their care.

Cleaning Wounds. Not all wounds require cleaning, but nurses usually clean wounds with significant amounts of drainage and wounds that are healing by secondary intention as part of a dressing change. Effective cleaning requires correct technique. Box 24–6 and Procedure 24–15 provide information about approaches to cleaning various types of wounds.

PROCEDURE 24–15. CLEANING A WOUND

☐ **PURPOSE:** To remove dead tissue and bacteria from wounds and promote healing.

☐ **EQUIPMENT:** Cleansing or antiseptic solution, receptacle for solution, sterile gloves, sterile gauze squares, sterile forceps, and waterproof bag for disposal of used swabs. May substitute commercially packaged antiseptic swabs according to medical order or agency policy.

ACTION

1. Remove dressings as described in Procedure 24–16. Prepare solution, gauze pledgets, and forceps or commercially packaged swabs.

   Preparing solution, gauze squares, and forceps:

   a. Pour solution (Box 22–13), open forceps and gauze packages (Box 22–12), use sterile field, if desired (Procedure 22–3).

(continued)

PROCEDURE 24–15. (continued)

b. Don sterile gloves (see Procedure 22–4) and pick up the forceps with dominant hand.

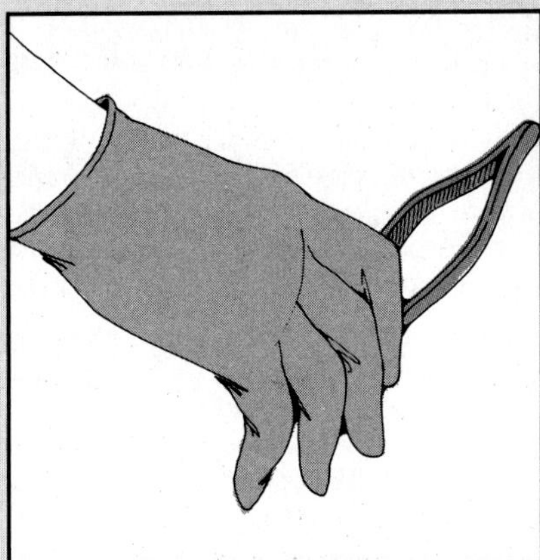

c. Fold a sterile gauze square in quarters with nondominant hand; transfer to forceps with folded edge out.

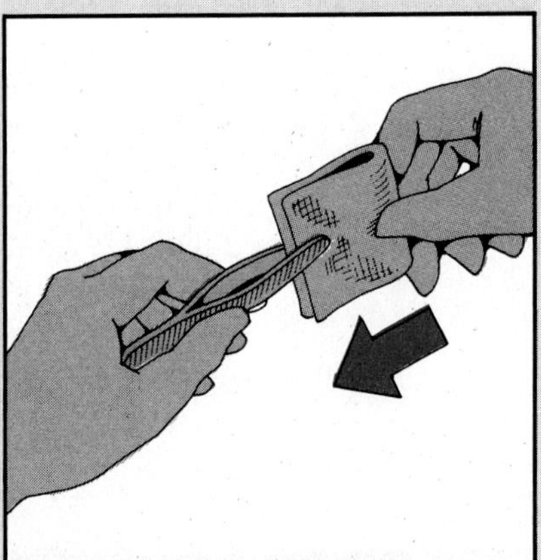

d. Dip gauze in solution until it is wet, but not dripping, keeping tip of forceps pointing down at all times, because gravity causes movement of liquid. If hand is lower, liquid may contact hand, then flow back to tip, which would contaminate tip.

e. When discarding gauze swabs, use care not to touch trash receptacle with forceps, which will be used for entire procedure.

NOTE: The nondominant hand may be ungloved at nurse's preference providing the option of touching unsterile items (eg, pouring additional solution) during the procedure, which would contaminate a glove if both hands were gloved.

Preparing commercially prepared antiseptic swabs: Open packet, remove one swab by grasping handle. Keep wet end of swab pointed downward at all times.

2. Cleaning vertical incision.
   a. Cleanse the incision line first. For vertical incision, cleanse from the top of the incision downward. Use more than one swab if the wound is long.

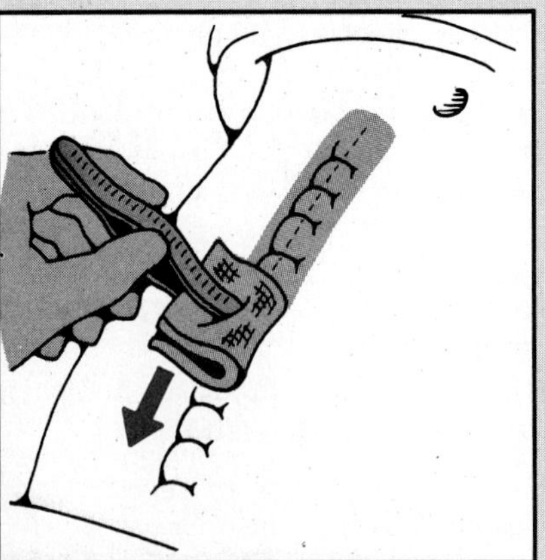

(continued)

PROCEDURE 24–15. (continued)

b. Cleanse the proximal skin on either side of the incision, working away from the incision, cleaning 3–4 inches of surrounding skin, and using a new swab for each stroke. This method prevents inoculating the incision with normal skin flora (because of the surgical skin prep, the incision has the lowest bacterial population, and drainage that harbors microorganisms flows downward).

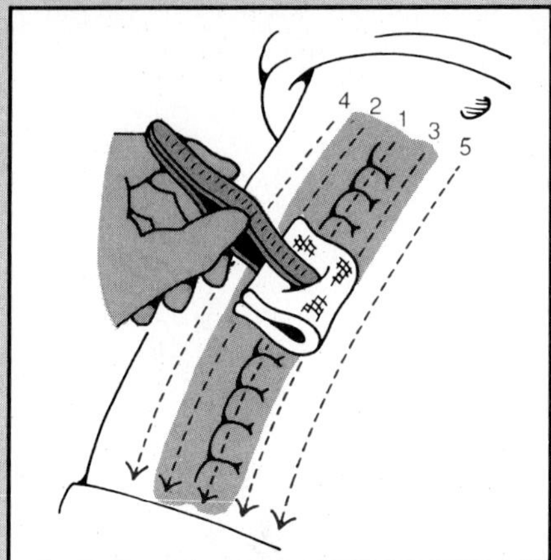

3. Cleaning a large horizontal incision.
   a. Cleanse the incision first from the center of the wound outward to either end, using separate swabs for each stroke.[a] For a small incision, clean from one end to the other.

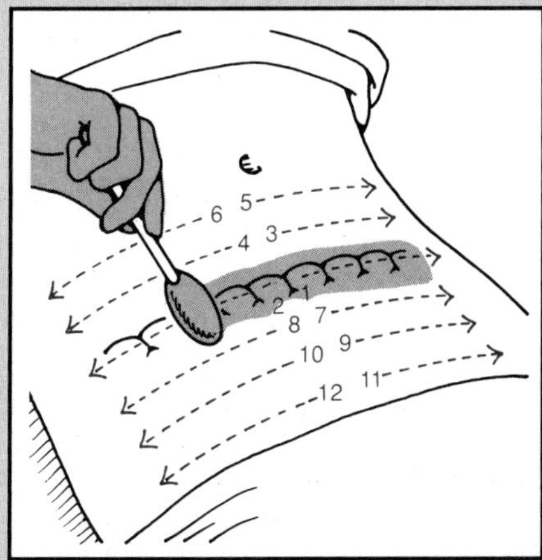

   b. Clean the skin above the wound, cleansing from the center outward, or from one side to the other, depending on the amount of drainage. Use a fresh swab for each stroke.

   c. Clean the skin below the wound in the same way.

4. If the wound has a drain, clean around it last to avoid inoculating the wound with organisms from the drain. Cleanse the skin around the drain, using circular strokes, working outward from the drain. Use fresh swabs as needed, depending on the amount of drainage.

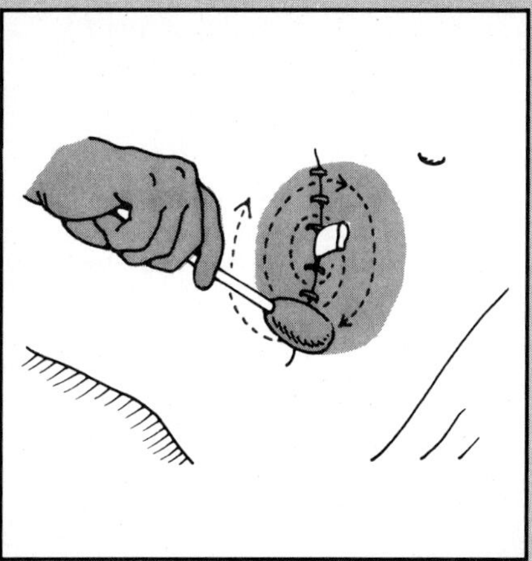

5. Cleanse circular or irregularly shaped wounds, such as pressure ulcers in the same manner: Cleanse from the center outward, using fresh swabs as needed. Clean wound and surrounding skin 3–4 inches around wound (or more if drainage is copious).

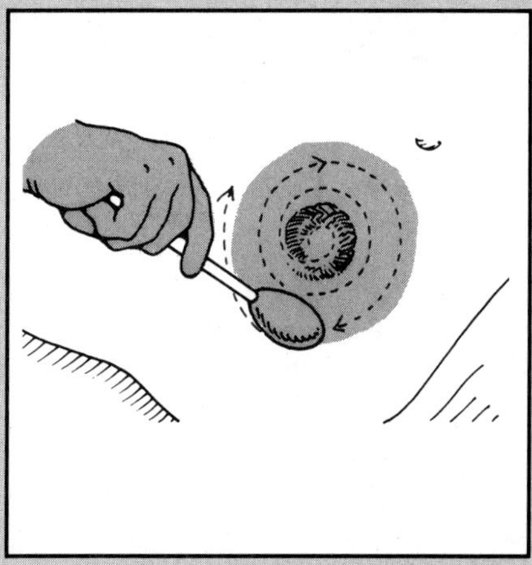

[a] Meshelaney CM. Post-op wound dressings: Your guide is impeccable technique. *RN*. 1979;42:22–33.

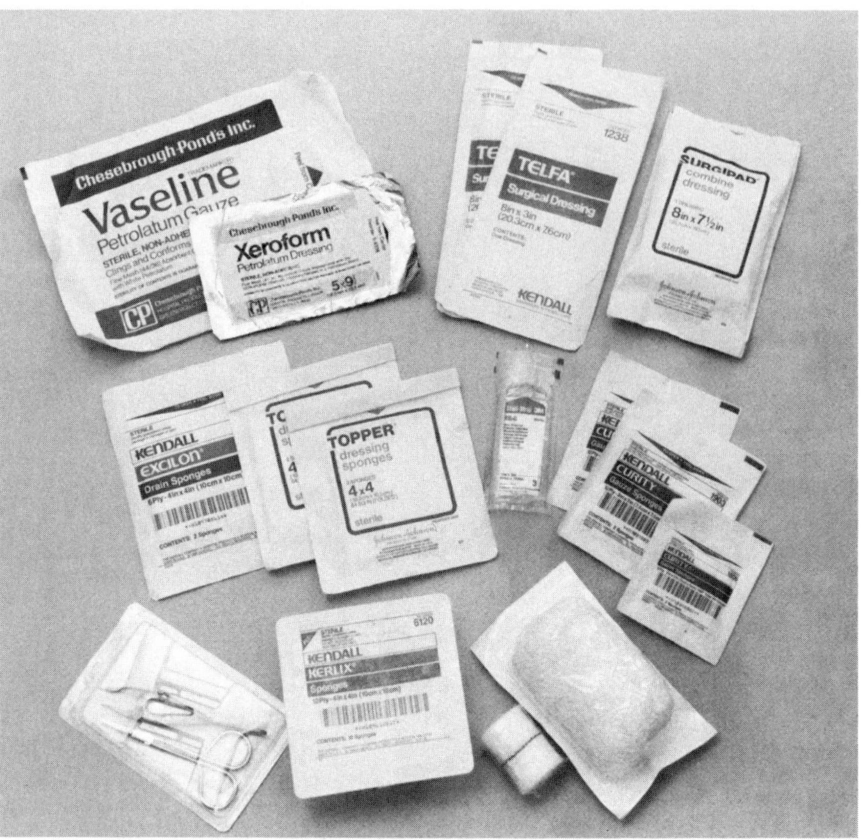

Figure 24–6. Supplies for wound care.

Common cleaning solutions include topical antiseptics such as povidone–iodine, hydrogen peroxide, sodium hypochlorite, and acetic acid. Sometimes physicians' orders or agency policy specify a solution or the nurse giving care may select one based on the type and status of the wound. Nurses should be aware that each of these solutions is contraindicated in some types of wounds and that all of them are cytotoxic in certain concentrations.[6,17] Some experts recommend isotonic solutions, such as normal saline or Ringer's lactate, particularly in wounds that are not infected.[21] The following discussion highlights recommended uses and cautions for common antiseptics.

Povidone–Iodine. Iodine kills bacteria, spores, viruses, and fungi. Povidone–iodine (Betadine) is effective as a preoperative skin disinfectant for clients and as a surgical scrub for operating room personnel. However, numerous studies have demonstrated that it is toxic to granulation tissue even in low concentrations and a systemic toxin if used in concentrations of 10 percent or greater.[21,22] It is best to use povidone–iodine only for infected wounds, and in a maximum concentration of 1 percent for wound care.

Hydrogen Peroxide. This agent is effective in mechanically debriding open wounds, but is broken down too rapidly to have sustained antiseptic action. **Debride** means to remove foreign material and dead or damaged tissue. Hydrogen peroxide is not safe to use in deep penetrating wounds or wounds that extend laterally under the surface of the skin because its effervescent action causes tissue trauma in enclosed spaces.[45] It removes blood clots, so is not useful in fresh bleeding wounds. It is usually dispensed in a 3-percent solution; one-half or one-fourth strength is most often recommended for wound care.

Sodium Hypochlorite. This chlorine compound, commonly called Dakin's solution, is locally irritating to intact skin and granulation tissue and inhibits blood clotting. Its principal use is debridement. Apply zinc oxide or petroleum jelly to skin around a wound being treated with Dakin's solution to protect it from irritation. The correct concentration for use on tissue is 0.5 percent. A 5-percent solution is used to disinfect utensils.

Acetic Acid. In a 0.12-percent solution, acetic acid is effective against pseudomonas aeruginosa, trichomonas, and candida. It is irritating to tissue, so protect the skin as with Dakin's. Acetic acid is toxic to cells in 0.25 percent strength or greater.

Isotonic Solutions. Sterile normal saline and Ringer's lactate have no antibacterial action, but are useful for removing exudates and moisturizing wound surfaces.

Applying Dressings. Ideally, dressings should create an optimum environment for wound healing. In reality, dress-

BOX 24–7. COMMON SUPPLIES USED FOR WOUND CARE

Solutions		Povidone–iodine Hydrogen peroxide Dakin's solution Acetic acid Sterile normal saline
Instruments		Dressing scissors Thumb forceps Straight hemostat (Kelly clamp)
Dressings	**Nonocclusive:**	Filled sponges Gauze sponges (unfilled) Drain sponges Fluffs Roller gauze Combination pads
	Occlusive:	Petrolatum gauze Furacin gauze Telfa
	Semi-occlusive:	Hydrocolloid Semipermeable polyurethane film
	Nonadhering:	Petrolatum gauze Telfa Medicated fine mesh gauze
	Synthetic:	Spray-on Semipermeable polyurethane film Hydrocolloid Hydrogels Hydrophilic gels
Tape		Cotton-backed Rayon taffeta Paper Plastic Elastic foam Waterproof Strapping Montgomery straps
Miscellaneous		Sterile gloves Sterile container (basin, cup) Sterile barrier towel Sterile tongue blades Sterile swabs Sterile applicators Antibiotic ointments Skin protectant (petroleum jelly, zinc oxide) Moisture-proof trash bag

ings sometimes interfere with healing, especially if caregivers select incorrect materials or apply them improperly. Dressings should protect the wound from microbial contamination and trauma, absorb drainage, and yet maintain a sufficiently moist environment to promote healing. Some kinds of dressings also mechanically debride wounds, maintain hemostasis, and promote wound contraction. Covering wounds is also helpful to clients' adaptation to the emotional stress of wounds, because it enables clients to decide when they wish to look at the wound. Many products are available for dressing and caring for wounds. Some of them are illustrated in Figure 24–6; more are listed in Box 24–7. The choice of supplies depends on the individual wound and client situation. In fact no single dressing can produce an optimum healing environment for all types of wounds or for all stages of healing of one wound.[46] For example, dry sterile dressings are a good choice for closed surgical wounds that are healing well (Procedure 24–16). Wet-to-dry dressings are sometimes used for mechanical debriding (Procedure 24–17). Hydrocolloid dressings, discussed in a later section, enhance healing of pressure ulcers. Sometimes improvising may be necessary to achieve the best environment for healing. Nurses' personal experience, consulting with experts such as clinical nurse specialists or enterostomal therapists (whose expertise with skin problems associated with stoma care is often applicable to problem wounds), and consulting professional literature such as that cited in the chapter references and bibliography, are good resources for answers to difficult wound-care problems.

Dressings must be properly secured over wounds with tape or bandages to allow air circulation and prevent slipping or dislodging with movement. Correct taping and bandaging are described in Box 24–8 and Table 24–6, respectively. Montgomery straps, which enable replacement of dressings without removing tape, are useful for situations requiring frequent dressing changes (Fig. 24–7). Elderly clients are especially vulnerable to skin damage from tape removal, which can actually cause extension of a wound.[9,47]

Special Wound Care Procedures. Some wounds require care in addition to cleansing and dressing. For example, many surgical wounds have drainage systems that nurses must manage. Wounds with thick eschar and necrotic tissue may need chemical debriding. These and other special procedures are discussed below.

Wound Drainage Systems. Wound drainage is a source of complications of healing. It creates dead space between wound edges, delaying healing, and provides an excellent medium for microorganism growth. To avoid these complications, surgeons often place soft latex drains called Penrose drains (Fig. 24–8C) or self-contained drainage systems such as the Hemovac (Fig. 24–8A) or Jackson-Pratt (Fig. 24–8B) to facilitate evacuation of wound exudates. One end of the drains is placed near the surgical site. The tubing is brought out of the body through a separate incision adjacent to the surgical incision to reduce the risk of wound infection.[48] Procedure 24–18 discusses management of wound drainage systems.

(Text continues on page 1053.)

TABLE 24–6. TECHNIQUES FOR BANDAGING

Illustration	Instructions	Use
Circular turns 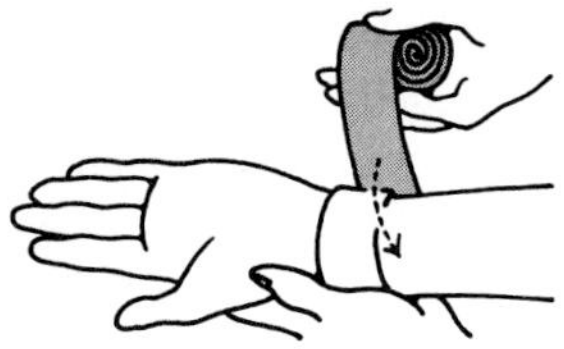	Place flat surface of bandage against extremity, anchor with thumb. Wrap two overlapping layers of bandage over same area.	To cover small cylindrical areas and to anchor bandage for other types of wraps.
Spiral turns 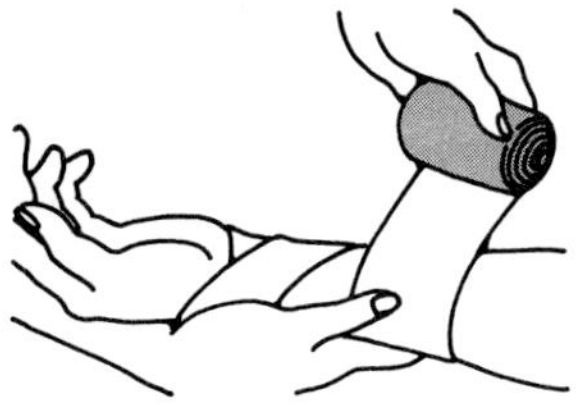	Anchor bandage with circular turns. Wrap bandage on ascending angle, with each turn overlapping previous by 1/3 to 2/3 of bandage width.	Secure dressing or wrap an extremity whose contour does not vary significantly.
Spiral reverse turn 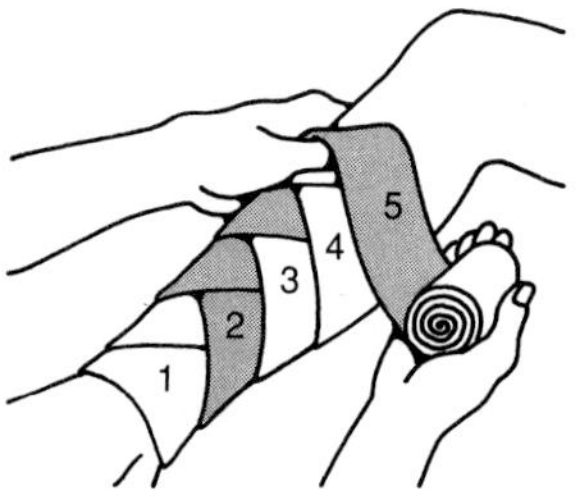	Anchor bandage with circular turns. Start ascending wrap as with spiral, but fold the bandage onto itself halfway through the turn and wrap downward. Overlap 2/3 of the previous turn to secure each layer.	Secure dressing or wrap an extremity that has a significantly larger circumference at one end than at the other.
Figure-eight wrap 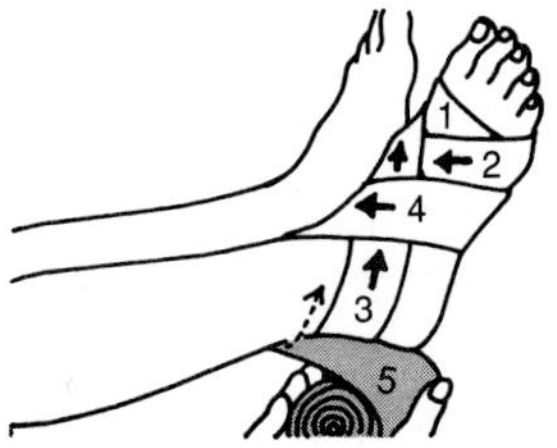	Anchor bandage with circular turns. Wrap around joint in alternately ascending and descending turns, as if to draw an "8."	Secure a dressing or wrap an extremity on or near a joint.
Recurrent bandage (scalp wrap) 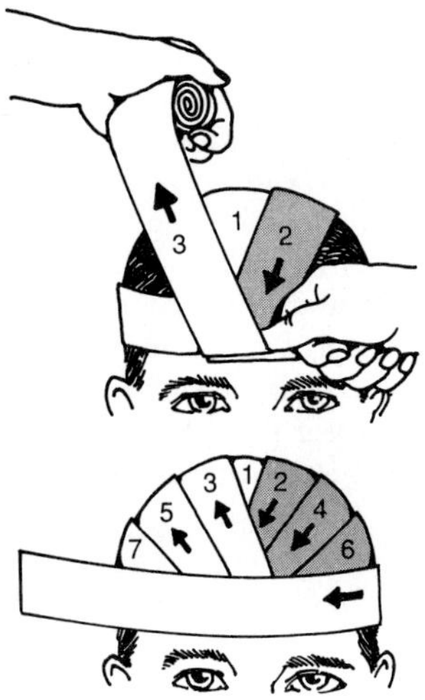	Anchor bandage with circular turns. At center front, make a perpendicular turn, bringing the bandage over the center of the head, until it meets the circular wrap at the back of the head. Reverse directions, bringing the next turn over the head from back to front. Continue wrapping in alternating directions until the head is covered, and then secure with circular turns. Note: Assistance in holding turns will be needed from client or another nurse. Circular turns may be interspersed with perpendicular turns to secure wrap.	Secures dressings on the scalp.

TABLE 24–6. (continued)

Illustration	Instructions	Use
Stump wrap 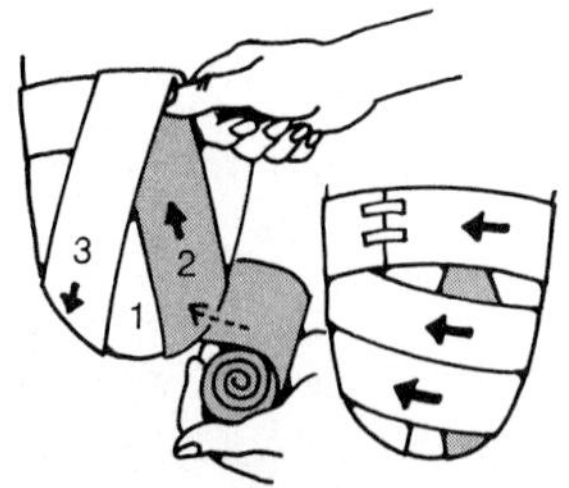	Anchor with circular turns at about 6 to 12 inches above the tip of the stump. Wrap as for scalp above, except after 4 to 5 lengthwise turns, finish with spiral turns in an ascending direction.	Secure dressings or provide compression for stump.

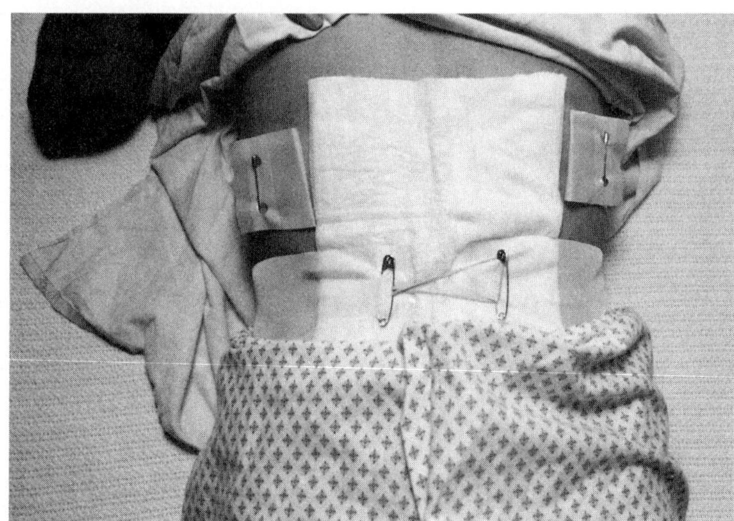

Figure 24–7. Montgomery straps with dressing.

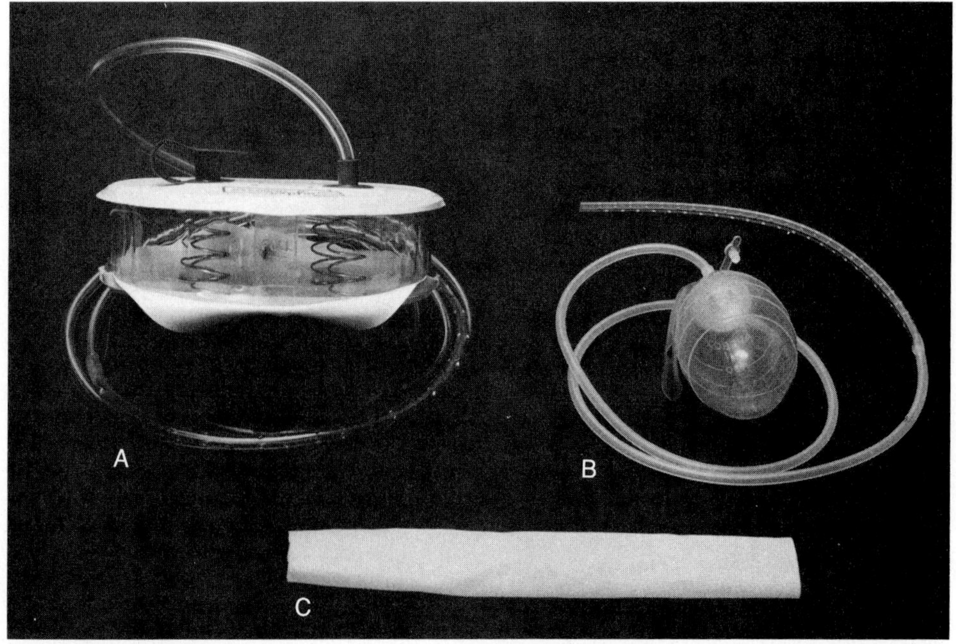

Figure 24–8. Wound drainage systems. **A.** Hemovac. **B.** Jackson-Pratt. **C.** Penrose.

PROCEDURE 24–16. CHANGING A DRY STERILE DRESSING

PURPOSE: To protect a wound from injury and microorganisms, absorb drainage, and promote healing.

EQUIPMENT: Sterile gloves, clean gloves, dressing materials, tape, waterproof bag for soiled dressings, and sterile barrier (optional). If wound cleansing is ordered, see Procedure 24–15.

ACTION	RATIONALE
1. Verify medical order; check operative report or nursing and medical progress notes to determine if a surgical drain is in place and current condition of wound. Gather supplies. NOTE: Many surgeons prefer to do the initial dressing change.	1. Wound care requires a medical order; many surgeons specify solutions or dressing materials desired. Information about wound status assists in the selection of supplies (type and amount), if none are specified in the order. Refer to Box 24–7.
2. Discuss the procedure with the client, including the expected benefits, usual sensations, desired participation, and the timing of the procedure. Determine the need for prior pain medication. NOTE: Some clients are anxious or fearful about looking at their surgical incision. Consider this when discussing and planning care. If medication is desired, administer so peak effect can be expected at the time wound care is planned. (See Chap. 22.)	2. The client will be likely to participate and less anxious if this information is shared. The procedure may be painful or emotionally traumatic so it is advisable not to plan it just prior to meals, scheduled therapy or expected visitors.
3. Wash your hands. Screen client, close door. Raise bed to your waist level. Ask or assist client to assume a comfortable position that allows exposure of dressing. Fold back covers so they cannot contact wound or surrounding skin when dressing has been removed. Provide additional drapes if necessary for warmth or modesty. If wound is to be cleansed and/or is draining profusely, protect the bed with a waterproof pad.	3. Screening and draping show respect for client's needs for privacy; closing door also minimizes air currents which could transmit airborne organisms to exposed wound. Hand washing and moving covers away from dressing prevent wound contamination by direct contact.

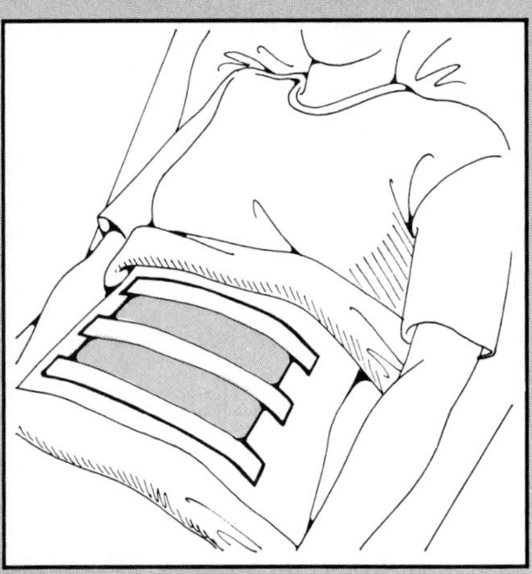

(continued)

PROCEDURE 24–16. (continued)

4. Prepare a working area large enough to accommodate all sterile supplies and located so it will not be at your back while you cleanse and dress the wound:
   a. Create a sterile field using a sterile barrier towel (see Procedure 22–3).
   b. Open sterile supplies and place them on the sterile field (Box 22–12).

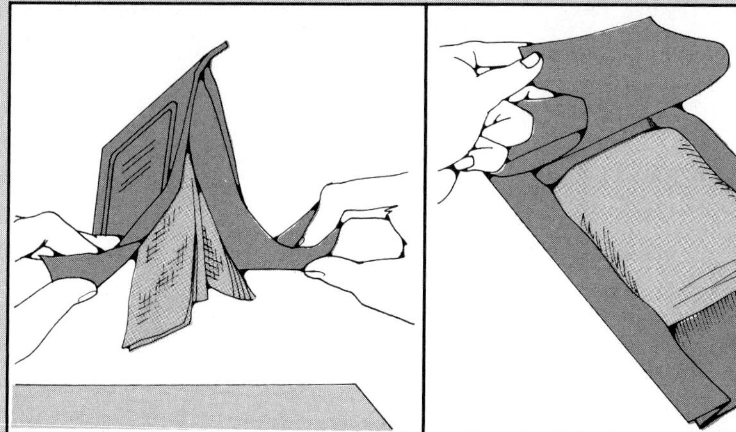

NOTE: A simple dressing change may be accomplished without a separate sterile field. The wrappers of sterile items may be used to make a sterile field if items are opened carefully. The opened wrappers and their contents are placed on the working area.

   c. Pour sterile solution for wound care if ordered (see Box 22–13).
   d. Make a cuff at the top of the waterproof bag and place it so used dressing materials can be discarded without reaching over opened sterile supplies. It may be taped to the siderail for convenience.

4. All items needed for a sterile procedure must be available in one area which is in view at all times. Because one would be unaware of contamination of items out of one's view, they must be considered contaminated.
   a, b. A sterile field creates a barrier between a clean surface and sterile items, preventing contact with microorganisms.
   d. Moving soiled items over a sterile field can contaminate the field because microorganisms on the items are aerosolized when they are manipulated. A cuff protects the outside of the trashbag so it is not contaminated by items that touch its top edge as they are being discarded. The outside of the bag must remain free of organisms from the wound to prevent transmitting them to the environment.

(continued)

PROCEDURE 24–16. (continued)

5. Loosen the tape holding the dressing in place. Pull the tape toward the wound while stabilizing the skin under the tape. Wetting the adhesive surface of the tape with an alcohol swab as you lift the tape facilitates removal. Adhesive remover may also be used, if necessary. Montgomery straps (see Fig. 24–7) are not removed unless wet. Release tie or band closure and fold straps away from the dressing.

5. Pulling toward the wound prevents disruption of healing. Stabilizing the skin reduces discomfort as the tape is removed. Leaving Montgomery straps in place reduces damage to epithelium caused by frequent removal and replacement of tape.

6. Remove the dressing carefully. If the dressing is dry, it may be removed with the bare hand. Don a clean glove to remove a dressing that is damp. All dressing layers may be removed at once if inner dressing does not adhere to the wound and if there is no drain in place. Remove one layer at a time when a drain is present. Use a sterile glove or forceps to remove inner dressings which are not removed with the outer dressing.

6. The outside of a dry dressing is clean, not sterile nor contaminated, therefore no protection is needed to remove it. A wet dressing is likely to be contaminated; the clean glove prevents contamination of the hand. Layer-by-layer removal of dressings around a drain reduces the possibility of dislodging the drain. Removal of inner dressings may involve contact with the wound; therefore, a sterile glove or forceps is used to prevent transfer of microorganisms from the hand to the wound.

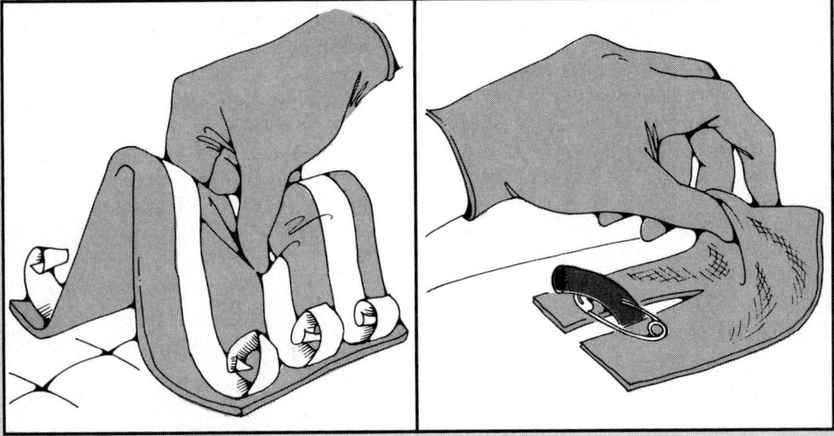

NOTE: If the inner dressing adheres to the wound, moisten with sterile normal saline to prevent disruption of healing.

(continued)

7. Note the amount, odor and character of drainage as you remove the dressing. Discard dressings and glove or forceps, if used, in bag.

NOTE: Report purulent, foul-smelling drainage or increased amount of drainage. Obtain culture (see Procedure 24–19).

7. Changes in the amount and character of drainage are cues to nursing action. Glove or forceps that has contacted the soiled dressing is contaminated and cannot be used to cleanse wound or apply new dressing.

8. Visually assess the wound (see also Box 24–3). Note approximation of wound edges, presence of granulation tissue, amount, character, and location of drainage. Don 1 sterile glove (see Procedure 22–4) on dominant hand, palpate wound site. Note areas that are warm or tender or have increased drainage. Palpate drain site last. Discard glove. Palpation is not necessary if wound appears dry with well-approximated edges. Report signs of infection or delayed healing. Obtain culture if infection is suspected.

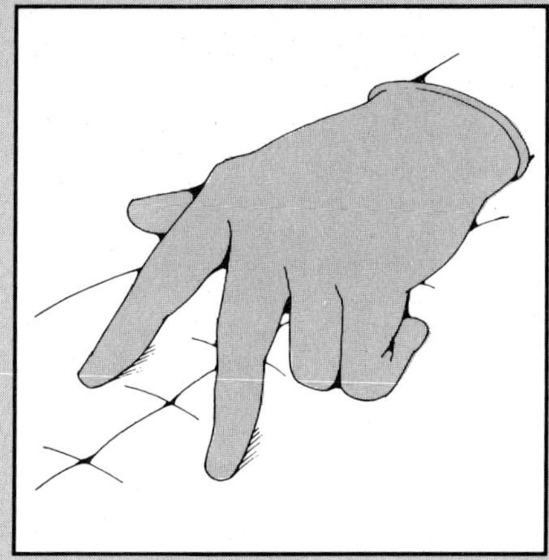

8. Approximation of edges of a surgical wound or granulation tissue in an open wound indicate healing. Warmth, tenderness, or gaping areas may indicate infection. See also step 7. Drain site is assessed last because accumulated drainage there increases the possibility that microorganisms may be present.

9. If necessary, cleanse the wound as described in Procedure 24–15, following physician's order or agency policy.

9. Wounds are cleaned to remove exudate, dead tissue, and bacteria. Wounds that are healing well may not need cleaning.

10. Cover wound with topper sponges, gauze squares, and/or nonadhering dressing as appropriate, using sterile gloved hand. Apply sufficient absorbent dressings for the drainage being produced. If copious drainage is produced and client is ambulatory, place extra dressings at the lowest portion of the wound. Hydrocolloid dressings are often used on decubitus ulcers instead of gauze squares or similar dressing materials. (See text section *Decubitus Care.*)

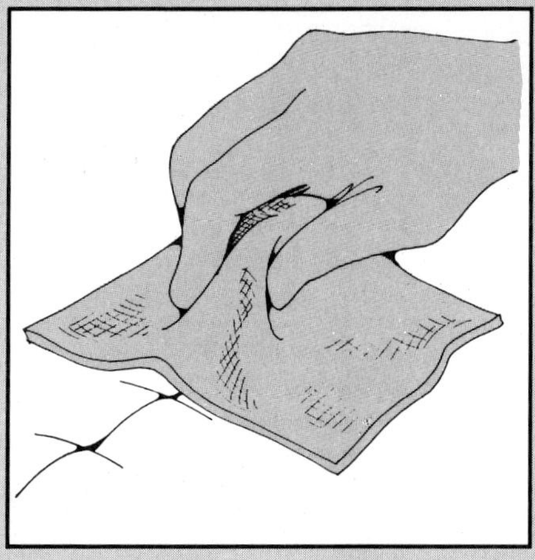

10. Nonadhering dressings prevent disruption of healing in wounds producing sticky exudate, which often causes gauze or toppers to adhere to the wound site. Nonadhering dressings neither absorb drainage nor wick it away from the wound, so absorptive dressings must be added. Wicking is important to prevent drainage accumulating at the wound surface, which macerates skin and slows healing. Gravity will pull drainage toward the bottom of the wound site when client ambulates. Placing extra absorbent materials there prevents drainage leaking onto gown or floor.

(continued)

PROCEDURE 24–16. (continued)

NOTE: Use the minimum amount of dressing materials that will accomplish the purpose for which the dressing is being applied. An unnecessarily bulky dressing is uncomfortable and using excessive supplies is not cost effective.

11. If there is a drain, don a second sterile glove and place 2 drain sponges around the drain in opposite directions.

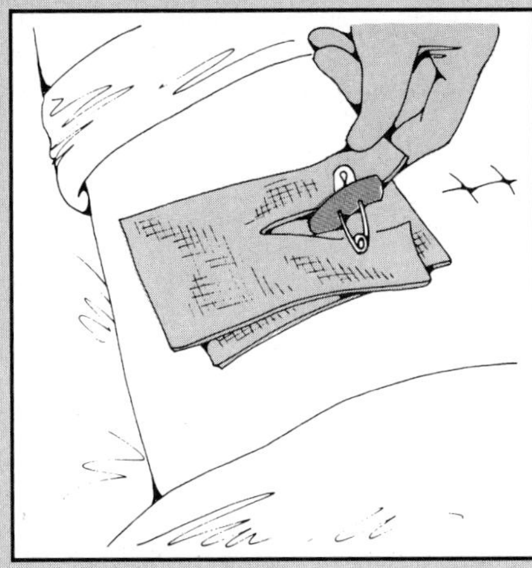

If drain sponges are not available, fold 2 toppers or 4 × 4s as follows:

a. Unfold to 4 × 8 size.
b. Refold in half lengthwise.
c. Fold at right angle, place next to drain.
d. Place second folded sponge on other side of drain with right angle in opposite direction.

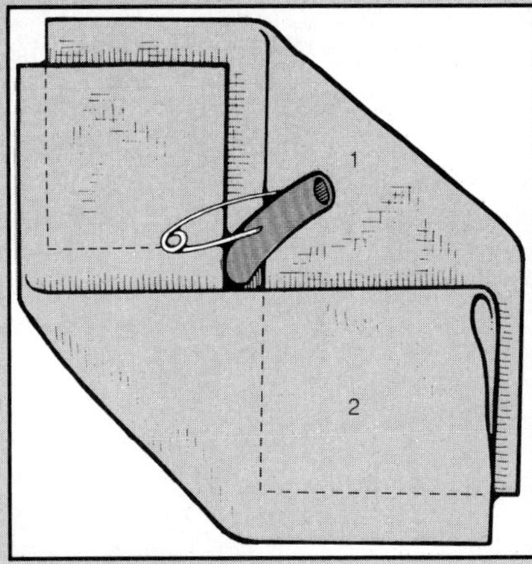

Cover with necessary amount of absorbent dressings.

NOTE: Cutting toppers or 4 × 4s to fit around a drain is not recommended, because cut fibers may adhere to or be imbedded in healing tissue.

11. Drainage is irritating to skin and slows healing. This arrangement of sponges protects skin around drain. Drain site is dressed last because it is more likely to be contaminated (see step 8 above).

(continued)

PROCEDURE 24–16. (continued)

12. If needed, place an outer dressing, such as a combipad over all layers of inner dressings. If glove is wet from touching drain, remove and discard it before placing outer dressing. Touch only the outside of the pad with ungloved hands. Wounds with little drainage may require only a topper(s) or gauze square(s).

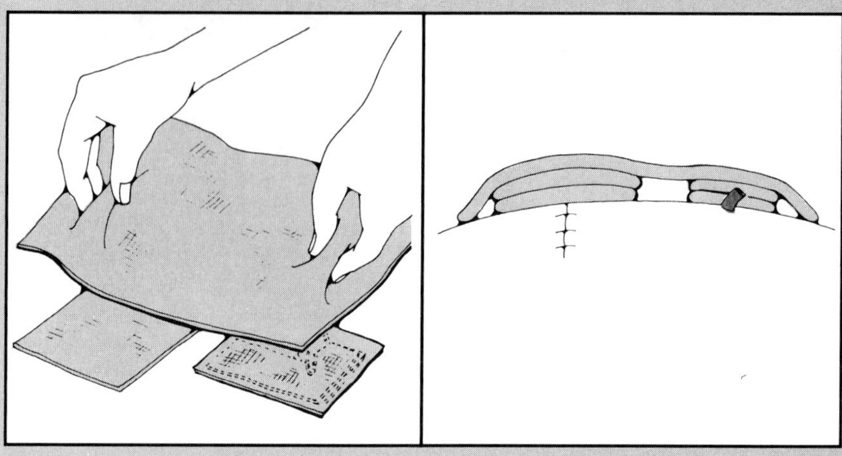

12. A single thick absorbent pad wicks and absorbs drainage, and holds all dressing materials in place with a minimum of tape. Glove is removed to prevent transferring potentially pathogenic organisms from drain site to outside of the dressing and, hence, the environment. Touching only the outside of the dressing maintains the sterility of the wound site.

13. Tape the outer dressing in place as described in Box 24–8.

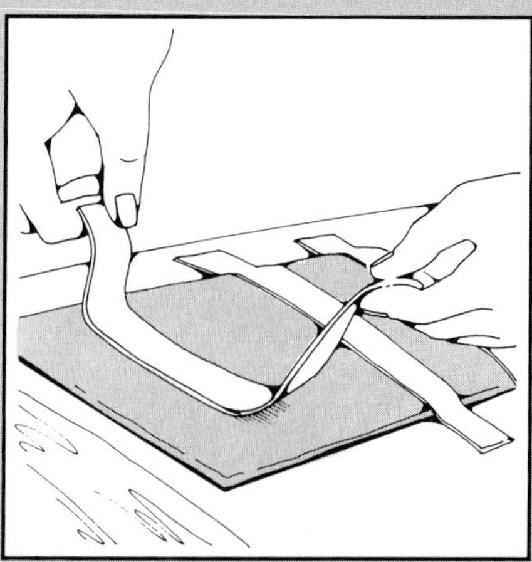

13. Correct taping secures the dressing while allowing air circulation to evaporate moisture from dressing, preventing maceration and delayed healing.

14. Rearrange client's gown and covers. Assist client with repositioning if needed and place bed in low position. Be sure all disposable items used in wound care are in waterproof waste bag. If items are too bulky to fit, they can be discarded in room trash container, if plastic-lined. Liner and contents must then be removed. (Dry wrappers may be left in trash can.) Close waste bags securely and dispose according to agency policy. In many agencies, a covered waste container for disposal of biohazardous waste, such as soiled dressings, is placed in each client room rather than transporting the wastes to a central disposal site after each procedure.

14. Shows respect for client's comfort and personal space. Soiled dressings and items used in wound care provide a medium for bacterial growth and create unpleasant odors. Removing from client's room and disposing in sealed waste containers reduces environmental hazards, both in and outside of hospital.

☐ **RECORDING:** Note initial appearance of dressing, condition of wound; amount, location, and nature of drainage; specific wound care provided; problems encountered, if any, and action taken to correct them; and client's response to care.

PROCEDURE 24–17. APPLYING WOUND PACKING OR WET-TO-DRY DRESSINGS

PURPOSE: To promote wound healing by debriding and to control bacterial growth in infected wounds. Packing or wet-to-dry dressings are commonly used on traumatic wounds, pressure ulcers, or infected surgical wounds.

EQUIPMENT: Clean gloves; sterile gloves, sterile barrier towel; wound-cleansing supplies, if ordered (see Procedure 24–15) or sterile irrigation kit, if ordered (see Procedure 24–18); unfilled wide-mesh gauze squares to pack and cover wound (roller gauze, plain or impregnated with antibacterial agent such as nitrofurazone may be ordered for packing); wetting solution as ordered; sterile basin; tissue forceps or sterile applicators (for small wound); tape or Montgomery straps; and waterproof trash bag.

ACTION	RATIONALE
1. Verify medical order; check operative report or nursing and medical progress notes to determine current condition of wound. Gather supplies.	1. Wound care requires a medical order; many surgeons specify solutions or dressing materials desired. Information about wound status assists in the selection of supplies (type and amount), if none are specified in the order. Refer to Box 24–7.
2. Discuss the procedure with the client, including the purpose and benefits, usual sensations, desired client participation and timing of the procedure. Determine the need for prior pain medication. NOTE: If pain medication is desired, administer so its peak effect can be expected at the time wound care is planned (see Chap. 22).	2. Clients will be less anxious and more likely to participate if adequate information is provided for informed decision making. The procedure may be painful or emotionally traumatic so it is advisable not to plan it just prior to meals, scheduled therapy or expected visitors.
3. Position client and prepare sterile field as in Procedure 24–16, steps 3–4. Place sufficient gauze squares or roller gauze to pack and/or cover the wound in sterile basin. Pour ordered wetting solution over gauze so it is completely saturated. Plastic container in which gauze is packaged may be used as sterile basin. Place it next to the sterile field, as the outside is contaminated.	3. See Procedure 24–16. Surgical asepsis is practiced even when wound is infected, to prevent additional infection by other organisms.

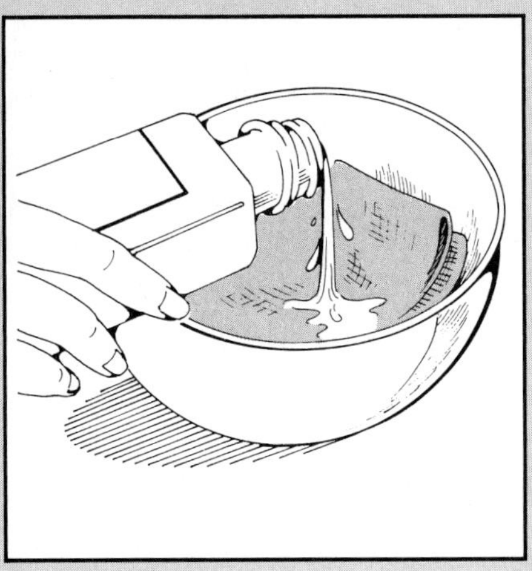

(continued)

PROCEDURE 24–17. (continued)

4. Loosen tape or Montgomery straps as in Procedure 24–16, step 5. Don clean gloves. Carefully grasp the outer dressing and underlying packing material. Cue client of possible discomfort. Pull dressing and packing away from the wound, pulling toward the center if the wound is large. Dressing will stick, but do not moisten unless dressing sticks to pink granulation tissue. If any packing remains in wound, do not remove it while wearing nonsterile glove.

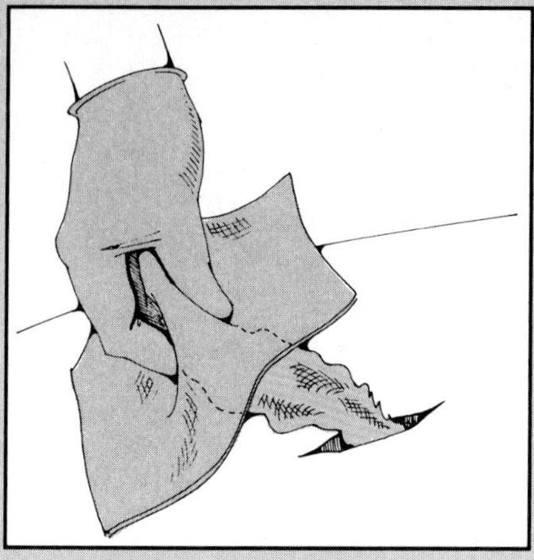

NOTE: It is not unusual for a small amount of bleeding to accompany the removal of the packing. If a wound is deep, all packing cannot be removed by grasping through outer dressing.

4. See Procedure 24–16, steps 5 and 6. Necrotic tissue interferes with granulation and epithelialization. Moistened gauze traps superficial necrotic tissue in its mesh as it dries. Necrotic debris is then removed with the dried gauze. Some associated discomfort is unavoidable, but is better tolerated if client is warned. Premedication will decrease pain.

5. Inspect the dressing, packing and wound as in Procedure 24–16, steps 7 and 8, noting also presence of necrotic debris on dressing and in wound. Discard dressings and glove in bag. Don sterile glove to remove any remaining packing material, inspect and discard as above. Discard glove.

NOTE: If the dressing is dry, but with little trapped debris, it was probably too dry when applied. If it is very wet, outer dressings or tape may have been too thick to allow drying.

5. See Procedure 24–16, steps 7 and 8. Assessment provides information about the effectiveness of the treatment and amount of healing. Necrotic tissue is gray to black. When most of the wound surface is covered with fresh pink granulation tissue, debridement is complete. Consult with physician regarding change in wound care.

6. Cleanse wound (Procedure 24–15) or irrigate (Procedure 24–18), if ordered.

6. Loosened necrotic debris may be removed by cleansing or irrigation. Irrigation is more common for deeper wounds.

(continued)

PROCEDURE 24–17. (continued)

7. Don sterile gloves. Designate one hand "contaminated," to be used for packing the wound, designate the other "sterile" to be used to obtain materials from the sterile field. Remove one gauze square and squeeze out excess moisture. It should be wet, but not dripping. Unfold the gauze (use both hands, but do not bring hands into contact with one another) (i) and place it into the wound cavity (ii). If wound is small, a sterile applicator or forceps may be used to pack gauze into crevices (iii). For a large wound, add additional squares until packing contacts all wound surfaces and cavity is filled. Some clinicians stipulate that roller gauze rather than several gauze squares be used to pack large wound cavities to prevent individual pieces of packing material being left in the cavity inadvertently. If roller gauze is used, unroll as wound is packed rather than placing roll in cavity (iv). Packing should be slightly fluffed to fill cavity, and completely, but not tightly, packed.

i ii

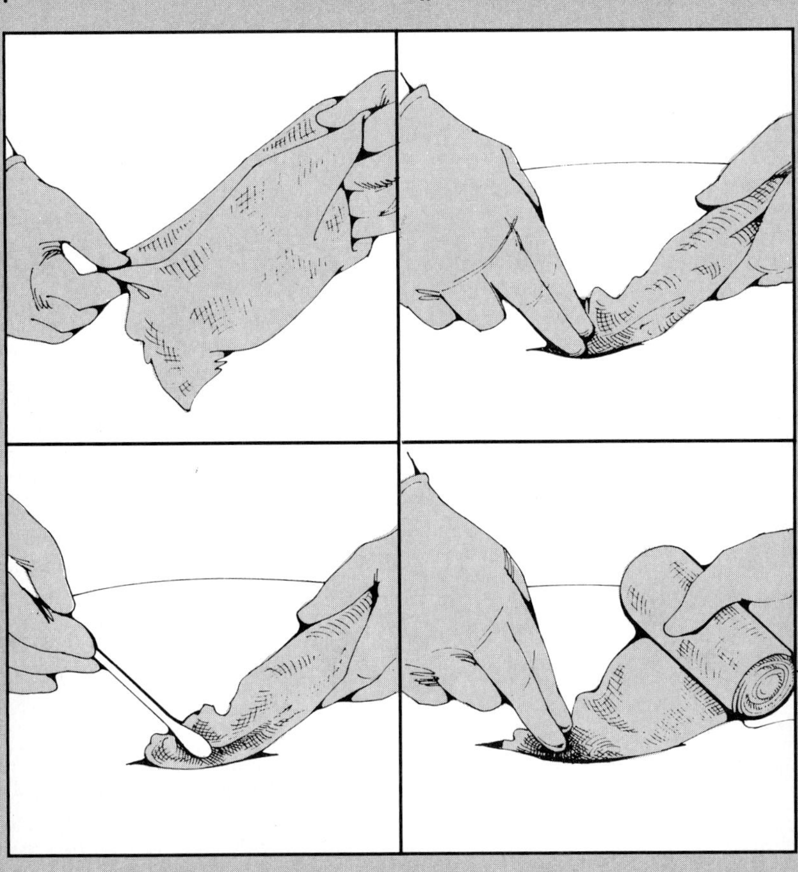

iii iv

7. Touching the sterile field with the hand that has contacted the wound transfers organisms to the field. Debridement occurs only if there is direct contact between tissue and moist gauze; therefore packing must touch all wound surfaces. Saturated or tightly packed gauze will not dry, so will not debride wound and may also cause tissue maceration. Packing the wound tightly may also impair circulation to the wound.

(continued)

PROCEDURE 24–17. (continued)

8. Using "sterile" hand, cover wound and packing with a sufficient number of dry sterile gauze squares to keep outermost dressing from becoming wet. Remove and discard gloves. A final unfolded gauze square may be applied to provide a continuous surface for taping the dressing. Do not touch inner surface with bare hands.

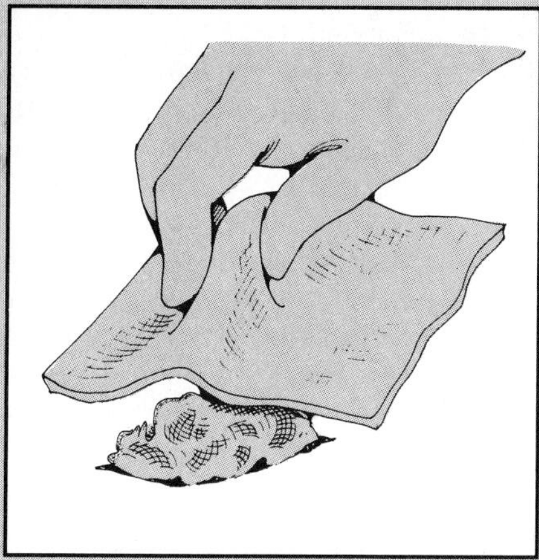

NOTE: Use of thick outer dressings like combipads is contraindicated, because thick dressings prevent air circulation and drying of packing.

8. Using hand that has contacted wound cavity to place outer dressings would transfer organisms to the outside of the dressing and to the environment. If outermost dressing becomes wet, cross-contamination between the wound and the environment is possible by capillary action. Outer dressing should allow air circulation to facilitate drying and debridement.

9. Secure dressings as described in Box 24–8 or Table 24–8. Montgomery straps are often used for wet-to-dry dressings because they are usually changed every 4–6 hours.

9. A correctly secured dressing will protect the wound without retarding drying.

10. Reposition client, remove equipment and replace client's personal belongings as in Procedure 24–16, step 14.

10. See Procedure 24–16, step 14.

RECORDING: Note initial appearance of dressing, condition of wound, including amount of necrotic and granulation tissue; amount, location, and nature of drainage; specific wound care provided; problems encountered, if any, and action taken to correct them; and client's response to care. In some agencies, it is recommended that the number of gauze squares used to pack a large wound be included in nurse's note.

PROCEDURE 24–18. MANAGING WOUND DRAINAGE SYSTEMS

PURPOSE: To maintain functioning of closed wound drainage systems and assess quantity and quality of drainage.

EQUIPMENT: Clean gloves, antiseptic swabs, measuring receptacle, and waterproof pad. For irrigation, solution and syringe to fit tubing.

ACTION

1. Assess amount of drainage in portable closed wound suction systems at least every 4 hours. Suction is significantly reduced and potential for clogging of tubing increased when device is more than one-third full, so it should be emptied whenever fluid approaches this level. Note presence of clots or kinks in tubing. Correct kinks by repositioning reservoir. See step 5 for clot removal. Fig. 24–8 illustrates two closed-wound suction systems and a soft latex (Penrose) drain. A Penrose drain does not contain drainage, so dressings must be assessed frequently and changed when wet.

(continued)

PROCEDURE 24–18. (continued)

2. To empty collection reservoir: Don gloves to protect your hands from exudate. Place waterproof pad on bed under reservoir. Unpin tubing from client's gown. Open reservoir port that is not connected to drainage tubing and pour contents into measuring receptacle. A medicine cup, disposable drinking glass, or any appropriately sized graduated container may be used. Capacity of graduate should be similar to that of reservoir.
3. To reestablish suction:
   a. *Disc-shaped unit:* Place unit on a firm surface with port open. Compress unit completely with palm of your hand. Close port before releasing pressure.

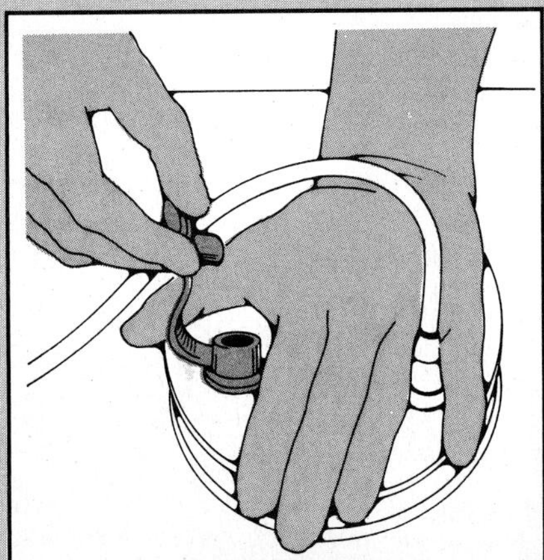

   b. *Bulb-shaped unit:* With port open, squeeze unit with one or both hands until all air is evacuated. Close port. Reattach unit to client's gown below level of wound with safety pin.

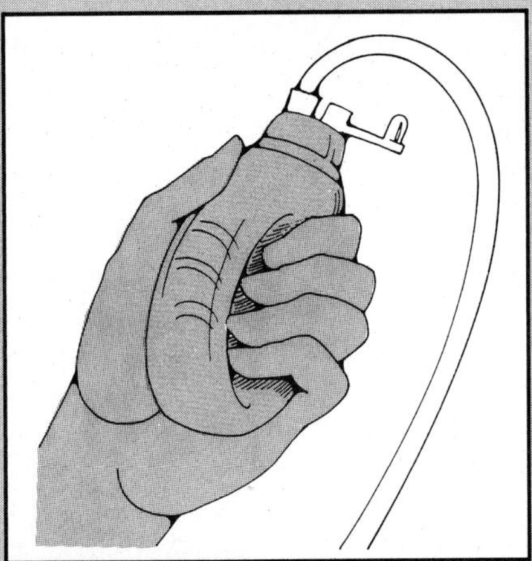

Either system will now exert mild negative pressure, pulling wound exudate into reservoir.

4. If tubing is occluded by clots, check agency policy or physician's order for irrigation. Milking or stripping tubing to dislodge clots is usually contraindicated.
5. To irrigate:
   a. Obtain syringe that will create a seal with tubing attached to unit. Tubing varies in size with size of unit. For very small units, a blunt needle may be required to connect syringe snugly to tubing.
   b. Obtain ordered solution. Sterile normal saline is the usual solution. Fill syringe aseptically.
   c. Place waterproof pad on bed under unit. Clean junction of tubing and reservoir with firm twisting motion.
   d. Detach tubing. Disc-shaped unit can remain on bed; bulb-type unit must be held upright to prevent contamination. Hold tubing in nondominant hand, attach filled syringe.

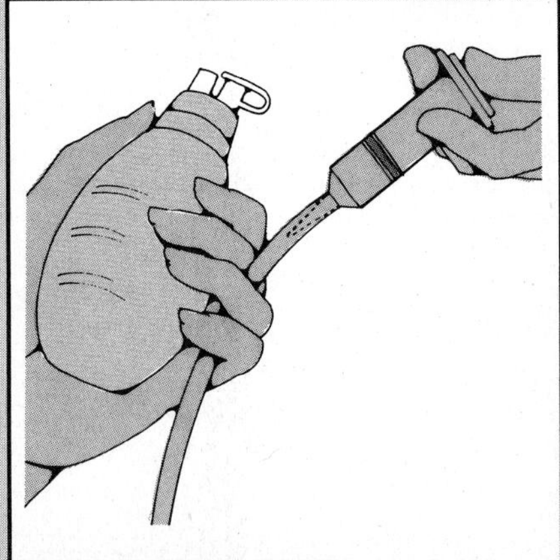

   e. Inject fluid slowly until clot is dislodged. If additional fluid is needed, refill syringe and repeat.
   f. Reestablish suction as in point 3 above.
   g. Reattach unit to cient's gown as above.

☐ **RECORDING:** Routine emptying is recorded on Intake and Output record. Note character of drainage in narrative notes. If irrigation is necessary, state reason for irrigation, amount and type of solution used, and functioning of unit after irrigation. Record irrigating solution as intake, return as output.

Wound Culture. A wound culture should be obtained whenever a nurse is suspicious that a wound infection is developing. See Box 24–3 and *Wound Infection* in Section 1 of this chapter for signs and symptoms. Remember to cleanse the wound before taking a culture specimen so the sample is of fresh drainage.[21,49] Drainage that has been in contact with the skin for some time is likely to have high populations of skin flora, which may mask the causative organism of an infection. Figure 24–9 illustrates several types of culture tubes. Procedure 24–19 outlines the procedure for getting the sample.

Wound Packing. Wound packing is a means of debriding and disinfecting contaminated wounds. Sterile wide-mesh gauze soaked in physiological or antibacterial solution is placed into a wound cavity so it contacts all wound surfaces. If used as a wet-to-wet dressing, wound packing maintains a moist environment and dilutes viscous exudates, but does not debride a wound.[28,29,50] When allowed to dry before removal, the packing acts as a debriding agent, as discussed in Procedure 24–17. When no more necrotic tissue remains, wounds healing by second intention are often packed with fine-meshed gauze (Fig. 24–10). This maintains a moist environment and absorbs exudate, but does not damage granulation tissue when removed.[6]

Wound Irrigation. Irrigation is another means of removing exudate and necrotic tissue from a wound cavity to create an environment for optimal healing. It is detailed in Procedure 24–20. In some settings, nurses use dental irrigation devices (eg, Water Pic) to irrigate wounds.[51,52]

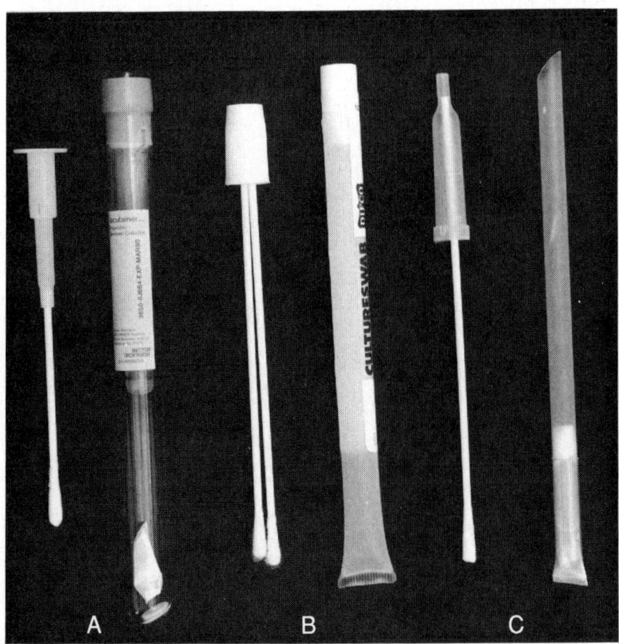

Figure 24–9. Types of culture tubes. **A.** Tube for anerobic culture. **B** and **C.** Tubes for routine culture.

BOX 24–8. GUIDELINES FOR TAPING DRESSINGS

1. Use porous hypoallergenic tape to prevent skin irritation. Occlusive tapes (eg, adhesive tape) trap moisture and cause maceration.[a]
2. Width of the tape should be sufficient to prevent its coming loose with client movement, but not so wide that it interferes with air circulation through the dressing. One-inch tape is generally effective; 2-inch tape may be needed for large dressings.
3. Use the minimum amount of tape that will secure the entire dressing and prevent it from moving over the surface of the wound. Length of the tape extending beyond the edge of the dressing should be approximately one third the width of the dressing. Apply strips of tape near both ends of the dressing. Use additional strip(s) of tape in the center if dressing is large or is applied over a joint.
4. Apply tape so air circulation is not occluded, unless occlusive dressing is ordered. Taping around the edges of a dressing occludes air circulation. Taping too tightly may compromise circulation and cause tension blisters.
5. Rotate sites where tape is applied whenever possible.
6. A skin sealant such as Skin-Prep or Protective Barrier Film before applying tape, or a solid skin wafer barrier around the wound edges (tape is applied to wafer), prevents skin damage from excessive drainage. Do not use sealants on damaged skin, as the alcohol will sting raw skin. Do not use tincture of benzoin. It is drying and causes irritation. Petrolatum-based ointment can also be used to protect wound edges, but apply only to edges to prevent interference with tape adherence.[a]
7. If dressing must be changed frequently, securing the dressing with Montgomery straps will decrease skin irritation from repeated tape removal (Fig. 24–7):
   - Cut straps of appropriate width (material comes in 8 by 10-inch sheets).
   - Remove protective film from adhesive portion, apply to skin adjacent to dressing. Apply a second strap on the opposite side of the dressing.
   - Apply a sufficient number of paired straps to hold dressing in place. (See item 3, above.)
   - Secure straps over dressing with twill tape or rubber bands and safety pins.
8. If tape is used to secure a dressing over a joint, apply tape in the opposite direction of body movement: across the joint, not lengthwise. Elastic tape may secure dressing over joints more effectively than standard tapes; tubular roller bandages may be preferable (see Table 24–6).
9. Do not apply tape around the entire circumference of an extremity.
10. Support skin while removing tape to prevent injury. If hair is present, peel tape in the direction of hair growth. Adhesive remover may be used, but residue should be washed off.

[a] *Bryant RA. Saving the skin from tape injuries.* Am J Nurs. *1988; 88:189–191.*

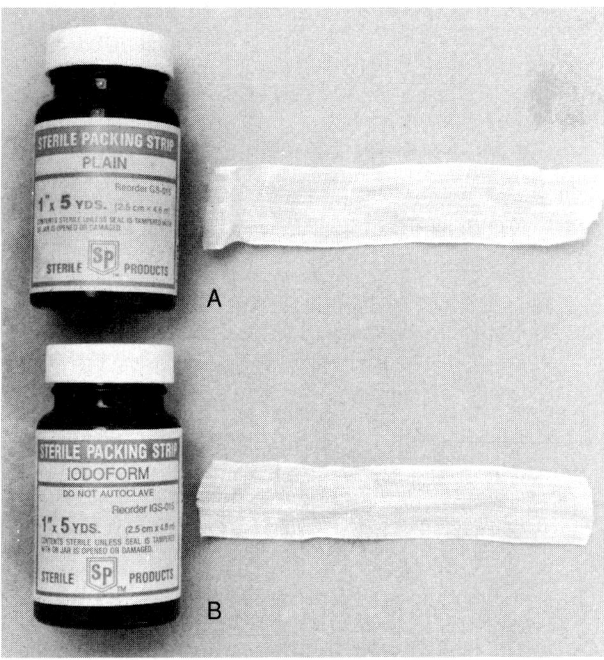

Figure 24–10. Fine-meshed gauze for moist wound packing. **A.** Plain packing. **B.** Medicated packing.

Pressure Ulcer Care. Pressure ulcers, or pressure sores, are a challenge to treat, for they often occur in debilitated or immobilized clients. The treatment of pressure ulcers, therefore, requires a holistic approach to support healing, discussed below, as well as local treatment of the wound itself.

The pathophysiology of pressure ulcers involves tissue necrosis, and so debriding by wound packing, wet-to-dry dressings, irrigation, or whirlpool baths is a common aspect of care. Chemical debridement using proteolytic enzymes is another alternative for debriding pressure sores. Hydrophilic products in the form of beads, gels, and powders also aid the debriding process.[50]

Microorganisms can always be cultured in pressure ulcers.[35] If the organisms are able to proliferate, this can lead to complications such as cellulitis (infection in adjacent tissue), osteomyelitis (infection of bone), or bacteremia (bacteria in the bloodstream). Synthetic semi-occlusive dressings, in particular the hydrocolloid type, are very effective in promoting phagocytosis, enhancing healing, and also may be used to debride wounds.[6,14,23,50,53] These dressings promote liquefaction of necrotic tissue. They absorb exudate and maintain a moist wound environment. This characteristic may be mistaken for signs of a wound infection by caregivers who are not familiar with hydrocolloid dress-

(*Text continues on page 1060.*)

PROCEDURE 24–19. OBTAINING AN AEROBIC OR ANEROBIC WOUND CULTURE

PURPOSE: To detect and identify wound pathogens so that definitive therapy can be instituted. Culture is usually obtained during wound care when suspicious drainage or appearance is noted.

EQUIPMENT: Culture tube with rayon- or polyester-tipped swab and culture medium (aerobic and anerobic tubes are available) and/or sterile syringe with needle for anerobic culture. Plastic bags for specimens. Supplies to cleanse and dress the wound.

ACTION	RATIONALE
1. Discuss the procedure with the client, including the purpose and benefits, usual sensations, desired client participation.	1. Clients will be less anxious and more likely to participate if this information is provided.
1. Position client and prepare sterile field as in Procedure 24–16, steps 3 and 4. Culture tubes or syringes may be removed from peel pack and placed on sterile field with other supplies or placed adjacent to the field on opened wrappers.	2. See Procedure 24–16. Culture may be obtained before or after donning sterile gloves.
3. Assess and cleanse the wound. If exudate does not flow spontaneously from the wound, don a sterile glove and press gently on the wound to express fresh drainage. Remove and discard glove.	3. Wound is cleansed to remove skin flora. Fresh drainage is most likely to be uncontaminated by skin flora and contain the causitive organism. Glove would contaminate outside of culture tube.

(continued)

PROCEDURE 24–19. (continued)

4. If exudate seems to be coming from deep within the wound, obtain anerobic culture first. Don clean gloves. Remove needle from syringe, withdraw fresh exudate, expel air from syringe, and quickly replace and tape needle. Place in bag, seal. If anerobic culture tube is used, follow manufacturer's directions. Systems used to remove air vary.

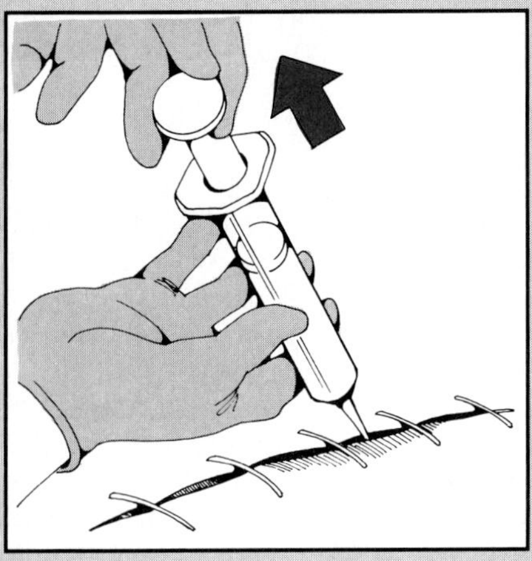

4. Organisms growing in deep wounds or poorly perfused tissue are most likely to be anerobes and so must be protected from air. Taped, capped needle and syringe plunger act as plugs, keeping air away from specimen. Bag protects environment from organisms on syringe.

5. Also obtain aerobic culture:
   a. Remove cap and attached swab from aerobic culture tube without touching swab.

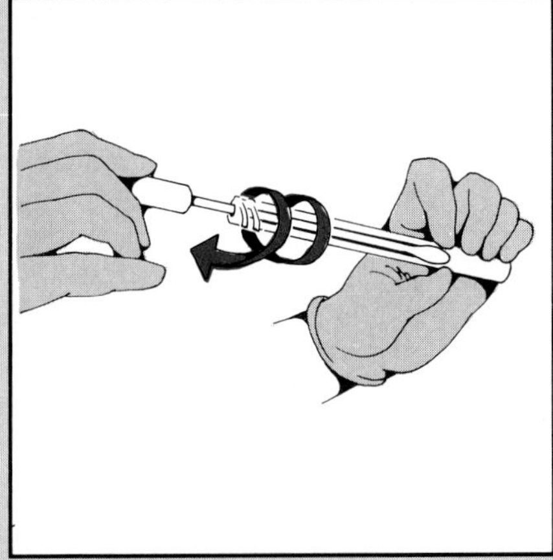

   b. Roll the tip of the swab in fresh exudate.
   c. Replace it in the culture tube without touching the outside, close tightly, and crush the ampule at the base of tube to release culture medium. Place tube in bag, seal.

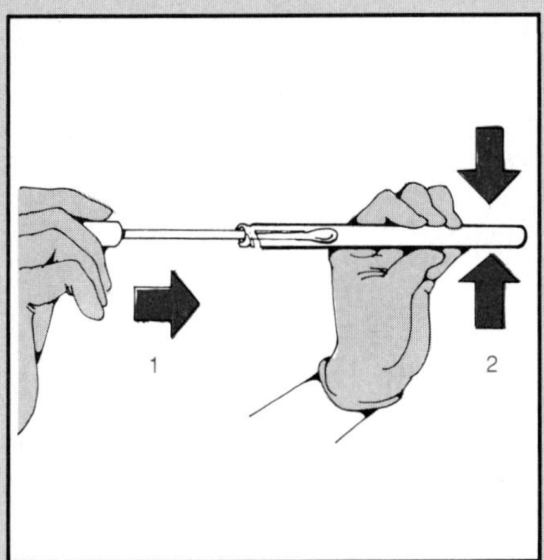

5. Aerobes may also infect wounds.
   a. Contact between the swab and nurse's hand transfers organisms to the swab and the wound.
   b. Rolling coats swab with exudate.
   c. If the swab with exudate touches the outside of the tube or the tube is not closed correctly, environmental or specimen contamination could result.

(continued)

PROCEDURE 24–19. (continued)

6. If a wound has a combination of inflamed, necrotic and/or purulent areas, obtain additional specimens from each area in a separate tube. Insert swabs as deeply as possible into wound crevices, abscess pockets, or eroded areas to obtain best specimen. Remove and discard gloves.

   6. Organisms with different sensitivity to antibiotics may be present within the same wound. All pathogens must be identified to successfully treat the infection.

7. Complete ordered wound care; dress wound, reposition client and dispose of supplies as in Procedure 24–16.

   7. See Procedure 24–16.

8. Label each specimen with client's name, room number, diagnosis, source of specimen, and test desired. If antibiotic therapy has been initiated prior to specimen, note name of drug.

   8. Facilitates prompt and accurate results. Lab personnel can take measures to prevent undergrowth of culture because of antibiotic in the specimen, if drug is identified.

9. Assure that the specimen is delivered to the lab within 20 minutes.

   9. Some organisms die quickly and others multiply rapidly, creating a potential for false diagnosis of the actual causitive organisms if lab cannot assess specimen promptly.

10. Inform client that test results take 48 hours or more. Inform client and physician of test results as soon as they are available.

    10. Positive identification of causitive organisms can only occur after sufficient number have multiplied. Physicians need accurate information to plan therapy. Clients have a right to information about their health status. Correct information facilitates positive coping.

RECORDING: Note conditions in wound that prompted obtaining culture, number, and type of specimens obtained, and disposition of specimen. See also Procedure 24–16.

PROCEDURE 24–20. IRRIGATING A WOUND

PURPOSE: To clean and debride a wound to promote healing. Irrigation is commonly used for traumatic wounds, pressure ulcers, or infected surgical wounds.

EQUIPMENT: Sterile irrigation set or sterile syringe, sterile basin and clean curved basin; irrigation solution as ordered; waterproof pad(s); clean gloves; equipment for wound packing (Procedure 24–17), if ordered; equipment for sterile dressing change (Procedure 24–16); and extra sterile glove and gauze squares to dry skin around wound. For deep wounds, a sterile catheter and additional sterile glove may be added; if irritating solution is used, add sterile tongue blades, sterile protective ointment, additional irrigation set, and sterile normal saline for rinsing.

(continued)

PROCEDURE 24–20. (continued)

ACTION	RATIONALE
1. Verify medical order; check operative report or nursing and medical progress notes to determine current condition of wound. Gather supplies. Check expiration date on irrigating solution.	1. Wound irrigation requires a medical order; information about wound status assists in the selection of dressing supplies (type and amount), if none are specified in order. Refer to Box 24–7. Many irrigation solutions have a short shelf life. Some must be refrigerated.
2. Discuss the procedure with the client, including the purpose and benefits, usual sensations, desired client participation, and timing of the procedure. Determine the need for prior pain medication. NOTE: If pain medication is desired, administer so its peak effect can be expected at the time wound care is planned (see Chap. 22).	2. Clients will be less anxious and more likely to participate if adequate information is provided for informed decision making. The procedure may be painful or emotionally traumatic so it is advisable not to plan it just prior to meals, scheduled therapy, or expected visitors.
3. Wash your hands. If work area is large enough, prepare sterile field with supplies for dressing (Procedure 16, step 4) and if ordered, packing the wound (Procedure 17, step 3), leaving adjacent space for irrigation equipment. If space is limited, defer sterile field until irrigation is complete; prepare trash bag as in Procedure 24–16, step 4d. NOTE: If rinsing with sterile normal saline is ordered, a second irrigation setup will be needed. Rinsing is not common, unless irritating irrigation solution is used (eg, Dakin's).	3. Preparing all equipment to complete wound care in advance limits the amount of time the wound is exposed to the environment, decreasing the possibility of airborne contamination and chilling the client, but if workspace is limited, sterile field is likely to be contaminated while irrigation equipment is being used. See also Procedures 24–16 and 24–17.
4. Loosen cover on irrigation solution. Unwrap irrigation set. Take solution container out of collection basin. Remove container cover and syringe as a unit, being careful not to touch syringe below cover. While holding syringe and cover, pour irrigation solution into container. (Amount depends on the size of the wound.) Remove protective tip from end of syringe and replace cover and syringe on container. If not using irrigation set, unwrap sterile basin and pour solution. Leave syringe in package until after donning gloves (see step 7).	4. Irrigation equipment is ready for use. Solution and distal end of syringe remain sterile, having contacted nothing unsterile and are protected by cover. Outside of container and proximal end of syringe need not remain sterile, as they will not contact wound.

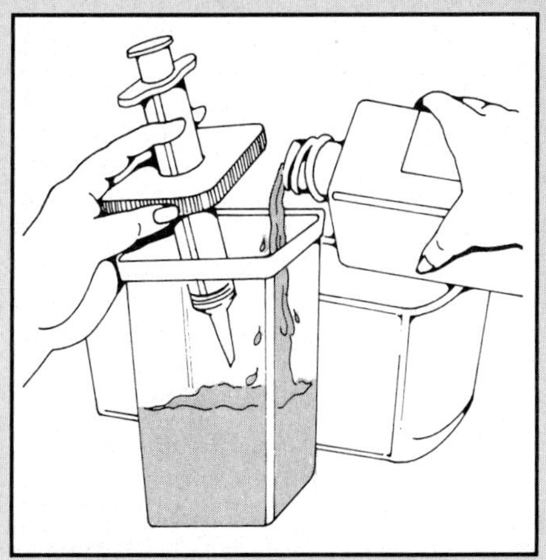

(continued)

PROCEDURE 24–20. (continued)

NOTE: Irrigation solution may be warmed by placing the bottle in a basin of hot tap water for 10–15 minutes before pouring into irrigation container. Warm solution promotes comfort and causes local vasodilation, hence facilitates healing.

5. Position client and expose dressing as in Procedure 24–16, step 3. Remove dressing; assess wound and dressing as in Procedure 24–16, steps 5–8. Palpatory assessment is usually not necessary.

5. See Procedure 24–16. Palpatory assessment is used to detect healing or complications in a sutured incision. Wounds needing irrigation are usually not sutured, but are healing by secondary intention.

6. Assist client to turn, if necessary, so solution will run by gravity to collection basin with least possible contact with intact skin. Tuck waterproof pad(s) under client, extending to edge of bed; place collection basin next to client on pad. If irritating solution is used, apply sterile protective ointment to wound edges with sterile tongue blade.

6. Solution flowing out of wound will contain debris and microorganisms. Minimizing its contact with skin and bed limits possibility of contamination. Protective ointments create a barrier over skin, so solution cannot contact and damage it. Wound healing is enhanced when surrounding skin is optimally healthy.

7. Don clean gloves. Fill irrigating syringe and flush wound with steady pressure from highest to lowest part of the wound. Do not touch wound with syringe. Direct stream so all crevices and wound surfaces are contacted by irrigant. (For deep wounds, see step 8, below.) Refill syringe and continue to flush wound until all areas have been cleansed. If possible, hold the collecting basin tightly against the skin below the wound with the nondominant hand while irrigating. Some clients may desire to help by holding collection basin.

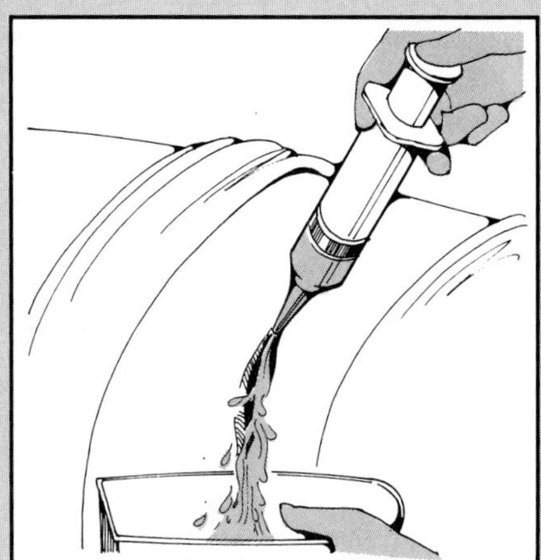

NOTE: Greater pressure is generated if a syringe with a small tip is used. This is preferable if debris is tenacious. Still greater pressure can be achieved by attaching a blunt needle to the syringe.

7. Gloves protect nurse's hands from organisms in irrigation return. Sterile gloves are not needed at this time because nurse's hands do not contact wound. Pressure of the flowing liquid physically removes superficial debris from wound so all surfaces must be flushed to completely clean the wound. Some solutions also have antibacterial action. Body contours make collecting return in a basin difficult, but close contact with the body will minimize spilling.

(continued)

PROCEDURE 24–20. (continued)

8. If wound is very deep, or has pockets which cannot be reached with fluid flowing from syringe, attach sterile catheter to filled syringe:
   a. Open peel pack, allow catheter to rest on sterile package. Don sterile glove on nondominant hand. Attach catheter to syringe with sterile gloved hand.
   b. Direct irrigant to wound pockets or crevices by moving catheter tip with sterile gloved hand.

8. Debris cannot be removed from a deep wound unless stream of liquid can be focused on all wound surfaces. Catheter acts as an extension of the syringe. Contact with wound and/or adjacent skin during irrigation contaminates glove, so it cannot be used to dress the wound.

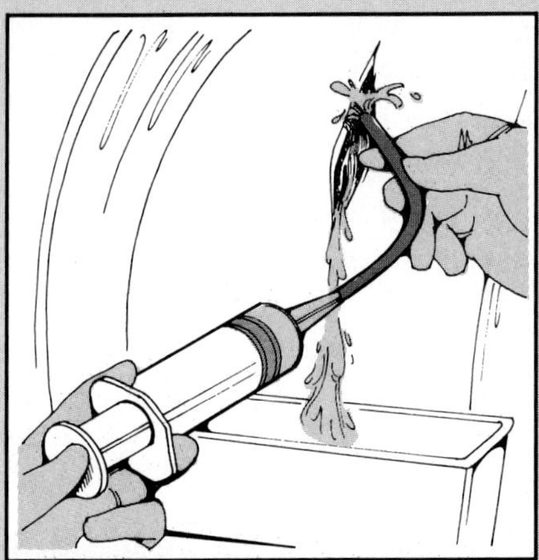

   c. Remove catheter to refill syringe (catheter may be placed on wrapper so both hands can be used to refill syringe).
   d. Repeat as above, discard catheter and glove, unless rinse is ordered.

9. Repeat step 7 or 8 using normal saline if Dakin's solution is used to irrigate wound. Remove and discard gloves.

9. Dakin's solution (0.5% sodium hypochlorite) is an effective debriding agent, but is irritating to healthy tissue and delays the clotting process, so residual solution must be removed.

10. Don sterile glove on dominant hand and blot residual irrigant from skin around wound. Discard glove.

10. Excessive moisture causes maceration, which interferes with healing. Glove has been contaminated by contact with skin, so it cannot be used to dress the wound.

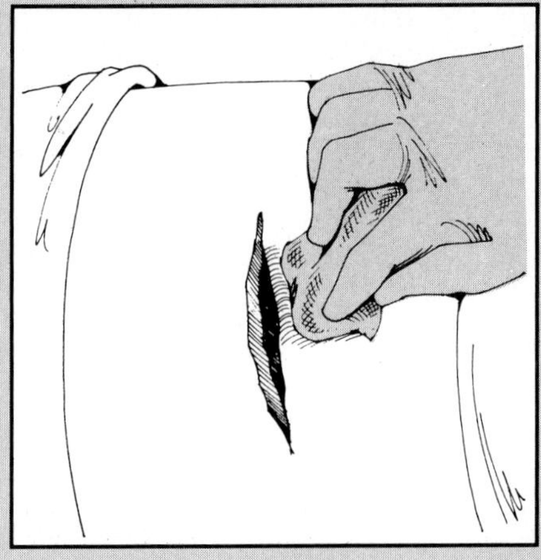

(continued)

PROCEDURE 24–20. (continued)

11. Pack and/or dress the wound as described in Procedures 24–16 and 24–17.	11. See Procedures 24–16 and 24–17.
12. Reposition client, remove equipment, and replace client's personal belongings as in Procedure 24–16, step 14. Irrigation set may not be reused for a subsequent procedure.	12. See Procedure 24–16, step 14. Liquid (even an antibacterial solution) in irrigation set may support growth of microorganisms.

RECORDING: Note initial appearance of dressing; condition of wound before and after irrigation, including amount of necrotic and granulation tissue; amount, location, and nature of drainage; specific wound care provided (including type of irrigation solution); problems encountered, if any, and action taken to correct them; and client's response to care.

ings.[53] Thorough cleaning or irrigation of the wound when changing the dressing will help to rule out this possibility. Application procedure and duration of application vary with specific products, so it is important to follow manufacturers' directions. Figure 24–11 illustrates application of a transparent polyurethane film type dressing. Table 24–7 provides guidelines for the selection of approaches for the care of pressure ulcers.

Researchers are testing various other treatments for treatment of pressure ulcers, such as topical application of cell-specific growth factors,[14,17,54,55] electrical stimulation,[17,56] CO_2 lasers,[57] and silicone implants over bony prominences.[17] Hyperbaric oxygenation also is used to promote healing. Although these are not nursing measures, nurses may assist in their application and assess the results.

The best treatment for pressure ulcers is prevention. Promoting mobility; supporting nutrition and fluid intake; preventing pressure, friction, and shearing; and controlling moisture (eg, from diaphoresis or incontinence) are important preventive measures. They are discussed in greater detail in Chapter 30.

Measures to Support Healing. Supportive care that promotes comfort and well-being enhances healing of wounds of all types. Hygiene measures such as oral care, baths, and shampoos; comfort measures such as positioning and massage; stress reduction techniques such as music therapy, imagery, and meditation; and exercise contribute to healing and support natural defenses against infection. Promoting intake of protein, vitamins A and C, zinc, and adequate fluids is critical to these efforts. Emotional support including active listening and discussion of treatment options and progress of healing is important. Soliciting client input in planning and carrying out treatment also supports well-being and therefore enhances healing.

Rehabilitative Care

Rehabilitative skin and tissue care involves supporting adaptation to chronic skin conditions and encouraging self-care or family member care of slow-healing or chronic wounds.

Chronic skin diseases are often debilitating because of

BUILDING NURSING KNOWLEDGE

Does the Amount of Care Make a Difference in Preventing Pressure Ulcers?

Clarke M, Kadhom HJ. The nursing prevention of pressure sores in hospital and community patients. *J Adv Nurs.* 1988; 13:365–373.

Clarke and Kadhom review research indicating that a long period of low pressure can be more harmful than a short period of high pressure in the generation of pressure ulcers. Thus, duration of pressure is an important factor in generation of pressure ulcers, and relief of pressure is important to prevention. Relief of pressure requires the careful attention of caregivers.

The investigators designed a study to determine the amount of time devoted to preventive pressure-area care for individuals cared for in two settings, hospital and community, and the outcome of that care. The criterion of success was whether or not pressure ulcers developed. To be admitted to the study, subjects had to be restricted to bed and without existing ulcers. Nurses were asked to keep a diary on the care of 88 hospitalized clients, while relatives were asked to do the same for 30 family members cared for at home. The diary was used to record each occasion of pressure-area care, the time of starting and finishing care, method used, and the state of the skin at the site. Data collection lasted 6 weeks or until the client developed an ulcer, resumed mobility, was discharged, or died.

The findings were that 26 of 88 (29.5 percent) hospitalized clients developed ulcers, while 6 of 30 (20 percent) clients cared for at home developed ulcers. Of the 13 community clients who were totally reliant on nurses for their care, 5 developed ulcers. The frequency of care was greater for community clients who did not develop ulcers than for those who did. Moreover, the amount of time devoted to pressure-area care was significantly greater on the average for clients in the community than for those in the hospital.

Among the hospitalized clients, those who developed ulcers received less time on average and received care less frequently than those who did not develop ulcers. The difference in amount of time was statistically significant. The investigators concluded that study findings show time and frequency of care to be significantly related to the prevention of pressure ulcers.

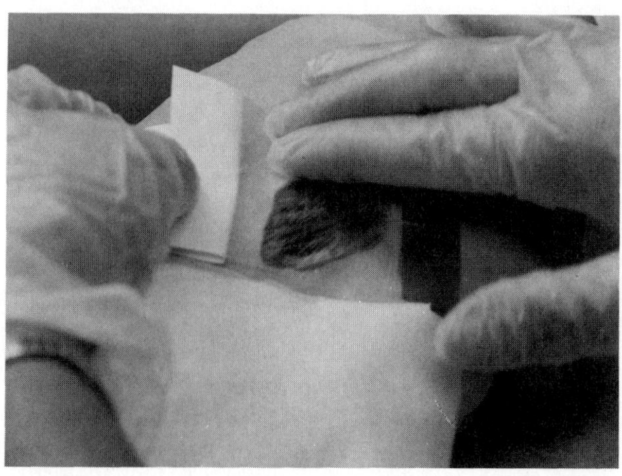

Figure 24–11. Application of a transparent polyurethane film type dressing. (*From Smith S, Duell D.* Clinical Nursing Skills: Nursing Process Approach; Basic to Advanced Skills, *2nd ed. Norwalk, CT: Appleton & Lange; 1988:596).*

their impact on appearance. Skin condition has considerable influence on self-concept and body image. Lesions on exposed parts of the body, especially the face, generate self-consciousness and lack of self-regard. Often individuals with skin alterations become extremely sensitive to others' responses and may even avoid social situations. The anticipation of stares or revulsion from others may be so emotionally stressful that clients perceive actual interactions as too difficult to deal with.

Skin diseases also alter communication. Fearing rejection because of their lesions, clients may limit communication through touching, thereby depriving themselves of a primary means to convey caring, intimacy, and sexuality.

Supporting adaptation to skin alterations begins with listening and encouraging expression of feelings. Many clients feel anger, frustration, and powerlessness. Venting these feelings is an effective prelude to learning about treatment alternatives and participating in planning management of the disease and related problems. Using touch, eye

TABLE 24–7. GUIDELINES FOR WOUND CARE OF PRESSURE ULCERS

Wound	Suggested Care	Action	Tips/Comments
Stage 1 ulcer	a. Transparent dressing.	a. Traps exudate containing macrophages and leukocytes against wound, promoting natural defenses (autolysis).	a. Adhesive backed, change when loose or fluid builds up; some advise not to use on infected wounds.
	b. Hydrocolloid dressing.	b. Maintains moist environment, promotes autolysis, absorbs exudate.	b. Adhesive, may be hard to remove, water resistant, client can bathe.
	c. Antibiotic, saline, or vaseline-impregnated dressing.	c. Maintains moist environment.	c. Absorptive outer dressing needed.
Stage 2 ulcer	a. Same as stage 1.	a. See stage 1.	a. See stage 1.
	b. Absorptive wound fillers (pastes, granules).	b. Absorbs exudate, nonocclusive, used with other dressings.	b. Do not use on deep, tunnelled wounds; may remain in place several days unless excessive exudate.
	c. Hydrogels.	c. Stimulates cellular activity, provides moist environment, debrides.	c. Change daily, dries out, may macerate surrounding skin, must be secured in place, do not use with undermining wounds.
	d. Polyurethane foam.	d. Absorbs exudate.	d. Used with wound fillers, do not use if minimal exudate.
Stage 3 ulcer	Same as stage 2.		
Stage 3, 4, yellow	High-pressure irrigation, hydrocolloids, hydrogels, fillers	Keeps wound clean and moist.	Document changes in color, depth, diameter of wound.
Stage 3, 4, pink to red	Transparent films, hydrocolloid, hydrogel.	Protects from trauma, promotes continued healing.	See stage 3, 4, yellow.
Stage 4, black wound	Proteolytic enzymes, whirlpool, high-pressure irrigation, surgical debridement, wet gauze.	Softens and/or removes dead tissue.	Use only until eschar is gone.

Braden BJ, Bryant R. Innovations to prevent and treat pressure ulcers. Geriatr Nurs. *1990;11:189–191. Fowler E, Cuzzell JZ, Papen JC. Healing with hydrocolloid.* Am J. Nurs. *1991; 91:63–64. Stotts NA. Seeing red and yellow and black: The three color concept of wound care.* Nursing 90. *1990;20: 59–61.*

contact, and accepting facial expressions—important aspects of effective care in most situations—are especially meaningful to clients with disfiguring skin lesions, because of the positive regard these behaviors convey.[51]

As with any chronic condition, successful adaptation involves progress toward self-acceptance and periods of apparent regression and discouragement. Clients unable to adapt constructively often benefit from a referral to a psychiatric clinical nurse specialist or other mental health professional.

Rehabilitative management of lesions involves many of the same approaches used in preventive, supportive, and restorative care. Good hygiene, maintaining healthy nutritional and fluid intake, regular exercise, and stress-management strategies contribute to general health and well-being and support healing of lesions. Therapeutic baths and other measures to reduce pruritus provide symptomatic relief of discomfort. Some conditions require special skin care and dressings.

Clients with chronic or slow-healing wounds are often candidates for home care. These clients need a holistic approach to care that takes into consideration social and financial variables, as well as those related to the physical care of the wound.[58] Establishing a trusting relationship through effective communication is pivotal. Teaching basic asepsis and techniques for wound assessment and care promotes transition to self-management of the wound and appropriate consultation with health care providers. Attention to nutritional status is also of primary importance. A recent study of clients receiving home care for wounds found many indicators of nutritional deficiencies. Nearly all of the clients had insufficient calorie intake for optimum healing, over half had less than the recommended daily allowance of protein, many had inadequate intake of vitamin C, and more than two thirds had lost weight.[59] Significantly delayed healing is a certain consequence of nutritional deficiencies such as this.

Despite the challenges clients with serious wounds and chronic skin diseases must face, sensitive nursing care with an emphasis on collaborative management can make a significant difference in client outcomes.

IMPLICATIONS FOR PROFESSIONAL COLLABORATION

Wound Healing

The expertise of many health professionals is sometimes needed to promote healing of chronic wounds. Nurses, enterostomal therapists, surgeons, diabetologists, social workers, and infectious disease specialists are among the many providers who may be involved in developing approaches to resolve difficult wounds. A holistic program emphasizing nutrition, exercise, hygiene, and stress management as well as innovative wound care strategies can achieve success.

EVALUATION

Evaluating outcomes of client care is a collaborative responsibility as well. Clear and reasonable outcomes with measurable or observable evaluation criteria make evaluation straightforward and uncomplicated. Nurse and client can easily evaluate progress toward healing during the course of care using measurements of wound or lesion size and depth as criteria. Other concrete evidence such as a change in tissue color from black (necrotic tissue) or yellow (fibrous debris or viscous exudate) to red (healthy granulation tissue) is also useful for evaluation.[23] Making a chart or graph keeps visual evidence of progress at hand. The need for changes in approaches as well as satisfactory improvement will be apparent.

The many variables (eg, nutrition, hydration, perfusion, immune status, infection, presence of dead or damaged tissue) that influence healing create the need for a multifaceted approach to care, making altering the plan when progress is unsatisfactory a potentially complex undertaking. Assuring that implementation addresses as many variables as possible and revising one element of the plan at a time is effective.

SUMMARY

Skin, mucosa, and associated appendages are important to health and well-being. They carry out many important functions, including protection, temperature regulation, sensation, excretion, and lubrication.

Factors such as age, nutritional status, sun exposure, personal hygiene, and general health status alter skin and mucosal integrity. Skin lesions, pigmentation changes, wounds, and mucosal disruptions result from mechanical, chemical, biological, and thermal trauma. The process of healing altered skin and tissue includes inflammation, proliferation, and maturation. Clotting, phagocytosis, fibroplasia, angiogenesis, collagen synthesis and lysis, and epithelialization occur to a greater or lesser degree, depending on whether a wound is healing by primary or secondary intention. Many of the same variables that affect skin integrity also influence healing. Complications such as hemorrhage, infection, and wound separation delay healing.

Assessment of integumentary health encompasses a history and examination of skin and mucosa in all parts of the body, as well as attention to cardiovascular functioning and nutritional, hydration, and emotional status.

Client and nurse collaboratively address nursing diagnoses including Impaired Skin Integrity, Impaired Tissue Integrity, Altered Oral Mucous Membranes, and Potential for Impaired Skin Integrity through care planning and management strategies.

Collaborative nurse–client management of skin and mucosal problems focuses on hygiene, comfort measures, wound care, and measures that support healing and general health such as optimum nutrition, fluid intake, regular exercise, and stress reduction. Teaching and effective communication contribute to positive outcomes. Evaluation of progress toward outcomes is also a mutual responsibility.

REFERENCES

1. Cuzzell JZ. Clues: Bruised, torn skin. *Am J Nurs.* 1990;3:16–18.
2. Hazen P. Basal cell carcinoma. *Hosp Med.* 1987;23:71.
3. Colburn L. Preventing pressure ulcers. *Nursing 90.* 1990;20:60–63.
4. Bruno PM. Injury: Inflammatory response and resolution. In: Patrick ML, Woods SL, Craven RF, et al, eds. *Medical-Surgical Nursing: Pathophysiological Concepts.* Philadelphia: Lippincott; 1991:155–166.
5. Hunt TK, Goodson WH. Wound healing. In: Way LW, ed. *Current Surgical Diagnosis and Treatment.* Norwalk, CT: Appleton & Lange; 1991.
6. Messer MS. Wound care. *Crit Care Nurs Q.* 1989;11:17–27.
7. Whitney JD. Physiologic effects of oxygen on wound healing. *Heart Lung.* 1989;18:466–474.
8. Garvin G. Wound healing in pediatrics. *Nurs Clin North Am.* 1990;25:181–192.
9. Jones PL, Millman A. Wound healing and the aged patient. *Nurs Clin North Am.* 1990;25:263–277.
10. Williams SR. *Essentials of Nutrition and Diet Therapy.* 5th ed. St. Louis: Times Mirror/Mosby College Publishing; 1990.
11. Young ME. Malnutrition and wound healing. *Heart Lung.* 1988;17:60.
12. Ruberg RL. Role of nutrition in wound healing. *Surg Clin North Am.* 1984;64:7.
13. Arbeit JM, Way LW. Surgical metabolism and nutrition. In: Way LW, ed. *Current Surgical Diagnosis and Treatment.* Norwalk, CT: Appleton & Lange; 1991.
14. Hotter AN. Wound healing and immunocompromise. *Nurs Clin North Am.* 1990;25:193–203.
15. Sheffield PJ. Tissue oxygen measurements. In: Hunt TK, Davis J, eds. *Problem Wounds: The Role of Oxygen.* New York: Elsevier; 1988.
16. Reese JL. Nursing interventions for wound healing in plastic and reconstructive surgery. *Nurs Clin North Am.* 1990;25:223–233.
17. Cuzzell JZ, Stotts NA. Trial and error yields to knowledge. *Am J Nurs.* 1990;90:53–60.
18. West JM. Wound healing in the surgical patient: Influence of the perioperative stress response on perfusion. *AACN Clin Issues Crit Care Nurs.* 1990;1:595–601.
19. Holden-Lund C. Effects of relaxation with guided imagery on surgical stress and wound healing. *Res Nurs Health.* 1988;11:235–244.
20. Robson MC. Disturbances of wound healing. *Ann Emerg Med.* 1988;17:1274.
21. Thomason SS. Front-line antiseptics. *Geriatr Nurs.* 1989;10:235–236.
22. Cooper DM. Optimizing wound healing. *Nurs Clin North Am.* 1990;25:165–180.
23. Cuzzell JZ. The new RYB color code. *Am J Nurs.* 1988;88:1342–1346.
24. Martin MM. Wound management and infection control after trauma. *Crit Care Nurs Q.* 1988;11:43–49.
25. Hunt TK. Infection, inflammation and antibiotics. In: Way LW, ed. *Current Surgical Diagnosis and Treatment.* Norwalk, CT: Appleton & Lange; 1991.
26. Pelligrini CA. Postoperative complications. In: Way LW, ed. *Current Surgical Diagnosis and Treatment.* Norwalk, CT: Appleton & Lange; 1991.
27. Roy LB, Edwards PA, Barr LH. The value of nutritional assessment of the surgical patient. *J Ent Parent Nutr.* 1985;9:170–172.
28. Iverson-Carpenter MS. Impaired tissue integrity. *J Gerontol Nurs.* 1988;14:25–29.
29. Demling RH, Way LW. Burns and other thermal injuries. In: Way LW, ed. *Current Surgical Diagnosis and Treatment.* Norwalk, CT: Appleton & Lange; 1991.
30. Colburn L. Preventing pressure ulcers. *Nursing 90.* 1990;20:60–63.
31. Bergstrom N, Braden BJ, Laguzza A, Holman V. The Braden scale for predicting pressure sore risk. *Nurs Res.* 1987;36:205–210.
32. Husian T. An experimental study of some pressure effects on tissues, with references to the bedsore problem. *J Pathol Bacteriol.* 1953;66:347–358.
33. Kosiak M. Etiology and pathology of ischemic ulcers. *Arch Phys Med Rehabil.* 1959;40:62–69.
34. Newson T, Rolfe P. Skin surface Po_2 and blood flow measurements over the ischial tuberosity. *Arch Phys Med Rehabil.* 1982;63:553–556.
35. Dimant J, Francis ME. Pressure sore prevention and management. *J Gerontol Nurs.* 1988;14:18–25.
36. Vasconez LO, Vasconez HC. Plastic and reconstructive surgery. In: Way LW, ed. *Current Surgical Diagnosis and Treatment.* Norwalk, CT: Appleton & Lange; 1991.
37. Weston WL. Skin. In: Hathaway WE, Groothuis JR, Hay WW, Paisley JW, eds. *Current Pediatric Diagnosis and Treatment.* Norwalk, CT: Appleton & Lange; 1991.
38. Fu KK, Phillips TL. Radiation therapy: Basic principles and clinical applications. In: Way LW, ed. *Current Surgical Diagnosis and Treatment.* Norwalk, CT: Appleton & Lange; 1991.
39. McHenry LM, Salerno E. *Pharmacology in Nursing.* St. Louis: Mosby; 1989.
40. De Witt S. Nursing assessment of the skin and dermatologic lesions. *Nurs Clin North Am.* 1990;25:235–245.
41. Van Slyke KK, Michel VP, Rein MF. Treatment of vulvovaginal candidiasis with boric acid powder. *Am J Obstet Gynecol.* 1981;141:145.
42. Flores AM, Zohman LR. Energy cost of bedmaking to the cardiac patient and the nurse. *Am J Nurs.* 1970;70:1264–1267.
43. Palmer EM, Griffith EW. Effect of activity during bedmaking on heart rate and blood pressure. *Nurs Res.* 1971;20:17–25.
44. Lane LD, Winslow EH. Oxygen consumption, cardiovascular response, and perceived exertion in healthy adults during rest, occupied bedmaking, and unoccupied bedmaking. *Cardiovasc Nurs.* 1987;23:31–36.
45. Neuberger GB. Wound care: What's clear, what's not. *Nursing.* 1987;17:34–37.
46. Turner TD. The development of wound management products. *Wounds.* 1989;3:155–171.
47. Bryant RA. Saving the skin from tape injuries. *Am J Nurs.* 1988;88:189.
48. Pellegrini CA. Postoperative care. In: Way LW, ed. *Current Surgical Diagnosis and Treatment.* Norwalk, CT: Appleton & Lange; 1991:15–25.
49. Marchiondo K. The very fine art of collecting culture specimens. *Nursing.* 1979;9:34–43.

50. Cuzzell JZ. Artful solutions to chronic problems. *Am J Nurs.* 1985;85:162–165.
51. Dunn LM. Nursing strategies for common integument problems. In: Patrick ML, Woods SL, Craven RF, Rokosky JS, Bruno PM, eds. *Medical-Surgical Nursing: Pathophysiological Concepts.* Philadelphia: Lippincott; 1991.
52. Diekmann JM, Smith JM, Wilk JR. Wound care forum: A double life for a dental irrigation device. *Am J Nurs.* 1985;85:1157.
53. Shannon ML, Miller BM. Pressure sore treatment: A case in point. *Geratr Nurs.* 1988;9:154–157.
54. Hudson-Goodman P, Girard N, Jones MB. Wound repair and the potential use of growth factors. *Heart Lung.* 1990;14:379–386.
55. Doucette MM, Fylling C, Knighton DM. Amputation prevention in a high-risk population through a comprehensive wound-healing protocol. *Arch Phys Med Rehabil.* 1989;70:780–785.
56. Itoh M, Montemayor JS Jr, Matsumoto E, Eason A, Lee MHM. Accelerated wound healing of pressure ulcers with pulsed high peak power electromagnetic energy (Diapulse). *Decubitus.* 1991;4:24.
57. Braden BJ, Bryant R. Innovations to prevent and treat pressure ulcers. *Geriatr Nurs.* 1990;11:182–186.
58. Tubman C. Holistic approach to healing, part 1. *Home Healthcare Nurse.* 1988;6:31–34.
59. Stotts NA, Whitney JD. Nutritional intake and clients in the home with open surgical wounds. *J Commun Health Nurs.* 1990; 7:77–86.

BIBLIOGRAPHY

Carpenito LJ. *Nursing Diagnosis: Application to Clinical Practice.* 3rd ed. Philadelphia: Lippincott; 1989.

Clarke M, Kadhom H. The nursing prevention of pressure sores in hospital and community patients. *J Adv Nurs.* 1988;13:365–373.

Cooper DM. Human wound assessment: Status report and implications for clinicians. *AACN Clin Issues Crit Care Nurs.* 1990;1: 553–565.

Cuzzell JZ. Choosing a wound dressing: A systematic approach. *AACN Clin Issues Crit Care Nurs.* 1990;1:577.

Fowler E, Cuzzell JZ, Papen JC. Healing with hydrocolloid. *Am J Nurs.* 1991;91:63–64.

French ET, Ledwell-Sifner K. A method for consistent documentation of pressure sores. *Rehabil Nurs.* 1991;16:204–207.

Fuller J, Schaller-Ayers J. *Health Assessment: A Nursing Approach.* Philadelphia: Lippincott; 1990.

Ganong WF. *Review of Medical Physiology.* 15th ed. Norwalk, CT: Appleton & Lange; 1991.

Hardy MA. The biology of scar formation. *Physical Ther.* 1989;69: 1014–1024.

Hathaway WE, Groothuis JR, Hay WW, Paisley JW. *Current Pediatric Diagnosis and Treatment.* Norwalk, CT: Appleton & Lange; 1991.

Ignevitius DD, Bayne MV. *Medical-Surgical Nursing: A Nursing Process Approach.* Philadelphia: Saunders; 1991.

Kee JL. *Handbook of Laboratory and Diagnostic Tests With Nursing Implications.* Norwalk, CT: Appleton & Lange; 1990.

Norris SO, Provo B, Stotts NA. Physiology of wound healing and risk factors that impede the healing process. *AACN Clin Issues Crit Care Nurs.* 1990;1:545–552.

North American Nursing Diagnosis Association. *Taxonomy I, Revised, 1990.* St. Louis: NANDA; 1990.

Pagana KD, Pagana J. *Diagnostic Testing and Nursing Implications.* 3rd ed. St. Louis: Mosby; 1990.

Patrick ML, Woods SL, Craven RF, Rokosky JS, Bruno PM. *Medical-Surgical Nursing: Pathophysiological Concepts.* Philadelphia: Lippincott; 1991.

Pernoll ML, ed. *Current Obstetric and Gynecological Diagnosis and Treatment.* 7th ed. Norwalk, CT: Appleton & Lange; 1991.

Stotts NA, Washington DF. Nutrition: A critical component of wound healing. *AACN Clin Issues Crit Care Nurs.* 1990;1:585–594.

US Department of Health and Human Services, Public Health Service. Update: Universal precautions for prevention of transmission of human immunodeficiency virus, hepatitis B virus, and other blood-borne pathogens in health care settings. *MMWR.* 1989;38:9–18.

Way LW, ed. *Current Surgical Diagnosis and Treatment.* 9th ed. Norwalk, CT: Appleton & Lange; 1991.

Yurik AG, Speir BE, Robb SS, Ebert NJ. *The Aged Person and the Nursing Process.* Norwalk, CT: Appleton & Lange; 1989.

CHAPTER 25

Nutrition

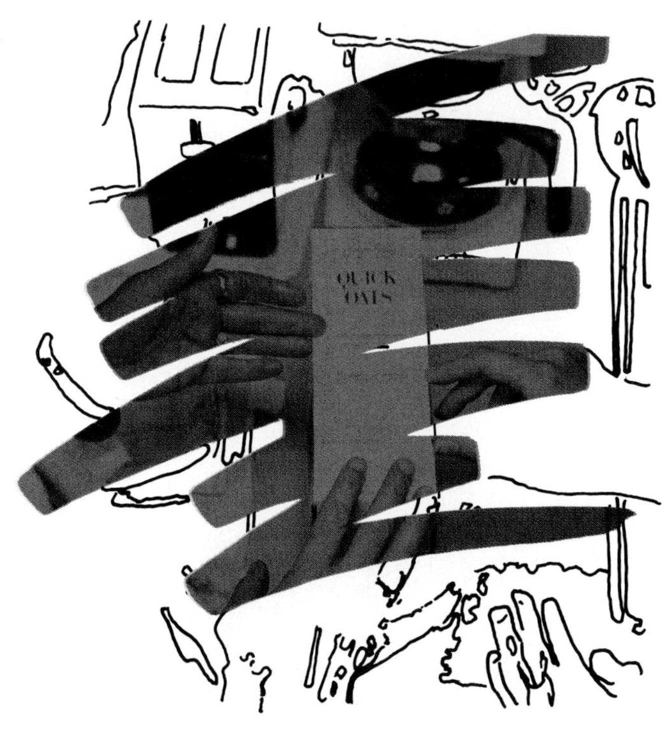

Behavioral Objectives

Upon completion of this chapter, the student will be able to:

1. Discuss the role of nutrition in the prevention of illness, restoration of health, and promotion of high-level wellness.
2. Define energy balance and identify the factors influencing energy input and output in the human energy system.
3. Define how to calculate the total daily energy requirement for a given client.
4. Describe the processes that are involved in the digestion and absorption of food.
5. Describe how the metabolism of carbohydrates, proteins, and fats occurs in the human system.
6. Describe the cultural dimensions of a client's nutritional needs, and discuss why nurses must consider these in assessing and planning care.
7. Describe the following guidelines and standards available to assist in nutritional planning: Recommended Dietary Allowances, four food groups, and Senate Select Committee Recommendations.
8. Describe the etiology and symptoms of selected nutritional deficiency diseases.
9. Outline the components of the nutritional history and suggest questions to obtain the needed information.
10. List and describe physical examination procedures useful to assess nutritional status.
11. Identify diagnostic tests that contribute information relevant to a nutritional assessment.
12. Identify at least three nursing diagnoses from the North American Nursing Diagnosis Association (NANDA) taxonomy that relate to nutritional problems.
13. Identify subjective and objective data suggestive of each diagnosis.
14. Describe nursing implementation appropriate for alleviating nutritional alterations.
15. Describe the importance of collaboration for optimum nutrition among the nurse, the client, and the dietitian, including the appropriate roles that can be taken by each.

KEY TERMS

absorption
amino acid
anabolism
anorexia nervosa
bulimia
cachexia
carbohydrate
catabolism
chyme
complementary protein
complete protein
complex carbohydrate
dietary fiber
digestion
energy balance
enteral
essential amino acid
essential nutrient
fat
fatty acid
gluconeogenesis
glycogen
glycogenolysis
insulin
intrinsic factor
kilocalorie
kwashiorkor
lipid
marasmus
metabolism
mineral
monosaturated fatty acid
nitrogen balance
nutrient
nutrition
obesity
overweight
peristalsis
polyunsaturated fatty acid
protein
protein–calorie malnutrition
Recommended Dietary Allowances
Recommended Nutrient Intakes
saturated fatty acid
simple carbohydrate
starch
total parenteral nutrition
vitamin

Nutrition is an essential process in all living organisms. **Nutrition** can be defined as the process by which the energy and chemical compounds necessary for the creation, maintenance, and restoration of body cells are made available to the body from food. There is an intimate relationship between the quality of a person's nutrition and his or her state of health. Further, nutritional needs vary in relation to specific health problems.

Nutrition has always been an important focus of nursing care. Nurses collaborate with dietitians as well as with pharmacists, physicians, and clients themselves in planning care to meet clients' nutritional needs. Nurses' participation in this collaboration is central, for it is usually nurses who are primarily responsible for the implementation of the plan of nutritional care.

In addition to the biological importance of food as the source of **nutrients**—the chemical elements and compounds necessary for the body's proper functioning—food has other aspects that are of enormous importance in human life. For organisms that are lower on the evolutionary scale, energy and nutrients are readily available in sun and soil. The accessibility of nutritional resources is not automatic for human beings. This is why, in all cultures and ages, food has received such interest and emphasis. Eating is also a source of great pleasure for human beings. What is for animals the pleasure derived from a life-giving activity is for human beings the pleasure derived from sensory stimulation, a social activity, and psychological reward.

Section 1. Understanding Nutrition

Human nutrition is a phenomenon that can be understood at many levels. At the chemical level, certain kinds of molecules and a certain amount of energy are necessary to keep the physical body functioning. At the organismic level, only certain foods are appropriate for ingestion by the human body. At the psychological level, foods and eating become colored by complex emotional associations. At the social level, food and its availability are connected with status, class, and privilege. At the cultural level, particular meanings and rituals related to food change from one culture to another. Finally, at the global level, nurses may be involved in analyzing the impact of food production and distribution patterns on client or community nutritional status. Quality nursing care includes all these aspects of nutrition in planning and providing for clients' nutritional needs.

Nutrition plays a major role in the promotion, maintenance, and restoration of health. No matter what a client's particular health care need, nutrition is an area that is always relevant. There are few situations in which dietary factors are not significant areas for counseling or intervention. When the client's status is on the wellness side of the health–illness continuum, nutritional counseling can assist the client to maintain wellness or to maximize it still further. When clients are experiencing illness, dietary factors may be the primary cause of the problem, and even if not so, they will play an important role in the restoration of health. For example, a client may be suffering from a viral infection of the gastrointestinal tract. A special diet would be an important part of the treatment even though diet was not the immediate cause of the problem.

Optimum health is the goal of collaborative nursing practice. Rarely are clients content to be merely free of disease. They usually seek a sense of maximum well-being, the fullest possible physical, emotional, and social functioning. Despite an absence of physical illness, a person may not feel truly well. He or she may lack energy or motivation and may view the world as dull and uninteresting. Minor physical discomforts may further dampen a person's spirits.

The role played by nutrition in the attainment of optimum health has been repeatedly acknowledged. The body is a highly complex and extremely sensitive organism, which can easily adapt to less-than-ideal nutritional states. But low-quality nutrition takes a subtle toll on people. There is a direct and causal relationship between quality of nutritional intake and overall sense of well-being. Subtle physical adjustments made to dietary habits have their effect on emotional, mental, and social aspects of people. Thus, the healthier, more high quality the diet, the higher one's level of well-being.

The link between dietary factors and a multitude of diseases has been firmly established. The list of diseases in which diet plays a causative role grows longer daily. Heart disease, certain forms of cancer, cerebral vascular disease, and diabetes are leading causes of death among American adults, and all of these have proven associations with dietary habits. For example, there is now widespread public awareness of research that has clearly linked a diet high in animal fat with incidence of heart disease, hypertension, and cerebral vascular disease. Because of increasing public awareness of the nutritional basis of many serious diseases, nurses must be prepared to meet the demand for current information.

IMPLICATIONS FOR NURSE–CLIENT COLLABORATION

Meeting the Client's Individual Needs

The collaborative approach to nurse–client interaction, in which the client is an active participant in dietary decisions, is helpful in meeting the client's individual as well as nutritional needs. Collaborative interaction may help to ease the sense of dependency and loss of control when clients must rely on others to supply nutritional intake. In the collaborative approach, nurses interact with clients to assist the selection of foods that both meet clients' nutritional needs and provide clients with a sense of satisfaction and well-being.

Perhaps in no other area of health care is the collaborative process so clearly necessary as in that of nutrition. Because of the highly individualized meanings, habits, and preferences surrounding eating, active involvement by clients in nutritional planning is of critical importance. Collaboration in meeting clients' nutritional needs also implies interprofessional collaborative activities. Dietitians are key figures in this process, as are nurses. A dietitian is formally educated and licensed to provide nutrition-related services to clients such as dietary assessment, teaching, and planning. Dietitians have a wealth of knowledge to assist clients in designing a suitable eating plan. Physicians may determine what kind of diet is appropriate as a primary or supportive therapy for a client's medical condition. Nurses, who have the most frequent and prolonged contact with clients in most settings, must be able to provide ongoing assistance and guidance in the implementation of the dietary regimen.

■ OPTIMUM NUTRITIONAL STATUS

Nutritional processes leave no part of the human being untouched. From the physical activities of food ingestion and digestion, through the physiological processes of absorption and metabolism, to the emotional and social aspects of eating, nutrition extends its sphere of influence. This section examines energy balance in the body, the basic nutrients involved in nutritional processes, and the phases of the process that begins with food ingestion and ends with the use of nutrients for energy production and cellular metabolism. This discussion of basic nutritional science pro-

IMPLICATIONS FOR NURSE–CLIENT AND PROFESSIONAL COLLABORATION

Teamwork to Meet the Client's Nutritional Needs

In many settings, the nurse is the only health care professional available to counsel the client on dietary questions. The nurse and client together collaborate to maximize the client's nutritional health. Frequently, however, teamwork is necessary. Teamwork is particularly important when clients have specific and complex problems; then collaboration includes other health care professionals. The physician, after conferring with the nurse, orders the diet that is appropriate to the client's medical condition; the dietitian helps the client to understand the physician's dietary recommendations and to plan for self-care. The nurse, who generally has the most frequent and prolonged contact with the client, collaborates with the physician in the initial assessment and consults with the dietician to design a suitable eating plan. The nurse assists the client to carry out the plan and monitors the client's nutritional progress, and supports the client's efforts to take personal responsibility.

vides an important knowledge base for nurses who must collaborate in the interdisciplinary team and provide expert care to clients.

Energy Balance

The concept of energy balance is fundamental to an understanding of nutrition. Energy is the power to do work, and fuel is any source of energy. The human being can be viewed as a single energy system in continuous interaction with the environment, which is a larger energy system. The human organism requires a constant input of energy in order to maintain its life processes and support its physical activities.

Energy balance refers to the amount of energy input in relation to the amount of energy output in a given system:

Energy balance = energy input − energy output.

A positive energy balance occurs when input exceeds output. A negative energy balance occurs when input is less than output.

Energy Input. Food provides the fuel for the human energy system. The energy of food is stored in the chemical bonds of protein, fat, and carbohydrate molecules, which will be discussed in more detail later in this section. The energy provided by food is measured in **kilocalories** (kcal) or joules. A calorie is a unit of heat energy and refers to the energy needed to raise the temperature of 1 g of water by 1C; a kilocalorie is the amount of heat needed to raise the temperature of 1 kg of water by 1C. Although some people use the words "kilocalorie" and "calorie" interchangeably, "kilocalorie" is the correct term when referring to nutritional energy intake and expenditure.

The body stores energy in several forms. When food is not available as a source of energy, the body must draw on its own energy stores in order to maintain its life processes. **Glycogen,** the stored form of carbohydrates, is most readily available. Fats are the next most easily recoverable energy stores and are stored in the adipose tissue of the body. Proteins are the last source of energy to be drawn upon when carbohydrate stores are exhausted and fat is being used. They are stored in body tissues such as muscles. Carbohydrates, proteins, and fats will be discussed in depth later in this section.

Energy Output. Energy output is the energy the body uses. The energy used in the body for support of tissues and organ functions is drawn from the high-energy phosphate bonds of ATP (adenosine triphosphate) molecules, which are generated by metabolic pathways to be discussed later. The amount of energy a person requires is primarily determined by two factors: the basal metabolic rate and the amount of physical activity. Energy expended for food use also plays a role. To maintain a daily energy balance, the energy intake in the form of food must equal the energy expenditure from basal metabolism, physical activity, and the energy used for food digestion, absorption, and transport.

Basal Metabolism. Basal metabolism refers to the chemical reactions occurring when the body is at rest. The basal metabolic rate (BMR) is the number of calories expended hourly in a resting state in relation to the surface area of the body:

BMR = calories/meter^2/hour.

General formulas have been developed to calculate the BMR of the average man and woman (Box 25–1).

Other Energy Expenditures. Table 25–1 lists the average energy used during some common daily activities. It can be used to estimate daily activity expenditure. Finally, the amount of energy used in the processing of ingested food can be calculated by taking 10 percent of the total kcal of food consumed. A client's total daily energy expenditure can then be determined using the formula in Box 25–1.

Energy Balance and Body Weight. The relation between energy input and output is reflected in a person's body

BOX 25–1. ESTIMATION OF DAILY ENERGY EXPENDITURE

Calculating Basal Metabolic Rate (BMR)

Women:
BMR = 0.9 kcal/kg body weight/hour.

Men:
BMR = 1.0 kcal/kg body weight/hour.

Calculating Daily Energy Expenditure

Daily energy expenditure = (BMR × 24) + (0.1 × daily kcal consumption) + energy of daily activities.

TABLE 25–1. AVERAGE ENERGY EXPENDITURE OF MEN AND WOMEN DURING COMMON DAILY ACTIVITIES

Activity	kcal/hour/kg	
	Men	Women
Very Light Dressing, washing, typing, writing, sewing, standing	1.5	1.3
Light Housekeeping, gardening, walking (slowly, level surface), light recreation	2.9	2.6
Moderate Digging, sexual activity, walking (small hills), stair climbing	4.3	4.1
Heavy Shoveling snow, climbing, jogging, swimming	8.4	8.0

From Green ML, Harry J. Nutrition in Contemporary Nursing Practice. 2nd ed. New York: Wiley; 1987.

weight. The energy output is the same value as the energy expenditure calculated by the formula in Box 25–1. If a state of energy balance or equilibrium exists (input = output), the body weight remains stable, unless a factor such as fluid imbalance causes a weight change. If a positive energy balance exists (input > output) over a long period of time, weight increases. If a prolonged negative balance occurs (input < output), a person experiences weight loss (Fig. 25–1). Many factors cause predictable changes in the basal metabolic rate of individuals, and thus change their energy requirements. These factors include age, the relative amounts of muscle and fat tissue in the body, endocrine influences, climate, illness, activity level, and malnutrition. These factors will be discussed fully later in this chapter.

Basic Nutrients

As mentioned earlier, food is the source of nutrients needed by the body for proper functioning. There are six major classes of nutrients: carbohydrates, proteins, fats (lipids), vitamins, minerals, and water. Each of these classes is described below. Carbohydrates, proteins, and fats are called "energy nutrients" because they provide kilocalories from food. Vitamins, minerals, and water are vitally important substances for the building, maintenance, and metabolic regulation of body tissues. **Essential nutrients** are nutrients that the human body cannot manufacture and that therefore must be supplied by food; current knowledge places the number of essential nutrients at about 50. Selected essential nutrients are identified in the discussion that follows.

Carbohydrates. **Carbohydrates** provide the most readily available and the most efficiently metabolized source of energy for the body. The two broad categories of carbohydrates are simple and complex.

Simple carbohydrates include monosaccharides (glucose, fructose, galactose) and disaccharides (maltose, sucrose, lactose). Sucrose is known as table sugar and is the principal ingredient of candies, cakes, and other concentrated sweets. Lactose is the principal carbohydrate found

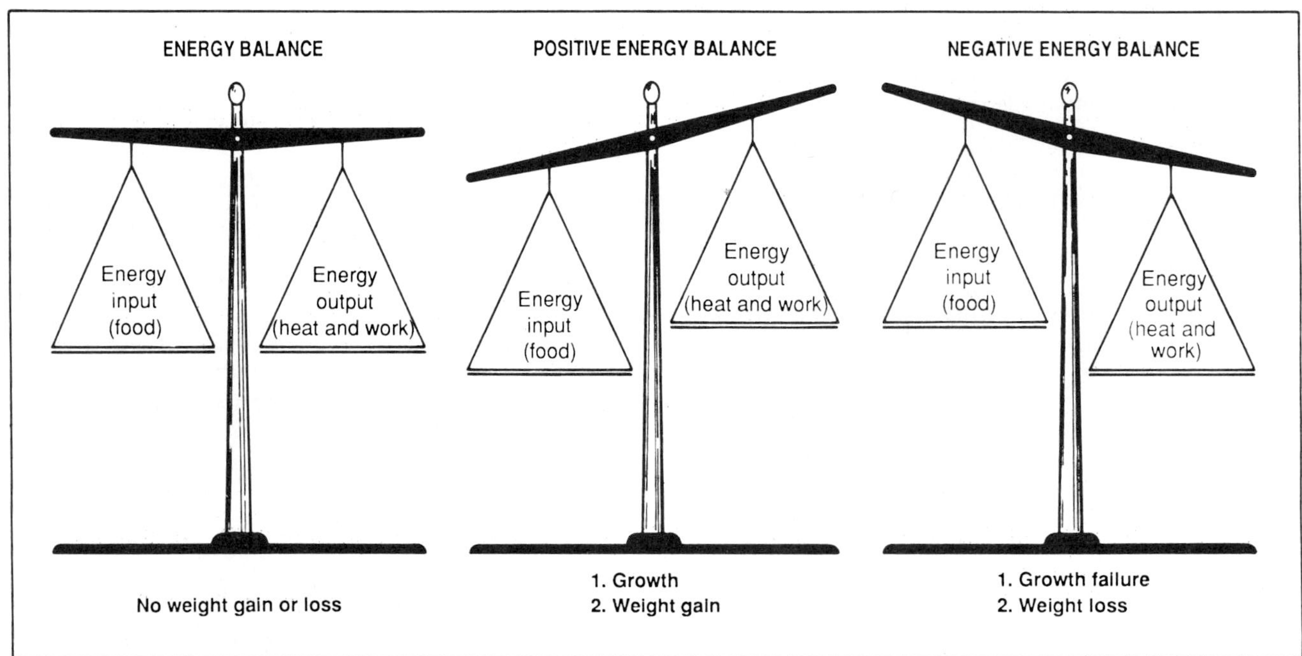

Figure 25–1. Concepts of energy balance. (*Adapted from Lewis CM.* Nutrition and Nutritional Therapy in Nursing. *Norwalk, CT: Appleton & Lange; 1986.*)

in milk. Some people lack the ability to digest lactose, particularly people from Native American, Asian, African, Mediterranean, and Middle Eastern populations.

Complex carbohydrates, or polysaccharides, are composed almost entirely of glucose molecules bonded together in varying ways. Some examples are glycogen, starches, and fiber. Glycogen is not found in food, but is the body's stored form of glucose. **Starches** consist of molecules of 300 to 1000 glucose units packed side by side in plant foods such as seeds, grains, potatoes and other roots, and legumes (beans). **Dietary fiber,** such as cellulose and pectin, is composed primarily of cell wall constituents of plant foods. In the digestive tract, food fibers absorb water, bind minerals and lipids, and exercise the intestinal muscles by adding "bulk."

Many dieters suffer from the misconception that carbohydrates (starches in particular) are fattening. Actually, one gram of carbohydrate provides 4 kcal of energy, far less than fats. Carbohydrate foods are important in the diet for many reasons: they are easily digested, absorbed, and metabolized; they are economical, tasty, and readily available. The most important reason for ensuring an adequate intake of carbohydrates is that a constant source of glucose is needed for brain and nerve function: a minimum of 100 g of carbohydrate per day is essential. Recent recommendations suggest that approximately 55 to 60 percent of the daily kilocaloric intake should come from complex carbohydrates.[1]

Increasing attention is being paid to the importance of dietary fiber in the management of a variety of digestive tract disorders and diseases (constipation, diarrhea, hemorrhoids, colon cancer), as well as in lowering of elevated blood lipids. There is no standardized recommendation for the optimum daily intake, but some recent sources suggest a daily intake of 25 g of dietary fiber.[2] Table 25–2 lists the fiber content of selected foods.

TABLE 25–2. FIBER CONTENT OF SELECTED FOOD PORTIONS

Food Portion	Fiber (g)
Fruits	
1 small apple	2
1 small banana	2
1 small orange	2
1 small pear	4
Breads/Cereals	
Whole-wheat bread, 1 slice	2
Dry oatmeal, 3 Tbsp	2
Corn Flakes, ⅔ cup	2
Wheat bran, 1 Tbsp	2
Grape Nuts, 6 Tbsp	4
Shredded Wheat, 2 biscuits	8
All Bran, 6 Tbsp	12
Vegetables	
Lettuce, raw, 1 cup	1
Carrots, ⅓ cup	2
Celery, 1 cup	2
Brussel sprouts, 4	2
Baked beans, canned, ½ cup	8

Proteins. A **protein** is a complex, long molecular chain made up of large molecules called **amino acids** (or peptides). Twenty-two different amino acids appear in human proteins in an astronomically large number of possible combinations. Most proteins are polypeptides containing 100 to 300 amino acids, folded and coiled elaborately. The human body contains tens of thousands of proteins, only a fraction of which have been identified. Although proteins can be used as sources of energy in the body, the other roles they play are so important that they are used as energy sources only when carbohydrates are not available.

Differences in body proteins distinguish one human chemically from any other. Amino acid sequences are determined by the genes inherited from one's parents. Some of the major kinds of proteins found in the body are enzymes, antibodies, and transport proteins. The latter help move molecules in and out of cells or carry molecules from organ to organ through body fluids. All body tissues and organs are made of proteins. Proteins also help to maintain fluid balance by increasing osmotic pressure, attracting water, and buffering acids.

Protein in food supplies the body with the amino acids it needs to make its own proteins. Although the body can make some amino acids itself, there are nine amino acids, called **essential amino acids,** that it cannot make. A body cell must have all the amino acids it needs for synthesis of a particular protein available at the same time, because amino acids are not stored. Thus, dietary sources of protein should supply all nine of the essential amino acids in a single meal. A **complete protein** is one containing all the essential amino acids in amounts adequate for use in the body. If one amino acid is absent, or present in an amount smaller than is needed, the use of all other amino acids for protein synthesis will be limited accordingly. The amino acids that cannot be used for synthesis are converted to fat. They cannot be stored (as amino acids) for future use. Box 25–2 lists the essential and nonessential amino acids found in human proteins.

Generally, animal sources of protein are complete proteins, whereas vegetable sources are incomplete. A vegetarian, however, can design a diet that will supply a complete set of essential amino acids in each meal by combining **complementary proteins,** that is, two or more incomplete proteins that together supply all the essential amino acids. Guidelines for vegetarian diets and meal planning will be discussed later in this chapter.

One gram of protein yields 4 kcal of energy. As mentioned earlier, however, dietary protein is not metabolized for energy efficiently; it takes more energy input than either carbohydrate or fat metabolism. A major reason why ample carbohydrate and adequate fat are necessary in the diet is to spare the body from the necessity of breaking down amino acids for energy production. If amino acids are used in this way, they cannot be used to build vital body proteins. It is currently recommended that approximately 10 percent of daily caloric intake, or 0.8 g/kg of body weight, should come from protein.[1]

BOX 25–2. ESSENTIAL AND NONESSENTIAL AMINO ACIDS

Essential Amino Acids	Nonessential Amino Acids
Histidine[a]	Alanine
Isoleucine	Arginine
Leucine	Aspartic acid
Lysine	Citrulline
Methionine	Cysteine
Phenylalanine	Cystine
Threonine	Glutamic acid
Tryptophan	Glycine
Valine	Hydroxylysine
	Hydroxyproline
	Proline
	Serine
	Tyrosine

[a] Histidine is essential for infants, and may be essential for adults.

Fats. Fats are also called **lipids,** a classification that includes fats, oils, and sterols. Fats yield more energy per gram than either carbohydrates or proteins—9 kcal. They also provide insulation of the body and protection of vital organs and tissues, are essential for nerve conduction, transport other molecules, and provide necessary components of many hormones. Chemically, simple fats are composed of triglycerides, which in turn consist of three fatty acids combined with glycerol. **Fatty acids** consist of a chain of carbon atoms with hydrogen attached.

Much attention has recently focused on the various types of fatty acids and their relation to cardiovascular disease. The primary variable of interest is the degree of saturation—that is, the number of hydrogen atoms a fatty acid chain is holding. A **saturated fatty acid** has a chain in which every available carbon bond is holding a hydrogen atom. If there is only one point on the chain where a hydrogen atom is missing, the molecule is called a **monounsaturated fatty acid. Polyunsaturated fatty acids** have more than one point of unsaturation.

Dietary saturated fats are now considered to play a major role in the development of cardiovascular diseases such as hypertension, coronary artery disease, stroke, and cerebral vascular disease. The common factor in these diseases is the laying down of fat deposits in the inner layer of arteries, which leads to narrowing and hardening (atherosclerosis). All animal foods contain varying amounts of saturated fats, with red meats having the highest proportion. Most vegetable fats and oils (except coconut and palm oils) are unsaturated. Current recommendations are that no more than 10 percent of total fat intake consist of saturated fats.[1]

Phospholipids and sterols are called compound fats because they combine simple fats with other compounds. They contribute about 5 percent of total dietary fat. Lecithin and cholesterol are of particular nutritional significance. Lecithin, a phospholipid, is an important constituent of cell membranes and also helps to keep other fats dissolved in body fluids. Cholesterol, a sterol, is metabolically a necessary nutrient, but is not essential because it is manufactured by the liver from either carbohydrate or fat.

Cholesterol performs important functions in the body. It may be transformed into sex or adrenal hormones or into bile. It can be packaged with other proteins and lipids (lipoproteins) for transport to and use by body tissues. It can also be deposited in arterial walls, where it can contribute to atherosclerosis. Two kinds of cholesterol-carrying lipoproteins have recently been associated with coronary heart disease. High-density lipoproteins (HDLs) lower the risk of this disease, whereas low-density lipoproteins (LDLs) increase the risk. To help consumers remember which lipoprotein is the desirable one and which one to avoid, it has been suggested to think of *H*DLs as "*h*ealthy" and *L*DLs as "*l*ousy."

In general, high blood cholesterol levels are associated with an increased incidence of heart attacks. However, it must be remembered that the body produces its own cholesterol, called endogenous cholesterol. Thus, controlling dietary (exogenous) cholesterol may not always lower blood cholesterol levels as expected. Some people may have a genetically determined high level of endogenous cholesterol, which persists despite severe limits on dietary cholesterol intake. Certain foods also affect blood cholesterol levels. For example, caffeine in excessive amounts has been linked to high serum cholesterol levels. Garlic, oat bran, and legumes (for example, beans) have a cholesterol-lowering effect.[3] Foods that contain high amounts of cholesterol are red meats, dairy products, and eggs.

Because of the risks associated with saturated fats and cholesterol, unsaturated fats are now recommended to comprise 20 percent of dietary fat intake. Polyunsaturated fats vary widely in their degree of unsaturation; generally, the harder a fat is at room temperature, the more saturated it is. A particular class of polyunsaturated fatty acids called omega-3 fatty acids (found primarily in fish oils) has received publicity as being of particular benefit in the prevention and/or management of heart disease, cancer, arthritis, and asthma.[1] Similar benefits are believed to be gained from the use of monounsaturated fatty acids (found in canola oil and olive oil), which tend to reduce blood cholesterol while maintaining optimum high-density lipoprotein levels. Thus, recent recommendations are that 10 percent of dietary fat be monounsaturated and 10 percent polyunsaturated.

A polyunsaturated fatty acid, linoleic acid, is the only essential fatty acid—that is, one that cannot be produced by the body. Linoleic acid must be obtained from dietary sources such as vegetable oils. It enhances skin and capillary integrity, lowers serum cholesterol levels, and prolongs blood clotting time.

Vitamins. Although they do not provide energy or building materials for the body, **vitamins** are indispensable organic nutrients that perform key roles in the metabolic processes that produce energy, the manufacture of red blood cells, and the building and repair of body tissues. Vitamins are often classified as to whether they are soluble in fat or in water. The fat-soluble vitamins are vitamins A, D, E, and K. They are found in dietary fats and oils and are stored in body fat tissues. Because they can be stored, an excessive intake of fat-soluble vitamins can lead to serious toxic effects.

The water-soluble vitamins include the B vitamins and vitamin C. They are found in the water portion of foods and are carried into water-filled body tissues. They can be readily excreted in the urine if their blood concentration rises too high, although toxic effects may still occur if taken in excessive amounts. The eight B vitamins play specific roles as parts of coenzymes, which combine with inactive proteins to make active enzymes. See Table 25–3 for a description of the Recommended Dietary Allowances, food sources, functions, and signs of deficiency and excess of each of the vitamins.

Minerals. Like the vitamins, **minerals** do not provide energy but are chemical elements that are involved in the maintenance of water and acid–base balance, the functioning of muscles and nerves, the composition of body cells and tissues, hormone production, oxygen transport, and other vital body processes. Although minerals can be classified as major or minor (trace) according to the quantities found in the body, this in no way should imply that trace minerals are less important. A lack of any trace mineral in the body may be fatal. Calcium, potassium, and sodium are major minerals that are so critical to vital body functions that they are carefully monitored and regulated in acutely ill clients. Other minerals may need the same careful adjustment in seriously ill persons with specific deficiencies or excesses. See Table 25–4 for the Recommended Dietary Allowances, food sources, functions, and signs of deficiency and excess of the minerals.

Water. Water provides more than a medium of transport for nutrients. It is itself a nutrient so essential to life that without it, the body can survive only a few days. Water is part of the molecules that form body cells, tissues, and organs. It is an active participant in numerous chemical reactions, a solvent for many small molecules and nutrients, a lubricant and shock absorber, and it plays a role in temperature regulation. Fluid and electrolyte balance is influenced by water intake. Water excretion is necessary to eliminate metabolic waste products from the body. Water is also produced as a by-product during energy metabolism. A daily minimum of 4 to 6 cups of water is needed to provide these functions. Complex renal and hormonal mechanisms adjust water excretion in accordance with water intake, so that an appropriate balance is maintained.

Effects of Storage, Processing, and Cooking. Nurses must be able to advise clients not only about the nutrient values of fresh or raw foods, but also should provide guidance regarding the effects of various methods of storage and preparation. In general, the longer fruits and vegetables are stored before being eater the greater the loss of vitamins. When storage is necessary, temperatures should be kept as low as possible without causing freezing, moisture in the produce should be maintained, and exposure to light should be minimized.

The more a food is divided or cut, the more surface area is exposed to oxygen in the air. Vitamin C is readily oxidized, and thus rendered nutritionally inactive. Therefore, fruits and vegetables should be cut as little and as close to eating time as possible. Soaking quickly depletes foods of water-soluble vitamins. The peels of fruits and vegetables have the most concentrated supplies of vitamins, so trimming or peeling will reduce their vitamin value.

Canning fruits and vegetables leads to approximately a 50 percent loss of vitamins, whereas freezing lowers the losses somewhat, particularly in fruits. Drying causes losses of vitamins A, C, and B_1 (thiamine). Boiling causes significant losses of minerals, vitamin C, and vitamin A. Steaming reduces these losses by about 50 percent, and pressure cooking greatly minimizes nutrient losses.

Digestion, Absorption, and Metabolism

The processes that enable the body to convert ingested food into energy available to body cells are digestion, absorption, and metabolism.

Digestion. Digestion is the breakdown of foods into smaller compounds that can be absorbed into body fluids. Digestion involves both mechanical activity and chemical activity.

Mechanical Digestion. Mechanical digestion involves neuromuscular processes that move food through the digestive tract so that it can be digested and absorbed. Through the interaction of several different types of muscles, two kinds of mechanical action occur in the digestive tract: (1) tonic contractions, which create a continuous muscle tone and facilitate the passage of food, and (2) periodic, rhythmic contractions, called **peristalsis,** which moves intestinal contents through the gastrointestinal tract.

Chemical Digestion. Chemical digestion is accomplished through the action of several secretions produced by the mucosal cells and accessory organs of the gastrointestinal tract. There are four types of secretions:

1. Enzymes specific for the breakdown of particular nutrients
2. Hydrochloric acid and buffers
3. Mucus
4. Water and electrolytes

Mucus is secreted by the mouth, stomach, and small intestine. It lubricates the food and protects the gastrointestinal mucosa. The secretions of the gastrointestinal tract are controlled by a number of factors: nerves, hormones, and the physical contact of food.

TABLE 25–3. ESSENTIAL INFORMATION ON VITAMINS

Vitamin	Adult RDA or RNI	Food Sources	Actions	Deficiency Symptoms	Excess Symptoms
Fat-soluble Vitamins					
A	**US**[a] F: 800 RE M: 1000 RE **Canada**[a] F: 800 RE M: 1000 RE	Dairy fats, yellow fruits and vegetables, dark green vegetables, tomatoes, liver, kidney, egg yolk.	Adaptation of eyes to light; epithelial and mucus membrane integrity; normal growth and bone development; role in reproduction.	Night blindness, keratinization of skin, dry eyes, retarded growth, sterility, decreased salivation, diarrhea, susceptibility to infection.	Hypervitaminosis A: *Early:* fatigue, anorexia, irritability, nausea, vomiting, inflamed and cracked lips, dry skin, pruritis. *Late:* liver and spleen enlargement, headache, subcutaneous swellings, bone pain, hair loss, ascites.
D	**US** 5 μg (age 19–24 years: 10 μg) **Canada** 2.5 μg (after age 50: 5 μg)	Fortified milk, eggs, butter, sunlight.	Essential for calcium and phosphorus metabolism.	*Children:* skeletal deformities (rickets), decreased muscle tone, constipation, decreased blood Ca^{++}. *Adults:* osteomalacia.	Hypervitaminosis D: elevated blood calcium, calcification of arteries and organs.
E	**US**[b] F: 8 mg α-TE M: 10 mg α-TE **Canada** F: 6–7 mg M: 7–10 mg	Polyunsaturated oils; whole grains; dark green, leafy vegetables; nuts; legumes.	antioxidant: cell membrane integrity.	*Infants:* hemolytic anemia, edema, skin lesions. *Adults:* muscular weakness.	Depression, fatigue, diarrhea with cramps, blurred vision, headaches, dizziness, increased clotting time, increased blood lipids, decreased thyroid levels.
K	**US** F: 65 μg M: 80 μg (M 19–24: 70 μg) **Canada** No RNI	Dark green, leafy vegetables, liver; eggs; cheese; wheat bran.	Essential for normal blood clotting.	Abnormal bleeding, hemorrhage.	*Infants:* hemolytic anemia, hyperbilirubinemia, brain damage.
Water-soluble Vitamins					
C	**US** 60 mg **Canada** F: 30 mg M: 40 mg (Smokers should increase intake by 50%)	Citrus fruits; papaya; cantaloupe; strawberries; cranberry juice; broccoli; brussel sprouts; cauliflower; cabbage; dark green, leafy vegetables; tomatoes; baked potatoes; green peppers.	Synthesis and maintenance of collagen: bone and teeth formation; blood vessel integrity; wound healing. Antioxidant: protects other nutrients; facilitates iron absorption; activates folic acid; synthesis of norepinephrine during stress; inflammation; resistance to infection.	Scurvy: follicular hyperkeratosis; skin hemorrhages; swollen, bleeding gums; soft tissue and joint hemorrhage; bone malformations; poor wound healing; weight loss; anemia; depression.	Increased urinary uric acid, kidney stones, hemolytic anemia, coagulation disorders, false-positive test for sugar in urine, diarrhea, rebound scurvy if massive doses suddenly withdrawn.
Thiamine (B_1)	**US** F: 1.1 mg M: 1.5 mg (age 51+: F: 1.0 mg M: 1.2 mg) **Canada** No RNI 0.4 mg ≠ 1000 kcal suggested	Brewer's yeast; wheat germ; whole grains; meat, especially pork; legumes; enriched cereals; nuts; enriched rice.	Essential for energy metabolism, especially of glucose; transmission of nerve impulses; conversion of tryptophan to niacin.	Beriberi: anorexia; muscle weakness; calf tenderness; palpitations; polyneuropathy (tingling and numbness of extremities, foot and wrist drop); constipation. "Wet beriberi": peripheral edema; hypertension; tachycardia; cardiac enlargement; heart failure; elevated blood pyruvic acid and lactic acid.	Unknown.

Riboflavin	**US** F: 1.3 mg M: 1.7 mg (age 51+: F: 1.2 mg M: 1.4 mg) **Canada** No RNI 0.5 mg/1000 kcal suggested	Brewer's yeast; organ meats; milk, dairy products; meats; poultry; fish; breads; pasta; enriched rice.	Energy metabolism; activates vitamin B_6; protein metabolism; formation of red blood cells; gluconeogenesis; glycogen formation; healthy skin and eyes.	Ariboflavinosis: dermatitis; cracks at corners of mouth; sore tongue; photophobia; corneal reddening.	Unknown.
Niacin	**US** F: 15 mg M: 19 mg (age 51+; F: 13 mg M: 15 mg) **Canada** No RNI 7.2 NE/1000 kcal suggested	Organ meats; brewer's yeast; meats; poultry; fish; peanuts; coffee; enriched grains; can be formed from tryptophan.	Energy metabolism; synthesis of carbohydrates, protein, fat; healthy skin, nerves, digestive tract.	Pellagra: dermatitis; diarrhea; dementia.	Unknown.
Pyridoxine (B_6)	**US** F: 1.6 mg M: 2 mg **Canada** No RNI 15 μg/g of protein suggested	Wheat, corn, wild rice, chicken (light meat), meat, liver, green beans, potatoes, bananas.	General metabolism of nutrients; synthesis of nonessential amino acids; converts tryptophan to niacin.	Anemia, weakness, dermatitis, gastrointestinal upset, irritability, convulsions.	Unknown.
Folic acid	**US** F: 180 μg M: 200 μg **Canada** F: 185–200 μg M: 215–230 μg	Liver; meat; green, leafy vegetables; whole grains; peanuts.	General metabolism of nutrients, especially amino acids; maturation of red blood cells.	Megaloblastic anemia: weakness; shortness of breath; sore tongue; diarrhea; edema; gastrointestinal upset.	Unknown.
Cobalamin (B_{12})	**US** 2.0 mg **Canada** 1.0 mg	Liver, meat, milk, cheese, eggs.	General metabolism of nutrients.	Megaloblastic anemia (see folic acid), pernicious anemia (symptoms similar to megaloblastic anemia), peripheral neuropathy.	Unknown.
Pantothenic acid	**US** No RDA 4–7 mg suggested **Canada** No RNI or suggested intake	Liver, eggs, milk, whole grains, legumes.	General metabolism of nutrients; synthesis of cholesterol.	Weakness, nausea, irritability.	Unknown.
Biotin	**US** No RDA 100–200 μg suggested **Canada** No RNI or suggested intake	Egg yolk, liver, milk, whole grains, legumes.	General metabolism of nutrients.	Dermatitis, muscle weakness, depression.	Unknown.

[a] RE = retinol equivalent.

[b] α-TE = alpha-tocepherol equivalent.

From Bureau of National Health and Welfare. Recommended Nutrient Intakes for Canadians. *Ottawa; 1990. Green, ML, Harry J. Nutrition in Contemporary Nursing Practice. 2nd ed. New York: Wiley; 1987. Subcommittee on the 10th Edition of the RDAs.* Recommended Dietary Allowances. *10th ed. Washington, DC: National Academy Press; 1989.*

TABLE 25–4. SELECTED ESSENTIAL MINERALS

Mineral	Adult RDA or RNI	Food Sources	Major Functions	Signs of Deficiency	Signs of Excess
Major Minerals					
Calcium	**US** 800 mg (age 19–24: 1200 mg) **Canada** F: 700 mg M: 800 mg	Milk, cheese, dark green vegetables, legumes.	Bone and tooth formation; blood clotting; nerve transmission; muscle activity; enzyme activator.	Stunted growth, tetany, osteoporosis, altered thyroid function.	Renal stones, constipation, blocks absorption of iron, zinc.
Phosphorus	**US** 800 mg (age 19–24: 1200 mg) **Canada** F: 850 mg M: 1000 mg	Milk, cheese, meat, poultry, fish, whole grains.	Bone and tooth formation; acid–base balance; component of coenzymes.	Weakness: demineralization of bone.	Tetany, rickets.
Magnesium	**US** F: 280 mg M: 350 mg **Canada** F: 200–210 mg M: 230–250 mg	Whole grains, green leafy vegetables, nuts.	Component of enzymes; regulates nerve and muscle activity.	Tremors, muscle spasms, muscle weakness, seizures.	Sedation.
Sulfur	No RDA, RNI, or suggested intake	Component of some amino acids and several B vitamins found in dietary proteins.	Component of cartilage, tendon, hair, nails.	Does not occur unless severe protein deficiency present.	Toxicity from nutritional intake unknown.
Sodium	**US** No RDA 1–3 g adequate **Canada** No RNI or suggested intake	Salt, milk, cured meats, pickles, canned soups, cheese, eggs.	Fluid balance; cell membrane permeability; muscle irritability.	Muscle cramps, nausea, anxiety.	Fluid retention, elevated blood pressure.
Potassium	**US** No RDA 1.9–5.6 g suggested **Canada** No RNI or suggested intake	Meats, milk, fish, whole grains, oranges, bananas, winter squash, legumes, potatoes.	Fluid balance; transmission of impulses; muscle contraction.	Muscular weakness, paralysis, loss of reflexes, heart block.	Nausea, diarrhea, muscular weakness, dyspnea, cardiac arrest.
Chloride	**US** No RDA 1.7–5.1 g suggested **Canada** No RNI or suggested intake	Salt, processed foods.	Fluid balance; acid–base balance; component of gastric juice.	Muscle cramps, anorexia.	Vomiting.
Trace Minerals					
Iron	**US** F: 15 mg (after 50: 10 mg) M: 10 mg **Canada** F: 13 mg (after 50: 8 mg) M: 9 mg	Liver, lean beef, legumes, whole grains, green leafy vegetables, dried fruit.	Constituent of hemoglobin and enzymes.	Iron-deficiency anemia: weakness, pallor, fatigue.	Acute poisoning: shock, death. Overload: liver damage.

TABLE 25–4. (continued)

Mineral	Adult RDA or RNI	Food Sources	Major Functions	Signs of Deficiency	Signs of Excess
Trace Minerals					
Iodine	**US** 150 mg **Canada** 160 mg	Saltwater fish and shellfish, iodized salt.	Constituent of thyroid hormones.	Goiter (enlarged thyroid).	Iodide goiter, skin lesions.
Fluoride	**US** No RDA 1.5–4 mg suggested **Canada** No RNI or suggested intake	Drinking water, tea, fish.	Strengthens tooth and bone structure.	Dental caries.	Mottling of teeth, bone deformation.
Zinc	**US** F: 12 mg M: 15 mg **Canada** F: 9 mg M: 12 mg	Meats, seafood, whole grains, legumes, nuts.	Cofactor for more than 70 enzymes; factor in protein metabolism; necessary for WBC functioning.	Growth retardation, impaired immune function, skin lesions, poor healing.	Anemia, vomiting, diarrhea, muscle pain, renal failure.
Selenium	**US** 150 mg **Canada** No RNI or suggested intake	Seafood, meat, whole grains.	Component of enzyme that functions as antioxidant.	Muscle pain, heart enlargement, heart failure.	Loss of hair, skin lesions, nerve damage.
Copper	**US** No RDA 2–3 mg suggested **Canada** No RNI or suggested intake	Shellfish, grains, nuts, legumes, meats.	Component of enzymes for energy production and hemoglobin synthesis; tissue maintenance.	Anemia, bone demineralization, neutropenia.	Liver and central nervous system damage, kidney malfunction.
Cobalt	No RDA, RNI, or suggested intake	Liver, meat, milk, cheese, eggs.	Constituent of vitamin B_{12}.	Not reported except as vitamin B_{12} deficiency.	Malformation of red blood cells.
Chromium	**US** No RDA 0.05–0.2 mg suggested **Canada** No RNI or suggested intake	Brewers' yeast, liver, oysters, wheat products, legumes.	Facilitates glucose uptake by cells; decreases serum cholesterol and triglycerides.	Impaired glucose metabolism.	Toxicity from nutritional intake unknown.
Manganese	**US** No RDA 2.5–5 mg suggested **Canada** No RNI or suggested intake	Nuts, wheat bran, leafy green vegetables, seeds, dried legumes.	Enzyme activator; catalyst for metabolic reactions.	Weight loss, skin lesions.	Inhalation of dust causes tremors; muscle weakness.
Molybdenum	**US** No RDA 0.15–0.5 mg suggested **Canada** No RNI or suggested intake	Organ meats, legumes, grains, dark green leafy vegetables.	Constituent of enzymes that catalyze oxidative reactions.	Deficiencies unknown.	Gout-like symptoms (joint inflammation).

From Subcommittee on the 10th Edition of the RDAs. Recommended Dietary Allowances. *10th ed. Washington, D.C. National Academy Press; 1989. Eschleman MM.* Introductory Nutrition and Diet Therapy. *Philadelphia: Lippincott; 1991. Green ML, Harry J.* Nutrition in Contemporary Nursing Practice. *2nd ed. New York: Wiley; 1987. Whitney EN, Cataldo CB, Rolfes SR.* Understanding Normal and Clinical Nutrition. *3rd ed. St Paul: West; 1991. Williams SR.* Essentials of Nutrition and Diet Therapy. *St Louis: Mosby; 1990.*

Organs Involved in Digestion. Digestion is accomplished by actions of several organs. Mechanical digestion as well as chemical digestion begins in the mouth with chewing and secretions of salivary amylase (ptyalin), an enzyme specific for starches. The food then moves down the esophagus into the stomach.

The stomach continues mechanical digestion and also secretes hydrochloric acid, enzymes, mucus, and intrinsic factor. Hydrochloric acid helps to uncoil proteins and converts pepsinogen to the gastric enzyme pepsin, which begins the process of protein breakdown. Lipase, the other major gastric enzyme, initiates fat breakdown. **Intrinsic factor** is a mucoprotein that combines with vitamin B_{12} in the stomach and facilitates its absorption in the terminal ileum of the small intestine.

The major part of digestion occurs in the small intestine. When the semiliquid mass of partly digested food called **chyme** is expelled by the stomach into the duodenum, complex neuronal and hormonal responses are initiated. In addition to parasympathetic and sympathetic regulation via the autonomic nervous system, the enteric nervous system (nerves in the intestinal wall that are capable of coordinating intestinal motor activity in the absence of autonomic innervation) also plays an independent role in neuronal control of small intestinal peristalsis. The pancreas, small intestine, and gallbladder together secrete nearly all of the enzymes responsible for the final breakdown of proteins, fats, and carbohydrates. Pancreatic and gallbladder enzymes are secreted into the duodenum. The small intestine also produces a number of important hormones, some of which delay gastric emptying and secretion so that the intestine is not overfilled.

Absorption. The small intestine is also the major site of nutrient **absorption,** in which the end products of digestion are transferred from the lumen of the intestine into the circulatory system. The large molecules of proteins, fats, and carbohydrates must be completely broken down into their smallest components before absorption can occur. To be absorbed, proteins must be in the form of amino acids; fats in the form of fatty acids or glycerides; and carbohydrates in the form of monosaccharides such as glucose or fructose. Vitamins and minerals are absorbed through the wall of the small intestine. The inner mucosal lining of the small intestine is uniquely designed to provide maximum surface area for absorption. Mucosal folds contain microscopic projections (villi and microvilli), which increase the inner surface area of the intestine several hundredfold.

A number of passive and active transport mechanisms are used to transfer substances from the inner wall of the small intestine into the blood or lymph vessels surrounding the intestine. All nutrients except for long-chain fatty acids directly enter the portal blood system after absorption. The fatty acids are absorbed into the lymph vessels, travel via the lymphatic system upward into the chest, and enter the blood where the thoracic duct empties into the left subclavian vein.

The primary function of the large intestine is the absorption of water, although minerals and electrolytes are also absorbed. It takes anywhere from 8 to 72 hours for food to complete its passage from the mouth to the rectum. The bacteria of the colon serve a number of important functions. They synthesize vitamin K and some of the B vitamins, break down bilirubin into bile pigments, and break down undigested proteins and carbohydrates. The gas present in the colon is partly due to this latter function. The characteristic odor of feces is due to amines that form from bacterial action on amino acids. Indigestible plant fiber remains as residue in the feces along with digestive solutions and mucous.

Metabolism and Storage. Metabolism refers to the cellular processes by which absorbed nutrients are used for cellular maintenance and energy production. The ultimate biological purpose of food ingestion is to support these metabolic processes, which are essential to the life of the organism. Anabolism and catabolism are the two basic metabolic activities. **Anabolism** consists of processes that construct body substances. **Catabolism** consists of processes that break down substances and lead to energy release.

Carbohydrate Metabolism. As noted earlier, carbohydrate metabolism is the primary source of energy for the body. The glucose available to body cells is obtained from dietary starches and sugars, certain amino acids, and glycerol. Excess glucose is stored as glycogen in limited amounts in the liver. After the body's energy requirements are met, any extra glucose is converted to fat and stored in adipose tissue. As the major storehouse and synthesizer of glucose, the liver also plays a central role in the regulation of blood glucose levels. These levels must be maintained within normal limits in order for the brain to function properly. Extreme alterations of blood glucose lead to convulsions, coma, and death.

The central pathway for the catabolism of glucose to energy is:

$$\text{Glucose} \leftrightarrow \text{Pyruvate} \rightarrow \text{Acetyl CoA} \rightarrow \text{Energy}$$

As shown by the two-way and one-way arrows, pyruvate can be reconverted to glucose but acetyl CoA cannot. This fact will become significant in the later discussion of metabolic interconversions.

Insulin is the major hormone involved in the regulation of blood glucose levels. Insulin lowers blood glucose. When it is absent, blood glucose levels increase. Six other hormones can cause blood glucose levels to rise by either directly or indirectly stimulating glycogenolysis or gluconeogenesis in the liver. **Glycogenolysis** is the breakdown of glycogen into glucose, which is then released from the liver into the bloodstream. **Gluconeogenesis** is the synthesis of glucose from amino acids or lipid breakdown products by the liver.

The actual cellular processes by which glucose is metabolized are exceedingly complex biochemical pathways. The Embden-Meyerhoff glycolytic pathway converts glucose into either glycogen or pyruvic acid/lactic acid. The

Krebs citric acid cycle, the final common pathway for all nutrients involved in energy production, provides nearly all of the body's energy in the form of adenosine triphosphate (ATP). The high-energy phosphate bonds of ATP are the major location of energy storage and release in all body cells.

Protein Metabolism. Understanding protein metabolism requires an understanding of the concepts of anabolism, catabolism, and nitrogen balance. In protein anabolism, proteins are synthesized by combining amino acids from dietary protein intake. Individual cells synthesize proteins specific for their own needs, using DNA as the template and regulator. Plasma proteins serve as storers of limited amounts of amino acids, and can quickly and readily transfer them to tissues in need; but unless these are replaced promptly by dietary intake, fluid balance and immune function are altered.

Protein catabolism occurs primarily in the liver by a process called deamination, in which the nitrogen unit is removed from an amino acid, resulting in ammonia and a carbon skeleton (or keto-acid). Ammonia is converted to urea and is excreted via the kidneys. Keto-acids can be used to make other amino acids, produce energy via the Krebs cycle, or make fatty acids for storage.

Nitrogen balance refers to the equilibrium between protein anabolism and catabolism. Nitrogen is the element that distinguishes proteins from carbohydrates and fats. Nitrogen is ingested as protein, but is excreted in the byproducts of protein catabolism (urea, creatinine, uric acid, ammonia salts). When a person is in a state of nitrogen balance, the intake of nitrogen is equal to its output. Situations characterized by nitrogen balance are those in which a person is healthy, ambulatory, not rapidly growing or replenishing tissue, and is consuming a diet adequate in essential amino acids and calories. A positive nitrogen balance exists when intake is greater than output, and is found during periods of rapid growth or tissue replacement. A negative nitrogen balance exists when output exceeds intake. It occurs when a diet is inadequate in essential amino acids or calories and during periods of immobility or severe physical trauma.

Fat Metabolism. Fat metabolism and storage occurs primarily in the liver and in adipose tissue. Remember that fats are made of glycerol and fatty acids. When absorbed from the intestine or released from storage in adipose tissue, glycerol is converted to pyruvate and fatty acids are converted to acetyl CoA in the liver. From either of these points, the Krebs cycle can be entered and energy produced.

Metabolic Interconversions. Metabolic interconversions are necessary because food intake is variable and intermittent. It is important that all foods be convertible to the same intermediate metabolites and that metabolism be able to continue in the absence of food. This is indeed the case. Recall that pyruvate can be reconverted to glucose but that acetyl CoA cannot. Now consider Figure 25–2, which describes the central pathways of energy metabolism. Only the glycerol portion of fats can be converted into glucose, if needed. But glycerol constitutes only about 5 percent of the

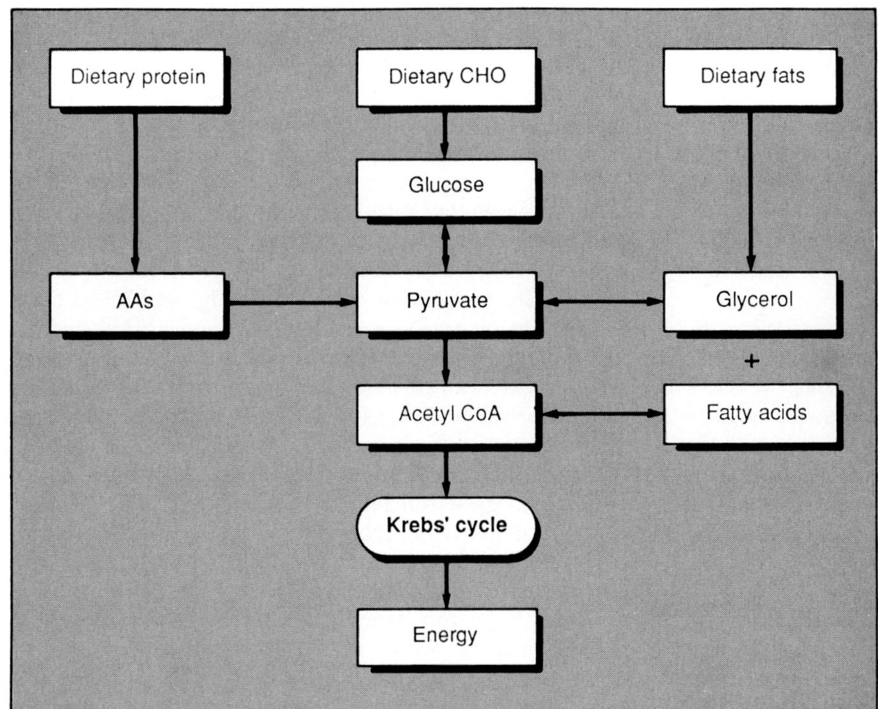

Figure 25–2. Pathways of energy metabolism.

weight of a triglyceride molecule. Amino acids, however, can be metabolized into substrates for glucose or fatty acid synthesis. Because fatty acids cannot be used for glucose synthesis, in periods of starvation amino acids are the principal source for gluconeogenesis and the maintenance of blood glucose levels. It should be remembered that neurons, the brain cells, do not store glucose and require a continuous supply for adequate energy and proper functioning. This is why it is crucial that a minimum blood glucose level be maintained at all times. Although amino acids and glycerol can be used for glucose synthesis, this is not desirable because toxic metabolites (ketones) accumulate and protein tissue is depleted. Therefore, the importance of adequate dietary intake of carbohydrate cannot be overemphasized. Such metabolic interconversions assume enormous clinical significance in conditions such as diabetes mellitus, when cells are unable to use glucose for energy production and turn to amino acids and fats for energy production.

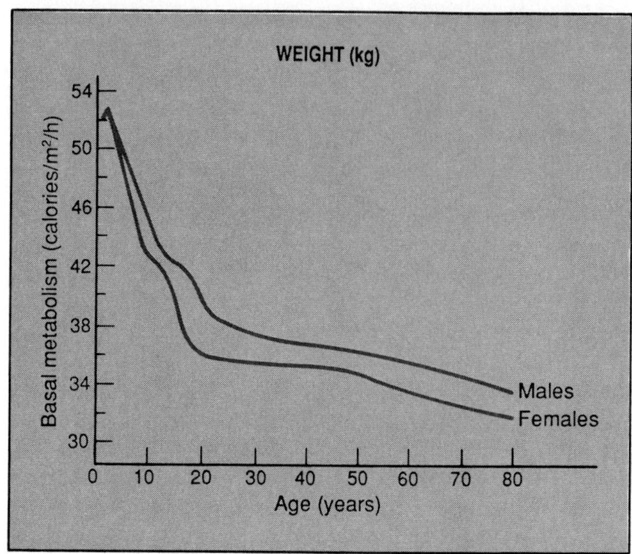

Figure 25–3. Age-related changes in basal metabolic rate. (*From Guyton A.* Textbook of Medical Physiology. *7th ed. Philadelphia: Saunders; 1986, with permission.*)

■ FACTORS AFFECTING NUTRITIONAL STATUS

Basal Metabolic Rate and Energy Requirements

Many factors can cause changes in the basal metabolic rate of an individual. Environmental temperature is rarely "neutral." A cool environment causes an increase in metabolic rate in order to generate more heat to maintain normal body temperature. A warm environment causes a lowering of metabolic rate to lower heat production by the body. In fever, the metabolic rate increases by about 7 percent for each increase of 1F (0.83C) in body temperature.[4] A person with a higher than normal proportion of muscle to fat tissue will have a higher metabolic rate. Developmental stages marked by rapid body growth (infancy, early childhood, puberty, and pregnancy) are characterized by an increase in metabolic rate. Aging is associated with a decreased rate (Fig. 25–3). Many diseases also cause alterations in metabolic rate. For example, cancer and hyperthyroidism involve increases in metabolic rate. Hypothyroidism and malnutrition cause a significant decrease in basal metabolic rate.

The relationship between changes in metabolic rate and daily energy requirements should be clear. When metabolic rate increases, energy requirements will also increase in order for an individual's weight to remain unchanged. If energy intake is not increased by adding additional calories, weight loss will occur. Conversely, if metabolic rate has decreased and energy intake is not decreased, weight gain will occur.

Age

In addition to variations in metabolic rate and hence general energy requirements, different age groups have varying requirements of specific nutrients. If these age-specific nutrient needs are not met, growth and development may be severely retarded or serious health problems may develop.

Infants. The first year of life is a critical period nutritionally. For example, brain development continues through the tenth month after birth. Rapid growth and metabolism require a large amount of energy in relation to body weight.

Protein requirements of newborns are higher than at any other stage of the life cycle because of rapid growth. Fats are also necessary, particularly the essential fatty acid linoleic acid. Fats contribute to nervous system development, especially myelinization of nerve fibers. Carbohydrates are also extremely important because of the high energy requirements of infancy. Because of their immature digestive systems, infants are not able to digest all forms of these three energy nutrients. The simpler proteins, fats, and carbohydrates found in human milk or formulas are generally easily digested.

Human breast milk has been clearly established to be superior to manmade formulas. It provides carbohydrate and protein in the form of lactose and lactoalbumin, both of which infants can easily digest. Its fat contains a generous proportion of linoleic acid. It contains ample amounts of vitamins and minerals that are easily absorbed, due to the presence of factors in the milk that facilitate absorption. In addition to these nutritional advantages, breast milk also contains maternal antibodies that can protect the infant from serious infections until the infant's own immune system matures. Another factor stimulates the development of the infant's gastrointestinal tract and its colonization with normal bacteria.

When a woman makes an informed choice or is unable to breastfeed, formula feeding may be used to provide adequate nutrition. National and international standards exist for the nutrient content of infant formulas. The Infant Formula Act of 1980 requires that the standards suggested by the American Academy of Pediatrics be met by commercial formulas. When an allergy to cow's milk is present, soy-based formula may be used.

The introduction of solid foods into the infant's diet is not recommended prior to approximately 6 months of age.[5] Rice cereal fortified with iron is a good first solid food, as allergic reactions to rice are rare and the starch is easily digestible. Then barley or oatmeal can be tried, followed by vegetables, and then by fruits. Egg yolk can be given at 6 months, but egg whites should be the last food added due to their allergic potential. Meats should be introduced late as well. Commercially prepared infant foods generally contain high amounts of sodium and sugar; parents should be warned not to season them additionally. Many parents prefer to prepare their own baby foods at home.

Water is a vitally important nutrient for infants for two reasons: their kidneys have not yet developed the ability to conserve water by concentrating the urine, and they lose more water through the skin than adults, due to their large body-surface-area-to-weight ratio. Therefore, infants require proportionally more water in relation to body weight than do adults. Water should be offered frequently between feedings.

Nutritional supplements for newborn infants are generally not needed, with three possible exceptions: vitamin D, fluoride, and iron. Breast milk does not contain vitamin D, so breast-fed infants who are not regularly exposed to sunlight will require vitamin D supplementation. If an infant is not receiving fluoridated water, the pediatrician may often prescribe appropriate supplementation because fluoride does not appear to be secreted into breast milk. As neonatal iron stores become depleted, starting at around 4 months of age, an iron supplement may be prescribed for breast-fed infants until adequate iron intake from solid foods can occur. Commercial formulas usually do not necessitate additional supplementation because they are fortified with required nutrients.

Children. Childhood is a critical period for the establishment of lifelong food habits. Desirable habits that parents should foster include the enjoyment of a wide variety of food types, openness to new foods, limitation of concentrated sweets, consumption of a balanced diet, and the establishment of regular eating times. Undesirable habits include random snacking on highly processed foods, and the use of food to meet emotional needs, to play out power struggles, or to provide reward and punishment.

After the age of 1 year, a child's growth rate slows, but body composition changes dramatically. In particular, a decrease in body fat and an increase in muscle and bone mass occurs. Growth typically comes in spurts, and food intake naturally increases due to an increase in appetite during these spurts. Generally a 1-year-old needs 100 kcal/day; a 3-year-old needs about 300 to 500 kcal more. Protein, calcium, phosphorous, magnesium, and zinc are important nutrients during childhood, and milk is still the most important food in the diet. For growing children, 3 cups of milk per day should be provided. For children over the age of 2, the use of low-fat or nonfat milk leaves more kcal available for consumption in the form of foods rich in other essential nutrients, such as iron.

School-age, preadolescent children experience a "latent period" of growth, with a relative decline in energy needs.

Adolescents. Adolescence involves another growth spurt in which caloric, protein, mineral, and B vitamin requirements are especially high. The onset of menarche in girls leads to an increase in basal metabolic rate and hence in energy requirements. Iron deficiency can also easily develop due to blood losses from menstruation unless foods high in iron are also consumed.

Fad foods and fad diets attain particular importance to adolescents. Fast food outlets often are popular places for social gathering, and the foods sold have great appeal largely because of high fat and salt content, which enhances taste. A high intake of fast foods at the expense of other foods results in serious nutritional imbalances: an excess of kilocalories, fat, salt, and sugar and deficiencies of vitamins, minerals, and complex carbohydrates.

Fad diets are also common among adolescents, especially girls. Changes in body composition associated with sexual maturation lead to an increase in body fat, which may be very distressing to the adolescent's changing body image. Fad diets to lose weight or change one's figure may precipitate severe malnutrition. Severe forms of this problem are the eating disorders anorexia nervosa and bulimia (discussed later in this chapter).

Young and Middle-aged Adults. Body maintenance and repair, rather than growth, are the processes that drive nutritional needs during adulthood. A notable exception to this is pregnancy, which is characterized by rapid growth and consequently greatly increased energy needs and specific nutrient requirements. An additional 300 kcal/day should be added to the pregnant woman's diet, or approximately 40 kcal/kg of prepregnant weight.[6] Weight gain during pregnancy is an important indicator of adequate kilocaloric intake. Total weight gain should be no less than 25 pounds. All nutrient intakes should be increased, with special attention paid to protein, iron, calcium, zinc, vitamin A, B vitamins, vitamin C, and vitamin D.

During lactation, nutritional demands exceed even those of pregnancy. An additional 500 to 600 kcal above nonpregnant levels is necessary. An extra quart of milk per day provides for increased protein and energy needs. Ample fruits and vegetables supply needed vitamins and minerals. A fluid intake of 2½ to 3 quarts per day is also necessary.

Nonpregnant and nonlactating young and middle-aged adults in good health must be particularly concerned with the type and quality, rather than the quantity, of their food intake. Caloric requirements generally are significantly lower once growth is completed, and they tend to steadily decline with age due to decreases in basal metabolic rate. Therefore, the calories that are consumed must be rich in essential nutrients so that adequate intake can be maintained. Women are at risk for iron and calcium deficiencies, and so particular attention is needed to assure adequate dietary intake of calcium- and iron-rich foods.

Older Adults. Food requirements for the elderly are influenced by reduced basal metabolic rates and reduced physical activity. Daily energy needs are reduced to approximately 1800 to 2200 kcal, although individual requirements are highly variable. Excessive fat should be avoided due to a decreased absorption capacity. Calcium intake for women should be at least 1200 mg daily, to prevent the development of osteoporosis. Iron supplementation may also be necessary if the diet is deficient in this mineral.

Loss of teeth, diminished senses of smell and taste, and reduced saliva production reduce some of the pleasure associated with eating and may influence food choices. Some older adults, therefore, prefer highly sweetened and strongly seasoned foods. Indigestion, constipation, and irritable colon, which are relatively common complaints because of decreased gastric secretions and reduced intestinal motility, sometimes suppress appetite. If elderly individuals must take several medications for chronic diseases, their side effects may enhance some of these problems or add others.

Personal and social factors also exert considerable influence on the nutritional status of elderly people. Many live alone, which decreases motivation to prepare well-balanced meals and eliminates the social pleasure associated with eating. Financial resources often limit affordable food choices. Loss of loved ones, relocation, and limited mobility—common life experiences among older adults—often produce emotional conditions that amplify these concerns.

BUILDING NURSING KNOWLEDGE

Can the Nurse Help Improve the Nutrition of Severely Ill Clients?

Taber J. Nutrition in HIV infection. *Am J Nurs.* 1989;89: 1446–1451.

In this article, Taber points out that malnutrition is a consequence of the symptoms of AIDS, a severe illness of the immune system. Unfortunately, malnutrition further weakens the already weakened body and hastens the complications of the disease. Nutritional intake among clients with this illness is reduced by persistent nausea, vomiting, and loss of appetite. These symptoms can be caused by the disease itself or by the drugs used to treat the disease. Psychological depression, physical weakness and fatigue, and mental disorientation often accompany the disease and exert profound effects on a person's appetite. Fever, which is a common feature of AIDS, also leads to weight loss and muscle wasting and raises the requirements for energy and protein. Thus, while the demands for nutrients increase, the ability to meet the demands is often severely reduced.

Taber stresses that nutrition therapy is as important as the drug therapy, and argues that nurses can facilitate improved nourishment by several means. One is to involve family and friends. This is important to create the atmosphere needed to stimulate appetite. Clients also benefit from counseling on strategies for nutritional self-care. For instance, clients might use times of peak energy for preparing foods to eat when energy wanes, or keep packaged or prepared foods on hand for those times. Hospitalized clients may need assistance in eating, may require frequent small meals, high-calorie snacks, soft foods, cold foods, or frequent oral hygiene care to overcome the many barriers to adequate intake.

Health Status

Major deviations from or threats to health usually create specific nutritional needs and serious nutritional problems if the needs are not met. Serious and chronic illnesses, surgery, injury, and emotional stress are some of the health-related factors influencing nutritional needs of clients.

Serious Illness. Acute major illnesses such as serious infections increase energy and specific nutrient requirements. This is in part due to the generalized stress response that is initiated during any physiological challenge (see Chap. 6). Specific aspects of the stress response that affect nutritional status are glycogenolysis, gluconeogenesis, and increased glucagon levels, which result in hyperglycemia; increased production of glucocorticoids and antidiuretic hormone, which result in sodium and water retention, potassium loss, and hyperglycemia; and sympathetic stimulation, which increases digestive secretions but decreases peristalsis, resulting in anorexia, loss of appetite, nausea, vomiting, and abdominal distention.[7]

These changes produce a hypermetabolic state in which protein catabolism, largely of skeletal muscle, to meet energy requirements may reach such intensity that, if untreated, a state of exhaustion and death may occur.

Chronic Illness. Individuals with chronic illnesses require consistently adequate diets in order to maintain a maximum quality of life as well as to prevent serious, potentially life-threatening complications. Loss of appetite is a common problem that makes it particularly difficult to maintain optimum intake. Appetite loss may be due to pain, depression, or the physical or metabolic effects of the disease and/or its treatment. Lack of energy or ability to prepare or eat food is another complicating factor. The nutritional hazards of immobility are another threat to clients with chronic illnesses. It is well known that immobility causes significant losses of calcium from bones, and stimulates protein catabolism.

Cancer serves as a good example of the problems described above. Loss of appetite is often the earliest symptom of an undiagnosed malignancy. This is felt to be due to metabolic by-products of tumor growth. These same by-products are also felt to alter taste perception so that meat, in particular, is usually no longer enjoyed. Difficulty with ingestion, digestion, or absorption may occur if the neoplasm is creating physical alterations in the digestive tract. Chronic pain and depression decrease the desire to eat. Cancer chemotherapy and radiation therapy are commonly associated with nausea and vomiting, mouth sores, diarrhea, and altered taste sensation. Thus, clients with cancer are in particular need of nonmeat, soothing sources of protein and calories.

Surgery. Food and fluids are generally withheld for at least 8 hours before surgery, and for many clients (particularly those undergoing gastrointestinal surgery) it may be several days or even weeks before a regular diet can be resumed. Loss of blood and body fluids during and after surgery can create severe fluid and electrolyte imbalances, as well as shock. The nutrient that the client recovering from surgery uses most is protein. It plays a pivotal role in antibody formation and wound healing. There is also a general increase in energy (calorie), zinc, and vitamin A, K, and C requirements.

Serious Injury. Burns are a clear example of the severe nutritional stresses that may occur after serious injury. A person with extensive burns undergoes intense stress and also has major damage to a vital organ, the skin. Protein demands are so high that vital body proteins are sacrificed. Protein and electrolyte losses from leakage into the burned area are extreme. Metabolic demands are also exceedingly high. Without nutritional support to supply protein, energy, and other nutrients, the client who is seriously burned cannot survive.

Emotional Stress. Emotional stress creates the same generalized stress response as does physical stress. Therefore, prolonged emotional stress can deplete protein stores and lower immunity by reductions in proteins available for antibody and white blood cell production. Loss of appetite may make replacement of protein stores difficult.

Sociocultural Influences

Culture of Origin. Dietary foods and eating habits are among the most deep-rooted aspects of culture. Cultural attitudes, values, beliefs, and practices about food exert a powerful internal influence over a person. Although they may seem strange to someone from a different culture, it is important to understand that culturally based food habits are often developed in response to the geographic and economic realities of a society. Additionally, the symbolic meaning of foods and eating may be intimately related to the culture's religious traditions, social organization, and history. Thus, the nutritional behavior of a culture is part of a complex web of many other dimensions.

It is essential that the nurse be familiar with the cultural dimensions of a client's eating behaviors. A collaborative relationship for nutritional planning is difficult without this understanding. Often the major obstacle to implementation of a dietary change will come from attitudes reflective of the client's cultural background. The plan of care must accommodate these attitudes. Box 25–3 describes the common food patterns of some cultural groups.

Religion. The influence of a client's religion on food habits may take the form of certain traditional ritual meals on specific days; for example, the seder on Passover for the Jewish faith, in which certain foods take on important symbolic value. Some religions prescribe food restrictions for their faithful. Catholics traditionally abstain from meat on Fridays during Lent. Mormons, Moslems, and Seventh-Day Adventists do not allow alcohol. Moslems and Jews allow only kosher meats, which are processed so that as much blood as possible is drained out. Jewish kosher laws prohibit the serving of meat and dairy products at the same meal or in the same set of dishes. Many Seventh-Day Adventists are vegetarian, as are virtually all Hindus and Buddhists. Food habits clearly can become highly symbolic of an individual's religious beliefs, which must always be respected by the nurse.

Knowledge About Nutrition. Ideally, an individual's knowledge of nutrition should come from educational programs provided by experts. In reality, people may be basing their food habits on beliefs acquired through competitive product advertising, peer groups, or family and cultural traditions. Misinformation may be propagated knowingly or unknowingly.

Food fads are common in the United States culture. They involve exaggerated claims about certain foods. It is undeniable that there is an important relationship between food and health. Extremes in dietary habits that lead to severe deficiencies in certain nutrients, however, can be dangerous. Many fraudulent food claims are made by people or businesses whose primary motive is profit. Individuals with severe or chronic health problems are particularly vulnerable to promises of instant cures, as are adolescents or young adults who are dissatisfied with their bodies.

The best defense against food faddism is an informed consumer. Nurses have an important role to play as information providers and dietary counselors. With a good understanding of basic nutritional principles, clients should be able to make informed choices that are personally satisfying and nutritionally appropriate.

It is important, however, that fad diets and healthy dietary changes not be equated. This can be illustrated by the recent increase in vegetarianism and "natural foods" in Western societies. This trend was initially labeled a fad by many observers; however, it is now acknowledged by medical and nutritional experts that vegetarians who include milk products in their diet are consuming highly nutritious diets, as long as they are carefully planned to include complementary protein sources in each meal.[2]

Life-style. Life-style exerts a major influence in the amount, type, and pattern of food ingested. Recent attention has

BOX 25–3. COMMON FOOD PREFERENCES OF SOME CULTURAL GROUPS

Southern Black

- Vegetables cooked with salt pork, ham, or bacon; served with liquid used in cooking.
- Salt pork and bacon.
- Hot breads, rice, and sweets.

Hispanic

- Foods are classified as "hot" or "cold" and are taken for certain illnesses.
- Chili peppers and hot sauces as seasoning.
- Tortilla (a flat, unleavened bread made from wheat or corn flour).
- Beans, cheese, and onions.
- Rice and lentils.
- Beef, salt pork, and chicken.

Asian (Chinese, Japanese)

- Foods are classified as "hot" or "cold" and are taken for certain illnesses.
- Large amounts of vegetables; lightly cooked in oil or steamed.
- Small amounts of meat or fish.
- Rice is the staple grain.
- Soups made with vinegar (extracts calcium from meat bones).
- Sweets in small quantities.

Indian

- Vegetables cooked in oil with numerous spices ("curried").
- Beans or legumes cooked with spices.
- Rice and wheat are staple grains.
- Chapati (a flat, unleavened bread made from wheat flour).
- Hindu Indians are lactovegetarian (no meat, fish, or eggs).
- Yogurt.

Jewish (Orthodox)

- No pork, ham, or bacon.
- Meat must be killed and prepared according to kosher laws, to remove all blood.
- Meat and dairy products are not eaten at same meal; are served with separate sets of dishes.
- Fish without fins or scales is prohibited.
- Challah (a leavened, braided white bread).

Middle Eastern

- Lamb and goat preferred as meats.
- Rice is the staple grain.
- Vegetables and legumes seasoned with herbs and spices.
- Homemade dark bread with every meal.
- Olive oil for cooking.
- Yogurt.
- Hot, sweet tea.

From Dudek SG. Nutrition Handbook for Nursing Practice. *Philadelphia: Lippincott; 1987, with permission.*

focused on life-style factors that can be changed to reduce the incidence of major chronic diseases such as cancer and heart disease. Dietary factors are major variables in these discussions and studies. Dietary guidelines for health promotion and disease prevention are discussed later in this section.

Frequently, a person's peer group is a major influence on dietary habits. Life-style factors influence what one eats, where one eats, with whom one eats, whether one cooks for oneself, how frequently food purchases are made, and how much time is allowed for eating.

The abuse of drugs and alcohol is a life-style of particular damage to a person's nutritional status. Drugs cause severe disturbances in appetite and can either raise or lower the basal metabolic rate. Alcohol abuse causes serious long-term effects such as elevated triglyceride levels, malabsorption, multiple nutrient deficiencies, anemia, gastritis, pancreatitis, organ damage, and potentially fatal liver disease.

Personal Preference. Many people make conscious decisions regarding how and what they will eat on the basis of their personal philosophy, beliefs, and values. Vegetarianism is a good example. Nurses must understand the many different forms a vegetarian diet may take and their nutritional implications so as to provide knowledgeable guidelines for clients who are vegetarian. Table 25–5 describes various types of vegetarian diets and nutritional considerations. Guidelines for vegetarian meal planning are discussed in the following section.

Economic Situation. In the United States more and more families and individuals are living below the poverty line. Hunger and malnutrition are serious problems for many people, not all of whom are economically deprived. The cost of food can become a major factor negatively influencing nutritional intake, unless knowledgeable choices are made. Living situations may prohibit the availability of time, space, or equipment necessary for even the most basic cooking. Such situations are encountered by the thousands of homeless people in our society. While this problem requires large-scale social planning, nurses can play an important role in helping people with limited food-purchasing power get the greatest possible nutritional return for every dollar spent on food. Strategies for purchasing economical and nutritious meals are discussed in Section 3. Nurses should also be aware that a person at a higher income level is not automatically protected from malnutrition. Much depends on the individual or family knowledge and habits, rather than on income alone.

■ GUIDELINES AND STANDARDS FOR NUTRITION

Numerous government and private organizations and groups have developed guidelines for healthy eating or standards for determining adequate intake of various nu-

TABLE 25–5. TYPES OF VEGETARIAN DIETS

Type	Description	Nutritional Considerations
Vegan or strict	Includes only foods derived from plants. No meat, dairy products, or eggs.	Requires careful planning to provide complementary proteins. Requires vitamin B_{12} supplement, possibly vitamin D.
Lactovegetarian	Includes dairy products along with plant foods. No eggs.	Dairy products complement plant products and provide important minerals such as calcium. Careful planning to include iron, vitamin B_{12}.
Ovolactovegetarian	Includes dairy products, eggs, and plant foods.	All nutrients can be provided in sufficient quantities.
Ovovegetarian	Includes eggs and plant foods.	All nutrients can be provided in sufficient quantities.

trients. Nurses should be familiar with as many of these guides as possible. At times the sheer number of guides available can create some confusion, as differences in recommendations can and do occur. It is important that nurses understand what population a set of guidelines is for, what its stated purpose is, and who developed the guidelines (for example, is there a hidden purpose such as the promotion of a particular industry's product?). Following are selected guidelines and standards that are widely recognized and that have relevance for the general population of healthy people, have been developed for health promotion and disease prevention, and have been compiled by reliable groups or agencies.

Recommended Dietary Allowances

Because it recognizes the importance of nutrition to the overall well-being and social productivity of its citizens, the United States government has delegated various aspects of nutritional research, education, and regulation to a number of federal agencies and groups. The **Recommended Dietary Allowances** (RDAs) are the guidelines regarding optimum nutrient intake for most normal, healthy people living in the United States. These recommendations are provided by the Food and Nutrition Board, National Academy of Sciences, and National Research Council, and are periodically updated in accordance with ongoing research.[8]

Specific RDAs have been established for protein, 11 vitamins, and 7 minerals. Variations are indicated for different developmental groups and for sex. For the essential nutrients not listed in the RDA table, too little information is felt to be available to establish a meaningful RDA.

The RDAs are used as standards for assessing and planning individual dietary intake, parenteral and enteral formulas, and food supplementation programs. It is important to understand that the RDAs do not designate *minimum* requirements; they are deliberately set *above* minimum nutrient needs (with the exception of kcal requirements) in order to encompass the needs of most people. It should also be recognized that specific individual needs even among healthy people may differ substantially from the RDAs.

To use the RDAs in determining the nutritional quality of a diet, one must first use a food table listing nutrient content of foods, and then add up the amount of individual nutrients consumed during a 24-hour period. The totals are then compared to the RDAs for the person's age and sex, adjusting if needed for diverse weights or heights.

Recommended Nutrient Intake (Canada)

Canada provides guidelines similar to the RDAs for its citizens, called **Recommended Nutrient Intakes** (RNIs). The guidelines are prepared by the Bureau of National Health and Welfare, and contain recommendations for protein, six vitamins, and six minerals, with variations for age and sex.

Standards for Food Labeling

The US RDA, used for food labeling, is a different set of standards than the RDAs, but was derived from the 1968 RDAs. The US RDA was developed by the Food and Drug Administration (FDA). For most nutrients, the US RDA value is the same as the highest RDA value for that nutrient (usually the RDA for adult males). By using the highest nutritional requirement as a labeling standard, the FDA felt that product label information could be generally applied, although individuals with lesser needs for that nutrient would receive a greater percentage of their daily requirement than that stated on the label. The US RDA labeling system includes selected nutrients only, so it is not useful for assessing total nutritional intake. However, comparing labels helps consumers differentiate the relative nutritional value of food products.

All food labels, by current law, must list the name of the product, name and address of the manufacturer, quantity of food provided, and a list of ingredients in descending order of predominance by weight. In addition, if any nutrition claim is made on a food package, the label must provide the following information: serving size; servings per container; kcal per serving; grams of carbohydrate, protein, and fat per serving; and protein, certain vitamins, and minerals as percentages of the US RDA per serving.

In November 1990, President Bush signed into law a new federal nutrition labeling and education act. The FDA was given 24 months to develop regulations to implement the law, which would then take effect 6 months later, in May 1993. The law requires that all food labels state the serving size; number of servings per container; number of calories per serving; number of calories derived from fat per serving; and the total amount of fat, saturated fat, cholesterol, sodium, sugars, dietary fiber, protein, total carbohydrates, complex carbohydrates, and certain vitamins and minerals. Beverage containers also must list the actual percentage of fruit or fruit juice.

In addition, retailers must post the same information about raw agricultural commodities, such as fruits, vegetables, and fish. There are additional specifications for foods making health or nutrition claims.

Meat and poultry products are not affected by this law, because they are regulated by the United States Department of Agriculture (USDA). The USDA has announced its intention to impose labeling requirements on these products, but current proposals identify serving sizes that differ from those used by the FDA, whose regulations will be used to enforce the new labeling law. Because this will make comparisons difficult between one product containing meat and another that does not (for example, a pepperoni pizza with a cheese pizza, or meat with seafood), a coalition of public health and consumer organizations, called the Nutritional Labeling Coalition, is lobbying the USDA to adopt serving sizes consistent with the FDA's. Because Americans consume a significant percentage of their meals in restaurants, this group is also working to have the labeling law apply to restaurants as well.

Because a healthy diet is critical to overall health and recovery from illness, nurses should help clients develop the ability to interpret and compare food labels for meal planning and purchase decisions. Figure 25–4 illustrates a sample label with nutritional information, plus optional information about fats and additional vitamins.

NUTRITION INFORMATION
(per serving)

Serving size = 8 oz — Servings per container = 2

Calories	560
Protein	23 g
Carbohydrate	43 g
Fat	33 g

(Percent of calories from fat = 53 percent)

Polyunsaturated*	22 g
Saturated*	9 g
Cholesterol* (18 mg, 100 g)	40 g
Sodium (365 mg 100 g)	310 mg

Percentage of U.S. Recommended Daily Allowance
(U.S. RDA)

Protein	35	Niacin	25
Vitamin A	35	Calcium	2
Vitamin C	10	Iron	25
Thiamine	15	Vitamin B_6	22
Riboflavin	15	Vitamin B_{12}	15

NOTE
* Information on fat and cholesterol content is provided for individuals who, on the advice of a physician, are modifying their total dietary intake of fat and cholesterol.

Figure 25–4. Sample food label with legally required nutritional information and optional information on fats and selected vitamins. (*From Lewis CM.* Nutrition and Nutritional Therapy in Nursing. *Norwalk, CT: Appleton & Lange; 1986.*)

Four Food Groups

Another frequently used nutritional guidance tool is the Daily Food Guide, which discusses the "four food groups." This guide is published by the USDA and the National Dairy Council. According to this framework, two portions per day from each of the milk and meat groups, and four portions from each of the fruits and vegetables and grains and cereals groups, will meet an "average" person's nutritional requirements (Fig. 25–5). The four food groups plan has received criticism on several points. It is quite easy to put together a food plan from these guidelines that does not meet minimum dietary standards for specific nutrients. It has also been claimed that unwanted weight gain by individuals with low metabolic rates is likely if the Daily Food Guide is used. The safest way of using the four food groups plan is to eat a variety of foods within each food group.

Other Dietary Recommendations

Many other groups have developed guidelines for food consumption that will promote health. Six selected examples are presented here.

Senate Select Committee Recommendations. In 1977, the Senate Select Committee on Nutrition and Health released a publication called Dietary Goals for the United States.[9] It recommended the following changes in food selection and preparation:

1. Increase consumption of fruits, vegetables, and whole grains.
2. Decrease consumption of refined and other processed sugars.
3. Decrease consumption of foods high in total fat and partially replace saturated fats with polyunsaturated fats.
4. Decrease consumption of animal fat and meats with a high proportion of saturated fat.
5. Except for young children, substitute low-fat and nonfat milk for whole milk and dairy products.
6. Decrease consumption of high-cholesterol foods such as butterfat and eggs.
7. Decrease consumption of salt and foods high in salt.

Surgeon General's Report. In 1988, the Public Health Service of the US Department of Health and Human Services released the first Surgeon General's Report on Nutrition and Health. This publication was the result of a review of a large body of scientific literature, particularly that regarding links between diet and chronic disease. The recommendations emphasize the importance of reducing intake of dietary fat, especially saturated fat, and increasing intake of foods high in complex carbohydrates, such as fruits, vegetables, and whole grains.

VEGETABLE AND FRUIT GROUP

Provides:
- Vitamin A
- Vitamin C
- Folic acid

Number of servings daily:
4 or more

Serving Size: ½ cup or 1 medium-sized

Lettuce	Beets
Cucumber	Grapes
†Cabbage	*Pumpkin
Mushrooms	Pineapple
Celery	*Peaches
‡Peppers	†Honeydew melons
*†Greens (all types)	*Apricots
†Cauliflower	‡Orange juice
Bean sprouts	Sweet corn
Green beans	‡Orange
Spinach	*Winter squash
†Asparagus	‡Cantaloupe
†Lemons	Apples
Plums	Pears
*‡Broccoli	Bananas
†Tomato	Prunes
*Carrots	†Potato
‡Brussels sprouts	*Sweet potato
*†Papayas	Raisins
‡Strawberries	†Avocado
	Canned fruit (in syrup)

* Vitamin A
† Good source of vitamin C
‡ Excellent source of vitamin C

MEAT GROUP

Provides:
- Protein
- Niacin
- Thiamin
- Iron
- Zinc
- Vitamin B_{12}

Number of servings daily:
2 or more

Serving Size	
2 oz	Chicken
2 oz	Lean beef
2 oz	Fish
1 oz	Turkey
2 oz	Lean pork chop
2 oz	Ham
2	Eggs
1 cup	Dry beans and peas
2 oz	Pork
2 oz	Refried beans
2	Hot dogs
4 Tbsp	Peanut butter
½ cup	Nuts

MILK GROUP

Provides:
- Calcium
- Protein
- Riboflavin
- Vitamin B_6
- Vitamin B_{12}

Number of servings daily:

Child, 2–9 yr 2–3	
Child, 9–12 yr	3 or more
Teenager	4 or more
Adult	2 or more
Pregnant or lactating woman	4 or more

Serving Size	
1 cup	Nonfat milk
1 cup	Buttermilk
1 cup	Low-fat milk
1 cup	Plain yogurt
1 cup	Whole milk
1½ oz	Processed cheese
1½ oz	Cheddar cheese
1 cup	Fruit-flavored yogurt
1 cup	Custard
1 cup	Milkshake
2 cups	Low-fat cottage cheese
1 cup	Pudding
1¾ cups	Ice cream
2 cups	Cottage cheese

BREAD AND CEREAL GROUP

Provides:
- Thiamin
- Niacin
- Iron
- Protein

Number of servings daily:
4 or more

Serving Size	
1 slice	Whole-wheat bread
1 slice	Rye bread
½ bun	Hamburger or hot dog
½ cup	Grits
1	Tortilla
1 slice	White bread
5	Crackers
½ cup	Cooked cereals
½ cup	Rice
½	Bagel
½ cup	Brown rice
1 cup	Dry cereal
½ cup	Macaroni
½ cup	Spaghetti
1	Pancake
1	Biscuit
1	Muffin
1	Cornbread
1 cup	Presweetened cereal

Figure 25–5. The four food groups with sample foods and principal nutrients provided by each group. (*From Burtis G, Davis J, Martin S.* Applied Nutrition and Diet Therapy. *Philadelphia: Saunders; 1988, with permission.*)

National Research Council Committee on Diet and Health. Many researchers have investigated the link between dietary factors and increased cancer risk. In 1989, the National Research Council made the following recommendations[10] about cancer risk and diet:

1. Reduce total fat to 30 percent or less of total calories. High-fat diets are associated with higher risks of colon, prostate, and breast cancer.
2. Eat five or more servings daily of vegetables and fruits, especially green and yellow vegetables and citrus fruits. Specific factors responsible for the protective action of these foods is not yet clear, but there is strong evidence that low intake of carotinoids (present in green and yellow vegetables) contributes to increased risk of lung cancer.
3. Maintain protein intake at moderate levels. Diets high in meat have been associated with increased risk of colon and breast cancer. It is unclear whether the adverse effects are due to the protein itself or to other factors, such as high fat content and low plant food levels in these diets.
4. Balance food intake and physical activity to maintain appropriate body weight. Excess weight is associated with increased risk of endometrial cancer.
5. Avoid alcohol. If consumed, limit consumption to less than one ounce of pure alcohol in a day (two cans of beer, two small glasses of wine, or two average cocktails). Alcohol consumption is associated with increased risk of cancers of the oral cavity, pharynx, esophagus, and larynx, especially when combined with smoking. There is some evidence that links alcohol with liver cancer and moderate beer intake with rectal cancer.
6. Consume salty, highly processed, salt-preserved, and salt-pickled foods sparingly. Frequent consumption may increase the risk of stomach cancer.

These recommendations are very similar to those made in 1982 by the Food and Nutrition Board of the National Academy of Sciences.

Dietary Guidelines for Americans. Published in 1980 by the federal government and updated in 1990, these guidelines emphasize prevention of obesity, cancer, and heart disease. They state not only what a person should eat, but also what should not be eaten. Box 25–4 details these guidelines.

Nutrition Recommendations for Canadians. The Canadian government is also concerned about how its citizens are eating. As can be seen from the summary in Box 25–5, there is similarity to the US dietary guidelines.

Vegetarian Dietary Guidelines. A modification of the traditional four food groups plan has been made for vegetarians.[2] The groups are as follows:

- Two servings of milk or milk products (or soy milk with vitamin B_{12}).
- Two servings of protein-rich foods (include 2 cups of legumes to meet iron needs of women; count 4 tablespoons of peanut butter as one serving).
- Four servings of whole-grain foods.
- Four servings of fruits and vegetables (include 1 cup of dark greens to meet iron needs of women).

BOX 25–4. DIETARY GUIDES FOR AMERICANS

1. *Eat a variety of foods daily.* Get the many nutrients your body needs by choosing different foods from these five groups daily: vegetables; fruits; grain products; milk and milk products; and meats (including poultry and fish) and meat alternatives (dry beans and peas, eggs, and nuts).
2. *Maintain a healthy weight.* Check to see if you are at a healthy weight. If not, set reasonable weight goals and try for long-term success through better eating and exercise habits.
3. *Choose a diet low in fat, saturated fat, and cholesterol.* Eat plenty of vegetables, fruits, and grain products; choose lean meats and poultry without the skin, and low-fat dairy products; use fats and oils sparingly.
4. *Choose a diet with plenty of vegetables, fruits, and grain products.* Vegetables, including dry beans and peas; fruits, and grain products including breads, cereals, pasta, and rice are emphasized in this guideline especially for their complex carbohydrates, dietary fiber, and other food components linked to good health.
5. *Use sugars only in moderation.* Sugars and many foods that contain them in large amounts supply calories, but are limited in nutrients. Sugars include sucrose (includes brown and raw sugar), glucose, dextrose, fructose, maltose, lactose, honey, syrup, corn sweetener, high-fructose corn syrup, molasses, and fruit juice concentrate. Read labels; a food is likely to be high in sugars if its ingredient list shows one of these first or second, or lists several of them.
6. *Use salt and sodium only in moderation.* Use salted snacks such as chips, crackers, pretzels, and nuts sparingly. Use salt sparingly if at all, in cooking and at the table. When planning meals, consider: fresh and plain frozen vegetables prepared without salt are lower in sodium than canned ones; cereals, pasta, and rice cooked without salt are lower in sodium than prepared cereals, pasta, and rice; milk and yogurt are lower in sodium than most cheeses; most frozen dinners and combination dishes, packaged dishes, canned soups, salad dressings, and condiments such as soy, pickles, olives, catsup, and mustard contain a considerable amount of sodium.
7. *If you drink alcoholic beverages, do so in moderation.* Alcoholic beverages supply calories, but little or no nutrients. Drinking them has no net health benefit, and is linked to many health problems. Moderate drinking is no more than one drink a day for women, two for men. Twelve ounces of beer, 5 ounces of wine, and 1.5 ounces of distilled spirits (80 proof) count as one drink.

From US Department of Agriculture, US Department of Health and Human Services. Dietary Guidelines for Americans. *3rd ed. Washington, DC: US Government Printing Office; 1990.*

BOX 25–5. CANADA'S GUIDELINES FOR HEALTHY EATING

- Enjoy a *variety* of Foods.
- Emphasize cereals, breads, other grain products, vegetables and fruits.
- Choose lower-fat dairy products, leaner meats, and foods prepared with little or no fat.
- Achieve and maintain a healthy body weight by enjoying regular physical activity and healthy eating.
- Limit salt, alcohol and caffeine.

From Canada's Guidelines for Healthy Eating (1991). *Ottawa: Department of National Health and Welfare; 1991.*

In order to ensure high-quality, complete protein intake, the concept of complementary proteins can be used. Research has identified specific combinations of plant foods that provide complete protein intake in a single meal:

- Legumes plus grains
- Legumes plus seeds
- Leafy vegetables plus grains

Vegetarian diets, if planned carefully, can be among the most healthful. They automatically reduce dietary risk factors for cancer and heart disease (particularly saturated fats) and provide generous amounts of fiber, vitamins, and minerals. For vegetarians who do not take milk products, the amounts of grains and legumes should be increased.

ALTERATIONS IN NUTRITION

Nutritional Disorders

Despite recent emphasis on optimum nutrition and prevention of nutritional deficiencies, the sad fact is that nutritional disorders are among the world's most serious health problems. It is the nurse's responsibility to recognize the early signs of such disorders so that prompt interventions may be instituted. Nutritional disorders tend to run an insidious and progressive course, but if treated early, can be completely cured in many cases.

Protein–Calorie Malnutrition. Protein–calorie malnutrition (PCM) or protein-energy malnutrition (PEM) is the tragic outcome of an overall lack of quality and quantity of food. The human suffering and waste of human life engendered by PCM is virtually inestimable. This is the most prevalent and most serious of the world's primary malnutrition syndromes.

Kwashiorkor is the original term used to describe the malnutrition that develops when babies are weaned from mother's milk without receiving a diet adequate in protein. The resulting protein deficiency creates a syndrome of retarded mental and physical growth, apathy, edema, muscular wasting, and skin depigmentation and dermatosis.

Marasmus is the syndrome resulting from a deficiency of both protein and calories. The result is a general emaciation, wasting of body tissues, gradual starvation, and gross underweight. Edema is minimal and diarrhea is frequent.

PCM is also the most common serious nutritional problem faced by clients in health care facilities. Some form of PCM affects one fourth to one half of the clients in acute care facilities. The irony of this is that "hospital PCM" is iatrogenic, caused by health care treatment itself. The problem is equally common in long-term care facilities. Three categories of PCM are encountered in health care agencies: (1) protein deficiency state (kwashiorkor type), (2) cachexia (marasmus type), and (3) mixed state.

Protein Deficiency State. Protein deficiency state occurs in clients experiencing short-term but severe disorders or stressors such as a major injury or surgery. They are often given nutritional support in the form of intravenous water, glucose, and electrolytes. Because one liter of this solution provides only 170 calories and the solution is totally without amino acids, protein malnutrition can develop after about 10 days if no other calorie source is provided. Clinical signs of this form of PCM include fatigue, apathy, edema, decreased serum protein levels, and, rarely, mild to moderate weight loss and muscle weakness and wasting. The effects of protein malnutrition pose serious hindrances to recovery from an acute stressor; for example, protein malnutrition may cause impaired wound healing and decreased immunity. This is because visceral protein, such as enzymes and blood protein (albumin, globulin, blood cells), are used as energy sources for metabolic processes when nutritional intake is suddenly drastically decreased. When serum levels of protein and blood cells decrease, immune function and healing are compromised.

Cachexia. A second type of hospital-related PCM is generalized **cachexia,** which develops from a more gradual but prolonged period of receiving an insufficient quantity of a nutritionally complete diet. The result is a marasmus-like syndrome of emaciation, tissue wasting, severe underweight, and sometimes diarrhea.

Mixed State. The third type of PCM seen among hospitalized clients is a mixed state in which a cachectic person is subject to an acute stress—for example, a person with cancer who develops pneumonia. This can create a life-threatening situation due to severe depletion of vital nutrients, such as the B-complex vitamins, iron, or vitamins A and C. Physiological changes can also occur in the gastrointestinal mucosa that impair nutrient absorption and aggravate the malnutrition still further. Aggressive nutritional restoration methods may be needed to save a client's life. Clinical signs of this form of PCM include specific indicators of nutrient deficiences—such as neurological deficits due to B vitamin deficiencies, skin changes, and visual disturbances—as well as the symptoms associated with the other forms of PCM.

Nurses play a critical role in the prevention of PCM in hospitalized clients. An assessment of every client's nutritional status upon admission is the essential first step. Clients at high risk for development of PCM should then be identified—for example, those scheduled for major surgery; those who are unable to ingest foods; those scheduled for multiple procedures requiring pre-fasting; those suffering from nausea and vomiting; and those experiencing major physiological or psychological stresses. Early dietary interventions such as careful menu selection and use of supplements should be initiated for those at high risk. Continuous monitoring of nutritional status and collaboration with dieticians and physicians to initiate enteral or parenteral feeding (see later section) early rather than late is also essential.

Vitamin and Mineral Deficiencies. Table 25–6 lists some of the major primary nutritional deficiency diseases. These are all called primary nutritional deficiencies because they are due to a dietary lack of the nutrient. Secondary deficiency diseases result from the body's inability to absorb or metabolize specific nutrients, and are encountered in a wide variety of disease states and situations. For example, surgical removal of a part of the gastrointestinal tract can easily lead to a secondary nutritional deficiency. The symptoms of a secondary deficiency of a specific nutrient will be the same as a primary deficiency.

Obesity. Obesity is defined as a body weight of 20 to 30 percent or more above the ideal weight; in other words, obesity is too much body fat. The National Center for Health Statistics reports that 26 percent of American adults are obese. The average fat content of a man's body is 14 percent and of a woman's body is 23 percent. This is not necessarily the optimal proportion; the ideal body weight and body fat distribution for sex, age, and height are still subjects of much debate and little consensus. **Overweight** is defined as a body weight of 10 percent above the ideal weight.

The most commonly used standards of ideal weight are the tables developed by the Metropolitan Life Insurance Company (see Chap. 16). The most recent revision of these tables occurred in 1983, and set forth values from 2 to 13 pounds higher than the earlier standards. There is increasing concern regarding the abuse of these tables.[11] The public and health care professionals alike have tended to follow these tables blindly, often acquiring a false sense of complacency if weight is within normal ranges, as well as a mistaken sense of concern if it is outside the norms. Research is still ongoing to determine what is the ideal weight for most people. It appears that there may not be a single ideal weight that applies to groups based on age, sex, or frame; the more likely case is that every person has a unique ideal weight at which he or she feels best, functions optimally, and is physically most healthy.

Despite the controversy over definitions of under- and overweight, it is still obvious that millions of Americans are unhealthily overweight or perceive themselves to be so. Weight loss has become an important goal for countless individuals, due partly to social pressures engendered by the ideal of thinness, especially affecting women in our society. Nurses must approach the subject of weight loss with both knowledge and sensitivity—knowledge of the various etiologies of obesity and of safe, effective means of weight reduction and sensitivity to the great personal distress or lowered self-esteem that often afflicts clients who have unsuccessfully attempted to lose weight.

Social undesirability is not the most important reason why health care professionals consider obesity to be a major health problem in our society. The risks associated with obesity appear to be numerous. The two health problems for which research has *conclusively* demonstrated a link to obesity are hypertension and diabetes.[4] Traditional medical opinion has also implicated obesity in the development of

TABLE 25–6. PRIMARY NUTRITIONAL DEFICIENCY DISEASES

Disorder	Nutrient Deficiency	General Symptoms
Vitamin Deficiencies		
Ariboflavinosis	Riboflavin	Dermatitis, eye lesions
Beriberi	Thiamine	Neuromuscular dysfunction
Hypovitaminosis A	Vitamin A	Corneal damage, blindness, night blindness, eye infections
Megaloblastic anemia	Folic acid	Weakness, shortness of breath, sore tongue, diarrhea, edema
Pellagra	Niacin	Gastrointestinal disturbances, stomatitis, dermatitis, neurological changes
Pernicious anemia	Folic acid, vitamin B_{12}	Weakness, pallor, fatigue, diarrhea, glossitis
Rickets	Vitamin D	Bone deformities
Scurvy	Vitamin C	Tissue and joint hemorrhages, impaired or delayed wound healing, anemia
Mineral Deficiencies		
Endemic goiter	Iodine	Enlarged thyroid gland
Iron deficiency anemia	Iron	Weakness, pallor, fatigue, headache, palpitations
Osteoporosis	Calcium	Curved spine, easy fracturing

hyperlipidemia, pulmonary and renal problems, and complications of pregnancy. Obese clients are considered to be higher surgical risks as well.

Currently, research regarding the etiology of obesity has focused on a number of different theories. Genetic, psychological, social, and physiological theories are under investigation. It appears that genetic inheritance influences a person's chances of becoming fat more than any other single factor. Although the high incidence of obesity within families may be partly due to socialization, studies of twins reared apart from each other have confirmed a strong genetic component.

A common misperception about individuals who are overweight or obese is that they have less control over their appetites and associate food with highly charged emotions. In fact, research has failed to support this characterization of overweight or obese people as a group. Other people exhibit the same psychological traits with about the same incidence;[12] however, there is no denying the critical role played by psychological factors in a client's efforts to lose weight.

Recent investigations have focused on physiological factors that may cause a predisposition to obesity. The "fat cell theory" maintains that every individual has a certain number of fat cells in the body. The number of fat cells determines how much body fat there will be. The fat cell quota is partly genetically determined, and is also influenced by eating patterns, particularly during infancy and childhood. There is a natural biological tendency to keep all of the fat cells filled with fat. Therefore, depletion of the cells' fat content by dieting simulates the experience of starvation within the organism, making weight loss extremely difficult to accomplish. It appears that exercise can exert an influence over fat cell metabolism so that the size of the cells is reduced.[13,14]

Another physiological theory that demonstrates the importance of exercise in treatment of obesity is set point theory. This theory takes an analogy from the home heater thermostat, which is set for a particular room temperature and will regulate the activity of the heater to maintain this temperature. Similarly, in each human body there is a "set point" for a certain amount of body fat. Weight loss will be difficult if this set point is violated. For example, some researchers have shown that after a few days of dieting, the body reacts by lowering the basal metabolic rate (BMR), thus making more efficient use of the calories available and making weight loss progressively more difficult; however, it does appear that the set point can be lowered by increasing the amount of physical exercise. This also raises the BMR, and "programs" the body to store less fat than it did before.[15]

The most effective approach to weight reduction appears to be a combination of an individualized reduced-calorie diet, regular exercise, and continuous social/psychological support. As indicated above, exercise clearly has physiological benefits that dramatically increase the effectiveness of dietary measures. Realistic goals, three or more balanced meals a day, and low-calorie snack foods also are helpful for the weight-reduction plan. See the section on nursing management for some specific approaches to healthful weight reduction.

Eating Disorders

Both anorexia nervosa and bulimia are severely destructive eating disorders attributed in large part to the American obsession with thinness. Common to both of these disorders is a deep-rooted insecurity, low self-esteem, dissatisfaction with one's body image, and extreme and pervasive fear of fatness. The actual behaviors associated with each of these disorders differ. However, many individuals manifest behaviors associated with *both* of these syndromes.

Anorexia Nervosa. Anorexia nervosa is, virtually, self-imposed starvation. It occurs primarily in adolescent and young adult females, but is also seen among women in their middle years. Usually, people with anorexia nervosa do not have any loss of appetite, but rigorously control intake. The typical client may be described as a perfectionistic, achievement-oriented adolescent or young woman who seeks control over her life by refusing to eat. Despite extreme emaciation, the disturbed body image of the person with anorexia nervosa will cause her to believe that she is too fat. The physiological effects of this long-term, slow starvation are drastic and frequently life-threatening. Brain shrinkage, endocrine disturbances such as amenorrhea, and severe nutritional deficiencies and metabolic imbalances result. Death is not unusual in prolonged, extreme cases.

Bulimia. Bulimia is characterized by a behavior pattern of uncontrollable binge eating of enormous amounts of food, followed by self-induced vomiting and use of laxatives or diuretics to control weight. The preferred foods are usually sweet, rich, and fatty. Most bulimic individuals maintain a thin appearance but do not *lose* weight; this factor makes their eating practices more difficult to detect. Tooth decay, menstrual irregularities, and severe electrolyte imbalances leading to life-threatening cardiac arrhythmias are the most common associated problems. Individuals with bulimia suffer from a double obsession—a craving for rich, tasty food and an obsessive fear of fatness. The cause is unknown, but theories include traumatic events involving loss, a history of being overweight, social pressures for thinness, and psychological depression as contributing to its onset.[16,17]

Anorectic and bulimic behaviors are often combined. For example, a person with anorexia may induce vomiting even without having consumed a large quantity of food. At times, individuals with bulimia may maintain periods of semistarvation in an attempt to control their weight, or induce vomiting after a normal-sized meal. Nurses must realize that these people often develop ingenious methods to hide their illness from others. Often, the physical effects of the disorder will be the first clues that a serious problem exists.

Section 2. Assessment of Nutrition

NUTRITIONAL DATA COLLECTION

All of the information discussed in the prior section must be applied through the nursing process to meet the client's nutritional needs. In the current section, the assessment phase of the nursing process will be discussed in relation to these needs. The importance of the assessment phase for nutritional planning and implementation cannot be overemphasized. Only through a thorough assessment can individualized client care be provided.

Nutritional assessment cannot be complete without full collaboration with clients. Because of the psychosocial meanings associated with food and eating, it is essential that the assessment take place within the context of a mutually developed nurse–client relationship. Clients must feel free to reveal all the details of their eating habits and nutritional state with full support, respect, and confidentiality on the part of the nurse. Data gathering for the assessment of nutritional status must include a nutritional history, physical examination, and a review of relevant laboratory and diagnostic test results.

Nutritional History

Taking the nutritional history elicits a wealth of subjective data concerning the client's eating habits, past nutritional problems, current or potential nutritional problems, and attitudes and knowledge about foods and nutrition. Family and social eating patterns are also of great significance in understanding the client's eating behaviors and for planning any changes. Without the client's collaboration, it is difficult to gain a complete or accurate history.

Primary Concern. The client history will reveal if a client's primary concern is related to nutrition. Some clients may refer directly to appetite, eating problems, body weight, or recent gains/losses in weight as a primary concern; however, many other stated concerns such as fatigue, skin problems, gastrointestinal problems, or generally diminished well-being may be nutrition related. Obtaining information about eating habits and nutritional status determines whether a client's primary concern can be corrected by nutrition-related approaches. The following example presents a nutrition-related primary concern.

- Debbie Ryan, a 15-year-old girl, comes to an outpatient clinic seeking help for her "horrible skin". The nurse notes that Debbie is quite obese and recognizes that the skin problem and the weight problem could both be related to nutritional habits. The nurse acknowledges Debbie's concerns and works with her to identify strategies that will both improve her skin and reduce her weight.

Current Understanding. If a client perceives that the current health problem is interfering with nutritional needs, review the Current Understanding as detailed in Chapter 16. As discussed above, illness or injury from almost any cause can create disturbances in a client's ability to meet nutritional needs. Treatments for many health problems likewise can cause nutritional problems for a client, as illustrated by the following example.

- Mrs. Anderson, a client undergoing chemotherapy after a modified radical mastectomy, complains that nausea has drastically reduced her food intake and caused her to lose 20 pounds of weight in 3 months. The nurse asks Mrs. Anderson for specific information about the degree of nausea; when exactly she experiences it in relation to administration of chemotherapy and how long it lasts; whether she has associated symptoms such as vomiting, diarrhea, and abdominal cramps; what makes the nausea better or worse; and what Mrs. Anderson has done to control the nausea. The nurse knows that cancer chemotherapy itself can cause nausea, and that people often experience anticipatory nausea prior to administration of chemotherapy. Obtaining a current understanding of the problem helps the nurse determine if this is anticipatory nausea, which will require different management than post-chemotherapy nausea.

Past Health Problems/Experiences. The nurse also needs to know if a client has experienced any health problems in the past that have altered nutritional status. Note the date, duration, treatment, and residual effects of any nutritional problems. Identify medications currently in use that could affect nutritional status, such as antibiotics, diuretics, and chemotherapy.

Personal, Family, and Social History. Ascertain any family history of obesity, eating disorders, food allergies, diabetes, hypertension, heart disease, cancer, colitis, or ulcers.

IMPLICATIONS FOR NURSE–CLIENT COLLABORATION

Nutritional Assessment

The nurse has an important role in promoting the health of every client. One of the ways nurses promote health is by discussing nutrition with their clients. This is done not only to identify clients' dietary habits, but also to assess clients' basic understanding of energy balance and the nutrient content of the foods they eat and beverages they drink. Questioning clients about their knowledge of basic nutrients and the caloric value of foods in their diet should be part of every health assessment. An exchange of information on dietary intake is an important part of a collaborative nurse–client relationship.

TABLE 25–7. NUTRITIONAL HISTORY: PERSONAL, FAMILY, AND SOCIAL HISTORY QUESTIONS

A. **Vocational**
1. What type of work do you do?
2. What hours do you work?
3. Does your work involve any physical activity?
4. Does your work ever cause you to skip meals or influence what you eat or drink?

B. **Home and family**
1. Do you live alone or with someone?
2. Does your family eat most meals together?
3. Do you like to cook?
4. Who buys food and cooks meals at home?
5. Do you eat alone much? Does that change what you cook? How much do you eat?

C. **Social, Leisure, Spiritual, and Cultural**
1. What kind of leisure activities do you enjoy?
2. Do you have time for leisure activities every week?
3. Do you eat with your friends often? What and where?
4. What kinds of foods do your friends prefer?
5. Do you eat out often?
6. Does your religion or culture of origin influence your food habits and preferences?

D. **Habits**

Exercise
1. Is your life-style active or sedentary?
2. Do you have a program of regular exercise? If so, what is it?
3. What kind of physical activity do you do in an average week?

Diet
1. Please write down everything that you have eaten or drunk in the last 24 hours. Is this a typical day's diet for you? If not, describe your usual pattern, if any.
2. Do you have regular meal times?
3. What times of the day do you eat?
4. Is your pattern at work the same as at home?
5. Under what conditions do you usually eat (noisy, relaxed, rushed, clean, dirty, etc)?
6. What special foods do you particularly enjoy?
7. What foods do you dislike?

Beverages
1. Do you usually drink liquids with meals? What type? How much?
2. What sorts of beverages do you drink between meals?
3. Do you drink alcohol?
4. Does alcohol intake ever influence what you eat?
5. Do you ever miss meals because of drinking?

Tobacco
1. Do you smoke? Use other forms of tobacco? Have you recently quit?
2. Do you notice a change in your appetite since you quit using tobacco?
3. Do you feel using tobacco changes the taste of foods you eat?

Other substances
1. Do you take any drugs not prescribed by a doctor? Any recreational drugs?
2. Have you noticed any change in your eating habits since you began taking _____?
3. Do you ever miss meals because of taking _____?

E. **Psychological**

Coping
1. What kind of situations either increase or decrease your appetite?
2. Do you ever eat when you aren't hungry? For example, because you are nervous? Stressed? Angry? Other reasons?
3. Do stress or emotions ever keep you from eating?
4. What is your overall feeling about food?

Self-image
1. Are you satisfied with your current weight?
2. Is there anything you would change about your body?
3. Do you ever skip meals or limit what you eat, even though you are hungry?
4. Have you ever made yourself vomit after eating?

These disorders are all associated with genetic etiologies, so a family history alerts nurses to the need for further evaluation and preventive measures. As discussed above, the psychological and sociocultural aspects of food and eating are of utmost importance in developing a collaborative approach to nutritional planning. Without a full understanding of the personal and sociocultural meaning of food, the nurse will be ineffective in working with the client. The questions in Table 25–7 are some suggestions for obtaining information about nutrition-related aspects of the client's life. It should be emphasized that questions and discussion related to culture and life-style must be approached in a sympathetic, nonjudgmental manner. The following example demonstrates the relevance of personal, family, and social history to health.

- Mr. Costello, a 46-year-old investment executive, is under treatment for chest pain of cardiac origin. The nurse asks Mr. Costello if anyone in his family has heart disease and if so at what age it was diagnosed. Because of the association of heart disease with a high-fat diet and stress, the nurse also pays special attention to Mr. Costello's personal and social nutritional history. Mr. Costello states that his father died of a heart attack at the age of 43. He states that he always has business lunches such as steak and french fries, and often does the same for dinner. His wife works also, and when they eat at home they often heat up commercial frozen foods in the microwave.

The fast pace and pressures of Mr. Costello's life become clear. The nurse realizes that he is particularly at risk for a heart attack because of his family history and life-style. The nurse knows that low-fat, low-salt meals are important dietary changes that Mr. Costello should make, and discusses with him low-fat foods that can be ordered at a restaurant. Mr. Costello is advised of the benefits of low-salt frozen foods and fresh fruits and vegetables. The nurse also discusses a program of regular exercise and relaxation techniques as stress-reducing measures.

BUILDING NURSING KNOWLEDGE

How Can the Nurse Identify Clients in the Hospital Who are at Risk for Malnourishment?

Karp RJ. The use of the "at-risk" concept to identify malnourished hospitalized patients. *Nutr Clin Practice.* 1988;3: 150–153.

The "at-risk" concept was developed from work in underdeveloped societies. It allows for early identification of clients in need of diagnostic and therapeutic services. An at-risk client is one with a predisposition to illness or one who has easily recognizable signs that illness is impending. Karp warns that early identification of malnourishment is important because of the serious complications that may develop, particularly among clients who have had surgery and who need nutrients to support tissue healing.

Karp reports that the sign found to be most effective as a screening indicator in identifying at-risk hospitalized clients is that of a 6 percent weight loss. This sign was found in studies to have a positive predictive value for nutrition-associated complications of surgery, and was valuable as a first step in identifying those clients who are at risk.

Subjective Manifestations. The nurse's questioning of a client regarding subjective manifestations is an extremely valuable tool for identifying related or hidden problems and for gaining a comprehensive view of a client's situation. Nurses make use of these findings in designing care plans with clients that address all of their nutritional problems and concerns. Chapter 16 provides sample questions for subjective manifestations.

Nutritional Examination

Areas of particular importance when conducting a physical examination for determining nutritional status are the client's general appearance, skin, mucus membranes, abdomen, and muscles. Certain physical measurements are also useful sources of data. Following are specific assessment areas for nutritional status.

Measurements. Measures of height, weight, and other anthropometric indicators are essential for making judgments about a client's nutritional status. A change in weight is an important indicator for diminished nutritional health. A 6 percent weight loss has been found to be a strong predictor of nutrition-associated complications of surgery, such as malnutrition, infections, and respiratory problems.[18] Height and weight should be measured with reliable scales and in a consistent manner. Compare the measurements to standard height and weight tables for the client's age and sex. Height and weight also can be used to compute body mass index (BMI), an index of a person's weight in relation to height. BMI is calculated by dividing weight in kilograms by the square of the height in meters. It is considered a more reliable indicator of obesity than weight alone. The desired range for women is 19.1 to 27.3, and for men 20.7 to 27.8. Obesity-associated health risks occur when BMI is in the range of 27 to 32; if BMI is more than 44.8, the individual is considered morbidly obese.

Other anthropometric measurements that dieticians use to make inferences about body fat and protein stores include the midarm circumference (MAC, MUAC), and the triceps skinfold (TSF). These two values can be used to compute the midarm muscle circumference (MMC). Although not routinely used by nurses, they are useful in collaborative assessment of high-risk clients.

Objective Manifestations

General Observations. General observations comprise the next aspect of the nutritional examination. Observe the client's overall appearance. Does the client appear over- or underweight? Does the client appear to be physically fit or unfit? What level of energy does the client appear to have? Do eyes appear dull or bright? Is there anything unusual about the client's breath and body odor? Do the client's movements, posture, or gestures indicate any abdominal pain? Does the client appear self-conscious or embarrassed about his or her body? Is clothing appropriate for age and climate, neat, and clean? What is the client's overall mood and quality of speech?

Any of the following findings suggest that nutritional problems may exist: excessive or inadequate body weight; flabby or wasted muscles; low energy level; dull or inflamed eyes; foul breath or body odor; appearance of abdominal pain; extreme self-consciousness about one's body; inappropriate, dirty, or disheveled clothing; slurred speech; poor posture; tremors or twitching; lack of alertness; irritability; and apathy.

Integument. Note any cracks in the corners of the mouth, the luster and quality of hair, the condition of the scalp, any rashes or petechiae (bruises) on the skin, and the overall condition of the skin, hair, and nails (see Chap. 16). The following findings indicate a possible nutritional problem: edema; pallor or jaundice; dermatitis or skin lesions; poor skin turgor; dull, brittle, or sparse hair; petechiae; dry or rough skin; and spoon-shaped, brittle, or rigid nails.

HEENT (Head, Eyes, Ears, Nose, and Throat). Note the clearness of the eyes, condition of the membranes, color of the sclera, and presence of any lesions on the eyelids. Assess vision. Eye findings that suggest possible nutritional problems include pale conjunctivae, redness of conjunctivae, dryness or inflammation, dullness of the cornea, and presence of infection or exudate. What is the number, condition, looseness of the teeth? If the client has dentures, are there any pressure areas visible on the gums? Are there any lumps or patches on the lips, mucosa, or tongue? If so, are the lumps fixed or movable? Is the thyroid gland palpable? Any of the following findings suggests the existence of a nutritional problem: swollen or spongy mucous membranes; red, inflamed, spongy, receding, or bleeding gums; swollen and inflamed tongue; unfilled caries, absent teeth; dry, cracked, or swollen lips; lesions at the corners of the lips; or an enlarged thyroid gland.

Abdomen. Note the presence or absence of symmetry, visible peristalsis (rhythmic intestinal contractions), masses, swellings, distention, ostomies, scars, striae (stretch marks), distended blood vessels, jaundice, and petechiae. Auscultate for the presence, frequency, and pitch of bowel sounds in all four quadrants. Lightly palpate for any muscle tenderness, distention, rigidity, or resistance. Findings suggestive of nutritional problems are hyper- or hypoactive bowel sounds; ascites; distention; palpable liver or spleen; presence of masses; jaundice, distended blood vessels, petechiae; and visible peristalsis.

Musculoskeletal. Assess the development of muscle tissue; muscle tone, strength, and size; presence of subcutaneous fat; and any skeletal malformations. Any of the following findings indicates a probable nutritional problem: poor muscle tone, muscle wasting, undeveloped muscles, decreased muscle strength (see Chap. 30), or muscle twitching.

Neurological. Assess reflexes, sensation, and the presence of any tremors or seizure activity (see Chap. 16). Vitamin deficiencies often alter neurological functioning. Table 25–8 summarizes the clinical signs of good and poor nutrition.

Diagnostic Tests

Laboratory tests, x-ray studies, and endoscopic exams are the most commonly used diagnostic approaches for diagnosis of nutritional problems. Nurses must be able to explain the purpose of these procedures and tests, prepare clients appropriately or ensure that clients have performed self-preparation appropriately, and monitor the results so that abnormalities are incorporated into the plan of client care.

Laboratory Tests. Laboratory tests are an important element of nutritional assessment. They are particularly useful in confirming malnutrition in an at-risk population;[18] however, one study showed that only 10 percent of nurses working on medical and surgical units of a large midwestern hospital routinely used laboratory data as part of their nutritional assessment.[19] Lymphocyte count, albumin, hemoglobin, and transferrin are especially useful. The blood and urine tests conducted to assess nutritional status may involve requirements that the client refrain from eating for a specified amount of time, or observe certain dietary specifications. See Table 25–9 for a description of laboratory tests that may be ordered for assessment of nutritional status. No single client will be subject to all of these tests; the physician will determine which are needed.

X-ray Studies. For abdominal x-rays and scans, often a bowel cleansing regimen and ingestion of a special radiopaque substance are needed. Clients must understand that observing the preparatory regimen is absolutely essential to the success of the test. If preparation has not been carefully completed, usually the entire regimen and test will need to be repeated. The nurse plays a key role in providing clients with a complete explanation of x-rays to be done and the specific self-preparation requirements (Table 25–9).

Endoscopic Examinations. Endoscopic examinations are invasive procedures in which a long, narrow tube with a light and magnifying lens on the distal end is inserted into the digestive tract, either through the mouth or the anus. Any portion of the digestive tract may be examined. Gastroscopy and colonoscopy are two common examples. Endoscopic procedures require that clients provide informed consent.

■ NURSING DIAGNOSIS OF NUTRITIONAL STATUS

The collaborative gathering of subjective and objective data provides the foundation for developing a nursing diagnosis of the client's nutritional status. It may be relatively easy to determine whether there is an excess or deficiency of calories or specific nutrients, but determination of the etiology of the problem requires the utmost skill on the part of the nurse and complete honesty on the part of the client. Clients need to be fully informed regarding the reasons for the assessment questions and diagnostic tests. The significance of all the information obtained through the assessment must also be explained.

The process of formulating the nursing diagnosis is likewise a collaborative venture. The nurse and the client should review the assessment data together, and should if possible develop the diagnosis and its etiology together. At the very least, the nurse's diagnostic judgment should be shared with clients or family so that the plan of care may be mutually developed and effectively implemented. Remember that initiating changes in a person's dietary regimen is

TABLE 25–8. CLINICAL SIGNS OF NUTRITIONAL STATUS

Body Area	Signs of Good Nutritional Status	Signs of Poor Nutritional Status
General		
Appearance	Alert, responsive.	Listless, apathetic, cachexia.
Vitality	Endurance, energetic, sleeps well, vigorous.	Easily fatigued, no energy, falls asleep easily, looks tired, apathetic.
Weight	Normal for height, age, body build.	Overweight or underweight.
Integument		
Hair	Shiny, lustrous, firm, not easily plucked, healthy scalp.	Dull and dry, brittle, loss of color, easily plucked, thin and sparse.
Face	Uniform skin color; healthy appearance, not swollen.	Dark skin over cheeks and under eyes, flaky skin, facial edema (moon face), pale skin color
Skin	Smooth, good color, slightly moist, no sign of rashes, swelling, or color irregularities.	Rough, dry, flaky, swollen, pale, pigmented, lack of fat under skin, fat deposits around the joints (xanthomas), bruises, petechiae.
Nails	Firm, pink.	Spoon shaped (koilonychia), brittle, pale, ridged.
HEENT		
Eyes	Bright, clear, moist, no sores at corners or eyelids, membranes moist and healthy pink color, no prominent blood vessels.	Pale eye membranes, dry eyes (xerophthalmia); Bitot's spots, increased vascularity, cornea soft (keratomalacia), small yellowish lumps around eyes (xanthelasma), dull or scarred cornea.
Lips	Good pink color, smooth, moist, not chapped or swollen.	Swollen and puffy (cheilosis), angular lesions at corners of mouth, or fissures or scars (stomatitis).
Tongue	Deep red, surface papillae present.	Smooth appearance, beefy red or magenta colored, swollen, papillae, hypertrophy or atrophy.
Gums	Firm, good pink color, no swelling or bleeding.	Spongy, bleed easily, marginal redness, recessed, swollen and inflamed.
Glands	No enlargement of thyroid, face not swollen.	Enlargement of thyroid (goiter), enlargement of parotid (swollen cheeks).
Cardiovascular	Normal heart rate and rhythm, no murmurs, normal blood pressure for age.	Cardiac enlargement, tachycardia, elevated blood pressure.
Gastrointestinal	No palpable organs or masses (liver edge may be palpable in children).	Hepatosplenomegaly.
Abdomen	Flat.	Swollen.
Musculoskeletal		
Skeleton	Good posture, no malformations.	Poor posture, beading of the ribs, bowed legs or knock-knees, prominent scapulas, chest deformity, deformity at diaphragm.
Teeth	Straight, no crowding, no cavities, no pain, bright, no discoloration, well-shaped jaw.	Cavities, mottled appearance (fluorosis), malpositioned, missing teeth.
Muscles	Well developed, firm, good tone, some fat under skin.	Flaccid, poor tone, wasted, underdeveloped, difficulty walking.
Extremities	No tenderness.	Weak and tender, presence of edema.
Neurological	Normal reflexes, psychological stability.	Decrease in or loss of ankle and knee reflexes, psychomotor changes, mental confusion, depression, sensory loss, motor weakness, loss of sense of position, loss of vibration, burning and tingling of hands and feet (paresthesia).

From Dudek SG. Nutrition Handbook for Nursing Practice. *Philadelphia: Lippincott; 1987, with permission.*

TABLE 25–9. TESTS OF NUTRITIONAL STATUS

Test	Findings/Implications: Normal	Findings/Implications: Abnormal	Client Preparation
Red blood cell count (RBC)	Male: 4.6–6.1 million/mm^3 Female: 4.2–5.4 million/mm^3	Decreased with iron deficiency, vitamin B_{12} deficiency. Mean cell volume (MCV) increased with B_{12} deficiency and decreased with iron deficiency. Mean cell hemoglobin concentration (MCHC) decreased with iron deficiency.	None
Hemoglobin (hgb or hg)	Male: 14–18 g/dL Female: 12–16 g/dL	Decreased if inadequate protein or Fe intake.	None
Hematocrit (hct)	Male: 40–54% Female: 37–47%	Decreased if inadequate protein or Fe intake.	None
Iron	50–150 g/dL	Decreased if inadequate iron intake and with protein malnutrition.	None
Total iron-binding capacity	250–450 μL/dL	Increased in iron deficiency anemia, decreased in protein deficiency. Sensitive indicator of protein malnutrition. 150–200: mild; 100–149: moderate; less than 100: severe.	None
Lymphocyte count	1700–3500/μL 25–35% of total WBCs	Decreased if inadequate protein intake. Sensitive indicator of nutritional state.	None
Protein serum urine	 6–8 g/dL 0–5 mg/dL	Decreased if inadequate protein intake or malabsorption syndrome.	Not after fatty meal
Albumin	3.5–5 g/dL	Decreased if inadequate protein intake; level of depletion implies degree of undernutrition. 2.8–3.4: mild; 2.1–2.7: moderate; less than 2.1: severe.	Not after fatty meal
Transferrin	20–50% saturation	Increased if iron stores low, decreased in protein malnutrition. TIBC is a quantitative measure of transferrin.	None
Calcium	4.5–5.5 mg/dL	Decreased if malabsorption or vitamin D deficiency.	None
Phosphorus	2.5–4.5 mg/dL	Decreased if vitamin D deficiency, undernutrition, starvation.	None
Fasting blood glucose	60–100 mg/dL	Increased if diabetic, in some infections.	Overnight fast
Fatty acids	25 mg/dL	Increase indicates high risk of heart disease.	Overnight fast
Cholesterol	120–220 mg/dL	Increase indicates high risk of heart disease: 200–240: moderate risk; greater than 240: high risk.	Overnight fast
HDL cholesterol	29–77 mg/dL	Less than 25: extreme risk for coronary heart disease (CHD); 26–35: high risk for CHD; 46–59: low risk for CHD.	Overnight fast
LDL cholesterol	60–160 mg/dL	Greater than 160: high risk for CHD; 130–159: moderate risk for CHD.	Overnight fast
Lipids	400–1000 mg/dL	Increase indicates high risk of heart disease.	Overnight fast
Triglycerides	20–190 mg/dL	Increase indicates high risk of heart disease.	Overnight fast
Creatinine serum urine	 0.5–1.5 mg/dL 85–135 mL/min	Decreased if inadequate protein intake, decreased in catabolic states when muscle mass depleted.	None
Urea nitrogen serum urine	 5–25 mg/dL varies with intake	Increased in catabolic state. 24-hour urine test can be compared to protein intake to assess nitrogen balance.	None
Barium x-ray	Normal organ structure and function	Abnormalities influence ingestion, digestion, or absorption.	Special diet and/or bowel cleansing (see Chap. 26)
Endoscopy	Normal organ structure and function	Abnormalities influence ingestion, digestion, or absorption.	Overnight fast and/or bowel cleansing (see Chap. 26)

From Collinsworth R, Boyle K. Nutritional assessment of the elderly. J Gerontol Nurs. *1989; 15:17–27. Eschleman MM.* Introductory Nutrition and Diet Therapy. *Philadelphia: Lippincott; 1991. Kee JL.* Handbook of Laboratory and Diagnostic Tests With Nursing Implications. *Norwalk, CT: Appleton & Lange; 1990. Pagana KD, Pagana TJ.* Diagnostic Testing and Nursing Implications. *3rd ed. St Louis: Mosby; 1990. Whitney EN, Cataldo CB, Rolfes SR.* Understanding Normal and Clinical Nutrition. *3rd ed. St Paul: West; 1991.*

an extremely difficult task. It becomes even more difficult if the problem-solving process is not a collaborative one.

Three nursing diagnoses related to nutrition have been identified by the National Conference Group for Classification of Nursing Diagnoses. These are: Altered Nutrition: Less than Body Requirements (specify deficit), Altered Nutrition: More than Body Requirements (specify excess), and Altered Nutrition: Potential for More than Body Requirements. These diagnoses are elaborated in the table Sample Nursing Diagnosis: Nutrition (below), which lists examples of subjective and objective data (defining characteristics) and sample etiologies. Other nursing diagnoses related to altered nutrition are listed in Box 25–6.

In addition to identifying the general nursing diagnosis, the specific excess or deficit must also be determined. Nurse must draw upon comprehensive knowledge of the signs of specific nutritional deficiencies to specify whether the alteration is related to calories, protein, carbohydrates, fats, particular vitamins, or minerals. For example, generalized overweight or underweight indicates an alteration in caloric intake. Inadequate muscular development or tone indicates a protein deficiency, as do the more severe signs of protein–calorie malnutrition discussed previously. An excess of carbohydrates may manifest as excess body weight, whereas a deficit will result in depletion of protein and fat reserves and a gradual weight loss. Inadequate intake of fats may lead to dryness of skin and hair and, if severe, hormonal alterations. Excessive intake of fats directly relates to an increase in body fat. Refer to Tables 25–3 and 25–4 for the signs of specific vitamin and mineral deficits. Often these deficits accompany calorie and/or protein deficiencies. The client's report about dietary patterns is crucial to accurate diagnosis of the specific deficiency or excess.

Altered Nutrition: Less Than Body Requirements

Altered Nutrition: Less than Body Requirements is an insufficient intake of nutrients to meet metabolic needs. This situation may result from conditions that interrupt the sup-

SAMPLE NURSING DIAGNOSES: NUTRITION

Nursing Diagnosis	Defining Characteristics/Manifestations		Etiology
	Subjective Data	Objective Data	
Altered Nutrition: More than Body Requirements for Calories *1.1.2.1.*	Reports chronic or sudden weight increase Reports sedentary life-style: "I usually don't like exercise"	Weight more than 20% above ideal Increased subcutaneous fat: triceps skin fold greater than norms	*Physical:* Excessive intake in relation to metabolic need: sedentary life-style
Altered Nutrition: Less than Body Requirements for Calories *1.1.2.2.*	None	Weight 20% below ideal 24-hour food intake less than 70% of RDA Not oriented to person, place, time or situation Progressive weight loss Poor muscle tone	*Cognitive:* Inability to ingest food: confusion
Altered Nutrition: Less than Body Requirements for Calories and Protein *1.1.2.2.*	States does not have enough money to buy food Reported food intake is less than RDA	Weekly food expenditures indicate inadequate money for food Steady weight loss Weight 20% below ideal 24-hour food intake less than 70% of RDA Poor muscle tone	*Sociocultural/Life Structural:* Inability to ingest food: insufficient income
Altered Nutrition: Less than Body Requirements for Protein *1.1.2.2.*	Reported intake of protein foods is less than RDA Unable to state importance of protein in diet Unable to list foods high in protein	Decreased muscle mass Poor muscle tone Generalized edema Decreased RBC count Decreased serum protein or albumin Decreased lymphocyte count	*Cognitive:* Inability to ingest protein: knowledge deficit

SAMPLE NURSING DIAGNOSIS NUTRITION (continued)

Nursing Diagnosis	Risk Factor
Altered Nutrition: Potential for More than Body Requirements for Calories *1.1.2.3.*	*Sociocultural/Life Structural:* Social/occupational situation encourages overeating and drinking

ply or use of nutrients or that increase the body's demand for nutrients. The nutritional deficit may be in calories, protein, fat, specific vitamins or minerals, or any combination of these. Height and weight tables will help to determine if a general caloric deficit exists. A body weight of 20 percent or more below the ideal is a major defining characteristic of this diagnosis. More specific assessment data are necessary to determine deficits of individual nutrients. The general etiologies of a nutritional deficit are briefly discussed below, along with more specific defining characteristics.

BOX 25–6. OTHER NURSING DIAGNOSES RELATED TO NUTRITION

Physical

Activity Intolerance
Constipation
Diarrhea
Impaired Physical Mobility
Ineffective Breathing Pattern
Fatigue
Fluid Volume Deficit
High Risk for Fluid Volume Deficit
Altered Oral Mucous Membranes
Self-feeding Deficit
Impaired Skin Integrity
High Risk for Impaired Skin Integrity
Impaired Swallowing
Impaired Tissue Integrity

Cognitive

Altered Health Maintenance
Knowledge Deficit
Altered Thought Processes

Emotional

Anxiety
Ineffective Individual Coping
Anticipatory Grieving
Dysfunctional Grieving
Spiritual Distress

Self-conceptual

Body Image Disturbance
Self-Esteem Disturbance

Sociocultural/Life Structural

Ineffective Family Coping: Compromised
Ineffective Family Coping: Disabling
Diversional Activity Deficit
Altered Family Processes
Impaired Home Maintenance Management
Social Isolation
Impaired Social Interaction

Etiology: Inability to Ingest Foods. A client may experience difficulty in ingesting foods due to a wide variety of possible factors. There may be a deformity of the oral cavity such as a cleft palate. There may be a medical problem such as cancer of the throat or an esophageal hernia. Such physical limitations on ingestion are often associated with protein deficiency, because of the difficulty encountered in eating meat. Psychological factors such as an obsessive fear of being poisoned or of becoming fat may be the cause of a severe limitation of food ingestion. Social and economic factors may place limits on the quantity and quality of food intake as serious and intractable as any physical causes.

Etiology: Inability to Digest Foods. Problems leading to an inability to digest foods are equally variable. There may be a congenital or surgically induced lack of one or more organs involved in digestion, such as the small intestine or the gallbladder. There may be a disease process, such as cancer or cystic fibrosis, that alters the gastrointestinal tract's secretion of enzymes or hormones essential for digestion. Psychological factors such as anxiety may interfere with digestion by causing severe diarrhea or vomiting. An inability to digest foods may be either complete, or specific for certain foods. For example, the client with celiac disease has particular difficulty with the digestion of fats. Many people experience allergies or enzyme deficiencies for particular foods, such as an inability to digest milk due to lactose intolerance.

Etiology: Inability to Absorb Nutrients. Structural alterations, disease processes, and other pathological processes may be responsible for problems with the absorption of nutrients. For example, a client who has undergone a total gastrectomy (removal of the stomach) will lack any supply of intrinsic factor, which is essential for the absorption of vitamin B_{12}. Thus, the client will not be able to absorb this particular nutrient. Inflammatory or infectious disease processes may alter the mucosal lining of the intestines so much that absorption will be impaired. Diarrhea due to psychological or physical factors may interfere with nutrient absorption because there is not enough contact time between the food and the mucosal lining.

Etiology: Knowledge Deficit. Knowledge deficits are among the most common etiologies of inadequate nutritional intake. One study investigating nutrient intake and knowledge about nutrition found that 70 percent of the population studied had intakes of less than 60 percent of the recommended dietary allowances for one or more nutrients. Most of them failed a simple test of nutrition knowledge. The average score was 58 percent; 70 percent had never sought nutrition information.[20] Many, perhaps most, people base their eating habits on peer pressure, personal preferences and aversions, or sociocultural traditions. Nutrition education, even when provided, is not effective unless a person is motivated to learn and the information is presented in a way that is easy to grasp. Knowledge deficits can lead to deficits in total energy or to deficits or excesses of any specific nutrient.

Altered Nutrition: More than Body Requirements

Altered Nutrition: More Than Body Requirements is an excessive caloric or nutrient intake relative to metabolic need. A body weight of 20 percent or more over the ideal is the general defining characteristic. The fundamental etiology of this alteration is a food intake that is greater than energy expenditure.

Etiology: Excessive Intake in Relationship to Metabolic Need. This imbalance may be due to a low energy expenditure because of, for example, a sedentary life-style, or due to a hypometabolic state that may occur in certain diseases such as hypothyroidism. Or it may be due to a large food intake due to compulsive eating, overfeeding, or social factors. A number of dysfunctional eating patterns have been associated with the development of obesity. Some of them are the pairing of food with other activities (such as studying, watching television), eating in response to external cues (such as social situations), and eating in response to internal cues (such as anxiety or depression). Usually, the excess intake will be of fats and sugars rather than of protein.

Altered Nutrition: Potential for More than Body Requirements

Because of the importance of preventive approaches to obesity, the diagnosis Altered Nutrition: Potential for More Than Body Requirements is included in the taxonomy. This diagnosis is defined as the presence of risk factors for excess caloric intake relative to metabolic need. The presence of any of the risk factors discussed in the following paragraphs, particularly when combined with a sedentary life-style and dysfunctional eating patterns (described in the previous paragraph), are predictive of a high risk for obesity.

Risk Factor: Hereditary Predisposition. Research has amply documented that obesity tends to occur in persons who have overweight family members, particularly one or both parents. Controversy exists, however, as to whether this pattern of occurrence is due to genetically controlled metabolic factors or to a family's attitudes toward food and its eating patterns. Body build and certain rare genetic disorders are clearly hereditary in nature and may exert a powerful influence in the development of obesity.

Risk Factor: Excessive Energy Intake During Late Gestational Life, Early Infancy, and Adolescence. The determination of this etiology is based on research regarding the development of adipocytes (fat cells) during the life span. Certain critical periods occur during which the adipocytes are most susceptible to proliferation or growth in size. These critical periods are the last half of pregnancy, the first two years after birth, and the adolescent years. If nutritional intake, especially of fats and sugar, exceeds energy requirements during these critical periods, fat tissue will be synthesized or increased and will be extremely difficult to remove or decrease afterward.

Risk Factor: Frequent, Closely Spaced Pregnancies. Because of the rapid and significant weight gain that normally occurs during pregnancy, women who have numerous pregnancies with only a short time interval in between will have difficulty returning to their normal nonpregnant weight. Each subsequent pregnancy therefore occurs at a higher baseline weight, compounding the overall weight gain and the problems associated with losing the excess weight.

Risk Factor: Dysfunctional Psychological Conditioning in Relationship to Food. Because of the tremendous symbolic importance of food in relation to human needs such as love, care, comfort, taste, variety, and prosperity, it is not surprising that food can easily become a substitute source of fulfillment. This is what is meant by dysfunctional conditioning: food becomes a replacement for the usual means of meeting these needs. Once such a cycle starts, it can be a very complex process to reverse.

Risk Factor: Membership in Lower Socioeconomic Group. Nutritionally imbalanced diets often occur among populations that must buy inexpensive foods, many of which are high in fat and low in protein. Fresh fruit and vegetables, dairy products, and lean meats tend to cost more than starchy, fatty "junk foods." Excessive calories but low quantities of nutrients are the typical content of low-cost diets. Furthermore, in families where both parents work, children are often left unsupervised, free to consume high-calorie snacks. For these reasons, members of lower socioeconomic groups have a higher incidence of obesity than members of higher socioeconomic groups.

Risk Factor: Knowledge Deficit. The earlier discussion of knowledge deficit as an etiology of inadequate nutritional intake applies to this diagnosis as well.

Stating the Nutritional Diagnosis

The nursing diagnosis of the client's nutritional status is the basis for mutual planning to correct nutritional problems. A diagnostic statement that is most useful for planning clearly identifies not only the problem but also its specific etiology and the major defining characteristics that the client exhibits.

The taxonomy of nursing diagnoses lists general etiologies that underlie excessive or inadequate calories or nutrients for body needs. These etiologies have been discussed above. To be useful in a clinical situation, these general etiologies must be refined—that is, the specific contributing factor(s) need to be identified, not only so nurses can ascertain whether nursing therapy can correct the problem but also so specific nursing implementation can be determined.

For example, a client who cannot ingest food because of a biological factor, paralysis of muscles needed for swallowing, requires medical intervention. In contrast, a client whose inability to ingest food is related to a different biological factor, ill-fitting dentures, can benefit from nursing measures to facilitate ingestion as a temporary measure until the denture problem is corrected.

There are multiple defining characteristics listed in the taxonomy that can be indicators of a nutritional problem. No one client would experience all of these signs and symptoms at the same time. Indicating those that a given client exhibits in the diagnostic statement facilitates later recognition of resolution of the problem, when these defining characteristics should no longer be evident.

The following are examples of complete nursing diagnostic statements of a nutritional problem:

1. Altered nutrition: less than body requirements for calories related to ill-fitting dentures, as evidenced by inability to ingest desired foods "because my upper plate slips" and "I can't chew right—makes me choke," sore inflamed buccal cavity, and body weight 20 percent less than ideal for height and frame.
2. Altered nutrition: more than body requirements for calories related to maintaining usual eating patterns while suspending regular exercise program, as evidenced by recent weight increase to 10 percent above ideal for height and frame, reports unable to attend exercise class because of schedule change, and description of typical daily intake "same as before," which is 500 kcal per day greater than calculated needs for current activity level.
3. Altered nutrition: potential for more than body requirements for calories and fat. Risk factors: 8-month-old child at 95th percentile of weight for age and height; mother reports continued intake of 30 ounces of formula daily while increasing intake of solid foods.

Section 3. Nurse–Client Management of Nutrition

PLANNING FOR OPTIMUM NUTRITION

After the assessment and diagnosis of nutritional status has been accomplished, the nurse and client must collaborate for the planning of desirable outcomes of care, strategies to attain these outcomes, and evaluation criteria to determine the extent to which the outcomes were achieved.

The more that desired outcomes are a reflection of the client's true wishes and expectations, as well as of the nurse's knowledge and experience, the greater will be the chances of successful accomplishment of the plan of care. For example, a diagnosis of altered nutrition: more than body requirements for calories due to excessive intake in relation to metabolic needs may have been made. The client may wish to lose 30 pounds in time for a vacation 1 month away. The nurse realizes that this is not a realistic expectation and sharing expertise in this matter will spare the client disappointment and frustration, and allow for realistically attainable goals and timeframes to be established. If the excessive intake is primarily due to emotional comfort derived from food, the holistic approach to outcome development focuses not on food intake alone but on resolving deeper emotional conflicts and on finding more enduring sources of emotional satisfaction. Appropriate outcomes would be: (1) client will ventilate emotions directly, (2) client will use support systems for emotional comfort, and (3) client will achieve a balance between calorie intake and metabolic needs.

The causes of nutritional alterations are complex and stem from all aspects of the person. Therefore, the desired outcomes of care must be equally holistic in scope. At the same time, evaluation criteria should be as specific as possible, with target dates for accomplishment.

Short-term outcomes are helpful to clients, as they are accomplished step by step in the direction of long-term goals. For example, a goal of increasing weight by 20 pounds for an anorexic will seem frightening and overwhelming. Identifying weekly goals of 1 or 2 pounds of weight gain will be easier to work with and more satisfying.

After determining specific desired outcomes for each nursing diagnosis, the next step in the collaborative planning of care for alterations in nutrition is determining effective measures to correct the alteration. The goal of planning client care is to maintain as high a level of client independence as possible, while promoting maximal nutritional benefit.

NURSING IMPLEMENTATION TO PROMOTE OPTIMUM NUTRITION

Nursing implementation to improve nutritional status encompasses a variety of approaches. The assessment data and desired outcomes direct clients and nurses to a general level of client care and to certain types of nursing approaches. The sample care plan Nurse–Client Management of Nutrition Problems on pages 1103–1105 describes examples of desired outcomes, nursing implementation, and evaluation criteria for sample diagnoses of nutritional alterations. These can be used as guidelines for individualized plans. In general, teaching activities and dietary counseling form an important part of a nutritional care plan. When clients cannot obtain foods or eat independently, more direct assistance—sometimes including specialized technical procedures—are required to provide a source of nutrition. These approaches are discussed in the following sections.

Preventive Care

The client requiring preventive care is in a healthy state, experiencing no obvious nutritional alterations; however, as mentioned earlier, high-level wellness depends on optimal nutrition, and is an appropriate goal of first-level nursing approaches. The identification of people at risk for nutritional alterations, either less than or greater than metabolic need, and nursing implementation designed to prevent nutritional alterations from occurring, are also important goals of preventive client care.

Life-style Analysis. Life-style analysis provides an important adjunct to the complete nutritional history and assessment for the identification of individuals at risk for nutritional alterations. A client's life-style provides important clues to potential nutritional problems. For example, a high-pressure, fast-paced career often predisposes an individual to caffeine and alcohol abuse, consumption of "junk foods," and inadequate relaxation for proper digestion. A sedentary life-style places a person at risk for nutrition intake greater than metabolic need. The etiologies for alterations in nutrition provide important clues about risk factors in apparently healthy individuals.

Life-style Counseling. Life-style counseling is indicated if the life-style analysis results in a client's decision to change to a healthier life-style. Counseling is a helping process in which clients define their needs and explore alternative solutions.[21] It is the client who determines the need for change and develops the plan of action. The nurse in the counseling role serves as a facilitator, rather than as a manager, of the process.

Values Clarification. Values clarification is another useful nursing approach for people at risk for nutritional alterations. Values are deep-seated, enduring beliefs about what is important in one's life. Clients will need to look within and at behavior to determine what kind of value they place on good nutrition in relation to other personal values. Does a client place more value on convenience and social conformity than on carefully prepared, healthy meals? Because nutrition is so directly related to health, how important is personal health in a client's scale of values? Does a client's money-spending patterns suggest that he or she values new clothes more than healthy food? Is time allowed for sharing relaxed, intimate meals with family or friends? Is cooking important? How important is it to the client to have a thin body? Does a client place more value on exercising or on reducing intake as a source of weight control?

Such questions and examination of behaviors and priorities are very useful in assisting clients to recognize what value they place on healthy eating. If clients recognize a contradiction between actual behavior and felt values, then they may be motivated to plan a change in life-style so that their actions are congruent with cherished values. Or, through discussion with the nurse, a client may decide to change priorities so that good nutrition is made a valued goal. Nutritional counseling can be effective only if clients value good nutrition.

Health Education. Basic nutritional knowledge is an essential tool that everyone should have in order to acquire and maintain optimum health. As the study previously mentioned pointed out, many people whose nutritional status is marginal have little knowledge of good nutrition.[20] Nurses are often in the position of being the providers of basic nutrition education. Chapter 20 provides a complete overview of the principles of teaching and learning. Nurses should assist clients to learn the following information: the names, functions, and food sources of the basic nutrients; appropriate dietary guidelines as discussed earlier in this chapter; and normal developmental needs for nutrients.

In addition to serving as a direct teacher, the nurse also serves an important role as provider of written information and audiovisual resources (Fig. 25–6). Numerous nutri-

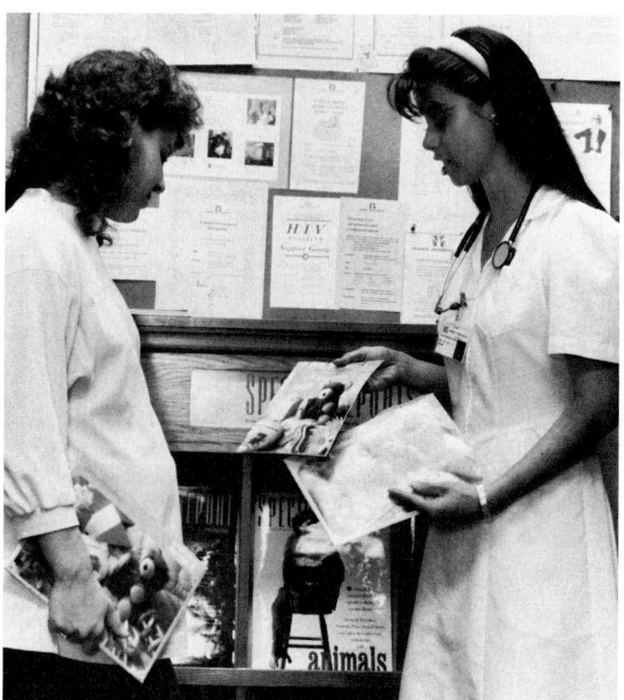

Figure 25–6. Women need to increase their intake of some nutrients during pregnancy. A nurse provides written guidelines to help this client achieve optimum intake.

NURSE–CLIENT MANAGEMENT OF NUTRITION PROBLEMS

Nursing Diagnosis	Desired Outcomes	Implementation	Evaluation
Altered Nutrition: More than Body Requirements for Calories R/T excessive intake in relation to metabolic need: sedentary life-style *1.1.2.1.*	1. Ideal body weight for height attained	1a. Review 24-hour food diary to identify patterns of excessive intake 1b. Teach principles and guidelines for good nutrition 1c. Provide food guide for use in menu planning 1d. Collaborate with client to plan a balanced and appealing low calorie diet 1e. Teach techniques to maintain diet plan: prepare small portions; eat slowly and chew thoroughly; eat low calorie snacks only at scheduled times; plan for a small weekly "splurge"; drink plenty of water	1a. Weight loss of 1-2 lb/week until ideal body weight attained 1b. Ideal body weight maintained
	2. Daily diet meets all RDAs	2a. Review 24-hour food diary to identify deficits of specific nutrients 2b. Teach principles and guidelines for good nutrition 2c. Provide food guide for use in menu planning 2d. Collaborate with client to plan a balanced and appealing low calorie diet	2a. 24-hour diary shows all RDAs met 2b. Physical exam: good muscle tone, skin, mucous membranes, and hair appear healthy; no edema; serum protein normal for age
	3. Engages in regular exercise	3a. Teach client ways that exercise promotes healthy weight loss 3b. Collaboratively develop a plan for increasing activity level and regular exercise that client enjoys	3. Client participates in aerobic exercise at least 30 min. 3–4 times per week
Altered Nutrition: Less than Body Requirements for Calories R/T inability to ingest food: confusion *1.1.2.2.*	1. Caloric and nutritional intake will meet RDAs	1a. Nurse, family or significant other to feed client. Meals planned by computing daily calorie and nutrient needs. 1b. Offer and assist with quality snacks between meals based on computation of daily calorie and nutrient needs	1a. 80% or more of each meal is ingested 1b. Progressive increase in or maintenance of weight at ideal value 1c. Progressive improvement in nutritional status as evidenced by: erect posture; good skin turgor; clear skin, eyes, and mucosa; firm muscles; prompt healing; mental alertness

NURSE–CLIENT MANAGEMENT OF NUTRITION PROBLEMS (continued)

Nursing Diagnosis	Desired Outcomes	Implementation	Evaluation
	2. No injury related to eating or ingestion	2a. Speak clearly to client when feeding, naming foods, describing texture and temperature 2b. Ensure upright positioning of client during eating	2. Client chews and swallows foods presented without aspiration
Altered Nutrition: Less than Body Requirements for Proteins and Calories R/T inability to ingest food: insufficient income *1.1.2.2.*	1. Knowledge of low cost foods with quality nutritional value	1a. Teach principles of good nutrition and shopping: ■ Avoid convenience foods ■ Use nonmeat protein sources ■ Buy in bulk when possible ■ Buy fresh, not canned, fruits and vegetables in season ■ Read labels for nutrient value of foods ■ Use complex carbohydrates rather than simple sugars ■ Compare prices 1b. Provide food guide for use in menu planning	1a. 80% or more of each meal is ingested 1b. Progressive increase in or maintenance of weight at ideal value 1c. Progressive improvement in nutritional status as evidenced by: erect posture; good skin turgor; clear skin, eyes, and mucosa; firm muscles; prompt healing; mental alertness
	2. Caloric and nutrient intake meets RDAs	2a. Provide food guide for use in menu preparation 2b. Collaborate with client to select menus that are appealing	2. 24-hour food diary shows balanced, adequate nutrient intake
	3. Knowledge of options to increase income	3. Consult with social worker to facilitate access to public assistance sources such as: programs for women and children, food stamps and job counseling	3. Client identifies and contacts community agencies for assistance
Altered Nutrition: Less than Body Requirements for Protein R/T inability to ingest protein: knowledge deficit *1.1.2.2.*	1. Knows importance of protein for optimum health	1a. Teach importance of protein for health 1b. Teach foods high in protein 1c. Provide food guide for use in menu planning; collaborate with client to select menus that are appealing	1. Correctly states roles played by protein in body functions
	2. Daily protein intake meets RDAs	2. Teach importance of protein for health	2a. Lists foods high in protein 2b. 24-hour food diary shows protein intake meets RDAs
	3. No signs of protein deficiency	3. Teach importance of protein for health	3. Physical exam shows good muscle tone, no edema, hair strong and shiny; serum protein RBCs and lymphocyte values normal for age

NURSE–CLIENT MANAGEMENT OF NUTRITION PROBLEMS (continued)

Nursing Diagnosis	Desired Outcomes	Implementation	Evaluation
Altered Nutrition: Potential for More than Body Requirements for Calories. Risk Factor: Social/Occupational Situation Encourages Overeating and Drinking *1.1.2.3.*	1. Caloric intake and metabolic demand are balanced	1a. Use 3-day food diary to assess current diet 1b. Teach principles of good nutrition 1c. Collaboratively develop a low fat diet plan and an exercise plan which are pleasing to client's needs and preferences	1. Achieves and maintains ideal weight
	2. Daily food intake meets RDAs	2a. Use 3-day food diary to assess current diet 2b. Teach principles of good nutrition 2c. Provide food guide for use in menu planning	2. Food diary shows diet meets RDAs
	3. Knowledge of strategies to avoid excessive intake in social situations	3. Discuss strategies to avoid intake related to social pressure including: ■ Choosing low calorie menu selections and nonalcoholic beverages for business lunches/socializing ■ Limiting snack intake in social settings—eat nutritious low calorie snack before event, drink water with lemon or lime during event ■ When eating with family, eating small portions of high calorie dishes, select larger portions of vegetables and salads ■ Avoiding social activities involving meals when possible ■ Joining support groups such as Weight Watchers	3. Identifies at least 3 strategies being used to decrease intake in social settings

tional education resources are available for consumer use from groups such as the USDA, National Cancer Institute, American Heart Association, and American Diabetes Association. Food tables list the nutrient values of foods, so that meal planning can be conducted in accordance with the RDAs. For clients who consume processed foods or who eat in restaurants, specialized food tables are available that give estimates of nutrient values of common restaurant foods. Diabetic clients who must plan their meals in terms of food exchange groups can be supplied with food exchange lists. It is helpful to collaborate with clients in planning meals for several days, to ensure that they understand how to use the food tables. Clients with special risk factors can be given special meal planning guides produced by various groups and agencies, such as the American Heart Association and the American Cancer Society. Collaboration with a dietician will help nurses gain access to a wealth of meal-planning resources.

Age-related Approaches. Children need to have a variety of foods available and should be given maximum freedom in selection of nutritious foods. Nutrition education should start during the late toddler or preschool period. School nurses have an important role in continuing children's education about good nutrition and providing nutritional counseling. As many as 25 percent of children and adolescents are obese, and the majority of these remain obese as adults.[22]

IMPLICATIONS FOR NURSE–CLIENT COLLABORATION

Health Education

At the core of the collaborative approach to client care is a value of self-responsibility and self-care. One of the most important contributions the nurse can make to support the client's personal responsibility for health is to promote and facilitate the health education of the client. In the course of collaborating with the client, the nurse becomes aware of the client's level of nutritional knowledge. When clients can benefit from dietary teaching, nurses are frequently in the best position to provide the necessary details on dietary guidelines and the names, functions, and sources of basic nutrients.

Adolescents and pregnant women, adults in their middle years, and the elderly are all at risk for nutritional problems and should be a special focus of teaching. For adolescents, nurses should emphasize the benefits of healthy food choices, such as fruits and vegetables, over the high-fat, empty calorie snack foods that are typical choices of this age group. Because weight control is often an issue, particularly with girls, a comparison of relative calorie density of fruits and vegetables versus milkshakes, french fries, and candy may be productive. Point out that meal skipping as a way of losing weight often backfires, because the amount of food meal-skippers consume at the next meal is often greater than if a regular meal schedule were followed.

Middle-aged adults are vulnerable to the negative nutritional impact of hectic life-styles and multiple responsibilities. They may believe they have too little time to prepare healthy meals or engage in regular exercise. Stress may curb appetite—or promote unhealthy eating as a form of relief. Nurses can point out the health benefits of meals prepared from fresh ingredients, compared to processed or convenience foods. Suggesting that adults purchase one of the many cookbooks now available that feature healthful, simple, quick-to-prepare recipes and microwave cooking as a means of achieving the goal of healthier eating habits is also a useful approach. Finally, nurses should complete the health picture by emphasizing the role of exercise in weight control, stress reduction, and increased productivity.

Older adults can benefit from practical tips that reduce food expenditures and the effort required for meal preparation.[23] Some examples follow.

- Buy only three pieces of various fresh fruits at a time: one ripe, one medium, one green. Eat the ripe one immediately, the second soon, and let the green one ripen on the window sill.
- Buy only what you can use. Don't be timid about asking a grocer to break open packaged vegetables or meats.
- Be creative when you must buy a larger quantity than you can use right away. Cut a head of cauliflower in thirds. Eat one part as a hot vegetable, marinate one part in vinegar and oil to use in a salad, and eat the other part raw as a snack.
- Make mixtures like stews and soups of whatever you have on hand. Bonus: a one-dish meal makes easier clean-up.
- If you cook a favorite dish, make enough to freeze several portions.
- If you have the space, buy large packages of meat and divide them for freezing. Wrap each in foil (which can line the cooking pan.) Don't label each one, but place them in a large brown labeled bag, so they are easier to find in the freezer and you'll know when your supply is low.
- Divide loaves of bread; keep half in the freezer to keep it fresher.

These tips do not address the problem of loneliness, at the root of many older adults' nutritional deficits. For this problem, nurses should encourage older adults to think of socializing when they think of food. Suggest that they schedule regular potluck meals with friends who are also alone. Or, tell them to consider arranging an exchange with a friend: invite the friend to eat once a week, and have the friend return the invitation once a week. Older adults should be encouraged to make new friends at the supermarket, church, or other social gatherings to expand possibilities for mealtime socializing. Volunteering at local hospitals or charitable organizations is another way to expand social contacts.

Knowledge may also be a means of preventing older adults from neglecting their nutritional needs. As mentioned earlier, many elderly do not understand basic nutritional facts or distinguish them from food fallacies. Being aware of the importance of good nutrition to well-being is a first step toward taking responsibility for eating well, despite social or economical concerns.

Social service programs, such as Meals-On-Wheels, group meals in senior centers, and public health department nutritional counseling, are also available to help the elderly attain and maintain healthy nutritional habits.

Supportive Care

The focus of nursing in supportive care is the client who is showing early signs of an alteration in nutrition, either more than or less than body requirements. Such individuals may require hospitalization, or may attempt to manage their problems while maintaining as normal a life-style as possible. The nurse's role in supportive care is to help clients assess the extent of the nutritional problem, determine the probable cause of the problem, choose appropriate interventions to restore maximum nutrition or to prevent further alteration, and to take action to prevent these alterations from developing.

Nursing implementation appropriate for supportive care of the client with an alteration in nutrition include those appropriate to preventive care. Life-style analysis and counseling, value clarification, teaching, and daily meal planning are all important means of assisting clients to cope with nutritional problems. Other appropriate measures are described below.

Nutritional Supplements. Nutritional supplements may be necessary for clients with early nutritional alterations. Such supplements are usually prescribed by the physician or dietician; the nurse's role is to monitor appropriate use and effectiveness of the supplement. The common view regarding use of nutritional supplements such as vitamins or minerals is that they are not needed for people able to consume normal, balanced diets in accordance with the RDAs. However, the client with an alteration in nutritional status may not be able to consume such a diet.

For a client whose nutritional intake is less than body requirements, weight gain may or may not be a desirable goal. If the nutritional deficit is of a specific nutrient rather than of total calories, a client's weight may be normal. For example, a deficit of thiamine is often associated with chronic alcoholism. A client may have a normal body weight because of the high calorie content of alcohol, but thiamine and other nutrients may be severely depleted. The nurse then assists the client to use appropriate nutritional supplements as well as dietary sources of thiamine.

Teaching. Teaching should include "smart shopping" for clients with early nutritional alterations. Learning to read the labels of food products and learning what foods are low-cost, high-nutrient values are important goals for most clients. A client who is experiencing an overall calorie deficit needs to learn what foods are high in calories and also high in nutrient value. A client who is overweight needs to recognize low-calorie, high-nutrition foods. The etiology of the nutritional problem determines the specific supportive teaching interventions.

Exercise. Exercise should be a key part of an overall program for weight reduction for clients who are overweight. Providing clients with the rationale for the inclusion of exercise may increase motivation to maintain a regular exercise program. Exercise should be individually planned in accordance with a client's capacity, body characteristics, interests, environment, and life-style. Aerobic exercise that maintains heart rate at 75 percent of the maximum rate for a 30-minute period has been shown to cause the body to turn to its fat stores for energy consumption.[24] (See Chap. 30 for a discussion of aerobic exercise.) A realistic schedule should be designed so that clients do not find it unduly difficult to observe. Initially, the exercise sessions can be planned for three times a week. Setting aside a specific time makes it easier to incorporate exercise into the schedule of activities.

Enhancing Eating Pleasure. If clients receiving supportive care are inpatients, nurses may be involved in preparing an environment conducive to eating. Clients receiving outpatient care can be counseled about environmental influences on intake. A relaxed atmosphere, clean and neat environment, social interaction, and adequate time are all helpful in promoting enjoyment of meals. Noxious smells and sights should be removed from the environment. Food presented in an attractive way, with manageable portions and needed utensils, is more appetizing. When possible, providing opportunities for clients to eat meals with other clients can enhance mealtime enjoyment.

BUILDING NURSING KNOWLEDGE

What is Food Refusal and How Do Caregivers Handle It?

Norberg A, Backstrom A, Athlin E, Norberg B. Food refusal among nursing home patients as conceptualized by nurses' aides and enrolled nurses: An interview study. *J Adv Nurs.* 1988;13:478–483.

Some clients seem to refuse food, a situation that causes anxiety among caregivers. The question about how clients who refuse food should be treated is especially difficult when clients are unable to make their own decisions. Moreover, the decision about what action to take and whether to use technical means to feed foods is often complicated by difficulty in deciding whether clients deliberately refuse food or are unable to eat. The caregiver's concept of food refusal is thus important to assessing the situation and to selecting the means to resolve the problem. The aim of this group of researchers was to elucidate how caregivers in nursing homes conceptualize food refusal.

The study was carried out in 23 nursing homes, with interviews of 193 caregivers. Interviews focused on food refusal, treatment of clients who seemed to refuse food, and feeding techniques.

Caregivers identified three categories of food refusal encountered among clients: (1) food refusal for physical reasons (too ill, unable to eat, has gastrointestinal symptoms); (2) food refusal for psychological reasons (wants to die, does not understand situation, has bizarre ideas, is having an emotional reaction; and (3) food refusal for cultural reasons (food taboos, unfamiliar with special food).

The findings indicated that few caregivers stressed the importance of identifying the cause of food refusal. Most described various techniques used to resolve the problem, such as offering clients different menus, and calming or persuading clients. Special methods to force clients to eat were also described, such as firmly commanding the client to eat or forcibly opening the client's mouth with a spoon. Caregivers defined "forced feeding" in two ways. Some defined it as any feeding that is against the client's will. Others described it as feeding techniques that are done in an unfriendly manner. Caregivers were against the use of force but expressed the difficulty of finding humane and effective feeding techniques. Often they were frustrated by an inability to differentiate a client's lack of desire to eat from an inability to eat. The investigators concluded that caregiver anxiety would be reduced and quality of care improved if more specific and precise nursing diagnoses of eating problems could be developed.

Assisting with Menu Selection. Clients may need or desire assistance from the nurse in selecting a nutritious meal plan from a hospital menu. A client may also need assistance in obtaining a special menu, such as one for kosher or vegetarian diets. The nurse can use this opportunity to provide individualized nutrition education as well as to ensure that high-quality foods are selected.

Restorative Care

Acute nutritional problems requiring complex nursing implementation are the focus of restorative care. Such problems may be related to severe primary nutritional deficiencies such as starvation, or may be due to a wide variety of disease processes. Examples of the latter are clients with complications of diabetes and clients with advanced cancer of the gastrointestinal tract or ulcerative colitis (chronic colon inflammation). Continuous assessment is necessary due to the unstable nature of such nutritional alterations. Often the nurse needs to serve as the primary provider of nutrition through feeding such clients orally or administering enteral or parenteral feedings. The physician or dietician may prescribe therapeutic diets, with the nurse's role being that of administration and evaluation. See Table 25–10 for a description of some commonly ordered therapeutic diets. Procedures 25–1 through 25–5 describe additional nursing techniques which may be necessary for restorative care.

Tray Presentation/Preparation. Assist clients to prepare for the meal as described in supportive care. Food should be served at the temperature intended—hot foods hot, cold foods cold. The tray should not be overly crowded, and all items should be within clients' reach. If clients cannot cut their own food, nurses should assist, but it is important that this is not done in a manner that is demeaning. Many adults find dependency of this kind humiliating.

Positioning for Safe Eating. Elevate the client's head as high as possible to minimize the risk of aspiration and provide access to the tray (Fig. 25–7). If at all possible, the

TABLE 25–10. DESCRIPTION OF STANDARD HOSPITAL DIETS

Diet	Indications for Use	Comment
Regular	Used for clients requiring no particular modification.	Based on the RDA and basic four food groups; foods that may cause digestive disturbances are omitted; can be increased in kcal and protein content by the addition of extra amounts of milk, meat, or high-protein supplements. Some hospitals may offer a prudent regular diet as a health-promoting measure (a prudent diet offers food low in saturated fat and cholesterol with substitution of polyunsaturated fat).
Soft Traditional	May be used during the transition phase in the progression from a liquid to a regular diet, in the convalescent phase of acute infections, and with mild gastrointestinal disturbances.	Based on the RDA and basic four food groups; modified in texture so as to include foods that are low in fiber and thus easy to chew, and foods that are simply prepared, mild in flavor, and easily digested; texture modifications for clients with chewing problems should be evaluated on an individual basis.
Mechanical or dental soft	May be used by clients who have chewing problems because of lack of teeth or suitable dentures.	
Liquid, full	May be used before and after surgery, in infectious diseases, in situations where chewing and swallowing problems are present, and with gastrointestinal problems.	Allows use of foods that are liquid at room or body temperature and low in fiber and easily digested and absorbed; may contain adequate kcal but is low in iron and other nutrients; can increase the kcal and nutritive value by addition of cream to milk, nonfat milk to beverages and soups, strained meat to soups, and sugar or Polycose to beverages; provide at least six feedings daily.
Clear	May be used before and after surgery or when illness is acute. Nausea, vomiting, distention, diarrhea, and anorexia are possible indicators for this diet.	Allows fluids that are transparent and consist primarily of carbohydrates that leave little residue after digestion; is nutritionally inadequate and should be used as the sole source of nutrition for no more than 24 to 48 hours; provide at least six feedings daily.

From Lewis CM. Nutrition and Nutritional Therapy in Nursing. *Norwalk, CT: Appleton & Lange; 1986.*

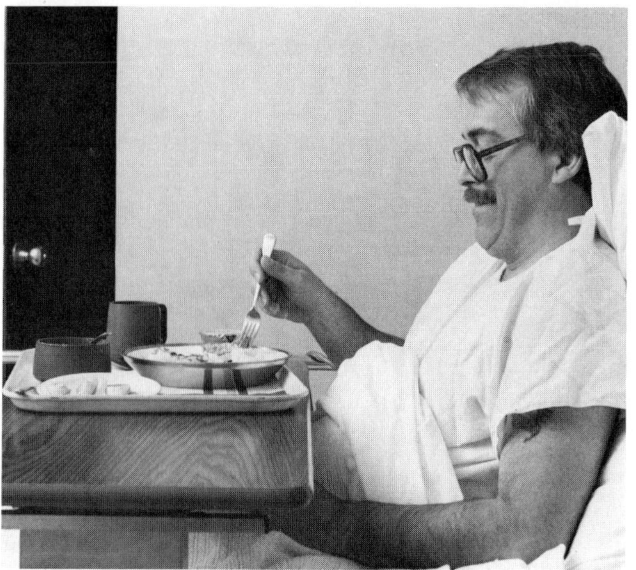

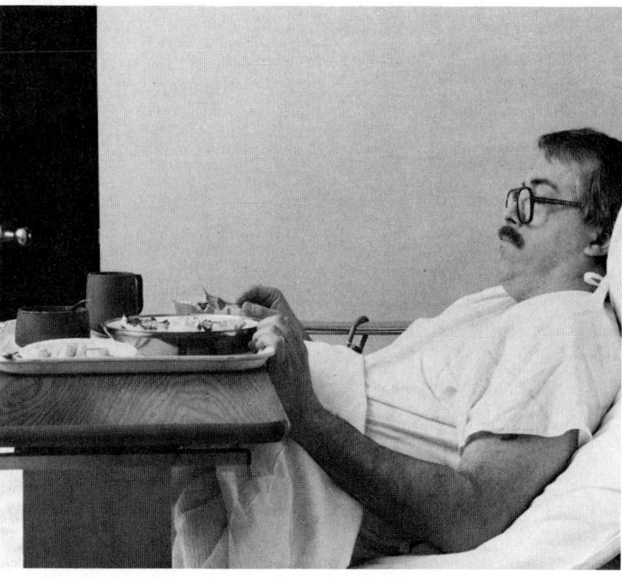

A B

Figure 25–7. **A.** Correct positioning for eating enhances comfort and eating enjoyment. **B.** A client who is not positioned correctly for eating has difficulty reaching food and is at greater risk for choking.

client should eat in a sitting position, either on the side of the bed or in a comfortable chair.

Assisting the Client With Dysphagia. Clients who have difficulty swallowing need to be provided foods that are easily swallowed. Bites should be small. Highly textured foods stimulate swallowing more than smooth foods. Lightly sweetened and seasoned foods are more easily handled. Foods to be avoided are milk, pulp fruits, hamburger patties, onions, thick soups, white bread, custards, crackers, and bitter or acidic foods. Provide ample time for swallowing each bite. Nurses may need to remain with clients so that in case choking occurs, they can give immediate assistance. Loss of lip function may also be a problem for clients with dysphagia. This often results in collection of food on the face and is a cause of distress and embarrassment. Assisting clients by focusing on rehabilitation of lip function can restore clients' enjoyment of eating.[25]

Feeding. Feeding clients unable to feed themselves is a skill and an art that takes diligence, patience, and a calm, pleasant atmosphere for maximum effectiveness. Perhaps in no other nursing care situation do clients feel so directly dependent on nurses for a function of such great symbolic importance. Feeding is a nurturing activity that should ideally take place within the context of a carefully developed therapeutic nurse–client relationship. Otherwise clients may have great difficulty in accepting a dependent role and may claim not to be hungry, or that they can feed themselves when in fact they cannot. Delegating feeding to nursing assistants is a common practice; however, a study of food refusal among nursing home clients revealed that this level of caregiver is often ineffective in dealing with clients' refusal to eat.[26] Refusal to eat may have complex etiologies that require professional-level intervention. Procedure 25–1 describes the procedure to be followed for feeding a client.

Use of Special Appliances and Utensils. Special appliances and utensils have been developed for people with specific physical disabilities that interfere with ingestion. Specially shaped spoons, forks, and knives allow easy grasping. Closed cups with no-spill straws and splints for support of hands or arms are also available. The nurse should consult with the dietician or occupational therapist when a special utensil is needed. Figure 25–8 illustrates some assistive devices.

Enteral Feeding. Enteral feeding has become an important means of feeding clients whose intake is less than body requirements. The types and number of enteral formulas have dramatically increased in the last few years. Table 25–11 describes some common types of enteral feedings. Equipment available for tube feedings and routes of administration have also become more sophisticated (Fig. 25–9). **Enteral** means, literally, via the gastrointestinal tract rather than by mouth. Enteral tubes are used to administer a liquid formula directly into the stomach, duodenum, and in some cases, the jejunum. The formulas are usually highly concentrated solutions of carbohydrates, fat, amino acids, vitamins, and minerals.

Because of their high osmolality, diarrhea is a common side effect of tube feedings. Osmolality refers to the con-

PROCEDURE 25–1. FEEDING A CLIENT

Purpose: To provide adequate nourishment to clients unable to feed themselves.

Equipment: Food selected by client, if possible; napkin or towel; instruments for cutting and eating; water; washcloth; towel; cup; and basin.

ACTION	RATIONALE
1. Wash hands.	1. Protect client from hospital-acquired infection.
2. Check tray: Foods ordered by client are delivered? Foods within prescribed diet?	2. Client involved in meal selection increases satisfaction; restricted foods may seriously harm client.
NOTE: If client unable to select foods, try to engage family/friends in selection. Use food selection as focus for teaching regarding healthy diets.	
3. Create a clean, quiet, and pleasant environment.	3. A cluttered, dirty, malodorous, or rushed atmosphere will decrease appetite.
4. Assist client to sitting position unless contraindicated. If client cannot sit, elevate head and shoulders.	4. Reduces risk of aspiration, facilitates swallowing.
5. Place a napkin or towel under client's chin.	5. Protects client and bed. Spilling is more likely when client is being fed by another.
NOTE: Many clients will feel demeaned by resemblance to bib. Acknowledge this and explain reason.	
6. Place tray where client can see and smell food. Encourage client to indicate what food is wanted for each bite. Serve hot and cold foods at intended temperatures.	6. Olfactory stimuli enhance appetite. Active participation reduces client's feelings of helplessness and/or loss of dignity.
NOTE: Conversing with the client about pleasant topics may stimulate appetite and ease anxiety.	

(*continued*)

PROCEDURE 25–1. (continued)

7. If client is unable to select foods, give a variety. Offer high-calorie, high-protein foods first.

7. If entire meal is not eaten, the most nourishing foods will have been ingested.

8. Offer quantities that can be easily chewed. Allow time for client to eat at own pace.

8. See rationale for step 4, above.

9. Offer liquids periodically.

9. Stimulates saliva, allowing improved digestion and easier swallowing.

10. When finished, offer materials for washing and mouth care and assist as needed. Leave in a position of comfort.

10. Hygiene and positioning enhance comfort and promote relaxation, which facilitates digestion.

RECORDING: Record type of diet client selects or is prescribed. Record percentage of meal consumed, client's response to eating, and any difficulties with chewing or swallowing. In many facilities, this information is recorded on a checklist rather than in narrative notes.

centration of particles in a solution. The greater the number of particles, the greater the osmolality. Fluids flow from lower to higher osmolality. Therefore, if a tube feeding formula with higher osmolality than blood (hypertonic) is administered, it will draw fluid into the lumen of the intestine from the bloodstream. The resulting increased volume in the intestine stimulates bowel motility and therefore causes diarrhea. To correct the diarrhea, solutions of lower osmolality can be used, or the solution can be diluted for administration and instilled at a lower rate. Another possible cause of diarrhea is a specific intolerance of one or more of the nutrients, such as lactose intolerance. Specially designed solutions are available for clients with particular intolerances. In regard to the type of solution to be used, collaboration among the physician, dietician, and nurse is of utmost importance. The nurse is the caregiver who critically observes and communicates the client's response to the formula. Diarrhea should never be accepted as a normal response to a feeding. Measures can and must be taken to prevent its occurrence.

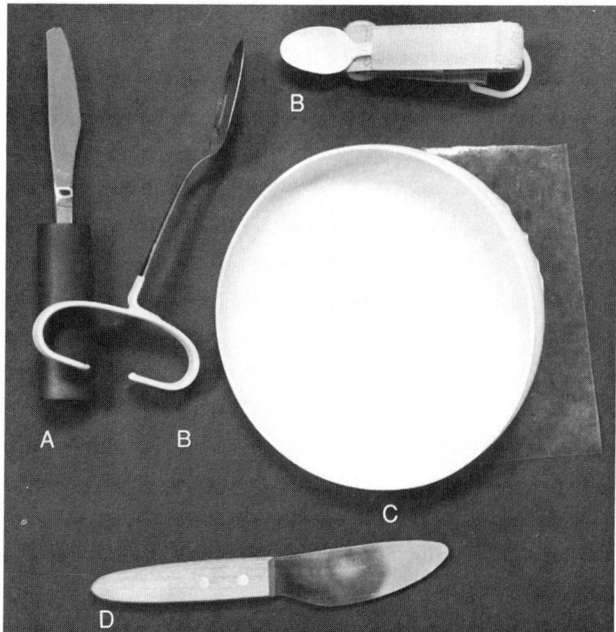

Figure 25–8. Special appliances to assist disabled clients to eat independently: **A.** Knife with large foam handle to facilitate grip. **B.** Spoons with modified handles to prevent dropping food. **C.** Plate with raised edge on nonslip pad to facilitate scooping food. **D.** Rocker blade knife to aid in cutting.

One way of preventing tube-feeding-related diarrhea is by continuous, rather than intermittent, feeding. A small amount of the formula is infused continuously, its rate maintained constant by use of a feeding pump. When intermittent feedings are used, a large quantity of formula is administered in a short time interval. This larger volume of high osmolality solution in the intestines is more likely to result in diarrhea. If intermittent feedings are in use or ordered, the nurse can discuss the possibility of changing to continuous feedings with a dietician and the client's physician, if the feedings produce diarrhea.

Insertion of a nasogastric feeding tube is usually the nurse's responsibility. A number of different types and brands of tubes are available. The tendency currently is to use tubes made of soft flexible material, with as small a diameter as possible to minimize client discomfort.

TABLE 25–11. CLASSIFICATION OF TUBE FEEDINGS

Type	Commercial Preparations	Comments
Blenderized	Compleat B (Doyle) Formula 2 (Cutter) Vitaneed (Biosearch)	Blended natural foods; ready-to-use.
Polymeric milk-based	Meritene (Doyle) Instant Breakfast (Carnation) Sustacal Powder (Mead Johnson)	Pleasant-tasting oral supplements; provide intact nutrients.
Polymeric lactose-free	Enrich with fiber (Ross) Ensure (Ross) Isocal (Mead Johnson) Osmolite (Ross) Precision Isotonic (Doyle) Nutri 1000 (Cutter) Renu (Biosearch) Sustacal (Mead Johnson) Travasorb (Travenol)	Used as tube feeding, meal replacement, or oral supplement; made with intact protein isolates, oligosaccarides and starches, and fats; provide 1 kcal/mL (others available providing up to 2 kcal/mL); in adequate quantities, meet RDAs for vitamins and minerals; ready to use (except Precision Isotonic); Isotonic (except Ensure, Sustacal, and Travasorb).
Elemental or monomeric formulas	Criticare (Mead Johnson) Vipep (Cutter) Vital (Ross) Vivonex (Eaton) Travasorb Standard (Travenol)	Partially digested nutrients for feeding; hypertonic; require reconstitution.

From Burtis G, Davis J, Martin S. Applied Nutrition and Diet Therapy. *Philadelphia: Saunders; 1988.*

For the client with a nasogastric feeding tube, mouth care is particularly important because there are no liquids being ingested orally to lubricate the oral mucosa. Also important is the protection of the skin surrounding the tube from pressure or other irritation. Tubes which are inserted surgically, such as jejunostomy tubes, require special skin care and sometimes dressings at the insertion site to prevent infection. Procedures 25–2 through 25–4 discuss the management of enteral tubes for feeding. Procedure 25–5 describes discontinuing an NG tube. Box 25–7 and Table 25–12 address nursing monitoring of clients receiving tube feedings, common problems associated with tube feedings, and possible causes, prevention, and treatment.

Total Parenteral Nutrition. When a client's digestive tract is unable to absorb nutrients, an alternate route for nutrient administration must be provided. **Total parenteral nutrition** (TPN) is the administration of a nutritionally complete solution intravenously. This process has revolutionized the nutritional care of clients many of whom would die of malnutrition were TPN not available. Any client who is unable to tolerate foods or fluids in the digestive tract should be considered a candidate for TPN if it is expected that the intolerance will persist for more than 1 or 2 weeks. If short-term nutritional support is expected, the solution can be given through a peripheral vein; if long-term support is anticipated, it must be given through a central vein, such as the subclavian. A full discussion of TPN and related nursing care is beyond the scope of this text. (*Text continues on page 1127.*)

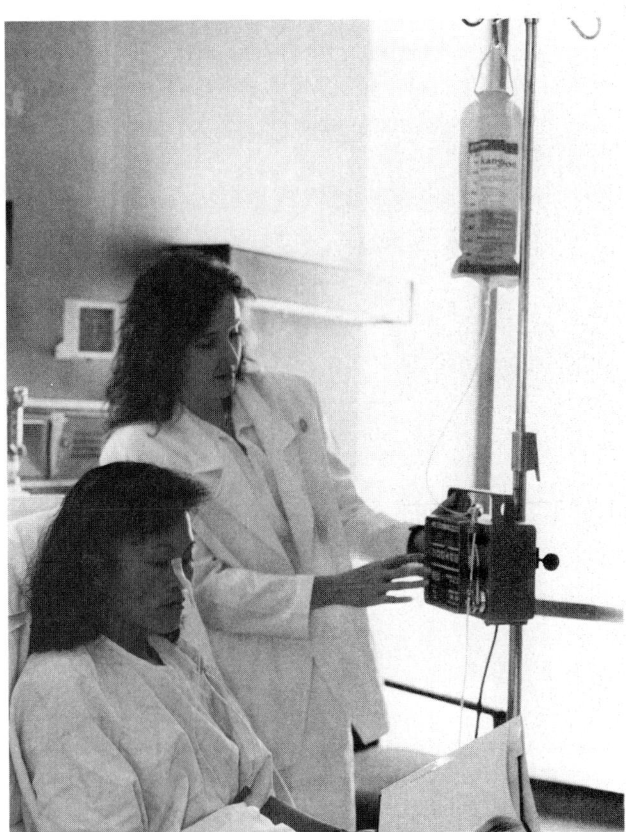

Figure 25–9. Nurse adjusts feeding pump to deliver enteral formula at correct rate. Client has soft, pliable small-bore feeding tube.

BOX 25–7. NURSING MONITORING OF CLIENTS RECEIVING TUBE FEEDINGS

Parameter	Frequency
Placement of nasogastric tube	Each time intermittent feeding is initiated At least every shift when feeding is continuous
Tolerance	
Nausea	At least every shift*
Abdominal distension	At least every shift*
Urine glucose and acetone	q8h, may discontinue after 48 hours if consistently negative in nondiabetic client
Residual feeding in stomach	Before starting intermittent feeding, every shift for continuous feeding*
Hydration	
Urine specific gravity	Every shift
Intake and output	Every shift
Weight	Daily
Skin turgor, moisture	Every shift
Nutrition Status (See Table 25–8)	Every 7–10 days
Lung sounds	Every shift

* Check q4h when continuous feeding first started or when rate is changed

TABLE 25–12. COMMON PROBLEMS ASSOCIATED WITH TUBE FEEDINGS

Problem	Possible Cause	Prevention/Treatment
Nausea, vomiting, abdominal distension	Administration too rapid, delayed gastric emptying	Avoid bolus feedings, administer by slow continuous drip Dilute formula, gradually increase concentration
Diarrhea, abdominal cramps	Intolerance to hypertonic formula	Dilute formula, gradually increase concentration
	Bacterial contamination	Refrigerate open containers of formula. Use medical sepsis when handling formula and equipment. Change bag and tubing at least q24h, rinse equipment used for intermittent feeding with each use
	Rapid administration of formula	Use slow continuous drip administration
	Lactose intolerance	Use lactose-free formula in high-risk clients
Clogged feeding tube	Medications not adequately flushed through tubing	Use liquid forms of drugs when available. Finely crush tablets and mix with water. Flush tube with water before and after medications
Dehydration	Diarrhea	See above
	Insufficient fluid intake	Calculate fluid needs, administer supplementary fluids to match needs
	Osmotic diuresis related to high carbohydrate concentration	See hyperglycemia
Hyperglycemia	High carbohydrate concentration	Assess blood and urine glucose, change to lower carbohydrate formula, dilute formula or slow rate of administration. Physician may consider giving insulin

PROCEDURE 25–2. INSERTING A NASOGASTRIC TUBE (FEEDING OR DECOMPRESSION TUBE)

PURPOSE: To provide a route for administration of liquid food or for removal of gastrointestinal fluid and air.

EQUIPMENT: Feeding tube (preferably small diameter, soft, plastic) or NG tube (usually a Levin or Salem sump tube); water-soluble lubricant; waterproof pad or towel; tissues; emesis basin; glass of water and straw, or ice chips; hypoallergenic adhesive tape, 50-mL syringe; stethoscope; penlight.

ACTION	RATIONALE
1. Wash hands.	1. Prevents the transfer of microorganisms from the nurse's hands to the client.
2. Discuss the procedure with the client, including its purpose and benefits, nurse's actions, desired client participation, and sensations commonly experienced.	2. Client will be less fearful and more willing to participate if the purpose, benefits, and procedure of the tube are clear.
NOTE: If client is unconscious, explain procedure to family, if present. Tell family tears are produced when nasal mucosa is irritated and they do not indicate client is in distress.	
3. Gather all equipment on overbed table. Raise bed to nurse's thigh level and lower siderail.	3. Provides for efficient performance of procedure with minimal strain to nurse and client.
4. Screen client. Place in high Fowler's position and place towel across chest.	4. Privacy is needed for invasive procedures. Tube will pass more easily in high Fowler's position because of gravity and client's effective swallowing.
NOTE: If client cannot sit up, lateral position may be used.	
5. Arrange a signal for client to indicate if feeling discomfort. Place tissues and emesis basis within client's reach.	5. Stimulation of throat may cause gagging or trigger emesis. Client will be less fearful if aware that nurse will respond to signal.

(*continued*)

PROCEDURE 25–2. (continued)

6. Determine the appropriate insertion length for the tube by measuring the distance from the client's nares to the earlobe and from the ear to the tip of the sternum. Mark this distance from the tube's end with a piece of tape. Many tubes are premarked to aid in noting distance to insert. The marks do not replace measuring as described, but eliminate need for marking with tape.

6. The tube must extend into the stomach to decrease risk of aspiration of tube feeding formula or to remove gastric contents. This measurement approximates the distance from the nose to the stomach cavity. Marking the length will decrease risk of the tube not being inserted far enough.

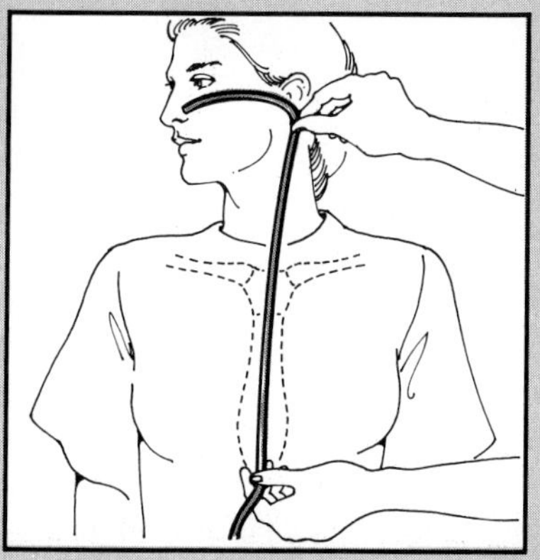

7. If inserting a small-bore feeding tube, lubricate *inside* of lumen (included in kit). Insertion stylet may have been placed inside feeding tube by manufacturer. If not, insert stylet now and secure with luer-lock connector.

7. Small-bore tubes are very soft and flexible. Stylet provides stiffness necessary for insertion of tube. Liquid reduces friction inside the small tube facilitating stylet insertion and removal.

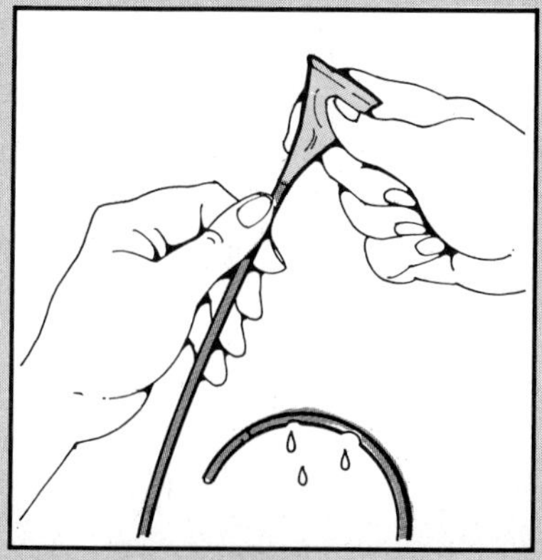

8. Lubricate the first 15 to 20 cm (6–8 in) of the outside of the tube with a water-soluble lubricant.

8. Reduces friction and irritation to mucosa, facilitating insertion. Water-soluble lubricant will dissolve without causing respiratory irritation if the tube accidentally enters the trachea.

9. Inspect nostrils to determine which one is most patent. Ask client about previous nose fracture or deviated septum.

9. Previous trauma to the nose may leave scar tissue, making the canal too narrow for the tube. Attempt to introduce tube in other nostril.

PROCEDURE 25–2. (continued)

10. Ask the client to hyperextend neck. Gently insert the tube into most patent nostril, advancing it straight back toward the posterior pharyngeal wall. Ask the client to open mouth. Slight pressure may be needed to advance tube.

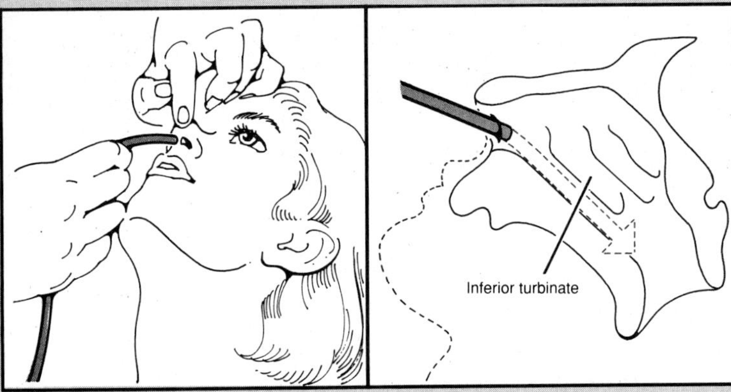

10. This direction follows the natural contour of the nasal passage, thereby decreasing mucosal irritation. Neck hyperextension straightens nasopharyngeal junction. Open mouth will help to keep the nares open.

11. If resistance is met, slightly withdraw the tube, rotate it, and readvance until it reaches the nasopharynx. If obstruction persists, relubricate tube and try the other nostril.

11. Rotating the tube alters its direction slightly, allowing its curvature to follow the nasal canal to the nasopharynx.

NOTE: If the tube coils up or advances into the mouth, withdraw it back into the nasopharynx.

12. If client gags, suggest panting for a few breaths. Then ask the client to flex the neck forward and swallow sips of water through a straw. Advance the tube with each swallow until premarked length is reached. Inserting tube too rapidly or out of synchrony with swallowing may cause tube to coil in oropharynx.

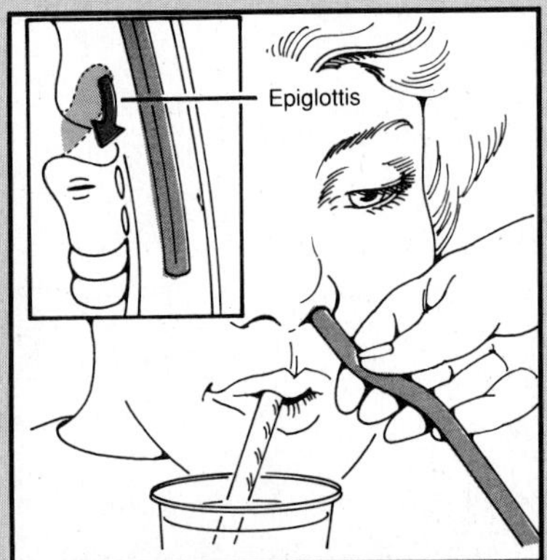

12. Flexing the neck directs the tube toward the esophagus and away from the trachea. Panting and swallowing suppress the gag reflex. Swallowing closes the epiglottis and assists passage of tube over the glottis and into the esophagus.

PROCEDURE 25–2. (continued)

13. If the client coughs or gasps for air, the tube has entered the trachea. Immediately withdraw the tube back into the nasopharynx.

13. The cough reflex is stimulated by the presence of a foreign body in the trachea. The tube will continue to interfere with O_2 exchange until it is removed.

NOTE: Some comatose clients may not retain this cough reflex. See step 14.

14. Confirm placement of tube in the stomach by either (*left*) aspirating gastric contents or (*right*) injecting 5 to 10 cc of air from the syringe into tube, and listening with stethoscope over the epigastric region for the sound of air entering the stomach.

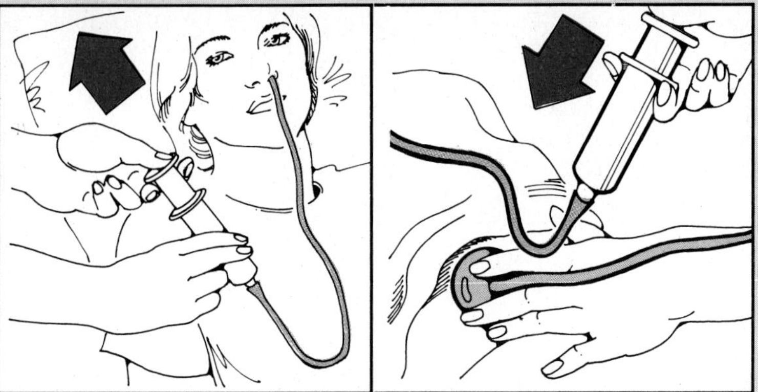

14. Placement in stomach must be confirmed to avoid risk of aspiration of liquid into the lungs.

NOTE: Recent research has indicated that the auscultatory method is not a reliable means of distinguishing among gastric, duodenal, and respiratory placement. The authors suggest that x-ray or assessing pH of tube aspirates are the only reliable means of determining tube placement. Mean gastric aspirate pH is 3.02, compared with 6.57 for intestinal and 7 or greater for lung aspirates.[a]

15. If tube inserted is small-bore feeding tube, remove stylet prior to testing for placement.

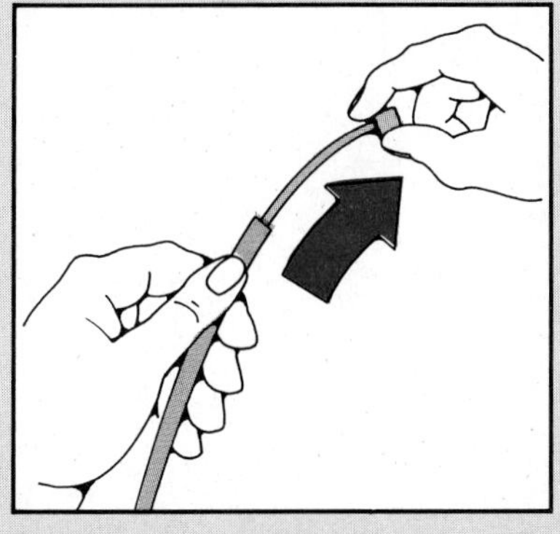

15. Lumen of these tubes is very small and is nearly obstructed by the stylet. Also the luer-lock device securing the stylet prevents attachment of a syringe for aspiration or instillation of air.

[a] Metheny N, McSweeney M, Wehrle MA, Wiersma L. Effectiveness of the auscultatory method in predicting feeding tube location. *Nurs Res.* 1990;39: 262–267.

(*continued*)

PROCEDURE 25–2. (continued)

NOTE: Small-bore soft tubes may make aspiration impossible because negative pressure causes them to collapse. If gastric contents cannot be aspirated, x-ray confirmation of feeding tube placement should be obtained.

16. Secure tube to prevent displacement and rubbing, which can erode nasal mucosa: Split a 2-inch piece of 1-inch wide hypoallergenic tape halfway down its length. Attach unsplit end of tape to nose and wrap split ends around tubing in opposite directions. For small-bore tubing, tape need not be split.

16. Displacement increases risk of aspiration. Rubbing against nasal and pharyngeal mucosa or traction from the tube being inadvertently pulled are very uncomfortable.

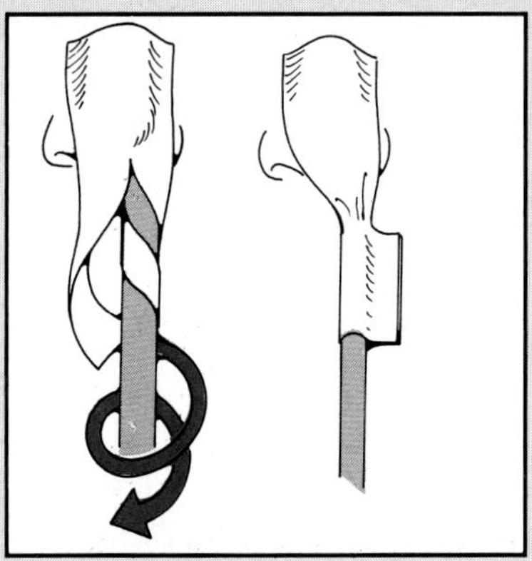

NOTE: Tape may need daily replacement as skin oils decrease adhesion. Clean residual adhesive from nose before applying new tape (acetone, nail polish remover, or tape remover can be used). Recheck placement after retaping.

17. Anchor tubing to client's gown with tape or rubber band and safety pin taking special care to keep the tube from rubbing against nasal mucosa.

17. Pressure of tubing can cause tissue ulceration and necrosis as well as discomfort.

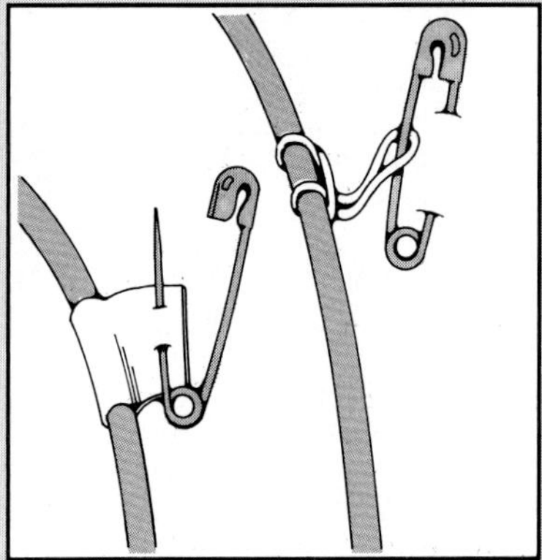

(*continued*)

PROCEDURE 25–2. (continued)

18. Connect distal end of tubing to suction machine (see Procedure 22–17) or to tube feeding apparatus (see Procedure 25–3) as ordered or plug end with catheter plug.

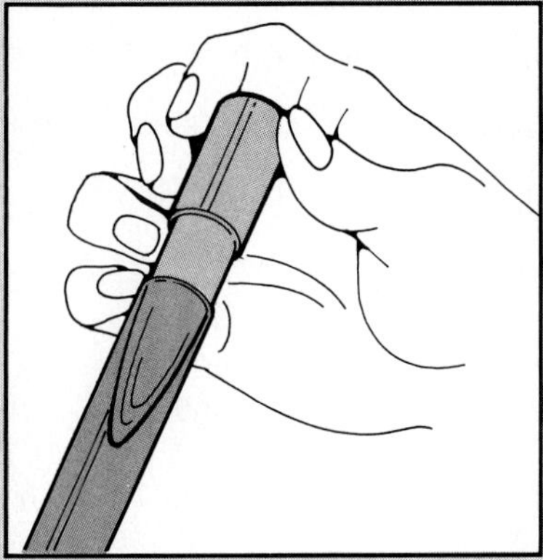

18. Intubation is ordered for a specific purpose, which should be promptly carried out. Gastric contents may leak from proximal end of tubing if it is not plugged or connected to appropriate apparatus.

19. Provide oral hygiene with mouthwash and/or lemon glycerine swabs q2–3 hours. Lip balm may be applied. Clean nares at least q shift with moist cotton-tip applicator. Apply water-soluble lubricant to nostril p.r.n.

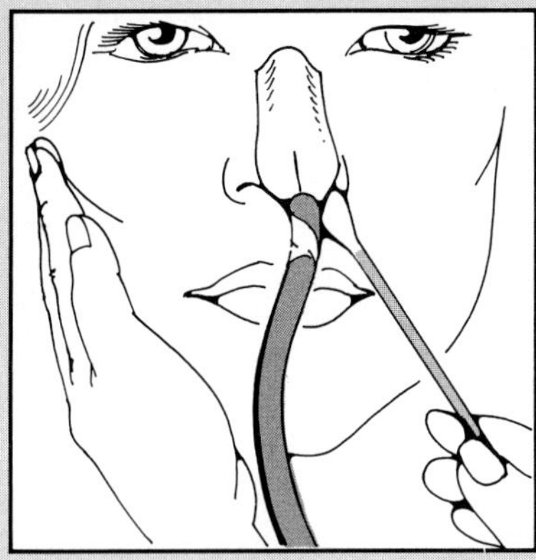

19. NG tubes often stimulate mouth breathing, which causes oral mucous membranes to become dry and uncomfortable. Nasal mucus production is stimulated by the tube and may become encrusted around tube.

NOTE: If NG tube is being used for decompression (see Procedure 22–3), some physicians allow ice chips, hard candy, or chewing gum to stimulate saliva and lubricate mouth.

RECORDING: Chart the time of insertion, which nostril was used; the quantity of fluid returned, if any; problems encountered, if any; associated actions taken; and client's response to the procedure.

PROCEDURE 25–3. ADMINISTERING TUBE FEEDING

PURPOSE: To provide nourishment to the client unable to ingest food by mouth.

EQUIPMENT: Feeding solution; feeding pump or drop regulator, or catheter-tip 60-mL syringe; cup of water.

ACTION	RATIONALE
1. Verify physician order for type, quantity, rate, and frequency of feeding.	1. Tube feeding formulas are considered medications. Nurses may not administer medications without a physician's order.
2. Discuss procedure with client, including purpose, anticipated benefits, nurse's actions, and desired client participation. Gather all equipment at bed- or chair-side.	2. Client will be less fearful and more willing to participate if the purpose, benefits, and procedure of tube insertion are clear.
3. Elevate head of bed 20 to 30 degrees.	3. Facilitates gastric emptying; prevents regurgitation or aspiration.
4. Verify placement of the feeding tube (see Procedure 25–2, step 14).	4. End of tube must be in the stomach. Aspiration pneumonia can occur if the formula is introduced into the trachea or flows there because of reflux from the esophagus.
NOTE: Soft feeding tubes collapse when negative pressure is applied. Use air instillation method or x-ray verification of placement.	
5. If residual from previous feeding is obtained, measure and record. Reinstill residual to stomach.	5. Residual formula is mixed with gastric secretions. It is returned to prevent electrolytic depletion.
NOTE: Residual of more than 150 mL suggests poor motility and absorption. Postpone feeding and notify physician.	

(*continued*)

PROCEDURE 25–3. (continued)

6. Continuous feedings.

a. Place a 4-hour supply of formula in feeding bag of bottle. Label container with date and time solution was added. Some institutions add food coloring to formula to aid in early detection of aspiration (mucus becomes colored if formula enters respiratory tract).

a. Milk-based formula is an excellent medium for bacterial growth. Potential increases with greater time at room temperature.

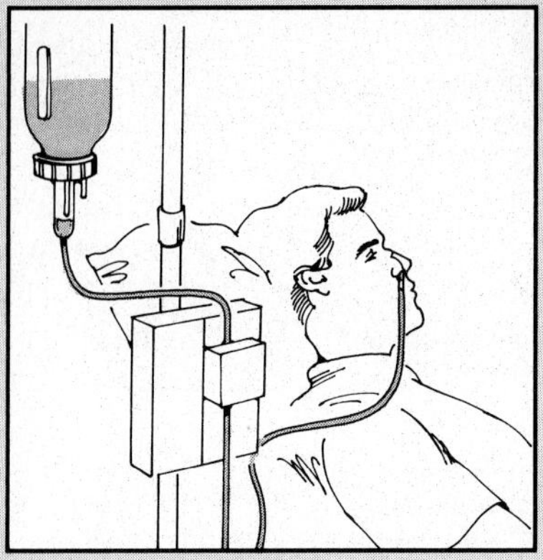

NOTE: Some agencies use prefilled, sealed containers, which can remain in use for 24 hours without risk of bacterial growth. Ice may also be used to slow bacterial growth, but not all clients tolerate iced formulas.

b. Hang container on IV pole, and clear air from tubing by allowing solution to flow through.

b. Air distends stomach, causing discomfort and possible vomiting.

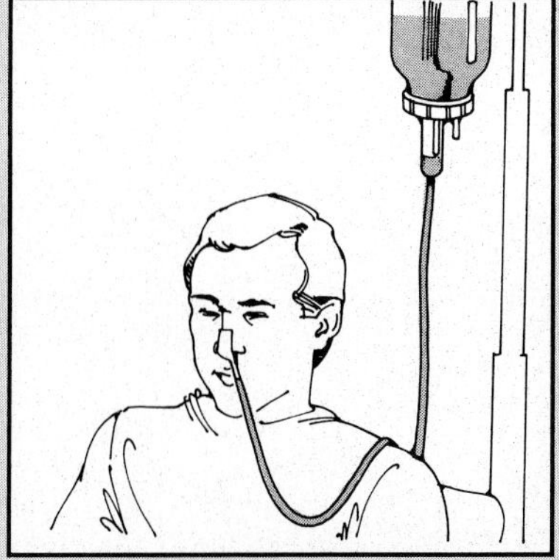

c. Regulate the infusion with the flow clamp or with an automatic pump.

c. Continuous slow drip is used to prevent complications related to highly concentrated formulas. Rapid uncontrolled infusion may cause diarrhea or vomiting. Small-bore tubes limit rate attainable by gravity drip, so positive peristaltic pumps must be used.

(*continued*)

PROCEDURE 25–3. (continued)

d. Assess lungs and abdomen every shift.

d. Lung congestion suggests aspiration. Check the placement. Distended abdomen or decreased bowel sounds suggest formula is not being absorbed. Consult with physician and/or dietician.

e. HOB should remain elevated to 20–30 degrees during infusions. If client care (such as linen change, chest physiotherapy) requires client to be flat, turn off feeding at least 30 minutes prior to positioning client flat.

e. Presence of tube affects efficiency of cardiac sphincter of stomach. Placing client flat while formula is infusing may allow reflux via esophagus to pharynx, causing aspiration.

f. Calculate 24-hour fluid requirements on all clients receiving continuous tube feedings. Interrupt feeding to administer water in 30–60 mL bolus via syringe attached to end of feeding tube (see step 7). Frequency varies with amounts of additional fluid required by client, but once per shift is common. Water may be given by mouth if client is conscious and able to swallow.

f. Continuous tube feeding orders are based on calorie needs, but may not supply adequate fluids.

g. Replace feeding bag and tubing at least every 24 hours.

g. See step 6a, above.

7. *Intermittent feedings*
Using a Prefilled Bottle:

a. Open the bottle and replace the cover with the tubing/screw-cap unit. Hang from IV pole and clear air from tubing as in step 6b.

a. Displacing air from the tubing prior to attaching it to the feeding tube prevents gastric distension and vomiting.

b. Attach tubing to feeding tube, remove or open clamp on feeding tube and regulate flow as ordered with screw clamp or feeding pump.

b. Careful regulation of flow prevents complications and discomfort. If bolus is given too rapidly, diarrhea, abdominal cramps, or vomiting may occur. If this happens, slow the rate of administration.

c. At completion of feeding, flush feeding tube with water as described under "Using a Syringe," below.

c. Flushing tubing helps prevent clogging and bacterial growth in tubing and provides fluid.

Using a Feeding Bag:

a. Add ordered amount of solution to feeding bag. Prepare and regulate flow as in steps 6a and b.

b. At completion of feeding, flush feeding tube with water as described under "Using a Syringe," below.

b. Flushing tubing helps prevent clogging and bacterial growth in tubing and provides fluid.

(*continued*)

PROCEDURE 25–3. (continued)

c. Rinse bag and tubing thoroughly and store for reuse. Discard and replace after 24 hours.

c. Rinsing removes residue of formula which is a medium for bacterial growth. Reusing equipment for more than 24 hours increases risk of contamination and related complications.

Using a Syringe:

Attach 50 mL syringe, without plunger, to clamped feeding tube.

a. Keeping tube clamped until syringe is filled with solution prevents air from entering stomach. (See step a, Using a Prefilled Bottle, above.)

b. Pour feeding solution into syringe, unclamp, and regulate flow of solution to approximately 30 mL/min by raising or lowering syringe. Refill syringe as necessary until ordered quantity has been administered. Do not allow syringe to empty completely before adding additional formula. If fluid does not flow by gravity, replace plunger and administer using positive pressure at no more than 30 ml/min.

b. Research has shown that this rate is tolerated by most clients. Refilling before syringe is empty prevents air from entering stomach.

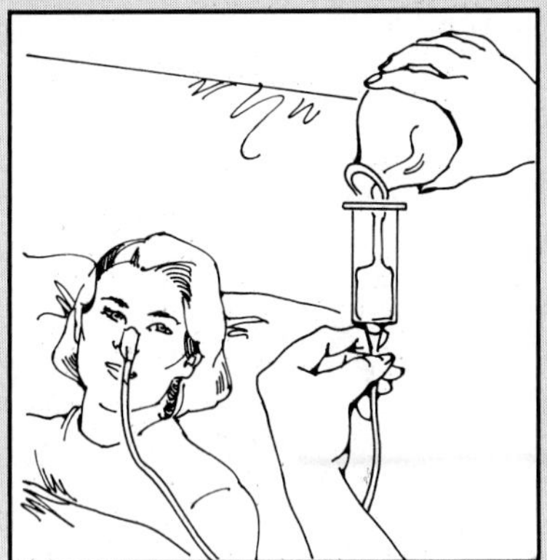

NOTE: Syringe administration is used most often for infants and children. It is an impractical method for the volumes required by adults.

c. When formula level reaches tip of syringe, flush feeding tube with 50 mL or prescribed amount of water; clamp tube before detaching syringe.

c. Flushing tubing helps prevent clogging and bacterial growth in tubing and provides fluid. Clamp prevents air from entering stomach or gastric contents from leaking out.

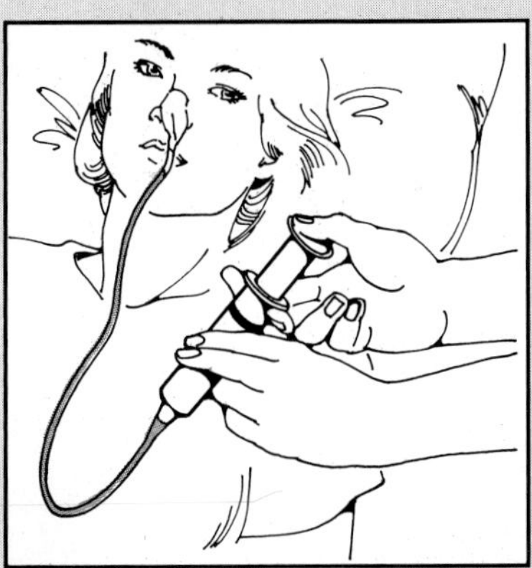

(*continued*)

PROCEDURE 25–3. (continued)

d. Position client or request client to keep head of bed elevated to 30 degrees for 30–60 minutes after feeding.

d. Facilitates gastric emptying; prevents regurgitation or aspiration.

RECORDING: Commonly charted on flowsheet. *Continuous feeding:* Document placement check, lung and abdominal assessment, type, concentration and rate of formula infusion. Note untoward effects and action taken. *Intermittent Feeding:* Document placement check, residual obtained. Note the time of feeding, amount of formula and water instilled and client response.

PROCEDURE 25–4. CARING FOR A GASTROSTOMY OR JEJUNOSTOMY TUBE SITE

PURPOSE: To prevent skin breakdown or infection and accidental tube removal.

EQUIPMENT: Catheter plug; 4 × 4-inch gauze dressing; tape; petrolatum; zinc oxide or other skin barrier; hydrogen peroxide; betadine or mild soap.

ACTION	RATIONALE
1. When tube is not in use for decompression or feeding, keep it sealed with a cap or clamp.	1. Prevents leakage of gastric or intestinal contents.
2. Check site of tube entry at least once per shift. Cleanse any leakage around the site as ordered and dry the skin. Use care not to disturb the suture securing the tube to the skin. Betadine, hydrogen peroxide, or soap and water are commonly ordered for skin care.	2. Leakage of gastric contents causes skin excoriation and possible subsequent infection.

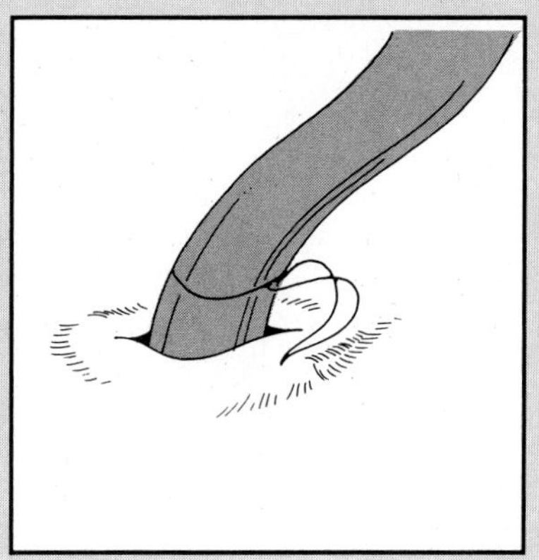

PROCEDURE 25–4. (continued)

3. Apply petrolatum or other skin barrier and cover with a 4 × 4-inch gauze dressing.

3. These substances are insoluble in water, and so will not dissolve in GI secretions and will therefore minimize skin irritation.

4. Tape tube to the outside of the dressing. Tube may be connected to feeding apparatus or, less commonly, to suction apparatus or gravity drainage.

4. Prevents tension on the tube causing possible widening of skin opening and/or accidental removal of tube.

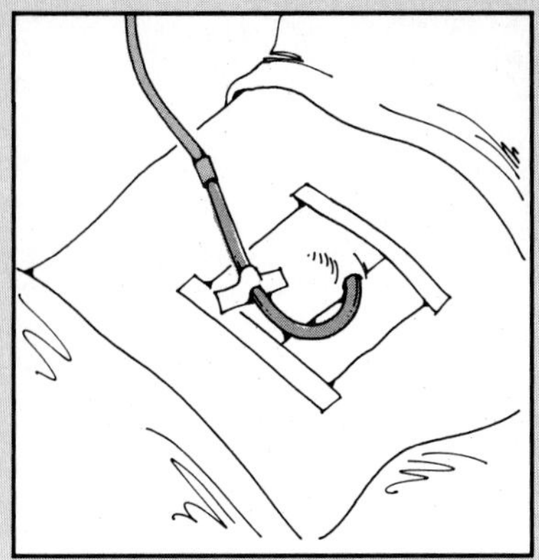

NOTE: If tube is accidentally pulled out, cover the opening with a sterile petrolatum dressing until tubing can be reinserted.

RECORDING: Record date and time of site check and/or dressing change. Record skin condition, any leakage of fluid or formula, skin care provided, and type of dressing applied.

PROCEDURE 25–5: REMOVING A NASOGASTRIC TUBE

PURPOSE: Discontinuing decompression or tube feeding.

EQUIPMENT: Waterproof pad, clean gloves, mouth care preparations of choice, fresh water, adhesive remover.

ACTION

1. Verify orders for removal of tube.

2. Assess abdomen for bowel sounds. If not audible, consult with physician.

NOTE: If used for administering liquid feedings, tubes are discontinued when client is able to resume oral intake. Bowel sounds should have been present throughout therapy.

RATIONALE

1. Medical order is required to discontinue a medically ordered treatment.

2. Decompression NG tubes are used postoperatively and are left in place until bowel sounds return. If removed before peristalsis resumes, pooled gastric secretions may cause nausea and vomiting.

PROCEDURE 25–5. (continued)

3. Discuss procedure with client. Provide information about desired participation and usual sensations associated with removal.
   a. Client should be in Fowler's position.
   b. Tube will be removed rapidly to minimize gagging.
   c. Exhaling as tube is removed will relax pharynx (decreasing irritation and preventing aspiration).
   d. Slight irritation of throat and nostril may accompany withdrawal. Eyes may water.
   e. Slightly bitter aftertaste is common; mouth care will relieve this effect.

   Rationale: 3. A clear understanding of the procedure will increase the effectiveness of client participation and reduce apprehension.

4. Free tubing from gown, carefully remove tape from nose, moving tube as little as possible.

   4. Movement of tube creates friction and erosion of mucous membranes of nose and throat. After several days of intubation, there is sufficient irritation that even a small amount of movement of the tube is painful.

5. Place waterproof pad over client's gown. Don clean gloves.

   5. Protects nurse and client from contact with secretions in or on tube.

6. Disconnect tube from suction machine or feeding pump. Firmly pinch tube or fold it back on itself to prevent fluid leaking.

   6. Leaking fluid from the tube during removal may cause aspiration.

7. Cue the client, then withdraw the tube steadily and rapidly while client exhales.

   7. Avoids startling client, enhances relaxation.

8. Wrap tube in waterproof pad; remove gloves; dispose of all according to agency policy.

   8. Prevents transfer of microorganisms to environment.

9. Provide tissues to blow nose; mouthwash, toothbrush, or lemon-glycerine swabs to freshen mouth. Provide opportunity (or assist) to wash face.

   9. Promotes comfort.

10. Offer fluids—encourage sipping, not rapid intake.

    10. Client with NG tube has been n.p.o. or receiving fluids by slow drip. Clients may be eager to drink, but rapid intake may cause nausea and vomiting.

RECORDING: Note completion of procedure, client's response, amount of drainage in suction container if tube was used for decompression, and complications (if any) and action taken.

Rehabilitative Care

Nutritional rehabilitation is the focus of this level of care. Here the aim is to maximize the client's nutritional status after an acute alteration from normal, and to facilitate self-care ability. The nurse uses strategies similar to those used in preventive and supportive care. Supporting life-style changes, counseling, and referral to support groups assume particular importance in the rehabilitation process.

Supporting Life-style and Habit Changes. After an acute nutritional alteration, clients are often highly motivated to implement life-style changes that will hasten their recovery and prevent further problems. Clients need specific guidelines and practical suggestions regarding new eating patterns and habits that will be of benefit. They also require encouragement and support as they initiate changes in previous patterns. Close follow-up and reinforcement are necessary.

Counseling. The same principles of counseling discussed earlier can be applied to rehabilitative care. The client's need for an attitude of optimism is particularly significant during the process of rehabilitation. Progress may be slow, so clients are vulnerable to discouragement. Nurses can provide a climate of realistic hope to support clients through these low points.

Referral to Support Groups. Adolescents, parents with children requiring long-term dietary regimens, and the elderly may find support groups particularly helpful in maintaining life-style changes. Dieticians may be of help in identifying local groups available for clients. In our society, support groups can usually be found for almost any major kind of health problem.

IMPLICATIONS FOR NURSE–CLIENT COLLABORATION

Evaluation

Evaluation of nutritional care is based on the many physical indicators of an adequate diet and intake of nutrients. Body weight, laboratory results, and physical signs such as the apparent energy shown in the client's behavior are important. The nurse uses all of these indicators in evaluating whether the client's nutritional status has improved with the care given.

Evaluating nutritional status also requires that the nurse is aware of the client's personal appraisal of the nutritional plan. Specifically, the nurse is concerned about whether the diet is meeting a client's emotional and social needs. An adequately nourished client has a sense of well-being. This aspect of evaluation can only be carried out by collaborating with clients and inviting them to share personal perspectives on how well the nutritional plan is working.

■ EVALUATION

The evaluation of nurse and client actions to promote optimum nutrition can only be as good as the desired outcomes that have been identified. If goals are specific and realistic, evaluation criteria, which also must be specific and measurable, easily flow from them. Many of the assessment criteria for nutritional status can be used as individual evaluation criteria. Clinical indicators of nutritional status—such as physical findings, anthropometric measures, and lab tests—are appropriate evaluation criteria. Nurses should attempt to be as specific and as individualized as possible when selecting criteria for the evaluation of nutritional care. Progress toward desired outcomes is monitored during the course of care as well as on specified target dates.

SUMMARY

Nutrition involves processes that are extremely complex and elaborately regulated in order to maintain a constant supply of nutrients to the cells of the body. The nutrients obtained from food are digested, absorbed, and metabolized for the production of energy necessary to sustain all the life processes of the body and to build and repair body tissues. The nursing diagnoses related to alterations in nutrition are derived from client problems of food intake, digestion, absorption, or metabolism.

Nutritional assessment must focus on all aspects of the client's nutritional activities and status, not only the physical dimensions. Because for the human being nutrition is intimately associated with emotional, social, and cultural factors, all of these must be thoroughly assessed. The entire process, including assessment and management of nutritional problems, must involve a fully collaborative relationship between the client and nurse in order to be effective. Nutritional alterations cannot be corrected without the client's active interest, motivation, and effort, and these can only be manifested in a collaborative nurse–client relationship.

Nursing implementation to promote clients' nutritional well-being may involve any of the four levels of client care. The spectrum of nursing skills ranges from teaching and counseling to complete responsibility for the feeding of a client. Feeding techniques include oral, enteral, and parenteral measures. The insertion of a tube into the alimentary tract is a frequently used technique to provide nutrition to clients unable to orally ingest food.

The nurse's role in a collaborative interprofessional effort to assist clients with nutritional alterations is of utmost significance. The primary caring relationship between nurse and client often places the nurse in the highly nurturing role of feeding the client. Even if this is not necessary, the nurse's continuous and intimate concern with the hour-to-hour nutritional needs of the client in the acute care setting places the nurse–client relationship in a central position.

REFERENCES

1. Newman CF. Americans: This is what you need to eat right. *NURSEweek*. June, 1989.
2. Cataldo CB, Nyenhuis JR, Whitney EN. *Nutrition and Diet Therapy: Principles and Practice*. 2nd ed. St. Paul: West; 1989.
3. Forde O. The Tromso heart study: Coffee consumption and serum lipid concentrations in men with hypercholesterolemia: A randomized intervention study. *Br Med J*. 1985;290:893.
4. Williams SR. Nutrition and Diet Therapy. 6th ed. St. Louis: Mosby; 1989.
5. Boynton RW, Dunn ES, Stephens GR. *Manual of Ambulatory Pediatrics*. 2nd ed. Glenview, IL: Scott, Foresman; 1988.
6. Green ML, Harry J. *Nutrition in Contemporary Nursing Practice*. 2nd ed. New York: Wiley; 1987.
7. Carrieri VK, Lindsey AM, West CM. *Pathophysiological Phenomena in Nursing: Human Responses to Illness*. Philadelphia: Saunders; 1986.
8. National Research Council, Committee on Dietary Allowances, Food and Nutrition Board. *Recommended Dietary Allowances*. 10th ed. Washington, DC: National Academy of Sciences; 1989.
9. Senate Select Committee on Nutrition and Health. *Dietary Goals for the United States*. 2nd ed. Washington, DC: US Govt Printing Office; 1977.
10. Committee on Diet and Health, National Research Council. *Diet and Health: Implications for Reducing Chronic Disease Risk (Executive Summary)*. Washington, DC: National Academy Press; 1989.
11. Williams SR. The use and abuse of height–weight tables. In: Williams SR, ed. *Essentials of Nutrition and Diet Therapy*. St. Louis: Mosby; 1990.
12. Hirsh J, Leibel RL. A new light on obesity. *N Engl J Med*. 1988;318:509.
13. Brownell KD. The psychology and physiology of obesity: Implications for screening and treatment. *J Am Dietetic Assn*. 1984; 84:406.
14. Williams SR. The control of body fat. In: Williams SR, ed. *Essentials of Nutrition and Diet Therapy*. St. Louis: Mosby; 1990.
15. Kemnitz JW. Body weight and set point theory. *Contemp Nutr*. 1985;10(2).
16. Rosenthal MB, Benson RC. Psychologic aspects of obstetrics and gynecology. In: Pernoll ML, ed. *Current Obstetric and Gynecologic Diagnosis and Treatment*. 6th ed. Norwalk, CT: Appleton & Lange; 1991.
17. Eschleman MM. *Introductory Nutrition and Diet Therapy*. Philadelphia: Lippincott; 1991.
18. Roy LB, Edwards PA, Barr LH. The value of nutritional assessment in surgical patients. *J Enteral Parenteral Nutr*. 1985;9:170–172.
19. Collinsworth R, Boyle K. Nutritional assessment of the elderly. *J Gerontol Nurs*. 1989;15:17–21.
20. Ryan VC, Gates AD. Nutrient intake status, knowledge, source of information and self-perceived health status among older adults in South Carolina. *J Nutr Elderly*. 1988;8:41–48.
21. Busse G. Nutritional counseling. In: Bulecheck GM, McCloskey JC, eds. *Nursing Interventions: Treatments for Nursing Diagnoses*. Philadelphia: Saunders; 1985.
22. Price JH, Desmond SM, Ruppert ES, Stelzer CM. School nurses' perceptions of childhood obesity. *J School Health*. 1987; 57:332–336.
23. Whitney EN, Cataldo CB, Rolfes SR. *Understanding Normal and Clinical Nutrition*. 3rd ed. St. Paul: West; 1991.
24. Pender NJ. *Health Promotion in Nursing Practice*. 2nd ed. Norwalk, CT: Appleton & Lange; 1987.
25. Carr EK, Hawthorn PJ. Lip function and eating after stroke: A nursing perspective. *J Adv Nurs*. 1988;13:447–451.
26. Norberg A, Backstrom A, Elsy A, Norberg B. Food refusal amongst nursing home patients as conceptualized by nurses' aides and enrolled nurses: An interview study. *J Adv Nurs*. 1988;13:478–483.

BIBLIOGRAPHY

American Institute for Cancer Research. *Dietary Guidelines to Lower Cancer Risk*. Washington, DC: American Institute for Cancer Research; 1982.

Burtis G, Davis J, Martin S. *Applied Nutrition and Diet Therapy*. Philadelphia: Saunders; 1988.

Carpenito LJ. *Nursing Diagnosis: Application to Clinical Practice*. 3rd ed. Philadelphia: Lippincott; 1989.

Committee on Diet, Nutrition, and Cancer, National Research Council. *Executive Summary: Diet, Nutrition, and Cancer*. Washington, DC: National Academy Press; 1982.

Dudek SG. *Nutrition Handbook for Nursing Practice*. Philadelphia: Lippincott; 1987.

Food and Nutrition Board, National Research Council. *Toward Healthful Diets*. Washington, DC: National Academy of Sciences.

Ganong WF. *Review of Medical Physiology*. 14th ed. Norwalk, CT: Appleton & Lange; 1991.

Green L, Harry J. *Nutrition in Contemporary Nursing Practice*. 2nd ed. New York: Wiley; 1987.

Hill L, Smith N. *Self-care Nursing*. 2nd ed. Norwalk, CT: Appleton & Lange; 1990.

Ignavicius DD, Bayne MV. *Medical-Surgical Nursing*. Philadelphia: Saunders; 1991.

Lappe FM. *Diet for a Small Planet*. 10th Anniversary Edition. New York: Ballantine; 1982.

McDougall JA. *McDougall's Medicine: A Challenging Second Opinion*. Piscataway, NJ: New Century Publishers; 1985.

Patrick M, Woods S, Craven R, Rokosky J, Bruno P. *Medical-Surgical Nursing: Pathophysiological Concepts*. 2nd ed. Philadelphia: Lippincott; 1991.

Spallholz JE. *Nutrition: Chemistry and Biology*. Englewood Cliffs, NJ: Prentice Hall; 1989.

US Department of Health and Human Services. *Diet, Nutrition, and Cancer Prevention: A Guide to Food Choices*. Pub. no. 87-2878. Washington, DC: National Institutes of Health; May 1987.

US Department of Health and Human Services, Public Health Service. *The Surgeon-General's Report on Diet and Health: Summary and Recommendations*. DHHS (PH) pub. no. 88-50210. Washington, DC: US Govt Printing Office; 1988.

CHAPTER 26

Elimination

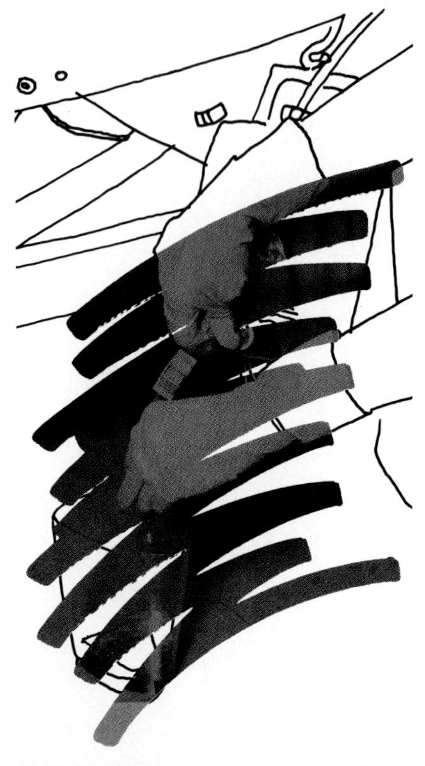

Objectives

Upon completion of this chapter, the student will be able to:

1. Name and describe the primary function of the major organs of bowel and urinary elimination.
2. Describe the normal patterns of elimination in an adult.
3. List four factors affecting bowel function and four factors affecting urinary function and describe their consequences.
4. Describe variations in elimination that may occur in the course of the life cycle.
5. Identify six alterations in bowel elimination.
6. Identify five alterations in urinary elimination.
7. List data to be obtained in an elimination history.
8. Identify essential elements of a nursing examination of bowel and urinary function.
9. Identify at least six diagnostic tests used in determining elimination status.
10. List three nursing diagnoses describing altered bowel elimination and identify an etiology for each.
11. List six nursing diagnoses describing altered urinary elimination and identify an etiology for each.
12. Describe two examples of preventive, supportive, restorative, and rehabilitative nursing implementation that promote bowel and bladder function and give the rationale for each.
13. Describe common learning needs of clients with an alteration in elimination.
14. Write a nursing care plan for a client with altered elimination.
15. Discuss the nurse's role in collaborating with the client to promote optimal elimination function.

KEY TERMS

adynamic ileus
anuria
constipation
diarrhea
duodenocolic reflex
dysuria
elimination
enema
enuresis
fecal impaction
fecal incontinence
flatulence
functional incontinence
gastrocolic reflex
glomerular filtration rate
Kegel exercises
melena
nephron
nocturia
oliguria
paralytic ileus
peristalsis
polyuria
proteinuria
stoma
stress incontinence
urinary frequency
urinary incontinence
urinary retention
Valsalva maneuver

Elimination is the process by which the body excretes waste products. Removal of body waste is a complex function that is vital to health. Elimination involves intricate physiological and psychological interrelationships and is affected by such factors as age, life-style, health status, and emotional state. This chapter discusses both bowel and urinary elimination. Bowel elimination rids the body of indigestible dietary matter after nutrients and water have been extracted for use by the body. Urinary elimination (urination) regulates fluid and electrolyte balance and rids the body of the end products of metabolism.

Alterations in elimination influence well-being and may indicate a change in health status. Examples of commonly experienced alterations in elimination include constipation when traveling away from home, and urinary frequency at times of stress. These and other alterations addressed in this chapter can be corrected by collaborative efforts of the client, nurse, and other members of the health care team.

Nurses need to acquire skill in collecting data about urinary and bowel function to identify alterations that can be corrected by nursing implementation. This data collection involves collaboration with the client and family in order to elicit comprehensive information. For effective data collection, nurses need to apply knowledge of basic anatomical structures and physiological functions related to elimination as well as communication and physical assessment techniques. Analysis of a comprehensive elimination data base yields nursing diagnoses of elimination alterations. Once nursing diagnoses are established, nurse and client mutually plan approaches to promote optimum elimination. Management approaches may include four levels of nursing implementation, as discussed in this chapter.

This chapter provides a basis for the understanding of elimination function, assessment of elimination, and management of common elimination problems. The nurse, in collaboration with the client and family, has a vital role in helping the client to achieve, maintain, and promote optimal elimination.

Section 1. Understanding Elimination

Many factors influence elimination, among them nutrition, exercise, emotions, and disease. Early toilet training often has a significant effect on elimination habits. Individuals highly value control of elimination, and being "wet" or "soiled" is very humiliating.

Healthy individuals often take for granted their ability to control elimination. Depending on a catheter for urinary drainage or soiling the bed with feces may embarrass a client and affect body image. An approach that demonstrates sensitivity and understanding is essential when caring for persons who are unable to manage elimination processes. A working knowledge of anatomy and physiology is basic to understanding elimination.

■ OPTIMUM BOWEL ELIMINATION

The function of bowel elimination is to rid the body of undigested waste once nutrients and water have been absorbed for use by the body. These functions are mainly carried out in the lower gastrointestinal (GI) tract, which consists of the colon, rectum, and anal canal. While the large intestine is primarily responsible for bowel elimination, the entire gastrointestinal tract plays a role.

Anatomy and Physiology

Upper GI Tract. Bowel elimination occurs after food has been processed throughout the entire gastrointestinal tract; therefore the entire tract is essential to the process of bowel elimination. Following ingestion of food, nutrients are mechanically and chemically broken down by enzymes in the mouth and stomach. The partially digested food then moves along the tract to the small intestine, where most nutrients are absorbed. (See Chap. 25 for a more detailed discussion of these processes.) The chyme (viscous, semifluid stomach contents) that has not been absorbed moves into the large intestine (colon) through the ileocecal valve. This valve, a circular muscle, prevents the contents of the colon from returning to the small intestine. The chyme enters the colon in a watery state and is concentrated into a soft formed mass as it moves through the colon.

Colon. The colon is a tubular structure of muscle lined with mucous membrane extending 1.5 m (5 ft) from cecum to anal canal (Fig. 26–1). It consists of the following divisions: cecum; ascending, transverse, and descending colon; sigmoid colon; rectum; and anus.

Colonic mucus is secreted to protect the lining of the colon. The mucus, which contains large numbers of bicarbonate ions, protects the intestinal wall from the acids formed in the feces. The mucus also serves as a binding agent to hold the fecal material together. Mucus secretion is stimulated by parasympathetic nerves. Therefore, an extreme emotional reaction can cause overstimulation of these nerves and an overproduction of mucus, resulting in stringy mucoid stools with little or no feces. The functions of the colon are (1) absorption of water and nutrients (2) fecal elimination.

The colon absorbs large quantities of water (as much as 2.5 L) in 24 hours. Up to 55 milliequivalents (mEq) of sodium and 23 mEq of chloride are absorbed daily. The speed at which the colonic contents move determines how much water is absorbed from the chyme.

Fecal elimination is accomplished by moving the chyme—normally a soft, formed mass—along the colon into the rectum and anal canal. This is accomplished by muscular actions called haustral shuffling, haustral contractions, and peristalsis. Haustral shuffling moves the chyme back and forth and aids in the absorption of water. Haustral contractions, also called segmentation, propel the contents along the colon. When one haustra (pouch-like section of

IMPLICATIONS FOR NURSE–CLIENT COLLABORATION

Personal and Social Meaning of Elimination

Elimination is a natural and normal body function, and one that is vital to health. Nevertheless, in modern society, there are strong social mores surrounding both the products and the process of human elimination. Individuals as members of society can be expected to share the conflicts of society, to appreciate the importance of healthy elimination, but also to fear a loss of control over their own elimination process. This fear is a powerful motivator and may significantly affect the client's capacity to collaborate when the health problem involves elimination. Even temporary problems with wetting or soiling can be humiliating; and when the problem is chronic or demands changes of a permanent nature, a person's body image and self-esteem can be profoundly affected. The nurse's sensitivity to the human emotions surrounding elimination is therefore essential to caring for persons who are unable to manage their own elimination.

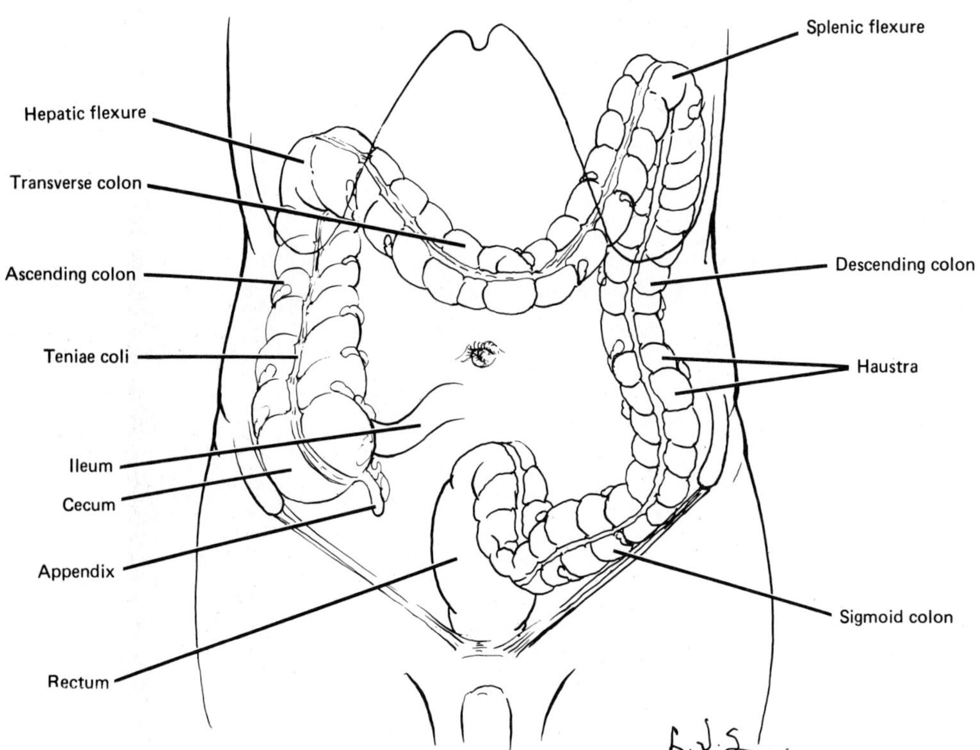

Figure 26–1. Anatomy of the colon. (*From Lindner HH.* Clinical Anatomy. *Norwalk, CT: Appleton & Lange; 1989. Modified from Way LW (ed).* Current Surgical Diagnosis and Treatment. *7th ed. Los Altos, CA: Lange; 1985.*)

the colon) is completely distended, it contracts and empties its contents into the next. **Peristalsis,** a wavelike muscular contraction along the length of the colon, also advances the colon contents. Mass peristalsis occurs about 1 hour after a meal. This knowledge should aid the nurse in planning elimination implementations for a client.

Rectum and Anal Canal. Waste products, now called feces, enter the sigmoid colon and are stored there until just before defecation (the act of having a bowel movement). The rectum is normally empty of feces until just before defecation. Rectum length varies according to age. In the adult, rectal length is about 10 to 15 cm (4 to 6 in). The distal portion of the rectum (3 to 5 cm or 1½ to 2 in long) is called the anal canal.

The rectum contains vertical and transverse folds of tissue that help retain feces. Each vertical fold contains a vein and an artery. The veins, when repeatedly distended either by pressure exerted during straining to defecate or by increased intra-abdominal pressure associated with pregnancy or heavy lifting, can become permanently dilated. This condition is called hemorrhoids. Hemorrhoids can make defecation painful and may cause varying amounts of blood loss (Fig. 26–2).

The anal canal contains internal and external sphincter muscles (Fig. 26–3). The internal sphincter is involuntarily controlled by the autonomic nervous system. While the ex-

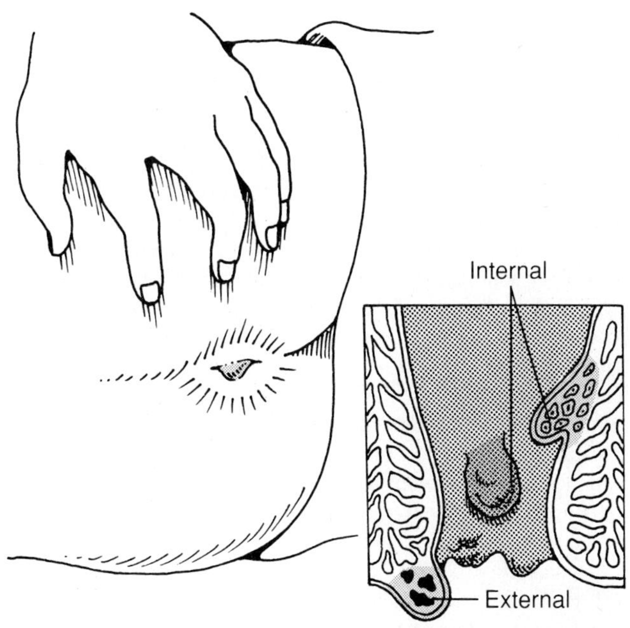

Figure 26–2. Hemorrhoids.

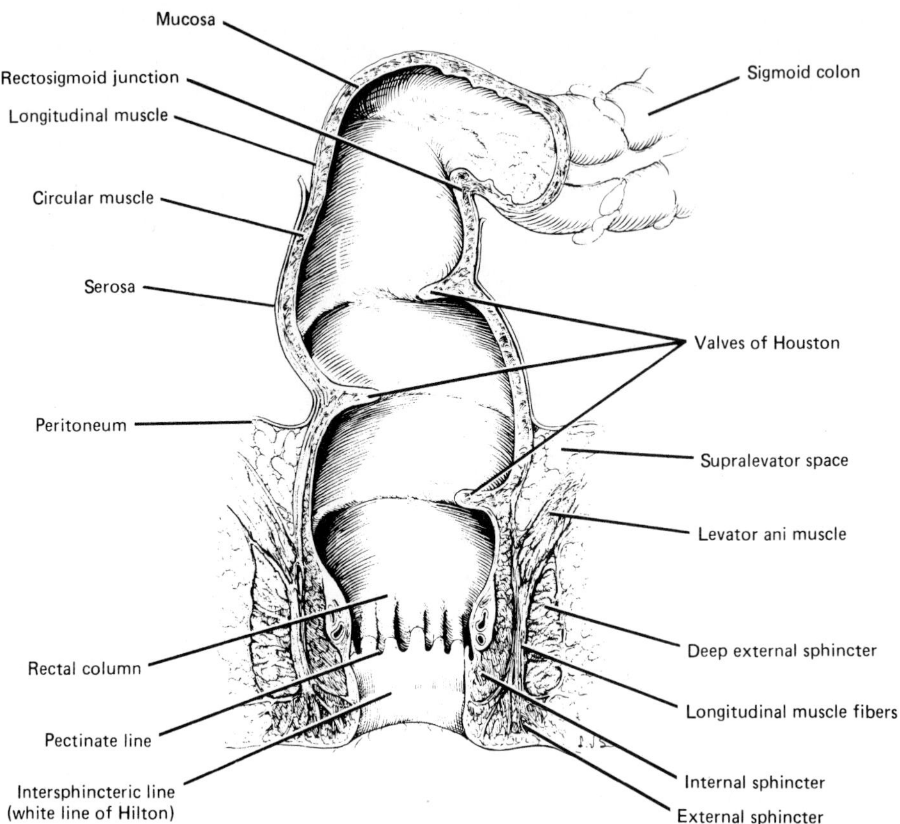

Figure 26–3. Anatomy of the rectosigmoid, rectum, and anus showing internal and external sphincters. (*From Lindner HH.* Clinical Anatomy. *Norwalk, CT: Appleton & Lange; 1989. Modified from Way LW (ed).* Current Surgical Diagnosis and Treatment. *7th ed. Los Altos, CA: Lange; 1985.*)

ternal sphincter is influenced by the internal sphincter, it is usually voluntarily controlled. When sensory nerves in the rectum are stimulated by the entrance of the fecal mass, the individual becomes aware of the need to defecate.

Defecation. Defecation is influenced by reflexes but is also under voluntary control. The **gastrocolic** and the **duodenocolic reflexes,** which occur in response to distension of the stomach and the duodenum, contribute to defecation by stimulating mass peristalsis along the entire length of the GI tract.[1] Mass peristalsis is most predominant within 15 minutes after eating breakfast.

The intrinsic defecation reflex occurs when feces distend the rectum, initiating the peristaltic waves in the descending and sigmoid colon and the rectum and forcing feces toward the anus. As these peristaltic waves approach the anus, the internal sphincter is inhibited from closing. The parasympathetic defecation reflex intensifies this intrinsic defecation reflex. It occurs when nerve fibers in the rectum are stimulated by the presence of fecal matter. Signals are sent to the spinal cord and back to the colon and rectum to intensify the peristaltic waves and relax the internal anal sphincter. When rectal pressure continues to increase, reflex relaxation of the external sphincter occurs, and the rectal contents are expelled.

Voluntary neuromuscular control can be used to delay or facilitate defecation. As the feces move into the anal canal and the internal anal sphincter relaxes, the individual feels the urge to defecate. Defecation is initiated by relaxing the external anal sphincter while contracting the abdominal muscles and the diaphragm. The increased abdominal pressure moves feces down the anal canal. The levator ani muscles of the pelvic floor are also voluntarily contracted to aid in fecal expulsion. The **Valsalva maneuver**—holding one's breath while exerting expiratory effort against a closed glottis, and then contracting the abdominal muscles—is also often used to help expel feces.

When an individual ignores the urge to defecate or consciously contracts the external sphincter muscles to delay defecation, the urge to defecate may disappear for several hours before reoccurring. Repeatedly ignoring the urge to defecate can result in an abnormally enlarged rectum and loss of rectal sensitivity. The individual's perception of the need to defecate becomes dulled, creating the potential for constipation, discussed below.

Normal Bowel Elimination

Normal Patterns. Normal patterns of bowel elimination vary widely. Some individuals defecate one to two times a day; others, two or three times a week. There are many techniques that individuals use to assist with bowel function, such as drinking a cup of hot water before breakfast, or prune juice at night, or reading while using the toilet.

Such measures may support physiological processes. Drinking warm fluids on arising, for example, stimulates the gastrocolic reflex and can create a desire to defecate.

Characteristics of Normal Stool. The nurse should observe feces for consistency, amount, color, shape, odor, and the presence of any unusual matter.

Consistency. Dietary intake and the quantity of fluid intake directly affect the stool's consistency; however, normal stool is soft and formed. Speed of peristalsis will determine the liquid content and the shape of the stool. Decreased peristalsis results in small, hard, dry stools; increased peristalsis causes liquid unformed stools.

Softer-than-normal stools are variously described as "soft," "semiformed," or "loose," if they are liquid with some solid material. "Liquid stools" consist of colored fluid only. Very solid stools can be described as "hard" or "constipated."

Amount. The amount of fecal material passed each day will vary depending on the dietary intake. Clients are the best source of information about their customary amounts of stool. The nurse should also observe and note any increase or decrease in the amount of stool.

Color. The color of adult stool is normally brown, because of the presence of bile pigments. If there is lack of bile or an obstruction to its flow, a clay-colored or white stool results. Formation of gallstones, which obstruct the biliary tract, is a common cause of clay-colored stools. Malabsorption syndrome also causes a pale-colored stool. Black stools may be a side effect of iron supplements or may be caused by upper gastrointestinal bleeding. Bright red blood in the stool is most commonly associated with bleeding hemorrhoids, but may also indicate lower GI bleeding. **Melena** is the term used to refer to blood in the feces.

Shape. The shape of a normal stool reflects that of the rectum. If an intestinal obstruction is present, the stool may become pencil-thin or ribbon-shaped as it squeezes by the obstruction. Pencil-thin stool can also be caused by rapid intestinal motility.

Odor. Stool usually possesses a characteristic fecal odor. Some foods may alter the stool odor. Foul-smelling stools are associated with malabsorption syndrome. Blood in the feces or intestinal infection may also change stool odor.

Components. Normal stool components include the end products of digestion. There should be no visible blood or mucus or any other unusual matter, such as undigested food or worms. Worms are common in some areas of the world and may occur occasionally in the United States. Pinworms, which resemble fine white threads, or tapeworms, which are ⅛ to ¼ inch wide and may grow 5 to 20 feet long, may be visible to the naked eye. Their eggs (ova) may be easily detected by microscopic survey of a strip of clear plastic tape that has been placed briefly over the anal opening. Tapeworms or segments of the worm can also appear in the stool.

Factors Affecting Bowel Function

Many factors may affect bowel function. Some common factors include age, life-style, health status, and emotional state. These factors produce the individual variation seen in bowel elimination.

Age. Fecal elimination patterns change throughout the life cycle. Some changes are caused by continued physiological development and aging.

Infants. The infant (birth to 1 year) is unable to control defecation due to lack of neuromuscular maturity. Stool frequency and characteristics depend upon feeding method. The infant who is breastfed has loose, seedy, golden yellow stools, often after every feeding. The stools are not irritating to the infant's skin. Stools of formula-fed infants are pale yellow, firmer, and irritating to the skin. Formula-fed infants usually have only one to two stools a day.

Toddlers. Toddlers (ages 1 to 3 years) become physically ready to control bowel elimination between 18 and 24 months of age; however, cognitive and psychosocial readiness, also essential, frequently is achieved later. Daytime bowel control, therefore, is usually accomplished around 30 months. Attempting to toilet train toddlers before they are ready, or punishing them for "accidents," may create significant stress and delay control. If toddlers are hospitalized, they often regress and temporarily lose control of elimination.

Preschool and School-Aged Children. Preschool (ages 3 to 5) and school-aged (ages 6 to 12) children exhibit a variety of defecation patterns, usually establishing an individual pattern that is characteristic. Constipation is a common problem in both age groups. It may be related to dietary changes, febrile illness, or emotional or environmental changes. Parents should be cautioned against indiscriminate use of laxatives to treat constipation; increasing fluids, fruits, vegetables, and grains is preferable.

Adolescents. Adolescents (ages 13 to 18) experience a period of rapid growth. Both the stomach and the colon enlarge to accommodate the greater food intake that accompanies this growth spurt, and stools often increase in size and number.

Young and Middle-Aged Adults. Young (ages 18 to 35) and middle-aged (ages 35 to 65) adults establish characteristic individual bowel elimination patterns that vary with dietary, life-style, and other variables discussed below.

Older Adults. Older adults (over age 65) frequently experience constipation. This can be attributed to several factors. Many elderly adults must take several medications for treatment of chronic diseases. Difficulties in chewing associated with loss of teeth or poorly fitting dentures lead to choosing soft foods, which decreases bulk in the stool. Diminished thirst sensation and reduced mobility contribute to limited fluid intake as well as to less activity. All of these factors, plus the loss of colon and abdominal muscle tone that frequently occurs with age, increase risk for constipation.[2] Many older individuals rely on laxatives to correct constipation, but laxative use often compounds the problem and may even result in dependency. Increasing exercise, fluids, and bulk-producing foods will reduce constipation risk and make laxatives unnecessary.

Loss of muscle tone may also affect the internal anal sphincter, and even though the external sphincter is still intact, some elderly persons experience difficulty controlling defecation. Older adults also may become less aware of the need to defecate because of impaired nerve impulse transmission. In addition, they may develop GI infections that may be difficult to identify because only vague symptoms are presented. In the elderly these infections can be life threatening.[3]

Life-style. Bowel function can be disrupted by a chaotic life-style of irregular meals, changing schedules, and increased stress. A sedentary life-style increases the risk of constipation, because peristalsis is stimulated by exercise. A regular pattern of intake and elimination is health promoting. Nurse–client collaboration can often help clients establish healthier patterns.

Diet. Diet plays an essential role in promoting healthy elimination. Eating meals at regularly scheduled times will help establish regular bowel patterns. Adequate intake of dietary fiber provides bulk that will keep the stool soft and increase the speed of passage through the intestines. This in turn limits the amount of water that is absorbed from fecal matter, thus producing a soft, formed stool. Foods that are valuable sources of fiber include whole grains (breads and cereals), fresh fruits (apples, oranges), root vegetables (carrots, turnips, celery), greens (lettuce, spinach), legumes (dried beans, peas), and cooked fruit (apricots, prunes).[4] These high-fiber or bulk-producing foods also stretch the bowel wall, stimulating peristalsis and initiating the defecation reflex. Some foods, such as beans, onions, and cabbage, are gas producing; the gas distends the bowel and may cause cramping or excessive bowel activity.

Certain foods are difficult for some people to digest and may cause digestive upsets and sometimes even watery stools (diarrhea). Foods that promote normal elimination in one person may create constipation or diarrhea in another. For example, milk and milk products should be avoided by people who are lactose intolerant. Milk contains lactose, a simple sugar, that is broken down in the body by the enzyme lactase. Individuals with lactose intolerance do not produce the enzyme lactase and are therefore unable to digest foods containing lactose. This can result in abdominal cramping, nausea, gaseous distension, and diarrhea.

Exercise. Exercise is important in maintaining the tone and strength of the abdominal and pelvic floor muscles that are used in defecation. A sedentary life-style decreases peristalsis. Conversely, regular exercise contributes to regular elimination patterns.

Weak muscles may result from severe illness, prolonged immobility, or neurological disease that impairs nerve function. Individuals with these conditions may benefit from special conditioning exercises to strengthen the muscles of the abdomen and pelvic floor to facilitate healthy elimination.

Elimination Habits. Elimination habits are influenced by a variety of factors, such as toilet training, type of toilet facilities, daily schedule, and attitude toward the body.

Bowel elimination is a private matter and most people prefer to use their own toilet facilities. Establishing a bowel pattern that permits use of home facilities at a convenient time is advantageous. Busy and changing work schedules can cause disruption of regular habits and increase risk for constipation.

Hospitalization often disrupts established elimination habits. Lack of privacy, change in routines, altered intake of food and fluids, diminished activity, and ingesting multiple medications all contribute to altered elimination patterns.

Health Status. A variety of health status factors can influence an individual's elimination patterns. These include hydration, pain, tissue integrity, and medications. Diagnostic procedures can also affect elimination, because many require fasting or enemas.

Hydration. Adequate hydration is crucial to healthy elimination. Six to eight glasses (1400 to 2000 mL) per day is the normal fluid requirement for an adult. Fluid is necessary for efficient movement of intestinal contents and for the absorption of nutrients and electrolytes. Fluids also enter the intestine from saliva, gastric secretions, pancreatic juices, and bile.

The gastrointestinal tract contributes to maintaining fluid balance. If alterations in other body systems cause a fluid loss or deficiency, the intestine will absorb more fluid, helping intra- and extracellular fluid volumes remain relatively constant. However, the resulting decrease in the amount of fluid within the intestine slows peristalsis and hardens the feces. Therefore, when assessing bowel function, nurses must be alert to any condition that causes fluid loss.

Pain. Pain also may influence bowel function. Hemorrhoids, rectal surgery, and abdominal surgery can cause discomfort during defecation. As a result, clients may suppress the urge to defecate and become constipated. Nurses should also be alert to other conditions that could create discomfort for clients during defecation. Position on the bedpan, decubiti (pressure ulcers), and pelvic and hip fractures are other possible causes of pain.

Tissue Integrity. Tissue integrity of the bowel and external anal area is another important nursing assessment consideration. For example, ulcerative colitis may result in diarrhea. Tissue integrity may also be compromised when hemorrhoids ulcerate and bleed. Ulcers and fissures sometimes develop in the anal area, causing excoriation and irritation. Excoriation of the perianal area in turn makes elimination painful and may lead to constipation. If a nurse discovers an alteration of tissue integrity, collaboration with the client is important to establish the most appropriate nursing diagnosis and approaches to care.

Medications. Many medications can alter bowel function. For example, antibiotics can produce diarrhea and abdominal cramping; narcotic analgesics and opiates decrease peristalsis and can create constipation. Diuretics, which cause the body to eliminate fluid, may predispose the individual to constipation. Iron preparations may also cause constipation. When clients have diarrhea or constipation it is important to evaluate the side effects of any medication they are taking.

Some medications aid in bowel elimination or relieve constipation. They are called laxatives or cathartics. These drugs act by softening the stool or by promoting peristalsis. Overuse of these drugs can cause dependency. Severe diarrhea can also result from overuse of laxatives, creating electrolyte imbalance and dehydration. Nurses should carefully assess clients' use of these medications, because they are readily available over the counter. Children may take large doses of gum or candy laxatives (such as Ex-Lax) if they are not kept out of reach, resulting in serious poisoning.

Eating high-fiber foods and avoiding highly refined breads and cereals can eliminate the need for laxative use. Drinking at least 2000 mL of water per day (8 glasses) can also prevent constipation. Daily exercise is also essential to regular bowel elimination. If a laxative is necessary, bulk laxatives or stool softeners are preferable.[5] These medications can be purchased over the counter or prescribed. Advise clients who use laxatives to carefully follow directions on the label to avoid any complications.

Anesthesia. Anesthesia and surgery also affect bowel elimination. General anesthetics produce temporary slowing or cessation of peristalsis, whereas regional or spinal anesthesia affects bowel activity minimally or not at all. Handling the bowel during surgery often leads to temporary loss of peristalsis. This is called **paralytic** or **adynamic ileus.** It can last for 24 to 48 hours, although some clients experience paralytic ileus for a longer period of time. Most surgeons order n.p.o. status (nothing by mouth) for postoperative clients until bowel sounds return. Therefore, auscultation for bowel sounds is an important aspect of care for all postoperative clients (see Chap. 16).

Diagnostic Procedures. Diagnostic procedures to evaluate gastrointestinal function usually require that the bowel be empty. Clients are expected not to eat or drink after midnight of the day preceding the examination and may be required to have a cathartic and an enema. After clearing the bowel for these tests, normal defecation will usually not occur until the client has resumed eating. If barium is used as a contrast medium for these procedures, constipation or fecal impaction may occur unless the barium is effectively cleared from the GI tract. Therefore, a posttest cathartic or enema is usually ordered.

Emotional State. Emotional stress can affect the function of all body systems; the GI system is particularly susceptible. Anxiety, fear, and anger accelerate the digestive process and increase peristalsis to provide nutrients for body defense. This acceleration can lead to gaseous distension and diarrhea. In contrast, some individuals experience sluggish peristalsis when under stress and may become constipated.

The symptoms and the course of diseases of the GI tract can be affected by emotional stress. Ulcerative colitis, gastric ulcers, and Crohn's disease all worsen with emotional stress, even though the primary cause of these diseases has been shown to be physiological.

Early toilet training can interfere with a child's later bowel elimination patterns. A child's bowel training should not begin until physical, cognitive, and psychosocial readiness has been developed. This usually occurs at about 2 to 3 years of age. Spanking or making a child sit on the potty chair for a long time will make this training extremely stressful. Continuous battles between parent and child may lead to chronic constipation in the child. The emotional stress usually results from the conflict between the child's desire both to please the parent and to retain control over his or her own body. Positive reinforcement and a relaxed atmosphere about toileting help reduce the child's emotional stress.

Some individuals are overly concerned, even preoccupied, by the need to have a daily bowel movement. Disruptions in regular habits related to illness or diagnostic tests may create significant concern. Nurses need to accept the level of anxiety that these individuals experience. Explanations of the physiological basis for the delay in bowel function may allay anxiety.

Clients reveal clues about their emotional state and elimination concerns in various ways. For example, some directly express concerns about elimination; others make multiple requests for laxatives or prune juice. Collaborative assessment and planning are effective in resolving bowel elimination problems.

■ ALTERATIONS IN BOWEL ELIMINATION

Alterations in bowel elimination include constipation, diarrhea, incontinence, flatulence, and fecal impaction. These problems may arise from physiological or psychological factors. Surgical alteration of the intestine also affects bowel elimination.

Constipation

Constipation is the passage of small, hard, dry stool, or the passage of no stool, for an unusually long period of time for that person. It is a common problem that nurses can help to prevent. Difficulty passing stool and straining accompany constipation. However, it is important to remember that some individuals defecate several times a week, others one to two times a day. Careful assessment of elimination habits, therefore, is necessary before making a diagnosis of constipation.

Constipation has many causes, including insufficient exercise, irregular defecation habits, overuse of laxatives, disease processes, inappropriate diet, medications, and increased emotional stress. Pregnant women may suffer from constipation because of increased progesterone levels, which cause smooth muscle relaxation and slow peristalsis.

Any condition that leads to slowing of intestinal peristalsis or causes excess absorption of water may result in constipation. For example, since insufficient exercise may lead to decreased peristalsis, a regular exercise pattern contributes to maintenance of optimal elimination patterns. Diets lacking in fiber also decrease the bulk and water-absorbing ability of the stool.

Constipation affects both healthy and ill individuals. The person who is constipated will have various complaints. Uncomfortable symptoms such as nausea, heartburn, back pain, headache, or distress in the rectum or intestines may be reported. The client will state that bowel elimination has been less frequent than usual or that there have been no stools. A feeling of abdominal distension or bloating is often described. Feelings of rectal fullness, pressure in the rectum, and a palpable mass may also be reported. Activities of daily living and appetite may be impaired. Clients often express difficulty in passing stools. Straining during defecation may lead to development of hemorrhoids and rectal bleeding.

Other threats to health occur with constipation when the client has had recent abdominal or rectal surgery. Sutures may rupture and wounds may open from the stress of straining at defecation, but this is a rare occurrence. Straining during defecation is accompanied by breath holding (the Valsalva maneuver), which can cause additional problems for the client with heart disease, brain injury, or respiratory disease. Breathing and exhaling through the mouth while straining can reduce the hazard, but it is best to avoid any straining.

Diarrhea

Diarrhea is the rapid movement of fecal matter through the intestine, resulting in frequent evacuation of loose and watery stools. The stools often contain mucus and may be blood streaked.

Food poisoning, food intolerance, infection, disease, and antibiotics and other drugs are among the causes of diarrhea. In addition, diarrhea can be caused by severe emotional stress. Some surgical procedures may result in diarrhea. The rapid passage of intestinal contents does not allow for the usual absorption of fluid and electrolytes, often resulting in serious fluid and electrolyte imbalances. This can be life-threatening, especially in infants or elderly and debilitated clients. Several causes of diarrhea, along with the body's physiological response, or alteration, are listed in Table 26–1.

The person with diarrhea is often disturbed and em-

TABLE 26–1. DIARRHEA: CAUSES AND PHYSIOLOGICAL RESPONSES

Cause of Diarrhea	Physiological Alteration or Response
Food poisoning/intestinal infection (streptococcal or staphylococcal enteritis)	Increased mucus secretion and rapid intestinal motility.
Food or fluid allergies	Food or fluid not digested completely.
Food intolerance (eg, lactose intolerance)	Increased mucus secretion and rapid intestinal motility.
Chemicals: medications, laxatives	Irritation of intestinal tissue and/or increased intestinal movement.
Antibiotics	Intestinal mucosa inflamed and irritated due to superinfection. Antibiotics suppress the normal bacterial flora and allow other bacteria normally limited by the presence of normal flora to multiply. Some of these bacteria are hydrophilic (water-attracting). They cause an influx of fluid into the colon, which stimulates excessive peristalsis.
Other chemicals ingested, or foreign substances (eg, food preservatives)	Irritation of intestinal mucosa.
Iron preparations	Irritation of intestinal tissue in some individuals.
Colon diseases	
Chron's disease, colitis	Ulceration, inflammation of intestinal walls, rapid intestinal motility.
Malabsorption syndrome	Fluid and nutrient absorption reduced.
Surgical procedures	
Gastrectomy	Stomach cannot hold as much food and food enters duodenum too rapidly for proper absorption.
Resection of colon	Loss of colon fluid absorption because colon length is reduced.
Emotional stress (anxiety)	Rapid intestinal motility.
Tapeworm	Irritation of intestinal tissue with increased motility of intestine.

IMPLICATIONS FOR NURSE–CLIENT COLLABORATION

Fecal Incontinence

One of the most difficult problems for nurse and client to manage is that of fecal incontinence. The social taboos surrounding fecal incontinence are strong, and the client's embarrassment is often proportional to the personal fear of social isolation that can accompany fecal incontinence. Even in the hospital, where the client has every right to expect tolerance and support for the problem, interpersonal messages too often reflect the attitudes of society. In collaborating with the client who suffers from fecal incontinence, the nurse will aid the client by communicating an understanding of and sensitivity to the client's situation, and then by establishing a plan to assist the client with personal hygiene and self-presentation until the problem is corrected or the client is able to resume self-care.

barrassed at having increased stool frequency and liquid stools. The odors and sounds of liquid stools and gas, and the possibility of not being able to get to the bedpan or commode in time, increase the client's anxiety. Frequent watery stools, abdominal cramps, and general weakness are the major symptoms reported. Nausea and vomiting often accompany diarrhea.

Diarrhea influences well-being by limiting activity and causing discomfort, loss of appetite, and weakness. Frequent trips to the bathroom may predispose weakened clients to injury from slipping or falling. Frequent liquid stools can cause skin breakdown of the anal and perineal areas and buttocks as a result of repeated contact by irritating intestinal contents.

Fecal Incontinence

Fecal incontinence is the loss of the voluntary ability to control the elimination of gas and feces. Comatose or confused clients are often incontinent of feces. Some neuromuscular diseases, spinal cord trauma, and tumors of the anal sphincter muscles interfere with the functioning of the anal sphincter or its nerve supply and cause fecal incontinence. Mental disorders such as dementia, Alzheimer's disease, schizophrenia, and severe depression may make the client unable to recognize the need to defecate.

Fecal incontinence can be severely damaging to an individual's body image. Odor, cleanliness, and staining are potential sources of embarrassment, and the person may not want to get out of bed or venture out of the house, causing social isolation.

Tissue breakdown in the perianal area may also result from incontinence. Acidic feces that contain digestive enzymes can cause excoriation, bleeding, and pain around the anal area. The client may then suffer physical discomfort as well as the psychosocial discomfort described above.

Flatulence

Flatulence or flatus is an accumulation of excessive amounts of gas in the gastrointestinal tract. If flatus is accompanied by increased motility, borborygmus (the sound made by the gas rumbling and being propelled through the intestines) results. When intestinal motility is decreased, gas accumulates and stretches and distends the bowel wall, causing abdominal fullness, pain, and cramping.

Normally gas formed in the GI tract by bacterial action on the chyme, and gas diffusing from the bloodstream, are expelled through the mouth or anus. It is not uncommon for an adult to form up to 10 liters of intestinal gas in 24 hours. However, certain foods (beans, cabbage, onions, and cauliflower) increase gas production and create flatulence. Carbonated beverages are another common cause of flatulence, as is swallowing large amounts of air. Air swallowing is sometimes associated with anxiety; gum chewing and using drinking straws also promote air swallowing.

Any of the factors that reduce intestinal activity have the potential for increasing flatulence, because the gas is not propelled out of the body. Narcotics, anesthetics, abdominal surgery, immobility, and tight-fitting clothing are some examples.

Clients with flatus complain of "gas pains" and "passing a lot of gas." They also may complain of fullness or a bloated feeling. Eructation (belching) is often present, along with the characteristic odor of gas that is expelled from the rectum, both of which may cause considerable embarrassment.

If gas accumulates and the bowel distends, cramping and pain may become pronounced and may limit activities of daily living. The resultant decrease in activity often exacerbates the problem. Some individuals also experience difficulty breathing and shortness of breath. This results when flatulence causes severe abdominal distension. Lung expansion is reduced because the diaphragm is pushed upward by the distension.

Fecal Impaction

A **fecal impaction** is a collection of putty-like or hard stool in the rectum that cannot be expelled. In severe cases the impacted feces may extend into the sigmoid colon. The stool must be removed to prevent serious illness.

In the well population, the elderly, children, and those with poor bowel habits are the most likely to develop fecal impaction. Others at risk for impaction include comatose, confused, or debilitated individuals and individuals who do not pass the barium contrast material after a barium enema.

Fecal impaction may cause great discomfort. People with a fecal impaction do not feel well; they often complain of a feeling of malaise. In spite of a frequent urge to defecate, people with an impaction are not able to do so. There may be diarrhea, caused by liquid feces draining around the impacted mass. Abdominal cramping, rectal pain, abdominal pain, and loss of appetite with nausea and vomiting may also occur.

Fecal Elimination Via an Ostomy

The term "ostomy" refers to the creation of an artificial mouth or opening. When cancer, other diseases, or trauma create conditions that will not allow the passage of fecal matter through the intestines and anus, an artificial opening or **stoma** may be constructed surgically in the abdominal wall (Fig. 26–4).

Description and Location of Ostomies. Ostomy procedures such as gastrostomy (opening through the abdominal wall into the stomach) and jejunostomy (opening through the abdominal wall into the jejunum) are often performed to provide an alternative feeding route. Bowel-diversion ostomies are performed to provide an alternative route for fecal elimination. There are two types: ileostomy (opening into the ileum); and ascending, transverse, and sigmoid colostomies (opening into the ascending, transverse, or sigmoid colon) (Fig. 26–5). Colostomies are further categorized according to (1) whether they are permanent or temporary and (2) the method of constructing the stoma or ostomy.

A temporary colostomy is often performed to allow the distal end of the bowel to rest or heal from injuries caused by trauma or disease. When the injury is healed, the colostomy is reanastomosed (the bowel is surgically sewn back together) and the regular fecal route is restored. When the rectum or anus is not functioning as a result of a birth defect or a disease, such as cancer of the bowel, a permanent colostomy is done. Diseased or injured bowel may or may not be removed when a permanent colostomy is created.

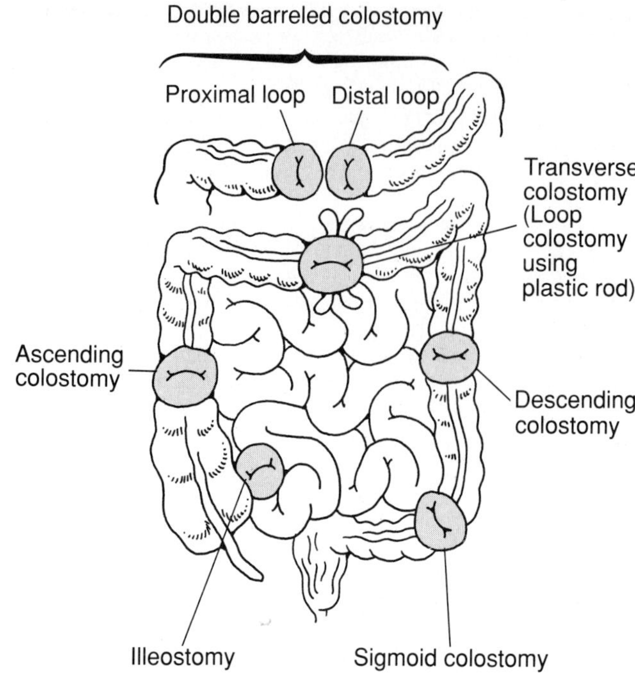

Figure 26–5. Ostomy locations.

Variations in the Characteristics of Stool. The site of the stoma determines the consistency of stool that is excreted. With an ileostomy, almost no water is absorbed because intestinal contents are excreted before they reach the colon. This results in frequent liquid stools. Liquid stools are also produced by an ascending colon colostomy for the same reason, but transverse colostomies have more solid formed stools. The stool from a sigmoid colostomy is very similar to that typically passed rectally.

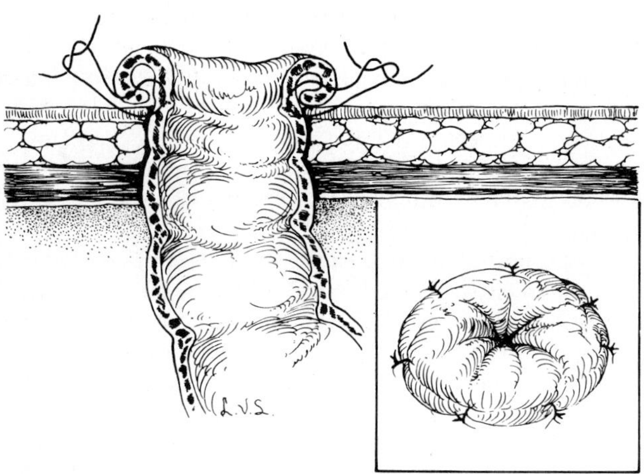

Figure 26–4. An intestinal stoma, showing the opening through the abdominal wall to the intestine (single-barreled end colostomy). (*From Way LW, ed.* Current Surgical Diagnosis and Treatment. *9th ed. Norwalk, CT: Appleton & Lange; 1991.*)

Variations in the Patterns of Elimination. Different ostomy sites result in varying patterns of elimination. A regular bowel elimination pattern cannot be established with ileostomies and ascending colostomies, because there is continuous drainage of liquid stool. Therefore, a bag or pouch must be worn all the time, and the bag must be emptied and washed several times a day. Skin care at the time the bag is changed, or when leakage occurs, is essential to prevent serious skin breakdown at the stoma site.

Descending and sigmoid colostomies generally allow a person to regain a regular bowel pattern. The client is taught to irrigate the colostomy, a procedure that is similar to an enema (see Procedure 26–9). This establishes a regular pattern of bowel emptying and eliminates the need to wear a pouch. Regulating the diet with selected foods at specific times also contributes to predictable bowel movements, usually once or twice a day. However, many clients choose to continue the use of a pouch in order to feel secure (Table 26–2 and Fig. 26–6).

Effect on Well-being. A person with a stoma for fecal elimination must adapt to a change in body image along with greatly altered bowel elimination patterns. Sexual functioning is often a major concern. Loss of self-esteem and an overwhelming sense of powerlessness may be created by spillage of liquid stool, foul odors, and inability to control and regulate bowel movements.

TABLE 26–2. ILEOSTOMY AND COLOSTOMY COMPARISONS

Ostomy	Drainage Type	Odor	Regulation	Skin Breakdown
Ileostomy	Semiliquid to liquid	Minimal	None—must wear plastic stoma bag or dressing[a]	Skin easily irritated because of high level of potent digestive enzymes
Ascending colostomy	Liquid to semisoft or soft	Need to use deodorant in bag	None—must wear plastic stoma bag or dressing[a]	Same as ileostomy
Transverse colostomy	Soft	Very strong odor	None—must wear stoma bag or dressing[a]	If exposed to stool, skin breakdown can occur
Sigmoid colostomy	Formed to soft	Odors usually can be controlled	May achieve control with irrigation—may not need bag or dressing over stoma	Same as transverse colostomy

[a] It has been reported that a few clients have achieved some control for these ostomies. The length of time an ostomy is in place may help the stool become more formed because the remaining colon compensates by increasing water absorption.

The client and significant others must deal with new equipment, odor control, scheduling bathroom time, sexuality, and adapting to and coping with an ostomy. Resources are often available to provide support and encouragement. For example, an enterostomal therapist, a nurse with additional education in stomal care, can help with teaching and coordinating care. Members of the United Ostomy Association can visit the client to explain how to live with an ostomy. Clients can join this organization and meet others who are dealing with ostomies. The American Cancer Society provides ostomy equipment and supplies for clients with financial need. (Refer to Box 26–4 later in this chapter for addresses of these organizations.)

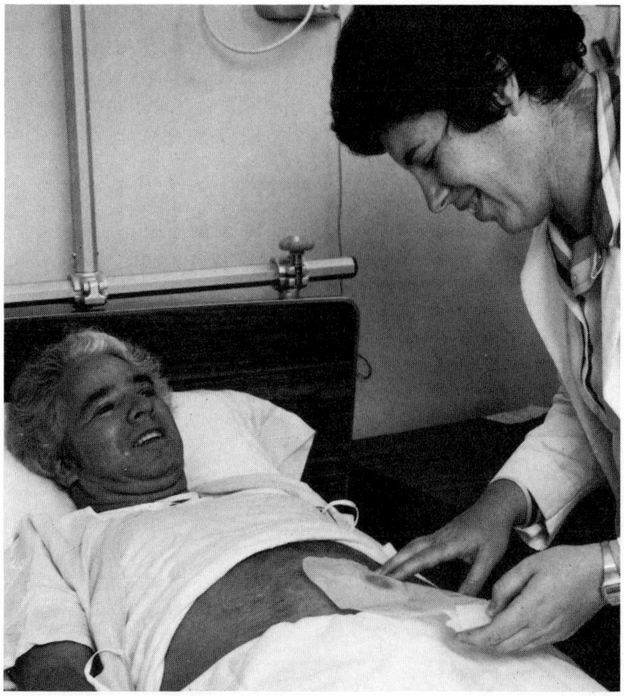

Figure 26–6. Colostomy with pouch. (*From Smith S, Duell D.* Clinical Nursing Skills: Nursing Process Model, Basic to Advanced Skills. *3rd ed. Norwalk, CT: Appleton & Lange; 1992.*)

■ OPTIMUM URINARY ELIMINATION

The purpose of urinary elimination is to replace fluid balance and rid the body of the end products of metabolism. This work is carried out primarily in the kidneys, where urine is formed, the end-products of metabolism are excreted, and control of fluid and electrolytes takes place. Each kidney contains over 1 million nephrons, the structures that collectively rid the body of wastes. The nephron is the functional unit of the kidney.

Although the kidneys are crucial to the filtration process, three other urinary tract structures—the ureters, bladder, and urethra—are vital to effective urinary elimination. Once urine is formed, it is drained by the ureters, which join the renal pelvis to the bladder. The bladder is the hollow organ that stores urine and serves as the organ of excretion. From the bladder, urine is transported to the outside of the body via the urethra (Fig. 26–7).

Urine formation and elimination depend on a number of physiological, sociocultural, and developmental factors. Blood volume and flow, and fluid and food intake affect the formation of urine. The urine elimination process, also called voiding, micturition, and urination, is affected by a person's neuromuscular status, position for voiding, privacy, cleanliness of surroundings, and age.

Anatomy and Physiology

Kidneys. The kidneys are positioned behind the peritoneum in the posterior aspect of the upper abdominal cavity, one on either side of the vertebral column. They lie in front of the 11th and 12th ribs and are well protected by the abdominal muscles, intestines, and a layer of fat. The right kidney lies slightly lower than the left because of the position and size of the liver, which lies above it. An adrenal gland is located above each kidney. An adult kidney is approximately 11 cm (4¼ in) long, 5 to 7.5 cm (2 to 2¾ in) wide, and 2.5 cm (1 in) thick; it weighs approximately 120 to 150 g (¼ to ⅓ lb) and is bean-shaped.

The medial margin of the kidney is concave; the other edges and surface areas are convex. The hilum originates from the medial side, and it is from the hilum that the ureters, lymphatics, nerves, and renal blood vessels enter and leave the kidney. The kidney is surrounded by a thin fibrous covering, the renal capsule, which is loosely attached to the underlying tissue. A longitudinal section shows the kidney is divided into three major areas: cortex, medulla, and pelvis (Fig. 26–8A).

The outermost layer, the cortex, lies under the renal capsule. It is here that urine formation begins. The medullary layer is divided into wedges or cone-shaped pieces called the renal pyramids, where the tubules and collecting ducts of the nephron are found. The apices of the pyramid form papillae, which have openings on the surface that empty urine into the renal pelvis. The renal pelvis connects to the ureter, which drains urine to the bladder. The renal pelvis only holds about 5 mL of urine. Approximately one to five times a minute, peristaltic waves move the urine in spurts down the ureters to the bladder. The urine is sterile when it reaches the bladder.

The **nephron** is the working unit of the kidney (Fig. 26–8B). The function of one nephron illustrates how the

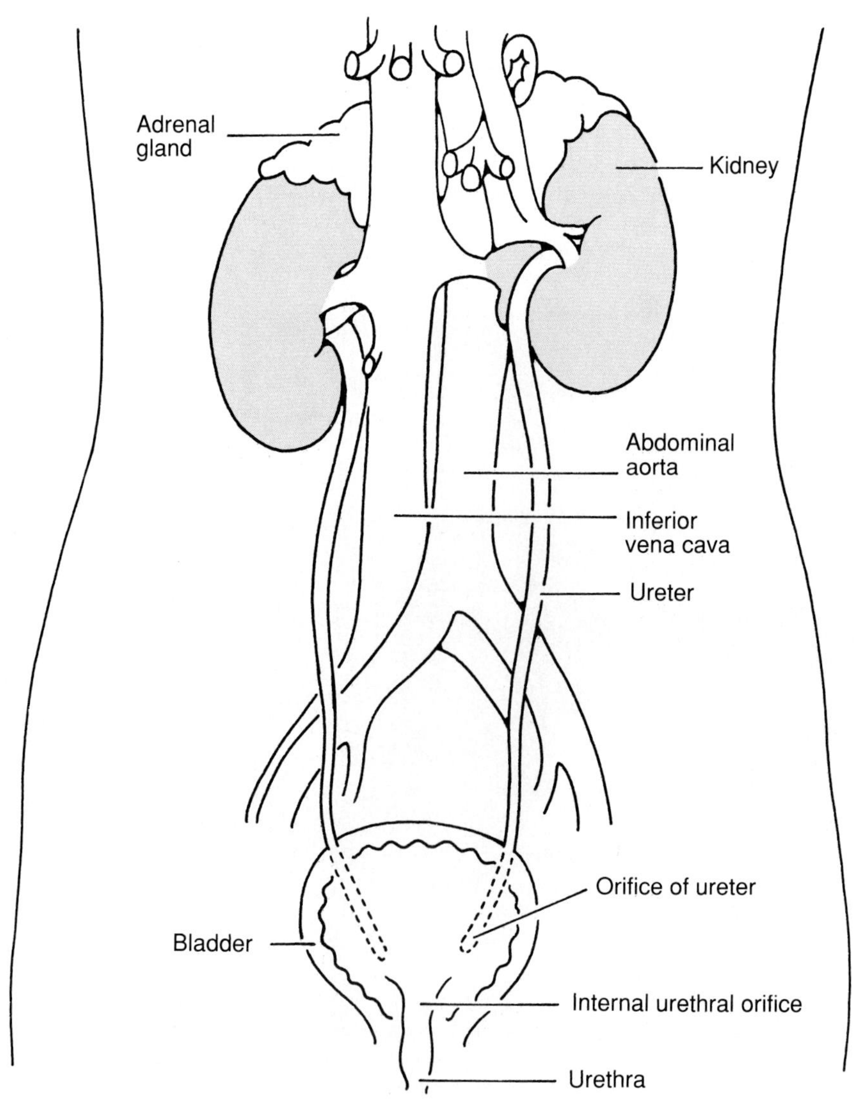

Figure 26–7. Major organs of urinary elimination.

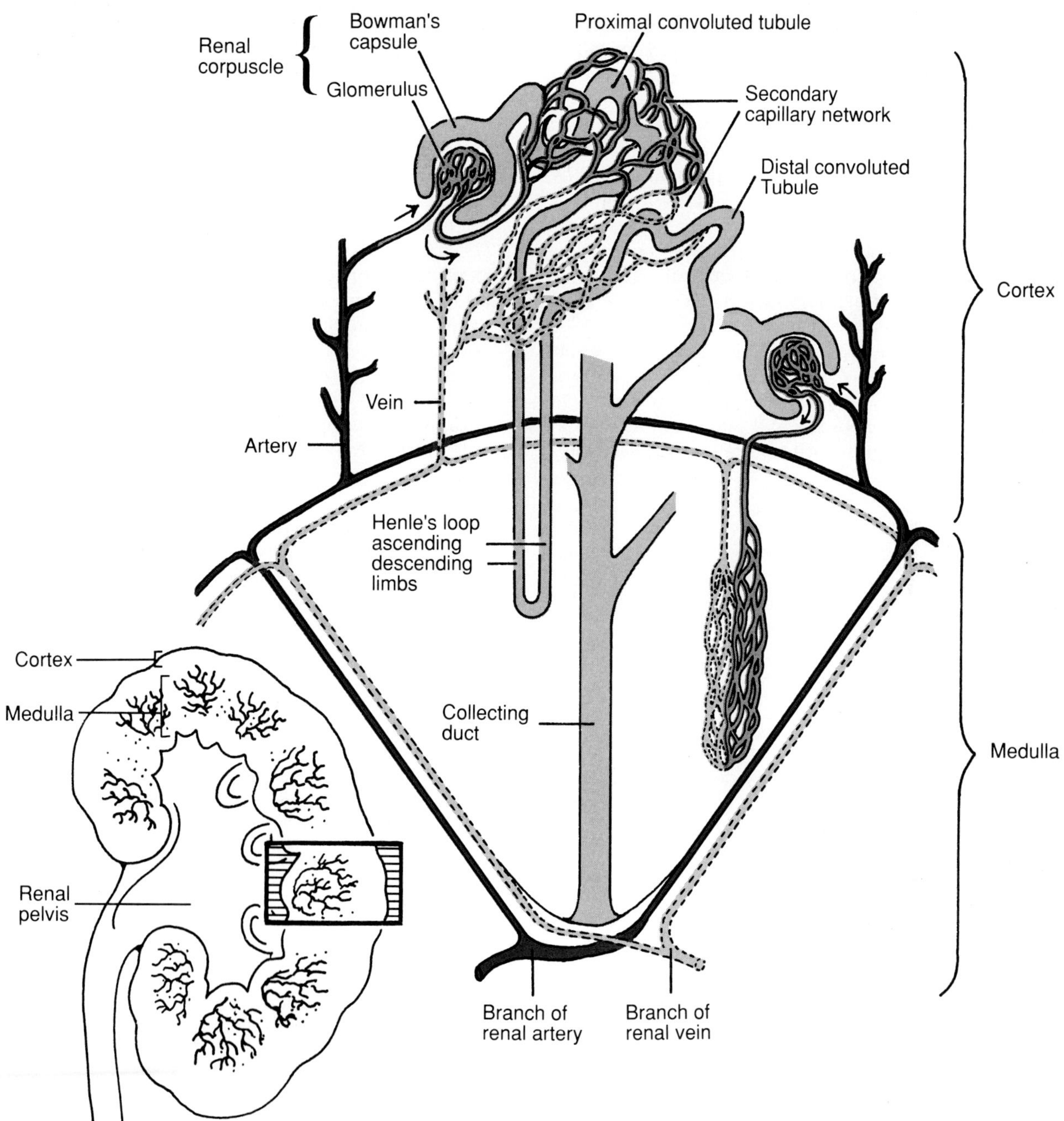

Figure 26–8. Cross-section of the kidney, with detail of the nephron.

kidneys rid the body of wastes. The processes of filtration, reabsorption, and secretion are carried out by the nephrons. Filtration occurs in the glomerulus, a group of capillary loops that create a semipermeable membrane that allows water and electrolytes to exit but not larger molecules. Glomerular filtrate is the term for the fluid that is filtered by the nephron unit. The **glomerular filtration rate** (GFR) indicates the amount of filtration that occurs within a given time. The average GFR for a normal adult is 125 mL per minute. An average of 180 L of glomerular filtrate is formed every day. Composition of the glomerular filtrate is basically the same as plasma, but without significant amounts of proteins. The appearance of protein in the urine (**proteinuria**) is often a sign of glomerular injury. Small amounts may normally appear after prolonged standing or heavy exercise.

Although the kidneys filter 180 L of fluid a day, the average urine output is only 1.2 to 1.5 L (1200 to 1500 mL) a day. This difference is explained by the reabsorptive functions of the renal tubular system, where approximately 99 percent of the filtrate, including water, electrolytes, and other compounds such as glucose, is reabsorbed.

In the tubular system, substances are also secreted and therefore excreted in urine. Some of these play a major role in the regulation of acid–base balance: potassium ions, hydrogen ions, and ammonia.

The usual composition of urine is 95 percent water and 5 percent solutes, which include electrolytes and organic solutes. The usual production of urine is 50 mL per hour; an hourly output of 30 mL or less suggests inadequate blood perfusion to the kidneys or kidney damage.

The rate of urine production is influenced by various factors: circulatory status, fluid intake, metabolic diseases such as diabetes, autoimmune diseases such as glomerulonephritis, congenital disorders and infections, drug or alcohol ingestion, and prescribed medications such as diuretics.

Ureters. Once urine is formed, it passes from the renal pelvis to the bladder via the ureter. The ureters are tubular structures that are 26 to 30 cm (10 to 12 in) long in the adult. The distal ends of the ureters connect to the bladder floor. A small flaplike fold at the junction of the ureters and bladder prevents the reflux of urine back into the kidneys. Small amounts of urine drain continuously from the kidneys into the ureters.

Bladder. The bladder usually holds 300 to 600 mL of urine. However, it is capable of holding twice that capacity because of folds in the lining and elasticity of the walls. When distended, the bladder may extend past the symphysis pubis and, in extreme cases, to the height of the umbilicus. When empty it lies posterior to the symphysis pubis. The bladder is located anterior to the uterus and vagina in women (Fig. 26–9); in men it can be found posterior to the prostate gland and anterior to the rectum (Fig. 26–10).

The bladder is composed mainly of two parts: the fundus or body, in which urine collects; and the neck, which is an extension of the urethra. At the base of the bladder is a triangular area called the trigone, where the ureters enter the bladder posteriorly and the urethra leaves the bladder. The bladder wall has four layers: an outer serous coat; a muscular layer known as the detrusor muscle, that has fibers that extend vertically, circularly, and obliquely; a submucosal layer; and an inner mucosal lining that is continuous with the inner lining of the urethra and ureters. The muscle within the bladder neck is frequently referred to as the internal sphincter. The tone of this muscle keeps the neck empty until the pressure in the fundus of the bladder rises. The internal sphincter is under the control of the autonomic nervous system.

Urethra. The urethra is the passageway through which urine leaves the body. It extends from the bladder to the urinary opening on the outside of the body (urinary meatus). Within the urethra is the second sphincter that controls urination, the external sphincter, which is under the control of voluntary skeletal muscle. The urethra contains a mucous lining that is continuous with that of the bladder and ureters. This lining is susceptible to trauma and infection, which can readily extend to the bladder, ureters, and kidneys. Women are more prone to these problems because the female urethra is very short, measuring about 3.7 cm (1½ in). Bacteria from the vagina and anal areas can easily travel this short distance to the bladder, where they can colonize and produce infection if natural defense mechanisms are not functioning optimally. In men, the urethra is approximately 20 cm (8 in) long. The male urethra also functions as a passageway for semen.

In women, the urinary meatus is located between the labia minora, below the clitoris, and above the vaginal orifice. In men, the opening is located at the distal end of the penis.

Micturition Reflex. The bladder is primarily innervated through pelvic nerves that connect mainly with the cord segments S-2 and S-3. The sensory nerves of the bladder send impulses to the spinal cord at the level of the second to fourth sacral vertebrae, where the micturition center is located. The stretch receptors in the bladder neck are particularly strong and are mainly responsible for starting the reflexes that control bladder elimination. Both the detrusor muscle and the internal sphincter are under parasympathetic control, which contracts the detrusor muscle and relaxes the internal sphincter in response to the signals sent to the micturition center. Unless the reflex is interrupted at this point by voluntary muscular control of the external sphincter, urination will occur.

The micturition reflex is present in infants and in small children who have not gained voluntary control of micturition. Spinal cord injury around the sacral area, or brain injury to the motor area of the cerebrum, cause loss of voluntary control of urination, but the micturition reflex may remain intact. Urination occurs reflexively in these individuals, as it does in the young child.

Voluntary Neuromuscular Control. After early childhood, urination is under voluntary control. Centers in the cerebral cortex and in the brainstem prevent or facilitate urination by sending signals to the external bladder sphincter, which remains contracted until the person chooses to void (empty the bladder). When a person is ready to void, the centers in the cortex can help initiate a micturition reflex and inhibit the contraction of the external sphincter. Voluntary urination usually occurs as follows: the abdominal muscles are contracted, which increases pressure in the bladder. Simultaneously, the muscles of the pelvic floor are relaxed, which allows more urine to enter the neck of the bladder, further stretching its walls. The micturition reflex is then initiated and the external urethral sphincter is relaxed. Under these

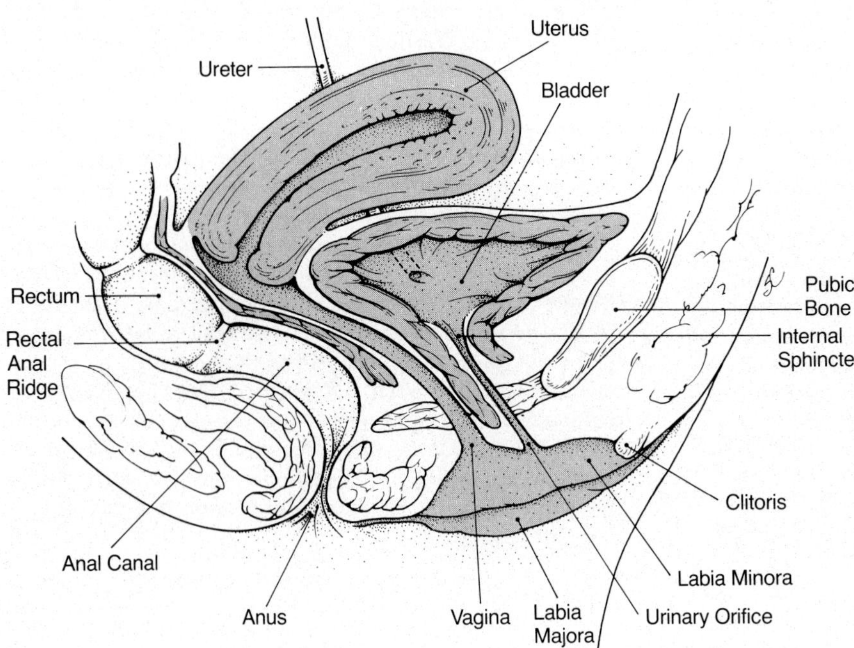

Figure 26–9. Normal position of the bladder in the female. (*From Smith S, Duell D.* Clinical Nursing Skills: Nursing Process Model, Basic to Advanced Skills. *3rd ed. Norwalk, CT: Appleton & Lange; 1992.*)

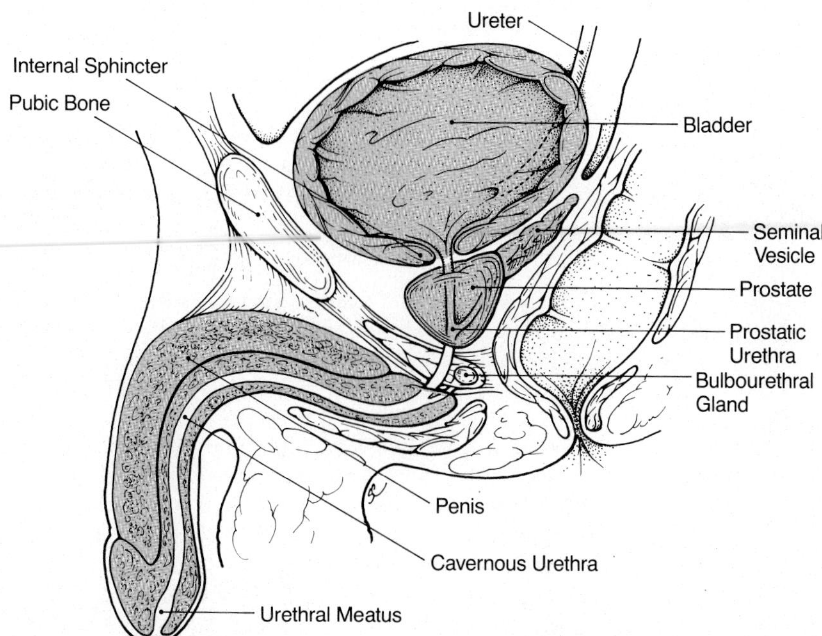

Figure 26–10. Normal position of the bladder in the male. (*From Smith S, Duell D.* Clinical Nursing Skills: Nursing Process Model, Basic to Advanced Skills. *3rd ed. Norwalk, CT: Appleton & Lange; 1992.*)

conditions the bladder is emptied. Usually, no more than 10 mL of urine remains in the bladder after voiding. Urine that is left in the bladder after voiding is called residual urine.

Normal Urinary Elimination

Normal Patterns. Patterns of urinary elimination vary among individuals, but most people void about five times a day while they are awake. They usually void initially upon waking, after meals, and at bedtime. Normally, voiding at night is minimal because of the reduced renal blood flow during rest, the kidney's ability to concentrate urine, and the decreased fluid intake as bedtime approaches. Urination is considered a private matter in North America.

Characteristics of Normal Urine

Color. Urine is usually light yellow due to the presence of the pigment urochrome. Depending on the specific gravity, normal urine may range from pale to deep yellow. Urine should be clear; the waste products are not usually visible, unless the urine is alkaline, which causes some phosphates and urates to settle out. Medications, disease, diet, and fluid intake may alter the color and clarity of urine.[6]

Many drugs can alter the color of urine; among these are multivitamins, iron preparations, and some diuretics. Color changes may range from pink, red, or orange to dark brown or black.

Odor. Freshly voided urine should have a slightly aromatic odor; a foul odor may be a result of drugs, food, or urinary tract infection. Stale urine smells of ammonia because bacteria convert urea to ammonia. Some genetic defects that cause metabolic abnormalities can cause specific odors in a newborn's urine.[7]

Amount. Daily urine production varies with age, fluid intake, and health status. Infants and children excrete large volumes of urine in relation to their size. A 6-month-old infant excretes between 400 to 500 mL of urine daily. In comparison, an adult normally voids 1200 to 1500 mL of urine a day, usually voiding 150 to 600 mL at a time. Urine output of less than 30 mL per hour should be reported immediately to a physician. Urine production of more than 55 mL per hour in an adult or more than 2000 mL a day is excessive. It may be caused by increased fluid intake, certain kidney disorders, endocrine diseases, or the use of diuretics.

Factors Affecting Urinary Elimination

Many factors affect urinary elimination. Among these are fluid intake, age, health status, medications, and emotional state.

Fluid Intake. Because the kidneys provide the main control for fluid homeostasis, fluid intake influences urine production and thus micturition. Water-induced diuresis occurs when an individual drinks a large amount of liquid. The fluids increase the circulating plasma volume and thus the amount of glomerular filtrate, resulting in increased urine production. Decreasing fluid intake will decrease urine output. Clients who complain of urinary frequency (voiding an increased number of times during the day or night) often cut back their fluid intake so as to decrease the need for urination. However, this requires client teaching on the nurse's part, because decreasing fluid intake can cause problems such as dehydration.

Certain fluids, such as alcohol and caffeine-containing drinks, inhibit the release of antidiuretic hormone (ADH), thereby directly influencing urine output. Cells in the renal tubules do not reabsorb water when ADH release is inhibited. Cola, cocoa, tea, and coffee all increase diuresis and micturition. Additionally, some foods high in water content, such as fruits and vegetables, may also increase urine output. If the body becomes depleted of fluid through perspiration, respiration, or digestion, water is reabsorbed by the glomeruli, urine becomes more concentrated, and output is decreased.

Age. Age influences both urinary production and urine excretion. Changes associated with age occur in the kidneys, bladder, and muscles and nerves that affect micturition.

Infants. Infants (birth to 1 year) cannot concentrate urine effectively. Therefore, they excrete large volumes of urine in relation to their size. The kidneys start excreting urine in utero between the 11th and 12th week of development, but the placenta carries out fetal regulatory and excretory function until birth.

Children. Between 1 and 2 years of age, a child's kidneys can concentrate as much urine as an adult's and urine takes on the characteristic yellow-amber color. Control of urination begins between 2½ to 3 years of age, but nighttime control may not be achieved until age 4 or 5. Girls are often able to gain urine control sooner than boys. During childhood, the kidneys and bladder grow in proportion to the rest of the body.

Adolescents and Adults. Renal filtration of the blood and micturition are usually maintained at full capacity through age 50. Diseases of the urinary tract and metabolic and cardiovascular problems can alter kidney function in the adult, as can other factors discussed below.

Older Adults. Older adults (above 65) frequently experience changes in urinary elimination. Age-related changes in the kidney result in a decreased adaptive capacity. Changes in the nephrons, proximal and distal convoluted tubules, and renal blood vessels produce diminished renal blood flow and glomerular filtration rate, as well as decreased ability to concentrate urine. The elderly therefore require greater amounts of fluid intake to excrete a given amount of metabolic waste. In healthy elderly people, control of fluid volume and excretion is usually effective, in spite of these changes. However, older adults are susceptible to kidney and urinary problems when stressed by injury or disease.

The ureter, bladder, and urethra also reflect the aging

process.[8] Urination often becomes a concern for the elderly, because decreased bladder capacity, combined with poor ability to concentrate urine, leads to more frequent urination. This can disrupt sleep patterns and create risks for injury when elderly people walk to the bathroom in semidarkness or when not fully awake. Vision or mobility problems, also common among older individuals, compound the problem.

Elderly women are also at risk for bladder infections and stress incontinence, because relaxation of perineal support structures interferes with complete emptying and external sphincter control. Periodic dribbling of urine may also be related to these changes. In men, prostatic hypertrophy (enlargement) often causes difficulties initiating urination. Incontinence does not occur because of aging, although some diseases may compromise urinary control. Other urination problems in the elderly are related to chronic diseases of other body systems. For example, arthritis may make getting to the bathroom and getting on and off the toilet difficult.

Health Status. Disease, surgical procedures, medications, and diagnostic examinations often alter urinary elimination patterns.

Diseases. Pathology involving the urinary system may affect urinary elimination or urine production. Hereditary anomalies, infection, cancer, and obstruction can all occur in the renal system. They may produce changes ranging from production alterations, such as release of large amounts of poorly concentrated urine, to blockages that result in obstruction of urinary outflow.

Cardiovascular, respiratory, and neuromuscular system pathology may alter urine production or affect a person's ability to void or to get to the toilet. Neuromuscular diseases may lead to loss of bladder tone and inability to control urination. Cardiovascular disease such as hypertension may cause changes in the blood flow to the kidneys, which can lead to decreased production of urine. Since the respiratory system and the renal system together maintain acid–base balance, diseases of the respiratory system affect the renal system. If both systems are impaired, acid–base balance may be severely compromised. (See Chap. 31 for discussion of acid–base balance.)

Surgery. Surgery alters urinary elimination in several ways. First, surgery initiates a stress response in which vasopressin (ADH), epinephrine, and renin levels are increased. These hormones increase vascular resistance, promote fluid retention, and therefore decrease urine output. Surgery also contributes to reduced urine output for two reasons: hypovolemia resulting from the n.p.o. (nothing by mouth) state prior to surgery, and blood and fluid loss during surgery. Anesthetics, anticholinergics, narcotics, and sedatives used before, during, and after surgery may interfere with voiding in the postoperative period. Anesthesia and other drugs such as narcotics and sedatives, which alter levels of consciousness, may make it difficult for an individual to realize the bladder is full, resulting in retention or incontinence. These same medications may also make it difficult to get on a bedpan or stand to void in a urinal.[9] To help reduce these problems, an indwelling (Foley) catheter is often placed before surgery.

Surgical or diagnostic procedures that involve instrumentation of the urinary tract, lower abdomen, or pelvic region may impair urination because of trauma and inflammation to tissues. Aftereffects of surgery include obstruction of urine flow, interference with the relaxation of sphincters and muscles, pain during voiding, and bleeding from the urinary tract.

Medications. A number of medications can alter normal urinary function, causing, for example, changes in urine characteristics, production, and elimination from the bladder. Diuretics are medications that increase urine excretion.

Because of its waste excretion, the kidney is especially vulnerable to toxicity from drugs. Although some drugs rarely cause nephrotoxicity, antibiotics (especially aminoglycocides, cephalosporins, tetracyclines, and sulfonamides); uricosurics; diuretics; and anesthetics are frequently toxic to the kidney.[10] Signs of nephrotoxicity include increased blood urea nitrogen (BUN) and serum creatinine levels, decreased urine output, edema, weight gain, hematuria, and albuminuria.

Emotional State. Individuals under acute stress often experience urinary urgency and frequency. The sympathetic nervous system promotes internal sphincter relaxation, therefore stimulating the urge to void even though the bladder is not full. Paradoxically, acute stress may also interfere with relaxation of the external sphincter and perineal muscles. When this occurs, complete emptying of the bladder is difficult or impossible, despite the frequent urge to void. If stress is prolonged (for several hours, for example), urine production is suppressed because of decreased circulation to the kidneys. In this situation, the urge to urinate may be delayed until the stress is resolved.

For some individuals, lack of privacy or anxiety associated with illness and hospitalization may disrupt normal voiding patterns. Incomplete emptying of the bladder or inability to initiate voiding is common

■ ALTERATIONS IN URINARY ELIMINATION

Alterations in urinary elimination comprise a broad category of problems, such as incontinence, retention, dysuria, anuria, and oliguria. Some alterations in elimination result from alterations in urine production. These include conditions such as anuria and oliguria, which nurses monitor but for which the physician prescribes specific treatments.

Urinary Incontinence

Urinary incontinence is the loss of control over voiding. The individual is unable to stop the passage of urine from the bladder. The problem may be temporary, as in the acutely ill client who is unconscious, or permanent because of neuromuscular damage. The flow of urine may be almost continuous or it may occur sporadically. Incontinence can be treated and in most cases controlled through nursing and medical interventions. The impact of incontinence is immense; it affects not only the client and family but also health care workers and the health care industry as well.

There are several types of incontinence, each with a different etiology (see the discussion of nursing diagnoses for Altered Patterns of Urinary Elimination in Section 2 of this chapter). Risk factors include infection of or trauma to the urinary tract; change in tissue and muscle tone after childbirth, with aging, and after weight loss or gain; neuromuscular conditions that interfere with the transmission of sensory or motor impulses for urination; medications that increase urinary frequency or change sensory input; and psychological factors such as anxiety, fear, confusion, or disorientation.

Incontinence can be devastating to clients and their families personally, socially, and financially. The individual may suffer from embarrassment, social isolation, depression, anxiety, or impaired skin integrity. The family responsible for the physical care of the incontinent client often experiences physical strain and mental worry. If the client is institutionalized, the family may be torn about the decision, and the client may feel betrayed.

Although incontinence may affect individuals at any age—a 33-year-old with multiple sclerosis, an 8-year-old with a head injury, or an 88-year-old with bladder cancer—it is most often seen in the elderly. Palmer[11] notes that incontinence is one of the major reasons cited for institutionalization of the aged. Women are more likely than men to suffer from incontinence and it becomes more severe as age and health problems increase. Palmer also comments that certain conditions, such as confusion and impaired mobility,[11] are often associated with incontinence. Many clients who have suffered strokes are incontinent, especially when cortical function is impaired. However, although incontinence affects the elderly more than other groups, it is not invariably associated with the aging process.

Enuresis and Nocturia

The involuntary loss of urine while sleeping, or bedwetting beyond the age when bladder control is usually achieved, is called **enuresis.** Most children can control nighttime voiding by age 4 or 5. Enuresis may be typified as primary or secondary. Primary enuresis indicates that the individual has never experienced a dry period; secondary enuresis is a reoccurrence of bedwetting after a period of dryness. Enuresis is further defined as nocturnal, diurnal, or both.[12]

Nocturnal enuresis is the loss of urine during sleep. This condition may continue into the teen years and, rarely, into adulthood. Diurnal enuresis is the loss of urine during the day. This latter condition often occurs because a child delays voiding too long because of play or other distractions.

Nocturia, in contrast, is excessive voiding at night; the individual is aware of the need to urinate and gets up to void. It is not unusual for some people to get up once at night to void, but when an individual's pattern changes, so that awakening for urination repeatedly occurs several times per night, the change should be assessed.

Age, stress, disease, and medications can play a role in both enuresis and nocturia. Heredity seems to play a role in enuresis, because there is an increased incidence of bedwetting among close relatives of those who have experienced bedwetting. Other physiological, psychological, and environmental factors thought to contribute to enuresis include food allergies, small bladder capacity, urinary tract infection, fluid intake after dinner, and inaccessibility to toilet facilities. Common causes of nocturia include pregnancy, urinary tract infections, stress, diuretics and increased fluid intake.

Age plays a role in both enuresis and nocturia. Enuresis is more common in young children between the ages of 5 and 8 years. In men past 50 years old, prostate enlargement contributes to nocturia. It is also felt that decreased bladder tone, chronic diseases such as congestive heart failure and diabetes, and use of diuretics play a significant role in nocturia that occurs with aging.

Safety is a concern for both adults and children who awake at night to go to the bathroom. Many accidents occur when sleepy individuals get up to go to the bathroom. Additionally, enuresis is often a source of embarrassment. Bedwetting may create feelings of isolation and altered self-concept.

It is important that the family be understanding of the alteration, because it can be a source of frustration, anxiety, isolation, and behavioral problems for the child.

Frequency, Urgency, and Dysuria

Normally, urination occurs painlessly and effortlessly about five times a day, and most people can hold about 150 mL of urine in the bladder without feeling a strong desire to void. **Urinary frequency** refers to urination at more frequent intervals. The amount voided may be either large or small; the term refers only to the number of times one voids in 24 hours. Urgency is a sudden strong desire to urinate. The urge to void may be so strong that it leads to incontinence. **Dysuria** means difficult or painful urination. Individuals may complain of discomfort during, before, or immediately after voiding. Frequency, urgency, and dysuria may occur separately or in combination.

Pregnancy, increased fluid intake, diuretics, and urinary tract infections are common causes of frequency. Urgency is a common complaint during stress or urinary tract infections, when it is associated with weak external sphincter control. Dysuria is common in any condition that causes trauma or inflammation to the bladder or urethra. When an individual complains of any of these symptoms, it is important to question him or her about other concerns, such as hesitancy (difficulty in initiating voiding), hematuria (blood in the urine), and pyuria (pus in the urine).

Frequency, urgency, and dysuria may cause minor problems for a client or they may be a main source of concern. These problems may disrupt activities of daily living and lead to embarrassment. Clients often attempt to reduce fluid intake to control these problems, but usually this does not solve the problem and may even make it worse.

Oliguria, Anuria, and Polyuria

Urine production of less than 30 mL an hour is termed **oliguria. Polyuria** is the production of large amounts of urine in relation to fluid intake; it does not refer to the frequency or time interval of urination. However, polyuria may accompany frequency. **Anuria,** the suppression of urine, refers to a production of urine of less than 100 mL in a day. Oliguria and anuria are signs that the kidneys are not working or are not adequately perfused.

A variety of metabolic, urological, and cardiovascular disorders manifest themselves as disturbances in the normal output of urine. Kidney disease, heart failure, severe burns, and shock can cause anuria or oliguria. Oliguria may also be present in dehydration. Causes of polyuria include diabetes mellitus, diabetes insipidus, kidney disease, diuretics, and increased fluid intake, especially fluids containing alcohol and caffeine.

Persons experiencing anuria or oliguria are often acutely ill. Fluid and electrolyte and acid–base imbalances, along with retention of metabolic wastes, cause edema, respiratory difficulty, and confusion. Renal failure may be present or impending. Shock or dehydration may also be present. The individual in shock appears pale and weak; the skin is usually cool and clammy. In dehydration, the skin feels hot and dry with decreased turgor. Anuria is a grave sign indicating that death may ensue if circulatory status or waste product removal is not improved.

The individual with polyuria may appear healthy or may have few complaints, but the nurse should assess for thirst and weight loss and determine whether excessive fluid intake is a factor.

Retention

Urinary retention is a state in which the individual cannot initiate or complete evacuation of accumulated urine from the bladder. Urinary retention may be acute or chronic. Chronic retention may persist over a period of months and may be irreversible. Chronic retention is sometimes referred to as "overflow incontinence" or "paradoxical incontinence," because clients are unable to void until the intra-abdominal pressure increases to such a degree that urine is involuntarily voided.

Acute retention may occur after surgery, diagnostic procedures involving the urinary tract, delivery of a baby, and with obstruction in the urinary system. Medications that may cause retention include anesthesia, opiates, sedatives, antihistamines, and anticholinergics. Social factors or emotion may also play a part in retention. Fear, stress, and pain may produce anxiety and tension, resulting in urinary retention.

Chronic retention is classified according to one of two causes: (1) weak or absent detrusor contraction or (2) bladder outlet obstruction. Factors that contribute to altered detrusor muscle contraction include chronic bladder distension, as with prostate enlargement, or impairment of the sensory and motor branches of reflex arc, as found after spinal cord damage. Factors that contribute to bladder outlet obstruction include strictures and prostatic hypertrophy.

Urinary retention can be a significant threat to well-being. In some cases of chronic retention, bladder-training programs can restore near-normal elimination patterns; however, some clients with chronic retention require a permanent indwelling catheter or must learn intermittent self-catheterization. These latter interventions may create significant body-image alterations.

The nurse's understanding of bowel and urine elimination is essential to providing quality care and to effective collaboration with the client. Helping the client understand elimination function will aid the process of collaboration. Understanding of elimination also is essential to more accurate and efficient assessment of elimination by the nurse.

Section 2. Assessment of Elimination

■ ELIMINATION DATA COLLECTION

Elimination data collection incorporates data about the process and products of elimination as well as factors that may influence elimination. An individual's elimination habits are a personal and private concern. Sensitivity, understanding, and the establishment of trust will help the nurse collect the data necessary to determine whether a nursing diagnosis related to elimination is appropriate. To lessen embarrassment during the assessment, it is important to provide privacy and to put the client at ease. The nurse must also avoid demonstrating embarrassment and must be able to discuss the client's elimination needs and problems openly. Most beginning nursing students will find this difficult, because of their own socialization about the privacy of elimination. Sharing these concerns in small groups or clinical conferences may help students develop a more relaxed and open attitude about this body function.

Elimination History

The elimination history should focus on the many factors that may affect this vital function. For example, normal elimination patterns may be altered by the home environment, number of bathroom facilities, number of family members, and any condition that might impair a client's ability to eat regularly, maintain a healthy fluid intake, or walk to the bathroom. Special dietary requirements, work schedules, and medications also may impede the establishment of elimination patterns.

Bowel and urinary elimination patterns are unique to each individual and are influenced by physiological, psychological, social, and cultural elements. Elimination problems have an impact on the client's life-style, self-concept, and activities of daily living. Information related to any change in bowel habits is especially significant because this may be one of the seven warning signs of cancer. Changes in urine characteristics and patterns signal possible urinary tract, metabolic, cardiovascular, or neuromuscular problems.

Primary Concern. Explore the client's primary concern to determine whether it is related to or has affected the client's elimination patterns. Some complaints—such as constipation, diarrhea, burning, and dribbling—are directly related to elimination. Other complaints—such as headache, nausea, and abdominal pain—may also be related to elimination. Abdominal trauma may affect elimination. Circulation or breathing problems may cause weakness and decreased mobility, which can interfere with elimination. Therefore an elimination assessment is necessary both for clients whose primary concern involves urination or bowel elimination and for those whose complaint suggests that elimination may be affected.

Current Understanding. If the primary concern is an elimination alteration it is helpful to obtain information about the nature of the problem, what the client believes may have caused it, what makes it better or worse, and what the client has done to correct it. If another health problem has contributed to altered elimination, find out how the problem interferes. Often this information suggests possible nursing diagnoses and topics for later health teaching. The following example illustrates the current understanding.

- Mrs. Elias, age 63, is being treated for joint pain and stiffness, especially in her hips and knees. She reports that sitting on the toilet is painful, so she has decreased her fluid intake "so I don't have to urinate so often." The nurse realizes that limiting fluid intake increases Mrs. Elias's risks of constipation and urinary tract infection and makes a note to discuss this further with her before she leaves the clinic.

Past Health Care Experiences/Problems. Determine whether past health care experiences have caused short-term or residual effects on bowel or urine elimination. Explore whether the client routinely takes medications that may alter urinary elimination (e.g., antihypertensives, steroids, or cardiac medications) or influence bowel elimination (e.g., laxatives or iron). If radiological studies of the urinary tract are planned, determine whether there is a history of allergies to iodine, because many contrast materials used in these studies contain iodine. The following example illustrates a past health care experience.

- Monica Flynn has delivered her second baby and is being admitted to the postpartum ward. She says, "I hope I don't have the same trouble I had with my first baby. It hurt so much to have a bowel movement because of my hemorrhoids and my stitches, so I kept holding back—and then I got constipated and it hurt even more." Monica's nurse resolves to encourage fluids and to teach Monica how high-fiber foods will contribute to soft, formed stools that are easier to pass.

Personal, Family, and Social History. Life-style affects elimination. Regularity of meals, fluid intake, and exercise routines are some examples. Besides personal activities, elimination patterns may be related to vocational or home and family factors. Conversely, alterations in elimination patterns affect feelings of well-being and therefore interfere with the quality of daily life. Current stressors and inadequate coping mechanisms may indicate why a client has developed diarrhea, urinary frequency, or retention. See Table 26–3 and the following example.

- Jeannette James is a young professional woman who seeks health care for urinary burning and frequency. She states that she feels like she has to empty her bladder often, but that "very little urine comes out." When the nurse questions her about her usual urinary patterns and typical fluid intake, Ms. James says that she doesn't drink much water because she rarely leaves her desk except for lunch and that on many days she empties her bladder only at lunch and after work. The nurse recognizes that these symptoms suggest a urinary tract infection and that Ms. James' habits increase the risk that this will be a recurrent problem.

Subjective Manifestations. A review of subjective manifestations helps nurses identify clients' usual patterns and recognize actual or potential abnormalities.

Chapter 16 provides sample questions for subjective manifestations related to elimination concerns. The following case illustration provides an example of the nurse's use of subjective manifestations data in planning client care.

- Mr. Jones, 75 years old, comes to the clinic because of abdominal pain. He states that his last bowel movement was 3 days ago and describes the stool as hard, formed, dry, and dark brown. He also states that he can't understand why he hasn't gone to the bathroom as he took a double dose of the laxative he usually uses. Upon further questioning, Mr. Jones reveals that he has used an over-

TABLE 26–3. ELIMINATION HISTORY: PERSONAL, FAMILY, AND SOCIAL HISTORY QUESTIONS

A. **Vocational**
  1. What type of work do you do?
  2. Do your working hours influence your urine or bowel elimination?

B. **Home and Family**
  1. Describe a typical day.
  2. Do you ever have to suppress elimination urges due to lack of facilities, time, or privacy?
  3. Are there any family members with past or current health problems affecting elimination?

C. **Social and Leisure**
  1. What are your favorite leisure activities?
  2. Do your elimination patterns have any effect on your leisure activities?

D. **Sexual**
  1. Has your sexual relationship been satisfactory?
  2. Have you noticed any symptoms of urinary problems after sexual intercourse?

E. **Habits**

  Exercise
  1. Do you exercise regularly? How often and what types of exercise?
  2. Have your elimination patterns influenced your exercising?
  3. Has your exercising had an effect on your elimination patterns?

  Diet
  1. How many meals do you eat per day?
  2. Are you on a special diet of any kind? Prescribed by a physician? Someone else? Self?
  3. Describe a typical day's menu at home and when you eat out.
  4. What are the types and amounts of bulk and fiber foods you eat most every day?
  5. Do any foods or fluids cause you elimination difficulties? List these.
  6. Do you use any foods and fluids to keep bowels regular?
  7. Are there any foods you don't eat? Why?

  Beverages
  1. How much fluid do you have each day? What types of fluids?
  2. Do you use alcohol? How much do you drink in a day? A week?
  3. Do you use caffeine? Tea? Coffee? Soft drinks? Do any beverages affect urination or bowel elimination?

  Sleep
  1. How many hours do you sleep at night?
  2. Are you awakened in the night by the urge to eliminate? How often? For bowel elimination? For urine?

  Other Substances
  1. What medications do you take regularly? Occasionally?
  2. Do any medications affect your elimination patterns?

F. **Psychological**
  1. Are you experiencing any stress currently?
  2. Do your elimination habits change when you become stressed?
  3. Has the recent change in elimination patterns been stressful?

the-counter laxative every day for the last 6 months. The nurse believes that Mr. Jones' constipation may be related to his reliance on laxatives. The nurse then further assesses Mr. Jones' definition of constipation, understanding of bowel function, usual diet, and fluid intake.

Elimination Examination

Physical assessment data obtained using measurement, inspection, auscultation, and palpation complete the picture of client elimination status suggested by the elimination history.

Measurements. Measurements that reflect elimination status include intake and output, weight, body surface, abdominal girth, and blood pressure.

Intake and Output. Accurate intake and output measurement is vital to determining fluid status and efficiency of kidney function. Comparing intake and output measurements provides clues to abnormalities such as oliguria, polyuria, frequency, and anuria. For comparisons of intake and output to be valid, all forms of output—including liquid stool, emesis, and wound and other drainage—must be measured and recorded. When there is excessive fluid loss via abnormal routes, urine output usually decreases to compensate. Refer to Chapter 31 for a more detailed discussion of intake and output measurement.

Weight. Short-term weight changes reflect fluid gains and losses. Clients with severe cardiac or renal disease may demonstrate consistent rapid weight gain over weeks or even months. Daily monitoring of weight provides data about trends and changes in status. For accurate comparisons, it is recommended that daily weights be measured at the same time each day, using the same scale. Many health care facilities schedule daily weights in the morning before breakfast.

Body Surface Area Calculation. Calculation of body surface area (BSA) to determine basal fluid requirements is frequently necessary for clients with compromised elimination, because fluid intake must be restricted to minimize fluid retention or increased to facilitate bowel elimination. Chapter 31 presents instructions for calculating BSA and measuring body weight on various types of scales.

Abdominal Girth. Abdominal girth may be part of the elimination examination, because it is one indicator of abdominal distension. Abdominal girth may increase because of abnormal fluid retention in the peritoneal cavity (ascites) or because of altered bowel elimination, such as constipation, excessive flatulence, or bowel obstruction. The circumference of the abdomen is measured with a tape measure at the level of the umbilicus. The girth may be measured daily or more frequently to detect increases or decreases. Consistent placement of the tape measure is essential for comparison of successive values to be valid.

Blood Pressure. Blood pressure measurement is also related to elimination status, particularly kidney function. When blood pressure is abnormally low, kidney perfusion may be inadequate for efficient filtration, and urine output falls. Elevated blood pressure is usually associated with vasoconstriction, which also reduces renal perfusion and therefore urine output. Moreover, many clients being treated for hypertension are given medications that influence kidney function, and some medications used for treatment of kidney problems influence blood pressure.

Objective Manifestations. The elimination examination also includes general observations and assessment of the skin, abdomen, genitalia, and perianal area, as well as inspection of urine and feces. If general observations point out problems with mobility or orientation, then mobility and neurological assessment is also relevant.

General Observations. General observation of the client may provide clues that elimination processes are altered or at risk. The client's overall appearance (general movement, facial expression, and posture) may indicate the presence of an elimination problem. For example, a client who grimaces, holds the stomach, and curls up in a fetal position often has acute abdominal pain. Abdominal pain is often associated with elimination problems such as diarrhea or intestinal obstruction. Dry skin and mucous membranes imply altered fluid status, which influences both urine and bowel elimination.

Confusion may indicate that the client is at risk for incontinence or it may be a manifestation of severe kidney failure. Odors may be another indicator of problems. An ammonia-like or feces-like smell may indicate incontinence. The nurse must verify the significance of general observations by collecting additional data relevant to the elimination status of the client.

Integument. The integument also provides information suggestive of elimination problems. (Refer to Chap. 16 for components and techniques of assessment.) Dry skin and mucous membranes, coated tongue, ropey saliva, and sluggish capillary refill imply fluid volume deficit. This may be caused by abnormal fluid losses in stool (diarrhea) or urine. Conversely, individuals with fluid volume deficit often become constipated because of increased reabsorption of water by intestinal mucosa.

Edema is another indicator of elimination problems. It often occurs with altered kidney function. The nurse should palpate all tissue, particularly dependent areas, for fluid collection. (Refer to Chap. 31 for technique and grading of edema.) In the ambulatory client, dependent areas are the lower legs and feet, but in the bedridden client, dependent areas include the sacrum and lower back.

Abdomen. Abdominal examination is an important component of the elimination assessment. As discussed in Chapter 16, this examination includes inspection, auscultation, and palpation. Inspection may reveal distension (a protuberant abdomen with a rounded contour). Although there are several causes of abdominal distension that are not related to elimination, generalized symmetrical distension may be caused by intestinal gas or constipation. Asymmetrical distension may be related to bowel obstruction. If obstruction is suspected, observe for the presence of visible peristaltic waves. Sit next to the client and gaze across the profile of the abdomen for several minutes. Observe for elevated oblique bands starting in the upper left quadrant and moving downward to the right. Distension that is limited to the area between the symphysis pubis and the umbilicus may be caused by a full bladder. Findings during auscultation may support or rule out these possible causes of distension.

Inspection also includes assessment of stomas and peristomal skin in clients who have had urinary or bowel diversion surgery. The stoma itself should be assessed for color, edema, and bleeding. A well-perfused stoma is deep pink to brick red, whereas a dark red to purple color suggests impaired circulation to the stoma or bowel. Stomal edema or bleeding is abnormal except during the immediate postoperative period. A small amount of oozing in a fresh stoma is not uncommon, but if frank, bright red blood is seen, the cause must be determined and corrected. Common peristomal skin alterations requiring attention include erythema, weeping, edema, erosion, itching, and burning. All of these may be caused by allergic reaction to products used in ostomy care or by irritation from fecal matter or urine.

Crusting, scaly patches, erosion, and bleeding commonly result from mechanical trauma—for example from vigorous or frequent removal of adhesives used to affix a stoma pouch. Folliculitis, evidenced by reddened, raised hair follicles around the stoma, may also result from trac-

BUILDING NURSING KNOWLEDGE

Is Constipation a Single Entity, or Are There Different Types?

McShane RE, McLane AM. Constipation: Impact of etiological factors. *J Gerontol Nurs.* 1988;14:31–34.

Although the complex nature of constipation has been recognized for some time, the use of the same word to apply to related but different problems is questionable. McShane and McLane argue that nursing diagnoses should reflect the differences. They describe several types of constipation in an effort to differentiate them and note that research identifies three patterns: imagined constipation, colonic constipation, and rectal constipation.

Imagined constipation is a state in which an individual self-diagnosis constipation and then overuses laxatives, enemas, and suppositories to ensure a daily bowel movement. Such individuals expect a daily stool and often are inactive physically. Lack of privacy, impaired thought processes, and environmental constraints are contributing factors. Management includes confronting the erroneous health belief about the need for daily defecation, teaching helpful diet and toileting habits, and substituting dietary bulk and fiber for use of laxatives.

In colonic constipation there is a slow passage of food residue, resulting in hard dry stool. Characteristics include decreased stool frequency, straining, painful defecation, abdominal distension, and a palpable mass. There may be a feeling of rectal pressure, increased flatus, abdominal pain, headache, appetite impairment, and blood with stool. Causative factors include inadequate fluid, dietary, or fiber intake; lack of availability of certain foods; change in daily routine; immobility; stress; lack of privacy; metabolic problems; little social support; and chronic use of medications and enemas. Correcting intake problems, establishing helpful activity schedules, repatterning bowel habits, reducing the use of laxatives and enemas, and reducing social isolation are important implementations.

Rectal constipation is characterized by normal stool consistency but delayed elimination. Characteristics are reduced stool frequency, abdominal discomfort, rectal fullness, change in flatus, decreased appetite, and headache. Causative factors include altered mobility, impaired communication, and emotional disturbances, all of which reduce the individual's capacity for self-care; and weak pelvic floor muscles; painful lesions in the anus; environment constraints; and lack of social support. McShane and McLane did not address management objectives for this type of constipation, which would center presumably on compensating for self-care deficits, diminishing environment constraints, facilitating social support, and referring clients for medical evaluation of rectal lesions and pelvic floor weakness.

tion when adhesives and pouch are removed. Some clients develop a fungal infection around a stoma site, which is manifested by patchy erythematous areas intermixed with dry, scaly itching areas. A bacterial infection may also occur, resulting in large weeping erythematous areas, crusting, and purulent sores. Clients with stomas benefit from teaching by the enterostomal therapist, as many of these complications can be avoided with appropriate stoma care.

When abdominal inspection is complete, auscultate for bowel sounds as discussed in Chapter 16. Absent bowel sounds are expected immediately after surgery, but absent or hypoactive bowel sounds (faint sounds occurring 30 seconds or more apart) in clients who are not postoperative suggest decreased intestinal motility or other pathology requiring further investigation. Borborygmus (loud rumbling, gurgling bowel sounds) are also abnormal and suggest increased motility. The cause may be gastroenteritis or recent laxative use.

Palpate the abdomen after auscultating. Light palpation (see Chap. 16) may detect generalized tenseness suggestive of excessive gas. Soft, boggy rounded masses may be felt across the two upper quadrants or along the left lateral border of the upper and lower left quadrants. These masses are feces within the transverse and descending colon. Although presence of fecal material in the descending colon is not abnormal, in the right transverse or ascending colon it suggests bowel elimination problems. Some clients may complain of cramping after bowel segments are palpated.

A distended bladder may also be confirmed by palpation. Palpate above the symphysis pubis for a smooth, round, rather tense mass. It may extend as high as the umbilicus. Often the client will complain of a desire to empty the bladder because of pressure caused by palpation.

Genitalia. Proceeding in a head-to-toe fashion, the next aspect of the elimination examination is assessment of the genitalia. Although this part of the examination is often uncomfortable for beginning students, particularly with clients of the opposite sex, it should not be omitted. Carrying out the assessment while providing perineal care may reduce embarrassment. A respectful, matter-of-fact approach is helpful to both client and nurse (see also Chap. 16). Findings that may be of significance to the client's elimination status include discharge from the urethra (or in the periurethral area in women) and redness, swelling, or excoriation of tissues. A urinary tract infection may be the cause of these symptoms, particularly if the client history includes complaints of frequency, urgency, and dysuria. Clients with indwelling catheters are at risk for periurethral irritation and discharge, as well as for bladder infections, and so more frequent assessments are warranted.

Perianal Area. Assessment of the perianal area is the next component of the elimination examination. Hemorrhoids may cause slight bleeding and pain with defecation. Some clients with hemorrhoids have frequent constipation as a result of suppressing defecation to avoid pain. Redness and excoriation in the perianal area may be caused by incontinence and will be exacerbated if incontinence continues.

Neurological and Mobility Assessment. Neurological and mobility assessments are relevant for any client whose ability to walk independently is compromised. Generalized

TABLE 26–4. REFERENCE CHART FOR URINE CHARACTERISTICS

Parameter	Usual Character	Common Alterations	Possible Cause
Color	Pale yellow (straw-colored to amber)	Dark amber	Decreased fluid intake, medications
		Colorless, pale	Large fluid intake; diuresis (caffeine, alcohol, other drugs); kidney disease; diabetes insipidus
Clarity	Clear	Cloudy	Infection: bacteria, pus, or white blood cells in urine; diet (increased protein)
Odor	Faint aromatic	Malodorous	Infection, medications, tannins in wine, diabetic acidosis

weakness, poor balance, lower extremity contractures, or a need for assistive devices (canes, crutches, wheelchair) imply difficulty getting to toilet facilities, particularly in a strange environment such as a health care institution. Confusion and disorientation may contribute to mobility problems and increase a client's risk for incontinence and subsequent skin breakdown related to poor hygiene. Paralysis, whether partial or complete, may compromise urinary and bowel elimination. Many paralyzed clients require indwelling urinary catheters and are incontinent of stool; some benefit from bowel training (see Rehabilitative Care later in the chapter) to facilitate management of bowel elimination. Comatose clients cannot control urine or bowel elimination and therefore require complete elimination care.

Urine and Stool Characteristics. Assessment of urine and stool characteristics completes the elimination examination. Tables 26–4 and 26–5 summarize usual characteristics of urine and stool, as well as common alterations and their causes.

TABLE 26–5. REFERENCE CHART FOR STOOL CHARACTERISTICS

Parameter	Usual Character	Common Alterations	Possible Cause
Color	Brown	Clay or white	Obstruction or absence of bile
		Light green	Enteric infection
		Black or tarry	Iron compounds; upper GI bleeding
		Pale with fatty-appearing substance	Fat malabsorption
		Red/blood-streaked	Lower GI bleeding, hemorrhoids, or some foods such as beets
Consistency	Moist, soft, and formed	Hard, dry	Slowed peristalsis, poor hydration
		Liquid, unformed	Intestinal irritants such as enteric pathogens, some foods, some medications; all promote hypermotility of the intestine and decreased water absorption
Odor	Characteristic pungent fecal odor, affected by food eaten	Aromatic, extremely pungent, foul	Blood or infection in intestinal tract, malabsorption of fat
Shape	Diameter and contour of the rectum	Narrow, pencil-shaped, ribbon-like	Obstruction with resulting hypermotility of the intestine
		Round, small	Poor hydration, slowed peristalsis
Amount	Varies with intake and diet (100–400 g daily)	Bulky (pale, frothy)	Fat malabsorption
Constituents	Dead bacteria, undigested food, fat, bile pigment, remains of digestive enzymes, sloughed intestinal mucosal cells, water	Blood, pus, mucus, foreign bodies, worms	GI bleeding, infection, intestinal parasites, swallowed objects, inflammation, irritation

Diagnostic Tests

Diagnostic examinations and laboratory tests provide additional data about the functioning of organs related to elimination. The nurse can use this information to support certain nursing diagnoses. Diagnostic tests include laboratory tests (blood, urine, and feces), x-rays, nonradiological examinations such as scans and sonography, and direct visualization. Most of these procedures are done in special departments by specially trained personnel. Refer to Tables 26–6 to 26–8. Nurses make independent decisions about performing some diagnostic tests. For example, nurses commonly check for the presence of blood in stool and assess the pH, specific gravity, sugar, ketones, blood, and protein in urine. See Preventive Care later in the chapter.

■ NURSING DIAGNOSIS OF ELIMINATION STATUS

The final step in the elimination assessment is analyzing the subjective and objective data to generate nursing diagnoses. These diagnoses then form the basis for collaborative planning with the client to promote optimum urinary and bowel elimination. The beginning student will find the

TABLE 26–6. COMMON LABORATORY TESTS OF URINE AND STOOL

Test/Description	Findings	Nurse's Responsibility
Urinalysis Gross and microscopic analysis for diagnosis of urinary tract infections, renal and other metabolic disease.	pH: 4.5–8.0 Specific gravity: 1.003–1.035. Protein: 2–8 mg/dL. Glucose: negative. Ketones: negative. RBCs: 1–2/low-power field. WBCs: 3–4/low-power field. Casts: 3–4/low-power field. Identifies causative organism of urinary tract infection and antibiotics to which the organism is susceptible.	Send a freshly voided, labeled specimen (see Procedure 26–3) of at least 50 mL to the lab in a clean, dry container. Specimen may be refrigerated 6–8 hours. Midstream specimen preferred.
Urine Culture and Sensitivity Analysis for presence of organisms in urine and drugs to treat the infection.	Identifies causative organism of urinary tract infection and antibiotics to which the organism is susceptible.	Send a freshly voided, labeled clean catch specimen (or obtain via catheterization) of 2–10 mL to the lab in a sterile container. Note time specimen was obtained on label.
24-Hour Urine Collection Measures 24-hour urine clearance of specific substances. Creatinine clearance is commonly measured to assess kidney function.	Identification of quantity of specific component(s) excreted in urine in a 24-hour period. Used to diagnose disease states that alter production and/or excretion of specific substances (eg, protein, electrolytes, metabolites).	Have client empty bladder at the time the test is to begin. Discard specimen and note time. Collect all urine produced for the next 24 hours in a clean container and transfer to collection bottle supplied by lab. Keep bottle cool. Label collection bottle with client name, time period of collection, and name of test(s) to be completed.
Stool Culture Analysis for causative organism of enteric infection.	Identifies organisms other than normal intestinal flora that are present in stool.	Collect fecal sample about 1 inch long. (See Procedure 26–2). Place in sterile container, label with client name and suspected organism. Do not administer barium or mineral oil 24 hours prior to test.
Stool for Ova and Parasites (O & P) Analysis for parasites or their eggs in client's intestine.	Identifies parasites such as protozoa or worms that are growing in intestinal tract.	Send serial specimens collected over a 3-day period. Take all specimens to the lab within 30 minutes. Identify countries client has visited within 1 year on lab slip. If tapeworm is suspected, send entire stool. Do not administer barium, antacids, or mineral oil for 1 week prior to test.
Stool for Occult Blood	See Procedure 26–3.	

TABLE 26–7. COMMON DIAGNOSTIC TESTS OF BOWEL FUNCTION

Test/Description	Client Preparation	Posttest Nursing Care
Upper GI Series X-ray of esophagus, stomach, and small intestine using contrast media such as barium or water-soluble agent such as Gastrographin. Used to diagnose obstructions, changes in mucosa and altered motility.	Discuss: ■ Purpose of test. ■ Need to drink 16–20 oz of contrast media (barium is chalky). ■ Test may take up to 6 hours. ■ Discomfort minimal. ■ Position changes necessary on rotating x-ray table. ■ n.p.o. 8–12 hours before test. ■ Need for laxative or enema after test if barium used; stool will be light-colored for a few days. Encourage questions. Check/obtain signed consent. Administer contrast media immediately before test.	Do not offer food or fluids until X-ray Department verifies all views have been completed. Encourage fluids to 2 L to facilitate elimination of barium. Administer laxatives as ordered; assess stool to verify excretion of barium. If client not hospitalized, request client notify physician if barium not excreted within 2 days. Provide opportunities to discuss concerns regarding test results.
Barium Enema X-ray of large intestine after administration of barium or barium and air via rectal tube. Used to diagnose obstructions and changes in bowel mucosa.	Discuss: ■ Purpose of test. ■ Colon must be free of fecal material for this test, so a clear liquid diet is required for the 24 hours prior to test, a laxative may be ordered the day before, and cleansing enemas are given before barium is administered. ■ Increased fluid intake is recommended the day before the test to maintain hydration. ■ Barium instillation may cause cramping; deep breathing/relaxation may relieve. ■ Retention of the barium during the test is important but rectal tube may have an inflated portion to assist retention. ■ X-ray table will be tilted; various positions will be necessary; test takes ½–1 hour. Encourage questions. Check/obtain signed consent. Administer enemas as ordered on day of test.	Assist client to toilet facilities to expel barium; all barium should be expelled immediately if possible. Encourage fluids to 2 L and administer a laxative to facilitate excretion of any residual barium. Provide opportunities for uninterrupted rest after test; most clients find it extremely tiring. Provide opportunities to discuss concerns regarding test results.
Sigmoidoscopy Visualization of the anus, rectum, and sigmoid colon. **Colonoscopy** Visualization of the colon. Used to evaluate and/or biopsy suspicious bowel lesions (tumors, inflammation).	Discuss: ■ Purpose of test. ■ Nature of test preparation (varies—usually involves clear liquid diet, cathartics, and enemas). ■ Position for sigmoidoscopy is knee chest or Sims; for colonoscopy Sims. ■ Insertion of well-lubricated flexible tube into the rectum will create pressure, urge to defecate. Air may be insufflated to aid visualization, which may cause cramping during and after the test. Relaxation/deep breathing helps; sometimes sedative given. ■ Sigmoidoscopy takes 15–30 minutes; colonoscopy, 30–90 minutes. Encourage questions. Check/obtain signed consent. Administer enema, sedative as ordered.	Assess vital signs every 30 minutes for 2 hours. Encourage expulsion of gas; large amounts expected. Provide opportunities for uninterrupted rest. Observe for signs of bowel perforation: rectal bleeding, abdominal pain, fever. Confer with physician if symptoms present (small amount of bleeding is expected if polyp removed). If client discharged, inform client to report these symptoms to physician. Provide opportunities to discuss concerns regarding test results.
CT/CAT Scan See Table 26–8.		

TABLE 26–8. COMMON DIAGNOSTIC TESTS OF URINARY FUNCTION

Test/Description	Client Preparation	Posttest Nursing Care
Blood Urea Nitrogen (BUN) Assessment of levels of nitrogenous wastes in the bloodstream. Reflects efficiency of glomerular filtration. Normal limits: 5–25 mg/dL.	Discuss purpose of test. No physical preparation required.	No physical care required. Compare with creatinine values; if both elevated, suggests kidney disorder. If kidney disorder is not suspected, encourage increased fluid intake; dehydration is a possible cause of elevated BUN.
Serum Creatinine Assessment of creatinine, a byproduct of muscle metabolism in serum. Excreted by kidneys; considered a more sensitive indicator of kidney function than BUN. Normal limits: 0.5–1.5 mg/dL.	See BUN, above.	No physical care required. Compare with BUN value, as above. Assess urine output.
KUB X-ray of kidneys, ureters, bladder. Reveals size, calculi, and bladder masses.	Discuss: ■ Purpose of test. ■ No pretest restrictions of food/fluid. ■ Position for test is supine, table may be tilted. Encourage questions.	No special care required. Provide opportunities to discuss concerns regarding test results.
Intravenous Pyelogram (IVP) X-ray of entire urinary tract after intravenous administration of contrast media. A series of x-rays is taken as kidney clears a contrast media and it is excreted via the bladder. X-ray taken after voiding (excretory urography) determines if residual media is in bladder. Used to detect calculi, masses, changes in kidney size or function.	Discuss: ■ Purpose of test. ■ Previous reaction to iodine, contrast dye, or seafood (may contraindicate test). ■ Need for n.p.o. 12 hours before test, laxative, and enema to prevent bowel contents from interfering with visualization. ■ Transient flushing, metallic taste associated with dye injection. ■ Supine position for test. ■ Length of test about 20–30 minutes; requires 5 or more x-rays, possibly one during voiding. Encourage questions. Check/obtain signed consent. Check BUN; confer with physician if over 40 mg/dL. Administer enema. Encourage client to empty bladder.	Monitor vital signs and urine output. Observe for delayed reaction to contrast media: urticaria (itchy rash), flushing, tachycardia, dyspnea. Confer with physician if allergic reaction or oliguria noted. Observe injection site for irritation, hematoma; apply warm or cold compresses if present. Offer food and fluids. Provide opportunities to discuss concerns regarding test results.
Retrograde Pyelogram X-ray of bladder, ureters, and kidney after contrast media is introduced via a ureteral catheter. Used to detect calculi, masses, and kidney hypertrophy, especially when IVP contraindicated (allergy to media or poor kidney function). May be combined with cystogram, in which bladder is filled to capacity with contrast media. This reveals bladder fistulas, tumors, or calculi, and prostate hypertrophy.	Discuss: ■ Purpose of test. ■ Need for laxative, enema as for IVP. ■ Use of cystoscope for placement of catheters (see discussion points on next page). ■ Lithotomy position for test. ■ Length of procedure 30–90 minutes. ■ Need for increased fluid intake before and after test to facilitate excretion of contrast media.	Assess as for cystoscopy (see below). Assess drainage from ureteral catheters if left in place. Provide food and fluids as soon as recovered from anesthesia. Provide opportunities to discuss concerns regarding test results.

(continued)

TABLE 26–8. (continued)

Test/Description	Client Preparation	Posttest Nursing Care
	Encourage questions. Check/obtain signed consent. Encourage client to empty bladder. Administer enema, sedatives, analgesics, as ordered.	
Cystoscopy Direct visualization of bladder, urethra, and prostate using a cystoscope. Used to detect calculi, tumors, urethral strictures, and prostate hypertrophy. Can also be used to remove calculi, perform biopsy, and resect excessive prostatic tissue.	Discuss: ■ Purpose of test. ■ Liquid diet day of test unless anesthesia planned, then n.p.o. ■ Use of anesthesia (local or general) or sedatives and analgesia for test. ■ Possible need for IV. ■ Possible use of antibiotics to prevent infection. ■ Use of cystoscope, a thin telescopic tube that is introduced via the urethra. Client may feel pressure if not anesthetized. ■ Lithotomy position for test. ■ Length of procedure 30–60 minutes (longer if tissue removal anticipated). ■ Possibility of retention catheter after procedure. ■ Possibility of swelling, blood in urine (hematuria), burning on urination (dysuria) after procedure. Encourage questions. Check/obtain signed consent. Administer premedications as ordered.	Assess vital signs according to postanesthesia policy. Assess urinary output (amount, character) for 48 hours after procedure. Confer with physician if urinary retention, gross hematuria (bright red urine), tachycardia, hypotension, or fever noted. Provide increased fluids. Provide pain relief measures (see Chap. 29). Provide opportunities to discuss concerns regarding test results.
CT (Computerized Tomography) **or CAT** (Computerized Axial Tomography) **Renal/Pelvic Scan** Uses a narrow x-ray beam to produce multiple-angle views of target organ, resulting in a three-dimensional picture. Used to detect structural bowel or urinary tract abnormalities, tumors, stones, abscesses, and cysts.	Discuss: ■ Purpose of test. ■ Use of oral contrast media (about 15 oz) evening before and day of scan for pelvic examination (bowel, bladder) or 1 hour before scan for kidney scan. ■ Allergies—see IVP. ■ Usual n.p.o. status 8 hours before exam. ■ Possible need for IV. ■ Scanner is a large circular machine (doughnut-shaped); client will be strapped to a narrow table, scanner will surround and revolve around body, making clicking noises. Test is not painful, but may be necessary to hold breath several times during test. ■ Length of procedure 30–90 minutes. Encourage questions. Check/obtain signed consent. Administer contrast media as ordered.	Assess for delayed allergic reaction to contrast (see IVP, above). Provide food and fluids. Provide opportunities to discuss concerns regarding test results.

BOX 26–1. OTHER NURSING DIAGNOSES RELATED TO ELIMINATION

Physical

- Impaired skin integrity
- High risk for impaired skin integrity
- High risk for infection
- Fluid volume deficit
- Activity intolerance
- Fatigue
- Impaired physical mobility
- Toileting self-care deficit
- Sleep pattern disturbance

Cognitive

- Sensory–perceptual alterations
- Pain
- Altered thought processes
- Knowledge deficit
- Dysreflexia

Emotional

- Anxiety
- Fear

Self-conceptual

- Body image disturbance
- Self-esteem disturbance
- Hopelessness

Sociocultural/Life Structural

- Social isolation

Developmental

- Altered growth and development

Sexual

- Altered sexuality patterns
- Rape-trauma syndrome

taxonomy of nursing diagnoses a helpful guide for clustering data and stating nursing diagnoses. The following sections discuss nursing diagnoses related to bowel and urinary elimination and their etiologies. The diagnoses have been approved by the North American Nursing Diagnosis Association (NANDA).

Three nursing diagnoses related to bowel elimination will be addressed here: constipation, diarrhea, and bowel incontinence. Examples of subjective and objective data, defining characteristics, and established or suggested etiologies for these diagnoses are presented in the table Sample Nursing Diagnoses: Bowel Elimination, below. Other nursing diagnoses that are related to altered bowel elimination but are not covered in detail here are listed in Box 26–1.

SAMPLE NURSING DIAGNOSES: BOWEL ELIMINATION

	Defining Characteristics/Manifestations		
Nursing Diagnosis	**Subjective Data**	**Objective Data**	**Etiology**[a]
Constipation *1.3.1.1* *1.3.1.2*[b]	Reports decreased frequency of bowel movement. Reports abdominal fullness, rectal pressure. Reports straining at stool. "I don't drink liquids much except with meals."	Hard, dry stools. Abdominal distension.	*Physical:* Less than adequate fluid intake.
Constipation	Reports decreased frequency of bowel movement. Reports abdominal fullness, rectal pressure. Reports straining at stool. "It's embarrassing to have a BM when someone else is in the room."	Hard, dry stools. Abdominal distension.	*Emotional/environmental:* Lack of privacy.
Diarrhea *1.3.1.2*	Reports frequent, loose, liquid stools since ingesting meal of "leftovers."	Hyperactive bowel sounds. Watery, brown stool with particles of fecal matter.	*Physical:* Intestinal irritation.

[a] Sample etiologies only; see text discussion and taxonomy for other etiologies and defining characteristics.
[b] Etiologies and defining characteristics for 1.3.1.1 and 1.3.1.2 are combined in this table.

Constipation

Constipation is defined in the taxonomy of nursing diagnoses as a change in normal bowel habits characterized by a decrease in frequency and/or passage of hard, dry stools. Many clients worry a great deal about their inability to defecate, which may cause additional emotional stress. There are many possible etiologies for this diagnosis. Therefore, collaboration with the client is important to determine the most appropriate one.

Etiology: Less Than Adequate Fluid Intake. If fluid intake is less than body requirements, extra water is absorbed from the colon to meet metabolic needs. Many factors may contribute to insufficient fluid intake. Addressing these factors will correct the immediate elimination problem and decrease the likelihood that it will recur.

Etiology: Less Than Adequate Dietary Intake. Excessive dieting, immobility, illness, and lack of interest in food sometimes found among the elderly population are among the reasons for diminished dietary intake. The volume of chyme one produces is proportional to the amount of food ingested; less food generates less chyme and therefore less peristalsis.

Etiology: Less Than Adequate Fiber. As discussed previously, fiber promotes peristalsis because it increases bulk of intestinal contents. A preference for highly processed convenience foods is a common reason for lack of fiber in the diet. Recent media emphasis on increasing dietary fiber to prevent colorectal cancer and heart disease has increased public awareness of the importance of fiber, but many individuals need assistance in determining the amount they need and recognizing the best sources.

Etiology: Less Than Adequate Physical Activity; Immobility. As discussed in an earlier section, activity promotes peristalsis. Whether related to general life-style or to illness and its treatment, minimal physical activity promotes constipation. Prudent nurses anticipate this risk factor when caring for clients whose illness or treatment involves limiting activity, and when possible take measures to offset the risk, such as increasing fluids and fiber.

Etiology: Lack of Privacy. Because most people consider defecation a private activity, they may suppress defecation when private toilet facilities are not available. This results in absorption of moisture from fecal matter and therefore more difficult elimination. As nursing students become accustomed to assisting others with elimination, they may forget the importance of privacy for most people. However, the simple act of providing privacy for elimination when clients are in health care facilities can prevent their becoming constipated.

Etiology: Emotional Disturbance, Stress. As discussed previously, the gastrointestinal system is particularly susceptible to alterations related to emotional status. Often the experience of seeking health care or concerns about the seriousness of a health problem or its treatment creates sufficient stress to interfere with normal bowel elimination. Therefore, constipation may accompany many health alterations.

Etiology: Chronic Use of Enemas and Laxatives. The effects of dependency on laxatives have been discussed above. Because a client's use of laxatives implies that bowel elimination is a real concern, nurses need to be sensitive in their approach to assisting the client to correct the laxative dependency.

Etiology: Change in Daily Routine. Having a bowel movement at the same time each day is one way to promote bowel regularity. As discussed earlier, the gastrocolic reflex stimulates mass peristalsis approximately 15 minutes after breakfast. Many people, therefore, have a pattern of regular bowel elimination after breakfast. If circumstances prevent elimination at this time, particularly over the course of several days, constipation may result. Illness, treatments, and diagnostic procedures are among the many life events that can change daily routines and so interfere with bowel elimination.

Diarrhea

Diarrhea is described in the taxonomy of nursing diagnosis as frequent passage of loose, fluid, unformed stool. Diarrhea is usually accompanied by cramping and abdominal pain and frequently limits daily activities. No etiologies for diarrhea have been included in the taxonomy to date; however, three generally accepted etiologies for diarrhea are presented here.

Etiology: Intestinal Irritation. Toxins, whether produced by contaminated foods or pathogens gaining entry into the GI tract, are irritating to the intestinal mucosa. Some individuals are allergic to certain foods. The natural defense of the body against this irritation is to increase peristalsis to hasten the exit of the offending substance from the body. The outcome is diarrhea and the accompanying loss of fluid and electrolytes. It should be noted that many laxatives are intestinal irritants and therefore can produce diarrhea if used incorrectly.

Etiology: Emotional Stress. Although for some people, stress produces constipation, others experience parasympathetic dominance of bowel function under stress. This results in increased motility and increased frequency of bowel movements. Often mucus production in the intestines increases as well, so stools may contain obvious mucus.

Etiology: High-osmolality Enteral Nutrition Formulas. Individuals who are unable to consume solid foods for an extended period of time are often given specially formulated liquids that contain all of the necessary calories for metabolic needs. The formulas may be given orally or via tube feedings. Many of these formulas have a high osmolality (concentration of molecules in a solution), and are therefore hypertonic. When in the intestine, the hypertonic liquid causes water to be drawn into the intestine from the mucosa of the intestines, increasing the volume of the intestinal contents and stimulating peristalsis. (See also Chap. 25 for further discussion of enteral feedings.)

Bowel Incontinence

The taxonomy of nursing diagnoses defines bowel incontinence as a change in normal bowel habits characterized by involuntary passage of stool. Bowel incontinence is a cause of physical, emotional, and social distress to individuals experiencing it and to their family members.

Etiologies of Bowel Incontinence. No accepted etiologies are included in the taxonomy. A review of the physiology of bowel elimination suggests that interference with neurological functioning, including problems that alter mental status, are most often responsible for bowel incontinence. Most of these cannot be influenced by nursing therapies. However, in some cases, bowel training programs, discussed below under Rehabilitative Care, are effective. Although nurses usually cannot correct bowel incontinence, they can help clients avoid some associated complications, such as skin breakdown, emotional distress, and social isolation.

Altered patterns of urinary elimination are also of concern to nurses. Nursing diagnoses related to urinary elimination include urinary incontinence and urinary retention. Although the taxonomy of nursing diagnosis includes five types of urinary incontinence (functional, reflex, stress, total, and urge incontinence), only functional and stress incontinence are addressed in this text. The table Sample Nursing Diagnoses: Urinary Elimination presents these diagnoses with sample etiologies and defining characteristics. Box 26–1 lists nursing diagnoses related to altered urinary elimination patterns.

IMPLICATIONS FOR NURSE–CLIENT COLLABORATION

Diagnosis of Incontinence

Several types of urinary incontinence are recognized in the taxonomy of nursing diagnosis. These varieties are differentiated by their nature and their etiologies. Because the nursing measures needed to assist a particular client will differ with the type of incontinence, a careful assessment of the client's specific subjective and objective manifestations is vital. Collaboration with the client to bring out the subtleties that may differentiate one type of incontinence from another is thus very important.

Functional Incontinence

The taxonomy of nursing diagnoses defines **functional incontinence** as the involuntary, unpredictable loss of urine. For example, the aged person who has limited mobility because of arthritis and must climb stairs to go to the bathroom may have a problem with this type of incontinence.

SAMPLE NURSING DIAGNOSES: URINARY ELIMINATION

Nursing Diagnosis	Defining Characteristics/Manifestations: Subjective Data	Defining Characteristics/Manifestations: Objective Data	Etiology[a]
Functional Incontinence *1.3.2.1.4*	Reports inability to control urine elimination at night: "I just can't find the way to the BR when I wake up in the night. It's only been a problem since I've been in here."	Newly admitted to skilled nursing facility. Bed or floor near bed wet at night on several occasions since admission.	*Environmental:* Altered environment.
Stress Incontinence *1.3.2.1.1*	Reports loss of small amounts of urine when laughs or sneezes.	Weight more than 20% over ideal for height.	*Physical:* High intra-abdominal pressure.
Urinary Retention *1.3.2.2*	Reports increasing bladder discomfort. "I got up to go twice, but I can't—I'm afraid it will hurt my stitches." "When you press there (lower abdomen), I really feel like I have to go!"	Spontaneous vaginal delivery 3 hours ago. Midline episiotomy; intact, no swelling. Bladder palpable above symphysis pubis.	*Emotional:* Fear or pain inhibiting reflex arc.

[a] Sample etiologies only; see text discussion and taxonomy for other etiologies and defining characteristics.

Etiology: Altered Environment. Causes of functional incontinence include barriers that interfere with timely access to toilet facilities. Environmental barriers may include lack of privacy, unfamiliarity with surroundings, or distance to the facilities.

Etiology: Sensory, Cognitive, or Mobility Deficit. These might include such variables as fear, anxiety, confusion, leg weakness, or severe pain, any of which may compromise an individual's ability to get to toilet facilities before the urge to void becomes too strong to repress.

Stress Incontinence

Stress incontinence is defined in the taxonomy of nursing diagnoses as the loss of urine of less than 50 mL that occurs when there is a sudden increase in intra-abdominal pressure. These sudden pressure increases may be caused by sneezing, laughing, lifting, or vomiting. When intra-abdominal pressure is increased, the bladder is compressed. If the urinary sphincters and pelvic floor muscles do not maintain sufficient tone, urine is squeezed out of the bladder. Stress incontinence is most common in women.

Etiology: Weakness or Degenerative Changes in Pelvic Muscles and Structural Supports. Degenerative changes in pelvic muscles and structural supports is a common reason for stress incontinence. This is most often related to the aging process, although obesity and multiple vaginal births contribute. Pelvic muscle weakness at middle age may also result from multiple vaginal deliveries.

Etiology: High Intra-abdominal Pressure. High intra-abdominal pressure may result from obesity or the increased size of the uterus during pregnancy. In some women, both are etiologic factors. With this etiology, muscle tone in sphincters and pelvic floor is adequate to contain urine under usual circumstances, but with the high baseline intra-abdominal pressure, even small unexpected pressure increases cause loss of urine.

Etiology: Overdistension. The individual who ignores the signal to urinate and consistently overdistends the bladder between voidings may develop stress incontinence. When the bladder is overdistended, pressure on the sphincters is increased. It then becomes increasingly difficult to control the external sphincter against leakage of urine with the added activity produced in sneezing, coughing, laughing, or lifting objects.

Urinary Retention

Urinary retention occurs when an individual is unable to empty the bladder completely. Typically, residual urine remains in the bladder after attempts to void. Eventually the bladder may become overdistended. Some of the etiologies of urinary retention, such as weak detrusor muscle tone (which causes continual constriction of the external sphincter, because detrusor contraction is the stimulus for sphincter relaxation); inhibition of reflex arc because of neurological pathology; and urethral blockage (which may be the result of trauma, prostate enlargement, or tumors); are not readily treatable by nursing therapies. Two etiologies, inhibition of reflex arc because of anxiety or fear and blockage because of swelling, can be treated by nursing implementation, and so are addressed here.

Etiology: Inhibition of Reflex Arc. Fear of pain during voiding or generalized anxiety can result in inability to relax the external sphincter, despite signals initiated by contraction of the detrusor muscle as the bladder distends. Even though the individual consciously attempts to relax the per-

BUILDING NURSING KNOWLEDGE

Can Nurses Alleviate Urinary Incontinence?

Tunink PM. Alteration in Urinary Elimination. *J Gerontol Nurs.* 1988;14:25–30.

In this article, Tunink notes that 50 percent of institutionalized elderly clients are incontinent. Despite the prevalence of incontinence, many health care professionals are unaware of the various types and causes of incontinence and their treatment. Nursing diagnoses identify six distinct types of incontinence, each of which requires different types of nursing intervention. This article focuses on two of the most common.

Functional incontinence refers to the inability to reach the toilet due to barriers or disorientation. The bladder and urethral functions are normal, but other physical, cognitive-perceptual, or psychosocial factors limit the individual's control of urinary elimination. The individual voids completely and in large amounts, and may display signs and symptoms of more than one etiology. An individual may fail to accomplish toileting because of mental disorientation *and* an inability to manipulate clothing. Both problems must be addressed.

Urge incontinence is characterized by involuntary urination that occurs soon after a strong sense of urgency to void. There are three common etiologies: (1) bladder irritation (from infection, concentrated urine, caffeine or alcohol intake); (2) decreased bladder capacity (from frequent voiding or use of an indwelling catheter); and (3) bladder overdistension (from increased urine production and increased fluid intake). The individual has a feeling of urgency followed by the involuntary loss of urine.

Tunink presents a case study of a 78-year-old man in a long-term care facility who had surgery for cancer of the prostate. The client wore disposable undergarments all day and used a urinal at night. He stated that he could tell when he needed to urinate, but would rather wear the undergarments than return to the nursing unit to toilet himself. At night he complained that he awoke from sleep but was incontinent before he could reach his urinal. He was able to use both his call-light and urinal. The diagnoses established were (1) Alteration in Urinary Elimination: Urge Incontinence Related to Overdistension of the Bladder; and (2) Alteration in Urinary Elimination: Functional Incontinence Related to Lack of Motivation to be Continent. The client was consulted about the importance of reduced fluids before bedtime and scheduled toileting, and became more interested in toileting himself as staff members began to spend time with him. He eventually achieved continence.

ineum and external sphincter, the sphincter remains contracted because of stronger sympathetic nervous system signals limiting relaxation.

Etiology: Blockage. The urethra and perineum may become inflamed and swollen due to irritation during urinary diagnostic procedures such as cystoscopy, surgery involving the bladder or prostate, or pressure of the fetal presenting part during childbirth. This swelling may present a physical barrier to the passage of urine as well as make sphincter relaxation difficult.

Stating the Elimination Diagnosis

The nursing diagnosis is the basis for a collaborative individualized client care plan. The more precisely it describes the etiology and defining characteristics a particular client presents, the more effectively it can guide the selection of nursing implementations. When possible, general etiologies and defining characteristics should be made more specific by using the signs and symptoms in the data base.

For example, a client complains of intermittent difficulty passing stools, stating that he often goes 4 days without a bowel movement and that his stools are hard, marblelike pieces. The nurse also learns that he works long hours at a desk job. He says, "I get a little exercise on the weekends, but I'm usually too tired to do anything after work but have a drink and watch TV. That's often the first liquid I'll have except for breakfast coffee and a soft drink at lunch." An appropriate nursing diagnosis for this client may be: Constipation related to lack of regular exercise and less than adequate daily fluid intake as evidenced by reported straining at stool; hard, small stools every 4 days; daily fluid intake of less than 1000 mL, and lack of regular physical exercise.

Another client complains of "wetting" herself at night as she is walking to the bathroom. She says she has recently been fitted with a leg brace that "helps me get around pretty good. When I take it off at night to sleep, I just can't get to the bathroom fast enough." The nurse determines that the leg brace was prescribed to assist the client with weight bearing on a weakened left leg. This client's elimination diagnosis might be: Functional nighttime incontinence related to lower extremity weakness as evidenced by reported loss of urine when walking to the bathroom without corrective brace.

This method of stating nursing diagnoses makes the exact nature of the client's elimination problem clear to all caregivers and provides guidelines for developing realistic desired outcomes and nursing implementation. When a client's primary concern is an elimination problem, or the nature of the problem suggests that elimination may be affected, a thorough data base that includes subjective and objective elimination data will facilitate nursing diagnosis. Then collaborative nurse–client management to bring about resolution of the problem can begin.

Section 3: Nurse–Client Management of Elimination

Collaborative management of altered elimination patterns begins with planning strategies that will help meet the client's elimination needs. Then implementation is carried out and evaluated for effectiveness in meeting the outcomes.

■ PLANNING FOR OPTIMUM ELIMINATION

The planning phase includes collaborating with the client to establish desired outcomes, identifying implementation that will help accomplish the outcomes, and selecting evaluation criteria. All components of the plan should be congruent with the client's wishes and resources.

Mutual consideration of the nursing diagnosis statement should generate desired outcomes that are realistic and agreeable to the client. An appropriate outcome for the client with constipation discussed above might be: Bowel elimination pattern of one soft, formed bowel movement at least every other day within 2 weeks. Short-term outcomes for increased fluid intake and regular exercise could also be established to assist in achieving the overall outcome. A client with functional incontinence of urine might strive for a desired outcome of: No incidents of nighttime urinary incontinence within 1 week. Such specific desired outcome statements help the nurse document progress toward outcome attainment and guide selection of implementations.

■ NURSING IMPLEMENTATION TO PROMOTE OPTIMUM ELIMINATION

Effective nursing implementation is specific to the individual client. As nurse and client collaborate to select implementation to promote optimum elimination, they consider the elimination data base and the client's developmental level as well as the client's preferences and the nurse's conceptual knowledge of elimination.

Nursing measures to promote elimination are divided into four levels of care: (1) preventive care—activities related to promoting healthy elimination, screening, and preventing elimination problems, (2) supportive care—assisting clients with early signs of elimination problems; (3) restorative care—assisting with acute elimination problems, and (4) rehabilitative care—facilitating adjustment to chronic alterations in elimination patterns. Descriptions of these nursing measures follow, providing the nurse with guidelines and approaches to use in caring for clients with elimination problems. The table Nurse–Client Management

NURSE–CLIENT MANAGEMENT OF ELIMINATION PROBLEMS

Nursing Diagnosis	Desired Outcomes	Implementation	Evaluation Criteria
Constipation related to less than adequate fluid intake *1.3.1.1.* *1.3.1.1.2*	1. Healthy bowel elimination pattern 2. Daily fluid intake at least 2000 mL	1. Teach client the relationship between fluid intake and bowel functioning. 2a. Discuss factors inhibiting adequate fluid intake. 2b. Devise fluid intake schedule with client to provide minimum of 2 L fluids/day 2c. Assist as necessary (provide fluids of choice, remind client to drink).	1a. Daily or q.o.d. stool of soft-formed consistency. 1b. No abdominal distension. 1c. States relief of rectal pressure, straining. 2. Daily fluid intake 2000 mL.
Constipation related to lack of privacy	1. Healthy bowel elimination pattern	1a. Transfer to private room, if possible. 1b. Discuss ways in which suppressing defecation contributes to constipation, and importance of regular bowel elimination to health. 1c. If private room unavailable, discuss ways client may enhance feelings of privacy when using bathroom (eg, changing beds so client's bed is nearer to bathroom, playing radio to mask noises associated with elimination). 1d. Provide high-fiber foods, adequate fluids as needed to correct current problem.	1a. Daily or q.o.d. stool of soft-formed consistency. 1b. No abdominal distension. 1c. States relief of rectal pressure, straining.
Diarrhea related to intestinal irritation secondary to contaminated food *1.3.1.2*	1. Healthy bowel elimination pattern 2. Understanding of strategies to prevent recurrence	1a. Suggest discontinue solid food for 12–24 hours. 1b. Encourage frequent sips of bland fluids at room temperature, particularly potassium-rich fluids such as broth, orange juice. Increase fluids if diarrhea abates. 1c. If liquids do not exacerbate diarrhea, suggest intake of small amounts of bland foods such as soda crackers, banana, rice, applesauce. Avoid milk products, whole grains until symptoms resolved. 2a. Teach relationship between "spoiled" food and diarrhea. 2b. Discuss safe food handling, cooking, and storage methods. 2c. Emphasize that bacteria or toxins do not always change color or odor of food.	1a. Daily or q.o.d. stool of soft-formed consistency. 2. Correctly verbalizes safe food handling and storage methods.
Functional Incontinence related to unfamiliar environment *1.3.2.1.4*	1. Urinary elimination without incontinence	1a. Place bedside commode near client's bed. 1b. Keep siderails down at foot end of bed to facilitate getting out of bed. 1c. Keep nurse call light in reach, encourage client to call for nurse if having difficulty getting up or getting to commode. 1d. If incontinent only at night, encourage spacing fluid intake so daily fluid needs met without fluid intake after 7–8 PM. 1e. Keep night light on when client asleep.	1. Client able to void in bedside commode without incidents of incontinence.

NURSE–CLIENT MANAGEMENT OF ELIMINATION PROBLEMS (continued)

Nursing Diagnosis	Desired Outcomes	Implementation	Evaluation Criteria
Stress Incontinence related to high intra-abdominal pressure *1.3.2.1.1*	1. Freedom from stress incontinence	1a. Discuss causes of stress incontinence. 1b. Teach exercises to strengthen pelvic floor muscles. 1c. Discuss benefits of frequent urination to prevent internal bladder pressure from full bladder. 1d. Discuss how obesity increases abdominal pressure. 1e. Collaboratively plan weight-reduction diet (see Chap. 25) and exercise plan (see Chap. 30) if client desires to lose weight.	1. Client reports no further incidents of stress incontinence.
Urinary Retention related to fear of pain inhibiting reflex arc *1.3.2.2*	1. Complete emptying without catheterization	1a. Discuss how emotions can inhibit perineal and external sphincter relaxation that is necessary for voiding. 1b. Apply topical anesthetic ointment to stitches, explain how this will prevent urine from irritating stitches. 1c. Explain how fluid intake facilitates bladder elimination. 1d. Encourage fluid intake of 2 L day. 1e. Explain that you must measure urine to assess for complete emptying; use "hat" collector (Fig. 26–14). 1f. Assist voiding by: Pouring measured amount of warm water over perineum. Providing basin of warm water to immerse hands. Running water in sink next to client. Encouraging client to visualize/imagine sight and sound of running water. Providing a glass of water and a straw; ask client to blow through the straw to produce bubbles in water. Breaking spirits of ammonia ampoule in "hat" collector (Fig. 26–14). 1g. Suggest client take warm shower and allow urine to flow during shower (subsequent voids must be measured to assess emptying). 1h. Assess for abdomen for bladder distension after voiding. 1i. Assess 3 consecutive voids for volume greater than 200 mL. 1j. If unable to void or residual urine suspected, confer with physician for order to catheterize.	1a. Client voids at least 200 mL. 1b. Abdomen nondistended. 1c. Continued independent voiding.

of Elimination Problems on pages 1164–1165 provides examples of appropriate outcomes, approaches, and evaluation criteria for bowel and urinary elimination problems.

Preventive Care

First-level nursing implementation for elimination is focused on promoting normal micturition and defecation in healthy clients. The most important first-level nursing activity is teaching clients to take time for elimination. Not taking the time to defecate or ignoring the urge to void are common causes of constipation and urinary tract infections. Teaching is thus an important part of preventive care.

Health Education. Areas to consider in client teaching are dietary habits and regular exercise. It is especially important that clients have an adequate fluid intake. Drinking eight glasses of water a day helps keep both bowel and urine elimination regular and effortless. Tea, coffee, colas, and alcohol have a diuretic effect; their use should be reduced or avoided if frequency or incontinence is a problem. Nutrition also plays a role in keeping elimination regular. Eating adequate amounts of fiber and eating foods from all the basic food groups is important in maintaining bowel elimination. Foods high in fiber stimulate peristalsis. High-fiber foods include whole grains and nuts, raw vegetables, and fresh fruits. Gum chewing and drinking carbonated beverages may contribute to flatulence, and the client may be advised to avoid these habits.

Helping the client determine the time when the urge to defecate usually occurs will help to establish regular bowel habits. Setting aside the same time each day for bowel elimination will help the client develop a pattern. Advising the client to avoid tight-fitting clothing may also be helpful. Tight clothing interferes with the ability to bear down using the abdominal muscles and thus hinders elimination.

In women, defecation and urination are promoted by assuming a squatting position. Toilet facilities should help provide an effective position for defecation. A squatting position with the thighs flexed will increase abdominal pressure and aid stool expulsion. Most adults achieve this by leaning forward while sitting on the toilet. Children and short people can gain a more functional position by using a footstool. Elderly clients and those with joint diseases may find it difficult to sit down and rise from a standard toilet seat and will benefit from the use of an elevated toilet seat (Fig. 26–11). Men commonly stand to urinate. All clients should be reminded of the importance of washing hands after elimination, and women should be taught to wipe the perineal area from front to back to avoid carrying microorganisms from the vagina or rectum to the urinary meatus. Those who change infants' diapers may need reinforcement about the importance of washing hands after diaper changes.

The nurse can also guide parents in managing effective and appropriate toilet training. The child should be physically, cognitively, and psychosocially ready before training begins. There is a wide age variance in attainment of readiness and in the length of time toilet training takes. Bowel control is usually achieved first, followed by daytime bladder control, and then by nighttime bladder control. At about the age of 2 years, many toddlers develop a desire to please significant others, so this is a good time to attempt use of the potty. Because eating stimulates bowel activity, children often defecate shortly after a meal at approximately the same time every day. Advise parents to observe their toddler's habits and to place the child on the potty at the time of the expected movement. A child-size potty that allows the child to sit comfortably with feet on the floor may be less threatening to the child than a standard-size toilet. As the toddler is placed on the potty, state the purpose in a positive manner. If the desired outcome of a bowel movement in the potty occurs, express pleasure and praise the child. The child should not sit on the potty too long. If the child shows resistance, delay further attempts for a few days, but do not make negative comments. Punishment and extreme sternness should be avoided. Do not use enemas or medications without the guidance of a pediatrician.

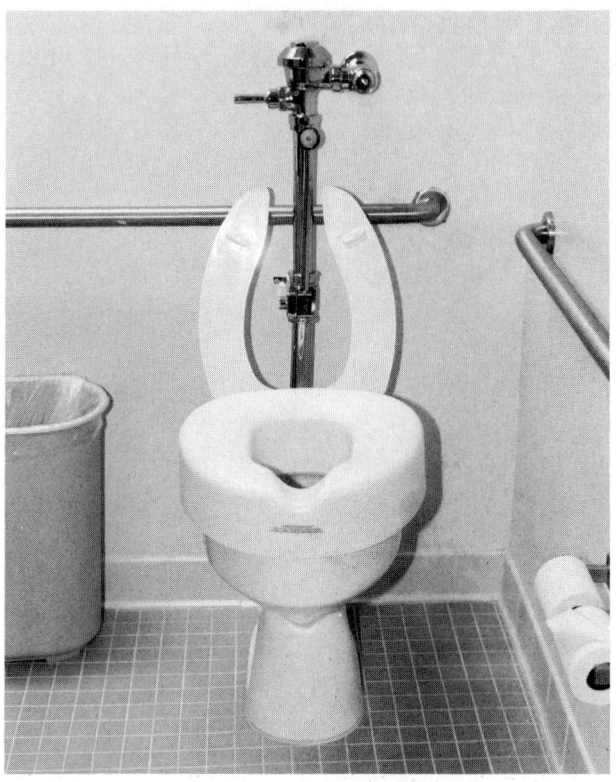

Figure 26–11. Elevated toilet seat.

Bladder control begins at the same time as bowel training but will take longer to achieve. At about 2 to 2½ years of age, children may begin to notify the caretaker that they are already wet. Soon, they interpret the full bladder as a need to "go" and begin to tell the caretaker before they are wet. Even when trained, children are sometimes too busy to notice a full bladder or the urge to defecate and therefore have accidents.

Nighttime bladder control is achieved after daytime

PROCEDURE 26–1. COLLECTING A RANDOM OR CLEAN-CATCH URINE SPECIMEN

PURPOSE: To collect urine for testing.

EQUIPMENT: Clean urinal, bedpan, or specimen hat (Fig. 26–14), specimen container with lid (sterile if specimen is for culture), nonsterile gloves, plastic bag, and twist tie. For clean catch, also need antiseptic wipes or antiseptic solution/ sterile cotton balls in sterile cup. (Commercial kits are available for clean-catch specimens.)

ACTION	RATIONALE
1. Discuss with the client the reason for the procedure, expected client participation, and expected benefits.	1. Client will be more willing to participate and less anxious if reasons and benefits are clear.
2. Assist the client to the bathroom or commode, if needed. Provide specimen container and, if specimen is to be clean catch, antiseptic wipes or antiseptic-soaked cotton balls.	2. Ambulatory, alert clients can independently obtain specimens and usually prefer to do so.
NOTE: If testing is to be completed by the nurse, specimen can be collected in a urinal or specimen hat rather than a specimen container.	
3. For a clean-catch specimen, instruct clients to: a. clean themselves prior to voiding, using the wipes or antiseptic soaked cotton. *Male client:* clean tip of penis from center outward using a circular motion, repeating three times (if uncircumcised, retract foreskin). *Female client:* spread labia minora with one hand, cleanse each side, and then center from front to back, using three separate cotton balls or wipes for each stroke. Keep labia spread during voiding.	a. Clean-catch urine is used to detect presence of bacteria inside the bladder. Friction and antiseptic action remove normal flora, which would contaminate specimen, from meatal area.
NOTE: This cleansing is unnecessary for random sample.	
b. Initiate voiding, then place the container in the stream of urine, filling it about half full, and then complete voiding into the toilet. Avoid touching the inside of the container. (Midstream sample is not needed for random urine.) Discard toilet tissue in toilet, not in specimen hat. NOTE: Females may find collecting the specimen is easier when sitting facing the back of the toilet.	b. Initial stream of urine flushes remaining microorganisms from the meatus. Midstream sample is most free of external contamination. Touching inside of the container would contaminate contents with normal flora from client's hands or genitalia.

(continued)

PROCEDURE 26–1. (continued)

c. Cover container tightly without touching inside of cover.	c. Prevents contamination of specimen or environment.
4. If assisting the client to obtain a specimen, don nonsterile gloves.	4. Body fluids may contain pathogenic organisms. Gloves prevent skin contamination by direct contact.
5. Provide privacy and place the female client on a bedpan (see Procedure 26–4), with legs spread so urine flow does not contact legs. Male client may use urinal for random (unsterile) sample or void directly into specimen container.	5. Elimination activities are considered private in most cultures. Respecting this need promotes trust and minimizes embarrassment.
NOTE: Male clients unable to stop the flow of urine in midstream can be placed on a bedpan to collect volume of urine greater than capacity of clean-catch container.	
6. For clean-catch specimen, cleanse labia or penis as described in step 3, above.	
7. Ask the client to void into the bedpan/urinal. If sample is to be clean catch, obtain a midstream sample as the client voids.	7. See step 3b.
8. Remove bedpan or urinal. Remove gloves to assist to position of comfort, if needed, then reglove to transfer specimen.	8. See Procedure 26–4.
9. Transfer urine to a specimen container if client has voided into a bedpan or specimen hat; cover tightly. Discard remaining urine.	9. See step 3c.
10. Clean the outside of the specimen container, remove gloves by turning inside out. Discard in biohazardous waste can. Wash hands. Place container in plastic bag and close with twist tie.	10. Prevents transfer of organisms from urine to environment.
11. Label specimen and send to lab as soon as possible.	11. Accuracy of some tests is compromised if urine stands at room temperature.
NOTE: Urine may be refrigerated without affecting some tests. Check with lab personnel.	
12. When laboratory report is returned to the client's chart, inform client of result.	12. Client has a right to information about personal health status.
NOTE: Encourage client to also discuss test results with the physician.	

RECORDING: Note date, time, and purpose of specimen; characteristics of urine; and complaints of dysuria, if any.

control, often simply because the child's bladder can hold a larger amount. Occasional lapses in control during toilet training are common and should be handled in a positive manner that will promote the child's self-esteem. A crisis in the family, such as a new baby or moving to a new home, may interrupt or delay toilet training. The caretaker's positive attitude and calm, patient reassurance helps the child attain successful toilet training.[2]

PROCEDURE 26–2. OBTAINING A STOOL SPECIMEN

PURPOSE: To obtain a sample for testing.

EQUIPMENT: A clean dry bedpan or specimen hat (Fig. 26–14), nonsterile gloves, plastic or waxed cardboard specimen cup with lid and/or culture tube, two tongue blades, plastic bag, and twist tie.

ACTION

1. Discuss the procedure with the client, emphasizing:
    a. The reason for the specimen.
    b. The importance of preventing mixing of urine with stool.
    c. That nurse should be notified as soon as defecation is complete.
2. Provide privacy. Assist client as needed to bathroom or commode or onto bedpan, and to place specimen hat.
3. When defecation is complete, assist client as needed with hygiene and/or returning to bed. (Gloves are needed to clean client.)
4. Don gloves. Assess feces for blood, mucus, or other abnormal constituents.
5. Using tongue blades, transfer a midportion of the sample, including any blood or other abnormal constituents, to specimen container and close tightly. If stool culture is ordered, dip applicator swab into feces and place in culture tube according to package directions. Use care not to contact outside of container with fecal matter.
6. Empty and clean bedpan or specimen hat and return it to its place (used for one client only). Specimen hat may be discarded after cleaning if no further samples are needed.
7. Remove gloves by turning them inside out over tongue blades and discard in leakage-resistant trash container. Wash hands.
8. Place specimen container in plastic bag, close bag, label according to agency policy, and send to lab within 1 hour.
9. When laboratory report is returned to client's chart, inform client of results.

RECORDING: Note date, time, and disposition of specimen; appearance of stool.

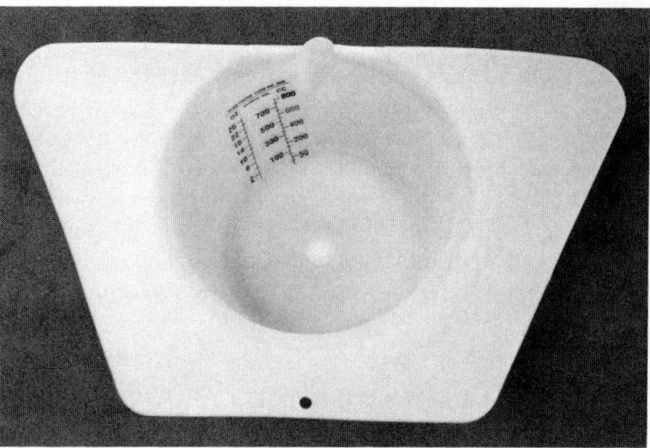

Figure 26–12. Specimen collector, often called "fireman's hat" or "top hat."

Routine Health Screening. Routine screening to detect elimination problems often involves testing of urine and stool specimens. The accuracy of some tests may be affected by collection and storage methods, and so it is helpful to know which tests are planned so that proper techniques can be used. See Table 26–6 for specific guidelines relating to common urine and stool tests.

Most clients prefer to obtain their own specimens; in some cases, the nurse may assist. Procedures 26–1 and 26–2 provide guidelines for collecting specimens, as well as appropriate client instructions for self-collection of specimens. Figure 26–12 illustrates a collector commonly called a "fireman's hat" or "top hat" that can be placed under the toilet seat to catch urine or stool. Figure 26–13 shows a pediatric

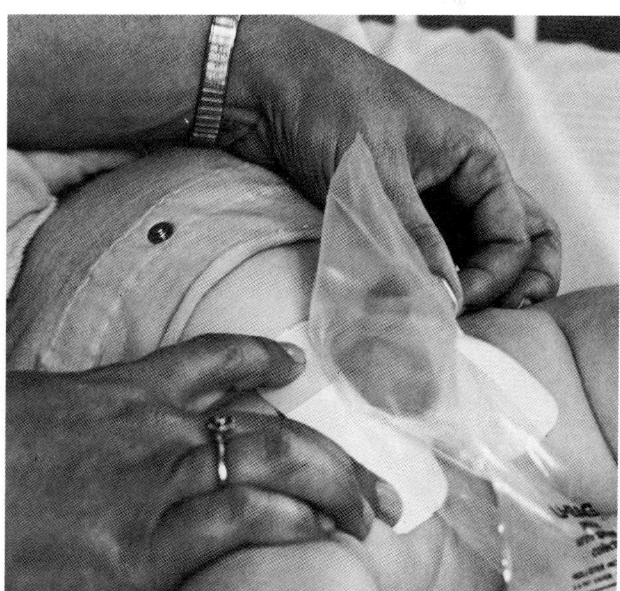

Figure 26–13. Pediatric urine collection bag. (*From Smith S, Duell D.* Clinical Nursing Skills: Nursing Process Model, Basic to Advanced Skills. *3rd ed. Norwalk, CT: Appleton & Lange; 1992.*)

urine-collection bag that is used to obtain urine samples from infants and children not yet toilet trained.

Sometimes nurses test specimens. Table 26–9 lists and describes techniques for urine tests. Measuring urine specific gravity requires a urinometer, illustrated in Figure 26–14.

The most common test of stool done by nurses is determining the presence of blood, often an early sign of colon cancer or other intestinal pathology. Refer to Procedure 26–3. The Hemoccult slide and developer, one of the methods described in that procedure, is illustrated in Figure 26–15.

Nurses may also instruct clients how to perform simple screening tests at home. It is particularly important to emphasize that accuracy depends on use of reagents before the expiration date stamped on the package and on precisely following manufacturers' directions. Sometimes different brands of reagents require slightly different steps to achieve a correct reading.

TABLE 26–9. COMMON URINE TESTS PERFORMED BY NURSES

Name, Range of Normal Limits	Procedure	Additional Information
Specific gravity 1.003–1.040	All urine specimens should be at room temperature. Fill the clean calibrated container (see Fig. 26–14) with urine, twirl the urinometer and allow it to float freely and stop. Read the number at the meniscus at eye level. Electronic monitors requiring only one drop of urine, that are also more accurate, are available in many settings.	Specific gravity of urine is a test of concentration and depends upon hydration status in the healthy person; thus, a dehydrated (and/or a hyperosmolar) client would have a high specific gravity. A fixed specific gravity indicates that the client's kidneys do not vary the concentration of urine.
Blood (occult blood, hemoglobin) Negative to 1000 RBC/mL	Follow the manufacturer's directions for dipstick, tablet, or other product.	Hematuria or hemoglobinuria can be detected by tests using a chemical that is sensitive to the presence of RBCs, hemoglobin, or myoglobin.
pH 4.5–8	Dip reagent-impregnated dipstick into urine sample or place a drop of urine on test tape. Pay particular attention to: (1) the time in which the reagent reacts and should be read, and (2) identification of the particular color chart for the test.	Maximum urine acidity is 4.5; maximum alkalinity is 8–9.
Protein Negative (trace in isolated sample)	Same as for pH, above.	Proteinuria or albuminuria merit further investigation; 24-hour quantitative collections are often ordered upon a repeated positive finding. Increase in glomerular permeability is often a cause of albuminuria.
Ketones (acetone, diacetic acid) (Acetest tablets, Ketostix) Negative	Dipstick (see pH, above) is most common method. If using tablets, follow manufacturer's directions	Excessive fat metabolism coupled with starvation state or diabetic ketoacidosis are common causes of ketonuria. Other diseases or ingestion of alcohol or drugs can also cause ketonuria.
Glucose (Clinistix, Diastix, Tes-tape, Clinitest tablets) Negative	Same as ketones, above.	Glycosuria (glucose in urine) occurs when the renal threshold for glucose (180–200 mg/dL) is exceeded. Most common cause is diabetes mellitus. Urine testing is not a precise method for diabetes control. Assessment of blood sugar using electronic monitors or reagent sticks has replaced urine testing in most health centers. Screening for glycosuria is routinely done during pregnancy and may be done on clients receiving hyperalimentation or high-carbohydrate tube feedings.

Adapted from Ashervath J, Blevins D. Handbook of Clinical Nursing Practice. *New York: Appleton-Century-Crofts; 1986:284–285.*

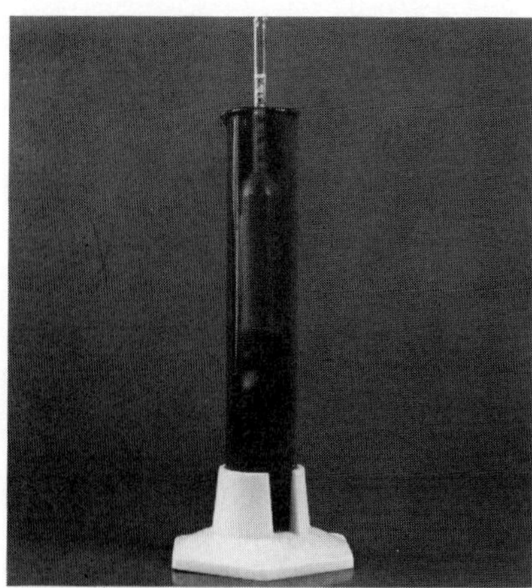

Figure 26–14. Urinometer for measurement of urine specific gravity. (*From Smith S, Duell D.* Clinical Nursing Skills: Nursing Process Model, Basic to Advanced Skills. *3rd ed. Norwalk, CT: Appleton & Lange; 1992.*)

Supportive Care

Clients who require supportive care generally demonstrate early signs of elimination alterations. The nurse will need to help the client evaluate the extent and nature of the elimination problem and determine whether nursing or medical treatment is indicated. If the problem is treatable by nurses, the client and nurse can discuss various approaches and develop outcomes aimed at restoring healthy elimination patterns and preventing other elimination problems.

Correcting Mild Constipation. Nursing implementation for clients with mild constipation includes some techniques that were discussed under Preventive Care. Other nursing measures focus on dietary and exercise measures.

Diet. Diet and adequate fluids continue to be important at this level of care. For the client who tends to be constipated, an increased intake of high-fiber foods and fluids will be helpful. Mild laxatives or a Fleet Enema may be prescribed to correct the immediate problem; however, teaching is an important part of care so that the constipation does not recur and the client does not learn to rely on laxatives or enemas.

Exercise. Exercise can be an important approach at this care level. Swimming, riding a stationary or regular bicycle, and walking stimulate peristalsis. Clients with sedentary employment are usually most in need of regular exercise to regain and maintain regular bowel patterns.

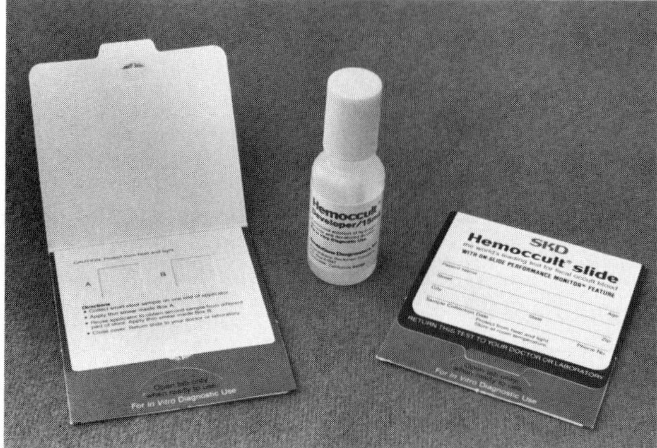

Figure 26–15. Hemoccult slide and developer.

PROCEDURE 26–3. TESTING STOOL FOR OCCULT BLOOD

☐ **PURPOSE:** To determine if gastrointestinal bleeding is occurring as indicated by hidden blood in the stool.

☐ **EQUIPMENT:** Materials to obtain stool specimen (Procedure 26–2). Testing products: reagent, hemoccult slide (Fig. 26–17) or hematest tablet, and filter paper.

ACTION

1. Discuss the procedure with the client, emphasizing:
   a. Purpose of the test
   b. That certain medications as well as meat, turnips, and horseradish may cause false-positive results, in which case a repeat test may be necessary after 48 to 72 hours without ingesting these substances.
   c. That vitamin C tablets may mask bleeding and must therefore be discontinued for 48 to 72 hours for accurate results.
   d. That up to three serial tests may be done.
2. Obtain the specimen according to Procedure 26–2.
3. Perform test according to manufacturer's directions. For example:
   Guaiac: Place a thin smear of feces on filter paper, place tablet in the middle of smear, and place 2 drops of water on tablet.
   Hemoccult: Open cardboard envelope and smear stool from two different parts of the sample on the circles indicated, close cover, turn over, and place 2 drops of reagent on indicated areas.
4. Read results. A dark blue reaction within 5 minutes is a positive reaction; pale blue indicates a retest on another specimen is desirable; no color change is negative.
5. Dispose of used test materials, gloves, and tongue blades in leakage-resistant trash container. Wash hands.
6. Inform client of test results, answer questions regarding significance.

☐ **RECORDING:** Note test performed and result.

Weakened abdominal and pelvic floor muscles can create difficulty passing stools. Two simple exercises to correct this are:

1. While lying supine, tighten abdominal muscles as though pushing them to the floor. Hold muscles tight to count of three and relax. Repeat five to ten times as tolerated.
2. Flex and contract thigh muscles by raising the knees one at a time slowly toward the chest. Repeat five times for each leg. Increase as tolerated.

These exercises often help clients who have been unable to get out of bed and have had to use a bedpan for a considerable time.

Correcting Mild Diarrhea. When mild diarrhea and cramping are present, food intake should be reduced or avoided. The healthy adult with mild diarrhea may avoid food for 12 to 24 hours with no serious side effects. The diet should be confined to bland, easily digested foods such as bananas, white rice, applesauce, and tea; avoiding foods, such as milk, that are high in fat. Clients should be taught that if symptoms persist for more than 24 hours, especially in children, assessment by a health care provider is necessary.

The client with recurrent mild diarrhea should avoid foods that exacerbate intestinal irritation and cramping. Limiting foods with high fiber content, such as raw fruits and vegetables, is helpful, because fiber stimulates peristalsis.

Preventing Recurring Urinary Tract Infections. Urinary tract infection (UTI) is relatively common, especially among women. This is because the proximity of the urinary meatus to the anus makes transfer of bowel flora likely and the short urethra allows bacterial migration to the bladder. Research indicates that some women have defects in the cells lining the bladder, which may be a significant variable increasing their vulnerability. Supportive care involves helping clients reduce their risks for recurrence. Techniques such as scrupulous hygiene, increased fluid intake, avoiding bladder distension, and urinating after intercourse are useful.

Hygiene. Hygiene practices include washing hands before and after urination. Instructing women to wipe the perineum from front to back is also an important teaching point.

Fluid Intake. Fluid intake promotes optimum urine flow, reducing opportunities for bacterial growth. A client with normal renal and cardiovascular states should drink 1500 to 2000 mL of fluid daily. The individual who is prone to UTI may need to increase the fluid intake to 3000 mL daily. The increased fluids may wash out any bacteria at the lower third of the urethra, thus reducing the chance of infection. The nurse may suggest strategies to increase daily intake despite the client's busy work schedule. Fluids should be limited before bedtime to prevent nocturia.

Preventing Bladder Distension and Urinary Stasis. To prevent bladder distension and urinary stasis, the nurse should teach the client to act upon the initial urge to void, not to hold the urine. The longer urine stays in the bladder, the more bacteria can multiply. Urinating more frequently helps prevent bacteria from multiplying.

Preventing Nocturia. Behaviors that help prevent nocturia or maturational enuresis include limiting fluids in the evening, avoiding fluids containing caffeine or alcohol, and voiding before bedtime. Sometimes waking a child during the night to void prevents nocturnal bedwetting. This temporary measure can contribute to the child's self-esteem, although it will not directly correct the problem.

Preventing Stress Incontinence. Strengthening the abdominal and perineal muscles helps promote complete bladder emptying and can prevent or correct stress incontinence. Abdominal exercises discussed previously as an aid to correcting constipation will also facilitate complete emptying of the bladder. Additionally, instructing clients to use the abdominal muscles during urination will help. Teach the client to lean forward, contract the abdominal muscles, and "bear down" (strain or push with the muscles while relaxing the perineum).

Pelvic-floor-strengthening exercises, also called **Kegel exercises,** are suggested to prevent loss of perineal muscle tone, and rarely may correct stress incontinence that has already developed.[13] These exercises entail tightening the perineal muscles as if to stop the passage of urine, and then relaxing them. Combinations of brief, rapid contractions (one or two per second) and maximal contractions held for 10 seconds are most effective. Gradually increasing the number of repetitions of each technique to 40 to 50 contractions per exercise session is recommended. Repeat each cycle at least twice a day so the total exercise period averages 15 minutes daily.[14] These exercises are useful to both women and men. Among women, 30 to 90 percent report improvement with exercise.[15] The client can also be instructed to stop and start the urine flow several times while voiding.

If the client is overweight, a weight-loss program to reduce intra-abdominal pressure may be helpful. Avoiding bladder stimulants such as caffeine or alcohol also decreases episodes of stress incontinence.

Restorative Care

Restorative care focuses on acute elimination problems. Providing assistance and correct positioning on the bedpan, administration of enemas and irrigations, insertion of urinary catheters and rectal tubes, removing fecal impactions, providing incontinence care, and colostomy care all are important aspects of this level of care.

Assisting With Elimination. Clients who require restorative care are often confined to bed and may therefore need to use the bedpan and urinal for elimination. The nurse should provide as much privacy as possible and help the

PROCEDURE 26–4. ASSISTING THE CLIENT WITH THE BEDPAN

PURPOSE: To facilitate elimination in nonambulatory clients.

EQUIPMENT: bedpan, toilet tissue, nonsterile gloves, damp washcloth or antiseptic towelette, and air freshener (optional).

1. Discuss with the client the reason for the procedure, expected client participation, and expected benefits.
   - Client will be more willing to participate and less anxious if there is an opportunity to clarify concerns and the reasons and benefits for the procedure are clear.
2. Close door, pull curtains around bed.
   - Elimination activities are considered private in most cultures. Respecting this need promotes trust and minimizes embarrassment.
3. Don nonsterile latex gloves.
   - Body fluids may contain pathogenic organisms. Gloves prevent skin contamination by direct contact.
4. Raise bed to nurse's waist level, fold top linen so placement of bedpan can be visualized.
   - Prevents nurse backstrain; facilitates correct placement of bedpan.
5. Raise head of bed 30–40°. Ask client to flex knees and raise buttocks off bed.
   - Use of client's muscles facilitates maintenance of muscle tone and strength.
6. Slide bedpan under buttocks so rounded seat is under buttocks. Avoid pressure on sacrum. Pan may be padded with a small towel to protect bony prominences if client is very thin.
   - Correct placement prevents discomfort and skin injury as well as preventing spills.

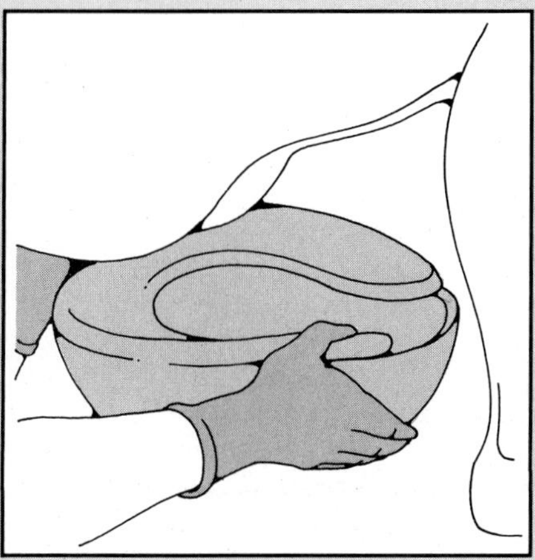

NOTE: If metal bedpan is used, rinse with warm water prior to placing it, to eliminate discomfort from cold bedpan.

(continued)

PROCEDURE 26–4. (continued)

7. If client cannot raise self, assist by placing your hand under client's lower back, with your elbow on the bed. Your arm can then act as a lever to assist in raising buttocks.

7. Leverage produces greater energy output with less effort than lifting directly.

8. If client is very weak or too large to lift, place bedpan by rolling. With bed flat and opposite siderail up, roll client away from you onto side; place pan against buttocks while pushing side of pan toward mattress; roll client onto back while stabilizing pan. Pan position may need slight adjustment. Some nurses prefer to roll client toward them. This is also permissible, but may make stabilizing the pan more difficult as the client rolls. Cornstarch may be used on the pan to promote sliding for repositioning pan.

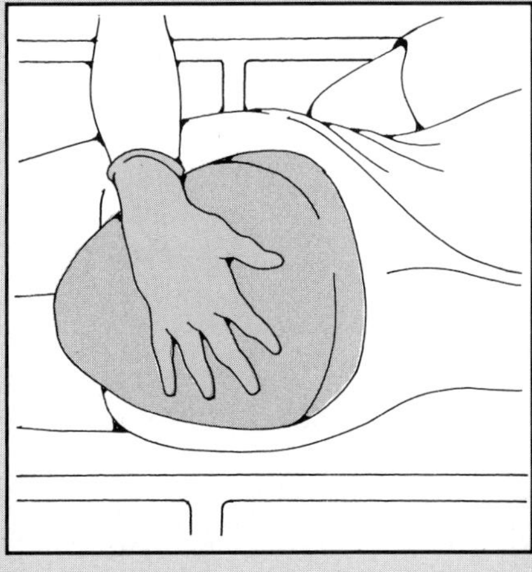

8. Lifting a client unable to assist is likely to cause injury to nurse. Rolling takes less energy and allows one nurse to safely position a large or helpless client.

9. Raise head of bed and knee gatch if not contraindicated. If head of bed cannot be raised, use fracture pan (Fig. 26–16).

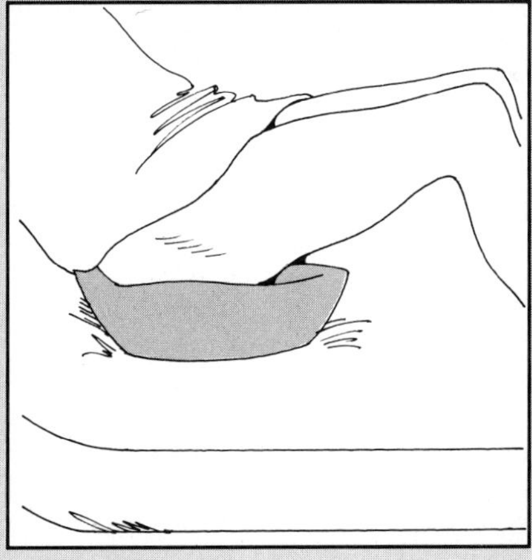

NOTE: Knee gatch should remain flat for clients with vascular stasis, vascular surgery, or hip injury/repair.

9. This position more closely approximates physiological position for defecation.

10. Replace covers, place tissue and call light in reach, and return bed to low position. Leave alert client to complete elimination. If specimen is needed or output is to be measured, provide alternate receptacle for discarding tissue. Remove gloves. Wash hands.

10. See steps 2 and 3 above.

(continued)

PROCEDURE 26–4. (continued)

NOTE: Remain in room or at bedside if there is any question about client's alertness. Do not leave any client on pan for more than 15 min.

11. When client has finished, provide towelette or warm damp washcloth for handwashing.

11. Removes perineal flora from client's hands, promotes comfort.

12. Reglove. Remove bedpan carefully as client raises buttocks. Note whether perineum was cleaned thoroughly by client. (See step 13 if further cleaning is needed.) Take pan to bathroom or dirty utility room to measure contents, obtain specimen, and empty. Some agencies provide bedpan covers—especially recommended if bathroom does not adjoin client's room.

12. See step 2. Contents of pan may easily spill. Immediate removal of contents reduces client embarrassment. Self-cleaning is awkward with bedpan and even alert clients may be unable to accomplish it. (See step 13.)

13. To assist client with perineal cleaning, ask client to roll to side, while you stabilize bedpan. Wrap toilet tissue around your gloved hand several times and wipe perineum from urinary meatus toward anus. Repeat as necessary with new tissue until perineum and anus are free of urine and feces. In some situations, warm soapy water may be needed to thoroughly clean clients after defacation in bedpan.

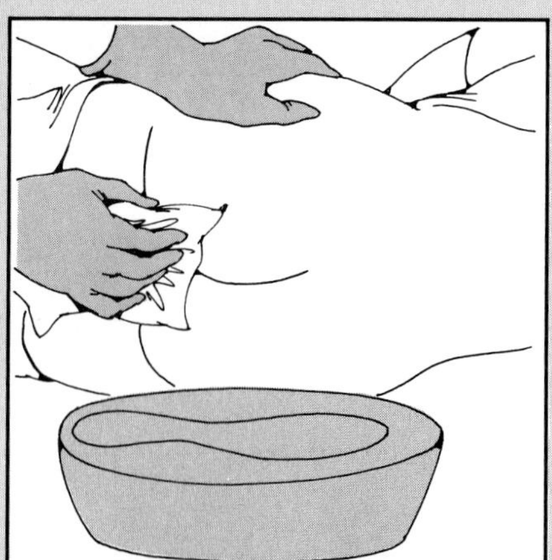

13. Urethral contamination with fecal organisms, which promotes urinary tract infection, is prevented by cleaning in this manner. Thorough cleaning is critical to prevent skin breakdown and odor/discomfort from residual feces or urine.

14. If client needs assistance with positioning and replacement of covers, place bedpan on bedside chair or near foot of bed, remove gloves, and assist. Then obtain new gloves to empty pan.

14. Gloves are contaminated with perineal and/or fecal organisms that would be transferred to other areas unless gloves are removed.

NOTE: Do not place pan on floor, to prevent transfer of bacteria from floor to bedpan, then to client's bed.

(continued)

PROCEDURE 26–4. (continued)

15. Empty bedpan into toilet or hopper and rinse with bedpan flusher. Return to storage. Remove and discard gloves in leak-resistant trash receptacle. Wash hands.	15. Prevents transfer of organisms from urine to environment.

NOTE: Bedpan should not be left on floor of bathroom (see step 14.)

RECORDING: Use of bedpan need not be recorded. If output is being measured, record on I&O record. If a specimen has been obtained and/or tested, record the test and results on appropriate flowsheet.

client position the pan correctly. Clients are often embarrassed and uncomfortable using the bedpan and may try to avoid its use. Some clients risk injury or falls to try to get to the bathroom themselves. It is therefore imperative that the nurse be acutely aware of the client's elimination needs to avoid accidents or falls. When the nurse does not offer the bedpan or urinal frequently to clients who are immobile or confused, accidental soiling of the bed is not unusual.

If the client is unable to position the urinal, the nurse should position it. Place the urinal between the client's legs, with the head of the penis directed into the urinal. It may be necessary for the nurse to hold the urinal in place. For incontinent bedridden male clients, the urinal is sometimes propped in place between the client's legs.

Children who are hospitalized may also need assistance with elimination. Like adults, some children are uncomfortable in strange surroundings and find they have difficulty with urination or bowel elimination. A change in surroundings may cause children to regress in their toilet habits. See the earlier discussion of toilet training under Health Education in the section on Preventive Care.

Two types of bedpans are available: a standard bedpan and a smaller type called a fracture pan. The fracture pan is used for the client who has musculoskeletal disorders that make it difficult or impossible to raise the buttocks off the bed. Figure 26–16 shows both types of bedpans and a urinal. Procedure 26–4 describes helping a client to use a bedpan.

Many clients who are unable to get to the bathroom but can bear weight can use a bedside commode. The bedside commode allows the client to assume a more effective po-

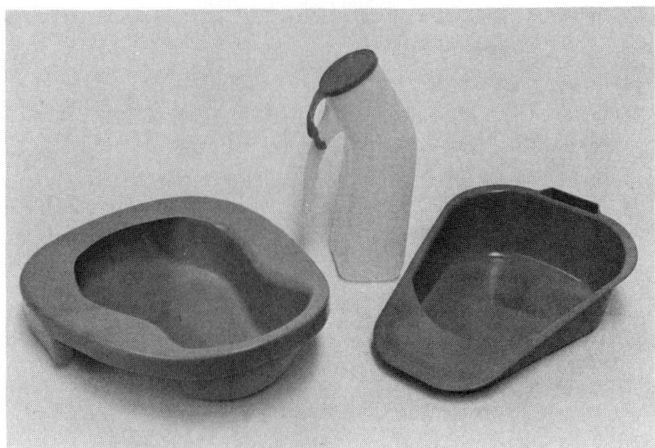

Figure 26–16. Standard bedpan, fracture pan, and urinal. (*From Smith S, Duell D.* Clinical Nursing Skills: Nursing Process Model, Basic to Advanced Skills. *3rd ed. Norwalk, CT: Appleton & Lange; 1992.*)

sition for elimination than a bedpan and usually is easier for nurse and client than placing and removing a bedpan. It can be left in place at the bedside, and many clients can use it without assistance from a nurse.

Administering Medications. Physicians often prescribe medications to aid bowel and urinary elimination. The nurse administers these drugs and checks for side effects in hospitalized clients.

Cathartics and laxatives promote emptying of the bowel and have short-term effects. These medications assist elimination by providing bulk or lubrication, causing chemical irritation, or softening stools. The nurse should teach the client about the potential harmful effects of these drugs. The action of laxatives ranges from harsh to mild, and these drugs affect different people in different manners, therefore the nurse will need to document in detail how these drugs are affecting the client.

Suppositories (bullet-shaped cylinders of medication administered into the rectum) are also used to promote bowel evacuation and require a physician's order. Suppositories are helpful in bowel retraining and generally act within 30 minutes. They may act by softening the stool, distending the rectum, or stimulating rectal mucosa nerve endings. Again, the nurse must be aware of any side effects and the action the suppository drug has on the client. Refer to Chapter 22 for discussion of the technique for administration of suppositories.

Antidiarrheal medications are also prescribed by physicians. These medications alleviate diarrhea by protecting irritated bowel mucosa, absorbing toxic substances and gas, or shrinking inflamed and swollen tissues.

Medications used to promote healthy urinary elimination include diuretics and antimicrobials. Diuretics influence water and electrolyte balance. They have a wide variety of mechanisms of action and frequently affect other body functions, such as blood pressure. Careful monitoring for effectiveness and side effects is critical. Antimicrobials are used to treat urinary tract infections. Usually the drug of choice is determined by the organism causing the infection. These drugs also produce side effects that should be monitored.

Administering Enemas. Enemas are used to remove feces and flatus and must be prescribed by a physician. The **enema** consists of a solution that is instilled into the rectum and sigmoid colon for the purpose of stimulating peristalsis and causing defecation to occur. Besides relief of constipation, enemas are used for:

1. Removal of impacted feces.
2. Bowel preparation for x-rays, endoscopic examinations, and surgical procedures.
3. Clearing the bowel so that a bowel training program can begin (see Table 26–10 and Procedure 26–5).

Enema equipment is available in disposable prepackaged units, some of which may be reused for the same client (Fig. 26–17). Some institutions use stainless steel enema cans, which are not disposable.

When the enema order states "Enemas until clear," the nurse repeats the enema until the client passes only fluid containing no fecal material. The fluid may be yellow-brown in color. Usually only three consecutive enemas are given. If the return still contains particles of feces after three enemas, notify the physician and request further directions, as repeated enemas can cause serious fluid and electrolyte depletion. If a client cannot control the external rectal sphincter, the nurse can administer the enema with the client positioned on the bedpan. Administering enemas with the client seated on the toilet is not effective because the solution does not enter enough of the rectal and colon area, and insertion of tubing when the client is seated can injure the rectal wall.

Because enema administration may be embarrassing to clients, nurses should provide for privacy by draping them. If the client uses the bathroom after the enema has been administered, instruct the client not to flush the toilet so that the enema results can be assessed and documented.

Relieving Flatus. The Harris flush, or colonic irrigation, is similar to an enema except that the fluid is repetitively instilled and withdrawn from the rectum. This procedure will trap accumulated gas in the fluids as it is instilled. The gas is then carried out with fluid as it is siphoned out when the bag is lowered. Refer to Procedure 26–6.

Another procedure to help expel flatus is the insertion of a rectal tube. To insert a rectal tube, provide privacy, position the client, and don unsterile gloves. Lubricate a rectal tube of appropriate size (22-24 French for adults, 12-18 French for children), separate the client's buttocks to visualize the anal opening, and gently insert the tube 4 to 6 inches toward the umbilicus. If hemorrhoids are present, especially cautious insertion is indicated. Enclose the open end of the tube in an absorbent pad or attach to a drainage receptacle such as a plastic bag. Remove the rectal tube after 20 to 30 minutes and document the client's response.

Caring for Fecal Impaction. When enemas and laxatives fail to promote the complete evacuation of fecal material, digital removal of impacted stool is the next alternative. Agency policies may specify the level of health care personnel permitted to remove stool digitally, and a physician's order may be required. Assist the client to a side-lying position, screen for privacy, and don clean gloves, lubricating the index finger. Slowly insert the lubricated finger and gently break up the fecal mass. Pull out small bits of fecal material with the curved index finger.

This procedure is usually uncomfortable for the client and can create irritation and bleeding. Observe the client for signs of fatigue, pallor, or change in pulse rate, and stop the procedure if these occur. Digital stimulation can induce the urge to defecate and the nurse may need to assist the client onto a bedpan or commode. Follow-up measures such as enemas or suppositories may be used for a few days after removal of the impaction to facilitate restoration of the usual defecation pattern.

TABLE 26–10. TYPES OF ENEMAS

Type of Enema	Mode of Action	Undesired Effects	Nursing Responsibilities
Cleansing			
1. Tap water enema (500–1000 mL) *Note:* Administer no more than three consecutive enemas without consulting physician. "Clear" does not mean without color. Infants and children should not be given tap water enemas because they are at risk for fluid and electrolyte imbalance.	Volume of fluid distends bowel and stimulates peristalsis.	Sodium deficit. Potassium deficit resulting from osmotic transfer of Na and K from cells lining the bowel to the water (hypotonic solution) in the bowel.	Observe client for symptoms of hyponatremia, hypokalemia, water intoxication, particularly when giving multiple enemas. *Hyponatremia* evidenced by decreased blood pressure, lethargy, stomach cramps. *Hypokalemia* evidenced by generalized muscle weakness, cardiac arrhythmias, shallow respirations. *Water intoxication* evidenced by: nausea and vomiting, tachycardia, increased blood pressure, headache, dizziness, confusion.
2. Normal saline (500–1000 mL) Infant (150–250 mL) Toddler (250–350 mL) Child (300–500 mL)	Same as above isotonic solution, so minimal disruption of fluid and electrolyte balance.	Minimal.	
Irritant 1. Bisacodyl or Fleet: (prepackaged 30 mL) 2. Soap solution (500–1000 mL: 5 mL mild soap to 100 mL water)	Hypermotility of the bowel is created by irritating the bowel mucosa. The contact laxative acts directly on the mucosa of colon by stimulating sensory nerve endings to produce peristalsis and evacuation.	Persistent mucosal irritation, can last for 3 weeks.	For soap solutions, put water in bag first to prevent soap from foaming; mix gently.
Hypertonic 1. Magnesium sulfate (Epsom salts)	Water is drawn into the bowel from the extracellular fluid. The bowel becomes distended and produces mechanical stimulation, leading to evacuation of large amounts of fluid and bowel contents.	Magnesium excess. Fluid volume deficit, caused by the hypertonic solution drawing water from interstitial spaces, especially in children and other susceptible persons.	Observe for symptoms of hypermagnesemia: flushing, hypotension, bradycardia, depressed deep tendon reflexes.
2. Sodium biphosphate and sodium phosphate (prepackaged 118 mL)	Same as above.	Increased sodium absorption: Should be avoided for client requiring sodium restriction, or with impaired renal function. Hyperphosphatemia and hypocalcemia.	Observe for symptoms of hypernatremia, such as red flushed skin, dry sticky mucous membranes, thirst, decreased urine production.
Lubricating Oil retention enema (mineral oil, prepackaged 133 mL)	Softens and lubricates hard stool without irritating mucosa of colon. Stimulates normal bowel movement, as only rectum, sigmoid, and part of the descending colon are evacuated.		Instruct client that holding the enema for 30 minutes to 1 hour will increase its effectiveness.
Carminative 1. 1-2-3 (30 g magnesium sulfate: 60 mL glycerine: 90 mL water) 2. Milk and molasses (equal parts of 80–100 mL) 3. Mayo (240 mL water: 60 mL sugar: 30 mL sodium bicarbonate)	Carminative enema solutions release gas, distend rectum and colon, and stimulate peristalsis.		

Adapted from Asheervath J., Blevins DR. Handbook of Clinical Nursing Practice. *Norwalk, CT: Appleton-Century-Crofts; 1986; 258–259.*

PROCEDURE 26–5. ADMINISTERING A CLEANSING ENEMA

PURPOSE: To empty the lower bowel in clients who are constipated, are being prepared for surgery or diagnostic studies, or who need bowel training.

EQUIPMENT: Enema setup including bag or can with attached rectal tube and clamp, water-soluble lubricant, and waterproof underpad; ordered solution; nonsterile gloves; and bath blanket (optional). If client cannot ambulate: bedpan or commode, toilet tissue, and damp washcloth or towelette. Prepackaged enema solutions may also be used as ordered (see end of Procedure).

ACTION	RATIONALE
1. Check physician's order.	1. Medical order is required for instillation of solutions into the rectum.
2. Discuss with the client the reason for the procedure, expected client participation, usual sensations and expected benefits.	2. Client will be more willing to participate and less anxious if there is an opportunity to clarify concerns and the reasons and benefits for the procedure are clear.
3. Clamp tubing. Prepare solution as ordered in enema container. Usual amount prepared is 1500 mL. 500–1500 mL may be administered (250–500 mL for children). See Table 26–10 for common additives in cleansing enemas.	3. Greater volumes may overdistend the bowel causing cramping pain.
4. If tap water is used to make solution, use water from the tap that feels warm (*not hot*) to the inner aspect of the wrist (105–110F). Small-volume commercial solutions are used at room temperature.	4. Warm water stimulates peristalsis, hot water will burn bowel mucosa, although client will not feel burning because bowel has no temperature-sensitive nerves.
5. Expel air from tubing by allowing solution to flow to tip. Reclamp.	5. Air may cause cramping if introduced into the bowel.
6. Identify client.	6. Administering an enema to the wrong client is considered a medication error. Serious harm to the client could result.

(continued)

PROCEDURE 26–5. (continued)

7. Close door and pull curtains around bed.

7. Elimination activities are considered private in most cultures. Respecting this need promotes trust and minimizes embarrassment.

8. Raise bed to nurse's waist height.

8. Prevents backstrain and fatigue from bending to bed in low position.

9. Ask/assist client to assume left lateral position.

NOTE: Position is not critical and may be altered for comfort to dorsal recumbent or right side.

9. Allows gravity to facilitate the flow of fluid along the curve of the sigmoid colon, and retention of fluid if sphincter is weak.

10. Arrange bed covers or bath blanket so only client's buttocks are exposed.

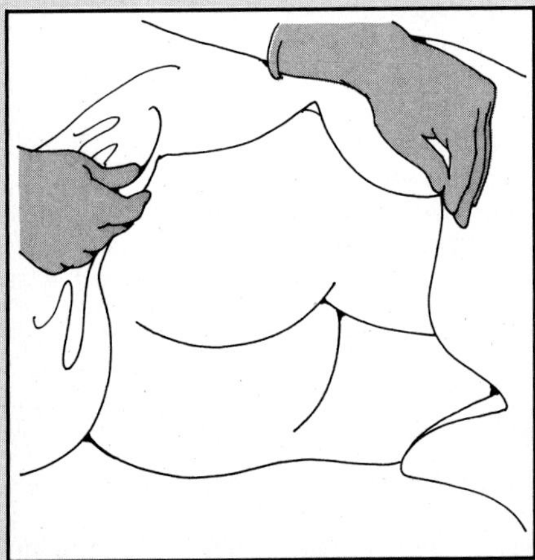

10. Unnecessary exposure is demeaning and may chill client.

11. Don nonsterile gloves.

11. Gloves are a barrier preventing contact with fecal material, which may contain pathogens.

12. If client is not ambulatory, place bedpan on bed or bedside commode next to bed. Some ambulatory clients may also prefer to have a pan or commode near. Clients with very poor sphincter control may be placed on bedpan to give enema.

12. Relieves anxiety about soiling the bed if enema cannot be retained.

13. Place waterproof pad under buttocks.

13. Protects bed linens from leakage that may occur while client is retaining enema.

(continued)

PROCEDURE 26–5. (continued)

14. Lubricate distal 8–10 cm (3–4 in) of tube. Lubricate 2–5 cm (1–2 in) for a child.

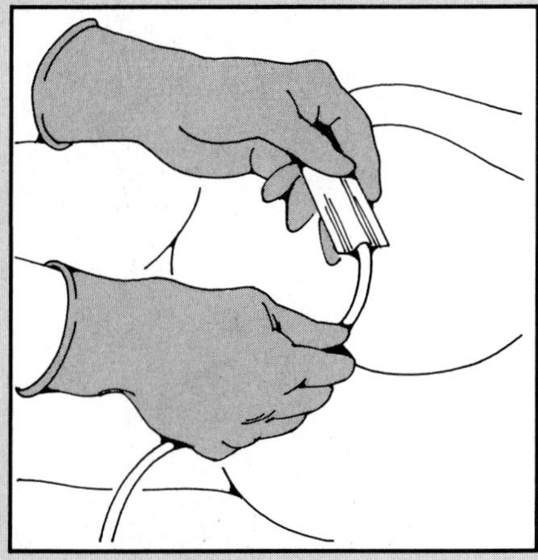

14. Reduces friction between tube and rectal mucosa. Friction damages tissue.

15. Lift the client's buttock to expose the anus. Ask client to take a deep breath and exhale slowly through the mouth while relaxing gluteal and sphincter muscles. Tell client you will introduce tube during exhalation.

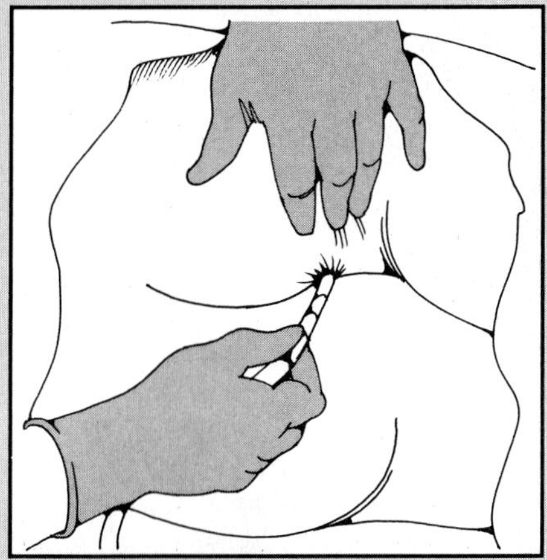

15. Breathing facilitates relaxation, thereby reducing discomfort from insertion of the tube. If client is alerted when tube will be inserted, reflex contraction of sphincter can be inhibited.

16. Slowly insert the tube into the rectum toward the umbilicus, advance about 3–4 inches (1–2 in for children).

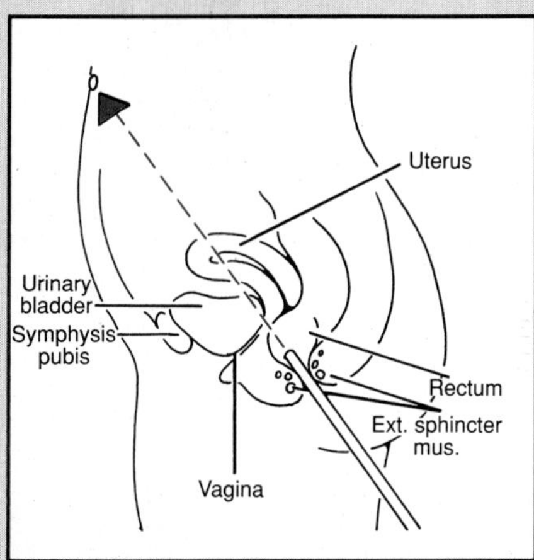

16. Follows the contour of rectum, minimizing risk of bowel perforation or abrasion, and locates tip of the tube above internal sphincter so enema can be retained.

(continued)

PROCEDURE 26–5. (continued)

NOTE: If hemorrhoids are noted, extra gentleness is necessary to reduce discomfort.

17. If tube meets resistance during insertion, recheck insertion direction. If correct, allow a small amount of fluid to flow while attempting to advance the tube. If resistance persists, assess for impaction. Do not force tube.

17. If insertion direction is correct, resistance is most likely caused by fecal material. Flow of liquid may allow tube to bypass feces.

18. Hold the tube in place, open the clamp and raise the container 30–45 cm (12–18 in) above the rectum. Container may be hung on IV pole adjusted to correct height.

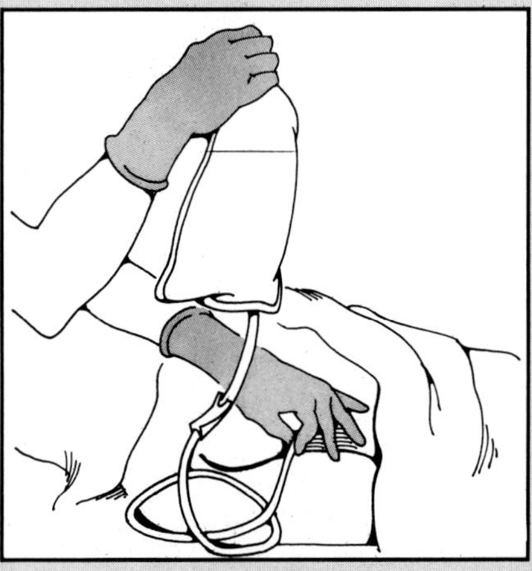

18. This height will introduce the fluid slowly so rapid distension and cramping are prevented.

19. If client complains of cramping, an urgent need to defecate, or if fluid flows out around the tube, lower container slightly or partially close clamp. If these actions do not correct situation, stop fluid flow.

19. These indicate distension of bowel was too rapid. Lowering container or constricting tube will slow flow and decrease this effect.

20. When cramping passes, continue to administer fluid until client complains of fullness or all solution has infused. Then clamp tubing and remove tube.

NOTE: Clients with poor sphincter control cannot retain large amounts of solution.

20. Attempting to administer more fluid than the client can tolerate will cause premature expulsion.

(continued)

PROCEDURE 26–5. (continued)

21. Tell the client that retaining the fluid for 5–10 min will increase the effectiveness of the enema, because the longer the solution is retained the stronger the resulting peristalsis.

NOTE: Holding a folded tissue firmly against the anus will assist the client to retain the enema.

21. Client is more likely to accept moderate discomfort if a clear benefit will result.

22. When client has a strong urge to defecate, assist as needed to bathroom, commode, or bedpan. Provide tissue and call light, then leave client to complete expulsion.

NOTE: Assess client for weakness and dizziness before leaving. Stay with client showing these symptoms.

22. Elimination activities are considered private in most cultures. Respecting this need promotes trust and minimizes embarrassment.

23. When client has expelled enema, assess amount and character of output.

NOTE: Rarely enema cannot be expelled and must be siphoned. Reposition client, reinsert lubricated tube. Introduce about 50 mL of fluid, then lower container below rectum, so negative pressure pulls fluid into container. Repeat until all fluid is returned.

23. Evaluation of effectiveness of procedure is necessary to determine the need for further treatment.

24. Assist as needed with hygiene, clean bedpan or commode, and discard enema supplies in leak-resistant trash receptacle. Remove gloves by pulling them off inside out and discard similarly. Wash hands.

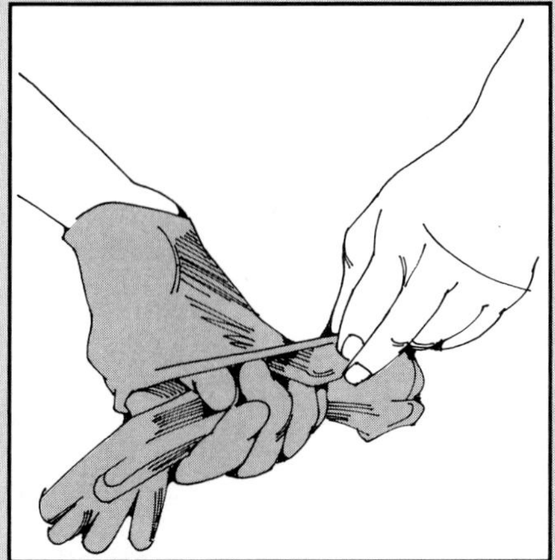

NOTE: If a series of enemas is needed, equipment may be reused, but should be disposed of correctly when series is complete.

24. These activities prevent transfer of fecal organisms to environment.

(continued)

PROCEDURE 26–5. (continued)

25. Assist as needed with repositioning in bed. Replace any soiled or damp linen.

25. Promotes comfort and well-being. Enemas are exhausting for most clients.

Prepackaged Enemas

1. Prepare the client as in steps 1 and 2, and 6–15, above.

See steps 1–15, above.

2. Remove cap and insert prelubricated tip into rectum toward umbilicus.

2P. Follows the contour of rectum, minimizing risk of bowel perforation or abrasion, and locates tip of tube above internal sphincter so enema can be retained.

3. Roll container (as with a tube of toothpaste) to expel all of the contents into the rectum.

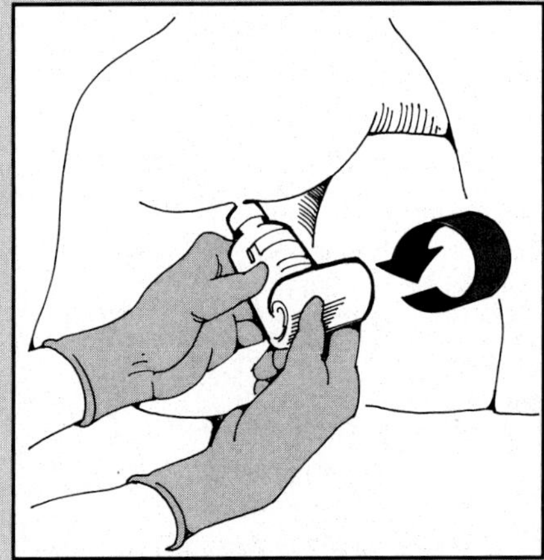

3P. Prepackaged enemas usually contain 200 mL or less. Because most of them are hypertonic, only small amounts are needed to stimulate defecation (see also Table 26–10).

NOTE: Some clients are able and prefer to self-administer this type of enema.

4. Continue with steps 21–25, above.

4P. See steps 21–25 above.

RECORDING: Note type of enema and results: amount, color, consistency, any abnormal constituents of return; state of abdomen (soft, distended); client response and condition of client after procedure.

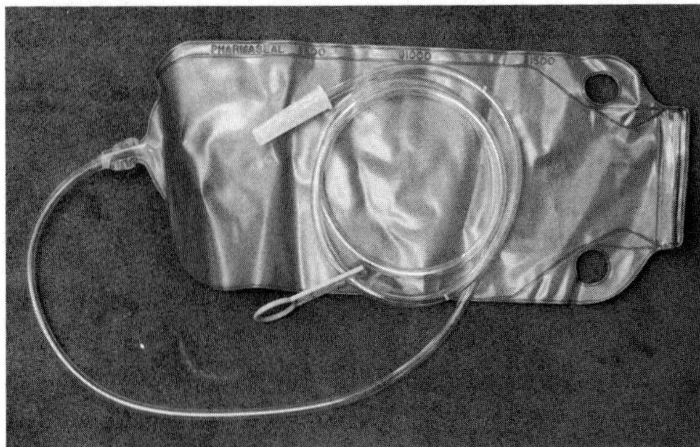

A

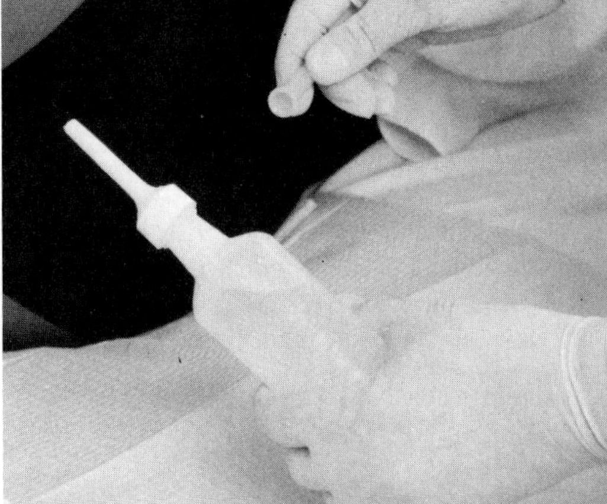

B

Figure 26–17. A. Disposable enema set. **B.** Prepackaged enema. (*From Smith S, Duell D.* Clinical Nursing Skills: Nursing Process Model, Basic to Advanced Skills. *3rd ed. Norwalk, CT: Appleton & Lange; 1992.*)

Assisting Clients Who are Incontinent of Feces. As discussed in the nursing diagnosis section above, most causes of fecal incontinence are not treatable by nurses. Offering a bedpan or assisting the client to toilet facilities within 20 to 30 minutes after breakfast, when the gastrocolic reflex is most active, may prevent accidental soiling. However, timing of bowel evacuation is difficult to predict in incontinent clients who do not eat regular meals or who are receiving liquid nutrient formulas. Fecal incontinence collectors are used in some health care facilities to alleviate soiling and prevent associated skin irritation. Figure 26–18 illustrates one type of collector; application and emptying of fecal in-

PROCEDURE 26–6. PERFORMING COLONIC IRRIGATION (HARRIS FLUSH)

▭ **PURPOSE:** To relieve and expel flatus and to stimulate peristalsis.

▭ **EQUIPMENT:** Disposable enema set (Fig. 26–19): container, tube with clamp, lubricant, waterproof underpad; nonsterile gloves; bath blanket (optional); and bedpan or commode for nonambulatory client.

ACTION

1. Discuss the procedure with the client, then prepare client and solution, as in steps 1–18 of Procedure 26–5, except prepare only 500 mL of solution.
2. Administer 100–200 mL of solution, then lower container below the level of the rectum to siphon solution into container.
3. Repeat inflow-outflow, observing for bubbles in solution, indicating gas is being trapped in the liquid and removed from colon. Continue until client reports relief of distension or until no more bubbles are seen in return.
4. If fecal matter is returned into bag and blocks the flow of fluid, discard return in toilet, rinse enema set, and prepare new solution.
5. If client feels an urge to defecate, remove tubing and provide assistance to bathroom, commode, or bedpan.
6. When irrigation is complete, discard returns in toilet, dispose of equipment (including gloves) in leak-resistant trash container. Wash hands. Enema kit may be reused for same client if procedure is repeated within 24 hours. Clean thoroughly and hang to dry in client's bathroom.
7. If client requires assistance with perineal hygiene, provide assistance before discarding gloves.

▭ **RECORDING:** Note procedure and results, including relief of abdominal distension, client response, and general condition after irrigation.

continence collectors are detailed in Procedure 26–7.

Routine Colostomy Care. Ostomy care requires that the nurse be knowledgeable about each type of ostomy, as discussed in Section 1 of this chapter (Table 26–2). Assessment of the stoma and surrounding area, as discussed under abdominal inspection, is essential to maintaining stomal integrity. Early recognition of potential problems assures prompt treatment.

Client collaboration in ostomy care helps the client ad-

PROCEDURE 26–7. APPLYING AND EMPTYING A FECAL INCONTINENCE COLLECTOR

PURPOSE: Used to collect feces with clients having no anal sphincter control, thereby preventing excoriation of skin and soiling of bed.

EQUIPMENT: Fecal incontinence collector, blunt-tip scissors, mild skin cleanser, water, washcloth and towel, waterproof underpad, nonsterile gloves, and spray adhesive or porous tape (optional). Drainage bag and tubing optional for liquid stool. Bedpan or graduate to empty collector.

ACTION

1. Discuss procedure, including purpose and benefits. Explain procedure, even if client appears unresponsive.
2. Screen client, raise bed to nurse's waist level, assist client to lateral or Sims' position. Arrange covers so only buttocks are exposed.
3. Don gloves, place underpad beneath client's buttocks. Thoroughly wash and dry perineal and anal area. Trim hair around anal opening so none will be under adhesive portion of collector.
4. Following manufacturer's directions, prepare collector to fit client. It may be necessary to cut a larger opening in the collector. Some brands may require use of skin prep or additional adhesive to improve adherence of device.
5. Fold adhesive portion in half to facilitate correct positioning on client, then remove paper backing to expose adhesive barrier.

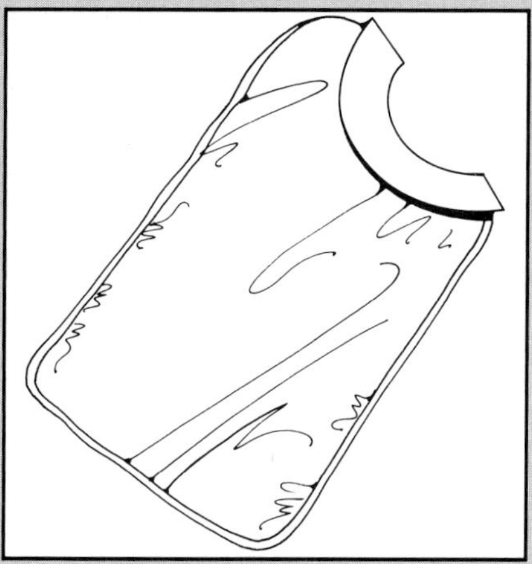

6. Lift client's buttock to expose anus. Press narrowest part of barrier between the anus and scrotum or vaginal opening, opposite end against coccygeal area. Release buttock and press sides of barrier so collector adheres to perianal skin without creating pressure or pulling of tissue.

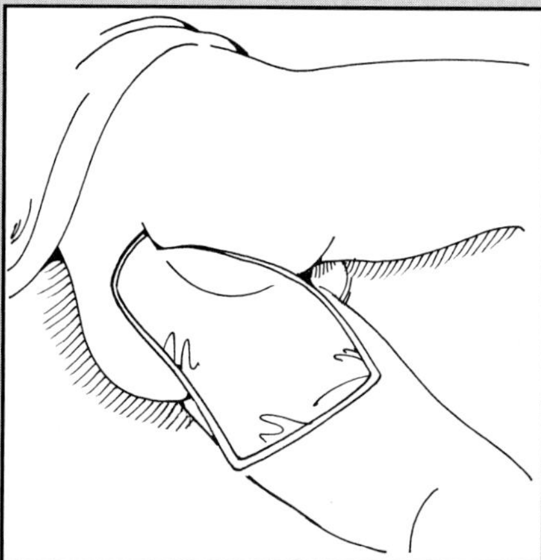

7. Check to see that drainage cap is securely closed. If client has frequent liquid stools, cap may be replaced with drainage tubing and collection bag similar to that used with indwelling catheters. For solid stools, drain may be cut off and bag sealed with pouch clamp (see Procedure 26–8).
8. Remove gloves and position client comfortably. Wash hands. Check collector several times each shift or whenever client is turned and repositioned. Empty frequently to prevent skin irritation, diminish odors, and prolong adhesive contact.
9. To empty collector: don gloves; with client sidelying, open drainage cap and squeeze contents into bedpan or large graduate. Discard gloves. Wash hands.
10. Replace collector whenever seal to skin is broken. Remove carefully and discard as with body wastes.

RECORDING: Note that collector is in use, and describe condition of perianal skin and amount and character of output.

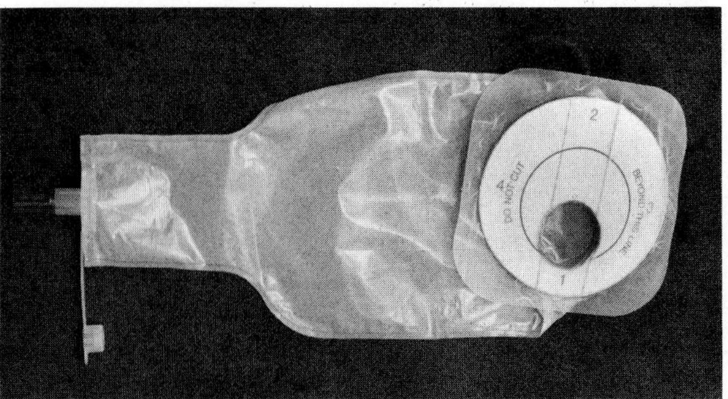

Figure 26–18. Fecal incontinence collector.

just to changes in defecation patterns, body image, and life-style. The nurse's attitude and knowledge can be an essential component in helping the client adapt. In addition, the expertise of a specialist in this field, the enterostomal therapist, should be used if available (Fig. 26–19). Procedures for changing and fitting ostomy appliances are not addressed in this text, but are included in most textbooks of medical-surgical nursing and nursing procedure books.

A great many products for ostomy care are on the market. Several examples are shown in Figure 26–20. These include skin care products, appliances to fit over the stoma, and special irrigating sets. The stoma therapist will know what a particular client needs and what is available. Selection of the appropriate appliances helps the client to become physically and socially active.[16] Appliances may be either disposable or reusable. Appliances used in hospitals tend to be disposable, whereas clients who have had a colostomy for some time usually use reusable appliances. Temporary appliances are made of transparent plastic with a peel-off adhesive square around the opening. This opening can usually be cut to fit closely around the stoma to prevent leakage and skin irritation. Disposable pouches should be drainable so they can be emptied without being removed (see Procedure 26–8).

Odor control, very important to the client, can be ensured by using the most appropriate type of appliance, emptying it frequently, and cleaning it well before reapplying. Some clients use special odor-absorbing products inside their ostomy appliance.

A colostomy irrigation distends the bowel and stimulates peristalsis, thereby causing bowel evacuation to occur via the stoma. Not all types of colostomies require routine irrigation. Descending and sigmoid colostomies are commonly irrigated, while ileostomies and ascending colostomies are not irrigated because feces are liquid and drain from the stoma continuously.

Daily irrigations can sometimes control the time of elimination. Therefore, irrigation should be done at the same time each day. Clients need to select a time for the irrigation that will allow this activity to fit into their schedule. Colostomy irrigation is detailed in Procedure 26–9. Since colostomy irrigation can take up to an hour to complete, clients often decide to control elimination by a rigid dietary regimen instead. Even with the use of irrigations, however, dietary factors are important. Laxative foods should be avoided as they may cause unexpected evacuation; gas-forming foods should also be avoided.

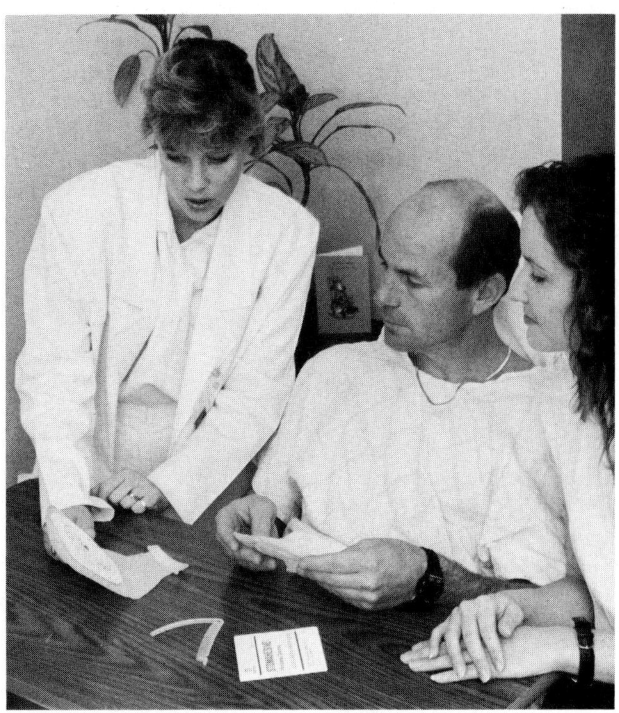

Figure 26–19. Enterostomal therapist with client and support person.

Inserting a Urinary Catheter. Urinary catheterization is the passage of a tube into the bladder through the urethra. Catheterization may be done for the diagnosis, treatment, or prevention of problems associated with the urinary tract. Some diagnostic reasons for insertion of a catheter include monitoring urine output and obtaining specimens. Catheterization can also be used to treat such problems as urinary obstruction or retention associated with surgery, medications, or childbirth. Catheters are often inserted before procedures that may result in urinary complications.

The purpose of the procedure determines the type of catheterization. A straight catheterization (intermittent) is often done for diagnostic purposes, such as measuring residual urine (the urine left in the bladder after voiding) or obtaining a sterile urine specimen. This type of catheterization may also be used in cases of simple postoperative retention. Some clients use intermittent self-catheterization as part of a bladder training program (see the section on bladder training later in this chapter).

When a catheterization is performed before surgery or for a urinary obstruction, such as benign prostatic hypertrophy, the catheter is left in place for hours or days. This

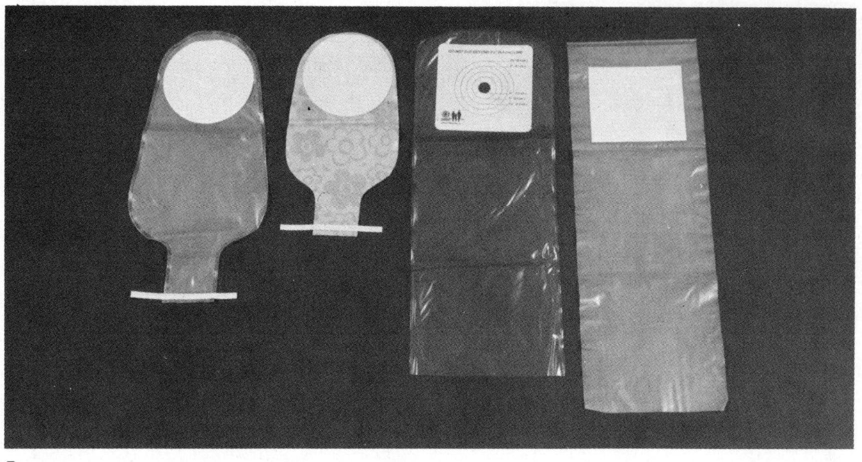

A

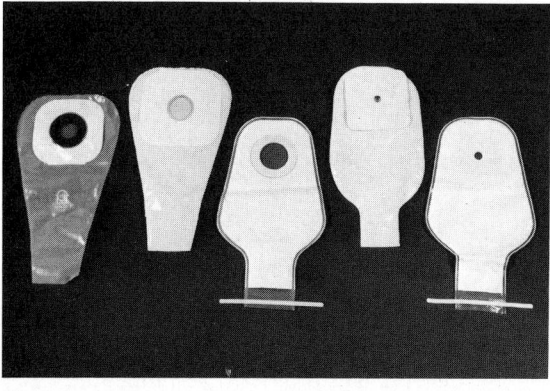

B

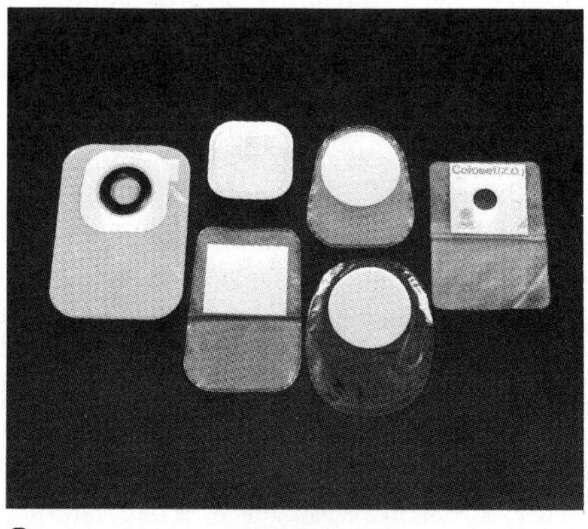

C

Figure 26–20. Examples of colostomy and ileostomy appliances. **A.** Styles of ileostomy pouches. **B.** Open-ended or drainable pouches for colostomies. **C.** Nondrainable pouches for colostomies. (*From Smith S, Duell D.* Clinical Nursing Skills: Nursing Process Model, Basic to Advanced Skills. *3rd ed. Norwalk, CT: Appleton & Lange; 1992.*)

is called an indwelling (or retention) catheter (sometimes the term Foley catheter is used). An indwelling catheter has a small inflatable balloon near the tip to hold it in place inside the bladder. Figure 26–21 shows the balloon both inflated and deflated. The balloon is deflated for insertion and removal of the catheter.

The steps for catheterization are essentially the same for both intermittent and indwelling catheters. The technique for inserting a catheter is described in Procedure 26–10. Figure 26–22 shows a complete kit for indwelling catheter insertion.

The purpose of the catheterization, the length of time the catheter will be in place, and the client's urinary tract anatomy determine the size and type of catheter to use. The most common catheters are straight or retention catheters in sizes 14-18 French gauge for adults and sizes 8-14 French gauge for children. Figure 26–23 shows catheters from 10 French to 18 French.

As with any procedure, catheterization carries risks. Therefore, it should be done only when it is in the client's best interest. If bladder control is an issue, it is better to use other methods first to promote bladder function. Complications of catheterization include urinary tract infection, mucosal trauma, and hydronephrosis (collection of urine in the renal pelvis). Urinary tract infections are a major concern. These infections account for 40 percent of all nosocomial infections.

Caring for the Client With an Indwelling Catheter. The care of the client with an indwelling catheter is a nursing responsibility. Monitoring for problems and preventing complications are the nurse's main roles. Positioning the catheter, maintaining sterility, obtaining specimens, monitoring urinary output, client teaching are some of the approaches nurses uses with catheterized clients.

Handwashing prior to and after contact with any part of the catheter is mandatory. Research has shown that personnel who fail to wash their hands between manipulating

PROCEDURE 26–8. EMPTYING AN OSTOMY POUCH

☐ **PURPOSE:** To remove fecal drainage, promote stoma and skin integrity, and reduce odor.

☐ **EQUIPMENT:** Nonsterile gloves, waterproof underpad, damp cloth, and bedpan or large graduate.

ACTION

1. Discuss procedure with client regarding needs for assistance, teaching, and scheduling of procedure. Pouches should be emptied when ⅓ to ½ full of drainage or when full of gas to prevent breaking seal on pouch due to increased weight of contents. When ostomy is fresh, disposable pouches are usually used. They are not removed until adhesive fails, as frequent removal damages underlying skin. Eventually most clients select reusable pouches. Some clients are able to empty ostomy pouches without assistance; others, especially if ostomy is a new one, will require teaching and support. Ultimately self-care of an ostomy is desirable. The enterostomal therapist is a resource for clients and nurses in selection of equipment and care of the stoma.
2. Screen client, and adjust bed to nurse's waist height and to semi-Fowler's position. Adjust covers so bag is exposed.
3. Don gloves. Place waterproof pad under pouch so client's body and bed linens are protected from spills.
4. Place bedpan or graduate on bed so clamped end of pouch extends over it. Holding pouch so clamped end is higher than stoma, open pouch clamp (sometimes rubber band may be used to close pouch).

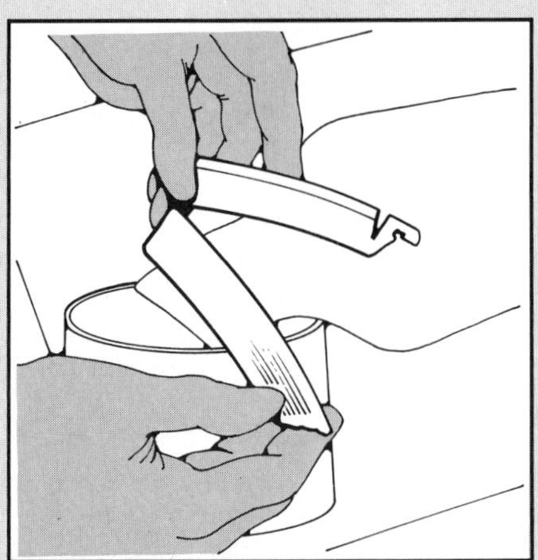

5. Unroll pouch end, and then fold back to make a cuff. This will prevent end from contacting fecal drainage, making cleaning end unnecessary before resealing bag. Drain pouch into collection container, flattening so all drainage is removed. Note character and amount of drainage.

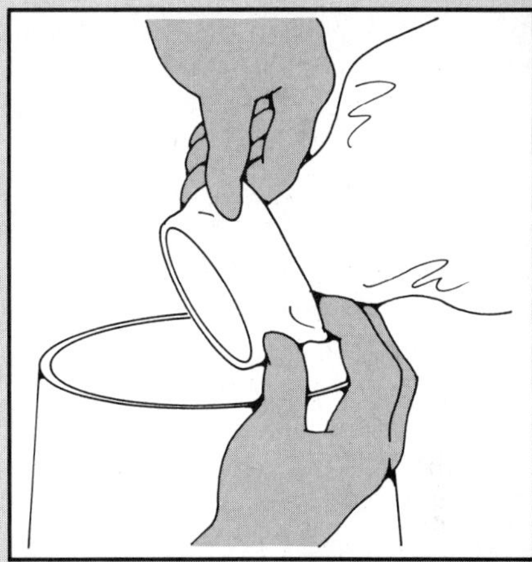

6. Raise pouch above level of stoma, unfold cuff, and then reroll end and apply clamp. Rinsing disposable pouches after emptying is usually unnecessary, but may be done by pouring water from a paper cup into the distal (draining) end. Some clients may desire that a pouch deodorant be placed in the pouch prior to closing it.

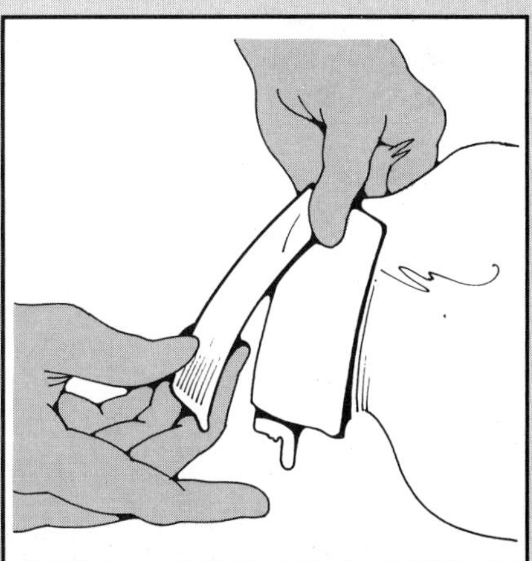

7. Discard drainage in toilet. Remove gloves by turning inside-out and discard in leak-resistant trash receptacle. Wash hands.

☐ **RECORDING:** Note character and amount of drainage, condition of stoma (may not be observable if bag is opaque), nature of teaching, and client response.

PROCEDURE 26–9. IRRIGATING A COLOSTOMY

▭ **PURPOSE:** To regulate time of colon elimination, prevent unexpected evacuation or leakage, or cleanse colon in preparation for visualization or surgery.

▭ **EQUIPMENT:** Colostomy irrigation set including irrigation bag with tubing, cone, clamp, and irrigation sleeve; prescribed irrigant; lubricant; nonsterile gloves, IV pole or wall hook to suspend bag; bath blanket; and bedpan and waterproof pad if client is to remain in bed.

ACTION

1. Discuss procedure with client, including timing and amount of assistance required. Optimal time is within 1 hour after a meal. Consultation with an enterostomal therapist may also be necessary to determine if modifications of equipment or procedure are necessary. Clients with long-standing colostomies usually manage irrigation independently.
2. If assistance is needed, prepare client and solution as for enema (see Procedure 26–5, steps 1–8, and 12). Client should be in semi-Fowler's position if irrigation is to be done in bed. Most clients prefer to do irrigation while seated on the toilet.
3. Arrange bed covers and gown to expose stoma. Place waterproof pad to protect bottom sheet. Clients seated on toilet may desire blanket to cover knees. Hang irrigating container so bottom is level with seated client's shoulder (12–18 in above stoma).
4. Don gloves. Remove and empty ostomy appliance, if necessary. Many clients who irrigate their colostomies to regulate elimination need only a gauze pad to cover the stoma between irrigations. Place drainage sleeve over stoma, secure around waist with belt. Karaya washer may be used around stoma to minimize leaking during procedure. Distal end of sleeve should extend between client's legs into toilet or into bedpan if client is in bed.

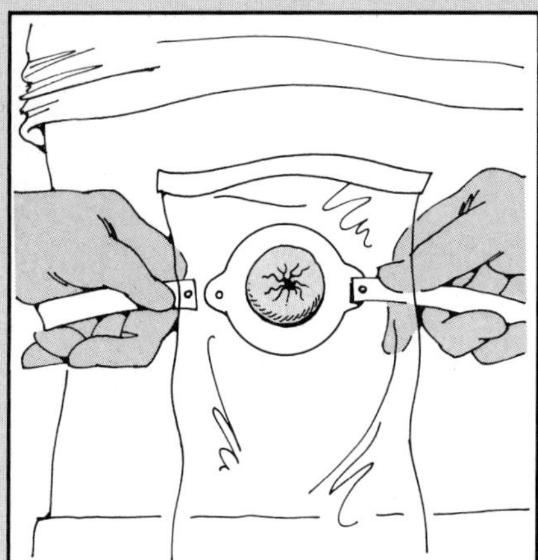

5. Lubricate end of tubing and cone. Insert both through opening at top of sleeve, and then into stoma, using rotating motion. Tubing should be carefully advanced 2–3 inches into bowel. Do not force tubing or colon perforation or abrasion could occur.

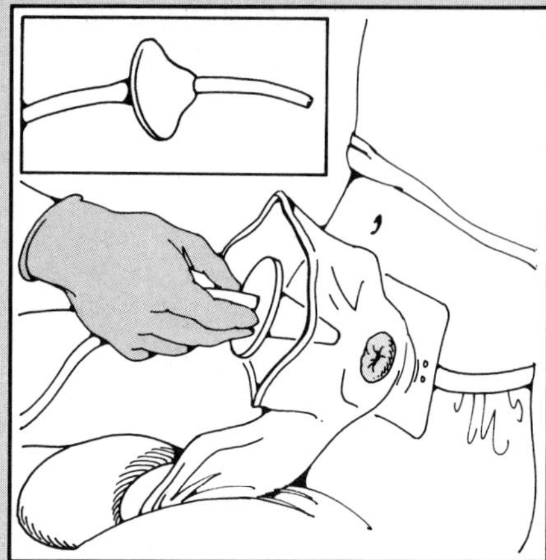

6. Open clamp to allow fluid to enter bowel using same precautions as with enema (Procedure 26–5, steps 19 and 20). Maintain pressure on cone or stoma to prevent backflow out of stoma.

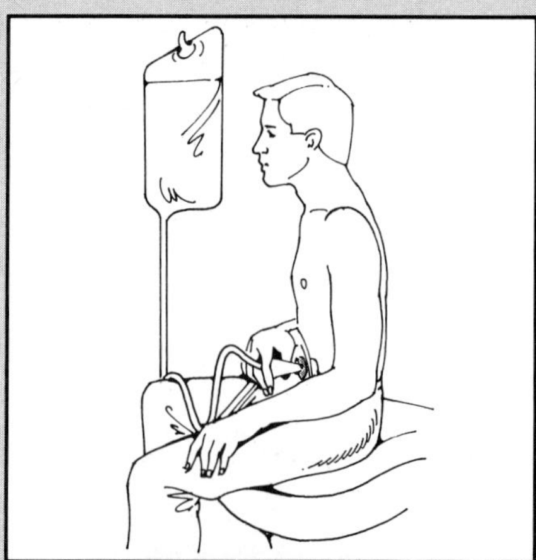

7. When fluid has been instilled, remove cone and catheter (some prefer to keep cone in place 5–10 min). When cone is removed, fluid and feces will flow into toilet or bedpan via sleeve in intermittent bursts.

(continued)

PROCEDURE 26–9. (continued)

8. After 15 min, or when flow of fluid ceases, clean bottom of sleeve, fold to waist, and secure with clamp. Remove and discard gloves in leak-resistant trash container. Wash hands. Encourage ambulatory client to move about for 20–30 min to facilitate elimination of any remaining feces and liquid.

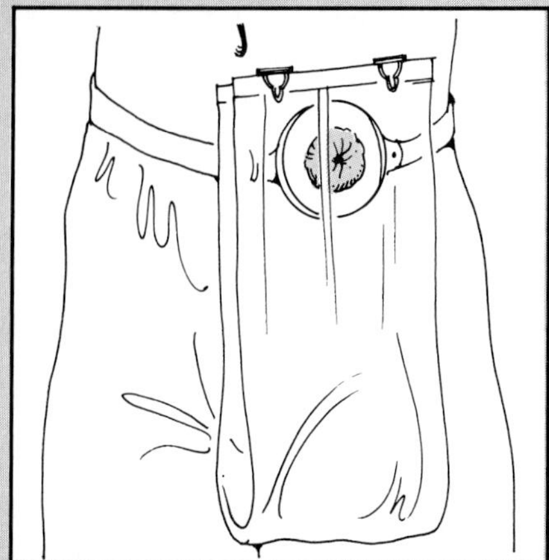

9. When evacuation is complete, reglove, and rinse sleeve with cool water from irrigation container while client is seated on toilet or bedpan. Cleanser such as Peri-Wash can also be used. Then remove sleeve, store for future use, clean around stoma, dry well, and replace appliance or gauze pad. Remove and discard gloves as above. Wash hands.

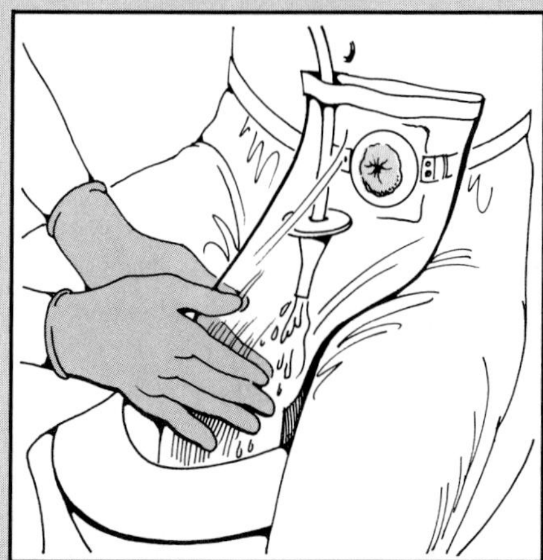

☐ **RECORDING:** Note time of procedure, volume instilled, nature of return, client response. Describe condition of stoma and peristomal skin, and note replacement of appliance or gauze. If teaching was done, document content of teaching and response.

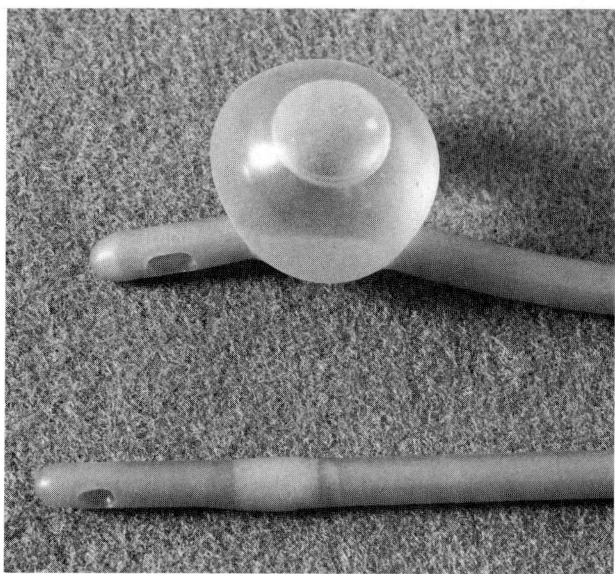

Figure 26–21. Indwelling catheter with balloon inflated, deflated.

catheters can cause cross-contamination among clients. Gloving alone is not sufficient to prevent this problem. For example, hands should be washed and then gloved before the catheter drainage bag is emptied. Once the emptying is done, gloves should be removed and the hands washed once again.[17] Some experts recommend that clients with catheters not be roomed together because of the high rate of cross-contamination.[18]

Perineal care is recommended at least twice daily when a client has an indwelling catheter. This care should include cleaning the first 1 to 2 inches of tubing as it leaves the meatus. Secretions are a good medium for bacterial growth and should be removed gently with soap and water (see Chap. 24).

Correct positioning of the drainage bag and tubing is another important aspect of indwelling catheter care. The tubing should hang freely at all times and be kept free of kinks or compression. The drainage bag should be kept below the level of the bladder at all times, and the drainage tubing should not drape below the level of the bag. Urine in the collection bag is a medium for bacterial growth; reflux of this contaminated urine into the bladder is a cause of urinary tract infections. When the client is in bed, the bag should hang on the bedframe; when the client is in a chair, the bag should hang on the side of the chair below the level of the bladder. The bag should be carried below the waist when the client is ambulating, and it should never be placed on the floor. Figure 26–24 illustrates correct and incorrect positioning for the urine collection bag.

PROCEDURE 26–10. INSERTING A STRAIGHT OR INDWELLING (FOLEY) URINARY CATHETER

PURPOSE: To remove urine from the bladder. Straight catheters are used to relieve retention, measure residual urine, or obtain a sterile urine specimen. Indwelling catheters are used to decompress the bladder during surgery, to maintain drainage in the postoperative period, and as a temporary remedy for incontinence. In some cases indwelling catheters are long term.

EQUIPMENT: Urinary catheterization set, nonsterile gloves, damp washcloth, towel, bath blanket, and extra light source.

ACTION	RATIONALE
1. Discuss with the client the reason for the procedure, expected client participation, and expected benefits.	1. Client will be more willing to participate and less anxious if there is an opportunity to clarify concerns and the reasons and benefits for the procedure are clear.
2. Provide privacy: close door, pull curtains around bed.	2. Genital exposure is considered invasive in most cultures. Client will feel less vulnerable in protected space.
3. Wash hands.	3. Prevents transfer of transient microorganisms on nurse's hands to client's environment.
4. Raise bed to nurse's waist level.	4. Allows nurse to complete procedure with optimal posture, thereby preventing backstrain.
5. Assist female client to dorsal recumbent position, drape with bath blanket: place over client with one corner directed toward her head, opposite corner over perineum. Wrap remaining corners around legs—over thigh, then under knee, anchor under heel. (Corner over perineum will be folded toward chest during procedure). Male client should be in supine position with thighs slightly abducted and covers arranged so penis is exposed but legs are covered. Bath blanket can be placed over chest and abdomen if desired.	5. Position provides access to urinary meatus without straining nurse's back. Draping diminishes feeling of exposure, prevents chilling.

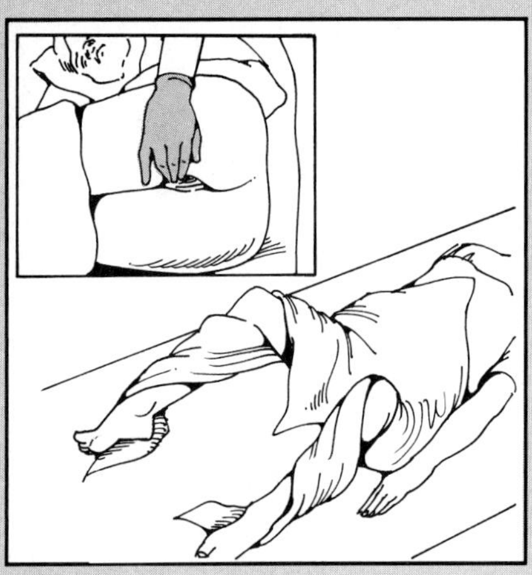

(continued)

PROCEDURE 26–10. (continued)

NOTE: If client prefers, cover torso only, omit drape over legs. Some elderly or arthritic females are unable to abduct thighs as required in dorsal recumbent position. Sidelying position with upper leg flexed toward shoulder may be used in this case.

6. Don nonsterile gloves. Wash perineal area with warm damp washcloth, dry thoroughly. If male client is not circumcised, retract foreskin during washing. Remove gloves by turning inside-out and discard in leak-resistant trash container.

6. Pericare reduces number of microorganisms around meatus. Gloves provide a barrier against perineal organisms, which may be pathogenic.

NOTE: Changes in perineal muscle tone associated with childbirth and aging may alter meatal location in females. Locating meatus during perineal care facilitates correct insertion of catheter.

7. Adjust extra light source so beam is directed on perineum. If free-standing lamp is not available, assistant may be needed to hold a flashlight.

7. Normal room lights may not provide sufficient focused light to locate female client's meatus.

8. Expose perineum. Place catheter set between client's legs and unwrap, touching corners only, creating sterile field. (See Procedure 22–3.) Most sets are packaged in a plastic bag, which can be taped to siderail for disposal of used supplies.

8. Facilitates carrying out procedure with minimal reaching over sterile field, thereby reducing possibility of contamination.

9. Unfold sterile underpad by grasping one corner with fingertips, lifting it away from sterile field and shaking it. Then grasp opposite corner. *Female client:* Ask client to raise buttocks, then slide drape about 2 inches under buttocks. *Male client:* slip drape under penis, covering thighs.

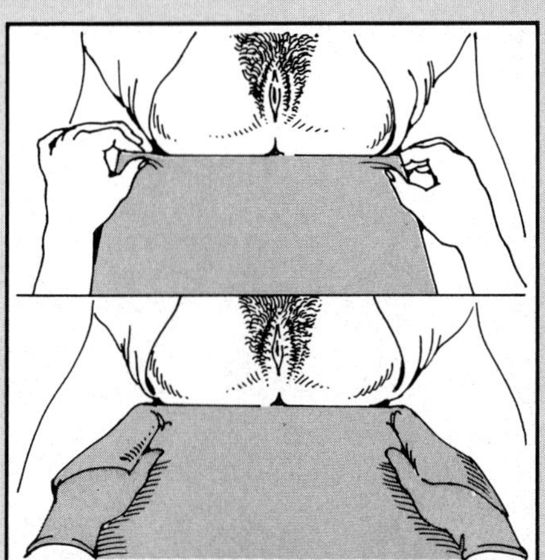

9. Drape and wrapper now create a continuous sterile field that acts as a barrier to microorganisms. Nurse has not touched portion of field on which sterile supplies will be placed.

(continued)

PROCEDURE 26–10. (continued)

NOTE: In some sets, sterile gloves are the first item. If so, don gloves (see Procedure 22–4). Pick up drape as described, then fold corners over your hands so gloves are covered while placing drape under female.

10. Don sterile gloves and prepare sterile field as follows. (For straight catheterization, omit steps a and b.)

    a. Close clamp at base of collection bag attached to catheter. In most sets, bag and catheter are beneath tray holding lubricant, cotton, etc.

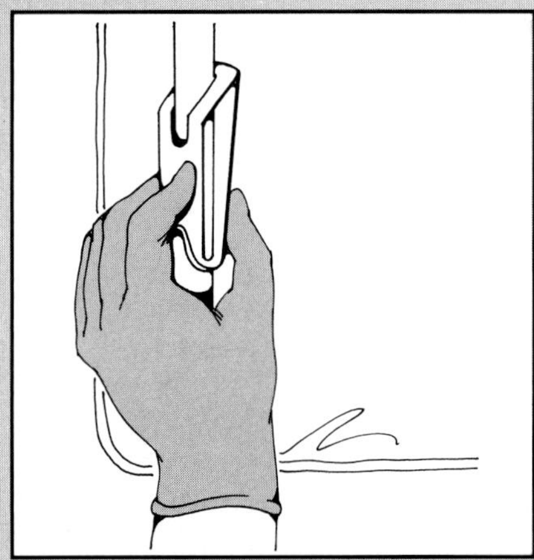

    b. Coil catheter around hand and pull off plastic covering. Test balloon: connect prefilled syringe to port, inject fluid; withdraw fluid, leaving syringe attached. If balloon leaks or does not inflate, obtain new catheter.

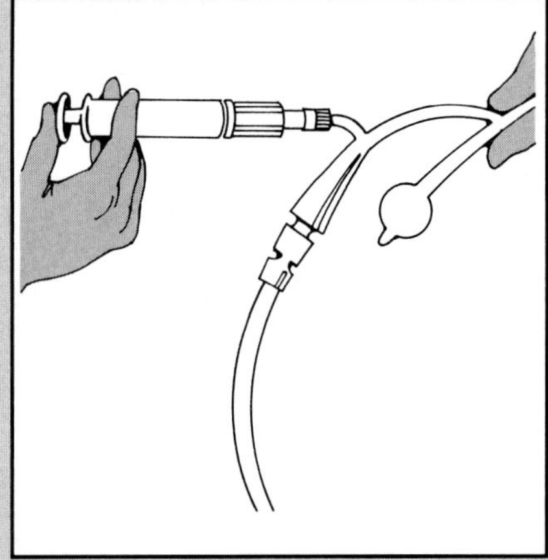

10. Sterile gloves act as a barrier preventing transfer of organisms from the nurse's hands to objects that will contact or enter sterile body cavity (bladder). Preparation of field requires two hands, so must be completed before nurse begins cleansing perineum. Gloved hands should touch only sterile items when preparing field.

(continued)

PROCEDURE 26–10. (continued)

c. Place fenestrated drape so opening exposes labia or penis.

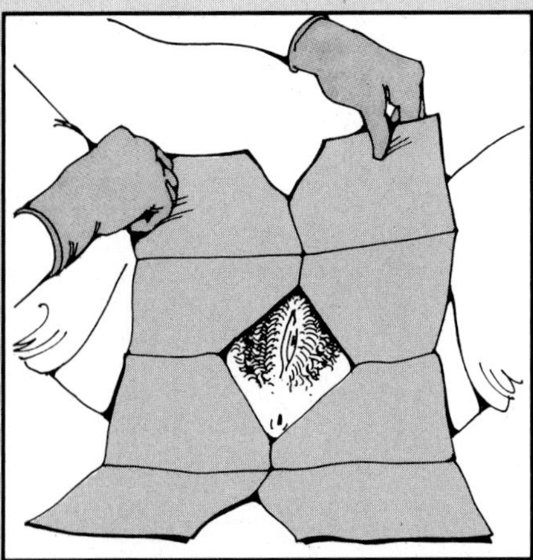

NOTE: Often omitted as it may slip, risking contamination.

d. Pour antiseptic over cotton balls, squeeze lubricant on tray, open specimen container.

NOTE: Lubricant is in a syringe in some kits.

11. Cleanse client as follows.

Female client:

a. Expose the meatus by spreading labia minora outward and upward: place the thumb and index or middle finger of your non-dominant hand about midway down the labia, between the labia minora; spread your fingers then pull tissue gently upward.

11a. Promotes cleansing of meatus and surrounding skin folds, reducing possibility of introducing organisms into the bladder.

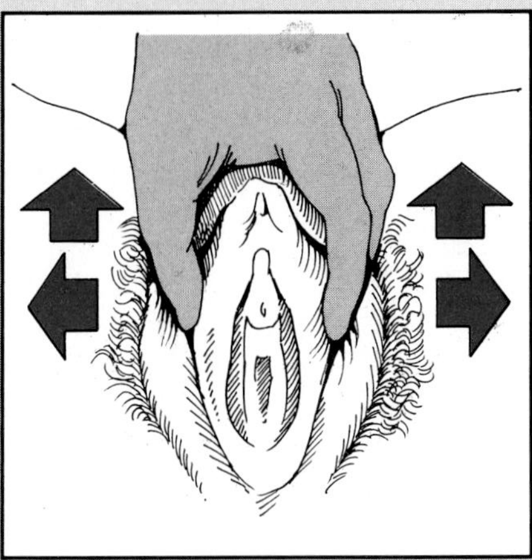

NOTE: Placing the fingers on the upper half of the labia majora to expose meatus is a frequent error. Poor cleansing and visualization of meatus results.

(continued)

PROCEDURE 26–10. (continued)

b. Holding one cotton ball with forceps for each stroke, cleanse the labia and meatus. Clean from labia majora inward, as shown in figure, using downward strokes. Labia should not be allowed to close until catheter is inserted.

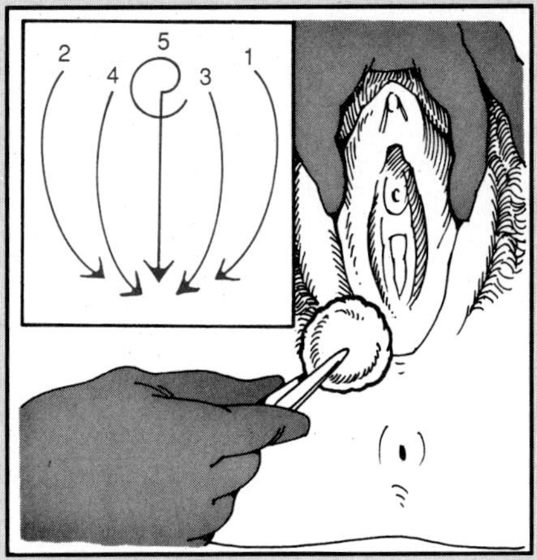

NOTE: Using a twisting motion when cleaning over the meatus may cause it to open slightly, facilitating visualization.

b. Friction and chemical action reduce bacterial population around meatus. Using new swab for each stroke and maintaining labia in open position prevent transfer of microorganisms from contaminated to cleaned area.

Male client:

a. Hold the penis up by grasping the shaft just below the glans.

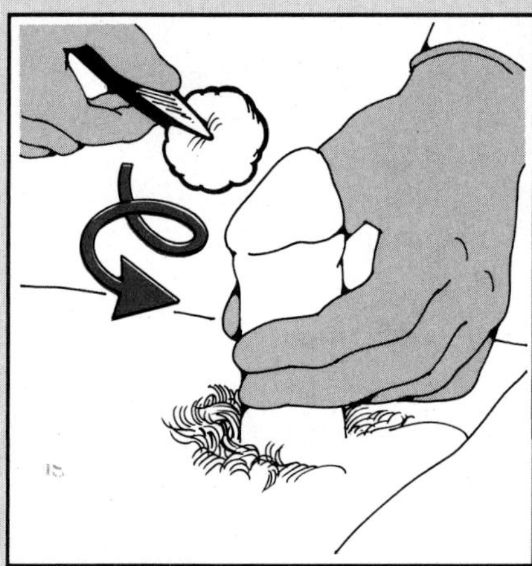

b. Clean the glans in a circular motion from meatus outward. Repeat three times using separate swab for each stroke. Continue to hold penis in this position until catheter has been inserted.

NOTE: If foreskin has not remained retracted, it must be retracted prior to cleansing to remove organisms beneath it.

a, b. Friction and chemical action reduce bacterial population around meatus. Using new swab for each stroke and maintaining penis in upward position prevent transfer of microorganisms from contaminated to cleaned area.

(continued)

PROCEDURE 26–10. (continued)

12. Generously lubricate catheter tip: 2–3 inches for female, 6–7 inches for male.

12. Lubrication reduces trauma to urethra from friction. Male urethra is longer, so more lubrication is needed.

NOTE: Some experts advocate instilling lubricant directly into the male urethra to improve lubrication.

13. If inserting a straight catheter, place the collection basin near the meatus and place distal end of catheter in it.

13. Urine will flow out of catheter as soon as bladder is entered.

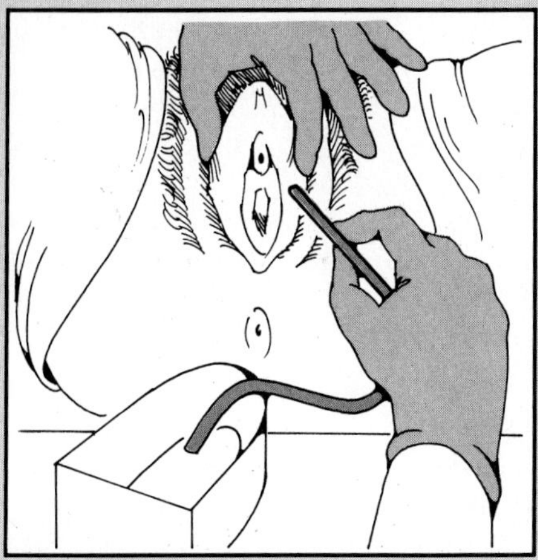

14. Tell client you are ready to insert the catheter, which will create a sensation similar to voiding; or rarely, pressure and mild burning; and that the sensation will cease when catheter is in place. Suggest that client take a deep breath, then exhale.

14. If the client knows what to expect, anxiety is decreased, trust increased. A deep breath facilitates sphincter relaxation, minimizing irritation.

15. As client exhales, insert the catheter in the direction of the urethra: in females parallel to the plane of the bed, then slightly downward, 2–3 inches; in males toward the abdomen, 8–9 inches. Slight resistance is commonly felt when catheter passes external and internal sphincters. Twist catheter slightly, and then pause or change the angle of the penis slightly to relax sphincters. Do not try to force catheter.

15. Following the anatomical direction reduces discomfort and irritation.

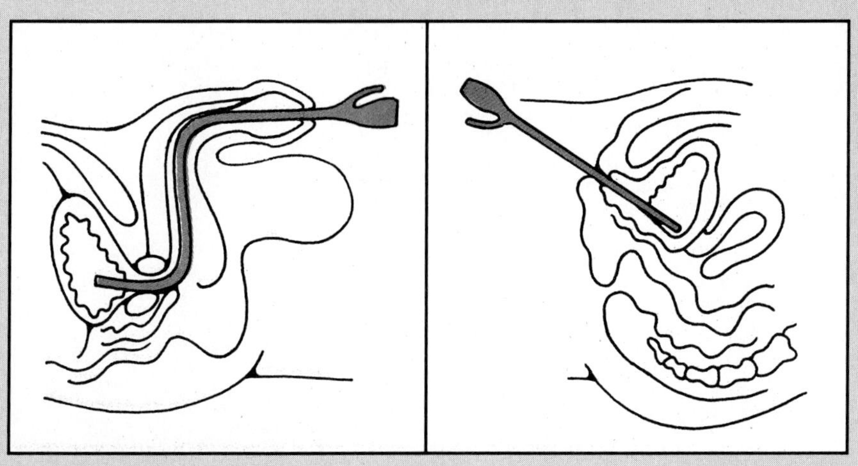

(continued)

PROCEDURE 26–10. (continued)

NOTE: If catheter has been advanced 4–5 inches in a female client with no urine return, it is likely that the catheter is in the vagina. Leave it in place to assist in correct location of meatus, obtain a new catheter set, and begin again. In males, unusual resistance may be caused by strictures, prostate enlargement, or other abnormality. If a smaller diameter-catheter cannot be inserted, consult with physician.

16. When urine flow is noted advance catheter 1–2 inches, then hold it in place with nondominant hand.

16. Advancing catheter well into bladder facilitates emptying and prevents trauma to bladder neck when retention balloon is inflated. Forcing catheter may cause urethral trauma.

17. For a straight catheter, hold catheter in place until urine flow ceases. (If specimen is required, pinch catheter after several mL have drained, direct flow of urine into specimen cup, then redirect to collection basin to complete emptying of bladder.) Tell client you are ready to remove catheter, then pinch catheter and withdraw in same direction as insertion.

17. Withdrawing in this manner minimizes irritation. Sterile midstream specimen is least likely to be contaminated by perineal organisms. Telling client before withdrawing catheter will facilitate relaxation (see step 14).

NOTE: Some sources indicate that no more than 750 mL should be drained from bladder at one time. Rapid decrease in intra-abdominal pressure may cause reflex dilation of pelvic vessels, which decreases venous return to the heart, lowering blood pressure.

18. For retention catheter, inject all liquid in syringe to inflate balloon, then tug gently to assure catheter is anchored.

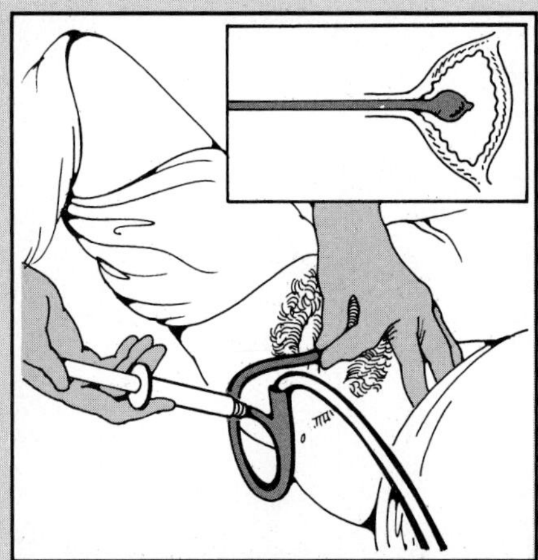

18. A 5-mL balloon requires 8 mL of liquid because 3 mL remains in the lumen of the catheter. A partially inflated balloon may traumatize bladder neck.

19. Clean client's perineum of residual lubricant and antiseptic. If foreskin was retracted, replace it over glans. Remove used equipment, including drapes and gloves, and discard in leak-resistant trash container. Wash hands.

19. Promotes client comfort and prevents transfer of microorganisms to environment.

(continued)

PROCEDURE 26–10. (continued)

20. Hang drainage bag on bedframe. Coil drainage tubing so downward flow of urine to collection bag is facilitated. Secure tubing to bottom sheet with safety pin or clamp.

20. Urine that has pooled in tubing may flow back into bladder if urine flow is impeded by kinks or loops in tubing below the level of the collection bag. Bacteria growing in this urine is a cause of catheter-induced urinary tract infections.

21. Tape catheter, allowing slack between perineum and tape to allow for changes in position without creating tension on balloon in bladder.
    Female clients: tape catheter to inner thigh.

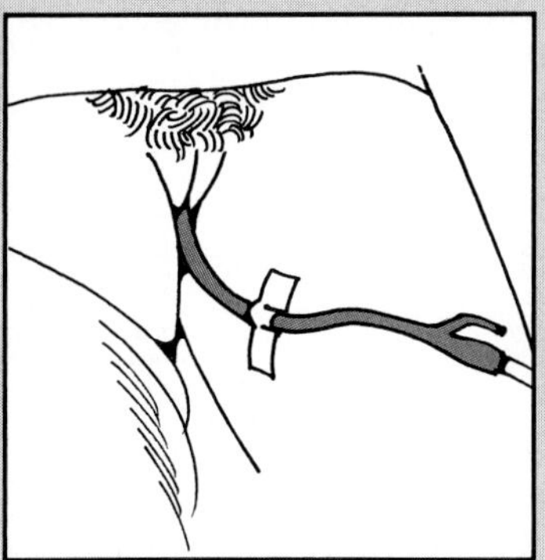

21. Pulling on the catheter as a result of movement or tangling will be directed against the tape, not the bladder neck, as would be the case were the catheter not taped securely.

Male clients: tape catheter to abdomen or to anterior thigh depending on agency policy.

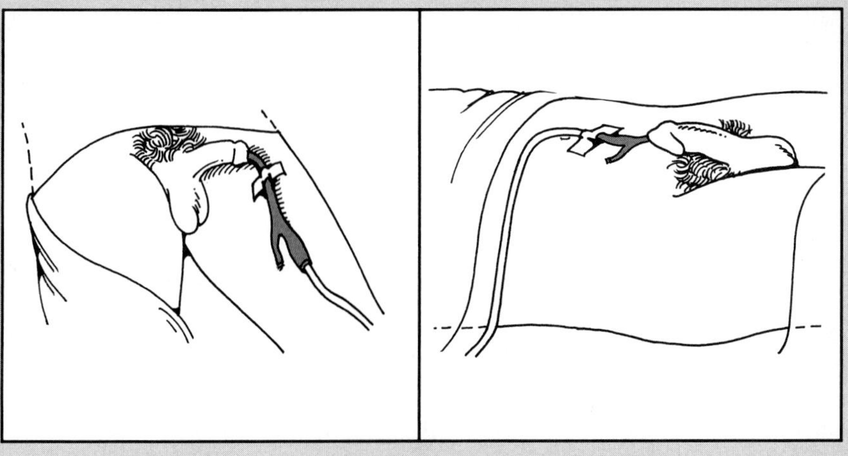

Pressure at the penile–scrotal junction caused by bending the catheter, which some urologists feel increases potential for tissue necrosis, is eliminated if the catheter is secured to the abdomen.

NOTE: Taping must be rechecked frequently. Some facilities use commercially prepared catheter straps to secure catheters.

22. If specimen is needed, it may be obtained from drainage bag. Don nonsterile gloves to obtain specimen. Label and send to lab (see Procedure 26–12).

22. Because catheter has just been inserted, bag contains fresh urine. Gloves protect nurse's hands from any organisms in client's urine.

(continued)

PROCEDURE 26–10. (continued)

NOTE: Subsequent specimens must be obtained via special port (see Procedure 26–12).

23. Inform client that lying on drainage tube will impede urine flow, pulling on catheter may cause pain and injury, and raising drainage collector above the level of the bladder is a cause of infections in the bladder.

23. An informed client can assume responsibility for health-related behaviors and can protect self from errors by uninformed providers.

RECORDING: Note type (straight or indwelling) and size of catheter inserted; amount and character of urine obtained; problems, if any, and action taken; client's response to procedure; and type, reason, and disposition of specimen.

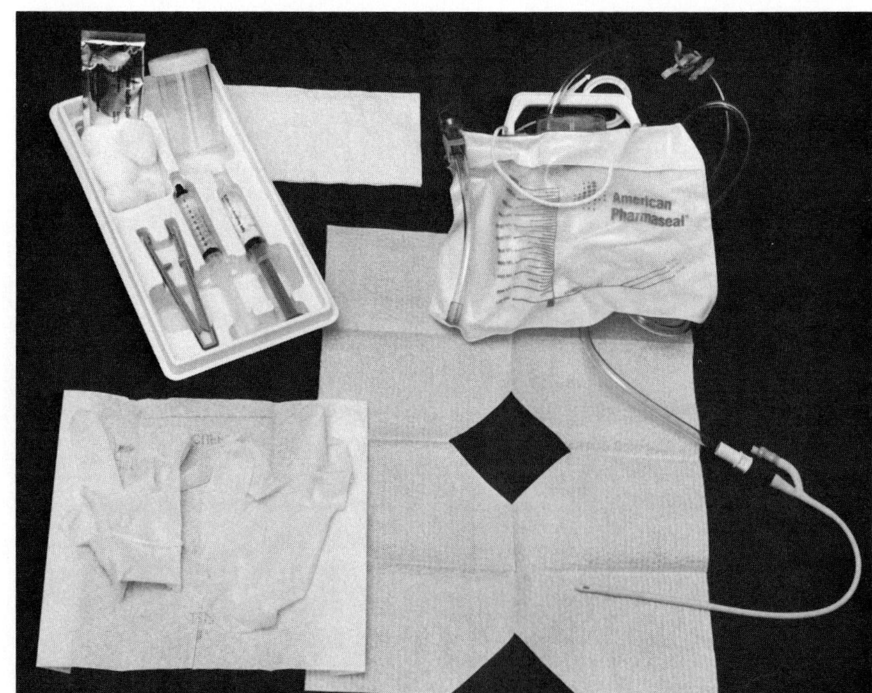

Figure 26–22. Equipment found in disposable kit for insertion of indwelling catheter.

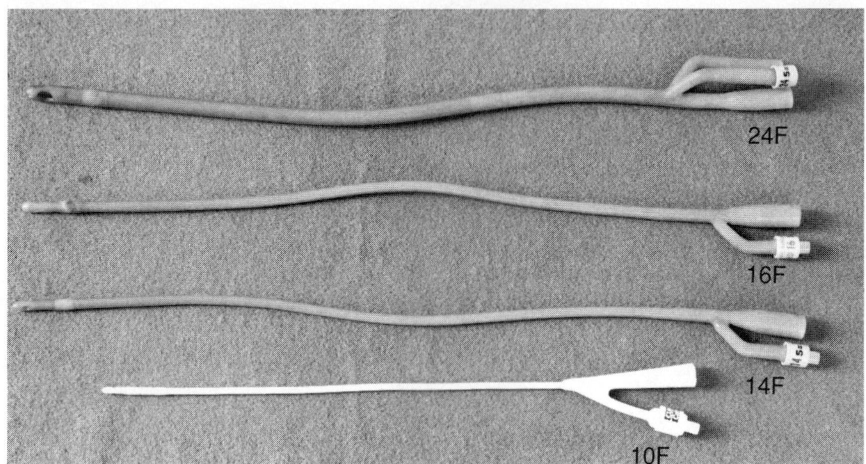

Figure 26–23. Comparison of urinary catheters showing sizes.

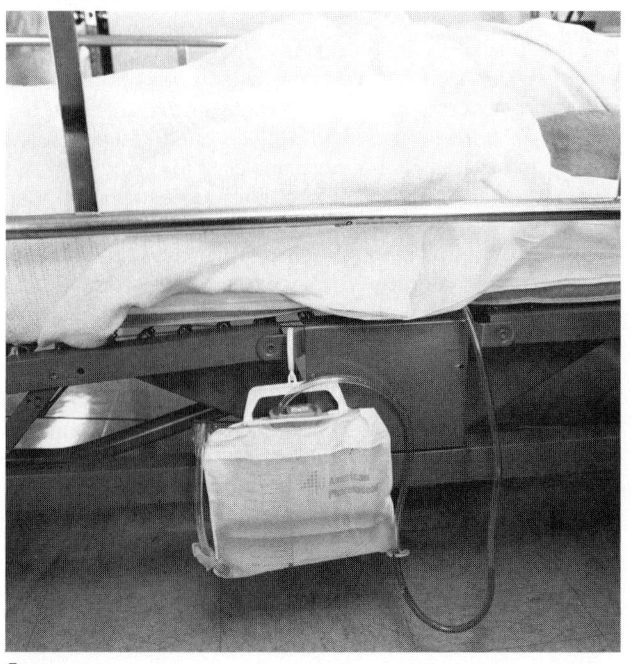

A

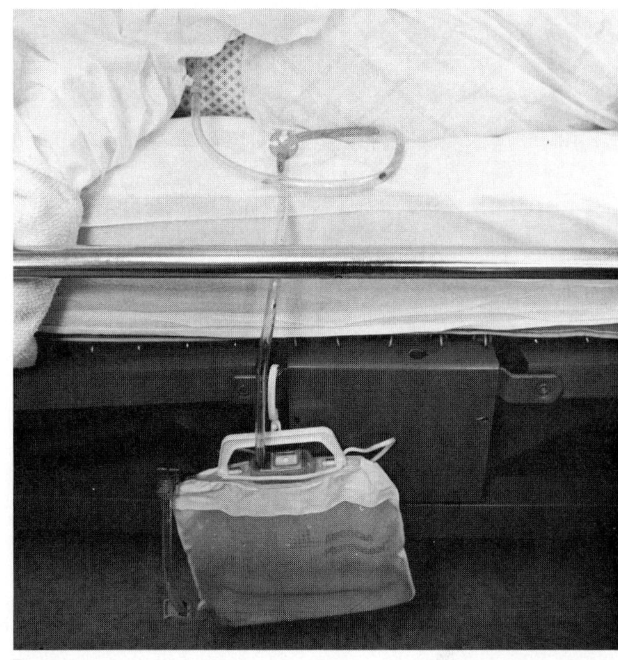

B

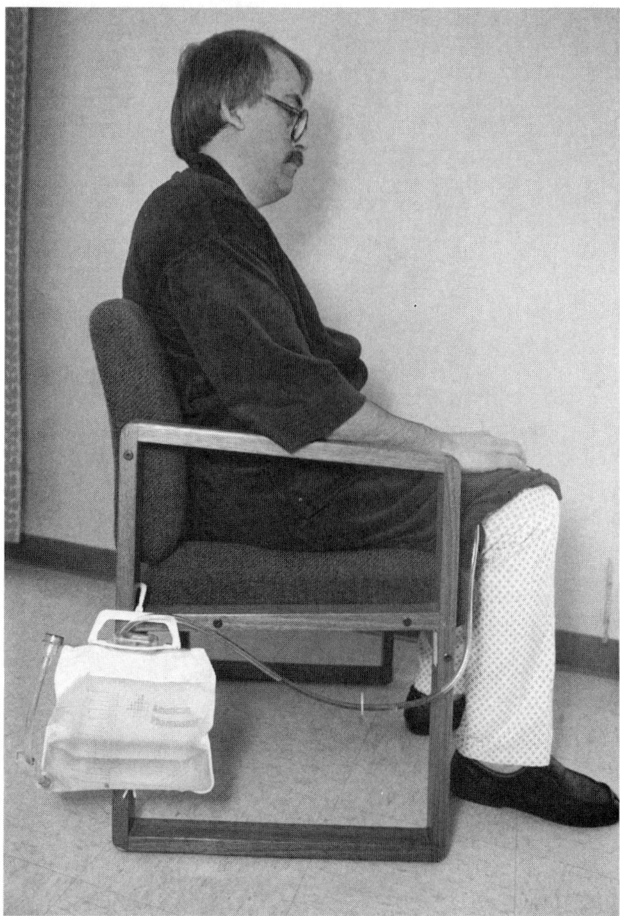

C

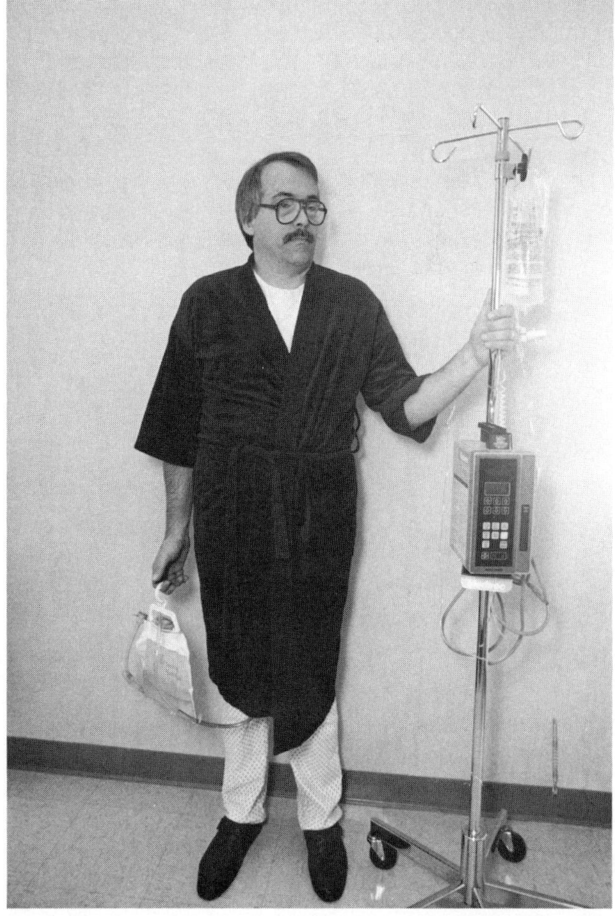

D

Figure 26–24. A–D. Incorrect (**A**) and correct (**B–D**) positions for urine drainage bag with indwelling catheter.

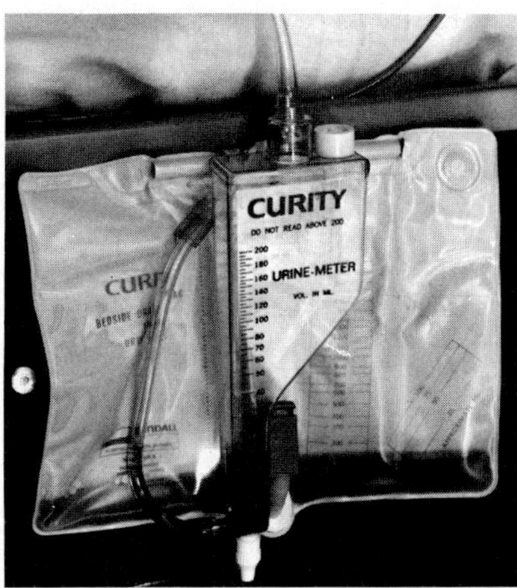

Figure 26–25. Urinary drainage bag with attached urine meter. (*From Smith S, Duell D.* Clinical Nursing Skills: Nursing Process Model, Basic to Advanced Skills. *3rd ed. Norwalk, CT: Appleton & Lange; 1992.*)

Emptying the urine collection bag must be done in such a way that contamination is avoided. At the bottom of the bag is a tube that drains the bag; this is always clamped, except when emptying. This drainage tube is housed in a protective covering that is connected to the drainage bag (Fig. 26–25). The urine should be emptied and measured using a graduated container that is used for urine only and that is used for only one client. Bags are usually emptied once every shift or when full.

Monitoring urine output is another nursing responsibility. Urine is monitored for color, amount, clarity, and odor. The frequency of monitoring depends on the client's condition. Some drainage bags have calibrated auxiliary containers, which allow for relatively precise hourly output readings without opening the system (Fig. 26–25). The nurse should question the client about discomfort, such as pain or burning around the catheter, when the urine is assessed. Urine draining from a catheter should be clear, yellow, and odorless.

If a urine specimen is needed from a client with an

PROCEDURE 26–11. OBTAINING A SPECIMEN FROM AN INDWELLING CATHETER

PURPOSE: To collect sterile urine for testing when a catheter is in place.

EQUIPMENT: Clamp or rubber band, nonsterile gloves, sterile alcohol wipes, a 3- to 10-mL sterile syringe with a 1-inch 21- to 25-gauge needle, and specimen cup (must be sterile if sample is for culture).

ACTION

1. Discuss the reason for the procedure, including expected client participation and benefits. Screen client, and place clamp or rubber band on drainage tubing, just distal to the aspiration port.

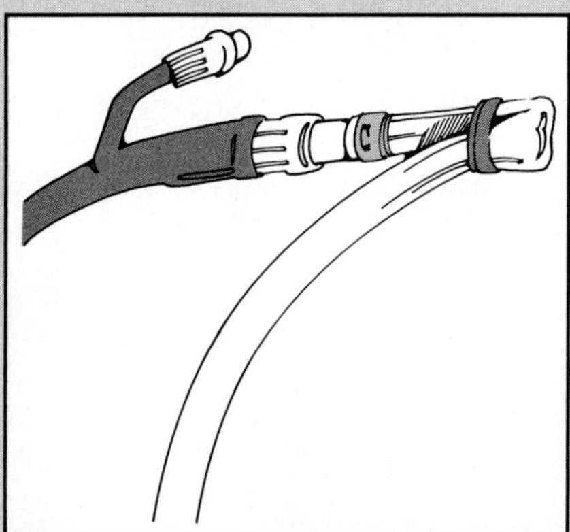

2. Return in 10–15 min, don gloves. Cleanse aspiration port with alcohol swab and insert needle into port at a 30° angle. (See A and B). If drainage system has no port, cleanse distal end of catheter and insert needle distal to balloon inlet at a 30° angle toward drainage tube. (C).

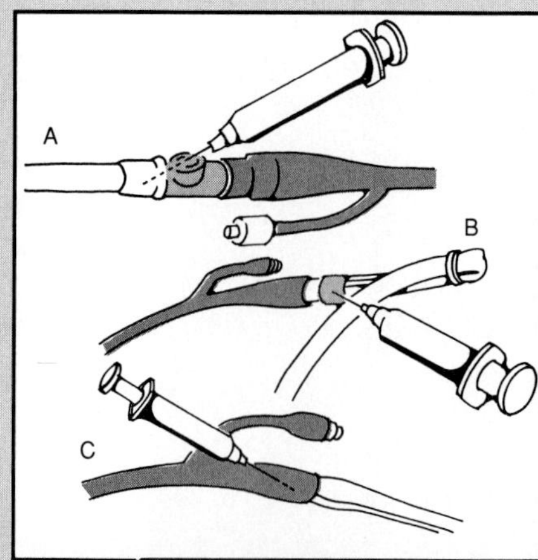

3. Withdraw 3–20 mL of urine (varies with number and type of tests ordered). Transfer urine to appropriate specimen container, label, and arrange for transport to lab within 30 min. May refrigerate sample for up to 1 hour without affecting accuracy of most tests.
4. When laboratory result is returned to client's chart, inform client of result.

RECORDING: Note character of urine, reason for specimen, and date and time sent to laboratory.

indwelling catheter, it should be obtained from a specific area near the proximal end of the catheter tubing where fresh sterile urine can be aseptically obtained. This portion of the tubing is made of resealable rubber and is often called a cathport. The urine is removed using sterile technique (see Procedure 26–11).

Removing a Retention Catheter. Removing a retention catheter is a relatively simple procedure. Wearing nonsterile gloves, remove the tape anchoring the catheter and then place a waterproof pad between the legs of a female client or over the scrotum and thighs of a male client. Insert the appropriate-size syringe, without a needle, into the valve at the end of the balloon arm and draw out fluid until negative pressure is felt. Remove the syringe from the valve. Instruct the client to take a deep breath and to release it slowly. Smoothly withdraw the catheter as the client exhales. After the catheter is removed, the nurse should discuss measures to promote normal elimination. Encourage fluid intake and emphasize the importance of responding promptly to the urge to void. Clients are also asked to urinate into a container in which the urine can be measured so urination patterns can be monitored.

An indwelling catheter may be left in place for days, weeks or months, depending on physician's orders. Catheters are not changed on a routine basis, but only as needed. Catheter bags and tubing should be changed if there is an excess of built-up sediment, leakage, or contamination. Sylastic catheters are reported to need changing less frequently than latex catheters and therefore are recommended for clients who need long-term catheter placement.

Applying an External Catheter. An external or condom catheter is a device that fits over the penis and is then attached to a drainage collection system. It is most frequently used for clients with total urinary incontinence, although it may be used for bladder training or collection of a urine specimen. External catheters are also called Texas catheters. Although an external catheter can be made from a condom, tape, tubing, and a collecting bag, commercially made catheters are readily available. Figure 26–26 illustrates various samples.

Applying the external catheter is not an invasive procedure, so there tends to be less trauma to the urinary tract and less potential for infection than with an indwelling catheter. However, skin excoriation and necrosis may occur, and external catheters may be difficult to keep in place. Careful monitoring of the catheter and perineum is mandatory, and the catheter should be replaced at least once every 24 hours (see Procedure 26–12).

Irrigating a Urinary Catheter. Catheter irrigations are usually done to maintain or restore patency when sediment, such as pus or blood, interferes with drainage. Sodium chloride is the most common solution used for urinary irrigation. Use of sterile technique is vital.

When irrigations are anticipated on a regular basis, the closed irrigation method should be used (Fig. 26–27).

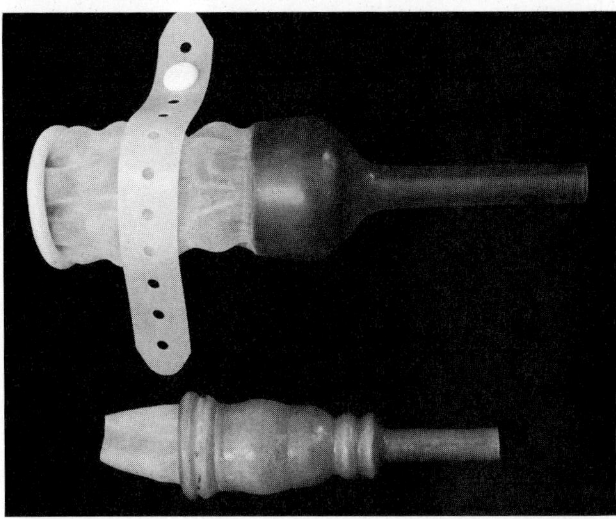

Figure 26–26. Condom catheters.

Closed irrigations may be continuous or intermittent. The closed technique is the preferred method of maintaining catheter patency because it minimizes the possibility of introducing microorganisms during irrigation. Open irrigation (also called hand irrigation) is sometimes used to restore patency of a urinary drainage. Hand irrigation involves separating the drainage tubing from the catheter and irrigating the catheter via a syringe (Fig. 26–28). Open irrigation is less desirable because there is a high likelihood of introducing microorganisms when the opened system is manipulated. Therefore, infection is more common when open irrigation is done.

Rehabilitative Care

Rehabilitation and the reestablishment of near-normal elimination patterns are the major concerns of fourth-level client care. This care should be initiated before the client is discharged from a health care facility. Home management of care requires the understanding and collaboration of the client, the client's family, and significant others.

The nurse collaborates with the client in planning bowel and bladder training or retraining. These programs involve monitoring fluid intake and diet, positioning techniques, muscle strengthening exercises, and habit formation. The goal is to retrain the bladder or bowel to empty periodically after injury or disruption of normal routines. The program can be supplemented by aids such as external catheters, intermittent self-catheterization, electrical stimulation of the micturition reflex, laxatives, or stool softeners.

Bowel Training. Through bowel training, some clients who are incontinent of stool can achieve normal defecation. Those who have some control of abdominal muscles and the anal sphincter are most likely to be successful. By setting up a daily routine for elimination and using measures

PROCEDURE 26–12. APPLYING AN EXTERNAL (CONDOM OR TEXAS) CATHETER

PURPOSE: To prevent soiling and skin excoriation from urinary incontinence. To collect a urine specimen from a client lacking voluntary control of urination.

EQUIPMENT: External catheter with adhesive (cloverleaf or spiral to apply directly to penis, or elastic tape or Velcro strap to apply outside the catheter sheath); nonsterile gloves, warm damp washcloth and towel; drainage collection bag (leg bag or indwelling catheter type); blunt scissors; and skin protector/tincture of benzoin (optional).

ACTION	RATIONALE
1. Discuss with the client the reason for the procedure, expected client participation, and expected benefits.	1. Client will be more willing to participate and less anxious if there is an opportunity to clarify concerns and the reasons and benefits for the procedure are clear.
NOTE: This device is often used on clients who seem unable to comprehend explanation; but explanation should not be omitted as clients may understand even though they do not respond.	
2. Close door, pull curtains around bed.	2. Genital exposure is considered invasive in most cultures. Client will feel less vulnerable in protected space.
3. Wash hands.	3. Prevents transfer of transient microorganisms on nurse's hands to client's environment.
4. Raise bed to nurse's waist level.	4. Allows nurse to complete procedure with optimal posture, thereby preventing backstrain.
5. Assist client to supine or semi-Fowler's position with thighs slightly abducted and covers arranged so penis is exposed but legs are covered. Bath blanket can be placed over chest and abdomen if desired.	5. Position provides access to urinary meatus without straining nurse's back. Draping diminishes feeling of exposure, prevents chilling.
6. Don nonsterile gloves. Wash perineal area with warm washcloth, dry thoroughly. If client is not circumcised, retract foreskin during washing, then replace. Assess penis and scrotum for skin irritation or edema. Document nature of lesions and action taken.	6. Gloves provide a barrier against perineal organisms, which may be pathogenic. Perineal care removes organisms and secretions that may cause skin irritation under catheter sheath.
7. If penis is free of lesions, gloves may be removed after peri care.	7. Adhesive materials are difficult to apply when wearing gloves. Barrier against microbes is unnecessary if no lesions are present.

(continued)

PROCEDURE 26–12. (continued)

NOTE: Catheter should not be applied over irritated skin unless skin barrier type of adhesive such as cloverleaf is used.

8. Clip hairs at base of penis. If using adhesive inside sheath apply as follows.
   Cloverleaf: Carefully pull the glans through the opening in the cloverleaf, remove protective backing on underside, press each "leaf" against shaft of penis, taking care to push away any hairs. Remove backing from outside of cloverleaf. Adhesive surface is now exposed to secure catheter.

8. Hairs easily adhere to adhesive, causing discomfort upon removal. Cloverleaf device is stretchable, so will accommodate changes in size of penis, such as an erection.

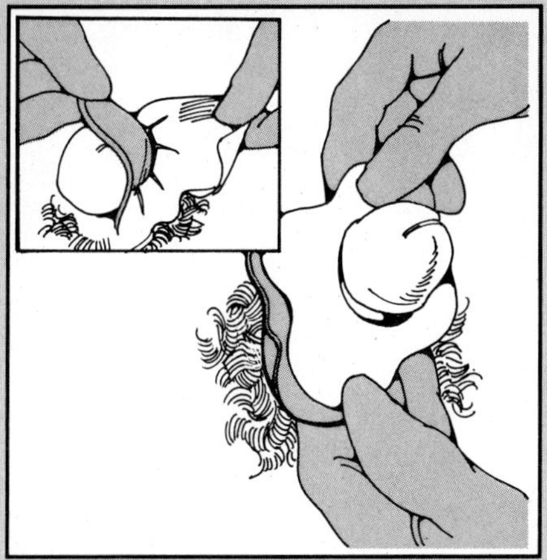

Spiral: Remove backing from foam adhesive strip and wrap it around the shaft of the penis in spiral fashion. Ends of strip should not overlap. Tincture of benzoin or protective skin spray may be used under strip. Remove backing from outside of foam strip.

If ends of adhesive overlap, circulation to penis would be impeded if size of penis increases. Spiral strips are not made from skin-protective barrier material, so benzoin or spray may be needed to protect sensitive skin from adhesive-related irritation.

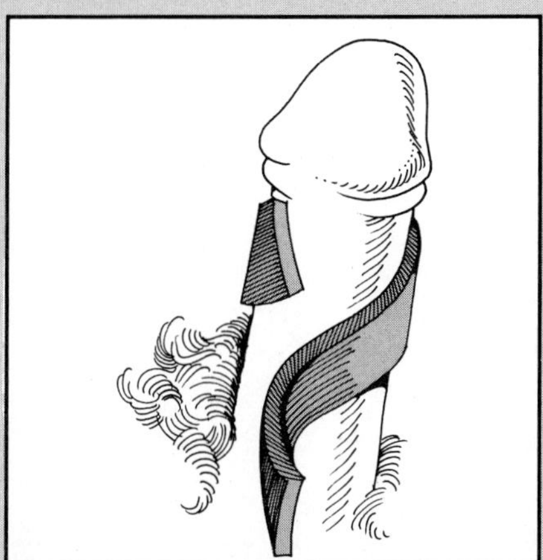

(continued)

PROCEDURE 26–12. (continued)

9. If sheath is not rolled, roll the top downward. Some types have an inner flap to prevent reflux, which should be exposed by rolling as in figure.

9. Rolled sheath is easier to fit smoothly over penis.

10. Position sheath so inner flap is centered around meatus. If there is no flap, place sheath over glans so there is a space of 1–2 inches (2.5–5 cm) between the tip of the glans and the tip of the sheath. Roll catheter smoothly up shaft of penis until adhesive is covered. Sheath usually covers ¾ of the length of the penis.

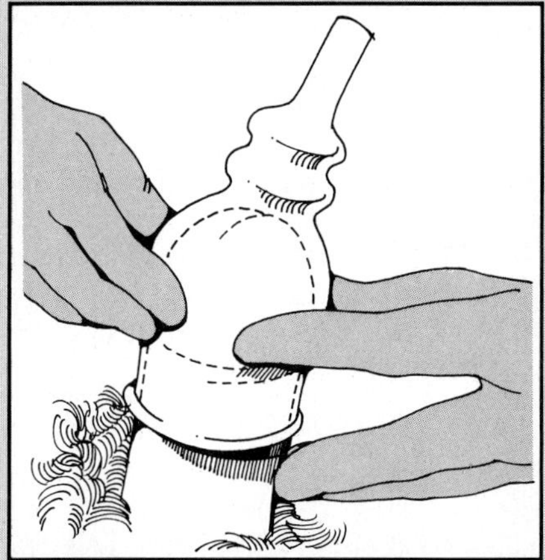

10. Inner flap must fit around meatus to prevent reflux. Sheath must be wrinkle free to diminish pressure or pulling on skin. Leaving space at end of sheath prevents irritation due to friction on glans and allows for free drainage of urine.

(continued)

PROCEDURE 26–12. (continued)

11. If no adhesive was used prior to applying, secure sheath with a strip of elastic tape wrapped over sheath in a close spiral or in a circular fashion with ends abutted, not overlapping. Velcro strap may be used. Follow manufacturer's directions.

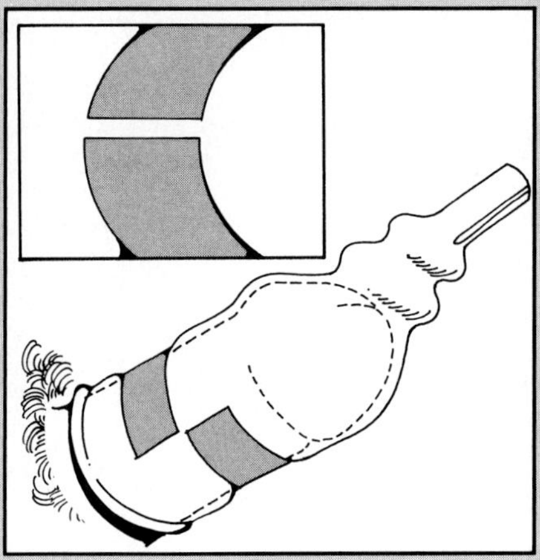

    Overlapping tape will cut off circulation to the penis if increase in size occurs.

NOTE: Nonelastic tape should never be used to secure catheter.

12. Attach drainage system securely to end of sheath.

    Provides conduit for urine, keeping client and bed dry.

NOTE: Leg bag is preferred for active client.

13. Hang drainage bag on bedframe. Coil drainage tubing so downward flow of urine to collection bag is facilitated. Secure tubing to bottom sheet with rubber band and safety pin or clamp.

    Urine that has pooled in tubing may flow back toward penis if urine flow is impeded by kinks or loops in tubing below the level of the collection bag. Bacteria growing in this urine is a cause of catheter-induced urinary tract infections. Moisture macerates skin.

NOTE: Leg bag has two elastic or rubber straps that secure it to lower leg. Tubing should be long enough to prevent pulling on catheter with movement.

14. Assess the condition of the penis 15 min after application, then hourly X2. Routine assessment is necessary whenever position is changed or at least twice per shift.

    If tape is too tight, circulatory stasis will be evidenced by discoloration, then edema. This must be corrected immediately to prevent necrosis. Position changes may cause twisting of the drainage tube, causing pressure on penis.

(continued)

PROCEDURE 26–12. (continued)

15. Remove catheter daily to assess skin condition and provide peri care.

15. Moisture from perspiration or urine that cannot evaporate make skin under sheath particularly vulnerable to breakdown.

NOTE: If breaks in skin are noted, an alternative method of applying catheter, or alternative method of collecting urine, is indicated.

16. To remove sheath, remove tape and roll or slip sheath off penis. If adhesive was applied directly to penis, use adhesive remover or alcohol swabs to moisten adhesive surface before removing. Protective skin spray peels off readily; benzoin may be washed off.

16. If adhesive is not removed carefully, skin may be damaged.

RECORDING: Note condition of perineal area, type of device and adhesive applied, and amount and character of urine collected. Document daily replacement of catheter and skin condition at the time catheter is changed.

to promote elimination, bowel reflexes may become controlled. Box 26–2 outlines the components of a bowel training program.

Home Management of Ostomies. The client with an ostomy should be given information about the anatomic changes caused by the surgery. The use and care of the ostomy equipment and the use of correct techniques for draining and irrigating ostomies are important considerations for this level of care. Other important areas are odor control, preservation of periostomal skin integrity, maintaining fluid and electrolyte balance, and identifying ways to prevent stoma blockage.

The client should know the signs and symptoms to report to the health care provider. Instructions for appropriate activity levels and precautions related to participa-

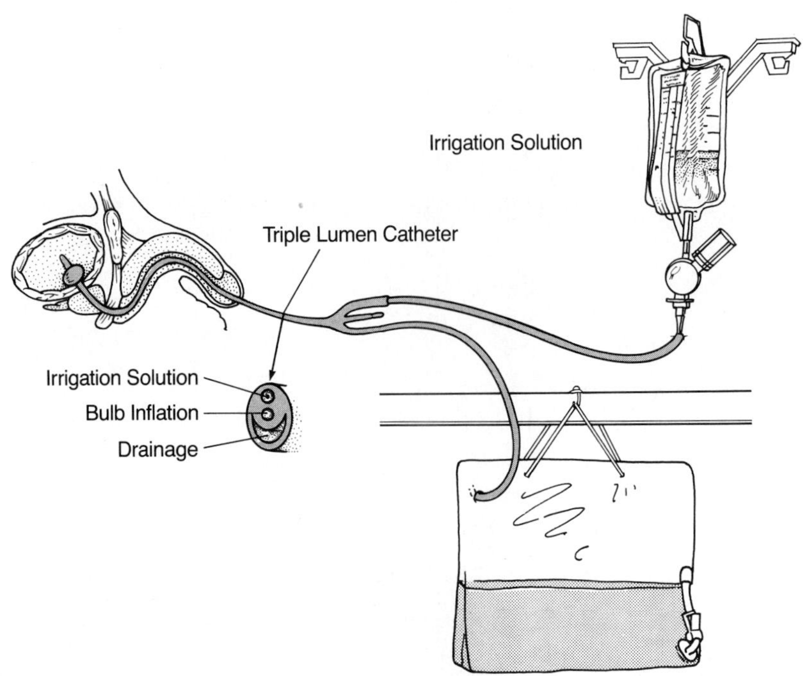

Figure 26–27. Setup for closed bladder irrigation using a triple-lumen catheter. (*From Smith S, Duell D.* Clinical Nursing Skills: Nursing Process Model, Basic to Advanced Skills. *3rd ed. Norwalk, CT: Appleton & Lange; 1992.*)

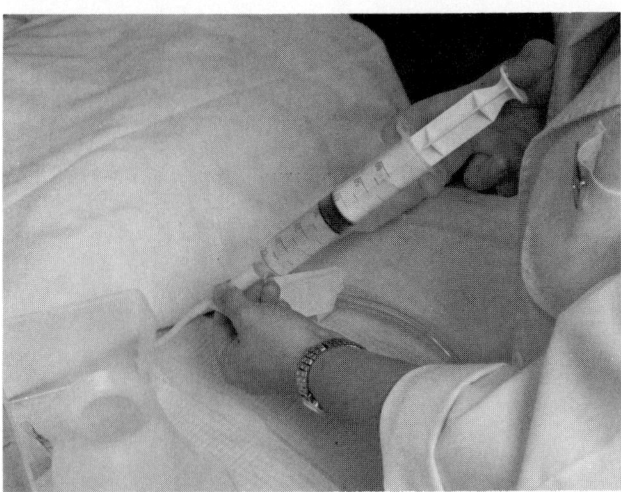

Figure 26–28. Hand irrigation of an indwelling catheter. (*From Smith S, Duell D.* Clinical Nursing Skills: Nursing Process Model, Basic to Advanced Skills. *3rd ed. Norwalk, CT: Appleton & Lange; 1992.*)

tion in contact sports are also important. Clients should be informed that they should not take enteric-coated tablets or time-released capsules because absorption may not take place before the medication is excreted if there is a bowel diversion ostomy.

Information also is needed about available community resources that can help the client and family with home management and adjustment to the changes that result from an ostomy. Some resources include the United Ostomy Association, ostomy support groups, community health agencies, enterostomal therapists, home health agencies, the Visiting Nurses' Association, as well as individual, family, and financial counseling services. These resources can help the client obtain equipment and supplies and work out financial and family problems.

BOX 26–2. COMPONENTS OF A BOWEL TRAINING PROGRAM

1. Determine what the client's usual elimination pattern is and document the incontinent episodes.
2. Collaborate with the client to determine the best time to initiate bowel control measures.
3. Obtain physician's order for oral stool softener or suppository if necessary to facilitate defecation.
4. Assess what fluids normally stimulate defecation for the client and administer before the time for bowel evacuation.
5. Provide assistance to the bathroom for the client at the selected times.
6. Maintain privacy for the client and limit elimination time to 15 to 20 minutes.
7. Instruct the client to lean forward at the hips while sitting on the toilet, place hands over the abdomen and apply some manual pressure, and bear down without straining to stimulate bowel evacuation.
8. Provide acceptance and encouragement even if the client is not able to defecate at the selected time.
9. Collaborate with the client to develop and carry out an exercise program that is within the client's ability.
10. Regular mealtimes and adequate intake of fiber and fluids are essential to bowel control. Work with the client to develop a plan that the client will follow.

IMPLICATIONS FOR NURSE–CLIENT COLLABORATION

Home Management of Ostomies

Whether or not a client is able to achieve optimal health after an ostomy will depend on the quality of home management. Although the procedure of caring for an ostomy requires the client's psychomotor skills, it is not nearly so difficult as the personal adjustment that may be required. New patterns necessitated by an ostomy may or may not be easily integrated into family life and daily living. The ability of client and significant others to manage the ostomy can be enhanced by caring support from the nurse. Frequently a client will benefit by collaborating with the nurse in the home setting, which provides the nurse with an opportunity to observe the supports and constraints—personal, social, and environmental—that the client faces every day in managing an ostomy. Collaborating with the client in his or her own surroundings can help to reduce external barriers and promote the client's confidence that the ostomy need not interfere with valued activities.

Bladder Training. Bladder retraining is often used for clients with a reflex bladder. These clients have an intact voiding reflex arc, but no sensory input from the bladder; therefore, the bladder empties without warning when it is full. The principles of bladder training are useful for any client who is incontinent of urine. Box 26–3 outlines the components of a bladder training program.

BOX 26–3. COMPONENTS OF A BLADDER TRAINING PROGRAM

1. Collaborate with the client to plan a regular daily fluid intake pattern that includes 2000 to 3000 mL of fluid.
2. Identify the usual voiding pattern of the client.
3. Plan a voiding schedule with regular attempts to void about 30 minutes prior to usual time bladder empties.
4. Assist the client to develop an association between a particular activity and emptying the bladder. Some effective "tricks" include concentration, stroking the inner thighs, drinking water, pulling the pubic hair, or manual pressure over the bladder.
5. Identify with the client factors that aggravate incontinence, such as medications or caffeine, and determine whether they can be reduced.
6. If the client is able, teach perineal exercises (see Second-Level Client Care earlier in the chapter).
7. Discuss the use of perineal pads or adult diapers to maintain dryness during the development of control.

BUILDING NURSING KNOWLEDGE

How Can Nurses Help Clients to Deal With the Problems of Bowel Dysfunction at Home?

Ellickson EB. Bowel management plan for the homebound elderly. *J Gerontol Nurs.* 1988;14:16–19.

Bowel dysfunction is one of the most frequently encountered problems of the elderly at home. Many complaints appear to be related to poor habits or to a preoccupation with eating and elimination. Isolation at home can increase a person's tendency to focus on bowel dysfunction. If not assisted, an elderly client may develop a feeling of hopelessness that will worsen the dysfunction of the bowel, according to Ellickson.

Bowel management begins with bowel assessment. Laxative abuse has been shown to be one of the main contributing factors to bowel disorders. Limited mobility and inactivity from various causes, decreased fluid intake, and inadequate or restricted diets are also factors, as is psychological depression. Many medications contribute to altered bowel function. The health examination should focus on such characteristics as dry skin, poor skin turgor, the presence of decubitus ulcers, abdominal distension, abdominal masses, and diminished bowel sounds. All can indicate bowel dysfunction. A rectal examination may reveal painful hemorrhoids or fissures that lead to bowel dysfunction.

Laxatives and enemas are *not* part of a bowel management program; laxatives actually promote constipation by disrupting intrinsic innervation of the colon. Diets need to be high in fiber. The highest source of fiber is in minimally processed cereal. Fresh fruits and vegetables, especially with the skins, are rich sources of fiber. Milk and milk products should be avoided if a client has a history of lactose intolerance, because they cause bloating and gas. Prune juice has little fiber, but produces catharsis. Adequate fluid intake is important, at least six 8-ounce glasses of fluid per day. Coffee, tea, and grapefruit juice, which contain diuretics, should be avoided.

Regular exercise is an important part of bowel management. Increasing activity to tolerance stimulates GI motility; but for the elderly, activity may be difficult. Even modest activity, such as sitting up in bed or turning or twisting in a chair, may help, according to the author. Steps to alleviate a client's psychological depression are important to successful management. Depression depletes the psychological energy necessary to eat, move about, and maintain proper elimination. It is also important to examine the medication profile to identify medications that might be contributing to bowel dysfunction.

In the rehabilitative stage of adapting to elimination problems, clients assume progressively greater responsibility for management of elimination. Rather than focusing on direct care or active collaboration, the nurse acts as a consultant. Resources such as those listed in Box 26–4 can provide clients with additional support and strategies for maintaining optimum elimination.

Some clients use intermittent self-catheterization as part of a bladder training program. Self-catheterization is scheduled so that continence is achieved and bladder distension is prevented; initially, it is usually performed every 4 hours. Although urinary catheterization is a sterile nursing procedure, studies have demonstrated the effectiveness and safety of clean technique for self-catheterization at home.[19] Important teaching points for self-catheterization include the following:

1. Emphasize the importance of clean equipment, proper handwashing, and thorough washing of the perineum before inserting the catheter.
2. Discuss techniques and rationale for lubricating the catheter adequately.
3. Demonstrate methods for correctly identifying the urinary meatus (women may find a mirror helpful).
4. Explain how far to insert the catheter.
5. Provide a list of signs and symptoms of urinary tract infection.

BOX 26–4. RESOURCE LIST FOR ELIMINATION CONCERNS

United Ostomy Association
1111 Wilshire Boulevard
Los Angeles, CA 90017

American Cancer Society
3340 Peachtree Road, NE
Atlanta, GA 30326
(404) 320-3333
(Local chapters may be found in local phone books.)

International Association For Enterostomal Therapy
27241 La Paz Road, Suite 121
Laquana Niquel, CA 92656
(714) 476-0268
This organization provides a directory listing clinics staffed by certified enterostomal therapists.

Hollister Incorporated
2000 Hollister Drive
Libertyville, IL 60048
Manufactures a drainable fecal incontinence collector, ostomy equipment, and urinary collecting products.

National Organization for Incontinence
The Simon Foundation
P.O. Box 835
Wilmette, IL 60091
(800) 23–SIMON

Help for Incontinent People (HIP)
P.O. Box 544
Union, SC 29379
(803) 579-7900

EVALUATION

Evaluation of client care related to elimination is the final component of nurse–client management of elimination. It is based on the desired outcomes and evaluation criteria that the nurse and client collaboratively developed. Client and nurse observe for the behaviors described in desired outcome statements or evaluation criteria. Evaluation of the desired outcome should be done at the time stated in the outcome, but the nurse and client should also monitor the progress made toward the goal. If the evaluation indicates that desired outcomes are not being achieved, reassessment and reconsideration of outcomes and implementation are needed.

As the outcomes are achieved, the progress is documented in the client's record. If outcomes are not met, the reassessment data and additional plans are also recorded.

Management of elimination concerns is a sensitive, sometimes difficult endeavor, because clients often hesitate to collaborate due to the intimate nature of the elimination process. Clients may find speaking about urination and defecation embarrassing or unpleasant. The nurse who demonstrates a concerned and professional approach will gain the client's trust and enhance his or her willingness to collaborate in managing elimination functions. The result will be achievement of greater autonomy and more healthful elimination.

SUMMARY

The lower gastrointestinal tract and the kidney with its associated structures are responsible for the excretion of the majority of the body's waste products. Understanding these organs' structure and function is necessary to carrying out nursing responsibilities related to promoting healthy elimination.

These responsibilities include collaborative assessment (data gathering, data analysis, and nursing diagnosis) and collaborative nurse–client management (planning, implementation, and evaluation) of elimination as well as carrying out elimination-related care ordered by physicians.

Elimination, particularly if altered, affects other body functions; therefore, the elimination assessment described in this chapter addresses not only the bowel and urinary tract but also selected aspects of integumentary, cardiorespiratory, neuromuscular, and psychological functioning.

The nursing diagnoses detailed in this chapter include only those directly related to elimination. These diagnoses and their etiologies are presented as a basis for identifying, understanding, and providing client care to promote optimum elimination. The discussion of nursing implementation focuses on independent nursing measures and medically ordered procedures that are directly supportive of elimination. These include health promotion and prevention, supportive care, restorative (or acute) care, and rehabilitative care.

Elimination alterations can be disruptive, uncomfortable, and embarrassing to clients. Nurses who are cognizant of this and who are sensitive about the distress that elimination assessment and implementation may cause can help alleviate client concerns and facilitate nurse–client collaboration to correct or minimize the impact of elimination problems.

REFERENCES

1. Guyton A. *Textbook of Medical Physiology.* 8th ed. Philadelphia: Saunders; 1990.
2. Schuster C, Ashburn S. *The Process of Human Development: A Holistic Approach.* Boston: Little, Brown; 1986:209–212, 801.
3. Ignatavicius DD, Bayne MV. *Medical-Surgical Nursing: A Nursing Process Approach.* Philadelphia: Saunders; 1991.
4. Whitney EN, Cataldo CB, Rolfes SR. *Understanding Normal and Clinical Nutrition.* St. Paul, MN: West Publishers; 1990.
5. Phipps WJ, Long BC, Woods NR, Cassmerry ZL. *Medical Surgical Nursing: Concepts and Clinical Practice.* 4th ed. St. Louis: Mosby; 1990.
6. Frank A, Murray S. A no-guess guide for urinary color assessment. *RN.* 1988;51:46–51.
7. Corbett J. *Laboratory Tests and Diagnostic Procedures With Nursing Diagnoses.* 3rd ed. Norwalk, CT: Appleton & Lange; 1991.
8. Matteson MA, McConnell E. *Gerontological Nursing.* Philadelphia: Saunders; 1988:280–285.
9. Fraulini K. *After Anesthesia: A Guide for PACU, ICU, and Medical-Surgical Nurses.* Norwalk, CT: Appleton & Lange; 1987:228–230.
10. Brenner MB, Rector F, eds. *The Kidney.* Philadelphia: Saunders; 1986:740.
11. Palmer M. Incontinence: The magnitude of the problem. *Nurs Clin North Am.* 1988;23:139.
12. Whaley LF, Wong DL. *Nursing Care of Infants and Children.* 4th ed. St. Louis: Mosby; 1990.
13. Newman DK, Lynch K, Smith DA, Cell P. Restoring urinary continence. *Am J Nurs.* 1991;91(1)-28–34.
14. Britton B, Kiesling S. The little muscle that matters. *Am Health.* 1986;5:59–61.
15. Reaching a consensus on incontinence. *Geriatr Nurs.* 1989;10: 78–80.
16. Erickson P. Ostomies: The art of pouching. *Nurs Clin North Am.* 1987;22:311–320.
17. Larson E. Handwashing: It's essential—even when you use gloves. *Am J Nurs.* 1989;89:934–941.
18. Ludwick R. Urethral catheterization. In: Asheervath J, Blevins D, eds. *Handbook of Clinical Nursing Practice.* Norwalk, CT: Appleton-Century-Crofts; 1986:278.
19. Ludwick R. Intermittent self-catheterization. In: Asheervath J, Blevins D, eds. *Handbook of Clinical Nursing Practice.* Norwalk, CT: Appleton-Century-Crofts; 1986:311–313.

BIBLIOGRAPHY

Alterescu KB. Colostomy. *Nurs Clin North Am.* 1987;22:281–289.

Alterescu V. The ostomy: What do you teach the patient? *Am J Nurs.* 1985;85:1250–1253.

Bates P. A troubleshooter's guide to indwelling catheters. *RN.* 1981; 44:63–68.

Beaman E. I'll never take bladder catheters for granted again. *RN.* 1985;48:30–32.

Birdsall C, Brassi O, et al. How do you use renal irrigations? *Am J Nurs.* 1987;87:909–910.

Broadwell DC. Peristomal skin integrity. *Nurs Clin North Am.* 1987; 22:321–322.

Clarke B. Bowel preparations for diagnostic procedures. *Nurs Times.* 1989;1:46–47.

Colling J. Educating nurses to care for the incontinent patient. *Nurs Clin North Am.* 1988;23:279–289.

Erickson PJ. Ostomies: The art of pouching. *Nurs Clin North Am.* 1987;22:311–320.

Ganong WF. *Review of Medical Physiology.* Norwalk, CT: Appleton & Lange; 1991.

Groth K. Age-related changes in the gastro-intestinal tract. *Geriatr Nurs.* 1988;9:278–280.

Hahn K. Think twice about diarrhea. *Nursing 87.* 1987;17:78–80.

Hahn K. Think twice about urinary incontinence. *Nursing 88.* 1988; 18:65–67.

Hardy M, Votava K, Stubbings M. Managing indwelling catheters in the home. *Geriatr Nurs.* 1985;6:280–285.

Henderson J, Taylor K. Age as a variable in an exercise program for the treatment of simple urinary stress incontinence. *J Obstet Gynecol Neonatal Nurs.* 1987;16:266–272.

Kaltreider DL, et al. Can reminders curb incontinence? *Geriatr Nurs.* 1990;11:17.

Kuhns-Hastings J. Management of female incontinence with Kegel exercises. *AAOHN.* 1988;36:78–83.

Maresca J, Stringari S. Assessment and management of acute diarrhea illness in adults. *Nurs Practitioner.* 1986;11:15–28.

McConnell E. Assessing the bladder. *Nursing 85.* 1985;15:44–46.

Miller J. Assessing urinary incontinence. *J Gerontol Nurs.* 1990;16: 15.

Newman DK, Smith DA. Incontinence, the problem patients won't talk about. *RN.* 1989;52:42.

O'Connor EM. How to identify and remove fecal impactions. *Geriatr Nurs.* 1984;5:158–161.

Pieper B, et al. Inventing urinary incontinence devices for women. *Image.* 1989;21(4):205.

Preshlock K. Detecting the hidden VTI. *RN.* 1989;vol?:65–69.

Robb S. Urinary incontinence verification in elderly men. *Nurs Res.* 1985;34:278–282.

Roe B. Catheter care: An overview. *Int J Nurs Studies.* 1985;22:45–55.

Roe B, Reid F, Brocklehurst J. Comparison of four urine drainage systems. *J Adv Nurs.* 1988;13:374–382.

Rogers W. Urinary tract irritation from shampoo. *Am J Nurs.* 1986; 86:66–67.

Ruge C. Catheter-related VTIs: What's the best way to prevent them? *Nursing 87.* 1987;17:50–51.

Smith C. Assessing bowel sounds. *Nursing 88.* 1988;18:42–43.

Smith D. The ostomy: How is it managed? *Am J Nurs.* 1985;85: 1246–1249.

Touch DC. Pelvic floor musculature exercises in treatment of anatomical urinary stress incontinence. *Phys Ther.* 1988;68:652.

Watt R. The ostomy: Why is it created? *Am J Nurs.* 1985;85:1242–1245.

Wright B, Staats D. The geriatric implications of fecal impaction. *Nurs Practitioner.* 1986;11:53–65.

Wyman J. Nursing assessment of the incontinent geriatric outpatient population. *Nurs Clin North Am.* 1988;23:169–187.

CHAPTER 27

Oxygenation

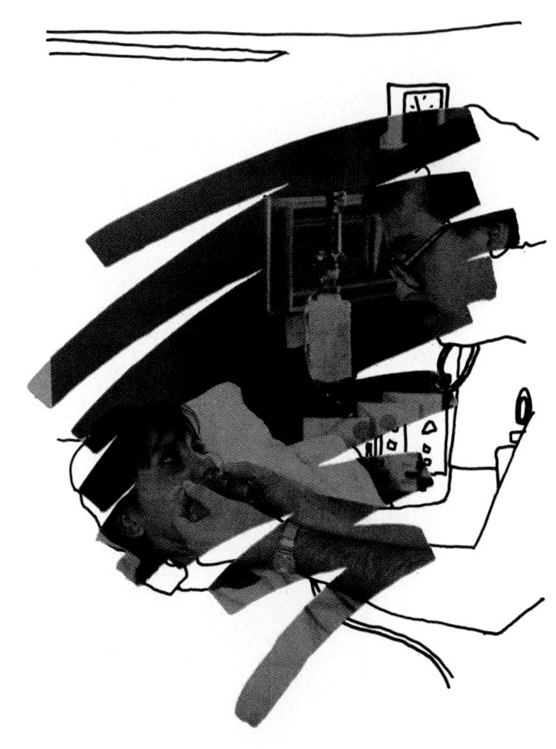

Behavioral Objectives

Upon completion of this chapter, the student will be able to:

1. Discuss the major organs involved in each of the following processes: ventilation, diffusion, perfusion, and cellular respiration.
2. Define and describe the processes of ventilation, diffusion, perfusion, and cellular respiration.
3. Discuss the impact of general health, development, and the environment on oxygenation.
4. Discuss at least two factors that cause alterations in ventilation, diffusion, perfusion, and cellular respiration.
5. Discuss how these factors can cause hypoventilation, hyperventilation, or tissue necrosis.
6. List data that are important in an oxygenation history.
7. Describe essential elements of an oxygenation examination.
8. List at least five laboratory tests or diagnostic examinations relevant to oxygenation.
9. Define three nursing diagnoses describing altered oxygenation and identify and explain at least two etiologies for each nursing diagnosis.
10. Describe at least two examples of nursing implementation for preventive, supportive, restorative, and rehabilitative oxygenation care.
11. Discuss nurses' responsibilities associated with oxygen administration.
12. Identify strategies to evaluate effectiveness of nursing implementation to support oxygenation.
13. Write a client care plan to promote optimum oxygenation for a specific client.

KEY TERMS

anatomical dead space
atelectasis
diastole
diffusion
expiration
expiratory reserve volume
functional residual capacity
hematocrit
hemoglobin
hyperpnea
hyperventilation
hypoventilation
hypoxia
inspiration
inspiratory capacity
inspiratory reserve volume
oxygenation
perfusion
residual volume
splinting
surfactant
sustained maximal inspiration
systole
tachypnea
tidal volume
total lung capacity
ventilation
vital capacity

Oxygen is fundamental to all life processes. Cells require oxygen to carry out their metabolic processes. Therefore, a steady supply of oxygen to each body cell is a primary bodily need. Airway, breathing, and circulation are always the first priorities for life. Oxygenation, the process of supplying the body cells with oxygen, is a multistep process. After air is inhaled and its oxygen extracted, the oxygen must be delivered to the cells. In addition, breathing and circulation work to remove the waste products of cellular metabolism and transport these to the proper organs for excretion or chemical breakdown.

Since oxygenation is so fundamental to life, any compromise of oxygenation can be a serious problem. Nurses can prevent some oxygenation problems and can teach clients how to prevent others. Nurses must also be able to intervene when oxygenation problems occur. Some clients who are at special risk for oxygenation problems include preoperative and postoperative clients, people who are sedentary or immobile, those with chronic illness, individuals with active respiratory disease, the very old and the very young, those with cardiovascular risk factors or disease, smokers, people exposed to heavy air pollution, and those exposed to respiratory hazards in the workplace.

Diseases affecting oxygenation are major causes of disability in North America. In the United States, mortality from lung disease is increasing faster than that for any other disease category,[1] while diseases of the heart and blood vessels are the leading cause of death.[2] In addition to those who die, many more people suffer the consequences of these diseases each year. Death caused by these diseases is often preceded by a long period of disability, suffering, and lowered quality of life.

Section 1. Understanding Oxygenation

THE PROCESS OF OXYGENATION

Oxygenation is the process of supplying oxygen to the body cells to support their metabolic processes. The three major processes of oxygenation are:

- **Ventilation:** Moving air into and out of the lungs.
- **Diffusion:** The process of gas exchange between alveoli and capillaries and between capillaries and tissues.
- **Perfusion:** Delivery of blood to the body for cellular gas exchange.

Perfusion involves the pumping action of the heart, the vascular delivery system of the blood, and the hemoglobin that carries most body oxygen and carbon dioxide.

The body oxygenates itself by drawing in air from the environment, carrying it through a series of passageways in the lungs, and exchanging the oxygen across an alveolar–capillary membrane to the blood. The heart pumps the oxygenated blood to all body cells to supply their energy and oxygenation needs. The waste product of cellular oxygen metabolism is carbon dioxide, which moves out of the cells and into the blood to be carried to the lungs for excretion. Other cellular waste products are delivered by the blood to the appropriate organs for breakdown and excretion.

Ventilation

Ventilation is accomplished through respiration, or the inhaling and exhaling of air via the respiratory tract. The respiratory tract has two divisions: (1) the upper airways and (2) the lower respiratory tract, which lies within the thoracic cavity.

Upper Airways. The upper portion of the respiratory tract consists of the nose, pharynx, larynx, and trachea. These structures have several functions. First, they form the passageway for air to enter the body. Because the entering air comes directly from the environment, many foreign substances can enter the body with the incoming air. To protect the body from harmful substances, there are several respiratory defense mechanisms (Table 27–1), the first of which, air filtration, occurs in the upper airway.

Normally, air enters the nose through the nares and moves to the pharynx on its way to the trachea. However, air may enter through the mouth rather than the nose. When this occurs, the conditioning and protective functions of the nose are lost, and dry, unfiltered air passes to the lungs. This can allow drying and irritation of the lung tissues as well as the entry of foreign particles.

The pharynx also allows for the passage of food and is the site of the larynx. In the back of the pharynx, at the base of the tongue, is the epiglottis, a small flap that closes over the airway to prevent food or foreign matter from entering the airway during swallowing. When the epiglottis is open, air moves down to the larynx, where the vocal cords are located, and on into the trachea.

The trachea, a passageway for air, is a cylindrical tube about 10 to 15 cm long and 1.5 cm in diameter in an adult. It is composed of C-shaped rings of cartilage that are incomplete on the posterior side. The cartilage supports the airway and keeps it stable and open. The rings are held together by elastic ligaments, connective tissue, and smooth muscle. The trachea divides (or bifurcates) into the right and left mainstem bronchi at a point called the carina.

Lower Respiratory Tract. The lungs, which lie inside the thoracic cavity, make up the lower respiratory tract. They are separated from each other by the mediastinal structures (the structures that are in the middle of the chest). The lungs are cone-shaped organs with narrow ends (apices) at the top and wide bases at the bottom. The right lung is divided into three major divisions or lobes, while the left lung has two lobes. Each lobe is divided into smaller compartments, or lobules, which are further divided into still smaller segments, acini. The final division is into alveoli (air sacs), which are the site of air exchange.

Air is supplied to the lungs via the trachea and the right and left mainstem bronchi. The right mainstem bronchus is shorter, straighter, and wider than the left. Each bronchus divides several times to form the lobar, segmental, and subsegmental bronchi, and finally the bronchioles. The most distant bronchioles are called the terminal and respiratory bronchioles. The pattern in which these airways branch is like an upside-down tree. Therefore, the structure is often called the respiratory tree (Fig. 27–1).

The diameter of each successive generation of branches of the respiratory tree is smaller than that of the preceding generation, and there are more branches in each generation. As a result, the surface area of each successively smaller section is larger than that of the section preceding it. There are about 16 generations of bronchi from the trachea. There is no gas exchange up to this point; the bronchi act solely as passages for air. The bronchi must, however, be filled with air with each breath. Because the air that fills the respiratory tree is not available for exchange, it is essentially wasted air and is called **anatomical dead space.** It comprises a volume of about 1 mL/lb normal body weight or about 150 mL in a 150-lb adult.[4]

Each terminal bronchiole supplies its own unit of several alveoli, called an acinus. The alveoli within the acinus do not have separate connections with the terminal bronchiole that serves them, but are of various shapes and interconnected to each other (see Fig. 27–1). The openings that connect them are called the pores of Kohn. These pores allow air to circulate among the alveoli so that, with a second or less after inspiration, all alveoli in the acinus have the same gas concentration. The individual alveolus is one layer of cells thick and is built on a structure of elastin and muscle fibers.

TABLE 27–1. RESPIRATORY DEFENSE MECHANISMS

Mechanism	Description	Factors That Reduce Defense
Air filtration	Nasal hairs, sharp angles of inside of nose, and nasal mucous membrane trap most large foreign particles that are inhaled.	Chronic, prolonged mouth breathing.
Mucociliary clearance	Mucus in the lower airways traps incoming particles and debris. Mucus contains secretory immunoglobulin A (IgA), which helps protect against bacteria and viruses. Many cilia (hairlike projections) beat rhythmically to move the mucus and trapped debris to the mouth for swallowing and expectoration.	Thickened sputum; dehydration; smoking; high oxygen levels; infection; drugs such as atropine, alcohol, anesthetics.
Cough	Clears airway by high-pressure, high-velocity airflow.	Lung disease; neuromuscular disease, intubation, thickened sputum.
Sneeze	Irritation to the nose stimulates trigeminal reflex to clear nose.	
Reflex bronchoconstriction	Inhalation of irritants (dust, allergens, aerosols, fumes, smoke) triggers immediate bronchoconstriction to shut out the irritant. Protection is most effective if the dose of irritant is small and exposure time brief.	Airways may be excessively irritable and overreact to inhalation of irritants, as in asthma.
Alveolar macrophages	Primary defense in alveoli. Macrophages rapidly phagocytize inhaled foreign particles. Debris from phagocytic process is moved to airways or to lymphatic system for removal from body. Nonphagocytized particles may remain in lungs for indefinite periods and stimulate tissue changes. Examples: asbestos, coal dust, silica, debris from smoking.	Smoking cigarettes or marijuana, air pollution, drugs such as alcohol, and steroids.
Immunologic defenses	T and B lymphocytes and certain phagocytes function in complex pattern to defend against foreign invasion. IgA is contained in airway mucus. This helps defend against sinus and respiratory infections.[3]	Certain lung and systemic diseases, such as AIDS; thickened sputum; infection; drugs such as atropine.
Sieve and filtering mechanisms	Pulmonary capillaries filter out large bacteria, blood clots, and fat globules to protect the heart, brain, and other body areas. If particles filtered out are small, they are handled by macrophages or immunologic defenses. If large, they may obstruct a pulmonary vessel and cause clinical symptoms.	

Thoracic Cavity. The chest wall structures include the rib cage, intercostal muscles, and diaphragm (Fig. 27–2). The chest is lined with parietal and visceral pleura (see Fig. 27–1). These pleural membranes are joined at the edges to form a potential space (intrapleural space). Their function is to secrete small amounts of pleural fluid, which lubricates the pleura and causes them to work as a single unit while sliding over each other during respiration. In other words, the lungs stick to the chest wall because of the pleural fluid. Anything (fluid, air, and so forth) that intervenes in the intrapleural space has the potential to reduce the adhesiveness between the two pleural membranes and to take up space, so that the lung volume is decreased. This then decreases oxygenation.

The sternum, spine, and 12 pairs of ribs shape, support, and protect the thorax. Several muscles are attached to the ribs. The major muscle of respiration is the diaphragm, a dome-shaped muscle that separates the chest and the abdomen. When the diaphragm contracts, it descends, increasing the size of the thoracic cavity. The abdominal contents are pushed downward by the diaphragmatic movement. Conditions such as obesity, abdominal distension, and pregnancy limit the downward movement of the diaphragm and thus may limit the depth of respiration. Upward movement of the diaphragm may be impeded by conditions that trap excess air in the lungs (such as asthma). When diaphragmatic action is limited or breathing is labored, the accessory muscles, including the scalene, sternocleidomastoid, and intercostal muscles, are used to increase the size of the chest cavity so that air may enter. The external intercostal muscles and parasternal muscles normally raise the rib cage and increase the size of the thoracic cavity. When a deep inspiration is forced, the scalene muscles and sternocleidomastoid muscles aid in the extra expansion and raising of the rib cage, thereby increasing the size of the thoracic cavity. Forced exhalation is accomplished by a squeezing action of the intercostal muscles.

Mechanics of Breathing. Breathing consists of two phases: **inspiration** (moving air in) and **expiration** (moving air out). Air movement results from changing intrathoracic pres-

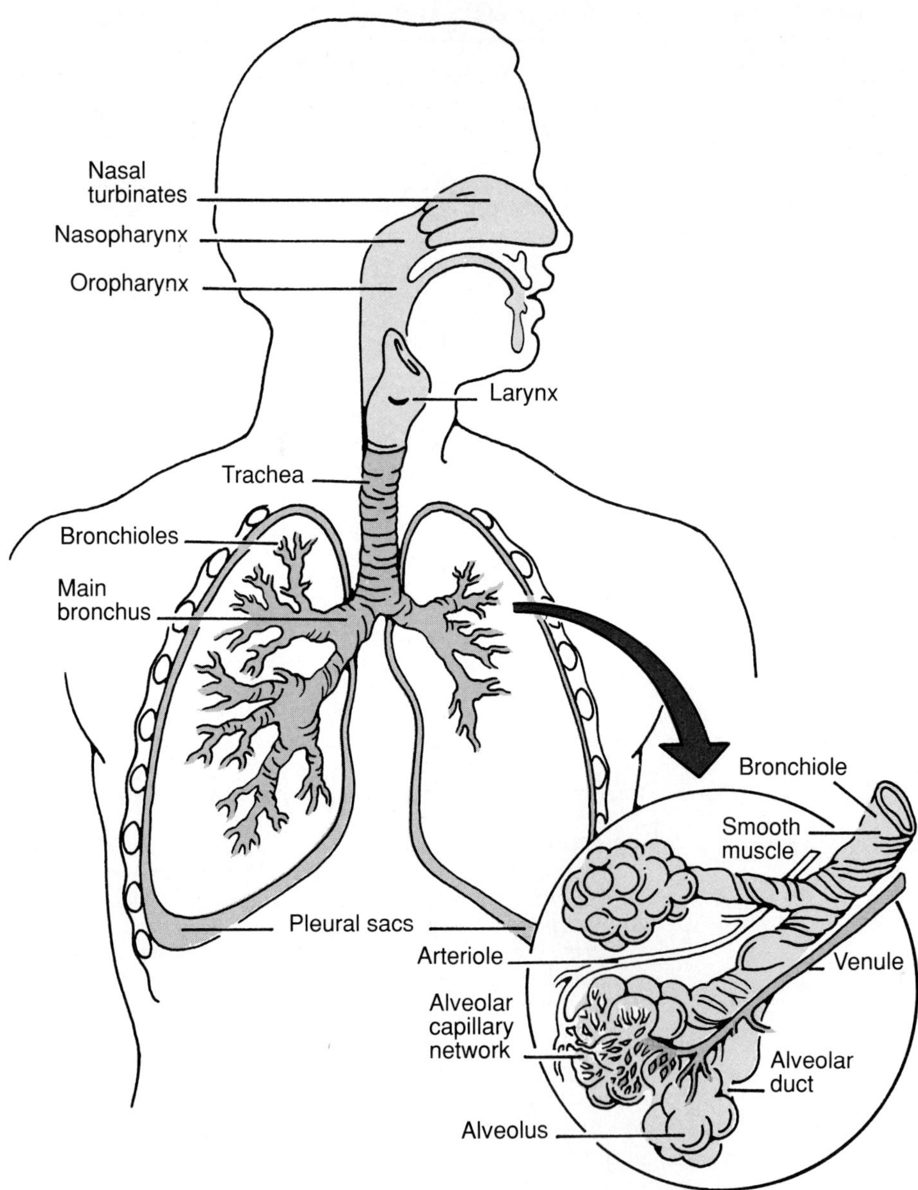

Figure 27–1. The respiratory tract.

sures in relation to atmospheric pressure, because gases always flow from an area of greater pressure to one of lesser pressure. When the pressure inside the chest is lower than atmospheric pressure, outside air flows into the chest. When the pressure inside the chest is greater than outside atmospheric pressure, air flows out of the chest.

The body lowers intrathoracic pressure by enlarging the thoracic cavity—the diaphragm contracts (lowers) and the chest wall expands. In quiet respiration, the diaphragm moves only about 1 cm. However, in forced inspiration, the diaphragm can move about 10 cm. To stimulate exhalation, the thorax and diaphragm relax and allow the chest cavity to decrease in size. This increases internal pressure and causes exhalation of air into the atmosphere.

Air movement, and thus ventilation, is facilitated by an upright or seated posture. The airways are larger in the upright position than in the supine. Normally, the bases of the lungs are better ventilated than the apices when a person is in an upright position.[4]

Control of Ventilation. Respiration is one of the few bodily functions that may be under either automatic or partial voluntary control.

Automatic Control. When control of respiration is automatic and unconscious, respiration is precisely regulated to supply appropriate amounts of oxygen to the body cells and to rid them of carbon dioxide (CO_2). Respiratory rate

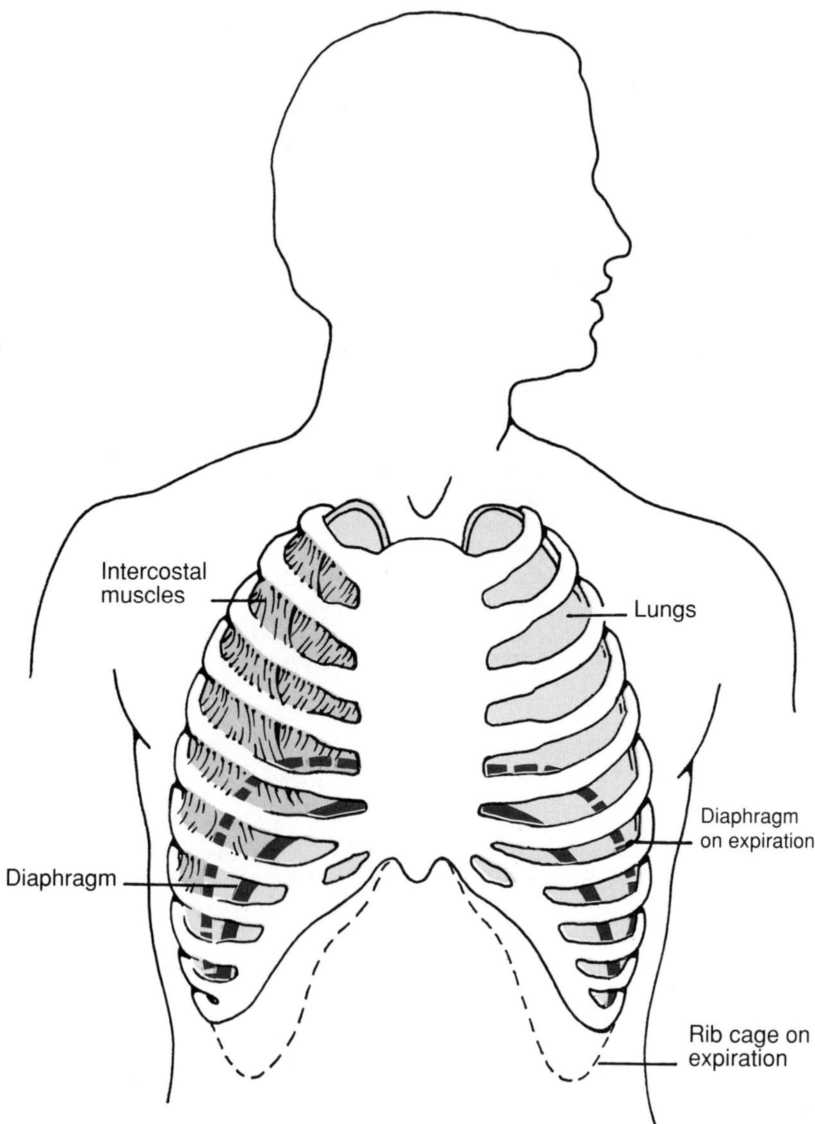

Figure 27–2. Chest wall structures.

and depth change quickly to accommodate varying metabolic needs. Respiration is ultimately controlled in the respiratory center, a collection of nerve fibers and cells located bilaterally in the medulla and pons sections of the brain. This respiratory center receives peripheral signals, both chemical and mechanical, from the body. In response, it sends impulses to the diaphragm and accessory muscles via the spinal cord and the phrenic nerves, which exit the spinal column at C-4. The respiratory center contains both chemoreceptors and mechanical sensors.

The chemoreceptors in the respiratory center respond to changes in the chemical composition of the blood and body fluids. The central chemoreceptors, which are located in the medulla, respond primarily to changes in acid–base balance or hydrogen ion concentration (pH). Increases in hydrogen ion concentration (decreased, or acid pH) stimulate ventilation, whereas decreases in body acids (increased, or alkaline pH) inhibit it.

The carbon dioxide level (Pco_2) in the blood is a primary regulator of ventilation because it affects the pH (acid–base level) of the cerebral spinal fluid and therefore the respiratory center. When a person breathes very rapidly or deeply, more CO_2 is excreted than usual, which elevates the pH of the blood. When the respirations are slower or more shallow, CO_2 builds up, reducing blood pH.

Under normal circumstances, Pco_2 is much more important than Po_2 (oxygen level) in regulating respirations; but if disease has rendered the cerebral chemoreceptors insensitive to higher than usual Pco_2 levels, a decrease in Po_2 can stimulate respiration via the peripheral chemoreceptors instead. This is called the **hypoxic respiratory drive.** The peripheral chemoreceptors are located in the carotid bodies, which are found at the bifurcation of the common carotid arch. These respond to decreases in arterial Pco_2 and to increases in arterial Pco_2. The perceived oxygen changes are conveyed to the respiratory center as a secondary regulator of respirations.

Mechanical sensors also play a part in regulating respirations. These are located in the lungs, upper airways, chest wall, and diaphragm. They are stimulated by such physical factors as airway obstruction, irritants, muscle stretching, and alveolar wall distortion. These are often minor everyday occurrences, such as inhaling noxious fumes or pollens. Pulmonary stretch receptors, a type of mechanical sensor, activate as the lungs inflate, causing the inspiratory center to prevent further expansion of the lungs and chest. This is called the Hering-Breuer reflex. If irritant receptors are stimulated, rapid, shallow breathing and bronchoconstriction result, preventing the irritant from reaching the gas-exchange surfaces.

The impulses from the mechanical sensors, including the Hering-Breuer reflex, are sent to the brain via the vagus nerve, which is part of the parasympathetic nervous system. As noted above, stimulation of the vagus nerve can cause bronchoconstriction (narrowing of the airways), which increases the work of breathing. If drugs are used to stimulate the sympathetic nervous system, the airways will relax and open somewhat (bronchodilation). The result will be easier breathing.

Pain and emotional stimuli also affect respiration, indicating that there must be afferent fibers from the limbic system and the hypothalamus to the respiratory neurons in the brainstem.[5] Typically, breathing becomes more rapid and shallow when a person is experiencing pain or a strong emotion. This response can be overridden by voluntary control, discussed in the next section.

Voluntary Control. Respiration can also occur under voluntary control. If a person wishes to breathe rapidly or slowly, this can be done for a certain period of time. A person cannot, however, voluntarily cease to breathe long enough to cause death. Ultimately, the brain will supersede voluntary control to keep the person alive. Respirations may also be consciously controlled for short periods of time by a person with respiratory problems. These methods of voluntary control can be taught as breathing exercises.

Lung Volumes and Capacities. There are anatomic measurements for the various amounts of air that can be contained in the lungs. The standard terminology for lung volumes and capacities and their definitions are given in Box 27–1. The simple lung volumes are listed first. The capacities, which are combinations of the volumes, are listed last. Anything that affects the volume of air contained in the lung can affect lung volumes and capacities. For example, a person with asthma or emphysema tends to retain air in the chest. This increases the residual volume, which in turn increases the functional residual capacity and lowers the tidal volume, the inspiratory reserve volume, and the expiratory reserve volume. The volumes and capacities are diagrammed in Figure 27–3.

BOX 27–1. STANDARDIZED TERMINOLOGY FOR LUNG VOLUMES AND CAPACITIES

Tidal volume (VT). The volume of gas that is moved with each breath. Composed of the volume entering the alveoli plus the volume remaining in the airway (about 500 mL in an adult).

Expiratory reserve volume (ERV). The maximum amount of gas that can be expired with a forced expiration.

Residual volume (RV) The volume of gas that remains in the lungs at the end of a forced expiration.

Inspiratory reserve volume (IRV). The maximum volume of gas that can be inhaled with a forced inspiration.

Inspiratory capacity (IC). Tidal volume plus inspiratory reserve volume.

Functional residual capacity (FRC). Expiratory reserve volume plus residual volume.

Vital capacity (VC). Inspiratory reserve volume plus tidal volume plus expiratory reserve volume.

Total lung capacity (TLC). Maximum volume of gas that the lungs can contain. Inspiratory capacity plus functional residual capacity or vital capacity plus residual volume. TLC is not a volume of air that can be exchanged.

Derived from data contained in Slonim NB, Hamilton LH. *Respiratory Physiology*, 3rd ed. St. Louis: Mosby; 1976.

Surfactant. **Surfactant** is a lipoprotein that decreases alveolar surface tension and thus increases alveolar stability. The alveolus is unstable and has a natural tendency to collapse. If the alveoli collapsed or closed at the end of each breath, a very high inspiratory pressure would be needed to force them open again to receive the next breath. Surfactant prevents the alveoli from collapsing with each breath and decreases the pressure needed to inflate the alveoli on the next breath. Surfactant thus reduces the work of breathing.[6] Surfactant also helps keep the alveoli dry by preventing movement of fluid from the capillaries into the alveoli. Surfactant is short acting, and so it must be continually replenished. Normal ventilation seems to be the most important factor in replenishment of surfactant. Hypoventilation may therefore lead to **atelectasis** (collapse of alveoli which may be limited to a small area or involve the whole lung) due to the diminished renewal of surfactant. To summarize, decreased oxygenation leads to decreased surfactant, which leads to decreased surface tension and widespread alveolar collapse. Cigarette smokers also have decreased levels of surfactant.

Diffusion

Diffusion, the process of oxygen–carbon dioxide exchange, occurs via the alveolar–capillary membrane, located in the lungs.

Alveolar–Capillary Membrane. The respiratory zone of the lung, where air exchange occurs, consists of the most distal

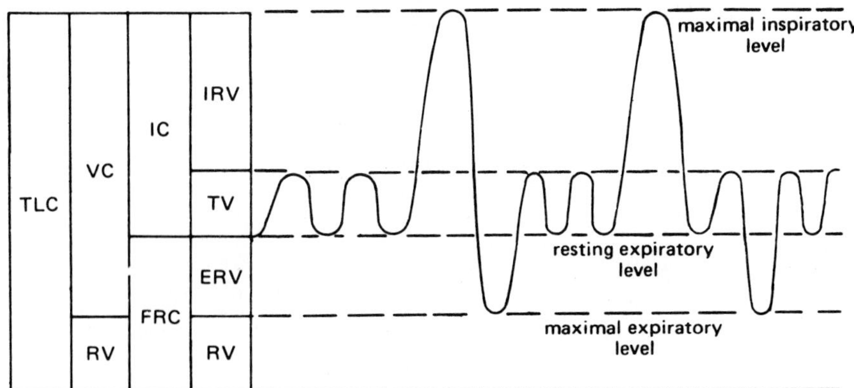

Figure 27–3. Lung volumes. (*From Hunsinger DL, Lisnerski KJ, Maurizi JJ, Phillips ML.* Respiratory Technology. *Reston, VA: Reston; 1980: 456.*)

respiratory bronchioles and the alveoli. An adult has about 300 million alveoli, with a total volume of about 2500 mL and a surface area for diffusing that is about the size of a tennis court. The alveoli are separated from the pulmonary capillaries by a membrane that is only one cell thick. This is the actual site of gas exchange[5] (Fig. 27–4). Conditions that increase the distance between the alveolus and the pulmonary capillary reduce gas exchange. Such conditions include pulmonary edema, where there is fluid in the interstitial space between the alveolus and the capillary. An infection such as pneumonia reduces gas exchange because inflammatory exudate inside the alveolus prevents oxygen from getting to the alveolar–capillary interface.

The Lung's Circulation. The lung has two circulatory systems: the pulmonary circulation, which provides blood for gas exchange with the alveoli, and the bronchial circulation, which supplies the metabolic needs of the pulmonary tissues.

The pulmonary circulation begins with the pulmonary artery, which arises from the right ventricle of the heart and branches so that each alveolus is in direct communication with a pulmonary capillary. This is where gas exchange (diffusion) occurs. The oxygenated blood is then pumped to the left side of the heart for distribution to the body. The pulmonary circulation also serves the oxygenation needs of the bronchi and alveoli.

The other lung tissues are oxygenated by blood from the bronchial circulation, which branches off from the bronchial arteries. These arteries arise from the thoracic aorta. The bronchial circulation supplies the lung's supporting tissues, nerves, and the outer layers of the pulmonary arteries and veins. In the event of interruption of the pulmonary circulation, the bronchial circulation can support the metabolic needs of the alveoli and bronchioles as well. This prevents an obstructed pulmonary capillary from causing the death of these tissues.[3]

Movement of Gases. Dalton's Law states that any one gas in a mixture of gases behaves as though it were the only gas present. Therefore, gases other than oxygen and carbon dioxide that are in the air do not have to be considered when studying the gases of respiration. The various respiratory gases are measured as partial pressures, or the pressure exerted by any single gas in a mixture of gases.[5] When these gases are discussed, the capital letter P is used before the chemical abbreviation for the gas (for example, Po_2). If the partial pressure in the alveolus is being discussed in particular, a small capital A is added after the P (for example, PAO_2). Further definitions are found in Box 27–2.

As previously stated, the alveolar–capillary membrane is only one cell thick. Oxygen and carbon dioxide move easily across this membrane by diffusion from areas of higher pressure to areas of lower pressure. As the alveoli fill with air on inhalation, the oxygen concentration is higher in the alveoli than in the capillary blood. Therefore, oxygen diffuses into the blood. In contrast, the pulmonary capillary blood returning from the body is high in carbon dioxide, which diffuses into the alveoli for excretion by exhalation. Carbon dioxide is 20 times more diffusible than oxygen, so Pco_2 is a better measure of ventilation, or the amount of air being moved by the lungs, than is Po_2.

The actual Po_2 of inhaled air depends on the barometric pressure of the environment. Po_2 is lower at high altitudes than at sea level. Therefore, living at a high altitude for about 6 weeks will cause the body to manufacture extra red blood cells (mild polycythemia) to compensate for the lower Po_2 in the outside air.

Once oxygen enters the body, some of its partial pressure is lost as it moves through the various body membranes and structures and as it is used by the cells. The body's oxygen level can be changed by administering oxygen therapy. This increases the amount of oxygen in the inhaled air and thus raises oxygen levels in every area of the body without a change in respiration.

Perfusion

Perfusion is accomplished via the action of the heart, the circulatory system, and the blood that is moved through the circulatory system.

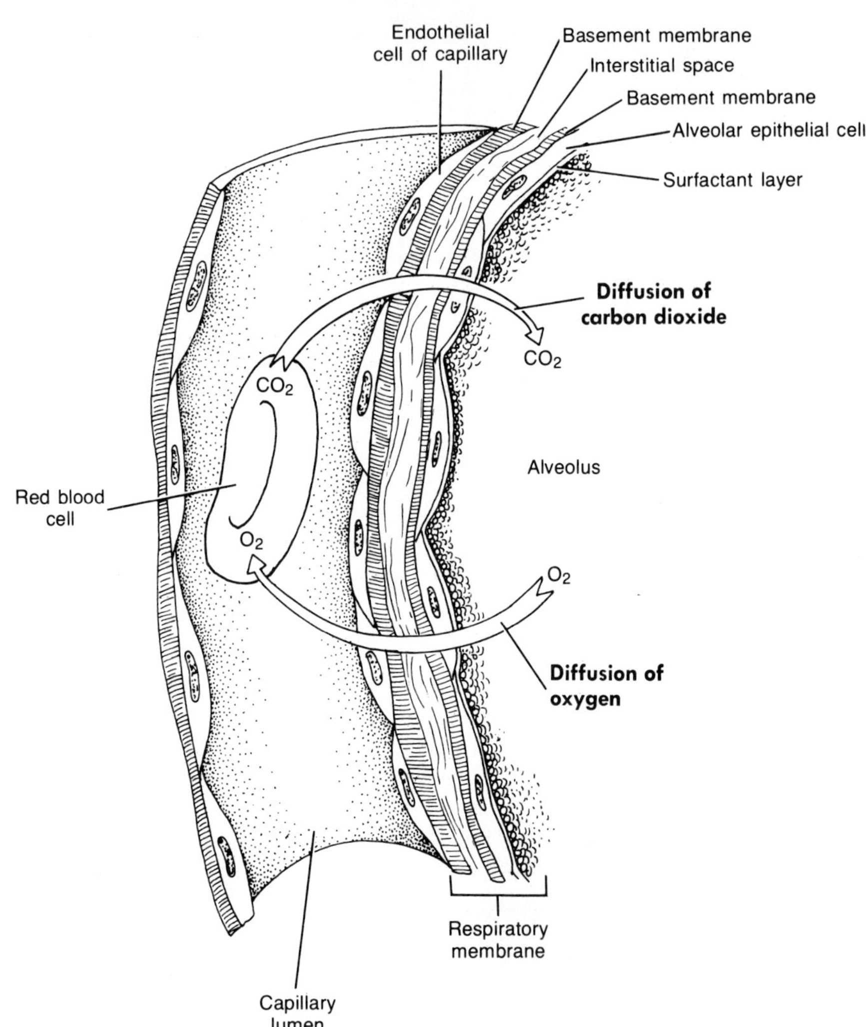

Figure 27–4. Alveolar capillary membrane. (*From Sexton DL.* Nursing Care of the Respiratory Client. *Norwalk, CT: Appleton & Lange; 1989: 14.*)

The Heart. The heart is a double pump that keeps the body alive by circulating the blood. It has the ability to adjust the rate and force of its contraction as the body's needs for blood supply change.

Anatomy. The heart is composed of four chambers: the right and left atria and the right and left ventricles (Fig. 27–5). Each side of the heart is composed of one atrium and one ventricle. The atria are storage areas and passageways for the blood to reach the ventricles. The ventricles are muscular structures that create the pumping force to move the blood: the right ventricle to the lungs and the left ventricle to the rest of the body. Ordinarily, the pressure in the pulmonary vessels is low, so relatively little force is required to move the blood to the lungs. As a result, the right ventricle is a relatively thin and weak muscle. The left ventricle, which must generate considerably greater force to pump blood to the entire body, is a heavier, stronger muscle.

The two atria and the two ventricles are each divided by a heavy wall called a septum. The ventricular septum also houses the tissue for conducting the electrical impulses that stimulate the ventricles to contract. Inside the ventricles are bundles of muscle and strong fibers, the chordae tendinae, which are attached to the margins of the valves separating the atria and ventricles. These fibers help the valves to open and close. The four valves of the heart are

BOX 27–2. SYMBOLS DESCRIBING PARTIAL PRESSURES OF SELECTED RESPIRATORY GASES

Po_2	Partial pressure of oxygen in the blood
PAo_2	Partial pressure of oxygen in the alveoli
Pco_2	Partial pressure of carbon dioxide in the blood
$PAco_2$	Partial pressure of carbon dioxide in the alveoli
Pao_2	Partial pressure of oxygen in the arteries
$Paco_2$	Partial pressure of carbon dioxide in the arteries
Pvo_2	Partial pressure of oxygen in the veins
$Pvco_2$	Partial pressure of carbon dioxide in the veins

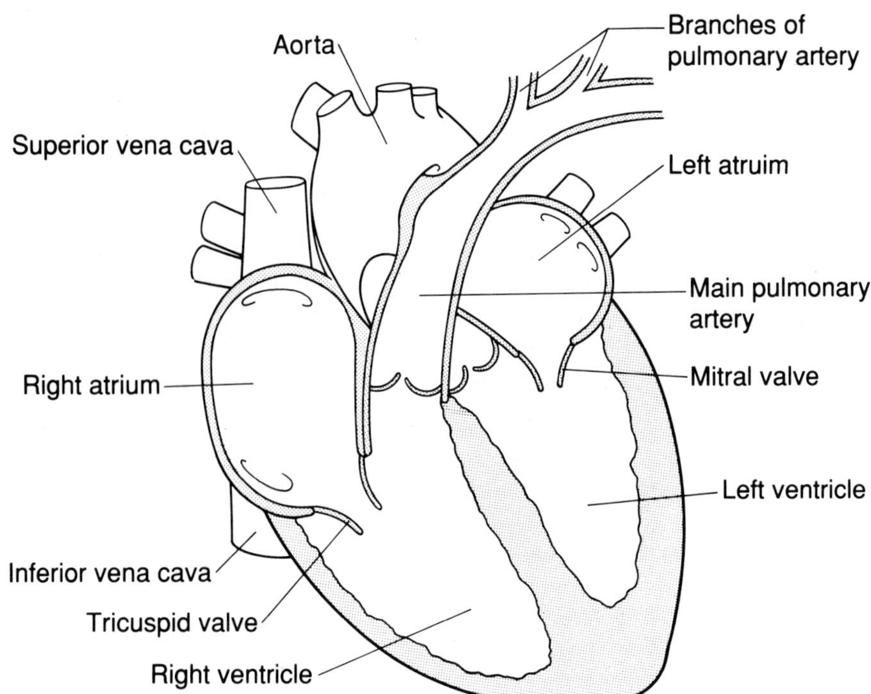

Figure 27–5. Heart: chambers and major vessels. (*From Chesnutt M, Dewar T.* Office and Bedside Procedures. *Norwalk, CT: Appleton & Lange; 1992.*)

the openings between the chambers and the portals of exit for blood leaving the heart. All of the valves are supported by strong fibrous tissue called valve rings.

Cardiac Cycle. The job of the heart is to pump blood. For maximal effect, all of the parts of the heart must act in a synchronized, rhythmic fashion. Several complex mechanisms act to achieve this synchronization. The myocardial, or heart muscle, cells are positioned in such a way that impulses generated in one cell quickly pass to the others, causing the entire group of cells in the atria or ventricle to contract as a unit. Nowhere else in the body are cells grouped in this manner. Each atrium and each ventricle acts as a separate unit. The atria fill simultaneously and they contract simultaneously to empty blood into the ventricles. After they have filled, the ventricles contract simultaneously to eject blood into the pulmonary artery and the systemic circulation. The mechanical events of the cardiac cycle are called systole and diastole. **Systole** refers to the time of ventricular contraction, when blood is being ejected from the heart to the lungs and the rest of the body. **Diastole** is the time of ventricular relaxation, or rest, repolarization, and refilling.

Control of the Heart. The heart has the property of automaticity, or the ability to contract in a regular rhythm. Cardiac action is regulated by a complex electrical conduction system (Fig. 27–6). Normally, this is paced by the Sinoatrial (SA) node, which is located in the right atrium. The SA node is controlled by the vagus nerve, a part of the parasympathetic nervous system. The vagus nerve exerts a slowing action on the SA node to prevent it from discharging electrical impulses too rapidly. The body has other mechanisms for regulating heart activity. These include changes in the systolic blood pressure and changes in blood pH, carbon dioxide, and oxygen levels.

Cardiac function may be affected by sympathetic nervous system stimulation, electrolyte imbalances, drugs, hypoxia, and cardiac injury or disease. These problems may cause the heart to be excitable or irritable, resulting in an irregular or rapid heartbeat. Conversely, the heart may be stimulated too infrequently, resulting in a slow heart rate. A compromised heart may be unable to tolerate excess work or to supply its own oxygen needs and, as a result, may fail.

Circulation. Blood leaves the heart through the arteries. Generally, arteries carry newly oxygenated blood to the tissues, and veins carry deoxygenated blood from the tissues back to the heart and lungs. The pulmonary artery, which carries blood from the heart to the lungs, is the only place in the body where unoxygenated blood is carried by an artery. The pulmonary artery branches into the pulmonary capillary bed for oxygen and carbon dioxide exchange. The oxygenated blood returns from the lungs to the left atrium via the pulmonary vein. This is the only vein in the body that carries newly oxygenated (arterial) blood. Blood leaves the left ventricle via the major artery in the body, the aorta. The aorta branches numerous times into smaller and smaller arteries that supply the entire body with blood. The smallest arterial structures, which branch into the capillary beds, are the arterioles. The junction of the arterioles and

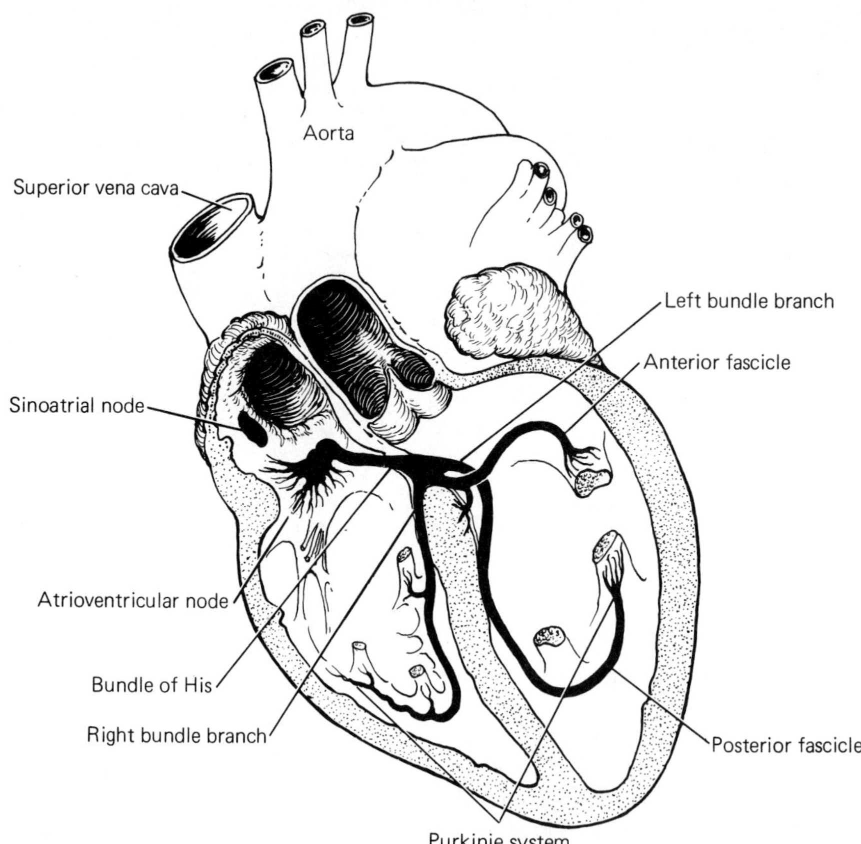

Figure 27–6. Conduction system of the heart. (*From Junqueira LC, Carneiro J.* Basic Histology, *4th ed. Los Altos, CA: Lange; 1983. In: Lindner HH, Clinical Anatomy. Norwalk, CT: Appleton & Lange; 1989: 245.*)

capillaries contains precapillary sphincters that can constrict or relax as necessary to control the flow of blood to a specific capillary bed.

Blood circulating through the capillary bed exits via the venules, or smallest veins in the body. Gradually, these drain the blood into larger veins until the superior vena cava and inferior vena cava drain the collected blood into the heart. Veins in the legs and skeletal muscles contain a series of flaps or folds (valves) to prevent backflow of blood due to gravity and thus aid in the movement of blood returning to the heart.

IMPLICATIONS FOR NURSE–CLIENT COLLABORATION

General Health and Life-style

Oxygen is fundamental to life, and therefore it is not surprising that diseases affecting oxygenation would be a major cause of long-term disability in the United States. Collaboration with clients to help them understand the relationship of life-style factors to oxygenation, and to the quality and length of life, is one of the most significant contributions a nurse can make to a client's care. A healthy life-style, one that promotes fitness, is one of the most important ways to ensure adequate oxygenation and to achieve one's life expectancy.

The Blood. Body oxygenation depends on the transport of oxygenated blood to the body tissues. When the blood leaves the tissues, it carries away the waste products of cellular metabolism, especially carbon dioxide. The blood cells that transport oxygen and carbon dioxide are called erythrocytes, or red blood cells (RBCs). Erythrocytes are small biconcave discs. There are about 5 million of them in each milliliter of blood. Their size and shape enhance their gas exchange ability and enable them to travel within the capillaries. The erythrocytes are formed in the bone marrow of long bones and large flat bones and complete their maturation in the circulatory system. There is rapid turnover of erythrocytes and hence a constant need for new cells. Each erythrocyte lives about 120 days.[7] Because of the rapid turnover, a relatively constant supply of nutrients is required to maintain a stable quantity of erythrocytes. The components of a balanced diet that are essential to erythrocyte synthesis include amino acids, iron, copper, vitamin B_6 (pyridoxine), cobalt, vitamin B_{12} (cobalamin), and folic acid.[8]

The **hematocrit** is a measure of the relationship of erythrocytes (or solids) to liquids in the blood. It is found by taking a blood sample and spinning it rapidly in a centrifuge to force the heavier solid elements (RBCs) to collect at one end of the tube and the lighter, liquid portion of the blood to collect at the other. The relationship between the two portions is then measured. If 40 percent of the length of the tube of blood is solids and 60 percent is liquids, then the hematocrit is said to be 40 percent. Normal hematocrit levels by age are shown in Table 27–6.

The essential component of the erythrocyte for oxygen transport is **hemoglobin,** which is made up of an iron-containing pigment (heme) and a protein (globin). Oxygen is loosely bound to the iron in the heme for distribution to body cells. This combination is called oxyhemoglobin. Each heme molecule can combine with a maximum of four oxygen molecules. A heme molecule that is carrying four oxygen molecules is considered to be 100 percent saturated. When heme is 100 percent saturated, oxygen transfer to tissue is optimal.

If the hemoglobin level is low, or if it is of poor quality and unable to take up normal amounts of oxygen (as in sickle cell anemia), the total amount of oxygen delivered to the tissues will be lower than normal. Normal oxygen transport is also compromised if the iron bound to the heme molecule does not remain in the ferrous state. Certain toxins and oxidizing agents convert ferrous iron to ferric iron, forming methemoglobin, which cannot carry oxygen.

Cellular Respiration

Cellular respiration, or internal respiration, consists of the use of oxygen and production of carbon dioxide by cells and the gaseous exchanges between the cells and their fluid medium.[5] All of the processes discussed thus far exist to support cellular respiration.

Plasma-to-cell Transfer. Hemoglobin-bound oxygen is not directly involved in the gas exchange with tissues. Oxygen diffuses from the hemoglobin molecule into the plasma, and then into the interstitial fluid, and finally into cells. For oxygen to be released from hemoglobin, a gradient must be established. This occurs when the small amount of free oxygen dissolved in plasma diffuses out of the bloodstream as the blood flows through the capillaries. The reduction in plasma Po_2 relative to erythrocyte Po_2 causes hemoglobin to release its oxygen to the plasma. Because the Po_2 of plasma is higher than that of the interstitial fluid or the cells, oxygen diffusion is a continuous process.

Several factors affect the release of oxygen from hemoglobin to the tissues. It is facilitated by an increase in $Paco_2$, greater production of metabolic acids (decreased pH), and an increase in body temperature. Conversely, hemoglobin's affinity for oxygen is greater, and oxygen is therefore less likely to be released, when body temperature falls, pH falls, or $Paco_2$ falls.

The loss of oxygen from the heme molecule increases its affinity for carbon dioxide, for which there is a gradient in the opposite direction. Hence, as oxygen moves into the cells, carbon dioxide moves from cells, to interstitial fluid, to plasma, to erythrocytes for transport to the alveoli, from which it is excreted from the body in the exhaled air.

Oxygen Use. Oxygen is essential to body cells because it is a major component of the reactions that produce cellular energy. The energy, which is produced in the form of adenosine triphosphate (ATP), is essential for the metabolic activities of the body cells. A continuous supply of oxygen is essential if the cells are to be able to carry on their activities.

Cellular oxygen requirements vary according to the demands placed on the cell. The body at rest normally requires about 250 mL of oxygen per minute and produces about 200 mL of CO_2 per minute. Factors that increase oxygen need are fever, exercise, and shivering. Heavy exercise increases muscular oxygen needs and CO_2 production by as much as 20 times. Factors that decrease cellular oxygen need are relaxation and hypothermia.[7]

Anaerobic Metabolism. If the blood is not adequately oxygenated, the diffusion gradient to the tissues is less, so the heme gives up oxygen less readily. A decrease in the oxygen supply to a cell or group of cells leads to a state of partial or total hypoxia. **Hypoxia** is oxygen deficiency at the tissue level. Anaerobic metabolism is the term for the cellular activities that take place when oxygen is not being supplied. Depending on the severity of the hypoxia, the cells may adapt, be injured, or die. With hypoxia occurs, production of ATP is impaired. Glycolysis, or the breaking down of glucose, can continue anaerobically for a time, but this produces only very small amounts of ATP. The waste product of anaerobic metabolism is lactic acid, not carbon dioxide. The lungs cannot rid the body of lactic acid, so it builds up in the body and causes metabolic acidosis.[5] The compensatory response by the lungs, hyperventilation, is discussed in a later section. However, respiratory compensation can be sustained only if there is a sufficient supply of oxygen to the body. Without oxygen, death ensues.

■ FACTORS AFFECTING OXYGENATION IN HEALTH

If the body is well oxygenated, its various organs should function well. A client whose body is well oxygenated should be able to carry out the usual activities of daily living without excess fatigue or dyspnea. There is a range of levels of oxygen need both among healthy individuals and within a given individual at different times and circumstances. Many of the factors that affect oxygenation in healthy or relatively healthy individuals could be considered life-style factors. Others are physiological, developmental, or environmental.

General Health and Life-style

Fitness. Exercise and conditioning, which are closely related, contribute to fitness.

Exercise. Exercise increases the metabolic rate of several major organs, thereby increasing their oxygen requirements. During exercise, skeletal muscles demand and receive a much larger blood supply than they do during rest.

The heart contracts more rapidly and forcefully and the person breathes more deeply and rapidly to supply the extra oxygen needed for exercise. The vessels that supply the exercising muscles dilate to receive the extra blood. Because the heart works harder during exercise, it must supply more oxygenated blood to its own tissues. To accomplish this, the coronary arteries dilate. If they cannot dilate, the lack of adequate oxygen will cause chest pain, limiting the person's ability to exercise.

Conditioning. Conditioning is the improvement in oxygen utilization that occurs in response to regular exercise. Consider the person who is beginning an aerobic exercise program. At first, this person can walk but does not have the stamina to run or jog any significant distance; however, after a few weeks of regular exercise, the person can run farther than he or she could walk originally and has more stamina as well. Why? A conditioned muscle requires less oxygen per unit of work than an unconditioned muscle. In other words, the more conditioned a muscle becomes, the less oxygen it needs to accomplish a given task. Hence the cardiopulmonary workload is reduced for all activities when a person is well conditioned. This is why aerobic exercise and conditioning programs are an important part of maintaining good health. The effect of conditioning on oxygenation is further explained in Chapter 30.

Nutrition. Two nutrition-related factors influence oxygenation: weight and nutrient intake.

Weight. Individuals who are overweight sometimes experience compromised oxygenation, because the heavy lower thorax and abdomen reduce the capacity of the lungs to expand. This is a particular problem when the person is lying down. Moreover, the extra muscular work required for body movement when a person is overweight increases oxygen demand. This effect may be magnified if the person is poorly conditioned, which is often the case, as a sedentary life-style is a common contributing factor to obesity. It is not unusual, therefore, for an overweight individual to experience shortness of breath with mild physical exertion.

Nutrient Intake. To produce the quantity and quality of erythrocytes needed for optimum oxygen transport, individuals must consume the nutrients needed to synthesize erythrocytes and hemoglobin (see The Blood, earlier in this chapter). A well-balanced diet should supply sufficient nutrients for healthy individuals to produce adequate erythrocytes. (See also Chap. 25.)

Smoking. Smoking is a life-style choice that is a direct cause of decreased oxygen availability to the body tissues. When a person smokes cigarettes, some of the oxygen in the lungs—and consequently in the blood—is replaced by carbon monoxide from the cigarette smoke. Therefore, bodily oxygenation is reduced. Chronic smokers always have a high level of carbon monoxide in their blood. This is also true of people who live and work with smokers. Smoking in a closed space, such as an automobile, leads to rapid accumulation of carbon monoxide in the enclosed air and a high carbon monoxide level in the blood of everyone inside, whether they are actually smoking or not.

Substance Abuse. Substance abuse is a major problem physiologically, psychologically, and socioeconomically. Various substances can cause diverse oxygenation problems. For example, opiates such as meperidine (Demerol), heroin, and morphine can cause (among other effects) slow, shallow respirations; hypoxia (oxygen deficiency); or even respiratory arrest, hypotension, cardiac dysrhythmias, and thrombophlebitis. The use of alcohol impairs judgment, which can result in drowning, and impairs the protective reflexes of the airway, which increases the risk of aspiration of food or emesis. Barbiturates produce bradycardia (slowed heart rate), hypotension, changes in respiratory rate and depth, and respiratory paralysis and circulatory collapse. Stimulants such as cocaine, amphetamines, and benzene can cause serious tachycardia (increased heart rate), hypertension, tachypnea (rapid shallow breathing), and even cardiac arrest. Hallucinogens such as LSD and PCP can cause tachycardia, hypertension, respiratory paralysis, and hyperthermia (which elevates metabolism). Withdrawing from drugs has serious consequences for oxygenation. Tachycardia, hypertension, respiratory changes, fever, and cardiovascular collapse have been reported.[9]

Emotional Stress. Stress can affect oxygenation by increasing the body's metabolic rate. When a person is upset or under acute stress, the adrenal medulla releases hormones called catecholamines, which act to prepare the body to protect itself. This increases the oxygen need of many body tissues and therefore increases the work of the heart and lungs, which must pump more oxygenated blood to meet the higher oxygen demands.

Development

Although the same general principles apply, there are some differences in the anatomy and physiology related to oxygenation of the body at various age levels, particularly at extremes of age.

Premature Infants, Infants, and Toddlers. Oxygenation is often compromised in premature infants for several reasons. Respiratory distress syndrome (RDS) is common. RDS occurs because premature infants often lack surfactant, which is necessary to maintain alveolar patency. Not only is the work of breathing increased dramatically in RDS, but insufficient oxygen–carbon dioxide exchange results in hypoxia. Premature infants are also at risk for irregular breathing patterns and apnea. There are many possible reasons for this, although general immaturity of body systems, especially respiratory and neurological, is the most common. Respiratory problems are exacerbated if the premature infant is chilled, which occurs readily if adequate measures are not taken to maintain body temperature. Premature infants have poorly developed thermoregulation mechanisms and no immediate way to raise body temperature if the environmental temperature is low.[10]

Term infants may also suffer from respiratory distress if chilled. Infants of diabetic mothers may have delayed lung maturation, which increases their risk for RDS.[11] In the first 3 months of life, infants are obligate nasal breathers due to the large size of the tongue and the shape of the epiglottis.[12] Therefore, it is critical that at least one nostril be kept clear at all times.

There are other anatomical differences that distinguish oxygenation in the newborn from that in adults. For example, the adult chest wall can expand downward, so its size is increased by lowering the diaphragm. Infants do not have this capability. Instead, their chest walls expand outward or horizontally to enlarge the chest cavity for inspiration. Normally, the infant's chest and abdomen are raised and lowered together in this process. In some cases, the infant's nonrigid chest wall may be drawn in during inspiration, creating mild retractions (or indentations of the chest wall). This is considered normal in the neonate. Retractions should disappear as the child becomes older and the chest becomes more rigid. The diaphragmatic-abdominal breathing continues until the child is about 5 years old. If the infant or young child has a respiratory problem, a state of respiratory insufficiency may be reached more quickly than in an older child or adult because the accessory muscles of breathing are not yet well developed.[12]

Infants are susceptible to airway obstruction or collapse because the airway is small and relatively straight and the cartilage that supports it is still soft. This area is susceptible to edema or trauma that would compromise the airway. The risk of airway obstruction continues through toddlerhood. At this age, aspiration of food or small objects is relatively common as well.

The respiratory rate of the infant is rapid, ranging from 30 to 70 breaths per minute; the sleeping respiratory rate is usually less than 40 per minute. The infant's normal pulse is 120 to 160 per minute. The toddler's respiratory rate averages 20 to 30 per minute; pulse rate is 100 to 110.

Preschool and School-aged Children and Adolescents. The cardiorespiratory physiological processes mature throughout childhood. By 7 years of age the transition to thoracic breathing is complete. The normal respiratory and pulse rates decline with age. For example, a preschool child might have a respiratory rate of 20 to 30 and a pulse rate of 90 to 120, while an elementary school age child might have a respiratory rate of 20 to 26 and a pulse rate of 70 to 110. Teenagers' pulse and respiratory rates, and their anatomy and physiology, are the same as that of adults.[12] Preschoolers, school-aged children, and adolescents are frequently exposed to respiratory infections, but these do not usually cause serious problems. Many adolescents try smoking. If this becomes a lifelong habit, serious health risks are likely, as discussed previously.

Older Adults. As a person ages, connective tissue changes cause some loss of lung elasticity. Some individuals also experience postural changes related to osteoporosis, which decrease the capacity for lung expansion. Normal Po_2 gradually declines with age. Healthy people in their 80s, for example, have some measure of alveolar deterioration, even if they have never smoked. This is called physiological emphysema. As a result, the normal Po_2 for an elderly person is somewhat lower than for a younger adult. The exact Po_2 that is normal for each elderly person is an individual matter, but anything above 80 mm Hg is considered acceptable. A low Po_2 may increase the cardiac workload and reduce exercise tolerance somewhat, but for the healthy aging person, it should not compromise the normal activities of daily life. Conditioning and individual factors such as genetics and smoking history affect the elderly person's oxygenation and exercise status far more than do physiological changes.

Environment

Air Quality. Clean air is essential to optimum oxygenation. Today air pollution is either a continuous or intermittent problem in many urban areas and is even a problem in some rural areas. Air stagnation worsens the effects of pollution. Air pollution interferes with oxygenation because some of the noxious gases in the air take the place of oxygen in the lungs and in the blood. Although the amount of pollution necessary to cause disease is not yet known, it is known that low levels of pollution may contain a variety of cancer-causing agents. These include such substances as asbestos and cigarette smoke. Air pollution can also cause beryllium poisoning, acute pneumonitis, and chronic lesions in the alveolar walls. People who drive in very heavy traffic for long periods of time can have a high level of carbon monoxide in their blood.

Air pollution can be either an additive or synergistic risk for cardiopulmonary disease. An additive risk means that a person who is exposed to two risk factors has the same statistical risk for disease as that caused by the two risks added together. A synergistic risk means that when a person is exposed to two risk factors for disease, that person's statistical risk of having the disease is multiplied by many times.

Altitude. The effect of altitude on bodily oxygenation was briefly addressed earlier. Because barometric pressure decreases as altitude increases, the oxygen content of the environmental air is lower at high altitudes than at sea level. If a person travels to a higher altitude and stays there for 6 weeks, extra red blood cells will be produced in order to carry more oxygen to the body cells. Therefore, the person will have increased fatigue and a reduced exercise tolerance for about 6 weeks; only after that time will he or she regain the previous energy level. High altitudes may have a particularly detrimental effect on a person with cardiac or pulmonary disease. Such a person's already compromised bodily Po_2 can fall low enough to cause serious respiratory distress.

Climate. Weather extremes also tend to increase bodily oxygen needs. Oxygen consumption increases in very hot weather as well as in very cold weather. Going out into very cold weather is stressful to the body and should be avoided by people with cardiopulmonary compromise. Individuals with oxygenation problems should not attempt to work outside in excessively hot or cold weather.

ALTERATIONS IN OXYGENATION

Interrelatedness of Oxygenation Processes

The processes that support oxygenation are interrelated. Therefore, a change in one of the processes often affects the others. Without adequate ventilation, for example, diffusion, perfusion, and cellular respiration will not be normal. Interference with diffusion across the alveolar–capillary membrane will compromise perfusion and cell function, unless compensatory changes in ventilation overcome interfering factors. If perfusion problems such as inadequate pumping by the heart or decreased oxygen-carrying capacity persist, ventilation will change to compensate. The compensatory changes are usually adaptive, but they occasionally complicate oxygenation problems.

Alterations in oxygenation may be divided into four categories: (1) altered ventilation, (2) altered diffusion, (3) altered perfusion, and (4) altered cellular respiration.

Altered Ventilation

Altered ventilation refers to changes in the movement of air from the atmosphere to the alveoli. There are two types of altered ventilation: hypoventilation and hyperventilation.

Hypoventilation. **Hypoventilation** is the condition of inadequate movement of air into and out of the lungs. Typically, this is detected by a rise in the P_{CO_2}. It *cannot* be accurately assessed by watching a person breathe. The signs and symptoms of hypoventilation include alterations in respiration (either slow and shallow or deep and labored due to efforts to move additional air), dyspnea (difficulty breathing), orthopnea (difficulty breathing unless sitting or standing), tachycardia, and anxiety. Neurological changes, such as altered judgment, coordination, or level of consciousness, also may be present. Factors contributing to hypoventilation may include airway obstruction, lung or chest pathology, and inappropriate administration of oxygen.

Airway Obstruction. Airway obstruction blocks movement of air into and out of the lungs. As the work of breathing increases, oxygenation may be compromised. Airway obstruction may be caused by a foreign body or by excess secretions, among other factors.

A foreign body is not an uncommon cause of airway obstruction. Children often place small objects or food in their mouths and aspirate them (ie, the object or food goes down the trachea to the lung). Adults aspirate food, fluids, or oral secretions. Once in the lung, the foreign body may partially or completely occlude a small or large airway. The more complete the obstruction and the larger the airway occluded, the more serious the client's respiratory distress will be.

Excessive respiratory secretions may also obstruct the airway when lung pathology is present. For example, a person with pneumonia or chronic bronchitis, both of which cause large amounts of secretions, may be unable to cough effectively to clear the secretions out of the airway. If a large airway or many smaller airways are affected, serious respiratory distress and compromised oxygenation can result.

People who are extremely fatigued, generally debilitated, or who have a neuromuscular disease that affects the chest may retain even moderate amounts of secretions because they are unable to cough well enough to clear them out of the chest. These individuals may also be unable to sustain the increased work of breathing caused by the obstructed airways and so are unable to move air into and out of the lungs effectively. As a result, oxygenation will be compromised.

Decreased Lung Capacity. If lung expansion is restricted, the volume of air that can be exchanged is also limited. Pregnancy is a common cause of decreased lung capacity. As pregnancy advances and the uterus expands, the diaphragm is pushed upward. Therefore, deep breathing is difficult and a subjective sensation of shortness of breath is common. Usually the loss of capacity is not severe enough to cause compromised oxygenation.

A full stomach can compromise respirations in a similar fashion. It is more likely to reduce oxygenation or cause respiratory distress in a person who already has cardiopulmonary disease. This is why those with oxygenation problems are encouraged to eat small meals rather than large ones and to avoid gas-forming foods.

Lung capacity can also be reduced by other circumstances. For example, if a person has pneumonia, many of the alveoli are filled with exudate and are not available for gas exchange. If a person has a chest injury and cannot expand the chest wall normally, the lung capacity is diminished. Diseases causing bony deformity of the thorax may limit lung expansion. These are only a few examples of disorders that can reduce lung capacity and increase the risk for hypoventilation.

Inappropriate Administration of Oxygen. Normally, the body is stimulated to breathe by the buildup of carbon dioxide, which stimulates the respiratory center. If a person has a chronic high CO_2 level, the respiratory center can lose its sensitivity to excess CO_2. When this happens, the peripheral chemoreceptors stimulate the body to breathe by their response to hypoxia or a low oxygen level. If a client who normally retains CO_2 excessively is given a high level of oxygen, the P_{O_2} will not fall to a level low enough to stimulate the peripheral chemoreceptors, and the person will cease to breathe. This sometimes happens to clients with chronic lung disease who turn their oxygen levels up too high in response to dyspnea or respiratory distress.

Hyperventilation. **Hyperventilation** means that a person moves more air through the lungs than normal. This can be assessed by a low Pa_{CO_2} when the arterial blood gases are measured. It cannot be assessed by watching the client breathe. A person's breathing may appear to be deep and rapid when, actually, the individual is simply working very hard to move an abnormally small amount of air. That person may have **tachypnea** (rapid, shallow respirations) or **hyperpnea** (increased rate and depth of respirations), but not necessarily hyperventilation. Some possible causes of hyperventilation are anxiety, pain, reduced atmospheric oxygen, lung pathology, and metabolic acidosis. Some of these are discussed below.

Decreased Atmospheric Oxygen. The body responds to reduced atmospheric oxygen on a short-term basis by hyperventilating. For example, if a person moves to a high altitude or is in a closed space with little available oxygen, the tendency is to breathe more rapidly in order to move more oxygen into the body and improve oxygenation.

Anxiety, Fear, and Pain. Anxiety, fear, and pain are stressors that can cause hyperventilation. Direct stimulation of the respiratory center from the limbic system (activated with strong emotions) may contribute to hyperventilation associated with fear and pain.[5] Conscious voluntary efforts to slow and deepen respirations can overcome stress-induced hyperventilation.

Acid–Base Balance. Metabolic status affects oxygen need in a variety of ways. The body cells must maintain a pH between 7.35 and 7.45 to function correctly. If metabolic acids build up in the body, the cells function less effectively and need more oxygen. In addition, the lungs attempt to reduce the total acid load in the body by eliminating more CO_2 than usual. Hence, hyperventilation can be a physiological response to metabolic acidosis as the lungs work to reduce the body's acid load. Conversely, in a person with metabolic alkalosis, or too little acid in the body, the lungs attempt to conserve acid by depressing ventilation. (Acid–base balance is discussed in detail in Chap. 31.)

Altered Diffusion

In altered diffusion, the ability of the respiratory gases to diffuse from the alveoli to the pulmonary capillaries and back again is impaired. Usually, the problem is one of extra barriers in the diffusion path, either fluid accumulation or excessive secretions, or of altered anatomy of the alveolar–capillary structure.

Fluid Accumulation. Many conditions may cause fluid accumulation in the diffusion path. One is failure of the left ventricle. When the left side of the heart cannot pump effectively, the blood then backs up into pulmonary circulation. The pulmonary capillaries are distensible and can accept a great deal of the blood; however, when they reach their capacity, the fluid is pushed out into the pulmonary interstitium. This results in a layer of fluid between the alveoli and capillaries, which greatly reduces the ability of the gases to diffuse between the alveoli and the pulmonary capillaries. As the condition progresses, fluid seeps into the alveoli as well, so that there are two layers of fluid between the gas in the alveoli and the pulmonary capillaries. As a result, the movement of oxygen and carbon dioxide between the air and the blood is seriously impeded.

Excessive Secretions. Secretions can accumulate in the alveoli for a variety of reasons, such as a chest cold or pneumonia. These secretions cover some of the alveolar surfaces so that the diffusing membrane becomes much thicker. As a result, gaseous movement is hampered.

Alveolar Pathology. Abnormalities of the alveoli may reduce the surface area available for gas exchange. For example, in emphysema, there is destruction of alveolar and capillary tissues. As a result, less surface area is available for gas exchange.

Altered Perfusion

Altered perfusion refers to problems with the delivery of oxygenated blood to the body tissues. A variety of problems can cause altered perfusion. Several of the major ones are discussed here.

Decreased Cardiac Output. The delivery of adequate oxygen to the tissues depends on a normally functioning heart. The left ventricle in particular must pump regularly and energetically to deliver blood to the body. If the functioning of the left ventricle is impaired, the body will not receive an adequate blood supply. This leads to fatigue and impaired organ function. In addition, blood can back up into the lungs, as described above under Fluid Accumulation.

Hypovolemia or Low Hemoglobin Level. For gas exchange to take place, adequate blood volume and adequate numbers of red blood cells must be available to carry the oxygen and nutrients. A serious blood loss (hypovolemia), a low hemoglobin level, or a low red blood cell count could leave the client with too few functioning red blood cells to carry the oxygen needed to nourish the body.

Vascular Occlusions. Delivery of blood to a localized area of the body can be interrupted by a variety of vascular occlusions. The occlusions may be divided into two types: internal and external.

Internal Occlusions. Internal occlusions may be caused by excessive clotting of the blood, stasis of the blood, or excessive viscosity of the blood. If an arterial blood vessel is totally or partially occluded by a clot, the area served by that vessel will not be properly perfused and oxygenated. The effects may be local, such as when the clot is in a leg or an arm, or they may be more widespread, such as when the clot is in the lung or the brain. A clot in the lung would cause hypoxia and its general effects, while a clot in the brain would cause a cerebral vascular accident (stroke).

Conditions of the vessels themselves can also impair the delivery of blood. Conditions involving thickening, loss of elasticity, and calcification of the arterial walls are not uncommon. There may also be deposits of fats, cholesterol, and debris on the inner walls of the arteries. Any of these conditions reduces the size of the involved vessels and reduces their ability to increase in diameter when an increased blood supply is needed in the area. Spasm of the arteries sometimes also occurs. This reduces the blood supply to the area served by the vessel. If it occurs in a vessel that supplies a skeletal muscle, the result is usually pain and reduced exercise tolerance.

External Occlusion. External occlusion of a vessel can result from factors within or outside the body. Either way, the compressed vessel cannot supply the needed amount of blood to body tissues. Within the body, the most common causes of pressure on a vessel are edema (swelling) or tumors. Pressure from outside the body can result from poor positioning (as when one leg is lying directly on top of the other), or from constricting bandages, casts, braces, antiembolism stockings, or clothing (such as garters). Signs and symptoms distal to the compression may include edema, discoloration, discomfort, coolness of the extremity, and diminished pulses. It is always important to check for indicators of external compression if any risk factor (such as a cast) exists and to take all possible measures to prevent external compression of the vessels.

Altered Cellular Respiration

Altered cellular respiration refers to a change in the oxygen–carbon dioxide exchange between the cells and the fluid medium surrounding them. Any of the above alterations may compromise cellular respiration on a local or generalized basis. In addition, fever, edema, toxic substances, or conditions that alter metabolism may influence cellular respiration directly.

BOX 27–3. TERMINOLOGY RELATED TO ALTERATIONS IN OXYGENATION

Hypoxia

- The lack of adequate oxygen supply at the tissue level. Reflected in low Po_2.
- *Signs and symptoms;* Increased respiratory rate and depth, impaired judgment, drowsiness, disorientation, headache, tachycardia, hypertension.

Hypercapnia

- Retention of CO_2 in the body. Reflected by high Pco_2.
- *Signs and Symptoms:* Initially stimulates respiration. If accumulates, produces central nervous system depression (confusion, diminished sensory acuity, coma, respiratory depression).

Hypocapnia

- Low concentration of CO_2. Reflected by low Pco_2. Usually caused by hyperventilation.
- *Signs and symptoms:* Lightheadedness, dizziness, and altered sensation (paresthesias).

Tissue Necrosis

- Tissue death due to low oxygenation.
- *Signs and symptoms:* Pain, darkened color, progressing to white; swelling; liquefaction.

IMPLICATIONS FOR NURSE–CLIENT COLLABORATION

Hypoxia

Although a careful history is a critical component of any assessment, there are times when the health interview must be postponed. Collaborating with a client who is severely hypoxic can be extremely taxing to the client and even inappropriate when hypoxia renders the client breathless or confused. Such manifestations significantly diminish the client's capacity to participate in a health interview, and it may be necessary to shift the focus of collaboration to the client's significant others until the client's condition is improved.

Fever. Fever is the most common condition that has a direct effect on cellular respiration. When the body temperature rises, the rate of metabolic activity increases, creating an increased demand for oxygen throughout the body. As previously discussed, more oxygen is released from hemoglobin when body temperature is elevated, which helps to meet cellular needs.

Some other problems that elevate metabolism are drugs such as steroids and adrenalin, and diseases of the adrenal glands or the thyroid. Metabolic increases can be particularly damaging to persons who have heart disease or compromised brain tissue. These tissues are easily damaged if their oxygen needs are not met.

Edema. In edema, fluid occupies space in interstitial fluid and thereby increases the distance between the cells and the capillaries that bring them oxygenated blood. The increased distance slows diffusion of oxygen from the capillaries to the cells and carbon dioxide from the cells into the bloodstream. Severe edema can significantly alter cellular respiration and result in cellular hypoxia.

Toxins. Toxic substances may prevent tissues from receiving adequate oxygen, even when perfusion is adequate. For example, carbon monoxide (CO) interferes with oxygen transport, because it binds more readily and tightly to heme, displacing oxygen. Even though the number of circulating red blood cells is adequate, many will be carrying CO, not O_2. CO does not diffuse from RBCs as blood passes through capillaries, so fewer RBCs are available to take up oxygen when the blood returns through the pulmonary circulation. Furthermore, the heme that is carrying oxygen releases it less readily in the presence of carbon monoxide.

Consequences of Alterations in Oxygenation

The consequences of alterations in oxygenation may include hypoxia, hypercapnia, hypocapnia, and tissue necrosis (Box 27–3). Further discussion of the signs and symptoms of oxygenation dysfunctions is found later in the chapter. Understanding the major causes and pathologies of alterations in oxygen provides a basis for assessment and management of related client health problems.

Section 2. Assessment of Oxygenation

■ OXYGENATION DATA COLLECTION

Because oxygenation is one of the most basic of human needs, the assessment of oxygenation status is a critical nursing activity. The nurse can obtain many clues to oxygenation status by skillful assessment. This section focuses on aspects of history and physical examination that are pertinent to oxygenation status. It should be used in addition to the other history and physical examination information contained in Chapter 16.

Oxygenation History

A careful history is a critical component of any assessment. However, taking a detailed history may be inappropriate for the newly admitted client with oxygenation problems. For example, the client who is severely hypoxic or in severe pain may be unable to talk except for very brief phrases and remarks. The hypoxic client also may be too confused to give an accurate history. In these instances, the client's energy is best saved for life processes. A history may be obtained from a family member or deferred until the client is better able to converse. Only the physical examination would be done at this time.

The historical information is organized according to the typical health history format. Following a specified format helps nurses collect data systematically without overlooking significant items. Using the same format consistently also enables nurses to record data systematically. A common organizational format also strengthens the collaboration among all health care team members.

Primary Concern. The primary concern is the focus of the client history and examination. Sometimes a client states the primary concern as a problem related to oxygenation—for example, "I can't catch my breath" or "I have a lot of congestion in my chest." In this case, immediately proceed with the oxygenation data collection. However, some statements of primary concern may be less direct; for example, "I'm too tired all of the time" or "I can't get around like I used to—don't even have the energy to keep my house clean." Such concerns may indicate a variety of problems, but because they can signal alterations affecting oxygenation, the prudent nurse would conduct an oxygenation assessment to verify or rule out a nursing diagnosis related to oxygenation.

■ Ann Seymore, a 35-year-old single professional woman, complains of audible wheezing and tightness in her chest. She states that she has been generally healthy throughout her life with no noticeable allergies or respiratory distress. Within the last few weeks, she has developed a tightness in her chest and her exercise tolerance is reduced. She had been running 2 miles a day. Now, she is unable to complete the 2 miles without one or two rest periods. Her friends have also commented that they can hear her wheezing. She did not notice the wheezing until they pointed it out. She wheezes audibly even at rest in an upright position. She is sleeping poorly at night but cannot point to any particular reason for awakening frequently and having to sit up for a while before she goes back to sleep. She has continued her usual work and household activities, but this is becoming increasingly difficult.

As a result of the discussion about Ms. Seymore's problem, the nurse recognizes that pursuing the oxygenation history and examination is relevant. He notes that Ms. Seymore's regular exercise can be an asset to her overall health status.

Current Understanding. Begin the interview by asking about the client's current understanding of the problem. Ask about the mode of onset, precipitating events, the client's view of the severity of the symptoms, their relation to daily activities or changes in them, and the effect of various treatments. Such questions tell the nurse what to look for in the detailed history and physical examination and give an idea of the client's expectation for care. They also can give clues about the client's understanding of the basis for the problem and possible health teaching that may be indicated.

For example, many smokers deny that they smoke enough to affect their health. They also may feel that they are unable to stop smoking and that as a consequence there is no point in trying. Therefore, heavy smokers commonly either deny that smoking is related to their present symptoms or make statements such as "coughing is normal for me."

Past Health Experiences/Problems. Find out if the client has had past health problems that have affected oxygenation, such as respiratory infections, allergies, coughs, dyspnea, wheezing, heart problems, or circulatory problems, and whether there are any residual effects. Because many medications influence cardiac or respiratory function, ask clients to list medications they take regularly or intermittently. The following case example illustrates the importance of past health experiences and problems in the oxygenation assessment.

■ Interviewing Mrs. Solomon, who was admitted to a medical unit after an acute asthma attack, the nurse learns that Mrs. Solomon has been treated with an iron preparation for "low blood" (ie, anemia) but that she stopped taking the medication because it caused constipation. Checking the client's current hemoglobin and hematocrit reports, the nurse finds that both hemoglobin and hematocrit are abnormally low. The nurse communicates with the physician about the possible need for iron therapy and devises a teaching plan to help Mrs. Solomon minimize the constipation associated with iron preparations.

Personal, Family, and Social History. Impaired cellular oxygenation can affect nearly all aspects of a person's life. Helping clients to minimize or cope effectively with the deficit is a primary nursing responsibility. The personal and social history provides information about clients' habits and preferences that can be used in collaborative planning of nursing approaches for the current health problem. See Table 27–2 and the following case example.

- Mrs. Jenkins, age 48, is referred to the pulmonary clinic after participating in a public health screening program that found her pulmonary function to be below normal limits. During the interview, she states that she has smoked three to four packs of

TABLE 27–2. OXYGENATION HISTORY: PERSONAL, FAMILY, AND SOCIAL HISTORY QUESTIONS

A. **Vocational**
1. What jobs have you had?
2. When was each and for how long?
3. Were you exposed to chemicals or other breathing hazards in any job (eg, asbestos, formaldehyde, pesticides, silica, etc)?

B. **Home and family**
1. Where do you live? How long have you lived there?
2. Where have you lived in the past?
3. Is environmental pollution a problem where you live?
4. Have your breathing problems interfered with your home and family responsibilities? How have you dealt with this?
5. Can you bend over and tie your shoes, carry a bag of groceries, walk uphill, climb stairs, make a bed, and vacuum? If you stopped any of these activities, when and why?

C. **Social and leisure**
1. What are your favorite leisure-time activities?
2. Who do you usually share these activities with?
3. Do you belong to clubs or groups?
4. Have you had to limit social or leisure activities because of breathing difficulties?
5. What are your hobbies?
6. Do any of your leisure activities involve exposure to dusts, fumes, or other irritants?

D. **Sexual**
1. Has your sexual activity been affected by your breathing problems? In what way?
2. If yes, have you and your partner been able to adapt in a way that both of you can accept?

E. **Habits**

Exercise
1. Approximately how much exercise do you get each week? What exercise do you do?
2. Do you have to stop and rest frequently during the activity?
3. Do you get short of breath or wheeze during exercise?

Diet
1. What do you eat during a typical day?
2. Do any foods cause you particular problems?
3. Are you able to prepare your meals without difficulty?
4. Do you ever skip meals because of breathing difficulty after eating?
5. Do you have any problems obtaining groceries?

Beverages
1. What kinds of beverages do you drink each day?
2. Do you drink caffeinated drinks? How many?
3. Do you use alcohol? How much?
4. How much milk do you drink per day?
5. What would you estimate to be the total number of 8-ounce glasses of all liquids that you drink on most days?

Sleep
1. In what position do you sleep?
2. Can you breathe comfortably when lying flat on your back? If not, how high do you prop up to breathe?
3. Do you ever wake up at night coughing or short of breath?

Tobacco use
1. Have you ever smoked cigarettes, cigars, or pipes? If so, when and how many?
2. Have you ever used smokeless tobacco (snuff)?
3. If you used any of these and stopped, when and why?
4. If you did smoke, did the amount you smoked change at different times during your life?
5. How many packs per day or cigars per day did you smoke during each of those time periods?

Other substances
1. Have you used marijuana, cocaine, pills, or other drugs at any time during your life?
2. What did you use and how long did you use it?
3. What symptoms did you get from it?
4. When and why did you stop?

F. **Psychological**

Coping
1. Have you experienced stress in your life recently?
2. What has been helpful to you in dealing with stress?
3. Has stress caused increased breathing difficulty?

Self-image
1. Has your illness affected the way you feel about yourself?
2. Would you say that your self-respect has been altered?

Sick role
1. Is there anything that is particularly difficult about being in the hospital (or, being sick right now)?
2. Is there anything that you feel could be done to make this experience easier?

cigarettes a day for about 30 years. She admits to increasingly frequent "colds" accompanied by the production of large amounts of yellow or green sputum. In the last 10 years, she has stopped hiking with her family and now leaves chores such as carrying groceries, bedmaking, and vacuuming to her teenage children. When asked why she has given up these activities, she attributes her loss of exercise tolerance to aging.

As a result of this history, the nurse recommends medical evaluation of Mrs. Jenkins's condition based on data regarding heavy smoking, increasing respiratory infections, reduced pulmonary function, and reduced exercise tolerance. She advises Mrs. Jenkins that with treatment, her condition will probably improve. Particularly important, she explains to Mrs. Jenkins that her problems are not solely due to aging.

Smoking history deserves special emphasis in a discussion related to oxygenation. Tobacco use is one of the most important risk factors for cardiopulmonary disease. If the client smokes or has smoked in the past, a specific smoking history is essential to the oxygenation assessment. Ask when the client began smoking, how many years he or she smoked, and how many packs per day. Inquire if the number of packs smoked per day has varied at different times (see Table 27–2). If so, find out how many years the client smoked each number of packs per day. A pack-year history can then be calculated by multiplying the number of packs per day times the number of years smoked. For example:

1 ppd × 10 years = 10 pack-years.

2 ppd × 10 years = 20 pack-years.

Refer to Box 27–4, which provides an example of calculating a smoking history using a case illustration. Ask when the client stopped smoking (if he or she has stopped) and why. People often stop smoking when symptoms become intolerable. The client's reason for stopping smoking gives an idea of the point at which the client acknowledged the seriousness of the symptoms.

Subjective Manifestations. A thorough review of the client's subjective manifestations, using clues found in the discussion of past health problems and the history of present problems, will help the nurse focus on pertinent areas of subjective manifestations. See Chapter 16 for sample questions to elicit information about subjective manifestations that are relevant to oxygenation. An explanation of the symptoms that frequently accompany oxygenation imbalances also is included in Table 27–3 as a guide to the nurse in directing these questions.

BOX 27–4. CALCULATING A SMOKING HISTORY

Mr. Garcia states that he started smoking at the age of 12 and smoked one pack of cigarettes per day until he was 16. At that time, he increased his smoking to one and one-half packs per day for 6 years. At age 22, he increased to three packs per day, and has smoked at that level since. He is now 48. What is his pack-year history?
1 ppd × 4 years = 4 pack-years.
1½ ppd × 6 years = 9 pack-years.
3 ppd × 26 years = 78 pack-years.
TOTAL: 4 pack-years + 9 pack-years + 78 pack-years = 91 pack-years total smoking.

Oxygenation Examination

The oxygenation examination focuses on areas of the body that are particularly affected by cardiovascular or respiratory pathology. It includes observation and assessment of vital signs, the chest, integument, HEENT (head, eyes, ears, nose, and throat), cardiovascular system, respiratory system, and abdomen. The information described below should be integrated with the basic physical examination, as described in Chapter 16. When rapid assessment of oxygenation status is needed, the practitioner can focus on the four areas outlined in Box 27–5.

Measurements. Every physical examination should include measurement of the vital signs, temperature, pulse, respiration, and blood pressure (see Chap. 16). Blood pressure should be measured with the client supine, standing, and sitting. Height and weight should also be measured and compared with a table of norms. Discuss recent changes in weight with the client.

Objective Manifestations. General observation and examination of the integument, HEENT, chest, cardiovascular system, abdomen, and neurological system supply data relevant to oxygenation status.

General Observations. The nurse can make some general observations relevant to oxygenation status while taking the health history or getting the client admitted and settled into the hospital. An observant nurse can gain a great deal of information before asking a single question. Is the client alert, oriented, and behaving appropriately? Confusion or lethargy may be due to hypoxia. Can he or she speak in complete sentences, or does shortness of breath limit expression to very short phrases? Does the client have frequent coughing, wheezing, swallowing, or sniffing?

Note and describe the client's general appearance. For example, does the client appear well groomed and clean, or disheveled, dirty, and unkempt? Poor hygiene may result from a low energy level or poor activity tolerance because of insufficient oxygenation. Does the client appear healthy or unhealthy? Are the nailbeds discolored from smoking?

During the initial contact, draw some conclusions regarding the client's apparent age. Oxygenation problems often cause individuals to appear much older than their biological age. This might be charted as "appears older than stated age."

The client's posture, movement, and apparent energy level can give more clues to oxygenation status. If a client is unable to move about at a healthy pace, his or her muscles

TABLE 27–3. SUMMARY OF SIGNS AND SYMPTOMS THAT FREQUENTLY ACCOMPANY ALTERATIONS IN OXYGENATION

Symptom	Definition	Explanation
General		
Fatigue	Feeling of tiredness, weariness.	Hypoxia, cardiac insufficiency, faulty dietary habits.
Reduced exercise tolerance (dyspnea on exertion [DOE])	Reduced capacity for activity.	May be due to impaired tissue oxygenation from cardiac or respiratory insufficiency.
Chills	Attacks of shivering, feeling of excessive coldness.	Often accompany infections or fever.
Sudden weight gain	As described.	May be due to fluid retention secondary to heart disease; may compromise ventilation.
Integument		
Coldness of extremities	As described.	May be due to poor circulation to extremity because of lowered cardiac output or vascular compromise.
HEENT		
Pain, itching of eyes or nose, nasal congestion, sneezing	As described.	Often due to allergy; may be due to infection of eyes, nose, sinuses.
Respiratory		
Orthopnea	Must sit or stand in order to breathe comfortably.	May be due to fluid accumulation in the lungs resulting from cardiac failure. May be due to poor diaphragmatic function or to lung pathology.
Dyspnea	Subjective or objective shortness of breath or difficulty in breathing.	May accompany lung or cardiac pathology. May result from inhaling fumes. May be due to allergy.
Hyperpnea	Increase in the rate and/or depth of breathing.	Exercise, partial airway obstruction, excessive lung secretions, hypoxia, early hypercapnia.
Tachypnea	Rapid, shallow breathing, usually defined as greater than 20 per minute.	Decreased lung capacity (obesity, pregnancy), anxiety, pain, shock, cocaine or amphetamine use, pulmonary disease, neurological disease, drug withdrawal.
Bradypnea	Decreased respiratory rate.	Hypercapnia, metabolic alkalosis, inappropriate administration of oxygen, opiate use, drug overdose, central nervous system dysfunction.
Apnea	Cessation of breathing.	Cardiac arrest, airway occlusion, injury to respiratory center.
Cheyne-Stokes respiration (periodic breathing)	Episodes of apnea interspersed with periods of rapid, deep breaths and then slow, shallow breaths.	Deep sleep, congestive heart failure, brain disease, drug overdose, renal failure.
Kussmaul respiration	Abnormally deep, often rapid, sighing-type respirations.	Diabetic ketoacidosis, metabolic acidosis.
Ataxic respiration	Short bursts of irregular breathing with periods of apnea.	Brain damage.
Pain during breathing	As described; worsens with inspiration.	May be due to chest wall injury, pleural irritation, or strained chest muscles.
Cardiovascular		
Paroxysmal nocturnal dyspnea (PND)	Sudden attacks of respiratory distress during sleep.	Usually due to cardiac failure.
Chest pain	Pain in the chest that may or may not radiate to the arm, shoulder, or jaw. Does not worsen with inspiration.	Usually due to insufficient oxygenation of the heart muscle.
Intermittent claudication	Pain in legs or hips when walking; relieved by rest.	Inadequate oxygenation of leg muscles on exercise, usually due to cardiovascular disease.
Neurological/Psychological		
Memory problems, confusion, anxiety	As described.	May be due to insufficient oxygenation to the brain as a result of cardiac or pulmonary insufficiency.

BOX 27–5. A QUICK GUIDE TO ASSESSING OXYGENATION

Because major body organs alter their function quickly in the presence of a low blood supply, assessment of these organs can provide information about oxygenation status.

Neurological function:

- Client should be alert and oriented, not unduly anxious or restless.
- Altered level of consciousness, irritability, poor judgment, or disorientation may reflect a low blood supply.

Cardiac function:

- Heart rate should be regular, and within normal limits for age and sex.
- Pulses should be present and of healthy quality.
- Continuous monitoring, if available, should reveal no arrhythmias.
- Capillary refill should be prompt.
- Extremities should be warm, dry, of healthy color, and without edema.

Blood pressure:

- Blood pressure should be within normal limits for age and sex with no abrupt changes related to changes in body position (eg, supine to standing).

Respiratory function

- Breathing should be quiet, regular, and unlabored.
- There should be no cough, shortness of breath, or orthopnea.

may be inadequately oxygenated. Often, simple activities of daily living can cause such a person to become dyspneic. Posture can also give clues to possible respiratory problems. If the client is unable to lie down, the orthopnea should be carefully assessed and noted.

The client's facial expression can convey a great deal of information. Does the client's face convey feelings of fear or panic? If the client's face or body language seems to convey a different emotion than the client's words, ask for clarification: "I notice that you are gritting your teeth and frowning. Are you feeling any discomfort?"

Integument. Integumentary assessment is also relevant to oxygenation. Oxygenation disorders may lead to a variety of changes in the skin color. Some people become ashen, pale, gray, or cyanotic (bluish color). Cyanosis may be generalized or it may be limited to certain areas, such as the lips and nailbeds. Document and describe the severity and location of the cyanosis. However, if a person does not appear cyanotic, do not take this as evidence of adequate oxygenation. Some people with pulmonary disease do not move air out of the lungs very well. As a result, they retain carbon dioxide, which is a vasodilator, and have a very pink, red, or ruddy skin color. This red color is also characteristic of carbon monoxide poisoning.

Another abnormality of skin color is the presence of excessive bruising or of purpura, which are tiny purple spots. These are most prevalent on the extremities and usually signal a bleeding disorder or long-term use of steroids.

Inspect the fingers closely. Persons with long-term oxygenation problems (such as cystic fibrosis and lung cancer) often have clubbing of the fingers (Fig. 27–7). In clubbing, the profile of the fingernails flattens out and the base of the fingernail becomes soft and spongy. Discoloration of the fingertips can be a clue to cigarette smoking.

The skin of the feet and lower legs displays characteristic changes in individuals with inadequate circulation. Poor peripheral oxygenation causes thin, darkly discolored, or purplish skin in the lower legs and feet.

Also, inspect the legs for edema or abnormal hair distribution. Individuals with insufficient arterial circulation may have no hair below their knees. They may have breaks in the skin or skin ulcers as well. Observe for varicose veins, which are large gnarled veins that are prominent on the surface of the legs. The feet may also feel much cooler than the rest of the body.

Note capillary refill time by depressing the skin over the sternum and the nailbeds of the fingers and toes and watching for return of the pink color. Normally the refill takes less than one second. Sluggish refill, greater than one second, indicates possible perfusion problems, often related to body fluid volume. Poor capillary refill in the toes can be related to vascular disease.

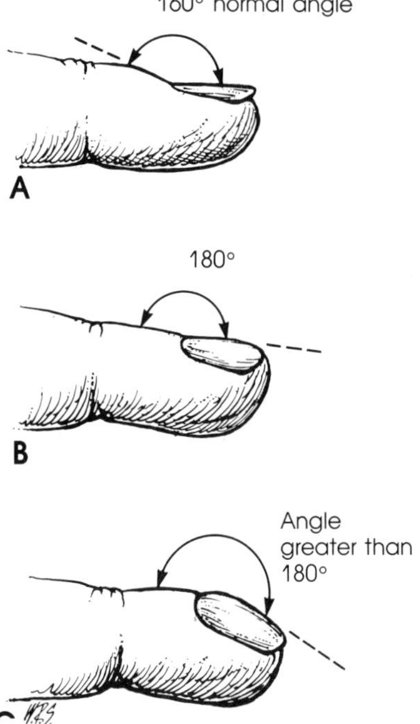

Figure 27–7. Clubbing of the fingers. **A.** Normal. **B.** Early clubbing. **C.** Late clubbing. (*From Block GJ, Nolan JW.* Health Assessment for Professional Nursing: A Developmental Approach. *2nd ed. Norwalk, CT: Appleton & Lange; 1986: 93.*)

HEENT. Several portions of the head, ear, eye, nose, and throat examination can yield important data about oxygenation. Particulars on how to conduct this portion of the examination, as well as more complete information about examination of these organs, may be found in Chapter 29.

Check the pupils for size, equality, and speed of reaction to light, which can give clues as to oxygenation of the brain. If there is cerebral edema (swelling of the brain) or lack of oxygen to the brain, the pupils tend to be large and less reactive. One or both pupils that are fixed (nonreactive to light) and dilated signal a neurological or oxygenation emergency.

Observe the form and symmetry of the nose. Note whether there are changes in the shape of the nostrils during breathing. Nasal flaring (enlargement of the nares on inspiration) indicates air hunger, suggesting serious respiratory distress. Carefully inspect the inner surfaces of the nose in good light for signs of inflammation. In healthy people, the nasal mucosa will be pink and moist, with no evidence of edema, bogginess, exudate, drainage, or bleeding. The nasal septum should be straight. There should be no polyps, which are fingerlike projections of nasal mucosa. Asthmatics are especially prone to nasal polyps.

Note the position of the mouth during breathing. Pursed-lip breathing, slow exhalation through puckered lips, is often used by individuals with chronic oxygenation problems to slow and control respiration and achieve better oxygen–carbon dioxide exchange with less respiratory effort. Note also whether this maneuver occurs only on exertion or during quiet sitting as well.

Carefully inspect the interior of the mouth and pharynx. Note the color and moisture of the mucosa. The pharyngeal and oral mucosa should be smooth, moist, and pink with no evidence of exudate, ulcerations, or discoloration. Cyanotic mucous membranes suggest hypoxia.

Inspect the neck for distension of the veins. Venous distension indicates increased venous pressure, which is often related to cardiac problems.

Chest and Cardiovascular System. Techniques for examining the chest and descriptions of the landmarks that guide the examination are discussed in Chapter 16. The discussion here addresses changes in the chest examination that suggest oxygenation problems.

Begin with inspection. First, expose the chest and inspect for shape. Some people with pulmonary disease have an increased distance from the front to the back of the chest (increased anterior-posterior [A-P] diameter), or barrel chest. This is a result of air trapping within the lungs; however, not all individuals who trap air have an increased A-P diameter. Some who have chronic obstructive pulmonary disease (COPD) may trap air by flattening their diaphragms. In this case, the chest contours do not change. The diaphragmatic flattening can easily be seen on a lateral chest x-ray. In contrast, some perfectly healthy people, such as singers, trap enough air to increase their A-P diameter. They may develop severe barrel chests. It is important to note whether an increased A-P diameter exists, but its presence or absence is not considered diagnostic. It is simply one piece of objective data.

Clients may have abnormally shaped chests for a variety of reasons. Some of the more severe abnormalities have major consequences for oxygenation because of pressure on the heart or lungs. Abnormal chest shapes, except for barrel chest and abnormalities related to spinal curvature, are relatively uncommon. Abnormalities of chest shape are illustrated in Figure 27–8.

Inspection also includes observing chest movements during the respiratory cycle to assess respiratory rate, rhythm, depth, quality, and type of breathing. Also consider the following: Are the respirations regular? Labored? Are they associated with use of the accessory muscles, such as the sternocleidomastoid and shoulder girdle? People in respiratory distress often sit upright and lean on their arms or elbows to aid in pushing up on the shoulder girdle. This position of resting on the arms to breathe is called the tripod position (Fig. 27–9). When the diaphragm, the major muscle of respiration, is not moving normally due to air trapping or pushing up from the abdomen, the only way the person can enlarge the chest to lower intrathoracic pressure and take a breath is to raise the shoulder girdle and upper chest. Often, the person who is using accessory muscles to breathe also purses the lips, as discussed above.

Retractions are another consequence of difficult air exchange. Intercostal retractions are indentation, or pulling in, of the intercostal muscles as the individual breathes in. Retractions are also sometimes evident above the clavicle and below the sternum. Bulging of the intercostal spaces during expiration may accompany retractions. In young infants, substernal retractions are common with only moderately increased inspiratory effort because the chest structures are very pliable.

When breathing is painful, many clients splint their respirations. They attempt to hold the chest as still as possible with each breath. Very little respiratory movement will be observed as the chest is held stiff, still, and rigid.

If the client is coughing, note whether the cough is productive or nonproductive. A nonproductive cough is often related to upper respiratory irritation or infection, whereas a productive cough often indicates lower respiratory problems. If the cough is productive, note the character of the sputum. Thick yellow-to-greenish sputum may signal an infection that could threaten oxygenation.

Inspect the precordium, the area of the chest just over the heart, for bulging or pulsations. These are abnormal signs that indicate cardiac enlargement or unusually forceful contractions of the cardiac muscle. These signs suggest the potential for perfusion problems.

Next, palpate the precordium for lifts, heaves, or thrills. Lifts or heaves indicate forceful heart contractions. Thrills, which feel like vibrations, are usually caused by turbulent blood flow through the heart valves. These abnormal signs indicate cardiac pathology that could compromise perfusion.

Palpation of the posterior chest for fremitus (vibration of the chest wall associated with speaking; see also Chap.

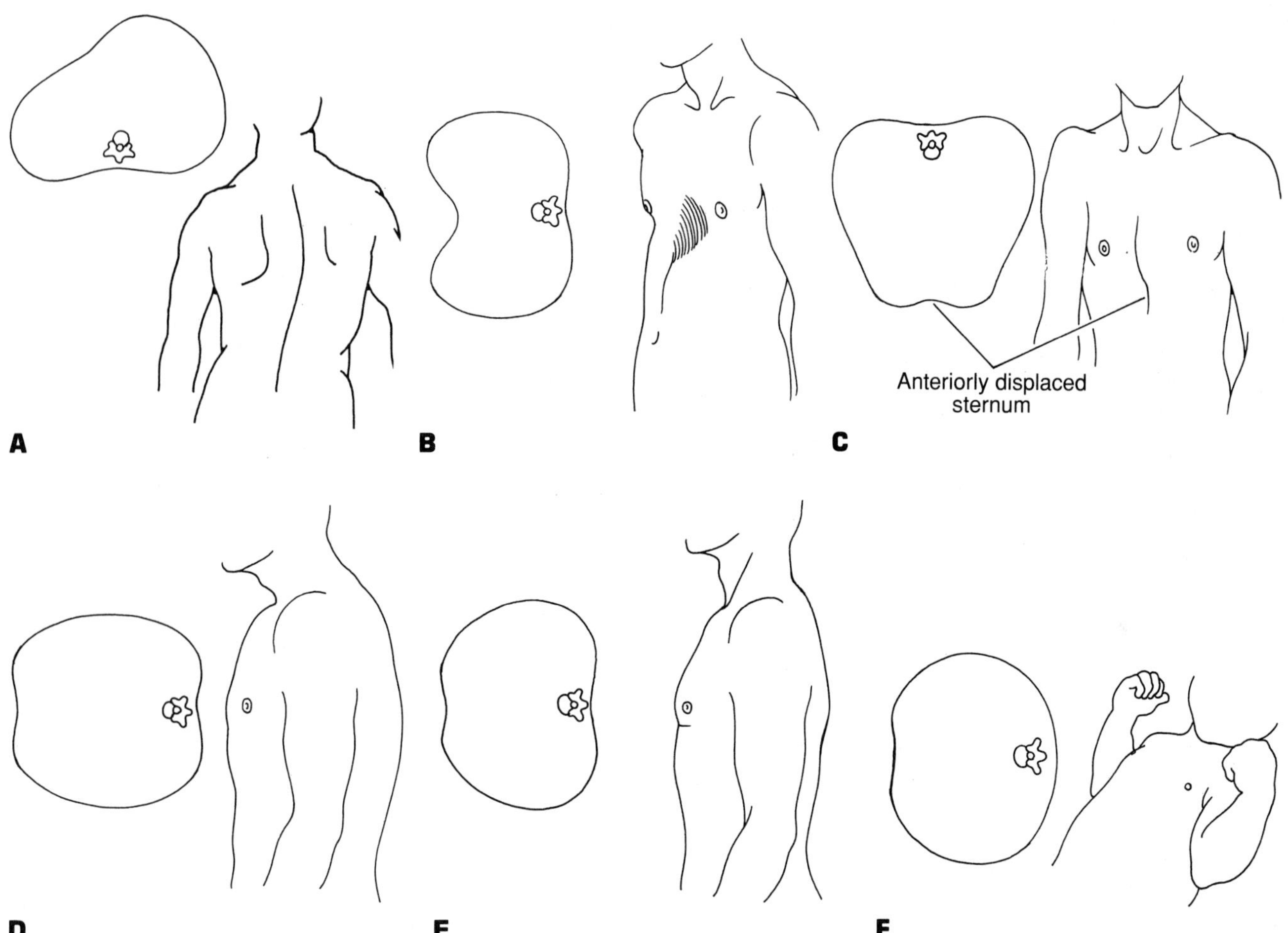

Figure 27–8. Normally and abnormally shaped chests. **A.** Thoracic kyphoscoliosis. **B.** Funnel. **C.** Pigeon. **D.** Barrel. **E.** Normal adult. **F.** Normal infant.

16) contributes more data about possible interferences with oxygenation. Conditions that increase lung density, such as pneumonia or tumors, increase fremitus, while airway obstruction decreases fremitus by interfering with the transmission of sound. It is more difficult to assess fremitus of the anterior chest because of interference by muscles and breast tissue. Therefore, examination of the anterior chest may be performed at the nurse's discretion.

Palpation of peripheral pulses provides information about perfusion of body tissues. (Pulse locations and techniques for palpating pulses are covered in Chap. 16.) Weakness or absence of a peripheral pulse implies impaired perfusion to the body parts distal to it. For example, a weak carotid pulse suggests diminished brain perfusion. Assess the femoral, posterior tibial, and dorsalis pedis pulses to evaluate circulation to the legs and feet. Box 27–6 lists and defines descriptive terms for pulses.

Auscultation of the chest is the next step in the oxygenation examination. Breath sounds indicate the movement of air in the lungs, obstructions to air flow, and the presence of secretions. Follow the guidelines for auscultation of breath sounds discussed in Chapter 16. Abnormal breath sounds and their causes are summarized in Table 27–4.

Heart sounds provide data about cardiac rhythm and blood flow through the heart. See the discussion in Chapter 16. Auscultate the heart with both the diaphragm and the bell of the stethoscope, because some abnormal heart sounds are low pitched and therefore are more audible through the bell.

Although normally only the S_1 and S_2 heart sounds are heard, it is sometimes possible to hear a third (S_3) or a fourth (S_4) heart sound. Some healthy children, teenagers, and adults under 30 have an S_3, especially if the chest wall is thin. Many pregnant women develop an S_3 by the 13th week of pregnancy. If a person is over 30 and not pregnant, the S_3 should be investigated as it may be an early sign of heart failure. A nurse can mimic the cadence of the S_1, S_2, and S_3 by silently sounding out "Kentucky" as the heart sounds are auscultated. The presence of an S_4 is not by

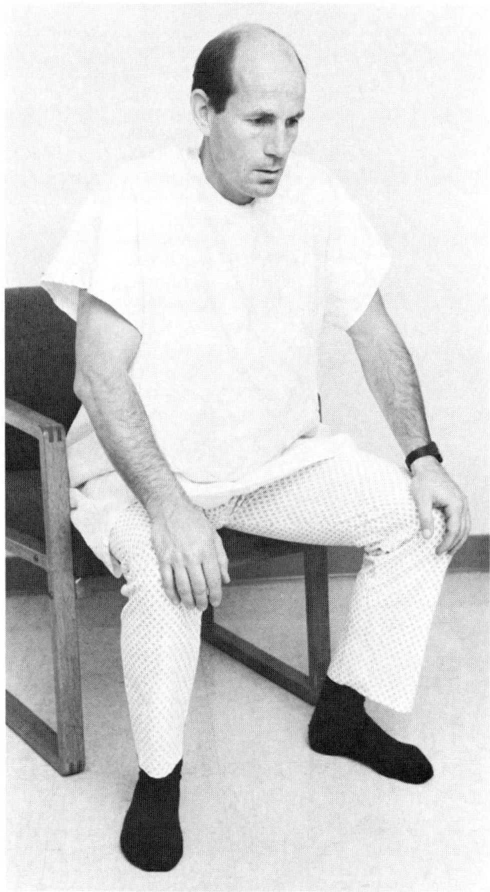

Figure 27–9. Tripod position.

BOX 27–6. DESCRIPTIVE TERMS FOR PULSES

Pulse rate

Tachycardia: Rate persistently greater than 100 beats per minute.
Bradycardia: Rate less than 50 beats per minute.

Pulse volume

Normal: Full, strong, easily palpable.
Thready: Weak throughout stroke.
Bounding: Unusually full, pounding.
Collapsing: Normal upstroke, fades immediately.
Bigeminal: Alternating amplitude: full beat followed by weak beat.

Quantifying volume

4+: Full, bounding, such as during or immediately after strenuous exercise.
3+: Normal.
2+: Slightly weaker than normal, such as in dehydration.
1+: Can be obliterated with pressure.
0 : Absent.

Pulse rhythm

Regular: Evenly spaced beats.
Irregular: Spaces between beats are of different lengths, may seem to be "regularly irregular" (a pattern can be noted) or completely irregular (spaces between beats erratic, unpredictable).

itself diagnostic of heart disease, although it is very often the result of pathology. The sound of "Tennessee" mimics the cadence of the S_4, S_1, and S_2.

A heart murmur is a swishing or whooshing noise caused by partial obstruction of the blood flow by one or more heart valves, increased flow across a valve, backward flow through a valve, or flow through a hole in the septum of the heart. Evaluation of murmurs is reserved for advanced practitioners.

Auscultation of blood vessels may be part of the oxygenation assessment. If plaque has built up within a vessel so that blood has to rush around it, a swishing noise can be heard on auscultation. This is called a bruit. Evaluation of the major arteries such as the abdominal aorta, carotids, and femoral artery may include auscultating for bruits; however, this is not part of routine assessment.

Blood pressure is evaluated as part of the oxygenation assessment. The techniques for blood pressure measurement and normal values are found in Chapter 16.

Abdomen. Any condition that increases the abdominal contents can cause abdominal organs to push up on the diaphragm and obstruct breathing. These include obesity, pregnancy, fluid accumulation in the abdomen such as ascites (fluid that accumulates due to liver disorders), and large tumors. Conditions that lead to abdominal guarding, a conscious attempt to limit abdominal muscle movement, can also affect chest movement and thus interfere with breathing. Such conditions include abdominal surgery incisions, peritonitis (inflammation of the abdominal lining), and other conditions that cause abdominal pain. Abdominal assessment is described in more detail in Chapter 16.

Neurological/Psychological. Interference with the oxygen supply to the brain can cause confusion, impaired judgment, compromised coordination, and altered levels of consciousness. Clients with difficulty breathing often are anxious or irritable. Increased levels of carbon dioxide in the blood diminish sensory acuity, whereas decreased levels cause abnormal sensations (paresthesias) such as numbness and tingling of the extremities. If any of these are noted, a more complete assessment of mental status, coordination, and sensation may be appropriate. These are detailed in Chapter 16.

Diagnostic Tests

A wide variety of diagnostic tests are used to evaluate oxygenation status. Laboratory tests of blood and sputum; and diagnostic examinations, including pulmonary function tests, vascular Doppler studies, and visualization via endoscope, x-rays, and scans; provide information about ventilation and perfusion that may be useful in diagnosing and treating oxygenation problems.

TABLE 27–4. SUMMARY OF ABNORMAL BREATH SOUNDS

Sound	Description	Location/Causes
Crackles (formerly called rales)	Diffuse, discontinuous crackling sounds. Usually heard during inspiration and don't generally clear with coughing. Can mimic by listening to soda fizz or by rubbing hairs together beside ear.	Localized or generalized throughout chest. Caused by movement of fluid in small airways or sudden popping open of alveoli or small airways that had been closed/deflated. Sounds that clear after a few deep breaths are known as atelectatic rales (crackles), an early sign of impending **atelectasis** (collapsed alveoli).
Gurgles and rumbles (formerly called rhonchi)	Heavy, continuous snoring or rattling sounds. Can often clear by coughing or suctioning.	Over-large airways. Sometimes diffuse throughout chest. Caused by air turbulence as air moves through large airways partially obstructed by secretions, swelling, or tumors.
Wheezing	High-pitched, continuous whistling sounds. Usually occur in a specific progression, which gives clues to severity of narrowing of airways. Often may be heard without a stethoscope. Does not clear with coughing.	Air rushing through a narrowed airway. Due to obstruction or bronchospasm (spasm of muscles surrounding the airways; asthma). Heard all over lung fields. Usually more prominent on expiration.
Pleural friction rub	Localized grating or clicking noises, associated with pain on breathing. Rub is not heard if breath is held. Does not clear with coughing.	Localized at any point of pleural irritation. Caused by inflamed pleura and chest wall.
Abnormal spoken breath sounds		
Egophony (E to A change)	When stethoscope is placed over localized area of consolidation and client says "E," it sounds like "A" through stethoscope. As the consolidation clears, the sound will become more like "E."	May be heard anywhere in lung fields. Consolidation or presence of infectious debris in alveoli (pneumonia) alters transmission of voice sounds through the chest wall.
Whispered pectoriloquy	Whispered syllables are heard more distinctly than usual through the stethoscope.	As above for egophony.
Absent or diminished	Normal vesicular sounds become distant or disappear.	May occur anywhere in lung fields. Diminished sounds caused by atelectasis; absent sounds by airway obstruction or pneumothorax (collapsed lung).

Nurses should understand the reasons for these procedures to be able to prepare the client for them. Nurses must also understand the basic nursing care related to each test. Tables 27–5 and 27–6 present an overview of information needed by the beginning nursing student about common tests of oxygenation.

NURSING DIAGNOSIS OF OXYGENATION STATUS

The data obtained in the oxygenation history and physical examination may indicate problems related to oxygenation status. The use of the taxonomy of nursing diagnoses can help beginning students identify relationships between pieces of data and to associate these data with specific nursing diagnoses. See the table Sample Nursing Diagnoses: Oxygenation. on page 1245. The diagnostic statement provides the basis for planning individualized care. For a nursing diagnosis to be most useful, it should include the cause, or etiology, of the problem if known.

Several nursing diagnoses are directly related to oxygenation status. These include Ineffective Airway Clearance, Ineffective Breathing Pattern, and Alterations in Tissue Perfusion. Other nursing diagnoses related to altered oxygenation status but not covered in detail here are listed in Box 27–7. Although the nursing diagnoses are distinct, there is a great deal of overlap among them. This will be clarified as the diagnoses are discussed.

Ineffective Airway Clearance

Ineffective Airway Clearance is a state in which the individual is unable to clear secretions in the respiratory tract or to protect and maintain the patency (openness) of the airways. The extent to which this interferes with oxygenation varies with the degree of obstruction.

There are several potential causes of Ineffective Airway Clearance. Accurate identification of the underlying cause of the problem is necessary, because the etiology often determines what type of nursing implementation is appropriate.

Etiology: Decreased Energy or Fatigue. Lack of energy may prevent coughing that is effective enough to clear the airways, even if the client is motivated to learn effective

TABLE 27–5. COMMON LABORATORY TESTS TO ASSESS OXYGENATION

Test/Description	Findings/Implications: Normal	Findings/Implications: Abnormal	Nurse's Responsibility
Hemoglobin (Hgb or Hb) Measures oxygen-carrying capacity of blood. Used to monitor client's response to treatment.	Neonate: 14–24 g/dL. Infant 1 month: 11–20 g/dL. 2 months to 1 year: 10–15 g/dL. Child: 11–16 g/dL. Adult male: 14–18 g/dL. Adult female: 12–16 g/dL. Elderly male: 12.4–15 g/dL. Elderly female: 11.7–13.8 g/dL.	*Low* hemoglobin indicates inadequate oxygen-carrying capacity of blood if less than 12 g/dL (male) or 10.2 g/dL (female). Caused by blood loss, RBC destruction, insufficient dietary iron or folic acid. *Effects:* Weakness, dizziness, tachycardia, fatigue, dyspnea. If extreme: cardiac failure.	Discuss: ■ Purpose of test. ■ Venipuncture required. ■ No food/fluid restrictions. Encourage questions. Request client to maintain pressure to site for 5 minutes after venipuncture. Discuss implications of test results. Teach nutrients necessary to maintain normal hemoglobin levels; food sources; and daily servings needed.
Hematocrit (Hct) Measures percentage by volume of red blood cells in whole blood. Used to evaluate anemia and oxygen-carrying capacity.	Neonate: 50–68%. Infant 1 month: 37–49%. 2 months to 1 year: 29–40%. Child: 31–45%. Adult male: 40–54%. Adult female: 36–46%. Elderly male: 36–56%. Elderly female: 30–54%.	*Increased* hematocrit caused by disease, severe dehydration, high altitude. *Effects:* Elevated hematocrit increases blood viscosity; therefore, creates risk for vascular congestion, elevated cardiac workload, thrombus formation. *Decreased* hematocrit caused by anemia, other diseases, hemodilution, reaction to blood transfusions. *Effects:* Fatigue, shortness of breath, dyspnea, increased cardiac workload.	Same as for hemoglobin. May use fingerstick to obtain. Do not obtain from arm with an IV running—will be diluted. If a tourniquet is on for over a minute, will elevate hct due to hemostasis.
Red blood cell count (RBC) A determination of the number of circulating erythrocytes in whole blood. Used to diagnose and evaluate anemias.	Neonate: 4.8–7.2. Infant 2 months to 1 year: 4.1–6.4. Child: 3.8–5.5. Adult male: 4.5–6.0. Adult female: 4–5 (all values in millions/μL).	Dehydration may mask anemia. *Increased* RBCs caused by disease, severe dehydration, shock. *Effects:* See Hematocrit, above. *Decreased* RBCs caused by impaired RBC production, increased RBC destruction, dietary deficiency of folic acid, B vitamins, pregnancy. *Effects:* See Hematocrit, above.	Same as for Hemoglobin, above.
Serum potassium (K+) Measures circulating K+. Most K+ in body is intracellular and cannot be measured. Is essential for maintenance of electrical conduction in heart and function of other muscles.	3.5–5.5. mEq/L.	Life-threatening values: below 2.5 or above 6.5 mEq/L. *Increased* K+ level caused by acidosis, cell damage, renal failure, excessive K+ therapy, IV K+ therapy when urine output is low. *Effects:* Weakness, malaise, nausea, vomiting, muscle irritability, cardiac arrhythmias. *Decreased* K+ levels caused by diarrhea, vomiting, nasogastric suction, diuretic therapy, IV therapy without K+ replacement. *Effects:* Decreased reflexes; rapid, irregular pulse; muscle weakness; hypotension; confusion.	Discuss: ■ Purpose of test. ■ No food/fluid restrictions. ■ Venipuncture required. Encourage questions. Avoid prolonged tourniquet. Deliver specimen to lab promptly. Standing leads to hemolysis which alters K+ values. Discuss results of test. Teach dietary sources of K+, number of daily servings. Discuss medications client takes that affect or are affected by K+ levels.

TABLE 27–5. (continued)

Test/Description	Findings/Implications: Normal	Findings/Implications: Abnormal	Nurse's Responsibility
Arterial blood gases (ABGs) Implies effectiveness of gas exchange in lungs. Assessment for disturbances of acid–base balance in body. Po_2: Amount of oxygen dissolved in blood. Pco_2: Amount of CO_2 dissolved in blood. pH: Measure of acid concentration in blood. HCO_3: Measure of bicarbonate or base in blood.	Po_2: 80–100 mm Hg. Pco_2: 35–45 mm Hg. Do not vary significantly with age except Po_2 is lowered in those over 80 and those living at high altitudes. pH: 7.35–7.45. HCO_3: 22–28 mEq/L.	*Low* Po_2, *high* Pco_2, caused by conditions that impair respiratory function: neurological, respiratory, or muscular disease; drug overdose; airway obstruction; lung damage. *Effects:* Respiratory distress, tachycardia, reduced level of consciousness, restlessness, anxiety. May result in cyanosis or death. *Low* Pco_2: Hyperventilation, fever, asthma. *Effects:* Tingling fingers and face, tachycardia, anxiety, dizziness, diaphoresis, tetany. *Low* pH (<7.35) indicates acidosis. May be caused by impaired oxygenation, or metabolic conditions (diabetes, severe diarrhea). *High* pH (>7.45) indicates alkalosis. May be caused by extreme anxiety, fever or metabolic conditions (severe vomiting, $K+$ loss). *Low* HCO_3 indicates primary base deficit (metabolic acidosis). *High* HCO_3 indicates base excess (metabolic alkalosis). HCO_3 fluctuates to compensate for Pco_2 imbalances.	Discuss: ■ Purpose of test. ■ Need for resting state 10–30 minutes before test. ■ The sample must be arterial, which causes discomfort. ■ Local anesthetic sometimes used. Encourage questions. Place specimen on ice and take to lab immediately. Apply firm pressure to site for 5–10 minutes and then apply firm dressing. Observe and report numbness, tingling, swelling at puncture site. Record amount of oxygen being administered and method used on lab request. Discuss implications of results.
Sputum tests Analyze sputum for presence of pathogens or malignant cells. Common tests include: ■ Culture and sensitivity. ■ Gram stain. ■ Acid-fast bacillus (TB). ■ Fungal studies. ■ Cytologic studies (for cancer cells).	Sputum should be relatively free of microorganisms, but there will be some contamination by oral flora. Small numbers of alpha-hemolytic streptococci, staphylococci, diphtheroids may be present.	Pathogenic bacteria, fungi, parasites, cancer cells, viral inclusions.	Discuss: ■ Purpose of test. ■ Specimen must be sputum, not saliva; deep cough or suction required. ■ Discuss implications of results. Encourage questions. Use sterile specimen container. Send specimen to lab immediately. Refer to Procedure 27–1 for more information.

Data in this table were adapted in part from Foster R, Hunsberger M, Anderson J. Family-centered Nursing Care of Children. *Philadelphia: Saunders; 1989. Treseler KM.* Clinical Laboratory and Diagnostic Tests. *2nd ed. Norwalk, CT: Appleton & Lange; 1988. Kee JL.* Handbook of Laboratory and Diagnostic Tests With Nursing Implications. *Norwalk, CT: Appleton & Lange; 1988.*

TABLE 27–6. COMMON DIAGNOSTIC EXAMINATIONS TO ASSESS OXYGENATION

Examination/Description	Client Preparation	Posttest Nursing Care
Chest x-ray Radiographic views of chest. Usually includes PA (back to front), AP (front to back), and lateral views. Can detect structural abnormalities, heart size, abnormal air accumulation, fluid in lung, atelectasis, tumors, abscesses.	Discuss: ■ Purpose of test. ■ Position of test: standing or lying down. ■ Need to remove clothing and jewelry above waist, wear hospital gown. ■ Need to take deep breaths during procedure. ■ Exposure to radiation is miminal. ■ X-ray results may reveal need for further tests. Encourage questions.	Assist as needed. Provide opportunities to discuss results of x-ray.
Pulmonary function tests A group of tests that measure various lung volumes and amount and rate of air movement. Used to diagnose and track progression of lung disease, discriminate between restrictive and obstructive disorders, determine the effects of medication.	Discuss: ■ Purpose of test. ■ Position for test: sitting or standing. ■ Breathing as directed through a mouthpiece is necessary; nose clip may be used. ■ Nonrestrictive clothing is advised. ■ Test may be repeated after bronchodilator spray used. ■ Need to avoid smoking 4–6 hours before test. ■ Need to avoid a heavy meal before test. Encourage practice of deep breathing, forced deep breathing, and rapid breathing techniques before test. Assess vital signs, note signs and symptoms of respiratory distress; delay test if distress present. Note client use of bronchodilators and steroids on test request slip. Note client age, height, and weight on request slip.	Assess for signs and symptoms of respiratory distress, report if present. Provide opportunities to discuss results of tests.
Bronchoscopy Direct visualization of airways with fiberoptic bronchoscope. May include fluoroscopy (direct projection of x-ray-type image on a screen). Can detect lesions, bleeding, secretions, mucus plugs. Suction, biopsy, or removal of foreign bodies may be done during procedure.	Discuss: ■ Purpose of test. ■ Position for test: sitting or lying down with neck hyperextended. ■ Bronchoscope is inserted through mouth or nose. It may create a feeling of being unable to breathe, but airway remains open. ■ Local anesthetic is sprayed on throat. ■ Sedation may be used. ■ Test takes about 1 hour. ■ Techniques and benefits of deep breathing and relaxation during procedure. ■ Keep npo 6–12 hours before test. ■ May have sore throat, hoarseness, and/or blood-tinged sputum after test. Encourage questions. Inquire if client has loose or capped teeth; note on chart. Check/obtain informed consent. Request or assist with removal of dentures. Check for allergies to local anesthetic.	Assess vital signs until stable. Assess for respiratory difficulty, cardiac arrhythmias, laryngeal edema, bronchospasm, bleeding. Report frank bleeding, respiratory distress, or major changes in vital signs. Check gag reflex with tongue blade (may be obliterated by local anesthetic). Keep npo until gag reflex returns. If sedated, position on side for drainage of oral secretions. Encourage client to avoid talking, smoking, coughing for 6–8 hours to reduce possibility of bleeding. Offer lozenges, ice bag for throat. Provide opportunities to discuss results of test.

TABLE 27–6. (continued)

Examination/Description	Client Preparation	Posttest Nursing Care
Lung scan (VQ scan) Provides a comparison of perfusion and ventilation. IV and inhaled radionuclides are used. Used to determine adequacy of blood flow to lungs and completeness of ventilation. Comparison of perfusion (P) and ventilation (Q) determines nature of pulmonary pathology. Can detect pulmonary embolism, distinguish between disease involving lung tissue versus vascular obstruction.	Discuss: ■ Purpose of test. ■ Position for test: lying down, sitting, several position changes necessary. ■ P-scan takes 30 minutes; V-scan 10–15 minutes. ■ Minimal discomfort except for injection of IV radionuclide and nose clip. ■ Exposure to radiation less than with x-ray, no danger to client or visitors; excreted in 6–24 hours. ■ Need to remove clothing and jewelry above waist, wear hospital gown. ■ For P-scan, a scanning device will move over chest to detect presence of radionuclide in pulmonary circulation. ■ For Q-scan, client will inhale oxygen with a small amount of radionuclide gas; need to take deep breath and hold briefly; scanner used during inspiration, holding, and exhalation to detect pattern of inflation. Encourage questions.	No specific test-related care. Provide opportunities to discuss results of test.
Electrocardiogram (ECG) Records electrical activity in heart; detects arrhythmias. Variations: stress test (ECG while client walks on treadmill) or over 24-hour period using portable Holter monitor device).	Discuss: ■ Purpose of test. ■ Position for test: supine unless treadmill or 24-hour test. ■ ECG is not painful or dangerous; no electricity is applied to body. ■ Need to remove clothing and jewelry above waist, remove nylon hosiery, wear hospital gown. ■ 12 electrodes (leads) are applied to the body using straps or suction device; conductive paste applied under electrode. ■ If exercise test is to be done, eat lightly (no coffee, tea, alcohol) 2 hours before test, wear loose comfortable clothing not made of nylon, rubber-soled shoes. Encourage questions.	Assist client to wash off conductive paste if needed. Provide opportunities to discuss results of test.
Vectorcardiogram Records electrical impulses, like ECG, but produces three-dimensional picture of cardiac activity, useful in diagnosis of myocardial infarction (heart attack).	Same as ECG, above.	Same as for ECG, above.
Cardiac catheterization Insertion of a long catheter into a vein or artery of the arm or leg and threading it to the chambers of the heart or coronary arteries. Contrast dye injected to visualize heart chambers, activity, or arteries. Can detect abnormal heart structure, size, valves; measure pressure in pulmonary circulation; detect coronary occlusions.	Discuss: ■ Purpose of test. ■ Position for test: supine on tilting table, ECG leads attached to chest. ■ Takes about 2 hours. ■ No food or fluids 6–8 hours before test. ■ IV will infuse during procedure; hot flushing sensation likely as dye injected; lasts 1–2 minutes.	Monitor vital signs q 15 min for 1 hour, then q 30 min until stable. Assess for arrhythmias on monitor or apical pulse. Observe catheter-insertion site for bleeding. Change dressings as needed; report continued bleeding. Assess peripheral pulses distal to insertion site q 15 min for 1–2 hours, then q 1–2 hours until stable.

(continued)

TABLE 27–6. (continued)

Examination/Description	Client Preparation	Posttest Nursing Care
Cardiac catheterization (continued)	■ Allergies to dye, seafood, iodine (if present, may use antihistamine night before test). ■ Possibility of palpitations as catheter is passed into heart. ■ Need to cough and deep breathe frequently during procedure. ■ Need to discontinue oral anticoagulants; IV heparin may be used, if needed. ■ Sedative given 30–60 minutes prior to procedure. ■ Need for bedrest 8–12 hours after test, cardiac monitoring may be used. Encourage questions. Check/obtain informed consent. Assess and record vital signs.	Assess for coolness, paleness, pain, numbness, tingling of insertion site extremity; report signs of circulatory insufficiency. Assess and report chest pain. Administer pain medications as ordered for site pain. Encourage fluids unless contraindicated. Provide opportunities to discuss results of test.
Vascular Doppler studies Evaluates blood flow in arteries and veins to arms, legs, neck, and abdomen using an ultrasound transducer placed over the skin. Can detect altered blood flow, arterial occlusion, deep vein thrombosis.	Discuss: ■ Purpose of test. ■ Position for test: supine. ■ Takes 10–30 minutes. ■ Test is not painful or uncomfortable. ■ Need to perform Valsalva maneuver at intervals during test. ■ Intermittent occlusion of extremity circulation manually or using blood pressure cuff. ■ External probe placement at several sites on affected extremities; opposite extremity also tested for comparison; conducting gel applied under probe. Encourage questions.	Assist client to remove gel, if needed. Provide opportunities to discuss results of test.

From Kee JL. Handbook of Laboratory and Diagnostic Tests. *Norwalk, CT: Appleton & Lange; 1988. Patrick ML, Woods SL, Craven RF, et al.* Medical-Surgical Nursing. *Philadelphia: Lippincott; 1991. Treseler KM.* Clinical Laboratory and Diagnostic Tests. *Norwalk, CT: Appleton & Lange; 1988.*

coughing techniques. Strong contraction of the abdominal and respiratory muscles is required to build sufficient intrapulmonary pressure to expel secretions from airways. An effective cough requires pressures of 100 mm Hg or more, creating an explosive outflow of air at velocities up to 965 km (600 miles) per hour.[5]

Etiology: Tracheobronchial Infection, Secretions, or Obstruction. Tracheobronchial infection often produces such copious secretions that coughing efforts cannot clear the airways. Also, these secretions are often viscous and may form mucus plugs that obstruct airways and add to the difficulty in clearing them. If the underlying cause of increased secretions is an infection, collaboration with a physician is necessary to achieve resolution because some infections require treatment with antibiotic therapy.

Obstruction can also be the result of aspiration of small pieces of food or small objects. Irritants such as smog or general anesthesia are another possible cause of excessive secretions.

Etiology: Trauma. Injuries or incisions in the chest, shoulder, back, or abdomen make coughing painful, because they often involve the muscles used in coughing. Contraction or stretching of the damaged muscles causes pain, and so individuals often suppress or abort coughing despite the presence of secretions that obstruct airways.

Etiology: Perceptual or Cognitive Impairment. Individuals whose cognitive processes have been impaired by injury or disease may have the physical ability to cough, but may have difficulty learning or remembering to cough effectively. In some cases, prompting can result in an effective cough, but prompts may be necessary each time coughing is expected.

Ineffective Breathing Pattern

Ineffective Breathing Pattern is a state in which a person's inhalation or exhalation does not bring about adequate inflation or emptying of the lungs. Examples include such respiratory patterns as hypoventilation, asymmetrical breathing, and excessively rapid or shallow breathing. A

SAMPLE NURSING DIAGNOSES: OXYGENATION

Nursing Diagnosis	Defining Characteristics/Manifestations: Subjective Data	Defining Characteristics/Manifestations: Objective Data	Etiology[a]
Ineffective Airway Clearance *1.5.1.2*	Reports inability to cough Reports fatigue	Gurgles, rumbles on chest auscultation. Decreased respiratory rate (RR). Weak, ineffective cough.	Physical: Decreased energy/fatigue.
	Severe dyspnea	Harsh cough. Diminished breath sounds. Excessive mucus. Wheezing or inspiratory stridor. Rumbles. Shallow respirations. Use of accessory muscles. Weak cough.	Physical: Bronchial obstruction: mucus plug.
Ineffective Breathing Pattern: Hypoventilation *1.5.1.3*	Reports incisional pain with deep inspiration	Decreased chest excursion. Shallow respirations. Diminished breath sounds. Hypercapnea Atelectatic crackles.	Physical: Acute pain: abdominal surgical incision.[b]
Ineffective Breathing Pattern: Hyperventilation *1.5.1.3*	Reports feeling nervous, being "on edge" Reports feeling lightheaded, faint	Tachypnea. Nasal flaring. Hypocapnea. Shallow respirations. Tremors. Sweaty palms. Clenched fists, jaw. Random repetitive movements.	Emotional: anxiety.
Altered Peripheral Tissue Perfusion *1.4.1.1*	Reports coldness of extremity Reports numbness/tingling of extremity	Skin locally reddened or pale, cool to touch. 4 + edema in legs.	Physical: Exchange problems 2° edema[b]
	Reports tightness of treatment modality (eg, bandage) Reports coldness of extremity Reports numbness/tingling in extremity	Skin locally pale or bluish, cool, edematous. Peripheral pulse in affected extremity weaker than in other extremity.	Physical: Interruption of arterial flow by constricting cast, bandage, poorly fitted TED hose.[b]

[a] Sample etiologies, only; see text discussion and taxonomy for other etiologies and defining characteristics.

[b] Example only. Many other specific examples of altered functioning with this general etiology are relevant to nursing diagnosis. Defining characteristics, desired outcomes, and nursing implementation would differ for each specific etiology.

client who has chronic lung disease may panic easily when minor dyspnea occurs and his or her breathing pattern may become ineffective.

Several conditions, including Ineffective Airway Clearance (discussed above), can produce an ineffective breathing pattern. The discussion that follows addresses the etiologies listed in the taxonomy of nursing diagnoses.

Etiology: Neuromuscular Impairment. Neuromuscular impairment implies that nervous control of the respiratory muscles is altered. Depending on the specific underlying problem, hyperventilation, hypoventilation, or asymmetrical breathing may result. Some of the underlying problems cannot be treated by independent nursing implementation; nevertheless, nursing care frequently contributes to improvement.

Etiology: Musculoskeletal Impairment. Examples of this etiology include fractures or changes in muscle functioning, such as weakness or contractures. Often, pain is a contributing factor. As in the previous etiology, nursing implementation alone may not always be sufficient to correct the underlying problem.

PROCEDURE 27–1. COLLECTING A SPUTUM SPECIMEN FROM A CLIENT ABLE TO COUGH

PURPOSE: To obtain a sample specimen of sputum for analysis for the presence of microorganisms or abnormal cells.

EQUIPMENT: Sterile specimen container with cover, nonsterile gloves, facial tissues, toothbrush and/or mouthwash, cup, and water.

ACTION	RATIONALE
1. Check medical orders for purpose of specimen and other specified conditions (amount of specimen, number of specimens, time of collection, purpose). NOTE: Bronchial secretions accumulate during sleep. It may be easier for client to produce sputum in early morning. Another good time to collect sputum is just after a bronchodilator treatment or postural drainage and percussion.	1. Specifications may vary with test. Obtaining the smallest amount of sputum sufficient for test will minimize stress on client.
2. Discuss the procedure and its purpose with the client.	2. Active participation is more likely if the client understands the expected behavior, its purpose, and anticipated benefits.
3. Provide privacy by closing the door or bedside curtains.	3. The procedure may be embarrassing to the client or offensive to others.
4. Ask the client to cleanse the mouth with mouthwash or by brushing the teeth.	4. Cleansing the mouth reduces possible contamination by oral flora.
5. Assess the client's ability to cough deeply and expectorate sputum. If client has a nonproductive cough and/or severe chest or abdominal pain, suctioning may be necessary (see Procedure 27–2).	5. A deep cough is essential to obtain mucus from the tracheobronchial tree. Simple clearing of the throat or spitting out saliva is inadequate.
6. Assess client's respiratory status: RR, depth, rhythm, skin color. NOTE: Do not attempt to obtain specimen from client in respiratory distress.	6. Active coughing may alter status. Baseline data can help determine impact of coughing.
7. Request client to assume upright position: high Fowler's, dangling, or standing. Assist to sit up if necessary. Clients who are able may prefer to take cup to bathroom after instruction on how to produce an acceptable specimen.	7. Upright position facilitates lung expansion and cough effort.
8. Instruct client to hold sputum container without touching inside of container or cover. If client is weak, or needs to splint an incision while coughing, don gloves and hold cup for client.	8. Normal flora from hands would contaminate inside of container, altering results of test.

(continued)

PROCEDURE 27–1. (continued)

9. Ask client to cough deeply (Procedure 27–6) and expectorate into container, repeating as necessary until the necessary quantity of sputum is obtained.

   9. Deep cough is necessary to bring up sputum from lower respiratory tree. Lower respiratory tract specimen is necessary for accurate test.

10. While wearing gloves, secure the cover on the container.

   10. Prevents contamination of specimen by environmental organisms, or transfer of organisms from specimen to environment.

11. Offer client facial tissues to wipe mouth or mouthwash or toothbrush as necessary. Assist client to a comfortable position.

   11. Promotes client comfort, reduces oral microorganisms.

12. Reassess client's respiratory status as above.

   12. The effort of coughing may cause oxygen deficit in clients with serious respiratory impairment.

13. Label container and send to lab according to agency policy.

   NOTE: Specimen may require special bagging or refrigeration.

   13. Facilitates prompt analysis of specimen and receipt of results to assist in treatment plan.

14. When laboratory report is filed in client's chart, share results with client.

   14. Client has a right to information about personal health status.

RECORDING: Describe respiratory status before and after specimen obtained, method used to obtain specimen, quantity and character (viscosity, color, odor) of sputum, and disposition of specimen. When results are obtained, notify physician and place result in client's record.

PROCEDURE 27–2. OBTAINING A SPUTUM SPECIMEN FROM A CLIENT UNABLE TO COUGH

PURPOSE: To obtain sample of sputum for analysis for presence of organisms (culture and sensitivity—C & S; or acid-fast bacilli—AFB) or abnormal cells (cytology).

EQUIPMENT: Suction device (wall or portable); sterile suction kit (includes catheter, glove, container for liquid), sterile water or saline; sterile sputum trap; towel or moisture-resistant pad; facial tissues; and mouthwash or toothettes.

ACTION

1. Refer to Procedure 27–1 for assessment and preparation of client.
2. Explain that suctioning should not cause great discomfort, but that it may stimulate gagging or coughing. This will diminish fear of the unknown and assist client to participate rather than resist procedure. Remember that unconscious clients may retain hearing and comprehension abilities. Do not omit explanation.
3. Request or assist conscious client to assume semi-Fowler's position with head turned toward nurse to facilitate insertion of the catheter while diminishing feelings of helplessness of client and minimizing risk of aspiration. Position unconscious client in lateral position facing nurse to allow tongue to fall forward and facilitate drainage of secretions with decreased risk of aspiration.
4. Attach suction tube to adapter on sputum trap to fa-

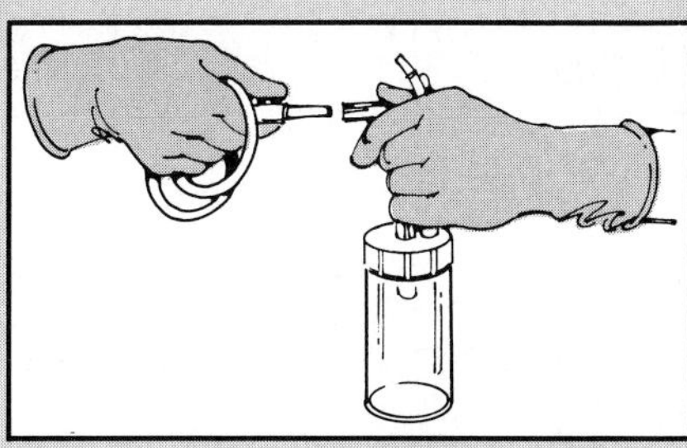

(continued)

PROCEDURE 27–2. (continued)

cilitate direct collection of sputum in container without risk of contamination of specimen or nurse.

5. Suction as described in Procedure 27–7. Repeat as necessary until sufficient amount of sputum obtained.
6. Provide for rest periods between catheter insertions to minimize stress.
7. Detach suction tubing from sputum trap. Seal trap with attached rubber tubing to prevent contamination of specimen and transfer of microorganisms to environment.

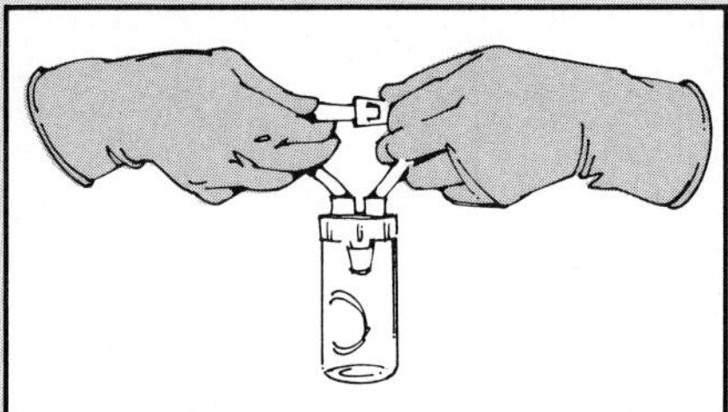

8. Assist client as needed and send specimen to laboratory as detailed in Procedure 27–1. When results obtained, discuss with client, notify MD, and place report in client's record.

▭ **RECORDING:** Describe respiratory status before and after specimen obtained, method used to obtain specimen, quantity and character of sputum, and disposition of specimen.

BOX 27–7. OTHER NURSING DIAGNOSES RELATED TO OXYGENATION

Physical

Activity Intolerance
Altered Cardiac Output: Decreased
Pain
Altered Fluid Volume: Excess or Deficit
Fatigue
High Risk for Infection
Impaired Gas Exchange
Impaired Home Maintenance Management
Potential for Infection
Potential for Injury
Potential for Aspiration
Impaired Physical Mobility
Altered Nutrition: More or Less Than Body Calorie Requirements
Self-care Deficit
Impaired Skin/Tissue Integrity
Sleep Pattern Disturbance
Altered Tissue Perfusion: Cerebral, Cardiopulmonary, Renal, or Gastrointestinal

Cognitive

Altered Thought Processes
Knowledge Deficit
Impaired Verbal Communication

Emotional

Anxiety
Fear
Hopelessness

Self-conceptual

Ineffective Individual Coping
Powerlessness
Body Image Disturbance
Altered Role Performance
Self-esteem Disturbance

Sociocultural/Life-structural

Ineffective Family Coping
Altered Family Processes
Impaired Social Interaction
Social Isolation
Ineffective Individual Coping

Developmental

Diversional Activity Deficit

Sexual

Altered Sexuality Patterns
Sexual Dysfunction

Etiology: Pain. Severe, acute pain frequently causes hyperventilation because the sympathetic nervous system response to pain causes increases in heart rate and oxygen demand. Conversely, localized pain in the abdomen, chest, shoulders, or back may result in hypoventilation because of shallow breathing. As discussed above, stretching of injured muscles stimulates pain receptors; therefore, shallow breathing to avoid this is a common response.

Etiology: Perceptual or Cognitive Impairment. Perceptual or cognitive deficits play similar roles in Ineffective Breathing Pattern to those discussed above under Ineffective Airway Clearance.

Etiology: Anxiety. The role of anxiety in the development of ineffective breathing patterns relates to sympathetic nervous system response to stress as well as possible limbic system influence on the respiratory center. The most common anxiety-related alteration in breathing pattern is hyperventilation.

Etiology: Decreased Energy, Fatigue. The work of breathing can become burdensome to extremely debilitated individuals. Paradoxically, bed rest, the common treatment for individuals in this state, increases the amount of energy needed to expand the lungs. This is because in the recumbent position, abdominal organs impinge upon the thoracic cavity and must be displaced by the diaphragm to create space for full lung inflation.

Etiology: Obesity. Obesity creates the same impediment to full lung expansion as recumbency. Increased adipose tissue deposits on the chest and abdomen make full lung expansion more difficult. Hypoventilation is a common result.

Altered Tissue Perfusion

Altered Tissue Perfusion is a state in which the supply of oxygenated blood to the legs, arms, hands, or feet is decreased. This can be the result of inadequate pumping action by the heart, decreased circulating blood volume, exchange problems, or interference with arterial blood flow. Only the latter two conditions will be addressed here.

Etiology: Interruption in Arterial Flow. Interruption in arterial flow is a major cause of impaired tissue perfusion. External pressure over bony prominences related to immobility is one cause of interrupted blood flow. Treatments such as casts, anti-embolism stockings, or improperly applied bandages on an extremity can interrupt arterial flow locally. Diseases that cause narrowing of arteries also impair perfusion. Although these require medical treatment, collaboration by nurses, such as teaching about dietary changes, can contribute to correcting the problem.

Etiology: Exchange Problems. Exchange problems refer to interference with the exchange of oxygen and carbon dioxide. Exchange problems can occur between alveoli and pulmonary capillaries (such as caused by secretions or fluid) or between peripheral capillaries and tissue cells, usually resulting from edema. Edema interferes with efficient diffusion of oxygen to the cells and carbon dioxide from the cells. In either case tissues receive insufficient oxygen.

Stating the Oxygenation Diagnosis

A complete nursing diagnosis statement includes the etiology and defining characteristics. Examples of nursing diagnoses related to oxygenation with sample etiologies and defining characteristics are presented, earlier, in the table Sample Nursing Diagnoses: Oxygenation, page 1245.

A nursing diagnosis statement is most useful as a basis for planning client care if it is individualized by specifying the problem statement, etiology, and defining characteristics as they are manifested by a particular client. For example, a client who remains in semi-Fowler's position for extended periods of time is noted to have a 2-inch-diameter reddened area over her sacrum; she states that "sometimes my tailbone feels a little numb." The redness is not relieved after lying on her side for 15 minutes. "Altered Peripheral Tissue Perfusion related to interrupted arterial flow" is an appropriate nursing diagnosis, but the statement "Altered perfusion of tissue over sacrum related to interruption of arterial flow from prolonged periods in semi-Fowler's position as evidenced by erythema, 5-cm diameter over sacrum, and localized numbness" communicates the nature of the problem more clearly and gives stronger guidance for corrective action.

A thorough oxygenation assessment is warranted whenever a client's primary concern or other risk factors suggest the possibility of compromised oxygenation. Precisely stated nursing diagnoses based on the oxygenation assessment provide a foundation for collaborative management, discussed in Section 3.

Section 3. Nurse–Client Management of Oxygenation

PLANNING FOR OPTIMUM OXYGENATION

An effective nursing care plan clearly communicates measurable outcomes for client care, related evaluation criteria, and nursing implementation to attain the outcomes. Desired outcome statements provide realistic goals for the client and the nurse, guidelines for client care, and are the basis for evaluation criteria.

Oxygenation outcomes, like other outcomes of care, are best determined through mutual goal setting. Assessment data helps nurses make nursing diagnoses and determine the reasonableness of the desired outcomes. Nurse and client should work together to established desired outcomes that both understand and accept. The desired outcomes for nursing care should also be compatible with the goals for medical treatment. Collaboration with the physician is necessary if the nursing and medical goals are to be complimentary and compatible.

Setting oxygenation outcomes can be difficult when a client is in an extremely debilitated state with little or no awareness of the quality of life that may be possible if these problems are well managed. In this case, the family may collaborate with the nurse and other caregivers if possible, or the nurse and other members of the health care team may need to establish outcomes and plan care until the client is well enough to participate in decision making.

Once desired outcomes are set, they should be stated clearly for mutual understanding. For example, an outcome for the sample nursing diagnosis in Section 2 might be: "improved tissue perfusion within 24 hours, as evidenced by progressive decrease in size of erythema and full return of sensation to area." Another sample oxygenation outcome might be "within 2 days, the client will walk 50 feet while correctly using pursed-lip breathing techniques." Another might be "at the end of 3 days, the client will correctly describe the structure and functions of normal lungs and how his or her own lungs differ from normal."

■ NURSING IMPLEMENTATION TO PROMOTE OPTIMUM OXYGENATION

Collaborative planning for oxygenation needs involves selecting nursing implementations to attain the desired outcomes. The appropriate level of care is suggested by the assessment data and the desired outcomes. Specific implementation is best derived collaboratively by nurse and client. Nursing measures should allow the client to draw on his or her strengths and provide supportive care where needed.

Sample nursing management of oxygenation, including appropriate outcomes, implementation, and evaluation criteria, is presented in the table Nurse–Client Management of Oxygenation Problems on pages 1251–1252. This table provides guidelines for the development of individualized nursing care plans in which outcomes, nursing implementation, and evaluation criteria are tailored to the strengths, needs, and life-style of a specific client and family.

Preventive Care

Nurses have an important role in the management of oxygenation status in all levels of care. A nurse can do many things to assist a client toward optimal oxygenation and to prevent oxygenation problems. Many oxygenation problems stem from life-style factors such as smoking, exposure to air pollution, failure to use masks during exposure to fumes and dusts, stress, improper diet, and lack of exercise. Preventive measures must begin early in life if long-term oxygenation problems are to be avoided. It is not enough to wait until symptoms occur and then change one's life-style. Nurses should be teachers and role models of how to keep healthy. Preventive care includes both screening and health education to facilitate life-style changes.

Screening. Nursing approaches to assist the client toward an optimal oxygenation status should include a life-style analysis as a method of identifying problems or planning preventive strategies. Factors to be considered relative to the client's life-style are discussed under "General Health and Life-style" in Section 1.

Health Education. Health education is a major nursing responsibility. Nurses should not assume that clients are aware of the hazards of smoking, exposure to air pollution, stress, lack of exercise, or improper diet. In addition, many people are unaware of simple everyday activities that will help them stay healthy.

Discouraging Smoking. Smoking is the most important preventable cause of disease and disability in the United States.[13] The US Department of Health and Human Services estimates that 30 to 40 percent of smokers do not believe that smoking increases the risk of certain diseases or that quitting smoking decreases the risk. Yet after 1 year off cigarettes, the excess risk of heart disease from smoking is reduced by half. Ten years after quitting, risk from lung cancer is halved and stroke risk returns to the level of those who have never smoked.[14]

Each year, 20 percent of all cardiovascular deaths, 35 percent of cancer deaths (including 87 percent of lung cancer deaths), and about 62,000 deaths from respiratory diseases are attributed to smoking.[13,15] In 1988, smoking caused about 434,000 deaths.[15] In addition, smoking shortens a person's projected life span by about 5 to 8 years.[16] Lung cancer has long been the number one cancer killer of men. It is now the top cancer killer in women as well, because cigarette smoking is increasing among women in general, particularly young women.[13]

Smoking may also lead to emphysema, chronic bronchitis, heart and blood vessel diseases, bladder and pancreatic cancers, and worsening of existing cardiopulmonary

IMPLICATIONS FOR NURSE–CLIENT COLLABORATION

Smoking

Smoking is a significant client care problem because of its well-documented systemic and addictive effects. In collaborating with adolescent clients, nurses can make a significant contribution by discouraging them from smoking, preferably before they start. When the client is already a smoker, education is essential, and a straightforward message that advocates quitting and points out the risks is most effective. Chronic smokers usually know they should stop smoking, and frequently they have tried several times. Such individuals may already have symptoms related to smoking; nevertheless they may still benefit from the nurse's patience, support, and encouragement.

NURSE–CLIENT MANAGEMENT OF OXYGENATION PROBLEMS

Nursing Diagnosis	Desired Outcome	Implementation	Evaluation Criteria
Ineffective Airway Clearance R/T decreased energy/fatigue *1.5.1.2*	1. Effective airway clearance	1a. Explain importance of effective coughing to reduce shortness of breath, DOE. 1b. Teach correct coughing technique (see Procedure 27–6). 1c. Encourage and positively reinforce effective coughing. 1d. Teach importance of refraining from smoking. 1e. Teach diaphragmatic breathing (Procedure 27–3) and pursed-lip breathing (Procedure 27–4). 1f. Administer oxygen in collaboration with physician. 1g. Tracheobronchial suctioning PRN.	1. Airway clear, AEB: ■ No gurgles, rumbles on chest auscultation ■ RR and depth within expected range for age and health status.
	2. Decreased fatigue	2a. Reduce metabolic demands: space activities requiring exertion; no bathing, ambulating, eating, etc, during periods of acute distress. 2b. Plan regular rest periods, especially after coughing, meals, exercise. 2c. Collaborate with physician to treat cause of fatigue.	2. Progressive energy level improvement AEB increased participation in regular activities without reports of fatigue, DOE.
Ineffective Airway Clearance R/T bronchial obstruction: mucus plug[a] *1.5.1.2*	1. Clear airway with unlabored respiration	1a. Assist with effective coughing techniques. 1b. Perform chest physiotherapy and postural drainage. 1c. Perform tracheobronchial suctioning if obstruction persists. 1d. Administer oxygen in collaboration with physician.	1a. RR and depth within expected range for age and health status. 1b. Stridor, adventitious breath sounds absent. 1c. Progressive decrease in cough, mucus. 1d. Client reports decreased dyspnea.
Ineffective Breathing Pattern: Hypoventilation R/T acute pain: abdominal surgical incision[a] *1.5.1.3*	1. Effective RR, rhythm, and depth	1a. Assess RR, rhythm, depth, lung fields at least q shift. 1b. Teach diaphragmatic pursed-lip breathing (Procedure 27–3).	1,2. Airway remains free of secretions AEB: ■ No gurgles, rumbles, crackles, or diminished breath sounds on chest auscultation. ■ RR and depth within expected range for age and health status.
	2. Lungs remain free of atelectasis and/or secretions	2a. Assist with coughing (Procedure 27–6) whenever secretions are present. 2b. Assist client to use sustained maximal inspiration device (Procedure 27–5) qh.	

NURSE–CLIENT MANAGEMENT OF OXYGENATION PROBLEMS (continued)

Nursing Diagnosis	Desired Outcome	Implementation	Evaluation Criteria
		2c. Encourage splinting of incision when performing deep breathing and coughing. 2d. Teach importance of not smoking.	
	3. Alleviation or elimination of pain	3. Provide pain-relief measures (see Chap. 29).	3. Client states that pain is diminished or gone.
Ineffective Breathing Pattern: Hyperventilation R/T anxiety[a] *1.5.1.2*	1. Effective RR, rhythm, and depth	1. Teach diaphragmatic and pursed-lip breathing.	1. RR and depth within expected range for age and health status.
	2. Decreased anxiety	2a. Teach breathing and relaxation techniques (see Chap. 22). 2b. Use active listening techniques to assist client to resolve feelings of anxiety (see Chap. 14). 2c. Collaborate with other health care team members (social worker, counselor, psychiatrist) as needed.	2. Anxiety decreased AEB: ■ Decreased tremors. ■ No sweaty palms. ■ Hands and jaw relaxed. ■ Decreased random movements. ■ Client reports not feeling edgy, nervous.
Altered Peripheral Tissue Perfusion R/T exchange problems: 2° edema[a] *1.4.1.1*	1. Peripheral tissue perfusion appropriate to client's health status	1a. Teach importance of qh position changes. 1b. Assist with position changes if client unable to perform independently (see Chap. 30). 1c. Elevate legs. 1d. Use protective devices as needed to decrease pressure (see Chap. 30).	1. Peripheral tissue adequately perfused AEB: ■ Skin over all bony prominences appropriate color for client. ■ No lesions related to pressure.
Altered Peripheral Tissue Perfusion R/T interruption of arterial flow by constricting cast, bandage, or poorly fitted TED hose[a] *1.4.1.1*	1. Peripheral tissue perfusion appropriate to client's health status	1a. Assess extremity on which cast, bandage, or TED hose has been newly applied qh ×4, q4h ×12h, then q shift for pallor, pulselessness, ischemic pain, paresthesia (abnormal sensation), poikilothermia (coolness), decreased capillary refill. 1b. When reapplying TED hose or bandages around an extremity, apply smoothly and snugly, but not tightly (see Procedure 27–15 and Chap. 22). 1c. Elevate extremity with cast, bandage, or TED hose.	1. Optimum peripheral perfusion AEB distal parts of extremity remain warm, appropriate color for client, without abnormal sensation or pain, with strong peripheral pulse and immediate capillary refill.

[a] Example only. Many other specific examples of altered functioning with this general etiology are relevant to nursing management. Defining characteristics, desired outcomes, and nursing implementation would differ for each specific etiology.

conditions such as asthma. Chronic smokers and those who are exposed to large amounts of smoke have a high blood level of carbon monoxide and consequently a reduced level of oxygen in their blood. Statistically, there are changes in the airways after only 20 pack-years of smoking, though clients at this level of smoking usually are not yet symptomatic.[17] The fact that smoking leads to changes in both oxygenation and in the cardiovascular system becomes even more problematic in view of the fact that smoking elevates heart rate. The heart, therefore, needs more oxygen to support the extra work it is doing at the same time that less oxygen is available to it.

Smoking seems to have a synergistic effect with other risk factors for cardiopulmonary disease. For example, diabetes is a major risk factor for cardiovascular changes. The vascular changes are increased many times if the diabetic is also a smoker. Asbestos workers who smoke are 90 times more likely to die of lung cancer than people who neither smoke nor work with asbestos.[16] A woman who uses oral contraceptives and smokes increases her risk of heart attack 39 times and her risk of stroke 22 times compared with a woman who does neither.[2]

Those who share the smoker's environment are also at risk. Up to 85 percent of the smoke from a cigarette, pipe, or cigar may be sidestream smoke, or smoke that simply goes into the environment. This smoke contains a higher concentration of dangerous gases than the smoke that is exhaled by the smoker. An estimated 30,000 to 80,000 deaths each year are attributed to passive smoking.[1]

The best solution to the problem of smoking is never to start. Therefore, educational programs for adolescents in the schools and other community settings are important. Nurses who work with adolescents should discourage smoking in health teaching and client care. Because adolescents are present-oriented, they are less likely to respond to discussions of long-term health risks than to emphasis on immediate negative effects, such as bad breath, stained fingers and teeth, and diminished performance in sports.

Education for those who already smoke is also important. A straightforward message advocating quitting and pointing out risks is most effective. Avoid scare tactics, guilt trips, or preaching.[18] Provide information about resources such as local offices of the American Lung Association, American Heart Association, and American Cancer Society, and about various smoking cessation methods, such as self-help strategies, aversion techniques, hypnosis, acupuncture, and behavior modification. Group programs as well as individual approaches are available. Selection of a program is an individual decision based on individual needs and preferences.

Nurses working with smokers who are trying to quit should remember that patience and support from those around the smoker are essential. Relapse is common. Many smokers try several times before quitting for good. Stress, being around other smokers, and weight gain are common causes of relapse. It is also important for individuals to know that when they stop smoking, their cough and sputum may remain for 3 to 6 months. Ex-smokers who do not understand this phenomenon may start smoking again to stop the cough. Actual tissue damage, such as emphysema, cannot be reversed by stopping smoking. However, the condition can be better treated and the client's general health improved if he or she stops smoking.

Air Pollution. Air pollution may be a continuing or an intermittent problem in any area of the United States. It can be either an additive or potentiating risk factor with smoking for cardiopulmonary disease.[19] Air pollution may cause increased morbidity and mortality, exacerbate existing cardiopulmonary disease, and cause sensory, neurological, and behavioral changes. The relationship between air pollution and lung cancer has not been proven, nor has the exact level of air pollution that is hazardous been determined. Vulnerable individuals (such as those with cardiopulmonary disease) should stay indoors and quiet during times of air stagnation or severe pollution. Even people who are at low risk should not play or exercise outdoors during severe air pollution.

Occupational Hazards. Unlike most other body systems, the respiratory tract is in direct contact with the outside environment. It can, therefore, be injured directly by exposure to noxious materials. Occupational respiratory hazards include dusts, fumes, silica (glass, sandstone, other rocks), coal dusts, asbestos, beryllium, and chemicals such as formaldehyde and glutoraldehyde. Workers who are exposed to occupational hazards should always wear appropriate protective masks. Sometimes special gloves and clothing and showering after exposure are also required. Necessary protective measures should be strictly enforced by plant management. Occupational health nurses have a special mandate to be certain that workers understand safety regulations and adhere to them to prevent disability and disease.

Preventing Aspiration. Aspiration is what happens when foods, fluids, saliva, foreign objects, or other matter enters the nose, throat, or lower airways. The best way to deal with aspiration and the resulting asphixiation or aspiration pneumonia is to prevent it.

Aspiration in young children frequently occurs because they put small objects, such as toys or coins, in their mouths. Small toys or toys with small removable parts should not be given to children under age 3. For example, children often pull or bite off the eyes or noses of some stuffed animals, so parents need to check these and other toys before allowing children to play with them.

Sometimes, aspiration or airway obstruction occurs when a person chokes on a piece of food during a meal. To some extent, such aspiration can be prevented. Children under 3 years old should not be given foods such as peanuts or pieces of chewy meats. Thorough chewing should be encouraged. In adults, aspiration of food may occur when the person has been drinking alcoholic beverages and the gag reflex and judgment are consequently impaired.

Heimlich Maneuver and CPR. The Heimlich maneuver is a technique for removing a foreign body that has lodged in the trachea or pharynx. It is effective and easy to learn.

BUILDING NURSING KNOWLEDGE

Do Clients Who Have Vascular Disease and Quit Smoking Differ from Those Who Continue?

Ronayne R, O'Connor A, Scobie TK. Smoking: A decision-making dilemma for the vascular patient, *J. Adv Nurs.* 1989; 14:647–652.

Vascular disease is a chronic disabling illness that affects primarily middle-aged to elderly people. Although it seldom causes death, it can result in disability and loss of limbs. The risk of developing vascular disease is two to nine times greater among smokers than nonsmokers. Although many individuals stop smoking after learning of their illness, the majority continue to smoke despite counseling. Ronayne and associates endeavored to identify factors that influence clients' decisions to quit, reduce, or continue smoking.

The study employs the "reasoned action model," which asserts that an individual is more likely to stop smoking if he or she (1) values living as a nonsmoker more than living as a smoker, (2) believes that the action will reduce the progress of the disease and prevent amputation, and (3) perceives that stopping smoking is worthwhile to the people he or she wishes to please.

The sample consisted of 20 subjects with vascular disease who quit smoking at least 6 months or more prior to entering the study, and 22 who elected to continue. Subjects were interviewed about the outcomes of quitting or continuing smoking and filled out surveys on their beliefs about smoking risks.

No significant differences were found between quitters and nonquitters in terms of age, sex, past surgical history, or illness severity. Subjects in both groups believed that quitting had more benefits for the respiratory system than for the circulatory system. The perceived respiratory benefits were related to "breathing better" and "coughing less." Other advantages cited were "increased appetite" and "feeling less tired." Quitters were more confident than nonquitters that stopping smoking would increase the likelihood of walking better and feeling less tension. Nonquitters, on the other hand, felt more concerned about weight gain and feared increased feelings of tension. Quitters more than nonquitters believed the risk of amputation to be substantially reduced by quitting. Almost all quitters (94 percent) perceived the risk of amputation to be unacceptable, whereas 47 percent of the nonquitters believed the risk of amputation to be unacceptable but felt powerless to do anything about the risk. Quitters and nonquitters reported that their physician, family, and friends encouraged them to stop smoking, suggesting that social pressure is not a significant factor in decision making.

Ronayne and colleagues concluded that the factor that differentiated the quitters from the nonquitters was their attitude toward risk. Subjects who perceived little or no risk continued to smoke. In clinical practice, clients who perceive no risk may benefit from individual counseling to increase their awareness of the harmful effects of smoking. Those who believe there is risk, but who feel powerless to change, require assistance to help translate their goals into action.

Teaching this maneuver to parents and others who care for individuals at risk for aspiration can prevent injury and save lives. CPR (cardiopulmonary resuscitation) is used when choking or another insult causes respiratory or cardiac arrest. Agencies such as the American Heart Association and the American Red Cross also provide classes for the general public on CPR and the Heimlich maneuver. These techniques are discussed later in this chapter. See Procedures 27–8 to 27–10.

Supportive Care

Supportive care is aimed at supporting clients' physiological and psychosocial adaptations so illness-related disruptions are minimal. As with preventive care, life-style modification and health education can often prevent mild health problems from becoming more serious. Three examples of supportive care related to oxygenation are discussed here: caring for clients with mild upper respiratory infections, assisting clients who have respiratory allergies, and providing preoperative care.

Caring for Clients with Mild Upper Respiratory Infections. Clients often self-diagnose and self-treat upper respiratory infections such as colds, laryngitis, and mild influenza. Although these infections do not usually seriously compromise oxygenation, they do make breathing more difficult. Individuals having frequent colds can benefit from help in identifying contributing factors and ways to reduce discomfort.

Reducing Incidence. Colds are caused by viruses. The mode of transmission is via droplet nuclei, although direct transmission of the virus from the hands to mucous membranes also occurs. Avoiding crowded places during the cold and flu season is one way to reduce one's incidence of colds. Individuals with respiratory allergies have heightened susceptibility to colds and should take preventive measures.

Advise individuals who have mild upper respiratory infections to avoid crowds and, in particular, contact with very young children, the elderly, or those with chronic disease because these groups are particularly vulnerable to the negative effects of colds.[20] Covering the mouth and nose when coughing or sneezing, frequent handwashing, and appropriate disposal of facial tissues also help prevent transmission of the virus.

Smokers are at greater risk for upper respiratory infections than nonsmokers because of damage to the respiratory tract mucosa. Pointing this out to a smoker who has frequent colds may be an incentive to quit.

Managing Symptoms. The minor discomforts of colds are often greatly relieved by over-the-counter medications such as decongestants (phenylephrine, pseudoephedrine) and analgesics (aspirin, acetaminophen). Clients should be cautioned to read package inserts about side effects and necessary precautions. Generally, if symptoms persist despite self-medication, consultation with a health care provider is advised. Increasing fluid intake is advisable during a cold.

Many clients find gargling with salt water and sucking on throat lozenges relieve sore throat and cough.

Clients should be advised that symptoms such as a fever over 100F, very sore throat, rash, or thick copious secretions suggest the possibility of a bacterial infection that requires medical treatment. Individuals with heart or lung disease should seek care for even mild influenza, because they are at risk for extension of the infection to the lower respiratory tract and other more serious complications.

Assisting Clients with Respiratory Allergies. Many people have allergies that are manifested by respiratory symptoms. Most can lead normal lives with little change in life-style. Others need support from health care providers to make life-style changes that will enable them to remain healthy and active.

Allergic rhinitis is a reaction of the nasal mucosa to specific allergens. An allergen is a substance that can produce a hypersensitive (allergic) reaction in the body. These may include inhaled allergens (such as pollens), food allergens, or systemic allergens (such as drugs). The manifestations of allergic rhinitis include nasal drainage or obstruction and stuffiness; sneezing; headaches; itching of the nose, eyes, throat, or ears; mouth breathing; and redness of the eyes. These manifestations usually do not interfere with oxygenation, although breathing may be difficult if nasal and pharyngeal mucosa become swollen and congested. Asthma, which is characterized by airway inflammation, hypersecretion, and contraction of airway smooth muscles, occurs in response to exposure to allergens. This is a potentially serious condition and requires more intensive treatment.

In general, therapy for allergies includes use of mild antihistamines and identification of the offending allergens. If the allergens can be identified, it may be enough for the person simply to avoid the allergens as much as possible. In other cases, desensitization (allergy shots) may be recommended.

Nurses can be instrumental in helping clients identify possible allergens and eliminate them from their environment. Discussion should focus on timing and frequency of symptoms and possible exposure to common allergens at the time symptoms appear.

Some examples of substances that often stimulate allergic reactions include cigarette smoke, molds, perfume, fumes from certain household cleaners, propellants from common aerosol products, pollens, and animal dander (the dry scales that are shed from the fur of animals and the feathers of birds). A dusty environment entraps allergens and therefore tends to exacerbate allergies.

Preoperative Teaching. Nursing care given before surgery to prevent postoperative oxygenation problems is also supportive care. Postoperative clients are at risk of developing oxygenation problems because of general anesthesia, postoperative pain, pain medications, and immobility.

General anesthesia sometimes depresses respirations in the postoperative period, which may result in hypoventilation and atelectasis. Moreover, some inhalation anesthetics irritate the respiratory mucosa, causing increased production of mucus, which can obstruct airways and inhibit air exchange if it is not effectively cleared.

Postoperative pain, particularly from abdominal or flank incisions, promotes shallow respirations and suppression of coughing, as discussed earlier. The narcotic analgesics usually prescribed to treat postoperative pain may also depress respirations.

Many clients are reluctant to move and change positions because of postoperative pain. As discussed in Chapter 30, the venous stasis associated with immobility increases the risk of thrombophlebitis. Thrombophlebitis is the inflammation of a vein wall in conjunction with the formation of a clot. The clot adhering to the inflamed vein wall can compromise circulation locally.

Other factors related to surgery increase the risk of thrombophlebitis. Surgery stimulates the clotting mechanism because blood vessels are cut during the surgical procedure. Vein walls in the lower extremities are sometimes damaged during surgery, because of body positioning for optimal surgical access. Also, the extended immobility during the operation precipitates venous stasis.

Thrombophlebitis can lead to a more serious complication, pulmonary embolus. This occurs when a clot breaks free of the vein wall and becomes entrapped in lung circulation. It can cause serious interference with lung perfusion. Pulmonary embolus is a serious postoperative complication whose management is beyond the scope of this text.

People with preexisting oxygenation problems have a higher than normal risk of postoperative respiratory or circulatory complications. In the preoperative period, particular attention should be given to the client's smoking history and to symptoms of cardiopulmonary problems such as dyspnea on exertion, wheezing, cough and sputum production, chest pain, or symptoms of right- or left-sided heart failure. Even if there is no evidence of long-term oxygenation problems, an acute respiratory disease as minor as the common cold can predispose to postoperative pulmonary problems. Other problems that may be associated in some measure with postoperative pulmonary or circulatory complications include advancing age, obesity, and varicose veins.

Some of the techniques to promote postoperative oxygenation are initiated in the immediate postanesthesia recovery period. Because clients' level of alertness is likely to be diminished at this time, preoperative teaching to orient clients to the techniques and equipment is beneficial. Nurses should consider the clients' level of anxiety regarding surgery when planning teaching sessions (see also Chap. 20).

Techniques to promote optimum oxygenation after surgery include leg exercises to enhance venous return, breathing exercises to maximize lung expansion, and effective coughing to maintain airway patency.

Leg Exercises. Several simple exercises that can be done in bed will stimulate venous return and reduce the risk of thrombophlebitis (Fig. 27–10):

- Calf pumping: Alternate plantar flexion and dorsiflexion (Fig. 27–10A).
- Foot circles: Rotate the forefoot as if to draw a circle with the great toe (Fig. 27–10B).
- Hip rotation: Alternate inward and outward rotation of the hip (Fig. 27–10C).
- Leg spread: Alternate abduction and adduction of the hip (Fig. 27–10D).
- Knee flexion: Alternately flex and extend the leg at the knee (Fig. 27–10E).

The optimum frequency and number of repetitions of these exercises vary from client to client and are best decided postoperatively. The longer the period of postoperative bed rest, the more important it is to schedule these exercises several times a day. Clients should be cautioned to avoid holding their breath or using a Valsalva maneuver when doing these exercises.

Breathing Exercises. Exercises that enhance lung expansion and therefore prevent atelectasis and hypoventilation include diaphragmatic breathing (Procedure 27–3), pursed-lip breathing (Procedure 27–4), and use of an incentive spirometer (Procedure 27–5). Diaphragmatic and pursed lip breathing are also effective for relief of respiratory distress.

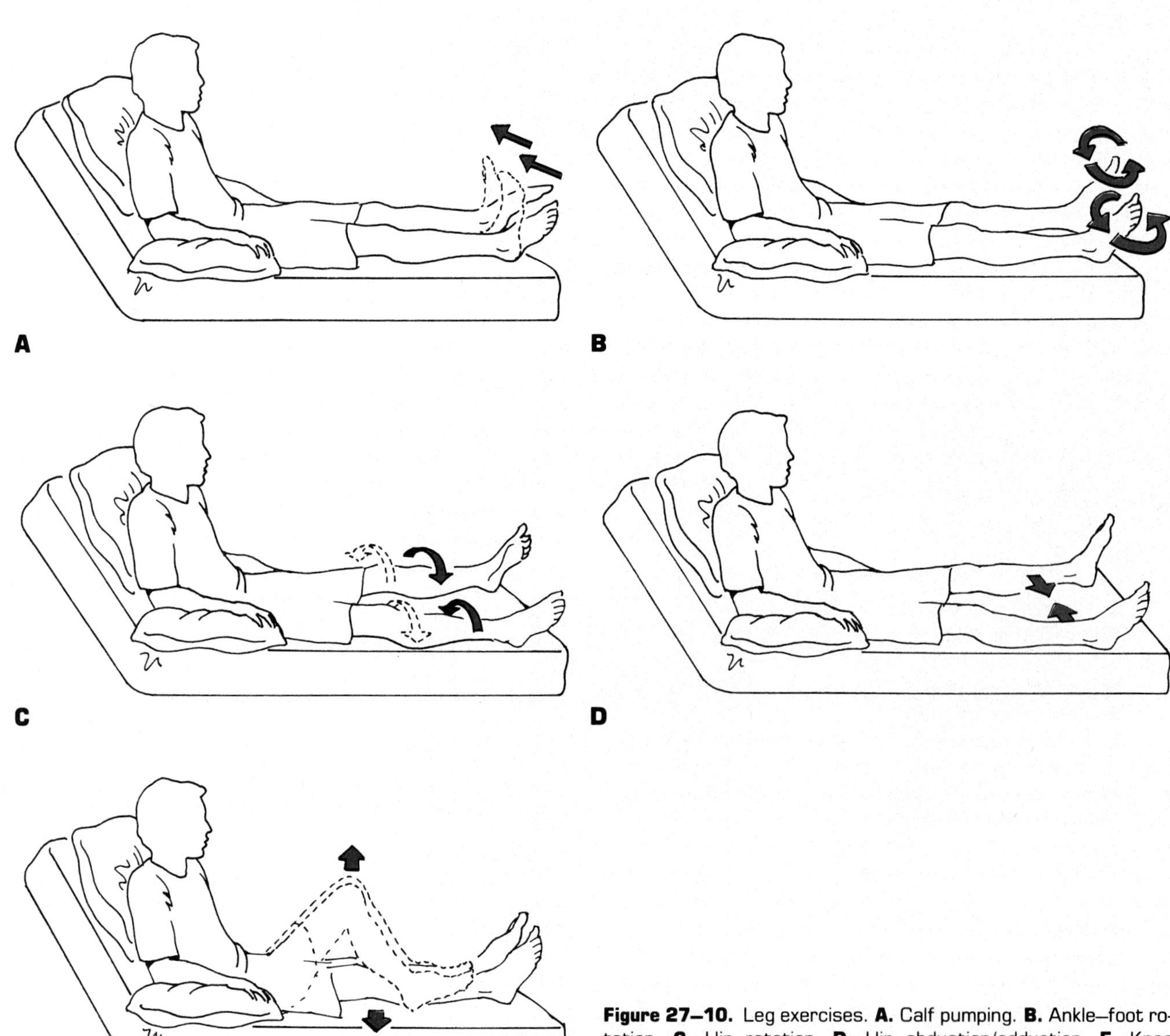

Figure 27–10. Leg exercises. **A.** Calf pumping. **B.** Ankle–foot rotation. **C.** Hip rotation. **D.** Hip abduction/adduction. **E.** Knee flexion/hyperextension.

PROCEDURE 27–3. TEACHING DIAPHRAGMATIC BREATHING

PURPOSE: To increase ventilation in the lower lobes, strengthen the diaphragm, and promote relaxation.

EQUIPMENT: None.

ACTION	RATIONALE
1. Select a time and setting that is mutually acceptable to you and the client.	1. Learning is facilitated when attention is focused. High anxiety levels interfere with learning; therefore, teaching should not be attempted when the client is uncomfortable, stressed, or dyspneic.
2. Discuss the procedure with the client, including desired client participation and anticipated benefits.	2. Active participation is more likely if the client understands the expected behaviors and the anticipated benefits.
3. If client has nasal congestion, suggest blowing the nose.	3. A clear airway is necessary for effective airflow.
4. With the client in a low Fowler's or sitting position, instruct the client to place one hand lightly on the abdomen, just over the umbilicus; and the other hand at mid-chest. Knees should be flexed to relax the abdominal muscles.	4. This hand placement enhances awareness of correct use of muscles during the exercises.
5. Describe and demonstrate to the client how to inhale slowly and deeply through the nose, while using the abdominal muscles to elevate the hand resting upon it. The client should feel as if the abdomen is gradually filling with air during inhalation. The chest should not move during this exercise.	5. Using multiple teaching modalities (in this case, auditory and visual) enhances learning. Use of the abdominal muscles facilitates relaxation and expands the chest cavity, inflating more alveoli.

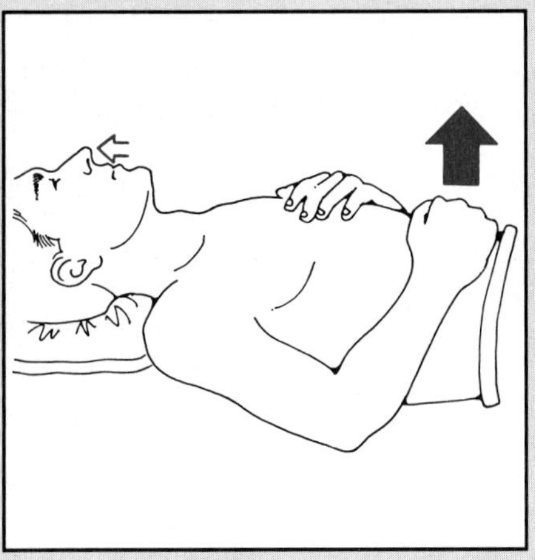

(continued)

PROCEDURE 27–3. (continued)

6. Describe and demonstrate slow and complete exhalation through pursed lips, while tightening the abdominal muscles. The abdomen should contract. Complete exhalation can also be facilitated by tightening the abdominal muscles and exerting light pressure with the hand on the abdomen.

6. See step 5, above. Exhaling through pursed lips slows collapse of small airways by maintaining higher bronchiole pressure, allowing slower and more complete exhalation (see Procedure 27–4).

7. Assess the client's response during several repetitions of the exercise to determine the number of repetitions per session to suggest as a short-term goal.

7. Clients with oxygenation problems fatigue easily. Several short exercise periods each day will promote maximum benefit with minimal fatigue.

8. Give positive feedback for correct performance of the exercise.

8. Positive reinforcement increases likelihood that the behavior will be repeated.

9. Instruct the client to rest 1 to 2 minutes after each minute of the breathing exercise.

9. Rest delays the onset of fatigue, allowing longer practice sessions.

10. Instruct the client to increase to about four 10-minute exercise sessions daily.

NOTE: If dizziness or shortness of breath occurs during the exercise, the client should rest and decrease the intensity or length of the exercise.

10. Improved pulmonary function should result from regular exercise, so the client will be able to tolerate longer exercise periods.

11. As the client gains competence in the technique, suggest performing the exercise in alternate positions, such as lying or standing, and during simple activities such as walking and stair climbing.

11. Facilitates transfer of learning so the client can use this technique to relieve respiratory distress if it occurs during regular daily activities.

RECORDING: Note the specific exercise taught, the degree of proficiency demonstrated by the client, the length of the exercise session, any problems noted, and mutual plans for continued practice. The exercise plan should be incorporated into the client care plan and posted at the client's bedside.

PROCEDURE 27–4. TEACHING PURSED-LIP BREATHING

PURPOSE: To provide a means of controlling respirations during exercise, dyspnea, or panic situations; to increase tidal volume and prevent air trapping by maintaining patency of small airways; to reduce unintentional breath holding during activity.

EQUIPMENT: None.

ACTION	RATIONALE
1. Select a time that is mutually acceptable to you and client.	1. Learning is facilitated when attention is focused. Low stress levels facilitate concentration. High anxiety or panic interferes with learning; teaching should not be attempted when client is uncomfortable, stressed, or dyspneic.
2. Discuss the exercise and its purpose with the client.	2. Learning is facilitated when the individual sees the relevance of what is being learned to the personal situation.
3. Request client to assume a sitting position in bed or chair. After client has mastered the technique, it can be performed in any position.	3. Upright position reduces pressure of abdominal organs on the diaphragm, creating more space for lung expansion.
4. Ask client to inhale deeply through the nose while you count slowly to two. When the breathing technique has been learned, ask the client to count with respirations.	4. Learning is facilitated when the learner can focus on one behavior at a time.
5. Ask client to form pursed lips as if to whistle, then exhale evenly while you count to four. Tell the client to listen for a soft whooshing sound as air is exhaled.	5. It takes about twice as long to exhale a given volume as to inhale it because small airway collapse retards expiratory airflow. Whooshing sound indicates correct lip position.
6. Ask the client to repeat the exercise several times while you count. Give positive feedback for correct performance.	6. Repetition enhances learning. Behavior that is positively reinforced is likely to be repeated.
7. When client can correctly perform the exercise as you count, ask him or her to breathe and count simultaneously, using the same rhythm as before. Reinforce correct performance.	7. Client must be able to perform the exercise independently for it to be useful in daily situations.
8. Work with the client to develop a regular practice schedule with increasing frequency of sessions per day until five sessions lasting 5–10 minutes a day are tolerated.	8. Repetition is necessary for the acquisition of a motor skill. The client is more likely to adhere to a schedule that he or she participates in developing. Short practice sessions are better tolerated by clients with respiratory dysfunction.

(continued)

PROCEDURE 27–4. (continued)

9. Encourage use of the technique during exercise, and activities such as shaving, dressing, carrying light loads, climbing stairs, and housework, or when stressed. Sample instructions: Shave only while exhaling. Tie shoes by first inhaling, then bending to tie one shoe while exhaling. Use similar inhalation–exhalation rhythm while making beds, vacuuming, climbing stairs.

   Rationale 9. The client with respiratory dysfunction becomes short of breath after very short periods of breath holding. Breath holding is common during exercise, shaving, and other activities listed. Stress tends to cause tachypnea, which results in decreased oxygen intake and possible hypoxia.

RECORDING: Document the specific exercise taught, the degree of proficiency demonstrated by the client, length of the exercise session, any problems noted, and mutual plans for continued practice. The exercise plan should be incorporated into the client care plan and posted at the client's bedside.

PROCEDURE 27–5. TEACHING USE OF THE INCENTIVE SPIROMETER

PURPOSE: To facilitate sustained maximal inhalation (SMI); and to prevent atelectasis, especially in clients who inhibit deep breathing because of postsurgical incisional pain or respiratory dysfunction.

EQUIPMENT: Incentive spirometer.

ACTION	RATIONALE
1. Discuss volume goals for spirometry with physician or respiratory therapist. (If using Tri-flow or similar type spirometer, volume goals are not necessary.) NOTE: Postsurgical clients may simply be encouraged to take as deep a breath as possible; clients with respiratory dysfunction may need to increase volume goals gradually.	1. Specific client variables will determine appropriate volumes.
2. Select a time and place that are mutually acceptable to you and the client. NOTE: It may be appropriate to give analgesia ½ hour before exercise for postsurgical clients.	2. Learning is facilitated when attention is focused. Pain, high anxiety, and distractions interfere with learning, so teaching should not be attempted when client is anxious, or during episodes of respiratory distress or pain.
3. Assess respiratory status: rate, depth, breath sounds, chest wall expansion, and symmetry.	3. Provides a baseline for assessing treatment effectiveness.
4. Discuss the procedure and its expected benefits with the client.	4. Active participation is more likely if the client understands the expected behaviors and anticipated benefits.

(continued)

PROCEDURE 27–5. (continued)

5. Instruct the client to:
   a. Hold the spirometer in an upright position (less critical in a flow-oriented spirometer).
   b. Exhale normally.
   c. Seal the lips tightly around the mouthpiece.

5a. Less negative pressure is required to move the balls or discs in a flow-oriented spirometer.
   c. If air leaks around the mouthpiece, less negative pressure will be generated inside the device. Feedback about performance will be inaccurate.

6. Ask the client to:
   a. Take a slow, deep breath through the mouth only, until the preset goal is reached; then hold the breath for 2 seconds, increasing to 6 seconds as tolerance increases.

6a. Greater lung expansion is achieved with slow inspiration. Holding the breath after maximal inspiration facilitates lung expansion.

NOTE: If incisional pain interferes with effective deep breathing, assist the client to splint the incision (see Fig. 27–12). The client should avoid rapid, shallow breaths; these do not inflate the alveoli effectively. If the client has difficulty inhaling only through the mouth, a nose clip may be used.

   b. Take the mouthpiece out of the mouth and exhale normally.
   c. Repeat the exercise five to ten times with normal breaths in between.

   b. The spirometer is not designed to allow expiratory flow through the chambers.

NOTE: If the client becomes dizzy or lightheaded, the exercise should be terminated and the number of repetitions decreased in subsequent sessions.

   c. Repetition increases inspiratory volume and improves alveolar ventilation.

7. If lung secretions are present, instruct the client to cough at the completion of each series of deep inhalations (see Procedure 27–6).

7. Deep breathing loosens secretions; coughing facilitates their removal.

8. Reassess respiratory status to compare with baseline data.

9. Instruct the client to repeat the exercise every hour.

9. Alveoli not being inflated tend to collapse within 1 hour.

RECORDING: Note the type of spirometer, number of repetitions, the volume or flow achieved, presence of secretions, any problems noted. Some institutions use a flowsheet or checklist to document use of an incentive spirometer.

An incentive spirometer encourages clients to breathe deeply and to hold the inspired breath briefly before exhaling. This is called **sustained maximal inspiration.** It is an effective way to prevent alveolar collapse. Different incentive spirometers are illustrated in Figure 27–11.

Effective Coughing. Coughing is often necessary postoperatively to clear secretions and maintain airway patency. Postoperative clients are often reluctant to cough and therefore cough ineffectively, which causes pain but does not move secretions. Procedure 27–6 assists the nurse in teaching effective coughing. Formerly, regular coughing concurrent with deep breathing was recommended as part of postoperative prevention of respiratory complications. However, current practice is to recommend postoperative coughing only when secretions are present. Routine coughing in the absence of secretions has been found to cause atelectasis and, because of associated pain, to decrease motivation for effective deep breathing. Splinting while coughing decreases the pain that postoperative coughing typically generates. **Splinting** is supporting the incision with

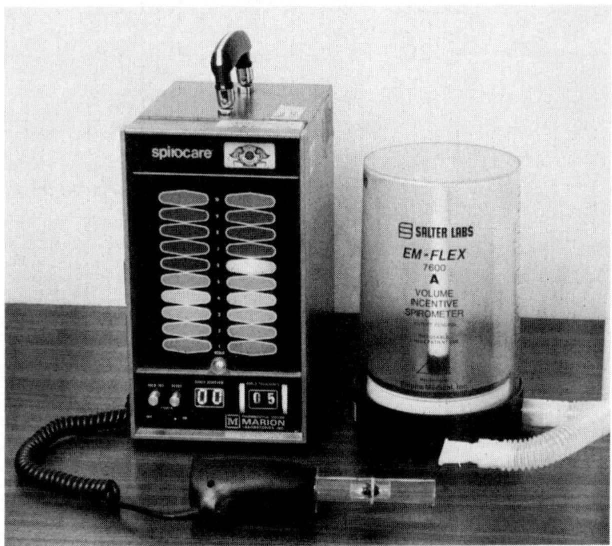

Figure 27–11. Electronic (left) and volume-type (right) spirometers.

interlaced hands and fingers and/or a pillow. As Figure 27–12 illustrates, splinting can be done by clients themselves or by a nurse.

Restorative Care

Clients who experience major interferences with oxygenation or perfusion of body tissues need restorative care. This care may take the form of nursing implementation to reduce oxygen demands, mobilize secretions, maintain airway patency, administer ordered therapy, and promote circulation.

Reducing Oxygen Demands. One of the most important things a nurse can do for a client with oxygenation problems is to help the client reduce the body's demands for oxygen. Many activities increase metabolism and consequently increase the body's oxygen need. When the client is in an oxygenation crisis, these activities should be kept to a minimum so that energy is available for the life-sustaining activities of breathing and circulation.

Reducing Activity. The client in respiratory distress should be encouraged to rest. Eating, entertaining visitors, ambulating, and bathing add to the body's oxygen demands. Planning nursing care so that a client has uninterrupted rest periods is an effective way to reduce oxygen demands. Because of the amount of care seriously ill clients require, they may not have a single hour of uninterrupted sleep for many days. Developing a schedule for essential care collaboratively with the client and other health care team members is necessary to support optimum oxygenation in those clients.

Digestion increases metabolic rate considerably. Therefore, many clients with oxygenation problems tolerate a light diet with frequent meals more readily than three large meals a day. Another reason for diet modification is that a full stomach presses upward on the diaphragm and tends to compromise its motion. This can lead to dyspnea or shortness of breath.

The client who is acutely ill with oxygenation problems should be taught to avoid the Valsalva maneuver. The Valsalva maneuver increases intrathoracic pressure. This reduces or occludes the return of blood to the heart, which temporarily reduces cardiac output so that the coronary tissues are inadequately perfused. Then, when the person stops straining, all the backed-up blood rushes into the heart quickly and can overwhelm it. Serious consequences, including a myocardial infarction (heart attack), can follow.

Reminding family members and other visitors of a client's need for rest is also helpful. Making sure they are aware that the client should not be awakened unnecessarily will help the client conserve oxygen. Sometimes restricting visiting privileges to a few selected close family members is necessary.

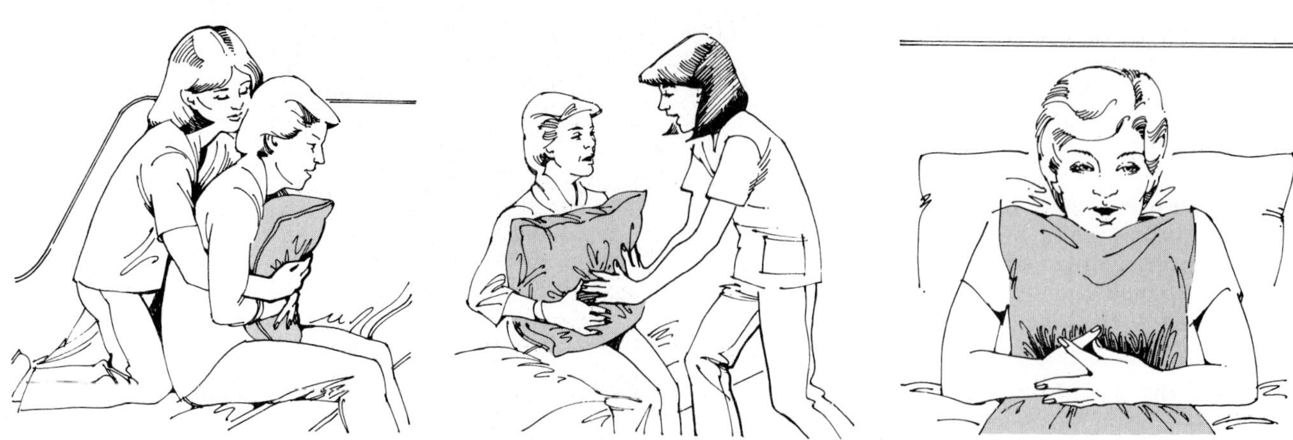

Figure 27–12. Splinting incisional chest pain to assist coughing.

PROCEDURE 27–6. TEACHING CASCADE COUGHING

PURPOSE: To raise respiratory secretions from large and small airways, facilitating optimum oxygenation in clients at risk for airway occlusion (postoperative clients; clients with restrictive lung disease, laryngeal disease, central nervous system disease, neuromuscular disease; clients on prolonged bedrest; and clients being treated with restrictive binders/dressing or with artificial airways).

EQUIPMENT: None.

ACTION	RATIONALE
1. Assess client to determine respiratory status and need for scheduled and PRN coughing. NOTE: Pain associated with unnecessary coughing in postoperative clients may decrease motivation to cough correctly when coughing is needed.	1. Regularly scheduled coughing (q 1–2 h) is necessary for immobile clients and those with diseases listed above, because secretion production interferes with oxygen exchange. Postoperative clients should cough PRN (only when secretions are present) because coughing when there are no secretions present can cause alveolar collapse and causes unnecessary pain.
2. Discuss the procedure and its expected benefits with the client. NOTE: Discussing the technique and having a practice session preoperatively increases likelihood of postoperative participation.	2. Active participation is more likely if client understands the expected behavior and its anticipated benefits.
3. Assist or instruct client to assume sitting position leaning slightly forward with feet on floor. Alternate positions for client confined to bed: high or semi-Fowler's, or side-lying with legs flexed, HOB slightly elevated.	3. Allows maximal lung expansion by diminishing pressure of abdominal organs on diaphragm and maximizes use of diaphragm and abdominal muscles to increase intrathoracic pressure by stabilizing torso.
4. Verbalize and demonstrate each of the following:	4. Use of multiple sensory modalities (visual and auditory) enhances learning.
a. Take a slow, deep breath (clients with severe airway disease may be able to take only more shallow breaths).	a. Slow, rather than quick, inhalation is less likely to pull secretions more deeply into the lungs.
b. Exhale, then repeat the deep inhalation. If first deep breath stimulates coughing, encourage the client to go ahead and cough.	b. Deep inhalations build up a volume of air behind the mucus, which will effectively propel it upward; inhaling deeply also stimulates the cough reflex.

(continued)

PROCEDURE 27–6. (continued)

c. Hold breath for 2 seconds; then exhale against closed glottis by contracting diaphragm. Telling the client to try to exhale with the throat closed may be easier for some to understand.

c. Builds up intrathoracic pressure. Combination of maximal air volume and pressure creates bolus of air, which moves secretions.

d. Open mouth and cough repeatedly without inhaling until nearly out of breath. The object is several small coughs rather than a few large coughs.

d. Cough with large lung volumes (immediately after inhalation) clears trachea and mainstem bronchi; later coughs at small volumes tend to milk mucus out of smaller airways.

NOTE: To assist clients with weak or paralyzed respiratory muscles, use quad coughing technique. If client cannot accomplish cascade cough, try "huff" cough (see Box 27–9).

e. Pause, then inhale slowly.

e. Pause prevents uncontrollable coughing, which may be stimulated by quick inhalation.

f. Rest, then repeat cough up to three times to clear airway.

f. Excessive coughing can cause hypoxia, airway collapse, and discomfort.

5. If paroxysmal coughing occurs, ask client to attempt slow, regular respirations until the urge to cough passes. Offer sips of water. Pursed-lip breathing may assist some clients to suppress cough (see Procedure 27–4).

5. Controlled breathing may suppress cough reflex. Water decreases mucusal irritation.

6. Assess secretions produced and respiratory status after coughing. Alert and oriented clients can be taught to self-evaluate secretions produced.

6. Evaluates effectiveness of coughing.

7. After completing coached cascade cough, ask client to verbally describe the steps. Repeat instruction as necessary.

7. Reinforces learning, allows nurse to evaluate understanding.

8. Collaborate with client to establish a coughing schedule if appropriate. Post schedule at client's bedside and record it in the care plan.

8. Clients are more likely to adhere to a schedule that is mutually developed. Posting a schedule will increase likelihood of adherence.

9. Assist client with coughing as scheduled. Intermittently observe client who is coughing independently to reinforce correct technique and/or suggest improvements.

9. Positive reinforcement increases likelihood that behavior will be repeated. Incorrect technique is ineffective and wastes energy.

RECORDING: Initial note should describe what was taught, accuracy of client performance, and plans for further teaching if needed. Describe client's respiratory status before and after coughing, effectiveness of cough, and amount and character of secretions produced, if any, on initial and routing charting.

Relieving Anxiety. Anxiety increases metabolism and therefore escalates bodily oxygen demands. A nurse can often reduce a client's anxiety by honest explanations and answers to questions. Listening as clients vent feelings and fears can also decrease their anxiety. Sometimes, the nurse need only stay in the room with a client to reduce anxiety. Encouraging a significant other to stay with the client often has a calming effect. Relaxation techniques (discussed in Chap. 22) can also promote feelings of tranquility and reduce oxygen demand. Clients with chronic lung disease often panic when dyspnea occurs. Remind them that panic increases dyspnea and suggest using pursed-lip breathing to gain control and improve oxygen intake (see Procedure 27–4).

Alleviating Pain. Pain triggers a stress reaction that stimulates the metabolism and increases the need for oxygenation. Nursing measures aimed at both preventing and relieving pain are important. For example, preventing pain includes techniques such as teaching postoperative clients how to turn in bed and cough effectively without causing incisional pain. Chapter 30 details techniques for helping clients move in bed; coughing was discussed previously.

Pain relief can be accomplished in several ways, depending on the cause and nature of the pain. Changing positions in bed, massage, and other noninvasive techniques are often effective for mild pain. Severe acute pain usually requires analgesic medications prescribed by the physician. To be most effective, analgesics must be administered before pain reaches its peak intensity, so prompt response to complaints of pain are particularly important when oxygenation is compromised.

Pain medications and tranquilizers are ordered cautiously for clients who have pulmonary disease, because these medications may reduce ventilatory drive. Some pulmonary clients suffer respiratory arrest because of this respiratory depression. Sometimes imagery, relaxation, or other noninvasive pain relief measures (discussed in Chap. 9) can relieve these clients' pain without compromising oxygenation.

Lowering Body Temperature. Each Fahrenheit degree of fever increases metabolism about 7 percent. This increases the body's need for oxygen by a like amount. The client with oxygenation problems may be unable to meet the extra oxygen and circulation demands caused by fever. Methods to reduce body temperature may be as simple as removing excess covers, improving room ventilation, or providing a sponge bath. Infection as a causative factor of fever must be ruled out or treated in collaboration with the physician. Antipyretic medications such as aspirin or acetaminophen may also be ordered.

BUILDING NURSING KNOWLEDGE

Is Getting Out of Bed During Bedmaking Safe for the Client Who Has Had a Heart Attack?

Lane LD, Winslow EH. Oxygen consumption, cardiovascular response, and perceived exertion in healthy adults during rest, occupied bedmaking, and unoccupied bedmaking activity. *Cardiovasc Nurs.* 1987; 23:31–36.

The seriously ill client who has had a heart attack is often prohibited from sitting beside the bed while the bed is made, and instead, is asked to turn from side to side as the nurse makes the occupied bed. Is this a safe procedure?

Lane and Winslow endeavored to measure the physiological stress in terms of energy costs and cardiovascular responses imposed by these approaches to bedmaking. The study employed a sample of 18 healthy subjects, 11 women and 7 men who ranged in age from 20 to 42 years. None of the subjects smoked or was pregnant; subjects consumed no food or caffeinated beverages prior to the study and engaged in no strenuous physical activity for 8 hours before the study.

Subjects' oxygen consumption during bedmaking was measured by open-circuit, indirect calorimetry. Expired air was tested for volume and composition by a gas analyzer. Electrocardiograms were recorded during rest and bedmaking, and peak heart rate was measured at intervals during the procedures. Blood pressure was measured using a cuff sphygmanometer. Following each bedmaking activity, subjects rated the perceived exertion they experienced using a special standardized scale. Bedmaking procedures for the study were standardized by the use of protocols.

Oxygen consumption during occupied and unoccupied bedmaking activities was significantly higher than during rest, but did not vary significantly between the two types of bedmaking. Heart rate after bedmaking did not differ significantly between rest and unoccupied approaches. Peak rates during both occupied and unoccupied bedmaking were significantly higher than rates at rest. No significant differences were measured in systolic blood pressure, diastolic blood pressure, or mean arterial pressure during rest and before and after bedmaking activities. No significant difference was found in subjects' ratings of perceived exertion. Lane and Winslow concluded that because both occupied and unoccupied bedmaking methods produced only small increases in energy cost over resting levels, the oxygen consumption findings provide no basis to restrict either bedmaking method. Because both methods produced low energy costs, clients should be able to tolerate either bedmaking method.

Mobilizing Secretions. Excessive respiratory tract secretions are produced as a result of mucosal irritation associated with respiratory illnesses or immobilization (see Chap. 30). These secretions can interfere with ventilation and diffusion across the alveolar–capillary membrane. Facilitating movement of these secretions so that they can be easily removed by coughing promotes optimum oxygenation. Nursing measures to mobilize secretions include improving hydration, humidification of air, frequent turning, and chest physiotherapy.

Improving Hydration. Adequate hydration keeps the sputum thin and easy to expectorate. If the sputum is sticky and difficult to cough up, this is a good indication that the client needs a higher fluid intake. In general, clients with chronic oxygenation problems need at least 64 ounces (1900 mL or 8 full glasses) of fluid daily (excluding milk, which thickens secretions). More fluid is necessary if the client has a respiratory infection. Strategies for assessing hydration status and increasing fluid intake are further discussed in Chapter 31.

Humidification. Even well-hydrated clients with copious secretions can benefit from breathing moist air rather than dry air. Dry air causes loss of moisture from mucosa by evaporation, creating thick, tenacious secretions that are difficult for cilia to clear or for the client to expectorate. Bubbling air or oxygen through water enables it to carry more moisture, which in turn hydrates rather than dehydrates respiratory mucosa. Sometimes aerosolized (liquid transformed into a fine mist) water or saline is introduced into the respiratory tree to produce the same effect. In the past humidified air was also warmed, but the benefits of this practice have recently been questioned.[21]

Frequent Turning. If a client with copious respiratory secretions remains in the same position for several hours, the secretions pool in the dependent portion of the airway. At the same time, the mucosa in the uppermost portion of the airway tends to become dry. This compromises the ability of the cilia to clear mucus. To prevent negative outcomes, the nurse should encourage or assist the client to turn frequently from side to side and to the supine position. The client should change positions at least every 2 hours; hourly is even better. Often deep-breathing and coughing exercises are done at the same time.

Chest Physiotherapy. Chest physiotherapy (CPT), also called postural drainage and percussion, may also be used to mobilize secretions. This method is used by nurses, physical therapists, and respiratory therapists who have been trained in its use. The client assumes specific positions selected to use gravity to drain lung segments in which secretions have accumulated. Percussion and vibration are then applied to physically loosen and mobilize pooled secretions. Percussion is clapping the chest wall with cupped hands. Vibration is application of rapid oscillating pressure, either with the hands or with a mechanical vibrator. The client is expected to cough in each position to remove secretions. If the client is unable to cough effectively after CPT, tracheobronchial suctioning may be used. This is discussed in a later section.

Maintaining Airway Patency. Nursing implementation to maintain airway patency includes encouraging clients to perform the coughing and deep-breathing exercises discussed above, teaching clients positions that facilitate ventilation, administering medications to dilate bronchioles, performing pharyngeal and tracheal suctioning, and using artificial airways, the Heimlich maneuver, and CPR.

Breathing Exercises. Pursed-lip breathing, discussed under *Supportive Care* earlier in the chapter (see Procedure 27–4), is effective in maintaining the patency of small airways because the resistance created by pursing the lips during expiration preserves a low level of pressure throughout the respiratory tree. It is particularly effective when combined with exercise or with resting positions as described below. The incentive spirometer (see Procedure 27–5) also enhances airway patency, particularly if the sustained maximal inspiration technique is used.

Positioning. Generally, airways are most patent when a person is upright. Clients who have difficulty breathing therefore breathe most comfortably when sitting in a chair, with the head of the hospital bed raised, or when propped up on pillows in a regular bed. These positions also lower the abdominal contents and reduce pressure on the diaphragm. Clients in respiratory distress find that resting their arms on the overbed table or the arms of a chair enables them to use the tripod position in order to breathe more effectively (Fig. 27–13 Left). In a standing position, leaning on a wall as shown in Figure 27–13 Right works well. Using pursed-lip breathing in these positions adds to their effectiveness in maintaining airway patency.

Unconscious or partially conscious clients should never be positioned on their backs. In the supine position, the tongue tends to fall backwards, blocking the airway, and aspiration of oral secretions is likely. For these reasons, anyone with a low level of consciousness or who has trouble swallowing oral secretions should be placed in a lateral position with the head to the side so that oral contents can drain out. Placing a towel or pad that can be changed frequently under the head will keep the client dry and comfortable. Often, oral suction is advisable to clear the mouth of secretions. Frequent turning, as discussed above, is particularly important for these clients, as their spontaneous movement is extremely limited.

Facilitating Effective Coughing. If secretions are present, a productive cough is the least traumatic way to clear airways. The cascade coughing technique shown in Procedure 27–6 generates optimal intrathoracic pressure to move secretions upward out of the respiratory tree. If clients are unable to cough effectively with this technique, try to determine the reason. Clients with pain from abdominal incisions or chest pain may need pain medication before they can cough effectively. Splinting the incision also helps, as discussed earlier. A client with severe airway disease may cough more effectively at low inspiratory volumes. Follow the steps in Procedure 27–6, but suggest that the client inhale less deeply before coughing. Other variations to enhance coughing are presented in Box 27–8.

Administering Bronchodilator Medications. Bronchodilators relax and open the airways. Using an inhaled bronchodilator before coughing can open the airways and enable the cough to clear the deeper, smaller airways more effectively. Bronchodilators may be delivered topically by hand-held cartridge inhalers; in nebulized form, in which the client breathes a mist of bronchodilator and air; or by intermittent positive pressure, in which the mist is delivered by a machine that blows air and mist in by positive pressure.

Use of bronchodilators is usually managed by a respiratory therapist; however, the nurse can collaborate by making sure that the client is in an upright position so that the drug will be delivered into the airways as deeply as possible and by monitoring the client's participation and comfort during the treatment.

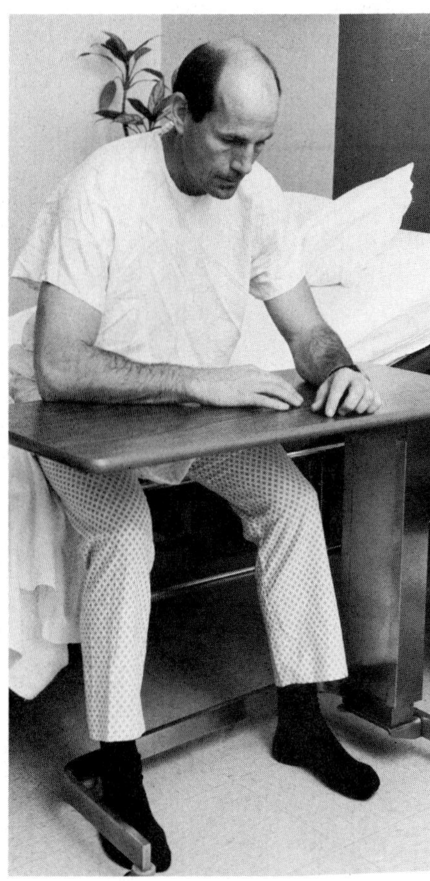

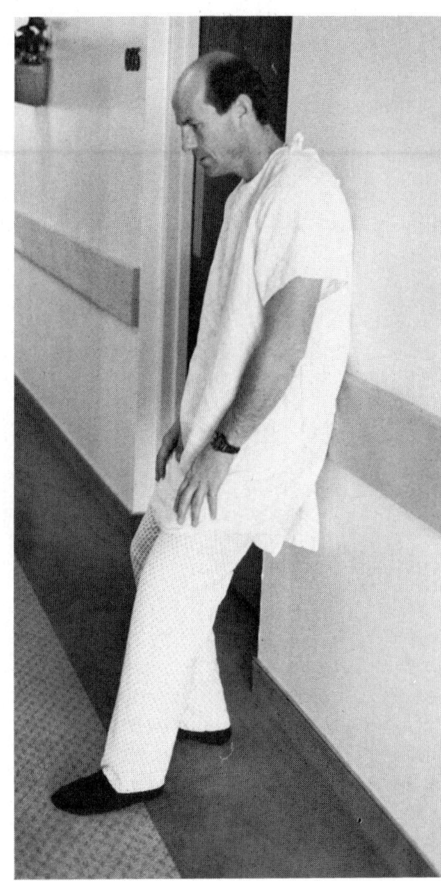

Figure 27–13. Resting positions.

The use of inhaled bronchodilators is usually combined with the use of systemic bronchodilators. In clients who are in acute distress, these medications are given intravenously. Otherwise, they are given orally. Some clients will also need oral or intravenous steroids. All of these medications require a physician's prescription.

Suctioning. If bronchodilators, steroids, and coughing exercises are ineffective in clearing the airway, or if clients are unable to cough, oropharyngeal or nasopharyngeal suctioning may be used (Procedure 27–7). Nasotracheal suctioning, in which the suction catheter is passed from the nose down into the trachea and airways is used in unconscious clients. This method is dangerous in the hands of an untrained person as it can cause laryngeospasm, closing the vocal cords and cutting off the air supply. Nasotracheal suctioning should be reserved for respiratory therapists and registered nurses who have been trained in its use. It is not described in this text, but is addressed in most textbooks of medical–surgical nursing.

Artificial Airways. If a client needs assistance in keeping the airway open, an oral airway or a nasal airway may be used. These are most often used in postanesthesia recovery rooms or other situations in which the need for airway assistance is short term. Some practitioners use artificial airways when doing cardiopulmonary resuscitation to avoid contact with another person's oral secretions. (See Universal Precautions, Box 22–7 and Procedure 27–9).

The oral airway helps to hold the tongue in place so it will not fall back and occlude the airway; however, conscious or partly conscious clients will gag and spit it out. These clients tolerate a nasal airway much better. This is a soft rubber airway that fits in the nose and extends into the pharynx so that even if the tongue falls back, there is an open airway. Airways are illustrated in Figure 27–14.

A tracheostomy is an artificial opening into the trachea. It may be created to treat a respiratory emergency or for other therapeutic purposes, such as long-term mechanical ventilator use. A curved plastic or metal airway is placed into the opening to maintain its patency. Tracheostomy care is an advanced clinical skill that is not addressed in this text.

Heimlich Maneuver. If a person aspirates an object or piece of food that is large enough to obstruct the airway, he or she will immediately begin gasping for breath and coughing. The person with an obstructed airway will be unable to speak. It is imperative to take measures to relieve the obstruction immediately. Put a baby or young child over your lap in the head-down position and give several quick thumps on the back. This will often dislodge the object. Do not use back thumps for someone who is not in the head-down position, as they may drive the object further down into the airway. A person of any age, including a young child, can have the airway cleared by the use of the Heim-

PROCEDURE 27–7. OROPHARYNGEAL AND NASOPHARYNGEAL SUCTIONING

PURPOSE: To relieve respiratory distress caused by upper airway secretions that client is unable to expectorate.

EQUIPMENT: Wall suction set-up cannister with filter, regulator, connecting tubing (portable suction machine may also be used); sterile suction kit containing catheter with thumb port, glove, water-soluble lubricant, and container for liquid; sterile water or normal saline; moisture-resistant bag; towel or disposable drape; nonsterile gloves, tongue blade, facial tissues; mouthwash; and toothbrush or toothettes.

ACTION	RATIONALE
1. Determine need for suctioning by assessing respiratory rate, depth, quality, presence of gurgles or rumbles on auscultation or signs of acute distress: gasping, grasping throat, cyanosis. If secretions are present, encourage coughing.	1. Presence of respiratory secretions interferes with optimum oxygenation. Clients who cannot cough effectively may need suctioning even if they are not in acute respiratory distress.

NOTE: It is common practice to keep a suction set-up ready for use and a supply of suction kits and appropriate-sized catheters in the room of a client who may need assistance to clear the airway. The correct sized catheter is about ½ the diameter of the client's nostril: large enough to move secretions, but not so large as to block the airway. If client is in acute distress, begin suctioning (see step 7) without delay. If able to cough, may still need assistance to completely clear the airway.

ACTION	RATIONALE
2. Discuss the procedure and its expected benefits with the client. Indicate that it may be uncomfortable, but is not painful, and that client relaxation will decrease difficulty for client and nurse. Let client know that gagging or coughing may occur. If client is expected or known to be uncooperative, have a second person available to restrain client movement.	2. Active participation is more likely if client understands the expected behavior and anticipated benefits. Fear is diminished if honest explanation of what client will experience is provided.
3. Check cannister to see that connecting tubing attached to the vacuum port is clear, that it has a regulator and is securely attached to wall outlet.	3. System must be intact to remove secretions effectively and safely. If cannister is full, it may overflow or automatic shutoff valve will make suctioning impossible. Regulator controls amount of negative pressure transmitted to client.
4. Close door or bedside curtains.	4. Provides privacy. Procedure may be embarrassing to client or offensive to others.
5. Assist client to semi-Fowler's position, with head turned toward you. Unconscious clients should be in lateral recumbent position, facing nurse, to minimize aspiration.	5. Facilitates coughing to assist in removal of secretions without aspiration; aids insertion of catheter.
6. Cover client's pillow with towel or disposable drape.	6. Protects from possible contamination by sputum.

(continued)

PROCEDURE 27–7. (continued)

7. Turn on and set regulator to appropriate setting:
   Infant: 60–100 mm Hg
   Child: 80–115 mm Hg
   Adult: 80–120 mm Hg
   Use lowest setting that will move secretions. If tip of connecting tubing has gauze covering, remove it.

   7. Excessive amounts of negative pressure can damage respiratory mucosa by drawing it into catheter.

8. Prepare suction kit: open package, pour sterile liquid into container; squeeze lubricant onto sterile surface; open catheter package, if separately wrapped, maintaining catheter's sterility by preventing contact with unsterile objects. If unfamiliar with principles of asepsis, refer to Procedure 22–3.

   8. Aseptic technique is important because clients needing suctioning often have reduced pulmonary function and are more vulnerable to infection. If client's resistance is low, it is recommended that each catheter be inserted only once.

9. Oxygenate client: instruct alert client to take several deep breaths; use resuscitation bag with mask to hyperinflate lungs of unconscious client. If client is receiving nasal oxygen, it should be continued while suctioning.

   9. Suctioning removes oxygen from client. Less distress occurs if client is well oxygenated before suctioning.

10. Don clean glove on nondominant hand, sterile glove on dominant hand. Some kits contain a pair, rather than a single glove, for nurse's convenience.

    10. The sterile gloved hand will be used to manipulate catheter, which is kept sterile to avoid introducing microorganisms into client's respiratory tract. Clean glove is to protect nurse from contamination by sputum.

11. Holding coiled catheter in dominant hand and connective tubing in the other, attach catheter to connective tubing. Catheter should not contact any other objects during connection.

    11. Maintains sterility of catheter, provides pathway for secretions to travel to collection cannister.

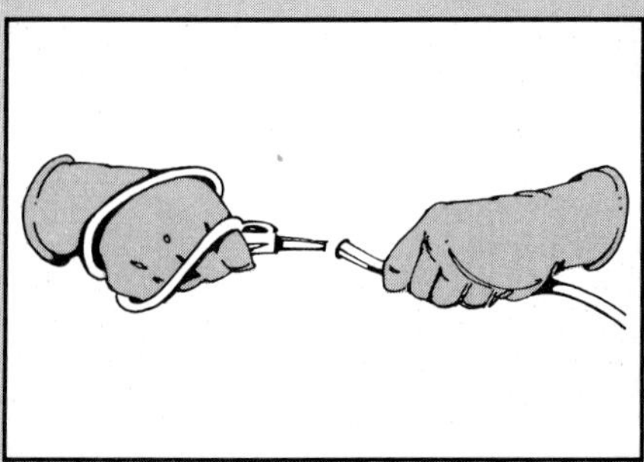

12. Place distal end of catheter into sterile liquid and cover thumb port; liquid should move into collection catheter. If liquid does not move through tube, check that all connections are secure and that regulator is set correctly.

    12. Demonstrates if equipment is working; facilitates movement of secretions by lubricating lumen of catheter.

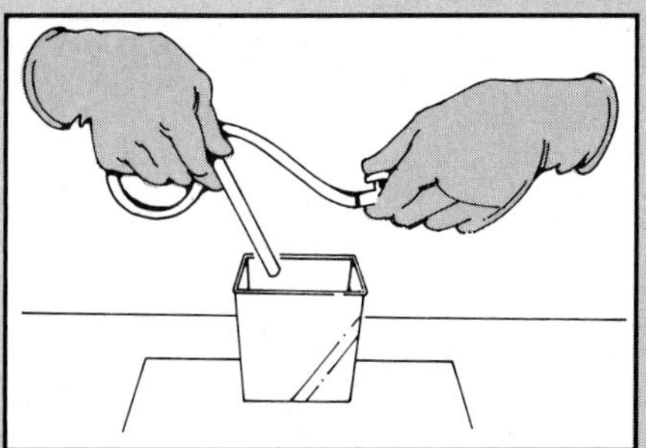

(continued)

PROCEDURE 27–7. (continued)

Nasopharyngeal Route

13. Dip distal tip (6–8 cm or 3–4 in) into sterile lubricant.

13. Lubricant reduces friction between catheter and mucosa, preventing mucosal injury and irritation. Mucosal trauma increases infection risk.

14. Note several markings on the catheter, which indicate average distances for insertion. Estimate the distance between the client's nose and earlobe and note which marking most closely approximates this distance.

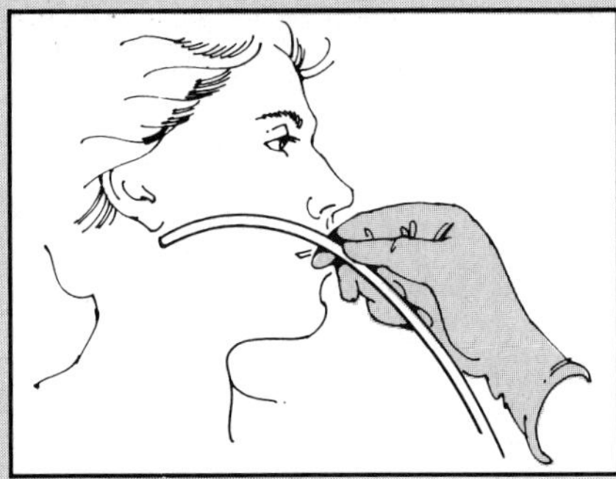

14. The distance between nose and earlobe is similar to the distance from nostril to the distal pharynx. Advancing the catheter to this point will decrease the likelihood of inserting it too deeply, causing gagging or laryngeal spasm.

15. Gently insert catheter into nares directing it along the floor of the nasal cavity, not upward. Thumb port should be open so no negative pressure is produced. Obtain client preference for which nostril is to be used.

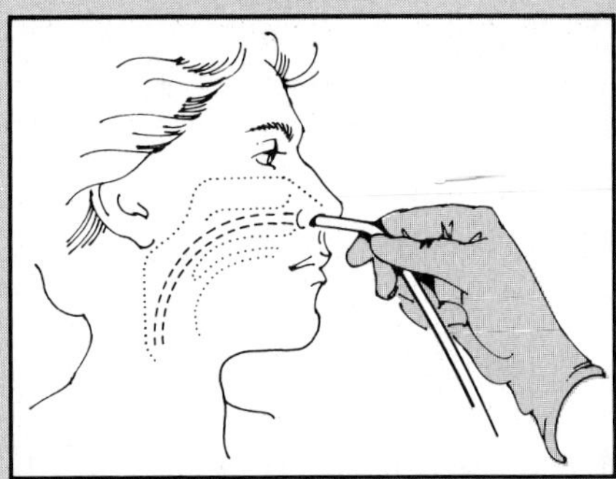

15. Following the natural curve of the nasal floor reduces mucosal damage due to friction or pressure from the catheter tip. Lack of negative pressure during insertion minimizes oxygen depletion and prevents trauma from mucosa being drawn into catheter as it advances.

16. Advance the catheter smoothly and rapidly to the mark selected in step 14.

16. Airway should be cleared as rapidly as possible to optimize oxygenation and minimize discomfort.

NOTE: Do not force catheter. If mucus plug is encountered, briefly cover thumb port to apply suction. Then advance catheter. If resistance is met, try opposite nostril.

17. If client coughs, pause, but do not remove catheter. Usually, it is not necessary to advance the catheter farther if effective cough occurs. If client coughs uncontrollably, remove and reinsert catheter if needed to clear remaining secretions.

17. Suction will remove coughed secretions. Removal and reinsertion increases mucosal trauma.

18. If crowing noise (stridor) is heard, remove catheter quickly.

18. Stridor indicates laryngeal spasm which interferes with breathing.

(continued)

PROCEDURE 27–7. (continued)

19. When catheter has been advanced to pharynx, cover thumb port intermittently while withdrawing the catheter with a twisting motion, in 10 seconds or less. (Count to 10 or hold your breath during suctioning to remind you to limit suctioning time.)

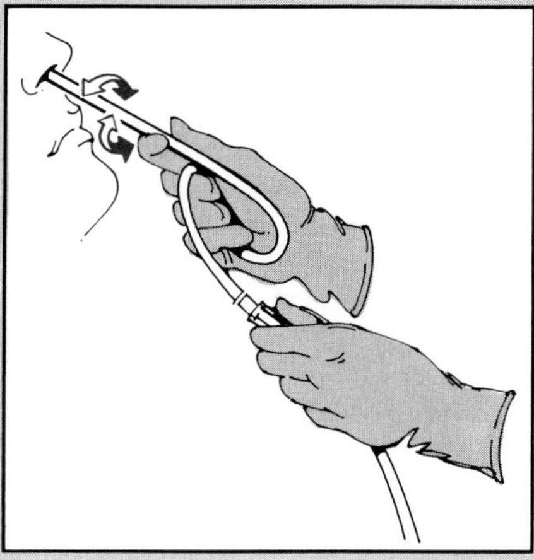

19. Intermittent negative pressure reduces mucosal trauma; twisting rotates catheter tip, so all surfaces are cleared of mucus. Prolonged suctioning (greather than 10 seconds) can cause hypoxia.

NOTE: Do not move catheter up and down while suctioning, as this injures mucosa. Suction children for 5 seconds only.

20. Rinse catheter in sterile liquid until all tubing is clear of secretions.

20. Flushes secretions into collection cannister for disposal.

21. Assess respiratory status to determine need for further suctioning. Repeat suctioning until pharynx is clear, allowing several minutes of rest and deep breathing between suction passes.

21. Hypoxia is prevented by allowing client time to take in oxygen between suction passes.

NOTE: Hypoxia is more common with deep tracheal suction, but can occur if pharyngeal suctioning is repeated without rest periods.

22. Check mouth for secretions, suction as above if needed. Most alert clients will be able to mobilize and expectorate oral secretions without assistance. Yankauer suction tip may be used to clear oral cavity, if desired.

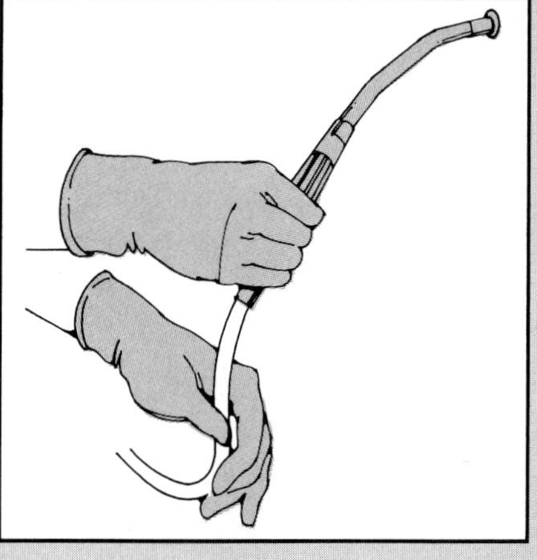

22. Mouth should be suctioned last, as it has more organisms than nose. Yankauer tip is rigid and more easily directed to all parts of oral cavity.

(continued)

PROCEDURE 27–7. (continued)

23. Assess secretions for color, amount, and odor. Complete procedure according to steps 27–33.

23. Assists in determining change in client's condition.

NOTE: Bloody secretions suggest mucosal trauma; gray-green secretions, infection; thick, viscous secretions, dehydration.

Oropharyngeal Route

24. Prepare suction kit as for nasal route, except for lubrication of catheter.

24. Saliva provides sufficient lubricant for oral cavity.

25. Ask client to open mouth and stick out tongue; if client is unconscious or weak, tongue blade may be used to hold tongue down.

25. Allows visualization of pharynx and easy passage of catheter.

26. Insert catheter over tongue to pharynx, then proceed with suctioning. (See steps 17–23 above.)

26. Pharynx should be cleared before mouth to optimize oxygen exchange.

27. When airway is cleared, coil catheter in sterile gloved hand and remove glove so it turns inside out over catheter. Remove second glove in same fashion. Auscultate lungs to ascertain that airways are clear.

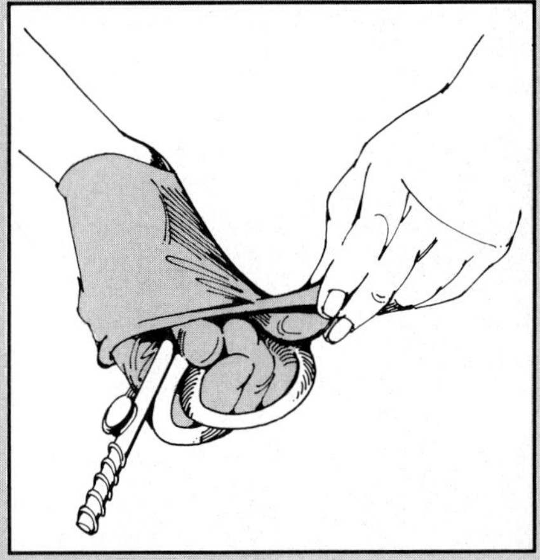

27. Provides barrier to prevent transfer of microorganisms from catheter by direct contact with objects in environment.

28. Place both gloves in moisture-proof bag. Turn off suction device.

28. Secretions are considered contaminated; see step 27 above.

29. Provide mouth care if desired by client.

29. Promotes comfort and well-being.

30. Discard remaining sterile liquid in sink, disposable equipment in trash, towel in laundry.

30. Promotes clean environment for client.

NOTE: If client is on isolation precautions, follow institutional guidelines for disposal of equipment.

(continued)

PROCEDURE 27–7. (continued)

31. Reposition client in correct alignment.

NOTE: Many clients with oxygenation problems may be placed in semi-Fowler's position, but prolonged use of this position increases risk of pressure sores and contractures (see Chap. 30).

31. Supports optimum oxygenation, motor function, and skin integrity.

32. Check cannister; if full, dispose and replace. Cover end of connecting tubing with sterile gauze so tip points away from floor. Assure that ample supply of suction kits is readily available for future use.

NOTE: Some cannisters are completely disposable, others have disposable liners. Do not empty cannister in room or attempt to reuse a disposable cannister. Cannister and tubing must be changed every 24 hours.

32. Prepares unit for prompt suctioning if respiratory distress occurs.

33. Collaborate with physician for revised treatment plan if sputum characteristics suggest change in condition.

33. Suctioning treats symptom of airway occlusion, but not underlying cause.

RECORDING: Describe client status before and after suctioning, response to procedure, nature and amount of secretions, and additional nursing actions taken, if any.

lich maneuver (Procedure 27–8). This maneuver is included as part of the American Red Cross and American Heart Association Cardiopulmonary Resuscitation (CPR) courses.

Cardiopulmonary Resuscitation. Cardiopulmonary resuscitation (CPR) is the act of giving mouth-to-mouth breathing and cardiac compressions (external pressure on the heart to circulate blood) to a person who has no pulse or respirations (cardiopulmonary arrest). Cardiac or respiratory arrest is a life-threatening problem that every member of the health care team must be prepared to handle at any time. Effective CPR must be begun within 4 minutes of cessation of respiration if brain death is to be prevented. The techniques for relieving airway obstruction and providing rescue breathing and external cardiac compressions are summarized in Procedures 27–9 and 27–10. A person should not attempt to use these techniques until he or she has completed a certification course. If the techniques are not used correctly, they will be ineffective and may cause harm, especially to infants and small children. Every nurse should complete a course in basic life support and recertify yearly. Nurses who work with critically ill and injured clients can also complete advanced cardiac life support (ACLS) courses.

An ambu-bag (hand-compressible breathing bag) may be used in the health care setting to aid in the resuscitation of a person who has suffered a cardiopulmonary arrest (Procedure 27–11).

Oxygen Therapy. Oxygen is commonly administered to people who are acutely or chronically ill with oxygenation problems. It improves cellular oxygenation while reducing cardiopulmonary workload. Oxygen therapy requires a physician's order. Orders for oxygen therapy should specify the type of delivery system or device and the rate of flow or oxygen concentration. Oxygen is not a "PRN" (as needed) therapy. The client should use the amount of oxygen that is prescribed and not adjust the oxygen flow rate up or down.

A device for determining the amount of oxygen in the blood, called a pulse oximeter, is useful for assessing the effectiveness of oxygen therapy (Fig. 27–15). The oximeter uses a noninvasive oxygen sensor that is clipped to a client's earlobe or finger. Monitoring can be continuous or intermittent. The sensor determines the level of oxygen saturation with sufficient accuracy for monitoring most clients who are not critically ill. Some physicians order oxygen therapy with the flow rate dependent on pulse oximetry readings (for example, "Oxygen via nasal prongs, 2 to 4 L per minute, to keep oxygen saturation at 90 percent").

The safest way to administer oxygen is to give the lowest flow or concentration that will maintain acceptable arterial blood gases or oximeter readings. Forty percent is a safe concentration for most clients. Some clients require up to 60 percent. Very high oxygen concentrations should be given for as short a time as possible, because they may damage lung tissue.

BOX 27–8. ALTERNATIVE STRATEGIES FOR EFFECTIVE COUGHING

Low inspiratory volume

- Useful for clients with severe airway disease.
- Use techniques in Procedure 27–6, but inhale less deeply.

Splinting

- Useful for clients with incisional or chest wall pain.
- A pillow, folded bath blanket, or interlaced fingers are placed over the painful area. Even pressure is then applied over the painful area when the client inhales prior to cough and during forced expiration. This technique can be done by a client or nurse. (See Fig. 27–12.)

Huff coughing technique

- Can stimulate a cough reflex and raise secretions in clients who cannot perform the cascade cough. Progressive inhalations and exhalations in this technique gradually increase the lung volume and pressure to aid in producing a forceful cough.
- The client (1) holds his or her breath for 2 seconds, and then exhales in short puffs (with enough velocity for the air to be felt by a hand 2 inches from mouth); (2) again inhales slowly, holds the breath, and exhales in slightly more forceful puffs as if to blow out a candle; (3) repeats this process, this time saying "huff" on exhalation (the "huff" should have a breathy quality); and (4) repeats the process again, this time coughing once or twice on exhalation.

Quad coughing technique

- Useful for clients with muscle weakness or paralysis.
- The nurse or client should do a modified Heimlich maneuver (push upward at the base of the sternum) as the client coughs. The nurse can place the base of the two hands at the base of the sternum (same position as for CPR, but lower). The client can make a fist and lean over onto it if he or she has little arm strength or control. This makes the cough more forceful and improves clearance of secretions.

In clients with chronic hypoxia, high concentrations of oxygen are particularly dangerous. As discussed earlier, clients who retain carbon dioxide are insensitive to the normal respiratory stimulus of elevated CO_2. Instead, their stimulus to breathe is a decrease in blood oxygen (hypoxia). Thus high concentrations of oxygen may eliminate such clients' stimulus for breathing and they may cease to breathe. Such clients are usually treated with oxygen at low concentrations or flow rates.

Oxygen supports combustion, and so certain precautions are required when it is being used. Box 27–9 summarizes safety information related to oxygen administration.

Oxygen Supply. Most health care agencies use oxygen piped to wall outlets from large, low-pressure storage reservoirs. When oxygen must be delivered in a setting that has no central oxygen supply system, such as in the home, oxygen cylinders containing compressed oxygen are used. Both large and small cylinders are available. The small cylinders, called E cylinders or portable oxygen tanks, can be mounted on small wheeled carriers or on holders attached to wheelchairs or gurneys.

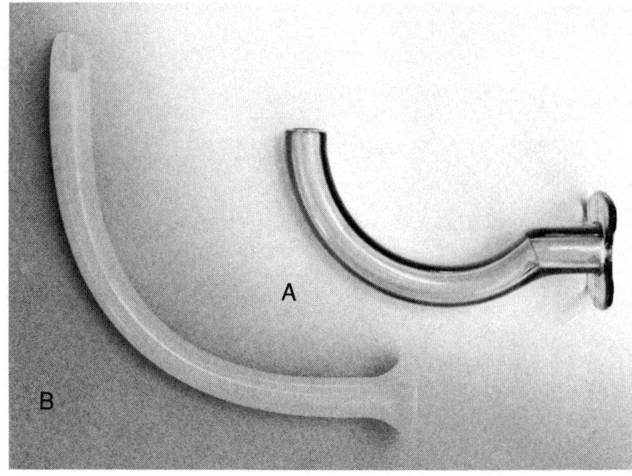

Figure 27–14. Oropharyngeal (**A**) and nasopharyngeal (**B**) airways.

Because compressed oxygen is stored under very high pressure in cylinders, a pressure regulator must be used in conjunction with a flowmeter when using oxygen from a cylinder. The regulator has a pressure-reducing valve that limits the rate of release of oxygen from the cylinder. A content gauge that indicates the amount of oxygen in the cylinder is part of the regulator. This gauge is calibrated in pounds per square inch (psi). Figure 27–16 illustrates an E cylinder on a stand with an attached regulator, content gauge, and flowmeter. Procedure 27–12 summarizes nursing responsibilities when administering oxygen from an E cylinder.

Measuring Oxygen Delivery. Oxygen used for oxygen therapy is measured in liters per minute (L/min). This unit is the flowrate, that is, the rate at which oxygen is flowing to the client. Flowrate is one way that oxygen therapy is prescribed. A device called a flowmeter is used to adjust and measure the flowrate. Two kinds of flowmeters are used: the Thorpe tube, which has a vertical flow indicator gauge; and the Bourdon gauge, which has a round flow indicator gauge. They are illustrated in Figure 27–17.

Oxygen dosage can also be ordered as a concentration, or percent of oxygen. Oxygen concentration is expressed as Fio_2, or fraction of inspired oxygen. All oxygen delivery devices mix supplemental oxygen from the supply source with room air (which is 21 percent oxygen). The Fio_2 indicates what fraction of the room air–oxygen mixture a client is receiving as oxygen. Fio_2 is expressed as a percentage.

Oxygen delivery systems that can precisely control the Fio_2 delivered to the client are called high-flow systems. If a specific oxygen concentration is critical for a given client, the physician will order a high-flow delivery device and specify the Fio_2 at which the device should be set (for example, "O_2 per Venturi mask at 28 percent").

(Text continues on page 1296.)

PROCEDURE 27–8. HEIMLICH MANEUVER (ABDOMINAL THRUSTS)

PURPOSE: To clear an obstructed airway.

EQUIPMENT: None.

ACTION / **RATIONALE**

SKILL A: Conscious Victim

1. Upon observing a person who has apparently choked, but who is not coughing, ask, "Are you choking?" If client speaks, take no action except encouraging coughing. The universal signal for choking is grasping the throat with one or both hands.

   Rationale: 1. Normal defenses of coughing are often more effective in clearing airway obstruction than external measures, which can actually interfere with a person's efforts to clear the airway.

2. If person is unable to speak, explain that you will try to assist in removing the foreign body. Emphasize the importance of relaxation during the maneuver, then initiate abdominal thrusts.

   Rationale: 2. A person unable to breathe will be anxious and may tense the chest and abdominal muscles, which may reduce the effectiveness of the thrusts.

NOTE: If client is pregnant, use Skill B, below; is a child, use Skill C.

3. Stand behind the victim. Make a fist, place it so thumb side is against victim's abdomen in the midline, just above umbilicus.

   Rationale: 3. Pressure will be exerted below the obstruction.

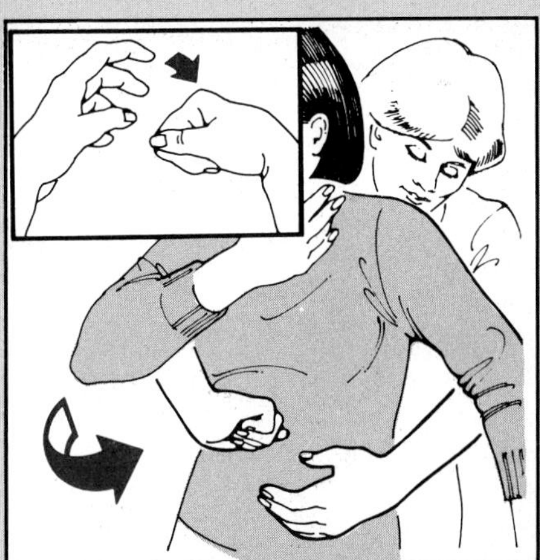

(continued)

PROCEDURE 27–8. (continued)

4. Grasp your fist with your other hand, then thrust it upward vigorously, as if to push out the obstructing object. Repeat several times.

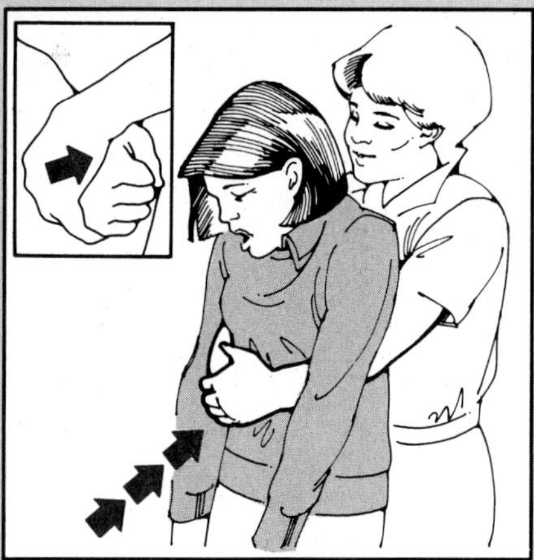

NOTE: Do not squeeze rib cage with forearms or exert pressure on xyphoid process or ribs.

4. Force of thrusts creates changes in air pressure producing a rush of air which will carry the obstructing object upward for expulsion.

5. Repeat until object is expelled or victim starts coughing or becomes unconscious. See Skill D for removing airway obstruction in an unconscious victim.

5. Object may be too deep to be expelled with one to two thrusts. It must be removed to prevent brain damage due to anoxia. Coughing indicates client is working to expel object.

SKILL B: Chest Thrusts

(Used if conscious choking client is pregnant or so obese that the rescuer cannot reach around the abdomen.)

1. Reach around client from behind, make a fist, place thumb side against sternum at the level of the armpits, explaining your intentions as you position your arms.

1. See steps 2 and 3, above.

2. Grasp your fist with your other hand and pull straight back sharply with a quick thrusting motion.

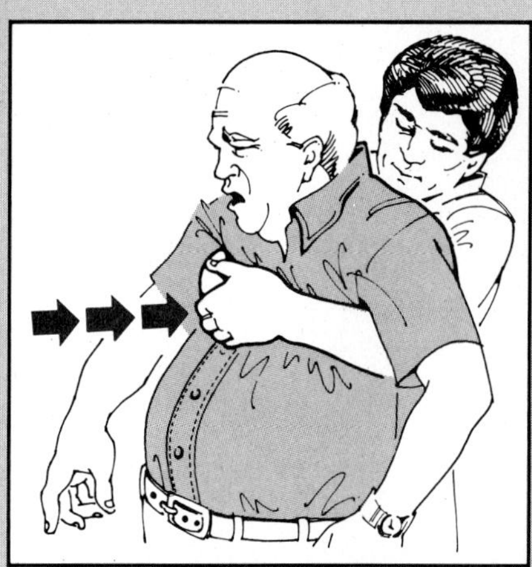

2. See step 4, above.

3. See step 5, above.

3. See step 5, above.

(continued)

PROCEDURE 27–8. (continued)

SKILL C: Back Blows
(Used when choking victim is an infant or small child.)

1. Place victim face down with head lower than chest. An infant should be held as follows: Support head and neck with your hand, the trunk with your forearm, then rest your forearm on your thigh. A small child can be positioned across your lap, with head down, because head support is not critical.

1. Adds gravity to assist the movement of the obstruction while minimizing injury to victim.

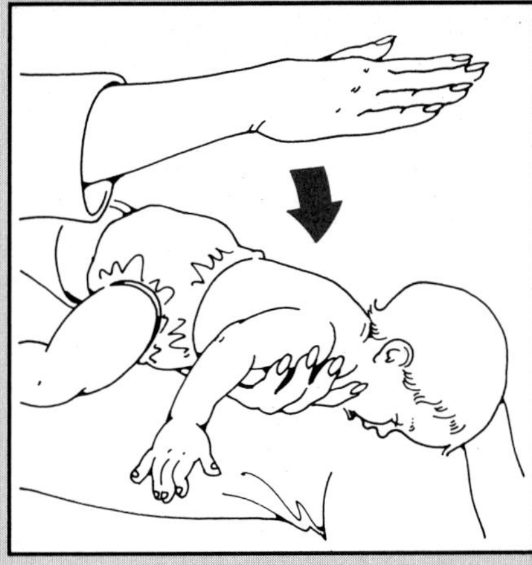

2. Deliver four sharp blows between the scapulae with the heel of the hand.

2. Jarring of blows may dislodge object.

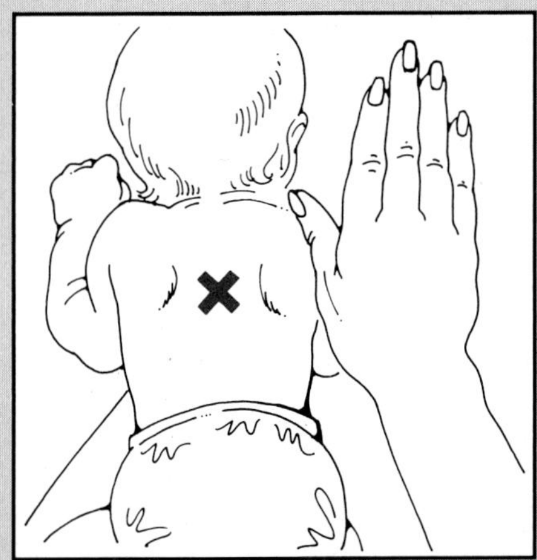

(continued)

PROCEDURE 27–8. (continued)

3. Turn infant over for chest thrusts as follows: Place your free hand on the back of the infant's head, with your arm extending down the infant's back. With the infant sandwiched between your arms, turn your arms over so the infant is supine.

3. The infant lacks muscle strength to support the head. Injury can occur if head is not supported when infant is turned.

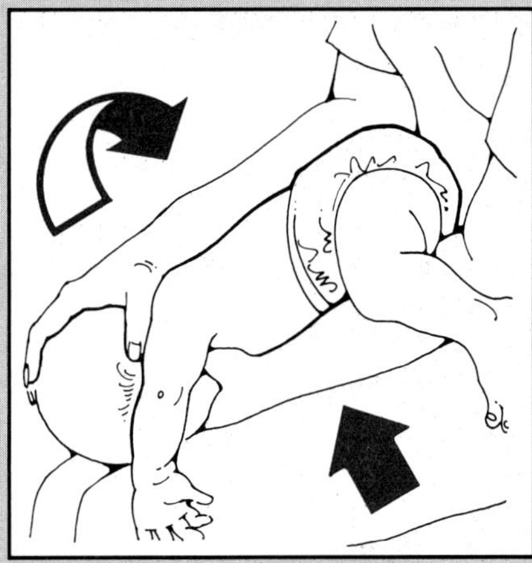

4. Deliver four sharp chest thrusts as described above, but with two or three fingers of one hand. Locate the correct position by placing your index finger on the sternum one finger-breadth below the nipple line; then placing your ring and middle fingers in a vertical line beside the index finger.

4. The use of two hands by an adult might create enough force to injure the infant. The thrusts should dislodge the object.

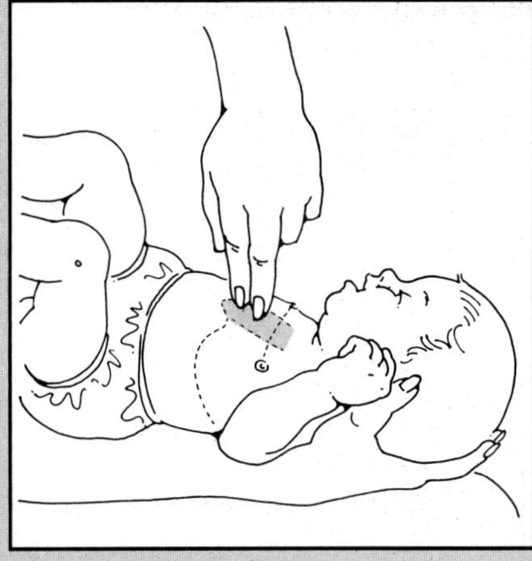

5. Alternate back blows and chest thrusts until spontaneous air exchange occurs or victim loses consciousness.

5. See Skill A, step 5.

SKILL D: Unconscious Victim (Adult)

1. Place victim in supine position.

1. Allows correct placement of hands for abdominal thrusts.

2. Shout for help or ask any available person to call 911 or comparable number. Activate client emergency call light if client is in hospital room.

2. Assistance with CPR may be needed to prevent anoxia and brain damage.

(continued)

PROCEDURE 27–8. (continued)

3. Perform a finger sweep: place thumb in victim's mouth over tongue; grasp chin and pull lower jaw upwards. Slide index finger of other hand along inside of cheeks, deep into throat, using a hooking motion across base of tongue.

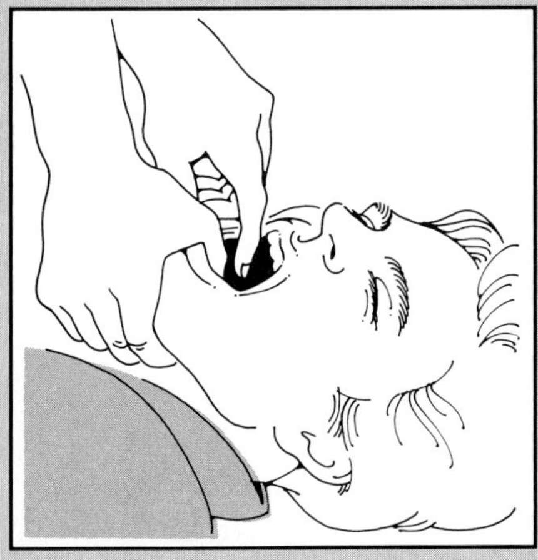

3. Hooking finger sweep may dislodge an obstruction that is not deep in airway. Avoid straight poking motion of finger, which may push obstruction deeper.

4. Attempt to ventilate victim (see Procedure 27–9). Make no further attempts to dislodge object if ventilation is possible.

4. Relaxation of throat muscles due to anoxia may allow passage of air even though obstruction is not dislodged.

5. If ventilation fails, initiate abdominal thrusts.

5. Airway must be patent to deliver oxygen and prevent brain damage.

a. Straddle victim. Place heel of one hand at the midline slightly above the umbilicus; place the other hand on top of the first, pointing fingers of both hands upward, away from chest wall.

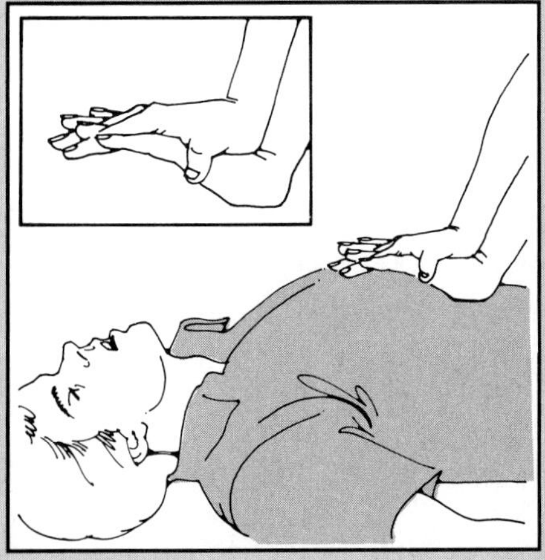

a. Locates upward force below obstruction while avoiding injury to victim's ribs or lungs.

(continued)

PROCEDURE 27–8. (continued)

b. With elbows straight and your shoulders over victim's lower abdomen, press inward and upward sharply, six to ten times. Avoid thrusts on either side of midline to prevent injury to victim.

b. Force of thrusts creates changes in air pressure, producing rushes of air which will carry the obstructing object upward for expulsion.

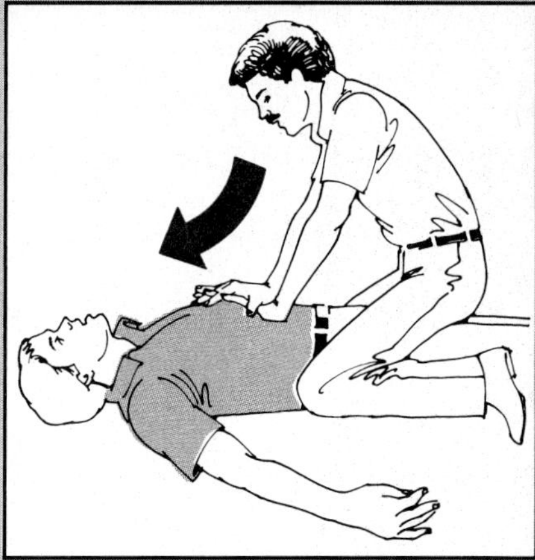

NOTE: For pregnant or obese victims, place your hands on the lower one-third of the sternum, above the xyphoid process, and administer downward thrusts.

6. If victim does not begin to breathe, repeat sequence of finger sweep, ventilation attempt, thrusts until airway is opened.

6. Relaxation of throat muscles after a period of anoxia may permit removal of object with subsequent attempts.

RECORDING: If cessation of breathing occurs in a client who is admitted to a health care facility, precise description of all events observed that could have contributed to cessation of respirations, or the state of the client when first noted to have stopped breathing, as well as all actions taken and their results, should be noted on the client's chart.

PROCEDURE 27–9. RESCUE BREATHING (ORAL VENTILATION)

PURPOSE: To ventilate an unconscious person until spontaneous breathing resumes or an oxygen delivery system is available.

EQUIPMENT: None.

ACTION	RATIONALE
1. Assess whether victim is unconscious by grasping the shoulder, shaking, and shouting, "Are you OK?"	1. Oral ventilation is contraindicated in a conscious victim.

(continued)

PROCEDURE 27–9. (continued)

2. If victim is unresponsive, check for respirations by:
   a. Placing the rescuer's cheek next to victim's nose to feel air movement.
   b. Listening for air escaping from nose, and
   c. Observing the chest and abdomen for rising and falling movement.

2. Oral ventilation is unnecessary if victim is breathing. If victim is not breathing, immediate ventilation is needed to prevent brain damage, which may occur within 4 minutes.

3. If victim is not breathing, call for help. Assistant should be prepared to call 911 or Code Blue if spontaneous breathing does not resume immediately.

3. Victim may also require external cardiac compressions and the assistance of specially trained resuscitation team.

4. Perform a finger sweep (see Procedure 27–8) and reassess for breathing.

4. This may clear airway to allow spontaneous breathing to resume.

5. If there is still no breathing, place the victim in supine position.

NOTE: If there is evidence of injuries, use care to reposition victim so injuries are not aggravated.

5. Allows visualization of chest to assess for breathing and facilitates external cardiac compressions, if necessary.

6. Open airway by *head-tilt, chin-lift:*
   a. Place palm of one hand on victim's forehead.
   b. Place fingers of opposite hand under victim's chin. Use care to avoid pressure on the soft tissue of the throat.
   c. Simultaneously push down on forehead and lift upward on chin.

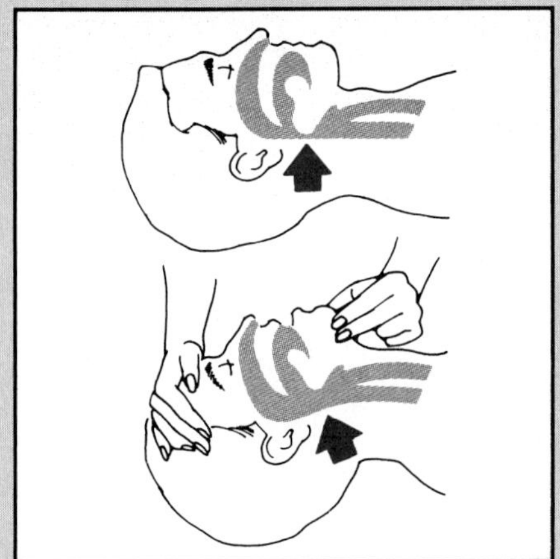

6. Loss of muscle tone due to unconsciousness causes tongue to fall backward, obstructing the pharynx. Head-tilt/chin-lift or jaw thrust move the jaw and attached tongue so pharynx is opened.

(continued)

or *jaw thrust:*
Pull upward on both mandibular angles (corner of jaw directly below ears) with tips of fingers; neck will hyperextend.

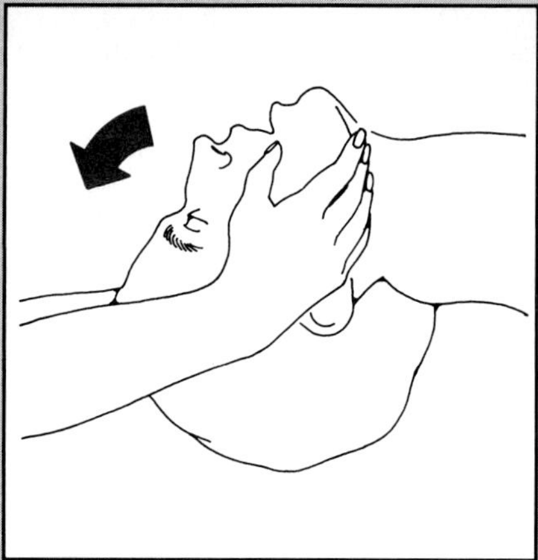

NOTE: If neck injury is suspected, do not hyperextend neck. Instead put thumb into the mouth and grasp lower jaw and pull jaw upward. For infants, see step 10, below.

7. Reassess for breathing (see step 2, above). If no breathing is noted, give two full slow breaths using one of the following methods.

7. Opening airway may restore breathing. If not, ventilation is needed to prevent brain damage or death.

8. Mouth-to-mouth resuscitation:
   a. Pinch nostrils together.
   b. Take a deep breath and place mouth over the victim's mouth forming a tight seal.
   c. Blow two full breaths, 1–1.5 seconds each, pausing between breaths to allow passive deflation of lungs.

8a. Prevents escape of air from nostrils.
   b. Deep-breathe to deliver sufficient oxygen to victim; seal to avoid loss of air.
   c. Provides sufficient oxygen and reduces the possibility of gastric distension due to excessive rate or pressure.

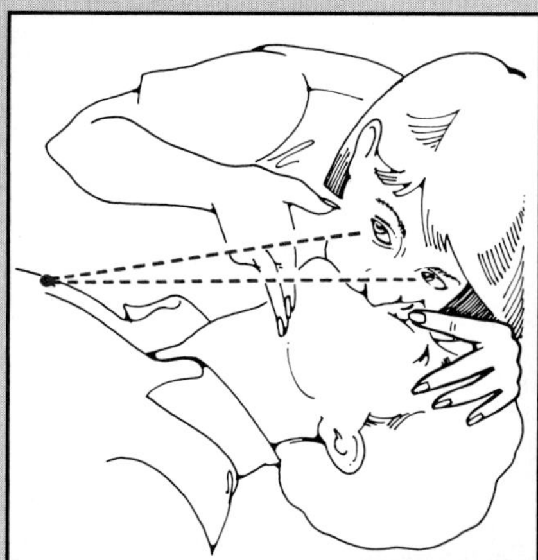

   d. Observe for chest expansion as ventilations are done.
   e. If chest does not rise, reposition head and ventilate again. If unsuccessful, repeat abdominal thrusts (see Procedure 27–8) and try again.

   d. Filling of lungs will cause chest to rise if ventilation is adequate.
   e. Failure to ventilate may be due to obstructed airway, which must be corrected to oxygenate victim.

NOTE: Oral airway may be used if readily available. Do not delay ventilation to obtain one. If victim has mouth injuries or is without teeth and an airtight seal cannot be made, refer to step 9, below. If an infant, refer to step 10.

(continued)

PROCEDURE 27–9. (continued)

9. Mouth-to-nose resuscitation:
   a. Hold victim's mouth closed while maintaining hyperextension of neck.
   b. Place mouth over victim's nose, making a seal on cheeks, and place your cheek over victim's lips.

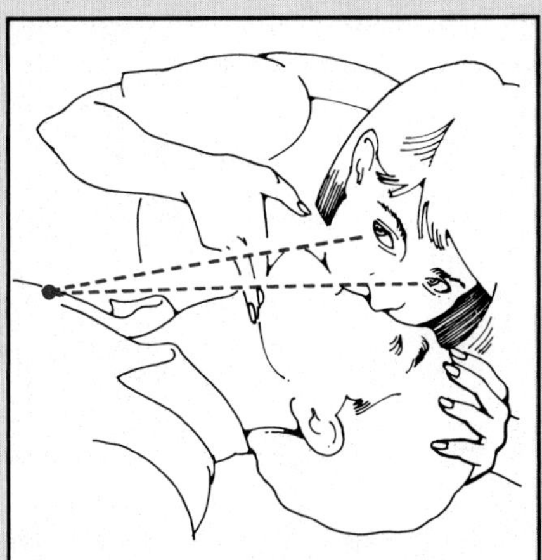

   c. Continue with steps 8c–e, above.

9a. Prevents loss of air via mouth.
b. Directs oxygen to victim's lungs.

10. Mouth-to-mouth-and-nose resuscitation:
   a. Do not use fingersweep on infants unless object can be seen; place thumb over tongue and pull jaw upward while looking in mouth. Carefully remove visible object with fingers. Assess for breathing after fingersweep.

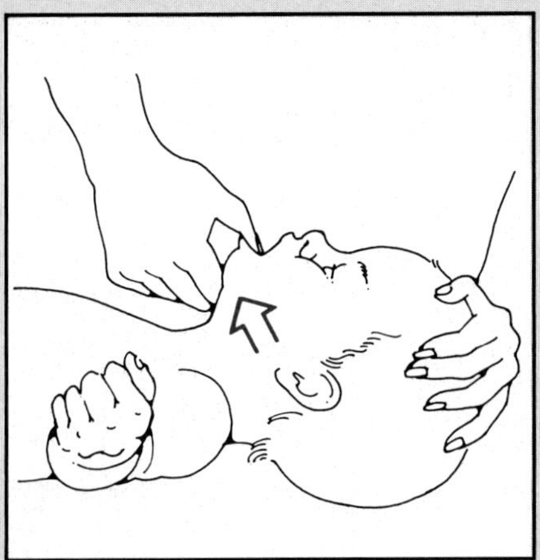

   b. Open airway as in step 5, above, but do not hyperextend neck as for adult victim.

10a. Infant's mouth is so small that fingersweep is more likely to push object further down than to remove it.
b. Infant has less muscle tone, so complete hyperextension of infant's neck may cause tracheal collapse or neck injury.

(continued)

c. Place mouth over infant's nose and mouth to form a seal.

c. The infant's face is too small to enable a tight mouth-to-mouth seal.

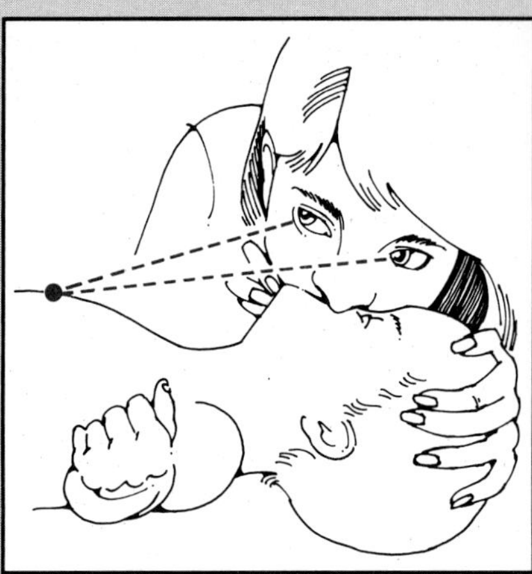

d. Gently blow two breaths of 1–1.5 seconds each into infant, pausing for passive deflation of lungs. Breaths should have just enough pressure to cause chest to rise.

d. Inflates lungs at lowest possible pressure, avoiding gastric distension.

e. If chest does not rise, repeat steps to clear airway until able to ventilate.

e. See step 8e, above.

11. After administering two full breaths, check the carotid pulse for 5–10 seconds by sliding fingers from chin along the groove of the neck toward the ear. The carotid pulse is just below the angle of the mandible (jawbone). For an infant, assess the brachial pulse midway between the axilla and the elbow on the medial aspect of the arm.

11. Cause of cessation of breathing may be a cardiac arrest. The victim will then need chest compressions, as well. If the heart is beating, the carotid pulse is most likely to be palpable as it carries one fourth of the person's total blood volume.

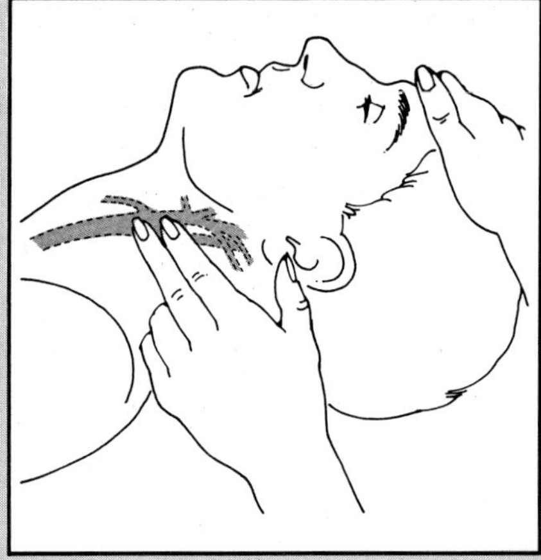

12. If there is no pulse, initiate cardiac compressions (see Procedure 27–10).

12. Lack of pulse signifies lack of circulation to vital organs.

13. If there is a pulse, continue to ventilate victim at rate of one breath every 5 seconds, removing your mouth from victim's mouth after each breath. Watch chest rise and fall and feel escape of air with your cheek. Ventilate an infant at a rate of one breath every 3 seconds.

13. This rate and volume of air will provide sufficient oxygen to prevent damage to vital organs as long as heart is beating. Continued observation of chest movement verifies continued ventilation.

(continued)

PROCEDURE 27–9. (continued)

14. Check pulse again after 2 minutes (12 breaths in an adult; 20 in an infant). Continue ventilation if pulse is present and add compressions if pulse is absent.

14. Palpable pulse verifies continued cardiac function.

15. If ventilations become impossible to administer, check the stomach for distension.

NOTE: Ventilation should not be interrupted. Remove gastric air only if pressure makes ventilation impossible.

15. Some of the air you are breathing into the victim may travel to the stomach via the esophagus. As the stomach fills with air, pressure increases and is transmitted to the mouth, causing resistance to incoming air.

16. If distended stomach prevents ventilation, remove the air as follows:
    a. Turn victim on side with back toward you.
    b. Place hand between victim's rib cage and waist and push on the stomach.

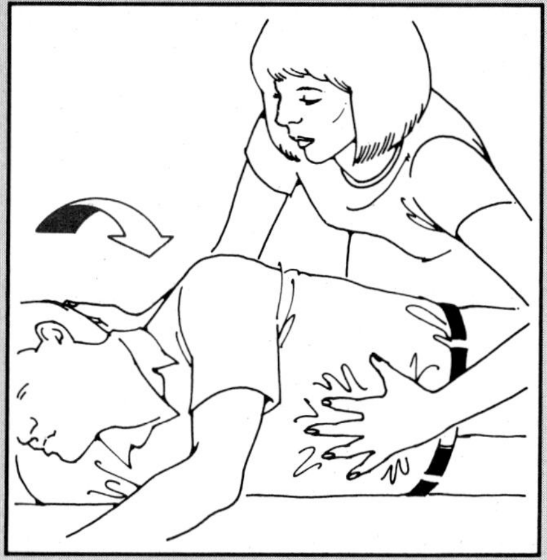

    c. Clear the mouth of emesis if vomiting occurs.
    d. Return victim to supine position and continue ventilation, checking carotid pulse every few minutes, until spontaneous breathing begins or trained resuscitation team arrives, or victim is pronounced dead by physician.

16a. Air removal could cause vomiting. If supine, victim could aspirate emesis.
  b. Pressure should push air out via the path of least resistance, the esophagus.
  c. Emesis could obstruct the airway or be pushed into the lungs with subsequent ventilations.
  d. Efforts to maintain ventilation and perfusion should continue until known to be futile.

17. If breathing resumes, observe carefully to verify continued spontaneous respiration.

17. Airway may still be partially occluded and may easily become obstructed again.

18. Maintain victim in a supine position with head and shoulders raised. Keep at a comfortable temperature.

NOTE: Do not raise head or shoulders of a potential spinal cord injured victim.

18. This position facilitates ease of respiration. Neutral temperature minimizes metabolic demands for oxygen.

(continued)

PROCEDURE 27–9. (continued)

19. Call a physician or ambulance for further assessment and treatment.

19. Complete assessment to determine and treat cause of respiratory arrest and any resulting complications is necessary to protect victim's health and well-being.

RECORDING: If victim is a client in a health care facility, the following should be documented: complete description of the precipitating events, if observed; the state in which the client was found; all actions taken by health care providers; and client's response to interventions. Many institutions provide a form for such documentation.

PROCEDURE 27–10. EXTERNAL CARDIAC COMPRESSIONS

PURPOSE: To circulate oxygenated blood to vital organs when cardiac function has been interrupted.

EQUIPMENT: Emergency "crash" cart, if available.

ACTION	RATIONALE
1. Confirm loss of consciousness and cessation of breathing and cardiac function as described in Procedure 27–9.	1. Cardiac compression and artificial ventilation are contraindicated if victim is conscious with cardiac and respiratory function.
2. If victim is not breathing, call for help, open airway, initiate rescue breathing (see Procedure 27–9); assess carotid pulse for 5 seconds after giving two ventilations; if absent, begin circulation (cardiac compressions) using one of the following methods. Using the mnemonic ABC (airway, breathing, circulation) will assist you in remembering the steps for CPR.	2. If respiration and circulation are absent, CPR must be initiated promptly to prevent brain damage or death.
SKILL A: Adult Victim/One Rescuer	
1. Place victim supine on a firm surface, head level with heart. A person in bed must be moved to the floor, or a cardiac board or similar large, flat, firm object must be placed beneath the back. The head- or footboard of some hospital beds may be removed for use as a cardiac board.	1. A firm surface facilitates the compression of the victim's heart between the sternum and spine. A soft surface absorbs the force of compressions so insufficient force is available to compress the heart. If head is higher than heart, the brain will not be perfused.

(continued)

PROCEDURE 27–10. (continued)

2. Locate the position for compression by using the fingers of your hand nearest the victim's legs to follow the lower edge of the rib cage toward the costalsternal notch where the ribs join the sternum.

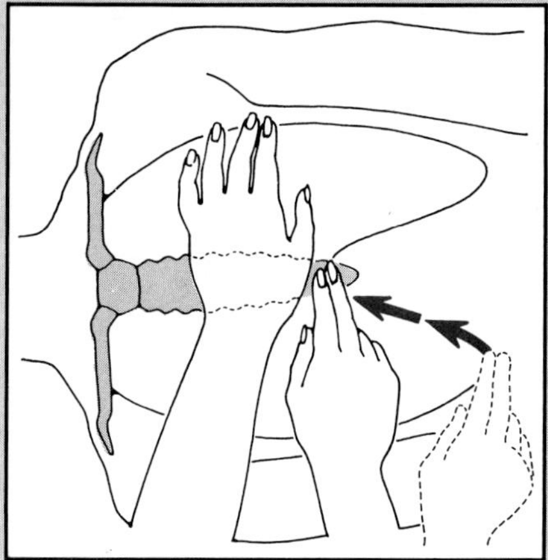

NOTE: Liver lacerations may occur if compressions are administered too low.

2. Correct hand placement is critical if injury is to be avoided. This method is a rapid and accurate way to avoid exerting pressure too low.

3. Place the heel of your other hand on the sternum, two finger breadths above the notch, then place the heel of the opposite hand over it, interlacing and holding fingers off the chest. Fingers should be perpendicular to the sternum; heels of the hands directly over lower half of sternum.

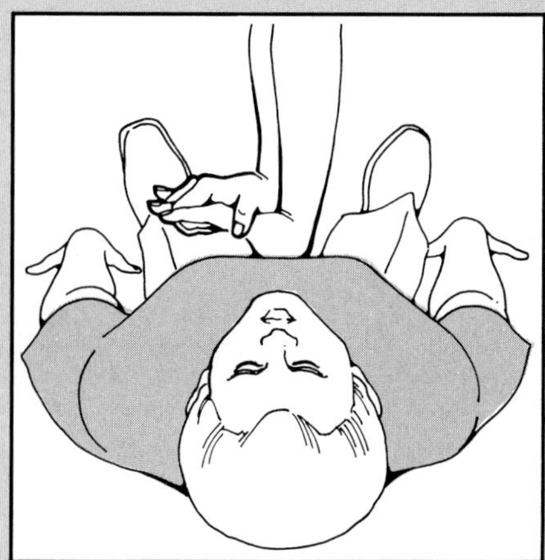

NOTE: Pressing on the ribs or the edge of the sternum could fracture the ribs.

3. This hand position will direct the force of compressions directly downward toward the heart without injuring the ribs.

(continued)

PROCEDURE 27–10. (continued)

4. Support your weight on your knees, then rock forward, bending at the hips, so shoulders are directly over victim's sternum, keeping arms straight and elbows locked.

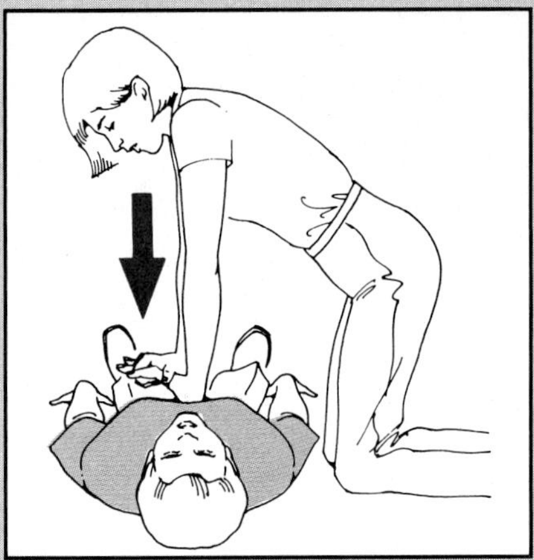

4. This motion uses the rescuer's weight to compress the heart in a smooth, regular pattern, similar to the rhythmic action of a functioning heart. Locking the hips or flexing the elbows results in less forceful or uneven compressions.

5. Press straight down on the sternum, compressing the chest 1½ to 2 inches.

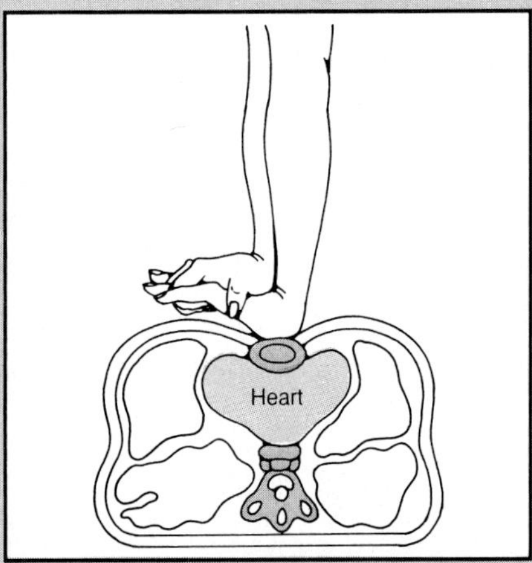

5. The pressure squeezes the blood out of the heart.

6. Rock back slightly, releasing pressure, but maintaining contact with body.

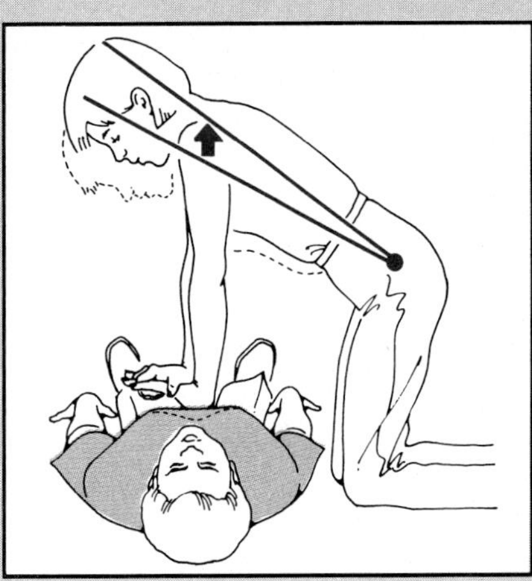

6. Release of pressure allows heart to refill with blood. Maintaining contact prevents malpositioning of the hands and possible injury on subsequent compressions.

(continued)

PROCEDURE 27–10. (continued)

Action	Rationale
7. Give compressions at rate of 80–100 per minute, counting "one and two and," etc, up to 15.	7. This rate will produce sufficient cardiac output to perfuse vital organs.
8. After each group of 15 compressions, give two full ventilations (Procedure 27–9). Use method in step 3, above, to reposition hands correctly after ventilations.	8. Blood must be oxygenated periodically.
9. After the first minute of CPR, check carotid pulse and resume CPR if pulse is absent. Recheck pulse every few minutes, but do not interrupt CPR for more than 5 seconds to do so. NOTE: Pulse should also be checked if signs of recovery such as movement, swallowing, or returning facial color occur.	9. Return of cardiac function signals that compressions may be discontinued. Continue ventilations without compressions if ventilations do not also resume.
10. If it does not seem likely that help will arrive, call 911 after several minutes of CPR.	10. The purpose of CPR is to keep a victim alive until medical help is available. EMS can be activated very quickly, assuring that help will arrive.
11. Continue CPR until heartbeat and breathing are restored, EMS team arrives, you are exhausted, or victim is pronounced dead by a physician.	11. Efforts to maintain life must be maintained until a thorough assessment can be made by a qualified person.
12. If heartbeat and breathing resume, continue to observe and arrange for transport of victim to health care facility.	12. Determination and treatment of the cause of cardiac arrest are necessary for victim's well-being.
SKILL B: Adult Victim/Two Rescuers	
1. When second rescuer arrives, ask that EMS be activated if you have not already done so.	1. EMS team is equipped with drugs, oxygen, and transport vehicle so victim can receive definitive treatment.
2. If second rescuer knows CPR, initiate two-person CPR.	2. Two-person CPR is more effective because more breaths per minute can be delivered. It can usually be maintained for a longer period of time because it is less fatiguing.
3. First rescuer should communicate to second whether to assume ventilations or compressions.	3. Prevents confusion and possible lengthy interruption of CPR.

(continued)

PROCEDURE 27–10. (continued)

4. If second rescuer ventilates:
   a. First rescuer assesses for pulse and breathing while second takes a position near victim's head.
   b. First rescuer states: "No pulse, continue CPR" and gives five compressions while second reopens airway and prepares to ventilate after fifth compression.
   c. Second rescuer checks pulse during compressions.

4a. Determines actual need for continued CPR.
b. Maintains cardiac output of oxygenated blood and allows for assessment of effectiveness of compressions.
c. Determines whether compressions are moving blood.

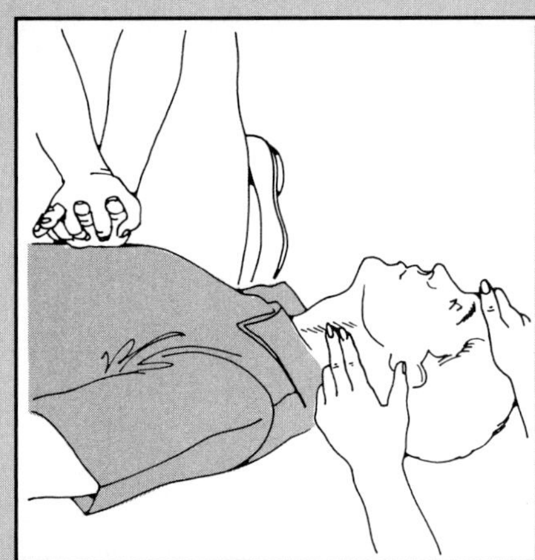

d. CPR continues at a ratio of one ventilation to five compressions, and a rate of 80–100 compressions/minute with first rescuer counting aloud. A 1–1.5-second pause is allowed after the fifth compression to allow time for a full ventilation.

d. Provides sufficient circulation to perfuse major organs while allowing enough time for full ventilation to oxygenate blood.

5. If second rescuer does compressions:
   a. First rescuer assesses pulse and breathing, second takes position near chest and locates xyphoid process (Skill A, step 2).
   b. First rescuer states "No pulse, continue CPR," and gives one ventilation.
   c. Second rescuer begins compressions as above.
   d. CPR is maintained as previously described.

5. See step 4, above.

6. When either rescuer tires, a clear signal is given to change positions.

6. Prevents lengthy interruption of CPR.

7. Switch is done after a ventilation:
   a. Ventilator moves to chest, locates xyphoid process, and awaits signal to begin.
   b. Compressor simultaneously moves to head, then opens airway, assesses pulse and breathing, verbalizes whether pulse and breathing are present or absent, and gives one slow, full ventilation if needed. If pulse and/or breathing is noted on assessment, compression and/or ventilation are discontinued.
   c. Compressor begins compressions at previous rate if told pulse is absent.

7. Maintains oxygenation of blood during switch.
   a–c. Coordinated movement and rapid assessment facilitate continuous ventilation and perfusion of victim's vital organs.

   d. CPR continues as above with rescuers switching as needed until EMS team arrives, victim is pronounced dead by a physician, or rescuers are exhausted.

   d. Efforts to maintain life must be maintained until a thorough assessment can be made by a qualified person.

(continued)

PROCEDURE 27–10. (continued)

SKILL C: Infant Victim/One Rescuer

1. Assess consciousness, breathing, and circulation, as described above, initiate ventilations if infant is not breathing.

2. If there is no brachial pulse, place the infant on a firm surface with your hand under the back.

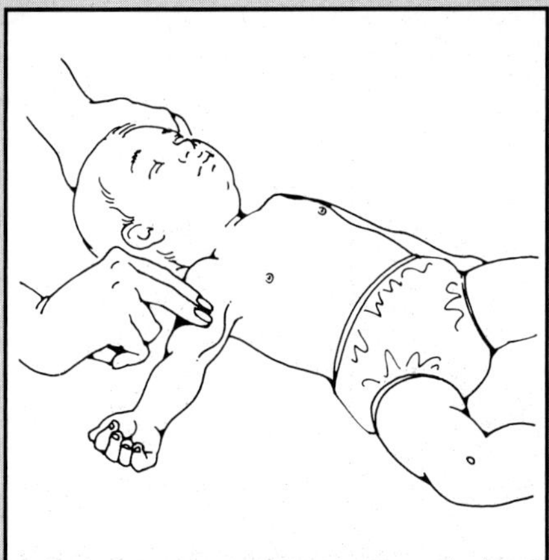

2. Firm surface is needed to compress the heart. Hand position maintains head tilt for ventilation. Head must be at same level as or lower than heart to adequately perfuse the brain.

3. Place the fingers of your other hand along the infant's sternum, one finger-breadth below nipple line.

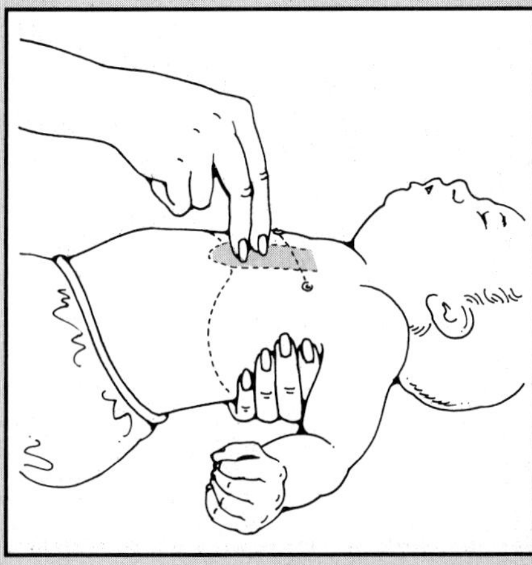

3. This is the location of the infant's heart.

4. Compress the chest ½ to 1 inch using two or three fingers at a rate of 100 compressions per minute. Do not press on the xyphoid process.

4. Greater pressure could cause injury; faster rate is nearer infant's normal heart rate.

(continued)

PROCEDURE 27–10. (continued)

5. Continue to provide ventilations and compressions at a ratio of one ventilation every five compressions, pausing 1–1.5 seconds for ventilation as with adult victim.

5. Maintains adequate oxygenation and perfusion.

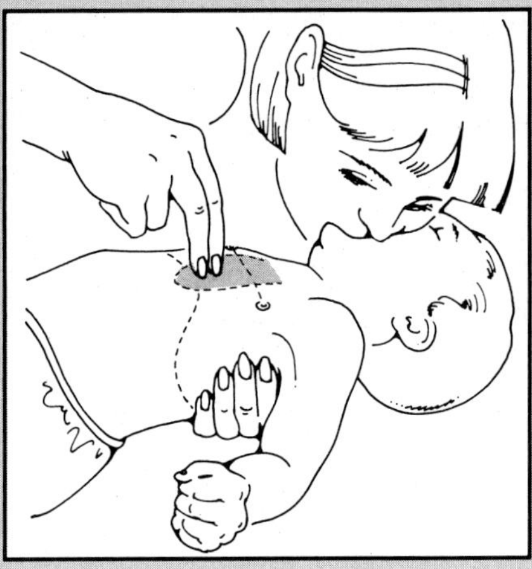

NOTE: Keeping your face very close to the infant's during compressions facilitates giving ventilation quickly.

6. Reassess breathing and brachial pulse after first minute of CPR and every few minutes thereafter, as with adult victim.

6. Verifies continued need for CPR.

7. Continue CPR until EMS team arrives, infant is pronounced dead by a physician, or you are exhausted.

7. Efforts to maintain life must be maintained until a thorough assessment can be made by a qualified person.

SKILL D: Child Victim (Less Than 8 Years Old)/One Rescuer

1. Assess consciousness, breathing, and circulation, as described above; initiate ventilations if no respiration.

2. Position child supine on a firm surface, head level with heart.

2. A hard surface facilitates the compression of the victim's heart between the sternum and spine. Head and heart must be on same level to perfuse brain.

3. Locate position for compressions as in Skill A, step 2.

3. See Skill A, step 2.

(continued)

PROCEDURE 27–10. (continued)

4. Give compressions with heel of one hand, depressing chest 1–1.5 inches at a rate of 80–100 per minute. For a child older than 8, use two hands for compressions.

   4. Creates sufficient pressure to squeeze blood out of heart without injuring child.

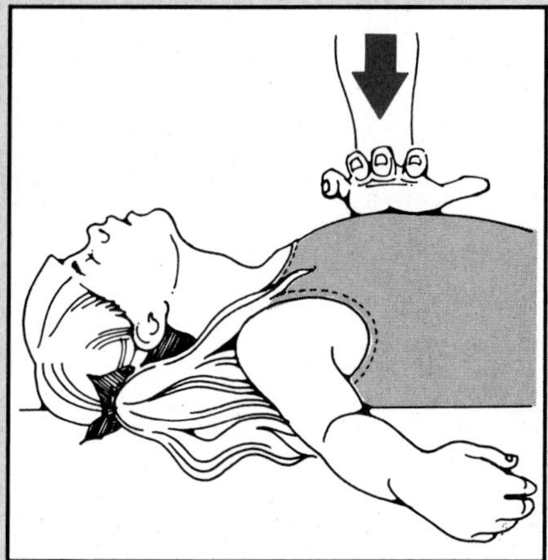

5. Continue CPR at a ratio of five compressions for each ventilation, pausing 1–1.5 seconds for ventilation.

   5. Maintains adequate oxygenation and perfusion.

6. Reassess breathing and carotid pulse as with adult victim.

   6. Verifies need for continued CPR.

7. Continue CPR until EMS team arrives, child is pronounced dead by a physician, or you are exhausted.

   7. Efforts to maintain life must be maintained until a thorough assessment can be made by a qualified person.

RECORDING: If victim is a client in a health care facility, the following should be noted on the client's record: events occurring before the arrest, if observed; condition of client when found if arrest was not witnessed; and all actions taken by health care providers, and client's response to interventions.

PROCEDURE 27–11. USING A HAND-COMPRESSIBLE BREATHING BAG (AMBU BAG)

PURPOSE: To ventilate an unconscious person who is not breathing.

EQUIPMENT: Hand-compressible breathing bag with mask to fit client. May be kept at bedside of client experiencing frequent respiratory difficulty or be kept on the emergency "crash" cart.

ACTION	RATIONALE
1. Assess consciousness and breathing as described in Procedure 27–9. If client is not breathing, open airway using one of the methods described in Procedure 27–9.	

(continued)

PROCEDURE 27–11. (continued)

2. Apply mask securely over client's nose and mouth, holding it in place and maintaining client's head position with one hand to keep airway open.

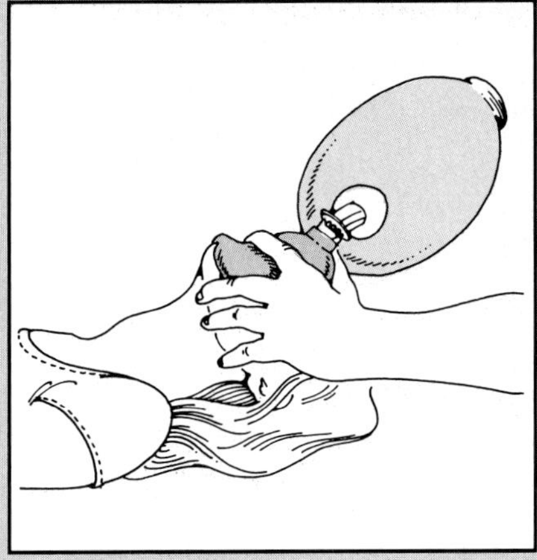

2. If airway is closed by client's head changing position, no oxygen will be delivered to lungs. If air escapes from sides of mask, less oxygen will be delivered.

3. Compress bag forcefully with your free hand while observing chest for elevation. Allow bag to self-reinflate by relaxing hold on it.

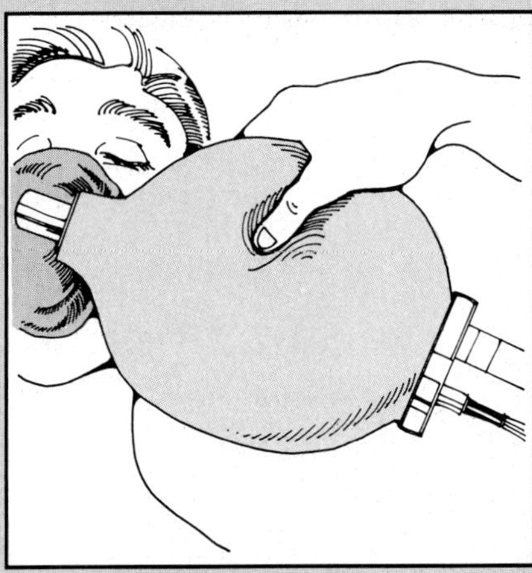

3. Compression of bag should inflate lungs and cause chest to rise. Exhaled air will be released into room via an exhaust valve; bag will refill with room air.

4. If no evidence of lung inflation is noted, reposition head and squeeze bag again. If still unable to verify lung inflation, attempt to remove possible foreign body obstruction using abdominal thrusts (Procedure 27–8). If tracheal suctioning equipment is available, suction to clear airway (Procedure 27–7).

4. Rapid attempts to open airway and deliver oxygen are necessary to prevent brain damage and death.

5. Assess for spontaneous breathing. If none, call for help. Give two full inflations, then assess carotid pulse for 5 seconds (Procedure 27–10).

NOTE: Many health care facilities have an emergency call button on wall to alert code team.

5. Opening airway and ventilation may restore breathing. If cardiac and respiratory arrest has occurred, CPR must be initiated and code team called.

(continued)

PROCEDURE 27–11. (continued)

6. If there is a pulse, continue to ventilate by squeezing bag at a rate of 12 breaths/minute (one per 5 seconds). If an oxygen source is available, connect it to the nipple at the top or bottom of the bag, set liter flow at 12–15 L/min, and ventilate at same rate.

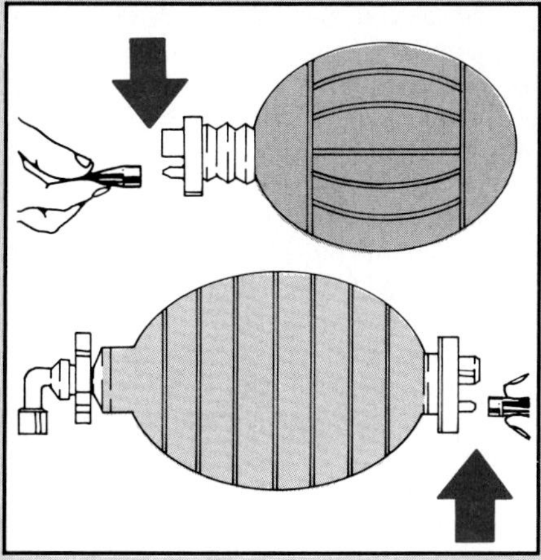

NOTE: Do not increase rate of inflations; bag must refill and be firmly squeezed to sufficiently inflate lungs.

6. Optimum perfusion is maintained by administering oxygen, as the apneic client has an oxygen deficit. If oxygen source is not available, room air will provide adequate perfusion until code team arrives.

7. If there is no pulse, initiate CPR (Procedure 27–10).

7. Ventilation is ineffective without circulation.

8. Be alert for vomiting, turning client to one side immediately should it occur, and clearing mouth before continuing to ventilate.

8. Ambu bag may deliver some air to stomach, causing distension and reflex vomiting. Side-lying position facilitates flow of emesis out of mouth. Emesis will cause pneumonia if aspirated or forced into lungs.

9. Continue resuscitation until client breathes spontaneously or until relieved by code team.

9. Health care facility policy usually designates code team to be responsible for immediate definitive treatment of client suffering cardiac and/or respiratory arrest. Nurse initiating ventilation may be asked to assist in this process.

10. Notify client's primary physician of respiratory arrest.

10. Primary physician is responsible for ongoing medical treatment of client.

RECORDING: Note events precipitating arrest, if observed; condition of client when found; and action taken by all health care providers, and client's response.

Most oxygen delivery systems cannot regulate the exact amount of oxygen a client receives, because the device supplies only the supplemental oxygen. The room air with which the oxygen is mixed enters the device as the client inhales. Therefore, the client's rate and depth of respiration influence the amount of room air that mixes with the oxygen coming from the delivery system and affects the percentage of oxygen the client takes in. These kinds of delivery systems are called low-flow systems. The approximate Fio_2 that low-flow devices supply can be predicted based on the oxygen flowrate being used (Table 27–7). Many clients who require oxygen therapy do not require precise concentrations of oxygen. In this situation, a physician orders a low-flow device, with a specified flowrate rather than a concentration (for example, "O_2 2 LPM via nasal prongs").

Humidifying Oxygen. Oxygen stored in cylinders or central reservoirs is dry. At all but the lowest flowrates (eg, 2 to 3 L/min) it can dry respiratory tract mucosa and thus compromise airway patency. Disposable or reusable humidifiers can be attached to oxygen delivery systems to prevent mucosal drying and irritation (see Procedure 27–14).

Oxygen Delivery Devices. Several kinds of oxygen delivery devices are available, each having advantages and disadvantages. Some, such as the oxygen hood and the croupette, or oxygen tent, are used only for pediatric clients.

Oxygen Hood. The rigid plastic hood, which covers only the head, is effective for neonates and premature infants. Because they do not move independently, the stationary hood provides a continuous supply of oxygen.

Croupette. The croupette is a large clear plastic tent that is placed inside a crib, providing sufficient space for a young infant or small child to move around. The entire tent is flooded with humidified oxygen. The croupette is useful for a child who will not wear a mask, but it has several disadvantages. It is difficult to maintain oxygen levels because the tent must be opened to give care. Moreover, the child may feel isolated within the tent. The humidity creates a mist that interferes with visual monitoring of the child and makes the child's clothing and bed linen damp. Pediatric-

BOX 27–9. SAFETY PRECAUTIONS DURING OXYGEN THERAPY

1. Post "NO SMOKING, OXYGEN IN USE" signs on the door of any room in which oxygen is being used and near the bed of a client who is receiving oxygen.
2. Explain to the client and significant others why open flames, ungrounded electrical appliances, volatile materials, or any item capable of creating sparks may not be used in a room in which oxygen is in use.
3. Show significant others the location and correct operation of the nearest fire extinguishers.
4. Help the client store personal effects that could support combustion in a secure but inaccessible place during oxygen therapy. These include:
   a. Smoking materials such as lighter and matches.
   b. Ungrounded electrical devices, such as radios, shavers, and hair dryers.
   c. Items that can generate static electricity, such as blankets or clothing made of wool or synthetic fabrics.
   d. Volatile toiletry products such as alcohol-based perfumes or colognes and nail polish remover.
   e. Petroleum-based products such as petroleum jelly.
5. Make sure that all hospital electrical equipment—such as beds, monitors, infusion pumps, and portable suction machines—is properly grounded. Notify hospital engineering or maintainance departments of any faulty electrical equipment.
6. Remove all volatile and petroleum-based hospital products from the room. Replace with water-soluble products when possible.

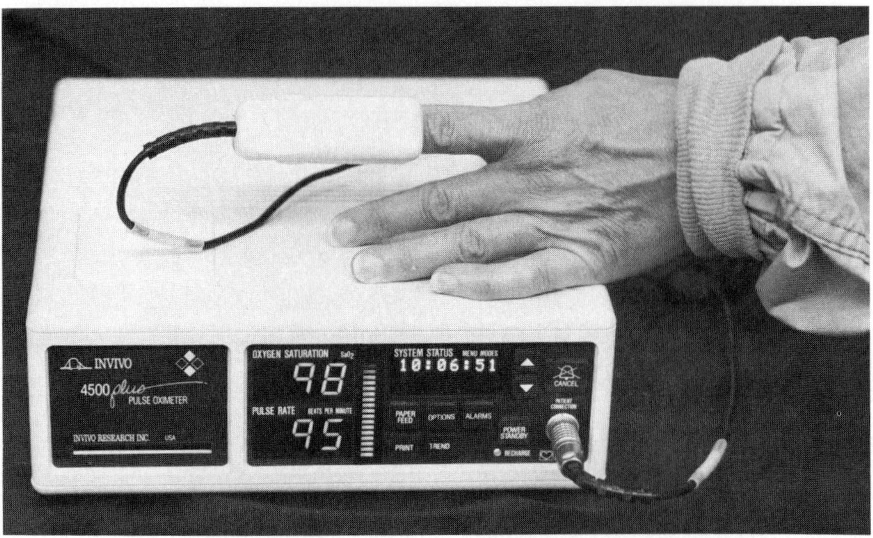

Figure 27–15. A pulse oximeter.

PROCEDURE 27–12. ADMINISTERING OXYGEN FROM A PORTABLE OXYGEN TANK

PURPOSE: To supply oxygen continually while client is ambulating or being transferred between departments (eg, treatments or tests).

EQUIPMENT: Portable oxygen tank (E cylinder), regulator with flowmeter, and client's oxygen delivery device with humidifier and connecting tubing.

ACTION

1. Explain the procedure and its expected benefits to the client. Obtain a portable tank.
2. Check the gauge for the amount of oxygen (psi) in the tank. Compute the length of time this amount will last using the following formula:

   $$\frac{\text{psi} \times 0.28}{\text{L/min ordered}} = \text{minutes of oxygen available.}$$

   Obtain a new tank if insufficient quantity remains for projected length of planned activity.
3. For a new cylinder:
   a. "Crack" the cylinder—turn the handwheel at the top slowly clockwise, then close it quickly to clear the valve opening of any dust or particles. Cracking the cylinder produces a loud hissing noise; this does not indicate malfunction.
   b. Attach a regulator with flowmeter to the cylinder outlet. A wrench is attached to the tank for this purpose. Tank oxygen is stored under pressure. The regulator controls the *pressure* at which the oxygen exits the tank. A flowmeter is needed to regulate the *rate* of flow.
   c. Open the cylinder valve by slowly turning the handwheel until it is fully open, to start the flow of oxygen, then turn it back one quarter turn.
4. Set the flowmeter at the ordered rate.
5. If the client is receiving humidified oxygen, remove the humidifier with the connecting tubing from the wall source and attach it to the portable tank below the flowmeter to prevent drying of mucous membranes. Humidifiers should not be used by more than one client. If left on tank from previous use, discard to prevent cross contamination.
6. If no humidifier is in use, remove the connecting tubing from the wall source and attach it to the portable tank below the flowmeter. Turn the wall flowmeter to zero.
7. Remind the client not to be around smokers while using portable oxygen.
8. After the client has returned to the room, reconnect the delivery system to the wall source and reset the flowmeter to the ordered rate. Turn off the flow of oxygen from the portable tank by setting its flowmeter at zero.
9. Store the portable tank so that it cannot fall or be easily tipped over, which could damage the regulator, resulting in rapid escape of gas under pressure from the tank and making the tank a projectile.

RECORDING: Document the use of portable oxygen, the specific activity, and the client's response.

sized masks or nasal cannulae are preferred delivery methods, if the child will tolerate them.

Nasal Cannula. For older children and adults, the nasal cannula (also called nasal prongs) is the best tolerated form of oxygen therapy. It consists of two soft plastic prongs, curved to fit into the nostrils, attached to a plastic tube (see Fig. 27–18A and Procedure 27–13). The nasal cannula delivers oxygen effectively regardless of whether the client breathes through the nose or the mouth. It does not interfere with eating or speaking or cause a closed-in feeling, which is a common complaint with oxygen masks. Nasal prongs deliver 24 to 44 percent FiO_2, depending on flowrate and respirations. Flowrates of 1 to 6 L/min are recommended.

Oxygen Masks. If mist or a higher oxygen flow is desired, there are several types of masks available (Fig. 27–18). Masks require flowrates of at least 5 L/min to flush exhaled CO_2 from the mask. The major disadvantage of masks is that clients find them uncomfortable and tend to remove them often. The masks must also be removed for eating, drinking, expectorating, and shaving. Oxygen should be supplied via nasal cannula during these activities. The masks should be removed and cleaned and the face washed and dried about every 2 hours. Procedure 27–13 presents nursing considerations for each of the types of masks discussed below.

- *Simple mask.* The simple mask can deliver FiO_2s of 40 to 60 percent. Room air is mixed with oxygen and exhaled air expelled via small perforations on either side of the mask.
- *Partial rebreather mask.* The partial rebreather mask delivers 35 to 60 percent FiO_2. It has an attached reservoir bag at its base that collects the first one third of the client's exhaled air. Because this air comes from the pharynx and trachea where no air is exchanged, its oxygen and CO_2 content approximate room air. Perforations on either side of the mask allow entry of room air and escape of the rest of the exhaled air.
- *Nonrebreather mask.* The nonrebreather mask has the same appearance as the partial rebreather, but a rubber one-

way valve at the base of the mask prevents exhaled air from entering the reservoir bag and another on the side of the mask limits intake of room air. This mask can deliver Fio_2s of 60 to 90 percent if it fits snugly on the face.

- *Venturi mask.* The Venturi mask is the only mask that can deliver specific concentrations of oxygen. Adapters are attached to the base of the mask that cause a predictable amount of room air to mix with the incoming oxygen at a given flowrate (refer to Table 27–7). The mask has large ports on each side to allow exhaled air to escape. Venturi masks can deliver Fio_2s of 24 to 40 percent, or if used with a nebulizer and high flowrate, up to 100 percent.

Face Tent. A face tent is a modified mask that is designed to deliver high-humidity oxygen. It does not fit closely against the face as oxygen masks do, and so it may be tolerated better than a mask. Because of its design, Fio_2 delivery is less predictable with the face tent than with other delivery devices. The face tent is illustrated in Figure 27–18C and discussed in Procedure 27–13.

Chest Tubes. When air has entered a client's pleural space (pneumothorax) or body fluids have accumulated in the pleural space (hemothorax), the lung may be completely or partially collapsed. As a result, oxygenation status is severely compromised. The air is removed from the pleural space by placing one or more chest tubes through the skin and into the pleural space, allowing the lung to reexpand. The distal ends of chest tubes are connected to a water-sealed drainage system to prevent air from reentering the pleural cavity. Clients who need chest tubes are usually seriously ill and require advanced nursing care that is beyond the scope of this text.

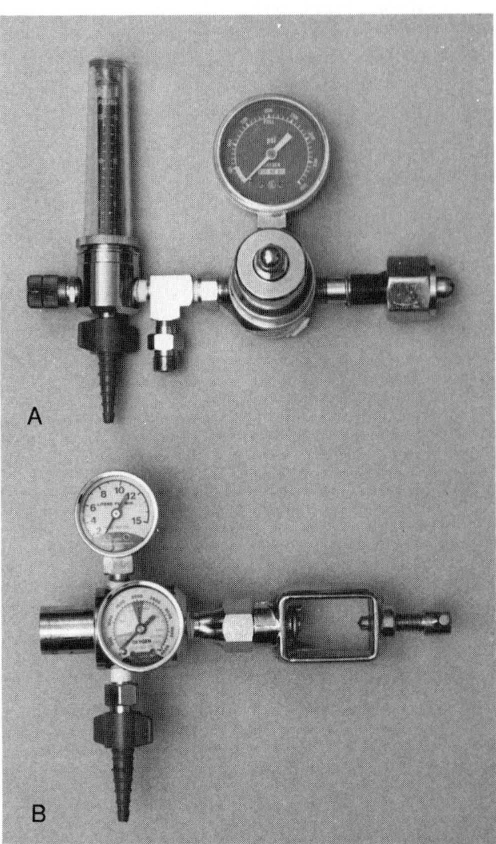

Figure 27–17. Thorpe (**A**) and Bourdan (**B**) flowmeters with content (quantity) gauge.

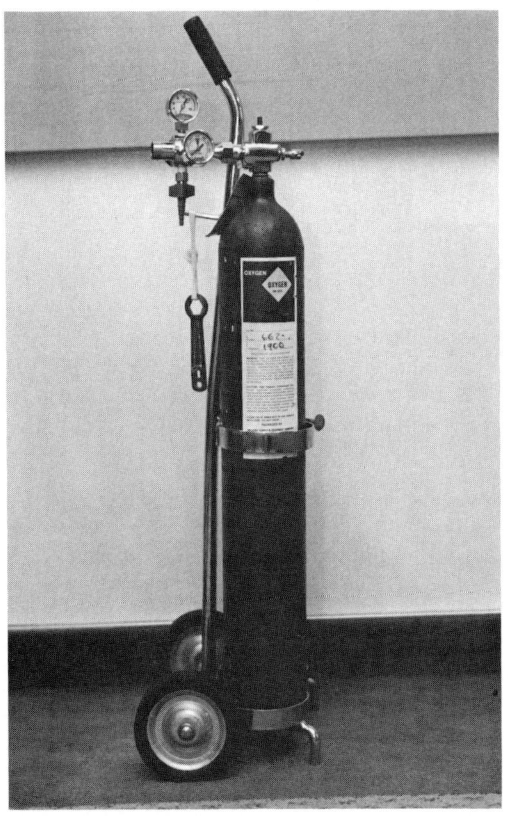

Figure 27–16. "E" tank on stand.

Supporting Circulation. Restorative care for oxygenation problems may also involve support of circulation. Examples include anti-embolism stockings, special exercises to promote circulation, positioning, and external cardiac compressions. These techniques result in improved oxygenation to various tissues of the body.

Anti-embolism Stockings. Anti-embolism stockings are used to enhance venous return, which improves peripheral circulation, reduces orthostatic hypotension, and reduces the risk of clot formation in the legs. There are two types of anti-embolism stockings. The elastic type is much like support hose. Procedure 27–15 describes their application. These stockings are supplied in knee-high and thigh-high styles. It is important to measure the client's leg carefully and apply the right size stocking.

Another type of anti-embolism stocking is the pulsatile

TABLE 27–7. FIO_2 Delivered by Various Devices at Various Flowrates

Device[a]	Flow	Flowrate (L/min)	FIO_2
Nasal cannula (prongs)	Low	1	24%
		2	28%
		3	32%
		4	36%
		5	40%
		6	44%
		(Higher flowrates not recommended)	
Simple mask	Low	5–6	40%
		6–7	50%
		7–8	60%
Partial rebreather mask	Flowrates <6 not recommended		
		6	60%
		7	70%
		8	80%
		9	90%
		10	99%
Nonrebreather mask	Low	6	55–60%
		8	60–80%
		10–15	80–90%
Face tent	Low	8–10	35–50%
Venturi mask	High	4	24%
		6	28%
		8	35%

[a] With low-flow devices, precise FIO_2 cannot be regulated. It is dependent upon respiratory rate and pattern. The figures here assume regular respiratory rate between 16 and 20 breaths per minute.

anti-embolism stocking (PAS). These stockings have an inflatable sleeve that fits into a pocket running along the length of the stocking or a series of inflatable cuffs that wrap around the calf. They are rhythmically inflated and deflated by a pneumatic pump, creating pulsations that stimulate leg circulation and improve venous return. As with the elastic stockings, it is important to apply the right size stockings and to assess circulation in the legs carefully before application and periodically during use. The stockings may be deflated for ambulation, but should not be disconnected for more than 1 hour at a time. They should be removed for 30 minutes each shift to provide skin care and assess skin and circulation.

Buerger-Allen Exercises. These exercises were developed for clients with compromised arterial circulation to the feet and legs. They can also be used to promote peripheral circulation in clients whose activity is limited because of illness or its treatment. The exercises discussed above (under Preoperative Teaching in the Supportive Care section) can also be used in conjunction with Buerger-Allen exercises for clients who are gradually increasing their activity level. Both can be continued into the rehabilitation phase of care, in combination with walking. Clients who use the exercises for severe peripheral vascular disease should follow the advice of the physician.

To perform Buerger-Allen exercises, clients should:

1. Lie flat on the back and elevate both legs and feet on a padded surface for 1 to 3 minutes. A large cushion or a chair tipped so its back creates an incline work well. The purpose of this step is to drain stagnant blood from the feet and lower legs, so feet should remain elevated until blanching occurs.
2. Sit in a chair or on the edge of the bed and repeat alternating flexion and extension of the feet, first with the feet in a normal position, then with the feet everted, and finally with the feet inverted. Each position should be held for 30 seconds. By this time the feet should be very pink, indicating that circulation has improved.
3. Conclude the exercise by lying flat in a supine position for 3 to 5 minutes. The entire set may then be repeated three to six times.

If at any time during the exercises the legs or feet become blue and painful, clients should lie down immediately with the feet elevated as in step 1 for as long as necessary to reverse the symptoms. These exercises usually are done three to four times a day.

Positioning. Positioning to promote circulation and avoid pressure on bony prominences is important for all clients whose mobility is limited. It is particularly important for clients with oxygenation problems.

When the client is lying in the lateral position in bed, support the nondependent leg on pillows so that it does not put pressure on the dependent leg and compromise circulation in both legs. Frequent repositioning will also help combat venous stasis. The client's hands should be supported so that they are at or above heart level. When a person with compromised circulation lies in bed for a prolonged period with the hands even slightly dependent, the hands can swell significantly. Placing the hands on pillows can prevent this. Refer to Chapter 30 for more information about positioning clients.

External Cardiac Compression. External cardiac compression, discussed above, is an emergency method to support circulation when the cardiac function has ceased. The steps of basic life support (CPR) as outlined in Procedures 27–9 and 27–10 should be closely followed, including verification that CPR is necessary.

Monitoring. Monitoring clients for adequacy and changes in oxygenation is part of restorative care. Several methods are used to monitor oxygenation status. These include vital signs and other special measurements such as arterial blood gases, central venous pressure (CVP), and pulmonary artery monitoring.

Vital Signs. Vital signs, specifically pulse and blood pressure, are important indicators of both circulatory status and the effectiveness of the pumping action of the heart.

(Text continues on page 1311.)

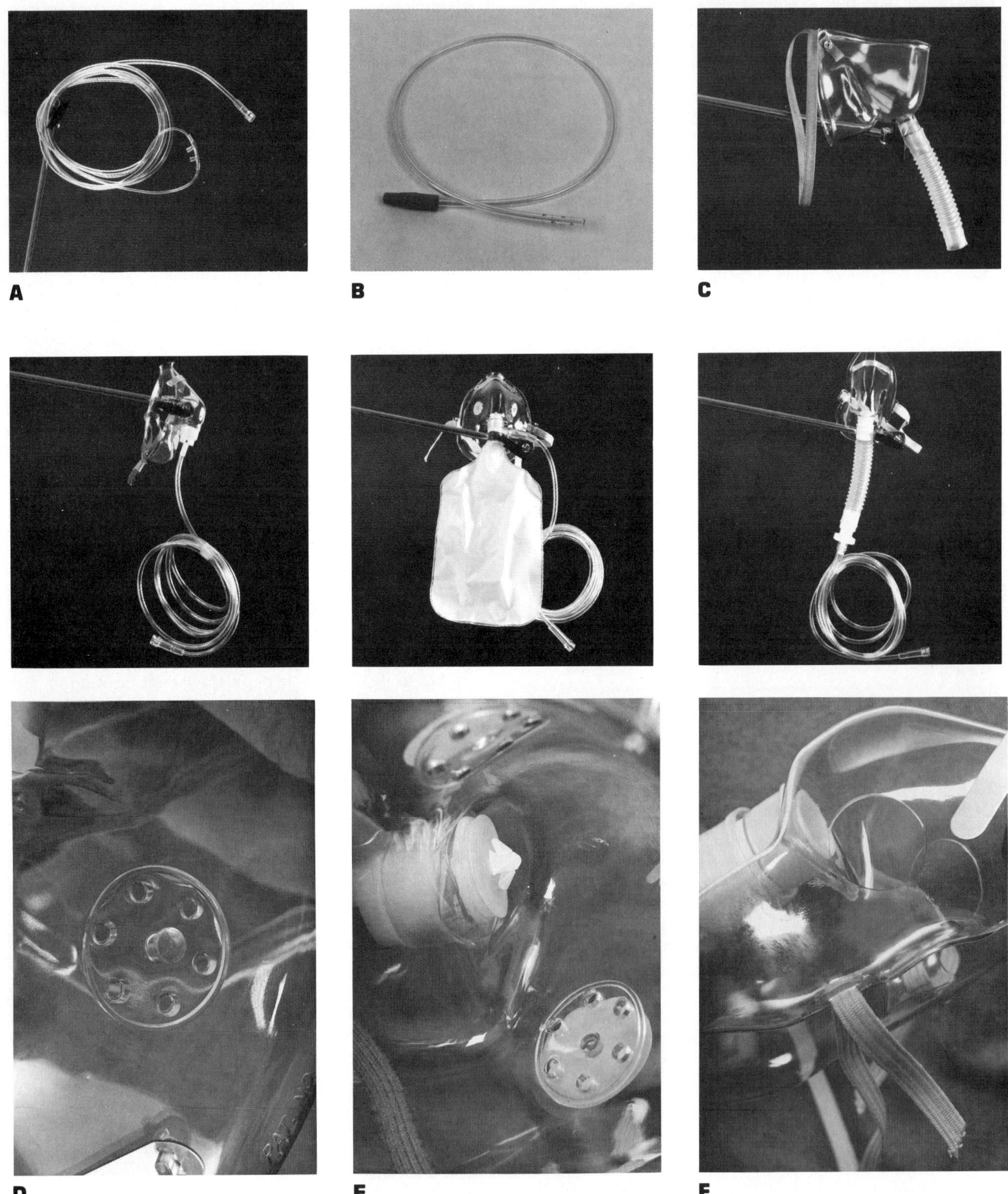

Figure 27–18. Oxygen-delivery devices. **A.** Nasal prongs. **B.** Nasal catheter. **C.** Face tent. **D.** Simple mask. **E.** Rebreather bag (inside view). **F.** Venturi mask. (*Top illustrations from Smith S, Duell D.* Clinical Nursing Skills: Nursing Process Model, Basic to Advanced. *3rd ed. Norwalk, CT: Appleton & Lange; 1992.*)

PROCEDURE 27–13. ADMINISTERING OXYGEN VIA NASAL CANNULA, FACE TENT, OR VARIOUS MASKS

PURPOSE: To maintain optimum oxygenation status in clients unable to maintain sufficient oxygen concentration when breathing room air, thereby decreasing the work of respiration and improving oxygenation of body tissues.

EQUIPMENT: Oxygen source; flowmeter; humidifier; oxygen tubing to be used with the specified device; oxygen delivery device specified in medical order; and "No Smoking, Oxygen in Use" signs.

ACTION	RATIONALE
1. Check the medical order for specific delivery device and oxygen flowrate or percent. Discuss the procedure and its expected benefits with the client.	1. Active participation is more likely if the client understands the expected behaviors and anticipated benefits.
2. Obtain baseline data regarding client's oxygenation status: level of consciousness; vital signs (BP, P, R); airway patency; color; activity tolerance; respiratory pattern.	2. Provides basis for evaluating effectiveness of oxygen therapy.
3. Check to see that the control on the flowmeter is in the "off" position. Then push the flowmeter into the wall outlet, exerting very firm pressure.	3. If the flowmeter control is in the "on" position, oxygen will escape when the flowmeter is attached to the wall outlet. Firm pressure is needed to secure the flowmeter.

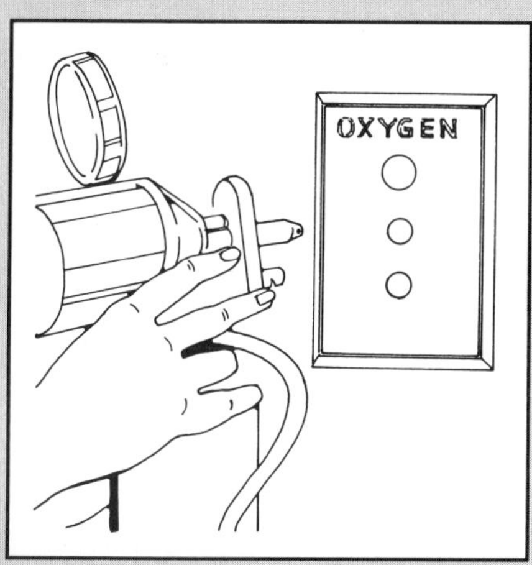

ACTION	RATIONALE
4. Attach the humidifier to the flowmeter if this is institutional policy (see Procedure 27–14). Some institutions do not humidify oxygen at low flowrates.	4. Unhumidified air often causes mucous membranes to dry out and sputum to become thick and tenacious.
5. Securely attach one end of connecting tubing to nipple on humidifier, the other to the oxygen-delivery device.	5. Provides a continuous leakfree system for oxygen delivery.
6. Set flowmeter at ordered flowrate. Caution client and others not to adjust the flowmeter under any circumstances.	6. Oxygen is prescribed specific to client condition. Rates higher or lower than ordered could result in danger to the client.

NOTE: Decreasing oxygen flow will deliver insufficient oxygen to maintain desired blood oxygen concentration (Po_2). Increasing flowrate could cause respiratory arrest in clients with a hypoxemic breathing drive.

(continued)

PROCEDURE 27–13. (continued)

7. Observe for bubbling in the humidifier as oxygen flows through the water.

7. If no bubbles appear, no oxygen is flowing through the humidifier nor is it being supplied to the client.

8. Place the oxygen delivery device on the client as follows:

SKILL A: Nasal Prongs (Cannula)

1. Position the prongs so they curve toward the nares, then place tubing over client's ears and under the chin. Adjust the tubing comfortably so oxygen is directed upward into nose, then pull up on slide until tubing is comfortably snug. Pad the tubing over the ears with gauze, if desired. Some models are secured by an elastic headband instead of a chinstrap.

1. If the prongs are not properly positioned, the oxygen flow may be blocked. If device is too snug, client may remove it, or it may cause pressure sores on the face or ears.

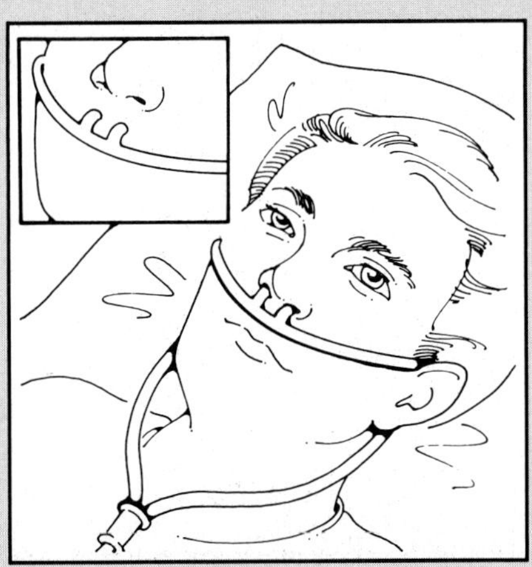

2. Instruct client to breathe in the pattern that is most comfortable.

2. Mouth breathing is acceptable and still produces adequate bodily oxygenation because oxygen is heavier than air and tends to go down into lungs along with air inhaled through the mouth.

3. Check the prongs at least q shift for occlusion by mucus and irritation of nares. Check frequently for correct prong placement.

3. Mucus will impede oxygen flow. Irritation from prongs may stimulate mucus production. The prongs tend to be displaced easily.

NOTE: Water-soluble lubricant may be used to reduce irritation, but petroleum-based products are contraindicated because they support combustion.

(continued)

PROCEDURE 27–13. (continued)

SKILL B: Simple, Partial Rebreather, or Nonrebreather Mask

1. Place mask so it covers client's nose and mouth. Adjust the elastic strap and the nose clip so mask fits snugly. Apply padding if strap irritates client's ears.

1. To deliver maximum oxygen, the mask must be sufficiently snug so that oxygen cannot escape at edges of mask.

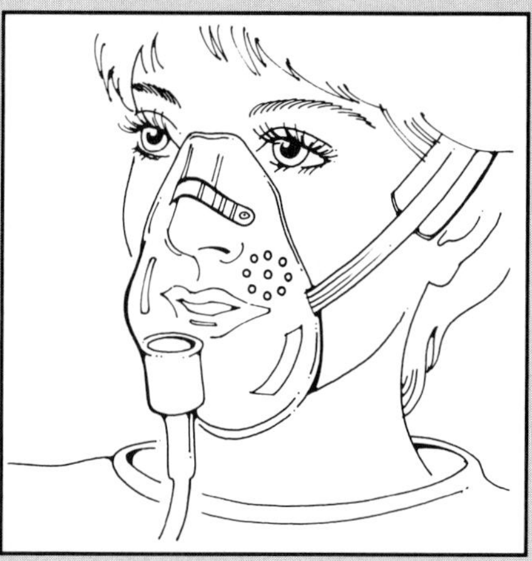

2. Observe for correct functioning of partial rebreather and nonrebreather masks as follows:
   a. *Partial rebreather:* Reservoir should fill on exhalation, and nearly collapse on inspiration.
   b. *Nonrebreather:* No change in reservoir on exhalation; slight deflation on inspiration.

2a. If the reservoir on a partial rebreather mask does not fill on exhalation, air is escaping via another route and the rebreather function is not operating.
 b. No exhaled air should flow into the reservoir of a nonrebreather mask, so the bag inflation should not change on exhalation. If the reservoir on either mask collapses on inspiration, flowrate is too low. A collapsed reservoir indicates no oxygen is flowing into mask.

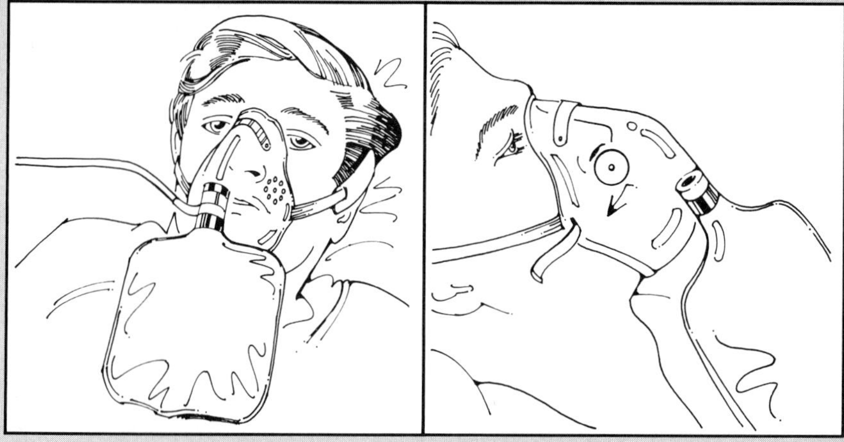

3. Stay with client until he or she adjusts to the sensation of breathing with mask on face.

3. Some clients feel claustrophobic with mask on until hypoxia is relieved and even afterward.

4. Check skin under mask several times per shift for signs of pressure or excessive moisture. Sputum may collect on the inside of the mask. Adjust, clean, and dry mask as necessary.

4. Moisture from condensation and perspiration collects under mask. It may cause irritation and/or skin breakdown and discomfort. Oral mucosa may become dry if client is mouth breathing.

(continued)

SKILL C: Venturi Mask

1. Set dial on mask or select the jet adapter that delivers the percent of oxygen specified in the medical order. Connect it to the distal end of the wide-bore tubing attached to the mask.

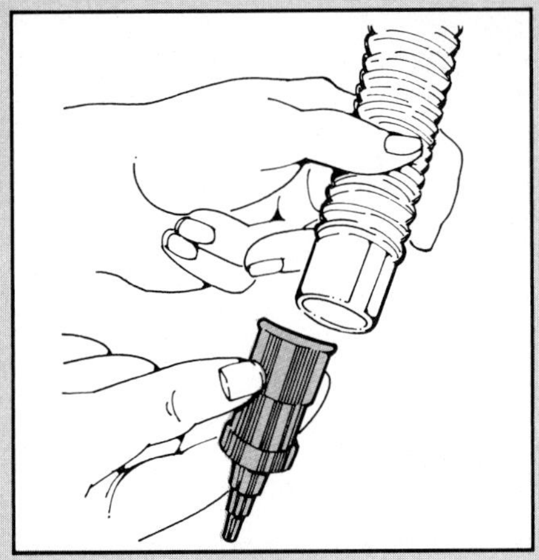

1. The jet adapter restricts the flow of oxygen so it mixes with air to deliver precise concentration of oxygen. Respiratory rate does not change the flowrate. A Venturi mask is used when precise oxygen concentrations are necessary.

2. Attach the humidity adapter (clear plastic sleeve) to the jet adapter to prevent blocking of the entrainment ports. Then attach the connecting tubing from the oxygen source to the jet adapter.

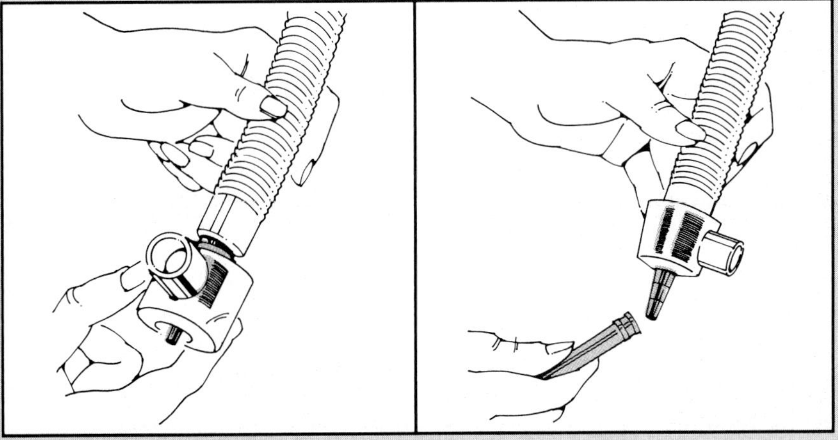

2. If the mask's ports are blocked (eg, by bed linen), room air will not flow into the ports and higher concentrations of oxygen will be delivered.

3. Use wide-bore tubing to attach a humidifying device to this sleeve if oxygen concentration of 30 percent or greater is ordered.

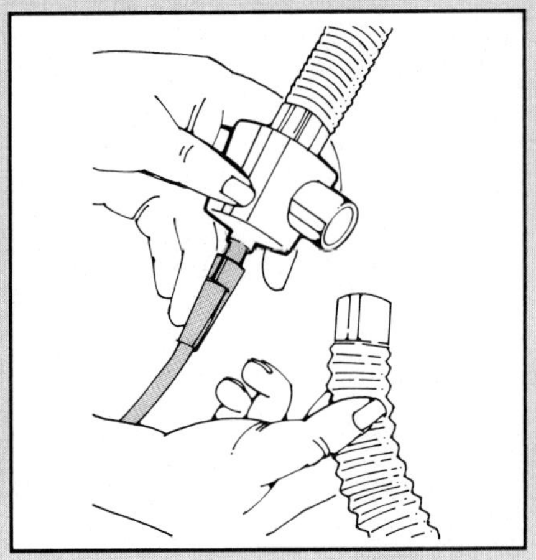

3. At flowrates required for delivery of these oxygen concentrations, significant drying of mucosa occurs.

(continued)

4. Apply mask as described above. Continue with other steps as for other masks.

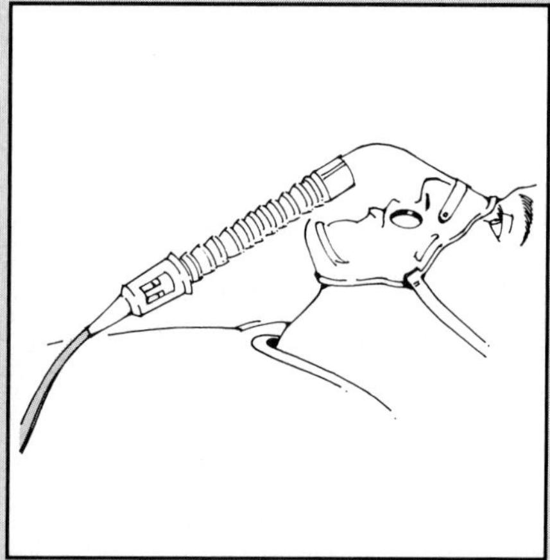

5. Check wide-bore tubing for condensation several times per shift. If present, separate tubing from humidity adapter and drain liquid into a container for disposal. Take care to prevent backflow of the liquid into the humidifier reservoir.

5. Velocity of gas in wide-bore tubing is slower, hence moisture supplied by humidifier condenses. It is a potential source of contamination, so must be removed. If liquid is left in wide-bore tube, it impedes oxygen flow.

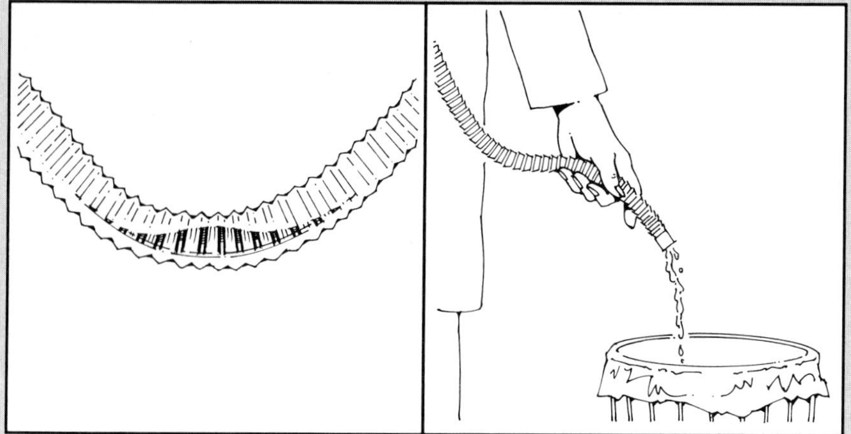

SKILL D: Face Tent

1. Apply the tent so it fits under chin and sweeps around face. Secure the strap behind head to keep the device in place. It does not fit snugly over nose and cheeks.

1. A face tent is used to deliver aerosolized gas for treatment of thick secretions. It is also better tolerated by clients who find conventional masks cause a feeling of claustrophobia.

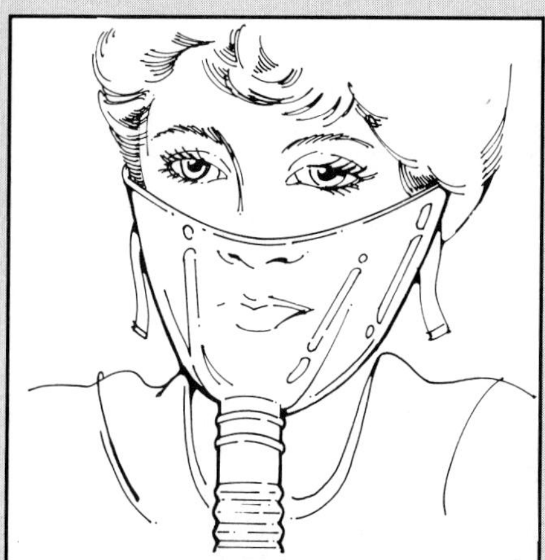

(continued)

PROCEDURE 27–13. (continued)

2. Use wide-bore tubing to connect face tent to humidifying device. An adapter may be needed.

   2. Wide-bore tubing transmits highly humidified gas more effectively.

3. Check for presence of mist inside face tent.

   3. Mist indicates humidified gas is being delivered.

4. Assess skin under tent, provide skin and mouth care, and clean mask as for conventional masks.

   4. Excess moisture could cause discomfort or skin irritation. Mucus from coughing could build up inside mask.

5. Check wide-bore tubing for condensation, and dispose of as described for Venturi mask; Skill C, step 5, above.

   5. See Skill C, step 5, above.

For All Devices:

A. Instruct client to keep the delivery device in place at all times and to call for assistance if problems occur.

   A. Interruption of oxygen therapy may result in decreased Po_2, and deterioration of condition.

NOTE: Clients receiving oxygen via mask or face tent should use nasal prongs while eating so no interruption of therapy occurs.

B. Discuss safety precautions outlined in Box 27–10. Discuss with client and significant others.

   B. Oxygen supports combustion so any situation that could create sparks must be prevented.

C. Instruct client to notify nurse if dyspnea, dizziness, or shortness of breath occurs.

   C. These symptoms suggest insufficient oxygen.

NOTE: Physician should be notified if respiratory problems occur so oxygen therapy prescription can be reevaluated.

D. If client is ambulatory, be sure connecting tubing is long enough to allow movement about the room without disconnecting oxygen. Proximal end of oxygen tubing can be secured to the client's clothing with a rubber band and safety pin to reduce pulling on prongs or mask when client moves.

   D. If movement is restricted by tubing that is too short, client may remove device while walking to bathroom or moving about the room.

E. Ask ambulatory client to obtain assistance to ambulate outside the room.

   E. A portable oxygen source must be used for ambulation outside the room (Procedure 27–12).

F. Post signs indicating that oxygen is in use on door to client's room and at bedside.

   F. Alerts visitors of necessary precautions.

G. Assess client's oxygenation status as described above.

   G. Determines effectiveness of oxygen therapy. Frequency of assessment is determined by client condition.

RECORDING: Note assessment findings, mode of oxygen delivery, flowrate, client's response to therapy, any adverse effects noted, and corresponding nursing action. This data should be recorded when oxygen therapy is initiated, and at least every shift thereafter.

PROCEDURE 27–14. USING A HUMIDIFIER FOR OXYGEN THERAPY

PURPOSE: To prevent drying of respiratory mucosa with high-liter-flow oxygen delivery.

EQUIPMENT: Disposable or reusable humidifier, adapter to connect to oxygen source.

ACTION

1. Discuss the procedure and expected benefits with the client. Assure client that interruption in oxygen flow will be temporary.
2. Attach the adapter to the top of the humidifier bottle to secure humidifier to oxygen flowmeter. Adapter is usually packaged with disposable humidifier.

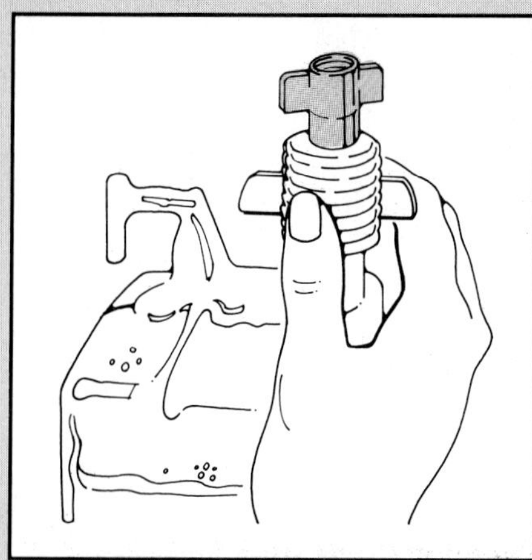

3. Snap off seal from outlet port of prefilled disposable humidifier. Reusable units will be enclosed in sterile wrap, but must be filled before use.
4. Attach humidifier to flowmeter by turning the adapter in a clockwise direction until it is tight. If not securely attached, oxygen could leak at connection and cause a fire hazard.

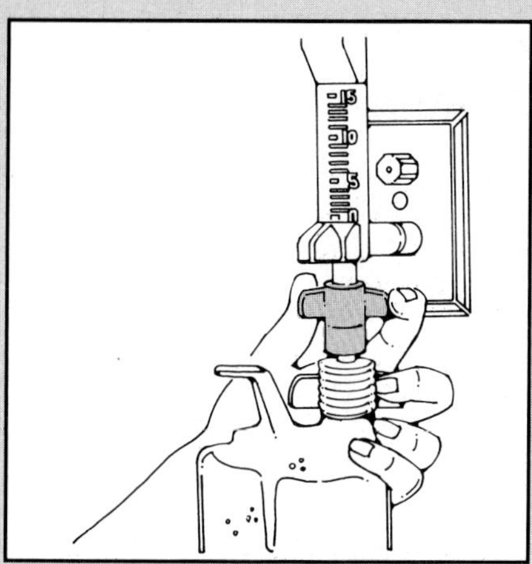

5. Attach the small-bore oxygen tubing connected to the oxygen delivery device to the outlet port of the humidifer.

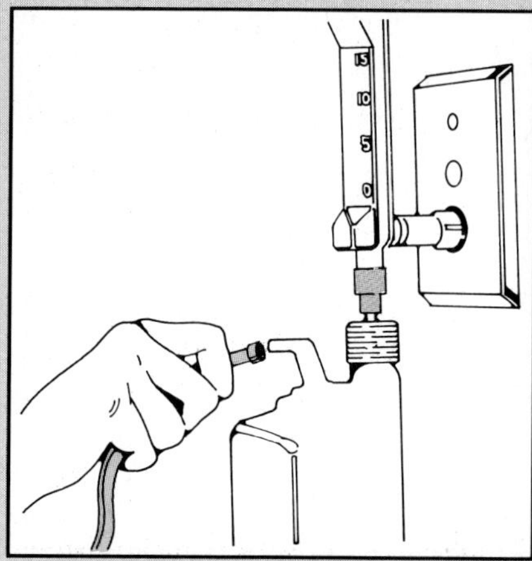

6. Adjust the flowmeter to the ordered flowrate and observe for bubbles as oxygen flows through the water in the humidifier. If there are no bubbles, no oxygen is flowing. Obtain assistance from respiratory therapist if flow cannot be initiated.
7. If delivery device is not already in place, apply to client (Procedure 27–13) and complete assessment of client's response to oxygen therapy.

RECORDING: In most health care facilities, humidification is routinely included when oxygen is delivered at flowrates above 4 L/min, so no specific entry related to humidifier is needed. If humidifier was added to a system at low flowrate, document reason for addition in client's progress notes. It may also be useful to post a sign for respiratory therapist that client needs humidifier, despite usual policy, and note same in the Kardex.

PROCEDURE 27–15. USING ANTI-EMBOLISM STOCKINGS (THROMBO-EMBOLI DETERRENT OR TED HOSE)

PURPOSE: To enhance venous return, thereby improving peripheral circulation, minimizing orthostatic hypotension, and reducing the risk of clot formation. Indicated for postoperative clients or clients who are immobilized.

EQUIPMENT: Stockings, tape measure.

ACTION	RATIONALE
1a. Be sure there is a valid medical order for hose. b. Discuss the procedure and its expected benefits with the client.	1a. Anti-embolism stockings require a physician's order b. Active participation is more likely if the client understands the expected behaviors and anticipated benefits.
2. Assess the circulation in the client's legs by: a. Palpating posterior tibial and dorsalis pedis pulse, rhythm, and volume. b. Noting signs of arterial insufficiency (skin cool, shiny, taut, pale), or venous insufficiency (ankle pigmentation, thickened skin, pitting edema). c. Observing for positive Homans' sign (calf pain on ankle dorsiflexion). d. Noting varicosities (distended leg veins when supine).	2. This assessment establishes a baseline against which to compare assessment data on circulation status obtained in periodic checks when stockings are in use.

NOTE: If previously unreported circulatory deficits or new skin lesions are detected, consult the physician before applying hose.

ACTION	RATIONALE
3. Measure the client's legs as follows: *For knee-high hose:* Midcalf circumference, heel to popliteal space.	3. Stockings must fit properly to achieve therapeutic effect. If they are too large, they will not provide adequate support. If they are too small, circulation may be impeded.

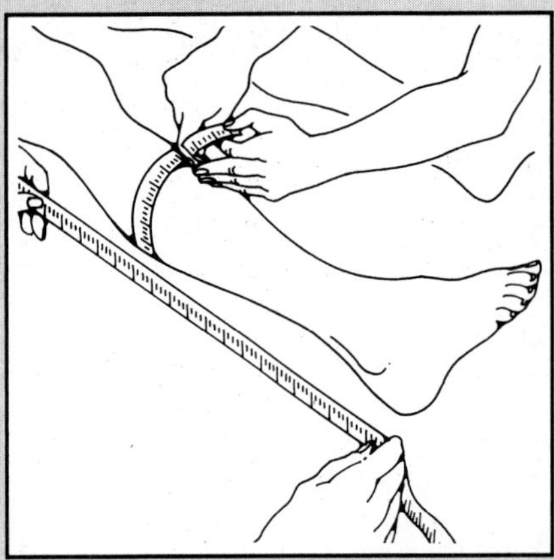

For thigh-high hose: Midcalf and midthigh circumferences, heel to gluteal fold.
Compare measurements to size chart to select correct size. Order two pairs.

NOTE: The best time to measure and apply hose is in the morning before client arises or after at least 1 hour of bedrest, to prevent dependent edema.

(continued)

4. Apply stockings:
   a. Turn leg portion of the stocking inside out over the foot portion by placing one hand into the stocking and holding the toe while inverting the stocking to its heel over your arm. The leg of the stocking should extend past the foot, rather than being bunched or rolled. The leg should be dry. Talcum powder may be applied sparingly to reduce irritation.

4a. Inverting, rather than rolling or bunching the stocking prevents constrictions in the stocking which would make its application difficult or even painful to the client.

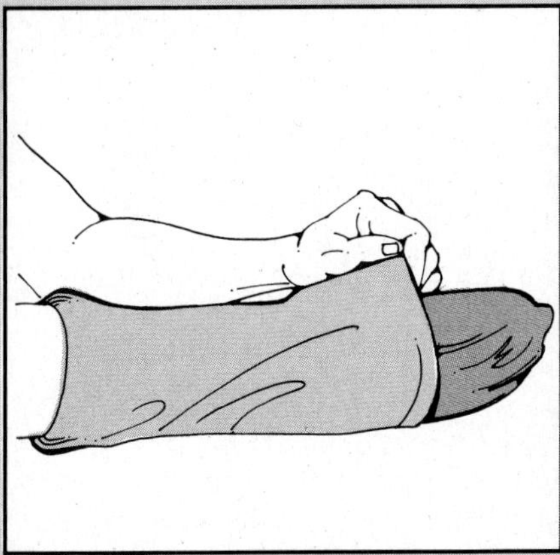

   b. Grasp each side of the stocking and slip it smoothly over the client's foot. The stocking should fit snugly without wrinkles or ripples.

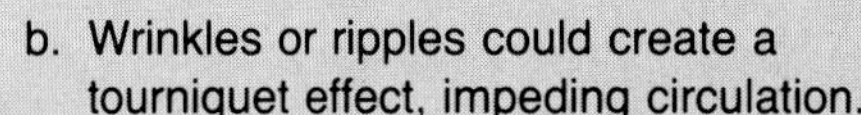

b. Wrinkles or ripples could create a tourniquet effect, impeding circulation.

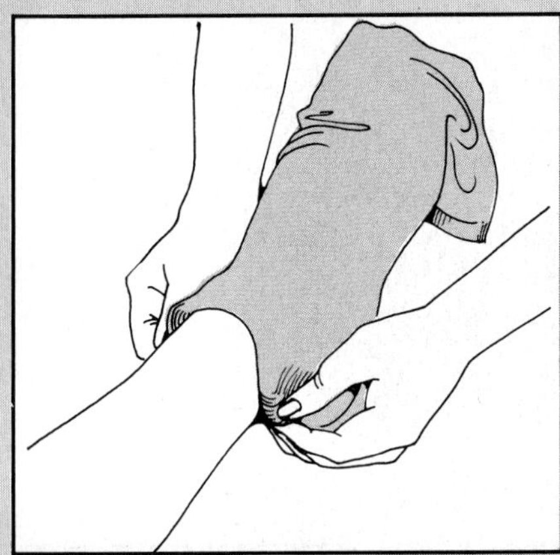

   c. Slide the remainder of the stocking up the client's leg, smoothing ripples if they develop.

c. See b, above.

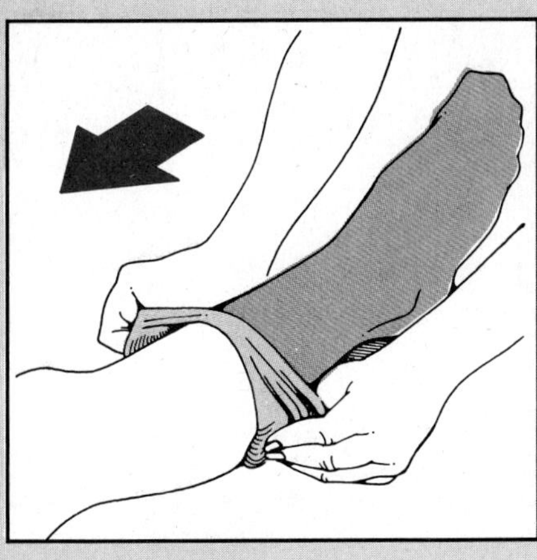

(continued)

PROCEDURE 27–15. (continued)

d. Check to see that the client's toes are covered, not extending out of the open area of the stocking, and that the stocking is correctly aligned for its entire length.

d. If the toes extend out of the opening, circulation may become constricted. The opening is provided for periodic assessment of the toes. (See action in step 6, below.)

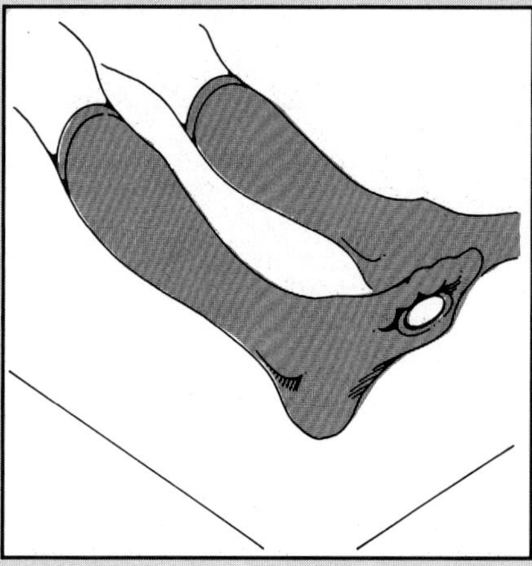

5. Repeat for second leg.

6. Discuss with the client how to assess for proper application, and ask client to notify the nurse to correct problems. Dangers of rolling stockings should be emphasized. Inspect the legs periodically to see that the stockings remain properly applied, that the legs above the stockings are not swollen, and that the toes remain warm and pink with good capillary refill.

6. Stockings may roll or twist as the client moves with resulting constricting areas.

7. Remove the stockings 30 minutes each shift, assess circulation, and provide skin care as needed.

7. Provides client comfort and opportunity for complete circulation assessment.

8. To remove stockings, grasp the top of the stocking on each side and pull it off. The stocking will be inside out. Avoid rolling to remove stocking.

8. Rolling or bunching even for a short time will cause constriction with resulting discomfort and temporary impairment of circulation.

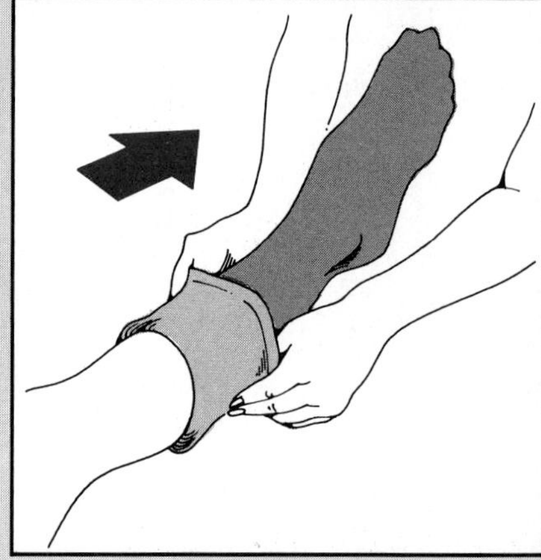

9. Launder hose about every 2–3 days in mild soap and water. Dry flat and away from direct heat. Use spare pair of hose during drying.

9. This care will prolong the life of the hose.

(continued)

PROCEDURE 27–15. (continued)

10. If signs of venous or arterial insufficiency or thrombophlebitis are noted, notify the client's primary nurse or physician.	10. These are complications that may require additional treatment.

RECORDING: Record the data and time of application of hose, the circulatory status, and the condition of the skin before application. When hose are removed, record skin and circulatory status and length of time hose remain off.

Respiratory rate and quality is an indicator of oxygen exchange. These measurements are discussed in detail in Chapter 16.

Special Measurements. The measurement of arterial blood gases (ABGs) can be an essential part of the assessment of oxygenation status. The tests that are included in the ABGs are: pH, Po_2, Pco_2, and HCO_3 (bicarbonate level). Sometimes base excess (a measurement of buffers in the bloodstream), oxygen saturation (how much oxygen the hemoglobin is carrying), and $CaPo_2$ (Pao_2 plus hemoglobin, which reflects total plasma oxygen concentration) are included. ABGs can help health care providers determine if there are disturbances of acid–base balance related to respiratory or metabolic function. (For further discussion of acid–base balance, refer to Chap. 31).

If ABGs are to be drawn, the client must be stabilized beforehand. The client should rest in bed without stimulation for about 30 minutes so that the metabolism will be at its lowest level before the gases are drawn. This is to allow comparison among successive readings. Once the metabolism is stabilized, a specially trained health care provider draws the blood sample via an arterial puncture. The nurse or person who drew the blood then applies firm pressure to the puncture site for 5 to 10 minutes to prevent the formation of a hematoma. Pressure is applied directly with the hand, not simply by placing a dressing on the site. An adhesive bandage or similar dressing is applied after the 5- to 10-minute period of pressure.

Hemodynamic monitoring such as central venous pressure and pulmonary artery pressure assessment also provide data about oxygenation. CVP reflects the pressure in the circulatory system as the blood is returned to the right atrium. One cause of a high CVP is ineffective pumping of the blood to the peripheral circulation, causing blood to back up into the right side of the heart. A low CVP may be caused by low blood volume. Either situation can compromise perfusion.

CVP is assessed using a glass manometer attached to an intravenous catheter. The intravenous catheter, often called a central line, goes from the subclavian vein to the right atrium. For an accurate reading the manometer must be held at heart level when a reading is taken. CVP is measured in centimeters of water (cm H_2O). The usual range is 5 to 10 cm H_2O. The central line insertion site requires a sterile occlusive dressing. Meticulous aseptic technique is required when the dressing is changed, because of the risk of introducing organisms into the subclavian vein and subsequently to the heart.

More sophisticated indicators of cardiac function and fluid load, such as pulmonary artery pressure (PAP) and pulmonary artery wedge pressure (PAWP), are often necessary for critically ill clients. These measurements directly reflect the functioning of the left side of the heart. They are done only in intensive care units and are addressed in advanced nursing courses.

Rehabilitative Care

Fourth-level client care focuses on rehabilitation. Clients with chronic lung disease can improve their quality of life and their well-being with an effective rehabilitation program; however, the use of the program and of standard therapy for the disease does not statistically prolong life.

Client Education. Client education plays a significant role in rehabilitative care (see also Chap. 20). The rehabilitation program for a client with a chronic oxygenation problem involves teaching about the problem and how to manage it.

Pathophysiological Process. A good place to begin is to describe normal physiology of the heart and lungs. Then, provide information about the pathophysiology of the client's condition; that is, how the client's lung or heart function is altered.

Medications. Many clients with chronic oxygenation dysfunction must take medications; teaching about prescribed

IMPLICATIONS FOR NURSE–CLIENT COLLABORATION

Education for Self-care

To assume self-responsibility, clients with long-term oxygenation problems need to learn to be alert to changes in their own physical status. Exchanges between nurse and client that focus on common subjective and objective manifestations of altered oxygenation can help prepare the client to take responsibility for health care decisions. Many times clients who are unprepared will ignore worsening symptoms that signal a deterioration in their condition. The nurse can make a significant contribution to the client's welfare by reviewing before discharge the critical factors for clients to monitor, once they return to their home setting.

medications is therefore essential. Clients should be taught the expected therapeutic effects, side effects, toxic effects, and pertinent information about medication administration. They should also know whether medications are to be taken with food or on an empty stomach. For example, bronchodilators can cause gastric irritation if they are taken on an empty stomach, so they should be taken with food. Clients must also be made aware of any specific combinations of food and drugs to be avoided. If a client has a cartridge inhaler for medications, he or she should know how to use it and how to clean the mouthpiece. Clients should be instructed not to use over-the-counter medications without consulting their physicians first.

Clients who are using oxygen at home must know why they are using it, when to use it, how much to use, and how to clean and care for the equipment. They must learn how to recognize when the oxygen supply is low. They must be encouraged to keep up usual activities while using oxygen and may also learn how to travel with oxygen. Clients should learn breathing techniques and exercises, as previously described.

Signs and Symptoms. Clients who have oxygenation problems should learn to be alert to changes in physical status so that they can contact the physician when such changes occur. Individuals with chronic conditions often ignore signs of increasing illness or are unaware of which symptoms to report. Pulmonary clients should be advised to notify the physician if the cough is worse, sputum is thicker and more difficult to cough up or a different color, or they are dyspneic or orthopneic. Both cardiac and pulmonary clients should monitor their weight at least three times a week and report any sudden weight gain, which may signal heart failure with fluid retention.

Changes in Daily Routines. The nurse should also discuss with the client changes in self-care or daily routines that may prevent further complications. For example, the importance of hydration must be taught to those with pulmonary problems. The client must know how much to drink and what types of fluids to drink. Most clients need at least 2000 mL of fluids per day. Milk and beverages containing caffeine or alcohol should be avoided or consumed only on a limited basis.

Measures to promote circulation can also be made part of daily routine. These are especially important for clients with chronically compromised circulation. The use of antithromboembolic stockings, as discussed under Restorative Care, is often continued into the rehabilitation phase of care. If a client has had or is at risk for thrombophlebitis, the legs should be inspected and the calves measured to see that they are of equal size (assuming that they were equal to begin with). Ask clients to report any change in size, redness, heat, or discomfort to their physician. A positive Homans' sign (pain in the calf when flexing the foot) may be a sign of thrombophlebitis and should also be reported.

There are several cautions that a client with compromised circulation can use when sitting or standing. People with vascular compromise should not sit with the legs crossed at the knees or stand in one position for long periods of time. Sitting with legs crossed at the ankles is acceptable. Sitting with the legs elevated on a footstool is better than allowing the legs to be dependent. Whenever extended periods of sitting are necessary, walking around for about 5 minutes each hour will help combat venous stasis.

BUILDING NURSING KNOWLEDGE

How Can Nurses Help Clients With Oxygenation Problems Make Necessary Life-style Changes?

Comoss PM. Nursing strategies to improve compliance with life-style changes in a cardiac rehabilitation population. *Cardiovasc Nurs.* 1988;2:23–36.

Rehabilitating clients with heart disease requires a complex regimen of physical and psychosocial life changes involving diet, exercise, regular medication, habit changes, and even new ways of handling stress. How to motivate clients to make the needed changes is the question that Comoss addresses in this article.

Comoss reports that studies comparing clients who complete cardiac rehabilitation programs with those who drop out show important differences between groups. Those who drop out have five times more fatal and nonfatal recurrences of their disease; however, half of those clients who start a program never finish. Dropout rates are low in the first 3 months, but increase dramatically after 6 months and average around 50 percent. One study reviewed by Comoss showed that the best adherence was to nonsmoking (74 percent), followed by low-cholesterol diet (58 percent) and exercise (43 percent), while the least was to stress management (35 percent).

Personal characteristics associated with a greater likelihood of dropping out included continued smoking, overweight, a preference for inactive leisure pursuits, lack of support from the spouse, low self-motivation, depression, anxiety, and an introverted personality.

Approaches to improve motivation include giving incentives to remain in the program. Barriers to participation such as transportation, distance, and schedule are minimized. Small-group programs are more successful because the social relationships that develop among program participants provide incentives and foster peer support. The ultimate goal is ongoing self-regulation. Clients do better if they examine their rationale for continuing new behavior and if they are involved in selecting their own learning priorities such as choosing when, where, and how to exercise, or deciding what to eat to maintain a low-fat, low-cholesterol diet. Commitment is reinforced by having clients write down the benefits and costs of continuing and by establishing written behavior contracts. Throughout cardiac rehabilitation, nurses have an important role to play as client motivators.

Assisting With Life-style Modification. Clients need information about modifiable risk factors. They need assistance and encouragement in modifying these risk factors as well as education about dietary modifications and other life-style modifications.

Quitting Smoking. If a client still smokes, teaching should be directed at why smoking is harmful and providing encouragement and support to stop smoking. See also Discouraging Smoking in the Preventive Care section earlier in the chapter.

Graded Aerobic Exercise Programs. Individually tailored exercise programs are important for people who have oxygenation problems. Graded aerobic exercise improves circulation and reduces the oxygen need per unit of work that a muscle does. A person with oxygenation problems who exercises appropriately will be able to accomplish more activities and have a better quality of life than one who does not exercise. Exercise is usually prescribed by the physician or multidisciplinary health care team. Often, in the early stages of rehabilitation, clients are asked to exercise in a setting where their activity can be closely observed and the heart and blood oxygen levels monitored during exercise. Clients with obstructive lung disease should use pursed-lip breathing while exercising and should use oxygen if it has been prescribed. Teach these clients how to decide if they need to rest during exercise, and give helpful tips for resting positions.

Isometric exercises should generally be avoided by those with oxygenation problems. These exercises—which include activities like weight lifting and using many of the machines at traditional exercise studios—increase the cardiac workload, promote the use of the Valsalva maneuver, and cause reflex hypertension. The physician should usually be consulted even about mild isometrics such as quadriceps setting, as most clients hold their breath during such exercises and they tend to increase blood pressure.

Energy Conservation Techniques. Energy conservation techniques can be helpful for the person with compromised oxygenation. The client should do as many tasks as possible while sitting down. For example, the client could assemble all items needed for food preparation and then sit to prepare the food. At the grocery store, the client should ask that groceries be divided into several lightweight bags. The use of a long-handled dustpan will enable the client to sweep floors without bending over. Long-handled tongs can be used to retrieve items from hard-to-reach shelves (Fig. 27–19). Men can sit rather than stand while shaving. Many men habitually hold their breath while shaving with a razor. Using pursed-lip breathing techniques during shaving will eliminate the shortness of breath problems related to this. The client can sit during a shower. Nurses and clients can collaborate to discover safe and effective methods to minimize the client's energy expenditures.

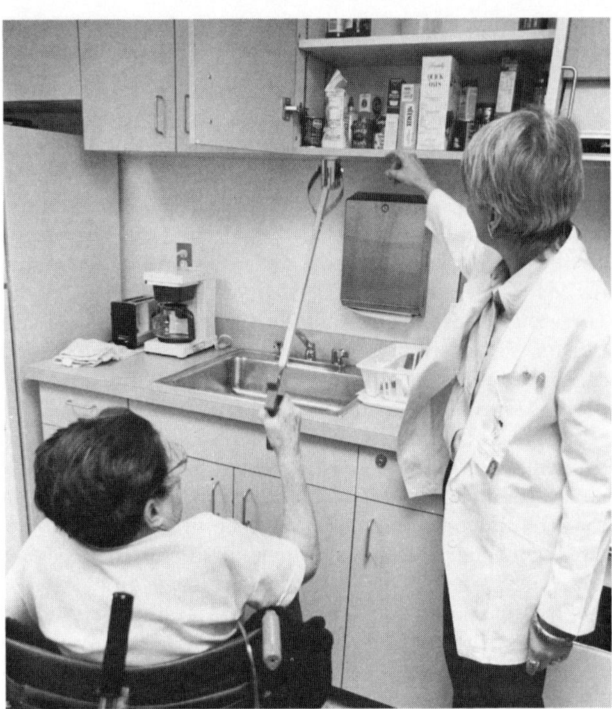

Figure 27–19. Long-handled tongs.

Counseling and Emotional Support. The life-style changes required to maintain adequate oxygenation may be difficult for clients to make. Often, they involve restrictions on recreational activities and activities of daily living. Sometimes occupational changes are also required. Often clients' independence is compromised.

Adaptation to these changes may be stressful and may cause economic hardship. Health care providers may inadvertently add to clients' stress by implying that modifications are easy to accomplish. In fact, the effects of the oxygenation problem itself and the reorganization in life-style that it demands are usually quite complex. Clients need empathy and support from health care providers and significant others. Many clients benefit from professional counseling to help them explore the implications of the oxygenation problem and associated life-style modifications. Counseling can help a client accept the condition, decide which life-style changes are possible, and make a commitment to accomplish them.

■ EVALUATION

When the nurse and client have stated precise, measurable outcomes or specific evaluation criteria in the planning phase of care, both ongoing and terminal evaluation are straightforward. To evaluate accomplishment of the outcomes, the nurse and client look for evidence that the criteria identified were attained. An example of a specific measurable outcome for a client who has altered ventilation due to a postoperative atelectasis might be that within 3 days, the client's lungs will be free of secretions, as evidenced by absence of adventitious breath sounds and regular, unlabored respirations at about 20 per minute. To evaluate, the nurse would auscultate the client's lungs and assess respirations regularly, informing the client if the lung sounds seemed to be improving. Thus, ongoing evaluations can be an incentive for the client to participate in activities that will promote progress toward the agreed-upon outcomes.

Another possible outcome might be that the client will be able to use the incentive spirometer effectively to a specified volume. The nurse can teach the client the technique and both can observe at intervals to see if the desired volume is being achieved. If the client has not achieved the desired volume on the specified date, the possible reasons can be examined and the desired outcome or technique revised as necessary. Perhaps on further discussion the nurse finds that the client modified the technique because of pain. The client may need more teaching about how to use the spirometer without causing incisional pain. Additional pain relief measures may also be needed. The date set might have been too soon. In this case, the same implementations might be continued but a new date for evaluation would be chosen. If the client is using the technique correctly, the outcome may have been unrealistic.

Evaluation is essential if the nurse and client are to know what outcomes have been achieved and whether modifications are necessary. As these examples indicate, the nursing process is circular. Once evaluation is done, the decision about whether to continue implementations or to change them can be made.

SUMMARY

Competent nursing care can make a difference to clients with oxygenation problems. Working collaboratively, nurses and clients can greatly improve the quality of the client's life. An understanding of the physiology of healthy oxygenation, including the functioning of the heart, lungs, and blood vessels, is required to ensure competent and knowledgable nursing care of oxygenation problems. Ventilation, diffusion, perfusion, and cellular respiration mechanisms in oxygenation are essential for optimum health.

Factors that affect oxygenation include developmental stage, general health and life-style, and environment. Alterations in oxygenation may involve ventilation, diffusion, perfusion, or cellular respiration and may result in hypoxia, hypercapnia, hypocapnia, and tissue necrosis.

Nurses can assess body oxygenation by examining the functioning of various body systems. The oxygenation history and physical examination includes the integument, chest and cardiovascular systems, abdomen, and mental status as they relate to oxygenation, as well as selected diagnostic and laboratory tests. Nursing diagnoses for clients with oxygenation problems include Ineffective Airway Clearance, Ineffective Breathing Pattern, and Altered Tissue Perfusion.

Nurse–client management of oxygenation problems—including planning, nursing implementation, and evaluation—assists clients to maintain or regain optimal functioning. Nursing implementation addresses four levels of care: preventive, supportive, restorative, and rehabilitative. Oxygenation is a fundamental life process. When oxygenation is compromised, many other functional dimensions are threatened as well. Therefore, client care to improve and maintain optimal oxygenation contributes significantly to clients' well-being.

REFERENCES

1. American Lung Association. *Statistical Update on Lung Disease—March 1991.* New York: American Lung Association; 1991.
2. American Heart Association. *1991 Heart and Stroke Facts.* Dallas: American Heart Association; 1991.
3. Bullock BL, Rosendahl PP. *Pathophysiology: Adaptations and Alterations in Function.* 2nd ed. Boston: Scott, Foresman; 1988.
4. West JB. *Pulmonary Pathophysiology: The Essentials.* 3rd ed. Baltimore: Williams & Wilkins; 1987.
5. Ganong WF. *Review of Medical Physiology.* 15th ed. Norwalk, CT: Appleton & Lange; 1991.
6. Slonim NB, Hamilton LH. *Respiratory Physiology.* 5th ed. St Louis: Mosby; 1987.
7. Des Jardins TR. *Cardiopulmonary Anatomy and Physiology: Essentials for Respiratory Care.* Albany: Delmar; 1988.
8. Williams SR. *Essentials of Nutrition and Diet Therapy.* St Louis: Mosby; 1990.
9. McHenry LD, Salerno E. *Pharmacology in Nursing.* St Louis: Mosby; 1989.
10. Sherwen LN, Scoloveno MA, Weingarten CT. *Nursing Care of the Childbearing Family.* Norwalk, CT: Appleton & Lange; 1991.
11. Avery ME, First L, eds. *Pediatric Medicine.* Baltimore: Williams & Wilkins; 1989.
12. Foster RLR, et al. *Family-centered Nursing Care of Children.* Philadelphia: Saunders; 1989.
13. US Department of Health and Human Services. *Reducing the Health Consequences of Smoking: 25 Years of Progress.* DHEW pub no. 623-880; 1989.
14. US Department of Health and Human Services. Public Health Service, Centers for Disease Control, Center for Chronic Disease and Health Promotion, Office of Smoking and Health. *The Health Benefits of Smoking Cessation.* DHHS pub no. 90-8416; 1990.
15. Centers for Disease Control. Smoking-attributable mortality and years of potential life lost—United States, 1988. *MMWR.* 1991;40:4.
16. McNaull RW. Tobaccoism in America. *Am J Nurs.* 1987;11:1430–1433.
17. West JB. *Pulmonary Pathophysiology—The Essentials.* Baltimore: Williams & Wilkins; 1987.
18. Osterud H. *Dealing with the Nicotine Addiction.* Portland: Oregon Health Sciences University; 1989.
19. American Lung Association. *Breath in Danger.* New York: American Lung Association; 1989.
20. Hall CB. Respiratory syncitial virus. In: Mandell GL, Douglas RG Jr, Bennett JE, eds. *Principles and Practices of Infectious Diseases.* New York: Wiley; 1989:489–493.
21. Chatburn RL, Primana RP Jr. A rational basis for humidity therapy. *Resp Care.* 1987;32:249.

BIBLIOGRAPHY

American Red Cross. *Cardiopulmonary Resuscitation.* Berkeley, CA: American Red Cross; 1987.

Anderson S. ABGs: Six easy steps to interpreting blood gases. *Am J Nurs.* 1990;90:42–46.

Beller LC, Neunaber KL. The "simple" Valsalva maneuver. *Am J Nurs.* 1986;86:398–399.

Canobbio MM. *Cardiovascular Disorders.* St. Louis: Mosby; 1991.

Casewit CW. *The Stop Smoking Book for Teens.* New York: Messner; 1980.

Dennison RD. Understanding the four determinants of cardiac output. *Nursing 90.* 1990;20:34–42.

Ehrhardt BS, Graham M. Pulse oximetry: An easy way to look at oxygen saturation. *Nursing 90.* 1990;20:50–54.

Fishbach F. *A Manual of Laboratory Diagnostic Tests.* Philadelphia: JB Lippincott; 1988.

Folta A, Metzger BL. Exercise and functional capacity after myocardial infarction. *Image.* 1989;21:215–219.

Gershwin ME, Klingelhofer EL. *Asthma: Stop Suffering, Start Living.* Reading, MA: Addison-Wesley; 1986.

Grandstrom D, Wierzbicki LA. A better way to deliver long-term oxygen therapy. *RN.* 1989;52:58.

Harrington G. *The Asthma Self-care Book.* New York: HarperCollins; 1991.

Hoffman LA, Wesmiller SW. Home oxygen—transtracheal and other options. *Am J Nurs.* 1988;88:464–471.

Hogshead N, Couzens GS. *Asthma and Exercise.* New York: Holt; 1991.

Kee JL. *Laboratory and Diagnostic Tests with Nursing Implications.* Norwalk, CT: Appleton & Lange; 1988.

McMahon A, Maibusch RM. How to send quit-smoking signals. *Am J Nurs.* 1988;88:1498–1499.

Mims BC. Interpreting ABGs. *RN.* 1991; 42.

Miracle VA, Allnutt DR. How to perform basic airway management. *Nursing 90.* 1990;20:55–60.

Morrissey MJ, Baldwin J. Exercise and chronic heart disease? *Geriatric Nurs.* 1987;8:138–140.

Openbrier DR, Fuoss C, Mall CC. What patients on home oxygen therapy want to know. *Am J Nurs.* 1988;88:198–201.

Openbrier DR, Hoffman LA, Wesmiller SW. Home oxygen therapy: Evaluation and prescription. *Am J Nurs.* 1988;88:192–197.

Patrick ML, Woods SL, Craven RF, et al. *Medical-Surgical Nursing.* Philadelphia: JB Lippincott; 1991.

Rogers J. *You Can Stop.* New York: Simon & Schuster; 1977; Pocket Books revision, 1986.

Sergi NA. When your patient needs a stress test. *RN.* 1991;vol 54:26–31.

Treseler KM. *Clinical Laboratory and Diagnostic Tests.* Norwalk, CT: Appleton & Lange; 1988.

Weinstein AM. *Asthma: The Complete Guide to Self-Management.* New York: McGraw-Hill; 1987.

Wilson SF, Thompson JM. *Respiratory Disorders.* St Louis: Mosby; 1990.

CHAPTER 28

Sleep–Rest Patterns

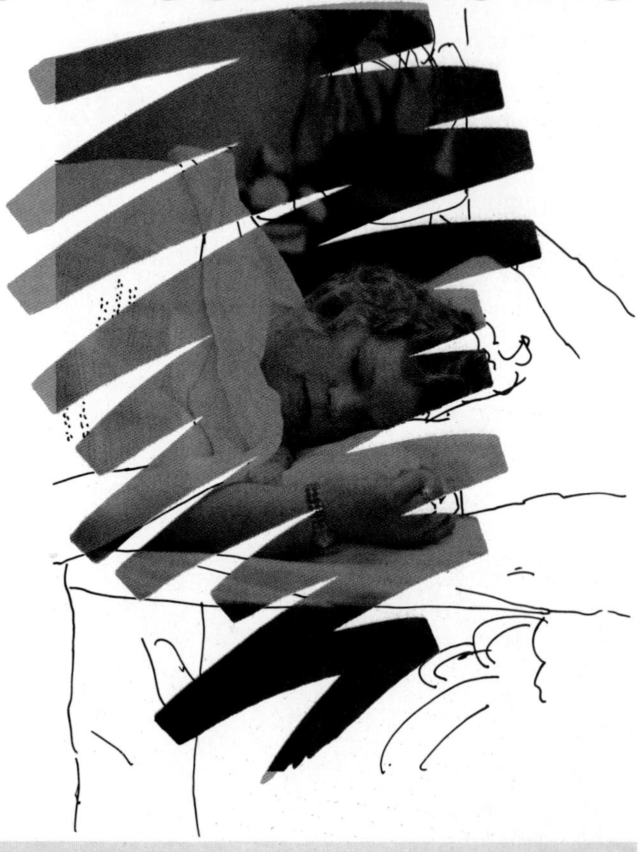

Behavioral Objectives

Upon completion of this chapter, the student will be able to:

1. Differentiate between the functions and characteristics of REM and NREM sleep.
2. List the consequences of REM sleep deprivation.
3. List the factors affecting sleep.
4. Summarize how sleep–rest patterns differ in each of the following age groups: infants, toddlers, children, adolescents, young adults, middle-aged adults, and older adults.
5. Describe at least five disorders of initiating and maintaining sleep found during the life cycle.
6. Describe at least two causes of excessive somnolence during the life cycle.
7. Describe at least three causes of disorders of arousal in individuals under 20 years of age.
8. State four causes of sleep problems in the elderly.
9. Explain the purpose of the following in assisting the client with sleep problems: polysomnography, sleep history, observation of the client, sleep nursing diagnosis, and sleep care plan.
10. State at least 10 nursing diagnoses related to the diagnosis of sleep–rest patterns.
11. List data to be obtained in a sleep–rest history.
12. List at least five nursing implementations useful in the promotion of sleep and rest.
13. Discuss the importance of collaboration in the management of sleep–rest problems.

KEY TERMS

ascending reticular activating system
fatigue
insomnia
narcolepsy
nocturnal myoclonus
nocturnal polysomnogram
nonrapid eye movement sleep
obstructive sleep apnea
parasomnias
rapid eye movement sleep
rest
sleep
sleep apnea
sundown syndrome

Sleep is a normal and complex physiological rhythm that involves altered states of consciousness from which the individual can be aroused by appropriate stimuli. Through the evolutionary process, humans have inherited the function of sleep as a behavior to enhance their survival by reducing sensory input, activity, and energy output. Sleep, then, is both an instinctive behavior and an inherent biological system that permits periods of nonresponding to the environment.[1]

Approximately one third of our lives is spent in sleep. Yet sleep remains a very individual experience. Some people sleep more at certain times of the day or night than others. Some people sleep for shorter periods of time than others. Some people consistently report more satisfactory sleep than others. Sleep is affected by such factors as age, emotions, noise, shift work, drugs, illness, diet, exercise, travel, and sex. Furthermore, sleep is intimately associated with other body functions and biological rhythms, including biochemical and neuroanatomical processes; nerve cell activity; changes in heart rate, blood pressure, and temperature; and bodily movement. In spite of these complexities, sleep varies within only three dimensions during a 24-hour period: sleep length, sleep onset, and sleep termination. These variations are usually interactive, and depend largely on an individual's personal and social habits, circadian rhythm, and age.[1]

The relationship between sleep and wellness is complex. Sleeping well is related to a sense of well-being and wellness. Loss of part or all of a night's sleep results in daytime sleepiness, alteration in one's mood, and an inability to concentrate. In essence, one's sense of well-being is somewhat diminished. The loss of sleep is an unpleasant experience that has led people to seek various remedies through the ages. The quest for a "good night's sleep" is a common reason for which individuals seek the advice of health care professionals.

The effects of prolonged sleep loss are serious. After 48 hours, hormone production is altered, psychomotor performance decreases, and perceptual abilities diminish.[2] The affected individual does not feel as well as when sleep patterns were maintained. With continued sleep loss, hallucinations, nervousness, irritability, and loss of concentration occur. Conversely, dysfunction of other body systems disrupts the normal sleep–wake cycle, and one's sense of wellness may be further decreased.

This chapter discusses healthful sleep patterns, factors affecting sleep–rest patterns, alterations in sleep–rest patterns, sleep–rest assessment, nursing diagnoses related to sleep–rest status, and nursing implementation to promote optimum sleep–rest. Because sleep is essential to one's physiological and psychological wellness and basic to the quality of life, it is not surprising that the nurse plays a key role in the maintenance of a client's sleep–rest patterns and in the assessment and management of sleep problems. A collaborative approach is the key to the success of this process. Through collaboration, the nurse and client share information and ideas about the client's sleep patterns and problems, and ways in which healthful sleep can be maintained or sleep problems handled. The collaborative process is discussed in more detail later in this chapter.

Section 1. Understanding Sleep and Rest

OPTIMUM SLEEP AND REST

To accurately assess and plan for the sleep-rest needs of clients, it is necessary to understand the concepts of sleep and rest. A basic understanding of the regulation of sleep–wakefulness and healthful sleep patterns is also needed. Factors that influence rest and sleep and common sleep–rest alterations should also be considered when assessing and planning for the client's sleep–rest needs.

Rest versus Sleep

Although rest and sleep are basic human needs, they are not the same. An individual may sleep well at night yet be unable to rest during the day because of the need for constant care. Similarly, a person may rest during the day but be unable to sleep at night due to noise or discomfort.

Rest is frequently defined as a period of inactivity during which one is free from fear or anxiety (Fig. 28–1). It offers the body and mind a chance to restore energy and resume optimal functioning.[3] Without rest, irritability, depression, feelings of tiredness, and loss of control may develop.[4]

When rest is prescribed for a client, its meaning should be clarified with the physician. It may be necessary to determine whether or not the entire body should be rested (as with a myocardial infarction) or just a specific body part (such as a broken arm). In order to recover from one activity before beginning another, rest and activity should be alternated.[3]

Even though rest and sleep are not the same, resting prepares a person for sleep because it involves mental and physical relaxation.[3] Sleep is commonly defined as a period during which bodily functions are partially suspended and consciousness is partially or completely interrupted.[4] Temperature, pulse, blood pressure, and respirations decrease; the kidneys are less productive; and digestive secretions diminish. As muscles relax, the basal metabolic rate declines and most reflexes disappear or weaken, except for the cough reflex.[3]

Sleep helps one to feel rested and renews the body's energy. Without sleep, concentration diminishes, energy decreases, activity declines, the body's sensitivity to discomfort increases and the individual may experience fatigue.[5] **Fatigue** is a subjective sensation associated with discomfort, decrease in motor and mental skill, productive incapacity, and sometimes feelings of weakness and futility.[5]

Regulation of Sleep–Wakefulness

Circadian Rhythms. Circadian rhythms refer to those events that occur at approximately 24-hour intervals. These rhythms include the sleep–wake cycle, core body temperature changes, and fluctuations in hormonal secretions. They are interrelated and coincide with given external events, such as day and night and light and dark. For example, a person's body temperature is at its highest while

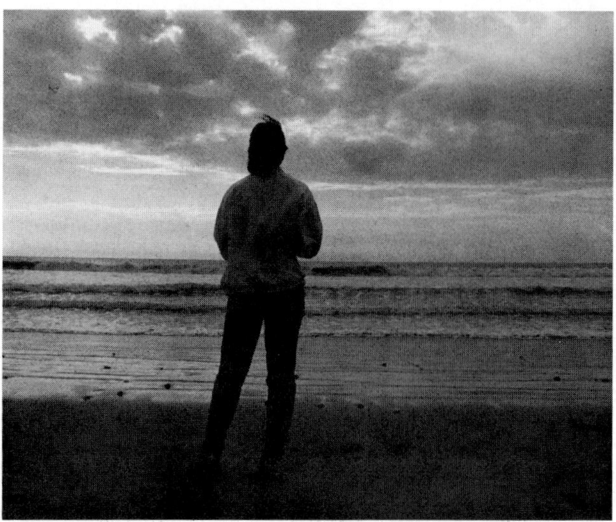

Figure 28–1. By giving oneself time to think and meditate, a person achieves rest for mind and body.

awake and is at its lowest while asleep. A change in the timing of the circadian rhythms may be precipitated by a change in the environment. For example, people who fly across several time zones must adjust to sleeping at a different time than they do at home. That is, their inherent circadian rhythms must change to accommodate the new environment. This process may require several days, and some people never adjust.

Neuroendocrine activity—growth hormone secretion, adrenocorticotropic hormone (ACTH) release, adrenal cortical secretion, and antidiuretic hormone release—has been linked to the 24-hour sleep–wake cycle.[6] A disruption in the individual's inherent sleep–wake cycle alters the secretion and release of these hormones. As a result, many target organs and body systems are affected by the changing levels of these hormones.

Circadian rhythms are subject to individual variation. Consequently, people differ in the time of day at which they function their best and in the times they prefer to go to bed, a fact that is too often overlooked in hospitals where staff organize routines around work flow rather than individual client sleep needs and preferences.[7]

Neurological Regulation of Sleep–Wakefulness. The **ascending reticular activating system** (RAS) is responsible for awareness, consciousness, wakefulness, and arousal. Increased activity in this part of the brain results in wakefulness, while decreased or inadequate activity causes sleep. Irreversible coma may occur when the reticular activating system is destroyed.[8]

In order for the RAS to regulate wakefulness, it must be stimulated from external sources. Pain impulses, visual and auditory signals, visceral sensations, and proprioceptive signals from the muscles will cause arousal. Once arousal occurs, RAS excitation is maintained through three feedback systems:

1. The RAS increases activity in the cerebral cortex. In turn, the cerebral cortex enhances RAS activity.
2. Increased RAS activity enhances muscular activity throughout the body. This increased muscle response promotes greater RAS response.
3. The RAS stimulates the release of the chemical epinephrine from the adrenal medulla, which increases RAS activity.[5]

After a period of wakefulness, RAS cells system become less excitable and activity of the feedback systems decreases. As a result, the reticular activating system is further depressed and sleep occurs. After a period of inactivity or sleep, RAS excitability is reestablished, and wakefulness occurs and is maintained for a period of time.[5]

Chemical Regulation of Sleep–Wakefulness. The role of epinephrine in maintaining the sleep–wake cycle was mentioned in the previous section. In addition to this substance, other chemicals have been identified as influencing sleep–wakefulness. High concentrations of norepinephrine, dopamine, serotonin, indoleamine, and the catecholamines are also found in the brainstem. Dopamine and norepinephrine have been associated with wakefulness and REM (rapid eye movement) sleep, while serotonin has been linked to NREM (nonrapid eye movement) sleep. However, the exact mechanism by which these chemicals influence sleep is unclear.[6]

BUILDING NURSING KNOWLEDGE

What Are the Factors That Affect Clients' Sleep?

Closs J. Patients' sleep–wake rhythms in hospital. *Nurs Times.* 1988;84:48–55.

Closs reports on the importance of normal sleep and the impact on sleep of hospitalization. The author reviewed a large body of literature on sleep that shows that sleep aids healing and that disruption of sleep leads to numerous adverse physiological and psychological consequences.

Closs reports that sleep deprivation results in clear signs of central nervous system impairment. Daily fluctuations in the levels of anabolic (metabolic buildup) and catabolic (metabolic breakdown) hormones suggest that anabolic processes occur during sleep. Thus, in sleep deprivation, people experience signs and symptoms including irritability, suspiciousness, speech slurring, visual misperceptions, and confusion.

According to this article, factors affecting sleep include age (there is less total sleep and reduction in stage IV sleep in the elderly); gender (more adult men than women have sleep disturbances); anxiety and depression (both are associated with changes in blood chemistry that interfere with sleep); diet (foods high in tryptophan promote sleep onset; withdrawal from alcohol or hypnotic drugs promotes disturbed sleep); respiration (insufficient blood oxygen and excessive blood carbon dioxide interfere with normal sleep); temperature (even slight changes in room temperature can change the sleep cycle; high and low temperatures reduce REM sleep); genetics (sleep requirements are partly genetic and sleep disturbances seem to occur more frequently in certain families); and position (poor sleepers spend more time lying supine and change positions more frequently; long periods of bed rest disrupt body rhythms).

Closs argues that many of the factors that alter sleep may be part of the hospital experience. Research reviewed showed that hospitalized clients experience sleep deprivation. In one study, clients who had undergone heart surgery were disturbed approximately 14 times each hour in the immediate period after surgery. Another study showed that 8-hour sleepers who had their sleep reduced to 6 hours experienced no significant effects, suggesting that some reduction of sleep is not harmful.

Healthful Sleep Patterns

Healthful sleep patterns are composed of nonrapid eye movement sleep and rapid eye movement sleep. These patterns change throughout the life cycle (Fig. 28–2). **Nonrapid eye movement (NREM) sleep** may be defined as that period of sleep during which no eye movements can be observed and the eyelids are still. There are four stages of NREM sleep. These are discussed in the following section.

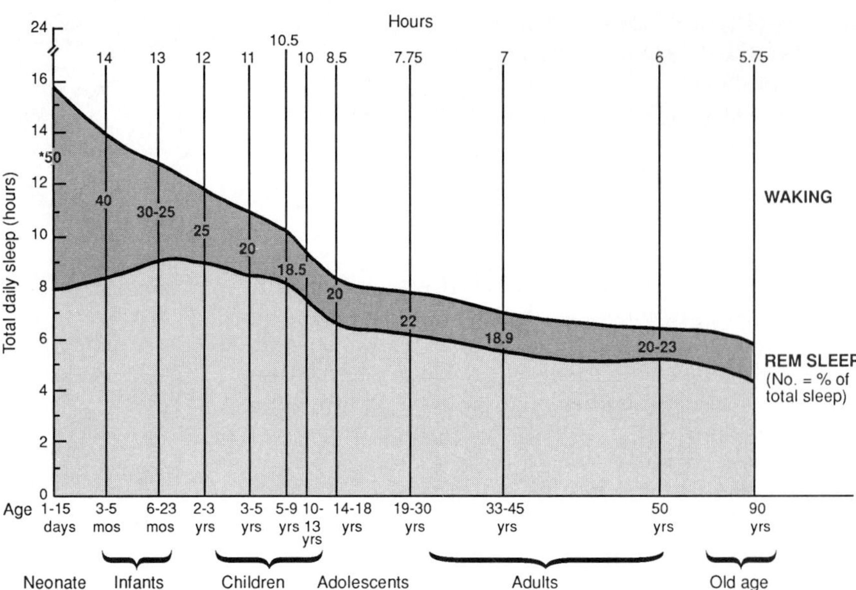

Figure 28–2. Changes with age in total amounts of daily sleep, daily REM sleep, and percentage of REM sleep. Note sharp diminution of REM sleep in the early years. REM sleep falls from 8 hours at birth to less than 1 hour in old age. The amount of NREM sleep throughout life remains more constant, falling from 8 hours to 5 hours. However, these NREM data do not show the large decreases in stage IV sleep, which decreases from 1.2 hours in young adulthood to 0 to 0.5 hours in old age. (*From Roffwarg HP, Muzio JN, Dement WC. Ontogenetic development of the human sleep–dream cycle.* Science. *1966; 152:604–619.*)

NREM sleep is a time of energy conservation and tissue repair.[9]

Rapid eye movement (REM) sleep may be defined as that period of sleep during which eye movements occur and the eyelids twitch. REM sleep serves the following functions: it restores one mentally; is important for memory, learning, and psychological adaptation; provides a review of the day's events; and allows information to be categorized and assimilated into the brain's storage system. The need for REM sleep increases when one is faced with new experiences and psychological stress.[10, 11] The consequences of REM sleep deprivation include irritability, apathy, increased sensitivity to pain, and a lack of alertness. A repeated loss of REM sleep results in increased anxiety, decreased coping abilities, confusion, and disorientation.[9, 10]

The basic physiological mechanisms underlying the stages of sleep are complex and much is still unknown about them. It is believed that a minimum of three major neurotransmitters are associated with the sleep stages. These include serotonin, acetylcholine, and norepinephrine. Each neurotransmitter is active in a different anatomical site in the brain and is associated with different sleep stages.[12]

Because serotonin is responsible for sleep onset and sleep maintenance, it initiates the physiological mechanism involved in stage I, stage II, stage III, and stage IV (NREM) sleep. It is also responsible for the onset of REM sleep. In spite of its major role in the sleep process, nothing is known about the causes of serotonin activation.[12]

The neurotransmitter acetylcholine is responsible for maintaining REM sleep. Norepinephrine is thought to be involved in maintaining wakefulness.[4]

NREM Sleep Stages

Stage I. Stage I of NREM sleep lasts only a few minutes and is the lightest of the sleep levels. It is characterized by decreases in temperature and in respiratory, pulse, and metabolic rates. A slight decrease in blood pressure occurs and the muscles relax. The individual may be easily aroused in this stage.[11]

Stage II. During stage II, the individual becomes more relaxed, but continues to be easily awakened. This stage lasts approximately 5 to 10 minutes.[11]

Stages III and IV. Stages III and IV comprise the deepest levels of sleep and last from 15 to 30 minutes. During this time the sleeper is not disturbed by sensory stimuli and seldom moves. In stage III, there is loss of muscle tone, reflexes diminish, and snoring may occur. The person may be aroused by touch only. Stage IV sleep rests, relaxes, and physically restores the body.[11] During this stage, the muscles are most relaxed.

REM Sleep

Following approximately 90 minutes of sleep, the individual returns from stage IV up through the lighter stages of sleep to stage I. Rather than entering stage I or awakening, one enters REM sleep. This stage is characterized by frequent bursts of rapid eye movements, dreams, muscular twitching, and profound muscle relaxation. Erections may occur in men. During this stage, the sleeper is more difficult to awaken than in any other stage.[12]

Following the period of REM sleep, the sleeper again descends through stages II to IV. Everyone averages 4 to 5 of these sleep cycles per night, each lasting approximately 90 to 100 minutes. With each cycle, stage IV sleep decreases and REM sleep increases. Thus, the major portion of stage IV sleep occurs early in the night, while the majority of REM sleep takes place in the last several hours before awakening. When awakened during any stage of this cycle, one must resume sleep at stage I and progress through the stages to REM sleep.[6]

■ FACTORS AFFECTING SLEEP–REST PATTERNS

Some common factors affecting sleep include age, environment, nutrition, stress, exercise, illness, medications, and alcohol and stimulants.

Age

Age may be the most important factor influencing sleep and rest needs. As discussed below, sleep changes from one developmental stage to another.[13]

Infants. Infants sleep an average of 14 to 18 hours per day. This sleep occurs in six or more short periods, and is distributed fairly evenly over a 24-hour period. Sleep episodes last from 20 minutes to 5 or 6 hours.[14] Infants usually awaken to be fed.[4]

By the age of six months, infants experience three to four sleep periods per 24 hours. Typically, this pattern occurs as a long period of nighttime sleep, with shorter morning and afternoon naps. About 80 percent of all infants are sleeping through the night at 6 months of age.[1]

Toddlers. By 2 years of age, toddlers sleep about 12 to 13 hours in a 24-hour period. Children in this age group give up morning naps and sleep 1 to 2 hours in the afternoon. Most children stop napping completely by the age of 3.[14] Sleep problems may develop if efforts are made to continue these nap periods beyond the child's need for them.

Children and Adolescents. Between 4 years of age and adolescence, there is a very slow decrease in total sleep time, from about 11 hours to approximately 8 hours per day. While the 4-year-old sleeps about 11 hours a night, the 12-year-old sleeps 8 hours. Most children in this age group do not nap, so all sleep occurs at night.[14]

Young Adults. The sleep of the normal young adult is the most simple and most common form of sleep. The individual usually sleeps from 7 to 8 hours per night. Young adults spend less time in bed and have a decrease in total sleep time from earlier years. Most young adults do not nap except in cultures where a siesta is the norm (as in tropical climates).[14]

Middle-aged and Older Adults. Throughout this period, sleep becomes increasingly fragmented. During middle age, the adult begins to experience an increased amount of time for sleep onset, an increased number of nocturnal awakenings, and less total sleep time.[14] These trends continue with advancing age. Men show greater changes in these sleep patterns than women. However, women report a higher incidence of sleep complaints than men.[15]

The older adult has a tendency to return to the polycyclic sleep patterns of earlier life. There is a significant tendency for older men to nap more than older women.[11] An increase in the number and length of daytime naps may compensate for a decrease in nocturnal sleep time. Conversely, daytime napping may decrease the need for nighttime sleep in older adults.[14]

Environment

Many environmental factors can encourage or interfere with sleep. Among these are room temperature, noise level, light-

---

IMPLICATIONS FOR NURSE–CLIENT COLLABORATION

Factors Affecting Sleep and Rest

Although the body's physiological processes normally support optimal cycles of sleep and rest, many factors can alter the internal mechanisms that regulate those cycles. Stress and illness, for instance, can interfere with rest. Nutrition and exercise changes may occur independent of illness or may be associated with it; in either case, these factors also alter the ability to sleep. The nurse endeavors to support the client's sleep by helping the client to maximize the factors promoting sleep and to minimize the factors that interfere with it. Through collaborative interaction, the nurse invites an exchange of information with the client that is valuable in promoting an optimal sleep pattern.

BUILDING NURSING KNOWLEDGE

How Can Nurses Facilitate Sleep for the Hospitalized Child?

Slota MC. Implications of sleep deprivation in the pediatric critical care unit. *Focus Crit Care.* 1988;15:35–43.

The conditions in an intensive care unit—the equipment, tubes, lines, wires, and the generally tense atmosphere—can result in sleep deprivation in children that are severe enough to cause repercussions even after discharge from the hospital, according to this author. Many variables exert an effect. These include noise levels, decreased environmental light–dark cycles, disruption of home sleep rituals, pain, discomfort, isolation and separation from significant others, immobilization induced by drugs and restraints, anxiety, and depersonalization.

According to Slota, when a child's sleep is continually disrupted, sleep becomes desynchronized and results in fatigue, restlessness, disorientation, combativeness, reduced sense of well-being, apathy, anorexia, inability to concentrate, and decreased stress tolerance.

Slota suggests nursing measures to promote sleep among hospitalized children. They include providing for uninterrupted periods of sleep by grouping procedures when possible to minimize the need to awaken the child; incorporating home rituals before the sleep time; dimming the lights, pulling the drapes, and making the child's security toy accessible; encouraging adults to read to the child; playing soft music and using headphones if the environment is noisy; arousing the child gently before beginning intrusive procedures; changing the immobilized child's position periodically and using massage and warm blankets to promote comfort; providing for privacy; and establishing trust so that the child does not have to be constantly on guard against threat.

ing, type of bed, size of bed, and unfamiliar surroundings.[6] For example, excessively warm or cold rooms inhibit sleep, while a temperature comfortable to the individual promotes sleep. Loud or unexpected noises—such as increased television volume, airplanes landing or taking off, or the telephone ringing—also disrupt sleep. Soft music may encourage sleep.

Diet

Certain foods and individual's weight influence sleep patterns. Although weight loss is associated with sleep loss, weight gain is related to uninterrupted sleep. Foods containing the amino acid L-tryptophan, such as cottage cheese, milk, poultry, tuna fish, and cashews, are a natural sedative and promote sleep.[4] Nurses should suggest these foods to individuals who are having difficulty sleeping. It is also important to determine recent weight loss in clients who express sleep problems.

Psychological Stress

Life changes that result in anxiety, depression, or nervousness lead to disrupted sleep patterns.[6] For example, the death of a loved one, divorce, birth of a child, or impending surgery may cause sleep loss. Nurses should remain alert to the possibility of stress when clients report changes in usual sleep patterns.

Exercise

Regular physical exercise performed early in the day promotes sleep. Excessive exercise done late in the day usually interferes with sleep. Exercise promotes the release of the hormone adrenaline, which causes the body to become alert and active.[6] For example, jogging 3 miles at 6 AM will enhance nighttime sleep, while the same activity done at 7 PM will interfere with sleep.

Illness

Numerous illnesses interfere with sleep[11] (see the section that discusses nursing diagnosis of sleep–rest status). For example, pain from arthritis may delay sleep onset or cause nocturnal awakenings. The need to urinate because of bladder infection or decreased bladder capacity often results in frequent nocturnal wakenings. Individuals with gastric ulcers may have difficulty falling asleep and increased gastric acid secretion during REM sleep may contribute to difficulty staying asleep.

Medications

Routine use of certain medications, such as sedatives, barbiturates, antidepressants, and anxiolytics, alters the sleep–wake cycle due to increasing tolerance to the pharmacological properties of the drug.[6] For example, if a sedative is taken for more than 10 to 14 days, the individual becomes used to the drug and again has difficulty falling asleep. The use of a sedative for 4 to 5 days does not result in this problem.

Drugs used to treat other health problems may also interfere with sleep due to their secondary effects. Amphetamines, antihistamines, and antihypertensives commonly impair sleep.[11]

Alcohol and Stimulants

Alcohol intake contributes to sleeplessness, but its effects may be difficult to assess, because initially it acts as a sedative and induces sleep. After several hours of sleep, the individual may awaken and be unable to return to sleep. Because of falling asleep readily, it is difficult for the individual to associate the use of alcohol with nighttime awakenings.[6]

Stimulants such as chocolate, coffee, tea, and cola drinks with high caffeine disturb sleep by making it difficult to fall asleep. Many individuals find it helpful to exclude these items for 8 to 10 hours before bedtime because it takes the body a minimum of 8 hours to metabolize caffeine.[6]

Comfort and Pain

Comfort enhances sleep, and discomfort often interferes with it.[7] Many sources of discomfort interfere with sleep, especially in the hospital. Hospital beds, for example, tend to be more firm than those used in homes, are often covered in plastic, and are usually of a different size than the beds with which clients are familiar. Illness, invasive procedures, and disturbance from the hospital routines may also interfere with sleep.

Clients in pain will not sleep. Jones and associates found that pain ranked second to discomfort as a contributory factor to sleep loss.[16] Pain relief generally enhances the individual's ability to go to sleep and may include a variety of measures (as discussed in Section 3 of this chapter).

■ ALTERATIONS IN SLEEP–REST PATTERNS

Disorders in Initiating and Maintaining Sleep

Infants and Toddlers. Colic is the primary cause of sleep dysfunction during the first 6 months of life. Infants with colic are irritable and cry frequently, particularly in the afternoon and evening. Due to extreme discomfort, sleep onset is delayed or attained only after infants are held or rocked for a prolonged period of time. Although colic usually improves after 3 months of age, infants may continue to exhibit disturbed sleep patterns out of habit. Parents who have become accustomed to providing comfort for the colicky infant may also have difficulty being realistic about the significance of the infant's cries when distress is no longer present. Limit-setting becomes a problem, and may set a pattern for sleep difficulties as the child grows.[17] Slota[13] recommends that parents use a gradual approach for training the child to fall asleep again by intervening with comforting words at planned intervals but not continuing the other behaviors such as rocking and feeding. Infants should be picked up only if a problem exists, such as a wet diaper. If such approaches are used, infants will gradually learn to decrease crying time and will learn to fall asleep when put to bed.

Children between the ages of 6 months and 3 years may awaken once or twice during the night. However, frequent awakenings, difficulty returning to sleep, or the need for outside assistance in returning to sleep are classified as sleep disturbances in this age group. Factors that may contribute to these problems include naps that are too long or too late in the day, failure of the child to learn to fall asleep without help, parents who have had little experience with children, and children who have physical or emotional problems. Acute illnesses (such as flu or colds) or chronic illnesses (such as otitis media) may temporarily disturb sleep in infants and toddlers. It is important to remember that illness that frequently disrupts sleep may lead to long-term sleep problems.[17]

Infants and toddlers frequently associate transitions to sleep with certain comfort measures (for example, a doll, blanket, or bottle). They may also have learned to fall asleep somewhere other than their crib (such as in a parent's lap or bed). Under these circumstances, children fall asleep without difficulty but if awakened during the night, cannot return to sleep without help. Excessive crying may result. Children must be taught to fall asleep initially under the same conditions used to return to sleep during the night. Parents must be taught to prolong the period of time they allow children to cry before checking on them.[17]

Excessive nocturnal fluid intake has also been identified as a cause of sleep disturbances in infants and toddlers.[17] The child's demand for water or other liquid before going to bed often leads to awakening during the night due to wetness, an upset stomach, or further demands for fluid. Gradual weaning and consistent limit setting by the parents usually solves the problem.

Other causes of difficulty in initiating and maintaining sleep in infants and toddlers include inconsistent limit setting by parents at bedtime, fear and anxiety on the part of the child, irregular schedules, and medication. Children in this age group are often afraid of the dark and fantasized monsters. Underlying these fears may be sibling rivalry, parental arguing, or fear of separation. If the source of the fear is developmental, the problem usually resolves itself. If not, parents may need professional help to change their patterns of interaction and to establish a firm bedtime routine.[17]

When fear or anxiety is present, toddlers may use various tactics to delay bedtime (such as requests for a glass of water, a need to use the bathroom, requests for "one more story"). These tactics may also be used by children without any obvious fear. Such requests seem small, and parents find it difficult to deny them. This lack of limit setting becomes a part of the bedtime routine, and though the child is able to fall asleep, it is easy to avoid doing so. The solution to the problem includes the institution of a bedtime routine that is consistently followed.

Infants and toddlers with irregular daytime schedules include those who eat, awaken, and nap at different times each day. Because these irregularities disrupt circadian rhythm, their nocturnal sleep is disturbed. The institution and reinforcement of a regular daily routine alleviates the problem.[17]

Finally, the use of medications can cause sleep disturbances in young children. Hyperactivity is a common side effect when using drugs with sedative properties (eg, antihistamines, tranquilizers) for even a brief time. Nonsedatives may also disrupt sleep due to unwanted side effects such as nausea or diarrhea. If the offending medication cannot be discontinued, the nurse should suggest to the physician that a different drug or a change in dosage may be helpful in reestablishing normal sleep patterns.[17]

Children. Problems in initiating and maintaining sleep are much less prevalent for children aged 3 to 12 years for two reasons: There is an actual decline in problems and parents may become less aware of existing difficulties as children mature.[17] For example, when the older child is put to bed and has difficulty falling asleep or awakens during the night, the child may continue to read or play quietly without parents' knowledge. Thus, sleep problems may go unrecognized unless the child is questioned directly. If children are experiencing sleep problems, it is usually due to worry or fear, such as the fear of dying while asleep.

Adolescents. During adolescence, problems in initiating and maintaining sleep increase. Factors implicated in the cause of these sleep problems include anxiety over impending adulthood; family problems, sexual problems, and school problems; drug abuse; alcohol abuse; menstrual problems; thyroid problems; and irregular sleep–wake patterns.[17]

Adults. As individuals age, complaints concerning the initiation and maintenance of sleep, or **insomnia,** increase dramatically. Difficulty with sleep usually begins in the 30s. By the 60s, 50 percent of the population reports some problem with sleep.[6]

Insomnia may be acute or chronic. Acute insomnia refers to difficulty in initiating and maintaining sleep for approximately 1 week to 3 months. After 3 months of poor sleep, insomnia becomes chronic.[4] Insomnia is also classified according to its timing in the sleep cycle. Initial insomnia describes difficulty falling asleep. Intermittent insomnia refers to periods of wakefulness that interrupt sleep cycles. Terminal insomnia means awakening earlier than desired.

The cause of insomnia may be an emotional or stress-related disturbance, physical illness, or medication. Anxiety, depression, and excess tension are the most common psychiatric causes of chronic insomnia.[18] Common medical causes of insomnia include arthritis, allergies, chronic pain, chronic brain syndrome, Parkinson's disease, hypothyroidism, diabetes, and nocturnal dyspnea.[11] Individuals with nocturnal myoclonus and sleep apnea may also complain of disturbed sleep.

Nocturnal myoclonus is characterized by a twitching of the legs that occurs at 20- to 60-second intervals and lasts from a few minutes to several hours. This twitching alternates with periods of undisturbed sleep, and the individual is usually not aware of its occurrence; however, there are frequent complaints of inadequate and restless sleep. Nocturnal myoclonus is frequently detected when the client's sleep partner describes its symptoms or complains of being kicked during the night. The incidence of nocturnal myoclonus increases with age. The cause is unknown.[18]

Sleep apnea is usually caused by a failure in the neural control of respiration (central apnea), an obstruction of the airway (obstructive apnea), or a combination of these two. It is characterized by periods of loud snoring or gasping for air alternating with periods of quiet sleep. Although breathing ceases briefly during these periods, the individual is usually unaware of these apneic episodes. Because of insomnia, the individual with sleep apnea commonly complains of daytime sleepiness.[18]

Older Adults. There are several causes of insomnia in the elderly. Anxiety over finances, living arrangements, or health may be the reason for sleeplessness. Depression may cause early morning awakenings or, in some instances, excessive sleepiness. It may be related to isolation, loneliness, or grief.[9]

Physical discomfort may either be the cause of sleep difficulties or aggravate preexisting sleep problems.[9] Pain may keep the elderly individual from falling asleep or cause nighttime awakenings. Other sources of physical discomfort include respiratory problems, an uncomfortable bed, excessive heat, cold, or noise.

Acute confusion is often responsible for reversal of day and night activities. The person may sleep during the day and remain awake all or part of the night.[9]

Sundown syndrome or nocturnal delirium is particularly distressing to families of the elderly. The elderly person who experiences **sundown syndrome** functions normally during the day, but suffers from hallucinations, delusions, and disorientation at night. This syndrome usually occurs in individuals with mild-to-moderate chronic brain disease. Because such episodes are frightening and disruptive to the family, sundown syndrome often leads to the institutionalization of the aged family member.[15]

Disorders of Excessive Somnolence

Children and Adolescents. The most common disorder of excessive somnolence in these age groups is obstructive sleep apnea.

Obstructive sleep apnea occurs in children and adolescents of all ages and is characterized by loud snoring and restless sleep. It is more common in males, and is usually associated with enlarged adenoids and tonsils. Marked daytime sleepiness is also present in adolescents. However, it may be masked in children by hyperactivity, lack of attention, decreased school performance, or behavior problems.[17]

In addition to sleep apnea, there are other causes of daytime sleepiness in childhood and adolescence. Depression in adolescents and the use of drugs and alcohol are characteristic examples. Complaints of daytime sleepiness may also be early symptoms of mononucleosis, hepatitis, leukemia, and anemia.[17] Thus, it is important to refer children and adolescents with excessive sleepiness to the appropriate health care provider for further evaluation.

Adults. The two most common disorders of excessive somnolence in adults are sleep apnea and narcolepsy. Sleep apnea in the adult was discussed under Disorders in Initiating and Maintaining Sleep. It is also classified as a disorder of excessive somnolence due to the daytime sleepiness that results from the loss of nocturnal sleep.

Narcolepsy is a chronic condition characterized by repeated, uncontrollable episodes of sleep and drowsiness from which the individual may be easily awakened. Onset is usually in the second or third decade of life. It occurs in both men and women equally, and has a tendency to run in families. Daytime sleepiness is a common symptom of narcolepsy.[11]

Disorders of Arousal (Parasomnias)

Disorders of arousal or **parasomnias** are rarely seen in those over 20 years of age. Common disorders in this category include sleepwalking, sleeptalking, confusional arousals, and enuresis.[17]

Children and Adolescents. Sleepwalking, sleeptalking, and confusional arousals occur at the end of an episode of deep sleep. The child arouses, the eyes are opened with a glassy appearance, and confusion occurs. Any verbalizations are not coherent, and the child may become frightened and cry. The child may also walk around without purpose. Efforts to restrain or comfort the child usually intensify the attack. It is also difficult to awaken the individual.[17]

These episodes may last as long as 30 minutes in the young child, while in the adolescent they last only a few minutes. Upon awakening, the child will not recall the episode, while the adolescent may have a vague recollection of it. During childhood, the etiology of these arousals is usually developmental in nature or related to stress. In adolescence, arousals usually have a psychological cause.[17]

Most enuresis (bedwetting) occurs during the first one third of the night. There is a higher incidence among boys, as well as an inherited tendency toward this disorder. Enuresis may occur in conjunction with a sleep terror or confusional arousal. Treatment for this problem depends on the child's age, frequency of occurrence, and the response of the child and the family to the problem[11] (see Nursing Implementation to Promote Optimum Sleep and Rest later in the chapter).

Rest and sleep are distinct from one another, yet each is necessary to the individual's physical and psychological well-being. Sleep patterns change throughout the life cycle. The amount of sleep time gradually decreases throughout childhood. While the newborn sleeps 14 to 18 hours per day, the preschooler sleeps 12 to 13 hours and usually takes only one nap per day. By adolescence, the individual usually sleeps 7 to 8 hours a night. This pattern continues into middle and old age, when sleep becomes fragmented and the individual tends to return to the napping patterns of earlier years. Many factors influence sleep. Among these are age, environment, nutrition, physical and psychological stress, exercise, illness, medications, alcohol, and stimulants. Certain sleep dysfunctions are also common to specific age groups. The information in this section can be used to assess and meet the sleep–rest needs of clients.

Section 2. Assessment of Sleep–Rest Patterns

SLEEP–REST DATA COLLECTION

The nurse uses knowledge of sleep patterns and sleep dysfunctions—such as difficulty in initiating and maintaining sleep, disorders of excessive somnolence, and disorders of arousal—in conjunction with the nursing process to assist the client to meet sleep–rest needs. For example, a toddler's parents state that their 2-year-old son has difficulty falling asleep at night. The nurse knows that this difficulty is often caused by allowing toddlers to go to bed at a different time each night. The nurse uses the first component of the nursing process, assessment, to determine if the toddler has a regular bedtime. The assessment information reveals that the toddler has an irregular bedtime and napping schedule. The nurse uses this information to collaborate with the parents in establishing a regular nap and bedtime schedule for their son.

As illustrated by the above example, an assessment of the client's sleep status is necessary in order to plan individualized and comprehensive nursing care. Assessment entails gathering information related to the client's sleep–rest history and the performance of a sleep–rest examination. Collaboration with the client, family, and health care team members is essential to ensure accurate assessment. The nurse begins the assessment by gathering data in collaboration with the client. Collaboration is characterized by the free exchange of ideas and information concerning sleep between the nurse and client or significant others. The nurse and client need to share information concerning the client's usual bedtime routines, sleep patterns, and sleep problems, and how healthful sleep–rest patterns can be maintained or sleep–rest problems alleviated. Thus, the client is actively involved in developing the plan of care, and the possibility of successful sleep management is enhanced. Collaborative assessment facilitates the establishment of a trusting, productive, and ongoing relationship between nurse and client as they work together, by mutual consent, to improve the client's sleep.

A complete history, physical examination, and review of pertinent laboratory reports are essential to the assessment of sleep–rest patterns. The nurse may gather the necessary information from the client, family members, the physician's report of the medical examination, and the medical history. The assessment process should begin with the initial nurse–client contact.

IMPLICATIONS FOR NURSE–CLIENT COLLABORATION

Sleep–Rest Data Collection

Collaboration with the client is essential to assure that the nurse understands the many factors—physical, emotional, and social—that converge to influence the client's ability to sleep. Collaboration on sleep problems involves the free exchange of ideas and information concerning sleep. In the hospital setting, the nurse and client may need to discuss the client's usual activity and bedtime routines to determine how an optimal sleep–rest pattern can be maintained. In the hospital setting and in other settings, the nurse and client may also need to identify new approaches for the client to use in solving rest and sleep problems.

Sleep–Rest History

Primary Concern. The client's primary concern may be directly or indirectly related to sleep. Some complaints directly related to sleep include excessive daytime fatigue and loss of appetite as well as narcolepsy, sleep apnea, insomnia, bedwetting, and sleepwalking. Concerns indirectly related to sleep are discussed below.

Current Understanding. The client may perceive that a current health problem interferes with obtaining satisfactory sleep. For example, a respiratory or cardiovascular problem (such as pneumonia or congestive heart failure) may be the client's primary concern. Yet, shortness of breath associated with the problem may inhibit sleep. Similarly, a sudden onset of acute chest pain may cause difficulty falling asleep or remaining asleep. The same is true for someone experiencing chronic pain such as from arthritis. The treatment of the problem may also interfere with the client's usual sleep patterns, as when diuretics given for congestive heart failure increase the need to void at night. Therefore, it is important that the nurse ask about the client's current understanding of the health problem and treatment in relation to any possible impact on the client's sleep. For example, the nurse should discuss any recent changes in sleep patterns with the client. It is important to assess when these changes occurred, what precipitated the changes, and how significant the changes are to the client. The nurse should also ascertain the onset, duration, and exacerbating and relieving conditions of the current health problem. In assessing the impact of the health problem on the client's sleep, it is also appropriate and necessary for the nurse to discuss any alterations in sleep patterns with the client's sleep partner. The partner can often identify disturbances that the client is not aware of, such as snoring, muscle twitching, and restlessness. The following example illustrates the importance of the current understanding.

- Ms. Orkin is admitted to the hospital with congestive heart failure. While obtaining the history, the nurse discovers that Ms. Orkin noted marked shortness of breath and some swelling of her fingers and ankles 48 hours prior to admission. These symptoms have become progressively worse over the past 24 hours. Ms. Orkin believes they were brought on by the fact that she forgot to take her "heart" medicine several times during the past week. Ms. Orkin states that oxygen, sleep, and her medicine usually help relieve the symptoms. Through further assessment, the nurse determines that since the onset of symptoms, Ms. Orkin has had difficulty falling asleep and remaining asleep due to her shortness of breath. Ms. Orkin states that these changes have been upsetting to her because she has difficulty carrying out her daily activities when she is tired. The nurse uses this information by reducing environmental stimuli to encourage rest, implementing nursing measures to decrease shortness of breath, and carrying out the physician's orders related to drug and oxygen therapy.

Past Health Problems/Experiences. The client's past health problems/experiences may disclose chronic problems or treatments related to sleep. Ask if the client has experienced any problems with sleep or other illnesses or injuries in the past that have affected sleep. If so, determine the date, severity, treatment, and any residual effects of the illness or treatment. The current use of any prescription or over-the-counter medications that could affect sleep should be noted (ie, those that act on the neurological, endocrine, respiratory, cardiovascular, or gastrointestinal systems). It is important to ask if any drugs are used to induce or maintain sleep, how long they have been taken, how often they are used, and whether any changes in usual sleep patterns have been noted since taking the medication. The following example illustrates the importance of past health problems/experiences.

- A nursing student is paying a home visit to 3-year-old Karen and her mother in order to complete a developmental screening for class. As part of the screening, the student must obtain Karen's past history. Upon questioning Karen's mother, the student learns that Karen has had frequent upper respiratory infections followed by otitis media. Karen's pediatrician has recommended that her mother administer antihistamines to Karen at the onset of an upper respiratory infection in an attempt to prevent the otitis. Karen's mother states that she tried this several times, but after several days Karen woke up screaming at night. The mother also states she becomes frightened because she doesn't know what is wrong with Karen. Because the nursing student knows that antihistamines may cause children to become restless and interfere with their usual sleep patterns, she decides that educating Karen's mother about the medication is in order. She also decides to recommend that the mother ask the pediatrician to change Karen's medication in an attempt to alleviate her sleep problems.

Personal, Family, and Social History. The client's personal, family, and social history can provide information for making nursing diagnoses about sleep status. Altered sleep patterns usually affect many areas of the client's daily life and sense of well-being. Necessary information includes the client's usual bedtime, approximate amount of time it takes to fall asleep, number of nocturnal awakenings, time of morning arousal, feelings of daytime drowsiness, and number and length of daytime naps. It is also important to ask the client for any subjective perceptions of how much movement occurs during sleep, how sound the sleep is, and how satisfying it is. The use of any special bedtime routine by the client should also be noted. Anything that the individual does on a nightly basis in preparation for sleep should be considered a bedtime routine. For example, many people have a snack, watch television, listen to the radio, bathe, brush their teeth, pray, or read before bedtime. The nurse should also inquire about the importance of these activities to the client and what happens to the sleep pattern if they are omitted from bedtime preparation. When feasible, routines should be incorporated in the client's plan of care. Nurses also need to gather information about the client's family. Are there any changes in the family relationships that could adversely influence sleep? For example, the presence in the home of a newborn baby, confused elderly adult, fearful child, or unsatisfactory marital relationship may alter sleep patterns. Close family members may also be able to contribute to the client's sleep history when direct communication with the client is difficult. Table 28–1 provides suggested questions for obtaining this information. The following example illustrates the use of this information.

- Mr. Warren is admitted to the medical floor for treatment of a gastric ulcer. While gathering his personal, family, and social history, the nurse notes that Mr. Warren follows a very specific bedtime routine. He brushes his teeth, takes a warm bath, listens to the radio, and likes to use two pillows. He states that this routine is extremely important to him. He also indicates that he usually retires at 10:30 PM and awakens at 6:30 AM. The nurse uses this information to plan collaboratively with the health care team to maintain Mr. Warren's bedtime routine during his hospital stay. The

TABLE 28–1. SLEEP–REST HISTORY: PERSONAL, FAMILY, AND SOCIAL HISTORY QUESTIONS

A. **Vocational**
1. What type of work do you do?
2. What hours do you usually work?
3. Does your work involve any physical activity?
4. Have you noticed any problems doing your work due to drowsiness or inability to concentrate?

B. **Home and Family**
1. Are you married?
2. Any difficulties with a relationship that disturbs your sleep? How?
3. Do you have children? Ages? How do they sleep at night?
4. Do you have any other family members living with you? Who? Ages?
5. What type of care, if any, do they require? How do they sleep at night?
6. Describe a typical day.

C. **Social and Leisure**
1. What are your favorite leisure activities?
2. Do drowsiness or feelings of tiredness ever interfere with these activities?
3. Have you given up any of these activities due to tiredness or lack of energy?

D. **Sexual**
1. Has your sexual relationship been satisfactory?
2. Have you noticed any changes related to your current illness? If so, what?
3. Does tiredness interfere with this relationship?
4. Do you have any sexual concerns that disturb your sleep? How?

E. **Habits**

Exercise
1. Do you exercise regularly? How often?
2. What time of day do you exercise?
3. Have you given up exercising due to tiredness or feeling sleepy?
4. Do you notice any changes in your sleep when your exercise pattern changes?

Sleep
1. Describe a typical night's sleep.
2. How many hours do you sleep at night?
3. Do you feel rested in the morning?
4. Do you nap? How often? How long?
5. Do you feel rested after napping?
6. Have you ever been told that you snore? That you're a restless sleeper?
7. How often do you awaken at night?
8. Do you have difficulty returning to sleep?
9. Do you have a bedtime routine? If so, what is it?
10. Do you need assistance with any bedtime routines?
11. Have you had difficulty sleeping since becoming ill?
12. Has this illness altered your sleep patterns?
13. If so, how? Do you think you sleep too much? Too little?
14. Describe any factors in the environment that are interfering with your sleep (eg, noise, room temperature, being awakened for treatments or medication, roommate).

Diet
1. How many meals do you eat per day?
2. Do you snack? When?
3. Do you ever have trouble sleeping due to indigestion?

Beverages
1. Do you use alcohol?
2. What do you usually drink?
3. How much do you drink in a typical week?
4. Have you ever noticed any difficulty sleeping after using alcohol?
5. Do you use caffeine? Tea? Coffee? Soft drinks?
6. How much of each per day?
7. What time do you have your last cup of coffee? Tea? Soft drink?
8. Do you notice any sleep changes when you use caffeine at night?

Other Substances
1. Do you use sleeping pills? How often?
2. What other medications do you take?
3. Do you use diet pills? Marijuana? Tobacco? Water pills? How often?

F. **Psychological/Coping**
1. Do you feel "blue" or downhearted? How often?
2. Do you feel like crying? How often?
3. Do you feel restless? Nervous? Irritable? How often?
4. Do you have problems making decisions?
5. Do you still enjoy things you used to?
6. Do you get upset easily? How often?
7. What do you usually do when you are "blue" (substitute "nervous," "irritable," "restless," "upset" as needed) to feel better?
8. Are you able to talk with anyone when you are "blue" (nervous, irritable, restless, upset)?
9. How do you sleep when you are "blue" (nervous, irritable, restless, upset)?

nurse also consults with the physician regarding the ordering of medication that does not need to be administered during the nighttime hours.

Subjective Manifestations. A review of subjective manifestations furnishes a complete picture of the symptoms the client perceives as related to sleep problems. Chapter 16 provides sample questions for subjective manifestations. The nurse must be aware that some individuals react to stress, emotional problems, or physical illness by having difficulty sleeping. Others respond by increasing their sleep time. Stress-reduction activities may counteract these responses by encouraging relaxation. These activities are very individual, but may include exercise, hand crafts, listening to music, or reading.

Sleep–Rest Examination

Assessment of the integument, head, neck, eyes, chest, abdomen, musculoskeletal system, and neurological system are major components of the sleep–rest examination.

Abnormalities in any of these areas can precipitate sleep disturbances or complicate existing sleep problems. Many clues regarding sleep status can be obtained from general observation of the client. These observations may indicate other areas needing more detailed assessment later in the examination.

Objective Manifestations

General Observations. General observation of the client's overall appearance should be made as an indication of states of rest and alertness. Note the client's posture. Is it slumped forward? Is the body properly aligned? Poor posture can indicate tiredness caused by poor sleep. Correct posture can indicate feeling rested and alert.

In conjunction with observing the client's posture, gait and motor activity should be noted. Clients who move with vigor and perform tasks with enthusiasm are indicating that they have energy provided by adequate sleep and rest. Loss of sleep may cause uncoordinated movements even when performing simple tasks.

During this general observation period, the nurse should also assess the client's facial features. Eyes that appear dull or puffy, have darkened areas under or around them, accompanied by a masklike facial expression, may indicate a lack of sleep.

The client's general physical condition and state of psychological well-being should be observed. The nurse will want to assess orientation to time, place, and person; anxiety level; and general mood. Prolonged loss of sleep often leads to disorientation, nervousness, and mood swings. A distinct personality change in someone who is sleep-deprived may be noted. For example, a usually cheerful person may look unhappy and cry without provocation. Upon questioning, this individual may admit to feeling anxious, a sense of not being "real," or feeling as if the head is going to explode. Individuals who are not sleeping well often have vague complaints of not feeling well in general. Mental status is usually assessed throughout the sleep examination. If the client is inattentive to the nurse, disoriented, anxious, uncooperative, or has vague physical complaints, further examination is warranted. Methods for further assessment are discussed in the section on the neurological examination later in this chapter.

Personal observation during sleep provides another objective means of examining the client. It is also important for the nurse to observe whether or not the client appears rested after sleeping.

Integument. During the sleep examination the integument should be observed for color, texture, and integrity. Healthy-appearing skin indicates adequate rest. Cyanotic skin may indicate a cardiac or pulmonary problem, such as bronchitis, that may interfere with sleep. Impaired skin integrity (such as painful sores or pruritic rashes) may interfere with the ability to obtain adequate sleep due to discomfort.

HEENT. In addition to the assessment of facial features discussed above, a head, eyes, ears, nose, and throat (HEENT) examination should be completed. The nurse should determine whether the client experiences any difficulty breathing through the nose when lying down. Obstruction of the nasal passages can be disruptive to sleep. Any neck vein distension should be noted, as it may indicate congestive heart failure (CHF). Clients with CHF typically have difficulty sleeping in a flat position. The client should also be assessed for distorted vision. Prolonged sleep loss causes the individual to see halos around lights or a webbing effect on the floor.

Chest. Chest inspection may disclose conditions that have potential for interfering with sleep. Observations include the "barrel-shaped chest" of chronic obstructive pulmonary disease (COPD) or the arrhythmia of a cardiac abnormality. The respiratory rate, depth, rhythm, and quality should also be assessed by inspection. Shallow breathing, labored breathing, coughing, or rapid breathing may disrupt sleep.

Chest auscultation will detect heart rate, rhythm, and any abnormal closure of the valves. Disturbances in any of these areas may interrupt sleep either through physical symptoms or from psychological distress due to fear or anxiety over one's cardiac status.

Abnormal breath sounds, such as crackles or wheezes caused by secretions or obstructions, may also be detected upon auscultation. If they are present, it is necessary to assess whether these respiratory problems interfere with the client's rest or sleep. Refer to Chapter 16 for a detailed discussion of the chest assessment.

Abdomen. In addition to the questions asked about gastrointestinal function, the nurse should auscultate the abdomen for the presence of hyperactive or hypoactive bowel sounds. Such sounds may indicate abnormalities that interfere with sleep, such as diarrhea or constipation. Percussion and palpation of the abdomen may reveal an enlarged liver, spleen, or areas of flatus in the intestines. If either is present, inquire about symptoms that may affect sleep, such as pain, tenderness, generalized itching, or the need to pass flatus at night. Chapter 16 provides more detail about the abdominal examination.

Musculoskeletal. For the sleep examination, the musculoskeletal system should be assessed for joint mobility and muscle tone and strength (see Chap. 30). The results of this assessment indicate how much activity the client can tolerate. Also ask how much physical activity is engaged in on a weekly basis. Moderate amounts of exercise several hours before bedtime enhances sleep.

Neurological. If information gathered during the general observation period of the client's mental status indicates a problem, further neurological assessment is necessary. Additional assessment of mental status is part of the neurological examination and involves determining the client's state of awareness, reaction time in performing motor activities, and the capacity for recall of recent and remote memories. The nurse also needs to assess the client's attention span, ability to understand what is being said, and degree of cooperation during the examination. With progressive loss of sleep, the client's state of awareness and attention span decrease while reaction time increases. The individual may exhibit difficulty in recalling the timing of recent events as one day blends into the next. Remote memory remains intact. Such a client also has difficulty understanding what is being said and may become less cooperative in the plan of care. The individual with severe sleep deprivation may even be unable to understand and carry out simple commands, such as "Please be seated" or "Take a deep breath."

Other neurological symptoms may develop with sleep loss. The client should be assessed for skeletal muscle strength, evidence of muscle tremor, and degree of coordination while performing motor tasks (see Chaps. 29 and 30). Lack of sleep results in loss of muscle strength, tremor, and uncoordination.

Diagnostic Tests

Objective methods for examining the client with a sleep dysfunction include the administration of a **nocturnal polysomnogram.** This test involves measuring the sleeping client's brain waves through an electroencephalogram (EEG), eye movements through an electrooculogram (EOG), and muscle movements through an electromyogram (EMG). As part of this examination, the client's respiratory rate, oxygen saturation, and leg movements while asleep are also measured.

The nocturnal polysomnogram reveals how long it takes the client to fall asleep, shows progress through the stages of NREM and REM sleep through the night, and indicates the soundness of sleep. Although the test is performed by someone other than the nurse, the results can be used as part of the assessment data.

■ NURSING DIAGNOSIS OF SLEEP–REST STATUS

Analyzing the data obtained in the sleep–rest history and examination indicates whether the client is experiencing a sleep problem that could be corrected by nursing treatment: a Sleep Pattern Disturbance. This nursing diagnosis and associated etiologies are discussed below and in the Sample Nursing Diagnoses: Sleep–Rest Patterns table, which presents examples of defining characteristics and etiologies for the diagnosis of sleep pattern disturbance. The data may also suggest other nursing diagnoses that may result from disturbed sleep–rest patterns or be caused by sleep disruptions. These diagnoses are listed in Box 28–1.

Sleep Pattern Disturbance

A Sleep Pattern Disturbance is defined as a condition in which individuals are either at risk for or are experiencing actual changes in their sleep patterns that cause discomfort or interfere with their desired life-style. The quality or quantity of sleep is altered for a prolonged time period. Often the reason for the disturbed sleep is an emotional response or a physical illness.

The loss of sleep for 1 to 2 nights followed by restored healthful sleep patterns does not constitute a sleep pattern disturbance. The diagnostic pattern emerges when periods of disturbed sleep continue without restoration of healthful sleep patterns. Unsatisfactory sleep occurs on a nightly basis and may interfere with the individual's emotional and physiological functioning. Performance of usual daytime activities is adversely affected. There are several etiologies of Sleep Pattern Disturbance.

BOX 28–1. OTHER NURSING DIAGNOSES RELATED TO SLEEP–REST PATTERNS

Physical

- Activity Intolerance
- Diarrhea
- Decreased Cardiac Output
- Fluid Volume Deficit
- Hypothermia
- Hyperthermia
- Impaired Physical Mobility
- Altered Nutrition: Less than Body Requirements
- Ineffective Airway Clearance
- Ineffective Breathing Pattern
- Impaired Gas Exchange
- Impaired Skin Integrity
- Altered Tissue Perfusion
- Altered Urinary Elimination Patterns
- Potential for Injury

Cognitive

- Pain
- Sensory Perceptual Alteration

Emotional

- Anxiety
- Ineffective Individual Coping
- Fear
- Grieving

Self-conceptual

- Disturbance in Self-esteem
- Powerlessness
- Hopelessness

Sociocultural/Life Structural

- Ineffective Coping
- Diversional Activity Deficit
- Altered Family Processes
- Social Isolation
- Impaired Home Maintenance Management
- Spiritual Distress

Sexual

- Altered Sexuality Patterns
- Sexual Dysfunction
- Rape-trauma Syndrome

SAMPLE NURSING DIAGNOSES: SLEEP–REST PATTERNS

Nursing Diagnosis	Defining Characteristics: Subjective Data	Defining Characteristics: Objective Data	Etiology
Sleep Pattern Disturbance *6.2.1*	States pain causes difficulty falling asleep. States awakens frequently during night because of pain. Reports not feeling rested.	Frequent yawning Increasing irritability Restlessness Lethargy Listlessness Expressionless face Slight hand tremor Drooping eyelids Dark circles under eyes	*Physical:* Illness: Pain/ discomfort[a]
Sleep Pattern Disturbance *6.2.1*	Reports not feeling rested. States newborn baby interfering with sleep—awakened early AM and throughout night.	Frequent yawning Increased irritability Listlessness Dark circles under eyes	*Developmental:* Social cues: Awakening to feed newborn[a]
Sleep Pattern Disturbance *6.2.1*	Reports not feeling rested. Reports difficulty falling asleep. States awakens earlier than desired. States has used a sleeping pill every night for 2 months so should be sleeping without problems.	Restlessness Lethargy Expressionless face Drooping eyelids Dark circles under eyes Thick speech with mispronunciation and incorrect words	*Cognitive:* Knowledge deficit: Inappropriate use of sleeping medication[a]
Sleep Pattern Disturbance *6.2.1*	Reports not feeling rested. States has difficulty falling asleep—"too much on my mind," "on edge." States hard to get back to sleep if awakened—"feel tense." Reports unfamiliar noises and roommate's need for frequent care cause frequent awakening.	Frequent yawning Increasing irritability Listlessness Dark circles under eyes Halls are noisy Roommate requires 24h care Observed awake 4 or 5 times at night	*Environmental:* Environmental changes: Recent hospitalization[a]

[a] Example only. There are other examples of Sleep Pattern Disturbance with this general etiology. Defining characteristics, desired outcomes, and nursing approaches would differ for each impairment.

Etiology: Illness. Potentially, all types of illness can lead to a diagnosis of sleep pattern disturbance. Individuals with cardiac, pulmonary, renal, gastrointestinal or urological disorders may be particularly vulnerable to disturbed sleep. For example, a client who has decreased circulation of oxygen to the heart may have chest pain at night, or a client with a bladder or kidney infection may need to urinate several times during the night. Other factors that relate to illness and disrupt sleep may include pain, diarrhea, nausea, and vomiting.

Etiology: Psychological Stress. Psychological stress—such as anxiety, grief, depression, tension, and changes in life-style—may disturb sleep for varying periods of time. For example, a student who is experiencing anxiety due to a final examination may not sleep well until the grade is known. Once the grade is received, usual sleep patterns return. On the other hand, an individual who is experiencing grief over the death of a loved one may have difficulty sleeping for several weeks.

Etiology: Environmental Changes. An individual may believe that a satisfactory night's sleep is possible only at home. A certain type of bed, such as a water bed, may be necessary in order for the person to obtain a good night's sleep. Other environmental factors influencing sleep include room temperature, noise level, lighting, time zone changes, changes in bedtime routine, and whether the individual is used to sleeping alone. Changes in any of these variables can disrupt sleep. A move from home to a hospital or nursing home is an example of an environmental change that many people find disrupts their sleep. For some people, any change in sleeping environment, even sleeping at the home of a friend or in a hotel, creates sleep disruptions.

Stating the Sleep–Rest Diagnosis

Analysis of the data to determine the exact nature of the sleep problem and its etiology should result in a precise statement regarding the client's sleep status. The assessment data provides clues that may be used to refine broad statements from the taxonomy (such as "Sleep Pattern Disturbance Related to Impaired Bowel Function") into concise statements with defining characteristics. These defining characteristics support the selection of the particular diagnosis. For example, the broad diagnosis cited above becomes "Sleep Pattern Disturbance related to diarrhea as evidenced by eight liquid stools from 1 AM to 3 AM, complaints of the continued need to use the bathroom during the night, and complaints of not feeling rested."

Complete assessment of the client's sleep patterns is an important aspect of comprehensive client care. A complete sleep–rest history includes the current understanding; past health problems/experiences; personal, family, and social history; subjective manifestations; and the results of diagnostic tests. The findings of the objective sleep–rest examination, or polysomnogram, to identify sleep dysfunctions should also be considered in the assessment process. The results of the assessment lead nurses to an accurate diagnosis of Sleep Pattern Disturbance and its etiology. After arriving at an accurate diagnosis, nurses collaborate with clients, family, and other health care professionals to manage the identified sleep disturbance.

Section 3. Nurse–Client Management of Sleep–Rest Patterns

Nurse–client management of sleep problems involves collaborative planning to meet the client's assessed sleep needs. Appropriate nursing implementation to enhance, promote, or reestablish sleep patterns is determined by the client's level of care and the cause of disrupted sleep.

PLANNING FOR OPTIMUM SLEEP AND REST

In addition to communicating the desired outcomes for client care, an effective client care plan also communicates the methods for achieving these outcomes. In an individualized care plan, the statements of desired outcomes should describe the amount of uninterrupted sleep the client should receive as a result of nursing care. These statements provide a guide to specific implementation that can be used and criteria by which the effectiveness of these implementations can be evaluated.

Sleep outcomes are best determined by mutual goal setting. From the assessment data, the nurse formulates perceptions of what factors are disrupting the client's sleep and what can realistically be done to alleviate the problem. The nurse should then share these perceptions with clients and ask for their input. In this way, the client can contribute to setting goals that are acceptable and important to individual care. The nurse may also need to consult with other health care professionals involved in the client's care (eg, the physician, physical therapist, and respiratory therapist) in order to establish realistic desired outcomes.

For example, Mr. Torcello and the nurse note that his sleep is interrupted every 4 hours during the night for medication. Mr. Torcello also states that physical therapy interrupts his morning nap and he feels "exhausted." After consulting with the physician, the nurse determines that Mr. Torcello's medication schedule cannot be changed. However, after talking with physical therapy, the therapist agrees to change his session to early afternoon. Thus, Mr. Torcello is able to nap for 3 hours in the morning.

When planning to reach a long-term outcome, it may be necessary to first set short-term outcomes. In the example given above, the long-term outcome would be: "The client will receive 8 hours of uninterrupted nocturnal sleep within 2 weeks." A short-term outcome would be: "The client will receive 2 hours of uninterrupted morning nap time every 24 hours." As the client's medication schedule changes, it will be possible to meet the long-term outcome with appropriate planning. In the meantime, it is possible to attain the short-term outcome. It is important to remember that the individualized outcome statement describes specific client behavior and establishes a time period within which the outcome should be attained. Thus, it is possible to measure and document progress toward outcome achievement.

IMPLICATIONS FOR NURSE–CLIENT COLLABORATION

Sleep–Rest Planning

Planning for a client's individual needs means determining what measures should be used to achieve the desired outcomes related to sleep and rest. Collaborative planning usually provides the most realistic and workable approaches to care, because it ensures that the choices will be compatible with the client's concerns and values as well as with the scientific principles that ground the nurse's recommendations.

NURSING IMPLEMENTATION TO PROMOTE OPTIMUM SLEEP AND REST

The next part of planning for clients' sleep needs is determining what nursing measures should be used to achieve

NURSE–CLIENT MANAGEMENT OF SLEEP–REST PROBLEMS

Nursing Diagnosis	Desired Outcomes	Implementation	Evaluation
Sleep Pattern Disturbance R/T pain, discomfort *6.2.1*	1. Progressive decrease in time between going to bed and sleep onset.	1a. Assist client into comfortable sleeping position. 1b. Teach client progressive relaxation. 1c. Offer a back massage. 1d. Reduce environmental distractions. 1e. Suggest bedtime snack containing tryptophane and carbohydrates, such as milk with fruit or cookie. 1f. Maintain client's usual bedtime routine. 1g. Suggest warm bath before bedtime.	1. Client reports falls asleep within 15 minutes after going to bed.
	2. Progressive increase in amount of uninterrupted sleep each night to 8 hours.	2. Consult with physician regarding an analgesic to be given before bedtime.	2. Client reports sleeps 6–8 hours each night without interruption.
	3. Progressive improvement in quality of rest each night.	3. Client reports sleeps 6–8 hours each night without interruption.	3a. Client reports feels rested in AM; is less irritable. 3b. No dark circles under eyes. 3c. No yawning noted.
Sleep Pattern Disturbance R/T social cues: awakening to feed newborn *6.2.1*	1. Increase in total sleep time per 24-hour period to total of at least 8 hours sleep per 24 hours.	1a. Suggest client feed and change infant immediately before retiring at night. 1b. Suggest client nap when infant naps during day. 1c. Teach client progressive relaxation, suggest warm bath before bedtime.	1. Client reports receiving 2 more 4-hour periods of uninterrupted nighttime sleep and napping 2 hours a day.
Sleep Pattern Disturbance R/T knowledge deficit: inappropriate use of sleeping medication *6.2.1*	1. Client aware of risks of long-term use of sleeping medications.	1a. Teach client the adverse effects on sleep of routine use of medication. 1b. Collaborate with physician and client to schedule gradual decrease in drug dosage until discontinued.	1. Client correctly states risks associated with use of sleeping medications.
	2. Progressive decrease in time between going to bed and sleep onset.	2a. Teach client progressive relaxation. 2b. Reduce environmental distractions. 2c. Suggest bedtime snack containing tryptophane and carbohydrates, such as milk with fruit or cookies. 2d. Maintain client's usual bedtime routine. 2e. Suggest warm bath before bedtime.	2. Client reports falls asleep within 15 minutes after going to bed.

Nursing Diagnosis	Desired Outcomes	Implementation	Evaluation
	3. Progressive increase in amount of uninterrupted sleep each night to 8 hours. 4. Progressive improvement in quality of rest each night.	3,4a. Discuss value of regular exercise in promoting healthy sleep patterns. 3,4b. Suggest limiting evening fluid intake, especially of alcoholic beverages and beverages containing caffeine.	3. Client reports sleeps 6–8 hours each night without interruption. 4a. Client reports receiving 6–8 hours of restful sleep 10 days after discontinuing sleeping medication. 4b. Dark circles under eyes/drooping eyelids absent. 4c. Speech clear. 4d. Facial expression animated.
Sleep Pattern Disturbance R/T recent hospitalization *6.2.1*	1. Progressive decrease in time between going to bed and sleep onset.	1a. Teach client progressive relaxation. 1b. Offer a back massage. 1c. Suggest warm bath before bedtime. 1d. Assess client's usual bedtime routine and incorporate into care.	1. Client reports falls asleep within 15 minutes after going to bed.
	2. Uninterrupted nighttime sleep.	2a. Reduce environmental distractions (close door to room, reassign to another room, reduce lighting). 2b. Give treatments, medications at same time when possible and time other than when client usually sleeps.	2a. Client reports sleeps 6–8 hours each night without interruption. 2b. Noted to be asleep when checked by night shift nurses.

the desired outcomes. The assessment data and selected outcomes suggest the appropriate client care. Again, collaborative or mutual planning among nurse, client, and other health care professionals provides the most realistic and workable approaches to care.

A complete sleep care plan addresses all of the problems stated in the nursing diagnoses and the implementation to be used to attain each outcome. The nursing treatment is then carried out, and its effectiveness is evaluated in terms of what progress the client is making in achieving the desired outcome. If this ongoing or day-to-day evaluation reveals that progress is slow or nonexistent, it is necessary to reassess the desired outcome and the treatments for their appropriateness to the client's needs. Revisions in the plan of care are made as needed.

Specific nursing approaches to assist the client with sleep needs involve a variety of nursing skills and depend upon the etiology of the sleep pattern disturbance and the related nursing diagnoses. The Nurse–Client Management of Sleep–Rest Problems table describes standardized management of sleep pattern disturbance for various etiologies. Age-appropriate implementation for each level of care is shown in Table 28–2.

Preventive Care

Preventive care focuses on the individual who is at risk for developing sleep pattern disturbances. Nursing implementation is formulated to prevent the development of these problems with the knowledge that clients are responsible for their care. Some factors that place an individual at risk for developing sleep pattern disturbance were described earlier in this chapter.

Screening and Risk Assessment. For the healthy individual at risk for developing disturbed sleep, screening and risk assessment are appropriate nursing actions. The nurse should explore any variables in the client's life-style that may disrupt sleep. These may include shift work, regular use of alcohol and/or stimulants, inappropriate timing of exercise in relation to bedtime, and inappropriate use of sleeping medication. Situational stressors should also be assessed. These may include job tension, interpersonal problems, or being responsible for a newborn or chronically ill family member.

Health Education. Health education is an important part of preventive care. Clients at risk should be taught the im-

TABLE 28–2. AGE-APPROPRIATE NURSING IMPLEMENTATION FOR SLEEP PATTERN DISTURBANCE

	Level of Client Care			
Developmental Stage	**Preventive**	**Supportive**	**Restorative**	**Rehabilitative**
Infant/Toddler	Screening and risk assessment with parents. Health education with parents regarding usual sleep patterns of developmental stage; reduction of environmental distractions and use of bedtime routines and comfort measures to induce sleep.	See preventive care. Initiate a daily schedule to incorporate sleep opportunities.	See preventive and supportive care. Use of any ordered medications and treatments for underlying illness interfering with sleep. Comfort measures, such as rocking, singing; appropriate room temperature, clothing, and bed covers.	See preventive and supportive care. Referrals to other health care professionals to reestablish healthful sleep patterns. Health teaching on ways to induce and maintain sleep.
Preschooler	Screening and risk assessment with parents. Health education with parents regarding usual sleep patterns of developmental stage; reduction of environmental distractions and use of bedtime routines and comfort measures to induce sleep.	Preventive care. Initiate a daily schedule to incorporate sleep opportunities. Have parents keep a sleep log of child's sleep patterns. Have parents complete assessment tool of child's sleep patterns.	Preventive and supportive care. Use of any ordered medications and treatments for underlying illness interfering with sleep. Comfort measures, such as rocking, singing; appropriate room temperature, clothing, and bed covers; reading a bedtime story; offering a bedtime snack; warm bath.	Preventive and supportive care. Referrals to other health care professionals to reestablish healthful sleep patterns. Health teaching on ways to induce and maintain sleep.
Child	Screening and risk assessment with parents. Health education with parents regarding usual sleep patterns of developmental stage; reduction of environmental distractions and use of bedtime routines and comfort measures to induce sleep. Routinely scheduled exercise to promote sleep.	Preventive care. Initiate a daily schedule to incorporate sleep opportunities. Have parents keep a sleep log of child's sleep patterns. Have parents complete assessment tool of child's sleep patterns. Initiate an exercise program.	Preventive and supportive care. Use of any ordered medications and treatments for underlying illness interfering with sleep. Comfort measures, such as appropriate room temperature, clothing, and bed covers; reading a bedtime story; offering a bedtime snack; warm bath, back rub; allowing older children to read, listen to music.	Preventive and supportive care. Referrals to other health care professionals to reestablish healthful sleep patterns. Health teaching on ways to induce and maintain sleep.
Adolescent/Young adult	1. Screening and risk assessment related to life-style and stressors that interfere with sleep. 2. Health education on reduction of environmental distractions and use of bedtime routines and comfort measures to induce sleep, and routinely scheduled exercise to promote sleep, as well as relaxation techniques.	1. Preventive care. 2. Initiate a daily schedule to incorporate sleep opportunities. 3. Initiate an exercise program. 4. Have client complete a sleep log. 5. Have client complete a self-assessment tool.	1. Preventive and supportive care. 2. Use of any ordered medications and treatments for underlying illness interfering with sleep. 3. Comfort measures, such as appropriate room temperature, clothing, and bed covers; bedtime snack; warm bath, back rub; listening to music; positioning.	1. Preventive and restorative care. 2. Referrals to other health care professionals to reestabish healthful sleep patterns. 3. Health teaching on ways to induce and maintain sleep. 4. Use of restorative care.

TABLE 28–2. (continued)

Developmental Stage	Level of Client Care: Preventive	Supportive	Restorative	Rehabilitative
			4. Limited use of sedatives. 5. Use of noninvasive pain relief, such as imagery, distraction.	
Middle-aged/Older adult	1. Screening and risk assessment related to life-style and stressors that interfere with sleep. 2. Health education on reduction of environmental distractions and use of bedtime routines and comfort measures to induce sleep, and routinely scheduled exercise to promote sleep, as well as relaxation techniques.	1. Preventive care. 2. Initiate a daily schedule to incorporate sleep opportunities. 3. Initiate an exercise program. 4. Have client complete a sleep log. 5. Have client complete a sleep self-assessment tool.	1. Preventive and supportive care. 2. Use of any ordered medications and treatments for underlying illness interfering with sleep. 3. Comfort measures, such as appropriate room temperature, clothing, and bed covers; bedtime snack; warm bath, back rub; listening to music; positioning. 4. Limited use of sedatives. 5. Use of noninvasive pain relief, such as imagery, distraction.	1. Preventive supportive and restorative care. 2. Referrals to other health care professionals to reestablish healthful sleep patterns. 3. Health teaching related to ways to induce and maintain sleep.

portance of maintaining a bedtime routine, remaining active during the day, and reducing or eliminating environmental distractions at bedtime. For example, the nurse may suggest that the client close the bedroom door, unplug the telephone, or request that others in the home reduce the volume of radios or televisions. The nurse should emphasize that regular physical exercise promotes sleep when carried out well before bedtime, and preferably in the early afternoon. Vigorous activity immediately before bedtime may delay sleep onset. Many people find that quiet activity such as reading or listening to soft music promotes relaxation and facilitates sleep.

The nurse can also teach clients the importance of certain comfort measures to induce sleep. These may include the use of an extra pillow or blanket or a freshly made bed. Some clients may find a warm bath a useful relaxation technique. Progressive relaxation (a combination of rhythmic, slow breathing and progressive relaxation of the body's muscle groups) may reduce anxiety and tension that delays sleep onset and/or interferes with sleep maintenance. (See Chap. 22 for further discussion of the use of progressive relaxation for hospitalized and nonhospitalized individuals.)

Many people experiencing occasional sleep problems view over-the-counter (OTC) sleep medications as a quick, easy solution. Teaching about the dangers associated with the use of OTC sleep preparations is therefore another focus for health education related to sleep problems. Inform clients that these drugs alter normal sleep cycles, especially REM sleep, and that prolonged use can result in dependency. Rebound insomnia and vivid dreams, even nightmares, often occur when OTC sleep medications are discontinued after regular use. Clients who are aware of the risks associated with inappropriate use of OTC preparations to induce sleep are more likely to select noninvasive approaches to enhance sleep and to use any medication for sleep with caution.

Supportive Care

Supportive care for sleep focuses on clients who are experiencing mild problems with sleep, such as a frequent traveler with jet lag or new parents experiencing sleep disruptions due to an infant's sleep–wakefulness cycle. This care usually occurs in a nonhospital setting, such as a community-health agency, physician's office, or the client's home; however, supportive implementation may also be appropriate for use with hospitalized clients. The primary goal is to prevent further disruption of sleep patterns. The nurse and client should collaborate to determine the cause of the sleep problems and make a daily schedule that incorporates adequate opportunities for sleep.

Sleep Log. The use of a sleep log in which clients record sleep periods can be used to identify sleep patterns. To keep a sleep log, clients can take a blank piece of paper and write down each time they sleep in a 24-hour period. They should include the approximate time they fall asleep and

PROCEDURE 28–1. PROVIDING EVENING (PM) CARE

☐ **PURPOSE:** To assist the client in preparing for bed and to promote sleep.

☐ **EQUIPMENT:** Basin of warm water; wash cloth; towels; dental care items; cup; emesis basin; skin lotion or powder; deodorant; urinal, bedpan, bedside commode, toilet paper.

ACTION

1. Gather equipment.
2. Discuss the purpose of evening care with the client.
3. Provide privacy.
4. Wash hands.
5. Adjust bed to a comfortable working position, with siderail farthest from nurse in up position.
6. To reduce possibility of interrupted sleep, if client is unable to walk to the bathroom, assist with bedpan, urinal, or bedside commode (see Procedure 26–4).
7. Provide basin with warm water and soap to wash face and hands. Assist as needed.
8. To promote comfort and relaxation, assist with dental and mouth care as needed (see Procedure 24–1).
9. If desired, assist with hair care.
10. If needed or requested by client, assist with bath (see Procedure 24–10).
11. Clean and store reusable equipment; discard disposables according to agency policy.
12. Replace any soiled linens. Straighten unsoiled linen and fluff pillow.
13. To promote muscle relaxation and minimize RAS activation, provide back rub (see Procedure 28–2).
14. Assist client into comfortable position for sleep.
15. Straighten top covers. Provide additional covers as needed.
16. Provide sleep medication if ordered.
17. To promote client safety, place bed in low position. Place call light within reach. For some clients, raise side rails to up position.
18. Wash hands.
19. Turn lights off or low to decrease RAS stimulation.

☐ **RECORDING:** Note specific care provided and client's response. Many agencies use a checklist for procedures such as evening care.

awaken for each sleep period. Finally, they total the number of hours slept for the past 24 hours. The sleep log should be kept for at least 7 days.

Self-assessment Tool. A self-assessment tool to be completed by clients is useful in identifying risk factors that can be altered to promote sleep. Such risk factors have been discussed previously in this chapter. Most self-assessment tools ask clients to record the time they go to bed, how calm they feel at bedtime, how tired they feel at bedtime, and to estimate the time they fall asleep. Clients indicate their bedtime routines; illnesses; exercise routines; and use of medications, alcohol, and caffeine-containing products, including the times these substances are ingested. In the morning, clients record the number of nighttime awakenings they experienced, their perceived movement during sleep, the time they awakened in the morning, and how satisfied they feel with the previous night's sleep. Sleep assessment tools should be used for at least 3 to 4 nights so that any patterns can be noted.

Supportive approaches to promote sleep include reestablishing the client's usual bedtime routines, exercising vigorously 6 to 8 hours before bedtime, reducing or eliminating environmental distractions, providing comfort measures, and teaching the client a relaxation technique. Several relaxation techniques are available (see Chap. 22). All of them reduce anxiety and tension that delay sleep onset and/or interfere with sleep maintenance. If the client is already familiar with a technique, encourage its use. Progressive relaxation may also be used in second-level care.

Restorative Care

Restorative care for sleep focuses on acute sleep pattern disturbances. Here, lack of sleep has become so pronounced that the client's physical and psychological well-being is threatened.

Noninvasive Measures. Nursing implementation for acute sleep disturbance includes treating the underlying cause of the sleep problem. In some cases, the cause of the client's sleep disturbance may be treatable by nurses using noninvasive pain measures (see Chap. 22) or assisting with positioning for comfort (see Chap. 30). Evening care, including a back rub, is a planned part of the client's care and can assist in the promotion of sleep. Procedure 28–1 presents the routine evening or PM care that should be given by the nurse. Procedure 28–2 outlines the correct procedure for a back rub.

Administering Medications. Sometimes correcting the cause of the sleep problem involves collaborating with other health care providers, such as administering medications and treatments ordered by the physician. When the underlying illness is resolved, healthier sleep patterns return. For example, clients with acute congestive heart failure often experience disturbed sleep due to difficulty breathing. Giving diuretics according to the physicians's order, cardiac medications, and oxygen often relieves the breathing difficulties, allowing the client to sleep more comfortably. The use of preventive and supportive implementation to promote comfort and reduce environmental stimuli is also appropriate during the acute phase of most illnesses if sleep is disturbed.

The nurse may also administer sedative–hypnotic or

PROCEDURE 28–2. GIVING A BACK RUB

PURPOSE: To promote relaxation and induce sleep.

EQUIPMENT: Skin care lotion, bath blanket, and bath towel.

ACTION	RATIONALE
1. Discuss the purpose and expected benefits of the back rub and ask the client if one is desired.	1. Client is more likely to agree to the activity if its purpose is clearly explained, and if the opportunity to provide consent is given.
NOTE: Use language that is easily understood. Some clients may view the back rub as an invasion of privacy or place it in a sexual context. A clear explanation of benefits of back rub can prevent misinterpretation.	
2. Provide privacy. Use low lighting.	2. Personal care is considered a private activity in most cultures; client relaxation is facilitated if need for privacy is respected. Low light reduces RAS activation.
3. Wash hands.	3. Removes transient microorganisms from nurse's hands, preventing transfer to client.
4. Adjust bed to a comfortable working position, with siderail farthest from nurse up.	4. Raising bed prevents nurse's backstrain. Raising side rail prevents client falling out of bed.
5. Assist or request that client assume prone or semiprone position. Pillow under head is optional. Pregnant clients, and those with recent abdominal surgery, may be unable to assume these positions. Use sidelying position instead.	5. These positions provide greatest exposure of back and buttocks.
6. Using a bath blanket, drape client so that back, shoulders, and upper buttocks are exposed. In some agencies, bed covers are used instead of bath blanket to cover abdomen (if sidelying) and legs.	6. Provides warmth, minimizes feelings of exposure.
7. Pour a moderate amount of lotion onto the palm of your hand. Rub your hands together to warm lotion. Lotion may also be warmed by placing bottle in a basin of warm water during preceding care activities.	7. Lotion reduces friction between nurse's hands and client's skin. Cold lotion is uncomfortable and may cause chilling.
8. Tell client you are ready to begin. Warn that lotion may feel a bit cool at first.	8. Avoids startling client.

(continued)

PROCEDURE 28–2. (continued)

9. Using firm, steady pressure, move your hands slowly up either side of the spine from the buttocks to the base of neck, across the shoulders, and down the lateral aspects of the back, returning to the buttocks. Repeat 3–5 times.

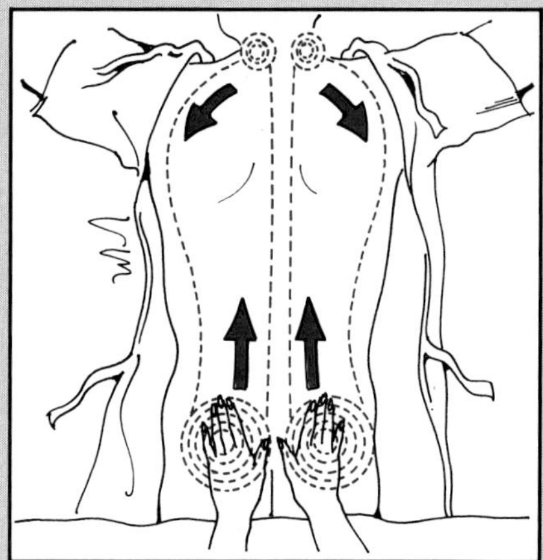

9. Firm pressure is relaxing and reassuring. Light pressure may be perceived as a tickling sensation. Rapid movements are stimulating rather than relaxing.

10. Next, using a kneading motion, rub your hands over the scapulae and upper shoulders. Work down to the sacrum and posterior illiac spines. Kneading should be done gently to avoid pinching the client. Obtain more lotion as needed.

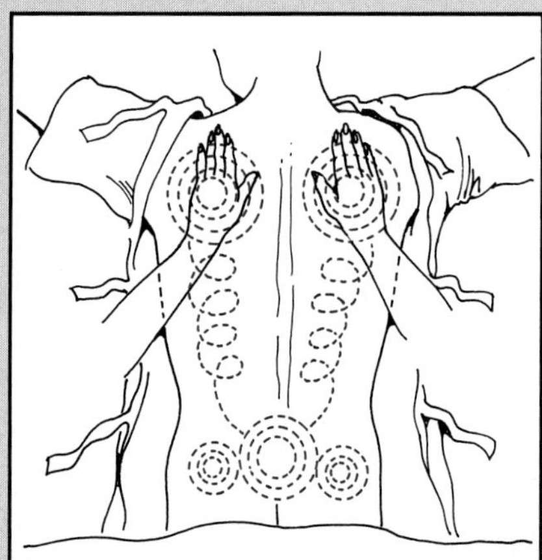

10–12. These movements promote muscle relaxation in all major muscle groups of posterior trunk, many of which may become tense and/or sore from bedrest. Tense or sore muscles may cause RAS activation, promoting wakefulness. Circulation over boney prominences (scapulae, sacrum, posterior illiac spines) is also stimulated, thereby reducing the risk of pressure ulcers (see Chap. 30).

(continued)

PROCEDURE 28–2. (continued)

11. Using a figure-8 motion, massage from the sacrum over each buttock. Repeat 3 times.

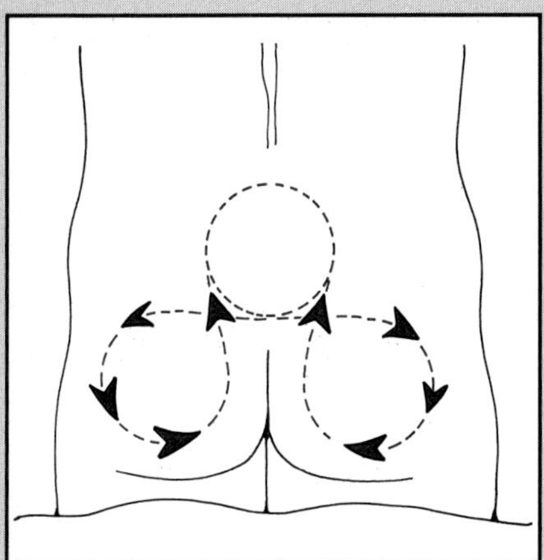

12. Rub up and down the back with a long, stroking motion. Repeat 3 times.

13. Repeat steps 9–12 for 5–10 minutes.

13. Time required to achieve relaxed state is variable.

14. Wipe excess lotion off the client's back with the bath towel, close gown, and remove and store bath blanket.

14. Excess lotion may cause skin, gown, or sheets to feel damp or sticky, interfering with relaxation.

15. Assist client into desired position and adjust bed covers.

15, 16. Promotes client comfort and safety, which reduces cortical activity, thereby minimizing RAS activation.

16. Place bed in low position with both siderails up. Place call light within reach.

17. Wash hands.

17. Removes transient microorganisms, preventing transfer to other clients.

RECORDING: Note procedure, condition of skin, degree of relaxation reported by client, and any complaints of discomfort. If skin lesions noted, record associated action taken.

tranquilizer drugs ordered by the physician to induce sleep directly. Examples of sedative–hypnotics include flurazepam (Dalmane), temazepam (Restoril), and triazolam (Halcion). Examples of tranquilizers include diazepam (Valium), chlordiazepoxide HCl (Librax), oxazepam (Serax), lorazepam (Ativan), and alprazolam (Xanax). These medications should be used only on a short-term basis while the client's normal sleep patterns are being restored. Prolonged use of these medications (over 2 weeks) may cause rebound sleep pattern disturbance, restlessness, depression, and drug dependency. Table 28–3 compares the various medications for sleep (see Chap. 22 for guidelines on administering controlled substances).

Reassessment of sleep during drug therapy is an important nursing function. If medication has been used every night for 10 to 14 nights, the nurse should discuss discontinuation of the medication with the physician. The client will also need information concerning these drugs and their actions and side effects so that they will not be used on a routine basis.

TABLE 28–3. COMPARISON OF MEDICATIONS USED FOR SLEEP

Medication	Mode of Action	Duration of Action	Side Effects	Nursing Implementation
Barbiturates pentobarbital (Nembutal) secobarbital (Seconal)	Produce all levels of CNS depression.	PO = 1–4 h IM = 1–4 h IV = 15 min Rectal = 1–4 h	*CNS:* drowsiness, lethargy, hangover, depression, delirium, excitation, restlessness. *Dermatological:* urticaria, rashes. *GI:* nausea, vomiting *Misc.:* hypersensitivity reactions, psychological dependence, tolerance to increasing doses, physical dependence at high doses.	■ Assess sleep patterns before and during drug therapy. ■ Caution client of possibility of increased dreaming upon discontinuing therapy. REM sleep is suppressed by barbiturates. ■ Limit amount of drug available to client, especially if suicidal, depressed, or has history of addiction. ■ Caution client to avoid daytime activities requiring alertness until effect of medication is known. ■ Advise against concurrent use of alcohol or CNS depressants. ■ Use side rails and place call light within reach after drug administration. ■ Assist with ambulation after administration. ■ Monitor respirations, pulse, and blood pressure during IV administration.
Benzodiazepines Sedative–hypnotics flurazepam (Dalmane) temazepam (Restoril) triazolam (Halcion)	Act on CNS to produce general depression.	flurazepam: 7–8 h temazepam: unknown triazolam: unknown	*CNS:* dizziness, drowsiness, lethargy, hangover, confusion, mental depression, headache, paradoxical excitation. *Dermatological:* rashes. *GI:* nausea, vomiting, diarrhea, heartburn. *Misc.:* psychological dependence, physical dependence, tolerance.	■ Assess sleep patterns before and during drug therapy. ■ Limit amount of drug available to client, especially if suicidal, depressed, or has history of addiction. ■ Caution client to avoid daytime activities requiring alertness until effect of medication is known. ■ Advise against concurrent use of alcohol or CNS depressants. ■ Use side rails and place call light within reach after drug administration. ■ Assist with ambulation after administration ■ For *triazolam* and *temazepam,* do not administer within 1 h of antacids, as they impair absorption. May administer with food to prevent gastric irritation.

TABLE 28–3. (continued)

Medication	Mode of Action	Duration of Action	Side Effects	Nursing Implementation
Tranquilizers alprazolam (Xanax) Chlordiazepoxide HCl (Librax) diazepam (Valium) lorazepam (Ativan) oxazepam (Serax)	Produce CNS depression and skeletal muscle relaxation. Have antianxiety properties.	alprazolam: up to 24 h chlordiazepoxide HCl: 4–8 h diazepam: up to 24 h lorazepam: up to 48 h oxazepam: 6–12 h	*CNS:* dizziness, drowsiness, lethargy, hangover, confusion, mental depression, headache, paradoxical excitation. *Dermatological:* rashes. *GI:* nausea, vomiting, diarrhea, heartburn. *Respiratory:* respiratory depression. *Misc.:* psychological dependence, physical dependence, tolerance.	■ Assess sleep patterns before and during drug therapy. ■ Limit amount of drug available to client, especially if suicidal, depressed, or has history of addiction. ■ Caution client to avoid daytime activities requiring alertness until effect of medication is known. ■ Advise against concurrent use of alcohol or CNS depressants. ■ Use side rails and place call light within reach after drug administration. ■ Assist with ambulation after administration. ■ Assess degree of anxiety before and during therapy. ■ Caution that abrupt withdrawal of medication may cause insomnia, nervousness, irritability. ■ May administer with milk to reduce gastric irritation.
Chloral hydrate Aquachloral, Noctec, Oradrate	Generalized CNS depression.	4–8 h	*CNS:* excess sedation, hangover, disorientation. *Dermatological:* rashes. *GI:* nausea, vomiting, diarrhea, flatulence. *Respiratory:* respiratory depression. *Misc:* tolerance, psychological dependence, physical dependence.	■ Assess sleep patterns before and during drug therapy. ■ Caution client to avoid daytime activities requiring alertness until effect of medication is known. ■ Use side rails and place call light within reach after drug administration. ■ Assist with ambulation after administration. ■ Advise that concurrent use of alcohol may cause vasodilation, flushing, tachycardia, hypotension, headache. ■ Caution that abrupt withdrawal may result in anxiety, CNS excitement, tremor, hallucination, delirium. ■ Advise client to swallow capsules whole with a full glass of water to avoid gastric irritation.

From Deglin JH, Vallerand AH. Davis' Drug Guide for Nurses. *Philadelphia: Davis; 1988. Gerald MC, O'Bannon FV.* Nursing Pharmacology and Therapeutics. *Norwalk, CT: Appleton & Lange; 1988. Karch AM, Boyd EH.* Handbook of Drugs and the Nursing Process. *Philadelphia: Lippincott; 1989.*

In addition to monitoring the client's use of sleep medication, the nurse should also assess the drug's effectiveness in treating the sleep problem. If the client's sleep is improved, the drug is serving its purpose. The client also needs to be assessed for side effects of the particular sleep medication being used. If any are present, the physician should be notified and the sleep medication discontinued or changed. Safety factors, such as keeping the bed in a low position and using siderails, must also be observed while sleep medication is in use.

Other nursing measures for acute sleep disturbances depend on the client's age and developmental stage. For example, if a toddler is experiencing disturbed sleep due to inadequate parental limit setting, the nurse and parents must plan together to establish appropriate and consistent bedtime limits for the child. Many times, these plans are similar to those for rehabilitative care.

Rehabilitative Care

Rehabilitative care is focused on reestablishing the client's usual sleep patterns or on establishing new habits because of health alterations or their treatment. Appropriate health teaching and referrals comprise the key implementation in this stage. The nurse should acquaint clients with the type and amount of sleep appropriate for their ages, assist in reducing stress that interferes with sleep, explain the causes of sleep pattern disturbances and ways to avoid them, and explain measures that can be used to relieve symptoms of disturbed sleep, such as relaxation exercises, physical exercise, and a glass of warm milk before retiring. Once again, the use of preventive and supportive implementations is appropriate in this stage and may be discussed with the client.

EVALUATION

In evaluating the effectiveness of the client care plan, the nurse and client consider progress toward the desired outcomes and the influence of current sleep patterns on physical and psychological well-being. If the evaluation reveals that satisfactory sleep has not been achieved, reassessment and replanning must be undertaken in collaboration with the client in another attempt to reach that outcome.

When the desired outcome has been achieved, a notation should be made in the chart. If it has not been achieved by the time indicated in the outcome statement, a notation of reassessment findings and alternative plans should be given.

IMPLICATIONS FOR NURSE–CLIENT COLLABORATION

Evaluation

Evaluation of sleep and rest is a collaborative process. One phase of evaluating the client's rest is to gain the client's subjective appraisal of how rested he or she feels. This requires that the nurse and client communicate directly about the amount of sleep or rest the client has had, the quality of the rest, and the energy level that the client experiences as a result. The nurse should also observe how well the client appeared to rest as well as observations on the client's mood and apparent energy. Based on this mutual assessment, care plan approaches are revised when it is clear to both the client and the nurse that they have not achieved desired sleep and rest outcomes.

SUMMARY

Sleep and rest are basic human needs essential to the individual's physical and psychological well-being and wellness. The sleep–wakefulness cycle is one of the circadian rhythms. It is regulated by neurological and chemical processes.

Healthful sleep patterns are composed of nonrapid eye movement (NREM) and rapid eye movement (REM) sleep. The four stages of NREM sleep conserve the body's energy and repair tissue. Most dreaming occurs during REM sleep. Healthful sleep patterns change throughout the life cycle and are affected by age, environment, nutrition, stress, exercise, illness, medications, alcohol, and stimulants.

Sleep dysfunctions are categorized into three major classes. Although specific disorders within these categories differ by developmental stage, there are some commonalities in these disorders across the life span. For example, Disorders in Initiating and Maintaining Sleep are characterized by difficulty in falling asleep, frequent awakenings, and difficulty returning to sleep regardless of age. Disorders of Excessive Somnolence are characterized by increased daytime sleepiness and include sleep apnea and narcolepsy. Disorders of Arousal are usually seen in those under 20 years of age and include sleepwalking, sleeptalking, confusional arousals, and enuresis.

Providing for adequate rest and sleep is a primary nursing responsibility. Collaboration with client, family members, and the health care team is essential to the success of this function. Assessment of sleep–rest patterns includes obtaining a complete sleep–rest history. The assessment data are used to formulate a nursing diagnosis of Sleep Pattern Disturbance with a specific etiology, that may be physical, emotional, developmental, cognitive, environmental, sociocultural/life structural, sexual, or self-conceptual.

Management of sleep pattern disturbance is also a collaborative effort. Specific nursing implementation depends on the client's level of care. Appropriate nursing implementation is selected on the basis of the client's identified level of care. Evaluation of the desired outcome—an adequate amount of restful sleep—is an essential part of this process.

REFERENCES

1. Webb WB. *Sleep: The Gentle Tyrant.* Englewood Cliffs, NJ: Prentice-Hall; 1975.
2. Glenville M, et al. Effects of sleep deprivation on short duration performance measures compared to the Wilkinson auditory vigilance task. *Sleep.* 1978;1:169–176.
3. Ellis JR, Nowlis EA. *Nursing: A Human Needs Approach.* Boston: Houghton-Mifflin; 1985.
4. Anch MA, et al. *Sleep: A Scientific Perspective.* Englewood Cliffs, NJ: Prentice-Hall; 1988.
5. Hart LK, Freel MI & Milde FK. Fatigue. *Nurs Clin North Am.* 1990;25(4):967–976.
6. Mendelson WB. *Human Sleep: Research and Clinical Care.* New York: Plenum; 1987.
7. Webster RA. Sleep in hospital. *J Ad Nurs.* 1986;11:447–457.
8. Guyton AC. *Textbook of Medical Physiology.* 8th ed. Philadelphia: Saunders; 1990.
9. Ebersole P, Hess P. *Toward Healthy Aging: Human Needs and Nursing Response.* St. Louis: Mosby; 1985.
10. Closs SJ. Assessment of sleep in hospital patients: A review of methods. *J Adv Nurs.* 1988;13:501–510.
11. Hayter J. The rhythm of sleep. *Am J Nurs.* 1980;80:457–461.
12. Robinson C. Impaired sleep. In: Carrieri VK, Lindsey AM, West CM, eds. *Pathophysiological Phenomena in Nursing: Human Responses to Illness.* Philadelphia: Saunders; 1986.
13. Slota MC. Implications of sleep deprivation in the pediatric critical care unit. *Focus Crit Care.* 1988;15(3):35–43.
14. Riley TL, Ferber R. Behavioral aspects of sleep. In: Riley TL, ed. *Clinical Aspects of Sleep and Sleep Disturbance.* Boston: Butterworth; 1985.
15. Carskadon MA. Insomnia and sleep disturbances in the elderly. *J Geriatr Psych.* 1980;13:135–151.
16. Jones J., Hoggart, B., Withey, J., et al. What patients say: A study of reactions to an intensive care unit. *Int Care Med.* 1979; 5:89–92.
17. Ferber R. Sleep disorders in infants and children. In: Riley TL, ed. *Clinical Aspects of Sleep and Sleep Disturbance.* Boston: Butterworth; 1985.
18. Hauri PJ. Primary sleep disorders and insomnia. In: Riley TL, ed. *Clinical Aspects of Sleep and Sleep Disturbance.* Boston: Butterworth; 1985.

BIBLIOGRAPHY

Becker PT, et al. Correlates of diurnal sleep patterns in infants of adolescent and adult single mothers. *Res Nurs and Health.* 1991; 14:97–108.

Carrier VK, Lindsey AM, West CM. *Pathophysiological Phenomena in Nursing: Human Responses to Illness.* Philadelphia: Saunders; 1986.

Closs J. Patient's sleep-wake rhythms in hospital. Part I. *Nurs Times.* 1988;84(1)48–50.

Closs J. Patient's sleep-wake rhythms in hospital. Part II. *Nurs Times.* 1988;84(2)54–55.

Deglin JH, Vallerand AH. *Davis's Drug Guide for Nurses.* Philadelphia: Davis; 1988.

Ellis JR, Nowlis EA. *Nursing: A Human Needs Approach.* Boston: Houghton-Mifflin; 1985.

Floyd JA. Interaction between personal sleep-wake rhythms and psychiatric hospital rest-activity schedule. *Nurs Research.* 1984; 33(5)255–259.

Goldson RL. Management of sleep disorders in the elderly. *Drugs.* 1981;21:390–396.

Greenberg R. Insomnia and sleep disturbances in the aged: Introduction. *J Geriatr Psychiatry.* 1980;13:131–134.

Harris E. Sedative-hypnotic drugs. *Am J Nurs.* 1981;81:1329–1334.

Karacan I, et al. Dose-related effects of flurazepam on human sleep–wake patterns. *Psychopharmacol.* 1981;73:332–339.

Lerner R. Sleep loss in the aged: Implications for nursing practice. *J Gerontol Nurs.* 1982;8:323–326.

Pacini CM, Fitzpatrick JJ. Sleep patterns of hospitalized and nonhospitalized aged individuals. *J Gerontol Nurs.* 1982;8:327–332.

Richards KC. A description of night sleep patterns in critical care unit. *Heart and Lung.* 1988;17(1)35–42.

Riley TL. *Clinical Aspects of Sleep and Sleep Disturbance.* Boston: Butterworth; 1985.

Shirmer MS. When sleep won't come. *J Gerontol Nurs.* 1983;9:16–21.

White JA. Touching with intent: Therapeutic massage. *Holistic Nurs Pract.* 1988;2(3)63–67.

CHAPTER 29

Neurosensory Integration

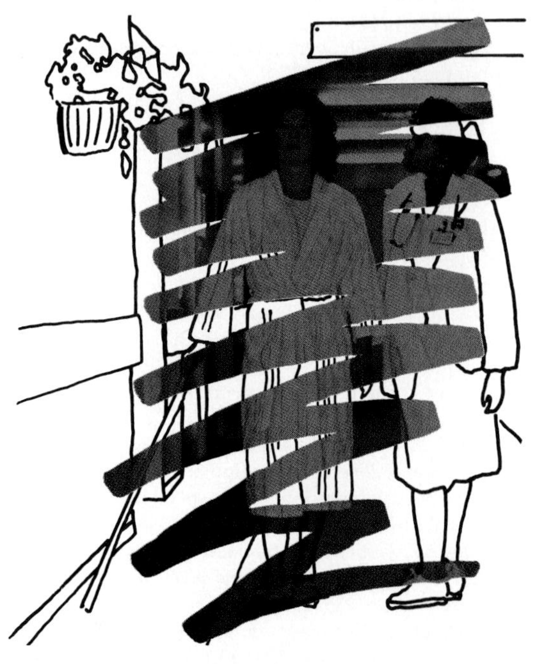

Behavioral Objectives

Upon completion of this chapter, the student will be able to:

1. Describe functions served by neurosensory integration.
2. Identify and describe the anatomical components, pathways, and components and the physiological mechanisms involved in pain.
3. Discuss the importance of neurosensory integration for the collaborative nurse–client relationship.
4. Identify factors affecting neurosensory integration.
5. Identify protective structures and processes involved in neurosensory functioning.
6. List and describe the basic causes of neurosensory alterations.
7. List and describe alterations in consciousness, memory, speech and language, and movement.
8. Describe alterations in perception, emotion, and memory.
9. Identify essential components of a neurosensory history and examination.
10. Explain the purpose of selected neurological diagnostic tests.
11. State three nursing diagnoses for clients experiencing an alteration in neurosensory integration.
12. Identify appropriate nursing implementations that reflect preventive, supportive, restorative, and rehabilitative levels of care for clients experiencing alterations in neurosensory integration.

KEY TERMS

affect
anesthesia
aphasia
arousal
central vision
classical conditioning
cognition
communication
consciousness
content
emotion
feeling
habituation
hyperesthesia
hypoesthesia
immediate memory
involuntary movement
language
long-term memory
memory
mood
movement
neurons
pain
paresthesia
perception
peripheral vision
sensitization
sensory deprivation
sensory overload
short-term memory
speech
thought
tone
voluntary movement

The neurosensory system is a complex entity incorporating the central nervous system (CNS), consisting of the brain and spinal cord, and the peripheral nervous system, consisting of the nerves that connect the CNS to other parts of the body (Fig. 29–1).

The nerve tissue of the brain and spinal cord is made up of masses of nerve cells known as **neurons** (Fig. 29–2). The millions of neurons in the neurosensory network serve as pathways for impulse conduction. Different types of neurons carry different messages. Afferent neurons transmit sensory stimuli from the periphery to a more central location for interpretation. Efferent neurons transmit impulses from more central locations in the neurosensory system to the peripheral nerves, which results in a motor response from muscles or glands.

The CNS and the peripheral nervous systems perform three general functions: a sensory function, a conscious or integrative function, and a motor function. The sensory function is to gather data from sensory receptors at the ends of the peripheral nerves. These receptors convey information regarding changes in and around the body including temperature, noise, light, and oxygen concentration in the blood.

All information that is gathered is converted into nerve impulses that are transmitted to the brain via the peripheral nerves. These impulses are brought together—or integrated—creating sensations, forming perceptions, adding to memory, or aiding formation of thoughts. The integrative function of the brain produces conscious and subconscious thoughts and decisions, enabling a person to see, hear, respond, eat, think, and move. The decisions made by the

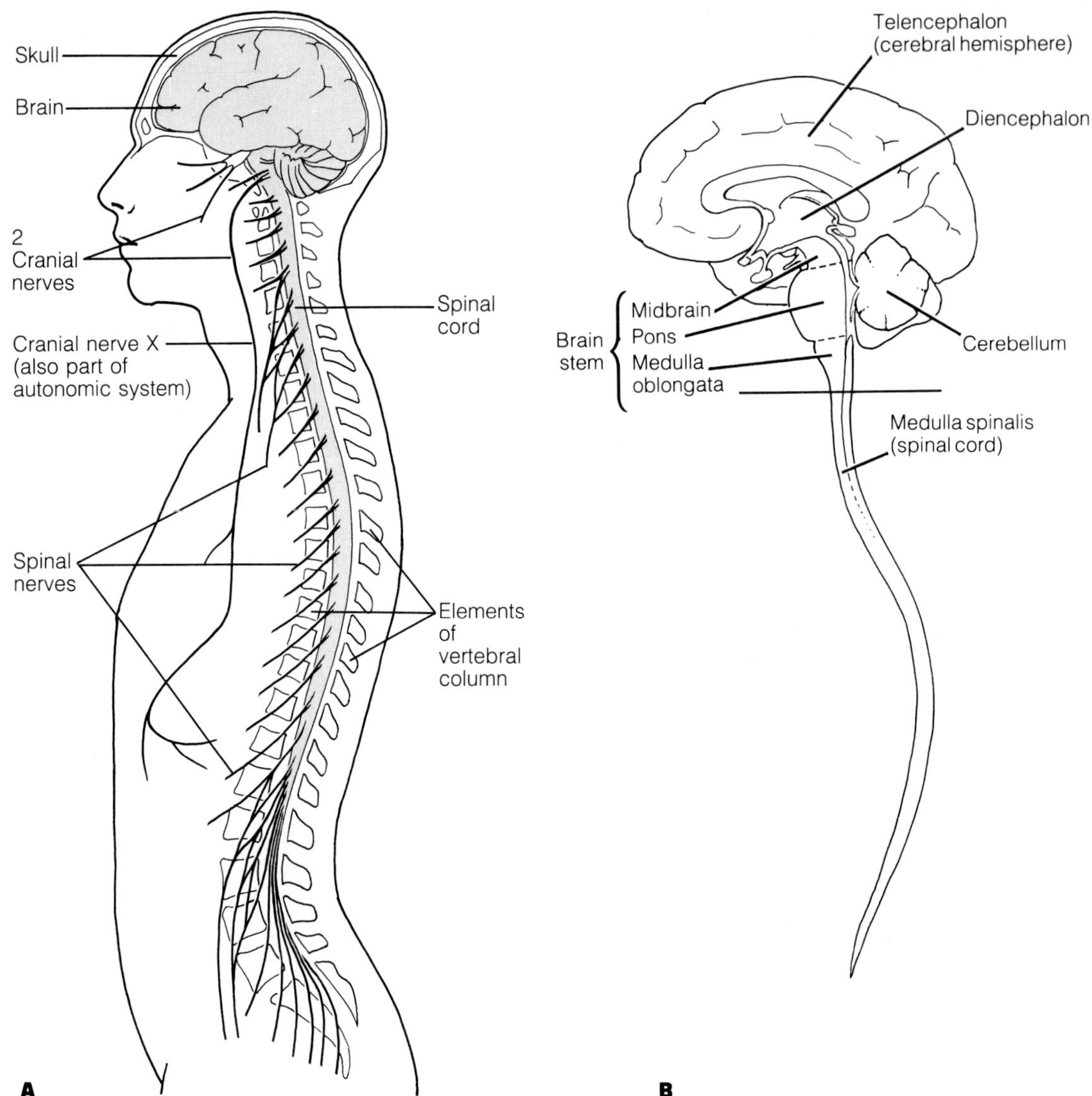

Figure 29–1. A. The structure of the central nervous system and the peripheral nervous system. **B.** The two major divisions of the central nervous system, the brain and the spinal cord. (*From deGroot J.* Correlative Neuroanatomy. *21st ed. Norwalk, CT: Appleton & Lange; 1991.*)

CNS enable the motor functions of the body to act. Neurosensory integration is a result of the networks and circuits of the neurosensory system blending information from all other systems into a unified whole so that each human being can function and think.

The motor functions of the nervous system occur as a result of CNS action. The peripheral nerves carry impulses from the brain to responsive parts in the body known as effectors. Effectors outside the nervous system include muscles that contract and glands that produce hormones or secretions when stimulated by nerve impulses.

Neurosensory integration is fundamental to individuality and responses to illness. Neurosensory integration enables clients to cope and, therefore, influences their requirements for nursing care. Coping is particularly important in illness because it affects the capacity to interact with others. Successful coping can support the healing process. Collaboration between the client and health care providers can be a crucial part of recovery. Without a significant level of neurosensory integration, a client's capacity to engage in a collaborative relationship may be seriously impaired, or the client may only be able to function in a limited capacity. Nursing assessment of the neurosensory system thus is essential to determine to what extent clients will be able to participate in care. Important nursing management decisions are derived from the nurse's impressions about the client's level of neurosensory function and ability to engage in a collaborative nurse–client relationship.

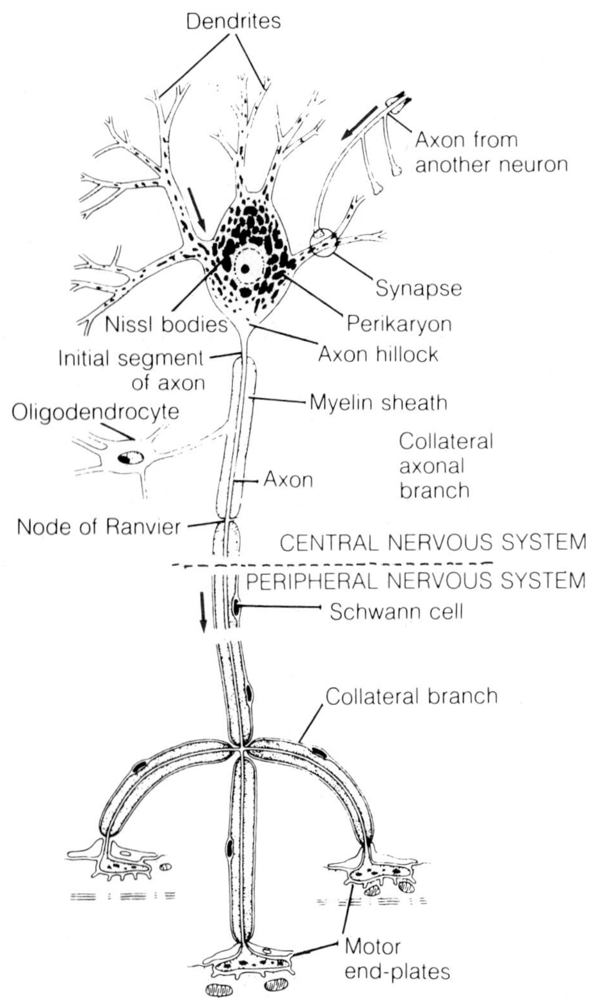

Figure 29–2. Neurons are present in the entire nervous system and serve as the information processors. Each neuron is specialized to react to physical and electrochemical changes occurring in its environment. It interprets the information and conducts nerve impulses through nerve networks to other nerves and to cells outside the nervous system. Neurons are capable of condensing information and spreading it considerable distances throughout the body. Alteration in impulse conduction can result in a neurosensory alteration. (*From Junqueira LC, Cameiro J, Kelley RO.* Basic Histology. *6th ed. Norwalk, CT: Appleton & Lange; 1986.*)

Section 1. Understanding Neurosensory Integration

The neurosensory network is an intricate collection of communication circuits that transmits sensory information, in the form of electrical and chemical energy, to central control centers in the brain. All of the aspects of the network work together to coordinate behavior. The circuits of the neurosensory network reach out to the sense organs and muscles, extend up and down the spinal cord, and bind the very different parts of the brain into an interlocking, coordinated control unit. The information processed produces perception, channels attention, creates thought and emotion, and initiates motor responses involved in carrying out effective action.

■ OPTIMUM NEUROSENSORY INTEGRATION

Neurosensory Functions

The functions served by neurosensory integration are consciousness; perception; memory; thought; speech, language and communication; and movement. Although the following discussion deals with each neurosensory function separately, these functions in actuality are closely interrelated, each function serving and supporting the others.

Consciousness. Consciousness (awareness) is the state of being aware of one's self and one's surroundings. It is the responsiveness of the mind to impressions made by the senses. Consciousness includes the ability to interpret sensory information, to react critically with thoughts and movements, to take appropriate action, to permit the accumulation of memory traces, and to develop an intellect.[1]

Consciousness has two components, arousal and content. **Arousal** corresponds to wakefulness. It is a state in which an individual attends to people, things, and events in the environment and is ready for activity. Wakefulness is not a constant state, but fluctuates normally with the state of sleep. Cycles of sleep and wakefulness allow for periods of activity followed by periods of rest and inactivity. These permit the body to restore energy reserves. (More about sleep and rest cycles can be found in Chap. 28.)

Changes in consciousness, from sleep to wakefulness and back again, are the most visible manifestations of the body's circadian (daily) rhythms and, in fact, are accompanied by changes in several physiologic processes. For example, a sharp reduction in the formation of urine occurs during sleep. The basal metabolic rate is decreased as well. Heart rate slows, pulse and blood pressure decrease, as does body temperature. There is a release of anabolic hormones, especially growth hormone, during sleep. Growth hormone assists in tissue repair.

Content, the second component of consciousness, is also controlled by and involves broad areas of the brain. **Content** is what is contained in the consciousness; the ideas, feelings, and sensations of which the individual is aware. Content is the sum of cognitive and affective (emotional) processes; the result of awareness, judgment, and emotional reaction.

The generation of mental content is a particularly complex aspect of neurosensory integration. It incorporates several vital mental operations, including perception of the environment and the capacity for thought, learning, and memory. Content is represented by what the individual communicates through language and behavior. Content is dependent on arousal. If a person is not alert, information cannot be received and fully perceived, leading to disorientation or confusion.

Neurosensory Basis of Consciousness. Arousal level is controlled by the reticular formation of the brain stem, which enables the body to shift from states of alertness to states of lethargy and sleep. The reticular formation consists of neurons distributed in the medulla oblongata, pons, mesencephalon, and portions of the diencephalon (Box 29–1). Responding to sensory information, the reticular formation screens messages to the brain, activating consciousness and responsiveness or protecting a restful state as appropriate to normal daily patterns and needs.

BOX 29–1. CONSCIOUSNESS AND THE RETICULAR FORMATION WITHIN THE RAS

Within the reticular formation there is a diffuse neural structure called the reticular activating system (RAS). The RAS is centered in a cone-shaped maze of nerves in the brain stem. The RAS is believed to control sleep and wakefulness, including activities such as attention, consciousness, and perception of sensory input. The RAS also selectively diverts information to other deep cerebral structures of the neurosensory system where it is processed automatically. Only information that requires attention is permitted to enter the cerebral cortex for conscious attention. Without the RAS, individuals would be overwhelmed with sensory information. When the RAS is inhibited (by the serotonin-secreting cells of the brain stem core) sleep results. When an alteration occurs within these structures, inappropriate cycles of sleep and wakefulness result. The result of such an alteration could be minimal, such as a lapse in attention, or serious, such as a comatose state.

Relationship of Consciousness to Other Neurosensory Functions. Consciousness depends on the interaction between the intact cerebral cortex and the upper brain stem. The cerebral cortex is responsible for consciousness and higher mental processes such as speech, language, memory, abstract reasoning, and learned responses to stimuli. It is comprised of two hemispheres joined by the corpus callosum. One hemisphere is dominant. The brain stem is involved in arousal and vital body functions such as breathing. Consciousness is required for voluntary activities such as interacting with others, walking, playing tennis, and other conscious activities, but not for autonomic processes such as breathing.

Perception. **Perception** is the ability of the mind to interpret and analyze input from the senses in order to understand the internal and external environment. Perception requires experience. Multiple stimuli must be evaluated, organized, and integrated to provide meaning. Human life, in fact, depends on successful and accurate relaying and interpretation of body signals and cues from the environment. Neurosensory organs regulating sensory input and perception are described in Box 29–2.

Sensory Input. Perception depends on sensory input. Stimuli are received by the sensory organs—eyes, ears, nose, tongue, and skin—which relay these signals to the brain for interpretation. In addition, spatial sensors in muscles, tendons and joints, and visceral organs relay information about body position and balance, enabling the person to carry out purposeful movements.

These sensors send a barrage of internal and external stimuli to support consciousness and arousal. Cutaneous stimuli assist in maintaining consciousness while visual, acoustic, and psychic stimuli influence arousal, attention, and perception. Because the brain cannot react completely to a barrage of incoming stimuli, the incoming messages are sorted and screened. Thus, a person will generally only react to meaningful stimuli.

Sight. Sight is the most important of the human senses. People receive 90 percent of their information about the world using the sense of sight. Through vision, color can be appreciated. Spatial and object discrimination are distinctive features of vision that allow the detection of shapes and the movement of objects. Both central and peripheral vision are important.

Central vision is vision that results from images falling on the macula of the retina. It is the vision people use to see when focusing on an object. **Peripheral vision** is the ability to see objects that reflect light waves falling on areas of the retina other than the macula. It is the vision people use to see out of the corners of their eyes. Peripheral vision is important because it contributes to depth perception and assists in detecting objects and sensing movement. These very complex functions of the sense of vision enable people

BOX 29–2. PERCEPTION AND NEUROSENSORY ORGANS REGULATING SENSORY INPUT

Cerebral Cortex

The cerebral cortex has four lobes that convert sensory information into perception:

1. *Frontal Lobes:* The frontal lobes comprise the part of the brain that is integrally involved with humanness. They are responsible for the intellect and for the functions of the brain that serve the intellect: memory, learning, thought, and judgment. The frontal lobes are responsible for individual personality. Each frontal lobe has an area called the motor cortex, which transmits motor messages to the skeletal muscles on the opposite side of the body and coordinates the motor activity of several cranial nerves.
2. *Parietal Lobes:* The parietal lobes contain the primary sensory cortex, which receives sensory transmissions from the opposite side of the body and interprets these incoming impulses. Functions of these areas include recognition of size, shape, texture, and consistency of objects; recognition of one's own body parts; discrimination of skin contacts; and written word comprehension.
3. *Temporal Lobes:* The temporal lobes function to interpret hearing, taste, smell, balance, and speech. The temporal lobe plays a critical role in the perception, discrimination, and interpretation of sensory data for the neurosensory network. The processing of these sensory inputs affect how the individual interacts with the environment. The temporal lobe also serves as a repository of long-term memory. It affects intellectual ability, sight, balance, language, and mobility.
4. *Occipital Lobes:* The primary function of the occipital lobes is visual reception and recognition of visual inputs.

Cerebellum

The cerebellum regulates muscle activity and influences balance. It may operate by comparing sensory information from the periphery with motor output from the cerebral cortex and brain stem, and continually correcting the efferent output to produce a precise, coordinated motion.

Brain Stem

The brain stem bridges the cerebral cortex and the spinal cord. The midbrain affects auditory and visual reflexes and serves as a conduction pathway between the cerebral cortex and other parts of the body. Cranial nerves III and IV originate from the midbrain. The pons is responsible for respiratory control centers, motor and sensory pathways from the cerebral cortex, parts of the RAS, and the neuronal links to the cerebellum. Cranial nerves V through VIII originate in the pons. The medulla oblongata connects the brain to the spinal cord. Cranial nerves IX through XII are joined at this point. The medulla has a prominent respiratory control center.

Spinal Cord

The spinal cord serves as the link from higher neurosensory functions to the rest of the body and vice versa.

Peripheral Nervous System

The peripheral nervous system comprises all nerve tissue in the body except the brain and spinal cord. These nerves gather data from the environment and telegraph them to the brain for interpretation. Sensory pathways carry information about temperature, touch, and pressure. Sensory perception begins with a stimulus that triggers a receptor. That receptor passes the stimuli along a neuron (sensory neuron I) to the central nervous system (CNS). From the spinal cord or brain stem, the impulses travel along sensory neuron II to the thalamus. These neurons synapse with sensory neuron III, which conducts the impulses from the thalamus to the parietal lobe.

to perceive objects and events surrounding them in the context of their environment, assigning meaning to the events.

The visual sense develops from birth as newborn infants begin to see light and recognize familiar objects, such as the mother's face, shapes, colors, and toys. Learning, whether cognitive, affective, or psychomotor, is dependent on sight.

Hearing. Hearing is important for protection, survival, and communication. Being able to converse and hear is vital to social skills and development of meaningful relationships. Hearing can be crucial to survival. Accuracy of perceptions, communication, and quality of life are also affected by one's sense of hearing.

Smell. The sense of smell is the least developed of the human senses. With the sense of smell, pleasant odors such as flowers, perfumes, freshly brewed coffee, and soups, and less pleasant odors, such as soured milk, exhaust fumes, smoke, and sewer gases, are detected.

The limbic system of the brain is closely associated with the area perceiving smell and may have developed from it. Because the limbic system serves the functions of memory, emotion, and learning, smell can awaken strong memories that can be perceived as good or bad. Smell is also a component in heightened sexual awareness. All of these effects of smell greatly enhance perception of stimuli.

Taste. Taste is an unrefined sense that detects only four qualities: sweet, sour, salty, and bitter. Chemical receptors, located separately on the tongue, enable individuals to taste foods. Taste is a major factor in selection of foods, leading people to form opinions of foods and thus influencing nutritional habits. The sense of taste is also protective. People are less likely to ingest harmful substances if they have a foul taste. Enjoyment of the flavors of food is not a function of taste, however, but rather of the smells associated with food.

Touch, Other Body Awareness Senses, and Temperature. Touch alerts people to the differences between hot and cold, pennies and quarters, cotton and wool, caresses and pinches. Touch and related sensory modalities, temperature and pain, are the last senses to vanish in unconsciousness, and the first to reawaken.

COMPONENTS OF TOUCH AND BODY AWARENESS. The sense of touch is comprised of several sensory modalities, each of which is detected by special receptors and sent to several relay stations and finally to the brain via special nerve tracts. These modalities include the tactile senses of vibration, pressure, and touch; stereognosis; and the kinesthetic sense of proprioception. Stereognosis allows people to identify objects by touch alone, through texture, size, and shape. Kinesthesia refers to the ability to perceive movement of muscles and joints. This ability is used to control and refine movements, posture, and equilibrium.

TEMPERATURE. The sense of temperature transmits information about hot and cold. The ability of the brain to interpret this information, identifying extremes of temperature, protects the individual from injury.

Balance. The last of the special senses is balance or equilibrium. Equilibrium provides sensory information about gravity and rotation of the body. Receptors are located in the vestibular apparatus in the ear. Several higher brain centers and the sensory association areas make interpretations about the body's upright position and execute careful reflex adjustments to maintain balance. Persons are unaware of the operation of these reflexes when standing, sitting, and walking.

Sensory Interpretation. The senses provide the input that is the basis of perception. However, perception also depends on the ability of the brain to integrate and interpret this input.

Cognition, the act or process of knowing, plays an important role in perception. Integration and interpretation are cognitive activities. Through cognition, various stimulus sensations are coordinated and united into a whole for complete awareness. For example, when one sees and smells a pizza, the brain interprets this and responds by causing salivation and stomach rumbling. Sensory integration refers to the assembly of this sensory input in a perceptual unit.

Sensory interpretation involves comparison of a meaningful event to previous experience. It allows for the significance of an event to be shaped. This interpretative capacity also enables the brain to recognize incoming sensations as gustatory, tactile, visual, olfactory, or auditory; to recognize body parts; and to recognize objects correctly through multiple senses. An example of multisensory interpretation is using vision, touch, and shape to correctly identify a set of car keys.

Several variables affect sensory interpretation, among them emotions, moods, motivations, memories and past life experiences, and coping styles. These are all part of personality. The role of emotion is complex and is discussed below. Sensory interpretation allows for the significance of an event to be shaped uniquely for each individual through mental activities of comparison and analysis that are unique to each personality. Individual differences in perception occur as a result of the cognitive process in perception. No two persons have the same life experiences; thus, no two persons perceive events in the same way. Hospitalization may mean confinement to some persons, danger and a threat to life for others, and a source of comfort and healing for still others.

Relationship of Perception to Other Neurosensory Functions

Role of Emotion. Emotions play an important role in sensory interpretation. **Emotion** is an affective state of consciousness in which joy, fear, anger, rage, and pleasure are experienced. Strong emotions are usually accompanied by physiological changes (such as increased heart rate) in the body. An example of a strong emotional response is the fight-or-flight response. (Refer to Chap. 6 for more detail.) Mild emotions, such as appreciation, affection, or irritation, may not have such apparent bodily changes.

Emotions color people's perceptions and ultimately help shape their behavior. Emotions affect a person's determination to persist in difficult tasks, to feel the weight of successful actions, and to reconsider plans of actions or behaviors if previously unsuccessful.

Emotions can lend many responses in an individual. Emotions seem to be linked to and inform the brain of an undefined sense of disruption or upset. Upsets can be pleasant, such as getting an A grade in a course, or unpleasant, such as failing a course or hearing footsteps from behind while walking alone in a dark alley. Emotions influence the ability to respond to stress, to take corrective action, and to restore equilibrium. To restore equilibrium, the brain's corrective action might be to fight (eg, to celebrate; to study harder; to turn around to see the person following in the dark alley) or flight (eg, to drop out of school; to flee from the stranger).

Emotion has subjective and objective components. The subjective component is the feeling state of an individual, described in terms of feeling, mood, affect, or tone. **Feeling** refers to the cognitive awareness of emotions such as happiness, fear, pleasure, anger, and irritability. When feeling is prolonged, a mood occurs. **Mood** refers to one's subjective description of feelings. In contrast, **affect** is the outward appearance of an emotional state to others. **Tone** describes the character or style in which a person communicates. Tone is influenced by affect and feelings (eg, "she spoke with a friendly tone in her voice").

An affect or mood is generally accompanied by an active expression. This expression is the objective component of emotion. The expression can be a change in bodily function manifested by an increase in heart rate, sweating, enlarged pupils, or blushing; or increased muscle activity such as fidgeting, shivering, or fleeing; or any of a number of verbal or nonverbal behaviors that correspond to a particular emotion.

The limbic system plays an essential role in processing the sensory input that produces emotions and accompanying physiological expressions. The deep cerebral structures of the limbic system form a loop or circuit around vital structures in the center of the brain, linking these structures and drawing on resources of the brain (eg, perceptions, memory, and cognition) to interpret or analyze stimuli and, subsequently, to produce an emotional expression (Box 29–3). Emotional expression is mediated by information stored in memory about past events.

As sensory input flows through this loop or circuit, brain chemicals known as neurotransmitters are released. Neurotransmitters influence emotional behavior and have tranquilizing and mood-elevating properties.

Pain. Pain is a naturally occurring phenomenon, a warning device to alert the individual of injury or illness. Sternbach describes pain as an "abstract concept that refers to (1) a personal, private sensation of hurt; (2) a harmful stimulus which signals current or impending tissue damage; (3) a pattern of responses which operate to protect the organism from pain."[2] This is a theoretical definition. A more useful definition for nurses has been developed by McCaffery, who defines **pain** as "whatever a person says it is, existing wherever the person says it does."[3]

Pain is a prevalent symptom and a universal human experience. It is the most common reason that people seek health care. Pain is a warning that something is wrong. It serves as an adaptive mechanism that alerts individuals of a potentially harmful situation.

The Pain Response. There are three components of the pain response: reception, perception, and response.

Reception. Reception is the neurological component of the pain response. Special receptors receive the painful stimulus and transmit it along afferent fibers in the peripheral nerves to the spinal cord. There, the simplest neurological response—reflex—occurs, resulting in a contraction of the muscle that leads to a protective withdrawal from the source of the pain (see Fig. 30–4). Pain impulses travel quickly to the brain where the stimulus is processed.

Perception. Perception involves the interpretation of the painful stimulus. It begins when the individual first becomes aware of the pain. Both physiological and psychological factors contribute to an individual's pain perception.

PHYSIOLOGICAL FACTORS. Pain impulses travel up the spinothalamic tract, activating the reticular formation, before proceeding to the higher brain centers in the cerebral cortex. The interpretation of data from all of these neurological centers provides perceptual information on the location, severity, and probable cause of the painful stimulus.

For pain to be perceived, the individual must have an intact neurological system. Factors that alter alertness lower pain perception; for example, anesthetics, pain medication, spinal cord trauma, or brain dysfunction cause an alteration in the way an individual perceives pain. On the other hand, factors that heighten awareness to stimuli will increase pain perception. Examples of this are stress and fatigue.

PSYCHOLOGICAL FACTORS. Psychological factors also affect how people perceive pain. Individuals do not perceive pain in the same way. A lifetime of events contributes to the way a person experiences pain. Interpretation of pain is influenced by past experiences. If a person has had severe pain without relief in the past, present pain may be viewed with anxiety and fear. On the other hand, if past experiences in coping with pain have been successful, the person may be better prepared to deal with another pain event.

Anxiety increases a person's perception of pain. A person who is anxious, apprehensive, or has used a great deal of psychological energy in coping may not be able to deal with pain as well as a person who is not as anxious. Other emotions also contribute to pain perception. Loneliness, depression, boredom, fear, hopelessness, and anger can cause heightened pain perceptions.

Cultural background regarding the meaning and significance of pain is an important aspect of pain perception. Cultural background influences how people think about pain, how they show pain, and decisions they make about

BOX 29–3. DEEP CEREBRAL STRUCTURES AND THEIR FUNCTIONS

Structures lying deep within the cerebral hemispheres include the limbic system, reticular activating system, amygdala, hippocampus, thalamus, and hypothalamus. These deep cerebral structures play an integral role in emotion, memory, and certain physiological functions.

Limbic System

The limbic system surrounds the head of the brain stem and contains portions of the amygdala, hippocampus, thalamus, and hypothalamus. It regulates subconscious reaction to emotions and aspects of memory related to these emotions. Its function includes feeling states, mood, instincts, primitive behaviors, self-preservation, interpretation of smell, and expression of libido. As one experiences an emotion, the limbic system modulates that emotion through a variety of endocrine, physiological, or psychological reactions, much as a circuit breaker modulates electrical current entering a building.

Amygdala

The amygdala interprets new situations. It can amplify or dampen the intensity of an emotional response. The amygdala, in conjunction with the hypothalamus, conveys the level of the emotion for activation of autonomic response.

Hippocampus

The hippocampus plays a role in long-term memory of past emotions experienced by a person. Storage of memories by the hippocampus is based on their importance, usefulness, or vividness. The hippocampus helps evaluate an event based on past experiences. If this structure is destroyed, new information cannot be recalled.

Thalamus

The thalamus serves as a station that receives the impulses from the senses, integrates the input, and relays the integrated messages to the cerebral cortex. It focuses attention and creates awareness of pain, touch, and temperature.

pain. People of one culture may take pride in not recognizing pain while others may view pain as something to endure. Values about pain include the perception that pain is punishment for past deeds.

Age is another factor in pain perception. Young children and the elderly may experience more pain than other clients. Because they are often unable to communicate their needs, these clients may not receive adequate pain relief measures.

Response. Response to pain has physiological and behavioral components. Physiological and behavioral responses may appear to conflict. For example, although the objective data may indicate the presence of pain (eg, elevated pulse, blood pressure, a gaping wound), a client may demonstrate behaviors indicating that pain does not exist.

PHYSIOLOGICAL RESPONSES. As the pain stimulus ascends the spinal cord, the autonomic nervous system is alerted as a part of the stress response. Pain of low to moderate severity or superficial pain evokes the fight-or-flight response (see Chap. 6). Responses evoked include: increased respiratory and pulse rate, increased blood pressure, increased muscle tension, dilated pupils, sweating, pallor, and nausea and vomiting. Unrelenting, severe pain or visceral pain causes the parasympathetic nervous system to act to protect the individual, as the physical symptoms of a sustained pain response would otherwise have serious effects. Therefore, clients with severe sustained pain may reach a state of equilibrium where they do not show any signs of pain.

BEHAVIORAL RESPONSES. There are many behavioral responses to pain. Most of these are observable. Clients may grind their teeth, clench their hands, rock side-to-side, pace, hug themselves, cry or moan, hold the painful area, or tense groups of muscles.

Pain Theories. In spite of numerous research studies, the exact mechanisms of the pain response remain a mystery. However, several theories of how people experience pain have been advanced.

Specificity Theory. Specificity theory postulates that there are specific nerve endings in the body that receive input only from certain painful stimuli. Once the pain receptors receive this stimulus, an impulse is transmitted along specific pain pathways until it is registered in the pain center (thalamus). This theory has undergone much research which has demonstrated that the specific receptors of pain also receive other stimuli and that many other areas of the brain also are involved in a pain response.

Pattern Theory. Pattern theories speculate that certain types of stimuli acting on nonspecific receptors appear to cause groups of impulses in neuronal pathways to produce a pattern that is interpreted by the brain as pain. It is speculated that these impulses are combined in the dorsal horn of the spinal cord to produce a relative intensity of the painful stimuli. Examples of pattern theories include: peripheral pain theory, central summation theory, and sensory interaction theory.

Gate-Control Theory. The gate-control theory, proposed by Melzack and Wall in 1965, describes how neurons in the dorsal horn of the spinal cord act as gates that regulate the transmission of pain impulses to the brain.[4] This is the most commonly accepted pain theory today.

Gate-control theory speculates that an area in the dorsal horn of the spinal cord known as the substantia gelatinosa acts as a gate that can increase or decrease the number of nerve impulses from the peripheral nerves to the brain. The gate is opened or closed depending on the input from small and large nerve fibers. Increased activity in the small fibers opens the gate, allowing the pain sensation to enter the brain. Conversely, increased activity in the large fibers closes the gate so that pain stimuli do not get through to the brain. Pain is perceived when the stimuli reaching the brain have surpassed a certain threshold limit.

Melzak and Wall also describe a cognitive influence on pain perception.[4,5] Age, anxiety, previous experiences, attention, expectation, sex, cultural background, and socioeconomic status all play a role in perception of pain. The overall pain recognition in the brain is modulated by input received from the spinothalamic tract, reticular formation, limbic system, and certain cerebral areas that control memory retrieval of past pain experiences. Thus, pain is determined by a combination of sensory input and impulses from the higher brain centers.

Endorphins and Other Endogenous Opioids. The brain is capable of producing chemical regulators, called endogenous opioids, that modify pain. It is thought that these regulators bind with opiate receptor sites that exist throughout the body and, in particular, in the dorsal horn of the spinal cord. The release of these endogenous opioids closes the gate by decreasing the number of pain impulses that are transmitted to the brain. To date three types of endogenous opioids have been discovered: endorphins, dynorphins, and enkephalins.

Endorphins are large polypeptides that supply the body with opiate-like substances. Endorphins probably modulate pain by binding with opiate receptor sites throughout the nervous system, inhibiting release of neurotransmitters, and thereby altering pain perception. It is thought that endorphins are made and stored in the pituitary gland. Receptor sites are found in the hypothalamus, midbrain, amygdala, pons, medulla, raphe nuclei, substantia gelatinosa, and the limbic system. The abundance of opiate receptor sites in the limbic system supports the assumption that opiates relieve pain by altering, rather than preventing, pain perception. Several subgroups of endorphins have been identified, including beta-endorphin, which is found in high concentration in the hypothalamus.

Dynorphins are found in the hypothalamus, pituitary gland, and spinal cord. They are 50 times as potent as beta-endorphin.

Enkephalin, a small polypeptide, binds to opiate receptor sites in the dorsal horn of the spinal cord where it acts to inhibit the release of a neurotransmitter referred to as substance P. Substance P acts to enhance pain transmission across synapses. By reducing pain transmission, enkephalins serve as an analgesic. Outside the spinal cord enkephalins are found in the brain stem, limbic system, hypothalamus, adrenal glands, and gastrointestinal tract. Subgroups of this endogenous opioid include levenkephalin and metenkephalin.

Classification of Pain. Pain is classified as acute or chronic. Acute pain serves as a protective mechanism and lasts up to 6 months. This may be reflected physiologically with an increase in heart rate, respiratory rate, blood pressure, peripheral blood flow, muscle tension, palmar sweating, and pupil size. Chronic pain is disabling and serves no useful purpose. This type of pain lasts longer than 6 months and can be a result of fractures, amputations, peripheral neuropathies (disease of one or more peripheral nerves), certain cancers, and herniated disc (protruding intervertebral disc that impinges on spinal cord). Persons with chronic pain frequently exhibit signs of psychological depression, whereas persons with acute pain often exhibit anxiety symptoms.

Pain can also be categorized according to its origin. Peripheral pain originates in the peripheral nervous system. Causalgia, a burning type of pain, results from injury to the peripheral nerves. Central pain originates in the central nervous system and occurs with brain tumors, multiple sclerosis, and spinal cord injury.

Cutaneous or superficial pain is felt at the site of injury or noxious stimulus. Blisters, stubbed toes, knocked elbows, and bumped heads are examples of cutaneous pain. Cutaneous pain that is abrupt in onset has a sharp, stabbing, burning quality; slower onset cutaneous pain has a dull, burning, or aching quality.

Pain that is deep and difficult to identify is characteristic of deep somatic pain or visceral pain. Deep somatic pain originates from bone, nerve, and muscle tissue; visceral pain from organs. Visceral pain occurs with appendicitis, gastric ulcers, and the heart pain associated with myocardial disease.

Memory. **Memory** is the mental capacity of receiving, registering, encoding, consolidating, storing, and retrieving information, impressions, or experiences. Memory function allows people to express feelings; to execute complex acts; to name similarities and differences of people, items, or things; to have a sense of who they are; to retain concepts about the world; and to know and understand the past. Without memory, people would only be able to experience stimuli, sensations, and events of the moment. Information would only be stored for seconds. The information would not be registered, and thus could not be retrieved.

Types of Memory. Memories are distinguished by their duration and purpose.

Immediate Memory. **Immediate memory,** which occurs in the sensory registers, refers to activity at the site of sensory registration. Information enters the system through the senses and is held briefly in the sensory form in which it was received (for example, a sound is heard in auditory form). There is a sensory register for each of the senses. Information stays only briefly in the sensory registers. The longer it stays, the weaker it becomes, until decay occurs. Information remains in the sensory registers from milliseconds to about 20 seconds.[6]

While the information is in the sensory register, it undergoes pattern recognition. Pattern recognition is a complex process that results when a group of pieces or elements is associated with previously acquired knowledge. It is a way of encoding the stimulus in a combined form; for example, a friend's face is stored as a face, not just a nose, eyes and mouth. Once encoded, the stimuli can be moved to short-term memory.

Short-term Memory. **Short-term memory** (STM), or working memory, is the site of ongoing cognitive activities such as word meaning and symbol manipulation as is used in mental arithmetic, and reasoning. These processes are carried out under the immediate awareness of the individual.

STM stores information in a processed form. This information can be called up at the individual's choice. The role of STM is to store and process significant information. STM is capable of holding five to nine pieces of information for a short amount of time. Information is generally held in STM for minutes to hours, but can be held there indefinitely by using a process called rehearsal.

Rehearsal is an overt or covert practicing or repetition of information, such as in reciting a grocery list or phone number. For example, STM allows one to remember a phone number just found in the telephone directory. The STM will hold the telephone number long enough to enable the person to dial the number. Then the number is forgotten. If that telephone number is significant and the individual needs to remember it, or if the number is dialed many times (rehearsed), the memory trace becomes permanent and is transferred to long-term memory.

Long-term Memory. **Long-term memory** (LTM) is the storage of information that lasts for hours to a lifetime. Without long-term memory, learning could not occur, and the brain would not have past experience with which to compare current events. Long-term memory provides permanent storage of information, memories, and events so that long-term learning and thought can occur.

As memories move from short-term memory to long-term memory, sensory associations are made that become a part of the memory trace. For example, words and ideas are one mechanism by which information is categorized before it is sent to LTM. These associations serve as a factor in retrieval. Visual memories of past similar stimuli are another possibility. The categorizations of certain memories are arranged by subject. This can be likened to a great library where books are organized by subject. The memories associated with seeing a lake are categorized by the senses: vision, smell, sound. Another feature of memory, besides categorization of information, is cross-indexing, again like the library that permits one to find a book cataloged under various categories. In the case of the ocean or lake memory, the memory could be evoked by a similar picture, a tape recording of waves sounding off a harbor, or the smell of lake or ocean water on clothing.

Once information is transferred to long-term memory, it is there forever. Retrieval of information then becomes the challenge. Memory is complex. Information is not stored in isolation; it is related to previous memory stores, put in a certain framework or file of knowledge, and these frameworks are organized. Memory is an active process. Knowledge and information are always changing and always being reexamined and reformulated as new facts and other data are gathered, processed, and stored.

Process of Memory. To successfully remember, three things must occur: reception, storage, and retrieval of information.

Retrieval of information depends on attention and how memories are stored. People remember by concentrating. They remember by relating information in elaborate ways, such as mnemonics; by noting similarities and differences; or by noting a relationship of the information to something already known. People recall information when they are given a stimulus or a cue to retrieve stored information.

Much research has been conducted to discover the memory center in the brain. To date no study has been able to pinpoint an exact location. Several areas of the cerebral cortex and related brain structures contribute to recall, revival, and recognition of information.

Scientists have long pondered and investigated the neurological basis of memory. It is believed that the sensory system stimulates neurons in such a way that a pattern is fired over millions of neurons, producing an imprint or memory trace. Because of the vast pattern of interconnections between nodes or neurons, the memory trace becomes the memory. When people remember, many nodes refire to allow recall.

One neuron can be a part of several memory traces, thus memory is represented in many neural networks and can be evoked or reached through several inputs. It is also believed that memories are not static, but constantly restructured in the neural networks as the brain receives new information and as learning occurs. Once the new information or learning occurs and becomes permanent, consolidation, or a permanent trace of the memory over the neurosensory network, occurs. This consolidation of memory can again be restructured with new information or learning.

Retrieval of Memories. Sensory input is involved in evoking memories. The sense of smell, in particular, is known to evoke strong memories. Consider how the scent of a pine tree might evoke memories of Christmas, or how the smell of cinnamon rolls baking reminds one of a grandmother baking those special treats. Not only is a scent pattern recalled, but scents can be remembered as well. This may occur as the neurons fire in long-term memory over broad areas. Anderson calls this notion spreading activation.[7] As a stimulus causes a few neurons to fire in long-term memory to cause an individual to remember an event or fact, those neurons fire other neurons and the recall becomes greater.

Emotions may well underlie memory imprinting, especially in long-term memory. Emotions associated with significant events evoke memories of those events; they become part of the neuronal circuit and engram.

Memory and Learning. Learning and memory are interrelated. The initial contact with a stimulus causes it to be processed and stored in long-term memory. Once there it can be recalled. The simplest kind of learning implies that something has been remembered. Learning has been defined in many ways. Psychologists view learning as a relatively permanent change in behavior as a result of experience, practice, or training. Physiologists define learning as the ability of the nervous system to store memories for future retrieval.

Importance of Learning. Learning helps human beings know and recognize their environment and surroundings. It is important for the development of thought and knowledge. It is involved in the development of physical skills and fine-tuned motor responses. Thus, learning is essential for actualization of the growth potential of human beings.

People who cannot remember cannot learn, and because of this, lack the ability to store or to recall facts and items of information. Without learning, there could be no change in an individual's responses, behaviors, or thoughts; life would be a moment-to-moment existence, lacking meaningfulness and connections to the past or future. An example might be the client who has a stroke damaging half of the brain. As a result, learning is impaired. The client forgets how to dress himself. Because the client cannot learn, directions from others will not help him learn to dress himself again. The act of instruction on dressing occurs as a single-moment experience for the client and lacks meaning.

Types of Learning. People learn by simple and complex means. Chapter 20 discusses theories on human learning. The reader is referred to that chapter for additional information.

SIMPLE LEARNING. There are three kinds of simple learning: (1) habituation, (2) sensitization, and (3) classical or Pavlovian conditioning.

Habituation is a form of learning that occurs when a stimulus that originally produced a response is presented so often that the individual stops responding to it.[8] Nurses observe learning by habituation in clients who must learn to give themselves injections. The individual gradually comes to view the pain from injections as nonthreatening and insignificantly painful and thus through habituation learns to deal with the pain.

Sensitization, a form of nonassociative learning, occurs when a person attends to a previously neutral stimulus.[8] Sensitization has the opposite effect of habituation. It arouses human interest. Through sensitization, people can determine noxiousness or dangerousness of events or stimuli. Persons who usually experience shortness of breath when they exercise, for example, may consider this a normal response to exercise. However, if a healthy individual becomes ill with a chest cold, and consequently experiences shortness of breath, he or she may become sensitized, viewing it as abnormal or potentially threatening.

Classical conditioning is a form of learning in which an individual learns to link two separate stimulus elements.[9] This occurs when a primary stimulus (a stimulus that naturally yields a certain reaction) is paired a number of times with another neutral stimulus and ultimately becomes conditioned. Eventually when the neutral stimulus is presented, it elicits the reaction formerly elicited only by the primary stimulus. The classic example is that of Pavlov's dogs. Pavlov discovered that dogs became conditioned to salivate (a normal reaction to the primary stimulus of food) in reaction to the presence of white-coated attendants (neutral stimulus) who brought the food.[8] Because Pavlov defined classical conditioning, it is also known as Pavlovian conditioning.

Humans learn by conditioning. Infants and children who experience pain in a visit to clinics become conditioned to view the physicians and nurses with fear. The health care professional (neutral stimulus) becomes associated with needle injections or other procedures (primary stimulus) that evoke fear (response) in the child. Because physicians and nurses are paired with the primary stimulus, eventually the child reacts with fear to the sight of the physician or nurse, even when the primary stimulus is absent. Similarly, people may learn to associate hospitals with death, after experiencing the death of a loved one there.

COMPLEX LEARNING. Complex learning is voluntary. It requires the use of cognitive (thinking) skills. Complex learning skills involve learning facts and rules, developing concepts, classifying objects, making associations to previously learned material, analyzing data, and evaluating.

Complex learning is associated with the ability to transfer information from short-term memory to long-term memory. How information is stored depends on a number of variables, such as age, attentiveness, motivation, positive and negative consequences, verbal ability, cognitive skills, and an intact neurosensory system.

Age determines how much an individual can learn. For example, a small child will learn differently than an adolescent or adult. Attention to material will enhance the transfer into long-term memory. Rewards for learning and punishments for not learning contribute to learning. A person's verbal level may affect the way the information is transferred to memory. Cognitive skills relate to the ways in which individuals regulate their own internal process such as attention, learning, remembering, and thinking.[10] It is these strategies that allow people to solve new problems, perform mathematical calculations, and carry out self-management behaviors.

Thought. **Thought** is the mental process that assigns meaning to and designs actions in response to the integration and interpretation of sensory input. It is the process whereby the brain sorts and integrates every relevant piece of information gathered throughout each day. The term *thought* is applied to that which is intellectual—having to do with logic and reason. It is distinguished by the capacity of reasoning. Mere perceiving, feeling, or willing are mental activities that do not require reasoning.

Thought comprises several mental functions. They are comprehension, reasoning, judgment, problem-solving, and conception (Table 29–1). The combination of these structured mental activities is also referred to as the cognitive capacities or the ability to think.

Importance of Thought. Humans have the ability to construct ideas in sequential fashion, to reason logically, to have insight into situations, to make appropriate judgments, to make decisions, to solve problems, to calculate, to demonstrate reality-based thoughts, to produce appropriate behaviors, to construct memories, and to formulate concepts. Thought allows individuals to make careful adjustments in order to adapt to their environment and work toward the goal of health. Through thought, individuals generate long-range goals and take action in light of those goals. A blending of sensory impressions and input from memory stores allows people to assign meaning to these specific events or goals and determine subsequent behaviors or thoughts.

Process of Thought. Thought is a complex, integrative mental activity involving many areas of the brain. For example, the frontal lobe of the cerebral cortex is responsible for emotions, intellect, learning, concentration, focusing attention, problem-solving and the ability to follow instructions. All of these functions are requisites of thought.

It is difficult to pinpoint where thought occurs. Neuroscientists have been researching this phenomenon for many years. It appears that for any task requiring thought, there are specific neural pathways that perform that task.[8] Moreover, the pathways may differ depending on the nature of the thoughts. It is known that certain parts of the thought process occur in a somewhat sequential fashion.

- *Phase I.* Perception, or attending to sensory stimuli, produces a conscious awareness of a particular stimulus. For example, when one experiences soft rubbing sensations on the skin, the sensory system sends information that produces awareness that something is there. This aware-

TABLE 29–1. FUNCTIONAL CAPACITY OF THOUGHT

Function	Definition
Comprehension	The act of understanding.
Reasoning	The drawing of inferences or conclusions using the power of comprehension.
Judgment	The capacity of the brain to form an opinion of an idea or event.
Problem-solving	The mind's ability to determine an action or solution based on judgment of a particular internal or external event.
Conception	The capacity, or function, of forming concepts or understanding ideas or abstractions; reflective thinking.

ness is general and nonspecific. An intact sensory system, an appropriate attention span, and the ability to recognize and interpret the incoming stimuli are necessary to discern what is causing the sensation.

- *Phase II.* The integration of stimuli results in interpretation and pinpointing the event. This information is interpreted in terms of words, concepts, and relationships. This step is dependent on language. The fuzzy creature might be a cat or a bear.
- *Phase III.* Phase II is the symbolic association, the assigning of symbols, particularly linguistic symbols, to a given perception. Phase III also involves an expressive thought or execution of motor activity, or change in mood and action based on the symbols attached to the perception. One pets the cat, talks to it, and feels pleasure, or one sees the bear, runs away, and feels intense fear.

Relationship of Thought to Other Neurosensory Functions. Thought is an integrative neurosensory function that is related to, dependent upon, and necessary for other functions. Perception and consciousness are necessary initially in the process of thought. Memory and memory retrieval and the ability to learn contribute to the store of neurosensory resources the brain uses during the analysis phase of thought. And lastly, thought is necessary for speech, language, communication, and movement. The brain is highly dependent on language in order to process conscious brain events.

The networks of neurons that produce thought are vast, complex, and highly ordered. This network lies on the outer surface of the brain and is dependent on input from neural pathways. Thought is produced in lightning-like fashion over these interconnections, and at a speed much faster than a person's consciousness can keep pace with.

Communication, Language, and Speech. Communication, language, and speech are intertwined. **Communication** is the act of sending and receiving messages by the use of verbal and nonverbal language. **Language** is a formal system of signs and symbols used for communication. **Speech** can be defined as the articulation or expression of thoughts and ideas using language.

Neurosensory Basis for Communication, Language, and Speech. Communication is a complex neurosensory process involving the entire brain. Language function is widely distributed throughout the dominant side of the brain. It relies on information stored in the front of the brain, as well as the touch, auditory, and visual interpretative areas that contribute comprehension of concepts, people, and thoughts.

Neurosensory Processes of Communication. The neurosensory processes involved in communication and the understanding of messages are complex. They involve reception, perception, conceptualization, formulation, and expression of verbal and written speech.

In reception, spoken words are converted into neural signals in the cochlea of the ears. Further transmission conveys the neural signal to an area of the brain where perception takes place. Visual information is also telegraphed to the brain. One generally looks at another person when speaking, or looks in the direction of a sound. Perception is the awareness of the stimuli. At this point, the message or idea is reconstructed through language into symbols or thought in areas of the brain. This is known as conceptualization. Knowledge, past experience, feelings, attitudes, and emotions that provide a frame of reference influence the perception and conceptualization of a message. Formulation is the detailed, coordinated plan for vocalization. It occurs as a result of the neural signal sent to the brain area that tells facial muscles, lips, and tongue to move in a specific pattern and sound sequence so that a particular sound is expressed. Expression is the articulatory and mechanistic vocalization known as speech. In order for articulation or speech to occur, the neurosensory network for communication must be intact.

Sensory and Motor Aspects of Communication. Communication involves both sensory and motor aspects. The sensory aspect includes the use of ears, eyes, and touch for reception and the ability to understand both the written and spoken word, which is used in perception, conceptualization, and formulation. The motor aspect involves the muscles used in vocalization and its control as well as the ability to produce speech and to write words.

Process of Speech. The process of speech is thought to occur according to the following model. Speech sounds and meaning arise in the dominant hemisphere of the brain and travel along bundles of nerve fibers, to an area of motor cells in the frontal brain. This neural impulse evokes a detailed and coordinated program for vocalization, containing details of how each lip, tongue, and throat muscle is to move. The program is then transmitted to adjacent motor cells that control the facial muscles. When words are read, the back of the brain where vision cells are located is activated, and the brain must work to match the visual input with the sounds those words have when spoken.

Relationship of Communication, Language, and Speech to Social Interaction. Communication is an individual's way of expressing himself or herself and relating his or her needs. Communication occurs throughout life. Relationships, whether casual or intimate, are established through communication. Communication is necessary for intellectual, spiritual, and physical growth.

Language and speech are prerequisites to communication. They allow humans to express knowledge that is learned, to describe events and happenings never before experienced, and to share emotions, such as pleasure or anger, in addition to needs and desires. Language and speech influence role behaviors, life-styles, and social interaction.

The social impact of problems of communication, language, and speech can have dramatic consequences for clients and their significant others. Poor communication can cause feelings of fear, frustration, anger, anxiety, hostility, depression, confusion, and isolation.

Relationship of Communication, Language, and Speech to Other Neurosensory Functions. Communication is related to all of the other functions of the neurosensory system, both supporting them and depending on them. In order to use language, for example, one must be conscious; in turn, language provides much of the content of conscious awareness. Language is dependent on information retention, recall, and the integration of symbols. Language is necessary for thought and, as a consequence, is intimately involved in the capacity to interpret the sensory stimuli that comprise perceptions.

Much of the content of memory and learning is structured around language. The capacity to use language in thought and speech is also dependent on memory and learning. Moreover, language has the capacity to evoke emotions that become associated with ideas embedded in the memory.

Speech depends on the interpretation of auditory and visual images that reach the higher intellectual centers during differing states of consciousness. To use speech, one must initially formulate the thought to be expressed, choose appropriate words, and then control the motor activity of the muscles of speech.

Movement. **Movement** can be defined as a change of place, position, or posture of any portion of the body. Movement, whether it be the wink of an eye or the outstretching of a hand, may appear to be a simple maneuver, but in actuality it is a highly complex neurosensory function. Controlled, purposeful movement as a result of neurosensory integration brings great fulfillment and joy to people's lives. Consider the independence, physical release and emotional response felt through exercise, and the expressions of written thought, art, dance, and speech achieved as a result of movement. To be effective, movement must be purposeful, controlled, balanced, upright, fluid, and smooth.

Types of Movement. Movement includes various activities such as walking and running, blinking, sphincter release of the bowel or the bladder, chewing, swallowing, tracking an object with the eye, handwriting, singing, and talking, to name a few. There are over 600 muscles in the human body, which are used in a large number of movements.

Movement can be classified as voluntary or involuntary. **Voluntary movement** is movement carried out consciously and intentionally under a person's will or volition. Brushing the teeth, walking, piano playing, and driving a car are examples of movements that are consciously and intentionally performed. **Involuntary movement** is movement performed unconsciously, without the person's will, or unintentionally. The quick release of the hand from a hot stove, stretching out the hands when falling, the unconscious blinking of the eye, and excursion of the chest during respiration occur spontaneously, quickly, and usually without conscious control.

Neurosensory Basis for Movement. The motor system controls movement. In contrast to the sensory system, which relays signals from the periphery (skin, visual field) upwards to specific brain sites, the motor system originates in specialized brain cells, called the motor cortex (see Fig. 30–3), and ends at the periphery, with the movements of muscles. The motor cortex is like a map with regions (brain cells) specialized to move each muscle of the body (Box 29–4 and Fig. 29–3).

Relationship of Movement to Other Neurosensory Functions. The pathway for movement outlined above provides a limited description of the complex process of movement. Some movements are under conscious control; others operate largely without conscious awareness. It is not known exactly how the brain comes to a decision to perform a particular action or in what area of the brain the decision originates. It is apparent, however, that movement is interrelated with other functions of the neurosensory system.

- *Movement and Perception.* Movement and perception might seem to be very separate systems, yet very few of the sensory signals sent to the brain end without initiating and modifying muscle action in some way. The pleasant smell of fresh flowers often stimulates the sensory system in such a way that one is drawn toward the smell and to find the flowers. The interaction between perception and movement remains incompletely understood; however, perception and movement rarely occur as isolated events.
- *Movement and Thought.* Interrelationships are necessary in order for purposeful movement to occur. The brain operates in lightning-like fashion in response to stimuli. Because people have the ability to analyze and judge, they also have the capacity to control movement.
- *Movement and Learning.* Movement and learning are linked in the achievement of skilled activities, as well as in dexterity of movement. Movements such as handwriting comprise a learned sequence of refined motions. Dexterity, coordination, and sequencing of movements are part

BOX 29–4. FUNCTIONAL ANATOMY OF MOVEMENT

The pathway for movement follows an orderly fashion from the motor cortex to the spinal cord to the muscle. Just below the motor cortex and before the spinal cord are two parallel brain areas that affect the integration of neural impulses sent to the muscles. These specialized areas fine-tune and regulate the performance of specific, directed voluntary movements. This is done, in part, by controlling and coordinating the pull and push forces of opposing muscle groups. Without this input, the rapid, consecutive, simultaneous motion involved in such gross movement as walking, standing, or sitting upright, or such fine movement as playing the piano and fingering a computer keyboard would not be possible. Movements in these activities would be awkward and erratic. Specialized areas that fine-tune movement are always at work during movement providing precision and control without the person's conscious awareness.

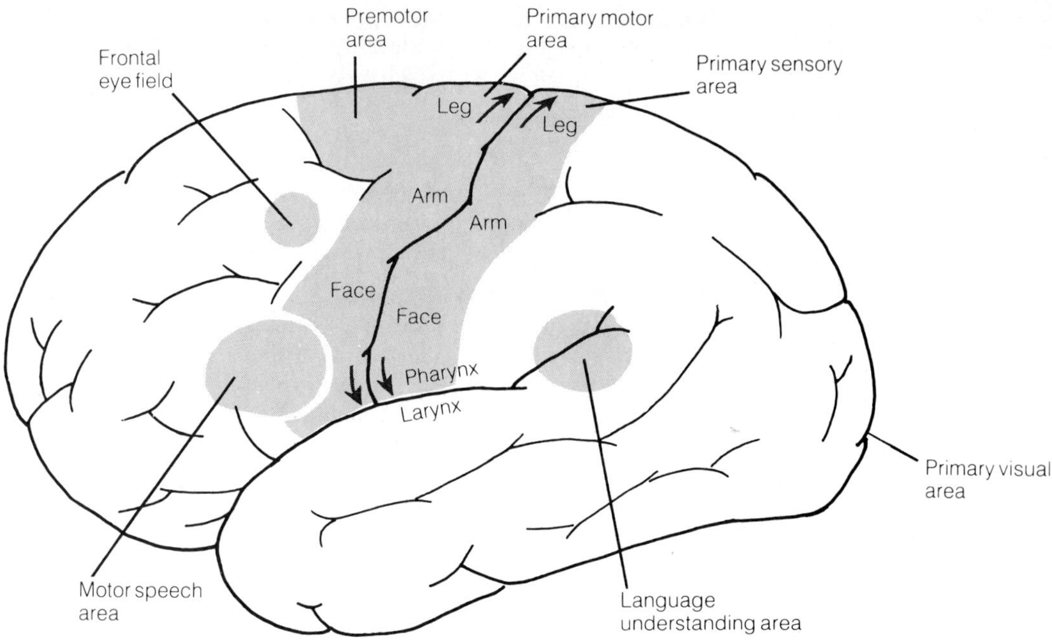

Figure 29–3. Cerebral cortex areas devoted to body areas for feeling and movement.

of skilled activities. Their efficiency increases and skill improves with learning.

- *Movement and Emotion.* Emotion and movement are linked in important ways. Emotions, such as anger and fear, activate the autonomic nervous system. The fight-or-flight response initiates a cascade of physiological responses that are automatic.
- *Movement and Communication.* Communication is so closely associated with movement that if one cannot communicate either verbally or in written word, the outer world becomes shut out.

Importance of Movement. One of the benefits of movement is clearly independence. Movement is a highly prized capability of human beings. All parents share the thrill of their baby's first steps. Athletes, dancers, and skaters embrace movement in highly skilled performance. Exercise, through activities such as walking, running, and bicycling, for example, diminishes tension and promotes mental rejuvenation. Society values both independence and movement. Individuals who can move are able to take care of their own self-care needs and thus preserve independence.

The integration of thought and movement is also linked to social functioning. Purposeful, controlled actions are necessary socially. Smiling, shaking hands and laughter control are some examples of "thoughtful" action.

Movement also allows expression of the self. Dancers express thoughts, emotions, and stories. Each person has certain movements that accompany various emotions. A happy smile, drooped shoulders, or raised eyebrows characterize differences in emotions. Sexuality is another form of expression that is influenced by movement. To touch, kiss, and express and receive love are integral to human behavior and growth.

Overall health is affected tremendously by movement. Exercise strengthens the heart, brings oxygen to the tissues, and relieves mental tension. Skin and bone breakdown, decreased mental stimulation, and increased dependence on others are examples of the negative health effects of immobility.

Implications of Neurosensory Functions for Collaboration

Consciousness. Consciousness serves the individual's capacity for social interaction. Without consciousness, the ability to think and to communicate are drastically diminished. Collaboration with clients is dependent on the client's state of consciousness, as altered states of consciousness place the client in a dependent condition. When a client's consciousness is diminished, it may become necessary for the nurse to shift the focus of collaboration from the client to others in the client's family who can communicate with the nurse.

Perception. Because no two individuals perceive any single event in the same way, it becomes essential in the collaborative process for the nurse to assess the client's reaction to the event, or cognitive perception, rather than the actual event itself. For example, a night nurse who admits two women for labor and delivery may find that they interpret their situations differently despite the fact that they are undergoing the same birthing process. A mother delivering her third baby may have a much different perception based on past experience and personality than a mother delivering her first child. Understanding the unique perceptions of each client enhances the care of each client.

Pain. Clients experiencing pain present an important challenge to nurses. To effectively collaborate with clients in pain, nurses must examine their own attitude toward pain, and their attitude toward the client's pain. Many times nurses underestimate clients' pain. When this occurs, clients generally receive insufficient medication for pain.[12] Awareness of these subjective elements along with careful, objective assessment of the nature of the pain and its meaning for the client will enable a nurse to collaborate with the client to effectively manage the client's pain.

Memory. Clients experiencing memory problems present challenges to the collaborative nurse–client relationship. Memory loss can mean inability to recall or store memories. This, in turn, means clients may have difficulty remembering explanations or instructions, and hence have trouble with learning. They may be unable to carry out tasks and to function independently and may be confused and disoriented. Such clients may require nursing interventions directed at safety and self-care. Clients with memory problems are thus placed in a more dependent role, shifting the focus of the collaborative nurse–client relationship.

Thought. Organized thinking, accurate perceptions of reality, an intact neurosensory network, and the higher cognitive functions of comprehension, reasoning, judgment, problem-solving, and conception are necessary for a collaborative nurse–client relationship. When altered thought processes occur, they become apparent in almost every aspect of an individual's behavior. In many cases, the client will be dependent on the nurse for guidance, safety, instruction, and interpretation of reality in order to accomplish activities of daily living and achieve a satisfactory and safe level of independence.

Communication. Communication is vital to the development of a collaborative nurse–client relationship. Through communication, nurse and client establish a relationship, share thoughts and feelings, and validate the clarity of messages and information exchanged. Communication is the tool by which nurses validate their inferences and judgments with clients in order to develop nursing diagnoses that clearly reflect clients' needs. The delivery of nursing care is most effective when clients can communicate their needs and desires. When there is insufficient communication or lack of client input, the nature of the nurse–client relationship changes from one of collaboration to a relationship in which the nurse must anticipate the needs of the client. Eye contact, voice intonation, and facial expression are a few of the ways in which nurses demonstrate caring and increase effectiveness of communication with clients experiencing impaired communication.

IMPLICATIONS FOR NURSE–CLIENT COLLABORATION

Neurosensory Functions

Collaboration as an interpersonal process is impossible without the support of the neurosensory functions: consciousness, perception, memory, thought, and communication. These functions of the nervous system comprise the anatomical and physiologic foundation of humanness and social interaction. When any one of these functions is altered or impaired, collaborative exchanges become difficult. In essence, neurosensory integration is a necessary condition for collaboration.

Emotions and Collaboration. Every human being experiences emotions. For nurses engaging in a collaborative nurse–client relationship, it becomes important to try to understand the emotions linked to the perceptions of clients who are experiencing illness. These emotions have a physiological as well as a psychological basis. Nurses administer drugs that act to affect moods or calm the body in the same way as the brain's own chemicals, the neurotransmitters. These drugs may influence the nature of the nurse's collaboration with the client.

Movement. One of the effects of the inability to move is dependence. Clients unable to move a part or all of their body become dependent on the nurse to assist them in activities of daily living. They may require assistance in transfers and in transportation from one area to another. They may also need assistance when walking or standing. The collaborative nature of the nurse–client relationship is shifted to focus on safety and protection under these conditions and the client becomes temporarily dependent on the nurse for mobility and interpretation of the surrounding environment. The nurse's roles in the collaborative relationship will be those of supporter and promoter of independence. Including the family and monitoring the client's needs is of prime importance.

FACTORS AFFECTING NEUROSENSORY INTEGRATION

Many factors influence neurosensory integration. Some are physical, others are psychological. Some factors can be controlled or regulated by the individual, others cannot.

Genetic Heritage

Genetic heritage is an important influence on neurosensory integration. Through the genes, genetic information is conveyed that shapes both the characteristics of the neurosensory apparatus common to humans and the unique features that are characteristic of the individual. Features of the neurosensory apparatus that in health protect neurosensory functions include the following.

- *Skull.* The skull is a bony structure composed of several bones that fuse after birth to form a rigid vault. This vault absorbs trauma to the head, protecting the brain.
- *Vertebral (Spinal) Column.* The vertebrae form a protective covering for the spinal cord and a support for the cranium and trunk. Each vertebra is cushioned from the next by a structure called the intervertebral disc, which has a high water content. When the core of the disc herniates through the outer layer, the disc loses its protective function. Further movement of the damaged disc can actually cause injury by compressing the spinal cord or spinal nerves.
- *Meninges.* The meninges are protective membranes covering the brain and spinal cord. Meningeal layers also provide blood supply and act as a cushion to the brain. There are three layers: the dura mater, the pia mater, and the arachnoid.
- *Cerebrospinal Fluid.* The cerebrospinal fluid (CSF) provides a cushion to prevent damage to the brain from blows, helps regulate intracranial pressure, and provides a mechanism for nutrient supply and waste removal. The CSF is produced by the filtration that occurs between the circulatory system and the choroid plexus. It filters out and coats the brain and spinal cord as it travels through the subarachnoid space. About 800 mL of CSF is secreted every day, although only approximately 150 mL is present at any one time in an adult. Reabsorption of CSF occurs through the arachnoid mater. CSF and molecules such as protein, glucose, and certain waste products are released back into the circulatory system. If the arachnoid villi are blocked, CSF cannot be reabsorbed and may result in injury.
- *Blood–Brain Barrier.* The blood–brain barrier is a unique protective structure of capillaries that supplies blood to the brain. These capillaries form a continuous wall that prevents many substances from entering the brain.[13] Water, oxygen, carbon dioxide, and glucose easily pass through this barrier. The membrane selectively also allows electrolytes, such as sodium, potassium, and chloride, to pass, and filters out extra nutrients and waste products of cell metabolism. If this barrier is injured, molecules that are normally excluded may be allowed to enter the brain, disrupting fluid and electrolyte balance.
- *Cerebral Circulation.* The cerebral circulation transports elements that are vital for central nervous system survival. Essential elements include oxygen and glucose, which the brain is unable to store. When arterial circulation ceases, the brain is depleted of oxygen in 4 to 6 minutes and is depleted of glucose in less than 1 minute. Arterial blood enters the CNS by two internal carotid arteries and two vertebral arteries.

Ordinarily the individual differences in genetic information create variation within certain limits that allows one individual to be differentiated from another but is nevertheless consistent with neurosensory integration. For example, skull shape and size may differ somewhat between individuals. Occasionally, however, the genetic information results in structural malformation that is inconsistent with integration. For example, the meninges may be malformed, interfering with the free flow of cerebrospinal fluid. This causes intracranial pressure to rise, thus interfering with brain activity. A detailed discussion of the various ways structural abnormalities impinge on neurosensory integration is beyond the scope of this text. However, it is important for the reader to understand that genetic heritage influences neurosensory integration through its capacity to cause malformation.

Age

Children. Young children have immature neurosensory systems. As they grow and learn, neurosensory functioning matures. Perception also changes with age. Infants and children need stimulation and parental affection to grow and develop. Too little stimulation can lead to the inability to conceptualize in later years. Too little affection can develop into failure to thrive in infants.

Many childhood diseases can affect the sensory organs. For example, measles can affect sight, resulting in blindness. Chronic ear infections, mumps, measles, or rubella can cause impaired hearing or deafness.

Older Adults. Cortical size and blood flow to the brain diminish with aging. The decrease in blood flow may result in a decrease of the oxygen supply, thereby compromising neurosensory function.

The senses also diminish with aging. Most elderly people develop some sight loss, hearing loss, loss of taste and smell, and loss of sensation. Balance may be affected, as well, as the muscles become weaker, or the neurosensory system degenerates.

Emotional changes may result from these neurosensory changes. The elderly may become depressed because of these changes. Sleep deprivation may cause delirium. Deprivation of NREM sleep (see Chap. 28) results in a reduction of hormones and produces lethargy and depression. Sensory deprivation may occur from the loss of sensory function.

Memory can be altered with the aging process. Decreased blood flow to the brain, atherosclerosis, and Alzheimer's disease are a few examples of aging changes contributing to altered memory. In addition, ability to learn may be altered and the speed of central processing is slowed.

Gait changes such as the slowing of step, widening of the base of support, and shuffling are related to a decrease in muscle mass and loss of large motor nerve fibers regulating nerve function.

General Health Status

Certain alterations in health can affect neurosensory functioning. Diseases or conditions that reduce blood circulation to the brain result in decreasing awareness and slowed responses. Diseases that alter brain tissue, such as Alzheimer's disease, result in a decreasing awareness. Diseases of the central nervous system can produce varying degrees of paralysis and sensory loss.

Physical alterations in other body systems can have an impact on neurosensory functioning. Decreased respiratory or cardiac function can lead to confusion, as can an imbalance in fluids and electrolytes. Renal alterations can result in a buildup of body toxins that can lead to an altered level of consciousness, as can liver dysfunction. An alteration in almost any body system can have an impact on neurosensory function.

Diet

Deficiencies in certain nutrients can influence sensory functioning. For example, semineural deafness is thought to be related to dietary deficiencies in vitamin D and calcium, which may affect the action potentials generated by the cochlea. Thiamin is essential for neurosensory integration (see Chap. 25). Electrolytes (chiefly sodium and potassium) are essential for nerve conduction and cellular integrity (see Chap. 31).

Environment

Stimuli. The environment is a major factor influencing conditions such as sensory deprivation or sensory overload. Too little meaningful stimuli can result in altered neurosensory integration, as can too much stimuli.

Excessive noise in the work environment can lead to diminished hearing, as can very loud music. Teenagers are at risk for hearing loss because of this.

Hazards. The word *toxin* means poison. Many substances in the home, workplace, and environment are toxic agents and act like poison in the body. Some have toxic effects, particularly on neurosensory integration, and the risk of accidental exposure is considerable.

Toxic agents are commonly found in solvents, paints, pesticides, and chemicals used in industry; in auto-engine emissions; and in industrial waste. In the hospital workplace, there is added risk of accidental exposure to mercury, a heavy metal.

Bacteria are another source of toxins that affect neurosensory integration. Tetanus and diphtheria are diseases produced by bacterial toxins. Both can be prevented with proper immunization. Another disease, botulism, is produced by a toxin that is potentially present in unrefrigerated foods, such as mayonnaise or salad dressings, and in meats, particularly chicken or pork, that are improperly cleaned or cooked. Simple prevention through proper preparation of food and refrigeration eliminates the potential harm from botulism toxin.

Toxins interfere with the transmission of impulses over the neurosensory network. A primary mechanism by which toxins exert their harmful effects is by interfering with the production, transfer, or release of neurotransmitters that relay signals from one neuron to another. The effects can be slight to overwhelming in nature. The functions of consciousness, memory, perception, speech, and movement may be affected.

The effects of toxic agents or chemicals on neurosensory integration can result in reversible or irreversible loss of function. Partial return of neurosensory function is also possible. Treatment is aimed at removal of the toxic agent and initiation of supportive and rehabilitative interventions. The extent of reversibility is evaluated as functions return.

Psychosocial Factors

Alterations in mental health can produce neurosensory alterations. Depression or withdrawal, for example, can in turn lead to further sensory deprivation.

Stress can affect behavior and thought. An individual's reaction to a stressful event will depend on the amount of stimulus presented by the stressful event and the number of other stressful events simultaneously occurring. When an individual does not cope well with stress, this in itself perpetuates the stress. Eventually stress may become overwhelming, and the individual may become disoriented, or confused.[14]

Medications and Other Substances

Many medications can affect neurosensory function. Sedations and tranquilizers may reduce alertness or lead to lethargy, drowsiness, or confusion. Antibiotics, such as streptomycin, neomycin, and gentamicin, can cause injury to the auditory nerve.

Alcohol and drugs can also result in toxicity to the neurosensory system. Ingestion of large amounts of alcohol and drugs is like ingesting a poison. While each drug interferes with the neural cell in its own destructive way, the effect is the same: neurosensory dysfunction. Altered consciousness, perception, movement, thought, or memory can occur with alcohol and drug toxicity.

■ ALTERATIONS IN NEUROSENSORY FUNCTIONING

Overview

Alterations in neurosensory functioning represent a common category of health problems for which clients may require supportive, restorative, and rehabilitative health care. Altered neurosensory functions can lead to serious long-term disability and frequently interfere with the client's quality of life and capacity to cope with the problems of life and living.

There are many causes of altered neurosensory functioning. The preceding discussion of factors affecting neurosensory integration suggests some of the etiologies involved in altered functioning. For example, genetic factors may cause illnesses that directly or indirectly affect neurosensory function. Genetic anomalies of the brain and spinal cord alter the structure and electrochemical processes of the central nervous system. These alterations can seriously interfere with the integration of neurosensory functions.

Deterioration of general health from nongenetic causes also can have pathophysiological consequences for neurosensory functions. Chronic kidney and liver disease, for example, can produce derangements in body chemistry that affect the whole body, including the nervous system. Wide fluctuations in the body's internal environment can disrupt the metabolism of cells in the neurosensory network, which interferes with neurosensory functions.

Alterations in neurosensory functions may also result from advancing age, poor nutrition, or environmental hazards. Accidents and trauma are common causes of neurosensory alterations. Motorcycle, bicycle, and automobile accidents too often result in serious, permanent disability.

Moreover, a number of diseases attack the neurosensory system itself and change its functioning. Disease processes can develop in virtually any aspect of the central or peripheral nervous systems and, depending on their location and severity, can alter an individual's consciousness, perception, memory, thought, communication, or movement. These processes include tumors, infection, toxicity, vascular lesions that disrupt circulation to the brain or spinal cord, and impaired neurosensory transmission.

Alterations in Consciousness

Alterations in consciousness result in decreased wakefulness (arousal) or decreased orientation or awareness of the environment (content). Causes of these altered states of consciousness can be physical damage to the brain tissue or metabolic abnormalities that interfere with the metabolism of the nerve cells.

Unconsciousness is a state in which people become unresponsive to external stimuli (noises, voices, pain). The unconscious state may be characterized by varying reductions in degree of arousal. Ambiguous terms, such as *disorientation, semi-consciousness,* and *coma,* are often used to describe altered levels of consciousness, or unconsciousness. It is not always important to find a label for a client's loss of consciousness so much as to describe the client's best response to verbal or painful stimuli.[15] Specific behavioral descriptions allow for less subjective interpretation (see the discussion of the Glasgow Coma in Section 2). However, several terms are commonly used to describe levels of consciousness. These are listed in Box 29–5.

IMPLICATIONS FOR NURSE–CLIENT COLLABORATION

Memory

Memory is a neurosensory function that many people take for granted; yet it underlies even the most basic human activity or social exchange. Chronic illnesses often have a harmful effect on memory, both in a direct way by their primary and secondary effects on the central nervous system, and by the severe stress they cause. Current population dynamics suggest that more and more older people with chronic illnesses will need health care in the future. Skill in assisting people with memory difficulties will determine whether or not nurse–client collaboration is successful. Supportive implementation that is constantly focused on bridging the cognitive gap created by a memory deficit will be a prominent feature of the care of many clients.

Alterations in Perception

The capacity of any sensory modality can be impaired with damage to the brain tissue or cells in the sensory pathway.

Altered Vision. Clients experiencing visual impairments or sight loss are handicapped, at least to some extent. Loss of vision may create a threat to safety, result in incomplete perceptions of events, limit educational and occupational opportunities, and limit mobility, as well as social and recreational activities. The nurse's role will involve assisting clients to adapt in various ways to their environment and sense of perception.

BOX 29–5. TERMS COMMONLY USED TO DESCRIBE ALTERATIONS IN CONSCIOUSNESS

- An **alert** individual is one who is fully aroused and fully oriented to person, place, and time. An alert client is fully conscious. Responses include appropriate acknowledgement of persons in the environment, turning the head or body in the direction of persons in the environment (unless impaired motor function is present), and an ability to focus attention on the environment.
- A **confused** individual has difficulty correctly interpreting and attending to stimuli. The individual may need some encouragement to focus on persons or things in the environment. The confused individual becomes disoriented first to time, then to place, then to person. He or she has difficulty following commands and remembering, and is easily distracted.
- A **delirious** individual is restless, incoherent, agitated, and may have alterations in thought patterns, such as delusions, illusions, or hallucinations. Delirious individuals may be loud and physically abusive. Prevention of harm to the individual and those around him is of special importance.
- An **obtunded** individual is sleepy or drowsy, but arouses easily. The individual's speech may be limited to the use of two- to three-word sentences, and may be inappropriate in nature.
- A **stuporous** individual is usually lethargic, slow to arouse, and drowsy. Painful stimuli are required to arouse the individual in this state and repetition of the painful stimulus is often required. Withdrawal from the painful stimulus occurs in response to stimulation.
- An individual in a state of **semi-consciousness** is unresponsive and does not move spontaneously unless a noxious stimulus is applied superficially. Moaning or groaning are brief responses observed to such noxious stimuli.
- **Coma** is a state of unarousability to deep noxious stimuli. Comatose clients usually lack withdrawal to the noxious stimulus, but slight muscle movement may be observed. Corneal, pupillary, and gag reflexes are present.
- An individual in a **deep coma** is completely unresponsive, lacks any response to deep noxious stimuli, and also lacks corneal, pupillary, gag, tendon, and plantar reflexes.

Visual alterations occur when there is external damage to the structure of the eye and its muscles, or internal damage to the optic nerve and nerve pathway. The result is decreased or absent visual capacity that manifests as refractive errors, dystopia, or blindness.

Refractive errors include such conditions as myopia, hyperopia, and presbyopia. Myopia, or nearsightedness, occurs from elongation of the eyeball. Only objects held close to the eye can be viewed without distortion. Objects that are distant are out of focus. Glasses with concave lenses correct this problem. Hyperopia, or farsightedness, is a condition in which persons have difficulty focusing on close objects, but can see distant objects clearly. Glasses with convex lenses correct this problem. Presbyopia occurs with aging. It is usually noticed around age 40 and occurs when the lens of the eye loses elasticity. Because of this loss of lens elasticity, persons cannot focus on close objects and must hold newspapers and other reading materials farther and farther away from the eye in order to read. Bifocals, trifocals, or reading glasses may be prescribed to correct the problem.

Diplopia is double vision or seeing two objects at one time. It usually occurs as a result of damage to the oculomotor nerve (cranial nerve III), but can involve dysfunction of the trochlear (cranial nerve IV) or abducens (cranial nerve VI) nerves, which control the movements of the eye. Dysfunction of these nerves usually interferes with up, down and lateral movements of the eye, and causes muscle weakness and uncoordinated eye movements, resulting in diplopia.

Cataracts, common in older persons, are opacities of the lens of the eye. In this condition, the amount of light reaching the retina is diminished because the cataract or opaque area is impervious to light. This results in diminished vision.

Glaucoma is a condition of increased intraocular pressure that can lead to blindness. It is related to an imbalance in production and drainage of the aqueous humor. Increased pressure from accumulating drainage damages the eye, producing visual field defects. This results in a person seeing only what is straight ahead of her, a situation that is referred to as tunnel vision.

A detached retina occurs when the sensory layer of the retina separates from the pigment layer, depriving the sensory layer of a blood supply. Clients may complain of partial blindness manifested as flashes of light, blurred or sooty vision, blank spots of vision, or complete loss of vision.

Alterations in color vision happen as a result of a defect in the visual color receptors of the retinal cones. The inability to distinguish certain colors is referred to as color blindness and is most commonly manifested as the inability to distinguish between red and green.

Blindness is the loss of ability to see. It may occur as a result of congenital malformation or may result from detachment of the retina, the visual reception area of the eye. Partial blindness is a condition in which persons have loss of vision in limited areas of the visual field. Hemianopsia is a form of partial blindness that occurs as a result of damage to the optic nerve behind the optic chiasm. A client with hemianopsia will experience blindness in one-half of the visual field of each eye.

Complete blindness is the total loss of vision from both eyes. Not all blind persons have a total loss of vision. The term *legal blindness* is used to describe severe, but incomplete, blindness. Legal blindness is defined as central visual acuity of 20/200 or less in the better eye, even when corrective lenses are worn.

Since sight is so important to functioning, its loss or absence represents an enormous loss to clients and has the potential to present a serious impairment.

Altered Hearing. Clients who have hearing loss present a special challenge to the nurse. Accurate assessment of the hearing loss, its meaning to the client, and adaptations for communicating with the client (hearing aid, sign language), influence the ability of the nurse and client to collaborate effectively. Changes in the structure and function of the ear can impair an individual's ability to hear. There are several types of hearing loss. Almost every type of hearing loss can be classified into one of three areas: conductive hearing loss, sensorineural or perceptive hearing loss, or mixed hearing loss.[16]

Conductive hearing loss can result from obstruction of the external canal by cerumen or a foreign body; a damaged eardrum (tympanic membrane); or immobility of the tympanic membrane or ossicles.[11] When sound vibrations are not adequately transmitted to the inner ear through the eardrum, middle ear, and ossicular chain, partial hearing loss results. This type of hearing loss can be treated. If the basic cause cannot be corrected, the client can use hearing aids to enhance hearing.

Sensorineural hearing, or perceptive hearing loss, occurs when there is a disorder of the inner ear,[11] for example, as a result of certain drugs; damage to the hair cells of the cochlea[17]; or pathology in the acoustic nerve (cranial nerve VIII) or the brain. In this type of hearing loss, vibrations are transmitted to the inner ear, but an impairment of the cochlea or acoustic nerve weakens the nervous impulses from the cochlea to the brain. Sensorineural hearing loss can also result from damage to the auditory pathways or auditory center of the brain. This type of hearing loss may be helped with hearing aids. Recently, devices known as cochlear implants have been designed to assist individuals with this type of hearing loss. The implants are inserted directly into the ear and compensate for damage to the sound-producing hair cells by sending out electrical signals to the hearing center in the brain.

Mixed hearing loss is a combination of conductive and sensorineural loss in the same ear. Mixed losses reduce both hearing sensitivity and discrimination, but because part of the loss is conductive, the ability to discriminate among sounds is reduced less than in sensorineural loss. Hearing losses may also result in speech deterioration, irritability and fatigue, social withdrawal, insecurity, indecision, suspiciousness, paranoia, and anger.

BUILDING NURSING KNOWLEDGE

Are Hearing Loss and Loneliness Related?

Christian E, Dluhy N, O'Neill R. Sounds of silence: Coping with hearing loss and loneliness. *J Gerontol.* 1989;15(11):4–9.

Studies have implicated that diminished auditory information results in withdrawal, depression, and social restriction. One study showed that 20 percent of those with hearing difficulties have feelings of loneliness some of the time. In this study, the researchers sought to determine the relationship of hearing loss and loneliness in an elderly population.

The study was conducted in three New England communities. Sixty-three subjects were 65 years of age or older and mentally clear. Subjects were interviewed to gain data on age, culture, marital status, financial status, mobility, and social interactions. All were tested for hearing acuity using a tetratone audiometer. Subjects were then categorized into two groups, normal-to-mild loss (response at 25 to 40 decibels), and serious-to-severe loss (response at 60 decibels or no response), and were asked to complete a self-administered standardized loneliness scale.

The average loneliness scores for the two groups were statistically compared. A definitive and statistically significant difference between the groups existed on their loneliness scores, confirming that elders who have greater hearing impairment experience more loneliness.

Altered Smell and Taste. Most people are born with the ability to smell. Alterations in the ability to smell can be caused by the common cold, strokes, head trauma, brain tumor, specific viral infections, cancer, nasal polyps, or heavy smoking, and frequently occur as a result of damage to cranial nerves II or V.

Clients sometimes experience impaired smell (hyposmia) or a distorted sense of smell (parosmia) from congestion. The complete absence of smell (anosmia) can be an important symptom of a brain tumor.

Damage to cranial nerves V or IX, which innervate the tongue, can result in alterations in taste. The effects of certain drugs also cause taste alterations. The partial, complete, or impaired sense of taste is called ageusia.

Loss of smell may be a barrier to occupational choices and pleasure, or a major health concern. For instance, a person who cannot smell will have difficulty detecting smoke or fire. Individuals employed in the preparation of foods, such as cooks and bakers, may not be able to pursue their occupations without their sense of smell.

Altered Touch. Alterations in tactile sensation or touch can result from damage to the peripheral sensory pathway or to the brain cells or pathways associated with sensation. Many of the sensations of altered touch are the same sensations that are perceived as pain, or lack of feeling. These sensations—paresthesia, hyperesthesia, and anesthesia—are discussed below under *Alterations in Pain.*

Loss of position sense is referred to as altered proprioception. Sensory nerve endings in muscles, tendons, and the labyrinth of the ear give individuals a sense of position. Proprioception also includes the sense of movement, the sense of vibration, deep pressure, and touch. With loss of proprioception, clients are susceptible to falls and injury, and may experience dizziness.

A client's inability to detect or accurately gauge temperature sensations cutaneously results in altered thermoreception. This loss of sensation can make the client vulnerable to accidental freezing or burning of the skin and subcutaneous tissue. The nose, ears, fingers, and toes are the first areas to freeze with exposure to cold. Prolonged exposure to cold results in frostbite, with sequelae of painful inflammation, blistering, ischemia, and gangrene.

Altered Sensory Input. Perceptual alterations occur as the result of the inability to interpret and integrate incoming sensory stimuli and messages into a meaningful whole. They frequently occur as a result of brain injury or stroke, and especially with damage to the right cerebral hemisphere, since it is concerned with perception, especially of spatial proportion, distance and rate; ability to recognize faces and familiar objects; perception of time; and ability to follow visual instructions. When perceptual deficits are compounded by other neurological deficits, interpreting the environment can become very difficult for the client.

Perceptual alterations include alterations in body awareness and visual–spatial relationships, apraxias, agnosias, sensory deprivation, and sensory overload.

One-sided neglect is an alteration in body awareness in which clients are not able to integrate and use perceptions from the affected side of the body and/or from the environment on the affected side. It often occurs in clients with right brain damage. One-sided neglect is manifested when clients simply deny the existence of one side of the body and pay no attention to the environment on the affected side. It may accompany one-sided blindness and interferes with self-care and safety.

Alterations in visual–spatial relationships involve difficulties in perceiving the position of two or more objects in relation to one's self and in relation to one another. Depth and distance perception may be affected and clients may have difficulty differentiating in–out, front–behind, or up–down. Clients may bump into objects, hit doorways with their wheelchairs, knock objects over on a table, have balance problems, and demonstrate confusion.

Inability to conceptualize, plan and execute skilled or nonhabitual motor activity despite adequate muscle power, sensation, and coordination is called apraxia.[18] This is a complex problem, a result of left or right cerebral hemisphere damage. A client with apraxia is able to understand the voluntary act required, but either is unable to carry out the act or does so incorrectly or inconsistently.

Inability to recognize objects or faces through the senses is called agnosia. There are different varieties of agnosia, which are usually labeled according to the sensory function that is impaired (Table 29–2).

Perceptual alterations include two other phenomena, sensory deprivation and sensory overload. **Sensory depri-**

TABLE 29–2. TERMS RELATED TO AGNOSIA

Term	Definition
Visual agnosia	The inability to name or recognize common objects by sight; damage is usually present in the visual cortex.
Auditory agnosia	The inability to name or recognize the meaning of environmental sounds. Clients can hear the sounds, but not put meaning to them. Lesions of the temporal lobe are associated with auditory agnosia.
Tactile agnosia	The inability to recognize common objects through the sense of touch. Inability to recognize car keys, pencils, combs with the eyes closed is a result of parietal lobe lesions.
Autotopagnosia	The inability to identify body parts and/or their relationships. This is a result of posterior-inferior parietal lobe damage.
Prosopagnosia	The inability to recognize familiar faces.
Unilateral asomatognosia	The inability to recognize or unawareness of one side of the body and its visual space (usually left asomatognosia due to right hemisphere damage).

vation occurs when there is a lack of input from the senses; this may alter a person's sense of reality and result in irritability, restlessness, confusion, boredom, sleepiness, decreased attention span, false sense of reality (hallucination), or false beliefs (delusions). Manifestations of sensory deprivation vary with an individual's adaptation ability and also vary at different times for any individual.

Sensory deprivation may occur when there is an interruption of sensory input. Blindness, deafness, or paralysis can result in sensory deprivation. Lack of environmental stimulation may precipitate sensory deprivation when a person is confined to a hospital room or is on bed rest. Socialization and conversation stimulate thought and emotions. When social input is lacking whether from mobility restrictions, communication problems, or confinement from hospitalization, sensory deprivation may occur.

Darkness may also contribute to sensory deprivation. The lack of light and lack of visual stimulation from a lighted room can decrease sensory input and alter perceptions of reality. This situation is common in older persons. They may be fully oriented during daytime hours, but with the onset of night and darkness, confusion, hallucinations, and irritability may set in. This condition is sometimes referred to as "sundowners syndrome."

Sensory overload occurs when there is too much sensory input impinging on the sensory network and brain, which also alters a person's sense of reality and results in slowed thinking, distractibility, impaired memory, confusion, irritability, difficulty sleeping, inability to concentrate, fear, anxiety, hallucinations, and delusions. The symptoms or results of sensory overload are very similar to those of sensory deprivation. Again, a person's ability to adapt and the timing of events influence that person's reaction to sensory overload.

Factors contributing to sensory overload are altered sleep patterns, pain, hospital or health care facility routines, an unfamiliar environment, and a different culture or language barrier. Any combination of one or more of these factors predisposes clients to sensory overload.

Sensory overload, which can be viewed as sensory bombardment, originates in the external environment. For hospitalized clients, sensory overload usually occurs in the intensive care unit. There, clients are subjected to a vast array of noises coming from beeping machines and alarms. Frequent nurse checks and physician rounds interrupt clients' rest and sleep schedules. Consequently, their sleep patterns are altered and/or shortened, producing irritability and anxiety.

Alterations in Pain

Pain is a naturally occurring phenomenon that protects the body from serious injury and alerts an individual to an alteration in health. If individuals did not experience pain when exposed to painful stimuli, they would not instinctively withdraw or be able to identify pain, allowing for more cellular damage to occur. Absence of the sense of touch or absence of pain is known as **anesthesia.** Reduced pain sensation can also result in injury or tissue damage. This condition is known as **hypoesthesia.**

Abnormal or strange sensations of pain are called **paresthesias.** These sensations may include burning, itching, tingling, or the feelings of an electrical shock.

More distressing than the feeling of pain is **hyperesthesia,** a heightened sense of touch or pain. A sheet covering a person who experiences hyperesthesia can produce severe pain.

Alterations in Memory and Learning

Memory and learning are integrally related, thus their manifestations of altered dysfunction are related. Brain injury, sensory overload or sensory deprivation, impaired neural transmission, and altered perception states interfere with the input of sensory stimuli and/or their reconstruction into meaningful patterns.

Alterations in memory involve difficulty with the ability to retain or store thoughts, information, and learned experiences. The loss of memory is termed amnesia. Three aspects of retrieval of information and experiences may be affected in amnesia. Sometimes with a concussion or mild head injury, a person loses consciousness momentarily and, upon awakening, cannot remember the events following or surrounding the head injury. Loss of recent memory is referred to as anterograde amnesia. New information or events cannot be stored and the client may demonstrate difficulty in learning.

Another aspect of information retrieval that may be lost with amnesia is immediate recall. In this case, the ability to remember events of the day or past minutes or hours is impaired. Loss of remote memory—difficulty remembering long-term memories of events and experiences of several years pasts—is referred to as retrograde amnesia. The person who sustains a head injury and has problems with remote memory would be unable to remember his birth date, names of family members, or the schools attended.

Forgetfulness involves disrupted retrieval, rather than storage, of information or experiences. It is usually seen as an inability to recall certain dates, peoples' names, or an item on the mental list. Forgetfulness differs from amnesia in that amnesia usually involves some brain tissue damage, major loss of information, and difficulty learning, whereas forgetfulness is a functional problem (rather than brain tissue damage) in the process of retrieving information, involves single items of information lost, and a person can be prompted to remember an item of information. Etiologies associated with forgetfulness include depression, disorientation, the aging process, and certain organic brain disorders.

Alterations in Thought

Thought is closely related to memory and learning. Impaired thinking involves the inability to carry out activities of logic, reasoning, insight, calculations, judgments and decision-making, dealing with reality, and abstract thought. External traumatic events as well as alterations in internal neurological structure or process may disrupt this complex process. Alterations in thought present problems in orientation, memory, and perception, and may also manifest in agnosias and apraxias (Table 29–3). Emotional disturbances can also result in disturbances in thought processes and neurosensory integration.

Alterations in Communication, Language, and Speech

Language is closely linked to thought and requires the abilities of concentration and attentiveness. Any alteration to the higher cerebral speech structures or to the cranial nerves that conduct nerve impulses can result in an altered ability to communicate. Consider, for example, the impact of a communication alteration when there is a loss of sensory function—hearing loss, blindness, inability or deficiency in intellectual thought, poor attention span, or memory deficit. The limitation on the person's ability to articulate needs and desires in turn creates feelings of frustration, anger, and isolation.

Persons with motor communication alterations experience mechanical difficulties in articulation of thought; for example, the lips, throat, or facial muscles may be paralyzed or damaged in some way. Inability to express needs and desires is impaired, the consequence of which is feelings of frustration and anger.

Whether communication problems are the result of unclear messages or of problems with reception and expression, clients will experience interference in interpersonal relationships and satisfaction of human needs. Alterations in language and speech production are thus related to alterations in thought and are manifested as aphasias and dysarthrias. These dysfunctions interfere with interper-

---

BUILDING NURSING KNOWLEDGE

How Does the Nurse Recognize When the Client's Thought Processes are Altered?

Hall GR. Alterations in thought process. *J Gerontol Nurs.* 1988;14(3):30–37.

Hall notes that alteration in thought process is a common nursing diagnosis among older clients. One study reported that 63 percent of nursing home clients were disoriented or had memory loss severe enough to impair performance of activities of daily living.

Altered thought process may be associated with a number of physiological changes affecting the brain including trauma, brain tissue degeneration, disease of other organs that alters brain metabolism, and the physiological stress of surgery. Hall points out that the most difficult physiological change results from the permanent and progressive organic degeneration of the cerebral cortex.

Assessment of altered thought process is often difficult because the client is generally unable to give reliable information and the nurse must validate data with family members, who are sometimes reluctant to discuss symptoms with the client.

Typical features of this diagnosis include memory loss and loss of time sense; inability to perform abstract thinking, to make decisions, to problem-solve, and to plan; poor judgment; altered perceptions; decreased attention span; and loss of language abilities. There is also loss of emotional expression (affect); inhibitions are diminished as manifested in temper displays and inappropriate behavior; there is loss of recognition of others, social withdrawal, self-preoccupation, suspiciousness (paranoia), and sometimes false ideas (delusions); lowered stress threshold may be manifested in belligerence, compulsive repetitive behavior, purposeless behavior, and wandering. Many of the characteristic behaviors worsen late in the day (sundowners syndrome) or follow a stimulating event that makes the client uncomfortable or distressed.

Nursing assistance focuses on reducing stress and providing safety and nutrition to aid coping. Clients are asked to do only things that are within their capabilities. Stimuli are monitored. Stressors that aggravate altered thought process include fatigue; change of environment, caregiver, or routine; misleading or overwhelming stimuli; or demands for achievement that exceed the client's functional capacity. It is important to facilitate the client's ability to respond appropriately by providing structure and routine to reinforce pattern and meaning. Routines reduce the need for the client to think and plan, and thus eliminate frustration for the client. Activities appropriate to the client's energy level and frequent rest periods may be helpful. Changes of pace are made only when they are within the client's level of tolerance.

TABLE 29–3. TYPES OF ALTERATIONS OF THOUGHT

Alteration	Definition
Impaired thought content	The inability to interpret internal and external stimuli accurately and meaningfully in one's environment. May be manifested as doubting and indecision, feelings of unreality and control by others, and compulsive phenomena, such as obsessions, phobias, or repetitive thinking about issues.
Illusions	A false interpretation of external, usually visual or auditory, sensory stimuli. For example, a client who is restrained in bed may falsely interpret the external environment as a department store in which she is tied to a playpen, with many people around that the client does not recognize.
Delusions	Fixed, irrational beliefs not consistent with cultural mores. May be persecutory, grandiose, nihilistic, or somatic. For example, a client receiving medication might have delusions that he is part of a drug ring and is being forced to take drugs.
Hallucinations	False sensory perceptions occurring without any external stimuli. Clients can see, feel, hear, smell, or taste things not apparent to the observer. For example, an alcoholic client experiencing drug withdrawal may see insects crawling on the wall; a confused elderly client may see deceased relatives in a familiar setting unreal to the client's current environment.
Impaired attention span	The inability to attend to incoming stimuli. The client will appear to be distracted, unable to engage in a conversation or to concentrate on activities, and will require assistance in nursing activities. Etiologies contributing to impaired attention span may include confusion, depression, sensory overload, or sensory deprivation.
Loss of abstract thinking	Client retains only the ability to deal with the concrete. Clients can manipulate objects correctly and deal with the here-and-now, but unfamiliar events and concepts pose problems. Problem-solving ability is decreased because the abstract representations cannot be used for making decisions. Implications are in the arena of social relations. A limited, dependent life-style will result with loss of interpretative abilities, sense of humor, and limited conversational abilities.
Confusion	A state in which a person's thoughts are disorganized and incongruent with reality. Although found in many metabolic and psychologic disorders, it is very characteristic of brain damage. It is manifested by misinterpretation of stimuli, paranoia, illusions, delusions, hallucinations, and confabulation.
Confabulation	Occurs when persons make up stories or explanations to correctly explain surrounding events or situations.
Emotional liability	Emotions that transition quickly from laughter to crying. Emotional outbursts may occur in response to ordinary activities, such as receiving a glass of water.

sonal relationships and the satisfaction of human needs, and cause severe emotional and communication problems.

Aphasia is an impairment of language in which there is loss of ability to communicate. Expressive aphasia, also known as Broca's aphasia, or motor aphasia, is the inability to transfer words into articulation. Damage to Broca's area (the speech motor association cortex in the dominant cerebral hemisphere) results in slowness of speech, difficulty in forming words for speech, and use of simple phrases. Clients with expressive aphasia alteration understand written and spoken words and know what they want to say but cannot utter the words to express themselves. Clients may resort to using only main ideas to convey wants and needs.

Receptive aphasia or sensory aphasia involves difficulty in comprehension of incoming messages. Damage occurs in Wernicke's area, the area of the cortex that involves interpretation of the spoken and written word. The incoming message makes no sense to the client, but the client is able to speak easily and to formulate words without difficulty. After a time, the listener becomes aware that even though speech is fluent, coherence and logic are missing. Clients may also have difficulty naming objects correctly.

Global aphasia is the combination of both expressive and receptive aphasia whereby all systems for communication are damaged. This has the poorest prognosis and causes the greatest problems for clients. Clients cannot understand what they see or hear, nor can they convey thought in speech or writing.

Dysarthria is a language disorder in which there is defective articulation caused by motor deficit of the tongue or the speech muscles (cranial nerves V, VII, IX, X). Clients have slurred speech and difficulty pronouncing the letters m, b, p, t, d, and the number one. However, the content of speech is intact.

Alterations in Movement

Alterations in body movement may occur as a result of injury to the neurons and pathways in the central nervous system or as a result of injuries to the peripheral nervous system. The reader is referred to Chapter 30 for a discussion of alterations in movement related to loss of strength, mobility, and flexibility.

Mobility can be altered in a variety of ways. Paralysis is the loss of voluntary muscle movement. Hemiplegia, paraplegia, and quadriplegia are types of paralysis. Hemiplegia refers to loss of motor function in one half of the body; paraplegia involves loss of motor function to the lower extremities; quadriplegia, loss of lower extremity function plus varying amounts of loss of upper extremity function, depending on the spinal cord level involved.

Loss of balance and coordination can result from diseases of the cerebellum. Ataxia, the incoordination of voluntary muscle action (especially the walking muscles), is the result of impaired balance and cerebellar function. With an ataxic gait, the feet are lifted high and then hit the floor heavily. There may also be a lurching walk. Another problem of balance and coordination may be the inability to maintain normal or desired body posture.

Change in muscle tone is another alteration of movement. Spasticity or hypertonic muscle tone is the result of damage to neural pathways or cells in the central nervous system, and results in undue resistance of the muscle to passive lengthening (the muscle is tight and resists stretching). Flaccidity or hypotonic muscle tone is caused by neuron damage in the peripheral nervous system, and results in muscle that is soft, floppy, and without tone. Rigidity involves a constant state of resistance. The dysfunction involves the extrapyramidal system and is seen in Parkinson's disease.

Tremors are involuntary muscle movements of the body or limbs resulting from contraction of opposing muscles. Resting tremors are tremors that occur when the person is at rest and are diminished by purposeful activity. Intentional tremors are tremors that are increased or precipitated by purposeful activity. These involuntary, abnormal movements interfere with clients' coordinated movement.

Tics are involuntary, compulsive stereotyped movements. Some tics are viewed as "nervous habits"; others are hereditary conditions.

Seizures are sudden, brief, jerky contractions of a muscle, muscle group, or the whole body. They occur because of uncontrolled and excessive electrical impulses in the brain cells; some are localized to the motor strip. A seizure is a phenomenon or symptom of a health alteration, not a disease.

Seizures are classified as generalized and partial. Generalized seizures involve both hemispheres of the brain. Generalized seizures are further classified as grand mal (tonic–clonic), petit mal (absence attacks), tonic, clonic, myoclonic, atonic, and akinetic seizures.

Grand mal seizures involve major motor activity and loss of consciousness. They are characterized by four phases: preictal (aura), tonic, clonic, and postictal phases. In the preictal phase, an aura may occur. An aura is a peculiar sensation experienced prior to the appearance of the more definite symptoms of seizures. Cognitive effects of the aura include feelings of deja vu, and of time standing still. In the tonic phase, which lasts 15 to 60 seconds, the muscles become rigid, the back arches, the jaw clamps shut, and sudden loss of consciousness occurs. Respirations also cease, and the pupils dilate. The tonic phase ends abruptly as the clonic phase begins. The clonic phase is characterized by rapid, violent, bilateral jerks lasting from 2 to 5 minutes. Rapid breathing occurs. Other symptoms include incontinence, clenching the teeth, sweating, changes in heart rate (raised or lowered), and pupil changes. In the postictal phase, muscle flaccidity occurs. Consciousness slowly returns, but often drowsiness, confusion, headaches, muscle aches, and fatigue occur. These seizures may be seen in persons of any age.

Petit mal seizures are characterized by loss of awareness but not of consciousness. The person appears to be staring but does not lose muscle tone. Seizures last for 10 to 30 seconds and may occur infrequently or up to hundreds of times daily. There is no aura or postictal phase. Petit mal seizures usually begin between the ages of 4 and 8. They may resolve spontaneously during adolescence or may develop into tonic–clonic seizures. When petit mal seizures continue into adulthood, they remain unchanged.

Tonic seizures are rare. They are characterized by sudden rigidity of muscles and loss of consciousness, flushing, increased heart rate and blood pressure, sweating, and pupil changes. No clonic jerks are seen.

Clonic seizures present with a brief generalized spasm followed by asymmetrical bilateral jerks. They can last up to several minutes. They do not have the phases of the tonic–clonic seizures. These seizures are generally restricted to children between the ages of 4 and 8.

Myoclonic seizures are brief, sudden muscle contractions in the arms and legs or the trunk. There is little or no loss of consciousness. This type of seizure may be associated with biochemical alterations, fevers, or spinal cord lesions.

Atonic and akinetic seizures display a loss of body tone associated with falling. Individuals with this seizure disorder may catch themselves before hitting the ground and do not lose consciousness.

Partial seizures occur when the electrical discharge involves only a part of the brain. Partial seizures may occur with a wide variety of symptoms, depending on which section of the cerebral cortex is involved. Partial seizures are further classified into elementary seizures, complex (temporal lobe or psychomotor) partial seizures, and partial seizures that are secondarily generalized.

Elementary partial seizures are caused by localized cortical electrical stimulation. Elementary seizures may demonstrate motor, sensory, or autonomic symptoms. Motor symptoms consist of focal jerks of any muscle but particularly the face and hands. The person loses control of the affected areas during the 5 to 15 second time period of the seizure. Sensory symptoms include hallucinations, sensory illusions, and sensations of numbness, burning, tingling, or crawling. Autonomic symptoms include signs of flushing, increased heart rate, sweating, increased or decreased blood pressure, and pupillary changes.

Complex partial seizures are focal seizures that arise from the anterior temporal lobe. These seizures generally present with an aura. Effects include fear and paranoia. Psychomotor symptoms include inappropriate activities, such as smacking the lips, chewing, swallowing, grimacing, or picking at the clothing.

Partial seizures that are secondarily generalized, complex partial seizures, may generalize into tonic–clonic seizures if both hemispheres are involved.

Causes of Altered Neurosensory Functioning

Trauma. Neurosensory integration can be dramatically impaired by traumatic events. Trauma is the leading cause of death for persons under 45 years of age. The major types of trauma that affect neurosensory integration include head trauma, spinal cord trauma, and peripheral nerve injury. Approximately 7 to 10 million head injuries occur in the United States each year. Most head injuries occur among males age 16 to 25. Spinal cord trauma also occurs in young, healthy adults. Approximately two thirds of clients with new spinal cord injuries each year are younger than 36 years of age. Approximately 100,000 Americans are presently paralyzed, and there are 7,500 to 10,000 new cases each year. Peripheral nervous system trauma occurs with knife wounds, assault and battery, falls, and industrial and sports-related accidents.

Major alterations in neurosensory integration are associated with traumatic injuries. Mobility, independence, health maintenance, skin integrity, bowel and bladder elimination, respiratory functions, thermoregulation, and self-care abilities can all be affected. These effects can be overwhelming to clients and their families or significant others. They also have economic consequences for society. The social impact of traumatic events disrupts every aspect of the injured person's life. Interpersonal relationships can become strained by overwhelming dependence for activities of daily living. For some individuals, the injury may mean the end of a career. Life-style may be drastically altered.

If trauma results in sequelae such as memory loss, speech disturbances, or personality changes, individuals have to cope with new, limited personal potential. Body image may change drastically with injuries such as paralysis, gunshot wounds, amputations, and scars from lacerations. Any of these disturbances can affect the ability to communicate with significant others, and loss of the ability to communicate effectively results in anger, frustration, and humiliation. Sexuality may undergo changes for individuals suffering from disfigurements, paralysis, or personality changes. The person's view of self is changed.

The families or significant others of injured clients experience disruptions in their patterns of living and life-style, as well. They are challenged to cope with the consequences of their loved one's altered physical or psychological makeup, as well as to meet his or her demands of support during hospitalization and at home.

The potential for recovery for clients experiencing the various types of trauma is dependent on the location, extent, and severity of damage to the brain, spinal cord, and peripheral nerves and muscles. While some injuries may be permanent, such as the inability to move the legs from a spinal cord injury, others result in full recovery. A minor head injury may have only temporary consequences.

Tumors. Tumors are a spontaneous new growth of tissue, resulting in an abnormal mass that interferes with the function of normal tissue. Tumors can develop in any area of the neurosensory system, but occur particularly in the brain and, occasionally, the spinal cord. Although many neurosensory tumors are malignant, and carry a poor prognosis, others are benign and can be treated effectively.

The impact of a tumor is similar to that of head and spinal trauma and may include (1) destruction of nerve cells by infiltration or compression, resulting in interrupted transmission of neural signals, (2) pressure on nerve tracts in the spinal cord or brain, interrupting transmission of neural signals, (3) irritation or destruction of specific brain tissues or structures, causing functional alterations (for example, thought and intellectual impairment), and (4) increased intracranial pressure as the tumor swells, grows, and enlarges. Any of the effects can be devastating to neurosensory function and can result in altered functions of consciousness, perception/sensation/vision, emotions, speech/language/communication/memory, thought and movement depending on what areas of the brain or spinal cord are involved.

Infection. Infections can alter neurosensory function. Commonly, infections of the nervous system result when some other area of the body has become infected and the infection spreads. Infections of the ear, sinuses, and tonsils are the most common initial sites for infections that spread to the neurosensory system. The brain or parts of the brain, the meninges, the spinal cord, spinal nerves, and peripheral nerves are all susceptible to infection.

Infections can affect the neurosensory network in one of two ways. The infection can remain a localized process, affecting a small area of neurosensory tissue, or it can become a widespread generalized condition involving substantial tissue. Whether localized or generalized, infections of the nervous tissue are very dangerous and require prompt medical treatment.

The impact of infection on neurosensory integration depends on the location of the infection in brain tissue and the function of the affected brain tissues. A localized infection may produce very specific altered neurosensory functions, such as speech impairment, or weakness or paralysis of an extremity. If the infection is widespread, the result may be generalized manifestations, such as loss of consciousness and alteration in vital functions.

Infections of the nervous system are dangerous because even when they are temporary, they can cause serious interference with functions of the nervous system and with other systems of the body, and because they can lead to permanent loss of function. Infections are more prevalent among the very old, the very young, clients with nutritional deficiencies, and those whose immune defenses are impaired by illness or medication.

Vascular Lesions. In the United States, vascular lesions of the brain strike more than half a million people each year and remain in third place (after heart disease and cancer) as a cause of death. These lesions represent an interruption to the blood supply to brain tissue (ischemia). They result in lack of oxygen and glucose to the neurons and the accumulation of end products from metabolism. These ischemic events are commonly referred to as a stroke.

Vascular lesions include blood clots and rupture of a blood vessel (hemorrhage). Blood clots occur when blood cells collect in the wall of a cerebral artery (thrombosis) or when a clot or foreign material dislodged from another site (embolism) travels to a brain vessel and lodges in the vessel causing a blockage. Rupture of a blood vessel, on the other hand, causes blood to surround brain tissue and cells, and disrupts the blood supply and available oxygen to the surrounding brain tissue. This may occur when the client has high blood pressure, when disease weakens the walls of a cerebral artery, or when a congenitally malformed vessel finally breaks open. Vascular lesions can adversely affect consciousness, perception, sensation, memory, thought, learning, language/speech/communication, emotions, and movement.

Impaired Neurosensory Transmission. Alterations in neurosensory functions can also result from impaired nerve impulse transmission. This can accompany trauma, clots, or lack of oxygen, or it can result from a host of degenerative conditions, such as Parkinson's disease, muscular dystrophy, and amyotrophic lateral sclerosis, which result in severe, progressive loss of muscle movement.

Another class of diseases, called demyelinating conditions, also affect impulse transmission. These conditions involve a defect that results in destruction of the protective sheath (myelin) around neuronal axons and dendrites in the central nervous system. With destruction of this myelin sheath, neural messages to move a muscle or organ cannot be relayed, resulting in movement problems. An example of a demyelinating condition is multiple sclerosis.

The neurosensory functions affected by neurosensory transmission disorders can include perception, memory, thought, emotion, language/speech/communication, and movement. Because the impact on movement and thought functions is so devastating, clients suffer severe economic and social costs. The economic costs of home care and rehabilitation can be overwhelming. The social costs include the consequences of restricted mobility, and the decreased socialization and recreational opportunities for clients. Families also suffer in having to deal with the changed personality and altered, deteriorating physical condition, of a loved one.

Because of the resulting impaired mobility, mental incapacitation, and dependency on others, the collaborative relationship between nurse and client is often affected by illnesses of the neurosensory system. Clients with unimpaired perceptual and cognitive function can collaborate with nurses in determining care. In cases of perceptual and cognitive impairment, or disorders of consciousness, however, nurses assume greater direction in the nature of the client–nurse relationship.

Section 2. Assessment of Neurosensory Integration

NEUROSENSORY DATA COLLECTION

Assessment of neurosensory integration enables the nurse, with client or family collaboration, to gather data on the client's condition and functional ability. Specifically, the nurse performs a neurosensory assessment to gain data about alterations in neurosensory function such as level of consciousness, altered memory and learning, altered perception, altered thought, altered communication, and/or altered movement; altered functions of body systems other than the neurosensory system that may lead to or result from loss of neurosensory integration; and pain.

Sharing information between nurse and client is essential to the assessment process. Neurosensory assessment incorporates a client history, client examination, and review of relevant diagnostic tests. Important nursing questions such as the following can be answered as the result of a neurosensory assessment:

- Can the client see and hear adequately?
- Will sensory losses impede the client's ability for self-care?
- Does the client have the balance necessary for safe ambulation?
- Is the client's judgment adequate for safe performance of activities of daily living?
- Can the client communicate sufficiently to make needs known?
- Does the client have the coordination needed for bathing and eating?
- Is the client alert enough to perceive dangers in the environment?
- Is the client aware of limitations?

Neurosensory assessment is extremely important to planning client care and to identifying the type of nursing assistance clients may want and need.

Neurosensory assessment need not always be a formal process. In a sense, every time a nurse interacts with a client, a neurosensory assessment is being performed. In the course of a conversation with a client, for instance, a nurse will make observations about how alert the client appears, the clarity of the client's speech, the coherence of the ideas the client is expressing, or the coordination of the client's gestures or movements. For the most part, neurosensory assessment does not require taking the client to an examination room but occurs during the course of other activities, such as the bed bath.

The formal neurosensory assessment is presented here in its entirety because it is the most thorough, systematic approach to gathering clinical data about the client's neurosensory functions, and because it is appropriate that the reader learn to perform a complete assessment. Once all aspects of the assessment are mastered and the clinical uses are understood, the nurse may elect to carry out a full neurosensory history and examination or select aspects according to the demands of particular client situations. A thorough assessment is especially important when initially establishing the client care plan. Thereafter, select observations may be sufficient to make an evaluation of the client's progress.

Neurosensory History

The neurosensory history provides vital information about losses in neurosensory integration that may interfere with the client's adaptation and ability to perform activities of daily living. It may be necessary to include family members in this process, particularly when the client's memory and thought are impaired. The level of neurosensory deficit can vary markedly and may affect clients' ability to complete a history, particularly if family members or significant others are not present. History-taking also provides the nurse with an opportunity to begin a working relationship with client and family.

Primary Concern. The primary concern is the first step in establishing a collaborative relationship because it allows the client to identify and prioritize reasons for seeking care and make them known to the nurse. The primary concern is the aspect of the problem for which the client seeks health care. For example, a woman with weakness in her right arm may be most concerned, not about an underlying disease state that the weakness may represent, but rather about her ability to work to earn money to support her family. By gathering this type of data, the nurse is able to identify areas of client needs and validate them with the client. Moreover, the nurse can use this information to make clinical appraisals not only of client concerns, but also of neurosensory functions. The integrity of the following neurosensory functions may become apparent as the client responds to the nurse's questions.

- *Consciousness:* Is the client alert enough to identify the primary concern?
- *Perception:* Does the client's concern relate to the problems the nurse sees?
- *Emotion:* Does the client express that concern with appropriate emotion?
- *Memory:* Does the client remember what the concern is?
- *Thought:* Does the client's statement of concern indicate difficulty in evaluating the seriousness of his condition?
- *Communication:* Does the client have problems with speech or understanding speech?

The following example illustrates a primary concern related to neurosensory functioning.

- Erin, a 13-year-old girl, has injured her right arm while swimming butterfly during swim practice. She is unable to fully raise her arm. The nurse who is interviewing Erin in the emergency department confirms that Erin's primary concern is being unable to swim in an upcoming swim event. Erin is not aware that there may be underlying damage to the neurosensory system, although the nurse recognizes this possibility. This data is used to establish initial nursing diagnoses that will be used in developing a plan of care for Erin.

Current Understanding/Pain History. The current understanding relates to the client's interpretation of the health problem and understanding of the causes and consequences of the problem. The nurse obtains this information by establishing the client's own understanding of the causes and effects of his or her health problem. The nurse may also help define the onset, sequence, and duration of the problem.

Pain History. Pain history is an essential component of the client's current understanding. Problems often arise in taking a pain history because of the subjectivity of the pain experience. Clients should be encouraged to describe pain in their own words. A pain history should be modified to fit the client's need; for example, questions asked a postoperative client would differ from those asked a client in chronic pain. Several factors that are relevant to pain include location, intensity, onset, duration, and quality.

Location. Pain may be generalized or quite regional. Asking the client to accurately identify or trace location may require repeated questioning to obtain a necessary level of specificity. The description should include the extent and spread of the pain, as well as identification of pain-free areas. The client may be entirely focused on the pain, or may be unable to adequately describe it because of neurosensory involvement. Anatomical diagrams may be useful if clients cannot adequately locate their pain or if there are multiple areas of pain interspersed with pain-free areas (see Fig. 29–4).

Terms that can be used to identify and describe pain location include: *localized*—confined to the area of focus; *radiating*—extending beyond the focus of the pain; *projected*—transmitted along nerve pathways; and *referred*—occurring in an area other than the source. When gathering data on pain location, the nurse should determine if the pain is superficial or deep, and if the pain location remains constant or if it moves. If location changes, ask the client to identify related factors. For example, does the location of the pain change when the client sits up?

Intensity. Intensity is probably the most subjective characteristic of pain. Certain types of pain are obviously more severe (eg, chest pain), or more annoying (eg, low back pain) than others. Pain intensity can reflect the intensity

Patient's name: ______ Diagnosis: ______
Pain medication(s): Date: ______ Time: ______ a.m./p.m.
______ Dosage: ______ Time given: ______ a.m./p.m.
______ Dosage: ______ Time given: ______ a.m./p.m.

PRI: S ______ (groups 1-10) A ______ (groups 11-15) E ______ (group 16) M ______ (groups 17-20)

NWC: ______ Comments: ______

PPI: ______

PRI

SENSORY (S)

1 1. FLICKERING — 2. QUIVERING — 3. PULSING — 4. THROBBING — 5 BEATING — 6. POUNDING —

2 1. JUMPING — 2. FLASHING — 3. SHOOTING —

3 1. PRICKING — 2. BORING — 3. DRILLING — 4. STABBING —

4 1. SHARP — 2. CUTTING — 3. LACERATING —

5 1. PINCHING — 2. PRESSING — 3. GNAWING — 4. CRAMPING — 5. CRUSHING —

6 1. TUGGING — 2. PULLING — 3. WRENCHING —

7 1. HOT — 2. BURNING — 3. SCALDING — 4. SEARING —

8 1. TINGLING — 2. ITCHY — 3. SMARTING — 4. STINGING —

9 1. DULL — 2. SORE — 3. HURTING — 4. ACHING — 5. HEAVY —

10 1. TENDER — 2. TAUT — 3. RASPING — 4. SPLITTING —

TOTAL ______

AFFECTIVE (A)

11 1. TIRING — 2. EXHAUSTING —

12 1. SICKENING — 2. SUFFOCATING —

13 1. FEARFUL — 2. FRIGHTFUL — 3. TERRIFYING —

14 1. PUNISHING — 2. GRUELLING — 3. CRUEL — 4. VICIOUS — 5. KILLING —

15 1. WRETCHED — 2. BLINDING —

TOTAL ______

EVALUATIVE (E)

16 1. ANNOYING — 2. TROUBLESOME — 3. MISERABLE — 4. INTENSE — 5. UNBEARABLE —

MISCELLANEOUS (M)

17 1. SPREADING — 2. RADIATING — 3. PENETRATING — 4. PIERCING —

18 1. TIGHT — 2. NUMB — 3. DRAWING — 4. SQUEEZING — 5. TEARING —

19 1. COOL — 2. COLD — 3. FREEZING —

20 1. NAGGING — 2. NAUSEATING — 3. AGONIZING — 4. DREADFUL — 5. TORTURING —

TOTAL ______

PPI

1. MILD — 2. DISCOMFORTING — 3. DISTRESSING — 4. HORRIBLE — 5. EXCRUCIATING —

CONSTANT — PERIODIC — BRIEF —

Mark E if pain is external; I if internal. If pain is both external and internal, mark EI.

ACCOMPANYING SYMPTOMS

NAUSEA — HEADACHE — DIZZINESS — DROWSINESS — CONSTIPATION — DIARRHEA — COMMENTS

SLEEP

GOOD — FITFUL — CAN'T SLEEP — COMMENTS:

FOOD INTAKE

GOOD — SOME — LITTLE — NONE — COMMENTS:

ACTIVITY

GOOD — SOME — LITTLE — NONE — COMMENTS:

Figure 29–4. McGill–Melzack pain questionnaire. (*Courtesy of R. Melzak. Copyright R. Melzak, 1970.*)

of the stimulus, the extent of tissue damage, the amount of psychological distress, or any combination of these factors.

It is difficult to gather objective data on pain intensity. Descriptive scales have also been created to assist in this effort. Clients are asked to point to the place on the scale where they perceive their pain intensity is.

Onset. Information about onset of pain includes mode of onset, pattern of pain, and history of pain. Was onset sudden or gradual? What was the client doing at the time? Is the pain steady or intermittent? If intermittent, does it follow a pattern? How frequently does pain occur? Has this type of pain occurred before? If so, what caused its onset?

Duration. Duration pertains to the length of time the pain is felt. How long does the pain last with each occurrence? When did the client last experience the pain? How frequently does it recur?

Quality. Assessing pain quality may require extensive questioning, as many clients experience difficulty in articulating the pain experience. The nurse can begin by asking, "How does your pain feel?" After giving the client enough time to think and respond, the nurse may suggest such words as stabbing, burning, aching, throbbing, and the like. The McGill–Melzak Pain Questionnaire was designed to assist health care providers to assess the dimensions of pain (Fig. 29–4).[19,20] The questionnaire has five basic sections:

- *Pain rating index.* This consists of 20 word groups used to determine pain quality. The groups are divided into subgroups: 1–10—sensory(S); 11–15—affective (A); 16—evaluative (E); 17–20—miscellaneous (M). Words in these categories aid clients in choosing a verbal description of their pain.
- *Present pain intensity.* A 5-point pain scale. The client points to the pain location on the scale.
- *Number of words chosen.* The total of pain rating index words chosen by the client.
- *Line drawing of the body.* The client points to areas of pain and describes whether pain is superficial or deep.
- *List of symptoms.* The client indicates associated symptoms.

Although this assessment tool was developed to be used in conjunction with pain medication administration, it is useful in general pain assessment as well.

Past Health Problems/Experiences. Past health problems may directly relate to the client's present problem or may alert the nurse to begin assessment of other pertinent areas. For instance, a client may reveal having had a traumatic injury to one of the peripheral nerves in the left lower extremity. This information would indicate to the nurse that careful assessment of neurosensory integration of that extremity and mobility is necessary.

Questions about prior drug therapy may contribute additional assessment data. For example, when a client who is admitted for a foot ulceration reveals he is diabetic and requires insulin injections, the nurse would assess the client's compliance with his diabetic management and would ask the client about the sensory perception from his feet, which can be reduced in diabetes contributing to ulcer-causing foot injuries.

Prior hospitalizations and prior interactions with the health care system can also affect the client's expectations and attitudes. Positive interactions lend a positive trustful attitude, while a previous negative experience may tend to make the client wary and more difficult to establish a trusting relationship. This is particularly true with clients with neurosensory alterations. They may have had many past interactions especially as a result of loss of function. These many interactions change the client's outlook and expectations.

The past health history provides a wealth of valuable data to use in client assessment, as illustrated by the following example.

- Paul Williams is a 39-year-old factory worker who is admitted to an orthopedic floor from the emergency room for diagnostic tests to determine the cause of low back pain incurred at work. He reports bending over to lift a large, heavy box and feeling his "back go out." Mr. Williams states that this has never happened to him before. He relates that he once had a kidney stone and when he passed it, the pain was horrible. He states that he hopes the current pain that he is experiencing can soon be relieved because he can't stand it. He also reports he has had a past health problem with hypertension, controlled with an antihypertensive medication.

  The nurse understands that Mr. Williams' current health problem, involving the neurosensory network, may enhance his stress and aggravate his hypertension. In addition, Mr. Williams has experienced severe pain in the past and is apprehensive about the present pain. As a part of the plan of care, the nurse decides to collaborate with the physician to assure that Mr. Williams' hypertensive medication is ordered and to monitor his blood pressure. Keeping Mr. Williams free of pain should reduce some of his anxiety. The nurse should also be alert to the fact that he has had kidney stones in the past and since he will be immobilized with back pain, he should drink a great deal of fluids to prevent recurrence of stones.

Personal, Family, and Social History. Obtaining the personal, family, and social history is very important for clients experiencing a neurosensory alteration, as any alteration in function will affect all of these aspects of clients' lives. Alterations in neurosensory function can cause changes in the client's ability to perform self-care and can also strain family and social relationships.

The personal, family, and social history also provides pertinent data about life-style patterns that may have contributed to the client's neurosensory function. For example, if the client has injured the spinal cord in a motor vehicle accident and is unable to work, the nurse would assess the client's personal, family, and social history to determine whether the client has support systems, coping mechanisms, and necessary personal habits to aid in recovery. If the client's history indicates he or she does not have sufficient resources, the nurse would determine to collaborate with other health professionals to address long-term needs.

Table 29–4 provides sample personal, family, and social history questions related to neurosensory assessment.

Subjective Manifestations. The neurosensory history includes subjective manifestations, which are the symptoms the client reports. Chapter 16 outlines a systematic approach for collection of this data. This information assists the nurse in planning approaches that will benefit the client, as the following example illustrates.

TABLE 29–4. NEUROSENSORY HISTORY: PERSONAL, FAMILY, AND SOCIAL HISTORY QUESTIONS

A. **Vocational**
1. What type of work do you do?
2. Does your work require mental concentration or coordinated physical activities?
3. Have you noticed any problems doing your work lately? If so, what? How long?
4. How do you usually get around? Drive? Ride the bus? Walk?

B. **Home and Family**
1. Are you married? Single? Involved in a relationship?
2. How long have you been in that relationship?
3. Do you have children? Ages?
4. If older children or other family members, do they live with you? Or near by?
5. How will they assist you in this situation?
6. Tell me about where you live. Stairs?
7. Describe a usual day.

C. **Social and Leisure**
1. What are your favorite leisure activities?
2. With whom do you do these?
3. Have these changed in the past because of a change in your health? If so, how?
4. Has your home life changed because of your health? If so, how?

D. **Sexual**
1. Has your sexual relationship been satisfactory?
2. Any changes related to this illness? What changes have occurred?

E. **Habits**

Exercise
1. How often do you exercise? Weekly? More or less often?
2. What types of exercise/activity do you enjoy?
3. Has your exercise pattern changed because of a change in health status? If so, how?
4. Is regular exercise an important part of staying healthy for you?

Sleep
1. How much sleep do you get? At night? From naps?
2. Do you feel rested?
3. Do you have sleep problems? How long? How have you dealt with them?
4. Describe a typical night's sleep.
5. Has this health concern affected your sleep? How?

Diet
1. How many meals do you eat every day? Are weekends different? Snacks?
2. Describe your appetite. Has it changed? If so, how?
3. What is a healthy diet? Is it important to you?
4. Has this health problem changed your eating habits?

Beverages
1. How much alcohol do you usually drink each week? What types?
2. Has this amount changed recently? Why?
3. Do you drink coffee, tea, or cola? How much?
4. Has your alcohol or other beverage intake changed recently because of your health status? How?

Drugs
1. Do you use any medications, such as aspirin, sleeping pills, diet pills, nerve pills? What are their names? How many do you take?
2. What other drugs do you use? Do you use marijuana, cocaine, or other drugs of this type? If so, what types and how often?
3. Do you find a difference in your health after you take these drugs? How so?
4. Has your use of these drugs changed since your health concerns became evident? How so?

F. **Psychological/Coping**
1. Have you noticed a change in how you feel about yourself?
2. Does this worry or concern you?
3. How have you dealt with this?
4. Has it been effective?
5. Do you feel your health has had something to do with this? How?
6. How do you feel about your health change? Are you coping? How so?
7. Do your past experiences with health changes help you cope?
8. What assistance do you think you will need during your hospital stay? At home?

■ Thomas White, a 68-year-old engineer, has sought care for headaches. He states that he is under a great deal of pressure at his job and is experiencing headaches once a week which last over 8 hours. Mr. White reports that when he has a headache, bright lights hurt his eyes. He also experiences pain aggravated by moderately loud noise and feels very nauseated. Further, he says he has a great deal of muscle tension in his shoulders and neck. The nurse develops the plan of care to include environmental measures to decrease noxious stimulation if the problem recurs. The nurse also collaborates with other health care team members and the physician to define other interventions, such as analgesic and antiemetic medications that may benefit Mr. White during his headaches. The nurse also educates Mr. White about stress reduction techniques, such as imagery and muscle relaxation, that may help him to cope with the pressures he has been experiencing at work.

Neurosensory Examination

The neurosensory assessment is carried out by the nurse to gain data about clinical manifestations of loss of neurosensory or neurosensory-related functions. It is by identifying these alterations that nurse and client are able to determine mutual goals of care to assist the client to attain a higher or a stable health state.

The neurosensory assessment is a purposeful collection of data as it relates to the client's health state. The assessment can be a complete neurosensory examination or it can be an ongoing assessment that the nurse conducts with each client encounter. A nurse should always be alert for content of thought, level of consciousness, balance, gait, motor ability, and similar neurosensory functions. The neurosensory examination requires keen assessment skills. The data obtained are interpreted and used to formulate nursing diagnoses.

Measurements. Temperature, pulse, blood pressure, and respirations are a necessary part of a neurosensory assessment as all of these vital parameters may be affected by the sensory system. Measurements of height and weight may also be made (refer to Chap. 16).

Temperature. Temperature is regulated by the hypothalamus and brain stem. A client with an injury or lesion to these areas may lose the ability to regulate body temperature. An increase in temperature may also indicate infection.

Temperature may also affect the CNS. Decreases in body temperature below 97 F (hypothermia) results in decreased metabolic rate, causing a decrease in cerebral blood flow and oxygen concentration. Increases in body temperature above 101 F (hyperthermia) increase the metabolic rate and cerebral metabolism, thereby placing an additional demand for oxygen and glucose on the body. Further, CNS function is impaired when body temperature varies 9 F either above or below the normal range.

Pulse and Blood Pressure. Changes in vital signs are usually a late sign of increasing intracranial pressure. More than transitory changes in pulse and blood pressure represent neurological deterioration. The rise in pulse and blood pressure is a compensatory mechanism. As edema, hemorrhage, blockage of cerebrospinal fluid, or lesion growth increase, pressure is exerted on the blood vessels that supply the brain. This causes ischemia of the brain tissue. Blood is pumped to the brain under increased pressure so that the ischemic tissue can receive both blood and glucose, resulting in an increase in blood pressure. At the same time, a slowing of the pulse occurs because of stimulation of the vagal nerve.

Respirations. Assessment of respiratory patterns assists the nurse to determine the client's level of brain functioning. A complete discussion of respiratory pattern changes associated with neurological damage is beyond the scope of this text; however, an overview of several key changes is necessary.

CNS respiratory failure results when neurons of the medulla become damaged. Severe bilateral hemisphere dysfunction may result in Cheyne-Stokes respirations (rapid, deep respirations alternating with no respirations). Involvement of the posterior hypothalamus and midbrain produces rapid respirations. Damage at or below the pons is manifested by irregular breathing patterns. Lesions in this area produce various patterns such as cluster breathing, gasping, or ataxic breathing. Extensive damage to the medullary reticular formation usually destroys central control of respiration leading to apnea and death.

Objective Manifestations

General Observations. General observations of the client's overall appearance are really an informal neurosensory assessment. They give the nurse an overview of the client. General observations can be made quickly as the client enters a room or interacts with the nurse. A more detailed assessment can then be completed as a part of the complete neurological examination; however, general observations continue throughout the examination. In some instances, the initial impression may set the focus of the interview and examination. For example, the client may have ptosis of the eyelid. This could indicate paralysis of the facial nerve.

The client's general health status, sex, race, and apparent age are noted. Much initial information can be gathered regarding the client's neurosensory function. Do the eyes track? Limited movement may indicate a problem with the cranial nerves that enervate the eyes. Does the client look alert? Do the muscles of the face move appropriately? Paralysis of the facial nerve will produce altered facial movement. Note the client's facial expression. Does the client appear to be in pain? Pain can indicate a wide variety of neurosensory alterations, such as lesions, pinched nerves, tumors, or pressure ulcers. Is the client dressed appropriately? Are the clothes clean? What is the client's level of hygiene? Inappropriate dress can indicate mental disorders or confusion. Dirty clothing and poor hygiene may indicate the inability to perform self-care as a result of neurosensory dysfunction, such as Alzheimer's disease, paralysis, pain, or weakness.

Assessment of mental status includes the apparent level of consciousness and orientation. Level of consciousness is one of the first parameters to deteriorate if the client is experiencing central neurological problems, such as brain tumors, hemorrhages, or degenerative neurological diseases. Orientation provides data regarding the client's perception of who he or she is, where he or she is, and what time it is. Memory and thought content are also assessed by the nurse in this process.

Station, posture, and body movement are assessed. Limited or fixed station or posture or involuntary body movement may indicate neurosensory network dysfunction, such as Parkinson's disease, tremors, or seizure activity.

Both sides of the body are observed for symmetry. Usually the dominant side is slightly larger because it is used more. However, a marked asymmetry may indicate cranial or peripheral nerve dysfunction.

Gait patterns affect client mobility and are regulated by the neurosensory network. Is the client's gait fluid and coordinated? Deficits in gait are manifested by short steps, wide-based gait, loss of arm movement, or dragging of feet. Neurosensory deficits such as stroke or peripheral nerve injury often result in problems with gait.

Handedness indicates cerebral dominance. Assess

whether the client is left- or right-handed. In states of neurosensory dysfunction, the client may lose the ability to use only one side of the body. If this is the dominant side, the client will have difficulty in performing activities of daily living.

Energy level reflects the client's ability to function in a consistent manner appropriate to the situation. Fatigue may accompany neurosensory problems, such as multiple sclerosis, head injury, or infection.

The nurse continually notes the client's speech. Is the speech fluent, well-articulated, and appropriate to age? Dysarthria and aphasia are commonly associated with neurosensory dysfunctions (see Section 1).

Odors from a client's breath may indicate that a health problem is present. Scents such as acetone, alcohol, or ammonia may be signs of a disease process or personal or social habits causing a change in neurosensory status.

Pain may be apparent as the nurse observes the client. Although pain is a subjective manifestation, the client may demonstrate observable signs. Pain behavior encompasses changes in facial expression, mental status, posture, gait, and energy level—virtually every aspect of general observation.

When clients are in severe pain, their mental status may change. In chronic pain, clients may appear older than their chronological age. Posture, movement, and gait may be altered. Energy level may also be diminished. Clients in pain demonstrate diffuse general observation alterations.

Integument. Skin is observed for skin integrity or defects such as areas of breakdown, discoloration, or lesions. Healthy skin generally is associated with neurosensory integration. Persons with healthy skin usually are able to feel pressure and pain and to change position when pressure gets uncomfortable. Intact skin, free of bruises, cuts, and burns, therefore generally indicates that individuals can feel pain and have intact pain reflexes.

HEENT

Head. The head is assessed for facial nerve function. This nerve has both motor and sensory function. Motor functions include maintenance of facial symmetry at rest and facial expressions such as smiling, frowning, or raising the eyebrows. Spasms, tremors, weakness, or atrophy are unusual findings that should be noted. The sensory function of this nerve involves the sense of taste on the anterior two-thirds of the tongue. The tastes of sweet, salty, sour, and bitter should be tested on each side of the protruded tongue with water given between each side and each taste. Loss of taste can lead to a loss of appetite.

The trigeminal nerve has both motor and sensory components. The nurse observes motor strength during mastication (chewing). The jaw reflex is elicited by tapping the jaw with a reflex hammer while the jaw is slightly open. The normal response, although weak, is closure of the mouth. The sensory component of this nerve is responsible for sensation on the skin of the face. The nurse asks the nurse to close the eyes and assesses both sides of the face for the sensations of temperature, light touch, and light pain.

Eye. The eyes provide sensory data for the brain to process. Any alteration in eye function results in a decrease in this ability. Thus, clients who experience a loss of vision often demonstrate alterations in balance, gait and ability to perform self-care, in addition to losing one of the main senses of the body.

The structural components of the eye allow those sensory inputs to enter and protect the eye from injury and are part of this assessment (see Chap. 16). Several special structures provide protection to the eye; these include the lashes, lids, and brow. The conjunctiva, a thin, clear membrane, has two distinct subdivisions: the bulbar (ocular) conjunctiva covers the white portion (sclera) of the eye; the palpebral conjunctiva deeply lines the eye socket and continues until it reaches the margin of the eye.

The visual fields of the client are tested as a part of the neurosensory assessment using a confrontation test. This test reveals gross abnormalities in visual fields. Blind spots may be due to loss of a portion of the visual field from strokes, carotid artery pathology, optic nerve interruptions, or tumors pressing on the optic pathways. Blurred vision may be caused by disturbances in the optic pathways in the brain. Diplopia (double vision) may result from cranial surgery or multiple sclerosis. Visual changes may result from past head injuries, altered sleep patterns, or abnormal ocular physiology. Loss of peripheral vision may result in injury as the client is unable to see out of the "corner" or outer portion of the eye.

The ophthalmoscopic examination is performed to view the inside of the eye by shining a light into the eye. It is an advanced technique, which students learn to perform later in the nursing curriculum. The normal disc is round with a clear distinct margin. A swollen optic disc (papilledema) is indicative of increased intracranial pressure.

Pupil size and reactivity is an indicator of neurosensory integration. It is therefore essential to observe the pupils of clients with neurosensory alterations.

Pupil size is determined by the balance of activity between the sympathetic and parasympathetic nervous systems. Checking the pupils involves first observing the size of one pupil and then observing its size in relation to the other pupil. Pupils should be equal in size and are measured in terms of millimeters (Fig. 29–5).

The pupils are also assessed for response to light. Response should be brisk; sluggish response or no response

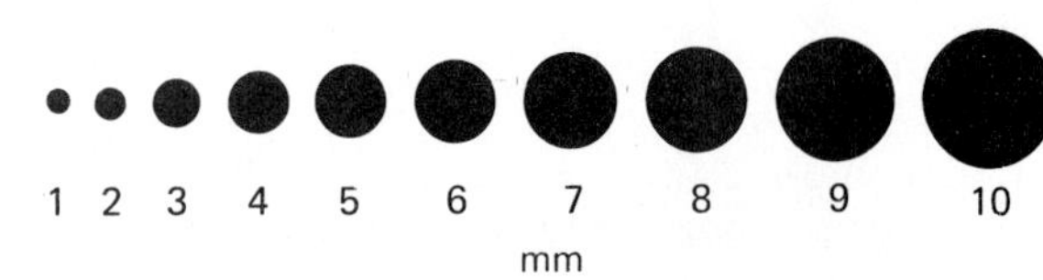

Figure 29–5. The pupils are measured in terms of millimeters.

should be noted since this can indicate a serious alteration in function of the third cranial nerve or the brain stem. The other pupil should also respond when the light is shined into one eye, but to a lesser degree. This is called the consensual response. Pupils should be round and equal in size. Unequal pupils may indicate brain damage.

The unconscious person may be assessed for the oculocophalic reflex, also called the doll's eyes phenomenon. In this procedure the head is rotated briskly from side-to-side while the examiner watches for movement of the eyes relative to head movement. The normal finding is for the eyes to move in the direction opposite that of the head, hence the name "doll's eyes." Eyes that do not move, but merely follow the motion of the head may indicate brain stem injury.

Ear. The ear provides necessary input for hearing and equilibrium. The acoustic nerve (cranial nerve VIII) is involved with the sensory functions of hearing and equilibrium. The cochlear nerve branch is responsible for hearing. Damage to these nerves causes diminished hearing.

The ear canal may be examined with an otoscope to determine if structural abnormalities exist. Hearing tests are routinely performed and include the watch ticking test, the lateralization test (Rinne test), and the bone-air conduction test (Weber test). These tests are described in Chapter 16.

The nurse should assess for pain in the ear caused by otitis media, which may cause inner ear damage. Altered hearing has many causes, including use of certain medications. Difficulty in hearing may be due to the aging process, obstruction of the ear canal by cerumen (ear wax), or congenital anomaly.

Nose. The sense of smell (cranial nerve I) is assessed. Damage to this nerve results in diminished smell. Because smell is closely related to taste, the client who has a diminished capacity for smell will also have a decreased sense of taste. Generally this results in loss of appetite, as well.

Mouth and Throat. The glossopharyngeal and the vagal nerves (cranial nerves IX and X) are tested together because of their similar functions. The nurse performs motor examination of these nerves by assessing the muscles of the pharynx and larynx for symmetry of movement, by watching how effectively the client swallows, and by listening to the client speak (phonation). Dysarthria occurs as a result of altered speech due to a motor deficit of the tongue and other speech muscles. Dysphonia is due to a disruption of the larynx which manifests as vocal hoarseness. Aphonia is also due to injury to the larynx or its innervation and results in whispering. Abnormality of these nerves may limit the client's ability to communicate and make his or her needs known.

The pharyngeal (gag) reflex is assessed by touching each side of the posterior soft palate with a tongue depressor. Loss of the gag reflex places clients at risk to aspirate foods and fluids. The palatal reflex is tested by stroking each side of the mucous membrane of the uvula. The uvula should rise and deviate to the side stimulated. The sensory component of these nerves involves the interpretation of pain, touch, and temperature in the pharynx, larynx, trachea, lungs, and esophagus. Taste on the posterior one-third of the tongue is also regulated by these cranial nerves. The autonomic functions include slowing of heart and bronchial constrictions.

The hypoglossal nerve (cranial nerve XII) is also assessed. The hypoglossal nerve controls tongue movement. The nurse should note tongue movement and strength. Fibrillations, indicating muscle atrophy, should be noted. Weakness or paralysis of the tongue will not allow the client to swallow correctly or speak.

In assessing the neck, the nurse assesses the spinal accessory nerve (cranial nerve XI), which innervates two large muscle groups, the sternocleidomastoid and the trapezius muscles. Its effect on those muscles is purely motor. The nurse assesses the first muscle group by asking the client to turn the head sideways. The trapezius muscle is assessed when the client shrugs the shoulders while the nurse places resistive pressure down with the hands. Both of these muscles should be inspected and palpated for symmetry of muscle mass, equality of strength, and any wasting or spasm. Nerve damage in this area may result in limited movement of the head.

Chest and Cardiovascular. The chest and cardiovascular systems are assessed for neurosensory function. Alterations in neurosensory function are generally related to pulse, blood pressure, and respiratory changes (see *Measurements*, above).

Abdomen. Examination of the abdomen and gastrointestinal system includes the techniques of inspection, palpation, auscultation, and if appropriate, percussion. Chapter 26 reviews these techniques in detail.

If innervation to the abdomen is altered, the contents of the gastrointestinal system will move through the system slower than normal, leading to fecal retention. The abdomen, especially the colon, should be palpated for extreme firmness or tenderness and auscultated for quantity and quality of bowel sounds to detect the presence of fecal retention. Normal bowel sounds occur every 3 to 5 seconds. The client may experience fecal retention as a result of spinal cord injury, a degenerative disease, or the aging process.

The nurse should also observe for signs and symptoms of fecal retention or fecal incontinence. Skin around the anus should be observed. Skin integrity may be disrupted if fecal incontinence is chronic.

Genitourinary. The client who has neurosensory deficit may demonstrate urinary retention or incontinence. The nurse should ask when the client last voided. If the client cannot provide this information, the nurse should palpate the bladder and percuss for normal position, slightly above the symphysis pubis bone. If the bladder is palpated much above this level, urinary retention may be present. The skin of the perineal region should also be assessed for redness and possible breakdown, which may indicate problems with urinary incontinence.

Musculoskeletal. The musculoskeletal examination is discussed in Chapter 30. Refer to that chapter for discussion of musculoskeletal findings.

Neurological. The first portion of a neurological assessment is the mental status examination, which includes the general observation portion of the examination. Other areas that are assessed include level of consciousness, orientation, mood and behavior, knowledge and vocabulary, judgment and abstraction, memory, language and speech, sensory and motor function, and reflexes.

Level of Consciousness. Level of consciousness is the key indicator of brain function. Altered states of consciousness indicate some level of brain failure.

The nurse first checks for response to auditory commands. Depending on the level of functioning, the client may respond appropriately, may answer with only a simple response, may appear unsure of what to do, or may not respond.

The level of consciousness is noted. This is important because it gives the nurse baseline data for comparison if changes occur in the client. A simple, consistent, and well-accepted guide for grading level of consciousness is the Glasgow Coma Scale (Fig. 29–6).[21]

If the client is unconscious, the nurse may need to use painful stimuli to elicit a response. Painful stimuli may include compression of the nail beds, pressure on the trapezius muscle, sternal rubbing, or pressure on the Achilles tendon of the lower leg. Responses to these stimuli may include purposeful actions (grimacing and pushing the examiner away), nonpurposeful actions (withdrawal from source of pain or inappropriate flexion or extension of arms), and no action (no reaction to stimuli).

The Glasgow Coma Scale focuses on cognitive behaviors.[22] However, individuals with significant brain injury may demonstrate behavioral, cognitive, and long-term memory deficits beyond the scope of the scale.[22] Any decrease in the level of consciousness of these clients must be compared to baseline data. Decrease in level of consciousness is a serious sign and must be reported to the physician immediately.

Best eye opening	
Spontaneous	= 4
To voice	= 3
To pain	= 2
None	= 1
	= 1–4
Best motor response	
Obeys commands	= 6
Localizes to pain	= 5
Flexor withdrawal	= 4
Abnormal flexion	= 3
Extension	= 2
Flaccid	= 1
Best verbal response	
Oriented	= 4
Confused conversation	= 3
Inappropriate words	= 2
Incomprehensible sounds	= 1
Best response	= 3–15

Figure 29–6. The Glasgow Coma Scale.

Orientation. Orientation is the client's awareness of person, place, and time. Orientation to person means the client knows his or her own name, family names, or names of health care professionals. Place is awareness of present location and address of home. Time consists of knowledge of hour, date, day of week, month, year, and noteworthy events, such as current season or recent holidays. Confusion may indicate brain deterioration. Confused clients will need to be reoriented consistently.

Mood and Behavior. Mood and behavior are actions that indicate the client is attentive to the examiner without being hostile, agitated, hypoactive, or bizarre. Delusions, illusions, or hallucinations indicate psychological dysfunctions. It is very difficult to establish a good nurse–client relationship with clients who are suffering from delusions, illusions, or hallucinations. Mood and behavior are assessed throughout the neurological assessment and should be continually assessed and compared for changes.

Knowledge and Vocabulary. Overall knowledge and vocabulary may be affected by cerebral hemorrhages, brain tumors, psychiatric disorders or by mental retardation. The nurse assesses the client for common knowledge, taking into account cultural differences.

Judgment and Abstraction. Judgment and abstraction are tested to determine the integrity of higher cerebral functions. The nurse assesses judgment by asking the client to describe common plausible life occurrences, such as what to do if one is locked out of one's house. Abstraction is assessed by asking the client to describe the meaning of proverbs.

Memory. Memory tests evaluate immediate recall, recent memory, and remote memory.

Immediate recall should occur within 3 to 5 minutes of initial information presentation. Note if the answer is correct, indicating intact immediate memory; incorrect, indicating some memory deficit; or contrived, indicating a psychological deficit. Clients with impaired memory can be difficult to teach. They cannot remember information about medications and their health requirements. Family members should be taught significant facts regarding care.

Recent memory is assessed by evaluating clients' recall of events that happened hours to several days ago. Loss of recent memory can be very frustrating for clients and can lead to anxiety. Good communication technique is essential, as is frequent reinforcement of who the client is, how the client got to the hospital, and health teaching.

Remote memory is memory of things long passed. The nurse questions the client about place of birth or names of family members, then verifies this information with family members.

Language and Speech. Language and speech assessment provides necessary information regarding how the client is processing and relating to the environment. The inability to communicate by language is termed aphasia. Speech is the ability to articulate sounds and words.

The client is asked to repeat the days of the week or months of the year (automatic speech), and then to repeat sounds and words of increasing difficulty (speech motor qualities). The nurse should listen to the quantity and quality of speech occurring. The amount and the pace of the speech may indicate abnormalities. Little speech, paced very slowly or with many silences, may indicate anxiety, depression, or organic brain disorders. The quality of speech includes how clear it is, how loud it is, and the inflections used. A very loud speech pattern, poor enunciation, or inappropriate inflection warrant further assessment.

Organization of speech and how coherent it is assist the nurse with assessment of level of consciousness and orientation. Clients who change words in mid-sentence or speak in a confused manner need further assessment. There may be other reasons however for altered language and speech besides a neurosensory problem.

Sensory and Motor Function. Assessment of special cortical functions includes the client's ability to recognize common objects by using the senses of sight, hearing, and touch. Assessment for neurosensory alterations in vision is usually performed during the neurological examination. The nurse may point to an object, ask the client to listen to a familiar sound or ask the client to touch a familiar object with eyes closed; the client is then asked to identify the sound or the object. An incorrect response to visual stimuli reflects occipital lobe alterations. Inability to interpret sounds indicates a temporal lobe deficit. Inability to identify items by touch suggests alterations in the parietal lobe. If clients are unable to perform a skilled act, such as writing their names or buttoning a shirt, in the absence of paralysis (apraxia), the deficit may be caused by injury to several areas in the dominant hemisphere.

Cerebellar function is determined by assessing balance and coordination. Balance can be assessed by performing Romberg's test and by evaluating gait (see Chap. 30). Gait is one of the first observations a nurse makes when meeting a client and should be assessed while the client is walking independently back and forth in the room. Posture, movement of body parts, stance of feet, and the types of steps taken should be noted. (See Chap. 30 for further details on normal gait.) Coordination can be assessed through a series of activities, which are described in Table 29–5. Abnormalities include lack of coordination between muscle groups, over- or underexaggeration of movements, alteration in rapid alternating movements, or incoordination of large muscle groups.

TABLE 29–5. COORDINATION SKILLS TEST

Component	Action
1. Finger to nose	1. With outstretched arms, client touches nose with index finger. Speed is increased with each successive attempt. Eyes are open at first, then are closed.
2. Finger to finger	2. Client is asked to touch examiner's index finger with client's index finger. The examiner moves the finger each time to change position. Repeat with client's opposite index finger.
3. Hand tapping	3. While sitting, the client is asked to supinate and pronate the left hand on the left knee and the right hand on the right knee.
4. Heel to shin	4. In a sitting or lying position, the client is asked to run the heel of one foot down the opposite leg. Repeat procedure for other foot.
5. Figure 8	5. While sitting, the client is asked to use the foot to draw a figure 8 in the air. Repeat procedure for opposite foot.
6. Tandem walking	6. With the client standing, arms at side, and eyes open, ask client to walk heel to toe across the room.

Motor function involves an assessment of the muscles and their movements. Muscles are examined for size and symmetry. Muscle tone is evaluated comparing muscles on one side of the body to those on the other side. The nurse should palpate the muscles and joints of each extremity at rest. Abnormal muscle tone findings include spasticity, manifested by undue resistance of the muscles to passive lengthening; rigidity, a constant state of resistance; and flaccidity, extreme fixing of muscles.

Muscle strength is tested by placing the joints through passive range of motion, against gravity and with active resistance from the nurse (see Box 30–4). The nurse may perform these tests in the initial examination but may also integrate them into daily interactions with the client, such as daily self-care activities.

Muscle movements should be observed (see Chap. 30). Abnormal muscle movements indicate an abnormality of nerve impulse transmission to or from the motor cortex. The nurse should note whether abnormal movements occur at rest or with motion, where they are located, what causes them, and whether they cease. Abnormal movements include tics, tremors, chorea, athetosis, and tonic–clonic movements. See discussion in Section 2.

Sensory assessment provides data on how the client perceives various sensory stimulation (refer to Chap. 16 for assessment technique). The primary sensory stimulation tests are superficial touch, temperature, position, vibration, superficial pain, and deep pressure pain. These assessments are performed when there are symptoms of numbness, tingling or loss of sensation, loss of motor function, areas of tissue breakdown, or muscle atrophy. Loss of sensation may indicate lesions in the posterior column of the spinal cord or the sensory cortex. Bilateral sensory loss in both lower extremities is indicative of peripheral neuropathy.

The secondary (cortical or discriminative sensation) stimulation tests assess two-point discrimination, extinction, graphesthesia, stereognosia, and texture. Alterations in function of the cortex results in loss of these cortical-integrating functions.

Reflexes. Assessment of deep tendon reflexes allows the nurse to obtain information regarding the function of the reflex area and spinal cord segments. Five common deep tendon reflexes are the biceps, triceps, brachioradialis, patellar, and achilles reflexes (see Chap. 30).

Reflexes may be altered in physiological changes involving the sensory pathways from the muscles and tendons or the motor components (upper motor neurons), or the anterior horn cells or their axons (lower motor neurons). Deep tendon reflexes are graded by the following scale:

Grade	Reflex Activity
0	0 = Absent
1	+ = Diminished
2	+ + = Normal
3	+ + + = More Brisk Than Normal
4	+ + + + = Hyperactive

The superficial reflexes are skin movements caused by stroking the skin rapidly with a blunt object, such as the end of a reflex hammer or pen. These reflexes include the umbilical reflex, cremasteric reflex, anal reflex, and plantar reflex. Although these reflexes provide information about the innervation from various spinal nerves, nurses do not perform these reflex tests routinely.

Several abnormal (pathological) reflexes generally denote deficits in the pyramidal tract, which assists with control of gross motor movements. The pathological reflexes are assessed in the following manner.

- *Babinski's reflex:* Stroke the lateral side of the sole of the foot and underneath the toes. Do *not* stroke the center of the foot.
- *Chaddock's reflex:* Stroke the foot below the lateral malleolus.
- *Oppenheim's reflex:* Stroke the anterior and medial portion of the tibia.
- *Gordon's reflex:* Squeeze the gastrocnemius.

A normal (negative) response of all four reflexes is flexion of the toes. An abnormal (positive) response is dorsiflexion of the big toe with fanning of the other toes.

Diagnostic Tests

A review of the findings of diagnostic tests of the neurological system can aid the nurse in understanding the underlying cause of a client's loss of neurosensory function. Thus, it is helpful to understand what the various tests reveal.

Nurses play a vital role in preparing clients for diagnostic tests. Providing necessary information in a professional way with appropriate depth is important. Many clients desire to know what the test is, why it is being done, what they will experience, and when they may be obtaining results. Teaching is individualized to meet clients' needs. Too much or too little information may cause anxiety about the procedure. Listening to clients' concerns and answering clients' questions are priorities.

A variety of tests may be performed. Each procedure involves different client preparation, but all procedures have some similar nursing actions. These common actions can be found in Box 29–6. Box 29–7 outlines client teaching for neurosensory tests.

Lumbar Puncture. The lumbar puncture is performed for a variety of therapeutic and diagnostic purposes. Therapeutically, it is administered to give medications and anesthesia, and to remove blood, pus, and cerebrospinal fluid

BOX 29–6. COMMON NURSING ACTIONS FOR NEUROSENSORY TESTS

Before Procedure:

1. Discuss procedure with the client (see Box 29–7).
2. Invite the client to ask questions.
3. Attempt to reduce anxiety and fear.
4. Instruct the client to lie very still and maintain position.
5. Monitor vital signs.
6. Assess general health status.
7. Assess neurological status.
8. Ascertain drug allergies particularly those related to local anesthetics and skin preparation.
9. Premedicate as needed, as per physician order.

Immediately Before Procedure:

1. Instruct the client to empty the bladder.
2. Administer muscle relaxants or sedatives, as per physician order, to decrease anxiety and reduce movement.
3. Assemble required equipment or obtain disposable tray.

During Procedure:

1. Assist the client to maintain position.
2. Assess respiratory function.
3. Provide comfort as needed.
4. Assist the physician as needed.

Following Procedure:

1. Position the client.
2. Obtain vital signs and compare to preprocedure vital signs.
3. Monitor neurosensory status.
4. Monitor for complications.
5. Document procedure as to date, time, client response, physician, any measurements made (eg, opening and closing pressures during lumbar puncture), appearance of samples taken, medications administered, etc.

BOX 29–7. CLIENT TEACHING FOR NEUROSENSORY TESTS

Before procedure, review the procedure with the client, even if client is semi-conscious or unconscious. Review the following areas. Additional information may be added if needed.

1. **Purpose:** Provide information that is relevant to specific indication for this test.
2. **Procedural Information:**
   a. *Client Position:* Inform the client to remain still during the procedure, since movement may cause injury in invasive procedures.
   b. *Client-specific Information:* Time of procedure; location where procedure will occur; health professionals in attendance during procedure; length of time for completion.
3. **After-Care Information:**
   a. *Positioning:* Advise client to maintain this position for specified amount of time because it may lessen chances for developing a headache.
   b. *Reporting:* Report anything unusual (dizziness, difficulty breathing, abnormal sensations, headache, numbness, tingling, or pain).

(CSF). Diagnostically, it allows for removal of CSF for inspection, measurement, and laboratory evaluation. A physician performs this test with the nurse assisting.

Complications of lumbar puncture include leakage of CSF, infection, damage to the spinal cord, damage to the vertebrae, respiratory failure, postpuncture headache, difficulty in voiding, backache, numbness, and tingling or pain radiating to the legs. Contraindications include local tissue infection, increased intracranial pressure, broken vertebrae, neck trauma, and anticoagulation therapy.

Clients often seek information about what the experience will be like. A description of the general procedure and possible sensations that may be experienced can help to allay client anxiety. Nurses should advise that the procedure may be slightly painful but may feel more like pressure. The physician will administer a local anesthetic to reduce discomfort. Brief shooting pains in the legs may be experienced if the needle touches the nerves to the legs. However, the needle is inserted below the level of the spinal cord, so there is little danger of the needle entering the spinal cord.

The procedure is performed with the client lying on the side in a knee-to-chest position (Fig. 29–7). This position allows easy passage of the needle into the subarachnoid space of the lumbar vertebrae. In adults, the needle is inserted into the lower lumbar vertebrae (L3 or L4) below the level of the spinal cord. In children, the spinal cord may end in the sacral area necessitating an even lower needle insertion. Placing the client's back close to the edge of the bed may facilitate needle insertion.

Aseptic technique is essential throughout the procedure to prevent contamination of the puncture site. Infection is a serious complication of the procedure in the normally sterile subarachnoid space.

After the procedure, the nurse instructs the client to remain supine and monitors the client's position. Often clients are restricted to bed rest for 6 to 24 hours with the head of the bed flat or slightly elevated. Standing or sitting up too early may cause a "spinal" headache. This can be treated with oral or intramuscular analgesics. Headaches may also result from CSF loss during the procedure, from CSF leakage at the insertion site after the procedure, or from meningeal irritation. The insertion site is monitored for edema or hemorrhage. Fluids should be encouraged to assist with replenishment of CSF.

Cerebral Angiography. Cerebral angiography assesses the status of cerebral vessels—their size, position, and integrity. The procedure involves the injection of radiopaque dye into a carotid or vertebral artery while radiographic exposures are taken of the blood vessels of the brain. Indi-

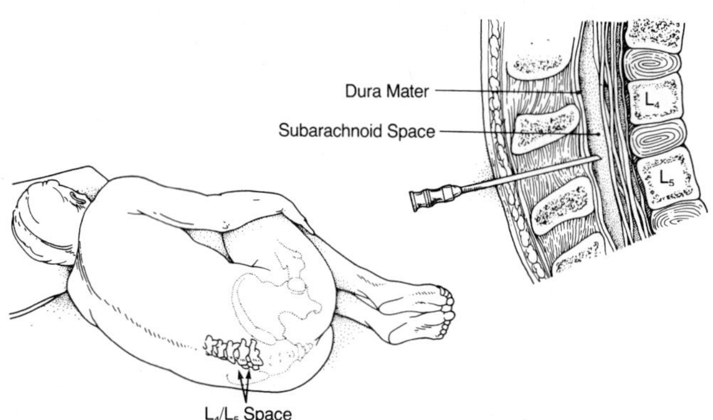

Figure 29–7. Client position for lumbar puncture. (*From Smith S, Duell D.* Clinical Nursing Skills: Nursing Process Model; Basic to Advanced Skills. *3rd ed. Norwalk, CT: Appleton & Lange; 1992.*)

cations for this procedure include visualization of cerebral arteries and veins and detection of intracranial lesions (abscesses, aneurysms, hematomas); however, the introduction of computerized axial tomography and magnetic resonance imaging has largely replaced this procedure.

Computerized Axial Tomography. Computerized axial tomographic (CAT) scans combine radiographic imaging with detailed analysis of tissue density by a computer. Radiographs of thin cross-sections of the brain are analyzed by the computer to discern tissue density differences that cannot be visualized by conventional x-ray films. Radiopaque contrast dye may be used to highlight small differences in tissue densities. The primary indication for CAT scan is diagnosis of intracranial lesions. Because a contrast medium may be used in this procedure, a contraindication is client sensitivity to the medium.

Before the procedure, clients require little physical preparation. The CAT scan does not produce pain and is noninvasive. However, the physical appearance of the CAT scan equipment may be intimidating; therefore, clients should be informed of its appearance and that the CAT machine will make humming and clicking sounds. In addition, clients must remain still for 15 to 30 minutes until the test is finished. This may seem like a long time to some clients, who become anxious and fearful. Results will show the areas of change that have caused neurosensory alterations.

During the procedure, the client is placed on a table in the Medical Imaging Department and the head is strapped into a rigid head support. During the CAT scan, the head is exposed 180 times to a narrow x-ray beam that penetrates through the various types of brain tissue. If a radiopaque dye is injected, the client may sense a warm feeling or a metallic taste in the mouth. The client should be monitored for anaphylactic or allergic reactions to the dye.

After the procedure, the client may return to the unit. The nurse continues to monitor for adverse reactions to the contrast medium. The nurse should also monitor the client's fluid status, as the hypertonic medium may increase blood volume and cause eventual diuresis.

Magnetic Resonance Imaging. Magnetic resonance imaging (MRI) is similar to the CAT scan, but uses magnetic polarity fields instead of x-rays. A computer is used to differentiate tissue densities. Indications for the test include detection of lesions and analysis of central nervous system structures. Foreign metal objects in the body, such as cardiac valves or orthopedic devices, may be disturbed because of the electromagnetic force fields applied during the procedure and serve as contraindications to the procedure.

No specific preprocedure preparation is needed, but clients should be told that they will be placed in a chamber similar to that used for CAT scans. The machine will sound like the beating of a drum and clients may be given earplugs if they wish. A consent may be obtained. All metal must be removed and the client is placed in a hospital gown. After the procedure, the client may resume normal preprocedure activities.

Electroencephalography. Electroencephalography assesses the brain's electrical activity by recording activity from the surface of the brain. The purposes of the test are assessment of overall brain activity, detection of abnormal brain activity, and determination of extent of abnormal impulses. The electroencephalogram (EEG) provides a visible record in the form of brain wave patterns of the electrical potentials generated by the brain. Because the test is noninvasive, contraindications are rare.

Client preparation involves discontinuing all anticoagulants, tranquilizers, and stimulants (alcohol or caffeine) for 24 to 48 hours before the test. Clients may also be fearful that the electrode placement will hurt, and that they might receive an electric shock. The need for scalp electrodes should be explained. No meals should be missed as hypoglycemia can alter brain wave patterns. The client's hair should be clean and dry and without oils, sprays, or lotions. It is best if the client goes to sleep late and arises early because this may increase the likelihood of abnormalities being recorded.

The procedure may be performed in an EEG laboratory or at the bedside. Adhesive surface scalp electrodes or subdermal needle electrodes may be used to detect the brain's electrical output. A baseline EEG will be documented in a dim, quiet environment. Three maneuvers may be performed. In the first, the client is asked to hyperventilate after the initial EEG is performed. This allows the blood pH to become alkalotic (pH>7.45), which increases excitability of the nerves and the client's potential of seizure activity. The client may feel faint or experience tingling, but this will cease as soon as hyperventilation is stopped. The second maneuver involves viewing a flickering light with the eyes closed. This helps to identify abnormal brain wave patterns that may indicate seizures. The third maneuver is performed when the client is drowsy or sleeping.

After the procedure, the hair may need cleansing. Necessary medications are resumed and vital and neurosensory assessments are completed. Results of the test aid in evaluating clients who have seizure disorders and in localizing brain tumors. Conditions such as meningitis, encephalitis, infection and drug overdose produce irregular EEGs.

NURSING DIAGNOSIS OF NEUROSENSORY INTEGRATION

The neurosensory assessment provides nurses with data that leads to development of nursing diagnoses. These diagnoses then form the basis for collaborative planning with clients to promote optimum neurosensory functioning. The following discussion focuses on nursing diagnoses representative of neurosensory dysfunction and their respective etiologies. These diagnoses have been approved by the North American Nursing Diagnosis Association (NANDA). Examples of subjective and objective data, defining characteristics, and etiologies for these diagnoses are presented in the table Sample Nursing Diagnoses: Neurosensory Integration, page 1384. Other nursing diagnoses related to neurosensory alterations are listed in Box 29–8.

Altered Thought Processes

The diagnosis of Altered Thought Processes describes a state in which a person experiences a disruption in mental activities and cognitive processes; for example, the ability to evaluate reality, to have conscious thought, to judge and problem-solve accurately, to be oriented to person, time, and place, and to comprehend incoming stimuli. Defining characteristics include inaccurate interpretation of the environment, distractibility, difficulty remembering, focus on the self (egocentricity), disorientation to person, place, or time, delusions (fixed false beliefs), and hallucinations. Clients who have difficulty conceptualizing, who think slowly, misinterpret events, or are confused reflect the diagnosis of Altered Thought Process. While NANDA has not yet developed specific etiologies for this diagnosis, other writers have proposed several possible etiologies.[23]

Etiology: Physical Changes. Many physical conditions can cause an alteration in thought processes.[24] Injury to the brain, brain tumors, or increased intracranial pressure can produce an altered level of consciousness or damage to the brain cells needed to think and respond. Other factors such as decreased cardiac output resulting in hypoxia cause alterations in thought because of lack of oxygen to the brain. Dehydration can cause brain cells to shrink, whereas alteration in electrolytes can result in disruption of the sodium–potassium pump. All of these conditions can result in altered thinking.

Etiology: Psychological Stress. Psychological stress such as anxiety, fear, depression, or acute grief may produce temporary changes in a client's thought processes. Some clients become so overwhelmed with the changes in their lives that they become disoriented.[23,25]

Etiology: Environmental Changes. Individuals who are admitted to a hospital may experience sensory overload or sensory deprivation. This results in upsetting the balance of the reticular activating system. Sensory overload results when clients receive more sensory stimuli than they can process. Sensory deprivation occurs when sensory input is less than the client needs to function. An example of environmental changes that result in sensory overload includes IV alarms, loudspeakers, paging systems, mechanical noises, and new smells, all bombarding the client at once. An example of sensory deprivation is a client who is placed alone in a room with minimal or no meaningful stimuli; for example, the client in isolation.

Etiology: Medications, Drugs, or Alcohol. Many medications can cause confusion. Examples include excess or deficiency in insulin, digitalis toxicity, narcotics, sedatives, and tranquilizers. Use of illegal drugs may lead to altered awareness, as well as alcohol abuse.

BOX 29–8. OTHER DIAGNOSES RELATED TO NEUROSENSORY ALTERATIONS

Physical

Altered Nutrition
Altered Oral Mucous Membrane
Bowel Incontinence
Constipation
Dysreflexia
Impaired Physical Mobility
Impaired Skin Integrity
Impaired Swallowing
Ineffective Airway Clearance
Ineffective Breathing Pattern
Ineffective Thermoregulation
Potential for Aspiration
Reflex Urinary Incontinence
Self-care Deficit
Sexual Dysfunction
Sleep Pattern Disturbance
Total Urinary Incontinence
Urinary Retention

Cognitive

Knowledge Deficit

Emotional

Anxiety
Ineffective Individual Coping
Grieving
Powerlessness
Social Isolation
Spiritual Distress
Post Trauma Response

Self-Conceptual

Altered Role Performance
Body Image Disturbance
Hopelessness
Personal Identity Disturbance
Self-Esteem Disturbance

Sociocultural/Life-Structural

Altered Family Processes
Altered Role Performance
Diversional Activity Deficit
Impaired Adjustment
Impaired Social Interaction
Social Isolation

Developmental

Altered Growth and Development

Sexual

Altered Sexuality Patterns
Sexual Dysfunction

Environmental

Impaired Home Maintenance Management

SAMPLE NURSING DIAGNOSES: NEUROSENSORY INTEGRATION

Nursing Diagnoses	Defining Characteristics/Manifestations: Subjective Data	Defining Characteristics/Manifestations: Objective Data	Etiology
Altered Thought Processes *8.3*	Reports inability to remember events, people prior to car accident.	Retains new information in short-term memory for 3–4 minutes. Oriented to person only; disoriented to place and time. Unable to carry out directions unless cued verbally with each step. Inappropriate answers to questions.	*Physical:* Head trauma.
Impaired Verbal Communication *2.1.1.1*	No subjective data. Client is unable to speak.	Indicates understanding and written communication. Unable to speak. Grunts, attempts to vocalize. Able to communicate by pointing to pictures, diagrams. Gestures to indicate requests.	*Physical:* Decrease in circulation to the brain
Pain *9.1.1*	Reports fell off ladder 30 minutes ago, twisting knee. Sharp, piercing, shooting pain in knee. States pain is constant, and worsened by movement.	Left knee bruised; diameter slightly greater than right knee. Holds and leans over knee, rocks back and forth. Intermittent crying, moaning. Contorted facial expression.	*Physical:* Traumatic injury to left leg.
Sensory–Perceptual Alteration: Auditory *7.2*	Reports inability to hear voices. Requests other people to speak louder. Reports humming or ringing in the ears.	Does not respond when cannot see persons speaking in a normal conversational tone. Increases volume of radio and TV beyond normal hearing levels. Neurosensory examination for hearing (ticking clock and tuning fork test) indicates hearing loss.	*Physical:* Altered auditory reception, transmission.

Acute Pain

Acute Pain describes temporary encounters with pain and is limited by time. Acute pain may last from a moment up to 6 months. McCaffery describes acute pain as pain that subsides as healing takes place or pain that has a predictable end.[3] Acute pain is generally characterized by being associated with a specific event, including: (1) fractures of bones, muscle spasms associated with injuries or accidents; (2) migraine headaches, gout, sickle cell crisis, or myocardial infarction; and (3) health treatments such as biopsies, surgery, diagnostic procedures, or dental procedures.[26]

Etiology: Injuring Agents. Agents causing pain are categorized as biological, chemical, physical, or psychological. Biological agents, such as bacterial or viral agents, can disrupt tissue integrity resulting in pain. Chemical agents are toxins within the environment, such as pesticides, ingested chemicals or drugs, that can disrupt neurosensory integration. For example, they can cause burn injuries, tissue breakdown, damage the respiratory tract if inhaled, or destroy the esophagus if swallowed.

Physical agents exacerbating an episode of acute pain are broadly categorized under trauma. Whether trauma occurs as an assault by another person, or an injury sustained from a moving object, such as a baseball bat, or from collision with an immovable object, such as the ground, acute pain is likely to develop.

Etiology: Psychological Factors. Psychological factors contributing to episodes of acute pain can arise within or outside the person. Fears regarding the nature and intensity of anticipated pain, for example dental procedures or discomfort associated with an angiogram, can contribute to an individual's episode of pain. External psychological factors, such as suggestions from health care workers about the nature of a diagnostic procedure, may alert the client to the potential for pain, causing fear and anxiety which may then interact with actual pain to enhance the pain response.

Chronic Pain

Prolonged pain that occurs continuously, pain that has active and inactive states over a lifetime, or pain that is acute for a lengthy, time-limited period are variations of pain that characterize the diagnosis of Chronic Pain. There is controversy regarding how long pain must occur before being termed chronic; however, pain existing longer than 6 months is considered chronic pain.[27]

Chronic pain can be described as pain that is limited, intermittent, or persistent.[27] Individuals with chronic pain may have adapted so that physical manifestations may not be obvious, such as grimacing or guarding of a painful area. Behaviors like depression, anger, withdrawal, or manipulation may characterize individuals who suffer with long-term pain.[28] These behaviors can be frustrating for family, clients, and health care personnel.

Etiology: Chronic Physical or Psychosocial Disability. Chronic pain is any pain, whatever its region, that recurs or persists over an extended period of time and that interferes with functioning. It may be a result of persistent diseases, such as low back pain, rheumatoid arthritis, or degenerative diseases of the joints; progressive diseases, such as cancer; or processes that are not clearly understood.

After an injury, pain receptors may become sensitized and continue to fire even after the injury has healed. This results in sending pain messages to the brain even when no new damage is present. It appears that the cellular damage as a result of degeneration or injury causes changes in the central processing system of the brain resulting in self-sustaining neural activity that sends impulses without pain stimulation. It is also hypothesized that chronic pain results from a series of biochemical changes that cause depletion of serotonin.[29] Serotonin affects sleep, mood, and perception of pain. Still other theories suggest that chronic pain may be a result of abnormal functioning of the endogenous opiate system.

Psychosocial disabilities refer to situations in which persons who experience chronic pain become overwhelmed with the pain. Anxiety and depression, as a result of loss of locus of control, are seen.

Impaired Verbal Communication

Impaired Verbal Communication reflects an individual's inability or decreased ability to send and/or receive messages. Individuals have difficulty relating thoughts, needs, and desires. Inability to communicate verbally can be experienced as (1) an inability to express oneself despite intact ability to understand words and formulate messages, or (2) an inability to understand and formulate messages resulting in incoherent messages and inability to communicate.

Behavioral characteristics of this diagnosis include inappropriate or absent speech response, confusion, weak or absent voice, and stuttering or slurring. Individuals may have difficulty finding the correct word when speaking, or have decreased hearing comprehension or deafness.

Etiology: Impaired Circulation to the Brain. Impaired circulation to the brain can result from occlusion of blood vessels, brain tumors, and blood clots. Any impairment of circulation results in tissue damage and cell death. If the impairment involves the brain areas responsible for speech or for motor control of speech organs, loss of ability for verbal expression results, as discussed earlier under alterations in neurosensory integration. The local inflammatory reaction often exaggerates the loss of function immediately after the injury; partial return of function is therefore possible after inflammation resolves in many clients.

Etiology: Cultural Differences. Impaired verbal communication can be a result of not being able to speak English. Although the client may be able to express thoughts and needs verbally, the nurse may not be able to understand the client's language. In addition, it is very difficult for the nurse to assess the client's content of speech.

Etiology: Physical Barriers, Tracheostomies, Intubation, or Laryngectomy. Some clients require a tracheostomy to allow them to breathe. Since air cannot pass the vocal cords, the client cannot speak without plugging the tracheostomy. Tracheal intubation has the same effect. Laryngectomy (removal of the vocal cords) presents an irreversible loss of capacity for normal speech, but artificial aids and speech therapy make verbal communication possible.

Sensory–Perceptual Alterations

Sensory–Perceptual Alterations refer to alterations in visual, auditory, kinesthetic, gustatory, tactile, and olfactory modes of perception. It is defined as the change in the amount or patterning of incoming stimuli and subsequent diminished, exaggerated, distorted, or impaired response to stimuli.

Defining characteristics of this diagnosis include disturbed sense of time, place, or person; a change in usual response to stimuli; change in behavior patterns; report of or measured change in sensory acuity; and change in ability to problem-solve and communicate. Restlessness, irritability, fear, anxiety, apathy; and auditory, visual, or other perceptual hallucinations are examples of behavioral characteristics also associated with this diagnosis.

Etiology: Altered Environmental Stimuli. Environmental stimuli can be experienced as excessive or insufficient amounts of sensory input. Excessive stimuli from the hospital environment might include such things as beeps and noises from machines (eg, suction machines and IV pumps), extraneous devices such as drainage tubes and intravenous lines, and various monitors. Many health care personnel assisting one client, multiple treatments or frequent assessment of vital signs, and sleep interruptions are other examples of excessive stimuli. The extremely ill, the critically ill, and the elderly are most likely to experience sensory overload or sensory deprivation. For clients who have diminished perceptual input, normal amounts of environmental stimuli may be too much, since they are not accustomed to what others would consider normal stimulation. Astute nursing assessment and discussion with clients can result in diagnosis statements that accurately reflect nurse–client collaboration in problem identification.

Insufficient environmental stimuli includes diminished sensory perceptual input, darkness, or simply lack of naturally occurring stimulating activities in a specific location. Consider being in a closed room with no windows, bare walls, and no furniture or extraneous materials. The lack of environmental stimuli might result in a sensory–perceptual alteration as a result of understimulation of the reticular activating system.[25] Sensory deprivation is characterized by auditory or visual hallucination, restlessness, and anxiety. Nurses who collaboratively assess and plan for clients' needs for sensory stimulation achieve optimal interventions.

Etiology: Altered Sensory Reception, Transmission, and Integration. This etiology describes a wide range of causes of neurosensory dysfunction. Whether the dysfunction involves reception, transmission, or integration, the end result is lost communication between the sensory input and the brain.

When the sensory receptors or their respective pathways to the brain become damaged, altered sensory reception occurs. Damage to a specific sensory organ will also result in altered sensory reception. This damage can happen as a result of a traumatic event, or as a result of some internal degenerative process to the sensory organ. The inability to send neural signals or impulses to the brain for interpretation results in altered sensory transmission. One factor causing impaired transmission is trauma or damage to sensory pathways that interrupts the transfer of neural messages. Lack of neurotransmitters, the neural chemicals necessary for communication between neurons, impairs the sending of neural signals. Another cause of altered sensory transmission is degenerative changes to the components of the neurosensory network.

Altered sensory integration can be described as disorganized or ineffective processing of sensory input. It is characterized by decreased cognitive abilities and by memory alterations. Causes include traumatic events, such as head injury, intracranial tumors, lack of neurosensory chemicals (eg, neurotransmitters), and abnormal firing of neural impulses from highly active neurons. The cells or structures necessary for integrative function are not properly functioning, whether from the results of direct pressure, cell death, or anoxia, and as a result do not process input into meaningful ideas or thoughts. Nurses can assist clients by providing sensory input for the unaffected senses, by providing reality orientation, protecting clients from injury, and providing emotional support.

Etiology: Chemical Alterations. Chemical alterations can be endogenous or exogenous alterations. Endogenous chemical alterations are changes within a cell or organism that are harmful to neurosensory integration. Examples of cellular changes include impaired oxygen transport and electrolyte disturbance within the cells. For example, lack of oxygen may cause the accumulation of hydrogen ions resulting in brain cell damage, leading to confusion or brain death.

Exogenous chemical alterations are changes introduced to the neurosensory network or cells that cause damage and impair sensory–perceptual function. Ingestion of drugs, toxins, and growth of bacteria in the neurosensory network can produce such chemical alterations. For example, some drugs bind to neurotransmission cells and the body's own neural transmitters cannot communicate with the system, resulting in impaired message reception and transmission.

Etiology: Psychological Stress. In this state, a person experiences a changed perception of events; that is, certain stimuli are viewed as stressful. This state may be accompanied by altered coping mechanisms in response to sensory–perceptual alterations from the senses or the environment.

Psychological stress causing altered sensory–perceptual function can be experienced as actual or perceived threats to self, anticipation of pain, or misinterpretation of persons or situations in the environment.

Stating the Neurosensory Diagnosis

Once the assessment is completed, analysis of the data regarding the client's neurosensory functioning culminates in the formulation of nursing diagnoses. Nursing diagnoses are formulated when the data are clustered in a meaningful way.

Complete assessment of the client's neurosensory status is essential so that the nurse, with client collaboration, can actively plan individualized client care. Collaboration with other health care professionals who would assist in overall comprehensive client care may be required in an attempt to assist the client in overcoming neurosensory deficits.

Nursing diagnoses are most meaningful and relevant to the care of a particular client when they include specific descriptions of the way that client exemplifies the diagnosis. General etiologies such as physical injuring agent, for the diagnosis of pain, are not as helpful as a statement that identifies the type of injury or event causing the pain. Likewise, defining characteristics can be made more descriptive to assist in identifying appropriate evaluation criteria and recognizing the absence of symptoms that originally validated that the diagnosis applied. "Moaning and restlessness" as defining characteristics of pain more clearly explains the client's situation than "distraction behaviors," for example, and "rigid shoulder and arm muscles" is preferable to "alteration in muscle tone." The diagnosis: Pain related to uterine contractions as evidenced by withdrawal from social contact, moaning and restlessness, and rigid arm and shoulder muscles provides more guidance for planning and providing care than the more general statement: Pain related to biological injuring agent as evidenced by narrowed focus, distraction behaviors, and altered muscle tone.

The same kind of individualization of etiologies and defining characteristics is appropriate for other neurosensory integration diagnoses as well.

Section 3. Nurse–Client Management of Neurosensory Integration

Once the nursing diagnosis of a neurosensory deficit has been made, the management phase begins. This involves collaboration with other health care providers, and with the client and the client's family. Appropriate implementation is instituted to prevent further alteration, or to promote, support, or restore optimal functioning.

■ PLANNING FOR OPTIMUM NEUROSENSORY INTEGRATION

Planning includes formulating desired outcomes; these outcomes are goals that determine priorities of care and are an important step in assuring that the client's care will be effective. Mutual goal setting is the ideal approach in determining neurosensory outcomes. Clients who share their perceptions are more likely to participate and progress toward achieving the mutually-determined goals.

Some clients experiencing alterations of neurosensory function have conditions that impair cognition and thought. When this is the case, it may be difficult to engage in mutual goal setting with the client. The nurse should then include family members who are close to the client or significant others in the goal-setting process to determine desirable goals for the client. At other times, particularly when the client is unconscious, the nurse may be required to assume full responsibility for decisions on client goals and approaches.

In addition to family members, nurses may need to consult other members of the health care team; physicians, physical therapists, occupational therapists, respiratory therapists, clinical nurse specialists, and others. The care of the client with a neurosensory problem can be complex and frequently necessitates professional collaboration.

■ NURSING IMPLEMENTATION TO PROMOTE NEUROSENSORY INTEGRATION

Nurse–client management involves implementation of planned goals. Measures to alleviate client problems should focus on the client's strengths, as well as needs, and provide support where needed. The plan of care for the client addresses all of the identified nursing diagnoses.

Specific nursing approaches are available for clients experiencing neurosensory problems. The table Nurse–Client Management of Neurosensory Integration Problems on pages 1388–1389 summarizes appropriate outcomes, approaches, and evaluation criteria for neurosensory problems.

Preventive Care

Preventive care includes health education, and health promotion and maintenance. Health education focuses on safety and accident prevention, whereas health maintenance involves encouraging clients to participate in or schedule hearing and vision checks, blood pressure monitoring and control, and exercise programs.

Health Education. Health education focuses on safety issues and accident prevention regarding risks associated with automobiles and motorcycles. Nurses may instruct clients to wear seat belts when driving or riding in cars; drive without consumption of alcohol or drugs; turn on lights when darkness descends; and avoid driving if experiencing night blindness. These measures, along with careful driving, can help prevent vehicular accidents which cause head injuries, spinal cord injuries, and cerebrovascular bleeding. Young adults and teenagers are at increased risk for motor vehicle accidents because of inexperience and risk taking.

Motorcycle accidents are a common cause of spinal cord and head injuries. Controversy exists regarding the wearing of helmets, but the protection to the head is far greater if helmets are worn.

Diving accidents are another cause of cervical spine injury, and result from diving into shallow water. Teenage males are frequent victims, along with persons under the influence of alcohol.

Other areas that are a focus for health education and prevention are smoking, nutrition and diet (especially the importance of lowered fats and cholesterol), and drug and alcohol use.

Health Maintenance. Screening for health problems is another preventive nursing activity. Vision screening to detect nearsightedness, farsightedness, and vision loss should be done on a yearly basis or as prescribed by an ophthalmologist or optometrist. Teaching clients to protect and preserve their eyesight is an important nursing role. Individuals should be taught measures to protect their eyes; for example, to wear goggles when using power tools. Individuals with eye disorders should be taught about their condition and about how to prevent further alterations.

IMPLICATIONS FOR NURSE–CLIENT COLLABORATION

Health Education

Many permanent neurosensory alterations are caused by accidents and trauma to the nervous system that could have been prevented or avoided. Motor vehicle, motorcycle, and bicycle accidents are frequently causes of severe head and spinal cord injury. Drug overdose is another way that individuals suffer a severe assault to neurosensory functions. Nurses are in a good position to educate the public on the tragic and costly consequences of preventable accidents. Part of each collaborative relationship should center on health education and providing information that individuals might need to understand the risks they face. Nurses can benefit clients by routinely asking them about their activities and their safety practices such as wearing helmets and seat belts.

NURSE–CLIENT MANAGEMENT OF NEUROSENSORY INTEGRATION PROBLEMS

Nursing Diagnosis	Desired Outcomes	Implementation	Evaluation
Altered Thought Process R/T head trauma *8.3*	1. Improved orientation (within limitations of physical condition).	1a. Give stimuli to achieve/maintain orientation: ■ Call client by preferred name. ■ Remind client of location. ■ Keep clock and calendar in client's view. ■ Encourage family involvement in care and activities to stimulate client. ■ Encourage family to bring photos and personal items from home. 1b. Speak slowly and clearly; allow ample response time. 1c. Establish and maintain a routine for personal care and other activities. 1d. Encourage client choice-making and participation in care.	1a. Client able to: state name, location, and time; identify family members and regular caregivers; remember recent events.
	2. Freedom from injuries	2a. Maintain adequate lighting. 2b. Keep bed in low position; use siderails if necessary, but avoid restraints, if possible. 2c. Assist with ambulation.	2. Client remains free of injury.
	3. Improved ability to respond to environment (within limitations of physical condition).	3a. Involve client in conversations about surroundings and daily events. 3b. Provide opportunities for interactions outside client's room.	3a. Responds appropriately to questions, events. 3b. Performs activities of daily living with assistance relative to physical condition.
Impaired Verbal Communication R/T decrease in circulation to the brain secondary to CVA (stroke) *2.1.1.1*	1. Needs communicated by alternate means.	1a. Speak to client in a normal conversational tone. 1b. When communicating, position yourself so client can readily see you; maintain eye contact. 1c. Provide alternate means of communication for client to use to express needs: magic slate, pictures or flashcards of common objects, pad/pencil, magnetic board with alphabet. 1c. Encourage use of gestures, nods, eye blinks to respond to questions. 1d. Provide sufficient time for client to express needs; meet needs promptly. 1e. Verbalize empathy and acceptance of anger, frustration. 1f. Explain the cause of speech loss to client; share prognosis for recovery, if known. 1g. Encourage and positively reinforce attempts to speak. 1h. Encourage family to engage in frequent communication with client.	1a. Client consistently uses alternative method of choice to communicate needs. 1b. Client indicates needs are met.
	2. Improved ability to communicate verbally commensurate with medical diagnosis.	2. Consult with speech therapist for collaborative plan to maximize speaking ability.	2. Comprehensible verbal communication at level permitted by medical condition.
Pain R/T traumatic injury to left leg *9.1.1*	1. Pain remains at tolerable level until definitive treatment of injury commences.	1a. Speak to client in soothing monotone voice. 1b. Position in good alignment; support and elevate left leg so it is above heart level. 1c. Apply ice bag to knee. 1d. Suggest and assist client with noninvasive pain relief measures: deep breathing/relaxation, guided imagery.	1a. States pain is tolerable. 1b. Cessation of crying, moaning. 1c. Facial and torso muscles relaxed.

Nursing Diagnosis	Desired Outcomes	Implementation	Evaluation
Sensory–Perceptual Alteration: Auditory R/T altered auditory reception/ transmission *7.2*	1. Communication with others via measures to support/augment hearing to aid independent functioning in the community.	1a. Collaborate with client to select preferred hearing support strategies: lip reading, hearing aid. 1b. If client has hearing aid, encourage its use; teach and assist as necessary with care, cleaning (see Procedure 29–2). 1c. Speak slowly and clearly to client with voice slightly louder than normal conversational level; keep messages short and concise. 1d. Use tactile and visual stimuli to compensate for auditory sensory loss. 1e. Make sure other caregivers are aware of hearing loss: post sign with preferred communication methods on client's bed. 1f. Teach client and family safety measures to compensate for hearing loss: increased visual vigilance; amplifier on telephone. 1g. Refer to appropriate community resources (eg, Teletype for Hearing Impaired, American Organization for the Education of the Hearing Impaired).	1a. Uses hearing aid and/or lip reading to help receive messages. 1b. Responds appropriately when others communicate with him/her. 1c. Makes contact with at least one community resource for hearing impaired.

Hearing screening helps detect types of hearing loss. Preschools and secondary schools schedule periodic hearing checks to detect abnormalities in children. Environmental precautions should be taken to reduce noise levels that might injure hearing.

Blood pressure screening is important for detecting high blood pressure and hypertension. Hypertension can precipitate cerebrovascular accidents (strokes) if prolonged and if blood pressure is very high (eg, 200/100).

Supportive Care

Supportive care focuses on care for clients who experience mild to moderate interruption in neurosensory integration. These clients require some assistance with self-care. The primary goals of care are to alleviate the neurosensory dysfunction and to prevent further loss of neurosensory integration.

Supporting Clients' Vision. Supporting clients' vision enhances optimal vision, promotes comfort, hygiene, body image, and prevents infection (see Chap. 24 for eye hygiene).

Approaches to Help Clients with Impaired Visual Acuity. Supporting impaired or reduced vision in clients entails proper knowledge and use of eye supports, and care of eye glasses, contact lenses, and glass eyes.

Eye Supports. Eye supports are devices or environmental modifications that enhance vision. Ensuring proper lighting for reading and providing adequate night lights provide optimal environmental lighting for comfort and safety. When caring for clients with reduced vision, collaboration in arrangement of bedside materials may enhance access to water, reading materials, and personal items. Large-print reading materials and magnifying glasses may assist clients in reading and are especially helpful for those without glasses who have myopic vision. In planning care, daily schedules, or medication schedules, bedside marker boards, or other paper and pen designs can facilitate clients' visual access to necessary information.

Eyeglasses. Clean eyeglasses enhance optimal vision. Eyeglasses require daily cleansing and special care when handling to prevent damage and scratching of lenses.

Eyeglasses with glass lenses should be cleaned with soap and warm water, and dried with a tissue or cloth that will not scratch lenses. Plastic lenses scratch easily and require specific cleaning solutions and drying tissues. Do not use fingernails or sharp objects to remove debris. Clients may request that nurses not cleanse their eyeglasses. Ask clients if they plan to clean the eyeglasses, or if it is necessary for the nurse to do so. Clients should be asked not to wear secondhand glasses or old glasses. Use of improper corrective lenses can lead to eye fatigue and contribute to vision problems.

If clients require assistance in removal of eyeglasses, gently grasp each side of the frame in front of the ears. (Avoid grasping only one side as this movement may bend frames if one bow remains behind the ear during removal.) Gently raise the curved ear portions up from the ear and direct the lenses downward and away from the face. Reverse the process when placing eyeglasses on clients.

Label eyeglasses and cases with the client's name. Store

eyeglasses in bedside units when not in use. Determine with the client where glasses are to be stored.

Contact Lenses. Contact lenses are thin curved plastic discs that fit on the cornea of the eye directly over the iris and pupil. There are two basic types of lenses, hard and soft. Lenses float on the fluid layer of the eye and, in most cases, offer better vision than eyeglasses.

Contact lenses are relatively easy for clients to insert and remove but are difficult for nurses to insert and remove. Hard nonpermeable lenses can be worn for up to 18 hours. Gas-permeable lenses can be worn for 1 to 3 days without damage to the eye. Soft contact lenses can be worn from 1 to 30 days depending on the brand.

Insertion and removal of contact lenses is usually done by clients themselves. If clients are temporarily unable to perform this task independently, most prefer to use glasses until they are again able to use their lenses without assistance. Soft lenses, in particular, are easily torn if handled improperly, and incorrect manipulation can injure clients' eyes, so it is difficult for another person to assist with this.

Nurses are sometimes called upon to help with the care of clients' contact lenses. There are several cleaning and care systems available for both hard and soft lenses. Most involve cleaning and disinfection. Both types of lenses should be cleaned with the solution of clients' choice each time they are removed and reinserted. Place a small amount of solution in the palm of your hand, then place the lens in the solution with the tip of a finger on the opposite hand and rub gently. Use care not to scratch the lens with your fingernails. It is a good idea to clean lenses over a towel placed either on a table or in the sink to avoid dropping the lens down the drain. Rinse lenses according to manufacturers' directions after cleaning. Saline or tap water are most often used.

Lens disinfection is most often accomplished by soaking in an enzyme solution, although some hard lens wearers prefer heat disinfection. Frequency of disinfection and length of time of soaking vary with the type of lens and solution used. Follow clients' or manufacturers' directions carefully to avoid damage to lenses or incomplete disinfection.

Assisting Clients who are Blind. Lack of vision, especially in the newly blind, is an anxiety-producing situation. Hospitalization for a person who is blind can also be frightening. When a blind person is placed in an unfamiliar environment, usual coping methods and adaptations for performing daily activities may no longer be successful. Blind individuals find dependence on others and asking for help the hardest part of being blind.[30] All of these factors can lead the person who is blind to experience high levels of stress during hospitalization.

A trusting nurse–client relationship can be established by spending time with the client and allowing the client to express apprehension and fears. Always introduce the client to yourself and to roommates, if applicable. It is also helpful to place the blind client closest to the bathroom and to walk the client around the room and bed, describing placement of bathroom and furniture. The nurse should allow time for the client to touch the furniture to understand the spatial scheme of the room.

Blind individuals can be aided in adjusting to visual alterations by contact with other visually impaired per-

BUILDING NURSING KNOWLEDGE

What Does the Loss of Vision Mean to Those Affected by It?

Allen MN. The meaning of visual impairment to visually impaired adults. *J Adv Nurs.* 1989;14:640–646.

This study explores the subjective meaning of visual impairment. Reactions of clients vary based on the personal meaning of the events surrounding the problem. Clients attempt to give meaning to the loss, to explain and thus control it. The meanings they derive condense their fears about illness, the social reactions of important others, and their therapeutic experiences and life stresses.

Allen examined the social and symbolic context of visual impairment. Data were obtained through observations and interviews with 25 individuals whose vision had been seriously impaired for 1 to 20 years. The etiologies for subjects' visual loss varied. The researcher's initial request of the subjects was to "tell me about your eye problems." This was an effort to gain insight into the context of the problem rather than to obtain clinical information. Interview data were coded, categorized and interpreted by the researcher.

Adjustment to visual impairment was found to occur in stages. The first stage, "preimpact/early loss," occurred when the loss had not yet caused major changes in the person's activities. The individual was not consciously aware of the implications of loss. The next stage, "impact/realization," involved the individual's awakening to the loss that had occurred. This was followed by a period of depression, self-pity, and withdrawal. Subjects became fearful and worried about going out alone and whether they could cope with the future. At some point, they made a conscious or unconscious decision to live with the impairment and learned new ways of doing things.

Adjustment was an ongoing process. New situations evoked frustration and annoyance. Being dependent on others and having to ask for help were most difficult, and tended to create a sense of being obligated or indebted, and of being unable to maintain a balance of give and take in a relationship. Contact with other visually impaired persons helped subjects to cope.

The meaning of visual impairment varied with the phase of adaptation. In the first stage, the condition seemed insignificant and relatively unimportant. In the second stage, the meaning changed to threat; subjects recognized that their life would have to change. As the implications became clear, the meaning changed again to one of punishment and loss, not just of vision but of valued activities. Some blamed other people or God. A few felt that life no longer had meaning. For some, who adjusted well, loss of vision also came to mean a value of positive effects that occurred as a result of their blindness.

sons.[30] Factors that hinder adjustment include lack of social support.

If planning to touch the client or perform a procedure, inform the client of your intentions. Move slowly and smoothly, and provide information on each step of the procedure to be performed. When talking with clients, face toward them when speaking and use words to describe events or situations that are occurring around them. If you are talking to a person who is blind in a group of people, address the person directly, stating his or her name first. Guidelines for care of clients who are blind are presented in Box 29–9.

Whether clients are mobile or immobile, it is important to collaborate with them on positioning of items and belongings in the room. Blind persons depend on routine placement of items and objects. Any person changing the location of items should inform the client and describe the changes made. A familiar environment increases a blind person's sense of security and independence.

Capitalizing on touch, nurses can guide clients around the room and have them touch their surroundings; for example, the bed, bedside chair, bathroom, sink, call light, and other important items in their surroundings. Walking sticks and canes, when tapped against various hard surfaces, reveal various pitched sounds of different objects. These sounds are useful for the blind client when becoming familiar with a new environment or when walking.

Most blind persons have a keen sense of hearing and touch and are sensitive to spatial perception. These senses become more developed and assist blind persons in adapting to their condition. Nurses can orient clients who are blind to unfamiliar sounds in the environment, such as noises at the nurses' desk, the beeps on certain machines, and other unfamiliar noises.

Blind persons may be sensitive to breezes. This use of spatial–perceptual abilities gives them information about location of doors and windows. When voices, music, and sounds reverberate against walls or other objects, there is an effect of an echo. Blind persons are sensitive to this and use this spatial–perceptual sense to note solid walls, fences, or other high objects.

Safety is of great importance for hospitalized clients who are blind. Precautions include keeping one siderail up, supervising smoking, and assisting clients when ambulating. Razors, scissors, or other hospital instruments should be removed from the bedside area.

Seeing eye dogs and canes are supports for the blind person. Blind persons who cannot have their seeing eye dogs with them feel helpless, lonely, and less organized. The nurse can explore with the client alternative methods for promoting independence and orientation to surroundings, as previously outlined. Walking canes provide clients who are blind with a sense of spatial perception; alert them to steps, curbs, and obstacles; and complement their increased acuity in hearing.

The newly blind client requires sensitivity and understanding on the part of caregivers. Loss of vision can be a traumatic loss; nurses can facilitate the grieving process by supporting clients' expressions of emotion—be it anger, sadness, or grief (see Chap. 23 for discussion of clients who are grieving a loss).

For clients who are newly blind, learning activities of daily living is the first step toward independence. Guidelines in assisting the newly blind to eat include the following.

- Have clients practice with an empty spoon or fork to gauge the distance between the plate and mouth. Clients may want to practice with an empty cup or glass, as well.
- Establish a routine placement for utensils and foods to provide a similar arrangement at every meal.
- Inform client of any changes in location of items listed above.
- When meal trays arrive, describe foods to the client. Identify liquids and their location on the tray. Use the hours on the clock, for example "3 o'clock" or "6 o'clock position" to identify location of foods, fluids, and other items.
- Glasses and cups should be two-thirds filled to prevent spilling.

BOX 29–9. GUIDELINES IN CARING FOR CLIENTS WHO ARE BLIND

1. Introduce yourself to clients each time you enter the room.
2. Speak to the clients before touching them or performing a procedure. Prepare clients for what is going to happen next.
3. Introduce clients to their surroundings. Allow blind persons to touch objects in the environment.
4. Always make sure call lights are available for clients.
5. Encourage independent activities of daily living; grooming, hygiene, eating, dressing.
6. Keep personal items and other important objects (eg, water pitcher, cup) in the same place.
7. Notify and describe to clients any changes made in the placement of items in the environment.
8. Inform clients when you are leaving the room.
9. When in a group of people, call the client out by name when speaking specifically to him or her.
10. When walking with a client, do not grasp the client's elbow, rather allow the client to hold onto your forearm as you stay one-half step ahead of him when moving. Describe stairs, doorways, obstacles, and other key elements in the environment.
11. Move slowly and smoothly. Do not rush or hurry with blind clients.
12. Gently inform clients of any facial grimaces or postures that call unnecessary attention to the client.
13. Place food on meal trays in a similar location, or inform clients of the specific location and layout of foods and items on the meal tray.
14. Keep doors wide open or completely shut to avoid bumping into doors.
15. Be alert to objects on floor and notify clients as to location of temporary objects, such as cleaning equipment.
16. Provide sensory stimulation for the other senses.
17. Orient client to time of day and date.

- Maintain privacy until clients feel comfortable eating with others present.

The assistance of other occupational therapists, physical therapists, social workers, and psychiatrists can facilitate adjustment and rehabilitation of the newly blind client. Agencies and other resources for clients who are blind are listed in Box 29–10.

Supporting Clients' Hearing. Many persons over 65 years of age experience some degree of hearing loss. Because these persons have difficulty communicating with persons who hear normally, they are at risk of being misunderstood as mentally incompetent.

The person experiencing hearing loss demonstrates inattentiveness to sounds and voices, may respond inappropriately in conversations because of "unheard" phrases or misinterpretation of words. Inappropriate shouting occurs when people lose the ability to hear their own voices.

Compensatory measures that supplement hearing acuity or offset the loss of hearing include lip reading, sign language, gestures, and hearing aids.

Ear Hygiene. Ear hygiene, performed daily, aids in preventing debris build-up and infection. Simple cleansing of the ear is carried out using a wash cloth folded over the tip of an index finger and carefully wiping out the ear canal. Cerumen, or ear wax, also may be removed in this manner. Build-up of cerumen is a common cause of diminished hearing. Cotton swabs and hair pins should never be used to clean ears or remove cerumen. In some cases, ear irrigations with warm tap water may be done to cleanse the ear canal. Ear drops for cerumen removal (Debrox) can be inserted into the ear canal to help dissolve large accumulations of cerumen. Procedure 29–1 describes irrigation of the ear.

BOX 29–10. RESOURCES FOR CLIENTS WHO ARE BLIND

American Foundation for the Blind, Inc.
15 West 16th Street
New York, NY 10011

The National Society for the Prevention of Blindness
79 Madison Avenue
New York, NY 10016

State Welfare Department:
Contact the Division of the Blind

Library of Congress
National Library Service for the Blind and Physically Handicapped
1291 Taylor Street, NW
Washington, DC 20542

Recordings for the Blind
212 East 58th Street
New York, NY 10022

Local Library: for books, magazines, and newspapers in braille, or for audio tapes

Lip Reading. Lip reading involves understanding speech by carefully observing lip movements, facial gestures, and body movements. Lip reading may be used by clients in combination with hearing aids. It is, therefore, very important to face directly persons who lip read and to maintain good eye contact during conversations. Lip reading requires a great deal of skill and concentration. Clients experiencing a great deal of pain, stress, or fatigue may therefore have difficulty using lip reading.

Sign Language. Sign language, although most commonly used by the deaf, may be used by hearing-impaired clients to supplement their communication. Sign language is communication by hand signals. Various hand signals represent the letters of the alphabet, certain phrases, and words.

Hearing Aids. Hearing aids are used by the hearing-impaired to improve or maintain communication. A hearing aid is a battery-operated, mechanical device that improves hearing by amplifying or intensifying the level of sound reaching the ear.

Over 700 types of hearing aids are currently available,[31] enabling a hearing aid to be tailored to the particular client's need. For example, a client with a conductive hearing loss may benefit from amplification alone if it can overcome the blockage or damage that prevents sound from reaching the inner ear. A client with a sensorineural hearing loss may need to have low tones depressed and high tones enhanced, rather than needing to have all sound amplified.

Hearing aids are most useful when hearing loss is conductive rather than sensorineural in origin. An otologist and or an audiologist will determine type of loss and assist the client in choosing the most appropriate hearing aid.

Before getting a hearing aid, clients should be told that using a hearing aid does not guarantee perfect hearing, and that not every person is a candidate for a hearing aid. Persons with middle ear problems benefit the most from hearing aids. Persons with nerve damage or sensorineural hearing loss may have more problems with hearing aids. This is related to lost ability to hear high frequencies, personal tolerance for loud noises, or cognitive inability to understand speech. Hearing aids amplify background noise as well as conversation, and some people find this distracting and annoying. In addition, as sound becomes louder, it does not necessarily become clearer. Individuals may require auditory training in addition to the hearing aid. Hearing aids, therefore, require careful selection and use.

Types of Hearing Aids. The amount and type of hearing loss determines the types of hearing aids that a client may choose. Smaller, less visible hearing aids tend to be most desired. Unfortunately their small size and the proximity of the hearing aid and the receiver limit the amount of amplification that can be achieved. Therefore, individuals with severe hearing loss cannot use them. Three common types of hearing aids are shown in Figure 29–8.

PROCEDURE 29–1 EAR IRRIGATION

PURPOSE: To remove excess cerumen or foreign body.

EQUIPMENT: Ordered solution (usually 500 mL is needed), 50-mL syringe or rubber bulb syringe (some agencies use a mechanical irrigation device such as that used to clean teeth), curved (emesis) basin, waterproof pad, towel.

ACTION

1. Review the medical order. Wash your hands. Discuss the procedure with the client, including the usual sensations, and desired participation.
2. Warm the ordered solution to body temperature to prevent vertigo or discomfort from cold solution stimulating the vestibular apparatus. Tap water, normal saline, or 50% hydrogen peroxide solution are commonly used irrigants.
3. Request or assist the client to a sitting position with the head tilted away from the affected ear. Protect the client's clothing with a towel and waterproof pad. Inspect the external auditory canal with an otoscope to assess the location and amount of cerumen or foreign body and to assure that the tympanic membrane is intact. Note the condition of the outer ear.
4. Place the basin with the concave side facing the client's cheek, directly below the ear. If the client holds the basin tightly against the cheek, more of the return will be collected in the basin.
5. Fill the syringe (or turn on the mechanical irrigation device). Straighten the ear canal to facilitate cleansing the entire canal: for adults, pull the pinna upward and backward; for young children, pull the pinna slightly downward.
6. Carefully position the syringe so that the tip is directed toward the top or side of the auditory canal to prevent solution from flowing directly onto the tympanic membrane. Administer solution until foreign body is removed or until returned solution is clear. Stop if client complains of dizziness or a sudden pain in the ear. For dizziness, warm solution slightly and administer slowly. Pain suggests rupture of the tympanic membrane. Assess immediately with the otoscope. If rupture is confirmed, report this to the physician; if membrane is intact, continue with irrigation, using care to avoid irritating the membrane.

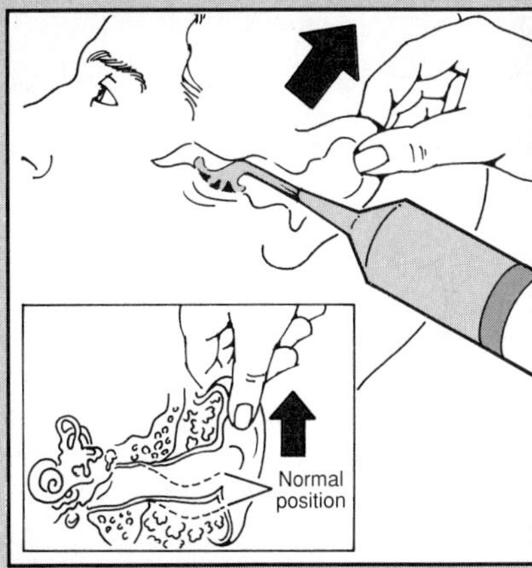

7. Reassess external auditory canal to assure that it is clear. Dry client's ear, cheek, and neck. Dispose of or clean equipment according to agency policy.

Recording: Note type and amount of solution, character of return, condition of external auditory canal and external ear before and after procedure, and client's response to irrigation.

BEHIND-THE-EAR HEARING AID. The behind-the-ear (BTE) hearing aid is the most commonly used hearing aid. It is shaped like a half-moon, fits behind the ear, and is connected by a short, clear plastic tube to an ear mold inside the ear. This device is comfortable and has cosmetic appeal, especially for clients with long or abundant hair, because it can be hidden. It is useful for clients with hearing loss in the range of 20 to 80 decibels (dB).[32]

IN-THE-EAR HEARING AID. The in-the-ear (ITE) hearing aid is also popular and commonly used. This device is a one-piece design and is the smallest of the hearing aids. With the ITE all components—hearing aid, receiver, and battery—fit directly into the ear. Because of its small size, it has aesthetic appeal. Unfortunately, it cannot be used by individuals with severe hearing loss. This device is useful for clients with hearing losses in the 25 to 55 dB range.[32]

EYEGLASSES HEARING AID. The eyeglasses hearing aid is similar to the BTE unit, but the receiver, tubing (which is connected by a tube to the microphone that fits into the ear canal) are hidden within the eyeglasses frame, and the earpiece of the glasses frame conceals the battery. A limitation of this type of hearing aid is that the eyeglass style is somewhat limited and must be fairly bulky to disguise the hearing aid equipment. This type of hearing aid is used for individuals with hearing loss in the 20 to 70 dB range.[32]

BODY AID. The body aid is a device used for individuals with severe hearing loss. It consists of a fitted ear mold connected to a round receiver that attaches to a transmitter the size of a cigarette case that can be concealed in clients' clothes. The body aid is used for clients with hearing losses in the 40 to 110 dB range.[32]

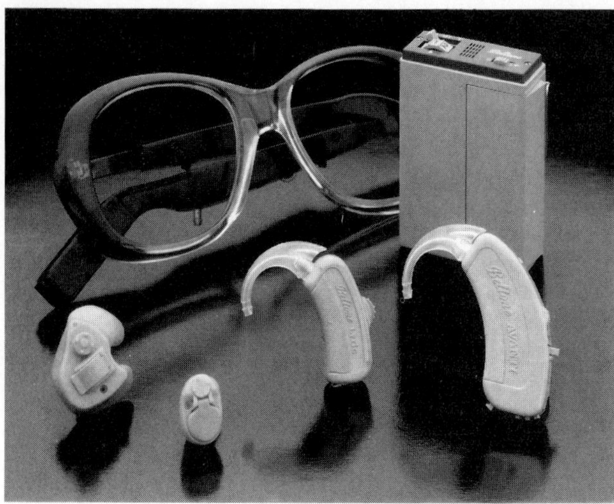

Figure 29–8. Types of hearing aids. Clockwise from top: Eyeglass aid, body aid (earpiece and cord to aid not shown), two behind-the-ear aids, canal aid, and in-the-ear aid. (*Courtesy of Beltone Electronics Corporation, 4201 West Victoria Street, Chicago, IL 60648.*)

COCHLEAR IMPLANT. The cochlear implant is a device that is surgically implanted into the ear. It has sometimes been referred to as the "artificial ear." The cochlear implant is intended for clients with sensorineural deafness; in these clients, the hair cells of the cochlea are impaired. The cochlear implant bypasses the damaged hair cells to stimulate the intact nerve fibers, which then send auditory impulses to the brain.

Caring for Hearing Aids. Hearing aids require delicate care and protection from moisture, heat, and breakage. Procedure 29–2 outlines the correct insertion, removal, and cleaning of hearing aids.

Volume control and tone can be individually adjusted for clients. Clients may require practice and many trials before an optimal setting is achieved. When hearing aids are turned on too loud, a high-pitched noise will come from the unit. Do not assume that clients whose hearing aids are in place have correct volume settings or properly functioning hearing aids.

Communicating with Hearing-Impaired Clients. Special considerations of the hearing impaired involve sensitivity on the part of nurses and others to the consequences of hearing loss. A first and most vital consequence is the lost ability to communicate with others and to detect environmental sounds. Lost ability to communicate effectively may result in lack of information and orientation to reality along with decreased touch and social isolation. Persons may find themselves treated as incompetent or receiving undeserving irritation from others who cannot understand them. Environmental sounds provide pleasure sensations as well as cues regarding warning signals or danger and orientation to the environment. The loss or impairment of hearing leaves persons socially and environmentally deprived and at risk for injury.

Communication with clients who are hearing impaired involves approaches that reduce social and environmental sensory deprivation and enhance effective communication. The following approaches are helpful.

- Make sure your presence is known.
- Avoid startling the client.
- Position yourself in front of the client so that he or she can lip read or near the client's good ear or hearing aid.
- Assure proper lighting so the client can see you.
- Speak normally or in a slightly raised voice; do *not* shout.
- Speak slowly, distinctly, and evenly so your voice does not trail off at the end of sentences.
- Use longer sentences so the client may understand the gist of the conversation; short phrases may not be heard or understood.
- Listen intently and focus on the client.
- Turn off television or radio, fan or other machinery (if possible).
- Supplement conversations with nonverbal gestures, cues, and pictures.
- Write out portions of conversations, if necessary.
- Communicate with the client by talking about the major topic first, then ask for details: "Bath time—do you want a shower or to wash up in your room?"
- Repeat phrases, when necessary.
- Use a calm reassuring manner when repeating phrases to facilitate communication.
- Use different words to communicate the same phrase, as an alternative.

Supporting Clients with Loss of Smell or Taste. Several concerns pertain to care of clients experiencing loss of smell or taste. The desire to eat involves taste and smell. Some persons may experience flat-tasting foods as a result of a loss of smell, and may subsequently lose their appetites. This places them at risk for food poisoning.

The focus of collaboration is on assisting clients in making meaningful adjustments to compensate for a temporary or permanent loss of smell. Specific approaches include the following.

- Monitor the diet to be sure the client is getting enough trace minerals, such as zinc, and adequate vitamins.
- Encourage the labeling of all foods with the type and date, as clients will be unable to smell spoiled food.
- Encourage thorough cooking of all foods.
- Additionally, all clients who have a smell alteration should have a smoke detector with active batteries.

Supporting Clients with Loss of Sensation. Loss of sensation can be rapid or slow and insidious depending on the cause. Loss of sensation may be the result of disease of one or more peripheral nerves, termed peripheral neuropathy. Common causes of peripheral neuropathy include: decreased perfusion due to decreased circulation; deficiency of B vitamins; alcoholism; and as a complication of diabetes

PROCEDURE 29–2. INSERTING, REMOVING, AND CLEANING A HEARING AID

☐ **PURPOSE:** To improve client's hearing function and maintain optimal functioning of hearing aid.

☐ **EQUIPMENT:** Hearing aid, soap and water, hearing aid case, towel or drying cloth, basin.

ACTION

1. Wash hands thoroughly.
2. Insertion:
   a. Check the hearing aid batteries.
   b. Turn the volume down and the hearing aid off to prevent sudden, high-pitched sounds directed in the ear during insertion.
   c. Check with the client for proper ear location and position of hearing aid.
   d. Place earmold in the external ear and gently press and rotate hearing aid into place. For behind-the-ear device, bring the connecting tubing and battery device up-over-and behind the ear; for body device, attach housing for microphone and battery pack to client's gown.
   e. Turn the hearing aid on and adjust the tone and volume to client preference.
3. Trouble-shooting if hearing aid does not function properly:
   a. Adjust volume.
   b. Check earmold for debris buildup.
   c. Assess ear canal for buildup of cerumen.
   d. Check the battery: remove hearing aid, turn volume to maximum. A continuous whistling indicates the battery is working. To replace a dead battery, place a towel over the working area. Open battery unit, replace battery and be sure (+) and (−) signs of battery match the hearing aid.
   e. If the client reports hearing a whistling sound, turn down the volume and check earmold placement.
4. Removal:
   a. Turn the hearing aid off and decrease the volume to prevent sudden, high-pitched sounds directed in the ear during removal.
   b. Turn the earmold slightly forward and pull outward.
   c. Remove batteries if hearing aid is not to be used for several days, as battery may corrode the hearing aid if left in the unit.
   d. Store the hearing aid in its case to protect it from damage due to moisture, heat, or cold.
5. Cleaning:
   a. Remove the earmold from the receiver if detachable. (An earmold secured by a small metal ring or glued cannot be detached.)
   b. Soak detachable earmolds in soap and water, wipe nondetachable earmold with a damp, soft cloth.
   c. Wash and dry earmold.
   d. Check the earmold for patency and cerumen buildup. Blow through the tube or remove wax with a pipe cleaner.
   e. Do not use alcohol. It can dry and crack the plastic.

☐ **RECORDING:** Describe assistance and care, any difficulties experienced, corrective measures taken, and client response.

mellitus or renal failure. Loss of all sensation occurs below the area of a severely damaged spinal cord.

Peripheral nerve degeneration begins with temporary episodes of pain, tingling, burning, prickling, or numbness in the lower extremity. Varying degrees of sensory, motor, and reflex loss typically occur in the feet before the hands and arms. As the degenerative process continues, muscle weakness, wasting, and diminished sensation occur, characterized by an ataxic (unsteady), wide-based gait. Clients may also develop foot drop and paraplegia.

Clients who experience peripheral neuropathies and loss of sensation are at risk for injury. These injuries include: falls, cuts, bruises, and burns. Clients at risk should be taught to carefully bathe their feet, dry between each toe, use talcum powder and lotions. Never use alcohol since it tends to dry skin and may result in breakdown. They should be encouraged to wear cotton socks and well-fitting shoes. A method to reduce the risk of burns is to have the client use a bath thermometer to measure the temperature of the bath, shower, or foot tub water.

Clients should be encouraged to seek a podiatrist for removal of corns, calluses and trimming the toenails. Further, clients should be told not to perform these procedures themselves because they may cut themselves and may develop an infection.

Supporting Clients with Altered Body Image. Loss of body parts or functions or a change in body image activates a period of grief and mourning for the lost part or body image. This period may be accompanied by feelings of helplessness, sadness, anger, guilt, or loneliness. Stages of grieving include shock and disbelief (denial), anger, depression, and eventual resolution which includes recognition and acceptance of the new body image. Chapter 23 discusses nursing approaches for clients who experience an alteration in body image.

Assisting Clients With Mild to Moderate Pain. Approaches to support clients who are experiencing mild and moderate pain are essential parts of client care. Nurses need to be sensitive to clients' pain. Often, nurses underestimate the level of pain a client is experiencing.[33] Further, there are some types of pain that caregivers can do little to alleviate,[34] such as intractable pain.

Little research has been performed to study how nurses determine how to medicate clients for pain. This may be because of the subjective nature of pain; the lack of measurement tools for accurate pain assessment; and the attitudes of nurses in measuring the presence and severity of pain.[35]

Clients tend to be undermedicated for pain. There are several reasons for this. The most prominent is the clients' fear of addiction. In reality, there is little chance for addiction to narcotics over the course of a hospitalization for acute pain.

Several methods may be used to alleviate pain in clients with mild to moderate pain. These include supportive approaches, noninvasive pain-relief measures, and medication.

Supportive Approaches. Sociocultural beliefs, childhood experiences, and misconceptions may influence the meaning clients place on pain. It is important for nurses to determine factors influencing the pain experience. Specific factors that may augment or worsen the pain experience for a client include the disbelief of others, fatigue, fear, knowledge of the event, misconceptions, and monotony.

Disbelief. Disbelief about a client's pain when displayed by others can frustrate and anger the client. Consequently, the client may focus on the pain in an effort to gain understanding. It is important, therefore, for nurses and others to acknowledge, with the client, the presence of pain, and to be responsive to the client's descriptions of the pain. Client's family members or significant others may have disbeliefs about the client's pain. It is also important to listen to the family's concerns and provide support for them so that they can restore their ability to support the client. The following approaches may be helpful in alleviating the factor of disbelief.

- Acknowledge the client's pain to the client. Effective approaches are, "Tell me about your pain." "You mentioned you had a headache. Could you specifically describe it for me?" "How are you handling this pain you have just described?"
- Listen responsively to client statements about pain.
- Respond to client needs surrounding the pain experience. Provide a quiet environment for rest, or distractions, such as television, games, books.

These will help the client understand that the nurse is interested and concerned about the pain.

Approaches that may be useful with the family members or significant others include the following.

- Relate that pain is a subjective, individual experience for human beings.
- Provide opportunities for family members to share concerns privately.

Fatigue. Fatigue influences clients' perceptions of pain. Individuals who are overly tired focus on the self. Consequently, with fatigue, clients will focus on the pain experience. Providing adequate rest, assessing sleep patterns for adequate intervals of sleep, and evaluating with client and physician the need for nocturnal sleep medications are approaches to fatigue reduction. It is important for clients to understand that pain itself can cause fatigue. Fatigue, in turn, can heighten the perception of pain.

Fear. Suffering may influence the amount of pain felt or perceived by clients. Fear increases the apprehension and physical tension of clients, thereby increasing the pain and anxiety, which further increases fear. An endless cycle thus becomes established.

The fear, as experienced by the client, needs to be explored. Fear of addiction, fear of constant pain, and fear of revealing to others how one handles pain are examples of different fears that may contribute to a client's pain experience.

In providing supportive care, the nurse should observe the following guidelines.

- Discuss the pain experience and what it means for the client.
- Share with the client the various methods for handling pain.
- Reassure the client that everything possible will be done to alleviate or reduce the pain.
- Educate the client about addiction to drugs.
- Tell the client it is important to request pain medication before the pain becomes too intense.
- Protect the client; the therapy should not cause more distress than the pain itself.

Knowledge of the Event. The client's knowledge of the painful event will contribute to the way the client responds to pain. Nursing approaches to address this factor include the following.

- Inform the client of the source of the pain.
- Teach the client about pain medication.
- Use measures that the client believes are effective from prior knowledge.
- Allow the client to participate in pain relief.
- Use pain relief measures that are based on the client's behavior.
- If therapy is ineffective at first, encourage the client to try it again before abandoning the therapy.

Misconceptions. Misconceptions can intensify the pain experience, for example, when clients believe false information or incorrectly relate their pain to other events. To avoid misconceptions, nurses should carefully explain to clients that pain is a very individual experience for each person. Mutual exploration with clients about why pain intensifies or occurs at certain times of the day can help nurses identify misconceptions about pain. For example, a client whose pain intensifies upon returning home from work may attribute the pain to the car ride home when, in fact, the pain intensifies as a result of fatigue.

Monotony. Monotony intensifies the pain experience because the focus of attention is on the pain. Therefore, distraction, which draws attention to an alternative focus such as reading, television, visitors, craft projects, or completion of a sports game, is often effective in minimizing pain. Perhaps you can remember doing a project, such as letter stuffing or sewing a garment. In the course of the particular work, you cut your finger, but you were unaware of the cut until after the work was done. Distracted by the work at hand, the pain went unnoticed.

Noninvasive Pain-alleviating Approaches

Cutaneous Stimulation. Cutaneous stimulation is stimulation of the skin for the purpose of relieving pain.[36] Massage, vibration, heat and cold therapy, transcutaneous electrical neurostimulation (TENS), and external analgesic treatments are superficial forms of pain relief accessible to nurses. These methods have highly variable and unpredictable results; however, they have added potential to distract and relax. They also enhance pain relief by means of therapeutic use of touch.

MASSAGE. Massage is commonly performed to relieve pain and tenseness in the back and shoulders, but can be applied to head, scalp, neck, arms, hands, and feet, as well. Massage results in relaxed muscles, relief of tension, and increased circulation. Massage can be performed for generalized pain or for pain localized to a particular area, for example, the lower back. Massage stimulates the large nerve fibers in the skin to prevent painful sensations in small nerve fibers from reaching the brain. (See the earlier discussion of gate-control theory in Section 1). For this reason, the pain experience can be modified or the client's perception can be altered using this intervention. (See Chap. 28 for guidelines on how to give a therapeutic massage.)

VIBRATION. Vibration is a form of cutaneous stimulation. It involves electrical massage with moderate pressure using a vibrator applied to the neck, face, shoulders, or to any body part. The vibrator produces sensations of numbness or decreased sensation to the body area stimulated, thus providing pain relief. Most vibrators may be hand-held or stationary.

Vibration is effective in relieving headache pain, muscle aches or spasms, itch, rheumatoid arthritis pain, phantom limb pain, or as a substitute for TENS (see *Rehabilitative Care*).

HEAT. Heat therapy involves the use of heat as a form of cutaneous stimulation. Heat has been employed historically to relieve aches and pains. Heat has many physiologic effects, such as vasodilation and increased metabolic activity in tissue and cells. Heat therapy can improve oxygen transport and blood flow to tissues. This also allows for metabolic end products to be transported away from injured tissue, accelerating the inflammatory response. Heat provides pain relief by the physiological mechanism of raising the pain threshold and promotes joint mobility by decreasing stiffness.

Heat therapy must be used judiciously, because extremes of temperature can cause burns and expose clients to risk of tissue injury. Heat therapy may involve the use of dry or moist heat (Table 29–6). Both dry and moist heat require careful monitoring. Heat applications are used to increase circulation to a local area, decrease pain, increase warmth, and as a mechanism for removal of infectious material.

Aquathermic pads are a source of dry heat and, when used with warm, moist compresses, the Aquathermic pad and moist compress together provide moist heat. Procedure 29–3 discusses the application of an aquathermic pad (see Chap. 24 for guidelines on the application of moist heat compresses).

Another form of heat therapy is the sitz bath. Commonly used for persons with hemorrhoids and for women following pelvic surgery or vaginal deliveries, this method promotes cleansing of perianal areas, along with healing, drainage promotion, pain relief and comfort, relaxation, and voiding (see Chap. 24, Procedure 24–3).

COLD. Cold therapy can produce desired effects of cutaneous stimulation. Moist cold compresses, ice bags or ice collars, and hypothermia blankets are all methods of applying cold therapy. Cold therapy is used to reduce inflammation and swelling and effectively alleviates pain. Types of cold application include: ice massage, aerosol sprays, cold soaks, ice bag or collar, ice glove, cold pack, cooling sponge bath, and full body hypothermia.

Cold therapy is effective because of its vasoconstrictive effect. Vasoconstriction reduces blood flow to an injured or

TABLE 29–6. TYPES OF HOT APPLICATIONS

Mode of Heat Transfer	Dry	Moist
Conduction (heat from warmer object transferred to cooler object by contact)	Hot water bottle or bag Electric heating pad Aquathermic, aquamatic, or Aqua K-pad Disposable heat pack	Hot compresses Hot packs Sitz bath Warm soaks
Radiation (heat transferred by electromagnetic waves)	Heat lamp Bed heat cradle	

From Stevens K. Thermal applications. In: Flynn JBMc, Hackel R (eds). Technological Foundations in Nursing. *Norwalk, CT: Appleton & Lange; 1990:534.*

PROCEDURE 29–3. AQUATHERMIC PAD APPLICATION

PURPOSE: Application of dry or moist heat to reduce muscle spasm, provide comfort to painful tissue, and reduce or eliminate localized areas of inflammation and swelling.

EQUIPMENT: Aquathermic pad (also called Aqua K-Pad) and control unit, moisture barrier—waterproof disposable pad, plastic (Saran wrap), tape, Kerlex, gauze, petroleum jelly (for moist heat), normal saline, bath thermometer

ACTION

1. Check physician's order for type of application, area to be treated, and length of time of treatment.
2. Assess condition of the skin over which pad is to be applied (aquathermic pads are rarely applied to open wounds); level of discomfort of area receiving aquathermic pad treatment; and sensitivity to temperature, pain, and light touch.
3. Prepare equipment and supplies:
   a. Check the control unit. Temperature setting should be between 40.5C and 43C (105 and 115F).
   b. Check the reservoir to see that it is two thirds full of water. Use only distilled water to refill.
   c. Connect the waterproof plastic pad with (attached) two hoses to the control unit.
4. Discuss the procedure and goals for treatment with the client, including nurse's action and behavior expected of client. Explain sensations to be felt or reported.
5. Application:
   a. Provide privacy and position client comfortably.
   b. For dry heat, cover the plastic pad with a pillowcase or soft covering, then apply to the body part and secure with tape, gauze or ties. (Do not use pins.)
   c. For moist heat:
      - Apply a thin layer of petroleum jelly on the body part to protect the skin.
      - Moisten gauze, washcloth, or towel, wring out, and apply to affected area.
      - Cover with Saran wrap, then apply and secure.
   d. Monitor:
      - Temperature of aquathermic pad.
      - Skin condition.
      - Time elapsed in treatment.
   e. Discuss importance of calling nurse if pad becomes too warm, cools off, or creates other discomfort, rather than removing pad.
6. Evaluation:
   a. Evaluate color, temperature, and intactness of skin exposed to aquathermic pad treatment.
   b. Assess pain relief or level of discomfort.

RECORDING: Identify site of application. Describe temperature setting; duration of therapy; client's responses; skin condition; evaluation of relief provided; problems, if any, and action taken.

painful area. The result of decreased blood flow is reduced inflammation and swelling, a local anesthetic effect. As cold therapy decreases tissue temperature, cell metabolism and need for oxygen and nutrients is reduced as well.

When applying cold therapy, it is important for the nurse to remember three points.

1. Skin temperatures fall quickly. Subcutaneous tissue and muscle cool more slowly, depending on the amount of fatty subcutaneous tissue. Direct application of cold applications for 2 to 3 minutes causes frostbite of the skin, although underlying cutaneous layers are not yet cooled. Thus, direct cold therapy must be applied, removed, and reapplied for a period of 15 to 30 minutes to produce effective results without danger of frostbite. (Frostbitten skin appears white, pale, blue, mottled, is pulseless and feels firm to the touch.)
2. Knowledge of the stages of sensation experienced with cold therapy is necessary in order to properly evaluate client responses (Table 29–7). This knowledge assists nurses in explaining the effects of the different stages of cold therapy to clients before initiating treatment. Expla-

TABLE 29–7. STAGES OF RESPONSE TO COLD THERAPY

Stage	Time	Response
Initial stage	1– 3 minutes following application	Feeling of cold may be uncomfortable
Stage 2	2– 5 minutes following application	Sense of burning and aching
Stage 3	5–12 minutes following application	Local numbness and decreased pain
Stage 4	12–15 minutes following application	Deep tissue changes, including alternating vasodilation and increased metabolism

nation of the therapy and assurance that the period of discomfort is short enhances clients' participation in the therapy.

3. When applying cold therapy to the skin, use of a towel or flannel cloth provides an insulating layer between the skin and the source of cold (Fig. 29–9). The insulating layer absorbs moisture and slows the effects of frostbite, enabling the cold to penetrate more deeply into the tissue. Table 29–8 identifies various types of cold therapy and summarizes their uses. Procedure 29–4 provides guidelines for application of ice packs.

EXTERNAL ANALGESIC MEDICATION. External analgesic medications are topically applied substances containing menthol, which acts as a counterirritant. Their mechanism of action is to create a sensation of coolness or warmth on the skin. This sensation serves to relieve the pain or draw attention away from the pain.

Menthol preparations are nonprescription, over-the-counter gels or lotions. Ben-Gay and Tiger-Balm are two such over-the-counter products. Menthol products provide continuous stimulation to the site of application. Intensity increases with the amount of menthol.

Menthol preparations may be applied topically to relieve muscle, joint, and tendon aches; sports injuries; neck and shoulder pain; gas pain and menstrual cramps; or sore throat. Menthol is contraindicated for use on open wounds, mucous membranes, and painful or uncomfortable skin areas. If menthol increases pain, it should be discontinued.

Relaxation. Relaxation is another category of noninvasive pain relief. Although particularly effective for clients with chronic pain, it can benefit those with mild to moderate acute pain.[37] Relaxation can be defined as the state in which an individual decreases anxiety and skeletal muscle tension and calms the mind, thereby interrupting the spiraling process of increased pain, anxiety, and muscle tension. The body responds physiologically by decreasing the respiratory rate and heart rate, decreasing muscle tension, decreasing blood pressure (in clients with hypertension), and decreasing oxygen consumption of the tissues.

Relaxation can be achieved by a variety of methods including meditation, progressive relaxation, and biofeedback. Most relaxation strategies necessitate a quiet environment, a comfortable position, a passive attitude, and a mental device or focus of concentration.[3] The reader is referred to Chapter 22 for details on methods of relaxation.

Distraction. A third category of noninvasive pain relief is distraction. Distraction can be simply defined as focusing on another source of attention other than pain. Although distraction cannot make the pain go away, it takes the client's attention away from the pain. Benefits include: (1) increased pain tolerance; makes pain more bearable; (2) offers clients a "sense of control" over pain; (3) improved affect or mood; (4) decreased intensity or quality of pain; and (5) allows clients to rest.

Distraction does not remove all sensations of pain, although persons who successfully use distraction techniques may appear temporarily as though they are not experiencing any pain. When the distraction ceases, clients may focus on the painful sensation again and exhibit irritability, complaints of pain, and fatigue.

To be effective, the distraction technique should have the following characteristics.

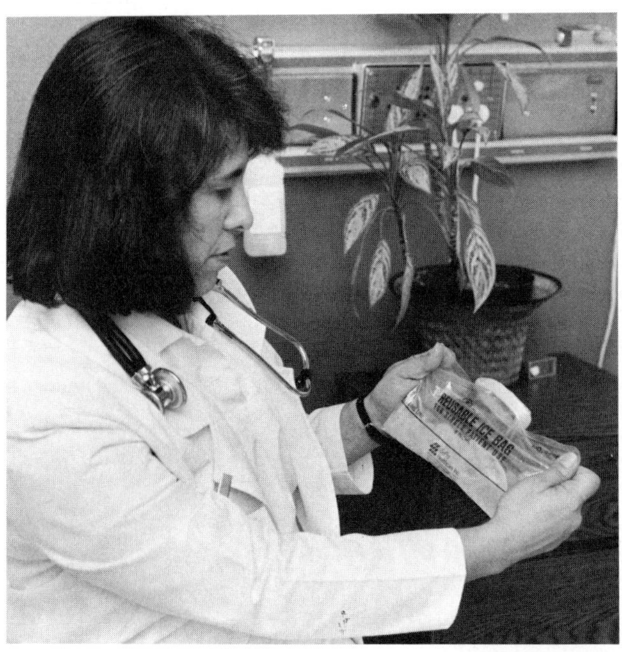

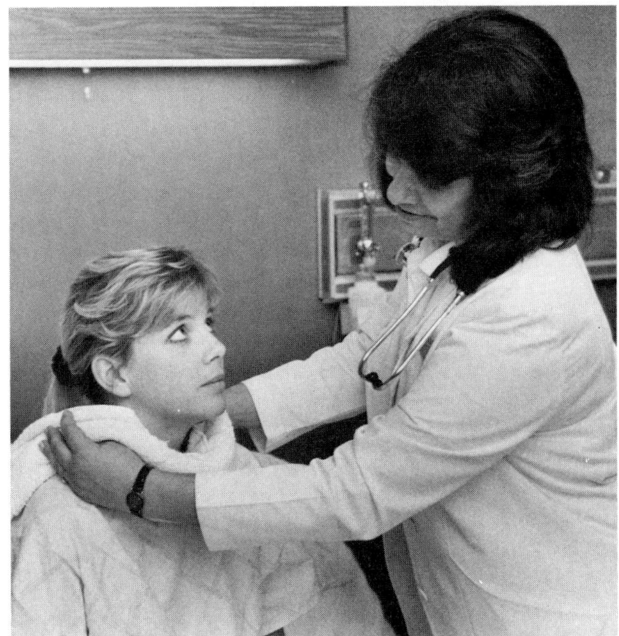

Figure 29–9. An ice collar aids in pain relief.

TABLE 29–8. VARIATIONS AND USES OF COLD THERAPY

Description	Uses
Cold Packs: Cold packs come in various forms, among them commercial products, frozen gels, chipped ice in a bag, chemical ice envelopes, ice massage (rubbing a block of ice over the skin).	Useful in effective cooling of deeper tissues, reducing inflammation, and swelling, and in relief of headaches.
Cold Compresses: A gauze dressing or washcloth soaked in ice water, wrung out, and applied to skin or injured area. This sequence needs to be repeated several times to maintain cool temperature. Open wounds may require sterile application.	Useful in reducing inflammation and edema, decreasing local bleeding and in creating localized numbness (see Chap. 24).
Hypothermia Blankets: A large, rectangular body-sized aquathermic pad. Also referred to as a cooling blanket. Distilled water flows through the pad and produces desired temperature via preset control unit.	Useful in lowering body temperature from high fevers or during surgery. Decreases intracranial pressure, bleeding, and severe pain by decreasing metabolic activity.
Alcohol Sponge Bath, Ice Massage, Cool Tepid Bath	Useful in reducing elevated body temperatures, especially in children.
Aerosol Spray	Useful in cooling the skin through evaporation. Does not penetrate deep tissue.

- Is interesting to the client.
- Is consistent with client's energy level and ability to concentrate.
- Rhythm is used and emphasized; for example, keeping time to music.
- Stimulates the major sensory modalities: hearing, vision, touch, and movement.
- Can provide a change in stimuli when the pain changes; for example, stimulus can be increased when pain increases.

GUIDED IMAGERY. Guided imagery is a specific distraction technique. It involves the structured use of the imagination and mental images to reduce pain. As persons engage in pleasant mental images, the images are stimuli to the autonomic nervous system and replace painful stimuli. Pleasant mental imagery activates calming responses of the autonomic nervous system, such as decreased heart rate, normal blood pressure, decreased respiratory rate, and warm skin.[38] As a well-chosen image activates the autonomic nervous system in this manner, it supersedes the effects of painful stimulations, which cause increased heart rate, increased blood pressure, increased respiratory rate and cool skin. Guided imagery techniques are discussed in Chapter 22.

MUSIC THERAPY. Music therapy is another method of distraction. The purpose of music therapy is to reduce anxiety by distracting the client, thereby reducing the client's perception of pain.

Therapeutic music is usually placed in a cassette player, and earphones are placed over the client's ears (Fig. 29–10). Tapes may contain soothing background music or the client's favorite music. Clients may use music therapy as a distraction as they wish, but should listen for at least 20 minutes twice a day.[3]

Besides its use as a pain relief measure, music therapy has been prescribed as an intervention to: (1) increase orientation in the elderly and psychiatric clients; (2) decrease anxiety and relieve the pain of burns, cancer, childbirth, and surgery; (3) increase stimulation for clients who are comatose, elderly, and blind; and (4) increase or improve movement in those with impaired neurosensory function from cerebral palsy, Huntington's chorea, Parkinson's, and speech disorders.[37]

Placing a radio beside a client's bed is not music therapy. Nurses must assess the type and kind of music to be used, its particular effects, when to use it, and for how long.

Medication for Mild and Moderate Pain. Relief of mild to moderate pain, using pharmaceutical drugs, focuses on nonnarcotic analgesics. Nonnarcotic analgesics include over-the-counter (OTC) drugs used in pain relief. They are also referred to as nonsteroidal antiinflammatory drugs (NSAIDS). The three main characteristics of nonnarcotic analgesics are antiinflammatory, analgesic, and antipyretic properties. An antiinflammatory drug is one that counteracts or reduces inflammation; an analgesic is a drug that reduces pain perception; and an antipyretic effect is one that reduces fever. Aspirin (ASA), and salicylic derivatives such as acetaminophen (Tylenol) and ibuprofen (Advil, Nuprin), are OTC drugs used in treatment of mild to moderate pain. Their effectiveness is enhanced when they are administered before pain becomes severe. Nonnarcotic analgesics act on the thalamus and cerebral cortex to alter the perception and interpretation of pain.

Use of Nonsteroidal Antiinflammatory Agents. Indications for the use of NSAIDS include pain of peripheral origin such as low back pain, ordinary headaches, muscle strains; inflammatory conditions such as rheumatoid arthritis; trauma; surgery; cancer; bone metastasis; dysmenorrhea; or when clients desire to avoid narcotics and request to be

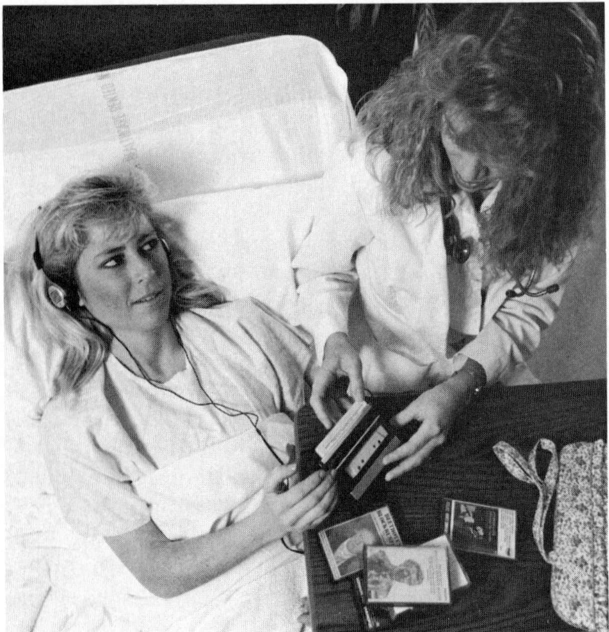

Figure 29–10. Music therapy is useful as a distraction technique for hospitalized clients.

alert and in control. Contraindications to the use of NSAIDS include intolerance or allergy to the drug. Stomach ulcers or bleeding disorders may limit the use of aspirin.

The oral or (p.o.) route medications in the form of capsules or tablets are preferred (see Chap. 22 for considerations in medication administration). If clients are unable to ingest pills or capsules because of decreased consciousness, natural difficulty swallowing pills, or impaired ability to swallow, nurses can crush pills and give them with apple sauce or yogurt, or seek a physician's order for a liquid or rectal form of the drug, if available. These drugs generally need to be taken every four hours.

The analgesic effect of nonnarcotic analgesics occurs in approximately 2 hours,[3] but the antiinflammatory effect is more variable, and can take up to a week. Nurses must carefully evaluate a client's pain, the purpose for giving such drugs, and common side-effects (see Chap. 22 for a discussion of medication administration).

Considerations in using nonnarcotic drugs as analgesics include the following.[3]

1. Acetaminophen is the easiest drug to take; it has fewer side-effects than other nonnarcotic agents but may be less effective for relief of more than mild pain.
2. Aspirin (salicylic acid) is an effective analgesic for mild to moderate pain, but is one of the most difficult drugs to take; it has many side-effects that may be intense enough to limit its use in some individuals.
3. Some of the other NSAIDS, such as ibuprofen, are likely to be better analgesics than acetaminophen, and at least equal to aspirin in analgesic ability, but they are usually

PROCEDURE 29–4. COLD APPLICATION

☐ **PURPOSE:** To decrease pain, reduce inflammation and edema.

☐ **EQUIPMENT:** Ice, ice bag, ice collar, or disposable glove, or chemical cold generation pack; disposable waterproof underpad; bath towels or washcloth.

ACTION

1. Check physician's order for type and length of treatment. If not specified, cold treatments are applied for 20–30 minutes. If used to treat an injury, cold is effective for the first 24–26 hours postinjury.
2. Assess:
   - Condition of the skin at site of application.
   - Level of discomfort at site of application.
   - Sensitivity to temperature, pain, and light touch. To avoid frostbite injury, do not apply cold to an area of diminished sensitivity.
3. Discuss procedure with the client, including expected sensations, desired client participation, and sensations to be reported to nurse.
4. Prepare and apply ice:
   - Fill ice bag, collar, or glove two thirds full of chipped ice.
   - Remove excess air to promote bag comforming to body contours and reduce interference to conduction of cold.
   - Ask or assist client to assume a comfortable position.
   - Apply a layer of cloth (towel or washcloth) over site of application to reduce risk of skin injury.
   - Apply ice, shaping for close contact with affected part.
   - For chemical cold generation pack, squeeze to activate; then apply as above.
   - Hold ice application in place with towels or pillowcase; tape as needed.
   - Place waterproof disposable underpad under part being treated.
5. Monitor affected part in 10 minutes for color, temperature, and sensation. Skin should be cool and slightly pale with reduced sensitivity to touch. Redness indicates reflex vasodilation; lack of sensation and whiteness indicate frostbite. If no negative effects noted, leave ice in place 20–30 minutes. May be reapplied 30 minutes later.
6. Evaluate effectiveness of therapy: assess comfort, swelling, and skin condition.

☐ **RECORDING:** Identify site of application. Describe site condition before and after treatment; client response; degree of relief obtained; problems, if any, and action taken.

easier to take than aspirin; that is, they have fewer or less intense side-effects.

Individuals may respond more favorably to one drug than to another. Thus, it may require some experimentation to determine the most effective drug for a particular client.

Side-Effects. Side-effects of nonnarcotic analgesics include decreased clotting time (bleeding), impaired liver and kidney function with chronic use, gastrointestinal irritation and gastric ulcers, fluid retention, and decreased growth of new bone. Aspirin may cause gastric irritation, tinnitus, and decreased clotting time, whereas acetaminophen in large doses impairs kidney function. Laboratory values and clients' physical status need to be monitored to observe for any changes indicating these side-effects.

Selecting Approaches. There are many considerations in selecting appropriate approaches for clients with mild to moderate pain. Nursing implementation for a person in pain involves more than giving a medication. Careful assessment of the nature of the pain, how it is experienced, the anatomy and physiology of pain, the kind of pain, relevant surgical or medical procedures, factors influencing pain, and sociocultural, personal, and past experiences with pain is needed in developing an appropriate management approach. Other considerations include the following.

- Nurses must examine their own feelings about pain and their own reactions to a client's pain.[33] This will make them more receptive and understanding of the client's pain.
- Careful listening and paraphrasing is essential in communicating with the client in pain. This will assist the nurse in performing an accurate pain assessment and aid in directing the pain management strategy.
- Any client reporting pain is having pain; the challenge is to help the client identify the source of the pain and manage it effectively.
- Once the source of the client's pain has been identified, consider simple comfort measures that might relieve the pain; for example, turning or repositioning, use of cool cloth, back rub, or other noninvasive approaches, either in conjunction with pain medication or alone.
- Know the action, purpose, and side-effects of all pain medications. Plan for potential side-effects; for example, monitor laboratory values, offer fluids if constipation is a side-effect.
- Identify and manage factors that influence pain: disbelief, fatigue, fear, knowledge, misconceptions, and monotony.
- Collaborate with clients in management of their pain. Nurses can offer alternatives and, when clients try new relief measures with a nurse's guidance, effective intervention can be accomplished.

Supporting Clients' Memory, Learning, and Thought. Many of the problems for clients with memory loss and impaired learning and thought relate to their inability to evaluate reality. Inability to concentrate, distractibility, disordered thinking, and poor judgment are problems for these clients.

Sensitivity to effective communication is required to facilitate a therapeutic relationship with clients. By engaging in open, honest conversation with clients, nurses can enhance clients' sense of integrity. Nursing strategies include approaching clients in a calm manner, being an attentive listener, and recognizing one's own body position, facial gestures, and tone of voice. Nurses should talk directly to clients and explain expectations required of them. They should *not* talk about clients in front of family members or health care personnel.

Reality orientation is essential to aid clients who have memory loss or misconceptions about reality. Asking clients to state where and who they are and to identify the date and time gives information about their orientation. Nurses should correct any misunderstood aspects of reality. Clients with head injuries who are recovering from memory loss, or other clients experiencing memory loss from brain damage, may require reality orientation many times in one day. This should be done in a patient, reassuring manner.

Large numbered calendars provide visual aids for orientation (Fig. 29–11). Daily schedules posted in large print or on grease boards facilitate recognition of daily patterns of activity. Pictures of family posted on walls may help stimulate clients' memories of significant others and past events. Cues such as family albums and favorite toys, books, clothing, and music can also provide stimuli to enhance memory in clients.

Focusing on the present is important for any client experiencing thought alterations, such as hallucinations. Nurses should also validate meanings of conversations with clients who experience disordered or altered thinking.

Breaking tasks into small steps often aids clients who

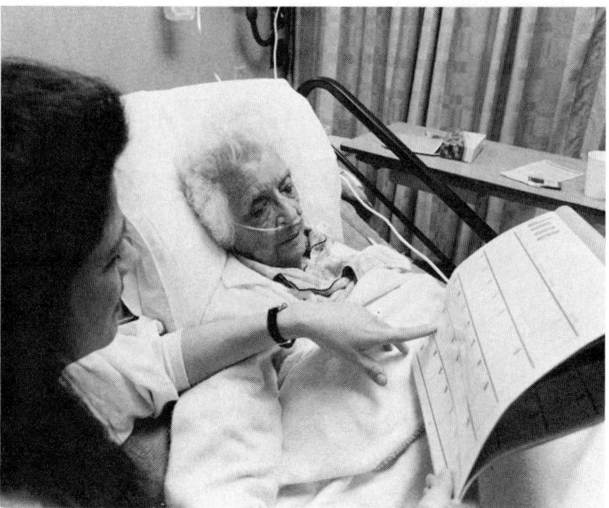

Figure 29–11. Use of a large calendar for reality orientation.

experience distractibility and shortened attention span. Accomplishing small steps increases self-esteem and feelings of success along with achievement of goals.

Measures to promote safety are necessary for clients who exhibit poor judgment or an inability to reason correctly. Clients may need careful supervision to prevent accidents. Client conversation may need to be monitored to ensure clients are not bothering others.

Validation of client teaching is essential. Clients should be asked to repeat material, using examples and their own words. Reading materials can be supplied to reinforce learning. It is also important to reduce pain and stress prior to teaching, as these are barriers to learning.

Supporting Clients' Communication, Language, and Speech. To work effectively with clients experiencing impaired communication, it is important to assume a calm, reassuring, and supportive manner that conveys a sense of caring and acceptance. Providing adequate time for communication and return responses by clients is essential for their self-esteem and the process of communication.

Supporting Clients with Expressive Aphasia. Nursing approaches for care of clients experiencing expressive aphasia include encouraging conversation and asking open-ended questions. Allow time for clients to find the right word, disregard incorrect word choices, and encourage pointing and pantomime for self-expression. Provide pictures of common activities or objects to stimulate conversation or choice of words. Acknowledging clients' frustration lets clients know their feelings are recognized. If appropriate, reassure clients that their speech will improve over time and that speech skills can be relearned.

For clients with expressive aphasia who cannot speak at all, it is helpful to ask closed, yes–no questions. Instead of asking "How was your visit with your family?", one could ask several yes–no questions, such as "Did your family visit last night?" and "Did you enjoy seeing your family?" Yes–no questions can thus enable clients to communicate. If clients' writing ability and expression are not impaired, be sure to provide paper and pen to facilitate written communication. Pictures can also be used to convey basic requests and needs. For example, clients can point to a picture of a glass of water to indicate that they are thirsty. Another method to facilitate effective communication is through use of a picture board (Fig. 29–12).

Supporting Clients with Receptive Aphasia. Receptive aphasia necessitates nursing approaches that address clients' comprehension problems. Clients may be unaware of a speaker's facial expressions, body position, or tone of voice. They may understand only fragments of conversation, and consequently answer inappropriately or incorrectly.

Comprehension can be facilitated by reducing environmental noise; for example, by turning off radio, television, and vibrating machines. Excessive environmental stimulation should also be eliminated. Too much clutter may be distracting to clients.

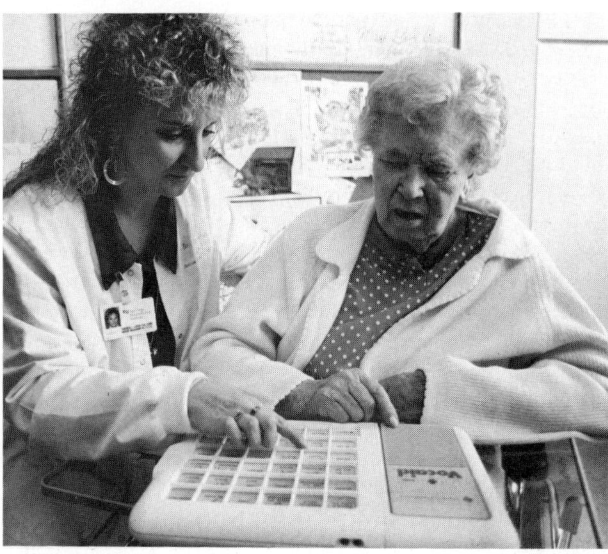

Figure 29–12. A speech therapist helps an aphasic client to communicate by using a picture board.

Approaching the client slowly and speaking distinctly in short phrases facilitates comprehension. Do not shout. Use gestures, touch, and lip movements as cues in speaking. The client's understanding of speech can be augmented by repeating and rephrasing statements calmly and without signs of irritation. To facilitate accomplishment of tasks, it is essential to divide each task into small units. The client's level of understanding and comprehension is best suited for achieving small steps.

Supporting Clients with Dysarthria. For clients with dysarthria, the speech difficulty is motor weakness; thus, clients generally have unimpaired thought processes. Although the client's speech may not be amenable to therapy, facial exercises such as pursing the lips, smiling, whistling, sticking out the tongue, and grimacing can assist clients to keep remaining muscles of speech. Reading aloud several times a day also exercises muscles and encourages breath control.

Articulation can be improved by having clients speak more slowly and exaggerate each spoken word. Encouraging clients to rephrase and shorten messages can facilitate articulation and improve communication. Use of gestures and written messages increases the likelihood that clients' communications will be understood by others. A simple alphabet or picture board can also facilitate communication. Clients point to letters on the board to spell a word, or point to pictures that communicate their need.

Supporting Clients' Movement. Chapter 30 discusses specific approaches that are concerned with increasing limb mobility with range of motion, proper positioning and body alignment, procedures for transfers, and assisting ambulation. The reader is referred to that chapter for discussion of those topics.

For many people experiencing an inability to move, the impact is devastating. Suddenly, people become dependent on others. For example, people who suffer brain damage to one side of the brain, through stroke, may become paralyzed on one side of the body and experience an impaired ability to communicate. This translates into dependence on others for (1) self-care activities (brushing teeth, dressing); (2) transfers from bed to wheelchair to car; (3) social activities, and (4) exercise. The impaired ability to communicate complicates expression of needs and desires and may precipitate emotions of depression, anger, hostility, and loneliness. Rehabilitation strategies are designed to help such individuals gain independence, but this requires much effort and energy expenditure.

Special appliances or modified devices may assist clients with impaired movement to carry out activities of daily living (Fig. 29–13). The purpose of assistive devices is to maintain or increase independence in self-care and activities of daily living.

For clients with impaired functioning of the hands, either from a stroke (brain damage) or spinal cord injury or peripheral nerve injury, the following assistive devices and measures may be helpful.

- Clothing that can be easily donned. Velcro closures can be substituted for buttons and zippers.
- Button hook and zipper pulls can be used for closing buttons and zippers.
- Plate guards, or metal half-circles, can be attached to plates to aid clients with impaired hand functioning. The client uses the guard to prevent spilling of food and to provide an edge on which to push or secure food onto the fork.
- Hand utensils can be built up with foam to improve the grip for persons with limited hand grasp.
- Hand straps or molds with clasps can be used to secure utensils or toothbrushes for those lacking any hand grasp.
- Knives with curved blades that rock back and forth can be used to cut meat.
- Long-handled brushes or sponges are useful in washing hard-to-get body areas.
- Sophisticated equipment is continually being developed to promote independent living and occupational work for clients with quadriplegia. Such devices as mouth-operated wheelchairs, electric wheelchairs, and computers with laser beam pointers and correctable displays and line printers offer new opportunities to enhance living for clients with complex neurosensory and mobility problems.

Activities of daily living (ADLs) become complicated for clients with mobility problems. With various modifications, nurses can assist clients to perform activities independently.

To assist with brushing the teeth, a person with only one strong hand can stabilize the toothbrush on a flat surface with the affected hand while squeezing out the toothpaste with the strong hand. Independent hair combing and brushing is a straightforward procedure if the hairstyle is simple. Other hairstyles may require assistance from the nurse or significant others. Electric razors are safe for shaving and can be used by persons with only one strong hand.

For dressing, the following approaches can assist the client who has only one strong hand and leg. When putting on a shirt, the client should sit on the edge of the bed and spread the shirt out on the lap. Insert the weak arm into the

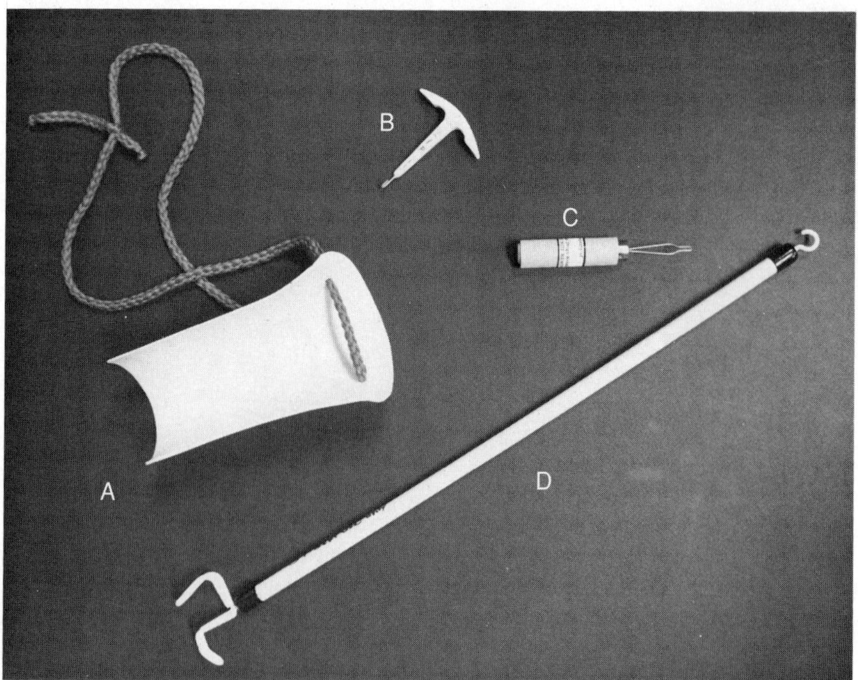

Figure 29–13. Assistive devices. **A.** Sock puller. **B.** Zipper pull. **C.** Button hook. **D.** Pants puller.

correct armhole, pull up the sleeve and throw the garment over the back. Use the strong arm to get into the remaining sleeve. The client should pull the pants leg over the weak foot first. The other pants leg should then be put on the strong leg as far as possible. In the standing or lying position, the pants can be pulled up over the hips and fastened.

Assistance with feeding may be required for persons with weak or paralyzed upper limbs or for persons with severe tremors. Approaches that facilitate independent eating are discussed in Chapter 25.

Collaboration with occupational and physical therapists is often a component of rehabilitation of clients with impaired mobility. Nurses can facilitate rehabilitation by understanding the goals and approaches in ADL training, dressing, hygiene, and exercises offered by physical and occupational therapists.

Restorative Care

Restorative care focuses on several acute disturbances in neurosensory dysfunction that are most often related to consciousness, movement, and pain. Clients who require nursing approaches that focus on physiological restoration are comatose clients, clients experiencing seizures, clients with sensory overload or sensory deprivation, and clients with severe pain.

Caring for Comatose Clients. When caring for the comatose client, the nurse must undertake all those functions that the client would normally carry out. Care of comatose clients is a challenge because they are completely dependent on the nurse for all of their care. Prioritization of client needs is essential, and the client's first priority is oxygenation.

The brain is highly dependent on oxygen. Proper oxygenation is important to cerebral function, prevention of increased intracranial pressure, and tissue healing. Assuring that the client's airway is clear is essential. Proper use of oxygen support devices, whether nasal cannulas, masks, or ventilators assists the client in meeting the oxygen requirements. Suctioning may be necessary to clear obstructed airways of sputum and other secretions and allow proper oxygenated air flow. Maintaining proper head position is important so that airways do not become obstructed. Turning clients from side-to-side allows for lung expansion and for settled lung secretions to be dislodged (see Chap. 27 for more on supporting and restoring the oxygenation function).

Circulation must be adequately maintained. Assessment of vital signs, and drawing of blood as well as blood gases as per physician's order, provides information about the client's circulatory status. Clients may be attached to a cardiac (ECG) monitor to monitor cardiac rhythm.

Fluid status must be carefully managed in the comatose client. The client may require supplemental IV fluids and electrolytes. The nurse must carefully infuse IV fluids (as per physician's order) to prevent rises in intracranial pressure, while still providing adequate hydration (see Chaps. 27 and 31 for more on restoring fluid balance and supporting circulation).

Monitoring of comatose clients is essential, as client status can change quickly. Assessment of vital signs and neurochecks may range from every 15 minutes, if the client is unstable, to every 2 to 4 hours, for a stabilized (noncritical) client (refer to Section 2 for additional information on vital signs and neurochecks).

Nutrition for the comatose client is one of the greatest challenges for health care providers.[33] A nasogastric or feeding tube may be inserted in order to feed the client liquid supplemental feedings (see Chap. 25). Adequate nutrition is essential for recovery of any client. Supplemental liquid feedings will provide the nutrition and calories necessary for client needs. If not contraindicated, a high-vitamin, high-protein feeding with 2500 to 3500 calories is recommended for an adult. For clients receiving liquid feeding, it is important to note the character and consistency of stools. Diarrhea is a frequent problem, and may indicate a need for a change in the formula of liquid nutrition used. Clients receiving supplemental tube feedings may also require supplemental water feedings to assure proper hydration. Nutritionists should be consulted for assessment of nutritional needs and problems associated with feedings. The reader is referred to Chapter 25 for discussion of nutrition and fluids.

Activities of daily living need to be performed for the client. Nurses should discuss with the family the client's pre-illness schedule and preferences. This information can be adapted for inclusion in the client care plan, if feasible. For example, the family may report the client likes a particular kind of music or bedtime routine; this can be incorporated into the client's care.

Hygiene measures include daily bathing and frequent back care and hair washing as appropriate. Mouth care can be performed at least every 4 hours. This includes applying petroleum jelly to the lips to avoid drying and cracking. Hair should be combed every shift, if possible, and at least daily. Long hair can be braided. Range-of-motion can be performed conveniently during the bath.

Skin and tissue care can be part of the hygiene routine and should be performed every 2 to 4 hours with vital sign checks (Box 29–11).

Bowel and bladder regimens need to be initiated and maintained to promote adequate functioning and prevent complications. Most comatose clients have a Foley catheter in place. Proper cleansing around the meatus or urethra aids in prevention of infection (see Chap. 26). Urine output and the nature and color of urine should be monitored, and any cloudiness, blood, or infectious material reported.

To maintain bowel evacuation, clients may require daily or every-other-day suppositories. It is important to assess for and prevent stool impactions. Chapter 26 provides additional information on bowel and bladder management.

Safety. Comatose clients must be protected against injury. If the client has seizures, the siderails should be padded

BOX 29–11. SKIN CARE FOR THE COMATOSE CLIENT

1. Assess skin for color, temperature, dryness, pressure ulcers, and reddened areas.
2. Cleanse skin daily and as needed. Skin may become dry and require frequent application of lotion. (See Chap. 24 for skin care.)
3. Provide back care with repositioning every 2 hours or more frequently if needed. Frequent repositioning minimizes pulmonary congestion and musculoskeletal deformities.
4. Perform massage to reddened areas. Check ears, heels, and elbows for skin breakdown. Place a pillow between knees and behind back when positioned on the side, and elevate heels off bed with a pillow.
5. Turn frequently. To prevent an increase in intracranial pressure by initiation of Valsalva maneuver, turn client while client is exhaling, if possible.
6. Cleanse eyes daily. Use eye lubricants and patches, if appropriate, to reduce dryness and corneal abrasions.

and kept up at all times. Immobility and its complications, such as contractures, skin breakdown, and decubitus ulcers, require attention. Contractures, such as wrist drop and foot drop, can be prevented with range-of-motion exercises (ROM), proper positioning, and appropriate use of splints (refer to Chap. 30 for additional information).

Communication is an area of special need. While clients are comatose, it is important to talk to them while performing care. Many times these clients are aware of their surroundings and can hear but not respond. Nurses, physicians, and other health care personnel should refrain from talking at the client's bedside. Touching and stroking clients during care, and encouraging family members to do so as well, promotes communication and provides stimulation for the client.

During the day, appropriate stimulation should be offered. Tuning the radio to the client's favorite station, or setting the television to a favorite program, is one way to provide stimulation. Calm reassuring talk to the client is another. Family members can relate the day's events, tell the client about friends and family members, and read stories.

At night, nurses should dim lights and coordinate nursing activities to promote a somewhat normal daily body rhythm, and to promote sleep.

Environmental Considerations. Most clients with alterations in consciousness are initially placed in an intensive care unit. This is a stressful and high-tech environment. Equipment is noisy and can fill the client's immediate environment with meaningless stimuli that can contribute to sensory overload or deprivation.

The client's dignity and humanity should be maintained by providing privacy when giving care, administering medications, and performing invasive techniques. If clients recover from the comatose state, it will become very important to reorient them to person, place, and time, and to help them understand what has happened.

Caring for Clients With Seizures. Clients who are comatose, who have brain injury or brain tumors, or who have internal excitability of brain cells may develop seizures. Seizures are the sudden discharge of electrical activity in brain cells, manifested in bizarre, jerking movements of the body, loss of consciousness, possible staring, inappropriate behaviors, and unusual visual, auditory, and gustatory sensations. Some persons may experience an aura, or warning signal, before the seizure occurs. Seizures that last a long time can be potentially life-threatening; however, most seizures last a few seconds up to several minutes.

Nursing management of clients experiencing seizures is an advanced skill and is directed toward accurate data gathering based on observation of the client, protecting the client from injury during a seizure, and employing seizure precautions. Box 29–12 summarizes key points of observation and management during a seizure. Seizure precautions are detailed in Box 29–13. Priorities during a seizure include: (1) staying with the client; (2) calling for help; (3) protecting

BOX 29–12. NURSING OBSERVATIONS AND MANAGEMENT DURING SEIZURES

Observations:

1. Determine whether there were any warning signs or an aura.
2. Assess where the seizure began and how it proceeded.
3. Note the type of body movements and what parts of the body were involved.
4. Note any changes in the size of pupils.
5. Assess for urinary and bowel incontinence.
6. Determine the duration of the seizure and phases, if any.
7. Assess client consciousness level throughout the seizure.
8. Describe the behavior of the client after the seizure.
9. Note any weakness or paralysis of extremities after the seizure.
10. Note lethargy and amount of sleep required after the seizure.

Management

1. If the client is in a chair at the onset of a seizure, ease to the floor.
2. Provide for privacy by pulling curtains or closing doors. Encourage onlookers to leave if there are no privacy measures.
3. Maintain a patent airway to ensure adequate ventilation. Constrictive clothing around the neck should be loosened.
4. Guide the client's movements so that the head or extremities do not bang against hard surfaces or the floor.
5. Always stay with the client during a seizure. Observation and prevention of injury cannot occur if the nurse is looking for help.
6. Turn the client on one side to allow for drainage of secretions when the seizure is completed.
7. Allow the client to sleep after a seizure.

BOX 29–13. SEIZURE PRECAUTIONS

1. Padded siderails are kept in the up position to protect client from injury.
2. An artificial airway is available at the head of bed, easily visible to protect client's tongue and keep airway open.
3. Suction is available at the bedside in the event client chokes or airway becomes blocked.
4. Beds are kept in low position for client safety.
5. Clients may be required to wear protective head gear or helmets for uncontrolled seizures.
6. Supervised ambulation may be required to prevent falls.

the client's head and arms and providing safety; (4) careful observation; and (5) ensuring a patent airway.

It is important to obtain any history of seizures during the neurosensory assessment. Clients who suffer head trauma may not have a seizure at the time of injury. Years later, however, seizures can develop spontaneously. Being alert to past traumatic events to the head, to the presenting diagnosis of clients, and carefully assessing for seizures when taking the client history will identify clients at risk for seizures.

Caring for Clients with Sensory Deprivation or Sensory Overload. Changes in the amount of sensory stimulation clients receive may result in altered functioning. Sensory deprivation occurs when stimulation is insufficient; sensory overload when clients receive more stimuli than they can effectively manage.

Sensory deprivation may occur in clients with brain damage or conditions that decrease input through the senses (blindness, deafness), in clients with spinal cord injury (loss of touch), and in aphasic clients who experience altered reception or expression of language and, occasionally, decreased sensation and movement in one-half of the body. Clients who suffer from severe pain may be vulnerable to sensory overload. It is also common in clients in an intensive care unit, and in clients who cannot process incoming stimuli at their previous speed. An unfamiliar environment with many machines and items may enhance sensory overload.

IMPLICATIONS FOR NURSE–CLIENT COLLABORATION

Sensory Overload and Sensory Deprivation

An optimal amount of sensory input is necessary for healthy functioning of neurosensory mechanisms. Both excessive sensory input (sensory overload) and deficit sensory input (sensory deficit) contribute to altered neurosensory functioning and stress. Individuals vary in their need for and capacity to handle sensory input. What may be stressful in some may be pleasant to others. Nurse–client collaboration is necessary to determine the optimal amount of sensory input—visual, auditory, tactile, olfactory, and gustatory—for individual well-being.

Nursing Approaches for Clients with Sensory Deprivation. Visual aids include use of pictures, calendars, or posters. Auditory stimuli include talking with the client and playing music, radio, or television. Tactile stimulation is important, and may include the use of touch, back rubs, or hand-holding. Social stimulation—encouraging visitors, sitting with clients, or encouraging group activities—is also beneficial to clients. Environmental stimulation may include providing proper lighting; opening or closing of drapes; or providing reading materials, such as books, magazines, or newspapers. Informing clients and significant others of the deprivation state can facilitate their interaction with others and generate other ideas for stimulation.

Nursing Approaches for Clients with Sensory Overload. Approaches to minimizing sensory overload involve altering the environment to reduce stimuli by dimming lights at night, and covering blinking lights. Reducing noise stimuli to alter the environment involves shutting off nonessential alarms and unnecessary equipment, using earplugs, avoiding loud noises and encouraging personnel to hold conversations away from the client's room. Explaining equipment, routines, and procedures may facilitate client's understanding of the surroundings. Promoting movement (turning, chair activity, and ambulation) and providing reorientation also reduces sensory overload for clients.

Planning rest periods and providing privacy reduce excess stimuli. Excessive activities should be eliminated. Grouping procedures and care activities reduces the continuous incoming pattern stimuli or interruptions. Orientation to daily activities and schedules of care or treatment assists clients in realistic expectations of their daily routine. Again, involvement of the client, family, and health care team in management of sensory overload facilitates common understanding for restrictions on visits and activities, and generates collaborative efforts toward reducing sensory overload.

Caring for Clients with Severe Pain. Clients who can experience severe pain include those who have had recent surgery, sustained some form of trauma, or are experiencing some acute, painful disruption in the neurosensory network. Care of clients in severe pain requires skill and sensitivity by nurses. Often clients cry out loudly, moan, or communicate in an angry manner. At first, inexperienced nurses may find such behavior can be intimidating or frightening. In time, however, nurses become expert at assessing and responding to the psychological and physiological needs of the client who experiences pain as they recognize the behaviors associated with severe pain and a variety of approaches that relieve pain.

Pain is a very stressful experience for clients. It can be fatiguing, and can make individuals irritable and tense. Prevention of pain is of primary importance for client comfort. Using a variety of pain-relief methods is useful. Incorporating the client's beliefs about pain and pain relief enables the client to collaborate in pain relief. Medications used in conjunction with alternate measures of pain relief may be required.

Methods of Pain Relief. Transcutaneous electric nerve stimulation (TENS) is used during and after minor painful procedures such as dressing changes and suture removal, and to control postoperative pain. The TENS unit is a noninvasive battery-powered device that transmits a low-voltage electrical impulse to the body through electrodes attached to the skin. TENS units are an alternative to narcotic analgesia. The exact mechanism of pain relief is not known, but it is hypothesized that electrical stimulation of large nerve fibers serves to "close the gate" so that painful stimuli cannot get through.[40] Another theory is that nerve stimulation triggers the release of endorphins causing inhibition of the transmission of noxious stimuli.

The advantages of using TENS units for pain control are that they are noninvasive, nonnarcotic, and nonaddicting. They enable clients to have some control over pain. Elderly clients are good candidates for TENS.

Clients who are not candidates for TENS units include those who have a cardiac pacemaker, especially the demand type since the electrical impulse from the TENS unit could interfere with pacing. It also should not be used with clients who have a significant cardiac dysrhythmia or present with recent or impending myocardial infarction. Further, TENS should not be used on pregnant women during the first trimester.

The primary adverse effect of TENS is skin irritation. This can be fairly serious, resulting in blisters at attachment sites.

Acupuncture is another method of pain relief. Acupuncture involves the placing of slender, solid needles in specific points around the body. These specific points are associated with areas where nerves enter muscles (over 800 motor points) or where nerves lie close to the surface of the skin.

Comfort measures are helpful in reducing pain. These include positioning clients comfortably; keeping bed linens free of wrinkles; eliminating as many environmental stressors as possible in order to reduce clients' stress; and keeping noise to a minimum.

Client teaching about pain includes informing clients to ask for medication before they are in severe pain. Once pain is severe, it may take from 20 minutes to several hours to obtain pain relief. If clients take medication prior to being in severe pain, they may obtain pain relief much faster.

Many clients have personal methods of pain relief or methods for comforting themselves. These include sitting in a certain position, pacing, drinking warm beverages, self-hypnosis, or taking hot baths or showers. Nurses should always ask clients about any personal pain relief methods and incorporate them in the pain-relief protocol.

Medication for Severe Pain. Narcotics are drugs that bind to multiple opioid receptor sites at the ends of nerves.[3] These drugs are referred to as opioid analgesics. Narcotics, when bound to receptor sites, provide pain relief or analgesia, and euphoria, even though pain may still persist. This occurs mainly because these drugs cause changes in mood, feeling, and attitude, thereby altering pain perception and providing pain relief. Narcotics are controlled substances that can only be prescribed by a physician. Refer to Chapter 22 for procedures and legal aspects of narcotics administration.

Types of Narcotics. There are two main groups of narcotics. Pure narcotic agonists are drugs such as morphine, codeine, methadone, dilaudid, and meperidine. The receptor site they occupy causes cognitive effects such as euphoria, analgesia, respiratory depression, physical dependence, tolerance for the drug, and constipation.[3] These drugs bind tightly to receptor sites and stop or block activity at that site. Narcotic agonist–antagonists are a second group of narcotics that occupy a different receptor site for pain relief but, in addition, antagonize the effects of the pure narcotic drugs (eg, respiratory depression and physical dependence).[3] Thus, the effects of these drugs are analgesia and sedation. Butorphanoe (Stadol), nalbuphine (Nubain), and pentazocine (Talwin) are agonist–antagonist narcotics. In addition, the agonist–antagonists are also capable of blocking the analgesic effect of pure narcotics similar to the narcotic antagonist effects of naloxone (Narcan).[41]

Administration of Narcotics. Narcotics are available in pure or synthetic form. They can be administered by intramuscular (IM) or intravenous (IV) routes. IV narcotics are recommended postoperatively to manage severe pain because (1) smaller doses can be given, and (2) severe pain is managed quickly and effectively. IM narcotics provide 3 to 4 hours of pain relief for most postoperative pain (2 to 3 days after surgery).

Narcotics in combination with nonnarcotics can be helpful in relieving severe pain. Narcotics are given with nonnarcotics because each enhances or contributes to the effect of the other in pain relief: narcotics alter the central nervous system (CNS) receptor sites, whereas analgesics alter the peripheral nervous system. Thus, narcotics plus nonnarcotics equal peripheral nervous system and central nervous system pain relief.[3] This combination results in an additive effect and reduces the narcotic dose needed for pain relief, thereby decreasing narcotic side-effects.[3] Common narcotic–nonnarcotic combinations are Empirin #3, Tylenol #3, and Percodan.

Patient-controlled-analgesia (PCA) is a new method of pain management that is commonly used postoperatively. PCA is self-administered by the client to manage pain. PCA operates with a pump and a timing device hooked up to an intravenous line. The client presses a button on the PCA unit whenever pain is experienced. The PCA unit controls the dosage and delivers a preset amount of analgesic, usually morphine.[42,43] Overdosage is prevented because of an inactivation period on the PCA unit. The major advantage of this system is that it gives clients some control over pain and pain relief, and eliminates having to wait for a pain medication.

Side-Effects of Narcotics. Common side-effects of narcotics are sedation, constipation, nausea and vomiting, dry mouth, and respiratory depression.

- *Respiratory depression* is always a concern with narcotic pain relief, but particularly so with large doses of morphine. Monitoring respiratory status while clients are resting is important. Encouraging coughing and deep breathing while clients are awake stimulates breathing and encourages good lung ventilation.
- *Sedation* is common for most narcotics. Inform clients that the drowsiness may subside after 2 to 3 days. If sedation seems excessive, consult the physician regarding a reduced dosage.
- *Constipation* occurs as a result of decreased peristalsis. Encourage clients to increase roughage (fruits, vegetables) in their diet, and increase water intake. A physician may need to write an order for a stool softener. Encourage exercise if clients are mobile.
- *Nausea and vomiting* may occur as a result of pain or from the narcotic itself. An antiemetic may be given intramuscularly or rectally to relieve nausea. It may be necessary to change the narcotic given if nausea and vomiting persist. Reduce unpleasant odors and sights that might stimulate vomiting.
- *Dry mouth* occurs as narcotics reduce saliva production. Instruct clients to rinse the mouth frequently, suck on sugarless candies, eat pineapple or watermelon, and drink plenty of fluids to enhance moisture in the mouth. Good oral hygiene and dental care are essential.

Care of Clients Receiving Narcotics. Fears and misconceptions exist regarding the use of narcotics in pain relief. The primary fear is that narcotic use will result in addiction or psychological dependence on narcotics. Research is revealing this to be an unfounded fear. Appropriate use of narcotics does not result in addiction. For clients with prolonged pain, it is important to differentiate between psychological and physiological dependence on narcotics.

Physical dependence or withdrawal symptoms from discontinuing narcotic drugs is another fear. Because most acute pain gradually subsides along with dosage and frequency of narcotic analgesics, physical dependence rarely occurs.

Tolerance to narcotics is a third area of concern to clients and health care personnel. This is based on a fear that increasing a dose of medication too quickly or in too large a dose will reduce effectiveness of the drug. True drug tolerance occurs when clients need more frequent, rather than larger, doses of pain relief, as is seen in intractable or chronic pain. It is important to explain to clients that it is appropriate to take whatever is needed to control pain.[3] Tolerance can be handled as it arises.

Respiratory depression is always a concern to all nurses. While this is a legitimate concern, McCaffery[3] states that no narcotic dose is automatically safe or fatal. The only safe way to administer a narcotic is to watch the first dose given to an individual. Subsequent doses tend to be safe unless the drug accumulates or the client's condition changes.

The nurse's responsibility in administering narcotic analgesics is an active one. Important choices to be made by nurses include: (1) choosing the appropriate analgesic or narcotic, as prescribed by the physician; (2) deciding whether to give a narcotic based on accurate pain assessment; (4) evaluating effectiveness of the narcotic; (3) determining if a change in pain medication is needed; (5) monitoring for side-effects of medications; and (6) educating clients about drugs, dosage, side-effects, and an effective schedule for taking the drug, and addressing fears or misconceptions.

Summary of Pain Management. Key points in the management of acute pain are as follows.

- Clients should be medicated before pain occurs, or before pain increases. This may mean medicating clients around the clock or every 3 to 4 hours. This prevents severe pain from worsening and not being effectively treated by medication.
- Narcotics can be used for severe pain without addiction. This does not mean that nurses should give clients the maximum dosage of pain medication, but rather that they should evaluate pain carefully with the client and provide maximum dosage of narcotics for severe pain when indicated.
- PRN (or as needed) pain medications should be given before pain worsens or increases. This facilitates management of pain so that pain does not become unnecessarily severe. When pain becomes severe, it takes longer for pain medication to be effective.
- General comfort measures should always be considered in conjunction with administration of narcotics. These measures may be effective in reducing severe pain or altering the pain experience in some way. Supportive approaches include keeping clients comfortable, dry, and warm (or cool, if preferred). Provide back rubs and massages as requested by clients. Repositioning clients can greatly affect comfort levels, or remove a source of pain.
- Rest periods are essential as they combat fatigue, which can worsen pain. Rest can also enhance the effectiveness of pain medications as they begin to work in the body.
- Coordinate care and pain-producing activities with the schedule for pain medications. Providing medication to clients before transferring to a chair or turning may enhance the ease of such activities.
- Immobilization and elevation of painful extremities or body parts will reduce swelling and pressure, and decrease jarring movements that send sharp signals of pain. Indirectly, as swelling is reduced, blood supply increases. This facilitates removal of waste products, which can cause pain and discomfort.
- Exercise is an important part of pain reduction when clients are able to ambulate. Exercises increases oxygenation to tissues, distracts the client, and facilitates sleep and rest, again taking the focus away from the pain.

- Noninvasive comfort measures, as described under *Supportive Care,* earlier, can be used in conjunction with narcotics or alone to provide relief of pain.
- When providing clients pain relief with prescribed analgesics and narcotics, nurses can use the guidelines found in Box 29–14.

Rehabilitative Care

Rehabilitative care focuses on reestablishing client life-style to adapt to or incorporate neurosensory alterations, if present. The optimal outcome is achieving the highest level of independence possible. For some clients, major life-style changes may occur.

Life-style Changes. Life-style changes may require adjustment in clients' level of independence. Many clients experience disabilities that leave them dependent on others for help in the home. Use of attendant help in the homes of paralyzed clients allows them to maintain independence with a minimal amount of assistance. Services such as day-care clinics or volunteers in the home can provide much needed relief for clients' families or significant others from the day-to-day responsibility of client care.

Occupational changes may be necessary for paralyzed clients or clients with impaired communication, memory, or thought. Vocational retraining may provide assistance in some cases. Social workers can serve as resources in planning home and occupational referrals. Local and state agencies can be consulted to inform clients and their families of services they provide for special needs.

Environmental Adaptation. Special appliances may be required as clients adjust to different levels of independence. Use of special appliances should be encouraged. Some clients will view adaptive devices negatively. Encourage expression of such emotions, but gently remind clients that special appliances can enhance independence, which enhances self-esteem.

Modified telephones with large printed numbers are effective for persons with visual acuity changes. For some clients, telephones that have prerecorded telephone numbers for frequently called numbers are useful. The client has only to touch the correctly labeled digit once, and the telephone number is automatically dialed.

Environmental adaptations in client homes can be made as rehabilitation in hospitals or other facilities is completed. Ramps for wheelchairs, flat door handles for persons with rheumatoid arthritis, or modified doorways for the wheelchair-bound are examples of modifications that provide adaptation in homes for clients with permanent neurosensory deficits. Bathroom fixtures with flat control bars and shower stalls with seats are other adjustments that can be made.

Approaches to Clients With Chronic Pain. For some clients, the outcome of a neurosensory dysfunction is chronic pain. Chronic pain, as previously defined, is pain that lasts 6 months or longer. Persons with chronic pain usually adapt to the pain and, consequently, may show no acute signs of grimacing or guarding. However, depression, withdrawal, decreased socialization, anger and hostility, and manipulative behavior are other indicators displayed by clients who experience chronic pain. Approaches in the management of clients with chronic pain include use of analgesics, medical treatment measures, and noninvasive approaches to pain control.

Analgesics. Analgesics are useful for acute episodes or flare-ups of pain in clients with chronic pain. When using nonnarcotic or narcotic analgesics as pain relief measures for clients, analgesics should be administered orally, if at all possible. It is essential to give high enough doses to provide sufficient pain relief. When using narcotics, use them effectively: administer maximum doses when needed and around the clock if necessary. Once acute pain subsides, reduce dosages and intervals of narcotics. Collaborating with clients in this adjustment of narcotics can facilitate the effectiveness of the drug therapy during acute flare-ups. Trust on the part of the client will be enhanced if he/she understands the pain relief plan.

Long-acting time-released oral preparations are available to treat chronic pain. Rectal and sublingual preparations are also available for clients who cannot take oral preparations.

Opiate cocktails (eg, Brompton's mixture) are effective in assisting the client to achieve a pain-free state. These preparations allow clients to remain alert and oriented while obtaining freedom from pain. They allow for pain relief without requiring repeated injections. If taken regularly, the cocktail prevents the reoccurrence of pain. This type of analgesia is generally reserved for clients with cancer.

BOX 29–14. GUIDELINES FOR ADMINISTRATION OF PRESCRIBED ANALGESICS

1. Determine the appropriate choice of medication for the client from among analgesics prescribed by the physician, being knowledgeable of client's despair, requests for pain relief, and of the basic action, dosage, side effects, and precautions of the prescribed narcotic or nonnarcotic analgesic.
2. Assess the client's response to medication. Return one-half hour after administration to evaluate the effectiveness of the narcotic or nonnarcotic analgesic.
3. Request the client to inform you of the relief received and to rate the severity of pain before and after medication administration.
4. Encourage the use of nonnarcotic and oral medications, if they can effectively relieve pain.
5. Reduce or eliminate side effects of narcotics.
6. Record the administration of narcotics, client response, and pain relief provided. Side effects and other concerns should be reported and recorded.
7. Approach the relief of pain individually for each client. Each time carefully assess the situation, as individual needs may vary.

Morphine administered by continuous IV drip is used to relieve pain for clients with cancer, clients with severe vomiting, clients who cannot tolerate the IM route, and clients who cannot swallow.[44] It provides more uniform and better pain relief because lower doses of pain medication are used over a shorter amount of time. This type of medication administration can be administered in the hospital or at home.

Given orally, a good portion of morphine never reaches the opiate receptors because it cannot cross the blood–brain barrier.[45] When given directly into the epidural space, however, this is no longer a problem. Pain, therefore, can be relieved with smaller doses of medications and less severe side-effects.[45]

Fentanyl lollipops are useful in managing chronic, severe pain without oversedation. Fentanyl is a short-acting synthetic opioid. These lollipops can be used by both adults and children and at present have been used to control the pain of terminal cancer clients.[46]

Medical Treatment Measures. Medical treatment measures may include nerve blocks or the cutting of sensory nerves to eliminate pain. Such measures require education and understanding of the potential benefits and disadvantages associated with the medical treatment that is being considered.

The dorsal column stimulator (DCS) is a new implantable device used to manage severe, chronic pain when other methods have failed. The device consists of four electrodes implanted into the spinal epidural space. The electrodes are connected to an external transmitter, which uses a battery device to block pain impulses to the spinal cord. The device is surgically implanted into a surgically created percutaneous sac in the lower abdomen or under the clavicle.

With dorsal column stimulation, pain control can be extended over large areas of the body. DCS does not cure the basic underlying problem; it only controls the symptoms. DCS has also been used to treat clients who have motor disturbances such as cerebral palsy, dystonia, post-traumatic brain injury, spinal cord injury, and degenerative diseases of the neurosensory system. DCS is most successful in the treatment of pain that results from injuries to the spinal cord and peripheral nerves.

TENS for chronic pain may be useful. Proper external placement of electrodes is essential for successful application. They should be placed: directly over the pain site, over pain trigger points along nerve pathway, at trigger points in same dermatome as pain, or at points distal to pain. The client then adjusts the amplitude setting that feels most comfortable and that provides the best pain relief.

Nerve blocks are another approach for treating chronic pain. In this procedure, specially trained anesthesiologists inject solutions into the nervous structure, such as nerve trunks, nerve roots, sympathetic ganglion, or the spinal cord. The procedure destroys or anesthetizes nerves that carry the pain messages to the brain. This procedure carries the risk of neurological injury and systemic side-effects. Nerve blocks can be temporary or permanent.

A cordotomy is an extensive surgical procedure designed to alleviate pain. It involves resecting the thoracic or cervical spinal cord at various levels. This procedure is used to relieve unrelenting or intractable pain. The higher the focus of the pain, the higher the site for the cordotomy. The procedure is not curative since the stimulus for the pain remains, but the stimulus does not reach the higher cerebral structures to be identified as pain. The client will have permanent loss of both pain and temperature sensation in the areas in which the resected nerves lie. Clients do, however, retain sense of touch and position. Clients should be cautioned to measure temperature of bath water and any warming devices (such as hot water bottles) to avoid burns to those areas.

A posterior rhizotomy entails the resection of the dorsal roots of a spinal nerve. This type of surgery is effective for relieving localized acute pain in the area supplied by the nerve root and deep visceral pain. As with a cordotomy, this procedure is not curative but only provides for pain relief.

Noninvasive Treatment Measures. Noninvasive measures of pain relief, as detailed in the discussion of *Supportive Care,* can be used for chronic pain relief or in conjunction with analgesic therapy. Nurses are encouraged to explore with clients which technique, whether relaxation, biofeedback, imagery or others, is preferable to them. Determine which methods, if used in the past, are effective. The use of noninvasive therapy is widely used in the treatment of chronic pain.

■ EVALUATION

Evaluation of client care is the final component of nurse–client management of neurosensory integration. Specific neurosensory outcomes identified in the client care plan provide the framework for monitoring the client's progress. If the desired outcomes have been met, the problem is resolved and a notation is made in the client's chart. If the desired outcomes have not been achieved, reassessment and replanning are necessary.

SUMMARY

Neurosensory integration represents the coordinated and unified functions that are essential to humanness, wholeness, and individuality. Consciousness, perception, memory, learning, thought, communication and movement—functions that form the basis of human personality—are only possible through neurosensory integration and are dependent upon the complex, interconnected circuitry of the nervous system for their elaboration. Together these functions make it possible for individuals to sense their environments, to respond to stimuli in appropriate ways, and to address the problems that people face in everyday life.

Each of the major neurosensory functions contributes

to individual coping, self-care, and capacity for collaborative interaction. Consciousness is the state of being aware of one's self and one's surroundings and perception is the ability of the mind to interpret and analyze input from the senses. Without these functions individuals become dependent on others to assist them in problem-solving. Pain, a natural phenomenon related to perception, serves a protective function, alerting the individual to the possibility of injury or illness. Theories of pain postulate various ideas on the neurological basis of pain with differing ideas on the role of receptors, pathways, patterns of stimulus, and stimulus transmission. Memory, the mental capacity for receiving, registering, encoding, consolidating, storing, and retrieving information, is essential to virtually every aspect of mental functioning and is closely associated with learning, which is a permanent change in behavior related to memory. Memory is vital to the accomplishment of even the simplest of human tasks. Thought is a complex set of mental processes that assigns meaning to sensory input and designs actions in response to interpretations of sensory input. Communication, closely related to thought, is the act of sending and receiving messages through the use of speech. Speech, in turn, is the vocal articulation of thoughts using language, a formal system of signs and symbols for communication. Movement is a change in place, position, or posture of any portion of the body, and is vital for engaging in activities of daily living. All of these functions, alone or in combination, are essential for a person's independence and for individuals to meet the demands of their environments.

Many factors act as variables to neurosensory integration. Genetic heritage, age, health, nutrition, environment, psychosocial factors, and medication act as influences on neurosensory integration. There are many alterations of neurosensory integration that act to disrupt neurosensory functions. Certain deficits and disabilities, catalogued in the preceding discussion, correspond to changes in consciousness, perception, memory and learning, thought, communication and movement. Such deficits interfere with self-care, independence, and collaboration. Trauma, tumors, infection, vascular lesions, and impaired neurosensory transmission are common causes of altered neurosensory integration.

Nurses are interested in neurosensory integration as it affects their clients' health. Nurses assess clients' neurosensory functions by conducting a thorough health history and health examination with emphasis on the subjective and objective manifestations of the neurosensory system and on the health of other body systems that contribute to maintaining neurosensory integration. Data collected clinically is correlated with the results of neurosensory diagnostic tests the client may undergo, and nursing diagnoses of the client's neurosensory status are derived.

Frequently, nurses find that their clients manifest some disturbance to neurosensory integration that requires nurse–client management. When the client's condition includes needs related to neurosensory functioning, there are a variety of implementations available to the nurse that may be useful, depending upon the nature and level of the client's need or problem. Most clients will have a need for preventive neurosensory care and will benefit from related health education and health screening. Many clients will also have a need for supportive care to assist them with common problems of sensory perception, including vision and hearing, mild to moderate pain, or communication difficulties. Preceding sections of this chapter have comprehensively reviewed a variety of approaches appropriate to the supportive care of clients with such problems.

Some clients will have a need for restorative care that addresses several problems of neurosensory integration such as coma, severe pain, and seizures. Preceding sections have also catalogued the fundamental approaches that are appropriate to caring for clients who require implementations to promote the restoration of neurosensory integration. Finally, some clients will have ongoing needs related to neurosensory integration that are exemplified by the client who experiences chronic pain. Ongoing medical treatment and alterations of the client's life activities are frequently required to cope with chronic pain. Rehabilitative care addresses the mediation of chronic problems through adjustments of life-style and life structural choices and through rehabilitative therapy. Collaboration in problems of neurosensory integration is sometimes limited by disruption to neurosensory function, but nevertheless is important not only to the assessment of the resulting problems, but also to the planning of implementations that are health enhancing.

REFERENCES

1. Rudy EB. *Advanced Neurological and Neurosurgical Nursing*. St. Louis: C.V. Mosby; 1984:81.
2. Sternbach R. *Pain: A Psychophysiological Analysis*. New York: Academic; 1963:12.
3. McCaffery M, Beebe A. *Clinical Manual for Nursing Practice*. St. Louis: C.V. Mosby; 1989.
4. Melzack R, Wall PB. Pain mechanisms: A new theory. *Science*. 1986;150:971.
5. Melzack R, Wall PB. *The Challenge of Pain*. New York: Basic Books; 1983:208–215.
6. Klatzky RL. *Human Memory*, 2nd ed. San Francisco: W.H. Freeman; 1980.
7. Anderson J. *The Architecture of Cognition*. Cambridge, MA: Harvard University Press; 1983:18.
8. Berne RM, Levy AN. *Physiology*, 2nd ed. St. Louis: C.V. Mosby; 1988.
9. Alkon DL. Memory storage and neural systems. *Sci Am*. 1989; 261(1):42–50.
10. Gagne R. *The Conditions of Learning*, 3rd ed. New York: Holt, Rinehart and Winston; 1977.
11. Bullock BL, Rosendahl PP. *Pathophysiology: Adaptations and Alterations in Function*, 2nd ed. Boston: Scott, Foresman/Little, Brown; 1988.
12. Ketovuori H. Nurses' and patients' conception of wound pain and the administration of analgesics. *J Pain Symptom Manage*. 1987;2(4):213–218.

13. Goldstein GW, Betz AL. The Blood-brain barrier. *Sci Am.* 1986; 255(3):74–83.
14. Manglass L, Flynn J-B McC. Ineffective coping requiring crisis intervention. In: Flynn J-B McC, Bruce NP, eds. *Introduction to Critical Care Nursing Skills.* St. Louis: C.V. Mosby; in press.
15. Ondra C, DeLoach P. Disturbance in sensory–perceptual integrity requiring intracranial pressure monitoring, seizure control, and skeletal traction. In: Flynn J-B McC, Bruce NP, eds. *Introduction to Critical Care Nursing Skills.* St. Louis: C.V. Mosby; in press.
16. Malasanos L, Barkauskas V, Moss M, Stoltenberg AK. *Health Assessment,* 4th ed. St. Louis: C.V. Mosby; 1991:213.
17. Hudspeth AJ. The hair cells of the inner ear. *Sci Am J.* 1983; 248:54–73.
18. Hickey JV. *The Clinical Practice of Neurological and Neurosurgical Nursing,* 2nd ed. Philadelphia: J.P. Lippincott; 1986:169–170.
19. Melzack R. McGill Pain Questionnaire: Major properties and scoring methods. *Pain.* 1:277–299.
20. Wilke DJ, Savedra MC, Holzemer WL, et al. Use of the McGill Pain Questionnaire to measure pain: A meta-analysis. *Nurs Res.* 1990;39(1):36–41.
21. Crosby L, Parsons LC. Clinical neurologic assessment tool: Development and testing of an instrument to index neurologic status. *Heart Lung.* 1989;18(2):121–128.
22. Hilton G. Review of neurobehavioral assessment tools. *Heart Lung.* 1991;20(5):436–442.
23. Roberts SL. *Nursing Diagnosis and the Critically Ill Patient.* Norwalk, CT: Appleton & Lange; 1987.
24. Manglass L, Flynn J-B McC. Ineffective coping. In: Flynn J-B McC, Bruce NP, eds. *Critical Care Nursing Skills.* St. Louis: C.V. Mosby; in press.
25. Flynn J-B McC. Sleep. In Flynn J-B McC, Heffron PB, eds. *Nursing: from Concept to Practice.* Norwalk, CT: Appleton & Lange; 1988.
26. Donovan MI. Acute pain relief. *Nurs Clin North Am.* 1990;25(4): 851–861.
27. Burkhardt CS. Chronic pain. *Nurs Clin North Am.* 1990;25(4).
28. Walding MF. Pain, anxiety and powerlessness, *J Adv Nurs.* 1991;16:388.
29. Sternbach RA. What is the most pressing problem we face today in the area of clinical pain management? *Am Pain Soc News.* 1988;11(4).
30. Allen MN. The meaning of visual impairment to visually impaired adults. *J Adv Nurs.* 1989;14:640–646.
31. Personal Communication. *Washington Hearing Aid Society.* October 9, 1991.
32. Kneisl CR, Ames SW. *Adult Health Nursing.* Reading, MA: Addison-Wesley; 1986:207.
33. Ketovuori H. Wound pain. *J Pain.* 1987;2(4):213–218.
34. Melzack R. The tragedy of needless pain. *Sci Am.* 1990;262(2): 27–33.
35. Holm K, Cohen F, Dudas S, et al. Effect of personal pain experience on pain assessment. *Image.* 1989;21(2):72–75.
36. Wallace KG, Hays J. Nursing management of chronic pain. *J Neurosurg Nurs.* August 1982;14(4):185–191.
37. Guzzetta CE. Effects of relaxation and music therapy on patients in a coronary care unit with presumptive acute myocardial infarction. *Heart Lung,* 1989;18(6):609–616.
38. Durham E, Frost-Hartzer P. Relaxation therapy works. *RN.* 1991; (8):40–43.
39. Varella L. Nutritional support and head trauma," *Crit Care Nurs.* 1989;9(6):28–34.
40. Hargreaves A, Lander J. Use of transcutaneous electrical nerve stimulation for post-operative pain. *Nurs Res.* 1989;38(3):159–161.
41. McGuire L. The power of non-narcotic pain relievers. *RN.* 1990; 54(4):28–36.
42. Ward LK, Pauli M, Serafin MB. Patient-controlled analgesia. *NITA.* 1987;10(1):34–39.
43. Gaysek SJ. IV team management of patient-controlled analgesia. *NITA.* 1987;10(2):142–144.
44. Pelin NJ. Intractable pain management with intravenous narcotic administration at home. *J IV Nurs.* 1990;12(4):228–232.
45. Chatupka S, Gillon-Allard B. When your patient has an epidural catheter. *RN.* 1989;52(12):70–77.
46. Ashburn MS, et al. Oral transmucosal fentanyl citrate for the treatment of breakthrough cancer pain. *Anesthesiology.* 1989; 71(10):615–617.

BIBLIOGRAPHY

Brady BA, Nesbitt SN. Using the right touch. *Nurs 91.* 1991;21(5): 46.

Bishop BS. Pathologic pupillary signs: Self-learning module, Part 3. *Crit Care Nurse.* 1991;11(8):30.

Cupp LA. The spectrum of suffering. *Am J Nurs.* 1990;90(8):35.

Dossey B. Awakening the inner healer. *Am J Nurs.* 1991;91(8):31.

Drummond BL. Preventing increased intracranial pressure: Nursing care can make the difference. *Focus Crit Care.* 1990;17(2):116.

Ferrell BR. Managing pain with long-acting morphine. *Nurs 91.* 1991;21(10):34.

Hall GR. The hospitalized patient has Alzheimer's. *Am J Nurs.* 1991;91(10):45.

Hilton G. Review of neurobehavioral assessment tools. *Heart Lung.* 1991;20(5):436.

Howie JN. Hypothermia and rewarming after cardiac operation. *Focus Crit Care.* 1991;18(5):414.

Kroeger LL. Critical care nurses' perceptions of the confused elderly patient. *Focus Crit Care.* 1991;18(5):395.

Lee ST. Intracranial pressure changes during positioning of patients with severe head injury. *Heart Lung.* 1989;18(4):411.

McCaffery M, Ferrell BR. Patient age. Does it affect your pain-control decisions? *Nurs 91.* 1991;21(9):44.

Morgan SP. A passage through paralysis. *Am J Nurs.* 1991;91(10):70.

Neundorfer MM. Coping and health outcomes in spouse caregivers of persons with dementia. *Nurs Res.* 1991;40(5):260.

Pace K, Emerich M. Keeping track of confused patients. *Nurs 90.* 1990;20(6):64.

Rasin JH. Confusion. *Nurs Clin North Am.* 1990;25(4):909.

Reimer M. Head-injured patients. How to detect early signs of trouble. *Nurs 89.* 1989;19(3):34.

Sisson R. Effects of auditory stimuli on comatose patients with head injury. *Heart Lung.* 1990;19(4):373.

Stewart-Amidei C. What to do until the neurosurgeon arrives. *J Emerg Nurs.* 1988;14(5):296.

Thelan LA, Davie JK, Urden LD, Kritek PB. *Textbook of Critical Care Nursing.* St. Louis: Mosby, 1990.

Watling SM. Continuously infused morphine. *Focus Crit Care.* 1991; 18(5):258.

CHAPTER 30

Mobility

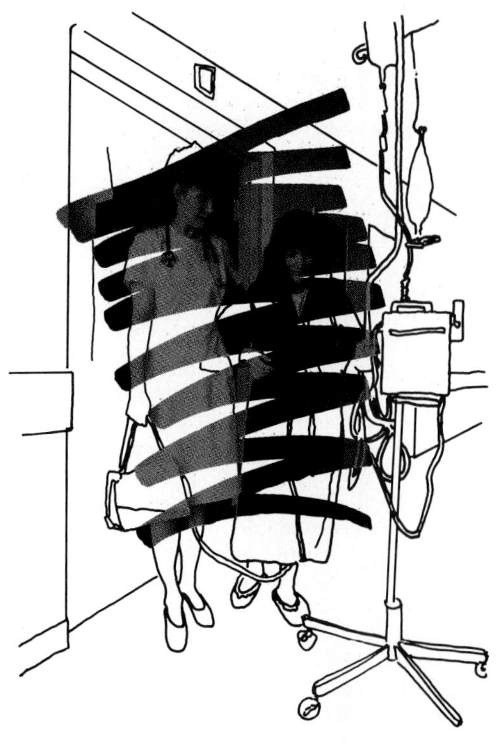

Behavioral Objectives

Upon completion of this chapter, the student will be able to:

1. Describe how each of the following affect mobility: musculoskeletal functioning, cardiopulmonary functioning, metabolic efficiency, and emotional status.
2. Briefly summarize the physiological response to increased muscular activity.
3. List and define the four components of fitness, and describe the type of activity required for optimum development of each component.
4. List at least six benefits of regular aerobic exercise and explain how exercise brings about these effects.
5. State two risks associated with exercise.
6. Describe how age, disability, general health, self-concept, and values affect mobility.
7. Describe at least three examples of problems in each of the following functional dimensions that result from decreased mobility: activity/mobility, rest/sleep, oxygenation, nutrition, fluid and elimination, sexuality, and psychological dimensions.
8. Describe essential elements of a mobility history.
9. Describe essential elements of a mobility examination.
10. Name three diagnostic tests useful in diagnosing mobility problems.
11. Define four nursing diagnoses that describe altered mobility.
12. Identify and explain at least two etiologies of each of the above diagnoses.
13. Describe at least three examples of preventive, supportive, restorative, and rehabilitative nursing implementation to promote, maintain, or enhance mobility.
14. List and explain seven basic guidelines for effective body mechanics.
15. Identify strategies to evaluate the effectiveness of client care related to mobility.
16. Discuss the relevance of a collaborative approach to client care related to mobility.
17. Write an individualized client care plan for a client experiencing mobility problems.

KEY TERMS

active range of motion
activities of daily living
aerobic exercise
anaerobic glycolysis
antagonist
dangling
disuse phenomenon
disuse syndrome
eggcrate mattress overlay
endurance
exercise tolerance
fitness
flexibility
footboard
hand roll
heel and elbow protectors
isokinetic exercise
isometric exercise
isotonic exercise
orthostatic (postural) hypotension
passive range of motion
pressure reduction device
pressure relief bed
prosthesis
strength
synergist
trochanter roll
valsalva maneuver

Human mobility is the movement of the body as a whole and the movement of body parts in relation to one another. The movement can be symbolic and elegant. The ancient oriental art of t'ai chi is a form of moving meditation that synthesizes the spiritual, intellectual, and physical aspects of the practitioner. Mobility in the form of dance reveals the human capacity for grace, which at times reaches a level of perfection that we laud as a form of art.

Although we tend to think of communication in terms of language, expression through the line and flow of body movement is a particularly direct and powerful form of human communication. The pristine purity of the ballet dancer and the exotic, sensual appeal of the belly dancer illustrate the contrast in symbolism possible through movement forms. Not all movement is poetic or beautiful, however, and in fact much of it is utilitarian and awkward, purely functional in nature, allowing us to accomplish the mundane activities of everyday life. This movement becomes precious to us when the capacity for mobility is interrupted and the same mundane activities become difficult or impossible.

That humans seem to have an innate need to move just for the sheer joy of it seems to be confirmed by the number of forms of movement that the public pursues as recreation. Hiking, jogging, skating, skiing, swimming, tennis, golf, and bowling, to name a few, are popular sports enjoyed by hundreds of thousands of individuals who actively participate in them. All are forms of movement and rely on the basic human capacity for mobility. These sports are pursued because people feel good doing them; humans need to move!

This need to move is so intrinsic, in fact, that we unconsciously express our inner experience and sometimes our innermost feelings with movements. We tap our toes to the beat of a tune, wrinkle our noses at an obnoxious odor, drum our fingers and pace across the floor when worried and upset. Thus, the physical aspects of movement have a deeper, psychological significance and our patterns of body movement are closely tied to our ability to establish and maintain a psychological equilibrium. Mobility is a part of the wellness of our person as well as our body.

The relationship of movement to wellness is complex. Scientific research documenting the importance of movement to physical health is vast and still mounting. Judging from the recent surge in the public's interest in physical fitness, public acceptance of exercise as necessary to physical well-being is a fact. Yet the physical integrity of body organs in turn is also essential for optimum mobility. Just as decreased physical activity can have a detrimental effect on organ function, the malfunction of one or more organs interferes with mobility. Thus, there is a physiological balance between organ function and body movement that determines the capacity for mobility.

There is also a balance between movement and psychological integrity that is related to one's level of self-esteem. Psychologically, we relate mobility to a sense of independence and power. To move one's body through space is liberating. To be unable to move, on the other hand, is profoundly frustrating and discouraging. Curtailment of movement is often associated with punishment. Parents discipline children by restricting activity. Criminals are punished by incarceration in a small cell. Governments refuse travel privileges to suspicious individuals.

The limitation of mobility may well be a fundamentally displeasurable human experience. When the capacity for movement is lost or diminished through illness, as it frequently is, discouragement is not only often evident, but can be severe. When the loss is temporary, we may adapt by patiently working toward a return of function. When it is permanent, the adaptation requires a change in self-concept, which can make extremely expensive demands on psychological energy. Grieving for the lost function—and the lost part of self—is not uncommon.

Considering that mobility is so important to human wellness and the quality of human life, and recognizing that disease is a common factor in mobility dysfunction, it is not surprising that nurses have a significant role in assisting clients with mobility problems. This chapter addresses optimum mobility, including physiological integration of mobility and fitness; factors that alter mobility and the effects of diminished mobility on other body functions; and nurse–client assessment and management of mobility.

Section 1. Understanding Mobility

OPTIMUM MOBILITY

Optimum mobility refers to the ability to willfully execute all of the many movements of which humans are capable. The concept suggests maintaining peak physiological functioning, for all body systems support mobility and are in one way or another affected by mobility or the lack of it. An understanding of the physiological integration of mobility and its exemplification in fitness, as well as an awareness of how to attain and maintain fitness, are basic to recognizing and supporting optimum mobility.

Physiological Integration of Mobility

Musculoskeletal, neurological, cardiorespiratory, and metabolic functioning underlie the physiological integration of mobility. Each has a distinctive role, yet all are interdependent.

Musculoskeletal Functioning. The skeleton provides a rigid framework for the body and protection for the major body organs. Bones afford maximum supportive strength with a minimum of weight because of their unique structure. Long bones are composed of a network of cancellous, lattice-like tissue. This tissue is porous, which makes it light, but the greater density at points of stress provides the durability required for weight bearing and activity.

Bones articulate in several types of joints, which facilitates a wide range of possible movements (Table 30–1).

IMPLICATIONS FOR NURSE–CLIENT COLLABORATION

The Meaning of Movement

The capacity to move has always been important to human survival and adaptation and, in today's complex society, is vital for accomplishing the tasks of daily living. The adaptive value of movement is accompanied by an expressive value. Humans seem to have an innate need to move just for the sheer joy of it. Movement is related to wellness and physical fitness, but just as importantly, to self-actualization. When the capacity to move is lost through illness, the adaptation may require many changes in the client's pattern of living. Preserving movement, regaining or enhancing it, or assisting clients in adapting to its loss, is a traditional and extremely important nursing responsibility. Working in partnership with the client to reach mobility outcomes addresses more than the function itself: It also promotes self-esteem and affirms the client's personal identity.

TABLE 30–1. TYPES OF JOINTS

Joint	Description	Movement
Ball and socket	Ball-shaped head fitting into a concave socket formed by another bone or bones. *Examples:* Shoulder, hip.	360 degrees: Flexion–extension, adduction–abduction, circumduction, hyperextension.
Hinge	One convex surface articulating with the concave surface of another bone or bones. *Examples:* Humerus/ulna at elbow, knee, finger, toe.	180 degrees: Flexion–extension in one plane only.
Pivot	Ring-shaped bony structure rotates on the rounded surface of another bone. *Examples:* Atlas, axis joints of spine, humerus/radius at elbow.	Rotation only.
Condyloid	Ovoid bony projection fits into elliptical cavity. *Examples:* Carpo/metacarpal, tarsal/metatarsal.	All movements except axial rotation.
Saddle	Convex–concave surface of one bone fits into concave–convex surface of another. *Examples:* Carpo/metacarpal at thumb.	Flexion, extension, circumduction, hyperextension abduction–adduction.
Gliding	Two flat/slightly curved bony surfaces articulate. *Examples:* Wrist, ankle, fibula/tibia, intervertebral.	Flexion–extension, hyperextension, rotation, adduction–abduction, circumduction.

Characteristically, joints are surrounded by ligaments, which provide stability and enclose the joint capsule. The capsule is lined with synovial membrane, which secretes synovial fluid to lubricate joint surfaces. The articulating bone surfaces are covered by cartilage for smoothness of movement over one another.

There are six distinct types of joints in the human skeleton, each capable of different kinds of movement. Table 30–1 lists and describes each type and identifies the movements that are possible. The movements are defined in Box 30–1.

The muscles directly responsible for movement are the skeletal or striated muscles. Each is composed of many contractile fibers bound together by connective tissue called fascia. The fascia attaches the muscle to bone by forming a tendon that fuses to the periosteum. Tendons are relatively inelastic tissue with high tensile strength, which makes them resistant to injury.

BOX 30–1. DEFINITIONS OF JOINT MOVEMENT

Movement	Definition
Flexion	Bending, reducing the angle at a joint.
Extension	Straightening, increasing the angle at a joint.
Hyperextension	Movement beyond normal joint alignment.
Abduction	Movement of a body part away from the midline.
Adduction	Movement of a body part toward the midline.
Rotation	Turning in a medial or lateral direction, pivoting on an axis.
Supination	Turning the palm of the hand upward.
Pronation	Turning the palm of the hand downward.
Inversion	Turning the sole of the foot inward.
Eversion	Turning the sole of the foot outward.
Circumduction	Movement of a body part so its distal portion describes a circle.

The arrangement of muscle fibers affects function. When maximum flexibility is required, the muscle fibers are parallel, arranged in spindles with a tendon at each end (Fig. 30–1A). This is called fusiform arrangement. The biceps and triceps brachii are examples of fusiform muscles. A pennate arrangement occurs when power is necessary (Fig. 30–1B). The muscle fibers are short and at an angle to the tendon, which is on one side. The vastus lateralis and vastus medialis are pennate muscles. An even stronger muscle results with the bipennate form (Fig. 30–1C). Here, the fibers are placed at an angle on either side of a central tendon. The gain in power due to the greater number of fibers results in a loss of range of motion compared to the fusiform type. Examples of bipennate muscles are the deltoid, the rectus femoris in the thigh, and the gastrocnemius in the calf.

When a muscle contracts, it shortens in length. One end, called the origin, remains relatively stable during the contraction, while the other end, the insertion, moves toward the origin. The shortening of the muscle results from structural rearrangement of the muscle proteins, actin and myosin in the myofibrils, the fine elements making up the muscle fiber. Figure 30–2 illustrates the structural arrangement. The actin and myosin lie entwined around one another in the myofibrils.

Myosin has been determined to be an enzyme that splits adenosine triphosphate (ATP), the compound in which a muscle's energy is stored. When the muscle is relaxed, myosin is inactive because of the presence of inhibitors. When a muscle is stimulated by impulses from the nervous system, calcium is released from muscle cells and surrounds the myofibrils. Calcium initiates the contraction process. The myosin inhibitors are temporarily bound and myosin splits ATP, liberating energy that moves the central

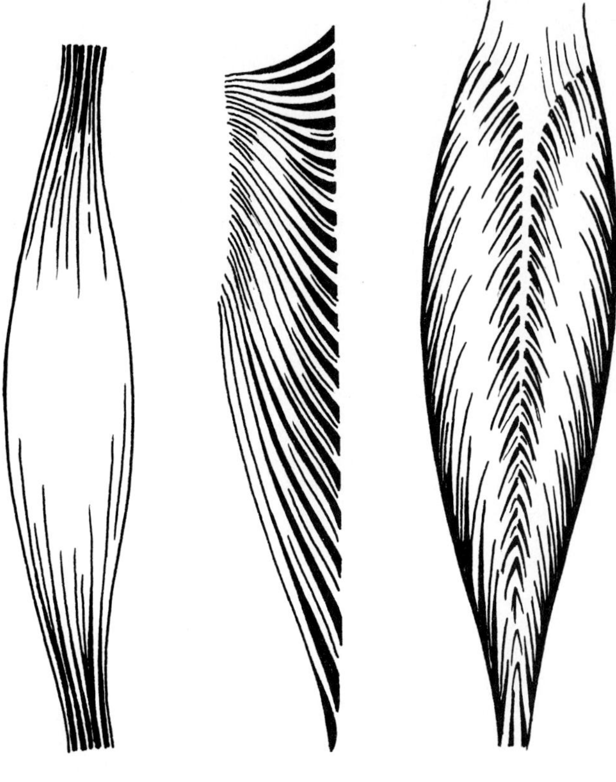

Figure 30–1. Varied muscle fiber arrangements: fusiform, pennate, bipennate.

ends of the actin filaments toward each other until they meet. This reduces the length of the muscle. Further contraction requires actual shortening of the actin fibers. If their length is reduced so much that the myosin fibers reach the Z bands, the myosin crumples. The structural changes that accompany contraction are illustrated in Figure 30–2.

During the recovery phase, the high-energy bonds are resynthesized. Without adequate oxygen for the recovery phase, ATP cannot be resynthesized and fatigue ensues. Normally, the energy to sustain muscular contraction comes from the oxidation of glycogen stored in the muscle. When muscular work is prolonged, liver glycogen and, ultimately, fat are metabolized for fuel.

Movement is the result of coordinated muscle activity. When two or more muscles interact together to accomplish a given movement, they are called **synergists.** The biceps brachii and the brachialis, which flex the elbow, are among many synergistic muscles in the body. Another type of coordination is required between muscles whose contraction results in opposite movements of the same body part. These muscle pairs, called **antagonists,** must contract and relax reciprocally for movement to be accomplished. For example, the triceps brachii, which extends the forearm at the elbow, must relax when the elbow is flexed by the biceps. During extension, the triceps contracts while the biceps relaxes. This complexity of function is controlled by the central nervous system, which plays a significant role in all movement.

Neuromuscular Integration. Many complex cerebral mechanisms underlie voluntary movement. Automatic responses (reflexes) are controlled by the reflex arc involving spinal neurons. Complete mobility depends upon CNS integration of both reflex and voluntary movement.

The cerebrum is responsible for imitating all purposeful movement. The motor cortex plays a key role, but the motor planning necessary to perform complex tasks originates in the premotor area. Sensory input is also needed. When afferent (sensory) fibers are eliminated, voluntary movements cease even though efferent (motor) fibers are intact. The sensory information comes from visual stimulation and from proprioceptors (receptors that respond to stimuli originating within the body, eg, stretch, position) located in the semicircular canals of the inner ear and in muscle spindles, tendons, and joints (Fig. 30–3). Once received, this information is interpreted by the higher centers in the brain to facilitate intentional coordinated movement. The cerebellum has an important role in this process. It receives proprioceptive signals and influences the amount of neural activity in the motor cortex. When the afferent signals have been interpreted by the cerebellum and the

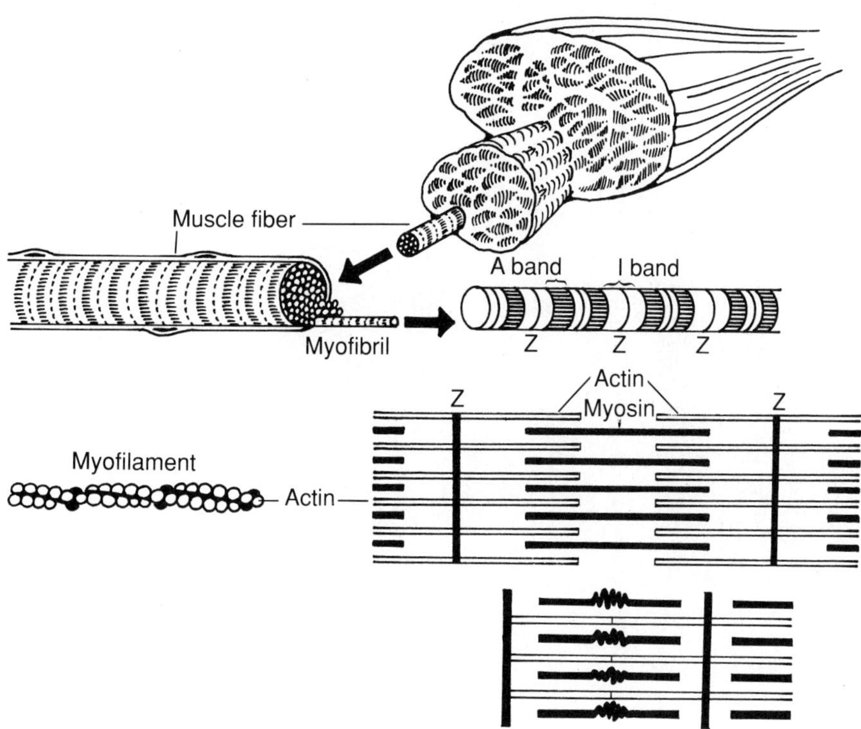

Figure 30–2. Structure of skeletal muscle.

premotor cortex, efferent impulses from the motor cortex travel down the pyramidal tract to the brainstem, cross to the opposite side, and then synapse with lower motor neurons in the ventral horn of the spinal cord. Each motor neuron sends an axon to a skeletal muscle, where it divides to innervate single muscle fibers. When the electrical impulse crosses the motor end plate, contraction results. Separate motor fibers carry inhibitory impulses that result in relaxation. The nerve cell with its associated branches and muscle fibers is called a motor unit. The average skeletal muscle has approximately 300 motor units. Because most of the efferent fibers cross in the area of the brainstem, the muscular activity on one side of the body is governed by the cortex on the opposite side. For this reason, a brain injury affecting the motor cortex of the left cerebral hemisphere interferes with movement on the right side of the body. This complex integration of brain, nerve, and muscle activity is necessary for all intentional movement.

Another category of movement, reflexes, are also essential for normal mobility. The reflex arc (Fig. 30–4) is composed of afferent and efferent neurons with interneurons between them in most cases. These interneurons are located in the spinal cord. No cortical interpretation or integration occurs in reflex movement. Because the response is automatic, it is predictable. A stimulus exciting a particular type of receptor will result in an invariable response. A familiar example is the withdrawal of a body part from a painful stimulus. Reflexes are also responsible for the maintenance of positive muscle tone. Reflexes undergo developmental changes; some disappearing with growth, others emerging. Pathological conditions affecting the nervous or muscular system alter reflexes, causing sluggish responses, brisk responses, or a return of infantile reflexes. For this reason, testing of reflexes is part of the nursing and medical assessment of motor functioning.

Cardiovascular–Respiratory Functioning. One of the most immediate needs of an exercising muscle is an increase in blood circulation. It is an essential phenomenon, for muscle contractions cannot be sustained for a significant length of time without it. The increased circulation accomplishes several important things. First, oxygen and metabolic fuel are supplied to provide energy for the contraction. Waste products—carbon dioxide and lactic acid—are removed. If these accumulated, muscle function would be impaired. Finally, the heat produced by the working muscles is dissipated by the increased circulation.

The cardiopulmonary system must be able to accomplish a series of steps when increased demands are made on it to supply oxygen to the muscles. First, environmental air must be inspired and mixed with lung gases. This occurs with the contraction of the respiratory muscles. It is important that the inspired air be sufficient in amount and be uniformly distributed to the alveoli, where oxygen enters capillary blood and carbon dioxide is retrieved. This diffusion of oxygen and carbon dioxide comprises the second step. Competent pulmonary circulation, adequate lung surface area to which the blood can be exposed, and sufficient

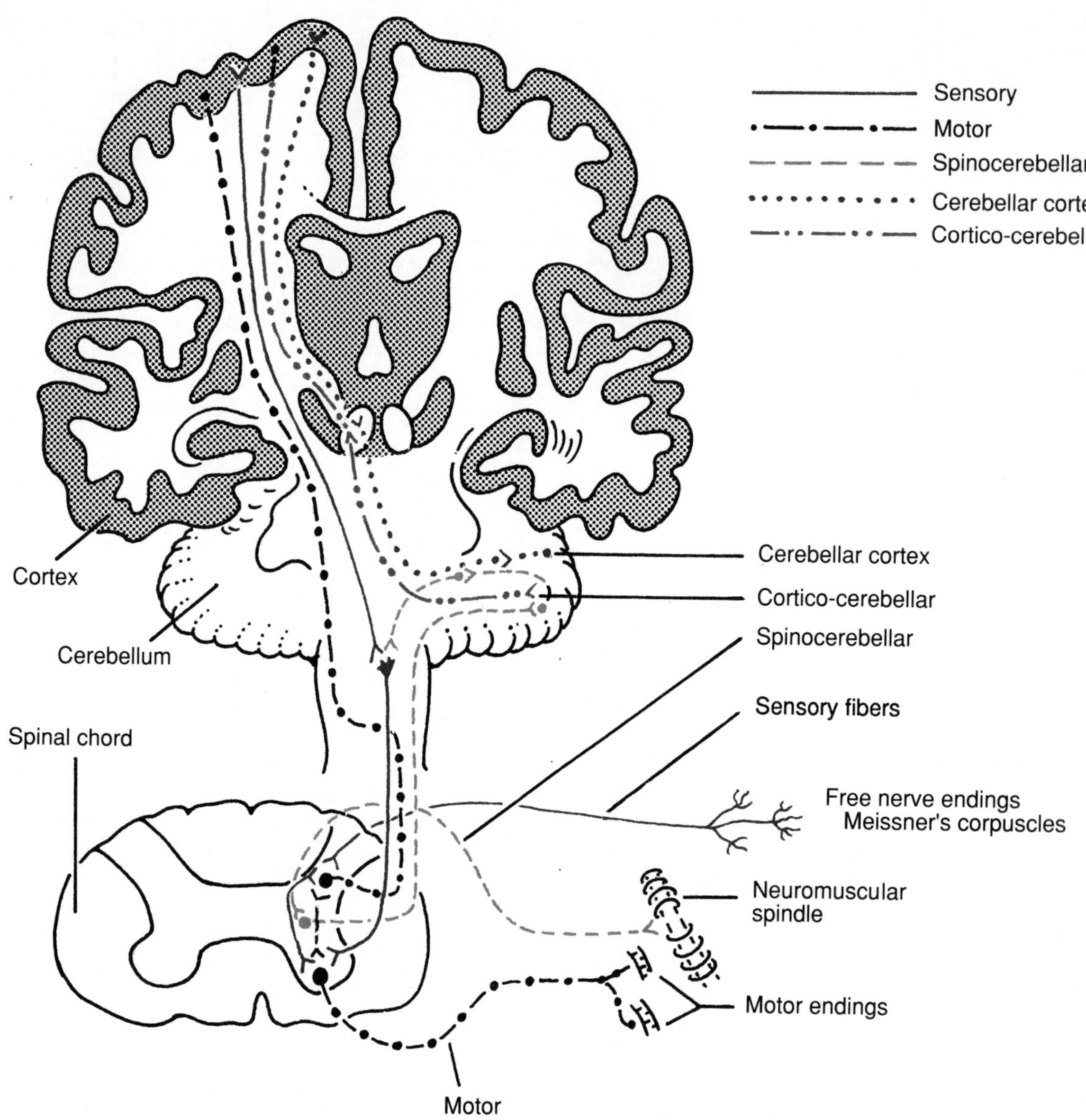

Figure 30–3. Neurological pathways controlling voluntary movement.

hemoglobin to carry the oxygen are necessary for optimum diffusion to occur.

The third step involves expanding the supply of oxygen-rich blood to the exercising muscles. Vasodilation in muscles, corresponding vasoconstriction in other organs, and a rise in cardiac output brings this about. The elevated cardiac output is accomplished by accelerated heart rate and greater stroke volume. Venous return is enhanced by muscular contraction. Sympathetic stimulation causes stronger ventricular contraction, and therefore, more blood is ejected from the heart with each beat.

The fourth step again involves diffusion, this time between blood and muscle tissue. It is believed that this process is facilitated by the contraction of the muscle. The final step requires the ability of the muscle to use the oxygen it has received. The key to this step is the proper functioning of the complex enzyme systems that bring about the breaking and reforming of the high-energy bonds in the muscle cells, discussed previously. It is only when all of these physiological processes are carried out effectively that an individual can exercise at high levels of energy expenditure for a significant length of time.

Metabolism. Physical activity requires energy, which is usually derived from oxidation of foods. Although the amount of food ingested affects performance, effective di-

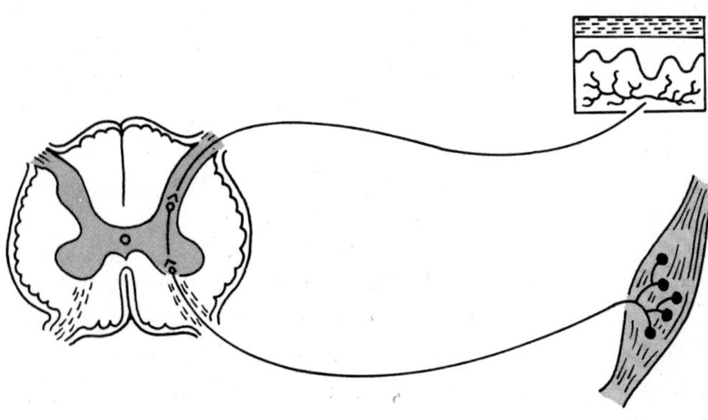

Figure 30–4. Reflex arc.

gestion, absorption, and excretion of wastes is critical for maintaining sufficient energy stores to support optimum mobility.

The stress of muscular work causes an increase in the production of adrenocortical hormones. These hormones stimulate the release of liver glycogen for use as metabolic fuel. The resulting rise in blood sugar levels is sustained until glycogen stores are exhausted. When blood sugar falls as a result of depletion of liver glycogen, symptoms of fatigue ensue. If continuing demands on the body are made, fat is oxidized to supply fuel for muscular work. These processes normally are aerobic and require a continuous supply of oxygen.

If the supply of oxygen is inadequate to allow oxidation of available glycogen, **anaerobic glycolysis** occurs. Although anaerobic breakdown of glycogen is a relatively quick source of energy, its end-product is lactic acid. When lactic acid accumulates in muscles, local fatigue ensues. The aerobic process is considerably more efficient. It produces almost 20 times more ATP than a comparable amount of anaerobic metabolism; it can use carbohydrate, fat, or protein as energy sources; and it avoids the fatiguing by-products. To use aerobic metabolic pathways for intense and prolonged activity, however, cardiorespiratory function must be optimum.

The heat produced by muscular work must be dissipated to prevent serious hyperthermia. This is accomplished chiefly by vasodilation and the production of perspiration. Considerable amounts of water and sodium can be lost in this way.

Kidney function is affected by these metabolic changes. Less urine is produced. This is due partly to increased tubular reabsorption of water to compensate for losses via perspiration and partly to a decrease in glomerular filtration rate because of decreased renal blood flow. The kidney is one of the organs from which blood is shunted to increase circulation to the muscles. The metabolic changes described above are reflected in the urine produced during exercise. It is more acidic due to higher lactic acid levels in the blood. Glucose may be present because the blood glucose concentration may increase faster than the tubules can reabsorb it. Sodium and chloride levels decrease, which partly compensates for increased losses via the skin.

The rate of metabolic processes is increased by exercise. More activity requires more energy. When overall exercise is increased without a corresponding increase in intake of nutrients, the additional energy required is obtained from body stores of adipose tissue. This state, in which energy expenditure exceeds energy (caloric) intake, is referred to as negative energy balance. It is a desirable state for a person who is overweight. However, it may also occur during illness, often interfering with recovery. When total caloric expenditure is equalled by caloric intake, a state of energy balance exists. This could be considered the ideal state for a healthy person. Positive energy balance occurs when more calories are ingested than are expended. This is the basic cause of obesity. A more detailed discussion of metabolism and digestion may be found in Chapter 25.

Body Response to Increased Muscular Activity. Any activity increases metabolism above the basal level. Movement that is part of activities of daily living does not usually cause noticeable change in bodily functioning, although homeostatic adjustments continually occur. When greater demands are made, the physiological responses are more dramatic.

The cardiovascular changes discussed above result in an acceleration in heart rate and increased systolic blood pressure. Ordinarily, the diastolic pressure does not increase, although if arteries have diminished elasticity secondary to arteriosclerosis, or if exercise is excessively vigorous, there may also be a rise in diastolic pressure.

A corresponding elevation in rate and depth of respiration occurs. A resting ventilatory rate of 6 liters per minute may increase to as much as 100 liters per minute if activity is strenuous. As the depth of breathing approaches the vital capacity, a sensation of being out of breath or "winded" is noted. The increased respiratory effort also gives rise to a stabbing pain in the side, commonly called a "stitch." This may be due to exhaustion of accessory respiratory muscles or to spasms of the diaphragm.

Increased demand for oxygen and nutrients in the muscles causes shunting of blood to the muscles and away from other organs. As a result, activity in organs of the digestive tract and kidneys is slowed. Intake of food or large amounts of fluid during or immediately before exercise is therefore not advisable. The presence of food in the stomach stimulates increased blood flow to the digestive organs, creating conflicting demands for circulatory and metabolic resources. The result can be nausea and sluggish muscular response.

Generalized warmth and increased perspiration result from the exertion. As vessels in the skin dilate to facilitate heat loss, flushing occurs. A sensation of fatigue will eventually be noted due to depletion of liver glycogen and accumulation of lactic acid in the muscles. The time of onset and degree of all of these responses is related to the strenuousness of the exercise and the level of conditioning of the individual. As will be seen in the next section, conditioning greatly increases one's capacity to engage in strenuous activity.

Fitness

The term physical fitness is frequently used to describe a state in which body systems functions optimally. **Fitness** is the ability to sustain vigorous physical exertion without overtaxing cardiopulmonary or muscular capacity. Many Americans are becoming involved in activities to improve their level of fitness (Fig. 30–5). Health spas and fitness centers have become a part of many neighborhoods.

It is estimated that 50 percent of adult Americans participate in some form of regular exercise, but many have no concept of what constitutes a safe and effective fitness program.[1] In recognition of the value of exercise to health, 11 of the 1990 health objectives for the United States addressed physical fitness and exercise.[2] The general thrust of the goals was greater awareness among adults of the duration and type of exercise necessary to promote cardiovascular fitness, and greater percentages of children, adolescents, and adults participating in that level of exercise on a regular basis.

In a summary of progress toward these goals through 1988, however, the US Public Health Service determined that only one goal had been met, and five were unlikely to be met. There were insufficient data available to predict achievement of the others. The only goal met related to increasing the number of companies offering employer-sponsored fitness programs. None of the goals for exercise awareness or exercise participation at the recommended level were predicted to be met.

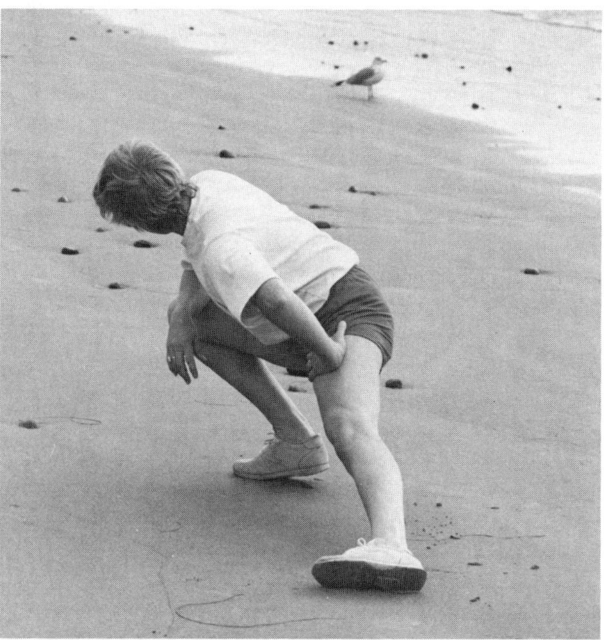

Figure 30–5. Stretching is an important element in an exercise program.

The 1990 goals recommended that exercise involving large muscle groups in dynamic contractions at a level of intensity that requires 60 percent or more of cardiorespiratory capacity be done at least three times per week in sessions lasting at least 20 minutes.[2] This was based on the belief that maximal fitness is necessary to reap the benefits of exercise.

There is growing evidence that regular exercise at lower levels than this also provides benefits.[3–5] For this reason, United States health objectives for the year 2000 address benefits from light- and moderate-intensity exercise and encourage greater participation at moderate as well as at vigorous levels. There is also greater emphasis on health care providers incorporating assessment and counseling regarding optimum physical activity into routine care.[6]

What is clear from these data is that more people need information about the benefits of exercise as well as encouragement to participate in exercise. Nurses have many opportunities to educate clients about fitness. Information about the components of fitness, the benefits of fitness, and types of exercise programs can be part of health teaching. Many people assume that fitness programs are unpleasant, strenuous, even boring. Emphasis on the variety of fitness programs and on social and recreational aspects of fitness can help to change these perceptions and attitudes.

Components of Fitness. Fitness has four components: body composition, strength, flexibility, and endurance. Different sorts of activity promote attainment of each component.

Body Composition. Body composition refers to maintaining a healthy body weight. It is impossible to be really fit if one is grossly overweight or underweight. Individuals who are physically fit have a lower percentage of body fat and greater lean body mass (body weight minus fat content) than individuals who are not. Height–weight tables are available that describe a healthy weight range for persons of both sexes of varying age and body build (see Chap. 25).

The concept of energy balance, discussed previously, is relevant here. People who maintain this state will remain at a stable weight. Overweight individuals should strive for a negative energy balance, one in which energy expenditure exceeds energy (caloric) intake, and underweight individuals should aim for the converse. A balanced diet is critical to achieving a healthy energy balance. Refer to Chapter 25 for more information about diet and nutrition.

Strength. **Strength** refers to force or power exerted by a muscle or group of muscles against resistance. Development of strength requires contraction of muscles in resistive exercises. Several types of exercises are effective for building strength. **Isotonic exercises,** such as lifting free weights, are exercises in which the tension within the muscle remains constant as its length changes to move the resistance (weight) through a range of motion. **Isokinetic exercise** maintains maximal tension on a muscle through full range of motion using computerized exercise equipment. **Isometric exercise** involves near-maximal contraction against a fixed object. The length of the muscle does not change, because there is no joint movement during the contraction. Strength training results in hypertrophy of individual muscle fibers, increases the number of active muscle fibers, and decreases the amount of fat within a muscle.[7,8]

Flexibility. The development of flexibility, by contrast, requires joint movement. The amount of movement possible at a given joint defines **flexibility.** Stretching, yoga, and calisthenics increase joint range of motion. Isokinetic exercise equipment can increase both flexibility and strength.

Endurance. **Endurance** pertains to a person's ability to persist in the performance of an activity without becoming fatigued. Endurance incorporates cardiorespiratory efficiency and muscular efficiency. It requires whole-body **aerobic exercise,** exercise that causes a sustained increase in heart rate and stroke volume. Activities such as jogging or swimming, and games such as basketball, which provide continuous cardiorespiratory demand, contribute to endurance. Isokinetic endurance training programs also are effective.[7] Aerobic activities lead to improved oxygen use by muscles, increased vascularity in cardiac and striated muscle, increased oxidation of fat for energy, and more effective aerobic metabolism of ATP.[7,8]

BOX 30–2. CRITERIA FOR EFFECTIVE EXERCISE

Mode

Large-muscle aerobic activity involving rhythmic repetitive motion. Examples: swimming, walking, cycling, rowing, jogging.

Intensity

60 to 90% of maximal heart rate.

Frequency

Minimum of three times per week, up to five times per week. Training more than five days a week may increase risk for injury and provides no additional improvement for most people.

Duration

Continuous activity for a minimum of 20 minutes, up to 60 minutes; lower-intensity exercise should be performed for longer time periods.

Benefits of Regular Exercise. Regular consistent aerobic exercise results in beneficial adaptations that contribute to overall well-being. Aerobic exercise increases the body's oxygen consumption for a sustained period of time. Sprinting, which immediately depletes the cardiorespiratory reserve, is not aerobic. Aerobic exercise increases heart rate significantly, but to a level that can be sustained for 5 minutes or more.

Although light and moderate exercise are beneficial, for maximal benefits certain criteria related to mode, intensity, frequency, and duration of exercise must be met.[2,8–11] Box 30–2 defines intensity of exercise in terms of a percentage of maximal heart rate (HRmax). Although the preferred method of determining one's HRmax is a graded exercise test,[5] it can be estimated by subtracting one's age from 220.[11,12] The training rate is then computed by multiplying the desired percentage at which one wishes to train times HRmax. Sedentary individuals beginning an exercise program should start at the lowest recommended level (60 percent HRmax) and gradually increase their target heart rate.

Individuals adhering to the guidelines in Box 30–2 can expect the following benefits:

1. Greater cardiac efficiency.[8,11–13] This is characterized by a lower resting heart rate and blood pressure, a smaller increase in heart rate with moderate activity, greater tolerance for near-maximum heart rate before fatigue onset, and a faster return to baseline heart rate and blood pressure after activity. These changes occur because stroke volume and therefore cardiac output increase due to regular exercise.
2. Improved pulmonary functioning,[8,11–13] including expansion of vital capacity, diminished "dead space," and increased maximal oxygen uptake. Well-conditioned individuals maximize the amount of oxygen they can take in during exhaustive exercise. Because of more efficient oxygen use, however (see numbers 3 and 5), their respiratory rate and depth do not increase significantly during moderate exercise.
3. Improved circulation throughout the body.[8,10] Aerobic demand during exercise multiplies capillaries in striated muscles.[7] More hemoglobin and red blood cells are produced to carry oxygen. Peripheral resistance lessens due to improved vascular tone. Fibrinolysin is produced in greater quantities, which diminishes the likelihood of pathological clotting.[8,11] These changes contribute to better delivery of oxygen and nutrients to body tissues as well as greater efficiency of waste elimination and heat dissipation.
4. Improved neuromuscular coordination.[14] Unnecessary movements are progressively eliminated and more complete relaxation of antagonists is achieved. Motions become simpler and more automatic. Training can therefore reduce the necessary energy expenditure to perform a particular skill.
5. Improved muscle tone and strength.[7,8,11] Conditioned people can produce more powerful contractions, repeat contractions more rapidly, and sustain activity for a longer period of time than before conditioning. Although the greater number of capillaries improves delivery of oxygen and metabolic fuel to muscles, studies have shown that conditioning also results in greater mechanical efficiency. That is, oxygen is taken up by muscles more rapidly, and for a given amount of work, less oxygen is consumed.[12,13] Furthermore, glycogen, ATP, and phosphocreatine are stored in larger amounts in the muscles themselves, and fatty acids are more efficiently used for energy during exercise, sparing glycogen.[7,8,12]

6. Increased bone density.[2,8,11] Weight-bearing, particularly against gravity, stimulates bone hypertrophy. Exercise transmits forces to bones, maintaining and even increasing bone strength. Bone mineral content is also increased with regular exercise.[12] Because of these factors, athletes have a greater bone mass than sedentary individuals. Postmenopausal women, at increased risk for osteoporosis, can reduce their risk for pathological fractures by exercising regularly.
7. Altered digestion and metabolism. Gastrointestinal motility is generally improved. Carbohydrate use is more efficient.[9] Alterations in fat metabolism result in lower serum levels of triglycerides and higher serum levels of HDL (high density lipoproteins), both of which are positive factors in the prevention of plaque deposits inside arteries (atherosclerosis).
8. Enhanced elimination of metabolic wastes. Lung and skin excretion increases.[8] Improved intestinal motility contributes to elimination of solid wastes. Circulatory efficiency reduces the amount of shunting to muscles; hence, kidney circulation can be maintained at more optimal levels, even during exercise. This facilitates excretion of urinary wastes.
9. Achievement and maintenance of appropriate body weight.[2,8,11] People who exercise regularly are most likely to remain in energy balance at a healthful weight. There is an increase in lean body mass and a reduction in body fat.[13] In contrast, a prolonged state of positive energy balance—a greater intake than expenditure of calories—produces obesity. The more energy expended through exercise, the higher can be the energy intake without risking obesity. Increasing activity is a health-promoting way for an overweight person to shift to a negative energy balance. Attempts to lose weight by reducing intake without increasing activity often fail and may rob individuals of essential nutrients.
10. Enhanced psychological well-being.[11,15] Endorphins, opium-like substances produced by the brain, are released in greater amounts during exercise in physically fit individuals.[8,14,15] Endorphins increase the pain threshold and produce a feeling of euphoria, sometimes called "the runner's high" because it was first identified in long-distance runners. Because regular exercise generally improves appearance, a more positive self-image results.[11,15–18] Regular physical activity reduces the prevalence and incidence of anxiety and depressive symptoms.[11,15,18–20] Maintaining an exercise program requires self-discipline and results in improved coordination, both of which contribute to self-esteem. Many people find exercise fun and diversionary, which in itself is valuable. Exercise also provides a satisfactory and nonthreatening outlet for expression of emotions, thus reducing stress levels.[15,18,20] Resting levels of catecholamines are lower after establishing a habit of regular exercise. Moreover, the levels of these hormones rise more slowly during exercise and during the alarm stage of stress in physically fit individuals.[18] Emotional or physical stress ordinarily results in the release of large amounts of catecholamines, with potentially pathogenic effects. Chapter 6 discusses the body's response to stress in greater detail.
11. Improved cognitive functioning. Several studies show a high correlation between exercise and improved cognitive function.[14,15,18] Appenzeller reports improved academic achievement in children after sustained programs for endurance training.[14] Several studies on elderly individuals showed significant improvement on cognitive tests in groups participating in exercise programs, while control groups who did not exercise did not show improvement.[18] Numerous studies on middle-aged adults report similar findings.[15]

Individuals can achieve these all-encompassing benefits by a commitment to a lifetime habit of regular exercise. It is the responsibility of nurses to teach all clients the benefits of regular, prudent exercise. Our credibility as teachers will be greater if we demonstrate at least a moderate level of fitness ourselves.

Risks Associated with Exercise. Despite all of the advantages and benefits associated with a life-style that includes regular exercise, physical training is not without risk. This is true for those participating at a recreational level as well as for elite athletes. Most exercise-related risks are associated with incorrect performance or inappropriate intensity of exercise for an individual's level of fitness. These injuries, although temporarily disabling, are not usually serious or life-threatening. The potential effects of exercise on those at risk for cardiovascular or other diseases is of greater concern, however.[21]

Apparently healthy active exercise participants under the age of 35, competitive athletes, children, and adolescents are currently considered to have no major risk factors that would prevent exercise participation.[22] These individuals need to use reasonable care, but with appropriate training technique are able to avoid significant injury. Sedentary individuals or recreational exercisers over 45 years old, and those of any age with symptoms of or known risk factors for liver, thyroid, or renal disease or diabetes, may risk complications associated with exercise and should undergo health assessment prior to beginning an exercise program. Those at highest risk include individuals with a known pulmonary, metabolic, or cardiovascular disease. These individuals not only require pre-exercise screening but should undergo periodic assessments as well. This latter group, in particular those with cardiovascular disease, is at the highest risk for sudden cardiac death related to exercise.[23] Despite substantial evidence that exercise training is beneficial for individuals with coronary artery disease and is likely to extend their life expectancy, careful screening and lower-intensity exercise is strongly suggested.[21,23]

Other risks associated with exercise that everyone who exercises regularly should consider include musculoskeletal injuries, psychological consequences, and trauma related to extremes of environmental temperature.

Musculoskeletal Injuries. There are two basic types of exercise-related musculoskeletal injuries: acute injuries and overuse injuries. Both should be distinguished from minor aches and pains associated with deliberately using muscles to increase their strength and endurance. The latter are manifested by stiffness after exercise and ischemic pain—the ache associated with a muscle having insufficient oxygen to continue work, but that stops when the exertion ceases—such as is common when extending the limits of ones' workouts. Accumulation of lactic acid or phosphate in muscles may contribute to this pain.[14] By contrast, an exercise-related injury causes actual tissue damage.

Strains and sprains are the most common types of acute injuries related to exercise. They are most common in "weekend" athletes whose exercises most often occurs in bursts and without the benefit of warming up. Strains or "pulls" are injuries to muscles or tendon attachments. They occur when a muscle is vigorously overstretched, such as when forcefully throwing a ball, stroking a tennis racket, or lifting a heavy object. Depending on the number of muscle fibers involved, the injury may be mild to severe. Sprains involve ligaments and joint capsules. They most often occur with rapid changes of direction or sudden starts and stops. Sprains are usually more severe than strains. Bone fractures can also occur as a result of exercise, but are less common.

Overuse injuries develop gradually from a repetitive activity. They are most common among individuals who regularly perform the same types of exercise, such as running.[24] Often overuse injuries have no obvious cause. They are the result of gradual microscopic injuries due to pushing beyond the body's ability to absorb the force of exercise. If exercise is continued despite the injury, the damage is extended and an acute injury at the site of the weakness is likely.[24] Tendinitis (inflammation of a tendon) and stress fractures are examples of overuse injuries.

Negative Psychologic Consequences. Some people for whom regular exercise is a major life-style component experience exercise addiction, characterized by feelings of irritability, restlessness, and fatigue when unable to exercise.[1,14,15] Tolerance, the need to constantly increase the amount one exercises in order to feel good about oneself, is another characteristic of this condition. Experts are divided on whether the symptoms are principally related to other psychological events in one's life so that exercise becomes an escape, are a result of obsessive traits that drive other behaviors as well as exercise behaviors, or have other origins. Research has identified no risk factors for this condition. Individuals experiencing any of the symptoms suggestive of exercise addiction listed above generally benefit from counseling to identify potential stressors and assist in modifying responses. It is worth noting that the concept of positive addiction has also been applied to exercise. In this concept the enhanced well-being that regular exercisers derive provides continued motivation to participate in exercise, but does not generate symptoms of tolerance and withdrawal described above.

Trauma Related to Extremes of Temperature. Because exercise generates heat, efficient heat dissipation is necessary to maintain normal body temperature during strenuous exercise. Endurance training improves the ability to disperse heat via cutaneous vasodilation and increased perspiration while still maintaining adequate circulation to muscles.[25] Exercise in hot, humid weather makes efficient cooling more difficult, even for well-conditioned individuals, and is especially stressful for those who are less fit. Profuse perspiration leading to dehydration is likely.[1] More serious heat effects such as heat exhaustion and heat stroke (see Chap. 22) occur if exercise continues.

Hypothermia and frostbite can be a consequence of exercise in cold environments. They are more likely if protective clothing becomes wet and when wearing insufficient protective clothing. Prolonged exercise with little fluid intake leads to dehydration and increases the risk of hypothermia, even at relatively mild temperatures.[25] Hypothermia is discussed further in Chapter 22.

■ FACTORS AFFECTING MOBILITY

Because mobility is to a large degree under voluntary control, individuals' level of mobility is largely influenced by personal choices. Although physiological limitations and psychological attributes play a role, these can often be overcome or altered by determined efforts. Physiological factors that may limit mobility include age, disability, and health status. Self-concept, emotions, and motivation also play a role. Values and beliefs, including one's personal definition of health and life-style, are choices that influence mobility.

Age

Mobility develops rapidly during the infant and toddler periods, and is refined and expanded throughout childhood and adolescence. Strength, endurance, and coordination continue to increase throughout adolescence and into young adulthood. With efforts to maximize these attributes, gains can continue into middle adulthood and levels can be maintained into late adulthood. However, age-related changes ultimately create a constraining influence.[11] Muscle strength peaks at age 30 and declines thereafter.[26] This loss is related to a decrease in the size of muscle fibers and in the number of mitochondria and is also influenced by altered hormonal and metabolic function. Changes in the hormonal regulation of calcium metabolism play a major role in deteriorating muscle activity.[27] Neurological alterations including slowed conduction velocity and diminished amounts of neurotransmitter substances contribute as well. Joint changes interfere with mobility as individuals age. Cartilage thickens and its surface roughens due to the stress of long-term use. This causes joint irritation and risk for osteoarthritis. Bones lose density and strength and develop bone spurs, which increases the tendency for joint irritation.

Aging also affects cardiovascular and respiratory fitness.[11,28] The resting stroke volume falls gradually from ages 25 to 85, the maximum attainable heart rate falls, resting and exercise blood pressure rises due to loss of elasticity in major blood vessels, lung vital capacity decreases, and the length of time necessary for heart rate, blood pressure, and oxygen consumption to return to baseline after exercise is longer.[28]

The timing of all of these changes is highly variable. An active life-style and good general health can delay both their onset and progression, as well as reverse some age-related changes.[28] In fact some researchers believe that disuse or inactivity accounts for half of the decline in function generally associated with aging.[11]

Disability

Disability refers to restrictions in ability to perform usual activities expected for a given age. Congenital abnormalities, trauma, or disease may cause disability. Neurological, musculoskeletal, and cardiorespiratory handicaps are most likely to interfere with mobility.

Health Status

Acute and chronic illnesses can affect mobility. Most individuals curtail activity as a consequence of diminished well-being associated with illness. Some illnesses interfere with mobility by causing weakness, impaired oxygenation, or pain. Sometimes activity limitations are imposed as part of therapy. As detailed later in the discussion of mobility alterations, there are often as many risks associated with therapeutic rest as there are benefits.

Self-concept and Emotions

Mobility has a reciprocal relationship to self-concept. Development of a healthy self-image requires mastery of a variety of skills and tasks, many of which require coordinated movement (see Chap. 11). Participation in childhood games and sports develops muscle coordination and promotes a sense of accomplishment, both of which enhance a positive self-concept.[29] In adolescence, the importance of mobility to healthy self-concept continues to be evident. Not only is there renewed emphasis on athletic performance, but popular adolescent social activities such as dancing also require coordinated movements. Children or adolescents unable to match the performance of peers may retain a persistent image of themselves as clumsy and inadequate. This negative self-concept can actually limit mobility by causing these individuals to avoid participating in sports and exercise during adulthood, compromising physical, social, and emotional health.[29]

If individuals with a poor self-concept begin to increase their activity level and become regular exercisers, their self-concept often improves considerably, as discussed earlier in the Benefits of Regular Exercise section.

Emotional status also affects a person's ability to move about freely. One of the symptoms of depression is a low energy level with minimal or very slow movement. In some severe forms of mental illness, voluntary movement may cease. The catatonic state is an example: One posture may be maintained for long periods of time with no apparent response to the environment.

Another example of the relationship between emotions and mobility occurs with stress. Stress is often localized in the muscles. The setting of the jaw and tension in the neck muscles are characteristics of emotional strain. Alexander Lowen[30] has postulated that chronic muscular tension or "muscular armoring" results from continuing emotional conflict. This armoring can cause abnormal body posture and interfere with fluid movement.

The role of motivation and personality in determining the amount or type of mobility or exercise in which an individual engages deserves mention. C. L. Hull[31] believed that along with such commonly recognized drives as hunger and thirst, there also exists an activity drive. This drive is expressed in a variety of ways, from exploration of one's environment to participation in organized physical activity such as sports and games. Not all theorists accept the concept of an innate drive for activity, but most recognize the influence of motivation. The motivation to engage in activity may be complex and related to other anticipated benefits such as health, social experiences, or a shapely body rather than purely for the sake of activity itself.

Values and Beliefs

Values and beliefs influence motivation and behavior. As discussed in Chapters 22 and 23, what individuals consider important in their lives and the influence they perceive they have over life events governs many life choices. An individual's definition of health and the value placed on health strongly influences choices related to activity and mobility. For some, exercise is synonymous with health. They consider regular exercise essential to well-being and would not define themselves as healthy if unable to exercise. This definition of health and the high value placed on feeling fit would demand and enhance a significant level of mobility. Others place less emphasis on activity as a measure of health. They may place greater value on pursuits congruent with a sedentary life-style and feel no particular motivation to be physically active as well. They would be likely to be content with a lower level of mobility, requiring only that sufficient for basic activities of daily living to consider themselves healthy. Many individuals value balance among physical and other types of pursuits and strive for excellence or at least participation in many different life activities. The influence of health beliefs, and one's concepts about personal efficacy and locus of control on health and health-related choices, is discussed in greater detail in Chapters 5, 12, and 22.

Life-style

Health status, values, beliefs, motivation, and self-concept, among other factors, influence life-style (see Chap. 23). Life-style influences mobility. Pender[32] considers life-style an expression of health and activity one of the dimensions through which it is expressed. She defines activity as encompassing meaningful work, meaningful play, and positive life patterns such as eating well, exercising regularly, resting adequately, and managing stress. To the extent that individuals share these ideas, their life-style will be an active one, in which choices for leisure, social, and avocational endeavors will involve mobility. Their choice of an active life-style will even be evident in small ways, such as their walking or cycling on errands rather than driving, or using stairs rather than elevators. Likewise, life-style choices may be sedentary, reflecting other values and beliefs and not enhancing or emphasizing mobility.

■ ALTERATIONS IN FUNCTION ASSOCIATED WITH LIMITED MOBILITY

Diminution of mobility occurs at many levels and for diverse reasons. For example, a person may experience complete loss of motor functioning because of a serious spinal cord injury. This loss would be permanent. Mobility may be temporarily limited because of an acute illness. Some people with chronic disease must permanently restrict their level of activity. Pain associated with illness or injury often limits mobility. Or some individuals may choose to be inactive, preferring a sedentary life-style.

Whatever the reason for diminished activity, predictable deleterious effects occur. These effects, called **disuse phenomena** or the **disuse syndrome,** occur at all levels of inactivity. They are more serious and numerous when activity is greatly curtailed, inactivity is prolonged, or when the individual was in a debilitated state prior to the onset of reduced activity. For example, a healthy, active man of 23, who remains in bed for 5 days because of influenza, would be at lesser risk for disuse phenomena than a 60-year-old man already debilitated by a chronic disease who became ill with influenza. If the 23-year-old were to remain on bed rest for several weeks because of a more serious health problem, his risk for disuse problems would also increase. In fact, in a well-known study, well-conditioned young men subjected to 3 weeks of bed rest developed changes in function roughly equal to that caused by 30 years of aging.[33] Initiating preventive nursing care at the onset of immobilization reduces immobility risks for all age groups.

Disuse phenomena are discussed in detail in the following sections. Section 2, *Assessment of Mobility,* provides a framework for predicting a given individual's risk for developing these immobility-related problems and identifying actual mobility problems.

Activity and Mobility Problems

Inactivity limits options for activity. Greatly restricted exercise results in bone, muscle, and joint changes that inhibit return to normal mobility. Because the drive for motor activity is diminished after deconditioning, the problems are compounded. Persistent and consistent efforts may be required to obtain client participation in preventive and rehabilitative exercises. Even well-conditioned individuals who have experienced a short-term period of diminished activity may find returning to their former exercise routine requires considerable mental discipline. These individuals, however, will probably not experience the serious musculoskeletal problems associated with more extensive limitation of activity, discussed below.

Bone Changes. Bone integrity is normally maintained by complimentary functioning of osteoblasts and osteoclasts. In a state of wellness, weight bearing and activities involving the large muscles stimulate osteoblasts to generate new bone matrix. This new tissue replaces that destroyed by osteoclasts, keeping the living bone in a state of dynamic equilibrium. When bed rest or diminished muscle activity is prolonged, bone building ceases while destruction of bone continues, releasing calcium and phosphorus into the bloodstream. This demineralization results in osteoporosis—literally, porous bone,[8,34,35] The rate of loss of bone density is most rapid in weight-bearing bones and in younger individuals.[34]

Immobility-induced osteoporosis takes place in several stages. The initial stage, occurring in the first 12 weeks of immobility, is most rapid but is also rapidly reversible with return to weight bearing. If immobility continues, a second phase in which bone loss is slower ensues. Ultimately, people whose immobility is very long term or permanent lose bone tissue until they reach bone volumes of 40 to 70 percent of the original volume.[34] Bone loss associated with long-term immobility is irreversible. Bones weakened as a result of osteoporosis are easily deformed and fracture readily. In fact, osteoporosis is responsible for 1.3 million fractures per year in the United States.[35] Although osteoporosis also occurs as a normal aspect of aging, lack of exercise hastens the process.

Muscle Changes. Like bones, muscles depend on activity to function efficiently. The demands of exercise cause an increase in the size and strength of muscles, as discussed earlier. The converse occurs when activity is reduced. There is decreased circulation to muscles, and muscle protein is lost, resulting in shortened muscle fibers as well as diminished tone and strength. Endurance declines and muscles become stiff. The flabby appearance of inactive middle-aged adults represents a less severe form of this phenomenon.

Severe muscle wasting is associated with prolonged bedrest. A person on complete bedrest loses 10 to 15 percent of muscle strength per week and 50 percent of strength in 2 to 5 weeks.[34] The lower leg muscles that are ordinarily used to resist gravity are the first muscles to weaken and atrophy when recumbent.[34,36] Muscle bulk may shrink to one half its original size in 2 months.[34] Muscles also lose oxidative efficiency when they are inactive.[8,34] This means that when exercise is attempted, oxygen debt occurs sooner and lactic acid builds up more rapidly.

Joint Changes. Flexibility is also affected by diminished activity. Connective tissue changes involving ligaments, tendons, and the joint capsule, as well as muscle shortening, are present to some degree in healthy sedentary persons and are more severe with bedrest.[34] When confined to bed, individuals frequently assume flexed positions, favoring shortening of the flexor muscles. The position of comfort assumed by many clients fosters flexion contractures of the knees and hips and plantar flexion (foot drop). As the muscles become increasingly resistant to stretching, the range of motion (ROM) of the joints is diminished, compromising walking and self-care. Contractures may eventually become so severe as to require surgical intervention.

Rest and Sleep Problems

Rest implies a sense of tranquility or relaxation, a cessation of activity. Sleeping is a necessary form of rest. The prescription to curtail activity or to remain in bed is usually predicated upon the assumption that increased rest will be the result. This is not always the case.

Having limits placed on one's activity can be stressful and can actually compound the physiological stress associated with illness or injury. This state of tension may make relaxation and sleep difficult. If the prescribed rest is to be obtained in a hospital, the stress may be greater, for many people find sleeping in an unfamiliar environment difficult. Also, the usual sleep–wakefulness rhythm is disturbed when inactivity is imposed at a time during which a person is usually active. Clients desiring to overcome the sense of decreased well-being associated with illness may attempt to increase their sleeping during daytime hours. These naps may actually diminish the quality of nighttime sleep by decreasing the amount of deep (stages 3 and 4) sleep.

Regular physical exercise promotes restful sleep. Increased amounts of stage 3 and 4 sleep have been found to occur after exercise. Individuals deprived of regular exercise may find restful sleep difficult to attain. Sedentary people sometimes experience a chronic diminution of the deeper stages of sleep. A sleep period with less time in deep sleep is less restorative. One may awaken unrefreshed, with a lingering sense of fatigue. This complaint is not uncommon among sedentary individuals. Sleep and rest are discussed in greater detail in Chapter 28.

Oxygenation Problems

Oxygenation involves taking oxygen into the body (ventilation), moving it from the lungs into the bloodstream (diffusion), transporting it to the tissues (perfusion), and moving it into the tissues from the bloodstream. All of these processes are less efficient in sedentary individuals and are compromised in well-conditioned individuals by inactivity. A period of bed rest as short as 3 to 5 days leads to cardiovascular deconditioning.[34] This is because the efficiency of the cardiopulmonary response to muscle work depends on frequent demands approaching the muscles' maximum capacity. The initial cardiovascular effect of bed rest is increased cardiac workload. This occurs as a result of a greater circulating blood volume because of less capillary pooling when legs are not dependent.[37] After this initial increase, cardiac output and stroke volume progressively decrease and oxygen uptake diminishes. The loss of cardiopulmonary efficiency is manifested by a higher resting pulse. When muscles are not regularly stressed, their oxygen use deteriorates as well. The result is a considerably reduced physical work capacity.[12]

When inactivity involves bedrest, there are additional constraints to ventilation, diffusion, and perfusion. Decreased metabolic demands associated with limited activity cause reduction in depth of respiration. This effect is enhanced when recumbent, because abdominal organs exert pressure on the diaphragm, constricting the size of the chest cavity. Weakening of the skeletal accessory muscles used in respiration also contributes to decreased oxygen and carbon dioxide exchange. Shallow respirations promote alveolar collapse, reducing the functional lung surface area.

Another factor interfering with ventilation and diffusion when individuals are confined to bed is pooling of mucus. Mucus is normally distributed evenly around the lumen of the bronchi. The action of gravity in the supine position favors collection of secretions in the dependent portion of the tubes, and drying of the upper portion. The pooling and drying interfere with the functioning of the cilia, resulting in still more pooling.

Generalized weakness related to the primary disease process, or to bed rest itself, and the supine position decrease the effectiveness of coughing. The static secretions become obstructive and are an excellent medium for the growth of microorganisms. A resulting complication is pneumonia.

Clients confined to bed often use the valsalva maneuver when using the trunk and arm muscles to change positions. The **valsalva maneuver** is attempting a forced expiration with the glottis closed. No movement of air occurs, but intrathoracic pressure increases, thereby decreasing blood flow in the major thoracic and coronary blood vessels. When the breath is suddenly released, the thoracic pressure falls and a surge of blood flows into the heart. The myocardium stretches more to accommodate the larger blood volume and contracts more forcefully to eject it. This may strain cardiac capacity in debilitated clients, causing arrhythmias and temporarily compromised perfusion.

Orthostatic (postural) hypotension, a precipitous drop in blood pressure associated with standing, is another phenomenon related to bedrest that interferes with perfusion. When active individuals rise from a recumbent position, reflex vasoconstriction of peripheral arterioles maintains blood pressure and blood supply to the brain. This reflex is dulled with bed rest. Therefore, vessels remain dilated, blood pools in the legs upon standing, and central blood pressure falls. Clients feel dizzy and light-headed and may faint because less blood is delivered to the brain.

Perfusion may also be altered by pathogenic clotting. Increased coagulability, venous stasis, and damage to the intima of the vein walls contribute to thrombus (clot) formation. Bed rest induces two of these three factors and often plays a role in the third. Plasma volume decreases with bed rest.[34] This increases blood viscosity and therefore increases coagulability. If clients are not well hydrated, the increase in blood viscosity and therefore coagulability is further magnified. Venous stasis occurs because of the lack of pumping action of the calf muscles during bed rest. There is often additional interference with blood return because of improper positioning. For example, many clients favor a semi-Fowler's (sitting) position when on bed rest. They often adjust the bed so their knees are bent to prevent slipping toward the foot of the bed. This creates pressure on the superficial veins behind the knee and interference with venous return. A similar problem occurs when side-lying with the superior leg resting on the dependent leg. Moreover, pressure on vessels in each of these situations may irritate or damage the inside of the blood vessels, therefore establishing the third contributing factor to thrombus formation. Clots compromise local circulation or may become dislodged and move through the circulatory system. This is called an embolism. Pulmonary embolism, a clot that lodges in the pulmonary artery or one of its branches, is a life-threatening complication of pathological clotting.

Another serious result of decreased perfusion is pressure ulcers. When clients are improperly positioned or remain in one position for more than 1 hour, external capillary pressure at bony prominences may increase as much as tenfold, making the exchange of oxygen, nutrients, and wastes impossible. This ischemia brings about necrosis (tissue death) of skin and underlying tissues, a pressure ulcer or pressure sore (see discussion in Chap. 24). Figure 30–6 shows the pressure points at which pressure ulcers are most likely to develop in commonly assumed positions. Clients at high risk for developing pressure ulcers include:

1. Clients whose spontaneous movements are greatly decreased. Examples are clients who are unconscious, paralyzed, heavily sedated, and/or elderly.
2. Obese clients, whose increased weight and dense subcutaneous tissue creates greater external pressure on capillaries over bony prominences.
3. Clients with edema. Edematous tissue is more vulnerable to circulatory interference because the edema fluid creates a barrier to exchange of oxygen, nutrients, and wastes.
4. Poorly nourished clients. Meager amounts of subcutaneous tissue and weakened collagen and elastin diminish tissue capacity to absorb and tolerate pressure.[38] Diminished tissue perfusion secondary to nutritional anemia further compromises resistance to pressure.
5. Clients who are incontinent. Urine and feces are irritating to skin, and dampness causes tissue maceration. Inflamed and macerated tissue is more vulnerable to breakdown.
6. Clients favoring Fowler's position. Sitting upright against the raised mattress exposes the skin over the sacrum and heels to shearing force (see Fig. 24–5). Shearing force results from the simultaneous downward and forward pressures created as clients slide gradually toward the foot of the bed. It tears the skin surfaces and damages capillaries and deeper tissues.

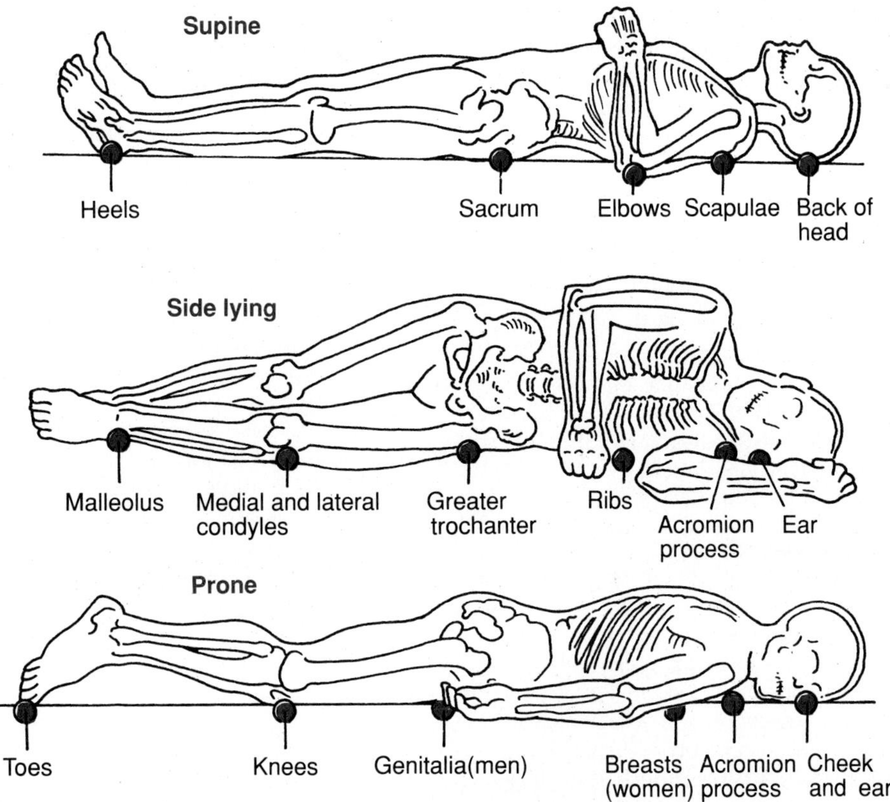

Figure 30–6. Pressure points in common positions.

Nutritional Problems

A healthy energy balance is difficult for inactive individuals to attain. More frequently, they remain in positive energy balance, which leads to weight gain. Sedentary individuals are frequently overweight.

Clients whose activity and environment are restricted by bed rest frequently experience diminution in appetite (anorexia). This may seem to be a beneficial effect, because caloric needs are diminished when activity is decreased. When bed rest is prescribed, however, it is usually to facilitate tissue repair. In this case, the body's demand for certain nutrients is greatly increased (see Chap. 24).

The anorexia is compounded by alterations in metabolism associated with decreased activity. When on bed rest, anabolic processes are slowed, while catabolic processes accelerate. Weight is lost, primarily lean body mass rather than fat. Inactive individuals on bed rest develop carbohydrate intolerance. Studies indicate that the release of insulin is normal, but that its effectiveness is diminished.[34] Inactivity seems to increase resistance to endogenous insulin (insulin produced within the body), so that even though serum levels are at or above normal, carbohydrate metabolism is not optimum.

Protein metabolism is also altered. Protein synthesis is reduced and protein breakdown is increased. The increase in nitrogenous wastes resulting from the breakdown of protein precipitates a state of negative nitrogen balance: excretion of nitrogenous products (from protein catabolism) exceeding their ingestion. Negative nitrogen balance causes diminished interest in food. If the lack of desire for food results in reduced intake and/or a nutritionally unbalanced diet, increasingly greater needs for nutrients in the face of a paradoxical decrease in appetite will prolong the recovery period.

Anorexia may also cause decreased fluid intake. Several changes in fluid metabolism discussed in the next section actually increase the client's fluid needs when on bed rest. As in the case of nutrients, the greater need accompanied by reduced desire may result in complications.

Fluid and Elimination Problems

All of the body's processes for elimination of waste products are altered by inactivity. The effect on carbon dioxide excretion via the lungs was discussed earlier. Skin, kidney, and bowel elimination are considered here.

Skin. There is no appreciable alteration in excretion of wastes by the skin associated with being sedentary. Although there is less obvious perspiration when one is not actively exercising, insensible losses continue. There is, however, increased loss of water and the electrolytes sodium, potassium, and chloride via the skin when confined to bed. Dilation of blood vessels occurs, which raises the skin temperature and therefore promotes perspiration, especially in areas where skin surfaces touch. Sheets and blankets prevent heat loss by radiation and conduction, and so also stimulate sweating. This profuse perspiration, called diaphoresis, contributes to skin breakdown and general discomfort.

Kidney. The physiological functioning of the kidney is not greatly altered by bed rest or inactivity; however, changes in the workload of the kidney occur with bed rest. The expanded circulating blood volume due to recumbency discussed under oxygenation problems gives rise to diuresis (increased urine output). This is because antidiuretic hormone (ADH) is suppressed when central blood volume increases and because the glomerular filtration rate (GFR) is greater secondary to increased renal blood flow. Diuresis causes significant loss of plasma volume.[34]

As a result of the catabolic processes previously discussed, serum levels of calcium, phosphorous, and nitrogenous wastes also increase significantly, intensifying filtration load in the glomeruli. Unless fluid intake is augmented, the combined effect of loss of plasma volume and higher levels of wastes is a rise in urine specific gravity. High urine specific gravity is related to another problem, renal calculi, discussed later in this section.

The supine position, frequently assumed on bed rest, is associated with two elimination problems, urinary stasis and overflow incontinence. In an erect position, drainage of urine from the kidney pelvis is facilitated by gravity. As the urine collects in the bladder, and the sensation of fullness is noted, elimination is initiated. This action involves voluntary relaxation of the external sphincter and perineal muscles, which triggers an autonomic reflex, causing contraction of the detrusor muscle. The ensuing increase in pressure within the bladder (intravesicular pressure) causes relaxation of the internal sphincter and the release of urine.

When confined to bed, clients may have difficulty with voluntary relaxation of the external sphincter. Also, using the bedpan or urinal may be embarrassing or uncomfortably awkward. Thus, clients may suppress the urge to void, causing urinary stasis. Gradually, the detrusor muscle becomes stretched and decreasingly sensitive. Bladder distension without the accompanying urge to void increases the intravesicular pressure, which can be transmitted to the kidney via the ureters, damaging the nephron, or result in overflow incontinence.

Urinary stasis predisposes clients to two further problems, urinary tract infection and renal calculi (stones). Ordinarily, the bladder is rather resistant to infection. Despite frequent exposure to microorganisms, most commonly from normal gastrointestinal flora, infection rarely occurs. This is due to the inherent antimicrobial properties of the bladder mucosa, phagocytosis, and to the mechanical flushing action of voiding. Distension of the bladder reduces mucosal blood flow, however. Ischemic tissue is less resistant to invasion by microorganisms. Additionally, due to the diminution of acid wastes usually produced by muscle activity, the urine of a person on bed rest becomes alkaline, favoring the growth of certain bacteria.

Static urine and the presence of bacteria enhance calculus formation. Formation of urinary calculi is also greatly facilitated by other circumstances resulting from bed rest. As noted previously, the serum level of calcium increases with inactivity. The high level of calcium promotes precipitation of crystals in the urine, which form the nucleus of stones, especially if the urine volume is decreased. Lithiasis (stones) may form anywhere in the urinary tract, but in the recumbent position, the renal pelvis is a common site. These stones become quite large, giving rise to a characteristic severe colicky pain. The presence of stones and damage to the mucosa caused by movement of the stones increases the risk of infection, creating a cycle of stone formation and bacterial proliferation.

Bowel. Bowel elimination requires normomotility of intestinal smooth muscle as well as voluntary contraction of skeletal muscles of the abdomen and pelvic floor in response to the pressure of fecal material in the rectum (see Chap. 26). Inactivity can interfere with both of these aspects of bowel elimination. Constipation is a common complication of bed rest and, not infrequently, a problem of sedentary individuals. Active exercise stimulates peristalsis and strengthens abdominal muscles. Conversely, intestinal motility is diminished with inactivity, and the loss of muscle tone associated with bed rest reduces the mechanical expulsive force created by the abdominal muscles. If use of the bedpan is necessary, the effectiveness of these muscles is further compromised, for the physiological squatting position cannot be assumed.

Dietary changes due to illness or lack of appetite and changes in daily schedules or routines interfere with usual bowel habits, increasing the risk for constipation. Lack of privacy also contributes to constipation in hospitalized clients. Individuals confined to bed may ignore the urge to defecate due to embarrassment associated with minimal screening and the unavoidable proximity of others. Repeated suppression of defecation diminishes sensitivity to rectal distension and produces a harder, drier stool that is more difficult to eliminate. A more serious complication, fecal impaction, may be the result (see also Chap. 26.)

Sexual Problems

There is no consistent relationship between sexual dysfunction and a physically inactive life-style. However, mobility restrictions that are related to illness, injury, or their treatment are potentially disruptive of satisfaction of sexual needs. The problem may be related to energy level. Being ill or depressed because of loss of independence may consume physical and emotional energy to such an extent that libido is diminished. This situation may be more stressful for the sexual partner than for the individual who is ill. Although illness does not always cause disinterest in sexual activity, some types of illness or injuries may make usual sexual relations physically impossible on a temporary or permanent basis. In these situations, counseling assistance may be warranted.

If immobility is imposed in a hospital or other institutional setting, achieving sexual satisfaction is directly inhibited. Any sexual expressions involving a partner are impossible. Rarely is there adequate privacy even for masturbation, which is a natural substitute under these circumstances. The resulting sexual frustration can add to the overall stress of being ill.

Self-concept alterations related to mobility (see next section) can also have a significant impact on sexuality and sexual expression. Feelings of inadequacy or dependency, or believing that one is no longer attractive, often result in fears of rejection by one's partner. These fears may diminish the sex drive and even cause impotence. As a result, clients often withdraw from their partner, even though their own sexual feelings are not diminished. Conflict and sexual tension between the partners often results.

Psychological Problems

As discussed above, being physically active and physically fit contributes to a positive self-image and increased self-esteem. Although the relationship is not simple and direct, it is also true that many people who choose a sedentary life-style, particularly if they are overweight, have less self-esteem and are less satisfied with their bodies than physically active people. These feelings sometimes produce social withdrawal, particularly from group activities that involve sports or exertion. Those who must restrict their activity because of a diminished level of wellness often experience a similar diminution of social options; however, prolonged restriction of mobility has even more far-reaching psychological effects.

Immobility alters identity. The complex components comprising who we are—self-concept, body image, relationships, perceptions, emotions, drives, roles, and choices—are modified when the ability to move about is partially or entirely curtailed. Moreover, physical mobility enhances psychological mobility. Moving through one's environment facilitates emotional contact with people and objects within it. Restriction of physical mobility limits individuals' control over their interactions with others. This loss of control is most dramatic for those confined to bed. Rather than seeking out or initiating exchanges with others, they must wait for others to initiate. There is a significant limitation of personal space when immobilized. This, too, is a potential stressor.

The American culture ascribes great significance to productivity and participation. Involuntary limitation of involvement in usual life-style behaviors is a major stressor. Valued roles are threatened in the family, workplace, and social contexts when mutual participation is reduced. When the ability to move about is critical for job performance, or being physically fit is central to self-concept, restricted movement may dramatically affect emotional status. This may occur even if the restriction is recognized as temporary.

Exercise is also a healthy way to dissipate pent-up energy caused by stress. When illness or injury interferes with opportunities to engage in exercise, the result is often more intense feelings of stress and an increase in stress-related behaviors. The restrictions and changes produce role conflict, altered body image, and disturbed self-concept. These alterations may cause immobilized individuals to experience a greatly diminished sense of worth.

Withdrawal and apathy, which delay recovery and compound the reduction in self-esteem, are potential manifestations. Conversely, anger, hostility, frustration, or even guilt may be responses to the loss of power to make choices. Mood changes are common. Many people become preoccupied with themselves and with bodily functions. When the disability is prolonged or permanent, these reactions are typically more intense. The behaviors characteristic of the grieving process—denial, anger, and bargaining—are common.

Immobility also affects perception.[34] A reduction in environmental stimuli (sensory deprivation), which occurs when a person is confined to a small space such as a bed, impairs the ability to interpret pattern, form, time, pressure, and temperature. Sensory deprivation compromises both motivation and capacity to learn cognitive and motor skills. The learning and perceptual deficits restrict problem-solving ability, further threatening independence and self-esteem.

The far-reaching effects of immobility on all body systems and on all human needs underline the need for client–nurse collaboration to identify creative, holistic approaches to care. Nurses must be alert to clues indicating immobility-related problems in clients with all levels of mobility curtailment, from inactivity to complete bed rest. Individual differences result in a wide range of reactions, not necessarily directly related to the degree of limitation. The following sections provide guides for nursing assessment and management of problems related to alterations in mobility.

IMPLICATIONS FOR NURSE–CLIENT COLLABORATION

The Problems of Immobility

The problems of immobility are far-reaching. Having one's activity curtailed can be stressful, physically and mentally. Besides the toll that is taken on the musculoskeletal system, immobility is also associated with oxygenation, nutritional, sleep–rest, and fluid balance changes and alterations in self-expression. Diligent care is needed to prevent the many complications of immobility. Collaborating with the client to assess for the subjective and objective manifestations of complications is thus essential as the nurse and immobile client begin to work together, and it continues to be important until mobility is reestablished. Ongoing monitoring, the assessment that occurs during implementation, is a central aspect of any plan of prevention for immobility complications.

Section 2. Assessment of Mobility

MOBILITY DATA COLLECTION

A complete assessment of a client's mobility status is necessary to plan comprehensive nursing implementation. This is best accomplished through a collaborative data-gathering process comprised of history, a clinical examination, and a review of relevant laboratory data. Nurses may obtain the needed information directly from clients and their families and also use data contained in the medical history and physical examination.

Mobility History

The mobility history provides important subjective data about a client's strengths and deficits relating to movement and activity. Sharing the purpose of the history with the client encourages full participation.

The mobility history includes information about a client's current level of mobility, usual exercise patterns, attitudes about mobility, and level of knowledge about related subjects such as rest and nutrition. If mobility has recently changed as a result of illness or injury, it is also important to determine how clients feel about their current situation. How significant is this change?

Level of understanding about the type of mobility or exercise that is appropriate during the acute, convalescent, and rehabilitation stages is also important to assess. For example, a client may resist attempts to increase activity after surgery because of erroneous fears that disruption of the incision could be caused by movement. A client who has suffered a stroke may not be aware that rehabilitation of currently nonfunctioning limbs can be facilitated by passive exercise in the period immediately following the stroke. A client being treated for cardiac problems may not realize the preventive and rehabilitative effects of prudent aerobic exercise.

The mobility history also encompasses clients' expectations for recovery. Determine anticipated changes in life-style, or needs for assistance from others, after leaving the hospital. Individuals' expectations about their level of functioning after the acute phase of illness affects mutual goal-setting. For example, clients who perceive that their mobility is permanently altered may feel a rehabilitation program is futile. Some clients make unrealistic plans for discharge life-style, based upon misunderstanding about the rate and degree of recovery possible.

Data about the family or other support persons are a necessary element in the mobility data base. Not only can these people contribute significantly to a client's recovery, they can also provide additional insights into a client's needs. The family is a primary source of data when a client is unable or unwilling to communicate.

The following sections present a description of each part of the mobility history, using a modification of the standard health history format. This model yields data useful to nurses in planning client care and also assists in collaborative planning with other members of the health team.

Primary Concern. Explore what aspect of a client's current health problem is most troubling. Loss of mobility is alarming to most individuals. Because many types of health problems threaten mobility, distress about real or anticipated mobility impairment is a frequent primary concern. Respiratory, circulatory, cardiac, neurological, and musculoskeletal problems interfere directly with ease or capacity for movement. Pain related to dysfunction anywhere in the body is a common cause of mobility limitations.

Sometimes it is the treatment of a health problem that produces mobility problems. Some medications cause side effects that alter mobility. Casts, splints, and braces change mobility. Prescribed rest and specific activity limitations are part of the therapy for many types of health problems.

For some clients, the results of altered mobility—such as time away from work or school, limited social and recreational activities, or the inability to carry out usual role functions in the home—are the primary concern. In all of these cases, a detailed mobility history is appropriate.

Current Understanding. Explore client perceptions about the relationship between the health problem for which clients sought care and their primary concern. Explore the course of the problem and consequences that have been troubling for the client. Determine what remedies a client has tried and whether relief was obtained. Find out if clients have other health problems that contribute to their concern and what role they see those problems playing in their present situation. The following example illustrates the importance of a client's current understanding in identifying appropriate client care.

- When discussing the reason for seeking care, Mr. Nelson states that he has been having acute epigastric pain that has been diagnosed as an ulcer. He is now scheduled for surgery after several weeks of taking medications without improvement in symptoms. During the hospital admission, Mr. Nelson expresses frustration about the interference his illness has caused in his usual physical fitness regimen, stating how much better he will feel after resuming regular jogging and weight lifting after his discharge from the hospital. The nurse makes a note of these apparently unrealistic expectations for postsurgical activity for later health teaching.

Past Health Problems/Experiences. Chronic conditions and their treatment, and past experiences with health care, are often relevant to current mobility status and related nursing care. Ask clients if they have ever had other illnesses, injuries, or operations that have affected mobility. Determine the date, severity, treatment, and residual effects, if any, of these. Note medications currently used that could affect mobility status, such as those acting on the cardiac, respiratory, circulatory, musculoskeletal, or neurological systems. The following example illustrates the relevance of past health problems and their treatment to mobility.

- Ms. Shapiro is admitted for observation because of apparently minor head injuries sustained when she fell at home as a result of having "blacked out." When questioned about medications used on a regular basis, Ms. Shapiro indicates that she has recently begun taking a new medication for high blood pressure (hypertension). The nurse is aware that this medication often causes transient dizziness, especially when rising quickly from supine to standing. He decides that the care plan for Ms. Shapiro should include safety measures such as dangling before ambulation and client education about side effects of the medication.

Personal, Family, and Social History. Personal, family, and social history provides significant data needed to make nursing diagnoses related to mobility status. Life-style choices, particularly diet and exercise habits, contribute to many of the health problems that cause limited mobility. Comprehensive exploration of daily routines and activities provides insights important to mobility care. Conversely, altered mobility potentially affects many facets of a person's life and often imposes life-style changes. Clues about resources and limitations affecting clients' ability to adapt to necessary changes come from the personal, family, and social history. The following example shows the relevance of this part of the history to mobility care. Table 30–2 lists sample questions to elicit appropriate information.

- Mr. Rothenberg is admitted to the surgical floor for a minor surgical procedure. The nurse notes that he appears to be overweight. When questioning him about his habits, she learns that his usual diet includes foods high in calories, both for meals and snacks. Mr. Rothenberg also reveals that he does not exercise regularly, preferring to watch television in his leisure time. The nurse decides that Mr. Rothenberg is in need of health teaching about exercise and nutrition to help him to make informed decisions about his overall health status. She plans to consult with the physician and dietitian to develop a collaborative education plan for Mr. Rothenberg.

Subjective Manifestations. An overview of subjective manifestations provides an overall picture of symptoms a client is experiencing. The questions in Table 30–3 focus on symptoms that may interfere with a client's mobility. The number and severity of symptoms experienced by a client determine the amount of nursing assistance needed for movement and daily care activities. The following example illustrates the use of subjective manifestations data.

- When interviewing Mrs. Johnson, an elderly client being admitted to the hospital, a nurse learns that

TABLE 30–2. MOBILITY HISTORY: PERSONAL, FAMILY, AND SOCIAL HISTORY QUESTIONS

A. **Vocational**

1. What type of work do you do?
2. Does your current work involve physical exertion? How much?
3. If yes, have you noticed any problems doing your work lately? How long has this been a problem?
4. What other job skills or interests do you have?
5. How do you usually get around—for example, to work, to shop? Do you drive? Ride the bus? Walk?
6. Have driving or walking become more difficult lately?

B. **Home and Family**

1. Are you married? In a relationship? How long?
2. Is the relationship satisfactory?
3. Do you have children? How many? Ages?
4. What other family members live with you? Nearby?
5. How do you see family members as helping you in this situation?
6. Do you perform many home maintenance tasks—cooking, cleaning, repairs?
7. Tell me about a typical day at home (tasks, activities).

C. **Social, Leisure, Spiritual, and Cultural**

1. What are your favorite leisure-time activities? With whom do you usually do these?
2. Are there other pastimes you enjoy or have enjoyed in the past?
3. Do you belong to any clubs or groups?
4. Has your illness affected your choice of leisure activities? How?
5. Has your social life been affected by the recent change in your health status? Tell me about it.

D. **Sexual**

1. Has your sexual relationship been satisfactory?
2. Any changes related to this illness?
3. What changes have occurred?

E. **Habits**

Exercise

1. Do you exercise regularly? Weekly? More often?
2. What type of exercise/activity do you enjoy most—games, individual sports, fitness activities?
3. Do you feel that regular exercise is an important part of staying healthy?
4. Has this illness affected your pattern of exercise? How?

Sleep

1. How many hours do you usually sleep each night?
2. Is this enough for you to feel rested?
3. Do you have any sleep problems? How have you dealt with these?
4. Do you notice any change in your sleep patterns when you increase or decrease your exercise? How does sleep change?
5. Has this illness affected your sleep? How?

Nutrition

1. How many meals do you usually eat daily? Any difference on weekends? Snacks?
2. What foods you do you eat most every day?
3. What kind of diet do you feel is necessary to stay healthy?
4. Describe your appetite.
5. Has this illness affected your eating habits? How?

Beverages

1. Do you drink coffee? Tea? Cola? How much of each per day?
2. Do you drink alcoholic beverages? What do you usually drink? Beer, wine, liquor?
3. How much alcohol do you drink in an average week?
4. Does your alcohol intake affect your activity? How?
5. Do you notice a change in your ability or motivation to exercise when you are drinking more?
6. Does alcohol intake affect your overall mobility? How?
7. Have you ever injured yourself as a result of your alcohol intake?
8. Has your alcohol intake changed since you became ill?

Tobacco

1. Do you smoke? Cigarettes, pipe, cigar?
2. How long have you been smoking?
3. How much do you smoke?
4. Have you ever quit? For how long?
5. Does smoking affect your activity? How?
6. Do you note a change in your ability to exercise when you are smoking more?

TABLE 30–2. (continued)

Drugs

1. Are there any drugs you use regularly, such as aspirin, sleeping pills, diet pills, nerve pills?
2. How frequently do you take these? For what reason?
3. Do any of these affect your ability or motivation to exercise as usual
4. Do they affect your overall mobility? How?
5. Have you ever injured yourself as a result of taking these? What was the injury?
6. Has your use of any of these changed recently? How?

Other Substances

1. Do you ever use marijuana? Cocaine? Crystal? Other drugs?
2. Do any of them influence your level of activity? Your motivation to exercise? Carry out usual home or work responsibilities?

F. **Psychological**

Coping

1. Has (current concern) caused any worries for you? For example, about your overall health? Possibility of improvement? Relationships with wife, family? Money?
2. How have you dealt with these concerns?
3. Has this been effective?

Self-image

1. Do you think the change in your mobility has changed the way you feel about yourself (for example, about the way you look, do your job, carry out your home responsibilities, parent, or relate to your spouse)?
2. How would you describe the change?

she has experienced joint stiffness in her back and legs, which is most severe when she first gets up in the morning. The symptom has sometimes been severe enough to make walking difficult, but it improved if Mrs. Johnson went about household activities at a slow pace. Mrs. Johnson has been bothered by this stiffness for about 5 years and occasionally takes aspirin for relief. The nurse realizes that lying in bed during the period of hospitalization will probably aggravate this symptom and resolves to include ROM and other in-bed exercises in Mrs. Johnson's care plan to prevent the stiffness from becoming more severe.

The mobility history should be initiated when a client is admitted to a hospital or seeks care for a concern related to mobility at an outpatient facility. It is important, however, for nurses to be sensitive to clients' ability to respond. Anxiety, fatigue, or pain may necessitate obtaining baseline data in several short interviews. Nurses must also review clients' medical records. Frequently, data gathered by other health care team members, such as the physician or dietitian, are useful in planning nursing care. Collaborative data gathering is efficient, conserving energy of clients and health care professionals.

Mobility Examination

The mobility examination provides critical information about a client's mobility status. The examination comprises measurements, inspection, palpation, and auscultation.

Measurements. Measure the client's height and weight and compare to normative charts. Is the client underweight? Overweight? Excess weight hints at a sedentary life-style. Lack of exercise and obesity can lead to a variety of health problems affecting mobility. Overweight people may have a significantly lower exercise tolerance than would be predicted for their age. Many have hypertension, cardiac problems, or respiratory difficulties that make activities of daily living or strenuous exercise difficult. When confined to bed, these clients have increased risk for such problems as decubitus ulcers, hypostatic pneumonia, and thrombophlebitis.

Conversely, underweight individuals may suffer from nutritional deficiencies and musculoskeletal weakness, both of which could affect endurance. They would have minimal energy reserve to withstand the stress of illness or injury and may require a prolonged period of convalescence. This could lead to many of the disuse phenomena discussed in Section 1.

Measure vital signs as discussed in Chapter 16. Resting pulse predicts activity tolerance and implies general activity level. Individuals who are physically active usually have a lower than expected resting pulse for their age. Pulse irregularities, respiratory difficulties, or hypertension suggest limitations in activity tolerance.

Objective Manifestations. Integument, eye and ear, chest, cardiovascular, musculoskeletal, and neurological examinations contribute to nursing diagnosis of mobility status. General observations at the beginning of the examination signal areas needing more detailed assessment later in the examination.

General Observations. General observations pertinent to mobility status include mental status, body proportions, energy level, skin color, posture, gait, and body movement.

Mental Status. Information about mental status and sensory capacity is necessary to determine whether indepen-

TABLE 30–3. SUBJECTIVE MANIFESTATIONS QUESTIONS

A. **General**
   1. Describe your overall state of health.
   2. Has there been a recent change?
   3. Do you require any help to move about, cook, shop, care for yourself?
   4. Has there been a recent change in these abilities?
   5. How much activity do you feel up to now? Sitting up? Walking to the door? In the hall? More strenuous activity?
   6. Do you ever experience difficulty walking due to problems with your eyesight? When does this happen?
   7. How about difficulty with transportation due to eyesight?
   8. Can you drive?
   9. Have you ever had difficulty orienting yourself because of hearing problems? When does this occur?

B. **Respiratory**
   1. Do you ever experience difficulty breathing? Coughing? Sneezing? Wheezing? Congestion?
   2. What precedes or aggravates these?
   3. Do you experience any of them when you are active?
   4. What kind of activity causes these symptoms—for example, walking, running, housework, stair climbing?
   5. How much can you do before these symptoms appear?
   6. Do you notice improvement when you rest?
   7. How much rest is necessary to relieve the symptoms?

C. **Chest, Cardiovascular**
   1. Do you ever experience a pounding sensation in the chest (palpitations)? A very rapid heart rate (tachycardia)? Sharp shooting pains in your legs (claudication)? Dizziness? Passing out (syncope)? Increased blood pressure (hypertension)?
   2. Do any of these occur or become worse with activity? What kind?
   3. How much of this activity can you do before these occur?
   4. Are they improved with rest?
   5. How long do you have to rest before they are better?

D. **Musculoskeletal**
   1. Do you ever experience muscle weakness? Cramps? Muscle aches and pains? Joint stiffness? Back pain or stiffness? Back pain that radiates to the legs (radicular pain)?
   2. What precedes or aggravates these?
   3. Are any of them caused or worsened by activity? What kind?
   4. How much activity before they appear?
   5. Do they get better with rest? How much rest?
   6. Do these symptoms keep you from being able to care for yourself?
   7. Have you ever experienced a fracture? Dislocation?
   8. Was it related to exercise? How did it happen?

E. **Neurological**
   1. Do you ever have headaches? A sense of confusion/disorientation? Loss of balance? Loss of coordination? Tingling in the arms, legs, fingers, toes? Numbness? Other changes in sensation or touch, such as "pins and needles" (paresthesia)?
   2. Are any of these related to activity? What kind of activity?
   3. Does rest or stopping the activity improve them?
   4. How long do you have to rest before they improve or disappear?
   5. Have you ever had convulsions? Are they associated with exercise or with a specific activity?
   6. Have you ever been injured as a result of a convulsion?

F. **Psychological**
   1. Do you notice mood swings associated with activity/exercise? When you don't exercise?
   2. How do these mood changes affect your interaction with others? Your job? Your interest in usual leisure activities?

dent mobility is safe for a client. Responses to questions during the history and client participation during measurements are general indicators of mental status. Clients who are confused or apparently unaware of their surroundings could injure themselves while ambulating or when getting out of bed without assistance. Clients who have trouble hearing questions during the history and examination, or difficulty seeing where they are going, may need help to ambulate safely.

Body Proportions and Energy Level. Body proportions and energy level of a client also suggests potential strengths and deficits pertaining to mobility. Note the general body build. Is the client slender? muscular? Do the muscles appear well toned? Overdeveloped? Flabby? Does the client seem fatigued? Lethargic? Energetic? Poor muscle tone implies a sedentary life-style. Fatigue or lethargy may point to nutritional deficits, oxygenation problems, or emotional problems, all of which can hinder mobility. Optimum tone, well-developed muscles, and a dynamic energy level suggest regular exercise habits. Individuals who exercise regularly usually have the capacity for optimum mobility, but often have difficulty adapting to restricted mobility during convalescence from illness, surgery, or injury.

Skin Color. Noting overall skin color is also part of general observations. A person who is unusually pale may be anemic (have an abnormally low concentration of circulating red blood cells). Not only would this client have a low energy level, but the ability to adequately perfuse cells, especially during increased activity, would be diminished.

Posture, Gait, and Body Movement. Posture, gait, and body movement are also important mobility indicators. Ideal standing posture consists of an erect position, with weight evenly distributed over both feet. The head is balanced midway between level shoulders. The shoulders are aligned directly above the hips, which are centered over the knees and ankles. The knees should be slightly flexed, not locked, and the pelvis level. Figure 30–7 contrasts ideal and incorrect posture.

Slumped posture or guarding of body parts could indicate pain or structural problems interfering with mobility. These can be more thoroughly investigated during the musculoskeletal and neurological assessments.

Gait can also provide clues about mobility status. Walking should be fluid and coordinated, with even weight bearing on each foot. The feet should be parallel. As a step is taken, the heel should strike the ground before the toe and the opposite arm should swing forward slightly. Shuffling, limping, or uncoordinated gait require further investigation later in the examination.

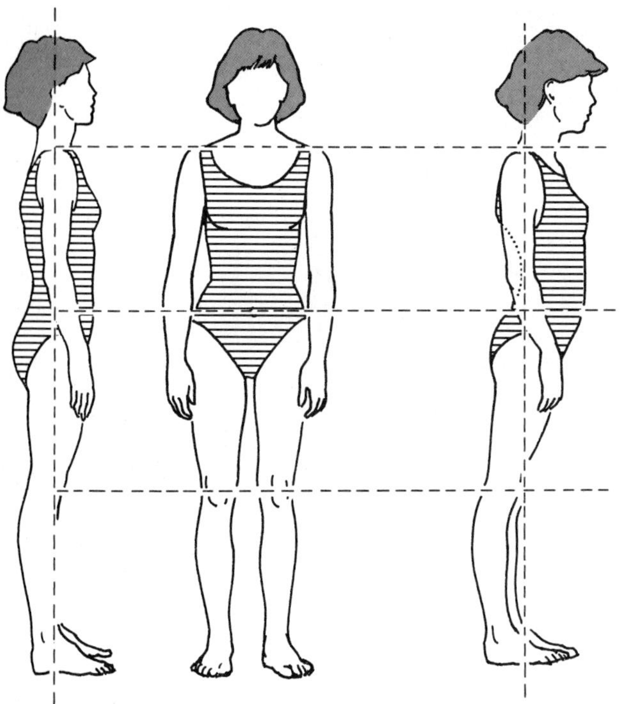

Figure 30–7. Ideal (left) versus incorrect (right) posture.

Gait assessment includes taking note of a client's need for a prosthesis (artificial replacement for a body part) or assistive device such as a cane or walker to walk. If possible, also assess walking without the assistive device and compare the assisted and unassisted gaits.

Observe clients' mode of sitting, lying, and rising from a sitting or lying position. Difficulty with these position changes may indicate a need for strengthening exercises or other nursing assistance with activity. Assess spontaneous body movements for coordination, speed, and symmetry. Uncoordinated, jerky movements; very slow, guarded movements; or marked differences between movements on one side of the body and the other may signal pain, injury, or a disease process that will interfere with mobility. Be aware, also, of apparently involuntary movements such as tics or tremors. Note whether the latter occur during movement or when the client is at rest. This information may be useful for later diagnosis.

If the client is not ambulatory, note the posture usually assumed in bed. Consistent use of one position, constant flexion of the extremities, or infrequent spontaneous movement increase the likelihood that problems related to disuse will develop.

Integument. Skin should be inspected for signs of vulnerability to pressure ulcers, as well as for actual skin breakdown. Skin changes indicating increased vulnerability to pressure ulcers include edema, circulatory stasis, and poor hydration. Edema fluid increases the distance between cells and the capillaries that supply them with nutrients and carry off wastes. Edematous tissue is thus more susceptible to further perfusion problems caused by increased external pressure. Skin that appears thin and shiny is indicative of poor circulation, which also enhances the risk for subsequent pressure ulcers. Skin that appears dry and cracked with poor turgor is poorly hydrated (see Chap. 31). When dehydrated, skin looses elasticity and is more vulnerable to damage from pressure and shearing.

Broken skin or redness over a bony prominence that does not resolve within 15 minutes after pressure is eliminated are indicators of a stage 1 pressure ulcer.[39] Chapter 24 presents a more detailed discussion of assessment for pressure ulcers and their characteristics.

HEENT (Head, Eyes, Ears, Nose, and Throat). If general observation indicates a possible hearing or vision deficit that could interfere with safe mobility, testing for visual and auditory acuity is indicated. Techniques for these examinations are discussed in Chapter 16.

Chest and Cardiovascular. Inspection of the chest reveals conditions that have potential for interfering with mobility. Is breathing labored at rest? With activity? Is the chest symmetrical? Rapid shallow breathing (tachypnea), rapid deep breathing (hyperpnea), or painful, difficult breathing (dyspnea) at rest or with moderate exertion imply a limited capacity for activity.

Abnormalities such as barrel chest or funnel chest, discussed in Chapter 27, are caused by pathological processes that limit air exchange. Abnormal spinal curves, discussed below, can decrease the size of the thoracic cavity, compromising respiratory function, which would also decrease activity tolerance.

Chest auscultation (see Chap. 16) may reveal abnormal breath sounds that are caused by secretions in the respiratory tract. Absence of breath sounds, which may be caused by pneumonia, atelectasis, or pneumothorax, is also significant. All of these conditions could be expected to limit mobility. Cardiac rate and rhythm can also be determined by auscultation of the chest. Additional data about cardiac function are provided by assessment of peripheral pulses (see Chap. 16). A later section, Exercise Tolerance, elaborates further on the assessment of cardiorespiratory function to determine mobility status. Chapters 16 and 27 presents a more detailed discussion of the chest and cardiovascular assessments.

Musculoskeletal. The musculoskeletal examination includes assessment of body alignment, joint mobility, and muscle strength and tone.

Body Alignment. Overall indication of body alignment is obtained during the general survey portion of the mobility examination, discussed earlier. Focused inspection and palpation of spinal curves provides more precise information. Normal spinal curvature is shown in Figure 30–8A: thorax—convex; lumbar—concave. Compare the normal curvature to the examples of abnormal curvature shown in the same figure. Lateral curvature (scoliosis) is more easily observable when a client bends at the waist. Figure 30–8B illustrates the prominent scapulae (winging) associated with scoliosis.

Joint Mobility. Inspection and palpation are also used to assess joint mobility (range of motion, or ROM). If a client is hospitalized, ongoing assessment of ROM is often carried out while assisting with hygiene care. All joints should be observed for swelling, tenderness, or deformity. Note whether temperatures in one or more joints is elevated in comparison to the rest of the body. This abnormal finding could indicate inflammation in the joints. Ask clients to move all joints through the normal ROM.

Normally, a person should be able to move all joints smoothly and without pain through the full range of motion. Inability to do so could be related to weakness, pain, contractures, or other pathology. If a client is unable to move any joint through the ROM independently, you should attempt to move that joint. Observe the approximate ROM active and/or passive, for each joint and compare it to the norms listed in Table 30–4. Do not attempt to force the joint if resistance or pain is felt. Table 30–5 illustrates the techniques for active and passive ROM that may be used as an assessment or a therapeutic measure. Further information about ROM appears in Procedure 30–1 (page 1450).

Muscle Strength and Tone. Muscle strength should also be assessed throughout the full ROM. This is subjectively assessed by applying resistance to clients' muscles as they perform active ROM.

To perform a comprehensive assessment of muscle strength on a client, support the extremities as described for each motion in Table 30–5, but ask the client to perform the corresponding active motion. At the same time, apply opposing pressure to the movement. For example if you have asked the client to adduct the arm at the shoulder, support the elbow and wrist as described for shoulder adduction in Table 30–5, and push on the inside of the arm at the elbow as he or she moves the arm toward the midline of the body. Figure 30–9 (page 1451) illustrates strength testing of some of the muscles of the shoulder girdle and the arm flexors and extensors. Figure 30–10 (page 1453) illustrates strength assessment of hip abductors and the flexors and extensors of the knee. Note that when testing lower extremity muscle strength, clients are asked to lie on an examining table or bed that supports the weight of the extremity. This conserves nurses' energy and enables both

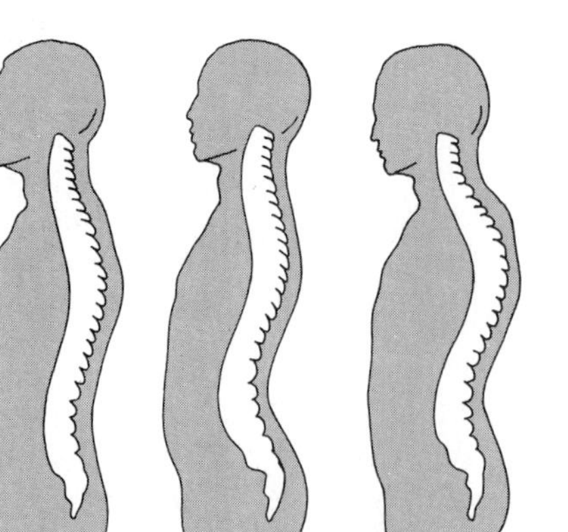

Scoliosis

Figure 30–8. Normal and abnormal spinal curves.

TABLE 30–4. NORMAL RANGE OF MOTION

Part/movement	Adduction	Abduction	Rotation	Flexion	Extension	Hyperextension	Other
Neck (head)	0	0	70°	45°	0	55°	Lateral flexion 45°
Spine-(trunk)	0	0	35°	80°	0	30°	Lateral flexion 35°
Shoulder	50°	180°	Internal 90° External 90°	180°	0° 0°	50° 50°	Elevation 30° Depression 20°
Elbow	0	0	0°	 160°	0	0	Supination 90° Pronation 90°
Wrist	35°	20°	0	90°	0°	70°	
Thumb	90°	90°	0	90°	70°	30–45°	Opposition
Finger	15°	15°	0	90	0	45°	
Hip	30°	45°	Internal 45° External 45°	120° (knee flexed) 90° (knee extended)	0	35°	
Knee	0	0	0	130°	0	10°	
Ankle	0	0	0°	Dorsi 20° Plantor 50°	 0	 0	Inversion 45° Eversion 30°
Toes	10°	10°	0	45°	0	70°	

nurse and client to use better body mechanics during the assessment. Box 30–3 summarizes an abbreviated test of muscle strength that is sufficient for assessing many clients without serious neuromuscular problems.

There are several scales for rating muscle strength, as indicated in Chapter 16. Some examiners use descriptive words such as paralysis; severe, moderate, or minimal weakness; and normal to describe muscle strength instead of the scale presented in Chapter 16. When testing muscle strength, the examiner must be mindful of differences related to age, sex, and level of conditioning. For example, an acutely ill 25-year-old athlete may complain of muscle weakness, but still exhibit a higher degree of resistance than a physically healthy 80-year-old.

Symmetrical response is expected. That is, resistance in the left arm should be about the same as in the right, although the dominant extremities are slightly stronger than those on the opposite side of the body in most healthy people. When a client has a disease or injury involving one extremity or one side of the body, using the healthy extremity as a basis for evaluating losses or gains in the involved extremity is useful.

You should be alert to such abnormalities as cramps, spasms, or increased muscle tone. Muscle cramps are observable as a knot in the belly of the muscle that feels hard when palpated. A spasm involves involuntary contraction of short duration with alternate periods of relaxation. Cramps or spasms can be associated with metabolic and electrolyte alterations, especially abnormal losses of sodium, calcium, and magnesium. They are more common in individuals who are sweating or dehydrated (see Chap. 31). Increased muscle tone can be noted when palpating or moving a relaxed extremity. When tone is increased, resistance is felt in the absence of active movement. Localized tension can be stress related, especially in the neck and jaw. Generalized or one-sided hypertonicity is often associated with neurological disorders.

Neurological. The mental status, balance, coordination, and deep tendon reflex (DTR) examinations are aspects of the neurological assessment that provide information needed for a mobility diagnosis. Much of the mental status assessment can be conducted during the interview. At this time, a nurse can determine a client's level of consciousness (LOC); orientation to time, person, and place; and ability to recall both recent and past events. The appropriateness of client responses to questions in the health history implies orientation and recall. Chapter 29 provides more information about assessing and describing LOC.

Observations of gait and overall movement, as well as assessment of muscle tone and strength, discussed earlier, provide evidence of the level of neurological functioning. If data gathered during these aspects of the examination indicate problems that could prevent safe mobility (eg, uneven, uncoordinated gait, decreased ROM, localized or generalized alterations in muscle strength and tone), a more specific assessment of the client's gait, balance, and coordination is warranted. Box 30–4 (page 1454) highlights elements to observe when assessing gait.

The Romberg test, a simple screening test for balance, is described in Chapter 16. Balance is essential for independent mobility. Balance deficits are a significant factor contributing to client falls, especially among the elderly.[40,41]

Chapter 29 discusses several tests for evaluating coordination. Clumsiness and irregularity of movement suggest the need for supervised or assisted ambulation to prevent injury. Whenever irregularities of movement are noted, it is useful to assess deep tendon reflexes (DTRs), as illustrated in Chapter 16. Abnormally slow or unusually brisk reflexes imply pathology that could interfere with safe ambulation.

Exercise Tolerance. **Exercise tolerance** refers to the amount (rate and duration) of a given exercise a person can perform before experiencing exhaustion or distress. Evaluating an individual's response to exercise demand is an important part of the mobility assessment. Prior to planning an exercise or activity regimen with clients, analyze baseline data about cardiopulmonary, neurological, and musculoskeletal functioning to predict the amount and type of activity that would provide sufficient stimulation to maintain or improve clients' level of fitness without overtaxing them. If a client is hospitalized, exercise is usually limited to ambulation, isometrics, and other stationary exercises described in a later section of the chapter, Nursing *Implementation to Promote Optimum Mobility.* Discharge or-

(Text continues on page 1449.)

TABLE 30–5. ASSESSING OR ASSESSING WITH RANGE OF MOTION

	Active		Passive	
Movement	**Illustration**	**Instructions for Client**	**Illustration**	**Description of Nurse's Action**
HEAD		Tell client to:		
Rotation	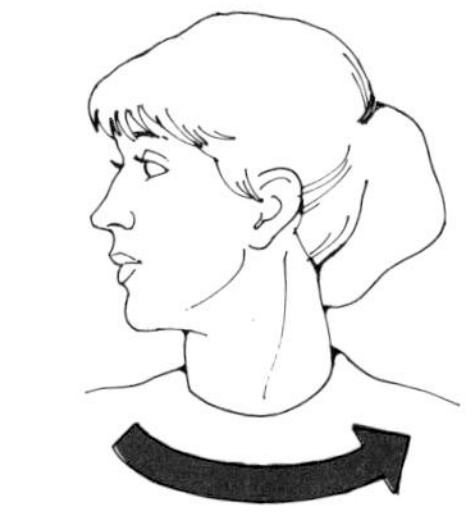	Turn head as far as possible to the left, then to the right.	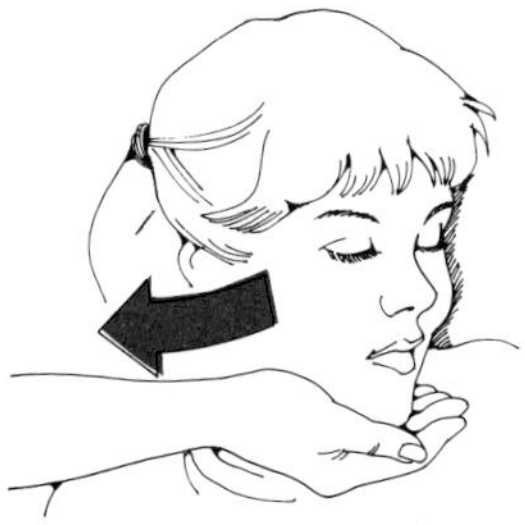	Cup the palm of your hand under the client's chin. Pull or push chin in an arc toward each shoulder and return. (Note: no pillow)
Forward Flexion	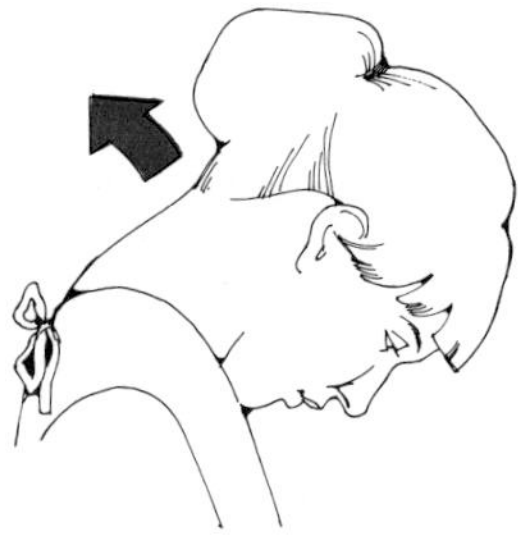	Move head as if to look at feet, then return to resting position.	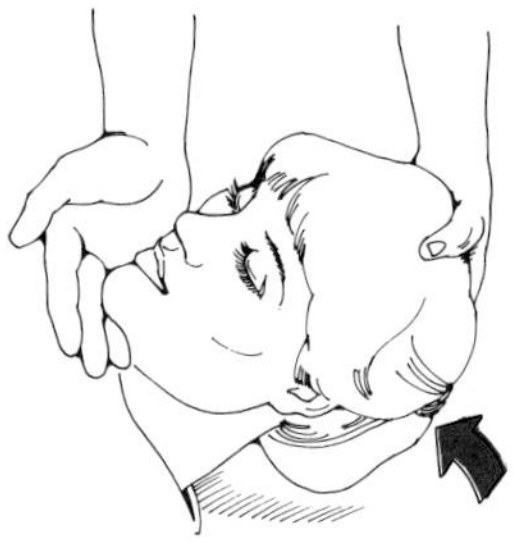	Cup hands behind client's head, pulling head upward toward chest.
Lateral Flexion	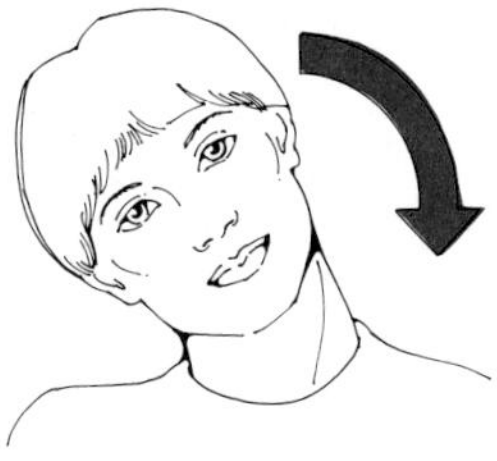	Tilt head so left ear moves toward left shoulder. Repeat for right.	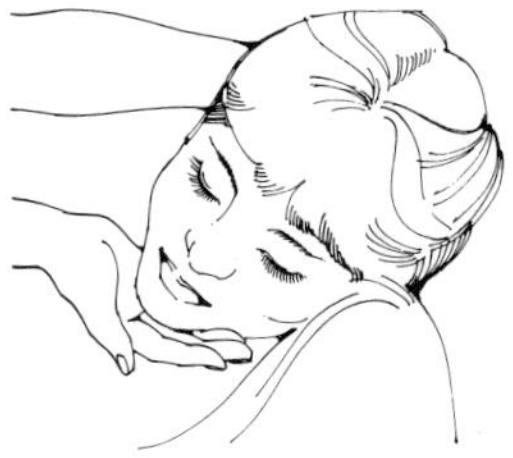	Supporting the head as above, tilt the head so left ear moves toward the left shoulder. Repeat for right.
Hyperextension	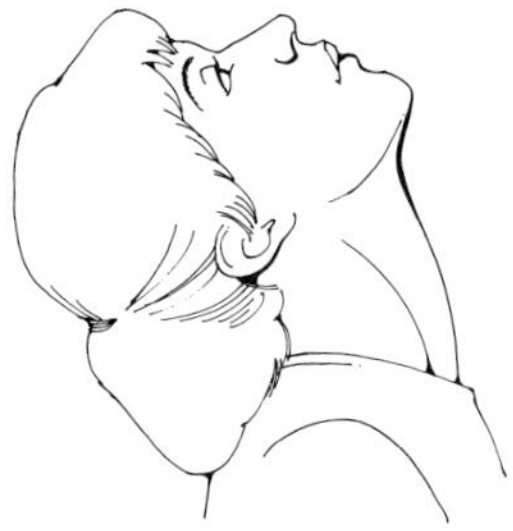	Tip head back as if looking up.	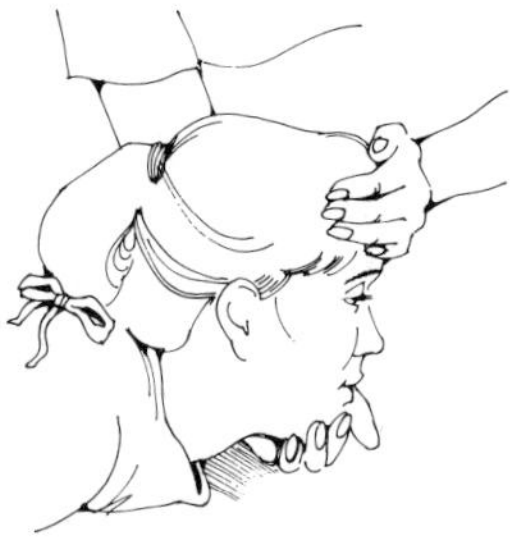	Seated or side-lying—done after all supine exercises. Place one hand on the client's forehead, the other under chin. Move the head in an arc toward the back.

TABLE 30–5. (continued)

Movement	Active: Illustration	Active: Instructions for Client	Passive: Illustration	Passive: Description of Nurse's Action
Circumduction	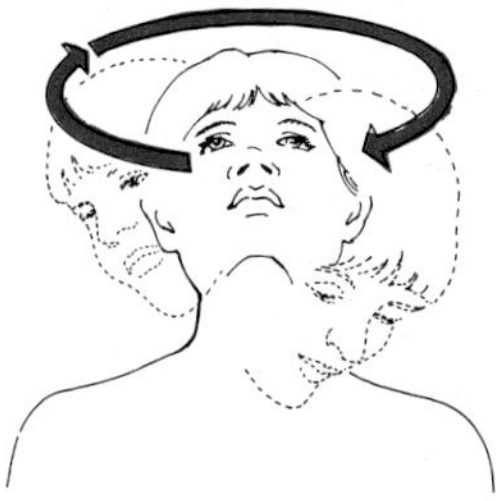	Roll head as if drawing a large circle with the top of the head, left to right, then right to left.	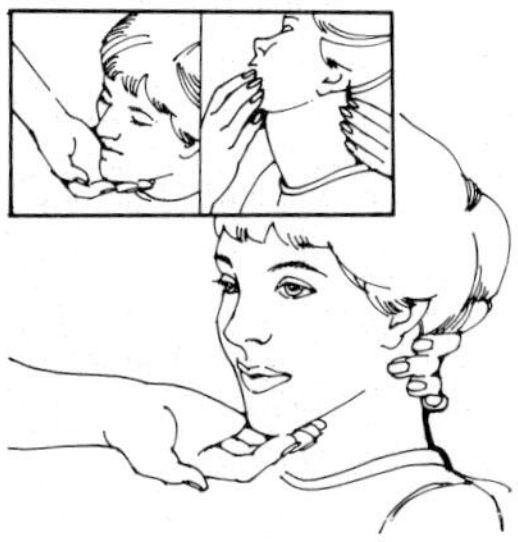	Support chin and occiput with palms of hands when client is sitting up. Rotate head in circular motion to right, then to left.
UPPER EXTREMITY				
Shoulder				
Flexion	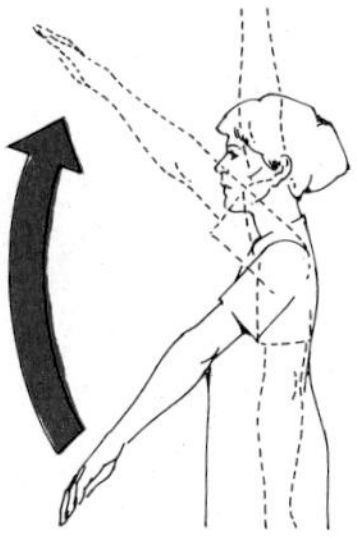	Start with arm at side or flexed so forearm is across chest. Move arm above head in a smooth arc. (Hand or elbow will make a half-circle in movement.)	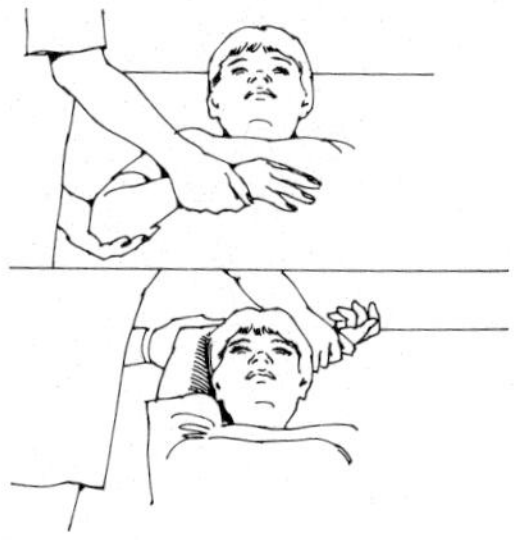	Flex arm across chest. Cup elbow in one hand, grasp wrist joint to support wrist and hand. Move arm above client's head so elbow describes 180° arc.
Adduction	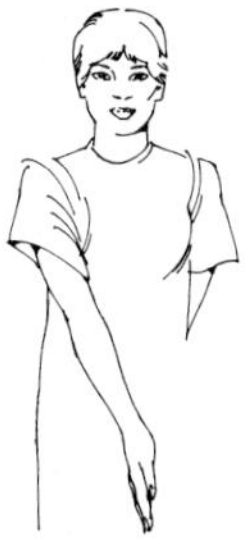	Bring arm across chest, moving elbow as close to middle of body as possible.	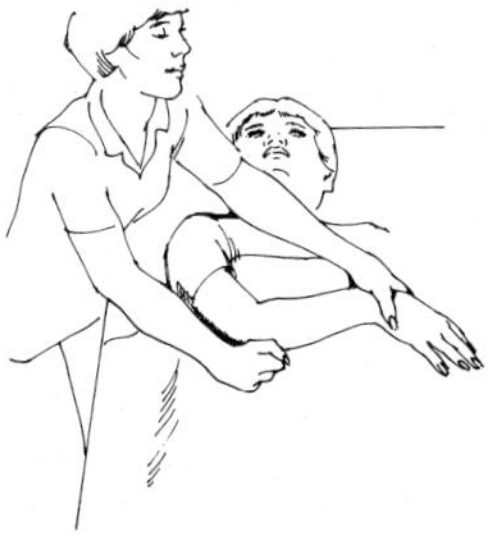	Bracketed movements are performed together: Grasping elbow and wrist joint as above, move elbow across chest toward midline.
Abduction	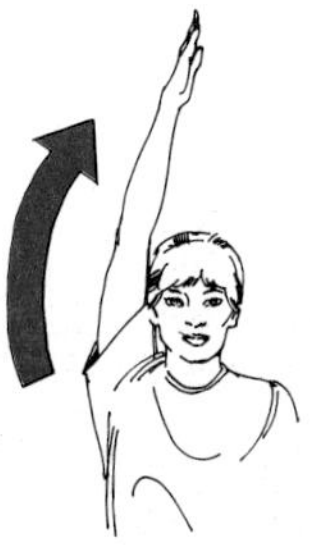	After the above, move arm outward, away from the body, then up over head.	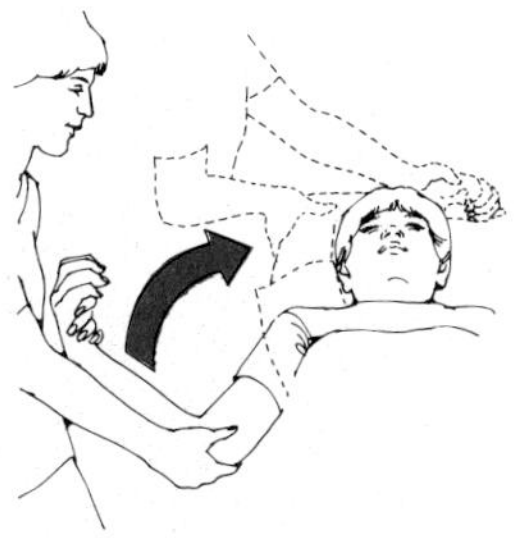	Starting in adduction and keeping arm flexed and supported as above, move arm away from the body, then over the head.
Internal rotation	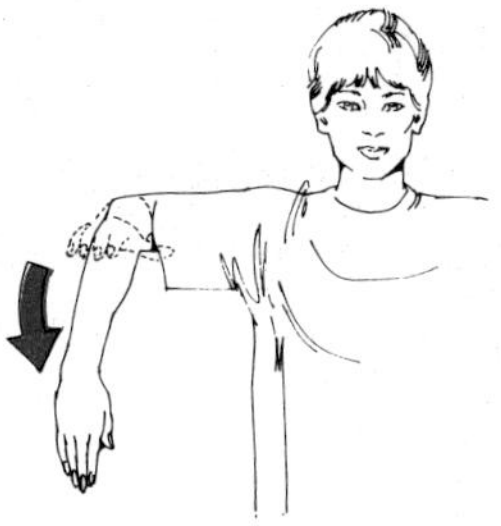	Start with arm straight out to the side from shoulder with palm facing front and elbow bent in 90° angle. Move hand downward so fingers point to floor. (If lying down, hand should be raised above body.) Move hand forward so palm touches bed next to hip. Upper arm remains on the bed.	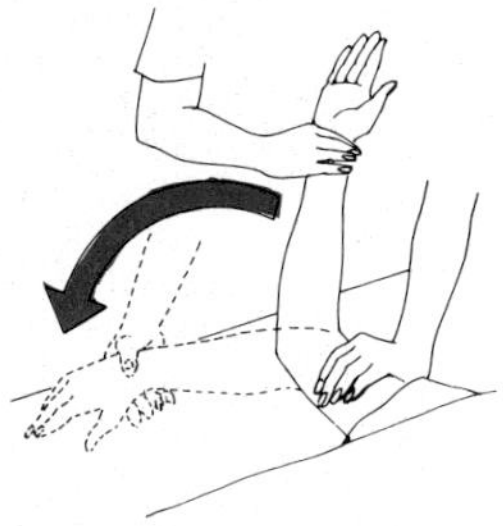	Move arm straight out from shoulder; flex elbow so hand is raised. Support wrist joint as above and stabilize upper arm. Press gently on shoulder with your other hand. With elbow as fulcrum, move the hand downward so hand describes an arc, touching bed next to client's hip if possible.

(continued)

TABLE 30–5. (continued)

	Active		Passive	
Movement	**Illustration**	**Instructions for Client**	**Illustration**	**Description of Nurse's Action**
External rotation	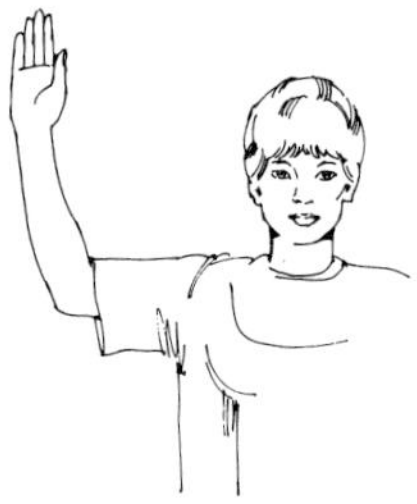	After completing internal rotation, move hand so fingers point up. (If lying down, keep upper arm on bed and move hand so back of hand touches bed next to head.)	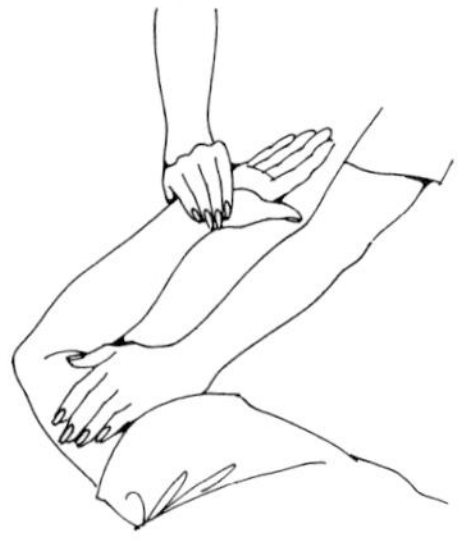	After above, move the hand upward so the back of the hand touches the bed next to client's head.
Circumduction	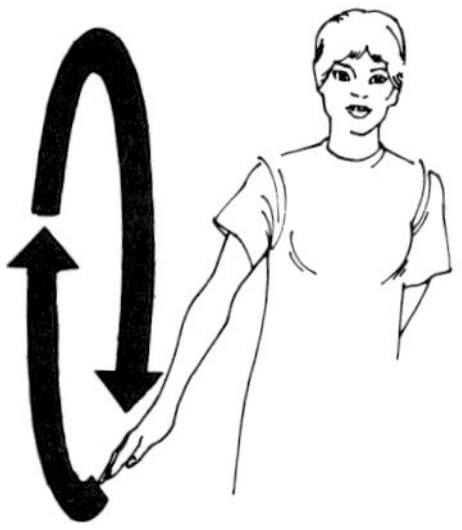	Extend arm straight out from body at shoulder. Move hand as if to draw a circle.	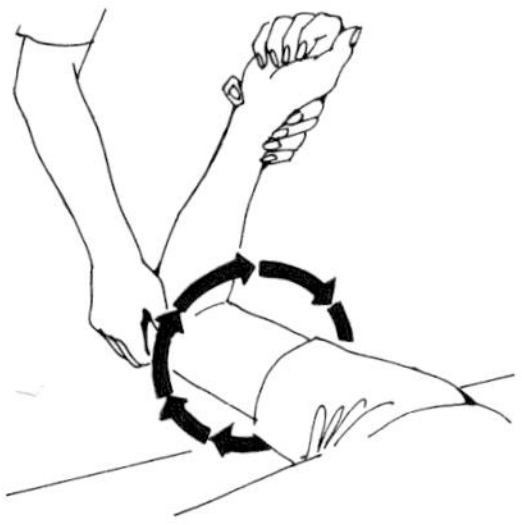	After above, extend the elbow so the arm points out from body. Cupping the elbow and supporting the wrist joint, move the arm in a circular motion.
Hyperextension	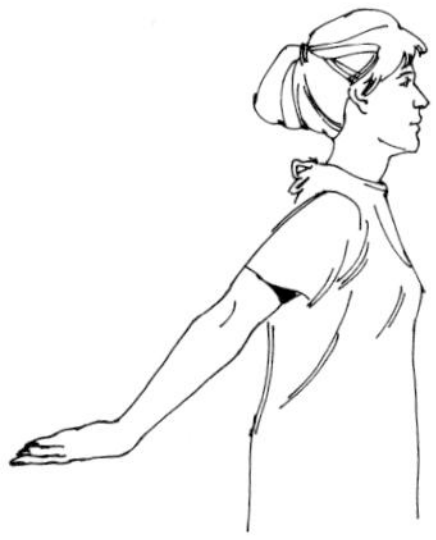	When standing or sitting with arm at side, swing arm backwards as far as possible without turning hand. May also be done lying on side.	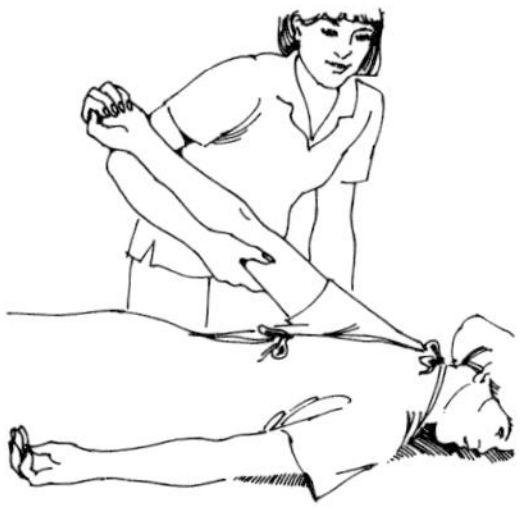	(Done at the completion of all exercises in the supine position.) With client prone or side-lying, arm at side, cradle arm to support elbow and wrist joints. Move the arm toward the back as far as possible, so the hand makes an arc.
ELBOW				
Pronation	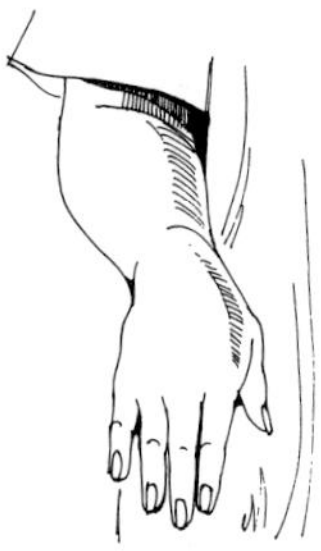	Starting with arms at sides, bend arm with palm facing upward, then turn palm toward floor.	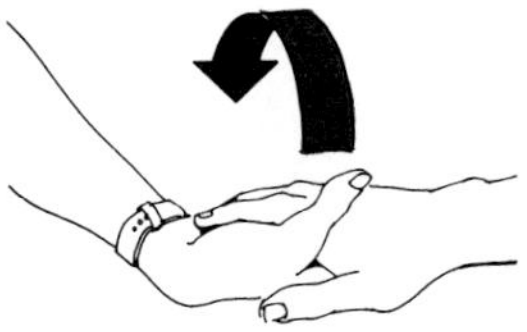	Hold client's hand as if to shake hands, elbow may rest on bed or be cupped by other hand. Turn your hand so client's hand faces the floor.
Supination	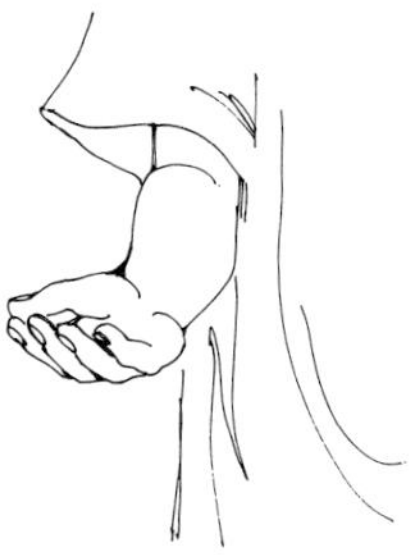	Starting in elbow pronation position, turn palm up toward ceiling.	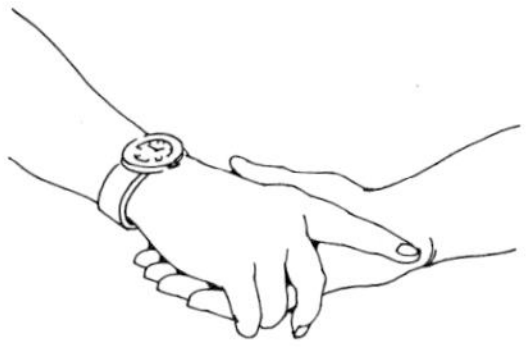	When above completed, turn palm up toward ceiling.

TABLE 30–5. (continued)

	Active		Passive	
Movement	**Illustration**	**Instructions for Client**	**Illustration**	**Description of Nurse's Action**
Flexion	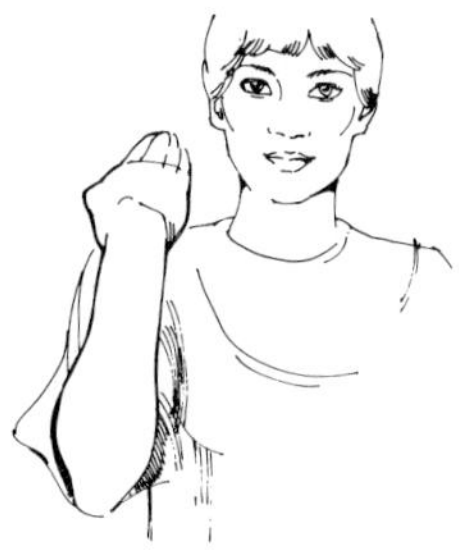	Starting with arm at side, bend elbow, moving hand toward shoulder.	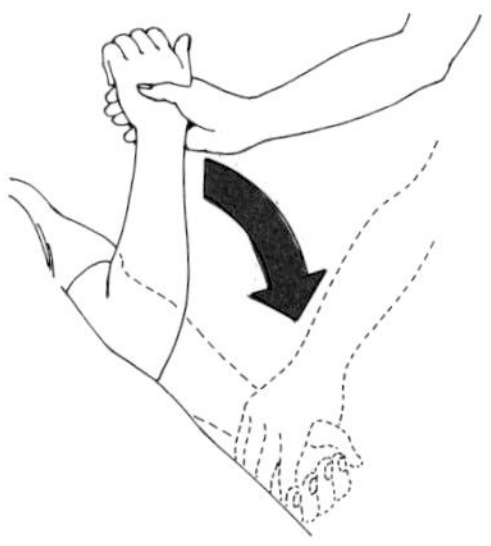	Place client's arm at the side, palm up or facing thigh. Grasp client's hand and wrist. With client's elbow resting on bed, move client's fingers toward the shoulder and return to straight position.
Extension	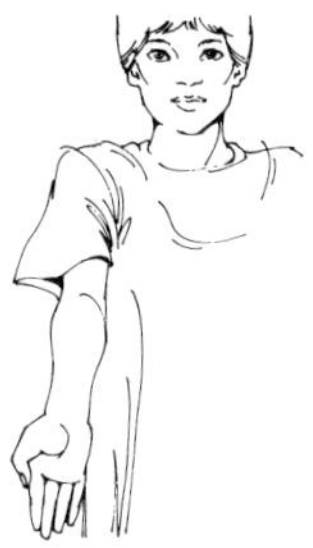	Return to starting position.		
Circumduction	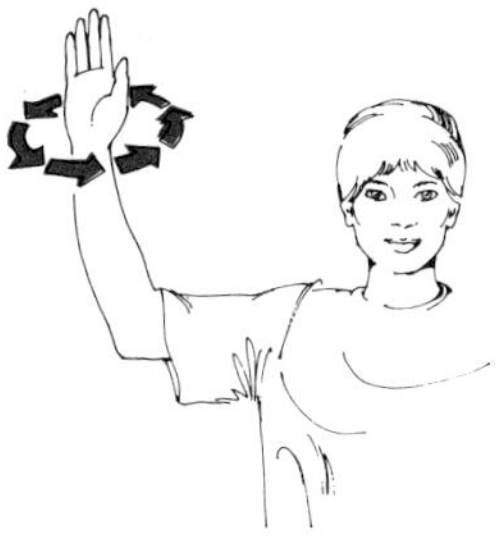	Place elbow out so it is level with shoulder. Move hand in a circle.	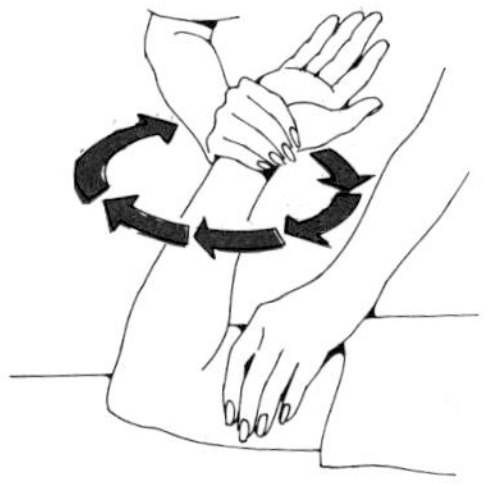	Rest elbow on bed. Grasp wrist and describe circle with hand while stabilizing upper arm with your other hand.
WRIST **Adduction (ulnar deviation)**	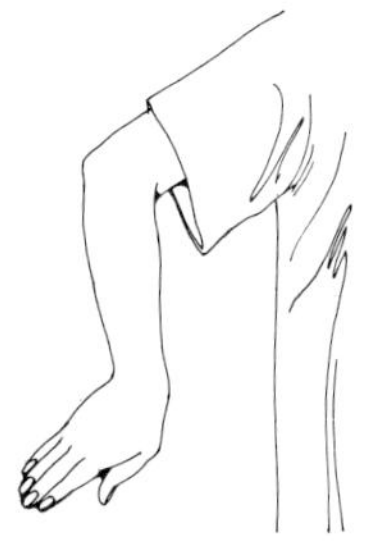	Tell the client Oto: With arm at side, bend wrist as if to touch side of arm with little finger.	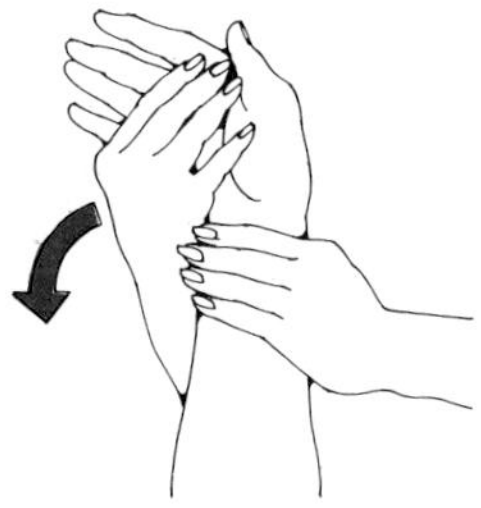	Place client's palm in yours. Grasp wrist with your other hand. Move client's hand from side to side as if to touch thumb (abduction) and little finger (adduction) alternately on either side of arm.
Abduction (radial deviation)	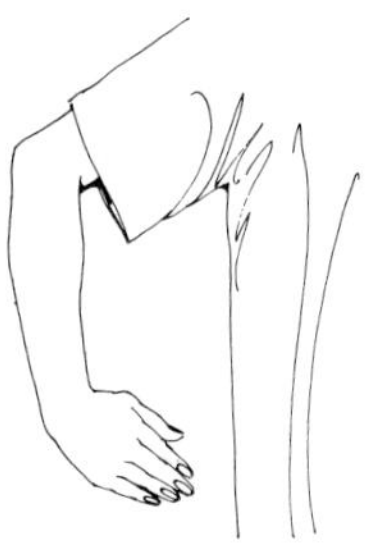	With arm at side, bend wrist as if to touch thumb on side of arm.	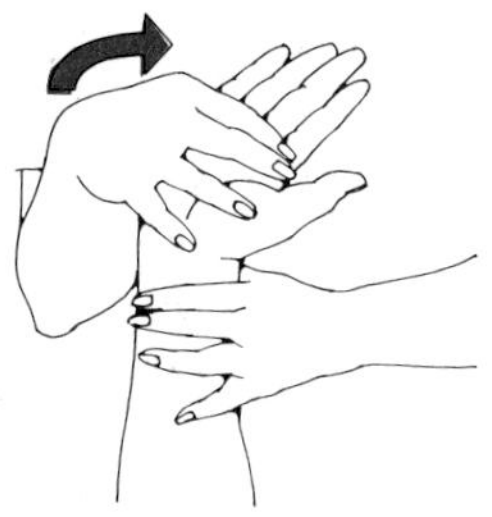	

(continued)

TABLE 30–5. (continued)

	Active		Passive	
Movement	**Illustration**	**Instructions for Client**	**Illustration**	**Description of Nurse's Action**
Flexion	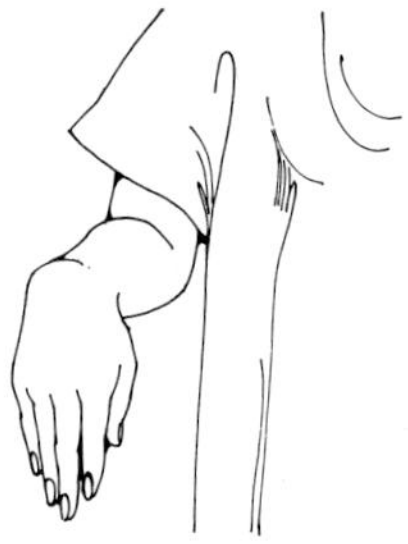	Bend wrist so palm moves toward it.	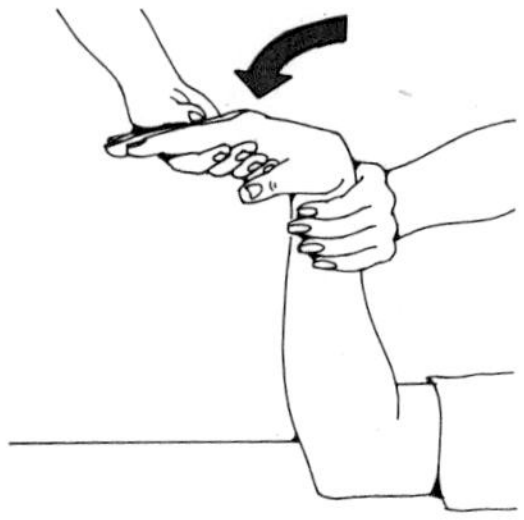	Rest elbow on bed, grasp wrist. Hold client's hand so yours and client's fingers are perpendicular. Flex palm toward wrist.
Hyperextension	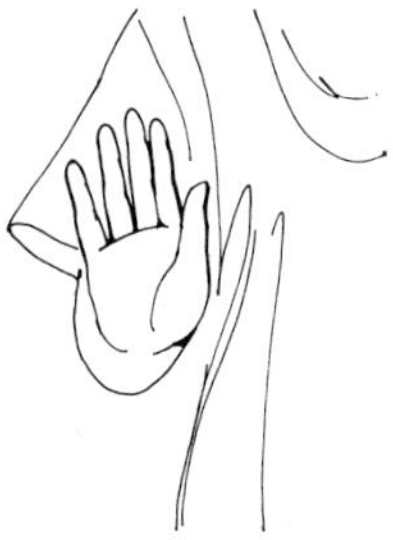	Bend wrist so back of hand moves toward it.	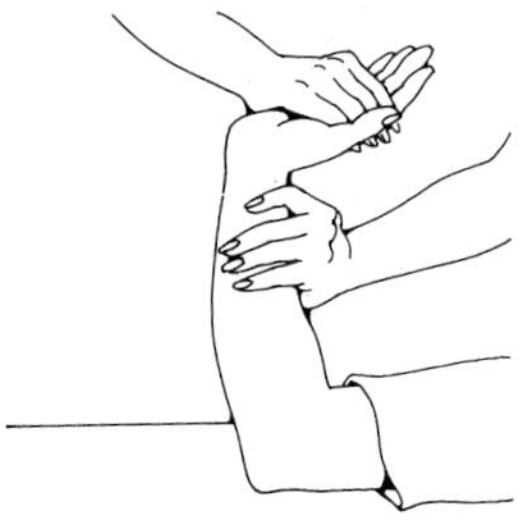	When wrist flexion completed, extend wrist, then move back of hand toward wrist.
Circumduction	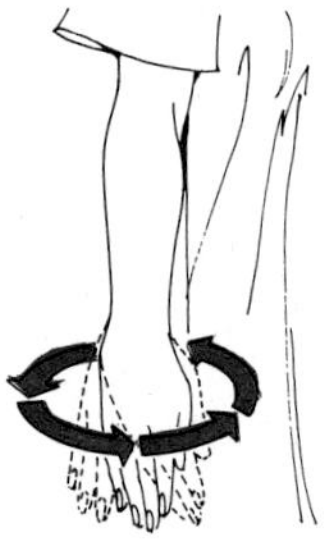	Move hand as if stirring—make a circle with hand.	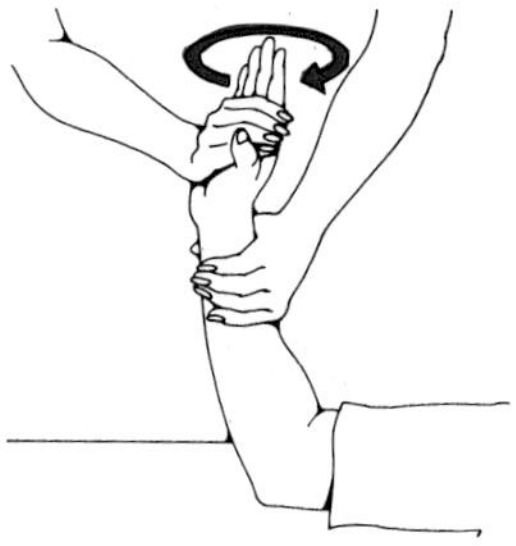	Supporting client's hand as above, move hand in circular motion.
FINGERS				
Adduction/ abduction	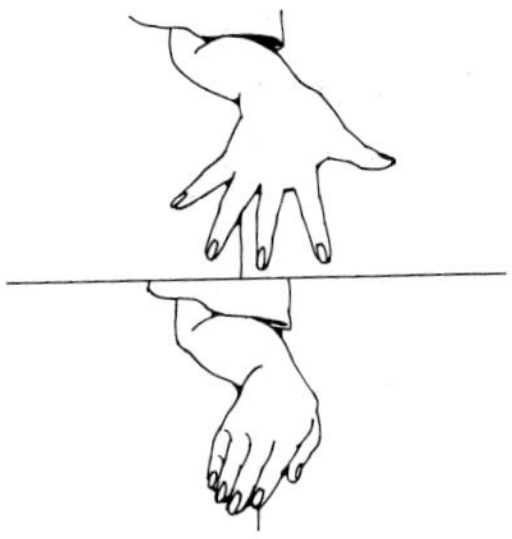	Spread fingers and thumb as far as possible, then bring together.	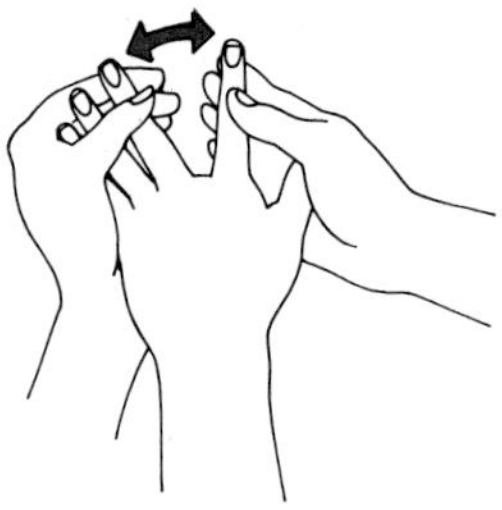	With arm resting on bed or across chest, move the thumb and each finger away from the adjacent finger and return.
Opposition	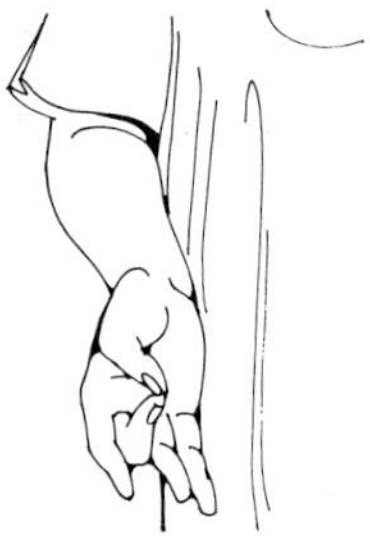	Touch each finger to thumb.	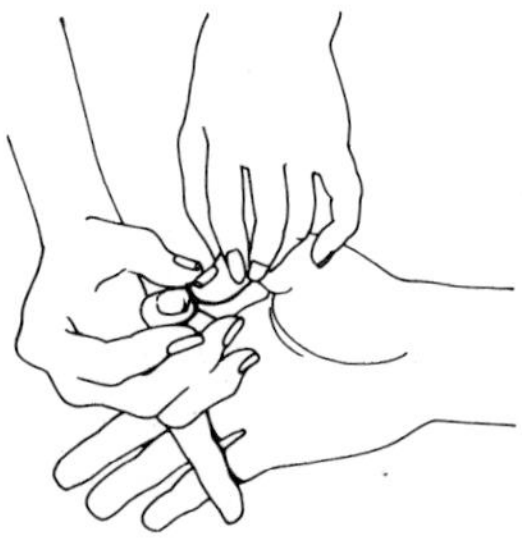	With hand still resting in bed, touch each finger to thumb.

TABLE 30–5. (continued)

	Active		Passive	
Movement	**Illustration**	**Instructions for Client**	**Illustration**	**Description of Nurse's Action**
Circumduction	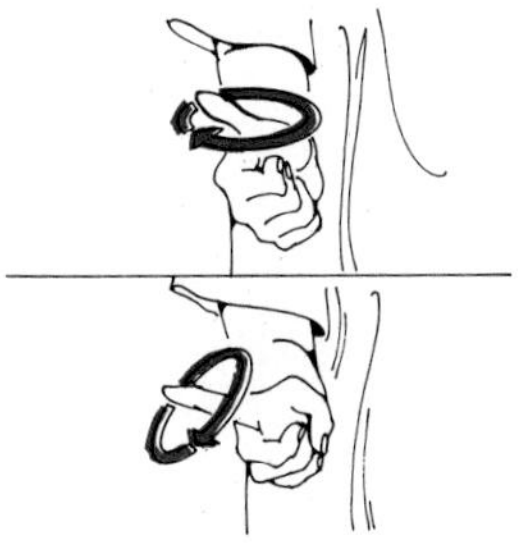	Make a circle with each finger and thumb.	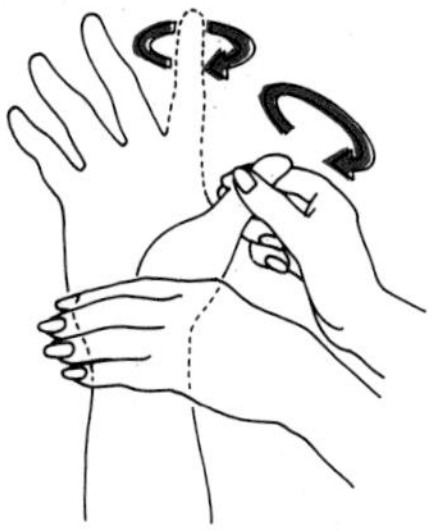	Move each finger and thumb in a circle while supporting wrist.
Flexion/ extension	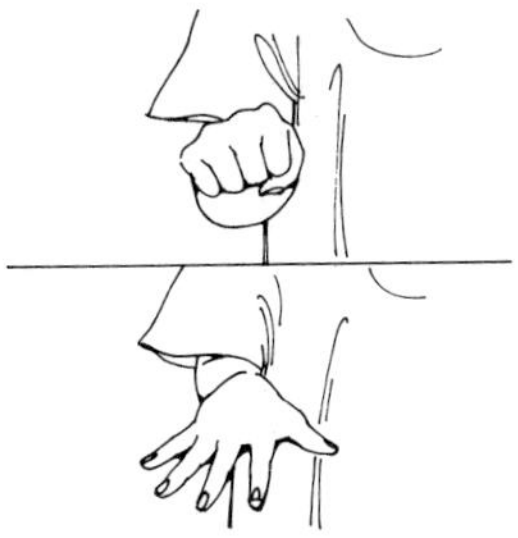	Make a fist, straighten and repeat.	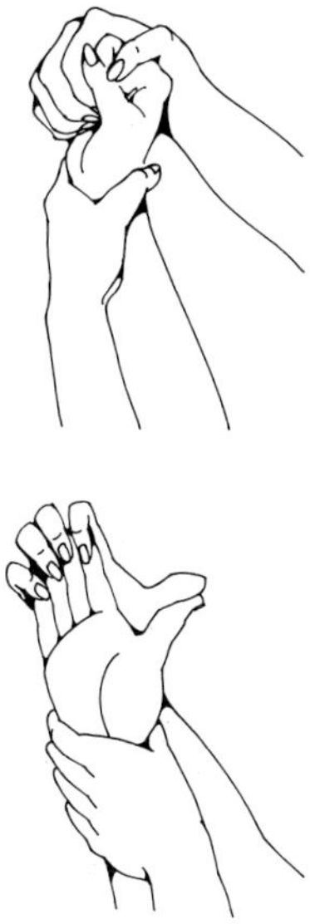	Flex elbow, grasp wrist. Place the palm of your other hand on the back of the client's hand and flex all fingers and thumb with yours. Hook your fingertips under client's flexed fingers and thumb and pull them to extension, *or* slide your palm under client's flexed fingers, extending the fingers and thumb as you do.
Hyperextension	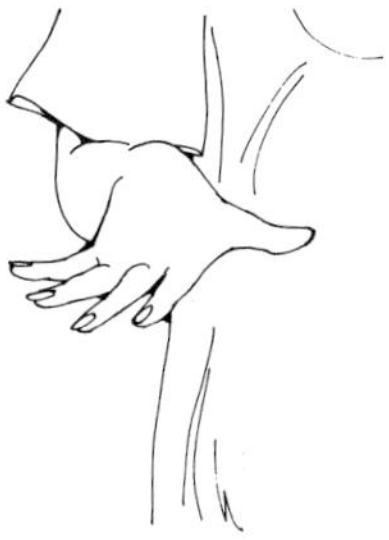	Stretch fingers and thumb toward the back of hand.	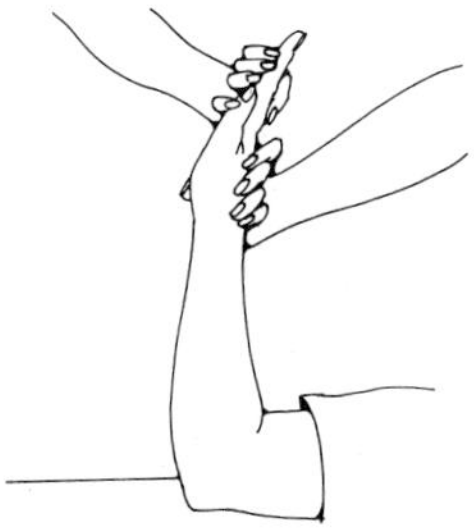	Continue to apply pressure on fingers and thumb to hyperextend them.
LOWER EXTREMITY				
HIP				
Internal rotation	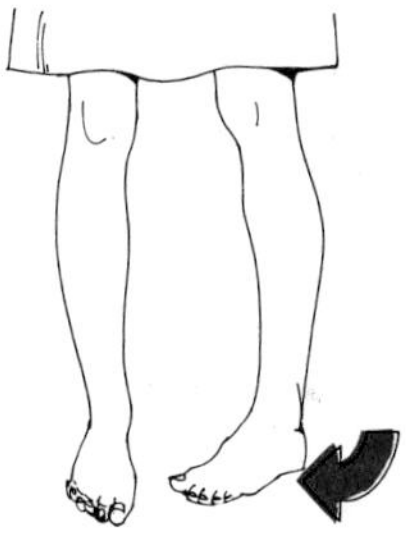	Keeping knee straight and foot perpendicular to leg, turn foot toward center of body.	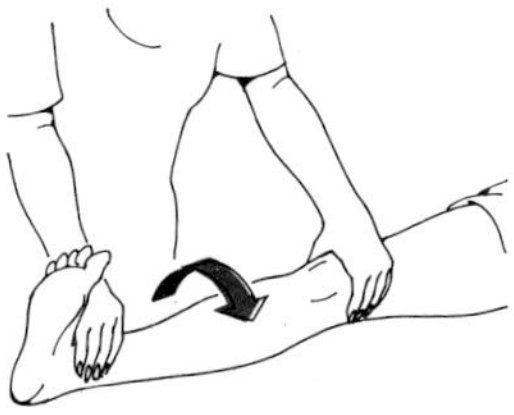	With leg resting on bed, rotate leg toward midline.

(continued)

TABLE 30–5. (continued)

	Active		Passive	
Movement	**Illustration**	**Instructions for Client**	**Illustration**	**Description of Nurse's Action**
External rotation	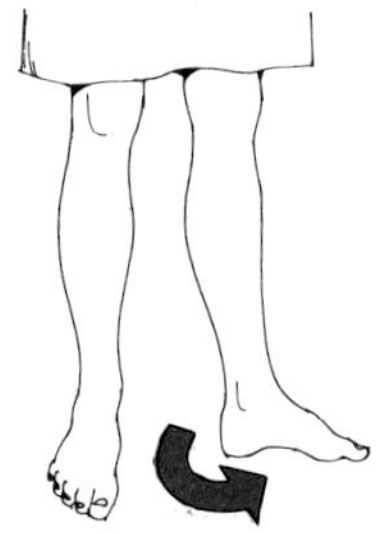	In same position as above, turn foot outward.	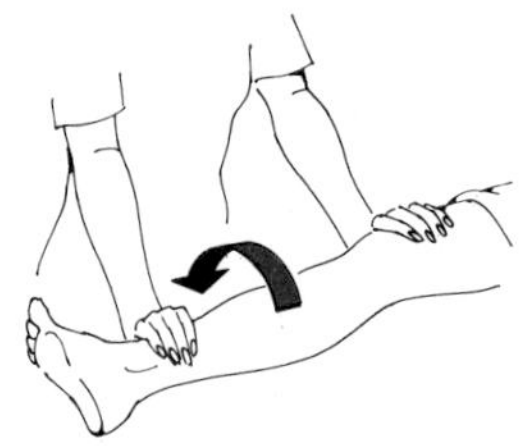	With leg resting on bed, rotate leg outward.
Adduction	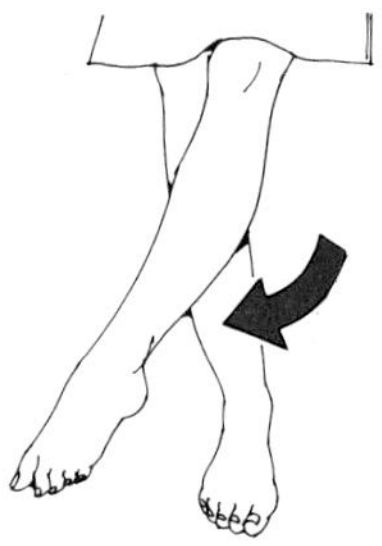	Bring one leg across and in front of the other leg.	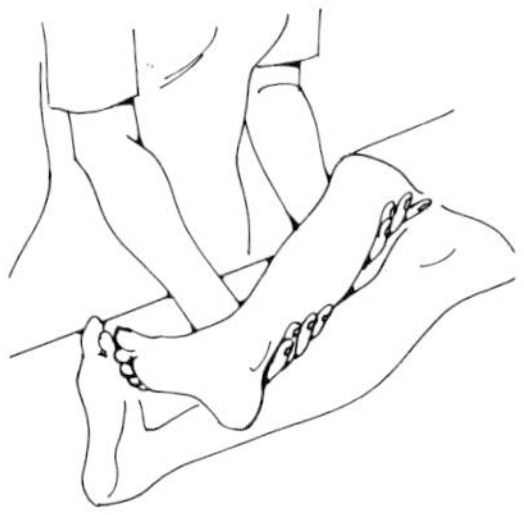	Support leg behind ankle and knee. Move leg toward midline.
Abduction	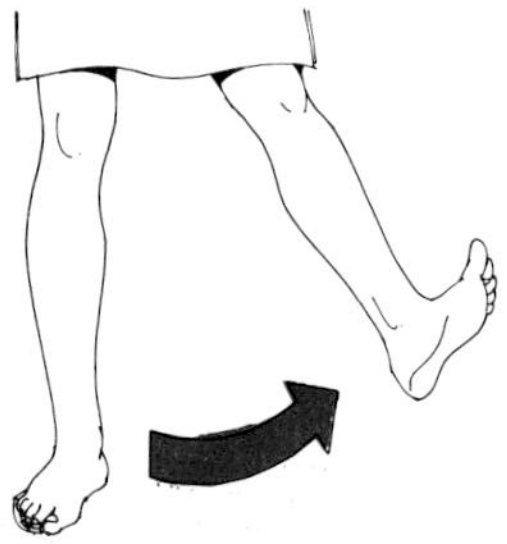	Move leg out to the side as far as possible.	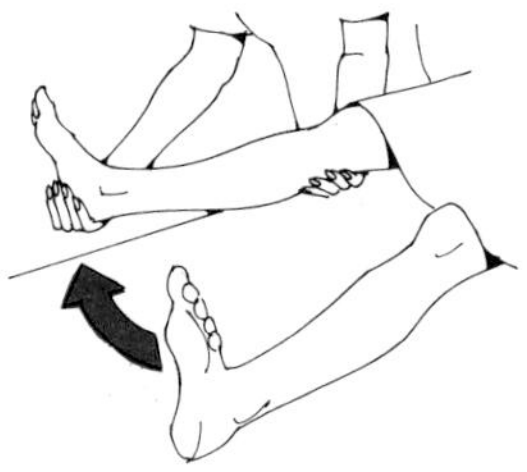	Support as above, move leg outward away from midline. Step away from side of bed to fully abduct hip.
Circumduction	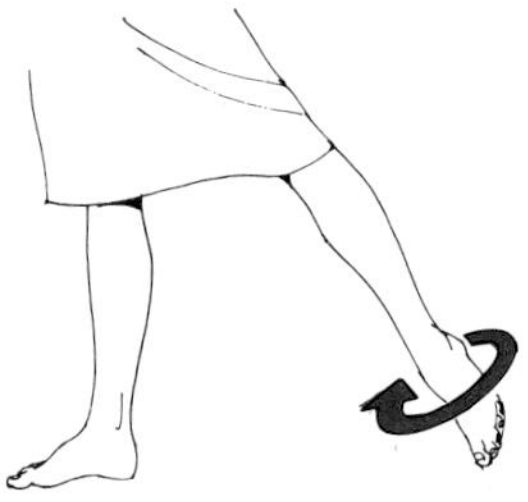	With leg straight, move foot in circular motion.	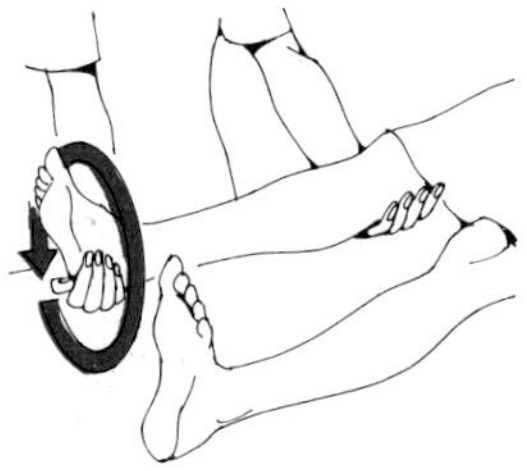	Supporting leg as above, move it in a circular motion, keeping leg straight.
Flexion	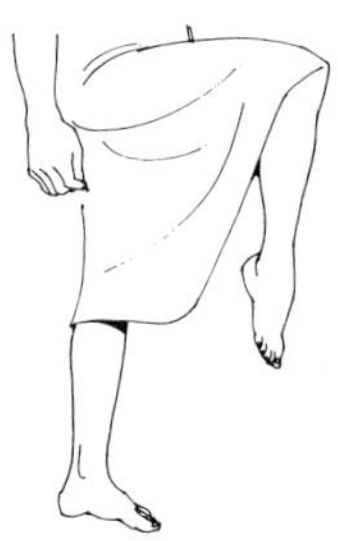	Bend hip and knee bringing knee close to chest. Can assist by grasping knee with arms (see knee flexion below).	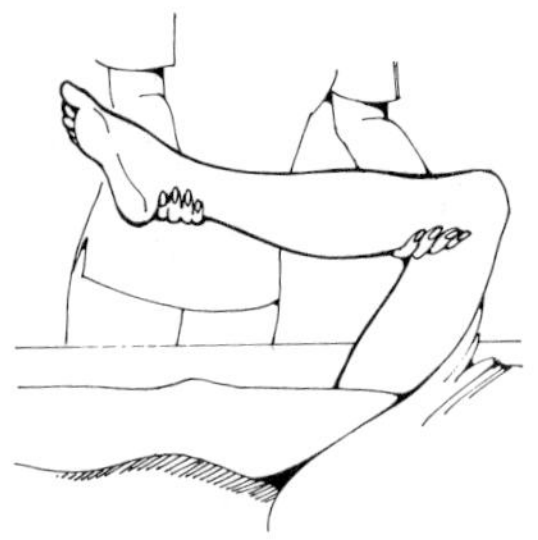	Support ankle and calf to flex knee and hip, pushing thigh toward abdomen.

TABLE 30–5. (continued)

Movement	Active: Illustration	Active: Instructions for Client	Passive: Illustration	Passive: Description of Nurse's Action
Hyperextension	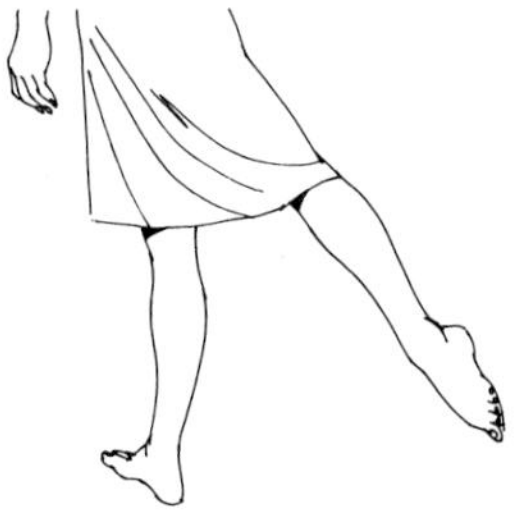	Point toe move leg backward with knee straight.	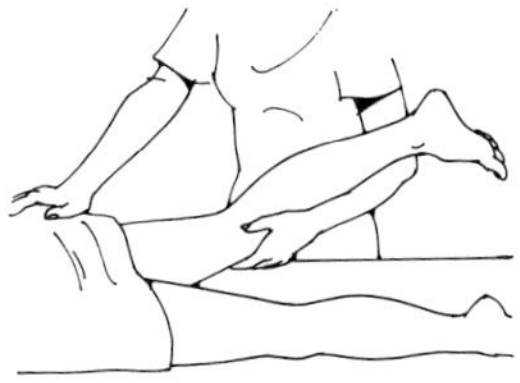	(Done after all leg exercises in supine position have been completed.) Place client on side or prone. Cradle lower leg with arm. Applying counterpressure on buttocks, raise leg off bed. (Move leg backward if lying on side.)
KNEE				
Flexion	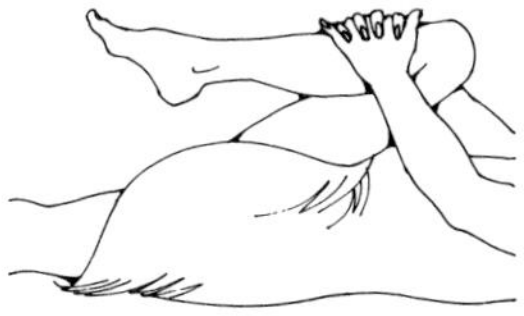	Lying on back, bend knee to chest and grasp with arms.		Done with hip flexion.
Circumduction	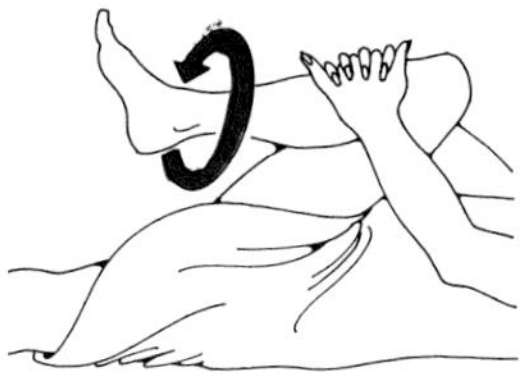	With knee flexed, move foot in circular motion.	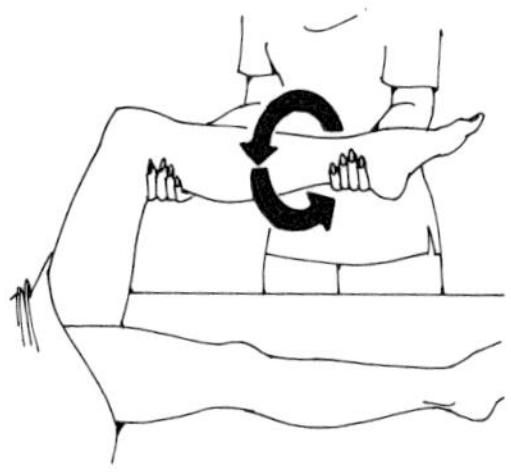	Support back of knee, ankle. With knee flexed, move lower leg in circular motion.
Hyperextension	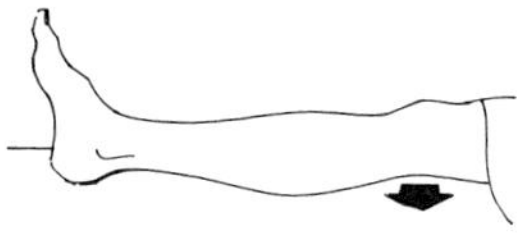	Sitting with leg extended, push back of knee against surface below.	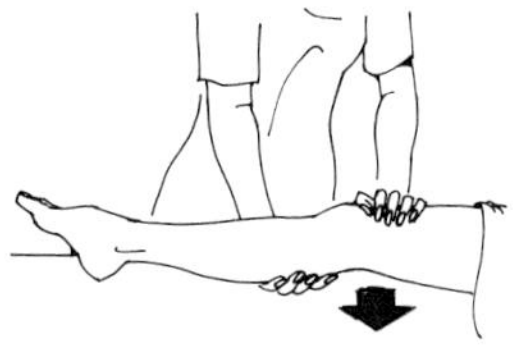	Cradle knee joint. Apply counterpressure above knee, gently raise lower leg until you feel resistance.
ANKLE				
Inversion		Tell the client to: Turn the sole of the foot toward the other leg.		With leg resting on bed, stabilize ankle, grasp forefoot with fingers on sole. Turn sole of the foot toward midline.

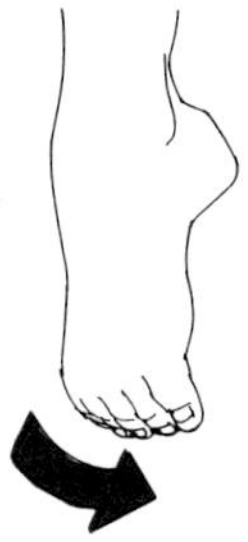

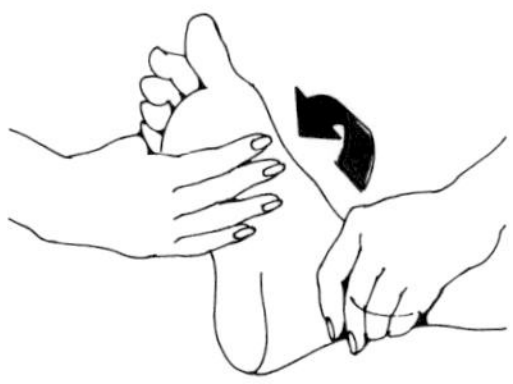

(continued)

TABLE 30–5. (continued)

	Active		Passive	
Movement	**Illustration**	**Instructions for Client**	**Illustration**	**Description of Nurse's Action**
Eversion	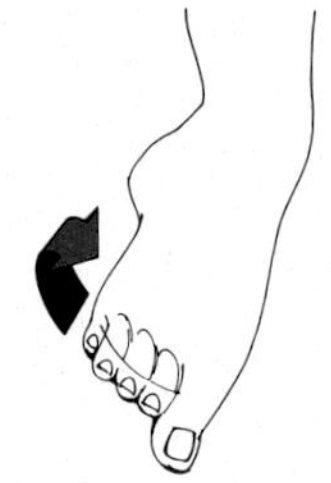	Turn the sole of the foot to the outside.	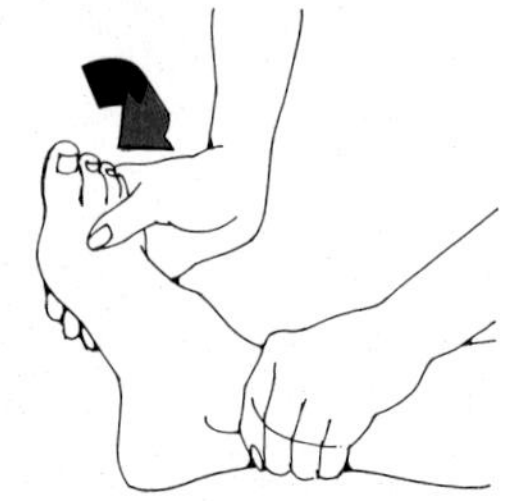	Holding forefoot as above, turn the sole away from the midline.
Dorsiflexion	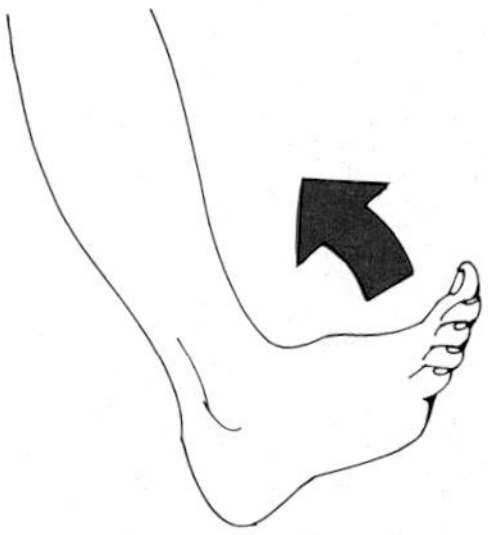	Bend the foot toward the shin.	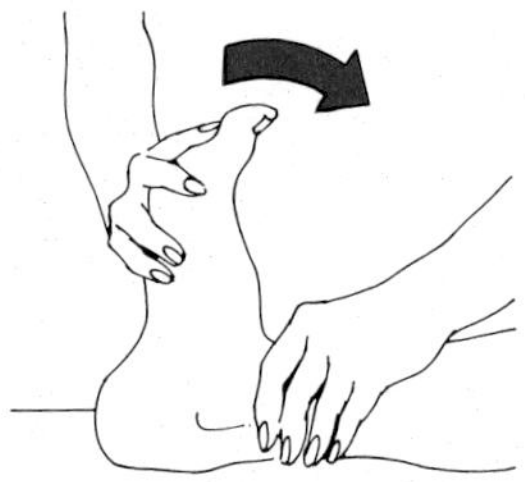	Holding foot as above, flex the foot toward the shin. (May also cup heel with hand and use forearm to flex foot.)
Plantar flexion	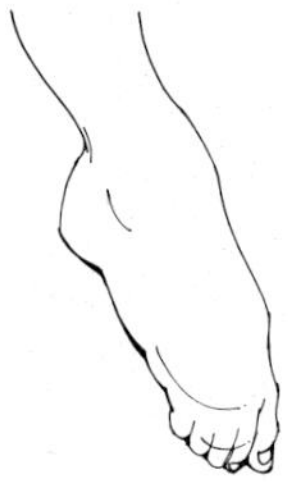	Point the toe.	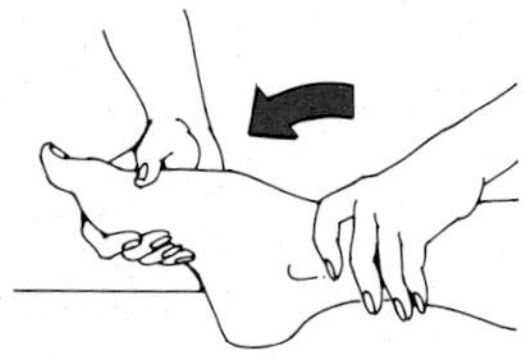	Holding foot as above, straighten foot as if to point toe.
Circumduction	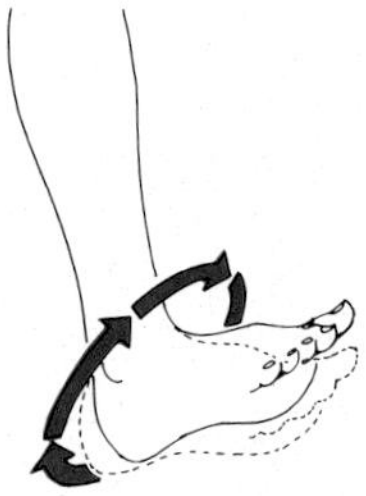	Move foot in circular motion at ankle without moving the knee.	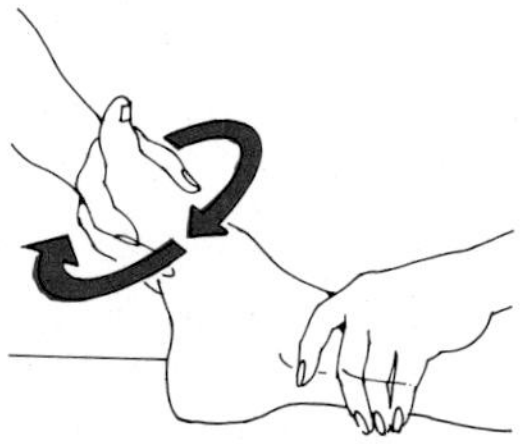	With foot in plantar flexion, rotate forefoot in circular motion.
TOES				
Flexion	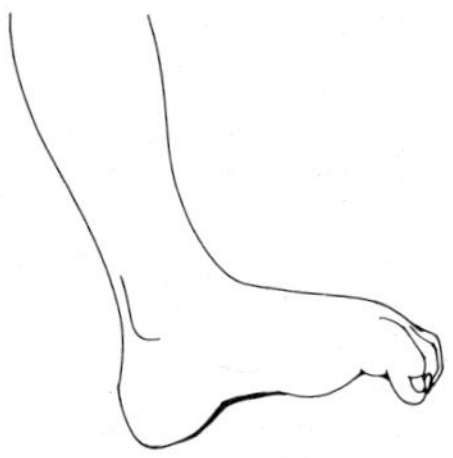	Curl toes.	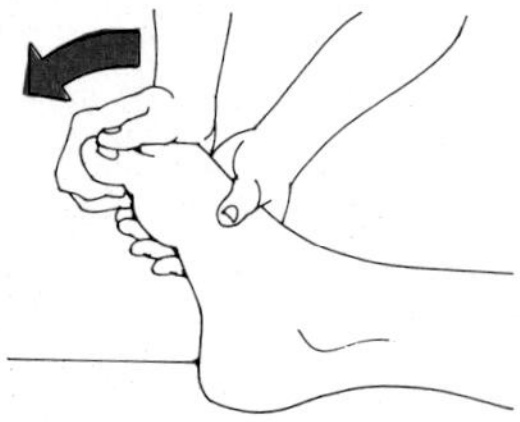	Flex toes toward sole of foot by applying pressure with fingers.

TABLE 30–5. (continued)

Movement	Active: Illustration	Active: Instructions for Client	Passive: Illustration	Passive: Description of Nurse's Action
Hyperextension		Raise toes off floor without raising foot.		Move one hand behind toes and the other hand to forefoot, apply hand pressure to more toes toward ankle.
Adduction/ abduction		Spread toes.		With leg resting on bed, separate each toe from the one adjacent.
Circumduction				Move each toe in a circular motion.

Document exercise as described in Proc. 30–1.

rehabilitation planning sometimes involves collaboration with other members of the health care team and the use of a more sophisticated testing protocol using standardized measures and special equipment. This kind of exercise testing is recommended for any sedentary individual over 45 years old who desires to begin an exercise program as well as clients having other risk factors discussed in Section. 1.[22]

Baseline data needed for activity assessment are shown in Table 30–6 (page 1455). If data in one or more categories indicate a caution, plan to initiate exercise at a mild level and increase the intensity gradually. Consultation with a physician or a physical therapist may be necessary prior to planning exercises for some clients.

Observations during exercise are a significant component of assessing activity tolerance. Many clients can assess themselves as they exercise; when assisting hospitalized clients with exercise, however, these observations are a nursing responsibility. Assess the following:

1. *Pulse rate and rhythm.* As discussed in Section 1, changes in pulse have been shown by research to be an accurate indicator of exercise tolerance. While higher target heart rates are desired to maximize exercise benefits, as noted in Section 1, increases of more than 20 to 25 beats per minute are not expected nor desired during exercises typical in a hospital setting. If a client's pulse increases more than 15 beats per minute or if alterations in pulse rhythm occur, the exercise session should be terminated. If no unusual circumstances can account for this change, the exercise plan should be reevaluated.
2. *Respiratory rate and depth.* An increase in both rate and depth of respiration is expected; however, dyspnea indicates overexercise. Diaphragmatic spasm may cause a pain in the side, commonly called a "stitch," when respiratory effort is increased, but this is not expected as a result of the level of exercise common in an acute care setting.
3. *Skin changes.* The vasodilation of skin blood vessels that occurs to dissipate the heat produced by increased muscular activity causes observable skin changes. Because the cheeks, lips, and nailbeds are highly vascular,

PROCEDURE 30–1. GUIDELINES FOR JOINT RANGE OF MOTION

PURPOSE: To assess current ROM, prevent joint contractures, and maintain muscle strength (active ROM only).

EQUIPMENT: None.

ACTION

1. Discuss the procedure and the purpose with the client, including the nurse's actions and client participation desired, using language the client can understand. Even apparently unconscious individuals may be able to hear and benefit from verbal communication.
2. Active ROM:
   a. Describe and demonstrate the desired movements for each joint (see Table 30–5 for details).
   b. Repeat demonstration/instruction as needed. Relate movements to usual activities of daily living—walking, sitting, eating, hygiene—to show how these contribute to mobility.
   c. Ask client to perform each exercise while you watch. Give immediate feedback to enhance learning and increase the likelihood of behavior being repeated.
   d. Provide positive reinforcement for correct performance. Give suggestions for change in technique, if exercise is performed incorrectly because incorrect performance of an exercise may result in minimal benefit or injury.
   e. Ask client to repeat each movement smoothly at least three to five times and to exercise three times every day. Remind client that pacing is important to prevent fatigue. Emphasize the importance of stopping the exercise if pain occurs and to report this immediately.
   f. Mutually developing a schedule for exercises based on client's usual daily pastimes will increase the likelihood that the exercise regimen will be accomplished.
3. Passive ROM:
   a. Support each extremity to prevent stress on all joints to avoid joint injury due to torsion or hyperextension. (See Table 30–5 for detail.)
   b. Move each joint through all possible movements smoothly and rhythmically. Do not force the joint if pain or resistance is felt. Gently stretching may facilitate increased ROM.
   c. Move each joint as far as it will go without forcing it, then hold at the point of maximum stretch for 15 to 30 seconds to stimulate Golgi tendon organs. This inhibits reflex muscle contractions in response to extension and therefore reduces soft tissue resistance to stretching.
   d. Repeat each movement three to five times. Opposing movements can be done together: flexion, extension; abduction, adduction.
   e. Provide ROM at least every 8 hours.
4. Assess the degree of mobility possible for each joint according to the frequency specified in the client care plan.
5. Document exercise as described in Table 30–5.

RECORDING: Note which joint or extremities were exercised; the number of repetitions for each; whether exercise was active, passive, or active with assistance; and whether pain or resistance was felt. Describe specific movement (in degrees) possible for each joint and compare to evaluation criteria.

changes can be readily observed in these areas. Mild exercise may produce slight flushing and noticeable perspiration. Generalized redness, diaphoresis, and increased skin temperature are noted with more strenuous exercise. Activity in the hospital would not be expected to cause these changes. If pallor, cyanosis, or coolness are noted, the exercise should be stopped immediately. These signs indicate vasoconstriction, poorly oxygenated blood, even impending shock. Though easily observed, skin changes are not conclusive indicators of activity tolerance. They are most useful when combined with other data.

4. *Rate and dexterity.* Onset of fatigue is frequently accompanied by a decrease in the rate and dexterity of an activity. If postural changes such as sagging shoulders or reaching out for support, or ataxic (uncoordinated) gait occur, the activity should be terminated.
5. *Pain or dizziness.* Dizziness or lightheadedness, brought on by maximal shunting of blood to the heart and muscles at the expense of the brain, indicates that rest is needed. Complaints of pain caused or aggravated by the activity may also indicate a need to change the exercise plan.

Many healthy individuals, exercising to increase fitness, tolerate some of the above symptoms and push themselves to higher levels of activity without harmful effects. Clients who are hospitalized have considerably less reserve and should be carefully monitored for signs that they are reaching or exceeding the limits of their exercise tolerance. Parameters that relate to the pathology for which a client is being treated deserve most careful attention.

Heart rate, rhythm, blood pressure, and respiratory rate should be assessed immediately after exercise and

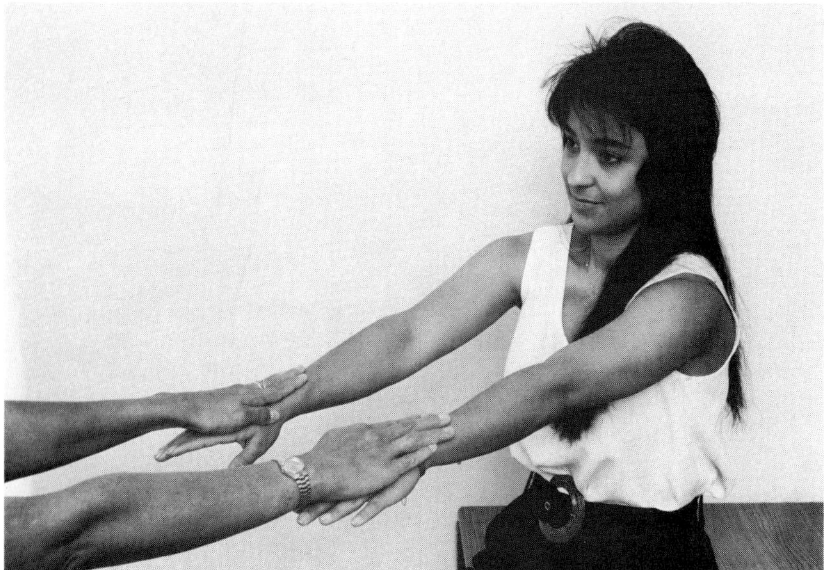

A

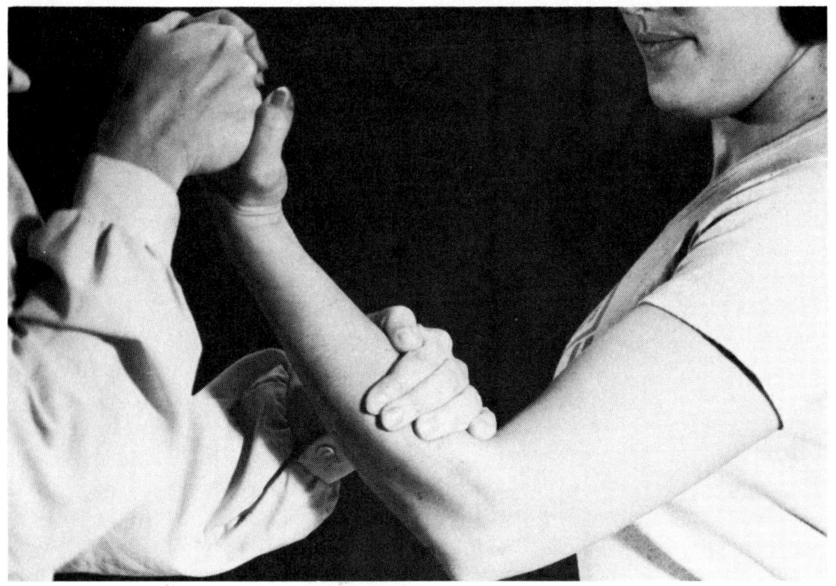

B

Figure 30–9. Strength testing of upper extremity. **A.** Shoulder and scapulae resistance. **B.** Elbow flexion. **C.** Elbow extension (*continued*). (**B** *and* **C** *from Block GJ, Nolan JW.* Health Assessment for Professional Nursing: A Developmental Approach. 2nd ed. *Norwalk, CT: Appleton-Century-Crofts; 1986.*)

again at 2 and 5 minutes postexercise. Pulse and respiration decrease rapidly after exercise ceases unless cardiac reserve has been exceeded. In relatively healthy individuals, these values should return to baseline in 1 to 2 minutes after exercise. Blood pressure usually continues to rise until approximately 30 seconds after exercise stops, then declines. Research by Barringer[42] showed that when peak blood pressure is reached as late as 50 to 90 seconds after exercise, the heart's reserve power has been overtaxed. Pulse, respiration, and blood pressure should return to baseline within 5 minutes after cessation of exercise in hospitalized clients. Should elevation be prolonged, less intense exercise, with a longer cool-down period, is recommended.

The mobility history and examination, obtained early in the nurse–client relationship, provide nurses with a data base for formulation of nursing diagnoses, discussed in a later section. Ongoing assessment throughout the course of care is necessary so that nursing diagnoses and management are current and appropriate.

Diagnostic Tests

Laboratory tests and diagnostic examinations provide useful information to support medical and nursing diagnoses and guide treatment plans. Tests relevant to mobility entail diagnostic examinations to assess joints, bones, and muscles including the arthrocentesis, arthrogram, arthroscopy,

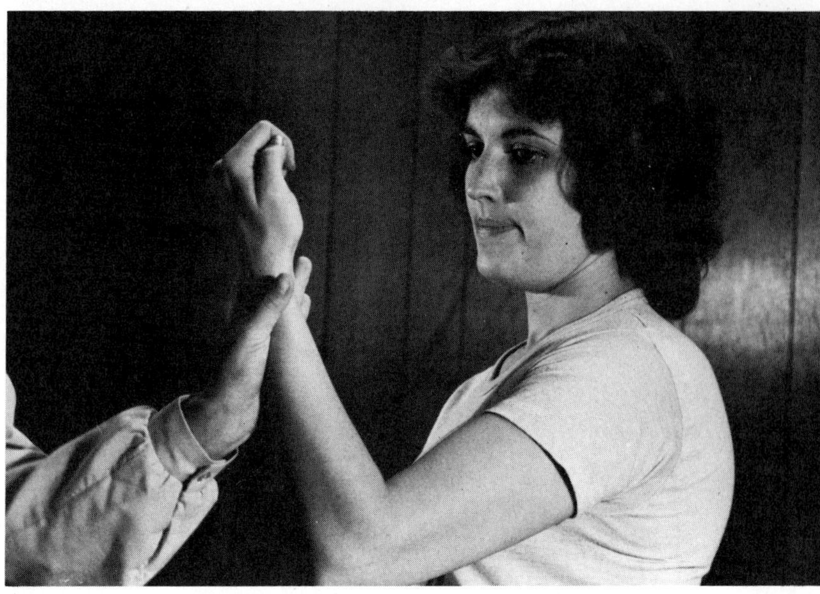

Figure 30–9. *(continued)* **C**

bone scan, and electromyogram, as well as the exercise stress test. Other tests of cardiac and pulmonary function that are also relevant to mobility status are discussed in Chapter 27.

Arthrocentesis. Arthrocentesis is the aspiration of synovial fluid from a joint. Ordinarily, joints have a very small amount of fluid, but a joint effusion (collection of fluid in a joint space) is an indicator of problems. Analysis of the aspirated synovial fluid provides clues about the cause of the effusion. Reassure clients that pain control is provided via local anesthesia. No food or fluid restrictions are necessary unless measuring synovial glucose concentration, which requires 6 to 8 hours of fasting prior to the test.

Arthrogram. This test is an x-ray of a joint space after it is injected with a contrast medium. It is done to determine the cause of joint pain. If the joint has excess fluid, it is usually aspirated prior to injecting the contrast medium. No food or fluid restrictions are required prior to the test. Client preparation includes alerting clients about the possibility of increased pain during and after the procedure. This is due to multiple position changes during the x-ray, and local reaction to the contrast media. Intermittent ice packs, and joint rest for 12 hours posttest provides adequate pain relief for most clients, although analgesics may also be prescribed.

Arthroscopy. This minor surgical examination is the direct visualization of the interior of a joint using a fiberoptic instrument that is surgically inserted into the joint. It is used to detect joint trauma and disease, as well as to facilitate the surgical removal of a damaged tissue. It may be done under local or general anesthesia. Clients must fast for 12 hours prior to general anesthesia. Swelling and pain are expected after arthroscopy. Tell clients to plan for limited activity for 2 to 3 days after the procedure. Ice and analgesia are used to relieve swelling and pain.

Bone Scan. A bone scan is a radionuclide imaging study of bones to detect conditions such as fractures, osteoporosis, cancer, or other causes of bone pain. The radionuclide is injected intravenously. After 1½ to 3 hours, a special camera (scintillation camera) is used to scan the involved area. Computers can be used to enhance and interpret the resulting image. Differences in the rate of uptake of the radionuclide in various parts of the bone result in varying intensities of shading in the image. "Hot spots" or areas of increased uptake, and "cold spots" or areas of decreased uptake, are diagnostic of certain conditions. There is no restriction of food or fluids before the test; often fluid is encouraged to hasten distribution of the radionuclide. The client will be required to lie relatively still during the 30- to 60-minute test. The radioisotopes used for scans have a very short half-life, and the dosages are small, so there is no radiation danger to clients and families. The isotope is excreted by the kidneys. Nurses should wear protective gloves when handling clients' urine after the test because repeated exposure to radioactive material increases risk.

Electromyogram (EMG). The electromyogram (EMG) measures the electrical activity of muscles at rest and during voluntary activity using small needle electrodes. It is used to detect muscle pathology. Usually a resting muscle demonstrates minimal electrical activity, whereas motor disorders produce abnormal electrical patterns in resting muscle. Clients must restrict intake of beverages containing

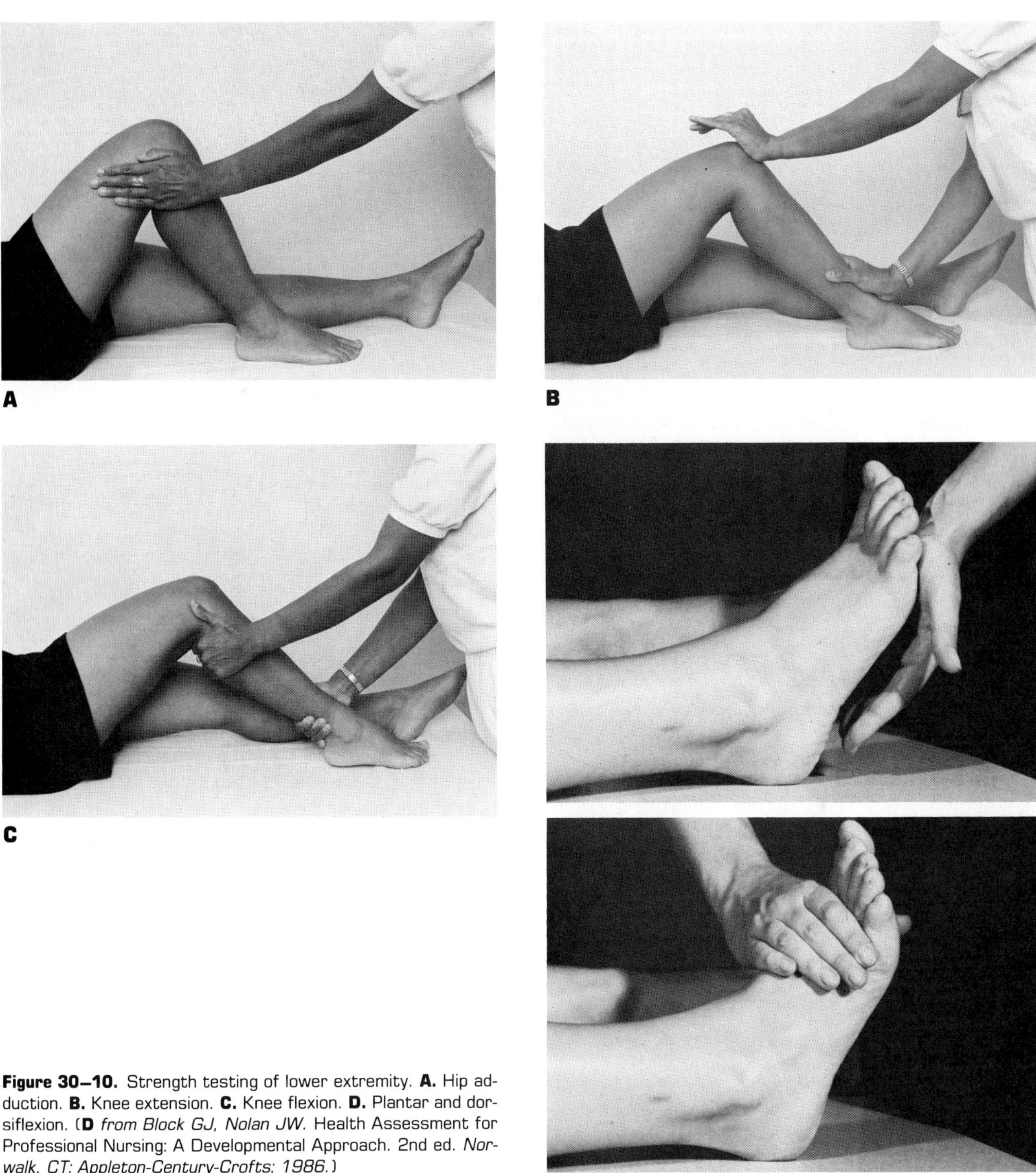

Figure 30–10. Strength testing of lower extremity. **A.** Hip adduction. **B.** Knee extension. **C.** Knee flexion. **D.** Plantar and dorsiflexion. (**D** *from Block GJ, Nolan JW.* Health Assessment for Professional Nursing: A Developmental Approach. 2nd ed. *Norwalk, CT: Appleton-Century-Crofts; 1986.*)

caffeine and abstain from smoking for 3 hours before the test. Reassure clients that the needles are very thin and Teflon coated so discomfort should be minimal. However, instruct them to report intense pain, which occurs if a terminal nerve is inadvertently struck. Should this happen, the needle is immediately removed. Relaxation facilitates testing, so instruction of effective technique is beneficial. Duration of the test varies with the number of muscle groups being tested. One extremity can be tested in 60 to 90 minutes.

BOX 30–3. ABBREVIATED TEST OF MUSCLE STRENGTH

Upper Extremities

1. *Grip strength:* Ask client to squeeze the first two fingers of each of your hands simultaneously. (Client grasps fingers of your left hand with his or her right hand, and vice versa). Grasp should be essentially equal; dominant hand may be slightly stronger.
2. *Arm and shoulder strength:* Ask client to extend arms to the front, palms down. Tell client to resist your pressure, then press downward on the backs of client's hands. Equal resistance against moderate pressure expected. (See Fig. 30–9a.)
3. *Shoulder and scapular strength:* Ask client to raise both arms above his or her head. Tell client to resist, then exert outward pressure on the medial aspect of both arms, just distal to the elbow, as if to push arms down to his or her sides. Equal resistance against moderate pressure expected.
4. *Finger strength:* Ask client to spread his or her fingers while you try to push them together. Test both hands together. Resistance should be essentially equal.

Lower Extremities

1. *Lower leg:* With client sitting or lying on examining table or bed, place your hand on the top of his or her foot and pull as if to point the toes while client resists (dorsiflexion). Then apply pressure to the ball of the foot and ask client to push the foot as if to point the toes while you apply opposing pressure. Test each foot/leg separately. Resistance should be equal. (See Fig. 30–10D.)
2. *Upper leg:* With client positioned as in step 1, hold one ankle and ask client to pull his or her heel towards buttocks. Repeat with other leg. Resistance should be equal.

BOX 30–4. KEY ELEMENTS OF GAIT ASSESSMENT

Head and neck mobility	Head and neck should turn side to side as needed, independent from trunk movement. If fixed in downward orientation, or movable only with trunk "all in one piece," could indicate neuromuscular abnormality.
Foot stance	Shoulder width expected. Wide stance can indicate neurological abnormality.
Pattern of steps	Steps should be even in length and pace with heel strike before toe. High step with slapping of the feet on the ground, wide waddling steps, shuffling, or short quick steps can indicate neuromuscular abnormality.
Equilibrium	No swaying or staggering is expected; can indicate neurological abnormality.
Trunk and arm movement	Body should move freely, arms should swing forward slightly as opposite heel strikes. Stiff trunk, asymmetrical, diminished, or unilateral arm swing could indicate neuromuscular abnormality.

Exercise Stress Test. This is an assessment of myocardial (heart muscle) perfusion. It is also called a thallium scan. It is used when an ECG (see Chap. 27) provides insufficient information about possible cardiac ischemia. Clients being tested must remain n.p.o. for at least 8 hours before the test. They should be instructed to wear comfortable clothing to the test. During the test, they are asked to walk on an exercise treadmill at a gradually increasing pace while cardiac function is monitored via ECG. Blood pressure and oxygen consumption are also monitored. The exercise is continued until a target heart rate or specified time span is reached. The test is terminated at any sign of distress. A radionuclide is intravenously injected 30 to 60 seconds before the cessation of exercise and imaging is done. Sometimes resting images prior to exercise and delayed images several hours after the exercise are taken.

NURSING DIAGNOSIS OF MOBILITY STATUS

Clustering of the data cues obtained in the mobility history and examination indicates whether a client has mobility problems that require nursing attention. Using a guide such as the list of nursing diagnoses approved by the North American Nursing Diagnosis Association (NANDA) assists beginning students to note relationships between cues and associate these cues with specific nursing diagnoses and their etiologies. See the table Sample Nursing Diagnoses: Mobility, page 1456. Box 30–5 presents a list of nursing diagnoses that may cause or be caused by mobility problems.

A diagnosis statement is important because it provides the basis for planning individualized care. For the diagnoses to be most useful in this regard, it should include the etiology of the problem. Four nursing diagnoses directly related to mobility are examined in this section: Impaired physical mobility, Activity intolerance, Potential for activity intolerance, and Potential for disuse syndrome.

Impaired Physical Mobility

Impaired physical mobility is a state in which an individual experiences a limitation of ability for independent physical movement.

Etiology: Activity Intolerance/Decreased Strength and Endurance. Decreased strength and endurance or activity intolerance diminishes ability and motivation to be mobile. Strength and endurance are two components of physical fitness, discussed earlier in this chapter. The relationship between fitness and mobility is reciprocal. Regular activity contributes to increased levels of fitness, while improved fitness allows a wider range of mobility. Inactive people,

TABLE 30–6. BASELINE DATA FOR ASSESSING EXERCISE TOLERANCE

Data	Caution
Age	Over 45
Usual activity level	Sedentary
Duration of activity reduction	Bed rest more than 3 days
Weight	More than 20 pounds overweight
Reclining/standing BP	Resting BP > 140/90 Standing systolic < reclining BP Dizziness on standing or sitting
Reclining/standing pulse, including rhythm strength	Standing pulse > 16 bpm faster than supine; arrhythmias; bounding or thready pulse
Resting respirations, including rhythm, depth, quality	R > 20, shallow, irregular, or labored; dyspnea; secretions in chest
Hemoglobin, hematocrit	< Normal or low normal
Joint ROM	Contractures of any major joint
Muscle strength	Generalized or local weakness, especially of lower extremities
Neurological status	Altered LOC, impaired balance, or coordination (see also Chap. 29)
Health history	Diagnosis or symptoms of cardiovascular, pulmonary, metabolic, liver, renal, or thyroid disease

therefore, have lower levels of fitness, less strength and endurance, and so a diminished capacity for mobility. Fitness is a component of optimal health.

The stress of illness can deplete one's energy stores, decreasing strength, endurance, and mobility. While a serious long-term illness would exhaust the energy reserve of even the healthiest individual, the person who is fit can withstand transient acute illness with minimal loss of mobility. This would not be true of marginally fit, sedentary, or debilitated individuals, who may experience severe energy depletion as a result of relatively minor illness or injury.

Etiology: Pain or Discomfort. Pain and discomfort are powerful inhibitors of mobility. Pain receptors are located throughout the body. They are activated by such stimuli as physical trauma, the presence of inflammatory exudates, and stretching or pressure such as occurs with swelling of a joint or distension of a hollow organ such as the bladder. Movement exacerbates the painful sensations relayed by these pain receptors. Therefore, a characteristic response to localized or generalized pain is to decrease movement. A person who has cut his or her finger may be able to perform most usual activities while immobilizing the finger and compensating for its loss of function by using other fingers. However, coping with some types of pain is more difficult. The pain of a severe headache, a surgical incision, or an inflamed major joint, for example, may be so aggravated by usual movements that the individual suffering from one of these may need to almost completely curtail movement to avoid increased pain. Even the generalized malaise of an infectious process can cause a person to limit movement.

Etiology: Neuromuscular Impairment. Neuromuscular impairment can severely alter movement. Neuromuscular functioning is essential for coordinated movement. The role of the central and peripheral nervous systems in mediating voluntary and reflexive movement was discussed earlier in this chapter. Interference with neuromuscular functioning can result from injury, illness, or a pathological process such as a cerebral vascular accident (stroke). Certain drugs may also alter the transmission of nerve impulses, as may imbalances of certain electrolytes (see Chaps. 29 and 31).

Etiology: Musculoskeletal Impairment. Musculoskeletal impairment can cause generalized or localized interference with movement. A person lacking the support of an intact skeleton or the contractile power of muscles would find movement difficult or impossible. The specific actions of muscles, bones, and related structures such as tendons and ligaments in mobility is discussed in Section 1. Disease, injury, and electrolyte imbalances are among the causes of musculoskeletal problems interfering with normal mobility.

Etiology: Perceptual/Cognitive Impairment. Perceptual/cognitive impairment encompasses a variety of problems. A person who is unable to receive or interpret signals from the environment may respond by decreasing voluntary movement. These individuals are often described as disoriented. They may actually be unable to initiate any purposeful movement because of the confusion resulting from misinterpreted stimuli. Hallucinations (sensory impressions having no basis in external stimulation) are another example of perceptual impairment that can affect mobility.

Psychological disorders, organic brain changes related to age or disease, electrolyte imbalance, and drug side effects or overdose are among the causes of perceptual/cognitive impairments that can result in mobility problems. Also, hearing loss and vision deficits alter or block perception of environmental cues needed for safe and effective

SAMPLE NURSING DIAGNOSES: MOBILITY

Nursing Diagnosis	Defining Characteristics/Manifestations		Etiology
	Subjective Data	Objective Data	
Impaired Physical Mobility 6.1.1.1	Reports pain increased by movement. Reports inability to perform specific movements.	Refuses to move. Grimaces when attempts to move.	*Physical:* pain.
Impaired Physical Mobility 6.1.1.1	None.	Does not follow simple commands. Cannot name or use common objects (eg, cup, pencil). Unable to correctly state name, location, or date. Does not perform spontaneous purposeful movement. Inconsistent response to environmental stimuli.	*Cognitive:* Perceptual/ cognitive impairment: confusion.
Activity Intolerance 6.1.1.2	Reports fatigue. Reports dyspnea on exertion.	Unable to resist moderate force in upper or lower extremities. HR increases 25 bpm with moderate activity. RR ↑ with labored respirations during moderate activity. HR, RR do not return to baseline until 8 minutes after moderate activity.	*Physical:* Generalized weakness.
Potential Diagnosis		**Risk Factors**	
Potential for Activity Intolerance 6.1.1.3		Deconditioned state; muscles soft; wt 20 lb above ideal for ht.	
Potential for Disuse Syndrome 1.6.1.5		Prescribed immobilization.	

mobility. Even lack of knowledge, which can be considered a cognitive impairment, can decrease mobility. A person lacking information about the benefits of exercise, for example, may choose a sedentary life-style, leading to diminished fitness and, therefore, diminished mobility.

Etiology: Depression. Depression depletes one's energy level. Expending the effort required to move may seem impossible or not worth attempting. Depressed people often desire to avoid interactions with others, which also can be accomplished by diminishing mobility. The etiology of depression is very complex. Mild depression may be caused by a situational stressor or a loss. Deeper or prolonged depression is considered to be related to psychopathology.

Etiology: Severe Anxiety. Severe anxiety is physically and emotionally immobilizing. The expression "frozen with fear" is an apt description of a person whose emotional state is so overwhelming that movement is impossible. The condition may be fleeting, or in some situations, persist, if an individual cannot resolve precipitating factors. The anxiety can interfere with problem-solving to the extent that any action, any movement cannot be attempted for fear of real or imagined consequences.

Activity Intolerance

Activity intolerance is a state in which an individual has insufficient physiological or psychological energy to endure or complete required or desired daily activities. Etiologies of activity intolerance are bed rest or immobility, generalized weakness, sedentary life-style, and imbalance between oxygen supply and demand.

Etiology: Bed Rest/Immobility. As discussed earlier under Alterations in Functioning Associated with Limited Mobility, there are many deleterious effects associated with bed rest or immobility that compromise individuals' ability to tolerate activity. Losses in muscle strength and efficiency and cardiopulmonary deconditioning have the greatest impact on activity tolerance. Changes in appetite associated with negative nitrogen balance contribute to insufficient nutrient and fluid intake. This can lead to dehydration and/or nutritional deficiencies that further strain physiological resources and deplete energy.

Etiology: Generalized Weakness. Even mild activity requires sufficient strength and endurance to move one's own body weight and the ability to effectively exchange and transport oxygen and metabolic wastes. Muscle weak-

BOX 30–5. OTHER NURSING DIAGNOSES ASSOCIATED WITH ALTERED MOBILITY

Physical

Altered Nutrition
Potential for Infection
Dysreflexia
Constipation
Altered Urinary Elimination
Reflex Incontinence
Functional Incontinence
Total Incontinence
Urinary Retention
Altered Peripheral Tissue Perfusion
Fluid Volume Deficit
Impaired Gas Exchange
Ineffective Airway Clearance
Ineffective Breathing Pattern
Potential for Injury
Impaired Tissue Integrity
Impaired Skin Integrity
Self-care Deficit
Sleep Pattern Disturbance
Fatigue
Altered Health Maintenance
Pain

Cognitive

Impaired Verbal Communication
Sensory Perceptual Alterations
Altered Thought Processes
Health-Seeking Behaviors
Knowledge Deficit

Emotional

Impaired Verbal Communication
Ineffective Individual Coping
Impaired Adjustment
Unilateral Neglect
Hopelessness
Powerlessness
Anxiety
Fear
Dysfunctional Grieving
Spiritual Distress

Self-conceptual

Altered Role Performance
Body Image Disturbance
Self-esteem Disturbance
Personal Identity Disturbance

Sociocultural-Life Structural

Impaired Home Maintenance Management
Impaired Social Interaction
Social Isolation
Altered Family Processes
Ineffective Family Coping

Sexual

Altered Sexuality Patterns
Sexual Dysfunction

Environmental

Diversional Activity Deficit

nesses, which may be caused by a sedentary life-style, bed rest, and many diseases, limits the capacity for movement and activity, because weak muscles cannot perform sustained activity. Weak muscles have a lower volume of mitochondria to metabolize ATP and fewer capillaries to transport oxygen to muscle cells for metabolic reactions.[7,43] Individuals who are weak experience feelings of muscle fatigue when attempting activity beyond their strength level. Muscle fatigue compromises dexterity. Movements become slower and less precise. Very weak individuals may fall or be physically unable to move further when pushed beyond their capacity.

Etiology: Sedentary Life-style. Sedentary individuals do not experience the positive physiological adaptations associated with regular exercise described in the earlier section on fitness. Moreover, many sedentary individuals are overweight because the limited activity in which they participate burns minimal calories. Although they may maintain a capacity for activity that is satisfactory for their daily routine, those who are sedentary have little aerobic or strength reserve for exertion beyond that level. Therefore, a decision to change life-style—for example to seek a job in which greater physical exertion is required, or to participate in a new leisure activity—can be difficult to carry out because their bodies' inability to sustain large-muscle activity generates activity intolerance.

Etiology: Imbalance Between Oxygen Supply and Demand. Because aerobic metabolism is considerably more efficient than anaerobic metabolism, insufficient oxygen supply cuts down a muscle's capacity to work. Exertion increases muscle oxygen uptake, and therefore increases oxygen demand. Inadequate oxygen prevents resynthesis of ATP; fatigue and exhaustion therefore follow. Moreover, the accumulated metabolic waste products from anaerobic metabolism, carbon dioxide and lactic acid, interfere with continued muscle function. If the supply of available oxygen is insufficient to support heart muscle function, arrhythmias and even cardiovascular collapse may occur.

Potential Activity Intolerance

Potential activity intolerance is a state in which an individual is at risk of experiencing insufficient physiological or psychological energy to endure or complete required or desired daily activities. Factors that place an individual at risk include deconditioned status, presence of circulatory of respiratory problems, and inexperience with the activity.

Risk Factor: Deconditioned Status. Deconditioned status refers to a state in which an individual lacks the capacity to sustain vigorous physical work without overtaxing cardiopulmonary of muscular capacity. The relationship between activity tolerance and conditioning is discussed in detail in Section 1. Planning and adhering to an individualized conditioning program will prevent individuals at risk from developing actual activity intolerance.

Risk Factor: Presence of Circulatory and Respiratory Problems. Circulatory or respiratory problems have the potential to compromise oxygen exchange and/or delivery. If the stress of the greater muscular demand for oxygen because of increased workload during activity overtaxes the limited respiratory or circulatory capacity, actual activity intolerance occurs. Pre-exercise testing, discussed above, can prevent serious problems.

Risk Factor: Inexperience with the Activity. Neuromuscular coordination during activity is improved with repetition of that activity.[14] Inexperience with a particular activity can be expected to cause individuals to expend greater energy in its performance than someone who is familiar with the required movements. The greater energy expenditure creates greater energy demand, potentially overtaxing them. Short practice sessions or breaking complex activities into several component parts to be mastered separately decreases inefficient energy expenditures.

Potential for Disuse Syndrome

Disuse syndrome refers to the collection of conditions discussed earlier under Alterations in Function Associated With Limited Mobility. The presence of risk factors such as paralysis, mechanical or prescribed immobilization, severe pain, and altered levels of consciousness creates a likelihood of developing disuse syndrome.

Risk Factor: Paralysis. Paralysis is a temporary or permanent loss of function, in particular the ability for voluntary motion. (See also Chap. 29.) It is most often a result of pathology or injury in the nervous system. The degree of risk for disuse syndrome is related to the extent of paralysis and the motivation of an individual to participate in preventive measures. Prevention of disuse syndrome in paralyzed individuals requires constant vigilance.

Risk Factor: Mechanical or Prescribed Immobilization. Mechanical immobilization—such as traction, braces, or casts—creates varying degrees of immobility. Prescribed immobilization that is not mechanical ranges from complete bed rest to restriction of only specific types of activity or movement. Some loss of function of immobilized body parts is inevitable, but attentive preventive care, discussed in Section 3, is effective in avoiding many immobility related problems.

Risk Factor: Severe Pain. Severe, intractable pain causes altered mobility and altered mobility is the basis for disuse syndrome (see discussion of Impaired Physical Mobility, above). Although there are many modalities for pain relief (see Chap. 29), some, such as narcotic analgesics, depress central nervous system function. This effect contributes to mobility problems. Pain also interferes with motivation to be mobile, so a multifocused approach to prevention of disuse syndrome associated with pain is necessary.

Risk Factor: Altered Level of Consciousness. One's state of awareness affects one's ability and desire to be mobile. Individuals who are lethargic or stuporous (slowed response to stimuli, little spontaneous movement) or comatose (unresponsive to stimuli, with some reflex movement) are at highest risk for disuse syndrome, because they make no spontaneous movements. See also Chapter 29.

Stating the Mobility Diagnosis

The analysis of the data to determine the precise mobility impairment and its specific etiology should result in a concise statement regarding the client's mobility status. The general statements from the taxonomy, such as "Impaired mobility related to pain," should be refined in the clinical setting when assessment data provide cues for a more exact statement. Examples might be:

- Impaired Mobility related to abdominal incisional pain, as evidenced by infrequent position changes, "I can't walk—it hurts too much," facial grimacing and guarding of abdominal incision whenever movement is attempted.

- Impaired Mobility: Inability to walk, related to muscle weakness in lower extremities; as evidenced by decreased muscle tone and muscle mass in legs and buckling of knees when standing is attempted.

Note that the defining characteristics (major manifestations) that support the selection of a given diagnosis and etiology are also included in a complete diagnostic statement. These detailed statements represent individualized diagnoses based on the taxonomy of approved nursing diagnoses. Because of their specificity, they can be useful in selection of nursing implementation.

A further refinement of the diagnosis Impaired physical mobility has been suggested. NANDA recommends that the following code for functional level classification, describing a client's degree of dependence/independence, be used as part of the diagnostic statement:

- 0 = Completely independent
- 1 = Requires use of equipment or device
- 2 = Requires help from another person for assistance, supervision, or teaching
- 3 = Requires help from another person and equipment or device
- 4 = Is dependent, does not participate in activity

As clients progress in level of independence, the level classification number can be changed to reflect the progress. In the sample nursing diagnoses above, the mobility impairment related to abdominal incisional pain might be initially designated level 2, while the client unable to bear weight might be considered to be at a functional level of 4.

The level numbers can be useful in predicting not only the specific client care that clients need, but also the amount of time needed to provide that care. This information could be used, both by charge nurses to determine the number and type of nursing personnel needed to care for a group of clients, and by the nurses providing care, who could use the data to organize and schedule care for the clients to whom they are assigned. The mobility diagnosis, therefore, when stated clearly and concisely, can provide the basis for management of client care, discussed in the next section.

Section 3. Nurse–Client Management of Mobility

■ PLANNING FOR OPTIMUM MOBILITY

A client care plan to promote optimum mobility can relate to concerns such as improving a client's level of fitness, supporting a client's plan for healthful weight reduction, assisting with activities of daily living during acute illness, or teaching self-care adaptations to accommodate residual disability. An effective client care plan communicates the desired outcomes of client care as well as the means for attaining the outcomes and evaluation criteria by which to judge outcome attainment. Statements of desired outcomes in a mobility care plan succinctly describe the level of mobility a client should attain as a result of nursing therapies, providing a guide to specific implementation and a basis for evaluation criteria.

Mobility outcomes, like other outcomes for client care, are best determined by a process of mutual goal-setting. Through analysis of assessment data, nurses develop a perception of the level of mobility a client can realistically attain. Nurses' sharing their perceptions with clients and requesting their input can contribute to setting goals that clients understand and accept. This collaborative effort should continue as clients and nurses work together to attain the mobility outcomes they have set.

The desired outcomes on the collaborative client care plan should also be compatible with the goals for medical treatment. In the example of the client who was unable to walk because of muscle weakness, a desirable long-term goal would seem to be that the client get stronger—if possible, strong enough to walk independently and be as active as before becoming ill. Analysis of the health assessment data and collaboration with the client and the physician would be necessary, however, to determine whether this goal is realistic. For example, the physician may have determined that the client's illness is serious and chronic and is therefore likely to cause long-term debilitation. Therefore, the desired outcome of regaining enough strength to return to the former level of functioning would be unrealistic. The client may desire to regain complete independence, and be unaware of the level of independence that is possible and the length of time rehabilitation may require. Or, the client may be discouraged by the diminished mobility and believe that recovery is impossible. Collaborative discussion among nurse, client, and physician would be useful in this situation. Through collaboration, each participant gains increased awareness of the others' perceptions and expectations. They could then set reasonable and compatible medical, nursing, and client goals.

The second part of planning for a client's mobility needs is deciding upon nursing implementation to attain the desired outcomes. The type of care that is appropriate is implied by the assessment data and the outcomes selected in the previous step. Client care should capitalize on client strengths and provide support where it is needed.

For the client with muscle weakness, a nurse might decide to begin by teaching the relationship between exercise and the development of muscle strength, unless the mobility history revealed that the client already knew this. Next might be planning a leg-strengthening exercise program and assisting the client to perform the exercises. The selection of exercises and their frequency would be determined by the information about the client's exercise tolerance obtained during the mobility examination.

A complete mobility care plan addresses all of the problem areas stated in the nursing diagnosis or diagnoses, including outcome(s) and implementation for each. The nursing implementation is then carried out and its effectiveness evaluated by comparing the client's progress to evaluation criteria derived from desired outcomes.

Evaluation of mobility status is both an ongoing and a terminal process. The final evaluation of a client's mobility is made at the end of the nurse–client relationship, often when the client is discharged from the hospital. At that time, nurses compare the client's status with the conditions described in the evaluation criteria. Observations made while providing client care indicate whether day-to-day progress is being made toward desired mobility outcomes. Documentation of a client's response to nursing treatment on the nursing progress notes in the client's medical record provides ongoing evaluation information. If clients demonstrate the desired level of mobility within the time frame indicated in the mobility care plan, the outcomes are considered to have been met. If the goals are not attained, reassessment is necessary to determine whether the goals were realistic and nursing treatment appropriate.

■ NURSING IMPLEMENTATION TO PROMOTE OPTIMUM MOBILITY

Nursing approaches to assist clients with mobility needs encompass a wide range. Clients whose mobility limitation is minimal may require assistance only with exercises to strengthen muscles or increase endurance. Others may need assistance with ambulation or teaching about healthy life-style habits to attain and maintain optimum mobility. More dependent clients may require assistance with all mobility, including changing positions in bed or transferring from a bed to a chair. These clients would also need nursing care to prevent disuse syndrome. The following sections provide detailed explanations of the nursing approaches to assist mobility for clients with needs for all levels of care.

The table Nurse–Client Management of Mobility, pages 1460–1461, presents sample outcomes, implementation, and evaluation criteria for nurse–client management of the nursing diagnoses related to mobility that are presented in this chapter. These are provided as examples only. Individualized plans of care should be developed for all clients based on their own particular needs and situation.

Preventive Care

Preventive mobility care includes health education about the benefits and risks of exercise, planning an individual exercise program, and the role of good nutrition and other positive life-style habits in enhancing optimum mobility. Screening to identify individuals at risk for compromised mobility or exercise-related injury is also part of preventive client care.

NURSE–CLIENT MANAGEMENT OF MOBILITY

Nursing Diagnosis	Desired Outcome	Implementation	Evaluation
Impaired mobility R/T pain 6.1.1.1	1. Resume former level of mobility without complaints of pain.	1a. Offer noninvasive pain relief measures (see Chap. 29). 1b. Offer analgesia as ordered if above unsatisfactory. 1c. Assist with movement, positioning, and ADL when pain is severe. 1d. Collaborate with client to develop an individualized exercise program to maintain strength, endurance, and flexibility to be used when pain relief is achieved.	1a. Progressive increase in self-care and freedom of movement without report of pain. 1b. ROM and muscle strength remain constant.
Impaired mobility R/T perceptual/cognitive impairment: confusion 6.1.1.1	1. Maintenance of current level of strength and flexibility. 2. Improved orientation appropriate to health status.	1a. Give verbal and visual cues to assist client in active ROM q3h whenever client is appropriately responsive. 1b. Incorporate resistance in above ROM whenever client is able. 1c. Attempt passive ROM at least q4h if client does not participate in active ROM. 1d. Attempt daily assisted walks of distance within client's tolerance. 2a. Speak distinctly explaining your actions and desired client participation. 2b. Correct inappropriate verbalizations or physical responses using a calm voice tone, explaining and repeating appropriate or correct response. 2c. Provide varied environmental stimuli, eg, conversation, music, change of location, group activity.	1a. Serial ROM measurement increases or remains same as initial measurement. 1b. Serial testing of muscle strength reveals no loss. 1c. Activity-related changes in P, R, BP remain same as initial assessment. 2a. Progressively increasing numbers of appropriate verbal and/or motor behaviors.
Activity intolerance R/T generalized weakness 6.1.1.2	1. Increased activity tolerance appropriate to age, sex, and health prognosis. 2. Increased strength appropriate to age, sex, and health prognosis	1. Collaborate with client to develop program for progressive ambulation. 2a. Collaborate with client to develop a muscle strengthening program that focuses on client's deficits. 2b. Assist in performance of ADL decreasing assistance as strength improves. 2c. Teach modified methods or provide assistive devices for ADL performance according to client need.	1. Progressive improvement in activity tolerance AEB: ■ Statements of improved energy level. ■ HR, RR, and BP return to baseline values after exercise within expected time frame for age and health status.

NURSE–CLIENT MANAGEMENT OF MOBILITY (continued)

Nursing Diagnosis	Desired Outcome	Implementation	Evaluation
			2a. Progressive increase in muscle tone and mass. 2b. Serial tests of muscle strength show progressive improvement.
Potential for activity intolerance: R/F deconditioned status 6.1.1.3	1. Improved exercise tolerance to 60% of HRmax.	1a. Teach client the health benefits of regular exercise. 1b. Collaborate with client to develop an exercise program that includes aerobic exercise of client's preference at least 3 days per week with gradually increasing duration and intensity. 1c. Teach client to assess pulse during and after exercise. 1d. Teach client how to compute HRmax.	1. No activity intolerance AEB able to participate in aerobic exercise at 60% HRmax without distress (no dyspnea, pallor, fatigue), with return to baseline HR within 1 minute after exercise ceases.
Potential for disuse syndrome: R/F prescribed immobilization 1.6.1.5	1. No evidence of disuse syndrome.	1a. Collaborate with client to develop a turning schedule in which no position is maintained for more than 2 hours. 1b. Maintain clean, wrinkle-free bed at all times. 1c. Teach client the benefits of fiber, fluids in maintaining bowel regularity and urinary function (see Chap. 26). 1d. Keep fluids of choice available at all times. 1e. Teach and encourage client to use deep-breathing exercises (see Chap. 27). 1f. Teach client leg exercises that are within the prescribed activity limitations (see Chap. 27). 1g. Collaborate with client to develop a program of exercises for strength and flexibility to be performed in bed that are within prescribed activity restriction. 1h. Involve significant others in planning activities with client to diminish boredom, isolation. 1i. Use therapeutic communication techniques to facilitate client coping with restricted activity (see Chap. 14). 1j. Offer choices and opportunities for decision-making about care regimen whenever possible.	1. Client remains free of symptoms of disuse syndrome, AEB: ■ Skin remains free of pressure ulcers. ■ Regular soft-formed BM. ■ Lungs remain free of secretions. ■ Extremities remain well perfused (see Chap. 27). ■ Regular urinary elimination without dysuria within expected range for intake. ■ ROM remains at expected measurements for age. ■ Maintains alert oriented mental status. ■ No indicators of disturbed body image (see Chap. 23). ■ Participates in planning and engages in measures to prevent disuse and treat primary health problems.

Health Education. Increasing the number of health care providers that routinely counsel clients about their specific needs for physical activity is one of the fitness goals cited in *Healthy People 2000*, the document by the United States Public Health Service.[6] Nurses can participate in this effort. Nurses have opportunities for health teaching about exercise in settings such as schools, workplaces, and communities, as well as in health care facilities.

Although school nurses are not usually responsible for curricular decisions, they can collaborate with educators in planning physical education activities that emphasize life-sports, such as tennis or cycling, as suggested in *Healthy People 2000*. School nurses can conduct classes or workshops on the benefits of exercise and safe approaches to exercise for students and parents.

Workplace health-promotion programs are becoming more common, particularly in large corporations. Corporations view these programs as having benefits for employees in terms of their improved health and fitness. The corporation also profits because healthier employees take fewer sick days, are more productive, and have decreased needs for illness care, thereby reducing benefit costs; moreover, sponsoring health-promotion programs improves a corporation's image.[44] Programs offered are diverse, but many have health education, activity, and life-style change components. Nurses can be involved in both the planning and execution of workplace programs such as these. Research has indicated that a major limiting factor in the success of workplace exercise programs is low employee participation.[45] This is a factor that occupational health nurses can correct by providing more effective education about the personal benefits of these programs.

Community-based efforts to educate the public, such as health fairs or public information classes, are other examples in which nurses can play a role in preventing health problems that limit mobility.

One-to-one teaching about the health benefits of exercise (discussed in Section 1) and related topics such as nutrition and smoking cessation (see Chaps. 22, 25 and 27), is probably the most effective means of promoting individual commitment to exercise. This teaching can be done during regular health assessment visits or when clients seek care for any health problem that affects activity. Besides providing general information, specific teaching about selecting an appropriate exercise program and reducing exercise risk as well as enhancing client's motivation to maintain the program, is important.

Selecting and Planning an Individual Exercise Program. Plans for an individual program should take into account a client's current level of health and fitness, as discussed in Section 2, and other personal factors such as time available, preferences for activity, and specific outcomes expected or desired from exercise. The *Canadian Standardized Test of Fitness Operations Manual* provides a useful approach to collaboration with individuals to plan an exercise regimen.[46] The following guidelines are adapted from the Canadian method:

1. *Build rapport.* Establish a positive climate by explaining the nature of the exercise assessment and addressing any anxiety a client expresses.
2. *Establish life-style goals.* Discuss other goals besides improving fitness that are important to a client, such as weight loss, stress reduction, or modification of personal risk factors for coronary artery disease.
3. *Conduct assessment.* Determine current fitness level and screen for the presence of risk factors (discussed in Section 1) that indicate a need for comprehensive assessment by specialists.
4. *Interpret results.* Discuss the assessment with clients in descriptive and understandable terms; give them a copy of the report for reference.
5. *Discuss activity preferences and interests.* Find out what kinds of activity a client enjoys, finds unpleasant, and for which the necessary equipment or facilities are readily available. Consider the amount of time the person can realistically commit to exercise every week.
6. *Match preferences and assessment results.* Determine whether a client's goals for exercise are realistic given current health and fitness, preferred activities, and time available. (Note that for anyone in a risk category, this determination would require collaboration with specialists.) See whether preferred activities are compatible with client's goals. Discuss the benefits and limitations of a client's preferred activities.
7. *Design a program.* Write out an action worksheet with progressive levels (eg, gradually increasing physiological demands) and reachable goals. If any activities require specialized equipment or skills (eg, weight training, specific sports), refer clients to resources for instruction. Schedule regular reevaluation.

Exercise programs that are most beneficial include components to improve aerobic fitness, flexibility, and strength; however, for many individuals a prudent plan to improve aerobic fitness provides sufficient benefits in strength and flexibility. Improvement in aerobic fitness involves integration of frequency, duration, intensity, and type of activity. Cox[13] recommends a prescription of "long, slow distance" (p. 27), particularly for a person who is currently sedentary. The distance selected depends on a client's energy level and time available. The pace can be governed by identifying a low (<65 percent HRmax), moderate (65 to 85 percent HRmax), or high (85 to 90 percent HRmax) intensity of exercise, depending on fitness level. This approach would apply to any aerobic activity, such as walking, jogging, rowing, cycling, swimming, or cross-country skiing. The long, slow distance program can be easily quantified, provides cardiorespiratory benefits, contributes to weight loss, and has a low risk of orthopedic injury and cardiovascular complications.[13]

Reducing Exercise Risks. Exercise-related injuries are one reason individuals become discouraged and lose commitment to an exercise program. Most exercise related injuries are preventable.

Selecting a program appropriate to an individual's current fitness level and gradually increasing the pace, duration, and intensity of exercise is an important injury-prevention strategy. Consistently warming up before exercise (for example, by stretching or beginning at a slow pace) and cooling down after exercise (ending the session with slower, less intense activity) is also effective.

Besides informing individuals about practices to prevent injury, educating them about the kinds of practices that increase their risk for injury enables them to make prudent choices. The editors of the *Berkeley Wellness Letter* have identified five factors that increase risk for exercise-related injury[24]:

1. *Overdoing it.* Dramatically increasing the intensity of duration of workouts, or performing a high-impact activity like running or aerobic dance more than four times a week, significantly increases risk.
2. *Inadequate footwear and equipment.* Athletic shoes are designed to provide support during the typical types of movement required for a specific sport or activity. Wearing worn-out shoes or the wrong shoes (eg, wearing running shoes for tennis) places stress on hips, knees, and ankles—where 90 percent of sports injury occur. A racket with a grip that is too large or a cycle that is too small also strains muscles and joints.
3. *Poor conditioning.* Exercising weak, tight muscles causes injury unless individuals take precautions to gradually increase stress. Muscle imbalance, such as occurs with participating in only one type of exercise or sport, creates a tendency for injury in the muscles that are not strengthened by that exercise. An example is shin splints, which result from strong calf muscles overwhelming weaker muscles in the front of the lower leg.
4. *Improper technique and training.* Poor form, such as an incorrect backhand stroke or improper footstrike in running, causes stress that leads to injury. Training on hard or uneven surfaces is another common cause of injury.
5. *Ignoring aches and pains.* "Running through" the pain or resuming exercise before an injury has fully healed worsens the current injury and increases the risk for reinjury. Taking note of unusual sensations and treating injuries as soon as possible prevents their becoming more serious.

Many exercise-related injuries are related to participation in competitive sports.[13] This is true even in informal, spontaneous games between friends. Individuals who enjoy competition tend to become so enthusiastic during the game that they may push themselves to greater intensity than their bodies are ready for, with resulting musculoskeletal injuries or even cardiovascular and pulmonary stress.

Enhancing Motivation. Many of the strategies that are effective for planning an exercise program also enhance client motivation to maintain an exercise program. Establishing a baseline, setting realistic goals, determining an appropriate exercise prescription, and selecting specific activities acceptable to the individual—all discussed above as part of establishing an exercise program—also strengthen motivation.[15] Other motivation-enhancing approaches include dispelling misconceptions about exercise, discussing obstacles to exercise and strategies to overcome them, emphasizing the value of play, providing feedback and positive reinforcement, and role modeling.[15]

Baseline and Goals. The fitness baseline established in the initial assessment provides a concrete means of measuring progress. Setting goals that are neither too easy nor too difficult makes goal attainment likely with reasonable effort. Anthony suggests that identifying several short-term goals to enable individuals to experience early successes contributes toward motivation to achieve long-term goals.[15]

Exercise Prescription and Activities. Using the goals and baseline assessment to identify the appropriate frequency, intensity, and duration of exercise; incorporating activities a client enjoys; and accommodating the client's time constraints should result in an exercise program that is likely to be continued. Success with this kind of program makes it more likely that a client will progress to a level of exercise that more closely approximates expert recommendations for ideal exercise (Box 30–2).

Dispelling Misconceptions. The "No pain, no gain" philosophy has received a lot of exposure in exercise self-help books and videos. Also, some people may interpret the ideal exercise criteria to mean that intense activity is necessary to achieve any health benefits. Moreover, many individuals' past experience with exercise has been with school competitive sports, wherein the typical message from coaches was in keeping with the concept of no pain, no gain. Informing clients about recent research findings supporting positive effects from mild to moderate activity levels will make exercise seem less formidable and benefits more achievable.

Another common misconception is that the health benefits ascribed to exercise are immediate and observable. In fact, 4 to 6 weeks of regular exercise is needed before most people experience noticeable improvement in performance.[13] Although feelings of improved well-being are common within 2 to 3 weeks of regular exercise, there may be no externally obvious evidence of improved health for many weeks. Many individuals embark on exercise programs in order to lose weight. Promises of fast, effortless weight loss made by many diet programs (although false and misleading) create unreasonable expectations of weight loss from exercise. Because a calorie deficit of 3500 calories is necessary to lose 1 pound of fat, a loss of 1 to 2 pounds per week is feasible.[47] A realistic perspective of the level of commitment to exercise needed to achieve the benefits prevents discouragement and disappointment from unmet expectations.

Miles[47] lists three other misconceptions that may dissuade individuals from making a commitment to a regular exercise program. The first is that exercise "wastes" heartbeats. This idea derives from a perspective of the heart as a pump with a finite life span and subject to mechanical failure. The anticipated increased demands during exercise are therefore thought to add strain and hasten mechanical failure. In fact the converse is true. Because of the decrease in resting heart rate secondary to endurance training, there is actually a net savings in heartbeats attributable to regular exercise. Decreasing one's resting heart rate from 80 to 70 beats per minute saves 14,400 beats a day, or 5,526,000 beats a year. The extra beats expended by exercise at 150 beats per minute for 30 minutes, 4 times per week total 8400 beats per week, or 436,800 beats a year. Therefore, the net savings is 5,089,200 beats a year![47]

A second misconception cited by Miles is that exercise increases appetite, causing increased intake that more than compensates for the energy expended during exercise. Although those who work and play hard tend to eat more than sedentary individuals, those who are active have more muscle mass and less body fat. Because muscle tissue is more metabolically active than fat, lean, active people burn calories more rapidly than those who are sedentary. Therefore, regular exercise usually results in a net decrease in calories stored.

Finally, Miles discusses the belief in spot reduction of body fat. This misconception is one that causes people to quit an exercise program because anticipated results did not occur. Proponents of the spot reduction theory state that fat stores in the muscles being exercised will be mobilized preferentially to other fat stores. Therefore, a person desiring to lose abdominal fat would be advised to do sit-ups, and one with excess fat on the thighs, leg lifts. There is no research to support spot reduction; rather, stored fat is mobilized equally from all areas of the body during exercise. Therefore, an extended period of balanced exercises would be needed to lose large local fat deposits.

Overcoming Obstacles to Maintaining an Exercise Program. Like any change, altering a sedentary life-style pattern can be difficult. Physical obstacles like transient muscle soreness during and right after exercise, rapid reversal of training effects if exercise is discontinued for a time, and injuries related to training cause some people to become disillusioned with an exercise plan. Environmental deterrents such as having to travel to an exercise facility or social obstacles, such as an unsupportive spouse or being unable to arrange child care, can make establishing and maintaining a regular exercise pattern difficult. Discussing potential obstacles in a general way, and exploring personal situations that could deter sticking to a commitment to exercise, is a good way to identify appropriate techniques for coping with obstacles. Belisle and colleagues[48] found that this kind of guidance as part of planning an exercise program increases adherence to the plan.

Emphasizing the Value of Play. In a discussion about expressing health through life-style patterns, Pender emphasizes the importance of balance between meaningful work and invigorating play throughout the life span.[32] The same philosophy is espoused in *Healthy People 2000*.[6] However, the life patterns of many adults exclude time for play. Our high-pressure, success-oriented culture causes many to devalue leisure, even to forget how to play. This perspective is at the root of many stress-related disorders. Dialogue with clients about the value of play, emphasizing that exercise is a form of play, can contribute to enhancing clients' awareness of imbalances in their lives. Awareness is the first step toward change. For some, seeing exercise as play also requires a shift in outlook. Stressing that selecting a form of exercise that is pleasurable is important in an effective exercise plan is helpful. A pleasurable activity is self-reinforcing and likely to be repeated.

Feedback and Positive Reinforcement. Although intrinsically pleasurable activities and generalized improvements in well-being are incentives to continue exercise, many formerly sedentary clients do not experience these feelings at the outset of an exercise program. The transition from an inactive to an active life-style is difficult for many. During the first several weeks of an exercise program, most clients need encouragement to continue. Commending clients for staying with the program shows recognition that continuing takes an effort. Giving feedback about progress toward goals and praise for gains are important incentives. When the exercise becomes incorporated into an individual's value system, and personal perceptions of gains are possible, external reinforcement ceases to be needed.

Role-Modeling. None of the strategies in which health care providers engage to encourage exercise have credibility with clients if it is obvious that a provider's personal life-style does not include regular exercise. Conversely, if we appear fit and can speak about exercise from the perspective of participants rather than observers, our efforts are more likely to be convincing and effective.

Screening for Risks for Compromised Mobility. Life-style choices create risk factors for compromised mobility. For example, smokers risk cardiopulmonary compromise that will eventually limit fitness and general mobility, even though they may feel capable of vigorous exercise at present. Clients whose weight exhibits a slow but steady increase are on a trajectory that exposes them to many health risks, including limitations in mobility. Obesity increases the risk for degenerative joint disease and limits cardiovascular capacity, among other problems. Sedentary women with low calcium intake and a positive family history are at greatly increased risk for developing osteoporosis. Alcohol and use of other substances, particularly while driving, or failure to use seatbelts, exposes individuals to accidents with potentially permanent mobility-altering consequences. Encouraging clients' examination of their risk for losing the capacity for optimum mobility is the first step in facilitating life-style changes. Tailoring health teaching to the particular risk factor and related variables that apply to a given individual is more effective than a broad general approach.

Supportive Care

Supportive care is appropriate for clients who are experiencing mild alterations in mobility. Examples include overweight individuals participating in an exercise program for weight control, well elderly individuals, and individuals with mild exercise-related injuries.

Supporting Overweight Individuals in Exercise Programs. Dropout rates from exercise programs are higher among obese individuals than among others.[16,47] Some have postulated that this relates to psychological factors, such as intimidation and self-consciousness.[49] Other research has shown that social factors such as group support influence exercise adherence.[16,50] These findings suggest that continued participation is more likely in programs tailored specifically for overweight clients. One study of overweight women found this to be true.[16] Nurses are often in a position to teach obese clients weight-control strategies and refer them to appropriate programs. Nurses who are well informed not only about dietary considerations to promote healthy weight loss, but also knowledgeable about the role of exercise in weight control and about programs specifically tailored to meet the needs of overweight clients, are in a better position to facilitate and support the positive efforts of clients to lose weight. Moreover, recognizing the possible effects of slow progress toward weight-loss goals and related discouragement, nurses should offer consistent positive reinforcement to these clients for continued participation and even minimal progress toward goals. Organizing multifocal programs for overweight clients that include nutritional, exercise, and interactional components would be an even more effective means of supporting weight loss in overweight individuals.

Enhancing Mobility in the Well Elderly. As discussed in Section 1, aging is a significant factor contributing to losses of mobility. Teaching elderly clients how they can retard loss of function and developing individual and group exercise programs specifically for older clients can greatly improve the quality of life of older individuals.[11,51–54] Activity is a major component in the health perception of the elderly.[52] Therefore participation in regular exercise not only maintains older adults' physical mobility but contributes to their image of themselves as healthy. The general guidelines for assisting in the planning of an exercise program discussed above are effective for older clients. A careful and complete pre-exercise assessment, including a drug and dietary history, evaluation for sensory deficits, musculoskeletal problems, and cardiovascular disease, is recommended prior to planning exercise.[28] Most experts recommend walking as an ideal aerobic activity for the elderly. Integrating social interaction with the exercise increases the overall benefits, because group support positively influences motivation. Moreover, the additional benefit of forming new friendships is important to this age group, who often experience losses of friends and loved ones. An example of a group program that integrates social activity and exercise is Mall Walking Clubs. Mall Walking Clubs were originally organized in a southwestern Virginia community as a means of assisting local senior residents to examine their health practices and promote positive health behaviors. These clubs, generally affiliated with community hospitals, in collaboration with shopping malls, now exist in communities throughout the country.[51] Nurses often provide health screening, teaching, and consultation for these clubs.

Fall prevention is another area in which nurses can promote optimum mobility in healthy elderly individuals. Because of changes in sensory acuity—particularly vision—and diminished strength, joint mobility, and balance, falls

BUILDING NURSING KNOWLEDGE

Do the Elderly Benefit from Taking Walks?

Gueldner SH, Spradley J. Outdoor walking lowers fatigue. *J Gerontol Nurs.* 1988; 14:6–12.

This article reports a survey of 32 ambulatory elderly showing that those who live in nursing homes walk less frequently than their counterparts who live in retirement villages. Although all of those in retirement villages spent some time out of doors, 36 percent of those in nursing homes said they never went outside. Of those who did, 81 percent never walked outside and most sat in rockers. Gueldner and Spradley suggest these findings are explained by the social expectation that persons living in nursing homes will be more passive than their counterparts who live independently. Fear of lawsuits resulting from client falls also may prevent institutional staff from actively encouraging residents to spend time outside.

The authors designed a protocol to test the benefit of outdoor walking for institutionalized elderly individuals. Their study looked at the affect of outdoor walking on fatigue. Fatigue was measured by asking subjects to rate their feelings on a rating scale. The 32 subjects were ambulatory, mentally alert individuals between 60 and 93 years of age; 16 were nursing home residents. The nursing home residents were placed together in group A, which was subdivided into three subgroups. Six were given an outdoor walking protocol consisting of short outdoor walks three times per week for a period of 3 weeks, and were pre- and posttested for fatigue self-perceptions. Five continued in their usual routines and were pre- and posttested. Another five were posttested only to identify whether extraneous variables introduced by the study erroneously changed study results. Group B, with 16 subjects from a retirement village, was also subdivided in the same manner as group A.

Nursing home residents who participated in the walking protocol reported significantly lower fatigue scores after 3 weeks of walking. Scores of those in the retirement village did not change appreciably, as expected by the fact that walking was already a part of their usual routine. Gueldner and Spradley concluded that outdoor walking is a readily accessible activity that may enable elderly individuals to enjoy an improved state of health.

IMPLICATIONS FOR NURSE–CLIENT COLLABORATION

Barriers to Mobility

Barriers to mobility take several forms, psychological, social, and environmental. The process of regaining mobility can be impeded by any of these barrier types. Clients may have personal fears, such as the fear of injury, or may be concerned about the burden their mobility problem places on others, or there may be actual physical barriers to be overcome in the environment that cause a client to be reticent. By collaborating with the client, the nurse may be able to identify the specific barriers that the client is experiencing, and thus to establish a plan that addresses these and that will enhance the client's feeling that mobility objectives are achievable.

are a potential cause of injuries for older adults. Collaborative assessment of elderly clients' homes for hazards that contribute to falls is a simple but effective means of preventing injury. Poor lighting, obstacles such as furniture and throw rugs, slippery surfaces in bathtubs and showers, and shoes that fit poorly or have very smooth soles create jeopardy for falls. Nurse–client discussions of possible environmental alterations while jointly conducting the assessment is an effective means of reducing or eliminating these hazards. Box 30–6 lists strategies to teach clients to prevent falls at home. Encouraging participation in exercise programs such as those discussed above is also a good fall-prevention strategy, because exercise improves strength, balance, and joint mobility.

Promoting Recovery from Mild Exercise-related Injuries. Cold, elevation, heat, massage, and rest are effective treatments for discomfort and minor muscle injuries related to exercise. Joint injuries often require more intensive treatment and should be assessed by a physician. Early stages of heat-related illness can be treated by rest and hydration.

Cold. Cold applications are appropriate immediately after an injury occurs. Ice or ice and water in plastic bags, or chemical cold generation packs, work well. Cold slows down local metabolic activity, decreases inflammation, and minimizes vasodilation.[55] Reducing venous dilation limits edema, because capillary bed hydrostatic pressure is lower when venous pressure decreases (see Chap. 31.) Cold applications can damage tissue, so the site should be checked periodically and the ice removed after 15 to 20 minutes or sooner if loss of local sensation occurs.[55] When the acute (red, warm, swollen) phase passes, heat therapy is recommended.

Elevation. Elevating an injured extremity prevents venous pooling, which is a contributing cause of edema after injury. Elevation used in conjunction with cold therapy inhibits inflammation and decreases pain.

Heat. Generalized soreness after exercise often improves with heat applications. Postexercise whirlpool promotes relaxation and comfort, but should not commence until heart rate and respirations have returned to resting values, be-

BOX 30–6. STRATEGIES TO TEACH CLIENTS TO REDUCE FALLS AT HOME

1. **General**

- Be sure all stairways have handrails.
- If vision is poor, mark step-up or step-down areas with bright colors.
- Use nonslip floorwax. Highly waxed floors invite falls.
- Use a sturdy stepstool to reach items in high places. Don't use a chair or unstable ladder. If balance is unstable, don't climb on any stool or chair; rather, store items so they can be reached when standing on the floor.

2. **Lighting**

- Use floor-level lighting to illuminate low obstacles.
- Use a dim nightlight to facilitate nighttime trips to the bathroom. A dim nightlight can make turning on regular lights unnecessary, eliminating the need for the eyes to accommodate a dark to bright to dark variation.
- Be sure all stairways are well lighted.

3. **Obstacles**

- Remove throw rugs, especially on waxed floors.
- Move furniture, especially small items, to provide ample walking space.
- Be sure magazines and newspapers are not left on floors; they are very slippery.
- Keep floors in traffic areas free of electrical cords.
- Do not leave items on stairs.

4. **Bathrooms**

- Apply nonskid adhesives to showers and tubs.
- Consider hold bars in the shower and next to the bathtub and the toilet.
- Consider a raised toilet seat to decrease the strain of sitting and rising from the toilet.

5. **Apparel**

- Use shoes and slippers with nonskid soles. Knitted or crocheted slippers and smooth leather or synthetic soles are very slippery and foster loss of footing.
- If shoes with laces are used, be sure the laces are securely tied.
- Avoid pants, skirts, robes, or nightgowns that are too long.

6. **Ambulation aids** (*See fig. 30–14*)

- Check that canes or walkers have intact rubber tips so they do not slip when used for support.
- Consider a walker, tripod, or quad cane if balance is slightly unstable.

7. **Avoiding postural hypotension**

- Avoid bending down to pick up low objects. Stoop, then rise to standing slowly.
- Be especially careful of abrupt position changes immediately after eating, when blood is shunted to the gastrointestinal tract.
- Sleep with the head of the bed elevated 8 to 12 inches (several pillows will accomplish this).
- Don't rise up suddenly. Sit up in bed for a minute, then at the edge of the bed for a minute, then stand still holding onto a stable piece of furniture for a minute.
- Wear elastic stockings at night.

cause high temperatures enhance vasodilation and therefore slow venous return to the heart.[55] Local hot packs are also effective in promoting healing after the acute phase of an injury, because of their vasodilating effect.

Massage. Massage is another modality that effects circulation, promoting muscle relaxation, faster muscle recovery, and pain relief. According to Kresge[56] and Knapp,[57] massage produces two different circulatory effects. The first is mechanical, a manual movement of venous blood, which is believed to promote more rapid emptying and refilling of vessels, improving removal of metabolic waste products. The second is reflex, caused by stimulation of peripheral receptors. The results of this stimulation are relaxation of muscles and release of acetylcholine and histamines, which cause sustained vasodilation. Massage counteracts the reflex muscle contraction and localized muscle splinting or guarding that occurs in response to pain. This splinting inhibits local circulation, causing ischemia and intensifying pain. Anxiety and stress aggravate secondary muscle contraction pain. Massage breaks the cycle by promoting relaxation. Because it increases lymph flow, massage also reduces edema.

Rest. Premature resumption of activity after an injury delays healing, stresses healthy fibers around the injured area, and predisposes an individual to further damage.[58] However, since deconditioning occurs rapidly when training ceases, experts recommend rest of the injured part, rather than total body rest. When possible injured individuals should continue aerobic activity at as close to preinjury levels as possible.[58] Advise selecting an activity that can be maintained continuously and that uses uninjured muscle groups. For example, someone with a lower leg injury can substitute swimming for running or cycling; an individual with an upper body injury can walk briskly.

Hydration. Exercising in hot weather causes heat-related illness. Mild forms of this can be treated by replacing lost fluids. Offer hypotonic liquids that are low in sugar, because glucose retards stomach emptying, delaying absorption.[1] Cold fluids are most effective because they pass through the stomach faster.

Restorative Care

Restorative mobility care is appropriate for clients with health problems causing significant interference with independent mobility. Assisting with exercise, transfers from bed to chair, moving and positioning in bed, and using protective devices and special beds are restorative client care measures to promote mobility. Most of these require the use of effective protective body mechanics.

Body Mechanics. Much of the client care related to acute problems involves lifting and moving clients. This creates potential for injury of both clients and nurses. Incorporating principles of protective body mechanics promotes safety as well as efficiency. Protective body mechanics involves using specific movements or techniques that result in maximum work output with minimum effort expended and with reduced possibility of injury. Principles of physics as well as anatomy and physiology apply. The following are basic guidelines for correct protective body mechanics.

1. *Start with correct posture.* Correct body alignment is described in Section 2 (see Fig. 30–7). It is fundamental to protective body mechanics. Muscles and joints function optimally when properly aligned. If work is attempted when posture is faulty (eg, with spine bent or twisted or with knees locked), injury to bones, muscles, and joints can result.
2. *Maintain a wide base of support.* Any object is unstable if its center of gravity is allowed to shift outside its base of support. In the standing position, the center of gravity of the body is located in the pelvic cavity, slightly anterior to the sacrum. Placing your feet at shoulder width with one foot slightly ahead of the other when lifting or moving heavy objects or clients provides the largest possible range of movement without straining to maintain balance.
3. *Use large muscles.* The muscles of the extremities are the largest and strongest muscles of the body. Their structure makes them able to perform strenuous work without injury (Fig. 30–1). Further protection from injury results when these muscles are contracted to stabilize joints prior to exertion. In contrast, the muscles of the back are smaller and more easily strained. Reaching and bending or twisting the spine while lifting or moving is likely to cause injury. For this reason, the working surface should be at or slightly above the waist and directly in front of the body. This will minimize reaching and twisting as well as allow maximum efficiency of large muscles (Fig. 30–11).

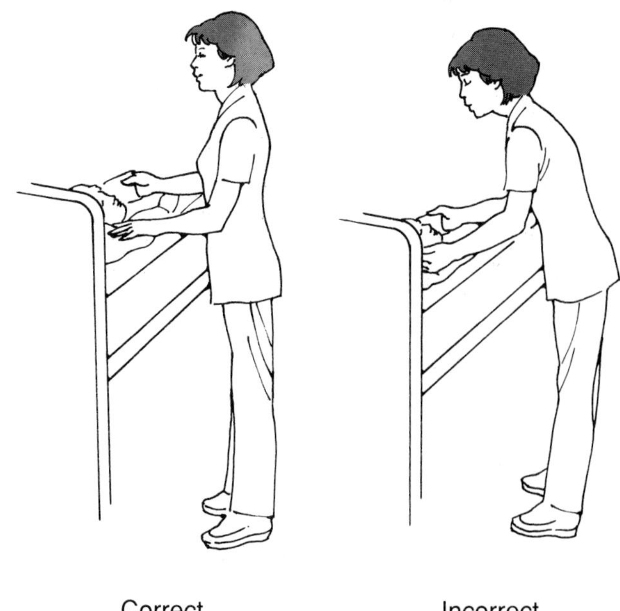

Figure 30–11. Correct versus incorrect height for working surface.

4. *Use your body as a counterweight.* A counterweight is a weight used to produce a force to move or balance another weight, called the resistance. When lifting or moving clients, your body weight can be used to counteract the weight of the client (the resistance) (Fig. 30–12). The added force of your body moving in the direction the resistance is to be moved reduces the force that must be generated by the muscles. This technique is useful for both pushing and pulling.
5. *Minimize friction.* Friction is the resistance created by a moving object on a surface. Friction is diminished when the surface is smooth and well-lubricated, when the area of contact between surface and object is decreased, or when an object is rolled.
6. *Incorporate leverage when possible.* A lever is a machine that uses a rigid bar that rotates around a fixed point called the fulcrum. A simple example is the teeter-totter. A lever accomplishes lifting or moving a weight (resistance) with much less force than with unassisted lifting. It is possible to use parts of one's body as the bar and/or fulcrum. Figure 30–13 illustrates one example of the use of leverage.
7. *Use mechanical aids for heavy objects.* Hydraulic lifts, pull sheets, and other devices discussed in the following section can greatly reduce muscle strain by incorporating leverage, reducing friction, and providing additional force. This not only saves nursing energy but also prevents injury to both client and nurse.

Use of these guidelines should become automatic during performance of client care involving lifting and moving. It is also useful to teach clients proper body mechanics to increase the safety and efficiency of independent client movement.

Exercise. Providing or assisting with exercise is a common nursing implementation for clients with mobility problems (see Procedure 30–2). Regular exercise is important for optimum health. To obtain the maximum benefit, exercise should be part of life-style, but any client experiencing mobility impairment has a special need for exercise to maintain intact function and to improve function that has been altered by disease or injury.

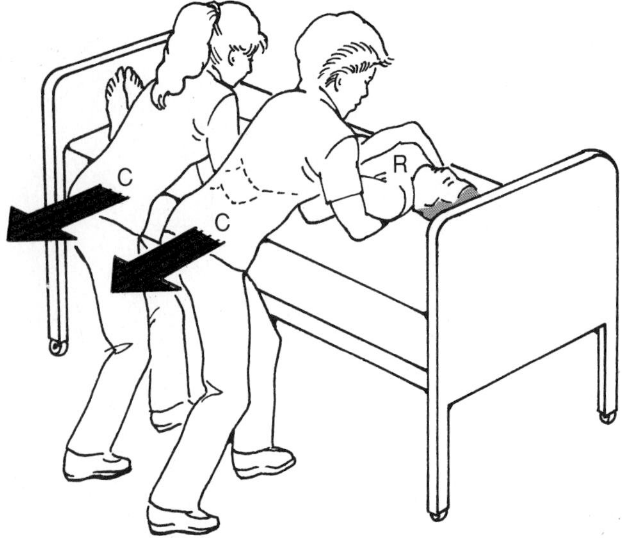

Figure 30–12. Use of the body as a counterweight.

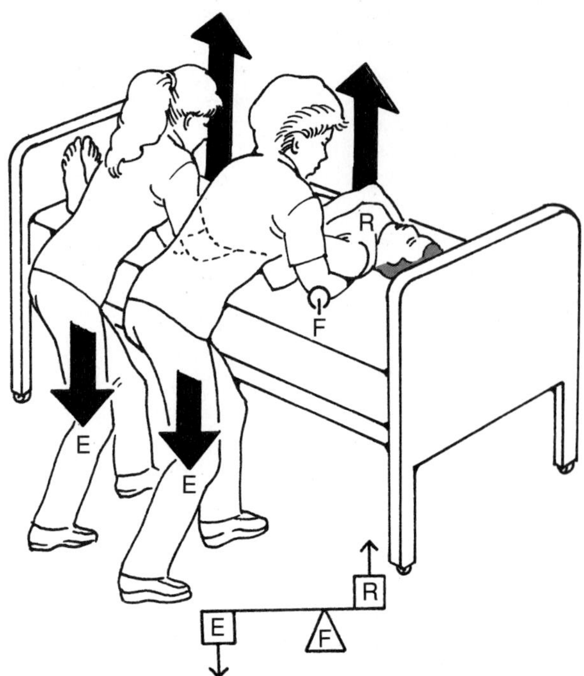

Figure 30–13. Use of leverage in lifting and moving clients.

Hospitalized clients often choose to remain in bed for most of the day, even though their condition might allow more ambulatory activity. There is limited space in which to ambulate, and few activities in which to participate in most acute care hospitals, so incentive to be active is limited. Establishing an exercise program for all clients not only is beneficial during hospitalization but may instill an awareness of the value of exercise for overall health and a sense of well-being. Table 30–7 includes types of exercise suitable for clients in acute care settings. Examples are listed for postdischarge exercise as well.

The type of exercise that is appropriate for a given client is dependent upon the medical and nursing diagnoses and upon the goals or expected outcomes for client care that nurse and client have formulated. Nurses should also collaborate with physicians and physical and occupational therapists in the selection of specific exercises for clients. Clients should be encouraged to continue the exercises after convalescence, augmenting them with more strenuous activities as strength and fitness improve.

Ambulation. Ambulation is usually the most strenuous aerobic exercise in which hospitalized clients can participate. Unless contraindicated by a client's condition, it should be a part of the exercise plan for every client. Ambulation promotes strength, endurance, and flexibility. The demands and benefits can be gradually increased as assess-

PROCEDURE 30–2. ASSISTING WITH ACTIVE EXERCISE

PURPOSE: To improve or maintain muscle tone, strength, and flexibility

EQUIPMENT: Varies with exercise; see also Tables 30–9 and 30–10 and Procedures 30–4 and 30–5.

ACTION	RATIONALE
1. Explain purpose of each exercise before beginning. Use language easily understood by the client.	1. Participation is facilitated when reasons or expected gain from an activity is clear and the relationship between the activity and the individual's needs or problems is explained.
2. Describe and demonstrate each exercise (see Table 30–9 and 30–10, and Procedures 30–4 and 30–5 for details).	2. Providing multiple modes for gaining information will increase likelihood of its being absorbed.
3. Assess pulse, respirations, and blood pressure before client attempts exercise.	3. Baseline data facilitate assessment of the effect of the exercise.
4. Assist or observe client's performance.	4. Active participation with immediate feedback enhances learning.
5. Provide positive reinforcement for correct performance.	5. Behavior that results in desirable consequences is likely to be repeated.
6. Give suggestions for change in technique if exercise is performed incorrectly.	6. Incorrectly performed exercise may result in minimal benefit or injury.
NOTE: If exercise is isometric, advise client that maximal benefit is obtained if muscles are contracted for 6 seconds, and rested for 2 seconds, then repeated.	
7. Assess pulse, respirations, skin color, temperature, and moisture as exercise is being performed. Ask client about subjective response to exercise (pain, fatigue, etc). Complete a similar assessment at the end of the exercise period.	7. These parameters indicate activity tolerance. Client will not benefit if overexercised. (See step 9, below.)
NOTE: Pulse increase of greater than 25 bpm, labored respiration, marked flushing, diaphroresis, pain, and severe fatigue are indications that exercise may be too strenuous or exercise period too long.	
8. Use above data to plan an exercise schedule with client participation.	8. Having control in a situation contributes to a sense of autonomy, which is necessary for self-esteem and motivation. A schedule promotes regular, consistent exercise, which results in beneficial adaptations contributing to well-being.

(continued)

PROCEDURE 30–2. (continued)

9. Periodically assess response (see step 7, above) to independent exercise program to determine readiness for a more strenuous program. (Assisted or passive exercises can be assessed continuously.)

NOTE: Changing the exercise program also prevents boredom. Even if tolerance increases slowly, selecting an alternate exercise that provides similar benefits is recommended.

9. The body responds to the physiological stress of overload by overcompensation. Therefore, by progressively increasing the intensity of effort, a series of compensatory adjustments will result in a gain in strength and/or endurance. Compensatory energy is limited. Exercise past the point of fatigue will overtax the client and delay recovery.

RECORDING: Indicate specific exercises performed, number of repetitions of each, duration of exercise, and assistance, if any. Describe specific response to exercise (refer to section on exercise tolerance).

TABLE 30–7. CATEGORIES OF EXERCISE APPROPRIATE FOR RESTORATIVE CARE

Type and Definition	Benefits	Examples
Aerobic: Exercise that increases the body's oxygen consumption for a sustained period of time (5 minutes or more).	Increases endurance, improves strength and flexibility in actively exercising parts of the body.	Walking,[a] running, bicycling, swimming.
Isotonic (same tone): Exercise in which the muscle tension is constant while the muscle moves through its range of motion (ROM).	Increases strength and flexibility.	Weight lifting, calisthenics, active ROM.[a]
Isometric (same length): Exercise in which muscle tension is increased, but the length of the muscle is not changed.	Maintain or improve strength.	"Setting" exercises,[a] pushing or pulling against an inmovable object.
Flexibility: Exercise that stretches muscles and joints to their maximum capacity.	Maintain or improve joint range of motion and muscle pliability.	Stretching, eg, to "warm up" prior to aerobic exercise, passive ROM[a]

[a] Suitable for clients in an acute care setting.

ment data demonstrate evidence of increased exercise tolerance.

Safe ambulation requires balance and adequate strength for weight bearing and maintenance of posture. Table 30–8 outlines parameters for selecting a safe ambulation method. Some clients require assistance from nurses to ambulate safely. Assessing for transient dizziness is an important precaution when preparing any client for ambulation. Even short-term bed rest, especially after injury or surgery, can be accompanied by orthostatic hypotension; orthostatic hypotension is a frequent complication of long-term bed rest. Moving too quickly from a recumbent to a standing position compromises brain perfusion because it allows insufficient time for the circulatory system to adjust. Asking clients to sit at the edge of the bed for several minutes before standing is usually sufficient to correct orthostatic hypotension. This activity is often called **dangling.** Nurses can perform several of the preambulation assessments described in Table 30–8 while a client is dangling. Procedure 30–3 discusses dangling.

Techniques for assisting clients to ambulate are described in Procedure 30–4 (page 1477). Some clients benefit from additional support in the form of walkers, canes, or crutches (Procedure 30–5, page 1482). Two types of walkers are illustrated in Figure 30–14 (page 1488). They allow body weight to be distributed between both upper and lower extremities and provide assistance in maintaining balance. The pick-up walker is generally preferred, as it is more stable. A rolling walker can be used for people with low endurance (fold-up seat can be used for resting), with inadequate bicep strength to lift a pick-up walker, and who can propel themselves with their legs while sitting (eg, to exercise legs). A walker does not encourage development of independent balance, so it is recommended that isometric and isotonic strengthening exercises, as well as supervised practice of unsupported standing, be included in client care to prepare clients for unassisted ambulation.

BUILDING NURSING KNOWLEDGE

What Can the Nurse Do to Maintain an Aging Client's Mobility?

Milde FK. Impaired physical mobility. *J Gerontol Nurs.* 1988; 14:20–24.

In this article, the author points out that almost all disease and recovery involves some degree of immobility. To explore the effect, Milde begins with a case study of a client and analyzes the impact of immobility and nursing intervention from a physiological perspective. The client was a 74-year-old woman, active prior to a hospitalization for an abdominal condition, who the nurse found to restrict the movement of one knee because of painful arthritis. The nurse established a nursing diagnosis of impaired physical mobility.

Milde notes that decreased physical mobility has serious affects on the musculoskeletal system. Research shows that aging produces changes in muscles and joints. After early adulthood, there is a marked and steady decline in muscle strength in leg and back muscles. Fast-twitch muscle fibers (fibers that produce power and strength) decline more than the slow-twitch fibers (fibers that serve endurance). This explains why strength is more affected than endurance. With aging, the length of muscle fibers decreases and the collagen content of connective tissue increases, causing an increase in the stiffness of the tissue and a decrease in joint mobility. Nursing assistance is directed toward maintenance of muscle strength and endurance, the maintenance of joint flexibility, and prevention of deterioration.

Outcomes, according to Milde, depend on instituting a regime of daily conditioning and the promotion of protein anabolism. Daily conditioning consists of isometric and isotonic muscle exercises. Isometric exercises increase muscle tension without changing muscle length or moving the joint. Muscles are tightened as hard as possible for 6-second periods. These exercises are helpful in maintaining the strength of the quadriceps, abdominal and gluteal muscles needed for upright mobility. According to Milde, isometric exercises are useful when the client has a heart condition and cannot tolerate strain. Isotonic exercises, in contrast to isometric exercises, change the length of a muscle without changing the tension. They involve pushing or pulling against a stationary object such as a trapeze used to lift one's body off of the bed. These exercises should be used with caution for clients with heart conditions because they increase strain, blood pressure, and cardiovascular load.

Promoting protein anabolism is done primarily through the intake of protein and calories to maintain body weight. Other nursing actions that are beneficial include positioning the client for proper body alignment, and passive range-of-motion exercises in which the nurse moves the client's joints through their full range of motion to maintain joint flexibility.

When clients have achieved independent balance and increased strength, they may progress to ambulation with crutches or a cane. A quad cane, a type of cane that offers greater stability than a standard cane, is illustrated in Figure 30–14B (page 1488). Assistance with crutch walking and safe use of canes is usually provided by the physical therapy department.

Isometric Exercise. Isometric exercises are useful for maintaining muscle tone and strength. They also protect against excessive bone loss, especially if they simulate weight bearing.[35] Physical therapists can offer help to formulate isometric exercises that simulate weight bearing.

Isometric exercises are not as strenuous as isotonic exercises, so they are suitable for initiating an active exercise program (see Table 30–9) Raising the number of repetitions increases both the effort expended and the strength gained. For maximum benefit, tell clients to hold muscle contractions for a minimum of 6 seconds, and extend the period of contraction to 10 to 15 seconds as strength improves. Studies have shown that isometric contractions can cause significant elevations in arterial blood pressure.[59] Although brief (5- to 6-second) repeated maximal contractions with 20-second rest periods between contractions usually result in no significant blood pressure changes, consultation with a physician is recommended before initiating isometric exercises with clients having a history of cardiac problems.

Isotonic Exercise. Even a short period of inactivity causes joint stiffness and weakness. Isotonic exercises involve movement and therefore can prevent these problems and promote flexibility and strength. They may be used as an adjunct to ambulation or in preparation for ambulation. As a client's strength improves, the exercises can be performed with small weights. Table 30–10 (page 1487) lists isotonic exercises that can be done by clients in bed and progressively more strenuous exercises that clients can use as their recovery advances.

Active range of motion (ROM) exercises are isotonic exercises. Performing active ROM with or without weights, therefore, maintains flexibility and strength. Daily systematic ROM is a good way to maintain flexibility and is especially helpful when a client spends all or a part of the day in bed. Some clients, either paralyzed or debilitated, are unable to participate in any active exercise program. These immobilized clients should receive **passive ROM** at least three times a day as soon as their condition permits. Although passive ROM does not prevent muscle atrophy because it involves no work by clients' muscles, it maintains joint flexibility. When performing passive ROM, observe the following guidelines:

1. Support all joints in the extremity being exercised.
2. Move extremities slowly and rhythmically.
3. Repeat each movement at least three times.
4. Do not force any joint beyond the point at which you feel resistance. Hold the position of maximum stretch for 15 to 30 seconds.
5. Encourage active participation to the degree possible.

General guidelines for active and passive ROM are found in Procedure 30–1. Correct technique for each joint movement is explained and illustrated in Table 30–5. As strength improves, clients can progress to active assisted ROM, in which they perform part of the movement without assistance from a nurse. Clients can also exercise their own

(*Text continues on page 1486.*)

TABLE 30–8. GUIDELINES FOR SELECTION OF AMBULATION OF TRANSFER METHOD

Parameter/Test	Evaluation			Associated Nursing Action
	Poor	Fair	Good	
1. Sitting balance: Ask or assist client to assume a sitting position at the edge of the bed.	1. Cannot hold sitting position without continuous maximal support.	1. Requires assistance to assume sitting position, but sits without assistance. Loses balance if resistance (ie, pushing on upper trunk) is applied.	1. Assumes sitting position with minimal or no assistance. Is able to maintain balance against resistance.	1. Client with poor sitting balance should not attempt ambulation. Use a transfer method requiring no client participation. If sitting balance is fair or good, proceed to test muscle strength.
2. Muscle strength	2. Extremity does not move, but muscle contraction can be seen or palpated.	2. Active movement is possible, but unable to move against resistance.	2. Active movement against moderate to maximal resistance is possible.	
a. *Quadriceps:* Ask client to extend the leg at the knee when seated at the edge of the bed.	a. Knees will buckle if standing is attempted.		a. Weight bearing is expected.	a. Client with poor or fair quadriceps strength in one or both legs cannot ambulate. Pivot transfer can be used if has good strength in one leg. If quadriceps strength in both legs and standing balance is good, can ambulate independently.
b. *Illiopsoas* (hip flexion): Ask client to raise the flexed knee toward ceiling when seated as above.	b. Client will be unable to advance affected foot when walking.		b. Independent steps expected.	b. Client with poor or fair illiopsoas strength can ambulate with two assistants and use pivot or walking transfer if quadriceps strength is good. If illiopsoas strength and balance are good, may ambulate independently.
c. Anterior tibialis (ankle dorsiflexion): Ask client to lift sole of foot while keeping heel on floor.	c. Sole of foot will not clear floor as client steps. Client may stumble.	c. Minimal or no problem with foot clearing floor expected.		c. If anterior tibialis strength is poor, ambulate with two assistants. One assistant is adequate if anterior tibialis strength is fair to good and quadriceps strength is good. If anterior tibialis and quadriceps strength and balance are good, can ambulate independently.

TABLE 30–8. (continued)

Parameter/Test	Evaluation: Poor	Evaluation: Fair	Evaluation: Good	Associated Nursing Action
3. Standing balance: After demonstration of good sitting balance, ask client to stand at bedside.	3. Support of one person required to maintain balance.	3. Can stand independently, but loses balance if resistance (see step 1, above) is applied.	3. Stands without support. Maintains balance despite resistance.	3. Client with poor standing balance requires support of one or two nurses (gait belt preferred). If quadriceps strength is only fair, use two assistants. Client with fair balance and good quadriceps strength can use a walker. If balance and muscle strength good, can ambulate independently.

PROCEDURE 30–3. ASSISTING A CLIENT TO A SITTING POSITION AT THE EDGE OF THE BED (DANGLING)

PURPOSE: To prepare clients for ambulation or transfer to a chair.

EQUIPMENT: None.

ACTION	RATIONALE
1. Discuss the procedure with the client, including nurse's actions, behavior desired of client, and signals to be used, if any.	1. Client will be more willing to participate if reasons and expected benefits of the activity are clear.
2. Raise the bed to your thigh level, lower siderail, lock wheels of bed.	2. Reduces nurse's backstrain, allows use of large muscles of arms and legs.
3. Screen the client, fanfold covers to foot of bed. Position IV or drainage tubes so no tension will be caused on them as client moves. NOTE: Tension on tubes could cause pain or disrupt IV or drainage system.	3. Provides privacy, prevents tubes and covers from becoming obstacles during movement.
4. Instruct or assist client to move near edge of bed (see Procedure 30–11). The distance between the edge of bed and the client's hips should be approximately two-thirds the length of the thigh.	4. Keeps client's weight close to nurse's center of gravity, reducing strain on nurse's back.

(continued)

PROCEDURE 30–3. (continued)

NOTE: If client is too close to the edge of the bed, lack of support for the thighs as client attempts to dangle could cause pain in an abdominal incision or cause client to slip off the bed.

5. Raise head of bed 60 to 80 degrees.

5. Conserves client's and nurse's energy by using mechanical power to achieve a sitting position.

6. Stand facing the side of bed next to the client's hips. Assume a broad stance with knees flexed, back straight. Most of your weight should be on the leg nearest the bed.

6. Facilitates using strong muscles of legs, not back muscles, as client is moved.

7. Slip one of your arms behind the client's back at level of scapulae, the other under the thighs.

7. Supports client near the center of gravity.

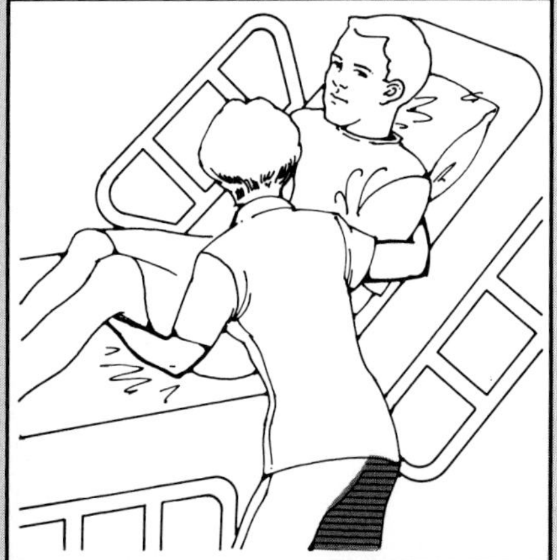

8. Pivot the client toward the edge of the bed by simultaneously swinging the client's legs over the side of the bed and pushing client's upper body to face side of the bed. Facilitate the client's pivot by stepping backward (toward the head of the bed) with your nonweight-bearing leg, shift your weight to that leg as you step, and pushing against the edge of the bed with your other thigh at the same time.

8. Movement of the nurse's body in the direction the client is to be moved and the use of the leverage created by pushing off the bed (thigh is fulcrum) reduces muscular energy expended.

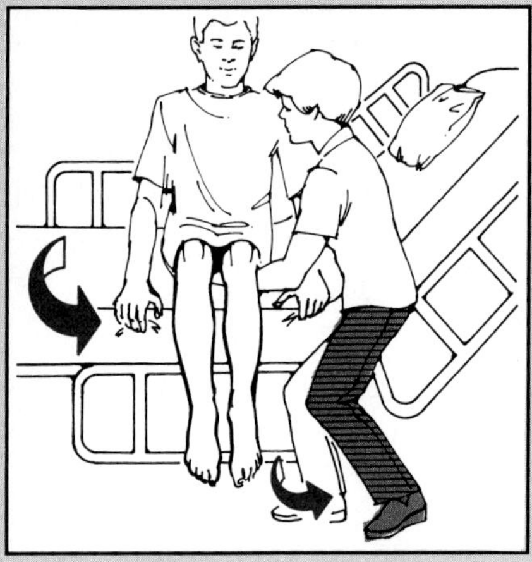

(continued)

PROCEDURE 30–3. (continued)

Or

If the client requires less assistance, replace steps 6 to 8 with the following instructions: Ask the client to roll to sidelying position, grasping the siderail for assistance, if needed. Then ask client to push torso off the bed with the uppermost arm while sliding legs over the edge of the bed. (If siderail extends whole length of bed, lower rail when client has rolled to side.) If client has an abdominal incision, assist the client to lower the legs to prevent incisional pain.

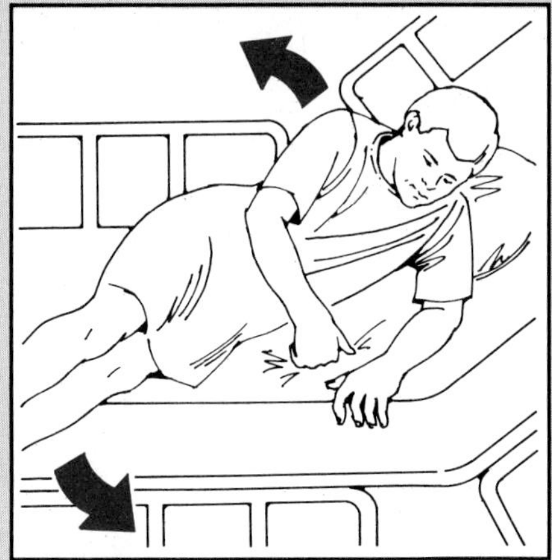

9. Lower height of bed so client's feet touch the floor. Assess client for increased pulse, shortness of breath, dizziness, and sitting balance.

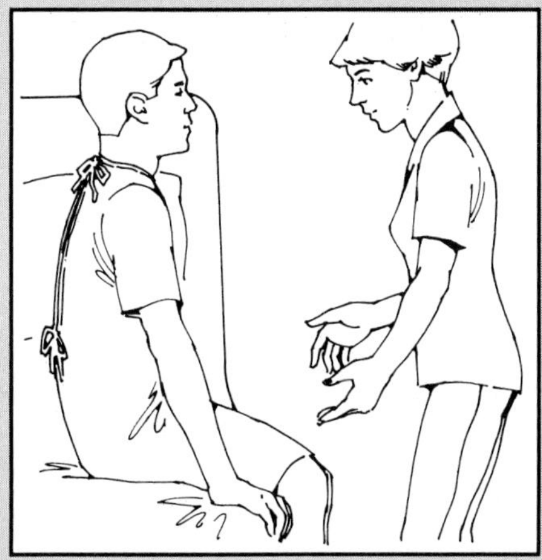

9. Prolonged recumbency causes sluggish response of arterial baroreceptors with subsequent pooling of blood in the dependent parts of the body, causing dizziness. Exertion causes increased pulse and respirations to supply greater O_2 requirements of working muscles. Dangling allows time for stabilization of both vital signs and perfusion.

10. If dizziness, increased pulse, or shortness of breath occurs and does not resolve within minutes, or if sitting balance cannot be maintained, return client to recumbent position.

10. These symptoms indicate that exertion of sitting up has used most of the client's available energy. The additional stress of ambulation or weight-bearing transfer to a chair is not likely to be tolerated.

(continued)

PROCEDURE 30–3. (continued)

11. To return client to supine position: Face the foot of the bed with a broad stance, knees flexed, back straight. Support client as in step 7, above.

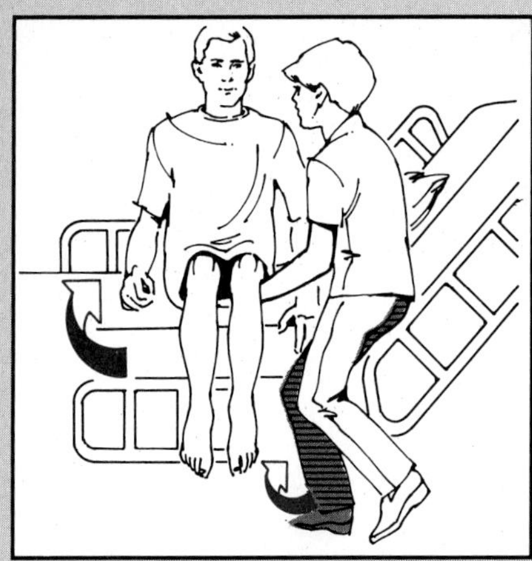

12. Turn client toward the bed, shifting your weight to your leg nearest the bed, placing the client's legs on the bed as you turn.

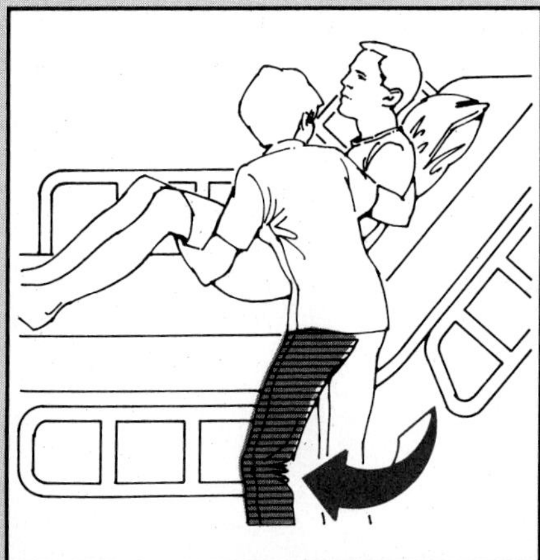

13. If there are no symptoms of overexertion, proceed with ambulation or transfer or continue to dangle for prescribed period before returning client to a supine position.

14. At completion of activity, leave client positioned comfortably in correct alignment, with bed in low position and siderails up.

11–14. See steps 6 to 8, above.

RECORDING: Indicate the amount of assistance needed to sit up. Describe tolerance in terms of vital sign changes, dizziness, sitting balance. Note length of time dangled or specific activity that followed.

PROCEDURE 30–4. ASSISTING WITH AMBULATION

PURPOSE: 1. To promote maintenance or restoration of endurance, muscle strength, and joint flexibility. 2. To provide environmental stimulation.

EQUIPMENT: Gait belt.

ACTION	RATIONALE
1. Obtain baseline pulse, respirations, and blood pressure. NOTE: If this is first ambulation of a client who has been on bed rest for several days, it is prudent to have one other person present to assist with ambulation.	1. Pulse, respirations, and blood pressure are indicators of the amount of stress caused by the exercise. Baseline values can be compared to values obtained during and after exercise to determine whether tolerance was reached or exceeded.
2. Discuss the procedure and its purpose with the client, including nurses' actions, and behavior desired of the client.	2. Active participation is more likely if client understands the procedure, desired behaviors, and anticipated benefits.
3. With bed at your waist level, assist client to a sitting position at the edge of the bed (see Procedure 30–3).	3. Correct working height reduces nurse's backstrain, allows use of large muscles. Back injury to nurse is possible if bed is too low.
4. Ask client to remain sitting at edge of bed ("dangle") while you assess for dizziness, increased pulse, shortness of breath, sitting balance. NOTE: If weight bearing is attempted before balance, vasomotor, and cardiovascular stabilization is established, orthostatic hypotension, syncope, or falls may occur.	4. Prolonged recumbency may cause sluggish response of arterial baroreceptors, with subsequent pooling of blood in dependent parts of the body, causing dizziness. Exertion causes increased pulse and respirations to supply increased O_2 requirements in muscle tissue. "Dangling" provides time for stabilization of both vital signs and perfusion.
5. If dizziness, increased pulse, or shortness of breath occurs and does not resolve within minutes, or if sitting balance cannot be maintained, return client to recumbent position and continue to prepare client for ambulation, using strengthening exercises and repeated dangling, to increase tolerance and improve balance.	5. These symptoms indicate that the exertion of sitting up has used most of the client's available energy. The additional stress of ambulation is not likely to be tolerated.
6. If balance is satisfactory, test quadriceps, iliopsoas, and anterior tibialis muscle strength (see Table 30–8) if there is any question about client's weight-bearing ability.	6. Adequacy of muscle strength determines whether client can ambulate, and indicates amount of assistance needed (see Table 30–8).

(continued)

PROCEDURE 30–4. (continued)

7. When client is stable, assist client to don nonslip footwear and robe. Footwear with open heel or high heel is not suitable. If client has no safe footwear, disposable slippers may be available on hospital supply cart.

NOTE: Ambulation without proper footwear predisposes client to falls and possible injury as well as promotes contamination of linen after return to bed. If client is not provided a robe, chilling, embarrassment, loss of self-esteem, and resistance to subsequent ambulation may occur.

7. Footwear is necessary to protect client from microorganisms on hospital floor and to prevent falls resulting from slipping. A robe prevents exposure of client's body.

8. Apply gait belt snugly but comfortably around client's waist (not needed for clients requiring minimal support (see Table 30–8). A belt-type restraint may be substituted if gait belt is not available.

NOTE: Ambulation without a gait belt can result in injury to client and nurse. If client becomes weak or dizzy, client may hold or lean on nurse for support, causing both to fall.

8. A gait belt provides a safe, sturdy means of support and allows the nurse to control the direction of a fall if loss of balance or syncope occurs without warning.

9. Lower bed so client can reach the floor without stretching or sliding.

9. Establishes firm footing prior to attempting weight bearing. Sliding or stretching to reach the floor from a high bed may cause client to slip, lose balance, possibly fall.

10. Face client, grasp belt on either side of client's spine. Instruct client to stand, using arms to assist in raising off the bed, while you assist by blocking client's knees with yours and pulling client to standing position. Nurse may reach under client's arms and place hands on client's scapulae if no gait belt is available.

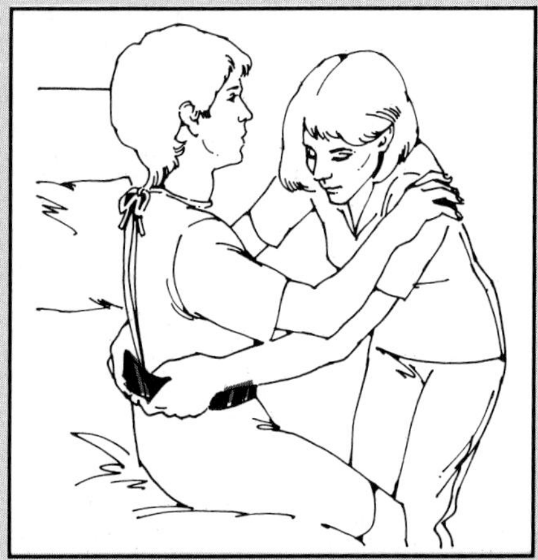

10. Enables active client participation, but the gait belt and blocking of the knees maintains control by the nurse so a fall can be prevented.

11. If client cannot maintain standing position without assistance, assist client to a sitting position at the edge of the bed, then return client to a recumbent position.

NOTE: Stand-up exercises (see Table 30–10) are indicated to increase strength for ambulation.

11. Ambulation requires independent weight bearing and balance.

(continued)

PROCEDURE 30–4. (continued)

12. When independent weight bearing is demonstrated, provide support for ambulation according to your assessment.

12. Enables clients to use their strength and balance to fullest extent, yet allows nurse to be aware of onset of weakness or decreased stability so immediate measures can be taken to provide client safety.

a. Minimal Support:
Stand next to client, slightly to the rear. Place one arm around client's waist, grasp the client's hand or forearm just below the elbow.

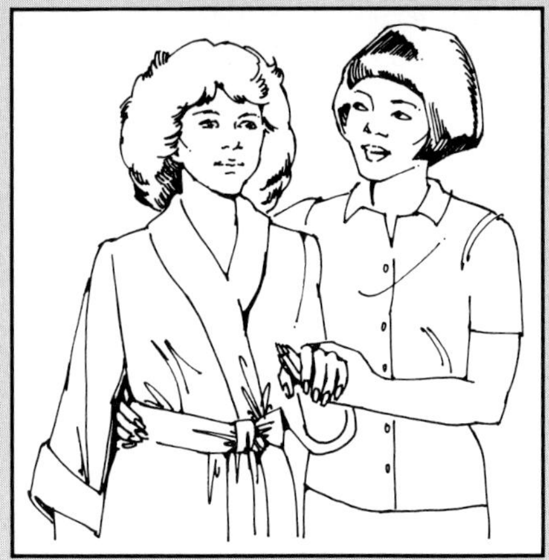

NOTE: If a client requires only reassurance, walk next to client. You may hold the upper arm lightly.

a. Holding client around the waist provides support and control if a fall is imminent (see step 16, below).

b. Moderate Support:
Stand next to the client's weaker side and slightly behind client. Grasp gait belt on either side of the client.

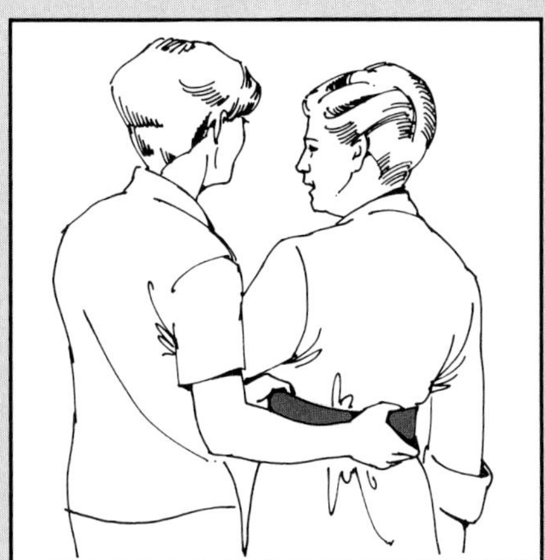

NOTE: Some clients lean toward the person assisting. In this case, standing on the strong side and slightly behind will help maintain better balance and prevent uneven weight shift to the weak side.

b. Most clients will fall toward their weaker side due to buckling of the weaker extremity. Standing at that side facilitates pulling the client toward you and controlling the fall.

(continued)

PROCEDURE 30–4. (continued)

c. Maximal Support:
Two nurses stand, one on either side and slightly behind the client, each grasping the belt at the back and the near side. Alternative support: Each nurse grasps belt on either side of the client's spine, holding client's near forearm with the other hand.

c. Provides balanced support and maximal control by nurses.

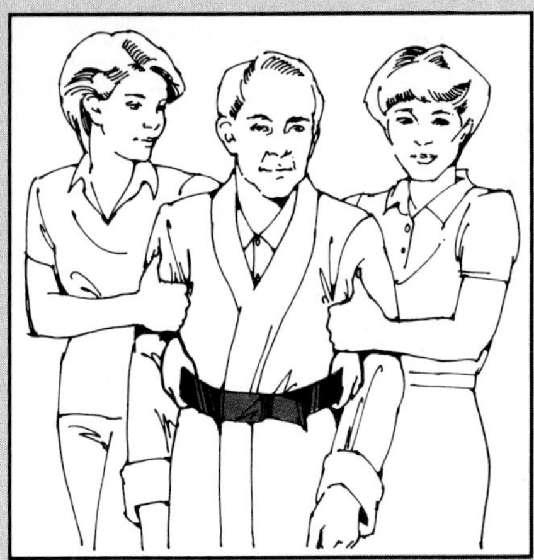

NOTE: One nurse attempting to assist a client needing maximal support risks injury to self and client.

13. Ambulate with the client the distance predetermined by prior assessment.

13. Prevents overexercise, fatigue, and/or injury.

14. Assess pulse, respirations, skin color, temperature, and moisture during ambulation and compare them to baseline data. Observe balance, stability of gait.

14. These are indicators of exercise tolerance.

15. If client reports weakness or dizziness or you note decreased stability, step close to client and support client by putting both arms around client's waist.

15. Provides temporary support for the client while a decision is made whether continued ambulation is possible.

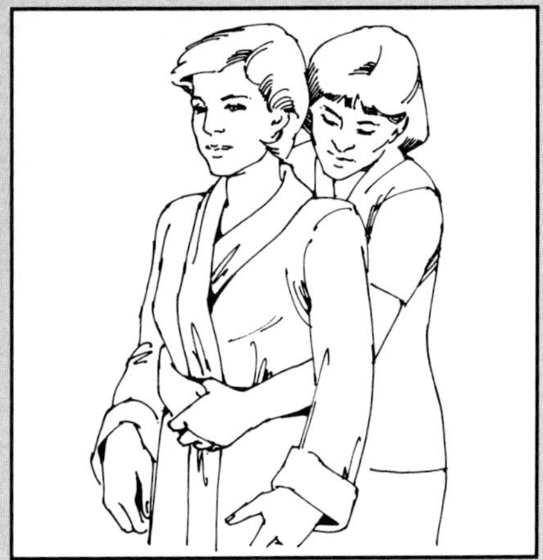

NOTE: Pulse increase of 20 to 25 bpm, labored respirations, diaphoresis, flushing, light-headedness, dizziness, or gait becoming uneven indicate that activity should be terminated.

(continued)

PROCEDURE 30–4. (continued)

16. If these symptoms occur, assist client to lean on nearby wall or sturdy furniture. For dizziness or light-headedness, have client inhale aromatic spirits of ammonia.

16. Support for a brief period may provide time for stabilization of pulse and respirations, allowing safe return to bed. Spirits of ammonia causes local irritation of respiratory membranes, resulting in increased respiratory rate and depth and therefore increasing O_2 delivery to the brain. May prevent fainting and can be used to arouse a person who has fainted.

17. If client is unable to continue ambulating, request another health care team member to obtain a wheelchair.

17. Provides a safe means of returning to bed without leaving the client unsupported.

18. If sudden loss of balance or syncope occurs while ambulating, pull the client toward you while stepping backward.

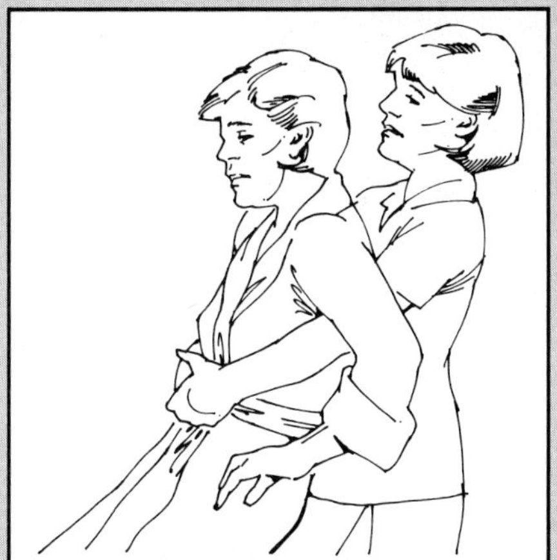

18. This action controls the direction of the fall by bringing the weight of the client to the nurse's center of gravity and into the nurse's base of support, therefore minimizing possibility of injury to the client or nurse. The weight of a falling client is too great for one or two nurses to support. Attempting to stop a fall will cause muscle strain or more serious injury.

19. Lower client to the floor by stepping backward and squatting or kneeling on one knee, keeping your back straight. Obtain assistance to place client in a wheelchair or on gurney and return client to bed.

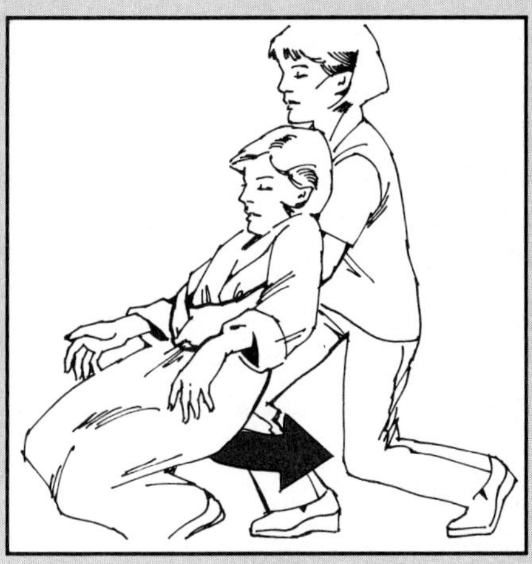

19. Uses larger stronger leg and arm muscles to control client movement.

NOTE: This incident should be reported to the team leader, head nurse, and physician. Immediately assess for injury.

(continued)

PROCEDURE 30–4. (continued)

20. If no symptoms of intolerance of exercise occur, complete ambulation as planned. Assess pulse, respirations, and blood pressure, and skin color, moisture, and temperature immediately after exercise and 5 minutes later. Question client about subjective sensations of fatigue. Compare values to preambulation baseline and previous postambulation data to determine progress. Exercise is appropriate if pulse increase is less than 20 bpm, respiration is not labored, diaphoresis is not excessive, and if pulse, respirations, and blood pressure return to baseline within 5 minutes. If skin and vital signs changes are absent or minimal, exercise may be increased.

    20. Comparison to preambulation data and assessment of time required for values to return to baseline provides a means to assess client's progress and plan for increases in exercise without causing undue stress.

21. Leave client resting comfortably in bed after exercise has been completed.

RECORDING: Indicate duration of ambulation, distance walked, amount and type of assistance needed, and specific response of client in nurse's notes. If a change in ambulation plan is indicated, record this on the client care plan.

PROCEDURE 30–5. ASSISTING WITH AMBULATION USING A WALKER

PURPOSE: To provide benefits of ambulation to clients with low endurance or poor balance.

EQUIPMENT: Pick-up or rolling walker.

ACTION	RATIONALE
1. Assess balance and shoulder, arm, and leg strength. NOTE: A walker is not stable enough to support a client with poor balance or without ability to bear weight in at least one leg. Falls could result.	1. A walker is suitable for a client with adequate arm and shoulder strength to support body weight, full weight-bearing ability in at least one leg, and the ability to balance with minimal support.
2. Measure walker and adjust so its height approximates distance between client's greater trochanter and floor, so client can stand between rear legs and grasp hand supports with arms flexed 20 to 30 degrees.	2. Allows efficient use of arm and leg muscles to support weight during ambulation. Early fatigue will result if walker is too high or too low.
3. Obtain baseline pulse, respirations, and blood pressure.	3. Changes in these values indicate amount of stress caused by exercise. Baseline values are compared to inter- and postexercise values to determine tolerance (see Table 30–6).

(continued)

4. Assist client to prepare for standing (see Procedure 30–4, steps 3 to 6). When rising to a standing position, chair arms or bed should be used for support, not walker.

4. See Procedure 30–4. Walker base of support is not broad enough to resist side and downard force without tipping.

5. Walk with client: Stand to the side of the walker (weaker side, if applicable) and slightly behind client.

5. Facilitates breaking a fall if sudden weakness, fainting, or loss of balance occurs.

6. Tell client to keep walker slightly ahead of him or her and to look ahead (not at floor) while walking.

6. Maintains a wide base of support over which to keep center of gravity during ambulation. Looking ahead facilitates maintenance of correct posture.

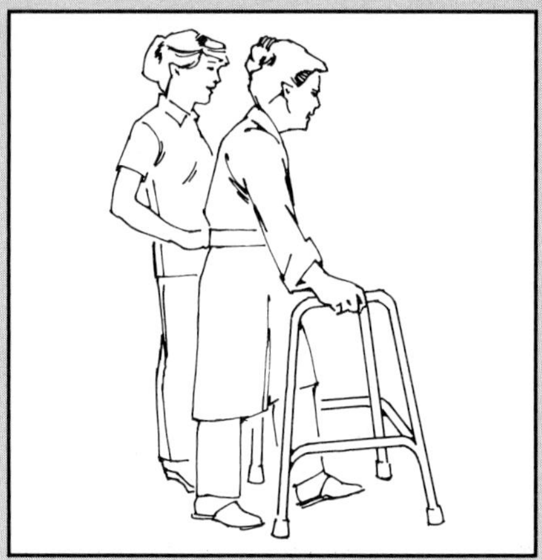

NOTE: if client steps too close to front bar of walker, his or her center of gravity may move so close to the edge of the base of support that walker may tip when client puts weight on hand supports.

7. Instruct client to keep weight forward when lifting walker and to set it down evenly, so all four legs touch floor simultaneously.

7. Maintains stable base of support, keeps client center of gravity over base of support.

NOTE: Bending and straightening the body as walker is lifted will cause client to shift weight backward when straightening, which may cause a backward fall.

8. Instruct client to use gait appropriate for abilities:

   a. Advance walker, then step with each foot, using arms for support.

8a. Weight-bearing gait for client too weak to walk unassisted, but with ability to bear weight on either leg.

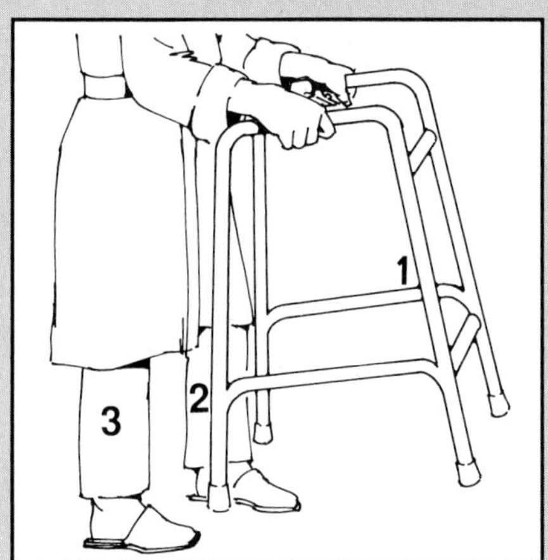

(continued)

PROCEDURE 30–5. (continued)

b. Advance walker and weaker leg simultaneously, then bring stronger leg forward.

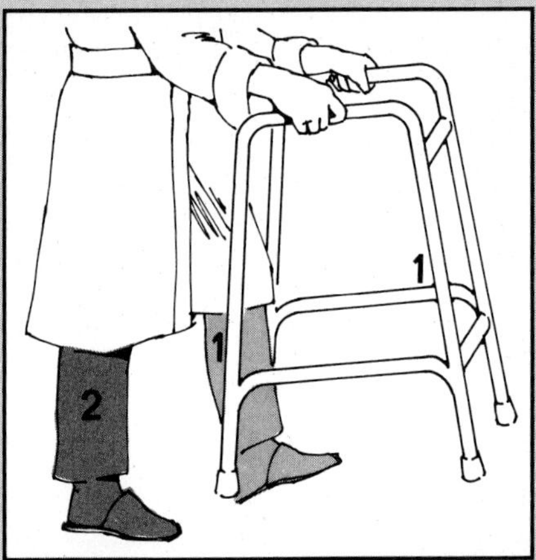

b. Allows partial or no weightbearing on weaker leg. Requires good balance and arm strength. Weight is concentrated on small base of support as walker is moved.

9. If turning is necessary during ambulation, instruct client to move toward the stronger side. Keep feet wide apart during turn to keep adequate base of support.

9. Weaker side then becomes center of a turning circle, requiring smallest amount of movement.

NOTE: Pivoting on either foot is not recommended, as fall is likely due to loss of balance. Pivoting creates very small base of support for wide mass of client and walker.

10. Assess activity tolerance during ambulation (see Procedure 30–4, steps 13 to 15).

10. See Procedure 30–4.

11. If sudden loss of balance or syncope occurs, step toward client. Grasp client around waist or under axilla and lower client to the floor by squatting or kneeling on one knee, keeping your own back straight. Obtain assistance to place client in a wheelchair or gurney to return to bed. Report fall to team leader, head nurse, and/or physician, so immediate assessment for injury can be done.

11. Controls direction of fall, minimizing possibility of injury to client or nurse. Provides safe means of return to bed.

NOTE: Attempting to stop the fall will result in muscle strain or more serious injury to nurse. Allowing the client to fall onto the walker could increase seriousness of the injury.

12. To return to a sitting position after successful ambulation:

a. Walk close to chair or bed, turning (see step 9) so back faces bed/chair. (Wheels must be locked.)

12a. Reduces risk of falls during turn to chair/bed (see step 9). Locked wheels prevent movement of bed/chair.

NOTE: Unlocked wheels are a major cause of falls as weight of client against unstable chair/bed causes movement and loss of support.

(continued)

b. Tell client to back up toward chair or bed as follows:
- Pull walker toward himself or herself.
- Place weight on hand supports, stepping back with strong leg. Then move weaker (shaded) leg back.
- Repeat until back of both legs touches bed/chair.

b. Maintains center of gravity over base of support, uses strongest muscles for effort of movement.

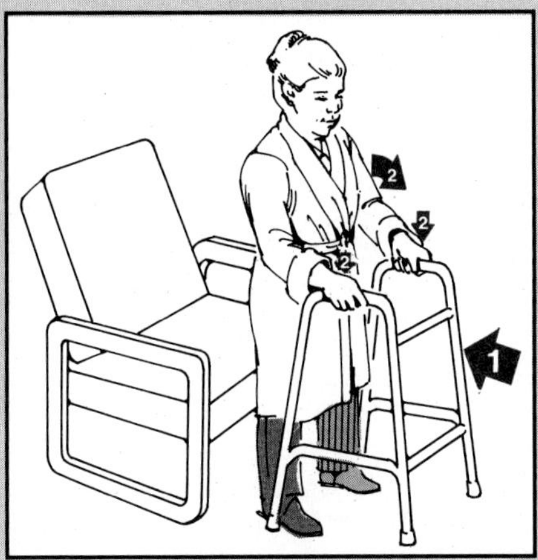

c. Reach back with one hand at a time, grasping chair arm or placing palm on surface of bed.

c. Creates widest support, demands minimal independent balance. Falls could result from loss of balance if client turns to see chair/bed or reaches back with both hands simultaneously.

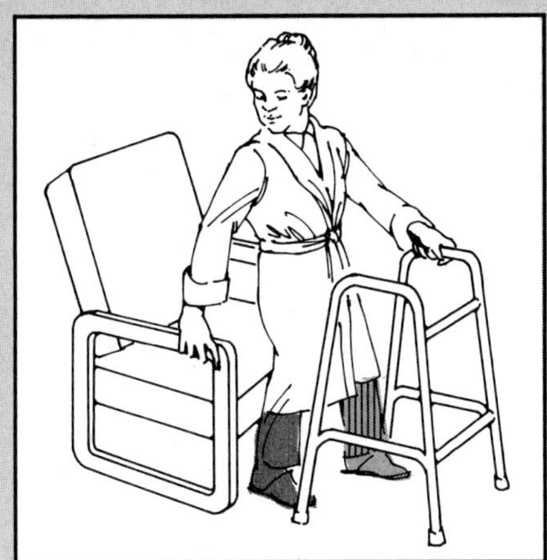

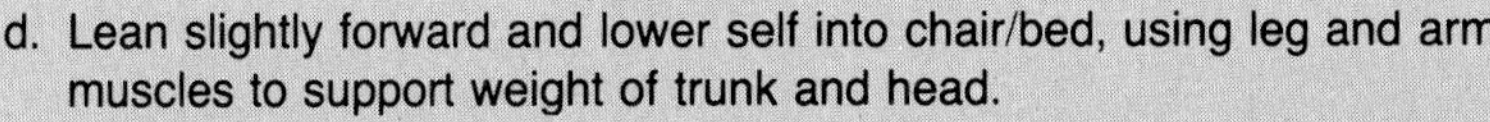

d. Lean slightly forward and lower self into chair/bed, using leg and arm muscles to support weight of trunk and head.

d. Until weight is centered over chair/bed, base of support is in front of chair/bed. Leaning back would allow nearly two thirds of body weight to be prematurely shifted beyond support of legs or arms.

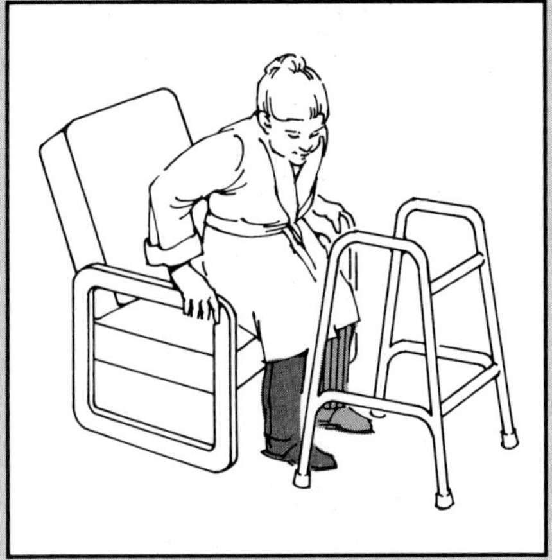

(continued)

PROCEDURE 30–5. (continued)

13. Assess exercise tolerance at completion of transfer to chair/bed. See Procedure 30–4, step 20. — 13. See Procedure 30–4.

14. Leave client resting comfortably.

RECORDING: Indicate distance walked; type of walker, skill in its use, amount and type of assistance needed, if any; and response of client, including any unusual occurrences (eg, falls) and action taken.

weak or paralyzed limbs using their stronger limbs, as illustrated in Figure 30–15.

Performing certain **activities of daily living** (ADL), self-care skills required for independent living, such as hygiene, grooming, and dressing, provides another opportunity for clients to actively exercise muscles and joints. Encourage clients to independently perform as many of these activities as possible to maintain their muscle and joint function. Gradually incorporate isometric and other isotonic exercises into the client exercise plan as well.

Transfers. Clients with mobility problems often need assistance moving from the bed to a chair, bedside commode, or gurney. These maneuvers are called transfers. It is beneficial for all but the most seriously ill clients to experience the change in environment and associated mental, social, and physical stimulation that transfers facilitate. As Figure 30–16 illustrates, being confined to bed surrounded by hospital equipment can be physically and psychologically confining. For the greatest physical benefit to clients, they should actively participate in the transfer maneuver to the maximum degree possible. This is an important step in progressive mobilization. To determine the type of transfer technique that is best for a particular client, use data obtained in the mobility assessment. The following factors are most relevant.

TABLE 30–9. ISOMETRIC EXERCISES

Exercise	Instruction	Purpose
	General: Hold each contraction 6 seconds. Repeat three times. Increase number of repetitions as strength increases.	
Quadriceps setting	Lie supine or sit with legs extended. Press the back of the knee against the surface of the bed.	Preparation for ambulation, prevention of flexion contracture of knee.
Abdominal setting	Supine: Attempt to "pull in stomach" or flatten abdomen. Prone: Pull abdomen up from surface of the bed without lifting shoulders or hips.	Preparation for ambulation, improve muscle tone.
Gluteal setting	Squeeze buttocks together. May be done lying prone, supine or sitting.	Preparation for ambulation.
Footboard exercise	Push against footboard with plantar surface (bottom) of foot while sitting with HOB elevated and knees slightly flexed.	Preparation for ambulation, prevention of foot drop.
Hand squeeze	Tightly clench fist. May also squeeze small rubber ball.	Increase hand strength for ADL or crutch walking or other ambulation aids.
Hand pulls	Flex fingers of both hands, interlock with one palm facing toward chest, the other away. Pull as if to separate hands.	Increase upper arm, shoulder, and grip strength.
Biceps setting	Push down on surface of mattress with palm of hand while lying prone.	Increase tone and strength of the biceps.
Triceps setting	Push down on surface of mattress with palm of hand while lying supine. Or, raise arms above chest, pushing palms together.	Increase tone and strength of the triceps.
Kegel exercises	Contract muscles of the pelvic floor as if to stop the stream of urine.	Improve tone of muscles of pelvic floor to diminish stress incontinence or to increase sexual pleasure.

TABLE 30–10. ISOTONIC EXERCISES

Exercise	Instruction	Purpose
Pelvic tilt	Lying supine, knees flexed, alternately arch and press small of back against surface of bed.	Relieves lower back stiffness, strengthens abdominal and back muscles.
Knee lift	Lying supine, legs extended. Bring one knee to flexed position on chest, grasping with arms. Return to extended position, repeat with other leg. May progress to flexing both legs simultaneously. Single leg flexor may be done standing.	Strengthens abdominals, quadriceps, and muscles of lower back. Increases flexibility of spine, hip and knee joints. When done in standing position, also improves balance.
Leg raiser	Lying supine, knees flexed. Extend one lower leg so leg forms a straight line from hip to toe. Return to start position and repeat with other leg. May progress to raising extended leg from hip.	See knee lift.
Knee extender	While seated in a chair, slide one foot back as far under the chair as you can reach, then straighten the leg so it extends out from the chair. Lower the leg halfway to the floor and hold 3 to 6 seconds. Repeat with other leg.	Strengthens quadriceps; good preparation for weight bearing, walking.
Head and shoulder curl	Lying supine, tuck hands under small of back, palms down. Contract abdominal muscles, raise head off mattress. May progress to raising head and shoulders, then head, shoulders, and elbows, then to full sit up.	Strengthens abdominals, neck muscles. Increases neck and upper spine flexibility.
Lateral leg raiser	Lying on side, arm extended above head, palm down, rest head on arm and raise leg off bed. Repeat on other side. As strength increases, increase height to which leg is raised.	Strengthens muscles of lateral thigh, increases hip flexibility.
Prone arch	Lying prone, arms at sides, palms up. Raise head from mattress. Return to resting position. May progress to raising head and shoulders, then head, shoulders, and legs, arching back.	Strengthens neck and abdominal muscles. Increases flexibility of spine, hip joint. When legs are also raised, hamstrings and calf muscles are also strengthened.
Trapeze pull-ups	Grasp overbed trapeze firmly in both hands. Flex elbows to pull up to sitting position, lower by extending arms. May progress to raising buttocks off bed.	Strengthens upper arms and shoulder girdle. Useful for preparation for ambulation with walker, cane, or crutches and improving flexibility of all upper extremity joints.
Knee push-ups	Lying prone, knees flexed, hands on mattress under shoulders, palms down. Push upper body off mattress until arms are fully extended and body forms a straight line from head to knees. Return to resting position.	Strengthens triceps, pectorals, muscles of shoulder girdle. Increased flexibility of wrist, elbow, shoulder, knee joints.
Sitting stretch	Sit with legs extended and apart, hands on knees. Bend forward at waist, extending arms as far as possible. Variation: Stretch first toward dorsiflexed right foot, return to sitting position, then stretch to left foot, pulling feet toward head.	Strengthens hamstrings, calf muscles. Increases flexibility of spine, hip and shoulder joints. Variation stretches heel cords.
Stand-ups	Begin with bed or chair seat raised (using books or catalogs) to a height equal to 1½ × length of a client's knee-to-foot measurement. Obtain a table (without wheels or with brakes) high enough to reach client's midthigh. Have feet on the floor (shoes on) and sit on the edge of chair or bed facing table, hands flat on table. Lean forward slightly, straighten legs and back until erect. Use table for balance, not to assist in standing. Stand 10 seconds, sit down 15 seconds, repeat 10 to 20 times. Do this set of stand-ups four times a day. As strength increases, lower the chair or bed to a level from which standing is moderately difficult. Continue to repeat 10 to 30 times, four times a day. Lower bed or chair until client can stand independently from a chair of standard height.	Increases strength of quadriceps, conditions autonomic reflexes controlling blood flow to the head. Prepares for independent ambulation.

(continued)

TABLE 30–10. (continued)

Exercise	Instruction	Purpose
Shoulder stretch	Stand erect, clench fists in front of chest with elbows at shoulder height. Keeping head erect, thrust elbows back without arching back. Return to starting position.	Reduces tension in neck and upper back.
Body bender	Stand erect, feet at shoulder width. Interlace fingers behind neck. Bend to right as far as possible, return to erect and bend to left. Variation: Extend arms above head. Bend side to side as above, sliding left arm down side of left leg and right arm down side of right leg.	Stretches muscles of lateral chest, lower back. Increases flexibility of shoulders, sacroiliac joint and spine. Variation stretches trapesius.
Torso twist	Stand erect, feet at shoulder width, arms extended laterally, level with shoulders. Without moving feet (twist at the waist), bring right arm and shoulder across chest and as far to the left as possible. Return to start and repeat with left arm.	Strengthens shoulder girdle muscles of back and lateral trunk. Increases flexibility of iliosacral joint, spine.
Half knee bend	Stand erect, feet at shoulder width, hands on hips. Bend knees halfway while extending arms forward, palms down. Return to start. May progress to full knee bends.	Strengthens biceps, shoulder girdle, quadriceps, and calf muscles. Increases flexibility of ankle, knee, hip joints.
Ankle stretch	Stand erect, feet together, arms extended forward at the shoulder. Raise up on tiptoe, return to start. Variation: Stand on large book, weight on balls of feet. Lower heels, then raise up on tiptoe. Return to start.	Strengthens shoulder girdle hamstrings, calf and foot muscles. Increases flexibility of foot and ankle joints. Variation also stretches heel cords and improves balance.
Toe toucher	Stand erect, feet at shoulder width, arms extended above head. Bend down, touching toes without bending knees. Return to start. Variation: Spread feet about 30 inches apart, arms extended laterally at shoulder height. Alternating sides, touch left hand to right toe, right hand to left toe, standing erect between toe touches.	Strengthens biceps, shoulder girdle, back muscles, gluteals, hamstrings, calf muscles. Increases flexibility of spine, hip joint.

1. *Strength.* A client's ability to support his or her own weight is a critical factor in the selection of a transfer method. Active standing transfers require good quadriceps strength in at least one leg. Guidelines for leg strength assessment appear in Table 30–8. Upper extremity strength should also be assessed. To assist even minimally in transfers, clients need sufficient upper extremity strength to move independently in bed.

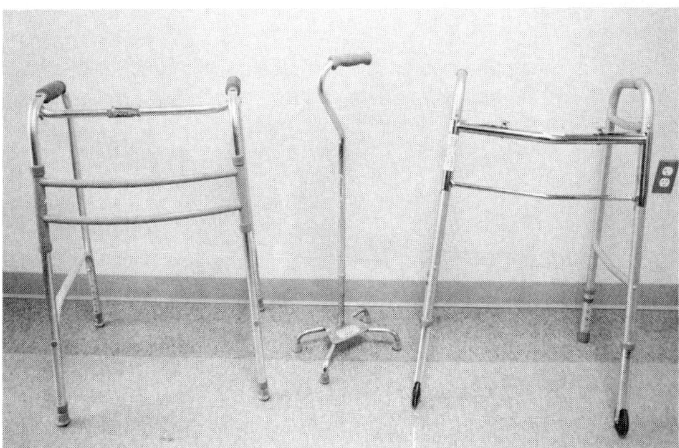

Figure 30–14. Two types of walkers and quad cane. **A.** Pick-up walker. **B.** Narrow-based quad cane. **C.** Rolling walker.

2. *Endurance.* Endurance can also be assessed by watching activity in bed. A client who can perform isotonic exercises for several minutes without fatigue has adequate endurance for an active transfer. Nurses must remember, however, that simply being up in a chair after a period of recumbency can be taxing. Assess clients for signs of fatigue at short intervals and offer assistance to return to bed before a client becomes exhausted.
3. *Balance.* Do not attempt an active standing transfer if a client's sitting balance is poor. Table 30–8 provides guidelines for determining both sitting and standing balance.
4. *Joint mobility.* Limitations in ROM of spine or extremities can interfere with or even preclude weight bearing and active participation in a transfer. The degree of interference depends upon other parameters, especially strength. Some alterations in transfer technique can be made to accommodate diminished ROM, but principles of body mechanics must be maintained.

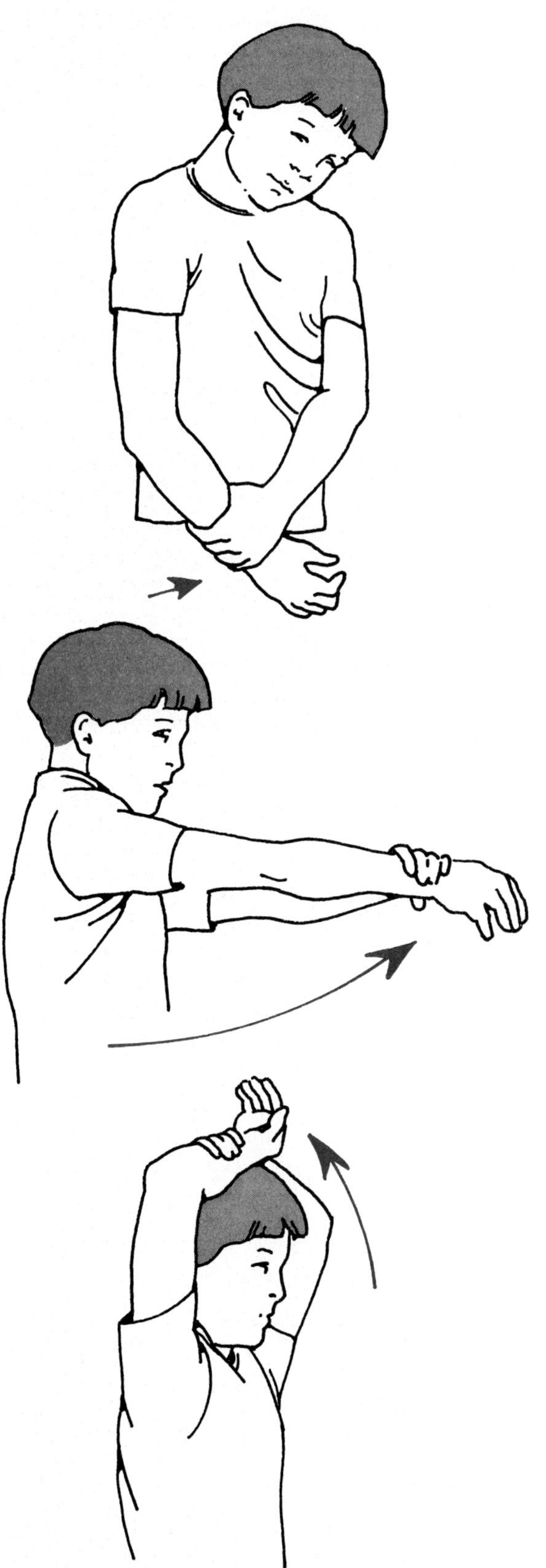

Figure 30–15. Active self-assisted shoulder exercise.

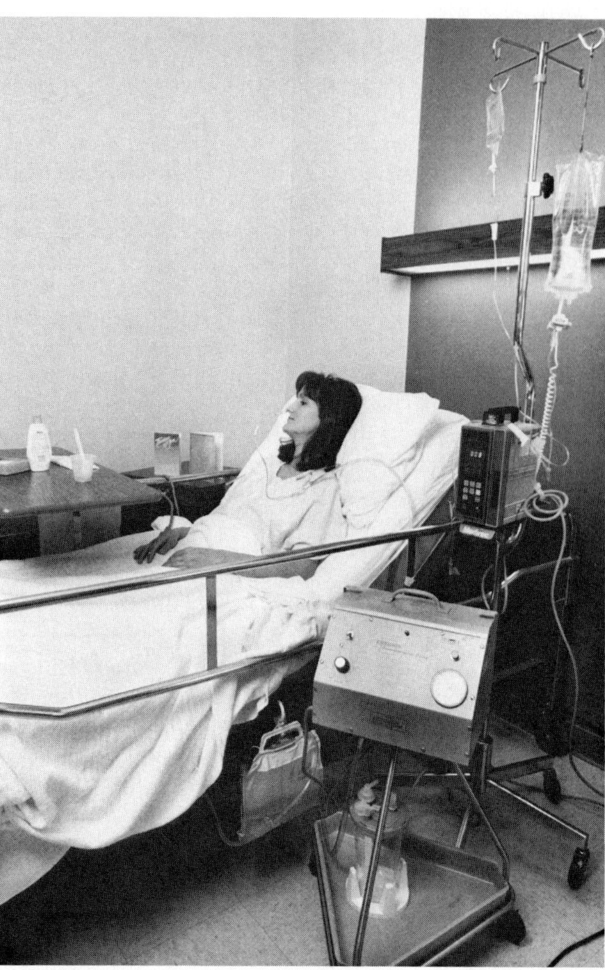

Figure 30–16. Hospital equipment creates physical and psychological barriers to mobility.

5. *Comprehension.* Clients must be able to understand and carry out simple verbal instructions to participate actively in a transfer. A client who is confused or disoriented requires maximum assistance during transfers to prevent injury to self and health care personnel. Visual and hearing deficits may also interfere with comprehension, although alternative methods of conveying signals may alleviate this problem. Take precautions to assure that a client can understand and respond appropriately to any signals to be used during an active transfer.
6. *Motivation.* A desire to become more independent is needed for active participation in transfers. Anxiety, pain, and misconceptions may contribute to poor motivation for independent activity. Inability to accept the sick role or body image changes may also inhibit participation. If you note lack of motivation or resistance to attempt progressive mobilization, take time to explore the possible contributing causes. Although positive reinforcement and a gradual increase in activity can be effective motivators, these strategies will not be sufficient for clients whose participation is limited because of

underlying attitudes that prevent them from using their available physical potential.

If the assessment indicates that independent transfer is appropriate, place a chair that promotes correct posture in the location the client desires. Cover the seat and back of the chair with a bath blanket. If the chair has wheels, be sure to lock the brakes before the client begins the transfer. The bed should be in the lowest position and wheels of the bed locked as well. Support the client if necessary while walking to the chair, as described in Procedure 30–4. When the client is seated, cover with a blanket if the client desires and secure the nurse call light within reach. For some clients, moving the chair to a location outside of the client's room provides needed stimulation and opportunities for communication.

For independent transfer to a gurney (for example, to transport a client to a diagnostic test or therapy), place it parallel to the bed so the head ends of bed and gurney are next to each other. Lock the brakes on both the bed and the gurney and adjust the height of the bed so it is even with the gurney. Screen the client and fold the covers out of the way. If the client has an IV or a urinary drainage system, move the containers and tubing so they will not be obstacles during the move. Often they can be secured on the side of the gurney farthest from the bed. Raise the head of the bed or ask the client to sit up and move to the edge of the bed. Have the client place one foot and hand on the gurney, then raise his or her hips to shift them onto the gurney and repeat this movement until centered on the gurney. Moving in a sitting position rather than shifting the body in segments while lying down is preferred for most clients because the former uses the larger, stronger limb muscles rather than the back and abdominal muscles. Rolling clients onto a gurney is also an effective means of transfer. This works well for alert clients who have received regional anesthetic blocks and do not have full use of all extremities. Position the gurney as described above. Stand next to the gurney and assist the client to roll toward you as described in Procedure 30–11. Cover the client and secure siderails or safety belt before moving. Procedures 30–6 and 30–7 describe transfer techniques for clients needing more assistance. The techniques for transfers to a chair can also be used to transfer clients to a bedside commode.

Devices to Facilitate Transfers. Although use of effective body mechanics can accomplish the safe transfer of many clients, assistive devices can enhance body mechanics or facilitate moving clients who are too heavy or too weak for nurses to move safely without extra support for clients' weight. A gait belt facilitates nurses' use of correct mechanics. Two other transfer devices to move heavy clients that are available in most acute care and rehabilitation facilities are a sliding board and a hydraulic lift.

Gait Belt. Gait belts have long been routinely used by physical therapists for transfer and gait training in rehabilitation

(*Text continues on page 1499.*)

PROCEDURE 30–6. TRANSFERRING A CLIENT FROM A BED TO A GURNEY

PURPOSE: To move a dependent client from bed to gurney to facilitate transport to treatment or diagnostic test or to provide environmental stimulation.

EQUIPMENT: Pull-sheet, gurney with brakes and siderails or safety belt, sliding board (if available); large plastic trash bag if no sliding board.

ACTION	RATIONALE
1. Discuss the procedure with the client, including nurse's actions, behavior desired of client, and signals to be used to synchronize actions. Screen client.	1. Client will be more willing and able to participate if expected behavior, reasons, and benefits of the procedures are clear.
2. Using pull-sheet method described in Procedure 30–11, move the client near the edge of the bed. NOTE: Using a sliding board or plastic trash bag under the pull-sheet reduces friction and therefore the effort needed to move client.	2. Shortens distance client must be moved after gurney is in position. The gurney lengthens the distance nurse(s) must reach, therefore increasing risk of back injury if the gurney were positioned prior to moving the client to the edge of the bed.

(continued)

3. Position the gurney so it is parallel to the bed with the head end of the gurney next to the head end of the bed. Adjust the height of the bed so it is level with the gurney. Lock wheels of bed and gurney.

3. Facilitates transfer with minimum effort and maximum safety.

4. Screen client, fanfold sheets to foot of bed. Move IV bottles or drainage bags, if any, and secure them on gurney so tubing does not become entangled as client moves.

4. Covers, IVs, drainage bags, and tubing are moved so they are not obstacles to smooth movement; screening maintains client's privacy.

NOTE: Heavy, helpless clients will require four nurses for transfer. If the number of available assistants is limited, alternate method, such as a hydraulic lifter, is recommended (see Procedure 30–8). Lighter clients can be moved by two to three nurses. The third nurse can assist by moving client's legs.

5. All nurses roll the pull-sheet so edges are close to client's body and grasp firmly so client is supported at the hips and shoulders. Nurse nearest head of bed can grasp corner of pillow so it will move with client, supporting the head.

5. Maximizes control during transfer, improves leverage.

6. Nurse(s) next to the gurney (side 1) assume a broad stance: Feet shoulder width apart with one foot next to the bed, the other foot about 2 feet from the bed, with weight on the foot nearest the bed.

6. This stance provides a stable base of support during shifting of nurses' weight as client is transferred.

7. Nurse(s) on opposite side (side 2) kneel on the bed with knees shoulder width apart and one knee slightly forward.

7. Allows nurse(s) to keep client's weight near their center of gravity during transfer.

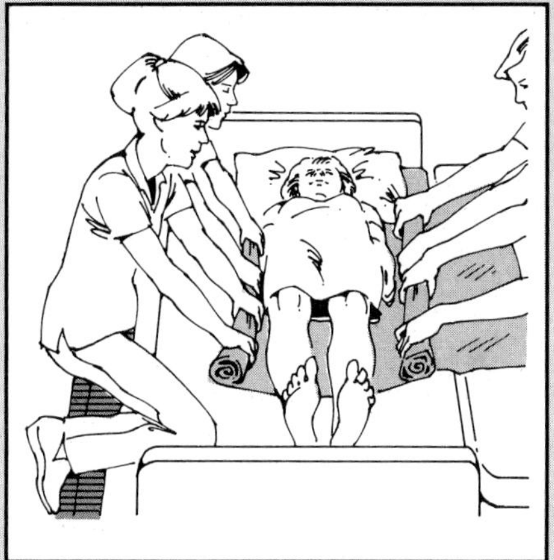

(continued)

PROCEDURE 30–6. (continued)

8. On signal, all nurses contract pelvic muscles, then side 1 nurse(s) shift to back foot, pulling on pull-sheet as weight is shifted. Side 2 nurse(s) lift up slightly on pull-sheet while shifting their weight to their forward knee.

8. Contracting pelvic muscles reduces potential for joint injury. Simultaneous weight shifts accomplish smooth transfer with least expenditure of nurses' energy. Slight lifting by side 2 nurse(s) reduces friction, but causes minimal strain as nurses are above the level of the client.

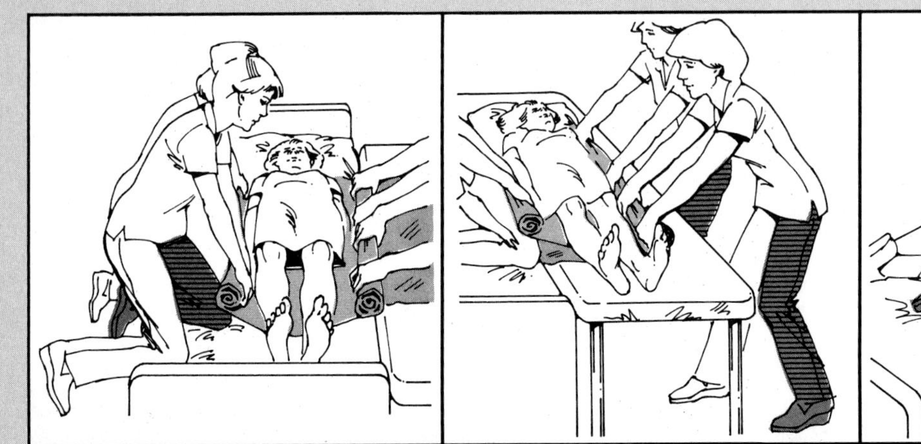

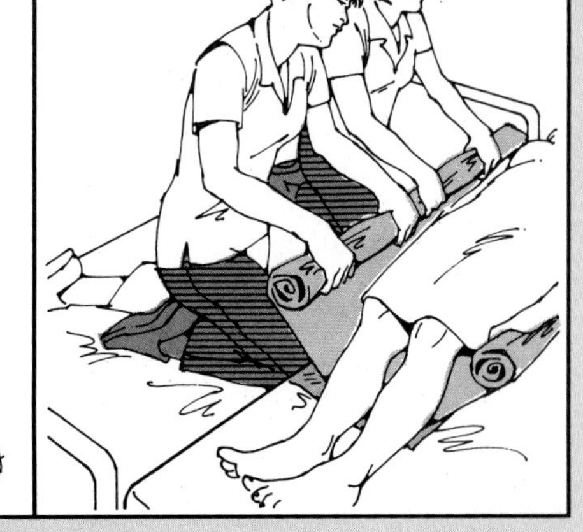

9. Repeat as necessary until client is centered on the gurney.

9. Several short moves expend less energy than one longer move.

10. At completion of transfer, provide pillows, cover client with sheet, secure safety belt, and/or raise siderails. Release brake and push gurney to intended destination in a feet-first direction.

10. Promotes client comfort and safety.

RECORDING: Method of transfer need not be documented in progress notes; however, it is common practice to note trips off the ward and indicate the purpose. Location of this entry varies with mode of record-keeping. It is helpful to indicate most effective method for transferring a client on the Kardex or client care plan.

PROCEDURE 30–7. TRANSFERRING A CLIENT FROM A BED TO A CHAIR

PURPOSE: *Pivot transfer:* To assist a client with weight-bearing ability in one leg only to move safely from bed to chair.
Two-person lift: To move a lightweight client unable to bear weight from bed to chair.

EQUIPMENT: Transfer belt, wheelchair, or other stable chair.

ACTION	RATIONALE
Method A: Pivot Transfer	
1. Discuss procedure and its purpose with the client, including nurse's actions, signals to be used, and behavior desired of the client.	1. Active participation is more likely if client understands expected behaviors, and anticipated benefits.
NOTE: If client's participation is not certain, another method of transfer should be selected, as cooperative weight bearing on the part of the client is required for a safe pivot transfer.	
2. Place a chair next to bed, adjacent to client's stronger (pivot) leg. Place a folded sheet or bath blanket over seat and back of chair. If wheelchair is used: Remove or reposition leg supports to provide leg room for you and client during pivot; secure brakes and swing front casters forward for maximum stability.	2. Provides shortest distance between client's weight-bearing leg and chair. Covering protects the chair from drainage or secretions and reduces the client's discomfort due to skin contact with plastic surface of the chair.
NOTE: If transfer is attempted in the direction of client's non-weight-bearing leg, the distance will be too great for a safe pivot. The client's weight must then be borne by the nurse, which may cause muscle strain, or more serious injury.	
3. Instruct or assist client to dangle (see Procedure 30–3).	
4. If assessment during dangling indicates client is stable enough for transfer, apply transfer belt, shoes, and robe.	4. Belt provides safe, sturdy means of support during pivot. Shoes minimize contamination of feet and bed from microorganisms on floor and provide stable footing; robe prevents exposure of client's body.

(continued)

PROCEDURE 30–7. (continued)

5. Lower the bed so the client's feet are firmly planted on the floor with the knees slightly lower than the hips. Client's lower legs should be angled back slightly toward the bed. (Strong leg is shaded.)

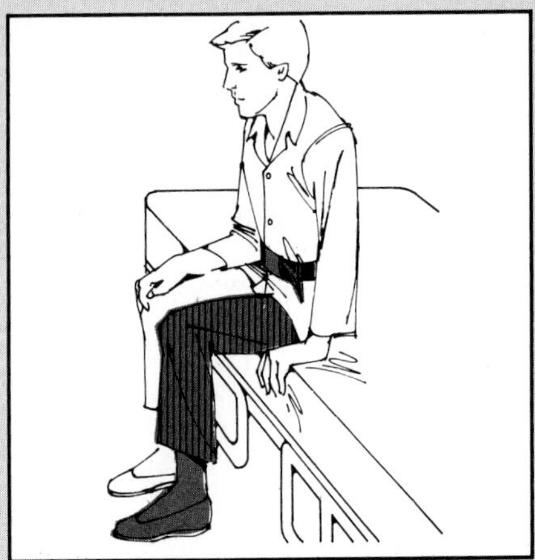

5. In this position, the least effort is required to attain a standing position. Higher level of hips reduces the distance the client must raise the body weight. Angle of the legs keeps base of support directly below client's center of gravity.

6. If client has an IV, Foley catheter, or other drainage bag, move them before attempting pivot, positioning them to prevent tension or tangling during transfer.

NOTE: Foley catheter drainage bag should be positioned below level of the bladder when client is seated to prevent reflux of urine into bladder, which creates risk for urinary infection.

6. Tension or tangling of tubing could cause disruption of IV or drainage system, pain, or injury to client. If client or nurse becomes entangled in tubing, a fall could result.

7. Face the client. Contract your pelvic muscles and assume the following stance:

   a. Place your foot nearest the chair outside the far front leg (or caster) parallel to the side of the chair.

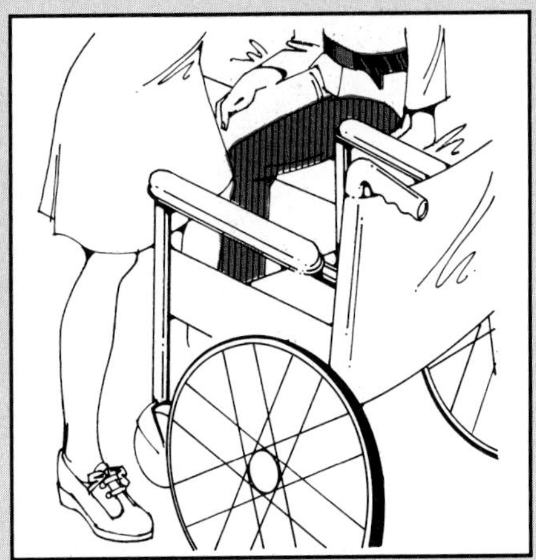

7. Protects nurse's hip joints, provides a wide base of support.

(continued)

PROCEDURE 30–7. (continued)

b. Place your other foot *inside* the client's pivot foot so your feet touch. Then move your knee so it is *outside* the client's knee. Both of your knees should be slightly flexed, your back straight.

b. Nurse's leg position blocks client's pivot leg, preventing buckling during pivot. Flexed knees facilitate use of stronger leg muscles to assist client to stand, protects nurse's back.

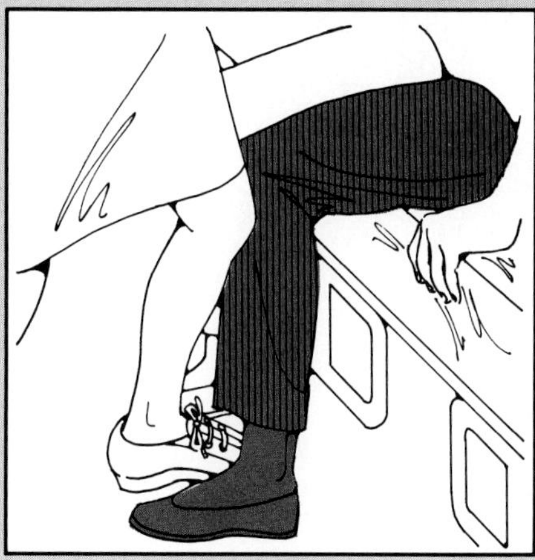

NOTE: Failing to correctly block client's weight-bearing leg could cause both client and nurse to fall if client is unable to support the weight as expected.

8. Ask the client to place one hand on your shoulder or on the arm of the wheelchair nearest the bed in preparation for standing. Grasp the transfer belt at the client's hips. If no transfer belt is available, reach under the client's arms and place your hands on the client's scapulae. Client may push self up from the bed if desired, then reach for arm of chair.

8. Provides support and guidance for client's upper body during pivot.

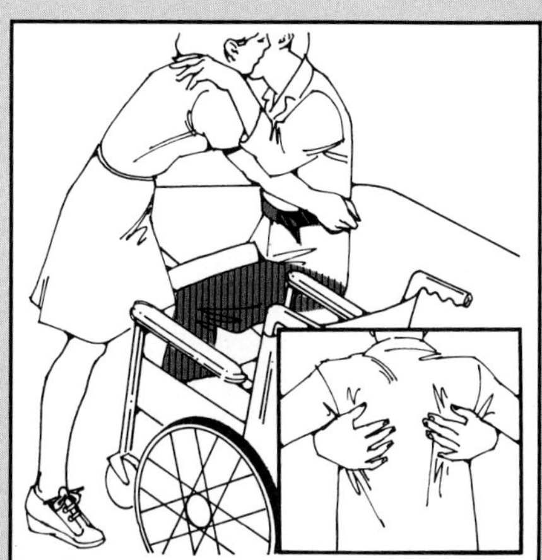

NOTE: It is important that the client be prevented from placing the arms around the nurse's neck. This will pull nurse toward client, moving the center of gravity outside the base of support, thereby increasing risk of falling and backstrain.

(continued)

PROCEDURE 30–7. (continued)

9. On signal, client stands while nurse assists by straightening own legs and shifting weight to back leg.

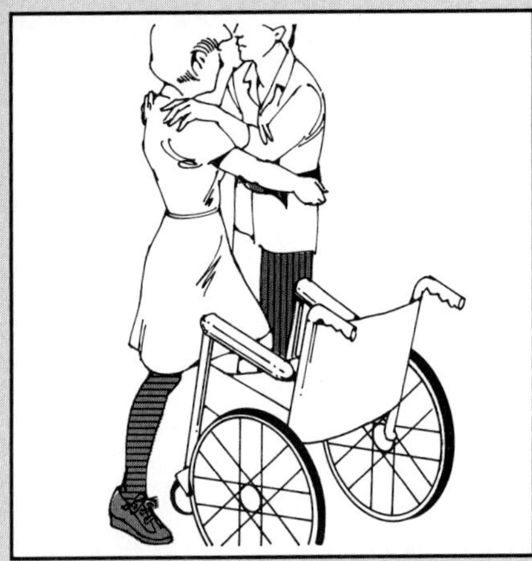

9. Work is accomplished by stronger leg muscles, not back muscles.

10. Nurse and client pivot toward chair simultaneously; client pivots on the ball of the pivot foot, nurse on the heel. Nurse's forefoot assists client's pivot.

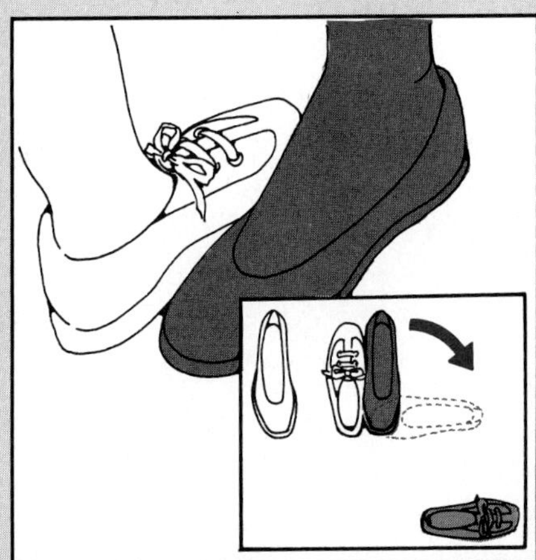

11. Ask client to reach back for arms of chair and sit down. Nurse assists by flexing own knees, not back, to lower client to a sitting position.

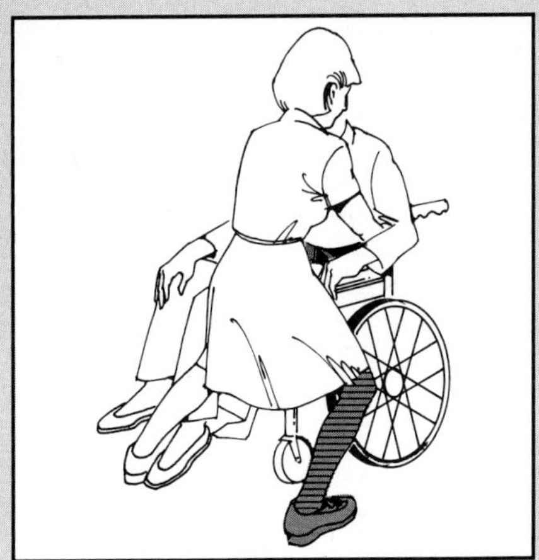

11. Client's arms will support part of the weight as client is seated. Nurse's knee flexion prevents leaning toward client, which would move nurse's center of gravity outside base of support. This may cause nurse to be pulled down onto client as client sits down.

(continued)

PROCEDURE 30–7. (continued)

12. Position client correctly in wheelchair (see Procedure 30–9). Apply safety belt or restraint if necessary (see Procedure 30–17).

NOTE: If client remains in room after transfer to a chair, it is critical to secure the nurse call light control within reach.

13. To return client to bed, reverse procedure. Chair must be moved so client's stronger leg is next to bed.

13. Pivot can only be accomplished safely when client's strong leg is near object to which client is moving.

METHOD B: Two-Person Lift

1. Discuss procedure and its purpose with the client, including nurse's actions, signals to be used, and behavior desired of client.

1. Awareness of how transfer will be accomplished will prevent or reduce clients' anxiety/fear of being injured.

2. Lock the wheels of the bed. Move the client close to the edge of the bed (see Procedure 30–11). Raise the head of the bed 60 degrees. Assess client for dizziness.

2. Reduces distance client must be lifted. Dizziness may be caused by pooling of blood in dependent parts of the body.

NOTE: Failing to secure brakes on bed and chair could result in client or nurse falling.

3. When dizziness subsides, place wheelchair next to the bed, facing the foot of bed. Adjust the height of bed so it is even with arms of the chair; lock the wheels of the chair.

3. More energy would be required to lift the client over the arms of the chair than to lower client to the chair seat from the height of the chair arms.

4. First nurse stands behind the backrest of chair, second nurse faces the chair. Both assume a broad stance with near foot perpendicular to plane of bed, far foot parallel to the side of wheelchair. Second nurse should place far foot outside foot supports of wheelchair if they are not removable.

4. This stance provides a wide, stable base of support and eliminates the need to pivot or twist nurses' upper bodies.

5. First nurse flexes knees and reaches under client's axilla. Client then folds the arms across the chest and the nurse grasps client's left forearm with the right hand, and the client's right forearm with the left hand.

5. Provides secure support for client's upper body without placing stress on muscles of client's shoulder girdle.

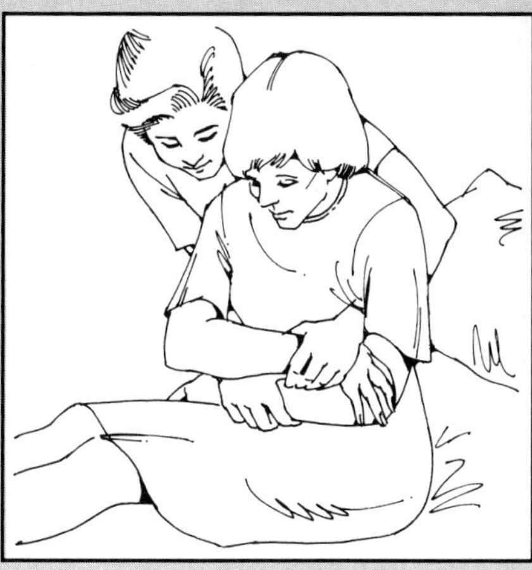

(continued)

6. Second nurse flexes knees and reaches under the client's thighs just above the knees, locking hands. (May interlock fingers or grasp wrist with opposite hand.) Client's knees should be flexed.

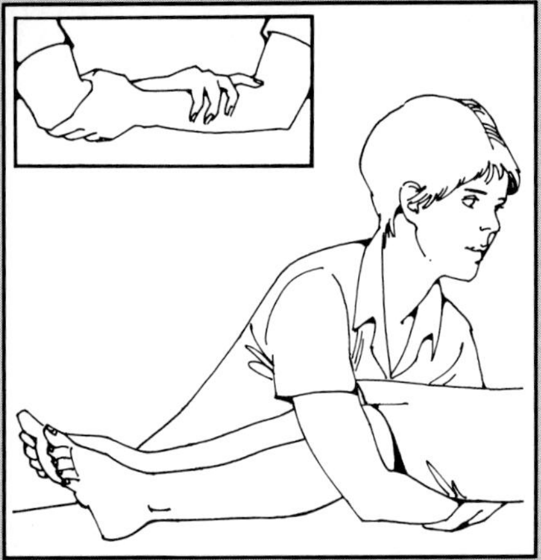

6. Provides secure support without pressure on vessels of popliteal space. Popliteal pressure can cause injury to large, superficial vessels and interfere with venous return.

7. Nurses contract their pelvic muscles and, on signal, extend knees to raise the client's buttocks from the bed, then both shift their weight to align the client over the seat of the chair.

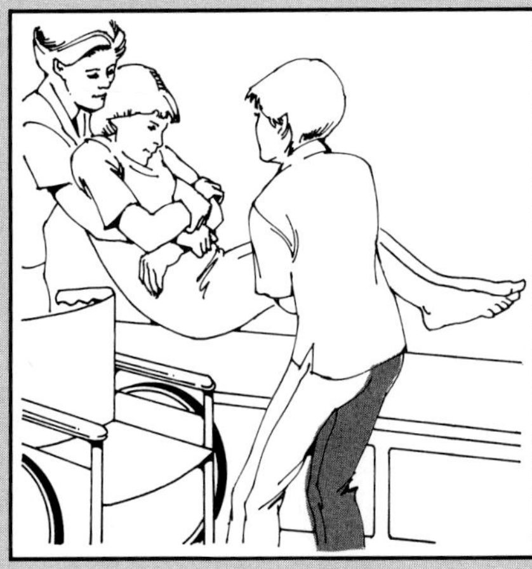

7. Protects nurses' back muscles by using stronger arm and leg muscles to move client. Flexing back rather than knees to seat client may strain nurses' backs.

NOTE: Additional force can be generated by using nurse's knee as a fulcrum against the edge of bed as client is moved toward chair.

8. Nurses flex their knees to seat the client.

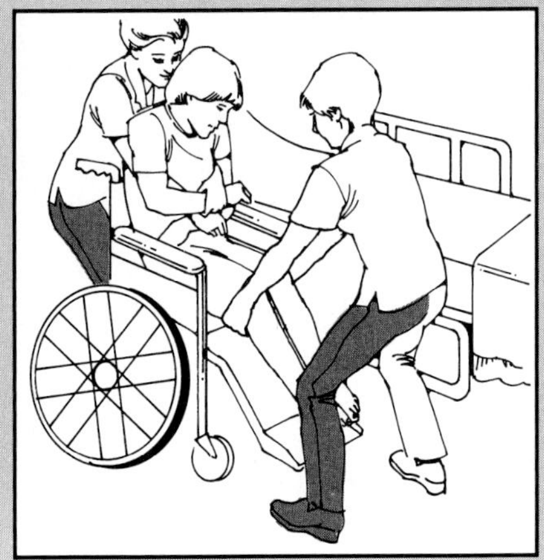

8. See step 7.

(continued)

PROCEDURE 30–7. (continued)

9. Position client correctly in the chair (see Procedure 30–9). Use safety belt if necessary.

NOTE: If client remains in his or her room after transfer to a chair, it is critical to secure the nurse call light control within reach.

10. To return client to bed, reverse the procedure:

a. If arms of wheelchair are removable, remove the arm nearest the bed and adjust the height of the bed so it is even with the seat of the chair. If the arm cannot be removed, the client must be lifted over it. Bed height should be even with the chair arm in this case.

10a. Removing the chair arm alleviates the need to lift the client, therefore conserving the nurses' energy.

b. Second nurse's legs should be positioned outside the client's legs. The nurse should step toward the bed as the client is moved.

b. Straddling the client's legs may cause them to become tangled between the nurse's legs as the client is moved toward the bed.

RECORDING: Pivot transfer: Indicate method of transfer, amount of client participation, amount of time in sitting position, and symptoms of overexertion, if any.
Two-person lift: Indicate type of transfer, amount of time client remained seated, and symptoms of overexertion, if any.

programs. Many nurses and nursing assistants working in acute and extended care facilities now recognize that gait belts are equally appropriate for helping clients with mobility at all stages of illness. Although several styles of belts are available, the simplest is a 2-inch-wide belt made of pliable heavy-duty cotton webbing that secures with a slip-proof buckle. Procedures 30–4, and 30–7 illustrate and describe using a gait belt for transfer and ambulation.

Sliding Board. There are several types of sliding boards, but all of them act as a bridge between the bed and chair or gurney. They are usually made of a thin layer of rigid plastic with a smooth, friction-reducing surface. After brakes have been secured on the bed and chair or gurney, the board is placed so its weight is supported on one side by the bed, on the other by the chair or gurney. Two or more nurses slide the client across the board using a pull sheet (see Procedure 30–6). To use a sliding board for a transfer to a chair, the chair's armrest must be removable. Because most hospital wheelchairs have armrests that are not removable, an alternative transfer method must be used. Some acute care and extended care facilities use chairs (sometimes called "geri" chairs) that convert to a flat configuration to facilitate transfers. Sliding boards work well with these chairs. A sliding board can also be used by clients for independent transfers to a chair with removable armrests.

Hydraulic Lift. A hydraulic lift is appropriate to move heavy, helpless clients to a chair, bedside commode, gurney, or bathtub. The lift has a detachable sling that is placed under the client and then reattached to the lift apparatus. When the lift is activated, it raises the client to a sitting position, and then off the surface of the bed. Using a hydraulic lift is a safe and efficient method for transfers, especially to a chair or bedside commode, which do not accommodate sliding board transfers. Attempting to transfer weak, heavy clients without the help of a lift is a common cause of back injuries to nurses. Procedure 30–8 describes the use of a hydraulic lift.

Positioning Clients in a Chair. Clients must be properly positioned when seated to prevent fatigue, contractures, and pressure ulcers. Figure 30–17 illustrates correct sitting posture. Note that the buttocks and spine should contact the backrest of the chair. The client's feet should rest on the floor and there should be no pressure on the popliteal space. A footstool can be used to assist clients whose legs are too short to reach the floor to maintain correct posture. If elevation of the client's lower extremities is indicated, provide support for the entire leg, not just for the feet (Fig. 30–18). Pillow supports can also be used to prevent leaning laterally, as shown in Figure 30–19. Placing a pillow behind a client's back is not recommended, because this

PROCEDURE 30–8. USING A HYDRAULIC LIFTER

PURPOSE: To move a heavy or helpless client from bed to chair or stretcher and back to bed. May also be used to transfer such clients to bathtub.

EQUIPMENT: Hydraulic (mechanical) lifter, chair or gurney.

ACTION	RATIONALE
1. If unfamiliar with sling design, obtain expert assistance. Practice with the sling and lift, using a staff member or mannequin as client stand-in before attempting to transfer a client. NOTE: Improperly applied sling could result in client slipping out during transfer.	1. Several styles of slings are available. Slings are intended to support the client in a semi-sitting position when raised off the bed.
2. Discuss the procedure with the client, including nurses' actions, behavior desired of the client, and signals to be used, if any. Clients may need reassurance that the device is strong enough to support their weight.	2. Client will be less anxious and more willing and able to participate if expected behavior and anticipated benefits are clear.
3. Place fabric sling under the client, aligning it carefully to provide even support.	3. If support is uneven, discomfort or injury is possible.

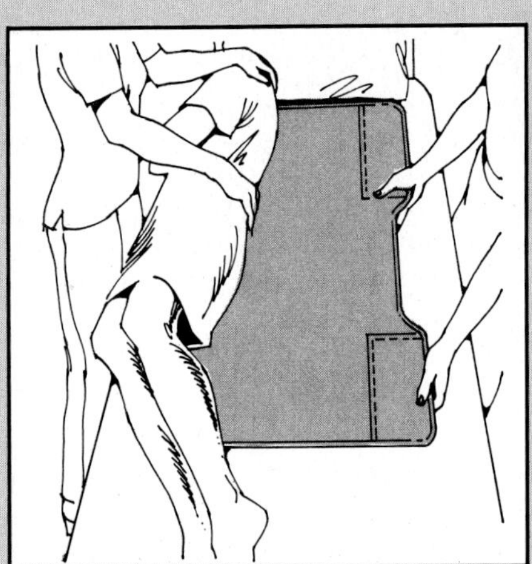

(continued)

PROCEDURE 30–8. (continued)

4. Place the lift next to the bed so the base bars are under the bed at right angles to the long axis of the bed. Center the overhead support bar across the bed about even with the client's chest. If lower bars are adjustable, adjust them to the widest possible position.

4. Provides maximum stability during transfer.

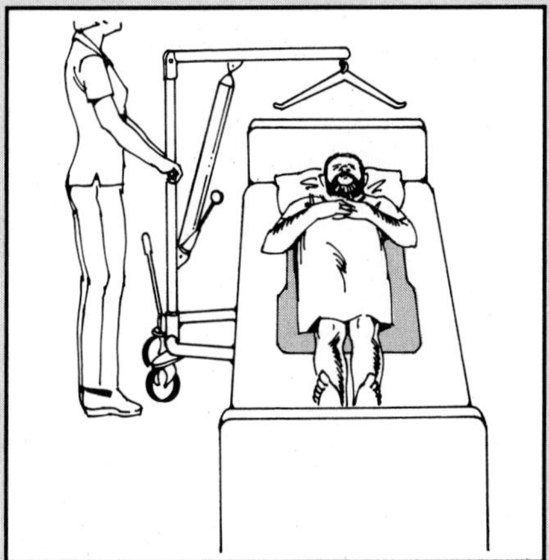

5. Insert "S" hooks from the overhead support into the grommets of the sling so the hooks point away from the client.

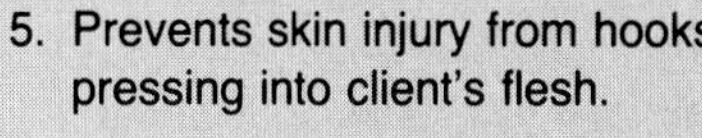

5. Prevents skin injury from hooks pressing into client's flesh.

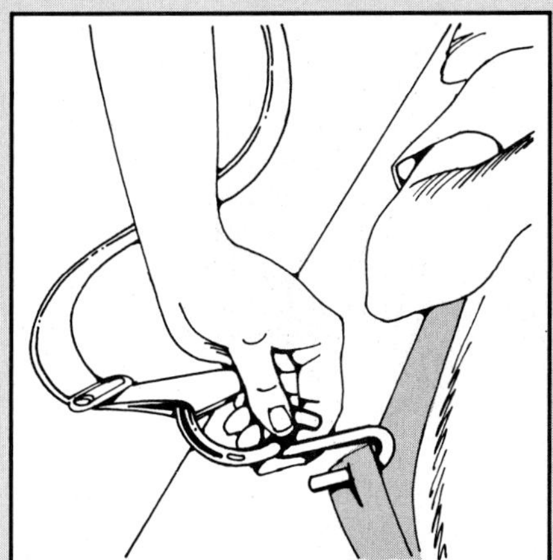

6. Ask the client to fold hands in lap or to grasp the overhead bar during the transfer. If the client has an IV or a Foley catheter drainage bag, these should be moved first and secured to the gurney, and tubing arranged to prevent tangling during transfer. If the tubing of the urinary drainage system is not long enough to allow the drainage bag to be moved before the client is transferred, the tubing can be clamped and the bag placed on the client's abdomen during the transfer. Drainage must be facilitated by opening the clamp and placing the bag below the level of the organ being drained at the completion of the transfer.

6. Pulling or tangling tubing may cause discomfort or dislodge it. Placing a drainage bag on the client's abdomen without clamping it will allow reflux of the contents into the client's body, which could cause infection or other complications. Failing to reopen the clamp at the completion of the transfer may cause distension of the organ being drained.

(continued)

PROCEDURE 30–8. (continued)

7. Close the pressure valve and pump the lift until the client attains a semi-sitting position clear of the bed.

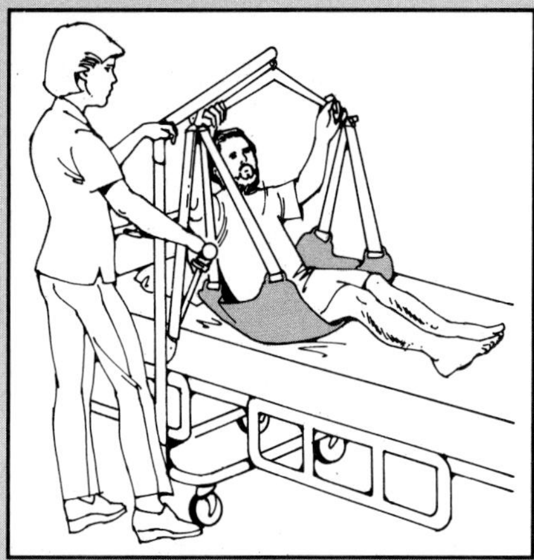

7. Pumping action creates pressure on the fluid in the cylinder of the lift, therefore the movable portion moves upward, raising the client off the bed.

8. The nurse operating the lift contracts his or her pelvic muscles and pulls the lift away from the bed, then turns it so the lower bars are under the gurney and the client is centered over it. If the client is being moved to a chair, the lower bars should straddle the chair.

8. Protects nurse from injury by stabilizing joints. Positioning the lift in this way maintains its stability and accomplishes the transfer without injury to the client.

9. Second nurse stands at the head of the bed and guides the client during the move so client does not swing and to assist in centering client before lowering to the gurney or chair. Third nurse may be needed to support legs of large or helpless client.

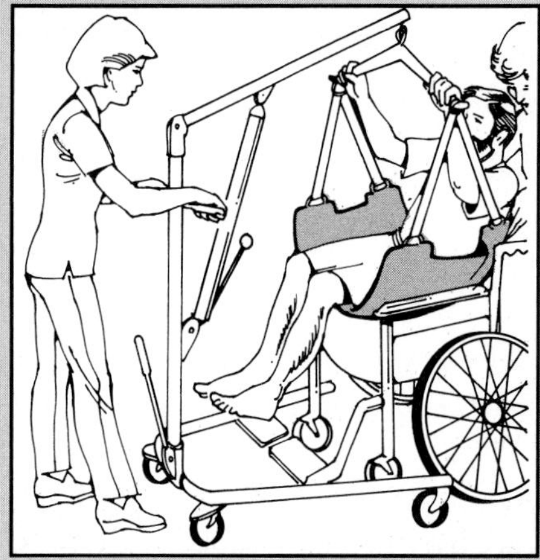

9. The movement of the lift shifts the client's weight, promoting swinging of the suspended client. Most clients find this movement unpleasant, and may fear falling.

10. Release pressure valve gradually so client is lowered slowly. Close valve as soon as client is resting on the chair or gurney.

10. Rapid downward movement may frighten client. Abrupt contact with chair or gurney could jar client.

11. Second nurse should support client's upper body as client is lowered from sitting to supine position if being moved to a gurney.

11. There is no back support from sling or gurney. Weak clients may be unable to change positions independently.

(continued)

PROCEDURE 30–8. (continued)

12. Release "S" hooks, leaving sling under client. If wrinkles are present, pull sling taut.	12. Leaving sling in place conserves time and energy and facilitates returning client to bed. Wrinkles in sling may cause pressure areas, increasing risk for ischemia.
13. At completion of transfer, position client in correct alignment; secure safety belt or siderails.	13. Maintains client comfort and safety.

RECORDING: It is not usually necessary to document use of a hydraulic lifter in nurse's progress notes, but including this information on the Kardex or client care plan is helpful.

contributes to slipping down in the chair, which causes back strain and contributes to skin breakdown due to shearing force. Slipping may occur even when clients are correctly supported. Procedure 30–9 outlines techniques to correctly reposition seated clients.

Moving Clients in Bed. Most clients who are alert and able to move spontaneously change positions when in bed just as you might shift in your seat during a lengthy classroom lecture. These movements occur even when asleep. Some clients, however, are unable to move independently due to weakness or disability, putting them at high risk for developing the disuse phenomena discussed in an earlier section. Nurses need to assist these clients to change positions at least every 2 hours. Correct positions and protective devices that facilitate maintaining proper alignment are discussed in the following sections.

Slipping toward the foot of the bed when using Fowler's (semi-sitting) position is a frequent problem. Even clients who are able to turn easily from side to side often require assistance to pull themselves to the head of the bed. A client having had recent abdominal surgery is an example. Techniques for assisting with this movement, as well as facilitating other position changes, are detailed in Procedures 30–10 through 30–14.

Using protective body mechanics is essential when performing these nursing procedures to prevent injury to cli-

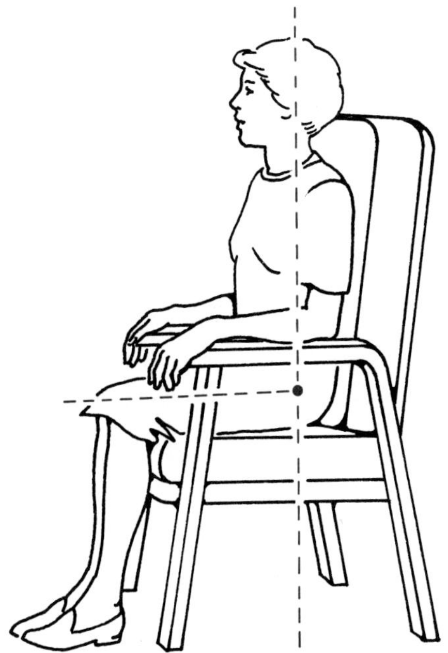

Figure 30–17. Correct sitting posture.

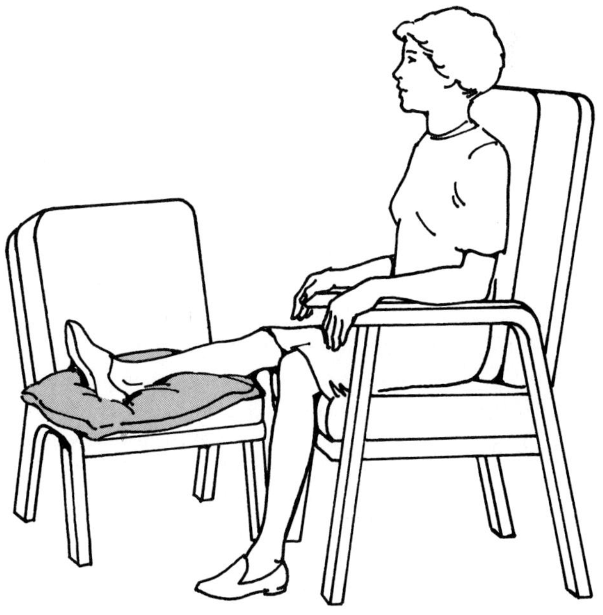

Figure 30–18. Correct leg support for elevating legs when seated.

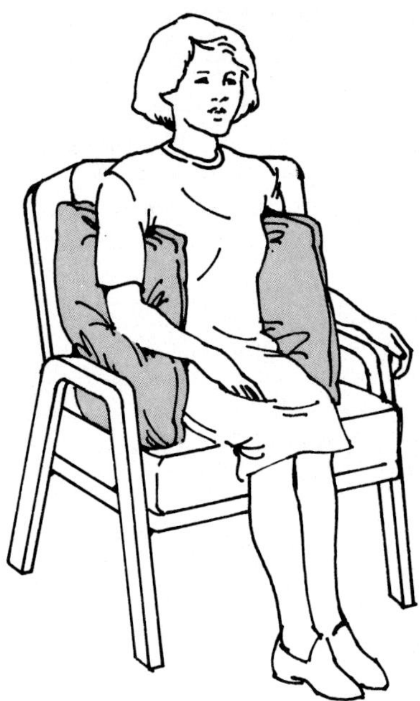

Figure 30–19. Pillow supports to prevent leaning in a large chair.

ents and nurses. Moving and positioning heavy clients or clients with limited ability to assist often requires two or more nurses. An overbed trapeze is a useful appliance to facilitate client participation or independent repositioning. The trapeze is suspended above a client's torso from a sturdy frame that extends the full length of the bed. Clients can use it to raise their hips off the bed so they can easily move toward the head or side of the bed. A trapeze is also useful for upper body exercise (see Table 30–10).

Positioning Clients in Bed. Effective positioning of clients unable to move is critical to preventing complications of bed rest. Four therapeutic positions are most commonly used: supine (Fig. 30–20), lateral (Fig. 30–21), prone (Fig. 30–22), and Fowler's (Fig. 30–23). Variations such as Sims', also called semiprone (Fig. 30–24), or low Fowler's, also called semi-Fowler's, are appropriate as well. Refer to Procedure 30–15 for nursing considerations associated with positioning.

When positioning clients who cannot move, nurses must pay particular attention to protecting joints from contractures and skin from pressure injuries. The joints most vulnerable to contractures associated with bed rest are those of the hip, knee, and ankle.[60] Full extension of the hip is difficult unless one is standing. Even in the prone position, there is 10 to 20 degrees less hip extension than when standing upright.[61] Fowler's position, elevating the head or legs when supine, and the lateral position involve even greater degrees of hip flexion. The knees are almost always flexed when in bed as well, except in the prone position. Ankle (plantar) flexion occurs because of the relative strength of the plantar flexion muscle group over the muscles used for dorsiflexion. When a client is supine, there is added force from gravity, which tends to pull the front of the foot downward; the weight of covers is another contributing factor. Correct positioning, frequent repositioning, and regular exercise are necessary to prevent joint contractures.

Pressure ulcers occur when external pressure exceeds capillary pressure, as discussed earlier. Pressure related to body position is diminished when a client's weight is distributed over a large area, rather than concentrated on a small surface such as occurs on the sacrum, coccyx, and ischial tuberosities in Fowler's position or when clients legs are positioned incorrectly when side-lying (Fig. 30–25). Frequent position changes, individualized to a client's tolerance, also prevent pressure ulcers. Meticulous assessment (see Chap. 24) of all vulnerable pressure points whenever a client's position is changed is critical to early detection and treatment of pressure ulcers. Massaging reddened areas over bony prominences, once a common practice, is no longer recommended.[62] Blood vessels surrounding the ischemic area are already dilated, so massage offers no therapeutic effect; moreover, massage may force exudate from damaged tissue into adjacent healthy tissue.[62] The best treatment for reddened areas is to avoid positions creating pressure over the affected area until it resolves. Special beds, discussed below, are also effective.

A schedule is useful to alert both client and nurses of the timing of position changes. When devising such a schedule, consider a client's daily activities and special needs. For example, mealtime or visiting hours are not ideal times to schedule "proning." If a client is unable to remain comfortable in a given position for 2 hours, reduce the scheduled time for that position rather than eliminating it from the schedule.

Prone position is one that many clients resist, because it limits their field of vision and their social interaction and makes some clients feel vulnerable. Some clients complain of difficulty breathing when prone. It is a useful position, however, because it counteracts flexion contractures of the lower extremities, which commonly develop in clients who remain in bed for long periods. The extra effort required for chest expansion in prone position can be minimized by using rolled towels under the shoulders or by using Sims' position. Sims' position also eliminates excessive flexion of the lumbar curve, which can occur when prone.

Many clients prefer to spend the longest time periods in Fowler's position. Sitting up allows greater visualization of one's surroundings and facilitates interaction with others. It also may diminish the association with illness created by being "flat on one's back" in bed.

Despite these advantages, there are several hazards associated with use of Fowler's position of which nurses and clients should be aware. The skin over the sacrum, scapulae, and heels is frequently damaged by the shearing force creased by a client slipping down in bed when the head of the bed is at an angle greater than 30 degrees (see Fig. 24–5). Also, the client's weight is concentrated on the ischial tuberosities. The shearing force and the excessive pressure on the ischial tuberosities can be reduced if low

(Text continues on page 1525.)

PROCEDURE 30–9. POSITIONING A CLIENT IN A CHAIR

PURPOSE: To achieve correct sitting posture after transferring a client to a chair or when client has slipped down in a chair.

EQUIPMENT: *Method A:* One pillow. *Methods B and C:* None.

ACTION	RATIONALE
METHOD A: Pushing a Client Toward the Back of a Chair	
1. Discuss the procedure and its purpose with the client, including nurse's actions, signals, if any, to be used, and behavior desired of the client.	1. Active participation is more likely if the client understands expected behaviors and anticipated benefits. Clarifying signals enhances cooperation.
2. Face the client. Place the pillow in front of client's knees and hold it in place with your knees. 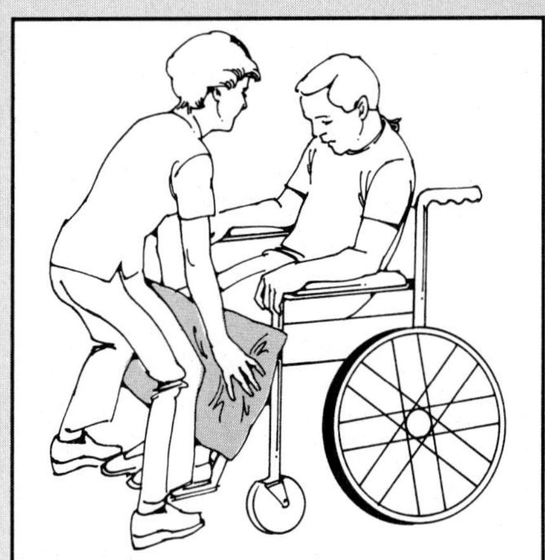	2. Pillow cushions contact point between bony portions of nurse's and client's knees.
3. Grasp the armrests of the chair. Plant your feet firmly and flex your knees and hips as if to sit down. 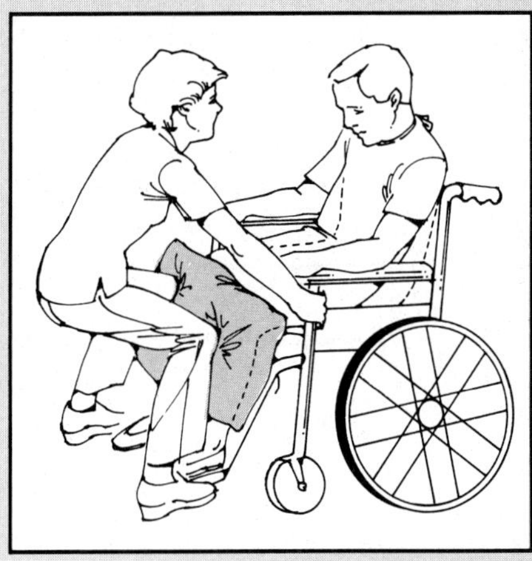	3. Grasping chair arms assists to maintain nurse's balance and directs the force created by nurse's knee and hip flexion toward client's knees, moving client back in the chair.

(continued)

PROCEDURE 30–9. (continued)

NOTE: Skin damage from friction may occur as client slides over the surface of the chair. This can be prevented by placing a layer of cloth (bath blanket or clothing) between client's skin and the surface of the chair, before transfer to the chair.

4. Repeat as necessary until client's buttocks and spine are in contact with the back of the chair.

   4. Heavy clients may move only small distance, even with the help of leverage.

5. Support trunk and extremities as needed to maintain correct alignment.

   5. Poor alignment causes discomfort and muscle and joint strain.

METHOD B: Pulling a Client Toward the Back of a Chair[a]

1. Discuss the procedure and its purpose with the client, as described for Method A, above.

2. Stand behind the chair. Reach under the client's axillae and grasp client's left forearm with your right hand and the right forearm with your left hand.

   2. Wide base of support prevents loss of balance as nurse pulls client's weight.

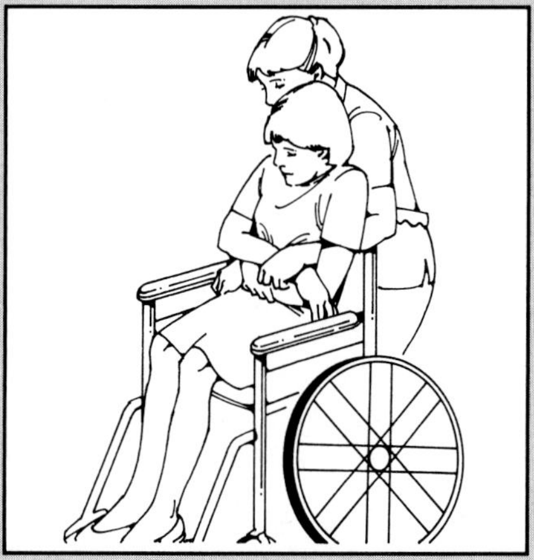

3. Ask the client to push with the legs as you pull.

   3. Decreases nurse's energy expenditure, provides active exercise for the client.

NOTE: If client is heavy and unable to assist, use two nurses. See footnote [a] and Method C. One nurse attempting to move a heavy client, even using correct body mechanics, will be ineffective and may result in injury.

[a] Methods A and B can be combined to move a heavy client: One nurse performs Method A (*pushing*) while a second nurse performs Method B (*pulling*).

(continued)

PROCEDURE 30–9. (continued)

4. Flex your knees; contract your pelvic muscles. Then, on signal, extend your legs, shifting your weight to your back leg and pulling the client backward. Repeat as necessary.

4. Uses strong muscles of the extremities and force of the nurse's weight to move the client.

5. Support trunk and extremities as needed to maintain correct alignment.

5. Poor alignment causes discomfort and muscle and joint strain.

METHOD C: Two-nurse Lift

1. Discuss the procedure and its purpose with the client, as described for Method A, above.

2. Nurses stand one on each side of the chair, facing client. Each places the arm nearer the client under the client's axilla. Nurses flex their arms so the antecubital space is under the client's axilla.

2. Provides a secure method to support the client.

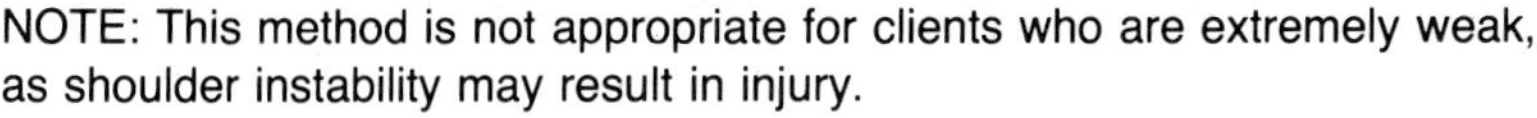

NOTE: This method is not appropriate for clients who are extremely weak, as shoulder instability may result in injury.

(continued)

PROCEDURE 30–9. (continued)

Action	Rationale
3. Both nurses assume a broad stance: Feet shoulder width apart; the foot nearer the chair should be in line with the client's hips, outside foot 24 inches ahead. (Outside foot will be behind the plane of the chair back.)	3. Provides a wide base of support to prevent loss of balance as nurses shift weight to move the client.

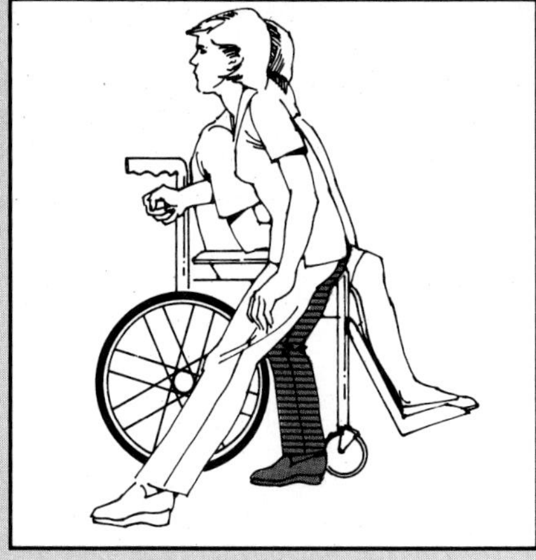

Action	Rationale
4. Both nurses flex their knees, contract pelvic muscles, and on signal shift their weight forward, pulling the client toward the back of the chair. Repeat as necessary.	4. Uses strong muscles of the nurses' extremities and force of their weight to move the client.

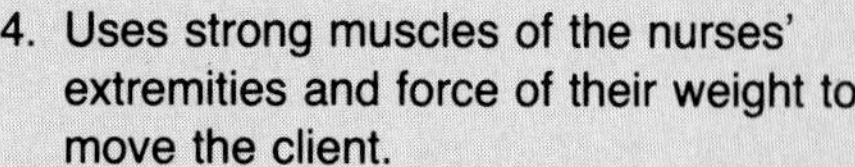

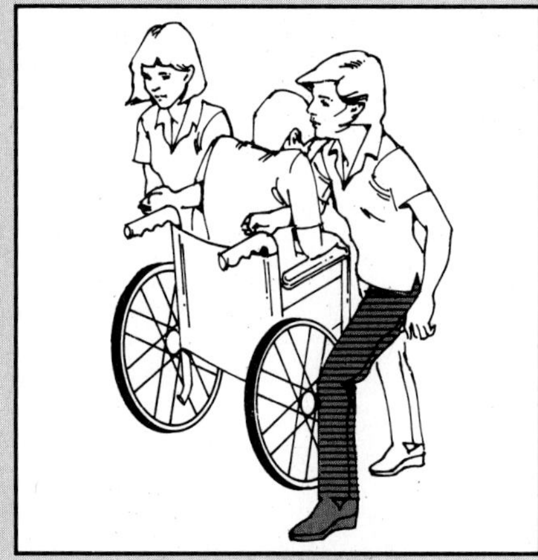

Action	Rationale
5. Support trunk and extremities as needed to maintain correct alignment.	5. Poor alignment causes discomfort and muscle and joint strain.

RECORDING: No recording is necessary.

PROCEDURE 30–10. ASSISTING A CLIENT TO MOVE TOWARD THE HEAD OF THE BED

PURPOSE: *Methods A and B:* To assist a heavy or weak client to achieve correct alignment and alleviate discomfort from cramped position caused by slipping toward the foot of the bed.
Method C: To assist a client unable to tolerate the supine position to achieve correct alignment and alleviate discomfort from the cramped position caused by slipping toward the foot of the bed. Also appropriate to assist any other client with moderate to optimum shoulder girdle strength who desires to remain in semi-Fowler's position.

EQUIPMENT: *Methods A and B:* Drawsheet. *Method C:* none.

ACTION	RATIONALE
METHOD A: Drawsheet (Pull-sheet) Method, Two to Four Nurses	
1. Discuss the procedure with the client, including nurse's actions, behavior desired of client, and signals to be used to synchronize efforts.	1. Client will be more willing and able to participate if the reasons and anticipated benefits of the activity are clear. Clarifying signals enhances cooperation.
2. Raise the bed to nurse's midthigh level, lower near siderail, and lock wheels of the bed.	2. This height facilitates use of major muscles of the extremities.
3. Fold drawsheet in half lengthwise, place under client so it extends from shoulder to hips.	3. Sheet will support bulk of client's weight for moving and positioning, reducing friction, and so decreasing energy expenditure.
NOTE: If client is known to require assistance with moving, including a pull-sheet in foundation linen when making the bed saves time and energy. If client cannot support the head, place sheet high enough to do so.	
4. Ask client to fold arms across the chest and flex knees.	4. Prevents squeezing client's arms between pull-sheet and client's torso. Reduces friction from pulling client's legs across sheets during move.
5. Roll sheet so edges are close to client's body and grasp firmly next to client's shoulders and hips.	5. Maximizes control during movement, improves leverage.

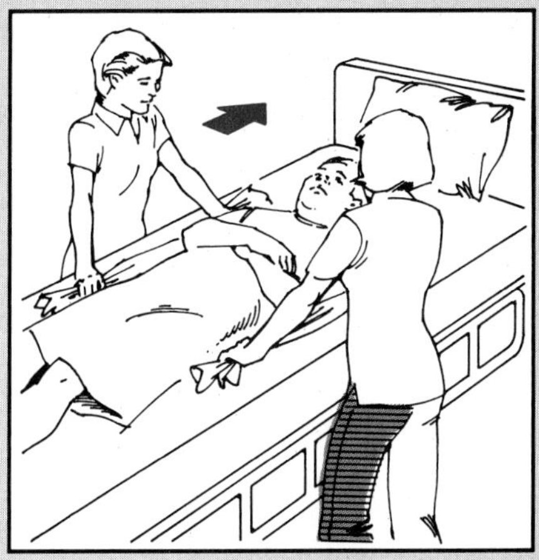

(continued)

PROCEDURE 30–10. (continued)

6. Face head of bed. Assume broad stance with legs slightly flexed. Outside foot is forward. Weight is on inside leg (shaded).

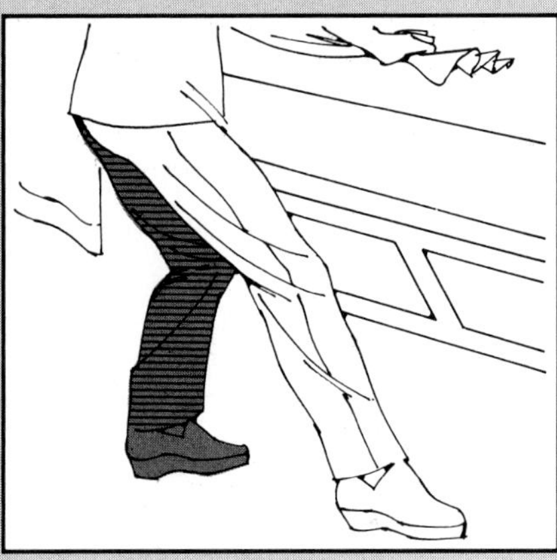

6. Broad stance increases base of support. Flexion allows smooth weight shift, with force exerted by arms and legs, not back.

NOTE: If client is very heavy, two nurses on both sides of the bed may be needed to prevent injury to nurses and client.

7. Ask client to raise head and exhale during the move.

7. Reduces weight and friction, thus conserving energy. Exhaling prevents Valsalva maneuver, which, if used, can stress the heart.

8. Contract your pelvic muscles. On signal, shift your weight to your forward leg, keeping your back straight, moving your arms and the client toward head of bed. Repeat, if necessary.

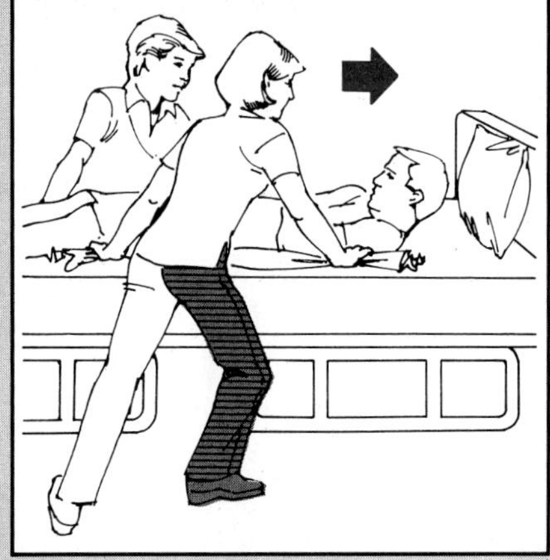

8. Shifting weight provides additional force of your body weight, decreasing work of muscles.

9. Replace pillows and other positioning aids to maintain correct alignment. Raise siderails.

(continued)

PROCEDURE 30–10. (continued)

METHOD B: Cradling Method, One or Two Nurses

One Nurse:

1. Discuss the procedure, and position bed and IV Foley tubing as in Method A. Ask client to flex knees.

NOTE: This technique is suitable for weak, lightweight clients; for heavier clients, use two nurses or select another method.

2. If client cannot assist in move, fold client's arms across client's chest.

2. Reduces friction from client's arms and legs being pulled across sheets as client is moved.

3. Slide one arm under the client's shoulders, the other under the small of client's back.

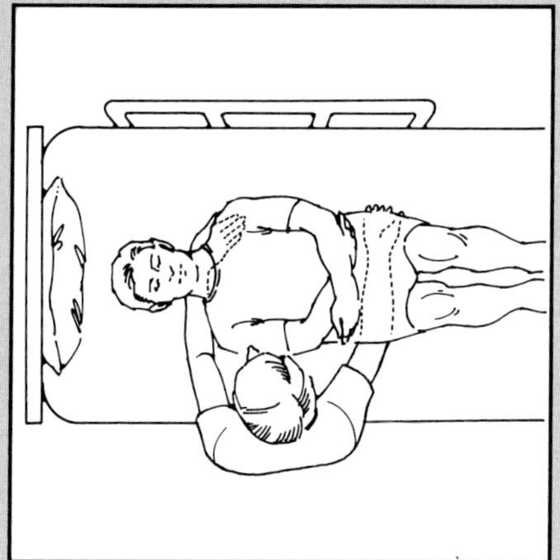

3. Provides support for weak clients unable to tolerate pressure on shoulder girdle.

4. Face head of bed. Assume broad stance with legs slightly flexed. Outside foot is forward. Weight is on inside leg (shaded).

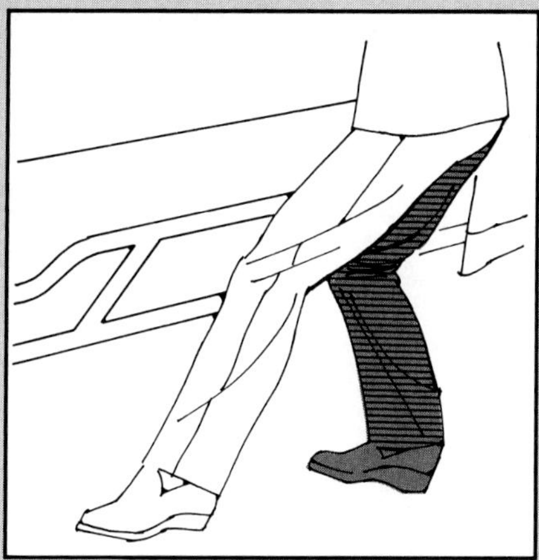

4. Broad stance increases base of support. Flexion allows smooth weight shift, with force exerted by arms and legs, not back.

(continued)

NOTE: Some nurses prefer to face foot of bed so effort is a pull rather than a push. Location of the bedside table or other furniture and equipment may make pulling method difficult.

5. Ask client to raise head and exhale during move. If client can assist, ask to push with the arm and legs on signal. (Flex legs at the knee.) Emphasize to client not to arch back while pushing with legs. If client has long hair, check to see that client is not lying on it.

   Rationale 5. Lifting head reduces weight and friction, thus conserving energy. Exhaling prevents Valsalva maneuver, which, if used, can stress the heart. Active assistance by the client provides benefits of exercise to client, reduces energy expenditure of nurse. Arching the back directs force into the mattress, rather than to head of bed.

6. Contract your pelvic muscles. On signal, shift your weight to your forward leg, keeping your back straight, moving the client toward the head of the bed. Repeat as necessary.

   Rationale 6. Shifting weight provides additional force of your body weight, decreasing work of muscles.

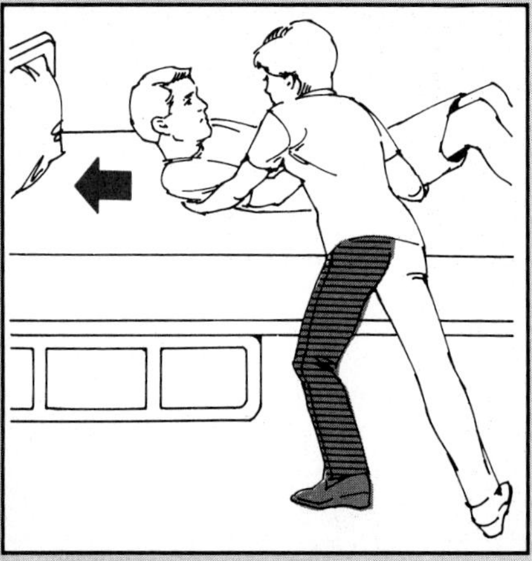

7. Replace pillows and other positioning aids to maintain correct alignment. Raise siderails.

Two Nurses:

1. Discuss the procedure and position bed, equipment, and client as above. First nurse slides one arm under client's shoulders, the other under the small of client's back. Second nurse stands on opposite side of bed and places arms under client, one above and one below the hips. If client is unable to raise the head, first nurse can support it by flexing upper arm and cradling head with elbow.

   Rationale 1. Bulk of client's weight is evenly distributed between two nurses.

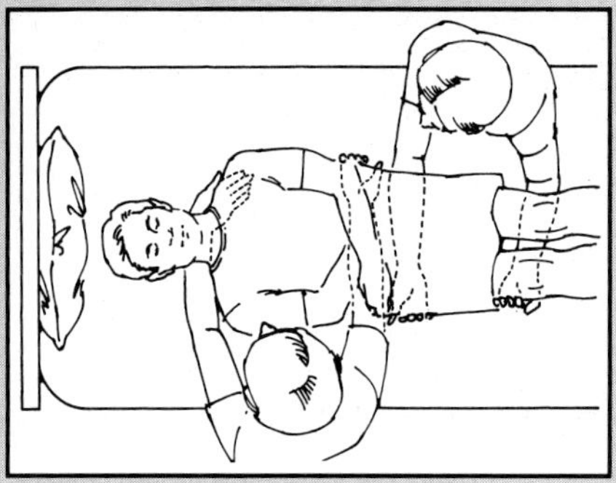

(continued)

PROCEDURE 30–10. (continued)

2. Complete the procedure as in steps 5 to 7, page 1512.

METHOD C: Sitting Method, Two Nurses

1. Discuss the procedure, as in previous techniques. Raise the bed to nurses' midthigh level, lock wheels of bed. Be sure IV or drainage tubing is positioned to prevent tension or tangling.

2. Face head of bed. Place your inside knee (knee nearest client) on the bed next to client's hip. Your weight should be on this knee. Place your other foot on the floor, slightly forward of knee.

2. Prepares for weight shift to assist client's movement, uses large muscles of the extremities.

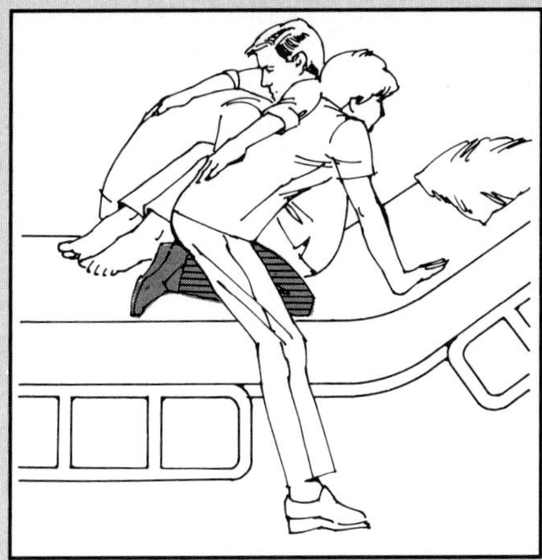

3. Place your near shoulder under client's axilla so the client's arm rests on your back. Then slide your near hand under the client's thigh in a medial-to-lateral direction.

3. Client's weight is supported by the muscle of the nurses' arms and legs; protects weaker back muscles.

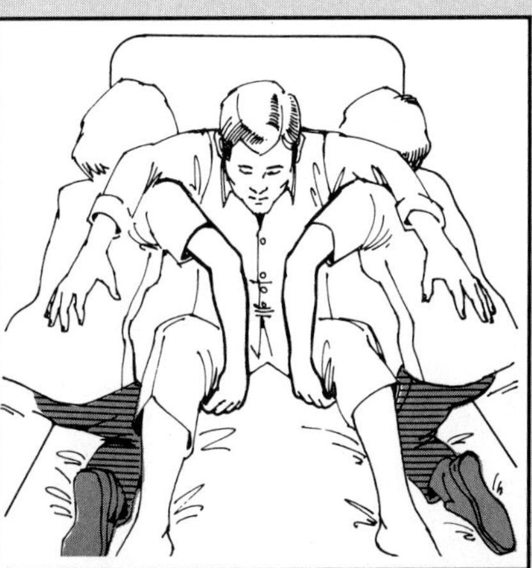

4. Place your other hand about 18 inches forward of your knee, with elbow extended.

4. The forward arm acts as a lever with the hand as fulcrum, as the nurses shift their weight to move client.

(continued)

PROCEDURE 30–10. (continued)

5. Contract your pelvic muscles. Rock forward on signal, stepping toward head of bed and partially extending knee on bed. Repeat as necessary.

5. Protects nurses' joints, adds the force of your body weight to move the client.

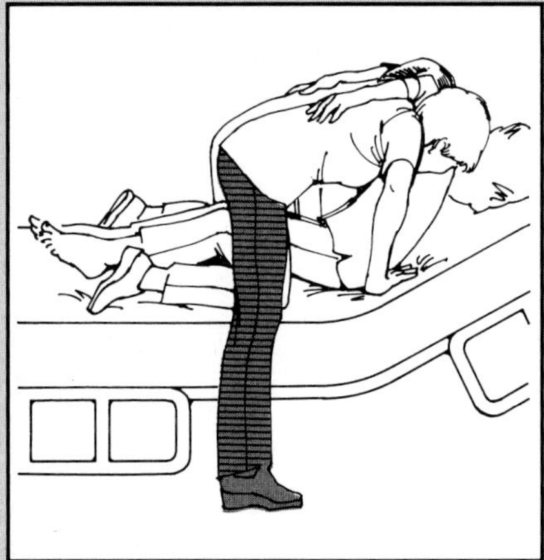

6. Replace pillows and other positioning aids to maintain correct alignment. Raise siderails.

RECORDING: It is not necessary to record having moved a client up in bed; however, it is helpful to indicate the most effective method for assisting a given client on the Kardex, client care plan, or turning schedule.

PROCEDURE 30–11. MOVING A CLIENT TOWARD ONE SIDE OF THE BED

PURPOSE: To prepare to: (1) reposition a supine client in a lateral or prone position, (2) assist a client to sit at the edge of the bed ("dangle"), or (3) make an occupied bed. (Method A is efficient for client needing frequent assistance.)

EQUIPMENT: *Method A:* Drawsheet. *Method B:* None.

ACTION	RATIONALE
METHOD A: Pull-sheet Method, Two to Four Nurses	
1. Discuss the procedure with client, including nurse's actions, behavior desired of the client, and signals used to synchronize efforts, if any.	1. Client will be more willing and able to participate if the reasons and anticipated benefits of the activity are clear. Clarifying signals enhances cooperation.
2. Raise bed to your hip level, lower near siderail, lock wheels of bed.	2. Maintains client safety, allows nurse to use major muscles of extremities and avoid back strain. Nurse may strain back if bed is left in low position during the move. If wheels are not locked, bed rather than client will move.

(continued)

PROCEDURE 30–11. (continued)

3. Lower head of bed, remove pillows used for positioning. Head pillow can be placed against head of bed.

3. Client's weight is more evenly distributed when bed is flat. Pillows would block client's movement.

4. Screen client. Fanfold covers to foot of bed. Arrange hospital gown to cover client as much as possible. Arrange IV or drainage tubing so it will not be pulled or entangled as client is moved.

4. Provides privacy. Moving tubing and covers keeps them from interfering with smooth movement. Tension or tubing could cause pain and/or disruption of IV or drainage system.

5. Ask client to fold arms across the chest.

5. Prevents injury to arms during move.

6. Fold drawsheet in half, place under client's body from shoulders to hips.

NOTE: If a client is known to require assistance with moving and positioning, including a drawsheet in foundation linen when making the bed will save time and energy.

6. Sheet will support bulk of the client's weight for moving and positioning, reducing friction and so reducing energy expenditure.

7. Roll sheet so edges are close to client's body and grasp firmly next to client's shoulders and hips.

NOTE: Nurse on side to which client is being moved can grasp corner of pillowcase with drawsheet, so pillow moves with client, supporting the head. Two nurses on each side of the bed may be necessary if client is heavy.

7. Maximizes control during movement, improves leverage.

8. Nurse on side of bed to which client is being moved (nurse 1) assumes a broad stance (feet shoulder width apart) with forward foot next to the bed, back foot about 2 feet from the bed. Knees should be slightly flexed with weight on leg nearest the bed.

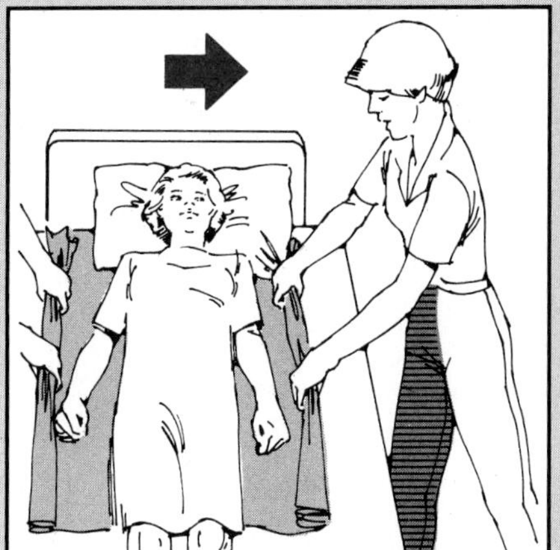

(continued)

PROCEDURE 30–11. (continued)

9. Nurse on opposite side (nurse 2) places one knee on bed, keeping other foot on the floor for stability. If client is large, third nurse may be needed to support client's feet and lower legs.

9. Keeps client's weight close to nurse's center of gravity during move, reducing potential for back injury to nurse.

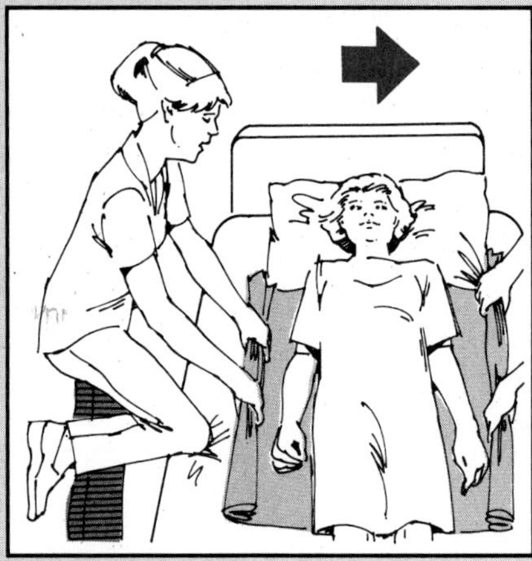

10. Nurses contract their pelvic muscles and, on signal, nurse 1 shifts weight to back foot while pulling on drawsheet. At the same time, nurse 2 pulls upward on drawsheet while shifting weight forward onto knee on the bed. If a third nurse is assisting, she or he should stand next to nurse 1 and support client's legs, assume same stance as nurse 1, and shift weight at same time.

10. Simultaneous weight shifts accomplish smooth movement with least expenditure of nurses' energy. Slight lifting by nurse 2 causes minimal strain as he or she is above client. The lifting reduces friction during move.

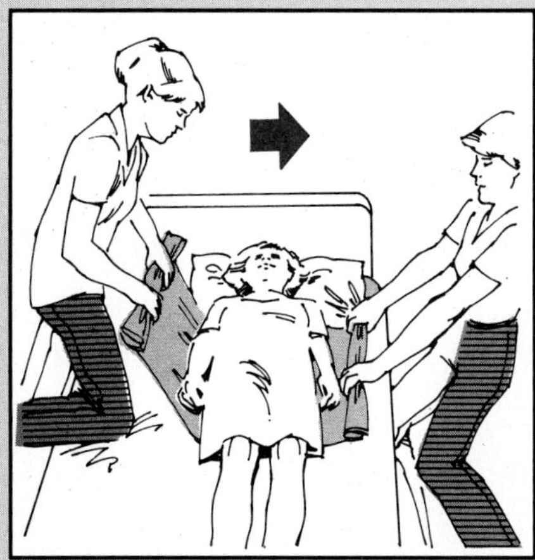

11. Repeat as necessary until client is at desired location.
12. Proceed with bedmaking or positioning client.
13. Replace covers, raise siderails, return bed to low position.

METHOD B: Segmental Method, One or Two Nurses

One Nurse:

1. Begin by discussing procedure and preparing client and beds as in Method A, steps 1 to 5.

1. Head pillow can remain in place to support client's head as he or she is moved.

(continued)

2. To move the client's upper body: Slide one of your arms under client's shoulders, supporting the head with your flexed elbow; the other arm under the upper back just below the level of the scapulae.

2. Provides safe support for upper segment of client's body.

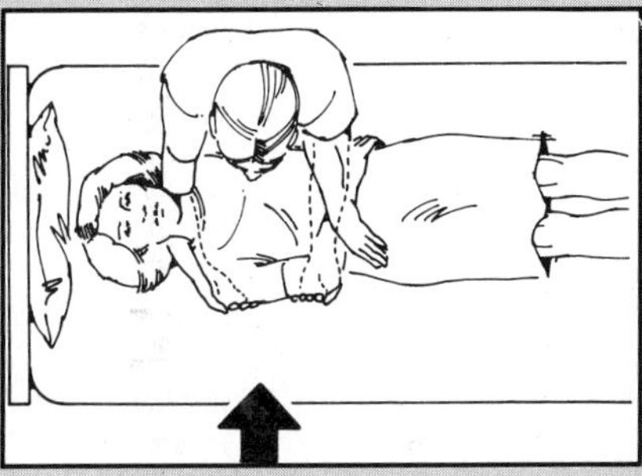

NOTE: Clients who are able can raise their heads during move, which decreases nurse's energy expenditure and provides client with small amount of active exercise.

3. Assume a broad stance (feet shoulder width apart) with forward foot next to the bed, back foot about 2 feet from the bed. Knees should be slightly flexed with weight on leg nearest the bed.

3. This stance provides a stable base of support during shifting of nurse's weight to move client.

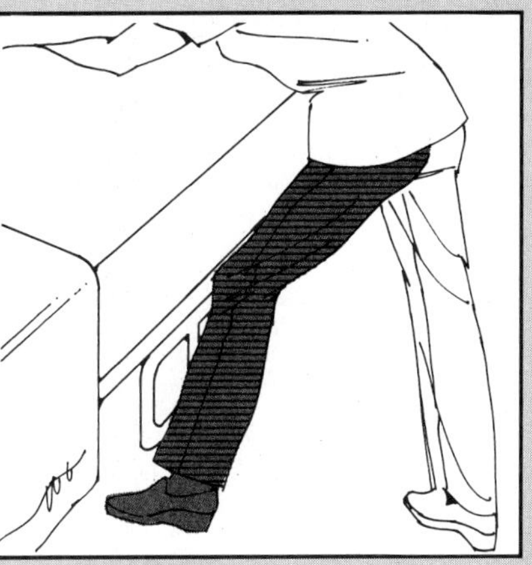

4. Contract your abdominal and gluteal muscles.

4. Provides pelvic joint stability, reducing potential for injury to the nurse.

5. Shift your weight to your back leg, pulling client's head and shoulders, as weight is shifted.

5. Shifting your weight provides additional force of your body weight, decreasing work of muscles.

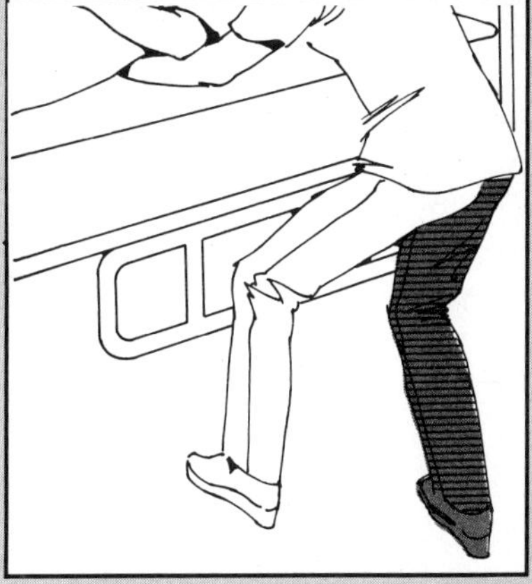

(continued)

6. Slide one of your arms under client's back at the waist, the other just below buttocks at the level of the greater trochanter.

   6. Nurse's arms are close together to provide support for heaviest part of the client's body.

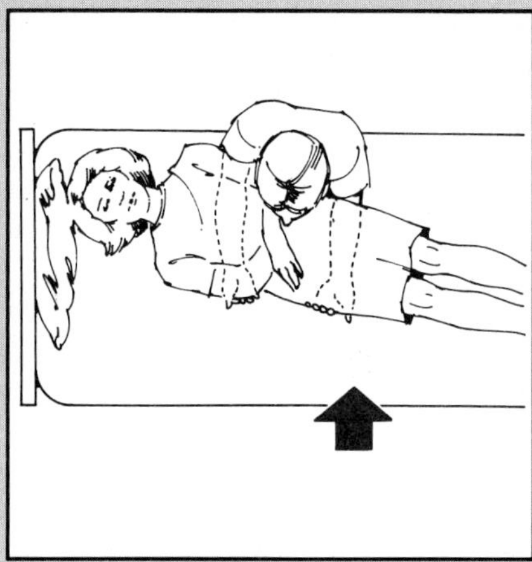

7. Move client's trunk by shifting your weight as described in steps 3 to 5 above.

8. Slide one of your arms under client's thighs, the other under the calves.

   8. Supports legs without stressing knee joint.

9. Move client's legs by shifting your weight as described in steps 3 to 5, above.

10. Repeat maneuver described above until client is as near side of bed as necessary.

    10. Several short moves expend less energy than one longer move.

11. Proceed with bedmaking or positioning client.

12. Replace covers, raise siderails, return bed to low position.

    12. Promotes client's safety and privacy.

Two Nurses:

1. Begin by discussing procedure and preparing client and bed as described in steps 1 to 5, above.

2. Nurses stand on same side of bed. Nurse nearest head of bed places her arms under client's shoulders and back as described in step 2 of Method B, the other under client's waist and buttocks as described in step 6.

   2. Provides simultaneous support for areas of client's body in which weight is concentrated.

(continued)

PROCEDURE 30–11. (continued)

3. Both nurses assume stance described in step 3 of Method B.

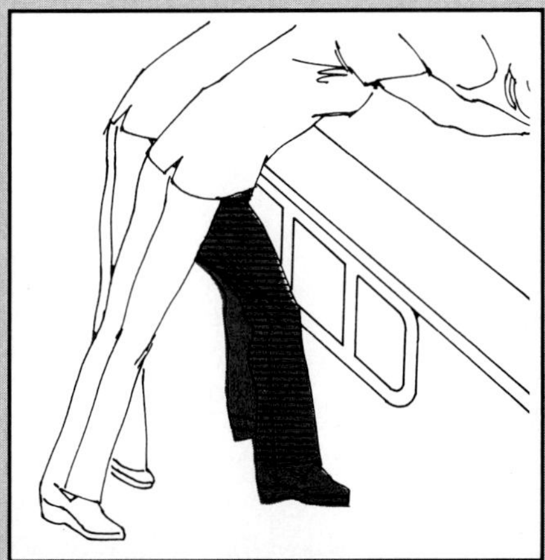

4. Each nurse stabilizes pelvis.

5. On signal, both nurses shift weight to back leg, pulling client as weight is shifted. Repeat as necessary.

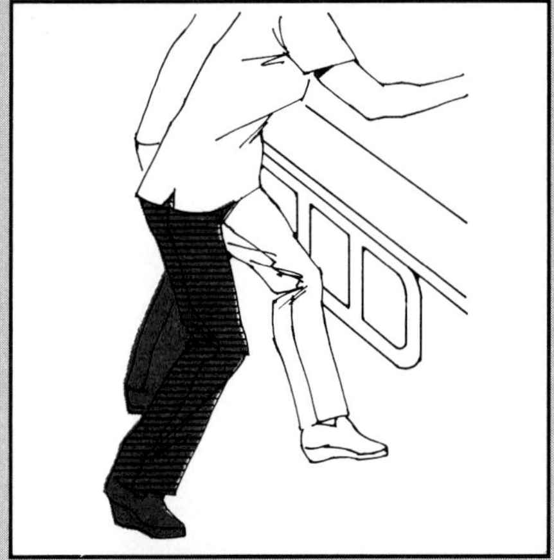

6. Proceed with bedmaking or positioning client.

7. Replace covers, raise siderails, return bed to low position.

RECORDING: No recording is necessary. Position changes should be documented on flowsheet or narrative notes.

PROCEDURE 30–12. TURNING A CLIENT FROM SUPINE TO PRONE OR LATERAL POSITION

PURPOSE: To facilitate repositioning of a client in correct alignment.

EQUIPMENT: None.

ACTION	RATIONALE
1. Discuss the procedure and its purpose with the client, including nurse's actions, desired client behavior, and anticipated benefits.	1. Client participation is more likely if expected behaviors and anticipated benefits are clear.
2. Move client near the edge of the bed (see Procedure 30–11).	2. Client will be too close to the edge of the bed when the roll is completed if the roll is commenced with the client in the center of the bed.
3. Standing at the side of the bed to which the client is to be turned, place the client's near arm on the bed, palm up next to body, or flexed on chest. The opposite arm should be placed next to client's body, with palm facing thigh. NOTE: Placing the client's near arm over the chest is preferred if the client is to be repositioned on the side. However, this arm position will cause client to roll onto arm if being rolled to the prone position.	3. Client will be rolled toward the nurse so speed and amount of roll can be controlled. Client will roll over near the arm if it is placed on the bed. Either arm position minimizes torque on arm when client is rolled.
4. Cross client's far leg over near leg, or flex far leg. 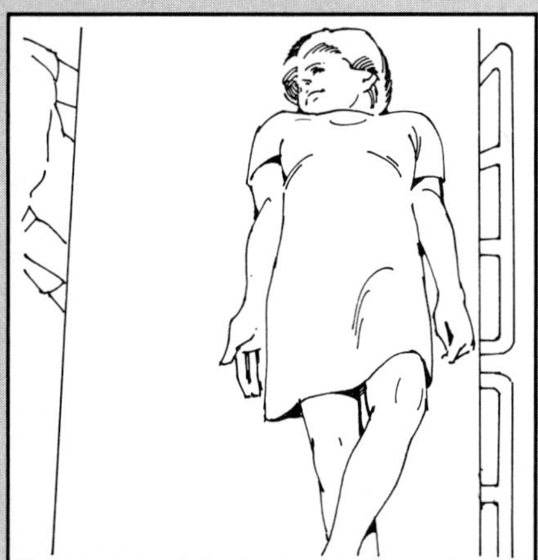	4. Either method will facilitate movement of far leg during roll.
5. Ask client to turn head away from you during the roll or position client's head if client is unable.	5. Prevents client from rolling onto the face.

(continued)

PROCEDURE 30–12. (continued)

6. Place your hands on the client's far shoulder and hip or, if the knee is flexed, on the shoulder and just above the knee, holding client's far arm next to the body with your wrist.

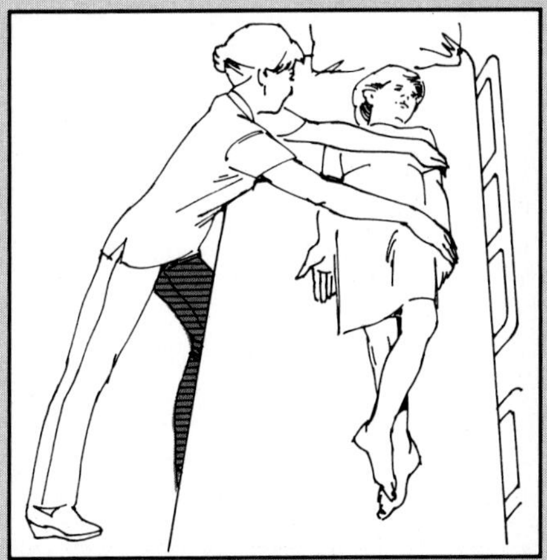

6. Provides turning force at area of greatest weight. Avoids torque on client's joints. Grasping arm or knee to turn client could cause injury to client's joints.

7. Assume a broad stance (feet shoulder width apart) with one foot next to the bed, the other foot about 2 feet from the bed. Knees should be slightly flexed with weight on leg nearest the bed.

7. This stance provides a stable base of support during shifting of nurse's weight to move client.

8. Contract your pelvic muscles. Shift your weight to your other leg (shaded), rolling client toward you as you move.

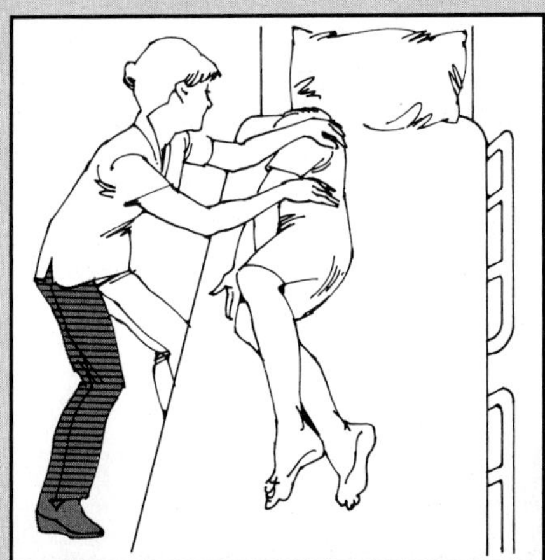

8. Shifting your weight provides additional force of your body weight, decreasing work of muscles.

(continued)

PROCEDURE 30–12. (continued)

9. When client is lying on the side, support extremities in proper alignment (see Fig. 30–21).
   OR:
   If client is to be placed in prone position, shift your hand position to the front of the shoulders and hips. Continue rolling until client is prone.

   Rationale 9. Client will be in the center of the bed. Client's hips or shoulders may require slight repositioning before placing pillow supports to assure correct alignment.

   This hand position controls speed and force of roll to abdomen.

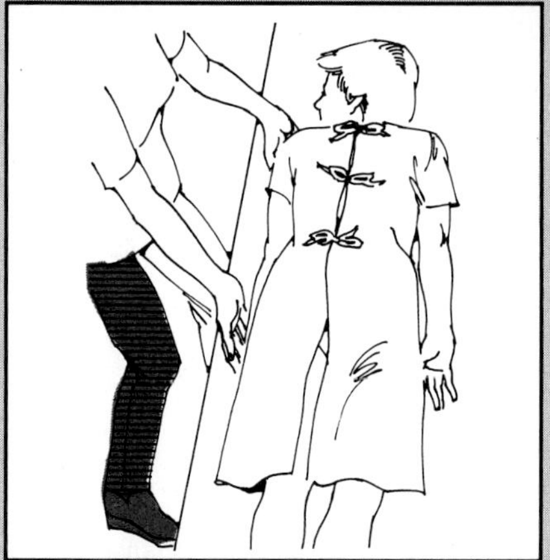

10. Move client's arm and head so client is comfortable.

    Rationale 10. Weak or paralyzed clients cannot adjust their position independently, nor maintain optimal positioning while being turned.

11. Move client to center of bed using techniques described in Procedure 30–11. Support in proper alignment (see Fig. 30–21).

    Rationale 11. Turning a client 180 degrees results in the client being near the edge of the bed. Correct positioning of extremities is difficult if a client is too near one side of the bed.

12. Replace covers, raise siderails, return bed to low position.

    Rationale 12. Promotes client's safety and privacy.

RECORDING: Note frequency of position changes; presence of reddened, macerated, or broken skin, including location, size, and description of lesion; and action taken if lesion noted.

PROCEDURE 30–13. LOG-ROLLING, SUPINE TO LATERAL POSITION, TWO OR THREE NURSES

PURPOSE: To facilitate repositioning of a client who cannot tolerate torsion of the spine (eg, clients having had spinal injury or surgery).

EQUIPMENT: None or drawsheet.

ACTION	RATIONALE
1. Discuss the procedure and its purpose with the client, including the nurse's actions, desired client behavior, and anticipated benefits.	1. Client participation is more likely if reasons and benefits of procedure are clear.

(continued)

2. Move client near the edge of the bed. At least two nurses are needed. See Procedure 30–11.

   2. One nurse cannot safely move a client whose spine must remain straight.

NOTE: Assistance of third person is needed for large clients.

3. Place client's arm across abdomen.

   3. Prevents lying on arm at completion of roll to side.

4. Place pillow(s) between client's legs to support the far leg during roll.

   4. Prevents torsion on spine caused by unsupported weight of leg.

5. Position a pillow under the client's head so head will be supported throughout roll.

   5. See step 4, above.

6. Standing on side of bed to which client is to be rolled, first nurse places hands on client's far shoulder and waist; second nurse places hands on client's far hip and thigh. If three nurses assist, second nurse places hands above and below hip, third nurse on thigh and calf.

   6. Will provide support for smooth turning without twisting spine.

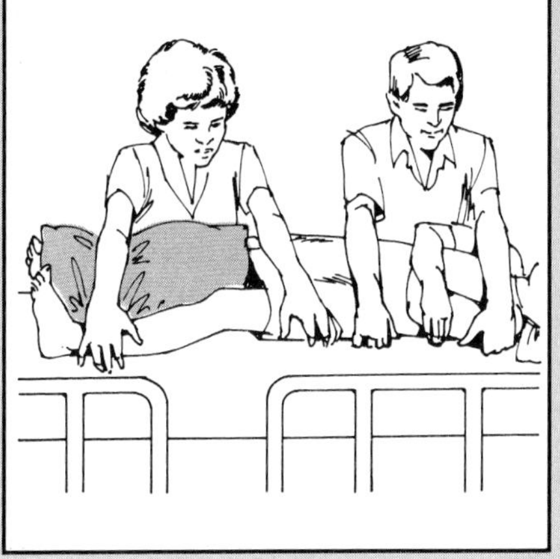

Or

Turning sheet can be used: Nurses reach over client, one grasping sheet at shoulder and waist, the other at hip and knee.

7. Both nurses assume broad stance with knees flexed as described in step 7 of Procedure 30–12.

   7. Provides a stable base of support.

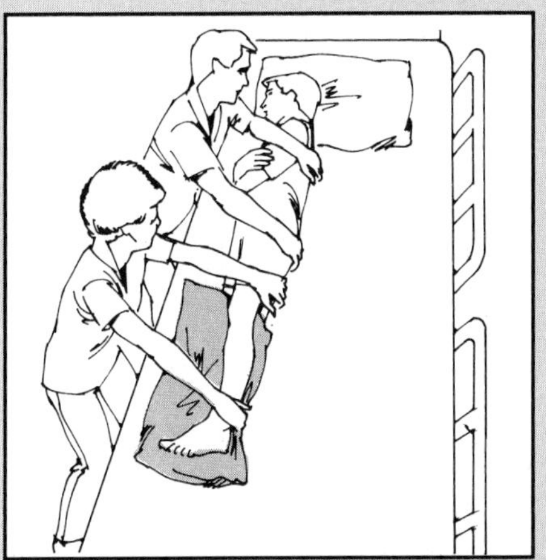

(continued)

PROCEDURE 30–13. (continued)

8. On signal, both nurses shift weight to back foot while rolling client toward them.

NOTE: All nurses must move at the same time to prevent strain on client's spine.

8. Weight shift provides force to move client, preventing nurse's muscle strain.

9. Position and support extremities in side-lying position (see Fig. 30–21).

10. Replace covers, raise siderails, return bed to low position.

RECORDING: Note method of turning, reason log-rolling is being used, client's responses, problems (if any), and corresponding action taken.

PROCEDURE 30–14. TURNING A CLIENT FROM PRONE TO SUPINE OR LATERAL POSITION

PURPOSE: To facilitate positioning in correct alignment.

EQUIPMENT: None.

ACTION

1. Discuss the procedure and its purpose with the client, including nurse's actions, desired client behavior, and anticipated benefits.

2. Move client near the edge of the bed (see Procedure 30–11). Standing at the side of the bed to which the client is to be turned, place client's near arm over the head if ROM in shoulder is sufficient to allow this. If not, place client's near arm, palm up, next to the body. The other arm is placed next to the body with palm facing thigh.

3. Cross client's far leg over the near leg.

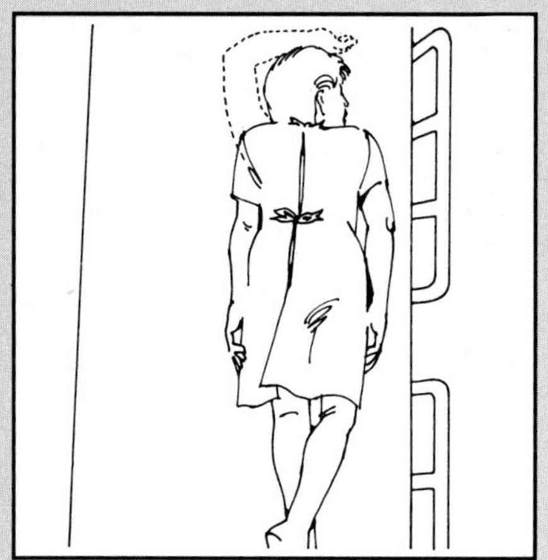

RATIONALE

1. Client participation is more likely if response and expected benefits of the procedure are clear.

2. Rolling is easier with arm above the head but this placement of the arm during and after the roll requires full ROM of shoulder and may be difficult or painful for some clients.

3. Facilitates movement of far leg.

(continued)

PROCEDURE 30–14. (continued)

4. Placing hands as for turning from supine to prone and assuming same stance, roll client toward you. Client's back will be toward you when client is in lateral position.

   4. See Procedure 30–12, steps 6 and 7.

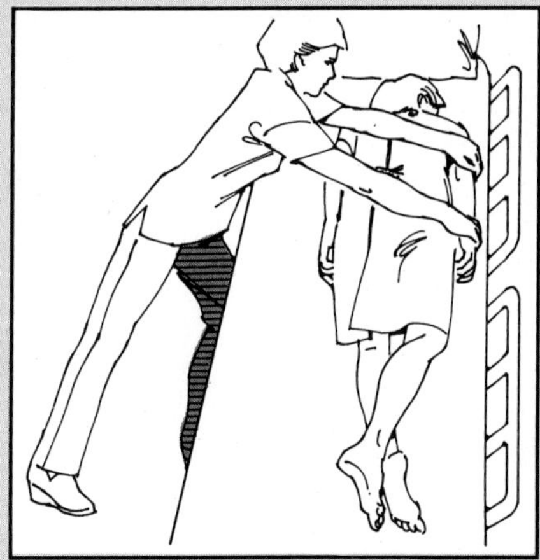

5. If moving client to supine position, shift your hands to the back of the shoulders and hips. Continue rolling until client is supine.

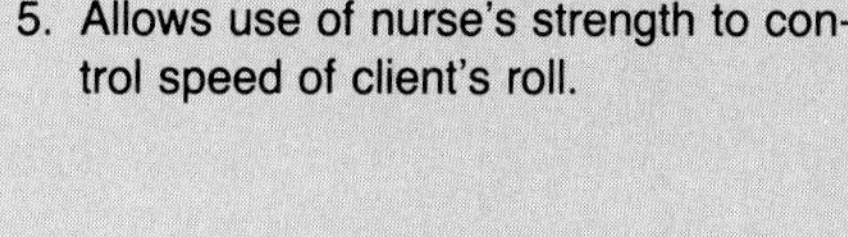

   5. Allows use of nurse's strength to control speed of client's roll.

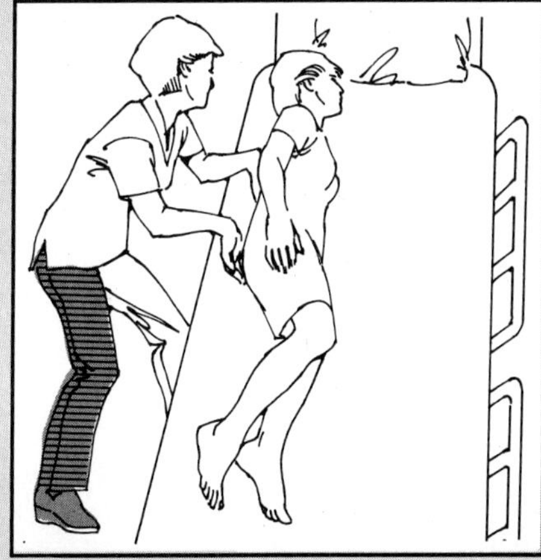

6. At completion of roll, move client to center of bed and position in correct alignment.

7. Replace covers, raise siderails, return bed to low position.

   7. Promotes client's safety and privacy.

RECORDING: Note frequency of position changes; presence of reddened, macerated, or broken skin, including location, size, and description of lesion; and action taken if lesion noted.

Fowler's (20 to 30 degrees) is used. Placing a footboard (see below) where the client can push against it further counteracts shearing.

Another problem associated with Fowler's position is caused by adjusting the bed to bend at the knee. The resulting pressure on the popliteal space interferes with circulation to the lower leg and may damage the intima of the vessels. This increases the risk of thrombus formation. Inform clients of this hazard, so that they refrain from adjusting the bed in this way to prevent their slipping down in bed.

Using Protective Devices. Special aids for maintaining correct alignment or reducing the pressure of the mattress on bony prominences are prudent whenever bedrest is pro-

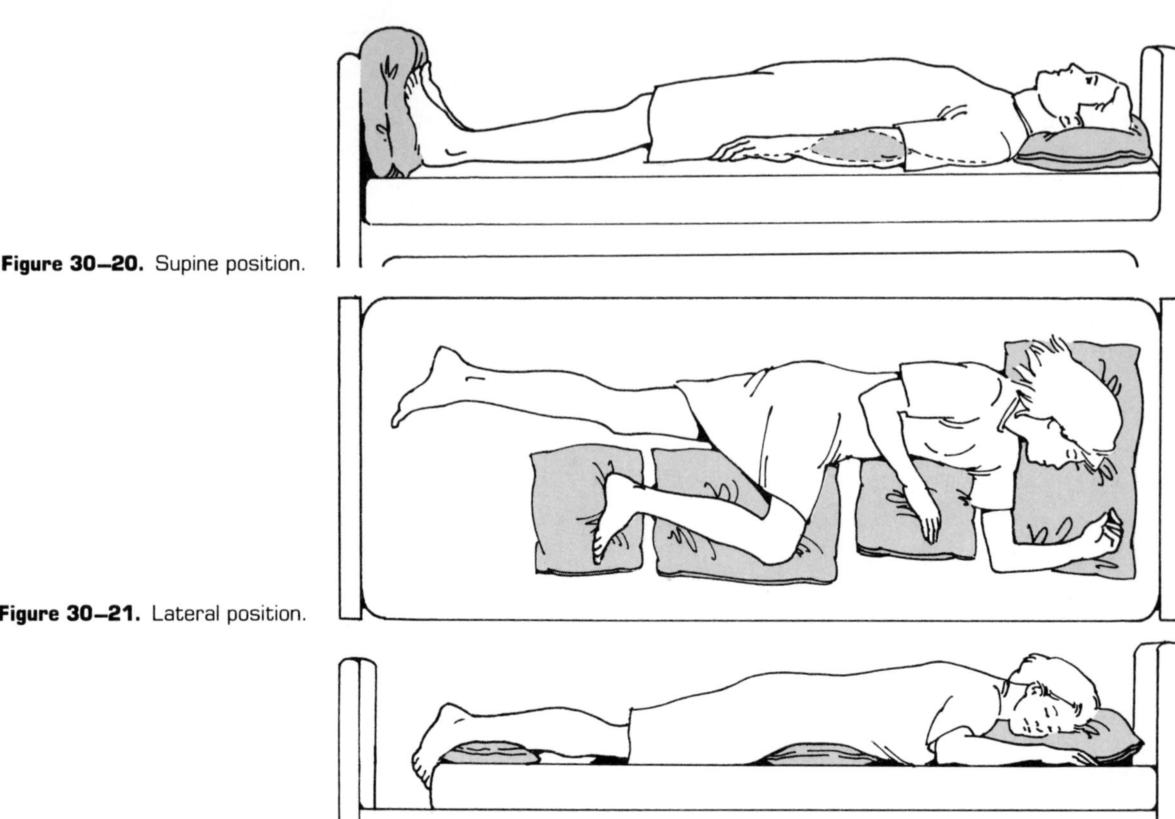

Figure 30–20. Supine position.

Figure 30–21. Lateral position.

Figure 30–22. Prone position.

longed or when diminished wellness creates increased risk for problems associated with positioning in bed. Most of these devices, discussed below, can be obtained for client use as an independent nursing judgment, although it is wise to check hospital policy to determine if collaboration with the client's physician is necessary.

Footboards. **Footboards** prevent heel cord contractures (plantar flexion, footdrop), and counteract shearing. Ellwood[63] suggests that to prevent decubiti on the heels and facilitate prone positioning without promoting knee or plantar flexion, a footboard should be installed with a 4-inch space between it and the end of the mattress. This footboard location allows space for the feet between the mattress and the footboard in prone position and for the heels to extend past the end of the mattress in supine position, maintaining the feet in correct anatomical position in both cases. However, this footboard placement cannot prevent shearing in Fowler's position because when a client's back is correctly supported, his or her feet cannot reach the footboard. Some footboard designs allow easy placement in various positions, either resting on the mattress for Fowler's position or secured as described above for other positions.

Individual Foot Supports. Rigid plastic supports that strap on to each foot are another alternative for preventing heel cord contractures. They conform to the shape of the foot and are padded to prevent pressure points. Because they are not attached to a fixed position on the bed, they do not protect clients against shearing. They must be removed several times a day for skin inspection and care. Although most are designed with ventilation ports, they tend to increase perspiration.

Bed Cradles. Bed cradles support the weight of the covers but provide no support for the feet. Therefore, although cradles are useful when skin problems such as burns, infections, or other pathology make contact with the sheets and blankets painful, they have minimal value in prevention of foot drop.

Trochanter Rolls. External rotation of the hip occurs when clients with poor muscle tone or paralysis are placed in supine or Fowler's position. **Trochanter rolls,** placed to extend from just above the iliac crest to midthigh, maintain correct hip alignment. They can be easily made by folding and rolling a bath blanket, as shown in Procedure 30–16.

Heel and Elbow Protectors. **Heel and elbow protectors** prevent damage from friction, pressure, and shearing force. Studies have shown that the calcaneus (heel), malleoli (ankles), and olecranon (elbow) are vulnerable to injury from these forces during bedrest. Heel and elbow protectors are commercially manufactured to conform to the structure of the heel and elbow joints. They are padded with foam or lined with synthetic sheepskin similar to the pads discussed

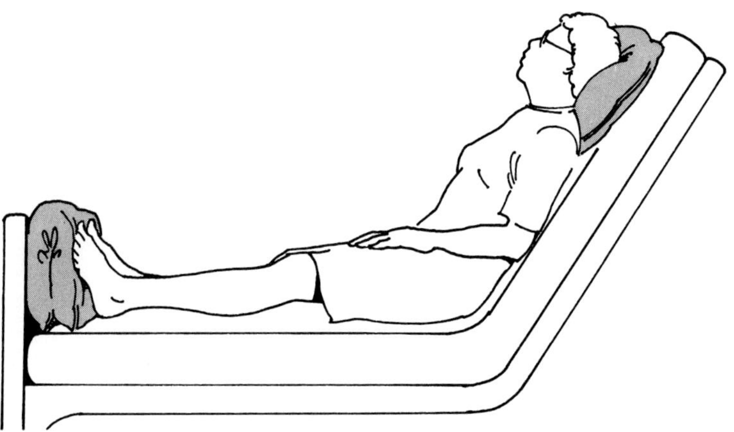

Figure 30–23. Fowler's position.

below, therefore providing cushioning to the bones as well as protecting the skin (Fig. 30–26). The protectors should be removed several times a day for inspection of the skin and skin care. They can be laundered if they become soiled or wet.

Sheepskin. The sheepskin is a synthetic pad with a thick nap, used to cushion bony prominences, thereby reducing pressure on them. It should be placed directly under the client over foundation bed linen. Placing incontinent pads over the sheepskin reduces the cushioning effect. Sheepskin pads can be laundered if they become soiled.

Hand Rolls. The use of a **hand roll,** made by folding, rolling, and taping one or more washcloths, will prevent contractures and spasticity of the fingers and thumb in paralyzed clients. The roll should be placed in the palm with fingers curved around the roll and the index finger opposite the thumb. Foam arm and hand supports are an alternative to hand rolls (Fig. 30–27).

Special Beds and Mattresses. There have been many innovations in pressure management techniques in the past decade. Perhaps the greatest progress has been made in the design of pressure reduction and pressure relief beds, mattresses, and mattress overlays. **Pressure relief beds** maintain interface pressure (the pressure between the bed surface and the client) below capillary closing pressure.[62] These specialty beds use an air-fluidized system (technology that suspends microparticles in moving air to simulate fluid support) or are air-filled with sophisticated pressure sensors and controls (Fig. 30–28A). **Pressure reduction devices** maintain interface pressures that are lower than standard mattresses, but not necessarily below capillary closing pressure.[62] These are primarily mattress overlays or pads that redistribute pressure over a large surface area. They use dense convoluted foam, gel, air, water, or combinations of these (Fig. 30–28B and C). Still another category of beds, the kinetic bed, combines pressure relief with constant slow turning, eliminating virtually all of the physiological complications of bed rest (Fig. 30–28D).

Many of these beds are very expensive and therefore are used only for very-high-risk clients, such as clients with several serious pressure ulcers, multiple orthopedic injuries, or severe burns; however, pressure reduction devices made of high-density convoluted foam, such as the example in Figure 30–28C, and the **eggcrate mattress overlay** (named for its appearance), are relatively inexpensive and are used routinely in acute care facilities. These mattress

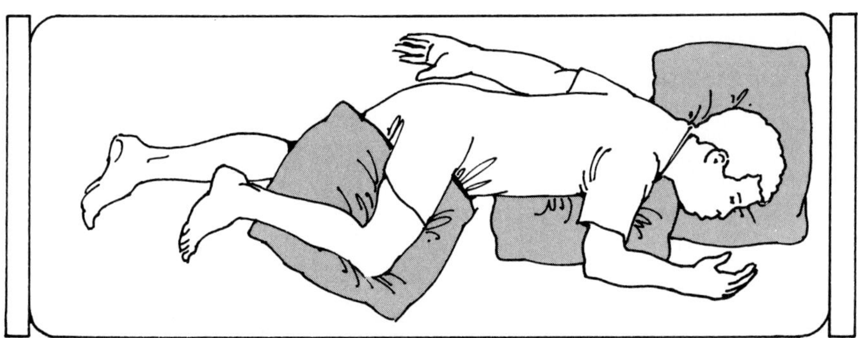

Figure 30–24. Sims' position.

PROCEDURE 30–15. POSITIONING A CLIENT IN BED

PURPOSE: 1. To maintain functional alignment of joints.
2. To prevent disuse syndrome secondary to prolonged use of one position

EQUIPMENT: Varies with client needs; may require pillows, pull-sheet, footboard, handroll, sheepskin, heel or elbow protectors, special mattress, trochanter roll.

ACTION	RATIONALE
1. Discuss procedure with client, including nurse's actions, behavior desired of client, and signals used to synchronize efforts, if any.	1. Client will be more willing and able to participate if reasons and expected benefits of the procedure are clear. Clarifying signals enhances cooperation.
2. Raise bed to your hip level, lower near siderail, lock wheels of bed. NOTE: Nurse may strain back if bed is left in low position during the move. If wheels are not locked, bed, rather than client, will move.	2. Maintains client safety, allows nurse to use major muscles of extremities and avoid back strain.
3. Lower head of bed, remove pillows used for positioning. Head pillow can be placed against head of bed.	3. Avoids working against gravity, diminishes friction from pillows.
4. Screen client. Fanfold covers to foot of bed. Arrange IV and drainage tubing so it will not be pulled or entangled as client is moved.	4. Provides privacy. Moving tubing and covers keeps them from interfering with smooth movement. Tension on tubing could cause pain and/or disruption of IV or drainage system.
5. Support joints in anatomical position, using pillows, folded bath blankets, or towels. Support is required above and below joints. Enclosing towels in pillowcases will reduce skin irritation from rough surface.	5. Contractures or injuries can result if there is torsion on joints or extremities extend beyond supportive devices.
6. Avoid skin-to-skin contact when alternate position is possible.	6. Increased local skin temperature due to contact results in increased perspiration, leading to loss of electrolytes and loss of skin integrity.
7. Check linen and gown for dampness whenever position is changed.	7. Maceration leads to increased possibility of skin breakdown causing discomfort and allowing microorganism invasion.

(continued)

PROCEDURE 30–15. (continued)

8. Distribute client's body weight over as large an area as possible, supporting extremities so they are not resting upon one another. Additional cushioning may be used for bony prominences so weight is not concentrated on them.	8. Pressure is inversely proportional to the area of the base of support. Capillary pressure ranges from 12 to 22 mm Hg. When this pressure is exceeded, perfusion is diminished or eliminated. Additional weight (eg, of extremity) increases likelihood that this pressure will be exceeded with resulting ischemia.
9. Turn and correctly reposition clients at least q2h. Individualize the amount of time in each position according to client tolerance and preference. Do not exceed 2 hours without a position change.	9. The longer the period of ischemia, the greater the possibility for tissue damage or necrosis.
NOTE: Writing a turning schedule in the client care plan listing the amount of time for each position and the hour of the day for each change will facilitate timely position changes.	
10. Inspect weightbearing bony prominences when position is changed.	10. Capillary pressure is more easily exceeded over bony prominences, because they lack cushioning of subcutaneous tissue and dense muscles, so pressure is concentrated on the small surface of the bony prominence.
11. If a reddened area that does not resolve by the time of the next position change or a break in skin is noted, avoid positions causing pressure on that area until skin returns to normal.	11. Redness or broken skin indicates ischemia; a stage 1 pressure ulcer. Continued pressure promotes progression to a more serious stage (see Chap. 24.)

RECORDING: Note frequency of position changes; positions used; presence of reddened, macerated, or broken skin, including location, size, and description of lesion; and action taken if lesion noted.

overlays do not replace consistent turning and positioning, but do provide protection from pressure sores. One drawback to the popular eggcrate mattress is that its effectiveness is significantly reduced when multiple layers of linen or incontinent pads are placed over it, because these tend to fill the cavities in the foam that disperse the pressure.

Another specialty bed (Fig. 30–28E) is used to assist clients to adapt to a vertical position after prolonged recum-

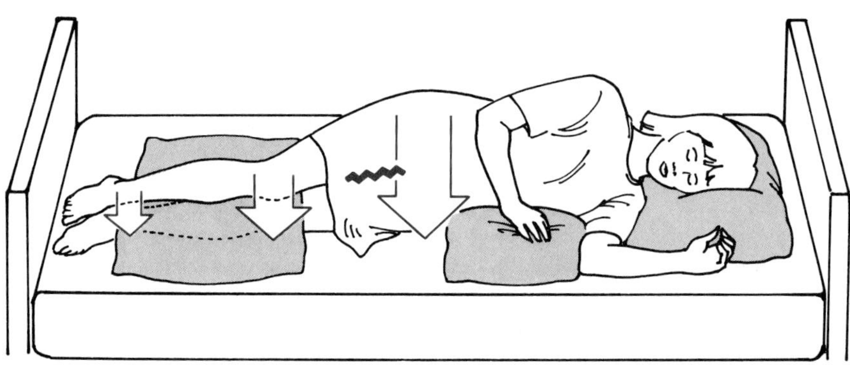

Figure 30–25. Incorrect lateral position. Indicates areas of additional pressure and of contact between skin surface when the dependent leg supports the other leg.

PROCEDURE 30–16. PLACEMENT OF TROCHANTER ROLLS

PURPOSE: Prevention of external hip rotation in supine and Fowler's position.

EQUIPMENT: 1 or 2 bath blankets.

ACTION

1. Fold bath blanket(s) in thirds or fourths lengthwise to create a roll of adequate length and diameter to fit client. The roll should extend from the iliac crest to midthigh and be about one-third the diameter of the thigh. One blanket is needed for each side, unless the client is very small.
2. Roll the client to one side (see Procedure 30–11) and place the folded blanket so it extends from the small of the back to midthigh and well under the client, so the client will not rest on the far edge when returned to supine position. Repeat for the opposite side if needed.

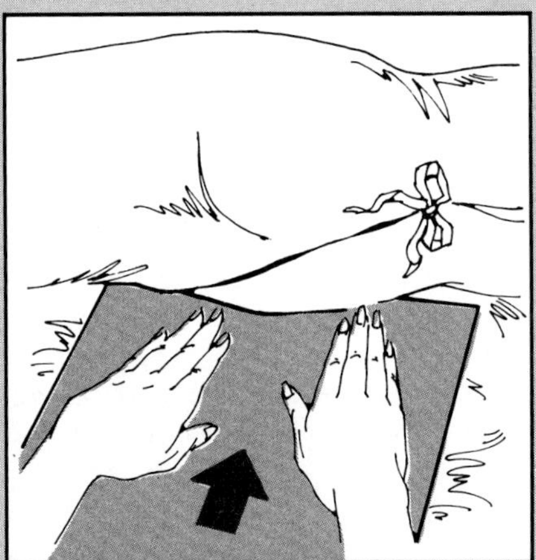

3. When the client is supine, roll the end of the blanket downward in a tight roll until the roll fits snugly against the client's hip. You will see the hip and leg return to correct anatomical position if the roll is properly placed. The roll needs no anchoring, as friction between the roll and the bed holds it in place. Repeat for opposite side if necessary.

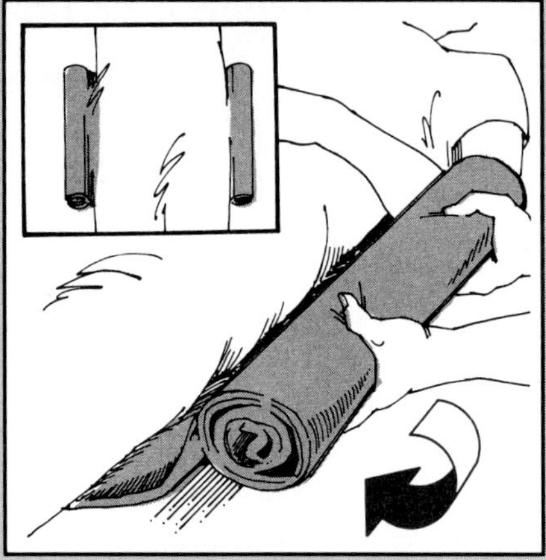

RECORDING: Indicate the use of uni- or bilateral trochanter rolls whenever a notation verifying a position change to supine or Fowler's position is made on flowsheet or narrative notes. Indicating a need for trochanter rolls on the client care plan and turning schedule is helpful.

bency. The stand-up bed can be gradually tilted toward a completely upright position, so clients need not be ready for independent weight bearing to stimulate vascular system adjustments to being upright.

Restraints and Fall Prevention. Restraints are devices that are used to decrease client mobility. There are many kinds of restraints available. The types most commonly used are vests, belts, and limb restraints. Procedure 30–17 illustrates these restraints and details their correct application. Improvised limb restraints and mitten restraints are also presented there.

The use of restraints originated to control the behavior of mentally ill clients who were considered a danger to themselves or others.[64] Elderly clients at risk for falling constitute another population for whom many care providers believe restraints are necessary and appropriate;[64–67] however, research indicates that the use of restraints does not reduce falls.[40] In fact, evidence suggests that the risk of injury from falls actually increases when restraints are applied.[64,67] This is because restraints tend to increase agitation and combative behavior as clients struggle to free themselves. Moreover, restraints increase risk for complications related to immobility. Serious injuries and even death have in fact been attributed to the use of restraints.[64,68]

Evans and Strumpf[64] discuss other erroneous beliefs that many care providers hold about restraints, including the beliefs that failure to restrain certain clients puts individual caregivers and institutions at risk for legal liability, that it doesn't really bother old people to be restrained, that restraints are necessary because of inadequate staffing, and that alternatives to physical restraints are not available. Other authors have reported similar beliefs among nurses and nurse's aids.[67–70]

Although lawsuits charging negligence for failure to use restraints have resulted in damages against profession-

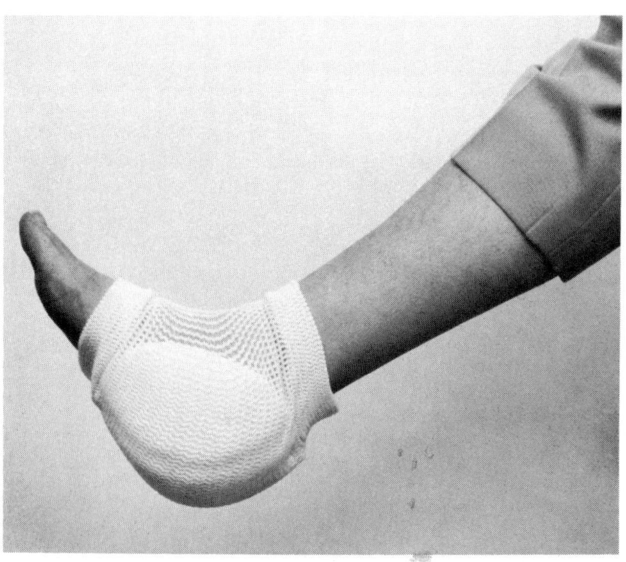

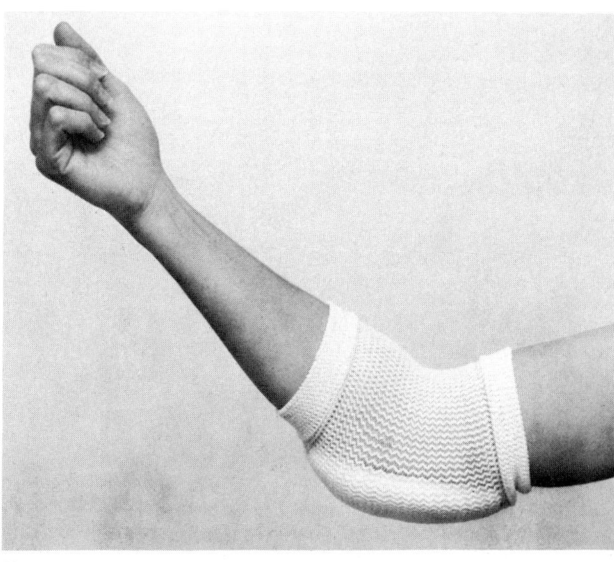

Figure 30–26. A. Heel protector. **B.** Elbow protector.

als and institutions, lawsuits involving improper use of restraints have been equally successful.[64] Federal legislation on the use of restraints (OBRA—the Omnibus Budget Reconciliation Act of 1987) became effective in October 1990. Rather than mandate conditions under which restraints must be used, it insures the right of all residents of nursing home facilities to be free from physical or pharmacological restraints unless they represent a specific treatment for a diagnosed condition. It also guarantees the right to refuse to be restrained. Under this law, nursing homes may be found liable for using restraints for staff convenience or in place of surveillance. This law does not currently apply to acute care facilities, such as hospitals, where broader discretion on the part of caregivers still applies. However, the use of restraints raises many serious ethical and moral questions. Questions related to informed consent, quality of life, and autonomy are examples.[71] Nurses contemplating use of restraints need to consider factors such as the emotional impact of restraints on clients and families and the effect on a client's self-concept, as well as the possible physical and legal ramifications. Being restrained is in fact deeply disturbing and personally demeaning to many clients.[64,71] If nurses use restraints, they must consider this a short-term solution until more effective action can be planned. There are many alternatives to restraints, as the following section indicates.

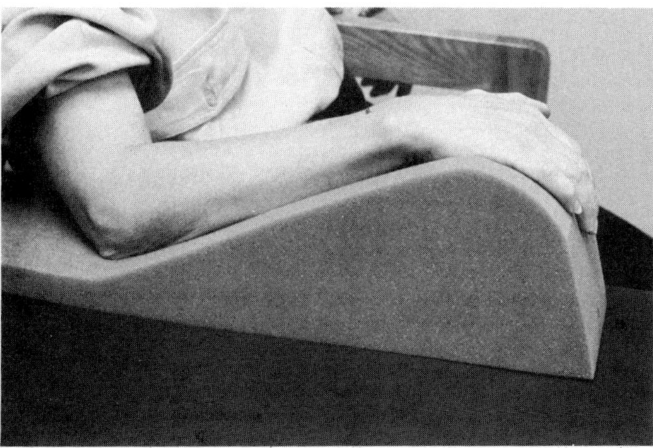

Figure 30–27. Foam arm support.

Identifying High-risk Populations. Several studies report significant reductions in client falls by clearly identifying clients at risk for falls.[40,41,65,66,72] Screening for fall risk can be incorporated into the admission assessment and periodically reassessed. Highly visible labels can then be used to maintain caregiver's awareness of clients' fall risk. Facilities have found several different approaches for identifying high-risk clients effective, such as placing the labels on client's wristbands, doorways, above client's beds, and on the Kardex and nursing care plans.

Environmental Modifications. Evans and Strumph,[64] Cutchins,[66] and Rader[73] identify environmental causes of falls that are easily modified, such as glare or poor lighting, unsteady furniture in common areas such as patient lounges, too much inappropriate environmental stimulation, and inappropriate wheelchair use. Besides modifying the physical environment, these authors suggest increasing appropriate environmental stimulation, such as more frequent staff communication with clients, providing companionship, and organizing quiet group activities with staff supervision.

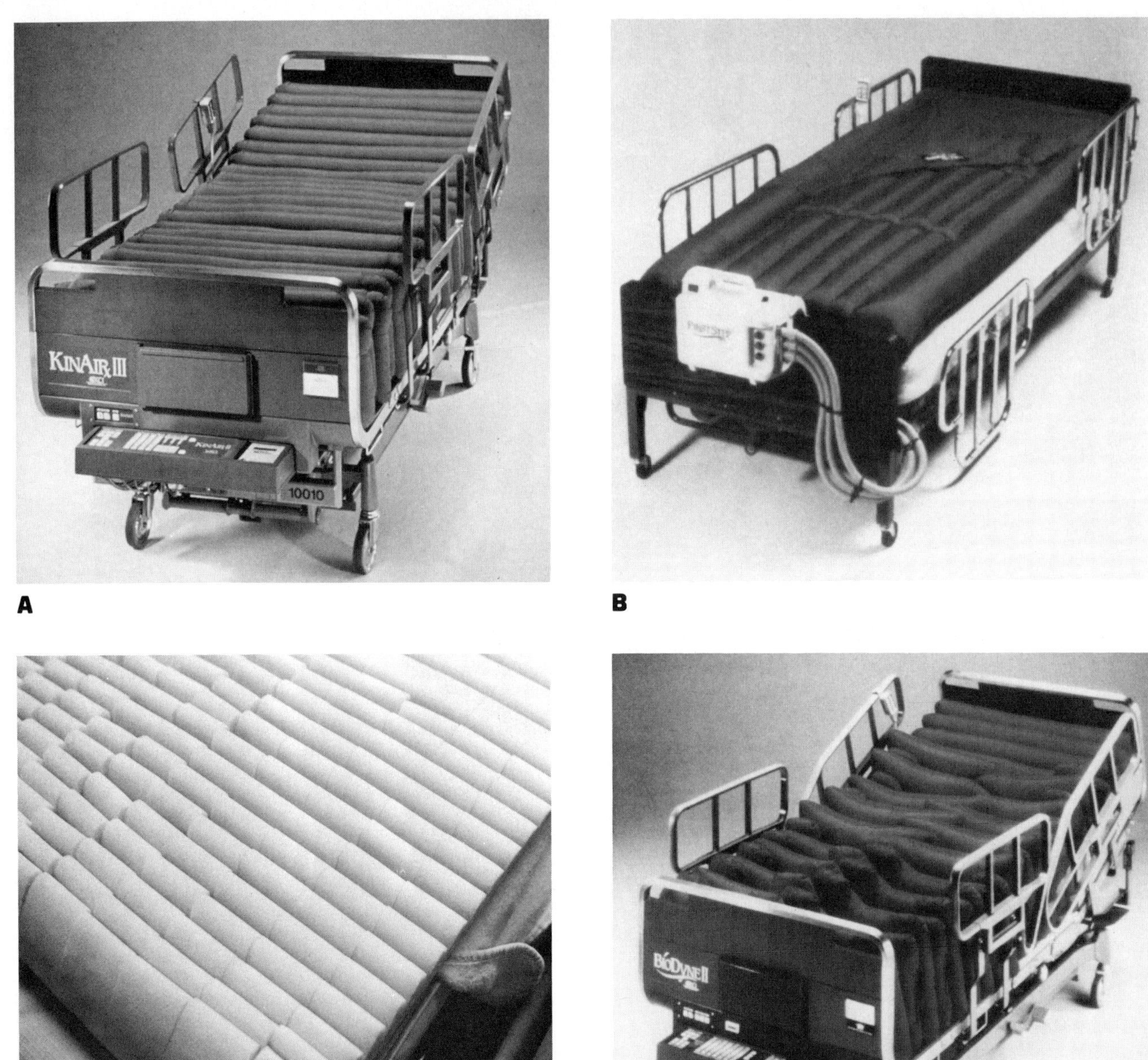

Figure 30–28. Special beds. **A.** Pressure relief bed. **B.** Pressure reduction mattress overlay. **C.** Foam mattress overlay. **D.** Kinetic bed. **E.** Stand-up bed (*continued*).

Individualizing Care. Certain clients have unique reasons for higher fall risks, such as unusual responses to certain environmental stimuli or habitual early awakening with personal care needs when staff are busy with change of shift activities.[66] Investigating underlying causes for individual client responses to the environment can help staff identify ways to modify a client's environment or help clients modify responses that lead to falls. Staff responsibilities can sometimes be restructured to increase their availability to clients at times of peak client needs. Some clients

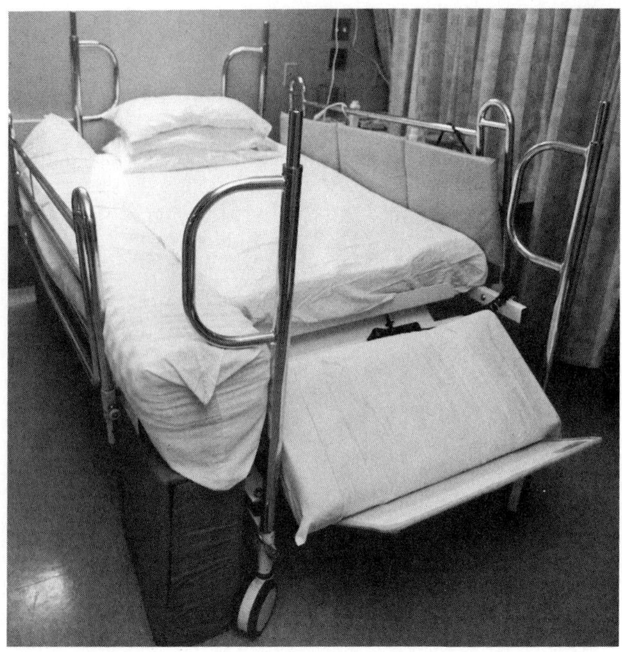

E

Figure 30–28. (*continued*)

display characteristic cues before engaging in behaviors leading to falls.[40,66] Identifying these cues on care plans alerts staff to intervene to prevent the risk behaviors whenever the cues are displayed.

Providing Frequent Assistance with Elimination. Many dependent clients fall while attempting to meet elimination needs independently rather than ask for assistance.[40,65,66,74] Offering help with toileting early in the morning, periodically throughout the day, and immediately before settling for the night, and establishing bowel and bladder programs to assist clients to more effectively regulate elimination, reduces falls related to elimination needs.

Educating Staff. Addressing caregiver attitudes and misconceptions about the use of restraints and exploring viable alternatives are critical to effective restraint-free fall prevention programs.[64,68–70,75,76] Basic nursing education, staff conferences, continuing education, and support for staff attempting new fall prevention approaches are some of the means that are effective in bringing about change in caregiver knowledge and attitudes about restraints.

Rehabilitative Care

The primary focus of rehabilitative mobility care is promoting self-care and a return to the community as a functioning, contributing member. Residual disabilities that interfere with mobility often compromise capacity for independent functioning. This is a significant loss that frequently precipitates a crisis and strains coping abilities. A holistic approach to rehabilitation addresses physical adaptation to specific deficits and focuses on motivating behavior change. Client collaboration with nurses, physical therapists, occupational therapists, social workers, and other care providers accomplishes the most satisfactory results. Nurses often coordinate collaborative planning throughout clients' rehabilitation.

Physical Adaptation. Strategies to enhance physical mobility, and adapted techniques for self-care and home management, facilitate physical adaptation to disability.

Enhancing Physical Mobility. Helping clients to become mobile is one of the most essential aspects of a rehabilitation program. Physical therapists have a major role in gait training and teaching clients to use mobility aids such as canes, walkers, braces, prostheses, and wheelchairs. Nurses have an important supportive role in reinforcing correct techniques, offering encouragement, and assisting with exercises to improve strength, flexibility, and endurance to maximize clients' abilities to use mobility aids. Early mobilization via exercises during the acute phase of the mobility problem lays the foundation for successful rehabilitation, and as such is really part of rehabilitative care.

Ongoing physical activity has an important place in the lives of individuals with handicapping conditions. Total-person rehabilitation for individuals with spinal cord injuries, introduced in the 1940s by Sir Luttwig Guttmann, is based on the premise that physical rehabilitation is of no avail unless handicapped individuals can find purpose in life. For many individuals, sports is integral in this process.[77] Guttman[78] believed that sport has the same meaning for handicapped individuals as for others, but that for individuals with handicaps, sport also plays an essential role in physical, psychological, and social rehabilitation.

Many communities offer a wide variety of organized sports and exercise programs for disabled individuals, including water sports, track and field, golf, weight training, basketball, skiing, and even rugby.[79] One rehabilitation center found that wheelchair karate classes improved client strength, transfer capacity, and self-esteem.[80] Some exercise classes focus on specific health problems or disabilities, such as stroke (Fig. 30–29), spinal cord injury, amputation, pulmonary problems, cardiac problems, and arthritis.[20,81,82] Nurses are instrumental in educating clients about the kinds of group programs that are available and in identifying suitable programs for a particular client.

Self-care and Home Management Techniques. Dressing, hygiene, and elimination are often challenges for clients with mobility impairments. Assessment of deficits and strengths to determine a client's self-management capacity is a nursing responsibility.[83] Teaching self-care techniques is a collaborative responsibility, shared with physical and occupational therapy. Assistive devices for dressing, such as button hooks, zipper pulls, long-handled reachers, and sock pullers, as well as clothing modifications such as velcro closures, enable clients to dress independently.[84] See also Chapter 29.

Adaptive equipment is often needed for personal hy-

(*Text continues on page 1540.*)

PROCEDURE 30–17. APPLYING BELT-TYPE RESTRAINTS

PURPOSE: *Method A:* To prevent a client from falling out of a chair. May also minimally restrict a client in bed (eg, to prevent an intermittently confused, forgetful, or pediatric client from attempting to get out of bed without assistance).

Method B: To prevent a client from getting out of bed or chair, yet allow movement of extremities. Controls upper body to a greater degree than belt restraint.

Methods C and D: To restrict movement of extremities, preventing disruption of treatment modality (IV, drainage tube) or preventing unsupervised mobility.

Method E: To restrict client's ability to use hand grasp, so pulling on tubes or dressing is not possible; also used to prevent scratching.

EQUIPMENT: *Method A:* Belt-type restraint. *Method B:* Vest or jacket restraint. *Method C:* Commercially manufactured limb restraints. *Method D:* 3 to 4 feet of 2- to 3-inch-wide cloth webbing, and soft washcloth for padding for each restraint. *Method E:* 1 or 2 mitten restraints.

ACTION	RATIONALE
METHOD A: Applying Belt-type Restraints	
1. Discuss the type of restraint and its purpose with the client and family.	1. Cooperation is more likely if client and family understand the purpose of and expected gains from restraints. Well-meaning family may release restraints if purpose is not clear to them.
2. With client sitting up, apply widest part of belt across client's abdomen. Cross ties in back, threading one tie through slot. Avoid twisting ties. 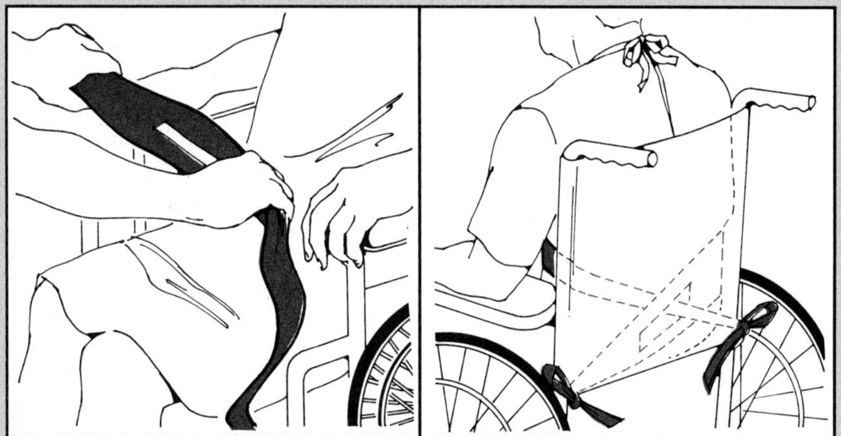	2. Will allow belt to be secured so client cannot easily slip out, yet permit rolling from side to side. Twists in the ties create pressure areas. Failing to thread tie through slot allows client to slip out of restraint with possibility of injuring self.

(continued)

PROCEDURE 30–17. (continued)

3. Allowing space for 2 fingerbreadths between restraint and client's body when chest is fully expanded, secure restraint to both sides of the bedframe or chair out of client's reach using a half-bow knot.

3. Prevents restriction of chest cavity, which could interfere with breathing; prevents circulatory stasis because of constriction. Half-bow knot, when correctly tied, will neither tighten nor loosen if client pulls against it, but can be easily released.

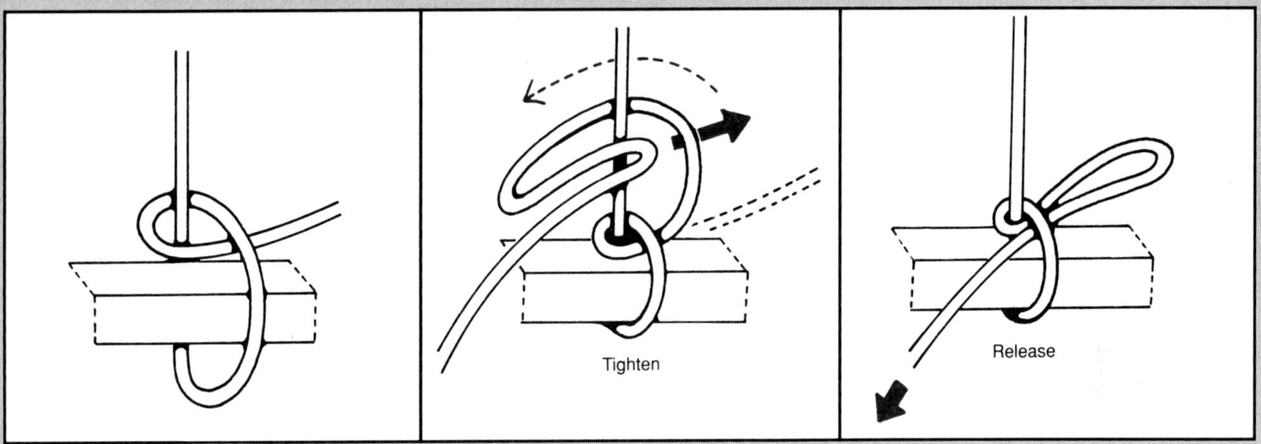

NOTE: Do not attach restraint to siderail or to an immovable part of the bed or chair. This could injure client if rail or bed is moved before releasing restraints.

4. Release restraint and inspect underlying skin for chafing at least q2h.

4. Increased perspiration caused by the restraint and friction from client movement predisposes client to skin damage under restraint.

5. Provide skin care with lotion and massage if redness is noted under restraint. If redness is not improved or reappears, select another type of restraint.

5. Continued pressure and friction causes tissue damage.

METHOD B: Applying Vest or Jacket-type Restraint

1. Discuss purpose of restraint, as described in Method A.

2. Place the vest over the hospital gown with opening in front.

2. Visibility of vest will alert health care personnel to release it prior to repositioning. Attempts to reposition client without releasing restraint could cause injury.

(continued)

PROCEDURE 30–17. (continued)

3. Apply so vest and gown are free of wrinkles.

3. Wrinkles create pressure areas, which may interfere with circulation. Pressure areas that result in restriction of circulation cause tissue damage due to ischemia.

4. Thread one tie through the slot, crossing open halves of vest front over one another.

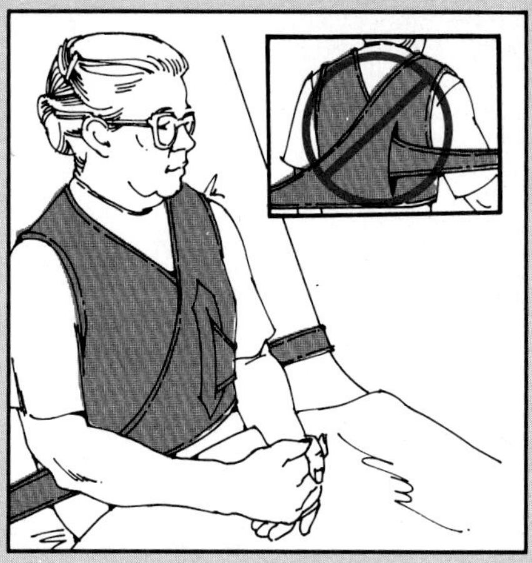

4. Keeps restraint securely in place. Restraint may slip upward if ties are not properly threaded, causing chafing or decreased circulation, especially in axillary area.

5. Complete procedure by performing steps 4 and 5 of Method A.

METHOD C: Applying Commercially Manufactured Limb Restraints

1. Discuss purpose of restraint, as described in Method A.

2. Place widest part of restraint around ankle or wrist with padded surface next to skin. If restraint is not padded, fold and wrap a soft washcloth around extremity before applying restraint.

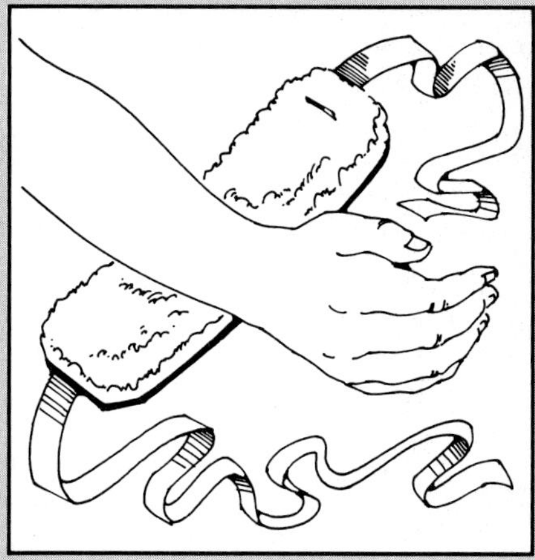

2. Padding dissipates pressure so bony prominences do not receive brunt of pressure when resistance is applied to restraint. Pressure, especially over bony prominences, causes tissue damage due to ischemia.

(continued)

PROCEDURE 30–17. (continued)

3. Secure restraint on extremity, using Velcro, buckle, or by threading one tie through the slot and bringing the other tie around the extremity to meet the first tie on the lateral aspect of the extremity.

   3. Restraint will then be too snug to slip off, yet will not restrict circulation.

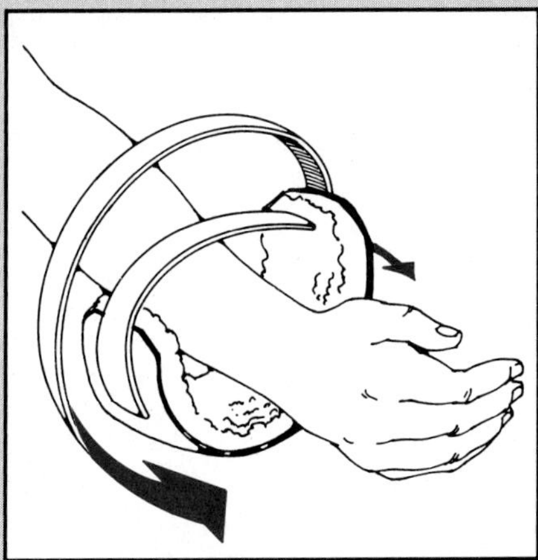

4. Tie half-hitch (single knot) to secure restraint on extremity. Allow space for one fingerbreadth between extremity and secured restraint.

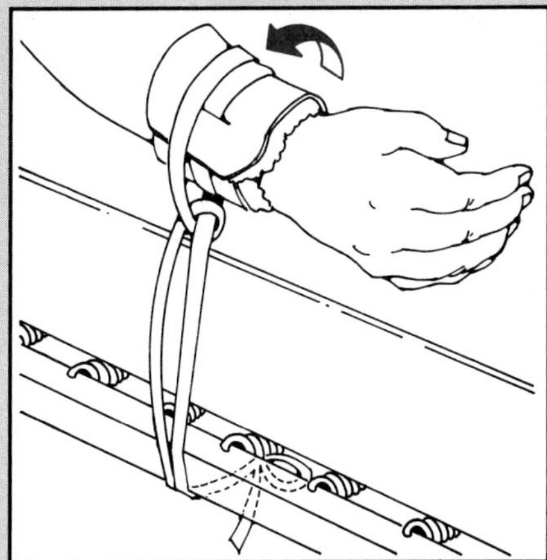

5. Position the extremity in slight flexion and secure both ties to the same side of the bed using a half-bow knot.

   5. Slight flexion allows for a small amount of joint movement without compromising effectiveness of the restraints.

NOTE: Do not tie to siderail or immovable part of bed. This could injure client if rail or bed is moved before releasing restraints.

6. Assess skin, circulatory status, and nerve integrity at least q2h.

   6. Coolness, pallor, tingling, or decreased sensation in restrained extremity indicate possible compromised circulation and/or nerve damage.

(continued)

PROCEDURE 30–17. (continued)

7. Provide range of motion or encourage active exercise to the degree possible for client at least q2h.

   7. Restriction of joint movement causes joint stiffening due to shortening of ligaments and tendons around joint capsule. Failure to provide ROM may result in contractures.

METHOD D: Applying Clove-hitch Limb Restraints

1. Discuss purpose of restraint as described in Method A.
2. Lay restraint material on a flat surface. Make two loops by bringing ends over the center so ends extend in opposite directions. If ends extend in the same direction, the restraint will tighten if resistance is applied.

   2. Creates loops to hold the extremity that will not tighten when resistance is applied. Circulatory stasis may result if the restraint tightens.

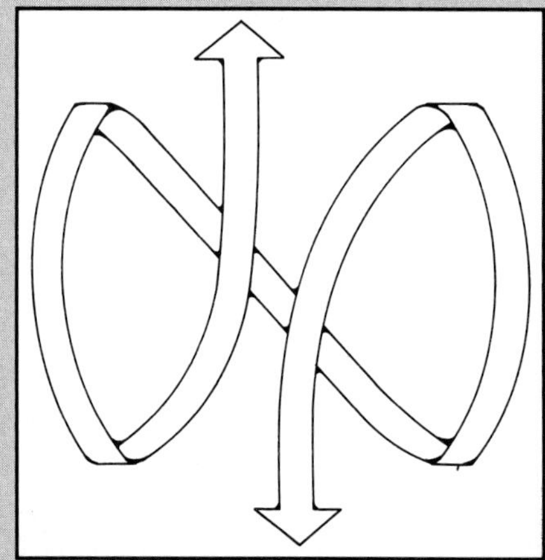

3. Pad extremity with folded washcloth.

   3. Prevents damage to skin and underlying tissue because of pressure from restraint.

4. Bring the loops together. Slip the loops over the padded extremity and adjust to allow one fingerbreadth between extremity and secured restraint.

   4. Restraint will then be too snug to slip off, yet will not restrict circulation.

(continued)

PROCEDURE 30–17. (continued)

5. Position the extremity in slight flexion and secure both ties to the same side of the bed using a half-bow knot (shown with step 3 of Method A).

5. Slight flexion allows for small amount of joint movement without compromising effectiveness of the restraint.

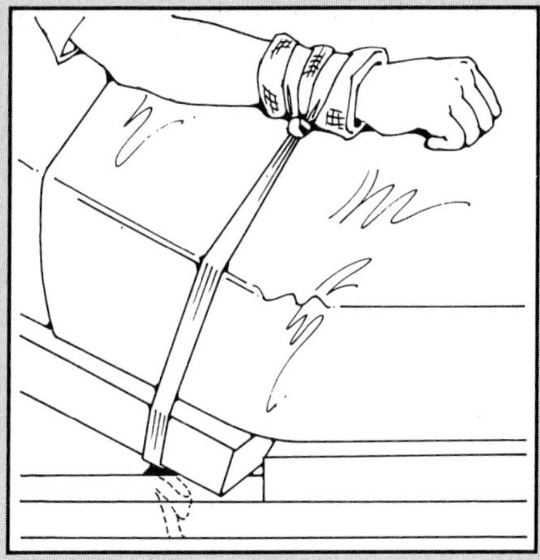

6. Provide range of motion or encourage active exercise to the degree possible for client at least q2h.

METHOD E: Applying Mitten Restraint

1. Discuss purpose of restraint as described in Method A.

2. Select a mitten of such a size as to allow full extension of fingers inside, but that prevents pincer grasp.

2. Too small a mitten will promote flexion contractures of fingers. If grasp is possible, restraint will not prevent pulling on tubes.

3. Place one padded mitten over each hand. Secure ties at the wrist, allowing one fingerbreadth between ties and wrist.

3. Prevents mitten from slipping off without interfering with circulation.

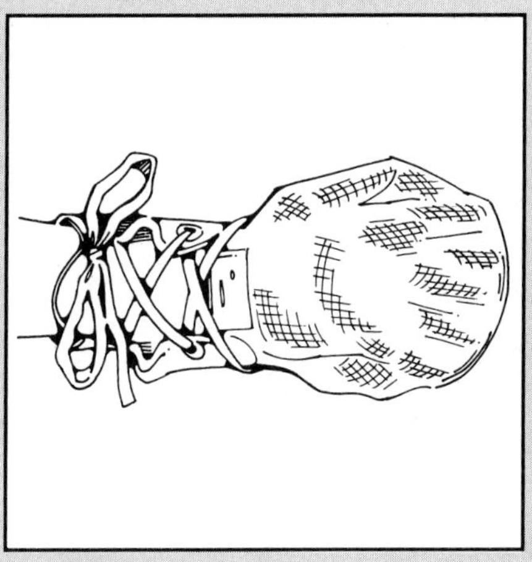

NOTE: May also be secured to bed frame, but this restriction of motion is usually unnecessary because mitten limits dexterity.

(continued)

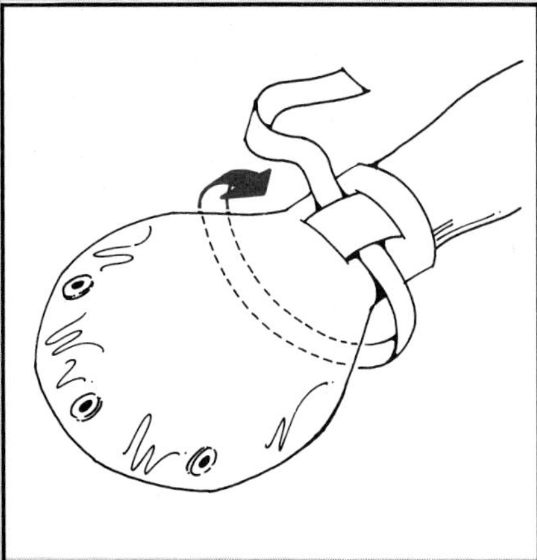

4. Release restraint and inspect underlying skin for chafing at least q2h.

4. Padding greatly increases perspiration and, therefore, the risk for maceration.

NOTE: Removing mitten for 20 minutes q1h is advisable, if possible.

RECORDING: Note type of restraint; reason for application, if not previously documented; amount of time secured and released; description of client behavior during periods of restraint and release; condition of skin and underlying tissue, and care provided, if any.

giene and grooming. Special handles for combs, brushes, toothbrushes, and razors can be designed to accommodate specific losses of hand and arm function. Shower chairs facilitate bathing with fewer risks than tub transfers, although some clients prefer using a stool with nonskid rubber tips on the legs in the bathtub.[84]

Many handicapped clients experience elimination challenges including loss of voluntary control and learning safe transfers to the toilet. For some clients, permanent indwelling catheters or intermittent self-catheterization are necessary. Bowel and bladder training programs, (Chap. 26) are successful for many others. Nurses play a primary role in teaching these elimination related skills.

The capacity for home management activities such as cleaning, laundry, and cooking is necessary for independent living. Multidisciplinary collaboration is most effective for teaching home-management skills. Some rehabilitation facilities have simulated apartments in which clients can

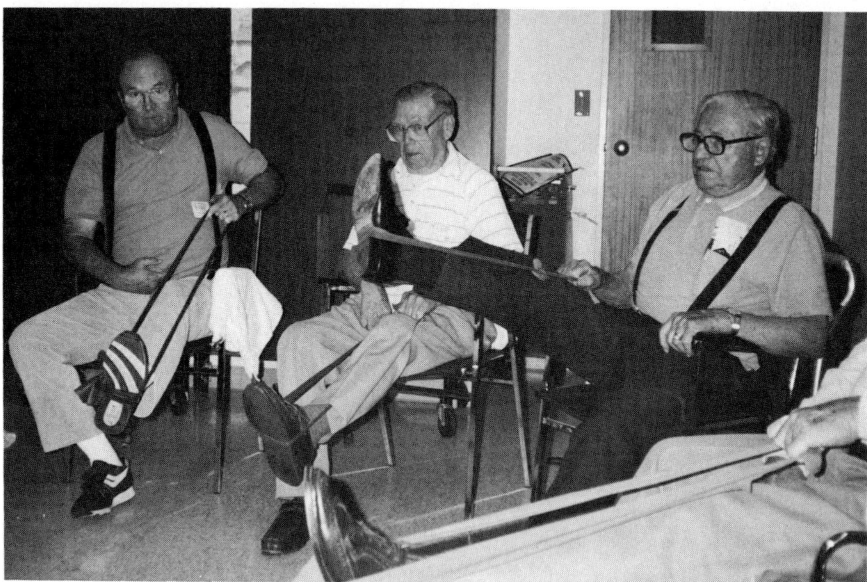

Figure 30–29. These men are participating in an exercise class for stroke rehabilitation. (*Courtesy of Sharp Cabrillo Hospital, San Diego.*)

learn home-management skills in preparation for discharge to their own homes. Adaptive equipment for home maintenance tasks promotes autonomy. See also Chapter 29.

Motivating Behavior Change. As discussed in Chapter 20, individuals' health beliefs, locus of control, and self-efficacy influence their motivation and accordingly, learning and capacity for behavior change. Rehabilitation involves significant behavior changes in almost every area of life. Consequently, rehabilitation is dependent on motivation; lack of motivation is particularly disruptive to rehabilitation.[85]

Concepts related to assessing health beliefs, locus of control, and self-efficacy are discussed in Chapters 20, 22, and 23. Clients who place a high value on independence, believe they are in control of their own lives, and see themselves as capable of change are intrinsically motivated. They are likely to participate actively in rehabilitation activities with little need for motivating strategies by nurses and other care providers. For many clients, however, external incentives reinforce participation, especially in the early stages of rehabilitation.[81]

Many of the strategies for enhancing participation in an exercise program, discussed under supportive care, apply to motivating behavior change in a rehabilitation population. Active participation by clients in goal-setting is especially significant in rehabilitation.[20,81] Comoss[81] asserts that fostering self-management of a rehabilitation program through stressing self-responsibility and teaching self-monitoring skills is crucial. This approach enables clients to continue the desired behaviors without reliance on health care professionals. She suggests that a concrete expression of commitment, such as a written contract, strengthens self-responsibility. A taped or written diary facilitates self-monitoring. Clients can readily track their progress and digression from the planned rehabilitation course by reviewing the diary and use this information to modify goals and approaches.

Positive social support is beneficial, some would say vital, to sustaining motivation for rehabilitation.[20,81] Social support comes from family and significant others, nurses, and often from other clients participating in the same program. Support from family and significant others frequently takes the form of direct involvement in the rehabilitation program. They, along with nurses, are an important source of positive reinforcement as well. Group support from peers is one of the most important advantages of a structured group rehabilitation program.[81] The group interaction decreases social isolation and provides a forum for addressing concerns, evaluating choices, and comparing decisions. The concept of "mutual aid" is a creative approach to group social support.[85] It proposes matching people of differing abilities and dissimilar handicaps in community placement—for example, an able-bodied blind person with a physically handicapped person. This approach would capitalize on the strengths of each individual and theoretically build self-esteem. Although there may be logistical problems, proponents of the mutual aid approach feel the problems are outweighed by the possible benefits.

Rehabilitation is a demanding phase of recovery from health problems. Strong commitment from clients and health care professionals is the basis for successful rehabilitation. The commitment is expressed through collaborative planning and implementation. A broad-minded and imaginative approach to the problems of clients with disabilities has the most potential for maximizing their functioning at home and in the community.

■ EVALUATION

Evaluation of nursing implementation to promote mobility completes the cycle of the nursing process. Examples of evaluation criteria for mobility can be found in the table Nurse–Client Management of Mobility on pages 1460–1461. The goal of any mobility care plan is to promote or return clients to the highest level of functioning possible. The determination of the level of functioning that is possible and realistic is complex. It requires nurses' diligent application of their body of knowledge and active collaboration with clients and other health care professionals. Clear concise evaluation criteria that describe evidence of that level of functioning are the key to monitoring progress and verifying outcome attainment.

SUMMARY

Mobility is a complex function that influences other realms of human functioning. It is a significant component of wellness. Optimum mobility creates nearly limitless options for life choices. On the other hand, altered mobility can be profoundly limiting.

The musculoskeletal, cardiopulmonary, and neurological systems play important roles in mobility. Understanding the interrelated functioning of these organs is necessary for nurses to promote optimum mobility.

Altered mobility frequently influences other body functions. Oxygenation, rest and activity, nutrition, elimination, sexual, and psychological functioning are affected by diminished mobility. Consequently, assessing and evaluating mobility includes a collaborative history and examination of integumentary, pulmonary, cardiovascular, musculoskeletal, neurological, and psychological functioning.

Impaired physical mobility, activity intolerance, potential activity intolerance, and potential for disuse syndrome and their etiologies are discussed in detail in this chapter to assist beginning students to formulate nursing diagnoses related to mobility and plan client care to improve or maintain mobility.

Preventive nursing implementation related to mobility includes health education about the benefits of exercise, collaborating with clients to develop individualized plans, and screening for clients at risk for altered mobility. Supporting clients who are participating in exercise programs to correct risk factors, including elderly clients, and treating minor exercise-related injuries, are examples of supportive mobility care. Restorative care encompasses assisting clients with exercise such as range of motion and ambulation, transfer techniques, moving and positioning clients in bed, and the judicious use of restraints. Using effective body mechanics underlies restorative mobility care. Rehabilitative mobility care requires a multidisciplinary approach to promote physical, social, and psychological adaptation to disability. Approaches to strengthen motivation are integral to fruitful rehabilitation.

Optimum mobility makes possible functional participation in the home, community, and society. Nurses make critical contributions to this outcome.

REFERENCES

1. Dunn MM. Guidelines for an effective fitness prescription. *Nurse Practitioner.* 1987; 12:9.
2. Progress toward achieving the 1990 health goals. *MMWR.* 1989; 38:449–453.
3. Powell KE, Spain KG, Christenson GM, Mollencamp MP. The status of the 1990 objectives for physical fitness and exercise. *Pub Health Rep.* 1986; 101:15–21.
4. Leon AS, Connett J, Jacobs DR Jr, Rauramaa R. Leisure-time physical activity levels and risk of coronary heart disease and death. *JAMA.* 1987; 258:2388–2395.
5. Pollack ML, Wilmore JH. *Exercise in Health and Disease.* Philadelphia: Saunders; 1990.
6. Physical activity and fitness. In: *Healthy People 2000: National Health Promotion and Disease Prevention Objectives.* Washington, DC: United States Department of Health and Human Services, Public Health Service; 1990.
7. Tursky EA. Muscle training: Physiology and practical applications of training for strength versus endurance. *Orthopaed Nurs.* 1991; 10:27–32.
8. Astrand PO. Exercise physiology and its role in disease prevention and in rehabilitation. *Arch Phys Med Rehabil.* 1987; 68: 305–309.
9. American College of Sports Medicine. The recommended quantity and quality of exercise for developing and maintaining cardiorespiratory and muscular fitness in healthy adults. *Med Sci Sports Exerc.* 1990; 22:265.
10. Larson EB. The benefits of exercise in an aging society. *Arch Inter Med.* 1987; 147:353–356.
11. Webster JA. Key to healthy aging: Exercise. *Gerontol Nurs.* 1988; 14:8–15.
12. Braun LT. Exercise physiology and cardiovascular fitness. *Nurs Clin North Am.* 1991: 26:135–147.
13. Cox MH. Exercise training programs and cardiorespiratory adaptation. *Clin Sports Med.* 1991; 10:19–32.
14. Appenzeller O. Neurology of endurance training: In: Appenzeller O, ed. *Sports Medicine.* 3rd ed. Baltimore: Urban & Schwarzenberg; 1988:35–69.
15. Anthony J. Psychologic aspects of exercise. *Clin Sports Med.* 1991; 10:171–180.
16. Gillett PA. Self-reported factors influencing exercise adherence in overweight women. *Nurs Res.* 1988; 37:25–29.
17. Bonheur B, Young SW. Exercise as a health promoting lifestyle choice. *Applied Nurs Res.* 1991; 4:2–6.
18. Kellner RK. Physical health, mental health, and exercise. In: Appenzeller O, ed. *Sports Medicine.* 3rd ed. Baltimore: Urban & Schwarzenberg; 1988:73–81.
19. Farmer ME, Locke BZ, Moscicki EK, Dannenberg AL, Larsen DB, Radloff LS. Physical activity and depressive symptoms: The NHANES 1 epidemiologic follow-up study. *Am J Epidemiol.* 1988; 6:222–227.
20. Parchert MA. Simon JM. The role of exercise in cardiac rehabilitation: A nursing perspective. *Rehabil Nurs.* 1988; 13:11–14.
21. Van Handel PJ. The preparticipatory fitness test. *Clin Sports Med.* 1991; 10:1–18.
22. Despres JP, Bouchard C, Malina RM. Physical activity and coronary heart disease risk factors during childhood and adolescence. *Exerc Sports Sci Rev.* 1990; 18:243–248.
23. Goss JE, Shadoff B. Sudden cardiac death in sports. In: Appenzeller O, ed. *Sports Medicine.* 3rd ed. Baltimore: Urban & Schwarzenberg; 1988:209–220.
24. University of California, Berkeley. Exercise without injury. *Berkeley Wellness Letter.* 1990; 6:4–5.
25. Appenzeller O. Temperature regulation in sports. In: Appenzeller O, ed. *Sports Medicine.* 3rd ed. Baltimore: Urban & Schwarzenberg; 1988:11–33.
26. Timaris PS. Aging of skeleton, joints, and muscle. In: Timaris PS, ed. *Physiological Basis of Geriatrics.* New York: Macmillan; 1988.
27. Davis-Sharts J. The elder and critical care. *Nurs Clin North Am.* 1989; 24:755–767.
28. Elia EA. Exercise and the elderly. *Clin Sports Med.* 1991; 10:141–155.
29. McKeag DB. The role of exercise in children and adolescents. *Clin Sports Med.* 1991; 10:117–130.
30. Lowen A. *Bioenergetics.* New York: Penguin; 1975.
31. Hull CL. *Principles of Behavior.* New York: Appleton-Century-Crofts; 1943.
32. Pender NJ. Expressing health through lifestyle. *Nurs Sci Q.* 1990; 3:115–122.
33. Taylor HL, Henschel A, Porozek J, Keys A. Effects of bedrest on cardiovascular function and work performance. *J Appl Physiol.* 1949; 2:223–229.
34. Halar EM, Bell KR. Rehabilitation's relationship to inactivity. In: Kottke FJ, Lehmann JF, eds. *Krusen's Handbook of Physical Medicine and Rehabilitation.* 4th ed. Philadelphia: Saunders; 1990; 1111–1133.
35. Holm K, Hedricks C. Immobility and bone loss in the aging adult. *Crit Care Nurs Q.* 1989; 12:46–51.
36. Carpenito LJ. *Nursing Diagnosis: Application to Clinical Practice.* 4th ed. Philadelphia: Lippincott; 1992.
37. Olson EV, Johnson BJ, Thompson LF. The hazards of immobility. *Am J Nurs.* 1990; 90:43–48
38. Bergstrom N, Braden BJ, Laguzza A, Holman V. The Braden scale for pressure sore risk. *Nurs Res.* 1987; 36:205–210.
39. Dimant J, Francis ME. Pressure sore prevention and management. *J Gerontol Nurs.* 1988; 14:18–25.
40. Gross YT, Shimamoto Y, Rose CL, Frank B. Why do they fall? Monitoring risk factors in nursing homes. *J Gerontol Nurs.* 1990; 16:20–25.
41. Berryman E, Gaskin D, Jones A, Tolley F, MacMullen J. Point by point: Predicting elders falls. *Geriatr Nurs.* 1989; 9:199–201.
42. Barringer TB. Studies of the heart's functional capacity. In: Brown RC Jr, Kenyon GS, eds. *Classical Studies of Physical Activity.* Englewood Cliffs, NJ: Prentice-Hall; 1968. (Reproduced from *Ann Inter Med.* 1917; 20:830–839.)
43. Wood SC. Oxygen transport during exercise at sea level and high altitude. In: Appenzeller O, ed. *Sports Medicine.* 3rd ed., Baltimore: Urban & Schwarzenberg; 1988:291–310.
44. Pencak M. Workplace health promotion programs. *Nurs Clin North Am.* 1991; 26:233–240.
45. Shephard RJ. Exercise and employee-wellness initiatives. *Health Ed Res.* 1989; 4:233–243.

46. *Canadian Standardized Test of Fitness Operations Manual.* Ottawa: Government of Canada Fitness and Amateur Sport; 1986:1–57.
47. Miles DS. Weight control and exercise, *Clin Sports Med.* 1991; 10:157–169.
48. Belisle M, Roskies E, Levesque JM. Improving adherence to physical exercise. *Health Psychol.* 1987; 6:159–172.
49. Brownell KD. Obesity: Understanding and treating serious, prevalent, and refractory disorder. *J Consult Clin Psychol.* 1982; 50:820–940.
50. Wankel LM. Decision making and social support strategies for increasing exercise involvement, *J Cardiac Rehabil.* 1984; 4:124–135.
51. Moore SR. Walking for health: A nurse-managed activity, *J Gerontol Nurs.* 1989; 15:26–28.
52. Gueldner SH, Spradley J. Outdoor walking lowers fatigue, *J Gerontol Nurs.* 1988; 14:6–12.
53. Amundsen LR, DeVahl JM, Ellingham CT. Evaluation of a group exercise program for elderly women. *Phys Ther.* 1989; 69:475–483.
54. Howze EH, Smith M, DiGilio DA. Factors effecting the adoption of exercise behavior among sedentary older adults. *Health Ed Res.* 1989; 4:173–180.
55. O'Brien WJ. Physical therapy in the maintenance of athletic performance. In: Appenzeller O, ed. *Sports Medicine.* 3rd ed. Baltimore: Urban & Schwarzenberg; 1988:481–487.
56. Kresge C. Massage and sport. In: Appenzeller O, ed. *Sports Medicine.* 3rd ed. Baltimore: Urban & Schwarzenberg; 1988:419–431.
57. Knapp ME. Massage. In: Kottke FJ, Lehmann JF, eds. *Krusen's Handbook of Physical Medicine and Rehabilitation.* 4th ed. Philadelphia: Saunders; 1990:433–435.
58. Croce P, Gregg JR. Keeping fit when injured. *Clin Sports Med.* 1991; 10:181–195.
59. DiNuble NA. Strength training. *Clin Sports Med.* 1991; 10:33–62.
60. Milde FK. Impaired physical mobility. *J Gerontol Nurs.* 1988; 14:20–24.
61. Kottke FJ. Therapeutic exercises to maintain mobility. In: Kottke FJ, Lehmann JF, eds. *Krusen's Handbook of Physical Medicine and Rehabilitation.* 4th ed. Philadelphia: Saunders; 1990: 436–451.
62. Braden BJ, Bryant R. Innovations to treat and prevent pressure ulcers. *Geriatr Nurs.* 1990; 12:182–186.
63. Ellwood PM Jr. Bed positioning. In: Kottke FJ, Lehmann JF, eds. *Krusen's Handbook of Physical Medicine and Rehabilitation.* 4th ed. Philadelphia: Saunders; 1990:528–520.
64. Evans LK, Strumpf NE. Myths about elder restraints. *Image.* 1990; 22:124–127.
65. Whedon MB, Shedd P. Prediction and prevention of patient falls. *Image.* 1989; 21:108–114.
66. Cutchins CH. Blueprint for restraint-free care. *Am J Nurs.* 1991; 91:36–42.
67. Sloane PD, Mathew LJ, Scarborough M, et al. Physical and pharmacologic restraint of nursing home patients with dementia: Impact of specialized units. *JAMA.* 1991; 265:1278–1282.
68. Neary MA, Kanski G, Janelli L, Scherer Y, North N. Restraints as nurse's aides see them. *Geriatr Nurs.* 1991; 12:191–192.
69. Scherer YK, Janelli LM, Kanski GW, et al. The nursing dilemma of restraints. *J Gerontol Nurs.* 1991; 17:14–17.
70. Bower HT. The alternatives to restraints. *J Gerontol Nurs.* 1991; 17:18–22.
71. Strumpf NK, Evans LK. The ethical problems of prolonged physical restraint. *J Gerontol Nurs.* 1991; 17:27–30.
72. Killpack V, Boehm J, Smith M, Mudge B. Using research based interventions to decrease patient falls. *Appl Nurs Res.* 1991; 4:50–56.
73. Rader JR. Modifying the environment to decrease the use of restraints. *J Gerontol Nurs.* 1991; 17:9–14.
74. Garcia RM, Cruz M, Reed M, et al. Relationship between falls and patient attempts to satisfy elimination needs. *Nurs Management.* 1988; 19:79–81.
75. Stilwell EM. Nurses' education related to the use of restraints. *J Gerontol Nurs.* 1991; 17:23–26.
76. Blakeslee JA, Goldman BD, Papougenis D, Torell CA. Making the transition to restraint free care. *J Gerontol Nurs.* 1991; 17:4–8.
77. Stein JU. The role of activity in handicapping conditions. *Clin Sports Med.* 1991; 10:211–221.
78. Guttman L. In: Maddox S, ed. *Spinal Cord Injury: A Primer—Spinal Injury Through History.* Boulder: Spinal Network; 1987; 22–25.
79. Sharp Memorial Rehabilitation Services. Sharp Momentum. *Sharp Healthcare.* Vol. 9, 1991.
80. Portnoy FL, Richards C, Roberts R. Wheelchair karate. *Geriatr Nurs.* 1989; 10:76–77.
81. Comoss PM. Nursing strategies to improve compliance with lifestyle changes in cardiac rehabilitation. *J Cardiovas Nurs.* 1988; 2:23–36.
82. Minor MA, Hewett JE, Webel RR, et al. Efficacy of physical conditioning exercise in patients with rheumatoid and osteoarthritis. *Arthritis Rheum.* 1989; 32:1396–1404.
83. Snyder M, Brugge-Wiger P, Ahern S, et al. Complex problems: Clinically assessing self-management abilities. *J Gerontol Nurs.* 1991; 17:23–27.
84. Leslie LR. Training for functional independence. In: Kottke RJ, Lehmann JF, eds. *Krusen's Handbook of Physical Medicine and Rehabilitation.* 4th ed. Philadelphia: Saunders; 1990:564–570.
85. Dacher JE. Rehabilitation and the geriatric patient. *Nurs Clin North Am.* 1989; 24:225–237.

BIBLIOGRAPHY

Appenzeller O, ed. *Sports Medicine.* 3rd ed. Baltimore: Urban & Schwarzenberg; 1988.

Block GJ, Nolan JW. *Health Assessment for Professional Nursing.* 2nd ed. Norwalk, CT: Appleton-Century-Crofts; 1986.

DiNubile NA, ed. *Clinics in Sports Medicine.* Philadelphia: Saunders; 1991.

Fuller J, Schaller-Ayers J. *Health Assessment: A Nursing Approach.* Philadelphia: Lippincott; 1991.

Ganong WF. *Review of Medical Physiology.* 15 ed. Norwalk, CT: Appleton & Lange; 1991.

Heeschen SJ. Getting a handle on patient mobility. *Geriatr Nurs.* 1989; 10:146–147.

Ignatavicius DD, Bayne MV. *Medical–Surgical Nursing: A Nursing Process Approach.* Philadelphia: Saunders; 1991.

Kee JL. *Handbook of Laboratory and Diagnostic Tests With Nursing Implications.* Norwalk, CT: Appleton & Lange; 1990.

Kottke FJ, Lehmann JF, eds. *Krusen's Handbook of Physical Medicine and Rehabilitation.* 4th ed. Philadelphia: Saunders; 1990.

McHenry LM, Salerno E. *Pharmacology in Nursing.* St. Louis: Mosby; 1989.

Olson EV. The hazards of immobility. *Am. J Nurs* 1967; 780–797.

Patrick ML, Woods SL, Craven RF, Rokosky JS, Bruno PM. *Medical–Surgical Nursing: Pathophysiological Concepts.* New York: Lippincott; 1991.

Rudy EB, Gray VR. *Handbook of Health Assessment.* 3rd ed. Norwalk, CT: Appleton Lange; 1991.

Treseler KM. *Clinical Laboratory and Diagnostic Tests: Significance and Nursing Implications.* Norwalk, CT: Appleton & Lange; 1988.

CHAPTER 31

Fluid and Electrolyte Balance

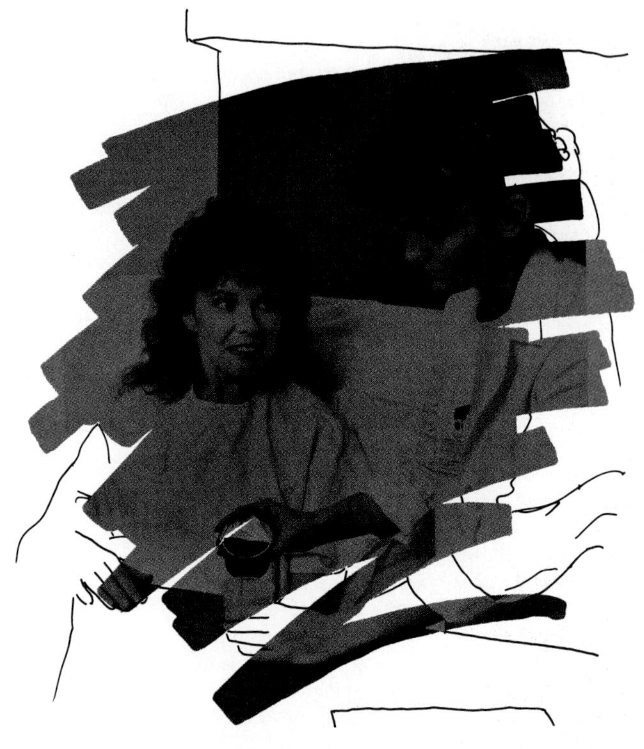

Behavioral Objectives

Upon completion of this chapter, the student will be able to:

1. Define key terms associated with fluid, electrolyte, and acid–base balance.
2. Describe the physiological processes involved in the maintenance of fluid balance.
3. Discuss at least four variables that influence the movement of fluid between body fluid compartments.
4. State the quantities and functions of major electrolytes in body fluids and describe clinical manifestations of electrolyte imbalances.
5. Describe how the body maintains acid–base balance.
6. Identify the major buffering systems controlling acid–base balance.
7. Compare and contrast the four acid–base abnormalities.
8. Identify appropriate history questions designed to gain information regarding a client's fluid and electrolyte balance.
9. Describe health examination observations useful in assessing a client's fluid and electrolyte balance.
10. Identify the subjective and objective manifestations suggestive of fluid and electrolyte imbalances.
11. Identify the nursing diagnoses associated with fluid balance problems.
12. Specify nursing implementation designed to alleviate fluid and electrolyte imbalances.
13. Discuss the oral and parenteral replacement of fluids with respect to type, indications, maintenance, and discontinuation.
14. Discuss the nurse's role in collaborating with the client to promote, maintain, or restore body fluid, electrolyte, and acid–base balance.

KEY TERMS

anions
buffers
cations
edema
hemolytic reaction
hypertonic
hypertonic dehydration
hypotonic dehydration
hypotonic
hypovolemia
insensible loss
intravenous infusion
isotonic
isotonic dehydration
metabolic acidosis
metabolic alkalosis
nasogastric gavage
obligatory urine output
pH
respiratory acidosis
respiratory alkalosis
serum osmolality
shock
third spacing
total body water
total parenteral nutrition
venipuncture

The human body is a collection of cells, each of which is similar to the primitive single-celled organisms that inhabited the ancient oceans. Human cells bathe in body fluid that is similar in composition and character to seawater. This internal fluid protects the structure and metabolic balance of each cell.

The body, as a whole, can adapt to a wide range of conditions, but the internal environment must be maintained within narrow physiological limits. Equilibrium is maintained by corrective biological reactions. Under normal conditions, individuals are unaware of the body's fluid adjustment processes. When these processes fail, the effects may be innocuous or totally debilitating, depending on the degree of fluid and electrolyte imbalance. The key to normal functioning is to return the individual to a state of fluid and electrolyte balance.

Collaboration with clients to promote, maintain, or restore fluid balance is one of the most important nursing responsibilities. As nurses' partners in decision making, clients share control over the environment, which helps them to actively involve themselves in care in order to reach the goal of fluid balance. Through collaboration, nurses can tailor client care to meet specific needs.

Body fluid balance is challenged repeatedly by conditions in everyday life. It is also threatened periodically by disease. The development of an understanding of fluid balance theory and nursing activities to preserve the client's well-being in the face of these threats is the aim of this chapter.

Section 1. Understanding Fluid and Electrolyte Balance

OPTIMUM FLUID AND ELECTROLYTE BALANCE

The Nature and Function of Body Fluid

Cellular functions require a system of circulating body fluids that transports nutrients and removes metabolic wastes. There are several types of body fluids, which vary in function, consistency, composition, and location. Collectively, these fluids regulate body temperature, cushion the joints and organs from injury, aid in the digestion of nutrients, transport gases to and from the cells, and maintain the cardiovascular system. Box 31–1 summarizes the functions of body fluid.

Water is the most abundant constituent of all body fluids. Water, the universal solvent, is the body's chief medium for chemical reactions, transportation of nutrients, and excretion of metabolic wastes. So crucial is water to sustaining the internal environment that, without it, life ceases to exist in a matter of days.

Volume and Distribution of Body Fluid

Volume. The total amount of water that exists in the body at any given time is referred to as **total body water** (TBW). This volume represents approximately 60 percent of body weight in adult men and 50 to 55 percent in adult women.[1] The percentage of body water varies substantially from individual to individual, depending on several factors.

Two of the most important factors determining the proportion of body water to weight are body fat content and age. Fat tissue cells contain very little fluid and, therefore, contribute little to total body water. As women tend to have a higher proportion of body fat than men, their percentage of body water is less. There is also a continual decrease in the percentage of TBW from birth to old age. In newborns, for example, the volume of body water may account for as much as 75 percent of weight.[2,3] By the age of 60, the percentage has dropped to between 50 and 55 percent as the result of a decrease in the number of body cells and an increase in fat tissue.[3] These statistics are illustrated in Table 31-1.

Distribution. Body fluid is distributed between two compartments, one intracellular and the other extracellular. Intracellular fluid (ICF), as the term implies, is the fluid located inside the cells. This compartment accounts for 40 percent of body weight in the lean adult male[1] (Fig. 31–1).

Extracellular fluid (ECF) is the fluid contained outside the body's cells. The extracellular fluid compartment is further divided into the intravascular fluid, or plasma; the interstitial fluid, consisting of lymph and fluid in the tissue spaces between cells; and the transcellular fluid, a specialized portion of the ECF that includes urine, bile, saliva, sweat, cerebrospinal fluid, and the aqueous humor of the eye.[1] The ECF accounts for approximately 20 percent of body weight in a lean adult male (Fig. 31–1).

BOX 31–1. COMMON FUNCTIONS OF BODY FLUID

- Dispersal of and regulation of body temperature
- Transport of nutrients to cells
- Transport of waste products away from cells
- Transport of hormones to activity sites
- Lubrication of joint spaces
- Maintenance of hydrostatic pressure in the cardiovascular system

Water Balance

The ICF and ECF compartments have dynamically changing volumes. Fluid moves relatively freely between compartments, with the intravascular fluid responding most to intake and elimination. The interstitial fluid and intracellular fluid, in turn, respond to changes in the intravascular fluid.[1] Normally, the net volume of each compartment is maintained in balance by several physiological processes which are described in the next section.

Gains. As water is the main constituent of body fluid, a balance between water gain and loss is essential to maintain the composition of body fluids. This balance is achieved by roughly matching the intake and output of body water over a 24-hour period.

In the healthy adult, the most significant fluid gains come from oral intake of fluids and foods. Suggested oral intake requirements for maintaining fluid balance vary between 1800 and 2500 mL/d.[1,3,4] Approximately 1200 mL/d is ingested in fluids and 1000 mL/d in food. Water is also produced inside the body through the oxidation of nutrients. This amounts to approximately 300 mL/d.[3]

The requirements for replenishment of fluids vary greatly with age, weight, temperature of the body and environment, and activity. For example, a fullterm infant re-

TABLE 31–1. TOTAL BODY FLUID AS A PERCENTAGE OF BODY WEIGHT IN RELATION TO AGE AND SEX

Age	Total Body Fluid (% body weight)
Fullterm newborn	70–80
1 year	64
Puberty to 39 years	Men: 60 Women: 52
40–60 years	Men: 55 Women: 47
More than 60 years	Men: 52 Women: 46

From Metheny NM. Fluid and Electrolyte Balance: Nursing Considerations. *Philadelphia: JB Lippincott; 1987, with permission.*

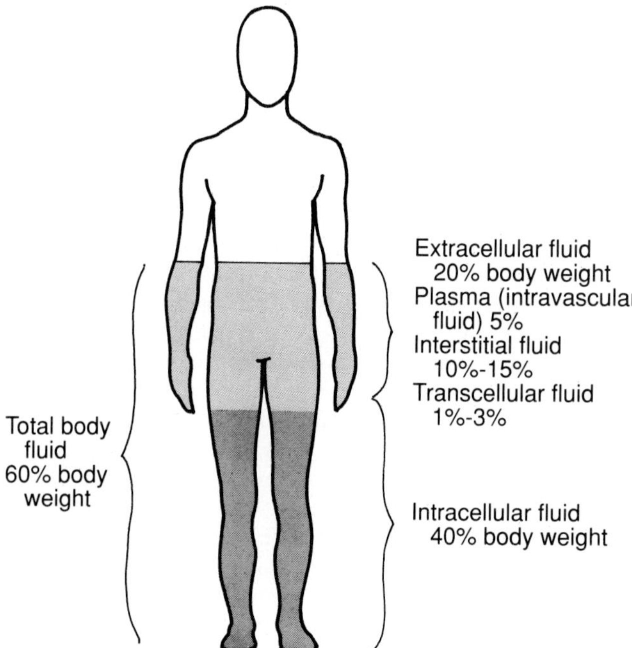

Figure 31–1. Total body fluid is equivalent to 60 percent of body weight.

quires 70 to 100 mL/kg per 24 hours to maintain adequate fluid balance, whereas an elderly adult may require 20 to 50 mL/kg per 24 hours. Of course, many other factors must be considered in calculating these requirements. An elderly client, for example, may require increased fluid intake because of losses from inadequate kidney function or insufficient intake resulting from a declining thirst mechanism. See Table 31–2 for a summary of fluid requirements by age and weight.[3,4]

The treatment procedures for ill clients contribute some unusual sources of water. For example, enteral (tube) feeding formulas contain a large quantity of water and therefore are a significant part of fluid intake. Likewise, intravenous fluids represent a large source of water for some ill clients.

TABLE 31–2. DAILY FLUID REQUIREMENTS BY AGE AND WEIGHT

Age	Amount by Weight (mL/kg)	Total Amount (mL/24h)
Newborn	60–100	200–300
6 months	130–140	900–1200
1 year	120–140	1100–3000
5 years	100–110	1500–2000
15 years	50–70	2200–2800
Adult	20–30	2400–2600
Over 65 years	20–50	2500–3000

From Masiak MJ, Naylor MD, Hayman LL. Fluids and Electrolytes Through the Life Cycle. *Norwalk, CT: Appleton-Century-Crofts; 1985.*

Losses. The body has several routes for water output. Generally, losses are divided into obligatory losses, or those necessary to carry out body waste elimination, and facultative losses, which depend on the body's need to conserve or eliminate water through the urine or to regulate internal temperature.

In normal circumstances, the kidneys eliminate the greatest volume of water. This amount varies according to the body's need to conserve or eliminate water and the individual's intake. Typically, an adult eliminates between 1200 and 1500 mL of water per day in the urine. The kidneys require a minimum volume of water to eliminate waste materials. This volume of water, referred to as **obligatory urine output,** amounts to between 500 and 900 mL/d.[3] An additional obligatory loss of approximately 100 mL/d is part of fecal elimination. (See also Chap. 26.)

Insensible loss is the moisture that continuously evaporates from the lungs and skin. This amount is usually estimated at 800 to 1000 mL/d but it varies in the presence of disease states or changes in environmental temperature. Fever and increased respirations increase insensible loss, as does a rise in the outside air temperature or increased exercise. These variations can increase insensible loss to 1400 mL/d or more.[4]

For dynamic fluid balance to be maintained, fluid loss must be offset by an equivalent intake. Measurements of these gains and losses are essential nursing interventions in aiding the client to maintain fluid balance. Simple but rapid assessment of fluid gains and losses can avoid serious illness. Box 31–2 presents average gains and losses for a 24-hour period.

BOX 31–2. AVERAGE FLUID GAINS AND LOSSES PER DAY

Fluid Gains

Ingested liquids	1200–1500 mL
Ingested food	1000 mL
Metabolic H_2O	300 mL
Total	2500–2800 mL

Fluid Losses

Urine	1200–1500 mL
Stool	100 mL
Lungs	300–500 mL
Skin	600–800 mL
Total	2200–2900 mL

Considerations

1. Liquid gains will usually match losses as long as the thirst mechanism is intact, and the client is able to ingest fluids.
2. Insensible losses are extremely variable because of the outside air temperature, client's exercise level, elevations in body temperature, and so on.

Chemical Composition of Body Fluids

Body fluid dynamics depend on the balance of body fluid constituents across the fluid compartments. Three types of substances are responsible for this balance: electrolytes, nonelectrolytes, and colloids.

Electrolytes. Certain chemical compounds break down when placed in solution. The products of this breakdown carry electrical charges, and are referred to as ions. The ions dissolved in body water are called electrolytes, primarily because they lend the characteristic of electrical conductance to body water. Acids, bases, and salts are examples of electrolytes found in body fluid.

Electrolytes are classified by the charge they carry. Positively charged electrolytes are referred to as **cations.** Negatively charged electrolytes are called **anions.** The most important cations in body fluid are sodium (Na^+), potassium (K^+), calcium (Ca^{2+}), and magnesium (Mg^{2+}). Physiologically important anions are chloride (Cl^-), bicarbonate (HCO_3^-), and phosphate (PO_4^-).

At any given time, the cation and anion concentrations of the body fluid compartments must be balanced to maintain physiological stability. Increases in cations are always offset by increases in anions. Thus, conversely, decreases in cations are balanced by decreases in anions. Body regulatory mechanisms depend on an overall balance. They also depend on the presence of specific amounts of the various types of cations and anions that go into creating an electrochemical balance. Too much or too little of one or another cation or anion can result in serious signs and symptoms such as cardiac irregularities, respiratory depression, muscular weakness, or even a decreased level of consciousness. Further discussion about the effects of specific electrolyte disturbances is presented below.

Electrolytes in body fluids are normally measured in terms of their chemical combining power rather than their weight. Chemical combining power is expressed in equivalents and refers to the ability of cations and anions to form molecules. Therefore, electrolytes are measured in terms of the number of charged particles that are available for combination, regardless of their size and weight. For example, on equivalent of sodium (23 g) contains the same number of ions as one equivalent of chloride (35.5 g). In solution, sodium and chloride in one equivalent measure combine fully and no free ions remain. This results in a state of electrochemical balance. One equivalent of any electrolyte is thus chemically equal to one equivalent of any other electrolyte.

Because the ion concentration of body fluid is small, concentrations are expressed as milliequivalents. One milliequivalent (mEq) equals 0.001 equivalent. The common practice is to define the concentration of physiological fluids in terms of milliequivalents per liter of solution (mEq/L).

Table 31–3 shows the ion concentrations present in the compartments of body fluid. Concentrations vary from compartment to compartment. Sodium is the major extracellular cation, with average concentrations of 140 mEq/L in the ECF and 10 mEq/L in the ICF. The opposite holds true for potassium, making it the major intracellular cation.

TABLE 31–3. ION CONCENTRATION BY BODY FLUID COMPARTMENT

Cation	mEq/L	Anion	mEq/L
Extracellular Compartment			
Intravascular Subcompartment (Plasma)			
Sodium (Na^+)	142	Chloride	103
Potassium	4	Bicarbonate	26
Calcium	4	Phosphate	2
Magnesium	2	Sulfate	1
		Organic acids	5
		Proteinate	17
Interstitial Subcompartment			
Sodium	145	Chloride	116
Potassium	4	Bicarbonate	27
Calcium	3	Phosphate	3
Magnesium	2	Sulfate	2
		Organic acids	5
		Proteinate	1
Intracellular Compartment (approximate)			
Sodium	10	Chloride	5
Potassium	150	Bicarbonate	10
Calcium	2	Phosphate } Sulfate }	150
Magnesium	40		
		Proteinate	40

From Metheny NL. Fluid and Electrolyte Balance: Nursing Considerations. *Philadelphia: JB Lippincott; 1987.*

Electrolyte balance within the fluid compartments is as important as balance between the compartments. Thus, within the ECF, cation concentration is balanced with anion concentration. When balance is maintained, such functions as optimal neuromuscular irritability and proper distribution of fluids are protected. The electrolyte concentrations typically vary within extremely limited ranges. Disturbances in concentrations of electrolytes have important physiological consequences, which will be discussed later in this chapter.

Nonelectrolytes. Some of the particles dissolved in body fluid are not electrolytes; nor do they break down into charged particles. Nevertheless these substances, called nonelectrolytes, are important components of body fluid and contribute to fluid movement between compartments. One such substance is glucose. Absorbed through the gastrointestinal (GI) tract and produced in the liver, glucose is vital to cellular metabolism. It is the chief source of cellular energy; however, when glucose accumulates in excessive amounts in the ECF, it pulls body water with it as it exits in the urine, creating a fluid volume deficit. Ultimately, the ICF may also lose fluid, creating a critical state of fluid volume deficit.

Colloids. Proteins in the intravascular compartment are important constituents of body fluid. They occur not as electrolytes but as large molecules called colloids. Because of their size, colloids cannot easily diffuse between compartments. Albumin and globulins are examples of colloidal, or plasma, proteins. The concentration of colloids in the intravascular compartment is important in regulating fluid movement in and out of the intravascular space. Although most proteins are colloids, one form, proteinate, carries an anionic charge. Proteinate is an important constituent of the intracellular compartment and participates in the electrochemical balance of the ICF.

Composition of Blood

Blood is a vital portion of the extracellular fluid. It consists of two components. Plasma is the liquid, noncellular portion, accounting for approximately 55 percent of blood volume. The second component, which is largely composed of cells, accounts for the remaining 45 percent of blood volume.

Plasma is a straw-colored watery substance comprising water and plasma proteins (albumin, fibrinogen, and gamma globulin). Antibodies, various nutrients, metabolic wastes, dissolved gases, enzymes, and electrolytes are also contained within plasma. Basically, plasma serves as a vehicle of transport for nutrient and waste exchange. The cellular components of blood, which travel in the plasma, are the red cells, the white cells, and the platelets. Blood is a complicated substance carrying immunologically essential antibodies. The antibody component makes blood typing possible. The particular antibodies vary with each individual, thus creating the differing blood types. (See the section on Transfusion Therapy later in this chapter.)

Body Fluid Dynamics

Movement of Body Fluids. Cell life is preserved and supported by the movement of fluid and solutes between the intracellular and extracellular compartments. The compartments are separated by membranes that are capable of selective permeability. In other words, body water and certain solutes pass with relative ease through the membranes, whereas some large-particle solutes and proteins cannot. Several critical processes, including diffusion, osmosis, active transport, and filtration, regulate the movement of body fluids.

Diffusion. Diffusion is the process by which solutes in the form of ions and molecules move among each other in liquids and gases, conducting themselves from an area of high concentration to an area of low concentration.[5,6] Ions, molecules, and colloids all diffuse in the same manner: by a random movement in which there is a transfer of energy from moving particles to stationary particles. In the body, the cell membrane constitutes a barrier for the movement of most water-soluble substances between the extracellular and intracellular fluid compartments. Some substances, however, penetrate the barrier, either to enter the cell or leave it, by diffusing directly through the membrane openings. This is referred to as simple diffusion; it contrasts with facilitated diffusion in which substances must combine with a carrier protein present within the membrane in order to move across the barrier.

Certain substances, like water, diffuse more easily than others. Factors that affect diffusion are the concentration gradient, the electrical gradient, and the pressure gradient. The concentration gradient refers to the fact that there is more available solute on one side of the membrane than the other. The electrical gradient is the inequality of electrical charges existing on either side of the membrane. The pressure gradient is a pushing force that is greater on one side of the membrane than the other, forcing electrolytes and water across. Generally, higher concentration, electrical, and pressure gradients for any given solute support more rapid diffusion.

Diffusion is involved in the balance of electrolytes between the ICF and ECF compartments, the absorption of nutrients across the GI tract membrane and into the bloodstream, and the passage of molecules from the bloodstream across the tubular membrane into the urine for elimination.

Osmosis. Osmosis is the process by which a solvent, such as water, moves through a selectively permeable membrane from an area of high water concentration to an area of low water concentration.[5] Osmosis is usually referred to in the physiological context as passive water movement.

A simple experiment illustrates the principle of osmosis. If a pouch made of a selectively permeable membrane is filled with a salt solution and submerged in a container of distilled water, it will expand. Water crosses the membrane into the pouch, seeking to dilute the concentration of salt and to balance the concentration of water on either side of the membrane. If the solutions are reversed so that the distilled water is inside and the salt solution outside, the pouch will shrink for the same reason.

The osmolality of fluid is an important concept in understanding body fluid balance. Chemically, osmolality refers to the number of gram molecular weights of a solute per liter of water in a solution. In simple terms, however, osmolality refers to the measure of active particles in a volume of solution. As a measure of concentration of body fluids, osmolality is expressed in milliosmoles (mOsm).

Tonicity, a term related to osmolality, refers to the capacity of a fluid for osmotic activity. Solutions of the same concentration are said to be **isotonic** to one another; that is, they create no osmotic movement of water across a selectively permeable membrane. Physiological fluids can be classified on the basis of their tonicity. In the body, plasma is the standard of concentration with which other fluids are compared. Fluids that have the same concentration as plasma are said to be isotonic to plasma. Should a body cell be placed in a bath of isotonic solution, no osmotic activity would take place: there would be no net movement of fluid into or out of the cell. No change in cell size would occur. Thus, an isotonic physiological solution, such as 0.9 percent sodium chloride, infused into the circulation, will not adversely affect the structure of body cells.[1]

Hypertonic solutions carry a greater concentration of solutes than plasma and thus have a higher osmolality. If a blood cell were suspended in a hypertonic solution, it would rapidly lose its internal cellular fluid to the solution and shrivel (a process known as crenation). Hypertonic solutions, such as 3 percent sodium chloride, are not infused into the body unless a deficit of solute exists or the pulling of excess fluid from one compartment to the other is desired.

Hypotonic solutions, on the other hand, have lower osmolality than plasma; they are more dilute than plasma. A blood cell suspended in a very hypotonic solution would swell and burst, because the intracellular solutes would attract the water from the solution. This condition is known as hemolysis. Clinically, hypotonic solutions are infused into the body to replace the fluid lost in dehydration states. See Figure 31–2 for illustrations of the effects on cells of fluids of varying tonicity.

Movement of fluid between the intracellular and extracellular compartments is generally governed by the osmolality of the fluids on either side of the cell membrane. An increase in the osmolality of the ECF can result in ICF dehydration and leads to cell crenation. Conversely, a decrease in ECF osmolality, or dilution of the ECF, may result in intracellular fluid congestion and thus produce hemolysis. Since osmolality is difficult to measure inside the cell, the osmolality of blood serum is measured to determine the fluid state of the ECF. From the serum measurement, inferences can be made as to the condition of the ICF, since a state of electrochemical balance is assumed to exist between the compartments. The reader should note that blood serum measurements are used because they closely approximate the values of plasma, which is a part of the ECF.

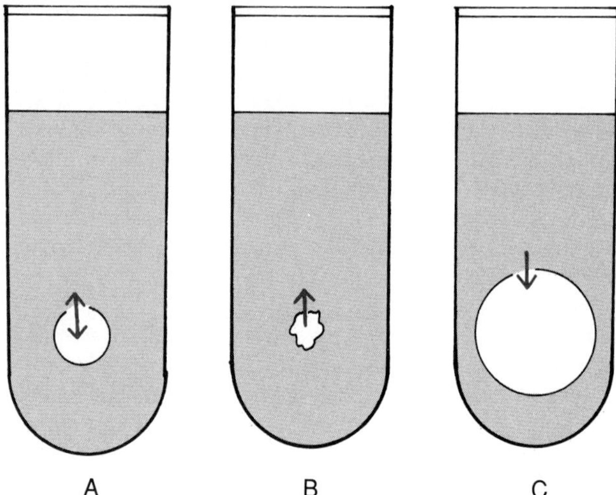

Figure 31–2. Tonicity: **(A)** Cells undergo no change in size in isotonic solutions. They decrease in size in hypertonic solutions **(B)** and increase in size in hypotonic solutions **(C)**.

Serum technically is the noncellular aspect of blood remaining after the cells are clotted and is used in laboratory analysis; plasma, as stated earlier, is the noncellular part of unclotted whole blood. Laboratory sample clotting results in some cellular breakdown; cells release their electrolytes, altering slightly the osmolality of the serum. Thus, serum measurements are somewhat different from actual plasma values.

Active Transport. Active transport is the mechanism by which ions travel against a concentration gradient. In other words, ions travel from areas of low concentration to areas of high concentration. This requires a substance to carry the ions, but unlike facilitated diffusion, it also requires energy to fuel the process.

For instance, when nerve impulses are transmitted, sodium moves into the cell and potassium out of the cell to the ECF. For the nerve cells to be able to continue transmitting impulses, the intracellular sodium concentration must be kept low. The so-called sodium pump accomplishes the necessary exchange by active transport. Sodium inside the cell attaches to a lipoprotein carrier substance and moves outside the cell, where it is released. The lipoprotein then chemically changes to accept potassium, which is moved to the inside of the cell. The energy substance that fuels the process is adenosine triphosphate (ATP), which is contained within the cell.[1]

Filtration. Filtration is the movement of body fluids through a selectively permeable membrane in response to pressure. Fluids have a natural tendency to move from an area of high pressure to an area of low pressure. In the body, opposing pressure forces between fluid compartments maintain a dynamic balance. Two forces, hydrostatic pressure and colloid osmotic pressure, maintain this balance.

Hydrostatic pressure is the force generated against the

vascular walls by the pumping of the blood through the circulatory system. If left unopposed, it would continuously push fluids and dissolved substances into the interstitial compartment. Colloid osmotic pressure is the force exerted by proteins contained in the intravascular and interstitial compartments.

Hydrostatic and colloid osmotic pressures coexist in the body fluid compartments. The interplay of these two forces is illustrated by the fluid exchanges that occur across the capillary membrane. Hydrostatic pressure is greater than colloid osmotic pressure at the arterial end of the capillary. This tends to force fluid out of the capillary and into the interstitial spaces. At the venous end of the capillary, however, the colloid osmotic pressure exceeds the hydrostatic pressure. This pulls fluid and solutes from the interstitial spaces into the capillary (Fig. 31–3). The opposing forces maintain a dynamic balance and also allow for the continuous movement of solutes, wastes, and other critical substances between body fluid compartments.

Electrolytes in Body Fluid

Sodium. As the most prevalent electrolyte in the ECF, sodium (NA^+) is the major contributor to the osmotic force. The saying "where salt goes, water follows" defines the primary role of sodium in water distribution and maintenance of ECF volume. In addition, sodium participates in neuromuscular excitation, transmission of nerve impulses, and acid–base balance.[6]

The sodium concentration in the ECF ranges between 135 and 145 mEq/L. Substantial quantities of sodium are found in gastric, intestinal, and pancreatic secretions and bile. Therefore, significant losses of these fluids may quickly deplete the ECF of sodium. To maintain body stores of sodium, daily intake must approach 2 to 4 g of sodium chloride.[5] Maintenance of sodium stores to ensure body fluid balance is so important that the body has safety mechanisms to conserve sodium. These are discussed later in this chapter. Table 31–4 lists the functions of sodium and other common electrolytes.

Potassium. Potassium (K^+) is the predominant intracellular electrolyte. Although it continuously moves in and out of the cells, approximately 98 percent remains in the ICF. Therefore, potassium plays an important role in maintaining the intracellular osmolality. Only the remaining 2 percent of the body's potassium, in the ECF, can be measured. It is maintained within very narrow limits at 3.5 to 5.0 mEq/L.

Potassium's most important role is in influencing neuromuscular excitability. Potassium also contributes to acid–base balance by exchanging with hydrogen ions (H^+) between the ICF and ECF. This shift helps maintain the balance of electrical charges between the compartments (electroneutrality), and frees the H^+ ions (acids) for elimination.

As with sodium, potassium stores must be replenished daily by an intake of 40 to 60 mEq. Because potassium is present in large quantities in most foodstuffs, daily intake is usually closer to 50 to 100 mEq per day.[7] Ordinarily, when the dietary intake of potassium is maintained and there is no other source of loss, the output of potassium balances the intake through a combination of renal tubular secretion and reabsorption mechanisms; however, when there is an added source of loss, such as when the renal mechanisms are altered through the use of diuretics, potassium supplements often become necessary. Likewise, when potassium excretion is diminished, such as when the kidneys fail to produce urine, it is often necessary to restrict potassium intake.

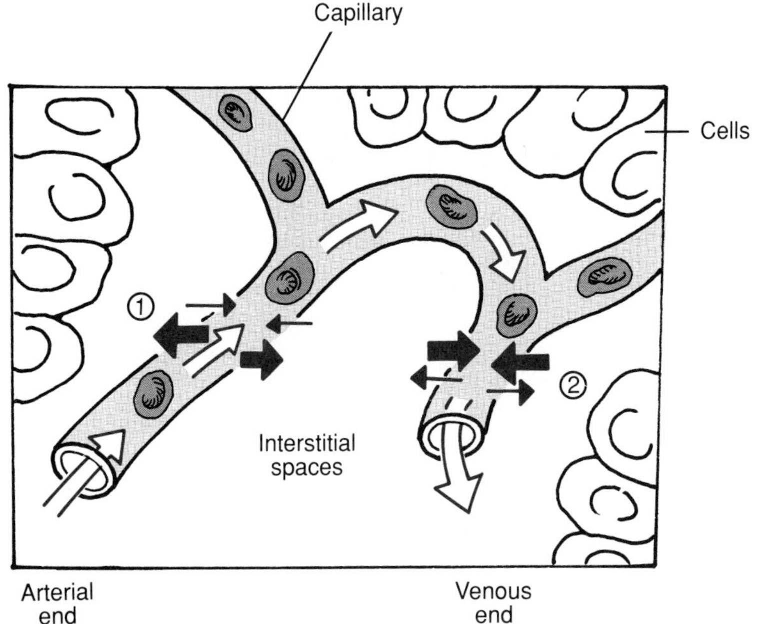

Figure 31–3. Interplay of hydrostatic pressure and colloid osmotic pressure at the capillary level: (1) at the arterial end, fluid tends to move predominantly from the bloodstream into the interstitial spaces; (2) at the venous end, fluid moves predominantly from the interstitial spaces into the bloodstream.

TABLE 31–4. SERUM ELECTROLYTES AND THEIR FUNCTIONS IN THE BODY

Electrolyte	Function
Sodium (Na^+)	Transmission and condition of nerve impulses Regulation of osmolality of ECF Sodium pump regulation Acid–base balance (in combination with buffers)
Potassium (K^+)	Neuromuscular function—nerve impulse transmission Muscular contractility (smooth, skeletal, and cardiac) Regulation of osmolality of ICF Maintenance of acid–base balance by exchanging with H^+ ions (acids) to maintain electroneutrality and free H^+ ions for elimination
Calcium (Ca^{2+})	Maintenance of cell permeability Neuromuscular function—nerve impulse transmission to myocardium and skeletal muscle Combines with various clotting factors to promote blood coagulation Maintenance of bone and tooth strength and durability
Magnesium (Mg^{++})	Neural transmission (CNS) Neuromuscular activity—myocardial Enzyme activator Maintenance of carrier substances for sodium pump Protein and carbohydrate metabolism
Phosphorus (PO_4^-)	Involved in formation of ATP, the main source of cellular energy Maintenance of neuromuscular function Maintenance of bone and tooth strength Utilization of B-complex vitamins Maintenance of cell membrane structure Acid–base buffering; combines with Na^+ and H^+ to provide for acid–base and electrolyte balance in the kidney tubules
Chloride (Cl^-)	Competes with bicarbonate for combination with Na^+, and exchanges with bicarbonate ions in red blood cells, to maintain acid–base balance Maintenance of ECF osmolality

From Metheny NL. Fluid and Electrolyte Balance: Nursing Considerations. *Philadelphia: JB Lippincott; 1987.*

Calcium. Calcium (Ca^{2+}) is the most abundant electrolyte in the human body, but all except 1 percent occurs in an inactive form as bone. The remaining 1 percent is contained in the cells or ECF. The calcium in the plasma is either bound to proteins as a reserve or is in the active ionized form. Total serum calcium, which reflects both the free calcium in the blood and the calcium bound to proteins, varies from 8.8 to 10.5 mg/dL. The serum value for ionized calcium is 4.5 to 5.8 mEq/L.

Calcium serves several important functions in the body. For example, calcium maintains bone strength and durability. It serves an important role in the transmission of nerve impulses, in particular affecting cardiac electrical conduction. Calcium maintains cellular permeability and promotes blood clotting by combining with the various clotting factors.

The maintenance of calcium levels depends not only on intake but also on the physiological mechanisms governing calcium absorption. Vitamin D must be present in sufficient quantities for adequate absorption to take place from the GI tract. Parathyroid hormone (PTH) and calcitonin influence liberation and deposition of calcium from the bone and thus affect daily need for the electrolyte.[8] The recommended daily calcium intake for adults is 1000 to 1200 mg.

Magnesium. The greatest percentage of magnesium (Mg^{++}) is located in the bone. The remaining magnesium is found in the ICF. Only 1 percent of the body's magnesium occurs in the ECF. Hence, the serum value of magnesium is only 1.5 to 2.5 mEq/L in the ECF.

Magnesium is responsible for the functioning of the intracellular carrier substances used in active transport. As a result, magnesium contributes significantly to neuromuscular transmission in the cardiac and skeletal muscle.

There is an interplay between magnesium, potassium, and calcium. Insufficient magnesium intake results in K^+ leaving the cell and being excreted in large quantities in the urine, thereby creating electrolyte imbalance. Magnesium competes with calcium for absorption from the GI tract. Generally, the electrolyte in most abundance at any one time will be absorbed in the greatest quantity. Maintenance of magnesium levels requires intake of approximately 300 mg each day in adults.[4]

Phosphorus. Phosphorus in the form of phosphate (PO_4^-) is a critically important intracellular anion. It occurs in the ICF and ECF in relatively small quantities and is maintained in an inactive form in the bone. Serum phosphorus levels are usually 2.5 to 4.5 mg/dL. An intake of 800 to 1500 mg/d in adults is required to maintain adequate levels.[4]

Phosphorus is important primarily in the formation of ATP, the main source of cellular energy. It plays a part in all cellular function, including neuromuscular excitability, maintaining cellular membrane structure, and combines with sodium and hydrogen to provide for acid–base and electrolyte balance in the kidney tubules.

Phosphorus and calcium have an inverse relationship in the body: When calcium levels are low, phosphorus levels are high, and vice versa. The feedback mechanism that governs this relationship is discussed in more detail under *Endocrine Glands*.

Chloride. Chloride (Cl^-) is an anion found abundantly in the ECF. The normal serum value for chloride is 98 to 108 mEq/L.[5] Chloride exists most often in combination with sodium and therefore acts to maintain ECF osmolality. Chloride also competes with bicarbonate for combination with sodium, thereby affecting acid–base balance. In addition, chloride exchanges with bicarbonate ions in the red blood cells to maintain acid–base balance. Recommended daily intake of chloride varies from 275 to 700 mg for infants to 1700 to 5100 mg for adults.

Body Fluid Regulation

Organs that Regulate Body Fluids. In healthy persons, closely coordinated physiological functions provide for a balance in the composition, volume, and distribution of body fluids. Through a series of physical and chemical feedback responses, most of the body's major organs continuously correct deviations in fluid balance. (See Chap. 6 for more on feedback responses.) The activation of any of these processes depends on the particular deviation. The roles of several of the body organs in body fluid regulation are described in the following paragraphs.

Brain. The brain exercises central control of body fluid balance. It regulates the intake and secretion of water and salt centrally. For example, areas in the medulla control plasma volume. Information from stretch receptors in the atria of the heart and pressure receptors in the atria and pulmonary arteries is fed to the brain centers. In turn, the brain triggers compensatory adjustments in the heart's rate and contractile force.

In addition, the brain monitors body fluid osmolality through osmoreceptors in the hypothalamus. The thirst sensation and the circulating level of antidiuretic hormone (ADH) is adjusted through this mechanism, resulting in the intake of fluids as well as changes in renal filtration and urine formation. (ADH is discussed in more detail under *Endocrine Glands*.)

Skin. The skin is involved in body fluid balance through the action of water and salt removal. Through sweating and evaporation, body water is lost and body temperature is regulated. The skin is thus primarily an organ of water elimination; however, it also serves as a protective barrier to conserve body water. Widespread loss of the skin, such as in third-degree burns, results in the loss of excessive quantities of body fluid.

Unobservable loss of moisture from the skin is referred to as insensible loss. Visible perspiration is referred to as sensible loss. The amount of fluid lost from the skin, both sensible and insensible, depends on environmental air temperature and an individual's level of hydration and rate of exercise.

One of the most important factors contributing to fluid loss through the skin is the humidity of the environmental air. Saturated air cannot pick up additional moisture, but dry air increases the rate of water evaporation. Thus when the surrounding air is hot and dry, the loss of water through the skin increases.

Lungs. Under normal conditions, the lungs are a site of insensible water loss. Moisture from the pulmonary membranes is picked up and removed, in droplet form, in expired air. The amount of fluid lost depends on the rate and depth of ventilation and the humidity of the environmental air. Fast, deep ventilation increases insensible loss, as does low environmental humidity.

Heart. The heart's hydraulic action plays a critical role in fluid balance. The pumping action of the heart supplies fluid to the peripheral tissues and maintains the blood supply to organs that maintain and modify the body's fluid and solute balance. Heart failure interrupts circulation, which results in underperfusion and congestion of blood in body organs. This can lead to widespread shifts in fluid between body compartments. Conversely, cardiovascular performance depends on fluid balance to provide for a sufficient blood volume.

Endocrine Glands. Three glands play central roles in regulating extracellular fluid composition: the pituitary, the adrenals, and the parathyroid. The secretion of hormones from these glands alters the reabsorption of body water and electrolytes.

The posterior part of the pituitary gland, the neurohypophysis, secretes antidiuretic hormone (ADH). ADH is secreted primarily in response to changes in serum osmolality but may also be secreted as a consequence of lowered blood volume and stress factors such as trauma, pain, and anxiety. ADH alters renal tubular permeability, thus adjusting water output from the kidney. An increase in the secretion of ADH helps conserve body water. As balance is restored, neurochemical signals (osmotic and pressure) are fed back to the pituitary, resulting in the cessation of ADH production.

The adrenal glands produce several hormones that help adjust extracellular fluid concentration. The primary adrenal hormone affecting fluid balance is aldosterone. Aldosterone is secreted in response to the powerful vasoconstrictive substance angiotensin II as part of a sophisticated mechanism for maintaining blood volume and controlling blood pressure. Aldosterone is also excreted in response to an elevation of potassium ions in the ECF and, in turn, acts on the kidneys to promote excretion. Aldosterone causes the renal tubules to conserve sodium ions, resulting in a corresponding secondary water retention.

Other adrenal hormones, such as cortisone and corticosterone, may also produce sodium and water retention. Under certain pathological conditions, increased levels of adrenal hormones cause excessive water and sodium retention. Conversely, insufficient levels of the hormones result in excessive sodium and water loss.

Finally, the parathyroid glands secrete parathyroid hormone (PTH), which controls the extracellular concentrations of calcium and phosphorus ions. PTH secretion results initially in calcium resorption from the bone, as well as absorption of calcium from the intestines and renal tubules. This raises the level of ionized calcium in the serum.

Stimulation of the parathyroid gland often results not only from low serum calcium levels but also from elevated serum phosphorus levels. Calcium and phosphorus levels are inversely related, through a feedback mechanism governed by circulating serum levels of the two electrolytes. High calcium levels suppress PTH release, and high phosphorus levels depress serum calcium, which eventually leads to PTH secretion. Elevated PTH levels raise serum calcium levels and lower serum phosphorus levels; decreased PTH levels lower serum calcium and raise serum phosphorus levels.

Kidneys. Through control of water reabsorption and excretion, the kidneys play a central role in maintaining blood volume (Fig. 31–4). The kidneys, composed of approximately two million working units known as nephrons, receive and filter the plasma portion of the blood at the rate of 180 L a day. Unless most of this fluid were reabsorbed, the body would quickly dry out, and would lose electrolytes and other essential compounds. In fact, only an average of 1200 to 1500 mL of urine is produced each day. This filtration begins at the part of each nephron known as the glomerulus, and produces fluid, called filtrate, from which urine is eventually produced. Under normal conditions, filtrate is produced at a rate of 125 mL/min, which is commonly referred to as the glomerular filtration rate (GFR). The GFR changes under the influence of several factors, such as water and solute intake, blood flow through the kidneys, and hormonal secretion, thus changing the rate of reabsorption and excretion of body water. (See Chap. 26 for further discussion.)

Urine is produced and concentrated by the tubular portions of the nephrons. Here the waste products of metabolism are removed. The nitrogenous end products of protein breakdown, such as urea, creatinine, and uric acid, are filtered and excreted, along with foreign substances, such as drugs and toxins. The kidneys also play an important role in maintaining the balance of acids, bases, and salts, primarily through renal tubular reabsorption and excretion.

Gastrointestinal Tract. Fluid and solutes are ingested through the mouth and absorbed by the stomach and intestines. Thus, replenishment of body water and electrolytes is a vital gastrointestinal function. The intestinal tract not only absorbs fluid ingested orally but also reabsorbs glandular and GI secretions. Table 31–5 summarizes the secretions produced by the GI tract.

Gastrointestinal fluids pass rapidly through the membranes of the gastric and intestinal membranes by passive diffusion and active transport. This rapid turnover of fluids, estimated at 3 L every 90 minutes, renders body fluid balance extremely vulnerable to excessive loss caused by dysfunctions of the GI tract.

Liver. Plasma proteins produced in the liver are essential to maintaining the circulating blood volume. These proteins maintain an osmotic pressure in the intravascular compartment that favors the retention of fluid. When the liver is diseased and insufficient plasma proteins are produced, this osmotic pressure cannot be maintained. The loss of pressure results in fluid shifts from the intravascular compartment, which affect the other fluid compartments as well.

Lymphatics. The lymph channels serve to return fluid from the interstitial spaces to the venous circulation. The flow of lymph occurs as lymph channels are squeezed by contracting skeletal muscles. When lymph channels become blocked, fluid builds up in the interstitial spaces. The increased pressure within the interstitial compartment results in increased fluid in the intravascular compartment, restoring equilibrium.

Homeostatic Mechanisms. The functions of the body's organs in regulating body fluid homeostasis are finely coordinated. Multiple mechanisms complement one another to regulate the intake, conservation, and excretion of water and salt.

Water and Salt Intake. Thirst, a conscious, subjective desire to take in fluids, plays an essential role in regulating fluid intake. When extracellular fluid osmolality exceeds 295 mOsm/L, receptors in the hypothalamus activate the cerebral cortex to create the sensation of thirst.[3] Although changes in ECF osmolality are the prime stimulus for thirst, decreased blood volume, increased salt intake, and mouth dryness may activate the thirst mechanism.[9]

Water and salt intake is also influenced by depletion of body fluids through excessive sweating or dysfunction of

TABLE 31–5. DAILY FLUID SECRETION IN THE GASTROINTESTINAL TRACT

Upper GI Fluids	
Saliva	1000 mL/24 h
Gastric fluid	2500 mL/24 h
Lower GI Fluids	
Bile	1500 mL/24 h
Pancreatic fluid	1000 mL/24 h
Intestinal fluid	3500 mL/24 h
Total	6500–9500 mL/24 h

From Metheny NM. Fluid and Electrolyte Balance: Nursing Considerations. *Philadelphia: JB Lippincott; 1987.*

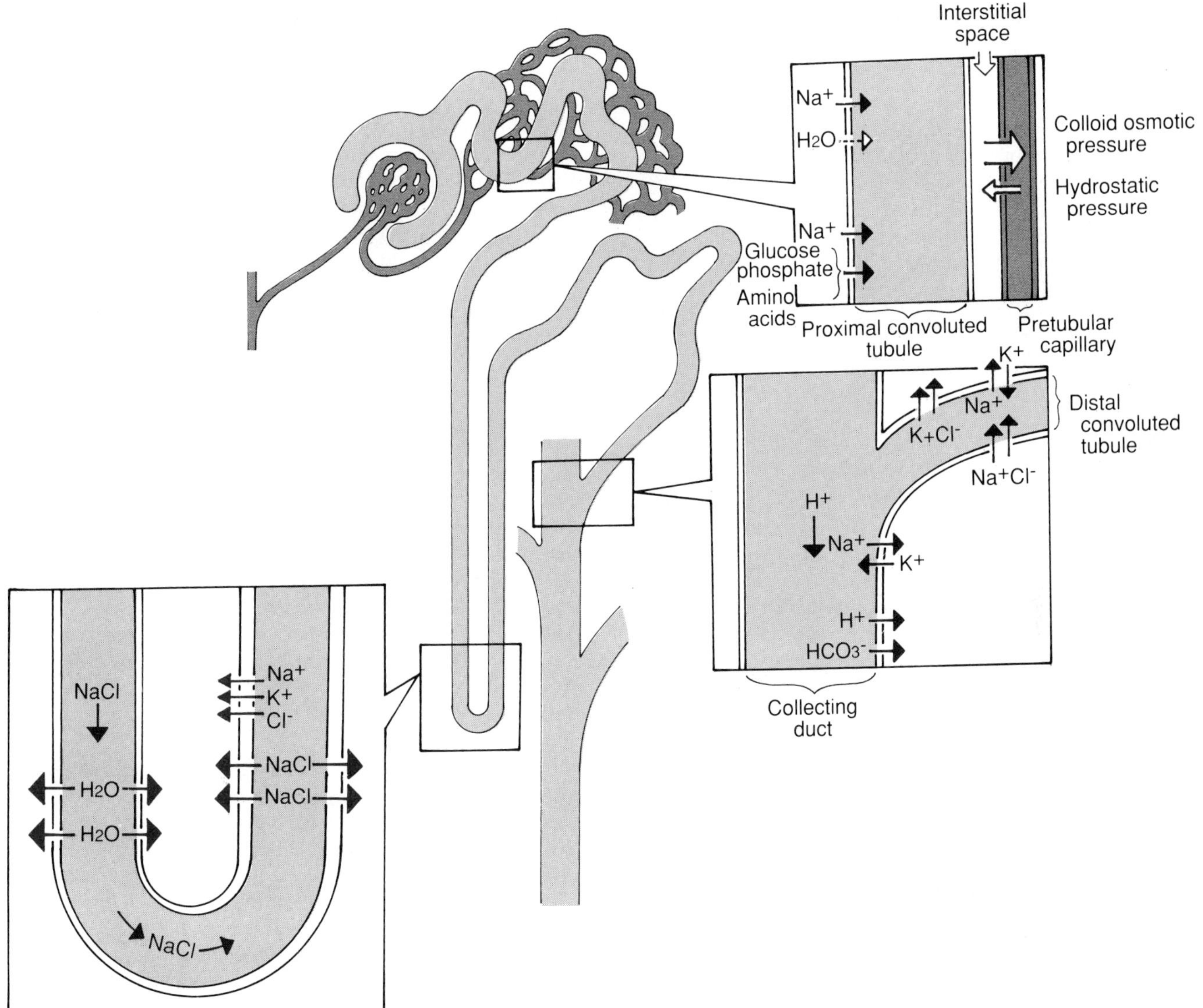

Figure 31–4. Renal regulation of the extracellular fluid. Arrows indicate the net direction of fluid in three key regions of the nephron, the proximal tubule, the loop of Henle, and the distal tubule and collecting duct.

the renal mechanism for salt conservation. Although little is know about the mechanism that governs salt intake, much is known about the link to salt excretion and the individual's resultant craving for it. Aldosterone, the adrenal mineralocorticoid responsible for sodium conservation, is linked to salt intake. Without sufficient amounts of aldosterone, the kidneys excrete sodium. This depletes the extracellular fluid of sodium and creates a desire for salt.

Water and Salt Conservation. The conservation of water and salt in the body results from the interplay of several physiological mechanisms, including fluid shifts between the intravascular and interstitial compartments, vasoconstriction, hormone release, and renal concentrating mechanisms.

Depletion of the extracellular fluid through sweating or severely decreased fluid intake is accompanied by a shift of fluid from the intravascular compartment to the dehydrated interstitial compartment. Conversely, if fluid is lost from the intravascular compartment, through hemorrhage for example, a shift of fluid from the interstitial compartment helps restore the losses. This, however, is a transient mechanism.

Another conservation mechanism involves the flow of plasma through the glomeruli of the kidneys. Vasoconstriction of renal blood vessels, a complex response involving the sympathetic nervous system as well as feedback mechanisms within the nephron itself, assists conservation by reducing blood flow through the kidneys. As body fluid losses accumulate to reduce the volume and pressure of plasma flowing through the glomeruli, a corresponding reduction in the amount of filtrate passing into the renal tubules occurs. Through various complicated mechanisms, the kidney responds by increasing its conservation of sodium and water, thus helping the body to maintain blood pressure and the perfusion of vital organs.

The primary mechanism regulating water and salt conservation is the renal tubule's ability to concentrate urine, thus conserving water and salt. Renal tubular reabsorption of water is regulated by ADH. A rise in ADH, triggered by the pituitary's response to an increase in osmolality of the serum bathing the pituitary cells and a decrease in plasma volume, results in increased permeability, and hence reabsorption of water, in the cells of the distal tubules and collecting ducts of the kidney.

Salt conservation goes hand in hand with water conservation. Sodium is actively pumped out of the proximal renal tubule and is also reabsorbed, along with chloride and potassium, in the ascending loop of Henle. Most of the sodium in the filtrate has been reabsorbed by the time it reaches the distal tubule; however, cells in the distal tubule, in response to the hormone aldosterone, also act to fine-tune sodium conservation by reabsorbing sodium in exchange for potassium.

Highly concentrated filtrate undergoes many changes as it travels through the various parts of the renal tubule. The final water and salt conservation depends on the osmotic forces at play in the collecting ducts, which are the end structures of each nephron. Filtrate passing through each collecting duct is less concentrated than the surrounding interstitium of the kidney. As a result, water is drawn through the pores in the ducts to the interstitium of the kidney. The permeability of the collecting duct wall is influenced by the secretion of ADH. Thus, under conditions of ECF volume deficit, the duct walls are highly permeable, leading to the retention of water by the kidney interstitium. The water is then returned to the renal capillaries surrounding each tubule for reentry into the general circulation.

Water and Salt Excretion. Water and salt excretion occurs essentially through the reversal of several of the conservation mechanisms. Excretion, like conservation, is automatically regulated, so that excessive intake is offset by acceleration of the feedback mechanisms controlling output. Thus water and salt are excreted at higher rates as a result of

- increases in blood pressure and glomerular filtration rates
- suppression of ADH secretion through detection of lowered serum osmolality
- a reduction in collecting duct permeability and water reabsorption
- increased renal tubular flow rate, producing increased filtrate
- increased fluid intake stimulating the appropriate hormone feedback mechanism for excretion

Through the mechanisms regulating water and salt intake, conservation, and excretion, the body maintains a dynamic balance. Reductions in intake of sodium, other electrolytes, or water trigger appropriate conservation. Conversely, excessive intake of water and solutes leads to the initiation of feedback mechanisms, which result in excretion.

Acid–Base Balance

To novice and experienced nurses alike, acid–base balance can be confusing and technically complicated. Yet, an understanding of the balance between acids and bases in the body fluids is critical because of the rapidity with which the balance can be interrupted, requiring swift intervention.

Definition of Acid and Base. In simple terms, an acid is a substance that breaks down and relinquishes hydrogen ions (H^+). A base is a substance that accepts hydrogen ions. The strength of acids and bases is expressed in terms of **pH,** the measure of the acidity or alkalinity of a fluid.

Basically pH represents the negative logarithm of H^+ ion concentration of a solution. As H^+ concentration increases, the pH decreases (becomes more acidic), and as H^+ concentration decreases, the pH increases (becomes more alkaline). A neutral pH, such as that of water, is 7.0, so bases have a pH higher than 7.0 and acids a pH lower than 7.0.[10] Because pH symbolizes a log or power of ten, a shift in pH by one unit, for instance from 7.4 to 6.4, actually signifies a tenfold change in hydrogen ion concentration. The body cannot tolerate a tenfold shift; thus, a pH below 7 or above 8 is not compatible with life for long.

pH of Body Fluids. The pH of various body fluids fluctuates constantly because different amounts of carbon dioxide and metabolic acids are present at any one time; however, these fluctuations are maintained within narrow parameters. For example, arterial blood pH is held within a narrow range of 7.35 to 7.45. Blood is thus slightly alkaline.[3]

The pH of specific body fluids reflects the acid concentrations necessary to carry out specific physiological roles (Table 31–6). For example, acid is necessary to facilitate the digestive processes in the stomach. Lower in the GI tract, however, the alkaline pancreatic fluid is necessary to neutralize the highly acidic gastric fluids. This prevents corrosion of the fragile intestinal mucosa. Optimal H^+ concentrations are also necessary for proper cell function and the efficient operation of enzyme systems. When cellular acid content becomes too high, enzyme proteins are denatured,

TABLE 31–6. pH OF VARIOUS BODY FLUIDS

Fluid	pH
Urine	4.5–8.0
Cerebrospinal fluid	7.36–7.44
Gastric fluid	1.0–3.5
Bile	5.0–7.8
Pancreatic fluid	8.0–8.3

From Guyton AC. Textbook of Medical Physiology, *8th ed. Philadelphia: WB Saunders; 1990.*

rendering the cell dysfunctional. Plasma hydrogen ion concentration is involved in the binding and release of oxygen and hemoglobin and hence plays a critical role in the transport of oxygen to the cell.

Buffer Systems. Acid–base balance is maintained in a dynamic balance by the constant activity of buffers. **Buffers** are substances that combine with acids and bases to prevent excessive changes in pH. Acids formed in the body, or introduced into it, combine with buffer bases and become weaker acids. Bases combine with the buffer acids and become weaker bases. In other words, buffers partially neutralize excessive acids or bases in the body. Four basic buffering systems provide either immediate control or continual fine-tuning of acid–base balance: the bicarbonate system, the phosphate system, the protein system, and the hemoglobin system.

Carbonic Acid–Bicarbonate System. Carbonic acid and bicarbonate constitute the buffer pair in highest concentration in the ECF. They are held at a ratio of 20:1 for bicarbonate (HCO_3^-) to carbonic acid (H_2CO_3), primarily as a result of the reabsorption of bicarbonate by the kidneys and the body's ability to transform any base and carbon dioxide into bicarbonate.[3]

Metabolism creates many strong organic and inorganic acids. Bicarbonate combines with these acids to form carbonic acid and a neutral salt. The carbonic acid further splits into carbon dioxide and water, which are eliminated, in varying quantities, from the lungs. Conversely, should a strong base be added to the body, carbonic acid combines with it to form sodium bicarbonate ($NaHCO_3$) and water (H_2O), both used in maintaining body fluid balance.[3] The following equation illustrates this process:

NaOH	+ H_2CO_3 ⟶	$NaHCO_3$	+	H_2O
sodium	+ carbonic ⟶	sodium	+	water
hydroxide	acid	bicarbonate		
(strong base)	(weak acid)	(weak base)		(neutral compound)

This system reacts rapidly to alter respiratory rate for increased carbon dioxide removal. It is, however, a temporizing system that requires the support of other buffering systems to maintain overall, ongoing acid–base balance in the body.

Phosphate System. The phosphate buffering system operates primarily in the red blood cells and the kidney tubules to release H^+ ions (acids) for elimination from the body and to return bicarbonate ions to the plasma. Excess hydrogen ions combine with disodium phosphate in the renal tubular cells, forming monosodium phosphate, which breaks down into sodium and phosphate. Sodium and bicarbonate ions are reabsorbed by combining with one another, and the remaining hydrogen ions are eliminated in the urine.[3,5,10]

Protein System. The protein buffer system operates primarily in the plasma, but may also work in the ICF. Proteins exist as either acids or bases and, therefore, bind with or release hydrogen ions.

Hemoglobin System. The hemoglobin buffer system operates in the plasma and inside the red blood cells to maintain hydrogen ion concentration and return carbon dioxide to the lungs for elimination. Cellular processes continuously produce CO_2. As the CO_2 concentration in the plasma rises, CO_2 travels into the red cells and is converted to carbonic acid. The carbonic acid breaks down into hydrogen ions and bicarbonate ions. The hydrogen attaches to hemoglobin and the bicarbonate to potassium. As the number of bicarbonate ions increases, they diffuse into the plasma and are replaced by chloride. The reduced hemoglobin in the blood cells acquires oxygen and reacts with bicarbonate to form carbonic acid, which causes the chloride to leave the cells. The carbonic acid is again split to release CO_2 and water.[11]

Respiratory Regulation of Acid–Base Balance. Should the chemical buffer systems fail, the second line of defense is the respiratory system. Increased hydrogen ion concentration in the cerebrospinal fluid stimulates the medulla to alter respiratory rate. As the cerebrospinal fluid becomes more acidic, the medulla responds by increasing the respiratory rate to eliminate the excess CO_2 and thereby normalize pH.[12]

Renal Regulation of Acid–Base Balance. The renal regulation of acid–base balance is much slower than respiratory regulation, which reacts immediately. Changes mediated by the kidneys may take from hours to 1 to 2 days to accomplish the fine-tuning of acid–base balance.

Regulation is accomplished by increasing or decreasing the amount of bicarbonate reabsorbed and by releasing hydrogen ions into the tubular fluid for elimination or replenishment of buffer substances. Bicarbonate is reabsorbed with sodium, which serves the dual purpose of regulating acid–base balance and conserving sodium.[1] Box 31–3 summarizes homeostatic mechanisms regulating acid–base balance.

FACTORS AFFECTING FLUID AND ELECTROLYTE BALANCE

Age

To help clients maintain fluid balance, it is essential for the nurse to understand the varying requirements for fluid replacement throughout the life span. Body weight, body surface area, renal filtration capacity, and metabolic rate influence required fluid intake at differing ages.

As previously noted, the ratio of body water to weight in infants is high. In the fullterm newborn, approximately 70 percent of weight is represented by body water; in the preterm infant, the percentage of water can be as high as 90 percent. Normal losses occur through rapid respirations, perspiration, and dilute urine from immature kidneys.[3] In

BOX 31–3. SUMMARY OF ACID–BASE HOMEOSTASIS

The slightly alkaline character of arterial blood and the neutral pH of most body cells is protected, moment to moment, primarily by the chemical reactions that occur between acids, bases, and buffer substances in the body fluid. It is also protected over short periods by adequate respiratory ventilation and over longer periods by the renal excretion of nonvolatile acids.

The body is always vulnerable to drastic shifts in pH. Homeostasis is maintained, moment to moment, primarily by buffer control. Buffers are capable of split-second chemical reaction. They immediately combine with any acid or alkali and thereby prevent excessive changes in H^+ concentration.

If H^+ concentration does change measurably, the respiratory center is immediately stimulated to alter the rate of pulmonary ventilation. A change in ventilatory rate automatically changes the rate of carbon dioxide removal from body fluid. Although this is not instantaneous, it is nevertheless a rapid reaction, requiring only 1 to 3 minutes to alter ventilation.

The kidney also responds to a change in H^+ concentration by changing the acidity of the urine through the reabsorption of bicarbonate and the excretion of hydrogen ions. Through the renal mechanism, acid–base balance is adjusted over several hours or days.

addition, infants have a high metabolic rate, resulting in a large quantity of metabolic wastes. Therefore, higher fluid intake is required for the kidneys to remove this extra load of metabolites.[3]

As individuals age, the kidneys lose nephrons, resulting in decreased renal concentrating ability and increased loss of water and salt. Aging may also be accompanied by a muting of the thirst response, leading to decreased intake. Chronic diseases such as cardiac disease, renal and hepatic disease, and diabetes can result in either severe losses of water and salts or retention of fluids, which can alter normal physiological functions.[3,13]

Climate

High heat and low environmental humidity increase sweating and fluid loss. Heavy sweating accompanies exertion and hot, dry atmospheric conditions. Exercise on a hot day may result in loss of up to 5 L of fluid and 10 to 20 times the usual amount of salt lost in a day. Failure to replace body fluids can result in heat exhaustion, which is characterized by decreased vascular volume and low cardiac output.

Stress

Physiological stressors are important in body fluid balance. Stress leads to stimulation of the pituitary gland and release of ADH. This causes the body to retain water and sodium and reduce urine output. This is a short-term defense mechanism for maintaining blood volume in the face of a physiological threat.

BUILDING NURSING KNOWLEDGE

What Determines How Much Fluid the Elderly Drink?

Gaspar PM. What determines how much patients drink? *Geriatr Nurs.* July/August 1988, pp. 221–224.

Noting a paucity of research, Gaspar designed a study to identify factors that affect intake volume among the elderly. The study, conducted in two rural Midwestern nursing homes, observed 67 elderly subjects ranging in age from 75 to 95 years. Observers randomly selected the 24-hour periods over 1 week. For each subject, the observers recorded data on food and fluid intake and the environmental circumstances at the time. Other data, particularly weight, height, and urine output, were obtained from medical records. A standardized rating scale was used to measure subjects' functional abilities.

The average fluid intake was 1893 mL per day with a range of 833 to 2863 mL. When the data for subjects were compared against an adult intake standard, the average intake was only 76 percent of the required amount. Age was inversely associated with water intake adequacy; as age increased, water intake decreased. Gaspar suggests that as people age, they may have a decrease in thirst resulting from diminished renal urinary concentration.

Four variables were found to be associated with water intake: speaking ability, visual capacity, opportunities for water ingestion, and time that water is in reach. The findings suggest that subjects who are functionally dependent actually have a greater chance of meeting water intake requirements than those who are more independent. Subjects who were immobile were offered water more frequently and drank more than subjects who were able to reach it for themselves; however, those who were most independent had more adequate water intakes than other subjects. The conclusion was that the subjects who were mobile but cognitively unaware of their needs were most at risk for inadequate water intake.

Diet

Adequate intake of fluid and nutrients is crucial to the maintenance of body fluid and electrolyte balance. Starvation causes the body to metabolize its own tissue for energy. As fat stores are consumed, ketones, which are strong acids, are produced. This additional acid load creates a shift in the acid–base balance toward the acidotic state.

Starvation also leads to a decrease in available proteins. The proteins are metabolized to provide the body with energy and are not replaced. Therefore, new proteins, particularly albumin, cannot be synthesized. The result is an inability to maintain intravascular osmotic pressure. Fluid will then shift from the intravascular to the interstitial compartment, decreasing vascular volume and pressure.

Illness

Several common clinical conditions are associated with fluid and electrolyte imbalances. A knowledge of these conditions helps nurses anticipate clients' fluid and salt replacement needs.

Nausea and Vomiting. Nausea and vomiting affect both intake and output. Nausea frequently results in insufficient intake of food and free fluids. Vomiting results in the expulsion of electrolyte- and hydrogen-rich fluids from the stomach and intestines. As the GI tract produces approximately 6 L of fluid per day, prolonged vomiting can result in rapid fluid depletion. Additionally, vomiting of gastric contents results in the loss of hydrogen ions, which over a period may lead to elevated bicarbonate levels, shifting the acid–base balance to alkalosis.

Diarrhea. As with vomiting, the loss of fluids and electrolytes through diarrhea can quickly lead to fluid volume deficit, serum electrolyte abnormalities, and shifts in acid–base balance. Because of the relatively high bicarbonate ion content in intestinal fluid, severe diarrhea can result in metabolic acidosis, from bicarbonate loss and relative hydrogen ion excess. Sodium and potassium deficits also accompany diarrhea, exacerbating the client's dehydration.

Increased Metabolism. Insensible fluid loss is increased by any influence that speeds the metabolism. Thus a rise in body temperature, which accelerates the metabolic rate, results in increased losses through the lungs and skin. Fevers between 101F and 103F increase the fluid requirements of adults by 500 mL per day; those above 103F increase requirements by 1000 mL.[4] Fever also increases the respiratory rate, which leads to further water loss through the expired air.

Wounds and Burns. Large wounds and burns provide avenues for the loss of considerable quantities of body water, electrolytes, and protein. Wound drainage, or transudate, is similar to plasma but contains a greater portion of water and electrolytes. Burn exudate, on the other hand, is actual plasma loss from the damaged extracellular compartment.

Burns represent a more complex fluid problem than simple ECF depletion. Compensatory fluid shifts between the intravascular and interstitial compartments often occur within 48 hours of a burn injury. Sodium and calcium deficits commonly accompany these large fluid losses. Potassium ions are lost as a result of liberation from the damaged cells. Because potassium levels in the body are tightly controlled by the kidneys, potassium liberated from damaged cells is excreted as long as the kidneys are functioning normally. Thus, as the tissue damaged by a large burn begins to heal, the client may require potassium supplements.

Medications

The excessive use of cathartics (agents that stimulate bowel elimination) and enemas can have effects similar to those of diarrhea on fluid and electrolyte balance. Some types of cathartics and enemas stimulate bowel evacuation by irritating the smooth muscle of the intestine. This can result in fluid volume deficit from excessive water and electrolyte loss.

Diuretics are agents that are used in the treatment of generalized fluid volume excesses. They affect the renal tubules' reabsorption and excretion of water, sodium, potassium, and chloride. All diuretics increase urine volume and thus may cause fluid volume deficit. Diuretics are classified according to their effect on potassium ion loss: potassium-wasting diuretics maintain the body's conservation of sodium, but result in increased loss of potassium; potassium-sparing diuretics act to conserve potassium but may create dangerously high serum potassium levels.

The adrenal cortical hormones, or steroids, are some of the body's chief regulators of water and salt balance. These hormones affect water retention by altering renal tubular reabsorption of sodium. When the adrenal glands are removed or become dysfunctional, excessive sodium and water may be lost in the urine. Serum potassium levels often rise as potassium ions are saved in the place of sodium. Conversely, when the adrenals are overactive or when ste-

BUILDING NURSING KNOWLEDGE

What Are the Risk Factors for Electrolyte Imbalance?

Felver L, Pendarvis JH. Electrolyte imbalances: Intraoperative risk factors. *AORN J.* 1989;49(4):992–1008.

Electrolyte imbalances are a threat to the well-being of clients who undergo surgery. This article presents information on risk factors that help identify clients who may develop electrolyte imbalance. The general risk factors identified for electrolyte excess are increased electrolyte intake or absorption, decreased electrolyte excretion, and electrolyte shift from a pool (intracellular compartment) to the extracellular fluid. The general risk factors for electrolyte deficit are the opposite, and relate to loss by an abnormal route.

The authors focus on three electrolytes: potassium, calcium, and magnesium. For example, they note that the administration of blood (packed cells or whole blood) during surgery is a significant source of potassium. When blood is stored, potassium leaks out of the red blood cells and into the plasma. The longer the blood is stored, the higher is the concentration of potassium in the plasma. Warming blood stems this process, according to the authors, and drives some of the potassium back into the red blood cells; however, if blood is stored for more than 3 days, plasma potassium will be high. This is one reason blood banking procedures require that the oldest blood on hand be used first. Nevertheless, clients who receive multiple transfusions are at risk for hyperkalemia and benefit from receiving freshly stored blood.

Conversely, preoperative anorexia, nausea, pain, or weakness, and n.p.o. status before diagnostic tests and surgery often limit the potassium intake of preoperative clients unless potassium-containing intravenous fluid is infused. Thus, the authors stress that nurses should check a client's serum potassium concentration before surgery. If no value is posted, the nurse should consult with the surgeon about the client's electrolyte status, notifying the surgeon of risk factors observed. Another cause of hypokalemia during surgery is hypothermia, which results in a release of epinephrine into the blood, causing potassium to shift into body cells. Using warming blankets during surgery and increasing the operating room temperature can help prevent this problem.

roids are given for their antiinflammatory or immunosuppressive effects, increased sodium and water are retained, often creating edema. This accelerates the loss of potassium ions in the urine.

Medical Treatments

Many medical treatments may result in secondary losses of fluids and electrolytes. Although the particular treatment may be necessary to accomplish therapeutic objectives, the health care team must prevent fluid and electrolyte problems through replacement therapy or other means.

Continuous gastric and intestinal suctioning usually produces many of the imbalances seen with persistent vomiting. To prevent fluid imbalances, intravenous fluids are given to replace the lost water and electrolytes. While intravenous therapy is not an independent nursing action, the nurse must be alert to body fluid problems to collaborate with the physician to ensure that replacement is instituted.

One practice that increases the potential for fluid and electrolyte imbalances is that of irrigating the suction tubing with hypotonic solutions such as distilled water. Distilled water is rapidly absorbed from the stomach into the interstitium and leads to the dilution of serum electrolytes. To avoid this situation, only isotonic solutions should be used for gastric irrigation.

Gavage feedings (described in Chap. 25) may result in fluid and electrolyte depletion. Although gavage feedings are given to prevent starvation, many solutions are several times more concentrated than blood serum. Introducing these solutions repeatedly into the GI tract can draw excessive fluid from the interstitium of the intestinal wall, causing osmotic diarrhea. Recently, however, the formulas of many of the commercially prepared foods have been adjusted to avoid the potential for diarrhea.

ALTERATIONS IN FLUID AND ELECTROLYTE BALANCE

Many diseases and pathological conditions upset normal fluid and electrolyte balance. In addition, many diagnostic and therapeutic interventions can temporarily upset this balance. The following discussion of the common imbalances of body fluid composition and volume will help the beginning practitioner to develop a clearer picture of the complexity of this topic. Terminology used in labeling fluid, electrolyte, and acid–base balance problems can be confusing. For clarity, synonyms that are commonly used to refer to fluid and electrolyte alterations are included in the discussion that follows.

Fluid Volume Alterations

Alterations in fluid volume include fluid volume deficit, fluid volume excess, and fluid shifts between compartments. Table 31–7 lists manifestations and causes of these alterations.

Fluid Volume Deficit. Fluid volume deficit, also known as *dehydration,* refers to the loss of water and/or electrolytes from extracellular fluid. This loss may be proportional, that is, the ratio of water to electrolytes is unchanged, or disproportional, with either water loss occurring in excess of electrolyte loss or electrolyte loss occurring in excess of water loss.

The term *extracellular fluid deficit* applies to either proportionate or disproportionate losses. Proportional losses of water and electrolytes are referred to as isotonic losses; thus then water and electrolytes are lost in the same measure, a condition of **isotonic dehydration** exists. On the other hand, when losses are disproportionate, two condi-

TABLE 31–7. FLUID VOLUME ALTERATIONS

Alteration	Signs and Symptoms	Causes
Fluid volume deficit		
Isotonic dehydration	Hypotension; low cardiac output; poor skin turgor; tachycardia; decreased urinary output; shock	Increased fluid output (vomiting; diarrhea; hemorrhage)
Hypertonic dehydration	See above	Increased solute intake Thirst mechanism failure Decreased renal concentrating ability Decreased fluid intake Diabetes insipidus; diabetic ketoacidosis
Hypotonic dehydration	See above	Renal regulatory failure Excessive thiazide diuretic use Adrenal insufficiency
Fluid volume excess	Pulmonary edema; peripheral edema; full bounding pulse; venous distension; ascites	Excessive volumes of dietary sodium and water intake Cardiac and renal disease Liver disease
Plasma-to-interstitial fluid shift	Generalized and pulmonary edema; ascites	Congestive heart failure Renal failure Burns, infection, and anaphylactic reactions

tions may result: **hypotonic dehydration,** in which electrolyte loss is proportionately greater than the loss of water, or **hypertonic dehydration** (also known as "true" dehydration) in which water loss is proportionately greater than electrolyte loss. Hypovolemia is a related term that often appears in discussions of fluid deficit and dehydration. **Hypovolemia** refers to a reduction in blood volume.

Sources and Causes. These categories of dehydration vary in the sources and causes of water and electrolyte loss.

Isotonic Dehydration. Isotonic dehydration occurs when losses are acute and of short duration so that the tonicity of the ECF remains unchanged. It may follow episodes of vomiting, diarrhea, losses from burns, wounds, intestinal fistulas, hemorrhage, or when GI suction is done with inadequate fluid replacement.[14] Probably the most common cause of fluid volume deficit is loss of gastrointestinal fluid, 8 to 10 L of which are produced each day. Since this fluid is also rich in electrolytes, sodium, potassium, and hydrogen ion or bicarbonate are also lost.[15]

Hypertonic Dehydration. Because thirst is the principal body defense mechanism for guarding against the overconcentration of body fluid, hypertonic dehydration usually occurs in those rare instances in which the thirst mechanism fails for some reason or when persons cannot voluntarily ingest fluid. Infants and immobilized or comatose persons are particularly vulnerable to this type of dehydration.[15] In such individuals, loss of dilute body fluid progressively elevates body fluid osmolality.

Individuals with diabetes insipidus (DI) are also vulnerable to hypertonic dehydration, but for a different reason. These individuals lose copious amounts of dilute urine from the kidneys because of an abnormal reduction in antidiuretic hormone from the posterior pituitary gland. This causes the output of dilute urine and can leave the ECF hypertonic. As long as individuals with diabetes insipidus are alert and able to drink, however, the thirst mechanism usually prevents dehydration.[15]

Still another cause of hypertonic dehydration is diabetic ketoacidosis, a complication of diabetes mellitus. Diabetes mellitus is a condition in which the pancreatic hormone insulin is lacking, and body cells are consequently unable to metabolize glucose. When diabetes mellitus is inadequately controlled, large amounts of glucose are filtered through the glomeruli of the kidneys creating an osmotic diuresis. The result is not only a loss of body water, but also a corresponding accumulation of sodium in the ECF. Hypertonic dehydration is most likely when the condition becomes so severe that coma develops, rendering the individual unable to ingest fluid.[15]

Hypertonic dehydration can also be caused by profuse sweating. Sweat is always hypotonic; thus it depletes extracellular water while leaving sodium behind to increase body fluid osmolality.[15] This type of dehydration may occur in individuals who fail to ingest sufficient replacement fluid while exercising strenuously.

Hypotonic Dehydration. In hypotonic dehydration, the tonicity of the ECF decreases. The most common causes are renal and endocrine regulatory failure and diuretic therapy, all of which cause disproportionate water and sodium loss.[15] Hypotonic dehydration occurs in the so-called "salt-wasting" renal diseases such as pyelonephritis.[14] Excessive salt and also water are lost in the urine and the individual becomes volume depleted and hyponatremic.[14]

Diuretics, a commonly prescribed class of medication, cause this type of disproportionate loss when used to excess. They act by inhibiting sodium reabsorption in the renal tubules which can lead to hypotonic dehydration.[15] Diuretics are often prescribed for long-term use in the treatment of edema. When the client is no longer edematous, the medication continues its fluid and solute removal effect on the kidneys, resulting in losses beyond those intended.

Adrenal insufficiency, another cause of hypotonic dehydration, is characterized by decreased production of the adrenal hormones. Without the hormonal stimulus to conserve sodium, the renal tubules excrete it in increasing quantities; water then follows sodium out of the body, but in an amount that is proportionately less than sodium.[15]

Effects. The effects of fluid volume deficit may be readily observable or subtle, rapid in onset or insidious. Fluid loss in small volumes over a sustained period may produce subtle changes, while rapid or large-volume losses produce classic signs and symptoms. Fluid volume deficit may be classified as mild, moderate, or severe depending on the symptoms produced, the rate of loss, and the volume or percentage of body fluid lost.

Hypovolemia. Hypovolemia results when there is a significant loss of blood volume either through hemorrhage, or through a severe depletion of the ECF by another source that causes a corresponding reduction in plasma. Any of the types of dehydration described above, when severe, may be accompanied by hypovolemia.

Hypovolemia is a serious condition because it can lead to circulatory failure. Any reduction in blood volume reduces the venous return to the heart. When the venous return becomes so low that the efforts of the body to compensate are overwhelmed, cardiac output drops, perfusion to body tissues diminishes, and shock ensues. **Shock** is the suspension or failure of the regulatory mechanisms that maintain circulatory perfusion of the body tissues. The individual becomes pale, diaphoretic, cold, hypotensive, and lethargic. Failure to prevent further loss and rapidly replace body fluids will result in cellular death and eventual cardiac standstill.

Other Effects. Brain cells are the most sensitive to ECF deficit; consequently changes in the sensorium are usually the first to accompany fluid volume deficit. Other signs and symptoms include tachycardia, restlessness, dry mucous membranes and poor skin turgor, and decreased urinary output.

Decreased urinary output follows any significant decrease in perfusion to the kidney tissue. As the nephrons rely on high-pressure flow to maintain filtration capacity, the reduction of flow from hypovolemia results in oliguria, or urine output below 500 mL/24 h (see Chap. 26).

Fluid Volume Excess. When water and solutes are gained in proportionate amounts in the ECF, the result is fluid volume excess, also called *extracellular fluid excess* or *overhydration.* Fluid volume excess can be caused by the rapid administration of excessive volumes of intravenous fluids, cardiac or renal failure, or liver disease, all of which can lead to severe fluid retention.[16]

One of the outcomes of fluid volume excess is generalized edema, the widespread accumulation of fluid in the interstitial spaces and the pulmonary interstitium (see further discussion below). Most of the signs and symptoms of fluid volume excess result from this pulmonary congestion. They include coughing, dyspnea, moist crackles on auscultation, galloping heart sounds, bounding pulse, weight gain, and neck vein engorgement.[1,17]

The syndrome of inappropriate ADH secretion, which is a physiological response to severe stress, results in a continual renal retention of water and extremely hypotonic ECF. Extreme stress, such as that caused by major surgery; CNS disorders such as head trauma, meningitis, and encephalitis; or the ingestion of drugs such as chlorpropamide, vincristine, or thiazide diuretics, may also increase ADH secretion.[18] The brain cells swell and produce symptoms of water intoxication, such as lethargy, headache, disorientation, anorexia, nausea and vomiting, seizures, and coma.[9,15,19]

Fluid Shift. Shifts of body fluids between compartments accompany disorders in which either the hydrostatic pressure or the colloid osmotic pressure within a compartment becomes deranged. In addition, any condition that leads to a change in capillary membrane permeability will contribute to shifts of body fluid between compartments. Fluid shifts typically result in fluid volume excess in one compartment and fluid volume deficit in the other.

Edema. A shift of fluid from the plasma to the interstitium results in an abnormal accumulation of fluid in the interstitial spaces, producing tissue swelling and congestion. This abnormal accumulation, commonly referred to as **edema,** can collect in virtually any body tissue, including the skin, brain, lungs, liver, heart, and gastrointestinal walls. Edema may be localized and superficial, as with an insect bite, or widespread and generalized. Large amounts of fluid must accumulate for generalized edema to become apparent. As fluid accumulation is accompanied by increased body weight, there must be as much as a 10 percent increase in weight before generalized edema is in evidence.

A common cause of edema is congestive heart failure (CHF). In CHF, the heart is unable to pump the volume of blood it receives, resulting in backup or congestion of blood in the left side of the heart and the pulmonary vessels. The increased hydrostatic pressure in the vessels pushes fluid into the lung tissues and alveoli, creating pulmonary edema. The accumulation of fluid causes respiratory signs and symptoms including coughing, dyspnea, moist crackles on auscultation, and orthopnea.[14]

Renal failure also causes widespread edema. As the kidneys fail, fluid and electrolytes are retained in the intravascular compartment. The hydrostatic pressure rises and fluid is forced from the intravascular space to the interstitial space. The peripheral tissues expand, resulting in an observable "swelling" of body parts and, eventually, a buildup of fluids in the pulmonary interstitium.[15]

Burns, sepsis, and anaphylactic reactions allow fluid, solutes, and protein to shift from the intravascular space to the interstitium. Burns destroy the capillary membranes, allowing proteins to seep out of the plasma. The proteins pull water along to the interstitium; this results in the development of blisters with second-degree burns. Sepsis and anaphylaxis chemically attack the capillary membranes with bacterial toxins or histamines, changing their permeability.

Third Spacing. A particular form of edema resulting from a fluid shift from the plasma to the interstitium is known as third spacing. **Third spacing** is the sequestering of large amounts of fluid in body spaces from which exchange with ECF is difficult. These include the pleural and pericardial sacs and the peritoneum, which usually contain only minute amounts of fluid but expand and trap fluid shifted from the vascular system. Large volumes of fluid may also be trapped within the intestines during bowel obstruction.

In liver disease, fluid shifts from the intravascular spaces to the peritoneal cavity lead to a condition known as ascites. Ascites is the collection of a large amount of fluid in the abdominal cavity, often leading to severe distension of the abdomen. The scarring of liver disease creates obstruction in the portal vein, creating a localized increase in intravascular hydrostatic pressure. The scarred liver is also relatively incapable of producing sufficient plasma proteins, reducing intravascular colloid osmotic pressure. The net effect is the filtration of fluid and protein substances into the expandable peritoneal cavity.[20]

IMPLICATIONS FOR NURSE–CLIENT COLLABORATION

Electrolyte Balance

Electrolyte imbalance affects human functions in a variety of ways, depending on the specific imbalance present. Mental operations may be altered by states of confusion, lethargy, irritability, anxiety, and a variety of physical symptoms that frequently impinge on mental well-being. Any of these changes can significantly interfere with the client's ability to carry on a collaborative relationship and to assume the responsibility of participating in health care decisions. The nurse's alertness to impending electrolyte imbalance can be an important factor in preserving not only the client's internal homeostasis, but also the client's capacity to collaborate.

Electrolyte Alterations

Electrolyte imbalances are fluctuations in the ECF concentration of one or more electrolytes. Once the ECF electrolyte concentration is altered, compensatory mechanisms to maintain the dynamic balance between the compartments will also affect ICF concentrations of electrolytes. Specific electrolyte imbalances are identified by measuring the electrolyte concentrations in blood serum (ECF), as measurement in the ICF is impossible. The common alterations and etiologies are listed in Table 31–8.

Hyponatremia. Hyponatremia (sodium deficit) may be described as an absolute loss of sodium in excess of water or as a state in which the sodium in the ECF is diluted by severe water overload. Conditions contributing to hyponatremia include watery diarrhea, severe burns, large draining wounds, intestinal fistulas, and overuse of diuretics.[21] The signs and symptoms of hyponatremia include muscle weakness, fatigue, abdominal cramps, headache, apprehension, confusion, seizure, and hypotension.[21]

Hypernatremia. Hypernatremia (sodium excess) can be described as an absolute excess of sodium in the ECF, or a relative loss of water. This may involve the compensatory influx of fluid, if compensatory mechanisms are intact, but the sodium gains are greater than the fluid gains. Hypernatremia may follow excessive therapeutic treatment with hypertonic solutions or may result from excessive production of aldosterone or steroids, or from the water losses caused by diabetes insipidus, decreased fluid intake, osmotic diuresis accompanying diabetes mellitus, or insensible losses from mouth breathing or mechanical ventilation. Hypernatremia may also result from use of solute-laden formulas, when insufficient fluids accompany their administration.[7] Signs and symptoms characteristic of hypernatremia are primarily those associated with the altered central nervous system functioning that accompanies brain cell shrinkage. Confusion, neuromuscular excitability, seizures, or coma may result.[14] When hypernatremia results from water loss due to failure of renal water conservation, the client may produce a large amount of very dilute urine. When it is caused by some other source of water loss, hypernatremia will be accompanied by other signs such as vomiting, diarrhea, or excessive sweating.

Hypokalemia. In hypokalemia (potassium deficit), potassium ions have been lost from the ECF or shifted into the ICF. Hypokalemia results from either interference with potassium intake or increased potassium loss via the renal or GI routes, or movement of potassium into the cells. Hyperglycemia, metabolic alkalosis, hypoxemia, toxic levels of digitalis, use of thiazide diuretics, and insulin administration contribute to the development of hypokalemia.[22]

As potassium plays an essential role in maintaining neuromuscular function, most signs and symptoms of hypokalemia are related to abnormal cardiac, smooth muscle, and skeletal muscle function. The individual experiences muscle weakness of the extremities that progresses toward the trunk. Smooth muscle alterations result in hypotension and decreased GI peristalsis. Finally, cardiac arrhythmias appear (tachycardias and atrial and ventricular ectopic beats).[15]

Hyperkalemia. As the renal system is responsible for 90 percent of potassium excretion, hyperkalemia (potassium excess) usually results from decreased renal function. Other causes include metabolic acidosis, red blood cell hemolysis, decreased aldosterone production, and overuse of potassium-sparing diuretics.[23]

Signs and symptoms of hyperkalemia are muscle weakness, decreased sensation, tingling around the mouth (circumoral), depressed reflexes, and electrocardiographic changes. The end result of hyperkalemia may be ventricular fibrillation and cardiac standstill.

Hypocalcemia. Hypocalcemia (calcium deficit) is an excessively low concentration of calcium in the ECF. Common etiologies of calcium deficit are decreased calcium intake, GI losses, renal failure, excessive use of phosphate laxatives and antacids, and a deficiency of parathyroid hormone.[21,23]

The signs and symptoms of calcium imbalances include muscle tetany (twitching), spasms, or cramps; paresthesias (abnormal burning or prickling sensations); bradycardia (abnormally slow heart rate); hypotension; and respiratory spasms.[19,23]

Hypocalcemia must be considered if a client responds poorly to treatment for hypotension. In addition, drugs such as sedatives and anticonvulsants may mask the muscle tetany in hypocalcemic clients, making identification of the disorder more difficult.[19,23]

Hypercalcemia. Hypercalcemia (calcium excess) is excessive calcium concentration in the ECF. Hypercalcemia occurs in conditions that cause bone demineralization and subsequent mobilization of calcium to the serum. As the result of this demineralization, pathological fractures and soft tissue calcification may occur.[24]

Hyperactivity of the parathyroid gland, with excessive PTH production, is most often the cause of hypercalcemia. Renal failure may cause overstimulation of the parathyroid glands. The resultant bone resorption from the high PTH secretion eventually elevates and sustains the high serum calcium level.[25]

Malignant tumors, especially of the breast and lung, are the second most common cause of hypercalcemia. Some tumors are capable of producing PTH; the remainder of the alterations are the result of metastatic bone destruction.[25]

Individuals with hypercalcemia usually show signs and symptoms of weakness, fatigue, impaired memory, anorexia, pruritus, bone and joint pain, kidney stones, hypertension, bradycardia, and heart block.[25] Soft tissue calcification, as mentioned earlier, can occur in the corneas, GI tract, arteries, and kidneys, resulting in permanent damage to these organs.

Hypomagnesemia. Hypomagnesemia (magnesium deficit) results primarily from insufficient intake of magnesium in the diet. The deficient diet of chronic alcoholism, the intake of magnesium-deficient total parenteral nutrition (TPN) solutions, or starvation diets may lead to this deficit. Diarrhea and malabsorption conditions also contribute to the development of hypomagnesemia.[26]

Low magnesium levels seem to depress PTH function so that calcium cannot be mobilized. The kidneys also react to low magnesium levels by increasing excretion of potas-

TABLE 31–8. ELECTROLYTE ALTERATIONS

Alteration	Signs and Symptoms	Causes
Sodium		
Hyponatremia	Dizziness, vertigo, hypotension; tachycardia; oliguria	GI fluid loss Increased sweat loss Diuretic abuse Adrenal insufficiency
Hypernatremia	Thirst; fever; dry, sticky mucous membranes; confusion; headache	Heatstroke Diarrhea Increased insensible loss (lungs, skin) Diabetes insipidus Excess infusion of hypertonic or isotonic saline
Potassium		
Hypokalemia	Muscle weakness; cardiac arrhythmias; abdominal distension; paresthesias; anorexia; depressed deep tendon reflexes	Diarrhea Gastric suction Diuretic use Metabolic alkalosis Poor intake
Hyperkalemia	Irritability; anxiety; muscular weakness; cardiac irregularities; nausea and vomiting; diarrhea; circumoral and fingertip tingling	Renal failure Red blood cell hemolysis Tissue trauma Metabolic acidosis Transfusion of old blood Potassium-sparing diuretics
Calcium		
Hypocalcemia	Muscle tetany; muscle cramps; cardiac arrhythmias; decreased clotting; pathological fractures	Decreased intake Insufficient vitamin D Severe diarrhea Burns Decreased PTH release Protein malnutrition Increased PO_4^- levels
Hypercalcemia	Bone and joint pain; lethargy; anorexia; muscle weakness	Increased PTH release Breast and lung cancers Decreased PO_4^- intake Prolonged immobilization
Magnesium		
Hypomagnesemia	Muscle spasticity; cardiac arrhythmias; muscle tetany	Chronic alcohol abuse Diuretic abuse Malnutrition Diarrhea
Hypermagnesemia	Respiratory depression; lethargy; bradycardia; depressed reflexes	Renal failure Excess antacid and laxative use
Phosphate		
Hypophosphatemia	Nausea and vomiting; anorexia; bone destruction; bleeding	Diabetic ketoacidosis Malabsorption states Low PO_4^- diets and total parenteral nutrition
Hyperphosphatemia	Muscle tetany; muscle weakness; tachycardia; abdominal cramps; diarrhea	Decreased excretion of PO_4^- Lack of PTH
Chloride		
Hypochloremia	Irritability; hypotension; lethargy; tachycardia	Vomiting GI suction Diuretic use Diaphoresis Metabolic alkalosis
Hyperchloremia	Weakness; lethargy; deep, rapid breathing	Severe dehydration Head injury Steroid use

Data from Methany,[4] Levinsky,[15] and Guyton.[21]

sium. Hence, hypomagnesemia often occurs in tandem with hypocalcemia and hypokalemia.

The signs and symptoms of hypomagnesemia reflect magnesium's role in neuromuscular transmission. Tremors, facial grimacing, and myoclonic jerking may precede seizure activity in severe cases. Ventricular arrhythmias, atrial fibrillation, generalized muscle weakness, and decreased GI motility may also occur.

Hypermagnesemia. Hypermagnesemia (magnesium excess), a rare condition, is usually associated with retention of magnesium in renal failure; however, excessive use of magnesium-containing antacids or overzealous use of intravenous magnesium may also lead to increased ECF magnesium levels.

Magnesium excess results in sedation of the central nervous system. Depression of reflexes, muscle paralysis, respiratory depression, decreased level of consciousness, and eventual cardiac arrest are the potential effects.[21]

Hypophosphatemia. Hypophosphatemia (phosphate deficit), a deficiency of serum phosphorus, may occur as the result of poor dietary intake from chronic alcoholism or the infusion of phosphate-poor TPN solutions. The overuse of antacids and the serum loss associated with burns can also deplete phosphorus stores.[27]

Phosphate deficits are frequently overlooked because they are often masked by calcium and magnesium imbalances; however, phosphorus is important to red blood cell membrane integrity, platelet function, and bone durability. Hypophosphatemia also reduces the availability of ATP and affects all of the cellular processes that use energy.

Signs and symptoms of hypophosphatemia range from emotional irritability to marked muscle weakness, paresthesias, and cardiac and respiratory depression. Bone demineralization occurs in chronic deficiency of phosphorus, as phosphorus is released from the bone to support the serum levels.[27]

Hyperphosphatemia. Most cases of hyperphosphatemia (phosphate excess) result from poor excretion of phosphates resulting from kidney failure; however, the lack of PTH also results in a buildup of serum phosphorus. Overuse of phosphate laxatives or excessive oral or parenteral intake of phosphorus may contribute to hyperphosphatemia.[8,27]

Hyperphosphatemia is a serious condition, because the high levels of serum phosphorus prevent the secretion of PTH. Insufficient secretion of PTH subsequently results in a serious reduction in serum calcium levels. The maintenance of high phosphorus levels and low calcium levels eventually results in calcium reabsorption from the bone, creating the potential for fractures.

Many of the signs and symptoms of hyperphosphatemia mimic hypocalcemia, with muscle tetany, heightened reflexes, flaccid paralysis, muscular weakness, tachycardia, nausea, abdominal cramps, and diarrhea.[27]

Hypochloremia. Chloride is an anion frequently found in combination with sodium. Thus, conditions that result in alteration of sodium or potassium levels usually alter chloride level, as well. For example, sodium-depleting diseases, such as adrenal insufficiency, also result in hypochloremia (chloride deficit). As chloride is the chief constituent of hydrochloric acid in the gastric fluid, repeated vomiting or prolonged nasogastric suctioning may also lead to chloride losses. In addition, acid–base abnormalities such as alkalosis may lead to hypochloremia as the kidney eliminates chloride in larger quantities and reabsorbs bicarbonate ions.[11]

The signs and symptoms of hypochloremia are the same as those of the underlying sodium, potassium, or acid–base alteration, and include weakness, hyperirritability, muscle tetany, low blood pressure, and slow, shallow respirations.[5]

Hyperchloremia. Hyperchloremia (chloride excess) commonly occurs in individuals suffering from volume fluid deficit, as water loss concentrates the ions in the ECF. Excessive adrenal hormone production, as in Cushing's disease, increases sodium and chloride reabsorption, thereby increasing the concentration of chloride ions in the ECF. Hyperchloremia also results from metabolic acidosis.[28]

Again, the signs and symptoms of hyperchloremia are related to the underlying sodium, potassium, or acid–base alteration. Lethargy, weakness, and deep, rapid respirations are common manifestations of hyperchloremia.[28]

Acid–Base Alterations

As discussed previously, the body has sophisticated respiratory and renal mechanisms to protect against acid–base alterations. Abnormal acid–base shifts are essentially exaggerations of the small normal shifts in acid–base balance. Disease states resulting in acid–base abnormalities, therefore, must be severe or prolonged to produce overt symptoms. Causes and manifestations of acid–base imbalances are summarized in Table 31–9.

Respiratory Acidosis. Respiratory acidosis, also called carbonic acid excess, is an accumulation of dissolved carbon dioxide in the blood, which, in combination with water, forms excessive amounts of carbonic acid. This increased acid load lowers serum pH. Any condition that causes hypoventilation leads inevitably to respiratory acidosis and may result in damage to the respiratory center of the brain or obstruction of the respiratory passages. These include trauma to the brain stem, cerebral tumors, emphysema, asthma, and chronic bronchitis. Narcotic overdose, neuromuscular diseases that weaken the respiratory muscles, and electrolyte alterations such as hypermagnesemia may also sufficiently reduce respirations as to cause respiratory acidosis.[11] The signs and symptoms of respiratory acidosis are dyspnea, lethargy, and disorientation.

Respiratory Alkalosis. Excessive excretion of carbon dioxide results in **respiratory alkalosis,** also called carbonic acid deficit. The most common cause of respiratory alkalosis is hyperventilation. The rapid, deep respirations may be vol-

TABLE 31–9. ACID–BASE ALTERATIONS

Alteration	Signs and Symptoms	Causes	Compensation
Respiratory acidosis	Dyspnea, lethargy, and disorientation	Respiratory depression as the result of narcotic or barbiturate overdose, inhalation of anesthesia, or chronic pulmonary disease	Renal compensation by retention of HCO_3^-
Respiratory alkalosis	Vertigo, lethargy, and tingling of fingers	Hyperventilation from anxiety, hysteria, high altitude, overuse of aspirin	Renal mechanism excretes HCO_3^-
Metabolic acidosis	Weakness, dizziness, rapid respirations, flushed skin, and restlessness	Renal, cardiac, or endocrine failure; excess acid produced or insufficient acid eliminated	Increased respiratory rate eliminates CO_2
Metabolic alkalosis	Hyperirritability, bradycardia, shallow respirations, and paresthesias	Vomiting, gastric suction, alkali ingestion (eg, baking soda)	Respiratory mechanism retains CO_2

Data from Mathewson and Mathewson[11] *and Levinsky.*[28]

untary or result from overstimulation of the respiratory center in the midbrain. Acutely anxious or hysterical individuals often hyperventilate. Mountain climbers or pilots in unpressurized planes may unconsciously increase the rate and depth of their respirations, thereby creating a mild respiratory alkalosis.

Metabolic Acidosis. There are two underlying causes of **metabolic acidosis** or plasma bicarbonate deficit. Metabolic acidosis occurs either from a rise in the hydrogen level, or a drop in the plasma bicarbonate level below the normal range.

Three essential mechanisms can bring about a rise in hydrogen ion level in metabolic acidosis: excessive intake, overproduction, or inadequate excretion of fixed acids. Fixed acids, sometimes referred to as nonvolatile or metabolic acids, are any acids other than carbonic acid, which is known as a volatile or respiratory acid.[6]

Excessive acid intake occurs when individuals use aspirin (acetylsalicylic acid) too frequently or in high doses. Overproduction of fixed acids, on the other hand, occurs in starvation, hyperthyroidism, severe infections, diabetic ketoacidosis, and cellular anoxia. In starvation, the accumulation of strong acids continues as long as cellular breakdown persists. Because the renal mechanism for correcting hydrogen ion accumulation involves a loss of sodium into the urine, water is excreted to maintain the tonicity of the ECF, and dehydration eventually results.[14] In severe tissue anoxia, another type of overproduction occurs. Cells are deprived of oxygen and convert to anaerobic metabolism. Lactic acid is formed as a by-product. Because respiratory or cardiac arrest often accompanies this condition, bicarbonate is given during resuscitation to reverse the metabolic acidosis.

Inadequate excretion of fixed acid, the third mechanism, occurs when the kidneys' mechanism for excreting hydrogen ions is impaired. This is often what happens in renal failure. The kidney no longer eliminates hydrogen ions, and the mechanism for reabsorption of bicarbonate ions is depressed, creating an increased plasma hydrogen ion concentration and a reduction in ECF pH.[11]

Metabolic acidosis can also result from a reduction of bicarbonate ions in relation to plasma hydrogen ion concentration. This usually happens when GI fluid is lost through suctioning, vomiting, or diarrhea. As previously described, the losses create a renal response whereby sodium and chloride are reabsorbed and large amounts of bicarbonate are eliminated, thus reducing the pH of the ECF.[29]

The objective manifestations of metabolic acidosis are flushing of the skin, deep and rapid respirations, restlessness, and dehydration.

Metabolic Alkalosis. Metabolic alkalosis is a plasma bicarbonate excess. There are two underlying mechanisms of metabolic alkalosis: a rise in serum bicarbonate levels or a drop in hydrogen ion concentration below the normal range. An abnormal rise in bicarbonate level may be caused by excessive ingestion of baking soda to treat an "acid stomach." Excessive loss of hydrogen ions may follow vomiting and GI suctioning of hydrogen-rich fluids.

The kidneys may complicate metabolic alkalosis when large GI fluid losses stimulate aldosterone production. As a result, sodium is reabsorbed along with massive amounts of bicarbonate, rather than chloride.[29] The typical signs and symptoms of metabolic alkalosis are shallow breathing and vomiting.

Alterations in body fluid balance are adaptations to body stressors. In themselves, these adaptations may also be threats to health. Therefore, nurses need a solid information base regarding body fluid composition, alterations, and regulatory mechanisms to identify and provide care for individuals who experience fluid alterations. This ensures that the nurse will identify problems swiftly and take preventive measures to avoid potential imbalances.

Section 2. Assessment of Fluid and Electrolyte Balance

FLUID AND ELECTROLYTE DATA COLLECTION

Nurses assess clients' requirements for fluids and electrolytes by analyzing information gathered from the history, physical examination, and laboratory and diagnostic studies. The nurse collects data and makes observations from a wide spectrum of physiological and psychosocial indicators that reflect the client's state of fluid and electrolyte balance. The nurse uses the information to formulate diagnoses of a client's fluid and electrolyte needs. The result is an effective client care plan to meet the individual's fluid and electrolyte needs. Some of the information collected by nurses helps in establishing medical diagnoses and is passed on to the physician as a part of the nurses' collaborative activity.

Through the assessment process, the nurse determines not only the nature and degree of the threat to the client's body fluid balance but also the effect of imbalances on the client's daily activities. This allows the nurse to collaborate with the client to improve the client's overall health.

Fluid and Electrolyte Balance History

Much of the information for the assessment is obtained from the client history. The nurse should gather information about the client's physiological and psychosocial functioning and current situational adaptation. Although the nurse may be able to use data collected by other health care providers, these data require augmentation through an expanded nursing interview to develop nursing diagnoses.

Because the symptoms of body fluid imbalances vary in severity, it is sometimes necessary to modify the techniques used in gathering historical information. A client may be unable to respond because of reduced consciousness or weakness and fatigue. In some cases, the nurse can collect information at intervals, while interspersing periods of rest; in other cases, friends and family members may provide information. Slurred speech, which sometimes accompanies body fluid imbalances, requires nurses to listen carefully and ask for restatements. Nervousness, anxiety, and general feelings of decreased well-being sometimes must be alleviated before clients can respond.

Primary Concern. Clients may seek health care for obvious fluid balance problems, such as prolonged diarrhea, severely diminished urine output, or edema of extremities; however, it is also important to consider other related concerns. For example, a client may be concerned about general malaise, muscle weakness, fatigue, dizziness, mild confusion, and apathy. Determining a link between fluid balance problems and the stated concern requires questioning about the client's physiological, mental, and emotional processes as well as daily habits such as fluid intake and elimination patterns. It is also important to determine the client's reason for concern and the way in which the problem affects the client's daily activities. The following example illustrates a fluid-related primary concern.

- The nurse asks what brought Mrs. Chin, a newly admitted elderly client, into the hospital. Mrs. Chin responds that she was suffering from weakness after an 8-hour episode of vomiting and diarrhea. When the nurse asks what about her problem troubles her most, Mrs. Chin begins to cry and responds, "This weekend is my grandson's graduation from high school. What a terrible time for this to happen." The nurse notes Mrs. Chin's concern and her desire to attend the important family occasion. The nurse's intention is to collaborate with the physician to establish a probable date for discharge.

Current Understanding. The client's understanding of the development of the fluid problem can help the nurse decide on nursing implementation. Clients often supply data about mode of onset, precipitating events, symptom severity, relationship to clients' activities, and the effects of treatments that provide valuable clues to possible nursing implementation. For example, when diarrhea is the problem, determining the rate and amount of fluid loss helps the nurse gauge the severity of fluid volume deficit and formulate plans for fluid replacement. An illustration of the current understanding follows.

- Mrs. Chin tells the nurse that she expects to reestablish her strength while in the hospital. She took baking soda the day before admission in the hope that it would "settle her stomach" and afterward experienced weakness to the point where she could not do her usual activities. She mentioned that others in her household had recently "had the flu." The nurse notes that the baking soda could have contributed to Mrs. Chin's severe weakness, and notes this as a topic for future collaboration with the client.

Past Health Problems/Experiences. Information about usual medications and treatments is important in determining body fluid balance. The abuse of laxatives, enemas, and diuretics can lead to severe fluid and electrolyte alterations. In addition, certain prescription drugs, such as steroids and antihypertensives, can disturb body fluid balance. Questioning clients about allergies can reveal liquids, foods, and medications to avoid in treatment. For example, milk and dairy products are common in hospital diets. Some clients, however, are highly allergic to or do not digest these products well.

Obtaining information about past health problems gives clues to deviations that may recur or cause current alterations. For example, diabetes mellitus can cause dehydration and other body fluid alterations. In addition, re-

TABLE 31–10. FLUID AND ELECTROLYTE BALANCE HISTORY: PERSONAL, FAMILY, AND SOCIAL HISTORY QUESTIONS

A. **Vocational**
1. What type of work do you do?
2. How much physical activity does your job involve?
3. Does your job involve exposure to high temperatures?

B. **Home and Family**
1. Do you or anyone in your family have a history of diabetes mellitus?

C. **Social, Leisure, Cultural, Spiritual**
1. Do you adhere to any food or beverage restrictions?
2. Do you use any home remedies or remedies prescribed by a religious or traditional healer?

D. **Habits**

Exercise
1. Do you exercise regularly? How often and what types of exercise?
2. Can you carry out your usual daily activities?

Diet
1. Have you noticed a weight gain or loss recently? How much?
2. What foods do you like to eat?
3. Are there any foods that you eat a lot of? What foods?
4. Are you on a restricted diet of any kind? What kind (eg, salt limitation, weight loss, fluid restriction)?
5. Do you salt your food at the table?
6. Are you fond of snack foods such as popcorn, nuts, and potato chips? How often do you eat these foods?
7. Do you use salt substitutes?

Beverages
1. How much fluid do you usually drink a day?
2. Do you drink fluids with meals? Between meals? Before going to bed?
3. What beverages do you like to drink?
4. Are there any beverages that you don't like?
5. Do you prefer hot or cold drinks?
6. Do you drink coffee, tea, or colas?
7. Do you drink extra fluid when the weather is hot?

Sleep
1. Do you experience any difficulty breathing while lying down to sleep at night?

Other Substances
1. Do you drink alcoholic beverages? Describe the amount you consume.
2. What medications do you take regularly? Occasionally?

E. **Psychological/Stress/Coping**
1. Have you experienced any unusual or particularly severe stress recently?
2. Have you had any major life changes recently?

sponses to past hospitalizations help nurses individualize client care and avoid recurrences of past problems. The following example illustrates a past health problem related to fluid balance.

- The nurse learns that Mrs. Chin has suffered from high blood pressure for several years and is taking a potassium-wasting diuretic and a potassium supplement. Because of her vomiting, Mrs. Chin has not taken her potassium supplement for 2 days. The nurse realizes that this may have contributed to Mrs. Chin's weakness and discusses this possibility with Mrs. Chin's physician.

Personal, Family, and Social History. The personal, family, and social history helps determine the influence of psychosocial factors on the client's fluid status. For example, the nurse might ask the parents of a dehydrated child whether the child has any significant handicaps that might interfere with the ability to take oral fluids. Determining the client's developmental level and physical capabilities guides caregivers in providing for fluid balance. Recent studies of the elderly point out that confusion, immobility, difficulty in communicating, and reluctance to ask for assistance can result in reduced fluid intake to the point of fluid volume deficit.[30] The following example underscores the relevance of the personal, family, and social history.

- The nurse discusses Mrs. Chin's health beliefs with her and discovers that Mrs. Chin uses a great many home remedies for various family health problems. An example is her use of baking soda for upset stomach. The nurse realizes that some of these remedies may be ineffective or even worsen the symptoms for which they are taken. She resolves to discuss the subject of home remedies with Mrs. Chin again before discharge to determine their importance to her and her receptiveness to additional information on self-care.

One of the key contributions the nurse can make to the client's health is to assist with the human problems of adapting to illness. The assessment of role and relationship patterns provides much information about the impact of symptoms on the client's life-style and life structure. Although fluid imbalances are often temporary and correctable, their symptoms can affect personal relationships and role fulfillment. The questions in Table 31–10 help the nurse obtain information about client values and life-style and therefore avoid approaches that clients are likely to reject.

Subjective Manifestations. Review of subjective manifestations can uncover information about the client's specific symptoms that, along with the observations made in the fluid and electrolyte examination, may help the nurse un-

IMPLICATIONS FOR NURSE–CLIENT COLLABORATION

Sick Role Behavior

Theory about human responses to health and illness indicates that one important factor in human coping is the individual's adoption of the sick role. A client may exhibit many signs and symptoms of fluid volume or electrolyte alteration and yet deny the presence of illness, thereby neglecting to seek help for a health problem. Did the client wait several days before going to a health care professional? A variety of factors may contribute to a client's hesitance to seek help. Holistic assessment, which looks not only at physical signs and symptoms or laboratory data but also at the client's behavior surrounding an episode of fluid imbalance, often enables the nurse to understand a dimension of the client's problem that previously has been unaddressed. The nurse's assessment is more thorough when issues surrounding the client's adaptation to the sick role are considered.

derstand the precise nature of the client's fluid needs. The questions in Table 31–11 can help to identify symptoms that are commonly associated with fluid imbalances of various types. Determining which symptoms the client experiences may help the nurse decide if a fluid imbalance exists and what nursing approaches may alleviate it.

Fluid and Electrolyte Balance Examination

Because so many organs are involved in protecting body fluid balance, the fluid and electrolyte examination must include almost every body system. The fluid and electrolyte examination also includes the laboratory and diagnostic data that reveal the chemical functioning of the body.

Measurements. Many of the observations on which diagnoses are based and plans for care are formulated vary slightly between observers. Height, weight, and vital signs provide numerical, factual evidence of the presence of fluid volume alterations and their extent.

Body Weight and Height. Body weight can help evaluate fluid gains and losses as well as the need for replacement. Body fat is gained or lost relatively slowly, but body water can be gained or lost quickly. Gains or losses of weight exceeding 0.5 to 1.0 pound per day usually indicate fluctuations in body fluids rather than fat stores.

The baseline weight obtained in the initial assessment provides a yardstick for evaluating fluid gains and losses. Thereafter, keeping in mind that every liter of fluid weighs 2.2 pounds, the nurse can correlate client weights to fluid intake. Body weights are of critical importance to the client with renal failure, as they are used in mathematical calculations to guide fluid removal during treatments. A 2 percent decrease in body weight represents mild fluid volume deficit, 5 percent a moderate change, and 8 percent a severe, debilitating alteration.[4]

TABLE 31–11. SUBJECTIVE MANIFESTATIONS OF FLUID AND ELECTROLYTE ALTERATIONS

A. **General**
   1. Have you noticed a weight gain or loss recently? How much?
   2. Have you noticed any unusual thirst?
   3. Have you noticed any change in your energy level recently? Have you felt unusually fatigued or tired?
   4. Have you felt anxious or irritable? Depressed, nervous, or restless?
   5. Have you had any problem with fever?

B. **Integument**
   1. Do you have dry skin?
   2. Have you noticed that your skin is unusually dry lately?
   3. Have you experienced any general itching?
   4. Have you noticed any puffiness of the skin of your hands, face, feet, or legs?

C. **HEENT**
   1. Do you have any problem hearing or seeing?
   2. Have you had a dry mouth or nose lately?
   3. Do you have any soreness or pain in your mouth or throat that affects your eating or drinking?
   4. Do you use dentures? Do they fit well?

D. **Chest/Cardiovascular System**
   1. Do you ever feel that your heart pounds or beats too rapidly?
   2. Do your ankles swell?
   3. Do you have chest pain?
   4. Have you experienced any recent difficulty breathing?
   5. Do you have difficulty breathing when lying down?
   6. Do you sit up or use extra pillows to get to sleep at night?
   7. Do you have a cough?

E. **Abdomen/Gastrointestinal Tract**
   1. Do you have trouble with indigestion?
   2. Have you been nauseated or vomited recently?
   3. Have you had diarrhea or constipation recently?
   4. Do you take enemas to defecate?

F. **Genitourinary System**
   1. Have you experienced an increase or decrease in urine volume recently?
   2. How often do you usually urinate? Have you noticed any changes in frequency?
   3. Has your urine changed in color?

G. **Musculoskeletal System**
   1. Have you noticed any weakness lately?
   2. Have you noticed any muscle twitching or spasms recently?
   3. Do you ever have muscle cramps? During exercise or at rest?

H. **Neurological System**
   1. Have you had any trouble remembering things lately? Are you ever confused?
   2. Have you had any unusual mood swings?
   3. Have you had any trouble with your speech?
   4. Do you have headaches?
   5. Have you felt any numbness or tingling in your face, hands, legs, or feet?

The client's height and weight are often used in combination on a nomogram (see page 817) to determine body surface area (BSA). Physicians and nurses use body surface area, in combination with body fat measurements and laboratory data, to determine fluid replacement.

Vital Signs. Vital signs are undoubtedly the most frequently observed parameters in physical assessment. Changes in body temperature, pulse rate, respirations, and blood pressure readily reflect body fluid changes. Alterations in vital signs may result from the imbalance or cause it.

For example, elevations in body temperature are associated with increases in sensible loss from perspiration and insensible loss from the lungs. In fever states, the normal requirements for adult fluid intake (1500 to 2500 mL/d) must be increased by 500 mL for a fever between 101F and 103F, and by at least 1000 mL for a sustained fever greater than 103F.[31]

Objective Manifestations. To understand the client's state of body fluid balance, the nurse must consider the whole range of clinical observations. Accurate diagnoses can be drawn only after considering the overall pattern of observation. The following paragraphs briefly describe the significance of many of the most common observations associated with body fluid assessment.

General Observations. Observations of mental and behavioral changes, as well as facial expression and overall appearance, are important indicators of fluid and electrolyte alterations.

Mental Status. Changes in level of consciousness, orientation, thought process, judgment, perception, and mood may accompany fluid balance alterations. When these functions are simultaneously but temporarily disturbed, a condition known as acute brain syndrome exists. Symptoms of acute brain syndrome include disorientation and confusion. This syndrome can accompany malnutrition, heart failure, stroke, pneumonia, or renal and liver disease. Elderly clients, because of declining organ function, are most vulnerable.

The nurse assesses cognitive pattern to determine if the client can understand the need for fluid intake, communicate the need, remember to take fluids, and decide the adequacy of body fluid balance. Cognitive alterations require support and collaboration from other health care team members.

LEVEL OF CONSCIOUSNESS. Level of consciousness is one of the most important indicators of fluid and electrolyte balance. Derangements of fluid and electrolytes may result in lethargy, stupor, or coma. In lethargy, the client is drowsy but is easily aroused. Stupor is a state of mental sluggishness and decreased responsiveness. Coma is the loss of consciousness. Alterations in water, sodium, potassium, and acid–base balance, in particular, cause changes in level of consciousness.

ORIENTATION. Orientation refers to the ability to recall person, place, time, and situation. Most of the fluid and electrolyte abnormalities that affect level of consciousness can also cause transient loss of orientation.

BEHAVIOR. In observing the client's behavior, the nurse should consider both response to surroundings and mood. For example, fluid volume alterations may not only render the client lethargic but also result in withdrawn, apathetic behavior.

Facial Expressions. A pinched or drawn expression, the appearance of emotional depression, apprehension, or anxiety can all indicate fluid loss and electrolyte alterations. For example, in fluid volume deficit states, the eyeball can seem to sink into the eye socket, a manifestation known as enophthalmos. In addition, the eyeball will feel unusually soft and mushy.

Appearance. Individuals with significant fluid and electrolyte imbalances become weak and fatigued, neglecting their hygiene and grooming as a result. Extremely poor nutrition can be readily observed in muscle wasting of the limbs and prominence of the facial bones.

Speech. In states of fluid imbalance, the quality, content, and formation of speech may change. Hoarseness, shrill pitch, slurring, and decreased volume can indicate fluid and electrolyte problems. Subtle changes, such as the client frequently moistening the mouth before talking, may reflect a change in the body fluid balance.

Integument. Clues to the client's fluid balance can be gained from observing the texture, moisture, turgor, color, and temperature of the skin.

Moisture/Texture. Normally, the skin has a smooth consistency and is slightly moist to the touch. The texture is not dry, scaly, or crusty; however, in fluid volume deficit, the skin becomes dry and scaly. Fluid volume excess may stretch the skin and give it a taut, shiny appearance. Changes in skin color may suggest underlying fluid and sodium problems. Pallor or flushing of the skin may indicate fluid losses or elevations of serum electrolyte levels.

Turgor. Skin turgor, or elasticity, is tested by lifting the skin over the dorsal surface of the hand (Fig. 31–5). As the skin is released, it should immediately fall into the normal position. In fluid volume deficit, the pinched skin remains elevated, or tented, for several seconds. This reflects a loss of turgor. Loss of turgor occurs normally with aging. In the elderly, loss of turgor over the hands is common, so an alternate site for assessment is the clavicular area.

In fluid volume excess, the skin can become too taut to pinch; however, pressing the skin over the pretibial area of the lower limbs may leave a characteristic indentation, which remains many seconds. This is called pitting edema. The degree of pitting generally correlates with the degree of fluid excess (Box 31–4). Remember that relatively healthy individuals may experience transient edema in normal circumstances, such as sitting for extended airline flights.

Color and Temperature. Skin color and temperature can suggest underlying fluid problems. Normal skin color is not

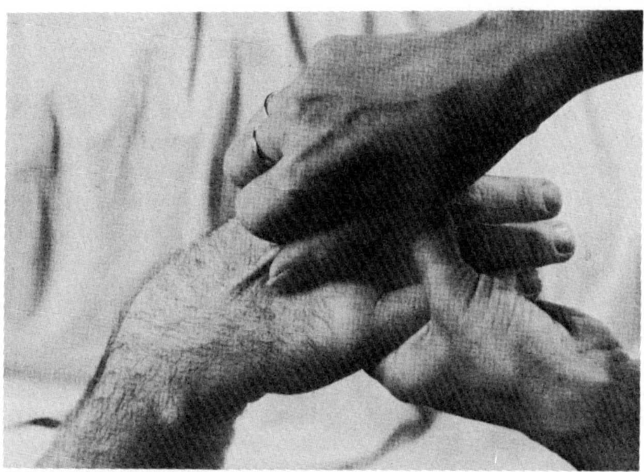

Figure 31–5. Testing skin turgor. (*From DeGroot KD, Damato MB.* Critical Care Skills. *Norwalk, CT: Appleton & Lange; 1987: 324.*)

pallorous or flushed; the skin should feel warm but not hot. Deviations can indicate fluid imbalance.

HEENT. The mucous membranes of the mouth readily demonstrate the effects of fluid depletion. Running a gloved finger along the surface between the cheek and gum may reveal dryness or stickiness indicative of fluid or sodium alterations. The surface of the tongue should be examined for the redness and swelling that accompany sodium imbalance. Shrinkage or fissuring of the tongue indicates fluid volume deficits. Excessive mouth breathing may also result in minor to moderate mucous membrane drying.[4]

In infants and very young children, a decreased or absent suck response indicates a moderate to severe fluid volume deficit.[4] In addition, the absence of tears in infants or very young children should arouse suspicion of fluid volume deficits.[32]

The appearance of the eyes also provides a useful assessment tool. The skin of the eyelid is thin and loosely attached to underlying tissue. Edema manifests itself in puffy eyelids. In normal individuals, the eyelid may become puffy after lying down for a few hours, but the puffiness diminishes after arising. Edema from fluid volume excess, on the other hand, persists.

BOX 31–4. ASSESSMENT OF PITTING EDEMA

Testing Scale	Depth	Excess Fluid Volume
+1	1 mm	5–7 lb
+2	2 mm	10–15 lb
+3	3 mm	20 lb
+4	4 mm and beyond[a]	>20 lb

Considerations

Not all individuals will harbor edema in the lower extremities. An alternate site for testing edema is the sacrum.

[a] 4+ edema takes at least 30 s to rebound.

Chest. Alterations in body fluid balance frequently cause changes in respiratory rate, depth, and character. In particular, acid–base changes, which set into motion respiratory compensatory mechanisms, result in observed changes in respirations. Fluid volume changes often result in observable changes in respiration as well.

In states of acid–base imbalance, the respirations may become abnormally rapid and deep (Kussmaul breathing), or slow and shallow. Some electrolyte abnormalities, such as magnesium changes, directly affect the respiratory center and slow the rate.

Congestion of the pulmonary tissue resulting from fluid volume excess produces a characteristic crackling sound when the lungs are auscultated. Coughing, labored breathing, and the production of pink, frothy sputum may also be associated with increased fluid volume. In addition, scratchy sounds, known as rubs, can be heard over the lung fields when a severe shift of plasma to interstitial fluid results in fluid collection in the pleural sacs. This is commonly referred to as a pleural rub (see Chap. 27).

Cardiovascular. Both fluid volume changes and electrolyte abnormalities result in cardiovascular changes. Auscultation of heart sounds, measurement of blood pressure and pulse, and observation of hand and neck veins provide important assessment data.

Heart Sounds/Rhythm. A change in heart sounds and rhythm often indicates fluid and electrolyte abnormalities. Any extra heart sound auscultated in the interval between two apical beats can signify fluid volume changes, particularly excesses. An irregular pulse may reflect changes in potassium, calcium, and magnesium concentrations.

Blood Pressure. Fluid volume excess, fluid volume deficit, fluid compartment shifts, and changes in ECF magnesium levels may all cause blood pressure changes. Characteristically, a decrease in ECF volume results in hypotension, whereas an increase is accompanied by hypertension.

Pulse. Pulse strength, rate, and rhythm changes may all indicate generalized or specific changes in body fluids and electrolyte levels. A bounding or thready pulse may appear in states of fluid volume deficit or excess. Weak pulses are often associated with potassium or calcium deviations of the ECF. A bounding pulse may reflect excess intravascular volume, as the result of fluid shifts.

Pulse strength is assessed by calculating the pulse pressure (the difference between systolic and diastolic blood pressures). Normal pulse pressure is 30 to 40 mm Hg. A widening of pulse pressure is associated with a bounding pulse, and is possibly indicative of fluid volume excess.[6] A narrowing of pulse pressure indicates possible fluid volume deficit and is frequently associated with a weak, thready pulse.[6,14,33]

Vein Filling. Peripheral vein fullness can indicate the adequacy of the client's hydration in relationship to the intravascular volume. Observations of the jugular veins of the neck and the peripheral veins on the dorsum of the hand are common indirect assessments of fluid balance. Commonly, elevation of the hand above ear level will empty and flatten the veins, while placing the hand in a dependent position will cause visible expansion of the vessels. Normal filling or emptying should occur in 3 to 5 seconds.

Jugular veins may normally be distended and visible if the client is lying flat or the head is lower than the heart; however, the veins should readily empty as the individual is brought to a sitting position. Measurement of the height of the jugular venous distension can be correlated to fluid volume excess (Fig. 31–6). Fluid volume excess usually results in venous distension, even though position change is achieved. Fluid volume deficit is usually reflected by a prolonged vein filling time.

Abdomen. The abdominal examination consists of abdominal inspection, auscultation, palpation, and percussion as well as observation of GI secretions, such as vomitus, drainage, and stool.

Abdominal Contour. Distension is the technical term for protrusion of the abdominal profile. Distension represents the outward stretching of the abdominal wall caused by the growth of a sizable internal mass, which may be composed of tissue or fluid. The accumulation of sizable amounts of fluid is known as ascites (see above). The degree of distension correlates with the volume of collected fluid, which may be as much as several liters.

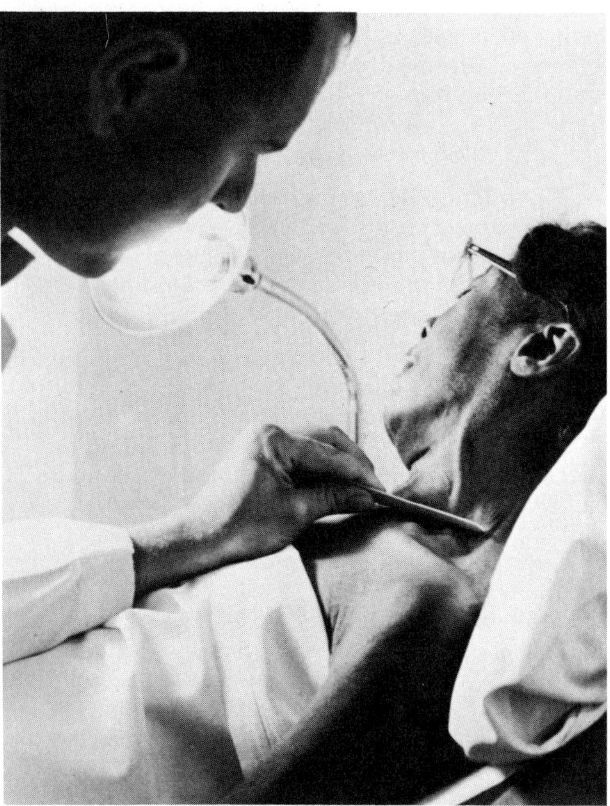

Figure 31–6. Jugular venous distension. (Reproduced with permission of the American Heart Association.)

Many conditions are associated with a protuberant abdomen, so determining when distension results from fluid accumulation requires skill. Ascites represents a generalized distension over the entire abdomen, whereas a full urinary bladder causes protrusion of the lower abdomen only. In ascites, no solid masses are palpable, and the umbilicus remains centrally located. The skin over the abdomen becomes shiny and taut, and the venous pattern becomes readily visible.

Striae, commonly called stretch marks, may develop as the abdomen becomes distended with fluid. Striae are shiny, vertical lines, usually near the flank areas. They result from severe thinning of the skin on the rapidly expanding abdomen. Striae often appear purple because the underlying vasculature of the skin shines through the severely stretched skin.

An examination referred to as "shifting dullness" helps the nurse verify that abdominal distension is due to fluid accumulation. With the client in a side-lying position, percuss from the midline to each flank, noting any areas of dullness. Then, placing the client supine, percuss again from midline to each flank. Changing areas of dullness will indicate shifting of fluid internally. Typically, fluid seeks the flank areas when the client is supine.

Bowel Sounds. A change in bowel sounds can accompany fluid imbalance. Hyperactive bowel sounds heard every 2 to 3 seconds, as opposed to the normal 3 to 5 seconds, are sometimes associated with diarrhea. The bowel sounds are also sustained and loud.[34]

Gastrointestinal Secretions. The volume and character of GI secretions are related to the client's state of hydration. Table 31–5 describes the relationship of GI secretions to fluid and electrolyte losses.

Genitourinary. The examination and measurement of the urine often provide valuable data for evaluating the client's fluid balance. Urine volume, specific gravity, pH, and color are commonly included in the assessment. Many assessments of urine are performed in the laboratory, and require collaboration between nurse and physician to obtain accurate assessment data.

Questions regarding elimination are also important in assessing intake and output. Ask the client to describe frequency and amount of urinary output, specific elimination habits, and problems with bladder function. Also ask about past bladder surgeries, past use of urinary catheters, and problems with incontinence.

Urine Volume. Urine volume normally varies with fluid intake: reduced fluid intake results in reduced urine output and vice versa. Urine output is roughly equivalent to intake over a 24-hour period. Significant disparity is cause to suspect fluid imbalance.

As a general rule, urine volume below 1000 mL in 24 hours may indicate a fluid volume deficit, and urine volume in excess of 2000 mL in 24 hours may indicate fluid volume excess; however, urine output can be influenced by increased insensible losses, increased solutes in the ECF, ADH and aldosterone production, and renal function.[4] The normal 40 to 80 mL/h output may shrink to as little as 30 mL/h during times of stress and ADH production.[4] Urine volume below 400 mL in 24 hours may indicate acute renal failure.[4]

Urine Color. The observation of urine color is often coupled with measurement of urine volume. Urine is usually a light amber or straw color. As the kidneys dilute the urine to excrete additional water, the urine becomes very pale. The pale urine may be associated with ingestion of large amounts of fluid, mobilization of fluid volume excesses or edema, or the ingestion of diuretics. Dark, amber urine indicates the kidneys' attempt to conserve extracellular water in the face of fluid deficit. Poor fluid intake or increases in fluid output relative to intake result in concentrated urine.

When evaluating urine color, the nurse should remember that the relationship between urine color and volume breaks down in the presence of certain disease states. For example, in renal failure, the kidneys produce a very dilute, pale urine, because they have lost the ability to concentrate the urine. In liver disease, dark bile pigments produce an intensely amber-to-brownish-colored urine.

Musculoskeletal. The musculoskeletal examination is included in fluid balance assessment to reveal changes associated with fluid loss and electrolyte abnormalities.

Muscle Tone and Strength. Muscle tone is the state of tension or responsiveness of the muscle to stimuli. Normally, muscles show slight resistance to passive movement, even when relaxed. There should be no spasticity (hypertensive, convulsive, jerking movement), rigidity (tension and stiffness preventing easy movement), or flaccidity (flabby, mushy response to stimulus). Changes in muscle tone are commonly seen in electrolyte abnormalities, particularly those associated with calcium and potassium.

Flabbiness and loss of muscle tone may indicate protein deficiency or electrolyte imbalance. Serum calcium, for instance, has an especially profound effect on muscle tone. Reduction in the serum calcium level may cause muscle rigidity or spasticity.

If an individual cannot flex and extend muscles against reasonable resistance, the muscles are considered weak. Decreased muscle strength is a common sign of electrolyte imbalance. Fluctuations in serum potassium levels may produce muscle weakness. This weakness may affect smooth muscle before it affects skeletal muscle, with the potential of causing vascular and intestinal motility problems.

Neurological. The nervous system's ability to evoke muscular response is often profoundly affected by electrolyte changes. In particular, changes in potassium, calcium, and magnesium levels may be tracked through the assessment of neurological signs or the use of diagnostic tests such as the electrocardiogram.

Neuromuscular Irritability. Chvostek's and Trousseau's signs are elicited to test neuromuscular irritability when imbalances of calcium or magnesium are suspected. Chvostek's sign is assessed by tapping the facial nerve located in front of the earlobe. A positive sign is a twitching of the facial muscles, producing a sneer and often a tremor of the eyelid (Fig. 31–7A). Trousseau's sign is tested by placing a blood pressure cuff on the arm and applying pressure slightly higher than the client's own systolic pressure for 3 minutes. A positive sign is pronounced palmar flexion with the thumb and small finger in opposition, commonly called carpal spasm (Fig. 31–7B).[4]

A particularly serious sign of heightened irritability of the neurological system is asterixis. Asterixis is elicited by asking the client to hyperflex both wrists, whereupon both hands of the client will exhibit an involuntary jerking tremor. This characteristic tremor, associated with hyponatremia and the buildup of metabolic wastes in clients with renal failure, is often referred to as the flapping tremor.

Reflexes. Normally, the biceps, triceps, bracheoradialis, patellar, and achilles deep tendon reflexes are present in

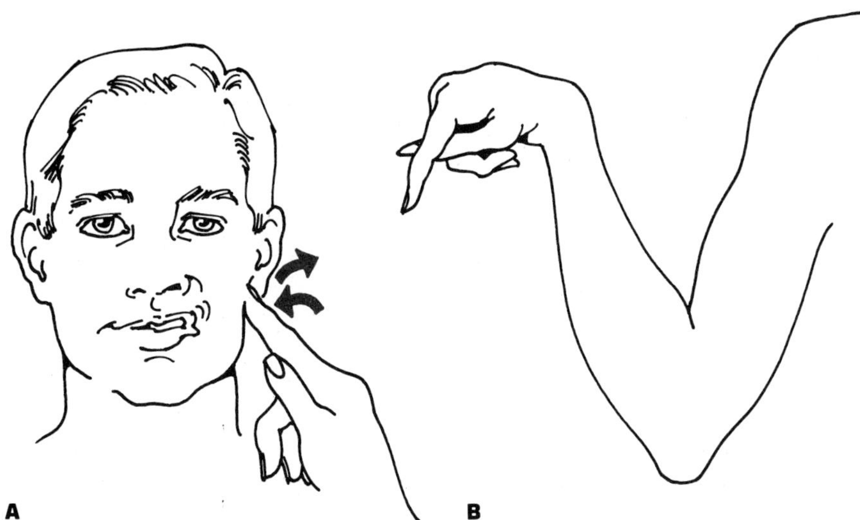

Figure 31–7. Checking for Chvostek's and Trousseau's signs. **A.** Chvostek's sign: Tap the client's facial nerve approximately 2 cm in front of the earlobe. Unilateral twitching of the facial muscles—a brief contraction of the upper lip, nose, or side of the face—is a positive sign. **B.** Trousseau's sign: Occlude the arterial blood flow of the client's arm with a blood pressure cuff. After 3 minutes, a carpopedal spasm—an adducted thumb and extended phalangeal joints—is a positive Trousseau's sign.

minimal to moderate intensity. In states of electrolyte and acid–base imbalance such as hypomagnesemia, hypernatremia, hyperkalemia, hypocalcemia, and respiratory and metabolic alkalosis, these reflexes may be hyperactive. The opposite conditions (hypercalcemia, hypermagnesemia, hyponatremia, hypokalemia, and acidosis) may result in diminished or absent reflexes.[4] Techniques to elicit deep tendon reflexes are specified in Chapter 29.

Senses. For the client to maintain self-care, intact senses are necessary. Changes in sight, smell, and taste, in particular, may alter the client's desire or ability to take in food and fluids. In addition, the nurse should determine whether the client uses glasses, hearing aids, or other sensory supports, as these devices may allow the client to participate in the plan of care for regaining body fluid balance.

The nurse should question the client about abnormal peripheral sensations. Prickling or burning sensations, known as paresthesias, often accompany electrolyte imbalances.

An explanation of common findings related to fluid and electrolyte assessment is presented in Table 31–12, grouped by body area.

Diagnostic Tests

Although the history and physical examination provide general clues to the state of the client's body fluid balance, laboratory and diagnostic tests are necessary to confirm clinical hypotheses. An understanding of the relationship between laboratory findings and fluid and electrolyte balance can help the nurse carry out the collaborative role. Often, the nurse is the first member of the health care team to receive laboratory and diagnostic findings. The nurse reviews and exercises judgment in their interpretation. Judgment is critical in determining whether an imbalance potentially or actually exists, whether immediate danger exists, and whether notifying the physician or changing the treatment is warranted.

PROCEDURE 31–1. MEASURING URINE SPECIFIC GRAVITY

PURPOSE: Rapid determination of the concentration of urine

EQUIPMENT: Glass cylinder, urinometer, specimen container, disposable gloves

ACTION

1. Don gloves and obtain a 10-mL sample of fresh urine. (See Procedure 26–3 or 26–11.)
2. Fill cylinder three-quarters full of urine.
3. Place the glass manometer in the cylinder and give it a gentle spin.
4. Position cylinder at eye level for reading. Read from the bottom of the meniscus across to the scale.

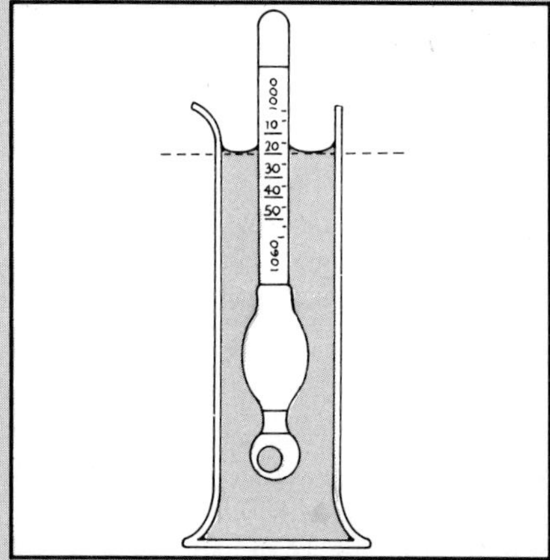

5. Rinse manometer with water, remove gloves, and wash hands.

RECORDING: Document the value obtained on the I&O (intake and output) sheet or other record, according to agency procedure.

Fluid Balance Tests. Tests that reflect fluid balance measure the degree of concentration of urine and blood. Serum osmolality, urine osmolality, and urine specific gravity reflect definitive changes in ECF fluid and electrolyte balance. Test descriptions and common values are listed in Table 31–13.

Serum Osmolality. **Serum osmolality** refers to the total concentration of dissolved particles in serum. Using the laboratory findings, the nurse can quickly compute an estimate of serum osmolality in one of two ways. First, a doubling of serum sodium provides a rough estimate. Second, the following formula, using serum sodium, glucose, and BUN measurements, can quickly determine serum osmolality.[35]

$$\text{Serum osmolality} = 2 \times \text{serum Na}^+ + \frac{\text{BUN}}{3} + \frac{\text{glucose}}{20}$$

Urine Specific Gravity. The urine specific gravity test is easily performed at the bedside by the nurse, by capturing fresh urine in a special graduated cylinder (see Procedure 31–1). A mercury-weighted glass dipstick is placed in the graduate. The urine supports the weight of the dipstick, according to the amount of solute in the urine. The more concentrated the urine, the higher the dipstick floats. A scale is read, at eye level, to determine the measurement.

Electrolyte Balance Tests. Tests reflecting electrolyte balance measure the concentration of the ionic solutes in the blood and urine. The values generally reflect concentrations in the ECF compartment; however, inferences regarding the ICF may be made on the basis of these measurements. Ranges for the normal and abnormal values of serum electrolytes are indicated in Table 31–13.

TABLE 31–12. SUMMARY OF FINDINGS RELATED TO FLUID BALANCE ASSESSMENT

Finding	Possible Significance
General	
Pinched or drawn facial expression	Fluid volume deficit
Rapid gain or loss in weight	Fluid volume excess or deficit
Apathy, restlessness, apprehension, and general behavioral changes	Electrolyte imbalances, especially hypernatremia, hyperkalemia, and hypercalcemia
Integument	
Dry, flaky skin	Fluid volume deficit
Tenting of skin	Fluid volume deficit
Pitting edema	Fluid volume excess of intravenous fluids, decreased renal function, decreased liver function, syndrome of inappropriate ADH secretion (SIADH), and compartmental fluid shifts from pressure changes
HEENT	
Dry, sticky oral mucous membranes	Fluid volume deficit Hypernatremia
Erythema and swelling of tongue	Hypernatremia
Fissuring of tongue	Fluid volume deficit Hypernatremia
Distended neck veins	Fluid volume excess
Sunken appearance of eyes	Fluid volume deficit
Cardiovascular System	
Rate changes (tachycardia, bradycardia)	Hypokalemia Hyperkalemia Hypovolemia Metabolic acidosis
Rhythm changes (gallops, missed beats)	Fluid volume excess Hypokalemia Hyperkalemia Hypocalcemia
Pulse pressure changes (increase or decrease)	Fluid volume excess or deficit
Blood pressure changes (hypertension, hypotension)	Fluid volume excess or deficit Hypomagnesemia Hypermagnesemia
Respiratory System	
Crackles on auscultation	Fluid volume excess
Decreased breath sounds	Fluid volume excess
Increased rate and depth	Metabolic acidosis Respiratory alkalosis Hypermagnesemia
Decreased rate and depth	Respiratory acidosis
Abdomen	
Ascites	Plasma-to-interstitial fluid shift—liver disease, starvation diet
Striae	Rapid development of plasma-to-interstitial shift
Nausea and vomiting	Hyperkalemia
Diarrhea	Hyperkalemia
Constipation	Mild fluid volume deficit
Genitourinary System	
Decreased output	Renal dysfunction SIADH Hyperaldosteronism
Increased output	Diuretic abuse Diabetes insipidus Hyperglycemia Hypoaldosteronism
Neurological System	
Decreased level of consciousness	Respiratory acidosis Hypermagnesemia Hyponatremia Hypernatremia
Disorientation	Hyponatremia Hypernatremia Hypomagnesemia
Tremors	
Paresthesias	Hypokalemia Hyperkalemia (face, tongue, feet and hands) Hypocalcemia
Tics, asterixis	Hyponatremia
Headache	Hyponatremia
Positive Chvostek's or Trousseau's sign	Hypocalcemia Hypomagnesemia
Deep tendon reflexes hyperactive	Hypocalcemia
Musculoskeletal System	
Muscle flaccidity	Hyperkalemia
Muscle weakness	Hypokalemia Hypercalcemia Hypermagnesemia
Muscular tetany	Hypocalcemia
Muscle cramps	Hyponatremia Hypocalcemia
Immunologic System	
Fever	Fluid volume deficit Hypernatremia

Data from Methany,[4] Levinsky,[15] Levinsky,[21] and Poyss.[34]

TABLE 31–13. COMMON LABORATORY TESTS TO ASSESS FLUID, ELECTROLYTE, AND ACID–BASE BALANCE

Test/Description	Normal Findings	Significance of Abnormal Findings
Fluid Balance Tests		
Serum osmolality: Measures total concentration of dissolved particles in serum; determined largely by Na^+ concentration	Child: 270–290 mOsm/kg Adult: 280–300 mOsm/kg	*Decreased* in dilutional states, decreased adrenal function, and SIADH *Increased* in hypernatremia, hyperglycemia, uremia, diabetes insipidus, and dehydration states
Urine osmolality: Measures concentration or number of solute particles, regardless of size, in urine	Newborn: 100–600 mOsm/kg Child/adult: 50–1200 mOsm/kg Average: 200–800 mOsm/kg	*Decreased* (<200 mOsm/kg) with excessive water intake or excess D5W infusion *Increased* (>800 mOsm/kg) in dehydration states and SIADH
Urine specific gravity: Measures density of water compared to distilled water; not as precise a measurement as urine osmolality	1.003–1.040	*Decreased* in water intoxication or fluid volume excess *Increased* in fluid volume deficit states NOTE: Heavy molecular solutes falsely elevate specific gravity; fixed low volume in renal failure
Hematocrit (Hct): Measures percentage by volume of red blood cells in whole blood; provides a relative indicator of fluid volume alteration	Adult male: 40–54% Adult female: 36–46%	*Decreased* in hypovovolemia, secondary to blood loss *Increased* in dehydration or hemoconcentration
Hemoglobin (Hgb or Hb): Measures oxygen-carrying capacity of blood; also an indicator of fluid balance	Adult male: 14–18 g/dL Adult female: 12–16 g/dL	*Decreased* in fluid volume excess from intravenous fluids *Increased* in dehydration states
Blood urea nitrogen (BUN): Measures levels of nitrogenous wastes in bloodstream; a relative indicator, affected by factors such as increased or decreased protein in diet, decreased renal clearance in elderly, catabolic drugs, and growth spurts in children	5–25 mg/dL	*Decreased* in fluid volume excess *Increased* in fluid volume deficit NOTE: If rehydration does not lower BUN, suspect renal damage
Electrolyte Balance Tests		
Serum electrolytes: Measures electrolyte levels in blood serum		NOTE: Prolonged storage of specimen or trauma to blood cells may result in elevated levels of certain electrolytes, particularly K^+
Sodium (Na^+)	135–145 mEq/L	*Decreased* in hyponatremia *Increased* in hypernatremia
Potassium (K^+)	3.5–5.0 mEq/L	*Decreased* in hypokalemia *Increased* in hyperkalemia
Calcium (Ca^{2+})	Ionized: 4.5–5.8 mEq/L Total: 8.8–10.5 mEq/L	*Decreased* in hypocalcemia *Increased* in hypercalcemia
Magnesium (Mg^{2+})	1.5–2.5 mEq/L	*Decreased* in hypomagnesemia *Increased* in hypermagnesemia
Phosphorus (PO_4^{2-})	2.5–4.5 mg/dL	*Decreased* in hypophosphatemia *Increased* in hyperphosphatemia
Chloride (Cl^-)	98–108 mEq/L	*Decreased* in hypochloremia *Increased* in hyperchloremia
Urine electrolytes: Measures electrolyte levels in urine; involves 24-hour collection of urine		
Sodium (Na^+)	40–220 mEq/L per 24 h	*Less than* 10 mEq/L indicates hypovolemia or hyponatremia *Between* 20 and 40 mEq/L indicates SIADH, diuretic abuse

TABLE 31–13. (continued)

Test/Description	Normal Findings	Significance of Abnormal Findings
Potassium (K^+)	40–80 mEq/L per 24 h	*Decreased* level indicates adrenal insufficiency or renal damage *Increased* level indicates hypersecretion of aldosterone or diuretic abuse
Calcium (Ca^{2+})	50–300 mg/24 h	*Decreased* in hypocalcemia *Increased* in hypercalcemia resulting from metastatic disease
Acid–Base Balance Tests		
Urine pH	4.5–8.0 (usually 6.0–6.5)	*Decreased* with use of vitamin C or certain antibiotics *Increased* in alkalotic states, except when K^+ lost in metabolic alkalosis; also increased in overuse of sodium bicarbonate as an antacid NOTE: Certain foods and fluids can acidify or alkalinize urine (cranberry juice, citrus fruits, etc)
Arterial blood gases (ABGs): Provides information on pressure exerted by gases dissolved in the blood	Po_2: 80–100 mmHg Pco_2: 35–45 mmHg pH: 7.35–7.45 HCO_3: 22–26 mEq/L Base excess: +2 to −2 mEq/L	NOTE: Altered values may indicate acidotic or alkalotic state (see Table 31–14; see also Chap. 27 and Table 27–6 for further discussion of ABG values).

Data from York[12] and Kee.[35]

Acid–Base Balance Tests. The tests involved in the determination of acid–base balance not only provide information regarding pH, bicarbonate, or the dissolved gases in the blood, but also serve to detect respiratory and renal compensation for acid–base imbalances. The most commonly performed test for acid–base balance, blood gas analysis, is usually performed using samples of arterial blood. The additional measurement of the anion gap, or total anions in the ECF, is not often obtained, but can serve to confirm acidosis.

Interpretation of acid-base alterations includes not only evaluations of the measurements in relationship to one another, but also interpretation of the mechanism at work to compensate for the alteration. An overview of blood gas analysis is presented in Table 31–14.

■ NURSING DIAGNOSIS OF FLUID AND ELECTROLYTE STATUS

Once the nurse has gathered the subjective and objective information, the data are analyzed for relationships and patterns that indicate a problem or client need. Client collaboration should be an integral part of this analysis.

The taxonomy of nursing diagnoses related to body fluid balance is still tentative. Because the nursing and medical aspects of fluid imbalance are so closely related, it is sometimes difficult to differentiate nursing problems from the realm of medical diagnosis and therapy. For this reason, it has been suggested that problems associated with electrolyte imbalance be designated collaborative problems, to indicate that they require interdependent care measures on the part of the nurse, physician, dietitian, and other team members. An example is the collaborative problem, "Potential Complication: Electrolyte Imbalance."[36]

This chapter adopts the framework of the taxonomy, discussing only those diagnoses of body fluid alterations that nurses diagnose independently. Electrolyte and acid–base imbalances are no longer included within these diagnoses. Because many of the etiologies of the diagnoses re-

TABLE 31–14. LABORATORY VALUES IN ACID–BASE IMBALANCES (ARTERIAL BLOOD GASES)

Respiratory Acidosis		**Metabolic Acidosis**	
pH	<7.35	pH	<7.35
Po_2	80 mm Hg	Po_2	Normal
Pco_2	50 mm Hg	Pco_2	Normal
HCO_3	Normal	HCO_3	22 mEq/L
		Base deficit	−2 mEq/L
Respiratory Alkalosis		**Metabolic Alkalosis**	
pH	>7.45	pH	>7.45
Po_2	Normal	Po_2	Normal
Pco_2	30 mm Hg	Pco_2	Normal
HCO_3	Normal	HCO_3	26 mEq/L
		Base deficit	+2 mEq/L

Data from Metheny[4] and York.[12]

quire therapy from the physician and other health care team members, the nurse is the critical link in ensuring collaboration and consensus regarding the client's problems and needs.

The North American Nursing Diagnosis Association (NANDA) has approved and classified three diagnoses related to body fluid balance: Potential Fluid Volume Deficit, Fluid Volume Deficit, and Fluid Volume Excess. The table of Sample Nursing Diagnoses contains subjective and objective defining characteristics and etiologies for the latter two diagnoses, and provides risk factors for Potential Fluid Volume Deficit. Box 31–5 lists other fluid balance-related diagnoses.

Diagnosing client problems demonstrates a nurse's concern for the prevention of illness and the maintenance or restoration of health. Early problem identification and intervention can ward off impending imbalances and often prevent secondary problems.

Potential Fluid Volume Deficit

Potential fluid volume deficit is the state in which an individual is at risk for developing an extracellular fluid volume deficit.[37,38] The defining characteristics of increased urinary output and altered intake are easily observed by client, family, or health care team members; however, the defining characteristic of thirst may be difficult to assess in very young or very old clients. Age itself is an etiology for potential fluid deficit.

Risk Factor: Extremes of Age. Very young and very old clients are at risk for developing a fluid volume deficit. Infants develop deficits rapidly because the majority of their fluid weight is located in the extracellular compartment. In addition, infants lose fluid rapidly from rapid respirations, dilute urine, and evaporation from the skin.[2] Insufficient intake or losses from conditions such as diarrhea can produce serious deficits in short periods.

The single greatest complicating factor for the infant is the need to rely on adults to meet intake needs or to recognize serious fluid losses. Nurses can avert great harm by educating parents about the importance of maintaining hydration and making appropriate referrals.

IMPLICATIONS FOR PROFESSIONAL COLLABORATION

The Taxonomy of Nursing Diagnosis

The characterization of problems associated with electrolyte imbalance as "collaborative problems" reflects the fact that decisions on how best to meet the client's fluid needs are often interdependent and involve the nurse, the physician, the dietitian, and other health care team members. Because many of the etiologies require confirmation from the physician and other team members as well as multidisciplinary input to the therapeutic plan, the nurse is the critical link in ensuring collaboration and consensus regarding the client's problems and needs.

Elderly clients are at risk for potential volume deficits as a result of normal physiological declines in renal function, integument, and the thirst mechanism. Kidney degeneration may cause decreased ability to concentrate urine and a higher waste and solute load in the ECF. Sweat gland function declines and subcutaneous fat is lost, making the elderly less able to withstand extreme environmental temperatures. Thirst sensation diminishes to the point that researchers have reported it can take 15 hours without sufficient intake before elderly clients complain of thirst.[3,30] Physiological and psychosocial factors, such as immobility, confusion, and fear of incontinence, lead to decreased fluid intake.[13,22,30]

Risk Factor: Excessive Losses Through Normal Routes (Vomiting, Diarrhea, Diuretic Use). Excessive losses of fluids and electrolytes in the urine or stool may not simply be related to physiological alterations. As elimination is a critical part of well-being, many individuals employ medications or other means to maintain regular bowel habits. Overuse of diuretics or laxatives and poor understanding of the effects of prolonged use may contribute to potential fluid deficit.

Physiologically, diarrhea produces copious fluid and electrolyte losses. Knowledge of the type of diarrhea can guide nurses in planning specific care to replace fluids, limiting the severity of losses, and educating the client about prevention. Osmotic diarrhea is created by nonabsorbable or high-molecular-weight materials passing through the intestine and creating extra pull on fluids in the intestinal lumen. This is usually transient and resolves with the passage of the material. A good example is the diarrhea that results from overingestion of fresh fruit or vegetables of high fiber and sugar content (peaches, pineapple, etc).[37]

Secretory diarrhea is caused by irritation of the intestine by bacterial toxins. A third type of diarrhea results from motility changes secondary to chemical or neurological alterations in the bowel. Diabetic neuropathy, a pathological reduction in nervous transmission secondary to diabetes, slows peristalsis, allowing for the collection of significant amounts of fluid surrounding the metabolized food. Disorders related to the blockage of bile flow, such as cholecystitis, may contribute to the inadequate breakdown of food in the intestine. The resulting coarse mass of partially digested food osmotically collects large amounts of fluid on the path through the intestinal lumen, predisposing the client to fluid losses.

Risk Factor: Loss of Fluids Through Abnormal Routes (Indwelling Tubes, Urinary and Small Bowel Diversions). Nasogastric intubation and urinary or small bowel diversions place clients at risk of fluid volume deficit and concomitant electrolyte loss. The potassium- and chloride-rich stomach fluid can be lost in quantities approaching 3 L/d with continuous suction. This results not only in fluid and electrolyte problems but also in acid–base alterations.[29] Ileostomy fluid output may range up to 600 mL/d, or more than five times the fluid in the normal fecal output.[29] Un-

SAMPLE NURSING DIAGNOSES: FLUID BALANCE

Nursing Diagnosis	Defining Characteristics/Manifestations		Etiology[a]
	Subjective Data	**Objective Data**	
Fluid Volume Deficit *1.4.1.2.2.1*	Reports fatigue Reports weakness Reports not feeling thirsty, has no desire for fluid	Mouth membranes dry Wets lips to speak Eyelids appear sunken Skin dry, flaky Intake 980 mL in previous 24 h; output 1500 mL Voids small amounts of dark urine Serum Na^+ increased Hemoconcentration (lab reports show increased BUN, Hct, Hgb) 4-lb weight loss in 3 days Makes no effort to drink Declines fluid when offered Seems confused (unable to state date, uncertain of location) Medical record indicates possible brain tumor	*Physical:* Failure of regulatory mechanisms—derangement of thirst mechanism[b]
Fluid Volume Deficit *1.4.1.2.2.1*	Reports recent diarrhea Reports feeling thirsty Reports mouth dry Reports recent fever, perspiration Reports feeling weak	Weight loss of 5 lb Decreased skin turgor Skin dry, flaky Oral mucous membranes dry Voiding small amount of concentrated urine Frequent liquid stools BP 104/70 24-h intake = 2300 mL, output = 1700 mL Urine specific gravity = 1.030 Hemoconcentration (increased BUN, Nct, Hgb)	*Physical:* Active loss—diarrhea[b]
Fluid Volume Excess *1.4.1.2.1*	Reports feeling "down" Reports "I went off my diet" Reports worried about business Reports fatigue after walking to bathroom	Facial expression sad, shoulders slumped, appears withdrawn (responds in short phrases; does not initiate conversation) 10-lb weight gain 3+ pitting ankle Jugular veins distended in sitting position Hemodilution (lab values show decreased BUN, Hct, Hgb) Medical record documents recent heart failure Medical treatment for 1000 mg/d restricted sodium diet	*Physical:* Excess sodium intake[b]

Nursing Diagnosis	Risk Factors
Potential for Fluid Volume Deficit *1.4.1.2.2.2*	Extremes of age: 79-year-old male Extremes of weight: Height = 60 in; weight = 210 lb Deviations reducing access to or absorption of fluids, eg, physical immobility Hypermetabolic states: Fever Altered intake: Averages 900 mL/24 h

[a] Sample etiologies only; see text discussion and taxonomy for other etiologies and defining characteristics.

[b] Example only. Many other specific examples of altered functioning with this general etiology are relevant to nursing diagnosis. Defining characteristics, desired outcomes, and nursing implementation would differ for each specific etiology.

BOX 31–5. OTHER NURSING DIAGNOSES RELATED TO BODY FLUID BALANCE

Physical

- Altered Nutrition: less than body requirements
- Impaired Swallowing
- Potential Impaired Skin Integrity
- Constipation
- Diarrhea
- Decreased Cardiac Output
- Sleep Pattern Disturbance
- Ineffective Breathing Pattern
- Impaired Gas Exchange
- Hyperthermia
- Altered Oral Mucous Membrane
- Altered Patterns of Urinary Elimination

Cognitive

- Altered Thought Processes
- Impaired Verbal Communication

Sociocultural/Life Structural

- Altered Role Performance
- Body Image Disturbance

fortunately, clients often fail to recognize a developing fluid deficit.

Risk Factor: Deviations Affecting Access to Intake or Absorption of Fluid. Limited mobility can place clients at risk of developing a fluid deficit. Simply placing fluids within reach of an immobile client increases the chance of preventing fluid deficit, but this is often overlooked. In addition, an immobile client may hesitate to ask for frequent assistance to satisfy thirst.[30]

ocial and environmental factors may complicate access to intake. Family members caring for a confused client may forget to encourage fluid intake. Institutionalized clients drink only what is given them, so that access must be increased to maintain sufficient intake. Access to a variety of fluids is often necessary to increase intake.[30]

Absorption of fluid may be influenced by diuretic use. Because these drugs cause fluid and potassium losses, clients must be taught that intake must match output.

Risk Factor: Factors Influencing Fluid Needs, Such as Hypermetabolic States. Fever, regardless of cause, significantly raises the body's metabolic demands and thereby requires extra water and solutes. The body's oxygen requirements increase 10 percent for every 1-degree rise in temperature.[33] As a result, strains are placed not only on the fluid stores but also on the acid–base regulation system and oxygen use. Nurses must recognize that the potential for loss is even higher for infants and elderly clients.

Risk Factor: Knowledge Deficit Related to Fluid Volume. Lack of knowledge regarding required fluid intake is often an important risk factor. Education in this area must be appropriate to the client's or family member's capacity to understand, include client preferences and cultural needs, and use familiar forms of measurement for the client. For example, the teaching plan should require the client to use an ordinary measuring cup or favorite glass, not complicated metric volumes.

Fluid Volume Deficit

Fluid volume deficit is defined as a state in which an individual experiences vascular, cellular, or intracellular dehydration. Etiologies for this diagnosis include derangement of regulatory mechanisms and active volume loss.

Etiology: Failure of Regulatory Mechanisms. Many pathological conditions alter the functioning of organs or feedback mechanisms that regulate fluid balance. Examples include brain injuries or tumors in the area of the hypothalamus, (which alter the thirst mechanism) and diabetes insipidus (which causes excessive urine output from insufficient ADH production in the hypothalamus or failure of the pituitary to release ADH.)[19] Although nurses do not treat the altered regulatory mechanism, careful monitoring of affected clients and support measures to maintain fluid balance are important nursing responsibilities when failure of regulatory mechanisms causes a fluid volume deficit.

Etiology: Active Loss. Active loss encompasses conditions that enhance fluid losses via normal routes to the point that a client cannot maintain sufficient intake to balance the loss, and conditions that cause fluid loss via abnormal routes. Diarrhea and profuse sweating associated with heat exhaustion are examples of excessive losses via normal routes. Vomiting, wound drainage, hemorrhage, and losses from burned tissue are examples of abnormal losses.

Hemorrhage is excessive blood loss. It often causes hypovolemic shock. Blood loss is not always overt; therefore careful assessment is required to prevent significant fluid deficit. Body cavities such as the abdomen and thorax can sequester large volumes of blood before the definitive signs and symptoms of hemorrhage appear. An abrupt change in mental status from alertness to confusion often signals impending shock. Postoperative clients or those with multiple trauma should be continuously observed for both the overt and covert signs of hemorrhage[39]

The massive fluid, electrolyte, and acid–base changes that accompany severe burns require a keen knowledge of basic physiological alterations and prompt intervention. The immediate problem facing these clients is a loss of fluid and solutes through burned areas and a fluid shift from intravascular to interstitial spaces. This leaves a severely depleted intravascular compartment. Blood and exudate losses ultimately contribute to the intravascular dehydration.[31]

Fluid Volume Excess

Fluid volume excess is the state in which an individual experiences an excess of volume in the extracellular compartment. Factors related to this diagnosis include compromised regulatory systems and excessive sodium collection in the ECF. Some of the manifestations of fluid volume excess are pitting edema, moist crackles in the lung fields, coughing and dyspnea, and hypertension.

Etiology: Fluid Volume Excess Related to a Compromised Regulatory Mechanism. One of the most serious regulatory mechanism failures involves the kidneys. Renal failure directly affects fluid, electrolyte, and acid–base balance. Sodium and potassium excesses and metabolic acidosis frequently accompany failure of the kidneys. Fluid volume excess develops as the kidneys are unable to filter the fluid load, resulting in the return of massive amounts of fluid to the intravascular volume.

Renal failure does not necessarily mean an immediate, complete cessation of urinary output. The kidney may produce a relatively normal volume of urine, or decreased urine (oliguria), or no urine (anuria), depending on the severity of the renal failure. Complete cessation of urinary production requires client care for fluid volume excess. As the kidney recovers, massive diuresis may ensue, requiring client care to avoid fluid and electrolyte deficits.

Etiology: Fluid Volume Excess Related to Excess Sodium Intake or Retention. Hypernatremia from excess oral sodium intake is a rare occurrence. Self-administration of salt tablets or use of salt far in excess of normal daily requirements or restricted allotments may result in sodium excess and fluid retention. This problem also commonly occurs when individuals on restricted sodium diets consume salty foods.

Intravenous intake of sodium is another cause of hypernatremia. Even isotonic saline (0.9 percent NaCl), given in excessive amounts, can increase ECF sodium levels temporarily, because it contains 150 mEq/L, which is slightly in excess of the normal levels. Retention of sodium may be seen in states of hypersecretion of aldosterone and in true water loss in excess of sodium, as in heat stroke.[31] Regardless of the cause, an increased ECF sodium load causes water to remain in the ECF in great quantities, creating a fluid volume excess.

Stating the Fluid and Electrolyte Diagnosis

Selection of the nursing diagnosis related to body fluid imbalance is the foundation for collaborative planning to resolve the client's problem. The diagnostic statement incorporates the general diagnostic label with the specific etiology underlying the diagnosis and the defining characteristics exhibited by the client. The following are examples of nursing diagnostic statements:

- Potential Fluid Volume Deficit; risk factors persistent diarrhea, elevated temperature, decreased fluid intake
- Fluid Volume Deficit related to persistent fever (102–103°F) as evidenced by concentrated urine, thirst, and dry skin and mucous membranes
- Fluid Volume Excess related to sodium intake in excess of prescribed diet as evidenced by increased arterial blood pressure, ankle edema, and 5-pound weight gain

NANDA lists several etiologies for the diagnoses related to fluid volume deficit and excess. To specifically plan goals and implementation to resolve the problem, the etiology must be defined by its contributing factors. This step helps the nurse ascertain the need for nursing care, the level of care required, and the need for collaboration with other health care team members.

Risk factors serve a twofold purpose: confirming the diagnosis and etiology and providing evidence of problem resolution. In other words, the disappearance of certain signs and symptoms of a particular disorder, the defining characteristics, indicates the eradication of the problem.

Section 3. Nurse–Client Management of Fluid and Electrolyte Balance

PLANNING FOR OPTIMUM FLUID AND ELECTROLYTE BALANCE

Once the nursing diagnosis is made, the nurse is ready to initiate nursing management. Management consists of planning, implementing, and evaluating care. Collaboration between nurse and client remains as important in planning as it was in the assessment phase. Exchanges between nurse and client regarding the client's beliefs, expectations, and pertinent life-style factors will improve the chances of successful implementation. For example, an elderly client with a diagnosis of fluid volume deficit secondary to insufficient fluid intake may not accept the teaching or suggestions of the nurse who does not take into consideration the client's fears of incontinence.

Planning involves setting desired outcomes and selecting implementations that are likely to achieve those outcomes. Body fluid balance ranks with oxygenation problems in degree of urgency, so desired outcomes in this area are a nursing priority. Desired outcomes should describe the client's condition, appearance, or behavior as the result of implementations. Two common desired outcomes related to fluid balance follow:

- Client will experience no thirst or dry mouth after oral rehydration.
- Client will experience increased urine output volume, corresponding to intake, after oral rehydration.

Realistic target dates for the achievement of goals should be included in the outcome statement as well.

Desired outcomes guide the nurse and client in choosing appropriate actions. Implementation should flow from discussion between nurse and client to decide on the specific approaches. The nurse offers guidance on the physiological requirements; the client gives input on habit patterns and personal preferences.

NURSING IMPLEMENTATION TO PROMOTE OPTIMUM FLUID AND ELECTROLYTE BALANCE

The following discussion of nursing implementation describes four levels of client care: prevention; supportive care; restorative or acute care; and rehabilitation. The table on Nurse–Client Management of Fluid Imbalance summarizes nursing care for each of the diagnoses related to fluid imbalance found in the table Sample Nursing Diagnosis related to Fluid Balance on page 1579. Desired outcomes, approaches, and evaluation criteria are listed for each diagnosis.

Preventive Care

Preventive client care involves ascertaining that the healthy client understands the principles of normal fluid balance in reference to healthful living. This level of care also includes identifying clients at risk for developing fluid imbalances.

Health Screening. The comprehensive fluid balance history (described in Section 2) and examination help nurses identify persons at risk for developing fluid, electrolyte, and acid–base problems. Those at risk include infants, the elderly, clients with chronic but controlled metabolic or endocrine disorders such as diabetes or adrenal disease, or clients taking medications associated with possible fluid balance problems, such as diuretics and steroids. Persons who are frequently exposed to high temperatures or who undertake strenuous exercise are also at risk (see Box 31–6).

Clients who are at risk should be given the opportunity to describe their habits and preferences for fluids, as well as exercise levels. The nurse then uses this information to suggest specific interventions or develop a teaching plan.

Individuals who fit into more than one risk category have greater potential for developing imbalances in body fluids. Those clients should be alerted to the risks and monitored carefully.

Life-style Analysis. The analysis of life-style factors is important to the prevention of body fluid imbalance. For example, clients who exercise vigorously may not appreciate the impact of climate on water balance and may therefore fail to increase intake. Sedentary elderly clients may fail to recognize the risk of fluid deficit in hot weather.

Family living is an important life-style factor. The presence of significant others often stimulates the client to maintain intake and becomes essential if the client has declining memory or mental acuity. Including family members in the plan of care often lends success to the plan.

An appraisal of the client's response to stress will point to interventions that avoid increasing the stress level. The nurse considers the potential effect of stress on fluid intake. For example, does the client's intake decline with increased stress? What specific stressors affect the client most? In what ways does the client usually respond to stress?

Life-style Counseling. Many life-style habits are related to fluid and electrolyte balance. Many people drink coffee, a diuretic that can create mild fluid volume deficit. Consumption of alcohol and of soft drinks in large quantities may disorder electrolyte balance. The nurse may help a healthy client make life-style changes by functioning as a life-style counselor. The client makes the decision to change and designs the plan, and the nurse confirms the appropriateness of the plan, provides referrals, and acts as a continuing resource person.

Values Clarification. Essential to any plan of care is assessment of values and health beliefs. Such beliefs tend to make behaviors hard to change. To accept a teaching plan, the client must be convinced that it will improve health. Thus, the nurse should determine whether the client views a given change in behavior as an improvement to the current state of health.

Health beliefs are also formed from cultural influences (see Chap. 9). If the nurse is careful to approach the client with cultural sensitivity, the client's motivation to change may be enhanced.

Health Education. Because of the critical need for fluids and electrolytes, it is important for clients to understand several basic factors related to body fluid maintenance. First, and most important, clients should know that it is not so much what they drink (with the exception of alcohol), but the amount they drink that determines fluid balance. In addition, fluids alone do not maintain balance: a diet containing the necessary solutes is just as important.

The client and family members should understand that not all of the water supplied to the body comes from the six to eight glasses of liquid recommended each day. Many foods, particularly those that melt at room temperature (Jello, ice cream), provide extra liquid (see Table 31–15).

Finally, individuals who care for infants or elderly persons should have basic information about risks to these individuals. This teaching may include some basic nursing measures, such as teaching a mother how to take an infant's rectal temperature or teaching a family member to measure an elderly client's intake and output.

BOX 31–6. FACTORS CREATING RISK OF FLUID IMBALANCE

- Exposure to high environmental temperatures
- Strenuous exertion
- Age (newborns, infants, young children, elderly)
- Physical disability (immobility, difficulty swallowing, etc)
- Psychosocial disability (confusion, psychoses, etc)
- Inadequate diet
- Therapeutic treatments (IVs, drainage tubes, catheters, enemas, irrigations, instillations, etc)
- Medications (diuretics, steroids, antacids, etc)
- Chronic disease states (diabetes, renal or liver disease, adrenal dysfunction, cardiac disease, pituitary dysfunction)

NURSE–CLIENT MANAGEMENT OF FLUID IMBALANCE

Nursing Diagnosis	Desired Outcome	Implementation	Evaluation Criteria
Potential for Fluid Volume Deficit, risk factor: physical immobility *1.4.1.2.2.2*	1. Maintains balanced intake and output	1a. Measure and record intake and output 1b. Monitor for new sources of fluid loss 1c. Observe urine concentration; monitor specific gravity periodically 1d. Monitor body temperature and respiratory rate 1e. Monitor body weight 1f. Involve client in self-monitoring, if appropriate	1. Intake equals output over 24 h
	2. Intake appropriate to body surface area	2a. Determine ideal intake in collaboration with physician 2b. Make fluids of client's choice easily available 2c. If compatible with diet order, provide electrolyte balanced solution (eg, Gatorade) for oral ingestion 2d. Assist client with oral fluid ingestion if necessary 2e. Devise a schedule for minimal hourly intake and post at bedside 2f. Discuss strategies with client to ensure minimal hourly intake	2. Maintains ideal daily intake
	3. Develops no manifestations of fluid volume deficit/hypovolemia	3a. Adjust thermostat to maintain comfortable environment 3b. Note onset of conditions that interfere with oral intake (eg, nausea, vomiting) and collaborate with physician on need for alternate intake route	3a. Does not exhibit dry skin; dry mucous membranes; tenting; enophthalomus; dark, concentrated urine; and other clinical signs of fluid volume deficit 3b. Laboratory values reflect state of fluid balance
	4. Demonstrates coping skills necessary to maintain fluid balance	4a. Discuss the risk factors of fluid imbalance with client 4b. Discuss healthful practices regarding fluid intake with client 4c. Provide opportunity for client to discuss personal concerns about fluid balance	4. Identifies risk factors and appropriate self-care

NURSE–CLIENT MANAGEMENT OF FLUID IMBALANCE (continued)

Nursing Diagnosis	Desired Outcome	Implementation	Evaluation Criteria
Fluid Volume Deficit related to deranged thirst mechanism *1.4.1.2.2.1*	1. Increases oral fluid intake	1a. Collaborate with physician on desired oral volume 1b. Discuss with client the importance of maintaining oral intake 1c. Encourage client to drink even though feels no thirst 1d. Monitor oral intake volume throughout day 1e. Measure and record all oral intake 1f. Provide favorite fluids compatible with diet order 1g. Discuss memory cues with client to ensure minimal hourly intake	1. Oral intake reaches desired volume
	2. Regains balance of intake and output	2a. Monitor oral intake 2b. Monitor parenteral intake 2c. Discuss with client need to measure output; measure urine output precisely 2d. Adjust thermostat to maintain comfortable environment 2e. Monitor client for new sources of fluid loss 2f. Monitor cardiovascular and neurosensory signs	2a. Urine output approximates intake 2b. Clinical signs of fluid volume deficit diminish: reports improved energy level; mucous membranes pink, moist; skin supple, turgor < 1 sec; urine amber; specific gravity 1.010; serum Na^+, Hgb, Hct, BUN normal for age
Fluid Volume Deficit related to diarrhea *1.4.1.2.2.1*	1. Maintains oral intake	1a. Collaborate with physician to establish desired oral volume 1b. Discuss with client importance of maintaining oral intake 1c. Make fluid easily accessible 1d. Encourage intake by offering fluid 1e. If compatible with diet order, provide electrolyte balanced fluid (eg, Gatorade) for oral ingestion 1f. Measure and record oral intake	1. Oral intake reaches desired volume
	2. Regains balance of intake and output	2a. Discuss with client need to measure all output, urine and fecal	2a. Total output approximates intake

NURSE–CLIENT MANAGEMENT OF FLUID IMBALANCE (continued)

Nursing Diagnosis	Desired Outcome	Implementation	Evaluation Criteria
		2b. Measure all output precisely and record 2c. Monitor cardiovascular and neurosensory signs 2d. Note trends in output and collaborate with physician if adjustments to intake volume seem indicated (oral and parenteral) 2e. Adjust thermostat to maintain comfortable environment 2f. Remove heavy blankets and clothing that might impede heat loss and promote perspiration 2g. Collaborate with physician to treat the cause of diarrhea	2b. Clinical signs of fluid volume deficit diminish: weight gain 2 lbs; skin supple, turgor < 1 sec; urine amber; specific gravity 1.010; serum Na^+, Hgb, Hct, BUN normal for age
Fluid Volume Excess related to excess sodium intake *1.4.1.2.1*	1. Maintains fluid and sodium restriction	1a. Provide client with opportunities to express feelings and concerns 1b. Review with client importance of maintaining fluid and diet restrictions 1c. Recognize and reinforce client's efforts to maintain restriction 1d. Discuss with client self-management strategies to prevent episodes of "going off diet" in future	1. Food and fluid ingested within prescribed limit
	2. Regains balance of intake and output	2a. Discuss with client importance of monitoring urinary output 2b. Measure and record all output 2c. Monitor body weight daily 2d. Monitor fluid, dietary intake 2e. Monitor respiratory, cardiovascular, and neurosensory clinical signs 2f. Note trends in intake and output and clinical signs and collaborate with physician if adjustment to diet, fluid order, or medications seems indicated	2. Output exceeds intake as clinical signs of fluid volume excess diminish, then approximates intake

TABLE 31–15. PERCENTAGE OF WATER IN COMMON FOODS

Food	Percentage
Eggs	75
Cooked meats	40–75
Hard cheeses	35
Breads	35
Dry cereals	4
Fats and oils	0
Sugars	0
Milk	88
Fruits and vegetables	75–95
Butter and margarine	16
Fish, cooked or canned	60–86
Nuts	2–5

From Williams SR. Essentials of Nutrition and Diet Therapy, *5th ed. St. Louis, MO: Mosby; 1990.*

Supportive Care

Clients with mild fluid and electrolyte imbalances may be seen by nurses in home care settings, physicians' offices, clinics, or hospitals. The nursing role is to help the client identify the problem and select approaches that will support the client's self-care. Thereafter, the nurse monitors the client's therapy and helps the client identify risk factors that may worsen the existing problem or create new ones. Because the levels of care overlap, teaching clients about intake and output or modifying intake patterns may be part of restorative care as well.

Diet and Fluid Counseling. At the heart of supporting clients' efforts to restore fluid balance is the teaching provided by the nurse. Clients suffering from mild edema or worsening hypertension may require teaching about the role of sodium, its relationship to edema, and the sodium content of foods and medications. In addition, clients may require counseling to prevent the overuse of diuretics. Some clients take extra doses to relieve increasing edema and fail to realize the danger of potassium loss.

Collaboration with the dietitian is often critical to enable clients to make necessary life-style changes. The dietitian can help to translate the various dietary controls into everyday practice and provide information about creative food preparation. Nurses can provide clients with information regarding over-the-counter drugs that affect fluid balance and demonstrate how fluid restrictions help control edema and hypertension and reduce weight.

Oral Rehydration. Oral rehydration is the process by which the client ingests therapeutic quantities of fluid to regain fluid balance. The physician may order the quantity of fluid a client requires, usually in conjunction with nurses' observations and professional opinions. The client's age, size (eg, BSA), and activity level are considerations. From these factors, the client's normal daily requirements will be estimated (baseline fluid intake). Then, losses of fluid caused by illness are calculated from the intake and output data and laboratory test results. Losses considered are of two types: prior losses, which occurred before institution of therapy; and current losses (eg, diarrhea, vomiting). Fluid losses may be calculated using the following equation:[3]

$$\text{Loss of fluids} = \text{current body weight} \times 60\% \text{ (in liters)} - \frac{\text{normal Na}^+}{\text{current Na}^+}$$

Example: $70\text{ kg} \times 60\% = 42\text{ L} - 140/168 \text{ or } 36.5\text{ L}$
$42\text{ L} - 36.5\text{ L} = 5.5\text{ L}$

Estimated daily amounts needed to achieve balance in a 150-pound adult appear in Box 31–7.

The phrase *force fluids* is used to refer to actions aimed at oral rehydration. This does not mean that clients are physically forced to consume fluids, but rather that they are encouraged to consume specific amounts of fluids on a fixed schedule. Approaches to assisting clients in need of oral rehydration are listed in Procedure 31–2.

For clients on regular hospital diets, choices of fluids are left to individual preference; however, some clients need counseling on the advantages and disadvantages of various fluids. For instance, an overweight client who selects milk shakes and sugary colas may be advised to choose fluids more compatible with weight reduction. Clients also can be counseled to choose foods with higher water content to help replenish body water.

Water is the fluid in most common use. The mineral content of tap water, particularly the sodium content, varies by region. Therefore, in certain circumstances, bottled or distilled water may be substituted.

In addition, fluids containing certain substances may not be suitable for special diets or physiological conditions. Although recent studies dispute the link between caffeine and cardiac problems, coffee, tea, and colas may not be suitable in large amounts for clients with cardiac disorders or neurological traumas. Once the fluid is selected, however, the nurse should keep containers, cups, straws, and other materials within reach and in plentiful supply. Fluids should also be maintained at the temperature the client prefers.

BOX 31–7. ESTIMATED FLUID VOLUMES FOR REHYDRATION (150-LB ADULT)

2% body weight loss (minimal fluid volume deficit)	2000–2500 mL/24 h
5% body weight loss (moderate fluid volume deficit)	2500–3000 mL/24 hr
8% body weight loss[a] (severe fluid volume deficit)	3000+ mL/24 h

[a] In severe dehydration states, oral and intravenous replacement fluids may be combined.

Oral Electrolyte Intake. In the ordinary course of care, the client receives electrolytes in the form of a well-balanced diet; however, increasing the client's intake of specific electrolytes is a common aspect of medical therapy. The nurse's role is to administer the prescribed supplements. The nurse must be knowledgeable about the client's condition, the properties of electrolytes, and side effects of supplements. For example, potassium is frequently administered to make up the amount lost by diuretic use; however, clients with renal failure usually should not be given potassium, because they cannot excrete it. In addition, intravenous solutions containing potassium should be volumetrically controlled to prevent severe cardiac arrhythmias or even cardiac standstill.

Oral electrolytes are provided in a variety of forms (powders, tablets, solutions). Some preparations, particularly potassium, must be mixed in juice to disguise the unpleasant taste. Clients who take calcium supplements must understand their tendency to cause constipation and flatulence.

Limitation of Oral Fluid Intake. Clients with conditions that lead to fluid volume excess often require restriction of oral fluid intake. The physician orders the basic restriction usually after collaboration with the nurse.

The calculation of fluid restriction takes into account all sources of output plus an arbitrary 500 mL per day for insensible loss.[7] Common restrictions range between 800 and 1000 mL per day. When the order for restriction is written, the nurse should clarify whether the prescribed amount includes fluids from the client's meals or is exclusive of those fluids. A total intake of 800 mL per day is much more restrictive than an intake of 800 mL plus dietary fluids.

Restriction of fluids is unnatural and stressful to clients. Explaining the reason usually helps, as does involving the client in establishing and implementing the intake schedule. Nevertheless, considerable understanding, encouragement, and support are usually required. Approaches to aid clients in restriction of fluids appear in Procedure 31–3.

Limitation of Oral Electrolyte Intake. Some clients must restrict their intake of certain electrolytes, usually because they have excessive blood serum levels. Sodium and potassium are the most commonly restricted electrolytes. The physician's order will specify the exact dietary allowance of the electrolyte by weight. For example, low-sodium diets may be ordered as 500 mg, 1000 mg, or 2000 mg. A dietary prescription is as important as any medication order, so it is important that the client, family, and all others in contact with the client understand the treatment plan (see Box 31–8). Collaboration between the health professionals caring for the client is important to ensure consistency and continuity of care.

The restriction of sodium or potassium in the diet can be even more challenging than fluid restriction. For most clients, attractive presentation of food and education in the use of alternative seasonings reduce the stress surrounding the restriction.

PROCEDURE 31–2. ORAL FLUID REHYDRATION

PURPOSE: To increase the intake of fluids in states of dehydration

EQUIPMENT: Cups, straws, liquid of choice

ACTION

1. Check physician's orders for amount prescribed.
2. Discuss with client and family the objective for the increased intake.
3. Assess client for dysphagia, vomiting, or oral lesions that may alter intake.
4. Establish comfortable environment if necessary.
5. Assist client with oral hygiene.
6. Keep fluids within reach, and offer small amounts frequently.
7. Help client to achieve optimal position for fluid intake (usually semi-Fowler's to Fowler's position).
8. Maintain sufficient cups, straws, and other items for intake.
9. Serve liquids at desired temperatures.
10. Offer choices of liquids and foods high in water content.
11. Offer frequently to assist client with toileting if necessary.

RECORDING: Maintain accurate intake and output records.

Aiding clients with electrolyte restrictions requires that nurses be knowledgeable about the electrolyte content of foods. Printed materials or dietary manuals can help nurses to provide accurate information to clients. Consultation with a dietitian is also often helpful in situations regarding fluid and electrolyte restrictions.

Intake and Output Monitoring and Recording. Indications for recording intake and output (I&O) appear in Box 31–9. The measurement of intake and output, although simple to accomplish, is comparable to the assessment of vital signs in importance. The intake and output record is only as accurate an assessment tool as the individual who measures it. Errors and omissions in measurement can render intake and output records useless as information regarding fluid balance.

Intake includes all fluids that enter the body, including oral fluids, intravenous solutions, irrigation solutions, tube feedings, enemas, and foods that are liquid at room temperature. Measurement is accomplished by transferring the liquid, prior to use, to a graduated container or syringe to assess volume. Premeasured volumes (from the client's meals, for example) may be ingested and then assessed, as these measurements are commonly listed on the contain-

PROCEDURE 31–3. ORAL FLUID RESTRICTION

PURPOSE: To limit the intake of fluids in states of overhydration

EQUIPMENT: None

ACTION

1. Check physician's order for amount prescribed.
2. Clarify order to determine if restriction is inclusive or exclusive of dietary fluid.
3. Discuss with client and family the therapeutic objectives of the restriction and some of the ways to maintain the restriction comfortably.
4. Alert staff, visitors, and family members to client's fluid restriction by posting signs at client's bedside or on door specifying amount of fluid allowed.
5. Develop a schedule with the client to spread allotment over 24 hours, with majority of fluids covering shifts that include meals.
6. Provide frequent oral hygiene and lip lubrication.
7. Encourage oral rinsing without swallowing.
8. Discuss reducing intake of dry, salty, or very sweet foods, which increase thirst.
9. Provide artificially sweetened hard candies and gum to stimulate salivation.
10. Provide fluids the client prefers unless contraindicated. Encourage noncaffeinated, nonalcoholic, isotonic beverages, which are more likely to quench thirst.
11. Encourage diversional activities.
12. Sips of water, ice chips, and small amounts of fluid given with medications must be accounted for in the restriction.

RECORDING: Enlist client's assistance to maintain strict intake and output records.

ers. A client who is alert, in no distress, and willing may be given recording materials and briefly instructed in the recording of intake and output.

The output record should include all measurable liquids that leave the body, such as urine, liquid feces, drainage from intestinal fistulas, wounds with drains or suction devices, urinary and small bowel diversions, suction drainage, and enema return. Perspiration, urinary incontinence, and drainage from large lesions should be estimated. Again, the client deemed capable of maintaining the output record should be taught and encouraged to do so.

Most intake and output records include the same parts, such as columns for oral and parenteral intake. Columns for output reflect urine and stool output, as well as drainage and other specific output. See Figure 31–8. Information may be recorded hourly or at wider intervals, or cumulative records may be kept over several hours. Grand totals of

BOX 31–8. MANAGEMENT STRATEGIES FOR SODIUM AND POTASSIUM RESTRICTION

Sodium Restriction

- Determine extent of sodium restriction (ie, mild, moderate, or severe).
- Clients with moderate to severe sodium restriction should avoid all products containing sodium as an ingredient.
- Clients should be encouraged to read food labels to avoid foods that contain the terms *salt, sodium,* and *soda.*
- Condiments such as mayonnaise and catsup contain sodium but may not have labeling to identify such an ingredient.
- Severe sodium restrictions may call for the use of low-sodium breads.
- Clients and family members should be encouraged to experiment with various herbs, vinegar, wine, sugar, honey, and onion to flavor meats and vegetables.
- Fruits may be consumed in moderation as they contain little sodium.
- Clients and family members should be aware that milk contains moderate amounts of sodium and may be discouraged for the client with a severe sodium restriction.
- Products labeled *sodium free* contain less than 5 mg of sodium, whereas low-sodium foods contain 140 mg or less.

Potassium Restriction

- All salt substitutes should be avoided.
- Vegetables should be sliced or diced and soaked in water that is discarded prior to cooking.
- Canned vegetables should be drained of the canning liquid and cooked in fresh water.
- Tea and coffee are high in potassium and should be avoided by the client with a potassium restriction.
- Fruits and deep green vegetables range from high (>10 mEq per serving) to moderate (5–10 mEq per serving) potassium content, which necessitates individual dietary counseling to educate the client and family in the moderation required of a potassium-restricted diet

Adapted from Eschleman MM. Introductory Nutrition and Diet Therapy, 2nd ed. Philadelphia: JB Lippincott; 1991.

BOX 31–9. INDICATIONS FOR RECORDING INTAKE AND OUTPUT

- Acute or chronic diseases of major organ systems (renal, cardiac, endocrine, neurological, hepatic, dermatological)
- Major trauma
- Surgery
- Draining wounds
- Altered intake or output
- Insufficient diet
- Nausea and vomiting
- Diarrhea or constipation
- Gavage treatments
- Intravenous therapy
- Oral fluid therapy
- Urinary catheters

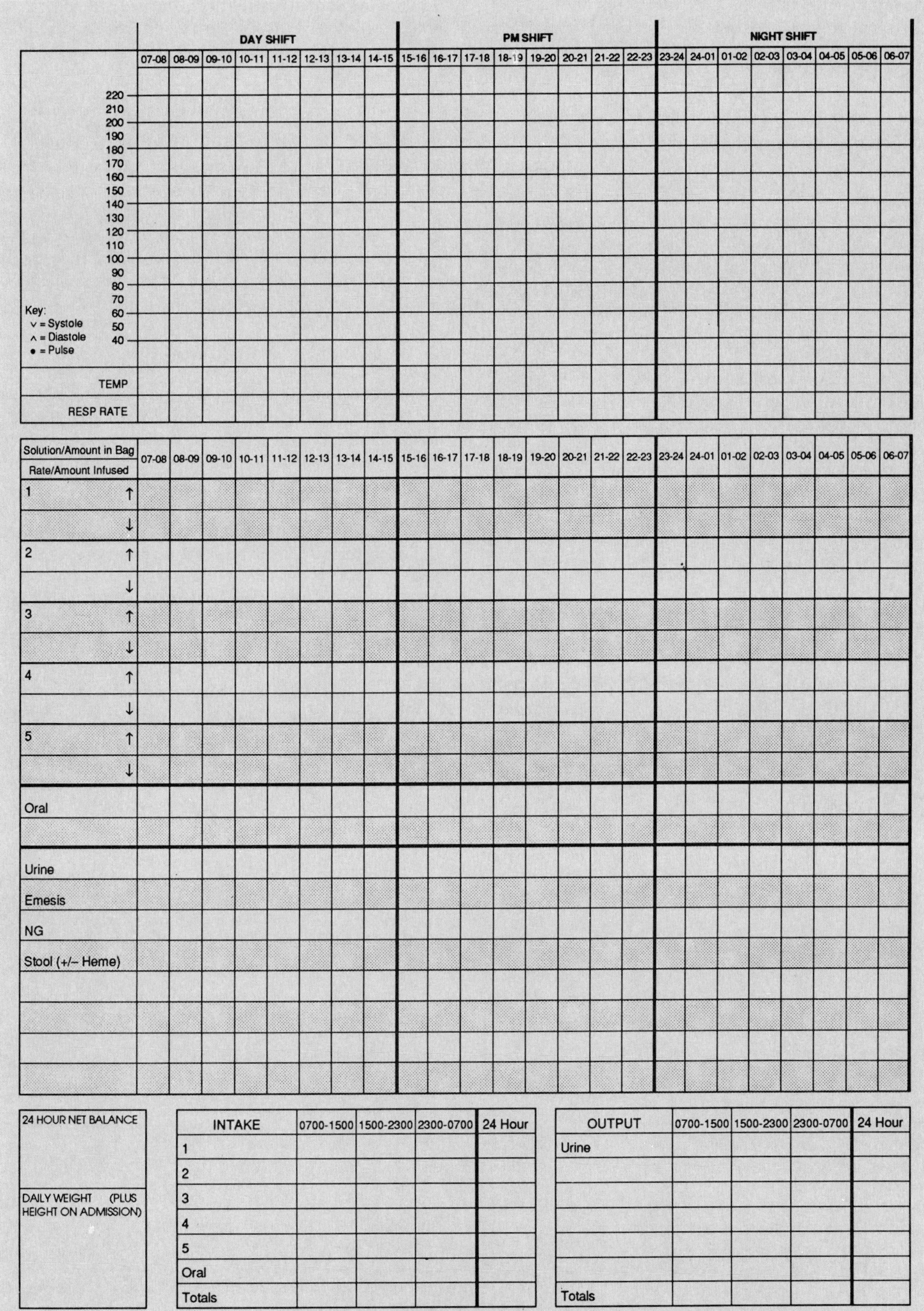

	DAY SHIFT								PM SHIFT								NIGHT SHIFT							
	07-08	08-09	09-10	10-11	11-12	12-13	13-14	14-15	15-16	16-17	17-18	18-19	19-20	20-21	21-22	22-23	23-24	24-01	01-02	02-03	03-04	04-05	05-06	06-07
220																								
210																								
200																								
190																								
180																								
170																								
160																								
150																								
140																								
130																								
120																								
110																								
100																								
90																								
80																								
70																								
60																								
50																								
40																								
Key: ∨ = Systole ∧ = Diastole • = Pulse																								
TEMP																								
RESP RATE																								

Solution/Amount in Bag Rate/Amount Infused	07-08	08-09	09-10	10-11	11-12	12-13	13-14	14-15	15-16	16-17	17-18	18-19	19-20	20-21	21-22	22-23	23-24	24-01	01-02	02-03	03-04	04-05	05-06	06-07
1 ↑																								
↓																								
2 ↑																								
↓																								
3 ↑																								
↓																								
4 ↑																								
↓																								
5 ↑																								
↓																								
Oral																								
Urine																								
Emesis																								
NG																								
Stool (+/– Heme)																								

24 HOUR NET BALANCE
DAILY WEIGHT (PLUS HEIGHT ON ADMISSION)

INTAKE	0700-1500	1500-2300	2300-0700	24 Hour
1				
2				
3				
4				
5				
Oral				
Totals				

OUTPUT	0700-1500	1500-2300	2300-0700	24 Hour
Urine				
Totals				

Figure 31–8. Form for recording intake and output.

intake and output should be calculated every 24 hours. If output consistently exceeds intake, then the potential for fluid volume deficit increases. If intake greatly exceeds output over time, then fluid volume excess should be suspected. Accuracy of intake and output may be enhanced by taking certain precautions and avoiding common pitfalls of measurement, as listed in Box 31–10.

Restorative Care

The client with moderate to severe fluid imbalance is the subject of restorative care. Such clients are commonly seen in the hospital with pathologies that promote or result from fluid imbalances. Collaborating with the client, family, physician, and other health care team members to correct the deviations and prevent further imbalance is an important part of nursing care.

The focus of restorative care is to replace fluid losses, decrease excesses, and prevent additional net change. Promoting client comfort, safety, and nutrition is an important contributory nursing objective.

Once it is determined that the client suffers from a fluid deficit or excess, common approaches are employed to correct the problems. Oral intake was discussed in the previous section. The client who requires restorative care often requires additional approaches, such as nasogastric gavage and intravenous infusion, to correct imbalances. Fluid restriction is employed in states of fluid excess.

BOX 31–10. IMPROVING INTAKE AND OUTPUT RECORDS

Communication/Collaboration

- Communicate to the entire staff that I&O recording is required for client.
- Discuss with client and family the need for I&O recording and reasoning behind the measurements.
- Post signs at client's bedside and in bathroom area as reminders.
- Clearly note the need for I&O recording on client's care plan.
- Update instructions for keeping accurate I&O records on a regular basis.
- Involve the alert, willing client and family in measurement and recording of I&O.

Equipment/Information

- Post a list of common volumes and measures for staff and at client's bedside (especially diet tray containers).
- Provide measuring containers at the bedside as soon as I&O measurement is instituted.

Precision/Pitfalls

- Whenever possible, measure, do not estimate.
- If measurement is not possible, estimate output volumes (incontinence, diarrhea, emesis).
- Estimate any increased perspiration loss.
- Weigh dry dressings; then weigh saturated dressings and subtract to find the weight. Convert to liquid measure.
- Consider ice as half the volume it occupies.
- Include irrigants as intake.
- Consider the difference between enema infusion and liquid output of enema results as intake.

Nasogastric Gavage. **Nasogastric gavage** involves the passage of a hollow, small-bore tube through the nasal passages into the esophagus and down into the stomach. Fluids and foods are then passed through the tube (see Procedures 25–2 and 25–3). Clients who require nasogastric gavage are either comatose or have impaired oral ingestion from dysphagia (difficulty swallowing), achalasia (esophageal obstruction), oral or esophageal tumors, or mouth trauma. The gavage method provides fluids directly to the GI tract and may be used in conjunction with intravenous infusion.

The principles that apply to oral therapy, as to the quantity and type of fluid, also apply to gavage fluids. Fluids from the regular hospital diet may be used, but specially prepared formulas are also used. (See Chap. 25 for more about special formulas.) These are rich solutions that provide nourishment as well as fluid. Most feeding solutions, however, are hypertonic and can draw additional fluids into the GI tract, leading to increased losses.[40] (See Table 31–16, which lists the tonicity of feeding fluids.) A client's ability to tolerate such a liquid diet must be individually assessed. It is common to administer these solutions in diluted forms, either quarter or half strength, to prevent fluid loss.

Medications may also be given via this route, as long as the tubing is thoroughly irrigated to maintain patency. The intake records for the gavage fluids should include any medications and irrigant used.

Intravenous Infusions. Administering solutions via peripheral or central veins is termed **intravenous infusion.** Intravenous infusion by gravity flow or pump method allows for the continuous, controlled delivery of fluids directly into the ECF.

Clients with moderate to severe fluid volume deficit usually require intravenous infusion in addition to oral replacement. Those with life-threatening hypovolemia require emergency intravenous infusions to support the cardiac out-

TABLE 31–16. TONICITY OF COMMONLY USED GAVAGE FORMULAS

Product	Strength (kcal/8 oz)	Tonicity (mOsm)
Ensure	250	470
Ensure Plus	355	690
Isocal	250	300
Osmolite	250	300
Sustacal	240	620
Vivonex	240	550

From Eschleman MM. Introductory Nutrition and Diet Therapy, *2nd ed. Philadelphia: JB Lippincott; 1991:496–497.*

put. Because the intestinal tract is bypassed, intravenous infusion is ideal for clients who are unable to ingest sufficient fluids orally. Calories, vitamins, and medications also can be delivered efficiently via the intravenous route.

Setting Up an Intravenous Infusion. A great number of setup components are available for assembling an intravenous apparatus. Generally, these components allow the clinician to vary the complexity of the setup to meet the therapeutic objectives. The basic setup, however, consists of a container and an administration set.

Solution Containers. Solution containers are of three types: glass bottles, soft plastic bags, and semirigid plastic containers. Each container is available in several sizes, ranging from 50 to 1000 mL in capacity (Fig. 31–9).

Glass bottles come in two varieties: those with a clear plastic airway within the bottle and those without. The airway, within the bottle, allows air to be drawn in to replace the fluid flowing out. This system prevents the development of a vacuum within the bottle, which prevents fluid flow. The bottle without the airway requires an administration set containing an air vent. Glass bottles commonly have volume calibrations, both upright and upside down, for easy inspection (see Fig. 31–9B).

Professional concern about the use of glass bottles arises because of the air required to displace fluid in the container to cause physical flow out of the container. There is still controversy about the sterility of room air, and whether it poses a possible risk of fluid contamination when drawn into the container.

The soft plastic bag is the most widely used container for solutions used in intravenous therapy. Because plastic bags are pliable, they collapse as the fluid flows out. The combination of gravity flow and the outside air pressing on the bag makes it unnecessary to have an air inlet port for the plastic bag.

Two ports are available, at the neck of the soft plastic bag. One is a resealable medication port; the other is for insertion of the administration set connector. The bag also contains calibrations of volume; however, the volume calibrations are difficult to use because plastic bags are often overfilled and collapse asymmetrically, and thus are unreliable. These calibrations, therefore, should be used only for cursory inspection.

The semirigid plastic container may be either cylindrical or square, and is composed of a semisoft compressible plastic. The advantage of these containers is that they collapse symmetrically, which allows for greater accuracy in

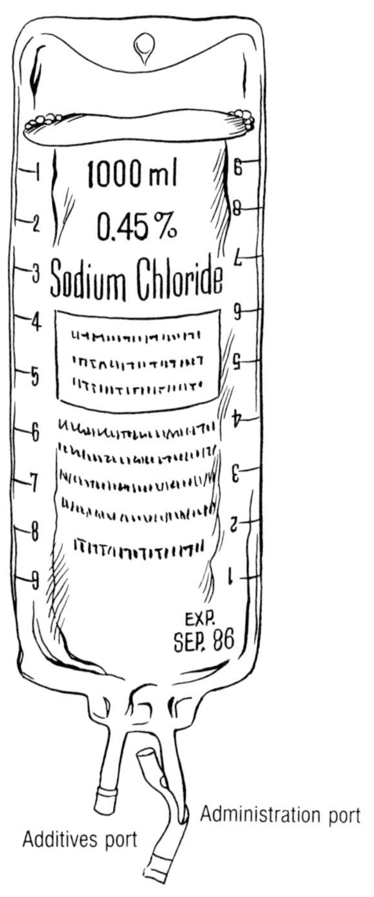

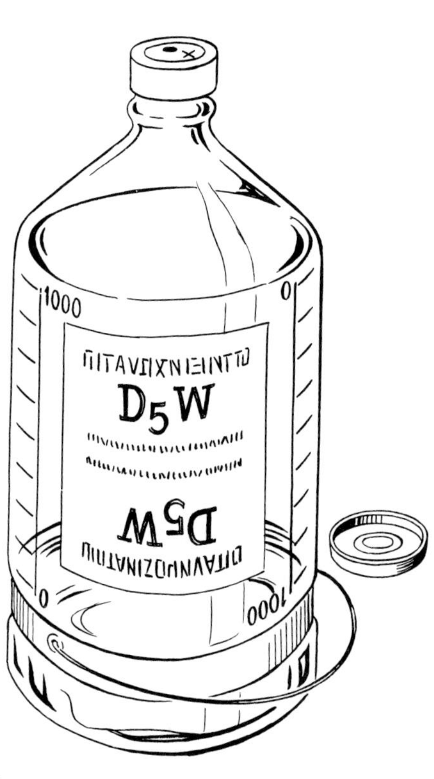

Figure 31–9. Types of IV solution containers: **A.** Plastic bag, **B.** glass bottle. (*From Norton BA, Miller AM.* Skills for Professional Nursing Practice: Communication, Physical Appraisal, and Clinical Techniques. *Norwalk, CT: Appleton-Century-Crofts; 1986:941.*)

observation of the infusing volumes of fluid. The plastic material is inert, so it is not reactive with the solutions or additives.

Intravenous Administration Sets. A basic intravenous administration set is illustrated in Figure 31–10. It consists of an insertion spike, a drip chamber, plastic tubing, a screw or roller clamp, a resealable injection site (often called a flashball), and a connector for attachment to the venipuncture device. The administration set provides a closed system for regulated flow from the solution container. Medications may be injected directly into the vein through the flashball.

The insertion spike is a pointed plastic cannula with a beveled end that is introduced into the entry port of the solution container. A short length of tubing leads from the insertion spike to the drip chamber. This small, flexible chamber, after being compressed and partially filled, allows the visualization of the drops of solution leaving the container. The drops are counted as a means of monitoring the rate of flow of the solution.

The roller clamp is a device that compresses the tubing that runs through it. By adjusting the clamp, the rate of flow of the solution is controlled. The flashball is a rubber hub with embossed circles that provide a guide to needle insertion. This hub is used for medication administration and can also serve as a temporary site for the addition of a second administration set from a different solution container.

The basic administration set ends with a plastic connector, often called the adaptor, to which the intravenous needle or cannula is attached. This connector may fit by friction or by a twisting lock system called a Luer lock.

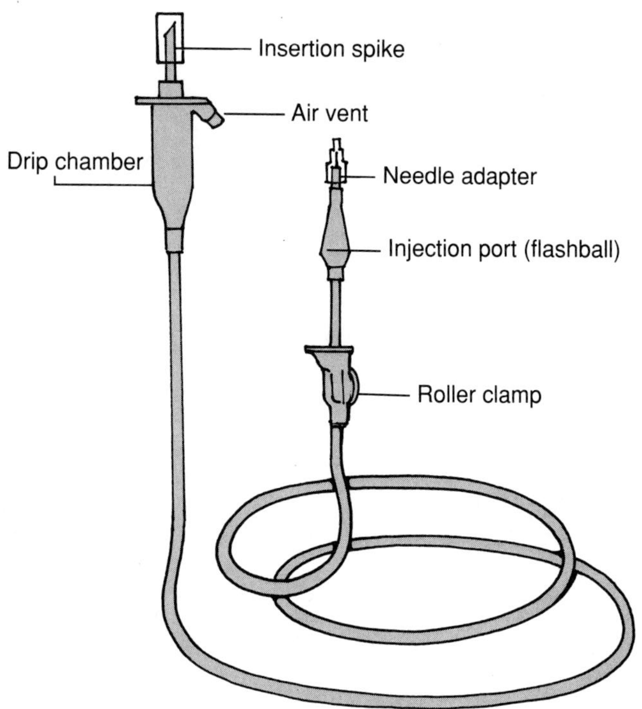

Figure 31–10. Basic intravenous infusion administration set.

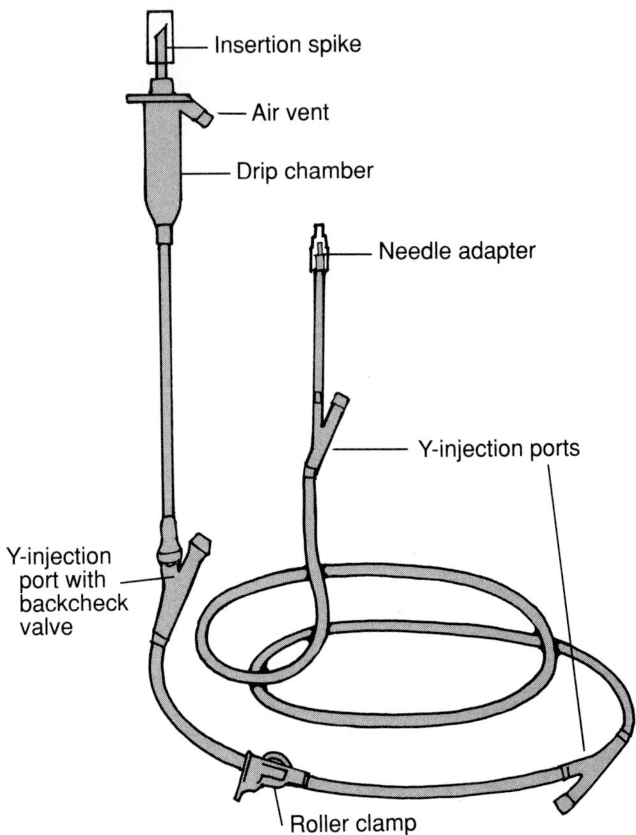

Figure 31–11. Intravenous tubing with Y injection site.

Additions to the basic administration set are numerous. Some of the more common devices are Y-type injection sets, check valves, in-line filters, and volume control sets. Many of these may be built in to different administration sets (Fig. 31–11), but are also available to add to the existing set should the need arise.

Administration sets are manufactured to deliver differing rates of flow. Common drip rates range from 10 to 20 drops per milliliter. Sets manufactured for pediatric use deliver 50 to 60 drops per milliliter. This information is provided on the packaging, and must be considered in calculating the rate of flow of the solution (Figs. 31–12 and 31–13). It is helpful to note that *drops* is frequently abbreviated as gtt. Where this abbreviation appears, it is accompanied by a number that designates the number of units per milliliter (the drip factor) delivered by the administration set, whether macrodrip or minidrip. The abbreviation may be found on the packaging or in the technical literature provided by administration set manufacturers.

The technique for preparing the solution container and administration set is outlined in Procedure 31–4. The ap-

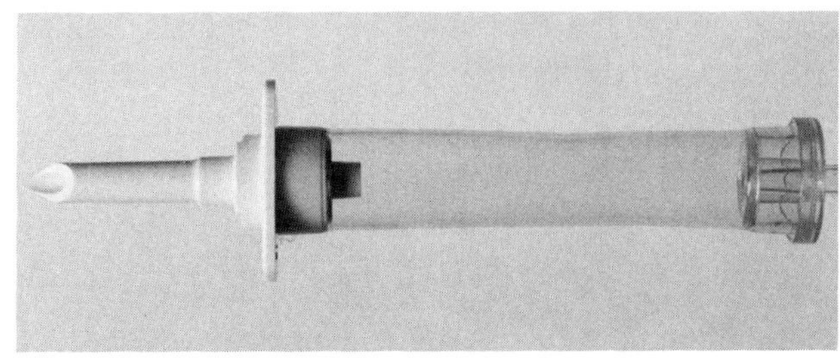

A

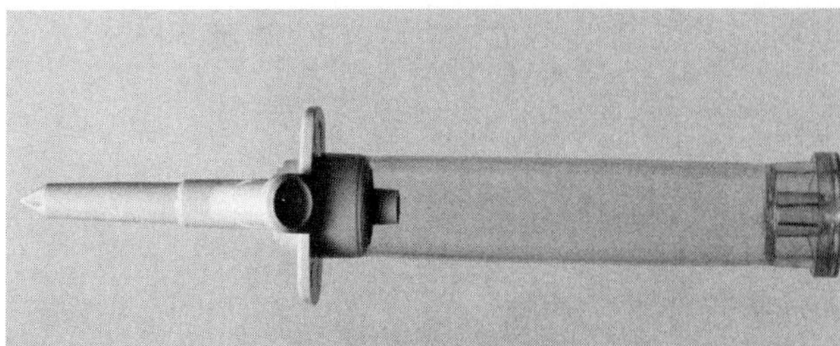

B

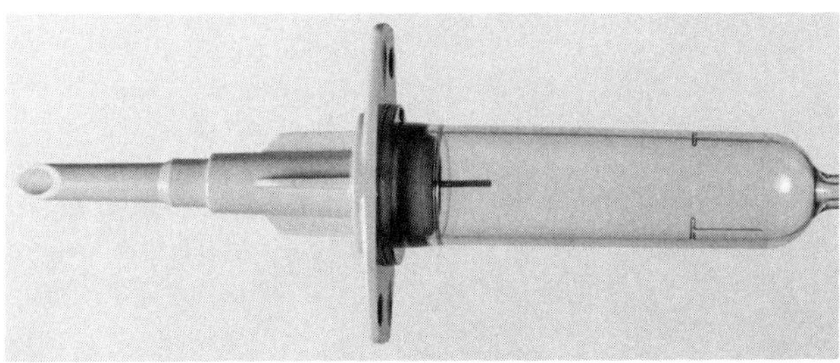

C

Figure 31–12. Vented and nonvented tubing: **A.** Nonvented macrodrip, **B.** vented macrodrip, **C.** microdrip.

paratus must be inspected, assembled, and filled before venipuncture.

Adjunctive Devices

IN-LINE FILTERS. In-line filters are devices designed to remove bacteria, fungi, and particulate matter from the solution before it enters the client (Fig. 31–14). The size of the pores, which filter contaminants, varies, but the most common size is 0.22 μm. Because of this microscopic pore size, they are often referred to as micropore filters. Filters are recommended for clients who are receiving total parenteral nutrition or heavily particulated solutions and for immunosuppressed clients.[31]

VOLUME CONTROL SETS. When a small volume of fluid, containing electrolytes or medications, is required, the use of a burette or a volume control set may be indicated. Burettes are small calibrated cylinders, with volumes of 50 to

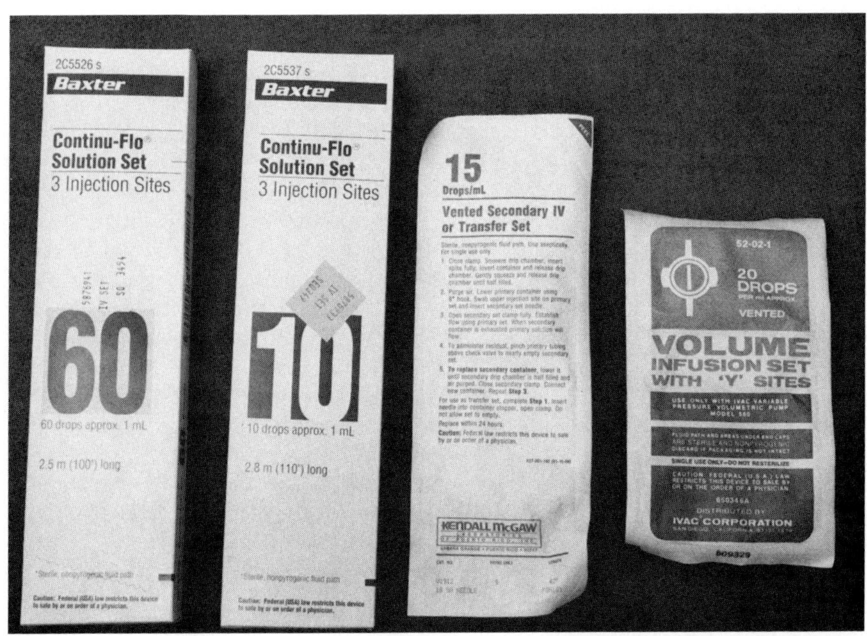

Figure 31–13. Intravenous tubing boxes showing various drip factors.

PROCEDURE 31–4. PREPARING AN INTRAVENOUS INFUSION SETUP

PURPOSE: To provide intravenous fluids and electrolytes to clients unable to ingest sufficient quantities orally; to treat fluid and/or electrolyte imbalances

EQUIPMENT: Ordered intravenous solution, basic IV administration set,[a] IV pole (if not available in room), label for tubing, in-line filter according to agency policy

ACTION	RATIONALE
1. Check physician's order for type and amount of solution, total time or flow rate of infusion, and additives, if any.	1. These are the components of a complete IV order; if elements are missing, confer with physician.
2. Wash your hands.	2. Transient organisms that could be pathogens are removed from hands, preventing transmission to the client.
3. Obtain the correct solution and administration set. NOTE: Select tubing with injection ports if IV piggyback medication is also ordered.	3. Incorrect solution can harm client and/or fail to achieve desired therapeutic effect. Incorrect tubing may prevent fluid flow.
4. Check container for leaks, cracks, or tears; solution for clarity, particles, and expiration date; set for cracks, crimps, or missing parts.	4. Any of these could allow contaminated solution to be administered to client.
5. Prepare container. **Plastic bag:** remove outer wrapping, leave ports covered. **Glass bottle:** remove metal ring and disk; leave latex disk in place.	5. Port covers and latex disk protect sterility of ports and contents until set is connected, by preventing direct contact with unsterile items.
6. Remove administration set from package and close roller clamp. NOTE: If in-line filter is required, attach it to tubing now, following manufacturer's directions.	6. Air is prevented from entering tubing and fluid from escaping through tubing.

[a] Unvented tubing is appropriate for plastic bags or bottles with airways; vented tubing for bottles without airways (see Figs. 31–12A and B).

(continued)

PROCEDURE 31–4. (continued)

7. Remove cap from spike end of tubing. Identify tubing port on container and insert spike. **Plastic bag:** pull off plastic cover and without touching spike to outside of port, insert spike with a firm twisting motion. Bag may be held on a flat surface or hung on IV pole.

Bag outlet is sealed before spiking, so no fluid will leak, even when bag is inverted. Touching spike to outside of port transfers organisms to spike, then to solution.

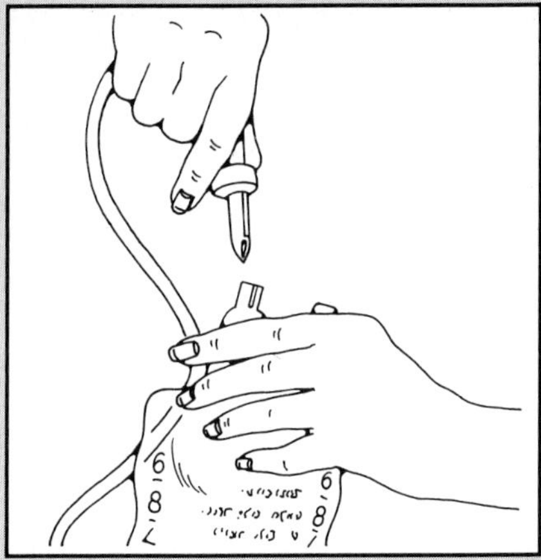

Glass bottle: remove latex disk (you should hear influx of air into bottle). With bottle standing on a secure surface, insert spike into larger of the two openings (not airway outlet) with a straight downward motion. Do not let spike contact rim of bottle.

There is no seal on bottle outlet once latex disk (which also seals vacuum) is removed, so it must remain upright. Secure surface allows force needed to insert spike into opening. Twisting spike into opening in bottle stopper may shear small shards of rubber and deposit them in IV solution. Touching spike to rim of bottle transfers organisms to spike, then to solution.

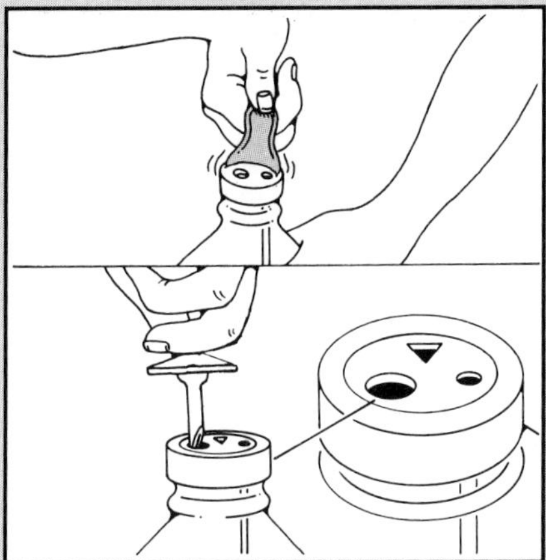

NOTE: Do not use bottle without vacuum seal (no "whoosh" of air). Without vacuum, contents may be contaminated.

8. Partially fill drip chamber: **Plastic bag:** squeeze chamber. **Glass bottle:** squeeze chamber, then invert bottle and hang on IV pole or wall hook. A small amount of liquid will escape from airway opening in vented bottles.

Squeezing chamber displaces air into container, allowing fluid to enter chamber. Overfilling drip chamber will make regulating IV impossible, as drips cannot be seen.

(continued)

PROCEDURE 31–4. (continued)

9. Remove and reserve protective cap from distal end of tubing. Hold tubing over sink, basin, or trash can and prime tubing by opening clamp and allowing fluid to displace all air in tubing. Do not allow end of cap or tubing to contact anything. Close roller clamp and replace cap.

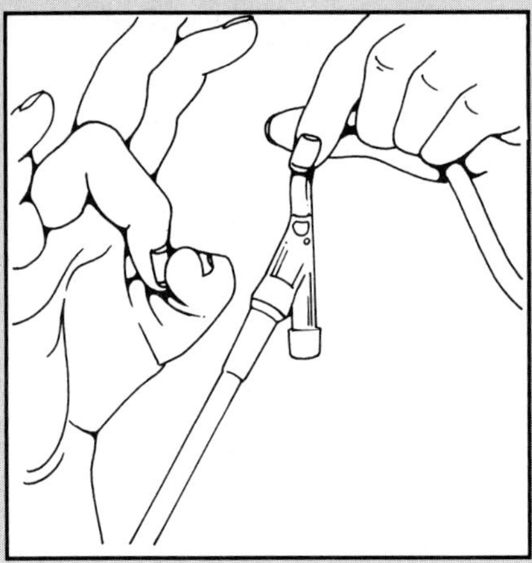

NOTE: If filter was added or tubing has injection ports, invert each one as tubing is primed and tap to remove air.

9. Air is removed from tubing to prevent air emboli (caused by entry of large amounts of air into bloodstream). Cap and tubing are prevented from contacting unsterile objects to prevent introduction of organisms into client's bloodstream.

10. Label tubing with date, time, and your initials. Time-tape container according to IV fluid order (see Procedure 31–9).

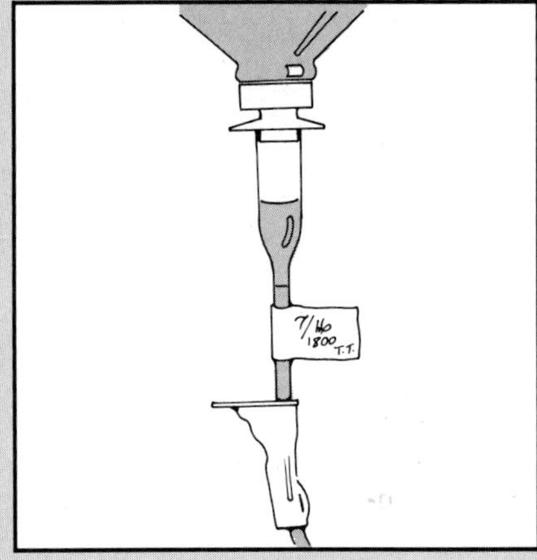

10. Permits changing tubing in accordance with agency policy and/or CDC guidelines to prevent fluid contamination secondary to prolonged use of IV equipment and readily assessing progress of infusion.

11. Take equipment to bedside and discuss anticipated venipuncture with the client.

11. Discussing procedure alleviates anxiety and concerns that may interfere with client participation.

RECORDING: Venipuncture (see Procedure 31–5) is recorded on nursing progress notes or daily care flowsheet. IV solution and flow rate may be documented on I&O sheet, flowsheet, or progress notes.

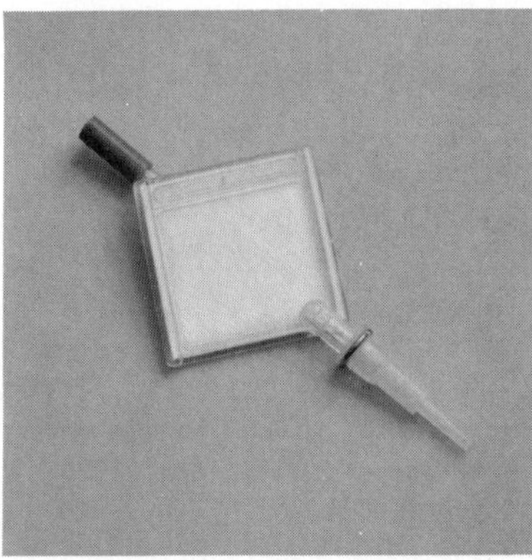

Figure 31–14. In-line filter. (*From Smith S, Duell D.* Clinical Nursing Skills: Basic to Advanced, *2nd ed. Norwalk, CT: Appleton & Lange; 1988:735.*)

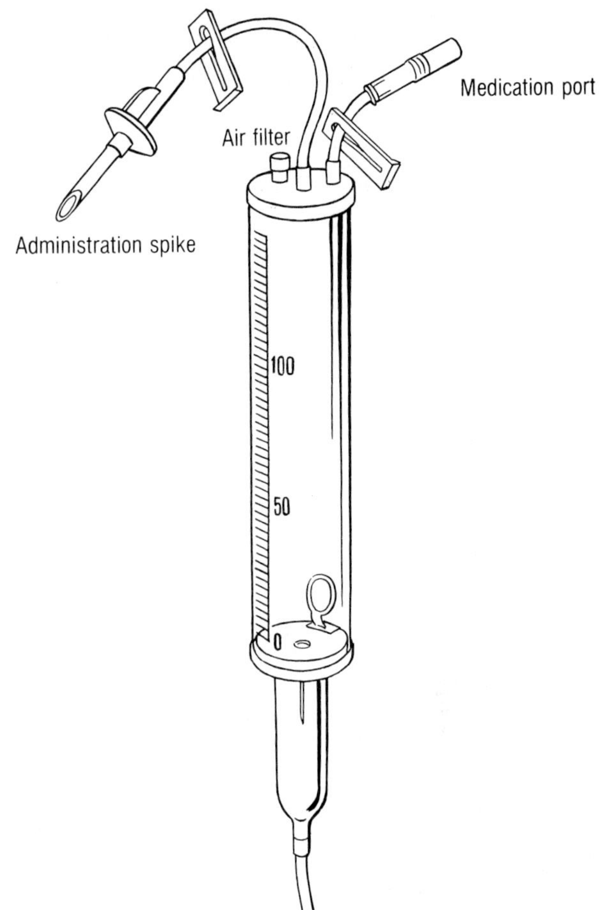

Figure 31–15. Burette style volume control container. (*From Norton BA, Miller AM.* Skills for Professional Nursing Practice: Communication, Physical Appraisal, and Clinical Techniques. *Norwalk, CT: Appleton-Century-Crofts; 1986:942.*)

150 mL, which are filled from the primary solution containers (Fig. 31–15). An additive port is usually located on top of the container. Roller clamps are located above and below the container for filling and control of flow. Drip rates varying from 10 to 60 drops per milliliter are provided.

HEPARIN LOCK. A heparin lock is a resealable injection port that can be attached to a venipuncture device (Fig. 31–16). It is used to administer intermittent medications via IV push or drip. It provides direct venous access, but allows clients much more mobility and freedom than a continuous IV infusion. It is called a heparin lock because a small amount of heparinized solution is injected into it after each use to maintain patency. Some agencies use a normal saline injection to maintain patency. Agency policies and procedures for infusing medications and maintaining patency of heparin locks vary. The SASH method (saline; administer medication; saline; heparin) is common. (See Procedure 22–18 for administration of an IV drip medication via a heparin lock.)

NEEDLELESS INJECTION SITE. In some agencies, the standard heparin lock is being replaced by a needleless injection site. Although similar in appearance to the heparin lock, its design permits puncture using a special plastic cannula (Fig. 31–17) rather than a needle. It reseals after puncture just as the standard heparin lock does. The manufacturer recommends that the needleless injection site be attached to the venipuncture device at the time of venipuncture, even when the purpose of the venipuncture is the administration of continuous intravenous fluids (see Procedure 31–4).

Attaching a companion device, a needleless cannula with threaded lock (Fig. 31–18), to the end of the intravenous tubing permits a secure connection between the injection site and the tubing; the system is then used exactly as standard IV equipment. However, if the course of the IV fluid therapy is sufficiently lengthy that the IV administration set (tubing) must be replaced, the threaded needleless cannula is easily separated from the injection site without loss of blood via the venipuncture device and new tubing with needleless cannula easily attached.

If a client no longer needs IV fluid therapy, but venous access is needed for administration of medications, disconnecting the threaded needleless cannula with attached tubing readies the injection site for IV push or IV piggyback medications (see Chap. 22). Patency of the injection site is maintained according to the same heparin flush protocol as for standard heparin locks. A needleless cannula without a threaded lock also is available for use on a standard syringe (Fig. 31–19), for administration of IV push medications or flushing with heparin.

Intravenous Solutions. Intravenous solutions are classified in three ways: according to their chemical nature (crystalloid or colloid), their tonicity, or their intended therapeutic use.

The physician's order for an intravenous solution should specify type of solution, amount to be infused, flow

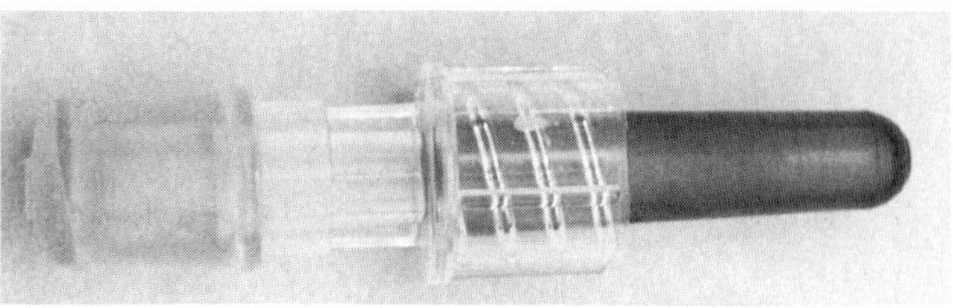

A

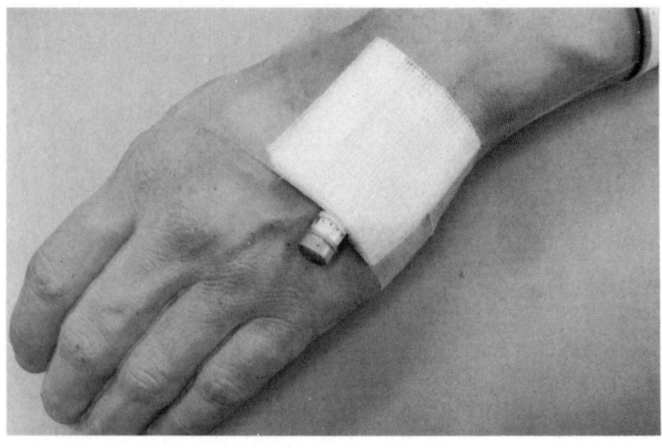

B

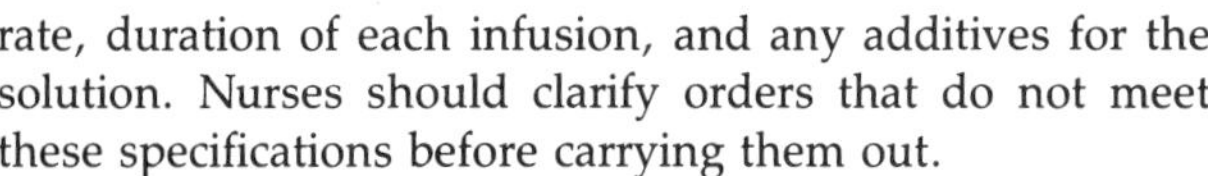

Figure 31–16. **A.** Heparin lock with Luer. **B.** Heparin lock on client. (**B** *from Smith S, Duell D.* Clinical Nursing Skills: Nursing Process Model; Basic to Advanced Skills, *2nd ed. Norwalk, CT: Appleton & Lange; 1988:766.*)

rate, duration of each infusion, and any additives for the solution. Nurses should clarify orders that do not meet these specifications before carrying them out.

Intravenous solutions are often divided into two classes: crystalloids and colloids. Crystalloid solutions are composed of water and solutes that tend to form crystals when the water is removed. Examples include 5 percent dextrose in water (D5W), lactated Ringer's (a solution containing sodium, potassium, calcium, chloride, and lactate), and normal saline (0.9 percent NaCl). Colloids are proteins, sugars, or starches suspended in fluid that exert the same type of osmotic force as plasma proteins.[41] Intravenous solutions are also designated as isotonic, hypotonic, or hypertonic in reference to plasma. Table 31–17 summarizes the types of available solutions, their tonicity, and their common therapeutic uses.

Isotonic solutions generally exert no net osmotic force in the intravascular compartment. Isotonic solutions tend to distribute between the intravascular and interstitial compartments the same way that body fluid does, thus hydrating both compartments.[41] Hypotonic solutions, which have less solute than water, dilute the plasma. As a result, fluid flows into the dehydrated interstitial compartment.[41] Hypertonic solutions, which have more solute than water, are generally used to replace solutes or to cause a net fluid shift into a dehydrated intravascular space.[41]

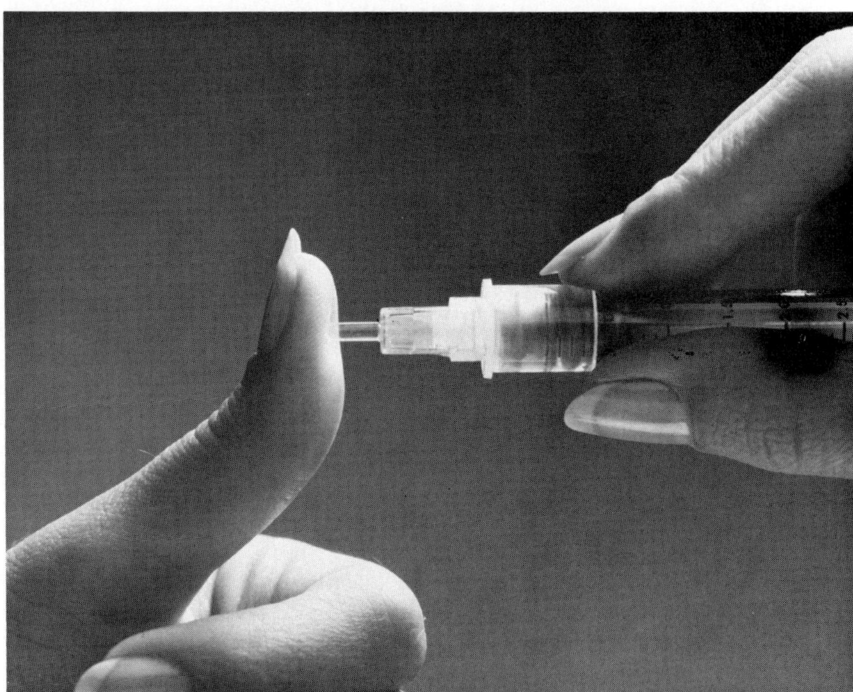

Figure 31–17. In the InterLink™ IV Access System, a blunt plastic cannula replaces the conventional sharp steel needle typically used. The InterLink™ cannula is used just like a sharp steel needle to pierce an injection cap, but the blunt cannula cannot cause an accidental needle stick. (*Courtesy of Baxter Healthcare Corporation, Deerfield, IL.*)

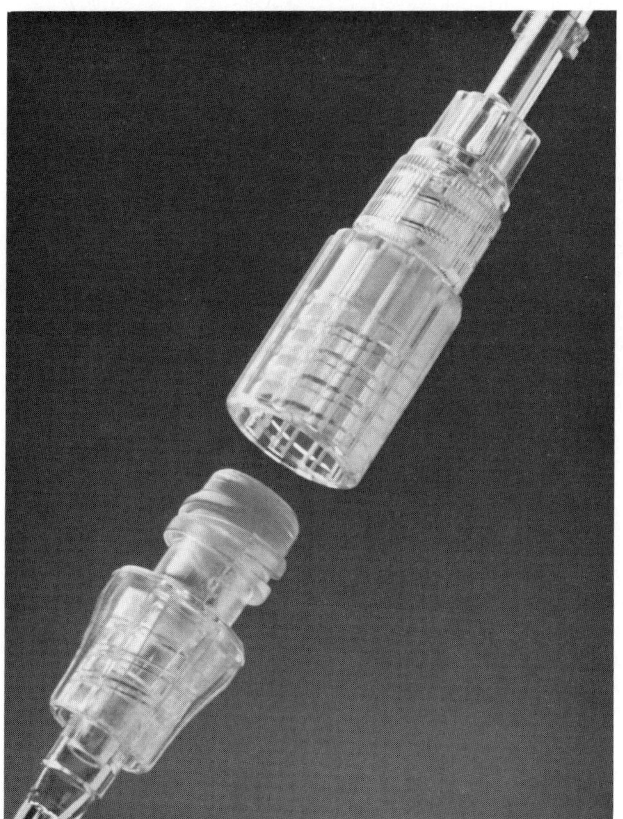

Figure 31–18. The InterLink™ Threaded Lock Cannula securely connects to an InterLink™ Injection Site without taping. This Luer locking feature provides a secure, sterile and leak-free connection between IV devices, that minimizes touch contamination. (*Courtesy of Baxter Healthcare Corporation, Deerfield, IL.*)

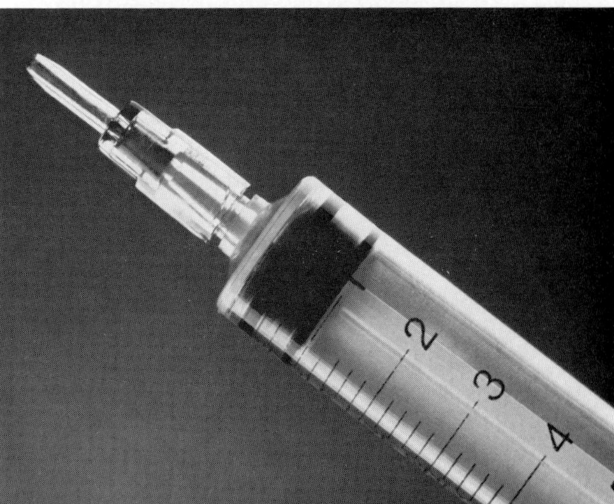

Figure 31–19. The InterLink™ Cannula can easily be fitted onto a standard syringe with the same technique used for traditional steel needles. (*Courtesy of Baxter Healthcare Corporation, Deerfield, IL.*)

Intravenous solutions are prepared to fulfill various therapeutic objectives. Rehydration, replacement of solutes and calories, correction of hypovolemia, and supporting nutrition are among the therapeutic values of the commonly used solutions.

Hydrating solutions are used to maintain or replace body water when there is no substantial solute loss. Hydrating solutions, in addition to supporting circulatory effort, reestablish urine flow reduced by dehydration.

Replacement solutions are used when there is a substantial loss of electrolytes and body water. Such fluids contain electrolytes, nonelectrolytes, acids, and bases to correct solute losses.

Plasma expanders expand the intravascular volume in hypovolemic states. They include actual plasma proteins in solution and large-molecule solutes, which contain roughly the same colloidal properties as plasma. As plasma expanders have osmotic properties, fluid shifts from the interstitial space, helping to further increase intravascular volume.

Nutrient solutions supply calories and prevent negative nitrogen balance. These solutions, such as total parenteral nutrition formulas (discussed below), may supply as much as 1000 calories per liter. Standard intravenous solution containing dextrose delivers minimum caloric content. One liter of D_5W provides only 177 calories.[31]

ADDITIVES. Nurses must sometimes add medications or solutes to intravenous fluid. These include electrolytes, antibiotics, and vitamins. Intravenous electrolytes, most often potassium, are usually prepared by the pharmacy, but it may be the nurse's responsibility to add specific amounts. It is therefore important to determine the solution suitable for mixing and delivering the supplement. Usually this information is available from a pharmacist or on the inserts that pharmacological companies supply with their medications.

Preparing the Intravenous Setup. The technique for preparing the intravenous setup is outlined in Procedure 31–4. Assemble the intravenous setup in the cleanest possible surroundings, to prevent contamination. Compare the solution container with the physician's order to ascertain the appropriate fluid. Before assembling the solution container with the intravenous tubing, compare any required additives with physician's orders and add them to the solution container. (See Chap. 22 for administration of IV additives.)

Venipuncture. **Venipuncture** is the act of puncturing a vein for any purpose. There are two major considerations in performing venipuncture: selection of appropriate equipment and selection of the best site for entering the vein. Policies regarding who is responsible for intravenous infusion and venipuncture, as well as care and maintenance of the sites and infusions, vary among institutions. The nurse

TABLE 31–17. COMMON INTRAVENOUS SOLUTIONS

Solution	Tonicity	Therapeutic Use
Crystalloids		
D5W (5% dextrose in water)	Isotonic	Hydration and minimal calorie replacement
D5NS (5% dextrose in normal saline)	Isotonic	Hydration, electrolyte and minimal calorie replacement
D5½NS (5% dextrose in 0.45% [half-strength] NaCl)	Hypotonic	Hydration
NS (normal saline; 0.9% NaCl)	Isotonic	Hydration and electrolyte replacement
½ NS (half-strength normal saline)	Hypotonic	Electrolyte replacement
3% NS[a]	Hypertonic	Electrolyte replacement
5% NS[a]	Hypertonic	Electrolyte replacement
Lactated Ringer's[b]	Isotonic	Hydration and electrolyte replacement
Isolyte R	Hypotonic	Hydration and multiple electrolyte replacement
Normosol M	Hypotonic	Hydration and multiple electrolyte replacement
Plasmalyte M	Hypotonic	Hydration and multiple electrolyte replacement
Colloids[c]		
Serum albumin 5%, 25%		Volume replacement in hemorrhage and hypovolemia Hypoproteinemia
Plasmanate 5%		Hypovolemia and hemorrhage
Dextran 6%, 10%		Hypovolemia and hemorrhage
Hetastarch		Hypovolemic states

[a] Hypertonic solutions are irritating to veins.
[b] Lactated Ringer's is not for use in clients with renal failure because of its potassium content.
[c] Colloids may predispose to allergic reactions.
Data from Sommers[41] and Rutherford.[42]

should be familiar with institutional policy before attempting venipuncture or intravenous infusion.

Venipuncture Equipment. There are four basic types of venipuncture devices. Each involves a slightly different technique for entering the vein. The devices include butterfly or wing-tipped needles, over-the-needle catheters, inside-the-needle catheters, and plastic indwelling catheters without needles (Fig. 13–20). All venipuncture devices share common features, such as variance in gauge and length, screw-lock adaptors, and various types of needle guards to protect sterility.

Butterfly needles are short and thin-walled, for entering very superficial veins. They vary from 27 to 16 gauge. Gauge refers to the inner diameter of the needle or catheter. The smaller the number, the larger the diameter. The short bevel, or diagonal cutting surface of the needle, prevents trauma to the opposite wall of the vein and leakage of blood into the tissue. Short needle lengths and large lumens allow for rapid fluid administration.

The butterfly device is well suited to short-term infusion into the small, peripheral veins (dorsum of hand, scalp, etc). Pediatric and elderly clients with small, fragile veins or sclerotic changes may benefit from the use of this type of device.

Over-the-needle and inside-the-needle catheters have similar components but are opposite in design. These plastic catheters are used when rapid or long-term infusion is required. They are better suited to the larger, sturdier peripheral veins.

The over-the-needle catheter consists of a catheter mounted over a needle, with the bevel of the needle protruding from the end of the catheter. Once the vein is pierced, the needle is withdrawn and the catheter inserted into the vein. The inside-the-needle catheter contains a catheter inside the needle lumen. As the vein is pierced, the needle is retracted back away as the catheter is inserted.

BUILDING NURSING KNOWLEDGE

What Are the Fluid Needs of the Client Who Is n.p.o.?

Kennedy-Caldwell C. Clinical triads: Water metabolism, the NPO patient, and parenteral nutrition. *Crit Care Nurs.* 1986;6(3):63–64.

The authors noted that one problem experienced by n.p.o. clients is body water imbalance. The normal rate of water turnover approaches 6 percent of body content per day in an adult and 15 percent per day in an infant. A reasonable water allowance is 1 mL (0.03 oz)/kcal for adults, or 1200 to 3300 mL/d. Water weight gain can be differentiated from true weight gain by assessing a client's total caloric intake and fluid intake and output. For a client who is on a refeeding (weight gain) regime, a weight gain of about 2 oz/d is desirable. Any greater rate probably reflects excess fluid.

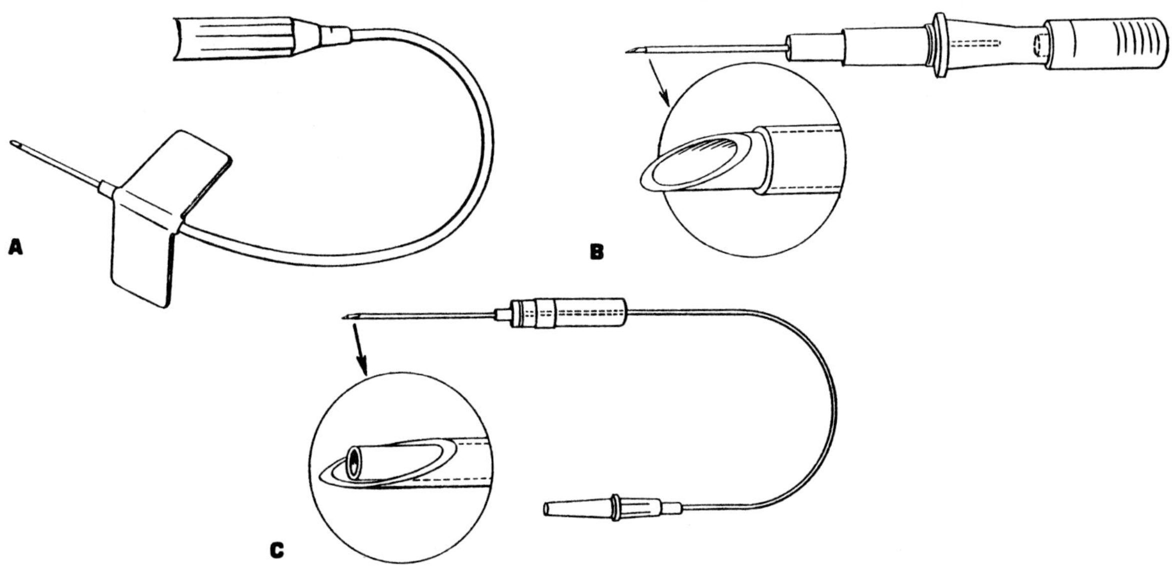

Figure 31–20. Various venipuncture devices: **A.** Double butterfly needle with attached heparin lockport; **B.** over-the-needle catheter, **C.** inside-the-needle catheter. (*Adapted from Norton BA, Miller AM.* Skills for Professional Nursing Practice: Communication, Physical Appraisal, and Clinical Techniques. *Norwalk, CT: Appleton-Century-Crofts; 1986:943.*)

In-the-needle catheters are typically longer and better suited to prolonged infusion, or the administration of particularly irritating solutions.

In situations of vascular collapse or severe sclerosis of the veins, it may become necessary for the physician to directly visualize and enter a vein. This procedure, known as cutdown, involves surgically entering the tissue and isolating a large vein. A plastic catheter, without a needle, is then inserted. Sutures are used to close and stabilize the area. This procedure is usually employed only in dire emergencies.

Intravenous Site Selection. Selection of the appropriate venipuncture site may often determine the success or failure of intravenous therapy. Factors to be considered in IV site selection include (1) purpose of the infusion, (2) condition of the veins, (3) type of solution and additives, (4) volume and rate of infusion, (5) duration of therapy, and (6) client activity level.

In general, veins should be selected that are elastic and apparently strong. As an additional rule of thumb, sites should be as distal as possible to preserve veins for a progressive proximal selection of sites, should the need arise. The most prominent veins are not always the most adequate; they may be sclerotic or have lumen obstruction. The veins commonly used for intravenous infusion are depicted in Figure 31–21.

The metacarpal veins on the dorsum of the hand are best suited to short-term infusions, because of their relative lack of stability and potential fragility. The larger veins of the forearm and antecubital fossa are best reserved for rapid, high-volume infusion or moderately prolonged therapy. These veins are usually employed for blood administration.

Veins of the lower extremities should be used only if no other sites are available, because of the risk of thromboembolism. They should never be used in diabetic clients, because of compromised circulation and potential for inflammation and tissue necrosis.[31]

The client's activity level is another important consideration. Although the dorsum of the hand may be an easy site to enter, the potential for movement and dislodgement is high. In the wrist or antecubital fossa, as well, flexion may require immobilization of the extremity, which may add to the client's discomfort.

The purpose of the infusion and the duration of therapy determine the type, volume, and rapidity of infusion. Highly viscous infusions, prolonged therapy, irritating drugs, large quantities of fluid, and fluid under pressure require large, strong veins.

Venipuncture Techniques. The technique for venipuncture is outlined in Procedure 31–5. Institutional policy will guide site preparation. In general, an antiseptic, such as alcohol or povidone–iodine, is used to cleanse the area. It is applied in a spiral pattern from site outward. Avoid povidone–iodine for clients allergic to iodine. A preparatory shave of the area is optional in clients with excessive hair growth at the selected site. This is not considered a routine measure.

Palpate the selected vein with two or three fingertips. Do not use the thumb, as it has a pulse and is less sensitive than the fingertips. Palpation should locate sufficient straight-vein area to accommodate the length of the catheter or needle from hub to tip.

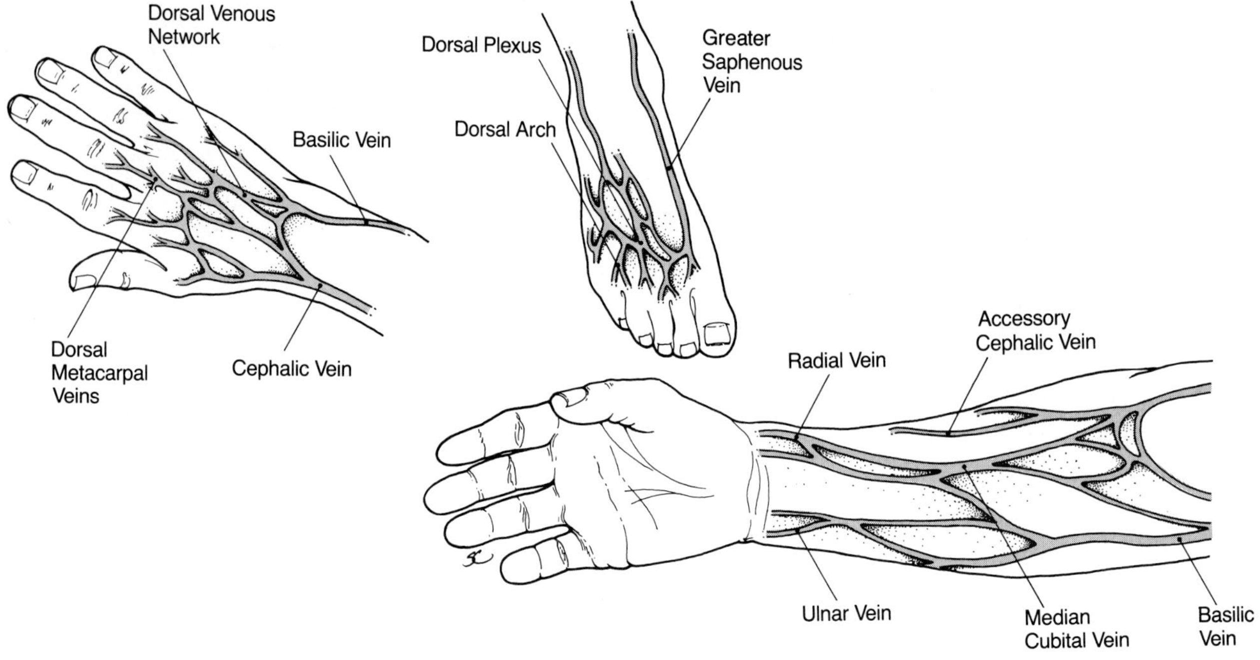

A

Internal jugular vein

Sternocleidomastoid muscle

External jugular vein

Clavicle

Sternum

Subclavian vein

B

Figure 31–21. Venipuncture sites: **A.** Peripheral sites (hand, arm, foot); **B.** central venous catheter sites (central venous catheters are inserted by physicians). (**A** *from Smith S, Duell D.* Clinical Nursing Skills: Nursing Process Model, Basic to Advanced Skills, *2nd ed. Norwalk, CT: Appleton & Lange; 1989:739.* **B** *from Chesnutt M, Dewar R.* Office and Bedside Procedures. *Norwalk, CT: Appleton & Lange; 1992: (Fig. 5–11.)*

PROCEDURE 31–5. STARTING AN INTRAVENOUS INFUSION

PURPOSE: To create access for administration of intravenous fluids, electrolytes, or medication

EQUIPMENT: Tourniquet, antiseptic cleanser, ½- and 1-in. tape, venipuncture device, assembled infusion set on overhead hanger or IV pole (see Procedure 31–4), gauze sponges or transparent dressing, disposable underpad, gloves, armboard (optional)

ACTION	RATIONALE
1. Discuss the procedure, desired client participation, and anticipated benefits with the client. Acknowledge discomfort associated with venipuncture.	1. Active participation is more likely if the client understands expectations and benefits and feels empathy from a nurse. Failure to recognize that the invasiveness and pain that occur with venipuncture are threatening to many individuals increases client's stress and distrust.
2. Wash your hands. Assemble equipment.	2. Removes transient organisms that could be pathogens from hands, preventing transmission to the client.
3. Palpate superficial veins of the nondominant hand or arm (dorsal foot veins used for infants/young children). Avoid veins that feel hard or ropey and veins near joint surfaces. If no suitable vein is found, assess other arm. Place disposable underpad under extremity selected for venipuncture.	3. Use of nondominant limb maximizes independence when IV is infusing. Vein sclerosis is possible cause of hard, ropey veins. Venipuncture near joint space limits client mobility and comfort and is more likely to infiltrate. Underpad under extremity protects bed linen in case of bleeding during venipuncture.
4. Ask the client to hold extremity in dependent position for a minute. Apply tourniquet proximal to the insertion site and ask client to pump the fist several times. 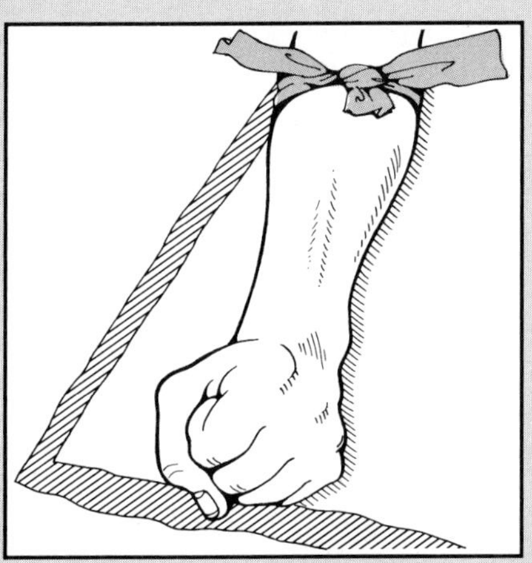	4. These measures dilate the vein. Dilation of vein facilitates venipuncture. If these measures are insufficient, tapping the vein or applying superficial heat for several minutes may help.

(continued)

PROCEDURE 31–5. (continued)

5. Cleanse the skin over the insertion site with antiseptic swabs, using a firm circular motion from the center outward.

5. Friction and outward cleansing motion, in addition to chemical antiseptic action, remove organisms from site, preventing their introduction into client's circulatory system.

6. Don gloves.

6. Body fluids, particularly blood, may contain pathogens that could infect nurse if introduced via breaks in skin, such as scratches and chapped skin.

7. Grasp the extremity, and apply traction to the skin distal to the insertion site.

7. Tension on the skin helps to stabilize the vein wall, and reduces the tendency of the vein to slip away from the needle tip.

8. Hold the needle, with the bevel up, and enter the skin at a 30- to 45-degree angle, over the intended site. Pierce the skin and subcutaneous tissue.

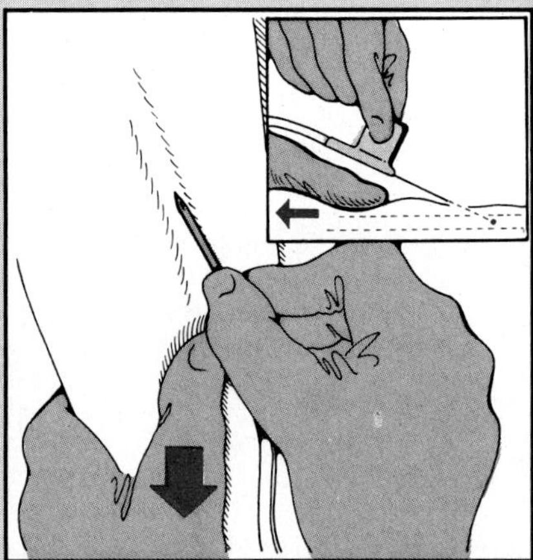

8. The angle of entry is varied with the depth of the vein: the deeper the vein, the wider the angle.

9. Once the needle has pierced the tissue, decrease the angle of the device closer to the client's skin and advance the needle in the direction of the vein until you feel a decrease in resistance to the needle.

9. Decreasing the angle places the venipuncture device in position to thread into the vein. Decreased resistance indicates needle has entered the vein.

(continued)

PROCEDURE 31–5. (continued)

10. Wait for a blood return into the butterfly tubing or catheter hub, then advance the device into the vein. If no blood return is noted immediately with over-the-needle catheter, partially withdraw needle. If catheter is in vein, blood should now flow into hub of needle. If so, advance catheter into vein.

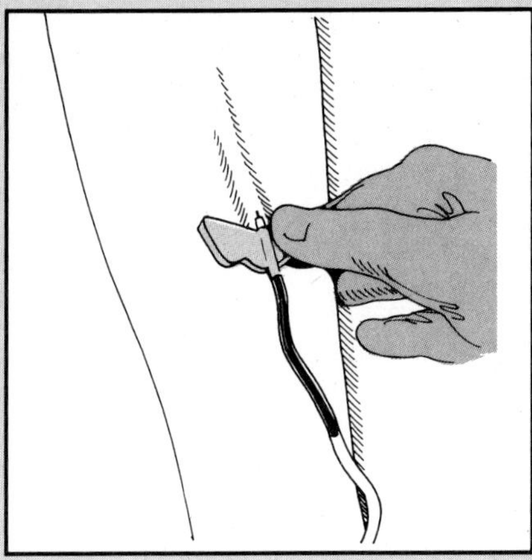

10. A blood return indicates successful entry into the vessel. If no blood return is noted, select a new site and attempt venipuncture with a new sterile device. With the over-the-needle catheter, needle inside plastic catheter may block blood flow until moved from catheter tip.

NOTE: Some practitioners advance the over-the-needle catheter only 0.6 cm (1/4 in.) before removing needle to decrease possibility of piercing vein wall (see step 11).

11. Attach the IV tubing:

a. *For butterfly:*
As blood is filling the butterfly tubing, remove protective cap from IV tubing without touching the end of the tubing or allowing it to contact client's skin. When blood reaches the end of butterfly tubing, connect IV tubing and butterfly tubing.

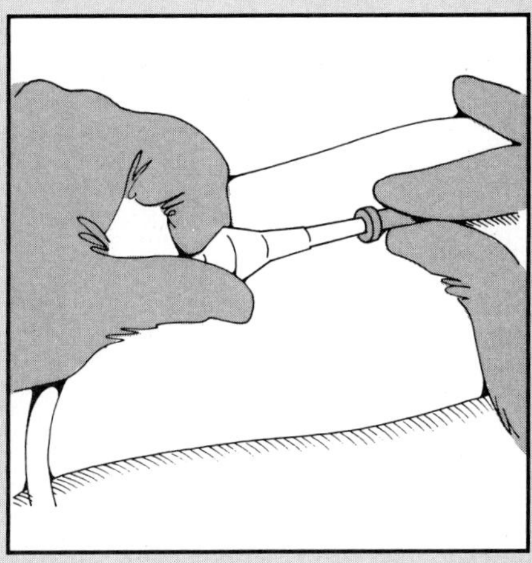

11a. Blood must displace air in butterfly tubing to prevent introducing air into client's bloodstream. Preventing contact of tip of tubing with unsterile objects prevents transfer of microorganisms into client's vein.

(continued)

PROCEDURE 31–5. (continued)

b. *For inside-the-needle or over-the-needle catheters:*
Place one finger or thumb firmly over skin above the tip of the catheter to temporarily occlude vein, and gently remove needle. Then remove cap from IV tubing and attach to catheter hub. Release finger pressure and advance catheter completely, if not advanced previously.

11b. Temporary occlusion of vein prevents blood loss while withdrawing needle and attaching tubing, thereby maintaining cleanliness and decreasing client's distress.

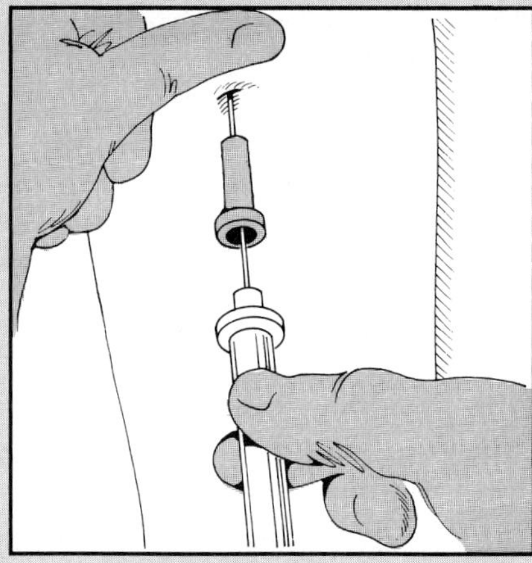

c. *For needleless injection systems:*
Before attempting venipuncture, attach needleless cannula with threaded lock to end of IV tubing, leaving protective cap in place. When venipuncture is accomplished, attach InterLink injection site to catheter hub or end of butterfly tubing. Then remove cap from needleless cannula (the channel for fluid escape) on tubing and attach to injection site, securing with threaded lock.

11c. Needleless system was designed to prevent needle-stick injuries and associated transmission of blood-borne diseases. Attachment of InterLink injection site at time of venipuncture makes conversion to a heparin lock (see Chap. 22) possible without breaking the continuity of the closed system, reducing infection risk to the client.

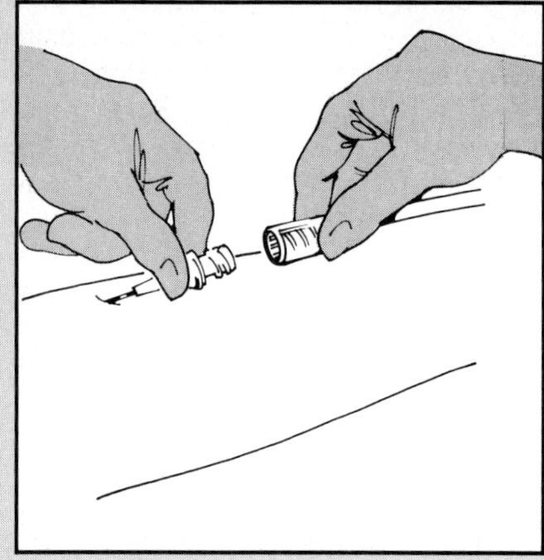

12. Release the tourniquet, and initiate flow of IV infusion.

12. Promotes normal blood flow and prevents clotting.

13. Stabilize the device and tubing with tape, and apply a sterile dressing over the venipuncture site (see Procedure 31–6).

13. Immediate stabilization of the area prevents dislodging the device.

(continued)

PROCEDURE 31–5. (continued)

14. Remove underpad and gloves, and dispose of them in receptacle marked infectious waste.

14. Labeling enables the staff to determine the schedule for dressing and site changes.

15. Label the site dressing with the date and time of insertion and the gauge of the venipuncture device, according to agency policy.

15. See step 6. These items may be soiled with blood.

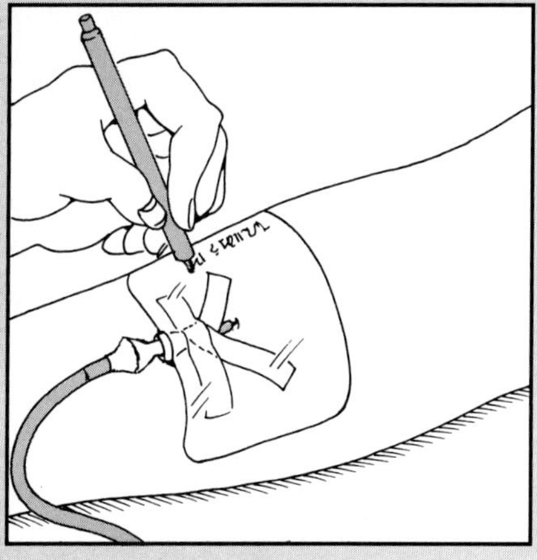

NOTE: Labeling is not done in some agencies.

16. Make sure client is clean and comfortable before leaving.

16. Promotes client well-being.

RECORDING: Note venipuncture location, size and type of device, type and rate of infusion, any problems with procedure, and associated actions in nursing progress notes. Record on IV or I&O records according to agency policy.

Maintaining the Venipuncture Site. Once the venipuncture has been completed and a connection made, it is essential to maintain stability of the device and prevent infection of the site. To accomplish these objectives, secure the venipuncture device against movement, apply appropriate site dressings frequently, monitor the infusion and site carefully, and immobilize the extremity, if necessary.

Securing the needle or catheter involves taping the device to the client's extremity. In taping the device, leave the injection ports uncovered for easy access. Specific considerations for securing the IV are discussed in Procedure 31–6.

The dressings used vary widely and are studied frequently in nursing research. Some institutions still use sterile gauze dressings and tape; others use transparent adhesive dressings. Sterile gauze dressings prevent direct visualization of the site and become soiled easily. Transparent adhesive dressings allow direct visualization of the area and form a bacterial barrier; however, they may irritate the skin and are more costly than sterile gauze. Dressings should be changed regularly, at least every 24 hours or sooner if wet or obviously soiled.

Immobilization of the extremity may become necessary to stabilize and protect the IV site. Application of an armboard can help secure a site at a flexion point. The armboard should be short, lightweight, well padded, and should allow for adequate circulation. Specific guidelines for applying an armboard are listed in Procedure 31–7.

Initiating, Regulating, and Monitoring the IV Flow Rate. Once venipuncture has been accomplished and the site stabilized, the flow of solution can begin. The nurse should check to see that air bubbles have been expelled from the tubing. Clients often fear that the tiniest air bubble is dangerous; however, most small bubbles are reabsorbed by the circulation. At least 10 mL of air is required to create an air embolus.

Initiating the IV Flow. To initiate the flow of solution, ensure that fluid fills the tubing, sterility has been maintained, and all necessary adjunctive equipment has been added. Check the solution again to make sure it is the correct type before beginning the infusion. Initiate the flow by slowly opening the roller clamp after connecting to the venipuncture device. The solution will begin to drip into the drip chamber. Next, regulate the flow according to the physician's pre-

PROCEDURE 31–6. SECURING AND DRESSING VENIPUNCTURE SITE

☐ **PURPOSE:** To prevent dislodging device and protect the site against infection

☐ **EQUIPMENT:** Sterile gauze square, adhesive bandage, or transparent dressing, ½ and 1-in. micropore tape, antibacterial ointment according to agency policy

ACTION

1. Secure venipuncture device:
   a. *To secure a butterfly needle:*
      "H" Method:
      Place a ½ × 2-in. piece of tape vertically over each wing.
      Place a ½ × 3-in. piece of tape across both wings.

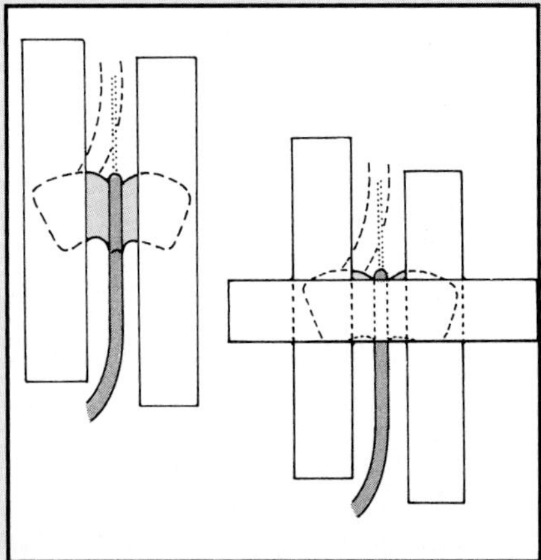

Chevron Method:
Place a ½ × 2-in. piece of tape across both wings.
Place a ½ × 3-in. piece of tape, sticky side up under butterfly tubing, just distal to wings.
Cross ends of tape diagonally across wings.

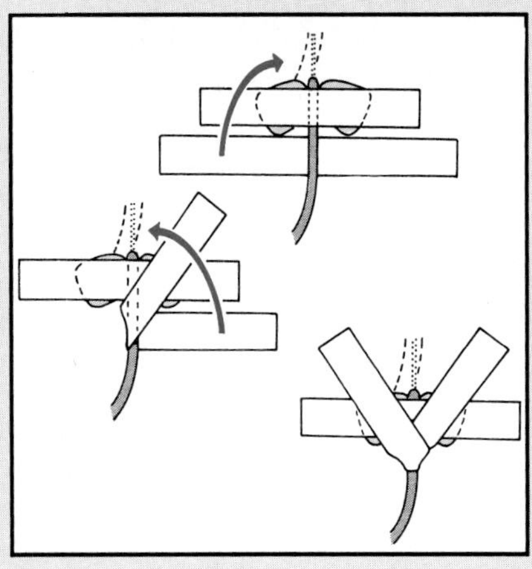

   b. *To secure over-the-needle catheter:*
      Place a ½ × 3-in. piece of tape sticky side up under hub.
      Cross ends of tape over one another in a "V" shape so the bars extend toward the heart.
      Place ½ × 2-in. piece of tape straight across hub.

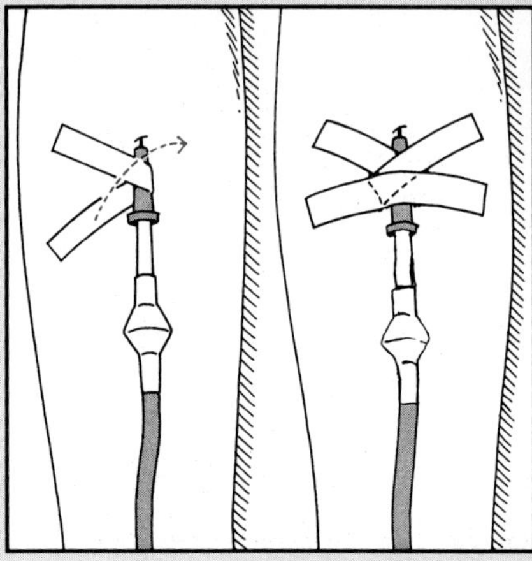

NOTE: if bandage or gauze dressing is planned (see step 3), place over puncture site before the above steps.

2. Place a small amount of antibacterial ointment on venipuncture site if agency policy so specifies.
3. Dress venipuncture site:
   a. *Transparent dressing*
      Remove smaller piece of paper backing; affix edge of dressing to skin so it will be centered over venipuncture site.
      Stabilize fixed edge of dressing with one hand. Smooth dressing over site by pulling remaining paper backing toward opposite edge of dressing.

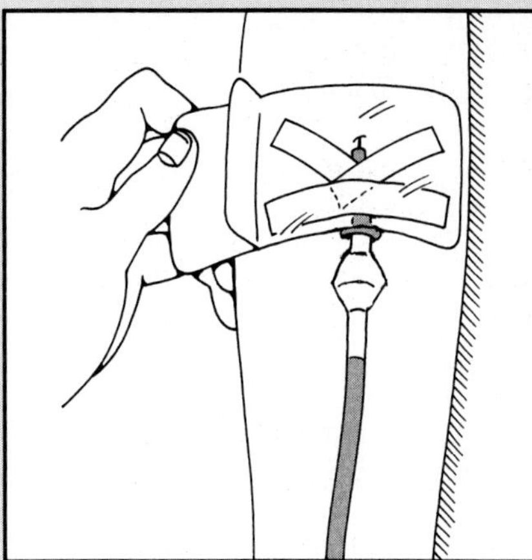

For window-type brands remove entire backing and use frame to center dressing over puncture site, smoothing dressing from center to edges.

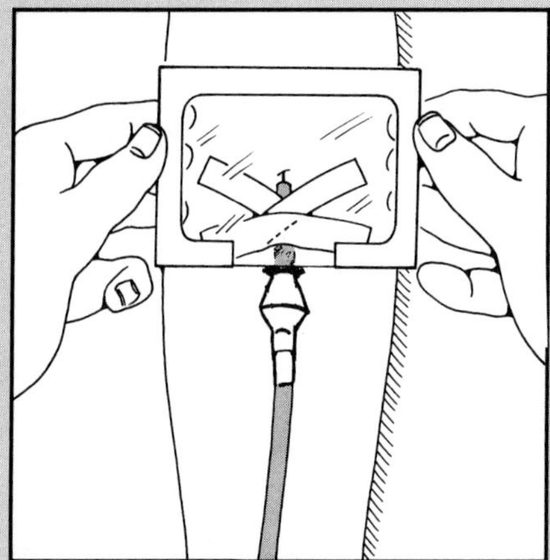

b. *Gauze dressing*
   Fold 2 × 2-in. in half, place over venipuncture site, and secure with 1-in. tape.
c. *Adhesive bandage*
   Center absorbent pad over venipuncture, and affix adhesive ends to skin.

4. Note current date and time on dressing, if agency policy.
5. Secure IV tubing. Make a loop using about 10 in. of tubing; secure loop above and below dressing with 1 × 4-in. pieces of tape.

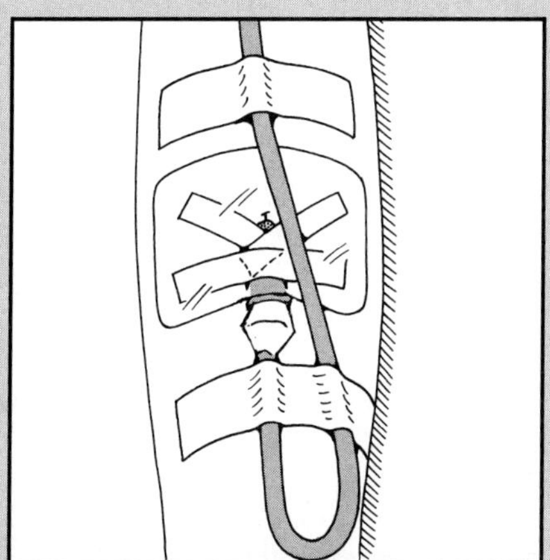

RECORDING: No separate recording is necessary, unless dressing on existing venipuncture site is being replaced. Then note date and time of dressing change and site condition on progress notes.

PROCEDURE 31–7. APPLYING AN ARMBOARD

PURPOSE: To limit flexion of a joint and provide stability to a venipuncture device located near the joint

EQUIPMENT: Padded armboard, 1-in. tape

ACTION

1. Cut two strips of 1-in. tape approximately one-half the circumference of the client's arm.
2. Cut two strips of tape long enough to nearly encircle the client's arm.
3. To "back" tapes, center the sticky side of the short tapes against the sticky side of the longer tapes, creating a nonadhesive band with two adhesive tails.

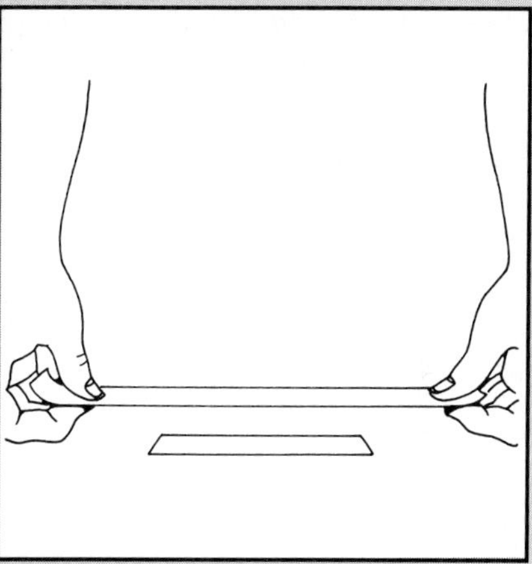

4. Place armboard under client's forearm, so that fingers flex over the end of the board and the thumb has full range of motion.
5. Place nonadhesive band over client's arm and affix sticky tape tails to underside of armboard. Do not overlap the ends of the tape to completely encircle the arm. This may constrict circulation. Apply at least one more tape to secure armboard.

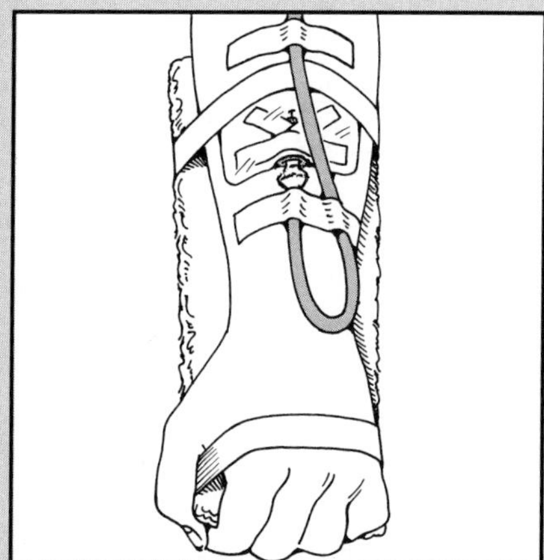

6. Assess circulatory status of fingers and client comfort.

RECORDING: No recording is required.

scription. The rate of flow is prescribed in milliliters per hour, and must be translated into drops per minute. Count the drops while adjusting the screw clamp to deliver the correct number of drops.

Calculating the IV Flow Rate. Box 31–11 shows the mathematical formula and guidelines for calculating and timing drip rates. Various types of intravenous tubing deliver different drop sizes, resulting in different numbers of drops per milliliter delivered. Check the package information to ascertain the drop factor of the tubing used.

Regulating the IV Flow Rate. Periodic checks of the drip rate are necessary because many variables can alter IV flow rate. Minor deviations often occur as the client changes positions. These may be of little consequence, if the IV does not require extremely precise regulation; however, to determine whether the rate of flow is adequate, monitor the solution level in the bottle as well as the drip rate. For precise control of volume delivered and drip rate, an in-line burette may be used. Procedure 31–8 describes how to fill an in-line burette.

BOX 31–11. CALCULATING AND ADJUSTING INTRAVEOUS DRIP RATES

Calculation Formulas

1. $\frac{\text{Total volume to be infused}}{\text{number of hours to run}} = \text{mL/h}$
2. $\frac{\text{mL/h} \times \text{gtt factor}}{\text{60 min/h}} = \text{gtt/min}$

Examples

1. $\frac{\text{1000 mL}}{\text{8h}} = \text{125 mL/h}$
2. $\frac{\text{125 mL/h} \times \text{15 gtt/mL}}{\text{60 min/h}} = \text{31.25 (32) gtt/min}$

Nursing Considerations

1. Check physician's order to verify flow rate.
2. Calculate drip rate, using formula.
3. Count drops for 15 seconds and multiply by 4 to determine actual IV flow rate.
4. Compare actual rate with prescribed rate.
5. Assess for any apparatus-related or client-related cause for flow discrepancy.
6. Remember that drip rates vary with quantity of fluid to be delivered and period of time for delivery. The larger the quantity of fluid, over the shorter the duration, the faster the drip rate.
7. Drip rates vary with size of droplets. The larger the droplet, the fewer drops necessary to deliver a given volume.
8. The "drop factor" indicates the caliber of the droplet dispensed. The packaging information for the various administration sets provides the information.
9. Reducing fraction to lowest common denominator results in a consistent ratio: if gtt factor is 10, divide mL/h by 6; if gH factor is 15, divide mL/h by 4; if gH factor is 20, divide mL/h by 3; if gtt factor is 60, divide mL/h by 1.

The solution level is easier to monitor when hourly levels are marked on the solution container. To do this, vertically align a strip of tape with the calibrations on the container and mark on the tape the level the solution should reach each hour. As the fluid level drops, the nurse can check whether the actual rate of flow corresponds with the desired rate. Procedure 31–9 outlines the steps in time-taping an intravenous container.

INFUSION CONTROL DEVICES. Unlike burettes, which control flow by limiting available volume, infusion control devices control the *rate* of fluid flow. Two problems with IV flow rates are (1) achieving precise control of volume delivered and (2) preventing uncontrolled, rapid delivery. Both problems may be minimized by the use of infusion control devices. Various types of devices are available; these include electronic pumps, infusion controllers, and devices that operate as both a pump and a controller (Fig. 31–22).

Infusion controllers control rate by the use of a photoelectric eye on the drip chamber. The tubing is enclosed in a clamping device inside the controller. The desired rate is set in milliliters per hour. Because a controller does not physically pump the solution, but acts with the use of gravity, it is necessary to maintain the solution container at least 36 in. above the venipuncture site.

Unlike controllers, which rely on gravity flow, infusion pumps create a positive pressure to direct flow. The rate-set pump relies on threading tubing through a series of clamps, which compress the tubing in wavelike form, creating peristaltic movement of the fluid. Volumetric pumps incorporate a piston, which fills and expels a precise amount of fluid, according to settings made on the face of the instrument.

Safety mechanisms, such as air bubble detectors and high-pressure clamps, are built into these devices. Most units also have electronic displays to guide the user in device setup, display total volumes infused, or warn of mechanical difficulties.

Client safety is maintained only if the nurse carefully checks the machine, the basic design, and the setup. The responsibility for correct operation, as well as monitoring the infusion, remains with the nurse. Use of the devices should not lure the nurse into a false sense of security.

Troubleshooting the Erratic IV. Despite the nurse's best efforts, some IVs require frequent adjustment. Many apparatus-related, solution-related, and client-related variables affect fluid flow and make control difficult. These factors are summarized in Table 31–18.

APPARATUS-RELATED VARIABLES. Variables related to the IV system involve the principles of fluid dynamics. The vertical distance between the solution container and the client is important in maintaining flow rate. The smaller the distance, the slower the flow. The recommended distance is at least 36 in. In addition, excessive tubing lengths, kinks in the tubing, or the use of very small gauge venipuncture devices will slow the flow rate.

SOLUTION-RELATED VARIABLES. The viscosity of the IV fluid affects the rate of flow. Blood, blood components, or

PROCEDURE 31–8. FILLING THE IN-LINE BURETTE

☐ **PURPOSE:** To closely control the volume of intravenous infusion

☐ **EQUIPMENT:** An in-place intravenous apparatus, inclusive of an in-line burette

ACTION

1. Assess for patency of the IV.
2. Open the airway and slide clamp on the top of the burette to allow for fluid flow.

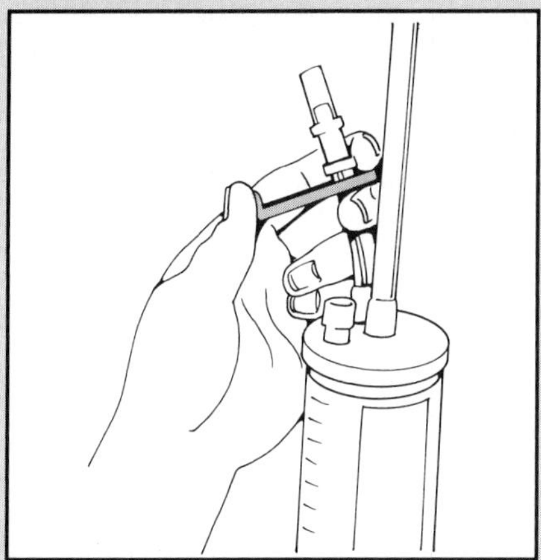

3. Open the roller clamp or slide clamp between the solution container and the burette and fill to desired level. Stop flow from solution container by closing the clamp.

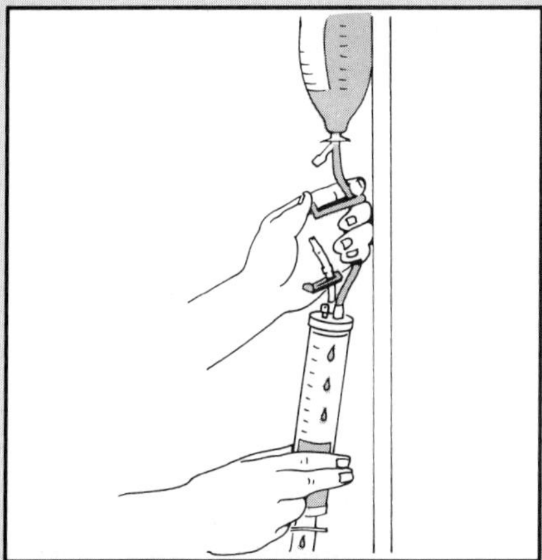

4. If burette is being used to administer medication, prepare medication in a syringe, cleanse medication port, insert needle, and inject medication into burette. Swirl burette or roll it between your hands to mix medication evenly in solution.

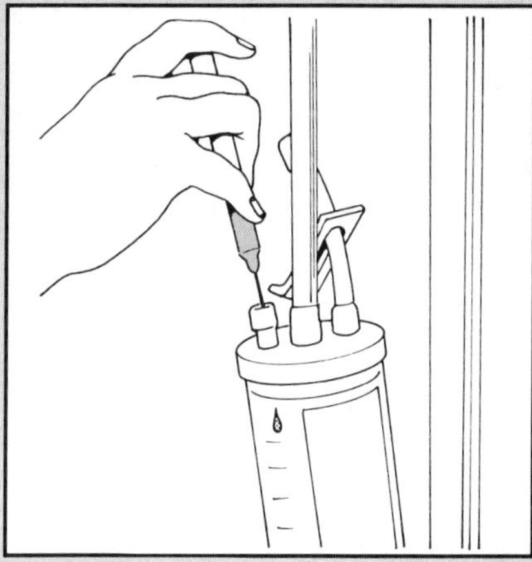

5. Start the infusion flow and adjust the rate of flow, using the roller clamp between the bottom of the burette and the venipuncture device.
6. Calculate the finish time of the volume contained in the burette.
7. Return prior to conclusion of the flow and assess for volume in the burette. Refill as necessary.

☐ **RECORDING:** Use of a burette need not be specifically recorded; however, hourly volume infused is recorded on I&O record and medication given is noted on medication administration record (MAR).

PROCEDURE 31–9. TIME-TAPING AN INTRAVENOUS CONTAINER

▭ **PURPOSE:** To provide rapid visible approximation of IV infusion flow

▭ **EQUIPMENT:** Commercial time-tape or 1-in. adhesive

1. Calculate the intravenous flow rate in mL/h.
2. Affix commercial time-tape to IV bottle or plastic bag so volume indications on time-tape line up with corresponding markings on container. If no commercial tape is available, affix 1-in. tape along the length of the container adjacent to the volume markings.

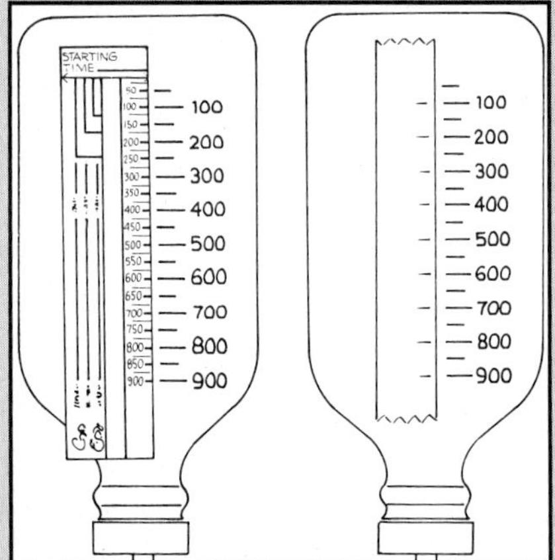

3. Make a mark on the tape at intervals representing the hourly volume to be infused. For example, if the rate is 100 mL/h, mark 100 mL, 200 mL, 300 mL, and so on.

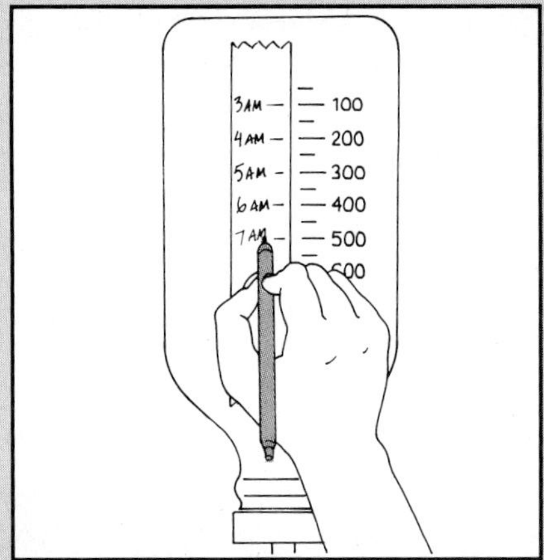

4. Write the current time at the top of the tape and the time at successive 1-hour intervals next to the marks along the length of the tape. The last time entry should approximate the time the infusion is expected to finish.

▭ **RECORDING:** No recording is required.

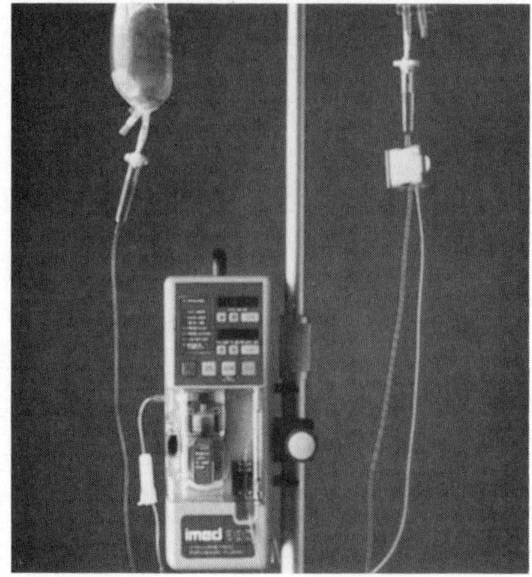

A

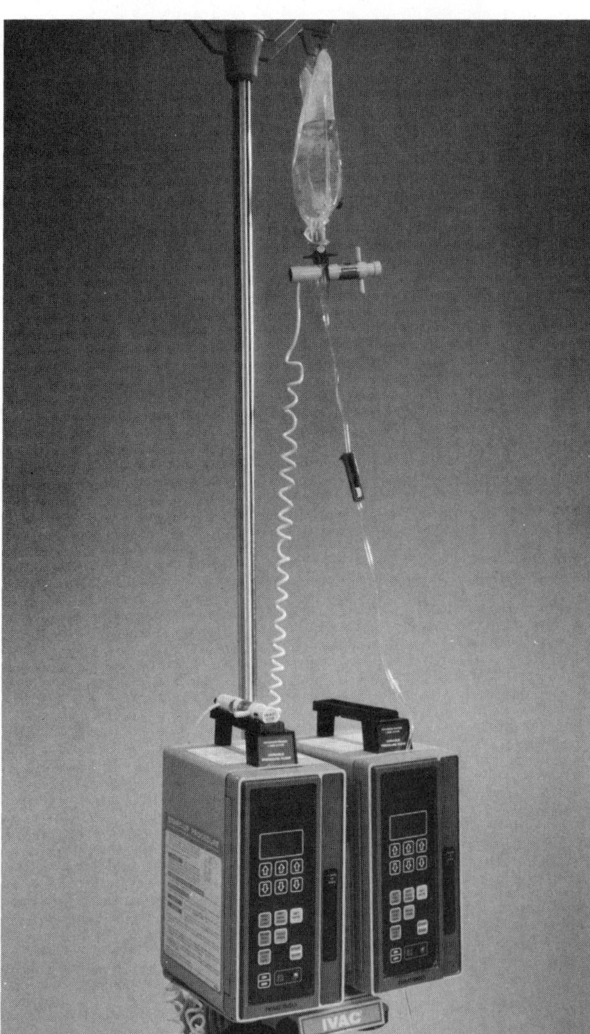

B

Figure 31–22. Infusion control devices: **A.** Volumetric pump. (Courtesy of IMED Corporation, San Diego, CA.) **B.** Volume controller. (*From Smith S, Duell D.* Clinical Nursing Skills: Nursing Process Model; Basic to Advanced Skills, *2nd ed. Norwalk, CT: Appleton & Lange; 1988:750.*)

TABLE 31–18. TROUBLESHOOTING THE INTRAVENOUS INFUSION

Problem	Approach
1. No flow is visible in tubing	Adjust height of container to achieve better gravitational flow
	Determine if the solution container or burette is empty, and refill or replace accordingly (see Procedure 31–10)
	Observe for clots or kinks in administration set
	Encourage client to rotate extremity gently to determine if flow resumes
	Observe for the signs of venous infiltration or phlebitis; if present, discontinue infusion, and restart according to physician's orders
2. Unable to see drops because drip chamber is full	Close roller clamp; remove solution container from pole and invert; squeeze drip chamber to depress half of contents back into solution container; rehang container and open clamp; readjust flow
3. Solution flow is slower than desired rate	Determine if tubing is too long and, if so, replace with shorter tubing or remove any added lengths of additional tubing
	Ask client to rotate extremity gently to determine if flow changes; if so, attempt to retape or secure device with additional tape
	Use infusion controllers or pumps with highly viscous solutions
	Assess if tape or armboard is constricting site, and loosen
	Observe for the signs of venous infiltration or phlebitis; if present, discontinue infusion, and restart according to physician's orders
	Assess for venous spasm; if present apply warm packs to area
4. Visible clots in tubing	Change the tubing; do not attempt to remove by irrigation
5. Client complaint of pain at venipuncture site and in extremity	Solution may be cold. Let solutions reach room temperature prior to infusion
	Assess the site for signs of infiltration or phlebitis; if present, discontinue infusion and resume with new venipuncture site and equipment, according to physician's orders
6. Large air spaces in tubing	Slow infusion rate. Insert a sterile 10–20 mL syringe with a 22–23 gauge needle into the additive port that is closest to the air space, but distal to it. As the air nears the port, crimp the tubing below the port and aspirate the air into the syringe.
	If most of the tubing is filled with air, change the tubing rather than attempting to remove the air. Small air bubbles have no pathological significance and can be ignored.

solutions with high solute content form smaller and fewer drops in a given period than less viscous solutions.

CLIENT-RELATED VARIABLES. Physiological parameters such as the client's blood pressure may affect the flow of the IV solution. Hypotension may predispose to clot formation or venous spasm. Client movement often repositions the venipuncture device within the vessel; the bevel may press against the wall of the vessel and occlude or markedly slow flow. The client who raises or lowers the extremity containing the IV changes the gravitational flow pattern by changing the height of the device in relation to the solution container.

Generally, it is best to begin problem assessment by starting at the solution container and working downward to the venipuncture site. Consider each component of the system, as well as the client's activity level and vital signs, when troubleshooting the intravenous infusion.

Replacing the Intravenous Container and Tubing. It is necessary to replace intravenous solution containers and tubing periodically to provide for continuous, unimpeded flow and prevent infection. To protect the client, the Centers for Disease Control (CDC) makes the following recommendations:

- Change the parenteral fluid container at least every 24 hours.
- Change administration sets to peripheral IV sites at least every 48 hours.
- Change peripheral IV site dressings at least every 24 hours.

- Rotate the peripheral IV needle or catheter insertions site at least every 48 to 72 hours.[43]

A recent study suggests that it is safe to keep intravenous burettes and tubings in place as long as 72 hours.[44] Because less frequent changes conserve supplies and professional time, many institutions are adjusting their policies to reflect this finding. Guidelines for replacing an intravenous container and tubing appear in Procedure 31–10.

Discontinuing an Intravenous Infusion. A physician's order is required for discontinuation of an IV. Guidelines for the removal of an IV are presented in Procedure 31–11.

Recording Intravenous Fluid Intake. The record of intravenous intake is important to the assessment of fluid balance. On the intake and output form, the nurse notes the time, type, and total amount of fluid started in the column for parenteral fluids. If a container is changed or the flow stopped before the container is empty, subtract the volume remaining from the total volume and record the actual volume infused.

Record the volume in the old container when a new container is started. In addition, record infusion volumes at the end of each shift and total them every 24 hours. The volume remaining at the end of each shift is carried over to the next shift's records.

Complications of Intravenous Infusions. Intravenous infusions carry the potential for many complications. Localized complications such as infiltration can cause discomfort. Systemic complications such as sepsis or air embolus can be life-threatening. All of the complications may be prevented through collaboration with the client and health care team. The most commonly observed complications are infiltration, thrombus formation, phlebitis, sepsis, air embolus, circulatory overload, and speed shock.

Infiltration. Infiltration is the internal puncture of the vein by the venipuncture device. This allows solution and blood to escape into the surrounding tissues. The result is slowing or stoppage of solution flow, edema, coolness and pallor of the site, and tenderness of the area. Infiltration may result in tissue necrosis if hypertonic or irritating solutions are being infused. Once the infiltration has been confirmed, the venipuncture device should be removed immediately.

Thrombus Formation. Thrombi are small blood clots that may occur if the venipuncture device traumatizes the vessel wall on entry. The resulting clot may eventually obstruct the needle or catheter. A clot also represents an accumulation site for bacterial growth in the vascular system, which may later predispose to sepsis.

Phlebitis. Phlebitis is inflammation of a vein. The signs are erythema (redness), tenderness, and heat. The erythema may extend along the course of the vein resulting in a characteristic streak of redness. The phlebitis may result from mechanical irritation from the venipuncture device or chemical irritation from the solution. Thrombus formation is often combined with phlebitis, resulting in thrombophlebitis. These conditions may limit the future use of the vessels for venipuncture.

Sepsis. Sepsis is the systemic invasion of the bloodstream by an infection source. Sepsis may lead to circulatory collapse and death. Suspect sepsis whenever a client develops fever, chills, and hypotension during an intravenous infusion. The entire solution container and administration set should be saved and scrutinized carefully for signs of contamination.

Air Embolism. An air embolism is a potentially deadly complication resulting from the entry of a large quantity of air forms into the systemic circulation. This air forms large bubbles that block the pulmonary circulation. Solution containers that require air venting predispose to this complication and should be monitored carefully.

The signs of air embolus are sudden hypotension, dyspnea, cyanosis, and eventual loss of consciousness. On seeing these signs, immediately clamp the administration set and place the client in the Trendelenberg position on the left side, which traps the air in the right atrium. Begin oxygen administration and seek immediate advanced medical treatment.

Measures to prevent air embolus include placing roller clamps below the client's chest level to avoid creating negative pressure (pulling) in the tubing, avoiding use of glass bottles, using longer infusion sets that drop slightly below the client's extremity, and keeping drip chambers partially filled to prevent air from entering the system.[31]

Circulatory Overload. Circulatory overload may result from rapid infusion of fluids into clients with impaired cardiac or renal mechanisms. Signs and symptoms include hypertension, dyspnea, and engorged neck veins. Preventive measures include maintaining prescribed flow rates, avoiding increased flow rates, and using volume-controlled administration sets.[31]

Speed Shock. Speed shock is a condition that develops when a medication or additive is infused too rapidly. The substances enter the circulation and collect, leading to a toxic effect. Signs and symptoms include hypotension, dyspnea, chest pain, facial flushing, and syncope. Use of pediatric infusion sets or electronically controlled infusion devices may control solution flow. If the medication is to be given by IV push, knowledge of the speed with which to give the medication and the potential effects of the medication is of paramount importance.

Assisting the Client With an IV to Perform Daily Activities. Clients with an IV in place may have difficulty changing gowns, eating, bathing, and ambulating. The insertion site should therefore be chosen with consideration of these activities. For most clients, the nondominant arm is best. If this is impossible, the client will require some help with

PROCEDURE 31–10. REPLACING INTRAVENOUS CONTAINER AND TUBING

PURPOSE: To prevent nosocomial infection

EQUIPMENT: Sterile solution container, sterile administration set, sterile gauze pads, gloves, label to date new tubing.

ACTION	RATIONALE
1. Discuss the procedure with the client, including the reason, the anticipated benefits, and the desired client participation.	1. Active participation is more likely if the client understands the expected benefits and desired behavior.
2. Wash your hands.	2. Removes transient organisms that could be pathogens from hands, preventing transmission to the client.
3. Prepare the new container and tubing and take to bedside. (See Procedure 31–4.) Remove dressing from venipuncture site. Remove tape securing tubing.	3. Dressing covers and secures needle adapter from existing tubing to venipuncture device.
4. Place a small sterile gauze pad under hub of venipuncture device; don gloves. Stabilize device with one hand. Carefully loosen existing tubing from device using a twisting motion, but do not disconnect. Close roller clamp on existing IV.	4. Gauze pad absorbs any blood that leaks during exchange; gloves protect nurse from pathogens that may be present in client's blood. Loosening tubing facilitates exchange without disrupting venipuncture device. Clamping tubing prevents leakage of solution during exchange.

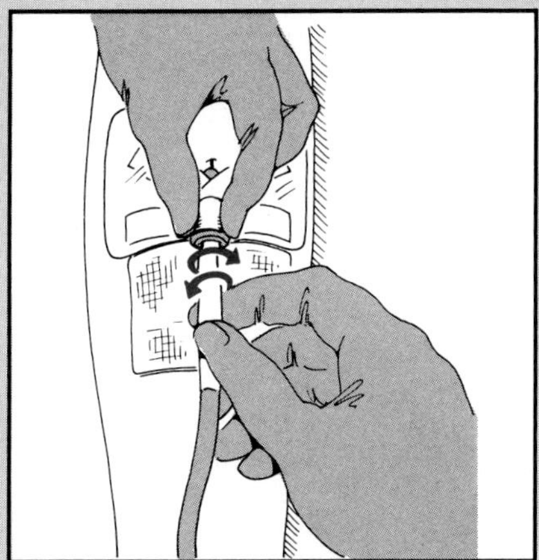

NOTE: Tubing may be difficult to loosen. If so, use hemostat to twist tubing while holding venipuncture device firmly with one hand.

(continued)

PROCEDURE 31–10. (continued)

5. Remove and discard protective cap from new tubing. Hold free end of tubing near venipuncture device. Remove old tubing, then quickly insert new tubing into device. Some nurses occlude the vessel proximal to the cannula with one finger of the hand holding the new tubing to prevent loss of blood during the exchange of tubing.

   Rationale: 5. Close proximity of tubing and device facilitates exchange with minimal loss of blood and minimal risk of introducing organisms into venipuncture device.

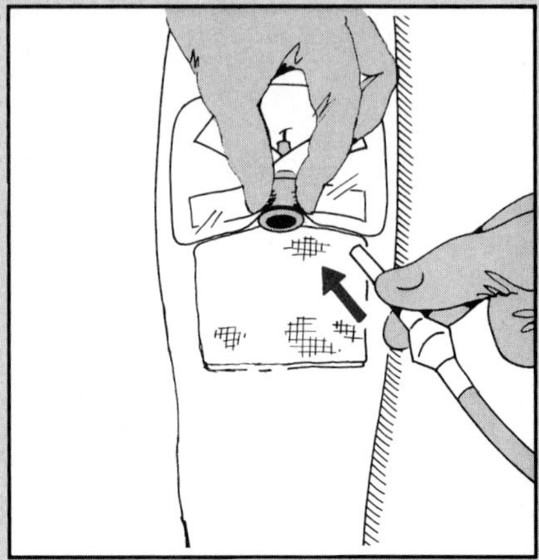

6. Stabilize venipuncture device with one hand and secure new tubing in device with twisting motion. Open roller clamp to KVO (keep-vein-open) rate.

   Rationale: 6. Tubing must be securely attached to venipuncture device to prevent accidental separation. Immediately initiating fluid flow prevents clotting at venipuncture site.

7. Cleanse skin around venipuncture site, if necessary. Remove gloves and discard in waste container marked infectious waste.

   Rationale: 7. Cleansing skin and properly disposing of materials that have contacted body fluids prevent infection.

8. Replace venipuncture dressing and secure tubing. Regulate IV flow to ordered rate and label tubing with time and date.

   Rationale: 8. Protects site from infection; achieves desired therapeutic effect. Alerts personnel to need for next tubing change.

RECORDING: Note amount of fluid infused from previous container and amount and type of solution in new container on I&O record. Document site assessment and dressing change on progress notes or daily care flowsheet according to agency policy.

PROCEDURE 31–11. DISCONTINUING AN INTRAVENOUS INFUSION

PURPOSE: To safely terminate an intravenous infusion when therapy has been accomplished

EQUIPMENT: Clean gloves, sterile gauze pads, adhesive tape or bandage, alcohol swabs

ACTION	RATIONALE
1. Check physician's order for termination of infusion.	1. IV may need to be restarted if infusion is discontinued in error.

(continued)

PROCEDURE 31–11. (continued)

NOTE: If IV is infiltrated, no order is needed to discontinue it.

2. Determine type of infusion (ie, peripheral, central venous, arterial).

   2. Central venous and arterial lines are removed only by personnel with special training.

3. Wash hands and don gloves.

   3. Handwashing removes transient flora from nurse's hands; gloves prevent contact with client's blood, which may contain pathogens.

4. Discuss the procedure with the client, including the reason, the anticipated benefits, and the desired participation.

   4. Active participation is more likely if client understands the expected benefits and desired behavior.

5. Close roller clamp on IV.

   5. Failing to clamp the IV allows solution to spill over linens, client, and caregiver.

6. Remove all outer tape from IV tubing and armboard, if present. Carefully remove inner tapes, which secure the device, while holding device stable with opposite hand.

   NOTE: Tape and transparent dressing can be removed more easily as follows: lift corner of tape or dressing; wipe interface between underside of tape and skin with an alcohol swab while lifting tape away from skin.

   6. Releasing the inner tapes close to insertion site can jerk device and cause vein trauma. Stabilizing the device prevents pain and site trauma as tape is being removed.

7. Cover insertion site with sterile gauze and apply gentle pressure to site, while carefully withdrawing the venipuncture device. Apply pressure at insertion site until bleeding stops, usually 2 to 3 minutes.

   NOTE: A longer period of pressure will be necessary if you are discontinuing a heparin lock and for clients who are on heparin therapy.

   7. Swab prevents contamination while pressure limits bleeding.

8. Discard soiled gauze in infectious waste container and apply dry, sterile gauze dressing or adhesive bandage, taping firmly into place.

   8. Blood on gauze may contain pathogens. Dressing protects puncture site during healing.

9. Dispose of IV equipment according to hospital policy.

   9. There are various policies for disposal of glass versus plastic supplies as well as various definitions about what materials must be handled as biohazardous wastes.

RECORDING: Record time IV discontinued, state of puncture site, and intactness of cannula in nursing records. Record volume of IV fluid absorbed from discarded container on I&O sheet.

these activities. Box 31–12 describes approaches for helping clients with IVs complete activities of daily living.

Transfusion Therapy. Some of the most serious body fluid deficits are caused by blood or fluid losses from the intravascular compartment. Losses of the various constituents of blood, such as albumin, platelets, plasma, and globulins, may have far-reaching consequences. Clotting abnormalities, immunological deficits, and tissue oxygenation problems often result from losses in the intravascular compartment. Therefore, transfusion of blood and its constituents is important not only to replace body fluids but also to restore function of other body mechanisms.

Blood is a living tissue and is often referred to as an organ. When this living tissue is transplanted, the possibility of grave reactions exists. Careful laboratory testing for matching the blood or blood product, as well as rigorous procedures for client and product identification, is essential to prevent these problems.

BOX 31–12. ASSISTING THE CLIENT WHO HAS AN INTRAVENOUS INFUSION

Gowning

1. Close the roller clamp on the infusion and crimp tubing near venipuncture site.
2. Remove solution container from IV pole and slide through sleeve of soiled gown and up sleeve of fresh gown.
3. Hang container on IV pole, uncrimping tubing and opening roller clamp.
4. Adjust flow to desired rate.

Bathing/Showering

1. Encourage clients who are unable to complete self care to do as much as possible; then assist them to complete the hygiene.
2. Take care to keep the IV site and dressing dry.
3. IV site dressing may be changed at the time of the bath or shower or covered with plastic wrap to protect it from water.

Feeding

1. Clients who have IV infusions in their upper extremities may have trouble preparing their food. Assist by opening containers, cutting meats, and spreading condiments.
2. If the client has trouble holding utensils, assist with feeding (see Chap. 25).

Ambulating

1. Provide client with a portable IV stand.
2. Assist client to the side of the bed and to a standing position.
3. Counsel client against putting traction on the tubing.
4. Secure the tubing before client begins to ambulate.
5. Assist the client in holding and moving the IV stand. Caution against using the IV stand for support and about the necessity for clearing door jambs.
6. Observe client on the first attempt to ambulate independently with the IV.

Blood Groups and Blood Matching. Human blood is classified into four blood compatibility groups based on immune reactivity. The four groups, A, B, O, and AB, are differentiated on the basis of polysaccharide antigens (called agglutinogens) on the erythrocyte surface. The presence or absence of A and B antigens on the cells is detected by using anti-A and anti-B reagents, but also by testing for agglutinins (antibodies) in the serum, known respectively as anti-A and anti-B antibodies.

Both cell typing and serum typing are performed routinely.[14] Type A blood reacts with anti-A reagent, and has anti-B antibodies present in the serum. Type B, on the other hand, reacts with anti-B reagent and has anti-A antibodies in the serum. Type AB reacts with both anti-A and anti-B reagents, and has no antibodies in the serum, whereas type O reacts with neither reagent and has both A and B antibodies in the serum.[14] As a rule blood selected for transfusion must be of the same type as that of the recipient. Blood transfusions, therefore, must be matched to the client's blood in terms of the compatibility of agglutinogens. Mismatched blood causes hemolytic reactions. In urgent situations, however, type O blood may be used for clients with other blood types.[14]

Rh typing is routinely performed along with ABO typing to determine the presence of the Rh factor. The Rh factor refers to the presence of Rh antibodies on the surface of the erythrocytes; these antibodies occur in about 85 percent of the population. The blood of persons with the factor is said to be Rh positive (+); the blood of persons without the factor is said to be Rh negative (−). Rh factor is an important cause of hemolytic reactions during transfusion. Clients with Rh negative blood should always receive Rh negative blood. Clients with Rh positive blood may receive either Rh positive or Rh negative blood.[14]

Whole Blood and Blood Products. Whole blood may be reduced to at least six different components for use in the human body. Whole blood, packed red cells, platelets, fresh or frozen plasma, serum albumin, and cryoprecipitate are used to correct various body fluid and clotting deficiencies.

Whole Blood. Whole blood is commonly used to replace blood lost to hemorrhage or major surgical intervention. Whole blood must contain an anticoagulant to prevent clotting in the container. It must also be used within 5 days of donation.[31] As blood ages, red cells die and potassium is released into the plasma, resulting in hyperkalemia. Coagulation factors also degrade as blood ages, lengthening the clotting time.

Packed Red Blood Cells. Packed red blood cells are a preparation of densely concentrated red cells resulting from the removal of plasma from the whole blood. Packed cells are used for clients who require red cells for increased tissue oxygenation but must have limited fluids.

Platelets. Platelets, or thrombocytes, aid in the clotting of blood. Platelets are obtained by centrifuging whole blood and removing the platelet component. Platelets should not be administered without compatibility tests, although the tests may be suspended in emergencies. Some plastics used in solution containers may cause platelets to adhere, so the container must be agitated frequently during administration.

Plasma. Plasma, the serous component of whole blood, is used to restore lost fluid and proteins in the intravascular compartment. Generally, plasma from a donor of the same blood group and type as the client is used.[31] Fresh-frozen plasma is treated by freezing to protect the clotting factors and thus must be warmed before it is used. Because rewarming can degrade the clotting factors, fresh-frozen plasma must be used within 6 hours of thawing.[31]

Serum Albumin. Serum albumin is used for specific plasma protein replacement. The osmotic characteristics of the albumin also help correct hypovolemia by causing a fluid shift from the interstitial to the intravascular compartment. Two strengths of serum albumin are available: 5 percent in saline and 25 percent solution.[31] The 25 percent solution will cause ICF dehydration if additional fluids are not supplied. Although some reactions have been noted to serum albumin, infusion compatibility testing is not usually required before use.

Cryoprecipitate. Cryoprecipitate is a solution containing clotting factor VIII, which is missing from the blood of hemophiliacs. It is removed from frozen plasma and administered in small quantities (approximately 50 mL). Treatment must be repeated frequently.[31]

Nursing Responsibilities in Transfusion Therapy. The nurse's responsibilities in transfusion therapy are to guard the client's safety and prevent side effects. To do this, the nurse carefully identifies the product and the client, follows approved administration techniques, and observes the client for reactions. General considerations and a step-by-step guide for the administration of blood appear in Procedure 31–12.

The first step in transfusion therapy is to obtain a blood specimen from the client for type and cross-matching. These compatibility tests identify the appropriate group and type of blood to infuse. Compatibility tests also determine if the client has immunological difficulties, such as difficult-to-match antibodies. When the specimen is drawn, the client is given a wristband with the same identification information that is printed on the specimen container. This is later used to identify the specific blood product to ensure that the client is not put at risk for hemolytic reactions.

Identification procedures should always be carried out before blood is transfused. Each unit volume of blood is checked separately. Cross-check the client's identification band with that on the unit for name, hospital number, unit identification number, group and type, and expiration date (Fig. 31–23). In general, most facilities require that two licensed, professional staff members check this information.

Inspect the blood component to be sure that the ports have not been opened and there are no leaks in the system. If there is evidence of clotting and serum separation, indicated by dark patches in the blood and amber serum separated from the cells, do not use the blood. The blood should have a uniform, deep crimson color.

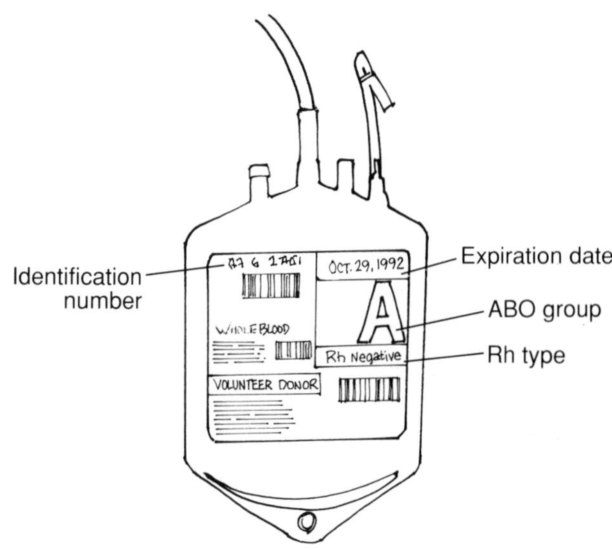

Figure 31–23. Administration of blood: blood identification.

Blood is commonly administered through a Y-tubing set (Fig. 31–24). Each arm of the Y-set has a separate drip chamber. One arm should be attached to a container of 0.9 percent saline, the other to the unit of blood. Maintenance of asepsis is essential, as blood is a prime medium for bacterial growth. If a micropore filter is not built into the set, add one between the unit and the administration set.

Normal saline is used to prime air from the system and to keep the vessel open while blood units are changed. It should not be infused simultaneously with the blood. Hypotonic or hypertonic solutions should not be used with blood, because of the possibility of cell damage.

The large veins of the upper extremities should be used for venipuncture for transfusion therapy. For adult clients, the venipuncture device should be no smaller than 19 gauge.[31]

To maintain the internal consistency of the unit, the blood should be used within 30 minutes of issue from the blood bank. Infusion times vary, but each unit should be infused over 1.5 to 2 hours.[34]

Complications of Transfusion Therapy. Complications of transfusion therapy are relatively rare; however, anaphylactoid, febrile, and hemolytic reactions, in addition to circulatory overload, may occur.[31] The nurse must know the signs and symptoms of these reactions and what actions to take on observing them (see Box 31–13).

Rare allergic or anaphylactoid reactions may occur in clients with multiple drug and food allergies. The client's hyperactive immune system reacts to the blood as foreign matter. Hives and temperature elevations are common. Treatment usually consists of antihistamine or steroid administration. The client may benefit from the prophylactic

PROCEDURE 31–12. ADMINISTERING BLOOD

PURPOSE: To safely infuse blood or blood products intravenously

EQUIPMENT: 1000 mL 0.9% normal saline (NS), in-line blood filter, blood administration set (Y-connection set) with attached filter, venipuncture device (19 gauge or larger), IV dressing, adhesive tape, clean gloves

ACTION	RATIONALE
1. Explain the procedure to the client and family. Take particular care to ask client to report any back pain, chills, itching, or respiratory changes. Signed consent may be required.	1. The necessity for transfusion is anxiety producing. Explanation gives the client and family an opportunity to express concerns and alleviate anxiety. Reporting of signs and symptoms aids the nurse in the decision to terminate the transfusion before significant harm comes to the client.
2. Wash your hands.	2. Handwashing removes transient flora and prevents transmission of microorganisms to client.
3. Prime the Y-infusion set with 1000 mL NS to ensure that air is removed from the main tubing and the short tubing to which unit of blood will be connected. Clamp short tubing after priming.	3. Normal saline is isotonic and does not interfere with the integrity of the red blood cells. Air in the tubing predisposes to clotting and the possibility of air in the client's bloodstream.
4. If client does not have an IV, don gloves and perform venipuncture with a 19-gauge or larger device. Connect the saline infusion to this device.	4. Viscous fluids, such as blood, require large-gauge devices to sustain flow. In addition, blood cells may sustain damage if forced to flow through small-bore devices.
NOTE: If existing IV device is less than 19 gauge, start a new IV.	
5. Take vital signs and record.	5. A baseline set of vital signs guides the nurse in determining significant changes in client condition during the transfusion.
6. Obtain the blood from the blood bank. Obtain only one unit of blood at a time, even if more than one unit will be required.	6. Blood must be used within a specific period to prevent cell hemolysis and clotting factor deterioration.

(continued)

PROCEDURE 31–12. (continued)

Action	Rationale
7. Complete all identification checks according to agency policy. The usual checks are done by two licensed personnel, and include unit ID number, group and type of blood, expiration date of unit, and the client's name and hospital ID number.	7. Hospital policies regarding the personnel responsible for the identification checks and the initiation of the transfusion may vary. The checks verify that the client is being given the same group and type of blood, and is not being given old blood.
8. Close the clamp on the saline infusion.	
9. Attach the unit of blood to the short tubing on the administration set. Invert the unit and squeeze it to fill the filter. Place the unit on IV pole and depress and release the drip chamber until it is filled with blood.	9. The filter captures clots and particulate matter that may have developed in processing or storing the blood product. Priming the filter promotes smooth flow and prevents air from entering the system.
10. Begin blood infusion at slow rate.	10. One unit of blood is generally infused over 1.5 to 2 hours. Rapid administration may lead to the development of transfusion reactions or circulatory overload.
11. Observe the client for any reactions to the infusion, and take vital signs according to agency policy.	11. Transfusion reactions usually occur early in the infusion, but some may be delayed. Vital signs are generally taken at least every 15 minutes during the transfusion.
12. Complete the transfusion and infuse NS to clear the tubing.	12. Infusing saline ensures that the entire amount of the blood product reaches the client.
13. Dispose of the used blood unit and administration set according to agency policy.	13. Many agencies require that all used units be returned to the blood bank. Others require different means of disposal.

RECORDING: Record the completion of the therapy, client response, complications, if any, and nursing action taken, and final nursing observations on the nursing progress notes. Record the total volume infused on the I&O record.

administration of antihistamines before beginning the infusion.[31]

By far the most serious reaction accompanying transfusion therapy is the hemolytic reaction. A **hemolytic reaction** involves the formation of antibodies in the recipient to the red cells in the donor blood, resulting in hemolysis, or destruction, of the cells. The release of hemoglobin from the destroyed red cells results in reduced oxygenation to the tissues. As a result, breakdown products collect in the kidneys and may lead to renal failure.

The signs and symptoms of hemolytic reactions develop rapidly after the transfusion is begun. Chills, fever, low back pain, chest pain, facial flushing, and hypotension characterize the reaction. The transfusion should be stopped immediately and the blood container saved for laboratory analysis. Treatment for hemolytic reaction often includes intravenous infusion of isotonic fluid to flush the kidneys and maintain urine flow, as well as administration of vasopressors to support the blood pressure.[31]

Careful preparation and frequent observation are es-

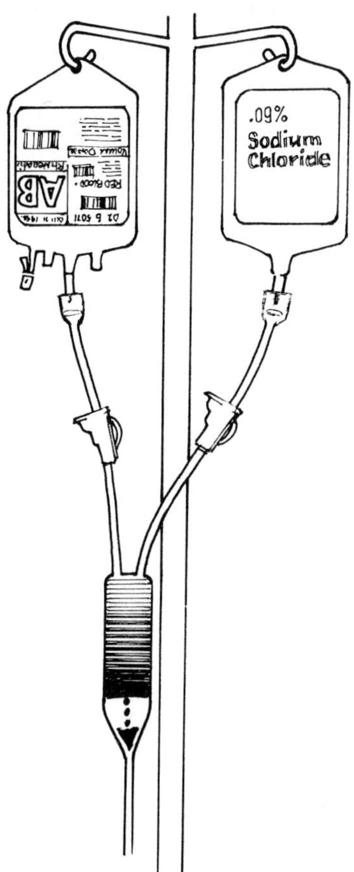

Figure 31–24. Blood transfusion setup.

sential during transfusion therapy. Vital signs are taken before and at frequent intervals during the procedure. The nurse is responsible for this care as well as for the careful identification procedures and continual monitoring of the client's well-being.

BOX 31–13. SIGNS AND SYMPTOMS OF TRANSFUSION REACTIONS

Manifestations Associated With Intravascular Hemolysis

- Restlessness
- Anxiety
- Flushing
- Chest or lumbar pain
- Tachypnea
- Tachycardia
- Nausea
- Shock
- Hives
- Chills
- Fever

Manifestations Associated With Circulatory Overload

- Dyspnea
- Chest pain
- Rales and rhonchi
- Anxiety
- Diaphoresis
- Blood-tinged sputum

From Ingram RH, Braunwald E. Dyspnea and pulmonary edema. In: Harrison TR, et al, eds. Principles of Internal Medicine, *12th ed. New York: McGraw-Hill; 1991.*

Total Parenteral Nutrition Therapy.

Total parenteral nutrition (TPN), or intravenous hyperalimentation, is the administration of nutrients intravenously to clients who cannot tolerate food via the GI tract. Although TPN does not directly correct body fluid imbalances, the electrolytes and proteins in the solutions often correct fluid shifts in the ECF compartment. Clients who may benefit from TPN are those with liver damage, renal failure, severe burns, multiple trauma, and metastatic cancer.[45] Post-surgical clients who experience complications that delay oral intake are also candidates for TPN.

TPN solutions are usually composed of water, 10 to 15 percent dextrose, and various additives, such as electrolytes, amino acids, vitamins, trace elements, and fatty acids. Some of the more common solutions are listed in Table 31–19.[45]

Administration of TPN. TPN solutions are hypertonic and thus are often administered over extended periods. Because of the character of TPN solutions, deep central veins are used for their delivery. The right subclavian vein and external and internal jugular veins are frequent sites for these infusions (see Fig. 31–17B).

Central Venous Catheters. Central venous catheters are used to access the deep veins for TPN administration. Central venous catheters are large-bore catheters that are inserted with a guidewire by the physician. After insertion, the guidewire is withdrawn and the catheter is sutured to the client's skin. During insertion, the client either lies flat or in the Trendelenberg position and is asked to perform the Valsalva maneuver as the catheter is introduced.[47]

Before using the central venous catheter, its position should be confirmed by x-ray. As the subclavian vein is quite close to the inferior vena cava and the right atrium, curling of the catheter or malposition can result in serious complications. On confirmation of position, the administration set may be attached and the infusion begun.[47]

Strict aseptic technique must be used not only in introduction of the catheter but also in subsequent dressing and tubing changes. Aseptic dressing changes are recommended every 48 hours and tubing changes every 24 hours with each new solution container. The aseptic handling of the solutions is mandatory, as the high glucose content of the TPN solution is a prime medium for bacterial growth.[47]

Nursing Responsibilities for TPN Therapy. Nursing care is integral to safe and successful administration of TPN. Nursing implementation for the client undergoing TPN therapy involves monitoring the TPN infusion and prevent-

BUILDING NURSING KNOWLEDGE

What Factors Should Be Considered in the Choice of Parenteral Fluids?

Rutherford C. Fluid and electrolyte therapy: Considerations for patient care. *Intravenous Nurs.* 1988;12(3):173–183.

In this article, Rutherford provides a comprehensive summary of the body's requirements for fluid to nourish and sustain body cell metabolism. The main focus is on parenteral fluid replacement. Rutherford notes that the primary purpose of parenteral fluid replacement is to restore previous and present fluid losses to reduce or prevent dehydration, and to provide nutrients. She advises that fluid loss may be estimated by determining loss of body weight; 1 L of body water equals 1 kg or 2.2 pounds of body weight.

The choice of parenteral fluid for treatment, according to Rutherford, depends on the fluid being lost. For example, if gastric fluid is lost in large amounts, either through vomiting or suctioning, then fluids resembling gastric fluid, called gastric replacement solutions, are used in parenteral therapy. They are constituted to correct the alkalosis that results from the loss of gastric acid. Likewise, lost intestinal fluids are replaced with intestinal replacement fluids. These are constituted to correct the acidosis that may occur as a result of an excessive loss of normally alkaline bile and pancreatic fluids.

Stress is another factor that must be accounted for in the choice of solutions. The stress of trauma and surgery has a profound effect on the body, causing an outpouring of adrenocortical steroids as an adaptive physiological response. This effects natural body water and sodium retention that is aggravated by the use of nonelectrolyte solutions (glucose in water). Hypotonic solutions administered at a time of water retention can cause serious hyponatremia, which may lead to expansion of the intracellular compartment and symptoms of water excess. The solution that is preferable for parenteral therapy during stress is 5 percent dextrose in 0.2 or 0.45 percent sodium chloride which prevents dilution while also preventing sodium excess.

Rutherford stresses that nutrition is a factor in the choice of parenteral fluid. Carbohydrates provide an indispensable source of calories, but they do not provide sufficient calories in prolonged therapy. One liter of 5 percent dextrose in water provides only 170 cal. Thus, to provide a day's nutrition, too much fluid would have to be given. When nutrition is required, a solution with a greater concentration of glucose (20 or 50 percent) is used.

When nutrition is insufficient, the body uses its own fat and protein to supply calories, creating a catabolic state. Amino acids help prevent catabolism; often they are combined with glucose and alcohol, which provide calories for metabolism, while amino acids help tissue repair. Such solutions are available in varying strengths and caloric values.

ing metabolic or apparatus-related complications. For example, the nurse must watch for signs and symptoms of inflammation at the catheter site and maintain the specified infusion rate to prevent rapid circulatory overload.

As TPN solutions contain high quantities of glucose, the monitoring of blood glucose levels to detect hyperglycemia often falls to the nurse. In addition, as the glucose in TPN solutions may result in osmotic fluid excesses or fluid shifts to the ECF, the nurse must closely monitor the client for signs and symptoms of fluid and electrolyte imbalance. Careful monitoring of intake and output, as well as daily weights, is a common nursing implementation for clients receiving TPN therapy.

Providing extra rest for clients receiving TPN therapy is an important nursing responsibility. Clients are often weak and debilitated. The nurse, in collaboration with the client and other caregivers, should schedule care to provide for extended periods of rest.

TABLE 31–19. CONTENTS OF TOTAL PARENTERAL NUTRITION FORMULAS

Additive	Amount
Amino acids	250 mL (4.25% concentration)
Dextrose	250 mL (25% concentration)
Electrolytes	
Sodium chloride	60 mEq
Potassium chloride	30 mEq
Potassium phosphate	30 mEq
Magnesium sulfate	8 mEq
Calcium gluconate	9 mEq
Trace minerals	
Zinc	Variable amounts, usually less than 5 mL
Copper	
Iron	
Manganese	
Multivitamins: B complex, A, C, D, E, and K	10 mL total
Fat emulsion formulas[a] (soybean or safflower derivatives)	
Intralipid 10% and 20%	500–1000 mL
Lyposin 10% and 20%	
Travmulsion 10% and 20%	
Soyacal 10% and 20%	

[a] Fat emulsions can be given separately or in tandem with the amino acid TPN formulas.

From Colley R, Duty VP. Total parenteral nutrition—Nursing practice. In: Plumer AL, ed. The Principles and Practice of Intravenous Therapy, *4th ed. Boston: Little, Brown; 1987:389–427.*

Complications of TPN Therapy. The complications of TPN therapy may be either apparatus related or client related (see Box 31–14). The nurse's careful observation for the signs and symptoms of these complications is essential to the client's well-being.

Rehabilitative Care

Rehabilitative care involves rehabilitation of clients with long-term fluid and electrolyte problems. Chronic illnesses such as renal failure, cardiac disease, and hypertension often require permanent life-style changes, including changes

BOX 31–14. COMPLICATIONS OF TOTAL PARENTERAL NUTRITION

Apparatus-related Complications

Pneumothorax, hemothorax, hydrothorax

- Observe for sharp chest pain, decreased breath sounds, asymmetrical chest expansion, and dyspnea on insertion of central venous catheter or commencing infusion of TPN.
- Firmly apply occlusive dressing when central catheter is discontinued.
- Ensure x-ray location of catheter prior to hookup.

Air embolism

- Place client in flat or Trendelenberg position prior to catheter insertion.
- Assess client's ability to hold breath and perform Valsalva maneuver prior to catheter insertion and thereafter, when changing tubing.
- Do not open closed system for tubing changes or capping the central line, unless client performs Valsalva or clamps are used on the catheter.

Client-related Complications

Hyperglycemia, hypoglycemia

- Test blood glucose at least every shift.

Osmotic diuresis

- Maintain strict intake and output records.
- Ensure that client is receiving sufficient fluids, in addition to TPN.

Circulatory overload

- Assess for neck vein distension, crakles in lungs on auscultation, and dyspnea.
- Maintain rate of TPN as ordered. Do not attempt to "catch up" for a rate slower than prescribed.

From Colley R, Duty VP. Total parenteral nutrition—Nursing practice. In: Plumer AL, ed. The Principles and Practice of Intravenous Therapy, *4th ed. Boston: Little, Brown; 1987:389–427.*

in fluid and dietary intake. To make the necessary changes, the client must go through a learning process.

Behavioral Changes. Principles of behavioral change and skills to assist the client are outlined in Chapters 6, 10, and 22. A client must express a willingness to change before collaboration is possible. In addition, the nurse must ascertain, through careful history taking, what physiological or psychosocial factors might preclude a successful behavioral change. The client and nurse should then discuss each factor and develop approaches to overcome them. The nurse must also help the client understand what behavioral change is expected. Ambiguity will inevitably lead to conflict between client and nurse.

Nursing implementations that can help the client to change behavior include encouraging the client to attend programs that improve self-esteem and coping skills, and referring the client to a support group of individuals with similar problems. For example, clients with chronic kidney failure face severe, long-term dietary and fluid restrictions. A discussion with other clients facing the same problems may demonstrate the importance of the restrictions and make them easier to accept.

One of the most critical aspects of nursing implementation during rehabilitative care is to maintain the nurse–client relationship. Clients often make life-style changes as the result of continued support, encouragement, and praise from a trusted nurse. Positive reinforcement for even a small step toward change can motivate the client to continue.

Self-monitoring Techniques. Simple self-monitoring techniques can help clients who must make long-term behavioral changes. The nurse might encourage the client on fluid restrictions to keep a log of fluid intake, including the time the fluid is ingested, the amount, the client's feelings at the time, and the client's activity level. The nurse and client can then review the log to identify situations that lead to excessive fluid ingestion.

Self-care Techniques. Many of the self-care techniques helpful to clients in maintaining long-term behavioral changes require stress management techniques, because motivation to maintain behavior changes often breaks down in time of stress. See Chapter 22 for more on self-management techniques. Nurses can encourage clients to change or control situations in which negative behaviors tend to arise. For instance, the client with a sodium restriction may suggest that his or her employer provide low-sodium beverages, such as fruit juices, in the workplace. This helps the client avoid the stress of temptation.

Finally, the client should attempt to incorporate exercise, rest, and relaxation techniques as life-style practices.

IMPLICATIONS FOR NURSE–CLIENT COLLABORATION

Rehabilitation

Rehabilitation is essential to self-care, particularly when the client has a fluid balance problem of long-standing nature. The problems on which nurse and client collaborate during rehabilitation are complex and may involve personal changes that, while improving the client's health, will nevertheless be difficult for the client to make. The nurse's support during rehabilitation is vital, as is the client's participation in the decisions that are made. The client's ultimate capacity to integrate changes may depend not only on how well he or she learns the skills involved, but also on whether those changes come to be valued as important to personal well-being. Collaboration between nurse and client can facilitate the exchange of information, opinions, and feelings that may ultimately influence the client to adopt values and behavior that support body fluid homeostasis.

Exercise strengthens the cardiovascular system and maintains fluid balance through a healthy cardiac output. Relaxation techniques help prevent the pituitary gland from oversecreting ADH. Even more important, rest and relaxation help the client cope physiologically and psychosocially with stress-producing behavioral changes.

■ EVALUATION

The evaluation of the collaborative care plan for body fluid management flows from the desired outcomes. The nurse and client review the desired outcomes as target dates are reached. Evaluation should be ongoing. Daily reviews of the client's weight and intake and output and frequent review of laboratory and diagnostic test results can provide much information to evaluate the success of the plan. A cursory daily physical examination of fluid indicators also may provide evaluation data.

SUMMARY

Body fluid disturbances are complex problems. Imbalances usually result from serious alterations in health or a prolonged assault by disease. Fluid intake and output are usually taken for granted, because regulatory mechanisms swiftly correct problems before the effects are noticeable.

Because of the high fluid content of the body cells, assessment of fluid balance and swift intervention when an imbalance occurs should be an integral part of any client's nursing care. The assessment must be thorough, to provide sufficient information for the development of a plan of care. Both physiological and psychosocial factors affect the intake and output of fluids.

The care plan for helping the client to adapt to body fluid changes flows from a collaboration between nurse and client. The client's input helps formulate a plan that is individualized and carries a high potential for success. The nurse can serve many roles, from observer to collaborator, to independent caretaker and supporter in helping the client identify and adapt to body fluid problems.

Most people take fluid balance for granted. When imbalance develops, the loss of function can be surprising and stressful for the client. The observant, knowledgeable, supportive nurse can help alleviate this stress and avert future problems.

REFERENCES

1. Chenevey B. Overview of fluid and electrolytes. *Nurs Clin North Am.* December 1987:749–759.
2. Hazinski MF. Understanding fluid balance in the seriously ill child. *Pediatr Nurs.* 1988;14(3):231–236.
3. Masiak MJ, Naylor MD, Hayman LL. *Fluids and Electrolytes Through the Life Cycle.* Norwalk, CT: Appleton-Century-Crofts; 1985.
4. Metheny NM. *Fluid and Electrolyte Balance—Nursing Considerations.* Philadelphia: JB Lippincott; 1987.
5. Kee JL. *Fluids and Electrolytes With Clinical Applications—A Programmed Approach,* 4th ed. New York: John Wiley & Sons; 1986.
6. Guyton AC, ed. *Textbook of Medical Physiology,* 8th ed. Philadelphia: Saunders; 1990.
7. Hoffart N. Nutrition in renal failure, dialysis, and transplantation. In: Lancaster L, et al, eds. *Core Curriculum for Nephrology Nursing.* Pitman, NJ: AJ Janetti, Inc; 1987:135–155.
8. Chambers JK. Metabolic bone disorders: Imbalances of calcium and phosphorus. *Nurs Clin North Am.* December 1987:861–872.
9. Germon K. Fluid and electrolyte problems associated with diabetes insipidus and SIADH. *Nurs Clin North Am.* December 1987:785–796.
10. Goldberger E. *A Primer of Water, Electrolyte, and Acid–Base Balance Syndromes,* 5th ed. Philadelphia: Lea & Febiger; 1975.
11. Mathewson M, Mathewson R. Establishing acid–base balance. *Crit Care Nurse.* 1987;7(5):77–85.
12. York K. The lung and fluid and electrolyte and acid–base imbalances. *Nurs Clin North Am.* December 1987:805–814.
13. Reedy DF. How can you prevent dehydration? *Geriatr Nurs.* July/August 1988:224–226.
14. Berkow R, Fletcher AJ, eds. *The Merck Manual of Diagnosis and Therapy,* 15th ed. Rahway, NJ: Merck Sharp & Dohme Research Laboratories; 1987.
15. Levinsky NG. Fluids and electrolytes. In: Harrison TR, et al, eds. *Principles of Internal Medicine.* New York: McGraw-Hill; 1991:278–289.
16. Folk-Lightly M. Solving the puzzles of patient's fluid imbalances. *Nursing 84.* 1984;14(2):33–41.
17. Ingram RH, Braunwald E. Dyspnea and pulmonary edema. In: Harrison TR, et al, eds. *Principles of Internal Medicine,* 12th ed. New York: McGraw-Hill; 1991.
18. Sheridan DP, Winograd IR. *The Preventive Approach to Patient Care.* New York: Elsevier; 1987.
19. Rice V. Problems of water regulation: Diabetes insipidus and SIADH. *Crit Care Nurse.* January/February 1983:64–73.
20. Adinaro D. Liver failure and pancreatitis: Fluid and electrolyte concerns. *Nurs Clin North Am.* December 1987:843–852.
21. Martof M. Electrolyte balance—Part II. *J Nephrol Nurs.* March/April 1985:49–55.
22. Stein J. Hypokalemia—Common and uncommon causes. *Hosp Pract.* March 30, 1988:55–68.
23. Felver L, Pendarvis J. Electrolyte imbalances: Intraoperative risk factors. *AORN J.* 1989;49(4):992–1013.
24. Coward DD. Cancer-induced hypercalcemia. *Cancer Nurs.* 1986;9(3):125–132.
25. Lancaster LE. Renal and endocrine regulation of water and electrolyte balance. *Nurs Clin North Am.* December 1987:761–772.
26. Flink EB. Causes of magnesium depletion. *Hosp Pract.* February 15, 1987:116I–116P.
27. Baker W. Hypophosphatemia. *Am J Nurs.* September 1985:999–1003.
28. Levinsky NG. Acidosis and alkalosis. In: Harrison TR, et al, eds. *Principles of Internal Medicine.* New York: McGraw-Hill; 1991:289–295.

29. Heitkemper MM, Bond E. Fluid and electrolytes: Assessment and intervention. *J Enterostomal Ther.* 1988;No.15:18–23.
30. Adams F. How much do elders drink? *Gerontol Nurs.* July/August 1988:218–221.
31. Plumer AL. *Principles and Practice of Intravenous Therapy,* 4th ed. Boston: Little, Brown; 1987:103–120, 137–186, 191–207, 269–291.
32. Tucker JA, Sussman-Karten K. Treating acute diarrhea and dehydration with oral rehydration solutions. *Pediatr Nurs.* 1987; 13(3):169–174.
33. Fuller J, Schaller-Ayers J. *Health Assessment—A Nursing Approach.* Philadelphia: Lippincott; 1990.
34. Poyss A. Assessment and nursing diagnosis in fluid and electrolyte disorders. *Nurs Clin North Am.* December 1987:773–784.
35. Kee JL. *Laboratory and Diagnostic Tests With Nursing Implications,* 2nd ed. Norwalk, CT: Appleton & Lange; 1987.
36. Carpenito LJ. *Nursing Care Plans and Documentation: Nursing Diagnosis and Collaborative Problems.* Philadelphia: JB Lippincott; 1991.
37. Binder HJ. The pathology of diarrhea. *Hosp Pract.* October 1984: 107–118.
38. Lederer JR, Marlescu GL, Mocnik B, Seaby N. *Care Planning Pocket Guide—A Nursing Diagnosis Approach.* Menlo Park, CA: Addison-Wesley Nursing; 1990.
39. Myers KA, Hickey MK. Nursing management of hypovolemic shock. *Crit Care Nurs Q.* 1988;11(1):57–67.
40. Eschleman MM. *Introductory Nutrition and Diet Therapy.* Philadelphia: JB Lippincott; 1991.
41. Sommers M. Rapid fluid resuscitation—How to correct dangerous deficits. *Nursing 90.* January 1990:52–59.
42. Rutherford C. Fluid and electrolyte therapy: Considerations for patient care. *J Intravenous Nurs.* 1988;13(3):173–183.
43. Centers for Disease Control. Guidelines for prevention of intravascular infections. *Infect Control.* 1982;3:61–72.
44. Snydman DR, Donnelly-Reidy M, Perry LK, Marvin WJ. Intravenous tubing containing burettes can be safely changed at 72 hour intervals. *Infect Control.* 1987;3(3):113–116.
45. Colley R, Duty VP. Total parenteral nutrition—Nursing practice. In: Plumer AL, ed. *The Principles and Practice of Intravenous Therapy,* 4th ed. Boston: Little, Brown; 1987:389–427.
46. Newman LN. A side-by-side look at two venous access devices. *Am J Nurs.* 1989;89(6):826–833.
47. Cosentino F. Central venous catheters. In: Plumer AL, ed. *The Principles and Practice of Intravenous Therapy,* 4th ed. Boston: Little, Brown; 323–364.

BIBLIOGRAPHY

Cogan MG. *Fluid and Electrolytes; Physiology and Pathophysiology.* Norwalk, CT: Appleton & Lange; 1991.

Earnest VV. *Clinical Skills and Assessment Techniques in Nursing Practice.* Glenview, IL: Scott, Foresman, and Co; 1989.

Enich M, Hinderer G. Performing venipuncture in elderly patients. *Nursing 91.* February 1991:32C–32H.

Gaspar PM. What determines how much patients drink? *Geriatr Nurs.* July/August 1988;221–223.

Holder C, Alexander J. A new and improved guide to IV therapy. *Am J Nurs.* 1990;90(2):43–47.

Hollenberg NK. The kidney in heart failure. *Hosp Pract.* January 1986:81–100.

Kennedy-Caldwell C. Water metabolism, the NPO patient, and parenteral nutrition. *Crit Care Nurse.* 1986;6(3):63–64.

Levine MM, Kleeman CR. Hypercalcemia: Pathophysiology and treatment. *Hosp Pract.* July 1987:93–110.

Rinard G. Water intoxication. *Am J Nurs.* December 1989:1635–1638.

Rose BD. *Clinical Physiology of Acid-Base and Electrolyte Disorders,* 3rd ed. New York: McGraw-Hill; 1989.

Sheridan DP, Winograd IR. *The Preventive Approach to Patient Care.* New York: Elsevier; 1987.

Watson JE. Fluid and electrolyte disorders in cardiovascular patients. *Nurs Clin North Am.* December 1987;797–804.

Yarnell RP, Craig MP. Detecting hypomagnesemia: The most overlooked electrolyte imbalance. *Nursing 91.* July 1991:55–57.

Zaloga GP, Chernow B. Hypocalcemia in critical illness. *JAMA.* 1986;256(14):1924–1929.

UNIT SEVEN
Scientific and Philosophical Foundations of Nursing Practice

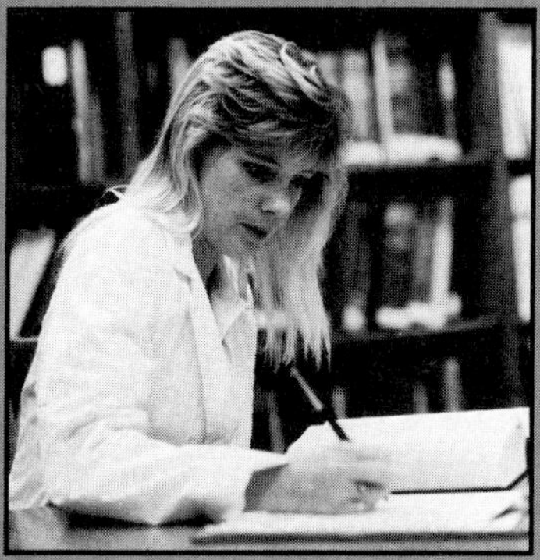

CHAPTER 32

Links Between Nursing Science and Nursing Practice

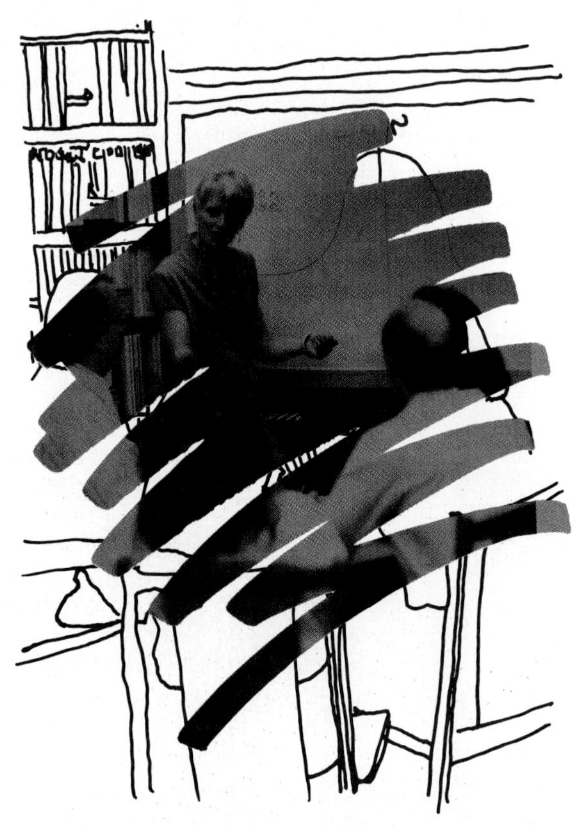

Behavioral Objectives

Upon completion of this chapter, the student will be able to:

1. Discuss the importance of science as a way of knowing in nursing.
2. Describe nursing science both as a body of organized knowledge and as an approach to problem-solving.
3. List and describe the steps in the research process.
4. Discuss the evolution of theory in nursing.
5. Describe four major nursing models.
6. Describe the major nursing research methods.
7. Discuss the relationship between nursing science and practice and the ways in which nurse scientists and clinicians collaborate to conduct research.

KEY TERMS

applied science
basic science
concept
conceptual framework
conceptual model
control
dependent variable
descriptive theory
design
experimental method
explanatory theory
holism
hypothesis
independent variable
logical positivism
manipulation
null hypothesis
operational definition
phenomenon
population
predictive theory
qualitative research method
quantitative research method
randomization
random sample
reliability
research
research hypothesis
research problem
research question
sample
sampling error
science
statistical method
subjectivity
theoretical framework
theory
validity
variable

Every profession, including nursing, exists to perform a needed service in society. To shape and direct its service, or practice, the nursing profession depends on a defined body of professional knowledge. Some of this professional knowledge is unique or specialized to nursing. Some is common to the practice of related professions, such as medicine.

Specialized nursing knowledge is largely what sets nursing apart from related professions. Specialized nursing knowledge is one parameter that sets the direction and limits of nursing practice. It does so by creating or defining the sphere in which the special expertise of nurses provides a basis for independent professional decision-making. For example, because of their close contact with clients and the responsibilities associated with nurses' roles, nurses have developed expert knowledge regarding methods of comforting, feeding, and bathing clients. Thus, nurses generally have the power to make independent decisions about these methods in practice situations.

However, specialized nursing knowledge is not the only parameter that sets nursing apart from related professions. Legal and political forces also shape the boundaries of nursing practice in society. Regardless of what a nurse may know or learn, a law or nurse practice act governs the functions that nurses can legally perform. (See Chaps. 3 and 4 for discussions of law and politics as they relate to nursing practice.) Nonetheless, because of the way knowledge defines and guides the practice of a profession, each profession is responsible for generating the specialized knowledge needed to support its service and advance its frontiers. Nursing is no exception.

Specialized nursing knowledge is historically scientific in nature; that is, it relies on systematic observation. By her pioneering writings, Florence Nightingale clearly established the importance of scientific knowledge to nursing practice. Her detailed accounts and statistics of conditions in the Crimea are the earliest known studies with implications for nursing care. From that beginning, the nursing profession, like other health care professions, has embraced the traditions of science as a way to generate knowledge for practice.

Because of the importance of scientific knowledge to

the nursing profession, this chapter aims to clarify the unique nature of nursing science and to specify ways in which nursing science and nursing practice are inextricably bound. Various types of knowledge that nurses use in practice are first discussed. Science and nursing science are then defined as both products and processes. Several widely used nursing theories and models are also presented and the major research methods nurses use are introduced. Finally, the connections between the roles of nurse clinicians and nurse scientists are examined and strategies for collaboration are discussed.

■ WAYS OF KNOWING IN NURSING

Throughout life, people come to know many things. Seldom in everyday life do people ask themselves how they came to know something, or question whether what they know is true or valid. However, when nurses depend on professional knowledge to guide their actions with clients, they must consider more directly and seriously the basis for and quality of that knowledge base. How can nurses know if available nursing knowledge is adequate to guide action?

An American philosopher, Charles Pierce,[1] can give direction to nurses in answering this question (Table 32–1). Pierce wondered how people come to know things. He reasoned that people know or "fix belief" by one of four methods: tenacity, authority, intuition, or science. Though all four methods rely on experience and contain a way to add to knowledge over time, only science has self-correcting features. None of these methods, however, is fail-proof; but because it attempts to find and expose its own errors, the method of science can yield the more dependable and transmittable knowledge base for nursing practice.

Other types of knowledge, such as philosophy and ethics (discussed in Chaps. 33 and 34), are also fundamental to nursing practice and enrich the body of professional knowledge. Carper,[2] a nurse philosopher, determined that four types of knowing are basic to nursing practice: empirics (science of nursing), esthetics (art of nursing), ethics (moral values of nursing), and personal knowledge (individual nurses' active comprehension of experience). Nonetheless, most nurse scholars would agree that the bulk of specialized knowledge needed to direct nursing practice is scientific. For example, facts about the normal range for physical functions such as blood pressure, pulse, and temperature are developed through scientific means. Likewise, scientific methods yielded knowledge of the most effective preoperative teaching strategies.

The question of whether nursing, as a *discipline* or body of specialized knowledge, ought to be exclusively a science is still an open one. A major problem in regarding nursing strictly as a science comes from the reductionistic nature of science. Reductionism refers to the way science examines only the objective aspects of experience. Scientists study only those parts of experience that can be accessed through the senses and thus verified publicly.

Many nurse scholars see the reductionistic nature of science as inconsistent with the holistic nature of nursing practice. **Holism,** a view that persons are more than and different from the sum of their parts, acknowledges the subjective aspects of experience that cannot be verified publicly and may be unique for each person. Information such as what it is like to be in pain, what it means to lose a child to fatal illness, or how a person adapts to life in a nursing home, is important to holistic nursing practice. If the discipline of nursing were a strict science, it would exclude the study of large areas of knowledge about human experience that are central to nursing practice. Some strict and traditional views of science do not include the study of these experiences; however, most nurse scientists accept as scientific those research methods that address such concerns. Nurse scholars continue to debate this dilemma and related issues as nursing strives to clarify its nature as a discipline.

Despite the absence of a final consensus on the relationship of nursing knowledge and science, nurse scholars agree that nursing is emerging as a distinct and primarily scientific discipline. Knowledge that is specific to nursing practice exists and nurse scholars generate more daily.

TABLE 32–1. PIERCE'S METHODS OF KNOWING

	Characteristic		
Method	**Source of Knowledge**	**Advancement of Knowledge**	**Limitation**
Tenacity	Innate, reinforced by personal history or experience.	Inferred from what is already known, circular.	False beliefs can be reinforced because evidence can be dismissed.
Authority	Knowledgeable others, authorities, higher powers.	Pools the knowledge of many, more open than tenacity.	Authority may be in error; authority consulted may be inappropriate to the problem.
Intuition	Self-evident, stands to reason, assumes humans are inclined toward truth.	Based on reason, logic, free discourse.	Derived knowledge may not agree with experience; conflicting, but equally logical conclusions may result.
Science	Objectified experience.	By verifying, replicating, and eliminating competing explanations.	Knowledge is always regarded as tentative; some experience cannot be objectified and cannot be known.

From Buchler J. *Philosophical Writings of Pierce.* New York: Dover; 1955.

■ THE NATURE OF SCIENCE AND OF NURSING SCIENCE

Scientific truth is the primary type of knowledge sought by nurse scholars, but it is not the only type. Because science is central to the discipline of nursing, it is especially important for nurses to understand both the strengths and limitations of this knowledge form. This section describes current ideas about the nature of science and summarizes the thinking of nurse scholars on the nature of nursing science.

What is Science?

Science and Theory. According to Kerlinger,[3] **science** is a form of discovery, the basic aim of which is to explain natural phenomena. In science, explanations are called theories. Thus, science is both a product—an organized body of knowledge in the form of theories—and a process. The process consists of systematized methods and procedures for making discoveries, verifying information, and solving problems.

Science and Common Sense. In distinguishing science from common sense, Kerlinger stressed that science uses concepts or terms more formally than they are used in common sense.[3] In science, concepts or terms have definite limited meanings. Scientists develop the meaning of a concept systematically and check their formulations against data. Further, in science, **hypotheses,** statements of tentative or alternate relationships among concepts, are tested. In common sense, hypotheses are not tested. Favored hypotheses are usually supported with selective evidence. People who reason with common sense often choose only that evidence that supports their argument. In addition, scientists systematically rule out competing causes or explanations rather than accept, as with common sense, the first fitting explanation. Finally, science concerns itself only with explanations that can be observed, while common sense can sometimes accept more metaphysical or mystical explanations.

Traditional Views of Science. Traditional science is rooted in a somewhat static view called **logical positivism.** Logical positivism is a philosophy that regards science as strictly objective, deduced from sensory data. **Subjectivity,** the involvement or infusion of the scientist's personal views into science, is denied. In this view, the general laws of nature, or the real world, exist "out there," apart from the scientist. The scientist, relying only on sensory data, aims to discover these laws. Knowledge acquired through this method accumulates. Each new discovery is added to this collection of laws or used to revise them with more adequate or encompassing theories and explanations.

Contemporary Views of Science. Contemporary views of science are more dynamic. The connection between sensory data and concept is as basic an idea in contemporary views of science as it has been in the traditional view; however, intuition, creativity, and inductive reasoning also play an accepted part in the scientific process. In this contemporary view, reality is constructed or invented, not discovered.[4] Scientists use existing knowledge as a base or model for generating new knowledge. As long as data support a theory, the theory represents a viable alternative view of reality. Like pieces of a puzzle or facets of a prism, competing theories illuminate different parts or aspects of a phenomenon. No one theory is regarded as giving the best, complete, or only true picture.

Theory: The Product of Science

Phenomena, Concepts, and Theories. Theory begins with an intriguing phenomenon. A **phenomenon,** the object of study, is the thing or event that attracts the scientist's attention. For example, phenomena could be reports and behaviors of a client that signify an uneasiness about the future or discomfort in some part of the body. Nurse scientists develop theories about phenomena like these, which they encounter in everyday nursing practice.

Theory advances as phenomena are labeled. A **concept** is a label applied to the sensory data (reports and observed behaviors) that tell the scientist the phenomenon is occurring. Once a label is applied, the scientist moves from the concrete world to the abstract realm of theory. Concepts are symbols for events in the real world, and as such they acquire special and precise meanings. Conceptual labels for the phenomena cited in the above example may be anxiety and pain. Concepts are then used to build theories.

Many authors have defined the term "theory" as it is used in science. Generally, scientists agree that a **theory** is a statement or set of statements that aims to describe, explain, predict, or control a phenomenon. One simple example of a theory is anxiety increases pain, where anxiety is a state of uneasiness about what may happen and pain is a state of physical discomfort. Theory asserts the existence of a concept, defines concepts, and specifies relationships among concepts. Developing theory is the goal of science.

Importance of Theory. Experience is the basis of all science. Experience alone, however, is blind. Data and facts have no meaning outside the context of a theory. That a client, John Smith, is grimacing has no meaning unless a nurse interprets his grimace as an indication of pain and, using the previous theory, validates his pain and, then, in an effort to reduce his pain, explores whether or not he is also anxious. Thus, theory allows scientists and clinicians to connect experience with larger, universal principles. Conversely, experience gives life to otherwise hollow concepts or ideas. Of what significance would the study of pain be if scientists and clinicians could not tell in the real world if and when they saw it? While theories help nurse scientists organize or structure knowledge for scientific testing, theories also help nurse clinicians organize observations and knowledge to direct nursing practice.

The Role of Measurement in Science. Scientists use the process of measurement to convert the raw experience into science and scientific theory. In science, measurement is the process that links experience (phenomena) and ideas (concepts). Through measurement, a concept is made concrete by applying rules or procedures that assign number values to observed phenomena. In the example of the theory of anxiety and pain, the scientist must devise a means to measure or quantify both concepts. A questionnaire may be used to determine how anxious a person is, or clients may be asked to rate the severity of their pain on a scale from one to ten. Though it may begin as simply as counting, measurement is the critical first step to the scientific study of any concept.

Strengths of Measurement. Measurement is a source of both strengths and limitations in scientific knowledge. Measurement is a strength because it provides a means to objectify, quantify, and standardize a phenomenon. Measurement reduces ambiguity in the meaning of concepts and enables scientists to verify and replicate experiments. Measurement aids by directing the scientist's attention to only those data signifying the phenomena of interest, thus paring away irrelevant information.

Limitations of Measurement. Measurement creates a limitation to scientific knowledge because, by its nature, measurement cannot capture the whole of experience. The resulting knowledge addresses only the particular, measurable aspects of phenomena. Measurement constricts what can be known about a phenomenon because not all aspects or dimensions of phenomena are measurable, especially in the human sciences.

As a simple example of measurement and its limitations, consider the following. Existing in the world is the experience (or phenomenon) of hotness or warmth. Observing hotness in a feverish client, the scientist invents the idea (or concept) of temperature. To study the phenomenon of hotness, the scientist devises a thermometer to measure temperature. The thermometer registers or objectifies hotness and gives it a number value.

Although there is much more to the feverish client's experience of hotness than is registered on a thermometer, the resulting scientific knowledge of hotness is limited to what thermometer readings can provide. Temperature, as measured by a thermometer, excludes other possible features of hotness such as color, odor, form, taste, feel, tingle, or glow. Thus, through measurement, hotness is reduced to a thermometer reading of temperature. Similarly, the scientific study of pain or other human experiences requires reducing them to a set of observable or objectified features such as frequency, location, and intensity. In practice, however, nurses may need to understand more about these phenomena than such measures can reveal.

Nonetheless, measurement is central to developing scientific theory. It provides a powerful way to focus attention on at least a portion of experience, to gain clarity and consistency in language, to apply statistics and test observations, and to generalize from many discrete observations to universal principles.

Characteristics of Effective Measuring Tools. Measurement is an important, and often the first, step in studying a phenomenon scientifically. Many important nursing phenomena remain unstudied because of the difficulty involved in measuring them. Consider, for example, the following clinical problems: loneliness in the elderly, self-image of women with mastectomies, or the strain of parents caring for chronically ill children. If loneliness, self-image, and strain could be measured as easily as temperature, scientific knowledge of these problems would advance more rapidly. Although clinical assessment tools, such as hospital admission forms, do have measurement potential, and scientific instruments such as thermometers have been applied to clinical uses, many phenomena seen in nursing practice, such as caring or clients' will to live, are lacking a means for measurement. The process of advancing nursing science and theory is often slowed by the need to first develop sound measuring tools. Nurse scientists have, however, already devised or adapted measures for many biophysical and psychosocial phenomena encountered in clinical nursing. How, then, can nurses evaluate the quality of their measuring instruments? Scientists rely on two primary characteristics of a measuring instrument to judge its quality or soundness: validity and reliability.

Validity. **Validity** is the extent to which an instrument measures what it is designed to measure. Consider, for example, a questionnaire intended to measure body image. It might include questions such as "How satisfied are you with the way you look?" or "When shopping, do you select clothes to try on that are too small?" At least on their face, these questions seem to fit the idea or concept of body image. The situation would be different, however, if the questionnaire included the following questions: "Are you displeased with yourself?" "When shopping, do you have a hard time selecting clothes?" Although these questions could indicate a problem with body image, they may also reflect a problem with the broader idea of self-concept. In other words, they are not specific enough to measure body image, and answers may be influenced by other aspects of self-concept. Measures can be invalid, as in this example, because they are imprecise and include things other than or irrelevant to that which the researcher intends to measure.

Measures are also invalid when they underrepresent a concept. For example, a sphygmomanometer without a stethoscope can indicate only systolic blood pressure. Because no information about diastolic blood pressure can be obtained with just a sphygmomanometer, it alone would not give a complete picture of blood pressure. Thus a blood pressure measurement taken without aid from a stethoscope would be considered invalid for studying blood pressure, but might be valid for studying the narrower concept of systolic blood pressure.

These examples illustrate the type of validity problems that commonly occur in nursing research; however, because many instruments used in nursing research are complex and new, validity problems may not be as obvious as in these examples. A published report of a nursing research study should contain some estimate, usually a statistical one, of how valid its measures were.

Reliability. **Reliability** is the extent to which repeated measurements, using an instrument under stable conditions, yield the same results. Imagine a scale designed to record weight in kilograms. In a study of infants receiving intravenous fluid, the scale is used to weigh clients once each shift. The nurse who weighs the infants notices that they are gaining weight faster than expected. In checking the scale, the nurse finds that the needle has drifted above the zero setting. After resetting the needle to zero, the nurse finds that infants' weight gains are now in the expected range. In this instance, the weighing procedure was unreliable because it yielded an artificially high reading.

Unreliable measures lead one to believe that change has occurred when it has not. Conversely, they can hide changes that are occurring. For example, a scale that has a 20-kilogram limit may be reliable at low weights, but would be unreliable for showing changes occurring over 20 kilograms. As with validity, problems in reliability of measures are not always obvious. Research reports should also contain reliability estimates for all measures.

Theory Construction. If measurement is the first step in developing scientific theory, subsequent steps involve describing phenomena and seeking and testing relationships among phenomena or concepts. Progress towards developing a scientific theory usually proceeds through several levels. The levels of scientific theory are summarized in Box 32–1.

At the first level, scientists develop descriptive theories. From multiple observations, **descriptive theories** summarize what is common among individuals, groups, events, or situations. Descriptive theories address the "What is . . ." of a phenomenon and lead to classification systems, types, and normal values. For example, with the phenomenon of vomiting, nurses could systematically record key features of numerous vomiting episodes observed in individuals representing many age groups and disease states, and develop a descriptive theory of categories or types of vomiting, such as vomiting during pregnancy or vomiting after surgery. Each type would have a set of defining features, physiology- or disease-related norms, and age-related norms.

Based on effective descriptive theory, scientists proceed to develop theory at the explanatory level. **Explanatory theories** link concepts together. Explanatory theories specify both which concepts are related and how they are related—for example, positively or negatively. In the example of the phenomenon of vomiting, nurses could next examine various types of vomiting in relation to nausea and fever. Such a study would reveal which types of vomiting occurred with nausea only, which with fever only, which with nausea and fever, and which with neither nausea nor fever.

The next level of theory is predictive. **Predictive theories** are about causes and effects or the "Why . . ." of a phenomenon. Predictive theories are developed from experiments that test the behavior of a phenomenon under varying conditions. Using the example above, predictive theory could be developed to inform nurses which clients under what conditions are likely to develop each type of vomiting, and which interventions would be most effective for treating each type.

BOX 32–1. LEVELS OF SCIENTIFIC THEORY

- Descriptive theories describe the features of a phenomenon common to multiple occurrences of it.
- Explanatory theories relate two or more concepts.
- Predictive theories stipulate which concepts are causes and which are effects.

BUILDING NURSING KNOWLEDGE

How Does the Research Process Differ from the Nursing Process?

Burns N. The research process and the nursing process: Distinctly different. *Nurs Sci Q.* 1989;2(4):157–158.

In this article, Burns is concerned about equating the research process with the nursing process, which some instructors do to make research more comprehensible to students. She takes issue with those who state that each time a nurse uses the nursing process, that nurse is conducting research, arguing that the analogy is limited.

Burns contends that the purpose, foundations, and implementation of research are different from those of the nursing process. For example, the purpose of research is to add to an existing body of knowledge. Thus the nature of research is abstract and general. The purpose of the nursing process, on the other hand, is to plan and give care that will improve the health of a single client, which is a specific and concrete endeavor.

Burns points out that the research process demands a degree of discipline and rigor that is not required by the nursing process, which is more flexible and less formal in its application. Although the nursing process is based on nursing theory, it does not have the strong, logical links to theory possessed by the research process. In addition, while the nurse may learn something by applying the nursing process, what the nurse learns is generally not incorporated into the body of general knowledge in the profession. This contrasts with the research process, which is both applicable to large numbers of clients and communicated to the profession through professional conferences and journals. Burns concludes that the research process and nursing process are distinctly different.

Research: The Organized Process of Science

As theory is the outcome or product of science, research is its process. Simply put, **research** is a systematic approach to solving a knowledge problem or of answering a scientific question. The problem may or may not relate directly to a practical concern. According to some scholars, scientists who research problems that have no immediately apparent practical application are basic scientists. Their research is known as **basic science.** Those who study problems that build on or test basic science for use in the world of practice are applied scientists. Their work is called **applied science.** Many nurse scholars characterize nursing research, as well as the clinical research of other professions, as applied science. However, when nurses study the progression of normal processes such as growth, dying, or adaptation, or examine phenomena such as fatigue, pain, or sleep under naturally occurring circumstances, their work can be characterized as basic nursing science.

The research process has many variations, with each discipline emphasizing particular methods and techniques. However, there is a logic common to all empirical research. This logic is often referred to as steps in the research process, as though each step were taken in sequence. However, in practice, scientists move back and forth between the steps, as ideas are refined or existing knowledge advances. For the purpose of clarity, the research process is summarized in steps in Box 32–2, and the steps are discussed below.

Step 1: Stating the Research Question. The point of a research study is to answer a question, usually to reveal something about a phenomenon or concept that is not yet known or to verify the findings of some earlier research. To produce meaningful answers, research questions must be posed precisely. A **research question** must be highly specific and must name at least the concepts and population of interest. Andersen and Briggs[5] give us examples of well-stated nursing research questions:

> Is there a difference in the number and quality of nursing diagnoses written when nurses use a nursing data base rather than a medical data base?
>
> What proportion of these diagnostic statements written by nurses are supported by the assessment data from which they were generated?

BOX 32–2. STEPS IN THE RESEARCH PROCESS

1. Stating the research question
2. Developing the research problem
3. Reviewing related research
4. Forming hypotheses and defining variables
5. Designing the research study
6. Selecting the sample
7. Collecting data
8. Analyzing data
9. Interpreting and communicating results
10. Protecting human subjects in research

IMPLICATIONS FOR PROFESSIONAL COLLABORATION

Research Questions Involving the Collaborative Approach

A critical step in subjecting the collaborative concept of client care to a scientific scrutiny is to develop research questions that reveal something about the concept. For instance, a researcher might ask, "What are the attitudes of clients toward engaging in necessary but potentially painful postoperative activities such as deep-breathing exercises and early ambulation when, in the preoperative period, they have had an opportunity to receive information about the purpose and value of those activities from the nurse, share their concerns about the possible discomfort, and participate in decisions about the conditions under which the activities will be performed?" The researcher might also inquire, "Are these attitudes different from the attitudes of clients who have not had the opportunity to collaborate?"

Sometimes, the research problem is stated as a declarative sentence, rather than as a question. Such a statement is referred to as the purpose, aim, or goal of a research study. An example of a well-stated purpose appeared in a study published by Sutton and Murphy:

> The purposes of this study were to: (a) determine the incidence and severity of selected stressors and the coping strategies used by a group of post-operative renal transplant patients; and (b) to explore the influence of time on stress and coping patterns.[6]

Some problems cannot be studied scientifically. Questions that are too vague or are ethical in nature cannot be researched empirically. This is an example of a vague question:

> Is it better for pregnant teenagers to have abortions, to surrender their children to adoption, or to keep and raise their children?

A scientist cannot measure "better," since its meaning is not explicit. Therefore, for a scientist to study this question, it must be restated to specify what is meant by better. The following is one possibility:

> What are the health consequences for three groups of teenage mothers (those who aborted, adopted, or are raising their children) at 1, 3, and 5 years postpregnancy?

An example of a question that is ethical in nature is:

> Should euthanasia be allowed for terminally ill elderly?

Though arguments for or against this question could be supported by data, this question is best answered using ethical, not scientific, reasoning.

Step 2: Developing the Research Problem. A research question is generally expanded and set in a context commonly called the **research problem.** In the problem statement, the researcher argues for the study's importance and sets the study in a theoretical context. The argument portion of the problem statement can be made on practical or theoretical grounds. A practical argument can be made in a study comparing the effectiveness of two treatments for pressure sores. A theoretical argument can be used to defend a study aimed at clarifying conflicting results of previous studies.

The second part of the problem statement is often called the **theoretical framework.** In this step of the research study, the scientist connects the research question to a theory. The theory is then used throughout the study to direct decisions about the research design and methods and to provide a context within which results can be interpreted. For example, using the theory about anxiety and pain cited earlier, the researcher might ask: Does fear of death (a specific form of anxiety) increase severity of traumatic pain (a specific form of pain) in victims of automobile accidents? Further, the scientist would measure fear of death (anxiety) in terms of accident victims' reports and behaviors, as opposed to their reports alone, because of the way anxiety is defined in the theory.

Step 3: Reviewing Related Research. A researcher further develops a study by connecting it to existing research on the same topic. The connection is made through literature review. An effective literature review summarizes and organizes what is known from previous studies, critiques the scientific quality of those studies, and uses the critique to strengthen the developing study. Scientists discover how others have measured the concepts of interest and addressed similar problems through literature review. A literature review strengthens the scientist's approach to answering the research question.

Step 4: Forming Hypotheses and Defining Variables. At this point in a study, the researcher uses the theoretical framework and literature review to make an educated prediction about the outcome of the study. Such predictions are called **research hypotheses.** Hypotheses link variables. **Variables** are those indicators of a concept that may assume differing values. Variables are of two main types: independent and dependent. **Independent variables** are those that the researcher thinks are causes. **Dependent variables** are those thought to be effects. In the nursing diagnosis research question example given under step 1, the dependent variable is the difference in the nursing diagnoses, the independent variable, the type of database used to generate the diagnoses. Hypotheses of a study are tested statistically to answer the research question.

Using the sample research question on teenage mothers, the following are some possible hypotheses:

> Teenage mothers who raise their children have better mental health but poorer physical health than teenage mothers in the other two groups.
>
> There is no difference in the health consequences among the three groups of teenage mothers at 1 year postpregnancy.

Many hypotheses could be developed from this sample question. Hypotheses can predict a definite outcome, as in the first hypothesis. Or a hypothesis can test the premise that an independent variable makes no difference on a dependent variable, as illustrated by the second hypothesis. Such hypotheses are called **null hypotheses.** In the second (null) hypothesis, the independent variable (group assignment reflecting a teenager's decision about her pregnancy) is predicted to have no effect on the dependent variable (health consequences). That is, the null hypothesis predicts that variations (differences in health status after birth) noted in a nonscientific observation of the population of interest (teenage mothers) are not real: caused by a specific external factor or factors (decision to abort, adopt or raise the child), but merely appear to be related to those factors and are instead related to intrinsic differences among the individuals (variations in the sample). The study aims to support the null hypotheses by carefully matching individuals in the sample, thus controlling for intrinsic differences in the population. The choice of which type of hypotheses to develop and test from a research question depends on a study's theoretical framework, the outcome of the literature review, and the design of the research.

Not all studies have hypotheses, however. Because they aim first to discover information about phenomena, some descriptive studies have only research questions. The outcome of these studies, which are often qualitative, may be used as hypotheses for testing in future studies.

In order to test a hypothesis, each variable in it must be measured or operationalized. An **operational definition** is a statement of the instruments or procedures that will be used to measure a variable. Some variables, such as stress, have many possible operational definitions. To strengthen the scientific merit of a study, a researcher develops operational definitions that fit the study's theoretical framework.

Step 5: Designing the Research Study. At this step of the research process, the scientist chooses a detailed plan, called a **design,** for conducting the study. The design of a study is an overall approach to the research. Several differ-

IMPLICATIONS FOR PROFESSIONAL COLLABORATION

Forming Research Hypotheses About Collaboration

A researcher who has posed research questions about the attitudes of clients who had a chance to collaborate with nurses preoperatively about necessary but potentially painful postoperative activities might hypothesize that: "Clients who have the opportunity to receive information from nurses about the purpose of potentially painful postoperative activities, share their concerns about discomfort, and participate in making decisions about the conditions under which these activities will be performed, will express fewer negative attitudes about postoperative activities than will those clients who do not collaborate with the nurse about their postoperative care."

ent types of research methods, or ways of obtaining and analyzing data, may be used to achieve the intended design. Major research designs used in nursing are listed and defined in Table 32–2. Research methods used in nursing are detailed in a later section.

The design includes general directions for structuring the overall study, choosing a sample, measuring variables, collecting data, analyzing data, and protecting the rights of human subjects, if any. For a study design to be valid, its components must be logically congruent, that is, they must relate to one another in a way that makes sense. For example, the methods selected to measure the variables must be consistent with the variables' operational definitions, which must also be consistent with the plans for data analysis. In addition, the design must flow logically from the research question and the theoretical framework. For example, research questions derived from descriptive and explanatory-level theory are usually built on survey designs, while those aimed at developing and testing predictive level theory often require some type of experiment. Further, if the research question calls for a survey design, a large, random sample is usually required. However, if the research question calls for an experiment, fewer subjects may be needed and it may not be necessary to choose them randomly, but random assignment to groups may be preferred.

The research question about teenage mothers requires a type of experiment. A true experiment could not be conducted because the rights of teenagers as human subjects in research studies prohibits the researcher from assigning them to a group at random.

The range of choices in planning a study's design, sample, data-collection procedures, and statistical analyses is vast and beyond the scope of this text. It is necessary, however, for beginning nursing students to recognize that criteria do exist for evaluating the strength of a scientist's study plan. These criteria are important when evaluating a research report for clinical application (see Evaluating the Scientific Merit of Research Studies, toward the end of this chapter).

Step 6: Selecting the Sample. From this point on in the research process, scientists move from planning a study to carrying it out. Researchers first identify the population from which the study's sample will be selected. The **population** refers to all individuals of a particular type; or in other words, a set of people with some characteristic in common. For example, one population commonly studied by nurses is that of pregnant women, from which samples of various types can be drawn. Because all people constituting the population of interest cannot feasibly be studied, the researcher must choose a sample. A **sample** is a small proportion of a population selected for study; for instance, pregnant teenagers might be a sample selected from the population of all pregnant women. In selecting the sample, possible subjects are included or excluded so that the final group is representative of the population of interest. Care must be taken to ensure that the sample is not biased (unrepresentative of the population).

In selecting a sample for a study of teenage mothers, a researcher would have to make many choices. These include specifying the age range representing teenagers, deciding whether to include those who have had multiple pregnancies or only those with a first pregnancy, determining the number of subjects needed in each group to support the statistical analyses, and selecting sites from which subjects would be recruited. Each of these choices can affect the quality and outcome of the study, and therefore must be carefully considered. If, for example, only low-income or Caucasian subjects were selected, the applicability of the study's results to all teenage mothers would be questioned.

One common approach to sample selection, particularly when statistical methods are incorporated in the research design, is that of randomization. A **random sample** is a sample chosen in such a way that each individual mem-

TABLE 32–2. MAJOR RESEARCH DESIGNS USED IN NURSING

Design	Description
Exploratory	A flexible research plan unique to the particular situation being investigated and allowing for the researcher to explore new clues as they present themselves. Assuring reliability and minimizing bias are key considerations.
Descriptive	A structured research plan that allows phenomena to be studied under naturally occurring conditions. Key features of descriptive designs include conceptual and operational definition of variables, systematic sampling procedures, valid and reliable instrumentation, and data-collection procedures that achieve some environmental control.
Correlational	A structured research plan that allows the study of relationships between two or more variables. A key feature of correlation studies is a sample that represents the population of interest and contains the full range of possible values for the variables of interest.
Quasi-experimental	A structured research plan that permits the limited study of causes and effects. Key features of quasi-experiments are nonequivalent control groups or repeated measures over time.
Experimental	A structured research plan that permits the study of causes and effects. Key features of experiments are manipulation of the independent variable; control of the experimental situation, including a control group; and random assignment of subjects to groups.

Adapted from Burns N, Grove SK. The Practice of Nursing Research Conduct, Critique and Utilization. *Philadelphia: Saunders; 1987: 241–276.*

ber of a population has an equal chance of being selected and each choice is independent of any other choice. This might be done by placing the names of population members in a container and, blindfolded, drawing out one name at a time until the desired number is obtained, or by using a computer-generated list of random numbers to select individuals from a consecutive list of names. Whatever the means, randomization eliminates sample bias, but is not always possible or even desirable in nursing research. Moreover, random samples are subject to **sampling error,** the effect of chance variation in sample selection. It is impossible to know, for instance, that even a randomly selected sample is truly representative of the population as a whole. Statistical methods have been developed to address this issue. **Statistical methods** are mathematical formulas that are applied to scientific experimentation. One variety, known as parametric or inferential statistics, is used specifically to identify sampling error. Inferential statistics enable the researcher to determine with greater certainty when study results are due to changes in the independent variable.

Step 7: Collecting Data. Once subjects have been chosen, researchers collect data from each according to the operational definitions and data-collection procedures specified in the design. Researchers may use people, documents, or laboratory tests as sources of data. Data-collection methods include interviews, questionnaires, psychological tests, physical and physiological measures, or direct observation of behavior. Data collection demands accuracy and organization. The best instruments and measures, if applied haphazardly, can introduce error, which may weaken an otherwise sound study.

In the study of teenage mothers, data could be collected by interviewing the teenagers about their health at 1, 3, and 5 years postpregnancy; by having them rate their health in questionnaires; by actually conducting physical and psychological examinations of the teens; or by reviewing their health records retrospectively. If all methods are valid and reliable and yield data that can be manipulated mathematically, the choice may depend on the researcher's time and material resources for conducting the study.

Step 8: Analyzing Data. Once collected, data must be organized and analyzed. This step of the process often entails use of a computer and knowledge of statistical procedures. Data are entered and defined in files, tabulated and summarized in tables and graphs, and manipulated to produce statistics. Statistics are then used to draw conclusions about the hypotheses and research question.

Step 9: Interpreting and Communicating Results. At this stage of the research process, the researcher has an obligation to interpret the results and to communicate them to relevant audiences. In interpreting results, researchers state the outcome of the study and explain why these results were achieved. Results are interpreted within the context of the theoretical framework and literature review. Sometimes results confirm the hypothesis, and researchers' original logic is upheld. At other times, results disprove the hypothesis, requiring researchers to reevaluate the methods, the theory, or both. Results that disprove the hypothesis may be more perplexing to researchers, but they often provide the clues or insights that lead to new scientific breakthroughs. In a study aimed to predict which nursing home residents might wander, for example, the researcher found that study variables were able to predict quite accurately those residents who did not wander, while chance was a better predictor of those who did. Consequently, these results led the researcher to reconsider whether wanderers constitute a group of residents with common characteristics or whether there could be several different types of wanderers.

This step in the research process involves public examination of the study. Researchers can accomplish this step

BUILDING NURSING KNOWLEDGE

How Well Are Nursing Research Results Disseminated to Practicing Nurses?

Luckenbill-Brett JL. Use of nursing practice research findings. *Nurs Res.* 1987;36:344–349.

The author of this article observes that little is understood about how well nursing research findings are disseminated. Only two studies reviewed by the author dealt with dissemination. These indicated that a small proportion of nurses had actually implemented important research findings on common nursing procedures into their practice.

Concerned about this, Luckenbill-Brett designed a study to determine the awareness of, opinions about, and use of research findings by practicing nurses. She collected data from 216 nurses working in hospitals of various sizes. The educational backgrounds of subjects were varied. Each subject completed a survey measuring awareness of research findings and attitudes toward adopting findings in practice. The survey presented 14 innovative findings identified from nursing research journals with national prominence.

The results indicated that the awareness of the subjects varied with the type of innovation. Between 34 and 95 percent reported having heard about any given item of those presented. Between 28 and 92 percent reported being persuaded that the various innovations should be put into practice. Ten of the innovations had actually been implemented by the majority of nurses in the sample.

Adoption of research findings was related to the number of hours in a week that subjects spent reading professional literature. No relationships were found between adoption of innovations and type and amount of nursing education, hours of continuing education, participation in research studies, or completion of a nursing research class. Nurses' perceptions about hospital policy on the various innovations were correlated strongly with adoption. The author concluded that this study shows research dissemination and use is occurring, but research is necessary on why certain findings are adopted more frequently than others.

BOX 32–3. RIGHTS OF HUMAN RESEARCH SUBJECTS

- Protection from harm
- Full disclosure of information
- Self-determination
- Privacy and confidentiality
- Protection of vulnerable subjects

by publishing the study in a journal or by presenting it verbally at scientific meetings. Disseminating the study publicly serves two purposes. First, dissemination allows the study to be scrutinized by members of the larger scientific community who judge the quality of the work and evaluate the strength of the results. This scrutiny is essential to preserving the integrity of scientific knowledge. Second, dissemination allows the results to reach audiences that can benefit from them. This second purpose is especially important in clinical research, where professional standards and practices may change on the basis of research findings.

Step 10: Protecting Human Subjects in Research. Researchers who study human subjects must protect their rights in the design and implementation of *every* step. Both the federal government and the American Nurses' Association have published guidelines to assist researchers in ensuring that the rights of the subject are protected and in obtaining informed consent of subjects (see Chap. 34 for further discussion of informed consent).

Institutions such as universities and hospitals, where research studies are often conducted, have special committees that review studies to ensure that researchers adhere to guidelines. However, as client advocates and potential participants in research activities, all nurses need to be aware of the rights of research subjects. Five rights specifically protected in these guidelines are the rights (1) not to be harmed; (2) to receive full disclosure; (3) to be free to participate or not; (4) to have privacy and confidentiality respected; and (5) in the case of vulnerable subjects, to have extra care taken in obtaining consent. These five rights are listed for quick reference in Box 32–3.

Protection from Harm. Protection from harm means that a subject must be advised of the risks involved in participating in a study and that researchers must take every reasonable precaution to reduce the likelihood of risk. Risks can be physical, psychological, emotional, financial, legal, or social in nature. Further, subjects must be advised of the recourse available should harm befall them.

Full Disclosure. Full disclosure means that subjects are given accurate and complete information about the study in terms they can understand. Subjects must receive information about the following aspects of a study:

- Its purposes, nature, and duration.
- Data-collection methods and procedures.
- Any and all potential risks, benefits, inconvenience, discomfort, side effects, or consequences that subjects may experience.
- How results will be used.
- Alternatives to participating.
- How to refuse or withdraw from a study.
- The identity of the investigator and how to contact him or her.

Self-determination. Self-determination means that subjects must be free of any undue influence or pressure to participate in a study. Although it is not unethical to provide some benefits to research subjects, the use of large incentives is coercive. People who tend to please authorities, particularly those who are dependent on them in some way, need special safeguards. Prisoners are an example of such dependent subjects.

Privacy and Confidentiality. Privacy and confidentiality require that the identity of subjects be protected and that information about a subject not be publicly revealed or available to others besides the research team. Specific techniques that ensure these rights must be used, and subjects must be informed of how these rights will be protected.

Vulnerable Subjects Protection. Vulnerable subjects are those whose ability to give informed consent is compromised in some way. Examples include mentally retarded people, children, confused elderly, and unconscious people. The population of interest in many nursing studies involves such subjects. In these cases, the researcher must take special care to afford the potential subject as much opportunity as possible for decision-making about the study and to obtain consent from a proxy, such as a legal guardian, parent, or spouse.

Nursing Science

Pursuit of theory and use of the research process are common to all sciences. However, each science is distinct from every other in some way. What makes a science distinct or unique? And how is nursing science distinct?

According to Schwab[7] and Foshay,[8] disciplines, including sciences, are distinguished from one another by seven characteristics: a community of scholars, a domain, a perspective, a set of persisting questions, history and traditions, a syntax, and a set of truth criteria. Though some disciplines share common characteristics, each discipline is unique in the way it defines itself on all characteristics together. Table 32–3 defines characteristics that distinguish disciplines.

As a discipline, nursing is just beginning to emerge and take shape (see Chap. 1). At this point in its development, a full or final consensus among nurse scholars in defining the discipline of nursing on important characteristics would be premature; however, to further clarify the nature of nursing as a discipline, nurse scholars engage in healthy and productive dialogue and debate in nursing literature and at scientific meetings. Some preliminary conclusions can be drawn from their work.

TABLE 32–3. CHARACTERISTICS DISTINGUISHING DISCIPLINES

Characteristic	Definition
Community of scholars	Group of thinkers and investigators concerned with generating and organizing knowledge within a discipline.
Domain	Subject matter of a discipline; the field of phenomena or range of events, occurrences, situations, or processes that scholars study. Because some subjects are so complex, there is considerable overlap in the domain of various disciplines.
Perspective	World view, orientation, focus, or outlook common to all or most members of a discipline.
Persisting questions	Central problems that perplex the scholars of a discipline over time; recurrent themes, ideas, or goals that are sought in the studies of a discipline's scholars.
History and traditions	Critical or significant events and practices that have shaped the discipline's evolution or course of development.
Syntax	Rules for or methods of inquiry; procedures, processes, research methods, or approaches to problem-solving.
Truth criteria	Standards used to evaluate or verify whether knowledge gained through research is valid to a discipline.

Adapted from Schwab JJ. The concept of the structure of a discipline. Educational Rec. *1964; 43:197–205. Foshay AW. Knowledge and the structure of disciplines. Unpublished paper; 1961.*

The Substantive Structure of Nursing. One major focus in discussions of nursing science has been on its substantive structure; in other words, the nature, substance, or content of its theories. What constitutes the perspective, domain, and persisting questions from which the theories of nursing science derive?

According to Donaldson and Crowley,[9] the uniqueness of a discipline stems from its perspective. Nursing's value orientation influences its perspective, which in turn influences its theorizing. Although many nurse scholars have analyzed value orientation and speculated about the nature of nursing as a discipline, few have attempted to state succinctly what nursing's perspective is. One common vantage point or recurrent theme that links many of these writings is nursing's concern with enabling humans to regulate themselves and their environments in pursuit of health. This theme is one way to express nursing's perspective.

More has been written concerning the domain of nursing. In the broadest sense, nurse scholars have identified four general concepts that encompass the domain: person, environment, health, and nursing.[10,11] Thus, at less abstract levels, nursing theories concern these four concepts and the relationships among them.

Donaldson and Crowley further specified the domain of nursing by identifying seven focal areas that characterize nursing phenomena. These areas are:

1. Distinctions between human and nonhuman.
2. Distinctions between living and nonliving.
3. Nature of environments and human–environment interactions from cellular to societal levels.
4. Illness versus health and well-being.
5. Functioning of whole organisms versus functioning of parts.
6. Hierarchy of levels of functioning of whole organisms.
7. Human characteristics and natural processes, such as healing, change, aging, and motivation.[9]

Although they are more specific than the four general concepts binding the domain of nursing, these focal areas are quite abstract and include a vast range of concepts and phenomena.

Scholars continue to clarify and refine nursing's domain. The work of the North American Nursing Diagnosis Association (NANDA) in generating a taxonomy of nursing diagnoses represents one more practical effort to identify and organize the domain of nursing.

Finally, several themes represent the recurring questions of the discipline of nursing. Donaldson and Crowley identified three such themes that have persisted in the studies of nurse scholars since Nightingale:

1. Principles and laws that govern life processes, well-being, and optimum functioning of human beings, sick or well.
2. Patterns of human behavior in interaction with the environment in critical life situations.
3. Processes by which positive changes in health status are effected.[9]

Together, perspective, domain, and persisting questions, along with the concepts and theories they generate, constitute the substantive structure of nursing. While nurses have accomplished much toward clarifying this structure, the work of defining the substance of nursing knowledge is just beginning.

The Syntactical Structure of Nursing. The other major focus in discussions of nursing science has been on its syntactical structure: the nature of its methods or rules for generating knowledge. In other words, what are the syntax, methods of inquiry, and truth criteria of nursing science?

Just as nursing's values influence its perspective, they also influence its scientific methods. Chief among these values is a respect for the uniqueness of individuals and a holistic orientation. Nursing's scientific literature contains many references to research methods and their appropriateness, or lack thereof, for nursing science.

For example, some nurse scholars argue that a research method appropriate for studying some subcellular process, even if it were important to healing or growth, is not a nursing research method. This argument stems from the holistic orientation, which puts the focus of nursing science at the level of the whole person in context, rather than at the level of body systems, organs, cells, or the like. A similar argument might be made against animal or other laboratory research, if ties to relevant phenomena in clinical nursing practice were not explicit and defensible. In determining if a method (or topic) is within the boundaries of nursing science, it is helpful to remember that the professional knowledge base encompasses much more than unique nursing science. Thus, some methods and topics are a legitimate part of the professional knowledge base but are not within the more circumscribed science of nursing. Knowledge of the leadership behavior of nurses or of methods to best teach nursing students are examples of professional nursing knowledge that lies outside the narrower boundaries of nursing science. All research conducted by nurses does not fall within the bounds of nursing science. Conversely, the research of non-nurses sometimes fits within the scientific purview of nursing.

Two major groups of research methods are most often used in nursing research: qualitative and quantitative. These methods are named for the type of data they yield. **Qualitative research methods** yield data that are more narrative than numerical. Data are analyzed by the techniques of coding, sorting, and grouping. **Quantitative research methods** yield numerical data. Data are analyzed using statistical techniques. Studies using quantitative methods result in numerical descriptions or tests of hypotheses. These two types of research methods, together with their differing truth criteria, are discussed in more detail in the Research Methods section later in the chapter.

Measurement, which is a way of making a concept concrete, is an aspect of the syntax of a science. Measurement is a difficult concept. Since many concepts of interest to nurse scientists are also studied by scientists in other health-related fields, nurses often "borrow" the measuring instruments of other sciences; however, borrowed measures often require adaptation to fit the view or perspective of nurses. In addition, by relying solely on the measures of other scientific fields, nurse scientists would be restricted to studying only a portion of the phenomena important to nursing practice. Phenomena primarily of interest to nurses would not be addressed.

Although borrowed measures have helped to give nursing science a head start, nurse scientists are now in the process of developing instruments specific to the science and practice of nursing. Concepts as diverse as social support, confusional states, hope, intracranial pressure, and the meaning of illness have been measured and studied by nurse scientists. The quality of the resulting scientific knowledge depends largely on the quality of measurement.

These comments on the substantive and syntactical structure of nursing science preface a more detailed discussion of nursing theories and nursing research methods. Though there is a need for more theory development in nursing, the discussion that follows on nursing theories and conceptual models can be seen as a sampling of nursing's substantive structure. The later discussion of nursing research methods is a representation of nursing's syntactical structure.

NURSING THEORIES AND CONCEPTUAL FRAMEWORKS

Theories are the core of every science. Theories represent the "truth," albeit tentative, that each science contributes to the collective wisdom of humankind. As a science, nursing also aims to contribute its truths and thus shape knowledge for the betterment of people. The body of theoretical knowledge in nursing is small when compared to some other sciences. This section provides an introduction to some of the major theoretical work in the discipline of nursing.

Development of Nursing Science and Theory

Disciplines take many years to develop a body of scientific theories. The science of physics, considered by some to be the "grandfather" of all sciences, dates back at least three centuries to the 1600s and the work of Isaac Newton. As an emerging discipline, nursing is very young. Serious and concerted scientific work within the discipline of nursing has been undertaken for approximately three decades. Thus, while progress in conceptualizing nursing as a scientific discipline has been impressive, much remains to be done in actually developing scientific theory in nursing.

As a first step in shaping nursing science, early scholars described nursing in abstract theoretical or conceptual terms. Dating back to Florence Nightingale,[12] whose *Notes on Nursing* constitutes the first conceptual nursing framework, over a dozen different descriptions have been developed, most since the late 1950s. These descriptions began to delimit or set the boundaries for nursing as a field of scientific inquiry. Each of these descriptions forms a sort of conceptual system, logic, or perspective that allows a person to "think nursing." Thus, they are useful in focusing the attention of budding nurse scientists on the substance, or proper content, of nursing research studies. Likewise, they are helpful to nurse clinicians in determining those matters in a clinical situation that are the appropriate object, focus, or goal of nursing care.

Theories Versus Conceptual Models. Some nurse scholars refer to these abstract descriptions as nursing theories. In a true scientific sense, this use of the term "theory" is a misnomer, as these works were not generally derived through systematic empirical approaches. More accurate terms for these works are **conceptual frameworks** or **conceptual models.** These terms acknowledge that the works are abstract, conceptual, or theoretical in nature and can be validated through research; however, they do not imply that these works were actually developed from research. Conceptual frameworks link groups of concepts into an entire perspective or view of a situation. Thus, conceptual frameworks or models are broader than theories.

Despite the fact that nursing's conceptual frameworks are not yet scientifically validated (and some may never be), they are quite influential in shaping the thinking of many modern nurses. In fact, many nursing schools use one or more conceptual models to structure their curricula. Thus, these frameworks represent a watershed or landmark in the rise of nursing as a science. Because of their significance, conceptual models are central to the study of nursing science.

Four of the more commonly used nursing conceptual frameworks are presented here. Because the concepts of person, environment, health, and nursing frame the domain of nursing as a discipline, the content of each framework is summarized around those general concepts. For further information on each model, refer to the original works of each theorist and to other published analyses and critiques of these models listed in the bibliography at the end of the chapter.

King's Theory of Goal Attainment

Summary of Model. King's basic thesis is that a client and nurse perceive each other and their situation, share information, set goals related to the client's health, explore means, and act to attain goals.[13–15] This interactive process is depicted in Figure 32–1. King framed nursing as a process using a set of three interlocking systems: personal, interpersonal, and social.

Person. King[13] described the individual, or personal system, as a "unified, complex whole self who perceives, thinks, desires, imagines, decides, identifies goals and selects means to achieve them" (p. 27). She further identified six concepts by which nurses could better understand persons: perception, self, growth and development, body image, space, and time. Table 32–4 lists and defines these concepts. King concluded that persons' perceptions of self, body image, space, and time influence their responses to other persons, objects, and life events. Also, changes in body structure and function occurring with growth and development further influence a person's perceptions of self.

Environment. King spoke of the environment as an open system that interacts with persons in exchanging matter, energy, and information. For example, the environment is a source of air that, when taken in by a person, is altered through a process of gaseous exchange occurring in the person's lungs. She also acknowledged an internal and external environment from which stressors could originate.

King's interpersonal and social systems can be viewed as components of the environment. Interpersonal systems are created when people interact in groups of two or more. Components of the interpersonal system are interaction, communication, transaction, role, and stress. All components are interrelated. Interactions, for example, are influenced by one's communication, role, and stress. These concepts are further defined in Table 32–5.

Groups of people are imbedded in social systems, which King[13] defined as "organized boundary system(s) of social roles, behaviors, and practices, developed to maintain values and the mechanisms to regulate the practices and rules" (p. 115). Social systems are characterized by the concepts of organization, authority, power, status, and decision-making. The social system, through its component concepts, provides the context that influences interpersonal and personal systems.

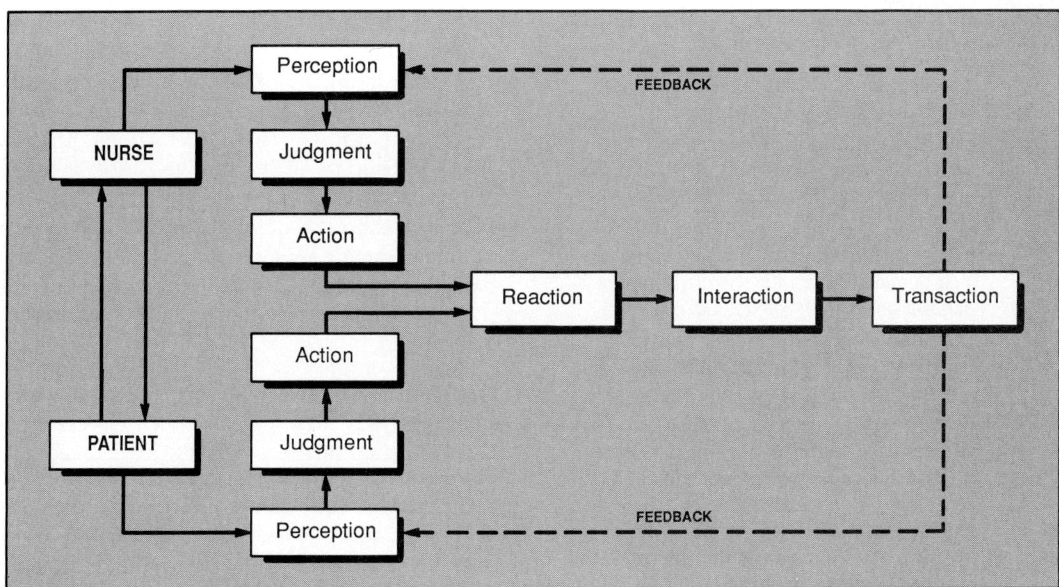

Figure 32–1. King's theory of goal attainment: A process of human interactions. (*From King IM.* A Theory for Nursing: Systems, Concepts, Process. *New York: Wiley; 1981; 145, with permission.*)

TABLE 32–4. KING'S CONCEPTS DESCRIBING PERSONAL SYSTEMS

Concept	Definition
Perception	A process of organizing, interpreting, and transforming information from sensory data and memory by which one gives meaning to experience, represents one's image of reality, and influences one's behavior.
Self	A composite of thoughts and feelings making up persons' awareness of who and what they are, including a system of ideas, attitudes, values, and commitments.
Growth and development	Physiological, cognitive, and behavioral changes occurring in people over time.
Body image	Persons' perceptions of their own body and of others' reactions to their appearance.
Space	The physical area called "territory," as defined by the behavior of its occupants.
Time	A sequence of events moving onward into the future and influenced by the past; duration between one event and another as uniquely experienced by each human being.

Adapted from King IM. A Theory for Nursing: Systems, Concepts, Process. *New York: Wiley; 1981.*

Health. King's framework adopts both adaptive and functional views of health. The adaptive view likens health to a process of adjusting or adapting. It is illustrated in King's[13] definition of health as "dynamic life experiences of a human being, which implies continuous adjustment to stressors in the internal and external environment through optimum use of one's resources to achieve maximum potential for daily living" (p. 5). Thus, a person could be seen as healthy, even with a diagnosis of diabetes mellitus, if he or she was able to keep blood sugar in control and allay development of complications enough to carry out a normal pattern of living. The functional view of health equates health with an ability to perform work and carry out roles. It was expressed when King[13] defined health more simply as "an ability to function in social roles" (p. 143).

TABLE 32–5. KING'S CONCEPTS DESCRIBING INTERPERSONAL SYSTEMS

Concept	Definition
Interaction	A sequence of verbal and nonverbal behaviors that are goal-directed.
Communication	A circular, irreversible, and unrepeatable process whereby information is given from one person to another either directly or indirectly.
Transaction	A process of interaction in which human beings communicate with the environment to achieve goals that are valued.
Role	A set of behaviors, defined by rules or procedures, that is expected when occupying a position in a social system.
Stress	A dynamic state whereby a human being interacts with the environment to maintain balance for growth, development, and performance, which involves an exchange of energy and information between the person and the environment for the regulation and control of stressors.

Adapted from King IM. A Theory for Nursing: Systems, Concepts, Process. *New York: Wiley; 1981.*

Nursing. King[13] viewed nursing as an interpersonal process the goal of which "is to help individuals maintain their health so they can function in their roles" (pp. 4–5). Thus, nursing is a special case of an interpersonal system, requiring nurse and client to collaborate. The domain of nursing[13] "includes promotion of health, maintenance and restoration of health, care of the sick and injured, and care of the dying" (p. 4).

The process of nursing is carried out through mutual goal setting. In mutual goal setting, nurse and client collaborate using an interpersonal process to define and attain the health goals of the client.

Analysis. King's framework is descriptive in that it provides a set of less abstract concepts that elaborate on the boundary concepts of person, environment, health, and nursing that define the domain of nursing science. Her framework is also process-oriented in that its focus is more on the flow of the nurse–client relationship than on its content or substance. Content is left for nurse and client to define. Thus, King's model offers a less clear distinction between nursing and other helping and health care professions than do some other nursing frameworks that focus on the content of nurse–client interactions. King's view of person is holistic in an integrative sense: it does not reduce people to parts or subsystems, but regards them in their entirety. Although quite abstract, King's notions of environment provide a way to examine stressors and forces that can affect a person's health. Further, her definition of health is dependent on social roles and is, therefore, culturally determined.

Orem's Self-care Deficit Theory of Nursing

Summary of Model. The main thesis of Orem's model is that people require nursing care when their needs for care exceed (or can be predicted to exceed) their own ability to meet these needs.[14,16–18] Orem called needs "self-care requisites" and ability "self-care agency." When individuals' needs exceed their ability, this situation is called a "self-care deficit."

Person. Within Orem's conceptual framework, a person is understood to be an integrated whole being who functions biologically, symbolically, and socially. Persons are viewed as agents with the potential power to meet their own needs for self-care.

According to Orem, self-care agency changes across individuals and within an individual over time. Factors that affect one's level of self-care agency are called basic conditioning factors. They include age, sex, developmental state, living conditions, family systems, sociocultural orientation, and health state. Self-care agency encompasses one's ability to recognize the need for, plan for, and provide one's own self-care. For example, evidence of self-care agency can be seen in a person's recognition of the need for food and in his or her actions to obtain, prepare, and ingest a balanced variety of foods in appropriate amounts.

People exercise self-care agency by taking action to meet their own needs for care arising from one or more of three sets of requisites: universal, developmental, or health deviation. Table 32–6 lists these requisites. Needs for care arising from self-care requisites are called "therapeutic self-care demands." For example, the universal requisite for balancing activity and rest creates a therapeutic self-care demand for the average adult to obtain 6 to 8 hours of sleep nightly.

Every person has a set of therapeutic self-care demands that are universal or common to all persons; however, each individual may also have self-care demands that are unique or particular. When an individual has insufficient self-care agency to meet a current or projected self-care demand, a self-care deficit exists. For example, an adult unable to obtain the 6 to 8 hours of sleep nightly will eventually become exhausted. Thus, exhaustion is a self-care deficit. Self-care deficits become the reasons a person needs nursing care.

Environment. Environment is a less developed concept in Orem's model than is person; however, Orem acknowledged environment in two ways. First, she viewed environment as having physical and psychosocial factors, elements, or conditions that give rise to self-care requirements. For example, an environment may pose special challenges, such as occupational hazards, that precipitate specific therapeutic self-care demands, such as the wearing of safety goggles or other protective equipment. Second, Orem considered the environment as having possible therapeutic value, which she termed "developmental environment." A developmental environment is one that uses specialized programs, routines, and physical structures to help persons establish goals and adjust behavior to reach them. A psychiatric unit of a hospital is one example of a developmental environment.

Health. According to Orem, health is a state of wholeness or of structural and functional integrity. She acknowledged physical, psychological, interpersonal, and social aspects of health, but viewed these as inseparable. Within this framework, health and illness are a continuum, and self-care is necessary to sustain or regain health.

Nursing. Orem viewed nursing as a helping service focused on assisting a person to achieve self-care. Nurses use a three-step process to provide this service; diagnosing therapeutic self-care demands, designing and planning needed self-care actions, and producing and managing appropriate nursing systems. Nursing care is aimed at meeting therapeutic self-care demands until a person's self-care agency (or the agency of a dependent caregiver) is adequate to meet those demands or until the demands are resolved.

Within this model, nurses use five modes of helping to meet therapeutic self-care demands: acting for/doing for another, guiding, supporting, teaching, and providing a developmental environment. Each of these modes can be applied in three types of nursing service systems: wholly compensatory, partially compensatory, and educative-supportive. In a wholly compensatory system, nurses perform all necessary self-care actions for a client. Such a system might be used in an intensive care unit or with an unconscious client. In a partially compensatory system,

TABLE 32–6. OREM'S UNIVERSAL, DEVELOPMENTAL, AND HEALTH DEVIATION REQUISITES

Universal Requisites	Developmental Requisites	Health-deviation Requisites
Maintaining a sufficient intake of air, water, and food. Providing care associated with elimination. Balancing activity and rest. Balancing solitude and social interaction. Preventing hazards to life, functioning, and well-being. Promoting normalcy as a functioning, developing, social human in accord with one's potentials and limitations.	Providing living conditions that support growth, development, and maturation throughout the life cycle. Preventing or overcoming the effects of situations that threaten or challenge continued development.	Knowing when and how to obtain appropriate medical help. Monitoring the effects of disease in one's self. Carrying out medically prescribed measures. Monitoring for ill-effects of medical measures. Adjusting self-concept to one's state of health. Learning to live constructively with the effects of disease.

From Orem DE. Nursing Concepts of Practice, *3rd ed. New York: McGraw-Hill; 1985.*

nurse and client collaborate to carry out the client's self-care actions. Many elderly residents in nursing homes require partially compensatory systems of nursing care because they are dependent in only some areas of self-care. In an educative-supportive system, nurses assist clients to perform their own self-care actions through teaching and encouragement. Much of the nursing care delivered in clinics or at health fairs illustrates an educative-supportive nursing care system.

Analysis. Orem's model is comprehensive in that it can apply to a wide range of nursing situations and health care settings. Supporters of the model hail its utility for defining a focus for nursing (self-care) that is distinct from medicine's focus (illness). However, critics of the model cite its complexity, detail, and cumbersome language. Further, her view of health is narrow and the role of environment is only vaguely described. Although Orem does espouse a holistic view of people, her view casts them as a compilation of needs, parts, or systems. This is in contrast to King's integrated view.

Roy's Adaptation Model

Summary of Model. The basic thesis of the Roy model is that nurses promote clients' adjustment to challenges that they encounter in that dimension of life relating to health and illness.[14,19,20] To Roy, adjusting is called "adaptation" and challenges are termed "stimuli."

Person. Like other theorists, Roy identified people as the focus of nursing. Roy defined people as bio-psycho-social beings. Within her model, a person is regarded as an adaptive system with regulator and cognator subsystems. A person is a system in that information, matter, and energy are taken in as inputs, processed as throughputs, and released as outputs. A person is adaptive in that constant adjustment to inputs is necessary for survival. Because Roy sees people as having biological, psychological, and social aspects, which function as subsystems, her view is holistic in an additive sense: the sum of the subsystem functions as the human system.

The regulator and cognator subsystems in Roy's model are mechanisms people use to adapt to or cope with stimuli (inputs). The regulator subsystem uses chemical, neural, and endocrine means to process system throughput. The cognator subsystem uses the higher-order cognitive processes of information processing, learning, judgment, and emotion. Perception links regulator and cognator subsystems. The regulator system input forms the basis for a perception, which is then modified by the cognator system; the modified perception then influences the regulator system response. For example, a person who has experienced a trauma (stimulus) and sustained a fracture will employ the regulator subsystem to control bleeding, announce pain, and release adrenaline; and the cognator subsystem to assess his or her level of danger or to obtain help.

People adapt by generating responses (outputs), which feed back as inputs into both subsystems. The output of regulator and cognator subsystems is coping behavior in one of four adaptive modes: physiological needs, self-concept, role function, and interdependence. In the trauma situation, an example of coping in the physiological-needs mode might be voluntarily immobilizing the fractured limb; coping in the self-concept mode could be thinking of oneself as strong enough to recover from the traumatic event; coping in the role-function mode might be arranging for a leave of absence from one's job until the acute phase of the fracture is stabilized; and coping in the independence mode could entail temporarily increasing one's dependence on others to accomplish tasks one can ordinarily do unaided. Roy's adaptive modes are summarized in Table 32–7.

Environment. In Roy's model, environments are of two types: internal and external. Both are always changing. Each environment is a source of stimuli to the adaptive system of person. Roy did not distinguish or relate the internal environment and the person as an adaptive system. This is a confusing point about her model.

Three classes of stimuli exist: focal, contextual, and residual. Focal stimuli are those of immediate importance. Contextual stimuli provide the relevant background of a situation and might include such things as genetic endowment, cultural orientation, and gender. Residual stimuli are other factors, which may or may not be relevant to the present situation, but whose effects cannot be known. Classification of stimuli as focal, contextual, or residual is determined by one's perception and situation. For example, a young girl darts onto the road in front of an oncoming motorist to retrieve her rolling ball. To the girl, a focal stimulus is the ball, a contextual stimulus may be her age, and

TABLE 32–7. ROY'S ADAPTIVE MODES

Mode	Description
Physiological needs	Encompass the needs for activity and rest, nutrition, elimination, fluid and electrolyte balance, oxygen and circulation, temperature regulation, sensory functioning, and regulation of the endocrine system.
Self-concept	Entails perceptions of the physical self, including physical attributes, functioning, sexuality, wellness–illness state, and appearance; and of the personal self, including moral-ethical self, self-consistency, self-ideal, and self-esteem.
Role function	Includes three types of roles: primary roles based on developmental level; secondary roles, related to autonomy; and tertiary roles, which are temporary and task-oriented.
Interdependence	Involves a balance between dependence and independence in relationships.

Adapted from Roy SC, Roberts SL. Theory Construction in Nursing: An Adaptation Model. *Englewood Cliffs, NJ: Prentice-Hall, 1981.*

a residual stimulus may be whether or not her mother was observing. To the motorist, a focal stimulus is the girl, a contextual stimulus is the level of alcohol in his or her blood, and a residual stimulus may be whether or not the girl's mother is observing.

Health. Roy viewed health, ranging from peak wellness to death, as the dimension of life of interest to nursing. Within this dimension, nursing's concern is to promote adaptation in each of the four modes. Adaptive responses are those promoting survival, growth, reproduction, and self-mastery.

Nursing. According to Roy, nursing is a theoretical knowledge system prescribing analyses and actions pertaining to the care of ill or potentially ill people. Nursing is required when unusual stresses or weakened coping mechanisms yield ineffective responses that threaten adaptation. Thus, as an outcome of a near accident (unusual stress), an alcoholic motorist who does not see himself or herself as an alcoholic (ineffective response) now recognizes alcoholism as a problem (weakened current coping in the self-concept mode) and seeks treatment, including nursing care, for alcoholism (threat to adaptation).

Roy proposed a six-step problem-solving process for nursing: assessing client behaviors, assessing influencing factors, identifying problems, setting goals, selecting interventions, and evaluating outcomes. Each step, described in great detail, follows from the subsystems and elements of her model. According to Roy, nursing acts to manipulate stimuli by increasing, decreasing, modifying, or maintaining them. For example, the nurse may aid the alcoholic through detoxification (decreasing the contextual stimulus for the alcoholic motorist) in the initial phase of care.

Analysis. Roy's model is complex and detailed, integrating information from many other disciplines and applying it from a nursing perspective. Her view of people is holistic in an additive sense. Unlike the previous two models, the Roy model conceptualizes the environment in more detail. Further, like Orem, she differentiates medicine from nursing by focusing the goals of nursing on adaptation, as opposed to health or illness in themselves.

Rogers' Science of Unitary Human Beings

Summary of Model. Rogers proposed a highly abstract conceptual model using terms not ordinarily applied to people.[14,21–24] The central thesis of her model is that people and their environment are integrated (inseparable), and that their mutual interaction produces the unfolding of a person's life process or development. The role of nurses is to support this process by promoting harmonious interaction of person and environment and strengthening the integrity of each.

Person. Rogers views people as energy fields that are four-dimensional (the three dimensions of space plus time) and negentropic (moving toward higher levels of order or organization). As energy fields, people are irreducible unified wholes who are more than and different from the sum of their parts. Thus, people cannot be known from their parts, like some aggregate of systems. People are continuously becoming or developing in the continuum of space-time. Development proceeds toward increasing complexity and diversity.

Within Rogers' model, a human field is characterized or known by its pattern, which is unique to each human. A pattern is perceived as a wave. Waves are thought to progress in specific directions. One example is the sleep–awake pattern of a person over a lifetime, which evolves through cycles of various frequencies and rhythms. Another is one's perception of time passing at various ages, where it drags as a child and races as an adult. Similar changes can be observed in many human rhythms, such as feeding patterns and activity levels. Pattern emerges from the mutual and continuous interaction of human and environmental fields.

Environment. Within Rogers' view, environment, like person, is a four-dimensional negentropic energy field. It encompasses all that is outside any given human field. It too is irreducible and perceived as a whole. Because an environment is all that is not person, the environment is unique for each person. For example, a nurse is in a client's environment, but the nurse is not in her own environment. Therefore, the environment is different for the nurse than it is for the client.

People and their environments are integral and cannot be separated from one another. Therefore, boundaries between a person and the environment are artificial or imagined, used for convenient thinking. Because they are integral, human and environmental fields cannot be fully understood apart from one another. For example, a person's sleep–wake pattern is a product of environmental factors, such as lighting, work schedule, and noise, and the person's energy field. Another person's pattern would be different because of a different merging of different energy fields.

Health. To Rogers, health is an expression of the life process that emerges from the mutual, simultaneous interaction of the human and environmental fields. Development and health are somewhat synonymous within Rogers' model. This developmental view of health, which focuses on change and growth, distinguishes Rogers from other theorists. Because Rogers considered terms such as "health" and "sickness," or "wellness" and "illness," to be value-laden, culturally infused, and arbitrarily defined, she did not focus on them.

Nursing. Rogers[25] defined nursing as both science and art. As a science, nursing's goals are "to study the nature and direction of unitary human development integral with the environment and to evolve the descriptive, explanatory, and predictive principles basic to knowledgeable practice in nursing" (p. 330). As an art, nursing's goals are[21] "to promote symphonic interaction between man and environment, to strengthen the coherence and integrity of the human field, and to direct and redirect patterning of human and environmental fields for realization of maximum health potential" (p. 122).

Like other theorists, Rogers acknowledged that nurses use a problem-solving process, but considered it only a means for implementing nursing knowledge and not nursing knowledge in itself. Fawcett[14] extracted the following elements of this process as Rogers saw it: assessment, diagnosis, goal setting, intervention, and evaluation.

Analysis. Rogers' model is very abstract and complex. It creatively synthesizes knowledge from many fields to yield a focus for nursing science that clearly differentiates it from any other science. Rogers presents a holistic view of people that is truly integrative. Within her framework, environment is as central a concept as person. In her view, health is synonymous with the life process or development.

Because the terms of Rogers' model reflect a high plane of abstraction, at times her model has been criticized as irrelevant to the everyday world of nursing. Nonetheless, among nurse scientists, Rogers' model has sparked more research than most other models. Rogers' model holds great potential for evolving a body of knowledge unique to nursing.

Williamson's Mutual Interaction Model

As early as 1981, Williamson[26] proposed the mutual interaction model of nursing practice. Although the mutual interaction model itself has not received the formal attention that other theoretical constructs in nursing, such as those described above, have received, and although little research that explicitly employs the model has appeared to date, it is nevertheless clear that there is wide interest in the ideas embodied in the model. Indeed, much has been written in the last decade about the importance of mutuality in person-centered client care, client self-determination, shared decision-making, and collaboration between nurse and client.[27–37]

Some authorities[30,33] who focus on collaboration between nurse and client, the central idea of the model, characterize it as a "style" of practice. A style is a distinctive or characteristic interactional manner or tone assumed by nurses in interacting with clients. Williamson, however, envisioned mutual interaction as something more than a style. She looked at mutual interaction as a framework for the structure of practice—that is, a plan for the basic pattern or organization of practice—in which nurses and clients jointly formulate care decisions. In the mutual interaction model, Williamson acknowledged clients' power within health care relationships by stressing the client's role as a mutual participant in outlining the goals and strategies of care and negotiating the care agenda.

Within the mutual interaction model, the person is viewed as instrumental, that is, capable of useful action and having the power to produce effects. This outlook is similar to the positions of King[13] and Orem.[16] Thus, individuals, according to Williamson, can use knowledge to make appropriate, self-determined decisions to influence the outcome of events that affect them. The person interacts with the environment as an open system, reflecting Rogers' ideas. Too often in Western health care, however, the environment is composed of dominant health care professionals who try to impose their priorities on health care "recipients"; the client's role in this system is to legitimize the professional's agenda by compliantly accepting the professional's judgments and is based on an implicit belief that only the professional understands health.

Mutual interaction rejects this idea. Under mutual interaction, health is achieved through a negotiated agenda for care in which nurse and client collaborate to assess the client's situation, determine priorities, and define outcomes. Health is thus a result of self-determination in which clients formulate private beliefs on the basis of information received, reconcile those beliefs with those of other important persons in their lives, and take control over the many factors that shape their behavior.[38] Nursing, under mutual interaction, is an interactive endeavor that facilitates this process and attempts to assist clients to understand the benefits of and resolve conflicts about health recommendations, but which also acknowledges clients' rights to reject recommendations. Nurses function as catalysts and guides, mutually interacting (again reflecting Rogers' open system concept of the environment) to assist clients to explore and understand the consequences of the various options open. Williamson outlines six steps in the joint negotiation of the client care agenda (see Table 37–1), but is less specific than Orem and Roy about the content of the agenda. Williamson's six-phase framework is discussed fully in Chapter 37.

IMPLICATIONS FOR PROFESSIONAL COLLABORATION

Collaboration As a Theoretical Formulation

This text espouses the philosophy that health care decision making is facilitated through exchanges of information, opinions, and attitudes between nurses and their clients. This exchange is known as collaboration.

A philosophy, while it may have intellectual and even emotional appeal, is not a theory but rather a statement of values or an expression of fundamental beliefs. Thus, a philosophy is an idea in which trust is placed but that is not necessarily tested in the scientific sense even though it may have an important influence on behavior. One hallmark of the health care professions is that they subscribe to the rigors of science, and therefore endeavor to challenge the beliefs that underlie their professional activities. For that reason, it is important to the development of theory in nursing that the concept of collaboration be subjected to scientific scrutiny.

For collaboration to be validated scientifically, the concept must first be operationally defined and hypotheses generated about its operation in specific situations. Scientific studies can then be designed to test whether or not collaboration benefits health care outcomes and under what individual and environmental conditions it best operates.

Implications for Nursing Science and Practice

Although similarities can be found among these conceptual models, each model focuses nursing thinking in a somewhat different way. A nurse using Orem's model, for example, would focus on the client's ability for self-care, while another nurse caring for the same client, but using Rogers' model, would focus on environmental and personal factors affecting the individual's development. As a result, nurse scientists observing the same situation through the "lens" of different models would focus on slightly different phenomena, apply diverse conceptual labels to what they observed, see differing aspects of a situation as related, and raise divergent questions from their observations. In these ways, conceptual models of nursing stand to strongly influence the substantive structure of the nursing discipline. In the long run, the use of a variety of conceptual frameworks by nurse scientists and clinicians may result in the proposing and testing of many competing theories concerning the clinical phenomena of interest to nursing. At this stage of nursing's scientific development, such diversity is needed. With time, those theories that best reflect empirical data will form the scientific basis for directing nursing practice. Those that fail this test will fade from use. Meanwhile, all nursing frameworks should be regarded as tentative pathways to nursing truths, each projecting a possible future world of nursing practice.

■ RESEARCH METHODS USED IN NURSING

Traditional thinkers characterize a discipline by its research methods. Some would say that it is their research methods that make disciplines distinct from one another. A more current view does not characterize disciplines by research method alone, but accepts diverse methods within a discipline. Changing views on this issue reflect contemporary views of science, as discussed earlier.

As an emerging discipline, nurse scientists use a variety of research methods. Several factors can explain this fact.

First, like other disciplines, nursing has traditional and contemporary thinkers. The most traditional thinkers regard only experimental methods as the mark of a true science. **Experimental methods** are those in which the independent variable is manipulated or controlled. Experimental methods are also quantitative, that is, they use numerical data. More liberal thinkers accept other quantitative approaches as scientific. Some contemporary thinkers also acknowledge qualitative methods as scientific. Qualitative methods are those that do not generally convert observations to numbers, but group or sort them to yield categories or labels. A study using an open-ended interview, where subjects are asked to tell as many techniques as they can think of to reduce fear, is one example. Subjects' answers would then be grouped or sorted into various categories.

Second, the perspective and values of a discipline also govern judgments on the appropriateness of research methods. As mentioned earlier, nurses' regard for holism and for the uniqueness and autonomy of individuals bears on the choice of research methods made by nurse scientists. Although science, by its nature, is reductionistic, some research methods preserve, capture, or encompass multiple dimensions of phenomena better than others. Thus, such methods may better fit a nursing perspective and value system.

Third, the nature of the phenomenon under study, the level of existing knowledge and theory regarding it, and the specific research question asked can also direct the scientist's choice of research method. Phenomena that have not been studied extensively lack well-developed measuring instruments or well-supported theories. Consequently, nurse scientists studying these phenomena are required to begin by asking questions at the descriptive level of theory development. At this level, qualitative methods may be most suitable. Experiments depend on a base of descriptive and explanatory theories and thus come later in the sequence of evolving scientific knowledge about a phenomenon. Because basic knowledge about so many clinical phenomena is yet undiscovered, research methods yielding descriptive-level theories are appropriate to nursing science.

The following discussion of research methods presents several examples of qualitative research methods, then proceeds to quantitative methods and finally to methods using experiments (Table 32–8). This organization was selected to emphasize the progressive nature of theory building and testing, based upon the phenomenon of interest, the level of existing knowledge, and the nature of the research question. Other organizational schemes for nursing research methods, based on statistical analyses or sampling techniques, do exist and can create terminology problems for the beginning student. Alternate names for various methods are mentioned, where appropriate, in the discussion that follows to reduce this confusion for students consulting other texts.

Clinical Observation Methods

Clinical observation methods are those that aim to define and describe a clinical phenomenon or situation, elucidating all dimensions, facets, or aspects of it. Some observational approaches also seek to distinguish the phenomenon from other related ones and to identify factors or variables associated with the phenomenon.[39] Clinical observation methods include the case study, phenomenological, participant-observer, and direct observation methods.

Observational methods can be applied to any phenomenon that can be sensed or is observable, either directly or indirectly by use of an instrument. Because they apply to a wide variety of phenomena and do not require a preexisting theory, observational methods represent a very important starting point in nursing science.

Observational methods generally require small samples or single cases, purposefully selected to illustrate, embody, or typify the phenomenon.[39] Thus, scientists usually do not generalize results of observational studies. Rather,

TABLE 32–8. RESEARCH METHODS USED IN NURSING

Clinical Observation Methods

Use one or more of the following approaches to study small samples of a given population.

Case study method: Client case example(s) is analyzed using a given theory.

Phenomenological method: Persons experiencing the phenomenon under study are observed and interviewed to determine the meaning of the phenomena to them.

Participant-observer method: Researcher experiences the phenomenon under study with the population being studied to determine the meaning of the phenomenon.

Direct observation method: Repeated observations of the phenomenon under study are made, with a focus on specific characteristics of the phenomenon.

Survey Method

Data are gathered via interviews, questionaires, and reviews of health and other records to describe the prevalence or distribution of a phenomenon among a large population group.

Cross-sectional Method

Uses large randomly selected samples to study a phenomenon in a specific developmental stage or age group over time.

Retrospective Method

Compares two groups of subjects: one with and one without the phenomenon under study, and/or one with and one without certain historical factors, to determine causative factors of the phenomenon.

Longitudinal Method

Examines a large random sample of subjects over time to determine causes, rates, and temporal relationships between the cause and effect(s) of a given phenomenon.

Experimental Methods

True experimental method: Randomly selected experimental and control groups are studied. The researcher manipulates the independent variable and/or controls intervening variables with the experimental group to determine whether or not the independent variable has the predicted effect. The control group is not exposed to the independent variable.

Quasi-experimental method: Control or randomization is not possible, so some or all of the subjects are exposed to the independent variable or exposed at different times. Comparison is made of those exposed and not exposed or of different times of exposure.

results serve more as a basis or point of departure for validation in later studies having random samples. Most observational methods are qualitative.

Case Study Method. A case study is an analysis—usually of a single case, subject, group, or institution—organized such that meaning or order is imposed on facts and data in a situation. For example, the facts and data describing the development of a client with an unusual health problem would be summarized and a theory or conceptual framework used to link the facts and data in an enlightening way. A small number of similar cases might also be compared and contrasted using this approach.[40] In case studies, facts or data are sorted and labeled according to a predetermined conceptual framework. Nursing conceptual frameworks have been useful for this purpose. Also, theories established to explain other phenomena can sometimes find new application within a case study.[41]

Phenomenological Method. The phenomenological method[42,43] is also an analysis drawn from one or a few persons aimed at discovering the *meaning* of a phenomenon or situation. Meaning here refers to significance or interpretation from the subject's point of view. The aim of this method is to uncover features of a phenomenon common to those who experience or live it: to get an insider's view of what it is like to be overweight, lonely, or pregnant for example. Phenomena most often studied by this method are human conditions or states, such as panic; or processes, such as dying.

Unlike a case study, this method is not used to organize data or facts according to a predetermined conceptual model. Rather, the researcher seeks natural order or meaning from the data themselves. Further, the phenomenological method permits nonobjective data, the subjective aspects of experience as reported by participants, to be recognized as valid data.

Participant–Observer Methods. This group of qualitative methods also seeks an insider's view of situations or processes by having the observer become part of the group observed. In general, the researcher in some way lives with the phenomenon or joins the population under study. By assuming such a relationship with the subject matter, the researcher gains access to information and develops insights into the data that are not accessible to scientists using more objective approaches. Phenomena most often studied by this method are natural processes, such as the transition to parenting, or cultural practices and life-styles, such as health practices of Navajo Indians.

Because researchers using this method embed themselves in groups, settings, or communities where the phenomenon is happening, participant-observer methods usually involve slightly larger samples than case or phenomenological approaches. Narrative data are recorded in extensive field notes or on audio- or videotape. Data are broken into units, coded, and sorted into conceptually meaningful categories. Categories are arranged into organized descriptions or explanations. Examples of participant-observer methods include grounded-theory[44] method and ethnography.[45]

Direct Observation Method. In direct observation, the scientist makes repeated observations of the focal phenomenon under naturally varying conditions. Specific characteristics of the phenomenon are recorded for each observation. Phenomena most often studied by this method are behaviors or behavior patterns that can be easily circumscribed or are naturally discrete, such as various types of movement, interactions between people, or eating behavior.

Unlike participant-observer methods, researchers who use this method maintain distance or objectivity. Objectivity is maintained by predetermining those features of the phenomenon to be noted and recorded. Features are chosen according to some conceptual framework. Because features of phenomena can be counted or quantified, direct observation is usually a quantitative method. Direct observation is one of the oldest scientific methods.

Survey Method

The survey method[46] aims to describe the prevalence and distribution of a phenomenon and related variables in a population. Children with leukemia or nursing home residents are examples. Phenomena that could be studied among leukemic children include their position in the family, blood type, or exposure to toxins. Surveys can establish norms concerning such phenomena in the population of interest.

The most common data-collection techniques employed in surveys are interviews, questionnaires, and reviews of records such as hospital charts or death certificates. Surveys are usually quantitative but may incorporate qualitative data.

A key difference between clinical observation methods and surveys is the selection of subjects. In clinical observation approaches, a few subjects are usually chosen expressly because they exemplify the phenomenon. In surveys, a sample is chosen to represent a population. Thus, surveys usually have large samples selected in a random fashion. A representative sample allows researchers to generalize findings of surveys.

Cross-sectional Method

The cross-sectional method studies various age groups or developmental stages at a single point in time to infer trends over time.[46] This method is used to narrow and isolate possible factors that may begin to explain why a phenomenon occurs. An example would be the study of coping skills of asthmatic children in various ages groups or at various stages of asthma.

Like surveys, cross-sectional studies ideally rely on large random samples. However, the sample is usually divided into groups that differ in regard to the phenomenon of interest. For example, immobile nursing home residents may be divided into those with and without pressure sores. Groups are then compared to identify other variables on which they differ. The results of earlier surveys and clinical observation studies generate the variables used for comparisons. Variables are measured quantitatively; a variety of data-collection techniques are possible in cross-sectional studies. Variables showing statistically significant differences between groups begin to form the basis of an explanation for the phenomenon and become the focus of later studies. The cross-sectional method and all methods that build from it are quantitative.

Retrospective Method

Retrospective studies[46] link subjects who presently demonstrate the phenomenon of interest to factors, presumed to be causes, that occurred in the past. In a way, retrospective studies are like reverse experiments: the result or effect is known and the cause is traced. For this reason, they are sometimes called "ex post facto" (after the fact) methods. An example is to compare obese persons and those of normal weight for factors in their past that vary, such as family history, exercise patterns, and birth weight.

Like cross-sectional studies, retrospective ones use at least two groups, generally those with and without the phenomenon. However, the groups are otherwise constructed to be as similar as possible. Groups are then compared on factors in their past that could account for the fact that they are now different with regard to the phenomenon of interest. Retrospective studies aim to further narrow and test the association of factors with a phenomenon.

Ideally, retrospective studies use random or matched samples. Matched samples reduce differences between experimental and control groups on the dependent variable so that results are less likely to be explained by sampling error. Again, results of previous studies direct the choice of variables used for matching and variables used for comparison. A variety of data-collection approaches are possible, but the "retrospective data" often come from historical sources such as census or school records. Therefore, data on factors that might explain the phenomenon, or effect, are not always available. Variables that continue to show significance in retrospective studies are retained for further investigation.

Longitudinal Method

Longitudinal studies are those that examine events or phenomena over time in order to determine time-ordered relationships. Longitudinal studies have three aims: to narrow and test associations between possible causes and effects, to establish incidence rates for phenomena, and to determine the temporal order between presumed causes and effects.[47] Phenomena that can be studied cross-sectionally or retrospectively can also be studied longitudinally.

Longitudinal studies begin with a large random sample, some of whose members are with and some without the presumed causal variables. Over time, the two groups are followed and measured for the effect or phenomenon of interest.[48] Incidence rates are compared to determine if those with the presumed cause are more likely to develop the effect. Longitudinal studies are also called prospective or causal comparative studies.

Because longitudinal studies establish the time order of events and allow for more control of confounding or intervening variables, they are stronger for inferring cause than are retrospective studies.[49] However, longitudinal studies are uncommon, primarily because they are expensive to carry out.

Experimental Methods

Experiments are considered the scientific ideal for establishing cause-and-effect relationships. Characteristics of experiments that permit this level of confidence are manipulation, control, and randomization. When any of these are not exercised, an experiment is weakened. **Manipulation** means that the presumed cause or treatment (independent variable) is varied by the researcher among the groups in the experiment. **Control** means that special procedures are followed to eliminate, distribute, consider, or measure the effects produced by variables other than the independent one. **Randomization** is a means to equalize groups or to distribute the effects of intervening variables. Though experiments involve groups, it is less important that subjects are randomly selected to represent a population (as in cross-sectional, retrospective, and prospective methods) and more important that subjects are randomly assigned to a group.[50]

In nursing research, as in other fields involving human subjects, true experiments are not always possible. Sometimes artificial manipulation of the independent variable or random assignment of subjects to groups is impossible or unethical. Consequently, researchers have developed two kinds of experimental methods: true experimental and quasi-experimental methods.

True Experimental Methods. True experiments are those in which the researcher is able to manipulate the independent variable or variables, control for the effects of intervening or confounding variables, and randomly select and assign subjects to groups.[51] The basic true experiment involves two equal groups. One (the experimental group) is exposed to the independent variable; the other (the control group) is not. Following exposure, both groups are tested for the effect (dependent variable). Results are compared to determine if the independent variable produced the hypothesized effect. This is called a posttest design. All other experimental designs are a variation of it. Variations are introduced to provide greater levels of control.

Quasi-experimental Methods. A quasi-experiment is a modified experiment, where either control or randomization are not fully possible. In quasi-experiments, some or all of the subjects are exposed to the independent variable; however, randomization or control is lacking. Thus quasi-experiments are weaker than true experiments for drawing causal inferences.

As for true experiments, quasi-experiments are all variations of the posttest design. Cook and Campbell[50] grouped quasi-experiments into nonequivalent control groups and time-series designs, each having a number of subtypes. Nonequivalent control group designs are generally hampered by lack of randomization. Thus, the groups may be fundamentally different in known or unknown ways, and this difference, rather than the independent variable, must be considered as a possible cause for any observed effects. Time-series designs are limited by lack of a control group. To compensate, subjects serve as their own controls. This is done by collecting data on the dependent variable at several points in time. During the course of data collection, the independent variable is introduced, and effects are observed and compared to the pretreatment pattern.

Other Research Methods Used in Nursing

The methods discussed above are those most commonly used for building theory from descriptive to predictive and control levels. However, there are several other research methods used in nursing that do not fit neatly into this progression. Among them are philosophical, historical, and methodological studies. The former two are most often used to clarify understanding of the roots or origins of the thinking on a subject. The latter method is most often used to determine the validity and reliability of measures.

Nursing research and science encompass a wide variety of research methods. Such variety is accepted within the nursing discipline because of the wide range of phenomena within the domain of nursing science and because of the need to develop theory about these phenomena in a progressive way, from descriptive- to predictive-level theories. In general, the following three principles characterize research methods appropriate to nursing science: both objective and subjective views of phenomenon are valued; systematic and progressive approaches are valued; and coherence between question, method, and perspective is necessary.

The wide variety of nursing research methods provides nurse scientists with many tools for the development of knowledge for nursing practice.

RELATIONSHIPS BETWEEN NURSING SCIENCE AND NURSING PRACTICE

Nurse scientists and clinicians are drawn together by a mutual interest in phenomena encountered in nursing practice, a common perspective from which those phenomena are viewed, and a shared professional value system. The task of the scientist is to generate knowledge of potential value to the clinician and to disseminate that knowledge for clinical use. The task of the clinician is to identify, evaluate, and apply knowledge relevant to clinical problems and to raise questions for investigation where nursing's knowledge base is inadequate. Nurse scientists and clinicians can benefit clients by sharing their ideas and collaborating to produce research studies. The following section describes in more detail the role of the clinician in advancing nursing practice through nursing science.

Identifying Knowledge for Practice

Knowledge is dynamic. Questions having no present answer may be answered in the near future, and what is thought to be true today may be proven false tomorrow. We live in the information age. The dynamic nature of knowledge implies a need for nurses to adopt an attitude of lifelong learning and to update their professional knowledge base continually.

Professional attitudes and an inquiring mind are easiest to cultivate during one's professional training, when support from peers and teachers is high and distractions from the work world may be few. Nurses who make the time to maintain active interest and involvement in the developments of nursing theory and research accrue many benefits to themselves, both personally and professionally, and to their clients. Personal benefits include increased satisfaction with work, recognition from peers and supervisors as a competent—even expert—clinician, and reduced frustration and burnout. Professional benefits include greater clinical efficiency and effectiveness and increased professional autonomy and control over clinical situations. Benefits to clients may be the most important of all. These benefits include more predictable outcomes of care, improved quality of care, and greater client satisfaction.

Nurses, beginning as students, need to know where and how to identify and locate relevant knowledge for nursing practice. Though textbooks can offer a comprehensive overview of a clinical topic, it is nursing journals and periodicals that offer the most in-depth and current information for practice.

In recent years, the number and quality of research-based nursing journals have increased substantially. Major nursing journals that regularly publish scientific advancements in nursing are listed in Box 2–1 in Chapter 2. Further, many general and specialized nursing journals emphasize the clinical application of research. Journals in related fields—such as psychology, physiology, gerontology, sociology, and medicine—can also provide valuable current information and ideas with relevance to nursing practice.

In fact, the field of nursing literature has grown so large and is advancing so rapidly that it is no longer possible to keep up with advancements in nursing science across all clinical specialties. To keep current, the professional nurse must select a focus or interest area within nursing practice. Interest in a specialized area of nursing practice often begins during a nurse's professional education and should be fostered through professional reading and scholarly activity.

Once a beginning nurse has selected a focus within nursing, one strategy for keeping current is to regularly review the two or three journals that relate most directly to that specialty area. This strategy can be achieved by reserving regular library time in one's personal schedule or by purchasing personal subscriptions to appropriate journals.

At times, when nurses are confronted or perplexed by a new or puzzling clinical situation, they may need to search out more information relating to that particular topic or problem than the journals they regularly read provide. The most useful tools for locating information on a specific topic are indexes or data bases. These references catalog articles published in major journals in a broad field of knowledge according to key words in the titles or abstracts (summaries) of articles. Articles are often cross-referenced under several related headings and can also be retrieved by author name or date of publication. Indexes may also identify whether an article is a research study, review, or case study.

Data bases are available in printed or electronic form, depending upon the library. Literature cataloged in electronic data bases usually can be searched quickly by computer. If an article has an abstract, electronic data bases often carry the abstract on-line. Major indexes of nursing and health literature include the *Cumulative Index to Nursing and Allied Health Literature* and the *Index Medicus.* Figure 32–2 shows an example of an article citation from *Paperchase,* a computerized version of the *Index Medicus.* Other related fields, such as psychology and physiology, also have major indexes. Further information on indexes and electronic literature searches can be found in Chapter 21.

Evaluating the Scientific Merit of Research Studies

Once nurses identify research articles relevant to their interests or questions, the next step is to read and evaluate the studies for their scientific merit. Most studies are reviewed by experts before they are chosen for publication. However, even published studies are not perfect. All research studies have both strengths and limitations. It is up to individual clinicians, as consumers of research, to evaluate the merit and applicability of research findings before incorporating new knowledge into their clinical practice.

To evaluate a research report for merit, the reader begins by reading the study and taking notes on it. The reader then attempts to summarize information about each step of the research process discussed earlier and outlined in Box 32–2. The reader looks for both strong points and weak points of the study, giving attention to what information the researcher has included in the report, as well as to information that was omitted. Once the study is summarized, the reader systematically evaluates each portion of the report, using a checklist of criteria or questions, such as those found in Table 32–9. The checklist can be modified to fit the type of research study being reviewed. Finally, it is a good idea for the reader to write a brief critique about the

(REFERENCE 9 OF 34)
89139077
1 McManus MA Newacheck PW
2 Rural maternal, child, and adolescent health.
3 HEALTH SERV RES 1989 Feb; 23(6):807–48

4 <CHILD HEALTH SERVICES> <MATERNAL HEALTH SERVICES> <RURAL HEALTH> <VITAL STATISTICS>

<ACUTE DISEASE> <ADOLESCENCE> <CHILD> <CHILD, PRESCHOOL> <CHRONIC DISEASE> <DELIVERY OF HEALTH CARE> <DEMOGRAPHY> <FEMALE> <HUMAN> <INFANT> <INFANT, NEWBORN> <MEDICAL ASSISTANCE, TITLE 19> <NATIONAL CENTER FOR HEALTH STATISTICS (U.S.)> <PREGNANCY> <REVIEW>
5 <*REVIEW,* TUTORIAL> <SUPPORT, NON-U.S. GOV'T>
<SUPPORT, U.S. GOV'T, NON-P.H.S.> <SUPPORT, U.S. GOV'T, P.H.S.> <UNITED STATES>

6 Authors cite recommendations for research in light of a general lack of current literature on health status, health services ulilization, organization and delivery of health services, and health care financing in this field.

7 Institutional address:
McManus Health Policy
Inc.
Washington
DC 20016.

Figure 32–2. Article citation from *Paperchase.* (Key: **1,** author; **2,** title of article; **3,** journal title, date, volume, (issue), page numbers; **4.** other terms under which the article is cross-referenced; **5,** indicates a review article; **6,** abstract; and **7,** address to contact author.)

soundness of the research, the credibility of the results, and the reasonableness of the researcher's conclusions, and keep a record of the critique for later personal reference.

Although a thorough review of a research study requires time, the benefits are well worth the effort. With each study reviewed, the clinician acquires a deeper understanding of a clinical problem, builds a reference file of clinically relevant information, comprehends more about the research and scientific processes, and develops greater sensitivity to the tentative nature and limits of scientific knowledge.

Applying Knowledge in Practice

The quest for empirical facts and scientific theories by nurse scientists is only an academic exercise unless such facts and theories are subsequently employed by practicing nurses to better the care of clients. Once a nurse has located and critiqued studies of clinical interest, the next step is to determine how valid research findings might be incorporated into practice.

Research frequently yields suggestions for nursing practice, and many published nursing research reports contain explicit implications for changing or introducing new clinical techniques. For example, a recent study[52] of the effects of circumvaginal muscle exercise demonstrated its effectiveness for increasing peak maximum pressure and thus increasing the mass of pelvic floor muscles. This finding may be useful in the treatment of urinary incontinence in women. Results of descriptive level studies, which are preliminary to developing tested interventions, can also sometimes be used to guide design of assessment protocols or selection of evaluation criteria. For example, several nurses[53] recently reported on a study characterizing the sucking patterns of preterm and full-term infants. Their method of observing sucking may become a clinical assessment tool for evaluating the neurobehavioral status of neonates and may have implications for feeding preterm infants.

Before applying research findings directly to a practice situation, the clinician must evaluate the study again. Such a review requires the nurse to judge the "fit" of the findings to the clinician's particular setting and the way in which the findings can be implemented. As when evaluating a study for scientific merit, a study can be evaluated for applicability by asking a number of questions. Questions to guide this evaluation are listed in Table 32–10.

In addition to applying research findings to clinical practice, Chinn and Kramer[54] described two approaches that clinicians can take to contribute more directly to the development and refinement of nursing theory itself: concept analysis and practical validation of theory. Concept analysis is a fundamental step in the process of theory development. In this process, experience is labeled and analyzed. Empirical indicators, or those aspects of the phenomenon with potential for measurement, are identified. The concept is then differentiated from similar ones by concrete example. Finally, criteria for nursing diagnoses related to the concept are isolated and related variables identified. Reed and Leonard[55] recently published a concept analysis of self-neglect, which refers to an intentional client pattern of neglecting prescribed self-care activities despite the availability of resources and knowledge. In their analysis, they described the behaviors that characterize self-neglect and differentiated it from related concepts such as suicidal be-

TABLE 32–9. QUESTIONS FOR EVALUATING THE SCIENTIFIC MERIT OF A STUDY

Problem Statement	Literature Review	Conceptual Framework
Is the problem stated clearly? Is the problem stated concisely? Can the question be answered empirically? Are important terms defined? Is the problem significant to nursing? Does the problem have relevance beyond the study setting?	Is the problem tied to previous related studies? Has the author consulted primary sources? Have important related studies been omitted? Does the review contain current studies? Does the review critically evaluate and compare key studies? Is the review logically organized? Does the review distill key information from all studies and relate it to the study problem?	Is the study linked to a theory? Would another theory be more appropriate? Are deductions from the theory logical?
Hypotheses	**Research Design**	**Research Procedures**
Are hypotheses stated? Does each hypothesis contain a relationship between two or more variables? Are hypotheses logically deduced from the theory or literature review? Are hypotheses testable? Are hypotheses stated concisely? Are hypotheses stated clearly? Do hypotheses identify the population of interest?	Is the design adequately described? Is the design the best approach to answering the research question? Does the design use adequate controls? Does the design rule out alternate explanations for results?	Are procedures described clearly enough for someone to duplicate? Are procedures for ensuring constancy of conditions described? Are procedures for preventing contamination of groups described? Is the setting appropriate to the question? Were the rights of subjects protected?
Subjects	**Data Collection**	**Data Analysis**
Is the target population identified? Does the sample represent the target population? Are sampling procedures described? Are potential biases identified for a nonprobability sample? Is the sample size adequate? Is the response rate adequate? Are characteristics of the sample adequately described?	Are data-collection instruments identified and described? Are the data-collection methods an appropriate way to measure the variables? Have instruments been pretested? Are the instruments reliable? Are the instruments valid?	How were the data analyzed? Was the type of analysis appropriate to the type of data? Are statistics used appropriately?
Findings	**Interpretation of Findings**	**Implications and Recommendations**
Are results clearly presented? Are tables and figures used effectively? Is there evidence of biased reporting?	Are all important findings discussed? Are results interpreted in light of each hypothesis? Are results interpreted in light of prior research studies? Are alternative explanations made? Are limitations considered?	Are implications discussed in relation to the guiding theory? Are practice implications discussed? Are implications appropriate? Are implications over-generalized? Are improvements in methods recommended? Are directions for further research made? Do recommendations match findings?

Adapted from Polit DF, Hungler BP. Nursing Research: Principles and Methods. *3rd ed. Philadelphia: Lippincott; 1987; 489–504.*

havior and noncompliance. Such work can aid in developing the self-care deficit theory of nursing as well as in clarifying the NANDA taxonomy of nursing diagnoses related to noncompliance. Clinicians can contribute much to concept analysis by formally sharing their clinical experiences with nurse researchers.

Practical validation of theory, another way clinicians can aid the advancement of science, is an effort to show how conclusions drawn from theory are false, thus forcing a restructuring of the theory to better fit clinical reality. The clinician can use an inductive approach, in which a concrete clinical example is used as a basis for generating modification of a theory; or a deductive approach, in which a theory is applied to describe a concrete clinical situation. Case studies that are analyzed using a nursing theory are good examples of the practical validation of theory. Case study

TABLE 32–10. QUESTIONS FOR EVALUATING THE CLINICAL APPLICABILITY OF A STUDY

Validation	Comparative Evaluation	Decision Making
Do the study's weaknesses invalidate the findings? Do the study's weaknesses invalidate the conclusions?	Can this study be used in the practice setting? How similar is the study's setting to the nurse's clinical setting? How similar are the study's subjects to the nurse's clinical population? Does the nurse's current practice really need to change? How feasible is it to implement study findings legally? ethically? What decisions or changes are needed to implement the findings? How do the study findings relate to policies and procedures in the nurse's setting? What resources are required to apply the study's findings?	Do results of the evaluation suggest that the study not be applied to practice at this time? Do results of the evaluation suggest that the study be used only to expand the nurse's understanding of the topic at this time? Do results of the evaluation suggest that the study can be applied in the nurse's current practice setting?

Adapted from Stetler C, Marram M. Evaluating research findings for applicability in practice. Nursing Outlook. *1976; 559–563.*

outcomes can act either to confirm or dissent from prevailing theory.

In the scientific tradition, clinicians should attempt to publish the results of projects that aim to apply theory and research findings clinically. Whether successful or not, attempts at application have value in advancing knowledge.

Raising Research Questions

Many research studies in nursing are rooted to a "clinical itch," a nagging clinical problem for which existing knowledge is inadequate. Nurses may experience this itch when existing knowledge is insufficient to explain a recurring situation, such as why a particular client with a chronic heart problem has many acute episodes requiring hospital treatment. In such instances, insufficient knowledge hampers the nurse from intervening effectively. Nurses may also experience this itch when existing knowledge is inadequate to explain unique situations, such as why a terminally ill client recovers against all odds. In such cases, existing knowledge disables nurses from replicating desirable outcomes. Because clinicians deal daily in the phenomena of nursing practice, they are intimately familiar with problems needing investigation. Scientists and researchers are often a step or more removed from clinical reality and thus may not be as aware of the most pressing needs for knowledge or the limitations of a clinical setting on the design of research studies. Consequently, clinicians are of enormous value in signaling the need for research.

In order for clinicians to convert a "clinical itch" to a researchable problem, collaboration with a nurse researcher is advisable. Many larger hospitals have a department of nursing research and development to foster in-house research projects that have practical meaning for the care of clients. Another approach to converting a "clinical itch" to a research problem is through collaboration with nurse researchers in a university-based school of nursing. Some hospitals and nursing homes have formal collaboration agreements with schools of nursing to facilitate development of research projects. Even where no formal agreement exists, university faculty are usually open to the research ideas of practicing nurses and encourage their participation in research projects. Clinicians with an interest in research should consider establishing and maintaining ties with nursing faculty in the community where they practice. Some ways to establish ties include participation in professional associations, attendance at continuing education offerings, and voluntary service to a school of nursing as a clinical preceptor or guest lecturer. These ties establish channels for communication and collaboration between cli-

IMPLICATIONS FOR PROFESSIONAL COLLABORATION

Raising Research Questions and the "Clinical Itch"

Many research studies in nursing are rooted in a "clinical itch," a nagging clinical problem for which existing knowledge is inadequate. Often practicing nurses are the ones who experience the frustration of being repeatedly confronted with a client problem for which they lack information and guidelines. Researchers may be a step removed from clinical reality and thus may not be aware of particular pressing needs for knowledge. One of the critical ways the practicing nurse can contribute to the building of nursing knowledge is to collaborate with nurse researchers by bringing important client care problems to their attention. Furthermore, clinicians can collaborate with nurse scientists to produce research by participating in data collection or assisting to identify subjects. Attending educational workshops on nursing research or requesting that local universities present such workshops is an effective way to become involved in nursing research.

nicians and researchers that are vital to the research endeavor.

Collaborating to Produce Research

Most research requires collaboration. Particularly in clinical investigations, a large team is often required. The composition of a research team varies according to the purpose and goals of the study; however, clinicians are often a vital part of the team. Clinicians may be involved in identifying appropriate research subjects, soliciting subjects' participation, insuring informed consent procedures, collecting data, or implementing a research protocol or intervention. They may also serve on review committees to evaluate studies for safeguards to human rights or act as design consultants regarding the feasibility of implementing a clinical study in a given setting. As managers, nurses may also control a researcher's access to the clinical setting and to potential research subjects.

The role of a clinician on a research team depends on both the individual's interest and research skills. The American Nurses' Association has developed guidelines that specify research functions of nurses with various levels of education.[56] Those functions appropriate to nurses with an associate degree in nursing include demonstrating awareness of the importance of research in nursing, identifying problem areas in nursing practice, and assisting with data collection according to a structured format. Functions appropriate to nurses with a baccalaureate degree in nursing include evaluating research for clinical applicability, identifying researchable problems, participating in the implementation of research studies, using nursing practice to refine and extend knowledge, applying well-founded research findings to practice, and sharing research findings with colleagues.

Important relationships exist between nursing science and nursing practice. Without nursing science, practice could not advance. Without nursing practice, nursing science would have no clear focus or practical purpose. Collaboration between nurse scientists and clinicians is foundational to advancing nursing knowledge and practice. To meet the social mandate for providing a needed service to society, it is essential that nurse scientists and clinicians understand, respect, and facilitate one another's efforts toward this end.

BUILDING NURSING KNOWLEDGE

How Can Research Be Promoted in Service Settings?

Rizzuto C, Mitchell M. Research in service settings: Consortium project outcomes. *J Nurs Admin.* 1988;18:32–37.

This article examines the problems practicing nurses encounter in becoming involved in research activities, given today's cost-conscious health care environment. It reports one successful effort. This case involved a group of eight nursing agencies that joined together to share resources to promote research by practicing nurses within their institutions.

The project was guided by the nursing research office of a major university, which provided a small staff comprised of nurse researchers, a project evaluator, a writer/editor, and a statistical consultant. This staff worked through staff nurses who acted as clinical coordinators in the participating institutions. The role of the coordinators was to promote and facilitate research by individual nurses in the institutions through organizing research committees and courses in their hospitals and providing consultation to other nurses.

The project was highly successful. A total of 200 practicing nurses attended educational workshops and courses on conducting research that were presented. Nurses who took the courses wrote 113 research proposals, three of which were submitted for funding by the project. A total of 27 studies were completed by nurses in the 3 years of the project and 13 more were in process. Ten research articles were accepted for publication, and 60 research-related papers were selected for presentation at a national research symposium.

Personal characteristics that differentiated practicing nurses who participated from those who did not were persistence, organization, confidence, and efficiency. Those who did studies were more logical, placed more value on intellectual matters, and perceived their work environment more positively than did the inactives. Educational background was not found to be a factor.

SUMMARY

Nursing science is a unique and necessary component of nursing's professional knowledge base. Though nurses rely on various sources of knowledge, such as ethics and personal knowledge, to provide high-quality care to clients, scientific knowledge offers the most reliable basis for nursing care. Although scientific knowledge is highly reliable, it is also reductionistic. At times, the reductionistic nature of science conflicts with the holistic perspective of nurses.

Science can be viewed as a product and a process. The product of science is an organized body of theories, built of concepts and the relationships among them. The process of science is research, a systematic approach to answering a scientific question. The product and process of science are united through the process of measurement.

As a discipline, nursing is a unique branch of science. Like other sciences, nursing science aims to generate theories using the research process. However, the uniqueness of nursing science stems from the perspective and value system of nurses, which hold the ideals of holism and individual autonomy in high regard. These views put the focus of nursing science on phenomena that nurses encounter in the context of caring for clients.

As theory, nursing science is concerned with relationships between the major concepts of person, environment, health, and nursing. Many conceptual nursing models have been developed to describe these concepts and their relationships in more detail and can aid in developing nursing theories. These theories can then direct the nursing care of clients.

As research, nursing science uses a variety of methods.

Nursing's perspective and value system necessitate such variety. Multiple research methods also are important within nursing science because of the breadth and diversity of the phenomena that nurse scientists study and the need to build theory from descriptive to predictive levels of understanding.

Nursing science and nursing practice are necessary to one another. Nurse scientists and clinicians concern themselves with the same domain of clinical phenomena and are united in perspective and values. However, scientists and clinicians play different roles in producing and using nursing knowledge. The clinician is vital to advancing nursing science through identification of knowledge for practice, evaluation of research for scientific merit, application of research findings in practice, generation of important research questions, and collaboration to produce research studies for the betterment of nursing care.

REFERENCES

1. Buchler J. *Philosophical Writings of Pierce.* New York: Dover; 1955.
2. Carper B. Fundamental patterns of knowing in nursing. *Adv Nurs Sci.* 1978;1:13–23.
3. Kerlinger FN. *Foundations of Behavioral Research.* 2nd ed. New York: Holt, Reinhart & Winston; 1973.
4. Polanyi M. *Personal Knowledge.* Chicago: University of Chicago Press; 1962.
5. Andersen JE, Briggs LL. A study of quality and supportive evidence. *Image.* 1988;20:141–145.
6. Sutton TD, Murphy SP. Stressors and patterns of coping in renal transplant patients. *Nurs Res.* 1989;38:46–49.
7. Schwab JJ. The concepts of the structure of a discipline. *Educ Record.* 1964;43:197–205.
8. Foshay AW. Knowledge and the structure of disciplines. Unpublished paper; 1961.
9. Donaldson SK, Crowley DM. The discipline of nursing. *Nurs Outlook.* 1978;26:113–120.
10. Fawcett J. Hallmarks of success in nursing theory development. In: Chinn PL, ed. *Advances in Nursing Theory Development.* Rockville, MD: Aspen; 1983:3–17.
11. Flaskerud JH, Halloran EJ. Areas of agreement in nursing theory development. *Adv Nurs Sci.* 1980;3:2.
12. Nightingale F. *Notes on Nursing.* London: D. Appleton; 1860.
13. King IM. *A Theory for Nursing Systems, Concepts, Process.* New York: Wiley; 1981.
14. Fawcett J. *Analysis and Evaluation of Conceptual Models of Nursing.* Philadelphia: Davis; 1984.
15. Gonot PJ, King IM. A theory for nursing. In: Fitzpatrick JJ, Whall AF, eds. *Conceptual Models of Nursing Analysis and Application.* Bowie, MD: Brady; 1989:271–283.
16. Orem DE. *Nursing Concepts of Practice.* 4th ed. New York: McGraw-Hill; 1990.
17. Nursing Development Conference Group. *Concept Formalization in Nursing Process and Product.* 2nd ed. Boston: Little, Brown; 1979.
18. Johnston RL. Orem self-care model of nursing. In: Fitzpatrick JJ, Whall AF, eds. *Conceptual Models of Nursing Analysis and Application.* Bowie, MD: Brady; 1989:165–184.
19. Roy SC, Roberts SL. *Theory Construction in Nursing: An Adaptation Model.* Englewood Cliffs, NJ: Prentice-Hall; 1981.
20. Tiedeman ME. The Roy adaptation model. In: Fitzpatrick JJ, Whall AF, eds. *Conceptual Models of Nursing Analysis and Application.* Bowie, MD: Brady; 1989:185–203.
21. Rogers ME. *The Theoretical Basis of Nursing.* Philadelphia: Davis; 1970.
22. Rogers ME. Nursing: A science of unitary human beings. In: Riehl-Sisca J, ed. *Conceptual Models for Nursing Practice.* 3rd ed. Norwalk, CT: Appleton & Lange; 1989:181–188.
23. Rogers ME. Science of unitary human beings. In: Malinski VM, ed. *Explorations on Martha Rogers' Science of Unitary Human Beings.* Norwalk, CT: Appleton-Century-Crofts; 1986:3–8.
24. Quillin SIM, Runk JA. Martha Rogers' unitary person model. In: Fitzpatrick JJ, Whall AF, eds. *Conceptual Models of Nursing Analysis and Application.* Bowie, MD: Brady; 1989:285–299.
25. Rogers ME. Nursing: A science of unitary man. In: Riehl JP, Roy C, eds. *Conceptual Models for Nursing Practice.* Norwalk, CT: Appleton-Century-Crofts; 1980.
26. Williamson J. Mutual interaction: A model of nursing practice. *Nurs Outlook.* 1981;29:104–107.
27. Caporeal-Katz B. Health, self-care and power: Shifting the balance. *Top Clin Nurs.* 1983;5:31–41.
28. Kim HS. Collaborative decision making in nursing practice: A theoretical framework. In: Chinn P, ed. *Advances in Nursing Theory Development.* Rockville, MD: Aspen; 1983.
29. MacElveen-Hoehn P. The cooperation model for care in health and illness. In: Chaska NL, ed. *The Nursing Profession: A Time to Speak.* New York: McGraw-Hill; 1983.
30. Kasch CR. Establishing a collaborative nurse–patient relationship: A distinct focus of nursing action in primary care. *Image.* 1986;18:44–47.
31. Sloan MR, Schommer BT. The process of contracting in community health nursing. In: Spradley B, ed. *Readings in Community Health Nursing.* 3rd ed. Boston: Little, Brown; 1986.
32. Sarvimaki A. Nursing care as a moral, practical, communicative and creative activity. *J Adv Nurs.* 1988;13:462–467.
33. Roberts SJ, Krouse HJ. Enhancing self-care through active negotiation. *Nurse Practitioner.* 1988;13:44–52.
34. Thorne SE, Robinson CA. Reciprocal trust in health care relationships. *J Adv Nurs.* 1988;13:782–789.
35. Kasch CR, Dine J. Person-centered communication and social perspective taking. *West J Nurs Res.* 1988;10:317–326.
36. Wheeler K. A nursing science approach to understanding empathy. *Arch Psychiatr Nurs.* 1988;2:95–102.
37. Pesznecker BL, Zerwekh JV, Horn BJ. The mutual participation relationship: Key to facilitating self-care practices in clients and families. *Pub Health Nurs.* 1989;6:197–203.
38. DiNicola DD, DiMatteo MR. Communication, interpersonal influence, and resistance to medical treatment. In: Wills TA, ed. *Basic Processes in Helping Relationships.* New York: Academic Press; 1982.
39. Lincoln YS, Guba EG. *Naturalistic Inquiry.* Beverly Hills: Sage; 1985.
40. Schultz PR, Kerr BJ. Comparative case study as a strategy for nursing research. In: Chinn PL, ed. *Nursing Research: Methodology, Issues and Implementation.* Rockville, MD: Aspen; 1986: 195–220.
41. Yin RK. *Case Study Research.* Newbury Park, CA: Sage; 1989.
42. Omery A. Phenomenology: A method for nursing research. *Adv Nurs Sci.* 1983;5:49–63.
43. Lynch-Sauer J. Using a phenomenological research method to

study nursing phenomena. In: Leininger MM, ed. *Qualitative Research Methods in Nursing*. Orlando: Grune & Stratton; 1985: 93–108.

44. Stern PN. Using grounded theory method in nursing research. In: Leininger MM, ed. *Qualitative Research Methods in Nursing*. Orlando: Grune & Stratton; 1985:149–160.
45. Leininger MM. Ethnography and ethnonursing: Models and modes of qualitative research data analysis. In: Leininger MM, ed. *Qualitative Research Methods in Nursing*. Orlando: Grune & Stratton; 1985:33–72.
46. Polit DF, Hungler BP. *Nursing Research: Principles and Methods*. 3rd ed. Philadelphia: Lippincott; 1987.
47. Clinton JF. Conceptual and technical issues in using time series methodology in clinical nursing research. In: Chinn PL, ed. *Nursing Research: Methodology, Issues and Implementation*. Rockville, MD: Aspen; 1986:275–283.
48. Given BA, Keilman LJ, Collins C, Given CW. Strategies to minimize attrition in longitudinal studies. *Nurs Res*. 1990;39:184–187.
49. Youngblut JM, Loveland-Cherry CJ, Horan M. Data management issues in longitudinal research. *Nurs Res*. 1990;39:188–198.
50. Cook TD, Campbell DT. *Quasi-experimentation: Design and Analysis Issues for Field Settings*. Boston: Houghton Mifflin; 1979.
51. Kirk RE. *Experimental Design: Procedures for the Behavioral Sciences*. Belmont, CA: Brooks/Cole; 1982.
52. Dougherty M, Bishop K, Mooney R, Gimotty P. The effects of circumvaginal muscle (CVM) exercise. *Nurs Res*. 1989;38:331–335.
53. Medoff-Cooper B, Weininger S, Zukowski K. Neonatal sucking as a clinical assessment tool: Preliminary findings. *Nurs Res*. 1989;38:162–165.
54. Chinn PL, Kramer MK. *Theory and Nursing: A Systematic Approach*. 3rd ed. St. Louis: Mosby; 1990.
55. Reed PG, Leonard VE. An analysis of the concept of self-neglect. *Adv Nurs Sci*. 1989;11:39–53.
56. American Nurses' Association, Commission on Nursing Research. *Guidelines for the Investigative Function of Nurses*. Kansas City: American Nurses' Association; 1981.

BIBLIOGRAPHY

Barrett EAM, ed. *Visions of Rogers' Science-Based Nursing*. New York: National League for Nursing; 1990.

Blalock HM. *Conceptualization and Measurement in the Social Sciences*. Beverly Hills: Sage; 1982.

Brink PJ, Wood MJ. *Basic Steps in Planning Nursing Research from Question to Proposal*. North Scituate, MA: Duxbury; 1978.

Burns N, Grove SK. *The Practice of Nursing Research: Conduct, Critique and Utilization*. Philadelphia: Saunders; 1987.

Chinn PL, ed. *Nursing Research: Methodology, Issues and Implementation*. Rockville, MD: Aspen; 1986.

Clayton GM, Baj PA. *Review of Research in Nursing Education*, vol. III. New York: National League for Nursing; 1990.

DeGroot HA. Scientific inquiry in nursing: A model for a new age. *Adv Nurs Sci*. 1988;10:1–21.

Dubin R. *Theory Building*. New York: Free Press; 1969.

Dzurec LC. The necessity for and evolution of multiple paradigms for nursing research: A poststructuralist perspective. *Adv Nurs Res*. 1989;11:56–68.

Fawcett J, Downs FS. *The Relationship of Theory and Research*. Norwalk, CT: Appleton-Century-Crofts; 1986.

Fowler FJ. *Survey Research Methods*. Newbury Park, CA: Sage; 1989.

Hogsdel MO, Sayner NC. *Nursing Research: An Introduction*. New York: McGraw-Hill; 1988.

Johnson MB. The holistic paradigm in nursing: The diffusion of an innovation. *Res Nurs Health*. 1990;13:129–139.

Leininger MM, ed. *Qualitative Research Methods in Nursing*. Orlando: Grune & Stratton; 1985.

Malinski VM, ed. *Explorations on Martha Rogers' Science of Unitary Human Beings*. Norwalk, CT: Appleton-Century-Crofts; 1986.

Manhart Barrett EA. *Visions of Rogers' Science-Based Nursing*. New York: National League for Nursing; 1989.

Meleis AI. *Theoretical Nursing: Development and Progress*. Philadelphia: Lippincott; 1985.

Moccia P, ed. *New Approaches to Theory Development*. New York: National League for Nursing; 1986.

Newman M. *Theory Development in Nursing*. Philadelphia: Davis; 1979.

Nicoll LH, ed. *Perspectives on Nursing Theory*. Boston: Little, Brown; 1986.

Nieswadomy RM. *Foundations of Nursing Research*. Norwalk, CT: Appleton & Lange; 1987.

Parker ME. *Nursing Theories in Practice*. New York: National League for Nursing; 1991.

Phillips LRF. *A Clinician's Guide to the Critique and Utilization of Nursing Research*. Norwalk, CT: Appleton-Century-Crofts; 1986.

Polit DF, Hungler BP. *Nursing Research: Principles and Methods*. 3rd ed. Philadelphia: Lippincott; 1987.

Reynolds PD. *A Primer in Theory Construction*. Indianapolis: Bobbs Merrill; 1971.

Sarter B, ed. *Paths to Knowledge: Innovative Research Methods for Nursing*. New York: National League for Nursing; 1988.

Sarter B. *The Stream of Becoming: A Study of Martha Rogers' Theory*. New York: National League for Nursing; 1988.

Tanner CA, Lindeman CA. *Using Nursing Research*. New York: National League for Nursing; 1989.

Walker LO, Avant KC. *Strategies for Theory Construction in Nursing*. 2nd ed. Norwalk, CT: Appleton & Lange; 1988.

Waltz CF, Srickland OL, eds. *Measurement of Nursing Outcomes, Measuring Nursing Performance: Practice, Education and Research*. New York: Springer; 1988.

Werley HH, Lang NM. *Identification of the Nursing Minimum Data Set*. New York: Springer; 1988.

CHAPTER 33

Philosophy and Nursing Practice

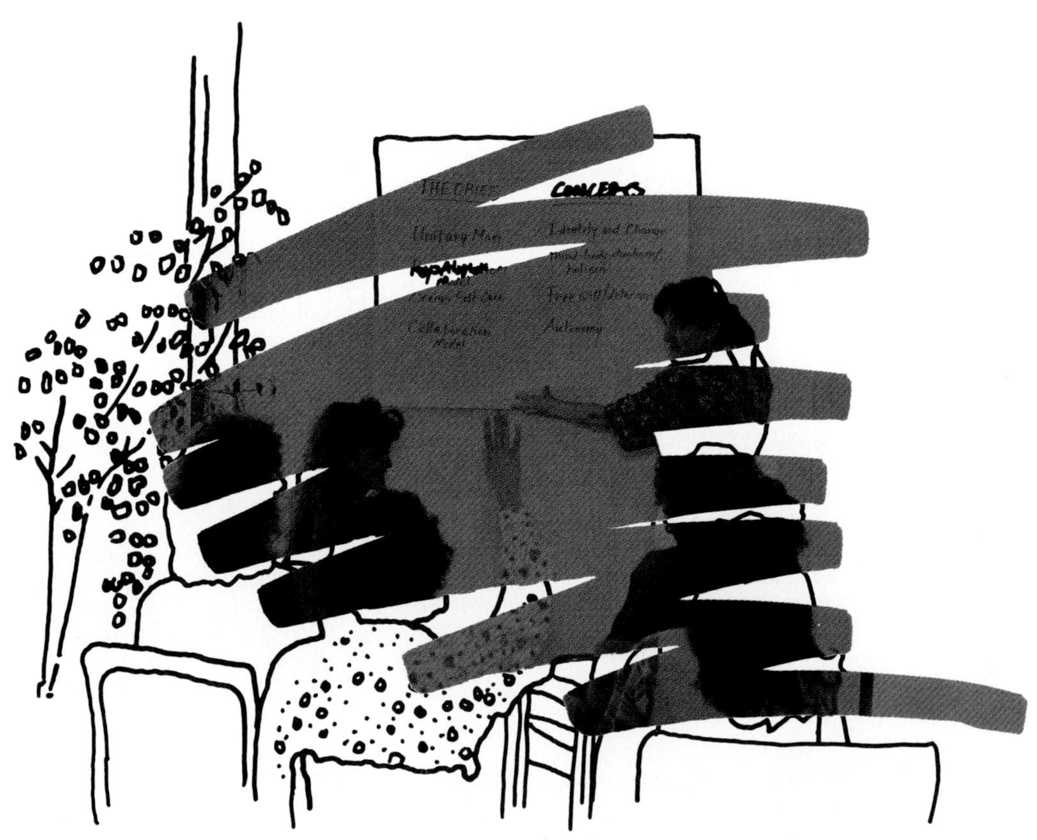

Behavioral Objectives

Upon completion of this chapter, the student will be able to:

1. Describe how philosophic skills may be used in nursing practice.
2. Differentiate between empiricism and rationalism as descriptions of how knowledge is obtained.
3. Discuss the relevance of epistemology to nursing.
4. Explain the importance of metaphysical questions to nursing.
5. Define ethics.
6. Identify key assumptions of the mutual interaction model.
7. Differentiate between decision-making for the competent client and the incompetent client.
8. Identify values common to all theories of nursing.
9. Explain the difference between "providing care" and the caring approach to the client.
10. Use philosophy to explore personal reasons for choosing to become a nurse.

KEY TERMS

best interest standard
caring
determinism
dualism
empiricism
epistemology
ethics
free will
holism
metaphysics
Natural Law
philosophic argument
philosophy
rationalism
substituted judgment
tacit assumption

Philosophy is a discipline that responds to human curiosity about the self, the world, and other people. Philosophy identifies and tries to answer fundamental questions about life: How do people discover knowledge and determine whether it is true or false? Are people free to choose their actions? What does it mean to have a body that functions in some respects as a machine, and a mind that seems totally free? If people are free to choose their actions, how do they determine what is right and wrong, and on what basis should their actions be decided? These persistent questions have been discussed and debated by philosophers for many centuries.

Philosophy is unique in that its questions and modes of analysis can be applied to many disciplines. The philosophy of nursing invites a reflective look at the foundational ideas, knowledge, methods, and values of professional nursing. A philosophic examination of nursing has two benefits: growth in self-knowledge for the individual nursing student, and continued development of nursing as a profession.

On an individual level, philosophic inquiry provides an opportunity for examination of one's own beliefs and values, the standards that influence life choices and goals.

Many persons go through life acting on the basis of values that are unexamined. It is important, however, for developing (and practicing) professionals to take time to examine personal and professional values in order to develop a thoughtful basis for practice. Nurses can begin this process by reflecting on ideas as they are expressed by others and then considering how these ideas fit or do not fit with their own. Philosophic inquiry assists developing nurses to clarify values and ideas, and to examine these ideas in light of views held by the nursing profession and by society as a whole.

On the professional level, nursing scholars over the past 10 to 15 years have recognized that the knowledge base of professional nurses should include not only technologies and professional science, but also liberal arts knowledge such as history, art and literature, and philosophy.[1,2] Gadow[3] observes that philosophic inquiry is an essential component of the forthcoming growth and self-examination of nursing as a profession:

> The direction in which nursing develops will determine whether the profession draws closer to the medical model, with its commitment to science, technology, and cure; reverts to historical nursing models, with their essentially intuitive approaches; or creates a new philosophy that sets contemporary nursing distinctively apart from both traditional nursing and modern medicine. . . . If nursing is to be defined as more than simply a set of care functions, then it must undergo self-examination and clarification of its major philosophic tenets (p. 79).

Personal and professional growth in nursing should also include an examination of the values implicit in nursing theories. The choice of a theory affects the nurse's approach to clients, as well as the organizing principles for nursing knowledge and research. The structure for nursing practice advocated in this text is one that is based on clients' rights to personal choice and shared decision-making for health care, a structure that has implications for client care as well as for nursing research. These ideas have been particularly emphasized in earlier chapters that dealt with planning and providing client care. In this chapter, the philosophy and values underlying nurse–client collaboration are examined.

■ PHILOSOPHIC METHODS

Asking Questions

Like nursing, philosophy is in part a set of skills or methods that are learned over time.[4] In its most general form, philosophy is the art of asking questions about situations one encounters. Asking questions enables one to find meaning in life experiences. For nurses, asking questions promotes more sensitive and higher quality care of clients. The following situation illustrates this point.

> SITUATION: The nurse caring for a client who has delivered a healthy infant by cesarean section senses that the client is disappointed. The client states that she feels she has "failed" because she had taken a prepared childbirth class and wanted to deliver vaginally. The client is upset, and the nurse asks the client's obstetrician about the client's concerns. The obstetrician responds that the client was adequately informed during her pregnancy about the possible need for cesarean delivery, and that the cesarean delivery was necessary.

After comforting the client, the nurse begins to wonder about the situation just encountered. Was the cesarean delivery necessary? How did the obstetrician make this determination? Was the client given appropriate opportunities to consider that vaginal delivery might not be possible for her? Was informed consent (client's free choice based on complete information) adequate in this client's situation? Should the nurse speak further with the obstetrician and possibly relay the client's feelings, with or without her explicit permission to do so? What is the nature of the nurse–client relationship: Is the nurse a comforter, an advocate, or an extension of the physician? The philosophic skill of asking questions can contribute to the nurse's initial analysis of this situation.

The nurse's initial questioning reveals that there are several issues to consider and possibly pursue in this situation: (1) the client's disappointment, (2) whether informed consent was adequate, (3) the nurse–client relationship, and (4) the nurse–physician relationship. Further analysis of these issues will assist the nurse to identify how to proceed. Asking questions is a skill that enables the nurse to identify key issues that affect client care in a particular situation.

Examining the Validity of Claims

Examining the validity of claims is a second philosophic skill relevant to the preceding situation of the nurse and the cesarean client. A claim is a statement that can be proven true or false. In the preceding example, several claims can be identified and examined: (1) the physician's assertion that cesarean delivery was necessary, (2) the physician's statement that the client was adequately informed, and (3) the client's opinion that delivery by cesarean section is inferior to vaginal delivery.

The first claim, the physician's assertion that cesarean delivery was necessary, depends to a large extent on medical knowledge and judgment; however, the nurse has expert nursing knowledge to use to examine whether cesarean delivery was necessary. Nursing education and experience provide information on the kinds of situations that usually require cesarean delivery. The nurse can compare this information to the client's situation and determine whether the client's situation seemed to fit within the usual indications for cesarean delivery. Such a comparison will assist the nurse in understanding the client's situation and enable the nurse to comfort the client by explaining why the surgery was necessary. If, on the other hand, the nurse does not understand why the physician decided on surgery, the nurse may decide to discuss the decision with the physician. The nurse and physician sharing points of view regarding indications for cesarean delivery is likely to contribute to mutual understanding and may influence how decisions are made in the future.

The second identified claim about informed consent can be accepted or rejected on the basis of standards for informed consent that have been proposed in the field of nursing ethics. In general, adequate informed consent includes information on a client's condition, a description of the health care procedure being considered, an explanation of the benefits and risks the procedure has for the client, and information on other treatments that could be used instead of the proposed procedure. Information should be provided in such a way that the client is free to consider and ask questions about health care procedures.[5] In an emergency, full explanations will not always be possible; however, in this client's situation, a possible need for cesarean delivery was discovered during prenatal care, and there was enough time to inform the client about this pos-

IMPLICATIONS FOR NURSE–CLIENT COLLABORATION

Examining the Validity of Claims

Collaboration, fundamentally, is a pattern for making health care decisions—a pattern of mutual influence among caregivers and between caregivers and their clients. In any interaction, people bring certain tacit assumptions—beliefs taken for granted as true—to the process. This is also true of the interactions nurses have with clients and colleagues. Methods of philosophy are designed to help nurses examine the truth of assertions people make and identify the assumptions behind them. It is helpful to examine these assumptions because they affect how people think, decide, and act. An understanding of philosophical methods can help nurses to identify the assumptions others and they themselves bring to health care decisions and to identify the ways in which these assumptions influence the interaction and the decisions that result.

sibility, other options, and risks and benefits of the surgery. The nurse can review with the physician and the client their understanding of the decision-making process that led to cesarean delivery. With this information, the nurse can assist the client to understand and, if possible, accept the need for delivery by cesarean section, and promote improved communication between the client and physician.

The third claim, the client's expression that delivery by cesarean section is inferior to vaginal delivery, is influenced by the client's feelings of inadequacy and disappointment. However, the nurse can assist the client to question the basis for her view and possibly arrive at a perception that the outcome (a healthy infant) was indeed satisfactory. Information about why the cesarean delivery was necessary and about the decision itself can assist the client in this process.

There are other elements in the example that are not stated claims, but tacit assumptions.[4] **Tacit assumptions** are beliefs and values that are taken for granted. It is important to examine tacit assumptions, because they can influence how people think, decide, and act. For example, the nurse, physician, and client have tacit assumptions about their roles. The obstetrician, acting out of tacit assumptions about duty to the mother and fetus, diagnosed the client's difficulties in delivering vaginally and decided that cesarean delivery was necessary. The nurse's role assumptions included assisting the physician, assessing the client's emotional state, and gathering information about the overall situation. The nature of the nurse's other responsibilities in this situation is not entirely clear. Should the nurse comfort the client, defend the physician, or act as a client advocate? The nurse can weigh these and other choices by analyzing personal assumptions about nurses' obligations to their clients and to fellow health care providers.

Examining the validity of claims and exploring tacit assumptions enables nurses to (1) support and educate clients, (2) participate in the delivery of appropriate care, and (3) raise the awareness of the obligations of health care providers toward one another and their clients.

Philosophic Argument

Philosophic argument is a third skill that may further assist nurses. Argument simply means providing good reasons for an idea or course of action. Perhaps the nurse in the preceding example, after careful consideration, resolves to assist the client to voice her concerns to the physician. Is this a good idea? The nurse should examine the personal reasons for this decision. These might include (1) providing help to the client, (2) assisting the physician to provide better care, and (3) ensuring that the client's wishes are taken into account. These are all good reasons, because they are consistent with the general goals of nursing. They support the course of action that the nurse has selected.

Courses of action that are not well supported by good reasons may not lead to good nursing care. For example, the nurse might consider simply ignoring the client's concerns, to avoid creating unnecessary work. But clearly this reason (desire to avoid unnecessary work) is not consistent with the goals of nursing. An essential part of nursing is comforting clients. Ignoring the client's concerns is not supported by good reasons and, therefore, is not acceptable.

Nurses should remember that philosophic skills are learned in dialogue with skilled thinkers and through reading, conversation, and reasoned argument. Philosophic argument can be highly useful to nurses, not only in discussions with clients and health care providers, but also in the analysis of clinical observations and nursing research (Table 33–1). This topic is considered in more detail later in the chapter. Finally, many of the decisions nurses make involve judgments of morality—that is, right and wrong. The study of philosophic argument as applied to moral decisions is included in the branch of philosophy called ethics, which is the topic of Chapter 34.

TABLE 33–1. PURPOSES OF SELECTED PHILOSOPHIC METHODS

Method	Purpose
1. *Asking questions.* What does the client think? How does the client feel about the situation? What further information would the client like to have?	To gather information, define issues for further exploration.
2. *Examining the validity of claims.* Are clients' beliefs true or false? Do others have true or false information regarding clients' knowledge?	To determine whether information is true or false. To explore differences of opinion regarding factual information. To identify beliefs that are tacitly held. To provide a basis for future action.
3. *Philosophic argument.* Making claims such as: Clients need accurate information, or nurses or physicians should provide information.	To provide good reasons for action. To communicate claims and requests to others for action.

■ FIELDS OF PHILOSOPHIC INQUIRY

The following discussion briefly considers the basic questions that philosophers ask. Philosophic methods are brought to bear on many areas of inquiry, including epistemology, metaphysics, and ethics. These areas of philosophy have many uses in personal and professional life.

Epistemology

Epistemology is the branch of philosophy that studies questions relating to knowledge. These questions include: (1) How is knowledge achieved? (2) How is the truth or falsity of knowledge determined? (3) Is it ever possible to be certain about knowledge? Epistemology attempts to reveal the thinking process that people use when they arrive at their convictions about the world. This can assist nurses in dealing with clinical situations. Professional nursing is not simply a practical activity, it is also a thinking one.

To use the earlier example, one could ask (1) How did the physician arrive at the belief that the client had been adequately informed about the need for cesarean delivery? Perhaps they discussed the situation at length, but because the client was so sure that she would not need surgery, she did not really pay attention. Were this the situation, one might conclude that the physician's belief was not supported by good evidence. This leads to the second question: (2) What would be good evidence for the claim that the client truly understood and consented to possible cesarean delivery? A simple and reasonable place to begin would be asking the client to repeat the information provided to her. (3) But is it ever possible to be sure that clients have given adequate informed consent? Perhaps many clients are too emotionally upset or too poorly educated to understand health care information. To counteract this concern, information should be presented clearly and at a level that is appropriate for the client. Along with asking clients to repeat information, nurses should present information in a nonthreatening way, perhaps on several different occasions.

In the earlier example, asking epistemological questions assisted the nurse to examine the reasons for the physician's claim about informed consent. Once the nurse had this information, she was able to approach the client, explore the client's understanding, and proceed to provide the client with more complete information, if necessary.

In another situation, sensitivity to epistemological concerns can assist a nurse to explore his views about a nursing colleague.

> SITUATION: Mr. Keil, RN, observes that a co-worker, Ms. Wheaton, has seemed tired and distracted lately. Mr. Keil has seen Ms. Wheaton drop a client's tray, and sometimes has not been able to find her for brief periods when she is needed. One day, Mr. Keil discovers a possible medication error involving narcotics. A client has requested pain medication and says he has not had any for 4 hours, but according to the chart, the medication was given recently by Ms. Wheaton. Mr. Keil begins to wonder whether Ms. Wheaton is using drugs intended for the clients. Perhaps this would explain Ms. Wheaton's distraction and the possible medication error. He wonders whether he should take his suspicion to their supervisor.

This is a serious accusation, and requires careful thought by Mr. Keil. Epistemological questions can assist him to explore the basis and validity of his suspicion. (1) How did he arrive at his suspicion? Upon reflection, Mr. Keil observes that he formed his opinion on the basis of unclear evidence. Ms. Wheaton has been tired and distracted, but there is no direct evidence that she is abusing drugs. Nevertheless, because client safety could be compromised if Ms. Wheaton's abilities were impaired, Mr. Keil should consider carefully what further evidence he needs to prove or disprove his suspicion. (2) What would provide evidence of substance abuse? If Mr. Keil observed Ms. Wheaton stealing drugs and ingesting them herself, he would have clear proof; however, waiting to observe such an action would take valuable time away from client care, and might expose clients to danger if Ms. Wheaton were, in fact, chemically impaired. A much better approach would be to speak privately with Ms. Wheaton at the earliest opportunity. This approach would demonstrate concern and respect for Ms. Wheaton, as well as primary concern for client welfare. The conversation should include discussion of Ms. Wheaton's fatigue, distraction, and possible medication error. The discussion also should remind Ms. Wheaton of peer assistance programs for impaired nurses, if she does admit to a drug problem. (3) Will it be possible for Mr. Keil to be certain about what Ms. Wheaton tells him? Suppose that she admits to a "slight drug problem" that started out when she began taking tranquilizers for stress; however, Ms. Wheaton promises to "shape up on the job." At this point, Mr. Keil must decide whether to trust her word. He might consider persuading Ms. Wheaton to discuss the situation with their supervisor, or he might tell her that unless her performance improves, he will go to the supervisor himself.

Epistemological questions have enabled Mr. Keil to reflect on the basis for his suspicion, the requirements for well-grounded beliefs, and the fact that it is sometimes not possible to be absolutely certain about observations. Despite uncertainty in this situation, the duty to protect clients required action on Mr. Keil's part. A discussion regarding ethical considerations when dealing with impaired colleagues follows in Chapter 34.

Epistemology in western culture has two main traditions: empiricism and rationalism. These two traditions offer different views of how knowledge is achieved and evaluated.

Empiricism. The prevailing philosophy of knowledge in the United States is **empiricism,** the view that knowledge of the world achieved by observation through the senses is most reliable. Physicians and nurses often use empirical assumptions about knowledge. Much of medical diagnosis and nursing diagnosis depends on the skilled gathering of observations about clients, through inspection, palpation, auscultation, and even olfaction. Furthermore, scientific research, which has been so successful in achieving modern advances in knowledge both of the world and of the human body, has depended for its success upon the view that people can skillfully observe and record their experiences of the world and discern regular patterns that can predict future events.

Empiricism is the basis for the scientific method, in which scientists begin with an observed relationship between events—for example, that handwashing seems to lower the incidence of infection. Having made that empirical observation, scientists can make a tentative proposal, or hypothesis, defining how handwashing and rates of infection are related. A controlled, experimental situation can then be devised to record further observation and determine whether the hypothesis is supported or rejected. Nursing and medical research often uses the empirical approach. For example, a study of clients in intensive care units showed that good communication between physicians and nurses improved clients' chances of recovery.[6] In this study, an empirical (observable) relationship between good physician–nurse communication and client recovery was demonstrated.

Many advances in modern science and technology—such as knowledge of human physiology, disease, and recovery—have been made through the use of the scientific method. Technological advances include heart-lung machines, incubators for newborns, and many others. Still, epistemologists have raised criticisms of empiricism as a description of knowledge. One is that the scientific method is not in itself strictly empirical—science could not proceed if scientists merely recorded experiences without interpreting what they observed.[4] In the example of the effects of good communication on client recovery, researchers had to have a tentative hypothesis in order to gather, organize, and interpret information. They had to have a belief about what "good" communication is. They had to suspect that this "good" physician–nurse communication might benefit clients; otherwise they would not have begun to gather information about communication.

A related problem with the scientific method is that people rely on many other ways of knowing (discussed below) in addition to empiricism, but because of the prevalence of the scientific method today, these other ways have not been recognized and developed to their full potential.[7]

BUILDING NURSING KNOWLEDGE

What Influence Has the Philosophy of Science Had on Nursing Practice?

Whall AL. The influence of logical positivism on nursing practice. *Image.* 1989;21:243–245.

This article looks at the prevailing philosophy of science and its impact on clinical nursing practice. Empiricism is the philosophy that emphasizes the need to subject all opinions or theories to the test of sensory experience. The author notes that in the 19th century, a form of empiricism called logical positivism arose, which became the prevailing influence on science for much of the 20th century. According to Whall, logical positivists sought to eliminate from science questions of a metaphysical nature—any proposition that could not be observed. They looked upon questions that could not be answered through observation, such as those about ethics and aesthetics or even emotional attitudes, as having no scientific meaning. The outcome of this position was a devaluing of subjective human experience in science.

Whall examined the impact of logical positivism on nursing practice during the peak of its influence on the profession, from the 1950s through the 1970s. This was a critical period for nursing, a period when several nursing theories were generated. To determine the impact of logical positivism on nursing practice, Whall reviewed the nursing textbooks, curricular guides, and standards of practice that were important during that period. Whall looked at their premises on the role of ethics, aesthetics, personal values, emotions, perceptions, and "introspective data" in nursing practice.

The author found that the major publications all recognized subjective aspects as having an important role in client care, although the same publications also emphasized the importance of observation and verification in nursing science. Whall found that none of the guides or standards suggested a strict logical positivist stance or denial of the place that values have in science. In concluding the report, Whall argues for the importance of "personal knowledge"—that is, knowledge gained by intuition—in nursing. The author's work illustrates the value of examining nursing's epistemological foundations.

Rationalism. Rationalism has its origins in Greek thought and attempts to find a basis for knowledge in the process of reasoning alone. **Rationalism** holds that philosophic claims should be supported by reasons and that philosophic argument should proceed on the basis of progressive clarification of agreed-upon definitions.

René Descartes (1596–1650), a French philosopher, used a rationalist method to respond to Copernicus' astronomical theory, which argued that the sun, not the earth, is at the center of the universe. Copernicus' theory called into question the human ability to observe and understand the world. To the naked eye, the sun appears to rise and set, and the earth appears to stand still. But Copernicus demonstrated that it is the earth that moves. Human observations thus appeared untrustworthy. This challenged the prevailing Biblical theories of creation, which held that people were the most important element in the universe. In response to this growing uncertainty about the validity of human knowledge, Descartes proposed his method of achieving certain knowledge. He proposed to reject all information based on experience because it seemed to be untrustworthy, as well as all of the previous knowledge and beliefs he had acquired. He subjected everything he seemed to know to a method of "radical doubt"; that is, Descartes refused to take at face value any knowledge based on experience. Only one thing was held as certain: "I think, therefore I am." From this one certainty, Descartes claimed to infer the existence of God, the validity of mathematics, and his own method of achieving certain knowledge.[8]

Descartes' method of philosophic doubt is useful because it teaches that any belief or proposition may be wrong and should be questioned. It highlights the importance of keeping an open, inquiring mind. The major criticism of Descartes' method is that it is, in practice, impossible to subject everything that one knows to doubt at the same time. In addition, people would not be able to think at all if they did not rely upon a taken-for-granted view of reality: their native language.[9] Furthermore, much of our modern knowledge in the fields of astronomy, chemistry, physics, biology, anatomy, sociology, and psychology rests on empirical observations. In the face of this evidence, Descartes' claim that experience is untrustworthy seems weak.

This discussion cannot resolve the debate between the empiricists and the rationalists. However, some modern epistemologists[4,6] argue that when one observes people as they actually go about investigating the world, they are seen to employ both thinking and observation. In actual life, then, people understand the world and other people through an integration of both empiricism and rationalism.[4,7,9]

The Relevance of Epistemology to Nursing. Familiarity with epistemological issues can assist nurses to develop and evaluate nursing knowledge in clinical practice and in research. Nurses in clinical practice are continually making observations. In the mutual interaction model, nurse and client first mutually explore expectations and reasons for requesting nursing services. Skills in thinking can assist nurses in keeping an open mind and understanding what a client is saying.

> SITUATION: A 65-year-old woman, Mrs. Carter, has been diagnosed with cancer and is being admitted for treatment in a large city hospital miles away from her home. The cancer can be successfully treated and Mrs. Carter has an excellent prognosis. The nurse conducting the admission interview observes that Mrs. Carter seems apprehensive, resigned, and unwilling to discuss plans for her future after discharge. Upon questioning, the nurse learns that Mrs. Carter believes that having cancer means that she will certainly die in the near future. Even more frightening to Mrs. Carter is her admission to the same hospital where a close relative recently died.

In this situation, it would be important for the nurse to assist Mrs. Carter in a tactful way, to explore the reasons for her beliefs and whether these reasons make sense in her particular situation. Skills in philosophic questioning and awareness that beliefs should be supported by good reasons can sharpen the nurse's ability to interact effectively with clients and to teach clients accurate information.

Familiarity with epistemology also benefits the development of nursing research and knowledge by assisting nurses to question ideas and practices that have been taken for granted. For many years, confused nursing home residents have been restrained in chairs or in bed to prevent possible falls. Some recent research indicates that the danger of falling increases with restraints because the residents can become even more confused and struggle to escape.[10] In addition, the residents' physical fitness, orientation to the environment, and emotional state may worsen with restraints.[10] Although research in this area is not yet conclusive, questioning the validity of restraining clients has yielded important information that may improve care of future clients.

Epistemology also encourages nurses to recognize that, while empirical research is highly important, other ways of achieving knowledge can make significant contributions to nursing practice. Carper identifies four patterns of knowing in nursing: empirical, personal, ethical, and aesthetic.[7] Empirical knowing has already been discussed. Personal knowing refers to the component of individual perception in each act of knowing. Ethical knowing refers to the perception of right and wrong. Aesthetic knowing refers to nurses' awareness of goodness or wholeness when investigating health care phenomena. According to Carper, all four patterns of knowing contribute to nursing knowledge.[7]

Awareness of different ways of knowing can lead to another type of empirical research that investigates the meaning of nursing experiences without the use of statistics or hypotheses: phenomenological research. Phenomenological research attempts to describe the essential nature of an observed event. An example is Drew's research on the meaning of caring.[11] Drew asked 35 hospitalized adults to describe situations in which they felt either depersonalized (alienated and excluded) or confirmed (respected and cared for) in their interactions with caregivers. Detailed interviews were transcribed by the researcher, and from them essential qualities of exclusion and confirmation began to emerge. Clients described a sense of exclusion when their caregivers lacked emotional warmth, or were cold, stiff, mechanical, bored, indifferent, or insensitive. In contrast, clients felt a sense of confirmation when caregivers liked their work, seemed to want to be with clients, had energy and enthusiasm, moved slowly, and leaned close to the clients.[11] This is invaluable information for nursing practice, yet it could not have been obtained using a cause-and-effect method. It is a descriptive study suggesting essential features of nurse–client interaction.

Metaphysics

Metaphysics is the branch of philosophy that studies the nature of existence. Metaphysics uses thinking and reasoning rather than empirical observation in its investigations. Many of the questions of metaphysics have an important bearing on the thinking of nurses today. Three of these issues will be considered in the following discussion: (1) identity and change, (2) mind and body, and (3) free will and determinism.

Identity and Change. Identity and change concerns the question of how objects or living things stay the same (retain their identity) despite change. An individual acorn will develop into an oak sapling and then a tree, exhibiting change. However, the acorn also possesses an identity leading to only one possible result: an oak tree. Over the centuries, many theories have been offered in an attempt to describe the relationship between identity and change.

The metaphysical theory of **Natural Law** proposes that changes occur in order to achieve a goal that is in the very nature of the object; hence change is purposeful. The acorn grows into an oak tree; this is its "nature" or "end." In the same way, a child grows into an adult. Natural Law theory has been influential in many ways, particularly in understanding biological processes and human life. Developmental theories of human beings are based on notions of identity and change. Natural Law theory also has fostered a major ethical theory that holds that a person should act to promote the natural ends of human life. (The ethical theory of Natural Law is discussed in Chap. 34.)

Natural ends include: (1) biological ends, such as growth, taking care of others, and reproduction; (2) social ends, such as working with others to improve the community, and (3) rational ends, such as learning and sharing knowledge. Nurses face many situations that can relate to Natural Law. They take care of other people, work to improve health care in society, and inform clients about their health care status. These nursing actions thus promote the general goals (biological, social, and rational ends) of Natural Law theory.

Mind and Body. Descartes addressed the relation between mind and body in developing his rationalist theory of knowledge.[8] He claimed that data from the senses were untrustworthy and began by systematically doubting all information received by experience of the world. The remaining thoughts and ideas were, according to Descartes, the product of the mind and not of the body. In Descartes' theory, the essential feature of human beings is that they are "thinking things." In contrast, for Descartes the body is merely a machine that is completely separate from the mind. This theoretical separation of mind and body is known as **dualism.** Mind–body dualism raises several issues. How can a physical event, such as illness, affect thinking? How can a thought process, such as a decision to seek nursing care, be acted out in the real world if mind and body are unconnected, as Descartes claimed? Despite these apparent contradictions, Descartes' theory has been influential. For example, his view of the body as a machine made possible the tremendous advances in understanding of human physiology and pathophysiology which we have today. Descartes' view of the body allowed people to examine and understand the body in a new way. We now know that most parts of the body have machine-like functions; the heart, kidneys, and digestive systems are examples.

Free Will and Determinism. Do people choose their actions freely, or are they merely machines? Philosophers explore this question when they discuss **free will** (choice) and **determinism** (the view that causal laws govern all events, including human action). The view that events in nature can be explained by causality was first applied to the physical sciences (astronomy, physics, and chemistry); and then to the biological and social sciences (sociology and psychology). The scientific success of the view that each event has a clear cause challenged human beings' sense of uniqueness and freedom in their actions.

Free will is the view that people are at liberty to make their own conscious decisions and choices. This view has much to support it. First is the ordinary experience of making choices in everyday life. Second, all cultures have religious beliefs and ethical standards. It would make no sense to expect people to obey moral rules if they were not free to do so. People experience remorse, regret, shame; and punish others who are found guilty. These and many other features of moral life assume that people are free agents who make choices.[12] Third, people are able to discover and invent new things and create realities that were not there before. Determinism, which proposes a strict cause-and-effect model of the world, cannot account for such innovation.

The Relevance of Metaphysics to Nursing. At first glance, it might not seem that abstract questions about identity and change, mind and body, and free will and determinism could have a bearing on nursing practice. Yet nursing practice relies on a set of beliefs and assumptions about people, the nature of health and illness, and the nurse–client relationship. Whether or not they are aware of it, nurses do hold beliefs that are metaphysical in nature. The next section of this chapter demonstrates how a number of nursing theorists have defined nursing practice. Each of these theories or conceptual models is based upon a set of beliefs about people and the nature of health and illness. Analysis and clarification of these beliefs are essential, as they influence nursing scholarship, practice, and individual nurses' self-understanding.

Questions of identity and change are of interest to nurses primarily because human beings grow and change through the life cycle. A fundamental assumption of many approaches to nursing is that people do change: through learning, maturation, and growth and development. Nurses assist individuals to change by helping them to examine the opportunities for personal growth and development in their experience of health and illness. An understanding of metaphysics reinforces that objective.

Theories incorporating growth and change must address human potential in extreme situations. Is an elderly man in a nursing home "the same" person he was when he was middle aged? Does he still subscribe to a value he expressed 10 years ago, that he does not want to be resuscitated if he has cardiac arrest? Is a young woman in an intensive care unit, who is hallucinating and asking to die, "the same" person she was before she was critically injured? Can we trust her expressions to be "her own"? Is she autonomous (free to choose her actions)? Is a fertilized ovum "the same" as a human being? Should it be transferred from one mother to another? May it be aborted? Is a brain-dead person who is being maintained on a ventilator still a person? What rights does he or she have? These questions have important implications for personal and professional ethics, as well as for public policy.

Mind–body issues are also crucially important to nurses. Descartes' view of the body as a machine has made possible tremendous technological advances in modern medicine and health care. However, an exclusive focus on the body as a machine can lead to a depersonalized view of the client that might be called "ICU metaphysics." Potentially depersonalized care is not the only problem to which a mechanistic view of the body can lead. Under this framework, one could overlook the mind–body, psychosomatic relations in health and illness: for example, the ways in which psychological stress can lead to illness, or illness and disability affect one's "body image"; the meaning of one's own body for oneself.

The issue of free will and determinism relates to the question of responsibility. Nurses often uncritically accept and express the view that clients are "responsible" for their illness. But what does this mean? Do clients always "cause" the illness they have? Or once they are sick, is it their "role" to get well? Alternatively, are they somehow liable or "to blame" for health deviations? Or finally, is one capable of directing one's own health care? These different senses of responsibility—causal-responsibility, role-responsibility, liability-responsibility, and capacity-responsibility—and their relationship to client care require clarification.[13] How, when, and whether one or more of these types of responsibility apply to a given health care situation is not a simple issue. Nurses applying them, appropriately or inappropriately, to a given health care interaction directly influence nurse–client relationships. For example, a nurse who believes that clients' life-style choices make them responsible for illnesses such as heart disease, lung cancer, or alcoholism, may approach all clients with these conditions in a negative, even accusing way. Even though the nurse's belief may be correct in certain circumstances, one might ask how the chosen approach to care benefits either the nurse or the client. Would an approach that emphasizes sharing information, taking responsibility for current choices, and "letting go" of past choices be more effective as well as being more compassionate? Exploration of the limits of capacity-responsibility is also relevant, particularly as it relates to collaboration. How do nurses facilitate mutuality? Should mutuality always be a goal? Nurses' thoughtful consideration of metaphysical questions and related issues will contribute to their being more caring and effective health care providers.

Ethics

Ethics is a branch of philosophy that analyzes whether actions are right or wrong. Nursing ethics, which is the subject of Chapter 34, attempts to clarify the principles (action guides) that should inform nursing practice. The ethical principles of respect for person, autonomy, veracity, beneficence, nonmaleficence, fidelity, confidentiality, and justice are commonly examined in the study of nursing ethics.

Respect of person means treating all clients—regardless of their age, mental status, or health care deviation—with concern and high regard. Autonomy means that competent adults can make their own decisions freely and on the basis of their own values. Closely related is veracity or truth-telling, which means providing accurate information to the client. Beneficence refers to the principle of doing good for another person. Nonmaleficence relates to avoiding or preventing harm. Fidelity means keeping promises. Under confidentiality, nurses safeguard the client's privacy, including personal information related to them by clients. Justice refers to the fair distribution of goods and services.

Understanding ethical principles is important because nurses will often find that two or more principles apply to a particular situation. The principles may even suggest conflicting actions. At this point, nurses need to question whether the reasons for upholding each principle are, in fact, good ones. This will assist nurses in deciding which principle or principles are most important. Chapter 34 discusses ethical analysis in greater detail. Table 33–2 summarizes the relevance of epistemology, metaphysics, and ethics for nursing.

■ PHILOSOPHY REFLECTED IN NURSING THEORY

Chapter 32 examined the relationship of nursing theory to nursing practice. The present discussion continues that examination by identifying some philosophic perspectives in selected nursing theories. Nursing theories provide ways of describing the practice of nursing. They specify when nursing care is needed, the nature of the nurse–client relationship, and the general goals of nursing care. Nursing theories are intended to enable practitioners to reflect on what nursing really is.

Students might have been surprised to learn, in Chapter 32, that there are differences of opinion regarding what nursing really is: Different theorists have described the reality of nursing in different ways. This variety is not a cause for concern, but is instead a sign of growth and development in the nursing profession. Asking "what is nursing?" is a way of becoming clear about the basic goals, values, and philosophic standpoints of the profession. Students can participate in professional growth by examining various theories and questioning whether the theories agree or disagree with their personal perception of reality.

Using a theory is like looking at reality through a particular lens. It will change the nursing encounter by highlighting some aspects, while others recede into the background. For example, Sister Callista Roy describes nursing as assisting with the client's adaptation to stimuli. Nurses alter the environment in order to promote client adaptation.[14] In Roy's theory, clients are seen as somewhat passive: acted upon, instead of acting with free will. In Williamson's mutual interaction model, however, the client is seen as a major figure in the nurse–client encounter.[15] Clients mutually determine, with nurses, what should be

TABLE 33–2. RELEVANCE OF EPISTEMOLOGY, METAPHYSICS, AND ETHICS FOR NURSING

Area of Philosophical Inquiry	Typical Question	Application to Nursing Practice
Epistemology	How is knowledge achieved? Is knowledge true or false? Is certainty possible?	Determination of a need for knowledge by self, clients, or colleagues. Identification of research questions, such as the relationship of frequent turning to skin integrity. Sensitivity to variety of research methods, such as cause-and-effect, descriptive, and phenomenological.
Metaphysics	What is the nature of reality? What is the nature of people?	
	Identity and change	Development of human beings through the life cycle.
	Mind and body	Holistic approach to client. Sensitivity to client's emotions and beliefs.
	Free will and determinism	Sensitivity to all clients despite reasons for health deviation.
Ethics	What is the right thing to do in this situation?	Principles guiding nurses in all areas of client care, such as confidentiality and respect of person.

done. Mutual interaction is consistent with the view that clients have free will. This example demonstrates that one's choice of a theory can lead to different views of nursing and of clients. These differences in turn affect nurses' approach to care.

Although nursing theories do not explicitly discuss philosophy, they do reflect philosophic positions. The following discussion uses the philosophical concepts of identity and change, mind and body, and free will and determinism to examine some aspects of selected nursing theories.

Identity and Change

Recall that the question of identity and change relates to the observation that people retain their unique identity despite change over time. The nursing theorist who considers this issue in greatest depth is Martha Rogers.[16] The theme of identity and change in Rogers' work applies to culture in general as well as to the individual person. Rogers begins her discussion of nursing by tracing the growth of human knowledge and culture from prehistoric times to the present. Rogers' theory also integrates perspectives from philosophy, religion, and the human sciences to underscore the view that past and present culture should be seen as an integral part of nursing. As a human activity, nursing has achieved its present identity by evolving over time.

Rogers then applies the notion of identity and change to the study of individuals. She regards people as unified, integral wholes who are different from the sum of their parts. All of human life is dynamic and creative, and persons respond to changes in their life by developing new patterns. According to Rogers, pattern and organization in one's life become more complex through time. For example, Daniel Williams is a 20-year-old college junior who has recently been diagnosed with diabetes. The diabetes will not require medication if Mr. Williams can manage his diet carefully at school. Because he eats in a cafeteria, and does not cook for himself, management of his diet is a challenge. Mr. Williams meets this challenge by discussing his needs and the cafeteria's recipes with the director of food services. On the basis of this information, he is able to maintain his health and manage his diabetes. In the example, Mr. Williams has responded with creativity to a change in his life. He has developed new knowledge, behaviors, and patterns of eating in order to control his diabetes. His patterns of living have become more complex, but he is still the same person: a college junior who can pursue his career and life goals.

In Rogers' theory, then, the issue of identity and change is clearly addressed. Rogers' theory is also compatible with the view that individuals have free will. In the example of Mr. Williams, this was shown by his decision to take steps to manage his diabetes. Rogers claims that people are able to think, imagine, and make decisions.[17]

Mind–Body Concepts

The mind–body issue emerges clearly in Roy's theory. Roy defines people as having biological, psychological, and social aspects.[14] Roy states that these aspects function in a holistic fashion: that is, all three components are unified. Individuals interact with their environment, and adapt to change. For Roy, change is presented to the individual in the form of stimuli. The person uses two adaptive mechanisms to respond to stimuli: (1) the regulator mechanism, which is the autonomic nervous system; and (2) the cognator mechanism, the central nervous system.[14] Roy's description of these two mechanisms in this way addresses the problem of mind–body dualism: one part of the brain controls bodily processes, and a second part controls choice. A possible drawback of Roy's approach is that it seems to be in conflict with a holistic view of the person. It places a heavy emphasis on biological aspects of human

BUILDING NURSING KNOWLEDGE

How Can the Nurse Select the Right Conceptual Model for Practice?

Buchanan BF. Conceptual Models: An Assessment Framework. *J Nurs Admin.* 1987;17:22–26.

In this article, Buchanan stresses the need to assist nurses to assess the value of the various models for practice and proposes an analytical framework for that purpose. The framework is composed of three general elements, context, process, and form, which are part of any model. Buchanan defines and illustrates the use of each.

A model places the client within the "context" of practice. Context refers to the environment in which nursing is practiced and experienced, for example, the hospital or community health care agencies. According to Buchanan, a model may be incompatible with certain contexts. For instance, a model that requires interaction between nurse and client may have limited use in contexts where clients are unable to interact, such as when they are unconscious or severely mentally disabled.

Models propose "forms" or concepts for collecting and analyzing data. These provide a guide by which to evaluate the relevance or irrelevance of data. According to Buchanan, a model that emphasizes the concept of social systems may be inadequate to describe the individual being acted upon.

"Process" differentiates the role of nurses from the role of clients. The process of a model deals with nurses' ways of thinking and reasoning and the procedures and behaviors nurses use as practitioners. A model that presents nursing as a transaction in which human beings participate together makes nurses' actions contingent on clients' participation. Such a model, Buchanan points out, may fail to distinguish between nurse and client, and may implicitly undermine standards of care.

Buchanan concludes that applying this framework enables nurses to evaluate biases and weaknesses and to make the assumptions underlying a model explicit. This aids in evaluating a model's appropriateness. Nurses can then select on the basis of a well-reasoned comparison.

behavior, and a lesser emphasis on psychological aspects of choice. In Roy's theory, the body is emphasized more than the mind.

Free Will and Determinism

Dorothea Orem's self-care theory raises the theme of free will.[18] Orem's view of people is holistic. Throughout life individuals engage in activities to take care of themselves. Orem calls this ability self-care agency (see Chap. 32). For example, an 18-year-old woman has asthma, and meets her requirement for air by regular use of a nebulizer with medication. In Orem's theory, that client has capacity and control in self-care. When clients can no longer meet health requirements, the goal of nursing is to help them regain self-care agency. The nurse–client relationship is contractual, and clients actively participate in their own care. This portion of Orem's description is clearly compatible with the notion of free will.

However, a question must be asked about the limits of free will in Orem's theory. If a client refuses to take self-care measures that a nurse recommends, what should the nurse do? This would occur if the 18-year-old woman with asthma refused to stop smoking. Would there be a conflict between the nurse's wish to benefit the client, and the client's free will? At issue is the question of whether the client or the nurse defines the meaning of appropriate self-care agency.

Nursing theories wrestle with philosophic issues, even though this is not always made explicit. Philosophic questions provide a starting point from which to begin comparing and questioning nursing theories. It is important for nursing students to study nursing theories with respect to philosophic issues in order to determine which theories seem compatible with their own views of professional practice. Table 33–3 summarizes philosophic themes in selected nursing theories.

VALUES REFLECTED IN NURSING THEORY

Despite philosophic differences among nursing theories, the majority of theories hold similar positions on certain basic values.

For example, most nursing theories would agree with the American Nurses' Association (ANA) definition of nursing as: "the diagnosis and treatment of human responses to actual or potential health problems."[19] In the ANA *Social Policy Statement*, nurses are called upon to meet health needs of people who are viewed as integrated beings rather than simply biological systems.

> Nurses are guided by a humanistic philosophy having caring coupled with understanding and purpose as its central feature. Nurses have the highest regard for self-determination, independence, and choice in decision making in matters of health (p. 18).

IMPLICATIONS FOR NURSE–CLIENT COLLABORATION

Free Will and Determinism in Nursing Theory

Orem's ideas about self-care agency have marked similarities to the assumptions made in Williamson's mutual interaction model of nurse–client collaboration. Both emphasize that throughout life, people engage in activities to take care of themselves; and both make assumptions about the philosophical issues of free will and determinism. In using these models, however, a question must be asked regarding the limits of free will. What should the nurse do if the client refuses to take self-care measures or to participate in planning care? Is that refusal an expression of free will? If so, what is the nurse's proper response to it? Chapter 37, Health Care as a Transaction, examines this question.

TABLE 33–3. PHILOSOPHIC THEMES IN SELECTED NURSING THEORIES

Philosophic Theme	Nursing Theory	Example
Identity and change	Martha Rogers: Theory of unitary man	Client incorporates the need to decrease serum cholesterol by joining a health club.
Mind and body	Sister Callista Roy: Adaptation model	A cook accidentally touches a hot skillet. The regulator automatically draws back his hand, and the cognator consciously moves the skillet with a potholder.
Free will and determinism	Dorothea Orem: Self-care deficit theory of nursing	The client's need for care arises when self-care agency is insufficient—an elderly client can no longer walk unaided and the nurse assists with walking.

Given this conceptual support, it is to be expected that nursing theories will reflect the value of self-determination. Health, holism, and caring are other essential values in nursing, and all major theories integrate these values into their discussion. Although these values receive different emphasis in various theories, it is beyond the scope of this discussion to outline these differences. The student is referred to the bibliography for further analysis.

Holism

Holism refers to the view that people are a unity of mental, physical, and social aspects. Nursing professes a holistic view of the individual. Despite that claim, in practice nurses often fall into a dualistic (mind–body) or even triadic (body–mind–spirit) approach. Examples include clients who are categorized as mentally ill who frequently find it difficult to have health care providers attend to their physical needs, and the emotional components of surgical procedures such as hysterectomies or vasectomies that are often disregarded or passed over lightly by health care providers. One might ask whether this occurs because nurses have not examined the philosophic basis of their practice deeply enough.

The belief in the holistic nature of individuals leads nurses to an approach to clients that is different from the physician's approach. For example, a surgeon may be satisfied when the client's colostomy is patent, and with the first bowel movement may believe that the client is ready for discharge. From the surgical perspective, this is accurate. Nurses, however, see clients as members of a family and community and attend to emotional and social concerns, as well as to physical needs. The person with the colostomy rather than the colostomy itself is the organizing focus. Psychological adaptation is so interwoven with the physical that, from the nursing perspective, both must be considered.

The holistic approach regards the person as the center of value. Individuals are not objects (are not acted upon) but are cared for and worked with. Most nursing theories address the holistic or unified nature of people, and it is expected that the practice of nursing will reflect that understanding. This does not mean that nurses must be all things to all people, but that they should be sensitive to the complexity of humans. Recognition of the holistic nature of people prompts nurses to work collaboratively with those in other disciplines, such as clergy and schoolteachers, as well as other health care providers, to more effectively address clients' complex needs.

Health

The justification for the profession of nursing and other forms of health care is the existence of health care problems. As with holism, nurses often verbally express a valuing of health, but at times other values may take precedence over health. For example, to promote efficient care of clients, nurses will sometimes adopt measures that may be easier initially, but that may work to the detriment of client health over the long term. These measures may include bathing or feeding clients instead of encouraging clients to perform these actions. Unnecessary restraints are another example. The value of efficiency seems to take a higher priority than long-term health in these circumstances. Nurses may find, as in this example, that the value of health may not always be a top priority, especially when nurses have a large number of clients.

For the health care provider, however, health should have high priority. Nurses are expected to have skills and knowledge that contribute to health, and must have a clear understanding of the broad meaning of the concept. Chapters 5 and 12 discuss concepts of health and illness in detail. Health–illness is described as a continuum and as a subjective state. Notions of health are important in any theory of nursing because, as the ANA states,[19] nursing exists to "diagnose and treat human responses to actual or potential health problems" (p. 9).

Health is a difficult concept to define, however, in part because it is used to describe a range of phenomena from a cellular level to a psychological and social level. It is easier to look at cellular function and say what is healthy. This is because at a biological level, human function is more mechanistic.[4] Thus, it is possible to state that an individual's hemoglobin is or is not in a healthy range. However, it is much more difficult to determine whether a person's social function is healthy. It should be noted that even on the biological level, people may attribute a wide range of meanings to findings that are outside of usual or normal boundaries.

While each nursing theory differs in its approach to health, all are similar with respect to themes of adaptation, wholeness, and integrity. All of the theorists address health as having a dynamic quality with biological and behavioral components. In other words, health is not static. It is ever changing and may involve things as diverse as enzymatic activity for glucose metabolism or working for nuclear disarmament in the interest of societal health.

Society holds nurses accountable for a body of knowledge and has certain expectations regarding health and health care practices. However, nurses cannot impose their own definition of health on clients; rather, this definition must be reached through a process of collaboration. This is a challenging requirement. Nurses also must first know what contributes to health with some certainty, and must also value clients' autonomy and the very subjective experience of health. From an ethical perspective, respect of autonomy is a primary principle that guides action. To be fully autonomous, however, clients must have information that is adequate to make informed decisions. Nurses, then, must have the knowledge and skill to provide information, to encourage deliberation, and to discern those situations in which clients' autonomy should be overruled in order to prevent harm. A more complete discussion of situations that may justify overruling client autonomy (paternalism) will be found in Chapter 34.

Caring

Caring refers to respectful and considerate relationships among persons. Caring is difficult to define because it is used in a variety of ways: as noun or verb; as feeling, attitude, or behavior. Gaylin describes caring as being an instinct that contributes to the human superiority to other species in the ability to survive. He believes it is the human capacity to care, not the tendency to be aggressors, that contributes to survival.[20] Caring is at the heart of the ethical principle of respect for person. To be caring is to be grounded or "rooted" in a sense of responsibility for protecting human dignity. It invokes a respect for the human dignity of all people, and is a universal phenomenon.[20–23]

Caring is an essential concept in nursing, because the basis of nursing practice is the helping relationship between nurse and client. Caring may be viewed as the basis for ethical behavior.[24]

It is important to distinguish "caring" from "providing care." In some client situations, such as a client who is permanently unconscious, providing care measures such as antibiotics or dialysis may not benefit the client. In other situations, such as the case of a seriously ill newborn who is not expected to live, continued treatment may be unethical because the treatment is painful or futile. In such situations, the caring response may be to stop providing treatment. However, even though *care measures* may be discontinued, caring itself is never withdrawn or withheld. Leininger[23] notes that "caring is the generic component of all nursing service, and without therapeutic caring attitudes, expressions, and activities, nursing services are incomplete, mechanistic, inadequate and questionable" (p. 137).

Caring does not require embracing all behavior as acceptable. Certainly abusive behaviors are wrong; but the person who is an abuser (whether of self or of others) is still a person. Nurses must be able to respect that person and acknowledge his or her pain. The behavior of abuse cannot be tolerated, but the person can be cared for in such a way as to foster hope that the behavior can be changed. In this example, genuine caring may indeed be the most therapeutic intervention possible. The person who is the abuser may be experiencing care for the first time. This caring does not negate calling the abusive behavior wrong, but it may involve supporting the person in bearing the consequences for having acted wrongly.

Caring for others also requires caring for self. In the development of caring there must be a notion of respect for self. However, in the therapeutic relationship the role of nurses is to be the one who is caring. It is clients who are in the more vulnerable position and it is clients who are seeking assistance and whose interest is to be served. Clients and their needs take precedence in nurse–client interactions. Table 33–4 summarizes values common to nursing theories.

IMPLICATIONS FOR NURSE–CLIENT COLLABORATION

Caring in Nursing Theory

The value of caring underlies the collaborative approach to client care. The mutual interaction model of nurse–client collaboration stresses the importance of equality and a sharing of perspectives between nurse and client. The nurse enters the situation as the caregiver, but both nurse and client have the capacity to negotiate the roles they will play. If the client is incapacitated, the nurse seeks out those who know the client best and who have legitimate relationships with the client, and engages them in planning the client's care. Collaboration is caring because the client's values are taken into account in all clinical decisions.

■ PHILOSOPHY AND VALUES REFLECTED IN THE MUTUAL INTERACTION MODEL

Philosophically, this text has adopted mutual interaction, or collaboration, as the model for the nurse–client relationship. The value of caring is consistent with the mutual interaction model. The mutual interaction model stresses the importance of equality, and a sharing of perspectives from both client and nurse. In the ideal situation, this caring would be mutual whether between nurse and client or between nurse and family. The nurse enters the situation pri-

BUILDING NURSING KNOWLEDGE

What Is Caring?

Forrest D. The experience of caring. *J Adv Nurs.* 1989;14: 815–823.

The author emphasizes that caring is traditional in nursing, but notes a lack of research on caring. Forrest designed a study to shed light on the nature of caring from the perspective of the practicing nurse. The purpose was to describe the meaning attached to caring by working nurses. The author used a research approach appropriate to the study of "lived experience." This approach sought to uncover the meaning of caring through an analysis of subjects' descriptions. Seventeen nurses were interviewed in taped sessions about what caring meant to them. Interviews varied in length from 50 minutes to 2 hours. The data were analyzed for recurring themes in subject statements.

Forrest found that for the practicing nurses in the study, caring was first and foremost a mental and emotional state that evolved from deep feelings for clients' experiences. Caring was characterized by putting clients before routine, by attending to clients' requests, and by encouraging client involvement in care even if it took more time. Being able to put oneself into the client's position was the source of the nurses' caring feeling.

Forrest found that a particular quality of interaction denoted caring. That quality developed from anticipating clients' needs and responding to subtle cues of which clients might be unaware. Part of caring involved "being firm" and "teaching," interactions that helped clients toward awareness, self-knowledge, and potential independence. Caring meant respect and closeness, being there, touching and holding, and coming to know clients well.

The nurses in Forrest's study reported that their capacity for caring was enhanced by comfort and support from immediate co-workers and from unit supervisors who alleviated daily frustration by recognizing the worth of each nurse. They also emphasized the influence of nursing educators who were caring in their interactions with clients, and the impact of certain instructors who were particularly caring in their qualities.

marily as the one who is caring; if the client has the capacity to interact, a negotiation takes place concerning roles and expectations. If clients lack this capacity nurses seek out those who know the client best or who have legitimate relationships with the client. Mutual interaction, or collaboration, involves genuine caring, as clients' views are taken into account in all clinical decisions. Clients' personhood is respected and their perspective is of primary importance in all decisions.

Another strength of the mutual interaction model lies in its emphasis on client autonomy (self-direction). There are at least two major assumptions in the model: (1) clients have the capacity and desire to participate actively in their own health care, and (2) clients are willing to accept the consequences of their choices.[15] Client and practitioner are seen as equal participants in the interaction. This valuing of an individual's autonomy is a primary expression of respect of person, which is an important value in nursing. The values of the mutual interaction model suggest three different approaches to nurse–client decision making. These approaches are consistent with the recommendations of the President's Commission Report, *Making Health Care Decisions.*[5]

First, if clients are competent, their right to self-determination is to be respected. The mutual interaction model expresses profound respect for an individual's right and need for self-control and self-direction; accordingly, respect for autonomy is the first approach to clients.

Second, clients who cannot speak for themselves require surrogate decision making. In this approach, people who know the clients best, usually the family, are asked to speak for them as they would have done if able. This approach, known as **substituted judgment,** will be discussed in more detail in Chapter 34. The surrogate can use a document such as a living will (see Chap. 3) or other communications in determining what should be done. On some occasions, if a family member is acting as the surrogate, family conflict may make the decision-making process difficult. On rare occasions, a family member may stand to benefit from a client's earlier death; obviously this situation must be avoided. Use of the wishes previously set forth by clients is very helpful.

Third, if incompetent clients have not provided clear advance directives, the surrogate decision-maker should approach decisions about health care using a **best interest standard.** That is, the decision-maker attempts to direct care decisions to those measures that will benefit the client. The decision-maker in this approach would consider benefits such as reducing discomfort, prolonging life, and improving quality of life.[5] The first two approaches to care decisions place greater emphasis on client autonomy, because clients' wishes are known. The third approach emphasizes beneficence (doing good for the client) or nonmaleficence (avoiding harm). All three approaches, however, focus on clients as the ones who are most important when decisions are made (Table 33–5).

At times, clients may be restricted from acting in ways that might harm themselves or others. Then, the principle of autonomy (self-direction) is temporarily set aside. Nurses need to bear in mind that there are ethical and societal obligations to protect clients or third parties from harm. Legally and ethically nurses cannot allow individuals to act against their own value systems. For example, a nurse counseling a pregnant woman seeking an abortion may discover that the woman herself feels uncertain about whether abortion is morally correct, but that pressure from her partner caused her to request the procedure. This situation calls for further exploration before proceeding, for in having the abortion, the client may be acting against personal values, to her potential harm. Given these exceptions (incompetence and special circumstances implying a need for protection), self-determination is to be respected. When incompetence is temporary, nurses adopt care measures designed to return clients to a competent state as soon as

TABLE 33–4. VALUES COMMON TO NURSING THEORIES

Value	Definition	Example
Holism	The person is a unity of mental, physical, and social aspects.	A nurse asks the client how he feels about his colostomy.
Health	A continuum, a subjective state.	An elderly person with controlled diabetes assists blood circulation with daily walks. The nurse regards her as healthy, despite her disease.
Caring	Considerate, respectful care of clients.	A nurse provides compassionate care to a client suspected of child abuse.
		A nurse uses simplified language in explaining care and procedures to a client with little education.

possible. This is consistent with respect for clients' autonomy, which is a primary value in the mutual interaction model.

USING PHILOSOPHY IN PERSONAL AND PROFESSIONAL LIFE

Philosophy Applied to Practice

This section of the chapter presents five hypothetical case histories of persons who chose nursing as a profession. Each has decided to pursue nursing as a career because of basic personal values. Each will find that these values are challenged, examined, and further expressed in a particular practice setting. In each situation, many values and philosophic issues are at work.

CASE STUDY 1: Maria Benavides enjoys technology. Ms. Benavides has chosen a career in nursing because she is fascinated by technological innovations in health care. Her dream of working in an adult intensive care unit is fulfilled when she begins her new position in the surgical intensive care unit (SICU) of a large city hospital. She quickly masters the challenges of her new position and gains the respect of her colleagues. However, some new experiences begin to challenge her view of technology as a consistently positive value. She observes that the relatives of her clients are often upset by seeing their loved ones "hooked up to machines." Visiting periods are 15 minutes in length, and there often is not enough time to assist families to deal with the level of technology required by clients. Ms. Benavides is also concerned about the possibility that the machines may sometimes receive more attention than the people in the beds. Ms. Benavides plans a discussion in her unit focused on the issue of caring. She and her colleagues plan ways to improve the care of clients and their families, so that the focus of nursing remains holistic and not mechanistic.

TABLE 33–5. APPROACHES TO NURSE–CLIENT DECISION-MAKING ABOUT HEALTH CARE

Type of Client	Approach to Care
Competent adult	Respect clients' own wishes as explored through informed discussion.
Incompetent adult who has provided advance directives (eg, living will)	Determine who will speak for the client. The surrogate should use clients' previously expressed wishes, or *substituted judgment.*
Incompetent adult who has provided no advance directives.	Determine who will speak for the client. The surrogate should use *best interests* as a guide to decision-making.

CASE STUDY 2: Elayne Rubenstein wants to work with young adults. Ms. Rubenstein believes in independent nursing practice and client autonomy. She is pleased when she is offered a position in a college student health service after completing her Master of Science degree in Nursing. She assists with many health assessments and counsels students on choices available to them when facing unplanned pregnancies. She also advises married students about the possibility of treatment for infertility when this is a problem. Several of her clients have attempted to become pregnant through in-vitro fertilization. One client in particular has spoken with Ms. Rubenstein at length about her experiences. She was able to become pregnant after several attempts, but the procedures were expensive and seemed to invade her privacy. Ms. Rubenstein begins to wonder whether client choice is always a positive value: choices can seemingly lead to abortion, single parenthood, or treatments that may not be in a client's best interest. Other questions that are raised include: When does human life begin? Is it acceptable to stop an unwanted pregnancy? Is pregnancy always a good thing? Ms. Rubenstein decides to examine her values on these issues.

CASE STUDY 3: James Kemper wants to work with terminally ill clients. Mr. Kemper gains personal satisfaction from helping people cope with life-threatening illness. Many of his clients have cancer and face surgical procedures as well as follow-up chemotherapy and radiation therapy. Many also are invited to participate in research studies to determine the effectiveness of treatment. Mr. Kemper starts to question whether adults facing serious illness are as autonomous as he thought they were. Are they able to make free decisions about therapy or being involved in research when their cancer is life-threatening? What about situations in which family members or physicians do not want clients to know they have cancer? Mr. Kemper values free will, but comes to believe that it must be carefully supported in hospital settings. He decides to work more closely with his clients to ensure that they have the information and emotional support they need to make informed decisions based on their own personal values. He also decides to find out more about the hospital ethics committee that protects human research subjects. Perhaps he will volunteer to serve on the committee.

CASE STUDY 4: Sharon Johns values helping people. Ms. Johns believes strongly in the right of all people to health care. She accepts a position at a community health clinic in a low-income neighborhood. After a few months, several issues begin to bother her. Many of the clients have very few financial resources and are unable to follow basic health guidelines for cleanliness and good nutrition, even though they are motivated to do so. What is the responsibility of nurses and the larger society if even basic needs cannot be met? Other clients are not motivated to help themselves. Ms. Johns cares for a man with lung disease who refuses to stop smoking. On occasion, persons who abuse drugs come to the clinic for treatment of infections at injection sites. These people raise the question of responsibility for one's own health. Are nurses obligated to care for persons who will not care for themselves? Ms. Johns decides that she will maintain respect for all clients, but will also set reasonable limits on what she personally can do for the most difficult clients. Caring for herself is also important, and she will focus on the positive changes she can make for many clients. She also supports local projects to assist disadvantaged persons in the community.

CASE STUDY 5: Lisa Kramer values independence in older adults. Because of positive experiences with her own grandparents, who remained active and independent until shortly before their death, Ms. Kramer decides to work with older adults in extended care facilities. She wishes to encourage a high level of independence in these clients. However, after she has worked a short time, she becomes discouraged. It does not seem possible for many of her clients to achieve a high level of health. Many of them have difficulty thinking or remembering, and are unable to make their own decisions. One older man cannot recognize his family when they visit. It seems regrettable that the identity of this man has undergone such profound change. With time, Ms. Kramer learns to accept that health may be on a continuum and may change throughout life. Even though her clients may have changed significantly in their later years, they deserve respect and high quality care. Ms. Kramer also determines that living wills or other advance directives would help in decision making for her incompetent clients, and she begins to review the policies of the extended care facility regarding this issue.

Developing a Personal Philosophy of Nursing

In the preceding examples, each nurse began with a particular belief. There was a complex interplay between personal philosophy and values, the practice setting, and the nurse–client relationship. Each nurse's professional experience made values clarification necessary. That is, each nurse was challenged to examine the assumptions that had been the basis of a career choice. (Values clarification, a process by which one discovers what one truly believes or values, is discussed further in Chap. 34.)

Having considered the concepts related to philosophic inquiry and values reflected in nursing theories, readers are invited to begin a process of self-examination. Box 33–1 lists several questions to aid readers in examining their own values. Answers to these questions provide a foundation for establishing personal views about nursing.

BOX 33–1. DEVELOPING A PERSONAL PHILOSOPHY OF NURSING

Ask Yourself:

- Why do I want to be a nurse? What are the reasons?
- What personal experiences have influenced my decision?
- Have my personal encounters with the health care system affected my decision? My attitudes about client care? In what way?
- Who are the nurses I admire? What are their qualities?
- How do those nurses benefit clients? What is their focus in giving client care?
- What do the actions of the nurses I admire say about their professional values and priorities?
- What would I do differently from those nurses?
- What institutional settings would I like to work in? What attracts me to them?
- What settings am I less interested in? Why?
- What is my definition of health? Caring? Nursing?
- What are my beliefs about identity? Holism? Free will?
- What conditions or limitations, if any, should be put on respect for the client? Are all clients (or people) worthy of respect? Does their mental capacity, motivation to care for themselves, or type of health problem make a difference?
- What is my definition of respect?

SUMMARY

The overview of philosophy given in this chapter has invited students to participate in personal and professional growth. Philosophic methods such as asking questions, examining claims, and presenting arguments can assist students to identify personal values, interact with clients, and function as effective client advocates.

Epistemology, metaphysics, and ethics are discussed as three areas of philosophical inquiry. Epistemology studies questions relating to knowledge, such as how knowledge is achieved. Empiricism and rationalism are two epistemological traditions. Empiricism views knowledge attained through the senses as most reliable. Rationalism, on the other hand, holds that knowledge should be supported by reason. Metaphysics studies the nature of existence through thinking and reasoning, rather than empirical observation. Ethics analyzes whether actions are right or wrong.

Awareness of how knowledge is developed and validated can assist nurses to question practices that have been taken for granted and to develop scientifically based knowledge. In addition, the study of epistemology can encourage the pursuit of alternative research methodologies, such as qualitative and phenomenological research, which can also provide meaningful insights into practice.

Metaphysical questions include the relationship of mind and body, free will and determinism, and identity and change. Nursing practice relies on a set of beliefs about people, the nature of health and illness, and the nurse–client relationship. The consideration of metaphysical issues allows clarification of the beliefs and opinions one holds, and critical awareness of values apparent in such documents as the American Nurses' Association Social Policy Statement.[19] Such a consideration also offers a historical perspective on beliefs and values.

The final section of the chapter provided an overview of three themes common to all theories of nursing: holism, health, and caring. It is appropriate to end this chapter with a philosophical consideration of the nurse–client relationship, because the act of caring for another is the essence of nursing. Gadow[3] distinguishes three options for the role of nurses, each implying a different kind of nurse–client relationship: (1) consumer advocacy, (2) paternalism, and (3) existential advocacy. As a consumer advocate, nurses merely provide clients with information and allow complete client decision making. In the paternalistic model, nurses tell clients what to do. As an existential advocate—the model Gadow defends—nurses' role is to help clients become clear about the meaning of illness. In this model, nurses are neither isolated from clients nor making decisions without the client's involvement. Instead, the nurse enters into clients' experiences with sympathy and assists clients to understand the personal meaning of illness and recovery. The reader is invited to reflect on this definition of the nurse–client relationship and its bearing on nurse–client collaboration and caring.

REFERENCES

1. Schlotfeldt R. The ND Program: Vision for the Future. The Schlotfeldt Lecture. Frances Payne Bolton School of Nursing, Case Western Reserve University, Cleveland, 1985.
2. Munhall P. Nursing philosophy and nursing research: In apposition or opposition? *Nurs Res.* 1982;37:176.
3. Gadow S. Existential advocacy: Philosophical foundation of nursing. In: Spicker S, Gadow S, eds. *Nursing Images and Ideals: Opening Dialogue With the Humanities.* New York: Springer; 1980: 79–102.
4. Polanyi M. *Personal Knowledge: Towards a Post-Critical Philosophy.* New York: Harper & Row; 1962.
5. United States President's Commission for the Study of Ethical Problems in Medicine and Biomedical and Behavioral Research. *Making Health Care Decisions: A Report on the Ethical and Legal Implications of Informed Consent on the Patient–Practitioner Relationship.* Washington DC: US Government Printing Office. 1982.
6. Knaus W, et al. An evaluation of outcome from medical care in major medical centers. *Ann Intern Med.* 1986;104:410–418.
7. Carper B. Fundamental patterns of knowing in nursing. *Adv Nurs Sci.* October, 1978; 13–23.
8. Descartes R; Haldane ES, Ross GRT, trans. *Meditations on First Philosophy: The Philosophical Works of Descartes.* Cambridge; 1934.
9. Merleau-Ponty M; Dreyfus HL, Dreyfus PA, trans. *Sense and Non-Sense.* Evanston: Northwestern University Press; 1964.
10. Evans LK, Strumpf NE. Tying down the elderly: A review of the literature on physical restraint. *J Am Geriatric Soc.* 1989;37: 65–74.
11. Drew N. Exclusion and confirmation: A phenomenology of patients' experiences with caregivers. *Image.* 1986;18:39–43.
12. Lewis CS. The humanitarian theory of punishment. In: Hooper W, ed. *God in the Dock.* Grand Rapids, MI: Eerdmans; 1970.
13. Hart HLA. Responsibility. In: Beauchamp T, Walters L, eds. *Bioethics.* Belmont, CA: Wadsworth; 1978;33–37.
14. Roy C. *Introduction to Nursing: An Adaptation Model.* 2nd ed. Englewood Cliffs, NJ: Prentice-Hall; 1984.
15. Williamson J. Mutual interaction: A model of nursing practice. *Nurs Outlook.* 1981;29:104–107.
16. Rogers ME. *The Theoretical Basis of Nursing.* Philadelphia: Davis; 1970.
17. Rogers ME. Nursing: A science of unitary human beings. In: Reihl-Sisca J, ed. *Conceptual Models for Nursing Practice.* 3rd ed. Norwalk, CT: Appleton & Lange; 1989.
18. Orem D. *Nursing Concepts of Practice.* 4th ed. New York: McGraw-Hill; 1990.
19. American Nurses' Association. *Nursing: A Social Policy Statement.* Kansas City, MO: ANA; 1980.
20. Gaylin W. *Caring.* New York: Knopf; 1976.
21. Noddings N. *Caring: A Feminine Approach to Ethics and Moral Education.* Berkeley: University of California Press; 1984.
22. Blevins D. Caring: A life force. In: Leininger M, ed. *Caring: An Essential Human Need.* Thorofare, NJ: Slack; 1981.
23. Leininger M, ed. *Caring: An Essential Human Need.* Thorofare, NJ: Slack; 1981.
24. Fry S. Toward a theory of nursing ethics. *Adv Nurs Sci.* 1989; 11:9–22.

BIBLIOGRAPHY

Benfield J. Two philosophies of caring. *Ohio Med J.* 1979; 508–511.

Benner P, Wrubel J. *The Primacy of Caring: Stress and Coping in Health and Illness.* Redwood City, CA: Addison Wesley; 1988.

Bernal E. Immobility and the self: A clinical-existential inquiry. *J Med Philosophy.* 1984;9:75–91.

Burr R, Goldinger M, eds. *Philosophy and Contemporary Issues.* 3rd ed. New York: Macmillan; 1980.

Cooper CC. Covenantal relationships: grounding for the nursing ethic. *Adv Nurs Sci.* 1988;10:48.

Davis AJ. Professional obligations, personal values in conflict. *Am Nurse.* 1990;22:7.

Erde EL. Free will and determinism. In: Reich W, ed. *Encyclopedia of Bioethics.* New York: Free Press; 1982;500–506.

Gadow S. Allocating autonomy: Can patients and practitioners share? In: Bell N, ed. *Who Decides? Conflicts of Rights in Health Care.* New York: Humana; 1982:95–106.

Gould JA, ed. *Classic Philosophical Questions.* 4th ed. Columbus: Merrill; 1982.

Jameton A, Fowler MDM. Ethical inquiry and the concept of research. *Adv Nurs Sci.* 1989;11:11–24.

Jones AH, ed. *Images of Nurses: Perspectives from History, Art and Literature.* Philadelphia: University of Pennsylvania Press; 1988.

Kass L. Thinking about the body. *Hastings Center Rep.* 1985;15:20–31.

Kestenbaum V. *The Humanity of the Ill: Phenomenological Perspectives.* Knoxville: University of Tennessee Press; 1982.

Ketefian S. Moral reasoning and ethical practice in nursing. *Nurs Clin North Am.* 1989;24:509–521.

Ketefian S, Ormond I. *Moral Reasoning and Ethical Practice in Nursing: An Integrative Review.* New York: National League for Nursing; 1988.

Reed P. Nursing theorizing as an ethical dilemma. *Adv Nurs Sci.* 1989;11:1–10.

Saladay SA, McDonnell Sr, MM. Spiritual care, ethical decisions and patient advocacy. *Nurs Clin North Am.* 1989;24:543–549.

Sontag S. *Illness as Metaphor.* New York: Farrar, Straus & Giroux; 1977.

Spicker S, Gadow S, eds. *Nursing Images and Ideals: Opening Dialogue With the Humanities.* New York: Springer; 1980.

Van Hooft S. Moral education for nursing decisions. *J Adv Nurs.* 1990;15:210–215.

Yeo M. Integration of nursing theory and nursing ethics. *Adv Nurs Sci.* 1989;11:33–42.

Zaner R. Embodiment. In Reich W, ed. *Encyclopedia of Bioethics.* New York: Free Press; 1982:361–366.

CHAPTER 34

Values and Ethics in Nursing

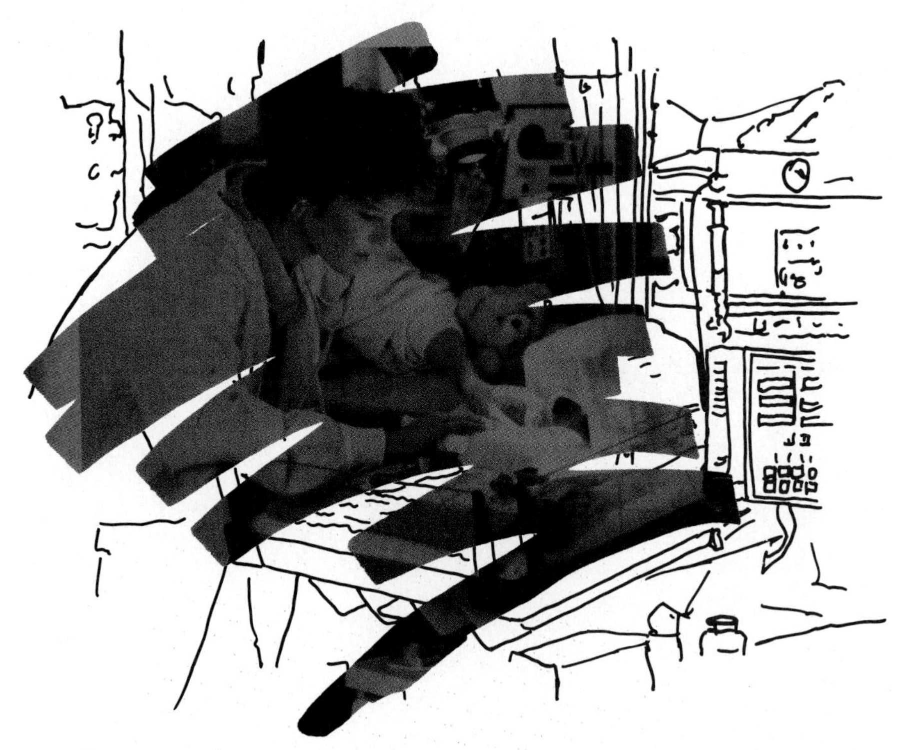

Behavioral Objectives

Upon completion of this chapter, the student will be able to:

1. Define ethics.
2. Distinguish between an ethical dilemma and an ethical problem.
3. Identify personal values that have an impact on ethical decision-making.
4. Discuss seven steps in the process of acquiring values.
5. Identify professional values as expressed in codes of ethics and selected professional documents.
6. Identify professional values inherent in the mutual interaction model of nurse–client collaboration.
7. Identify eight general ethical principles that influence nursing practice.
8. Differentiate between the ethical theories of teleology and deontology.
9. Discuss caring as the basis of ethical behavior.
10. Identify several common ethical issues of nursing practice.
11. Resolve an ethical dilemma using a framework for justification.
12. Identify the ethical responsibilities of the professional nurse.

KEY TERMS

beneficence
client advocacy
code of ethics
confidentiality
deontology
deception
ethical dilemma
ethical principle
ethical problem
ethical theory
ethics
fidelity
justice
maxim
nonmaleficence
paternalism
personal value
prima facie duty
professional value
respect of autonomy
respect of person
teleology
theory of virtue
value
values clarification
value system
veracity

Ethics is the branch of philosophy that attempts to discern which actions are right within a given situation. Ethics also deals with the principles that should promote action and the theories that justify those principles. The process by which one examines ethical concerns is known as ethical analysis.

This chapter emphasizes ethics that pertain to common concerns in everyday nursing practice. The ability to address and resolve common ethical concerns contributes to professional excellence as well as to personal satisfaction in nursing. Unlike the ethical questions involved in dramatic life-and-death situations, everyday ethical concerns are often not recognized because they are mundane. Yet it is the common issues encountered in daily practice that occupy the majority of nursing time and effort. These issues are important because an ethical basis established in ordinary activity can be applied to the more dramatic issues that nurses will encounter.

It is important for nurses to prevent ethical problems as well as to identify and resolve them. This requires an understanding of the foundations of ethical practice in addition to the development of decision-making skills that are based on relevant ethical concepts. This chapter presents an introduction to ethical issues in nursing practice and a framework for analysis of ethical problems and dilemmas. An individual's perception of a problem or dilemma arises from conflicts in personal values, professional ideals, ethical principles, or ethical theories. These four entities, along with values clarification, are examined, as they form a foundation for nursing ethics.

■ FOUNDATIONS FOR ETHICAL PRACTICE

The fundamental question in ethical decision making is "What, all things considered, ought to be done in a given situation?"[1] To answer this question, nurses need to be aware of personal and professional values that have a bearing on the situation and ethical principles and theories that might apply.

To begin, it is important to clarify the relationship of ethical to moral and legal concepts. Although the terms "ethics" and "morals" often are used interchangeably, a helpful distinction is to describe ethics as the rational or deliberate thinking about the moral. The nature of professional activity requires careful thought about what is moral—that is, good or right; such activity is described as ethical. To be ethical requires taking individual responsibility about particular matters. Legal requirements, on the other hand, are legislated by governing bodies or institutions and requires no individual deliberation. Ethical obligations extend beyond the legal. Excellence in practice cannot be legislated; it requires, among other things, individual and collective commitment to ethical principles. There is an obligation to know and abide by the law, but there is also an obligation to make judgments and seek to have laws changed when they do not agree with one's moral and ethical understanding of societal needs.

In thinking about ethical issues, it also is helpful to distinguish between an ethical problem and an ethical dilemma.[2] An **ethical dilemma** is a situation in which there are two or more alternatives for action based upon ethical principles, each of which has undesirable consequences. An **ethical problem,** on the other hand, is one in which the "right" or the "good" thing to do is clear, but accomplishing it is extremely difficult.

The following situation provides a starting point for examining the foundations of ethical practice.

> SITUATION: Sharon Miller, RN, is the primary nurse caring for Mrs. James, who had major abdominal surgery yesterday. Mrs. James is in a great deal of pain, although she has been taking her pain medication. Nurse Miller is attempting to convince Mrs. James that she needs to ambulate. She explains that walking will improve Mrs. James' circulation, breathing, and muscle tone and will help her get better faster. Mrs. James refuses. Nurse Miller wonders what she should now do to help Mrs. James. Should she try to "pressure" her to get up, or should she let the client make her own decision?

Personal Values

To deal effectively with the preceding situation, or any other situation in nursing practice, it is important for nurses to be aware of the personal values that influence individuals' actions. **Values** can be defined as standards of choice that provide meaningful direction for individuals and groups.[3] **Personal values** are those values held, or ascribed to, by an individual. Each person has his or her own set of values, sometimes referred to as a **value system.**[4] A value system reflects an individual's culture and society and is generally consistent over time. It represents an individual's sense of "the good life."[5] Values have both cognitive (thinking) and affective (feeling) dimensions. In other words, people not only think about and verbally defend what they value, but they also care deeply about things that they believe to be good and invest emotional energy to act in their defense.

Personal values are reflected in the way in which individuals spend time and money, in the choice of friends, and in risk taking and goal achievement. Values are apparent in all daily activities including health behavior and are represented in career choices. According to Raths and associates,[6] valuing is a process composed of seven steps and three levels of action (Box 34–1).

The first level of action in valuing is choosing one's beliefs and behaviors from among alternatives. Ordinarily, the alternatives available to any one person are presented by the person's culture, which includes family, community, school, society, and religion. Individuals must consider the consequences of various alternatives and be free to make a choice. For example, a nursing student who conforms to a dress code only because of external pressure from an instructor is not really choosing freely.

The second level in the valuing process is an identification with the belief or behavior. There is an affective (or feeling) state associated with the action, object, or idea. A person feels good about the choice and has a willingness to affirm this by public statement, if necessary. From the previous example, suppose the nursing student continues to maintain a professional appearance when no longer subject to the evaluation of the instructor. In this case, the nurse is proud of his or her appearance and publicly affirms its personal and professional value.

The third level is one of action. According to Raths and co-workers,[6] unless one acts repeatedly on an expressed belief, the belief is not really a personal value. The nursing student truly has adopted the value of professional appearance when it is consistently expressed in all situations. In summary, then, valuing includes a pattern of consistency in choice, expressed feeling, and action.

In a complex pluralistic society, a variety of values influence individual choice and action in any particular situation. Some values will be shared, but others will be highly specific to individuals. When values are shared there is cohesion and people can work together with ease. Differing values can contribute to dissonance, conflict, and difficulty in problem-solving. For example, a group of five students

BOX 34–1. LEVELS OF ACTION IN VALUING

Choosing one's beliefs and behaviors
1. Choosing from alternatives
2. Considering consequences
3. Choosing freely

Prizing one's beliefs and behaviors
4. Being proud of and cherishing
5. Publicly affirming when appropriate

Acting on one's beliefs
6. Acting
7. Acting consistently or with a pattern

From Raths L, Harmin M, Simons S. Values and Teaching. *Columbus, OH: Merrill; 1966.*

are working together on a project. Three of the students are interested in the topic and value the learning that can come in shared work. One of the students has a 4.0 grade-point average and values being in control because she doesn't want to risk her straight-A record in the group project grade. The fifth group member is happy to "get by" and values social life above academic achievement. This group will need to address these differences in values if they wish to work together effectively.

All health care endeavors require interpersonal interaction. In a given situation everyone acts from their individual value systems. Therefore, a part of growth for students of a profession is to learn how to be true to a personal value system, which is a mark of integrity, and at the same time to respond compassionately to those with very different values. In the context of care, nurses need to tolerate and affirm a diversity of religious and cultural beliefs and values. Persons who enter nursing with rigid or narrow religious or social perspectives need to step back and reflect on the meaning of personal freedom and choice. For example, the value of not receiving blood is as precious to a Jehovah's Witness as the value of baptizing an infant is to a Catholic. Each value is critical to the view of eternal life in their respective belief systems. An individual nurse may not hold to either of these values but can respond to them out of a personal valuing of the importance of respect for individual human choice in matters of religious belief. Personal values, then, must be examined from the perspective of broad ethical principles. These principles may become personal values and can be applied in caring for people who affirm diverse beliefs.

Just as it is inappropriate for nurses to impose their specific value system on a client, it would also be inappropriate for clients (or employers) to expect nurses to act against deeply held and carefully examined moral convictions. In such circumstances, which are rare, nurses may withdraw from care after ensuring that the client has access to another caregiver and does not feel abandoned. Nurses are obligated to inform the employer at the time of employment about any deeply held values that may prevent participation in certain procedures.[7]

It should be clear that personal values are a constant influence on individual choices and action. In the earlier situation of Mrs. James and Nurse Miller, any number of personal values may influence the interaction. The nurse may value providing comfort, being liked, being efficient, being in control, or having a coffee break with peers. If she acts on the value of having a coffee break with peers and manipulates Mrs. James into walking immediately, the nurse's action may be inconsistent with another personal value of providing comfort. In order to discover inconsistencies in personal value systems, individuals need to examine their actions as expressions of values.

IMPLICATIONS FOR PROFESSIONAL COLLABORATION

Pluralism

In a pluralistic society, some values will be shared, but others will be highly specific to individuals. When values are shared, there is cohesion and persons work together with ease. When values are not shared the door is open to conflict and difficulty in problem-solving. Collaboration among all who are party to a decision—nurses, other providers, clients, and their families—can reveal commonalities in belief and enhance cohesion. It can also reveal dissimilarities and signal a need for a special sensitivity to the various emotions people associate with ideas, objects, and actions.

Values Clarification

Values clarification is a conscious process of identifying and ranking personal values. Understanding and clarifying personal values is an important starting point in developing integrity, which is the basis for the ethical practice of nursing. Truly confronting the values that underlie one's behavioral choices can be a complex and sometimes threatening undertaking. There is merit in the process, however, because it can lead to increased understanding of self and more responsible autonomous decision making. The difficulty lies in being confronted with one's own inconsistent behavior and in coping with significant change.

Values clarification is important not only in the personal and professional growth of the nurse but in client–nurse interactions as well. Illness and injury may force individuals to discover or realign values. Nurses can be instrumental in this discovery. The athlete who loses the physical capacity to participate in sports can be helped to grieve the loss and also to discover and affirm something new or different. Even though a highly valued skill was lost, all that the individual valued was not lost.

Gadow emphasizes that values clarification is a part of advocacy and derives from a client–nurse relationship that is collaborative in nature. The collaborative relationship involves a sharing of perspective that encourages clients to reflect on and become clear about their own values.[8] This process of values clarification arises naturally within the collaborative relationship; it is not in any way contrived.

There is a large body of literature including many published exercises on the topic of values clarification. Steele and Harmon,[9] Pender,[10] and Uustal[11] are all excellent resources. A values clarification exercise also is included in the Study Guide. Many assumptions are made about the benefit of values clarification. However, there is little research to support that participating in the process leads to better or more satisfying action. This is an area rich in possibility for the nurse researcher.

As stated earlier, personal value systems are influenced by culture and society. Although some values are deeply rooted and consistent over time, others may change as individuals mature and acquire new knowledge and experience. For example, certain values will lead individuals to choose nursing as a professional goal. In the process of professional education, some values will be strengthened, some discarded, and others added. It is expected that professional values will become a part of the personal value system of the

BUILDING NURSING KNOWLEDGE

Are Values Involved in Clients' Health Decisions?

Gortner SR, Zyzanski SJ. Values in the choice of treatment: Replication and refinement. *Nurs Res.* 1988;37:220–244.

The authors note that values are important in clients' decisions about health care. However, even within families, individuals may apply different values to make important decisions. In this study the investigators endeavored to refine a questionnaire they devised for use with clients.

Items on the questionnaire reflected two ethical themes, autonomy and beneficence. Autonomy encompassed values on personhood, free choice, consent, competence, comprehension, and disclosure of information. This theme was reflected by the degree of subjects' agreement with statements such as the following: Clients and families need thorough descriptions of surgical risks and benefits in order to decide; Additional medical opinions should be obtained before undertaking the treatment; One should have complete details of risks and benefits of treatment even if they are frightening.

Beneficence dealt with values on the balance of benefits. Beneficence was reflected by agreement statements such as the following: Some would rather risk dying in surgery than to burden their family as an invalid; Quality of life can be so poor that it is worth running the risks of surgery; If a person has chosen a treatment for himself, it is the right choice.

The questionnaire was administered to 67 clients who had undergone major heart surgery and their spouses. The purpose was to determine the correspondence of values within families. The findings showed little difference between clients and their spouses on their scores for autonomy and beneficence. Family scores (client-spouse average) indicated autonomy was valued more strongly than beneficence. Clients under the age of 50 had significantly higher autonomy scores than did those over age 70. While this information is helpful for a general understanding, the investigators point out that the study was done after clients had crystallized their decisions, and another study is required to provide clues to the operation of values as clients weigh their decisions.

nurse. In the next section, discussing professional values, readers are encouraged to consider these choices.

Professional Values

All professions have a foundation of values that guide practice. **Professional values** are those concepts describing "right" or "good" practice that are affirmed publicly by official professional organizations. Nursing values come from the collective wisdom of past and present nurses; therefore, they represent a broad perspective and have a universal quality. It is important for nurses to study and internalize the publicly expressed values of the profession in addition to clarifying and examining personal values in light of these professional values. The American Nurses' Association (ANA) *Code for Nurses,*[7] the Canadian Nurses' Association (CNA) *Code of Ethics for Nursing,*[12] the American Nurses' Association *Social Policy Statement,*[13] and the American Association of Colleges of Nursing *Essentials of College and University Education for Professional Nursing*[14] provide a beginning for identifying these values. In addition to publicly expressed values, implicit values underlie the various nursing theories and the nurse–client relationship. An understanding of professional history and changing practice will illuminate present values and how values have changed. A historical perspective is beyond the scope of this chapter, but the reader is encouraged to consider this source of professional roots and growth.

Codes of Ethics. A **code of ethics** is an expression of professional values; of necessity it must be a broad statement to permit wide application. A code of ethics provides general, rather than specific, guidelines, and does not necessarily give answers to specific problems. At times, statements within the code itself may be in tension or conflict. Resolution or justification of dilemmas cannot come from the code itself, but must come from deliberation about underlying philosophic or ethical positions.

A portion of what society can expect of professionals is expressed in codes of ethics. These codes are not laws in the legal sense, but they are consistent with and uphold the law. They are a public statement of responsibility, and can therefore be seen as a public promise. It is important that professionals take these codes seriously because they serve as reminders that the power that comes from expert knowledge and privilege of practice must be tempered with moral considerations of good, bad, right, wrong, and respect for person. A code gives direction to individual nurses who are expected to practice in a way that upholds the values of the profession. The ANA *Code for Nurses* and the CNA *Code of Ethics for Nursing* are included in this chapter (Figs. 34–1 and 34–2).

The ANA *Code for Nurses*[7] was revised in 1976 and new interpretive statements were published in 1985. The first three statements of this code refer to the client and call for respect of person, including respect of the client's privacy and confidentiality and protection of the client from harm caused by others. These statements clearly establish that the primary obligation of nurses is to clients. Statements four, five, and six state that nurses should be accountable, competent, and collaborative in practice. Statements seven through ten speak to individual nurses' responsibility to the profession and also to collective professional responsibility (Fig. 34–1).

The CNA *Code of Ethics for Nursing*[12] was revised and published in 1985. This code is presented in four sections that "correspond to the sources of nursing obligations: clients, health team, the social context of nursing and responsibilities of the profession" (p. 11). In addition to the 12 statements (Fig. 34–2) that are referred to as values in the preamble, the document includes standards and limitations. The standards provide some specific directions for acting on the values, and the limitations "describe exceptional circumstances in which a value or standard cannot receive its usual application" (p. 9).

Values expressed in obligations to clients include respect of person, autonomy, confidentiality, dignity, profes-

AMERICAN NURSES' ASSOCIATION *CODE FOR NURSES*

Preamble

A code of ethics makes explicit the primary goals and values of the profession. When individuals become nurses, they make a moral commitment to uphold the values and special moral obligations expressed in their code. The Code for Nurses is based on a belief about the nature of individuals, nursing, health, and society. Nursing encompasses the protection, promotion and restoration of health; the prevention of illness; and the alleviation of suffering in the care of clients, including individuals, families, groups and communities. In the context of these functions, nursing is defined as the diagnosis and treatment of human responses to actual or potential health problems.

Since clients themselves are the primary decision makers in matters concerning their own health, treatment and well-being, the goal of nursing actions is to support and enhance the client's responsibility and self-determination to the greatest extent possible. In this context, health is not necessarily an end in itself, but rather a means to a life that is meaningful from the client's perspective.

When making clinical judgments, nurses base their decisions on consideration of consequences and of universal moral principles, both of which prescribe and justify nursing actions. The most fundamental of these principles is respect for persons. Other principles stemming from this basic principle are autonomy (self-determination), beneficence (doing good), non-maleficence (avoiding harm), veracity (truth-telling), confidentiality (respecting privileged information), fidelity (keeping promises), justice (treating people fairly).

In brief, then, the statements of the code and their interpretation provide guidance for conduct and relationships in carrying out nursing responsibilities consistent with the ethical obligations of the profession and with high quality in nursing care.

Code for Nurses

1. The nurse provides services with respect for human dignity and the uniqueness of the client, unrestricted by considerations of social or economic status, personal attributes, or the nature of health problems.
2. The nurse safeguards the client's right to privacy by judiciously protecting information of a confidential nature.
3. The nurse acts to safeguard the client and the public when health care and safety are affected by the incompetent, unethical, or illegal practice of any person.
4. The nurse assumes responsibility and accountability for individual nursing judgments and actions.
5. The nurse maintains competence in nursing.
6. The nurse exercises informed judgment and uses individual competence and qualifications as criteria in seeking consultation, accepting responsibilities, and delegating nursing activities to others.
7. The nurse participates in activities that contribute to the ongoing development of the profession's body of knowledge.
8. The nurse participates in the profession's efforts to implement and improve standards of nursing.
9. The nurse participates in the profession's effort to establish and maintain conditions of employment conducive to high quality nursing care.
10. The nurse participates in the profession's effort to protect the public from misinformation and misrepresentation and to maintain the integrity of nursing.
11. The nurse collaborates with members of the health professions and other citizens in promoting community and national efforts to meet the health needs of the public.

Figure 34–1. American Nurses' Association Code for Nurses. (*Source: American Nurses' Association. Code for Nurses with Interpretative Statements. Kansas City, MO: ANA; 1985. Reprinted with permission of the American Nurses' Association.*)

sional competence, advocacy, and nursing. Values that address obligation to the health care team are those of cooperation with other health care providers as well as responsibility to secure quality care for clients. Under the social context of nursing there is a valuing of professional satisfaction in the workplace and of collective action in order to ensure conditions of employment that contribute to the safety of clients. The final statement addresses responsibilities of the profession and expresses a valuing of ethical conduct as an organizational obligation to respond to the "rights, needs and legitimate interests of clients and nurses" (p. 32). There is an explicit value here that nurses should support nurses and also that education regarding ethics should extend throughout a nurse's career.

Social Policy Statement. *Nursing: A Social Policy Statement*[13] was published by the ANA in 1980. This document was drafted by a task force of the Congress for Nursing

CANADIAN NURSES' ASSOCIATION *CODE OF ETHICS FOR NURSING*

Clients

I. A nurse treats clients with respect for their individual needs and values.
II. Based upon respect for clients and regard for their right to control their own care, nursing care reflects respect for the right of choice held by clients.
III. The nurse holds confidential all information about a client learned in the health care setting.
IV. The nurse is guided by consideration for the dignity of clients.
V. The nurse provide competent care to clients.

Nursing Roles and Relationships

VI. The nurse maintains trust in nurses and nursing.
VII. The nurse recognizes the contribution and expertise of colleagues from nursing and other disciplines as essential to excellent health care.
VIII. The nurse takes steps to ensure that the client receives competent and ethical care.
IX. Conditions of employment should contribute in a positive way to client care and the professional satisfaction of nurses.
X. Job action by nurses is directed toward securing conditions of employment that enable safe and appropriate care for clients and contribute to the professional satisfaction of nurses.

Nursing Ethics and Society

XI. The nurse advocates the interest of clients.
XII. The nurse represents the values and ethics of nursing before colleagues and others.
XIII. Professional nurses' organizations are responsible for clarifying, securing and sustaining ethical nursing conduct. The fulfilment of these tasks requires that professional nurses' organizations remain responsive to the rights, needs and legitimate interests of clients and nurses.

Figure 34–2. Canadian Nurses' Association Code of Ethics for Nursing. (*Source: Canadian Nurses' Association.* Code of Ethics for Nursing. *Ottawa: CNA; 1991. © by the Canadian Nurses' Association. Reprinted with permission.*)

Practice and was accepted as a basis for ANA policy after review by many nurses and practice councils. Therefore, as with codes of ethics, it represents professional consensus and gives direction to individual practice as well as to collective concerns of the profession.

The *Social Policy Statement* affirms nursing as a public good. Not only does nursing provide a needed and valued service but "public good must be the overriding concern" of nursing. Health is a part of public good and nursing has a role in providing health care that is "available, accessible and acceptable" (p. 3).

In addition to the values expressed in the codes of ethics, the *Social Policy Statement* affirms self-help or self-care as being important to individual and public well-being as well as to cost-containment. Collaboration is affirmed as a desirable working relationship. Self-regulation and accountability are described as critical components of nursing's social contract with society.

American Association of Colleges of Nursing Values. The American Association of Colleges of Nursing (AACN), a group of professional educators, has identified seven essential values for professional nursing.[14] These are altruism, equality, esthetics, freedom, human dignity, justice, and truth. Table 34–1 gives the AACN definitions of each value as well as examples of personal qualities and professional behaviors that would reflect commitment to these values. The AACN essential values report states a belief that nurses guided by these values will provide "safe, humanistic care focused on health and quality of life."[14]

The ANA *Social Policy Statement*, CNA and ANA codes of ethics, and the AACN essential values report are public expressions of values and expectations that form a promise by nursing to society. The values expressed in these documents need to become the action guides for every nurse. A summary of these values is presented in Table 34–2. The way in which these values are acted out in practice will depend upon the nature of the client–nurse relationship. Several other sources of professional values need to be mentioned before discussing this relationship.

Other Sources of Professional Values. In addition to the previously mentioned documents, other sources that provide direction for nurses in ethical decision making are the ANA *Standards of Nursing Practice*,[15] ANA *Human Rights Guidelines for Nurses in Clinical and Other Research*,[16] *Patient's Bill of Rights*,[17] and ANA *Ethics in Nursing: Position Statements and Guidelines*.[18] Other documents also have been developed by various specialty groups in nursing. All of these documents articulate the principle of self-determination or autonomy for clients and emphasize that clients are central in the practice of nursing. In addition, they specify or imply

TABLE 34–1. AACN VALUES, ATTITUDES, AND PROFESSIONAL BEHAVIORS

Essential Values[a]	Examples of Attitudes and Personal Qualities	Examples of Professional Behaviors
ALTRUISM Concern for the welfare of others	Caring, commitment, compassion, generosity, perseverance	Gives full attention to clients when giving care. Assists other personnel in providing care when they are unable to do so. Expresses concern about social trends and issues that have implications for health care.
EQUALITY Having the same rights, privileges, or status	Acceptance, assertiveness, fairness, self-esteem, tolerance	Provides nursing care based on individuals' needs irrespective of personal characteristics.[b] Interacts with other providers in a nondiscriminatory manner. Expresses ideas about the improvement of access to nursing and health care.
ESTHETICS Qualities of objects, events, and people that provide satisfaction	Appreciation, creativity, imagination, sensitivity	Adapts the environment so it is pleasing to clients. Creates a pleasant work environment for self and others. Presents self in a manner that promotes a positive image of nursing.
FREEDOM Capacity to exercise choice	Confidence, hope, independence, openness, self-direction, self-discipline	Honors individuals' right to refuse treatment. Supports the rights of other providers to suggest alternatives to the plan of care. Encourages open discussion of controversial issues in the profession.
HUMAN DIGNITY Inherent worth and uniqueness of an individual	Consideration, empathy, humaneness, kindness, respectfulness, trust	Safeguards individuals' right to privacy. Addresses individuals as they prefer to be addressed. Maintains confidentiality of clients and staff. Treats others with respect regardless of background.
JUSTICE Upholding moral and legal principles	Courage, integrity, morality, objectivity	Acts as a health care advocate. Allocates resources fairly. Reports incompetent, unethical, and illegal practice objectively and factually.[a]
TRUTH Faithfulness to fact or reality	Accountability, authenticity, honesty, inquisitiveness, rationality, reflectiveness	Documents nursing care accurately and honestly. Obtains sufficient data to make sound judgments before reporting infractions of organizational policies. Participates in professional efforts to protect the public from misinformation about nursing.

[a] The values are listed in alphabetic rather than priority order.
[b] From *Code for Nurses,* American Nurses' Association, 1976.
From American Association of Colleges of Nursing. Essentials of College and University Education for Professional Nursing. *Washington, DC: AACN; 1986, with permission.*

that nurses are expected to serve as client advocates. (Client advocacy will be discussed later in the chapter.)

Professional values are also embedded in the various nursing theories, as discussed in Chapter 33. All major nursing theories support commitment to the values of holism, health, caring, and self-determination. Other values specific to individual theories can also be identified. Choice of a theory to guide nursing practice implies acceptance of the values underlying that theory. Adoption of a particular nursing theory as the basis for nursing practice by a health

TABLE 34–2. COMPARATIVE LIST OF PROFESSIONAL VALUES

Social Policy Statement	ANA Code for Nurses	CNA Code of Ethics	AACN Essential Values
Human dignity Quality of life	Respect of person Dignity, privacy, confidentiality	Respect of person Dignity, privacy, confidentiality	Human dignity
Individual freedom and choice Self-help, self-regulation, accountability	Self-determination Competence Accountability, responsibility	Autonomy Competence Accountability, responsibility	Freedom
Research	Research	Research	Truth
Continuing education	Continuing education	Continuing education	
	Informed consent	Informed consent	
Protection Prevention of disease	Nonmaleficence	Nonmaleficence	
Collaboration	Interdisciplinary cooperation, collaboration	Interdisciplinary cooperation	Equality
Health care Available, accessible, acceptable	Nondiscriminatory care, nonprejudicial care	Advocacy for clients Rights of nurses	Justice
Cost-containment	Conditions for quality care Adequate conditions of employment	Conditions for quality care Adequate conditions of employment	
Nursing Standards of practice	Integrity of nursing Standards of practice	Integrity of nursing Standards of practice	
Health—wholeness Care of sick	Beneficence	Beneficence	Altruism
Generativity	Improving environment	Improving environment	Esthetics
Public good			

care institution suggests a clear valuing of theory-directed practice in that setting. It indicates institutional support of nursing as both art and science. The result should be a consistent representation of the values underlying the particular theory in the care of individual clients and in testing of that theory through nursing research. Some nurses deliberately seek positions in institutions with a specific theory-based practice because of a commitment to the values of a particular theory.

The key to the effectiveness of theory-based practice is in the hands of individual nurses, and much depends upon the model of the nurse–client relationship to which an individual nurse subscribes. The nature of the nurse–client relationship is the critical link between the ideas and action. The relationship is very personal and has very subtle qualities. Therefore, it needs to be created carefully with attention to detail, much as an artist paints or a composer writes music. As nurses formulate their own professional style it is important for them to have a broad perspective of professional values. These values may result in varying actions in different circumstances, but they serve as a guide for professional decisions and behavior.

The Mutual Interaction Model as a Vehicle of Professional Values. Part of the philosophical foundation for this text, the mutual interaction model of nurse–client collaboration, serves as a vehicle for incorporating the professional values listed in Table 34–2. The model embodies professional values. In addition to incorporating self-determination, health, and caring (discussed in Chap. 33), the mutual interaction model provides a basis for **client advocacy.** Gadow[8] describes advocacy as follows:

> Advocacy is actively assisting patients in their free self-determination of treatment options. Advocacy not only safeguards but positively contributes to the exercise of self-determination. In concrete terms, it is an effort to help individuals become clear about what they want in a situation, to assist them in discerning and clarifying their values, and to help them in examining available options in light of their values (p. 137).

Curtin[19] notes that client advocacy is a philosophical foundation for nursing. She states that "it involves the basic nature and purpose of the nurse–patient relationship. It is proposed as a very simple foundation upon which the nurse and patient in any given encounter can freely determine the form that relationship is to have" (p. 3). Other descriptions of client advocacy in the nursing literature have been summarized by Donahue,[20] but Gadow[8] and Curtin[19] capture the conceptualization of client advocacy found in the mutual interaction model. Within this model, clients are respected as self-determining and are equal partners in planning and decision making. Even when clients cannot express their wishes their perspective must be foremost in considering treatment options. (See Philosophy and Values Reflected in the Mutual Interaction Model in Chap. 33.)

The values addressed above have been publicly acclaimed by official professional organizations. Practicing nurses will also encounter a host of other values in institutional settings, among them values of efficiency, cost-containment, guarding tradition, respect of authority figures, or product management. These values have importance to institutional goals and should not be discounted. It is quite likely, however, that conflicts of values will arise in the complexity of health care settings. Professionals must develop strategies to deal with these conflicts.

To conclude this discussion of professional values, the reader can return to the situation of Mrs. James and Nurse Miller to examine how professional values might influence action. There are three alternatives: (1) ambulate Mrs. James now, (2) wait until Mrs. James is ready to walk, and (3) share perspectives and negotiate walking.

First, Nurse Miller could insist that it is in Mrs. James' best interest to walk now. A certain amount of pain and suffering is bound to occur in the early convalescent period, and future harm of postoperative complications is to be avoided. The value of preventing harm is apparent here, but other values, such as time management and cost-containment, are likely influences as well.

Second, Nurse Miller could assume that Mrs. James is making a reasonable decision for herself. The nurse enables Mrs. James to remain in control by saying, "Okay, it's your decision, call me when you're ready to get up." This respects Mrs. James' self-determination, and it also frees the nurse to do other things. Therefore, in addition to self-determination, time management or efficiency may be influential values.

The third option represents collaboration. Here Nurse Miller encourages Mrs. James to share her perspective more fully and then explains the nursing perspective. This leads to mutual understanding, and increases client awareness of the benefits of walking. The likely outcomes of the collaboration would be better pain management and increased ambulation. The value of collaboration includes a respect for the perspective of clients and the judgment of nurses. The values of competence, responsibility, and accountability are also motivating factors. As Mrs. James acquires an increased understanding of the benefit of walking to her own recovery and as Nurse Miller responds empathically and competently to Mrs. James and her pain, nursing care will be effective.

It is important to observe that examination of personal and professional values does not provide any criteria for making choices when there is a conflict within a nurse's value system or between a nurse and others. As with other forms of conflict, becoming clear about the problem often leads to a solution. If persons can identify and discuss the values that are in conflict, compromise or mediation frequently is possible. It is helpful in this process to examine values in light of ethical principles that have a fundamental or universal quality.

IMPLICATIONS FOR PROFESSIONAL COLLABORATION

Principles of Ethics

The conceptualization of client advocacy found in the mutual interaction model holds that clients are to be respected as self-determining and equal partners in planning and decision-making. The mutual interaction model serves as a vehicle for incorporating these professional values into practice. Respect of person is a fundamental ethical principle. Under the mutual interaction model, respect of person is communicated by encouraging clients and clients' families to take part in health decisions. Such communication reflects the nurse's acknowledgment of the client's ability to determine a personal course of action (autonomy). Moreover, because of the understanding of the client's perspective that nurses gain through collaborating directly with clients, the likelihood is enhanced that nurses' subsequent actions will cause clients no suffering (nonmaleficence) and in fact will produce good consequences (beneficence).

Ethical Principles

Similar to personal and professional values, **ethical principles** are basic concepts that provide direction for making professional decisions. They are broad or general guides to action. These principles are applicable to all aspects of life; they are not exclusively the property of any profession, vocation, or culture. Principles have a universal quality in that there is widespread common agreement that following these concepts contributes positively to human relationships and thus to moral behavior; however, some differences in interpretation of principles may exist, as expressed in the rules or laws of a society or a profession. The general nature and universal quality of principles set them apart from the values discussed thus far, but these principles also become a part of individual personal and professional value systems. (See Chap. 37 for principles of consensus building.)

Respect of person is a fundamental principle in ethics and is the foundational or primary principle in the practice of nursing.[13] Other principles that represent components of respect of person are respect of autonomy, nonmaleficence, beneficence, justice, fidelity, confidentiality, and veracity.

Respect of Person. A basic ethical premise of individual and group interaction, **respect of person**, is the recognition of the dignity and unconditional worth of each person in the human community, including oneself. Among other things, respect is manifested in empathy (seeing the world from the perspective of the other person), in sensitivity to suffering, in respect of privacy, and in seeing people as potentially good rather than evil. Respecting people contributes to individual and common good. The general nature of this principle makes it necessary to examine other principles that add to an understanding of respect of person. First and foremost is respect of autonomy.

Respect of Autonomy. **Respect of autonomy** means to "recognize with due appreciation an individual's ability to determine his or her own course of action in accordance with a plan chosen by himself or herself."[21] Autonomy often is described as self-determination and requires the capacity to make choices.

The capacity for decision-making includes (1) the ability to understand choices, (2) the ability to recognize and weigh the risks and benefits of each alternative, (3) the ability to see these in light of one's own values and life plan, and (4) the freedom to act on these choices.[22] If people have these capacities, their choices concerning themselves ought to be respected.[23]

According to the President's Commission report, *Making Health Care Decisions*,[23] respect for another person's autonomy should be a fundamental value upheld in the health care setting. This principle has its basis in Western ethical traditions, and affirms the intrinsic worth of human beings. Respect for autonomy also is a basic principle in the law.

As noted previously, respect of autonomy is at the heart of the mutual interaction model. This principle is expressed as a value in actions of nurses such as seeking clients' perspectives, active listening, information giving, and advocacy.

It is important, however, to recognize some limitations on autonomy. If the request of a person violates professional or societal norms, this choice needs to be examined carefully with that person. Respect of autonomy needs to take into account the rights of other people because exercise of autonomy includes a responsibility not to infringe on another person's autonomy. Acting on this concern is critical in collaboration because very careful negotiation is required in order to respect the autonomy of all the individuals directly concerned with a particular decision. The Bouvia case[24] illustrates this issue well. In this situation Ms. Bouvia, a handicapped person, requested not to be fed but wanted the health care providers to provide comfort and relief of pain as she died. Ms. Bouvia was not terminally ill when she made this request. The debate surrounding this case weighed respecting Ms. Bouvia's autonomous choice against protecting her from harm or death. Situations such as this force a prioritizing of ethical principles as well as an examination of professional role when a client's request is infringing on professional autonomy. Discussion of this situation requires an understanding of other ethical principles, including nonmaleficence, which is frequently in tension with autonomy.

Nonmaleficence. **Nonmaleficence** is the duty to do no harm. Historically nonmaleficence has been regarded as the most compelling of ethical principles in medicine as expressed in the familiar phrase: "Above all, do no harm." Some direct actions that are generally seen as harmful are killing, abusing, injuring, inflicting suffering, and stealing. These actions are prohibited; in addition, they are to be avoided or prevented.

Some situations of nonmaleficence are discerned easily; for instance, nurses are advised that they ought not to participate directly in the act of capital punishment.[18] This direct involvement in killing is antithetical to professional goals. Nurses are also expected to assess for and report suspected abuse of children or the elderly.

However, interpretation of this principle becomes more difficult in discerning the meaning of refraining from inflicting suffering. It is clear that nurses should never participate in action where the intent is to inflict suffering; for example, the actions of the holocaust. An example of malicious intent that is closer to everyday practice would be delaying or withholding pain medication from a "complainer." There are two forms of maleficence here: the delay of needed care and the negative labeling of a person. Even more subtle would be the unconscious effect of prejudice on the giving or withholding of care. The issue becomes less clear when suffering must be inflicted in order to promote healing or recovery. Health care providers in burn units face this question daily in painful dressing changes. Invasive technical procedures do cause suffering; sometimes it is justifiable, sometimes not.

Avoidance of harm, then, requires constant vigilance. Particular situations need to be discussed from a variety of perspectives in order to find resolution.[25] In both the ANA and CNA ethical codes, the nurse's obligation to protect the client from harm is stated clearly.[7,12] This obligation includes taking action regarding incompetent practice of others as well as maintaining an environment for quality nursing care. The following situation describes a blatant example of maleficence.

> SITUATION: Mrs. Rose, a mentally alert 91-year-old woman who lives alone, is admitted to an acute care setting for a minor injury. About 36 hours following admission, her granddaughter visits and is distressed by her grandmother's confusion. Upon questioning Sue Prim, RN, the granddaughter is told, "This is expected in 91-year-old people. Just accept her as she is." The granddaughter's protests are unheard and her requests for information about her grandmother's medicine are answered deceptively: "She isn't getting anything." Mrs. Rose subsequently dies because of pharmacological mismanagement.

In this instance, not only would it have taken less nursing time to respond to the granddaughter's questions accurately than to argue with her and to deal with her anger, but had this been done it is also likely that Mrs. Rose would have lived. Had another nurse observed this incident between Ms. Prim and the granddaughter, that nurse would have been responsible for several actions: (1) intervening in the interest of Mrs. Rose; (2) addressing Ms. Prim directly; and (3) possibly following with an incident report. Ms. Prim is to be treated with respect, but she cannot be allowed to continue to practice in this manner, as is demonstrated clearly by the outcome of this incident.

The principle of nonmaleficence is closely associated

with the principle of beneficence, and the distinction between the principles varies among philosophers. Regardless of definition, the crossover from doing good to causing harm can occur all too easily in technologically complex health care settings.

Beneficence. **Beneficence** is the duty to do good or to produce good consequences. Beneficence, like respect of person, can be interpreted as a fundamental principle of ethical behavior. This discussion will direct attention to examples of doing good other than avoiding harm, which was considered with nonmaleficence. It is generally accepted that the obligation to avoid harm is of greater significance than the obligation to produce good consequences. Nevertheless, beneficence is an important ethical principle for health care providers. Values of life, health, and helping others are expressions of beneficence that underlie health professions.

Nursing as a profession is a societal good, and this good is expressed in nursing actions such as promoting and restoring health, assisting people to be self-care agents, caring for the sick, supporting the dying, and searching for knowledge through research. Much of the daily work of nurses has to do with doing good. The small expressions of kindness, actions of courage, cooperation, and the search for cost-effective ways of providing quality care all are examples of beneficence.

Technological advances generally are regarded as being good. The capacity to prolong life by artificial means, organ transplants, artificial organs, and in-vitro fertilization are examples of such advanced interventions. In the face of this capacity to extend life, the ethical question becomes, "Should we, in all circumstances?" Sometimes, what seems good becomes a harm. Another ethical consideration is how to decide who should benefit from these advances when they cannot be provided for all. This is a question of justice.

Justice. In the health care setting, **justice** is related to the fair distribution of scarce resources. Scarce health care resources include costly treatments such as kidney dialysis, heart transplants, and in-vitro fertilization; as well as measures that many would consider ordinary care: adequate nutrition, access to skilled nursing and medical personnel, eyeglasses. In the United States, excellent health and medical care are available, but not to everyone. Clearly, there is injustice in our present system. People without insurance may be denied admission to some institutions, and elderly people may expend all of their savings within a year of the onset of a catastrophic health problem. Questions are being raised about the exercise of two levels of health care: one for those with insurance and the ability to pay for care and the other for the poor. These are problems of distributive justice.

There are a number of ways that health care resources could be distributed: on the basis of ability to pay, social status, contributions to society, future potential, or need. Many nurses would regard the basis of need as the fairest way of distributing health care; however, deciding that need is the most important criterion does not always solve the problem of how resources should be allocated. For example, the federal government spends billions of dollars yearly to pay for the cost of hemodialysis for people with end-stage renal disease. Certainly, these people need the treatment, which no one would want to deny to them; however, it is worth considering whether the billions of dollars spent on dialysis treatment would be better spent in preventive measures: better education regarding kidney problems, screening programs designed to detect kidney disease in the earliest stage, and research.

Questions of justice arise not only for society as a whole, as just described, but also for individual nurses in their own practice. Nurses must decide each day how their time and skills can best be allocated. Who is treated first? Who gets the most time? Who requires the care of an RN? Are psychosocial needs always the last priority? How is the workload distributed in situations of short staffing? How can nurses contribute to more efficient and less costly health care? Although there are no easy answers to these questions, they deserve careful consideration and reflection. Otherwise care will be haphazard, and serious problems may not be addressed until there is a tragic incident.

Personal and professional values have an impact on individual approaches to justice. A values clarification approach is a first step in revealing the power of personal professional values to influence one's decisions. For example, a student or staff nurse might give thought to how time and energy were spent in the care of a group of clients and then identify the values reflected in these activities. Broad ethical questions can then be posed: All things considered, is this what ought to be done? What would be the result if all nurses acted in this way? More specific questions of what comprises justice also can be posed: Is justice providing the most good to the most people? Are care and attention given to the most vulnerable and powerless? Is justice giving people what they have earned and can afford? Is it providing a basic minimum care to all people?

Clearly the decisions that nurses make are influenced not only by their philosophy of care but by the financial resources allocated by the institutions for which they work and ultimately by society as a whole. The interplay between nursing practice and public policy is one reason why nurses must clarify their philosophy of nursing and seek ways to implement this philosophy within public policy. Some of these concerns were addressed in Chapter 4. The nursing profession is also confronted with serious issues related to control of nursing practice and defining the role of nurses in providing effective and cost-saving health care as discussed in Chapter 1. Some of these justice-related problems can be addressed at the institutional level but others will require concerted political action at the state and national levels.

Thus far, four primary ethical principles, in addition to respect of person, have been addressed: respect of autonomy, nonmaleficence, beneficence, and justice. Three related principles, which also are identified as important professional values, will be discussed now: fidelity, confidentiality, and veracity.

Fidelity. Keeping promises, or **fidelity,** is an ethical principle that means keeping one's word. Promises that nurses make to clients may be explicit and written, as in the ANA Code for Nurses.[7] In this code, nurses promise to care for all clients, regardless of the health care deviation the client is experiencing. Other promises made in the code relate to maintaining professional competence, safeguarding clients from professional misconduct observed in others, and improving health conditions in society through public education and participation in professional societies.

Promises to clients may be verbal, made in one-to-one interaction. In the Williamson model of mutual interaction,[26] nurse and client set forth the goals that they mutually agree to pursue through health care interventions. This "contracting" can be regarded as the establishment of a set of agreements that both client and nurse promise to keep.

Promises to clients may also be implicit—that is, not stated—but implied by generally accepted cultural values. In recent times, controversy has arisen over the question of whether clients must always be fed (implicit promise), or whether food and water may sometimes be forgone, for example, if a client so desires or if the treatment is futile. Many nurses regard food and water as basic human needs that should always be provided. This belief, akin to a fundamental promise, finds expression in many aspects of human culture, such as in religious ceremonies. Many religious traditions elevate the provision of food and water to a ceremonial and sacred status: the Roman Catholic Eucharist is one example. According to Meilaender, feeding is symbolic and should always be provided.[27]

Keeping promises, whether they are explicit or implicit, has a significant relationship to personal integrity. Along with keeping one's word, and being an honorable person, fidelity is foundational to trust within the nurse–client relationship—without fidelity the relationship is a sham. A part of fidelity is the promise of protecting or guarding personal information. This is expressed as the principle of confidentiality.

BUILDING NURSING KNOWLEDGE

What is the Best Foundation for a Nursing Ethic?

Cooper MC. Covenantal relationships: Grounding for the nursing ethic. *Adv Nurs Sci.* 1988;10:48–59.

A nursing ethic is a moral position for centering the nursing profession and guiding its actions. Cooper disagrees with the point of view that the ability of nursing as a profession to set its own moral agenda is constrained by the power structure of hospitals or the traditions of health care that give power to physicians and administrators. She disputes the argument that nursing can only implement standards of care for its own practice by reforming institutions or by acquiring a balance of controlling power in those institutions. According to Cooper, these ideas fail to address that nursing's primary concern should be the well-being of the client, not autonomy. In Cooper's view the nurse–client relationship should provide the foundation for a nursing ethic.

After reviewing several current paradigms of the nurse as contracted clinician, healer, client advocate, health educator, and physician surrogate, Cooper proposes an alternative view for a nursing ethic. She proposes the "covenantal relationship." This is a relationship between nurse and client characterized by mutuality, reciprocity, and caring, and is grounded on the concept of fidelity or promise keeping.

A covenantal relationship is based on sense of debt for the opportunity to practice. The provider enters the relationship promising implicitly or explicitly to safeguard the client by using skills mastered through the advantages of the education the provider has received. This promise gives rise to an obligation. The client's presence binds the provider in the duty of fidelity. The provider must remain true to the promise; however, the provider's need to be of service is met by the client's presence. Thus the client's presence is a gift to the provider.

Cooper emphasizes that a hallmark of covenantal relationships is that they are mutually beneficial. While some in health care would exclude the client from health care decision making because of professional, bureaucratic, or social concerns, Cooper notes that nursing has a long tradition of assuming that equal client input is important. This assumption represents nursing's commitment to protecting and enhancing human dignity and provides a further basis for a nursing ethic.

Confidentiality. **Confidentiality** is a principle that is based on an individual's right to privacy. In health care, confidentiality has to do with the protection of private information that is entrusted to the health care provider.

The person who enters a relationship with a health care provider risks revealing information about self which could be embarrassing. Nurses, then, must safeguard clients' privacy by keeping the shared information confidential,[7,12] and by requesting only information that is necessary to provide quality care. Information about clients should not be shared with other health care providers unless this is necessary for the client's welfare. The "lunchroom phenomenon" of talking about clients to make interesting conversation or to vent feelings is obviously inappropriate. Privileged information should not be shared, even with the client's family, without the client's expressed permission.

Ideally, then, control of information should be with clients. However, in this day of computerized records and numerous health care providers with access to these records, confidentiality becomes difficult to control. This increases the burden for health care providers to maintain diligence in protecting individual privacy.

Confidentiality is not an absolute principle, in that there are other principles which may take priority, particularly nonmaleficence. One circumstance under which confidentiality may be broken is when not sharing the information will cause serious harm to a third party. The legal requirement of reporting possible child abuse means that the nurse is breaking confidentiality in order to prevent serious harm to a child. There is also a legally based "duty to warn" if a client threatens to injure or kill another person.

Nurses need to help clients to understand the limits of confidentiality. For example, if a young teenager makes a request of "I want you to promise not to tell anyone what I am going to tell you," the nurse needs to express some reservations. Often, nurses may be able to help clients in sharing information with others when disclosure is indicated or required.

Nurses should not make promises that must be broken. If the promise of confidentiality has been made either implicitly or explicitly and then must be broken, nurses, as a general rule, have an obligation to be truthful with clients and explain the action that must be taken in the interest of avoiding harm. This, then, requires the understanding of another principle: veracity.

Veracity. Devotion to the truth, or **veracity,** is a compelling ethical principle. Without a basic premise that people will be truthful with one another there can be no trust, and trust is critical to sound, healthy interpersonal relationships at both individual and group levels. There is a societal expectation that people will be honest in all modes of communication whether written or spoken; it is also understood that the pursuit of what is true is a lifelong endeavor. Therefore, clients and health care providers have a mutual obligation to express what they believe to be true to one another and also to continue to seek to find the truth. In health care settings, veracity is particularly important in terms of clients' rights to information about themselves; the interaction of health care providers with one another; accuracy in communication of information; and a commitment to searching for the truth.

Health care providers or family members sometimes are concerned that being truthful with clients will cause harm or undue suffering; however, this consideration, if used as a reason for not disclosing information, must be examined carefully for accuracy. Considerable research supports the view that openness in relationships is healthy and that secrets may be harmful. In general, people deal better with the truth than with deception.

The seven major ethical principles discussed thus far are obligations in a nurse–client relationship that is philosophically grounded in the most basic ethical principle, respect of person. As individuals begin to act on these principles, the principles become personal and professional values. This is an important step because it moves the principle from a theoretical ideal to a reality of life and work. Table 34–3 summarizes these principles and provides clinical examples of professional behavior that demonstrates application of these principles at a very practical level.

Ethical Theories

The preceding discussion clarifies several ethical principles relevant to nursing practice. These principles are universally applicable as action guides for the human community but the principles alone do not give any direction for making choices or prioritizing. **Ethical theories** provide systematic approaches for establishing priorities. These theories are often used implicitly by health care professionals as they consider ethical questions, so it is important for nurses to be able to recognize and apply them in decision-making. It is also important to note that even though theories are helpful in organizing one's thinking about ethical problems, they do not provide specific answers.

Two major ethical theories are teleology and deontology. Each provides a different direction in answer to the question, "What, all things considered, ought I to do?" The teleologist regards the outcome or consequence of action as a primary concern. The deontologist views certain duties or actions as a primary moral obligation without regard to consequences. Theories of virtue, a third approach, ask the question, "Who should I be?"[21] Theories of virtue focus on the inner nature of being human, which is seen as the stimulus for ethical behavior. Although the question of who I

TABLE 34–3. ETHICAL PRINCIPLES

Principle	Definition	Nurse's Behavior
Autonomy	Exercise of free choice	Collaborates with clients in establishing client-centered goals. Respects client's wish to refuse care.
Nonmaleficence	To do no harm	Follows medication procedure meticulously. Reports colleagues incompetence appropriately.
Beneficence	To do good	Interacts empathically with clients. Spends time reminiscing with elderly clients.
Justice	Fair distribution of resources	Plans daily schedule to assure that the most vulnerable clients are given adequate care. Participates in professional efforts to provide health care to the homeless.
Fidelity	Faithfulness	Returns to spend time with a client after promising to do so. Supports colleague who is working to improve standards of nursing care.
Confidentiality	Protection of private, personal information	Refuses to discuss hospitalized colleague's condition with non-health-care providers. Does not obtain unnecessary information.
Veracity	Truthfulness	Reports and records accurately. Admits own errors immediately.

am cannot be separated from what I do, ethical theories differ in their perspective of which of these questions is primary.

The following discussion of these three theoretical approaches provides a general overview of very complex systems of thought. All health care providers are well advised to take courses in bioethics taught by philosophers who have specific skills in facilitating the learning of these thought processes.

Teleology. **Teleology** holds that good or right actions are measured by the consequences of those actions. Good consequences are described by various theorists as overall benefits, happiness, or pleasure. The two major teleological, or goal-based, approaches are act- and rule-utilitarianism. Act-utilitarianism analyzes individual actions according to the benefits they produce. It holds that individuals are obligated to examine their actions in order to produce the best or the least harmful consequences for the greatest number of people. Long-term or future consequences to everyone affected by the action must be predicted. Each situation is to be analyzed by calculating risks and benefits of each alternative for action. Theoretically the alternative of choice can be determined mathematically.

Critics of act-utilitarianism point out that it is very difficult to predict the long-term consequences of any action with certainty. More importantly, this approach runs the risk of subordinating the autonomy of clients to the needs of other persons. For example, act-utilitarianism could probably justify the use of human subjects in research that harmed the subjects, but provided a benefit for other members of society. Act-utilitarianism values autonomy only insofar as it produces benefits for all persons concerned.

Rule-utilitarianism attempts to answer these criticisms. Instead of basing the rightness of each individual action on the benefits that it will produce, rule-utilitarianism proposes a number of rules of conduct. These rules, in turn, are justified by determining which ones would promote the greatest good for the greatest number of people in a society. Rule-utilitarians regard principles such as respect for autonomy, beneficence, nonmaleficence, confidentiality, and justice as good because they promote the overall happiness, good, or balance of pleasure over pain for most people.

Under rule-utilitarianism, everyone in society is obligated to act on these moral rules. This universal application of rules requires that exemptions to rules must also be universalized as well. For example, suppose there is a rule that cardiopulmonary resuscitation (CPR) must be started in all cases of cardiopulmonary arrest. A nurse decides not to perform CPR based on a person's age of 85. The rule-utilitarians would ask, "What would the consequences be if all nurses refused to perform CPR on all people 85 years or older?" It is unlikely that age alone can be used as a criterion for exceptions to this rule. Therefore, this action would not be justifiable from a rule-utilitarian's perspective, but it could be justified from an act-utilitarian's perspective.

Objections to rule-utilitarianism include questions about how rules are to be determined. In any form of utilitarianism, the weighing of risks and benefits is somewhat arbitrary and prediction of outcomes is difficult. There is always danger of losing sight of the individual in the interest of the outcome or the larger group. Thus, utilitarianism can provide an important perspective when approaching ethical problems, but it does not satisfy all questions about moral interaction. Another mode of ethical thought, deontology, provides a different approach to ethical action.

Deontology. **Deontology** holds that a person ought to follow those actions that are in accordance with certain duties. Neither one's feelings nor the possible consequences are relevant. A nurse may not enjoy telling a client that surgery causes postoperative pain, and in the short term at least, this news may not make the client happy. But in deontology happiness or pleasure is not the ultimate "good." Most deontologists would agree that respect for autonomy, veracity, beneficence, nonmaleficence, and justice are fundamental duties. Natural law and the theories of Immanuel Kant and David Ross are examples of deontological theory.

Immanuel Kant (1724–1804). Kant contends that the duty of respect for person overrides all other duties—it is, in fact, an absolute duty. He believes that each person is an individual center of value, and no action that involves treating an individual as an object for other purposes is acceptable. No matter how worthwhile the goal and no matter what the other positive consequences, one's primary consideration must be respect for person. Accordingly, considerations such as efficiency, economy, or success would be irrelevant. Only the fulfillment of obligations is important, not the consequences of an action. A second element for guiding actions in Kant's theory is using a rational thought process to evaluate a potential course of action. If a given act can be "consistently willed," that is, carried out in all similar situations, it is an appropriate action.[28] An explicit statement describing that action can then be generated and used to guide actions in the future. This statement, or general guide to action, would then be called a **maxim**. A maxim can be considered a universal law.

Kantian theory has been highly influential in Western ethical thought, and is especially commendable for its emphasis on the value and autonomy of people. However, a fundamental task of nursing is to promote the health of clients. This is clearly a task which is goal-oriented; therefore, consequences must be taken into account. Other deontological approaches are less rigid than the Kantian perspective.

David Ross. David Ross[29] presents a deontological theory that outlines fundamental duties but, unlike Kant's theory, does not view these duties as being absolute. Ross holds that certain things are intrinsically good and that these are "self-evident" to an individual. Individuals' internal sense of what they ought to do creates a **prima facie duty,** that is, a moral obligation. This obligation is not absolute because of the complexity of human encounters that may bring moral duties into conflict. For example, in some situations one cannot both keep a promise and avoid harm. Although both of these are moral duties, a choice must be made usually based on predicted "general good." This approach allows for exceptions to a moral duty but "only when it is overridden by another moral duty."[30] Ross recognizes the importance of considering consequences but considers the primary concern to be the fulfillment of moral duty. Ross identifies three moral duties in addition to those generally accepted by deontologists: self-improvement, reparation, and gratitude. Self-improvement, particularly the development of virtue and acquisition of knowledge, is a moral obligation to self as well as to the human community. Reparation is a duty to "right a wrong" that has been committed against another. Gratitude is the obligation to be appreciative of what one has received from others.

Ross shows a particular sensitivity to relationships. He does not prioritize the duties of moral obligation, but believes that if there is a conflict, the duty that should take priority can be determined by reason and intuition.[30] He does assume a strong position that avoiding harm is a greater obligation than producing good consequences.

In approaching ethical problems from the perspective of Ross, a nurse would carefully analyze the obligations to others and self within the situation considering duty first, and then consequences. Critics see this process as cumbersome but there are really no easy answers to complex ethical situations. The major criticism of Ross' approach is that no direction is given for the prioritizing process.

Natural Law. Natural Law, which was also discussed in Chapter 33, is a third deontological approach. The basic premise of this theory is that the truest nature of human beings is good and that their basic duty is to seek that good. The natural ends to be promoted are rational, social, and biological. The individual's duty, then, is to be fully human and to act to the best of natural inclinations; thus promoting good over evil. This theory, like that of Ross, takes into account both duty and consequences.

Although modern expression of Natural Law is seen mainly in Roman Catholic theology, it has its origins in the work of Aristotle.[31] Parts of the constitution of the United States are based on Natural Law: the view that equal rights are due to all persons, because all persons are created equal.

Natural Law theory has been criticized because it seems difficult to determine which ends or goals truly are essential to human life.[32] A second difficulty relates to the problem of determining which ends should take precedence. For instance, the biological end of procreation might seem to conflict with rational choices of whether or not to bear children. Are people fundamentally biological, or are we rational creatures who can control our environment and our own bodies? Clearly these differing views of what it means to be human have implications for ethics and self-understanding. On the positive side, this theory has a high regard for the value of people, and considers both goals and duties in deciding the rightness of actions. It offers strong support for the principle of autonomy, and is widely used by bioethicists.

All of the theories discussed thus far place an emphasis on obligation: obligation to produce good consequences or obligation to perform certain moral duties. Although both Natural Law theory and Rossian theory hint at the inner nature of the ethical person, this is not stated as the basis of the theory. Theories that approach ethics by focusing on the characteristics of persons are described as theories of virtue.

Theories of Virtue. **Theories of virtue** are concerned with intrinsic qualities that enhance the capacity of people to be fully human and to live together within a moral community. These theories include basic assumptions about the innate ability of people to be good. It is this virtuous quality that leads to ethical behavior rather than an externally imposed system of obligation.

Although the theories of obligation and virtue might seem to be opposing perspectives, one might also propose that it is from the innate sense of wanting to be individuals of integrity that the questions of obligation are asked. This sensitivity to moral questions and problems and to the moral nature of the nurse–client relationship is critical to the practice of nursing.

Caring, which has been described as the philosophic basis of nursing and of nursing ethics by several nurse theorists,[33–37] provides an example of a theory of virtue. Caring, as a moral ideal,[33] "entails a commitment to the protection and enhancement of human dignity" (p. 32). But it is more than an ideal. Caring is a subjective, action-oriented expression within human relationships. As described by Noddings,[37] caring is an "approach that begins with a moral attitude or longing for goodness and not with moral reasoning" (p. 2). It is a state of being—a quality inherent in individuals, not an externally imposed norm. Thus caring demonstrates an approach analogous to the theories of virtue. Caring, viewed as a theory of virtue, provides a perspective for understanding self and others and, thus, a basis for ethical action.

In the world of nursing practice, a rigid adherence to either deontology or teleology has limitations. Deontology provides little direction for resolving conflicts between principles such as confidentiality and nonmaleficence. Teleology has the potential for treating people as objects or disregarding minority groups. However, neither theoretical perspective should be disregarded as each provides important direction for ethical behavior. Both approaches will be applied in the health care setting, and the counterbalance or tension between the obligations of duties and goals may lead to better decision-making than the reliance on either alone.[25]

In clinical situations, problems sometimes arise because people involved in decision-making are asking different questions about the meaning of the situation and may seem to be in irreconcilable positions. In approaching the situation from a perspective of caring, the questions of obligation also may be asked: What is my duty? What course of action seems to indicate the greatest benefit? This type of pluralistic approach gleans what is helpful from a variety of theories.

There is no perfect theory of ethics and there are no easy solutions to ethical problems. This chapter has described several prominent modes of ethical thinking. Others such as Rawls' theory of justice have not been included in this discussion but are nonetheless important to health care decisions.[38] As stated in the CNA code for nurses, professionals have an ongoing obligation to expand knowledge and understanding of ethical concerns.[12] This discussion is just the beginning of a lifelong endeavor for the professional nurse. Raising consciousness about issues is one way to assist individuals to examine values and take action. The following section examines some common ethical problems faced by nurses.

ETHICAL ISSUES IN NURSING PRACTICE

Ethical problems and conflicts are a part of everyday nursing practice. Many of these problems are very complex; others are beyond the scope of a text such as this. The discussion that follows is intended to present several examples of types of conflicts that must be confronted by nurses and to stimulate student thinking and discussion. These activities will enhance sensitivity to ethical issues, assisting beginning students to recognize when an issue exists, as well as emphasizing the need for effective strategies to deal with these issues. In some situations, it may be appropriate for an individual involved in an ethical conflict to come to an individual solution. More often, discussion with colleagues or referral to an institutional ethics committee is warranted.

Four issues related to health care are addressed here: Must personal privacy always be protected? Can paternalism be justified? What constitutes adequate protection of incompetent clients? And how can one best protect clients from professional misconduct?

Must Personal Privacy Always be Protected?

Protecting personal privacy derives from the basic ethical principle of respect for person. Nurses show respect for clients' privacy by simple acts such as knocking before entering a client's room, recognizing the needs of a client and family to have time alone, and assuring that physical care and examinations are conducted discreetly and respectfully. Respect for privacy also encompasses taking care that clients are not discussed in public places such as hallways, elevators, the hospital cafeteria, or in the presence of another client. In these situations, client privacy is not at issue—in fact it would almost universally be considered a right.

A more difficult situation related to a client's personal privacy arises when respecting that right causes potential conflict with another valued entity. Consider, for example, the current law in most states regarding reporting of AIDS test results. Test results may not be released to anyone (including health care providers) other than the client without the client's prior written consent. Among the reasons given for restricted access to test results are concerns that because of the extraordinary public concern about AIDS, individuals known to be infected, or even carriers, may be subjected to discrimination in employment or be denied insurance coverage. Nevertheless, many health care workers believe that this protection of client privacy violates the principle of nonmaleficence. These individuals feel their own rights to personal safety and those of society at large to protection from communicable disease are in jeopardy. Some concerned providers, therefore, advocate AIDS testing of all people admitted to health care institutions, for the purpose of informing providers which individuals are infected or are carriers. Laws requiring that cases of other communicable diseases be reported and that individuals identified as having been exposed be notified are given as additional validation for this proposal. Although the laws determine current policy, the ethical debate continues, and may result in attempts to change the law.

Another issue related to privacy is whether parents have a right to know when their teenaged children seek contraception or abortion. Does a teenager's right to privacy supersede the parents' obligation to protect their child from what the parents believe may be harmful? The principle of nonmaleficence as applied to society's responsibility to protect the teenager is also a consideration: Might the teenager be harmed if the parents were made aware of the teenager's choices? This issue also raises questions related to autonomy: Is a teenager competent to make an informed decision about contraception or abortion?

As nurses, you are likely to have to confront these issues, not only from a philosophic or theoretical viewpoint but from a concrete viewpoint—that is, involving yourself as a caregiver for actual clients. How will you act? What questions must you ask yourself to make an ethical decision?

When Can Paternalism Be Justified?

Paternalism characterizes situations in which an authority makes decisions or takes action for a competent adult without that adult's consent, as a parent would make such decisions for a child. In health care, paternalism relates to circumstances wherein health care providers assume that they know best and act accordingly without the consent of clients. Paternalism is regarded as an act of nonmaleficence and must always be justified. This means that health care providers should not assume that it is right to act paternalistically either to do good or to avoid harm. Such an action must always have substantial reasons because it denies respect for a client's own choices and values. Benjamin and Curtis describe this as showing contempt for persons and regarding them as objects rather than partners in their care.[1]

Three criteria are to be used to justify paternalism[1]:

1. Preservation of autonomy: a client is not capable of making sound judgments in this particular incident. Action is taken in order to preserve or restore autonomy.
2. Avoidance of harm: a client is in probable danger of serious harm or there is serious danger to an innocent third party.
3. Likely ratification: a client, at a later time, is likely to agree that paternalistic action was justified (p. 53).

For example, if there is immediate danger such as a fire, clients could be moved quickly, even forcibly, in the interest of preserving their lives and autonomy. The three conditions would be satisfied because (1) clients are not aware of the fire, so autonomy is temporarily limited; (2) there is immediate danger and potential for serious harm; and (3) clients will thank health care providers for the rescuing behavior once the emergency is past.

As a second example, Jack R., a college student, is coming to the emergency room frequently with complaints of pain and high anxiety. He requests medication with meperidine. The medical evaluation is essentially negative so the physician decides to treat with a placebo. Jack responds with a quick relief of symptoms. Several hours later the physician discusses the events and the positive effects of the placebo with Jack. Jack responds favorably, recognizing that he has some problems he needs to get under control and that his present coping style is not healthy. In this situation (1) Jack was temporarily out of control and not making sound decisions for himself; action is taken to restore his autonomy. (2) Jack is seeking the use of narcotics frequently and is demonstrating harmful coping mechanisms; there is high probability of harm to Jack if he is supported in his present behavior. (3) Jack acknowledges and thanks the health care provider for clearly demonstrating that he does not need meperidine.

Paternalistic action was justified in this situation, but there are significant details here that help with the justification. One is that the intent of the physician was to invoke limited paternalism. That is, the physician took action to restore Jack to a more rational state and then was truthful with Jack. The second factor is that Jack ratified the decision of the physician immediately. This does not always occur; frequently it requires a longer span of time for a client to see the good in what was done. Clients may be very angry about providers' actions. The criteria state that there is hope of ratification; it cannot be assured in advance. What is important in paternalistic action is that it is done in the best interest of clients and not for the convenience of care providers.

Deception, intentional concealment of the truth, is another action related to paternalism. It can take the form of providing partial truths, being silent, or misrepresenting the truth. Clients need accurate information about their health state in order to exercise autonomy—that is, to be active participants in health care decisions and in control of their daily activities. In the past, however, physicians and nurses often withheld information from clients "for their own good." It was widely believed that people with cancer, for example, would be emotionally devastated by the truth about their diagnosis and would "give up." The paternalistic model is becoming less acceptable to clients as they become more aware of their rights. Current practice is to provide clients with full information about their health and treatment options, although some providers still believe that "benevolent deception" can be justified in certain situations.

The dilemma here is a conflict between the principles of beneficence (doing good) and veracity (truth-telling). Providers who justify benevolent deception do so based on their perceptions about a client (and what would constitute "good" or "harm" for that client), but they also must recognize the influence of their own attitudes about sickness and death and of their roles in the health care system.[39]

Nurses may also be confronted with situations in which families wish to withhold information from loved ones. Nurses can be instrumental in assisting families to examine their values and to consider the possible negative effect of deception on family relationships. This issue is further analyzed in the clinical situation example later in the chapter.

Another situation involving paternalism is the decision to use physical restraints (such as vests or belts by which clients are tied to beds or chairs) on elderly clients. Reasons commonly given for this practice are beliefs that the elderly are more likely to fall and that nurses have a moral obligation to protect them from this risk (nonmaleficence). Furthermore, many nurses are convinced that "it doesn't really bother old people to be restrained."[40] Evans and Strumpf refute the accuracy of both of these ideas. Not only are the beliefs inaccurate, they are paternalistic and may actually violate the principle of nonmaleficence. The reasons given to support use of restraints deny the capacity of elderly individuals to control their mobility (autonomy) and the restraints may also inflict greater risks than those they purport to prevent.[40]

Because the policy of restraining elders is so pervasive in our health care system, discussions related to the ethics of such policy may indeed be intense. Nevertheless, readers are encouraged to thoughtfully question this practice on a case-by-case as well as an ethical basis.

What Constitutes Proper Protection of Incompetent Clients?

Thus far, discussion has centered on respect for autonomy for the competent client. It is important also to address the meaning of respect of autonomy for people who are no longer competent and therefore not fully autonomous.

Declaring people as incompetent to make decisions for themselves is problematic. The reader is encouraged to pursue this topic in the literature of both ethics and psychology. Suffice it to say that loss of rational capacity to make decisions in one's own best interest is a critical element of loss of competence.

The loss of competence may be temporary, as in a state of unconsciousness from which the person is expected to recover, or permanent, as in dementia. As discussed in Chapter 33, health care providers need to be sensitive to the personal perspective of clients even though they lack the capacity to communicate. This is accomplished best through a surrogate decision-maker: one who can speak for clients just as they would speak if it were possible. If a client has expressed advanced decisions, the respect of these decisions is respecting autonomy. Advanced decisions may be in the form of living wills or expressed through a durable power of attorney as discussed in Chapter 3.

If an individual has never been autonomous, as in infancy or profound mental retardation, or if there is no surrogate, there is no autonomy to respect. Direction then must be found from other principles such as nonmaleficence or beneficence, with the primary concern being the best interest of the client. Best interests include, but are not limited to, recovery, reduction of pain and suffering, increased life expectancy, and increased quality of life. The key is that the center of concern is the client, not the decision-maker.

Examples of adult clients lacking decision-making capacity include people with serious mental or emotional disorders, people who have recently been seriously injured, and people who are permanently comatose. It is important to remember that a particular health problem does not lead automatically to incompetence. A person who is elderly and confined to a wheelchair may be perfectly capable of making major decisions. A person with intermittent confusion may still be able to decide on many courses of action. It is the responsibility of health care providers to assess carefully and fairly the strengths and limitations of clients with respect to each decision, and to presume competence unless and until there is clear evidence that the person lacks decision-making capacity.

Earlier in this chapter a question was raised concerning the ordinary obligation of providing food and water. Lynne and Childress[41] draw a distinction between normal eating and drinking and the progressively more invasive intravenous line, nasogastric tube, and gastrostomy. They argue that under certain circumstances, feeding and hydration may cause more discomfort than they alleviate. The person who is dying from cancer may not wish to eat, and a nasogastric tube might only prolong the person's discomfort unnecessarily. Similarly, a gastrostomy entails other risks that must be weighed against the potential benefit of the procedure. It is justified to keep the competent client in control of these decisions, but it becomes more difficult to make these decisions for the incompetent. Decisions regarding these situations are frequently decided in the courts and vary from state to state.

Important questions to raise are: If we allow the competent person to make this decision to reduce pain and suffering, then why should we not make this same decision in the best interest of an incompetent client? Are we prolonging futile and sometimes painful life at great cost to the individual and to society? Are we obligated to do this, and who are we helping in these endeavors?

Protection from Professional Misconduct

The ANA and CNA codes of ethics address the obligation of nurses to safeguard clients from incompetent, unethical, or illegal practice. The earlier situation of Mrs. Rose pointed out an instance in which there was a duty to act to protect the client. A variety of types of situations call for this form of advocacy: chemical impairment of a health care provider; faulty, unsafe, or illegal techniques of practice; misrepresentation of information; abuse or neglect of clients. If it is clear that there is definite or significant risk of harm to clients, nurses are faced with an ethical problem, not a dilemma. Tension between loyalty to a friend or institution and the obligation to prevent harm may make it difficult to act, but the client or future clients who are vulnerable must be protected.

Critical factors in taking action in instances of suspected misconduct begin with gathering and accurately documenting facts. Documentation includes the objective recording of behaviors observed without accusatory language as, for example, "Slurred speech, unsteady gait, uncoordinated hand movements," not "Appears drunk." The codes of ethics[7,12] emphasize that nurses follow institutional guidelines in reporting professional misconduct. Protocols of recording and reporting should be established and followed carefully. Nurses taking action appropriately should be able to do so without fear of reprisal. Direct confrontation of the offender must occur early in the process, usually first. This requires effective communication skills and concern for the offender, as well as clarity of purpose. The primary obligation is protecting the client; vindictiveness does not have a place in the process. It is unfortunate that these situations often become a topic of gossip and the focus of a lot of complaining. The ethical approach, however, calls for respect of all people.

If nurses find themselves in situations in which they are not heard within the employing institution, they should seek guidance and assistance from state nursing associations or other legally constituted bodies. Going public with an issue is referred to as "whistle blowing." As a general rule it is advisable to garner support before going public. Nurses who find themselves standing alone on an issue need to seek wise and objective counsel. Incompetent practitioners place themselves in jeopardy as well as their clients. It is important to keep this in mind when faced with difficult decisions.

■ FRAMEWORK FOR ETHICAL ANALYSIS

Foundations of ethical practice in the form of personal and professional values, ethical principles, and ethical theories, plus a brief overview of some ethical issues in nursing, have been discussed thus far in this chapter. In this section, a framework for ethical decision-making is presented that will assist in showing how these foundational elements are influential and important.

A variety of frameworks for ethical decision-making are available in the literature.[1,2,42–44] All of these are variations of the problem-solving process already familiar to nursing students. In any ethical decision-making process, specific emphasis on the careful examination of alternatives and thoughtful justification of choice of action are required. Justification always includes an appeal to ethical principle. There is no cookbook approach to decision-making and there will be uncertainty in some ethical decisions. Health care providers are uncomfortable with uncertainty, but the reality is that good and reasonable people may come to different decisions in ethically complex situations. What is

BOX 34–2. STEPS IN ETHICAL DECISION-MAKING

1. Perceive problem
2. Gather data
3. Analyze data
4. Clarify problem or dilemma
5. List alternatives with ethical reasons for each
6. Weigh alternatives considering duties, goals, and priorities
7. Make a choice
8. Justify choice including anticipation of objections
9. Act on choice
10. Reflect on outcome

required is good decision-making that leaves people satisfied that the best possible action was taken.

Steps in ethical decision-making are listed in Box 34–2. Each of these steps will be discussed by analyzing a common clinical situation.

SITUATION: Mr. Martin is recovering from prostatic surgery. He has been making slow progress in his recovery. His wife and daughter have been informed that Mr. Martin has cancer that has spread throughout his body and his prognosis is grave with death expected within 6 months. The wife and daughter request that Mr. Martin should not be given this bad news. They tell the physician that such news will cause Mr. Martin to become depressed and that he will give up and die within the month. The physician, after some discussion with the wife and daughter, agrees to abide by their request. She states on the chart that the diagnosis of the metastasis (spreading of the cancer) and the prognosis are not to be revealed to the client in deference to the family wishes. A community health nurse is caring for Mr. Martin at home, seeing him twice a week. The nurse finds that Mr. Martin appears discouraged. He is questioning his slow recovery and wonders why he isn't very energetic. The nurse is uneasy and believes Mr. Martin should know the whole truth about himself.

Step	Application
1. Perceive problem	1. The perception of an ethical problem requires a sensitivity to moral components of nursing. The nurse feels "uneasy." A personal value of honesty and professional value of respect of person trigger a reaction to this situation. The nurse also approaches Mr. Martin with a deep sense of care, wanting him to have fulfillment and meaning in his life. The nature of their relationship is collaborative and that relationship appears to be jeopardized by the concealing of information that is highly significant to Mr. Martin.
2. Gather data	2. Discussion with the family and with the physician will give more information about facts, feelings, and values. Further discussion with Mr. Martin about his own perceptions about what is happening will add to the data base. It is revealed that Mr. Martin has been severely depressed in the past and has attempted suicide. He responded positively to psychotherapy. The family seems to understand the gravity of the diagnosis but doesn't want to deal with the emotional reality or with depression at this point. They do not want to contribute to anything that will cause Mr. Martin's death sooner. The physician is willing to accept the family perspective believing that the family must cope in their own way. She will wait until they are ready to share the diagnosis.
3. Analyze data	3. Where does the conflict lie? The conflict appears to be between the nurse and the family. The nurse is approaching the situation from a sense of duty to tell the truth. The family is intent on short-term goals of happiness or benefit. The family is assuming that there will be serious negative, even harmful consequences if the truth is divulged. The nurse may be acting from a Kantian deontological perspective; therefore, she may not be concerned with consequences but believes that being truthful with Mr. Martin is a universal duty in respect of person.
4. Clarify problem or dilemma	4. This is a dilemma concerning respect of autonomy (truth-telling) versus nonmaleficence (paternalism).
5. List alternatives with ethical reasons for each	5. The nurse could: a. Withhold the truth in accord with family wishes in order to avoid harm, such as an untimely death for Mr. Martin. This satisfies the physician's order and the family's desire and could be justified from an act-utilitarian perspective. This makes the assumption that there is a higher likelihood of harm from being truthful than from participating in deception. The greatest harm would be suicide and an untimely death. There is greater benefit and less harm to all concerned in acting on this alternative. b. Tell Mr. Martin the truth based upon the duty to be truthful as part of respect of person. This could be justified from a Kantian perspective. The truth should be told without regard for consequences. This position makes the assumption that Mr. Martin will then be in more control of his life. The integrity of the nurse–client relationship is upheld but there is a possibility that the relationship between the nurse and family will deteriorate and the nurse must be prepared to justify deliberate disregard of a physician's order. The nurse's own integrity is preserved. c. Withdraw from the situation by having another nurse assume Mr. Martin's care. This could be justified by an act- or rule-utilitarian perspective. In the rule-utilitarian perspective the rule would be "nurses may withdraw from care after assuring that the client is not abandoned in situations where there is a violation of the nurse's deeply in-

Step	Application
	grained moral values." This alternative may or may not be satisfying to the nurse or the client. The nurse is unlikely to take this alternative unless there is also a deep respect for the family. This alternative respects their perspective while removing the nurse from a compromising situation. d. Inform the family and the physician that the nurse will respond truthfully to all of Mr. Martin's questions. Try to help the family see this as a perspective of care for Mr. Martin. Help them to see that relationships are more natural when dealing with the truth than when dealing with deception. This is an assertive position but it allows Mr. Martin the control. The nurse is not imposing the truth on Mr. Martin but is respecting his right to the truth. There is a possibility in assuming this position that the family will request the nurse to refrain from caring for Mr. Martin.
6. Weigh alternatives considering duties, goals, and priorities	6. The priority for all concerned is to treat Mr. Martin with respect. He is the most vulnerable and all decisions must be made with his best interests in mind. He is mentally competent; therefore, his decisions about himself need to be respected. He cannot make autonomous decisions if significant information is being withheld from him. There is a duty to be faithful to the implicit promise of the relationships involved. There are goals of continuing productive family relationships, having Mr. Martin in as much control as he chooses, having a satisfactory life for Mr. Martin for as long as possible, and providing a chance for Mr. Martin to come to closure and to say good-bye to family and friends. There is no serious conflict with legal or societal expectations in the alternatives stated, although alternative b could raise some legal questions.
7. Make a choice	7. The nurse will act on alternative d by informing family and physician that Mr. Martin will have his questions answered truthfully by the nurse but the truth will not be imposed on Mr. Martin without his request.
8. Justify choice including anticipation of objections	8. The choice is justified from a Natural Law perspective. It comes out of a sense of care in human relationships, and it treats Mr. Martin with respect by giving due regard to his right to know about himself. This is in keeping with the natural rational and social ends of human beings. Relationships will be more natural if dealing with truth than with deception. Death is regarded as a natural end to life and, at this point, is not seen as the enemy. An empathic relationship with the family as they deal with grief and loss also is an expression of care. Mr. Martin can be supported in living to the fullest and in a peaceful death. The strongest objection probably will come from the duty to protect from harm through paternalistic action. This can be refuted by considering the three criteria of paternalism. (a) *Autonomy*—Mr. Martin's autonomy is not being preserved by withholding information critical to his own condition. (b) *Harm*—There is as much of a possibility of harm to Mr. Martin coming from not disclosing as disclosing. There is no evidence to support that serious harm will come to others by being truthful. (c) *Ratification*—There is no evidence to support that Mr. Martin will later thank the nurse for being deceptive, particularly since he is asking for information.
9. Act on choice	9. Action is taken. Mr. Martin requests information and it is given to him.
10. Reflect on outcome	10. Mr. Martin, indeed, did suspect that serious information was being withheld, both because of his physical state and the artificial way in which the family was responding to him. Once the truth was divulged, all relationships were less strained and the nurse–client relationship continued to be effective, as it was based on a continuing trust.

The preceding framework and analysis uses a pluralistic approach, examining the situation from a variety of ethical perspectives. Although this framework can be applied solely from a deontologic or a teleologic perspective, a pluralistic approach allows for greater diversity in thinking.[25] A desired use of the framework includes shared discussion among those directly concerned. Shared discussion increases the possibility for consciousness-raising and for cooperation and collaboration leading to more effective decision-making. One of the best methods for students to use in learning how to analyze ethical conflicts is to engage in discussion with professionals about the conflicts.

Another factor to consider when using this framework is the need to examine the chosen alternatives in light of social norms and legal requirements.[2] This becomes a part of the weighing of alternatives (Step 6) and anticipation of objections (Step 8). Societal norms and legal expectations cannot be disregarded, but they are not the basis of ethical reasoning. There are times when ethical examination of the law or social norms leads to questioning, consciousness-raising, and an impetus for change.

If free expression and active listening are combined and values are clarified by appeal to broad principles, ethical conflicts may be minimized. A desirable state is one in which individuals learn to function with integrity, being true to their own values, while accepting diversity within the limits of moral behavior.

ETHICAL RESPONSIBILITIES OF THE NURSE

The foundational knowledge and skills for assuming ethical responsibility have been discussed throughout this chapter and in Chapter 33. Nurses need to reflect on personal and professional values in view of ethical principles and theories in order to answer the basic question, "What, all things considered, ought I to do?" Nurses undertake this analysis because individually each nurse wishes to be a person of integrity, and because professionally nurses recognize that to be a professional includes being accountable for practice that is guided by ethical standards. Every nurse must acknowledge both an individual and a collective responsibility. Nurses must respond and speak out against practice that is unprofessional and must support one another in upholding professional standards.

The word *ETHICAL* encapsulates these basic ethical responsibilities providing a device for easy recall and an appropriate stimulus for foundation-building for beginning nurses. Professional nurses should demonstrate commitment to:

*E*xcellence—being clinically competent
*T*hinking—demonstrating critical reasoning
*H*olism—respecting person as a unified being
*I*ntegrity—having a sense of self as a moral agent
*C*ollaboration—being committed to mutual interaction
*A*dvocacy—standing with and for clients
*L*oyalty—fidelity in upholding professional standards

These qualities are in accord with a collaborative approach to the nurse–client relationship and also provide a substantive foundation for situations wherein nurses must draw upon their own resources to determine what the client's choice would be if it could be communicated. The professional practice of nursing requires a depth of understanding of self and others, a willingness to enter into the experience of joy and suffering with others, and an ability to make sound professional judgments serving the interests of individuals and society.

SUMMARY

This chapter has focused on the ethical dimensions of the nurse–client relationship, drawing for the most part on common clinical situations. Foundations for ethical practice include concrete personal and professional values and more abstract ethical principles. Ethical theories, including teleology, deontology, and theories of virtue, provide systems of reasoning about ethical behavior. Ethical principles: respect of person, respect of autonomy, nonmaleficence, beneficence, justice, fidelity, confidentiality, and veracity are applied in these theories and serve to guide ethical decision-making by nurses and other professionals. Applying these ethical principles is also consistent with a collaborative approach to client care.

Personal values that motivate behavior need to be examined in light of professional values and ethical principles. Professional values are embodied in codes of ethics and other documents published by professional organizations. Ethical principles are concepts that contribute to moral behavior, providing broad or general guides to right action. Doing the right or the good thing does not occur automatically in the complex and rapidly changing health care environment. It has been noted that our capacity to do things has moved ahead of our careful thinking about whether these things ought to be done in all situations. The framework for analysis of ethical problems presented in the chapter can assist students to develop a careful thinking process to guide clinical decisions.

Nursing students need to formulate personal standards of behavior that conform to the professional expressions of ethical nursing practice as a basis for their own practice. Being ethical is not just an exercise in thinking about abstract concepts; rather, it is a discipline that manifests itself in behavior that is critical to professional excellence.

REFERENCES

1. Benjamin M, Curtis J. *Ethics in Nursing.* New York: Oxford University Press; 1986.
2. Curtin LL, Flahesty MJ. *Nursing Ethics: Theories and Pragmatics.* Bowie, MD: Brady; 1982.
3. Morrill RL. *Teaching Values in College.* San Francisco: Jossey Bass; 1980.
4. Rokeach M. *The Nature of Human Values.* New York: Free Press; 1973.
5. Purtilo R. *Health Professional and Patient Interaction.* 4th ed. Philadelphia: Saunders; 1990.
6. Raths L, Harmin M, Simons S. *Values and Teaching.* Columbus, OH: Merrill; 1966.
7. American Nurses' Association. *Code for Nurses With Interpretive Statements.* Kansas City, MO: ANA; 1985.
8. Gadow S. Advocacy: An ethical model for assisting patients with treatment decisions. In: Wong C, Swazey J, eds. *Dilemmas of Dying.* Boston: Hall; 1981.
9. Steel S, Harmon V. *Values Clarification in Nursing.* 2nd ed. Norwalk, CT: Appleton-Century-Crofts; 1983.
10. Pender N. *Health Promotion in Nursing Practice.* 2nd ed. Norwalk, CT: Appleton & Lange; 1987:159–182.
11. Uustal D. *Values and Ethics in Nursing: From Theory to Practice.* East Greenwich, RI: Educational Resources in Nursing and Wholistic Health; 1985.
12. Canadian Nurses' Association. *Code of Ethics for Nursing.* Ottawa: CNA; 1985.
13. American Nurses' Association. *Nursing: A Social Policy Statement.* Kansas City, MO: ANA; 1980.
14. American Association of Colleges of Nursing. *Essentials of College and University Education for Professional Nursing.* Washington, DC: AACN; 1986.
15. American Nurses' Association Congress for Nursing Practice. *Standards of Nursing Practice.* Kansas City, MO: ANA; 1973.
16. American Nurses' Association. *Human Rights Guidelines for Nurses in Clinical and Other Research.* Kansas City, MO: ANA; 1975.
17. American Hospital Association. *A Patient's Bill of Rights.* AHA; 1973.
18. American Nurses' Association. *Ethics in Nursing: Position Statements and Guidelines.* Kansas City, MO: ANA; 1988.
19. Curtin L. The nurse as advocate: A philosophical foundation for nursing. *Adv Nurs Sci.* 1979;1:1–10.
20. Donahue MP. Advocacy. In Bulechek G, McCloskey J., eds. *Nursing Interventions.* Philadelphia: Saunders; 1985:338–351.

21. Beauchamp T, Childress J. *Principles of Biomedical Ethics.* 2nd ed. New York: Oxford; 1983.
22. Miller B. Autonomy and the refusing of life saving treatment. *Hastings Center Rep.* August 1981; 22–28.
23. United States President's Commission for the Study of Ethical Problems in Medicine and Biomedical and Behavioral Research. *Making Health Care Decisions: A Report on the Ethical and Legal Implications of Informed Consent on the Patient–Practitioner Relationship.* Washington, DC: US Government Printing Office; 1982.
24. Annas G. When suicide prevention becomes brutality: The case of Elizabeth Bouvia. *Hastings Center Rep.* 1984;14:20.
25. Boody BA. *Life and Death Decision Making.* New York: Oxford; 1988.
26. Williamson J. Mutual interaction: A model of nursing practice. *Nurs Outlook.* 1981;29:104–107.
27. Meilaender G. On removing food and water: Against the stream. *Hastings Center Rep.* 1984;14:11–13.
28. Mappes T, Zembaty J. Kantian deontology. In: Mappes T, Zembaty J, eds. *Biomedical Ethics.* New York: McGraw-Hill; 1986:17–22.
29. Ross WD. *The Right and the Good.* Oxford: Clarendon; 1930:21–22.
30. Edwards RB, Graber GC. *Bioethics.* San Diego: Harcourt Brace Jovanovich; 1988:1–28.
31. Aristotle; Ostwald M, trans. *Nichomachean Ethics.* Indianapolis: Bobbs-Merrill; 1962.
32. Carlson JW. Natural Law theory. In: Mappes T, Zembaty J, eds. *Biomedical Ethics.* New York: McGraw-Hill; 1981:37–43.
33. Gadow S. Nurse and patient: The caring relationship. In: Bishop A, Scudder J, eds. *Caring, Curing, Coping.* University, AL: University of Alabama Press; 1985:31–43.
34. Fry S. Toward a theory of nursing ethics. *Adv Nurs Sci.* 1989; 11:9–22.
35. Watson J. *Nursing: Human Science and Human Care.* Norwalk, CT: Appleton-Century-Crofts; 1985.
36. Benner P, Wrubel J. *The Primacy of Caring: Stress and Coping in Health and Illness.* Redwood City, CA: Addison-Wesley; 1988.
37. Noddings N. *Caring.* Berkeley: University of California Press; 1984.
38. Rawls J. *A Theory of Justice.* Cambridge: Belknap; 1971.
39. Schmelzer M, Anema MG. Should nurses ever lie to patients? *Image.* 1988;20:110–112.
40. Evans LK, Strumpf NE. Myths about elder restraint. *Image.* 1990;22:124–127.
41. Lynne J, Childress J. Must patients always be given food and water? *Hastings Center Rep.* 1983;13:17–22.
42. Aroskar M. Anatomy of an ethical dilemma. *Am J Nurs.* 1980; 80:658–660.
43. Payton RJ. Pluralistic ethical decision making. In: *Clinical and Scientific Sessions 1979.* Kansas City, MO: American Nurses' Association; 1979; 9–16.
44. Wright R. *Human Values in Health Care.* New York: McGraw-Hill; 1987:44–61.

BIBLIOGRAPHY

Annas G. The case of Elizabeth Bouvia. *Hastings Center Rep.* 1984; 14:20–22.

Aroskar M. A question of ethics: The patient's right to privacy. *Nurs Life.* 1982;2:35–38.

Beauchamp TL, Childress JF. *Principles of Biomedical Ethics.* 3rd ed. New York: Oxford; 1989.

Benjamin M, Curtis J. *Ethics in Nursing.* 2nd ed. New York: Oxford; 1986.

Callahan S. The role of emotion in ethical decisionmaking. *Hastings Center Rep.* 1988;18:9–14.

Chinn P, ed. Caring. *Adv Nurs Sci.* 1990;13:1.

Davis AJ. New developments in international nursing ethics. *Nurs Clin North Am.* 1989;24:571–577.

Davis AJ. Professional obligations, personal values in conflict. *Am Nurs.* 1990;22:7.

DeGroot KD, Damato MB. Attitudes and requirements of various religious groups. In: DeGroot KD, Damato MB. *Critical Care Skills.* Norwalk, CT: Appleton & Lange; 1987:389–395.

Fry ST. Toward a theory of nursing ethics. *Adv Nurs Sci.* 1989;12: 9–22.

Fry ST. Ethical issues in providing nursing care to human immunodeficiency virus-infected populations. *Nurs Clin North Am.* 1989;24:523–534.

The Hastings Center. Termination of life-sustaining treatment and care of the dying; 1987.

Jarczewski PH. What is an ethical decision? Ethics for contemporary nursing practice. *Adv Clin Care.* 1990;5:23.

Kaczorowski J. Refusing life-sustaining treatment. *J Psychosoc Nurs Mental Health.* 1988;26:8–12.

Ketefian S. Moral reasoning and ethical practice in nursing. *Nurs Clin North Am.* 1989;24:509–521.

Kiely M, Kiely D. Whistleblowing: Disclosure and its consequences for the professional nurse and management. *Nurs Management.* 1987;18:41–45.

Lund M. Conflict in ethics: Is giving pain relief always right? *Geriatr Nurs.* 1990;11:83–84.

Moody HR. Ethics and aging. *Generations.* 1985;10:5–9.

Mumma C. Withholding nutrition: A nursing perspective. *Nurs Admin Q.* 1986;10:31–38.

Murphy P. The role of the nurse on hospital ethics committees. *Nurs Clin North Am.* 1989;24:551–556.

Noddings N. *Caring: A Feminine Approach to Ethics and Moral Education.* Berkeley: University of California Press; 1984.

Pender N. Values clarification. In: Pender N, ed. *Health Promotion and Nursing Practice.* 2nd ed. Norwalk, CT: Appleton & Lange; 1987:159–182.

Smurl J. Making hard choices. *Nursing 88.* 1988;18:105–108.

Smurl J. The court and Nancy Cruzan. *Hastings Center Rep.* 1990; 20:38–50.

Steele S, Harmon V. *Values Clarification in Nursing.* 2nd ed. Norwalk, CT: Appleton-Century-Crofts; 1983.

Twomey JG Jr. Analysis of the claim to distinct nursing ethics: Normative and nonnormative approaches. *Adv Nurs Sci.* 1989; 11:25–32.

Veach RM, Fry ST. *Case Studies in Nursing Ethics.* Philadelphia: Lippincott; 1987.

Watson J. *Nursing: Human Science and Human Care.* Norwalk, CT: Appleton-Century-Crofts; 1985.

Winslow GR. From loyalty to advocacy: A new metaphor for nursing. *Hastings Center Rep.* 1984;14:32–40.

Wright R. *Human Values in Health Care: The Practice of Ethics.* New York: McGraw-Hill; 1987.

UNIT EIGHT
Nursing and Health Care as Business

CHAPTER 35

Health Care Delivery

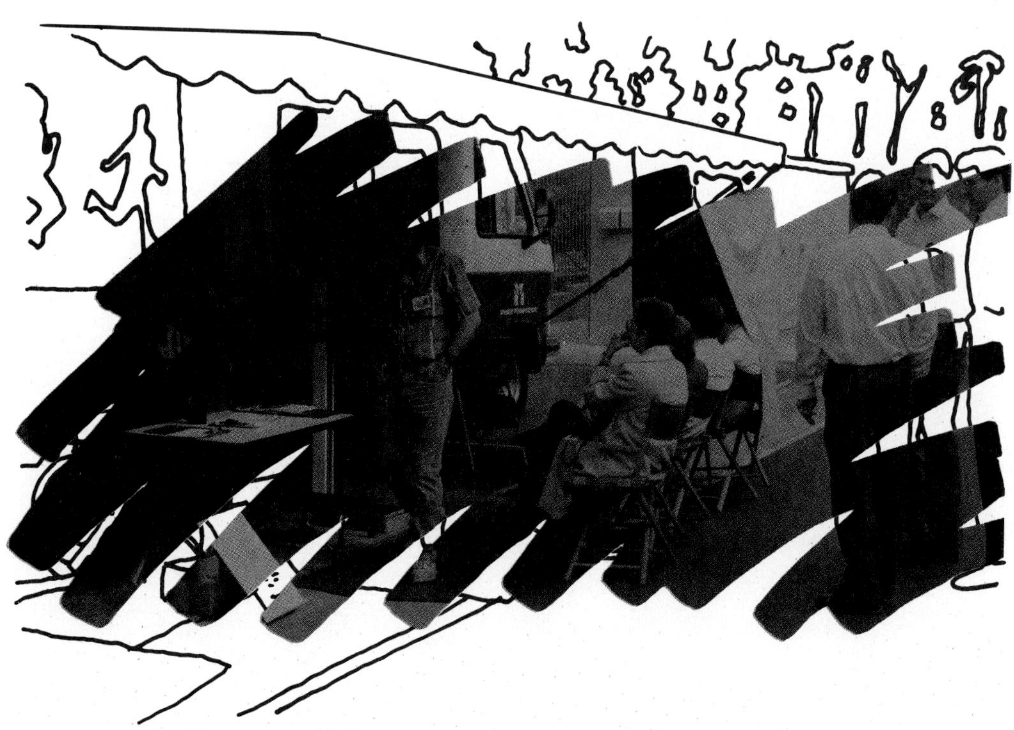

Behavioral Objectives

Upon completion of this chapter, the student will be able to:

1. Name at least three health-related functions carried out by the federal, state, and local governments.
2. Compare and contrast fee-for-service, capitation, and fee-for-diagnosis methods of health care payment.
3. Describe the third-party payment system currently used in the United States.
4. Define what is meant by a health maintenance organization.
5. Briefly discuss the original intent of the Medicare program and discuss one major factor that has altered the implementation of this program.
6. Discuss the original intent of the Medicaid program.
7. Define Medicare's prospective payment system and the diagnostic related group (DRG).
8. Discuss attempts by insurance companies, employers, community health care services, health care providers, and the federal government to reduce health care costs.
9. Discuss the effects of changing population demographics for the health care system.
10. Discuss factors that can encourage the client to become an active health care consumer.
11. Identify and explain two major challenges facing the nurse in promoting cost-conscious health care.
12. Identify two implications for the nursing profession resulting from the lack of third-party reimbursement for nursing services.

KEY TERMS

accreditation
ambulatory care
capitation
case managers
certification
employee medical benefits
fee-for-diagnosis
fee-for-service
health maintenance organization
home care
hospice care
managed care
Medicaid
Medicare
peer review
peer review organization
primary care
prospective payment system
quality of care
secondary care
self-monitoring review system
tertiary care
utilization review

The health care delivery system in the United States is a multilevel, multipurpose organizational structure designed to provide health care to consumers. This system, which developed in response to society's goal of providing care for the ill, traditionally has emphasized care for the most critical conditions, relying on medical science and technology to solve acute health care problems. A health care system that is more accurately described as an "illness care" system has evolved. Ideas about health promotion and illness prevention, which exert considerable influence on today's health care system, have not always played such a role. Changes in technology, consumer awareness, and the philosophy of health care professionals are generating a gradual shift of emphasis from illness care to wellness care, illness prevention, and health promotion. Chapters 5 and 22 also address these topics.

The health care financing system mirrors the health care system in complexity. It reflects the priorities of the health care system as a whole and has emphasized the handling of short-term, acute health problems rather than the prevention of chronic, degenerative diseases. The health care financing structure, which includes both government and private components, is increasingly challenged to meet the needs of a growing elderly population, the group most often faced with chronic illnesses requiring expensive health care, lifetime medications, and life-style adjustments.

Health care continually increases in cost and complexity as our society's attitudes toward health care mature and the technology of health care advances. The US Department of Commerce has estimated that spending on health care will exceed $756 billion in 1991.[1] If the health care system remains unchanged, expenditures will reach between \$2.1 and 2.7 trillion by the year 2000.[2] Affordability, availability, and accessibility of health care for those who need it, however, remain critical issues facing health care providers and consumers.

As the health care system expands and develops, so do the roles of nurses and other health care professionals. The health care delivery system is changing at such a rapid rate that health care professionals need to appraise their roles and the product they deliver. Although the federal government is placing more stringent controls on the delivery of health care, individual professionals are challenged to identify alternative, less expensive ways to deliver quality services to consumers. Traditional, fixed lines of authority and responsibility are beginning to erode in favor of a flexible, collaborative approach to meeting clients' health care needs.

These and other trends have a profound impact on the health care delivery system. They create a special opportunity for the nursing profession to educate the public and members of the health care team regarding nursing's role in improving the quality of health care available to the population. This chapter provides a broad overview of the health care delivery system in the United States, and its key aspects and trends, which can help students develop a clearer understanding of nursing's central role in a changing health care environment.

IMPLICATIONS FOR NURSE–CLIENT COLLABORATION

Government Organization

The nurse will frequently encounter clients who need assistance in obtaining and financing health care but who may not be aware of government services available to help them or how to gain access to those services. An understanding of the organizational structure of government and the roles played by the levels of government in facilitating and providing health care service enables the nurse to better assist such clients.

HEALTH CARE DELIVERY SYSTEM

The health care delivery system in the United States is charged with the responsibility of meeting the health care needs of more than 250 million people. This delivery system has been developed to provide care through programs at the federal, state, and local levels.

Health Care Delivery Structure

Role of the Federal Government. The federal government first assumed a role in the provision of health care in 1798, when President John Adams authorized the Marine Hospital Service to care for US merchant seamen. This was the beginning of the US Public Health Service. Since then, the federal government has assumed an ever-increasing role in the provision of health care services, and such responsibility has been recognized and accepted as a major obligation of the federal government.

Federal health care activities are implemented by the Department of Health and Human Services (DHHS). This department oversees four major agencies: the Office for Human Development Services, the Public Health Service, the Health Care Financing Administration, and the Social Security Administration (Fig. 35–1). Of these agencies the last three are most pertinent to this discussion.

The Public Health Service (PHS) is considered the primary health care agency within the federal government. It has the responsibility of protecting the physical and emotional health of US citizens. It attempts to meet this responsibility by collaborating with the states to identify health care needs and originate programs to meet these needs. The PHS also is involved in collecting statistics, conducting research, and providing financial assistance to educational institutions. The PHS provides grants, acts as a resource center, and performs a regulatory role by enforcing certain health-related laws. The major agencies within the PHS are the Alcohol, Drug Abuse, and Mental Health Administration; the Centers for Disease Control; the Agency for Toxic Substances and Disease Registry; the Food and Drug Administration; the National Institutes of Health; the Health Resources and Services Administration; and the Indian Health Services (Fig. 35–2).

The Health Care Financing Administration (HCFA) plays a principal role in the operation of the multi-billion-dollar federal health insurance programs, Medicare and Medicaid. Medicare is an insurance program covering some hospital, physician, and various related expenses for the disabled and those over age 65. Medicaid is a federally funded financial aid program operated by the states and offered to the poor. These programs will be discussed in detail later in this chapter. HCFA regulates the distribution of federal funds under Medicare and Medicaid. To ensure equitable distribution of these funds and promote quality care, HCFA applies both financial audit and quality assurance programs to providers requesting payment under Medicare or Medicaid. HCFA is responsible for monitoring the development and use of peer review organizations, which evaluate the quality of health care provided in a community. See also *Regulating the System* later in this chapter.

The Social Security Administration directs and manages the operation of the Social Security system, a self-supporting retirement plan co-financed by employers, employees, and tax revenue.

In addition to being responsible for the operation of specific federal health-related programs and agencies, DHHS also supplies money directly to the states to be used in state-operated health care programs. This federal money is distributed in the form of block grants. Block grants are designed to give community government agencies local control over the distribution of federal monies with a minimum of federal regulatory involvement. Since the Budget and Reconciliation Act of 1981, block grants have been given

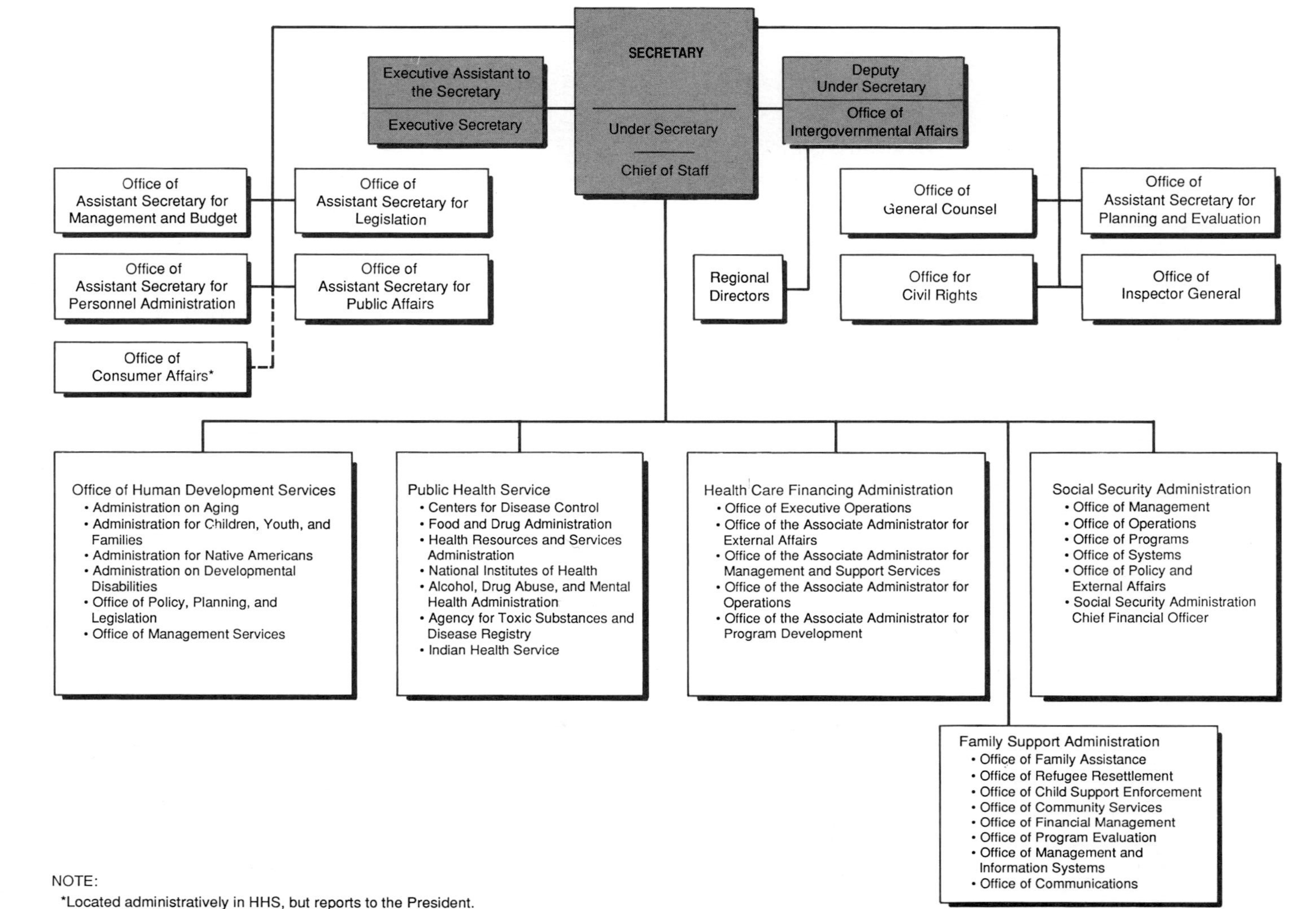

Figure 35–1. The Department of Health and Human Services is a large, complex agency of the federal government that regulates and monitors compliance with federal health policy. (*From* The United States Government Manual, 1990/91. Superintendent of Documents. US Government Printing Office, Washington, DC. Revised July 1990.)

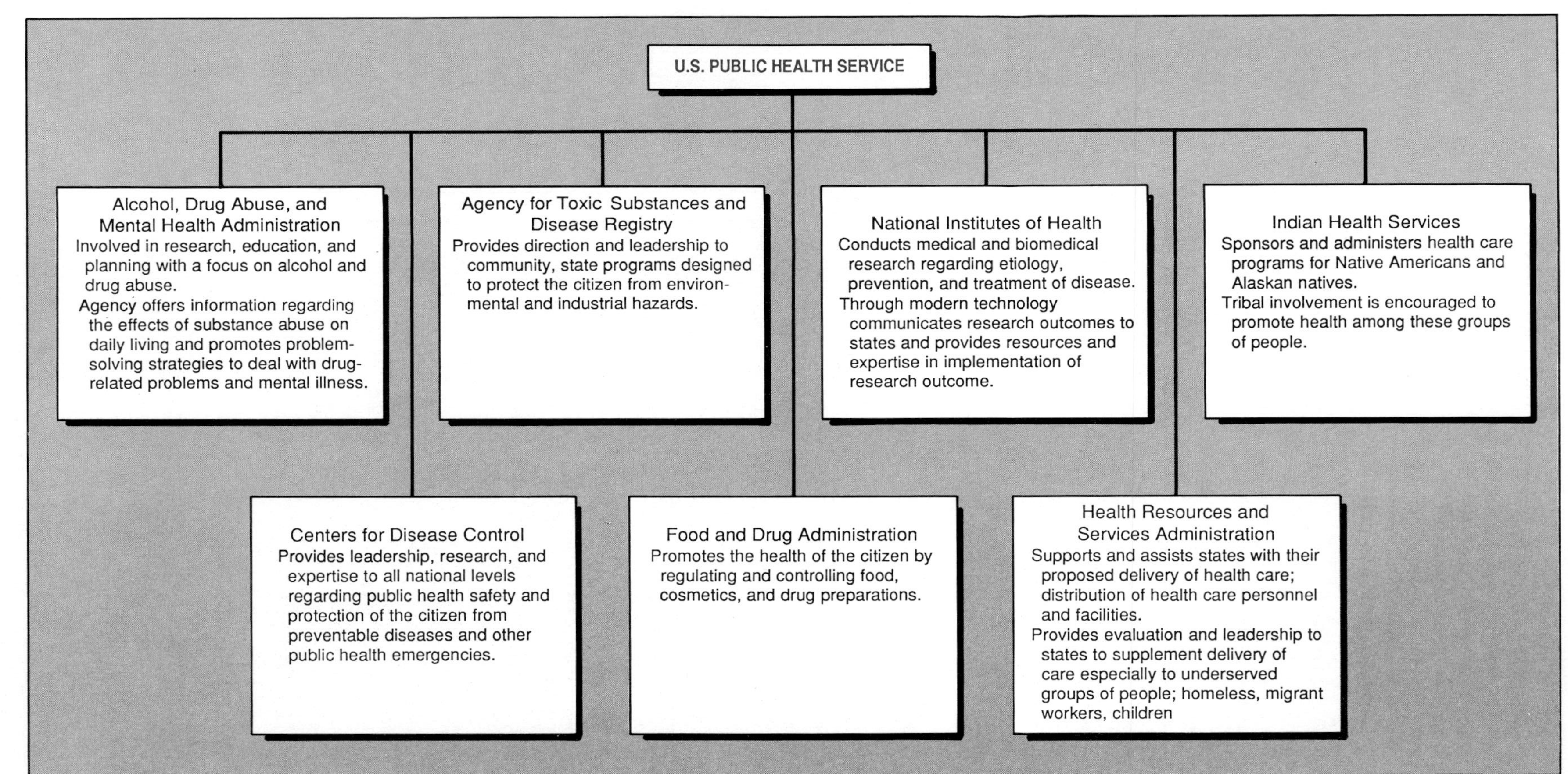

Figure 35–2. Major agencies within the US Public Health Service. (*Source:* US Government Manual 1988/89. *Washington, DC: US Govt Printing Office; 1988: 296–307.*)

to communities to be used for maternal and child health, preventive health, alcohol and drug abuse, and mental health.

Role of the States. Though the individual states' health care systems share similar goals, there is great variation among state programs. Today's state health departments work closely with the PHS, which administers grants and financial assistance to state public health departments and provides specialized technical personnel to states. The typical state health department addresses a wide range of health problems. Problems such as maternal and child health, infectious disease, epidemic control, and administration of food handling standards and sanitation regulations receive special emphasis on the state level. Most state health departments have licensing responsibility for local health care facilities. State-level health departments also assume responsibility for evaluating and regulating health care practices, evaluating and accrediting health education institutions, and granting professional licensure to health care professionals. States are also responsible for co-administering the Medicaid program with the federal government.

Role of Local Government. Services provided by local health departments commonly include control of infectious disease, management of school health programs, and immunization plans. Local health care agencies are frequently involved in enforcement of health codes and food establishment practices. The local-level health agencies frequently work closely with their state and federal counterparts in developing approaches and solutions to community health problems.

Health Care Delivery Services

Health care services are classified according to the complexity of care, as well as according to the setting in which clients receive care. The terms that describe levels of complexity of health care are primary, secondary, and tertiary.

Primary care is care given at an individual's first point of contact with the health care delivery system. Primary care providers offer health promotion, preventive care, and continuing care for common health problems and refer clients to specialists when the illness requires more sophisticated care. **Secondary care** is provided by specialists on referral from primary care providers. It is generally offered in larger medical centers. **Tertiary care** is the most highly technical health care available. There are a limited number of tertiary care facilities in the US; most are affiliated with large research centers or teaching hospitals. They offer advanced diagnostic and treatment care requiring personnel and equipment that are not economically feasible in smaller facilities.

Classifications of health care delivery related to the care setting include ambulatory or outpatient services and institutional or inpatient services. There are several kinds of health care facilities in each category (Fig. 35–3).

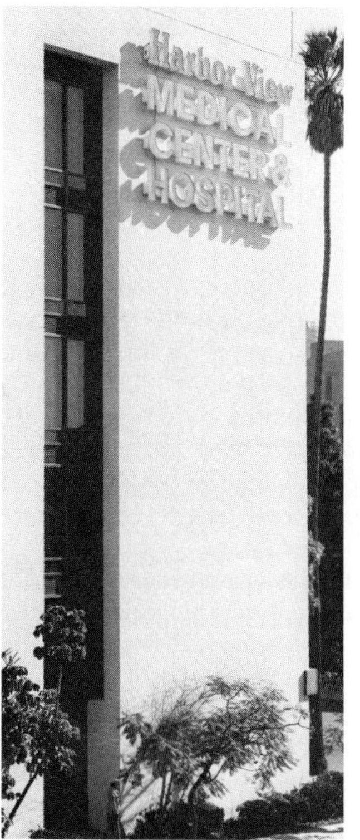

A

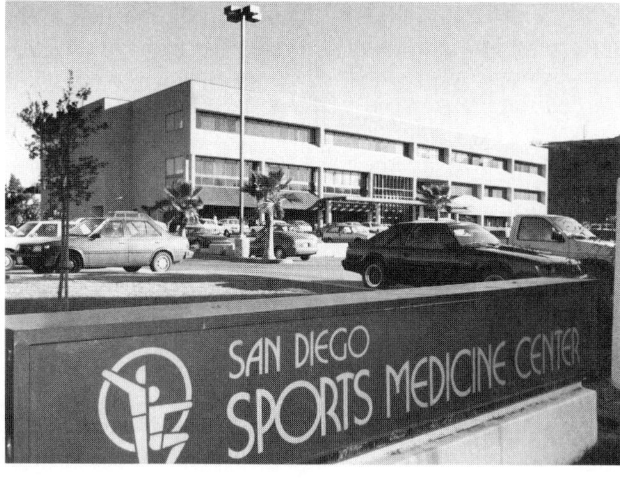

B

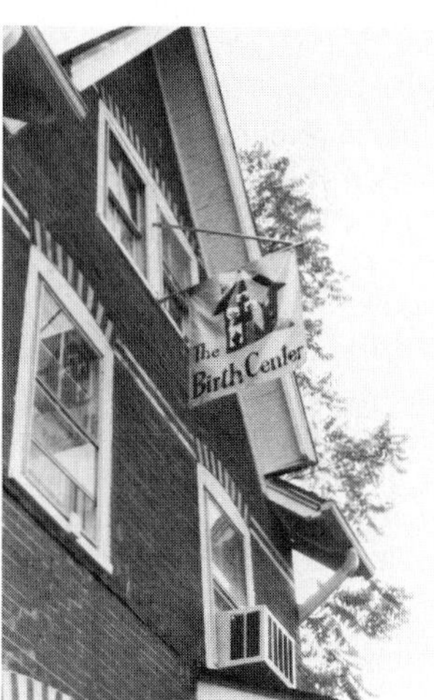

C

Figure 35–3. Health care delivery settings include **(A)** short-term private hospitals, **(B)** ambulatory care clinics, and **(C)** birth centers. (***C*** *courtesy of Carol Weingarten.*)

Ambulatory Care Services. Outpatient or **ambulatory care** facilities provide care for clients whose health problems do not require continued around the clock surveillance by a health care provider. Ambulatory care facilities are the usual setting for primary care. Settings include physician's offices, clinics, industrial health centers, ambulatory care centers, clients' homes, and hospices.

Traditionally, physicians in private or small group practices have provided most primary health care. The family physician was the cornerstone of health care in most small communities and often a trusted friend, as well. Demographic and economic changes have reduced the number of physicians in private solo or small group practices today.

Clinic is a term that refers to several kinds of ambulatory care facilities. Clinics may be privately owned, as by a group of physicians, affiliated with community hospitals, run by a governmental agency, or a combination of these. Some clinics offer care that is specific to a particular health problem, such as hypertension, chemical dependency, and diabetes, or to a specific population, such as well-child and prenatal clinics.

Industrial health centers are becoming more common as corporations strive to contain the costs of employee health care. Often nurse practitioners or community health nurses manage these clinics, providing health screening, health education, employee safety programs, and minor emergency care.

Neighborhood ambulatory care centers for diagnosis and treatment of acute illnesses and minor emergencies (emergicenters) often offer walk-in service and extended hours. These centers and others with a specific care focus, for example, minor surgery (surgicenters) and childbirth (birthing centers) are relatively new developments in health care. These ambulatory care centers offer care at lower cost than traditional in-hospital services.

Health care may also be delivered to clients in their homes. Supported in some instances by government tax-funded programs and provided by voluntary community groups as well as proprietary organizations, home health programs target specific groups at high risk for health problems. **Home care** services provided include health education, diagnostic screening, and therapeutic intervention, as well as rehabilitative support. Home health programs also provide follow-up physical care for clients who have been discharged from a hospital but who require some nursing care. Ideally, the home care team consists of physicians; nurses; nutritionists; occupational, speech, and physical therapists; social workers; and others.

Hospice care is a specific type of care designed for terminally ill clients who choose to spend their remaining days at home or in a homelike setting rather than in an institution (Fig. 35–4). A hospice team assists clients and family members to cope with the dying process and the stages of grief and bereavement. Hospice care includes pain control measures, nutritional planning, physical relaxation methods, and emotional support. Members of the hospice team include thanatology specialists or those who have studied the dying process, in addition to the various members of the home care team.

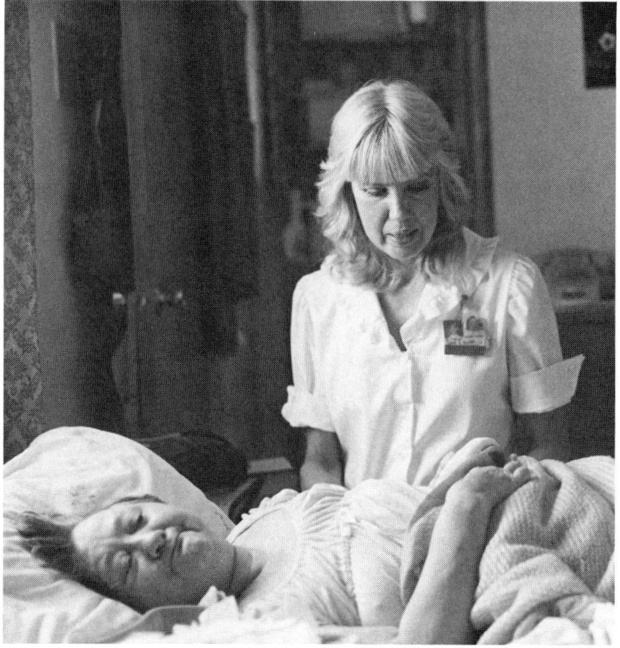

Figure 35–4. Hospice care.

Institutional (Inpatient) Services. The organizational structure at the core of the US health care system is the hospital. Originally designed to offer shelter and food to the poor and outcast, hospitals have evolved in their purpose, goals, and reputation. Today they are considered to be centers for care of the sick and for restoration of health and wellness. Although hospital organizations and operations vary widely, they are categorized according to two major classification systems: type of services provided and ownership.

Hospitals that provide mixed services, such as medical, surgical, obstetric, and psychiatric care, to various age groups are classified as general hospitals. Specialty hospitals are those that offer care only to specific client populations. Examples include specialization according to age (eg, pediatric hospitals), according to type of health problem (eg, cancer, psychiatric, and rehabilitation hospitals), and according to length of stay (eg, acute care or chronic care hospitals).

There are two principal modes of hospital ownership: private and public. Private hospitals are categorized by the use to which they put their surplus income. They may be investor-owned for profit (proprietary) or not for profit (voluntary). Public hospitals are categorized by the level of government jurisdiction that owns and operates them: federal, state, or local.

Nursing homes are long-term care facilities that render health care services to individuals who are unable to care for themselves independently but do not require the intensity of care a hospital provides. If these facilities comply with state and federal regulations, they may be eligible for financial reimbursement from Medicare or Medicaid.

In nursing homes, nursing care is the primary focus of treatment. The intensity and type of nursing care provided vary. Some facilities provide nursing care for persons discharged from an acute care hospital who require a period of convalescence before they are able to care for themselves at home. Other facilities provide limited nursing care to clients with an emphasis on assisting with activities of daily living. Still other facilities provide only room and board. In the past, the classification of nursing homes was based on the level of care the agency provided. Nursing homes were classified as skilled nursing facilities (SNFs) or intermediate-care facilities (ICFs). Skilled nursing facilities provided the highest or most intense level of nursing care. Intermediate-care facilities provided services to individuals with less critical needs for nursing care who required institutional care because of physical or mental limitations.

Federal legislation that merged ICFs and SNFs into one level of care went into effect in 1990. Staffing by licensed practical nurses, formerly allowed during certain hours of the day in ICFs, is no longer allowed. The new law requires 24-hour supervision by a registered nurse, although states may waive this requirement under certain circumstances.

Health Care Providers

Health care is provided by individuals with various educational backgrounds and varying credentials or state licensure. (See the later section, The Regulators.) The basic, fundamental structure of the health care team includes two groups of practitioners: professionals and support staff (Box 35–1).

BOX 35–1. MEMBERS OF THE HEALTH CARE TEAM

Clients

Professional Practitioners

- Physicians
- Registered nurses
- Dentists
- Pharmacists
- Social workers
- Dieticians
- Physical therapists
- Occupational therapists
- Optometrists
- Chiropracters

Support Staff

- Administrators
- Chaplains
- Clerical workers
- Licensed vocational/practical nurses
- Respiratory therapists
- Physician's assistants
- Dental assistants
- Nursing assistants/shift partners
- Laboratory and x-ray technicians

Professional practitioners have completed a standardized program and have demonstrated an ability to meet their profession's standards for practice. The professional's practice is based on a body of scientific and technical knowledge unique to his or her profession that is dynamic and continually being developed, expanded, and evaluated through ongoing research. Professionals are responsible for making judgments about health care and assisting clients in decision making about health as well as providing direct client care. (Refer to Chap. 19 for further discussion of roles and responsibilities of members of the health care team.) For every professional practitioner, there are many individuals in technical, administrative, and other support positions on whom the efficient delivery of health care depends.

■ REGULATING THE SYSTEM

A complex, multilevel health care delivery system brings with it the need for some degree of regulatory control. Although the direct assessment of health care is the primary concern of the regulatory agencies, other areas that receive attention are cost and accessibility of service and frequency of use of specific services. Continual evaluation, problem identification, and problem resolution form the basis of the regulatory process.

Defining the Standard

The quality of care offered by a particular health facility is a major area of concern of regulatory agencies. Yet quality in health care is difficult to define. Staff expertise, technical performance, and equipment, as well as a client's satisfaction with the outcome and overall impression of the facility are included in definitions of quality. Quality care does not require that health care procedures be successful. Donabedian defines **quality of care** as follows: "The highest quality of care is . . . that which yields the greatest expected improvement in health status, health being defined very broadly to include physical, physiological and psychological dimensions."[3] Oberst defines quality of care from the point of view of the recipient: "A client with a chronic, debilitating disease such as cancer needing continuous interventions from the health care team may liken the quality of health care interventions as synonymous with the resulting quality of life he's able to live."[4]

Current definitions of quality focus on the achievement of anticipated outcomes for clients as measured against generally recognized standards of practice.[5] Beyers[6] emphasizes the central role of clients in definitions of quality by referring to quality as the vehicle to ensure public trust in health care.

Regardless of the precise definition used by the observer, there is agreement on the importance of quality in health care. According to Haffner and others, "In a sense,

IMPLICATIONS FOR PROFESSIONAL COLLABORATION

Roles of Professional Colleagues

Nurses interact with providers of all types in the course of assisting clients. Understanding the various roles and contributions of health care professionals enables the nurse to help improve the client's health care in a variety of ways. Identifying the need for the services of other providers, initiating referrals, and coordinating communication between the client and other providers and among the providers themselves are all important nursing functions. These functions require a working knowledge of what other providers can do for the client.

quality care is like honesty. It must pervade the very fiber of the individual or the institution."[7]

Quality of care has been a continuing concern of the nursing profession. One of the first voices raised concerning the need to achieve a standardized quality of care was that of Florence Nightingale. According to Covell, the first recorded analytical approach to measuring the quality of care was "Florence Nightingale's effort to develop a reporting system to provide patient care data, profiles and outcomes (expressed as mortality rates) in an attempt to improve the care provided to casualties of the Crimean War."[8] These themes prevail in contemporary quality assurance programs.

The Regulators

"Regulators" are the public- and private-sector groups who, out of concern for the individual, have established rules, regulations, and policies to ensure standards of quality in health care. In the United States, these include Congress and federal administrative agencies, state and local government entities, private organizations, and health care professionals.

Federal Regulation. The federal government has increasingly become involved in health care delivery. This increased involvement brought demands for standardization of policies and procedures on the part of health care providers. It also brought increased awareness that quality was not something to be taken for granted and that providers must be accountable for the quality of their service.

One of the methods by which the federal regulatory role is exercised over health care facilities is the **utilization review** procedure. Utilization review evolved from the 1965 Social Security Act, which mandated that health care reimbursement under Medicare and Medicaid would be provided only for health care that was medically necessary. To implement this standard, legislation required that each institution seeking federal reimbursement for health care establish a utilization review committee. The committee was to review the necessity for client admissions, the reasons supporting the length of hospital stay, and the appropriateness of the treatment provided. These reviews were retrospective, that is, they occurred after the care was given and billed. Although there were some limits on reimbursement, this system created an incentive to provide more costly services.

The resulting alarming escalation in Medicare hospital expenditures during the 1970s and early 1980s led to the Tax Equity and Fiscal Responsibility Act of 1982 (TEFRA). TEFRA mandated that DHHS develop legislative proposals for prospective reimbursement. In 1983, the prospective payment bill mandating diagnosis related grouping (DRGs) as a basis for prospective reimbursement was passed. TEFRA also set a ceiling on certain costs and established **Peer Review Organizations** (PROs) to assess health care utilization and provide quality control. A PRO is a group of professionals such as physicians, nurses, medical records personnel, and others involved in providing health care. They are employed by a private organization that is under contract to the Health Care Financing Administration.[9] PROs establish a preadmission (prospective) program and conduct post-discharge (retrospective) reviews of the care given in the facility. PROs also encourage institutions to conduct their own review of the care in their facility.

The Food and Drug Administration (FDA), an agency within the US Public Health Service, has the responsibility of safeguarding the public from unsafe or hazardous consumer goods such as foods, drugs, and cosmetics. The FDA's regulatory role is to evaluate research data compiled by pharmaceutical companies on proposed new drugs. Collecting drug data and complying with governmental regulations are costly and time-consuming. Extensive research is required before permission to market a new drug is given. The research requirements are designed to ensure that manufacturers have thoroughly investigated the effectiveness, side effects, safety, and long-term effects of new compounds. Only after preliminary investigation indicates that the proposed drug is safe is permission given to use the drug on humans on an experimental basis and later to market it. Research regarding the safety and effectiveness of the drug continues after it is released for widespread public use.

State Regulation. State organizations exert considerable influence on the health care industry. State health departments provide for accreditation and licensing of health-related facilities and certain health care personnel. **Accreditation** is a process wherein an institution or educational program seeks the evaluation of an outside agency. Accrediting bodies may be part of a state government or private entities. The latter are discussed later in this section. The accrediting agency evaluates the standards of operation of the institution or educational program according to predetermined qualifications. Institutions and programs that meet the evaluation criteria are recognized and thereby accredited by that particular specialized agency. State accreditation is usually a mandatory process. Schools of nursing, for example, must be state accredited to operate.

Licensing is a mandatory, formal process through

IMPLICATIONS FOR NURSE–CLIENT AND PROFESSIONAL COLLABORATION

Standards of Practice

Each client care decision reflects the provider's understanding of standards of practice. Standards of practice are promulgated by government bodies and private agencies to protect clients from incompetent health care service. Licensing of providers and facilities is a significant way in which state governments set standards, just as certification and accreditation are important private-sector means of regulation. In collaborating with the client and other providers, the nurse is always cognizant of the need to uphold standards of practice and to have those standards represented in the plans for action that result.

which a governmental agency grants an individual or institution the right to provide certain services. Designated authorities within each state license the majority of health care professionals, including physicians, dentists, pharmacists, and nurses. The requirements for professional licensure are based on standards of care and are specific to each profession. Acceptance of professional licensure carries with it the requirement that the license holder provide a quality of care that equals or exceeds the minimum standard. The role of the Board of Registered Nursing, the state-level agency that regulates the licensure of nurses and the accreditation of nursing programs, is discussed in greater detail in Chapter 3.

The state also licenses health care facilities. The state monitors and evaluates the quality of care provided by health care institutions, such as community hospitals, specialty hospitals, and long-term convalescent homes. When reviewing a facility for licensure, the state agency focuses on the facility's structural capacity as well as its ability to provide a safe level of care.

Local Regulation. Formerly, regulation of health care on the local level was carried out primarily by federally mandated, community-based health planning agencies called health system agencies (HSAs). HSAs were created in 1975 by the National Health Planning and Resources Act. Their function was to examine the distribution of health care facilities within specific geographic areas and to prevent duplication.[10] Successes of the HSAs were limited and their existence became controversial. As a consequence, in 1986, Congress decided not to continue federal monies to support these agencies. Some states still use certificates of need (CONs), the mechanism used by HSAs to control development of new facilities, particularly for programs such as trauma, cardiac surgery, neonatal intensive care, and transplants.[11] In other states, no consistent local or regional regulatory system is in place; rather, free market competition prevails and supply and demand drive development of programs. Advocates of a return to regional control believe it is a way to assure appropriate allocation of scarce resources, by making high-cost services available, but limiting the number of facilities that provide those services.[12]

Private Sector Regulation. Because the standards set forth by state agencies are usually minimum standards, professionals and health care facilities may seek additional voluntary credentialing from professional organizations. Such credentialing may be either certification of individuals or accreditation of institutions. **Certification** is a procedure by which a nongovernmental entity recognizes an individual's competence through evaluation of educational preparation, performance, and professional skills. Private-sector accreditation refers to the recognition of an institution or educational program that has met predetermined qualifications and standards held by the accrediting body.

Many nursing organizations, including the national organization for professional nurses, the American Nurses' Association (ANA), formally certify nurses' advanced expertise in designated areas of nursing practice. The Organization for Obstetric, Gynecologic, and Neonatal Nurses (NAACOG) and the American Association of Critical Care Nurses (AACCN) are other examples of private-sector organizations that offer certification.

Hospitals and professional institutions have sought voluntary regulation since the early 1900s. The Joint Commission on the Accreditation of Healthcare Organizations (JCAHO) is held in high regard for this role in the medical and governmental communities.

The National League for Nursing (NLN) is the principal private-sector accrediting agency for nursing education programs. NLN focuses on the identification of the nursing needs of a community and the provision of the educational components necessary to prepare nurses to meet those needs. The League has been a serious proponent of consumerism and has sought to combine the efforts of professional education, citizen need, community agencies, and allied health professionals to provide consumers with quality care.

Self-regulation. Health care professionals have traditionally used a **self-monitoring review system,** or **peer review,** as a means of evaluating their professional performance. Over the years this process has become increasingly refined and respected. As outside regulating committees have assumed greater responsibility for monitoring the overall quality of care, there has been parallel development of nursing peer review systems. Properly organized nursing peer review is a way of identifying and correcting nursing care problems in an individual health care facility. Professional peer review reaches maximum effectiveness in attaining desired quality of care when health care professionals apply a collaborative approach. (See Chap. 18 for further discussion of quality assurance processes used by nurses.)

Enforcement

Effective regulatory procedures require methods to correct deviations from accepted standards. Both government and private organizations have established enforcement procedures.

State licensing agencies conduct ongoing programs designed to monitor the quality of health care provided by individuals. Because of limited resources, most states gear their investigative activities to following up on complaints received from consumers or local agencies.

State and private-sector accrediting bodies also engage in limited enforcement activities designed to protect the integrity of their accreditation. Agencies that accredit institutions generally reinspect each facility on a periodic basis as part of their effort to monitor quality of care. Serious deficiencies trigger a more detailed examination. If the deficiency is not corrected subsequently, this omission may lead to a loss of accreditation.

Violations of accepted standards may at first result only in written warnings or informal counseling, depending on the seriousness of the error. Serious or repeated lesser violations may prompt formal, direct action against the license holder or facility. Serious cases sometimes result in the suspension or revocation of the license or the accreditation. Accrediting bodies resort to such actions only when absolutely necessary; however, a credible regulatory system must be prepared to take such actions.

Although self-regulation (peer review) enforcement procedures are not subject to outside authority, health care consumers are taking growing interest in peer review within the health professions. Self-regulation is a privilege, and the public will not support professional self-regulation if it sees peer review as a system of self-protection rather than self-regulation.

FINANCING HEALTH CARE

Health care is one of the most expensive necessities of everyday life. Consequently, many approaches to financing the health care system have been developed.

Types of Billing

There are three types of billing for health care services: fee-for-service, capitation, and fee-for-diagnosis.

Fee-for-service. In **fee-for-service** billing, consumers pay for each health service as it is provided. In theory, health care consumers choose which services to use. In practice, however, not all consumers are willing or able to assume such a primary role in the selection of services, nor are all providers willing to relinquish their traditional prescriptive power. Nevertheless, collaboration to select mutually acceptable services is a viable option in a fee-for-service system.

Capitation. **Capitation** systems require that individuals or employers pay a negotiated fee, which pays for a package of health care services during a specific time period. This system is used by **health maintenance organizations** (HMOs). Today's HMO is an organized system of health care delivery whose members (subscribers) prepay a monthly fee that is guaranteed to cover all services named in the contract. Collaborative decision making about services to be used is also possible in capitation systems. More information about HMOs is found in a later section, Current Trends and Issues in Health Care.

Fee-for-diagnosis. **Fee-for-diagnosis** is a type of **prospective payment system** (PPS). Under this system, facilities are given a fixed dollar amount for the treatment of a client before services are provided. The fee amount is based on the client's principal diagnosis, secondary diagnoses, demographic data such as age and sex, and the usual treatment necessary for the client's health problem. The DRG classification system that was developed to regulate the amount that inpatient health care facilities could bill the government for health services they provide to Medicare clients is an example of a fee-for-diagnosis system.

Fee-for-diagnosis, like fee-for-service, does not provide incentives for preventive care or for cost reduction, because the system requires a client diagnosis to generate a fee for the provider.

Methods of Payment

In the US health care system, the main sources of payment for care are direct personal payment, private insurance

BUILDING NURSING KNOWLEDGE

What Are Some of the Effects of the Prospective Payment System and Its Implications for Nursing?

Jones KR. Evolution of the prospective payment system: Implications for nursing. *Nurs Econ.* 1989;7(6):299–305.

Despite the incentives of prospective payment for cost reduction, which have been in operation since 1982, economic and demographic forces continue to push health care costs up. Jones feels it is important for nurses to understand the effects of prospective payment on health care.

Alternatives to hospital care have proliferated, eroding the hospital industry's market. In response, hospitals are establishing satellite clinics to attract patients; they are also opening ambulatory care services to compete in the marketplace. Many hospitals are specializing in certain services and discontinuing unprofitable services; they are also doing more marketing to attract consumers.

A question of increasing importance is, "What is quality care?" Are all medical orders needed for high quality care? Jones points out that answering this question means confronting the values embedded in medical practice. Increasingly, hospitals are using case management, a system of case-by-case cost analysis, to keep costs down without sacrificing quality. Whether hospitals will cut back on necessary services as well as unnecessary care is a serious concern. Research, as yet, is inconclusive and further study is needed.

payment, and payment by government health plans. Figure 35–5 summarizes the distribution of payment in 1989.

Direct Personal Payment. Direct personal payment pays for health care costs that are not covered by insurance plans and so must be paid out of pocket by the consumer. In 1988, the average health consumer paid $503 for services not covered under insurance plans.[13] The proportion of health care expenses paid by direct personal payment has decreased in recent years, reflecting the increasing availability of private and government insurance plans.

In 1965, consumers paid 46 percent of health care costs out of pocket. By 1980, out-of-pocket expenses had dropped to 23 percent; by 1989 to 21 percent.[14] Even with these reductions in consumer costs, direct personal payment for health care by US consumers is considerably greater than that in most other countries. For example, in the United Kingdom, consumers paid only 3 percent out of pocket in 1989; in West Germany, consumers paid 7 percent.[14]

Private Insurance Payment. The majority of individuals seeking health care are covered by private voluntary insurance plans. In 1990, private insurance covered an estimated 85 percent of the population under age 65.[14] However, this leaves 33.1 million people without health insurance, and therefore essentially without access to care.[14] Eighty percent of these uninsured have some connection with the work force;[14] 50 percent have full-time jobs;[15,16] one-third have incomes below the poverty line.[17]

The large and growing numbers of uninsured are attributed to changes in the private insurance market, reductions in employer-sponsored health policies, and limited availability of dependent coverage.[17] Moreover, health insurance policies rarely assume all costs of health care. Most include a deductible, an amount the insured must pay in full before payments are made by the insurer. Policies also generally include a co-payment provision, which limits the percentage an insurer will pay for a covered service after the deductible has been reached. The insured individual usually pays a co-payment amount to the provider to pay for services not covered by the primary policy or takes out a co-insurance policy—a supplemental policy that covers such items.

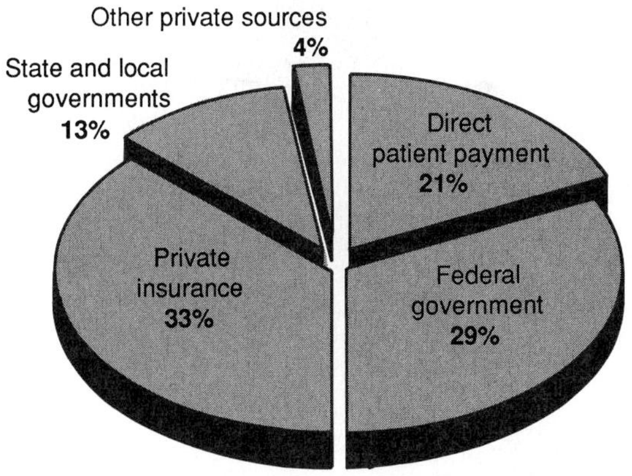

Figure 35–5. Payment sources for 1989 health care expenditures. (*Source: Congressional Budget Office.* Rising Health Care Costs: Causes, Implications, and Strategies. *Washington, DC: US Govt Printing Office; 1991.*)

Much of today's health insurance is provided by **employee medical benefits.** When health insurance is a fringe benefit of employment, the employer's cost of providing coverage is a deductible business expense. Essentially, then, part of the cost of employee medical benefits is subsidized by the federal government through a reduction in the employer's taxes. This tax benefit has not been sufficient to offset the rate of insurance cost expansion, so many companies are now more willing to raise salaries than to provide medical coverage benefits.[18]

Insurance premiums paid by employers have been steadily escalating since the 1970s. Between 1970 and 1980, the amount that US employers paid for employee insurance costs increased 352 percent; the rate of increase slowed in the mid-1980s, but has increased at double-digit rates annually since.[13] Small businesses are finding providing health insurance coverage for employees increasingly expensive; in the past five years the cost of premiums has doubled and in some cases tripled.[14]

Although voluntary insurance is beneficial to the insured individual seeking health care, it has the unfortunate effect of increasing health care costs. This is because a cost-reimbursement model encourages increased use of services, including costly hospital care.[19] Furthermore, when consumers are not responsible for immediate payment, they are less likely to shop for the best value. (See also Chaps. 36 and 37.)

Government Health Plans. The federal government plays an extensive role in financing health care, primarily through Social Security. The Social Security program is not a health insurance program per se; however, the program contains several health insurance components applicable to a limited class of beneficiaries that have significant impact on the health care delivery system. The two most recent additions to the Social Security benefit package, Medicare and Medicaid, have had the most profound impact.

Medicare was designed to provide health care to individuals 65 years of age and older, the group with the greatest health care needs and fewest resources. In the preamble to legislation mandating Medicare, Congress declared that "access to good health care was the right of all Americans and that there should be no discrimination with respect to access to the finest health care America has to offer based on a person's ability to pay for such care."[20]

Medicare is organized into two sections: Part A and Part B. Part A is available to the disabled and to individuals age 65 and over who are eligible for Social Security or Railroad Retirement. It provides insurance toward the cost of hospitalization. Medicare clients pay a deductible amount and have co-payment responsibilities. In 1990, Medicare's single annual deductible increased to $592, a cost the clients must pay out of their own pockets.[13] When the deductible has been paid, Medicare then pays most of the remaining hospital bills for that year. Medicare Part B is voluntary. It provides partial coverage for physician services to those eligible for Part A coverage, on payment of a monthly premium.

When Medicare was instituted, its purpose was to assist the elderly during periods of acute, episodic illness, rather than provide comprehensive health care coverage. As such, Medicare does not cover dental visits, dentures, eyeglasses, hearing aids, or examinations to prescribe or fit them. Similarly, preventive care, such as routine physical examinations, or diagnostic tests related to routine physical examinations are not covered. In 1989, approximately 95 percent of individuals over age 65 were enrolled in Medicare. In 1989, Medicare paid $99.9 billion for health services, which is an 11.4 percent increase and the largest annual increase since 1983.[21]

Despite cost-containment measures, experts predict that the amount of money paid for Medicare recipients will continue to spiral upward. This is largely because of growth in the eligible population. HCFA projects that in the year 2050, there will be 69 million people over the age of 65 eligible for Medicare, compared to the 33 million covered in 1988.[13] In spite of these payments for Medicare recipients and supplemental co-insurance plans held by some elderly, the average annual out-of-pocket expenditure for the elderly is $1000, more than their total average expenditure before Medicare was enacted.[22]

Medicaid is a financial aid program designed to provide medical assistance to low-income persons who are aged, disabled, blind, or members of families with dependent children. The program is jointly sponsored by the federal and state governments. The federal government established broad guidelines for the operation of the program and provides matching funds to states that meet the guidelines. Although these guidelines mandate certain basic services, states have wide latitude in determining eligibility and benefit criteria. Therefore, states can limit access to services by the way they define eligibility criteria. Currently, only 40 percent of the population with incomes below the poverty level is covered by Medicaid.[13,17] Moreover, reimbursement levels to providers are low.[23] In California, for example, they are so low that many hospitals choose not to contract with the state to provide services.[17] Fewer than 10 states reimburse physicians according to insurance company standards for usual, customary, and reasonable fees.[24]

The Department of Veteran Affairs (DVA) provides medical care and all related health care services to approximately 28.5 million individuals who have served in the armed services. DVA operates medical centers, over 200 clinics, and 100 nursing homes that provide general acute care and long-term care for veterans. In fiscal year 1987, the government spent approximately $9.7 billion providing medical care to those eligible.[25] It was projected that the VA health care expenditure for 1990 would be more than $18 billion.[26]

■ CURRENT ISSUES AND TRENDS IN HEALTH CARE

As the foregoing discussion makes clear, the health care system in the United States is not meeting the health care needs of all its citizens, despite constantly increasing expenditures. Growth in spending persists and is forecast to continue even in the face of efforts by government, businesses, and health care agencies to control costs. The percentage of the gross national product (GNP) spent on health care in 1989 was 11.6 percent. It is predicted to reach 15 percent of the GNP by the year 2000.[14] Per capita expenses are currently in excess of $2100 per year.[13] In 1990, health spending accounted for 14 percent of the federal budget and the Congressional Budget Office has projected that 19.5 percent will go to health spending by 1996.[14] The Medicare budget is the fastest growing among government programs; its growth rate exceeds that of the defense budget.[27]

Despite all of this spending, there are major barriers even to basic care for many Americans. These include lack of health care facilities in some regions, inadequate transportation, and lack of insurance or ineligibility for government programs resulting in the inability to pay.[14–19,28,29] According to Enthoven and Kronick, the present system of financing health care in the United States is inflationary, unfair and wasteful; a paradox of excesses and deprivation.[30] Expensive, high-tech diagnosis and treatments are available to some, while others have no care at all.[15,18,19,28] Thus, despite the exceptionally high level of spending for health care in the United States, health outcomes such as infant mortality rates and life expectancy at birth are no better than outcomes in other industrialized countries that spend substantially less on health care.[14,31] For instance, per capita expenditures on health are nearly 40 percent greater in the United States than they are in Canada and more than double those in Japan, yet both Japan and Canada have comparable or better health outcomes than the United States.[14,32]

Clearly, it is time for creative and concerted efforts by concerned individuals and groups to bring about change. The following sections explore conditions that have contributed to this state of crisis, adaptations that have occurred in the health care system in response, and proposals for further change. The final section of the chapter examines implications of the current health care situation for nurses.

Pressures for Change

The circumstances that have led to the present problems in health care, including the fragmented system of health care financing, changing patterns of health and disease, rising consumer expectations, and advances in technology are creating pressures for change in the health care delivery system.

Fragmented Health Care Financing. Health care financing in the United States has evolved incrementally without a plan or theme, in response to perceived needs and problems over the course of history. There are now multiple methods of billing and paying for health care and many possibilities for overlap and manipulation among them. According to Enthoven and Kronick,[30] health care in the United States today is dominated by fee-for-service payment to physicians, third-party payers (the insurance system, including the government) motivated to conserve their funds, and consumers who are largely unaware of costs. Each of these elements has contributed to the steadily rising cost of care and to limited access to care for certain segments of the population because of the lack of a focused plan for allocation of resources.

The fee-for-service payment system as it operates in the United States permits providers to set their own fee schedules.[14] Payers, particularly those representing large groups, can negotiate with individual providers for discounted fees. One consequence of this system is that different consumers may be charged markedly different prices for a given service, even by one provider. Third-party payers (insurance companies) reimburse providers based on the provider's fee schedule subject to the limitations set by state insurance commissioners. Medicare reimbursement for hospital care is an exception; the DRG prospective payment system controls that.

One advantage of the fee-for-service system is that it has provided consumers an opportunity to choose their own physician and type of coverage. Because Americans place a high value on freedom of choice, the fee-for-service system has persisted despite many flaws. Principal among these is that it encourages increased use of services, especially inpatient and other costly services.[14,19]

In a fee-for-service system, the more services used, the more money made. Physicians tend to prescribe more services when costs are at least partially paid by insurance than they would were clients paying out of pocket. Consumers visit physicians more frequently and agree to elective, sometimes marginally beneficial procedures when health insurance reimbursements reduce out-of-pocket costs. Few consumers comparison shop for health care or pay providers directly. They are frequently unaware of the actual costs of services and often think of the costs of health care only in terms of their own personal expenditures, especially if their coverage is an employee benefit. In this scenario, everyone seems to win—physicians and hospitals who make more money, and consumers who feel well cared for at what seems like reasonable cost.

Eventually, however, high use reimbursed by insurance drives up insurance premiums. High insurance costs are the main reason large numbers of citizens today are uninsured or inadequately insured. To be able to afford the premiums, consumers and employers funding insurance must opt for plans with sizable deductibles and copayments and, often, limited coverage. Consumers with this marginal insurance, like the uninsured, have diminished access to health services, particularly for preventive care or early treatment of illness when the cost of care would be lower.[18,28] Others cannot obtain insurance because insurance companies, seeking to protect themselves from increased costs, often exempt from coverage those individuals and groups considered high risk; in effect, those who need insurance most.[14,15]

Administrative costs of multiple competitive insurance companies and government programs also add to costs of care. In fact, the United States spends 18 percent of its total health care expenditures on overhead costs, such as marketing, itemized billing, collecting premiums, risk assessment, and reviewing claims for validity.[16] These costs are a result of the fragmented financing system in the United States. In countries with national health insurance, administrative costs are significantly lower.[14,15]

Another phenomenon associated with this fragmented system of paying for health care is cost shifting. Cost shifting is a method used by health care facilities to recoup the cost of providing care to those who cannot pay. To balance expenses incurred from providing care without reimbursement, providers increase charges to third-party payers, who pass these expenses on to the consumers who pay for insurance. These increased costs, in turn, limit the coverage options consumers can afford.

Prospective payment and other cost control measures discussed in a later section have now made cost shifting difficult. Without cost shifting, care for the medically indigent is a significant liability for physicians and hospitals. This situation has led to "dumping." Dumping refers to the transfer of nonpaying individuals needing emergency care to public health care facilities. A federal law against transferring medically unstable emergency clients for economic reasons was passed in 1986, but variations of dumping still occur.[19] Additionally, some community hospitals, fearing excessive monetary losses related to the care of medically indigent clients, have closed their emergency rooms, eliminating one of the few means for many uninsured to receive care.[30]

The inability of DRGs and other prospective payment systems to contain costs of health care is another problem. One reason costs have not abated is the increased volume of services that occurred when prospective payment placed a limit on the fee that could be charged for each service.[33] Data collected by the Congressional Budget Office shows that although many hospitals are closing because of financial difficulties, hospital margins (total revenues minus total costs) have increased since 1970.[14] Moreover, physicians' incomes, which historically have risen faster than incomes of many other groups, rose 10 percent in 1989.[13] There has also been a trend toward increased use of ambulatory care facilities, which peaked in 1988 when the number of outpatient visits (many to hospital outpatient departments) increased by 10 percent.[13] These facts, coupled with a 17 percent annual increase in charges for Medicare, Part B (the part that pays physicians), suggests service shifting. That

BUILDING NURSING KNOWLEDGE

What Can Be Done to Address the Needs of the Medically Indigent?

Murphy EK. Health care: Right or privilege? *Nurs Econ.* 1986; 4(2):66–68.

Statistics show that about 36 million Americans are uninsured or underinsured for health care. The medically indigent include those unqualified for various public programs, high-risk groups who cannot obtain insurance, and the underinsured. In one state, 65 percent of the medically indigent were families with incomes under $10,000; 10 percent were unemployed; and 25 percent were children under 18.

Murphy notes that the United States has always distributed health care funds with full knowledge that some people could not afford necessary medical attention. However, this effect has been tempered in the past by tax subsidies for public institutions, by welfare programs, by providers shifting costs from insured patients to cover the cost of the uninsured, and by charity care. This system is now under strain because of cuts in government health care budgets, reduction of charity by individual providers, and the effect of prospective payment. Unfortunately, the numbers of medically indigent are rising.

Murphy emphasizes that nurses can help alleviate this situation through an extension of the profession's historical emphasis on cost-effectiveness. Murphy states that nurses should lobby for and engage in clinical evaluations of the cost-effectiveness of health care practices. She points out that on the basis of their clinical research, nurses can help legislators avoid cutbacks in areas that have serious health implications. Murphy also states that nurses should be more visible in representing the medically indigent in the public policy arena.

is, many services previously offered in inpatient settings are now provided in ambulatory settings instead as a means of avoiding the prospective payment constraints on billing for inpatient care.

It seems apparent that controlling only one component of the health care delivery system invites increased costs in the segments that are not controlled. The government response has been to add a new element of control. To curb the growing escalation in physician costs, the Omnibus Budget Reconciliation Act (OBRA) of 1990 restricts substantially Medicare reimbursements for physician services.[34]

As this discussion emphasizes, a basic problem with health care financing in the United States is the lack of a sound plan. Rather than determining in advance what proportion of the national budget to spend on health care, costs are totalled at the end of each year. Each year, the costs climb. Furthermore, there is no real assessment of the effectiveness of dollars spent and therefore no plan for apportionment of expenditures to achieve the best possible health care outcomes.[15] The result is runaway expenditures for some types of service and inadequate funding for others.

Changing Patterns of Health and Disease. A decline in the death rate and a corresponding increase in longevity are having a significant impact on needs for health services. The 19th and early 20th centuries saw a tremendous improvement in longevity as people became aware of the importance of proper nutrition and sanitation. Antibiotics were introduced. Infant death rates fell significantly. Advances in technology and treatment technique curtailed the impact of infectious diseases and other illnesses that often claimed the lives of young adults. Fifty years ago young adults began to survive solely because of advances in medical treatment that were not available to the generation before them. These young adults are now grandparents and great-grandparents.

People in the United States today, including the elderly, can anticipate an increased life expectancy. Adults 65 years old in 1985 could expect to live another 16.7 years, to a life expectancy of 81.7 years. Those 75 years of age in 1985 could expect to live an additional 10.6 years, and those 85 and older in 1985, another 6.0 years.[35] In 1985, for the first time in US history, the number of persons over the age of 65 exceeded the number under the age of 18.[36] Between 1990 and 2010, the number of people 65 and older is projected to increase by at least 7 million, and the number of people between 15 and 44 years of age could decrease by 9 million.[37] Men and women 85 and older constitute the fastest growing age group in the United States.[35]

The shift in population has affected both the cost and the type of health care provided. The elderly have the greatest demands for expensive, long-term care for chronic, degenerative diseases. Fifty percent of all acute care admissions are for persons over age 75; 45 percent of critical care beds are filled by persons over 65.[38] Seventy-seven percent of Medicare costs are incurred by elderly clients in the last 6 months of their lives.[39] It has been predicted that in 2040, the elderly will make up 29 percent of the population and account for 45 percent of total health care expenditures.[35]

There also exists an increased demand for treatment of disorders related to societal problems. A variety of problems related to the social environment afflict people to a degree not seen by previous generations. For example, eating disorders such as anorexia nervosa and bulimia are all considered by many professionals to be physical manifestations of emotional problems related to the social environment. Alcoholism and drug abuse, previously thought to be indicators of personality disorders or character defects, are now recognized as disorders that require professional intervention as are child abuse and abuse of the elderly. Contemporary health care is challenged to treat clients with these disorders and to prevent underlying problems through health education.

Escalating numbers of clients with acquired immunodeficiency syndrome (AIDS) is another challenge affecting needs for health care. There is a growing concern that the costs of caring for persons with AIDS will overwhelm the system and compromise care needed by other segments of the population.[15] As of early 1990, more than 132,000 cases of AIDS had been reported to the Centers for Disease Con-

IMPLICATIONS FOR NURSE–CLIENT COLLABORATION

Mutual Interaction

The mutual interaction model for client care discussed in Chapter 37 and throughout this text directly addresses the trend for health consumers to participate in the health care decisions that affect their health and well-being. The mutual interaction model proposes that nurse–client interaction is most beneficial when it is collaborative. In collaborative interaction, nurses and clients join together and influence each other in making decisions about the client's health care.

trol.[40] The 1992 total is expected to be 192,000 cases.[41] Because many persons with AIDS lose their jobs and are denied private insurance coverage, Medicaid is assuming a heavy share of the cost burden for their care. In 1986, $2.3 billion was spent on AIDS; in 1992, the total is expected to be $47 billion.[42]

Rising Consumer Expectations. In 1945, President Truman proposed an "Economic Bill of Rights" in a special message to Congress. In this message he stated that the American people had "the right to adequate medical care and to the opportunity to achieve and enjoy good health." President Truman also stated his belief that every US citizen should have the right "to adequate protection from the economic fears . . . of sickness."[43]

The concept of a "right to health care" has become a fundamental belief of many Americans. It has led to rising expectations on the part of the public regarding the proper governmental role in the health care system. Many believe that the government should provide health care to all, regardless of ability to pay.

Furthermore, American consumers' expectations for health care now encompass prevention as well as treatment of illness. Many consumers are well informed about healthy life-styles and take more responsibility for their own health than consumers in the past. They are also more familiar with advances in health care technology, so when they become ill, they expect the best the system has to offer and are ready to play an active role in treatment decisions. They expect prompt treatment with no barriers to care. Since under the current system, many US consumers have substantial freedom to choose among insurance packages, providers, and treatment alternatives, these preferences are probably responsible, in part, for the high health care spending in this country.[13,14]

Besides having specific preferences for their own health care, Americans also have high expectations for the nation's health care system as a whole. The increasingly obvious inability of the system to meet the health care needs of its population has led to increasing public dissatisfaction with both the quality and costs of care.[31,44] Americans are also critical of physicians, attributing costs and availability of care to their influence.[45] In a study of satisfaction with health care in 10 countries, US respondents were the most dissatisfied with their health care system. Sixty percent indicated that fundamental changes are needed; 29 percent that the system needs complete rebuilding.[46]

One way that consumers are showing their dissatisfaction is by suing practitioners for malpractice. The incidence of malpractice litigation is increasing. As a consequence, health care providers are faced with higher malpractice insurance rates, which like any other component of health care costs are passed along to consumers. In 1988, providers spent $5 billion on malpractice insurance, directly accounting for 0.9 percent of all health spending for that year.[14] Many physicians practice "defensive medicine" to protect themselves against claims of negligence, ordering extra diagnostic studies, for example, which also drives up health care costs. Another consequence of the prohibitive costs of malpractice is the decision of many physicians to leave specialties with high litigation rates, such as obstetrics, or to leave private practice to work for organizations that offer employer-paid insurance premiums.

Advances in Technology. There is a bias in this country toward high technology, even without scientific evidence of superior results.[15] Whereas in most industries, managers and executives expect technology to provide a better product at a lower price, health care technology is a significant factor in runaway health care costs.[47] The development, purchase, and use of high-technology equipment all increase health care costs.

Research and development costs for new technologies are significant. In 1989, $10.2 billion in public funds and considerably more from private sources was spent on medical research.[14] Since health care research funds are becoming more difficult to obtain in the face of general budgetary problems in the United States, preferential spending to develop high-technology equipment can adversely affect progress on other health-related research, such as effective treatment for AIDS and resistant forms of cancer.

When new technology becomes available, there is great incentive to spend whatever it takes to obtain it. Hospitals see new technology as a welcome opportunity to elevate their standing in the community, an inducement in recruiting high-status specialized physicians, and a means of attracting clients. Because there are neither data nor guidelines for establishing the clinically necessary supply of specific technologies, there is no plan or limitation on their growth.[14] The competition for status and clients frequently leads to duplication of costly equipment in a given geographic area. Excess capacity can then lead to overuse of technologies. That this occurs is strongly supported by studies showing that a substantial portion of certain high-technology medical procedures performed are not clinically indicted.[14] Overuse leads to unnecessary exposure of clients to risks and side effects as well as to excess costs, as most insurance policies reimburse for diagnostic tests or procedures that are not considered experimental.

There are less obvious costs caused by implementation of technology. Technology is often used to extend life, but does not necessarily restore health or functional capacity.

Heaney[48] contends that for many physicians, prolonging life (or defeating death) is the ultimate purpose of medicine, and therefore they do not address difficult questions about quality of life. He suggests that a more responsible approach requires that these questions be primary for justifying all medical intervention, but in particular, the use of expensive high-technology care. The added costs to clients and society of extending life without restoring functional capacity go substantially beyond monetary considerations.

Health Care System Adaptations

There have been efforts on the part of the various components of the US health care delivery system to stem rising costs, and integrate health promotion more fully into the mainstream of health care services. Other adaptations include strategies to attract consumers such as marketing services and offering a wider variety of services and service locations.

Cost Control Strategies. The government has used many strategies during the last two decades to stem the rising costs of health care. The complexity of the problem has challenged all efforts, however, and to date, the varied approaches have slowed but have not arrested the dramatic rate of cost escalation. Several representative approaches are discussed here.

Price Controls. Legislation establishing the prospective payment system for federally subsidized health care was the first significant attempt to set limits on the prices that providers could charge for services. A temporary freeze on physicians' fees was imposed during the mid 1980s, and again at the close of fiscal year 1990. Also, most states limit reimbursements to physicians and hospitals under the Medicaid program. The most recent federal price control strategy was enacted as part of the Omnibus Budget Reconciliation Act (OBRA) of 1990. OBRA 1990 limits payments for hospital outpatient services and establishes a fee schedule for physician services based on the resource-based relative value scale (RBRVS).[49] This system uses the relative value of the resources used to provide the services as the basis for setting maximum allowable fees. Allowable fees for some procedures will be reduced as much as 15 percent. Price limits have not generally been as effective as desired because, typically, more services are provided when allowable prices are reduced, or more expensive services are substituted if all services are not uniformly controlled. Cost shifting, discussed above, also dilutes the efficacy of price controls.

Regulation of Market Services. Market regulation sets prescriptions, for example, on quality of services, who may provide services, and who must receive services. Some of these prescriptions have been applied to the entire health care market, rather than only the segment funded by the government. The law mentioned previously that prohibits patient "dumping" is an example. Other restrictions have been applied only to those programs receiving federal support. Health planning, in effect from 1974 to 1986, was an attempt to limit the expansion and proliferation of health care facilities and high-technology equipment; however, it was judged to be ineffective and, therefore, dropped. Some experts maintain that regulation can be very effective in containing costs, citing successes in other countries as examples.[50]

Competition. In the late 1970s, proposals to reduce restrictions on health care delivery and promote free market competition among providers and insurers were introduced with the expectation that competition would result in downward pressures on prices and greater efficiency in providing health care. (See also Chap. 36.) Encouraging competition led to the opening of urgent care centers and walk-in clinics and to advertising by physicians and other providers. For many reasons that discussed in Chapter 36, free enterprise does not operate in the health care industry as it does in more highly market-oriented industries. Some research suggests that greater competition has led to higher rather than lower costs.[14] Although some authorities feel that it is too soon to judge the effectiveness of the competition strategy, others feel it has been even less successful in containing health care expenditures than earlier regulatory attempts.[12,51]

Alternative Insurance Delivery Systems. The development and spread of insurance alternatives such as HMOs, PPOs, and group self-insurance have had a substantial effect on the insurance market. Although HMOs, that is, combined insurance delivery systems, have existed since the 1930s, federal legislation that mandated employers to include an HMO option in all employee benefit packages led to significant expansion in the numbers of HMOs and the options they offer. HMOs can offer services at substantially lower premiums because they have more control over use of services and the decisions of contracted providers. Preferred provider organizations (PPOs), like HMOs, achieve savings by directing consumers to specific providers contracted to provide care at predetermined cost-effective prices. PPOs contract with networks of private or group practice providers. The federal government currently uses HMOs and PPOs to provide care for some Medicare and Medicaid clients in an effort to curtail costs.[13]

Group self-insurance plans are those in which a group, usually a corporation with many employees, a consortium of similar smaller companies, or a union, assumes all or part of the responsibility for processing and paying health care claims for group members, rather than paying premiums to an insurance company for those services. Since self-insurance plans are exempt from certain premium taxes and fees that insurance companies must pay, they are usually able to provide employee coverage at less cost to the company than insurance companies.

Managed Care. **Managed care** refers to plans that coordinate a broad range of client services and monitor care to assure that it is appropriate and provided in the most efficient and inexpensive way.[13] Its thrust is intervening in the decisions made by providers of care in order to ensure that only necessary services are provided.[14] HMOs and PPOs are examples of managed care plans as are a variety of free-for-service plans. Many insurers currently operating under traditional reimbursement models have made commitments to develop and use comprehensive managed care plans because of their cost-saving benefits. Some health care providers see managed care plans as a means of restricting client options and saving insurers money;[28] however, managed care can be an effective means of meeting clients' health needs and saving costs if structured with those goals in mind.

One means of making managed care client oriented as well as cost conscious is by using **case managers.** Case managers assess clients' overall needs for different health services, delineate comprehensive client outcomes, identify and procure the most cost-effective means of meeting these outcomes, and evaluate the effectiveness of the procured services. Case managers oversee the complete episode of a client's care from preadmission through rehabilitation. There are many different models of case management; often, selection of a particular model depends on the setting. HMOs, acute- and extended-care facilities, and community health settings use case management.[52–57] Several different health care professionals are qualified to be case managers. Nurses, social workers, and physicians are the most common. Case managers in private practice offer services to individuals and families.[52] Agencies using case management report increased client and provider satisfaction, as well as significant cost savings.[53–55]

Alternative Professional Providers. Many of the primary care services traditionally provided by physicians are now being offered by alternative professional providers, such as nurse practitioners, certified nurse-midwives, and clinical nurse specialists. Their services include physical examination, diagnostic screening, and teaching, as well as traditional health care treatment. Care by nurse practitioners is high in quality, less expensive, and well accepted by clients. Researchers have evaluated the professional competence of nurse practitioners as compared with that of internists and family physicians in the areas of cost effectiveness, quality of treatment plans, diagnostic studies, prescription errors, consultant referrals, and treatment errors. In all areas, performance of the nursing personnel was found to be at least equal in quality to that of the physician groups studied.[58] Nurse practitioners, certified nurse-midwives, and clinical nurse specialists are now eligible for direct reimbursement for certain care under Medicare, Medicaid, and the Federal Employees Federal Health Benefits Program.[59]

Health Promotion. Preventive care and health promotion have significant potential to maximize individuals' well-being, reduce social ills, and decrease trauma from chronic disease. The US health care system is beginning to act on the general consensus among health care practitioners that merely curing disease does not guarantee health. Preventive care and health education have become a noticeable part of the total health care delivery system. There also is a trend toward interdisciplinary collaboration and teamwork in health promotion. Many hospitals, ambulatory care facilities, and community health centers offer health education about life-style changes to promote health and strategies to prevent specific illnesses.

Community centers have developed health awareness programs focused on the aging process. Adult day care centers offer nutritional counseling, mental health services, exercise classes, and social activities to ambulatory individuals (Fig. 35–6). These centers provide a caretaker staff to supervise activities and provide support for individuals who have no serious health problems but are unable to remain at home without assistance or social diversion when other family members are away at work.

Wellness centers whose only mission is health promotion are recognized as part of the contemporary health care system. Their popularity stems from greater consumer awareness about health and clients' motivation to seek providers who can support and promote their efforts to make life-style changes to improve and maintain their health.

Employer-sponsored wellness programs are a health promotion strategy that has demonstrated cost-reduction effectiveness as well.[18] These on-site programs offer services such as wellness counseling, risk assessment, exercise programs, and stress management classes.

Strategies to Attract Consumers. Increased awareness about options for care on the part of health care recipients

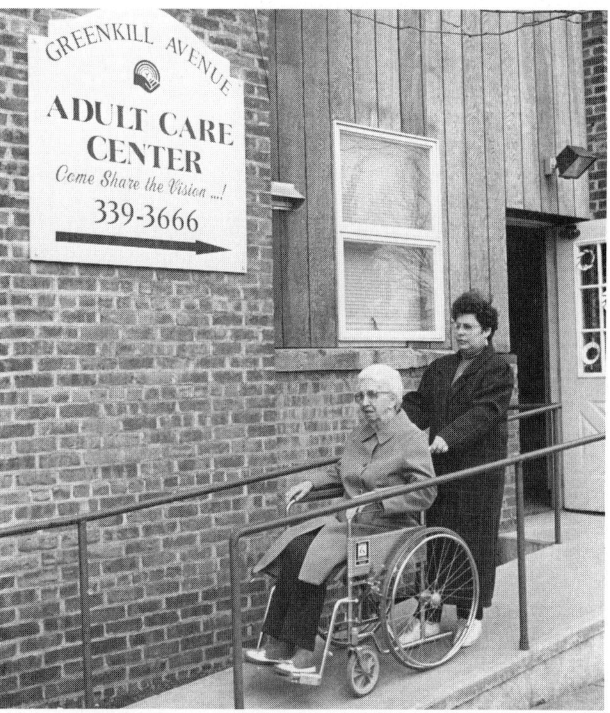

Figure 35–6. Trends in health care: an adult day care center.

has been accelerated by a marketing revolution in the health care industry. Hospitals have begun to advertise their services in daily newspapers and on television. Discount coupons for new community emergency centers appear in newspapers. Insurance plans are advertised with increasing frequency and are often promoted with celebrity endorsements. Health-related programs are now commonplace on both public and commercial television, and health-care products are advertised and promoted by celebrities. The mass media point out the problems associated with the misuse of drugs and dangers of defective health care products and certain forms of alternative treatment.

Intensified cost-containment efforts have prompted both hospitals and private health care agencies to target their services and their marketing to specific groups of consumers. Delivery of a specific service to a target group is believed to be cost effective, because it allows specialization and promotes the efficient use of resources. In one such plan a hospital attracts senior citizens by agreeing to pay the deductible on their Medicare insurance plan. Other facilities that often market to target groups are birthing centers, free-standing cancer care centers, wellness centers, pain control clinics, alcohol and drug abuse facilities, and rehabilitation centers.

Providers are offering more types and locations of services to consumers. Ambulatory care services such as birthing centers, surgicenters, and urgent care centers are relatively recent developments in health care. They serve a dual purpose of attracting consumers and avoiding fee limitations imposed by the DRG program. The Medicare prospective payment system has resulted in earlier discharges from acute care settings, often before clients are ready to assume independent self-care. As a consequence, many home care services—some affiliated with hospitals, others independent businesses—now exist to serve these clients. Medicare, Medicaid, and many major insurance companies provide coverage for home care.

Holistic health and alternative care providers have become more prominent in contemporary health care. Holistic health first gained public attention in the 1960s (see Chap. 5). Holistic health advocates view individuals as composites of physical, emotional, social, and spiritual components. For an individual to be in a state of health, each component must be functioning at its optimal level and in harmony with the whole. Holism emphasizes self-care, self-responsibility for health, and life-style approaches that enhance balance, centeredness, and serenity. Advocates of a holistic health philosophy prefer to use natural therapies, rather than invasive or chemical substances.

Alternative health care encompasses approaches further from Western medical philosophy. Techniques such as polarity therapy, reflexology, acupuncture, and herbal medicine have become increasingly popular. A discussion of specific alternative therapies is beyond the scope of this text; however, readers are encouraged to pursue further understanding of holistic and alternative health care to enhance their sensitivity to consumers who value these approaches.

These adaptations in the health care delivery system have not had the desired level of success in containing costs, satisfying consumers, or in improving access to care. Experts believe that without significant further changes, it is unlikely that the United States can achieve much greater control over spending or better address the needs of those who are underinsured than was evident in the 1980s.[14] There is a growing national demand for universal access to basic hospital and physician services, and growing speculation that some form of policy change to achieve it will be made in the 1990s.[60,61] Policy makers are currently considering various policy alternatives for the reform of US health care. Political candidates, moreover, are making health care reform one of the major issues in state and national election campaigns.

The key issue for health care in the 1990s is what role the federal and state governments will play in achieving the goal of health care access for all. The options for government involvement can be viewed on a continuum.[62] At one end is the laizzez-faire approach, unworkable in today's environment, in which the private sector—providers, technology and pharmaceutical suppliers, and the private insurance industry—handles the problems of delivery and distribution by charging prices that the market will bear and by giving free services to the indigent. At the other end is the option of a unified, government-run, national health insurance program. National health insurance, as yet untried in the US, is usually envisioned as a single, comprehensive, compulsory program financed through taxation that is made available to all citizens regardless of ability to pay. Such a program, if put into place, could be modeled after the Canadian system of national health insurance, described in Chap. 37, and would represent a radical restructuring of US health care. In between are various options for reworking the current system. These generally combine the resources of the private and public sectors in government programs designed to subsidize private health insurance for the underinsured and those without insurance or to expand health care coverage in existing government programs that target vulnerable populations. Such mixed programs are compatible with the pluralistic environment of American health care and with the traditional American preference for incremental change and democratic compromise. Nursing's approach can be viewed as a mixed or pluralistic approach.

Because it is likely that the debate on health care reform will occupy the political spotlight for some time to come, it is important that readers understand the various options being entertained, and particularly the plan proposed by nursing.

Nursing's Agenda for National Health Care Reform

The agenda for health care reform developed under the auspices of the American Nurses' Association (ANA) proposes significant change while preserving and building on the best elements of the existing US health care system.[63] This proposal is designed to achieve the goal of universal access. It has the endorsement of more than 40 nursing specialty organizations and several nonnursing, health-care related groups. Key features of this agenda include enhanced access to care by delivering primary care in community-based settings, emphasis on personal responsibility for individual health based on informed decision making, use of the most cost-effective providers, and a "Healthstart Plan" (on the concept of Headstart in education) that focuses on underserved, vulnerable populations.

The premises of nursing's agenda for change are the following:

- All citizens must have equitable access to essential health care services.
- Primary health care services must play a very basic and prominent role in service delivery.
- Consumers must be the central focus of the health care system. Assessment of health care needs must be the determining factor in the ultimate structuring and delivery of programs and services. Health care professionals must work in partnership with consumers to evaluate the full range of consumer needs and available services.
- Consumers must be guaranteed direct access to a full range of qualified health care providers who offer their services in a variety of delivery arrangements at community-based sites such as schools, workplaces, and homes which are accessible, convenient, and familiar to the consumer.
- Consumers must assume more responsibility for their own care and become better informed about the range of providers and the potential options for services. Working in partnership with providers, consumers must actively participate in choices that best meet their needs.
- Health care services must be restructured to create a better balance between the prevailing orientation toward illness and cure and a new commitment to wellness and care.
- The health care system must assure that appropriate, effective care is delivered through the efficient use of resources.
- A standardized package of essential health care services must be provided and financed through an integration of public and private plans and sources.
- Mechanisms must be implemented to protect consumers against catastrophic costs and impoverishment.[63]

Nursing's plan advocates a central role for the federal government in the form of federal minimum standards for essential services and federally defined eligibility requirements. At the same time it advocates decentralized decision making to permit local areas to develop specific programs best suited to local consumer needs. The cornerstone of the plan is to reform the delivery of primary health care services to households and individuals in convenient, familiar places. The essential services advocated by nursing are summarized in Box 35–2.

Financing mechanisms envisioned under nursing's plan include a public insurance plan administered by the states to provide coverage to the poor (those below 200 percent of the poverty level), high-risk populations, and the potentially medically indigent. Any employer or individual also would have the option of buying into this plan as their source of coverage. Private plans, employer-based benefit programs, and commercial health insurance covering the rest of the population would be required to offer, at a minimum, the nationally standardized package of essential services—a package that could be enriched by employer or individual purchase of additional services. Both public and private plans would use deductibles and co-payments to provide consumers with financial incentives for economy in their use of services, but limits would be placed on out-of-pocket payments for catastrophic illnesses (illnesses of unusual length and intensity). Nursing's agenda also ad-

BOX 35–2. KEY ELEMENTS OF NURSING'S AGENDA FOR HEALTH CARE REFORM

Services Covered

- Primary health care, hospital care, emergency treatment, inpatient and outpatient professional services, home care, hospice care, long-term care for a limited period, restorative services to prevent long-term institutionalization, mental health and substance abuse treatment and rehabilitation.
- Prevention services, including prenatal and perinatal care; well-child care; school-based disease prevention programs; speech therapy, dental, hearing, and eye care for children under 18; routine health screening procedures with proven effectiveness.
- Prescription drugs, medical supplies and equipment, laboratory and radiology services.
- Long-term care services of relatively short duration.

Coverage Options

- A public plan to be administered by states will provide coverage for anyone whose income is less than 200 percent of the poverty level and for high-risk populations. Any individual or employer can buy into this plan.
- Private plans (including employment-based health benefit programs and commercial plans) must match the nationally standardized plan, but may offer additional services.

Cost-reduction Strategies

- Use of alternate providers
- Consumer involvement in assessment of personal health care needs and treatments.
- Multidisciplinary clinical practice guidelines.
- State and local review bodies for resource allocation.
- Managed care and case management.

Sources of Revenue

- Consumer cost sharing.
- Employer health benefits.
- State governments.
- Alcohol and tobacco taxes, additional payroll taxes, raised or eliminated ceiling for FICA tax, possible value-added tax.

Box compiled from American Nurses' Association. *Nursing's Agenda for Health Care Reform.* Washington, DC: ANA Publishing; 1991.

vocates strengthened private insurance programs and innovative financing arrangements for long-term care.

Cost-containment measures in the nursing agenda include state and local review bodies from public and private sectors composed of payers, providers, and consumers operating under federal guidelines. Managed care is advocated to reduce costs and assure consumer access, along with case management for coordinating cost-effective caregiving to individuals, and wider use of a range of qualified health professionals, particularly in primary health care and in underserved regions to improve health care access.

Nursing's plan thus calls for implementation of universal coverage through combining public and private resources. Nurses are well positioned to assist in fulfilling the workforce needs for the expansion of services that universal access will require. As the next section emphasizes, nurses also can play a major role in achieving nursing's agenda for health care reform.

Implications for Nursing

The current state of the health care delivery system in the United States and the climate for change have many implications for nurses and nursing. How effectively nurses address issues such as access to care, collaboration with clients and other health professionals, cost and reimbursement for care, the current shortage of nurses, nursing education and research, and political activism will determine the future of nursing practice and its role in the health care delivery system.

Facilitating Access to Care. Access to care is the fundamental issue underlying the call for a national health insurance program. Nurses can contribute to improved access to care in several ways. Nurses with advanced practice credentials have demonstrated their ability to provide quality and cost-effective care in many ambulatory care settings that have traditionally relied upon more expensive physician care.[18,28] Lucille Joel, president of the American Nurses' Association (ANA), in remarks about new laws permitting direct reimbursement for nurses stated: "By enlarging the pool of providers, more people will have access to the health care system, and complications can be discovered in their early stages." (p. 34)[59] Other nursing leaders point out, however, that access to care does not assure use. Often creative outreach programs are necessary to make consumers aware that health services are available and to show them how these programs can help them.[18,63] Nurses, particularly community health nurses, could be instrumental in such efforts. In fact, some authorities believe that nurses are better able to serve certain client populations, such as the poor, the disadvantaged, and those from minority cultures, than physicians because nurses typically are less intimidating and better able to relate to these individuals.[64,65]

Nursing case managers in both inpatient and outpatient settings have been effective in promoting client access to the appropriate, cost-effective health care services. Several of the policy proposals for health care reform recommend universal case management. If implemented, nurses will have an opportunity to expand their professional roles, experience greater personal satisfaction, and improve quality of care for more consumers.

Greater Need for Collaboration. Health promotion and prevention, requisites for efficient, cost-effective health care services, demand client collaboration. Collaboration requires informed, involved consumers. Nurses, as the single largest health care provider group and the group with the most sustained contact with clients, have opportunities and responsibilities to use their communication and teaching skills to facilitate clients' collaboration in their care.

Some leaders in nursing and medicine have advocated nursing joint practice with physicians, through case management or other models.[56,57,66,67] Joint practice provides more effective care delivery and better use of resources and enhances job satisfaction.[66,67] This kind of collaboration also reduces conflict between physicians and nurses as both become more focused on client outcomes than on protecting their own "turf."[68] These outcomes are benefits as the health care system is operating today, and would be equally beneficial in a reformed system.

Cost and Reimbursement Issues. The advent of DRGs created an opportunity to identify the cost of nursing care.[17,27] Using the DRG patient classification system or modifications of it as a basis for comparison, nursing managers or consultants track and analyze nursing care hours. This process has been useful for several reasons. The analysis is a means of measuring nursing resources and productivity, both for staffing and budgetary considerations.[69,70] Attaching a monetary value to nursing services has also provided the ability to demonstrate that nursing generates revenue in health care facilities.[70,71] This is advantageous, considering the calls for setting practice standards to measure quality and efficiency of care. Moreover, it can provide a basis for extending direct reimbursement for nurses to care given in inpatient settings. Some nursing leaders feel this outcome is one means to achieve recognition for the nursing profession's autonomy and unique expertise.[18,70] Others cite the benefit to consumers, as it may serve to expand their options for cost-effective providers.

Assuring an Adequate Supply of Nurses. A gap between the supply and the demand for nurses has been growing for the past two decades. In 1988, the Secretary's Commission on Nursing officially documented the shortage and predicted a shortfall of 1 million nurses by the year 2000.[72] Most nursing leaders attribute the shortage to an increasing demand for nurses that has not been matched by numbers of new nurses entering the field. In light of goals to improve access to care through health policy changes, the demand for nurses can only be expected to escalate. The solution to the problem seems to lie in more efficient use of nurses and in empowering nurses to realize their full potential as members of the health care team.

Studies have alleged that nurses spend between 5 and

40 percent of their work time in tasks having nothing to do with nursing.[73–76] At a time when the need for nurses is so intense, restructuring of nurses' responsibilities can save cost, improve care, and increase nurses' job satisfaction.

It is the growing lack of job satisfaction that many believe is responsible for the numbers of nurses leaving the profession.[77] Insufficient autonomy, lack of respect from other providers, lack of opportunities for advancement, and inadequate resource allocation are among the reasons cited for nurses' dissatisfaction. Although advances such as direct reimbursement for nursing services and enhanced professional roles such as case management are improving many nurses' work environments, more changes still are needed. Nurses are intimately involved with the health of individuals. Although society has, in the past, placed a low value on health for all, proposed policy changes, discussed in Chap 37, promise to significantly improve access to health care. This creates an opportunity for nursing to gain the autonomy, respect, and resources it deserves through reemphasizing and actively demonstrating its commitment to health for all.

Changes in Nursing Education and Research. To support nursing's demands for autonomy in practice and an appropriate share of available resources, research is needed on comprehensive cost-benefit and cost-effectiveness analyses, the effects of technology and client care, evaluations of innovative client care delivery methods, and ethical issues related to the allocation of scarce resources.[78] Changes in the scope and focus of nursing education are also needed. In response to the growing numbers of nurse educators with master's, doctoral, and post-doctoral degrees, nursing curricula are becoming more sophisticated and diverse.[31] An understanding of economic concepts, the operation of the health care delivery system, and viable options for change is essential for nurses to achieve the role they desire in the health care system.[18,65]

Moreover, nurse educators need to model collegiality in their teaching approaches and emphasize greater self-responsibility for learning to enhance students' self-respect and independent thinking. Graduates with self-respect, who have learned collegial relationships, assertive communication skills, conflict management, and self-responsibility will be able to address successfully the critical issues facing nursing.[79] These skills, grounded on a foundation of caring, will enable nurses to be effective advocates for themselves and their clients.

Political Action to Influence Public Policy. Nursing's Agenda for Health Care Reform is an example of a public stand that unequivocally demonstrates the profession's value of health care for all. Unless all nurses actively and vocally support this document, the credibility of the profession is weakened. To gain the respect of health care colleagues, legislators, and the general public, nurses must back their words with action. This means communicating with legislators, seeking positions on policy-making boards, and engaging in informed dialogue with consumers and other health care providers.

SUMMARY

The US health care delivery system is a complex, fragmented system that is not yet meeting the needs of all of its citizens for care. Although health care is available in many different ambulatory and inpatient settings and from an increasing variety of providers, many citizens have inadequate access to care. The cost of care, whether paid directly by consumers, by employers, the government, or other third-party payers, continues to climb. Efforts such as prospective payment systems, increased government regulation, utilization review, alternative insurance delivery systems such as HMOs and PPOs, and alternative care delivery systems such as managed care and case management have failed to contain costs or improve access to care.

This climate has created impetus for policy changes that make care available to all. The nursing profession is among the groups that have offered a proposal for reforming the health care delivery system. Although this is an important step, difficult decisions about allocation of scarce resources will complicate the process of achieving consensus.

The nursing profession must be actively involved in the process of reforming the system. Nurses must make their vital role in health care known and act to attain an image commanding respect. Nursing as a profession has been gaining strength. Nurses must effectively use that strength to empower themselves and health care consumers to attain the goal of optimal health for all. The current climate of change provides opportunities for progressive nurses to advance progressive ideas.

REFERENCES

1. US Department of Commerce. Health and medical services. In: *US Industrial Outlook, 1991*. Washington, DC: US Govt Printing Office; 1991:1–6.
2. National Leadership Coalition for Health Care Reform. A comprehensive reform plan for the health care system, 1991:2. Cited in American Nurses' Association. *Nursing's Agenda for Health Care*. Kansas City, MO: ANA Publishing; 1991:7.
3. Donabedian A, Wheeler J, Wyszewianski L. An integrative model of quality, cost, and health. *Medical Care*, 1982;20(10). In: Pena JJ, Haffner AN, Rosen B, Light DW, eds. *Hospital Quality Assurance*. Rockville, MD: Aspen Systems Corp; 1984:66.
4. Oberst MT. Patients' perceptions of care. *Cancer*. 1984;53(10): 2366.
5. Patterson CH. Standards of patient care: The joint commission focus on nursing quality assurance. *Nurs Clin North Am*. 1988; 23(3):625–638.
6. Beyers M. Quality: The banner of the 1980's. *Nurs Clin North Am*. 1988;23(3).
7. Haffner AN, Jonas S, Pollack, B. Regulating the quality of pa-

tient care. In: Pena JJ, Haffner AN, Rosen B. Light DW, eds. *Hospital Quality Assurance.* Rockville, MD: Aspen Systems Corp; 1984:4.

8. Covell RM. The impact of regulation on health care quality. In: Levin A, ed. *Regulating Health Care: The Struggle for Control.* New York: Academy of Political Science; 1980:Vol. 30, No. 4, p. 133.
9. Department of Health and Human Services, Health Care Financing Administration. Medicare and Medicaid programs: Peer review organizations; final rules. *Fed Regis.* 1985;50(74): 15312–15330.
10. Koff S. *Health Systems Agencies: A Comprehensive Examination of Planning and Process.* New York: Human Sciences Press; 1988: 204–208.
11. Simpson R, Waite R. NCNIP's system of the future: A call for accountability, revenue control, and national data sets. *Nurs Admin Quart.* 1989;14(1):72–77.
12. Sampson LF. Economic perspective. In: Bertram DL, Wilson JL, eds. *Financial Management in Critical Care Nursing.* Baltimore: Williams and Wilkins; 1991:234–248.
13. Health Insurance Association of America. *Source Book of Health Insurance Data.* Washington, DC: Health Insurance Association of America; 1990.
14. Congress of the United States, Congressional Budget Office. *Rising Health Care Costs: Causes, Implications, and Strategies.* Washington, DC: US Govt Printing Office; 1991.
15. Starck PL. Health care under siege: Challenge for change. *Nurs Health Care.* 1990;12(1):26–30.
16. Woolhandler S, Himmelstein D. Resolving the cost/access conflict: The case for a national health program. *J Gen Intern Med.* 1989;4(1):54–60.
17. Gomez DS. Issues and trends: In: Bertram DL, Wilson JL, eds. *Financial Management in Critical Care Nursing.* Baltimore: Williams and Wilkins; 1991:264–274.
18. Johnson PA. A national health insurance program: A nursing perspective. *Nurs Health Care.* 1990;11(8):416–429.
19. Gaines BC. Health/illness care: Who pays? In: Lambert CF, Lambert VA, eds. *Perspectives in Nursing: The Impacts on the Nurse, the Consumer, and Society.* Norwalk, CT: Appleton & Lange; 1989:403–417.
20. US Congress, House Select Committee on Aging. *Medicare After 15 Years: Has it Become a Broken Promise to the Elderly?* Report before the Select Committee on Aging, the US House of Representatives, 96th Congress, 2nd session, November 1980:1.
21. Prospective Payment Assessment Commission. *Medicare Prospective Payment and the American Health Care System.* Report to the Congress. Washington, DC; June 1990:9–10.
22. Dimond M. Health care and the aging population. *Nurs Outlook.* 1989;37(2):76–77.
23. Thorpe K, Siegal J, Daily T. Including the poor: The fiscal impacts of Medicaid expansion. *JAMA.* 1989;261(7):1003–1007.
24. Friedman E. Medicare and Medicaid at 25. *Hospitals.* 1990; 64(15):38–34.
25. Cournoyer PR. The Veterans Administration's resource allocation system. *Nurs Clin North Am.* 1988;23(3):531–538.
26. Arnett RH. McCusick D, Sonnefeld S, Cowell C. *Health Care Financing Review.* Vol VII, No. 3: *Projections of Health Care Spending to 1990.* Washington, DC: US Department of Health and Human Services, Health Financing Administration, Spring 1986.
27. McGill P. Reimbursement analysis. In: Bertram DL, Wilson JL, eds. *Financial Management in Critical Care Nursing.* Baltimore: Williams and Wilkins; 1991:211–219.
28. American Nurses' Association. *Nursing's Agenda for Health Care.* Kansas City, MO: ANA Publishing; 1991:7.
29. Cardin S. Hospital organization. In: Bertram DL, Wilson JL, eds. *Financial Management in Critical Care Nursing.* Baltimore: Williams and Wilkins; 1991:249–263.
30. Enthoven A, Kronick R. A consumer-choice health plan for the 1990s, part I. *N Engl J Med.* 1989;320(1):29–37.
31. Moccia P. Toward the future. *Nursing Clinics of North America.* 1990;25(3):605–613.
32. Southby RF, Rakich JS. International healthcare expenditures. *Hosp Topics.* 1991;69(2):8–13.
33. Congress of the United States, Congressional Budget Office. *Physician Payment Reform Under Medicare.* Washington, DC: US Govt Printing Office; 1990.
34. Grimaldi PL. Congress slices medicare physician fees. *Nurs Manag.* 1991;22(1):22–24.
35. US Bureau of the Census. *Statistical Abstract of the United States: 1988,* 108th ed. Washington, DC. US Govt Printing Office; 1987: 72.
36. Callahan D. *Setting Limits: Medical Goals in an Aging Society.* New York: Simon & Schuster; 1987.
37. Spencer G. Projections of the population of the United States, by age, sex, and race: 1988 to 2080. In: Bureau of the Census. *Current Population Reports,* Series P-25, No. 1018. Washington, DC: US Govt Printing Office; 1989.
38. Disch JM. Future directions. In: Bertram DL, Wilson JL, eds. *Financial Management in Critical Care Nursing.* Baltimore: Williams and Wilkins; 1991:275–281.
39. Fulmer TT, Walker MK. Lessons from the elder boom in ICU's. *Geriatr Nurs.* 1990;7(3):23–27.
40. Zuercher A. A look at the latest AIDS projections. *Health Aff.* 1990;9(2):6–21.
41. Centers for Disease Control. *MMWR.* 1988;37:551–554.
42. Scitovsky AA. The economic impact of AIDS in the United States. *Health Aff.* 1988;7(4):32–35.
43. Sobel LA, ed. *Health Care: An American Crisis.* New York: Facts on File; 1976.
44. Blendon R. Three systems: A comparative survey. *Health Manag Quart.* 1989; First Quarter.
45. Hart P. National health issues: A report to the NLN Board of Governors, November, 1989. Cited in: Moccia P. Toward the future. *Nurs Clin North Am.* 1990;25(3):605–613.
46. Blendon RJ, Leitman R, Morrison I, Donelan K. Satisfaction with health care systems in ten nations. *Health Aff.* 1990;9(2): 185–192.
47. Frech HE. *Health Care in America.* San Francisco: Pacific Research Institute for Public Policy; 1988.
48. Heaney RP. Technological imperative and decision support. In: Lindeman CA, McAthie M, eds. *Nursing Trends and Issues.* Springhouse, PA: Springhouse Corp; 1990:303–307.
49. Grimaldi PL. Congress slices Medicare physician fees. *Nurs Manag.* 1991;22(1):22–24.
50. Reinhardt UE. Providing access to health care and controlling costs: Approaches abroad, options for US health care delivery. *Proceedings, ANNA Conference.* Washington, DC; April, 1990:1–17.
51. Evans RG, Lomas J, Barer M, et al. Controlling health expenditures—the Canadian reality. *N Engl J Med.* 1989;320(2):94–101.
52. Parker M, Secord LJ. Guiding the elderly through the health care maze. In: Lindeman CA, McAthie M, eds. *Nursing Trends and Issues.* Springhouse, PA: Springhouse Corp; 1990:271–274.
53. Knollmueller RN. Case management: What's in a name? *Nurs Manag.* 1989;20(10):38–41.

54. McKenzie CB, Torkelson NG, Holt MA. Care and cost: Nursing case management improves both. *Nurs Manag.* 1989;20(10):30–34.
55. McGill P. Reimbursement analysis. In: Bertram DL, Wilson JL, eds. *Financial Management in Critical Care Nursing.* Baltimore: Williams and Wilkins; 1991:211–220.
56. Zander K. Case management: A golden opportunity for whom? In: McClosky JC, Grace HK, eds. *Current Issues in Nursing.* St. Louis: CV Mosby; 1990:199–204.
57. Marriner-Tomey A. Assignment systems: The delivery of care in the acute care setting. In: Lambert CE Jr, Lambert VA, eds. *Perspectives in Nursing: The Impacts on the Nurse, the Consumer, and Society.* Norwalk, CT: Appleton & Lange; 1989: 81–92.
58. Light DW. Quality and competition. In: Pena JJ, Haffner AN, Rosen B. Light DW, eds. *Hospital Quality Assurance.* Rockville, MD: Aspen Systems Corp; 1984:135.
59. Sharp N. Direct reimbursement for nurses. *Nurs Manag.* 1991; 22(1):34–35.
60. Weil TP. The US healthcare system after NHI: Financial ramifications for providers and personnel. *Hosp Topics.* 1991;69(2): 36–40.
61. Curtain LL. Rube Goldberg and the great American healthcare system. Editorial opinion. *Nurs Manag.* 1991;22(5):9–11.
62. Kalish B, Kalish P. *The Politics of Nursing.* Philadelphia: JB Lippincott; 1982.
63. American Nurses' Association. *Nursing's Agenda for Health Care Reform.* Kansas City, MO: ANA Publishing; 1991.
64. Ginzberg E. *American Medicine: The Power Shift.* Totowa, New Jersey: Rowman & Allanheld; 1985.
65. Sweeney SS, Switt KE. Does nursing have the power to change the healthcare system? In: McClosky JC, Grace HK, eds. *Current Issues in Nursing.* St. Louis: CV Mosby; 1990:283–297.
66. Hamilton S. Collaborative practice is necessary in ICU. *Nurs Manag.* 1991;22(5):96J–96L.
67. Aiken LH, Mullinix CF. The nurse shortage: Myth or reality? *N Engl J Med.* 1987;317(10):641–645.
68. Ryan SA. A new decade of leadership: From vision to reality. *Nurs Clin North Am.* 1990;25(3):597–604.
69. Scherubel JC. Costing out nursing services. In: McClosky JC, Grace HK, eds. *Current Issues in Nursing.* St. Louis: CV Mosby; 1990:393–398.
70. Fralic MF, Brett JL. Nursing's newest mandate: The cost-quality imperative: In: McClosky JC, Grace HK, eds. *Current Issues in Nursing.* St. Louis: CV Mosby; 1990:398–404.
71. Trofino J. JACHO nursing standards: Nursing care hours and LOS per DRG—part II. *Nurs Manag.* 1989;20(1):33–35.
72. US Public Health Service, Office of the Secretary. *Secretary's Commission on Nursing: Final Report* (Vol. 1). Rockville, MD: The Division; 1988
73. Hamm-Vida DE. Cost of non-nursing tasks. *Nurs Manag.* 1990; 21(4):46–52.
74. Friedman E. Nursing: New power, old problems. *JAMA.* 1990; 264(23):2977–2982.
75. Watson PM, Lower MS, Wells SM, et al. Discovering what nurses do and what it costs. *Nurs Manag.* 1991;22(5):38–45.
76. Hay Group. *The Nursing Crisis.* Atlanta: Hay Group; 1989.
77. Hall JM, Stevens PE. The nursing shortage in the context of national health care. *Nurs Outlook.* 1991;39(2):69–72
78. Ingersol GL, Hoffort N, Schultz AW. Health services research in nursing: Current status and future directions. *Nurs Econ.* 1990;4:229–238.
79. Martin CE. A response from an educational perspective. *Nurs Clin North Am.* 1990;25(3):561–568.

BIBLIOGRAPHY

Bertram DL, Wilson JL, eds. *Financial Management in Critical Care Nursing.* Baltimore: Williams and Wilkins; 1991.

Beyers M. Quality assurance. *Nurs Clin North Am.* 1988;23(3):613–677.

DeLoughery G. *Issues and Trends in Nursing.* St. Louis: Mosby Yearbook; 1991.

Ferguson V, ed. The nursing shortage: Dynamics and solutions. *Nurs Clin North Am.* 1990;25(3):503–616.

Gale B, Stessl B. The long-term care dilemma: What nurses need to know about Medicare. *Nurs Health Care.* 1992; 13(1):34–41.

Lambert CE Jr., Lambert VA. *Perspectives in Nursing: The Impacts on the Nurse, the Consumer, and Society.* Norwalk, CT: Appleton & Lange; 1989.

Lee PR. *The Nation's Health: Delivery and Financing of Health Care: Role of the Nurse.* Boston: Jones & Bartlett; 1990.

Lindeman CA, McAthie M, eds. *Nursing Trends and Issues.* Springhouse, PA: Springhouse Corp; 1990.

Little C, ed. *Nursing and Health Care: The Supplement.* New York: NLN; 1990.

Long RE. *Crisis in Health Care.* New York: HW Wilson Co; 1990.

Maraldo PJ, Preziosi P, Binder I. *Talking Points: A Public Policy Guide to Key Issues in Nursing and Health Care.* New York: NLN; 1991.

McClosky JC, Grace HK, eds. *Current Issues in Nursing.* St. Louis: CV Mosby; 1990.

Natapoff JN. *Maternal–Child Health Policy: A Nursing Perspective.* New York: Springer; 1990.

National League for Nursing. *Indices of Quality in Long-term Care: Research and Practice.* New York: NLN; 1989

National League for Nursing. *Mechanisms of Quality in Long-term Care: Service and Clinical Outcomes.* New York: NLN; 1991.

National League for Nursing. *Nursing Centers: Meeting the Demand for Quality Health Care.* New York: NLN; 1989.

National League for Nursing. *Perspectives in Nursing—1989–1991.* New York: NLN; 1990.

Neil RM, Watts R, eds. *Caring and Nursing: Explorations in Feminist Perspectives.* New York: NLN; 1990.

Perkins C, Perkins K. Uncompensated care: The millstone around the neck of US health care. *Nurs Health Care.* 1992; 13(1):20–23.

Roberts N, Minnick A, Ginzberg E, Curran C. *What to Do About the Nursing Shortage.* New York: Commonwealth Fund; 1989.

Shaffer FA. DRG's, Nursing, and Health Care. *Nurs Clin North Am.* 1988;23(3):447–612.

Schramm C. Healthcare industry problems call for cooperative solutions. *Health Care Financ Manag.* 1990;44(1):54–61.

Winstead-Fry P, Shippee-Rice R, Tiffany J. *Rural Health Nursing.* New York: NLN; 1991.

CHAPTER 36

Economics in Health Care and Nursing

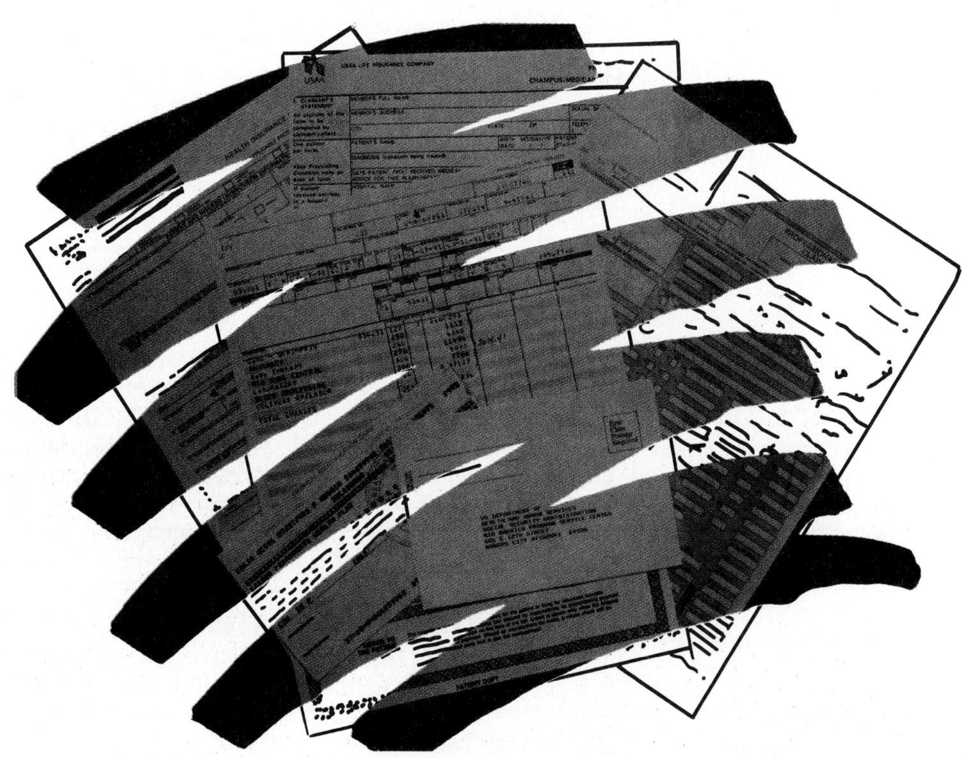

Behavioral Objectives

Upon completion of this chapter, the reader will be able to:

1. Define economics.
2. State the importance of economics in health care and describe its contribution to the functioning of the health care system.
3. Explain how resources are allocated within the economy and within the health care system.
4. Discuss the concepts of efficiency and effectiveness in producing health care services.
5. List the decisions that must be made by an economic system.
6. Describe the conflict that arises between individuals and society in the use of health care services.
7. State the fundamental conditions for a competitive market.
8. List factors that affect the demand for health care services.
9. List factors that affect the supply of health care services.
10. List the distinctive economic characteristics of the US health care system and discuss their implications.
11. Identify several differences between the way economics works in the health care system and in most other industries.
12. State the relevance of economics to nursing and nurses.
13. Describe how nurses can use economics in collaborating with clients in their care.

KEY TERMS

accountability
capitalism
capitation
case management
derived demand
economic resources
economics
economies of scale
effectiveness
efficiency
managed care
monopoly power
monopsony power
multi-institutional systems
price elasticity
productivity
rational economic behavior
socialism
utility
utilization management

Economics and economists have been called many things—some humorous, some not. Regardless of one's opinion about the value of economics or economists, the discipline of economics provides a useful framework for analyzing economic problems. When the economy takes a turn for the worse, when interest rates rise, or when health care costs soar out of control, economists are the first professionals to be asked for explanations and solutions.

Economics provides a unique approach to analyzing problems, because it is a particular way of looking at situations. Therefore, economics may be said to be a way of thinking. Indeed, this chapter attempts to expand the reader's thinking by challenging the reader to consider health care and nursing in economic terms.

The application of economics to problems in health care is a relatively new trend and a departure from the historical view that health care should not be subjected to the economic considerations applied to other human activities.[1] Only recently have policy makers, professionals, and consumers looked at health care as an industry and acknowledged that economic concepts are as relevant to health care as they are to any other industry. These new attitudes are a reaction to the troublesome spiral of cost inflation that has plagued health care delivery for the last three decades (refer to Chap. 35.)

Today, as a consequence of fundamental changes in the social and economic environment of health care, there is widespread recognition that economic judgment is essential at all levels of decision making. Economic analysis is needed not only at the level of social policy making or at the institutional level in the struggle to balance budgets, but also at the individual level, as providers make decisions about how best to use their time and energy to benefit clients. More and more, health care professionals are examining the services they provide to determine whether the benefits are worth the costs. Economic pressures demand this kind of self-scrutiny as part of the overall effort to improve the level of efficiency in health care delivery.

Thus, as health professionals collaborate to make decisions about how best to use health resources, they will rely increasingly on economic concepts to guide them. Economically speaking, nursing service is one of the largest components of health care. Thus, in the years to come, nurses can expect to play a central role in the economic decisions that face the health care industry.[2] To prepare themselves, nurses need a basic understanding of economic concepts. This chapter outlines the fundamental ideas of economics as they relate to health care and nursing. It also addresses the economic issues and decisions that face health care providers, particularly nurses, now and in the future.

ECONOMIC CONCEPTS

What is economics? One of the difficulties in trying to discuss what economics is and what it contributes is that to some extent everyone is an economist. Most people have an opinion about whether the United States is spending too much for national defense, whether the rate of inflation is too high, whether plumbers or physicians earn too much, or whether the government should provide health insurance for every citizen. These are all economic issues. They are also political issues, and given that economists reflect the political differences that characterize the general public, it is understandable that they are said to never agree on anything.

To the extent that economics is political, its development as a discipline is shaped by the political environment in which it operates. Economics, as it has evolved in the United States, is concerned primarily with the operations of a free-market economy in which competition determines the primary functions of the economic system; however, when competition fails to produce results that society deems appropriate, government attempts to provide a more equitable or, at least, a more acceptable solution. Indeed, it can be said that the United States manages the distribution of its resources by competition tempered with government intervention. Other types of systems, however, provide different approaches to the problem of how to distribute a society's resources.

In a broad sense, economics can be viewed as the science of economic systems. Economic systems are important because they profoundly affect the welfare of a society and all of its components. The economic system can enhance or impede the ability of a society to meet its needs. In the United States, the effect of the free-market system in the delivery of health care has been debated for several decades. Rising health care spending has begun to impede society's ability to achieve other desired goals, such as a better educational system, a cleaner environment, and housing for the homeless. One impact of rising costs is that the health care industry is being asked to justify its use of society's resources and to deliver services more efficiently.[3] With the mounting pressures for a more rational approach to the management of health care, public decision makers look to economics for ideas on how to regain control. The following text explains the basic concepts that economists use to understand and explain economic behavior.

Scarcity of Resources

In general, economics is concerned with three basic elements:

1. Desires (what people want)
2. Resources (what is available to meet the people's wants)
3. Choices (decisions that must be made because resources are almost always limited)[4]

Society as a whole and each of its citizens must decide which desires will be satisfied and which will not.

Resources are the means available to accomplish valued goals. **Economic resources** commonly refer to natural, man-made, and human resources used to produce material goods and services such as food, shelter, defense, and health care.[5] Many resources are necessary to a society. Energy, raw materials, and labor are all important resources that are necessary to produce the goods and services society needs and desires. Time and money are also important resources, as is the basic health of the population. Without resources, people, and therefore society, cannot function. When resources are scarce, society must ration those that are available.

Resources are scarce when the desire for them exceeds the quantity that is available or supplied.[4] Thus, a resource is scarce when there is not as much of it as people would like to have or feel that they need. For example, hospitals have limited amounts of dollars to spend. This fact prevents administrators from purchasing all the things they believe they need to provide the highest possible quality of services to anyone who needs or wants hospital care. Consequently, administrators must make choices about what to buy with their limited dollars (scarce resources). They must ask themselves whether hospital dollars should be spent on hiring more nurses, buying new technology, increasing unit supplies, making renovations, providing for staff education, or any of a number of other possibilities.

The idea of scarcity can be applied to every item produced or consumed in an economy. There is almost never enough of any given item to satisfy public wants. Thus, there is scarcity. If there were no scarcity, people could have what they wanted because there would be enough resources to go around; however, this is almost never the case, and because scarcity exists, difficult choices must be made.

Definition of Economics

If there were no scarcity, in fact, there would be no need for economists. Economists attempt to devise remedies for the problems created by scarcity and to help policy makers and the public make choices about how best to use scarce resources. Indeed **economics** can be defined as the study of the efficient allocation of scarce resources.[6]

Choice Making

Taking the desires of society as a given (so many automobiles, houses, universities, televisions, hospitals, and so on), the problem for society is to determine how to minimize the resources used in meeting those desires or, conversely, how to maximize the number of desires met with the limited resources available.[3] An individual must decide whether to buy a Mercedes or to buy a Volkswagen and spend the extra money on an education. Society must decide whether to spend money to build new hospitals or to upgrade the existing ones and use the savings on space exploration or the war against drugs. These allocations are decisions on which rational individuals can logically disagree.

Economics provides a way of systematically evaluating the alternatives that confront individuals and society. The role of economics is to help analyze the economic consequences of alternatives. Economics is not concerned with making value judgments about choices. It is not the role of economics, for example, to judge whether resources should go into health care instead of some other area.

Rather, economics is concerned with trying to make decisions as rational as possible by estimating the probable efficiency and effectiveness of various alternatives. How can society do all or most of the things it wants with the resources it has? The goal of applying economic principles is to satisfy as many of society's wants as possible within the limited resources available.[4]

Rational Economic Behavior

Economics provides society with analytic tools for making the difficult decisions created by resource scarcity. These tools are grounded on the idea of rational economic behavior.[4] **Rational economic behavior** is behavior that is consistent with the incentives provided by the economic system. The assumption is that when incentives are built into a system, people make decisions that allow them to avail themselves of the incentives. Theoretically, this creates the greatest good for society, provided that the incentives encourage an efficient and effective use of resources.

Efficiency and Effectiveness

With the scarcity of resources comes the need to determine how those resources are to be used and the responsibility to ensure that resources are used efficiently and effectively. In any economy, regardless of politics, the various industries—education, defense, food, housing, health care, and so forth—compete with one another for the resources available. Because an economy's ability to increase its production of goods and services is limited by the scarcity of its resources,[5] one sector can increase its share of the total production only by taking away from another sector.[1] As competition builds, so do pressures for efficiency.

This principle can be applied to health care cost inflation. Systems for third-party payment in health care, public and private, expanded rapidly after World War II and again during the mid-1960s.[7] Until recently, these systems have provided strong incentives for health professionals to expand the health care system and for consumers to use it.[7] (For more information on health care systems, refer to Chap. 35.) Before the reforms of the 1980s, third-party payers guaranteed payment for services rendered. Consumers were thus encouraged to use health services, and providers and institutions were free to pass along their costs to a bureaucracy that essentially put no cap on the amounts it would pay out.

In effect, government and private insurers said, "We will pay for whatever services are provided."[8] Under such an arrangement, it is difficult to establish whether the services are rendered efficiently or effectively.

Efficiency refers to the amount of resources used to achieve a desired result.[9] With no cost parameters to work from, third-party payers had no way of knowing whether the health services they paid for could have been rendered at a lower cost, or whether more services could have been provided at the same cost. As they assumed the financial risk for the decisions of consumers and providers, costs mounted. This created the impetus for the cost-controlling measures imposed in the 1980s.[7] For example, the prospective payment system instituted under the Tax Equity and Fiscal Responsibility Act of 1982 established binding cost parameters. It has been a landmark step in the direction of defining standards for efficiency in health care.[10] (See Chap. 35 for more on prospective payment.)

Productivity is a concept that is closely related to efficiency. **Productivity** is a measure of the efficiency with which labor, materials, and equipment are converted into goods and services.[11] It is usually expressed as a ratio of input to output. When health services are delivered more efficiently, the productivity of health professionals increases. Given the economic pressures in health care, nurses are increasingly concerned about their productivity.[11–13] The phrase "doing more with no more," found in the nursing literature, reflects that concern.[14]

Effectiveness is concerned with results. It is a measure of whether the services provided have the intended or desired outcome.[9] Like efficiency, effectiveness is difficult to judge when no criteria are established for the finished product. Is the health of the public better served by providing basic preventive and acute care services to a large number of people or by making the latest technology available to a few? Under economic pressure, health care decision makers are attempting to find answers. Health care spending increased 60 percent in one recent 5-year period, yet the average life expectancy at birth increased only 1 percent.[15] Moreover, research examining some accepted, widely practiced, expensive medical procedures casts doubt on whether the benefits always justify the costs.[16]

Accountability

For the past 30 years, health care has been viewed as the right of every individual.[17] Although the social desirability of that policy cannot be challenged, one of its implications is that cost is no factor. The policy assumes that there is no scarcity: when the cost of care increases, the government raises subsidies (and taxes) or the insurer raises premiums to cover the cost.

But scarcity exists, and the enormity of the economic obligation represented by that social policy became clear in the early 1970s when the Nixon administration warned the nation that it faced a crisis in health care finance.[18] Significant changes in the health care delivery system followed that warning.[18,19] Nevertheless, the cost of health care has continued to skyrocket, and it now jeopardizes the government's ability to do many other worthwhile and necessary things. Figure 36–1 demonstrates the extent to which health care costs are increasing.

Today, with an inflation rate for health care at twice the rate for the rest of the economy and with total expenditures exceeding half a trillion dollars,[17] together with soaring insurance premiums and increasing numbers of uninsured citizens,[10] policy makers are being forced to take another look at health care economics. Costs have thus become an urgent public issue.

One result is the increasing importance of accountability in health care. **Accountability** refers to the undertaking of practices to enable the tracking and explanation of the use of resources. For example, because the health care industry is using such a large proportion of our nation's limited resources, health care providers and managers are being asked to demonstrate that their procedures are efficient and effective and to show that their use of resources has proportionate benefits for society.[3] Cost accounting and financial management have become part of the day-to-day reality of health care. Health care providers are now required to answer for their financial decisions.

Individual Versus Social Economic Perspective

In the allocation of scarce resources, conflicts sometimes arise between the interests of the individual and the interests of society as a whole. This is true for any resource, including health care. When viewed from the individual's perspective, the objective of the health care system is to improve health or postpone death. Given the cost of health care, however, this perspective ultimately leads to inequities. Providing the maximum amount of service to some individuals means that others may receive minimal services or no services at all.[20] Although such a system may have tremendous benefits for those individuals who gain admittance, the exclusion of others can be detrimental to society.

Recognizing that the health care system cannot do everything for everybody, the societal alternative is to provide the greatest number of benefits to the greatest number of people. Under this approach, the welfare of society, not the welfare of the individual, is the goal. As a result, it is sometimes necessary to do less than the maximum for some individuals to provide minimum care for all.[21]

The societal approach requires setting priorities for the use of scarce resources—it forces us to ration scarce resources. Such decisions constitute difficult policy choices.[17] Alternative courses of action must be analyzed not only for their economic efficiency but also for their social acceptability. The problem of fairness in the use of public resources also must be addressed. One contemporary approach is to stress the value of health promotion and disease prevention over heroic treatment measures and other types of remedial care (care given once disease has occurred).[17,22] There is controversy, however, about this approach. Like remedial measures, health promotion programs are costly, the benefits are uncertain, and the link to positive outcomes has not been conclusively established.[22]

■ ECONOMIC SYSTEMS

Although economic concepts can help explain the current environment of health care, they do not tell the whole story.

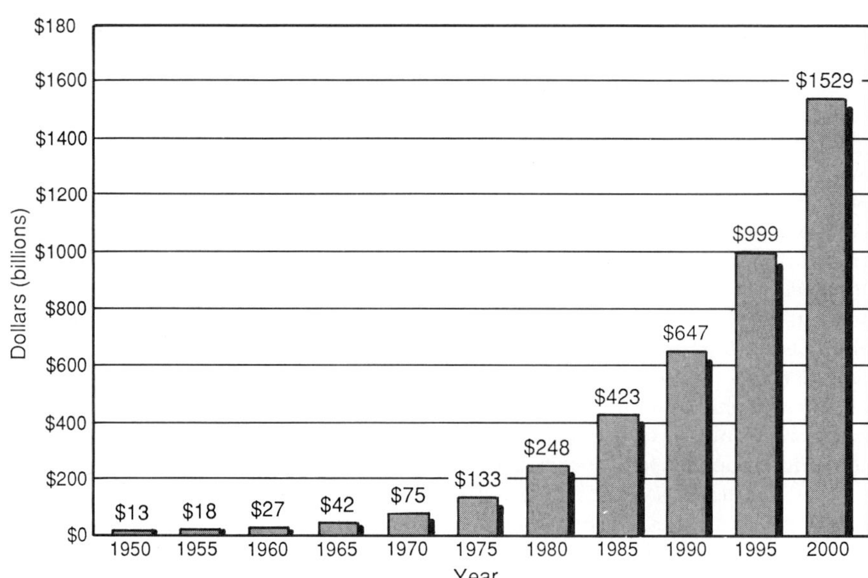

Figure 36–1. Rising health care expenditures, 1950–2000. (From Francis S. Health care forecasts: U.S. industrial outlook, 1988. *Med Benefits*, February 15, 1988, pp. 1–3.)

It is also necessary to understand the functions and practices of the economic system within which the health care industry operates. An economic system is a collection of institutions, guiding principles, and values that, taken together, answer the economic questions any society must confront. Different systems offer different approaches to resource allocation.

Types of Economic Systems

As defined earlier, the United States has a market economy. **Capitalism** is the term that applies to the political and economic system in which the market is allowed to determine resource allocation.[23] Capitalism relies on the principle of rational economic behavior, which holds that people make decisions consistent with their own economic advantage. Producers compete with one another to make and sell goods and services, and consumers seek out the goods and services that best meet their needs. Capitalism emphasizes private ownership and control over production and a minimum of government intervention in resource allocation.

Other economic systems approach resource allocation in different ways. **Socialism,** for example, disavows private ownership, competition, and profit. In socialist societies, a central authority, usually the government, allocates resources for society.[23] The linkage that is formed in a capitalist system between what people want (demand) and what producers provide (supply) is thus broken in a socialist system.

Most economic systems are neither purely socialist nor purely capitalist. The imbalances in resource allocation that normally occur lead to political reforms that result in a mixed system. Thus, in the United States, the largest part of the economy is free market, but important parts, such as the educational and postal systems, are under government control. In the United Kingdom, health care resources are controlled by the government. On the other hand, in socialist economies such as China and the Commonwealth of Independent States, where, until recently, all parts of the economy were under government control, features of the market system are now being introduced. The purpose of these reforms is to invigorate these relatively stagnant economies with market incentives to elicit rational economic behavior and enhance economic production.

Questions Answered by an Economic System

All societies need rules and guiding principles to help them decide how to allocate resources. An economic system provides these rules and decides four basic economic issues: what goods and services are produced, how the goods and services are produced, how the goods and services are distributed, and how much is to be consumed.[6]

In a market economy, the market manages society's resources. Thus the problem of how to allocate resources is decided by the exchanges between consumers and producers in the marketplace. In a centralized economy, these decisions are made by the government, which also determines how the goods and services will be produced and who will get them.

THE MARKET SYSTEM

The functions and practices of a market system are determined by the components of the system and described in theories about the system's operation.

Components

Any market system comprises certain basic components. These are (1) a market in which (2) economic exchanges occur between (3) producers and (4) consumers.

A market is the mechanism—a place, situation, or procedure—by which buyers and sellers get together to exchange goods and services.[9] Markets exist for almost anything that can be exchanged, including health care. Markets can be local, regional, national, or international, depending on the nature of the goods and services being exchanged.

In a so-called free-market economy, exchanges between producers and consumers shape three crucial conditions: demand, supply, and price. These conditions are vital to the operation of a market system and are largely responsible for how our society's resources are allocated.

Demand refers to the quantity and types of goods and services that each consumer desires and is able to purchase at various prices. The consumer has a limited amount of money to spend and must decide how to allocate it—for an automobile, an education, health insurance, or, more realistically, some combination of these and other things.

Supply refers to the quantity and types of the goods and services that each producer offers for sale at various prices. Producers attempt to provide only the supply from which they believe they can profit, that is, only as many automobiles or television sets as they believe they can sell or only as many hospital beds as they think they can fill profitably.

Price is the quantity of something that is required in exchange for something else. It is generally expressed as a monetary unit of exchange: the number of dollars it costs to buy a television or visit a physician. Producers and consumers must somehow reach an agreement about price. When agreement has been reached, a transaction takes place. Price is related to, but not the same as, value. Value reflects the scarcity of a good or service. Value measured in money is called price. Scarce resources generally carry higher prices than abundant ones. Value is related to, but is not the same as, usefulness or utility. In economics, **utility** refers to the satisfaction that a good or service can provide.

The Market System and Economic Questions

The market's answers to four crucial economic questions are determined through the dynamics of supply, demand, and price.

What Is Produced? The market determines the types of goods and services that are produced by assessing the types and quantities of goods and services people want.[6] In a market system, demand stimulates production. How many cars? How much health care? These questions are answered in the marketplace through the mechanism of demand.

How are Goods Produced? In a market system, the market influences not only what is produced but also how items are produced. It does this by determining the amount of labor, technology, and facilities that will be required for production. Production of health care, for example, requires a labor force of trained professionals, sophisticated technology, and special facilities. All of these factors of production are established by the market in response to a demand for health care.

How are Goods Distributed? The market also determines how goods and services are distributed. As goods and services are limited, everyone cannot have everything desired; consequently, a mechanism must exist by which the available goods and services can be rationed.[9] In a market economy, price is a primary influence in determining who gets what and in what quantity.

How Much is Consumed? A final question the market answers for society is how much of its resources are to be consumed and how much are to be saved. If an economic system is to grow rather than stagnate, it must devote some of its productive resources to increasing its ability to meet future needs: it must invest in new plants and equipment and in the education of its citizens. Again, the market determines how much can be consumed in the present and how much must be saved to avoid jeopardizing future needs.

Conditions for a Market System

The purpose of a market is to create the conditions necessary for exchanges to occur. Markets provide the following mechanisms[4]:

1. A mechanism by which individuals can determine the kinds and amounts of goods and services they wish to purchase
2. A way for individuals to communicate their preferences for goods and services to those who can satisfy them
3. A means by which resources needed for producing a good or service can be identified
4. A mechanism for identifying the individuals who might benefit from the good or service

When the market fulfills these conditions, the interaction of demand, supply, and price provides society with the combination of goods and services its members prefer. When the market fails to fulfill any of these conditions, society does not obtain the right combination of goods and services.

Competitive Market Model

An economic model is a theory used by economists to analyze economic behavior. Economists use economic models to forecast economic conditions in a society.[4] One model used to describe conditions in a market system is the competitive market model. The competitive market model describes a situation in which two or more producers seek to gain an advantage over each other for control of a market.

Characteristics of a Competitive Market. Economic theory states that a perfectly competitive system is good for consumers because sellers must offer their products at the lowest prices or lose business. It is good for producers because it provides incentive to improve the product, lower the cost of production, and thus earn more money. A perfectly competitive system has the following characteristics:[9]

1. Identical products are made by all producers
2. Perfect knowledge about alternative options is available to producers and consumers; therefore, there are no uninformed decisions
3. Profits are maximized by producers and satisfaction is maximized by consumers
4. There are enough buyers and sellers, acting independently, so that no one individual has a significant impact on prices
5. There are no barriers to the entry and exit from the market of either producers or consumers

A perfectly competitive system is desirable because, theoretically, it provides the most ideal allocation of goods and services. Imperfect competition creates imbalances. Without competition, sellers with **monopoly power,** the power gained when there is only one seller in a market, may take advantage of consumers. Likewise, buyers with **monopsony power,** the power gained when there is only one buyer in a market, may take advantage of their suppliers. Rarely, however, does perfect competition exist. Because competitive systems often fail to act in an ideal way, they require regulation and control to protect participants. Although perfect competition is uncommon, the model of pure competition provides a yardstick against which to measure the characteristics and efficiency of any particular market—agriculture, textiles, retail sales, or health care.

Competition and Health Care. Health care deviates substantially from the model of perfect competition. In fact, it has been said that consumers do not enter or leave the health care market at will. They are constrained by a variety of factors, such as lack of information, lack of well-defined health outcomes, and lack of service accessibility. Providers, moreover, are limited in number, provide nonidentical services, are burdened by heavy government regulations, and have little control over those who allocate health care resources.[24,25]

These are important deviations and they reflect the fact that the market for health care is not naturally competitive. Ever since the Nixon administration's warning of fiscal catastrophe, policy makers have been seeking ways to make compatible the economically contradictory goals of health care access and cost containment.[17] In principle, the mechanisms available to them have been those of central regulation or the strengthening of market forces. In most cases, government has chosen to strengthen market forces through competition.

The rationale for this reiterates the classic arguments in favor of capitalism. Proponents stress that competition encourages innovation, promotes greater diversity of services, provides the incentives needed for production efficiency, and increases consumer choice.[25] Regulation, they fear, would stifle these effects. Thus most legislative approaches have been efforts to increase competition within health care in one way or another so that the market might correct the system's ills.[18,19,26–28]

Limitations of the Competitive Model. An important limitation of the competitive market model, however, is that it does not guarantee equity or equality in the distribution of resources.[4] Competition makes no value judgments about social desirability. In a competitive market, exchanges in the marketplace determine who receives a good or service. This can result, for example, in only 10 percent of the population receiving 90 percent of the goods and services available. For some products, such as automobiles, unequal distribution might be acceptable to society. For other products, such as health care, unequal distribution might be unacceptable. Thus, debate about social goals is necessary even when competition is strong.[20] Indeed, opponents of the market approach stress that competition will do little to advance the national commitment to an equitable distribution of health care. They advocate expanded government control over health care resources.[25]

Theory of Demand and Supply

Theory of Demand. To economists, demand has a precise definition: demand is the quantity of a good or service that consumers are willing and able to purchase at a given price during a given time period.[4]

The theory of demand states that, under normal conditions, as the price of an item increases, consumers buy less of it, and as the price decreases, consumers buy more of it, all other things remaining the same.[9] For example, when the price of meat increases, people generally buy less meat (or cheaper meat). When the price decreases, people generally buy more meat (or more expensive meat). The implication of the theory of demand is that lower prices encourage consumption, and higher prices discourage consumption.

Determinants of Demand. Utility is an important factor in demand. In general, utility diminishes with consumption. As an individual consumes more units of an item, each additional unit generally provides less satisfaction or, in economic terms, has less utility, than the previous unit.[9] As each additional unit provides less satisfaction, an individual is generally unwilling to pay as much for additional units as for the original unit: the law of diminishing marginal utility.

This phenomenon applies to practically any item consumed: automobiles, appliances, houses, food. It seems logical that it would also apply to health care. In other words, an individual's willingness to pay for health care services should decrease as he or she consumes more services.

In any market, factors other than price can have a dramatic effect on demand. These include the urgency of the consumer's need; the consumer's tastes, preferences, and level of income; and the prices of other goods that can be substituted.[4]

Price elasticity reflects the responsiveness of demand to price changes.[29] Price and the quantity purchased do not always change in proportion to one another. Sometimes the quantity of a product sold is very responsive to price changes. When this happens, the demand is said to be elastic. For example, a 25 percent drop in the price of meat may elicit a 100 percent increase in meat sales. Sometimes, however, the quantity of a product sold is not responsive to price changes. When this happens, the demand is said to be inelastic. For example, the price of salt may increase 50 or 100 percent without a substantial decrease in sales.

Demand for a product or service usually becomes inelastic when (1) the product consumed is considered a necessity, (2) the outlay represents a small portion of the individual's or institution's budget, or (3) it is difficult to find a substitute.[29] A substitute is a product or service that performs the same function or meets the same need as another product or service. For example, over-the-counter medications or cheaper generic medications often can be substituted for expensive brand-name prescription drugs.

Because health care is often viewed as a necessity, the demand for health care is relatively inelastic. Additionally, most consumers require medical advice for making decisions on substitutes, which contributes to the price inelasticity of the demand for health care. Also, consumers do not pay directly for much of their health care, decreasing their sensitivity to price.

Demand and Health Care. The theory of demand provides a basic framework for analyzing the determinants of the demand for and price of health care in an economy. The demand for health care is hi¸hly complex. It requires an understanding of some additional factors that do not apply to other industries.[30] In addition to the normal factors that affect demand, discussed earlier, demand for health care is influenced by five other factors:[31]

1. Individual need for the health service
2. Recognition that the need exists
3. Availability of financial resources (private or public funding) for obtaining care
4. Motivation to obtain care
5. Availability of services

A primary factor in the demand for health care is the health status of the population. Although finance and service availability obviously have an important impact on the demand for health care, unless people have health problems there can be no demand for health care, regardless of price or the financial resources of the consumer.[30]

The demand for health care is also unique in that it is unpredictable and irregular. This reflects the fact that illness itself is unpredictable and irregular. Except for preventive services, health care provides satisfaction to the consumer only when the individual experiences a deviance from normal conditions (illness).

Determining the demand for health care is difficult for other reasons. First, the nature of the product is vague. In most markets, the product is relatively easy to define and measure. For example, the automobile industry produces cars and trucks. The demand for health care, however, arises out of the consumer's demand for another product, "good health."[1] Economically speaking, the demand for health care is a **derived demand:** it is derived from another demand.

It can thus be said that demand for health care is an unpredictable, derived demand for the commodity good health. Unfortunately, there are no tools for measuring good health. People vary considerably in their definitions of what constitutes good and poor health, as Chapters 5, 10, and 12 showed, and that makes direct measurement of the demand for health care difficult. As a consequence, the market system for health care can be established only indirectly by averaging the use of all individuals in a market. This is the only way to estimate demand and thus to determine how many hospitals, physicians, and nurses are necessary to meet society's needs.

The interaction of price and demand in health care is also complex, to a large extent because society looks on health care as a necessity, not as a privilege to be rationed by the marketplace like other commodities. Third-party payment, both public and private, represents a vast system of subsidizing health care that has undeniable social benefits. Economically, however, third-party payment also has the consequence of removing price as the determinant for allocating health care resources.[33]

Thus, price increases in health care do not have the same effect on demand that they have in other industries. In other markets, the consumer pays the seller directly for the item being purchased. In the health care market, a third party, often the insurer, pays the bills. Third-party payment reinforces price inelasticity because consumers are insensitive to price: they know that the insurer will pick up the cost.[34] Even in today's climate of consumer cost consciousness, people do not shop for a surgical procedure the way they shop for a pair of shoes, with price and efficiency in mind.[15]

Moreover, under third-party payment, demand itself increases, as the curb that price might place on consumption is absent. For people with adequate health insurance, desires for health care easily become needs.[17]

Given the scarcity of resources, attempts to counter the inflationary features of demand in the health care market are to be expected. In fact, a variety of rationing devices other than price have evolved.[17] For example, Medicare and most health insurance companies have instituted and gradually increased "copayments" and "deductibles," the out-of-pocket payments that the insured must make. Theoretically, these devices have the effect of price increases and operate to reduce demand.

Theory of Supply. Supply is the quantity of a good or service that producers would be willing and able to sell at any given price during a given time interval.[9]

The theory of supply states that, under normal conditions, as the price of an item increases, suppliers offer more of it for sale, and as the price of an item decreases, suppliers offer less, all other things remaining the same.[4] For example, if the price of meat increases, ranchers will make more livestock available for sale. Conversely, if the price of meat falls, ranchers will make less available. The implication of the theory of supply is that higher prices encourage production, and lower prices discourage production.

Determinants of Supply. As with demand, price is not the only determinant of the amount of a product offered for sale. Other factors that significantly affect supply include the technology available; the prices charged for other goods, especially for closely related products; the supply of the factors necessary for production (labor, capital, natural resources); and the suppliers' expectations about future prices.[9]

Generally, in a competitive market, the producer has little or no control over price. The amount a single producer produces is simply too little to influence market conditions. Therefore, to be able to offer a product at the market price and still generate profit, the producer must minimize the costs of production. In this way the competitive market stimulates efficiency.

Productivity is a major factor affecting the supply of a good or service. In accordance with the law of diminishing returns, as more economic resources are consumed in production, productivity increases, but only to a point. After that point, fewer additional goods are produced. Thus, for any product, there is an optimal combination of the various economic resources that tends to maximize efficiency. When that combination is exceeded, efficiency declines.

Skilled nursing service, for example, might best be provided with a hypothetical ratio of 10 nurse extenders to one registered nurse. If the number of registered nurses was maintained constant, and the number of nurse extenders increased to 11, 12, or 13, productivity would increase, but less dramatically with each additional worker. Finally, the addition of one more nurse extender would add nothing to the productive capacity of the facility.[35] When the last unit costs more than the value it creates, profits decline. Therefore, it is necessary for producers to analyze their use of resources carefully to determine the most efficient combination possible.

Just as budget-conscious consumers look for cheaper substitutes for products, producers also substitute one economic resource for another to reduce the cost of production. Substitution is also possible in health care. For instance, the same respiratory care procedures can be performed by a respiratory therapist or by a registered nurse. Likewise, nurse practitioners, trained to perform many of the functions of the physician, can act as physician substitutes in certain circumstances.[36] Nurses make good substitutes in the production of health care. They have a broad range of skills—technical, organizational, and managerial—that make them suitable substitutes for other classes of personnel.[14] A good substitute increases productivity and reduces the costs of production.[37]

Supply and Health Care. The economic theory of supply provides a basic framework for analyzing the determinants of the price and quantity of health services in a market system. As with demand, the supply of health care is complex. The general determinants of supply—price, technology, prices of substitute goods and services, availability of materials, and future expectations—are influenced by several other factors that are specific to the supply of health care services, including the following[3]:

1. Legal restrictions (licensing of providers, accrediting of institutions, regulation of services)
2. Regulation of the combination of resources that can be used in the production of services
3. Introduction of technology for reasons other than cost reduction
4. Production goals other than cost minimization and profit maximization

A number of legal restrictions (licensing, accrediting, regulations) limit the tasks or otherwise restrict the services that specific health care providers can perform. Those restrictions constrain producers from substituting one type of economic resource for another.[37] Producers' options for increasing productivity are thus limited, and costs increase.

For example, hospital accreditation standards require that a hospital maintain a certain number of registered nurses on staff. Licensing statutes also stipulate that certain tasks can be performed only by registered nurses. Neither nurse extenders nor licensed vocational nurses, both less costly, can be substituted. Although these standards protect the quality of care offered to the consumer, the hospital administrator's ability to control costs is nevertheless reduced.

Furthermore, a variety of restrictions are placed on the combinations of economic resources that can be used in the production of health care services. Those restrictions also limit the ability of producers to vary the types and amounts of economic resources they use in their attempts to achieve the lowest costs of production.[37] For example, many states limit the number of physician assistants a physician may supervise. The ability of health care providers to increase their own efficiency is thus restricted.

Technology is another factor. In most markets, technologies are introduced only if they allow goods and services to be produced at a lower cost. In health care, on the other hand, technologies are often introduced to improve treatment outcomes. New technologies may contribute very little to production efficiency or may actually increase the cost of production.[3]

BUILDING NURSING KNOWLEDGE

How Do Supply and Demand Affect Health Care Costs?

Bloch H, Pupp R. Supply, demand, and rising health-care costs. *Nurs Econ.* 1985; 3(2):119–123.

Bloch and Pupp analyzed some of the factors that have contributed to escalating health care costs in terms of supply and demand in the health care marketplace. They propose that supply and demand factors in health care, rather than counterbalancing one another to stabilize costs, instead have acted to fuel cost escalation over the past 20 years. The single most important aspect of the marketplace is the hospital. Of all the expenditures on health care (drugs, professional services, and so on) in the past 20 years, hospital room charges grew the fastest. The charge for a hospital room is related to the supply of rooms in a community. In the 1970s and 1980s, facilities were overbuilt. Duplication of facilities leads to underused facilities and inefficiency, which is costly. It would have been reasonable for hospitals to lower their room charges to encourage more use; however, the nonprofit financial structure of most hospitals provided no incentive to do that. Nonprofit institutions do not seek a profit and are not accountable to stockholders. In addition, Bloch and Pupp believe the strategy to reduce rates would have been unsuccessful because the third-party insurance payment system insulates the consumer from the effects of changes in health care prices.

Another factor influencing health care costs is technological advancement. Technology is costly. During the previous two decades, technology in hospitals exploded and created an inefficient use of resources. Consumers equated well-equipped hospitals with good care, and physicians wanted high-tech diagnostics to protect themselves from malpractice litigation. The advent of intensive care units, respiratory therapy departments, and radiotherapy and diagnostic units added greatly to hospital costs. Bloch and Pupp note, however, that the new technology did not lead to proportionate improvement in mortality rates.

The demand factor was also skewed. The single most important factor affecting demand is the way the costs of care are subsidized. As hospitals and technology increased the price of care, the demand for hospital services did not drop as might have been expected. Federal tax laws made employee group health plans an allowable business tax deduction, but did not treat the plans as taxable income to employees. Thus, there were strong incentives for higher levels of health benefits. With this form of tax subsidization, the price of care became irrelevant. The authors conclude that a rational realignment of supply and demand factors is needed to improve the efficiency of the hospital care system.

Finally, in the health care industry, producers often have goals other than cost minimization and profit maximization. There is a strong tradition in the United States of valuing heroic measures to extend and improve the quality of an individual's life, even if only slightly.[34] Thus, when an individual enters the health care system with a serious illness, the cost of treatment is usually not a determining factor in decisions about the therapeutic plan. The client expects that the provider will do everything possible to preserve life and to hasten the return of health. In fact, providers are legally obligated to meet that expectation. When they fail, they become vulnerable to the threat of malpractice litigation. (See Chap. 3 for more on malpractice.) Providers are consequently generous in their use of available technology.[34]

Third-party payment also affects health care supply. The constraint that cost places on supply in other markets is absent in health care to a large extent because of third-party payment. The effect of health insurance on health care supply is similar to the effect in other industries of a revolutionary new technology that substitutes for labor and markedly lowers production costs. The supply increases, even though price is unchanged. Until recently, third-party payment acted as an incentive for providers to generate rather than limit costs.[38] That distorts the market operation of supply, and as a result, the health care industry uses more resources than absolutely necessary.

Given the scarcity of resources, it is predictable that attempts would be made to counter the inflationary features of health care supply. The federal government took the lead by instituting the prospective payment system, which capped federal allotments to hospitals; however, there are an array of private-sector market responses, such as new types of insurance plans that limit the amounts paid to providers and alternative provider systems that emphasize efficiency (HMOs, PPOs, and IPAs). (See Chap. 35 for more on alternative provider systems.)

Putting Demand and Supply Together: How the Market Works

The preceding discussion has focused on demand and supply in the market. A market can function only when demand and supply interact to establish the price at which sellers offer just the amount that buyers wish to purchase. This is the point at which supply equals demand.

Market Equilibrium. If a market is working effectively, interactions between producers and consumers will establish equilibrium, the point at which the quantity supplied and the quantity demanded are in balance. At the equilibrium price, buyers can purchase the amount they desire and sellers can provide just that amount. No one is disappointed.[4] At equilibrium, for example, all nurses who wish to work in a hospital for the current wage are doing so. Likewise, hospitals are able to hire all the nurses they need and have no vacant positions. When equilibrium is achieved, it can be said that the market is working in an ideal fashion.

If no barriers interfere with the market's own internal adjustments, the competitive market will automatically move over time toward an equilibrium of price and quantity. In an unconstrained market, price is the primary factor that determines equilibrium. Once a market achieves equilibrium, there is no pressure for prices to change, as long as the other factors affecting the participants remain unchanged. Thus, at market equilibrium, there is neither excess demand (shortages) nor excess supply (surplus).

Surplus. When the price of a good or service increases, and no other changes take place, then the quantity that producers are willing to supply will exceed the quantity consumers are willing to purchase at the new price. The result is a market surplus. Wage increases in a field, for example, sometimes have the effect of creating a surplus supply of labor. When wages go up, more people may be willing to work than employers are willing to hire.

Shortage. On the other hand, when the price of the good or service decreases, the quantity that producers are willing to supply is less than consumers are willing to purchase at the new price. The result is a market shortage. At present, the shortage of nurses and the numerous vacant hospital nursing positions concern many in health care. The shortage indicates that the market for registered nurses is not in equilibrium. (Factors contributing to the nursing shortage are discussed in Chap. 35.)

Market Adjustments. One of the important features of the competitive market is that it is self-correcting. When the current market price rises above the market equilibrium level, producers become dissatisfied with market conditions. They can no longer sell as much of the product as they wish at that price. Under competitive conditions, producers' efforts to increase the quantity of their sales will result in a reduction in price.[6]

On the other hand, when the current price falls below the market equilibrium level, consumers become dissatisfied. They are no longer able to purchase as much of the product as they would like at that price. Under competitive conditions, consumers' efforts to increase the quantity of their purchases will result in an increase in price.

Any price that is different from the equilibrium price therefore affects both the quantity and the price of the product and initiates changes in the behavior of producers and consumers. These changes continue until the market reaches a new equilibrium.[6] That is how a competitive market allocates resources.

How the Market for Health Care Works

As shown earlier, health care demand and supply are distorted by unique features of the industry. The equilibration typical of other markets does not exist in the health care market. Consequently, prices and quantities of services offered and purchased are different from those that would be achieved in an unconstrained market. Deviations from the competitive model do not insulate the health care system from economic realities, however. The system must still determine answers to the most basic economic questions:

1. What health care services should be produced?
2. How can services best be produced?
3. Who should receive the health care services provided?
4. What proportion of health care resources should be used and what proportion should be saved to meet future needs?

5. How much of society's total resources should go into the production of health care?[39]

Given the peculiarities of supply and demand, these questions are difficult to answer.[40] Moreover, the costly inefficiencies that result have undesirable social effects, including high prices and decreased availability of services for many in society.

Characteristics of the Health Care Industry. In addition to those already mentioned, other characteristics of the health care industry interfere with market self-correction. The most distinctive are (1) fragmentation, (2) relative consumer ignorance, (3) selectivity in third-party payment, (4) provider–agent conflict, (5) skewed incentives, and (6) infinite expandability.

Fragmentation. One characteristic of a truly competitive market is the unity created by the many sellers in the market who act independently to offer similar products. The market for health care does not share that feature. Although there are over 6000 hospitals and 450,000 physicians in the United States, many areas have only one hospital or only a few physicians. As a result, the market for health care is fragmented into a number of local markets rather than unified in a single, large market. This creates geographic constraints that reduce client access to providers outside of the immediate market vicinity. Though competition may prevail in large, densely populated areas, providers outside of those areas often are not required to react to external market conditions, and thus are able to control the price and quantity of services delivered.[41] This reduces the overall efficiency of the market.[39]

Relative Consumer Ignorance. In a competitive system, information enhances competition. Because illness is periodic and infrequent, however, the interaction of most individuals with the health care system is sporadic.[2] Consumers thus have little opportunity to expand their understanding of health care options. The provider, on the other hand, must have substantial expertise to render care, and is far better informed about services than the consumer and better able to judge the efficiency and effectiveness of services. Consequently, the consumer usually must rely on the provider to make judgments about the need for services and what services to use. This places the provider at a competitive advantage.

Unfortunately, consumers' attempts to gain information are thwarted by certain market conditions, such as barriers to market entry by providers and restrictions on communication. Unlike most markets, whose entry is relatively unrestricted, in health care, academic standards, licensing requirements, and accreditation requirements make entry difficult.[42] These barriers restrict the supply of providers and, as a consequence, the potential sources for consumer information.

Provider ethics are another obstacle. Although producers in most markets are anxious to publicize their competitors' shortcomings, disparaging remarks by one health professional about another are considered unethical and are actively discouraged.[43] Ethical standards for provider communication are undoubtedly necessary, but they have the practical effect of reducing consumer information. Moreover, advertising, which in many markets is a major source of information about competing products, has been tolerated in health care only recently. To date most health care advertising has focused on aspects other than price competition.[44]

Consumer information is increasing slowly. The Health Care Financing Administration (HCFA), for instance, has begun publishing lists of hospitals showing higher than expected mortality rates for Medicare admissions.[45] Nevertheless, the large disparity between the consumer's knowledge and the provider's knowledge persists.[26] Consumers need to know which treatments work and which providers do them most efficiently and effectively.[34,45,46] It is no surprise that clients greatly appreciate providers who explain medical procedures and help them consider both the benefits and the costs of their care.

Selectivity in Third-party Payment. An important feature of health care insurance coverage is that it is selective and uneven in the services covered. This distorts demand and price. For example, a yearly physical examination is not covered, but a series of allergy shots is. Outpatient surgery is covered in full, but inpatient surgery is subject to a high deductible payment. Because insurance reduces the direct charges to the consumer, clients and providers tend to use covered services and avoid other services. This happens regardless of the effect on overall costs or the constraints it places on treatment choices.[37] Selective coverage thus results in an overproduction of covered services and an underproduction of uncovered services.[47]

Under current insurance regulations, for example, third-party payment covers the services of physicians.[22] Although the same services might cost less when provided by others, consumers will demand physician services if they are the ones covered by insurance. Until recently nurses unsuccessfully have sought to be included under third-party payment regulations as a way to increase the demand for their skills.[22] Third-party reimbursement allows nurse specialists to enter the market as primary care providers rather than as institutional employees. Experts believe expanded third-party payment for nurses might well lower overall health care costs and enhance market competition[22] (see Chap. 35). On the other hand, selective coverage that underwrites care only by those with the highest level of training contributes to increased costs and constrains competition.[22]

Provider–Agent Conflict. The market for health care is unique in another way. In most markets, the consumer directly decides what to purchase. To a large extent in the health care industry, it is the provider, not the consumer, who decides what services to use.[37] The provider acts as an agent for the consumer. That is, the consumer selects a provider, usually a physician, who decides whether the consumer is admitted to a hospital and what treatment he or she receives.

As agent for the consumer, the provider might be expected to consider not only the client's health needs in treatment decisions but also the client's financial resources.[37] This does not hold true in all cases, however. Providers, particularly physicians, often have a financial interest in the use of services. The monetary return on the provider's time is greater if a procedure is performed, which creates an incentive to act in a manner that is not solely in the interests of the consumer.[34] Until recently, third-party payment has provided economic rewards for overtreatment or unnecessary treatment, and this has driven up overall health care costs.

Skewed Incentives. The incentives for providers are biased toward the provision of specialized, high-technology, high-cost care. Specialization and specialized practice, in fact, are typical of the US system.[48] In comparison with other countries, the United States has a high ratio of specialists to general practitioners.[49] The large number of specialists reduces the average specialist's work load and reduces the productivity of the system. All of these factors support the provision of elaborate health care.[48]

The bias toward specialization stems from two factors. First, medical students are usually educated in facilities that contain the most advanced, most elaborate, and most sophisticated equipment. They learn to depend on elaborate procedures and equipment.[48] Second, specialized services are usually viewed by consumers and providers as the key to therapeutic success.

Infinite Expandability. All of these factors contribute to the expandable nature of health care. If curbs are not placed on it, some authorities believe that the demand for health care may be infinitely expandable.[50] That is, the health care industry may be able to consume almost any amount of resources made available to it. In response to the uncertainties in medicine, for example, physicians are likely to continue to look for greater and greater margins of safety in diagnostic procedures, offer more and more heroic lifesaving treatments, and screen for less and less probable diseases, all of which drive up the cost of care.[50] Hospitals, pinched for revenue, are likely to add more and more new services. These factors interfere with market self-correction and contribute substantially to the total consumption of resources.

Measures to Enhance Health Care Competition. Historically in health care, economic power, the power to control prices and quantities, has rested with providers, whereas economic risk, the responsibility for payment, has rested with third-party payers, public and private. Measures to cure the ills of the health care market by enhancing marketplace competition have thus centered on shifting power from providers to payers and shifting risk from payers to consumers and providers.[28]

Provider Competition. Efforts to unleash market forces have taken several forms. In 1971, the Nixon administration endorsed HMOs, a type of prepaid group medical practice, as the new national health strategy, and pressed Congress to enact laws to encourage development of HMOs.[51] HMOs assume economic risk by selling a package of services for a fixed fee. On the basis of their lower prices, HMOs can compete with independent providers. In fact, enrollment in HMOs has quintupled over the past 20 years, expanding from 6 million to 29.3 million enrollees.[51] Moreover, the success of HMOs encouraged independent providers to join together in various group arrangements (PPOs, IPAs) to stay competitive.

In today's market, HMOs and PPOs offer a variety of attractively priced benefit packages, and IPAs negotiate discounted physician fee schedules with insurance companies or offer their own benefit packages. All bid competitively for contracts with Medicare, insurance companies, large corporations, and unions.

Insurer Competition. Another development is the new managed-care policies offered by insurance companies.[52] These are fee-for-service plans that reduce premiums and costs by constraining treatment choices. Limitations are placed on the treatments covered and on the providers and institutions authorized to render care. Only cost-efficient providers and institutions are authorized.

Alternative provider systems and the new insurance plans are collectively referred to as the managed-care industry. **Managed care** aims to provide the most efficient packages of services at the most reasonable costs. Managed-care arrangements shift economic risk to the provider by various means, often employing a combination of devices. Mechanisms such as **capitation** fix payments to providers regardless of the amount of services they render. **Utilization management,** sometimes referred to as "prior authorization," is the case-by-case assessment by third-party payers of the appropriateness of care before it is provided.[53] Under this mechanism, which focuses on hospitalization, the need for medical procedures is reviewed before admission. Unnecessary procedures are denied authorization. **Case management,** on the other hand, is an institutional response to declining reimbursements.[54] It is a process of economic oversight conducted within the hospital that aims to provide quality care with reduced resources. Case managers (physicians and nurses) work collaboratively to eliminate unnecessary expenses and to prevent delays and cost overruns during a client's hospitalization. (See Chap. 2 for more on case management.)

Over the last several years, managed care has become a significant force in health care delivery and finance. By 1987, in fact, managed care was the mainstream of health care finance, with more than 60 percent of Americans enrolled in an HMO, PPO, IPA, or managed-care insurance plans.[55]

Hospital Competition. Efforts to enhance competition are also apparent in hospital services. Although hospital competition was not the purpose of the prospective payment system instituted in 1982, it has been one of its effects.[28] Reductions in hospital use that followed prospective payment stimulated new markets for outpatient and home care.

BUILDING NURSING KNOWLEDGE

What Is the Nurse's Role in Cost Containment?

Bair NL, Griswold JT, Head JL. Clinical RN involvement in bedside-centered case management. *Nurs Econ.* 1989; 7(3):150–154.

In the current health care system, there is often a gap between the cost of care provided to clients and the amount reimbursed to the institution under the prospective payment system. Additional revenue cannot be generated by increasing charges, so the institution's survival must be protected by decreasing costs. Bair, Griswold, and Head describe one hospital that was able to reduce this gap through the central role of the bedside nurse in cost containment that is fostered by the case management system. The overall approach is based on the belief that the bedside nurse is most familiar with the client and is trained to evaluate how cost-containment efforts affect the quality of care.

At this hospital, the bedside nurse is placed in charge of ensuring that care is efficient during the client's hospitalization. The nurse also makes sure that there is an effective discharge plan for the client's care after discharge. This is vital to decrease the likelihood of a need for further hospital care. The bedside nurse identifies necessary care and discharge needs, and develops a plan of care mindful of the need to economize. A care coordination team made up of other health professionals in the unit then reviews the plan, makes additional recommendations, and returns it to the nurse for evaluation. The team also assists the nurse in implementing the plan. During care, the nurse acts as client advocate to ensure quality as efforts are made to economize. The nurse reviews official reimbursement criteria and collaborates with physicians to keep them focused on tracking costs. Other health professionals are also informed. This team approach, with the bedside nurse as central coordinator, emphasizes problem solving and use of the resources that are best able to meet the client's needs.

To offset the loss of inpatient reimbursement, hospitals moved quickly to offer new services, including ambulatory surgery and diagnostics.[28] Not all institutions have succeeded, however. In the early and mid-1980s, investor-owned (for-profit) institutions were thought to be a significant force in the competitive market because of their innovative management, access to capital, and ability to generate profits.[28] Many of these institutions, however, have become financially strained under the pressure to discount their services.[28]

Still another market change has been the merging of hospitals, nonprofit and investor-owned, into large hospital chains, or **multi-institutional systems,** in connection with alternative provider organizations, home health agencies, long-term-care facilities, or hospices.[56] Mergers offer institutions **economies of scale,** that is, increases in efficiency made possible through consolidation. Administrative functions, advertising and other marketing operations, and equipment and supply procurement can all be centralized. Costs can be lowered by purchasing directly from manufacturers rather than through local distributors. Through consolidation, institutions enhance their ability to compete in the regional markets for clients.

The most important question currently, however, is whether enhancing competition can cure the ills of a market that is not naturally competitive.[57] The consensus is that, as yet, the strategies employed have failed to control costs and increase efficiency.[10,19,24,26,28] Although competition strategies, combined with regulatory efforts, have slowed the rate of inflation in the health care industry, they have not stopped the expansion of resources that health care consumes.

In addition, many hospitals and HMOs, strained by the competition, are in financial difficulty.[24,28] Overall hospital costs are rising despite the falloff in use.[29] Hospital productivity is falling, as reflected by increases in the number of employees per bed, and the rise in physicians' incomes continues to outpace inflation.[28] Meanwhile, the number of uninsured citizens is increasing, and of 243.1 million people in the United States, 31.5 million are without insurance coverage.[58] Some authorities point out that competition strategies take time to work and that the current problems at least partially reflect government policy, which has failed to support market forces.[10,52,57] Many agree, however, that further changes, market and regulatory in nature, are inevitable.[10,19,24,26,28,52,57]

To summarize, the dynamics of supply and demand in health care deviate significantly from those of the competitive market model. In important ways these deviations interfere with the market's determination of what is produced, how it is produced, how it is distributed, and how much of it is consumed.

Despite the strong new health care finance regulations introduced in the 1980s and despite the strengthening of market forces, the cost of health care is still expanding out of proportion to the general economy. There is a growing recognition, moreover, that spending more on medical services may not significantly improve the health of the population. Society is thus reexamining the unrestricted flow of resources to the health care system.[59]

■ MAKING ECONOMIC CHOICES

Levels of Decision Making

In any economic system, decisions about how to allocate resources are made at a number of levels, from the individual level on up to the level of society as a whole.[60] In general, the decisions made at each higher level have an increasingly wide impact. More people are affected by the decisions, and they are affected to a greater extent. Figure 36–2 depicts the various decision levels within the national economy and the health care industry.

Level 1. Level 1 decisions, at the top of the inverted pyramid, involve the systemwide resource allocations that are made through health care policy. At the broadest societal level, the primary concern is how to maximize society's

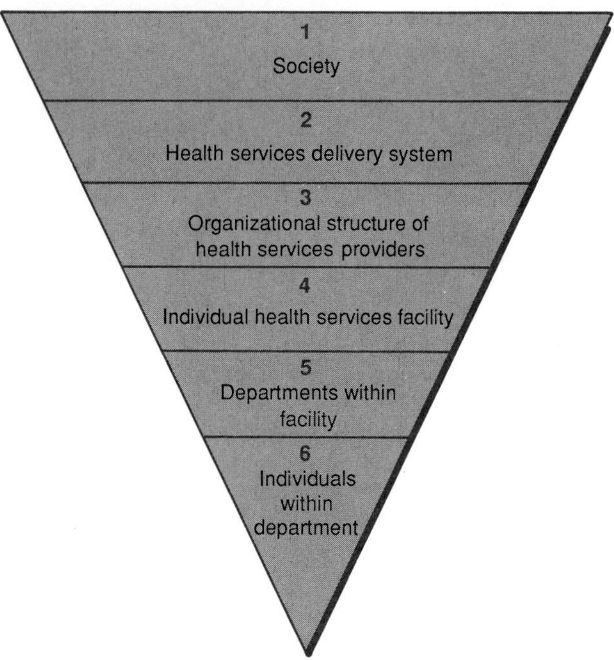

Figure 36–2. Decision-making pyramid. (*From Hicks LL, Boles KE. Why health economics.* NRG Economic J. *1984; 2 [May/June].*)

welfare. Health care must compete for resources with other social needs such as housing, food, law enforcement, defense, education, and the environment. Government structures and regulations used to administer resources are also established at this level.

The decisions made at Level 1 reflect the consensus among policymakers about what should be achieved. Those decisions take into account moral, ethical, social, and political factors[60] and are influenced by the voting patterns, letter writing, and other lobbying behavior of political constituents.

Level 2. Level 2 decisions deal with resource allocation within the health care industry. The decisions at this level represent industry responses to the social policy set at Level 1. Social policy creates the economic environment that shapes, to a large extent, the types of institutions and people that will be involved in the system. For example, a policy decision to expand Medicaid with a stringent emphasis on cost containment would place a premium on the use of efficient facilities, personnel, and technologies. Economic analysis could then help to determine the most efficient organizational structures and personnel for delivering health services industrywide.

Level 3. Level 3 decisions deal with the allocation of resources within multi-institutional systems such as hospital chains. Economic analysis by institutional leaders at Level 3 helps determine the most efficient combination of institutions and services to include within a multi-institutional system. It also helps to determine organizationwide policies for staffing, procedures, and supply procurement. Analysis at this level also determines the merged institution's policies on such issues as the provision of services to the medically indigent.

Level 4. Level 4 decisions deal with the allocation of resources within individual agencies and institutions. Single agencies must function within all of the constraints established at the previous three levels. Thus, they have less flexibility to make decisions that meet their own organizational goals. Institutional administrators use economic analysis to determine how to maximize the use of available funds.

Level 5. Level 5 decisions deal with the allocation of resources within the departments of a single institution. The major focus is on determining the most efficient methods of providing services. Department managers use economic analysis to decide what combinations of personnel and supplies to use in providing care.

Level 6. Level 6 decisions involve the priorities and practices of individual clinicians within a department. The decisions reached at Level 5 regarding personnel and equipment limit the choices made at Level 6 by individual practitioners; however, practitioners can still decide many issues. Clinicians use informal economic analysis to allocate personal time and energy, which are scarce resources.

Nursing, Nurses, and Economic Decision Making

Resources represent power. In any industry, the people who control the resources generally influence the decisions that are made. Health care faces some far-reaching economic decisions in the 1990s—decisions about the kinds of services that will be offered, how much service will be offered, who will provide and who will receive these services, and how the services will be paid for.[61] These are all decisions in which nursing has a vital interest. Nursing is, moreover, one of the most important scarce resources involved in the production of health care.[62] Therefore, it has a tremendous potential to shape the important decisions to come. In their own self-interest and, more importantly, in the interest of clients, nurses will want to participate in decision making and in resolving these basic questions about resource allocation in health care.

Level 1. Nurses have a vital interest in the economic decisions made at the broad societal level. Nurses are concerned, for instance, that all individuals have access to adequate health services. To the extent that individual nurses view access to health care as a right, they will be interested in the public policies at national, state, and local levels that address that issue.[60] The economic decisions related to health care access on which nurses have begun to focus include the following:

IMPLICATIONS FOR PROFESSIONAL COLLABORATION

Economic Issues in Nursing

Nurses have a vital interest in the access of all individuals to health care, regardless of ability to pay. To the extent that individual nurses have strong feelings about health care access they will be interested in public policies at the national, state, and local levels that address these issues, which include the structure of health care finance, third-party payment for nurses, government loans and scholarships to support nursing education and grants for nursing research, and government appropriations for public hospitals and public health agencies.

1. Revisions in the structure of health care finance that address the problem of the uninsured
2. Third-party payment to place nurses in the provider market
3. Government grants, scholarships, and loans to support nursing education and increase the supply of nurses
4. Federal budget appropriations to advance nursing research on the delivery of nursing services
5. Federal, state, and county appropriations for maintaining public hospitals and other public health agencies

As Chapter 4 establishes, nurses can act on these issues by being politically active. To participate, they can support nursing organizations, support candidates who have similar strong convictions, work in election campaigns, give campaign contributions, lobby legislators, and speak with friends and neighbors to inform them about health care policy issues. Membership in nursing organizations is particularly important, because in politics votes are a scarce resource, and those who control the votes have the influence. Nursing's professional organizations can wield influence only in proportion to the size of their voting membership.

Level 2. Level 2 decisions focus the attention and efforts of nurses on the structure and organization of health care institutions, given the constraints imposed by government policy. Decisions at this level require that nurses examine their health care objectives from an institutional perspective and consider the industrywide impact of government policy and regulations on health care and nursing services.

Legislation to reduce revenue for hospital acute care, for example, could be expected to create a new demand and market for home care. This is what happened in the period after the institution of the Medicare prospective payment system.[28] Concerned about the trend toward "quicker and sicker" hospital discharges, nursing leaders began to work toward expanding services into the home through their involvement in national and regional planning groups.

Another issue at Level 2 is the response of nurses to market forces and competition in the health care industry. Competition creates winners and losers, even among health care providers. To compete successfully, nurses are examining nursing services as a product.[63] This new view redefines nursing as a competitive, revenue-generating component in the manufacture of health care. Traditionally, nursing has been regarded as a "cost center," as part of the hospital's overhead costs included in the client's room charges. Nursing has not been looked on as a service that brings in revenue to the institution. Changing the way nursing is economically defined gives nursing economic power, but it involves changing accounting practices industrywide. For several years, nursing leaders have been devising ways to price the nursing product and establish the necessary accounting practices.[62]

Finally, nurses at Level 2 are concerned about the indirect impact of cost efficiency on nursing, particularly in these times of institutional mergers. To be competitive, health care institutions must keep their costs as low as possible. Theoretically, large health care institutions can exert monopsonistic (or single buyer) power over industry labor markets, including nursing. That means institutions are able to cut costs by keeping wages and salaries artificially low.[64] Low wages in turn reduce the supply of nurses and, ultimately, the enrollment in nursing education programs.[64] Understanding this, nurses support collective bargaining to protect not only their economic self-interest but also the interests of health care consumers and the nursing profession.

Level 3. Nursing administrators, clinical managers, and clinical nurses have an institutional policy role at Level 3. Nurses who work in multi-institutional systems are involved in setting policy for all facilities in the system. They influence the types of nursing services offered systemwide, including discharge planning and home care. They influence budgeting and staffing standards, including decisions about the mix of professionals, technicians, and ancillary personnel in individual institutions. They are also involved in finding producers for nursing supplies who ensure consistency, quality, and low cost.

Level 4. At Level 4, the level of the individual institution, nursing administrators, clinical managers, and clinical nurses influence decisions on the optimal number of nursing staff, the kinds and amounts of services to be offered, and the combination of nursing personnel and supplies needed to produce them.[60] Constraints established at the preceding level substantially limit the options of nurse managers at Level 4. It may be impossible, for example, to increase employee morale if the cause of low morale is the unfilled nursing positions that result from the budgets established at Level 3.

Under the conditions of a tight budget, however, nurses, working collaboratively with institutional administrators, can demonstrate their own cost efficiency. They are challenged to identify the activities that are unique to nursing—those activities that cannot be performed by other health professionals—to define nursing's economic base. Nurses also have the incentive to look at activities that are not exclusive to nursing, but that nurses might perform more cost effectively than others.[14] For example, they can scrutinize care given by specialized therapists to determine if it is more cost efficient when the hands-on procedures are done by nurses. To be successful, however, nurses must show that they can either (1) achieve better results than others or (2) achieve the same results at a lower total cost to the institution.[60]

Level 5. At Level 5, the departmental level, clinical managers and clinical nurses make decisions about the direct provision of nursing services. At this level, attention is focused on determining the best ratio of registered nurses to nurse extenders, given the department work load and the composition of the department staff. Other decisions at the department level involve determining staff assignments and deciding whether to use part-time personnel and substitutes for trained personnel to lower costs. Also at the department level, nurses are involved in establishing standard care plans for common nursing care problems. Standard care plans can substantially increase nursing productivity, and they provide a basis for the economic decisions that are made as part of the nurse's role in case management.[14] (See Chap. 18 for more on standard care plans.)

BUILDING NURSING KNOWLEDGE

What are Some of the Ways Nurses Can Work To Control Health Care Costs?

Smeltzer CH, Hyland J. A working plan to understand and control financial pressures. *Nurs Econ.* 1989; 7(4):208–214.

In most health care institutions, nursing constitutes the single largest expense. Smeltzer and Hyland argue that financial fluctuations in the health care environment will have an impact on nursing budgets and nursing. They stress that nursing must anticipate financial changes and respond aggressively to control costs and enhance the financial skills of clinical nurses who have management responsibility.

Smeltzer and Hyland suggest several ways to do this. Wages constitute about 90 percent of the typical nursing budget. Part-time nursing personnel hired from pools to fill in during the nursing shortage have proved expensive. The trend now is to save money by reducing the use of pool nurses by hiring more full-time nursing assistants. Another trend is to save money by reducing the number of nurses in administrative positions.

Supplies represent the remaining 10 percent of the typical nursing budget. Supply usage is thus important to cost containment. Nurses may object to supply controls because it is difficult to supervise all who have access to supplies. The authors feel that it is important for nurses to have a sense of ownership when it comes to supplies, as this results in careful scrutiny of their use, and recommend that nurses take over some of the functions of the supply department such as ordering, counting, and receiving supplies.

The authors recommend that clinical nurses who manage units participate in the budget development process so that they are aware of the overall goals. A basic fact is that nursing controls most of the institutional expenditures. If conditions call for reducing nursing hours allocated for each client day, clinical nurses need to be involved in budgeting and implementing the change.

Level 6. Finally, at Level 6, individual nurses make decisions about their priorities for providing direct client care. In spite of the constraints imposed at the preceding levels, nurses nevertheless make decisions at the bedside on the use of scarce resources. Any service provided to a client uses valuable resources, such as the nurse's time and energy. Those resources could be used to provide other services for the client or to care for other clients. Decisions on the allocation of the nurse's time and energy are thus economic decisions.

Priority Setting. Clinical priority setting involves difficult decisions. For example, how much time should the nurse spend comforting a distraught client while other clients are left unattended?[43] How much time should the nurse spend developing comprehensive nursing notes in a client's record if that activity reduces the time available for direct care? How much time should the nurse spend answering a client's questions about an upcoming operation if that means delaying a treatment for the client in the next bed?

Each of these situations forces the nurse to ration a scarce resource—time—in the course of clinical practice. Ultimately the answers to many of these questions lie in procedures and policies set at Levels 4 and 5. For example, a department may use group counseling and teaching or shift teaching activities to the preadmission phase of care. Such changes may be unavoidable as short hospital stays limit the nurse's time for addressing complicated problems.[14]

Use of Supplies. The use of expensive supplies is another area of concern to nurses at Level 6. Nurses frequently decide what products to use in performing their clinical responsibilities. Consider the problem of wound care. In deciding on a product, the nurse weighs economic factors such as a product's convenience of use, administration time, number of units required, and price per unit. Another economic consideration is the effect of the product on wound healing time.[65] Judicious decisions reduce not only costs but also the overall consumption of the nurse's and client's time and energy. At Level 6 nurses can examine routine procedures from the standpoint of cost and efficiency. They can often reduce or minimize the use of unnecessary supplies (Fig. 36–3).

Use of Personnel. As cost controls tighten, nurses are being pressured to improve their economic efficiency. Nurses must therefore ensure that they are being used efficiently. Understanding their own economic value, nurses are collaborating with physicians to establish clinical practice arrangements that maximize the use of nurses' clinical skills. Nurses are also requesting clerical help and computer systems to free their time for client care. (See Chap. 21 for more about computer systems in client care.)

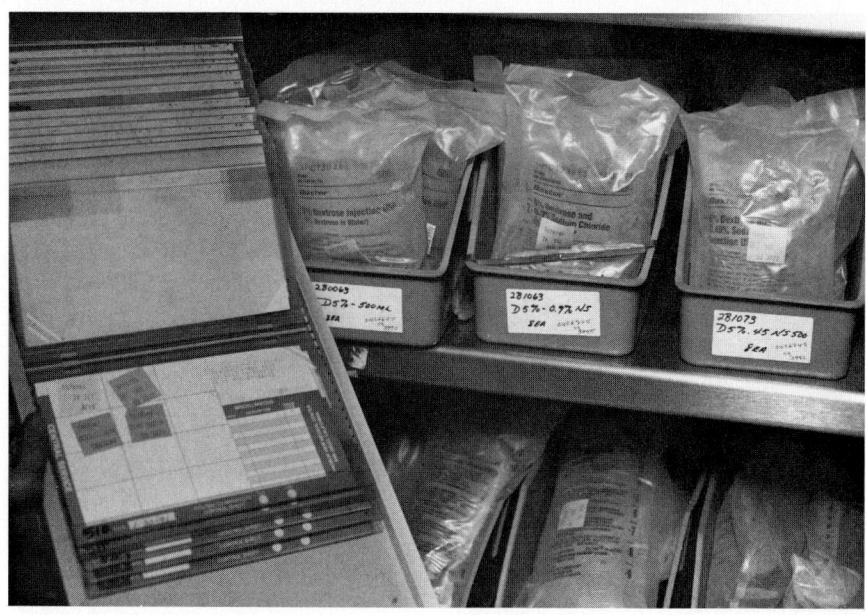

Figure 36–3. Nurses can help to control health care costs by becoming more aware of supply costs and minimizing use of expensive but nonessential supplies.

Economic Value of Collaboration. Increasingly, clinical nurses will be analyzing client care planning from an economic point of view. In making decisions about client care plans, nurses are recognizing that collaboration with the client has economic as well as professional value. Indeed, a plan designed to be cost efficient, one that is highly economic with respect to professional time and supplies, may turn out to be economically inefficient if the client fails to adhere to it. Therefore, nurses at Level 6 can influence the cost of care by considering their clients' values and expectations when devising care plans.

Finally, nurses at Level 6 help to reduce the total costs of care by educating clients to undertake self-care and to assume an active role in making health decisions. In recognition of this principle, nurses at Level 6 provide the client with the knowledge necessary to use health care resources appropriately and economically. Nurses at this level motivate clients to select healthier life-styles and help them obtain the skills necessary to make changes in their life-styles.[65] Resources spent on changing harmful life-styles generally reduce the need for expensive medical services.

Clinical Use of Economic Reasoning. Individual nurses make many economic decisions. Nurses should develop the mental habit of considering the benefits and costs of the clinical choices available. This type of reasoning is valuable for achieving clinical goals. It is also valuable for empowering nurses and nursing within the institutional context of health care.[66]

IMPLICATIONS FOR NURSE–CLIENT COLLABORATION

Economics of Nursing Care Planning

Collaboration with the client has value for economic as well as professional reasons. Client care plans must be effective to be efficient. Considering the client's desires, values, and expectations for health care increases the likelihood that the client will use the resulting plan. Conversely, misunderstandings from conflicts in values increase the total costs of care.

SUMMARY

Economics is the study of the efficient allocation of scarce resources. It is a way of thinking, and the tools of economics can be used to improve the production and distribution of health care services. When resources are scarce, choices have to be made about how they will be used and who will receive them. Along with choice comes the responsibility to use resources efficiently to maximize society's welfare.

Increasingly, health care services are being evaluated for economic efficiency. Because nursing care is one of the largest components of health service, nurses must help improve the operating efficiency of the health care industry. As health professionals collaborate to maximize the health of society, nurses must lead in minimizing the use of resources while maximizing the results. To do so, nurses must understand and apply economic tools at all levels of decision making.

As resources available to the health care industry are limited, conflicts between the needs of society and the needs of individuals will increasingly arise. As society decides who gets what resources, these conflicting needs must be accommodated and the benefits and costs must continuously be balanced. In the 1990s, nursing must consider economic values as well as humanistic values in selecting which needs to meet.

REFERENCES

1. Sorkin AL. *Health Care and the Changing Economic Environment.* Lexington, MA: DC Heath; 1986.
2. Sovie MD. Exceptional executive leadership shapes nursing's future. *Nurs Econ.* 1987;5(1):13–20, 31.
3. Rosko MD, Broyles RW. *The Economics of Health Care.* New York: Greenwood Press; 1988.
4. Dolan EG. *Economics,* 4th ed. Chicago: Dryden Press; 1986.
5. van der Gaag J, Neenan WB, Tsukahara T. *Economics of Health Care.* New York: Praeger; 1982.
6. Waud RN. *Economics.* New York: Harper & Row; 1980.
7. Fuchs VR. The "competition revolution" in health care. *Health Affairs,* summer 1988, pp. 5–8.
8. Russell LB. *Medicare's New Hospital Payment System: Is It Working?* Washington, DC: Brookings Institution; 1989.
9. Ruffin RJ, Gregory PR. *Principles of Economics,* 2nd ed. Glenview, IL: Scott, Foresman; 1986.
10. Cohodes DR. Competition and regulation redux. *Inquiry,* winter 1988, pp. 421–422.
11. Edwardson SR. Measuring nursing productivity. *Nurs Econ* 1985;3(1):9–14.
12. Strasen L. Standard costing/productivity model for nursing. *Nurs Econ* 1987;5(4):158–161, 198.
13. Smeltzer CH, Hyland J. A working plan to understand and control financial pressures. *Nurs Econ* 1989;7(4):208–214.
14. Sovie MD. Managing nursing resources in a constrained economic environment. *Nurs Econ* 1985;3(2):85–94.
15. US Department of Health and Human Services. *Health, United States, 1988.* Washington, DC: US Govt Printing Office; 1988.
16. Bloch H, Pupp R. Supply, demand, and rising health care costs. *Nurs Econ* 1985;3(2):119–123.
17. Callahan D. Meeting needs and rationing care. *Law, Medicine, & Health Care.* 1988;16(3/4):261–266.
18. Nutter DO. A hard look at cost-containment. *N Engl J Med* 1987;316(18):1151–1158.
19. Marone JA. The long rise and fast fall of health care competition. *Bull NY Acad Med.* 1988;64(1):101–116.
20. Hiatt HH. Protecting the medical commons: Who is responsible? *N Engl J Med* 1975;293(5):235–241.
21. Sloan FA, Blumstein JF, Perrin JM. *Cost, Quality, and Access in Health Care.* San Francisco: Jossey-Bass; 1988.
22. Higgins CW. The economics of health promotion. *Health Promotion* 1988;12(5):39–45.
23. Sorkin AL. *Health Economics: An Introduction,* 2nd rev ed. Lexington, MA: DC Heath; 1984.
24. Curtin LL. Economic competition: Has the "solution" become the problem? *Nurs Manage* 1989;20(5):7–8.
25. Boyar DA. Will a healthy dose of competition cure the health care system's ills? *Nurs Econ* 1985;3(4):234–237.
26. Fuchs VR. The "competitive revolution" in health care. *Health Affairs,* summer 1988, pp. 5–24.
27. Spitz B, Abramson J. Competition, capitation, and case management: Barriers to strategic reform. *Millbank Q* 1987; 65(3):348–370.
28. Goldsmith JC. Competition's impact: A report from the front. *Health Affairs,* summer 1988, pp. 162–173.
29. Gordon SD, Dawson GG. *Introductory Economics.* Lexington, MA: DC Heath; 1987.
30. Wirick GC. A multiple equation model of demand for health care. *Health Services Res* 1966;1(3):301–346.
31. Jacobs P. *The Economics of Health and Medical Care,* 2nd ed. Rockville, MD: Aspen; 1987.
32. Arrow KJ. Uncertainty and the welfare economics of medical care. *Am Econ Rev* 1963;53(5):941–973.
33. Eastaugh SR. *Financing Health Care: Economic Efficiency and Equity.* Dover, MA: Auburn House; 1987.
34. Mitchell SA. Defending the U.S. approach to health spending. *Health Affairs,* winter 1988, pp. 31–34.
35. Dougherty CJ. *American Health Care: Realities, Rights, and Reforms.* New York: Oxford University Press; 1988.
36. Phillips CY. Reimbursement for nursing services revisited. *Nurs Econ.* 1987;5(5):220–224.
37. Feldstein PJ. *Health Care Economics,* 3rd ed. New York: Wiley; 1988.
38. Glaser WA. *Paying the Hospital: The Organization, Dynamics, and Effects of Differing Financial Arrangements.* San Francisco: Jossey-Bass; 1987.
39. Fuchs VR. *The Health Economy.* Cambridge, MA: Harvard University Press; 1986.
40. Fuchs VR. *How We Live: An Economic Perspective on Americans from Birth to Death.* Cambridge, MA: Harvard University Press; 1983.
41. Menzel PT. *Medical Costs, Moral Choices: A Philosophy of Health Care Economics in America.* New Haven, CT: Yale University Press; 1983.
42. Frech HE III. *Health Care in America.* San Francisco: Pacific Research Institute for Public Policy; 1988.
43. Daniels N. *Just Health Care.* Cambridge, MA: Cambridge University Press; 1988.
44. Evans RG. *Strained Mercy: The Economics of Canadian Health Care.* Toronto: Butterworths; 1984.
45. Vladeck BC, Goodwin EJ, Myers LP, Sinisi M. Consumers and hospital use: The HCFA "death list." *Health Affairs,* summer 1988, pp. 122–125.
46. Brook RH, Kosecoff JB. Competition and quality. *Health Affairs,* summer 1988, pp. 150–161.
47. Fein R. *Medical Care, Medical Costs.* Cambridge, MA: Harvard University Press; 1986.
48. McClure W. The medical care system under national health insurance: Four models. *J Health Politics, Policy Law* 1976;1(1): 22–68.
49. Fuchs VR. Learning from the Canadian experience. *Health Affairs,* winter 1988, pp. 25–30.
50. Pellegrino ED. Medical morality and medical economics. *Hastings Center Report,* August 1978, pp. 8–11.
51. Gruber LR, Shadle M, Polich CL. From movement to industry: The growth of HMOs. *Health Affairs,* summer 1988, pp. 197–208.
52. Enthoven AC. Managed competition: An agenda for action. *Health Affairs,* summer 1988, pp. 25–47.
53. Field MJ, Gray BH. Should we regulate "utilization management?" *Health Affairs,* winter, 1989, pp. 103–112.
54. Bair NL, Griswold JT, Head JL. Clinical RN involvement in bedside-centered case management. *Nurs Econ.* 1989;7(3): 150–154.
55. Gabel J, Jajich-Toth C, de Lissovoy G, Rice T, Cohen H. The changing world of group health insurance. *Health Affairs,* Summer 1988, pp. 48–65.
56. Krampitz SD, Coleman JR. Marketing—A must in a competitive health care system. *Nurs Econ* 1985;3(5):286–289.
57. Quinn CC. Health care regulation and market forces. *Nurs Econ* 1984;2(3):204–209.
58. *Sourcebook of Health Insurance Data.* Washington, D.C.: Health Insurance Association of America, 1990.

59. Strosberg MA, Fein IA, Carroll JD. *Rationing of Medical Care for the Critically Ill.* Washington, DC: Brookings Institution; 1989.
60. Hicks LL, Boles KE. Why health economics? *Nurs Econ* 1984; 2(3):175–180.
61. Francis S. Health care forecasts: U.S. industrial outlook, 1988. *Med Benefits,* February 15, 1988, pp. 1–3.
62. Sovie MD, Smith TC. Pricing the nursing product: Charging for nursing care. *Nurs Econ* 1986;4(5):216–226.
63. Strong VL. Nursing products: Primary components of health care. *Nurs Econ* 1985;3(1):60–61.
64. Aiken LH, Mullinix CF. The nurse shortage, myth or reality? *N Engl J Med* 1987;317(10):641–645.
65. Fry SI. Moral values and ethical decisions in a constrained economic environment. *Nurs Econ* 1986;4(4):160–163.
66. Russell LB. *Is Prevention Better Than Cure?* Washington, DC: Brookings Institution; 1986.

BIBLIOGRAPHY

Altman SH, Brecher C, Henderson MG, Thorpe KE. *Competition and Compassion.* Ann Arbor, MI: Health Administration Press; 1989.

Bloom JR, Alexander JA, Flatt S. Organization turnover among registered nurses: An exploratory model. *Health Services Manage Res* 1988;1(3):156–167.

Eastaugh S. The impact of the Nurse Training Act on the supply of nurses, 1974–1983. *Inquiry* 1985;22(4):404–417.

Enthoven AC. Managed competition of alternative delivery systems. In: Greenburg W, ed. *Competition in the Health Care Sector: Ten Years Later.* Durham, NC: Duke University Press; 1989.

Feldman R, Dowd B. Is there a competitive market for hospital services. *J Health Econ* 1986;5(4):277–292.

Gabel J, Jajich-Toth C, Williams K, Loughran S, Haugh K. The commercial health insurance industry in transition. *Health Affairs* 1987;6(3):46–60.

Helmer FT, McKnight P. Management strategies to minimize nursing turnover. *Health Care Manage Rev* 1989;14(1):73–80.

Hicks LL. Increasing role of economic analysis in the health care industry. *J Am Phys Ther Assoc* 1986;66(10):1563–1566.

Melhado EM, Feinberg W, Swargz HM. *Money, Power, and Health Care.* Ann Arbor, MI: Health Administration Press; 1988.

Menzel PT. Economic competition in health care: A moral assessment. *J Med Philos* 1987;12:63–84.

Meyers JA. *Incentives vs Controls in Health Policy: Broadening the Debate.* Washington, DC: American Enterprise Institute; 1985.

Prescott PA. DRG prospective reimbursement: The nursing intensity factor. *Nursing Manage* 1986;17(1):43–46.

Reinhardt UE. Rationing the health-care surplus: An American tragedy. *Nurs Econ* 1986;4(3):101–108.

Rorem CR. A quest for certainty: Views, memoirs, and predictions on health care economics. *Inquiry* 1982;19(2):99–104.

Stewart DW, Hickson GB, Pechmann C, Koslow S, Altemeier WA. Information search and decision making in the selection of family health care. *J Health Care Marketing* 1989;9(2):29–39.

Weiner J, Steinwachs D, Williamson J. Nurse practitioner and physician assistant practices in three HMOs: Implications for future U.S. health manpower needs. *Am J Public Health* 1986;76(5):507–511.

CHAPTER 37

Health Care as a Transaction

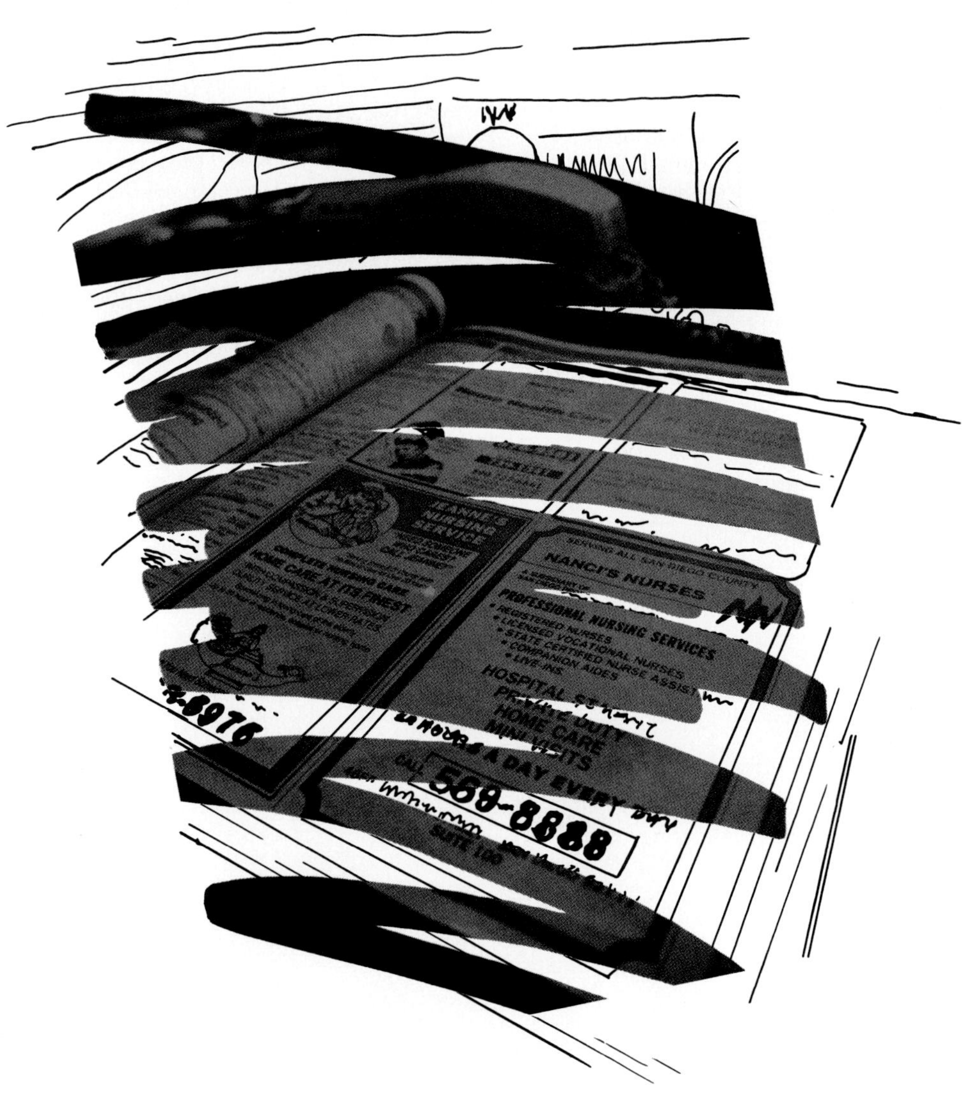

Behavioral Objectives

Upon the completion of this chapter, the student will be able to:

1. Define the transaction concept as it pertains to health care.
2. Summarize several factors that influence the delivery and cost of health care, and list the major barriers to health care access in the United States.
3. Describe the policy alternatives for achieving the goal of universal access to health care.
4. Describe four moral arguments for a right to health care.
5. Define consumerism, list several rights and obligations of consumers, and describe the place of consumerism in health care transactions.
6. List obstacles to consumer decision making in health care and discuss ways nurses can help clients to become successful consumers.
7. State the difference between a "disease paradigm" and an "illness paradigm" for viewing sickness and discuss the relevance of the transactional approach to provider–client relationships.
8. Define collaboration.
9. List the assumptions and describe the phases of the mutual interaction model of client care.
10. Discuss what is meant by a client contract and discuss its role in collaboration.
11. List client- and nurse-related variables influencing the use of the mutual interaction model.
12. State the relationship between mutual interaction, adherence, and caring.
13. Discuss the role of negotiation in collaboration, and define what is meant by consensus-building.
14. State several approaches to clients that promote principled negotiation.

KEY TERMS

adherence
agenda decisions
collaboration
collaborative decision-making
consensus building
consumerism
control
individualism
influence
leadership
management
management by objectives
mutual interaction
operational control decisions
power resource
principled negotiation
program decisions
shared governance
transaction
transformational leadership

The United States today is at a crossroads, confronting fundamental questions about its health care delivery system. Reform, in all likelihood, lies ahead. Not only is our approach to the financial transactions on which health care depends at issue, but along with that, the basic model for the organization and delivery of service and the nature of the services to be offered. At issue, too, is the even more fundamental question of the role that government will play in a revamped system.

This chapter builds on discussions in Chapters 35 and 36 of the current problems in US health care delivery and the obstacles to equitable health care distribution within a free-market economy. From the perspective of American values, it looks at the options for change currently under consideration, highlighting the essential features of various policy proposals, and pointing out the economic implications and political feasibility of major plans for reform.

This chapter also examines the importance of consumerism in health care, recognizing its potential role under those reform proposals that are likely to prevail, and it considers the importance of consumer needs to the role of the nurse. The transactional model for health care encounters presented in the chapter should prove useful under any new approach to health care delivery. Referred to as mutual interaction, the model is based on a collaborative philosophy that is uniquely appropriate to the traditional American value of individual self-determination and to the contemporary reality of individual and cultural diversity in an increasingly complex, pluralistic society.

Finally, the chapter presents a transactional view of

management and leadership in nursing that is well-suited to the transformational changes that appear to lie ahead and to nursing's role in influencing their direction.

■ HEALTH CARE AS AN ECONOMIC TRANSACTION

The United States has a long history of managing the distribution of its resources through competition and free-market transactions in the private sector tempered only as necessary by government intervention to balance the inequities that develop because of market imperfections. The United States, for historical and Constitutional reasons, distributes health care primarily through the private sector, leaving its purchase to the individual transactions that are used for any material good. **Transactions** can be viewed as acts of exchange—economic, political, and human, based on personal preference and means—into which people enter for their mutual benefit and welfare.

The American approach is grounded on a value of self-determination and a philosophy of economic individualism.[1] Individualism holds that individuals (in contrast to the government) are the best judge of their own interests in the marketplace. Our system, based on this philosophy, is premised on the idea that the free market will provide a range of options for health care as for any good or service from which individuals can select according to the immediacy and extent of their needs and their ability to pay. It is also premised on a theory of demand and supply under which consumers, through their purchasing power, have the market influence necessary to assure that at least some of the options are affordable.

However, the ability of the market to achieve distributive justice exists only when markets are working in an ideal fashion—a situation that almost never occurs in health care services industry, as Chapter 36 pointed out. The price of self-determination in the purchase of health care then is that it places the burden of responsibility on individuals. This ultimately leads to inequities because some people have greater needs than others and are less able than others to fend for themselves.

Current Mechanism for Achieving Distributive Justice in Health Care

Over the years, two systems have evolved to assist individuals with the burden of obtaining health care, both of which were detailed in Chapter 35. One is the system of private health insurance that emerged in the Great Depression and became popular as a fringe benefit of employment during World War II.[2] Aided by government tax incentives and labor union pressure, employer-paid private insurance expanded steadily over the years, until today it is firmly established as the primary means of health care finance, serving 57 percent of the US population,[3] and 85 percent of those under age 65.[4] The other system is our system of government health care entitlement programs comprised primarily of Medicare and Medicaid. Initiated in 1965 under the Great Society legislation of the Johnson Administration, these programs serve the health care needs of certain vulnerable populations, specifically, the elderly, the poor, and the disabled. They, too, have grown over the years, and today their combined enrollment numbers over 60 million people, or roughly 25 percent of the US population.[5]

Despite these vast systems, between 31 and 37 million people go unserved, the result of the unrelenting rise in health care costs and the price of insurance premiums that has plagued the nation for decades and continues today. People without coverage, many of whom are employed, are left to depend on the charity of others, often providers, or are forced to purchase what care they can afford out-of-pocket, using their limited disposable incomes.

Problems in Achieving Distributive Justice in Health Care

Many of the factors that drive up the cost of health care were detailed in Chapters 35 and 36, as was the effect of third-party payment on demand and supply in health care. The overall impact of runaway costs and high use, as indicated in those chapters, has been to drive up the price of health insurance premiums for both group plans and individuals. The workplace is no longer the guarantor of coverage it once was.

The high cost of care is a particular problem for large corporations, many of which are self-insured. It is well known, for example, that General Motors now pays more for the health care of its employees and their families than for the steel it uses in cars. To cope with cost pressures, large corporations have sought to reduce the typically generous benefits they provide.[6] Whereas to date, labor unions have successfully resisted employers' attempts at benefit reduction, declines in coverage for workers' dependents reflect, in part, the increased contributions to premiums employers now require from their employees.[6]

Job-based insurance is even more insecure for employees of small businesses than for those of large businesses, but for different reasons. In small businesses, the threat is not so much from the high cost of care, as from the high cost of health insurance premiums. Some describe the cause as a disintegration of the small-group insurance market.[6,7] Insurers generally consider small groups to represent a greater risk, a fact that puts upward pressure on the price of premiums.

Squeezed economically, small businesses have been forced to shop aggressively for lower premiums. In response, small-group insurers have offered plans, but to keep premiums down, have competed on the basis of **risk selection**. That means insurers avoid insuring workers or groups who have experienced illness, or who for various reasons, are thought to be at risk for illness and therefore likely to be high users of benefits.[6] Thus, insurers, to remain competitive, now focus more on ways to avoid risk than to share it.

The result is that employees who were once well insured now face the possibility that coverage will become unavailable when they need it most. Many feel trapped in jobs they would like to leave, fearing that they may not be included in the group plan provided by a new employer. Moreover, many small businesses (71 percent) simply do not provide health benefits, with cost cited as the major deterrent.[7] Only recently has the government reached out to assist the self-employed by offering them a temporary 25 percent tax-deduction for their health insurance premiums,[7] a figure that contrasts markedly to the 100 percent exclusion given to those employed by others. Thus, small business employees and the self-employed are two groups facing substantial insecurity in obtaining health care.

Another reason for the growth in the numbers of uninsured is the erosion of Medicaid over the years. Here again cost is a primary factor. Medicaid programs depend on state as well as federal contributions, with states setting the eligibility requirements. Some states are better able than others to fund health benefits for their poor citizens and adjust their eligibility requirements accordingly. Thus, coverage varies substantially from state to state, with the northern and western states offering more generous benefits than other areas.[8,9] Unlike Medicare, eligibility for Medicaid is said to be means-tested. That is, receipt of benefits depends on people's potential to provide for themselves as defined by their annual income. States usually define eligibility standards as a percentage of the federally defined poverty level, some states setting eligibility at 100 percent of the federal figure (currently defined as $13,400 for a family of 4), but many setting it at less.[10]

During the 1980s, both state and federal governments sought to reduce Medicaid expenditures, with a reduction of federal funds coming as a result of tax cuts made during the Reagan Administration. This led to reductions in eligibility and an expansion in the number of people without insurance, the largest group of which are people age 19 to 24, followed by children under 18 years.[11,12] This is a matter of great concern given the importance of preventive care and early intervention for this group. While the 1990 Budget Reconciliation Act contained provisions to expand eligibility, particularly for pregnant women and children under 19, states are expected to have difficulty financing these expansions.[5] Thus, the outlook for coverage of the poor is even more uncertain than for those with job-based insurance.

Medicare, which has no means test, has fared better than Medicaid over the years, covering more and more elderly each year for acute care and reaching most of the elderly in need. Nevertheless, out-of-pocket costs are growing, as Chapter 35 indicated, and this increases concerns about the continued ability of the elderly to obtain care.[9] Moreover, long-term care coverage is skimpy.[9]

The issue of long-term care is particularly important, given the expected growth in the elderly population. Estimates project that the demand for nursing home care will triple by the year 2000.[13] Given that figure, a serious question arises about how the nation will pay for long-term care in the future. Unfortunately, the present structure fails to meet the needs of those without the means to finance such care, and this contributes to the problem of the uninsured. For example, there is no mechanism comparable to the commercial insurance available for acute care. Less than 2 percent of long-term care, in fact, which is often required for catastrophic illnesses such as Alzheimer's disease and accidental brain damage, is financed through private insurance.[14] Furthermore, current public programs stringently limit the long-term care they provide. Medicare has restrictive conditions governing eligibility and pays only for 100 days of skilled nursing care per episode of illness.[15] Although asset protection mechanisms are being developed at the state and national level, Medicaid at present pays only for those who are without any financial means whatsoever; thus families must be impoverished before assistance is available. Given that long-term care is in ever-increasing demand and costly (in excess of $30,000 per year per client), the problem of payment is of great concern not only to aging individuals, but to the nation and has become a critical issue in health care delivery.

Finally, the financial base of Medicare may be at risk, a fact that threatens the future entitlement of the aging, baby-boom generation (those born between 1945 and 1960). Today, four workers' tax contributions are needed to support a single Medicare beneficiary. As the population continues to age, the ratio of taxpayers to beneficiaries may well decrease, perhaps to as low as 2:1 by the middle of the next century.[16] A shrinking taxpayer base means higher premiums in the future.[16] Without additional revenues, the system may well collapse, spurring authorities to call for a more actuarially sound, prefunded program that will avoid financial bankruptcy.[16]

In addition to the present inadequacies of the employer-paid insurance system and the public entitlement programs, other problems exist that threaten equitable distribution of health care more directly. These focus on provider availability. Hospital services account for 40 percent of total US expenditures on health care.[17] Because of falling revenues from various public and private sector cost-containment measures and the increasing barriers to cost-shifting mentioned in Chapter 35, hospitals today are struggling to provide quality care, both to those who can and cannot pay, with far lower margins between their expenses and operating revenue than in previous years.[18] While market strategies, described in Chapter 35, have helped to offset revenue reduction, they have not filled the gap completely.[19,20] Service shifting to ambulatory clinics and centers, not, as yet, reimbursed prospectively, also reduces hospital use and consequently hospital revenue.[18,21]

As a result hospitals are clearly being hurt. Lower revenue, poor cash flow, and the economic pressure of caring for the uninsured are creating operating losses resulting in an alarming number of hospital closures. Indeed, some 500 hospitals have closed nationwide since the early 1980s, and it is estimated that another 200 may close before 1995.[21,22] Three types of institutions seem to be particularly vulnerable: (1) public hospitals serving urban populations and a large percentage of the uninsured; (2) rural hospitals encountering not only falling revenues but difficulties finding qualified personnel for the range of services required for accreditation;[21] (3) investor-owned hospitals in highly competitive markets where the big discounts necessary to attract third-party health plans often jeopardize institutional finances.[20] Reduction in the number of hospitals serving urban and rural populations promises to further increase distribution inequities.

Physician services are another concern. Rate setting by Medicare insurers, pressures to become "participating physicians" in managed care plans with negotiated fee schedules, and recent reforms by the Health Care Financing Agency (UCFA) challenging the procedure-based reimbursement system are forces for substantial constraint of physicians' incomes.[23] It remains to be seen what impact HCFA's reforms, aimed at rewarding evaluation and management while reducing payments for procedures, will have in a litigious practice environment in which physicians are strongly motivated to perform procedures in the practice of defensive medicine. Moreover, there are increasing attempts by government and private insurers to regulate medical practice in the interest of cost-containment. Some authorities are concerned that these factors taken together—increased regulation and falling reimbursement in an environment that has yet to deal effectively with the spector of malpractice litigation faced by medical practitioners—will ultimately reduce the appeal of medicine as a potental profession among talented college students, threatening the number and quality of future practitioners.[24]

A severe shortage of nurses, however, already exists, as Chapter 35 indicated. This is complex phenomenon relating to both demand (increasing illness intensity) and supply (job satisfaction, wage structure) factors,[22] and it has very serious implications given its extent, and the demonstrated relationship between greater numbers and qualifications of nursing staff and reduction in hospital morbidity and mortality rates.[25] Compressed wage schedules for registered nurses have made it possible for hospitals to substitute nurses for nonnursing personnel, and to downsize their support staff infrastructures.[22] This means that nurses have been expected to absorb additional duties from such departments as pharmacy, central supply, housekeeping, transport, and clerical service, reducing nurses' time for clinical activities and contributing to job dissatisfaction.[22] Some authorities believe that the nursing shortage would be diminished significantly by improving job conditions and by improving nurses salaries which have failed to reflect the significant increases that labor shortages usually bring.[22,26] Unfortunately, both of these strategies are substantially more difficult to undertake now than in the past, given the current hospital reimbursement climate.

All of these factors, then, the high cost of health care, related problems in the health care financing system that contribute to the millions of uninsured, along with reimbursement conditions that fail to serve providers interests are the current focus of national attention. The nation is alert to the fact that advances in quality and efficiency are being overtaken by reimbursement constraints and that substantial distributive injustice exists in US health care. Citizens and health care professionals seem eager to take another look at US health care policy, as evidenced by attention to the topic in the popular media and professional journals and conferences. Policy makers, executive and legislative, and policy researchers (experts employed by universities or policy research institutes) are also paying a great deal of attention to health care, drafting various proposals for the nation to consider. It remains to be seen whether this national debate will result in incremental change, thus preserving vestiges of economic individualism, or whether a bold, new system will emerge that takes a more collective approach to human welfare.

Alternatives to the Current System

Chapter 35 described a continuum of policy options for confronting the nation's health care problems: the laizzez-faire option, unworkable under current conditions, that leaves access and distribution to be worked out in the private sector; the various intermediate options, involving degrees of policy change and system restructuring, that combine the resources of the private and public sectors to provide universal access; and the option of a totally new, comprehensive government-run system on the model of Canada's system of national health insurance. While current proposals seek to achieve the same goals, universal coverage and cost-containment, they vary considerably in the means proposed, and particularly on the role of government in achieving desired outcomes.

Market Proposals. Market proposals reject increased government regulation as an answer to our health care delivery problems, and stress that it is possible to achieve equitable distribution by making adjustments to correct health care market deficiencies.

Market proposals typically limit the role of government to making the necessary statutory changes, although they do not replace Medicaid and Medicare. Advocates point out that market deficiences in health care have to do with lack of direct consumer involvement under third-party payment. A tax-credit plan, they feel, would provide the means for low-income families to participate in the system, while using the dynamics of the market to achieve cost-containment. Critics, however, stress that health care consumers often encounter significant barriers to informed decision making, and are overwhelmed by the complexities of a system with multiple insurers. Countering such criticisms, advocates argue that groups of consumers (in unions, professional organizations, churches, or alumni associations) could act collectively, using agents to negotiate favorable rates and plans.[27]

Another market approach, one promoted by insurers, is to increase the number of people covered by reforming the small-group insurer market.[7] This would be done by creating a system of private reinsurance. Reinsurance means to insure again, and would create a way for small-group insurers to cover groups with high-risk individuals. Losses incurred in covering high-risk persons would be spread equitably across all insurers in the private marketplace. That way, additional reforms would be possible, including the elimination of the practice of risk-selection that today excludes entire groups of individuals. Limits could also be placed on variation in insurance carriers' rates.[7] Tax assistance to small-businesses, another idea, would enable employers of fewer than 25 employees to offer group plans. This approach also advocates the establishment of state risk pools to insure those high-risk individuals who are uninsurable under employer plans, with losses covered by tax revenue.[7]

While market reforms appeal to many, opposition to them as a sole approach comes from citizens, policy makers, and professionals who believe that the current piecemeal system of multiple payors is simply too inefficient to perpetuate, that the system of tax credits required would be too expensive, that the market approach will fail to contain costs, that the desired outcome of univeral coverage would not be achieved, or that market approaches fall short on important problems such as long-term care or reorienting the delivery system toward preventive care.

Play or Pay. Other proposals, put forth by those who believe the market alone cannot solve delivery problems, contain reforms of a more far-reaching nature, often including market features, but going beyond to propose broad new regulations or public finance structures. One popular approach would require employers by law to provide health benefits. Such proposals, commonly referred to as "play or pay" plans, typically advocate the development of new government insurance systems, to which employers would be required to make contributions through a payroll tax, if they chose not to provide private insurance benefit packages. Proposals vary on whether new systems would be run by federal or state governments, and on whether they replace or retain Medicare and Medicaid.

Typically, these proposals give new powers to the federal government to define minimum benefit packages for private and public insurers, relax eligibility requirements for an expanded Medicaid system to cover the unemployed, and devise stringent cost-containment strategies. Frequently such plans also contain tax assistance for small businesses and place emphasis on providing preventive services and correcting current inadequacies in long-term benefits.

Advocates of play or pay believe the play or pay strategy represents a definitive step toward health care reform and correcting the distributive injustice of the current system. Critics, on the other hand, state that play or pay simply mandates that employers will enter a seriously flawed system. They point out that given the high cost of premiums, many employers may opt to pay rather than play (a problem some plans attempt to remedy), thereby putting additional responsibility on the government to finance coverage.[28]

National Health Insurance. National health insurance proposals represent the most comprehensive, far-reaching, and some would say radical, approach to health care reform. Such a plan involves replacing the current delivery system with a new, tax-financed, government run system of health insurance.

National health insurance is not a new idea. Indeed, it was first mentioned as a US policy option as early as 1911,[29] and seriously considered in the early 1970s, being dropped only after strong lobbying by organized medicine and the insurance industry, groups that stand to lose power under such a system.

Essential features of a national health insurance program are that it is compulsory, covering everyone for medically essential services, replaces multiple private insurers with a single public insurer, uses global budgeting, planned allocation of resources and monopsony (single-buyer) power to contain costs, and employs utilization review to monitor the appropriateness of care, and is tax-funded.

Global budgeting refers to setting targets or caps on health care spending, commonly tied to the nation's gross national product (GNP). Such a system has worked well in the former West Germany and in Canada. Both countries use a system of negotiated regional or provincial spending caps, implemented through comprehensive hospital budgets and fee schedules for physician services that are reimbursed on a fee-for-service basis. If spending exceeds the expenditure target in a given time period, payments are reduced for the succeeding budget period.

Planned allocation of resources refers to the control of new facility construction and major capital improvements to existing facilities. Planned allocation is accomplished by exluding capital improvements from hospital budgets and subjecting capital spending proposals to stringent review procedures carried out by government agenices. This allows the regionalization of costly technology and the reduction of facility duplication. Planned allocation is thought to be an important reason for Canada's success in cost-containment.[30]

Monopsony power, dicussed in Chapter 36, also contributes to cost containment. The unified administration of a national health insurance plan means that the government acts as the monopsonistic purchaser of the goods and services necessary for delivering health care. It is therefore able to take advantage of economies of scale and to arrange favorable prices from suppliers and wage schedules from workers. This serves as a substantial constraint on cost-inflation.

Utilization review as it is employed in the United States refers to government-mandated peer review organizations (PROs) that review cases to determine whether health services were appropriately provided and are therefore reimbursable under government entitlement programs. Under national health insurance, however, utilization review often means the application of more comprehensive standards to minimize costs. One variation, used in Canada, is to substitute a review of physicians whose practice costs deviate from the norm for a case-based review system.

Proponents of national health insurance in the United States frequently point to the Canadian system as a model to follow. The Canadian system provides universal coverage and a uniform, comprehensive package of benefits to all its citizens with no cost-sharing or consumer billing, and does so expending proportionately less of its national resources than the United States.

Canada's system is administratively decentralized and relies primarily on tax-funding from the federal government and its 10 provincial and two territorial governments. Each province and territory maintains its own structure, comprised of a health ministry and public insurer operating under federal guidelines.[31] Three provinces charge premiums, Alberta, British Columbia,[32] and Ontario,[31] but these comprise a minor portion of provincial plan revenue (19 percent in the case of Ontario). Ontario employers, for example, pay premiums for workers; they and the self-employed pay premiums directly to the public insurer; those over 65 are required to pay no premiums, and those without resources are eligible for full or partial assistance.[33]

Under federal guidelines, all Canadians are entitled to the same coverage and eligible for the same benefits. Beneficiaries have free choice of providers. Reimbursement involves transactions between provider and public insurer; consumers receive no bills and there are no deductibles and copayments. Extra-billing (billing the consumer for charges in excess of government allottments for services) is illegal, so that once premiums are paid, consumers drop out of the payment system entirely. Private insurers are prohibited by law from offering services provided by a provincial plan, but may offer services not covered. Private plans provide consumers with options to which they are not entitled under the government plan, such as private and semiprivate hospital rooms.[33]

Benefits include an extensive array of services not unlike those of many US employer-paid private policies, including a broad range of hospital, therapeutic, and diagnostic services, but, unlike the United States, also including long-term care. Services *not* covered include dental work, eyeglasses, artifical limbs, crutches and braces, cosmetic surgery, psychological testing, and employment and insurance physical examinations.

Canada has been able to provide an impressive list of services to its entire population, and yet contain costs more successfully than the United States. In 1987, for example, Canada spent 8.6 percent of its GNP on health care while the United States spend 11 percent.[34] Authorities believe that Canada has been able to do this largely because its monopsony power, global budgeting, and planned allocation mentioned above, but also because of the administrative efficiency of a single-payer system. Indeed, some experts feel that lower administrative costs are one of the chief reasons that Canada has been able to stabilize its health care inflation rates.[35]

Nevertheless, problems are emerging in the Canadian system and these need to be considered in a decision on national health insurance in the United States. Canada now faces rising costs from high public use and the pressure to keep up with dramatic technological changes in virtually every field of health care. Despite universal coverage, consumers must often wait to receive elective procedures. In addition, Linton states that global budget caps are forcing rationing decisions at the local level, of which the public, as yet, is unaware.[36] Moreover, global budgeting is inhibiting institutional ability to develop new programs for communities' changing needs. Negotiations over physicians' fees are becoming more heated at the same time the government is entertaining the need to control the number of services for which it will pay. Linton suggests that these pressures ultimately may make health care rationing inevitable in Canada.[36]

Advocates of a Canadian-style system point to its success with universal coverage and cost-containment. Critics, however, stress the disadvantages identified above, and dispute whether such a system would transfer to the United States with a population 10 times larger than Canada's. While national health insurance has substantial support, some experts point to the potential economic disruption that abolishing the private health care system, a system that employs 7.7 million workers, would cause.[6,16]

A Canadian-Style System for the United States? Despite the many attractions of the Canadian system, its financial support requires that Canadians pay taxes at a higher rate than in the United States. It is estimated, for example, that $250 billion in new taxes would be required to run a Canadian-style program in the United States; and even though much of this amount would replace insurance or out-of-pocket payments, it would nevertheless be a highly visible expenditure and subject to intense political scrutiny.[37] To date, the United States has handled its problems with incremental policy changes. It thus seems likely that before a plan of national health insurance is adopted, further steps will be taken to modify the current system.

Consumerism in Health Care

Definition of Consumerism. In general, **consumerism** refers to the promotion of consumer interests. However, the term, as it is used in the literature, has at least two distinct meanings. One meaning views consumerism as the organized reaction of individuals to the perceived or real inadequacies of sellers and their products, to the marketplace or market mechanisms, or to government services or consumer policy.[38] This meaning highlights consumerism as a coordinated social movement and focuses on actions of consumer research and advocacy groups to advance people's preferences for economic, political, and social benefits to be derived from public decisions. Another meaning views consumerism as the direct, face-to-face challenges to sellers' claims that consumers make in their efforts to be discriminating buyers. This meaning focuses on promotion of individual self-interests within bargaining relationships and refers specifically to such consumer methods as comparison shopping, checking performance records, seeking the best quality, and bargaining to secure the most reasonable cost.[39]

Consumerism in health care, as in other areas, refers to the collective and individual acts by which people assert their economic interests. This may mean a collective challenge to government or an employer to secure health benefits; it may mean an individual challenge to a bureaucracy or institution to ascertain one's rights; or it may mean a challenge to an individual provider to voice one's point of view and to demand a share in decisions on the health diagnosis and plan of treatment and care.

Origins of Consumerism. Consumerism as a social movement arises when consumers sense an inequity between their own power and the consolidated power of the seller, which they perceive to threaten their interests in some way. Such conditions have existed intermittently in the United States since the beginning of the century, as documented by a series of books that have exposed adulteration, fraud, and unsafe practices to the American public.[40–42] One of those books, published in 1927, was entitled *Your Money's Worth*.[41] It highlighted many of the ways consumers were being exploited at the hands of the business interests.

Schlink, a coauthor of the book, went on to form Consumers' Research Corporation in 1929; this company continues today to do product testing for American consumers. The Consumers Union, founded in 1936, also continues to do consumer research and publishes *Consumer Reports*, a popular magazine covering consumer research, including research on nonprescription health care products. In 1933, the consumer movement became international with the presentation of the Canadian "Consumer Manifesto" at the Canadian Commonwealth Confederation in Winnipeg, and thereafter spread to Europe as European consumers struggled with problems of product availability in the aftermath of World War II.[38]

The focal event of the consumer movement in the United States, however, was John F. Kennedy's message to Congress in the spring of 1962 in which he outlined his well-known Consumer Bill of Rights (Fig. 37–1). That bill identified four consumer rights: the right to safety, the right to be informed, the right to choose, and the right to be heard.[38] Table 37–1 expands on the meaning of these rights. Subsequently, Ralph Nader, generally recognized as the leader of contemporary consumerism, has carried the banner of consumerism for the American public. With Nader's influence, significant gains were made in the 1960s, including the passage of several pieces of legislation to protect the American consumer, among them the Highway Safety Act

1. **The Right to Safety.**
   This refers to the consumer's right to be protected against the marketing of goods that are hazardous to health or life. It encompasses dangers to health and safety from voluntary use of a product. The US Food and Drug Administration is the government body that is foremost in protecting this right for the health care consumer.
2. **The Right to be Informed.**
   This refers to the right to be protected against fraudulent, deceitful, or grossly misleading information, advertising, labelling or other practices, and to be given the facts needed to make an informed choice. In health care it is synonymous with the right to informed consent. (See Chap. 3 for more about informed consent.)
   (*Note:* There is a basic question concerning this right about whether the right to information goes beyond the right not to be deceived. Those who take the seller point of view believe that the buyer should be guided by personal judgments about the manufacturer's reputation and the quality of the brand; whereas the consumer point of view is that information should be provided by impartial sources and reveal performance characteristics. In health care, the US government is moving toward the latter position by publishing information about the mortality rates in hospitals treating Medicare beneficiaries.)
3. **The Right to Choose.**
   This refers to the right to be assured whenever possible, access to a variety of products and services at competitive prices, and in those areas in which competition is not workable and government regulation is substituted, an assurance of satisfactory quality and service at fair prices. For many years this right has been clearly manifested in the structure of public and private health care reimbursement, but it is now threatened by strong economic pressures for cost-containment in health care.
   (*Note:* There is a basic question concerning this right about whether it should be limited by the need to protect consumers against themselves. The manipulation of preferences in the marketplace, in health care as well as in other areas, creates tension between individual freedom and the need to protect inexperienced, poorly educated, or disadvantaged consumers. This controversy centers on arguments about whether government paternalism, a system in which authority undertakes to supply needs and regulate conduct, is justified. See Chap. 34 for more about paternalism.)
4. **The Right to be Heard.**
   This refers to the right to be assured that consumer interests will receive full and sympathetic consideration in the formulation of government policy and fair and expeditious treatment by its administrative bodies. Most states have departments of consumer affairs to which consumers can appeal regarding their claims of unfair transactions. In health care, professional licensing boards are commonly the government agencies that accept consumer complaints about a professional's conduct.

Figure 37–1. The consumer's bill of rights. (*Adapted from Executive Office of the President.* Consumer Advisory Council, First Report. *Washington, DC: US Government Printing Office; 1963; and Day GS, Aaker DA. A guide to consumerism.* J Marketing. *1970; 34:15.*)

TABLE 37–1. RIGHTS AND RESPONSIBILITIES IN ECONOMIC TRANSACTIONS

	Rights	Responsibilities
Consumer	■ To be informed ■ To choose ■ To safety ■ To be heard	■ To seek product or services information ■ To use judgment and knowledge in choosing ■ To speak out and participate in establishing economic policy
Seller/ Provider	■ To offer products or services for sale ■ To set terms of sale ■ To be paid	■ To comply with industry laws and regulations ■ To follow a code of business ethics ■ To ensure production service safety

of 1966, the Truth in Packaging Bill of 1966, and the Truth in Lending Bill of 1968. However, because of a worldwide recession and intense pressures on public budgets, the trends changed to favor business interests in the late 1970s and 1980s. Nevertheless, the consumer movement in the United States has continued to mature and international networks of consumer groups continue to hone their research, organizational, and political skills.[38]

Consumerism is driven by consumer dissatisfaction. An old adage, *caveat emptor*—"let the buyer beware"—captures the essence of consumerism. While consumers, exercising their freedom of choice in the marketplace, may well be satisfied with the majority of their economic transactions, the potential nevertheless exists for some transactions to be dissapointing or even harmful to the consumer. Consumerism is the countervailing force to marketplace manipulation. Seeking to safeguard themselves against the disadvantages to which they can be placed, good consumers are ever watchful, budget-minded, rational, and mindful of their need to maximize the value received for resources expended.[38]

Consumerism in Health Care. The origins of consumerism in health care also reflect a desire for redress of power inequities; however, the inequities in this case often center on the paternalistic authority of physicians to control circumstances in health care encounters.[39] A rise of consumerism in health care began in the late 1960s in response to several influences, summarized below.

- *Antiauthority trends.* Antiauthority attitudes stemming from the Vietnam War resulted in significant challenges to authority of many types in the United States during the late 1960s. The "new careers" movement of the period, for example, questioned the ability of mental health professionals and social workers to comprehend the needs of the poor.[39] Antiprofessional attitudes spilled over into other groups who began to oppose physician power.[43] Feminists charged obstetricians and gynecologists, most of whom were male, with being oblivious to women's concerns.[44] One of their goals was to establish a woman's right to make decisions about her own body, including not only reproductive freedom but also freedom from the authority of physicians, through self-care.
- *Consumer education.* Higher educational levels also accounted for public willingness to question medical authority. By the 1960s, 50 percent of the population had some post-high-school training. To serve the needs of a more educated public, a literature developed that catered to the distribution of health information and offered guidelines for dealing with physicians and the health care establishment. Health magazines appeared and rapidly grew in popularity; today, they continue as an important source of consumer health education. Moreover, hundreds of consumer-oriented books with information and how-to guidelines have been written over the intervening years. Media attention undoubtedly has been an important factor in the growth of health care consumerism, both through providing the public with medical information and informing readers about medical mistakes and mishaps.[39] As a result, consumers have come to understand not only that mistakes occur but that there is disagreement over what constitutes error.[39]
- *Growth of allied health professions.* New professions, often extensions of the nursing profession, flourished in the 1970s, and demonstrated that for some conditions and types of care, physicians' services were unnecesssary. Originally viewed as compensations for physician shortages, nurse practitioners, nurse-midwives, and nurse anesthetists have taken over or been delegated functions formerly considered the prerogative of physicians.
- *Medical ethics.* The 1970s witnessed a burgeoning concern about medical ethics on the part of both the public and the government. People began to question the assumption that physicians could be relied upon to place the patient's interest above their own.[39] This called into question not only physician authority but also the service component and gave a substantial impetus to consumerism.

Challenges to physician authority were consequently expressed in other trends that further eroded this authority, including the following.

- *Self-care.* A trend to self-care emerged along with the challenge to physician authority.[39] Home remedies, always a part of health care, became a preferred mode of care for many Americans in the 1970s, linked to a reluctance to seek professional care.[39] Do-it-yourself books continue to encourage self-care, as does the ready availability of nonprescription medications, health foods, and "natural" remedies. The increase in chronic illness over the last three decades has also contributed to the use of self-care in conjunction with and sometimes in place of professional care.[39]
- *Physician accountability.* Partly in response to media accounts of physician performance and concerns about

medical ethics, public demand for physician accountability intensified in the 1970s.[39] This trend represented a rejection of the notion that physicians should be accountable only to their peers. It also articulated a strong underlying belief on the part of consumers that they need their own enunciated rights, such as the right to informed consent, and that even if they are not experts, consumers should have a say over what is done to them. Indeed, access to information since the 1970s has been central to client rights (see Chap. 3, Fig. 3–4).

Consumerism and the Sick Role. All of these trends expressed in the public desire for a redistribution of power in the health care market represented a reaction against the monopoly physicians held over medical information and the assymmetry that monopoly created in the physician–patient relationship.[39]

Frustration was at its high point in the late 1960s, when the prevailing sociological view was that illness was a form of deviance that interfered with the social order. Parsons' theory of the sick role, first published in 1951 (and discussed in Chapter 12) proposed the idea of illness as deviance, and identified the physician as the agent of social control whose rightful power over the ill person lay in the capacity to control the distribution of information on diagnosis and treatment.[45] Such attitudes, reflected in the behavior of physicians, met resistance from an increasingly educated and skeptical public in the 1960s and 1970s. Parson's functional concept of the sick role, in which society survives through shared values, interrelated functions, and accepted instruments of social control, was subsequently criticized and ultimately rejected by those who held a wider view recognizing the inherent conflict in culture, one expression of which is consumerism.

Freidson, a contemporary of Parsons, ultimately produced a conflict model of the sick role more consistent with a consumerist perspective. Freidson's model acknowledged differences in physician and consumer perspectives as a given in health care and advocated their resolution through negotiation rather than an imposition of authority.[46]

Consumerism in Health Care Relationships. By the late 1970s, consumerist values had largely replaced the passive acceptance of physician authority. A large study by Haug and Lavin produced strong evidence of a consumerist perspective among both consumer and physician subjects.[39] This perspective was defined as a point of view that accepted consumers' rights and encouraged negotiation among equals in health care encounters.

Consumers in the study expressed both a desire to share in decison-making about treatment and a willingness to raise questions that suggested a challenge to physician authority. Physicians, in turn, indicated their awareness of consumer attitudes in the clients they encountered in practice. Some physicians in the study rejected those attitudes; others (a majority) responded to consumer challenges by using persuasion to convince clients to accept the medical plan or by negotiating to achieve acceptable compromises.[39]

Expressions of Consumer Dissatisfaction. In the years since this study, physicians have remained the primary focus of consumers' dissatisfaction. Expression, however, has taken the form of malpractice litigation rather than the more common consumer forms of exit and voice. Exit is the consumer's option to try to change seller behavior by simply taking one's business elsewhere.[47] Exit fails to work in health care because it gives the provider an unclear message about the nature of the consumer's complaint, whether related to technical competence, communication, environment, or price. Voice is the expression of dissatisfaction through working for public policies to curb unsatisfactory seller behavior. Voice gives unambiguous messages, but requires altruism on the part of the disgruntled consumer. Having taken their exit, most consumers are simply uninterested in pressing for improvements that will benefit others.[48] Thus, in health care, malpractice litigation is the mode that has proliferated.

Some authorities have called for creating representation mechanisms for expression of consumer dissatisfaction,[48] and, in fact, at least one proposal for health care reform advocates quality assurance through consumer access to professional review organizations (PROs). Whether this will foster increases in the use of voice among consumers remains unclear.

Another issue is whether physicians will continue to be the primary focus of consumer dissatisfaction. Given the present degree of third-party control over health care, the focus of consumerism could expand to include the bureaucracies and institutions that increasingly make decisions about health care for individual consumers. The fact is that physicians no longer wield the power over the system that they once did. The economic forces of the last decade have effectively shifted power away from physicians and toward third party payers.[49]

For the consumer, then, the problem is no longer a lack of participative decision-making in the physician–client relationship, but rather rather whether or not the insurer will underwrite decisions reached jointly by physician and client. Unless a national health insurance plan is enacted to take health care out of the marketplace, it is likely that consumers will begin to challenge private health plan representatives as they seek to redress perceived power inequities.

Consumer Exchange Transactions. In a perfectly competitive market, consumers are sovereign because they initiate the marketplace dynamic of demand and supply. Sellers, eager for a sale, compete with one another for consumers' business. Consumers, by the same token, are free to choose the product and price that best serve their needs. Under these conditions, consumers occupy a position of power that ordinarily goes a long way toward assuring the realization of their interests in economic transactions.

Perfectly competitive markets, however, are rare in our economy and virtually absent in the market for health care services, as Chapter 36 established. Nevertheless, providers and payers in health care are not insensitive to the importance of consumer satisfaction; they recognize that their well-being is linked to that of consumers.[50] Thus, individual consumers have, whether they recognize it or not, a considerable amount of transactional power. Despite this, consumer transactions in health care may be more difficult than those in other economic areas. The reasons have to do with the nature of illness and the technological complexity of health care.

Health care consumers, even with competition working for them, experience several difficulties in realizing their interests in market transactions. These difficulties fall into three categories: (1) determining wants, (2) making product/service comparisions, and (3) identifying the best value.[51]

Determining wants is problematic because the need for health care is episodic and therefore difficult to predict with any degree of certainty. Although consumers are usually able to predict their needs for regular checkups, they cannot predict their needs for emergency services. Thus, consumers must weigh the options of various benefit plans without a clear idea of what they may ultimately need. Under these conditions it is easy to err either by purchasing too few or too many health care beneifts.

Making product or service comparisons is also difficult. Consumers may be able to judge quality and know price for services they use relatively frequently. For those they use infrequently, however, the problem is more complex; consumers must often depend on seller-provided information as opposed to information gleaned from observation. Although consumers may seek information from people and sources other than sellers, there remains a question of what standards of comparison to apply. Is it enough that one's neighbor was satisfied with the care she received? Does the fact that one's neighbor failed to be cured mean that her physician or hospital was at fault? Is advertising any indication of quality?

Acquiring the information necessary to compare services presents a large problem for most consumers. Sources of consumer information, while more plentiful than they once were, are often limited, at least for some topics; the time required to obtain and process medical information, moreover, is considerable, and there are often barriers presented by technical language that make the processing difficult. A natural tendency for consumers under these conditions is to hedge their bets and look for associations with people or institutions who are established and well-known. A consumer may be unfamiliar with Dr. Brown but familiar with General Hospital where Dr. Brown practices and may make a decision on that basis.

Lastly, determining value is also difficult because it requires a clear knowledge of wants and prices and a standard for appraising performance, all of which are difficult to achieve. Determining value requires that the consumer weigh the perceived benefits against the costs, which is virtually impossible when information is lacking. Most medical advertising ignores price competition. Thus, advertising fails to assist consumers in making value determinations. Furthermore, the circumstances surrounding the need for health care often do not allow for price comparison; for example, emergencies generally preempt opportunities for comparison shopping.

Health care consumers' major need in exchange transactions is for information and eduction; information about options and product or service comparisons, and education about how to use the information effectively to optimize consumption. Pauly, an analyst of consumer exchanges, characterizes health care services as "reputation goods." Reputation goods are goods whose value is judged by the experience of the consumer's friends.[52] Pauly estimates that as many as three fourths of consumer health care transactions are made on a reputation basis.

Growing competition in the health care market has made sellers aware of the power of information, and this may soon give rise to a new market in health care, a market for health information. Organizations are at present assembling outcome-based performance data for internal use that Pauly expects will ultimately be provided to the public as a way of maximizing providers' competitive advantages in the market.[52] The practice of publishing outcome data is not new; the Health Care Financing Agency has published mortality information on hospitals serving Medicare beneficiaries since 1986.[1] It is not clear yet whether such information is having an effect on consumer choices. Nevertheless, the emergence of an industry that furnishes consumers with measures of severity, outcome, and quality may mean the health care market is on the verge of remedying its information deficit.[52]

Assisting Consumers to Optimize Transactions. For the present, the health care consumer's most important need remains that of information. Only informed consumers can make intelligent health care decisions. Health care providers can do much to assist consumers in closing the information gap.[53]

Despite the information explosion in health care, consumers education is left largely to individual initiative, in part because of the financial constraints on the health care system as a whole.[54] Nevertheless, hospitals and other providers are reaching out to consumers by providing community-based consumer education programs on such topics as diet, exercise, fitness, disease risk factors, and new technology and treatments. Such programs benefit consumers and providers; consumers obtain needed information, and providers are able to introduce themselves and their services to consumers. Moreover, hospitals are increasingly offering their own co-insurance plans (plans that cover items not covered under regular plans). These are targeted to particular populations like the elderly as a way of enticing consumers to their institutions; often these have consumer education programs among their benefits. Such programs help to narrow the knowledge differences between consumer and provider.

One-to-one professional encounters are another vehicle for consumer education in health care. Health care professionals, particularly nurses, help clients become good consumers by being sensitive to client needs for health information. Almost every health care encounter presents opportunities to convey some kind of health information to the client (Fig. 37–2).

Nurses are often asked for professional opinions about providers, the pros and cons of various types of benefit plans, or the efficacy of treatment modalities. Nurses must be informed themselves so that they can respond to clients' questions in an enlighted manner. Sometimes client questions go beyond the scope of the nurse's knowledge, but even in those cases nurses can be helpful by referring clients to likely sources of the information needed. Making clients aware of the local opportunities for consumer education and information is another way nurses can be helpful. Clients may be unaware, for example, of the various consumer-oriented health information books and magazines available. The nurse's important role in assisting consumers is not new, and is recognized in the American Nurses' Association's Code for Nurses, section 10 of which directs nurses to participate in the profession's efforts to protect the public from misinformation and misrepresentation (see Fig. 34–1).

Consumer education is important to both consumers and providers. Information fosters consumer involvement in health care and thus helps to satisfy the consumer desire to exercise free choice in exchanges with providers. Consumer education, moreover, redistributes the responsibility for health care from provider to consumer, and this ultimately serves the interests of both by enlisting the consumer's partnership in the diagnostic process.[55] Involved consumers make early detection and therapy more likely and

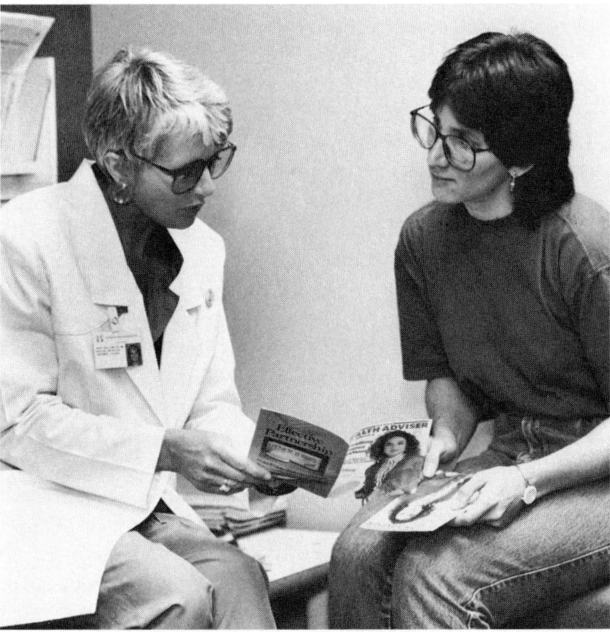

Figure 37–2. The nurse–client relationship is one vehicle for providing health care information to consumers.

enhance the probability of positive outcomes. Positive outcomes in turn foster consumer satisfaction.

Consumer education programs can significantly influence clients' acceptance of treatment and ultimately their adaptation to illness. Awareness of the risk factors for various chronic diseases, for example, helps consumers assume the role of self-regulating problem-solvers. Aware consumers are more likely to self-screen (monitor for the signs and symptoms of illness in one's own body), a complex process that is subject to many influences, internal and external.[56] Research has demonstrated individual differences in the extent to which people are attuned to body sensations, symptoms of illness, and side effects of treatments and medication.[57,58] Education serves to correct misunderstandings about sensations and symptoms.[56] Self-screening requires reliable indicators and methods of health appraisal; consumer education is a way of providing consumers with the indicators and methods they need.[56]

Consumers and Quality Assessments. Along with efficiency and equity, quality—fueled by concerns about the impact of cost-containment—is once again an important issue in health care. Today's competitive market focuses attention on quality as providers seek to improve their services and distinguish themselves from others. This in turn shifts the direction of quality assessment increasingly toward consumers' perceptions of quality. This is an ironic development, as a chief impediment to consumer satisfaction in the past has been consumers' perception that providers were concerned only about quality as a technical issue.[59] Today, however, hospitals and providers are responding to the competitive environment by struggling for definitions of quality that include the consumer's point of view.[50,60,61]

Despite current interest, the debate about the consumer's role in quality assessment is far from settled. Although there is a consensus that consumers are prepared to judge the interpersonal aspects of their health care encounters, there is by no means a consensus on their ability to judge the technical aspects of care. Opponents of consumer participation in quality assessment express concern that the average consumer is unable to evaluate technical interventions. Davies and Ware, however, reviewed an extensive literature showing that this concern may well be unfounded.[61]

Proponents of consumer participation in quality assessment argue that (1) consumers' assessments of quality predict their behavior in the marketplace; (2) consumers, even those lacking in technical qualifications, can render judgments about quality; and (3) data from consumers provide information otherwise unavailable.[61] The Davies and Ware review showed support for these arguments.

Studies showed that consumers who hold more favorable views toward technical and interpersonal features of care are significantly less likely to change providers.[61] Studies of the accuracy of consumer ratings of technical performance, moreover, correlated highly with physician ratings, particularly among younger and better-educated consumers.[61] Until recently, most methods for evaluating quality have focused on inpatient care and relied solely on examination of the medical record. Records are often incomplete, however, particularly with respect to interpersonal aspects of care. Thus, consumer quality assessment data can provide data that otherwise would be unavailable.[61]

Nurses, like other providers, are also concerned about quality. Chapter 18 discusses quality assessment as an occupational responsibility. Nursing has excelled in defining quality from a professional standpoint, but is only beginning to focus attention on monitoring quality standards from the client's perspective.[60] Strasen, a nurse executive, points out that clients who have less technical information upon which to base their judgments often substitute alternative standards to evaluate the quality of health care services. These standards often relate to the satisfaction of basic human needs, such as comfort; a clean, safe environment; good food; and friendly, courteous interpersonal interactions with providers. When these expectations are met, clients respond well to the other therapeutic implementations ordered by the physician and nurse.[60] When they are not met, clients become frustrated, stressed, and unable to maximally respond to complex implementations.

Many health care professionals, including nurses, resist measuring quality outcomes in terms of client satisfaction. They separate "professional services" from "hotel services" and seek to minimize the latter as menial or nonprofessional. Strasen argues, however, that staff professionals need to integrate services directed toward basic needs into an overall concept of therapeutic intervention that is oriented to returning clients to an optimal state of health.[60] One of the chief criteria by which clients evaluate services is how much staff professionals "care," which clients generally identify as how well nurses provide for basic client needs. Nursing, which defines its mission as caring, cannot afford to overlook client satisfaction in assessments of service quality.

Is Health Care a Right?

The purpose of any economic system, as Chapter 36 established, is to allocate scarce resources. In the United States, allocation of resources is accomplished through competition in the marketplace. The US system of economic individualism puts decison-making in the hands of the people. **Individualism** holds that each person should be the best judge of his or her own interests in the marketplace. However, this ultimately leads to injustice, because some people are less able than others to help themselves.[62] The question for society then becomes one of how to meet the needs of those who are unable to fend for themselves, particularly in areas of the basic necessities such as health care.

One answer to the problem of inequity would be for society to provide for the less fortunate by making basic necessities the right of every individual. Rights are serious entitlements that are derived from explicit rules of law or from implicit rules of morality.[63] Unfortunately, the United States has no constitutional entitlement to health care.[64] The right to health care is not guaranteed by the Constitution, nor does it appear to follow from any of the substantive rights set out in the Constitution.[63] Thus, any right to health care must be based on moral arguments.

Dougherty, in a book entitled *American Health Care: Realities, Rights, and Reforms,* considers four moral perspectives—utilitarianism, egalitarianism, libertarianism, and contractarianism—to examine whether there is a right to health care regardless of ability to pay.[63] All support, in full or in part, the right of access to a decent level of health care, as summarized below.

- Utilitarianism, or teleology (previously described in Chap. 34) judges the rightness or wrongness of an act based on its consequences. This perspective supports the right to health care because this right would maximize good consequences for society by alleviating unnecessary pain and suffering, disability, and premature death now experienced by disadvantaged Americans. This consequence is good, however, only as long as the cost of a policy of guaranteed access can be contained; otherwise good consequences for some might mean harmful consequences to others.
- Egalitarianism is a moral point of view that stresses the inherent worth and right to respect of each individual, and therefore requires that all people be treated as equals. This perspective supports the right to health care because health care is necessary to protect the incalculable and intrinsic worth of the individual. Thus, the fact that 37 million Americans are left without health insurance is implicitly condemned by egalitarianism. The question under egalitarianism is not whether there is a right to health care, but rather to what kinds and how much. These questions are answered under egalitarianism on the basis of procedural equality, so that health care is distributed in terms of the need for it. Where all basic needs cannot be met, people are to be treated equally in their chances for access to limited care.[63]
- Libertarianism is a point of view that demands that people's rational agency (transactional freedom) be protected, especially as it expresses itself in ownership. Libertarianism provides only partial support for a right to health care. Under libertarianism, special emphasis is placed on the right of noninterference in order to help assure personal liberty. The role of government is kept to a minimum and serves largely to prevent the use and threat of violence, fraud, and other harms. Nevertheless, Dougherty found libertarianism to guarantee access to at least some level of health care.[63]
- Contractarianism emphasizes people's rational agency, but only when freedom is limited through the self-imposed constraints characteristic of a truly free people. Because people are inherently social, living together in communities and producing a range of social goods, contractarianism asserts that self-imposed limitations must be established through the use of social contracts. Such contracts are unworkable on a massive social scale, however, and are replaced by institutional arrangements for

assuring social justice. Contractarianism supports a right to health care on the basis that health care would be essential to guaranteeing liberty and providing equal opportunity, and to improving the condition of the worst-off people in society.[63]

Dougherty concludes that the absence of health insurance experienced by so many Americans represents a violation of their rights and that health care reform is a moral necessity. These perspectives provide a pluralistic foundation for the right to health care comprising four elements: (1) the right to be free of health interference (from harmful conditions); (2) the right of access to a minimally decent standard of primary care, pegged to society's ability to afford it; (3) the right to curative health care to the extent that normal functioning can be preserved and restored; and (4) the right to purchase additional health care goods, services, and amenities in a free market.[63]

HEALTH CARE AS A HUMAN TRANSACTION

The spirit of democracy that gave rise to consumerism in health care has also contributed in recent years to scholarly and professional interest in the client's role in influencing the nature of health care. Both consumerist attitudes and the informed consent movement as expressions of a larger national interest in civil and human rights have been important influences on emerging ideas in health care, and have caused scholars and practitioners to reexamine the desirability of the one-sided distribution of power and knowledge that has characterized provider–client relationships in the past.

The first call for a more egalitarian approach to health care encounters was probably Szasz and Hollender's publication of a model that proposed mutual participation as the appropriate structure for relationships in cases of chronic illness (see Chap. 12).[65] Subsequently, a number of authorities in the fields of sociology, medicine, and nursing have contributed to the body of theory and research redefining the provider–client relationship along more egalitarian lines.[66–96] These authors vary in the emphasis they give to various issues and themes, but all recognize the desire of people to participate in the decisions that affect their health and the importance of mutual influence in provider–client interactions. These authors also acknowledge the differences that can and often do exist in the perspectives people bring to the health care encounter.

Many labels have been given to the outlook embodied in these works: negotiated consensus,[66,73,75] the customer approach,[73] collaboration,[80,82] mutual participation,[65,92] and mutual interaction.[79] Aside from the differences in labels, however, there is more that is similar than different in the ideas put forth.

In general, these authors reject the paternalistic position that professional authority is the only legitimate basis for health care decisions, although they also acknowledge the often crucial importance of professional input. What makes these approaches unique is their common view that professional contribution to health care decisions should never be made to the exclusion of considering the client's point of view and preferences; and, moreover, that differences between the professional viewpoint and the client's viewpoint should be resolved through working toward a mutually acceptable compromise that seeks to integrate the client's intentions with the professional's evaluation.

IMPLICATIONS FOR PROFESSIONAL COLLABORATION

A Transactional Model of Health Care

A transactional model looks at health care as a process of negotiation, and requires that the consumer (client) be involved in the process. Under a transactional model the consumer participates in planning, implementing, and evaluating decisions, and in the assessment process that precedes them. The egalitarian nature of the provider–client relationship puts the interaction on a more humanistic level: The provider and client become partners in the health care experience.

The theoretical underpinnings of this point of view are provided by interactionist theory, which suggests that in any relationship people are bound together by a mix of common and divergent goals and thus may have competing definitions of the situation and different interactional agendas.[68,72,76] Professionals and clients in a pluralistic culture thus may well have different rules, role expectations, and beliefs about what constitutes appropriate behavior in health care encounters or about what constitutes an appropriate solution to a given health problem. Thus a concept of the professional–client relationship is necessary that provides a mechanism for resolving differences.

Whereas the traditional approach to the sick role ignores differences and requires that clients passively comply with the professional's authority, a collaborative model of the helping relationship asks that clients adopt an expanded role and work jointly with the professional to determine goals and weigh alternative courses of action.[82] The collaborative model is based on the idea that equality among human beings is desirable, and that this should extend to health care relationships.[65] Consequently, the roles of professional and client under this model are viewed as a partnership in the joint venture of promoting or restoring the client's health.[65]

The nursing profession has a long history of interest in ideas that are related to this emerging framework for the sick role and the health care encounter. For example, two nursing theories—Orem's theory of self-care and King's theory of goal attainment—focus specifically on the client's capacity for self-care, the client's participation in care, and the importance of mutual planning of care.[97] Thus, it is consistent that nurses would favor a definition of the professional–client relationship that places the spotlight on collaboration. Nurses also are very much aware of the importance of the client's locus of control and sense of self-efficacy, two concepts that underscore self-regulation as a

BUILDING NURSING KNOWLEDGE

What is Therapeutic Reciprocity?

Marck P. Therapeutic reciprocity: A caring phenomenon. *Adv Nurs Sc.* 1990; 13:49–59.

Marck notes that there is a basic human motivation to reciprocate in relationships that is influenced by a person's perceptions of fairness and sense of give and take. She suggests that this motivation has relevance to the nurse–client relationship.

Marck reviews the works of nine theorists all of whom give support to the idea that reciprocity or mutuality is important in health care relationships. Through these works runs the theme of mutual exchange, which manifests as an accommodation of personal space between nurse and client in mutual self-disclosure, in exchanges of humor, or in efforts to enlist one another in making mutual decisions.

In a reciprocal relationship the nurse and client share meanings. When these are positive meanings—the kind that characterize therapeutic reciprocity—genuine caring occurs and nurse and client share control. They mutually participate in making decisions about care. Outcomes are not predetermined. They evolve in the exchange on the basis of knowledge that builds in the sharing process. Developing this knowledge demands skilled efforts by the nurse to understand the perspective of the client.

One important implication of shared control is that responsibility is also mutual, and this empowers both nurse and client. Neither the nurse nor the client holds sole accountability for the outcomes of their interaction, but their mutual effort creates meanings that change the outcome for the better.

Some nurses attempt to protect themselves from job burnout by remaining aloof from their clients, yet there is a danger, Marck notes, in nursing from an "emotional distance." Marck cites literature that indicates emotional numbing alienates the nurse from the humanity of self and client, while remaining open can actually promote coping. In fact, therapeutic reciprocity transforms the emotional "costs of care" into shared experiences that produce positive growth for nurse and client.

means to good health;[98,99] they understand the power of health beliefs as an influence on client behavior.[98] Thus, a model that affirms the usefulness of the client's perspective and centers on maximizing client involvement in decision-making would seem to fit well with the values of the nursing profession.

Indeed, nursing's use of language confirms that collaboration is compatible with nursing's professional values. Some years ago, nurses adopted the word "client" as a substitute for the word "patient."[100] The rationale for the exchange was that the term "client" connoted a view of the person as autonomous in its implication of an individual's rational agency in acts of engaging the professional advice or services of another. The term "patient," on the other hand, in its reference to "one who is acted upon"[101] (rather than one who acts), was thought to reflect a more Parsonian concept of the sick role. This text thus uses the word "client" and also incorporates other terminology as a way of emphasizing the importance of mutuality in the helping relationship. See Box 37–1 for a list of collaborative terms that may be applied in nursing practice. A profession's use of language is important because it reveals underlying assumptions that are likely to affect practitioner behavior.

A collaborative approach to practice has many advantages. Several studies have shown that client's active participation enhances outcomes.[78,102] Nevertheless, collaboration is far from easy. Each participant in the helping relationship must have the capacity for perspective-taking—the ability to look at a situation from another's point of view,[103] and at the same time each must engage in the complex process of identification—the ability to think of another in terms of oneself.[65] The following sections outline the concepts and skills of collaboration and detail one model that has been proposed for nursing practice.

Collaboration in Nursing Practice

Collaboration is an approach to professional–client relationships that requires moving beyond client dependency and professional dominance. Basic to this approach is the need for professionals to reevaluate the relative importance of expert (technical) knowledge and personal knowledge in making health care decisions. Emphasizing one type of knowledge to the exclusion of the other is a major source of conflict and misunderstanding in the helping relationship.

Kleinman and associates, for example, argue that professionals and clients bring two different paradigms (explanatory models) to the helping relationship.[72] The "disease paradigm" often held by professionals emphasizes the malfunctioning or maladaptation of biological and psychophysiological processes in the individual, and leads professionals to view the disease as the disorder. In contrast, the "illness paradigm" reflects the personal, interpersonal, and cultural reactions to disease and discomfort. It is the model the client is likely to hold, and often leads clients to view the difficulties in living with the disease as constituting the disorder. Because our culture is diverse, illness paradigms

BOX 37–1. TERMINOLOGY FOR A COLLABORATIVE MODEL OF THE HELPING RELATIONSHIPS

Collaborative Term	Traditional Term
Adherence	Compliance
Client	Patient
Client care	Nursing care
Client care planning	Nursing care planning
Discuss	Inform
Enable/empower	Allow
Joint decision-making	Nursing orders
Mutual evaluation	Nursing evaluation
Mutual learning	Patient teaching
Negotiate/bargain	Tell
Nurse–client implementation	Nursing intervention
Persuade	Prescribe
Recommend	Require

BUILDING NURSING KNOWLEDGE

How Can a Nurse Establish a Collaborative Relationship With a Client?

Kasch CR. Establishing a collaborative nurse–patient relationship: A distinct focus of nursing action in primary care. *Image.* 1986; 18:44–47.

Kasch notes that the trend in provider–client relationships is toward joint exploration of the client's experience. This involves negotiation and consensus-seeking rather than the traditional questioning and order-giving. Health care professionals and clients often have different beliefs about what is appropriate behavior in health care relationships. Thus, in Kasch's view, negotiation may be necessary to establish who exerts control in the relationship, who makes decisions, which goals are pursued, and what the level of client participation is. In fact, these aspects may have to be negotiated anew in each nurse–client encounter.

In a collaborative relationship, according to Kasch, clients adopt an expanded role and work jointly with the nurse to determine goals, weigh alternative courses of action, and approach their own health care as a problem-solving endeavor. To establish a collaborative relationship, therefore, the nurse may have to redefine the interaction. The formal interview may become a conversation in a collaborative relationship. The nurse's task changes from one of making decisions about the client's care to fostering joint decision-making. In a collaborative relationship the ideas of both the client and the nurse receive an equal hearing. Even though clients lack expert knowledge, they have their own ideas about health and illness. The nurse needs to understand these to be able to help the client.

differ. There is great variation across ethnic, class, and family boundaries in illness behavior.

Collaboration offers a way to reconcile disease and illness paradigms within the helping relationship. It promotes the management of conflicts between the two points of view on the basis of negotiations worked out through reciprocal, dynamic exchanges between professional and client that integrate personal and expert knowledge in decisions.

Definition of Collaboration. **Collaboration** is a process in which two or more individuals work together, jointly influencing one another, for the attainment of a goal. **Collaborative decision-making** is an act of selecting a choice among two or more possible alternatives for an action by a group of individuals mutually influencing the decision. These definitions suggest that collaboration is the use of persuasion or influence in situations where decision-making is a social venture (involves two or more parties) and is expressed by the degree to which mutual influence is achieved.[80]

Collaboration and Decision-making. Professional decisions in nursing are those that directly affect the client and that are independent of the scope of practice of other professionals. They fall into three categories: program decisions, operational control decisions, and agenda decisions.[80]

Program decisions involve care planning decisions and the consideration of the alternatives in dealing with a client's specific health problem.[80] Selecting goals and implementations such as teaching strategies are examples of program decisions. **Operational control decisions** are decisions that address how to do specific aspects of what has been planned. Such decisions address how to perform procedures, the materials to use, and the information needed to accomodate a unique situation. **Agenda decisions** are decisions on the priority of activities and involve sequencing planned events into some kind of temporal order.[128] Agenda decisions focus on the client's daily schedule, or the order of activities that will structure the client's time.

These decision types differ in their immediate and long-term relevance to client's health[80] and in the amount of time required to resolve a dilemma. Operational control decisions generally require immediate, on-the-spot decisions to satisfy a particular need at a particular moment. Such decisions often are not appropriate for lengthy discussion between nurse and client unless the nurse is acting in the role of a teacher, perhaps in the home setting, with the goal of having the client independently perform a particular activity. Program and agenda decisions, on the other hand, are likely to be subject to constraints that arise for the client's perspective and are often most appropriately handled through collaboration.

Thus, the context of decision-making is important in applying collaboration to client care situations. Not every decision requires or is appropriately resolved through collaborative interaction. Emergencies, for example, significantly alter the context of decision-making, because the urgent need for action generally precludes lengthy collaboration, particularly when the client's vital functions are under immediate threat. Thus, collaboration can be viewed as a prefered manner of approach in situations where no immediate threat to safety exists, and on decisions that are important to client health and likely to engage client desires for self-determination.

A Model of Collaboration. Williamson has proposed mutual interaction as a model that meets the objectives of limiting client dependency and professional dominance and maximizing client participation in the health care process.[79] **Mutual interaction** is a model of professional interaction that combines collaborative aims with the decision-making framework of the nursing process.

The model provides a method for simultaneously building consensus and solving problems by its integration of negotiation and decision making. Through the exchanges of mutual interaction, client and nurse come to an agreement on the desired outcomes and strategies to be employed for promoting and restoring the client's health. Agreements thus reached are equivalent to contracts, as they represent a promise to act according to a mutually agreed upon plan. The model not only endeavors to involve clients in their own care, it assures through their participation that clients assume a greater proportion of the responsibility for the outcomes of care than would be the case were they to take an entirely passive role.

Mutual interaction is not a theory of nursing in the sense that it defines the nature of client care problems to which nurses address themselves. It does, however, identify an approach to problem-solving that builds on societal values and public and professional interests in the health care encounter. Mutual interaction is thus compatible with and may be used in conjunction with theories of nursing such as those outlined in Chapters 32 and 33 that do define the nature of health and illness and nursing action.

Assumptions of Mutual Interaction. Williamson identifies the following assumptions of mutual interaction:

- The individual has a right to self-determination and to choose to participate or not in the process of decision-making.
- The client and the professional interact in a reciprocal relationship and are amenable to each other's influence.
- The responsibility for health is a personal one, not a professional one.
- Each individual's concept of health is legitimate for that person.[79]

Phases of Mutual Interaction. The mutual-interaction model closely parallels classical decision-making frameworks such as the nursing process. It characterizes collaborative decisions as evolving in six phases: the exploratory, information-sharing and analysis, mutual goal-setting, strategy-devising, alternative-implementing, and evaluation phases.[79]

Exploratory Phase. The exploratory phase consists of the initial period of contact between client and nurse during which information is exchanged. In this phase the nurse encourages the client to share the story of his or her illness (see Chap. 16), to state the reasons for seeking care, and to indicate personal expectations for the outcome of care.

During the exploratory phase, the nurse must determine not only the client's perspective but whether the proper foundations exist for further transactions. The nurse thus establishes whether he or she possesses the professional knowledge and skills needed to care for the client's wants and needs, and communicates to the client the range of services the nurse is prepared to give. This may be a fairly simple exchange in hospital situations where the scope of services is well defined and the nature of the client's needs is established prior to admission; it may not be so straightforward in ambulatory settings where clients may present a wide range of requests for assistance. If a client's desire is to deal with a problem of obesity, for example, the nurse must have skills and knowledge in approaches to weight control to be helpful. Otherwise, a referral to another professional is in order. Once the nurse is aware of the client's expectations, is satisfied that nursing services are appropriate to the client's needs, and sees that the client is aware of those services and desires them, advancement is made to the next phase.[79]

Information Sharing and Analysis. The goal of the information sharing and analysis phase is for nurse and client to clarify issues and share perceptions on their individual assessments of the client's health problem. The client is invited to share his or her ideas on the causes of the problem and the contributing factors that have served to relieve or worsen it. So that the assessment will be a mutual one, nurse and client work to reach an agreement by sharing the clues they find significant and by exchanging their rationales for their personal interpretations. For example, a client may be concerned about an unhealing foot sore and view it as the result of an ill-fitting shoe. The nurse, on the other hand, may recognize failure to heal as a sign not of chronic irritation but possibly of an internal metabolic or circulatory problem, and may redirect the client's attention to a generalized local skin discoloration that implicates circulation as the problem.

Through this process of sharing, the ideas of participants generally begin to converge, although in some cases there may be additional barriers to agreement that need to be addressed. Specific assessment skills are helpful in this phase, as are guidelines from compatible nursing theoretical models (those of King or Rogers, for example) and a thorough understanding of psychophysiological responses to illness.[79] Once the nurse and client reach a common definition of the problem, they can advance to mutual goal setting.

Mutual Goal Setting. This phase is oriented to determining with the client his or her current circumstantial and developmental state and the desired state to be achieved.[79] It involves collegial negotiation and compromise in a democratic manner, which contrasts with the more traditional approach in which the practitioner sets the goals and simply communicates them to the client. Outcomes are stated in precise terms so that progress can be monitored and evaluated in accordance with the specifications spelled out in Chapter 18. For goals to be attainable, they must be congruent with the client's values, belief system, resources, and capability. A client seeking a quick solution to a health problem will be unlikely to attain outcomes that require long-term measures. The nurse must evaluate the legal and ethical implications of differences in outcome perspectives when they exist.

Stragegy Devising. In this phase, nurse and client jointly select strategies to reach mutually defined outcomes. Exchanges focus on the benefits, costs, and risks of alternative strategies, and on the probable consequences of any given course of action in light of the client's particular situation. For example, the nurse and client might review the benefits, risks, and consequences of trying a new shoe style as a solution to the problem of a chronic foot sore. Although the cost of further laboratory testing needed to establish alternative etiologies might be saved, this short-term savings may be made at the expense of a poorer ultimate outcome if other types of strategies are delayed.

Here, professional input is particularly important. Generally clients will be persuaded by the logic of arguments based on the nurse's knowledge and experience. By exploring benefits and costs, the participants are able to reach an informed consent on the alternatives to be pursued. Once this is achieved, role delineation is addressed, and issues such as the timing and sequencing of approaches and the respective responsibilities of each participant can be resolved.

Negotiation of outcomes and strategies concludes the orientation phase of interaction and results in a contract between nurse and client.[104] Agreements are formalized in a written client care plan, and may be reinforced in situations where special emphasis is important (such as when outcomes involve life-style changes) through the use of a special contract form, signed by client and nurse, copies of which are distributed to both parties (Fig. 37–3). Although these forms as yet have no legal status in the sense that the client's failure to comply is not subject to legal redress by the nurse, they nevertheless do carry a psychological significance and have the therapeutic benefit of motivating the client to work toward desired outcomes.[105]

Implementation Phase. In the implementation stage, strategic action is taken to resolve the client's problem. Experiential feedback on the efficacy of the plan becomes available, which may either validate the plan or indicate that reassessment is necessary. This enables participants to correct and adjust the plan in a process of formative evaluation. Thus, corrective changes are made concurrently with the implementation of care. Again, both nurse and client perspectives are accommodated in plan modifications.[79]

Evaluation. While evaluation goes on throughout implementation (and indeed during the entire course of the encounter), it becomes the critical focus as the relationship nears its end. End-phase (or summative) evaluation examines whether or not desired outcomes were achieved and the process of collaboration was meaningful for the client. Nurse and client then determine the appropriate next step—termination or the formulation of additional plans.[79] Termination may be logical when the period of the contract has expired, the terms of the contract have all been met, or

SAMPLE CONTRACT

I, __(client)__, would like to achieve the following objective:

1. Walk three times per week for 30 minutes.

To achieve this objective, I, __(client)__, agree to the following responsibilities:

1. Arrange my weekly schedule to provide 30 minutes three times per week for walking.
2. Record dates and times spent walking.
3. Bring the record of the walking schedule to the next clinic appointment in 1 month.
4. Meet with the nurse monthly for counseling, support, and encouragement.
5. Reward myself for achieving the objective on a weekly basis by treating myself to a paperback book, movie, or long distance telephone call to a friend or relative.

Signature: __(client)__ Date: ______

I, __(nurse)__, agree to assist __(client)__ with the objective of walking 30 minutes three times per week. My responsibilities include:

1. Meet with __(client)__ on a monthly basis for 1 hour.
2. Review the walking record monthly.
3. Monitor __(client's)__ blood pressure on a monthly basis.
4. Listen to the achievement and/or disappointment in the accomplishment of the objective. Offer support and encouragement and assist in problem solving during monthly meetings.

Signature: __(nurse)__ Date: ______

Date of evaluation: ______

Results / Revisions:

Record brought to appointment. Thirty minutes of walking three or four times per week recorded. Walking time established as after work. Rewarded self with book or telephone call after achievement of weekly objective. BP 152/90. Nurse and client agree to continue the contract and reevaluate in 1 month.

Figure 37–3. A client care contract. (*From Christensen P. Planning, priorities, goals, and objectives. In: Griffith-Kenney, Christensen PJ, eds.* Nursing Process: Application of Theories, Frameworks, and Models. *St Louis: Mosby; 1986.*)

there are no additional problems for which the client needs or desires professional help.[104] Sometimes, termination results when unanticipated events make contract provisions impossible to meet; in this case, client and nurse agree to release each other from the contract.[104] Table 37–2 summarizes the phases of mutual interaction.

Options in Mutual Interaction. At the juncture of each phase of the mutual interaction process, nurse and client negotiate for three possible outcomes: agreement to proceed, referral, or termination.[79] Such decisions are made at the end of exploration, information sharing, goal setting, and strategy devising.

Most of the time the perspectives of participants coincide: The nurse is aware of the client's expectations and agrees the nurse's services will help; the client is aware of what the nurse can and cannot do and desires the nurse's assistance. Sometimes the expectations of the client are most appropriately met by another type of nurse or a professional in another field, and referral is appropriate. Occasionally, however, the nurse and client may be unable to reach coinciding ideas about caregiving, so that the client declines the nurse's services and offers of referral.

An intermediate course when disagreement exists is for nurse and client to pursue those objectives upon which they do agree and to limit their relationship to areas of agreement. For example, the nurse and client might agree to pursue the strategies of hygiene and pressure relief for a decubitus ulcer, while agreeing to eliminate a stringent weight reduction diet from the plan upon the client's insistence and refusal to adhere. Such decisions are always made on the basis of informed consent, and after full review of the options; their benefit, costs, and consequences; and of the client's reasons for declining. Sometimes the client will reverse an initial decision to decline, and so a certain amount of persistence and persuasion on the nurse's part is appropriate. (See the discussion below on Collaboration and Negotiation.)

Advantages of Mutual Interaction. Mutual interaction significantly broadens the issues considered in the helping relationship. In contrast to the disease paradigm and the biomedical approach, which attend solely to the client's signs and symptoms, mutual interaction, by involving the client, refocuses attention on the client's response to disease and the problems the client experiences in living with illness. Thus, mutual interaction requires participants to examine such issues as the effect of illness and health care on the client's family, leisure activities, and work, as well as the range of alternatives available to the client and their risks and costs in relation to the possible benefits.

Mutual interaction is a comprehensive and holistic approach to caregiving that redefines how health care decisions are made. It theoretically acknowledges the client's right of self-determination within a framework for achieving informed consent. This is important, because although the doctrine of informed consent is mandated by law for invasive procedures, too often it is omitted from the structure of the decision-making that pertains to the everyday problems of caregiving.

Limitations of Mutual Interaction. The preceding discussion identified the decision contexts for which collaboration and mutual interaction are most appropriate. Another consideration in the application of the model is the participant context—the context of the client and nurse.[80]

Although participation in decision-making that influences one's own affairs is a value held by most, individuals may not necessarily be willing—let alone happy—to participate in decision-making in all circumstances, and some may lack the capacity.[80] Capacity relates both to situational and developmental factors and is essential to the client's ability to give informed consent.[106] Clients who are extremely ill or mentally disabled generally lack the capacity, as do very young children, although there may be limited contexts in which people even in these categories may be able to collaborate. In client care situations, client partici-

TABLE 37–2. PHASES OF THE MUTUAL INTERACTION MODEL

Phase	Activity
Exploratory	The client states reasons for seeking care and expectations for general outcomes. The nurse states the services he or she is able to provide. Client and nurse decide whether client desires and expectations match with the nurse's skills; they explore the options to proceed, refer, or terminate.
Information sharing and analysis	The client and nurse define the client's problems and identify the available resources.
Mutual goal setting	The client and nurse each state their objectives for care and negotiate specific outcomes. Client and nurse define their respective roles in meeting client care outcomes.
Strategy devising	The client and nurse explore strategies, and discuss the risks and benefits of strategies considered. Client and nurse reach an agreement on strategies and arrive at a client care contract.
Implementation of alternatives	The client and nurse do a formative evaluation of care in progress; they exchange information needed in order to make ongoing adjustments in the plan.
Evaluation	The client and nurse review the client care experience; they share information needed to make a summative evaluation and prepare to terminate the contract.

Adapted from Williamson JA. Mutual interaction: A model for nursing practice. Nurs Outlook. *1981; 29:104–107.*

pation may be influenced by the following four types of client-related factors identified by Kim.[80]

- *Client role expectations.* Clients' sick role perceptions influence the role they expect to play in nurse–client encounters. Previous experience in traditional sick-role and professional authority situations give clients a sense of what to expect that may act as a strong influence on their behavior. Clients who have had no previous exposure may not be constrained by internalized role expectations. The professional may need to reeducate clients whose views are more traditional to accept a collaborative approach.
- *Client knowledge level.* Clients may be socialized to defer to technical knowledge, and thus may be inclined to take the dependent role in relation to the nurse's expert knowledge. This is particularly true when clients believe they lack the knowledge necessary for decision-making.[80] Once they are provided with the information they need and lack, however, many clients become willing and able to participate. Information, along with capacity, is essential to informed consent and is especially important to facilitate nurse–client collaboration.
- *Client personality characteristics.* Clients are individuals who differ from one another in their personal traits and characteristics, as recognized in psychological theory and research. Some clients naturally acquire or develop a stronger internal locus of control and a stronger sense of self-efficacy than others.[107,108] Clients with these characteristics may be more likely to seek out a collaborative arrangement in the health care encounter than those clients without them; clients who are more external in their locus of control, or who lack a belief in their capacity to participate, may require more encouragement and support in a collaborative role.
- *Client definition of the situation.* Clients are sensitive to the nuances of the environment and look for clues and symbols that indicate the social norms and sanctions for specific behavior. These normative forces define action within formal and informal situations; nevertheless no two people's definitions, expectations, or behavior are ever exactly the same. Interpretations of social clues vary. Client definitions will always be subject to individual differences in their perceptions of who will exert control in a situation, whose goals will be dominant, and what their level of participation will be; and these may shift from encounter to encounter. Thus it is necessary for professionals to understand the client's definition of the situation and whether that definition is compatible with collaboration.

These client factors influence initial client responses to collaboration, which may range from enthusiasm to bewilderment to distress. Often clients need no encouragement and enter the health care encounter with the expectation (or the demand) that they will participate. Some clients require little encouragement and quickly become comfortable with an active role. Others may display reticence and need a substantial amount of support and encouragement from the nurse. Still others may react with uneasiness when they are prompted to participate. Nurses must be prepared to respond to each of these client contexts.

Nurses also act to shape the interactional climate that supports or limits collaborative interactions. Although client characteristics determine the client's tendency to participate, nurse characteristics influence the degree to which the client is "invited" or "given permission" to participate. The following four types of nurse-related factors, as identified by Kim,[80] influence nurse communications in client care situations.

- *Nurse role expectations.* Nurses, like clients, have internalized role expectations, often reinforced over the long course of nursing education and career involvement. Nurses often reflect the expectations that are implicit in their institutional cultures; these may be more or less traditional or progressive. Internalized role expectations influence nurse behavior in obvious or subtle ways, including the way a nurse performs duties, exerts influence, or attempts decisional control. Kim emphasizes the specific importance of nurses' attitudes towards clients' rights for collaboration in decision-making.[80] Nurses who believe health care decisions are best made on the basis of authority are unlikely to invite the client to participate.
- *Nurse knowledge.* The level of knowledge affects the confidence with which nurses approach collaborative interaction. The effect of the nurse's knowledge can either increase or decrease the nurse's propensity for collaboration. Nurses with a high level of expertise, for example, may be confident of their knowledge and thus comfortable in "letting go" and assuming a more consultative role, or they may experience discomfort and prefer to retain control given the gap they perceive between the client's and their own knowledge level.
- *Nurse personality characteristics.* Similar to clients, nurse behavior in decision-making situations may also be influenced by personal traits such as locus of control, self-efficacy, self-confidence, or a need for dominance.[80]
- *Nurse definition of the situation.* Just as clients are sensitive to social nuances, so are nurses, and their perceptions of who will exert control in a situation and whose goals will be dominant may also vary from encounter to encounter. Nurses, moreover, are responsible for evaluating the decision context. Thus their own behavior may change with the nature of the decision to be made or the nature of the conditions for decision-making.

Thus, the participant context is a variable condition under which nurses and clients determine whether or not they will engage in collaborative interaction. Clients and nurses both vary in the traits required for collaboration, and will vary in their success in achieving a participative arrangement in interaction.

As with any new approach, mutual interaction requires time and experience to master, for nurses and clients. Nursing students who are struggling to learn the fundamentals of client care will certainly require practice to master not only the content on which decisions are based, but also how to use that content in a collaborative situation. Even experienced nurses, however, may experience some difficulty in their initial attempts to employ mutual interaction. Whenever difficulty in collaboration is experienced, it may be helpful to examine the interaction by considering the following questions:

1. Did I clearly communicate that I welcome the client's participation?
2. Is the client prepared to participate? Did I give the client enough information?
3. Does the client have the capacity to participate? Is the decision an appropriate one for collaboration? Does the situation require another approach?
4. Does the client desire to participate? Are the client's values compatible with the model?
5. Are my values compatible with the model?

Answers to these questions may assist nurses to identify client-related or nurse-related hindrances to adopting a collaborative mode of interaction.

What should the nurse do if the client seems unprepared to collaborate? The nurse may elect to discuss the collaborative approach directly with the client. Clients who have been socialized to expect an authoritarian provider role may have difficulty interpreting clues that contradict their expectations. Thus, the nurse may assist them by discussing the transactional expectations of collaboration and the advantages of participative decision-making for the client. This kind of informative exchange may be sufficient to encourage a reticent client.

For clients who lack the physical and mental capacity to collaborate, on the other hand, the nurse may well be advised to limit collaboration to those select areas where the client's participation will result in no harm to the client, although collaboration may be used with the guardians of those who lack capacity. As clients who are physically ill recover from illness, it may become appropriate to adjust the interactional mode to fit the client's improved condition. Collaboration can gradually be substituted for professional control of decision-making.

Occasionally, clients may prefer not to participate in decision-making and may wish to depend more substantially on their professionals.[69,78,86] Cassileth and associates recommend that in these situations, professionals be guided by the clients' verbal and behavioral clues that indicate their preferences.[78] Preference for a more traditional arrangement in such situations may be viewed as a form of self-determination.

Mutual Interaction and "Adherence." The difficulties and problems that cause people to seek professional assistance may diminish their sense of control, and they may feel a reduced sense of personal efficacy in dealing with the environment. Individual feelings of control may be further threatened by the helping relationship itself, given that the act of seeking help is an act of communicting one's inability to deal with difficulties on one's own. Diminished feelings of control induce stress and anxiety; conversely, greater feelings of control have a positive impact on psychological well-being and physical health.[109] A number of studies have documented the fact that those who believe they have more control, whether or not they choose to exercise it, exhibit reduced stress.[110,111]

IMPLICATIONS FOR NURSE–CLIENT COLLABORATION

Caring

Caring is accepted as the essence of the professional relationship in nursing. Caring has been defined as a commitment to protecting the dignity of clients. Dignity can be viewed as the condition of being worthy of basic rights and of being capable of the corresponding responsibilities. By encouraging the client's participation in health care decisions, the nurse respects the client's right to self-determination and thus affirms the client's dignity.

Control is the ability to have an impact on an outcome. Closely tied to the concept of control is the notion of predictability, that is, the ability to forecast that an outcome will occur. By having control over an outcome through personal action, an individual is usually better able to predict that an outcome will occur. Moreover, having control over a situation is likely to raise a person's perception of responsibility for the outcome.[109]

The perception of control is important in that it alters the client's psychological disposition toward the plan of care, raising adherence levels.[76,109] **Adherence** refers to a client's follow-through in carrying out professional recommendations. For example, clients with high blood pressure who perceive the process of their care and treatment as inviting them to be active participants in decision-making, have been shown to be more likely to adhere to the treatment plan and to achieve the desired outcome.[112] Furthermore, some authorities have argued that clients whose feelings of control are threatened by being given recommendations in an authoritarian manner (as indicated by the professional's use of terms such as "must" or "should") are unlikely to adhere to the plan of care, as a way of reexerting their control in a situation.[113]

Thus, many authorities emphasize the importance of a transactional approach to caregiving, such as that represented in collaboration and mutual interaction, as a way of improving adherence. Incorporating mutual interaction into the health care encounter increases the likelihood that:

1. The client will be approached in collaborative rather than an authoritarian manner.
2. The professional will explore the client's perspective.
3. Issues that concern the client will be addressed in the interaction.
4. Differences in outcome expectations will be resolved.
5. Strategies planned will fit with the client's values and life situation.
6. The interaction will support rather than threaten the client's sense of control.
7. Client self-efficacy will be enhanced through an exchange of information.

> **IMPLICATIONS FOR NURSE–CLIENT COLLABORATION**
>
> **Informed Consent**
>
> One meaning of informed consent in nursing practice rests in its application to transactions between nurse and client during care planning. Informed consent pertains to open, direct exchanges about the goals and strategies under consideration. When the client participates in decision-making, and in the negotiations to reach decisions, informed consent is implicit in the process.

8. Client motivation will be enhanced by giving the client a personal investment in the solutions.

As an architect of the plan, the client is more likely to be motivated to see that the plan is carried out. The plan becomes a personal document, not something that is superimposed by others but rather a solution that the client has participated in creating.

Mutual Interaction and Caring. Caring is largely accepted as a value that depicts the essence of the helping relationship in health care.[114] Gadow, an authority on caring, emphasizes that caring is a commitment to protecting and enhancing the client's dignity.[115] Webster's defines dignity as the quality or state of being worthy, honored, or esteemed.[101] One might presume that to mean the condition of being worthy of basic human rights, including the right to self-determination. Mutual interaction acknowledges client rights by bringing clients into the decision-making process, and thus can be viewed as grounded on a value of caring.

If caring is linked to dignity and self-determination, then it is also linked to informed consent. So far, two of the essential elements of informed consent, capacity and information, have been mentioned; a third is voluntariness. Voluntariness reflects on the client's participation in weighing the risks and benefits of the health care plan. Hogue points out that informed consent is meaningful only when it reflects a dialogue in which clients are able to ask questions and obtain complete, truthful answers that address their important concerns. Only then are choices freely made.[106]

One possible outcome of the client's participation, however, is that the client, fully informed, will take the option of "informed dissent." After assessing all of the pertinent information, the client may opt to decline care or to seek unorthodox care. This does not reflect negatively on the client's capacity to make an informed choice, but does necessitate that the practitioner be prepared to accept the client's preferences as an expression of self-determination. Increasingly, the link between dignity and self-determination is being recognized in law, most recently in the enactment of the Patient Self-Determination Act of 1991, which requires hospitals to inform clients that they have the right to decline care.

Collaboration and Negotiation. Although caring can be linked to dignity and self-determination, it is not linked to client appeasement. Nurses who embrace a collaborative approach with clients are not required to make concessions that will be harmful to the client. They are, however, required to negotiate differences.

Acknowledging that clients bring their own ideas to the nurse–client relationship, the problem for nurses becomes that of negotiating a successful resolution when differences exist. Finding the essential common ground with the client is the cornerstone of collaboration. Reaching a common ground involves a process of consensus building. **Consensus building** refers to the interpersonal approaches and techniques people use to resolve their differences on important issues. It is part of every step of the negotiation. Fisher and Ury describe consensus building as the process of "getting to yes."[116]

Consensus building is an art that is based on the skillful use of interpersonal diplomacy. Nevertheless, certain techniques can be helpful to anyone who endeavors to resolve interpersonal differences. Many of the techniques of consensus building are outlined in Table 37–3. Although this chapter focuses on nurses' relationships with clients, the guidelines presented in Table 37–3 are also applicable to relationships with peers, family, and friends, and can be taught to clients for their own use.

Negotiation emphasizes people, interests, options, and the use of objective criteria for reaching accord.[116] To negotiate effectively, it is necessary to understand each of those aspects and how to treat them.

People. The emphasis in negotiation is on the people first and the problem second. Successful consensus-building seeks to both strengthen relationships and find common ground through what Fisher and Ury call principled negotiation.[116] **Principled negotiation** is the alternative to giving in to the other person's position or to coercing the other person to accept one's own.

The first step in principled negotiation is to separate the people from the problem. This serves to protect the relationship between the parties to the negotiation. A working relationship where trust, understanding, respect, and friendship build up over time helps to make each negotiation easier and more efficient. People, including clients and nurses, desire to feel good about themselves; they care about what other people think. On the other hand, they have emotions and get angry, depressed, fearful, hostile,

> **IMPLICATIONS FOR NURSE–CLIENT COLLABORATION**
>
> **Negotiation**
>
> One of the essential elements of any transactional relationship is negotiation. In a collaborative approach to health care the nurse and client negotiate the goals to achieve and the strategies to reach them. They do this largely by sharing information, perspective, and values. Communication skill is essential to the success of the negotiations involved in caregiving, and lack of communication skill can impede the development of consensus on health care decisions.

TABLE 37–3. GUIDELINES FOR NEGOTIATING AND CONSENSUS-BUILDING

Guideline	Rationale
1. Separate the person from the problem.	Approach the situation from a perspective of working side by side as partners; invite client to be your partner; attack the problem, not the partner. Remember, negotiators are people first; people have emotions and egos; deal with emotions separately from the problem; make emotions explicit, acknowledge them as legitimate; convey that you respect client's emotions. Understanding client's feelings may help solve the problem; put yourself in client's shoes; do not assume that your feelings are client's feelings; discuss each other's perceptions. Give client a stake in the outcome by making sure client participates in the process; make your proposals consistent with client values whenever possible; allow partner to let off steam and do not react to outbursts; build a working relationship.
2. Separate the position from the person's interests.	Taking a position tells the other party what you want, provides an anchor in the bargaining, but also creates an incentive to stubbornly hold a position, and may endanger the relationship; positions are what people ask for—interests are why they want it. Behind opposite positions lie shared as well as conflicting interests; identify interests by asking "why?" and also ask what decision the client thinks you are asking him or her for. Remember the more powerful interests are basic human needs; make the client's interests and your interests explicit; acknowledge a difference in interests as part of the problem; talk about interests before making proposals; formulate options, but remain flexible.
3. Invent options for mutual gain.	Formulate several options; negotiators often feel only one option—theirs—is reasonable; avoid premature judgment; avoid searching for a single answer; avoid thinking that the differences between you and your partner are the partner's problem. Brainstorm with client before deciding; do not eliminate options that may be less than ideal from a professional point of view—some adherence to the health care plan may be better than no adherence. Look for win-win options; consider using an impartial arbiter; be sure to ask the client for his or her preferences; make choosing as painless as possible; look at problem from client's point of view—ask what client most fears, what client is hoping for. Consider client's social world and how enacting your options might have social consequences for the client—this will help you appreciate restraints on client; reflect your understanding of client's situation to the client—may help increase client's awareness and increase generation of feasible options.
4. Use objective decision criteria.	Avoid pitting your will against client's; use criteria based on fairness, efficiency, precedent, tradition, or scientific merit for deciding; frame each issue as a joint search for objective criteria. Remember, professional standard of legitimacy is only one standard; client's and nurse's paradigms for viewing problems frequently differ; be open to reason as to which standards are most appropriate; and how they should be applied; ask the client to propose standards—these can be used as a lever to persuade client. Do not yield to pressure in any of its forms (bribe, threat, manipulative appeal to trust, or refusal to budge)—ask client to state reasoning, suggest objective criteria you think apply, insist on the use of criteria for a final agreement. If the client truly will not budge and fails to advance a persuasive basis for position, there is no further negotiation.
5. Focus attention on the merits.	Concentrate on the merits of negotiating and emphasize interests, options, and criteria; focus the client's attention as well as your own on the merits; do not reject the client's position—treat it as one possible option, look for the interests behind it, talk to the client about the principles it reflects. Explore its benefits and risks and think about ways to improve it. Invite the client's criticism of professional proposals—ask the client: "What concern of yours does this plan fail to take into account?" Ask the client's advice—what he or she would do in your position: "If you were the nurse, what advice would you give to solve this problem?" Use questions instead of statements—questions educate, statements generate resistance—there is an important difference between "You should take your pills!" and "Do you know the benefits of taking these pills?" Ask questions and pause; silence is a good motivator, particularly when people have doubts about the merits of something they have said. Remain open to persuasion by cautiously treating objective facts as possibly inaccurate: "Mr. Jones, I've just learned—please correct me if I'm wrong—that you declined to take your medication earlier. Have I been misinformed?" This approach makes you and the client two colleagues who are trying to get at the facts. Give personal support to the client during negotiation—"Mr. Jones, I understand that you made a great effort to increase your intake of fluid today, and I appreciate that." This puts you and the client on the same side.

TABLE 37–3. (continued)

Guideline	Rationale
	Remind the client that your concern is the client's health; ask the client what considerations he or she thinks you should take into account in finding a solution; reflect your understanding of the client's position to the client and ask the client to correct any misunderstanding you might have.
	Take time to consider the client's position. Say "Let me get back to you, I want to think about it a little while." This lets the client know you are considering his or her position; also time and distance aid clear thinking. Show your openness to persuasion by presenting your concerns about the client's position; "Let me show you where I have trouble following your reasoning."

Adapted from Fisher R, Ury W. Getting to Yes: Negotiating an Agreement Without Giving in. *New York: Penguin; 1981.*

frustrated, and offended, particularly under the stressful conditions associated with illness. Failure to deal sensitively with human responses to stress can be disastrous to negotiations.[116]

A good relationship with the client does much to help the achievement of consensus. Nevertheless, there is a tendency when negotiations become frustrating to treat the person and the problem as one.[116] Frustration over a situation may cause a person to express anger toward the other party or to misinterpret. It is thus important to separate the relationship from the problem. This is done by considering perceptions, emotions, and communication.

Understanding the other person's perceptions helps to resolve differences. The ability to see a situation as the other person sees it enables the negotiator to feel the power of the other person's point of view and to feel the emotional force with which they believe in it. To do this, the negotiator must be prepared to withhold judgment until he or she is reasonably sure of how the other party perceives the problem. Asking clients for their point of view is therefore essential.[116]

For example, when a client declines to take medications, the nurse should respond by asking the client to share the reasons. This enables the nurse to understand the problem from the client's point of view. Perhaps the client has noticed certain side effects that suggest an adjustment in the dosage is necessary. Appreciating the other person's point of view does not mean one agrees with it; however, it does aid understanding, and that is often helpful in the quest for solutions.

A good technique for dealing with perceptions is to share one's own perceptions with the other person. This can help to create understanding, especially when done in a frank, honest manner that conveys respect.[116] For example, when clients decline their medication, it can be helpful for nurses to convey their personal point of view on the client's reasons. "I have the impression that you are afraid that this medication will make you feel worse somehow, am I wrong?" Sharing one's perception lets others know that their thoughts are important and it invites them to share what their thoughts are.

It is also important to recognize and understand emotions—the other person's and one's own. Just as it helps to make perceptions explicit, it also helps to make emotions explicit.[116] Moreover, it is important to let the other person express emotions without fear of reprisal. Psychological release achieved through expressing grievances often enables the other person to resume participation in productive problem-solving.

The most important aspect of principled negotiation, however, is communication. No consensus is possible if communication breaks down.[116] Good communication (as discussed in Chap. 14) depends upon active listening, acknowledging what is being said, demonstrating to the other person that he or she is understood, and clarifying misinterpretations. It is especially important to building good communication that one avoid blaming the other person either explicitly or implicitly for any difficulty in the negotiations.

Interests. Most people negotiate by taking positions. They announce what they want out of a situation (their position) and then argue for it. For example, the nurse taking a position might say to the client who declines medications, "I want you to take your medicines because you need them." Although this may not be an entirely unproductive strategy, it usually is not the most efficient means to reach an agreement, and it may have the undesirable side effect of damaging the relationship in the process.[116] Moreover, positions reduce a person's negotiating flexibility. The more people try to convince others they are serious about their position, the more difficult it becomes to be flexible. In other words, arguing for a position makes compromise more difficult. This can lead ultimately to a breakdown in negotiation.

Moreover, when more attention is paid to positions, less attention is usually devoted to the concerns that underlie those positions—to the interests the participants have in the negotiation.[116] Generally it is through understanding interests that breakthroughs in negotiation are achieved. Thus, arguing for a position or focusing on the other person's stated position is often inefficient because it may keep one from understanding the reasons behind the position.

For example, in taking a position on the medications the client declines to take, the nurse fails to pursue the client's reasons (interests) and alternatives that might be acceptable to both. Perhaps the medication with the side effect could be avoided by requesting the physician to substitute another medication. The real object of negotiating is not to press for one's position, but to find a solution that satisfies the underlying interests of both parties.

Thus, the second step of principled negotiation is to separate peoples' positions from their interests.[116] This is very important for problem-solving. Consider the following example. A client with chronic respiratory disease suddenly refuses to accept his respiratory therapy treatment—a treatment that requires the client to assume an awkward head-down position. A nurse taking a position-oriented approach would insist that the client undergo the treatment, arguing on the basis of its importance to the client's overall respiratory status.

The position-oriented approach could be successful, but it nevertheless ignores the client's interests and reasons for refusal. With an interest-oriented approach, on the other hand, the nurse would avoid taking a position, and instead ask the client to identify his interests. Perhaps the client finds that the head-down position constrains his breathing during the procedure, making him feel breathless and anxious. Knowing this, the nurse might be able to suggest an alternative position that would make it possible for the client to accept the procedure. In taking an interest-oriented approach, the nurse seeks to open communication and get the client's point of view. The benefit is that options frequently open up that may ultimately promote a consensus.

To identify another person's interests, it is helpful to ask oneself why the other person wants his or her position or what the person hopes to gain from it. Another approach is to ask why the person does not want to do what he or she thinks is being requested.[116] What client interests stand in the way of client agreement? In the case of the client's refusal of the respiratory treatment, the client's interest was to feel comfortable during the procedure. It is important to remember that the most powerful interests are often basic human needs.[116] When basic needs are met, agreements are often easier to reach.

Talking with one another about interests generally serves the purpose of negotiation.[116] It may help the client, for example, to hear the nurse's interests verbalized. For instance, communicating to the client that the nurse's interests include making therapy as easy as possible for the client may relieve some of the client's anxiety and make it easier for him to participate in problem-solving.

Options. It is valuable in a negotiation to have as many options as possible, although clinical circumstances sometimes make it difficult to spend the time needed. In any situation there are likely to be obstacles that inhibit option invention. These obstacles often include (1) premature judgment, (2) searching for a single answer, (3) the assumption that the problem is an either–or situation, and (4) thinking that solutions are the other person's problem.

Premature judgment means that people are ready to discount ideas before they have examined them on their merits. Premature judgment is very damaging to creativity in a negotiating relationship.[116] Judgment hinders imagination. The client's ability to accept the respiratory procedure, for example, requires creative ideas for how to achieve the desired results through alternative means. Solving the problem requires imagination that would be stifled if the nurse dismissed alternatives out of hand. Premature judgment cuts off the process of finding acceptable alternatives, as does looking at the problem as an either–or situation, or searching for a single best answer. All of these approaches narrow the field of options and prevent the negotiators from broadening the possibilities for problem-solving.

Criteria. There are always situations in which it becomes impossible to reach consensus because the underlying interests are conflicting. For example, a nurse may want to bathe a client before she goes to x-ray because the unit will be too busy later to take the time necessary for the client's bath. The client, on the other hand, may be tired and may wish to rest, preferring to bathe before her husband is scheduled to visit. In such situations principled negotiation requires that the two sides identify objective critreria by which to make a decision.

Developing objective criteria for deciding involves finding principles that are independent of the will of the negotiators. Examples of acceptable criteria might include using standards of fairness, merit, or precedent. Taking turns is an example of a standard of fairness. Reciprocity is another standard of fairness—getting something for what one gives. Perhaps the client would be willing to accept an earlier bath today, in exchange for having a later supper that allowed her more time to visit with her husband. Other categories of standards might include tradition, scientific merit, or efficiency.

Objective criteria are identified by framing the issue as a joint search for criteria.[116] The nurse asks the client to identify ways that might be used to reach agreement on the problem. "We seem to have come to an impasse. How do you think we might resolve this problem?" It is important to be open to reason and to be open to the other person's criteria when this approach is taken. Insisting that the decision be based solely on one's own criteria is not a characteristic or principled negotiation.[116] Shifting the discussion from the question of what the other side is willing to do, to how the matter ought to be decided, may not end the problem, but it will provide a strategy that can be vigorously pursued without the potentially high cost of positional bargaining.

■ LEADERSHIP AND MANAGEMENT AS TRANSACTIONS

Nursing is at a crossroads in its professional history. Never before has the climate been so right as it is now for society's full recognition of the contribution nurses make to health care and to people. Times and conditions have changed. The economic dynamics of the 1980s have effectively altered the power equation that once favored physicians.

Nurses are now moving ahead to achieve the long-standing goals of the nursing profession. Moreover, cost-containment, the dominant policy of the 1980s, will in all likelihood persist through the 1990s and into the 21st century, giving nurses an extended period of time in which to take advantage of the opportunities that accrue to a profession that is well positioned to help society meet its objective of affordable health care.

Nursing also faces important problems, however, and these too will continue into the foreseeable future. Some of them, like the need to do more with fewer resources in virtually every practice setting, and the dwindling infrastructure of support personnel in many health care institutions, can be mediated, if not solved, by excellent management. Thus nurses in the years to come will need to understand what management is and what differentiates excellent management from not-so-excellent management. Nurses also will need to examine their roles at the bedside, in the unit, and in the institution from a management perspective, and to integrate principles of management into the everyday performance of their duties, whether or not they occupy a management position.

Other problems that face nursing—like the shortage of nurses, turnover in the workplace, impact of time constraints and technology on relationships with clients, or restructuring nursing reimbursement—go beyond the scope of management to resolve and require effective leadership at the institutional, regional, and national level. Thus nurses also will need to understand what leadership is and what differentiates effective leadership from not-so-effective leadership. Additionally, nurses will need to examine their own actions and attitudes from a leadership perspective, recognizing that each and every nurse, regardless of personal ambitions or position in the organization, will be called upon to participate in deciding nursing's direction for the future.

Management in Nursing

Management is the effective use of human and material resources to achieve a person's or an organization's objectives. Management is not something that is unique to business or to the corporate world, but rather is something that all people experience and do in their everyday lives. Every individual is a manager in one way or another. Whenever an activity is planned, a schedule made, or resources budgeted, the people conducting those activities are acting as managers.

Characteristics of Management. What characterizes management and, particularly, what differentiates management from leadership, are issues that have been debated for many years. Many people consider management and leadership to be the same thing; they argue that one cannot be an effective leader without being a good manager, and vice versa. Other people argue strenuously that the two are different, and that there are important distinctions to be made.

Rost,[117] a contemporary leadership scholar, strongly differentiates management from leadership. He identifies four essential characteristics of management:

1. Management is an authority relationship.
2. Management involves at least one manager and one subordinate.
3. Manager(s) and subordinate(s) coordinate their activities.
4. Manager(s) and subordinate(s) produce and sell particular goods and services.

The hallmark of management, according to Rost, is that it is a relationship based on contractual authority (formally written or spoken, or informally implied) in which people accept superordinate and subordinate responsibilities in an organization; thus, management requires at least two people.[117]

Contractual authority in hierarchical organizations, such as in hospitals and many other health care agencies, is arranged so that people are ranked one above another according to the amount of authority they are contractually authorized to exercise. Thus superordinate personnel have contractual authority over subordinate personnel to monitor and control subordinate behavior, while subordinate personnel are contactually obligated to report to and obey their managers. It is on the basis of contractual authority, for example, that the director of nursing (DON) is able to control the behavior and activities of nurses at the unit level, or that charge nurses are able to control the behavior of nurses working at the bedside (Fig. 37–4). Contractual authority, then, allows managers to tell subordinates what to do. Usually this does not mean that a manager's behavior is coercive or that he or she adopts a military approach to discipline. It simply means that the influence of managers derives primarily from the power of their position, and secondarily from the force of their ideas, although their ideas may have merit on their own.[117]

Management, according to Rost, is a relationship.[117]

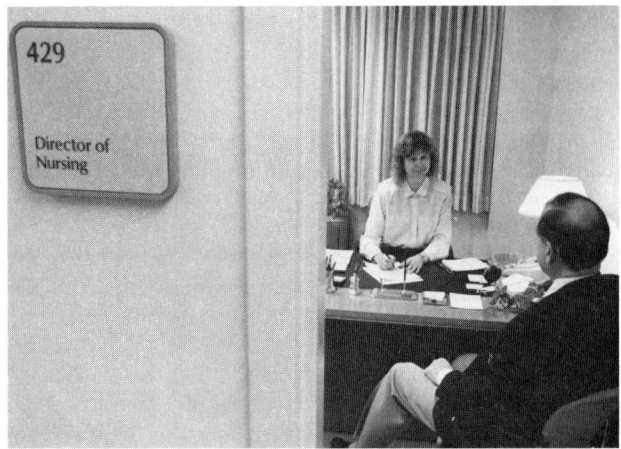

Figure 37–4. The director of nursing has contractual authority in a hierarchical organization, the hospital.

Therefore, managers and subordinates both contribute to management through their relationship to each other, although not necessarily in the same way or to equal degrees. In fact, the relationship may be inherently unequal, with the manager (in the person of the hospital administrator, director of nursing, or unit manager) playing the more dominant and influential role than the subordinate (bedside nurse). Despite the inherent power inequities between managers and subordinates, management is nevertheless a two-way relationship. In traditional organizations, managerial directives generally flow down the organizational hierarchy, and subordinate responses flow up. In organizations that are more democractic, however, the hierarchical structure of authority, typically pyramidal in traditional organizations, tends to be flattened. Contractual authority is decentralized, distributed horizontally among unit leaders, and is shared to a greater degree with subordinates.[117]

For management to achieve its purposes, managers and subordinates must coordinate their activities. Without such coordination, the organization's services cannot be produced or delivered. In health care, medical and nursing services are the services for which institutions exist. Managers and subordinates enter into the management relatioship so that services can be rendered to clients. Unless services are successfully delivered, the management relationship is incomplete.[117]

Manager Roles. The manager of an organization or an organization subunit is responsible for assuring that services are produced and distributed efficiently. This is a rather open-ended job that often leaves managers feeling there is always something more to do to assure that things will go well. It is also a job that requires the manager to play many roles. Mintzberg, a management theorist, has outlined the roles that managers play. These roles fall into three categories: interpersonal, informational, and decisional.[118]

Managers, first of all, are figureheads, which is necessitated by their responsibility to carry out a number of social, inspirational, legal, and ceremonial duties. Managers must be available to those people who request to deal with them because of their status and authority. For example, in nursing service, unit managers are often the people to whom clients complain about unsatisfactory service, not because the manager has made a mistake but because it is the manager's role as head of the unit to resolve difficulties. Thus, the role of figurehead often involves the role of disturbance handler.[118]

Managers act as liaisons in dealing with people outside of the organizational unit. Nursing unit managers, for example, usually have contact with the managers of other hospital services such as pharmacy, accounting, or outpatient clinics. Managers thus develop and maintain the network of contacts that are required to assure that a unit will function efficiently. In nursing service, such roles are often paramount to achieve an optimal scheduling of the work flow through the unit and through the organization. Successful managers, on the basis of their contacts in the organization, gain ways of circumventing bottlenecks in the organization's processing of certain client services. This requires that they monitor information from internal and external sources to develop a thorough knowledge of the organization. Managers also transmit information to those who need it to assure that their own unit functions efficiently and effectively. Thus the manager is the spokesperson and chief communicator for the organization or unit.[118]

Managers are also resource handlers and oversee the allocation of the organization's or unit's resources. This role is very important at the unit level in nursing service, where supplies are numerous and expensive. Successful unit cost-containment often depends upon the effectiveness of the system enacted by the manager to assure that supplies are available, accounted for, and used with discretion.[118]

To summarize, managers must design the work of the unit so as to be able to monitor the environment, initiate change when desirable, and renew stability when something threatens the equilibrium of unit functions.[118]

Management Functions. Management consists of a number of tasks or functions that are carried out by managers and generally are viewed as making up a managerial process.[119] The success with which managers carry out these functions, in hospitals and health care agencies as well as in other types of organizations, determines how effectively the organization operates. Management functions generally include planning, organizing, staffing, influencing, and controlling.

Planning. Planning refers to the strategic decisions managers make from which unit objectives, policies, programs, and procedures logically follow. Planning is a primary function of nursing managers, beginning with the director of nursing, including unit managers, head nurses, and also encompassing unit nurses who plan care for individual clients and who advise unit managers. Subordinates frequently participate in organization planning, particularly in organizations that are run democratically. Planning is important because people are generally unable to work effectively without a plan, and plans generally need to be revised and adjusted on an ongoing basis to accommodate the dynamic relationship that most organizations have with their environment. Budgeting is a big part of planning. Budgets are forecasts of projected revenue (income) and anticipated expenses (outgo) in dollars and cents over a specified planning period. Budgets are necessary for the realization of plans; no plan can be enacted without the resources to underwrite it. A plan to reduce nurse–client ratios in a nursing unit, for example, cannot be implemented without budgeting for the extra personnel such a plan is likely to require.[119]

Organizing. Organizing refers to the development of a work structure—the framework within which the tasks necessary to an organization's objectives are carried out. Organizing involves assigning activities, dividing work into jobs, and delegating the authority necessary to complete those jobs. In organizations such as hospitals, which are staffed primarily by professionals whose functions are mandated by licensing laws, there are certain commonalities in the assignment of tasks and jobs and in the allocation of authority. Hospital organization charts (graphic depictions of personnel relationships) and job descriptions (policies defining personnel duties) show marked similarities from institution to institution.[119]

Staffing. Staffing refers to the recruitment and scheduling of workers, selection and training of managers, establishment of procedures for promoting and replacing employees and evaluating and compensating performance. Staffing is particularly important in nursing, where services center on around-the-clock responsibility for the welfare of ill people. Thus, one of the unit manager's most important functions is to see that there are enough qualified personnel at all times to meet the needs of clients for care. Those needs vary with the number of clients and the intensity of their problems, so that staffing is a fluid, dynamic problem—one that often changes from week to week, day to day, and shift to shift. Staffing, moreover, is a difficult function to carry out in this era of cost-containment, rapid personnel turnover in nursing, and the need to rely on part-time personnel.[119]

Influencing. Influencing involves shaping motivation to create a work environment that satisfies employees, maintains the necessary degree of organizational flexibility, and promotes the organization's objectives. A good manager is able to engage employees toward the organization's objectives so that both the employees' and the organization's needs are met. In fulfilling this function, managers are concerned with morale, employee satisfaction, productivity, communication, and leadership. Morale is a special problem for many nurse managers who are trying to cope with their employees' frustrations in regard to lack of support personnel and a compressed wage structure.[119]

Controlling. Controlling is the process through which managers ensure that organization plans are being followed. Control involves internal accounting and auditing functions, from supervision of the budget on an ongoing basis, to auditing procedures at the unit level, to controlling the use and handling of supplies, to engaging in quality assessment procedures to assure the quality of the services rendered by the unit.[119]

These functions, then—and the success with which managers carry them out—determine how effectively an organization operates. If an organization is viewed as an instrument developed to perform certain tasks (such as rendering health care), the manager's job becomes that of wielding the instrument so as to perform those tasks as effectively as possible.[119]

Managerial Skills. Regardless of the level of their authority, or the goals they are obligated to meet, managers need certain common skills, among them, human skills, conceptual skills, specialized skills, and general skills.[119] Human skills are the skills managers use to motivate each other and their subordinates. These involve interpersonal communication and consensus-building techniques, and the ability to apply motivation theory to practical situations. Table 37–4 summarizes some of the important theories of motivation that managers apply.

Conceptual or mental skills are skills that help managers use general principles to solve specific organizational

TABLE 37–4. THEORIES OF MOTIVATION

Content Theories	(Theories based on concepts of human needs)
Maslow's hierarchy of needs	A theory of motivation that indicates people are motivated by unsatisfied human needs—physiological, safety, belonging, love, esteem, and self-actualization.
McClelland's trio	A theory of motivation that relates motivation to a need for achievement, affiliation, and power. In some societies, like the United States and Canada, culture, tradition, and socialization patterns emphasize achievement motivation.
Hertzberg's factors	A theory of motivation that relates motivation to satisfiers and hygiene factors. Satisfiers are elements that increase job satisfaction (opportunities for recognition, duties of the job). Dissatisfiers reduce it (lack of recognition, menial tasks). Satisfaction increases productivity through reduced absenteeism and employee turnover rates. Hygiene factors are environment elements that include administrative policy, salary, supervision, and work conditions. Their primary impact is not on satisfaction but on dissatisfaction and they are not viewed as strong motivators.
Process Theories	(Theories based on concepts of individual decision-making)
Equity theory	A theory that relates motivation to evaluation, comparison, and behavior. Social relationships are evaluated as any other economic transaction: by measuring investment against returns. People respond positively when they perceive their relationships to be equitable. They compare their own evaluations against those of others. Thus, people not only want to know what they got for their investment, but what others got for theirs. They will reduce their effort when underpaid.
Expectancy theory	A theory that says people are motivated by their expectations and by how effective they expect their efforts to be. People are motivated by situations wherein they perceive that their performance will result in a desired outcome.

From Haimann T, Scott WG, Conner PE. Management. *Boston: Houghton Mifflin; 1985.*

problems. For example, a manager must know how to apply organization theory to the needs of a specific unit in order to design a plan of organization that will work for that unit. Organization theories can be classed into three categories: systems, contingency, and human values.

Systems theory deals with the interdependencies between the organization and its environment and recognizes that a change in the environment will cause a corresponding change in the organization.[119] For example, a fluctuation in the supply of nurses will usually cause a change in the staffing patterns of a hospital. Systems theory also recognizes the interrelationship between organizational units, and recognizes that by making changes in one subunit, changes are almost always required in others.[119] It is difficult to change the hospital pharmacy schedule, for instance, without creating a need to make corresponding changes in nursing unit procedures to accomodate the modifications in the pharmacy's operation. Managers use systems theory to help them plan for appropriate organizational change. Good managers appreciate the relationships between their organization or subunit and its environment.

Contingency theory, on the other hand, emphasizes the contingent factors—factors over which the manager may have no control—that influence what managers are able and unable to do, and that define their limitations and opportunities. Contingency factors in health care services include patterns of disease in a community, the occurrence of disaster that places sudden burdens on health service institutions, government policy changes for institutional reimbursement, changes in other organizational subunits, employee absenteeism, and so on. Understanding the contingency factors in an organization's operations helps managers to forecast and anticipate some of the major elements with which they may have to deal. Good managers are aware of the contingencies that place pressure on their organization or subunit and endeavor to accommodate them through contingency planning.[119]

Human values is another conceptual approach needed by managers. People have certain expectations they try to fulfill by working in organizations, and managers, to be socially responsible, must be sensitive to these expectations. Organizations affect people's lives in a multitude of ways, and managers must be aware of how their organization or subunit affects people to advance the well-being of those within and outside of the organization.[119]

Specialized or general skills are skills that enable managers to cope with the unique requirements of their organizational unit. The need for general and specialized skills varies with the manager's position. Nursing services differ in the type of client problem they serve. Some units provide fundamental general services; managers in these units must be well prepared to deal with a wide range of general health problems. Other units are highly specialized, for example, burn treatment units. Managers of these units must be specially prepared in the techniques of burn treatment and be prepared to supervise and educate staff in a variety of specialized techniques. Thus, managers to be effective must have a range of knowledge and skill that is uniquely tailored to the needs of the services their units provide.[119]

Managers' Styles. Chapter 19 reviewed the nature, advantages, and disadvantages of various styles of group leadership that are also applicable to managerial styles. Those were the authoritarian, democratic, and laissez-faire modes. The reader is referred to Chapter 19 for a full discussion.

Participative Management and Shared Governance. Governance refers to the exercise of power in an organization. **Shared governance** is a democratic approach to organization governance in which there is participation by people at all levels of an organization in the control and determination of the direction of the organization.

Participative management is a synonymous term. Participative management is a transactional approach to management in which managers and subordinates share management responsibilities to a higher degree than in traditional organizations. Participative management generally refers to forms of group decision-making, decentralized authority, and management by objectives.[120] **Management by objectives** is an approach that seeks to obtain subordinate commitment to employee performance objectives through participative goal-setting. Mutually set objectives are converted to action plans that set out a clear path for successful subordinate performance.[120]

Under systems of participative management and shared governance, subordinates and managers act as partners in addressing the problems of the organization as a whole and those of the subunits in which they work. Participative management is thought to increase employee job satisfaction, reduce turnover, and increase the base of creativity in an organization. Creativity is essential for the organizational innovation that is necessary to accommodate to environmental change. By drawing subordinates into the decision-making process, authorities argue that the subordinates are more likely to contribute their ideas, and that these often have an influence on the level of excellence an organization achieves. Sovie contends that a professional work force such as that in the field of nursing expects to participate in organizational decisions, and that this expectation must be accommodated for an institution to excel.[121] Participative management does place responsibilities on subordinates to inform themselves about the organization as a whole, its various departments, and its fiscal status to be able to participate effectively.

Leadership in Nursing

Many definitions of leadership have been offered over the years. Rost,[117] in his book entitled *Leadership for the Twenty-first Century*, has listed various definitions that prevailed in the 1980s and that operate today. These are summarized in Table 37–5. **Leadership,** however, can best be viewed as an influence relationship among leaders and followers who intend real changes that reflect their mutual purposes.[117]

TABLE 37–5. DEFINITIONS OF LEADERSHIP

Definition	Explanation
Leadership as communicating expectations	Defines leadership as a process by which the leader makes clear what he or she wants done and then persuades followers to do it; goals are those of the leader.
Leadership as influencing organization goal achievement	Defines leadership as centered on meeting group or organizational goals; leader's goals and organization goals are the same.
Leadership as management	Defines leadership as planning, organizing, staffing, influencing, and controlling.
Leadership as influence	Defines leadership as interpersonal influence but ignores other components of management.
Leadership as traits	Defines leadership as a set of personality traits, such as decisive, forceful, persuasive, charismatic, charming, dedicated, visionary, energetic, trustworthy, goal-directed, empowering.
Leadership as a transformational process	Defines leadership as the pursuit of excellence through environmental transformation; a leader through willful acts is able to construct or reconstruct the social environment for others in ways that meet people's needs.

BUILDING NURSING KNOWLEDGE

What is a Clinical Leader?

Harper D. Clinical Leadership. *Nurs Connect.* 1988; 1:81–84.

The author's purpose in this report is to define clinical leadership, the kind of leadership that does not depend on having a specific job or position.

Harper stresses that clinical leadership is not synonymous with administration or management. Clinical leaders rise up from within an organization rather than through the administrative hierarchy. A clinical leader is any nurse who possesses exceptional clinical expertise and who uses interpersonal skills to facilitate the delivery of quality client care. Clinical leaders influence the organization not by the authority of their role but by their special ability to identify and manage clinical problems. They are pathfinders by virtue of their expertise. Moreover, clinical leaders are nurses who have a natural ability to weave theory and research into their practice as a way of adapting to change. They help to motivate others around them and to stimulate learning by serving as role models.

Characteristics of Leadership. Given this definition of leadership, it is possible to identify the essential elements of leadership and to distinguish it from management. Rost[117] identifies four fundamental characteristics of leadership:

1. Leadership is a relationship based on influence.
2. The leadership relationship includes at least one leader and one follower.
3. Leaders and followers purposefully desire certain changes, and these changes must be of a transforming nature.
4. The mutuality of purposes between leaders and followers is forged through their noncoercive influence relationship.

The hallmark of leadership, according to Rost, is that it is a relationship based on influence. **Influence** is the process of using persuasion to have an impact on other people.[122] Thus managers are leaders when they base their approaches to subordinates on influence rather than authority; when a manager uses influence, it means that subordinates have a choice as to whether they are or are not influenced.

Influence in a leadership relationship, however, amounts to more than having a reasoned argument; it involves other elements such as reputation, prestige, authority, personality, purpose, status, interpersonal and group skills, motivation, give-and-take behavior, and other features that Rost refers to as **power resources.** Leaders use their power resources to persuade and influence; nevertheless, leadership does not rest on the power of position. The leaders in an organization may or may not be those who occupy positions of authority.

The leadership relationship is multidirectional.[117] Interactions may be vertical, horizontal, diagonal, or circular, which means essentially that anyone can be a leader. Leadership in nursing service, for example, can be exerted by clinicians or by administrative personnel. Clinical leadership, however, is not synonymous with nursing management. Clinical leaders are those who lead on the basis of their expertise and knowledge in a particular practice area and who through their interpersonal skill influence other nurses to deliver quality client care.[123]

Leaders in a multidirectional relationship persuade followers and other leaders. Followers, however, also often persuade leaders. Leadership is entirely noncoercive; no contractual authority exists to obligate followers to follow in the same way subordinates are obligated to report to a manager. Indeed, coercion and authority as a basis of action are antithetical to leadership; in a leadership relationship, followers maintain the right to decline to behave in the ways leaders suggest. Unit nurses may recognize a clinical leader's expertise, but may not always agree with their methods; they are nevertheless free to choose when and when not to follow the clinical leader. In a leadership relationship, people are free to influence or not influence, to be influenced or not to be influenced.[117]

Followers in a leadership relationship are active rather than passive. Because influence patterns are unequal, relationships between leaders and followers are also unequal. The activity of followers thus will fall on a continuum from highly active to minimally active. Thus, leaders and followers are distinguished primarily by the relative amounts of time they spend influencing as opposed to being influenced. For example, clinical leaders spend more time influencing other nurses to practice in a certain way than they spend responding to the influence of others, for example. Leaders are leaders because they are generally willing to commit more of their power resources to the leadership relationship. Nevertheless, in a leadership relationship it is possible for followers to periodically seize the initiative and drive the relationship.[117]

One of the most important aspects of leadership is that it addresses real changes. By that it is meant that leaders and followers act on a transformational model of leadership. **Transformational leadership** refers to real changes, initiated by a leadership process, that carry through "from decision making stages to the point of concrete changes in people's lives, attitudes, behaviors, institutions" (p. 414).[124]

In transformational leadership, people are transformed through the leader–led interactions and become able to engage in higher levels of functioining, and organizations are transformed to higher levels of excellence.[124,125] Leaders, along with followers, mobilize resources—economic, political, and motivational—in order to realize goals that are mutually held. Intended changes do not, and need not, always materialize. However, the intentions of leaders and followers must be demonstrated by action.[117]

A leader's most important function under a transformational model is to establish for followers a vision of desired outcomes, and to hold followers' focus on that vision until their common purposes are realized.[125] Activating and nurturing others' adoption of and focus on a certain result is necessary to catalyze movement beyond the status quo.[125]

Organizational change from the bottom up is possible when subordinates have leaders with an inspired vision of how the organization or unit might operate, and when their leaders have the requisite interpersonal skills to keep everyone's attention on the goals and to mobilize their power resources in the organization. Nurses, for example, who desire to institute participatory management in a hospital may organize themselves toward that objective and use their power resources to bring their ideas for change to administrative personnel. Such transformational changes are possible, however, only when there is sufficient leadership to keep followers motivated during the ups and downs of the power transformations that are inevitably involved.

BUILDING NURSING–KNOWLEDGE

What Makes for Exceptional Leadership?

Sovie MD. Exceptional executive leadership shapes nursing's future. *Nurs Econom.* 1987; 5:13–20.

In this article Sovie looks at the characteristics of exceptional leadership, the kind of leadership that she feels is needed in these turbulent times in health care. Sovie describes the position of J. M. Burns. Burns is an important theorist on leadership who believes that leadership is more than getting things done—leadership is transforming. Burns' major idea is that in transforming leadership, the leader and the led affect each other, raising one another to higher levels of performance, motivation, and morality. There is give and take between group and leader and a partnership develops.

In Sovie's opinion, exceptional leaders in nursing are transforming leaders. They empower other nurses to act, produce, create, and excel. The more nursing leaders empower, the more successful the whole enterprise becomes. Every professional nurse is knowledgeable. A culture of shared ownership or partnership recognizes the professional's expertise and enhances productivity. Exceptional leaders thus serve to unleash the energy in others. They act as coaches, cheerleaders, and developers. They invite the professional nurses practicing in the organization to share in the organization's decisions.

A Vision for Nursing. Nursing now faces and will continue to face many problems that are in need of transformational leadership. Vision is an indispensable ingredient for dealing with the dissatisfiers that currently exist in the workplace and that must be resolved for the good of the profession. Fortunately, nursing has many leaders at the local, regional, and national levels with a vision for the future. L. H. Aiken, Director for the Center for Health Services and Policy Research at the University of Pennsylvania School of Nursing, is a national leader who has outlined such a vision. Aiken looks for the transformation of nursing through the development of career tracts for nurses, particularly in hospitals, that approximate more closely the organization of medical care.[22] She outlines four possible career trajectories: attending nurses, intensivists, subspecialist consulting nurses, and nurse managers.

Attending Nurses. Noting that physicians are organized into clinical services that admit clients for care to many hospital units, Aiken suggests that nurses adopt such a mode rather than being constrained to activity on a single nursing unit. It is the difference in basic mode of organization that Aiken finds to be at the heart of much of the miscommunication and difficulties between physicians and nurses in practice settings.

Under current arrangements, Aiken points out, it is an accident when a physician responsible for a client encounters the nurse who knows the client best. Moreover, the current mode separates nurses and physicians so that they rarely come to know or appreciate each others' clinical judgment.

Thus, Aiken proposes organizing senior nurse clinicians into attending nurse services and integrating them into existing medical staff organization so that each clinical service consists of a nurse/physician practice group. Attending nurses would have 24-hour client care responsibility and would make decisions about client care for all clients on the service whatever their location in the hospital. Staff nurses would continue to cover specific nursing units on a shift basis to implement the plan of care developed by attending nurses and physicians.[22]

Intensivists. Aiken also proposes that career trajectories be developed for the most expert and knowledgeable nurses in clinical areas such as trauma and emergency care, surgery, recovery, and intensive care. In these highly specialized areas, attending nurses would delegate responsibility for the client's care to nurse intensivists for the duration of their stay in the specialized unit. Nurse intensivists would work closely with physicians in a joint practice model.[22]

Subspecialist Consulting Nurses. Aiken proposes a cadre of subspecialist consultants who would consult across clinical specialties and units of the hospital. Psychiatric nurses specializing in psychiatric manifestations of acute illness would consult with nurses on medical and surgical units who had clients with difficulties in the psychological adaptation to illness. Nurse subspecialists would hold an appointment on the clinical service of their specialty but would be available to consult on any service.[22]

Nurse Managers. Aiken proposes a fourth career tract for career managers. Nurse managers would be responsible for ensuring that the necessary staff nurse coverage and ancillary support personnel were available for the safety and well-being of clients around the clock. Nurse managers also would be responsible for communicating the needs of nurse clinicians to hospital management and for helping clinicians adapt to institutional priorities. The nurse manager would be responsible for supervising all nursing personnel at the staff nurse level and would share responsibility with attending nurses for nurturing the development of staff nurses in mentoring relationships.[22]

The Importance of a Vision. No change is possible in the absence of a vision for the future. Aiken's ideas represent one vision and are important because they represent a cohesive view from which plans for change might be structured. Nursing benefits by the promulgation of various views of how change might solve the problems of the profession. Any single vision, however, will have clear advantages or disadvantages. Alternative visions therefore must be conceived and drafted and various complementary and competing visions considered and weighed by members of the profession before action is taken.

Aiken's view is one that holds promise for integrating new satisfiers into the job structure of nursing; such a plan could have a positive affect on nurse recruitment and retention. Other visions might emphasize entirely different approaches to nursing's future. Nevertheless, the outcomes of the nursing profession's transactions with its environment will be determined by the quality of the visions for change that emerge from nursing's leaders. Every nurse is a creative resource and has a potential leadership role to play in the process of nursing's transformation.

SUMMARY

This chapter has explored health care as a transaction from an economic and human perspective. While the American system of health care is without equal in many respects, there are nevertheless problems and conflicts within it that prevent quality care for some and equitable distribution for others. Plans to revamp aspects of the current system in order to strengthen the system as a whole were reviewed; plans for alternatives to the current system were also examined. Moreover, the relationship of current trends to consumerism and the direction of consumerism in health care was identified.

This chapter also has explored a transactional approach to provider–client relationships. Collaboration and mutual interaction provide a model for nurses to use in engaging clients in a partnership for caregiving. It is a model that is compatible with social trends and with consumer interests, and one that ultimately promises to improve the satisfaction of both clients and nurses with the process and outcomes of care.

Finally, this chapter has reviewed definitions of management and leadership and identified their place in nursing now and in the future. Many problems confronting nursing and health care require transformational leadership at every level of the system. Political transactions undoubtedly will be crucial to the transformation of the health care system as a whole. Human and leadership transactions will be crucial to the transformation of nursing and to its realization of professional goals. Nursing has a leadership role to play in moving the health care system in the direction of assuring the necessary quality and quantity of health care for all Americans at a price that society can afford to pay. Nursing also has a leadership role to play in assuring that services are rendered in a manner that respects the human differences that typify our society and that acknowledges their importance to the achievement of optimal health.

REFERENCES

1. Vladeck BC, Goodwin EJ, Myers LP, Sinisi M. Consumers and hospital use: The HCFA "death list." *Health Affairs.* 1988;7:122–125.
2. Califano JA. *American's Health Care Revolution: Who Lives? Who Dies? Who Pays?* New York: Random House; 1986.
3. Davis K. Expanding medicare and employer plans to achieve universal health insurance. *JAMA.* 1991;265:2525–2528.
4. Congress of the United States, Congressional Budget Office. *Rising Health Care Costs: Causes, Implications, and Strategies.* Washington, DC: US Government Printing Office; 1991.
5. Wilensky GR. From the Health Care Financing Administration. *Journal of the American Medical Association. JAMA.* 1991;265:2461.
6. Rockefeller JD IV. A call for action: The Pepper Commission's blueprint for health care reform. *JAMA. 1991;265:2507–2510.*
7. Schramm CJ. Health care financing for all Americans. *JAMA.* 1991;265:3296–3299.
8. Thibaut JW, Kelley HH. *The Social Psychology of Groups.* New York: Wiley; 1959.
9. Friedman E. The uninsured: From dilemma to crisis. *JAMA.* 1991;265:2491–2495.
10. Department of Health and Human Services, Office of the Secretary. Annual update of HHS poverty income guidelines. *Federal Register.* 1991; 56(34):6859–6861.
11. Short PF, Monheit A, Beauregard K. National Medical Expenditure Survey: A Profile of Uninsured Americans: Research Findings 1. Rockville, MD: National Council for Health Services Research and Health Care Technology Assessment; 1989.
12. Short PF. *National Medical Expenditure Survey: Estimates of the Uninsured Population, Calendar Year, 1987: Data Summary 2.* Rockville MD: National Center for Health Services Research and Health Care Technology Assessment; 1990.
13. Division of Cost Estimates, Office of the Actuary, Health Care Financing Administration. National health expenditures, 1986–2000. *Health Care Financ Rev.* 1987;8:1–36.
14. Friedland RB. Financing long-term care. In: McArdle FB, ed. *The Changing Health Care Market.* Washington, DC: Employee Benefit Research Institute; 1987.
15. Jencks SF, Benedict MB. Accessibility and effectiveness of care under Medicaid. *Health Care Finac. Rev.* 1990; (suppl):47–56.
16. Todd JS, Seekins SV, Krichbaum JA, Harvey LK. Health access America—Strengthening the US health care system. *JAMA.* 1991;255:2503–2506.
17. Ginzberg E. A hard look at cost-containment. *N Engl J Med.* 1987;316:1151–1154.
18. Solovy A. Health care in the 1990s: Forecasts by top analysts. *Hospitals.* 1989;63:34–46.
19. Marone JA. The long rise and fast fall of health care competition. *Bull NY Acad Med.* 1988;64:101–116.
20. Goldsmith JC. Competition's impact: A report from the front. *Health Affairs.* 1988;7:162–173.
21. Wesbury SA. The future of health care: Changes and choices. *Nurs Econom.* 1988;6:59–62.
22. Aiken LH. Charting the future of hospital nursing. *Image.* 1990; 22:72–78.
23. Inglehart JK. The struggle over physician-payment reform. *N Engl J Med.* 1991;325:823–828.
24. Crowley AE, Etzel S, Peterson. Undergraduate medical education. *JAMA.* 1987;258:1013–1020.
25. Scott WR, Forrest WH, Brown BW. Hospital structures and postoperative mortality and morbidity. In: Shortell S, Brown M, eds. *Organizational Research in Hospitals.* Chicago: Blue Cross Association; 1976.
26. University of Texas Medical Branch. *National Survey of Hospital and Medical School Salaries.* Galvaston: University of Texas; 1989.
27. Butler SM. A tax reform strategy to deal with the uninsured. *JAMA.* 1991;265:2541–2544.
28. Enthoven AC, Kronick R. Universal health insurance through incentives reform. *JAMA.* 1991;265:2532–2536.
29. Kalisch B, Kalisch P. *The Politics of Nursing.* Philadelphia: JB Lippincott; 1982.
30. Inglehart JK. Canada's health care system. Part II. *N Engl J Med.* 1986;315:778–784.
31. Miserner JH. The impact of technology on the quality of health care. *QRB.* 1990; 16:209–213.
32. Rakich JS. Canada's universal-comprehensive healthcare system. *Hosp Topics.* 1991;69:14–19.
33. Inglehart JK. Canada's health care system. Part I. *N Engl J Med.* 1986;315:202–208.
34. Evans RG, Lomas J, Barer ML, et al. Controlling health expenditures—The Canadian reality. *N Engl J Med.* 1989;320: 571–577.
35. Grumbach K, Bodenheimer T, Himmelstein DU, Woolhandler S. Liberal benefits, conservative spending: The physicians for a national health program proposal. *JAMA.* 1991;265:2549–2554.
36. Linton AL. The Canadian health care system: A Canadian physician's perspective. *N Eng Med.* 1990;322:197–199.
37. Holahan J, Moon M, Welch WP, Zuckerman S. An American approach to health system reform. *JAMA.* 1991;265:2537–2540.
38. Forbes JD. *The Consumer Interest: Dimensions and Policy Implications.* London: Croom Helm; 1987.
39. Haug M, Lavin B. *Consumerism in Medicine: Challenging Physician Authority.* Beverly Hills: Sage; 1983.
40. Sinclair U. *The Jungle.* New York: Viking; 1946.
41. Chase S, Schlink FJ. *Your Money's Worth.* New York: Macmillan; 1927.
42. Nader R. *Unsafe at Any Speed.* New York: Pocket Books; 1965.
43. Haug M, Sussman M. Professional autonomy and the revolt of the client. *Social Problems.* 1969;17:153–161.
44. Zola IK. Structural constraints in the doctor–patient relationship: The case of non-compliance. In: Eisenberg L, Kleinman A, eds. *The Relevance of Social Science for Medicine.* Dordrecht, Holland: Reidel; 1981.
45. Parsons T. *The Social System.* New York: Free Press; 1951.
46. Freidson E. *Professional Dominance.* New York: Atherton; 1970.
47. Hirschman AO. *Exit, Voice, and Loyalty.* Cambridge, MA: Harvard University Press; 1970.
48. Klein R. Economic versus political models in health care policy. In McKinlay JB, ed. *Health Care Consumers, Professionals, and Organizations.* Cambridge, MA: MIT Press; 1980.
49. Congress of the United States, Congressional Budget Office. *Rising Health Care Costs: Causes, Implications, and Stragegies.* Washington, DC: US Government Printing Office; 1991.
50. Louden TL. Customer perception counts in quality assurance. *Hospitals.* 1989;63:84.
51. Forbes JD. *The Consumer Interest: Dimensions and Policy Implications.* London: Croom Helm; 1987.
52. Pauly MV. Is medical care different? Old, questions, new an-

swers. In: Greenberg W, ed. *Competition in the Health Care Sector: Ten Years Later.* Durham: Duke University Press; 1988.

53. Thorelli HB, Thorelli S. *Consumer Information Systems and Consumer Policy.* Cambridge, MA: Ballinger; 1977.
54. Madnick ME. *Consumer Health Education: A Guide to Hospital-based Programs.* Wakefield, MA: Nursing Resources; 1980.
55. Green LW. Health promotion policy and the placement of responsibility for personal health care. *Fam Community Health.* 1979;2:51–64.
56. Keller ML, Ward S, Baumann LJ. Processes of self-care: Monitoring sensations and symptoms. *Adv Nurs Sci.* 1989; 12:54–66.
57. Pennebaker JW, Watson D. Blood pressure estimation and beliefs among normotensives and hypertensives. *Health Psychol.* 1988;7:309–328.
58. Prohaska T, Keller M, Leventhal H. Influence of symptom characteristics and aging attribution on coping with illness. *Health Psychol.* 1987;6:496–515.
59. Fleming J. Consumerism and the nursing profession. In: Chaska N, ed. *The Nursing Profession: A Time to Speak.* New York: McGraw-Hill; 1983.
60. Strasen L. Incorporating patient satisfaction standards into quality of care measures. *J Nurs Admin.* 1988;18:5–6.
61. Davies AR, Ware JE. Involving consumers in quality of care assessment. *Health Affairs.* 1988;7:33–48.
62. Smith NC. *Morality and the Market.* London: Routledge; 1990.
63. Dougherty CJ. *American Health Care: Realities, Rights, and Reforms.* New York: Oxford University Press; 1988.
64. Curran WJ. The constitutional right to health care. *N Engl J Med.* 1989;320:788–789.
65. Szasz T, Hollender M. A contribution to the philosophy of medicine: The basic models of the doctor–patient relationship. *Arch Intern Med.* 1956;97:585–592.
66. Scheff TJ. Negotiating reality: Notes on power in the assessment of responsibility. *Social Problems.* 1963;16:3–17.
67. Bloom SW, Wilson RN. Patient–practitioner relationships. In: Freeman HE, Levine S, Reeder LG, eds. *Handbook of Medical Sociology.* Englewood Cliffs, NJ: Prentice-Hall; 1977.
68. Stimson GV. Obeying doctor's orders: A view from the other side. *Social Sci Med.* 1974;8:97–104.
69. Vertinsky IB, Thompson WA, Uyeno D. Measuring consumer desire for participation in clinical decision making. *Health Serv. Res.* 1974;vol:121–134.
70. McKinlay JB. Who is really ignorant—physician or patient? *J Health Soc Behav.* 1975;16:3–11.
71. Eisenthal S, Lazare A. Evaluation of the initial interview in a walk-in clinic: The patient's perspectives on a "customer approach." *J Nerv Mental Dis.* 1976;162:169–176.
72. Kleinman A, Eisenberg L, Good B. Culture, illness, and care: Clinical lessons from anthropologic and cross-cultural research. *Ann Intern Med.* 1978;88:251–258.
73. Lazare A, Eisenthal S. A negotiated approach to the clinical encounter: Attending to the patient's perspective. In: Lazare A, ed. *Outpatient Psychiatry.* Baltimore: Williams & Wilkins; 1979.
74. Lazare A, Eisenthal S, Frank A. A negotiated approach to the clinical encounter: Conflict and negotiation. In: Lazare A, ed. *Outpatient Psychiatry.* Baltimore: Williams & Wilkins; 1979.
75. Anderson WT, Helm DT. The physician–patient encounter: A process of reality negotiation. In Jaco EG, ed. *Patients, Physicians, and Illness.* New York: Free Press; 1979.
76. Eisenthal S, Emery R, Lazare A, Udin H. "Adherence" and the negotiated approach to patienthood. *Arch Gen Psychiatry.* 1979;36:393–398.
77. Barsky AJ, Kazis LE, Freiden RB, et al. Evaluating the interview in primary care medicine. *Social Sci Med.* 1980;14A:653–658.
78. Cassileth BR, Zupkis RV, Sutton-Smith K, March V. Information and participation preferences among cancer patients. *Ann Internal Med.* 1980;92:832–836.
79. Williamson JA. Mutual interaction: A model for nursing practice. *Nurs Outlook.* 1981;29:104–107.
80. Kim HS. Collaborative decision making in nursing practice: A theoretical framework. In: Chinn PL, ed. *Advances in Nursing Theory Development.* Rockville, MD: Aspen; 1983.
81. Boyar DC. Compliance and participation concepts in nursing practice. *Wash State J Nurs.* 1983;54;31–34.
82. Kasch CR. Establishing a collaborative nurse–patient relationship: A distinct focus of nursing action in primary care. *Image.* 1986;18:44–47.
83. Yuen FKH. The nurse–client relationship: A mutual learning experience. *J Adv Nurs.* 1986;11:529–533.
84. Molde S. Understanding patients' agendas. *Image.* 1986;18: 145–147.
85. Price B. First impressions: Paradigms for patient assessment. *J Adv Nurs.* 1987;12:699–705.
86. Dennis KE. Dimensions of client control. *Nurs Res.* 1987;36: 151–156.
87. Thorne SE, Robinson CA. Reciprocal trust in health care relationship. *J Adv Nurs.* 1988;13:782–789.
88. Sarvimaki A. Nursing as a moral, practical, communicative and creative activity. *J Adv Nurs.* 1988;13:462–467.
89. Morse JM. Reciprocity for care: Gift giving in the patient–nurse relationship. *Can J Nurs Res.* 1989;21:33–46.
90. Roberts SJ, Krouse HJ. Enhancing self-care through active negotiation. *Nurse Practitioner.* 1988;13:44–52.
91. Thorne SE, Robinson CA. Guarded alliance: Health Care relationships in chronic illness. *Image.* 1989;21:153–157.
92. Peznecker BL, Zerwekh JB, Horn BJ. The mutual participation relationship: Key to facilitating self-care practices in clients and families. *Pub Health Nurs.* 1989;6:197–203.
93. Dobson SM. Conceptualizing for transcultural health visiting: The concept of transcultural reciprocity. *J Adv Nurs.* 1989;14: 97–102.
94. Marck P. Therapeutic reciprocity: A caring phenomenon. *Adv Nurs Sci.* 1990;13:49–59.
95. Dennis K. Patients' control and the information imperative: Clarification and confirmation. *Nurs Res.* 1990;39:162–166.
96. Morse JM. Negotiating commitment and involvement in the nurse–patient relationship. *J Adv Nurs.* 1991;16:455–468.
97. Hanucharurnkul S. Comparative analysis of Orem's and King's theories. *J Adv Nurs.* 1989;14:365–372.
98. Shillinger FL. Locus of control: Implication for clinical nursing practice. *Image.* 1983;25:58–63.
99. Gortner SR, Miller NH Jenkins LS. Self-efficacy: Key to recovery. In: Jillings CR, ed. *Cardiac Rehabilitation Nursing.* Rockville, MD: Aspen; 1988.
100. MacElveen-Hoehn P. The cooperation model for care in health and illness. In: Chaska N. ed., *The Nursing Profession: A time to Speak.* New York: McGraw-Hill; 1983.
101. Woolf HB, *Webster's New Collegiate Dictionary.* Springfield, MA: Merriam; 1981.
102. Swain MA, Steckel SB. Influencing adherence among hypertensives. *Res Nurs health.* 1981;4:213–222.

103. Kasch CR, Dine J. Person-centered communication and social perspective taking. *West J Nurs Res.* 1988;10:317–326.
104. Griffith-Kenney JW, Christensen PJ. *Nursing Process: Application of Theories, Frameworks, and Models.* St. Louis: Mosby; 1986.
105. Steckel S. Contracting with patient-selected reinforcers. *Am J Nurs.* 1980;80:1596–1599.
106. Hogue E. *Nursing and Informed Consent.* Owings Mills, MD: National Health Publishing; 1985.
107. Rotter JB. *Clinical Psychology.* Englewood Cliffs, NJ: Prentice Hall; 1971.
108. Bandura A. Self-efficacy: Toward a Unifying Theory of Behavioral Change. *Psychol Rev.* 1977;84:191–215.
109. Schorr D, Rodin J. The role of perceived control in practitioner–patient relationships. In: Wills TA, ed. *Basic Processes in Helping Relationships.* New York: Academic Press; 1982.
110. Geer JG, Davidson GC, Gatchel RJ. Reduction of stress in humans through nonveridical perceived control of aversive stimulation. *J Personality Soc Psychol.* 1970;16:731–738.
111. Kanfer FH, Seidner ML. Self-control: Factors enhancing tolerance of noxious stimulation. *J Person Soc Psychol.* 1973;25: 381–389.
112. Schulman BA. Active patient orientation and outcomes in hypertensive treatment: Application of a socio-organizational perspective. *Med Care.* 1979;17:267–280.
113. Hayes-Bautista DE. Modifying the treatment: Patient compliance, patient control and medical care. *Soc Sci Med.* 1976;10: 233–238.
114. Bishop AH, Scudder JR. *Caring, Curing, and Coping.* Birmingham: University of Alabama Press; 1985.
115. Gadow SA. Nurse and patient: The caring relationship. In: Bishop AH, Scudder Jr, eds. *Caring, Curing, and Coping.* Birmingham: University of Alabama Press; 1985.
116. Fisher R, Ury W. *Getting to Yes: Negotiating an Agreement Without Giving In.* New York: Penguin; 1981.
117. Rost JC. *Leadership for the Twenty-first Century.* New York: Praeger; 1991.
118. Mintzberg H. A comprehensive description of managerial work. In: Rosenbach WE, Taylor RL, eds. *Contemporary Issues in Leadership.* Boulder: Westview; 1984.
119. Haimann T, Scott WG, Connor PE. *Management.* Boston: Houghton Mifflin; 1985.
120. Callahan CB. Participative management: A contingency approach. *J Nurs Admin.* 1987;17:9–15.
121. Sovie MD. Exceptional executive leadership shapes nursing's future. *Nurs Econom.* 1987;5:13–31.
122. Bell DJ. *Power, Influence, and Authority.* New York: Oxford University Press, 1975.
123. Harper D. Clinical leadership. *Nurs Connections.* 1988;1:81–84.
124. Burns JM. *Leadership.* New York: Harper & Row; 1978.
125. Adams JD. *Transforming Leadership: From Vision to Results.* Alexandria: Miles River; 1986.

BIBLIOGRAPHY

Boettcher EG. Nurse–client Collaboration: Dynamic Equilibrium in the Nursing Care System. *J Psych Mental Health Serv.* 1978; 16:7–15.

Budden MC, Griffin TF, Miller JH. Ten simple rules for improving advertising in health care institutions. *J Hosp Marketing.* 1988;3: 75–79.

Calnan M. Towards a conceptual framework of lay evaluation of health care. *Soc Sci Med* 1988;27:927–933.

Davis D, Hobbs G. Measuring patient satisfaction with rehabilitation services. *QRB.* 1989;15:192–197.

Freitag EM. Marketing in home health care. A practical approach. *Nurs Clin North Am.* 1988;23:415–429.

Fry ST. Toward a theory of nursing ethics. *Adv Nurs Sci.* 1989;11: 9–22.

George JE, Quattrone MS. Standardized care plans: Legal implications. *J Emerg Nurs.* 1988;14:183–184.

Hemelt MD, Mackert ME. *Dynamics of the Law in Nursing and Health Care.* Reston, VA: Reston; 1978.

Kane KM. A need to market nursing's usefulness as a profession. *Pediatric Nurs.* 1989;15:191–192.

MacStravic C. The patient as partner: A competitive strategy in health care marketing. *Hosp Health Serv Admin.* 1988;33:15–24.

Marsden C. Casegiver fidelity in a pediatric bone marrow transplant team. *Heart and Lung.* 1988;17:617–625.

Moss V, Webster JA. Marketing yourself as a professional. *AORN J.* 1986;43:345.

Quelch JA. Hospitals, consumers, and advertising. *Dimen Health Serv.* 1979;56:33–36.

Sporty L, Trembath P. Lizza P. Linking the public care system and private practitioner: A study in the use of contracts. *Hosp Community Psychiatry.* 1980;31:45–48.

Swain MA, Steckel S. Influencing adherence among hypertensives. *Res Nurs Health.* 1981;4:213–222.

Szasz T, Hollender MH. The basic models of doctor–patient relationship. In: Schwartz HD, Hart GS, eds. *Dominant Issues in Medical Sociology.* Reading, MA: Addison-Wesley; 1978: 100–107.

Weisman E, Koch N. Special patient satisfaction issue. *QRB.* 1989; 15:166–167.

Weiss GL. Patient satisfaction with primary medical care. Evaluation of sociodemographic and predispositional factors. *Med Care.* 1988;26:383–392.

Weiss SJ. The influence of discourse on collaboration among nurses, physicians, and consumers. *Res Nurs Health.* 1985; 8:49–59.

Zangari ME, Duffy P. Contracting with patients in day-to-day practice. *Am J Nurs.* 1980;80:451–455.

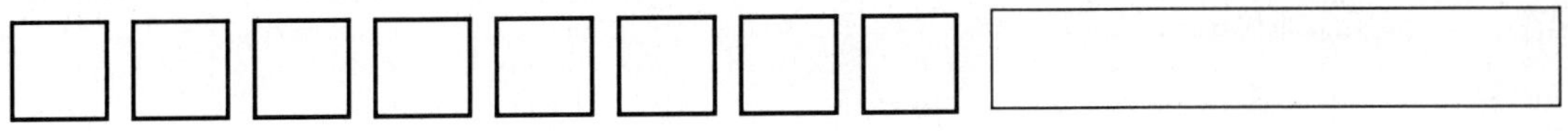

Glossary

absorption The process in which the end products of digestion are transferred through the walls of the intestines. The process by which a drug is transferred from its site of entry into the body to the circulatory system.
accommodation According to Piaget, the process of modifying old ways of thinking to fit new situations.
accountability Taking responsibility for one's actions. In economics, the undertaking of practices to enable the tracking and explanation of the use of resources.
accreditation A system for review and approval of institutions that meet professional standards.
acculturation The partial change of a group's or individual's culture as a result of contact with a different culture.
acquired immunity Immunity resulting from the presence in the blood of specific antibodies for certain communicable diseases.
action phase According to Gazda, the third phase of a helping relationship, in which helper and client collaborate on developing a plan to deal with the present problem and devise a method to deal with future problems.
active immunity Immunity developed by having an infectious disease that stimulates antibody production, by having a related disease that stimulates cross-immunity, or by immunization.
active range of motion The movement at a joint that a person can accomplish without assistance; therapeutic exercise used to maintain flexibility.
activities of daily living Self-care skills required for daily living.
acute illness Illness that can be recognized by a severe, rapid onset of pronounced symptoms, usually of short duration.
adaptation The process through which individuals accommodate changes in the environment in such a way that their functioning is preserved and their general goals can be pursued.
adherence A client's follow-through in carrying out professional recommendations.
administrative regulation Regulation enacted by the agencies of the executive branch of government to guide the implementation of statutes.
advocacy Health care professionals' focus on protecting clients' interests.
advocacy, client Actively supporting clients in their free self-determination of treatment options.
adynamic ileus See *paralytic ileus*.
aerobic exercise Whole-body exercise that causes a sustained increase in heart rate and stroke volume.
affect The outward appearance of an emotional state to others.
affective function In family theory, the process by which the family meets the needs of family members for affection and understanding.
agenda decisions Decisions on the priority of activities that involve sequencing planned events into some kind of temporal order.
agent In epidemiology, the cause of a health problem.
alarm stage The first stage of Selye's general adaptation syndrome, in which the central nervous system is aroused and the physiological defense is mobilized.
algor mortis Physical changes that occur gradually after death, causing a reduction of the body temperature and loss of skin elasticity.
ambivalence An emotional state in which a person holds conflicting emotions and opposing attitudes about his or her situation.
ambulatory care Outpatient facilities that provide care for clients whose health problems do not require continued around-the-clock surveillance by a health care provider.
amino acid Large molecules having an amino (NH_2) and a carboxyl (COOH) group that make up protein chains; also called peptides.
ampule A clear glass container with a constricted neck that holds a single dose of medication.
anabolism Metabolic process that constructs body substances.
anaerobic glycolysis Breakdown of glucose yielding lactate. Occurs when the supply of oxygen is inadequate for oxidation processes.
anaphylaxis A severe, life-threatening allergic reaction.
anatomical dead space Air that fills the respiratory tree, which is not available for exchange.
anesthesia Absence of the sense of touch or of pain.
anion Negatively charged electrolyte.
anorexia nervosa An eating disorder characterized by self-imposed starvation through a rigorously controlled diet.
antagonist Muscle pairs that contract and relax reciprocally to accomplish movement of a body part.
anticipatory grief Grief that is experienced before a loss occurs.
anuria Urine production of urine of less than 100 mL in a day.
anxiety A feeling of uneasiness or apprehension.
aphasia Loss of the ability to communicate through speech, writing, or signs.
applied science A discipline using knowledge to solve problems in a practice setting. Research that builds on or tests basic science for use in the world of practice.
appropriating legislation Legislation providing funds.
arithmetic/logical unit Component of the central processing unit of a computer that performs actual operations, such as addition, subtraction, and comparison of data.
arousal A state in which an individual attends to people, things, and events in the environment and is ready for activity; corresponds to wakefulness.
assault The apparent imminent threat of physical harm; threat to provide treatment without client consent.

assembly language Computer language that uses abbreviations or mnemonic codes rather than binary code.
assertive communication The presentation of facts and feelings in a rational emphatic way, but not in a way that devalues the listener.
assertiveness The expression of confidence and self-assurance that one's ideas and rights are important and should be recognized.
assessment phase The first phase of the nursing process; includes data collection, data analysis, and development of nursing diagnoses.
assimilation The process by which members of a group gradually give up traditional ways of life to conform to the standards of the dominant group. According to Piaget, the process of learning from new experience.
atelectasis Collapse of alveoli; may range from a small area to the whole lung.
at-risk role Role in which a client agrees to take steps to reduce known risk factors.
attachment behaviors Mutually responsive reactions and interactions between parents and child that indicate that the cues given by one person are accurately interpreted and acted on by the other person.
attending behavior Physical acts that a listener uses to communicate interest in a speaker.
audit See *quality assurance program.*
auscultation Technique of physical examination that employs the sense of hearing to assess naturally occurring body sounds.
authoritarian A type of working relationship in which the individual in the position of authority or power gives direction and makes all decisions for others.
authorizing legislation Legislation creating a program.
autocratic A style of leadership in which the leader makes all decisions for the group.
autonomy Independence or freedom to choose one's actions; the capacity for self-direction.

basal metabolic rate The rate at which an individual oxidizes nutrients under basal conditions (12 or more hours after eating, after sleep, with no intervening exercise).
basic science Research that has no immediately apparent practical application.
battery Touching with apparent intent to harm.
behavior A publicly observable activity.
behavioral objective An objective that describes learner behavior; see also *learning objective.*
beneficence An ethical principle concerned with the duty to do good or to produce good consequences.
bereavement A role transition that survivors undergo on the death of someone close.
best interest standard Approach to care of an incompetent client who has not provided advance directives, in which the decision-maker attempts to direct care decisions to measures that will benefit the client.
bias A subjective feeling that reflects a particular point of reference or point of view.
biotransformation Metabolism of a drug that converts it to an inactive form and produces byproducts for excretion.
bit Binary digit (0 or 1) used to represent data in computer memory.
blended family Family form consisting of a husband and wife, either or both of whom have been married before and bring one or more children from the previous marriage to the present family; also referred to as a stepfamily or reconstituted family.
blood pressure The pressure of the blood within the systemic arteries.
board A public regulatory body composed of appointed individuals who are charged with the responsibility of overseeing a specific activity.
body image The cluster of attitudes and beliefs one holds about one's body, including qualities such as appearance, functioning, and overall wellness.
body language Nonverbal behaviors that convey a message.
body of knowledge The collected information that defines a discipline's overall areas of interest and reflects its philosophy.
body temperature The level of hotness or coldness of the body measured in heat units called degrees.
boycott The organized refusal to deal with a person or organization to achieve certain goals.
buccal mucosa The membrane covering the interior surface of the cheeks.
buffers Substances that combine with acids and bases to prevent extreme changes in pH.
bulimia An eating disorder characterized by a behavior pattern of uncontrollable binge eating, followed by self-induced vomiting and use of laxatives or diuretics.
burnout A condition of emotional and physical exhaustion resulting from chronic job stress.
byte A group of eight bits.

cachexia Emaciation, tissue wasting, and severe underweight resulting from a gradual, prolonged period of insufficient nutritional intake.
capitalism The political and economic system in which the market is allowed to determine resource allocation.
capitation Billing system in which a fixed fee pays for a package of health care services during a specific time period regardless of the amount of services used.
carbohydrate A nutritional compound made up of carbon, hydrogen, and oxygen; the most efficiently metabolized source of energy for humans; includes simple (sugars) and complex (starches) carbohydrates.
caries Tooth decay; also known as "cavities."
caring Respectful and considerate relationships among persons; to feel concern about another.
carrier In epidemiology, an agent who has been infected by a pathogen but has no symptoms and is potentially capable of infecting others.
case management A process of need assessment and coordination of health care that aims to provide quality cost-effective care. A model of care involving collaborative physician-nurse joint practice.
case managers Individuals who assess clients' overall needs for health services, delineate comprehensive client outcomes, procure the most cost-effective means of meeting outcomes, and evaluate the effectiveness of services.
case nursing Model of nursing care in which one nurse is assigned to provide total care for one client for the period of a single work shift.
catabolism Metabolic process involving the breakdown of substances and energy release.
category label The problem component of a nursing diagnosis; see also *problem.*

catharsis The process of psychologically purging or getting rid of emotion.
cation Positively charged electrolyte.
central processing unit Component of a computer that controls operations and performs calculations.
cephalocaudal Principle of maturation that motor development progresses from head to feet.
certification A process by which a nongovernmental entity recognizes an individual's competence through evaluation of educational preparation, performance, and professional skills.
certified nurse-midwife A nurse certified to provide primary health care for women, with an emphasis on assessment and care during pregnancy, labor, and delivery.
chain of infection Concept that implies that communicability of disease rests on the connections between a series of necessary factors.
change The process by which the normal course of events is altered. In individuals, the process in which modifications in ways of being or functioning occur.
chemical name An exact description of the chemical composition of a drug.
chronic illness Illness characterized by long duration, frequent recurrence, or slow progression.
chyme The semiliquid mass of partly digested food.
civil law Law that protects the rights of a citizen of a state or country.
classical conditioning A form of learning in which an individual learns to respond to a formerly neutral stimulus through its being paired with a familiar stimulus.
client care plan Document that provides a guide for resolving health problems that client and nurse have identified through collaborative assessment.
client record A permanent, legal document that describes client health history and current health status; also called a medical record or chart.
clinical nurse specialist A master's prepared nurse who specializes in the care of specific types of clients, such as children, women, or clients with mental health problems.
clinical stage The stage of illness in which signs and symptoms of a health problem appear.
closed systems Systems that limit their interaction with the environment.
coalition A group of individuals or organizations that have temporarily come together for the purpose of collectively working toward a common policy goal.
code of ethics A formalized expression of professional values.
coercive power The use of punishment to achieve a desired result.
cognition The act or process of knowing.
cognitive appraisal Conscious recognition of an event as stressful.
cognitive reappraisal A method of stress management involving choosing alternate responses to stressful events.
cognitive development According to Piaget, the acquisition of the ability to think and reason in a logical manner.
cognitive style Thought processes and ways in which an individual ascribes meaning to symbols.
cohesiveness The degree of togetherness or bonding among group members.
collaboration A process in which two or more individuals work together, jointly influencing one another.
collaborative decision making Selecting a choice among two or more possible alternatives for action by two or more individuals mutually influencing the selection.
collaborative function See *interdependent function.*
collagen Fibrous protein component of connective tissue; gives the healing wound tensile strength.
collective bargaining The process by which an organized group of employees negotiates with an employer to define the conditions of employment.
collective power The ability to influence derived from the concerted efforts of groups of individuals.
commission See *board.*
common law The oldest and ultimate form of law; the body of judicial decisions rendered in specific cases; also referred to as case law.
communal family Family form made up of a group of unrelated adults and their children who make a commitment to each other to live together in a simulated family form.
communicable disease An infectious disease that spreads from person to person.
communication To make common, that is to exchange ideas or feelings such that sender and receiver perceive a common meaning; a dynamic process that occurs via many channels, eg, verbal, nonverbal.
community Any group of people who have common interests and problems and who work together to solve those problems.
community health The health status of the individuals, families, and groups within a community and the ability of the community to carry out certain necessary functions.
community health nursing Nursing specialty that involves health promotion of groups of people.
community/locality standards Standards of professional practice established within a community or locality; now largely replaced by national or regional standards.
comparator In a homeostatic control system, the component that determines whether there is a deviation of the input from the desired level.
complementary protein Two or more incomplete proteins that in combination supply all the essential amino acids.
complete protein A protein that contains all the essential amino acids in amounts adequate for use in the body.
complex carbohydrate Polysaccharides (starch, glycogen) composed of chains of monosaccharides, chiefly glucose molecules; one of the two broad categories of carbohydrates.
comprehensive family care Care directed to the integrated physical, emotional, social, cultural, and spiritual needs of individual family members and the family as a unit.
computer A machine that accepts input; stores, retrieves, and processes information; and generates output.
computer-assisted instruction A method of teaching that involves interaction between the learner and the computer, in which the computer takes the role of teacher.
concept A label applied to the sensory data (reports and observed behaviors) that tell a researcher a phenomenon is occurring.
conceptual framework Frameworks that link groups of concepts into an entire perspective or view of a situation.
conceptual model See *conceptual framework.*
concreteness Being specific when discussing a client problem.
conditioned response The response to a conditioned stimulus.
conditioned stimulus In classical conditioning, a new, formerly neutral, stimulus to which an organism learns to respond in the absence of the original stimulus.
conditioning The process of creating new relationships or associations between stimuli and responses.
conduction Heat loss from a warmer substance or object to a cooler substance or object with which it is in contact.

confidentiality An ethical principle concerned with duty to protect an individual's privacy.
confrontation The process of informing a client of the discrepancy between what the client has said and what the client has been doing.
conjunctiva The mucous membrane that lines the eyelids.
connotative meaning The personalized meaning of a word.
consciousness The state of being aware of one's self and one's surroundings; awareness.
consensus building The interpersonal approaches and techniques people or groups use to resolve their differences on important issues.
consolidated client record A record in which written communication by health care team members is documented on one common form rather than in several areas.
constipation The passage of small, hard, dry stool, or the passage of no stool, for an unusually long period of time.
constitutional law A system of fundamental laws that establishes the overall structure and powers of government and the rights of the citizenry under that government.
consultation The action of contacting an expert to help solve client problems; also called referral.
consumerism The promotion of consumer interests.
context One of the components of communication; refers to the setting and circumstances in which the interaction occurs.
contract In the helping relationship, the establishment of mutual expectations.
contributing factor See *related factor*.
control The ability to have an impact on an outcome. In research, special procedures followed to eliminate, distribute, consider, or measure the effects produced by variables other than the independent one.
control unit Component of the central processing unit of a computer that determines the sequence of operations and routes data between different parts of the computer.
contusion A blow from a blunt object that entails soft tissue damage, but no break in the skin.
convection Heat loss by means of currents to surrounding air or fluid.
coping The manner in which an individual attempts to make a stressful situation better.
cornea Part of the fibrous membrane of the eye, which is continuous with the sclera but is transparent and colorless.
crackles Abnormal breath sounds that are diffuse, discontinuous crackling sounds caused by the movement of fluid in small airways or the sudden opening of closed alveoli; formerly called rales.
credentialing The process whereby qualified agents certify that individual nurses or the institutions and programs that prepare them meet minimum standards.
criminal law Law concerned with punishing the perpetrator of a crime.
crisis The situation that exists when coping responses to stress fail, and an event is experienced as overwhelming.
critical periods Those periods of development during which a person is more vulnerable to physical, chemical, psychological, or environmental influences.
cue A piece of information; a raw fact.
cultural conflict Conflict that occurs when there is a lack of awareness, understanding, acceptance, or responsiveness between members of different cultural groups.
cultural relativism Perspective that any culture is different from, but not superior or inferior to, any other culture.
cultural sensitivity Individuals' awareness of which issues or concerns are important to their own culture and to the culture of others.
culture A pattern of learned behaviors and values that are shared among members of a designated group.
culture shock The difficulties that people experience in adjusting to life in a culture different from their own.
cyanosis A bluish-gray skin color that occurs when oxygen content of the intravascular hemoglobin is diminished or when blood flow rate is slowed; for example, when a person is chilled.

dangling Activity in which a client sits at the edge of the bed for several minutes before standing; used to correct orthostatic hypotension.
data anaylsis The process of analyzing and interpreting data.
data base Information gathered through the health history, examination, and subsequent diagnostic testing.
data collection The process of obtaining a data base.
debride To remove foreign material and dead or damaged tissue.
deception Intentional concealment of the truth.
decision analysis methods Systematic and deliberative techniques used to analyze problems.
decision environment The context (circumstances, conditions, and setting) in which decisions are made.
deductive reasoning Process of thinking that moves from general principles to the collection of specific data that confirm or negate a hypothesis.
defense mechanisms Emotional defenses that are commonly used by people to allay painful or stressful feelings.
defining characteristics Observed, reported, or measured findings that serve as supporting evidence of a nursing diagnosis; also called manifestations or signs and symptoms.
dehiscence Separation of the edges of a wound.
demand The quantity of a good or service that consumers would be willing and able to purchase at various prices during a given interval of time.
democratic Style of leadership in which the leader supports group members' active participation in decision making.
denial A stage of illness in which symptoms are ignored or minimized.
denotative meaning The relationship that exists between an object in the physical world and the word that stands for that object.
deontology Ethical theory that holds that a person ought to follow those actions that are in accordance with certain duties.
dependent function Nursing activities requiring that someone else, typically a physician, write an order for the activity that a nurse then carries out.
dependent variable In a research study, a variable thought to be an effect rather than a cause of a phenomenon.
depersonalization The feeling that one is observing what is happening rather than experiencing it.
derived demand A demand for a product derived from another demand.
dermatitis Inflammation of the skin characterized by redness and itchiness.
dermis The layer of the skin lying directly below the epidermis and containing the specialized cardiovascular, neurological, and lymphatic systems of the skin.
descriptive theory Theory that summarizes what is common among individuals, groups, events, or situations.
desired outcome Statement that describes the expected client status when a nursing diagnosis has been resolved.

detente In group dynamics, the type of relationship in which there is an accepted balance of authority between individuals with some degree of mutuality regarding goals.

determinism The view that causal laws govern all events, including human action.

development A qualitative term used to describe changes in psychosocial, cognitive, or moral functioning; a gradual change or expansion of a person's capabilities.

developmental crises See *maturational crises.*

developmental task A task that arises at or about a certain period in the life of an individual.

deviance Behaviors that depart from established social norms.

diagnostic label The problem component of a nursing diagnosis; see also *problem.*

diagnostic reasoning A process comprised of collecting and organizing data, clustering cues, and validating inferences by which a diagnosis is reached.

diarrhea The rapid movement of fecal matter through the intestine, resulting in frequent evacuation of loose and watery stools.

diastole In the cardiac cycle, the time of ventricular relaxation, repolarization, and refilling.

diastolic blood pressure The arterial blood pressure that is measured as the left ventricle relaxes and the heart is at rest.

dietary fiber Fiber, such as cellulose and pectin, composed primarily of cell wall constituents of plant foods.

diffusion The process of gas exchange between alveoli and capillaries and between capillaries and tissues.

digestion The breakdown of foods into smaller compounds that can be absorbed into body fluids.

direct question A question that seeks a yes or no answer, or other short response.

direct transmission Method of transmitting infection in which the infectious agent is transmitted immediately from the reservoir of the infected host to a new host without the intervention of intermediate objects; also referred to as contact transmission.

discharge planning A process that attempts to project client health status and needs for continuing care at the time of discharge from the health care agency.

discrimination Differential, unequal behavioral treatment based solely on ethnicity, race, religious affiliation, or sex.

disease A condition in which there is an observable disruption of structure or function.

disease prevention Activities undertaken to prevent a specific disease or disorder.

distress The state of mental or physical anguish that corresponds to stress.

distribution The process by which a drug is transported from the site of absorption to the site of action.

disuse phenomenon The debilitative effect of inactivity.

disuse syndrome See *disuse phenomenon.*

dominant culture In a multicultural society, the group that functions as guardian and sustainer of the controlling value system and allocates rewards and punishments.

drug See *medication.*

drug tolerance Condition that exists when an individual requires increasing dosages of a particular medication to maintain a given therapeutic effect.

dualism In philosophy, the theoretical separation of mind and body.

duodenocolic reflex Reflex peristalsis that occurs in response to distension of the duodenum.

durable power of attorney An option that delegates to a specific person the authority to make health care decisions if a client becomes unable to do so.

dysuria Difficult or painful urination.

ecchymosis Diffuse bleeding into surrounding tissue; a bruise.

economic resources Natural, man-made, and human resources used to produce material goods and services such as food, shelter, defense, and health care.

economics The study of the efficient allocation of scarce resources.

economies of scale Increases in efficiency made possible through consolidation.

edema Abnormal accumulation of fluid in the interstitial spaces, producing tissue swelling and congestion.

effectiveness In economics, a measure of whether services provided have the intended or desired outcomes.

effector In a homeostatic control system, the component that corrects its function to offset the error in the system.

efficiency In economic theory, the amount of resources used to achieve a desired result.

ego In psychoanalytic theory, one of three divisions of the psyche; serves as an organized conscious mediator between the individual self and reality.

elimination The process by which the body excretes waste products.

emollient A fatty or oily substance that soothes or softens dry skin or mucous membranes.

emotion An affective state of consciousness in which joy, fear, anger, rage, and pleasure are experienced.

empathy To recognize and accept the feelings of another.

empiricism The view that knowledge of the world achieved by observation through the senses is most reliable.

employment contract A legally binding document that describes rights and responsibilities of both employer and employee.

empowering response A response that acknowledges clients' verbal and nonverbal communication in a way that communicates acceptance.

enculturation The process by which one learns ways of acting and meeting one's needs that conform to the norms of one's cultural group.

endurance A person's ability to persist in the performance of an exercise activity without becoming fatigued.

enema A solution that is instilled into the rectum and sigmoid colon for the purpose of stimulating peristalsis and causing defecation to occur.

energy balance The amount of energy input in relation to the amount of energy output in a given system.

enteral Via the gastrointestinal tract.

enuresis The involuntary loss of urine while sleeping; bedwetting beyond the age when bladder control is usually achieved.

epidemiological triad Classic model of epidemiology that examines health problems in terms of three categories of contributing factors: agent factors, host factors, and environmental factors.

epidemiology The study of factors that affect the occurrence of disease.

epidermis The outer surface of the skin.

epistemology The branch of philosophy that studies questions relating to knowledge.

epithelialization Migration of epithelial cells to close a wound site.

erythema A generalized area of redness that blanches when palpated.
eschar The thick layer of dried protein and dead cells that produces a scab on a wound.
essential amino acid An amino acid that the body cannot manufacture and that therefore must be supplied by food.
essential nutrient A nutrient that the body cannot manufacture and that therefore must be supplied by food.
ethical dilemma A situation in which there are two or more alternatives for action based upon ethical principles, each of which has undesirable consequences.
ethical principle A fundamental standard that provides direction for making moral decisions.
ethical problem A situation in which the "right" or the "good" thing to do is clear, but accomplishing it is extremely difficult.
ethical theory Theory that provides systematic approaches for establishing priorities for good or right action.
ethics The branch of philosophy that attempts to discern which actions will produce good and avoid wrong.
ethnicity Affiliation with a group based on hereditary and cultural traditions, such as language and religion.
ethnocentrism The belief that one's culture or way of life is superior to that of other cultural groups.
etiology The cause of a problem (to the extent that cause and effect can be known or shown).
eudaimonstic Referring to happiness or well-being.
evaluation The final step of the management phase of the nursing process; determining the effectiveness of assessment and management strategies through a systematic comparison of a client's health status to standards mutually developed by the client and nurse.
evaluation criterion Statement that describes acceptable evidence that desired outcomes have been achieved.
evaporation The conversion of a liquid to a gaseous form, producing transfer of heat to the environment.
excretion The process by which metabolites and drugs are eliminated from the body.
exercise tolerance The amount (rate and duration) of a given exercise a person can perform before experiencing exhaustion or distress.
exhaustion stage The third stage of Selye's general adaptation syndrome, in which the individual's ability to adapt is exceeded or exhausted.
experimental method Research method in which the independent variable is manipulated or controlled.
expert power The ability to influence derived from professional knowledge and information.
expert witness A witness who possesses specialized knowledge of a profession; his or her testimony is used to establish standards of care against which the actions of an accused licensee can be judged in a court of law.
expiration One of the two phases of breathing: moving air out of the lungs.
expiratory reserve volume The maximum amount of gas that can be exhaled with a forced expiration.
explanatory theory Theory that links concepts together, specifying which concepts are related and how they are related.
extended family Family form that includes close relatives such as grandparents, aunts, uncles, cousins, and various other kinfolk who may, but do not necessarily, live with the family.
exudate The fluid that accumulates around the site of an injury.
facilitation phase According to Gazda, the first phase of a helping relationship, in which a helper facilitates a client's self-exploration of a problem.
family A small social system made up of individuals related to each other by reason of strong reciprocal affection and loyalties.
family assessment The collection and analysis of data relevant to family health.
family function What the family does; tasks performed by family members and their consequences for the family.
family life cycle The successive stages of growth and development that families undergo as a unit.
family of origin The family into which an individual is born or adopted and socialized.
family of procreation The family created by marriage, childbearing, and childrearing.
family power structure The relationships in a family through which family members influence each other.
family structure The family organization and the relationships between its members.
family value system The conscious and unconscious ideas, attitudes, and beliefs by which family members are bound together in a common culture.
fat A nutrient classification that includes a mixture of triglycerides; adipose body tissue which serves as an energy reserve; see also *lipid*.
fatigue A subjective sensation associated with discomfort, decrease in motor and mental skill, productive incapacity, and sometimes feelings of weariness and futility.
fatty acid A chain of carbon atoms with hydrogen and an acid group attached; may be saturated, monounsaturated, or polyunsaturated.
fear A state in which an individual experiences a feeling of physiological or emotional disruption related to an identifiable source that is perceived as dangerous.
fecal impaction A collection of putty-like or hard stool in the rectum that cannot be expelled.
fecal incontinence The loss of the voluntary ability to control the elimination of gas and feces.
feedback In communication, the message that the receiver returns to the sender in response to the sender's message. In teaching-learning, information given to the learner about the quality and accuracy of a response.
fee-for-diagnosis A type of prospective health care payment system in which facilities are given a fixed dollar amount for the treatment of an episode of illness based on a system of diagnosis-related groups (DRGs).
fee-for-service Billing system in which consumers are charged for each health service as it is provided.
feeling The conscious phase of nervous activity; the cognitive awareness of emotions.
felony A criminal wrong punishable by imprisonment in a penitentiary or by execution.
fibroblast One of the primary functioning cells of the dermis, which acts in the building and rebuilding of connective tissue.
fidelity An ethical principle concerned with observance of duty; keeping one's word.
field A term used by Gestaltists that encompasses a person, the person's environment, and the interaction between the two.
fine motor control Coordination of small muscle groups so that delicate, subtle, and precise motor activities are possible.
fitness A state in which body systems function optimally. The ability to sustain vigorous physical exertion without overtaxing cardiopulmonary or muscular capacity.

fixation According to psychoanalytic theory, blocks in an individual's development that may be caused by anxiety, threat, or frustration.

flatulence An accumulation of excessive amounts of gas in the gastrointestinal tract.

flexibility The amount of movement possible at a given joint.

formative evaluation In nursing process, ongoing evaluation that gauges progress toward desired outcomes.

free will The philosophical view that humans are free to make their own decisions and choices.

fremitus Vibrations that are felt over the chest wall when a client speaks.

functional incontinence According to NANDA taxonomy, the involuntary, unpredictable loss of urine.

functional nursing Model of nursing in which the major nursing care tasks are delegated by the nurse in charge to individual nurses.

gastrocolic reflex Peristaltic wave in the colon that occurs in response to distension of the stomach.

gay or lesbian family Family form in which two adults of the same sex share an intimate relationship with each other and live together with or without children.

gender Sex classification; can be biologically or behaviorally derived.

gender identity An individual's perception of himself or herself as masculine or feminine, a perception that may or may not correspond to the individual's biological sex.

gender role A person's characteristic behavior pattern associated with being male or female, usually associated with sexual preference.

general adaptation syndrome The physiological response to stress, described by Hans Selye, consisting of three successive stages: alarm, resistance, and exhaustion.

generic name The name given a drug by the manufacturer who first develops it; often derived from the chemical name.

genuineness In the helping relationship, the ability to communicate what one really feels.

Gestalt An organized configuration or pattern, a unified whole that cannot be defined by the summation of its components.

gingiva The gums.

gingivitis Inflammation of the gums.

glomerular filtration rate The amount of filtration by the glomerulus of the kidney that occurs within a given unit of time.

gluconeogenesis The synthesis of glucose in the liver from noncarbohydrate substances such as amino acids or fatty acids.

glycogen The stored form of carbohydrates in most humans; the most easily recoverable source of stored energy for the body.

glycogenolysis The breakdown of glycogen into glucose.

good samaritan laws Laws that provide that a health care professional who stops to give aid at an accident scene is ordinarily immune from being sued.

granulation tissue The new tissue that fills a large wound space or bridges the small gap between margins of a sutured wound.

grief The private experience of persons who are anticipating loss or who have sustained a loss of something that is critical to their sense of well-being.

gross motor control The ability to control the large muscle groups necessary for movement.

group dynamics The patterns and activities of interaction and communication among group members.

growth A qualitative term used to describe a physical change, such as an increase in size, height, or weight. In psychology, a personal response to change that leads beyond adaptation to the achievement of a healthier state of functioning.

gurgles Abnormal breath sounds that have a heavy snoring or rattling quality caused by turbulence as air moves through large airways partially occluded by secretions; formerly called rales.

habituation A form of learning that occurs when a stimulus that originally produced a response is presented so often that the individual stops responding to it.

hardiness According to Kobasa, a personality trait encompassing control, commitment, and challenge, characteristics likely to make an individual more resistant to stress and illness.

hardware The physical components of a computer.

health assessment The first phase of the nursing process; involves data gathering for the purpose of identifying, describing, and treating the client's health needs and problems.

health care team conference Formal mode of collaboration among health care providers that focuses on client problems and planning coordinated care.

health education The process that provides people with the knowledge and skills needed to make informed health care decisions.

health examination The hands-on portion of health assessment, in which caregivers use their observation skills to identify the physical signs of health and illness.

health history An organized body of information comprising a client's verbal reports about his or her own health state.

health-illness continuum A continuum that depicts health and illness as extreme elements of a unified concept.

health maintenance The preservation of the status quo—neutral or average health.

health maintenance organization An organized system of health care delivery whose members (subscribers) prepay a monthly fee that is guaranteed to cover all services named in the contract.

health promotion Health care strategies to maintain or enhance health through alteration of personal habits or the environment in which people live.

helping relationship A goal-directed professional relationship dedicated to facilitating clients' interpersonal growth through effective communication.

hematocrit The volume of packed erythrocytes in a given volume of blood, expressed as a percent.

hematoma Encapsulated bleeding; a bruise.

hemoglobin The essential component of the erythrocyte for oxygen transport, made up of an iron-containing pigment (heme) and a protein (globin).

hemolytic reaction Response to a blood transfusion of an incompatible blood type. Clumping and lysis of donor erythrocytes by agglutinens in the recipient's blood release free hemoglobin, which may cause jaundice and kidney damage. Produces flushing, back pain, and shock.

hemorrhage Excessive loss of blood.

heuristics Easy-to-use cognitive strategies, "rules of thumb," or procedures that simplify cognitive processing of information.

high-level language Computer language that closely resembles English.

high-level wellness An integrated level of functioning in which an individual maximizes the potential of which he or she is capable.

holism The view that an individual is a unity that cannot be reduced to the sum of its parts.

home care Health care services provided in the home; includes health education, diagnostic screening, therapeutic intervention, and rehabilitative support.
homeodynamics The human–environment interaction that continuously creates new and different ways of being in the world.
homeostasis A human response to change in which the desired outcome is the maintenance of a stable state of functioning.
hope An attitude that is characterized by a confident, yet uncertain, expectation of achieving a future good, which to the hoping person is realistically possible and personally significant.
hospice care Care designed for terminally ill clients who choose to spend their remaining days at home or in a homelike setting rather than in an institution.
hospital information systems Automated information systems that facilitate communication of relevant client care and administrative information within a hospital.
host In epidemiology, the person or group upon whom the causative disease agent acts and who, as a result, develops a health problem or contracts a specific disease.
human needs Physiological or psychological conditions that must be met in order for an individual to achieve well-being.
hyperesthesia A heightened sense of touch or pain.
hyperpnea Increased rate and depth of respirations.
hypertonic A solution having a greater concentration of solutes than plasma and thus a higher osmolality. A state in which a muscle has greater than normal tension.
hypertonic dehydration The condition in which water loss is proportionately greater than electrolyte loss; also called "true" dehydration.
hyperventilation The condition in which more air is moved through the lungs than normal.
hypoesthesia Reduced pain sensation.
hypothesis In science, a statement of tentative or alternate relationship among concepts.
hypotonic Having a lower concentration of solutes than plasma and thus a lower osmolality. A state in which a muscle has less than normal tone.
hypotonic dehydration The condition in which electrolyte loss is proportionately greater than water loss.
hypoventilation The condition of inadequate movement of air into and out of the lungs.
hypovolemia Diminished blood volume.
hypoxia Oxygen deficiency at the tissue level.

id In psychoanalytic theory, one of the three divisions of the psyche; serves as the unconscious source of psychic energy derived from instinctual drives and needs.
identity The conscious sense that an individual has about personal uniqueness and general continuity of character.
illness behavior According to Mechanic, a culturally and socially learned response pattern to altered wellness.
immediacy The communication between individuals in a helping relationship that focuses on their relationship as it exists at that moment in time.
immunity A state of being protected against a disease.
immunization The process of protecting people from infectious disease by inoculating them with immunity-producing vaccines.
implementation A step in the nursing process; refers to carrying out planned nursing care.
incidence In epidemiology, the number of new cases of a specific health problem that have occurred in a population in a given time period.
incision A clean-edged cut made with a sharp instrument.
incompetence Commission of an error by a licensed professional that has harmed or could have harmed a client.
incongruent communication Lack of agreement between literal communication and metacommunication; also known as a double message.
incremental change Change that occurs in a small, step-by-step fashion.
independent function Nursing implementation that nurses themselves are licensed to plan and carry out.
independent variable In a research study, a variable thought to be a cause of variations in indicators relevant to the subject being studied.
indirect transmission Method of transmitting human infection in which the agent is transmitted via an intermediary.
individualism Economic philosophy that holds that each person should be the best judge of his or her own interests in the marketplace.
individuality The total character peculiar to an individual that distinguishes that individual from all other people.
individuation A phase of emotional development that occurs by 7 to 9 months in which an infant becomes aware of self as separate from mother or father.
inductive reasoning A process of thinking that moves from particular facts to a general principle.
infectivity The ability of a microorganism to gain entry into the host.
inference The assignment of meaning to cues.
inferential leap A jump to a conclusion, based upon premature termination of the data-gathering/data-analysis phase of the nursing process.
inflammation A nonspecific defensive response to injury.
informed consent The right of a client, based on sufficient understandable information about the risks and benefits of and alternatives to proposed treatments, to *voluntarily* consent to or refuse treatment.
informed dissent The right of an informed, competent client to decline therapy regardless of the seriousness of the illness.
insensible loss Imperceptible loss of fluid from the body via the lungs and skin.
insight The mental ability to perceive and clearly understand concepts or events.
insomnia Difficulty in the initiation or maintenance of sleep.
inspection Technique of physical examination in which body parts are observed and examined.
inspiration One of the two phases of breathing: moving air into the lungs.
inspiratory capacity Tidal volume plus inspiratory reserve volume.
inspiratory reserve volume The maximum volume of gas that can be inhaled with a forced inspiration.
insulin A major hormone secreted by the pancreas essential for metabolism of glucose and the regulation of blood glucose levels.
intentional tort A violation of civil law that involves provable intent to harm.
interdependent function Activity performed jointly by nurses and other members of the health care team; also called a collaborative function.
interpersonal communication Communication between two persons.
interpersonal relationship A social relationship; or a relationship that occurs among people within a social context.
interview A structured conversation with a specific purpose.

intimite distance In communication theory, a distance of 18 inches or less between people.
intradermal Within the dermal layer of the skin.
intramuscular Within a muscle.
intrapersonal communication Communication with oneself; often reflects one's level of self-esteem.
intrapersonal relationship The relationship individuals have with themselves.
intravenous Within a blood vein.
intravenous infusion Administration of solutions via peripheral or central veins.
intrinsic factor A mucoprotein that combines with vitamin B_{12} in the stomach and facilitates its absorption in the terminal ileum of the small intestine.
involuntary movement Movement performed unconsciously, without the person's will, or unintentionally.
ischemia Local interference with circulation to body tissue.
isokinetic exercise Exercise that maintains maximal tension on a muscle through full range of motion; often requires computerized exercise equipment.
isometric exercise Exercise that involves near-maximal contraction of a muscle against a fixed object.
isotonic Having the same concentration; fluids that have the same concentration as plasma are said to be isotonic to plasma.
isotonic dehydration Proportional losses of water and electrolytes.
isotonic exercise Exercises in which the tension within the muscle remains constant as its length changes to move the resistance through a range of motion.

justice An ethical principle relating to equitableness and fairness in matters such as the use of scarce resources.

Kardex A filing system used in hospital and other inpatient facilities to compile data about individual clients and their care needs for quick reference by providers.
Kegel exercises Pelvic-floor strengthening exercises that entail tightening the perineal muscles as if to stop the passage of urine, and then relaxing them.
kilocalorie In nutrition, the unit used to measure the energy provided by food.
knowledge deficit A nursing diagnosis referring to the inability to state or explain information or demonstrate a required skill related to disease management procedures, or the inability to explain or use self-care practices recommended to restore health or maintain wellness.
Korotkoff sounds Characteristic sounds created when flow through an artery has been temporarily occluded; these sounds are heard during blood pressure measurement.
kwashiorkor Protein deficiency syndrome characterized by retarded mental and physical growth, apathy, edema, muscular wasting, and skin depigmentation and dermatosis.

laceration A tissue tear having uneven edges and often contaminated with dirt, grass, or other debris.
laissez-faire Style of leadership in which neither the leader nor the group takes specific responsibility for initiating decisions or actions.
language A formal system of signs and symbols used for communication.
law The written rules under which a society agrees to function.
leadership An influence relationship among leaders and followers who intend real changes that reflect their mutual purposes.
learning The modification of a behavioral tendency by experience.
learning disorder Behavior that indicates impaired neurological or intellectual processing.
learning domain A particular category, or class, of learning in which learning behaviors or abilities are defined and organized according to their relative complexity or difficulty.
learning objective A statement that describes the behavior a learner should be able to demonstrate after completing a learning experience; also called a behavioral objective.
legislative process The process through which policy ideas are converted into law.
legitimate power Power inherent in a particular role or position.
lesion A circumscribed area of pathologically altered tissue.
licensure A formal mandatory process through which a government agency grants an individual the right to provide certain services.
life structure According to Levinson, the basic pattern or design of a person's life at a given moment; it changes and evolves as an individual passes from one phase of growth and development to another.
life-style An individual's typical way of life, which emerges from the life structure.
lipid A class of nutritional compounds including triglycerides, phospholipids, and sterols.
literacy The ability to recognize words as well as comprehend their meaning in context.
living will A document prepared by clients who are of sound mind, directing that when death is inevitable, no unusual or extraordinary measures are to be taken to prolong life and delay a "natural death."
livor mortis Physical change occuring after death that causes a purple discoloration of the skin in the lowermost portions of the body as red blood cells begin to break down.
lobbying In politics, actions undertaken by individuals and groups to influence legislation.
locus of control Beliefs an individual holds about his or her control over events in his or her life. Internal orientation refers to belief in self-control; external orientation to beliefs that outside forces control events.
logical positivism A philosophy that regards science as strictly objective, deduced from sensory data.
loneliness A subjective feeling experienced in response to a deficit in meaningful social relationships.
long-term memory The storage of information that lasts for a period of several hours to a lifetime.
long-term outcome In client care planning, a desired outcome that describes complete resolution of a problem, often characterizing desired client status in broad, global terms.
loss The state of being deprived of or being without something one has had.

machine language Computer language that uses the binary numbers 0 and 1, representing on and off electronic impulses.
macrophage A reticuloendothelial cell whose primary function is phagocytosis.
magical thinking The belief that an event happens because of one's thoughts; characteristic of preschool children.
maladaptation A failure of adaptation (eg, to stress or change).

malpractice suit An assertion by a client (the plaintiff) that a wrong has been done against him or her by a professional (the defendant).

managed care Arrangement that aims to provide the most efficient package of health care services at the most reasonable cost.

management The effective use of human and material resources to achieve a person's or an organization's objectives.

management by objectives An approach that seeks to obtain subordinate commitment to employee performance objectives through participative goal-setting.

management phase The second phase of the nursing process; involves planning, implementation of the plan, and evaluation.

manifestations See *defining characteristics.*

manipulation The act of using another to meet one's own needs. In an experiment, the varying of the presumed cause or treatment (independent variable) among groups in the experiment.

marasmus Syndrome resulting from a deficiency of both protein and calories, and characterized by general emaciation, wasting of body tissues, gradual starvation, growth retardation, and gross underweight.

maturation A differentiation or increasing complexity of a person's capabilities that may come with age.

maturational changes Changes that occur as a result of the process of human development.

maturational crises Crises that occur as a result of failure to cope with the transition from one developmental stage to the next; also called developmental crises.

maxim A general truth or principle that serves as a guide to action.

maximizing strategy Strategy in which a decision maker searches for the best solution to a problem; also called an optimizing strategy.

Medicaid Financial aid program designed to provide medical assistance to low-income persons who are aged, disabled, blind, or members of families with dependent children.

medical asepsis Infection control measures that limit the growth and/or spread of microorganisms.

medical data base The body of information collected by physicians, nurse practitioners, physician's assistants, and nurses; it is generally focused on the client's disease process and the objective of its construction is to determine appropriate medical management.

Medicare Government health plan designed to provide health care to individuals 65 years of age and older.

medication A chemical substance used for therapeutic purposes (diagnosis, treatment, cure, or prevention of disease); also called a drug.

melena Black tarry stools resulting from intestinal secretions' action on blood in fecal material.

memory The mental capacity of receiving, registering, encoding, consolidating, storing, and retrieving information, impressions, or experiences.

message One of the components of communication; includes verbal and nonverbal behaviors and the total impact conveyed by these behaviors.

metabolic acidosis The condition of plasma bicarbonate deficit.

metabolic alkalosis The condition of plasma bicarbonate excess.

metabolism The cellular processes by which absorbed nutrients are used for cellular maintenance and energy production.

metacommunication The total impact of the verbal and nonverbal messages people send.

microchip An integrated circuit consisting of miniature transistors on a small piece of silicon, used in computers.

metaphysics The branch of philosophy that studies the nature of existence.

microprocessor A miniaturized central processing unit on a single silicon chip.

mineral A chemical element that is involved in the maintenance of water and acid–base balance, the functioning of muscles and nerves, the composition of body cells and tissues, and many other vital body processes; may be classified as major or minor (trace).

minority culture In a multicultural society, a group or groups that are singled out from the rest of society based on physical appearance or cultural practices.

misdemeanor A criminal wrong that is usually punished by fines or imprisonment in a jail.

monitoring Ongoing collection of data about a client's condition.

monopoly power The power gained when there is only one seller in a market.

monopsony power The power gained when there is only one buyer in a market.

monounsaturated fatty acid A fatty acid chain in which there is only one point on the chain where a hydrogen atom is missing.

mood One's subjective description of feelings.

moral development The term used to describe development of internal beliefs and attitudes of fairness, social justice, respect, and loyalty.

morbidity rate Statistic that reflects the number of people in a specific population who are ill with certain diseases.

mortality rate Statistic that reflects the number of deaths in a given population from a specific cause; usually broken down by age.

mourning The cultural patterning of expression of a bereaved person's grief.

multi-institutional systems Large hospital chains, in connection with alternative provider organizations, home health agencies, long-term-care facilities, or hospices.

multiple-causation theory Theory that suggests that disease is usually the result of the interaction of a number of factors.

mutual interaction A model of professional interaction that combines collaborative aims with a decision-making framework of the nursing process.

mutuality The process of sharing with another person.

narcolepsy A chronic condition characterized by repeated, uncontrollable episodes of sleep and drowsiness from which the individual may be easily awakened.

nasogastric gavage The passage of a hollow, small-bore tube through the nasal passages into the esophagus and down into the stomach for the purpose of providing fluids and foods.

Natural Law The metaphysical theory that proposes that changes occur in order to achieve a natural end. A deontological theory in ethics that holds that the basic nature of humans is good and their basic duty is to seek good.

negative feedback A series of changes to maintain physiological homeostasis initiated by a control system that cause a return to a more normal state.

negative reinforcement In operant conditioning theory, a stimulus whose withdrawal strengthens the desired response.

negligence Failure of a licensed professional to exercise the degree of care prescribed by law.

nephron The working unit of the kidney, which functions to help rid the body of wastes.

neurons Nerve cells; consistuents of the nerve tissue of the brain and spinal cord.

nitrogen balance The equilibrium between protein anabolism and catabolism.
nocturia Excessive voiding at night.
nocturnal myoclonus Condition characterized by a twitching of the legs that occurs during sleep.
nocturnal polysomnogram Diagnostic test that measures a sleeping client's brain waves through an electroencephalogram, eye movements through an electooculogram, and muscle movements through an electromyogram.
nonmaleficence An ethical principle concerned with the duty to do no harm.
nonrapid eye movement sleep That period of sleep during which no eye movements can be observed and the eyelids are still; incorporates deepest sleep stages.
nonverbal communication All forms of communication that do not involve words.
normal flora Nonpathogenic organisms that ordinarily exist in a specific organ or location in the body and protect the organism against invasion by pathogenic bacteria.
nosocomial infection A hospital-acquired infection.
nuclear family The traditional family form composed of mother, father, and children by birth or adoption.
null hypothesis In scientific research, a hypothesis that tests the premise that an independent variable has no effect on a dependent variable.
nurse anesthetist A registered nurse who is certified to administer surgical anesthesia under the supervision of an anesthesiologist and monitors clients' responses to anesthetic medications.
nurse–client relationship A shared learning experience between a nurse and a client in which health problems are explored, and attempts are made to resolve or adapt to the situation.
nurse practice act A law that defines and regulates nursing practice in a given state.
nurse practitioner A registered nurse with advanced preparation who provides primary care to clients across the lifespan.
nursing As defined by the American Nurses' Association, the diagnosis and treatment of human responses to actual or potential health problems.
nursing data base The body of information collected by nurses; focuses on a client's health habits and how illness and health care are affecting a client.
nursing diagnosis The final step of the assessment phase of the nursing process, whereby nurses interpret assessment data and apply standardized labels to health problems they identify and anticipate treating. A clinical judgment that describes a health alteration that nurses are capable and licensed to treat.
nursing implementation The collective activities of nurse and client that they jointly select to correct or alleviate a health problem identified in a nursing diagnosis statement.
nursing order Nursing implementation statement that contains subject, focus, action verb, time, quantity/condition, date, and signature.
nursing process A deliberative systematic method for identifying a client's health-related strengths and deficits and for planning and providing corresponding client care in collaboration with the client.
nutrient An element or chemical compound necessary for the body's proper functioning.
nutrition The process by which the energy and chemical compounds necessary for the creation, maintenance, and restoration of body cells are made available to the body from food.

obesity A body weight of 20 to 30 percent or more above the ideal weight.
objective data Data derived from clinical observation and testing.
object permanence The awareness that unseen objects do not disappear.
obligatory urine output The minimum volume of water required by the kidneys to eliminate waste materials.
obstructive sleep apnea See *sleep apnea*.
official name The name by which a drug is listed in official pharmacological publications; often the drug's generic name.
oliguria Urine production of less than 30 mL an hour.
open-ended question A question that does not restrict responses to a specific topic or theme.
open systems Systems that openly interact with, influence, and are influenced by their environment.
operational definition A statement of the instruments or procedures that will be used to measure a variable.
ophthalmoscope An instrument used to observe the internal structures of the eye.
optimal health The best health possible for a particular individual.
optimizing strategy See *maximizing strategy*.
organizational framework A system for separating and organizing data.
orientation phase The second phase of the helping relationship as described by Sundeen and associates, in which nurse and client get to know one another, share expectations for the relationship, and establish mutual goals.
orthostatic hypotension A precipitous drop in blood pressure associated with standing; also called postural hypotension.
otoscope An instrument used to observe the internal structures of the ear.
overweight A body weight of 10 percent above the ideal weight.
oxygenation The process of supplying oxygen to the body cells to support their metabolic processes.

pain A naturally occuring phenomenon that serves as a warning to alert an individual of injury or illness.
palpation The technique of examining by use of touch.
panic The level at which an individual's perception of a situation is distorted, leaving the individual unable to function.
paralytic ileus The temporary loss of peristalsis that often occurs after handling of the bowel during surgery; also called adynamic ileus.
parallel play A form of play characteristic of toddlers, characterized by playing "beside" but not "with" their playmates.
parasomnias Disorders of arousal from sleep.
paresthesia Sensation of numbness, prickling, or tingling; heightened sensitivity (eg, to pain).
passive immunity Form of acquired immunity in which the body itself is not involved in producing the antibodies to communicable disease.
passive range of motion Range of motion exercises in which the movement is carried out by a health care provider without active client participation.
paternalism An approach in which an authority makes decisions or takes action for a competent adult without that adult's consent, as a parent would make decisions for a child.
pathogenicity The ability of the agent to cause disease once it enters the host.
patient-controlled analgesia A drug delivery system that enables clients to administer pain medication as they need it.

peer review Evaluation of the performance of a particular category of health care providers in a facility performed by an organized group of their peers.
Peer Review Organization A group of professionals from an outside agency who assess health care utilization and quality of care in a health care facility.
perception The ability of the mind to interpret and analyze sensory input in order to understand the internal and external environment. A process in communication whereby one person discerns both the apparent and disguised behavior of another.
perceptions Mental images that individuals have of their environment, which serve as subjective interpretations of reality for the individual.
perceptual field The sum total of an individual's conscious experience at any given moment; composed of the individual's perceptions, beliefs, imaginings, and memories; also called a phenomenal field.
percussion The assessment technique of tapping the body surface with the fingers or with an instrument to produce sounds.
perfusion Delivery of blood to the body for cellular gas exchange.
perioperative nursing The name given to the nursing activities performed before, during, and after surgery.
peripheral vision The ability to see objects that reflect light waves falling on areas of the retina other than the macula.
peristalsis Periodic, rhythmic contractions that move intestinal contents through the gastrointestinal tract.
personal distance In communication theory, a distance of 18 inches to 4 feet between people.
personality The total character of an individual including attitudes, habits, values, motives, abilities, appearances, and psychic state.
personal power The ability to influence others derived from the force of an individual's personality.
personal value A value held, or ascribed to, by an individual.
PES format The conventional format for documenting nursing diagnoses; indicates the direction of the relationship between the health problem (P), its etiologic factors (E), and definining characteristics or signs and symptoms (S).
pH The measure of the acidity or alkalinity of a fluid; represents the negative logarithm of hydrogen ion concentration of a solution.
phagocytosis Ingestion and digestion of foreign cells and debris by phagocytes.
pharyngitis Inflammation of mucosa of the throat.
phase A particular period in a cycle of changes.
phenomenal self An individual's unique way of organizing myriad perceptions of self. The most stable part of an individual's perceptual field.
phenomenon In research, the object of study; the thing or event that attracts a scientist's attention.
philosophic argument An argument in which an individual examines reasons for ideas or a course of action.
philosophy A discipline that identifies and tries to answer fundamental questions about life.
pilomotor activity "Gooseflesh" caused by movement of body hairs in response to cold or emotion.
planned change Change that involves choices and allows individuals to make decisions prior to the time that the change is required.
planning The first step of the management phase of the nursing process; involves specifying desired outcomes, selecting nursing implementation, and determining evaluation criteria.
plaque (dental) A mixture of saliva, bacteria, and sloughed epithelial cells that grows on the crowns and spreads to the roots of teeth.
plural family Family form made up of a man, his wives, and their collective children; also known as a polygamist family.
point of maximal impulse The area, usually less than 2 cm in diameter, where the apex of the heart is in closest proximity to the chest wall.
policy A set of plans or a course of action designed to guide and determine present and future decisions.
policy evaluation The process by which a policy is examined to determine whether or not the regulations in force are adequately addressing the problem they were created to solve.
policy-making The process by which goals, purposes, and strategies are identified and priorities defined. In government, laws or regulations legitimize policy decisions.
political action committee A group of individuals who agree to work together to elect candidates who agree to support the policy interests of the group in return for its support.
politics Activities used by groups to exert control over their common affairs.
polyunsaturated fatty acid A form of fatty acid in which more than one carbon atom is missing a hydrogen atom.
polyuria The production of large amounts of urine in relation to fluid intake.
population In a research study, all individuals of a particular type; a set of people with some characteristic in common.
portal of entry In epidemiology, the route by which microorganisms gain access to the host.
portal of exit In epidemiology, the route by which microorganisms leave the reservoir.
positive feedback A series of changes that occur when effector mechanisms cause an error in a physiological system to increase.
positive reinforcement In operant conditioning, a stimulus whose presence strengthens the response.
postural hypotension See *orthostatic hypotension*.
potentiation Drug interaction in which the combined effect of two drugs is greater than the anticipated effects of each drug given alone.
power The ability to do or to act.
preclinical stage In the natural history of a disease, the period of time from exposure to a causative agent until the manifestation of a disease.
precordium The area of the chest overlying the heart.
predictive theory A theory that addresses causes and effects of a phenomenon.
preexposure stage The stage of illness that encompasses those factors that exist prior to an individual's or group's exposure to a health problem.
pre-interaction phase The first phase of the helping relationship as described by Sundeen and associates, in which a nurse becomes aware of personal thoughts, feelings, and preconceptions about a client.
prejudice A negative attitude acquired without any prior adequate evidence or experience with a group.
pressure ulcer Area of cellular necrosis that develops when soft tissue is pressed between a bony prominence and a firm surface; also called a pressure sore.
prevalence In epidemiology, the total number of cases of a disease in a particular population at any point in time.
preventive care Client care provided to clients having no signs or symptoms of a health problem. Focuses on promoting health and identifying risk factors for illness.
price elasticity The responsiveness of demand to price changes.

prima facie duty A moral obligation to do what one thinks is right.
primary care The care provided at a client's first contact with the health care system.
primary intention healing Healing of a wound in which there is no tissue loss.
primary lesion Lesion that appears in previously healthy skin.
primary memory The space within a computer that allows for immediate access.
primary nursing A model of nursing in which one nurse (the primary nurse) is accountable for planning and coordinating comprehensive 24-hour care for a client throughout his or her stay in a health care facility.
primary prevention Efforts aimed at improving general health and at specific protection from disease.
primary reinforcement In operant conditioning, reinforcement that strengthens a certain behavior because it satisfies a basic or biological need of the organism.
primary socialization The child's interaction within the family in which socialization occurs.
prime In teaching–learning interaction, a teacher stimulus that tells a learner the exact response that is desired.
principled negotiation The alternative to giving in to the other person's position or to coercing the other person to accept one's own.
priority setting In the nursing process, ranking the urgency or relative importance of nursing diagnoses, desired outcomes, and/or nursing implementation.
privacy The right of individuals to decide what personal information should be communicated to others and under what conditions.
PRN order Medical order that specifies that a medication or treatment is to be administered as the client needs it within certain limits.
problem A set of undesirable circumstances. In nursing process, a concise statement of a client's actual or potential health problem or health state.
problem-oriented record Client record in which client data are arranged according to identified client problems rather than the data entry source.
productivity In economics, a measure of the efficiency with which labor, materials, and equipment are converted into goods and services.
profession A vocation or discipline requiring specialized knowledge, having a code of ethics, dealing with matters of human urgency and assuming accountability for its practice.
professional decision making A methodical, systematic way of acquiring and combining information to make choices from among a set of alternatives.
professional values Beliefs or concepts that influence practice, are generally acclaimed as being important to the discipline, and are affirmed publicly by official professional organizations.
programs See *software*.
prompt In teaching–learning interaction, a hint or clue that helps the learner think of the correct response.
proprietary name Brand name of a drug; see also *trade name*.
prospective payment system System of health care financing in which facilities are given a fixed dollar amount for the treatment of a client before services are provided.
prosthesis Artificial replacement for a body part.
protein A nutritional compound made up of a long complex chain of large molecules called amino acids or peptides.
protein–calorie malnutrition A nutritional deficiency resulting from an overall lack of quality and quantity of food; also called protein–energy malnutrition.
proteinuria Protein in the urine.
protocol A collaboratively developed written institutional guideline that describes health care procedures to be carried out in specific situations. Generally, the specified procedures are not independently performed under usual conditions.
proximodistal In growth and development theory, the term used to describe development proceeding from the midline to the outside of the body.
psychosocial development In growth and development theory, the personality changes that occur as a result of interactions between people.
puberty The period during which children become physically capable of sexual reproduction; begins between the ages of 9 and 14 years of age in girls and between 12 and 16 years of age in boys.
public policy The culmination of society's decisions on how to allocate scarce resources for reaching common goals; usually embodies a plan for solving public problems.
pulse The elastic expansion and recoil of an artery in response to pressure waves created by the beating of the heart.
pulse pressure The difference between the systolic and diastolic blood pressure.
pulse rate The number of ventricle contractions or heartbeats that occur in a minute; indirectly reflects cardiac output.
pulse rhythm The cadence or pattern of the pulse.
pulse symmetry Equality of pulses on both sides of the body; also referred to as bilateral equality.
pulse volume The strength or quality of the pulse.

qualitative research method Research method that yields data that are more narrative than numerical.
quality assurance program A systematic, comprehensive institutional evaluation; also called an audit.
quantitative research method Research method that yields numerical data.

race A group of people (family, tribe, or nation) who are descended from a common ancestor and possess common interests, appearance, or habits.
racism Any ethnocentric activity that is based on the belief that one racial group is superior to another.
radiation The transfer of heat from one object to another via electomagnetic waves without the necessity of contact between those objects.
rales See *crackles*.
random-access memory The main memory of most computers.
randomization In a scientific experiment, a means to equalize groups or to distribute the effects of intervening variables.
random sample In a research study, a sample chosen in such a way that each individual member of a population has an equal chance of being selected and each choice is independent of any other choice.
range-of-motion Exercise or assessment that involves performing all of the movements of which a given joint is capable.
rapid eye movement sleep That period of sleep during which eye movements occur and the eyelids twitch; the phase of sleep in which dreaming occurs.
rate In epidemiology, statistic that reflects the number of occurrences of a specific event per 1000 people in the population (or 100,000 if the event occurs infrequently).

rationalism In philosophy, the view that philosophic claims should be supported by reasons and that philosophic argument should proceed on the basis of progressive clarification of agreed-upon decisions.

rational economic behavior Behavior that is consistent with the incentives provided by the economic system.

readiness Willingness to take action or to participate in a teaching–learning interaction.

read-only memory Memory that is permanently imprinted in a computer and can be read but not changed or written onto.

receiver One of the components of communication; refers to the person who sends the message.

receptor In a homeostatic control system, the component that receives and senses input.

reciprocity A situation in which two licensing agencies have mutually agreed to recognize and accept the licenses granted by the other.

recommended dietary allowances Guidelines regarding optimum nutrient intake for most normal healthy people living in the United States; see also *US Recommended Daily Allowances.*

recommended nutrient intakes Canadian guidelines containing recommendations for protein, six vitamins, and six minerals, with variations for age and sex.

reference groups The groups whose values and rules an individual adopts.

referrent power The power to influence others based on the force of a person's or an organization's reputation.

regression A return to a level of behavior appropriate for an earlier age or level of development; used as a coping mechanism. In psychoanalytic theory, a return to earlier forms of impulse gratification.

regulation In public policy implementation, a prescribed rule of conduct or procedure that implements and supplements legislation.

rehabilitative care Client care that assists individuals to return to the highest level of functioning possible after an illness. Often involves adaptation to permanent alterations in function and appearance.

related factor The etiology component of a nursing diagnosis; see also *etiology*.

relaxation response A state of heightened parasympathetic stimulation leading to decreased anxiety, tension, and pain, and an increased feeling of well-being.

reliability In scientific experiments, the extent to which repeated measurements, using an instrument under stable conditions, yield the same results.

religion An organized system of worship with central beliefs, rituals, and practices.

reproductive function In family theory, the process by which the family perpetuates itself.

research A systematic approach to solving a knowledge problem or answering a scientific question.

research design A detailed plan for a research study.

research hypothesis An educated prediction about the outcome of a study.

research problem A problem statement expanded from a research question, in which the researcher argues for the study's importance and sets the study in a theoretical context.

research question The object of a research study; a highly specific question that must name at least the concepts and population of interest.

reservoir In epidemiology, a habitat in which disease-causing agents can live and multiply for their perpetuation.

residual volume The volume of gas that remains in the lungs at the end of a forced expiration.

resilience A personality characteristic that embodies the ability to restore balance by integrating difficult life events into life experience.

resistance stage The second stage of Selye's general adaptation syndrome, in which the fight-or-flight response is carried out; the adaptation stage.

resolution stage The stage of illness in which the health problem has reached an outcome.

respect The demonstration of belief in another person's abilities and uniqueness.

respect of autonomy The ethical principle prescribing recognition of an individual's ability to determine a personal course of action; self-determination.

respect of person The ethical principle prescribing recognition of the dignity and unconditional worth of each person in the human community, including oneself.

respiration The exchange of oxygen and carbon dioxide in the lungs.

respiratory acidosis An acid–base alteration in which dissolved carbon dioxide accumulates in the blood and, in combination with water, forms excessive amounts of carbonic acid; also called carbonic acid excess.

respiratory alkalosis An acid–base alteration in which there is excessive excretion of carbonic acid; also called carbonic acid deficit.

respiratory depth The volume of air that is inhaled and exhaled.

respiratory rate The number of respiratory cycles that occur in one minute.

respiratory rhythm The cadence or pattern of respiration.

respiratory quality The distinctive traits or characteristics of respiration.

respondeat superior "Let the master answer"; relates to professional liability; under this approach, it is assumed that the "captain of the ship" or "master" (supervisor) is responsible for the physical acts of the crew or servant (subordinate).

response An organism's overt physical reaction to stimulation from the environment. In the stimulus-response model of stress, any of the physiological changes and behavioral manifestations of stress, such as fear, anxiety, or increased blood pressure.

response time As a component of communication, the promptness with which a speaker's presence or words are acknowledged.

rest A period of inactivity during which one is free from fear or anxiety.

restorative care Client care that focuses on management of acute health problems, prevention of complications, and return to a healthy state.

reticular activating system The portion of the brain that is responsible for awareness, consciousness, wakefulness, and arousal.

retractions Pulling of tissue over the lungs because of increased inspiratory effort; may be intercostal (between ribs), supraclavicular (above clavicles) or substernal (below the sternum).

retrospective evaluation In a health care quality assurance program, evaluation that occurs after the termination of care.

return demonstration A method of evaluating learning in which the learner performs a skill without coaching.

reward power The ability of the person in power to grant benefits to achieve a desired result.

rhinitis Inflammation of the nasal mucosa.

rhonchi See *gurgles*.

rigor mortis Physical changes that occur within 2 to 4 hours of death, causing stiffening of the body.
risk In epidemiology, the chance of exposure to a specific hazard or danger.
risk factor Factor that places a client at higher risk for a health problem than the general population.
risk taking Taking action or stating a value that is outside of the prevaling group norm.
role A set of behaviors, attitudes, beliefs, principles, and values that characterize the occupant of a given social position or status.
role complementarity Condition in which the performance of one member of a role set matches the expectations of other members, maintaining equilibrium.
role-modeling Teaching by demonstrating examples of new behaviors.
role performance The way an individual carries out a particular role in relation to societal expectations for that role.
role set A group of roles that are related to each other within a structured entity (eg, a family or a corporation).
role transition The process of moving from one set of values, responsibilities, and functions to another.
rumbles See *gurgles.*

sample In a research study, a small representative proportion of a population selected for study.
sampling error In a research study, the effect on the outcome of the study of chance (unplanned) variation in sample selection.
satisficing Strategy for decision making in which the decision maker searches for a solution only long enough to find one that works and meets the needs of the situation.
saturated fatty acid A form of fatty acid in which every available carbon bond is holding a hydrogen atom.
science A form of discovery, the basic aim of which is to explain natural phenomena.
sclera White, opaque portion of the fibrous membrane that covers the eye, extending from the optic nerve to the cornea.
screening The examination of subgroups in the population for specific illnesses or risk factors related to these illnesses.
secondary care Care provided by specialists on referral from primary care providers.
secondary intention healing Replacement of functional tissue with granulation tissue; the process by which tissue-loss wounds heal.
secondary lesion An alteration in a primary skin lesion.
secondary memory In a computer, the location where information can be stored on a long-term basis.
secondary prevention Activities aimed at early diagnosis and prompt treatment of disease.
secondary reinforcement In operant conditioning, reinforcement that has acquired value indirectly through learning; also called higher order reinforcement.
secondary socialization The socialization that older children, young adults, and adults receive as they progress through school, interact with others, and observe others who share a similar role.
self The union of elements, such as body, emotions, thoughts, and sensations, that constitute the individuality and identity of a particular person.
self-acceptance The ability to acknowledge and be comfortable with the various attributes one perceives about oneself.
self-care Concept of care in which individuals are encouraged to create their own health and are considered to be the best resource for achieving their own level of optimal wellness.
self-concept An organized pattern of beliefs about oneself encompassing one's collection of self-perceptions related to the multiple aspects of human experience.
self-disclosure Communication of inner thoughts and feelings that is uncontrived, spontaneous, and truly expressive of an individual's self-understanding.
self-efficacy An individual's belief that he or she can successfully execute a required behavior necessary to produce a desired result.
self-esteem The degree to which an individual likes or dislikes the self.
self-expression The process by which a person's self-understanding is shared with others.
self-monitoring review system See *peer review.*
self-presentation The conscious or unconscious attempts of individuals to control the images of themselves they convey to other people, imagined or real, or to themselves.
sender One of the components of communication; refers to the individual who is sending the message.
sensitization In learning theory, a form of simple learning in which a previously neutral stimulus elicits arousal and response.
sensory deprivation Condition characterized by confusion, irritability, restlessness, and hallucinations that occurs when there is a lack of or significantly diminished input from the senses.
sensory overload Condition characterized by poor concentration, confusion, sleep problems, and hallucinations that occurs when there is too much sensory input.
serum osmolality The concentration of dissolved particles per unit of serum.
sex An individual's anatomic differentiation as male or female; gender.
sexism The social domination and economic exploitation of members of one sex by the other.
sexuality The pervasive characteristic of personality reflected in the totality of a person's feelings, attitudes, beliefs, and behavior related to being male or female.
sexual orientation Individuals' preferences for the sex of their partners or for the means of expression of sexual thoughts and feelings.
shared governance A democratic approach to the exercise of authority and control in an organization. Involves participation by people at all levels of the organization in decisions about policy and use of resources.
shearing The mechanical stress created from the sliding of one load against another.
shock The suspension or failure of the regulatory mechanisms that maintain circulatory perfusion of the body tissues. Characterized by pallor; cyanosis; rapid, thready pulse; shallow rapid respirations; and falling blood pressure.
short-term memory The site of ongoing cognitive activities such as word meaning and symbol manipulation; working memory.
short-term outcome In nursing process, desired outcome that is precise, relates to immediate changes in client status, and often represents steps toward long-term outcomes.
sick role A social role that embodies a set of norms and values about health and illness behavior; the role that individuals take on when they define themselves as ill.
side effect An effect of a prescribed medication that is unintended and undesirable.
simple carbohydrate One of the two broad categories of carbohydrates; includes monosaccharides and disaccharides.

simultaneous mutual interaction In cognitive-field learning theory, the continuous exchanges between individual and environment through which each influences the other.
single-parent family Family form consisting of one parent, either father or mother, and one or more children.
situated identities Identities that reside neither in the person nor in the environment, but rather in the relationship between the two at any point in time.
situational changes Changes that arise from the interaction between individuals and the environment.
situational crises Crises that occur as a result of external events that are beyond individual control and cannot be anticipated.
sleep A normal and complex physiological rhythm that involves altered states of consciousness from which the individual can be aroused by appropriate stimuli.
sleep apnea Multiple, brief episodes of cessation of breathing during sleep. Usually caused by a failure in the neural control of respiration (central apnea), an obstruction of the airway (obstructive apnea), or a combination of these two.
slow code A situation in which a health care team goes through the motions of a cardiopulmonary resuscitation but responds slowly and with no expectation of success.
social distance In communication theory, a distance of 4 to 12 feet between people.
socialism The political and economic system that disavows private ownership, competition, and profit.
socialization The process of learning those behaviors that are appropriate for members of a particular status group.
socialization and social placement function In family theory, the process by which a child learns attitudes, behaviors, skills, and the interpretation of social norms from significant others.
social network A weblike structure comprising an individual's relationships.
social relationships A component of culture comprising behavior between and among people, behavior toward possessions, work, learning, worshipping. Also encompasses affect and emotions associated with these behaviors.
social structure The relationships that hold society together; also known as social organization.
social support The positive, need-gratifying consequences of interpersonal relationships, including affection, approval, belonging, identity, and security.
society A group of people in a specific locality whose members share a common culture and are dependent on each other for survival.
software Sets of instructions that control the operation of a computer; also called programs.
source-oriented record Client health record that contains a separate section for each discipline to record pertinent observations, care, or responses to care.
special interest group A group that has a vested interest in the outcome of public policy decisions.
speech The articulation or expression of thoughts and ideas using language.
sphygmomanometer A device used to measure blood pressure.
spirituality A belief in or relationship with a higher power, divine being, or creative life force.
splinting A method of limiting incisional pain during coughing and deep breathing. Involves applying pressure over an incision with interlaced hands and fingers and/or a pillow.
stability In change theory, rhythms of daily life that are characterized by firmly established or well-balanced functions or patterns.
standard care plan A preprinted plan based on a particular nursing diagnosis that provides general directions for desired outcomes and client care related to that diagnosis.
standard of care Standardized guideline used by nurses to organize care for clients with a specific medical diagnosis.
starch A form of complex carbohydrate, consisting of molecules of 300 to 1000 glucose units packed side by side in plant foods such as seeds, grains, potatoes and other roots, and legumes.
statistical method Using mathematical formulas to design a scientific experiment and interpret the results.
stat order A physician's order for a medication or treatment to be given immediately, but not repeated.
statutory law The statutes (laws) enacted by the legislative arm of government at the federal, state, or local level.
stereotyping A response to a person or group based on preconceived negative labels without an objective assessment of the individual or group.
sterile technique See *surgical asepsis.*
stimulus In behaviorism, an event or agent in the environment that acts upon an organism.
stoma (ostomy) An artificial opening of the intestine onto the abdominal wall to allow passage of digestive waste products.
stomatitis Inflammation of the mouth.
strength Force or power exerted by a muscle or group of muscles against resistance.
stress The nonspecific, systemic, adaptive response of the body to a stressor or multiple stressors. The situation that occurs when change is considered to be threatening, harmful, or overly challenging.
stress incontinence The loss of urine of less than 50 mL that occurs when there is a sudden increase in intra-abdominal pressure.
stressor An external situation that disrupts internal equilibrium within the human organism and interferes with the meeting of needs.
subculture Subgroups within a culure that share value differences and customs.
subcutaneous Beneath the skin; within the subcutaneous tissue.
subcutaneous fat A lipid layer lying below the dermis, containing major vascular networks, the lymphatics, and nerve fibers.
subjective data In a health assessment, information that the client verbally reports.
substituted judgment Approach to care of an incapacitated client in which people who know the client best are asked to speak for the client as he or she would have done if able.
summative evaluation In nursing process, evaluation that occurs on specific target dates identified in a client care plan and at the termination of care.
sundown syndrome Condition in which a person functions normally during the day but suffers from hallucinations, delusions, and disorientation at night; also called nocturnal delirium.
sunset laws Laws requiring licensing boards or other public agencies to justify their existence at regular intervals.
sunshine laws Laws requiring that certain governmental entities conduct meetings in public.
superego In psychoanalytic theory, one of three divisions of the psyche which is only partly conscious and represents internalization of parental conscience and rules of society.
supportive care Client care provided in the early stages of alterations in health state; aimed at managing the current problem and preventing complications.
surfactant A lipoprotein that decreases alveolar surface tension and thus increases alveolar stability.

surgical asepsis The method by which items and specific areas in the health care setting are kept free of all microorganisms; also called sterile technique.
sustained maximal inspiration The action of breathing deeply and holding the inspired breath briefly before exhaling.
sympathy To experience the same feelings another person is experiencing.
synergist One of two muscles that interact together to accomplish a given movement.
system An organized set of components or parts that mutually interact to form an integrated whole.
systole In the cardiac cycle, the time of ventricular contraction, when blood is being ejected from the heart to the lungs and the rest of the body.
systolic blood pressure The pressure exerted against the arterial wall as the left ventricle contracts and forces blood into the aorta.

tachypnea Rapid, shallow respirations.
tacit assumption In philosophy, a belief or value that is taken for granted.
target group In a community, a group of people with special needs for whom specific health programs are designed.
tartar (dental) A hard yellowish substance that forms on teeth along the gum line.
taxonomy A classification system that organizes known phenomena into a hierarchical structure and helps direct the discovery of new phenomena.
teaching Deliberately influencing learning toward specific goals.
team A number of persons who are associated together in a work activity.
team nursing Model of nursing in which a registered nurse serves as leader and manager for a group of nurses and allied health personnel who assume responsibility for meeting the health care needs of a group of clients through cooperation and collaboration.
teleology Ethical theory that holds that good or right actions are measured by the consequences of those actions.
termination phase The formal ending of the helping relationship as described by Sundeen and associates.
territoriality The innate need to claim control and to dominate various facets of one's existence.
tertiary care Advanced diagnostic and treatment care requiring specialized personnel and equipment.
tertiary prevention Activities designed to assist clients to deal with residual consequences of a health problem or to prevent its recurrence.
testimony A public means of sharing information with all persons or groups involved in the process of making public policy; may be written or oral.
theoretical framework In a research study, the explication of the link between the research question that is the focus of the study and an existing theory or theories.
theory A statement or set of statements that aims to describe, explain, predict, or control a phenomenon.
theory of virtue An ethical theory concerned with intrinsic qualities that enhance the capacity of people to be fully human and to live together within a moral community.
therapeutic effect The desired or intended physiological effect for which a drug is prescribed.
therapeutic play Specially designed play activities that help children to express fears, conflicts, and other feelings.
therapeutic use of self A caregiver's ability to use personality characteristics consciously and in full awareness in order to form a relationship and to structure interventions.
third spacing The sequestering of large amounts of fluid in body spaces from which exchange with extracellular fluid is difficult.
thought The mental process that assigns meaning to and designs actions in response to the integration and interpretation of sensory input.
thrombus A platelet and fibrin plug that seals off the site of an injury from further blood loss; also called a clot.
tidal volume The volume of gas that is moved with each breath.
tone In communication theory, the character or style in which a person communicates.
tort A violation of a civil right (a right established in civil, rather than criminal, cases).
total body water The total amount of water that exists in the body at any given time.
total lung capacity The maximum volume of gas that the lungs can contain.
total parenteral nutrition The administration of a nutritionally complete solution intravenously to clients who cannot tolerate food via the gastrointestinal tract; formerly called intravenous hyperalimentation.
toxic effect An adverse effect that results from a drug overdose or from abnormal accumulation of a medication in the body.
trade name The name under which a manufacturer markets a drug; also called the *proprietary name* or brand name.
transaction An act of exchange through which people negotiate with one another to carry out a give and take of valuable human resources.
transcultural reciprocity Collaborative interaction based on an exchange of cultural respect and understanding between members of different cultures.
transformational leadership Changes initiated by a leadership process that carry through from decision making to the point of concrete change.
transition phase According to Gazda, the second phase of a helping relationship, in which helpers work with clients to define the problem.
transmission A component of communication that involves the actual expression of the message from the sender to receiver.
turgor Skin elasticity.

unintentional tort A tort in which harm occurred, but there is evidence that the harm was unintentional.
universal precautions Series of precautions recommended by the Centers for Disease Control under which blood and certain body fluids of all clients are considered potentially infectious. Requires strict adherence to infection control measures for minimizing risk of exposure to organisms.
unplanned change Unpredictable change that occurs spontaneously and outside of an individual's control.
urethritis Inflammation of the urethra.
urinary frequency Urination at more frequent intervals than normal.
urinary incontinence The loss of control over voiding.
urinary retention A state in which an individual cannot initiate or complete evacuation of accumulated urine from the bladder.
US Recommended Daily Allowances A set of figures designed specifically for use on food labels in the United States. In most cases, they are the highest recommended daily allowance of a given nutrient for any age group or sex. See also *recommended dietary allowances*.

utility In economic theory, the satisfaction that a good or service can provide.

utilization management The case-by-case assessment by third-party payers of the appropriateness of care before it is provided; sometimes referred to as "prior authorization."

utilization review A retrospective review of health care provided in a particular facility to determine its appropriateness. Federally mandated in institutions seeking federal reimbursement for health care.

vaccine An antigenic substance deliberately introduced into the body to promote the development of antibodies, resulting in immunization.

vaginitis Inflammation of the vaginal mucosa.

validity In scientific experiments, the extent to which an instrument measures what it is designed to measure.

Valsalva maneuver The attempt to force an expiration with the glottis closed.

value A standard that provides meaningful direction for individual or group behavior. In ethics, that which is seen as intrinsically good or right.

values clarification A conscious process of identifying, clarifying, and ranking personal values.

value system An individual's own set of values.

variable In a research study, those indicators of a concept that may change under differing conditions.

vector In epidemiology, a living intermediary, usually arthropod, that mechanically transmits infectious agents.

vehicle In epidemiology, a nonliving intermediary that serves as a transmitter for microorganisms.

venipuncture The act of puncturing a vein for any purpose.

ventilation The process of moving air into and out of the lungs.

veracity An ethical principle prescribing devotion to truth.

verbal communication Communication through language, incorporating denotative and connotative meanings ascribed to words.

vial A glass container with a self-sealing rubber cap through which medication can be withdrawn.

virulence In epidemiology, the severity of disease caused by a microorganism.

vital capacity Inspiratory reserve volume plus tidal volume plus expiratory reserve volume.

vitamin An organic nutrient that is essential for normal metabolism, growth, and development.

voluntary movement Movement carried out consciously and intentionally under a person's will or volition.

warmth In communication theory, the emotional expression of nonverbal caring and love.

well-being An individual's subjective perception of his or her current level of functioning and satisfaction with life.

wellness An individual process or life-style that is oriented toward attaining an optimal level of physical fitness and physical–emotional harmony, that supports a sustained zest or joy of living, and that provides maximum resistance to disease.

wheezing Continuous abnormal, high-pitched whistling breath sound caused by air rushing through an airway narrowed because of bronchospasm or obstruction.

working phase The third phase of the helping relationship as described by Sundeen and associates, in which nurse and client engage in active problem solving.

wound An injury to tissue that disrupts normal cellular processes.

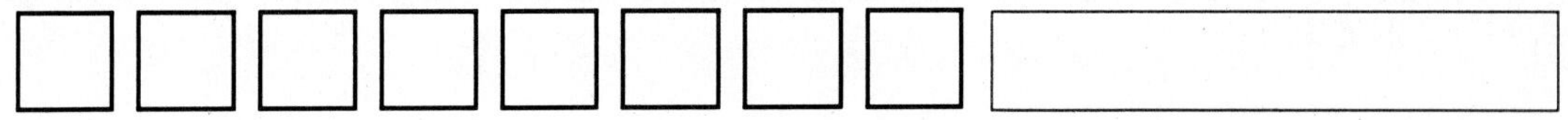

Index

Italicized numbers indicate material in Boxes, Tables and Figures.

PHYSICAL GROWTH FROM BIRTH TO 18 YEARS

Age	Percentile, Boys								Percentile, Girls						
	5th	*10th*	*25th*	*50th*	*75th*	*90th*	*95th*		*5th*	*10th*	*25th*	*50th*	*75th*	*90th*	*95th*
At birth	46.4	47.5	49.0	50.5	51.8	53.5	54.4	**Length (cm)**	45.4	46.5	48.2	49.9	51.0	52.0	52.9
	18¼	18¾	19¼	20	20½	21	21½	Length (in.)	17¾	18¼	19	19¾	20	20½	20¾
	2.54	2.78	3.00	3.27	3.64	3.82	4.15	**Weight (kg)**	2.36	2.58	2.93	3.23	3.52	3.64	3.81
	5½	6¼	6½	7¼	8	8½	9¼	Weight (lb)	5¼	5¾	6½	7	7¾	8	8½
	32.6	33.0	33.9	34.8	35.6	36.6	37.2	**Head C (cm)**	32.1	32.9	33.5	34.3	34.8	35.5	35.9
	12¾	13	13¼	13¾	14	14½	14¾	Head C (in.)	12¾	13	13¼	13½	13¾	14	14¼
3 months	56.7	57.7	59.4	61.1	63.0	64.5	65.4	**Length (cm)**	55.4	56.2	57.8	59.5	61.2	62.7	63.4
	22¼	22¾	23½	24	24¾	25½	25¾	Length (in.)	21¾	22¼	22¾	23½	24	24¾	25
	4.43	4.78	5.32	5.98	6.56	7.14	7.37	**Weight (kg)**	4.18	4.47	4.88	5.40	5.90	6.39	6.74
	9¾	10½	11¾	13¼	14½	15¾	16¼	Weight (lb)	9¼	9¾	10¾	12	13	14	14¾
	38.4	38.9	39.7	40.6	41.7	42.5	43.1	**Head C (cm)**	37.3	37.8	38.7	39.5	40.4	41.2	41.7
	15	15¼	15¾	16	16½	16¾	17	Head C (in.)	14¾	15	15¼	15½	16	16¼	16½
6 months	63.4	64.4	66.1	67.8	69.7	71.3	72.3	**Length (cm)**	61.8	62.6	64.2	65.9	67.8	69.4	70.2
	25	25¼	26	26¾	27½	28	28½	Length (in.)	24¼	24¾	25¼	26	26¾	27¼	27¾
	6.20	6.61	7.20	7.85	8.49	9.10	9.46	**Weight (kg)**	5.79	6.12	6.60	7.21	7.83	8.38	8.73
	13¾	14½	15¾	17¼	18¾	20	20¾	Weight (lb)	12¾	13½	14½	16	17¼	18½	19¼
	41.5	42.0	42.8	43.8	44.7	45.6	46.2	**Head C (cm)**	40.3	40.9	41.6	42.4	43.3	44.1	44.6
	16¼	16½	16¾	17¼	17½	18	18¼	Head C (in.)	15¾	16	16½	16¾	17	17¼	17½
12 months	71.7	72.8	74.3	76.1	77.7	79.8	81.2	**Length (cm)**	69.8	70.8	72.4	74.3	76.3	78.0	79.1
	28¼	28¾	29¼	30	30½	31½	32	Length (in.)	27½	27¾	28½	29¼	30	30¾	31¼
	8.43	8.84	9.49	10.15	10.91	11.54	11.99	**Weight (kg)**	7.84	8.19	8.81	9.53	10.23	10.87	11.24
	18½	19½	21	22½	24	25½	26½	Weight (lb)	17¼	18	19½	21	22½	24	24¾
	44.8	45.3	46.1	47.0	47.9	48.8	49.3	**Head C (cm)**	43.5	44.1	44.8	45.6	46.4	47.2	47.6
	17¾	17¾	18¼	18½	18¾	19¼	19½	Head C (in.)	17¼	17¼	17¾	18	18¼	18½	18¾
18 months	77.5	78.7	80.5	82.4	84.3	86.6	88.1	**Length (cm)**	76.0	77.2	78.8	80.9	83.0	85.0	86.1
	30½	31	31¾	32½	33¼	34	34¾	Length (in.)	30	30½	31	31¾	32¾	33½	34
	9.59	9.92	10.67	11.47	12.31	13.05	13.44	**Weight (kg)**	8.92	9.30	10.04	10.82	11.55	12.30	12.76
	21¼	21¾	23½	25¼	27¼	28¾	29½	Weight (lb)	19¾	20½	22¼	23¾	25½	27	28¼
	46.3	46.7	47.4	48.4	49.3	50.1	50.6	**Head C (cm)**	45.0	45.6	46.3	47.1	47.9	48.6	49.1
	18¼	18½	18¾	19	19½	19¾	20	Head C (in.)	17¾	18	18¼	18½	18¾	19¼	19¼
24 months	82.3	83.5	85.6	87.6	89.9	92.2	93.8	**Length (cm)**	81.3	82.5	84.2	86.5	88.7	90.8	92.0
	32½	32¾	33¾	34½	35½	36¼	37	Length (in.)	32	32½	33¼	34	35	35¾	36¼
	10.54	10.85	11.65	12.59	13.44	14.29	14.70	**Weight (kg)**	9.87	10.26	11.10	11.90	12.74	13.57	14.08
	23¼	24	25¾	27¾	29¾	31½	32½	Weight (lb)	21¾	22½	24½	26¼	28	30	31
	47.3	47.7	48.3	49.2	50.2	51.0	51.4	**Head C (cm)**	46.1	46.5	47.3	48.1	48.8	49.6	50.1
	18½	18¾	19	19¼	19¾	20	20¼	Head C (in.)	18¼	18¼	18½	19	19¼	19½	19¾
36 months	91.2	92.4	94.2	96.5	98.9	101.4	103.1	**Length (cm)**	90.0	91.0	93.1	95.6	98.1	100.0	101.5
	36	36½	37	38	39	40	40½	Length (in.)	35½	35¾	36¾	37¾	38½	39¼	40
	12.26	12.69	13.58	14.69	15.59	16.66	17.28	**Weight (kg)**	11.60	12.07	12.99	13.93	15.03	15.97	16.54
	27	28	30	32½	34¼	36¾	38	Weight (lb)	25½	26½	28¾	30¾	33¼	35¼	36½
	48.6	49	49.7	50.5	51.5	52.3	52.8	**Head C (cm)**	47.6	47.9	48.5	49.3	50.0	50.8	51.4
	19¼	19¼	19½	20	20¼	20¼	20¾	Head C (in.)	18¾	18¾	19	19½	19¾	20	20¼

From National Center for Health Statistics, Health Resources Administration, DHEW, Hyattsville, MD. Data from Fels Research Institute, Yellow Springs, Ohio; smoothed by least squares-cubic-spline technique. Conversion of metric data to inches and pounds by Ross Laboratories.